Williams
OBSTETRICS

Williams OBSTETRICS

23RD EDITION

F. Gary Cunningham, MD
Beatrice & Miguel Elias Distinguished Chair in Obstetrics and Gynecology
Professor, Department of Obstetrics and Gynecology
University of Texas Southwestern Medical Center at Dallas
Parkland Health and Hospital System
Dallas, Texas

Kenneth J. Leveno, MD
Jack A. Pritchard Chair in Obstetrics and Gynecology
Vice Chair for Maternal-Fetal Medicine
Professor, Department of Obstetrics and Gynecology
University of Texas Southwestern Medical Center at Dallas
Parkland Health and Hospital System
Dallas, Texas

Steven L. Bloom, MD
Mary Dees McDermott Hicks Chair in Medical Science
Professor and Chair, Department of Obstetrics and Gynecology
University of Texas Southwestern Medical Center at Dallas
Chief of Obstetrics and Gynecology
Parkland Health and Hospital System
Dallas, Texas

John C. Hauth, MD
Professor and Chair, Department of Obstetrics and Gynecology
University of Alabama at Birmingham
Chief of Obstetrics and Gynecology
University of Alabama Birmingham Hospital
Birmingham, Alabama

Dwight J. Rouse, MD
Director of UAB Center for Women's Reproductive Health
Professor, Department of Obstetrics and Gynecology
University of Alabama at Birmingham
University of Alabama Birmingham Hospital
Birmingham, Alabama

Catherine Y. Spong, MD
Bethesda, Maryland

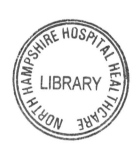

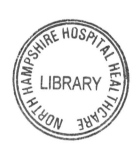

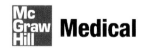

New York   Chicago   San Francisco   Lisbon   London   Madrid   Mexico City
Milan   New Delhi   San Juan   Seoul   Singapore   Sydney   Toronto

Williams Obstetrics, Twenty-Third Edition

1 2 3 4 5 6 7 8 9 0 DOW/DOW 14 13 12 11 10 9

ISBN 978-0-07-149701-5
MHID 0-07-149701-3

This book was set in Adobe Garamond by Aptara, Inc.
The editors were Alyssa Fried and Karen Davis.
The production supervisor was Phil Galea.
Production management was provided by Satvinder Kaur, Aptara, Inc.
The illustration manager was Armen Ovsepyan.
The designer was Alan Barnett.
The cover art director was Margaret Webster-Shapiro; the designer was Kiley Fusco.
Illustration by Marie Sena and Erin Frederikson.
The index was prepared by Maria Coughlin.
RR Donnelley was printer and binder.

This book is printed on acid-free paper.

Library of Congress Cataloging-in-Publication Data

Williams obstetrics. — 23rd ed. / [edited by] F. Gary Cunningham . . .
[et al.].
    p. ; cm.
  Includes bibliographical references and index.
  ISBN-13: 978-0-07-149701-5 (hardcover : alk. paper)
  ISBN-10: 0-07-149701-3 (hardcover : alk. paper)
 1. Obstetrics.   I. Cunningham, F. Gary. II. Williams,
J. Whitridge (John Whitridge), 1866–1931. III. Title: Obstetrics.
  [DNLM: 1. Obstetrics. WQ 100 W7283 2010]
  RG524.W7 2010
  618.2—dc22
                                                                    2009029027

ASSOCIATE EDITORS

Diane M. Twickler, MD
Dr. Fred Bonte Professorship in Radiology
Residency Director, Department of Radiology
Professor, Department of Radiology and
    Department of Obstetrics and Gynecology
University of Texas Southwestern Medical Center at Dallas
Medical Director of Obstetrics and Gynecology
    Ultrasonography
Parkland Health and Hospital System
Dallas, Texas

George D. Wendel, Jr., MD
Alvin "Bud" Brekken Professor of Obstetrics and Gynecology
Vice Chair for Education and Residency Director for
    Obstetrics and Gynecology
Professor, Department of Obstetrics and Gynecology
University of Texas Southwestern Medical Center at Dallas
Parkland Health and Hospital System
Dallas, Texas

CONTRIBUTING EDITORS

Jodi S. Dashe, MD
Professor, Department of Obstetrics and Gynecology
University of Texas Southwestern Medical Center at Dallas
Medical Director of Prenatal Diagnosis and Genetics
Parkland Health and Hospital System
Dallas, Texas

Barbara L. Hoffman, MD
Assistant Professor, Department of Obstetrics and Gynecology
University of Texas Southwestern Medical Center at Dallas
Parkland Health and Hospital System
Dallas, Texas

Mala S. Mahendroo, PhD
Associate Professor, Department of Obstetrics and
    Gynecology
University of Texas Southwestern Medical Center at Dallas
Dallas, Texas

James M. Alexander, MD
Professor, Department of Obstetrics and Gynecology
University of Texas Southwestern Medical Center at Dallas
Service Chief of Obstetrics
Parkland Health and Hospital System
Dallas, Texas

Jeanne S. Sheffield, MD
Fellowship Director, Maternal-Fetal Medicine
Associate Professor, Department of Obstetrics and
    Gynecology
University of Texas Southwestern Medical Center at Dallas
Parkland Health and Hospital System
Dallas, Texas

Brian M. Casey, MD
Professor, Department of Obstetrics and Gynecology
University of Texas Southwestern Medical Center at Dallas
Medical Director of Prenatal Clinics
Parkland Health and Hospital System
Dallas, Texas

ARTISTS

Marie Sena
Freelance Illustrator
Graduate, Biomedical Communications Graduate Program
University of Texas Southwestern Medical Center at Dallas

Erin Frederikson
Freelance Illustrator
Graduate, Biomedical Communications Graduate Program
University of Texas Southwestern Medical Center at Dallas

DEDICATION

These are the times that try men's souls.

—Thomas Paine, *The American Crisis,* 1776–1783

This 23rd edition of *Williams Obstetrics* arrives at a time of economic uncertainty for our country—indeed, for the world. There is especial anxiety provoked by the anticipated tumultuous reorganization of our healthcare system. We dedicate this book to those who are fair minded and who strive to bring about these changes with equanimity. We include all those who work to construct a system that is the best for all, includes those who are disadvantaged, but does not diminish the quality of healthcare for those who will ultimately finance the system—a tall order indeed. We echo the philosophy of the American College of Obstetricians and Gynecologists that all women and their unborn children should have access to obstetrical care and family planning services.

CONTENTS

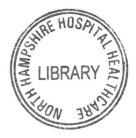

SECTION 1

OVERVIEW

SECTION 2

MATERNAL AND FETAL ANATOMY AND PHYSIOLOGY

SECTION 3

ANTEPARTUM

SECTION 4

LABOR AND DELIVERY

SECTION 5

FETUS AND NEWBORN

SECTION 6

PUERPERIUM

SECTION 7

OBSTETRICAL COMPLICATIONS

SECTION 8

MEDICAL AND SURGICAL COMPLICATIONS

APPENDIX

PREFACE

In this 23rd edition of *Williams Obstetrics*, we continue to emphasize the science-based underpinnings and evidence-based practices of our specialty. Most professional and academic organizations embrace these principles, and while some promulgate guidelines and recommendations, others provide funding for such investigations. Our policy is to cite these whenever possible. A major impetus for these studies comes from the *Eunice Shriver Kennedy* National Institute of Child Health and Human Development—also called the NICHD. For many decades, this Institute has supported basic and clinical research to improve healthcare for women and children. We especially rely on investigations performed through NICHD-sponsored Maternal-Fetal Medicine Units and Neonatal Units Networks. There is also fiscal support for young investigators in obstetrics and allied specialties that comes from a number of societies and organizations. Among others, these include the American College of Obstetricians and Gynecologists, the American Gynecological and Obstetrical Society, the Society for Maternal-Fetal Medicine, the Society for Gynecological Investigation, and the American Board of Obstetrics and Gynecology.

A major objective of this book is to provide a convenient source that will aid the busy practitioner—those "in the trenches." To this end, we summarize new data that has influenced evidence-based management to improve pregnancy outcomes. And while we cite numerous sources to accomplish this, we again mention some important caveats. For example, while we try to avoid—or at least soften—dogmatism that creeps into obstetrical practice, we often cite our combined clinical experiences drawn from large teaching services. We remain convinced that these are disciplined examples of evidence-based obstetrics. Importantly, we do not represent that these constitute the sole method of management.

To succeed in these self-imposed mandates, we have again added new editors with especial expertise in important areas to ensure accurate interpretation of recent scientific and clinical advances. To allow for this, two editors who have served with distinction for several editions of this book have passed their pens on to others. Dr. Larry Gilstrap has traded the Chair of Obstetrics, Gynecology, and Reproductive Sciences at the University of Texas-Houston Medical School to become Executive Director of the American Board of Obstetrics and Gynecology. Dr. Kathy Wenstrom has left the University of Alabama at Birmingham to become Chief of Maternal-Fetal Medicine at Brown University. We will miss them both and value their contributions. To fill their shoes, two associate editors have assumed their duties. Dr. Dwight Rouse from the University of Alabama at Birmingham continues to lend his expertise in many areas of obstetrics, maternal-fetal medicine, and epidemiology. He also has many years of experience as a leading investigator in the Maternal-Fetal Medicine Units Network.

Dr. Catherine Spong continues her ever-increasing duties as Chief of the Pregnancy and Perinatology Branch of the *Eunice Shriver Kennedy* National Institute of Child Health and Human Development. Cathy also serves as program scientist for the vitally important Maternal-Fetal Medicine Units Network cited above. A third vacancy in the associate editorship is Dr. William Rainey, who left UT Southwestern and is a Regents' Professor of Physiology at the Medical College of Georgia. Bill performed a fantastic job for the 22nd edition in dissecting basic science principles of human reproduction in a textbook written primarily for clinicians.

Dr. George Wendel remains on the team as associate editor. He is internationally recognized for his expertise in obstetrical, perinatal, and sexually transmitted infections. He is widely published in these fields and has mentored numerous fellows who have followed in his footsteps. Also joining us from UT Southwestern as associate editor is Dr. Diane Twickler, Professor of Radiology as well as Obstetrics and Gynecology. Her incredible wealth of knowledge and clinical and research experience with a variety of imaging techniques used during pregnancy have been unsung contributions for many previous editions of this book.

Reflecting the rapidly accruing knowledge in clinical obstetrics is the further addition of six extremely talented contributing editors, all from UT Southwestern Medical Center. Dr. Jodi Dashe uses her extensive experience and incredible skills with obstetrical sonography, fetal diagnosis, and prenatal genetics to provide input for this 23rd edition as she has namelessly done now for many previous ones. Dr. Barbara Hoffman has widespread clinical expertise with contraception and sterilization issues, embryology and anatomy, and especial interest in congenital and acquired genital tract anomalies. Equally importantly, she has served as the in-house production editor for the 22nd and 23rd editions and has spent countless evenings and weekends applying her considerable editorial talents and creative illustration production. Dr. Mala Mahendroo is a basic scientist who performs a magnificent job of providing a coherent clinical translational version of basic science aspects of human reproduction. To do so, she draws from her own research experience with cervical remodeling during pregnancy and initiation of human labor. Dr. Jim Alexander brings his expertise with the conduct of normal as well as abnormal labor and delivery, cesarean delivery, conduction analgesia, preeclampsia, and obstetrical hemorrhage. Dr. Brian Casey lends his in-depth clinical and research experience with diabetes, fetal growth disorders, and thyroid physiology. Dr. Jeanne Sheffield joins us as a vital member of the obstetrical infectious diseases group. In addition to her wealth of clinical and research experience with maternal, perinatal, and sexually transmitted infections, she also has extensive experience in managing drug dependency as well as a host of other medical and surgical disorders that complicate pregnancy.

We continue to rely heavily on other colleagues for their intellectual and clinical input and the use of photographs and other illustrations that improve immensely the readability of this 23rd edition. Although these colleagues are too numerous to mention individually, we attempt to thank those with especial contributions. From UT Southwestern and Parkland Hospital, we cite the entire faculty of the Maternal-Fetal Medicine Division, who, in addition to providing expert content, graciously helped us cover clinical duties when writing and editing were especially time consuming. These include Drs. Oscar Andujo, Morris Bryant, Susan Cox, Jennifer Hernandez, Robyn Horsager, Julie Lo, Mark Peters, Scott Roberts, Vanessa Rogers, Patricia Santiago-Munoz, Steve Shivvers, Ed Wells, Kevin Worley, and Mike Zaretsky. Also in the division, our special thanks go to Dr. Don McIntire, who retrieved and tabulated electronically stored data for Parkland Hospital obstetrical outcomes that are shown in numerous tables and figures throughout this book. Dr. Barry Schwarz shared his extensive knowledge of contraceptive management for preparation of that chapter. Dr. Kelly Carrick of the Department of Pathology contributed numerous photographs illustrating both normal and abnormal features of the female reproductive tract. Dr. Gerda Zeeman from the University of Groningen in The Netherlands—but who remains in Dallas in spirit—graciously provided magnetic resonance images from women with eclampsia. We also thank the fellows of our Maternal-Fetal Medicine Division and our many residents in obstetrics and gynecology. Their vigilant search for perfect examples of normal and abnormal findings has led to many of the photographs in this edition. We specifically thank Drs. Mina Abbassi-Ghanavati and Laura Greer for their time-consuming efforts to provide the first-ever appendix of normal values during pregnancy for common and uncommon laboratory tests. We predict that this will be a priceless resource for practitioners.

From the University of Alabama at Birmingham, Ms. Suzanne Cliver provided material for tables and figures from the perinatal database. Drs. Ona Marie Faye-Peterson and Michael Conner of the Department of Pathology generously contributed pictures and photomicrographs of placental pathology. From Bethesda, Dr. Rosemary Higgins of the Neonatal Units Network provided expert input for disorders of the fetus and newborn.

Thanks to generous funding from The McGraw-Hill Companies, this 23rd edition has full-color photographs and illustrations. Many were either replaced or redrawn for consistency of style. More than 200 of the new color illustrations were created by two talented medical illustrationists. Ms. Marie Sena was one of the major artist contributors to the inaugural edition of *Williams Gynecology*. To even further her experiences for the current book, she logged countless hours in labor and delivery, in the anatomy laboratory, and in model simulations. Ms. Erin Frederikson, also a veteran of our art team, added insightful images depicting cesarean delivery, peripartum hysterectomy, and fetal development. Additional artwork was generously provided by Mr. Jordan Pietz and Ms. Jennifer Hulsey. All of these talented artists trained on campus under the stimulating leadership of Mr. Lewis Calver, who is Chair of the Biomedical Communications Graduate Program. More artistic support came from Mr. Joseph Varghese and his team at Thomson Digital, who provided the full-color graphs and line art that completes this edition's art program. They were aided by medical content expert Dr. Anuradha Majumdar, who precisely translated our academic vision to each image. Both tirelessly coordinated efforts between our authors and their art team and graciously accommodated our numerous changes and tweaks. In addition to these artists, we were grateful for photographic contributions from academic giants in their field. We boast seminal placental images generously donated by a dear friend, Dr. Kurt Benirschke, laparoscopic images of ectopic pregnancies from Dr. Togas Tolandi, and fetal surgery images from Dr. Timothy Crombleholme.

Production of the 5,000-page typewritten manuscript would be impossible without a dedicated team to bring these efforts together. Once again, we are deeply indebted to Ms. Connie Utterback for her untiring efforts as production coordinator for Dallas, Birmingham, and Washington, D.C. She received able assistance with manuscript production from the Dallas group that included Ms. Minnie Tregaskis, Ms. Melinda Epstein, Ms. Mary Kay McDonald, Ms. Dina Trujillano, and Ms. Ellen Watkins. From Birmingham, production coordination and manuscript preparation were ably provided by Ms. Belinda Rials and Ms. Sue Capps. Ms. Cherry Neely coordinated database analysis and presentation with help from research nurses Ms. Allison Northen and Ms. Rachel Copper. Graphic illustration for the Birmingham group was provided by Ms. Jo Taylor.

It again has been a privilege and a pleasure to work with the dedicated personnel from McGraw-Hill. A number of individuals were crucial to the success of this 23rd edition. Dr. Anne Sydor helped us to conceive the project, and she provided the inspiration and obtained financial support to present this full-color edition. Ms. Marsha Loeb served as senior editor during the bulk of its production, and she was an efficient and steadfast advocate who frequently went above and beyond to accommodate our needs. Her responsibilities were assumed in the "home stretch" by Ms. Alyssa Fried, who has ably led us to completion. We appreciate her efforts and thank her for her help and her patience. Integral to a project of this scope and complexity is attention to detail. This 23rd edition would have never seen the light of day without the considerable talents of Mr. Phil Galea, Mr. John Williams, and Mr. Armen Ovsepan. They have been long-standing members of the *Williams* team and have lent their considerable talents to several editions. An especially warm thank you is extended to a long-time colleague, Ms. Karen Davis, who coordinated production of this edition. Karen has been a tireless and committed member of our *Williams* family. Over the many years that we have worked with her, she has always handled problems quickly and expertly as soon as they arose. Her dedication to creating the best textbook possible equaled our efforts, and we are in awe of her unflappable, gracious, and effective style. Finally, McGraw-Hill enlisted Aptara Inc. for composition. We thank Ms. Satvinder Kaur for her talents in coordinating and overseeing composition. Her attention to detail and organization skills were vital to completion of our project.

Our goal at the outset of this 23rd edition was to create a visual landmark to equal the written content. To this end, almost 90 percent of images in this edition have been upgraded or revised. Of these, 220 images were rendered by our medical illustrators cited above. It will also be apparent that almost all previous black-and-white photographs have been replaced by those in vivid color. This is supplanted by a thorough canvass of the literature with stated efforts to emphasize evidence-based management. To do this, almost 2000 new journal and textbook references were added, and more than 400 of these were published in 2009. All of this talent and hard work has come to fruition in what we hope is the best edition so far of *Williams Obstetrics*. We further hope that the reader will enjoy studying its content as much as we have enjoyed conveying it.

Williams
OBSTETRICS

SECTION 1
OVERVIEW

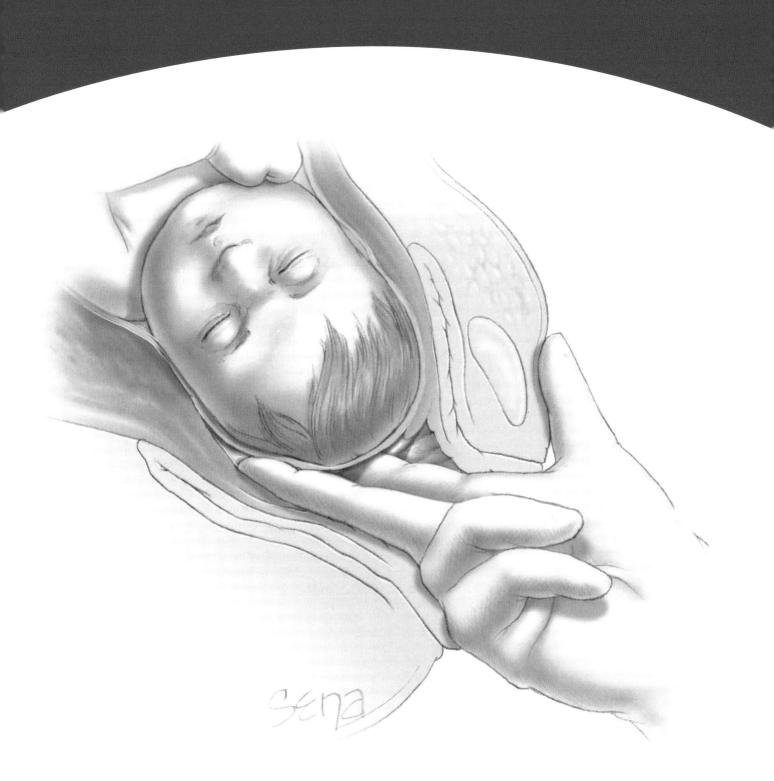

CHAPTER 1

Overview of Obstetrics

According to the Oxford English Dictionary, the word *obstetrics* is defined as "that branch of medicine that deals with childbirth and the care and treatment of the mother before and after birth." Its derivation is from the Latin *obstetrix*, meaning midwife—from "mid"—with, and "wif"—meaning woman. Petraglia (2008) describes evidence of midwifery from records found in ancient Egypt and the Roman Empire. The Egyptian Ebers Papyrus (1900 to 1550 BC) recognized midwifery as a female occupation concerned with obstetrics and gynecology, and specifically with the acceleration of parturition and the birth process. Petraglia further reports that midwifery services were described through the Middle Ages and into the 18th century, at which time the role of the surgeon superseded that of the midwife. It was at this time that medicine began to assert that its modern scientific processes were better for mothers and infants than those of folk-medical midwives.

In the contemporaneous sense, obstetrics is concerned with reproduction of humans. The specialty promotes health and well-being of the pregnant woman and her fetus through quality prenatal care. Such care entails appropriate recognition and treatment of complications, supervision of their labor and delivery, ensuring care of the newborn, and management of the puerperium to include follow-up care that promotes health and provides family planning options.

The importance of obstetrics is attested to by the use of maternal and neonatal outcomes as an index of the quality of health and life in human society. Intuitively, indices that reflect poor obstetrical and perinatal outcomes would lead to the assumption that medical care for the entire population is lacking. With those thoughts, we now provide a synopsis of the current state of maternal and newborn health in the United States as it relates to obstetrics.

VITAL STATISTICS

The National Vital Statistics System of the United States is the oldest and most successful example of intergovernmental data sharing in public health. The National Center for Health Statistics (NCHS) collects and disseminates official statistics through contractual agreements with vital registration systems operated in various jurisdictions legally responsible for registration of births, fetal deaths, deaths, marriages, and divorces. Legal authority resides individually with the 50 states; two regions—the District of Columbia and New York City; and five territories—American Samoa, Guam, the Northern Mariana Islands, Puerto Rico, and the Virgin Islands. Schoendorf and Branum (2006) provide a thoughtful review of the use of these statistics to conduct obstetrical and perinatal research.

Standard certificates for the registration of live births and deaths were first developed in 1900. An act of Congress in 1902 established the Bureau of the Census to develop a system for the annual collection of vital statistics. The Bureau retained authority until 1946, when the function was transferred to the United States Public Health Service. It is presently assigned to the Division of Vital Statistics of the NCHS, which is a division of the Centers for Disease Control and Prevention (CDC). The standard birth certificate was extensively revised in 1989 to include more information on medical and lifestyle risk factors and also obstetrical care practices.

Further revisions were initiated in some states in 2003, but full implementation in all states will not be completed for several more years. The 2003 revision focuses on fundamental changes in data collection aimed at improving accuracy.

Changes also include a format conducive to electronic processing, to collect more explicit parental demographic data, and to improve selection of information regarding antepartum and intrapartum complications. Some examples of new data to be collected include those related to uterine rupture, blood transfusion, and pregnancy resulting from infertility treatment.

Definitions

The uniform use of standard definitions is encouraged by the World Health Organization as well as the American Academy of Pediatrics and the American College of Obstetricians and Gynecologists (2007). Such uniformity allows comparison of data not only between states or regions of the country, but also between countries. Still, not all of these definitions are uniformly applied, as illustrated by the example of definitions of inclusive fetal birthweights. To wit, these two organizations recommend reporting to include all fetuses and neonates born weighing at minimum 500 g, whether alive or dead. But not all of the 50 states follow this recommendation. For example, 28 states stipulate that fetal deaths beginning at 20 weeks' gestation should be recorded as such; 8 states report all products of conception as fetal deaths; and still others use a minimum birthweight of 350 g, 400 g, or 500 g to define fetal deaths. To further the confusion, the National Vital Statistics Reports tabulates fetal deaths as those 20 weeks' gestation or older (Centers for Disease Control and Prevention, 2009). But the 50th percentile for fetal weight at 20 weeks approximates 325 to 350 g—considerably less than the 500-g definition. Indeed, a birthweight of 500 g corresponds closely with the 50th percentile for 22 weeks.

Definitions recommended by the NCHS and the CDC are as follows:

Perinatal period. The period after birth of an infant born after 20 weeks and ending at 28 completed days after birth. When perinatal rates are based on birthweight, rather than gestational age, it is recommended that the perinatal period be defined as commencing at 500 g.

Birth. The complete expulsion or extraction from the mother of a fetus after 20 weeks' gestation. As described above, in the absence of accurate dating criteria, fetuses weighing <500 g are usually not considered as births, but rather are termed abortuses for purposes of vital statistics.

Birthweight. The weight of a neonate determined immediately after delivery or as soon thereafter as feasible. It should be expressed to the nearest gram.

Birth rate. The number of live births per 1000 population.

Fertility rate. The number of live births per 1000 females aged 15 through 44 years.

Live birth. The term used to record a birth whenever the newborn at or sometime after birth breathes spontaneously or shows any other sign of life such as a heartbeat or definite spontaneous movement of voluntary muscles. Heartbeats are distinguished from transient cardiac contractions, and respirations are differentiated from fleeting respiratory efforts or gasps.

Stillbirth or fetal death. The absence of signs of life at or after birth.

Early neonatal death. Death of a liveborn neonate during the first 7 days after birth.

Late neonatal death. Death after 7 days but before 29 days.

Stillbirth rate or fetal death rate. The number of stillborn neonates per 1000 neonates born, including live births and stillbirths.

Neonatal mortality rate. The number of neonatal deaths per 1000 live births.

Perinatal mortality rate. The number of stillbirths plus neonatal deaths per 1000 total births.

Infant death. All deaths of liveborn infants from birth through 12 months of age.

Infant mortality rate. The number of infant deaths per 1000 live births.

Low birthweight. A newborn whose weight is < 2500 g.

Very low birthweight. A newborn whose weight is < 1500 g.

Extremely low birthweight. A newborn whose weight is <1000 g.

Term neonate. A neonate born anytime after 37 completed weeks of gestation and up until 42 completed weeks of gestation (260 to 294 days).

Preterm neonate. A neonate born before 37 completed weeks (the 259th day).

Postterm neonate. A neonate born anytime after completion of the 42nd week, beginning with day 295.

Abortus. A fetus or embryo removed or expelled from the uterus during the first half of gestation—20 weeks or less, or in the absence of accurate dating criteria, born weighing < 500 g.

Induced termination of pregnancy. The purposeful interruption of an intrauterine pregnancy with the intention other than to produce a liveborn neonate, and which does not result in a live birth. This definition excludes retention of products of conception following fetal death.

Direct maternal death. The death of the mother that results from obstetrical complications of pregnancy, labor, or the puerperium and from interventions, omissions, incorrect treatment, or a chain of events resulting from any of these factors. An example is maternal death from exsanguination after uterine rupture.

Indirect maternal death. A maternal death that is not directly due to an obstetrical cause. Death results from previously existing disease or a disease developing during pregnancy, labor, or the puerperium that was aggravated by maternal physiological adaptation to pregnancy. An example is maternal death from complications of mitral valve stenosis.

Nonmaternal death. Death of the mother that results from accidental or incidental causes not related to pregnancy. An example is death from an automobile accident or concurrent malignancy.

Maternal mortality ratio. The number of maternal deaths that result from the reproductive process per 100,000 live births. Used more commonly, but less accurately, are the terms *maternal mortality rate* or *maternal death rate*. The term *ratio* is more accurate because it includes in the numerator the number of deaths regardless of pregnancy outcome—for example, live births, stillbirths, and ectopic pregnancies—whereas the denominator includes the number of live births.

Pregnancy-associated death. The death of a woman, from any cause, while pregnant or within 1 calendar year of termination of pregnancy, regardless of the duration and the site of pregnancy.

Pregnancy-related death. A pregnancy-associated death that results from: (1) complications of pregnancy itself, (2) the chain of events initiated by pregnancy that led to death, or (3) aggravation of an unrelated condition by the physiological or pharmacological effects of pregnancy and that subsequently caused death.

PREGNANCY IN THE UNITED STATES

Data from diverse sources have been used to provide the following snapshot of pregnancy in the United States during the first decade of the 21st century.

Pregnancy Rates

According to the Centers for Disease Control and Prevention (2009), and as shown in Table 1-1, the fertility rate in 2006 of women aged 15 to 44 years was 68.5 live births per 1000 women. This rate began trending downward in 1990 and decreased even lower than that for replacement births, indicating a population decline (Hamilton, 2004). However, this was offset by considerable net migration into the United States that is discussed further on page 10. For example, there were more than 1 million migrants each year from 2000 to 2002.

There were nearly 4.3 million births in 2006, and this constituted a birth rate for the United States of 14.2 per 1000 population. This rate was up from that in 2002, which was the lowest rate ever recorded—13.9 per 1000 population. Hispanic women accounted for more than 1 in 5 births. The average American woman has 3.2 pregnancies in her lifetime, and 1.8 of these are considered wanted pregnancies (Ventura and colleagues, 1999). After exclusion of fetal losses and induced terminations, American women on average deliver 2.0 live births in a lifetime. By way of example, Table 1-1 includes more than 5.1 million pregnancies in the United States that were classified

TABLE 1-1. Some Statistics Concerning Reproductive Outcome for the United States in 2005 or 2006

Statistic	Number or Rate
Births	
Total	4,265,555
Birth rate	14.2 per 1000 population
Fertility rate	68.5 per 1000 women aged 15–44 years
Abortion	
Total	820,151
Birth rate	223 per 1000 live births
Fertility rate	15 per 1000 women aged 15–44 years

Data from Centers for Disease Control and Prevention (2008, 2009).

as live births or induced abortions. Assuming another 15 percent for spontaneous abortion, there are approximately 6 million pregnancies in this country each year.

Pregnancy-Related Care

This is a major component of health care. In 2001, delivery was the second leading cause of hospitalization behind heart disease (Hall and DeFrances, 2003). The average length of hospital stay for all deliveries was 2.5 days. Prenatal care was the fourth leading reason for office visits to physicians and accounted for nearly 20 million visits in 2001 (Cherry and associates, 2003). Nondelivery hospitalizations have decreased substantially since the late 1980s due to efforts to minimize expenditures. The leading indication for hospitalization unrelated to delivery is preterm labor. Nicholson and co-workers (2000) estimated that the total national cost of hospitalization for preterm labor that did not eventuate in delivery was $360 million in 1996 dollars. This sum increased to $820 million when women with preterm labor who actually delivered early were added.

MEASURES OF OBSTETRICAL CARE

There are a number of indices—several among the vital statistic definitions described above—that are used as a yardstick of obstetrical and perinatal outcomes to assess quality of care.

Healthy People 2010 and 2020

Objectives for maternal and infant health for the decade now ending were promulgated by the Centers for Disease Control and Prevention and the Health Resources and Service Administration (2000) and included in the nationwide goals termed *Healthy People 2010*. Progress toward some of these goals has been disappointing. Notably, one major objective was to lower the number of preterm births, but these have actually increased since 2000. Also, the disparity in pregnancy outcomes between whites and racial/ethnic minorities has persisted, and the infant mortality rate in African-American women is now almost twice that of white mothers. Other objectives were concerned with decreasing the rates of maternal, perinatal, and infant morbidity and mortality.

Planning for Healthy People 2020 began in 2008 guided by the Office of Disease Prevention and Health Promotion (2009). Goals are being determined using science-based findings that have accrued over the current decade with launch expected in 2010.

Perinatal Mortality

As previously defined, the perinatal mortality rate includes the numbers of stillbirths and neonatal deaths per 1000 total births. According to the National Vital Statistics Reports by MacDorman and Kirmeyer (2009), in 2005 there were 25,894 fetal deaths of 20 weeks' gestation or more. As shown in Figure 1-1, the fetal death rate declined gradually from 1999 but plateaued in 2003. Most of the improvement was a decrease in fetal deaths between 20 and 27 weeks.

Fetal deaths after 20 weeks are an important public health issue. Although there is appropriate concern concentrated on infant mortality—death in the first year of life—a focus on fetal mortality may provide further opportunities for prevention. For

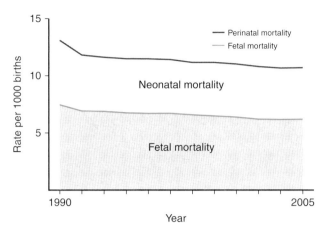

FIGURE 1-1 Fetal mortality rates from 1990 through 2005 in the United States are depicted by the blue line. Fetal mortality (*gray area*) and neonatal mortality rates (*yellow area*) are combined to reflect the total the perinatal mortality rate, which is shown by the red line. (Data points estimated from National Vital Statistics Reports by MacDorman and Kirmeyer, 2009.)

example, racial and ethnic disparity associated with fetal death is obvious as shown in Figure 1-2. In 2004, approximately a fourth of the 18,593 neonatal deaths were due to preterm delivery and approximately a fifth was caused by a congenital malformation (Heron, 2007). Worldwide, approximately 4 million babies are stillborn each year, and another 4 million die in the first 4 weeks of life (Lawn and colleagues, 2005).

Infant Deaths

There were 28,384 infant deaths in 2005, a rate of 6.9 per 1000 live births compared with 6.8 in 2001 (Mathews and MacDorman, 2008). The three leading causes of infant death—congenital malformations, low birthweight, and sudden infant death syndrome—accounted for 44 percent of all deaths. Infants born at the lowest gestational ages and birthweights have a large impact on these mortality rates. For example, 55 percent of all infant deaths in 2005 occurred in 2 percent of infants born before 32 weeks' gestation. Indeed, the percentage of infant deaths related

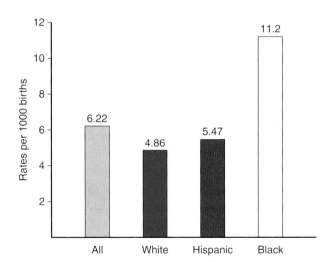

FIGURE 1-2 Fetal death rate for various populations in the United States in 2005. (Data from National Vital Statistics Reports by MacDorman and Kirmeyer, 2009.)

to preterm birth increased from 34.6 percent in 2000 to 36.5 percent in 2005. When analyzed by birthweight, two thirds of infant deaths were in low-birthweight neonates. Of particular interest are those birthweights less than 500 g, for which neonatal intensive care can now be offered. In 2001, there were 6450 live-born infants weighing less than 500 g, but 86 percent of these infants died during the first 28 days of life. Of the 1044 who survived the first 28 days of life, there were 934 who lived for at least 1 year. Thus, only 11 percent of all neonates weighing < 500 g survived infancy. Importantly, developmental and neurological sequelae are common in the survivors (see Chap. 36, p. 807).

St. John and associates (2000) have estimated the total cost of initial care in the United States for all newborns as $10.2 billion annually. Almost 60 percent of this expenditure is attributed to preterm births before 37 weeks, and 12 percent is spent on neonates born between 24 and 26 weeks.

Maternal Mortality

Pregnancy and childbirth have never been safer for women in the United States. In fact, pregnancy-related deaths are so uncommon as to be measured per 100,000 births. Still, some women die from early pregnancy complications related to ectopic pregnancy, miscarriage, and induced abortion and later complications such as hypertensive disorders, hemorrhage, and infection. Kung and colleagues (2008) reported for the National Vital Statistics System that there were 623 pregnancy-related deaths in the United States in 2005. Some of the more common causes of pregnancy-related maternal deaths are shown in Table 1-2. Hemorrhage and infection cause half of deaths associated with ectopic pregnancy and abortion. Taken together, embolism, hemorrhage, hypertension, and infection accounted for 65 percent of maternal deaths after midpregnancy. It is also important to consider the role that the increasing cesarean delivery rate has on maternal mortality risks (Clark and associates, 2008; Deneux-Tharaux and co-workers, 2006; Lang and King, 2008).

There are a number of other factors important to the discussion of maternal mortality. First, maternal deaths are notoriously underreported, possibly by as much as half (Koonin and colleagues, 1997). Even so, there is no doubt that a major accomplishment of obstetrical care is the markedly decreased risk of death from pregnancy complications. As shown in Figure 1-3, maternal mortality rates decreased by two orders of magnitude—almost 99 percent—in the United States during the 20th century. Still, it is unfortunate that mortality rates have plateaued since 1982 (Lang and King, 2008). This may be due in part to an artificial increase caused by a classification system change. For example, new International Statistical Classification of Diseases and Related Health Problems, 10th Revision (ICD-10) codes were implemented in 1999.

A second important consideration is the obvious disparity of increased mortality rates in indigent and minority women as shown in Figure 1-4. The disparity with indigent women is exemplified by the study of maternal deaths in women cared for in a third-party payer system, the Hospital Corporation of America. In this study of nearly 1.5 million pregnant women, Clark and associates (2008) reported an impressively low maternal mortality rate of 6.5 per 100,000.

TABLE 1-2. Causes of Pregnancy-Related Maternal Deaths in the United States[a] Compared with Those of Pooled Data from Developed Countries[b]

Cause of Death	United States 1991–1999[c] (n = 4200) Percent	Pooled Data for Developed Countries after 1990[d] (n = 2047) Percent
Embolism	19.6	20.5
Hemorrhage	17.2	18.5
Gestational hypertension	15.7	22.2
Infection	12.6	2.8
Other pregnancy-related	34.1	29.4
Cardiomyopathy	8.3	
Stroke	5.0	
Anesthesia	1.6	
Others[e]	19.2	
Unknown	0.7	6.6

[a]Data from Centers for Disease Control and Prevention reported by Chang and colleagues (2003).
[b]Data from the World Health Organization reported by Khan and associates (2006).
[c]Includes abortion and ectopic pregnancy.
[d]Excludes abortion and ectopic pregnancy.
[e]Includes cardiovascular, pulmonary, neurological, and other medical conditions.

The third important consideration is that many of the reported maternal deaths are considered preventable. According to Berg and colleagues (2005), this may be up to a third of pregnancy-related deaths in white women and up to half of those in black women. And even in the insured women described above and reported by Clark and co-workers (2008), 28 percent of 98 maternal deaths were judged preventable. Thus, although significant progress has been made, measures to prevent more deaths are imperative for obstetrics in the 21st century.

Severe Maternal Morbidity

The concept of "near miss" maternal mortality has led to development of statistical data systems that measure indicators of *severe maternal morbidities*. This evolution followed inadequacies in hospitalization coding to reflect the severity of maternal complications. Thus, coding indicators or modifiers are used to allow analysis of clinical "near misses." Such a system has been implemented in Britain and is termed the UK Obstetric Surveillance System—UKOSS (Knight and colleagues, 2005, 2008).

Ad hoc studies of severe maternal morbidity for the United States have been reported. From the Centers for Disease Control and Prevention, Callaghan and colleagues (2008) analyzed nearly 425,000 records from the National Hospital Discharge Summary (NHDS) from 1991 through 2003. *Selected International Classification of Diseases, Ninth Revision, Clinical Modification (ICD-9-CM)* codes were used to tabulate a number of severe morbidities, and some of those most commonly encountered are listed in Table 1-3. These investigators reported that 5 per 1000 of these 50.6 million pregnant women had at least one indicator for severe

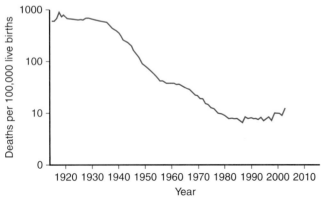

FIGURE 1-3 Maternal mortality rates for the United States from 1915 to 2003. (From the National Center for Health Statistics reported by Hoyert, 2007.)

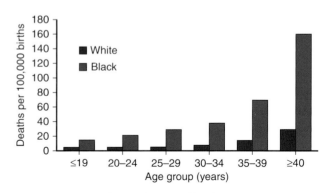

FIGURE 1-4 Maternal mortality ratio (deaths per 100,000 live births) by age and according to race for the United States, 1991 through 1999. (Data from the Centers for Disease Control and Prevention as reported by Chang and co-workers, 2003.)

TABLE 1-3. Severe Obstetrical Morbidities Identified[a] During Delivery Hospitalizations–United States, 1991–2003

Category	Percent of Morbidities[b]
Transfusions	48
Eclampsia	14
Hysterectomy	12
Cardiac events	7.6
Respiratory failure	6.7
Anesthesia complications	4.6
Mechanical ventilation	4.2
Septicemia	4.2
Renal failure	2.5
Stroke	2.5
Invasive monitoring	1.8
Hemorrhagic shock	1.5
Pulmonary embolism	0.8

[a]Identified by International Classification of Diseases, Ninth Revision, Clinical Modification (ICD-9-CM) codes.
[b]Percent exceeds 100 because some patients had multiple diagnoses.
Data from the Centers for Disease Control and Prevention reported by Callaghan and colleagues (2008).

morbidity. Said another way, for every maternal death, approximately 50 women experience severe morbidity.

A similar study was recently reported by Kuklina and associates (2009) from the National Institutes of Child Health and Human Development and the Centers for Disease Control and Prevention. They performed a cross-sectional study of severe obstetrical complications identified from the 1998–2005 National Inpatient Sample of the Healthcare Cost and Utilization Project that included more than 32 million discharges. Severe complications similar to those shown in Table 1-3 were identified with a rate of 6.4 per 1000 in 1998-1999 and 8.1 per 1000 for 2004–2005.

These rates of 5 to 8 per 1000 deliveries have been reported from other developed countries. From Canada, Wen and associates (2005) surveyed 2.54 million deliveries between 1991 and 2000 and reported an overall rate of severe morbidity of 4.6 per 1000 deliveries. From the Netherlands, Zwart and co-workers (2008) studied nearly 325,000 deliveries and reported an overall incidence of severe morbidity of 7.1 per 1000 deliveries. As with maternal deaths, these morbidities can be studied to discover and correct systemic errors and to improve substandard care (Pearlman, 2006).

TIMELY TOPICS IN OBSTETRICS

A variety of topics have been in the forefront for obstetrical providers in the 4 years since the last edition of this textbook. Our purpose here is to review some of these topics selected because of their likely impact on our specialty in the coming years.

Rising Cesarean Delivery Rate

In the preceding edition we noted that in 2002, the cesarean delivery rate climbed to the highest level ever reported in the United

States—26.1 percent. Since that time, this record has subsequently been broken each year with the new record of 31.1 percent in 2006 (Martin and colleagues, 2009). This rise in the total rate is a result of upward trends in both the primary and the repeat cesarean rate. Indeed, more than 90 percent of women with prior cesarean deliveries now undergo repeat procedures. The forces involved in these changes in cesarean delivery rates are multifactorial and complex. We cite a few examples:

1. As discussed in Chapter 20 (p. 465), the major indication for primary cesarean delivery is dystocia, and there is evidence that this diagnosis has increased.
2. As discussed throughout Chapter 26, the sharp decline in vaginal births after cesarean—VBAC—deliveries is likely related to the uterine rupture risk associated with VBAC.
3. As discussed in Chapter 25 (p. 548), a new and controversial factor is *cesarean delivery on maternal request—CDMR*. This is defined as a cesarean delivery at term for a singleton pregnancy on maternal request in the absence of any medical or obstetrical indications (Reddy and Spong, 2006). The magnitude of the CDMR phenomenon in American obstetrics has been difficult to quantify. Meikle and co-workers (2005) estimated that the rate of such elective procedures increased from 20 percent of all primary cesareans in 1994 to 28 percent in 2001. Thus, such elective cesarean deliveries constitute between 3 and 7 percent of all deliveries to women without a previous cesarean delivery (Menacker and colleagues, 2006). To address this issue, the National Institute of Child Health and Human Development (NICHD) convened a State-of-the-Science Conference in 2006 to provide an in-depth evaluation of the evidence, raise public awareness, identify research goals, and guide practitioners in assessing risks and benefits. According to Dr. James Scott, editor of *Obstetrics & Gynecology*, more than 500 people attended, and it was apparent that there were numerous advocacy groups concerned about and opposed to the direction that CDMR has taken. In a summary of the meeting—*NIH State-of-the-Science Conference Statement on Cesarean Delivery on Maternal Request (2006)*—it was concluded that there was insufficient evidence to evaluate fully the benefits and risks of CDMR versus planned vaginal delivery. Importantly, CDMR was not recommended for women desiring several children because the risks of placenta previa and accreta increase with each cesarean delivery. Moreover, it was concluded that CDMR should not be performed before 39 completed weeks' gestation or before verification of fetal lung maturity. It is hoped that some evidence-based guidelines will soon be available.

Measuring Healthcare Outcomes

Much publicity followed the report by the Institute of Medicine entitled *To Err Is Human* (Kohn and colleagues, 2000). The report greatly increased interest in measuring healthcare outcomes and adverse events (Grobman, 2006). Even the U.S. Congress has determined that reimbursements by Medicare and Medicaid should be indexed to selected healthcare outcomes. Specifically, wide and often dizzying spectra of benchmarks have

TABLE 1-4. Recommended Adjustments to Current ACGME Resident Guidelines for Work Hours

	2003 ACGME Guidelines	2008 IOM Recommendations
Maximum hours of work per week	80 hours, averaged over 4 weeks	No change
Maximum shift length	30 hours (admitting patients up to 24 hours then 6 additional hours for transitional and educational activities)	• 30 hours (admitting patients for up to 16 hours, plus 5-hour protected sleep period between 10 p.m. and 8 a.m. with the remaining hours for transition and educational activities) • 16 hours with no protected sleep period
Maximum in-hospital on-call frequency	Every third night, on average	Every third night, no averaging
Minimum time off between scheduled shifts	10 hours after shift length	• 10 hours after day shift • 12 hours after night shift • 14 hours after any extended duty period of 30 hours and not to return until 6 a.m. of next day
Maximum frequency of in-hospital night shifts	Not addressed	• 4 night maximum; 48 hours' off after 3 or 4 nights of consecutive duty
Mandatory time off duty	• 4 days off per month • 1 day (24 hours) off per week, averaged over 4 weeks	• 5 days off per month • 1 day (24 hours) off per week, no averaging • One 48-hour period off per month
Moonlighting	Internal moonlighting is counted against 80-hour weekly limit	• Internal and external moonlighting is counted against 80-hour weekly limit • All other duty hour limits apply to moonlighting in combination with scheduled work
Limit on hours for exceptions	88 hours for select programs with a sound educational rationale	No change
Emergency room limits	12-hour shift limit, at least an equivalent period of time off between shifts; 60-hour workweek with additional 12 hours for education	No change

ACGME = Accreditation Council for Graduate Medical Education; IOM = Institute of Medicine.
From the Institute of Medicine (2008).

been proposed for measurement of the quality and safety of obstetrical care. Pearlman (2006) reviewed the present state of quality outcome measures in obstetrics and provided an agenda for the future. In our view, the greatest impediment to deriving meaningful measures of obstetrical care is the continued use of administrative and financial data—instead of clinical data—to set benchmarks for outcomes such as rates of perinatal deaths, cesarean delivery, or third- or fourth-degree perineal lacerations.

Residency Training Work Hours

In 2003, the Accreditation Council for Graduate Medical Education (ACGME) set a national standard restructuring the resident physician workweek to a maximum 80 hours per week averaged over 4 weeks and limiting the longest consecutive period of work to 30 hours. These and other 2003 ACGME guidelines are shown in Table 1-4. Following this, the Institute of Medicine (IOM) (2008) commissioned a study to determine

factors of patient safety vis-a-vis resident work hours. The Institute recommended changes that are also listed in Table 1-4. These investigators concluded that costs incurred would range annually from $1.1 to $2.5 billion in 2006 dollars, but with unknown effectiveness.

As expected, some disagree with the IOM recommendation for swift implementation of these changes. Citing lack of evidence-based efficacy, inflexibility of the guidelines, and possible adverse effects on resident training, Blanchard and associates (2009) called for studies to determine factual effects before implementation. Indeed, there is evidence that the guidelines will likely adversely affect residency training in neurosurgery (Grady and colleagues, 2009; Jagannathan and co-workers, 2009).

At least in 2009, the plan is for the ACGME Duty Hours Congress to review available data as well as responses from various professional societies and boards. In 2010, the ACGME plans to revise Common Program Requirements. After this, individual Residency Review Committees will revise these for their own specialty specific requirements, which likely will be implemented in July 2011.

Electronic Medical Records

Rising costs and inconsistent quality are both significant challenges in the delivery of healthcare in the United States. Electronic health records have been identified as a means of improving the efficiency and effectiveness of healthcare providers (Jha and co-workers, 2009). Methods to speed the adoption of health information technology have received bipartisan support in Congress, and the American Recovery and Reinvestment Act of 2009 has made such a system a national priority. Jha and colleagues (2009) surveyed hospitals nationwide and found that only 1.5 percent had a comprehensive electronic records system. And only 17 percent of physicians reported using some type of electronic records system (DesRoches and colleagues, 2008). Obviously, implementation of an interconnected national system is a daunting task that will require many years.

Conflicts of Interest

According to Brennan and colleagues (2006), physician commitment to altruism, putting the interests of patients first, scientific integrity, and an absence of bias in medical decision making are regularly in conflict with financial interests. Although physician groups have instituted self-regulation, it is now widely per-

ceived that more stringent regulation is necessary. To this end, the American College of Obstetricians and Gynecologists (2008b) has published a *Committee Opinion* that details recommendations for relationships between physicians and industry.

Research

It has become increasingly recognized that although per capita healthcare expenditures in the United States are the highest in the world, healthcare outcomes not infrequently lag behind those in nations spending far less. A major factor in this disparity is thought to be expenditure overuse, underuse, and misuse driven by rationale- instead of evidence-based health care. To this end, the National Institutes of Health began a nationwide research program of Clinical and Translational Science Awards (CTSA) to enhance evidence-based health care. (National Center for Research Resources, 2009). The neutral premise of this approach is that successful healthcare interventions require systematic translation of developments from the basic sciences. We applaud this decision.

Medical Liability

The American College of Obstetricians and Gynecologists periodically surveys its fellows concerning the impact of professional liability on their practice. The 2006 Survey on Professional Liability is the ninth such survey since 1981 (Wilson and Strunk, 2007). The survey reflects experiences of more than 10,500 members, and some of these findings are listed in Table 1-5.

TABLE 1-5. 2006 Survey of Fellows on Professional Liability by the American College of Obstetricians and Gynecologists

Since 2003 Survey	Responses[a]
Practice change(s)	70 percent overall with one or more changes 30 percent increased number of cesarean deliveries 26 percent stopped performing VBACs 26 percent decreased number of high-risk patients 12 percent decreased number of deliveries 7 percent stopped all obstetrics
Open or closed claims	55 percent overall with one or more claim (62 percent obstetrics, 39 percent gynecology) • 31 percent—neurologically impaired infants • 16 percent—stillborn or neonatal death • 16 percent—shoulder dystocia • 11 percent—electronic fetal monitoring • 9 percent—resident physicians
Average paid claims	$505,000 all paid claims $1,150,000 for neurologically impaired infants $477,000 for other infant injury—major $259,000 for stillbirth or neonatal death
Co-defendants	42 percent—hospital 29 percent—partners 15 percent—residents 12 percent—nurses 11 percent—nonpartner OB-GYN 7 percent—anesthesiologists 4 percent—nurse midwives

[a]Percentages rounded off.
VBAC = vaginal birth after cesarean.
Data from Wilson and Strunk (2007).

Importantly, 70 percent of fellows responded that some aspect(s) of liability had changed their practice since last surveyed in 2003. Some of these changes undoubtedly were not positive.

Thus, by all accounts, there is still a "liability crisis" that is complex. Because it is largely driven by money and politics, a consensus seems unlikely. Although some interests are diametrically opposite, other factors contribute to its complexity. For example, each state has its own laws and opinions of "tort reform." Meanwhile, liability claims remain a "hot button" in obstetrics because of their inherent adversarial nature and the sometimes outlandish plaintiff verdicts that contribute to increasing liability insurance premiums. In some states, annual premiums for obstetricians approach $300,000—expenses that at least partially are borne by the patient, and certainly by the entire healthcare system. Liability issues are daunting, and in 2002, all tort costs in the United States totaled $233 billion—an astounding 2.2 percent of the *gross domestic product* and averaging $890 per citizen (Tillinghast-Towers Perrin, 2009).

Related to plaintiff awards, Hankins and co-workers (2006) reported that only 6 percent of premium payments will be used to underwrite medical expenses for a patient! This is in contrast to 22 percent for plaintiff lawyers' expenses and contingency fees. According to the *New York Times*, "The very phrase 'trial lawyer' has become associated with unadulterated greed; the Association of Trial Lawyers of America now calls itself the 'American Association for Justice'" (Glater, 2008). In their review, Berkowitz and colleagues (2009) compared them with Willie Sutton, the (in)famous bank robber who stole more than $600 million in his prolific career from the 1920s until the early 1950s.

The American College of Obstetricians and Gynecologists has taken a lead in adopting a fair system for malpractice litigation—or *maloccurrence litigation*. The Committee on Professional Liability has produced a number of related documents that help fellows cope with the stresses of litigation (2008a), provide advice for the obstetrician giving expert testimony (2007c), and that outline recommendations for disclosure of adverse events (2007b).

National liability reform likely will come in some form with the push for universal medical insurance coverage. President Obama, in his 2009 address to the American Medical Association, indicated that national malpractice liability reform was negotiable. U.S. Congressman Michael Burgess asked the president to reaffirm this commitment. We applaud their efforts and wish for their success.

Births to Immigrants

Persons born outside the United States comprised an estimated 11 percent of the population—more than 30 million people (Gold, 2003). Approximately a third are undocumented—here illegally or with an expired visa—and this proportion has increased tenfold over the past 30 years (Goldman and colleagues, 2006). According to the Pew Hispanic Center (2009), 57 percent of immigrants are from Mexico, 24 percent from Latin America, and the remainder from Asia, Europe, and Africa. The American College of Obstetricians and Gynecologists (2009a) has taken the position that all immigrants within our borders should receive basic health care.

Family Planning Services

Politics and religion over the years have led to a variety of governmental interferences with the reproductive rights of women.

These interferences have disparately affected indigent women and teenagers. An example from the recent past is the consideration by Congress in 1998 of the Title X Parental Notification Act to mandate parental notification for minors seeking contraception at federally funded clinics. Reddy and colleagues (2002) reported that this would have dissuaded almost half of girls younger than 17 years from seeking contraceptive services and testing or treatment for sexually transmitted disease. The increased number of unintended teenage pregnancies and abortions that would inevitably ensue are discussed subsequently.

A recent example is the tug-of-war over emergency contraception, and more specifically over the *morning-after pill* (see Chap. 32, p. 692). The 2004 decision by the Bush Administration to override the 23 to 4 vote to approve *Plan B* for over-the-counter sales to 17-year-old women was decried appropriately by editorials in the *New England Journal of Medicine* (Drazen and colleagues, 2004; Steinbrook, 2004). This was overturned in April 2009 by a federal district court in New York that ordered the Food and Drug Administration (FDA) to make emergency contraception available over the counter to women 17 years or older. The American College of Obstetricians and Gynecologists (2009b) lauded the decision, citing the more than 800,000 yearly teenage pregnancies in this country and the fact that many are terminated. Also cited were data showing that most adolescents have sex for the first time at age 17.

Perhaps the most egregious example of both federal and state governmental intrusion into women's reproductive rights is the often poor availability of federally funded family planning services for indigent women. This is despite all reports of the overwhelming success of such programs. According to the Guttmacher Institute (2009), publicly funded family planning services in 2006 prevented nearly 2 million unintended pregnancies and 800,000 abortions in the United States (Fig. 1-5). They conclude that without such funding the abortion rate would be nearly two thirds higher for all women, and nearly twice as high for poor women.

Teenage Pregnancy

In 2006, there were almost a half million births to women aged 15 to 19 years (Centers for Disease Control and Prevention, 2009). The national rate was 42 births per 1000 females aged 15 to 19 years. Although this rate is substantively reduced compared with 77 per 1000 in 1990, measures to lower it further should remain a

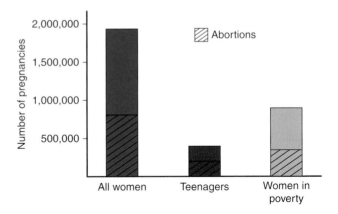

FIGURE 1-5 Number of unintended pregnancies including elective abortions prevented in 2006 by publicly funded clinics. (Data approximated from reports by the Guttmacher Institute, 2009.)

top priority. Like abortion, teen pregnancy is a complex situation and is influenced by strong opinions and religious ideology that have in some cases resulted in blocked access to family planning services for teenagers. Another confounding factor is that it is related to the prevalence of sex education in schools.

Despite the successes of family planning programs described above, and usually driven by sociopolitical concerns, a number of states have linked funding to "abstinence-only" counseling and to exclusion of family planning counseling that include abortion topics. Writing in *Newsweek*, Anna Quindlen (2009) concluded that "Congress has poured $1.5 billion into what is essentially anti-sex ed, abstinence-only programs, despite the following facts: They don't work. They're actually counterproductive."

Even worse, some states have diverted funds from family planning services and put them into programs for abstinence-only counseling. In this regard, Texas may serve as the worst-case example. According to the *Dallas Morning News* (2009), 96 percent of Texas school districts, yielding to pressure from the Board of Education, either teach abstinence-only counseling or avoid talking about sex entirely. It is thus not surprising to many that Texas has been ranked in the top five states for teenage-pregnancy rates over the past several years. In 2006, according to the Centers for Disease Control and Prevention as reported by Ventura (2009), Texas ranked number one with 63 births per 1000 females aged 15 to 19 years. This compared with the national average of 42 per 1000. And Alaska—another state that has recently showcased its abstinence programs—led the nation with a 19-percent increase in the teenage birth rate from 2005 to 2006.

Abortion

It continues to be a sad fact that up to a fourth of pregnancies in this country are terminated by elective abortion. According to the American College of Obstetricians and Gynecologists (2007a): "The most effective way to reduce the number of abortions is to prevent unwanted and unintended pregnancies." Importantly, the negative attitudes, beliefs, and policies toward family planning services and sex education discussed above have helped to contribute to the 1 million or so abortions performed yearly in the United States.

The history of legislative regulation and federal court decisions regarding abortions is considered in Chapter 9 (p. 227). At the time of the 22nd edition of this book, the *Partial Birth Abortion Ban Act of 2003* had been signed into law. In 2007, the United States Supreme Court ruled that the ban—officially known as *Gonzales v. Carhart*—is constitutional. This again caused editorialists in the *New England Journal of Medicine* to decry the intrusion of government in medicine (Charo, 2007; Drazen, 2007; Greene, 2007). Since that time, negative effects on abortion services and training have been reported (Haddad and colleagues, 2009; Weitz and Yanow, 2008).

Healthcare Reform

Many readers of this textbook can remember when the Clinton administration was unsuccessful in passing healthcare reform legislation. Now, more than 15 years later, healthcare reform once again has been made a priority by the Obama administration. By mid-2009, momentum was building for policies that would move the United States toward universal health insurance (Mello and associates, 2009, Oberlander, 2009).

TABLE 1-6. Four Key Factors Implicated in the High Costs of Health Care in the United States

1. Higher administrative costs
2. Higher wages for healthcare workers and professionals
3. Greater use of expensive technological interventions
4. Unnecessary or inappropriate care

From Sessions and Detsky (2009).

To put pregnancy-related health care into perspective, a fifth of the $875 billion charged by U.S. hospitals in 2005 was for treatment of five conditions: (1) pregnancy and childbirth, (2) infant care, (3) coronary artery disease, (4) heart attack, and (5) congestive heart failure (Andrews and Elixhauser, 2009). Health care is the largest industry in this country, employing 13.5 million workers—10 percent of the total workforce (Sessions and Detsky, 2009). And importantly, 5.5 percent of the gross domestic product (GDP) went to health care 50 years ago compared with 16 percent currently.

Four key driving forces considered responsible for the escalating cost of health care in the United States are shown in Table 1-6. Like other healthcare providers, we too have had to increasingly grapple with layer upon layer of bureaucracy. No wonder that 27 percent of the total jobs in the healthcare workforce are devoted to administrative functions! In the midst of all this, given its large role in the healthcare economy, it seems clear that perinatal care will figure prominently in any reform movement. Along with others, we nervously await implementation.

REFERENCES

American Academy of Pediatrics and the American College of Obstetricians and Gynecologists: Guidelines for Perinatal Care, 6th ed. Washington, DC, AAP and ACOG, 2007

American College of Obstetricians and Gynecologists: Abortion policy. Statement of policy reaffirmed. July 2007a

American College of Obstetricians and Gynecologists: Disclosure and discussion of adverse events. Committee Opinion No. 380, October 2007b

American College of Obstetricians and Gynecologists: Expert testimony. Committee Opinion No. 374, August 2007c

American College of Obstetricians and Gynecologists: Coping with the stress of medical professional liability litigation. Committee Opinion No. 406, May 2008a

American College of Obstetricians and Gynecologists: Relationships with industry. Committee opinion No. 401, March 2008b

American College of Obstetricians and Gynecologists: Health care for undocumented immigrants. Committee Opinion No. 425, January 2009a

American College of Obstetricians and Gynecologists: ACOG lauds court decision regarding emergency contraception. ACOG News Release, 2009b

Andrews RM, Elixhauser A: The national hospital bill: Growth trends and 2005 update on the most expensive conditions by payer. HCU Project Statistical Brief #43, December 2007. Rockville, MD, Agency for Healthcare Research and Quality. Available at: http://www.hcupus.ahrq.gov/reports/statbriefs/sb42.pdf. Accessed May 8, 2009

Berg CJ, Harper MA, Atkinson SM, et al: Preventability of pregnancy-related deaths. Results of a state-wide review. Obstet Gynecol 106:1228, 2005

Berkowitz RL, Hankins G, Waldman R, et al: A proposed model for managing cases of neurologically impaired infants. Obstet Gynecol 113:683, 2009

Blanchard MS, Meltzer D, Polonsky KS: To nap or not to nap? Residents' work hours revisited. N Engl J Med 360(21):2242, 2009

Brennan TA, Rothman DJ, Blank L, et al: Health industry practices that create conflicts of interest. A policy proposal for academic medical centers. JAMA 295:429, 2006

Callaghan WM, MacKay AP, Berg CJ: Identification of severe maternal morbidity during delivery hospitalizations, United States 1991–2003. Am J Obstet Gynecol 199:133.e1, 2008

Centers for Disease Control and Prevention: Abortion Surveillance-United States, 2005. MMWR 57(SS13):2008

Centers for Disease Control and Prevention: Births and natality. FastStats. Available at: http://www.cdc.gov/nchs/fastats/births.htm. Accessed May 8, 2009

Centers for Disease Control and Prevention and Health Resources and Service Administration: Maternal, infant, and child health. In: Healthy People 2010, conference ed. Atlanta, GA, CDC, 2000

Chang J, Elam—Evans LD, Berg CJ, et al: Pregnancy-related mortality surveillance-United States, 1991–1999. MMWR 52(SS-2):4, 2003

Charo RA: The partial death of abortion rights. N Engl J Med 356:2125, 2007

Cherry DK, Burk CW, Woodwell DA: National Ambulatory Medical Care Survey: 2001 Summary: Advance data from vital and health statistics, Vol 51, No 337. Hyattsville, MD, National Center for Health Statistics, 2003

Clark SL, Belfort MA, Dildy GA, et al: Maternal death in the 21st century: Causes, prevention, and relationship to cesarean delivery. Am J Obstet Gynecol 199(1):36.e1, 2008

Dallas Morning News: Get real about sex: Texas schools' reliance on abstinence fails teens. Editorial. March 3, 2009

Deneux-Tharaux C, Carmona E, Bouvier-Colle MH, et al: Postpartum maternal mortality and cesarean delivery. Obstet Gynecol 108:541, 2006

DesRoches CM, Campbell EG, Rao SR, et al: Electronic health records in ambulatory care—a national survey of physicians. N Engl J Med 359:50, 2008

Drazen JM: Government in medicine. N Engl J Med 356:2195, 2007

Drazen JM, Greene MF, Wood AJJ: The FDA, politics, and Plan B. N Engl J Med 350:1561, 2004

Glater JD: To the trenches: The tort war is raging on. New York Times, June 22, 2008

Gold RB: Immigrants and Medicaid after welfare reform. Guttmacher Rep Public Policy 6(2):6, 2003

Goldman DP, Smith JP, Sood N: Immigrants and the cost of medical care. Health Aff 25:1700, 2006

Grady MS, Batjer HH, Dacey RG: Resident duty hour regulation and public safety: Establishing a balance between concerns about resident fatigue and adequate training in neurosurgery. J Neurosurg 110(5):828, 2009

Greene MF: The intimidation of American physicians—Banning partial-birth abortion. 356:2128, 2007

Grobman WA: Patient safety in obstetrics and gynecology. The call to arms. Obstet Gynecol 108(5):1058, 2006

Guttmacher Institute: Facts on publicly funded contraceptive devices in the United States. Available at: http://www.guttmacher.org/pubs/fb_contraceptive_serv.html. Accessed May 8, 2009

Haddad L, Yanow S, Delli-Bovi L, et al: Changes in abortion provider practices in response to the Partial-Birth Abortion Ban Act of 2003. Contraception 79(5):379, 2009

Hall NJ, DeFrances CJ: 2001 National Hospital Discharge Survey: Advance data from vital and health statistics, Vol 51, No 332. Hyattsville, MD, National Center for Health Statistics, 2003

Hamilton BE: Reproduction rates for 1990–2002 and intrinsic rates for 1990–2001: United States. National Vital Statistics Reports, Vol 52, No 17. Hyattsville, MD, National Center for Health Statistics, 2004

Hankins GDV, MacLennan AH, Speer ME, et al: Obstetric litigation is asphyxiating our maternity services. Obstet Gynecol 107:1382, 2006

Heron MP: Deaths: Leading causes for 2004. National vital statistics reports; Vol 56, No 5. Hyattsville, MD, National Center for Health Statistics, 2007

Hoyert DL: Maternal mortality and related concepts. National Center for Health Statistics. Vital Health Stat 3(33):1, 2007

Institute of Medicine: Resident duty hours: Enhancing sleep, supervision, and safety. December 2, 2008

Jagannathan J, Vates GE, Pouratian N, et al: Impact of the Accreditation Council for Graduate Medical Education work-hour regulations on neurosurgical resident education and productivity. J Neurosurg 110(5):820, 200

Jha AK, DesRoches CM, Campbell EG, et al: Use of electronic health records in U.S. hospitals. N Engl J Med 360:1628, 2009

Khan KS, Wojdyla D, Say L, et al: WHO analysis of causes of maternal death: A systematic review. Lancet 367:1066, 2006

Knight M, Kurinczuk JJ, Tuffnell D, et al: the UK obstetric surveillance system for rare disorders of pregnancy. BJOG 112:263, 2005

Knight M on behalf of UKOSS: Antenatal pulmonary embolism: Risk factors, management and outcomes. BJOG 115:453, 2008

Kohn LT, Corrigan JM, Donaldson MS, editors. To err is human: Building a safer health system. Washington, DC, National Academy Press, 2000

Koonin LM, MacKay AP, Berg CJ, et al: Pregnancy-related mortality surveillance—United States, 1987–1990. MMWR 46:127, 1997

Kuklina EV, Meikle SF, Jamieson DJ, et al: Severe obstetric morbidity in the Unites States: 1998-2005. Obstet Gynecol 113:293, 2009

Kung HC, Hoyert DL, Xu J, et al: Deaths: Final data for 2005. National Vital Statistics Reports 56(10):1, 1008

Lang CT, King JC: Maternal mortality in the United States. Best Pract Res Clin Obstet Gynaecol 22(3):5117, 2008

Lawn JE, Cousens S, Zupan J et al: 4 million neonatal deaths: When? Where? Why? Lancet 365(9462):891, 2005

MacDorman MF, Kirmeyer S: Fetal and perinatal mortality, United States, 2005. National Vital Statistic Reports 57(8), 2009

Martin JA, Hamilton BE, Sutton PD, et al: Births: Final data for 2006. National Vital Statistics Reports; Vol 57, No 7. Hyattsville, MD, National Center for Health Statistics, 2009

Mathews TJ, MacDorman MF: Infant mortality statistics from the 2005 period linked birth/infant death data set. National Vital Statistics Reports; Vol 57, No 2. Hyattsville, MD, National Center for Health Statistics, 2008

Meikle SF, Steiner CA, Zhang J, et al: A national estimate of the elective primary cesarean delivery rate. Obstet Gynecol 105:751, 2005

Mello MM, Brennan TA: The role of medical liability reform in federal health care reform. N Engl J Med 361(1):1, 2009

Menacker F, Declercq E, MacDorman MF: Cesarean delivery: Background, trends, and epidemiology. Semin Perinatol 30:235, 2006

National Center for Research Resources: Clinical and Translational Science Awards. NCRR Fact Sheet, April 2009. Available at: http://www.ncrr.nih.gov/publications/pdf/NCRR_Fact_Sheet_CTSA_Final_2_508.pdf. Accessed May 9, 2009

National Institutes of Health State-of-the-Science Conference Statement: Cesarean delivery on maternal request. Obstet Gynecol 107(6):1386, 2006

Nicholson WK, Frick KD, Powe NR: Economic burden of hospitalizations for preterm labor in the United States. Obstet Gynecol 96:95, 2000

Nuckols TK, Bhattacharya J, Wolman DM, et al: Cost implications of reduced work hours and workloads for resident physicians. N Engl J Med 360(21):2242, 2009

Oberlander J: Great expectations—The Obama administration and health care reform. N Engl J Med 360(4):321, 2009

Office of Disease Prevention and Health Promotion: Healthy people 2020: The road ahead. U.S Department of Health and Human Services. Revised 31 Mar 2009

Pearlman MD: Patient safety in obstetrics and gynecology. An agenda for the future. Obstet Gynecol 108(5):1266, 2006

Petraglia F: President's Newsletter. Society for Gynecologic Investigation. September 2008

Pew Hispanic Center: Unauthorized migrants: Numbers and characteristics. Washington, DC, PHC, 2005. Available at: http://pewhispanic.org/files/reports/46.pdf. Accessed May 9, 2009

Quindlen A: Let's talk about sex. The Last Word. Newsweek, March 16, 2009

Reddy DM, Fleming R, Swain C: Effect of mandatory parental notification on adolescent girls' use of sexual health care services. JAMA 288:710, 2002

Reddy UM, Spong CY: Introduction. Semin Perinatol 30(5):233, 2006

Schoendorf KC, Branum AM: The use of United States vital statistics in perinatal and obstetric research. Am J Obstet Gynecol 194:911, 2006

Sessions SY, Detsky AS: Employment and U.S. health care reform. JAMA 301(17):1811, 2009

St. John EB, Nelson KG, Cliver SP, et al: Cost of neonatal care according to gestational age at birth and survival status. Am J Obstet Gynecol 182:170, 2000

Steinbrook R: Waiting for plan B—The FDA and nonprescription use of emergency contraception. N Engl J Med 350:2327, 2004

Tillinghast-Towers Perrin. U.S. tort costs: 2003 update. Trends and findings on the costs of the U.S. tort system. Available at: http://www.towersperrin.com/tillinghast/publications/reports/2003_Tort_Costs_Update/Tort_Costs_Trends_2003_Update.pdf. Accessed March 29, 2009

Ventura SJ: Changing patterns of nonmarital childbearing in the United States. National Center for Health Statistics Data Brief No. 18, May 2009

Ventura SJ, Mosher WD, Curtin SC, et al: Highlights of trends in pregnancies and pregnancy rates by outcome: Estimates for the United States, 1976–96. National Vital Statistics Report, Vol 47, No 29. Hyattsville, MD, National Center for Health Statistics, 1999

Weitz TA, Yanow S: Implications of the Federal Abortion Ban for Women's Health in the United States. Reprod Health Matters 16(31 Suppl):99, 2008

Wen SW, Huang L, Liston R, et al: Severe maternal morbidity in Canada, 1991–2001. CMAJ 173(7):759, 2005

Wilson N, Strunk AL: Overview of the 2006 ACOG survey on professional liability. ACOG Clinical Review 12(2):1, 2007

Zwart JJ, Richters JM, Ory F, et al: Severe maternal morbidity during pregnancy, delivery and puerperium in the Netherlands: A nationwide population-based study of 371,000 pregnancies. BJOG 115(7):842, 2008

SECTION 2

MATERNAL AND FETAL ANATOMY AND PHYSIOLOGY

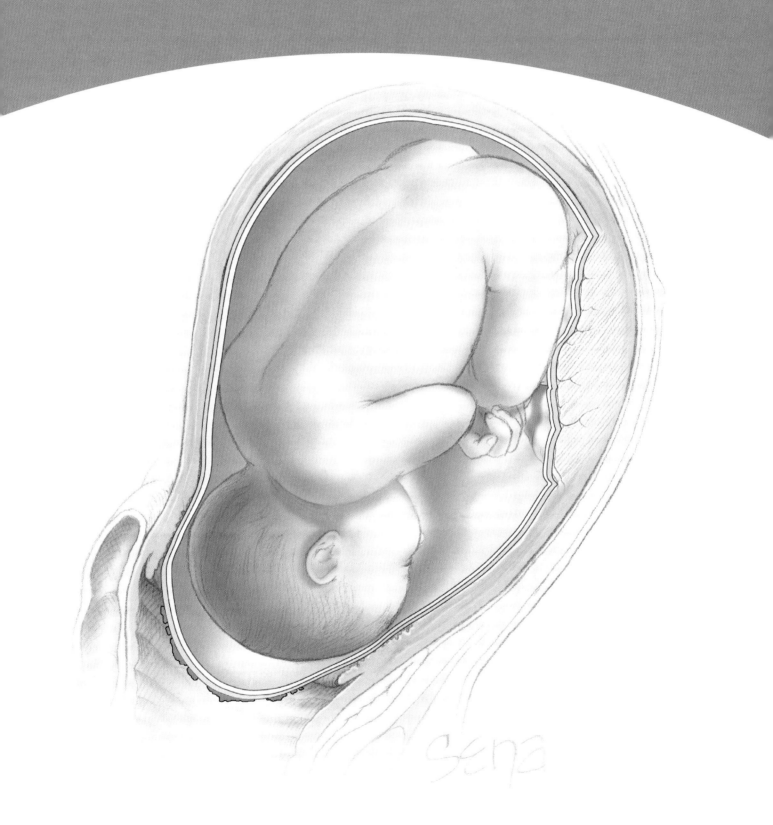

Maternal Anatomy

An understanding of the anatomy of the female pelvis and lower abdominal wall is essential for obstetrical practice. There may be marked variation in anatomical structures in individual women, and this is especially true for major blood vessels and nerves.

ANTERIOR ABDOMINAL WALL

The anterior abdominal wall confines abdominal viscera, stretches to accommodate the expanding uterus, and provides surgical access to the internal reproductive organs. Thus, a comprehensive knowledge of its layered structure is required to surgically enter the peritoneal cavity.

Skin

Langer lines describe the orientation of dermal fibers within the skin. In the anterior abdominal wall, they are arranged transversely. As a result, vertical skin incisions sustain increased lateral tension and thus, in general, develop wider scars. In contrast, low transverse incisions, such as the Pfannenstiel, follow Langer lines and lead to superior cosmetic results.

Subcutaneous Layer

This layer can be separated into a superficial, predominantly fatty layer—*Camper fascia,* and a deeper, more membranous layer—*Scarpa fascia.* These are not discrete layers but instead represent a continuum of the subcutaneous tissue layer.

Rectus Sheath

The fibrous aponeuroses of the external oblique, internal oblique, and transversus abdominis muscles join in the midline to create the *rectus sheath* (Fig. 2-1). The construction of this sheath varies above and below a demarcation line, termed the *arcuate line.* Cephalad to this line, the aponeuroses invest the rectus abdominis bellies above and below. Caudal to this line, all aponeuroses lie anterior to the rectus abdominis muscle, and only the thin transversalis fascia and peritoneum lie beneath.

In the lower abdomen, transition from the muscular to the fibrous aponeurotic component of the external oblique muscles takes place along a vertical line through the anterosuperior iliac spine. Transition from muscle to aponeurosis for the internal oblique and transversus abdominis muscles takes place more medially. For this reason, muscle fibers of the internal oblique are often noted below the aponeurotic layer of the external oblique during creation of low transverse incisions.

Blood Supply

Femoral Artery Branches

The *superficial epigastric, superficial circumflex iliac,* and *external pudendal* arteries arise from the femoral artery just below the inguinal ligament in the region of the femoral triangle (see Fig. 2-1). These vessels supply the skin and subcutaneous layers of the anterior abdominal wall and mons pubis. The superficial epigastric vessels course diagonally toward the umbilicus. During low transverse skin incision creation, the superficial epigastric vessels can usually be identified at a depth halfway between the skin and the rectus fascia, several centimeters from the midline.

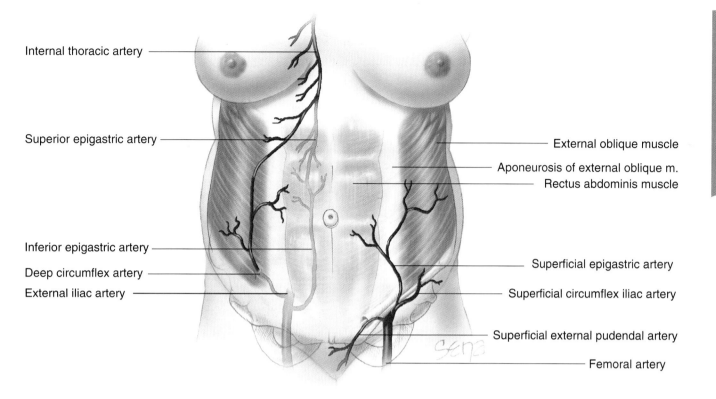

Internal thoracic artery

Superior epigastric artery

Inferior epigastric artery

Deep circumflex artery

External iliac artery

External oblique muscle

Aponeurosis of external oblique m.

Rectus abdominis muscle

Superficial epigastric artery

Superficial circumflex iliac artery

Superficial external pudendal artery

Femoral artery

FIGURE 2-1 Muscles and blood vessels of the anterior abdominal wall.

External Iliac Artery Branches

The *inferior "deep" epigastric vessels* and *deep circumflex iliac vessels* are branches of the external iliac vessels. They supply the muscles and fascia of the anterior abdominal wall. The inferior epigastric vessels initially course lateral to, then posterior to the rectus muscles, which they supply. They then pass anterior to the posterior rectus sheath and course between the sheath and the rectus muscles. Near the umbilicus, the inferior epigastric vessels anastomose with the superior epigastric artery and veins, branches of the internal thoracic vessels.

Hesselbach triangle is the region in the anterior abdominal wall bounded inferiorly by the inguinal ligament, medially by the lateral border of the rectus muscles, and laterally by the inferior epigastric vessels. Direct hernias protrude through the abdominal wall in Hesselbach triangle, whereas indirect hernias do so through the deep inguinal ring lying lateral to this triangle.

Innervation

The anterior abdominal wall is innervated by the abdominal extensions of the intercostal nerves (T_{7-11}), the subcostal nerve (T_{12}), and the iliohypogastric and the ilioinguinal nerves (L_1). The T_{10} dermatome approximates the level of the umbilicus.

The iliohypogastric nerve provides sensation to the skin over the suprapubic area. The ilioinguinal nerve supplies the skin of the lower abdominal wall and upper portion of the labia majora and medial portion of the thigh through its inguinal branch. These two nerves pass 2 to 3 cm medial to the anterior superior iliac spine and course between the layers of the rectus sheath (Whiteside and colleagues, 2003). The ilioinguinal and iliohy-

pogastric nerves can be entrapped during closure of low transverse incisions, especially if incisions extend beyond the lateral borders of the rectus muscle. These nerves carry sensory information only, and injury leads to loss of sensation within the areas supplied.

EXTERNAL GENERATIVE ORGANS

Vulva

The *pudenda*—commonly designated the *vulva*—includes all structures visible externally from the pubis to the perineal body. This includes the mons pubis, labia majora and minora, clitoris, hymen, vestibule, urethral opening, and greater vestibular or Bartholin glands, minor vestibular glands, and paraurethral glands (Fig. 2-2). The embryology of the external genitalia is discussed in Chapter 4 (p. 98).

Mons Pubis

Also called the *mons veneris*, this fat-filled cushion overlies the symphysis pubis. After puberty, the skin of the mons pubis is covered by curly hair that forms the *escutcheon*. In women, it is distributed in a triangular area, the base of which is formed by the upper margin of the symphysis. In men and in some hirsute women, the escutcheon is not so well circumscribed and extends onto the anterior abdominal wall toward the umbilicus.

Labia Majora

Embryologically, the labia majora are homologous with the male scrotum. These structures vary somewhat in appearance,

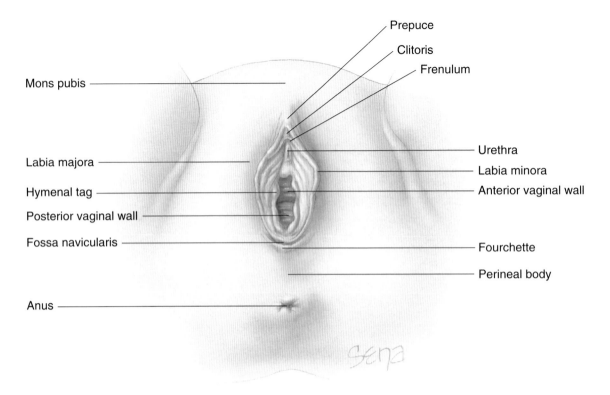

FIGURE 2-2 External female reproductive organs.

principally according to the amount of fat they contain. They are 7 to 8 cm in length, 2 to 3 cm in depth, and 1 to 1.5 cm in thickness. They are continuous directly with the mons pubis superiorly, and the round ligaments terminate at their upper borders. Posteriorly, the labia majora taper and merge into the area overlying the perineal body to form the *posterior commissure.*

The outer surface of the labia majora is covered with hair, whereas on their inner surface, it is absent. In addition, apocrine and sebaceous glands are abundant. Beneath the skin, there is a dense connective tissue layer, which is nearly void of muscular elements but is rich in elastic fibers and adipose tissue. This mass of fat provides bulk to the labia majora and is supplied with a rich venous plexus. During pregnancy, this vasculature commonly develops varicosities, especially in parous women, from increased venous pressure created by advancing uterine weight. They present as engorged tortuous veins or as small grapelike clusters but are typically asymptomatic.

Labia Minora

Each is a thin fold of tissue, which lies medial to each labia majora. In males, its homologue forms the ventral shaft of the penis. The labia minora extend superiorly, where each divides into two lamellae. The lower pair fuses to form the *frenulum of the clitoris,* and the upper pair merges to form the *prepuce.* Inferiorly, the labia minora extend to approach the midline as low ridges of tissue that fuse to form the *fourchette.*

Structurally, the labia minora are composed of connective tissue with many vessels, elastin fibers, and some smooth muscle fibers. They are supplied with a variety of nerve endings and are extremely sensitive. The epithelia of the labia minora vary with location. Stratified squamous epithelium covers the outer surface of each labium. The lateral portion of the inner surface is covered by stratified squamous epithelium to a demarcating line—the *Hart line.* Medial to this line, each labium is covered by squamous epithelium that is nonkeratinized. Although the labia minora lack hair follicles, eccrine glands, and apocrine glands, there are many sebaceous glands.

Clitoris

This principal female erogenous organ is the erectile homologue of the penis and is located beneath the prepuce and above the urethra. It projects downward between the branched extremities of the labia minora, and the free end points downward and inward toward the vaginal opening.

The clitoris rarely exceeds 2 cm in length and is composed of a glans, a corpus or body, and two crura. The *glans* is usually less than 0.5 cm in diameter, is composed of spindle-shaped cells, and is covered by stratified squamous epithelium that is richly innervated. The *clitoral body* contains two corpora cavernosa. Beneath the ventral surface of this body, homologues of the corpora spongiosa unite to form a commissure. These homologues are anterior extensions of the vestibular bulbs (O'Connell and DeLancey, 2006). Extending from the clitoral body, each corpora cavernosa diverges laterally to form the long, narrow *crura.* These lie along the inferior surface of the ischiopubic rami and deep to the ischiocavernosus muscles.

Vestibule

The vestibule is the functionally mature female structure derived from the embryonic urogenital membrane. In adult women, it is an almond-shaped area that is enclosed by Hart line laterally, the external surface of the hymen medially, the clitoral frenulum anteriorly, and the fourchette posteriorly. The vestibule usually is perforated by six openings: the urethra, the vagina, two Bartholin gland ducts, and at times, two ducts of the largest paraurethral glands—the Skene glands (see Fig. 2-2). The posterior portion of the vestibule between the fourchette and the vaginal opening is called the *fossa navicularis*. It is usually observed only in nulliparous women.

Vestibular Glands

The pair of *Bartholin glands,* also termed greater vestibular glands*,* are the major glands. They measure 0.5 to 1 cm in diameter. They lie inferior to the vestibular bulbs and deep to the inferior ends of the bulbocavernosus muscle on either side of the vaginal opening. Their ducts are 1.5 to 2 cm long and open distal to the hymenal ring at 5 and 7 o'clock. Following trauma or infection, either duct may swell and obstruct to form a cyst or if infected, an abscess.

The *paraurethral glands* are collectively an arborization of glands whose ducts open predominantly along the entire inferior aspect of the urethra. The two largest are called *Skene glands*, and their ducts typically lie distally near the urethral meatus. Inflammation and duct obstruction of any of the paraurethral glands can lead to urethral diverticulum formation. The *minor vestibular glands* are shallow glands lined by simple mucin-secreting epithelium and open along Hart line.

Urethral Opening

The lower two thirds of the urethra lie immediately above the anterior vaginal wall. The urethral opening or meatus is in the midline of the vestibule, 1 to 1.5 cm below the pubic arch, and a short distance above the vaginal opening.

Vestibular Bulbs

Embryologically, the vestibular bulbs correspond to the corpus spongiosum of the penis. These are almond-shaped aggregations of veins, 3 to 4 cm long, 1 to 2 cm wide, and 0.5 to 1 cm thick, which lie beneath the bulbocavernosus muscle on either side of the vestibule. The bulbs terminate inferiorly at approximately the middle of the vaginal opening and extend upward toward the clitoris. Their anterior extensions merge in the midline, below the clitoral body. During childbirth, the vestibular bulbs may be injured and may even rupture to create a vulvar hematoma.

Vaginal Opening and Hymen

The vaginal opening is rimmed distally by the hymen or its remnants. In adult women, the hymen is a membrane of varying thickness that surrounds the vaginal opening more or less completely. It is composed mainly of elastic and collagenous connective tissue, and both outer and inner surfaces are covered by stratified squamous epithelium. The aperture of the hymen ranges in diameter from pinpoint to one that admits the tip of one or even two fingers. *Imperforate hymen* is a rare lesion in which the vaginal orifice is occluded completely, causing retention of menstrual blood (see Chap. 40, p. 892).

As a rule, however, the hymen is torn at several sites during first coitus. Identical tears may occur by other penetration, for example, tampons used during menstruation. The edges of the torn tissue soon re-epithelialize. In pregnant women, the epithelium of the hymen is thick, and the tissue is rich in glycogen. Changes produced in the hymen by childbirth are usually readily recognizable. Over time, the hymen consists of several nodules of various sizes, also termed *hymenal caruncles.*

Vagina

This musculomembranous structure extends from the vulva to the uterus and is interposed anteriorly and posteriorly between the bladder and the rectum. The upper portion arises from the müllerian ducts, and the lower portion is formed from the urogenital sinus (see Fig. 40-1, p. 891). Anteriorly, the vagina is separated from the bladder and urethra by connective tissue— the *vesicovaginal septum.* Posteriorly, between the lower portion of the vagina and the rectum, there are similar tissues that together form the *rectovaginal septum.* The upper fourth of the vagina is separated from the rectum by the *recto-uterine pouch,* also called the *cul-de-sac of Douglas.*

Normally, the anterior and posterior vaginal walls lie in contact, with only a slight space intervening between the lateral margins. Vaginal length varies considerably, but commonly, the anterior and posterior vaginal walls are, respectively, 6 to 8 cm and 7 to 10 cm in length. During her lifetime, the average woman may have a shortening of her vagina by 0.8 cm (Tan and associates, 2006). The upper end of the vaginal vault is subdivided into anterior, posterior, and two lateral fornices by the cervix. These are of considerable clinical importance because the internal pelvic organs usually can be palpated through their thin walls. Moreover, the posterior fornix provides surgical access to the peritoneal cavity.

At the midportion of the vagina, its lateral walls are attached to the pelvic walls by visceral connective tissue. These lateral attachments blend into investing fascia of the levator ani muscles. In doing so, they create the anterior and posterior lateral *vaginal sulci.* These run the length of the vaginal sidewalls and give the vagina an H shape when viewed in cross section. There are numerous thin transverse ridges, known as *rugae*, found along the length of the anterior and posterior vaginal walls.

Histology

The vaginal lining is composed of nonkeratinized stratified squamous epithelium and underlying lamina propria. Below this there is a muscular layer, which consists of smooth muscle, collagen, and elastin. Beneath this muscularis lies an adventitial layer consisting of collagen and elastin (Weber and Walters, 1997). There are no vaginal glands. Instead, the vagina is lubricated by a transudate that originates from the vaginal subepithelial capillary plexus and crosses the permeable epithelial layer (Gorodeski, 2005). Due to increased vascularity during pregnancy, vaginal secretions are notably increased. At times, this may be confused with amnionic fluid leakage, and clinical differentiation of these two is described in Chapter 17 (p. 392).

After birth, fragments of stratified epithelium occasionally are embedded beneath the vaginal surface. Similar to its native tissue, this buried epithelium continues to shed degenerated cells and keratin. As a result, firm *epidermal inclusion cysts,* which are filled with keratin debris, may form.

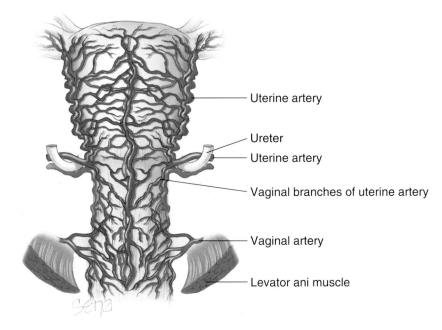

Uterine artery

Ureter

Uterine artery

Vaginal branches of uterine artery

Vaginal artery

Levator ani muscle

FIGURE 2-3 Uterine and vaginal blood supply. The origin of the vaginal artery varies and may arise from the uterine, inferior vesical, or internal iliac artery.

Vascular and Lymphatic Supply

The vagina has an abundant vascular supply (Fig. 2-3). The proximal portion is supplied by the cervical branch of the uterine artery and by the vaginal artery. The latter may variably arise from the uterine, inferior vesical, or directly from the internal iliac artery. The middle rectal artery contributes to supply the posterior vaginal wall, whereas the distal walls receive contributions from the internal pudendal artery. At each level, blood supply from each side anastomoses on the anterior and posterior vaginal walls with contralateral corresponding vessels.

An extensive venous plexus immediately surrounds the vagina and follows the course of the arteries. Lymphatics from the lower third, along with those of the vulva, drain primarily into the inguinal lymph nodes. Those from the middle third drain into the internal iliac nodes, and those from the upper third drain into the external, internal, and common iliac nodes.

Perineum

The perineum is the diamond-shaped area between the thighs. The anterior, posterior, and lateral boundaries of the perineum are the same as those of the bony pelvic outlet: the pubic symphysis anteriorly, ischiopubic rami and ischial tuberosities anterolaterally, sacrotuberous ligaments posterolaterally, and coccyx posteriorly.

Anterior Triangle

An arbitrary line joining the ischial tuberosities divides the perineum into an anterior triangle, also called the *urogenital triangle*, and a posterior triangle, termed the *anal triangle* (Fig. 2-4). The anterior triangle is bounded by the pubic rami superiorly,

the ischial tuberosities laterally, and the superficial transverse perineal muscle posteriorly.

The anterior triangle is further divided into superficial and deep spaces by the *perineal membrane*. This is a sheet of dense fibrous tissue and was previously known as the *inferior fascia of the urogenital diaphragm*. The perineal membrane attaches laterally to the ischiopubic rami, medially to the distal third of the urethra and vagina, and posteriorly to the perineal body. Anteriorly, it attaches to the arcuate ligament of the pubis.

Superficial Space of the Anterior Triangle. This space is bounded deeply by the perineal membrane and superficially by Colles fascia. It is a closed compartment, and infection or bleeding within it remains contained. The anterior triangle contains several important structures that include the ischiocavernosus, bulbocavernosus, and superficial transverse perineal muscles; Bartholin glands; vestibular bulbs; clitoral body and crura; and branches of the pudendal vessels and nerve (see Fig. 2-4).

The *ischiocavernosus muscle* attaches to the medial aspect of the ischial tuberosities inferiorly and the ischiopubic rami laterally. Anteriorly, it attaches to the crus of the clitoris. This muscle may help maintain clitoral erection by compressing the crus to obstruct venous drainage. The *bulbocavernosus muscles* overlie the vestibular bulbs and Bartholin glands. They attach to the body of the clitoris anteriorly and the perineal body posteriorly. The muscles constrict the vaginal lumen and aid release of secretions from the Bartholin glands. They also may contribute to clitoral erection by compressing the deep dorsal vein of the clitoris. The bulbocavernosus and ischiocavernosus muscles also pull the clitoris downward. The *superficial transverse perineal muscles* are narrow strips that attach to the ischial tuberosities laterally and the perineal body medially. They may be attenuated or even absent, but when present, they contribute to the perineal body (Corton and Cunningham, 2008).

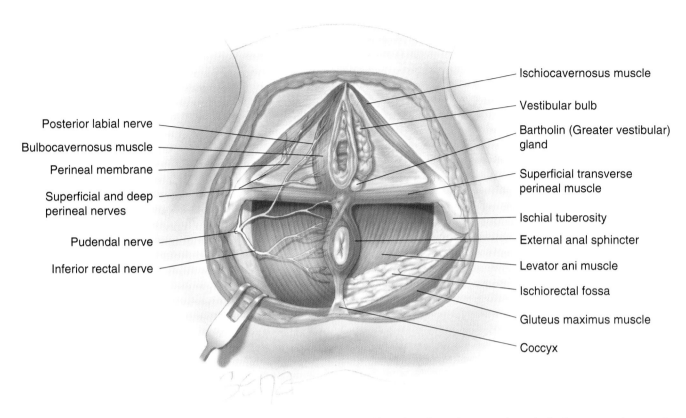

FIGURE 2-4 Perineal anatomy. Anterior and posterior triangles are defined by a line drawn between the ischial tuberosities. The superficial space of the anterior triangle and its contents are shown above this line.

Deep Space of the Anterior Triangle. This space lies deep to the perineal membrane and extends up into the pelvis (Mirilas and Skandalakis, 2004). In contrast to the superficial perineal space, which is a closed compartment, the deep space is continuous superiorly with the pelvic cavity (Corton, 2005). It contains the compressor urethrae and urethrovaginal sphincter muscles, external urethral sphincter, parts of urethra and vagina, branches of the internal pudendal artery, and the dorsal nerve and vein of the clitoris (Fig. 2-5).

Posterior Triangle

This triangle contains the ischiorectal fossa, anal canal, anal sphincter complex, and branches of the internal pudendal vessels and pudendal nerve (see Figs. 2-4 and 2-5).

Ischiorectal Fossae. These are two fat-filled wedge-shaped spaces found on either side of the anal canal and comprise the bulk of the posterior triangle (Fig. 2-6). Their structure reflects their function. They provide support to surrounding organs, yet allow distension of the rectum during defecation and stretching of the vagina during delivery.

The anal canal and sphincter complex lie in the center of these fossae. Deeply, there is no fascial boundary between the fossa and the tissues above the perineal membrane. Thus, the two fossae communicate posteriorly, behind the anal canal. This continuity of the ischioanal fossa across perineal compartments allows fluid, infection, and malignancy to spread from one side of the anal canal to the other as well as into the areas deep to the perineal membrane. This can be clinically important if episiotomy infection extends to involve either fossa.

Pudendal Nerve and Vessels

The pudendal nerve is formed from the anterior rami of the second through fourth sacral nerves. It courses between the piriformis and coccygeus muscles and exits through the greater sciatic foramen in a location posteromedial to the ischial spine (Barber and colleagues, 2002). This anatomy is important when injecting local anesthetic for a pudendal nerve block. The ischial spine serves an easily identifiable landmark for anesthetic infiltration around this nerve (see Chap. 19, p. 450).

The pudendal nerve then courses along the obturator internus muscle. Along this muscle, the nerve lies within the *pudendal canal*, also known as *Alcock canal*, which is formed by splitting of the obturator fascia (Shafik, 1999). The pudendal nerve leaves this canal to enter the perineum and divides into three terminal branches (see Fig. 2-4). The *dorsal nerve of the clitoris* supplies the skin of the clitoris. The *perineal nerve* serves the muscles of the anterior triangle and labial skin. The *inferior rectal* branch supplies the external anal sphincter, the mucous membrane of the anal canal, and the perianal skin (Mahakkanukrauh and associates, 2005).

The major blood supply to the perineum is via the internal pudendal artery and its branches. These include the inferior rectal artery and posterior labial artery.

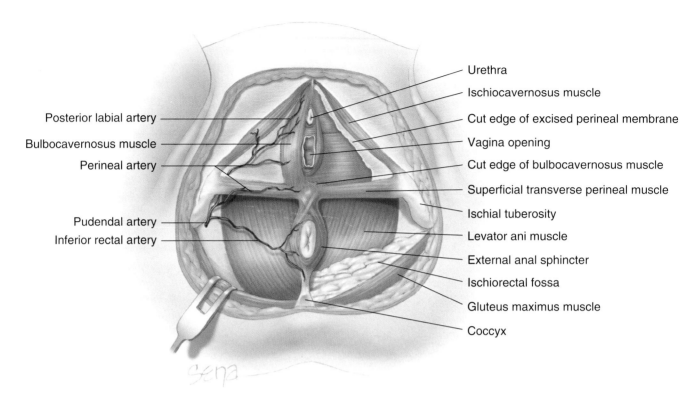

Posterior labial artery

Bulbocavernosus muscle

Perineal artery

Pudendal artery

Inferior rectal artery

Urethra

Ischiocavernosus muscle

Cut edge of excised perineal membrane

Vagina opening

Cut edge of bulbocavernosus muscle

Superficial transverse perineal muscle

Ischial tuberosity

Levator ani muscle

External anal sphincter

Ischiorectal fossa

Gluteus maximus muscle

Coccyx

FIGURE 2-5 Perineal anatomy. Anterior and posterior triangles are shown. Within the anterior triangle, the contents of the deep space are shown on the image's right, whereas those of the superficial space are on the left.

Anus

Anal Sphincters

Two sphincters surround the anal canal to provide continence—the *external* and *internal anal sphincter* (Fig. 2-6). Both lie proximate to the vagina, and one or both may be torn during vaginal delivery. Of these disruptions, many are not clinically identified at delivery. For example, Sultan (1993) performed endoanal sonography 6 weeks following delivery and found that 28 of 79 primiparas—35 percent—had sphincter defects, more

commonly involving the internal sphincter. Clinically, these defects can have functional consequences. Oberwalder and colleagues (2003) performed a meta-analysis of 717 women after a vaginal delivery and found that almost 80 percent of those with anal sphincter defects had impaired control of stool or flatus.

External Anal Sphincter (EAS). This ring of striated muscle attaches to the perineal body anteriorly and the coccyx posteriorly. It maintains a constant state of resting contraction that provides increased tone and strength when continence is

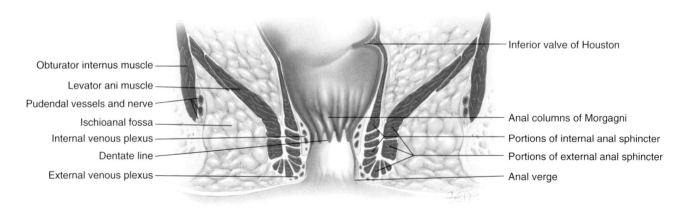

Obturator internus muscle

Levator ani muscle

Pudendal vessels and nerve

Ischioanal fossa

Internal venous plexus

Dentate line

External venous plexus

Inferior valve of Houston

Anal columns of Morgagni

Portions of internal anal sphincter

Portions of external anal sphincter

Anal verge

FIGURE 2-6 Anatomy of the anorectum, drawn to show relations of the internal anal sphincter, the external anal sphincter, and the levator ani muscles. The boundaries of the ischiorectal fossa are shown. The ischiorectal fossa is bounded deeply by the inferior fascia of the levator ani muscles, superficially by the perineal skin, anterolaterally by the fascia of the obturator internus muscles and ischial tuberosities, posterolaterally by the gluteus maximus muscles and sacrotuberous ligament, and medially by the anal canal and sphincter complex.

threatened, and it relaxes for defecation. Hsu and colleagues (2005) studied structure of the EAS using magnetic resonance (MR) imaging. They identified three structures: the main body—EAS-M, the subcutaneous sphincter—EAS-SQ, and the wing-shaped end—EAS-W, which has fibers with lateral origins near the ischiopubic ramus. The external sphincter receives blood supply from the inferior rectal artery. Somatic motor fibers from the inferior rectal branch of the pudendal nerve supply innervation.

Internal Anal Sphincter (IAS).

This sphincter contributes the bulk of anal canal resting pressure for fecal continence, and it relaxes prior to defecation. The sphincter is formed by distal continuation of the inner circular smooth muscle layer of the rectum and colon. The IAS measures 3 to 4 cm in length, and at its distal margin, it overlaps the external sphincter for 1 to 2 cm (DeLancey and co-workers, 1997; Rociu and associates, 2000). Thus, the IAS may be involved in fourth-degree lacerations, and reunion of this ring is incorporated in their repair (see Chap. 17, p. 400).

Anal Cushions

Within the anal canal, there are highly vascularized cushions, which when apposed aid complete closure of the anal canal and fecal continence. Increasing uterine size, excessive straining, and hard stools can increase venous engorgement within these cushions to form *hemorrhoids* (Fig. 2-7). External hemorrhoids are those that arise distal to the dentate line. They are covered by stratified squamous epithelium and receive sensory innervation from the inferior rectal nerve. Accordingly, pain and a palpable mass are typical complaints. Following resolution, a *hemorrhoidal tag* may remain and is composed of redundant anal skin and fibrotic tissue. In contrast, *internal hemorrhoids* are those that form above the dentate line and are covered by insensate anorectal mucosa. These may prolapse or bleed but rarely become painful unless they develop thrombosis and necrosis.

Hemorrhoids form commonly in pregnancy (see Chap. 8, p. 211). Abramowitz and colleagues (2002) evaluated 165

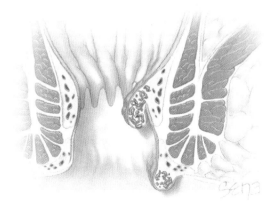

FIGURE 2-7 Veins within the anal cushions engorge to form hemorrhoids. Those above the dentate line are termed internal, whereas those below it are called external hemorrhoids.

TABLE 2-1. Perineal Body

Function
Anchors the anorectum
Anchors the vagina
Helps maintains urinary and fecal continence
Maintains the orgasmic platform
Prevents expansion of the urogenital hiatus
Provides a physical barrier between the vagina and rectum

Potential Morbidity
Episiotomy may injure the perineal body
Pudendal nerve injury may be associated with concurrent perineal body injury

Adapted from Woodman and Graney (2002).

consecutive pregnant women proctoscopically and found thrombosed hemorrhoids in 9 percent during their last 3 months of pregnancy and an even greater percentage postpartum.

Perineal Body

The median raphe of the levator ani, between the anus and the vagina, is reinforced by the central tendon of the perineum. The bulbocavernosus, superficial transverse perineal, and external anal sphincter muscles also converge on the central tendon. Thus, these structures contribute to the perineal body, which provides significant perineal support as shown in Table 2-1. The perineal body is incised by an episiotomy incision and is torn with second-, third-, and fourth-degree lacerations.

INTERNAL GENERATIVE ORGANS

Uterus

The nonpregnant uterus is situated in the pelvic cavity between the bladder anteriorly and the rectum posteriorly. Almost the entire posterior wall of the uterus is covered by serosa, that is, visceral peritoneum. The lower portion of this peritoneum forms the anterior boundary of the *recto uterine cul-de-sac*, or *pouch of Douglas*. Only the upper portion of the anterior wall of the uterus is so covered (Fig. 2-8). The peritoneum in this area reflects forward onto the bladder dome to create the *vesicouterine pouch*. The lower portion of the anterior uterine wall is united to the posterior wall of the bladder by a well-defined loose layer of connective tissue. This is the *vesicouterine space*. During cesarean delivery, the peritoneum of the vesicouterine pouch is sharply incised and the vesicouterine space is entered. Dissection caudally within this space lifts the bladder off the lower uterine segment for hysterotomy and delivery (see Chap. 25, p. 550).

Size and Shape

The uterus is described as being *pyriform* or pear-shaped, and as shown in Figure 2-9, it resembles a flattened pear. It consists of two major but unequal parts: an upper triangular portion—the

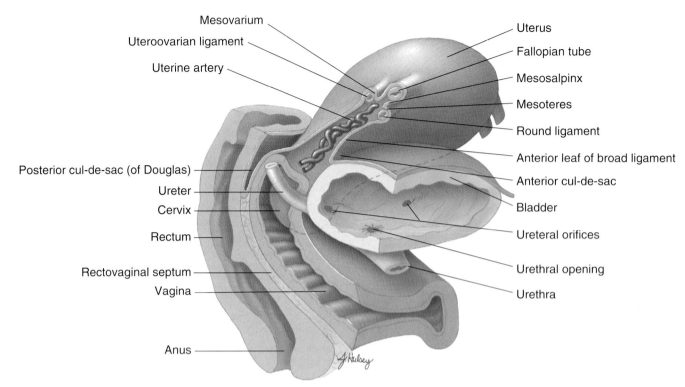

FIGURE 2-8 Vertical section through the uterine end of the right broad ligament. (Used with permission from Jennifer Hulsey.)

body or *corpus,* and a lower, cylindrical portion—the *cervix,* which projects into the vagina. The *isthmus* is that portion of the uterus between the internal cervical os and the endometrial cavity (Fig. 2-10). It is of special obstetrical significance because it forms the lower uterine segment during pregnancy (see Chap. 6, p. 142). The fallopian tubes, also called oviducts, emerge from

the *cornua* of the uterus at the junction of the superior and lateral margins. The fundus is the convex upper segment between the points of insertion of the fallopian tubes.

The bulk of the body of the uterus, but not the cervix, is composed of muscle. The inner surfaces of the anterior and posterior walls lie almost in contact, and the cavity between these

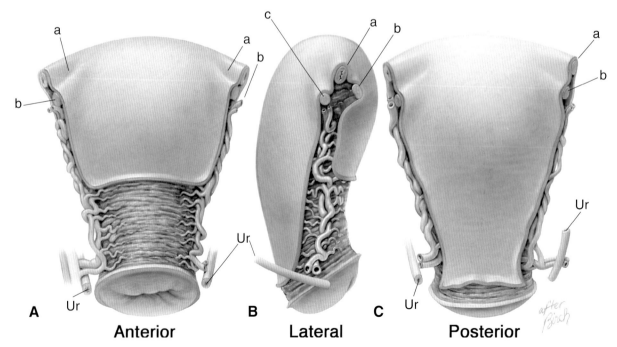

FIGURE 2-9 Anterior **(A)**, right lateral **(B)**, and posterior **(C)** views of the uterus of an adult woman. (a = oviduct; b = round ligament; c = ovarian ligament; Ur = ureter.)

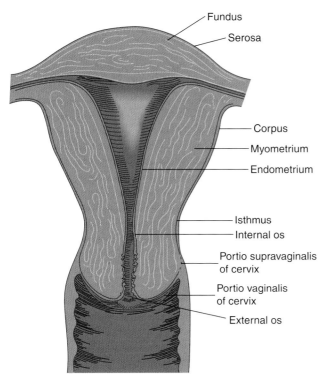

FIGURE 2-10 Uterine and cervical anatomy. Reprinted from Schorge J, Schaffer J, Halvorson L, et al: *Williams Gynecology*, p. 782. Copyright © 2008 The McGraw-Hill Companies, Inc.

walls forms a mere slit. The uterus of adult nulliparous women measures 6 to 8 cm in length as compared with 9 to 10 cm in multiparous women. In nonparous women, the uterus averages 50 to 70 g, whereas in parous women it averages 80 g or more (Langlois, 1970). In nulliparous women, the fundus and cervix are approximately equal length, but in multiparous women, the cervix is only a little more than a third of the total length.

Pregnancy-Induced Uterine Changes

Pregnancy stimulates remarkable uterine growth due to hypertrophy of muscle fibers. Uterine weight increases from 70 g to approximately 1100 g at term. Its total volume averages about 5 L. The uterine fundus, a previously flattened convexity between tubal insertions, now becomes dome shaped (Fig. 2-11). The round ligaments now appear to insert at the junction of the middle and upper thirds of the organ. The fallopian tubes elongate, but the ovaries grossly appear unchanged.

Congenital Anomalies

Abnormal müllerian fusion may give rise to a number of uterine anomalies that are discussed in Chapter 40 (p. 891).

Cervix

The cervical portion of the uterus is fusiform and open at each end by small apertures—the *internal* and *external os* (see Fig. 2-10). Anteriorly, the upper boundary of the cervix is the internal os, which corresponds to the level at which the peritoneum is reflected up onto the bladder. The upper segment of the cervix—the *portio supravaginalis*, lies above the vaginal attachment to the cervix. It is covered by peritoneum on its posterior surface, the cardinal ligaments attach laterally, and it is separated from the overlying bladder by loose connective tissue. The lower vaginal portion of the cervix is called the *portio vaginalis*.

Before childbirth, the external cervical os is a small, regular, oval opening (Fig. 2-12). After labor, and especially vaginal childbirth, the orifice is converted into a transverse slit that is divided such that there are the so-called *anterior* and *posterior lips* of the cervix. If torn deeply during delivery, the cervix may heal in such a manner that it appears to be irregular, nodular, or stellate. These changes are sufficiently characteristic to permit an examiner to ascertain with some certainty whether a woman

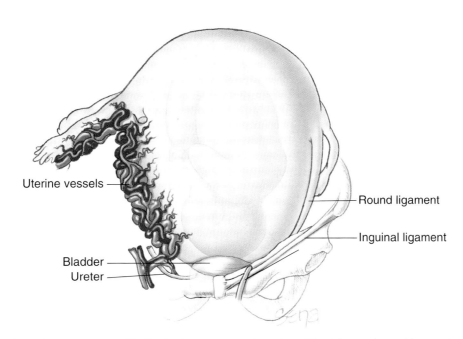

FIGURE 2-11 Uterus of near-term pregnancy. The fundus is now dome shaped, and the tubes and round ligaments appear to insert in the upper middle portion of the uterine body. Note the markedly hypertrophied vascular supply.

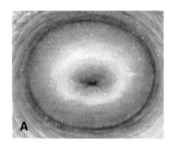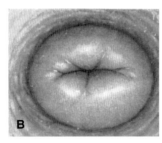

FIGURE 2-12 Differences in cervical os apperance due to labor and delivery. **A.** Nulliparous cervix. **B.** Parous cervix.

has borne children by vaginal delivery. If a woman undergoes cesarean delivery, however, then the postoperative cervical appearance reflects the degree of dilatation prior to surgery. Cervices without labor may appear nulliparous, whereas as those with intrapartum dilation may appear parous.

The portion of the cervix exterior to the external os is called the *ectocervix* and is lined predominantly by nonkeratinized stratified squamous epithelium. In contrast, the endocervical canal is covered by a single layer of mucin-secreting columnar epithelium, which creates deep cleftlike infoldings or "glands." Mucus produced by the endocervical epithelia changes during pregnancy. It becomes thick and forms a mucus plug within the endocervical canal.

Commonly during pregnancy, the endocervical epithelia moves out and onto the ectocervix during enlargement of the cervix in a process termed *eversion* (see Chap. 5, p. 109). As a result, a band of columnar epithelium may ring the external os. With time, this everted columnar epithelium, under the influence of vaginal acidity or during reparative healing, may be replaced by squamous epithelium in a process termed *squamous metaplasia*. This replacement with squamous epithelium may block endocervical clefts. If so, accumulated mucus from the underlying clefts forms *nabothian cysts*, which are benign, firm, smooth, rounded, opaque-yellow or groundglass gray elevations on the ectocervix.

The cervical stroma is composed mainly of collagen, elastin, and proteoglycans, but very little smooth muscle. Changes in the amount, composition, and orientation of these components lead to cervical ripening prior to labor onset (see Chap. 6, p. 138). In early pregnancy, increased vascularity and edema within the cervix stroma leads to the blue tint and softening characteristics of Chadwick and Hegar signs, respectively.

Endometrium

This mucosal layer lines the uterine cavity in nonpregnant women. It is a thin, pink, velvet-like membrane, which on close examination, is perforated by many minute ostia of the uterine glands. The endometrium normally varies greatly

in thickness. It is composed of surface epithelium, glands, and interglandular mesenchymal tissue in which there are numerous blood vessels (Fig. 2-13).

The epithelium is comprised of a single layer of closely packed, high columnar cells that rests on a thin basement membrane (see Fig. 3-2 p. 38). The tubular *uterine glands* are invaginations of the epithelium. The glands extend through the entire thickness of the endometrium to the myometrium, which is occasionally penetrated for a short distance. The connective tissue between the surface epithelium and the myometrium is a mesenchymal stroma. Histologically, the stroma varies remarkably throughout the ovarian cycle. Specifically, following ovulation, *decidualization* of the stromal compartment develops in the mid-luteal phase. As discussed further in Chapter 3 (p. 42), this process of endometrial remodeling prepares for pregnancy and includes secretory transformation of the uterine glands and vascular remodeling (Gellersen and colleagues, 2003, 2007).

The vascular architecture of the uterus and endometrium is of signal importance in pregnancy. The uterine and ovarian arteries branch and penetrate the uterine wall obliquely inward

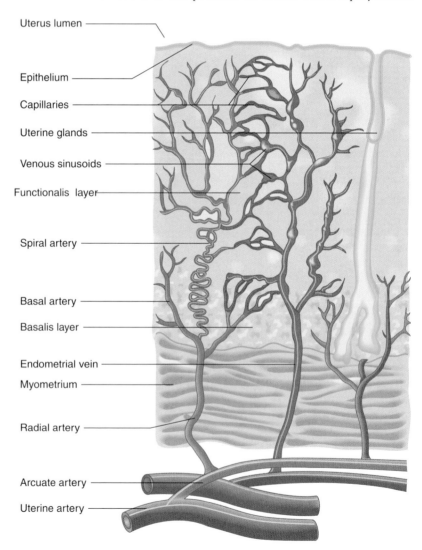

FIGURE 2-13 Vascular supply to the endometrium. (Reprinted from Schorge J, Schaffer J, Halvorson L, et al: *Williams Gynecology*, p. 177. Copyright © 2008 The McGraw-Hill Companies, Inc.)

and reach its middle third. They then ramify in a plane that is parallel to the surface and are therefore named the *arcuate arteries* (DuBose and colleagues, 1985). Radial branches extend from the arcuate arteries at right angles and enter the endometrium to become *coiled* or *spiral arteries*. Also from the radial arteries, *basal* or *straight arteries* branch at a sharp angle. The spiral arteries supply most of the midportion and all of the superficial third of the endometrium. These vessels respond—especially by vasoconstriction, to a number of hormones and thus probably serve an important role in the mechanism(s) of menstruation. The basal arteries extend only into the basal layer of the endometrium and are not responsive to hormonal influences.

Myometrium

This layer comprises most of the uterus. It is composed of bundles of smooth muscle united by connective tissue in which there are many elastic fibers. The interlacing myometrial fibers that surround the myometrial vessels are integral to control of bleeding from the placental site during the third stage of labor. As shown in Fig. 2-14, vessels are compressed by smooth muscle contraction. According to Schwalm and Dubrauszky (1966), the number of muscle fibers of the uterus progressively diminishes caudally such that, in the cervix, muscle comprises only 10 percent of the tissue mass. In the inner wall of the body

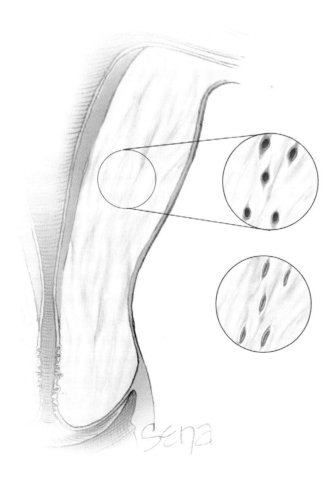

FIGURE 2-14 The smooth muscle fibers compress traversing blood vessels when contracted.

of the uterus, there is relatively more muscle than in the outer layers; and in the anterior and posterior walls, there is more muscle than in the lateral walls. During pregnancy, the upper myometrium undergoes marked hypertrophy, but there is no significant change in cervical muscle content.

Ligaments

Several ligaments extend from the lateral surface of the uterus toward the pelvic sidewalls and include the round, broad, and cardinal ligaments. The *round ligaments* originate somewhat below and anterior to the origin of the fallopian tubes (see Fig. 2-8). Each round ligament extends laterally and downward to the inguinal canal, through which it passes to terminate in the upper portion of the labium majus. *Sampson artery*, a branch of the uterine artery, runs within this ligament. The location of the round ligament anterior to the fallopian tube can help distinguish surgical anatomy such as with puerperal tubal sterilization (see Chap. 33, p. 698). This may be especially true if pelvic adhesions limit tubal mobility and thus, limit identification of fimbria prior to tubal ligation.

The round ligament corresponds embryologically to the gubernaculum testis of men. In nonpregnant women, it varies from 3 to 5 mm in diameter and is composed of smooth muscle (Ozdegirmenci and colleagues, 2005). During pregnancy, the round ligaments undergo considerable hypertrophy and increase appreciably in both length and diameter.

The *broad ligaments* are composed of two winglike structures that extend from the lateral uterine margins of the uterus to the pelvic sidewalls. They divide the pelvic cavity into anterior and posterior compartments. Each broad ligament consists of a fold of peritoneum termed the *anterior* and *posterior leaves*. This peritoneum drapes over structures extending from the cornua. Peritoneum that overlies the fallopian tube is termed the *mesosalpinx*, that around the round ligament is the *mesoteres*, and that over the uterovarian ligament is the *mesovarium* (see Fig. 2-8). Peritoneum that extends beneath the fimbriated end of the fallopian tube to the pelvic wall forms the *infundibulopelvic ligament* or *suspensory ligament of the ovary*, through which the ovarian vessels traverse. During pregnancy, these vessels, especially the venous plexuses, are dramatically hypertrophied.

The thick base of the broad ligament is continuous with the connective tissue of the pelvic floor. The densest portion is usually referred to as the *cardinal ligament*—also called the *transverse cervical ligament* or *Mackenrodt ligament*. It is composed of connective tissue that medially is united firmly to the supravaginal portion of the cervix. A vertical section through the uterine end of the broad ligament is triangular, and the uterine vessels and ureter are found within its broad base (see Fig. 2-8). In its lower part, it is widely attached to the connective tissues that are adjacent to the cervix, that is, the *parametrium*.

Each *uterosacral ligament* extends from an attachment posterolaterally to the supravaginal portion of the cervix and inserts into the fascia over the sacrum. Umek and colleagues (2004) used magnetic resonance imaging to describe anatomical variations of these ligaments. The ligaments are composed of connective tissue, small bundles of vessels and nerves, and some smooth muscle. They are covered by peritoneum and form the lateral boundaries of the pouch of Douglas.

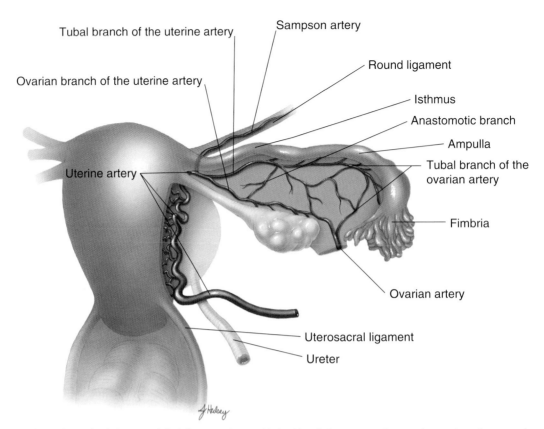

FIGURE 2-15 Blood supply to the left ovary, left fallopian tube, and left side of the uterus. The ovarian and uterine vessels anastomose freely. Note the uterine artery and vein crossing over the ureter that lies immediately adjacent to the cervix. (Used with permission from Jennifer Hulsey.)

Blood Vessels

The vascular supply of the uterus is derived principally from the uterine and ovarian arteries. The uterine artery, a main branch of the internal iliac artery—previously called the hypogastric artery—enters the base of the broad ligament and makes its way medially to the side of the uterus. Immediately adjacent to the supravaginal portion of the cervix, the uterine artery divides. The smaller cervicovaginal artery supplies blood to the lower cervix and upper vagina. The main branch turns abruptly upward and extends as a highly convoluted vessel that traverses along the margin of the uterus. A branch of considerable size extends to the upper portion of the cervix, and numerous other branches penetrate the body of the uterus. Just before the main branch of the uterine artery reaches the fallopian tube, it divides into three terminal branches (Fig. 2-15). The ovarian branch of the uterine artery anastomoses with the terminal branch of the ovarian artery; the tubal branch makes its way through the mesosalpinx and supplies part of the fallopian tube; and the fundal branch is distributed to the uppermost uterus.

Approximately 2 cm lateral to the cervix, the uterine artery crosses over the ureter. The proximity of the uterine artery and vein to the ureter at this point is of great surgical significance. Because of their close proximity, the ureter may be injured or ligated during a hysterectomy when the vessels are clamped and ligated.

The *ovarian artery* is a direct branch of the aorta. It enters the broad ligament through the infundibulopelvic ligament. At the ovarian hilum, it divides into a number of smaller branches that enter the ovary. Its main stem, however, traverses the entire length of the broad ligament and makes its way to the upper lateral portion of the uterus. Here it anastomoses with the ovarian branch of the uterine artery. There are numerous additional communications among the arteries on both sides of the uterus.

When the uterus is in a contracted state, its numerous venous lumens are collapsed. But in injected specimens, the greater part of the uterine wall appears to be occupied by dilated venous sinuses. On either side, the arcuate veins unite to form the *uterine vein,* which empties into the internal iliac and then the common iliac vein. Some of the blood from the upper uterus, the ovary, and the upper part of the broad ligament is collected by several veins. Within the broad ligament, these veins form the large *pampiniform plexus* that terminates in the ovarian vein. The right ovarian vein empties into the vena cava, whereas the left ovarian vein empties into the left renal vein. During pregnancy, there is marked hypertrophy of the uterine vasculature (see Fig. 2-11).

Blood supply to the pelvis is predominantly supplied from branches of the internal iliac artery (Fig. 2-16). These branches are organized into anterior and posterior divisions and subsequent branches are highly variable between individuals. The anterior division provides substantial blood supply to the pelvic organs and perineum, whereas the posterior division branches extend to the buttock and thigh. In some cases, branches of these vessels traverse close to the presacral space (Wieslander and associates, 2006). The surgical anatomy of the internal iliac artery is discussed further in Chapter 35, p. 796.

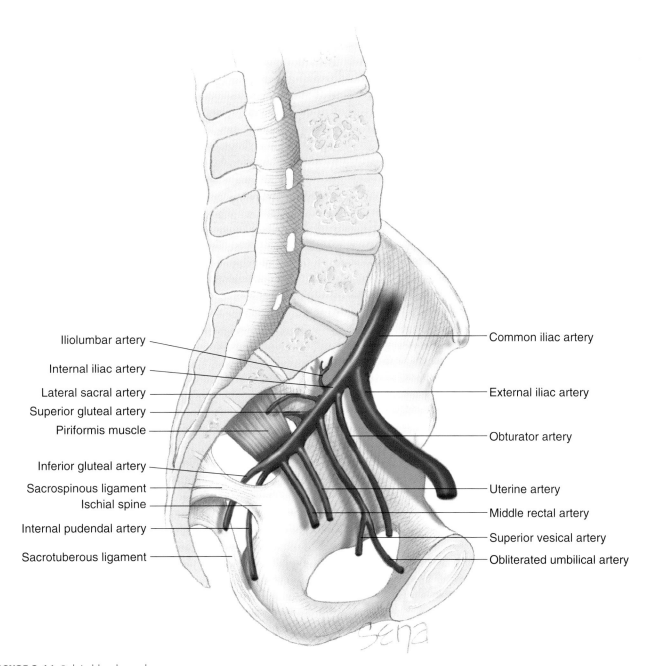

Iliolumbar artery

Internal iliac artery

Lateral sacral artery

Superior gluteal artery

Piriformis muscle

Inferior gluteal artery

Sacrospinous ligament

Ischial spine

Internal pudendal artery

Sacrotuberous ligament

Common iliac artery

External iliac artery

Obturator artery

Uterine artery

Middle rectal artery

Superior vesical artery

Obliterated umbilical artery

FIGURE 2-16 Pelvic blood supply.

The pelvis has extensive collateral circulation, and the internal iliac artery shares anastomoses with branches of the aorta and external iliac and femoral artery. As a result, ligation of the anterior division of the internal iliac artery can be performed without compromise to pelvic organ viability. For this reason, during internal iliac ligation to control obstetrical hemorrhage, many advocate internal iliac ligation distal to the posterior division to avoid compromised blood flow to the areas supplied by this division (Bleich and colleagues, 2007; Burchell, 1968).

Lymphatics

The endometrium is abundantly supplied with true lymphatic vessels that are confined largely to the basal layer. The lymphatics of the underlying myometrium are increased in number toward the serosal surface and form an abundant lymphatic plexus just be-neath it. Lymphatics from the cervix terminate mainly in the internal iliac nodes, which are situated near the bifurcation of the common iliac vessels. The lymphatics from the uterine corpus are distributed to two groups of nodes. One set of vessels drains into the internal iliac nodes. The other set, after joining certain lymphatics from the ovarian region, terminates in the para-aortic lymph nodes.

Innervation

The pelvic nerve supply is derived principally from the sympathetic nervous system, but also partly from the cerebrospinal and parasympathetic systems. The parasympathetic system is represented on either side by the pelvic nerve, which is made up of a few fibers that are derived from the second, third, and fourth sacral nerves. It loses its identity in the *cervical ganglion of Frankenhäuser*. The sympathetic system enters the pelvis by way of the internal iliac plexus that arises from the aortic plexus just below the promontory of the sacrum (Wieslander and colleagues, 2006). After descending on either side, it also enters the *uterovaginal plexus of Frankenhäuser*, which is made up of ganglia of various sizes, but particularly of a large ganglionic plate that is situated on either side of the cervix, proximate to the uterosacral ligaments and just above the posterior fornix in front of the rectum.

Branches from these plexuses supply the uterus, bladder, and upper vagina. In the 11th and 12th thoracic nerve roots, there are sensory fibers from the uterus that transmit the painful stimuli of contractions to the central nervous system. The sensory nerves from the cervix and upper part of the birth canal pass through the pelvic nerves to the second, third, and fourth sacral nerves. Those from the lower portion of the birth canal pass primarily through the pudendal nerve. Knowledge of the innervation of dermatomes and its clinical application to providing epidural or spinal analgesia for labor and vaginal or cesarean delivery is illustrated in Figures 19-1 and 19-3 (p. 447).

Fallopian Tubes

These tubular extensions from the uterus vary in length from 8 to 14 cm, and each tube is divided into an interstitial portion, isthmus, ampulla, and infundibulum. The *interstitial portion* is embodied within the muscular wall of the uterus. The *isthmus*, or the narrow portion of the tube that adjoins the uterus, passes gradually into the wider, lateral portion, or *ampulla*. The *infundibulum*, or fimbriated extremity, is the funnel-shaped opening of the distal end of the fallopian tube (Fig. 2-17). The fallopian tube varies considerably in thickness. The narrowest portion of the isthmus measures from 2 to 3 mm in diameter, and the widest portion of the ampulla measures from 5 to 8 mm. The fimbriated end of the infundibulum opens into the abdominal cavity. One projection, the *fimbria ovarica*, which is considerably longer than the other fimbriae, forms a shallow gutter that approaches or reaches the ovary.

Tubal smooth muscle is arranged in an inner circular and an outer longitudinal layer. In the distal portion, the two layers are

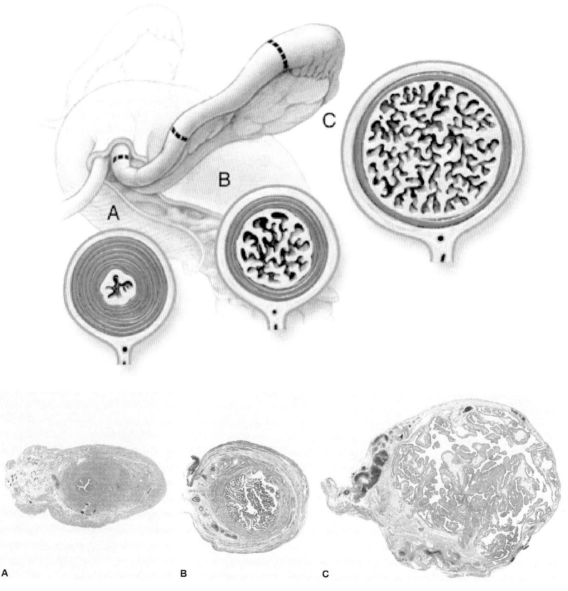

A   B   C

FIGURE 2-17 The fallopian tube of an adult woman with cross-sectioned illustrations of the gross structure in several portions: **(A)** isthmus, **(B)** ampulla, and **(C)** infundibulum. Below these are photographs of corresponding histological sections. (Used with permission from Dr. Kelley S. Carrick.)

less distinct and near the fimbriated extremity, are replaced by an interlacing network of muscular fibers. The tubal musculature undergoes rhythmic contractions constantly, the rate of which varies with ovarian cyclical hormonal changes. The greatest frequency and intensity of contractions is reached during transport of ova.

The fallopian tubes are lined by a single layer of columnar cells, some of them ciliated and others secretory. The ciliated cells are most abundant at the fimbriated extremity, elsewhere, they are found in discrete patches. There are differences in the proportions of these two types of cells in different phases of the ovarian cycle. Because there is no submucosa, the epithelium is in close contact with the underlying muscular layer. In the tubal mucosa, there are cyclical histological changes similar to those of the endometrium, but much less striking. The mucosa is arranged in longitudinal folds that are more complex toward the fimbriated end. On cross-sections through the uterine portion, four simple folds are found that form a figure that resembles a Maltese cross. The isthmus has a more complex pattern. In the ampulla, the lumen is occupied almost completely by the arborescent mucosa, which consists of very complicated folds. The current produced by the tubal cilia is such that the direction of flow is toward the uterine cavity. Tubal peristalsis is believed to be an extraordinarily important factor in ovum transport.

The tubes are supplied richly with elastic tissue, blood vessels, and lymphatics. Sympathetic innervation of the tubes is extensive, in contrast to their parasympathetic innervation.

Diverticula may extend occasionally from the lumen of the tube for a variable distance into the muscular wall and reach almost to the serosa. These diverticula may play a role in the development of ectopic pregnancy (see Chap. 10, p. 240).

Ovaries

Compared with each other, as well as between women, the ovaries vary considerably in size. During childbearing years, they are from 2.5 to 5 cm in length, 1.5 to 3 cm in breadth, and 0.6 to 1.5 cm in thickness. Their position also varies, but they usually lie in the upper part of the pelvic cavity and rest in a slight depression on the lateral wall of the pelvis. This *ovarian fossa of Waldeyer* is between the divergent external and internal iliac vessels.

The ovary is attached to the broad ligament by the *mesovarium*. The *utero-ovarian ligament* extends from the lateral and posterior portion of the uterus, just beneath the tubal insertion, to the uterine pole of the ovary. Usually, it is a few centimeters long and 3 to 4 mm in diameter. It is covered by peritoneum and is made up of muscle and connective tissue fibers. The *infundibulopelvic* or *suspensory ligament of the ovary* extends from the upper or tubal pole to the pelvic wall; through it course the ovarian vessels and nerves.

The ovary consists of the cortex and medulla. In young women, the outermost portion of the cortex is smooth, has a dull white surface, and is designated the *tunica albuginea*. On its surface, there is a single layer of cuboidal epithelium, the *germinal epithelium of Waldeyer*. The cortex contains oocytes and developing follicles. The *medulla* is the central portion, which is composed of loose connective tissue. There are a large number of arteries and veins in the medulla and a small number of smooth muscle fibers.

The ovaries are supplied with both sympathetic and parasympathetic nerves. The sympathetic nerves are derived primarily from the ovarian plexus that accompanies the ovarian vessels. Others are derived from the plexus that surrounds the ovarian branch of the uterine artery. The ovary is richly supplied with nonmyelinated nerve fibers, which for the most part accompany the blood vessels.

MUSCULOSKELETAL PELVIC ANATOMY

Pelvic Bones

The pelvis is composed of four bones: the sacrum, coccyx, and two innominate bones (Fig. 2-18). Each innominate bone is formed by the fusion of the *ilium, ischium,* and *pubis.* The innominate bones are joined to the sacrum at the sacroiliac synchondroses and to one another at the symphysis pubis.

The *false pelvis* lies above the *linea terminalis* and the true pelvis below this anatomical boundary (Fig. 2-19). The *false pelvis* is bounded posteriorly by the lumbar vertebra and laterally by the iliac fossa. In front, the boundary is formed by the lower portion of the anterior abdominal wall.

The *true pelvis* is the portion important in childbearing. It is bounded above by the promontory and alae of the sacrum, the linea terminalis, and the upper margins of the pubic bones, and below by the pelvic outlet. The cavity of the true pelvis can be described as an obliquely truncated, bent cylinder with its greatest height posteriorly.

The walls of the true pelvis are partly bony and partly ligamentous. The posterior boundary is the anterior surface of the sacrum, and the lateral limits are formed by the inner surface of the ischial bones and the sacrosciatic notches and ligaments. In front, the true pelvis is bounded by the pubic bones, the ascending superior rami of the ischial bones, and the obturator foramen.

The sidewalls of the true pelvis of an adult woman converge somewhat. Extending from the middle of the posterior margin of each ischium are the ischial spines. These are of great obstetrical importance because the distance between them usually represents the shortest diameter of the pelvic cavity. They also serve as valuable landmarks in assessing the level to which the presenting part of the fetus has descended into the true pelvis (see Chap. 17, p. 392).

The sacrum forms the posterior wall of the pelvic cavity. Its upper anterior margin corresponds to the promontory that may be felt during bimanual pelvic examination in women with small pelves. It can provide a landmark for clinical pelvimetry. Normally, the sacrum has a marked vertical and a less pronounced horizontal concavity, which in abnormal pelves may undergo important variations. A straight line drawn from the promontory to the tip of the sacrum usually measures 10 cm, whereas the distance along the concavity averages 12 cm.

The descending inferior rami of the pubic bones unite at an angle of 90 to 100 degrees to form a rounded arch under which the fetal head must pass.

Pelvic Joints

Symphysis Pubis

Anteriorly, the pelvic bones are joined together by the symphysis pubis. This structure consists of fibrocartilage and the superior and inferior pubic ligaments. The latter are frequently designated the *arcuate ligament of the pubis.*

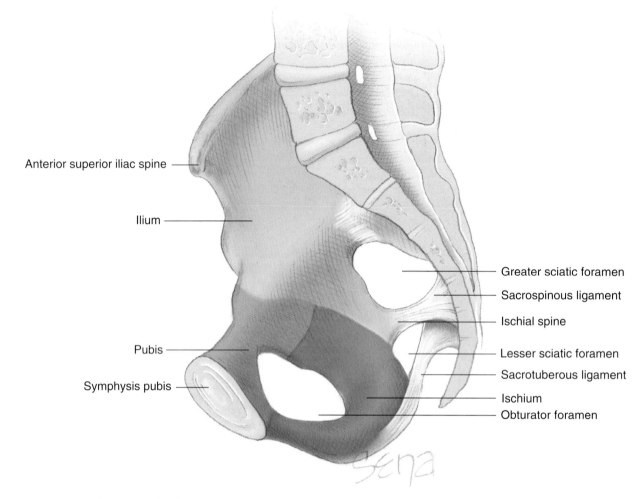

Anterior superior iliac spine

Ilium

Greater sciatic foramen

Sacrospinous ligament

Ischial spine

Lesser sciatic foramen

Pubis

Sacrotuberous ligament

Symphysis pubis

Ischium

Obturator foramen

FIGURE 2-18 Sagittal view of pelvic bones.

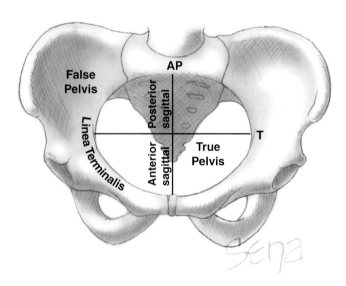

FIGURE 2-19 Anteroposterior view of a normal female pelvis. Anteroposterior (AP) and transverse (T) diameters of the pelvic inlet are illustrated.

Sacroiliac Joints

Posteriorly, the pelvic bones are joined by articulations between the sacrum and the iliac portion of the innominate bones to form the sacroiliac joints. These joints also have a certain degree of mobility.

Relaxation of the Pelvic Joints

During pregnancy, there is remarkable relaxation of these joints, although the cause(s) is unclear. It likely results from hormonal stimulation (see Chap. 5, p. 130). Abramson and co-workers (1934) observed that relaxation of the symphysis pubis commenced in women in the first half of pregnancy and increased during the last 3 months. They also observed that this laxity began to regress immediately after parturition and that regression was completed within 3 to 5 months. The symphysis pubis also increases in width during pregnancy—more so in multiparas than in primigravidas—and returns to normal soon after delivery.

There are important changes in sacroiliac joint mobility. Borell and Fernstrom (1957) demonstrated that the rather marked mobility of the pelvis at term was caused by an upward gliding movement of the sacroiliac joint. The displacement, which is greatest in the dorsal lithotomy position, may increase the diameter of the outlet by 1.5 to 2.0 cm. **This is the main justification for placing a woman in this position for a vaginal delivery.** But increase in diameter of the pelvic outlet occurs only if the sacrum is allowed to rotate posteriorly. Thus, it will not occur if the sacrum is forced anteriorly by the weight of the maternal pelvis against the delivery table or bed (Russell, 1969, 1982). Sacroiliac joint mobility is also the likely reason that the McRoberts maneuver often is successful in releasing an obstructed shoulder in a case of shoulder dystocia (see Chap. 20, p. 483). These changes have also been attributed to the success of the modified squatting position to hasten second-stage labor (Gardosi and co-workers, 1989). The squatting position may increase the interspinous diameter and the diameter of the pelvic outlet (Russell, 1969, 1982). These latter observations are unconfirmed, but this position is assumed for birth in many primitive societies.

Planes and Diameters of the Pelvis

The pelvis is described as having four imaginary planes:

1. The plane of the pelvic inlet—the superior strait.
2. The plane of the pelvic outlet—the inferior strait.
3. The plane of the midpelvis—the least pelvic dimensions.
4. The plane of greatest pelvic dimension—of no obstetrical significance.

Pelvic Inlet

The superior strait or pelvic inlet is bounded posteriorly by the promontory and alae of the sacrum, laterally by the linea terminalis, and anteriorly by the horizontal pubic rami and the symphysis pubis. The inlet of the female pelvis—compared with the male pelvis—typically is more nearly round than ovoid. Caldwell (1934) identified radiographically a nearly round or *gynecoid* pelvic inlet in approximately half of white women.

Four diameters of the pelvic inlet are usually described: anteroposterior, transverse, and two oblique diameters. The obstetrically important *anteroposterior diameter* is the shortest distance between the promontory of the sacrum and the symphysis pubis and is designated the *obstetrical conjugate* (Fig. 2-20). Normally, this measures 10 cm or more. This diameter is distinct from the anteroposterior diameter of the pelvic inlet that has been identified as the *true conjugate*. The obstetrical conju-

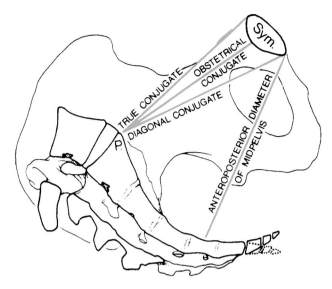

FIGURE 2-20 Three anteroposterior diameters of the pelvic inlet are illustrated: the true conjugate, the more important obstetrical conjugate, and the clinically measurable diagonal conjugate. The anteroposterior diameter of the midpelvis is also shown. (p = sacral promontory; sym = symphysis pubis.)

gate cannot be measured directly with the examining fingers. For clinical purposes, the obstetrical conjugate is estimated indirectly by subtracting 1.5 to 2 cm from the *diagonal conjugate*, which is determined by measuring the distance from the lower margin of the symphysis to the sacral promontory (Fig. 2-21).

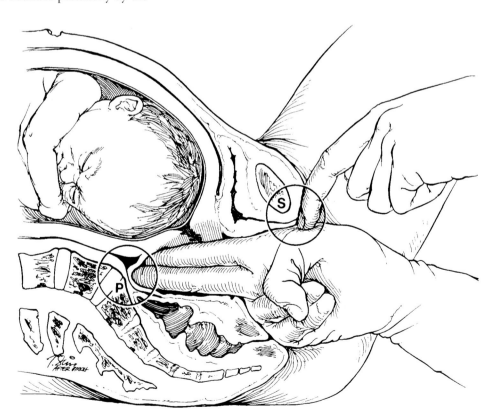

FIGURE 2-21 Vaginal examination to determine the diagonal conjugate. (p = sacral promontory; s = symphysis pubis.)

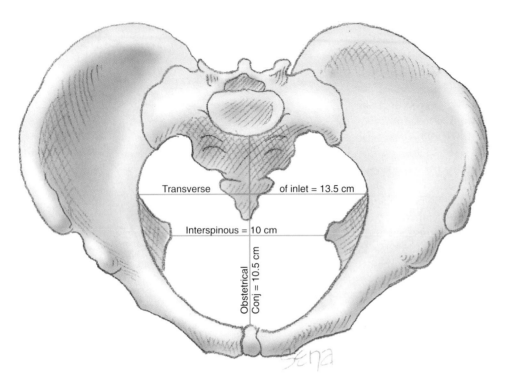

FIGURE 2-22 Adult female pelvis demonstrating the interspinous diameter of the midpelvis. The anteroposterior and transverse diameters of the pelvic inlet are also shown.

The *transverse diameter* is constructed at right angles to the obstetrical conjugate and represents the greatest distance between the linea terminalis on either side (Fig. 2-22). It usually intersects the obstetrical conjugate at a point approximately 4 cm in front of the promontory. Each of the two oblique diameters extends from one of the sacroiliac synchondroses to the iliopectineal eminence on the opposite side. They average less than 13 cm.

Midpelvis

The midpelvis is measured at the level of the ischial spines—the midplane, or plane of least pelvic dimensions (see Fig. 2-22). It is of particular importance following engagement of the fetal head in obstructed labor. The *interspinous diameter*, 10 cm or slightly greater, is usually the smallest pelvic diameter. The anteroposterior diameter through the level of the ischial spines normally measures at least 11.5 cm.

Pelvic Outlet

This consists of two approximately triangular areas that are not in the same plane. They have a common base, which is a line drawn between the two ischial tuberosities (Fig. 2-23). The apex of the posterior triangle is at the tip of the sacrum, and the lateral boundaries are the sacrosciatic ligaments and the ischial tuberosities. The anterior triangle is formed by the area under the pubic arch. Three diameters of the pelvic outlet usually are described: the anteroposterior, transverse, and posterior sagittal.

Pelvic Shapes

Caldwell and Moloy (1933, 1934) developed a classification of the pelvis that is still used. The classification is based on the shape of the pelvis, and its familiarity helps the clinician understand better the mechanisms of labor.

The *Caldwell-Moloy classification* is based on measurement of the greatest transverse diameter of the inlet and its division into anterior and posterior segments. The shapes of these are used to classify the pelvis as gynecoid, anthropoid, android, or platypelloid (Fig. 2-24). The character of the posterior segment determines the type of pelvis, and the character of the anterior segment determines the tendency. These are both determined because many pelves are not pure but are mixed types. For example, a gynecoid pelvis with an android tendency means that the posterior pelvis is gynecoid and the anterior pelvis is android in shape.

From viewing the four basic types in Figure 2-24, the configuration of the gynecoid pelvis would intuitively seem suited for delivery of most fetuses. Indeed, Caldwell and co-workers (1939) reported that the gynecoid pelvis was found in almost half of women.

Muscular Support

The *pelvic diaphragm* forms a broad muscular sling and provides substantial support to the pelvic viscera (Fig. 2-25). This

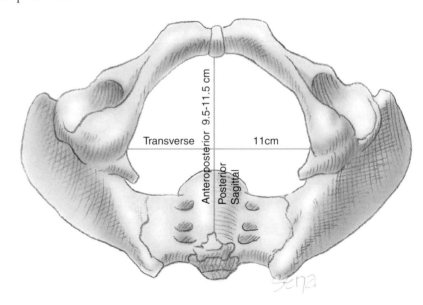

FIGURE 2-23 Pelvic outlet with diameters marked. Note that the anteroposterior diameter may be divided into anterior and posterior sagittal diameters.

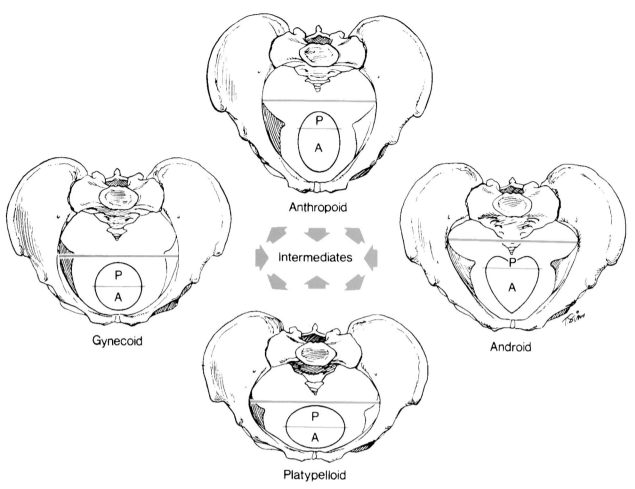

Anthropoid

Intermediates

Gynecoid

Android

Platypelloid

FIGURE 2-24 The four parent pelvic types of the Caldwell–Moloy classification. A line passing through the widest transverse diameter divides the inlets into posterior (P) and anterior (A) segments.

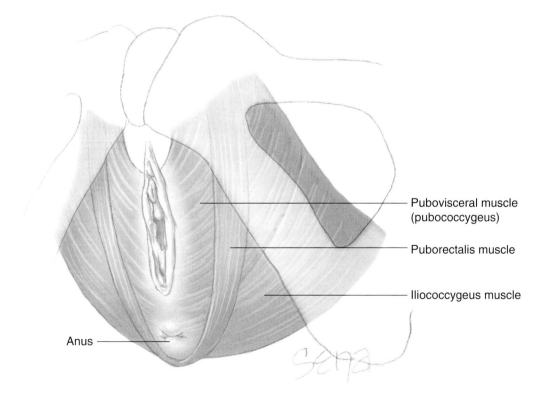

Puboviscceral muscle
(pubococcygeus)

Puborectalis muscle

Iliococcygeus muscle

Anus

FIGURE 2-25 Pelvic floor muscles.

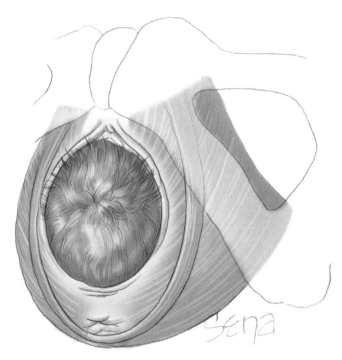

FIGURE 2-26 Illustration of levator ani muscle stretch during delivery.

muscle group is comprised of the *levator ani* and the *coccygeus muscle*. The levator ani is composed of the *pubococcygeus, puborectalis*, and *ileococcygeus muscles*. The pubococcygeus muscle now is preferably termed the *pubovisceral muscle* and is subdivided based on points of insertion and function. These include the *pubovaginalis, puboperinealis, and puboanalis muscles*, which insert into the vaginal, perineal body, and anus, respectively (Kearney and co-workers, 2004).

As shown in Figure 2-26, vaginal birth conveys significant risk for damage to the levator ani muscle or to its innervation (DeLancey and associates, 2003; Weidner and colleagues, 2006). Of these muscles, the pubovisceral muscle is more commonly damaged (Lien and associates, 2004; Margulies and colleagues, 2007). Evidence supports that these injuries may predispose women to greater risk of pelvic organ prolapse or urinary incontinence (DeLancey and associates, 2007a, b; Rortveit and co-workers, 2003). For this reason, current research efforts are aimed at minimizing these injuries.

REFERENCES

Abramowitz L, Sobhani I, Benifla JL, et al: Anal fissure and thrombosed external hemorrhoids before and after delivery. Dis Colon Rectum 45:650, 2002

Abramson D, Roberts SM, Wilson PD: Relaxation of the pelvic joints in pregnancy. Surg Obstet Gynecol 58:595, 1934

Barber MD, Bremer RE, Thor KB, et al: Innervation of the female levator ani muscles. Am J Obstet Gynecol 187:64, 2002

Bleich AT, Rahn DD, Wieslander CK, et al: Posterior division of the internal iliac artery: Anatomic variations and clinical applications. Am J Obstet Gynecol 197:658.e1-5, 2007

Borell U, Fernstrom I: Movements at the sacroiliac joints and their importance to changes in pelvic dimensions during parturition. Acta Obstet Gynecol Scand 36:42, 1957

Burchell RC: Physiology of internal iliac artery ligation. BJOG 75:642, 1968

Caldwell WE, Moloy HC: Anatomical variations in the female pelvis and their effect in labor with a suggested classification. Am J Obstet Gynecol 26:479, 1933

Caldwell WE, Moloy HC, D'Esopo DA: Further studies on the pelvic architecture. Am J Obstet Gynecol 28:482, 1934

Caldwell WE, Moloy HC, Swenson PC: The use of the roentgen ray in obstetrics, 1. Roentgen pelvimetry and cephalometry; technique of pelviroentgenography. Am J Roentgenol 41:305, 1939

Corton MM: Anatomy of the Pelvis: How the pelvis is built for support. Clin Obstet Gynecol, 48:611, 2005

Corton MM, Cunningham FG: Anatomy. In Schorge JO, Schaffer JI, Halvorson LM, et al (eds): Williams Gynecology, New York, McGraw-Hill, 2008, p. 798

DeLancey JO, Miller JM, Kearney R, et al: Vaginal birth and de novo stress incontinence: Relative contributions of urethral dysfunction and mobility. Obstet Gynecol 110:354, 2007a

DeLancey JO, Morgan DM, Fenner DE, et al: Comparison of levator ani muscle defects and function in women with and without pelvic organ prolapse. Obstet Gynecol 109:295, 2007b

DeLancey JO, Toglia MR, Perucchini D: Internal and external anal sphincter anatomy as it relates to midline obstetric lacerations. Obstet Gynecol 90:924, 1997

DeLancey JOL, Kearney R, Chou Q, et al: The appearance of levator ani muscle abnormalities in magnetic resonance images after vaginal delivery. Obstet Gynecol 101:46, 2003

DuBose TJ, Hill LW, Hennigan HW Jr, et al: Sonography of arcuate uterine blood vessels. J Ultrasound Med 4:229, 1985

Gardosi J, Hutson N, Lynch CB: Randomised, controlled trial of squatting in the second stage of labour. Lancet 2:74, 1989

Gellersen B, Brosens IA, Brosens JJ: Decidualization of the human endometrium: Mechanisms, function, and clinical perspectives. Semin Reprod Med 25:445, 2007

Gellersen B, Bronsens J: Cyclic AMP and progesterone receptor cross-talk in human endometrium: A decidualizing affair. J Endocrinol 178:357, 2003

Gorodeski GI: Aging and estrogen effects on transcervical-transvaginal epithelial permeability. J Clin Endocrinol Metab 90:345, 2005

Hoffman BL: Abnormal uterine bleeding. In Schorge JO, Schaffer JI, Halvorson LM, et al (eds): Williams Gynecology, New York, McGraw-Hill, 2008, p. 177

Hsu Y, Fenner DE, Weadock WJ, et al: Magnetic resonance imaging and 3-dimensional analysis of external anal sphincter anatomy. Obstet Gynecol 106:1259, 2005

Kearney R, Sawhney R, DeLancey JO: Levator ani muscle anatomy evaluated by origin-insertion pairs. Obstet Gynecol 104:168, 2004

Langlois PL: The size of the normal uterus. J Reprod Med 4:220, 1970

Lien KC, Mooney B, DeLancey JO, et al: Levator ani muscle stretch induced by simulated vaginal birth. Obstet Gynecol 103:31, 2004

Mahakkanukrauh P, Surin P, Vaidhayakarn P: Anatomical study of the pudendal nerve adjacent to the sacrospinous ligament. Clin Anat 18:200, 2005

Margulies RU, Huebner M, DeLancey JO: Origin and insertion points involved in levator ani muscle defects. Am J Obstet Gynecol 196:251.e1-5, 2007

Mirilas P, Skandalakis JE: Urogenital diaphragm: An erroneous concept casting its shadow over the sphincter urethrae and deep perineal space. J Am Coll Surg 198:279, 2004

Oberwalder M, Connor J, Wexner SD: Meta-analysis to determine the incidence of obstetric anal sphincter damage. Br J Surg 90:1333, 2003

O'Connell HE, DeLancey JO: Clitoral anatomy in nulliparous, healthy, premenopausal volunteers using unenhanced magnetic resonance imaging. J Urol 175:790, 2006

Ozdegirmenci O, Karslioglu Y, Dede S, et al: Smooth muscle fraction of the round ligament in women with pelvic organ prolapse: A computer-based morphometric analysis. Int Urogynecol J Pelvic Floor Dysfunct 16:39, 2005

Rociu E, Stoker J, Eijkemans MJC, et al: Normal anal sphincter anatomy and age- and sex-related variations at high-spatial-resolution endoanal MR imaging. Radiology 217:395, 2000

Rortveit G, Daltveit AK, Hannestad YS, et al: Vaginal delivery parameters and urinary incontinence: The Norwegian EPINCONT study. Am J Obstet Gynecol 189:1268, 2003

Russell JGB: Moulding of the pelvic outlet. J Obstet Gynaecol Br Commonw 76:817, 1969

Russell JGB: The rationale of primitive delivery positions. Br J Obstet Gynaecol 89:712, 1982

Schwalm H, Dubrauszky V: The structure of the musculature of the human uterus—muscles and connective tissue. Am J Obstet Gynecol 94:391, 1966

Shafik A, Doss SH: Pudendal canal: Surgical anatomy and clinical implications. Am Surg 65:176, 1999

Sultan AH, Kamm MA, Hudson CN, et al: Anal-sphincter disruption during vaginal delivery. N Engl J Med 329:1905, 1993

Tan JS, Lukacz ES, Menefee SA, et al: Determinants of vaginal length. Am J Obstet Gynecol 195:1846, 2006

Umek WH, Morgan DM, Ashton-Miller JA, et al: Quantitative analysis of uterosacral ligament origin and insertion points by magnetic resonance imaging. Obstet Gynecol 103:447, 2004

Weber AM, Walters MD: Anterior vaginal prolapse: Review of anatomy and techniques of surgical repair. Obstet Gynecol 89:311, 1997

Weidner AC, Jamison MG, Branham V, et al: Neuropathic injury to the levator ani occurs in 1 in 4 primiparous women. Am J Obstet Gynecol 195:1851, 2006

Whiteside JL, Barber MD, Walters MD, et al: Anatomy of ilioinguinal and iliohypogastric nerves in relation to trocar placement and low transverse incisions. Am J Obstet Gynecol 189:1574, 2003

Wieslander CK, Rahn DD, McIntire DD, et al: Vascular anatomy of the presacral space in unembalmed female cadavers. Am J Obstet Gynecol 195: 1736, 2006

Woodman PJ, Graney DO: Anatomy and physiology of the female perineal body with relevance to obstetrical injury and repair. Clin Anat 15:321, 2002

CHAPTER 3

Implantation, Embryogenesis, and Placental Development

All obstetricians should be aware of the basic reproductive biological processes required for women to successfully achieve pregnancy. A number of abnormalities can affect each of these processes and lead to infertility or pregnancy loss. In most women, spontaneous, cyclical ovulation at 25- to 35-day intervals continues during almost 40 years between menarche and menopause. Without contraception, there are approximately 400 opportunities for pregnancy, which may occur with intercourse on any of 1200 days—the day of ovulation and its two preceding days. This narrow window for fertilization is controlled by tightly regulated production of ovarian steroids. These hormones promote optimal regeneration of endometrium after menstruation ends in preparation for the next implantation window.

Should fertilization occur, the events that unfold after initial implantation of the blastocyst onto the endometrium and through to parturition result from a unique interaction between fetal trophoblasts and maternal endometrium-decidua. The ability of mother and fetus to coexist as two distinct immunological systems results from endocrine, paracrine, and immunological modification of fetal and maternal tissues in a manner not seen elsewhere. The placenta mediates a unique fetal–maternal communication system, which creates a hormonal environment that helps initially to maintain pregnancy and eventu-

ally initiates the events leading to parturition. The following sections address the physiology of the ovarian-endometrial cycle, implantation, placenta, and fetal membranes, and specialized endocrine arrangements between fetus and mother.

THE OVARIAN–ENDOMETRIAL CYCLE

The endometrium-decidua is the anatomical site of blastocyst apposition, implantation, and placental development. From an evolutionary perspective, the human endometrium is highly developed to accommodate endometrial implantation and a hemochorial type of placentation. Endometrial development of a magnitude similar to that observed in women—that is, with special spiral (or coiling) arteries—is restricted to only a few primates, such as humans, great apes, and Old World monkeys. Trophoblasts of the blastocyst invade these endometrial arteries during implantation and placentation to establish uteroplacental vessels.

These primates are the only mammals that menstruate, which is a process of endometrial tissue shedding with hemorrhage and is dependent on sex steroid hormone-directed changes in blood flow in the spiral arteries. With nonfertile, but ovulatory, ovarian cycles, menstruation effects endometrial desquamation. New growth and development must be initiated with each cycle so that endometrial maturation corresponds rather precisely with the next opportunity for implantation and pregnancy. There seems to be a narrow window of endometrial receptivity to blastocyst implantation that corresponds approximately to menstrual cycle days 20 to 24.

The Ovarian Cycle

The development of predictable, regular, cyclical, and spontaneous ovulatory menstrual cycles is regulated by complex interactions of the hypothalamic-pituitary axis, the ovaries, and the genital tract (Fig. 3-1). The average cycle duration is approximately

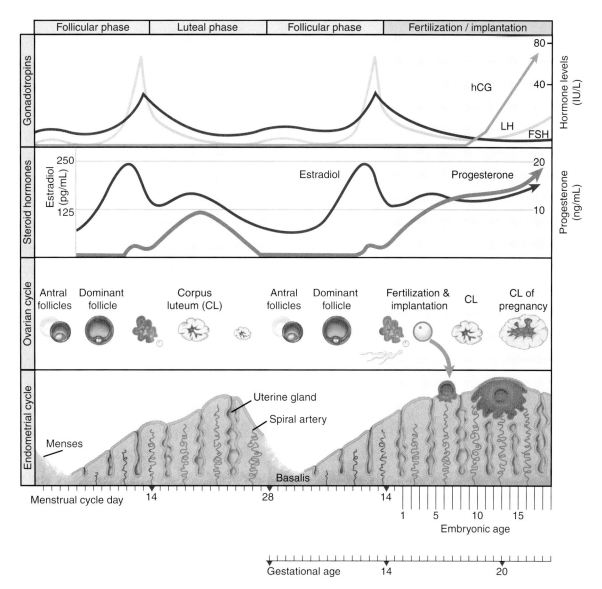

FIGURE 3-1 Gonadotropin control of the ovarian and endometrial cycles. The ovarian-endometrial cycle has been structured as a 28-day cycle. The follicular phase (days 1 to 14) is characterized by rising levels of estrogen, thickening of the endometrium, and selection of the dominant "ovulatory" follicle. During the luteal phase (days 14 to 21), the corpus luteum (CL) produces estrogen and progesterone, which prepare the endometrium for implantation. If implantation occurs, the developing blastocysts will begin to produce human chorionic gonadotropin (hCG) and rescue the corpus luteum, thus maintaining progesterone production. FSH = follicle-stimulating hormone; LH-luteinizing hormone.

28 days, with a range of 25 to 32 days. The sequence of hormonal events leading to ovulation directs the menstrual cycle. The cyclical changes in endometrial histology are faithfully reproduced during each ovulatory cycle.

In 1937, Rock and Bartlett suggested that endometrial histological features were sufficiently characteristic to permit "dating" of the cycle. These changes are illustrated in Figure 3-2. The follicular—proliferative—phase and the postovulatory-luteal or secretory—phase of the cycle are customarily divided into early and late stages.

Follicular or Preovulatory Ovarian Phase

There are 2 million oocytes in the human ovary at birth, and about 400,000 follicles are present at the onset of puberty (Baker, 1963). The remaining follicles are depleted at a rate of

approximately 1000 follicles per month until age 35, when this rate accelerates (Faddy and colleagues, 1992). Only 400 follicles are normally released during female reproductive life. Therefore, more than 99.9 percent of follicles undergo atresia through a process of cell death termed *apoptosis* (Gougeon, 1996; Kaipia and Hsueh, 1997).

Follicular development consists of several stages, which include the gonadotropin-independent recruitment of primordial follicles from the resting pool and their growth to the antral stage. This appears to be under the control of locally produced growth factors. Two members of the transforming growth factor-β family—*growth differentiation factor 9 (GDF9)* and *bone morphogenetic protein 15 (BMP-15)*—regulate proliferation and differentiation of granulosa cells as primary follicles grow (Trombly and co-workers, 2009; Yan and colleagues, 2001). They

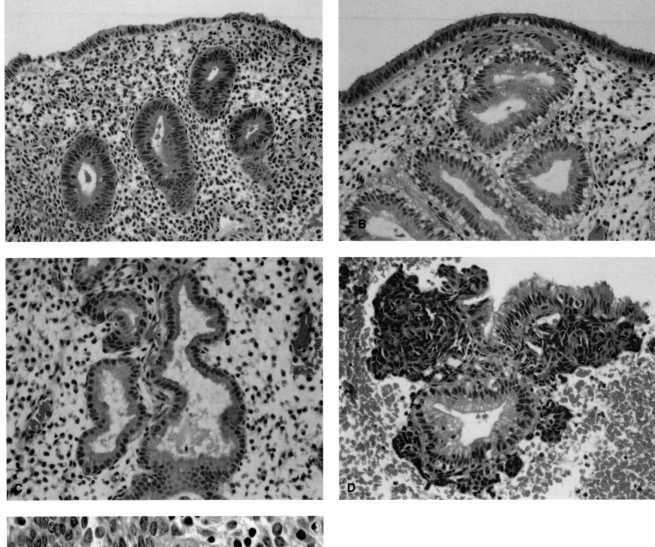

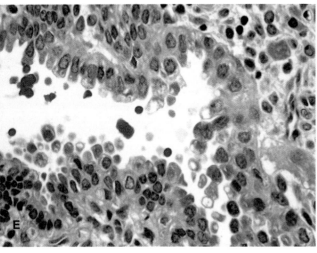

FIGURE 3-2 Photomicrographs illustrating endometrial changes during the menstrual cycle. **A.** Proliferative phase: straight to slightly coiled, tubular glands are lined by pseudostratified columnar epithelium with scattered mitoses. **B.** Early secretory phase: coiled glands with a slightly widened diameter are lined by simple columnar epithelium that contains clear subnuclear vacuoles. Luminal secretions are seen. **C.** Late secretory phase: serrated, dilated glands with intraluminal secretion are lined by short columnar cells. **D.** Menstrual phase: fragmented endometrium with condensed stroma and glands with secretory vacuoles are seen in a background of blood. (Courtesy of Dr. Kelley Carrick.) **E.** Early pregnancy: a hypersecretory effect demonstrated by cell clearing and cytoplasmic blebs is seen. (Courtesy of Dr. Raheela Ashfaq.)

also stabilize and expand the cumulus oocyte complex (COC) in the oviduct (Aaltonen and associates, 1999; Hreinsson and colleagues, 2002). These factors are produced by oocytes, suggesting that the early steps in follicular development are, in part, oocyte controlled. As antral follicles develop, surrounding stromal cells are recruited, by a yet-to-be-defined mechanism, to become thecal cells.

Although not required for early stages of follicular development, follicle-stimulating hormone (FSH) is required for further development of large antral follicles (Hillier, 2001). During each ovarian cycle, a group of antral follicles, known as a *cohort*, begins a phase of semisynchronous growth as a result of their maturation state during the FSH rise of the late luteal phase of the previous cycle. This FSH rise leading to

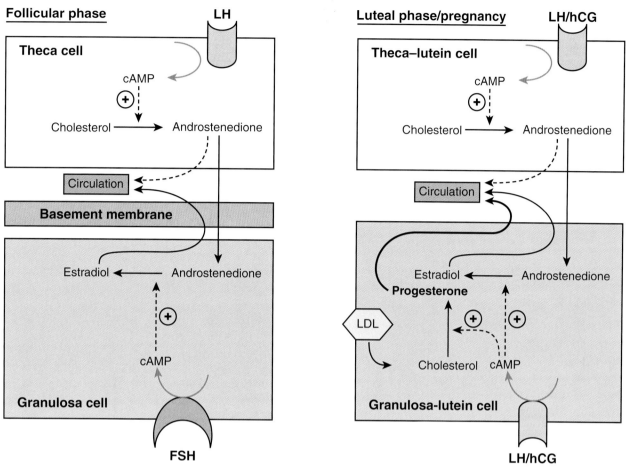

FIGURE 3-3 The two-cell-two-gonadotropin principle of ovarian steroid hormone production. During the follicular phase (*left panel*), luteinizing hormone (LH) controls theca cell production of androstenedione, which diffuses into the adjacent granulosa cells and acts as precursor for estradiol biosynthesis. The capacity for the granulosa cell to convert androstenedione to estradiol is controlled by follicle-stimulating hormone (FSH). After ovulation (*right panel*), the corpus luteum forms and both theca-lutein and granulosa-lutein cells respond to LH. The theca-lutein cells continue to produce androstenedione, whereas granulosa-lutein cells greatly increase their capacity to produce progesterone and to convert androstenedione to estradiol. If pregnancy occurs, the production of human chorionic gonadotropin (hCG) by the placenta rescues the corpus luteum through the LH receptor. Low-density lipoproteins (LDL) are an important source of cholesterol for steroidogenesis. cAMP = cyclic adenosine monophosphate.

follicle development is called the *selection window* of the ovarian cycle (Macklon and Fauser, 2001). Only the follicles progressing to this stage develop the capacity to produce estrogen.

During the follicular phase, estrogen levels rise in parallel to growth of a dominant follicle and the increase in its number of granulosa cells (see Fig. 3-1). These cells are the exclusive site of FSH receptor expression. The increase in circulating FSH during the late luteal phase of the previous cycle stimulates an increase in FSH receptors and subsequently, the ability of cytochrome P_{450} aromatase to convert androstenedione into estradiol. The requirement for thecal cells, which respond to luteinizing hormone (LH), and granulosa cells, which respond to FSH, represents the *two-gonadotropin, two-cell hypothesis* for estrogen biosynthesis (Short, 1962). As shown in Figure 3-3, FSH induces aromatase and expansion of the antrum of growing follicles. The follicle within the cohort that is most responsive to FSH is likely to be the first to produce estradiol and initiate expression of LH receptors.

After the appearance of LH receptors, the preovulatory granulosa cells begin to secrete small quantities of progesterone. The preovulatory progesterone secretion, although somewhat limited, is believed to exert positive feedback on the estrogen-primed pituitary to either cause or augment LH release. In addition, during the late follicular phase, LH stimulates thecal cell production of androgens, particularly androstenedione, which are then transferred to the adjacent follicles where they are aromatized to estradiol (see Fig. 3-3). During the early follicular phase, granulosa cells also produce inhibin B, which can feed back on the pituitary to inhibit FSH release (Groome and colleagues, 1996). As the dominant follicle begins to grow, the production of estradiol and the inhibins increases, resulting in a decline of follicular-phase FSH. This drop in FSH is responsible for the failure of other follicles to reach preovulatory status—*the Graafian follicle stage*—during any one cycle. Thus, 95 percent of plasma estradiol produced at this time is secreted by the dominant follicle—the follicle destined to ovulate. During this time, the contralateral ovary is relatively inactive.

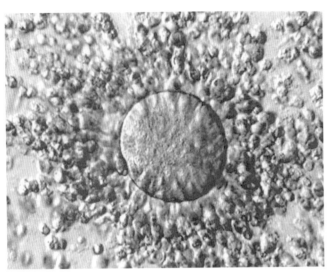

FIGURE 3-4 An ovulated cumulus-oocyte complex (COC). An oocyte is at the center of the complex. Cumulus cells are widely separated from each other in the cumulus layer by the hyaluronan-rich extracellular matrix. (Courtesy of Dr. Kevin J. Doody.)

Ovulation

The onset of the gonadotropin surge resulting from increasing estrogen secretion by preovulatory follicles is a relatively precise predictor of ovulation. It occurs 34 to 36 hours before release of the ovum from the follicle (see Fig. 3-1). LH secretion peaks 10 to 12 hours before ovulation and stimulates the resumption of meiosis in the ovum with the release of the first polar body. Current studies suggest that in response to LH, increased progesterone and prostaglandin production by the cumulus cells, as well as GDF9 and BMP-15 by the oocyte, activates expression of genes critical to formation of a hyaluronan-rich extracellular matrix by the COC (Richards, 2007). As seen in Figure 3-4, during synthesis of this matrix, cumulus cells lose contact with one another and move outward from the oocyte along the hyaluronan polymer—this process is called *expansion*. This results in a 20-fold increase in the volume of the complex. Studies in mice indicate that COC expansion is critical for maintenance of fertility. In addition, LH induces remodeling of the ovarian extracellular matrix to allow release of the mature oocyte with surrounding cumulus cells through the surface epithelium. Activation of proteases likely plays a pivotal role in weakening of the follicular basement membrane and ovulation (Curry and Smith, 2006; Ny and colleagues, 2002).

Luteal or Postovulatory Ovarian Phase

Following ovulation, the corpus luteum develops from the remains of the dominant or *Graafian follicle* in a process referred to as *luteinization*. Rupture of the follicle initiates a series of morphological and chemical changes leading to transformation into the corpus luteum (Browning, 1973). The basement membrane separating the granulosa-lutein and theca-lutein cells breaks down, and by day 2 postovulation, blood vessels and capillaries invade the granulosa cell layer. The rapid neovascularization of the once avascular granulosa may be due to angiogenic factors that include vascular endothelial growth factor (VEGF) and others produced in response to LH by theca-lutein and granulosa-

lutein cells (Albrecht and Pepe, 2003; Fraser and Wulff, 2001). During luteinization, these cells undergo hypertrophy and increase their capacity to synthesize hormones (see Fig. 3-1).

It has been well established in studies of hypophysectomized women that LH is the primary luteotropic factor (Vande Wiele and colleagues, 1970). The life span of the corpus luteum in these women is dependent on repeated injections of LH or human chorionic gonadotropin (hCG). In addition, LH injections can extend the life span of the corpus luteum in normal women by 2 weeks (Segaloff and colleagues, 1951). In normal cycling women, the corpus luteum is maintained by low-frequency, high-amplitude pulses of LH secreted by gonadotropes in the anterior pituitary (Filicori and colleagues, 1986).

The pattern of hormone secretion by the corpus luteum is different from that of the follicle (see Fig. 3-1). The increased capacity of granulosa-lutein cells to produce progesterone is the result of increased access to considerably more steroidogenic precursors through blood-borne low-density lipoprotein (LDL)-derived cholesterol (see Fig. 3-3)(Carr and colleagues, 1981b). It is also due to increases in the level of steroidogenic acute regulatory protein. This protein transports cholesterol from the outer to the inner mitochondria, where the enzyme that metabolizes cholesterol to progesterone is found (Devoto and colleagues, 2002). The important role for LDL in progesterone biosynthesis is supported by the observation that women with extremely low levels of LDL cholesterol exhibit low progesterone secretion during the luteal phase (Illingworth and colleagues, 1982). In addition, high-density lipoprotein (HDL) may contribute to progesterone production in granulosa-lutein cells (Ragoobir and colleagues, 2002).

Estrogen levels follow a more complex pattern of secretion. Specifically, just after ovulation, estrogen levels decrease followed by a secondary rise that reaches a peak production of 0.25 mg/day of 17β-estradiol at the midluteal phase. Toward the end of the luteal phase, there is a secondary decrease in estradiol production.

Ovarian progesterone production peaks at 25 to 50 mg/day during the midluteal phase. With pregnancy, the corpus luteum continues progesterone production in response to embryonic hCG, which will bind and activate luteal cell LH receptors (see Fig. 3-3).

The human corpus luteum is a transient endocrine organ that, in the absence of pregnancy, will rapidly regress 9 to 11 days after ovulation. The mechanisms that control luteolysis remain unclear. However, in part, it results from decreased levels of circulating LH in the late luteal phase and decreased LH sensitivity of luteal cells (Duncan and colleagues, 1996; Filicori and colleagues, 1986). The role of other luteotropic factors is less clear, however, prostaglandin $F_{2\alpha}$ ($PGF_{2\alpha}$) appears to be luteolytic in nonhuman primates (Auletta, 1987; Wentz and Jones, 1973). Within the corpus luteum, luteolysis is characterized by a loss of luteal cells by apoptotic cell death (Vaskivuo and colleagues, 2002). The endocrine effects, consisting of a dramatic drop in circulating estradiol and progesterone levels, are critical to allow the follicular development and ovulation during the next ovarian cycle. In addition, corpus luteum regression and decrease in circulating steroids signal the endometrium to initiate molecular events that lead to menstruation.

Estrogen and Progesterone Action

Estrogen Effects

The fluctuating levels of ovarian steroids are the direct cause of the endometrial cycle. Recent advances in the molecular biology of estrogen and progesterone receptors have greatly improved our understanding of their function. The most biologically potent naturally occurring estrogen—17β-estradiol—is secreted by granulosa cells of the dominant follicle and luteinized granulosa cells of the corpus luteum (see Fig. 3-3). Estrogen is the essential hormonal signal on which most events in the normal menstrual cycle depend. Estradiol action is complex and appears to involve two classic nuclear hormone receptors designated estrogen receptor α (ERα) and β (ERβ) (Katzenellenbogen and colleagues, 2001). These isoforms are the product of separate genes and can exhibit distinct tissue expression. Both estradiol-receptor complexes act as transcriptional factors that become associated with the estrogen response element of specific genes. They share a robust activation by estradiol. However, differences in their binding affinities of other estrogens and their cell-specific expression patterns suggest that ERα and ERβ receptors may have both distinct and overlapping function (Saunders, 2005). Both receptors are expressed in the uterine endometrium (Bombail and co-workers, 2008; Lecce and colleagues, 2001).

The interaction with steroid ligands brings about estrogen receptor–specific initiation of gene transcription. This in turn promotes synthesis of specific messenger RNAs, and thereafter, the synthesis of specific proteins. Among the many proteins upregulated in most estrogen-responsive cells are estrogen and progesterone receptors themselves. In addition, estradiol has been proposed to act at the endothelial cell surface to stimulate nitric oxide production, leading to its rapid vasoactive properties (Shaul, 2002). The ability of estradiol to work in the cell nucleus through classic ligand-regulated nuclear hormone receptors and at the cell surface to cause rapid changes in cell signaling molecules is one explanation for the complex responses seen with estrogen therapies.

Progesterone Effects

Most progesterone actions on the female reproductive tract are mediated through nuclear hormone receptors. Progesterone enters cells by diffusion and in responsive tissues becomes associated with progesterone receptors (Conneely and colleagues, 2002). There are multiple isoforms of the human progesterone receptor. The best understood isoforms are the progesterone receptor type A (PR-A) and B (PR-B). Both arise from a single gene, are members of the steroid receptor superfamily of transcription factors, and regulate transcription of target genes. These receptors have unique actions. When PR-A and PR-B receptors are co-expressed, it appears that PR-A can inhibit PR-B gene regulation. The inhibitory effect of PR-A may extend to actions on other steroid receptors, including estrogen receptors. In addition, progesterone can evoke rapid responses such as changes in intracellular free calcium levels that cannot be explained by genomic mechanisms. G-protein-coupled membrane receptors for progesterone have been identified recently, but their role in the ovarian-endometrium cycle remains to be elucidated (Peluso, 2007).

Expression patterns of PR-A and PR-B endometrial receptors have been examined using immunohistochemistry (Mote and colleagues, 1999). The endometrial glands and stroma appear to have different expression patterns for these receptors that vary over the menstrual cycle. The glands express both receptors in the proliferative phase, suggesting that both receptors are involved with subnuclear vacuole formation. After ovulation, the glands continue to express PR-B through the mid-luteal phase, suggesting that glandular secretion seen during the luteal phase is PR-B regulated. In contrast, the stroma and pre-decidual cells express only PR-A throughout the menstrual cycle, suggesting that progesterone-stimulated events within the stroma are mediated by this receptor.

Progesterone receptor expression has not been found in inflammatory cells or in endothelial cells of endometrial vessels. The role of these two receptor isoforms in the regulation of human menstruation is unclear, but they likely play distinct roles. Animal models suggest that PR-A regulates the antiproliferative effects of progesterone during the secretory phase.

The Endometrial Cycle

Proliferative or Preovulatory Endometrial Phase

Fluctuations in estrogen and progesterone levels produce striking effects on the reproductive tract, particularly the endometrium (Fig. 3-2). The growth and functional characteristics of the human endometrium are unique. Epithelial—glandular cells; stromal—mesenchymal cells; and blood vessels of the endometrium replicate cyclically in reproductive-aged women at a rapid rate. The endometrium is regenerated during each ovarian–endometrial cycle. The superficial endometrium, termed *functionalis layer*, is shed and regenerated from the deeper *basalis layer* almost 400 times during the reproductive lifetime of most women (Fig. 3-5). There is no other example in humans of such cyclical shedding and regrowth of an entire tissue.

Follicular-phase production of estradiol is the most important factor in endometrial recovery following menstruation. Although up to two thirds of the functionalis endometrium is fragmented and shed during menstruation, re-epithelialization begins even before menstrual bleeding has ceased. By the fifth day of the endometrial cycle—fifth day of menses, the epithelial surface of the endometrium has been restored, and revascularization is in progress. The preovulatory endometrium is characterized by proliferation of vascular endothelial, stromal, and glandular cells (see Fig. 3-2). During the early part of the proliferative phase, the endometrium is thin, usually less than 2 mm thick. The glands at this stage are narrow, tubular structures that pursue almost a straight and parallel course from the basalis layer toward the surface of the endometrial cavity. Mitotic figures, especially in the glandular epithelium, are identified by the fifth cycle day, and mitotic activity in both epithelium and stroma persists until day 16 to 17, or 2 to 3 days after ovulation. Although blood vessels are numerous and prominent,

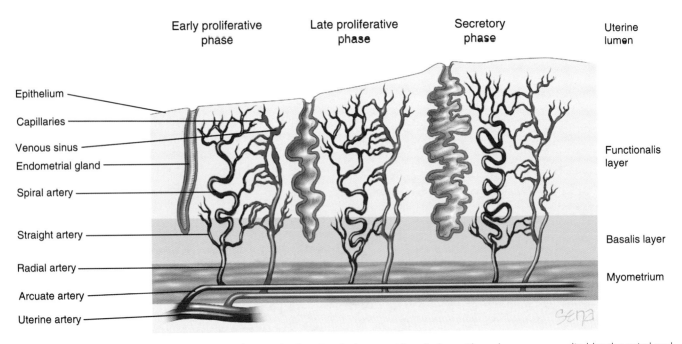

FIGURE 3-5 The endometrium consists of two layers, the functionalis layer and basalis layer. These layers are supplied by the spiral and straight arteries, respectively. Numerous glands also span these layers. As the menstrual cycle progresses, greater coiling of the spiral arteries and increased folds in the glands can be seen. Near the end of the menstrual cycle (day 27), the coiled arteries constrict, deprive blood supply to the functionalis layer, and lead to necrosis and sloughing of this layer.

there is no extravascular blood or leukocyte infiltration in the endometrium at this stage.

Clearly, re-epithelialization and angiogenesis are important to cessation of endometrial bleeding (Chennazhi and Nayak, 2009; Rogers and associates, 2009). These are dependent on tissue regrowth, which is estrogen regulated. Epithelial cell growth also is regulated in part by epidermal growth factor (EGF) and transforming growth factor α (TGFα). Stromal cell proliferation appears to increase through paracrine and autocrine action of estrogen and increased local levels of fibroblast growth factor-9 (Tsai and colleagues, 2002). Estrogens also increase local production of VEGF, which causes angiogenesis through vessel elongation in the basalis (Bausero and colleagues, 1998; Gargett and Rogers, 2001; Sugino and coworkers, 2002).

By the late proliferative phase, the endometrium thickens from both glandular hyperplasia and increased stromal ground substance, which is edema and proteinaceous material. The loose stroma is especially prominent, and the glands in the functionalis layer are widely separated. This is compared with those of the basalis layer, in which the glands are more crowded and the stroma is denser. At midcycle, as ovulation nears, glandular epithelium becomes taller and pseudostratified. The surface epithelial cells acquire numerous microvilli, which increase epithelial surface area, and cilia, which aid in the movement of endometrial secretions during the secretory phase (Ferenczy, 1976).

Determining the menstrual cycle day by endometrial histological criteria, termed *dating*, is difficult during the proliferative phase because of the considerable variation of phase length among women. Specifically, the follicular phase normally may be as short as 5 to 7 days or as long as 21 to 30 days. In contrast, the luteal or secretory postovulatory phase of the cycle is remarkably constant at 12 to 14 days.

Secretory or Postovulatory Endometrial Phase

During the early secretory phase, endometrial dating is based on glandular epithelium histology. After ovulation, the estrogen-primed endometrium responds to rising progesterone levels in a highly predictable manner (see Fig. 3-1). By day 17, glycogen accumulates in the basal portion of glandular epithelium, creating subnuclear vacuoles and pseudostratification. This is the first sign of ovulation that is histologically evident. It is likely the result of direct progesterone action through receptors expressed in glandular cells (Mote and colleagues, 2000). On day 18, vacuoles move to the apical portion of the secretory nonciliated cells. By day 19, these cells begin to secrete glycoprotein and mucopolysaccharide contents into the lumen (Hafez and colleagues, 1975). Glandular cell mitosis ceases with secretory activity on day 19 due to rising progesterone levels, which antagonize the mitotic effects of estrogen. Estradiol action is also decreased because of glandular expression of the type 2 isoform of 17β-hydroxysteroid dehydrogenase. This converts estradiol to the less active estrone (Casey and MacDonald, 1996).

Dating in the mid- to late-secretory phase relies on changes in the endometrial stroma (see Fig. 3-2). On days 21 to 24, the stroma becomes edematous. On days 22 to 25, stromal cells surrounding the spiral arterioles begin to enlarge, and stromal mitosis becomes apparent. Days 23 to 28 are characterized by predecidual cells, which surround spiral arterioles.

An important feature of secretory-phase endometrium between days 22 and 25 is striking changes associated with predecidual transformation of the upper two thirds of the functionalis layer. The glands exhibit extensive coiling and luminal secretions

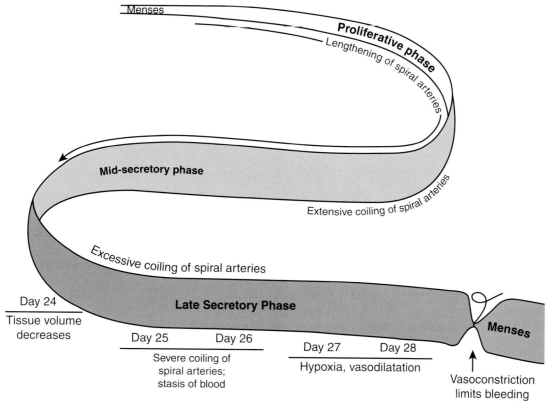

FIGURE 3-6 The spiral arteries of human endometrium are modified during the ovulatory cycle. Initially, changes in blood flow through these vessels aid endometrial growth. Excessive coiling and stasis in blood flow coincide with regression of corpus luteum function and lead to a decline in endometrial tissue volume. Finally, spiral artery coiling leads to endometrial hypoxia and necrosis. Prior to endometrial bleeding, intense spiral artery vasospasm serves to limit blood loss with menstruation.

become visible. Changes within the endometrium also can mark the so-called *window of implantation* seen on days 20 to 24. Epithelial surface cells show decreased microvilli and cilia but appearance of luminal protrusions on the apical cell surface (Nikas, 2003). These *pinopodes* are important in preparation for blastocyst implantation. They also coincide with changes in the surface glycocalyx that allow acceptance of a blastocyst (Aplin, 2003).

The secretory phase is also highlighted by the continuing growth and development of the spiral arteries. Boyd and Hamilton (1970) emphasized the extraordinary importance of the endometrial spiraling or coiled arteries. They arise from arcuate arteries, which are myometrial branches of the uterine vessels (see Fig. 3-5). The morphological and functional properties of spiral arteries are unique and essential for establishing changes in blood flow to permit either menstruation or implantation. During endometrial growth, spiral arteries lengthen at a rate appreciably greater than the rate of increase in endometrial tissue height or thickness (Fig. 3-6). This growth discordance obliges even greater coiling of the already spiraling vessels. Spiral artery development reflects a marked induction of angiogenesis, consisting of widespread vessel sprouting and extension. Perrot-Applanat and associates (1988) described progesterone and estrogen receptors in the smooth muscle cells of the uterus and spiral arteries. They further demonstrated that such rapid angiogenesis is regulated, in part, through estrogen- and progesterone-regulated synthesis of VEGF (Ancelin and colleagues, 2002; Chennazhi and

Nayak, 2009). This protein is secreted by stromal cells and glandular epithelium and stimulates endothelial cell proliferation and increases vascular permeability. Thus, steroid hormone influences on growth and vasculature are directed to a large degree through the local production of growth factors.

Menstruation

The midluteal–secretory phase of the endometrial cycle is a critical branch point in endometrial development and differentiation. With corpus luteum rescue and continued progesterone secretion, the process of decidualization continues. If luteal progesterone production decreases with *luteolysis*, events leading to menstruation are initiated. Many molecular mechanisms involving endometrial progesterone withdrawal, as well as the subsequent inflammatory response that causes endometrial sloughing, have been defined (Critchley and colleagues, 2006).

A notable histological characteristic of late premenstrual-phase endometrium is stromal infiltration by neutrophils, giving a pseudoinflammatory appearance to the tissue. These cells infiltrate primarily on the day or two immediately preceding menses onset. The endometrial stromal and epithelial cells produce interleukin-8 (IL-8), which is a chemotactic–activating factor for neutrophils (Arici and colleagues, 1993). IL-8 may be one agent that serves to recruit neutrophils just prior to menstruation. Similarly, monocyte chemotactic protein-1 (MCP-1) is synthesized by endometrium (Arici and colleagues, 1995).

Leukocyte infiltration is considered key to extracellular matrix breakdown of the functionalis layer. Invading leukocytes secrete enzymes that are members of the matrix metalloproteinase (MMP) family. These add to the proteases already produced by endometrial stromal cells. The rising level of MMPs tips the balance between proteases and protease inhibitors, effectively initiating matrix degradation. This phenomenon has been proposed to initiate the events leading to menstruation (Dong and colleagues, 2002).

Anatomical Events During Menstruation

The classic study by Markee (1940) described tissue and vascular changes in endometrium before menstruation. First, there were marked changes in endometrial blood flow essential for menstruation. With endometrial regression, coiling of spiral arteries becomes sufficiently severe that resistance to blood flow increases strikingly, causing hypoxia of the endometrium. Resultant stasis is the primary cause of endometrial ischemia and tissue degeneration (Fig. 3-6). A period of vasoconstriction precedes menstruation and is the most striking and constant event observed in the cycle. Intense vasoconstriction of the spiral arteries also serves to limit menstrual blood loss. Blood flow appears to be regulated in an endocrine manner by sex steroid hormone–induced modifications of a paracrine-mediated vasoactive peptide system as described subsequently.

Prostaglandins and Menstruation

Progesterone withdrawal increases expression of inducible cyclooxygenase 2 (COX-2) enzyme to synthesize prostaglandins and decreases expression of 15-hydroxyprostaglandin dehydrogenase (PGDH), which degrades prostaglandins (Casey and colleagues, 1980, 1989). The net result is increased prostaglandin production by stromal cells along with increased prostaglandin receptor density on blood vessels and surrounding cells.

A role for prostaglandins—especially vasoconstricting prostaglandin $F_{2\alpha}$ ($PGF_{2\alpha}$)—in initiation of menstruation has been suggested (Abel, 2002). Large amounts of prostaglandins are present in menstrual blood. $PGF_{2\alpha}$ administration prompts symptoms that mimic dysmenorrhea, which is commonly associated with normal menses and likely caused by myometrial contractions and uterine ischemia. $PGF_{2\alpha}$ administration to nonpregnant women also will cause menstruation. This response is believed to be mediated by $PGF_{2\alpha}$-induced vasoconstriction of spiral arteries, causing the uppermost endometrial zones to become hypoxic. This is a potent inducer of angiogenesis and vascular permeability factors such as VEGF. Prostaglandins play an important role in the cascade of events leading to menstruation that include vasoconstriction, myometrial contractions, and upregulation of proinflammatory responses.

Vasoactive Peptides and Menstruation

A number of peptides may comprise a hormone-responsive paracrine system in the endometrium to regulate spiral artery blood flow. One is the endothelin–enkephalinase system (Casey and MacDonald, 1996). The endothelins—ET-1, ET-2, and ET-3—are small, 21-amino-acid peptides. Endothelin-1 (ET-1) is a potent vasoconstrictor first identified as a product of vascular endothelial cells (Yanagisawa and colleagues, 1988). Endothelins are degraded by enkephalinase, which is localized in endometrial stromal cells. Its specific activity in these cells increases strikingly and in parallel with the increase in progesterone blood levels after ovulation. The specific activity of enkephalinase is highest during the midluteal phase and declines steadily thereafter as progesterone plasma levels decrease (Casey and colleagues, 1991).

Activation of Lytic Mechanisms

Following vasoconstriction and endometrial cytokine changes, activation of proteases within stromal cells and leukocyte invasion is required to degrade the endometrial interstitial matrix. And matrix metalloproteases—MMP-1 and MMP-3—are released from stromal cells and may activate other neutrophilic proteases such as MMP-8 and MMP-9.

Origin of Menstrual Blood

Menstrual bleeding is from both systems, but arterial bleeding is appreciably greater than venous. Endometrial bleeding appears to follow rupture of an arteriole of a coiled artery, with consequent hematoma formation. With a hematoma, the superficial endometrium is distended and ruptures. Subsequently, fissures develop in the adjacent functionalis layer, and blood, as well as tissue fragments of various sizes, are sloughed. Hemorrhage stops with arteriolar constriction. Changes that accompany partial tissue necrosis also serve to seal vessel tips.

The endometrial surface is restored by growth of flanges, or collars, that form the everted free ends of the endometrial glands (Markee, 1940). These flanges increase in diameter very rapidly, and epithelial continuity is reestablished by fusion of the edges of these sheets of migrating thin cells.

Interval between Menses

The modal interval of menstruation is considered to be 28 days, but there is considerable variation among women, as well as in the cycle lengths of a given woman. Marked differences in the intervals between menstrual cycles are not necessarily indicative of infertility. Arey (1939) analyzed 12 studies comprising about 20,000 calendar records from 1500 women. He concluded that there is no evidence of perfect menstrual cycle regularity. Among average adult women, a third of cycles departed by more than 2 days from the mean of all cycle lengths. In his analysis of 5322 cycles in 485 normal women, an average interval of 28.4 days was estimated. Average cycle length in pubertal girls was 33.9 days. Haman (1942) surveyed 2460 cycles in 150 women, and the distribution curve for cycle length is shown in Figure 3-7.

THE DECIDUA

The decidua is a specialized, highly modified endometrium of pregnancy and is a function of hemochorial placentation. The latter has in common the process of trophoblast invasion, and considerable research has focused on the interaction between decidual cells and invading trophoblasts. *Decidualization*—transformation of secretory endometrium to decidua—is dependent on estrogen and progesterone and factors secreted by the implanting blastocyst. The special relationship that exists between the decidua and the invading trophoblast seemingly defies the laws of transplantation immunology (Beer and

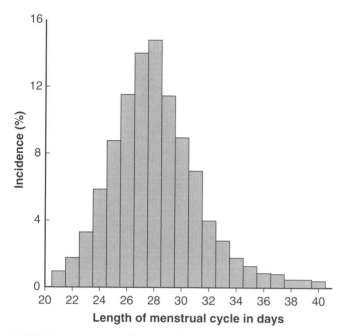

FIGURE 3–7. Duration of menstrual cycle. (Based on distribution data of Arey, 1939, and Haman, 1942.)

Billingham, 1971). The success of this unique semiallograft not only is of great scientific interest but may involve processes that harbor insights leading to more successful transplantation surgery and perhaps even immunological treatment of neoplasia (Billingham and Head, 1986; Lala and colleagues, 2002).

Decidual Structure

The first scientific description of the *membrana decidua* was in the 18th century by William Hunter. According to Damjanov (1985), *membrana* denoted its gross anatomical appearance, whereas *decidua* was an analogy to deciduous leaves to indicate that it is shed after childbirth. The decidua is classified into three parts based on anatomical location. Decidua directly beneath blastocyst implantation is modified by trophoblast invasion and becomes the *decidua basalis*. The *decidua capsularis* overlies the enlarging blastocyst, and initially separates it from the rest of the uterine cavity (Fig. 3-8). This portion is most prominent during the second month of pregnancy, consisting of decidual cells covered by a single layer of flattened epithelial cells. Internally, it contacts the avascular, extraembryonic fetal membrane—the *chorion laeve*. The remainder of the uterus is lined by *decidua parietalis*—sometimes called *decidua vera* when decidua capsularis and parietalis are joined.

During early pregnancy, there is a space between the decidua capsularis and parietalis because the gestational sac does not fill the entire uterine cavity. By 14 to 16 weeks, the expanding sac has enlarged to completely fill the uterine cavity. With fusion of the decidua capsularis and parietalis, the uterine cavity is functionally obliterated. In early pregnancy, the decidua begins to thicken, eventually attaining a depth of 5 to 10 mm. With magnification, furrows and numerous small openings, representing the mouths of uterine glands, can be detected. Later in pregnancy, the decidua becomes thinner, presumably because of pressure exerted by the expanding uterine contents.

The decidua parietalis and basalis, like the secretory endometrium, are composed of three layers. There is a surface, or compact zone—*zona compacta*; a middle portion, or spongy zone—*zona spongiosa*—with remnants of glands and numerous small blood vessels; and a basal zone—*zona basalis*. The zona compacta and spongiosa together form the *zona functionalis*. The basal zone remains after delivery and gives rise to new endometrium.

Decidual Reaction

In human pregnancy, the decidual reaction is completed only with blastocyst implantation. Predecidual changes, however, commence first during the midluteal phase in endometrial stromal cells adjacent to the spiral arteries and arterioles. Thereafter, they spread in waves throughout the uterine endometrium and then from the site of implantation. The endometrial stromal cells enlarge to form polygonal or round decidual cells. The nuclei become round and vesicular, and the cytoplasm becomes clear, slightly basophilic, and surrounded by a translucent membrane. Each mature decidual cell becomes surrounded by a pericellular membrane. Thus, the human decidual cells clearly build walls around themselves and possibly around the fetus. The pericellular matrix surrounding the decidual cells may allow attachment of cytotrophoblasts through

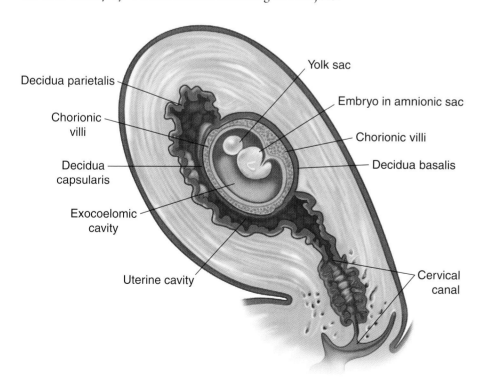

FIGURE 3-8 Decidualized endometrium covers the early embryo. Three portions of the decidua (basalis, capsularis, and parietalis) also are illustrated.

cellular adhesion molecules. The cell membrane also may provide decidual cell protection against selected cytotrophoblastic proteases.

Decidual Blood Supply

As a consequence of implantation, the blood supply to the decidua capsularis is lost as the embryo-fetus grows. Blood supply to the decidua parietalis through spiral arteries persists, as in the endometrium during the luteal phase of the cycle. The spiral arteries in the decidua parietalis retain a smooth muscle wall and endothelium and thereby remain responsive to vasoactive agents that act on their smooth muscle or endothelial cells.

The spiral arterial system supplying the decidua basalis directly beneath the implanting blastocyst, and ultimately the intervillous space, is altered remarkably. These spiral arterioles and arteries are invaded by cytotrophoblasts. During this process, the walls of vessels in the basalis are destroyed. Only a shell without smooth muscle or endothelial cells remains. Importantly, as a consequence, these vascular conduits of maternal blood—which become the uteroplacental vessels—are not responsive to vasoactive agents. By contrast, the fetal chorionic vessels, which transport blood between the placenta and the fetus, contain smooth muscle and thus do respond to vasoactive agents.

Decidual Histology

The decidua contains numerous cell types, whose composition varies with the stage of gestation (Loke and King, 1995). The primary cellular components are the true decidual cells, which differentiated from the endometrial stromal cells, and numerous maternal bone marrow–derived cells. The zona compacta consists of large, closely packed, epithelioid, polygonal, light-staining cells with round nuclei. Many stromal cells appear stellate, with long protoplasmic processes that anastomose with those of adjacent cells. This is particularly so when the decidua is edematous.

A striking abundance of large, granular lymphocytes termed decidual natural killer cells (NK) are present in the decidua early in pregnancy. In peripheral blood, there are two subsets of NK cells. About 90 percent are highly cytolytic and 10 percent show less cytolytic ability but increased secretion of cytokines. In contrast to peripheral blood, 95 percent of NK cells in decidua secrete cytokines. About half of these unique cells also express angiogenic factors. These decidua NK cells likely play an important role in trophoblast invasion and vasculogenesis.

Early in pregnancy, zona spongiosa of the decidua consists of large distended glands, often exhibiting marked hyperplasia and separated by minimal stroma. At first, the glands are lined by typical cylindrical uterine epithelium with abundant secretory activity that contributes to nourishment of the blastocyst. As pregnancy progresses, the epithelium gradually becomes cuboidal or even flattened, later degenerating and sloughing to a greater extent into the gland lumens. Later in pregnancy, the glandular elements largely disappear. In comparing the decidua parietalis at 16 weeks with the early proliferative endometrium of a nonpregnant woman, it is clear that there is marked hypertrophy but only slight hyperplasia of the endometrial stroma during decidual transformation.

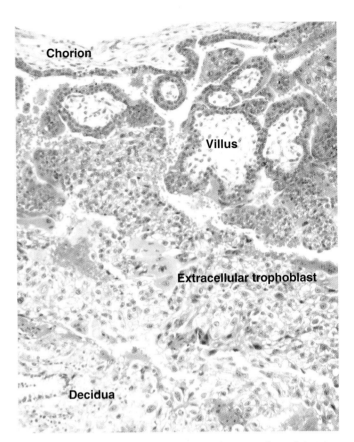

FIGURE 3-9 Section through junction of chorion, villi, and decidua basalis in early first-trimester pregnancy. (Used with permission from Dr. Kurt Benirschke.)

The decidua basalis contributes to the formation of the basal plate of the placenta (Fig. 3-9). It differs histologically from the decidua parietalis in two important respects. First, the spongy zone of the basalis consists mainly of arteries and widely dilated veins, and by term, the glands have virtually disappeared. Second, the decidua basalis is invaded by large numbers of interstitial trophoblast cells and trophoblastic giant cells. Although most abundant in the decidua, the giant cells commonly penetrate the upper myometrium. Their number and invasiveness may be so extensive as to resemble choriocarcinoma.

The *Nitabuch layer* is a zone of fibrinoid degeneration in which invading trophoblasts meet the decidua. If the decidua is defective, as in placenta accreta, the Nitabuch layer is usually absent (see Chap. 35, p. 776). There is also a more superficial, but inconsistent, deposition of fibrin—*Rohr stria*—at the bottom of the intervillous space and surrounding the anchoring villi. McCombs and Craig (1964) found that decidual necrosis is a normal phenomenon in the first and probably second trimesters. Thus, necrotic decidua obtained through curettage after spontaneous abortion in the first trimester should not necessarily be interpreted as either a cause or an effect of the pregnancy loss.

Decidual Prolactin

Convincing evidence has been presented that the decidua is the source of prolactin that is present in enormous amounts in amnionic fluid (Golander and colleagues, 1978; Riddick and co-workers, 1979). Decidual prolactin is not to be confused with placental lactogen (hPL), which is produced only by the syncytiotrophoblast. Rather, decidual prolactin is a product of the same gene that encodes for anterior pituitary prolactin. And although the amino acid sequence of prolactin in both tissues is identical, an alternative promoter is used within the prolactin gene to initiate transcription in decidua (Telgmann and Gellersen, 1998). The latter is thought to explain the different mechanisms that regulate expression in the decidua versus pituitary (Christian and colleagues, 2002a, 2000b).

The protein preferentially enters amnionic fluid, and little enters maternal blood. Consequently, prolactin levels in amnionic fluid are extraordinarily high and may reach 10,000 ng/mL during weeks 20 to 24 (Tyson and colleagues, 1972). This compares with fetal serum levels of 350 ng/mL and maternal serum levels of 150 to 200 ng/mL. As a result, decidual prolactin is a classic example of paracrine function between maternal and fetal tissues.

Role(s) of Decidual Prolactin

The exact physiological roles of decidual prolactin are still unknown. Its action is mediated by relative expression of two unique prolactin receptors as well as the amount of intact or full-length prolactin protein compared with the truncated 16-kDa form (Jabbour and Critchley, 2001). Receptor expression has been demonstrated in decidua, chorionic cytotrophoblasts, amnionic epithelium, and placental syncytiotrophoblast (Maaskant and colleagues, 1996). There are a number of possible roles for decidual prolactin. First, because most or all decidual prolactin enters amnionic fluid, there may be a role for this hormone in transmembrane solute and water transport, and thus, in maintenance of amnionic fluid volume. Second, there are prolactin receptors in a number of bone marrow-derived immune cells, and prolactin may stimulate T cells in an autocrine or paracrine manner (Pellegrini and colleagues, 1992). This raises the possibility that decidual prolactin may act in regulating immunological functions during pregnancy. Prolactin may play a role in regulation of angiogenesis during implantation. In this regard, intact prolactin protein enhances angiogenesis, whereas the proteolytic fragment can inhibit new vessel growth. Lastly, decidual prolactin has been shown in the mouse to have a protective function by repressing expression of genes detrimental to pregnancy maintenance (Bao and colleagues, 2007).

Regulation of Decidual Prolactin

Factors that regulate decidual prolactin production are not clearly defined. Most agents known to inhibit or stimulate pituitary prolactin secretion—including dopamine, dopamine agonists, and thyrotropin-releasing hormone—do not alter decidual prolactin secretion either in vivo or in vitro. Brosens and colleagues (2000) demonstrated that progestins act synergistically with cyclic adenosine monophosphate on endometrial stromal cells in culture to increase prolactin expression. This suggests that the level of progesterone receptor expression may determine the decidualization process, at least as marked by prolactin production. And arachidonic acid, but not $PGF_{2\alpha}$ or PGE_2, attenuates the rate of decidual prolactin secretion (Handwerger and colleagues, 1981). Conversely, a variety of cytokines and growth factors—ET-1, IL-1,

IL-2, and epidermal growth factor—decrease decidual prolactin secretion (Chao and colleagues, 1994; Frank and associates, 1995).

IMPLANTATION, PLACENTAL FORMATION, AND FETAL MEMBRANE DEVELOPMENT

Human placental development is as uniquely intriguing as fetal embryology. During its brief intrauterine passage, the fetus is dependent on the placenta for pulmonary, hepatic, and renal functions. These are accomplished through the unique placental anatomical association with the maternal interface. The placenta links mother and fetus by indirect interaction with maternal blood that spurts into the intervillous space from uteroplacental vessels. Maternal blood bathes the outer syncytiotrophoblast to allow exchange of gases and nutrients with fetal capillary blood within connective tissue at the villous core. Fetal and maternal blood are not normally mixed in this hemochorial placenta. There is also a paracrine system that links mother and fetus through the anatomical and biochemical juxtaposition of extraembryonic chorion laeve of fetal origin and maternal decidua parietalis. This is an extraordinarily important arrangement for communication between fetus and mother and for maternal immunological acceptance of the conceptus (Guzeloglu-Kayisli and associate, 2009).

Fertilization and Implantation

Ovum Fertilization and Zygote Cleavage

The union of egg and sperm at fertilization represents one of the most important and fascinating processes in biology. Ovulation frees the secondary oocyte and adherent cells of the cumulus-oocyte complex from the ovary. Although technically this mass of cells is released into the peritoneal cavity, the oocyte is quickly engulfed by the infundibulum of the fallopian tube. Further transport through the oviduct is accomplished by directional movement of cilia and tubal peristalsis. Fertilization normally occurs in the oviduct, and it is generally agreed that it must take place within a few hours, and no more than a day after ovulation.

Because of this narrow window of opportunity, spermatozoa must be present in the tube at the time of oocyte arrival. Almost all pregnancies result when intercourse occurs during the 2 days preceding or on the day of ovulation. Thus, the postovulatory and postfertilization developmental ages are similar.

Steps involved with fertilization are highly complex. Molecular mechanisms allow passage of spermatozoa between follicular cells, through the zona pellucida, and into the oocyte cytoplasm leading to the formation of the zygote. These are reviewed by Primakoff and Myles (2002).

The timing of events in early human development is described as days or weeks postfertilization, that is, postconceptional. By contrast, in most chapters of this book, clinical pregnancy dating is calculated from the start of the last menstrual period. As discussed earlier, the length of the follicular phase of the cycle is subject to more variability than the luteal phase. Thus, 1 week postfertilization corresponds to approximately 3 weeks from the last menstrual period in women with regular 28-day cycles.

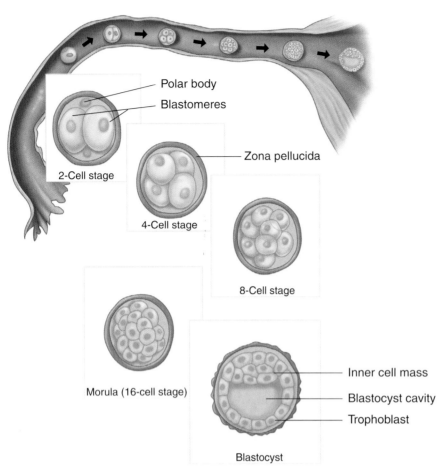

FIGURE 3-10 Zygote cleavage and formation of the blastocyst. The period of the morula begins at the 12- to 16-cell stage and ends when the blastocyst forms, which occurs when there are 50 to 60 blastomeres present. The zona pellucida has disappeared by the late blastocyst stage (5 days). The polar bodies, shown in the 2-cell stage, are small nonfunctional cells that soon degenerate.

After fertilization in the fallopian tube, the mature ovum becomes a *zygote*—a diploid cell with 46 chromosomes—that then undergoes cleavage into blastomeres (**Fig. 3-10**). In the two-cell zygote, the blastomeres and polar body are free in the perivitelline fluid and are surrounded by a thick *zona pellucida.* The zygote undergoes slow cleavage for 3 days while still within the fallopian tube. As the blastomeres continue to divide, a solid mulberry-like ball of cells—the *morula*—is produced. The morula enters the uterine cavity about 3 days after fertilization. Gradual accumulation of fluid between the cells of the morula results in the formation of the early *blastocyst.*

The Blastocyst

In the earliest stages of the human blastocyst, the wall of the primitive blastodermic vesicle consists of a single layer of ectoderm. As early as 4 to 5 days after fertilization, the 58-cell blastula differentiates into five embryo-producing cells—the *inner cell mass,* and 53 cells destined to form trophoblasts (Hertig, 1962). In a 58-cell blastocyst, the outer cells, called the *trophectoderm,* can be distinguished from the inner cell mass that forms the embryo (see Fig. 3-10).

Interestingly, the 107-cell blastocyst is found to be no larger than the earlier cleavage stages, despite the accumulated fluid. It measures about 0.155 mm in diameter, which is similar to the size

of the initial postfertilization zygote. At this stage, the eight formative, or embryo-producing cell, are surrounded by 99 trophoblastic cells. It is at this stage that the blastocyst is released from the zona pellucida as a result of secretion of specific proteases from the secretory-phase endometrial glands (O'Sullivan and colleagues, 2002).

Release from the zona pellucida allows blastocyst-produced cytokines and hormones to directly influence endometrial receptivity (Lindhard and colleagues, 2002). Evidence has accumulated that IL-1α and IL-1β are secreted by the blastocyst and that these cytokines can directly influence the endometrium. Embryos also have been shown to secrete human chorionic gonadotropin (hCG), which may influence endometrial receptivity (Licht and coworkers, 2001; Lobo and colleagues, 2001). The receptive endometrium is thought to respond by producing leukemia inhibitory factor (LIF) and colony-stimulating factor-1 (CSF-1). These serve to increase trophoblast protease production that degrades selected endometrial extracellular matrix proteins and allows trophoblast invasion. Thus, embryo "hatching" is a critical step toward successful pregnancy as it allows association of trophoblasts with endometrial epithelial cells and permits release of trophoblast-produced hormones into the uterine cavity.

Blastocyst Implantation

Implantation of the embryo into the uterine wall is a common feature of all mammals. In women, it takes place 6 or 7 days after fertilization. This process can be divided into three phases: (1) apposition—initial adhesion of the blastocyst to the uterine wall; (2) adhesion—increased physical contact between the blastocyst and uterine epithelium; and (3) invasion—penetration and invasion of syncytiotrophoblast and cytotrophoblast into the endometrium, inner third of the myometrium, and uterine vasculature.

Successful implantation requires receptive endometrium appropriately primed with estrogen and progesterone. As shown in Figure 3-1, uterine receptivity is limited to days 20 to 24 of the cycle (Bergh and Navot, 1992). Adherence to epithelium is mediated by cell-surface receptors at the implantation site that interact with receptors on the blastocyst (Carson, 2002; Lessey and Castelbaum, 2002; Lindhard and associates, 2002; Paria and colleagues, 2002). Development of a receptive epithelium results from the postovulatory production of estrogen and progesterone by the corpus luteum. If the blastocyst approaches the endometrium after cycle day 24, the potential for adhesion is diminished because synthesis of antiadhesive glycoproteins prevents receptor interactions (Navot and Bergh, 1991).

At the time of its interaction with the endometrium, the blastocyst is composed of 100 to 250 cells. The blastocyst loosely adheres to the endometrial epithelium by *apposition.* This most commonly occurs on the upper posterior uterine wall. In women, syncytiotrophoblast has not been distinguished prior to implantation. Attachment of the trophectoderm of the blastocyst to the endometrial surface by apposition and adherence appears to be closely regulated by paracrine interactions between these two tissues.

Successful endometrial blastocyst adhesion involves modification in expression of cellular adhesion molecules (CAMs). The *integrins*—one of four families of CAMs—are cell-surface receptors that mediate adhesion of cells to extracellular matrix proteins (Lessey and Castelbaum, 2002). Great diversity of cell binding to a host of different extracellular matrix proteins is possible by differential regulation of the integrin receptors. Endometrial integrins are hormonally regulated, and a specific set of integrins expressed at implantation (Lessey and colleagues, 1996). Specifically, αVβ3 and α4β1 integrins expressed on endometrial epithelium are considered a marker of receptivity for blastocyst attachment. Aberrant expression of αVβ3 has been associated with infertility (Lessey and coworkers, 1995).

Biology of the Trophoblast

The formation of the human placenta begins with the trophectoderm, which is first to differentiate at the morula stage. It gives rise to the layer of trophoblast cells encircling the blastocyst. And then until term, the trophoblast plays critical roles at the fetal-maternal interface. Trophoblast exhibits the most variable structure, function, and developmental pattern of all placental components. Its invasiveness provides for implantation, its role in nutrition of the conceptus is reflected in its name, and

its function as an endocrine organ is essential to maternal physiological adaptations and to maintenance of pregnancy.

Trophoblast Differentiation

By the eighth day postfertilization, after initial implantation, the trophoblast has differentiated into an outer multinucleated syncytium—primitive *syncytiotrophoblast,* and an inner layer of primitive mononuclear cells—*cytotrophoblast* (Fig. 3-11). The latter are germinal cells for the syncytium and are the primary secretory component within the placenta. Although the ability to undergo DNA synthesis and mitosis, a well-demarcated cell border, and a single nucleus characterize each cytotrophoblast, these characteristics are lacking in the syncytiotrophoblast (Arnholdt and colleagues, 1991). It is so named because it has no individual cells. Instead, it has an amorphous cytoplasm without cell borders, nuclei that are multiple and diverse in size and shape, and a continuous syncytial lining. This configuration aids transport across the syncytiotrophoblast, because control of transport is not dependent on the participation of individual cells.

After implantation is complete, the trophoblast further differentiates along two main pathways, giving rise to villous and extravillous trophoblast. As shown in Figure 3-12, both pathways give rise to populations of trophoblast cells that have distinct functions when in contact with maternal tissues (Loke and King, 1995). The *villous trophoblast* gives rise to the chorionic villi, which primarily transport oxygen and nutrients between the fetus and mother. The *extravillous trophoblast* migrates into the decidua and myometrium and also penetrates maternal vasculature, thus coming into contact with a variety of maternal cell types (Pijnenborg, 1994). The extravillous trophoblast is thus further classified as *interstitial trophoblast* and *endovascular trophoblast.* The interstitial trophoblast invades the decidua and eventually penetrates the myometrium to form placental bed

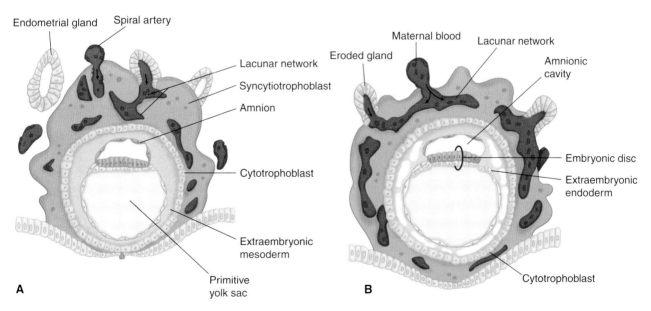

FIGURE 3-11 Drawing of sections through implanted blastocysts. **A.** At 10 days. **B.** At 12 days after fertilization. The stage of development is characterized by the intercommunication of the lacunae filled with maternal blood. Note in **(B)** that large cavities have appeared in the extraembryonic mesoderm, forming the beginning of the extraembryonic coelom. Also note that extraembryonic endodermal cells have begun to form on the inside of the primitive yolk sac. (Adapted from Moore, 1988.)

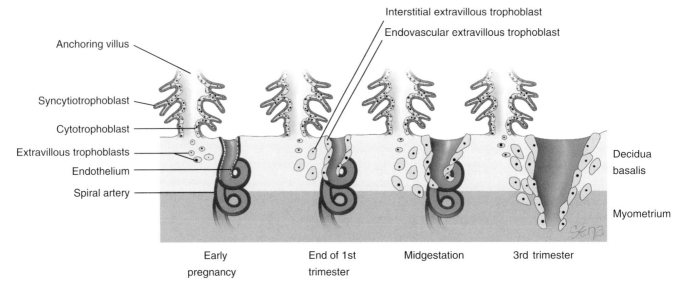

FIGURE 3-12 Extravillous trophoblasts are found outside the villus and can be subdivided in endovascular and interstitial categories. Endovascular trophoblasts invade and transform spiral arteries during pregnancy to create low-resistance blood flow that is characteristic of the placenta. Interstitial trophoblasts invade the decidua and surround spiral arteries.

giant cells. These trophoblasts also surround spiral arteries. The endovascular trophoblast penetrates the lumen of the spiral arteries (Pijnenborg and colleagues, 1983). These are both discussed in greater detail in sections that follow.

Embryonic Development after Implantation

Early Trophoblast Invasion

After gentle erosion between epithelial cells of the surface endometrium, invading trophoblasts burrow deeper, and by the 10th day, the blastocyst becomes totally encased within endometrium (Fig. 3-13). The mechanisms leading to trophoblast invasion into the endometrium are similar to the characteristics of metastasizing malignant cells. They are discussed further on page 53.

At 9 days of development, the blastocyst wall facing the uterine lumen is a single layer of flattened cells (Figs. 3-11 and 3–14). The opposite, thicker wall comprises two zones—the trophoblasts and the embryo-forming inner cell mass. As early as 7½ days after fertilization, the inner cell mass or embryonic disc is differentiated into a thick plate of

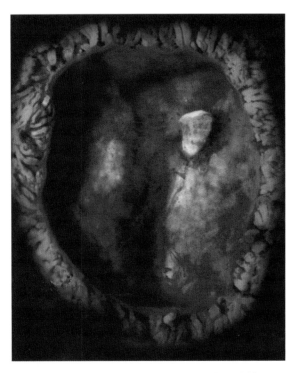

FIGURE 3-13 Photomicrograph of an early implanted blastocyst. (From Tsiaras, 2002, with permission; visualization is provided by www.theVisualMD.com.)

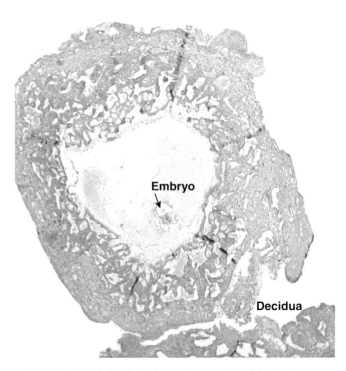

FIGURE 3-14 Early implantation of a conceptus. (Used with permission from Dr. Kurt Benirschke.)

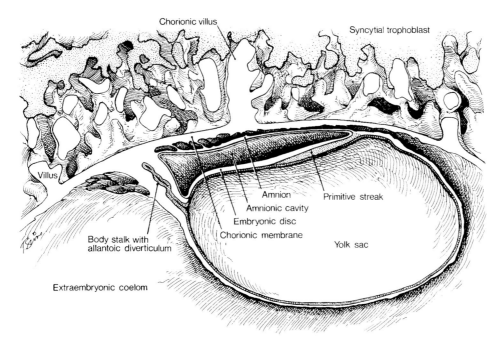

FIGURE 3-15 Median view of a drawing of a wax reconstruction of an 18-day-old Mateer-Streeter embryo shows the amnionic cavity and its relations to chorionic membrane and yolk sac (×500). (After Streeter, 1920.)

primitive ectoderm and an underlying layer of endoderm. Some small cells appear between the embryonic disc and the trophoblast and enclose a space that will become the amnionic cavity.

Embryonic mesenchyme first appears as isolated cells within blastocyst cavity. When the cavity is completely lined with mesoderm, it is termed the *chorionic vesicle,* and its membrane, now called the *chorion,* is composed of trophoblasts and mesenchyme. The amnion and yolk sac are illustrated in Figure 3-15. Mesenchymal cells within the cavity are the most numerous and eventually will condense to form the body stalk. This stalk joins the embryo to the nutrient chorion and later develops into the umbilical cord. The body stalk can be recognized at an early stage at the caudal end of the embryonic disc.

Lacunae Formation within the Syncytiotrophoblast

Beginning about 12 days after conception, the syncytiotrophoblast of the trophoblast shell is permeated by a system of intercommunicating channels called trophoblastic lacunae. As the embryo enlarges, more maternal decidua basalis is invaded by basal syncytiotrophoblast. After invasion of superficial decidual capillary walls, lacunae become filled with maternal blood (see Fig. 3-11). At the same time, the decidual reaction intensifies in the surrounding stroma, which is characterized by enlargement of the decidual stromal cells and glycogen storage.

Development of Primary Villous Stalks

With deeper blastocyst invasion into the decidua, the extravillous cytotrophoblasts give rise to solid primary villi composed of a cytotrophoblast core covered by syncytium. These arise

from buds of cytotrophoblast that begin to protrude into the primitive syncytium before 12 days postfertilization. As the lacunae join, a complicated labyrinth is formed that is partitioned by these solid cytotrophoblastic columns. The trophoblast-lined labyrinthine channels form the intervillous space, and the solid cellular columns form the primary villous stalks. The villi initially are located over the entire blastocyst surface. They later disappear except over the most deeply implanted portion, which is destined to form the placenta.

Placental Organization

The term *hemochorial* is used to describe human placentation. It derives from *hemo* referring to maternal blood, which directly bathes the syncytiotrophoblast, and *chorio* for chorion (placenta). The older term *hemochorioendothelial* takes into consideration that chorionic tissue is separated from fetal blood by the *endothelial* wall of the fetal capillaries that traverse the villous core.

Chorionic Villi

Beginning on approximately the 12th day after fertilization, chorionic villi can first be distinguished. Mesenchymal cords derived from extraembryonic mesoderm invade the solid trophoblast columns. These form *secondary villi*. After angiogenesis begins in the mesenchymal cores, the resulting villi are termed *tertiary.* Although maternal venous sinuses are tapped early in implantation, maternal arterial blood does not enter the intervillous space until around day 15. By approximately the 17th day, however, fetal blood vessels are functional, and a placental circulation is established. The fetal–placental circulation is completed when embryonic blood vessels are connected with chorionic vessels. In some villi, there is failure of angiogenesis from lack of circulation. They can be seen normally, but the most striking exaggeration of this process is seen with hydatidiform mole (see Chap. 11, p. 257).

Villi are covered by the outer layer of syncytium and inner layer of cytotrophoblasts, which are also known as *Langhans cells* (see Fig. 3-12). Cytotrophoblast proliferation at the villous tips produce the trophoblastic cell columns that form *anchoring villi*. They are not invaded by fetal mesenchyme, and they are anchored to the decidua at the basal plate. Thus, the base of the intervillous space faces the maternal side and consists of cytotrophoblasts from cell columns, the covering shell of syncytiotrophoblast, and maternal decidua of the basal plate. The base of the chorionic plate forms the roof of the intervillous space and consists of two layers of trophoblasts externally and fibrous mesoderm internally. The "definitive" chorionic plate is formed by 8 to 10 weeks as the amnionic and primary chorionic plate mesenchyme fuse together. This formation is accomplished by expansion of the amnionic sac, which also surrounds the connective stalk and the allantois and joins these structures to form the umbilical cord (Kaufmann and Scheffen, 1992).

Villus Ultrastructure

Interpretation of the fine structure of the placenta came from electron microscopic studies of Wislocki and Dempsey (1955). There are prominent microvilli on the syncytial surface that correspond to the so-called brush border described by light microscopy (Fig. 3-16). Associated pinocytotic vacuoles and vesicles are related to absorptive and secretory placental functions. Microvilli act to increase surface area in direct contact with maternal blood. This contact between the trophoblastic surface and maternal blood is the defining characteristic of the hemochorial placenta.

The human hemochorial placenta can be subdivided into hemodichorial or hemomonochorial (Enders, 1965). The di-

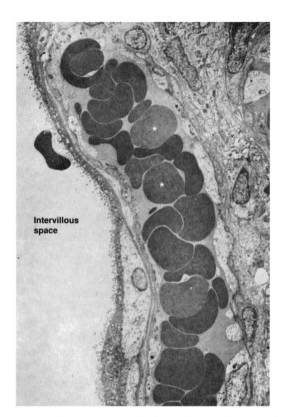

FIGURE 3-17 Electron micrograph of term human placenta villus. A villus capillary filled with red blood cells (*asterisks*) is seen in close proximity to the microvilli border. (From *The Human Placenta*, JD Boyd and WJ Hamilton (eds), p. 154. Copyright © 1970 Heffer & Sons, Ltd. Reproduced with permission of Blackwell Publishing Ltd.)

chorial type is more prominent during the first trimester of gestation. It consists of the inner layer of the cytotrophoblasts with the associated basal lamina, covered by a layer of syncytiotrophoblasts (see Fig. 3-16). Later in gestation the inner layer of cytotrophoblasts is no longer continuous, and by term there are only scattered cells present (Fig. 3-17). These create a narrower hemomonochorial barrier that aids nutrient and oxygen transport to the fetus.

Placental Development

Development of the Chorion and Decidua

In early pregnancy, the villi are distributed over the entire periphery of the chorionic membrane. A blastocyst dislodged from the endometrium at this stage of development appears shaggy (Fig. 3-18). As the blastocyst with its surrounding trophoblasts grows and expands into the decidua, one pole extends outward toward the endometrial cavity. The opposite pole will form the placenta from villous trophoblasts and anchoring cytotrophoblasts. Chorionic villi in contact with the decidua basalis proliferate to form the *chorion frondosum*—or leafy chorion—which is the fetal component of the placenta. As growth of embryonic and extraembryonic tissues continues, the blood supply of the chorion facing the endometrial cavity is restricted. Because of this, villi in contact with the decidua capsularis cease to grow and degenerate. This portion of the chorion becomes the avascular fetal membrane that abuts the decidua parietalis, that is, the chorion laeve—or

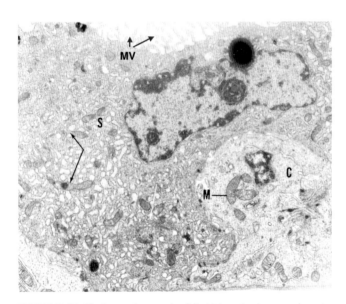

FIGURE 3-16 Electron micrograph of first-trimester human placenta showing well-differentiated syncytiotrophoblast (S) with numerous mitochondria (*black arrows*). Cytotrophoblast (C) has large mitochondria (M) but few other organelles. At the top, there is a prominent border of microvilli (*red arrows*) arising from the syncytium.

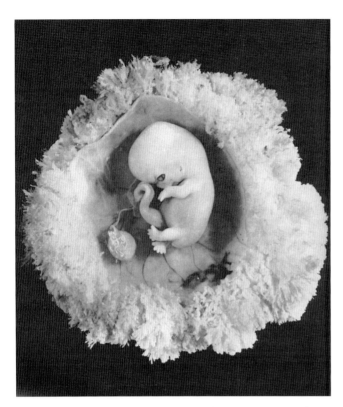

FIGURE 3-18 Photograph of an opened chorionic sac. An early embryo and yolk sac are seen. Note the prominent fringe of chorionic villi. (From *The Human Placenta*, JD Boyd and WJ Hamilton (eds), p. 84. Copyright © 1970 Heffer & Sons, Ltd. Reproduced with permission of Blackwell Publishing Ltd.)

smooth chorion. The chorion laeve is generally more translucent than the amnion and rarely exceeds 1-mm thickness. The chorion is composed of cytotrophoblasts and fetal mesodermal mesenchyme that survives in a relatively low-oxygen atmosphere.

Until near the end of the third month, the chorion laeve is separated from the amnion by the exocoelomic cavity. Thereafter, they are in intimate contact to form an avascular amniochorion. These two structures are important sites of molecular transfer and metabolic activity. Moreover, they constitute an important paracrine arm of the fetal–maternal communication system.

With continued expansion of the embryo–fetus, the uterine lumen is obliterated, and the chorion laeve becomes contiguous with the entire maternal decidua parietalis that is not occupied by the placenta. As the fetus grows, the decidua capsularis merges with the parietalis. The capsularis then is largely lost by pressure and the attendant loss of blood supply. The area of decidua where decidua capsularis and decidua parietalis merge is referred to as the *decidua vera*.

Maternal Regulation of Trophoblast Invasion and Vascular Growth.
Decidual natural killer cells (dNK) accumulate in the decidua during the first half of pregnancy and are found in direct contact with trophoblasts. As described on page 46, these cells lack cytotoxic functions as well as other unique properties that distinguish them from circulating natural killer cells and from natural killer cells in the endometrium prior to pregnancy (Manaster and co-workers, 2008). This is important because it prevents them from recognizing and destroying fetal cells as

"foreign." Hanna and associates (2006) have elucidated the ability of dNK cells to attract and promote invasion of trophoblast into the decidua and promote vascular growth. Decidual NK cells express both interleukin-8 and interferon-inducible protein-10, which bind to receptors on invasive trophoblast cells to promote their invasion into the decidua toward the spiral arteries. Decidual NK cells also produce proangiogenic factors, including VEGF and placental growth factor (PlGF), which promote vascular growth in the decidua. In addition, trophoblasts secrete specific chemokines that attract the dNK cells to the maternal-fetal interface. Thus, both cell types simultaneously attract each other to promote decidual population.

Trophoblast Invasion of the Endometrium.
The extravillous trophoblast of the first-trimester placenta are highly invasive. They form columns of cells that extend from the endometrium to the inner third of the myometrium. Recall that hemochorial placental development requires invasion of endometrium and spiral arteries. The invasive ability of trophoblasts results from their ability to secrete numerous proteolytic enzymes capable of digesting the extracellular matrix as well as activating proteinases already present in the endometrium. Trophoblasts produce urokinase-type plasminogen activator, which converts plasminogen into the broadly acting serine protease *plasmin*. This in turn both degrades matrix proteins and activates matrix metalloproteinases (MMPs), which are a family of structurally similar enzymes. One member of the family, matrix metalloproteinase-9 (MMP-9), appears to be critical for human trophoblast invasion. MMP-9 production is increased by trophoblast factors such as IL-1 and hCG as well as paracrine uterine factors such as leukemia inhibiting factor and colony-stimulating factor-1 (Bischof, 2002; Fitzgerald, 2008; Librach, 1991, and all their colleagues).

The relative ability to invade maternal tissue in early pregnancy compared with limited invasiveness in late pregnancy is controlled by autocrine and paracrine trophoblastic and endometrial factors. Trophoblasts secrete insulin-like growth factor II, which acts in an autocrine manner. It promotes invasion into the endometrium, whereas decidual cells secrete insulin-like growth factor binding protein type 4, which blocks this autocrine loop. Thus, the degree of trophoblast invasion is controlled by regulation of matrix degradation as well as by factors that cause trophoblast migration.

Integrin subunit expression also appears important to control trophoblast invasion and adhesive interactions between trophoblast cells during column formation. Recall that the decidual cell becomes completely encased by a pericellular extracellular matrix membrane. This "wall" around the decidual cell provides a scaffolding for attachment of the cytotrophoblasts of the anchoring villi. The cytotrophoblast first elaborate selected proteinases that degrade decidual extracellular matrix. Thereafter, expression of a specific group of integrins enables the docking of these cells. There are also integrin-mediated adhesive interactions of trophoblast cells with each other. In particular, the interaction of L-selectin with its carbohydrate ligands in the cytotrophoblast is important in formation and maintenance of cell columns (Prakobphol and colleagues, 2006). Trophoblasts are further secured by fetal fibronectin (Feinberg and colleagues, 1991). Fetal-specific fibronectin (fFN) is a unique glycopeptide of the fibronectin molecule. It is also called *trophoblast glue* to describe a critical role in the migration and attachment of trophoblasts to maternal decidua. And related, presence of fFN in cervical or vaginal fluid is used as a prognostic indicator for preterm labor (see Chap. 36, p. 816).

Invasion of Spiral Arteries

One of the most remarkable features of human placental development is the extensive modification of maternal vasculature by trophoblasts, which are by definition of fetal origin. These events occur in the first half of pregnancy and are considered in detail because of their importance to uteroplacental blood flow. They are also integral to some pathological conditions such as preeclampsia and fetal-growth restriction (see Chap. 34, p. 710). Modifications of spiral arteries are carried out by two populations of extravillous trophoblast—interstitial trophoblast, which surrounds the arteries, and endovascular trophoblast, which penetrates the spiral artery lumen (see Fig. 3-12). Although earlier work has focused on the role of the endovascular trophoblast, function of the interstitial trophoblast has more recently been investigated (Benirschke and Kaufmann, 2000; Pijnenborg and colleagues, 1983). These interstitial cells are now recognized to constitute a major portion of the placental bed, penetrating the decidua and adjacent myometrium. They aggregate around spiral arteries, and their functions may include vessel preparation for endovascular trophoblast invasion.

Endovascular trophoblast enters the lumen of the spiral arteries and initially forms cellular plugs. It then destroys vascular endothelium via an apoptosis mechanism and invades and modifies vascular media. Thus, fibrinoid material replaces smooth muscle and connective tissue of the vessel media. Spiral arteries later regenerate endothelium. Hamilton and Boyd (1966) report that Friedlander in 1870 first described structural changes in spiral arteries. Invading endovascular trophoblast can extend several centimeters along the vessel lumen, and they must migrate against arterial flow. These vascular changes are not observed in the decidua parietalis, that is, in decidual sites removed from the invading cytotrophoblasts. Of note, invasion by trophoblasts involves only the decidual spiral arteries and not decidual veins.

In their summary of anatomical studies of the uteroplacental vasculature, Ramsey and Donner (1980) described that development of these uteroplacental vessels proceeds in two waves or stages. The first wave occurs before 12 weeks postfertilization and consists of invasion and modification of spiral arteries up to the border between deciduas and myometrium. The second wave is between 12 and 16 weeks and involves some invasion of the intramyometrial segments of spiral arteries. The remodeling by this two-phase invasion converts narrow-lumen, muscular spiral arteries into dilated, low-resistance uteroplacental vessels. Molecular mechanisms of these crucial events, and their significance in the pathogenesis of preeclampsia and fetal-growth restriction, have been reviewed by Kaufmann (2003) and Red-Horse (2006) and their associates.

Establishment of Maternal Blood Flow

About 1 month after conception, maternal blood enters the intervillous space in fountain-like bursts from the spiral arteries.

Blood is propelled outside of the maternal vessels and sweeps over and directly bathes the syncytiotrophoblast. The apical surface of the syncytiotrophoblast consists of a complex microvillous structure that undergoes continual shedding and reformation during pregnancy.

Villus Branching

Although certain villi of the chorion frondosum extend from the chorionic plate to the decidua to serve as anchoring villi, most arborize and end freely in the intervillous space. As gestation proceeds, the short, thick, early stem villi branch to form progressively finer subdivisions and greater numbers of increasingly smaller villi (Fig. 3-19). Each of the truncal or main stem villi and their ramifications (rami) constitute a placental *lobule,* or *cotyledon.* Each lobule is supplied with a single truncal branch of the chorionic artery. And each lobule has a single vein so that lobules constitute functional units of placental architecture.

Placental Growth and Maturation

Placental Growth

In the first trimester, placental growth is more rapid than that of the fetus. But by approximately 17 postmenstrual weeks, placental and fetal weights are approximately equal. By term, placental weight is approximately one sixth of fetal weight. According to Boyd and Hamilton (1970), the average placenta at term is 185 mm in diameter and 23 mm in thickness, with a volume of 497 mL and a weight of 508 g. These measurements vary widely, and there are multiple variant placental forms and several types of umbilical cord insertions. These are discussed in detail in Chapter 27 (p. 577).

Viewed from the maternal surface, the number of slightly elevated convex areas, called *lobes,* varies from 10 to 38. Lobes are incompletely separated by grooves of variable depth that overlie *placental septa,* which arise from folding of the basal plate. Although grossly visible lobes are commonly referred to as cotyledons, this is not accurate. Correctly used, lobules or cotyledons are the functional units supplied by each primary villus.

The total number of placental lobes remains the same throughout gestation, and individual lobes continue to grow—although less actively in the final weeks (Crawford, 1959).

Placental Maturation

As villi continue to branch and the terminal ramifications become more numerous and smaller, the volume and prominence of cytotrophoblasts decrease. As the syncytium thins, the fetal vessels become more prominent and lie closer to the surface. The villous stroma also exhibits changes as gestation progresses. In early pregnancy, the branching connective-tissue cells are separated by an abundant loose intercellular matrix. Later, the stroma becomes denser and the cells more spindly and more closely packed.

Another change in the stroma involves the infiltration of *Hofbauer cells,* which are fetal macrophages. These are nearly round with vesicular, often eccentric nuclei and very granular or vacuolated cytoplasm. Hofbauer cells are characterized histochemically by intracytoplasmic lipid and by phenotypic markers specific for macrophages. They increase in numbers and

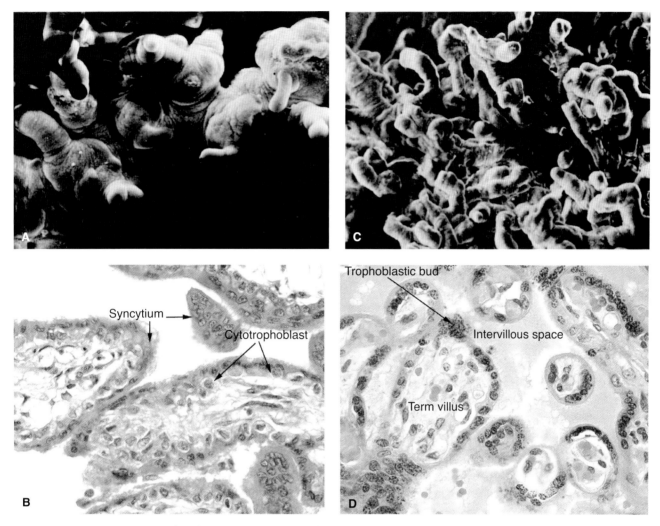

FIGURE 3-19 Electron micrographs **(A, C)** and photomicrographs **(B, D)** of early and late human placentas. **A** and **B.** Limited branching of villi is seen in this early placenta. **C** and **D.** With placenta maturation, increasing villous arborization is seen, and villous capillaries lie closer to the surface of the villus. (The electron micrographs were published in *American Journal of Obstetrics & Gynecology,* Vol. 122, No. 7, BF King and DN Menton, Scanning electron microscopy of human placental villi from early and late in gestation, pp. 824–828, Copyright Elsevier 1975. Photomicrographs used with permission from Dr. Kurt Benirschke.)

maturation state throughout pregnancy. These macrophages are phagocytic, have an immunosuppressive phenotype, can produce a variety of cytokines, and are capable of paracrine regulation of trophoblast functions (Cervar and colleagues, 1999; Vince and Johnson, 1996).

Some of the histological changes that accompany placental growth and maturation provide an increased efficiency of transport and exchange to meet increasing fetal metabolic requirements. Among these changes are decreased syncytiotrophoblastic thickness, significant cytotrophoblast reduction, decreased stroma, and increased number of capillaries with their approximation to the syncytial surface. By 16 weeks the apparent continuity of the cytotrophoblasts is lost. At term, the covering of the villi may be focally reduced to a thin layer of syncytium with minimal connective tissue in which thin-walled fetal capillaries abut the trophoblast and dominate the villi.

There are some changes in placental architecture that can cause decreased efficiency of placental exchange if they are sub-

stantive. These include thickening of basal lamina of trophoblast or capillaries, obliteration of certain fetal vessels, and fibrin deposition on the villi surface.

Fetal and Maternal Blood Circulation in the Mature Placenta

Because the placenta is functionally an intimate approximation of the fetal capillary bed to maternal blood, its gross anatomy primarily concerns vascular relations. The fetal surface is covered by the transparent amnion, beneath which chorionic vessels course. A section through the placenta includes amnion, chorion, chorionic villi and intervillous space, decidual (basal) plate, and myometrium (Figs. 3-20, 3-21, 3-22). The maternal surface is divided into irregular lobes by furrows produced by septa, which consist of fibrous tissue with sparse vessels. The broad-based septa ordinarily do not reach the chorionic plate, thus providing only incomplete partitions (Fig. 3-23).

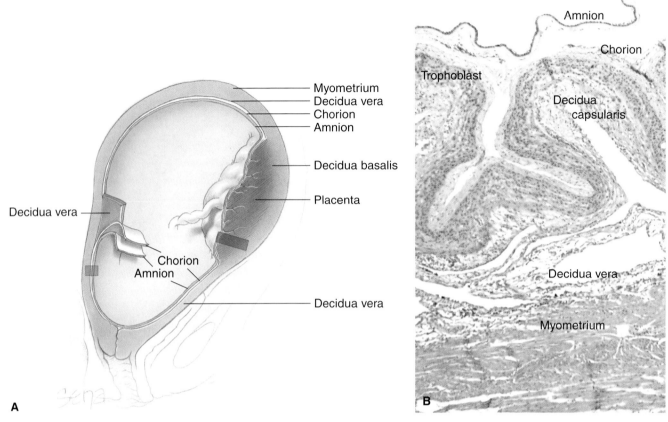

FIGURE 3-20 A. Uterus of pregnant woman showing a normal placenta in situ. **B.** Photomicrograph of a histologic section through amnion, chorion, and decidua vera that is depicted in **(A)** (*green slice*). (Used with permission from Dr. Kurt Benirschke.)

Fetal Circulation

Deoxygenated venous-like fetal blood flows to the placenta through the two umbilical arteries. As the cord joins the placenta, these umbilical vessels branch repeatedly beneath the amnion and again within the dividing villi, finally forming capillary networks in the terminal divisions. Blood with significantly higher oxygen content returns from the placenta via a single umbilical vein to the fetus.

The branches of the umbilical vessels that traverse along the fetal surface of the placenta in the chorionic plate are referred to as the *placental surface* or *chorionic vessels*. These vessels are responsive to vasoactive substances, but anatomically, morphologically, histologically, and functionally, they are unique. *Chorionic arteries always cross over chorionic veins.* Vessels are most readily recognized by this interesting relationship, but they are difficult to distinguish by histological criteria. In 65 percent of placentas, chorionic arteries form a fine network supplying the cotyledons—a pattern of disperse-type branching. The remaining 35 percent radiate to the edge of the placenta without narrowing. Both types are end arteries that supply one cotyledon as each branch turns downward to pierce the chorionic plate.

Truncal arteries are perforating branches of the surface arteries that pass through the chorionic plate. Each truncal artery supplies one cotyledon. There is a decrease in smooth muscle of the vessel wall and an increase in the caliber of the vessel as it penetrates through the chorionic plate. The loss in muscle continues as the truncal arteries and veins branch into their rami.

Before 10 weeks, there is no end-diastolic flow pattern within the umbilical artery at the end of the fetal cardiac cycle (Cole, 1991; Fisk, 1988; Loquet, 1988, and all their colleagues). After 10 weeks, end-diastolic flow appears and is maintained throughout normal pregnancy (Maulik, 1997). Clinically, these are studied with Doppler sonography to assess fetal well-being (see Chap. 16, p. 363).

Maternal Circulation

Because an efficient maternal–placental circulation is requisite, many investigators have sought to define factors that regulate blood flow into and from the intervillous space. An adequate mechanism must explain how blood can: (1) leave maternal circulation; (2) flow into an amorphous space lined by syncytiotrophoblast, rather than capillary endothelium; and (3) return through maternal veins without producing arteriovenous-like shunts that would prevent maternal blood from remaining in contact with villi long enough for adequate exchange. Early studies of Ramsey and Davis (1963) and Ramsey and Harris (1966) help to provide a physiological explanation of placental circulation. These investigators demonstrated, by careful, low-pressure injections of radiocontrast material, that arterial entrances as well as venous exits are scattered randomly over the entire base of the placenta.

The physiology of maternal-placental circulation is depicted in Figure 3-24. Maternal blood enters through the basal plate and is driven high up toward the chorionic plate by arterial

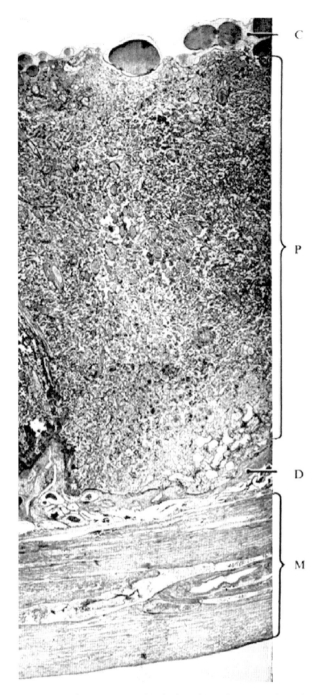

FIGURE 3-21 Photomicrograph of a histological section through amnion, chorion, and decidua basalis depicted in Figure 3-20A (*blue slice*). C = chorionic plate with fetal blood vessels; P = placental villi; D = decidua basalis; M = myometrium.

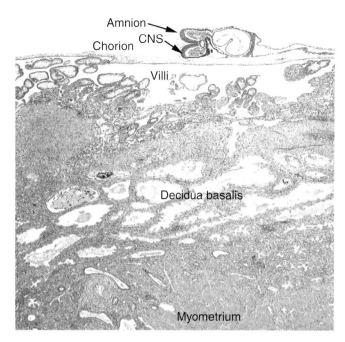

FIGURE 3-22 Photomicrograph of early implanted blastocyst. Trophoblasts are seen invading the decidua basalis. (Used with permission from Dr. Kurt Benirschke.)

arrangement aids closure of veins during a uterine contraction and prevents entry of maternal blood from the intervillous space. The number of arterial openings into the intervillous space becomes gradually reduced by cytotrophoblast invasion. According to Brosens and Dixon (1963), there are about 120 spiral arterial entries into the intervillous space at term. These discharge blood in spurts that bathes the adjacent villi (Borell and co-workers, 1958). After the 30th week, a prominent venous plexus separates the decidua basalis from the myometrium, thus participating in providing a plane of cleavage for placental separation.

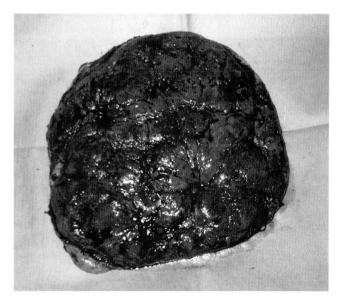

FIGURE 3-23 Photograph of the maternal surface of the placenta. Placenta lobes are formed by clefts on the surface that originate from placental septa. (Used with permission from Dr. Judith J. Head.)

pressure before laterally dispersing. After bathing the external microvillous surface of chorionic villi, maternal blood drains back through venous orifices in the basal plate and enters uterine veins. Thus, maternal blood traverses the placenta randomly without preformed channels. The previously described trophoblast invasion of the spiral arteries creates low-resistance vessels that can accommodate massive increase in uterine perfusion over gestation. Generally, spiral arteries are perpendicular to, but veins are parallel to, the uterine wall. This

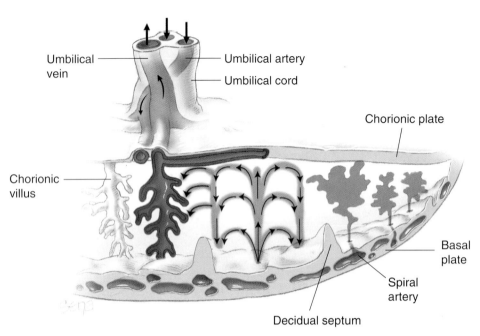

Umbilical
vein

Umbilical artery

Umbilical cord

Chorionic plate

Chorionic
villus

Basal
plate

Spiral
artery

Decidual septum

FIGURE 3-24 Schematic drawing of a section through a full-term placenta. Maternal blood flows into the intervillous spaces in funnel-shaped spurts. Exchanges occur with fetal blood as maternal blood flows around the villi. In-flowing arterial blood pushes venous blood into the endometrial veins, which are scattered over the entire surface of the decidua basalis. Note also that the umbilical arteries carry deoxygenated fetal blood to the placenta and that the umbilical vein carries oxygenated blood to the fetus. Placental lobes are separated from each other by placental (decidual) septa.

As discussed, both inflow and outflow are curtailed during uterine contractions. Bleker and associates (1975) used serial sonography during normal labor and found that placental length, thickness, and surface area increased during contractions. They attributed this to distension of the intervillous space as the consequence of relatively greater impairment of venous outflow compared with arterial inflow. During contractions, therefore, a somewhat larger volume of blood is available for exchange even though the rate of flow is decreased. Subsequently, by use of Doppler velocimetry, it was shown that diastolic flow velocity in spiral arteries is diminished during uterine contractions.

From these observations, it can be seen that principal factors regulating blood flow in the intervillous space are arterial blood pressure, intrauterine pressure, the pattern of uterine contractions, and factors that act specifically on arterial walls.

Breaks in the Placental "Barrier"

The placenta does not maintain absolute integrity of the fetal and maternal circulations. There are numerous examples of *trafficking* cells between mother and fetus in both directions. This situation is best exemplified clinically by erythrocyte D-antigen isoimmunization and *erythroblastosis fetalis* (see Chap. 29, p. 618). Desai and Creger (1963) found that, even under normal conditions, labeled maternal leukocytes and platelets crossed the placenta from mother to fetus. Although this likely is a small amount in most cases, occasionally the fetus exsanguinates into the maternal circulation. Indeed, in their recent review, Silver and colleagues (2007) found that fetomaternal hemorrhage accounted for 3 to 14 percent of stillbirths.

It is indisputable that fetal cells can become engrafted in the mother during pregnancy and can be identified decades later. Fetal lymphocytes and CD34+ mesenchymal stem cells reside in maternal blood or bone marrow (Nguyen and co-workers, 2006; Piper and colleagues, 2007). Termed *microchimerism*, such residual stem cells may participate in maternal tissue regeneration and have been implicated to explain the disparate female:male ratio of autoimmune disorders (Gleicher and Barad, 2007; Stevens, 2006). As discussed in Chapter 53 (p. 1127), they are associated with lymphocytic thyroiditis, scleroderma, and systemic lupus erythematosus.

Immunological Considerations of the Fetal–Maternal Interface

For more than 50 years, there have been many attempts to explain survival of the semiallogenic fetal graft. One of the earliest explanations was based on the theory of antigenic immaturity of the embryo-fetus. This was disproved by Billingham (1964), who showed that transplantation (HLA) antigens are demonstrable very early in embryonic life. Another theory posited diminished immunological responsiveness of the pregnant woman, but there is little evidence for this to be other than ancillary. In another explanation, the uterus (decidua) is proposed to be an immunologically privileged tissue site. However, this theory is challenged by cases of advanced ectopic pregnancies (see Chap. 10, p. 240). Thus, the enigma continues.

Clearly, there is no doubt that the lack of uterine transplantation immunity is unique compared with that of other tissues. Survival of the conceptus in the uterus can be attributed to an immunological peculiarity of cells involved in implantation and fetal-placental development. These include decidual natural killer cells with their inefficient cytotoxic abilities, decidual stromal cells, and invasive trophoblasts that populate the decidua (Hanna, 2006; Santoni, 2007; Staun-Ram, 2005, and all their co-workers). The trophoblasts are the only fetal-derived cells in direct contact with maternal tissues. Previous studies have suggested that maternal natural killer cells act to control the invasion of trophoblast cells, which have adapted to survive in an immunologically hostile environment (Thellin and associates, 2000). More recently Hanna and colleagues (2006) have reported a "peaceful" model of trophoblast invasion and maternal vascular remodeling. In this scheme, decidual natural killer cells work in concert with stromal cells. They mediate angiogenesis through production of proangiogenic factors such as VEGF and control trophoblast chemoattraction toward spiral arteries by production of interleukin-8 and interferon inducible protein-10.

Immunogenicity of the Trophoblasts

More than 50 years ago, Sir Peter Medawar (1953) suggested that survival of the fetal semiallograft might be explained by *immunological neutrality*. The placenta was considered immunologically inert and therefore unable to create a maternal immune response. Subsequently, research was focused on defining expression of the *major histocompatibility complex (MHC)* antigens on trophoblasts. *Human leukocyte antigens* (*HLAs*) are the human analogue of the MHC. And indeed, MHC class I and II antigens are absent from villous trophoblasts, which appear to be immunologically inert at all stages of gestation (Weetman, 1999). But invasive extravillous cytotrophoblasts do express MHC class I molecules, which have been the focus of considerable study.

Trophoblast HLA (MHC) Class I Expression

The HLA genes are the products of multiple genetic loci of the MHC located within the short arm of chromosome 6 (Hunt and Orr, 1992). There are 17 HLA class I genes, including three classic genes, *HLA-A, -B,* and *-C,* that encode the major class I (class Ia) transplantation antigens. Three other class I genes, designated *HLA-E, -F,* and *-G,* encode class Ib HLA antigens. The remaining DNA sequences appear to be pseudogenes or partial gene fragments.

Moffett-King (2002) reasoned that normal implantation depends on controlled trophoblastic invasion of maternal endometrium–decidua and spiral arteries. Such invasion must proceed far enough to provide for normal fetal growth and development, but there must be a mechanism for regulating its depth. She suggested that uterine decidual natural killer cells (uNK cells) combined with unique expression of three specific HLA class I genes in extravillous cytotrophoblasts act in concert to permit and subsequently limit trophoblast invasion.

Class I antigens in extravillous cytotrophoblasts are accounted for by the expression of classic HLA-C and nonclassical class Ib molecules of HLA-E and HLA-G. To elucidate the importance of HLA-C, HLA-E, and HLA-G expression, it is important to understand the unusual lymphocyte population of the decidua.

Uterine Natural Killer Cells (uNK)

These distinctive lymphocytes are believed to originate in bone marrow and belong to the natural killer cell lineage. They are by far the predominant population of leukocytes present in midluteal phase endometrium at the expected time of implantation (Johnson and colleagues, 1999). These uNKs have a distinct phenotype characterized by a high surface density of CD56 or neural cell adhesion molecule (Loke and King, 1995; Manaster and associates, 2008; Moffett-King, 2002). Their infiltration is increased by progesterone and by stromal cell production of IL-15 and decidual prolactin (Dunn and co-workers, 2002; Gubbay and colleagues, 2002).

Near the end of the luteal phase of nonfertile ovulatory cycles, the nuclei of the uterine NK cell begin to disintegrate. But if implantation proceeds, they persist in large numbers in the decidua during early pregnancy. By term, however, there are relatively few uNK cells in the decidua. In first-trimester decidua, there are many uNK cells in close proximity to extravillous trophoblast where it is speculated that they serve to regulate trophoblast invasion. These uNK cells secrete large amounts of granulocyte-

macrophage–colony-stimulating factor (GM-CSF), which suggests that they are in an activated state. Jokhi and co-workers (1999) speculate that GM-CSF may function primarily to forestall trophoblast apoptosis and not to promote trophoblast replication. Expression of angiogenic factors by uNK cells also suggests a role in decidual vascular remodeling (Li and colleagues, 2001). In this case, it is uNKs, rather than the T lymphocytes, that are primarily responsible for decidual immunosurveillance.

HLA-G Expression in Trophoblasts

This antigen is expressed only in humans, and it has a highly restricted tissue distribution. It is expressed in cytotrophoblasts contiguous with maternal tissues, that is, decidual and uNK cells. Indeed, HLA-G antigen expression is identified only in extravillous cytotrophoblasts in the decidua basalis and in the chorion laeve (McMaster and colleagues, 1995). During pregnancy, a soluble major isoform—HLA-G2—is increased (Hunt and colleagues, 2000a, b). Embryos used for in vitro fertilization do not implant if they do not express this soluble HLA-G isoform (Fuzzi and colleagues, 2002). Thus, HLA-G may be immunologically permissive of the maternal-fetal antigen mismatch (LeBouteiller and colleagues, 1999). Finally, Goldman-Wohl and associates (2000) have provided evidence for abnormal HLA-G expression in extravillous trophoblasts from women with preeclampsia.

The Amnion

At term, the amnion is a tough and tenacious but pliable membrane. This innermost avascular fetal membrane is contiguous with amnionic fluid and occupies a role of incredible importance in human pregnancy. The amnion provides almost all tensile strength of the fetal membranes. Thus, development of its components that protect against its rupture or tearing is vitally important to successful pregnancy outcome. Indeed, preterm rupture of fetal membranes is a major cause of preterm delivery (see Chap. 36, p. 817).

Structure

Bourne (1962) described five separate layers of amnion. The inner surface, which is bathed by amnionic fluid, is an uninterrupted, single layer of cuboidal epithelium believed to be derived from embryonic ectoderm (Fig. 3-25). This epithelium is attached firmly to a distinct basement membrane that is connected to the acellular compact layer, which is composed primarily of interstitial collagens. On the outer side of the compact layer, there is a row of fibroblast-like mesenchymal cells, which are widely dispersed at term. These are probably derived from embryonic disc mesoderm. There also are a few fetal macrophages in the amnion. The outermost layer of amnion is the relatively acellular zona spongiosa, which is contiguous with the second fetal membrane, the chorion laeve. The human amnion lacks smooth muscle cells, nerves, lymphatics, and importantly, blood vessels.

Development

Early during implantation, a space develops between the embryonic cell mass and adjacent trophoblasts (see Fig. 3-11). Small cells that line this inner surface of trophoblasts have been called

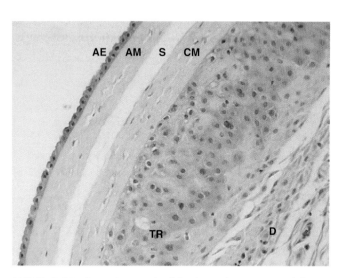

FIGURE 3-25 Photomicrograph of fetal membranes. From left to right: AE = amnion epithelium; AM = amnion mesenchyme; S = zona spongiosa; CM = chorionic mesenchyme; TR = trophoblast; D = decidua. (Used with permission from Dr. Judith R. Head.)

amniogenic cells—precursors of amnionic epithelium. The amnion is first identifiable about the seventh or eighth day of embryo development. It is initially a minute vesicle, which then develops into a small sac that covers the dorsal surface of the embryo. As the amnion enlarges, it gradually engulfs the growing embryo, which prolapses into its cavity (Benirschke and Kaufmann, 2000).

Distension of the amnionic sac eventually brings it into contact with the interior surface of the chorion laeve. Apposition of the chorion laeve and amnion near the end of the first trimester then causes an obliteration of the extraembryonic coelom. The amnion and chorion laeve, although slightly adherent, are never intimately connected and can be separated easily.

Amnion Cell Histogenesis. It is now generally accepted that the epithelial cells of the amnion are derived from fetal ectoderm of the embryonic disc. They do not arise by delamination from trophoblasts. This is an important consideration from both embryological and functional perspectives. For example, HLA class I gene expression in amnion is more akin to that in cells of the embryo than that in trophoblasts.

In addition to the epithelial cells that line the amnionic cavity, there is a layer of fibroblast-like mesenchymal cells that are likely derived from embryonic mesoderm. Early in human embryogenesis, the amnionic mesenchymal cells lie immediately adjacent to the basal surface of the epithelium. At this time, the amnion surface is a two-cell-layer structure with approximately equal numbers of epithelial and mesenchymal cells. Simultaneously with growth and development, interstitial collagens are deposited between these two layers of cells. This marks formation of the compact layer of the amnion, which also brings about a distinct separation of the two layers of amnion cells.

As the amnionic sac expands to line the placenta and then the chorion frondosum at 10 to 14 weeks, there is a progressive reduction in the compactness of the mesenchymal cells. These cells continue to separate and become sparsely distributed. Early in pregnancy, amnionic epithelium replicates at a rate appreciably faster than mesenchymal cells. At term, these cells form a continuous uninterrupted epithelium on the fetal amnionic surface. Conversely, mesenchymal cells are widely dispersed, being connected by a fine lattice network of extracellular matrix with the appearance of long slender fibrils.

Amnion Epithelial Cells. The apical surface of amnionic epithelium is replete with highly developed microvilli that are consistent with a major site of transfer between amnionic fluid and amnion. This epithelium is active metabolically, and these cells synthesize tissue inhibitor of metalloproteinase-1, PGE_2, and fetal fibronectin (Rowe and colleagues, 1997). In term pregnancies, amnionic expression of prostaglandin endoperoxide H synthase correlates with elevated fetal fibronectin (Mijovic and co-workers, 2000). By prostaglandin production, amnionic epithelium participates in the "final common pathway" of labor initiation. Epithelial cells may respond to signals derived from the fetus or the mother, and they are responsive to a variety of endocrine or paracrine modulators. Examples include oxytocin and vasopressin, both of which increase PGE_2 production in vitro (Moore and associates, 1988). They may also produce cytokines such as IL-8 during initiation of labor (Elliott and colleagues, 2001).

Amnionic epithelium also synthesizes vasoactive peptides, including endothelin and parathyroid hormone-related protein (Economos and associates, 1992; Germain and colleagues, 1992). The tissue produces brain natriuretic peptide and corticotropin-releasing hormone (CRH), which are peptides that are smooth muscle relaxants (Riley and colleagues, 1991; Warren and Silverman, 1995). It seems reasonable that vasoactive peptides produced in amnion gain access to adventitial surface of chorionic vessels. Thus, amnion may be involved in modulating chorionic vessel tone and blood flow. Amnion-derived vasoactive peptides function in other tissues in diverse physiological processes. After their secretion, these bioactive agents enter amnionic fluid and thereby are available to the fetus by swallowing and inhalation.

Amnion Mesenchymal Cells. Mesenchymal cells of the amnionic fibroblast layer are responsible for other major functions. Synthesis of interstitial collagens that comprise the compact layer of the amnion—the major source of its tensile strength—takes place in mesenchymal cells (Casey and MacDonald, 1996). These cells also synthesize cytokines that include IL-6, IL-8, and monocyte chemoattractant protein-1 (MCP-1). Cytokine synthesis increases in response to bacterial toxins and IL-1. This functional capacity of amnion mesenchymal cells is an important consideration in the study of amnionic fluid for evidence of labor-associated accumulation of inflammatory mediators (Garcia-Velasco and Arici, 1999). Finally, mesenchymal cells may be a greater source of PGE_2 than epithelial cells (Whittle and colleagues, 2000).

Anatomy of the Amnion

Reflected amnion is fused to the chorion laeve. Placental amnion covers the placenta surface and thereby is in contact with the adventitial surface of chorionic vessels. Umbilical amnion covers the umbilical cord. In the conjoined portion of membranes of diamnionic-dichorionic twin placentas, fused amnions are separated by fused chorion laeve. Thus, aside from the small area of the membranes immediately over the cervical os, this is the only site at which the reflected chorion laeve is not contiguous with decidua. With diamnionic-monochorionic placentas, there is no intervening tissue between the fused amnions.

Amnion Tensile Strength

More than 135 years ago, Matthew Duncan examined the forces involved in fetal membrane rupture. During tests of tensile strength—resistance to tearing and rupture—he found that the decidua and then the chorion laeve gave way long before the amnion ruptured. Indeed, the membranes are quite elastic and can expand to twice normal size during pregnancy (Benirschke and Kaufmann, 2000). The amnion provides the major strength of the membranes. Its tensile strength resides almost exclusively in the compact layer, which is composed of cross-linked interstitial collagens I and III and lesser amounts of collagens V and VI.

Interstitial Collagens. Collagens are the major macromolecules of most connective tissues and the most abundant proteins in the body. Collagen I is the major interstitial collagen in tissues characterized by great tensile strength, such as bone and tendon. In other tissues, collagen III is believed to make a unique contribution to tissue integrity, serving to increase tissue extensibility and tensile strength. For example, the ratio of collagen III to collagen I in the walls of a number of highly extensible tissues—amnionic sac, blood vessels, urinary bladder, bile ducts, intestine, and gravid uterus—is greater than that in nonelastic tissues (Jeffrey, 1991). Although collagen III provides some of the extensibility of this membrane, elastin microfibrils have also been identified (Bryant-Greenwood, 1998).

The tensile strength of amnion is regulated in part by interaction of fibrillar collagen with proteoglycans such as *decorin,* which promote tissue strength. Compositional changes at the time of labor include a decline in decorin and increase in hyaluronan resulting in loss of tensile strength (Chap. 6, p. 140)(Meinert and associates, 2007). Fetal membranes overlying the cervix have a reported regional decline in expression of matrix proteins such as fibulins. This change is suggested to contribute to tissue remodeling and loss of tensile strength (Moore and co-workers, 2009).

Metabolic Functions

From the foregoing, it is apparent that the amnion is clearly more than a simple avascular membrane that contains amnionic fluid. It is metabolically active, is involved in solute and water transport for amnionic fluid homeostasis, and produces an impressive array of bioactive compounds. The amnion is responsive both acutely and chronically to mechanical stretch, which alters amnionic gene expression (Nemeth and colleagues, 2000). This in turn may trigger both autocrine and paracrine responses to include production of matrix metalloproteinases, IL-8, and collagenase (Bryant-Greenwood, 1998; Maradny and colleagues, 1996). Such factors may modulate changes in membrane properties during labor.

Amnionic Fluid

The normally clear fluid that collects within the amnionic cavity increases as pregnancy progresses until about 34 weeks, when there is a decrease in volume. At term, the average volume is about 1000 mL, although this may vary widely in abnormal

conditions. The origin, composition, circulation, and function of amnionic fluid are discussed further in Chapter 21 (p. 490).

Umbilical Cord and Related Structures

Cord Development

The yolk sac and the umbilical vesicle into which it develops are prominent early in pregnancy. At first, the embryo is a flattened disc interposed between amnion and yolk sac (see Fig. 3-15). Because its dorsal surface grows faster than the ventral surface, in association with the elongation of the neural tube, the embryo bulges into the amnionic sac and the dorsal part of the yolk sac is incorporated into the body of the embryo to form the gut. The allantois projects into the base of the body stalk from the caudal wall of the yolk sac and later, from the anterior wall of the hindgut.

As pregnancy advances, the yolk sac becomes smaller and its pedicle relatively longer. By about the middle of the third month, the expanding amnion obliterates the exocoelom, fuses with the chorion laeve, and covers the bulging placental disc and the lateral surface of the body stalk. The latter is then called the *umbilical cord*—or *funis.* Remnants of the exocoelom in the anterior portion of the cord may contain loops of intestine, which continue to develop outside the embryo. Although the loops are later withdrawn into the peritoneal cavity, the apex of the midgut loop retains its connection with the attenuated vitelline duct.

The cord at term normally has two arteries and one vein (Fig. 3-26). The right umbilical vein usually disappears early during fetal development, leaving only the original left vein. In sections of any portion of the cord near the center, the small

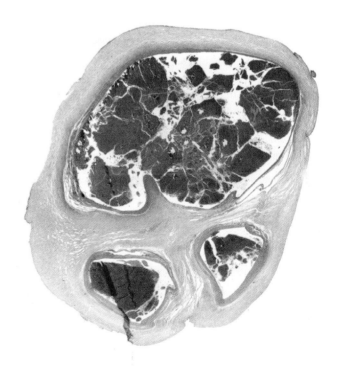

FIGURE 3-26 Cross-section of umbilical cord. The large umbilical vein carries oxygenated blood to the fetus *(above)*. Below it, are the two smaller umbilical arteries, carrying deoxygenated blood from the fetus to the placenta. (Used with permission from Dr. Mandolin S. Ziadie.)

duct of the umbilical vesicle can usually be seen. The vesicle is lined by a single layer of flattened or cuboidal epithelium. In sections just beyond the umbilicus, another duct representing the allantoic remnant is occasionally found. The intra-abdominal portion of the duct of the umbilical vesicle, which extends from umbilicus to intestine, usually atrophies and disappears, but occasionally it remains patent, forming the *Meckel diverticulum*. The most common vascular anomaly is the absence of one umbilical artery which may be associated with fetal anomalies (see Chap. 27, p. 582).

Cord Structure and Function

The umbilical cord, or funis, extends from the fetal umbilicus to the fetal surface of the placenta or chorionic plate. Its exterior is dull white, moist, and covered by amnion, through which three umbilical vessels may be seen. Its diameter is 0.8 to 2.0 cm, with an average length of 55 cm and a range of 30 to 100 cm. Generally, cord length less than 30 cm is considered abnormally short (Benirschke and Kaufmann, 2000). Folding and tortuosity of the vessels, which are longer than the cord itself, frequently create nodulations on the surface, or false knots, which are essentially varices. The extracellular matrix is a specialized connective tissue referred to as *Wharton jelly*. After fixation, the umbilical vessels appear empty, but normally the vessels are not emptied of blood. The two arteries are smaller in diameter than the vein. The mesoderm of the cord, which is of allantoic origin, fuses with that of the amnion.

Blood flows from the umbilical vein and takes a path of least resistance via two routes within the fetus. One is the ductus venosus, which empties directly into the inferior vena cava (see Fig. 4-12, p. 90). The other route consists of numerous smaller openings into the hepatic circulation. Blood from the liver flows into the inferior vena cava via the hepatic vein. Resistance in the ductus venosus is controlled by a sphincter situated at the origin of the ductus at the umbilical recess and innervated by a branch of the vagus nerve.

Blood exits the fetus via the two umbilical arteries. These are anterior branches of the internal iliac artery and become obliterated after birth. Remnants can be seen as the medial umbilical ligaments.

Anatomically, the umbilical cord can be regarded as a component of the fetal membranes. Vessels contained in the cord spiral or twist. Spiraling may occur in a clockwise (dextral) or anticlockwise (sinistral) direction. Anticlockwise spiral is present in 50 to 90 percent of fetuses. It is believed that the spiraling serves to prevent crimping, which occurs in all hollow cylinders subjected to torsion. Boyd and Hamilton (1970) note that these twists are not true spirals, but rather they are cylindrical helices in which a constant curvature is maintained equidistant from the central axis. Benirschke and Kaufmann (2000) reported that there is an average of 11 helices in a cord.

PLACENTAL HORMONES

The production of steroid and protein hormones by human trophoblasts is greater in amount and diversity than that of any single endocrine tissue in all of mammalian physiology. A compendium of average production rates for various steroid hormones in nonpregnant and in near-term pregnant women is given in Table 3-1. It is apparent that alterations in steroid hormone production that accompany normal human pregnancy are incredible. The human placenta also synthesizes an enormous amount of protein and peptide hormones. This includes nearly 1 gram of placental lactogen (hPL) every 24 hours, massive quantities of chorionic gonadotropin (hCG), adrenocorticotropin (ACTH), growth hormone variant (hGH-V), parathyroid hormone–related protein (PTH-rP), calcitonin, relaxin, inhibins, activins, and atrial natriuretic peptide. In addition, there are various hypothalamic-like releasing and inhibiting hormones such as thyrotropin-releasing hormone (TRH), gonadotropin-releasing hormone (GnRH), corticotropin-releasing hormone (CRH), somatostatin, and growth hormone–releasing hormone (GHRH).

TABLE 3-1. Steroid Production Rates in Nonpregnant and Near-Term Pregnant Women

Steroid[a]	Production Rates (mg/24 hr)	
	Nonpregnant	Pregnant
Estradiol-17β	0.1–0.6	15–20
Estriol	0.02–0.1	50–150
Progesterone	0.1–40	250–600
Aldosterone	0.05–0.1	0.250–0.600
Deoxycorticosterone	0.05–0.5	1–12
Cortisol	10–30	10–20

[a]Estrogens and progesterone are produced by placenta. Aldosterone is produced by the maternal adrenal in response to the stimulus of angiotensin II. Deoxycorticosterone is produced in extraglandular tissue sites by way of the 21-hydroxylation of plasma progesterone. Cortisol production during pregnancy is not increased, even though the blood levels are elevated because of decreased clearance caused by increased cortisol-binding globulin.

It is understandable, therefore, that yet another remarkable feature of human pregnancy is the successful physiological adaptations of pregnant women to the unique endocrine milieu as discussed throughout Chapter 6.

Human Chorionic Gonadotropin (hCG)

This so-called pregnancy hormone is a glycoprotein with biological activity similar to luteinizing hormone (LH). Both act via the plasma membrane LH-hCG receptor. Although hCG is produced almost exclusively in the placenta, it also is synthesized in fetal kidney. Other fetal tissues produce either the β-subunit or intact hCG molecule (McGregor and associates, 1981, 1983).

Various malignant tumors also produce hCG, sometimes in large amounts—especially trophoblastic neoplasms (Chap. 11, p. 257). Chorionic gonadotropin is produced in very small amounts in tissues of men and nonpregnant women, perhaps primarily in the anterior pituitary gland. Nonetheless, the detection of hCG in blood or urine is almost always indicative of pregnancy (see Chap. 8, p. 192).

Chemical Characteristics

Chorionic gonadotropin is a glycoprotein with a molecular weight of 36,000 to 40,000 Da. It has the highest carbohydrate content of any human hormone—30 percent. The carbohydrate component, and especially the terminal sialic acid, protects the molecule from catabolism. The 36-hour plasma half-life of intact hCG is much longer than the 2 hours for LH. The hCG molecule is composed of two dissimilar subunits. One is designated α and is composed of 92 amino acids, whereas the β subunit contains 145 amino acids. These are noncovalently linked and are held together by electrostatic and hydrophobic forces. Isolated subunits are unable to bind the LH receptor and thus lack biological activity.

This hormone is structurally related to three other glycoprotein hormones—LH, FSH, and TSH. The amino-acid sequence of the α-subunits of all four glycoproteins is identical. The β-subunits, although sharing certain similarities, are characterized by distinctly different amino-acid sequences. Recombination of an α- and a β-subunit of the four glycoprotein hormones gives a molecule with biological activity characteristic of the hormone from which the β-subunit was derived.

Biosynthesis

Both α- and β-chain synthesis of hCG are regulated separately. A single gene located on chromosome 6 encodes the α-subunit for hCG, LH, FSH, and TSH. There are seven separate genes on chromosome 19 for the β-hCG–β-LH family. Six genes code for β-hCG and one for β-LH (Miller-Lindholm and colleagues, 1997). Both subunits are synthesized as larger precursors, which are then cleaved by endopeptidases. Intact hCG is then assembled and rapidly released by exocytosis of secretory granules (Morrish and colleagues, 1987).

Site of hCG Synthesis

Before 5 weeks, hCG is expressed in both syncytiotrophoblast and cytotrophoblast (Maruo and colleagues, 1992). Later, when maternal serum levels peak, hCG is produced almost solely in syncytiotrophoblasts (Beck and associates, 1986; Kurman and colleagues, 1984). At this time, hCG mRNAs for both α- and β-subunits in syncytiotrophoblast are greater than at term (Hoshina and co-workers, 1982). This may be an important consideration when hCG is used as a screening procedure to identify abnormal fetuses.

Molecular Forms of hCG in Plasma and Urine

There are multiple forms of hCG in maternal plasma and urine. Some result from enzymatic degradation, and others by modifications during molecular synthesis and processing. These multiple forms of hormone vary enormously in bioactivity and immunoreactivity.

Free Subunits. Circulating free β-subunit levels are low to undetectable throughout pregnancy. In part, this is the result of its rate-limiting synthesis. Free α-subunits that do not combine with the β-subunit are found in placental tissue and maternal plasma. These levels increase gradually and steadily until they plateau at about 36 weeks. At this time, they account for from 30 to 50 percent of hormone (Cole, 1997). Thus, α-hCG secretion roughly corresponds to placental mass, whereas secretion of complete hCG molecules is maximal at 8 to 10 weeks.

Concentrations of hCG in Serum and Urine

The intact hCG molecule is detectable in plasma of pregnant women 7 to 9 days after the midcycle surge of LH that precedes ovulation. Thus, it is likely that hCG enters maternal blood at the time of blastocyst implantation. Plasma levels increase rapidly, doubling every 2 days, with maximal levels being attained at 8 to 10 weeks (Fig. 3-27). Appreciable fluctuations in levels for a given patient are observed on the same day—evidence that trophoblast secretion

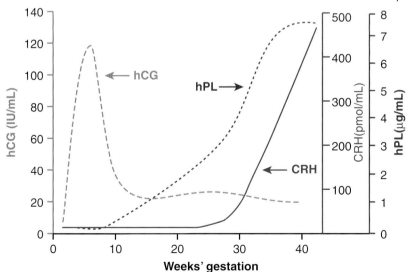

FIGURE 3-27 Distinct profiles for the concentrations of human chorionic gonadotropin (hCG), human placental lactogen (hPL), and corticotropin-releasing hormone (CRH) in serum of women throughout normal pregnancy.

of protein hormones is episodic (Barnea and Kaplan, 1989; Diaz-Cueto and colleagues, 1994).

Because hCG circulates as multiple highly related isoforms with variable cross-reactivity between commercial assays, there is considerable variation in calculated serum hCG levels among the more than 100 assays. Peak maternal plasma levels reach about 100,000 mIU/mL between the 60th and 80th days after menses (see Fig. 3-27). At 10 to 12 weeks, plasma levels begin to decline, and a nadir is reached by about 16 weeks. Plasma levels are maintained at this lower level for the remainder of pregnancy.

The pattern of hCG appearance in fetal blood is similar to that in the mother. Fetal plasma levels, however, are only about 3 percent of those in maternal plasma. Amnionic fluid hCG concentration early in pregnancy is similar to that in maternal plasma. As pregnancy progresses, hCG concentration in amnionic fluid declines, and near term the levels are about 20 percent of those in maternal plasma.

Maternal urine contains the same variety of hCG degradation products as maternal plasma. The principal urinary form is the terminal degradation hCG product—the β-core fragment. Its concentrations follow the same general pattern as that in maternal plasma, peaking at about 10 weeks. It is important to recognize that the so-called β-subunit antibody used in most pregnancy tests reacts with both intact hCG—the major form in the plasma, and with fragments of hCG—the major forms found in urine.

Significance of Abnormally High or Low hCG Levels.

There are a number of clinical circumstances in which substantively higher maternal plasma hCG levels are found. Some examples are multifetal pregnancy, erythroblastosis fetalis associated with fetal hemolytic anemia, and gestational trophoblastic disease. Relatively higher hCG levels may be found at midtrimester in women carrying a fetus with Down syndrome—an observation used in biochemical screening tests (see Chap. 13, p. 293). The reason for this is not clear, but it has been speculated that it is due to reduced placental maturity. Relatively lower hCG plasma levels are found in women with early pregnancy wastage, including ectopic pregnancy (see Chap. 10, p. 245).

Regulation of hCG Synthesis

Placental GnRH is likely involved in the regulation of hCG formation. Both GnRH and its receptor are expressed on cytotrophoblasts and syncytiotrophoblast (Wolfahrt and colleagues, 1998). Also, GnRH administration elevates circulating hCG levels, and cultured trophoblast cells respond to GnRH treatment with increased hCG secretion (Iwashita and colleagues, 1993; Siler-Khodr and Khodr, 1981). Pituitary GnRH production also is regulated by inhibin and activin. In cultured placental cells, activin stimulates and inhibin inhibits GnRH and hCG production (Petraglia and co-workers, 1989; Steele and colleagues, 1993).

Metabolic Clearance of hCG

Renal clearance of hCG accounts for 30 percent of its metabolic clearance. The remainder is likely cleared by metabolism in the liver (Wehmann and Nisula, 1980). Clearances of β- and α-subunit are about 10-fold and 30-fold, respectively, greater than that of intact hCG. By contrast, renal clearance of these subunits is considerably lower than that of dimeric hCG.

Biological Functions of hCG

Both hCG subunits are required for binding to the LH-hCG receptor in the corpus luteum and the fetal testis. LH-hCG receptors are present in a variety of tissues, but their role there is less defined. The best-known biological function of hCG is the so-called rescue and maintenance of function of the corpus luteum—that is, continued progesterone production. Bradbury and colleagues (1950) found that the progesterone-producing life span of a corpus luteum of menstruation could be prolonged perhaps for 2 weeks by hCG administration. This is only an incomplete explanation for the physiological role of hCG in pregnancy. For example, maximum plasma hCG concentrations are attained well after hCG-stimulated corpus luteum secretion of progesterone has ceased. Specifically, progesterone luteal synthesis begins to decline at about 6 weeks despite continued and increasing hCG production.

It is also known that hCG stimulates fetal testicular testosterone secretion, which is maximum approximately when peak levels of hCG are attained. Thus, at a critical time in sexual differentiation of the male fetus, hCG enters fetal plasma from the syncytiotrophoblast. In the fetus, it acts as an LH surrogate to stimulate replication of Leydig cells and testosterone synthesis to promote male sexual differentiation (see Chap. 4, p. 101). Before about 110 days, there is no vascularization of the fetal anterior pituitary from the hypothalamus. Thus, there is little pituitary LH secretion and hCG acts as LH before this time. Thereafter, as hCG levels fall, pituitary LH maintains a modest level of testicular stimulation.

The maternal thyroid gland is also stimulated by large quantities of hCG. In some women with gestational trophoblastic disease, biochemical and clinical evidence of hyperthyroidism sometimes develops (see Chap. 11, p. 260). This once was attributed to formation of *chorionic thyrotropins* by neoplastic trophoblasts. It was subsequently, however, shown that some forms of hCG bind to TSH receptors on thyrocytes (Hershman, 1999). And treatment of men with exogenous hCG increases thyroid activity. The thyroid-stimulatory activity in plasma of first-trimester pregnant women varies appreciably from sample to sample. Modifications of hCG oligosaccharides likely are important in the capacity of hCG to stimulate thyroid function. For example, acidic isoforms stimulate thyroid activity, and some more basic isoforms stimulate iodine uptake (Kraiem, 1994; Tsuruta, 1995; Yoshimura, 1994, and all their colleagues). Finally, the LH-hCG receptor is expressed by thyrocytes, which suggests that hCG stimulates thyroid activity via the LH-hCG receptor and by the TSH receptor (Tomer and colleagues, 1992).

Other hCG functions include *promotion of* relaxin secretion by the corpus luteum (Duffy and co-workers, 1996). LH-hCG receptors are found in myometrium and in uterine vascular tissue. It has been hypothesized that hCG may act to promote uterine vascular vasodilatation and myometrial smooth muscle relaxation (Kurtzman and colleagues, 2001).

Human Placental Lactogen (hPL)

Prolactin-like activity in the human placenta was first described by Ehrhardt (1936). The responsible protein was isolated from placental extracts and retroplacental blood (Ito and Higashi, 1961; Josimovich and MacLaren, 1962). Because of its potent lactogenic and growth hormone-like bioactivity, as well as an immunochemical resemblance to human growth hormone (hGH), it was called human placental lactogen or chorionic growth hormone. It also has been referred to as chorionic somatomammotropin. Currently, *human placental lactogen* (hPL) is used by most. Grumbach and Kaplan (1964) showed that this hormone, like hCG, was concentrated in syncytiotrophoblast. It is detected as early as the second or third week after fertilization. Also similar to hCG, hPL is demonstrated in cytotrophoblasts before 6 weeks (Maruo and associates, 1992).

Chemical Characteristics

Human placental lactogen is a single nonglycosylated polypeptide chain with a molecular weight of 22,279 Da. It is derived from a 25,000-Da precursor. There are 191 amino-acid residues in hPL compared with 188 in hCG. The sequence of each hormone is strikingly similar, with 96-percent homology. HPL also is structurally similar to human prolactin (hPRL), with a 67-percent amino-acid sequence similarity. For these reasons, it has been suggested that the genes for hPL, hPRL, and hGH evolved from a common ancestral gene—probably that for prolactin—by repeated gene duplication (Ogren and Talamantes, 1994).

Gene Structure and Expression

There are five genes in the growth hormone–placental lactogen gene cluster that are linked and located on chromosome 17. Two of these—*hPL2* and *hPL3*—both encode hPL, and the amount of mRNA in the term placenta is similar for each. In contrast, the prolactin gene is located on chromosome 6 (Owerbach and colleagues, 1980, 1981). **The production rate of hPL near term— approximately 1 g/day—is by far the greatest of any known hormone in humans.**

Serum Concentration

HPL is demonstrable in the placenta within 5 to 10 days after conception and can be detected in maternal serum as early as 3 weeks. Maternal plasma concentrations are linked to placental mass, and they rise steadily until 34 to 36 weeks. Serum concentrations reach levels in late pregnancy of 5 to 15 μg/mL— higher than those of any other protein hormone (see Fig. 3-27). The half-life of hPL in maternal plasma is between 10 and 30 minutes (Walker and co-workers, 1991).

Very little hPL is detected in fetal blood or in the urine of the mother or newborn. Amnionic fluid levels are somewhat lower than in maternal plasma. Because hPL is secreted primarily into the maternal circulation, with only very small amounts in cord blood, it appears that its role in pregnancy, if any, is mediated through actions in maternal rather than in fetal tissues. Nonetheless, there is continuing interest in the possibility that hPL serves select functions in fetal growth.

Regulation of hPL Biosynthesis

Levels of mRNA for hPL in syncytiotrophoblast remain relatively constant throughout pregnancy. This finding is supportive of the idea that the rate of hPL secretion is proportional to

placental mass. There are very high plasma levels of hCG in women with trophoblastic neoplasms, but only low levels of hPL in these same women.

Prolonged maternal starvation in the first half of pregnancy leads to an increase in the plasma concentration of hPL. Short-term changes in plasma glucose or insulin, however, have relatively little effect on plasma hPL levels. In vitro studies of syncytiotrophoblast suggest that hPL synthesis is stimulated by insulin and insulin-like growth factor-1 and inhibited by PGE_2 and $PGF_{2\alpha}$ (Bhaumick and associates, 1987; Genbacev and colleagues, 1977).

Metabolic Actions

HPL has putative actions in a number of important metabolic processes. These include:

1. Maternal lipolysis with increased levels of circulating free fatty acids. This provides a source of energy for maternal metabolism and fetal nutrition. In vitro studies suggest that hPL inhibits leptin secretion by term trophoblast (Coya and associates, 2005).
2. An anti-insulin or "diabetogenic" action that leads to increased maternal insulin levels. This favors protein synthesis and provides a readily available source of amino acids to the fetus.
3. A potent angiogenic hormone that may play an important role in the formation of fetal vasculature (Corbacho and co-workers, 2002).

Other Placental Protein Hormones

Chorionic Adrenocorticotropin

ACTH, lipotropin, and β-endorphin—all proteolytic products of proopiomelanocortin—are recovered from placental extracts (Genazzani and associates, 1975; Odagiri and colleagues, 1979). The physiological role of placental ACTH is unclear. Although maternal plasma levels of ACTH increase during pregnancy, they remain lower than those in men and nonpregnant women, except during labor (Carr and colleagues, 1981a). Placental ACTH is secreted into both maternal and fetal circulations, however, maternal ACTH is not transported to the fetus. Importantly, placental ACTH is not under feedback regulation by glucocorticoids, which may explain maternal partial resistance to dexamethasone suppression (Nolten and Rueckert, 1981). Placental corticotropin-releasing hormone (CRH) stimulates synthesis and release of chorionic ACTH. Placental CRH production is positively regulated by cortisol, producing a novel positive feedback loop. As discussed later, this system may be important for controlling fetal lung maturation and timing of parturition.

Relaxin

Relaxin expression has been demonstrated in human corpus luteum, decidua, and placenta (Bogic and colleagues, 1995). This peptide is synthesized as a single 105 amino-acid preprorelaxin molecule that is cleaved to A and B molecules. Relaxin is structurally similar to insulin and insulin-like growth factor. Two of the three relaxin genes—*H2* and *H3*—are transcribed in the corpus luteum (Bathgate and associates, 2002; Hudson and colleagues, 1983, 1984). Other tissues, including decidua, placenta, and membranes, express *H1* and *H2* (Hansell and colleagues, 1991).

The rise in maternal circulating relaxin levels seen in early pregnancy is attributed to secretion by the corpus luteum, and levels parallel those seen for hCG. The uterine relaxin receptor was cloned by Hsu and colleagues (2002). It has been proposed that relaxin, along with rising progesterone levels, acts on myometrium to promote relaxation and the quiescence observed in early pregnancy (see Chap. 6, p. 153). In addition, the production of relaxin and relaxin-like factors within the placenta and fetal membranes is believed to play an autocrine-paracrine role in postpartum regulation of extracellular matrix degradation (Qin and colleagues, 1997a, b).

Parathyroid Hormone-Related Protein (PTH-rP)

Circulating levels of PTH-rP are significantly elevated in pregnancy within maternal but not fetal circulation (Bertelloni and colleagues, 1994; Saxe and associates, 1997). Although not clear, many potential functions of this hormone have been proposed. PTH-rP synthesis is found in several normal adult tissues, especially in reproductive organs that include myometrium, endometrium, corpus luteum, and lactating mammary tissue. PTH-rP is not produced in the parathyroid glands of normal adults. Placental-derived PTH-rP may have an important autocrine–paracrine role within the fetal–maternal unit as well as on the adjacent myometrium. It may activate trophoblast receptors to promote calcium transport for fetal bone growth and ossification.

Growth Hormone Variant (hGH-V)

The placenta expresses a growth hormone variant that is not expressed in the pituitary. The gene encoding hGH-V is located in the hGH–hPL gene cluster on chromosome 17. Sometimes referred to as *placental growth hormone*, hGH-V is a 191 amino-acid protein that differs in 15 amino-acid positions from the sequence for hGH. Placental hGH-V presumably is synthesized in the syncytium, but its pattern of synthesis and secretion during gestation is not precisely known because antibodies against hGH-V cross-react with hGH. It is believed that hGH-V is present in maternal plasma by 21 to 26 weeks, increases in concentration until approximately 36 weeks, and remains relatively constant thereafter. There is a correlation between the levels of hGH-V in maternal plasma and those of insulin-like growth factor-1. Also, the secretion of hGH-V by trophoblasts in vitro is inhibited by glucose in a dose-dependent manner (Patel and colleagues, 1995). Overexpression of hGH-V in mice causes severe insulin resistance, and thus it is a likely candidate to mediate insulin resistance of pregnancy (Barbour and associates, 2002).

Hypothalamic-Like Releasing Hormones

For each of the known hypothalamic-releasing or -inhibiting hormones described—GnRH, TRH, CRH, GHRH, and somatostatin—there is an analogous hormone produced in human placenta (Petraglia and colleagues, 1992; Siler-Khodr, 1988). Many investigators have proposed that this is indicative of a hierarchy of control in the synthesis of chorionic trophic agents.

Gonadotropin-Releasing Hormone (GnRH).
There is a reasonably large amount of immunoreactive GnRH in the placenta (Siler-Khodr, 1988; Siler-Khodr and Khodr, 1978). Interestingly, it is found in cytotrophoblasts, but not syncytiotrophoblast. Gib-

bons and co-workers (1975) and Khodr and Siler-Khodr (1980) demonstrated that the human placenta could synthesize both GnRH and TRH in vitro. Placental-derived GnRH functions to regulate trophoblast hCG production, hence the observation that GnRH levels are higher early in pregnancy. Placental-derived GnRH is also the likely cause of elevated maternal GnRH levels in pregnancy (Siler-Khodr and colleagues, 1984).

Corticotropin-Releasing Hormone (CRH).
This hormone is a member of a larger family of CRH-related peptides that includes CRH, urocortin, urocortin II, and urocortin III (Dautzenberg and Hauger, 2002). CRH produced in nonpregnant women has relatively low serum levels of 5 to 10 pmol/L. During pregnancy, these increase to about 100 pmol/L in the early third trimester and to almost 500 pmol/L abruptly during the last 5 to 6 weeks (see Fig. 3-27). Urocortin also is produced by the placenta and secreted into the maternal circulation, but at much lower levels than seen for CRH (Florio and co-workers, 2002). After labor begins, maternal plasma CRH levels increase further by two- to threefold (Petraglia and colleagues, 1989, 1990).

The biological function of CRH synthesized in the placenta, membranes, and decidua has been somewhat defined. CRH receptors are present in many tissues: placenta, adrenal gland, sympathetic ganglia, lymphocytes, gastrointestinal tract, pancreas, gonads, and myometrium. Some findings suggest that CRH can act through two major families—the type 1 and type 2 CRH receptors (CRH-R1 and CRH-R2). Trophoblast, amniochorion, and decidua express both CRH-R1 and CRH-R2 receptors, as well as several variant receptors (Florio and colleagues, 2000). Both CRH and urocortin increase trophoblast ACTH secretion, supporting an autocrine-paracrine role (Petraglia and co-workers, 1999). Large amounts of CRH from trophoblast enter maternal blood, but there also is a large concentration of a specific CRH-binding protein in maternal plasma, and the bound CRH seems to be biologically inactive.

Other proposed biological roles include induction of smooth muscle relaxation in vascular and myometrial tissue and immunosuppression. The physiological reverse, however, induction of myometrial contractions, has been proposed for the rising levels of CRH seen near the end of gestation. One hypothesis suggests that CRH may be involved with parturition initiation (Wadhwa and colleagues, 1998). Prostaglandin formation in the placenta, amnion, chorion laeve, and decidua is increased with CRH treatment (Jones and Challis, 1989b). This latter observation further supports a potential role in the timing of parturition.

Glucocorticoids act in the hypothalamus to *inhibit CRH release*, but in the trophoblast, glucocorticoids *stimulate* CRH gene expression (Jones and colleagues, 1989a; Robinson and co-workers, 1988). Thus, there may be a novel positive feedback loop in the placenta by which placental CRH stimulates placental ACTH to stimulate fetal and maternal adrenal glucocorticoid production with subsequent stimulation of placental CRH expression (Nicholson and King, 2001; Riley and colleagues, 1991).

Growth Hormone-Releasing Hormone (GHRH).
The role of placental GHRH is not known (Berry and associates, 1992). *Ghrelin* is another regulator of hGH secretion that is produced by

placental tissue (Horvath and colleagues, 2001). Trophoblast ghrelin expression peaks at midpregnancy and is a potential regulator of hGH-V production or a paracrine regulator of differentiation (Fuglsang and associates, 2005; Gualillo and co-workers, 2001).

Other Placental Peptide Hormones

Leptin

This hormone is normally secreted by adipocytes. It functions as an anti-obesity hormone that decreases food intake through its hypothalamic receptor. It also regulates bone growth and immune function (Cock and Auwerx, 2003; La Cava and colleagues, 2004). Leptin also is synthesized by both cytotrophoblast and syncytiotrophoblast (Henson and Castracane, 2002). Relative contributions of leptin from maternal adipose tissue versus placenta are currently not well defined. Maternal serum levels are significantly higher than those in nonpregnant women. Fetal leptin levels are correlated positively with birthweight and likely play an important role in fetal development and growth. Recent studies suggest that leptin inhibits apoptosis and promotes trophoblast proliferation (Magarinos and associates, 2007).

Neuropeptide Y

This 36 amino-acid peptide is widely distributed in brain. It also is found in sympathetic neurons innervating the cardiovascular, respiratory, gastrointestinal, and genitourinary systems. Neuropeptide Y has been isolated from the placenta and localized in cytotrophoblasts (Petraglia and colleagues, 1989). There are receptors for neuropeptide Y on trophoblast, and treatment of placental cells with neuropeptide Y causes CRH release (Robidoux and colleagues, 2000).

Inhibin and Activin

Inhibin is a glycoprotein hormone that acts preferentially to inhibit pituitary FSH release. It is produced by human testis and by ovarian granulosa cells, including the corpus luteum. Inhibin is a heterodimer made up of an α-subunit and one of two distinct β-subunits, βA or βB. All three are produced by trophoblast, and maternal serum levels peak at term (Petraglia and co-workers, 1991). One function may be to act in concert with the large amounts of sex steroid hormones to inhibit FSH secretion and thereby inhibit ovulation during pregnancy. Inhibin may act via GnRH to regulate placental hCG synthesis (Petraglia and colleagues, 1987).

Activin is closely related to inhibin and is formed by the combination of the two β-subunits. Its receptor is expressed in the placenta and amnion. Activin A is not detectable in fetal blood before labor but is present in umbilical cord blood after labor begins. Petraglia and colleagues (1994) found that serum activin A levels decline rapidly after delivery. It is not clear if chorionic activin and inhibin are involved in placental metabolic processes other than GnRH synthesis.

Placental Progesterone Production

After 6 to 7 weeks' gestation, little progesterone is produced in the ovary (Diczfalusy and Troen, 1961). Surgical removal of the corpus luteum or even bilateral oophorectomy during the 7th to 10th week does not cause a decrease in excretion of urinary pregnanediol, the

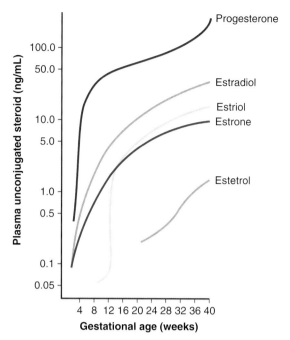

FIGURE 3-28 Plasma levels of progesterone, estradiol, estrone, estetrol, and estriol in women during the course of gestation. (From Mesiano, 2001. This figure was published in Yen SSC, Endocrine-metabolic adaptations in pregnancy, in *Reproductive Endocrinology: Physiology, Pathophysiology, and Clinical Management*, 3rd ed., SSC Yen and RB Jaffe (eds.), pp. 936–981, Copyright Elsevier/Saunders 1991, with permission.)

principal urinary metabolite of progesterone. Before this time, however, removal of the corpus luteum will result in miscarriage unless an exogenous progestin is given (see Chap. 40, p. 906). After approximately 8 weeks, the placenta assumes progesterone secretion, which continues to increase such that there is a gradual increase in maternal serum levels throughout pregnancy (Fig. 3-28). By the end of pregnancy, these levels are 10 to 5000 times those found in nonpregnant women, depending on the stage of the ovarian cycle.

Progesterone Production Rates

The daily production rate of progesterone in late, normal, singleton pregnancies is about 250 mg. In multifetal pregnancies, the daily production rate may exceed 600 mg/day. Progesterone is synthesized from cholesterol in a two-step enzymatic reaction. First, cholesterol is converted to pregnenolone within the mitochondria, in a reaction catalyzed by cytochrome P_{450} cholesterol side-chain cleavage enzyme. Pregnenolone leaves the mitochondria and is converted to progesterone in the endoplasmic reticulum by 3β-hydroxysteroid dehydrogenase. Progesterone is released immediately through a process of diffusion.

Even though the placenta produces a prodigious amount of progesterone, there is limited capacity for trophoblast cholesterol biosynthesis. Radiolabeled acetate is incorporated into cholesterol by placental tissue at a slow rate. The rate-limiting enzyme in cholesterol biosynthesis is 3-hydroxy-3-methylglutaryl coenzyme A (HMG CoA) reductase. Because of this, the placenta must rely on exogenous cholesterol for progesterone formation. Bloch (1945) and Werbin and co-workers (1957) found that after intravenous administration of radiolabeled cholesterol to pregnant women, the amount of radioactivity of urinary pregnanediol was similar to that of plasma cholesterol. Hellig and associates (1970) also found that maternal plasma cholesterol was the principal precursor—as much as 90 percent—of progesterone biosynthesis. The trophoblast preferentially uses LDL cholesterol for progesterone biosynthesis (Simpson and Burkhart, 1980; Simpson and colleagues, 1979). In studies of pregnant baboons, when maternal serum LDL levels were reduced, there was a significant drop in placental progesterone production (Henson and associates, 1997). Thus, placental progesterone is formed through the uptake and use of a maternal circulating precursor. This mechanism is unlike the placental production of estrogens, which relies principally on fetal adrenal precursors.

Progesterone Synthesis and Fetal Relationships

Although there is a relationship between fetal well-being and placental production of estrogen, this is not the case for placental progesterone. Fetal demise, ligation of the umbilical cord with the fetus and placenta remaining in situ, and anencephaly are all conditions associated with very low maternal plasma levels and low urinary excretion of estrogens. In these circumstances, there is not a concomitant decrease in progesterone levels until some indeterminate time after fetal death. Thus, placental endocrine function, including the formation of protein hormones such as hCG and progesterone biosynthesis, may persist for long periods (weeks) after fetal demise.

Progesterone Metabolism During Pregnancy

The metabolic clearance rate of progesterone in pregnant women is similar to that found in men and nonpregnant women. This is an important consideration in evaluating the role of progesterone in initiation of parturition (see Chap. 6, p. 154). During pregnancy, there is a disproportionate increase in the plasma concentration of 5α-dihydroprogesterone as a result of synthesis in syncytiotrophoblast from both placenta-produced progesterone and fetal-derived precursor (Dombroski and co-workers, 1997). Thus, the concentration ratio of this progesterone metabolite to progesterone is increased in pregnancy. The mechanisms for this are not defined completely but may be relevant to the resistance to pressor agents that normally develops in pregnant women (see Chap. 5, p. 120). Progesterone also is converted to the potent mineralocorticoid deoxycorticosterone in pregnant women and in the fetus. The concentration of deoxycorticosterone is increased strikingly in both maternal and fetal compartments (see Table 3-1). The extra-adrenal formation of deoxycorticosterone from circulating progesterone accounts for most of its production in pregnancy (Casey and MacDonald, 1982a, 1982b).

Placental Estrogen Production

The placenta produces huge amounts of estrogens using blood-borne steroidal precursors from the maternal and fetal adrenal glands. Near-term, normal human pregnancy is a hyperestrogenic state. The amount of estrogen produced each day by syncytiotrophoblast during the last few weeks of pregnancy is equivalent to that produced in 1 day by the ovaries of no fewer than 1000 ovulatory women. The hyperestrogenic state of human pregnancy is one of continually increasing

magnitude as pregnancy progresses, terminating abruptly after delivery.

During the first 2 to 4 weeks of pregnancy, rising hCG levels maintain production of estradiol in the maternal corpus luteum. Production of both progesterone and estrogens in the maternal ovaries decreases significantly by the seventh week of pregnancy. At this time, there is a luteal-placental transition. By the seventh week, more than half of estrogen entering maternal circulation is produced in the placenta (MacDonald, 1965; Siiteri and MacDonald, 1963, 1966). These studies support the transition of a steroid milieu dependent on the maternal corpus luteum to one dependent on the developing placenta.

Placental Estrogen Biosynthesis

The pathways of estrogen synthesis in the placenta differ from those in the ovary of nonpregnant women. Estrogen production in the ovary takes place during the follicular and luteal phase through the interaction of theca and granulosa cells. Specifically, androstenedione is synthesized in ovarian theca and then transferred to adjacent granulosa cells for estradiol synthesis. Estradiol production within the corpus luteum of nonpregnant women as well as in early pregnancy continues to require interaction between the luteinized theca and granulosa cells. In human trophoblast, neither cholesterol nor progesterone can serve as precursor for estrogen biosynthesis. A crucial enzyme necessary for sex steroid synthesis—steroid 17α-hydroxylase/17,20-lyase (CYP17)—is not expressed in the human placenta. Consequently, the conversion of C_{21}-steroids to C_{19}-steroids—the latter being the immediate and obligatory precursors of estrogens—is not possible.

Although C_{19}-steroids—dehydroepiandrosterone (DHEA) and its sulfate (DHEA-S)—often are called adrenal androgens, these steroids can also serve as estrogen precursors (Fig. 3-29). Ryan (1959a) found that there was an exceptionally high capacity of placenta to convert appropriate C_{19}-steroids to estrone and estradiol. The conversion of DHEA-S to estradiol requires placental expression of four key enzymes that are located principally in syncytiotrophoblast (Bonenfant and colleagues, 2000; Salido and co-workers, 1990). First, the placenta expresses high levels of steroid sulfatase (STS), which converts the conjugated DHEA-S to DHEA. DHEA is then acted upon by 3β-hydroxysteroid dehydrogenase type 1 (3βHSD) to produce androstenedione. Cytochrome P_{450} aromatase (CYP19) then converts androstenedione to estrone, which is then converted to estradiol by 17β-hydroxysteroid dehydrogenase type 1 (17βHSD1).

Plasma C₁₉-Steroids as Estrogen Precursors

Frandsen and Stakemann (1961) found that levels of urinary estrogens in women pregnant with an anencephalic fetus were only about 10 percent found in normal pregnancy. The adrenal glands of anencephalic fetuses are atrophic because of absent hypothalamic-pituitary function, which precludes ACTH stimulation. Thus, it seemed reasonable that fetal adrenal glands might provide substance(s) used for placental estrogen formation.

In subsequent studies, DHEA-S was found to be a major precursor of estrogens in pregnancy (Baulieu and Dray, 1963; Siiteri and MacDonald, 1963). The large amounts of DHEA-S in plasma and its much longer half-life uniquely qualify it as

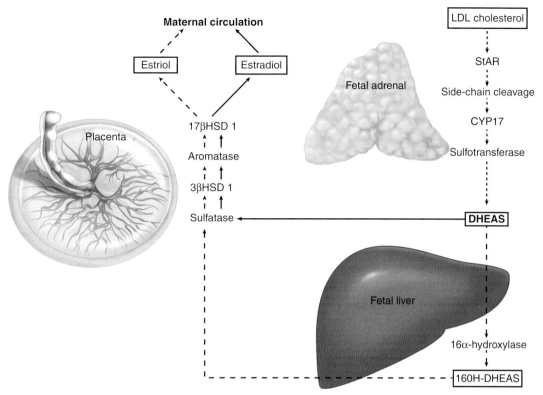

FIGURE 3-29 Schematic presentation of the biosynthesis of estrogens in the human placenta. Dehydroepiandrosterone sulfate (DHEA-S), secreted in prodigious amounts by the fetal adrenal glands, is converted to 16α-hydroxydehydroepiandrosterone sulfate (16αOHDHEA-S) in the fetal liver. These steroids, DHEA-S and 16αOHDHEA-S, are converted in the placenta to estrogens, that is, 17β-estradiol (E2) and estriol (E3). Near term, half of E2 is derived from fetal adrenal DHEA-S and half from maternal DHEA-S. On the other hand, 90 percent of E3 in the placenta arises from fetal 16αOHDHEA-S and only 10 percent from all other sources.

the principal precursor for placental estradiol synthesis. There is a 10- to 20-fold increase in the metabolic clearance rate of plasma DHEA-S in women at term compared with that in men and nonpregnant women (Gant and co-workers, 1971). This rapid use results in a progressive decrease in plasma DHEA-S concentration as pregnancy progresses (Milewich and co-workers, 1978). However, maternal adrenal glands do not produce sufficient amounts of DHEA-S to account for more than a fraction of total placental estrogen biosynthesis. **The fetal adrenal glands are quantitatively the most important source of placental estrogen precursors in human pregnancy.** A schematic representation of the pathways of estrogen formation in the placenta is presented in Figure 3-29. As shown, the estrogen products released from the placenta are dependent on the substrate available. Thus, estrogen production during pregnancy reflects the unique interactions between fetal adrenal glands, fetal liver, placenta, and maternal adrenal glands.

Directional Secretion of Steroids from Syncytiotrophoblast

More than 90 percent of estradiol and estriol formed in syncytiotrophoblast enters maternal plasma (Gurpide and co-workers, 1966) (see Table 3-1). And 85 percent or more of placental progesterone enters maternal plasma, with little maternal progesterone crossing the placenta to the fetus (Gurpide and co-workers, 1972).

The major reason for directional movement of newly formed steroid into the maternal circulation is the nature of hemo-

chorioendothelial placentation. In this system, steroids secreted from syncytiotrophoblast can enter maternal blood directly. Steroids that leave the syncytium do not enter fetal blood directly. They must first traverse the cytotrophoblasts and then enter connective tissue of the villous core and then fetal capillaries. From either of these spaces, steroids can reenter the syncytium. The net result of this hemochorial arrangement is that there is substantially greater entry of steroids into the maternal circulation compared with the amount that enters fetal blood.

FETAL ADRENAL GLAND HORMONES

Morphologically, functionally, and physiologically, the fetal adrenal glands are remarkable organs. At term, the fetal adrenal glands weigh the same as those of the adult. More than 85 percent of the fetal gland is composed of a unique fetal zone, which has a great capacity for steroid biosynthesis. Daily steroid production of fetal adrenal glands near term is 100 to 200 mg/day. This compares with resting adult steroid secretion of 30 to 40 mg/day. Thus, the fetal adrenal gland is a truly prodigious steroidogenic tissue.

The fetal zone is lost in the first year of life and is not present in the adult. In addition to ACTH, fetal adrenal gland growth is influenced by factors secreted by the placenta. This is exemplified by the continued growth of the fetal glands throughout gestation, but rapid involution immediately after birth when placenta-derived factors dissipate.

Placental Estriol Synthesis

The estrogen products released from the placenta are dependent on the substrate available. Estradiol is the primary placental estrogen secretory product at term. In addition, significant levels of estriol and estetrol are found in the maternal circulation, and they increase, particularly late in gestation (see Fig. 3-28). These hydroxylated forms of estrogen are produced in the placenta using substrates formed by the combined efforts of the fetal adrenal gland and liver.

There are important fetal-maternal interactions through the fetal liver (see Fig. 3-29). High levels of fetal hepatic 16α-hydroxylase act on adrenal derived steroids. Ryan (1959b) and MacDonald and Siiteri (1965) found that 16α-hydroxylated C_{19}-steroids, particularly 16α-hydroxydehydroepiandrosterone (16-OHDHEA), were converted to estriol by placental tissue. Thus, the disproportionate increase in estriol formation during pregnancy is accounted for by placental synthesis of estriol principally from plasma-borne 16-OHDHEA-S. Near term, the fetus is the source of 90 percent of placental estriol and estetrol precursor in normal human pregnancy.

Thus, the placenta secretes several estrogens, including estradiol, estrone, estriol, and estetrol. Because of its hemochorial nature, most placental estrogens are released into the maternal circulation. Maternal estriol and estetrol are produced almost solely by fetal steroid precursors. Thus, levels of these steroids were used in the past as an indicator of fetal well-being. However, low sensitivity and specificity of such tests have caused them to be discarded.

Enzymatic Considerations

There is a severe deficiency in the expression of the microsomal enzyme 3α-hydroxysteroid dehydrogenase, Δ^{5-4}-isomerase (3βHSD) in adrenal fetal zone cells (Doody and co-workers, 1990; Rainey and colleagues, 2001). This limits the conversion of pregnenolone to progesterone and of 17α-hydroxypregnenolone to 17α-hydroxyprogesterone, an obligatory step in cortisol biosynthesis. There is, however, very active steroid sulfotransferase activity in the fetal adrenal glands. As a consequence, the principal secretory products of the fetal adrenal glands are pregnenolone sulfate and DHEA-S. Comparatively, cortisol, which likely arises primarily in the neocortex and transitional zone of the fetal adrenal glands and not in the fetal zone, is a minor secretory product until late in gestation.

Fetal Adrenal Steroid Precursor

The precursor for fetal adrenal steroidogenesis is cholesterol. The rate of steroid biosynthesis in the fetal gland is so great that its steroidogenesis alone is equivalent to a fourth of the total daily LDL cholesterol turnover in adults. Fetal adrenal glands synthesize cholesterol from acetate. All enzymes involved in cholesterol biosynthesis are elevated compared with that of the adult adrenal gland (Rainey and colleagues, 2001). Thus, the rate of de novo cholesterol synthesis by fetal adrenal tissue is extremely high. Even so, it is insufficient to account for the steroids produced by these glands. Therefore, cholesterol must be assimilated from the fetal circulation. Plasma cholesterol and its esters are present in the form of very-low-density lipoprotein (VLDL), low-density lipoprotein (LDL), and high-density lipoprotein (HDL).

Simpson and colleagues (1979) found that fetal glands take up lipoproteins as a source of cholesterol for steroidogenesis. LDL was most effective, HDL was much less, and VLDL was devoid of stimulatory activity. They also evaluated relative contributions of cholesterol synthesized de novo and that of cholesterol derived from LDL uptake. These authors confirmed that fetal adrenal glands are highly dependent on circulating LDL as a source of cholesterol for optimum steroidogenesis (Carr and colleagues, 1980, 1982; Carr and Simpson, 1981).

Most fetal plasma cholesterol arises by de novo synthesis in the fetal liver (Carr and Simpson, 1984). The low level of LDL cholesterol in fetal plasma is not the consequence of impaired fetal LDL synthesis, but instead, it results from the rapid use of LDL by the fetal adrenal glands for steroidogenesis (Parker and colleagues, 1980, 1983). As expected, in the anencephalic newborn with atrophic adrenal glands, the LDL cholesterol levels in umbilical cord plasma are high.

Fetal Conditions That Affect Estrogen Production

Several fetal disorders alter the availability of substrate for placental steroid synthesis. A schematic representation of the pathways of placental estrogen formation is presented in Figure 3-29.

Fetal Demise

It has been known for many decades that fetal death is followed by a striking reduction in levels of urinary estrogens. It was also known that there was an abrupt and striking decrease in the production of placental estrogens after ligation of the umbilical cord with the fetus and placenta left in situ (Cassmer, 1959). These findings led to at least two interpretations. The first was that maintenance of the fetal placental circulation is essential to the functional integrity of the placenta. This was unlikely to be correct because placental production of progesterone was maintained after occlusion of the umbilical cord. A second explanation was that after umbilical cord ligation, an important source of precursors of placental estrogen—but not progesterone—biosynthesis was eliminated upon fetal death.

Fetal Anencephaly

In the absence of the fetal zone of the adrenal cortex, as in anencephaly, the formation rate of placental estrogens—especially estriol—is severely limited because of diminished availability of C_{19}-steroid precursors. Therefore, almost all estrogens produced in women pregnant with an anencephalic fetus arise by placental use of maternal plasma DHEA-S. Furthermore, in such pregnancies, the production of estrogens can be increased by the maternal administration of ACTH, which stimulates the rate of DHEA-S secretion by the maternal adrenal gland. Because ACTH does not cross the placenta, there is no fetal adrenal stimulation. Finally, placental estrogen production is decreased in women pregnant with an anencephalic fetus when a potent glucocorticoid is given to the mother. This suppresses ACTH secretion and thus decreases the rate of DHEA-S secretion from the maternal adrenal cortex (MacDonald and Siiteri, 1965).

Fetal Adrenal Hypoplasia

Congenital adrenal cortical hypoplasia occurs in perhaps 1 in 12,500 births (McCabe, 2001). There appear to be two primary forms. In the *miniature adult form*, which results from anencephaly or abnormal pituitary function, there is a very small adrenal cortical zone. The *cytomegalic form* is so called because of nodular formation of eosinophilic cells in the fetal zone. Estrogen production in pregnancies with either form is limited and suggests the absence of C_{19}-precursors. The cytomegalic form results from disruptive mutations in the gene known as the *dosage-sensitive sex reversal–adrenal hypoplasia congenita critical region on the X chromosome, gene 1(DAX1)* (McCabe, 2001).

Fetal-Placental Sulfatase Deficiency

Placental estrogen formation is generally regulated by the availability of C_{19}-steroid prohormones in fetal and maternal plasma. Specifically, there is no rate-limiting enzymatic reaction in the placental pathway from C_{19}-steroids to estrogen biosynthesis. An exception to this generalization is placental sulfatase deficiency, which is associated with very low estrogen levels in otherwise normal pregnancies (France and Liggins, 1969). Sulfatase deficiency precludes the hydrolysis of C_{19}-steroid sulfates, the first enzymatic step in the placental use of these circulating prehormones for estrogen biosynthesis. This deficiency is an X-linked disorder, and all affected fetuses are male. Its estimated frequency is 1 in 2000 to 5000 births and is associated with delayed onset of labor. It also is associated with the development of ichthyosis in affected males later in life (Bradshaw and Carr, 1986).

Fetal-Placental Aromatase Deficiency

There are a few well-documented examples of aromatase deficiency (Simpson, 2000). Fetal adrenal DHEA-S, which is produced in large quantities, is converted in the placenta to androstenedione, but in cases of placental aromatase deficiency, androstenedione cannot be converted to estradiol. Rather, androgen metabolites of DHEA produced in the placenta, including androstenedione and some testosterone, are secreted into the maternal or fetal circulation, or both, causing virilization of the mother and the female fetus (Harada and colleagues, 1992; Shozu and associates, 1991). Although pregnancies with aromatase deficiency and a male fetus may be uneventful, these estrogen-deficient males have delayed epiphyseal closure during puberty. As a consequence, affected men continue to grow during adulthood, becoming very tall and displaying deficient bone mineralization (Morishima and colleagues, 1995).

Trisomy 21—Down Syndrome

Second-trimester maternal serum screening for abnormal levels of hCG, alpha-fetoprotein, and other analytes has become universal (see Chap. 13, p. 292). As a result, it was discovered that serum unconjugated estriol levels were low in women with Down syndrome fetuses (Benn, 2002). The likely reason for this is inadequate formation of C19-steroids in the adrenal glands of these trisomic fetuses. This supposition is supported by reduced DHEA-S levels in both amnionic fluid and maternal serum in Down syndrome pregnancies (Newby and colleagues, 2000).

Deficiency in Fetal LDL Cholesterol Biosynthesis

A successful pregnancy in a woman with β-lipoprotein deficiency has been described (Parker and co-workers, 1986). The absence of LDL in the maternal serum restricted progesterone formation in both the corpus luteum and placenta. In addition, levels of estriol were lower than normal. Presumably, the diminished estrogen production was the result of decreased fetal LDL formation, which limited fetal adrenal production of estrogen precursor.

Fetal Erythroblastosis

In some cases of severe fetal D-antigen isoimmunization, estrogen levels in maternal plasma are elevated above normal. This is likely due to an increased placental mass from hypertrophy. This is seen with other causes of hyperplacentosis with a fetal hemocytic anemia, which occurs in such pregnancies (see Chap. 29, p. 618).

Maternal Conditions That Affect Placental Estrogen Production

Glucocorticoid Treatment

The administration of glucocorticoids in moderate to high doses to pregnant women causes a striking reduction in placental estrogen formation. Glucocorticoids act to inhibit ACTH secretion by the maternal and fetal pituitary glands, resulting in decreased maternal and fetal adrenal secretion of the placental estrogen precursor, DHEA-S.

Maternal Adrenal Dysfunction

In pregnant women with Addison disease, maternal urinary estrogen levels are decreased (Baulieu and colleagues, 1956). The decrease principally affects estrone and estradiol, because the fetal adrenal contribution to the synthesis of estriol, particularly in the latter part of pregnancy, is quantitatively much more important.

Maternal Ovarian Androgen-Producing Tumors

The extraordinary efficiency of the placenta in the aromatization of C_{19}-steroids may be exemplified by two considerations. First, Edman and associates (1981) found that virtually all of the androstenedione entering the intervillous space is taken up by syncytiotrophoblast and converted to estradiol, and none of this C_{19}-steroid enters the fetus. Second, it is relatively rare that a female fetus is virilized when there is a maternal androgen-secreting ovarian tumor. This finding also indicates that the placenta efficiently converts aromatizable C_{19}-steroids, including testosterone, to estrogens, thus precluding transplacental passage. Indeed, it may be that virilized female fetuses of women with an androgen-producing tumor are cases in which a nonaromatizable C_{19}-steroid androgen is produced by the tumor—for example, 5α-dihydrotestosterone. Another explanation is that testosterone is produced very early in pregnancy in amounts that exceed the capacity of placental aromatase.

Gestational Trophoblastic Disease

In the case of complete hydatidiform mole or choriocarcinoma, there is no fetal adrenal source of C_{19}-steroid precursor for trophoblast estrogen biosynthesis. Consequently, placental estrogen formation is limited to the use of C_{19}-steroids in the maternal plasma, and therefore the estrogen produced is principally estradiol (MacDonald and Siiteri, 1964, 1966). Great variation is observed in the rates of both estradiol and progesterone formation in molar pregnancies.

REFERENCES

Aaltonen J, Laitinen MP, Vuojolainen K, et al: Human growth differentiation factor 9 (GDF-9) and its novel homolog GDF-9B are expressed in oocytes during early folliculogenesis. J Clin Endocrinol Metab 84:2744, 1999

Abel MH: Prostanoids and menstruation. In Baird DT, Michie EA (eds): Mechanisms of Menstrual Bleeding. New York, Raven, 2002, p 139

Albrecht ED, Pepe GJ: Steroid hormone regulation of angiogenesis in the primate endometrium. Front Biosci 8:D416, 2003

Ancelin M, Buteau-Lozano H, Meduri G, et al: A dynamic shift of VEGF isoforms with a transient and selective progesterone-induced expression of VEGF189 regulates angiogenesis and vascular permeability in human uterus. Proc Natl Acad Sci U S A 99:6023, 2002

Aplin JD: MUC-1 glycosylation in endometrium: Possible roles of the apical glycocalyx at implantation. Hum Reprod 2:17, 2003

Arey LB: The degree of normal menstrual irregularity: An analysis of 20,000 calendar records from 1,500 individuals. Am J Obstet Gynecol 37:12, 1939

Arici A, Head JR, MacDonald PC, et al: Regulation of interleukin-8 gene expression in human endometrial cells in culture. Mol Cell Endocrinol 94:195, 1993

Arici A, MacDonald PC, Casey ML: Regulation of monocyte chemotactic protein-1 gene expression in human endometrial cells in cultures. Mol Cell Endocrinol 107:189, 1995

Arnholdt H, Meisel F, Fandrey K, et al: Proliferation of villous trophoblast of the human placenta in normal and abnormal pregnancies. Virchows Arch B Cell Pathol Incl Mol Pathol 60:365, 1991

Auletta F: The role of prostaglandin F2a in human luteolysis. Contemp Obstet Gynecol 30:119, 1987

Baker T: A quantitative and cytological study of germ cells in human ovaries. Proc R Soc Lond B Biol Sci 158:417, 1963

Bao L, Tessier C, Prigent-Tessier A, et al: Decidual prolactin silences the expression of genes detrimental to pregnancy. Endocrinology 148:2326, 2007

Barbour LA, Shao J, Qiao L, et al: Human placental growth hormone causes severe insulin resistance in transgenic mice. Am J Obstet Gynecol 186:512, 2002

Barnea ER, Kaplan M: Spontaneous, gonadotropin-releasing hormone-induced, and progesterone-inhibited pulsatile secretion of human chorionic gonadotropin in the first trimester placenta in vitro. J Clin Endocrinol Metab 69:215, 1989

Bathgate RA, Samuel CS, Burazin TC, et al: Human relaxin gene 3 (H3) and the equivalent mouse relaxin (M3) gene. Novel members of the relaxin peptide family. J Biol Chem 277:1148, 2002

Baulieu EE, Bricaire H, Jayle MF: Lack of secretion of 17-hydroxycorticosteroids in a pregnant woman with Addison's disease. J Clin Endocrinol 16:690, 1956

Baulieu EE, Dray F: Conversion of 3H-dehydroepiandrosterone (3b-hydroxy-D5-androstene-17-one) sulfate to 3H-estrogens in normal pregnant women. J Clin Endocrinol 23:1298, 1963

Bausero P, Cavaillé F, Meduri G, et al: Paracrine action of vascular endothelial growth factor in the human endometrium: Production and target sites, and hormonal regulation. Angiogenesis 2:167, 1998

Beck T, Schweikhart G, Stolz E: Immunohistochemical location of HPL, SP1 and beta-HCG in normal placentas of varying gestational age. Arch Gynecol 239:63, 1986

Beer AE, Billingham RE: Immunobiology of mammalian reproduction. Adv Immunol 14:1, 1971

Benirschke K, Kaufmann P: Pathology of the Human Placenta, 4th ed. New York, Springer, 2000

Benn PA: Advances in prenatal screening for Down syndrome: I. General principles and second trimester testing. Clin Chim Acta 323:1, 2002

Bergh PA, Navot D: The impact of embryonic development and endometrial maturity on the timing of implantation. Fertil Steril 58:537, 1992

Berry SA, Srivastava CH, Rubin LR, et al: Growth hormone-releasing hormone-like messenger ribonucleic acid and immunoreactive peptide are present in human testis and placenta. J Clin Endocrinol Metab 75:281, 1992

Bertelloni S, Baroncelli GI, Pelletti A, et al: Parathyroid hormone-related protein in healthy pregnant women. Calcif Tissue Int 54:195, 1994

Bhaumick B, Dawson EP, Bala RM: The effects of insulin-like growth factor-I and insulin on placental lactogen production by human term placental explants. Biochem Biophys Res Commun 144:674, 1987

Billingham RE: Transplantation immunity and the maternal fetal relation. N Engl J Med 270:667, 1964

Billingham RE, Head JR: Recipient treatment to overcome the allograft reaction, with special reference to nature's own solution. Prog Clin Biol Res 224:159, 1986

Bischof P, Meisser A, Campana A: Control of MMP-9 expression at the maternal-fetal interface. J Reprod Immunol 55:3, 2002

Bleker O, Kloostermans G, Mieras D, et al: Intervillous space during uterine contractions in human subjects: An ultrasonic study. Am J Obstet Gynecol 123:697, 1975

Bloch K: The biological conversion of cholesterol to pregnandiol. J Biol Chem 157:661, 1945

Bogic LV, Mandel M, Bryant-Greenwood GD: Relaxin gene expression in human reproductive tissues by in situ hybridization. J Clin Endocrinol Metab 80:130, 1995

Bombail V, MacPherson S, Critchley HO, et al: Estrogen receptor related beta is expressed in human endometrium throughout the normal menstrual cycle. Hum Reprod 23(12):2782, 2008

Bonenfant M, Provost PR, Drolet R, et al: Localization of type 1 17beta-hydroxysteroid dehydrogenase mRNA and protein in syncytiotrophoblasts and invasive cytotrophoblasts in the human term villi. J Endocrinol 165:217, 2000

Borell U, Fernstrom I, Westman A: An arteriographic study of the placental circulation. Geburtshilfe Frauenheilkd 18:1, 1958

Bourne GL: The Human Amnion and Chorion. Chicago, Year Book, 1962

Boyd JD, Hamilton WJ: The Human Placenta. Cambridge, England, Heffer, 1970

Bradbury J, Brown W, Guay L: Maintenance of the corpus luteum and physiologic action of progesterone. Recent Prog Horm Res 5:151, 1950

Bradshaw KD, Carr BR: Placental sulfatase deficiency: Maternal and fetal expression of steroid sulfatase deficiency and X-linked ichthyosis. Obstet Gynecol Surv 41:401, 1986

Brosens I, Dixon H: The anatomy of the maternal side of the placenta. Eur J Endocrinol 73:357, 1963

Brosens J, Hayashi N, White J: Progesterone receptor regulates decidual prolactin expression in differentiating human endometrial stromal cells. Eur J Obstet Gynaecol Surv 142:269, 2000

Browning HC: The evolutionary history of the corpus luteum. Biol Reprod 8:128, 1973

Bryant-Greenwood GD: The extracellular matrix of the human fetal membranes: Structure and function. Placenta 19:1, 1998

Carr BR, Ohashi M, Simpson ER: Low density lipoprotein binding and de novo synthesis of cholesterol in the neocortex and fetal zones of the human fetal adrenal gland. Endocrinology 110:1994, 1982

Carr BR, Parker CR Jr, Madden JD, et al: Maternal plasma adrenocorticotropin and cortisol relationships throughout human pregnancy. Am J Obstet Gynecol 139:416, 1981a

Carr BR, Porter JC, MacDonald PC, et al: Metabolism of low density lipoprotein by human fetal adrenal tissue. Endocrinology 107:1034, 1980

Carr BR, Sadler RK, Rochelle DB, et al: Plasma lipoprotein regulation of progesterone biosynthesis by human corpus luteum tissue in organ culture. J Clin Endocrinol Metab 52:875, 1981b

Carr BR, Simpson ER: Cholesterol synthesis by human fetal hepatocytes: Effect of lipoproteins. Am J Obstet Gynecol 150:551, 1984

Carr BR, Simpson ER: Lipoprotein utilization and cholesterol synthesis by the human fetal adrenal gland. Endocr Rev 2:306, 1981

Carson DD: The glycobiology of implantation. Front Biosci 7:d1535, 2002

Casey ML, Delgadillo M, Cox KA, et al: Inactivation of prostaglandins in human decidua vera (parietalis) tissue: Substrate specificity of prostaglandin dehydrogenase. Am J Obstet Gynecol 160:3, 1989

Casey ML, Hemsell DL, MacDonald PC, et al: NAD+-dependent 15-hydroxyprostaglandin dehydrogenase activity in human endometrium. Prostaglandins 19:115, 1980

Casey ML, MacDonald PC: Extraadrenal formation of a mineralocorticosteroid: Deoxycorticosterone and deoxycorticosterone sulfate biosynthesis and metabolism. Endocr Rev 3:396, 1982a

Casey ML, MacDonald PC: Metabolism of deoxycorticosterone and deoxycorticosterone sulfate in men and women. J Clin Invest 70:312, 1982b

Casey ML, MacDonald PC: The endothelin-parathyroid hormone-related protein vasoactive peptide system in human endometrium: Modulation by transforming growth factor-beta. Hum Reprod 11 Suppl 2:62, 1996

Casey ML, Smith JW, Nagai K, et al: Progesterone-regulated cyclic modulation of membrane metalloendopeptidase (enkephalinase) in human endometrium. J Biol Chem 266:23041, 1991

Cassmer O: Hormone production of the isolated human placenta. Acta Endocrinol (Suppl) 32:45, 1959

Cervar M, Blaschitz A, Dohr G, et al: Paracrine regulation of distinct trophoblast functions in vitro by placental macrophages. Cell Tissue Res 295:297, 1999

Chao HS, Poisner AM, Poisner R, et al: Endothelin-1 modulates renin and prolactin release from human decidua by different mechanisms. Am J Physiol 267:E842, 1994

Chennazhi, Nayak NR: Regulation of angiogenesis in the primate endometrium: vascular endothelial growth factor. Semin Reprod Med 27(1):80, 2009

Christian M, Pohnke Y, Kempf R, et al: Functional association of PR and CCAAT/enhancer-binding protein beta isoforms: Promoter-dependent cooperation between PR-B and liver-enriched inhibitory protein, or liver-enriched activatory protein and PR-A in human endometrial stromal cells. Mol Endocrinol 16:141, 2002a

Christian M, Zhang XH, Schneider-Merck T, et al: Cyclic AMP-induced forkhead transcription factor, FKHR, cooperates with CCAAT/enhancer-binding protein beta in differentiating human endometrial stromal cells. J Biol Chem 277:20825, 2002b

Cock T-A, Auwerx J: Leptin: Cutting the fat off the bone. Lancet 362:1572, 2003

Cole LA: Immunoassay of human chorionic gonadotropin, its free subunits, and metabolites. Clin Chem 43:2233, 1997

Cole LA, Kardana A, Andrade-Gordon P, et al: The heterogeneity of human chorionic gonadotropin (hCG). III. The occurrence and biological and immunological activities of nicked hCG. Endocrinology 129:1559, 1991

Condon JC, Hardy DB, Kovaric K, et al: Up-regulation of the progesterone receptor (PR)-C isoform in laboring myometrium by activation of nuclear factor-kappaB may contribute to the onset of labor through inhibition of PR function. Mol Endocrinol 20:764, 2006

Conneely OM, Mulac-Jericevic B, DeMayo F, et al: Reproductive functions of progesterone receptors. Recent Prog Horm Res 57:339, 2002

Corbacho AM, Martinez DLE, Clapp C: Roles of prolactin and related members of the prolactin/growth hormone/placental lactogen family in angiogenesis. J Endocrinol 173:219, 2002

Coya R, Martul P, Algorta J, et al: Progesterone and human placental lactogen inhibit leptin secretion on cultured trophoblast cells from human placentas at term. Gynecol Endocrinol 21:27, 2005

Crawford J: A study of human placental growth with observations on the placenta in erythroblastosis foetalis. Br J Obstet Gynaecol 66:855, 1959

Critchley HO, Kelly RW, Baird DT, et al: Regulation of human endometrial function: Mechanisms relevant to uterine bleeding. Reprod Biol Endocrinol 4 Suppl 1:S5, 2006

Curry TE Jr, Smith MF: Impact of extracellular matrix remodeling on ovulation and the folliculo-luteal transition. Semin Reprod Med 24(4):228, 2006

Damjanov I: Vesalius and Hunter were right: Decidua is a membrane! Lab Invest 53:597, 1985

Dautzenberg FM, Hauger RL: The CRF peptide family and their receptors: Yet more partners discovered. Trends Pharmacol Sci 23:71, 2002

Desai R, Creger W: Maternofetal passage of leukocytes and platelets in man. Blood 21:665, 1963

Devoto L, Kohen P, Vega M, et al: Control of human luteal steroidogenesis. Mol Cell Endocrinol 186:137, 2002

Diaz-Cueto L, Mendez JP, Barrios-de-Tomasi J, et al: Amplitude regulation of episodic release, in vitro biological to immunological ratio, and median charge of human chorionic gonadotropin in pregnancy. J Clin Endocrinol Metab 78:890, 1994

Diczfalusy E, Troen P: Endocrine functions of the human placenta. Vitam Horm 19:229, 1961

Dombroski RA, Casey ML, MacDonald PC: 5-Alpha-dihydroprogesterone formation in human placenta from 5alpha-pregnan-3beta/alpha-ol-20-ones and 5-pregnan-3beta-yl-20-one sulfate. J Steroid Biochem Mol Biol 63:155, 1997

Dong JC, Dong H, Campana A, et al: Matrix metalloproteinases and their specific tissue inhibitors in menstruation. Reproduction 123:621, 2002

Doody KM, Carr BR, Rainey WE, et al: 3b-hydroxysteroid dehydrogenase/isomerase in the fetal zone and neocortex of the human fetal adrenal gland. Endocrinology 126:2487, 1990

Duffy DM, Hutchison JS, Stewart DR, et al: Stimulation of primate luteal function by recombinant human chorionic gonadotropin and modulation of steroid, but not relaxin, production by an inhibitor of 3 beta-hydroxysteroid dehydrogenase during simulated early pregnancy. J Clin Endocrinol Metab 81:2307, 1996

Duncan WC, McNeilly AS, Fraser HM, et al: Luteinizing hormone receptor in the human corpus luteum: Lack of down-regulation during maternal recognition of pregnancy. Hum Reprod 11:2291, 1996

Dunn CL, Critchley HO, Kelly RW: IL-15 regulation in human endometrial stromal cells. J Clin Endocrinol Metab 87:1898, 2002

Economos K, MacDonald PC, Casey ML: Endothelin-1 gene expression and protein biosynthesis in human endometrium: Potential modulator of endometrial blood flow. J Clin Endocrinol Metab 74:14, 1992

Edman CD, Toofanian A, MacDonald PC, et al: Placental clearance rate of maternal plasma androstenedione through placental estradiol formation: An indirect method of assessing uteroplacental blood flow. Am J Obstet Gynecol 141:1029, 1981

Ehrhardt K: Forschung und Klinik. Ober das Lacttazionshormon des Hypophysenvorderlappens. Muench Med Wochenschr 83:1163, 1936

Elliott CL, Allport VC, Loudon JA, et al: Nuclear factor-kappa B is essential for up-regulation of interleukin-8 expression in human amnion and cervical epithelial cells. Mol Hum Reprod 7:787, 2001

Enders AC: A comparative study of the fine structure in several hemochorial placentas. Am J Anat 116:29, 1965

Faddy MJ, Gosden RG, Gougeon A, et al: Accelerated disappearance of ovarian follicles in mid-life: Implications for forecasting menopause. Hum Reprod 7:1342, 1992

Feinberg RF, Kliman HJ, Lockwood CJ: Is oncofetal fibronectin a trophoblast glue for human implantation? Am J Pathol 138:537, 1991

Ferenczy A: Studies on the cytodynamics of human endometrial regeneration. I. Scanning electron microscopy. Am J Obstet Gynecol 124:64, 1976

Filicori M, Santoro N, Merriam GR, et al: Characterization of the physiological pattern of episodic gonadotropin secretion throughout the human menstrual cycle. J Clin Endocrinol Metab 62:1136, 1986

Fisk NM, MacLachlan N, Ellis C, et al: Absent end-diastolic flow in first trimester umbilical artery. Lancet 2:1256, 1988

Fitzgerald JS, Poehlmann TG, Schleussner E, et al: Trophoblast invasion: the role of intracellular cytokine signaling via signal transducer and activator of transcription 3 (STAT3). Hum Reprod Update 14(4):335, 2008

Florio P, Franchini A, Reis FM, et al: Human placenta, chorion, amnion and decidua express different variants of corticotropin-releasing factor receptor messenger RNA. Placenta 21:32, 2000

Florio P, Mezzesimi A, Turchetti V, et al: High levels of human chromogranin A in umbilical cord plasma and amniotic fluid at parturition. J Soc Gynecol Investig 9:32, 2002

France JT, Liggins GC: Placental sulfatase deficiency. J Clin Endocrinol Metab 29:138, 1969

Frandsen VA, Stakemann G: The site of production of oestrogenic hormones in human pregnancy: Hormone excretion in pregnancy with anencephalic foetus. Acta Endocrinol 38:383, 1961

Frank GR, Brar AK, Jikihara H, et al: Interleukin-1 beta and the endometrium: An inhibitor of stromal cell differentiation and possible autoregulator of decidualization in humans. Biol Reprod 52:184, 1995

Fraser HM, Wulff C: Angiogenesis in the primate ovary. Reprod Fertil Dev 13:557, 2001

Fuglsang J, Skjaerbaek C, Espelund U, et al: Ghrelin and its relationship to growth hormones during normal pregnancy. Clin Endocrinol (Oxf) 62(5):554, 2005

Fuzzi B, Rizzo R, Criscuoli L, et al: HLA-G expression in early embryos is a fundamental prerequisite for the obtainment of pregnancy. Eur J Immunol 32:311, 2002

Gant NF, Hutchinson HT, Siiteri PK, et al: Study of the metabolic clearance rate of dehydroisoandrosterone sulfate in pregnancy. Am J Obstet Gynecol 111:555, 1971

Garcia-Velasco JA, Arici A: Chemokines and human reproduction. Fertil Steril 71:983, 1999

Gargett CE, Rogers PA: Human endometrial angiogenesis. Reproduction 121:181, 2001

Genazzani AR, Fraioli F, Hurlimann J, et al: Immunoreactive ACTH and cortisol plasma levels during pregnancy. Detection and partial purification of corticotrophin-like placental hormone: The human chorionic corticotrophin (HCC). Clin Endocrinol (Oxf) 4:1, 1975

Genbacev O, Ratkovic M, Kraincanic M, et al: Effect of prostaglandin PGE2alpha on the synthesis of placental proteins and human placental lactogen (HPL). Prostaglandins 13:723, 1977

Germain A, Attaroglu H, MacDonald PC, et al: Parathyroid hormone-related protein mRNA in avascular human amnion. J Clin Endocrinol Metab 75:1173, 1992

Gibbons JM Jr, Mitnick M, Chieffo V: In vitro biosynthesis of TSH- and LH-releasing factors by the human placenta. Am J Obstet Gynecol 121:127, 1975

Gleicher N, Barad DH: Gender as risk factor for autoimmune diseases. Autoimmun 28:1, 2007

Golander A, Hurley T, Barrett J, et al: Prolactin synthesis by human chorion-decidual tissue: A possible source of prolactin in the amniotic fluid. Science 202:311, 1978

Goldman-Wohl DS, Ariel I, Greenfield C, et al: HLA-G expression in extravillous trophoblasts is an intrinsic property of cell differentiation: A lesson learned from ectopic pregnancies. Mol Hum Reprod 6:535, 2000

Gougeon A: Regulation of ovarian follicular development in primates: Facts and hypotheses. Endocr Rev 17:121, 1996

Groome NP, Illingworth PJ, O'Brien M, et al: Measurement of dimeric inhibin B throughout the human menstrual cycle. J Clin Endocrinol Metab 81:1401, 1996

Grumbach MM, Kaplan SL: On placental origin and purification of chorionic growth hormone prolactin and its immunoassay in pregnancy. Trans N Y Acad Sci 27:167, 1964

Gualillo O, Caminos J, Blanco M, et al: Ghrelin, a novel placental-derived hormone. Endocrinology 142:788, 2001

Gubbay O, Critchley HO, Bowen JM, et al: Prolactin induces ERK phosphorylation in epithelial and CD56(+) natural killer cells of the human endometrium. J Clin Endocrinol Metab 87:2329, 2002

Gurpide E, Schwers J, Welch MT, et al: Fetal and maternal metabolism of estradiol during pregnancy. J Clin Endocrinol Metab 26:1355, 1966

Gurpide E, Tseng J, Escarcena L, et al: Fetomaternal production and transfer of progesterone and uridine in sheep. Am J Obstet Gynecol 113:21, 1972

Guzeloglu-Kayisli O, Kayisli UA, Taylor HS: The role of growth factors and cytokines during implantation: endocrine and paracrine interactions. Semin Reprod Med 27(1):62, 2009

Hafez ES, Ludwig H, Metzger H: Human endometrial fluid kinetics as observed by scanning electron microscopy. Am J Obstet Gynecol 122:929, 1975

Haman JO: The length of the menstrual cycle: A study of 150 normal women. Am J Obstet Gynecol 43:870, 1942

Hamilton W, Boyd J: Trophoblast in human utero-placental arteries. Nature 212:906, 1966

Handwerger S, Barry S, Barrett J, et al: Inhibition of the synthesis and secretion of decidual prolactin by arachidonic acid. Endocrinology 109:2016, 1981

Hanna J, Goldman-Wohl D, Hamani Y, et al: Decidual NK cells regulate key developmental processes at the human fetal-maternal interface. Nat Med 12:1065, 2006

Hansell DJ, Bryant-Greenwood GD, Greenwood FC: Expression of the human relaxin H1 gene in the decidua, trophoblast, and prostate. J Clin Endocrinol Metab 72:899, 1991

Harada N, Ogawa H, Shozu M, et al: Biochemical and molecular genetic analyses on placental aromatase (P-450AROM) deficiency. J Biol Chem 267:4781, 1992

Hellig H, Gattereau D, Lefebvre Y, et al: Steroid production from plasma cholesterol. I. Conversion of plasma cholesterol to placental progesterone in humans. J Clin Endocrinol Metab 30:624, 1970

Henson MC, Castracane VD: Leptin: Roles and regulation in primate pregnancy. Semin Reprod Med 20:113, 2002

Henson MC, Greene SJ, Reggio BC, et al: Effects of reduced maternal lipoprotein-cholesterol availability on placental progesterone biosynthesis in the baboon. Endocrinology 138:1385, 1997

Hershman JM: Human chorionic gonadotropin and the thyroid: Hyperemesis gravidarum and trophoblastic tumors. Thyroid 9:653, 1999

Hertig AT: The placenta: Some new knowledge about an old organ. Obstet Gynecol 20:859, 1962

Hillier SG: Gonadotropic control of ovarian follicular growth and development. Mol Cell Endocrinol 179:39, 2001

Horvath TL, Diano S, Sotonyi P, et al: Minireview: Ghrelin and the regulation of energy balance—a hypothalamic perspective. Endocrinology 142:4163, 2001

Hoshina M, Boothby M, Boime I: Cytological localization of chorionic gonadotropin alpha and placental lactogen mRNAs during development of the human placenta. J Cell Biol 93:190, 1982

Hreinsson JG, Scott JE, Rasmussen C, et al: Growth differentiation factor-9 promotes the growth, development, and survival of human ovarian follicles in organ culture. J Clin Endocrinol Metab 87:316, 2002

Hsu SY, Nakabayashi K, Nishi S, et al: Activation of orphan receptors by the hormone relaxin. Science 295:671, 2002

Hudson P, Haley J, John M, et al: Structure of a genomic clone encoding biologically active human relaxin. Nature 301:628, 1983

Hudson P, John M, Crawford R, et al: Relaxin gene expression in human ovaries and the predicted structure of a human preprorelaxin by analysis of cDNA clones. EMBO J 3:2333, 1984

Hunt JS, Jadhav L, Chu W, et al: Soluble HLA-G circulates in maternal blood during pregnancy. Am J Obstet Gynecol 183:682, 2000a

Hunt JS, Orr HT: HLA and maternal-fetal recognition. FASEB J 6:2344, 1992

Hunt JS, Petroff MG, Morales P, et al: HLA-G in reproduction: Studies on the maternal-fetal interface. Hum Immunol 61:1113, 2000b

Illingworth DR, Corbin DK, Kemp ED, et al: Hormone changes during the menstrual cycle in abetalipoproteinemia: Reduced luteal phase progesterone in a patient with homozygous hypobetalipoproteinemia. Proc Natl Acad Sci U S A 79:6685, 1982

Ito Y, Higashi K: Studies on prolactin-like substance in human placenta. Endocrinol Jpn 8:279, 1961

Iwashita M, Kudo Y, Shinozaki Y, et al: Gonadotropin-releasing hormone increases serum human chorionic gonadotropin in pregnant women. Endocr J 40:539, 1993

Jabbour HN, Critchley HOD: Potential roles of decidual prolactin in early pregnancy. Reproduction 121:197, 2001

Jeffrey J: Collagen and collagenase: Pregnancy and parturition. Semin Perinatol 15:118, 1991

Johnson PM, Christmas SE, Vince GS: Immunological aspects of implantation and implantation failure. Hum Reprod 14(suppl 2):26, 1999

Jokhi P, King A, Loke Y: Production of granulocyte/macrophage colony-stimulating factor by human trophoblast cells and by decidual large granular lymphocytes. Hum Reprod 9:1660, 1999

Jones SA, Brooks AN, Challis JR: Steroids modulate corticotropin-releasing hormone production in human fetal membranes and placenta. J Clin Endocrinol Metab 68:825, 1989a

Jones SA, Challis JR: Local stimulation of prostaglandin production by corticotropin-releasing hormone in human fetal membranes and placenta. Biochem Biophys Res Commun 159:192, 1989b

Josimovich JB, MacLaren JA: Presence in human placenta and term serum of highly lactogenic substance immunologically related in pituitary growth hormone. Endocrinology 71:209, 1962

Kaipia A, Hsueh AJ: Regulation of ovarian follicle atresia. Annu Rev Physiol 59:349, 1997

Katzenellenbogen BS, Sun J, Harrington WR, et al: Structure-function relationships in estrogen receptors and the characterization of novel selective estrogen receptor modulators with unique pharmacological profiles. Ann NY Acad Sci 949:6, 2001

Kaufmann P, Black S, Huppertz B: Endovascular trophoblast invasion: Implications for the pathogenesis of intrauterine growth retardation and preeclampsia. Biol Reprod 69:1, 2003

Kaufmann P, Scheffen I: Placental development. In Polin R, Fox W (eds): Fetal and Neonatal Physiology. Philadelphia, Saunders, 1992, p 47

Khodr GS, Siler-Khodr TM: Placental luteinizing hormone-releasing factor and its synthesis. Science 207:315, 1980

King BF, Menton DN: Scanning electron microscopy of human placental villi from early and late in gestation. Am J Obstet Gynecol 122:824, 1975

Kraiem Z, Sadeh O, Blithe DL, et al: Human chorionic gonadotropin stimulates thyroid hormone secretion, iodide uptake, organification, and adenosine 3′,5′-monophosphate formation in cultured human thyrocytes. J Clin Endocrinol Metab 79:595, 1994

Kurman RJ, Young RH, Norris HJ, et al: Immunocytochemical localization of placental lactogen and chorionic gonadotropin in the normal placenta and trophoblastic tumors, with emphasis on intermediate trophoblast and the placental site trophoblastic tumor. Int J Gynecol Pathol 3:101, 1984

Kurtzman JT, Wilson H, Rao CV: A proposed role for hCG in clinical obstetrics. Semin Reprod Med 19:63, 2001

La Cava A, Alviggi C, Matarese G: Unraveling the multiple roles of leptin in inflammation and autoimmunity. J Mol Med 82:4, 2004

Lala PK, Lee BP, Xu G, et al: Human placental trophoblast as an in vitro model for tumor progression. Can J Physiol Pharmacol 80:142, 2002

LeBouteiller P, Solier C, Proll J, et al: Placental HLA-G protein expression in vivo: Where and what for? Hum Reprod Update 5:223, 1999

Lecce G, Meduri G, Ancelin M, et al: Presence of estrogen receptor beta in the human endometrium through the cycle: Expression in glandular, stromal, and vascular cells. J Clin Endocrinol Metab 86:1379, 2001

Lessey BA, Castelbaum AJ: Integrins and implantation in the human. Rev Endocr Metab Disord 3:107, 2002

Lessey BA, Castelbaum AJ, Sawin SW, et al: Integrins as markers of uterine receptivity in women with primary unexplained infertility. Fertil Steril 63:535, 1995

Lessey BA, Ilesanmi AO, Lessey MA, et al: Luminal and glandular endometrial epithelium express integrins differentially throughout the menstrual cycle: Implications for implantation, contraception, and infertility. Am J Reprod Immunol 35:195, 1996

Li XF, Charnock-Jones DS, Zhang E, et al: Angiogenic growth factor messenger ribonucleic acids in uterine natural killer cells. J Clin Endocrinol Metab 86:1823, 2001

Librach CL, Werb Z, Fitzgerald ML, et al: 92-kD type IV collagenase mediates invasion of human cytotrophoblasts. J Cell Biol 113:437, 1991

Licht P, Russu V, Wildt L: On the role of human chorionic gonadotropin (hCG) in the embryo-endometrial microenvironment: Implications for differentiation and implantation. Semin Reprod Med 19:37, 2001

Lindhard A, Bentin-Ley U, Ravn V, et al: Biochemical evaluation of endometrial function at the time of implantation. Fertil Steril 78:221, 2002

Lobo SC, Srisuparp S, Peng X, et al: Uterine receptivity in the baboon: Modulation by chorionic gonadotropin. Semin Reprod Med 19:69, 2001

Loke YM, King A: Human Implantation. Cell Biology and Immunology. Cambridge, England, Cambridge University Press, 1995

Loquet P, Broughton-Pipkin F, Symonds E, et al: Blood velocity waveforms and placental vascular formation. Lancet 2:1252, 1988

Maaskant RA, Bogic LV, Gilger S, et al: The human prolactin receptor in the fetal membranes, decidua, and placenta. J Clin Endocrinol Metab 81:396, 1996

MacDonald PC: Placental steroidogenesis. In Wynn RM (ed): Fetal Homeostasis, Vol. I. New York, New York Academy of Sciences, 1965, p 265

MacDonald PC, Siiteri PK: Origin of estrogen in women pregnant with an anencephalic fetus. J Clin Invest 44:465, 1965

MacDonald PC, Siiteri PK: Study of estrogen production in women with hydatidiform mole. J Clin Endocrinol Metab 24:685, 1964

MacDonald PC, Siiteri PK: The in vivo mechanisms of origin of estrogen in subjects with trophoblastic tumors. Steroids 8:589, 1966

Macklon NS, Fauser BC: Follicle-stimulating hormone and advanced follicle development in the human. Arch Med Res 32:595, 2001

Magarinos MP, Sanchez-Margalet V, Kotler M, et al: Leptin promotes cell proliferation and survival of trophoblastic cells. Biol Reprod 76:203, 2007

Manaster I, Mizrahi S, Goldman-Wohl D, et al: Endometrial NK cells are special immature cells that await pregnancy. J Immunol 181:1869, 2008

Maradny EE, Kanayama N, Halim A, et al: Stretching of fetal membranes increases the concentration of interleukin-8 and collagenase activity. Am J Obstet Gynecol 174:843, 1996

Markee J: Menstruation in intraocular endometrial transplants in the rhesus monkey. Contrib Embryol 28:219, 1940

Maruo T, Ladines-Llave CA, Matsuo H, et al: A novel change in cytologic localization of human chorionic gonadotropin and human placental lactogen in first-trimester placenta in the course of gestation. Am J Obstet Gynecol 167:217, 1992

Maulik D: Doppler ultrasound in obstetrics. Williams Obstetrics, 20th ed. Stamford, Appleton & Lange, 1997, p 1

McCabe ERB: Adrenal hypoplasias and aplasias. In Scriver CR, Beaudet AL, Sly WE, et al (eds): The Metabolic and Molecular Bases of Inherited Disease. New York, McGraw-Hill, 2001, p 4263

McCombs H, Craig M: Decidual necrosis in normal pregnancy. Obstet Gynecol 24:436, 1964

McGregor WG, Kuhn RW, Jaffe RB: Biologically active chorionic gonadotropin: Synthesis by the human fetus. Science 220:306, 1983

McGregor WG, Raymoure WJ, Kuhn RW, et al: Fetal tissue can synthesize a placental hormone. Evidence for chorionic gonadotropin beta-subunit synthesis by human fetal kidney. J Clin Invest 68:306, 1981

McMaster M, Librach C, Zhou Y, et al: Human placental HLA-G expression is restricted to differentiated cytotrophoblasts. J Immunol 154:3771, 1995

Medawar PB: Some immunological and endocrinological problems raised by the evolution of viviparity in vertebrates. Symp Soc Exp Biol 44:1953

Meinert M, Malmström E, Tufvesson E: Labour induces increased concentrations of biglycan and hyaluronan in human fetal membranes. Placenta 28:482, 2007

Merlino AA, Welsh TN, Tan H, et al: Nuclear progesterone receptors in the human pregnancy myometrium: Evidence that parturition involves functional progesterone withdrawal mediated by increased expression of PR-A. J Clin Endocrinol Metab 92:1927, 2007

Mesiano S: Roles of estrogen and progesterone in human parturition. In Smith R (ed): The Endocrinology of Parturition. Basic Science and Clinical Application. Basel, Karger, 2001, p 86

Mijovic JE, Demianczuk N, Olson DM, et al: Prostaglandin endoperoxide H synthase mRNA expression in the fetal membranes correlates with fetal fibronectin concentration in the cervico-vaginal fluids at term: Evidence of enzyme induction before the onset of labour. Br J Obstet Gynaecol 107:267, 2000

Milewich L, Gomez-Sanchez C, Madden JD, et al: Dehydroisoandrosterone sulfate in peripheral blood of premenopausal, pregnant and postmenopausal women and men. J Steroid Biochem 9:1159, 1978

Miller-Lindholm AK, LaBenz CJ, Ramey J, et al: Human chorionic gonadotropin-beta gene expression in first trimester placenta. Endocrinology 138:5459, 1997

Moffett-King A: Natural killer cells and pregnancy. Nat Rev Immunol 2:656, 2002

Moore JJ, Dubyak GR, Moore RM, et al: Oxytocin activates the inositol-phospholipid-protein kinase-C system and stimulates prostaglandin production in human amnion cells. Endocrinology 123:1771, 1988

Moore RM, Redline RW, Kumar D, et al: Differential expression of fibulin family proteins in the para-cervical weak zone and other areas of human fetal membranes. Placenta 30(4):335, 2009

Morishima A, Grumbach MM, Simpson ER, et al: Aromatase deficiency in male and female siblings caused by a novel mutation and the physiological role of estrogens. J Clin Endocrinol Metab 80:3689, 1995

Morrish DW, Marusyk H, Siy O: Demonstration of specific secretory granules for human chorionic gonadotropin in placenta. J Histochem Cytochem 35:93, 1987

Mote PA, Balleine RL, McGowan EM, et al: Colocalization of progesterone receptors A and B by dual immunofluorescent histochemistry in human endometrium during the menstrual cycle. J Clin Endocrinol Metab 84:2963, 1999

Mote PA, Balleine RL, McGowan EM, et al: Heterogeneity of progesterone receptors A and B expression in human endometrial glands and stroma. Hum Reprod 15(suppl 3):48, 2000

Navot D, Bergh P: Preparation of the human endometrium for implantation. Ann N Y Acad Sci 622:212, 1991

Nemeth E, Tashima LS, Yu Z, et al: Fetal membrane distention: I. Differentially expressed genes regulated by acute distention in amniotic epithelial (WISH) cells. Am J Obstet Gynecol 182:50, 2000

Nguyen H, Dubernard G, Aractingi S, et al: Feto-maternal cell trafficking: A transfer of pregnancy associated progenitor cells. Stem Cell Rev 2:111, 2006

Newby D, Aitken DA, Howatson AG, et al: Placental synthesis of oestriol in Down's syndrome pregnancies. Placenta 21:263, 2000

Nicholson RC, King BR: Regulation of CRH gene expression in the placenta. Front Horm Res 27:246, 2001

Nikas G: Cell-surface morphological events relevant to human implantation. Hum Reprod 2:37, 2003

Nolten WE, Rueckert PA: Elevated free cortisol index in pregnancy: Possible regulatory mechanisms. Am J Obstet Gynecol 139:492, 1981

Ny T, Wahlberg P, Brandstrom IJ: Matrix remodeling in the ovary: Regulation and functional role of the plasminogen activator and matrix metalloproteinase systems. Mol Cell Endocrinol 187:29, 2002

Odagiri E, Sherrell BJ, Mount CD, et al: Human placental immunoreactive corticotropin, lipotropin, and beta-endorphin: Evidence for a common precursor. Proc Natl Acad Sci U S A 76:2027, 1979

Ogren L, Talamantes F: The placenta as an endocrine organ: Polypeptides. In Knobil E, Neill JD (eds): The Physiology of Reproduction. New York, Raven, 1994, p 875

O'Sullivan CM, Liu SY, Karpinka JB, et al: Embryonic hatching enzyme strypsin/ISP1 is expressed with ISP2 in endometrial glands during implantation. Mol Reprod Dev 62:328, 2002

Owerbach D, Rutter WJ, Cooke NE, et al: The prolactin gene is located on chromosome 6 in humans. Science 212:815, 1981

Owerbach D, Rutter WJ, Martial JA, et al: Genes for growth hormone, chorionic somatomammotropin, and growth hormones-like gene on chromosome 17 in humans. Science 209:289, 1980

Paria BC, Reese J, Das SK, et al: Deciphering the cross-talk of implantation: Advances and challenges. Science 296:2185, 2002

Parker CR Jr, Carr BR, Simpson ER, et al: Decline in the concentration of low-density lipoprotein-cholesterol in human fetal plasma near term. Metabolism 32:919, 1983

Parker CR Jr, Illingworth DR, Bissonnette J, et al: Endocrinology of pregnancy in abetalipoproteinemia: Studies in a patient with homozygous familial hypobetalipoproteinemia. N Engl J Med 314:557, 1986

Parker CR Jr, Simpson ER, Bilheimer DW, et al: Inverse relation between low-density lipoprotein-cholesterol and dehydroisoandrosterone sulfate in human fetal plasma. Science 208:512, 1980

Patel N, Alsat E, Igout A, et al: Glucose inhibits human placental GH secretion, in vitro. J Clin Endocrinol Metab 80:1743, 1995

Pellegrini I, Lebrun JJ, Ali S, et al: Expression of prolactin and its receptor in human lymphoid cells. Mol Endocrinol 6:1023, 1992

Peluso JJ: Non-genomic actions of progesterone in the normal and neoplastic mammalian ovary. Semin Reprod Med 25:198, 2007

Perrot-Applanat M, Groyer-Picard MT, Garcia E, et al: Immunocytochemical demonstration of estrogen and progesterone receptors in muscle cells of uterine arteries in rabbits and humans. Endocrinology 123:1511, 1988

Petraglia F, Florio P, Benedetto C, et al: Urocortin stimulates placental adrenocorticotropin and prostaglandin release and myometrial contractility in vitro. J Clin Endocrinol Metab 84:1420, 1999

Petraglia F, Gallinelli A, De Vita D, et al: Activin at parturition: Changes of maternal serum levels and evidence for binding sites in placenta and fetal membranes. Obstet Gynecol 84:278, 1994

Petraglia F, Garuti GC, Calza L, et al: Inhibin subunits in human placenta: Localization and messenger ribonucleic acid levels during pregnancy. Am J Obstet Gynecol 165:750, 1991

Petraglia F, Giardino L, Coukos G, et al: Corticotropin-releasing factor and parturition: Plasma and amniotic fluid levels and placental binding sites. Obstet Gynecol 75:784, 1990

Petraglia F, Sawchenko P, Lim AT, et al: Localization, secretion, and action of inhibin in human placenta. Science 237:187, 1987

Petraglia F, Vaughan J, Vale W: Inhibin and activin modulate the release of gonadotropin-releasing hormone, human chorionic gonadotropin, and progesterone from cultured human placental cells. Proc Natl Acad Sci U S A 86:5114, 1989

Petraglia F, Woodruff TK, Botticelli G, et al: Gonadotropin-releasing hormone, inhibin, and activin in human placenta: Evidence for a common cellular localization. J Clin Endocrinol Metab 74:1184, 1992

Pijnenborg R: Trophoblast invasion. Reprod Med Rev 3:53, 1994

Pijnenborg R, Bland JM, Robertson WB, et al: Uteroplacental arterial changes related to interstitial trophoblast migration in early human pregnancy. Placenta 4:397, 1983

Piper KP, McLarnon A, Arrazi J, et al: Functional HY-specific CD8+ T cells are found in a high proportion of women following pregnancy with a male fetus. Biol Reprod 76:96, 2007

Prakobphol A, Genbacev O, Gormley M, et al: A role for the L-selectin adhesion system in mediating cytotrophoblast emigration from the placenta. Dev Biol 298:107, 2006

Primakoff P, Myles DG: Penetration, adhesion, and fusion in mammalian sperm-egg interaction. Science 296:2183, 2002

Qin X, Chua PK, Ohira RH, et al: An autocrine/paracrine role of human decidual relaxin. II. Stromelysin-1 (MMP-3) and tissue inhibitor of matrix metalloproteinase-1 (TIMP-1). Biol Reprod 56:812, 1997a

Qin X, Garibay-Tupas J, Chua PK, et al: An autocrine/paracrine role of human decidual relaxin. I. Interstitial collagenase (matrix metalloproteinase-1) and tissue plasminogen activator. Biol Reprod 56:800, 1997b

Ragoobir J, Abayasekara DR, Bruckdorfer KR, et al: Stimulation of progesterone production in human granulosa-lutein cells by lipoproteins: Evidence for cholesterol-independent actions of high-density lipoproteins. J Endocrinol 173:103, 2002

Rainey WE, Carr BR, Wang ZN, et al: Gene profiling of human fetal and adult adrenals. J Endocrinol 171:209, 2001

Ramsey E, Davis R: A composite drawing of the placenta to show its structure and circulation. Anat Rec 145:366, 1963

Ramsey E, Harris J: Comparison of uteroplacental vasculature and circulation in the rhesus monkey and man. Contrib Embryol 38:59, 1966

Ramsey EM, Donner MW: Placental Vasculature and Circulation. Philadelphia, Saunders, 1980

Red-Horse K, Rivera J, Schanz A, et al: Cytotrophoblast induction of arterial apoptosis and lymphangiogenesis in an in vivo model of human placentation. J Clin Invest 116:2643, 2006

Richards JS, Genetics of ovulation. Semin Reprod Med 25(4):235, 2007

Richards JS: Ovulation: New factors that prepare the oocyte for fertilization. Mol Cell Endocrinol 234:75, 2005

Riddick DH, Luciano AA, Kusmik WF, et al: Evidence for a nonpituitary source of amniotic fluid prolactin. Fertil Steril 31:35, 1979

Riley S, Walton J, Herlick J, et al: The localization and distribution of corticotropin-releasing hormone in the human placenta and fetal membranes throughout gestation. J Clin Endocrinol Metab 72:1001, 1991

Robidoux J, Simoneau L, St Pierre S, et al: Characterization of neuropeptide Y-mediated corticotropin-releasing factor synthesis and release from human placental trophoblasts. Endocrinology 141:2795, 2000

Robinson BG, Emanuel RL, Frim DM, et al: Glucocorticoid stimulates expression of corticotropin-releasing hormone gene in human placenta. Proc Natl Acad Sci U S A 85:5244, 1988

Rock J, Bartlett M: Biopsy studies of human endometrium. JAMA 108:2022, 1937

Rogers PA, Donoghue JF, Walter LM, et al: Endometrial angiogenesis, vascular maturation, and lymphangiogenesis. Reprod Sci 16(2):147, 2009

Rowe T, King L, MacDonald PC, et al: Tissue inhibitor of metalloproteinase-1 and tissue inhibitor of metalloproteinase-2 expression in human amnion mesenchymal and epithelial cells. Am J Obstet Gynecol 176:915, 1997

Ryan KJ: Biological aromatization of steroids. J Biol Chem 234:268, 1959a

Ryan KJ: Metabolism of C-16-oxygenated steroids by human placenta: The formation of estriol. J Biol Chem 234:2006, 1959b

Salido EC, Yen PH, Barajas L, et al: Steroid sulfatase expression in human placenta: Immunocytochemistry and in situ hybridization study. J Clin Endocrinol Metab 70:1564, 1990

Santoni S, Zingoni A, Cerboni C, et al: Natural killer (NK) cells from killers to regulators: distinct features between peripheral blood and decidual NK cells. Am J Reprod Immunol 58:280, 2007

Saunders PTK: Does estrogen receptor β play a significant role in human reproduction? Trends Endocrinol Metab 16:222, 2005

Saxe A, Dean S, Gibson G, et al: Parathyroid hormone and parathyroid hormone-related peptide in venous umbilical cord blood of healthy neonates. J Perinat Med 25:288, 1997

Segaloff A, Sternberg W, Gaskill C: Effects of luteotrophic doses of chorionic gonadotropin in women. J Clin Endocrinol Metab 11:936, 1951

Shaul PW: Regulation of endothelial nitric oxide synthase: Location, location, location. Annu Rev Physiol 64:749, 2002

Short R: Steroids in the follicular fluid and the corpus luteum of the mare. A "two cell type" theory of ovarian steroid synthesis. J Endocrinol 24:59, 1962

Shozu M, Akasofu K, Harada T, et al: A new cause of female pseudohermaphroditism: Placental aromatase deficiency. J Clin Endocrinol Metab 72:560, 1991

Siiteri PK, MacDonald PC: Placental estrogen biosynthesis during human pregnancy. J Clin Endocrinol Metab 26:751, 1966

Siiteri PK, MacDonald PC: The utilization of circulating dehydroisoandrosterone sulfate for estrogen synthesis during human pregnancy. Steroids 2:713, 1963

Siler-Khodr TM: Chorionic peptides. In McNellis D, Challis JRG, MacDonald PC, et al (eds): The Onset of Labor: Cellular and Integrative Mechanisms. Ithaca, Perinatology Press, 1988, p 213

Siler-Khodr TM, Khodr GS: Content of luteinizing hormone-releasing factor in the human placenta. Am J Obstet Gynecol 130:216, 1978

Siler-Khodr TM, Khodr GS: Dose response analysis of gnRH stimulation of hCG release from human term placenta. Biol Reprod 25:353, 1981

Siler-Khodr TM, Khodr GS, Valenzuela G: Immunoreactive gonadotropin-releasing hormone level in maternal circulation throughout pregnancy. Am J Obstet Gynecol 150:376, 1984

Silver RM, Varner MW, Reddy U, et al: Work-up of stillbirth: A review of the evidence. Am J Obstet Gynecol 196:433, 2007

Simpson ER: Genetic mutations resulting in loss of aromatase activity in humans and mice. J Soc Gynecol Investig 7:S18, 2000

Simpson ER, Burkhart MF: Acyl CoA:cholesterol acyl transferase activity in human placental microsomes: Inhibition by progesterone. Arch Biochem Biophys 200:79, 1980

Simpson ER, Carr BR, Parker CR, Jr, et al: The role of serum lipoproteins in steroidogenesis by the human fetal adrenal cortex. J Clin Endocrinol Metab 49:146, 1979

Staun-Ram E, Shalev E: Human trophoblast function during the implantation process. Reprod Biol Endocrinol 3:56, 2005

Steele GL, Currie WD, Yuen BH, et al: Acute stimulation of human chorionic gonadotropin secretion by recombinant human activin-A in first trimester human trophoblast. Endocrinology 133:297, 1993

Stevens AM: Microchimeric cells in systemic lupus erythematosus: Targets or innocent bystanders? Lupus 15:820, 2006

Streeter GL: A human embryo (Mateer) of the presomite period. Contrib Embryol 9:389, 1920

Sugino N, Kashida S, Karube-Harada A, et al: Expression of vascular endothelial growth factor (VEGF) and its receptors in human endometrium throughout the menstrual cycle and in early pregnancy. Reproduction 123:379, 2002

Telgmann R, Gellersen B: Marker genes of decidualization: Activation of the decidual prolactin gene. Hum Reprod Update 4:472, 1998

Thellin O, Coumans B, Zorzi W, et al: Tolerance to the foeto-placental "graft": Ten ways to support a child for nine months. Curr Opin Immunol 12:731, 2000

Thomson A, Billewicz W, Hytten F: The weight of the placenta in relation to birthweight. Br J Obstet Gynaecol 76:865, 1969

Tomer Y, Huber GK, Davies TF: Human chorionic gonadotropin (hCG) interacts directly with recombinant human TSH receptors. J Clin Endocrinol Metab 74:1477, 1992

Trombly DJ, Woodruff TK, Mayo KE: Roles for transforming growth factor beta superfamily proteins in early folliculogenesis. Semin Reprod Med 27(1):14, 2009

Tsai SJ, Wu MH, Chen HM, et al: Fibroblast growth factor-9 is an endometrial stromal growth factor. Endocrinology 143:2715, 2002

Tsiaras A, Werth B: From Conception to Birth. New York, Doubleday, 2002, pp 75, 175, 189

Tsuruta E, Tada H, Tamaki H, et al: Pathogenic role of asialo human chorionic gonadotropin in gestational thyrotoxicosis. J Clin Endocrinol Metab 80:350, 1995

Tyson JE, Hwang P, Guyda H, et al: Studies of prolactin secretion in human pregnancy. Am J Obstet Gynecol 113:14, 1972

Vande Wiele RL, Bogumil J, Dyrenfurth I, et al: Mechanisms regulating the menstrual cycle in women. Recent Prog Horm Res 26:63, 1970

Vaskivuo TE, Ottander U, Oduwole O, et al: Role of apoptosis, apoptosis-related factors and 17 beta-hydroxysteroid dehydrogenases in human corpus luteum regression. Mol Cell Endocrinol 194:191, 2002

Vince GS, Johnson PM: Immunobiology of human uteroplacental macrophages—friend and foe? Placenta 17:191, 1996

Wadhwa PD, Porto M, Garite TJ, et al: Maternal corticotropin-releasing hormone levels in the early third trimester predict length of gestation in human pregnancy. Am J Obstet Gynecol 179:1079, 1998

Walker WH, Fitzpatrick SL, Barrera-Saldana HA, et al: The human placental lactogen genes: Structure, function, evolution and transcriptional regulation. Endocr Rev 12:316, 1991

Warren W, Silverman A: Cellular localization of corticotrophin releasing hormone in the human placenta, fetal membranes and decidua. Placenta 16:147, 1995

Weetman AP: The immunology of pregnancy. Thyroid 9:643, 1999

Wehmann RE, Nisula BC: Renal clearance rates of the subunits of human chorionic gonadotropin in man. J Clin Endocrinol Metab 50:674, 1980

Wentz AC, Jones GS: Transient luteolytic effect of prostaglandin F2alpha in the human. Obstet Gynecol 42:172, 1973

Werbin H, Plotz EJ, LeRoy GV, et al: Cholesterol: A precursor of estrone in vivo. J Am Chem Soc 79:1012, 1957

Whittle WL, Gibb W, Challis JR: The characterization of human amnion epithelial and mesenchymal cells: The cellular expression, activity and glucocorticoid regulation of prostaglandin output. Placenta 21:394, 2000

Wislocki GB, Dempsey EW: Electron microscopy of the human placenta. Anat Rec 123:133, 1955

Wolfahrt S, Kleine B, Rossmanith WG: Detection of gonadotrophin releasing hormone and its receptor mRNA in human placental trophoblasts using in-situ reverse transcription-polymerase chain reaction. Mol Hum Reprod 4:999, 1998

Yan C, Wang P, DeMayo J, et al: Synergistic roles of bone morphogenetic Protein 15 and growth differentiation Factor 9 in ovarian function. Mol Endocrinol 15:854, 2001

Yanagisawa M, Kurihara H, Kimura S, et al: A novel potent vasoconstrictor peptide produced by vascular endothelial cells. Nature 332:411, 1988

Yoshimura M, Pekary AE, Pang XP, et al: Thyrotropic activity of basic isoelectric forms of human chorionic gonadotropin extracted from hydatidiform mole tissues. J Clin Endocrinol Metab 78:862, 1994

CHAPTER 4

Fetal Growth and Development

Contemporary obstetrical research focuses on the physiology and pathophysiology of the fetus, its development, and its environment. An important result is that the status of the fetus has been elevated to that of a patient who, in large measure, can be given the same meticulous care that obstetricians provide for pregnant women. In the course of these studies, it has become apparent that the conceptus is a dynamic force in the pregnancy unit. Normal fetal development is considered in this chapter. Anomalies, injuries, and diseases that affect the fetus and newborn are addressed in Chapter 29.

DETERMINATION OF GESTATIONAL AGE

Several terms are used to define the duration of pregnancy, and thus fetal age, but these are somewhat confusing. They are shown schematically in Figure 4-1. *Gestational age* or *menstrual age* is the time elapsed since the first day of the last menstrual period, a time that actually precedes conception. This starting time, which is usually about 2 weeks before ovulation and fertilization and nearly 3 weeks before implantation of the blastocyst, has traditionally been used because most women know their last period. Embryologists describe embryofetal development in *ovulation age,* or the time in days or weeks from ovula-

tion. Another term is *postconceptional age,* nearly identical to ovulation age.

Clinicians customarily calculate gestational age as menstrual age. About 280 days, or 40 weeks, elapse on average between the first day of the last menstrual period and the birth of the fetus. This corresponds to 9 and 1/3 calendar months. A quick estimate of the due date of a pregnancy based on menstrual data can be made as follows: add 7 days to the first day of the last period and subtract 3 months. For example, if the first day of the last menses was July 5, the due date is 07-05 minus 3 (months) plus 7 (days) = 04-12, or April 12 of the following year. This calculation has been termed Naegele's rule. Many women undergo first- or early second-trimester sonographic examination to confirm gestational age. In these cases, the sonographic estimate is usually a few days later than that determined by the last period. To rectify this inconsistency—and to reduce the number of pregnancies diagnosed as postterm—some have suggested assuming that the average pregnancy is actually 283 days long and that 10 days be added to the last menses instead of 7 (Olsen and Clausen, 1998).

The period of gestation can also be divided into three units of three calendar months (13 weeks) each. These three *trimesters* have become important obstetrical milestones.

MORPHOLOGICAL GROWTH

Ovum, Zygote, and Blastocyst

During the first 2 weeks after ovulation, development phases include: (1) fertilization, (2) blastocyst formation, and (3) blastocyst implantation. Primitive chorionic villi are formed soon after implantation. With the development of chorionic villi, it is conventional to refer to the products of conception as an *embryo.* The early stages of preplacental development and formation of the placenta are described in Chapter 3 (p. 47).

Embryonic Period

The embryonic period commences at the beginning of the third week after ovulation and fertilization, which coincides in time with the expected day that the next menstruation would have started. The embryonic period lasts 8 weeks and is when organogenesis takes place (see Fig. 4-1). The embryonic disc is well defined, and most pregnancy tests that measure human chorionic gonadotropin (hCG) become positive by this time (see Chap. 8, p. 192). As shown in Figure 4-2, the body stalk is now differentiated, and the chorionic sac is approximately 1 cm in diameter. There is a true intervillous space that contains maternal blood and villous cores in which angioblastic chorionic mesoderm can be distinguished.

The schematic timeline is shown in Figure 4-3. During the third week, fetal blood vessels in the chorionic villi appear (Fig. 4-4). In the fourth week a cardiovascular system has formed, and thereby, a true circulation is established both within the embryo and between the embryo and the chorionic villi. By the end of the fourth week, the chorionic sac is 2 to 3 cm in diameter, and the embryo is 4 to 5 mm in length (Figs. 4-5, 4-6, and 4-7). Partitioning of the primitive heart begins in the middle of the fourth week. Arm and leg buds are present, and the amnion is beginning to unsheathe the body stalk, which thereafter becomes the umbilical cord.

At the end of the sixth week, the embryo is 22 to 24 mm in length, and the head is large compared with the trunk. The heart is completely formed. Fingers and toes are present, and the arms bend at the elbows. The upper lip is complete, and the external ears form definitive elevations on either side of the head.

Fetal Period

The end of the embryonic period and the beginning of the fetal period is arbitrarily designated by most embryologists to begin

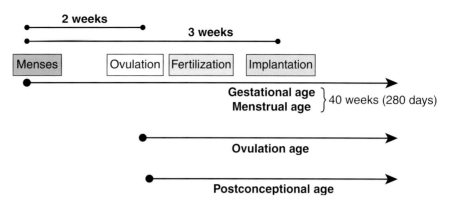

FIGURE 4-1 Terminology used to describe the duration of pregnancy.

8 weeks after fertilization—or 10 weeks after onset of last menses. At this time, the embryofetus is nearly 4 cm long (Fig. 4-8).

Referring back to Figure 4-3, development during the fetal period consists of growth and maturation of structures that were formed during the embryonic period. Because of the variability in the length of the legs and the difficulty of maintaining them in extension, crown-to-rump measurements, which correspond to the sitting height, are more accurate than those corresponding to the standing height (Table 4-1).

12 Gestational Weeks

The uterus usually is just palpable above the symphysis pubis, and the fetal crown-rump length is 6 to 7 cm. Centers of ossification have appeared in most of the fetal bones, and the fingers and toes have become differentiated. Skin and nails have developed and scattered rudiments of hair appear. The external genitalia are beginning to show definitive signs of male or female gender. The fetus begins to make spontaneous movements.

16 Gestational Weeks

The fetal crown-rump length is 12 cm, and the weight is 110 g. Gender can be determined by experienced observers by inspection of the external genitalia by 14 weeks.

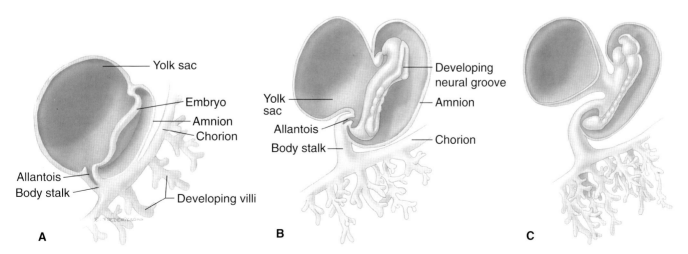

FIGURE 4-2 Early human embryos. Ovulation ages: **A.** 19 days (presomite). **B.** 21 days (7 somites). **C.** 22 days (17 somites). (After drawings and models in the Carnegie Institute.)

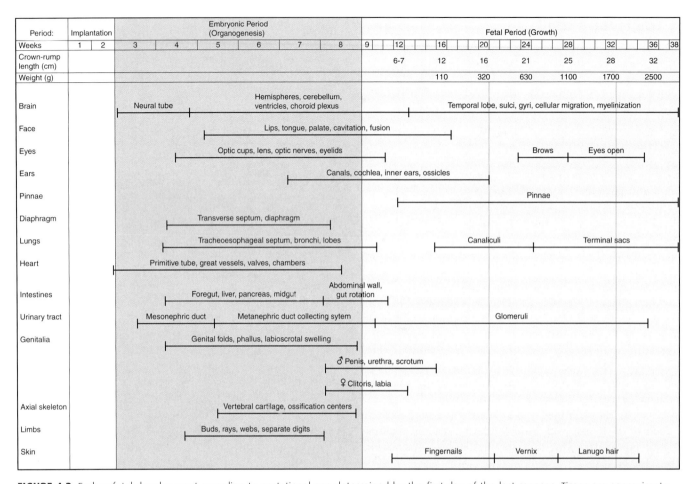

Period:	Implantation		Embryonic Period (Organogenesis)						Fetal Period (Growth)								
Weeks	1 2	3 4	5	6	7	8	9	12	16	20	24	28	32	36	38
Crown-rump length (cm)								6-7	12	16	21	25	28	32	
Weight (g)								110	320	630	1100	1700	2500		

Brain — Neural tube — Hemispheres, cerebellum, ventricles, choroid plexus — Temporal lobe, sulci, gyri, cellular migration, myelinization

Face — Lips, tongue, palate, cavitation, fusion

Eyes — Optic cups, lens, optic nerves, eyelids — Brows — Eyes open

Ears — Canals, cochlea, inner ears, ossicles

Pinnae — Pinnae

Diaphragm — Transverse septum, diaphragm

Lungs — Tracheoesophageal septum, bronchi, lobes — Canaliculi — Terminal sacs

Heart — Primitive tube, great vessels, valves, chambers

Intestines — Foregut, liver, pancreas, midgut — Abdominal wall, gut rotation

Urinary tract — Mesonephric duct — Metanephric duct collecting sytem — Glomeruli

Genitalia — Genital folds, phallus, labioscrotal swelling — ♂ Penis, urethra, scrotum — ♀ Clitoris, labia

Axial skeleton — Vertebral cartilage, ossification centers

Limbs — Buds, rays, webs, separate digits

Skin — Fingernails — Vernix — Lanugo hair

FIGURE 4-3 Embryofetal development according to gestational age determined by the first day of the last menses. Times are approximate.

20 Gestational Weeks

This is the midpoint of pregnancy as estimated from the beginning of the last menses. The fetus now weighs somewhat more than 300 g, and weight begins to increase in a linear manner. From this point onward, the fetus moves about every minute and is active 10 to 30 percent of the time (DiPietro, 2005). The fetal skin has become less transparent, a downy lanugo covers its entire body, and some scalp hair has developed.

24 Gestational Weeks

The fetus now weighs about 630 g. The skin is characteristically wrinkled, and fat deposition begins. The head is still comparatively large, and eyebrows and eyelashes are usually recognizable. The canalicular period of lung development, during which the bronchi and bronchioles enlarge and alveolar ducts develop, is nearly completed. A fetus born at this time will attempt to breathe, but many will die because the terminal sacs, required for gas exchange, have not yet formed.

28 Gestational Weeks

The crown-rump length is approximately 25 cm, and the fetus weighs about 1100 g. The thin skin is red and covered with *vernix caseosa*. The pupillary membrane has just disappeared from the eyes. The otherwise normal neonate born at this age has a 90-percent chance of survival without physical or neurological impairment.

32 Gestational Weeks

The fetus has attained a crown-rump length of about 28 cm and a weight of approximately 1800 g. The skin surface is still red and wrinkled.

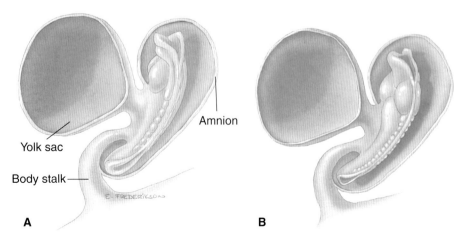

FIGURE 4-4 Early human embryos. Ovulation ages: **A.** 22 days. **B.** 23 days. (After drawings and models in the Carnegie Institute.)

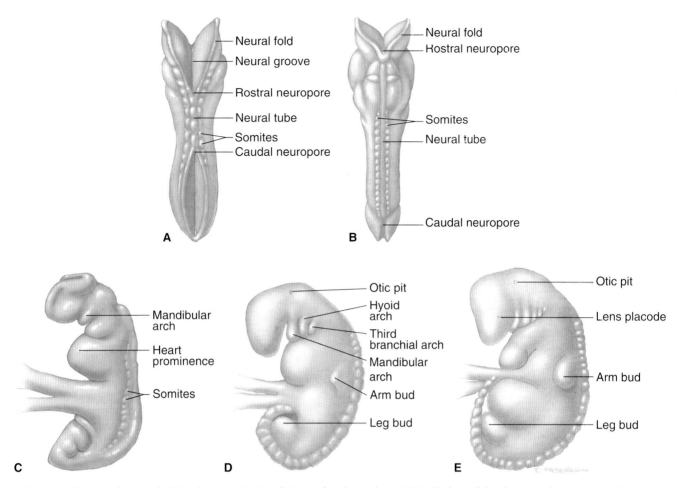

FIGURE 4-5 Three- to four-week-old embryos. **A, B.** Dorsal views of embryos during 22 to 23 days of development showing 8 and 12 somites, respectively. **C–E.** Lateral views of embryos during 24 to 28 days, showing 16, 27, and 33 somites, respectively. (Redrawn from Moore, 1988.)

36 Gestational Weeks

The average crown-rump length of the fetus is about 32 cm, and the weight is approximately 2500 g. Because of the deposition of subcutaneous fat, the body has become more rotund, and the previous wrinkled appearance of the face has been lost.

40 Gestational Weeks

This is considered term from the onset of the last menstrual period. The fetus is now fully developed. The average crown-rump length is about 36 cm, and the weight is approximately 3400 g.

Fetal Head

From an obstetrical viewpoint, the fetal head size is important because an essential feature of labor is the adaptation between the head and the maternal bony pelvis. Only a comparatively small part of the head at term is represented by the face. The rest of the head is composed of the firm skull, which is made up of two frontal, two parietal, and two temporal bones, along with the upper portion of the occipital bone and the wings of the sphenoid. These bones are separated by membranous spaces that are termed *sutures* (Fig. 4-9).

The most important sutures are the frontal, between the two frontal bones; the sagittal, between the two parietal bones; the

two coronal, between the frontal and parietal bones; and the two lambdoid, between the posterior margins of the parietal bones and upper margin of the occipital bone. Where several sutures meet, an irregular space forms, which is enclosed by a membrane and designated as a *fontanel* (see Fig. 4-9). The greater, or anterior, fontanel is a lozenge-shaped space that is situated at the junction of the sagittal and the coronal sutures. The lesser, or posterior, fontanel is represented by a small triangular area at the intersection of the sagittal and lambdoid sutures. The localization of these fontanels gives important information concerning the presentation and position of the fetus during labor.

It is customary to measure certain critical diameters and circumferences of the newborn head (see Fig. 4-9). The diameters include:

1. The *occipitofrontal* (11.5 cm), which follows a line extending from a point just above the root of the nose to the most prominent portion of the occipital bone.
2. The *biparietal* (9.5 cm), the greatest transverse diameter of the head, which extends from one parietal boss to the other.
3. The *bitemporal* (8.0 cm), which is the greatest distance between the two temporal sutures.
4. The *occipitomental* (12.5 cm), which extends from the chin to the most prominent portion of the occiput.

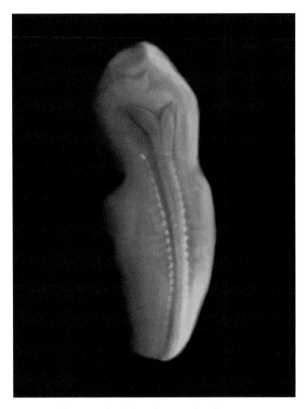

FIGURE 4-6 Photograph of dorsal view of embryo at 24 to 26 days and corresponding to Figure 4–4B. (Visualization is provided by www.theVisualMD.com.)

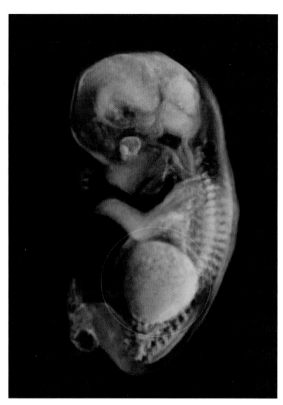

FIGURE 4-8 Lateral view of embryofetus at 56 days, which marks the end of the embryonic period and the beginning of the fetal period. The liver is within the dotted-line circle. (Visualization is provided by www.theVisualMD.com.)

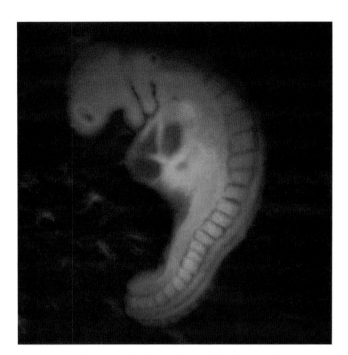

FIGURE 4-7 Photograph of lateral view of embryo at about 28 days and corresponding to Figure 4–4E. (Visualization is provided by www.theVisualMD.com.)

5. The *suboccipitobregmatic* (9.5 cm), which follows a line drawn from the middle of the large fontanel to the undersurface of the occipital bone just where it joins the neck.

The greatest circumference of the head, which corresponds to the plane of the occipitofrontal diameter, averages 34.5 cm, a size too large to fit through the pelvis without flexion. The smallest circumference, corresponding to the plane of the suboccipitobregmatic diameter, is 32 cm. The bones of the cranium are normally connected only by a thin layer of fibrous tissue. This allows considerable shifting or sliding of each bone to accommodate the size and shape of the maternal pelvis. This process is termed *molding.* The head position and degree of skull ossification result in a spectrum of cranial plasticity from minimal to great. In some cases, this undoubtedly contributes to fetopelvic disproportion, a leading indication for cesarean delivery (see Chap. 20, p. 472).

Fetal Brain

There is a steady gestational age-related change in the appearance of the fetal brain so that it is possible to identify fetal age from its external appearance (Dolman, 1977). Neuronal proliferation and migration proceed along with gyral growth and maturation (Fig. 4-10). Manganaro and colleagues (2007) have provided sequential maturation studies of the developing fetal brain imaged with magnetic resonance imaging. Myelination of the ventral roots of the cerebrospinal nerves and brainstem begins at

TABLE 4-1. Criteria for Estimating Age During the Fetal Period

Age (weeks)		Crown-Rump Length (mm)[a]	Foot Length (mm)[a]	Fetal Weight (g)[b]	Main External Characteristics
Menstrual	Fertilization				
11	9	50	7	8	Eyes closing or closed. Head more rounded. External genitalia still not distinguishable as male or female. Intestines are in the umbilical cord.
12	10	61	9	14	Intestines in abdomen. Early fingernail development.
14	12	87	14	45	Sex distinguishable externally. Well-defined neck.
16	14	120	20	110	Head erect. Lower limbs well developed.
18	16	140	27	200	Ears stand out from head.
20	18	160	33	320	Vernix caseosa present. Early toenail development.
22	20	190	39	460	Head and body (lanugo) hair visible.
24	22	210	45	630	Skin wrinkled and red.
26	24	230	50	820	Fingernails present. Lean body.
28	26	250	55	1000	Eyes partially open. Eyelashes present.
30	28	270	59	1300	Eyes open. Good head of hair. Skin slightly wrinkled.
32	30	280	63	1700	Toenails present. Body filling out. Testes descending.
34	32	300	68	2100	Fingernails reach fingertips. Skin pink and smooth.
38	36	340	79	2900	Body usually plump. Lanugo hairs almost absent. Toenails reach toe tips.
40	38	360	83	3400	Prominent chest; breasts protrude. Testes in scrotum or palpable in inguinal canals. Fingernails extend beyond fingertips.

[a]These measurements are average and so may not apply to specific cases; dimensional variations increase with age.
[b]These weights refer to fetuses that have been fixed for about 2 weeks in 10-percent formalin.
Fresh specimens usually weigh approximately 5 percent less.
Reprinted from *The Developing Human: Clinically Oriented Embryology,* 2nd ed., by KL Moore, Copyright 1977, with permission from Elsevier.

approximately 6 months, but the major portion of myelination occurs after birth. The lack of myelin and the incomplete ossification of the fetal skull permit the structure of the brain to be seen with sonography throughout gestation.

THE PLACENTA AND FETAL GROWTH

The placenta is the organ of transfer between mother and fetus. At the maternal-fetal interface, there is transfer of oxygen and nutrients from the mother to the fetus and carbon dioxide and metabolic wastes from fetus to mother. There are no direct communications between fetal blood, which is contained in the fetal capillaries of the chorionic villi, and maternal blood, which remains in the intervillous space. Bidirectional transfer depends on the processes that permit or aid the transport through the syncytiotrophoblast of the intact chorionic villi.

That said, there are occasional breaks in the chorionic villi, which permit escape of various numbers of fetal cells into the maternal circulation. This leakage is the mechanism by which some D-negative women become sensitized by the erythrocytes of their D-positive fetus (see Chap. 29, p. 618). It can also lead to *chimerism* from entrance of allogeneic fetal cells, including trophoblasts, into maternal blood. These are estimated to range from 1 to 6 cells/mL around midpregnancy, and some are "immortal" (Lissauer and colleagues, 2007). A clinical corollary is that some maternal autoimmune diseases may be provoked by such chimerism (see Chap. 54, p. 1146).

The Intervillous Space

Maternal blood in the extravascular compartment, that is, the intervillous space, is the primary biologic unit of maternal–fetal transfer. Blood from the maternal spiral arteries directly bathes the trophoblasts. Substances transferred from mother to fetus first enter the intervillous space and are then transported to the syncytiotrophoblast. Substances transported from the fetus to the mother are transferred from the syncytium into the same space. Thus, the chorionic villi and the intervillous space function together as the fetal lung, gastrointestinal tract, and kidney.

Circulation within the intervillous space is described in Chapter 3 (p. 55). Intervillous and uteroplacental blood flow increases throughout the first trimester of normal pregnancies (Mercé and associates, 2009). At term, the residual volume of

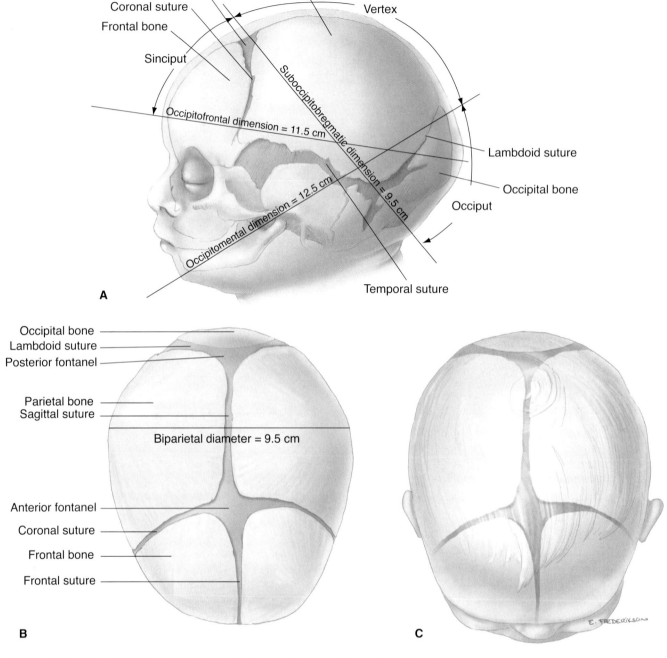

FIGURE 4-9 Fetal head **(A-C)** at term showing fontanels, sutures, and the various dimensions.

the intervillous space measures about 140 mL. Before delivery, however, the volume of this space may be twice this value (Aherne and Dunnill, 1966). Uteroplacental blood flow near term has been estimated to be 700 to 900 mL/min, with most of the blood apparently going to the intervillous space.

Active labor contractions reduce blood flow into the intervillous space, the degree of which depends on the intensity of the contraction. Blood pressure within the intervillous space is significantly less than uterine arterial pressure, but somewhat greater than venous pressure. The latter, in turn, varies depending on several factors, including maternal position. When supine, for exam-

ple, pressure in the lower part of the inferior vena cava is elevated, and consequently, pressure in the uterine and ovarian veins, and in turn in the intervillous space, is increased.

Placental Transfer

Chorionic Villus

Substances that pass from maternal blood to fetal blood must first traverse the syncytiotrophoblast, then stroma of the intravillous space, and finally the fetal capillary wall. Although this histological barrier separates the blood in the maternal and fetal

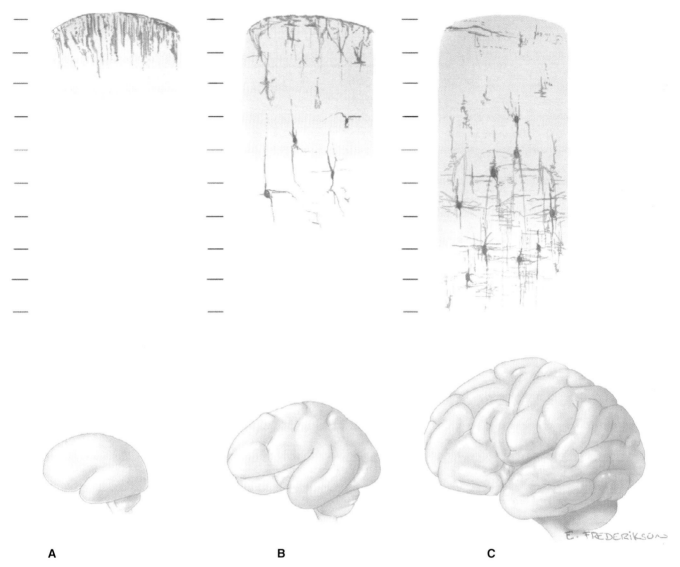

FIGURE 4-10 Neuronal proliferation and migration are complete at 20 to 24 weeks. During the second half of gestation, organizational events proceed with gyral formation and proliferation, differentiation, and migration of cellular elements. Approximate gestational ages are listed. **A.** 20 weeks. **B.** 35 Weeks. **C.** 40 Weeks.

circulations, it does not function like a simple physical barrier. In fact, throughout pregnancy, syncytiotrophoblast actively or passively permits, facilitates, and adjusts the amount and rate of transfer of a wide range of substances to the fetus.

Regulation of Placental Transfer

The syncytiotrophoblast is the fetal tissue interface. Its maternal-facing surface is characterized by a complex microvillus structure. The fetal-facing basal cell membrane of the trophoblast is the site of transfer to the intravillous space through which the fetal capillaries traverse. These capillaries are an additional site for transport from the intravillous space into fetal blood, or vice versa.

In determining the effectiveness of the human placenta as an organ of transfer, at least 10 variables are important.

1. The concentration of the substance in maternal plasma, and the extent to which it is bound to another compound, such as a carrier protein.
2. The rate of maternal blood flow through the intervillous space.
3. The area available for exchange across the villous trophoblast epithelium.
4. If the substance is transferred by simple diffusion, the physical properties of the trophoblastic tissue.
5. For any substance actively transported, the capacity of the biochemical machinery of the placenta for effecting active transfer, for example, specific receptors on the plasma membrane of the trophoblast.
6. The amount of the substance metabolized by the placenta during transfer.
7. The area for exchange across the fetal intervillous capillaries.
8. The concentration of the substance in the fetal blood.
9. Specific binding or carrier proteins in the fetal or maternal circulation.
10. The rate of fetal blood flow through the villous capillaries.

Mechanisms of Transfer

Most substances with a molecular mass less than 500 Da pass readily through placental tissue by simple diffusion. Also, some low-molecular-weight compounds undergo transfer facilitated by syncytiotrophoblast. These are usually those that are in low concentration in maternal plasma but are essential for normal fetal development. Simple diffusion appears to be the mechanism involved in the transfer of oxygen, carbon dioxide, water, and most electrolytes. Anesthetic gases also pass through the placenta rapidly by simple diffusion.

Insulin, steroid hormones, and thyroid hormones cross the placenta, but at very slow rates. The hormones synthesized in situ in the trophoblasts enter both the maternal and fetal circulations, but not equally (see Chap. 3, p. 62). Examples are concentrations of chorionic gonadotropin and placental lactogen, which are much lower in fetal plasma than in maternal plasma. Substances of high molecular weight usually do not traverse the placenta, but there are important exceptions, such as immunoglobulin G—molecular weight 160,000 Da—which is transferred by way of a specific trophoblast receptor–mediated mechanism.

Transfer of Oxygen and Carbon Dioxide

It has long been recognized that the placenta serves as the fetal lung. As early as 1674, Mayow suggested that the placenta served as the fetal lung (Morriss and associates, 1994). In 1796, Erasmus Darwin, only 22 years after the discovery of oxygen, observed that the color of blood passing through lungs and gills became bright red. He deduced, from the structure as well as the position of the placenta, that it likely was the source of fetal oxygen.

Placental oxygen transfer is blood-flow limited. Using estimated uteroplacental blood flow, Longo (1991) calculated oxygen delivery to be about 8 mL O_2/min/kg of fetal weight. And because fetal blood oxygen stores are sufficient for only 1 to 2 minutes, this supply must be continuous. Normal values for oxygen, carbon dioxide, and pH in fetal blood are presented in Figure 4-11. Because of the continuous passage of oxygen from maternal blood in the intervillous space to the fetus, its oxygen saturation resembles that in the maternal capillaries. The average oxygen saturation of intervillous blood is estimated to be 65 to 75 percent, with a partial pressure (Po_2) of 30 to 35 mm Hg. The oxygen saturation of umbilical vein blood is similar, but with a somewhat lower oxygen partial pressure.

In general, transfer of fetal carbon dioxide is accomplished by diffusion. The placenta is highly permeable to carbon dioxide, which traverses the chorionic villus more rapidly than oxygen. Near term, the partial pressure of carbon dioxide (Pco_2) in the umbilical arteries averages about 50 mm Hg, or approximately 5 mm Hg more than in the maternal intervillous blood. Fetal blood has less affinity for carbon dioxide than does maternal blood, thereby favoring the carbon dioxide transfer from fetus to mother. Also, mild maternal hyperventilation results in a fall in Pco_2 levels, favoring a transfer of carbon dioxide from the fetal compartment to maternal blood (see Chap. 5, p. 122).

Selective Transfer and Facilitated Diffusion

Although simple diffusion is an important method of placental transfer, the trophoblast and chorionic villus unit demonstrate enormous selectivity in transfer. This results in different con-

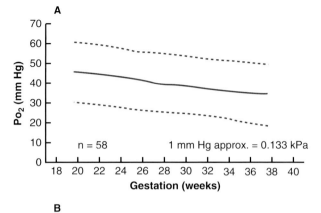

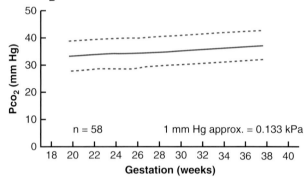

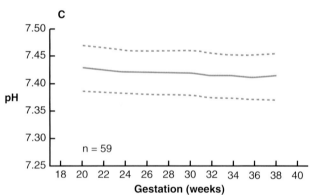

FIGURE 4-11 Umbilical venous oxygen pressure (Po_2) **(A)**, carbon dioxide pressure (Pco_2) **(B)**, and pH **(C)** from cordocentesis performed in fetuses being evaluated for possible intrauterine infections or hemolysis, but who were found to be healthy at birth and appropriately grown. (Reprinted from *Normal Values in Pregnancy*, by MM Ramsay, DK James, PJ Steer, and B Gonik, Fig. 75, p. 106, Copyright 1996, with permission from Elsevier Ltd. and MM Ramsay.)

centrations of a variety of metabolites on the two sides of the villus. The concentrations of a number of substances that are not synthesized by the fetus are several times higher in fetal than in maternal blood. Ascorbic acid is a good example. This relatively low-molecular-weight substance resembles pentose and hexose sugars and might be expected to traverse the placenta by simple diffusion. The concentration of ascorbic acid, however, is two to four times higher in fetal plasma than in maternal plasma (Morriss and associates, 1994). Another example is the unidirectional transfer of iron across the placenta. Typically, maternal plasma iron concentration is much lower than that in her fetus. Even with severe maternal iron-deficiency anemia, the fetal hemoglobin mass is normal.

FETAL NUTRITION

Because of the small amount of yolk in the human ovum, growth of the embryofetus is dependent on maternal nutrients during the first 2 months. During the first few days after implantation, the nutrition of the blastocyst comes from the interstitial fluid of the endometrium and the surrounding maternal tissue.

Maternal adaptations to store and transfer nutrients to the fetus are discussed in Chapter 5 and summarized here. The maternal diet is transferred into storage forms to meet her demands for energy, tissue repair, and new growth, including maternal needs for pregnancy. Three major maternal storage depots—the liver, muscle, and adipose tissue—and the storage hormone insulin are intimately involved in the metabolism of the nutrients absorbed from the maternal gut.

Insulin secretion is sustained by increased serum levels of glucose and amino acids. The net effect is storage of glucose as glycogen primarily in liver and muscle, retention of some amino acids as protein, and storage of the excess as fat. Storage of maternal fat peaks in the second trimester, and then declines as fetal demands increase in late pregnancy (Pipe and colleagues, 1979). Interestingly, the placenta appears to act as a nutrient sensor, altering transport based on the maternal supply and environmental stimuli (Fowden and colleagues, 2006; Jansson and Powell, 2006).

During times of fasting, glucose is released from glycogen, but maternal glycogen stores cannot provide an adequate amount of glucose to meet requirements for maternal energy and fetal growth. Augmentation is provided by cleavage of triacylglycerols, stored in adipose tissue, which result in free fatty acids. Lipolysis is activated, directly or indirectly, by hormones that include glucagon, norepinephrine, placental lactogen, glucocorticosteroids, and thyroxine.

Glucose and Fetal Growth

Although dependent on the mother for nutrition, the fetus also actively participates in providing for its own nutrition. At midpregnancy, fetal glucose concentration is independent of and may exceed maternal levels (Bozzetti and colleagues, 1988). Glucose is the major nutrient for fetal growth and energy. It is logical that mechanisms exist during pregnancy to minimize maternal glucose use so that the limited maternal supply is available to the fetus. It is believed that placental lactogen (hPL), a hormone normally present in abundance in the mother but not the fetus, blocks the peripheral uptake and use of glucose, while promoting the mobilization and use of free fatty acids by maternal tissues (see Chap. 3, p. 65).

Glucose Transport

The transfer of D-glucose across cell membranes is accomplished by a carrier-mediated, stereospecific, nonconcentrating process of *facilitated diffusion*. At least 14 separate glucose transport proteins (GLUTs) have been discovered (Leonce and colleagues, 2006). They belong to the 12-transmembrane segment transporter superfamily and are characterized further by tissue-specific distribution. GLUT-1 and GLUT-3 primarily facilitate glucose uptake by the placenta and are located in the plasma membrane of the microvilli of the syncytiotrophoblast (Korgun

and colleagues, 2005). GLUT-1 expression increases as pregnancy advances and is induced by almost all growth factors (Sakata and colleagues, 1995).

Glucose, Insulin, and Fetal Macrosomia

The precise biomolecular events in the pathophysiology of fetal macrosomia are not defined. Nonetheless, it seems clear that fetal hyperinsulinemia is one driving force (Schwartz and colleagues, 1994). As discussed in Chapter 38 (p. 842), insulin-like growth factor, as well as fibroblast growth factor, also is involved (Giudice and associates, 1995; Hill and colleagues, 1995). Therefore, a hyperinsulinemic state with increased levels of selected growth factors, together with increased expression of GLUT proteins in syncytiotrophoblast, may promote excessive fetal growth.

Leptin

Leptin was originally identified as a product of adipocytes and a regulator of energy homeostasis. However, this polypeptide also contributes to angiogenesis, hematopoiesis, osteogenesis, pulmonary maturation, and neuroendocrine, immune, and reproductive functions (Henson and Castracane, 2006; Maymo and colleagues, 2009).

During pregnancy, leptin is produced by the mother, fetus, and placenta. It is expressed in syncytiotrophoblasts and fetal vascular endothelial cells. Of placental production, 5 percent enters fetal circulation, whereas 95 percent is transferred to the mother (Hauguel de Mouzon and associates, 2006) As a result, the placenta greatly contributes to maternal leptin levels.

Fetal levels begin rising approximately at 34 weeks and are correlated with fetal weight. Abnormal levels have been associated with growth disorders and preeclampsia. Postpartum, leptin levels decline in both the newborn and mother (Grisaru-Granovsky and co-workers, 2008).

Lactate

Lactate is transported across the placenta by facilitated diffusion. By way of co-transport with hydrogen ions, lactate is probably transported as lactic acid.

Free Fatty Acids and Triglycerides

The human newborn has a large proportion of fat, which averages 15 percent of body weight (Kimura, 1991). This indicates that late in pregnancy, a substantial part of the substrate transferred to the human fetus is stored as fat. Neutral fat in the form of triacylglycerols does not cross the placenta, but glycerol does, and fatty acids are synthesized in the placenta. Lipoprotein lipase is present on the maternal but not on the fetal side of the placenta. This arrangement favors hydrolysis of triacylglycerols in the maternal intervillous space while preserving these neutral lipids in fetal blood. Fatty acids transferred to the fetus can be converted to triacylglycerols in the fetal liver.

The placental uptake and use of low-density lipoprotein (LDL) is an alternative mechanism for fetal assimilation of essential fatty acids and amino acids (see Chap. 3, p. 67). The LDL particles from maternal plasma bind to specific LDL receptors in the coated-pit regions of the microvilli on the maternal-facing side of the syncytiotrophoblast. The large—about 250,000

Da—LDL particle is taken up by a process of receptor-mediated endocytosis. The apoprotein and cholesterol esters of LDL are hydrolyzed by lysosomal enzymes in the syncytium to give: (1) cholesterol for progesterone synthesis; (2) free amino acids, including essential amino acids; and (3) essential fatty acids, primarily linoleic acid. Indeed, the concentration of arachidonic acid, which is synthesized from linoleic acid in fetal plasma, is greater than that in maternal plasma. Linoleic acid or arachidonic acid or both must be assimilated from maternal dietary intake.

Amino Acids

The placenta concentrates a large number of amino acids (Lemons, 1979). Neutral amino acids from maternal plasma are taken up by trophoblasts by at least three specific processes. Presumably, amino acids are concentrated in the syncytiotrophoblasts and thence transferred to the fetal side by diffusion. Based on data from cordocentesis blood samples, the concentration of amino acids in umbilical cord plasma is greater than in maternal venous or arterial plasma (Morriss and associates, 1994). Activity of the transport systems is influenced by gestational age and environmental factors including heat stress, hypoxia, under- and overnutrition, as well as hormones such as glucocorticoids, growth hormone, and leptin (Fowden and colleagues, 2006). Recent in vivo studies suggest an upregulation of transport for certain amino acids and an increased fetal delivery in women with gestational diabetes associated with fetal overgrowth (Jansson and colleagues, 2006).

Proteins

Generally, there is very limited placental transfer of larger proteins. There are important exceptions, for example, immunoglobulin G (IgG) crosses the placenta in large amounts via endocytosis via trophoblast Fc receptors. IgG is present in approximately the same concentrations in cord and maternal sera, but IgA and IgM of maternal origin are effectively excluded from the fetus (Gitlin and colleagues, 1972).

Ions and Trace Metals

Iodide transport is clearly attributable to a carrier-mediated, energy-requiring active process. And indeed, the placenta concentrates iodide. The concentrations of zinc in the fetal plasma also are greater than those in maternal plasma. Conversely, copper levels in fetal plasma are less than those in maternal plasma. This fact is of particular interest because important copper-requiring enzymes are necessary for fetal development.

Placental Sequestration of Heavy Metals

The heavy metal–binding protein, metallothionein-1, is expressed in human syncytiotrophoblast. This protein binds and sequesters a host of heavy metals, including zinc, copper, lead, and cadmium.

The most common source of cadmium in the environment is cigarette smoke. Cadmium levels in maternal blood and placenta are increased with maternal smoking, but there is no increase in cadmium transfer into the fetus. Presumably, the low levels of cadmium in the fetus are attributable to the sequestration of cadmium by metallothionein(s) in trophoblast. This

comes about because cadmium acts to increase the transcription of the metallothioncin gene(s). Thus, cadmium-induced increases in trophoblast metallothionein levels result in placental cadmium accumulation by sequestration. In the rat, data suggest that cadmium reduces the number of trophoblast cells, leading to poor placental growth (Lee and co-workers, 2009).

Metallothionein also binds and sequesters copper (Cu^{2+}) in placental tissue, thus accounting for the low levels of Cu^{2+} in cord blood (Iyengar and Rapp, 2001). A number of enzymes require Cu^{2+}, and its deficiency results in inadequate collagen cross-linking and in turn, diminished tensile strength of tissues. This may be important because the concentration of cadmium in amnionic fluid is similar to that in maternal blood. The incidence of preterm membrane rupture is increased in women who smoke. It is possible that cadmium provokes metallothionein synthesis in amnion, causing sequestration of Cu^{2+} and a pseudocopper deficiency.

Calcium and Phosphorus

These minerals also are actively transported from mother to fetus. A calcium-binding protein is present in placenta. Parathyroid hormone-related protein (PTH-rP), as the name implies, acts as a surrogate PTH in many systems, including the activation of adenylate cyclase and the movement of calcium ions (see also Chap. 3, p. 66, and Chap. 6, p. 149). PTH-rP is produced by the placenta as well as in fetal parathyroid glands, kidney, and other fetal tissues. Moreover, PTH is not demonstrable in fetal plasma, but PTH-rP is present. For these reasons, some refer to PTH-rP as the fetal parathormone (Abbas and associates, 1990). There is a Ca^{2+}-sensing receptor in trophoblast, as there is in the parathyroid glands (Juhlin and colleagues, 1990). The expression of PTH-rP in cytotrophoblasts is modulated by the extracellular concentration of Ca^{2+} (Hellman and co-workers, 1992). It seems possible, therefore, that PTH-rP synthesized in decidua, placenta, and other fetal tissues is important in fetal Ca^{2+} transfer and homeostasis.

Vitamins

The concentration of *vitamin A (retinol)* is greater in fetal than in maternal plasma and is bound to retinol-binding protein and to prealbumin. Retinol-binding protein is transferred from the maternal compartment across the syncytium. The transport of *vitamin C—ascorbic acid*—from mother to fetus is accomplished by an energy-dependent, carrier-mediated process. The levels of the principal *vitamin D—cholecalciferol*–metabolites, including 1,25-dihydroxycholecalciferol, are greater in maternal plasma than are those in fetal plasma. The 1β-hydroxylation of 25-hydroxyvitamin D_3 is known to take place in placenta and in decidua.

FETAL PHYSIOLOGY

Amnionic Fluid

In early pregnancy, amnionic fluid is an ultrafiltrate of maternal plasma. By the beginning of the second trimester, it consists largely of extracellular fluid that diffuses through the fetal skin and thus reflects the composition of fetal plasma (Gilbert and Brace, 1993). After 20 weeks, the cornification of fetal skin prevents this diffusion, and amnionic fluid is composed largely of fetal urine. Fetal kidneys start producing urine at 12 weeks, and by 18 weeks, they are producing 7 to 14 mL per day. Fetal urine contains more urea, creatinine, and uric acid than fetal plasma. Amnionic fluid also contains desquamated fetal cells, vernix, lanugo, and various secretions. Because these are hypotonic, the net effect is that amnionic fluid osmolality decreases with advancing gestation. Pulmonary fluid contributes a small proportion of the amnionic volume, and fluid filtering through the placenta accounts for the rest.

The volume of amnionic fluid at each week is quite variable. In general, the volume increases by 10 mL per week at 8 weeks and increases up to 60 mL per week at 21 weeks, then declines gradually back to a steady state by 33 weeks (Brace and Wolf, 1989).

Amnionic fluid serves to cushion the fetus, allowing musculoskeletal development and protecting it from trauma. It also maintains temperature and has a minimal nutritive function. Epidermal growth factor (EGF) and EGF-like growth factors, such as transforming growth factor-β, are present in amnionic fluid. Ingestion of fluid into the gastrointestinal tract and inhalation into the lung may promote growth and differentiation of these tissues. Animal studies have shown that pulmonary hypoplasia can be produced by draining off amnionic fluid, by chronically draining pulmonary fluid through the trachea, and by physically preventing the prenatal chest excursions that mimic breathing (Adzick and associates, 1984; Alcorn and colleagues, 1977). Thus, the formation of intrapulmonary fluid and, at least as important, the alternating egress and retention of fluid in the lungs by breathing movements are essential to normal pulmonary development. Clinical implications of oligohydramnios and pulmonary hypoplasia are discussed in Chapter 21 (p. 496).

Fetal Circulation

The fetal circulation is substantially different from that of the adult and functions until the moment of birth, when it is required to change dramatically. For example, because fetal blood does not need to enter the pulmonary vasculature to be oxygenated, most of the right ventricular output bypasses the lungs. In addition, the fetal heart chambers work in parallel, not in series, which effectively supplies the brain and heart with more highly oxygenated blood than the rest of the body.

Oxygen and nutrient materials required for fetal growth and maturation are delivered from the placenta by the single umbilical vein (Fig. 4-12). The vein then divides into the ductus venosus and the portal sinus. The ductus venosus is the major branch of the umbilical vein and traverses the liver to enter the inferior vena cava directly. Because it does not supply oxygen to the intervening tissues, it carries well-oxygenated blood directly to the heart. In contrast, the portal sinus carries blood to the hepatic veins primarily on the left side of the liver where oxygen is extracted. The relatively deoxygenated blood from the liver then flows back into the inferior vena cava, which also receives less oxygenated blood returning from the lower body. Blood flowing to the fetal heart from the inferior vena cava, therefore, consists of an admixture of arterial-like blood that passes directly through the ductus venosus and less well-oxygenated blood that returns from most of the veins below the level of the diaphragm. The oxygen content of blood delivered to the heart from the inferior vena cava is thus lower than that leaving the placenta.

In contrast to postnatal life, the ventricles of the fetal heart work in parallel, not in series. Well-oxygenated blood enters the left ventricle, which supplies the heart and brain, and less oxygenated blood enters the right ventricle, which supplies the rest of the body. The two separate circulations are maintained by the structure of the right atrium, which effectively directs entering blood to either the left atrium or the right ventricle, depending on its oxygen content. This separation of blood according to its oxygen content is aided by the pattern of blood flow in the inferior vena cava. The well-oxygenated blood tends to course along the medial aspect of the inferior vena cava and the less oxygenated blood stays along the lateral vessel wall. This aids their shunting into opposite sides of the heart. Once this blood enters the right atrium, the configuration of the upper interatrial septum—the *crista dividens*—is such that it preferentially shunts the well-oxygenated blood from the medial side of the inferior vena cava and the ductus venosus through the foramen ovale into the left heart and then to the heart and brain (Dawes, 1962). After these tissues have extracted needed oxygen, the resulting less oxygenated blood returns to the right heart through the superior vena cava.

The less oxygenated blood coursing along the lateral wall of the inferior vena cava enters the right atrium and is deflected through the tricuspid valve to the right ventricle. The superior vena cava courses inferiorly and anteriorly as it enters the right atrium, ensuring that less well-oxygenated blood returning from the brain and upper body also will be shunted directly to the right ventricle. Similarly, the ostium of the coronary sinus lies just superior to the tricuspid valve so that less oxygenated blood from the heart also returns to the right ventricle. As a result of this blood flow pattern, blood in the right ventricle is 15 to 20 percent less saturated than blood in the left ventricle.

Almost 90 percent of blood exiting the right ventricle is shunted through the ductus arteriosus to the descending aorta. High pulmonary vascular resistance and comparatively lower resistance in the ductus arteriosus and the umbilical–placental vasculature ensure that only about 15 percent of right ventricular output—8 percent of the combined ventricular output—goes to the lungs (Teitel, 1992). Thus, one third of the blood passing through the ductus arteriosus is delivered to the body. The remaining right ventricular output returns to the placenta through the two hypogastric arteries, which distally become the umbilical arteries. In the placenta, this blood picks up oxygen and other nutrients and is recirculated through the umbilical vein.

Circulatory Changes at Birth

After birth, the umbilical vessels, ductus arteriosus, foramen ovale, and ductus venosus normally constrict or collapse. With the functional closure of the ductus arteriosus and the expansion of the lungs, blood leaving the right ventricle preferentially enters the pulmonary vasculature to become oxygenated before it returns to the left heart. Virtually instantaneously, the ventricles, which had worked in parallel in fetal life, now effectively work in series. The more distal portions of the

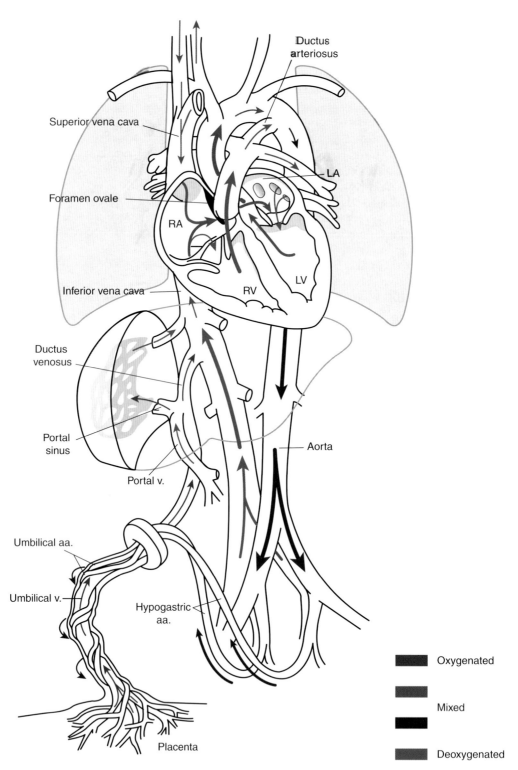

Ductus
arteriosus

Superior vena cava

LA

Foramen ovale

RA

Inferior vena cava

LV

RV

Ductus
venosus

Portal
sinus

Aorta

Portal v.

Umbilical aa.

Umbilical v.

Hypogastric
aa.

Oxygenated

Mixed

Deoxygenated

Placenta

FIGURE 4-12 The intricate nature of the fetal circulation is evident. The degree of oxygenation of blood in various vessels differs appreciably from that in the postnatal state as the consequences of oxygenation being provided by the placenta rather than the lungs and the presence of three major vascular shunts—the ductus venosus, foramen ovale, and ductus arteriosus. (aa = arteries; LA = left atrium; LV = left ventricle; RA = right atrium; RV = right ventricle; v = vein.)

hypogastric arteries, which course from the level of the bladder along the abdominal wall to the umbilical ring and into the cord as the umbilical arteries, undergo atrophy and obliteration within 3 to 4 days after birth. These become the umbilical ligaments, whereas the intra-abdominal remnants of the umbilical vein form the ligamentum teres. The ductus venosus constricts by 10 to 96 hours after birth and is anatomically closed by 2 to 3 weeks, resulting in the formation of the ligamentum venosum (Clymann and Heymann, 1981).

Fetal Blood

Hemopoiesis

In the very early embryo, hemopoiesis is demonstrable first in the yolk sac. The next major site is the liver, and finally the bone marrow. The contributions made by each site are depicted in Figure 4-13.

The first erythrocytes released into the fetal circulation are nucleated and macrocytic. Mean cell volumes are expressed in femtoliters (fL), and one femtoliter equals one cubic micrometer. The mean cell volume is at least 180 fL in the embryo and decreases to 105 to 115 fL at term. The erythrocytes of aneuploid fetuses generally do not undergo this maturation and maintain high mean cell volumes—130 fL on average (Sipes and associates, 1991). As fetal development progresses, more and more of the circulating erythrocytes are smaller and nonnucleated. As the fetus grows, both the volume of blood in the common fetoplacental circulation and hemoglobin concentration increase. Hemoglobin content of fetal blood increases to about 12 g/dL at midpregnancy and to 18 g/dL at term (Walker and Turnbull, 1953). Because of their large size, fetal erythrocytes have a short life span, which progressively lengthens to approximately 90 days at term (Pearson, 1966). As a consequence, red blood cell production is increased. Reticulocytes are initially present at high levels, but decrease to 4 to 5 percent of the total at term. The fetal erythrocytes differ structurally and metabolically from those of the adult. They are more deformable, which serves to offset their higher viscosity, and contain several enzymes with appreciably different activities (Smith and co-workers, 1981).

Erythropoiesis

This process is controlled primarily by fetal erythropoietin because maternal erythropoietin does not cross the placenta. Fetal erythropoietin production is influenced by testosterone, estrogen, prostaglandins, thyroid hormone, and lipoproteins (Stockman and deAlarcon, 1992). Serum levels of erythropoietin increase with fetal maturity, as do the numbers of responsive erythrocytes. The exact site of erythropoietin production is disputed, but the fetal liver appears to be an important source until renal production begins. There is a close correlation between the concentration of erythropoietin in amnionic fluid and that in umbilical venous blood obtained by cordocentesis. After birth, erythropoietin normally may not be detectable for up to 3 months.

Fetal Blood Volume

Although precise measurements of human fetoplacental volume are lacking, Usher and associates (1963) reported values in term normal newborns to average 78 mL/kg when immediate cord-clamping was conducted. Gruenwald (1967) found the volume of fetal blood contained in the placenta after prompt cord clamping to average 45 mL/kg of fetal weight. Thus, fetoplacental blood volume at term is approximately 125 mL/kg of fetal weight.

Fetal Hemoglobin

This tetrameric protein is composed of two copies of two different peptide chains, which determine the type of hemoglobin produced. Normal adult hemoglobin A is made of α and β chains. During embryonic and fetal life, a variety of α and β chain

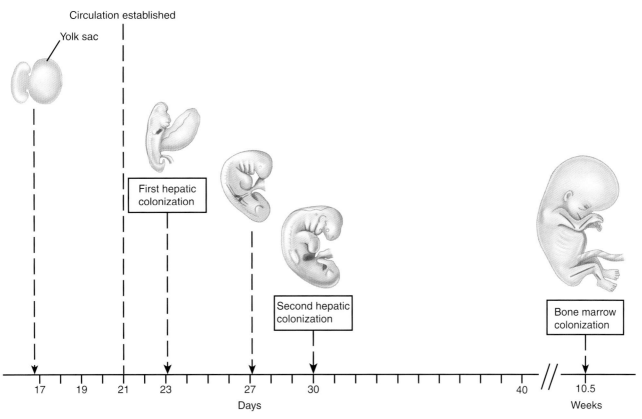

FIGURE 4-13 Chronological appearance of hemopoietic stem cells in the human embryo. (Modified from Tavian and Péault, 2005.)

precursors are produced, resulting in the serial production of several different embryonic hemoglobins. The genes that direct production of the various embryonic versions of these chains are arranged in the order in which they are temporally activated. Genes for β-type chains are on chromosome 11 and for α-type chains on chromosome 16. This sequence is shown in **Figure 4-14**. Each of these genes is turned on and then off during fetal life, until the α and β genes, which direct the production of hemoglobin A, are permanently activated.

The timing of the production of each of these early hemoglobin versions corresponds to changes in the site of hemoglobin production. As Figure 4-13 illustrates, fetal blood is first produced in the yolk sac, where hemoglobins Gower 1, Gower 2, and Portland are made. Erythropoiesis then moves to the liver, where fetal hemoglobin F is produced. When hemopoiesis finally moves to the bone marrow, adult-type hemoglobin A appears in fetal red blood cells and is present in progressively greater amounts as the fetus matures (Pataryas and Stamatoyannopoulos, 1972).

The final adult version of the α chain is produced exclusively by 6 weeks. After this, there are no functional alternative versions. If an α-gene mutation or deletion occurs, there is no alternate α-type chain that could substitute to form functional hemoglobin. In contrast, at least two versions of the β chain—δ and γ—remain in production throughout fetal life and beyond. In the case of a β-gene mutation or deletion, these two other versions of the β chain often continue to be produced, resulting in hemoglobin A_2 or hemoglobin F, which substitute for the abnormal or missing hemoglobin.

Genes are turned off by *methylation* of the control region, which is discussed in Chapter 12 (p. 278). In some situations, methylation does not occur, and in newborns of diabetic women, there may be persistence of hemoglobin F from hypomethylation of the γ gene (Perrine and associates, 1988). With sickle cell anemia, the γ gene remains unmethylated, and large quantities of fetal hemoglobin continue to be produced (see Chap. 51, p. 1085). Increased hemoglobin F levels are associated with fewer sickle-cell disease symptoms, and pharmacological modification of these levels by hemoglobin F-inducing drugs is one approach to disease treatment (Trompeter and Roberts, 2009).

There is a functional difference between hemoglobins A and F. At any given oxygen tension and at identical pH, fetal erythrocytes that contain mostly hemoglobin F bind more oxygen than do those that contain nearly all hemoglobin A (see Fig. 42-3, p. 931). This is because hemoglobin A binds 2,3-diphosphoglycerate (2,3-DPG) more avidly than does hemoglobin F, thus lowering the affinity of hemoglobin A for oxygen (De Verdier and Garby, 1969). During pregnancy, maternal 2,3-DPG levels are increased, and because fetal erythrocytes have lower concentrations of 2,3-DPG, the latter has increased oxygen affinity.

The amount of hemoglobin F in fetal erythrocytes begins to decrease in the last weeks of pregnancy so that at term, about three fourths of total hemoglobin is hemoglobin F. During the first 6 to 12 months of life, the proportion of hemoglobin F continues to decrease and eventually reaches the low levels found in adult erythrocytes. Glucocorticosteroids mediate the switch from fetal to adult hemoglobin, and the effect is irreversible (Zitnik and associates, 1995).

Fetal Coagulation Factors

There are no embryonic forms of the various hemostatic proteins. With the exception of fibrinogen, the fetus starts producing normal, adult-type procoagulant, fibrinolytic, and anticoagulant proteins by 12 weeks. Because they do not cross the placenta, their concentrations at birth are markedly below the levels that develop within a few weeks of life (Corrigan, 1992). In normal neonates, the levels of factors II, VII, IX, X, XI, and of prekallikrein, Protein S, Protein C, antithrombin, and plasminogen are all approximately 50 percent of adult levels. In contrast, levels of factors V, VIII, XIII, and fibrinogen are closer to adult values (Saracco and colleagues, 2009). Without prophylactic treatment, the vitamin K-dependent coagulation factors usually decrease even further during the first few days after birth. This decrease is amplified in breast-fed infants and may lead to hemorrhage in the newborn (see Chap. 29, p. 629).

Fetal *fibrinogen*, which appears as early as 5 weeks, has the same amino acid composition as adult fibrinogen but has different properties (Klagsbrun, 1988). It forms a less compressible clot, and the fibrin monomer has a lower degree of aggregation (Heimark and Schwartz, 1988). Plasma fibrinogen levels at birth are less than those in nonpregnant adults.

Levels of functional fetal *factor XIII—fibrin-stabilizing factor*—are significantly reduced compared with those in adults (Henriksson and co-workers, 1974). Severe deficiencies of *factors VIII, IX, XI, or XIII* are usually suspected after observing a continuous ooze from the umbilical stump. Nielsen (1969) described low levels of plasminogen and increased *fibrinolytic activity* in cord plasma compared with that of maternal plasma. *Platelet* counts in cord blood are in the normal range for nonpregnant adults.

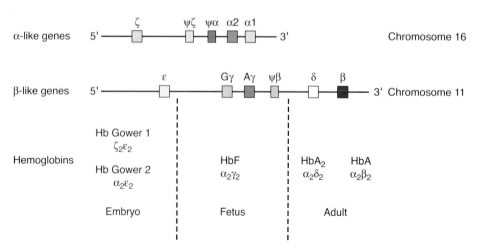

FIGURE 4-14 Schematic drawing of the arrangement of the α and β gene precursors on chromosomes 11 and 16 and the types of hemoglobin made from them. (Modified after Thompson and colleagues, 1991.)

Despite this relative reduction in procoagulants, the fetus appears to be protected from hemorrhage because fetal bleeding is a rare event. Excessive bleeding does not usually occur even after invasive fetal procedures such as cordocentesis. Ney and colleagues (1989) have shown that amnionic fluid thromboplastins and some factor in Wharton jelly combine to aid coagulation at the umbilical cord puncture site.

A variety of thrombophilias, such as protein C, S, antithrombin III deficiency, or the factor V Leiden mutation, may cause thromboses and pregnancy complications in adults (see Chap. 47, p. 1014). If the fetus inherits one of these mutations, thrombosis and infarction can develop. This is usually seen with homozygous inheritance, but Thorarensen and colleagues (1997) described three neonates with ischemic infarction or hemorrhagic stroke who were heterozygous for factor V Leiden mutation.

Fetal Plasma Proteins

Liver enzymes and other plasma proteins are produced by the fetus, and these levels do not correlate with maternal levels (Weiner and colleagues, 1992). Concentrations of plasma protein, albumin, lactic dehydrogenase, aspartate aminotransferase, γ-glutamyl transpeptidase, and alanine transferase all increase, whereas levels of prealbumin decrease with gestational age (Fryer and colleagues, 1993). At birth, mean total plasma protein and albumin concentrations in fetal blood are similar to maternal levels (Foley and associates, 1978).

Ontogeny of the Fetal Immune Response

Infections in utero have provided an opportunity to examine some of the mechanisms of the fetal immune response. Evidence of immunological competence has been reported as early as 13 weeks. Altshuler (1974) described infection of the placenta and fetus by cytomegalovirus with characteristic severe inflammatory cell proliferation as well as cellular viral inclusions. Fetal synthesis of complement late in the first trimester has been demonstrated by Kohler (1973) and confirmed by Stabile and co-workers (1988). In cord blood at or near term, the average level for most components is about half that of the adult values (Adinolfi, 1977).

Fetal Immunocompetence

In the absence of a direct antigenic stimulus such as infection, fetal plasma immunoglobulins consist almost totally of transferred maternal immunoglobulin G (IgG). Thus, antibodies in the newborn are most often reflective of maternal immunological experiences.

Immunoglobulin G

Maternal IgG transport to the fetus begins at about 16 weeks and increases thereafter. The bulk of IgG is acquired during the last 4 weeks of pregnancy (Gitlin, 1971). Accordingly, preterm neonates are endowed relatively poorly with protective maternal antibodies. Newborns begin to slowly produce IgG, and adult values are not attained until 3 years of age. In certain situations, the transfer of IgG antibodies from mother to fetus can be harmful rather than protective to the fetus. The classical example is hemolytic disease of the fetus and newborn resulting from D-antigen isoimmunization (see Chap. 29, p. 618).

Immunoglobulin M

In the adult, production of immunoglobulin M (IgM) in response to an antigenic stimulus is superseded in a week or so predominantly by IgG production. In contrast, very little IgM is produced by normal fetuses, and that produced may include antibody to maternal T lymphocytes (Hayward, 1983). With infection, the IgM response is dominant in the fetus and remains so for weeks to months in the newborn. And because IgM is not transported from the mother, any IgM in the fetus or newborn is that which it produced. Increased levels of IgM are found in newborns with congenital infection such as rubella, cytomegalovirus infection, or toxoplasmosis. Serum IgM levels in umbilical cord blood and identification of specific antibodies may be useful in the diagnosis of intrauterine infection. Adult levels of IgM are normally attained by 9 months of age.

Immunoglobulin A

Differing from many mammals, the human newborn does not acquire significant passive immunity from the absorption of humoral antibodies ingested in colostrum. Nevertheless, immunoglobulin A (IgA) ingested in colostrum provides mucosal protection against enteric infections. This may also explain the small amount of fetal secretory IgA found in amnionic fluid (Quan and colleagues, 1999).

Lymphocytes

The immune system begins to develop early and B lymphocytes appear in fetal liver by 9 weeks, and in blood and spleen by 12 weeks. T lymphocytes begin to leave the thymus at about 14 weeks (Hayward, 1983). Despite this, the newborn responds poorly to immunization, and especially poorly to bacterial capsular polysaccharides. This immature response may be due to either deficient response of newborn B cells to polyclonal activators, or lack of T cells that proliferate in response to specific stimuli (Hayward, 1983).

Monocytes

In the newborn, monocytes are able to process and present antigen when tested with maternal antigen-specific T cells.

Nervous System and Sensory Organs

The spinal cord extends along the entire length of the vertebral column in the embryo, but after that it grows more slowly. By 24 weeks, the spinal cord extends to S1, at birth to L3, and in the adult to L1. Myelination of the spinal cord begins at midgestation and continues through the first year of life. Synaptic function is sufficiently developed by the eighth week to demonstrate flexion of the neck and trunk (Temiras and co-workers, 1968). At 10 weeks, local stimuli may evoke squinting, opening of the mouth, incomplete finger closure, and flexion of the toes. Swallowing begins at about 10 weeks, and respiration is evident at 14 to 16 weeks (Miller, 1982). Rudimentary taste buds are present at 7 weeks, and mature receptors are present by 12 weeks (Mistretta and Bradley, 1975). The ability to suck is not present until at least

24 weeks (Lebenthal and Lee, 1983). During the third trimester, integration of nervous and muscular function proceeds rapidly.

The internal, middle, and external components of the ear are well developed by midpregnancy (see Fig. 4-3). The fetus apparently hears some sounds in utero as early as 24 to 26 weeks. By 28 weeks, the eye is sensitive to light, but perception of form and color is not complete until long after birth.

Gastrointestinal System

Swallowing begins at 10 to 12 weeks, coincident with the ability of the small intestine to undergo peristalsis and transport glucose actively (Koldovsky and colleagues, 1965; Miller, 1982). Much of the water in swallowed fluid is absorbed, and unabsorbed matter is propelled to the lower colon (Fig. 4-15). It is not clear what stimulates swallowing, but the fetal neural analogue of thirst, gastric emptying, and change in the amnionic fluid composition are potential factors (Boyle, 1992). The fetal taste buds may play a role because saccharin injected into amnionic fluid increases swallowing, whereas injection of a noxious chemical inhibits it (Liley, 1972).

Fetal swallowing appears to have little effect on amnionic fluid volume early in pregnancy because the volume swallowed is small compared with the total. Late in pregnancy, however, the volume appears to be regulated substantially by fetal swallowing, for when swallowing is inhibited, hydramnios is common (see Chap. 21, p. 492). Term fetuses swallow between 200

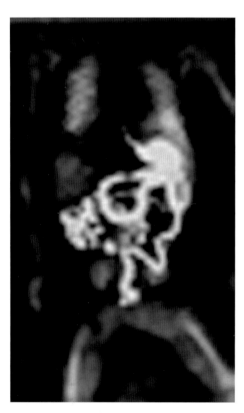

FIGURE 4-15 Radiograph of a 115-g fetus—about 16 weeks' gestational age—showing radiopaque dye in the lungs, esophagus, stomach, and entire intestinal tract after injection into the amnionic cavity 26 hours before delivery. These represent inhalation as well as active swallowing of amnionic fluid. (From Davis and Potter, 1946, with permission.)

and 760 mL per day—an amount comparable to that of the neonate (Pritchard, 1966).

Hydrochloric acid and some digestive enzymes are present in the stomach and small intestine in very small amounts in the early fetus. Intrinsic factor is detectable by 11 weeks, and pepsinogen by 16 weeks. The preterm neonate, depending on the gestational age when born, may have transient deficiencies of these enzymes (Lebenthal and Lee, 1983).

Stomach emptying appears to be stimulated primarily by volume. Movement of amnionic fluid through the gastrointestinal system may enhance growth and development of the alimentary canal. However, other regulatory factors likely are involved because anencephalic fetuses, in whom swallowing is limited, often have normal amnionic fluid volumes and normal-appearing gastrointestinal tracts. Gitlin (1974) demonstrated that late in pregnancy, about 800 mg of soluble protein is ingested daily by the fetus.

Several anomalies can affect normal fetal gastrointestinal function. *Hirschsprung disease*—known also as *congenital aganglionic megacolon,* prevents the bowel from undergoing parasympathetic-mediated relaxation and thus from emptying normally (Watkins, 1992). It may be recognized prenatally by grossly enlarged bowel during sonography. Obstructions such as duodenal atresia, megacystis-microcolon syndrome, or imperforate anus can also prevent the bowel from emptying normally. Meconium ileus, commonly found with fetal cystic fibrosis, is bowel obstruction caused by thick, viscid meconium that blocks the distal ileum (see Chap. 13, p. 298).

Meconium

Fetal bowel contents consist of various products of secretion, such as glycerophospholipids from the lung, desquamated fetal cells, lanugo, scalp hair, and vernix. It also contains undigested debris from swallowed amnionic fluid. The dark greenish-black appearance is caused by pigments, especially biliverdin. Meconium can pass from normal bowel peristalsis in the mature fetus or from vagal stimulation. It can also pass when hypoxia stimulates arginine vasopressin (AVP) release from the fetal pituitary gland. AVP stimulates the smooth muscle of the colon to contract, resulting in intra-amnionic defecation (DeVane and co-workers, 1982; Rosenfeld and Porter, 1985). Small bowel obstruction may lead to vomiting in utero (Shrand, 1972). Fetuses who suffer from congenital chloride diarrhea may have diarrhea in utero, which leads to hydramnios and preterm delivery (Holmberg and associates, 1977).

Liver

Serum liver enzyme levels increase with gestational age but in reduced amounts. The fetal liver has a gestational-age related diminished capacity for converting free unconjugated bilirubin to conjugated bilirubin (see Chap. 29, p. 625). Because the life span of normal fetal macrocytic erythrocytes is brief, relatively more unconjugated bilirubin is produced. The fetal liver conjugates only a small fraction, which is excreted into the intestine and ultimately oxidized to biliverdin. Most of the unconjugated bilirubin is excreted into the amnionic fluid after 12 weeks and is then transferred across the placenta (Bashore and colleagues, 1969).

Importantly, placental transfer is bidirectional. Thus, a pregnant woman with severe hemolysis from any cause has excess unconjugated bilirubin that readily passes to the fetus and then into the amnionic fluid. Conversely, conjugated bilirubin is not exchanged to any significant degree between mother and fetus.

Most fetal cholesterol is from hepatic synthesis, which satisfies the large demand for LDL cholesterol by the fetal adrenal glands. Hepatic glycogen is present in low concentration during the second trimester, but near term there is a rapid and marked increase to levels two to three times those in the adult liver. After birth, glycogen content falls precipitously.

Pancreas

The discovery of insulin by Banting and Best (1922) came in response to its extraction from the fetal calf pancreas. Insulin-containing granules can be identified by 9 to 10 weeks, and insulin in fetal plasma is detectable at 12 weeks (Adam and associates, 1969). The pancreas responds to hyperglycemia by secreting insulin (Obenshain and colleagues, 1970). Serum insulin levels are unusually high in newborns of diabetic mothers and other large-for-gestational age neonates, but insulin levels are low in those small-for-gestational age (Brinsmead and Liggins, 1979). This is further described in Chapter 38 (pp. 843 and 845).

Glucagon has been identified in the fetal pancreas at 8 weeks. In the adult rhesus monkey, hypoglycemia and infused alanine cause an increase in maternal glucagon levels. Although, in the human, similar stimuli do not evoke a fetal response, by 12 hours after birth, the newborn is capable of responding (Chez and co-workers, 1975). At the same time, however, fetal pancreatic α cells do respond to L-dopa infusions (Epstein and associates, 1977). Therefore, nonresponsiveness to hypoglycemia is likely the consequence of failure of glucagon release rather than inadequate production. This is consistent with findings of the developmental expression of pancreatic genes in the fetus (Mally and associates, 1994).

Most pancreatic enzymes are present by 16 weeks. Trypsin, chymotrypsin, phospholipase A, and lipase are found in the 14-week fetus at low levels, and they increase with gestation (Werlin, 1992). Amylase has been identified in amnionic fluid at 14 weeks (Davis and associates, 1986). The exocrine function of the fetal pancreas is limited. Physiologically important secretion occurs only after stimulation by a secretagogue such as acetylcholine, which is released locally after vagal stimulation (Werlin, 1992). Cholecystokinin normally is released only after protein ingestion and thus ordinarily would not be found in the fetus. Its release, however, can be stimulated experimentally. For example, Pritchard (1965) reported that radioiodine-labeled albumin injected into the amnionic sac was swallowed, digested, and absorbed from the fetal intestine.

Urinary System

Two primitive urinary systems—the pronephros and the mesonephros—precede the development of the metanephros (see Chap. 40, p. 890). The pronephros has involuted by 2 weeks, and the mesonephros is producing urine at 5 weeks and degenerates by 11 to 12 weeks. Failure of these two structures either to form or to regress may result in anomalous development of the definitive urinary system. Between 9 and 12 weeks, the ureteric bud and the nephrogenic blastema interact to produce the metanephros. The kidney and ureter develop from intermediate mesoderm. Greater maternal anthropometrics and fetal biometrics are associated with larger fetal kidneys, whereas preferential fetal blood flow to the brain is associated with smaller kidneys (Geelhoed and colleagues, 2009). The bladder and urethra develop from the urogenital sinus. The bladder also develops in part from the allantois.

By week 14, the loop of Henle is functional and reabsorption occurs (Smith and associates, 1992). New nephrons continue to be formed until 36 weeks. In preterm neonates, their formation continues after birth. Although the fetal kidneys produce urine, their ability to concentrate and modify the pH is limited even in the mature fetus. Fetal urine is hypotonic with respect to fetal plasma and has low concentrations of electrolytes.

Renal vascular resistance is high, and the filtration fraction is low compared with values in later life (Smith and colleagues, 1992). Fetal renal blood flow and thus urine production are controlled or influenced by the renin-angiotensin system, the sympathetic nervous system, prostaglandins, kallikrein, and atrial natriuretic peptide. The glomerular filtration rate increases with gestational age from less than 0.1 mL/min at 12 weeks to 0.3 mL/min at 20 weeks. In later gestation, the rate remains constant when corrected for fetal weight (Smith and colleagues, 1992). Hemorrhage or hypoxia generally results in a decrease in renal blood flow, glomerular filtration rate, and urine output.

Urine usually is found in the bladder even in small fetuses. The fetal kidneys start producing urine at 12 weeks. By 18 weeks, they are producing 7 to 14 mL/day, and at term, this increases to 27 mL/hr or 650 mL/day (Wladimiroff and Campbell, 1974). Maternally administered furosemide increases fetal urine formation, whereas uteroplacental insufficiency and other types of fetal stress decrease it. Kurjak and associates (1981) found that fetal glomerular filtration rates and tubular water reabsorption were decreased in a third of growth-restricted newborns and in a sixth of those of diabetic mothers. All values were normal in anencephalic neonates and in those with hydramnios.

Obstruction of the urethra, bladder, ureters, or renal pelves can damage renal parenchyma and distort fetal anatomy. With urethral obstruction, the bladder may become sufficiently distended that it ruptures or dystocia results. Kidneys are not essential for survival in utero, but are important in the control of amnionic fluid composition and volume. Furthermore, abnormalities that cause chronic anuria are usually accompanied by oligohydramnios and pulmonary hypoplasia. Pathological correlates and prenatal therapy of urinary tract obstruction are discussed in Chapter 13 (p. 307).

Lungs

The timetable of lung maturation and the identification of biochemical indices of functional fetal lung maturity are of considerable interest to the obstetrician. Morphological or functional immaturity at birth leads to the development of the *respiratory distress syndrome* (see Chap. 29, p. 605). The presence of a sufficient amount of surface-active materials—collectively re-ferred to as *surfactant*—in the amnionic fluid is evidence of fe-tal lung maturity. As Liggins (1994) emphasized, however, the structural and morphological maturation of fetal lung also is ex-traordinarily important to proper lung function.

Anatomical Maturation

Like the branching of a tree, lung development proceeds along an established timetable that apparently cannot be hastened by antenatal or neonatal therapy. The limits of viability, therefore, appear to be determined by the usual process of pulmonary growth. There are three essential stages of lung development as described by Moore (1983):

1. The *pseudoglandular stage* entails growth of the intrasegmental bronchial tree between the 5th and 17th weeks. During this period, the lung looks microscopically like a gland.
2. The *canalicular stage*, from 16 to 25 weeks, is when the bronchial cartilage plates extend peripherally. Each terminal bronchiole gives rise to several respiratory bronchioles, and each of these in turn divides into multiple saccular ducts.
3. The *terminal sac stage* begins after 25 weeks and during this, alveoli give rise to the primitive pulmonary alveoli—the terminal sacs. Simultaneously, an extracellular matrix devel-ops from proximal to distal lung segments until term. An extensive capillary network is built, the lymph system forms, and type II pneumonocytes begin to produce surfac-tant. At birth, only about 15 percent of the adult number of alveoli are present, and thus the lung continues to grow, adding more alveoli for up to 8 years.

Various insults can upset this process, and their timing de-termines the sequela. With fetal renal agenesis, for example, there is no amnionic fluid at the beginning of lung growth, and major defects occur in all three stages. A fetus with membrane rupture before 20 weeks and subsequent oligohydramnios usu-ally exhibits nearly normal bronchial branching and cartilage development but has immature alveoli. Membrane rupture af-ter 24 weeks may have little long-term effect on pulmonary structure.

Surfactant

After the first breath, the terminal sacs must remain expanded despite the pressure imparted by the tissue-to-air interface, and surfactant keeps them from collapsing. There are more than 200 pulmonary cell types, but surfactant is formed specifically in type II pneumonocytes that line the alveoli. These cells are characterized by multivesicular bodies that pro-duce the *lamellar bodies* in which surfactant is assembled. During late fetal life, at a time when the alveolus is character-ized by a water-to-tissue interface, the intact lamellar bodies are secreted from the lung and swept into the amnionic fluid during respiratory-like movements that are termed fetal breathing. At birth, with the first breath, an air-to-tissue in-terface is produced in the lung alveolus. Surfactant uncoils from the lamellar bodies, and it then spreads to line the alveo-lus to prevent alveolar collapse during expiration. Thus, it is the capacity for fetal lungs to produce surfactant, and not the

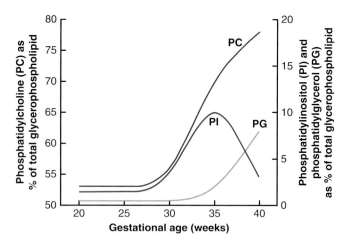

FIGURE 4-16 Relation between the levels of lecithin, or dipalmi-toylphosphatidylcholine (PC), phosphatidylinositol (PI), and phos-phatidylglycerol (PG) in amnionic fluid as a function of gestational age.

actual laying down of this material in the lungs in utero, that establishes lung maturity.

Surfactant Composition. Gluck and associates (1967, 1970, 1972) and Hallman and co-workers (1976) found that about 90 percent of surfactant dry-weight is lipid. Proteins account for the other 10 percent. Approximately 80 percent of the glyc-erophospholipids are phosphatidylcholines (lecithins). The principal active component of surfactant is a specific lecithin—*dipalmitoylphosphatidylcholine (DPPC or PC)*—which accounts for nearly 50 percent. *Phosphatidylglycerol (PG)* accounts for an-other 8 to 15 percent (Keidel and Gluck, 1975). Its precise role is unclear because newborns without phosphatidylglycerol usu-ally do well. The other major constituent is *phosphatidylinositol (PI)*. The relative contributions of each component are shown in Figure 4-16.

Surfactant Synthesis. Biosynthesis takes place in the type II pneumocytes. The apoproteins are produced in the endoplas-mic reticulum, and the glycerophospholipids are synthesized by cooperative interactions of several cellular organelles. Phospho-lipid is the primary surface tension-lowering component of sur-factant, whereas the apoproteins aid the forming and reforming of a surface film. The surface properties of the surfactant phos-pholipids are determined principally by the composition and degree of saturation of their long-chain fatty acids.

The major apoprotein is surfactant A (SP-A), which is a gly-coprotein with a molecular weight of 28,000 to 35,000 Da (Whitsett, 1992). It is synthesized in the type II cells, and its content in amnionic fluid increases with gestational age and fe-tal lung maturity. SP-A may also play a role in the onset of par-turition (Mendelson and Condon, 2005). Synthesis of SP-A is increased by treatment of fetal lung tissue with cyclic adenosine monophosphate (AMP) analogues, epidermal growth factors, and triiodothyronine. Increased apoprotein synthesis precedes surfactant glycerophospholipid synthesis.

SP-A gene expression is demonstrable by 29 weeks (Snyder and colleagues, 1988). There are two separate genes on chromo-some 10—SP-A1 and SP-A2—and their regulation is distinctive and different (McCormick and Mendelson, 1994). Specifically, cyclic AMP is more important in SP-A2 expression, whereas dexamethasone decreases SP-A2 expression.

Several smaller apoproteins such as SP-B and SP-C are likely important in optimizing the action of surfactant. For example, deletions in SP-B gene are incompatible with survival despite production of large amounts of surfactant.

Corticosteroids and Fetal Lung Maturation.

Since Liggins (1969) first observed lung maturation in lamb fetuses given glucocorticosteroids prior to preterm delivery, many suggested that fetal cortisol stimulates lung maturation and surfactant synthesis. It is unlikely that corticosteroids are the only stimulus for augmented surfactant formation, as clearly, respiratory distress syndrome is not universal in neonates with limited cortisol production. These include those with anencephaly, adrenal hypoplasia, or congenital adrenal hyperplasia. There is evidence, however, that glucocorticosteroids administered at certain critical times during gestation effect an increase in the rate of fetal lung maturation. The use of betamethasone and dexamethasone to accelerate fetal lung maturity, as well as neonatal replacement surfactant therapy, is discussed in Chapter 36 (p. 821).

Respiration.

Within a few minutes after birth, the respiratory system must provide oxygen as well as eliminate carbon dioxide. Respiratory muscles develop early, and fetal chest wall movements are detected by sonographic techniques as early as 11 weeks (Boddy and Dawes, 1975). From the beginning of the fourth month, the fetus is capable of respiratory movement sufficiently intense to move amnionic fluid in and out of the respiratory tract.

Endocrine Glands

Pituitary Gland

The fetal endocrine system is functional for some time before the central nervous system reaches maturity (Mulchahey and co-workers, 1987). The pituitary adenohypophysis develops from oral ectoderm—Rathke pouch, whereas the neurohypophysis derives from neuroectoderm.

Anterior Pituitary.

The adenohypophysis, or anterior pituitary, differentiates into five cell types that secrete six protein hormones: (1) lactotropes produce prolactin—PRL; (2) somatotropes produce growth hormone—GH; (3) corticotropes produce corticotrophin—ACTH; (4) thyrotropes produce thyrotropin or thyroid-stimulating hormone—TSH; and gonadotropes produce (5) luteinizing hormone—LH and (6) follicle-stimulating hormone—FSH.

ACTH is first detected in the fetal pituitary gland at 7 weeks, and GH and LH have been identified by 13 weeks. By the end of the 17th week, the fetal pituitary gland is able to synthesize and store all pituitary hormones. Moreover, the fetal pituitary is responsive to hormones and is capable of secreting these early in gestation (Grumbach and Kaplan, 1974). Levels of immunoreactive GH are high in cord blood, although its role in fetal growth and development is not clear. The fetal pituitary secretes β-endorphin, and cord blood levels of β-endorphin and β-lipotropin increase with fetal P_{CO_2} (Browning and colleagues, 1983).

Neurohypophysis.

The posterior pituitary gland is well developed by 10 to 12 weeks, and oxytocin and arginine vasopressin (AVP) are demonstrable. Both hormones probably function in the fetus to conserve water by actions largely at the lung and placenta rather than kidney. Levels of AVP in umbilical cord plasma are increased strikingly compared with maternal levels (Chard and associates, 1971; Polin and co-workers, 1977). Elevated fetal blood AVP appears to be associated with fetal stress (DeVane and co-workers, 1982).

Intermediate Pituitary Gland.

There is a well-developed intermediate lobe in the fetal pituitary gland. The cells of this structure begin to disappear before term and are absent from the adult pituitary. The principal secretory products of the intermediate lobe cells are α-melanocyte–stimulating hormone (α-MSH) and β-endorphin.

Thyroid Gland

The pituitary–thyroid system is functional by the end of the first trimester. The thyroid gland is able to synthesize hormones by 10 to 12 weeks, and TSH, thyroxine, and thyroid-binding globulin (TBG) have been detected in fetal serum as early as 11 weeks (Ballabio and colleagues, 1989). The placenta actively concentrates iodide on the fetal side, and by 12 weeks and throughout pregnancy, the fetal thyroid concentrates iodide more avidly than does the maternal thyroid. Thus, maternal administration of either radioiodide or appreciable amounts of ordinary iodide is hazardous after this time. Normal fetal levels of free thyroxine (T_4), free triiodothyronine (T_3), and thyroxin-binding globulin increase steadily throughout gestation (Ballabio and associates, 1989). Compared with adult levels, by 36 weeks, fetal serum concentrations of TSH are higher, total and free T_3 concentrations are lower, and T_4 is similar. This suggests that the fetal pituitary may not become sensitive to feedback until late in pregnancy (Thorpe-Beeston and co-workers, 1991; Wenstrom and colleagues, 1990).

Fetal thyroid hormone plays a role in the normal development of virtually all fetal tissues, but especially the brain. Its influence is illustrated by congenital hyperthyroidism, which occurs when maternal thyroid-stimulating antibody crosses the placenta to stimulate the fetal thyroid. These fetuses develop tachycardia, hepatosplenomegaly, hematological abnormalities, craniosynostosis, and growth restriction. As children, they have perceptual motor difficulties, hyperactivity, and reduced growth (Wenstrom and colleagues, 1990). Neonatal effects of fetal thyroid deficiency are discussed in Chapter 53 (p. 1126).

The placenta prevents substantial passage of maternal thyroid hormones to the fetus by rapidly deiodinating maternal T_4 and T_3 to form reverse T_3, a relatively inactive thyroid hormone (Vulsma and colleagues, 1989). A number of antithyroid antibodies—immunoglobulin G—cross the placenta when present in high concentrations. Those include the long-acting thyroid stimulators (LATS), LATS-protector (LATS-P), and thyroid-stimulating immunoglobulin (TSI). It was previously believed that normal fetal growth and development, which occurred despite fetal hypothyroidism, provided evidence that T_4 was not essential for fetal growth. It is now known, however, that growth proceeds normally because small quantities of maternal T_4 prevent antenatal cretinism in fetuses with thyroid agenesis (Vulsma and colleagues, 1989). The fetus with congenital hypothyroidism typically does not develop stigmata of cretinism until after birth. Because administration of thyroid hormone will prevent this, all newborns are tested for high serum levels of TSH (Chap. 28, p. 598).

Immediately after birth, there are major changes in thyroid function and metabolism. Cooling to room temperature evokes sudden and marked increase in TSH secretion, which in turn causes a progressive increase in serum T_4 levels that are maximal 24 to 36 hours after birth. There are nearly simultaneous elevations of serum T_3 levels.

Adrenal Glands

The fetal adrenal glands are much larger in relation to total body size than in adults. The bulk is made up of the inner or *fetal zone* of the adrenal cortex and involutes rapidly after birth. This zone is scant to absent in rare instances in which the fetal pituitary gland is congenitally absent. The function of the fetal adrenal glands is discussed in detail in Chapter 3 (p. 69).

DEVELOPMENT OF GENITALIA

Embryology of Uterus and Oviducts

The uterus and tubes arise from the müllerian ducts, which first appear near the upper pole of the urogenital ridge in the fifth week of embryonic development (Fig. 4-17). This ridge is composed of the mesonephros, gonad, and associated ducts. The first indication of müllerian duct development is a thickening of the

coelomic epithelium at approximately the level of the fourth thoracic segment. This becomes the fimbriated extremity of the fallopian tube, which invaginates and grows caudally to form a slender tube at the lateral edge of the urogenital ridge. In the sixth week, the growing tips of the two müllerian ducts approach each other in the midline. One week later, they reach the urogenital sinus. At that time, the two müllerian ducts fuse to form a single canal at the level of the inguinal crest. This crest gives rise to the gubernaculum, which is the primordium of the round ligament.

Thus, the upper ends of the müllerian ducts produce the oviducts, and the fused parts give rise to the uterus. The vaginal canal is not patent throughout its entire length until the sixth month (Koff, 1933). Because of the clinical importance of anomalies that arise from abnormal fusion and dysgenesis of these structures, their embryogenesis is discussed in detail in Chapter 40 (see also Fig. 40-1, p. 891).

Embryology of the Ovaries

At approximately 4 weeks, gonads form on the ventral surface of the embryonic kidney at a site between the eighth thoracic and fourth lumbar segments. The coelomic epithelium thickens, and clumps of cells bud off into the underlying mesenchyme. This circumscribed area of is called the *germinal epithelium*. By the fourth to sixth week, however, there are many large ameboid cells in this region that have migrated into the body of the embryo from the yolk sac (see Fig. 4-17). These *primordial germ cells* are distinguishable by their large size and certain morphological and cytochemical features.

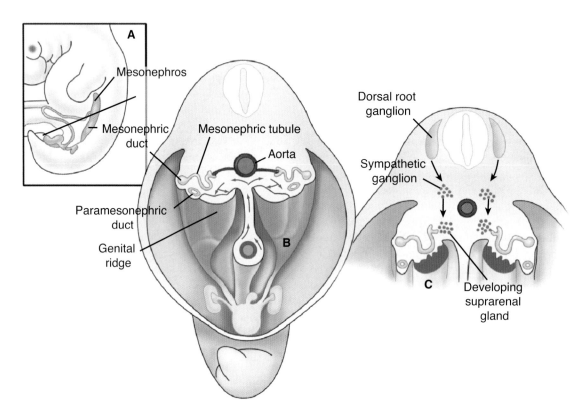

FIGURE 4-17 A. Cross-section of an embryo at 4 to 6 weeks. **B.** Large ameboid primordial germ cells migrate (*arrows*) from the yolk sac to the area of germinal epithelium, within the genital ridge. **C.** Migration of sympathetic cells from the spinal ganglia to a region above the developing kidney. (After Moore and colleagues, 2000.)

When the primordial germ cells reach the genital area, some enter the germinal epithelium and others mingle with groups of cells that proliferate from it or lie in the mesenchyme. By the end of the fifth week, rapid division of all these cell types results in development of a prominent *genital ridge*. The ridge projects into the body cavity medially to a fold in which there are the *mesonephric—wolffian* and *para-mesonephric—müllerian ducts* (Fig. 4-18). By the seventh week, it is separated from the mesonephros except at the narrow central zone, the future hilum, where blood vessels enter. At this time, the sexes can be distinguished, because the testes can be recognized by well-defined radiating strands of cells termed sex cords. These cords are separated from the germinal epithelium by mesenchyme that is to become the tunica albuginea. The sex cords, which consist of large germ cells and smaller epithelioid cells derived from the germinal epithelium, develop into the seminiferous tubules and tubuli rete. The latter establishes connection with the mesonephric tubules that develop into the epididymis. The mesonephric ducts become the vas deferens.

In the female embryo, the germinal epithelium proliferates for a longer time. The groups of cells thus formed lie at first in the region of the hilum. As connective tissue develops between them, these appear as sex cords. These cords give rise to the medulla cords and persist for variable times (Forbes, 1942). By the third month, medulla and cortex are defined (see Fig. 4-18). The bulk of the ovary is made up of cortex, a mass of crowded germ and epithelioid cells that show some signs of grouping, but there are no distinct cords as in the testis. Strands of cells extend from the germinal epithelium into the cortical mass, and mitoses are numerous. The rapid succession of mitoses soon reduces the size of the germ cells to the extent that these no longer are differentiated clearly from the neighboring cells. These germ cells are now called *oogonia*.

By the fourth month, some germ cells in the medullary region begin to enlarge. These are called primary oocytes at the beginning of the phase of growth that continues until maturity is reached. During this period of cell growth, many oocytes undergo degeneration, both before and after birth. A single layer of flattened follicular cells that were derived originally from the germinal epithelium soon surrounds the primary oocytes. These structures are now called *primordial follicles* and are seen first in the medulla and later in the cortex. Some follicles begin to grow even before birth, and some are believed to persist in the cortex almost unchanged until menopause.

By 8 months, the ovary has become a long, narrow, lobulated structure that is attached to the body wall along the line of the hilum by the *mesovarium*, in which lies the *epoöphoron*. The germinal epithelium has been separated for the most part from the cortex by a band of connective tissue—*tunica albuginea*. This band is absent in many small areas where strands of cells, usually referred to as cords of Pflüger, are in contact with the germinal epithelium. Among these cords are cells believed by many to be oogonia that resemble the other epithelial cells as a result of repeated mitosis. In the underlying cortex, there are two distinct zones. Superficially, there are nests of germ cells in meiotic synapsis, interspersed with Pflüger cords and strands of connective tissue. In the deeper zone, there are many groups of germ cells in synapsis, as well as primary oocytes, prospective follicular cells, and a few primordial follicles.

Fetal Gender

Theoretically, there should be a primary gender ratio of 1:1 at the time of fertilization because there are equal numbers of X- and Y-bearing spermatozoa. This is not the case, however, and many factors have been shown to contribute to gender ratios at conception. These include differential susceptibility to environmental exposures as well as medical disorders. Also, couples with a large age discrepancy are more likely have a male offspring (Manning and associates, 1997). Whatever the cause, it is impossible to determine the primary gender ratio because this would require gender assignment to zygotes that fail to cleave, blastocysts that fail to implant, and other early pregnancy losses.

The secondary gender ratio is that of fetuses that reach viability and is usually held to be about 106 males to 100 females. The unbalanced secondary gender ratio is explicable by the loss of more female than male embryofetuses during early pregnancy. However, Davis and colleagues (1998) report a significant decline in male births since 1950 in Denmark, Sweden, the Netherlands, the United States, Germany, Norway, and Finland. Allan and co-workers (1997) reported that live births in Canada since 1970 dropped by 2.2 male births per 1000 live births.

Gender Assignment at Birth

The first thing that parents in the delivery room want to know is the gender of their newborn. If the external genitalia of the newborn are ambiguous, the obstetrician faces a profound dilemma because it is not possible to assign proper functional gender by simple inspection in the delivery room. Assignment requires knowledge of the karyotypic sex, gonadal sex, hormonal milieu to which the fetus was exposed, exact anatomy, and all possibilities for surgical correction. In the past, most newborns with a small or likely insufficient phallus were often assigned to the female gender. Based on what is now known of the role of fetal exposure to hormones in establishing gender preference and behavior, it can be seen why such a policy may have caused *gender identity disorder* (Slijper and colleagues, 1998). Thus, it seems best to inform the parents that although their newborn appears healthy, the gender will need to be determined by a series of tests. To develop a plan that can assist in determining the cause of ambiguous genitalia, the mechanisms of normal and abnormal sexual differentiation must be considered.

Sexual Differentiation

Phenotypic gender differentiation is determined by the chromosomal complement acting in conjunction with gonadal development.

Chromosomal Gender

Genetic gender—XX or XY—is established at the time of fertilization, but for the first 6 weeks, development of male and female embryos is morphologically indistinguishable. The differentiation of the primordial gonad into testis or ovary heralds the establishment of gonadal sex (see Fig. 4-18).

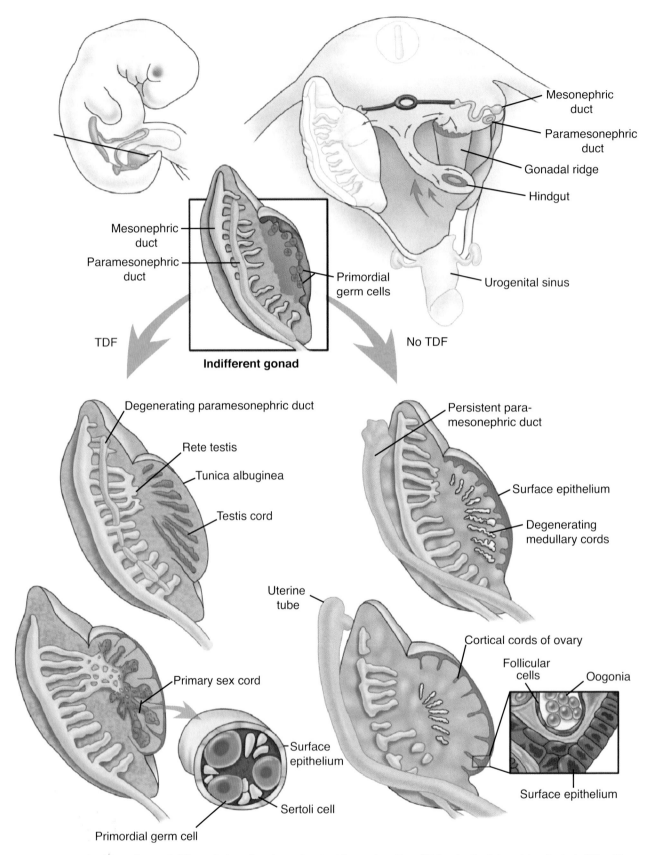

FIGURE 4-18 Continuation of sexual differentiation of embryo. See text for explanation. (TDF = testis-determining factor.) (After Moore and colleagues, 2000.)

Gonadal Gender

As described earlier and shown in Figure 4-17, primordial germ cells that originate in the yolk sac endoderm migrate to the genital ridge to form the indifferent gonad. If a Y chromosome is present, at about 6 weeks after conception, the gonad begins developing into a testis (Simpson, 1997). Testis development is directed by a gene located on the short arm of Y—*testis-determining factor (TDF),* also called *sex-determining region (SRY).* This gene encodes a transcription factor that acts to modulate the rate of transcription of a number of genes involved in gonadal differentiation. The *SRY* gene is specific to the Y chromosome and is expressed in the human single-cell zygote immediately after ovum fertilization. It is not expressed in spermatozoa (Fiddler and co-workers, 1995; Gustafson and Donahoe, 1994). In addition, testis development requires a *dose-dependent sex reversal (DDS)* region on the X chromosome, as well as other autosomal genes (Brown and Warne, 2005).

The contribution of chromosomal gender to gonadal gender is illustrated by several paradoxical conditions. The incidence of 46,XX phenotypic human males is estimated to be about 1 in 20,000 male births (Page and colleagues, 1985). These infants apparently result from translocation of the Y chromosome fragment containing *TDF* to the X chromosome during meiosis of male germ cells (George and Wilson, 1988). Similarly, individuals with XY chromosomes can appear phenotypically female if they carry a mutation in the *TDF/SRY* gene. There is evidence that genes on the short arm of the X chromosome are capable of suppressing testicular development, despite the presence of the *SRY* gene. Indeed, this accounts for a form of X-linked recessive gonadal dysgenesis.

The existence of autosomal sex-determining genes is supported by several genetic syndromes in which disruption of an autosomal gene causes, among other things, gonadal dysgenesis. For example, *camptomelic dysplasia,* localized to chromosome 17, is associated with XY phenotypic sex reversal. Similarly, *male pseudohermaphroditism* has been associated with a mutation in the Wilms tumor suppressor gene on chromosome 11.

Phenotypic Gender

After establishment of gonadal gender, phenotypic gender develops very rapidly. It is clear that male phenotypic sexual differentiation is directed by the function of the fetal testis. In the absence of a testis, female differentiation ensues irrespective of the genetic gender. The development of urogenital tracts in both sexes of human embryos is indistinguishable before 8 weeks. Thereafter, development and differentiation of the internal and external genitalia to the male phenotype is dependent on testicular function. The fundamental experiments to determine the role of the testis in male sexual differentiation were conducted by the French anatomist Alfred Jost. Ultimately, he established that the induced phenotype is male and that secretions from the gonads are not necessary for female differentiation. Specifically, the fetal ovary is not required for female sexual differentiation.

Jost and associates (1973) found that if castration of rabbit fetuses was conducted before differentiation of the genital anlagen, all newborns were phenotypic females with female external and internal genitalia. Thus, the müllerian ducts developed into uterus, fallopian tubes, and upper vagina.

If fetal castration was conducted before differentiation of the genital anlagen, and thereafter a testis was implanted on one side in place of the removed gonad, the phenotype of all fetuses was male. Thus, the external genitalia of such fetuses were masculinized. On the side of the testicular implant, the wolffian duct developed into the epididymis, vas deferens, and seminal vesicle. With castration, on the side without the implant, the müllerian duct developed but the wolffian duct did not.

Wilson and Gloyna (1970) and Wilson and Lasnitzki (1971) demonstrated that testosterone action was amplified by conversion to 5α-dihydrotestosterone (5α-DHT). They showed that in most androgen-responsive tissues, testosterone is converted by 5α-reductase to 5α-DHT. This hormone acts primarily and almost exclusively in the genital tubercle and labioscrotal folds.

Physiological and Biomolecular Basis of Gender Differentiation

Based on these observations, the physiological basis of gender differentiation can be summarized as follows. Genetic gender is established at fertilization. Gonadal gender is determined primarily by factors encoded by genes on the Y chromosome, such as the *SRY* gene. In a manner not yet understood, differentiation of the primitive gonad into a testis is accomplished.

Fetal Testicular Contributions to Male Sexual Differentiation

The fetal testis secretes a proteinaceous substance called *müllerian-inhibiting substance,* a dimeric glycoprotein with a molecular weight of about 140,000 Da. It acts locally as a paracrine factor to cause müllerian duct regression. Thus, it prevents the development of uterus, fallopian tube, and upper vagina. Müllerian-inhibiting substance is produced by the Sertoli cells of the seminiferous tubules. Importantly, these tubules appear in fetal gonads before differentiation of Leydig cells, which are the cellular site of testosterone synthesis. Thus, müllerian-inhibiting substance is produced by Sertoli cells even before differentiation of the seminiferous tubules and is secreted as early as 7 weeks. Müllerian duct regression is completed by 9 to 10 weeks, which is before testosterone secretion has commenced. Because it acts locally near its site of formation, if a testis were absent on one side, the müllerian duct on that side would persist, and the uterus and fallopian tube would develop on that side.

Female external genital differentiation is complete by 11 weeks, whereas male external genital differentiation is complete by 14 weeks (Sobel and colleagues, 2004).

Fetal Testosterone Secretion

Apparently through stimulation initially by human chorionic gonadotropin (hCG), and later by fetal pituitary LH, the fetal testes secrete testosterone. This hormone acts directly on the wolffian duct to effect the development of the vas deferens, epididymis, and seminal vesicles. Testosterone also enters fetal blood and acts on the anlagen of the external genitalia. In these tissues, however, testosterone is converted to 5α-DHT to cause virilization of the external genitalia.

Genital Ambiguity of the Newborn

Ambiguity of the neonatal genitalia results from excessive androgen action in a fetus that was destined to be female or from inadequate androgen representation for one destined to be male. Rarely, genital ambiguity indicates *true hermaphroditism*. Abnormalities of gender differentiation causing genital ambiguity can be assigned to one of four clinically defined categories that include: (1) female pseudohermaphroditism; (2) male pseudohermaphroditism; (3) dysgenetic gonads, including true hermaphroditism; and rarely (4) true hermaphroditism (Low and Hutson, 2003).

Category 1. Female Pseudohermaphroditism

In this condition, müllerian-inhibiting substance is not produced. Androgen exposure is excessive, but variable, for a fetus genetically predestined to be female. The karyotype is 46,XX and ovaries are present.

Therefore, by genetic and gonadal gender, all are predestined to be female, and the basic abnormality is androgen excess. Because müllerian-inhibiting substance is not produced, the uterus, fallopian tubes, and upper vagina develop.

If affected fetuses were exposed to a small amount of excess androgen reasonably late in fetal development, the only genital abnormality will be slight to modest clitoral hypertrophy, with an otherwise normal female phenotype.

With somewhat greater androgen exposure, clitoral hypertrophy will be more pronounced, and the posterior labia will fuse. If androgen levels increase earlier in embryonic development, then more severe virilization can be seen. This includes formation of labioscrotal folds; development of a urogenital sinus, in which the vagina empties into the posterior urethra; and development of a penile urethra with scrotal formation—the empty scrotum syndrome (Fig. 4-19).

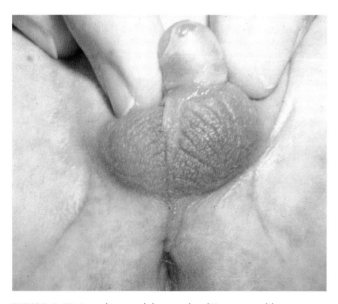

FIGURE 4-19 Female pseudohermaphroditism caused by congenital adrenal hyperplasia. Infant was 46,XX and has severe virilization with scrotal formation without a testis and has a penile urethra. (Used with permission from Dr. Lisa Halvorson.)

Congenital Adrenal Hyperplasia. This is the most common cause of androgenic excess in fetuses with female pseudohermaphroditism. The hyperplastic glands synthesize defective enzymes that cause impaired cortisol synthesis. This leads to excessive pituitary ACTH stimulation of the fetal adrenal glands with secretion of large amounts of cortisol precursors, including androgenic prehormones. These prehormones, for example, androstenedione, are converted to testosterone in fetal extra-adrenal tissues.

Mutations may involve any of several enzymes, but the most common are steroid 21-hydroxylase, 11β-hydroxylase, and 3β-hydroxysteroid dehydrogenase. Deficiency of the last prevents synthesis of virtually all steroid hormones. Deficiency of either 17β- or 11β-hydroxylase results in increased deoxycorticosterone production to cause hypertension and hypokalemic acidosis. These forms of congenital adrenal hyperplasia thus constitute medical emergencies in the newborn (Speroff and colleagues, 1994). Currently, 21-hydroxylase deficiency can be diagnosed in utero through molecular fetal DNA analysis. Prenatal maternal dexamethasone administration has shown to safely reduce fetal genital virilization (Nimkarn and New, 2009).

Excessive Androgen from Maternal Sources. Another cause of androgen excess in the female embryofetus is the transfer of androgen from the maternal compartment. This may arise from the ovaries with hyperreaction luteinalis or theca-lutein cysts or from tumors such as Leydig cell tumors and Sertoli-Leydig cell tumors (see Chap. 3, p. 71, and Chap. 40, p. 905). In most of these conditions, the female fetus does not become virilized. This is because during most of pregnancy, the fetus is protected from excess maternal androgen by the extraordinary capacity of the syncytiotrophoblast to convert most C_{19}-steroids, including testosterone, to estradiol-17β. The only exception to this generalization is fetal aromatase deficiency, which produces both maternal and fetal virilization (see Chap. 3, p. 71). Some drugs also can cause female fetal androgen excess. Most commonly, the drugs implicated are synthetic progestins or anabolic steroids (see Chap. 14, p. 321).

Importantly, except those with aromatase deficiency, all with female pseudohermaphroditism can be normal, fertile women if the proper diagnosis is made and appropriate and timely treatment initiated.

Category 2. Male Pseudohermaphroditism

This is characterized by incomplete and variable androgenic exposure of a fetus predestined to be male. The karyotype is 46,XY, and there are either testes or no gonads. In some cases, incomplete masculinization follows inadequate production of testosterone by the fetal testis. It also may arise from diminished responsiveness of the genital anlagen to normal quantities of androgen—including failure of the in situ formation of 5α-DHT in androgen-responsive tissue. Because testes were present for at least some time in embryonic life, müllerian-inhibiting substance is produced. Thus, the uterus, fallopian tubes, and upper vagina do not develop.

Fetal testicular testosterone production may fail if there is an enzymatic defect of steroidogenesis that involves any one of four enzymes in the biosynthetic pathway for testosterone synthesis. Impaired fetal testicular steroidogenesis can also be caused by an abnormality in the LH-hCG receptor and by Leydig cell hypoplasia.

With embryonic testicular regression, the testes regress during embryonic or fetal life, and there is no testosterone production thereafter (Edman and associates, 1977). This results in a spectrum of phenotypes that varies from a normal female with absent uterus, fallopian tubes, and upper vagina, to a normal male phenotype with anorchia.

Androgen resistance or deficiencies in androgen responsiveness are caused by an abnormal or absent androgen receptor protein or by enzymatic failure of conversion of testosterone to 5α-DHT in appropriate tissues (Wilson and MacDonald, 1978).

Androgen Insensitivity Syndrome. Formerly called *testicular feminization,* this is the most extreme form of the androgen resistance syndrome, and there is no tissue responsiveness to androgen. There is a female phenotype with a short, blind-ending vagina, no uterus or fallopian tubes, and no wolffian duct structures. At the expected time of puberty, testosterone levels in affected women increase to values for normal men. Nonetheless, virilization does not occur, and even pubic and axillary hair do not develop because of end-organ resistance. Presumably, because of androgen resistance at the level of the brain and pituitary, LH levels also are elevated. In response to high concentrations of LH, there is increased testicular secretion of estradiol-17β compared with that in normal men (MacDonald and colleagues, 1979). Increased estrogen secretion and absence of androgen responsiveness act in concert to cause feminization in the form of breast development.

Individuals with *incomplete androgen insensitivity* are slightly responsive to androgen. They usually have modest clitoral hypertrophy at birth (Fig. 4-20). And at the expected time of puberty, pubic and axillary hair develop but virilization does not occur. These women also develop feminine breasts,

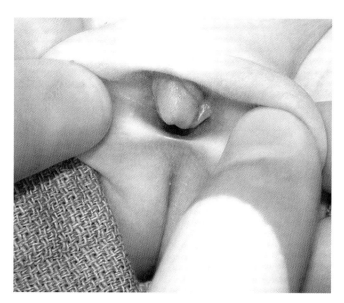

FIGURE 4-20 Male pseudohermaphroditism caused by incomplete androgen insensitivity syndrome. Infant is 46,XY with external genitalia demonstrating clitoral hypertrophy. (Used with permission from Dr. Lisa Halvorson.)

presumably through the same endocrine mechanisms as in women with the complete form of the disorder (Madden and co-workers, 1975).

Another group has been referred to as *familial male pseudohermaphroditism, type I* (Walsh and colleagues, 1974). Also commonly referred to as *Reifenstein syndrome,* it constitutes a spectrum of incomplete genital virilization. Phenotypes can vary from a phenotype similar to that of women with incomplete androgen insensitivity to that of a male phenotype with only a bifid scrotum, infertility, and gynecomastia.

The gene encoding the androgen-receptor protein is located on the X chromosome. More than 100 different mutations have been demonstrated. This accounts for the wide variability in androgen responsiveness among persons in whom the androgen-receptor protein is absent or abnormal, and for the many different mutations associated with one disorder (McPhaul and associates, 1991; Patterson and co-workers, 1994).

An alternate form of androgen resistance is caused by 5α-reductase deficiency in androgen-responsive tissues. Because androgen action in the external genitalia anlagen is mediated by 5α-DHT, persons with this enzyme deficiency have external genitalia that are female but with modest clitoral hypertrophy. But because androgen action in the wolffian duct is mediated directly by testosterone, there are well-developed epididymides, seminal vesicles, and vas deferens, and the male ejaculatory ducts empty into the vagina (Walsh and associates, 1974).

Category 3: Dysgenetic Gonads

In affected individuals, karyotype varies and is commonly abnormal. As the name describes, most have abnormally developed gonads, and streak gonads are typically found. As a result, müllerian-inhibiting substance is not produced and fetal androgen exposure is variable. The uterus, fallopian tubes, and upper vagina are present.

The most common form of gonadal dysgenesis is *Turner syndrome (46X)*. The phenotype is female, but secondary gender characteristics do not develop at the time of expected puberty, and genital infantilism persists. In some persons with dysgenetic gonads, the genitalia are ambiguous, a finding indicating that an abnormal gonad produced androgen, albeit in small amounts, during embryonic-fetal life. Generally, there is mixed gonadal dysgenesis—one example is a dysgenetic gonad on one side and an abnormal testis or dysontogenetic tumor on the other.

Category 4: True Hermaphroditism

In most cases, the guidelines for category 3 are met. External genitalia of such a case are shown in Figure 4-21. In addition, true hermaphrodites have both ovarian and testicular tissues with germ cells for both ova and sperm in the abnormal gonads.

Preliminary Diagnosis of the Cause of Genital Ambiguity

A preliminary diagnosis of genital ambiguity can be made at the birth of an affected child. By history, during physical and sonographic examination of the newborn, an experienced examiner

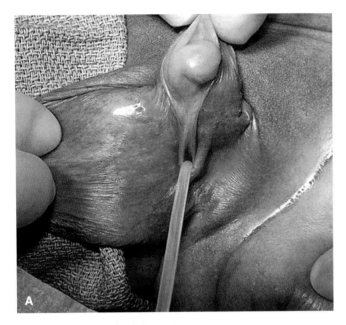

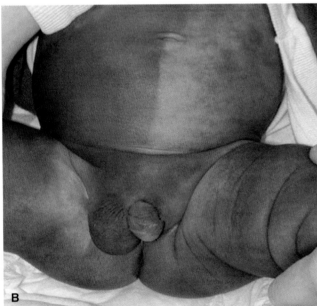

FIGURE 4-21 True hermaphroditism in infants with 46,XX/46,XY. **A.** The clitoris and hood are apparent, and the probe is in the urogenital sinus. **B.** A hemiscrotum is seen, and this infant shows different skin tones on each side. (Used with permission from Dr. Lisa Halvorson.)

can ascertain a number of important findings—whether gonads are palpable, and if so, where they are; phallus length and diameter; position of the urethral meatus; degree of labioscrotal fold fusion; and whether there is a vagina, vaginal pouch, or urogenital sinus (Speroff and associates, 1994). If the uterus is present, the diagnosis must be female pseudohermaphroditism, testicular or gonadal dysgenesis, or true hermaphroditism. A family history of congenital adrenal hyperplasia is helpful. If the uterus is not present, the diagnosis is male pseudohermaphroditism. Androgen resistance and enzymatic defects in testicular testosterone biosynthesis are often familial.

REFERENCES

Abbas SK, Pickard DW, Illingworth D, et al: Measurement of PTH-rP protein in extracts of fetal parathyroid glands and placental membranes. J Endocrinol 124:319, 1990

Adam PAJ, Teramo K, Raiha N, et al: Human fetal insulin metabolism early in gestation: Response to acute elevation of the fetal glucose concentration and placental transfer of human insulin-I-131. Diabetes 18:409, 1969

Adinolfi M: Human complement: Onset and site of synthesis during fetal life. Am J Dis Child 131:1015, 1977

Adzick NS, Harrison MR, Glick PL, et al: Experimental pulmonary hypoplasia and oligohydramnios: Relative contributions of lung fluid and fetal breathing movements. J Pediatr Surg 19:658, 1984

Aherne W, Dunnill MS: Morphometry of the human placenta. Br Med Bull 22:1, 1966

Alcorn D, Adamson TM, Lambert TF, et al: Morphological effects of chronic tracheal ligation and drainage in the fetal lamb lung. J Anat 3:649, 1977

Allan BB, Brant R, Seidel JE, et al: Declining sex ratios in Canada. Can Med Assoc J 156:37, 1997

Altshuler G: Immunologic competence of the immature human fetus. Obstet Gynecol 43:811, 1974

Ballabio M, Nicolini U, Jowett T, et al: Maturation of thyroid function in normal human foetuses. Clin Endocrinol 31:565, 1989

Banting FG, Best CH: Pancreatic extracts. J Lab Clin Med 1:464, 1922

Bashore RA, Smith F, Schenker S: Placental transfer and disposition of bilirubin in the pregnant monkey. Am J Obstet Gynecol 103:950, 1969

Boddy K, Dawes GS: Fetal breathing. Br Med Bull 31:3, 1975

Boyle JT: Motility of the upper gastrointestinal tract in the fetus and neonate. In Polin RA, Fox WW (eds): Fetal and Neonatal Physiology. Philadelphia, Saunders, 1992, p 1028

Bozzetti P, Ferrari MM, Marconi AM, et al: The relationship of maternal and fetal glucose concentrations in the human from midgestation until term. Metabolism 37:358, 1988

Brace RA, Wolf EJ: Normal amniotic fluid volume changes throughout pregnancy. Am Obstet Gynecol 161:382, 1989

Brinsmead MW, Liggins GC: Somadomedin-like activity, prolactin, growth hormone and insulin in human cord blood. Aust NZ J Obstet Gynecol 19:129, 1979

Brown J, Warne G: Practical management of the intersex infant. J Ped Endocrin Metab 18:3, 2005

Browning AJF, Butt WR, Lynch SS, et al: Maternal plasma concentrations of β-lipotropin, β-endorphin and α-lipotrophin throughout pregnancy. Br J Obstet Gynaecol 90:1147, 1983

Chard T, Hudson CN, Edwards CRW, et al: Release of oxytocin and vasopressin by the human foetus during labour. Nature 234:352, 1971

Chez RA, Mintz DH, Reynolds WA, et al: Maternal-fetal plasma glucose relationships in late monkey pregnancy. Am J Obstet Gynecol 121:938, 1975

Clymann RI, Heymann MA: Pharmacology of the ductus arteriosus. Pediatr Clin North Am 28:77, 1981

Corrigan JJ Jr: Normal hemostasis in the fetus and newborn: Coagulation. In Polin RA, Fox WW (eds): Fetal and Neonatal Physiology. Philadelphia, Saunders, 1992, p 1368

Davis DL, Gottlieb MB, Stampnitzky JR: Reduced ratio of male to female births in several industrial countries: A sentinel health indicator? JAMA 279:1018, 1998

Davis ME, Potter EL: Intrauterine respiration of the human fetus. JAMA 131:1194, 1946

Davis MM, Hodes ME, Munsick RA, et al: Pancreatic amylase expression in human pancreatic development. Hybridoma 5:137, 1986

Dawes GS: The umbilical circulation. Am J Obstet Gynecol 84:1634, 1962

DeVane GW, Naden RP, Porter JC, et al: Mechanism of arginine vasopressin release in the sheep fetus. Pediatr Res 16:504, 1982

De Verdier CH, Garby L: Low binding of 2,3-diphosphoglycerate to hemoglobin F. Scand J Clin Lab Invest 23:149, 1969

DiPietro JA. Neurobehavioral assessment before birth. MRDD Res Rev 11:4, 2005

Dolman CL: Characteristic configuration of fetal brains from 22 to 40 weeks gestation at two week intervals. Arch Pathol Lab Med 101:193, 1977

Edman CD, Winters AJ, Porter JC, et al: Embryonic testicular regression. A clinical spectrum of XY agonadal individual. Obstet Gynecol 49:208, 1977

Epstein M, Chez RA, Oakes GK, et al: Fetal pancreatic glucagon responses in glucose-intolerant nonhuman primate pregnancy. Am J Obstet Gynecol 127:268, 1977

Fiddler M, Abdel-Rahman B, Rappolee DA, et al: Expression of SRY transcripts in preimplantation human embryos. Am J Med Genet 55:80, 1995

Foley ME, Isherwood DM, McNicol GP: Viscosity, hematocrit, fibrinogen and plasma proteins in maternal and cord blood. Br J Obstet Gynaecol 85:500, 1978

Forbes TR: On the fate of the medullary cords of the human ovary. Contr Emryol Carneg Inst 30:9, 1942

Fowden AL, Ward JW, Wooding FPB, et al: Programming placental nutrient transport capacity. J Physiol 572 (1) 5 2006

Fryer AA, Jones P, Strange R, Hume R, Bell JE. Plasma protein levels in normal human fetuses: 13-41 weeks' gestation. Br J Obstet Gynecol 100:850, 1993

Geelhoed JJ, Verburg BO, Nauta J et al: Tracking and determinants of kidney size from fetal life until the age of 2 years: The Generation R Study. Am J Kidney Des 53(2):248, 2009

George FW, Wilson JD: Sex determination and differentiation. In Knobil E, Neill J (eds): The Physiology of Reproduction. New York, Raven, 1988, p 3

Gilbert WM, Brace RA: Amniotic fluid volume and normal flows to and from the amniotic cavity. Semin Perinatol 17:150, 1993

Gitlin D: Development and metabolism of the immune globulins. In Kaga BM, Stiehm ER (eds): Immunologic Incompetence. Chicago, Year Book, 1971

Gitlin D: Protein transport across the placenta and protein turnover between amnionic fluid, maternal and fetal circulation. In Moghissi KS, Hafez ESE (eds): The Placenta. Springfield, IL, Thomas, 1974

Gitlin D, Kumate J, Morales C, et al: The turnover of amniotic fluid protein in the human conceptus. Am J Obstet Gynecol 113:632, 1972

Giudice LC, de-Zegher F, Gargosky SE, et al: Insulin-like growth factors and their binding proteins in the term and preterm human fetus and neonate with normal and extremes of intrauterine growth. J Clin Endocrinol Metab 80:1548, 1995

Gluck L, Kulovich MV, Eidelman AI, et al: Biochemical development of surface activity in mammalian lung, 4. Pulmonary lecithin synthesis in the human fetus and newborn and etiology of the respiratory distress syndrome. Pediatr Res 6:81, 1972

Gluck L, Landowne RA, Kulovich MV: Biochemical development of surface activity in mammalian lung, 3. Structural changes in lung lecithin during development of the rabbit fetus and newborn. Pediatr Res 4:352, 1970

Gluck L, Motoyama EK, Smits HL, et al: The biochemical development of surface activity in mammalian lung, 1. The surface-active phospholipids; the separation and distribution of surface-active lecithin in the lung of the developing rabbit fetus. Pediatr Res 1:237, 1967

Grisaru-Granovsy S, Samueloff A, Elstein D: The role of leptin in fetal growth: a short review from conception to delivery. Eur J Obstet Gynecol Reprod Biol 136(2):146, 2008

Gruenwald P: Growth of the human foetus. In McLaren A (ed): Advances in Reproductive Physiology. New York, Academic Press, 1967

Grumbach MM, Kaplan SL: Fetal pituitary hormones and the maturation of central nervous system regulation of anterior pituitary function. In Gluck L (ed): Modern Perinatal Medicine. Chicago, Year Book, 1974

Gustafson ML, Donahoe PK: Male sex determination: Current concepts of male sexual differentiation. Annu Rev Med 45:505, 1994

Hallman M, Kulovich MV, Kirkpatrick E, et al: Phosphatidylinositol and phosphatidylglycerol in amniotic fluid: Indices of lung maturity. Am J Obstet Gynecol 125:613, 1976

Hauguel-de Mouzon S, Lepercq J, Catalano P: The known and unknown of leptin in pregnancy. Am J Obstet Gynecol 193(6):1537, 2006

Hayward AR: The human fetus and newborn: Development of the immune response. Birth Defects 19:289, 1983

Heimark R, Schwartz S: Cellular organization of blood vessels in development and disease. In Ryan U (ed): Endothelial Cells, Vol II. Boca Raton, FL, CRC Press, 1988, p 103

Hellman P, Ridefelt P, Juhlin C, et al: Parathyroid-like regulation of parathyroid hormone related protein release and cytoplasmic calcium in cytotrophoblast cells of human placenta. Arch Biochem Biophys 293:174, 1992

Henriksson P, Hedner V, Nilsson IM, et al: Fibrin-stabilization factor XIII in the fetus and the newborn infant. Pediatr Res 8:789, 1974

Henson MC, Castracane VD: Leptin in pregnancy: an update. Biol Reprod 74(2):218, 2006

Hill DJ, Tevaarwerk GJ, Caddell C, et al: Fibroblast growth factor 2 is elevated in term maternal and cord serum and amniotic fluid in pregnancies complicated by diabetes: Relationship to fetal and placental size. J Clin Endocrinol Metab 80:2626, 1995

Holmberg C, Perheentupa J, Launiala K, et al: Congenital chloride diarrhea. Arch Dis Child 52:255, 1977

Iyengar CV, Rapp A: Human placenta as a "dual" biomarker for monitoring fetal and maternal environment with special reference to potentially toxic trace elements. Part 3: Toxic trace elements in placenta and placenta as a biomarker for these elements. Sci Total Environ 280:221, 2001

Jansson T, Cetin I, Powell TL, et al: Placental transport and metabolism in fetal overgrowth—a workshop report. Placenta 27:109, 2006

Jansson T, Powell TL: Human placental transport in altered fetal growth: Does the placenta function as a nutrient sensor? A review. Placenta 27:S91, 2006

Jost A, Vigier B, Prepin J: Studies on sex differentiation in mammals. Recent Prog Horm Res 29:1, 1973

Juhlin C, Lundgren S, Johansson H, et al: 500-kilodalton calcium sensor regulating cytoplasmic Ca^{2+} in cytotrophoblast cells of human placenta. J Biol Chem 265:8275, 1990

Kimura RE: Lipid metabolism in the fetal-placental unit. In Cowett RM (ed): Principles of Perinatal-Neonatal Metabolism. New York, Springer-Verlag, 1991, p 291

Klagsbrun M: Angiogenesis factors. In Ryan U (ed): Endothelial Cells, Vol II. Boca Raton, Fla, CRC Press, 1988, p 37

Koff AK: Development of the vagina in the human fetus. Contr Embryol Carnegie Inst 24:59, 1933

Kohler PF: Maturation of the human complement system. J Clin Invest 52:671, 1973

Koldovsky O, Heringova A, Jirsova U, et al: Transport of glucose against a concentration gradient in everted sacs of jejunum and ileum of human fetuses. Gastroenterology 48:185, 1965

Korgun ET, Celik-Ozenci C, Seval Y, et al: Do glucose transporters have other roles in addition to placental glucose transport during early pregnancy? Histochem Cell Biol 123:621, 2005

Kurjak A, Kirkinen P, Latin V, et al: Ultrasonic assessment of fetal kidney function in normal and complicated pregnancies. Am J Obstet Gynecol 141:266, 1981

Lebenthal E, Lee PC: Interactions of determinants of the ontogeny of the gastrointestinal tract: A unified concept. Pediatr Res 1:19, 1983

Lee CK, Lee JT, Yu SJ, et al: Effects of cadmium on the expression of placental lactogens and Pit-1 genes in the rat placental trophoblast cells. Mol Cell Endocrinol 298(1-2), 2009

Lemons JA: Fetal placental nitrogen metabolism. Semin Perinatol 3:177, 1979

Leonce J, Brockton N, Robinson S, et al: Glucose production in the human placenta. Placenta 27:S103, 2006

Liggins GC: Fetal lung maturation. Aust NZ J Obstet Gynaecol 34:247, 1994

Liggins GC: Premature delivery of fetal lambs infused with glucocorticoids. J Endocrinol 45:515, 1969

Liley AW: Disorders of amniotic fluid. In Assali NS (ed): Pathophysiology of Gestation. New York, Academic Press, 1972

Lissauer D, Piper KP, Moss PA, et al: Persistence of fetal cells in the mother: Friend or foe? BJOG 114:1321, 2007

Longo LD: Respiration in the fetal-placental unit. In Cowett RM (ed): Principles of Perinatal-Neonatal Metabolism. New York, Springer-Verlag, 1991, p 304

Low Y, Hutson JM: Rules for clinical diagnosis in babies with ambiguous genitalia. J Paediatr Child Health 39:406, 2003

MacDonald PC, Madden JD, Brenner PF, et al: Origin of estrogen in normal men and in women with testicular feminization. J Clin Endocrinol Metab 49:905, 1979

Madden JD, Walsh PC, MacDonald PC, et al: Clinical and endocrinological characterization of a patient with syndrome of incomplete testicular feminization. J Clin Endocrinol 41:751, 1975

Mally MI, Otonkoski T, Lopez AD, et al: Developmental gene expression in the human fetal pancreas. Pediatr Res 36:537, 1994

Manganaro L, Perrone A, Savelli S, et al: Evaluation of normal brain development by prenatal MR imaging. Radiol Med 112:444, 2007

Manning JT, Anderton RH, Shutt M: Parental age gap skews child sex ratio. Nature 389:344, 1997

Maymó JL, Pérez Pérez A, Sánchez-Margalet V, et al: Up-regulation of placental leptin by human chorionic gonadotropin. Endocrinology 150(1):304, 2009

McCormick SM, Mendelson CR: Human SP-A1 and SP-A2 genes are differentially regulated during development and by cAMP and glucocorticoids. Am J Physiol 266:367, 1994

McPhaul MJ, Marcelli M, Tilley WD, et al: Androgen resistance caused by mutations in the androgen receptor gene. FASEB J 5:2910, 1991

Mendelson CR, Condon JC: New insights into the molecular endocrinology of parturition. J Steroid Biochem Molec Biol 93:113, 2005

Mercé LT, Barco MJ, Alcázar JL, et al: Intervillous and uteroplacental circulation in normal early pregnancy and early pregnancy loss assessed by 3-dimensional power Doppler angiography. Am J Obstet Gynecol 200(3): 315.e1, 2009

Miller AJ: Deglutition. Physiol Rev 62:129, 1982

Mistretta CM, Bradley RM: Taste and swallowing in utero. Br Med Bull 31:80, 1975

Moore KL: Before We Are Born. Basic Embryology and Birth Defects, 2nd ed. Philadelphia, Saunders, 1983

Moore KL: The Developing Human, 2nd ed. Philadelphia, Saunders, 1977

Moore KL: The Developing Human: Clinically Oriented Embryology, 4th ed. Philadelphia, Saunders, 1988

Morriss FH Jr, Boyd RDH, Manhendren D: Placental transport. In Knobil E, Neill J (eds): The Physiology of Reproduction, Vol II. New York, Raven, 1994, p 813

Mulchahey JJ, DiBlasio AM, Martin MC, et al: Hormone production and peptide regulation of the human fetal pituitary gland. Endocr Rev 8:406, 1987

Ney JA, Fee SC, Dooley SL, et al: Factors influencing hemostasis after umbilical vein puncture in vitro. Am J Obstet Gynecol 160:424, 1989

Nielsen NC: Coagulation and fibrinolysin in normal women immediately postpartum and in newborn infants. Acta Obstet Gynecol Scand 48:371, 1969

Nimkarn S, New MI: Prenatal diagnosis and treatment of congenital adrenal hyperplasia due to 21-hydroxylase deficiency. Mol Cell Endocrinol 300 (1-2):192, 2009

Obenshain SS, Adam PAJ, King KC, et al: Human fetal insulin response to sustained maternal hyperglycemia. N Engl J Med 283:566, 1970

Olsen O, Clausen JA: Determination of the expected day of delivery—ultrasound has not been shown to be more accurate than the calendar method. Ugeskr Laeger 160:2088, 1998

Page DC, de la Chapelle A, Weissenbach J: Chromosome Y-specific DNA in related human XX males. Nature 315:224, 1985

Pataryas HA, Stamatoyannopoulos G: Hemoglobins in human fetuses: Evidence for adult hemoglobin production after the 11th gestational week. Blood 39:688, 1972

Patterson MN, McPhaul MJ, Hughes IA: Androgen insensitivity syndrome. Bailleres Clin Endocrinol Metab 8:379, 1994

Pearson HA: Recent advances in hematology. J Pediatr 69:466, 1966

Perrine SP, Greene MF, Cohen RA, et al: A physiological delay in human fetal hemoglobin switching is associated with specific globin DNA hypomethylation. FEBS Lett 228:139, 1988

Pipe NGJ, Smith T, Halliday D, et al: Changes in fat, fat-free mass and body water in human normal pregnancy. Br J Obstet Gynaecol 86:929, 1979

Polin RA, Husain MK, James LS, et al: High vasopressin concentrations in human umbilical cord blood—lack of correlation with stress. J Perinat Med 5:114, 1977

Pritchard JA: Deglutition by normal and anencephalic fetuses. Obstet Gynecol 25:289, 1965

Pritchard JA: Fetal swallowing and amniotic fluid volume. Obstet Gynecol 28:606, 1966

Quan CP, Forestier F, Bouvet JP: Immunoglobulins of the human amniotic fluid. Am J Reprod Immunol 42:219, 1999

Ramsey, MM: Normal Values in Pregnancy. London, Saunders, 1996

Rosenfeld CR, Porter JC: Arginine vasopressin in the developing fetus. In Albrecht ED, Pepe GJ (eds): Research in Perinatal Medicine, Vol 4. Perinatal Endocrinology. Ithaca, NY, Perinatology Press, 1985, p 91

Sakata M, Kurachi H, Imai T, et al: Increase in human placental glucose transporter-1 during pregnancy. Eur J Endocrinol 132:206, 1995

Saracco P, Parodi E, Fabris C, et al: Management and investigation of neonatal thromboembolic events: Genetic and acquired risk factors. Thromb Res January 21, 2009

Schwartz R, Gruppuso PA, Petzold K, et al: Hyperinsulinemia and macrosomia in the fetus of the diabetic mother. Diabetes Care 17:640, 1994

Shrand II: Vomiting in utero with intestinal atresia. Pediatrics 49:767, 1972

Simpson JL: Diseases of the gonads, genital tract, and genitalia. In Rimoin DL, Connor JM, Pyeritz RE (eds): Emery and Rimoin's Principles and Practice of Medical Genetics, Vol I, 3rd ed. New York, Churchill Livingstone, 1997, p 1477

Sipes SL, Weiner CP, Wenstrom KD, et al: The association between fetal karyotype and mean corpuscular volume. Am J Obstet Gynecol 165:1371, 1991

Slijper FM, Drop SL, Molenaar JC, et al: Long-term psychological evaluation of intersex children. Arch Sex Behav 27:125, 1998

Smith CM II, Tukey DP, Krivit W, et al: Fetal red cells (FC) differ in elasticity, viscosity, and adhesion from adult red cells (AC). Pediatr Res 15:588, 1981

Smith FG, Nakamura KT, Segar JL, et al: In Polin RA, Fox WW (eds): Fetal and Neonatal Physiology, Vol 2, Chap 114. Philadelphia, Saunders, 1992, p 1187

Snyder JM, Kwun JE, O'Brien JA, et al: The concentration of the 35 kDa surfactant apoprotein in amniotic fluid from normal and diabetic pregnancies. Pediatr Res 24:728, 1988

Sobel V, Zhu Y-S, Imerato-McGinley J: Fetal hormones and sexual differentiation. Obstet Gynecol Clin N Am 31:837, 2004

Speroff L, Glass RH, Kase NG: Clinical Gynecologic Endocrinology and Infertility, 5th ed. Baltimore, Williams & Wilkins, 1994

Stabile I, Nicolaides KH, Bach A, et al: Complement factors in fetal and maternal blood and amniotic fluid during the second trimester of normal pregnancy. Br J Obstet Gynaecol 95:281, 1988

Stockman JA III, deAlarcon PA: Hematopoiesis and granulopoiesis. In Polin RA, Fox WW (eds): Fetal and Neonatal Physiology. Philadelphia, Saunders, 1992, p 1327

Tavian M, Péault B: Embryonic development of the human hematopoietic system. Int J Dev Biol 49:243, 2005

Teitel DF: Physiologic development of the cardiovascular system in the fetus. In Polin RA, Fox WW (eds): Fetal and Neonatal Physiology, Vol I. Philadelphia, Saunders, 1992, p 609

Temiras PS, Vernadakis A, Sherwood NM: Development and plasticity of the nervous system. In Assali NS (ed): Biology of Gestation, Vol VII. The Fetus and Neonate. New York, Academic Press, 1968

Thompson MW, McInnes RR, Willard HF: The hemoglobinopathies: Models of molecular disease. In Thompson MW, McInnes RR, Huntington FW (eds): Thompson and Thompson Genetics in Medicine, 5th ed. Philadelphia, Saunders, 1991, p 247

Thorarensen O, Ryan S, Hunter J, et al: Factor V Leiden mutation: An unrecognized cause of hemiplegic cerebral palsy, neonatal stroke, and placental thrombosis. Ann Neurol 42:372, 1997

Thorpe-Beeston JG, Nicolaides KH, Felton CV, et al: Maturation of the secretion of thyroid hormone and thyroid-stimulating hormone in the fetus. N Engl J Med 324:532, 1991

Trompeter S, Roberts I: Haemoglobin F modulation in childhood sickle cell disease. Br J Haemotol 144(3):308, 2009

Usher R, Shephard M, Lind J: The blood volume of the newborn infant and placental transfusion. Acta Paediatr 52:497, 1963

Vulsma T, Gons MH, De Vijlder JJM: Maternal-fetal transfer of thyroxine in congenital hypothyroidism due to a total organification defect or thyroid agenesis. N Engl J Med 321:13, 1989

Walker J, Turnbull EPN: Haemoglobin and red cells in the human foetus and their relation to the oxygen content of the blood in the vessels of the umbilical cord. Lancet 2:312, 1953

Walsh PC, Madden JD, Harrod MJ, et al: Familial incomplete male pseudohermaphroditism, type 2: Decreased dihydrotestosterone formation in pseudovaginal perineoscrotal hypospadias. N Engl J Med 291:944, 1974

Watkins JB: Physiology of the gastrointestinal tract in the fetus and neonate. In Polin RA, Fox WW (eds): Fetal and Neonatal Physiology. Philadelphia, Saunders, 1992, p 1015

Weiner CP, Sipes SL, Wenstrom K: The effect of fetal age upon normal fetal laboratory values and venous pressure. Obstet Gynecol 79:713, 1992

Wenstrom KD, Weiner CP, Williamson RA, et al: Prenatal diagnosis of fetal hyperthyroidism using funipuncture. Obstet Gynecol 76:513, 1990

Werlin SL: Exocrine pancreas. In Polin RA, Fox WW (eds): Fetal and Neonatal Physiology. Philadelphia, Saunders, 1992, p 1047

Werth B, Tsiaras A: From Conception to Birth: A Life Unfolds. New York, Doubleday, 2002

Whitsett JA: Composition of pulmonary surfactant lipids and proteins. In Polin RA, Fox WW (eds): Fetal and Neonatal Physiology. Philadelphia, Saunders, 1992, p 941

Wilson JD, Gloyna RE: The intranuclear metabolism of testosterone in the accessory organs of reproduction. Recent Prog Horm Res 26:309, 1970

Wilson JD, Lasnitzki I: Dihydrotestosterone formation in fetal tissues of the rabbit and rat. Endocrinology 89:659, 1971

Wilson JD, MacDonald PC: Male pseudohermaphroditism due to androgen resistance: Testicular feminization and related syndromes. In Stanbury JB, Wyngaarden JD, Frederickson DS (eds): The Metabolic Basis of Inherited Disease. New York, McGraw-Hill, 1978

Wladimiroff JW, Campbell S: Fetal urine-production rates in normal and complicated pregnancy. Lancet 1:151, 1974

Zitnik G, Peterson K, Stamatoyannopoulos G, et al: Effects of butyrate and glucocorticoids on gamma- to beta-globin gene switching in somatic cell hybrids. Mol Cell Biol 15:790, 1995

CHAPTER 5

Maternal Physiology

The anatomical, physiological, and biochemical adaptations to pregnancy are profound. Many of these remarkable changes begin soon after fertilization and continue throughout gestation, and most occur in response to physiological stimuli provided by the fetus and placenta. Equally astounding is that the woman who was pregnant is returned almost completely to her prepregnancy state after delivery and lactation.

Many of these physiological adaptations could be perceived as abnormal in the nonpregnant woman. For example, cardiovascular changes during pregnancy normally include substantive increases in blood volume and cardiac output, which may mimic thyrotoxicosis. On the other hand, these same adaptations may lead to ventricular failure if there is underlying heart disease. Thus, physiological adaptations of normal pregnancy can be misinterpreted as pathological but can also unmask or worsen preexisting disease.

During normal pregnancy, virtually every organ system undergoes anatomical and functional changes that can alter appreciably criteria for diagnosis and treatment of diseases. Thus, the understanding of these adaptations to pregnancy remains a major goal of obstetrics, and without such knowledge, it is almost impossible to understand the disease processes that can threaten women during pregnancy.

REPRODUCTIVE TRACT

Uterus

In the nonpregnant woman, the uterus is an almost-solid structure weighing about 70 g and with a cavity of 10 mL or less. During pregnancy, the uterus is transformed into a relatively thin-walled muscular organ of sufficient capacity to accommodate the fetus, placenta, and amnionic fluid. The total volume of the contents at term averages about 5 L but may be 20 L or more. By the end of pregnancy, the uterus has achieved a capacity that is 500 to 1000 times greater than in the nonpregnant state. The corresponding increase in uterine weight is such that, by term, the organ weighs approximately 1100 g.

During pregnancy, uterine enlargement involves stretching and marked hypertrophy of muscle cells, whereas the production of new myocytes is limited. Accompanying the increase in the muscle cell size is an accumulation of fibrous tissue, particularly in the external muscle layer, together with a considerable increase in elastic tissue. The network that is formed adds strength to the uterine wall.

Although the walls of the corpus become considerably thicker during the first few months of pregnancy, they actually thin gradually as gestation advances. By term, they are only 1 to 2 cm or even less in thickness. In these later months, the uterus is changed into a muscular sac with thin, soft, readily indentable walls through which the fetus usually can be palpated.

Uterine hypertrophy early in pregnancy probably is stimulated by the action of estrogen and perhaps that of progesterone. It is apparent that hypertrophy of early pregnancy does not occur entirely in response to mechanical distention by the products of conception, because similar uterine changes are observed with ectopic pregnancy (see Chap. 10, p. 242). But after approximately 12 weeks, the increase in uterine size is related predominantly to pressure exerted by the expanding products of conception.

Uterine enlargement is most marked in the fundus. In the early months of pregnancy, the fallopian tubes and the ovarian and round ligaments attach only slightly below the apex of the fundus. In later months, they are located slightly above the middle of the uterus (see Fig. 2-11, p. 23). The position of the placenta also influences the extent of uterine hypertrophy, because the portion of the uterus surrounding the placental site enlarges more rapidly than does the rest.

Arrangement of the Muscle Cells

The uterine musculature during pregnancy is arranged in three strata:

1. An outer hoodlike layer, which arches over the fundus and extends into the various ligaments.
2. A middle layer, composed of a dense network of muscle fibers perforated in all directions by blood vessels.
3. An internal layer, with sphincter-like fibers around the fallopian tube orifices and internal os of the cervix.

The main portion of the uterine wall is formed by the middle layer. Each cell in this layer has a double curve so that the interlacing of any two gives approximately the form of a figure eight. This arrangement is crucial because when the cells contract after delivery, they constrict the penetrating blood vessels and thus act as ligatures (see Fig. 2-14, p. 25).

Uterine Size, Shape, and Position

For the first few weeks, the uterus maintains its original pear shape, but as pregnancy advances, the corpus and fundus assume a more globular form, becoming almost spherical by 12 weeks. Subsequently, the organ increases more rapidly in length than in width and assumes an ovoid shape. By the end of 12 weeks, the uterus has become too large to remain entirely within the pelvis. As the uterus continues to enlarge, it contacts the anterior abdominal wall, displaces the intestines laterally and superiorly, and continues to rise, ultimately reaching almost to the liver. With ascent of the uterus from the pelvis, it usually undergoes rotation to the right. This *dextrorotation* likely is caused by the rectosigmoid on the left side of the pelvis. As the uterus rises, tension is exerted on the broad and round ligaments.

With the pregnant woman standing, the longitudinal axis of the uterus corresponds to an extension of the axis of the pelvic inlet. The abdominal wall supports the uterus and unless it is quite relaxed, maintains this relation between the long axis of the uterus and the axis of the pelvic inlet. When the pregnant woman is supine, the uterus falls back to rest on the vertebral column and the adjacent great vessels, especially the inferior vena cava and aorta.

Contractility

Beginning in early pregnancy, the uterus undergoes irregular contractions that are normally painless. During the second trimester, these contractions may be detected by bimanual examination. Because attention was first called to this phenomenon in 1872 by J. Braxton Hicks, the contractions have been known by his name. Such contractions appear unpredictably and sporadically and are usually nonrhythmic. Their intensity varies between approximately 5 and 25 mm Hg (Alvarez and Caldeyro-Barcia, 1950). Until the last several weeks of pregnancy, these *Braxton Hicks contractions* are infrequent, but they increase during the last week or two. At this time, the contractions may occur as often as every 10 to 20 minutes and also may assume some degree of rhythmicity. Correspondingly, studies of uterine electrical activity have shown low and uncoordinated patterns early in gestation, which become progressively more intense and synchronized by term (Garfield and associates, 2005). Late in pregnancy, these contractions may cause some discomfort and account for so-called *false labor* (see Chap. 17, p. 390). One clinical implication recently shown is that 75 percent of women with 12 or more of these contractions per hour were diagnosed with active labor within 24 hours (Pates and colleagues, 2007).

Uteroplacental Blood Flow

The delivery of most substances essential for growth and metabolism of the fetus and placenta, as well as removal of most metabolic wastes, is dependent on adequate perfusion of the placental intervillous space (see Chap. 3, p. 55). Placental perfusion is dependent on total uterine blood flow, which is principally from the uterine and ovarian arteries. Uteroplacental blood flow increases progressively during pregnancy, with estimates ranging from 450 to 650 mL/min near term (Edman and associates, 1981; Kauppila and co-workers, 1980).

The results of studies conducted in rats by Page and co-workers (2002) show that the uterine veins also undergo significant adaptations during pregnancy. Specifically, their remodeling includes reduced elastin content and adrenergic nerve density, which results in increased venous caliber and distensibility. Logically, such changes are necessary to accommodate massively increased uteroplacental blood flow.

Assali and co-workers (1968), using electromagnetic flow probes placed directly on a uterine artery, studied the effects of labor on uteroplacental blood flow in sheep and dogs at term. They found that uterine contractions, either spontaneous or induced, caused a decrease in uterine blood flow that was approximately proportional to the intensity of the contraction. They also showed that a tetanic contraction caused a precipitous fall in uterine blood flow. Harbert and associates (1969) made a similar observation in gravid monkeys. Uterine contractions appear to affect fetal circulation much less, and Brar and colleagues (1988) reported no adverse effects on umbilical artery flow.

Regulation of Uteroplacental Blood Flow. The progressive increase in maternal-placental blood flow during gestation occurs principally by means of vasodilation, whereas fetal-placental blood flow is increased by a continuing growth of placental vessels. Palmer and colleagues (1992) showed that uterine artery diameter doubled by 20 weeks and concomitant mean Doppler velocimetry was increased eightfold. It appears likely that vasodilation at this stage of pregnancy is at least in part the consequence of estrogen stimulation. For example, Naden and Rosenfeld (1985) found that 17β-estradiol administration to nonpregnant sheep induced cardiovascular changes similar to those observed in pregnant animals. Using measurements of the uterine artery resistance index, Jauniaux and associates (1994) found that both estradiol and progesterone contributed to the downstream fall in vascular resistance in women with advancing gestational age (see Chap. 16, p. 364).

Other mediators, in addition to estradiol and progesterone, modify vascular resistance during pregnancy, including within the uteroplacental circulation. For example, significant decreases in uterine blood flow and placental perfusion have been demonstrated in sheep following *nicotine* and *catecholamine* infusions (Rosenfeld and co-workers, 1976; Rosenfeld and West, 1977; Xiao and associates, 2007). The latter is likely the consequence of greater sensitivity of the uteroplacental vascular bed to epinephrine and norepinephrine compared with that of the systemic vasculature. In contrast, normal pregnancy is characterized by vascular refractoriness to the pressor effects of infused *angiotensin II* (see p. 120). This insensitivity serves to increase uteroplacental blood flow (Rosenfeld and Gant, 1981; Rosenfeld, 2001). More recently, Rosenfeld and associates (2005) have discovered that large-conductance potassium channels expressed in uterine vascular smooth muscle also contribute to uteroplacental blood flow regulation through several mediators, including estrogen and nitric oxide.

Cervix

As early as 1 month after conception, the cervix begins to undergo pronounced softening and cyanosis. These changes result from increased vascularity and edema of the entire cervix, together with hypertrophy and hyperplasia of the cervical glands (Straach and associates, 2005). Although the cervix contains a small amount of smooth muscle, its major component is connective tissue. Rearrangement of this collagen-rich connective tissue is necessary to permit functions as diverse as maintenance of a pregnancy to term, dilatation to aid delivery, and repair following parturition so that a successful pregnancy can be repeated (see Fig. 6-3, p. 139) (Timmons and Mahendroo, 2007; Word and associates, 2007).

As shown in Figure 5-1, the cervical glands undergo such marked proliferation that by the end of pregnancy they occupy approximately half of the entire cervical mass, rather than a small fraction as in the nonpregnant state. These normal pregnancy-induced changes represent an extension, or *eversion*, of the proliferating columnar endocervical glands. This tissue tends to be red and velvety and bleeds even with minor trauma, such as with Pap smear sampling.

The endocervical mucosal cells produce copious amounts of a tenacious mucus that obstruct the cervical canal soon after conception. As discussed on page 116, this mucus is rich in immunoglobulins and cytokines and may act as an immunological barrier to protect the uterine contents against infection from the vagina (Hein and colleagues, 2005). At the onset of labor, if not before, this *mucus plug* is expelled, resulting in a *bloody show*. Moreover, the consistency of the cervical mucus

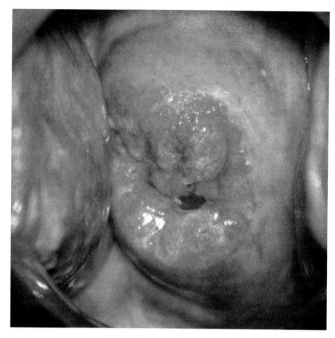

FIGURE 5-1 Cervical eversion of pregnancy as viewed through a colposcope. The eversion represents columnar epithelium on the portio of the cervix. (Used with permission from Dr. Claudia Werner.)

changes during pregnancy. In most pregnant women, when cervical mucus is spread and dried on a glass slide, it is characterized by crystallization, or *beading*, as a result of progesterone. In some women, arborization of the crystals, or *ferning*, is observed as a result of amnionic fluid leakage (see Figs. 8-3 and 8-4, p. 192).

During pregnancy, basal cells near the squamocolumnar junction are likely to be prominent in size, shape, and staining qualities. These changes are considered to be estrogen induced. In addition, pregnancy is associated with both endocervical gland hyperplasia and hypersecretory appearance—the *Arias-Stella reaction*—which makes the identification of atypical glandular cells on Pap smear particularly difficult (Connolly and Evans, 2005).

Ovaries

Ovulation ceases during pregnancy, and the maturation of new follicles is suspended. Ordinarily, only a single corpus luteum can be found in pregnant women. This functions maximally during the first 6 to 7 weeks of pregnancy—4 to 5 weeks postovulation—and thereafter contributes relatively little to progesterone production. These observations have been confirmed by surgical removal of the corpus luteum before 7 weeks—5 weeks postovulation—which results in a rapid fall in maternal serum progesterone and spontaneous abortion (Csapo and co-workers, 1973). After this time, however, corpus luteum removal ordinarily does not cause abortion. Indeed, even bilateral oophorectomy at 16 weeks has been reported to result in an otherwise uneventful pregnancy (Villaseca and associates, 2005). Interestingly in such cases, FSH levels do not reach perimenopausal levels until approximately 5 weeks postpartum.

A *decidual reaction* on and beneath the surface of the ovaries, similar to that found in the endometrial stroma, is common in pregnancy and is usually observed at cesarean delivery. These elevated patches of tissue bleed easily and may, on first glance, resemble freshly torn adhesions. Similar decidual reactions are seen on the uterine serosa and other pelvic, or even extrapelvic, abdominal organs. Although the development of such decidual reactions is incompletely understood, Taussig (1906) and others have deduced that these findings likely represent cellular detritus from the endometrium that has passed through the fallopian tubes.

The enormous caliber of the ovarian veins viewed at cesarean delivery is startling. Hodgkinson (1953) found that the diameter of the ovarian vascular pedicle increased during pregnancy from 0.9 cm to approximately 2.6 cm at term—recall that Poiseuille's law is that flow in a tubular structure is dependent on the product of its radius to the fourth power!

Relaxin

As discussed in Chapter 3 (p. 65), this protein hormone is secreted by the corpus luteum, decidua, and placenta in a pattern similar to that of human chorionic gonadotropin (hCG). It is also expressed in a variety of nonreproductive tissues, including brain, heart, and kidney. It is mentioned here because one of its major biological actions appears to be remodeling of reproductive tract connective tissue to accommodate pregnancy parturition (Park and colleagues, 2005). Relaxin also appears to be an important factor in the initiation of augmented renal hemodynamics (p. 123) and decreased osmolality (p. 112) associated with pregnancy (Smith and associates, 2006). Despite its name, serum relaxin levels do not correlate with increasing peripheral joint laxity during pregnancy (Marnach and co-workers, 2003).

Pregnancy Luteoma

In 1963, Sternberg described a solid ovarian tumor that developed during pregnancy and was composed of large acidophilic luteinized cells, which represented an exaggerated luteinization reaction of the normal ovary. These so-called *luteomas of pregnancy* are variable in size, ranging from microscopic to over 20 cm

in diameter (Fig. 5-2). Typical sonographic characteristics include a solid, complex-appearing unilateral or bilateral mass with cystic features that correspond to areas of hemorrhage. It is usually not possible to differentiate luteomas from other solid ovarian neoplasms, such as luteinized thecoma, granulosa cell tumor, or Leydig cell tumor, by sonographic characteristics alone (Choi and associates, 2000).

Pregnancy luteomas may result in maternal virilization, but usually the female fetus is not affected. This is presumably because of the protective role of the trophoblast with its high capacity to convert androgens and androgen-like steroids to estrogens (Edman and co-workers, 1979). Occasionally, however, a female fetus can become virilized (Spitzer and co-workers, 2007). Although luteomas regress after delivery, they may recur in subsequent pregnancies (Shortle and associates, 1987).

Theca-Lutein Cysts

These benign ovarian lesions result from exaggerated physiological follicle stimulation—termed *hyperreactio luteinalis*. Although the cellular pattern of hyperreactio luteinalis is similar to that of a luteoma, these usually bilateral cystic ovaries are moderately to massively enlarged. The reaction is associated with markedly elevated serum levels of hCG. And not surprisingly, theca-lutein cysts are found frequently with gestational trophoblastic disease (see Chap. 11, p. 259). They are also more likely to be found with a large placenta such as with diabetes, D-isoimmunization, and multiple fetuses (Tanaka and colleagues, 2001). Theca-lutein cysts have also been reported in chronic renal failure as a result of reduced hCG clearance, and in hyperthyroidism as a result of the structural homology between hCG and thyroid-stimulating hormone (Coccia and colleagues, 2003; Gherman and co-workers, 2003). But they also are encountered in women with otherwise uncomplicated pregnancies and are thought to result from an exaggerated response of the ovaries to normal levels of circulating hCG (Langer and Coleman, 2007).

Although usually asymptomatic, hemorrhage into the cysts may cause abdominal pain. Maternal virilization may be seen in up to 25 percent of women (Foulk and associates, 1997). Changes including temporal balding, hirsutism, and clitoromegaly are associated with massively elevated levels of androstenedione and testosterone. The diagnosis typically is based on sonographic findings of bilateral enlarged ovaries containing multiple cysts in the appropriate clinical settings. The condition is self-limited, and resolution follows delivery. In some women, increased ovarian responsiveness to gonadotropin can be confirmed by several weeks postpartum (Bradshaw and co-workers, 1986; Sherer and associates, 2006). Their management is discussed further in Chapter 40 (p. 904).

Fallopian Tubes

The musculature of the fallopian tubes undergoes little hypertrophy during pregnancy. The epithelium of the tubal mucosa, however, becomes somewhat flattened. Decidual cells may develop in the stroma of the endosalpinx, but a continuous decidual membrane is not formed. Very rarely, the increasing size of the gravid uterus, especially in the presence of paratubal or ovarian cysts, may result in fallopian tube torsion (Batukan and co-workers, 2007).

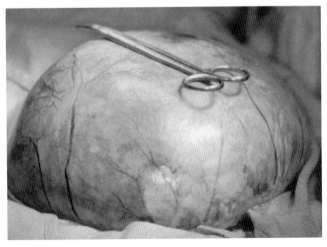

FIGURE 5-2 Large luteoma of pregnancy removed at laparotomy postpartum.

Vagina and Perineum

During pregnancy, increased vascularity and hyperemia develop in the skin and muscles of the perineum and vulva, with softening of the underlying abundant connective tissue. Increased vascularity prominently affects the vagina and results in the violet color characteristic of *Chadwick sign*. The vaginal walls undergo striking changes in preparation for the distention that accompanies labor and delivery. These changes include a considerable increase in mucosal thickness, loosening of the connective tissue, and hypertrophy of smooth muscle cells. The papillae of the vaginal epithelium undergo hypertrophy to create a fine, hobnailed appearance.

The considerably increased volume of cervical secretions within the vagina during pregnancy consists of a somewhat thick, white discharge. The pH is acidic, varying from 3.5 to 6. This results from increased production of lactic acid from glycogen in the vaginal epithelium by the action of *Lactobacillus acidophilus*.

SKIN

Blood Flow in Skin

Increased cutaneous blood flow in pregnancy serves to dissipate excess heat generated by increased metabolism (see Chap. 56, p. 1187).

Abdominal Wall

Beginning after midpregnancy, reddish, slightly depressed streaks commonly develop in the abdominal skin and sometimes in the skin over the breasts and thighs. These are called *striae gravidarum* or *stretch marks*. In multiparous women, in addition to the reddish striae of the present pregnancy, glistening, silvery lines that represent the cicatrices of previous striae frequently are seen. In a study of 110 primiparous patients, Osman and colleagues (2007) reported that 48 percent developed striae gravidarum on their abdomen; 25 percent, on their breasts; and 25 percent, on their thighs. The strongest associated risk factors were weight gain during pregnancy, younger maternal age, and family history.

Occasionally, the muscles of the abdominal walls do not withstand the tension to which they are subjected. As a result, rectus muscles separate in the midline, creating a *diastasis recti* of varying extent. If severe, a considerable portion of the anterior uterine wall is covered by only a layer of skin, attenuated fascia, and peritoneum. True fascial defects lead to ventral hernia, which uncommonly require antepartum surgical correction.

Hyperpigmentation

This develops in up to 90 percent of women. It is usually more accentuated in those with a darker complexion (Muallem and Rubeiz, 2006). The midline of the abdominal skin—*linea alba*—becomes especially pigmented, assuming a brownish-black color to form the *linea nigra*. Occasionally, irregular brownish patches of varying size appear on the face and neck, giving rise to *chloasma* or *melasma gravidarum*—the so-called *mask of pregnancy*. Pigmentation of the areolae and genital skin may also be accentuated. These pigmentary changes usually disappear, or at least regress considerably, after delivery. Oral contraceptives may cause similar pigmentation.

Very little is known of the nature of these pigmentary changes, although melanocyte-stimulating hormone, a polypeptide similar to corticotropin, has been shown to be elevated remarkably from the end of the second month of pregnancy until term. Estrogen and progesterone also are reported to have melanocyte-stimulating effects. These conditions are considered in greater detail in Chapter 56 (p. 1185).

Vascular Changes

Angiomas, called *vascular spiders,* develop in about two thirds of white women and approximately 10 percent of black women. These are minute, red elevations on the skin, particularly common on the face, neck, upper chest, and arms, with radicles branching out from a central lesion. The condition is often designated as nevus, angioma, or telangiectasis. *Palmar erythema* is encountered during pregnancy in about two thirds of white women and one third of black women. The two conditions are of no clinical significance and disappear in most women shortly after pregnancy. They are most likely the consequence of hyperestrogenemia.

BREASTS

In the early weeks of pregnancy, women often experience breast tenderness and paresthesias. After the second month, the breasts increase in size, and delicate veins become visible just beneath the skin. The nipples become considerably larger, more deeply pigmented, and more erectile. After the first few months, a thick, yellowish fluid—*colostrum*—can often be expressed from the nipples by gentle massage. During the same months, the areolae become broader and more deeply pigmented. Scattered through the areolae are a number of small elevations, the *glands of Montgomery,* which are hypertrophic sebaceous glands. If the increase in breast size is extensive, striations similar to those observed in the abdomen may develop. Rarely, breast enlargement may become so pathologically extensive—referred to as *gigantomastia*—that it requires surgical intervention (Pasrija and Sharma, 2006; Vidaeff and associates, 2003). Interestingly, prepregnancy breast size and volume of milk production do not correlate (Hytten, 1995). Histological and functional changes of the breasts induced by pregnancy and lactation are further discussed in Chapter 30 (p. 649).

METABOLIC CHANGES

In response to the increased demands of the rapidly growing fetus and placenta, the pregnant woman undergoes metabolic changes that are numerous and intense. Certainly no other physiological event in postnatal life induces such profound

TABLE 5-1. Analysis of Weight Gain Based on Physiological Events During Pregnancy

Tissues and Fluids	Cumulative Increase in Weight (g)			
	10 Weeks	20 Weeks	30 Weeks	40 Weeks
Fetus	5	300	1500	3400
Placenta	20	170	430	650
Amnionic fluid	30	350	750	800
Uterus	140	320	600	970
Breasts	45	180	360	405
Blood	100	600	1300	1450
Extravascular fluid	0	30	80	1480
Maternal stores (fat)	310	2050	3480	3345
Total	650	4000	8500	12,500

Modified from Hytten (1991).

metabolic alterations. By the third trimester, maternal basal metabolic rate is increased by 10 to 20 percent compared with that of the nonpregnant state. This is increased by an additional 10 percent in women with twin gestations (Shinagawa and associates, 2005). Viewed another way, additional total pregnancy energy demands are estimated to be as high as 80,000 kcal or about 300 kcal/day (Hytten and Chamberlain, 1991).

Weight Gain

Most of the normal increase in weight during pregnancy is attributable to the uterus and its contents, the breasts, and increases in blood volume and extravascular extracellular fluid. A smaller fraction of the increased weight is the result of metabolic alterations that result in an increase in cellular water and deposition of new fat and protein—so-called *maternal reserves.* Hytten (1991) reported that the average weight gain during pregnancy is approximately 12.5 kg or 27.5 lb (Table 5-1). Maternal aspects of weight gain are considered in greater detail in Chapter 8 (p. 200).

Water Metabolism

Increased water retention is a normal physiological alteration of pregnancy. It is mediated, at least in part, by a fall in plasma osmolality of approximately 10 mOsm/kg induced by a resetting of osmotic thresholds for thirst and vasopressin secretion (Heenan and colleagues, 2003; Lindheimer and Davison, 1995). As shown in Figure 5-3, this phenomenon is functioning by early pregnancy.

At term, the water content of the fetus, placenta, and amnionic fluid approximates 3.5 L. Another 3.0 L accumulates as a result of increases in the maternal blood volume and in the size of the uterus and breasts. Thus, the minimum amount of extra water that the average woman accrues during normal pregnancy is approximately 6.5 L. Clearly demonstrable pitting edema of the ankles and legs is seen in most pregnant women, especially at the end of the day. This accumulation of fluid, which may amount to a liter or so, is caused by increased venous pressure below the level of the uterus as a consequence of partial vena cava occlusion. A decrease in interstitial colloid osmotic pressure induced by normal pregnancy also favors edema late in pregnancy (Øian and co-workers, 1985).

Longitudinal studies of body composition have shown a progressive increase in total body water and fat mass during pregnancy. Both initial maternal weight and weight gained during pregnancy are highly associated with birthweight. It is unclear, however, what role maternal fat or water have in fetal growth. Studies in well-nourished women suggest that maternal body water, rather than fat, contributes more significantly to infant birthweight (Lederman and co-workers, 1999; Mardones-Santander and associates, 1998).

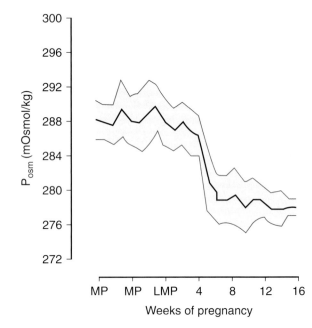

FIGURE 5-3 Mean values (*black line*) ± standard deviations (*blue lines*) for plasma osmolality (P$_{osm}$) measured at weekly intervals in nine women from preconception to 16 weeks. (LMP = last menstrual period; MP = menstrual period.) (From Davison and colleagues, 1981, with permission.)

3078

Protein Metabolism

The products of conception, the uterus, and maternal blood are relatively rich in protein rather than fat or carbohydrate. At term, the fetus and placenta together weigh about 4 kg and contain approximately 500 g of protein, or about half of the total pregnancy increase (Hytten and Leitch, 1971). The remaining 500 g is added to the uterus as contractile protein, to the breasts primarily in the glands, and to the maternal blood as hemoglobin and plasma proteins.

Amino acid concentrations are higher in the fetal than in the maternal compartment (Cetin and co-workers, 2005; van den Akker and associates, 2009). This increased concentration is largely regulated by the placenta, which not only concentrates amino acids into the fetal circulation, but also is involved in protein synthesis, oxidation, and transamination of some nonessential amino acids (Galan and colleagues, 2009).

Mojtahedi and associates (2002) measured *nitrogen balance* across pregnancy in 12 healthy women. It increased with gestation and thus suggested a more efficient use of dietary protein. They also found that urinary excretion of 3-methylhistidine did not change, indicating that breakdown of maternal muscle is not required to meet metabolic demands. Further support that pregnancy is associated with nitrogen conservation comes from Kalhan and colleagues (2003), who found that the turnover rate of nonessential serine decreases across gestation. The daily requirements for dietary protein intake during pregnancy are discussed in Chapter 8 (p. 202).

Carbohydrate Metabolism

Normal pregnancy is characterized by mild fasting hypoglycemia, postprandial hyperglycemia, and hyperinsulinemia (Fig. 5-4). This increased basal level of plasma insulin in normal pregnancy is associated with several unique responses to glucose ingestion. For example, after an oral glucose meal, gravid women demonstrate both prolonged hyperglycemia and hyperinsulinemia as well as a greater suppression of glucagon (Phelps and associates, 1981). This cannot be explained by a decreased metabolism of insulin because its half-life during pregnancy is not changed (Lind and associates, 1977). Instead, this response is consistent with a pregnancy-induced state of peripheral insulin resistance, the purpose of which is likely to ensure a sustained postprandial supply of glucose to the fetus. Indeed, insulin sensitivity in late normal pregnancy is 45 to 70 percent lower than that of nonpregnant women (Butte, 2000; Freemark, 2006).

The mechanism(s) responsible for insulin resistance is not completely understood. Progesterone and estrogen may act, directly or indirectly, to mediate this resistance. Plasma levels of placental lactogen increase with gestation, and this protein hormone is characterized by growth hormone–like action that may result in increased lipolysis with liberation of free fatty acids (Freinkel, 1980). The increased concentration of circulating free fatty acids also may aid increased tissue resistance to insulin (Freemark, 2006).

The pregnant woman changes rapidly from a postprandial state characterized by elevated and sustained glucose levels to a fasting state characterized by decreased plasma glucose and some amino acids. Simultaneously, plasma concentrations of

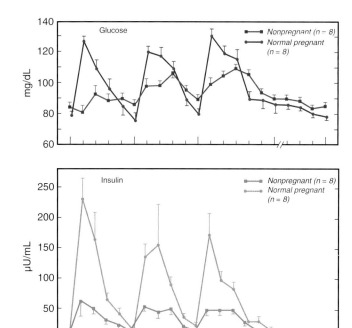

FIGURE 5-4 Diurnal changes in plasma glucose and insulin in normal late pregnancy. (This figure was redrawn from *American Journal of Obstetrics & Gynecology,* Vol. 140, No. 7, RL Phelps, BE Metzger, and N Freinkel, Carbohydrate metabolism in pregnancy. XVII. Diurnal profiles of plasma glucose, insulin, free fatty acids, triglycerides, cholesterol, and individual amino acids in late normal pregnancy, pp. 730–736, Copyright Elsevier 1981, with permission.)

free fatty acids, triglycerides, and cholesterol are higher. Freinkel and colleagues (1985) have referred to this pregnancy-induced switch in fuels from glucose to lipids as *accelerated starvation.* Certainly, when fasting is prolonged in the pregnant woman, these alterations are exaggerated and ketonemia rapidly appears.

Fat Metabolism

The concentrations of lipids, lipoproteins, and apolipoproteins in plasma increase appreciably during pregnancy. The storage of fat occurs primarily during midpregnancy (Hytten and Thomson, 1968; Pipe and co-workers, 1979). This fat is deposited mostly in central rather than peripheral sites. It becomes available for placental transfer during the last trimester when fetal growth rate is maximal along with essential fatty acids requirements (Herrera and colleagues, 2006; Innis, 2005). It may be that progesterone acts to reset a lipostat in the hypothalamus, and at the end of pregnancy, the lipostat returns to its previous nonpregnant level, and the added fat is lost (Hytten and Thomson, 1968). Such a mechanism for energy storage, theoretically at least, might protect the mother and fetus during prolonged starvation or hard physical exertion.

Maternal hyperlipidemia is one of the most consistent and striking changes to take place in lipid metabolism during late pregnancy. Triacylglycerol and cholesterol levels in very-low-density lipoprotein (VLDL), low-density lipoproteins (LDLs), and high-density lipoproteins (HDLs) are increased during the third trimester compared with those in nonpregnant women. The mechanisms responsible for these changes include increased lipolytic and decreased lipoprotein lipase activities in adipose tissue (Herrera and colleagues, 2006). The hepatic effects of estradiol and progesterone also play an important role (Desoye and associates, 1987).

During the third trimester, average total serum cholesterol, LDL-C, HDL-C, and triglyceride levels are approximately 267 ± 30 mg/dL, 136 ± 33 mg/dL, 81 ± 17 mg/dL, and 245 ± 73 mg/dL, respectively (Lippi and associates, 2007). After delivery, the concentrations of these lipids, as well as lipoproteins and apolipoproteins decrease. Lactation speeds the change in levels of many of these (Darmady and Postle, 1982).

Hyperlipidemia is of some concern because it is associated with endothelial dysfunction. From their studies, however, Saarelainen and associates (2006) found that endothelium-dependent vasodilation responses actually improved across pregnancy. This was partly because increased concentrations of HDL-cholesterol likely inhibit oxidation of low-density lipoprotein and thus protect the endothelium. Their findings suggest that the increased risk of cardiovascular disease in multiparous women may be related to factors other than maternal hypercholesterolemia.

Leptin

In nonpregnant humans, this peptide hormone is primarily secreted by adipose tissue. It has a key role in the regulation of body fat and energy expenditure. Maternal serum leptin levels increase and peak during the second trimester and plateau until term in concentrations two to four times higher than those in nonpregnant women. This increase is only partially due to pregnancy weight gain, because leptin also is produced in significant amounts by the placenta. Indeed, placental weight is significantly correlated with leptin levels measured in umbilical cord blood (Pighetti and co-workers, 2003). Hauguel-de Mouzon and associates (2006) have hypothesized that increased leptin production may be critical for the regulation of increased maternal energy demands. Leptin may also help to regulate fetal growth and play a role in fetal macrosomia as well as growth restriction (Gohlke, 2006; Grisaru-Granovsky, 2008; Henson, 2006, Lepercq, 2003, and all their associates). This topic is discussed further in Chapter 38 (p. 842).

Ghrelin

This is another hormone secreted by adipose tissue that likely has a role in fetal growth and cell proliferation. It is also expressed in placental tissue, and this hormone regulates growth hormone secretion. Maternal serum levels of ghrelin increase and peak at midpregnancy and then decrease until term (Fuglsang, 2008). This is explicable in that ghrelin levels are known to be decreased in other insulin-resistant states such as metabolic syndrome (Riedl and associates, 2007).

Electrolyte and Mineral Metabolism

During normal pregnancy, nearly 1000 mEq of *sodium* and 300 mEq of *potassium* are retained (Lindheimer and colleagues, 1987). Although the glomerular filtration of sodium and potassium is increased, the excretion of these electrolytes is unchanged during pregnancy as a result of enhanced tubular resorption (Brown and colleagues, 1986, 1988). And although there are increased total accumulations of sodium and potassium, their serum concentrations are decreased slightly because of expanded plasma volume (see Appendix). Still, they remain very near the range of normal for nonpregnant women (Kametas and colleagues, 2003b).

Total serum *calcium* levels decline during pregnancy, the reduction reflecting lowered plasma albumin concentration and, in turn, the consequent decrease in the amount bound to protein. Levels of serum ionized calcium, however, remain unchanged (Power and associates, 1999). The developing fetus imposes a significant demand on maternal calcium homeostasis. For example, the fetal skeleton accretes approximately 30 g of calcium by term, 80 percent of which is deposited during the third trimester. This demand is largely met by a doubling of maternal intestinal calcium absorption mediated, in part, by 1,25-dihydroxyvitamin D_3 (Kovacs and Fuleihan, 2006). In addition, dietary intake of sufficient calcium is necessary to prevent excess depletion from the mother (see Table 8-7, p. 201). This is especially important in pregnant adolescents, in whom bones are still developing (Repke, 1994).

Serum *magnesium* levels also decline during pregnancy. Bardicef and colleagues (1995) concluded that pregnancy is actually a state of extracellular magnesium depletion. Compared with nonpregnant women, they found that both total and ionized magnesium were significantly lower during normal pregnancy. Serum *phosphate* levels are within the nonpregnant range (Kametas and colleagues, 2003b). The renal threshold for inorganic phosphate excretion is elevated in pregnancy due to increased calcitonin (Weiss and colleagues, 1998).

With respect to most other minerals, pregnancy induces little change in their metabolism other than their retention in amounts equivalent to those needed for growth (see Chap. 4, p. 88, and Chap. 8, p. 202). An important exception is the considerably increased requirement for *iron,* which is discussed subsequently.

HEMATOLOGICAL CHANGES

Blood Volume

The well-known hypervolemia associated with normal pregnancy averages 40 to 45 percent above the nonpregnant blood volume after 32 to 34 weeks (Pritchard, 1965; Whittaker and associates, 1996). In individual women, expansion varies considerably. In some there is only a modest increase, whereas in others the blood volume nearly doubles. A fetus is not essential for this because increased blood volume develops in some women with hydatidiform mole (Pritchard, 1965).

Pregnancy-induced hypervolemia has important functions:

1. To meet the metabolic demands of the enlarged uterus with its greatly hypertrophied vascular system.
2. To provide an abundance of nutrients and elements to support the rapidly growing placenta and fetus.
3. To protect the mother and in turn the fetus, against the deleterious effects of impaired venous return in the supine and erect positions.
4. To safeguard the mother against the adverse effects of blood loss associated with parturition.

Maternal blood volume begins to increase during the first trimester. By 12 menstrual weeks, plasma volume expands by approximately 15 percent compared with that of prepregnancy (Bernstein and co-workers, 2001). As shown in Figure 5-5, maternal blood volume expands most rapidly during the second trimester. It then rises at a much slower rate during the third trimester to plateau during the last several weeks of pregnancy.

Blood volume expansion results from an increase in both plasma and erythrocytes. Although more plasma than erythrocytes is usually added to the maternal circulation, the increase in erythrocyte volume is considerable, averaging about 450 mL (Pritchard and Adams, 1960). Moderate erythroid hyperplasia is present in the bone marrow, and the reticulocyte count is elevated slightly during normal pregnancy. As discussed in Chapter 51 (p. 1079), these changes are almost certainly related to the increase in maternal plasma erythropoietin levels, which peak early during the third trimester and correspond to maximal erythrocyte production (Clapp and colleagues, 2003; Harstad and co-workers, 1992).

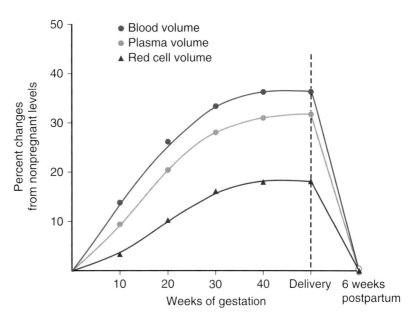

FIGURE 5-5 Changes in total blood volume and its components (plasma and red cell volumes) during pregnancy and postpartum. (From Peck and Arias, 1979, with permission.)

Hemoglobin Concentration and Hematocrit

Because of great plasma augmentation, hemoglobin concentration and hematocrit decrease slightly during pregnancy (see Appendix). As a result, whole blood viscosity decreases (Huisman and colleagues, 1987). Hemoglobin concentration at term averages 12.5 g/dL, and in approximately 5 percent of women, it is below 11.0 g/dL (Table 51-1, p. 1080). Thus, a hemoglobin concentration below 11.0 g/dL, especially late in pregnancy, should be considered abnormal and usually due to iron deficiency rather than due to hypervolemia of pregnancy.

Iron Metabolism

Storage Iron

The total iron content of normal adult women ranges from 2.0 to 2.5 g or about half the amount found normally in men. Importantly, the iron stores of normal young women are only approximately 300 mg (Pritchard and Mason, 1964).

Iron Requirements

Of the approximate 1000 mg of iron required for normal pregnancy, about 300 mg are actively transferred to the fetus and placenta, and another 200 mg are lost through various normal routes of excretion, primarily the gastrointestinal tract. These are obligatory losses and occur even when the mother is iron deficient. The average increase in the total volume of circulating erythrocytes—about 450 mL—requires another 500 mg because 1 mL of erythrocytes contains 1.1 mg of iron. Because most iron is used during the latter half of pregnancy, the iron requirement becomes large after midpregnancy and averages 6 to 7 mg/day

(Pritchard and Scott, 1970). This amount is usually not available from storage iron in most women, and the optimal increase in maternal erythrocyte volume will not develop without supplemental iron. Without supplementation, the hemoglobin concentration and hematocrit fall appreciably as the blood volume increases. At the same time, fetal red cell production is not impaired because the placenta transfers iron even when the mother has severe iron deficiency anemia. In severe cases, we have documented hemoglobin values of 3 g/dL and hematocrits of 10 percent.

It follows that the amount of dietary iron, together with that mobilized from stores, will be insufficient to meet the average demands imposed by pregnancy. As shown in Figure 5-6, if the

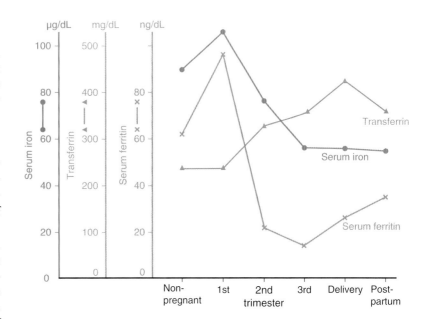

FIGURE 5-6 Indices of iron turnover during pregnancy in women without overt anemia but who were not given iron supplementation. (From Kaneshige, 1981, with permission.)

nonanemic pregnant woman is not given supplemental iron, which is discussed in Chapter 8, then serum iron and ferritin concentrations decline after midpregnancy. The early pregnancy increases in serum iron and ferritin are likely due to minimal iron demands early on combined with the positive iron balance from amenorrhea (see Fig. 5-6).

The Puerperium

Generally, not all the maternal iron added in the form of hemoglobin is lost with normal delivery. At the time of vaginal delivery, and through the next few days, only approximately half of the added erythrocytes are lost from most women. These normal losses are from the placental implantation site, episiotomy or lacerations, and lochia. On average, maternal erythrocytes corresponding to approximately 500 to 600 mL of predelivery whole blood are lost with vaginal delivery of a single fetus (Pritchard, 1965; Ueland, 1976). The average blood loss associated with cesarean delivery or with the vaginal delivery of twins is about 1000 mL (see Fig. 35-2, p. 760).

Immunological Functions

Pregnancy is thought to be associated with suppression of a variety of humoral and cell-mediated immunological functions to accommodate the "foreign" semiallogeneic fetal graft (Thellin and Heinen, 2003). This is discussed further in Chapter 3 (p. 58). One mechanism appears to involve suppression of T-helper (Th) 1 and T-cytotoxic (Tc) 1 cells, which decreases secretion of interleukin-2(IL-2), interferon-γ, and tumor necrosis factor-β (TNF-β). There is also evidence that a suppressed Th1 response is requisite for pregnancy continuation. It also may explain pregnancy-related remission of some autoimmune disorders. Examples include rheumatoid arthritis, multiple sclerosis, and autoimmune thyroiditis—which are Th1-mediated diseases (Kumru and colleagues, 2005). As discussed in Chapter 34 (p. 711), failure of Th1 immune suppression may be related to development of preeclampsia (Jonsson and co-workers, 2006).

Not all aspects of immunological function are depressed. For example, there is upregulation of Th2 cells to increase secretion of IL-4, IL-6, and IL-13 (Michimata and colleagues, 2003). In cervical mucus, peak levels of immunoglobulins A and G (IgA and IgG) are significantly higher during pregnancy. Similarly, the amount of interleukin-1β found in cervical mucus during pregnancy is approximately 10-fold greater than in nonpregnant women. Because oral contraceptives have been shown to induce similar changes, Kutteh and Franklin (2001) hypothesized that changes in the cervical mucus may be a result of estrogen and progesterone. Although these changes may be important for fetal protection, their actual clinical significance is unclear.

Leukocytes

Some polymorphonuclear leukocyte chemotaxis and adherence functions are depressed beginning in the second trimester and continuing throughout pregnancy (Krause and associates, 1987). Although incompletely understood, this may be partly related to the finding that relaxin (see p. 110) impairs neutrophil activation (Masini and co-workers, 2004). It is possible that these depressed leukocyte functions of pregnant women also ac-

count in part for the improvement of some autoimmune disorders and possible increased susceptibility to certain infections.

Although the leukocyte count varies considerably during pregnancy, usually it ranges from 5000 to 12,000/μL. During labor and the early puerperium, it may become markedly elevated, attaining levels of 25,000/μL or even more, however, it averages 14,000 to 16,000/μL (Taylor and co-workers, 1981). The cause for the marked increase is not known, but the same response occurs during and after strenuous exercise. It probably represents the reappearance of leukocytes previously shunted out of active circulation. Interestingly, increasing numbers of immune cells are also found in the uterine wall during normal pregnancy. Garfield and co-workers (2006) have found that these cells, especially mast cells, may play an important role in mediating uterine contractility.

In addition to normal variations in the leukocyte count, the distribution of cell types is altered significantly during pregnancy. Specifically, during the third trimester, the percentages of granulocytes and CD8 T lymphocytes are significantly increased along with a concomitant reduction in the percentages of CD4 T lymphocytes and monocytes. Moreover, circulating leukocytes undergo significant phenotypic changes including, for example, the upregulation of certain adhesion molecules (Luppi and associates, 2002).

Inflammatory Markers

Many tests performed to diagnose inflammation cannot be used reliably during pregnancy. For example, *leukocyte alkaline phosphatase* levels are used to evaluate myeloproliferative disorders and are increased beginning early in pregnancy. The concentration of *C-reactive protein,* an acute-phase serum reactant, rises rapidly to 1000-fold in response to tissue trauma or inflammation. Watts and colleagues (1991) measured C-reactive protein levels across pregnancy and found that median values were higher than for nonpregnant women. Levels were elevated further in labor. In women not in labor, 95 percent had levels of 1.5 mg/dL or less, and gestational age did not affect serum levels. Another marker of inflammation, the *erythrocyte sedimentation rate (ESR),* is increased in normal pregnancy because of elevated plasma globulins and fibrinogen (Hytten and Leitch, 1971). Lastly, *complement factors C3* and *C4* also are significantly elevated during the second and third trimesters (Gallery and colleagues, 1981; Richani and associates, 2005).

Coagulation and Fibrinolysis

During normal pregnancy, both coagulation and fibrinolysis are augmented but remain balanced to maintain hemostasis. They are even more enhanced in multifetal gestation (Morikawa and colleagues, 2006). Evidence of activation includes increased concentrations of all clotting factors, except factors XI and XIII, and increased levels of high-molecular-weight fibrinogen complexes (Table 5-2). The clotting time of whole blood, however, does not differ significantly in normal pregnant women. Considering the substantive physiological increase in plasma volume in normal pregnancy, such increased concentrations represent a markedly augmented production of these procoagulants. For example, plasma fibrinogen (factor I) in normal nonpregnant women averages about 300 mg/dL and ranges from 200 to 400 mg/dL.

TABLE 5-2. Changes in Measures of Hemostasis During Normal Pregnancy

Parameter	Nonpregnant	Pregnant (35–40 weeks)
Activated PTT (sec)	31.6 ± 4.9	31.9 ± 2.9
Thrombin time (sec)	18.9 ± 2.0	22.4 ± 4.1[a]
Fibrinogen (mg/dL)	256 ± 58	473 ± 72[a]
Factor VII (%)	99.3 ± 19.4	181.4 ± 48.0[a]
Factor X (%)	97.7 ± 15.4	144.5 ± 20.1[a]
Plasminogen (%)	105.5 ± 14.1	136.2 ± 19.5[a]
tPA (ng/mL)	5.7 ± 3.6	5.0 ± 1.5
Antithrombin III (%)	98.9 ± 13.2	97.5 ± 33.3
Protein C (%)	77.2 ± 12.0	62.9 ± 20.5[a]
Total Protein S (%)	75.6 ± 14.0	49.9 ± 10.2[a]

[a]Statistically significant difference.
Data shown as mean ± standard deviation.
PTT = prothrombin time; tPA = tissue-type plasminogen activator.
Reprinted from *European Journal of Obstetrics & Gynecology and Reproductive Biology,*
Vol. 119, EH Uchikova and II Ledjev, Changes in haemostasis during normal pregnancy,
pp. 185–188, Copyright 2005, with permission from Elsevier.

During normal pregnancy, fibrinogen concentration increases approximately 50 percent. It averages 450 mg/dL late in pregnancy, with a range from 300 to 600 mg/dL. The percentage of high-molecular-weight fibrinogen is unchanged (Manten and colleagues, 2004). This contributes greatly to the striking increase in the *erythrocyte sedimentation rate* as discussed previously. Some of the pregnancy-induced changes in the levels of coagulation factors can be duplicated by the administration of estrogen plus progestin contraceptive tablets to nonpregnant women.

The end product of the coagulation cascade is fibrin formation, and the main function of the fibrinolytic system is to remove excess fibrin. Tissue plasminogen activator (tPA) converts plasminogen into plasmin, which causes fibrinolysis and produces fibrin degradation products such as D-dimers. Studies of the fibrinolytic system in pregnancy have produced conflicting results, although most evidence suggests that fibrinolytic activity is actually reduced in normal pregnancy. For example, tPA activity gradually decreases over the course of normal pregnancy. Moreover, plasminogen activator inhibitor type 1 (PAI-2) and type 2 (PAI-2), which inhibit tPA and regulate fibrin degradation by plasmin, increase during normal pregnancy (Robb and co-workers, 2009). As reviewed by Holmes and Wallace (2005), these changes—which may indicate that the fibrinolytic system is impaired—are countered by increased levels of plasminogen and decreased levels of another plasmin inhibitor, α_2 antiplasmin. Such changes serve to ensure hemostatic balance during normal pregnancy.

Platelets

Normal pregnancy also involves changes in platelets (Baker and Cunningham, 1999). In a study of almost 7000 healthy women at term, Boehlen and associates (2000) found that the average platelet count was decreased slightly during pregnancy to 213,000/µL compared with 250,000/µL in nonpregnant control women. They defined thrombocytopenia as below the 2.5th percentile, which corresponded to a platelet count of 116,000/mL. Decreased platelet concentrations are partially due to the effects of

hemodilution. However, they also likely represent increased platelet consumption, leading to a greater proportion of younger, and therefore, larger platelets (Tygart and co-workers, 1986). Further supporting this concept, Hayashi and associates (2002) found that beginning in midpregnancy, production of thromboxane A_2, which induces platelet aggregation, progressively increases.

Regulatory Proteins

There are a number of natural inhibitors of coagulation, including proteins C, S, and Z and antithrombin. Inherited or acquired deficiencies of these and other natural regulatory proteins—collectively referred to as thrombophilias—account for many thromboembolic episodes during pregnancy. They are discussed in detail in Chapter 47.

Activated protein C, along with the co-factors protein S and factor V, functions as an anticoagulant by neutralizing the procoagulants factor Va and factor VIIIa (see Fig. 47-1, p. 1016). At the same time, resistance to activated protein C increases progressively and is related to a concomitant decrease in free protein S and increase in factor VIII. Between the first and third trimesters, levels of activated protein C decrease from about 2.4 to 1.9 U/mL, and free protein S decreases from 0.4 to 0.16 U/mL (Walker and colleagues, 1997). Oral contraceptives also decrease free protein S levels. *Protein Z* is a vitamin-K dependent glycoprotein that inhibits activation of factor X. Quack Loetscher and co-workers (2005) reported a 20-percent increase across pregnancy. Effraimidou and associates (2009) have speculated that low protein Z levels may prove to be a risk factor for otherwise unexplained recurrent early pregnancy loss. Levels of *antithrombin* remain relatively constant throughout gestation and the early puerperium (Delorme and associates, 1992).

Spleen

By the end of normal pregnancy, the splenic area enlarges by up to 50 percent compared with the first trimester. The echogenic appearance of the spleen remains homogeneous throughout gestation (Maymon and co-workers, 2007).

CARDIOVASCULAR SYSTEM

During pregnancy and the puerperium, the heart and circulation undergo remarkable physiological adaptations. Changes in cardiac function become apparent during the first 8 weeks of pregnancy (McLaughlin and Roberts, 1999). Cardiac output is increased as early as the fifth week and reflects a reduced systemic vascular resistance and an increased heart rate. The resting pulse rate increases about 10 beats/min during pregnancy (Stein and co-workers, 1999). Between weeks 10 and 20, plasma volume expansion begins and preload is increased. Ventricular performance during pregnancy is influenced by both the decrease in systemic vascular resistance and changes in pulsatile arterial flow. As discussed subsequently, multiple factors contribute to these changes in overall hemodynamic function and allow the cardiovascular system to adjust to the physiological demands of the fetus while maintaining maternal cardiovascular integrity. These changes during the last half of pregnancy are graphically summarized in Figure 5-7, which also shows the important effects of maternal posture on hemodynamic events during pregnancy.

Heart

As the diaphragm becomes progressively elevated, the heart is displaced to the left and upward and rotated somewhat on its long axis. As a result, the apex is moved somewhat laterally from its usual position, causing a larger cardiac silhouette on chest radiograph (Fig. 5-8). Furthermore, pregnant women normally have some degree of benign pericardial effusion, which may in-

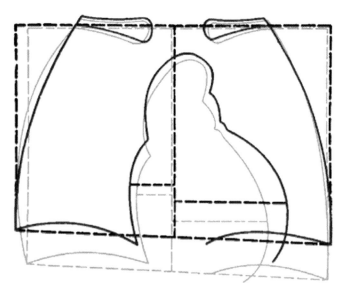

FIGURE 5-8 Change in cardiac outline that occurs in pregnancy. The blue lines represent the relations between the heart and thorax in the nonpregnant woman, and the black lines represent the conditions existing in pregnancy. These findings are based on radiographic findings in 33 women. (Redrawn from Klafen and Palugyay, 1927, with permission.)

crease the cardiac silhouette (Enein and colleagues, 1987). Variability of these factors makes it difficult to precisely identify moderate degrees of cardiomegaly by simple radiographic studies. Normal pregnancy induces no characteristic electrocardiographic changes other than slight left-axis deviation as a result of the altered heart position.

Many of the normal *cardiac sounds* are altered during pregnancy. Cutforth and MacDonald (1966) used phonocardiography and documented: (1) an exaggerated splitting of the first heart sound with increased loudness of both components; (2) no definite changes in the aortic and pulmonary elements of the second sound; and (3) a loud, easily heard third sound (Fig. 44-1, p. 960). They heard a systolic murmur in 90 percent of pregnant women that was intensified during inspiration in some or expiration in others, and disappeared shortly after delivery. A soft diastolic murmur was noted transiently in 20 percent, and continuous murmurs arising from the breast vasculature in 10 percent.

The increased plasma volume during normal pregnancy, which was discussed previously (p. 115), leads to several reversible morphological and functional adaptations. There is no doubt that the heart is capable of remodeling in response to stimuli such as hypertension and exercise. Cardiac *plasticity* likely is a continuum that encompasses physiological growth, such as that in exercise, as well as pathological hypertrophy—such as with hypertension (Hill and Olson, 2008). And although it is widely held that there is physiological hypertrophy of cardiac myocytes as a result of pregnancy, this has never been absolutely proven. For example, in one study, Schannwell and associates (2002) performed serial echocardiographic examinations across pregnancy and postpartum in 46 healthy women and found a 34-percent greater left ventricular muscle mass index during late versus early pregnancy. These and earlier studies with similar findings were derived with echocardiography but have not been verified with the more precise techniques of magnetic resonance

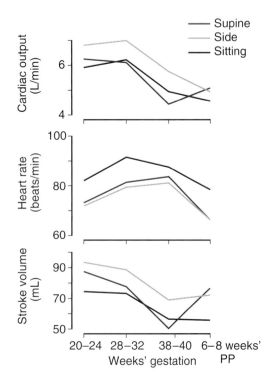

FIGURE 5-7 Effect of maternal posture on hemodynamics. PP = postpartum. (From Ueland and Metcalfe, 1975, with permission.)

imaging. Hibbard and colleagues (2009) concluded that any increased mass does not meet criteria for hypertrophy.

Cardiac Output

During normal pregnancy, mean arterial pressure and vascular resistance decrease, while blood volume and basal metabolic rate increase. As a result, cardiac output *at rest,* when measured in the lateral recumbent position, increases significantly beginning in early pregnancy (Duvekot and colleagues, 1993; Mabie and co-workers, 1994). It continues to increase and remains elevated during the remainder of pregnancy (Fig. 5-9).

During late pregnancy with the woman in the supine position, the large pregnant uterus rather consistently compresses venous return from the lower body. It also may compress the aorta (Bieniarz and associates, 1968). The results are that cardiac filling may be reduced with diminished cardiac output (see Fig. 5-7). Specifically, Bamber and Dresner (2003) found cardiac output at term to increase 1.2 L/min—almost 20 percent—when a woman was moved from her back onto her left side. Moreover, in the supine gravid patient, uterine blood flow estimated by Doppler velocimetry decreases by a third (Jeffreys and associates, 2006). Of note, Simpson and James (2005) found that fetal oxygen saturation is approximately 10 percent higher when a laboring woman is in a lateral recumbent position compared with supine. Upon standing, cardiac output falls to the same degree as in the nonpregnant woman (Easterling and associates, 1988).

In multifetal pregnancies, compared with singletons, maternal cardiac output is augmented further by another almost 20 percent because of a greater stroke volume (15 percent) and heart rate (3.5 percent). Left atrial diameter and left ventricular end-diastolic diameter are also increased due to augmented preload (Kametas and co-workers, 2003a). The increased heart rate and inotropic contractility imply that cardiovascular reserve is reduced in multifetal gestations.

During the first stage of labor, cardiac output increases moderately. During the second stage, with vigorous expulsive efforts, it is appreciably greater (see Fig. 5-9). The pregnancy-induced increase is lost after delivery, at times dependent on blood loss.

Hemodynamic Function in Late Pregnancy

To further elucidate the net changes of normal pregnancy-induced cardiovascular changes, Clark and colleagues (1989) conducted invasive studies to measure hemodynamic function late in pregnancy (Table 5-3). Right heart catheterization was performed in 10 healthy nulliparous women at 35 to 38 weeks, and again at 11 to 13 weeks postpartum. Late pregnancy was associated with the expected increases in heart rate, stroke volume, and cardiac output. Systemic vascular and pulmonary vascular resistance both decreased significantly, as did colloid osmotic pressure. Pulmonary capillary wedge pressure and central venous pressure did not change appreciably between late pregnancy and

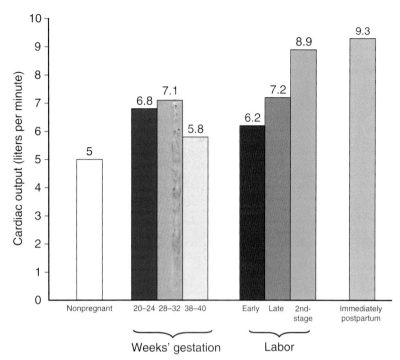

FIGURE 5-9 Cardiac output during three stages of gestation, labor, and immediately postpartum compared with values of nonpregnant women. All values were determined with women in the lateral recumbent position. (Adapted from Ueland and Metcalfe, 1975, with permission.)

the puerperium. Thus, as shown in Figure 5-10, although cardiac output is increased, left ventricular function as measured by stroke work index remains similar to the nonpregnant normal range. Put another way, normal pregnancy is not a continuous "high-output" state.

Circulation and Blood Pressure

Changes in posture affect arterial blood pressure. Brachial artery pressure when sitting is lower than that when in the lateral recumbent supine position (Bamber and Dresner, 2003). Arterial pressure usually decreases to a nadir at 24 to 26 weeks and rises thereafter. Diastolic pressure decreases more than systolic (Fig. 5-11).

Antecubital venous pressure remains unchanged during pregnancy. However, in the supine position, femoral venous pressure rises steadily, from approximately 8 mm Hg early in pregnancy to 24 mm Hg at term. Wright and co-workers (1950) demonstrated that venous blood flow in the legs is retarded during pregnancy except when the lateral recumbent position is assumed. This tendency toward stagnation of blood in the lower extremities during the latter part of pregnancy is attributable to the occlusion of the pelvic veins and inferior vena cava by the enlarged uterus. The elevated venous pressure returns to normal when the pregnant woman lies on her side and immediately after delivery (McLennan, 1943). These alterations contribute to the dependent edema frequently experienced and to the development of varicose veins in the legs and vulva, as well as hemorrhoids. They also predispose to deep-venous thrombosis (see Chap. 47, p. 1019).

TABLE 5-3. Central Hemodynamic Changes in 10 Normal Nulliparous Women Near Term and Postpartum

	Pregnant[a] (35–38 wks)	Postpartum (11–13 wks)	Change[b]
Mean arterial pressure (mm Hg)	90 ± 6	86 ± 8	NSC
Pulmonary capillary wedge pressure (mm Hg)	8 ± 2	6 ± 2	NSC
Central venous pressure (mm Hg)	4 ± 3	4 ± 3	NSC
Heart rate (beats/min)	83 ± 10	71 ± 10	+17%
Cardiac output (L/min)	6.2 ± 1.0	4.3 ± 0.9	+43%
Systemic vascular resistance (dyne/sec/cm^{-5})	1210 ± 266	1530 ± 520	−21%
Pulmonary vascular resistance (dyne/sec/cm^{-5})	78 ± 22	119 ± 47	−34%
Serum colloid osmotic pressure (mm Hg)	18.0 ± 1.5	20.8 ± 1.0	−14%
COP-PCWP gradient (mm Hg)	10.5 ± 2.7	14.5 ± 2.5	−28%
Left ventricular stroke work index (g/m/m^2)	48 ± 6	41 ± 8	NSC

[a]Measured in lateral recumbent position.
[b]Changes significant unless NSC = no significant change.
COP = colloid osmotic pressure; PCWP = pulmonary capillary wedge pressure.
Adapted from Clark and colleagues (1989), with permission.

Supine Hypotension

In about 10 percent of women, supine compression of the great vessels by the uterus causes significant arterial hypotension, sometimes referred to as the *supine hypotensive syndrome* (Kinsella and Lohmann, 1994). Also when supine, uterine arterial pressure—and thus blood flow—is significantly lower than that in the brachial artery. As discussed in Chapter 18 (p. 432), this may directly affect fetal heart rate patterns (Tamás and colleagues, 2007). This also occurs with hemorrhage or with spinal analgesia (see Chap. 19, p. 452).

Renin, Angiotensin II, and Plasma Volume

The renin-angiotensin-aldosterone axis is intimately involved in renal control of blood pressure via sodium and water balance. All components of this system are increased in normal pregnancy (Bentley-Lewis and co-workers, 2005). Renin is produced by both the maternal kidney and the placenta, and increased renin substrate (angiotensinogen) is produced by both maternal and fetal liver. This increase in angiotensinogen results, in part, from high levels of estrogen production during normal pregnancy. August and colleagues (1995) observed that stimulation of the renin-angiotensin system is important in first-trimester blood pressure maintenance.

Gant and associates (1973) studied vascular reactivity to angiotensin II throughout pregnancy. Nulliparas who remained

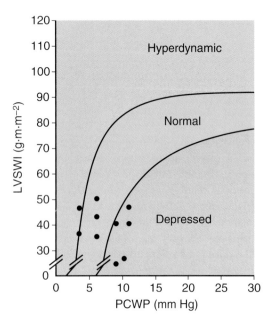

FIGURE 5-10 Relationship between left ventricular stroke work index (LVSWI) (cardiac output) and pulmonary capillary wedge pressure (PCWP) in 10 normal pregnant women in the third trimester. (Figure from Hauth and Cunningham, 1999; data from Clark and colleagues, 1989.)

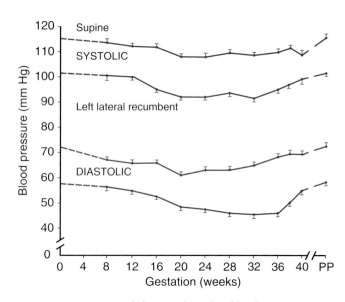

FIGURE 5-11 Sequential changes (±SEM) in blood pressure throughout pregnancy in 69 women in supine (*blue lines*) and left lateral recumbent positions (*red lines*). PP = postpartum. (Adapted from Wilson and colleagues, 1980.)

normotensive became and stayed refractory to the pressor effects of infused angiotensin II. Conversely, those who ultimately became hypertensive developed, but then lost, this refractoriness. Follow-up studies by Gant (1974) and Cunningham (1975) and their associates indicated that increased refractoriness to angiotensin II resulted from individual vessel refractoriness. Said another way, the abnormally increased sensitivity was an alteration in vessel wall refractoriness rather than the consequence of altered blood volume or renin-angiotensin secretion.

The vascular responsiveness to angiotensin II may be progesterone related. Normally, pregnant women lose their acquired vascular refractoriness to angiotensin II within 15 to 30 minutes after the placenta is delivered. Moreover, large amounts of intramuscular progesterone given during late labor delay this diminishing refractoriness. And although exogenous progesterone does not restore angiotensin II refractoriness to women with gestational hypertension, this can be done with infusion of its major metabolite—5α-dihydroprogesterone.

Cardiac Natriuretic Peptides

At least two species of these—*atrial natriuretic peptide (ANP)* and *B-type natriuretic peptide (BNP)*—are secreted by cardiomyocytes in response to chamber-wall stretching. These peptides regulate blood volume by provoking natriuresis, diuresis, and vascular smooth-muscle relaxation (Clerico and Emdin, 2004). In nonpregnant patients, levels of BNP as well as amino-terminal pro-brain natriuretic peptide—or Nt pro-BNP—may be useful in screening for depressed left ventricular systolic function and determining prognosis in chronic heart failure (Heidenreich and associates, 2004; Jarolim, 2006).

During normal pregnancy, plasma ANP levels are maintained in the nonpregnant range despite increased plasma volume (Lowe and co-workers, 1992). In one study, Resnik and co-workers (2005) found that median BNP levels are less than 20 pg/mL and are stable across normal pregnancy. However, these levels are increased in severe preeclampsia. Tihtonen and colleagues (2007) concluded that this resulted from cardiac strain caused by high afterload. It would appear that ANP-induced physiological adaptations participate in the expansion of extracellular fluid volume and the increase in plasma aldosterone concentrations characteristic of normal pregnancy.

A third species, *C-type natriuretic peptide (CNP),* is predominantly secreted by noncardiac tissues. Among its diverse biological functions, this peptide appears to be a major regulator of fetal bone growth. Walther and Stepan (2004) have provided a detailed review of its role during pregnancy.

Prostaglandins

Increased production of prostaglandins during pregnancy is thought to have a central role in control of vascular tone, blood pressure, and sodium balance (Gallery and Lindheimer, 1999). Renal medullary prostaglandin E_2 synthesis is increased markedly during late pregnancy and is presumed to be natriuretic. Prostacyclin (PGI_2), the principal prostaglandin of endothelium, also is increased during late pregnancy and regulates blood pressure and platelet function. It also has been implicated in the angiotensin resistance characteristic of normal pregnancy (Friedman, 1988). The ratio of PGI_2 to thromboxane in mater-

nal urine and blood has been considered important in the pathogenesis of preeclampsia (see Chap. 34, p. 714).

Endothelin

There are a number of endothelins generated in pregnancy. Endothelin-1 is a potent vasoconstrictor produced in endothelial and vascular smooth muscle cells and regulates local vasomotor tone (Feletou and Vanhoutte, 2006). Its production is stimulated by angiotensin II, arginine vasopressin, and thrombin. Endothelins, in turn, stimulate secretion of ANP, aldosterone, and catecholamines. As discussed in Chapter 6 (p. 161), there are endothelin receptors in pregnant and nonpregnant myometrium. Endothelins also have been identified in the amnion, amnionic fluid, decidua, and placental tissue (Kubota and colleagues, 1992; Margarit and associates, 2005). Vascular sensitivity to endothelin-1 is not altered during normal pregnancy (Ajne and associates, 2005). These investigators postulated that vasodilating factors counterbalance the endothelin-1 vasoconstrictor effects and produce reduced peripheral vascular resistance.

Nitric Oxide

This potent vasodilator is released by endothelial cells and may have important implications for modifying vascular resistance during pregnancy (Seligman and colleagues, 1994). As discussed in Chapter 34 (p. 714), abnormal nitric oxide synthesis has been linked to the development of preeclampsia (Baksu, 2005; Savvidou, 2003; Teran, 2006, and all their colleagues).

RESPIRATORY TRACT

The diaphragm rises about 4 cm during pregnancy (see Fig. 5-8). The subcostal angle widens appreciably as the transverse diameter of the thoracic cage increases approximately 2 cm. The thoracic circumference increases about 6 cm, but not sufficiently to prevent a reduction in the residual lung volume created by the elevated diaphragm. Diaphragmatic excursion is actually greater in pregnant than in nonpregnant women.

Pulmonary Function

The respiratory rate is essentially unchanged, but *tidal volume* and *resting minute ventilation* increase significantly as pregnancy advances. In a study of 51 healthy pregnant women, Kolarzyk and co-workers, (2005) reported significantly increased mean tidal volume—0.66 to 0.8 L/min—and minute ventilation—10.7 to 14.1 L/min—compared with nonpregnant women. The increase in minute ventilation is caused by several factors including enhanced respiratory drive primarily due to the stimulatory effects of progesterone, low expiratory reserve volume, and compensated respiratory alkalosis (Wise and associates, 2006). These are discussed in more detail subsequently.

The *functional residual capacity* and the *residual volume* are decreased as a consequence of the elevated diaphragm (Fig. 5-12). *Peak expiratory flow rates* decline progressively as gestation advances (Harirah and associates, 2005). *Lung compliance* is unaffected by pregnancy, but *airway conductance* is increased and *total pulmonary resistance* reduced, possibly as a result of

Nonpregnant | Term pregnancy

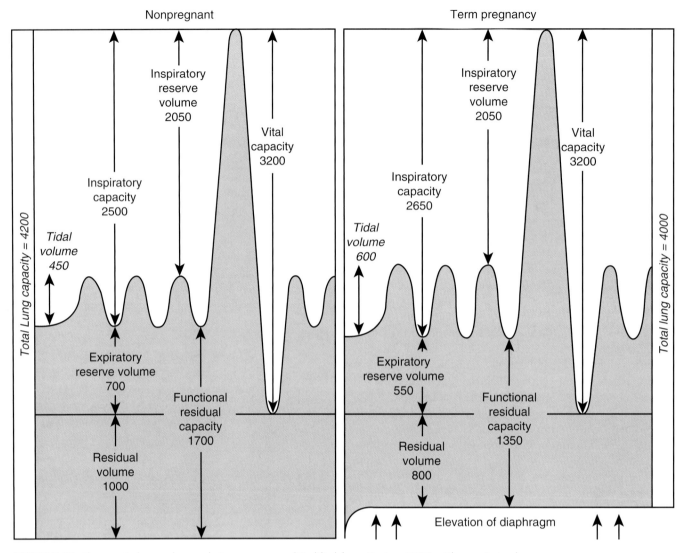

FIGURE 5-12 Changes in lung volumes during pregnancy. (Modified from Bonica, 1967, with permission.)

progesterone. The *maximum breathing capacity* and *forced* or *timed vital capacity* are not altered appreciably. It is unclear whether the critical *closing volume*—the lung volume at which airways in the dependent parts of the lung begin to close during expiration—is changed. It has been held that this is higher in pregnancy, but this is disputed (DeSwiet, 1991). The increased oxygen requirements and perhaps the increased critical closing volume imposed by pregnancy tend to make respiratory diseases more serious during gestation (see Chap. 46).

McAuliffe and associates (2002) compared pulmonary function in 140 women with a singleton pregnancy with that in 68 women with twins. They found no significant differences between the two groups.

Oxygen Delivery

The amount of oxygen delivered into the lungs by the increased tidal volume clearly exceeds oxygen requirements imposed by pregnancy. Moreover, the total hemoglobin mass, and in turn total oxygen-carrying capacity, increases appreciably during normal pregnancy, as does cardiac output. As a consequence, the *maternal arteriovenous oxygen* difference is decreased.

Acid–Base Equilibrium

An increased awareness of a desire to breathe is common even early in pregnancy (Milne and colleagues, 1978). This may be interpreted as dyspnea, which may suggest pulmonary or cardiac abnormalities when none exist. This physiological dyspnea is thought to result from increased tidal volume that lowers the blood P_{CO_2} slightly, which paradoxically causes dyspnea. The increased respiratory effort, and in turn the reduction in P_{CO_2}, during pregnancy is most likely induced in large part by progesterone and to a lesser degree by estrogen. Progesterone appears to act centrally, where it lowers the threshold and increases the sensitivity of the chemoreflex response to CO_2 (Jensen and associates, 2005).

To compensate for the resulting respiratory alkalosis, plasma bicarbonate levels decrease from 26 to approximately 22 mmol/L. Although blood pH is increased only minimally, it does shift the oxygen dissociation curve to the left. This shift increases the affinity of maternal hemoglobin for oxygen—the *Bohr effect*—thereby decreasing the oxygen-releasing capacity of maternal blood. This is offset because the slight pH increase also stimulates an increase in 2,3-diphosphoglycerate in maternal erythrocytes. This shifts the curve back to the right (Tsai and de Leeuw, 1982). Thus, reduced P_{CO_2} from maternal hyperventilation aids carbon dioxide (waste) transfer from the fetus to the mother while also facilitating oxygen release to the fetus.

URINARY SYSTEM

Kidney

A remarkable number of changes are observed in the urinary system as a result of pregnancy (Table 5-4). *Kidney size* increases slightly. Using radiographs, Bailey and Rolleston (1971) reported that the kidney was 1.5 cm longer during the early puerperium compared with 6 months later. The *glomerular filtration rate (GFR)* and *renal plasma flow* increase early in pregnancy. The GFR increases as much as 25 percent by the second week after conception and 50 percent by the beginning of the second trimester. Renal plasma flow increases are even greater (Davison and Noble, 1981; Lindheimer and co-workers, 2001). Animal studies suggest that both relaxin and neuronal nitric oxide synthase may be important for mediating both increased glomerular filtration and plasma flow during pregnancy (Abram and colleagues, 2001; Conrad and associates, 2005). As shown in Figure 5-13, elevated glomerular filtration persists until term, even though renal plasma flow decreases during late pregnancy. Primarily as a consequence of this elevated GFR, approximately 60 percent of women report urinary frequency during pregnancy (Sanhu and associates, 2009).

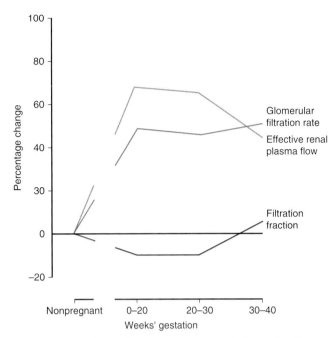

FIGURE 5-13 Relative changes in measures of glomerular filtration rate (GFR), effective renal plasma flow (ERPF), and filtration fraction during normal pregnancy. (Data from Davison and Dunlop, 1980, with permission.)

TABLE 5-4. Renal Changes in Normal Pregnancy

Alteration		Clinical Relevance
Kidney size	Approximately 1 cm longer on radiograph	Size returns to normal postpartum
Dilatation	Resembles hydronephrosis on sonogram or IVP (more marked on right)	Can be confused with obstructive uropathy; retained urine leads to collection errors; renal infections are more virulent; may be responsible for "distension syndrome"; elective pyelography should be deferred to at least 12 weeks postpartum
Renal function	Glomerular filtration rate and renal plasma flow increase ~50%	Serum creatinine decreases during normal gestation; >0.8 mg/dL (>72 μmol/L) creatinine already borderline; protein, amino acid, and glucose excretion all increase
Maintenance of acid-base	Decreased bicarbonate threshold; progesterone stimulates respiratory center	Serum bicarbonate decreased by 4–5 mEq/L; P_{CO_2} decreased 10 mm Hg; a P_{CO_2} of 40 mm Hg already represents CO_2 retention
Plasma osmolality	Osmoregulation altered: osmotic thresholds for AVP release and thirst decrease; hormonal disposal rates increase	Serum osmolality decreases 10 mOsm/L (serum Na ~5 mEq/L) during normal gestation; increased placental metabolism of AVP may cause transient diabetes insipidus during pregnancy

AVP = vasopressin; CO_2 = carbon dioxide; IVP = intravenous pyelography; P_{CO_2} = partial pressure carbon dioxide.
Modified from Lindheimer and colleagues (2000).

Kallikrein, a tissue protease synthesized in cells of the distal renal tubule, is increased in several conditions associated with increased glomerular perfusion in nonpregnant individuals. Platts and colleagues (2000) found increased urinary kallikrein excretion rates in women at 18 and 34 weeks, but excretion returned to nonpregnant levels by term. The significance of these fluctuations remains unknown.

As with blood pressure, maternal posture may have a considerable influence on several aspects of renal function. Late in pregnancy, for instance, urinary flow and sodium excretion average less than half the excretion rate in the supine position compared with that in the lateral recumbent position. The impact of posture on glomerular filtration and renal plasma flow is much more variable.

Loss of Nutrients

One unusual feature of the pregnancy-induced changes in renal excretion is the remarkably increased amounts of various nutrients lost in the urine. Amino acids and water-soluble vitamins are lost in the urine in much greater amounts in pregnancy (Hytten, 1973; Powers and associates, 2004).

Tests of Renal Function

The physiological changes in renal hemodynamics induced during normal pregnancy have several implications for the interpretation of tests of renal function (see Appendix). *Serum creatinine* levels decrease during normal pregnancy from a mean of 0.7 to 0.5 mg/dL. **Values of 0.9 mg/dL suggest underlying renal disease and should prompt further evaluation** (Lindheimer and associates, 2000). *Creatinine clearance* in pregnancy averages about 30 percent higher than the 100 to 115 mL/min in nonpregnant women (Lindheimer and associates, 2000).

Creatinine clearance is a useful test to estimate renal function provided that complete urine collection is made during an accurately timed period. If either is done incorrectly, results are misleading (Davison and colleagues, 1981). During the day, pregnant women tend to accumulate water as dependent edema, and at night, while recumbent, they mobilize this fluid with diuresis. This reversal of the usual nonpregnant diurnal pattern of urinary flow causes nocturia, and the urine is more dilute than in nonpregnant women. Failure of a pregnant woman to excrete concentrated urine after withholding fluids for approximately 18 hours does not necessarily signify renal damage. In fact, the kidney in these circumstances functions perfectly normally by excreting mobilized extracellular fluid of relatively low osmolality.

Urinalysis

Glucosuria during pregnancy may not be abnormal. The appreciable increase in glomerular filtration, together with impaired tubular reabsorptive capacity for filtered glucose, accounts in most cases for glucosuria (Davison and Hytten, 1974). For these reasons alone, Chesley (1963) calculated that about a sixth of pregnant women should spill glucose in the urine. That said, although common during pregnancy, the possibility of diabetes mellitus should not be ignored when glucosuria is identified.

Proteinuria normally is not evident during pregnancy except occasionally in slight amounts during or soon after vigorous labor. Higby and associates (1994) measured protein excretion in 270 normal women throughout pregnancy. Their mean 24-hour excretion was 115 mg, and the upper 95-percent con-

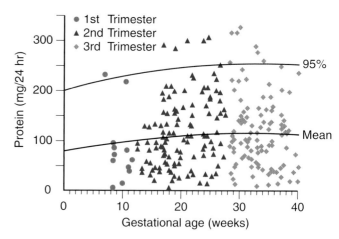

FIGURE 5-14 Scatter plot of all patients showing 24-hour urinary total protein excretion by gestational age. Mean and 95-percent confidence limits are outlined. (Data from Higby and colleagues, 1994, with permission.)

fidence limit was 260 mg/day without significant differences by trimester (Fig. 5-14). These investigators also showed that albumin excretion is minimal and ranges from 5 to 30 mg/day. Nomograms for urinary microalbumin and creatinine ratios during uncomplicated pregnancies have been developed by Waugh and co-workers (2003).

Hematuria is often the result of contamination during collection. If not, it most often suggests urinary tract disease as discussed in Chapter 48 (p. 1033). Hematuria is common after difficult labor and delivery because of trauma to the bladder and urethra.

Ureters

After the uterus rises completely out of the pelvis, it rests upon the ureters, laterally displacing and compressing them at the pelvic brim. This results in increased intraureteral tonus above this level (Rubi and Sala, 1968). Ureteral dilatation is impressive, and Schulman and Herlinger (1975) found it to be greater on the right side in 86 percent of women (Fig. 5-15). Unequal dilatation may result from a cushioning provided the left ureter by the sigmoid colon and perhaps from greater compression of the right ureter as the consequence of dextrorotation of the uterus. The right ovarian vein complex, which is remarkably dilated during pregnancy, lies obliquely over the right ureter and may contribute significantly to right ureteral dilatation.

Progesterone likely has some effect. Van Wagenen and Jenkins (1939) described continued ureteral dilatation after removal of the monkey fetus but with the placenta left in situ. However, the relatively abrupt onset of dilatation in women at midpregnancy seems more consistent with ureteral compression.

Ureteral elongation accompanies distention, and the ureter is frequently thrown into curves of varying size, the smaller of which may be sharply angulated. These so-called kinks are poorly named, because the term connotes obstruction. They are usually single or double curves, which when viewed in the radiograph taken in the same plane as the curve, may appear as acute angulations. Another exposure at right angles nearly always identifies them to be more gentle curves. Despite these anatomical changes, Semins and associates (2009) concluded, based upon their review of the literature, that complication

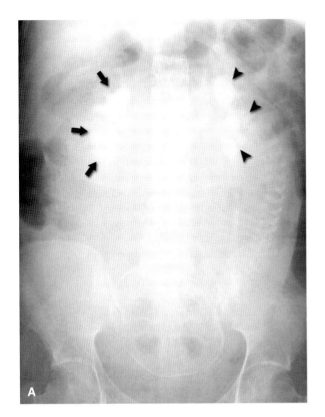

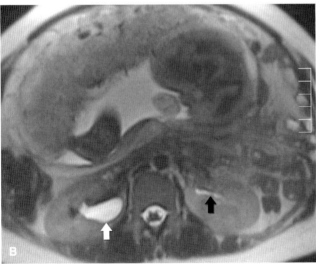

FIGURE 5-15 Hydronephrosis. **A.** Plain film from the 15-minute image of an intravenous pyelogram (IVP). Moderate hydronephrosis on the right (*arrows*) and mild hydronephrosis on the left (*arrowheads*) are both normal for this 35-week gestation. **B.** Axial MR image from a study performed for a fetal indication. Moderate hydronephrosis on the right (*white arrow*) and mild on the left (*black arrow*) are incidental findings.

rates associated with ureteroscopy in pregnant and nonpregnant patients do not differ significantly.

Bladder

There are few significant anatomical changes in the bladder before 12 weeks. From that time onward, however, increased uterine size, the hyperemia that affects all pelvic organs, and the hyperplasia of the bladder's muscle and connective tissues elevates the bladder trigone and causes thickening of its poste-

rior, or intraureteric, margin. Continuation of this process to the end of pregnancy produces marked deepening and widening of the trigone. There are no mucosal changes other than an increase in the size and tortuosity of its blood vessels.

Using urethrocystometry, Iosif and colleagues (1980) reported that bladder pressure in primigravidas increased from 8 cm H_2O early in pregnancy to 20 cm H_2O at term. To compensate for reduced bladder capacity, absolute and functional urethral lengths increased by 6.7 and 4.8 mm, respectively. At the same time, maximal intraurethral pressure increased from 70 to 93 cm H_2O, and thus continence is maintained. Still, at least half of women experience some degree of urinary incontinence by the third trimester (van Brummen and colleagues, 2006; Wesnes and co-workers, 2009). Indeed, this is always considered in the differential diagnosis of ruptured membranes.

Toward the end of pregnancy, particularly in nulliparas in whom the presenting part often engages before labor, the entire base of the bladder is pushed forward and upward, converting the normal convex surface into a concavity. As a result, difficulties in diagnostic and therapeutic procedures are greatly increased. In addition, the pressure of the presenting part impairs the drainage of blood and lymph from the bladder base, often rendering the area edematous, easily traumatized, and probably more susceptible to infection.

GASTROINTESTINAL TRACT

As pregnancy progresses, the stomach and intestines are displaced by the enlarging uterus. Consequently, the physical findings in certain diseases are altered. The appendix, for instance, is usually displaced upward and somewhat laterally as the uterus enlarges. At times, it may reach the right flank.

Gastric emptying time, studied using acetaminophen absorption techniques, appears to be unchanged during each trimester and during comparison with nonpregnant women (Macfie and colleagues, 1991; Wong and associates, 2002, 2007). During labor, however, and especially after administration of analgesic agents, gastric emptying time may be prolonged appreciably. As a result, a major danger of general anesthesia for delivery is regurgitation and aspiration of either food-laden or highly acidic gastric contents (see Chap. 19, p. 459).

Pyrosis (heartburn) is common during pregnancy and is most likely caused by reflux of acidic secretions into the lower esophagus (see Chap. 49, p. 1052). Although the altered position of the stomach probably contributes to its frequent occurrence, lower esophageal sphincter tone also is decreased. In addition, intraesophageal pressures are lower and intragastric pressures higher in pregnant women. At the same time, esophageal peristalsis has lower wave speed and lower amplitude (Ulmsten and Sundström, 1978).

The gums may become hyperemic and softened during pregnancy and may bleed when mildly traumatized, as with a toothbrush. A focal, highly vascular swelling of the gums, the so-called *epulis* of pregnancy, develops occasionally but typically regresses spontaneously after delivery. Most evidence indicates that pregnancy does not incite tooth decay.

Hemorrhoids are fairly common during pregnancy. They are caused in large measure by constipation and elevated pressure in veins below the level of the enlarged uterus (see Fig. 2-7, p. 21).

Liver

Unlike in some animals, there is no increase in liver size during human pregnancy (Combes and Adams, 1971). Hepatic blood flow, however, increases substantively as does the diameter of the portal vein (Clapp and colleagues, 2000). Histological evaluation of liver biopsies, including examination with the electron microscope, has shown no distinct morphological changes in normal pregnant women (Ingerslev and Teilum, 1946).

Some laboratory test results of hepatic function are altered during normal pregnancy, and some would be considered abnormal for nonpregnant patients. Total *alkaline phosphatase* activity almost doubles, but much of the increase is attributable to heat-stable placental alkaline phosphatase isozymes. Serum aspartate transaminase (AST), alanine transaminase (ALT), γ-glutamyl transferase (GGT), and bilirubin levels are slightly lower compared with nonpregnant values (Girling and colleagues, 1997; Ruiz-Extremera and associates, 2005).

The concentration of serum albumin decreases during pregnancy. By late pregnancy, albumin concentrations may be near 3.0 g/dL compared with approximately 4.3 g/dL in nonpregnant women (Mendenhall, 1970). Total albumin is increased, however, because of a greater volume of distribution from plasma volume increase. There is also a slight increase in serum globulin levels.

Leucine aminopeptidase is a proteolytic liver enzyme whose serum levels may be increased with liver disease. Its activity is markedly elevated in pregnant women. The increase, however, results from the appearance of a pregnancy-specific enzyme(s) with distinct substrate specificities (Song and Kappas, 1968). Pregnancy-induced aminopeptidase has oxytocinase and vasopressinase activity which occasionally causes transient diabetes insipidus (see Chap. 53, p. 1139).

Gallbladder

During normal pregnancy, the contractility of the gallbladder is reduced, leading to an increased residual volume (Braverman and co-workers, 1980). This may be because progesterone impairs gallbladder contraction by inhibiting cholecystokinin-mediated smooth muscle stimulation, which is the primary regulator of gallbladder contraction. Impaired emptying leads to stasis, which associated with increased bile cholesterol saturation of pregnancy, contributes to the increased prevalence of cholesterol gallstones in multiparous women.

The effects of pregnancy on maternal bile acid serum concentrations have been incompletely characterized despite the long-acknowledged propensity for pregnancy to cause intrahepatic cholestasis and pruritus gravidarum from retained bile salts. Intrahepatic cholestasis has been linked to high circulating levels of estrogen, which inhibit intraductal transport of bile acids (Simon and colleagues, 1996). In addition, increased progesterone and genetic factors have been implicated in the pathogenesis (Lammert and associates, 2000). Cholestasis of pregnancy is described in greater detail in Chapter 50 (p. 1073).

ENDOCRINE SYSTEM

Some of the most important endocrine changes of pregnancy are discussed elsewhere, especially in Chapter 3.

Pituitary Gland

During normal pregnancy, the pituitary gland enlarges by approximately 135 percent (Gonzalez and colleagues, 1988). Although it has been suggested that the increase may be sufficient to compress the optic chiasma and reduce visual fields, impaired vision due to physiological pituitary enlargement during normal pregnancy is rare (Inoue and associates, 2007). Scheithauer and colleagues (1990) have provided evidence that the incidence of pituitary prolactinomas is not increased during pregnancy. When these tumors are large before pregnancy—a macroadenoma is 10 mm or greater—then enlargement during pregnancy is more likely (see Chap. 53, p. 1139).

The maternal pituitary gland is not essential for maintenance of pregnancy. Many women have undergone hypophysectomy, completed pregnancy successfully, and undergone spontaneous labor while receiving glucocorticoids along with thyroid hormone and vasopressin.

Growth Hormone

During the first trimester, growth hormone is secreted predominantly from the maternal pituitary gland, and concentrations in serum and amnionic fluid are within nonpregnant values of 0.5 to 7.5 ng/mL (Kletzky and associates, 1985). As early as 8 weeks, growth hormone secreted from the placenta becomes detectable (Lønberg and co-workers, 2003). By approximately 17 weeks, the placenta is the principal source of growth hormone secretion (Obuobie and co-workers, 2001). Maternal serum values increase slowly from approximately 3.5 ng/mL at 10 weeks to plateau after 28 weeks at approximately 14 ng/mL. Growth hormone in amnionic fluid peaks at 14 to 15 weeks and slowly declines thereafter to reach baseline values after 36 weeks.

Placental growth hormone—which differs from pituitary growth hormone by 13 amino acid residues—is secreted by syncytiotrophoblasts in a nonpulsatile fashion (Fuglsang and co-workers, 2006). The regulation and physiological effects of placental growth hormone are incompletely understood, but it appears to have some influence on fetal growth as well as the development of preeclampsia (Mittal and co-workers, 2007). For example, placental growth hormone is a major determinant of maternal insulin resistance after midpregnancy. And maternal serum levels correlate positively with birthweight, and negatively with fetal-growth restriction and uterine artery resistance (Chellakooty and colleagues, 2004; Schiessl and associates, 2007). That said, fetal growth still progresses in the complete absence of placental growth hormone. Freemark (2006) concluded that the hormone, although not absolutely essential, may act in concert with human placental lactogen and other somatolactogens to regulate fetal growth.

Prolactin

Maternal plasma levels of prolactin increase markedly during normal pregnancy and concentrations are usually 10-fold greater at term—about 150 ng/mL—compared with nonpregnant women. Paradoxically, plasma concentrations decrease after delivery even in women who are breast feeding. During early lactation, there are pulsatile bursts of prolactin secretion in response to suckling.

The physiological basis of the marked increase in prolactin prior to parturition is still unclear. What is known is that estrogen stimulation increases the number of anterior pituitary lactotrophs and may stimulate their release of prolactin (Andersen, 1982). Thyroid-releasing hormone also acts to cause an increased prolactin level in pregnant compared with nonpregnant women, but the response decreases as pregnancy advances (Miyamoto, 1984). Serotonin also is believed to increase prolactin, and dopamine—previously known as prolactin-inhibiting factor—inhibits its secretion.

The principal function of maternal prolactin is to ensure lactation. Early in pregnancy, prolactin acts to initiate DNA synthesis and mitosis of glandular epithelial cells and presecretory alveolar cells of the breast. Prolactin also increases the number of estrogen and prolactin receptors in these cells. Finally, prolactin promotes mammary alveolar cell RNA synthesis, galactopoiesis, and production of casein, lactalbumin, lactose, and lipids (Andersen, 1982). A woman with isolated prolactin deficiency described by Kauppila and co-workers (1987) failed to lactate after two pregnancies, thus establishing prolactin as a requisite for lactation but not for pregnancy.

Prolactin is present in amnionic fluid in high concentrations. Levels of up to 10,000 ng/mL are found at 20 to 26 weeks. Thereafter, levels decrease and reach a nadir after 34 weeks. There is convincing evidence that the uterine decidua is the site of prolactin synthesis found in amnionic fluid (see Chap. 3, p. 46). Although the exact function of amnionic fluid prolactin is not known, it has been suggested that this prolactin impairs water transfer from the fetus into the maternal compartment, thus preventing fetal dehydration.

Thyroid Gland

Physiological changes of pregnancy cause the thyroid gland to increase production of thyroid hormones by 40 to 100 percent to meet maternal and fetal needs (Smallridge and associates, 2005). To accomplish this, there are a number of pregnancy-induced changes that are documented.

Anatomically, the thyroid gland undergoes moderate enlargement during pregnancy caused by glandular hyperplasia and increased vascularity. Glinoer and colleagues (1990) reported that mean thyroid volume increased from 12 mL in the first trimester to 15 mL at delivery. Total volume was inversely proportional to serum thyrotropin concentrations. Such enlargement is not pathological, but normal pregnancy does not typically cause significant thyromegaly. Thus, any goiter should be investigated.

A number of alterations in thyroid physiology and function during pregnancy are detailed in Figure 5-16. Beginning early in the first trimester, levels of the principal carrier protein—*thyroxine-binding globulin*—increases, reaches its zenith at about 20 weeks, and stabilizes at approximately double baseline values for the remainder of pregnancy. *Total serum thyroxine* (T_4) increases sharply beginning between 6 and 9 weeks and reaches a plateau at 18 weeks. *Free serum T_4* levels rise slightly

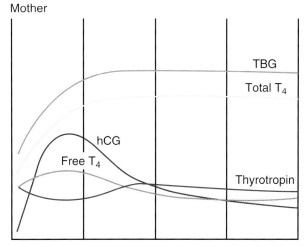

Mother

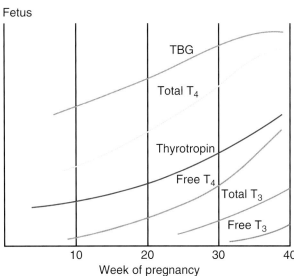

Fetus

FIGURE 5-16 Relative changes in maternal thyroid function during pregnancy. Maternal changes include a marked and early increase in hepatic production of thyroxine-binding globulin (TBG) and placental production of chorionic gonadotropin (hCG). Increased thyroxine-binding globulin increases serum thyroxine (T_4) concentrations, and chorionic gonadotropin has thyrotropin-like activity and stimulates maternal T_4 secretion. The transient hCG-induced increase in serum T_4 levels inhibits maternal secretion of thyrotropin. Except for minimally increased free T_4 levels when hCG peaks, these levels are essentially unchanged. (T_3 = triiodothyronine.) (Modified from Burrow and colleagues, 1994.)

and peak along with hCG levels, and then they return to normal. The rise in *total triiodothyronine (T_3)* is more pronounced up to 18 weeks, and thereafter, it plateaus. *Thyroid-releasing hormone (TRH)* levels are not increased during normal pregnancy, but this neurotransmitter does cross the placenta and may serve to stimulate the fetal pituitary to secrete thyrotropin (Thorpe-Beeston and associates, 1991).

Interestingly, the secretion of T_4 and T_3 is not similar for all pregnant women (Glinoer and associates, 1990). Approximately a third of women experience relative hypothyroxinemia, preferential T_3 secretion, and higher, albeit normal, serum thyrotropin levels. Thus, there may be considerable variability in thyroidal adjustments during normal pregnancy.

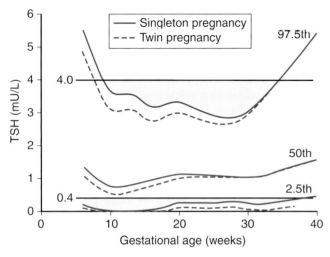

FIGURE 5-17 Gestational age-specific TSH nomogram derived from 13,599 singleton and 132 twin pregnancies. Singleton pregnancies are represented with solid blue lines and twin pregnancies with dashed lines. The nonpregnant reference values of 4.0 and 0.4 mU/L are represented as solid black lines. Upper shaded area represents the 28 percent of singleton pregnancies with TSH values above the 97.5th percentile threshold that would not have been identified as abnormal based on the assay reference value of 4.0 mU/L. Lower shaded area represents singleton pregnancies that would have been (falsely) identified as having TSH suppression based on the assay reference value of 0.4 mU/L. (From Dashe and colleagues, 2005, with permission.)

The modifications in serum *thyrotropin*—known also as thyroid-stimulating hormone (TSH)—and chorionic gonadotropin (hCG) as a function of gestational age also are shown in Figure 5-16. As discussed in Chapter 3 (p. 63), the α-subunits of the two glycoproteins are identical, whereas the β-subunits, although similar, differ in their amino acid sequence. As a result of this structural similarity, hCG has intrinsic thyrotropic activity, and thus, high serum levels cause thyroid stimulation. Indeed, thyrotropin levels decrease in more than 80 percent of pregnant women, whereas they remain in the normal range for nonpregnant women (see p. 1126).

As shown in Figure 5-17, normal suppression of TSH during pregnancy may lead to a misdiagnosis of subclinical hyperthyroidism. Of greater concern is the potential failure to identify women with early hypothyroidism because of suppressed TSH concentrations. To mitigate the likelihood of such misdiagnoses, Dashe and co-workers (2005) conducted a population-based study at Parkland Hospital to develop gestational-age-specific TSH nomograms for both singleton and twin pregnancies.

These complex alterations of thyroid regulation do not appear to alter maternal thyroid status as measured by metabolic studies. Although basal metabolic rate increases progressively during normal pregnancy by as much as 25 percent, most of this increase in oxygen consumption can be attributed to fetal metabolic activity. If fetal body surface area is considered along with that of the mother, the predicted and observed basal metabolic rates are similar to those in nonpregnant women. Fetal thyroid physiology is discussed in Chapter 4 (p. 97).

Parathyroid Glands

The regulation of calcium concentration is closely interrelated to magnesium, phosphate, parathyroid hormone, vitamin D, and calcitonin physiology. Any alteration of one of these factors is likely to change the others. In a longitudinal investigation of 20 women, More and associates (2003) found that all markers of bone turnover increased during normal pregnancy and failed to reach baseline level by 12 months postpartum. They concluded that the calcium needed for fetal growth and lactation may be drawn at least in part from the maternal skeleton.

Parathyroid Hormone and Calcium

Acute or chronic decreases in plasma calcium or acute decreases in magnesium stimulate the release of parathyroid hormone, whereas increases in calcium and magnesium suppress parathyroid hormone levels. The action of this hormone on bone resorption, intestinal absorption, and kidney reabsorption is to increase extracellular fluid calcium and decrease phosphate.

Parathyroid hormone plasma concentrations decrease during the first trimester and then increase progressively throughout the remainder of pregnancy (Pitkin and associates, 1979). Increased levels likely result from the lower calcium concentration in the pregnant woman. As discussed earlier, this is the result of increased plasma volume, increased glomerular filtration rate, and maternal-fetal transfer of calcium. Ionized calcium is decreased only slightly, and Reitz and co-workers (1977) suggest that during pregnancy a new "set point" is established for ionized calcium and parathyroid hormone. Estrogens also appear to block the action of parathyroid hormone on bone resorption, resulting in another mechanism to increase parathyroid hormone during pregnancy. The net result of these actions is a *physiological hyperparathyroidism* of pregnancy, likely to supply the fetus with adequate calcium.

Calcitonin and Calcium

The calcitonin-secreting C cells are derived embryologically from the neural crest and are located predominantly in the perifollicular areas of the thyroid gland. Calcium and magnesium increase the biosynthesis and secretion of calcitonin. Various gastric hormones—gastrin, pentagastrin, glucagon, and pancreozymin—and food ingestion also increase calcitonin plasma levels.

The known actions of calcitonin generally are considered to oppose those of parathyroid hormone and vitamin D to protect skeletal calcification during times of calcium stress. Pregnancy and lactation cause profound calcium stress, and during these times, calcitonin levels are appreciably higher than those in nonpregnant women (Weiss and co-workers, 1998).

Vitamin D and Calcium

After its ingestion or synthesis in the skin, vitamin D is converted by the liver into 25-hydroxyvitamin D_3. This form then is converted in the kidney, decidua, and placenta to 1,25-dihydroxyvitamin D_3, serum levels of which are increased during normal pregnancy (Weisman and co-workers, 1979; Whitehead and associates, 1981). Most likely this form is the biologically active compound, and it stimulates resorption of calcium from bone and absorption from the intestines. Although its control is unclear, the conversion of 25-hydroxyvitamin D_3 to 1,25-dihydroxyvitamin D_3 is facilitated by parathyroid hormone and by low calcium and phosphate plasma levels and is opposed by calcitonin.

Adrenal Glands

In normal pregnancy, the maternal adrenal glands undergo little, if any, morphological change.

Cortisol

The serum concentration of circulating cortisol is increased, but much of it is bound by *transcortin*, the cortisol-binding globulin. The rate of adrenal cortisol secretion is not increased, and probably it is decreased compared with that of the nonpregnant state. The metabolic clearance rate of cortisol, however, is lower during pregnancy because its half-life is nearly doubled over that for nonpregnant women (Migeon and associates, 1957). Administration of estrogen, including most oral contraceptives, causes changes in serum cortisol levels and transcortin similar to those of pregnancy.

During early pregnancy, the levels of circulating corticotropin (ACTH) are reduced strikingly. As pregnancy progresses, the levels of ACTH and free cortisol rise (Fig. 5-18). This apparent paradox is not understood completely. Nolten and Rueckert (1981) have presented evidence that the higher free cortisol levels observed in pregnancy are the result of a "resetting" of the maternal feedback mechanism to higher levels. They further propose that this might result from *tissue refractoriness* to cortisol. Keller-Wood and Wood (2001) later suggested that these incongruities may result from an antagonistic action of progesterone on mineralocorticoids. Thus, in response to elevated progesterone levels during pregnancy, an elevated free cortisol is needed to maintain homeostasis. Indeed, experiments in pregnant ewes demonstrate that elevated maternal cortisol and aldosterone secretion are necessary to maintain the normal increase in plasma volume during late pregnancy (Jensen and associates, 2002).

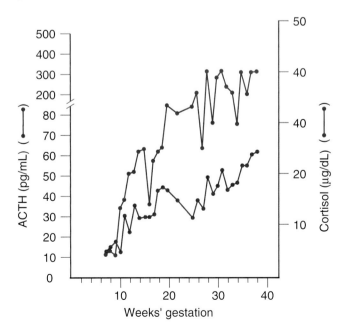

FIGURE 5-18 Serial increases in serum cortisol (*blue line*) and ACTH (*red line*) during pregnancy in normal controls throughout pregnancy. (From Carr and co-workers, 1981, with permission.)

Aldosterone

As early as 15 weeks, the maternal adrenal glands secrete considerably increased amounts of aldosterone. By the third trimester, about 1 mg/day is secreted. If sodium intake is restricted, aldosterone secretion is elevated even further (Watanabe and co-workers, 1963). At the same time, levels of renin and angiotensin II substrate normally are increased, especially during the latter half of pregnancy. This scenario gives rise to increased plasma levels of angiotensin II, which by acting on the zona glomerulosa of the maternal adrenal glands, accounts for the markedly elevated aldosterone secretion. It has been suggested that the increased aldosterone secretion during normal pregnancy affords protection against the natriuretic effect of progesterone and atrial natriuretic peptide.

Deoxycorticosterone

Maternal plasma levels of this potent mineralocorticosteroid progressively increase during pregnancy. Indeed, plasma levels of deoxycorticosterone rise to near 1500 pg/mL by term, a more than 15-fold increase (Parker and associates, 1980). This marked elevation is not derived from adrenal secretion but instead represents increased kidney production resulting from estrogen stimulation. The levels of deoxycorticosterone and its sulfate in fetal blood are appreciably higher than those in maternal blood, which suggests transfer of fetal deoxycorticosterone into the maternal compartment.

Dehydroepiandrosterone Sulfate

Maternal serum and urine levels of *dehydroepiandrosterone sulfate* are decreased during normal pregnancy. As discussed in Chapter 3 (p. 68), this is a consequence of increased metabolic clearance through extensive maternal hepatic 16α-hydroxylation and placental conversion to estrogen.

Androstenedione and Testosterone

Maternal plasma levels of both of these androgens are increased during pregnancy. This finding is not totally explained by alterations in their metabolic clearance. Maternal plasma androstenedione and testosterone are converted to estradiol in the placenta, which increases their clearance rates. Conversely, increased plasma sex hormone-binding globulin in pregnant women retards testosterone clearance. Thus, the production rates of maternal testosterone and androstenedione during human pregnancy are increased. The source of this increased C_{19}-steroid production is unknown, but it likely originates in the ovary. Interestingly, little or no testosterone in maternal plasma enters the fetal circulation as testosterone. Even when massive testosterone levels are found in the circulation of pregnant women, as with androgen-secreting tumors, testosterone levels in umbilical cord blood are likely to be undetectable and are the result of the near complete trophoblastic conversion of testosterone to 17β-estradiol (Edman and associates, 1979).

OTHER SYSTEMS

Musculoskeletal System

Progressive lordosis is a characteristic feature of normal pregnancy. Compensating for the anterior position of the enlarging uterus, the lordosis shifts the center of gravity back over the lower extremities. In a recent and interesting anthropological study, Whitcome and colleagues (2007) demonstrated that this curvature and reinforcement of the lumbar vertebrae have evolved in humans to permit bipedal posture and locomotion despite up to a 31-percent increase in the maternal abdominal mass by term.

The sacroiliac, sacrococcygeal, and pubic joints have increased mobility during pregnancy. As discussed earlier (p. 110), the increase in joint laxity during pregnancy does not correlate with increased maternal serum levels of estradiol, progesterone, or relaxin (Marnach and co-workers, 2003). Joint mobility may contribute to the alteration of maternal posture and in turn may cause discomfort in the lower back. This is especially bothersome late in pregnancy, during which time aching, numbness, and weakness also occasionally are experienced in the upper extremities. This may result from the marked lordosis with anterior neck flexion and slumping of the shoulder girdle, which in turn produce traction on the ulnar and median nerves (Crisp and DeFrancesco, 1964).

The bones and ligaments of the pelvis undergo remarkable adaptation during pregnancy. In 1934, Abramson and colleagues described the normal relaxation of the pelvic joints, and particularly the symphysis pubis, that occurs during pregnancy (Fig. 5-19). They reported that most relaxation takes place in the first half of pregnancy. However, pelvic dimensions measured by magnetic resonance imaging are not significantly different before compared with up to 3 months after delivery (Huerta-Enochian and associates, 2006).

Although some symphyseal separation likely accompanies many deliveries, those greater than 1 cm may cause significant pain (Jain and Sternberg, 2005). Regression begins immediately following delivery, and it is usually complete within 3 to 5 months.

Eyes

Intraocular pressure decreases during pregnancy, attributed in part to increased vitreous outflow (Sunness, 1988). Corneal sensitivity is decreased, and the greatest changes are late in gestation. Most pregnant women demonstrate a measurable but slight increase in corneal thickness, thought to be due to edema. Consequently, they may have difficulty with previously comfortable contact lenses. Brownish-red opacities on the posterior surface of the cornea—*Krukenberg spindles*—have also been observed with a higher than expected frequency during pregnancy. Hormonal effects similar to those observed for skin lesions are postulated to cause this increased pigmentation. Other than transient loss of accommodation reported with both pregnancy and lactation, visual function is unaffected by pregnancy. These changes during pregnancy, as well as pathological eye aberrations, were reviewed by Dinn and colleagues (2003).

Central Nervous System

Women often report problems with attention, concentration, and memory throughout pregnancy and the early postpartum period. Systematic studies of memory in pregnancy, however, are limited and often anecdotal. Keenan and colleagues (1998) longitudinally investigated memory in pregnant women as well as a matched control group. They found pregnancy-related memory decline, which was limited to the third trimester. This decline was not attributable to depression, anxiety, sleep deprivation, or other physical changes associated with pregnancy. It was transient and quickly resolved following delivery. Interestingly, Rana and associates (2006) found that attention and memory were improved in women with preeclampsia receiving magnesium sulfate compared with normal pregnant women.

Zeeman and co-workers (2003) used magnetic resonance imaging to measure cerebral blood flow across pregnancy in 10 healthy women. They found that mean blood flow in the middle and posterior cerebral arteries decreased progressively from 147 and 56 mL/min when nonpregnant to 118 and 44 mL/min late in the third trimester, respectively. The mechanism and clinical significance of this decrease is unknown. Pregnancy does not appear to impact cerebrovascular autoregulation (Bergersen and co-workers, 2006).

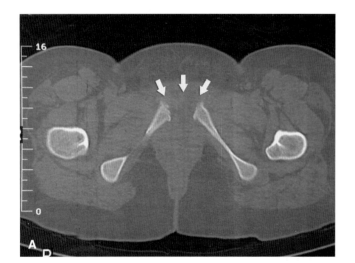 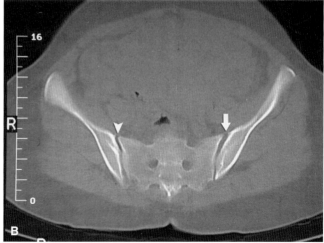

FIGURE 5-19 A. Symphyseal diastasis. Marked widening of the pubic symphysis (*arrows*) consistent with diastasis after vaginal delivery. **B.** Sacroiliac (SI) joint widening. Left (*arrow*) greater than right (*arrowhead*) widening of the anterior SI joints. (Courtesy of Dr. Daniel Moore.)

Sleep

Beginning as early as about 12 weeks and extending through the first 2 months postpartum, women have difficulty going to sleep, frequent awakenings, fewer hours of night sleep, and reduced sleep efficiency (Lee and colleagues, 2000; Swain and colleagues, 1997). The frequency and duration of sleep apnea episodes were reported to be decreased significantly in pregnant women compared with those postpartum (Trakada and coworkers, 2003). In the supine position, however, average PaO_2 levels were lower. The greatest disruption of sleep is encountered postpartum and may contribute to *postpartum blues* or to frank depression (see Chap. 55, p. 1176).

REFERENCES

Abram SR, Alexander BT, Bennett WA, et al: Role of neuronal nitric oxide synthase in mediating renal hemodynamic changes during pregnancy. Am J Physiol Regul Integr Comp Physiol 281:R1390, 2001

Abramson D, Roberts SM, Wilson PD: Relaxation of the pelvic joints in pregnancy. SGO 58:59S, 1934

Ajne G, Ahlborg G, Wolff K, Nisell H: Contribution of endogenous endothelin-1 to basal vascular tone during normal pregnancy and preeclampsia. Am J Obstet Gynecol 193:234, 2005

Alvarez H, Caldeyro-Barcia R: Contractility of the human uterus recorded by new methods. Surg Gynecol Obstet 91:1, 1950

Andersen JR: Prolactin in amniotic fluid and maternal serum during uncomplicated human pregnancy. Dan Med Bull 29:266, 1982

Assali NS, Dilts PV, Pentl AA, et al: Physiology of the placenta. In Assali NS (ed): Biology of Gestation, Vol I. The Maternal Organism. New York, Academic Press, 1968

August P, Mueller FB, Sealey JE, et al: Role of renin–angiotensin system in blood pressure regulation in pregnancy. Lancet 345:896, 1995

Bailey RR, Rolleston GL: Kidney length and ureteric dilatation in the puerperium. J Obstet Gynaecol Br Commonw 78:55, 1971

Baker PN, Cunningham FG: Platelet and coagulation abnormalities. In Lindheimer ML, Roberts JM, Cunningham FG (eds): Chesley's Hypertensive Diseases in Pregnancy, 2nd ed. Stamford, CT, Appleton and Lange, 1999, p 349

Baksu B, Davas I, Baksu A, et al: Plasma nitric oxide, endothelin-1 and urinary nitric oxide and cyclic guanosine monophosphate levels in hypertensive pregnant women. Int J Gynaecol Obstet 90:112, 2005

Bamber JH, Dresner M: Aortocaval compression in pregnancy: The effect of changing the degree and direction of lateral tilt on maternal cardiac output. Anesth Analg 97:256, 2003

Bardicef M, Bardicef O, Sorokin Y, et al: Extracellular and intracellular magnesium depletion in pregnancy and gestational diabetes. Am J Obstet Gynecol 172:1009, 1995

Batukan C, Tuncay-Ozgun M, Turkyilmaz C, et al: Isolated torsion of the fallopian tube during pregnancy: A case report. J Reprod Med 52:745, 2007

Bentley-Lewis R, Graves SW, Seely EW: The renin-aldosterone response to stimulation and suppression during normal pregnancy. Hyperten Preg 24:1, 2005

Bergersen TK, Hartgill TW, Pirhonen J: Cerebrovascular response to normal pregnancy: A longitudinal study. Am J Physiol Heart Circ Physiol 290:1856, 2006

Bernstein IM, Ziegler W, Badger GJ: Plasma volume expansion in early pregnancy. Obstet Gynecol 97:669, 2001

Bieniarz J, Branda LA, Maqueda E, et al: Aortocaval compression by the uterus in late pregnancy, 3. Unreliability of the sphygmomanometric method in estimating uterine artery pressure. Am J Obstet Gynecol 102:1106, 1968

Boehlen F, Hohlfeld P, Extermann P, et al: Platelet count at term pregnancy: A reappraisal of the threshold. Obstet Gynecol 95:29, 2000

Bonica JJ: Principles and Practice of Obstetric Analgesia and Anesthesia. Philadelphia, FA Davis, 1967

Bradshaw KD, Santos-Ramos R, Rawlins SC, et al: Endocrine studies in a pregnancy complicated by ovarian theca lutein cysts and hyperreactio luteinalis. Obstet Gynecol 67:66S, 1986

Brar HS, Platt LD, DeVore GR, et al: Qualitative assessment of maternal uterine and fetal umbilical artery blood flow and resistance in laboring patients by Doppler velocimetry. Am J Obstet Gynecol 158:952, 1988

Braverman DZ, Johnson ML, Kern F Jr: Effects of pregnancy and contraceptive steroids on gallbladder function. N Engl J Med 302:362, 1980

Brown MA, Gallery EDM, Ross MR, et al: Sodium excretion in normal and hypertensive pregnancy: A prospective study. Am J Obstet Gynecol 159:297, 1988

Brown MA, Sinosich MJ, Saunders DM, et al: Potassium regulation and progesterone–aldosterone interrelationships in human pregnancy: A prospective study. Am J Obstet Gynecol 155:349, 1986

Burrow GN, Fisher DA, Larsen PR: Maternal and fetal thyroid function. N Engl J Med 331:1072, 1994

Butte NF: Carbohydrate and lipid metabolism in pregnancy: Normal compared with gestational diabetes mellitus. Am J Clin Nutr 7:1256S, 2000

Carr BR, Parker CR Jr, Madden JD, et al: Maternal plasma adrenocorticotropin and cortisol relationships throughout human pregnancy. Am J Obstet Gynecol 139:416, 1981

Cetin I, Nobile de Santis MS, et al: Maternal and fetal amino acid concentrations in normal pregnancies and in pregnancies with gestational diabetes mellitus. Am J Obstet Gynecol 192:610, 2005

Chellakooty M, Vangsgaard K, Larsen T, et al: A longitudinal study of intrauterine growth and the placental growth hormone (GH)–insulin-like growth factor I axis in maternal circulation. J Clin Endocrinol Metab 89:384, 2004

Chesley LC: Renal function during pregnancy. In Carey HM (ed): Modern Trends in Human Reproductive Physiology. London, Butterworth, 1963

Choi JR, Levine D, Finberg H: Luteoma of pregnancy: Sonographic findings in two cases. J Ultrasound Med 19:877, 2000

Clapp JF III, Little KD, Widness JA: Effect of maternal exercise and fetoplacental growth rate on serum erythropoietin concentrations. Am J Obstet Gynecol 188:1021, 2003

Clapp JF III, Stepanchak W, Tomaselli J, et al: Portal vein blood flow—effects of pregnancy, gravity, and exercise. Am J Obstet Gynecol 183:167, 2000

Clark SL, Cotton DB, Lee W, et al: Central hemodynamic assessment of normal term pregnancy. Am J Obstet Gynecol 161:1439, 1989

Clerico A, Emdin M: Diagnostic accuracy and prognostic relevance of the measurement of cardiac natriuretic peptides: A review. Clin Chem 50:33, 2004

Coccia ME, Pasquini L, Comparetto C, et al: Hyperreactio luteinalis in a woman with high-risk factors: A case report. J Reprod Med 48:127, 2003

Combes B, Adams RH: Disorders of the liver in pregnancy. In Assali NS (ed): Pathophysiology of Gestation, Vol I. New York, Academic Press, 1971

Connolly TP, Evans AC: Atypical Papanicolaou smear in pregnancy. Clin Med Res 3:13, 2005

Conrad KP, Jeyabalan A, Danielson LA, et al: Role of relaxin in maternal renal vasodilation of pregnancy. Ann NY Acad Sci 1041:147, 2005

Crisp WE, DeFrancesco S: The hand syndrome of pregnancy. Obstet Gynecol 23:433, 1964

Csapo AI, Pulkkinen MO, Wiest WG: Effects of luteectomy and progesterone replacement therapy in early pregnant patients. Am J Obstet Gynecol 115:759, 1973

Cunningham FG, Cox K, Gant NF: Further observations on the nature of pressor responsivity to angiotensin II in human pregnancy. Obstet Gynecol 46:581, 1975

Cutforth R, MacDonald CB: Heart sounds and murmurs in pregnancy. Am Heart J 71:741, 1966

Darmady JM, Postle AD: Lipid metabolism in pregnancy. Br J Obstet Gynaecol 89:211, 1982

Dashe JS, Casey BM, Wells CE, et al: Thyroid-stimulating hormone in singleton and twin pregnancy: Importance of gestational age-specific reference ranges. Obstet Gynecol 106:753, 2005

Davison JM, Dunlop W: Renal hemodynamics and tubular function in normal human pregnancy. Kidney Int 18:152, 1980

Davison JM, Hytten FE: Glomerular filtration during and after pregnancy. J Obstet Gynaecol Br Commonw 81:588, 1974

Davison JM, Noble MC: Serial changes in 24-hour creatinine clearance during normal menstrual cycles and the first trimester of pregnancy. Br J Obstet Gynaecol 88:10, 1981

Davison JM, Vallotton MB, Lindheimer MD: Plasma osmolality and urinary concentration and dilution during and after pregnancy: Evidence that lateral recumbency inhibits maximal urinary concentrating ability. Br J Obstet Gynaecol 88:472, 1981

Delorme MA, Burrows RF, Ofosu FA, et al: Thrombin regulation in mother and fetus during pregnancy. Semin Thromb Hemost 18:81, 1992

Desoye G, Schweditsch MO, Pfeiffer KP, et al: Correlation of hormones with lipid and lipoprotein levels during normal pregnancy and postpartum. J Clin Endocrinol Metab 64:704, 1987

DeSwiet M: The respiratory system. In Hytten FE, Chamberlain G (eds): Clinical Physiology in Obstetrics, 2nd ed. Oxford, Blackwell, 1991, p 83

Dinn RB, Harris A, Marcus PS: Ocular changes in pregnancy. Obstet Gynecol Surv 58:137, 2003

Dunbar RP, Ries AM: Puerperal diastasis of the pubic symphysis. A case report. J Reprod Med 47:581, 2002

Duvekot JJ, Cheriex EC, Pieters FA, et al: Early pregnancy changes in hemodynamics and volume homeostasis are consecutive adjustments triggered by a primary fall in systemic vascular tone. Am J Obstet Gynecol 169:1382, 1993

Easterling TR, Schmucker BC, Benedetti TJ: The hemodynamic effects of orthostatic stress during pregnancy. Obstet Gynecol 72:550, 1988

Edman CD, Devereux WP, Parker CR, et al: Placental clearance of maternal androgens: A protective mechanism against fetal virilization. Abstract 112 presented at the 26th annual meeting of the Society for Gynecologic Investigation, San Diego, 1979. Gynecol Invest 67:68, 1979

Edman CD, Toofanian A, MacDonald PC, et al: Placental clearance rate of maternal plasma androstenedione through placental estradiol formation: An indirect method of assessing uteroplacental blood flow. Am J Obstet Gynecol 141:1029, 1981

Effraimidou S, Farmakiotis D, Topalidou M: Protein Z levels and recurrent pregnancy loss. Fertil Steril 91(5):e27, 2009

Enein M, Zina AA, Kassem M, et al: Echocardiography of the pericardium in pregnancy. Obstet Gynecol 69:851, 1987

Feletou M, Vanhoutte PM: Endothelial dysfunction: A multifaceted disorder (The Wiggers Award Lecture). Am J Physiol Heart Circ Physiol 291:H985, 2006

Foulk RA, Martin MC, Jerkins GL, et al: Hyperreactio luteinalis differentiated from severe ovarian hyperstimulation syndrome in a spontaneously conceived pregnancy. Am J Obstet Gynecol 176:1300, 1997

Freemark M: Regulation of maternal metabolism by pituitary and placental hormones: Roles in fetal development and metabolic programming. Horm Res 65:41, 2006

Freinkel N: Banting lecture 1980: Of pregnancy and progeny. Diabetes 29:1023, 1980

Freinkel N, Dooley SL, Metzger BE: Care of the pregnant woman with insulin-dependent diabetes mellitus. N Engl J Med 313:96, 1985

Friedman SA: Preeclampsia: A review of the role of prostaglandins. Obstet Gynecol 71:122, 1988

Fuglsang J: Ghrelin in pregnancy and lactation. Vitam Horm 77:259, 2008

Fuglsang J, Sandager P, Moller N, et al: Kinetics and secretion of placental growth hormone around parturition. Eur J Endocrinol 154:449, 2006

Galan HL, Marconi AM, Paolini CL, et al: The transplacental transport of essential amino acids in uncomplicated human pregnancies. Am J Obstet Gynecol 200(1):91.e1-7, 2009

Gallery ED, Raftos J, Gyory AZ, et al: A prospective study of serum complement (C3 and C4) levels in normal human pregnancy: Effect of the development of pregnancy-associated hypertension. Aust N Z J Med 11:243, 1981

Gallery EDM, Lindheimer MD: Alterations in volume homeostasis. In Lindheimer ML, Roberts JM, Cunningham FG (eds): Chesley's Hypertensive Diseases in Pregnancy, 2nd ed. Stamford, CT, Appleton and Lange, 1999, p 327

Gant NF, Chand S, Whalley PJ, et al: The nature of pressor responsiveness to angiotensin II in human pregnancy. Obstet Gynecol 43:854, 1974

Gant NF, Daley GL, Chand S, et al: A study of angiotensin II pressor response throughout primigravid pregnancy. J Clin Invest 52:2682, 1973

Garfield RE, Irani AM, Schwartz LB, et al: Structural and functional comparison of mast cells in the pregnant versus nonpregnant human uterus. Am J Obstet Gynecol 194:261, 2006

Garfield RE, Maner WL, MacKay LB, et al: Comparing uterine electromyography activity of antepartum patients versus term labor patients. Am J Obstet Gynecol 193:23, 2005

Gherman RB, Mestman JH, Satis AJ, et al: Intractable hyperemesis gravidarum, transient hyperthyroidism and intrauterine growth restriction associated with hyperreactio luteinalis. A case report. J Reprod Med 48:553, 2003

Girling JC, Dow E, Smith JH: Liver function tests in preeclampsia: Importance of comparison with a reference range derived for normal pregnancy. Br J Obstet Gynaecol 104:246, 1997

Glinoer D, de Nayer P, Bourdoux P, et al: Regulation of maternal thyroid during pregnancy. J Clin Endocrinol Metab 71:276, 1990

Gohlke BC, Huber A, Bartmann P, et al: Cord blood leptin and IGF-I in relation to birth weight differences and head circumference in monozygotic twins. J Pediat Endocrin Metabol 19:1, 2006

Gonzalez JG, Elizondo G, Saldivar D, et al: Pituitary gland growth during normal pregnancy: An in vivo study using magnetic resonance imaging. Am J Med 85:217, 1988

Grisaru-Granovsky S, Samueloff A, Elstein D: The role of leptin in fetal growth: a short review from conception to delivery. Eur J Obstet Gynecol Reprod Biol 136(2):146, 2008

Harbert GM Jr, Cornell GW, Littlefield JB, et al: Maternal hemodynamics associated with uterine contraction in gravid monkeys. Am J Obstet Gynecol 104:24, 1969

Harirah HM, Donia SE, Nasrallah FK, et al: Effect of gestational age and position on peak expiratory flow rate: A longitudinal study. Obstet Gynecol 105:372, 2005

Harstad TW, Mason RA, Cox SM: Serum erythropoietin quantitation in pregnancy using an enzyme-linked immunoassay. Am J Perinatol 9:233, 1992

Hauguel-de Mouzon S, Lepercq J, Catalano P: The known and unknown of leptin in pregnancy. Am J Obstet Gynecol 194:1537, 2006

Hauth JC, Cunningham FG: Preeclampsia–eclampsia. In Lindheimer MD, Roberts JM, Cunningham FG: Chesley's Hypertensive Disorders in Pregnancy, 2nd ed. Stamford, CT, Appleton & Lange, 1999, p 174

Hayashi M, Inoue T, Hoshimoto K, et al: The levels of five markers of hemostasis and endothelial status at different stages of normotensive pregnancy. Acta Obstet Gynecol Scand 81:208, 2002

Heenan AP, Wolfe LA, Davies GAL, et al: Effects of human pregnancy on fluid regulation responses to short-term exercise. J Appl Physiol 95:2321, 2003

Heidenreich PA, Gubens MA, Fonarow GC, et al: Cost-effectiveness of screening with B-type natriuretic peptide to identify patients with reduced left ventricular ejection fraction. J Am Coll Cardiol 43:1019, 2004

Hein M, Petersen Ac, Helmig RB, et al: Immunoglobulin levels and phagocytes in the cervical mucus plug at term of pregnancy. Acta Obstet Gynecol Scand 84:734, 2005

Henson MC, Castracane VD: Leptin in pregnancy: An update. Biol Reprod 74:218, 2006

Herrera E, Amusquivar E, Lopez-Soldado I, Ortega H: Maternal lipid metabolism and placental lipid transfer. Horm Res 65:59, 2006

Hibbard JU, Shroff SG, Lindheimer MD: Cardiovascular alterations in normal and preeclamptic pregnancy. In Lindheimer MD, Roberts JM, Cunningham FG (eds): Chesley's Hypertension in Pregnancy, 3rd ed. Elsevier, New York, 2009, p 249

Higby K, Suiter CR, Phelps JY, et al: Normal values of urinary albumin and total protein excretion during pregnancy. Am J Obstet Gynecol 171:984, 1994

Hill JA, Olson EN: Cardiac plasticity. N Engl J Med 358:1370, 2008

Hodgkinson CP: Physiology of the ovarian veins in pregnancy. Obstet Gynecol 1:26, 1953

Holmes VA, Wallace JM: Haemostasis in normal pregnancy: A balancing act? Biochem Soc Transact 33:428, 2005

Huerta-Enochian GS, Katz VL, Fox LK, et al: Magnetic resonance—based serial pelvimetry: Do maternal pelvic dimensions change during pregnancy? Am J Obstet Gynecol 194:1689, 2006

Huisman A, Aarnoudse JG, Heuvelmans JHA, et al: Whole blood viscosity during normal pregnancy. Br J Obstet Gynaecol 94:1143, 1987

Hytten FE: The renal excretion of nutrients in pregnancy. Postgrad Med J 49:625, 1973

Hytten FE: Weight gain in pregnancy. In Hytten FE, Chamberlain G (eds): Clinical Physiology in Obstetrics, 2nd ed. Oxford, Blackwell, 1991, p 173

Hytten FE: Lactation. In: The Clinical Physiology of the Puerperium. London, Farrand Press, 1995, p 59

Hytten FE, Chamberlain G: Clinical Physiology in Obstetrics. Oxford, Blackwell, 1991, p 152

Hytten FE, Leitch I: The Physiology of Human Pregnancy, 2nd ed. Philadelphia, Davis, 1971

Hytten FE, Thomson AM: Maternal physiological adjustments. In Assali NS (ed): Biology of Gestation, Vol I. The Maternal Organism. New York, Academic Press, 1968

Ingerslev M, Teilum G: Biopsy studies on the liver in pregnancy, 2. Liver biopsy on normal pregnant women. Acta Obstet Gynecol Scand 25:352, 1946

Innis SM: Essential fatty acid transfer and fetal development. Placenta 26:570, 2005

Inoue T, Hotta A, Awai M, et al: Loss of vision due to a physiologic pituitary enlargement during normal pregnancy. Graefe's Arch Clin Exp Ophthalmol 245:1049, 2007

Iosif S, Ingemarsson I, Ulmsten U: Urodynamic studies in normal pregnancy and in puerperium. Am J Obstet Gynecol 137:696, 1980

Jain N, Sternberg LB: Symphyseal separation. Obstet Gynecol 105:1229, 2005

Jarolim P: Serum biomarkers for heart failure. Cardiovasc Pathol 15:144, 2006

Jauniaux E, Johnson MR, Jurkovic D, et al: The role of relaxin in the development of the uteroplacental circulation in early pregnancy. Obstet Gynecol 84:338, 1994

Jeffreys RM, Stepanchak W, Lopez B, et al: Uterine blood flow during supine rest and exercise after 28 weeks of gestation. BJOG 113:1239, 2006

Jensen D, Wolfe LA, Slatkovska L, et al: Effects of human pregnancy on the ventilatory chemoreflex response to carbon dioxide. Am J Physiol Regul Integr Comp Physiol 288:R1369, 2005

Jensen E, Wood C, Keller-Wood M: The normal increase in adrenal secretion during pregnancy contributes to maternal volume expansion and fetal homeostasis. J Soc Gynecol Investig 9:362, 2002

Jonsson Y, Ruber M, Matthiesen L, et al: Cytokine mapping of sera from women with preeclampsia and normal pregnancies. J Reprod Immunol 70:83, 2006

Kalhan SC, Gruca LL, Parimi PS, et al: Serine metabolism in human pregnancy. Am J Physiol Endocrinol Metab 284:E733, 2003

Kametas NA, McAuliffe F, Krampl E, et al: Maternal cardiac function in twin pregnancy. Obstet Gynecol 102:806, 2003a

Kametas N, McAuliffe F, Krampl E, et al: Maternal electrolyte and liver function changes during pregnancy at high altitude. Clin Chim Acta 328:21, 2003b

Kaneshige E: Serum ferritin as an assessment of iron stores and other hematologic parameters during pregnancy. Obstet Gynecol 57:238, 1981

Kauppila A, Chatelain P, Kirkinen P, et al: Isolated prolactin deficiency in a woman with puerperal alactogenesis. J Clin Endocrinol Metab 64:309, 1987

Kauppila A, Koskinen M, Puolakka J, et al: Decreased intervillous and unchanged myometrial blood flow in supine recumbency. Obstet Gynecol 55:203, 1980

Keenan PA, Yaldoo DT, Stress ME, et al: Explicit memory in pregnant women. Am J Obstet Gynecol 179:731, 1998

Keller-Wood M, Wood CE: Pregnancy alters cortisol feedback inhibition of stimulated ACTH: Studies in adrenalectomized ewes. Am J Physiol Regul Integr Comp Physiol 280:R1790, 2001

Kinsella SM, Lohmann G: Supine hypotensive syndrome. Obstet Gynecol 83:774, 1994

Klafen A, Palugyay J: Vergleichende Untersuchungen über Lage und Ausdehrung von Herz und Lunge in der Schwangerschaft und im Wochenbett. Arch Gynaekol 131:347, 1927

Kletzky OA, Rossman F, Bertolli SI, et al: Dynamics of human chorionic gonadotropin, prolactin, and growth hormone in serum and amniotic fluid throughout normal human pregnancy. Am J Obstet Gynecol 151:878, 1985

Kolarzyk E, Szot WM, Lyszczarz J: Lung function and breathing regulation parameters during pregnancy. Arch Gynecol Obstet 272:53, 2005

Kovacs CS, Fuleihan GE: Calcium and bone disorders during pregnancy and lactation. Endocrin Metab Clin North Am 35:21, 2006

Krause PJ, Ingardia CJ, Pontius LT, et al: Host defense during pregnancy: Neutrophil chemotaxis and adherence. Am J Obstet Gynecol 157:274, 1987

Kubota T, Kamada S, Hirata Y, et al: Synthesis and release of endothelin-1 by human decidual cells. J Clin Endocrinol Metab 75:1230, 1992

Kumru S, Boztosun A, Godekmerdan A: Pregnancy-associated changes in peripheral blood lymphocyte subpopulations and serum cytokine concentrations in healthy women. J Reprod Med 50:246, 2005

Kutteh WH, Franklin RD: Quantification of immunoglobulins and cytokines in human cervical mucus during each trimester of pregnancy. Am J Obstet Gynecol 184:865, 2001

Lammert F, Marschall HU, Glantz A, et al: Intrahepatic cholestasis of pregnancy: Molecular pathogenesis, diagnosis and management. J Hepatol 33:1012, 2000

Langer JE, Coleman BG: Case 1: Diagnosis: Hyperreactio luteinalis complicating a normal pregnancy. Ultrasound Q 23:63, 2007

Lederman SA, Paxton A, Heymsfield SB, et al: Maternal body fat and water during pregnancy: Do they raise infant birth weight? Am J Obstet Gynecol 180:235, 1999

Lee KA, Zaffke ME, McEnany G: Parity and sleep patterns during and after pregnancy. Obstet Gynecol 95:14, 2000

Lepercq J, Guerre-Millo M, Andre J, et al: Leptin: A potential marker of placental insufficiency. Gynecol Obstet Invest 55:151, 2003

Lind T, Bell S, Gilmore E, et al: Insulin disappearance rate in pregnant and nonpregnant women, and in non-pregnant women given GHRIH. Eur J Clin Invest 7:47, 1977

Lindheimer MD, Davison JM: Osmoregulation, the secretion of arginine vasopressin and its metabolism during pregnancy. Eur J Endocrinol 132:133, 1995

Lindheimer MD, Davison JM, Katz AI: The kidney and hypertension in pregnancy: Twenty exciting years. Semin Nephrol 21:173, 2001

Lindheimer MD, Grünfeld J-P, Davison JM: Renal disorders. In Barran WM, Lindheimer MD (eds): Medical Disorders During Pregnancy, 3rd ed. St. Louis, Mosby, 2000, p 39

Lindheimer MD, Richardson DA, Ehrlich EN, et al: Potassium homeostasis in pregnancy. J Reprod Med 32:517, 1987

Lippi G, Albiero A, Montagnana M, et al: Lipid and lipoprotein profile in physiological pregnancy. Clin Lab 53:173, 2007

Lønberg U, Damm P, Andersson A-M, et al: Increase in maternal placental growth hormone during pregnancy and disappearance during parturition in normal and growth hormone-deficient pregnancies. Am J Obstet Gynecol 188:247, 2003

Lowe SA, MacDonald GJ, Brown MA: Acute and chronic regulation of atrial natriuretic peptide in human pregnancy: A longitudinal study. J Hypertens 10:821, 1992

Luppi P, Haluszczak C, Trucco M, et al: Normal pregnancy is associated with peripheral leukocyte activation. Am J Reprod Immunol 47:72, 2002

Mabie WC, DiSessa TG, Crocker LG, et al: A longitudinal study of cardiac output in normal human pregnancy. Am J Obstet Gynecol 170:849, 1994

Macfie AG, Magides AD, Richmond MN, et al: Gastric emptying in pregnancy. Br J Anaesth 67:54, 1991

Manten GTR, Franx A, Sikkema JM, et al: Fibrinogen and high molecular weight fibrinogen during and after normal pregnancy. Thrombosis Res 114:19, 2004

Mardones-Santander F, Salazar G, Rosso P, et al: Maternal body composition near term and birth weight. Obstet Gynecol 91:873, 1998

Margarit L, Griffiths A, Tsapanos V, et al: Second trimester amniotic fluid endothelin concentration: A possible predictor for pre-eclampsia. J Obstet Gynaecol 25:18, 2005

Marnach ML, Ramin KD, Ramsey PS, et al: Characterization of the relationship between joint laxity and maternal hormones in pregnancy. Obstet Gynecol 101:331, 2003

Masini E, Nistri S, Vannacci A, et al: Relaxin inhibits the activation of human neutrophils: Involvement of the nitric oxide pathway. Endocrinology 145:1106, 2004

Maymon R, Zimerman AL, Strauss S, et al: Maternal spleen size throughout normal pregnancy. Semin Ultrasound CT MRI 28:64, 2007

McAuliffe F, Kametas N, Costello J, et al: Respiratory function in singleton and twin pregnancy. Br J Obstet Gynaecol 109:765, 2002

McLaughlin MK, Roberts JM: Hemodynamic changes. In Lindheimer ML, Roberts JM, Cunningham FG (eds): Chesley's Hypertensive Diseases in Pregnancy, 2nd ed. Stamford, CT, Appleton and Lange, 1999, p 69

McLennan CE: Antecubital and femoral venous pressure in normal and toxemic pregnancy. Am J Obstet Gynecol 45:568, 1943

Mendenhall HW: Serum protein concentrations in pregnancy. 1. Concentrations in maternal serum. Am J Obstet Gynecol 106:388, 1970

Michimata T, Sakai M, Miyazaki S, et al: Decrease of T-helper 2 and T-cytotoxic 2 cells at implantation sites occurs in unexplained recurrent spontaneous abortion with normal chromosomal content. Hum Reprod 18:1523, 2003

Migeon CJ, Bertrand J, Wall PE: Physiological disposition of 4-^{14}C cortisol during late pregnancy. J Clin Invest 36:1350, 1957

Milne JA, Howie AD, Pack AI: Dyspnoea during normal pregnancy. Br J Obstet Gynaecol 85:260, 1978

Mittal P, Espinoza J, Hassan S, et al: Placental growth hormone is increased in the maternal and fetal serum of patients with preeclampsia. J Matern Fetal Neonatal Med 20:651, 2007

Miyamoto J: Prolactin and thyrotropin responses to thyrotropin-releasing hormone during the peripartal period. Obstet Gynecol 63:639, 1984

Mojtahedi M, de Groot LC, Boekholt HA, et al: Nitrogen balance of healthy Dutch women before and during pregnancy. Am J Clin Nutr 75:1078, 2002

More C, Bhattoa HP, Bettembuk P, et al: The effects of pregnancy and lactation on hormonal status and biochemical markers of bone turnover. Eur J Obstet Gynecol Reprod Biol 106:209, 2003

Morikawa M, Yamada T, Turuga N, et al: Coagulation-fibrinolysis is more enhanced in twin than in singleton pregnancies. J Perinat Med 34:392, 2006

Muallem MM, Rubeiz NG: Physiological and biological skin changes in pregnancy. Clin Dermatol 24:80, 2006

Naden RP, Rosenfeld CR: Systemic and uterine responsiveness to angiotensin II and norepinephrine in estrogen-treated nonpregnant sheep. Am J Obstet Gynecol 153:417, 1985

Nolten WE, Rueckert PA: Elevated free cortisol index in pregnancy: Possible regulatory mechanisms. Am J Obstet Gynecol 139:492, 1981

Obuobie K, Mullik V, Jones C, et al: McCune-Albright syndrome: Growth hormone dynamics in pregnancy. J Clin Endocrinol Metab 86:2456, 2001

Øian P, Maltau JM, Noddeland H, et al: Oedema-preventing mechanisms in subcutaneous tissue of normal pregnant women. Br J Obstet Gynaecol 92:1113, 1985

Osman H, Rubeiz N, Tamim H, et al: Risk factors for the development of striae gravidarum. Am J Obstet Gynecol 196:62.e1, 2007

Page KL, Celia G, Leddy G, et al: Structural remodeling of rat uterine veins in pregnancy. Am J Obstet Gynecol 187:1647, 2002

Palmer SK, Zamudio S, Coffin C, et al: Quantitative estimation of human uterine artery blood flow and pelvic blood flow redistribution in pregnancy. Obstet Gynecol 80:1000, 1992

Park JI, Chang CL, Hsu SY: New insights into biological roles of relaxin and relaxin-related peptides. Rev Endocr Metab Disord 6:291, 2005

Parker CR Jr, Everett RB, Whalley PJ, et al: Hormone production during pregnancy in the primigravid patients. II. Plasma levels of deoxycorticosterone throughout pregnancy of normal women and women who developed pregnancy-induced hypertension. Am J Obstet Gynecol 138:626, 1980

Pasrija S, Sharma N: Benign diffuse breast hyperplasia during pregnancy. N Engl J Med 355:2771, 2006

Pates JA, McIntire DD, Leveno KJ: Uterine contractions preceding labor. Obstet Gynecol 110:566, 2007

Peck TM, Arias F: Hematologic changes associated with pregnancy. Clin Obstet Gynecol 22:785, 1979

Phelps RL, Metzger BE, Freinkel N: Carbohydrate metabolism in pregnancy, 17. Diurnal profiles of plasma glucose, insulin, free fatty acids, triglycerides, cholesterol, and individual amino acids in late normal pregnancy. Am J Obstet Gynecol 140:730, 1981

Pighetti M, Tommaselli GA, D'Elia A, et al: Maternal serum and umbilical cord blood leptin concentrations with fetal growth restriction. Obstet Gynecol 102:535, 2003

Pipe NGJ, Smith T, Halliday D, et al: Changes in fat, fat-free mass and body water in human normal pregnancy. Br J Obstet Gynaecol 86:929, 1979

Pitkin RM, Reynolds WA, Williams GA, et al: Calcium metabolism in normal pregnancy: A longitudinal study. Am J Obstet Gynecol 133:781, 1979

Platts JK, Meadows P, Jones R, et al: The relation between tissue kallikrein excretion rate, aldosterone and glomerular filtration rate in human pregnancy. Br J Obstet Gynaecol 107:278, 2000

Power ML, Heaney RP, Kalkwarf HJ, et al: The role of calcium in health and disease. Am J Obstet Gynecol 181:1560, 1999

Powers RW, Majors AK, Kerchner LJ, et al: Renal handling of homocysteine during normal pregnancy and preeclampsia. J Soc Gynecol Investig 11:45, 2004

Pritchard JA: Changes in the blood volume during pregnancy and delivery. Anesthesiology 26:393, 1965

Pritchard JA, Adams RH: Erythrocyte production and destruction during pregnancy. Am J Obstet Gynecol 79:750, 1960

Pritchard JA, Mason RA: Iron stores of normal adults and their replenishment with oral iron therapy. JAMA 190:897, 1964

Pritchard JA, Scott DE: Iron demands during pregnancy. In: Iron Deficiency-Pathogenesis: Clinical Aspects and Therapy. London, Academic Press, 1970, p 173

Quack Loetscher KC, Stiller R, Roos M, et al: Protein Z in normal pregnancy. Thromb Haemost 93:706, 2005

Rana S, Lindheimer M, Hibbard J, Pliskin N: Neuropsychological performance in normal pregnancy and preeclampsia. Am J Obstet Gynecol 195:186, 2006

Reitz RE, Daane TA, Woods JR, et al: Calcium, magnesium, phosphorus, and parathyroid hormone interrelationships in pregnancy and newborn infants. Obstet Gynecol 50:701, 1977

Repke JT: Calcium homeostasis in pregnancy. Clin Obstet Gynecol 37:59, 1994

Resnik JL, Hong C, Resnik R, et al: Evaluation of B-type natriuretic peptide (BNP) levels in normal and preeclamptic women. Am J Obstet Gynecol 193:450, 2005

Richani K, Soto E, Romero R, et al: Normal pregnancy is characterized by systemic activation of the complement system. J Matern Fetal Neonat Med 17:239, 2005

Riedl M, Maier C, Handisurya A, et al: Insulin resistance has no impact on ghrelin suppression in pregnancy. Intern Med 262:458, 2007

Robb AO, Mills NL, Din JN, et al: Acute endothelial tissue plasminogen activator release in pregnancy. J Thromb Haemost 7(1):138, 2009

Rosenfeld CR: Mechanisms regulated angiotensin II responsiveness by the interoplacental circulation. Am J Physiol Regul Integr Comp Physiol 28:R1025, 2001

Rosenfeld CR, Barton MD, Meschia G: Effects of epinephrine on distribution of blood flow in the pregnant ewe. Am J Obstet Gynecol 124:156, 1976

Rosenfeld CR, Gant NF Jr: The chronically instrumented ewe: A model for studying vascular reactivity to angiotensin II in pregnancy. J Clin Invest 67:486, 1981

Rosenfeld CR, Roy T, DeSpain K, et al: Large-conductance Ca^{2+}-dependent K^{+} channels regulate basal uteroplacental blood flow in ovine pregnancy. J Soc Gynecol Investig 12:402, 2005

Rosenfeld CR, West J: Circulatory response to systemic infusion of norepinephrine in the pregnant ewe. Am J Obstet Gynecol 127:376, 1977

Rubi RA, Sala NL: Ureteral function in pregnant women, 3. Effect of different positions and of fetal delivery upon ureteral tonus. Am J Obstet Gynecol 101:230, 1968

Ruiz-Extremera A, López-Garrido MA, Barranco E, et al: Activity of hepatic enzymes from week sixteen of pregnancy. Am J Obstet Gynecol 193:2010, 2005

Saarelainen H, Laitinen T, Raitakari OT, et al: Pregnancy-related hyperlipidemia and endothelial function in healthy women. Circ J 70:768, 2006

Sandhu KS, LaCombe JA, Fleischmann N: Gross and microscopic hematuria: guidelines for obstetricians and gynecologists. Obstet Gynecol Surv 64(1):39, 2009

Savvidou MD, Hingorani AD, Tsikas D, et al: Endothelial dysfunction and raised plasma concentrations of asymmetric dimethylarginine in pregnant women who subsequently develop pre-eclampsia. Lancet 361:1511, 2003

Schannwell CM, Zimmermann T, Schneppenheim M, et al: Left ventricular hypertrophy and diastolic dysfunction in healthy pregnant women. Cardiology 97:73, 2002

Scheithauer BW, Sano T, Kovacs KT, et al: The pituitary gland in pregnancy: A clinicopathologic and immunohistochemical study of 69 cases. Mayo Clin Proc 65:461, 1990

Schiessl B, Strasburger CJ, Bidlingmeier M, et al: Role of placental growth hormone in the alteration of maternal arterial resistance in pregnancy. J Reprod Med 52:313, 2007

Schulman A, Herlinger H: Urinary tract dilatation in pregnancy. Br J Radiol 48:638, 1975

Seligman SP, Buyon JP, Clancy RM, et al: The role of nitric oxide in the pathogenesis of preeclampsia. Am J Obstet Gynecol 171:944, 1994

Semins MJ, Trock BJ, Matlaga: The safety of ureteroscopy during pregnancy: Abhoffm systematic review and meta-analysis. J Urol 181(1):139, 2009

Sherer DM, Dalloul M, Khoury-Collado F, et al: Hyperreactio luteinalis presenting with marked hyperglycemia and bilateral multicystic adnexal masses at 21 weeks gestation. Am J Perinatol 23:85, 2006

Shinagawa S, Suzuki S, Chihara H, et al: Maternal basal metabolic rate in twin pregnancy. Gynecol Obstet Invest 60:145, 2005

Shortle BE, Warren MP, Tsin D: Recurrent androgenicity in pregnancy: A case report and literature review. Obstet Gynecol 70:462, 1987

Simon FR, Fortune J, Iwahashi M, et al: Ethinyl estradiol cholestasis involves alterations in expression of liver sinusoidal transporters. Am J Physiol 271:G1043, 1996

Simpson KR, James DC: Efficacy of intrauterine resuscitation techniques in improving fetal oxygen status during labor. Obstet Gynecol 105:1362, 2005

Smallridge RC, Glinoer D, Hollowell JG, Brent G: Thyroid function inside and outside of pregnancy: What do we know and what don't we know? Thyroid 15:54, 2005

Smith MC, Murdoch AP, Danielson LA, et al: Relaxin has a role in establishing a renal response in pregnancy. Fertil Steril 86:253, 2006

Song CS, Kappas A: The influence of estrogens, progestins and pregnancy on the liver. Vitam Horm 26:147, 1968

Spitzer RF, Wherrett D, Chitayat D, et al: Maternal luteoma of pregnancy presenting with virilization of the female infant. J Obstet Gynaecol Can 29:835, 2007

Stein PK, Hagley MT, Cole PL, et al: Changes in 24-hour heart rate variability during normal pregnancy. Am J Obstet Gynecol 180:978, 1999

Sternberg WH: Non-functioning ovarian neoplasms. In Grady HG, Smith DE (eds): International Academy of Pathology monograph no. 3. The Ovary. Baltimore, Williams & Wilkins, 1963

Straach KJ, Shelton JM, Richardson JA, et al: Regulation of hyaluronan expression during cervical ripening. Glycobiology 15:55, 2005

Sunness JS: The pregnant woman's eye. Surv Ophthalmol 32:219, 1988

Swain AM, O'Hara MW, Starr KR, et al: A prospective study of sleep, mood, and cognitive function in postpartum and nonpostpartum women. Obstet Gynecol 90:381, 1997

Tamás P, Szilágyi A, Jeges S, et al: Effects of maternal central hemodynamics on fetal heart rate patterns. Acta Obstet Gynecol Scand 86:711, 2007

Tanaka Y, Yanagihara T, Ueta M, et al: Naturally conceived twin pregnancy with hyperreactio luteinalis, causing hyperandrogenism and maternal virilization. Acta Obstet Gynecol Scand 80:277, 2001

Taussig FJ: Ectopic decidua formation. Surg Gynecol Obstet 2:292, 1906

Taylor DJ, Phillips P, Lind T: Puerperal haematological indices. Br J Obstet Gynaecol 88:601, 1981

Teran E, Escudero C, Vivero S, et al: NO in early pregnancy and development of preeclampsia. Hypertension 47:e17, 2006

Thellin O, Heinen E: Pregnancy and the immune system: Between tolerance and rejection. Toxicology 185:179, 2003

Thorpe-Beeston JG, Nicolaides KH, Snijders RJM, et al: Fetal thyroid-stimulating hormone response to maternal administration of thyrotropin-releasing hormone. Am J Obstet Gynecol 164:1244, 1991

Tihtonen KM, Kööbi T, Vuolteenaho O, et al: Natriuretic peptides and hemodynamics in preeclampsia. Am J Obstet Gynecol 196:328.e1, 2007

Timmons BC, Mahendroo M: Processes regulating cervical ripening differ from cervical dilation and postpartum repair: Insights from gene expression studies. Reproductive Sciences 14:53, 2007

Trakada G, Tsapanos V, Spiropoulos K: Normal pregnancy and oxygenation during sleep. Eur J Obstet Gynecol Reprod Biol 109:128, 2003

Tsai CH, de Leeuw NKM: Changes in 2,3-diphosphoglycerate during pregnancy and puerperium in normal women and in β-thalassemia heterozygous women. Am J Obstet Gynecol 142:520, 1982

Tygart SG, McRoyan DK, Spinnato JA, et al: Longitudinal study of platelet indices during normal pregnancy. Am J Obstet Gynecol 154:883, 1986

Uchikova EH, Ledjev II: Changes in haemostasis during normal pregnancy. Eur J Obstet Gynecol Reprod Biol 119:185, 2005

Ueland K: Maternal cardiovascular dynamics, 7. Intrapartum blood volume changes. Am J Obstet Gynecol 126:671, 1976

Ueland K, Metcalfe J: Circulatory changes in pregnancy. Clin Obstet Gynecol 18:41, 1975

Ulmsten U, Sundström G: Esophageal manometry in pregnant and nonpregnant women. Am J Obstet Gynecol 132:260, 1978

van Brummen H, Bruinse HW, van der Bom J, et al: How do the prevalences of urogenital symptoms change during pregnancy? Neurourol Urodynam 25:135, 2006

van den Akker CH, Schierbeek H, Dorst KY, et al: Human fetal amino acid metabolism at term gestation. Am J Clin Nutr 89(1):153, 2009

Van Wagenen G, Jenkins RH: An experimental examination of factors causing ureteral dilatation of pregnancy. J Urol 42:1010, 1939

Vidaeff AC, Ross PJ, Livingston CK, et al: Gigantomastia complicating mirror syndrome in pregnancy. Obstet Gynecol 101:1139, 2003

Villaseca P, Campino C, Oestreicher E, et al: Bilateral oophorectomy in a pregnant woman: Hormonal profile from late gestation to post-partum: Case report. Hum Reprod 20:397, 2005

Walker MC, Garner PR, Keely EJ, et al: Changes in activated protein C resistance during normal pregnancy. Am J Obstet Gynecol 177:162, 1997

Walther T, Stepan H: C-type natriuretic peptide in reproduction, pregnancy and fetal development. J Endocrinol 180:17, 2004

Watanabe M, Meeker CI, Gray MJ, et al: Secretion rate of aldosterone in normal pregnancy. J Clin Invest 42:1619, 1963

Watts DH, Krohn MA, Wener MH, et al: C-reactive protein in normal pregnancy. Obstet Gynecol 77:176, 1991

Waugh J, Bell SC, Kilby MD, et al: Urinary microalbumin/creatinine ratios: Reference range in uncomplicated pregnancy. Clin Sci 104:103, 2003

Weisman Y, Harell A, Edelstein S, et al: 1α,25-Dihydroxyvitamin D_3 and 24,25-dihydroxyvitamin D_3 in vitro synthesis by human decidua and placenta. Nature 281:317, 1979

Weiss M, Eisenstein Z, Ramot Y, et al: Renal reabsorption of inorganic phosphorus in pregnancy in relation to the calciotropic hormones. Br J Obstet Gynaecol 105:195, 1998

Wesnes SL, Hunskaar S, Bo K, et al: The effect of urinary inconrinence status during pregnancy and delivery mode on incontinence postpartum. A cohort study. BJOG 116(5):700, 2009

Whitcome KK, Shapiro LJ, Lieberman DE: Fetal load and the evolution of lumbar lordosis in bipedal hominins. Nature 450:1075, 2007

Whitehead M, Lane G, Young O, et al: Interrelations of calcium-regulating hormones during normal pregnancy. BMJ 283:10, 1981

Whittaker PG, MacPhail S, Lind T: Serial hematologic changes and pregnancy outcome. Obstet Gynecol 88:33, 1996

Wilson M, Morganti AA, Zervoudakis I, et al: Blood pressure, the renin-aldosterone system and sex steroids throughout normal pregnancy. Am J Med 68:97, 1980

Wise RA, Polito AJ, Krishnan V: Respiratory physiologic changes in pregnancy. Immunol Allergy Clin North Am 26:1, 2006

Wong CA, Loffredi M, Ganchiff JN, et al: Gastric emptying of water in term pregnancy. Anesthesiology 96:1395, 2002

Wong CA, McCarthy RJ, Fitzgerald PC, et al: Gastric emptying of water in obese pregnant women at term. Anesth Analg 105:751, 2007

Word RA, Li XH, Hnat M, et al: Dynamics of cervical remodeling during pregnancy and parturition: Mechanisms and current concepts. Semin Reprod Med 25:69, 2007

Wright HP, Osborn SB, Edmonds DG: Changes in rate of flow of venous blood in the leg during pregnancy, measured with radioactive sodium. Surg Gynecol Obstet 90:481, 1950

Xiao D, Huang X, Yang S, et al: Direct effects of nicotine on contractility of the uterine artery in pregnancy. J Pharmacol Exp Ther 322:180, 2007

Zeeman GG, Hatab M, Twickler DM: Maternal cerebral blood flow changes in pregnancies. Am J Obstet Gynecol 189:968, 2003

CHAPTER 6

Parturition

The last few hours of human pregnancy are characterized by uterine contractions that effect cervical dilatation and cause the fetus to descend through the birth canal. Long before these forceful, painful contractions, there are extensive preparations in both the uterus and cervix, and these progress throughout gestation. During the first 36 to 38 weeks of normal gestation, the myometrium is in a preparatory yet unresponsive state. Concurrently, the cervix begins an early stage of remodeling termed *softening*, yet maintains structural integrity. Following this prolonged uterine quiescence, there is a transitional phase during which myometrial unresponsiveness is suspended, and the cervix undergoes ripening, effacement, and loss of structural integrity.

The physiological processes that regulate parturition and the onset of labor continue to be defined. It is clear, however, that labor onset represents the culmination of a series of biochemical changes in the uterus and cervix. These result from endocrine and paracrine signals emanating from both mother and fetus. Their relative contributions vary between species, and it is these differences that complicate elucidation of the exact factors that regulate human parturition. When parturition is abnormal, preterm labor, dystocia, or postterm pregnancy may result. Of these, preterm labor remains the major contributor to neonatal mortality and morbidity in developed countries (see Chap. 36, p. 804).

PHASES OF PARTURITION

Parturition, the bringing forth of young, requires multiple transformations in both uterine and cervical function. As shown in **Figure 6-1**, parturition can be arbitrarily divided into four overlapping phases that correspond to the major physiological transitions of the myometrium and cervix during pregnancy (Casey and MacDonald, 1993, 1997; Challis and associates, 2000; Word and colleagues, 2007). These phases of parturition include: (1) a prelude to—first phase; (2) the preparation for—second phase; (3) the process of—third phase; and (4) recovery from—fourth phase. Importantly, the *phases of parturition* should not be confused with the *clinical stages of labor,* that is, the first, second, and third stages—which comprise the third phase of parturition (Fig. 6-2).

Phase 1 of Parturition: Uterine Quiescence and Cervical Softening

Uterine Quiescence

Beginning even before implantation, a remarkably effective period of myometrial quiescence is imposed. This phase normally comprises 95 percent of pregnancy and is characterized by uterine smooth muscle tranquility with maintenance of cervical structural integrity. The inherent propensity of the myometrium to contract is held in abeyance, and uterine muscle is rendered unresponsive to natural stimuli. Concurrently, the uterus must initiate extensive changes in its size and vascularity to accommodate the pregnancy and prepare for uterine contractions in phase 3 of parturition. The myometrial unresponsiveness of phase 1 continues until near the end of pregnancy.

Although some myometrial contractions are noted during the quiescent phase, they do not normally cause cervical dilatation. They are characterized by their unpredictability, low intensity, and brief duration. Any discomfort that they produce usually is

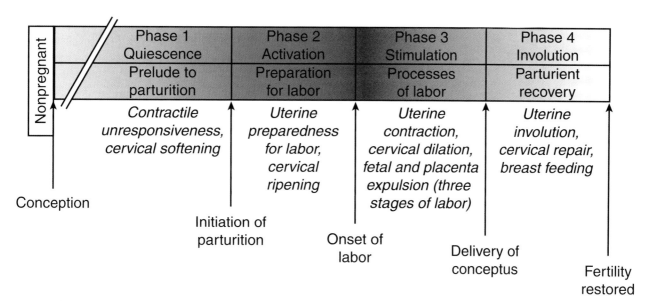

FIGURE 6-1 The phases of parturition.

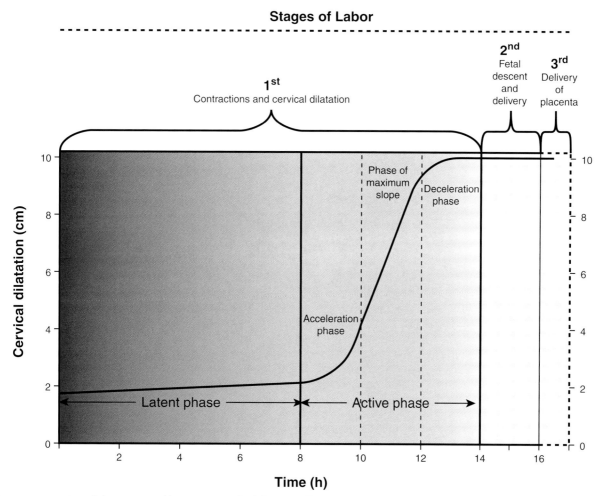

FIGURE 6-2 Composite of the average dilatation curve for labor in nulliparous women. The curve is based on analysis of data derived from a large, nearly consecutive series of women. The first stage is divided into a relatively flat latent phase and a rapidly progressive active phase. In the active phase, there are three identifiable component parts: an acceleration phase, a linear phase of maximum slope, and a deceleration phase. (Redrawn from Friedman, 1978.)

confined to the lower abdomen and groin. Near the end of pregnancy, contractions of this type become more common, especially in multiparous women. They are sometimes referred to as *Braxton Hicks contractions* or *false labor* (see Chap. 17, p. 390).

Cervical Softening

The cervix has multiple functions during pregnancy that include: (1) maintenance of barrier function to protect the reproductive tract from infection, (2) maintenance of cervical competence despite the increasing gravitational forces imposed by the expanding uterus, and (3) orchestrating extracellular matrix changes that allow progressive increases in tissue compliance in preparation for birth.

In nonpregnant women, the cervix is closed and firm, and its consistency is similar to nasal cartilage. By the end of pregnancy, the cervix is easily distensible, and its consistency is similar to the lips of the oral cavity. Thus, the first stage of this remodeling—termed *softening*—is characterized by an increase in tissue compliance, yet the cervix remains firm and unyielding. Hegar (1895) first described palpable softening of the lower uterine segment at 4 to 6 weeks' gestation, and this sign was once used to diagnose pregnancy.

Clinically, the maintenance of cervical anatomical and structural integrity is essential for continuation of pregnancy to term. Preterm cervical dilatation, structural incompetence, or both may forecast an unfavorable pregnancy outcome that ends most often in preterm delivery (see Chap. 36, p. 814). Indeed, cervical shortening between 16 and 24 weeks has been associated with an increased risk of preterm delivery (Hibbard and associates, 2000; Iams and colleagues, 1996).

Structural Changes with Softening. Cervical softening results from increased vascularity, stromal hypertrophy, glandular hypertrophy and hyperplasia, and compositional or structural changes of the extracellular matrix (Danforth and colleagues, 1974; Leppert, 1995; Liggins, 1978 ; Word and associates, 2007). Specifically, during phase 1 of parturition, the cervix begins a slow, progressive increase in turnover of matrix components. For example, in mouse models with deficiency of the extracellular matrix protein, thrombospondin 2, collagen fibril morphology is altered and there is premature cervical softening (Kokenyesi and co-workers, 2004).

Another change found in animal models is that physiological softening is preceded by an increase in collagen solubility (Read and associates, 2007). This reflects a change in collagen processing or a change in the number or type of covalent cross-links between collagen triple helices which are normally required for stable collagen fibril formation (Fig. 6-3) (Canty and Kadler, 2005). A reduction in cross-linking of newly synthesized collagen may aid cervical softening because decreased transcripts and activity of the cross-linking enzyme, lysyl oxidase, have been reported in the mouse cervix during pregnancy (Drewes and associates, 2007; Ozasa and colleagues, 1981).

In humans, the clinical importance of these matrix changes is shown by the greater prevalence of cervical incompetence in women with inherited defects in collagen and elastin synthesis or assembly—for example, Ehlers-Danlos and Marfan syndromes (Anum, 2009; Hermanns-Lê, 2005; Paternoster, 1998; Rahman, 2003; Wang, 2006, and all their colleagues).

Phase 2 of Parturition: Preparation for Labor

To prepare for labor, the myometrial tranquility of phase 1 of parturition must be suspended through what has been called *uterine awakening* or *activation*. This process constitutes phase 2 and represents a progression of uterine changes during the last 6 to 8 weeks of pregnancy. Importantly, shifting events associated with phase 2 can cause either preterm or delayed labor. Thus, understanding myometrial and cervical modifications during phase 2 provides a better understanding of events leading to normal and abnormal labor.

Myometrial Changes During Phase 2

Most myometrial changes during phase 2 prepare it for labor contractions. This shift probably results from alterations in the expression of key proteins that control contractility. These *contraction-associated proteins (CAPs)* include the oxytocin receptor, prostaglandin F receptor, and connexin 43 (Smith, 2007). Thus, myometrial oxytocin receptors markedly increase along with increased numbers and surface areas of gap junction proteins such as connexin 43. Together these lead to increased uterine irritability and responsiveness to *uterotonins*—agents that stimulate contractions.

Another critical change in phase 2 is formation of the lower uterine segment from the isthmus. With this development, the fetal head often descends to or even through the pelvic inlet—so-called *lightening*. The abdomen commonly undergoes a change in shape, sometimes described as "the baby dropped." It is also likely that the lower segment myometrium is unique from that in the upper uterine segment, resulting in distinct roles for each during labor. This is supported by baboon studies that demonstrate differential expression of prostaglandin receptors within myometrial regions. There are also human studies that report an expression gradient of oxytocin receptors, with higher expression in fundal myometrial cells (Fuchs, 1984; Havelock, 2005; Smith, 2001, and all their colleagues).

Cervical Ripening During Phase 2

Prior to the initiation of contractions, the cervix must undergo more extensive remodeling. This eventually results in cervical yielding and dilatation upon initiation of forceful uterine contractions in the third phase of parturition. Cervical modifications during this second phase principally involve connective tissue changes—so-called *cervical ripening*. The transition from the softening to the ripening phase begins weeks or days before onset of contractions. During this transformation, the total amount and composition of proteoglycans and glycosaminoglycans within the matrix are altered. Many of the processes that aid cervical remodeling are controlled by the same hormones regulating uterine function. That said, the molecular events of each are varied because of differences in cellular composition and physiological requirements. The uterine corpus is predominantly smooth muscle, whereas the cervix is primarily connective tissue. Cellular components of the cervix include smooth muscle, fibroblasts, and epithelia.

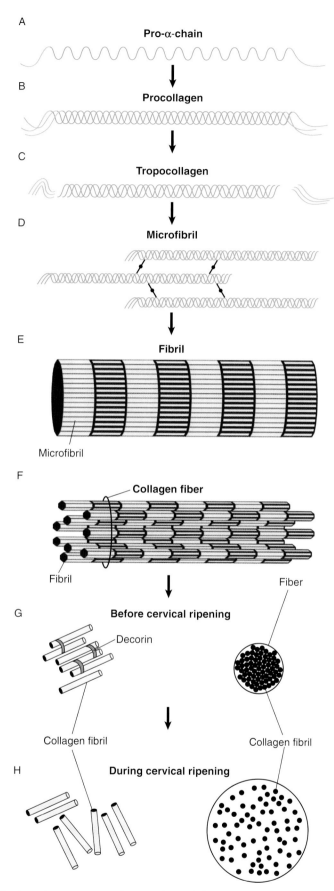

FIGURE 6-3 Fibrillar collagen synthesis and organization. Three α chains **(A)** are synthesized to form procollagen. **B.** Amino terminal and carboxy terminal propeptide (indicated in green) are cleaved from procollagen by specific proteases outside the cell. **C.** Tropocollagen results from this cleavage. **D.** Removal of these propeptides results in a decline in solubility of collagen and self-assembly of collagen α chains into fibrils. The enzyme lysyl oxidase catalyzes the formation of nonreducible cross-links between two triple helical regions to make stable collagen fibrils **(E). F.** Fibrils, in turn, are assembled into collagen fibers. **G.** Fibril size and packing are regulated in part by small proteoglycans that bind collagen such as decorin. Before cervical ripening, fibril size is uniform, and fibrils are well-packed and organized. **H.** During cervical ripening, fibril size is less uniform, and spacing between collagen fibrils and fibers is increased and disorganized.

Endocervical Epithelia. During pregnancy, endocervical epithelial cells proliferate such that endocervical glands occupy a significant percentage of cervical mass by the end of pregnancy. The endocervical canal is lined with mucus-secreting columnar and stratified squamous epithelia, which protect against microbial invasion. Mucosal epithelia function as sentinels that recognize antigens, respond in ways that lead to bacterial and viral killing, and signal to underlying immune cells when pathogenic challenge exceeds their protective capacity (Wira and co-workers, 2005). Recent studies in mice suggest that cervical epithelia may also aid cervical remodeling by regulating tissue hydration and maintenance of barrier function. Hydration may be regulated by expression of *aquaporins*—water channel proteins, whereas paracellular transport of ion and solutes and maintenance of barrier function is regulated by tight junction proteins, such as claudins 1 and 2 (Anderson and colleagues, 2006; Timmons and Mahendroo, 2007).

Cervical Connective Tissue. The cervix is made up of only 10 to 15 percent smooth muscle with the remaining tissue comprised primarily of extracellular connective tissue. Constituents of the latter include type I, III, and IV collagen, glycosaminoglycans, proteoglycans, and elastin.

Collagen. This material is the major component of the cervix and it is largely responsible for its structural disposition. Collagen is the most abundant mammalian protein, and it has a complex biosynthesis pathway including at least six enzymes and chaperones to accomplish maturation (see Fig. 6-3). Each collagen molecule is composed of three alpha chains, which wind around each other to form procollagen. Multiple collagen triple-helical molecules are cross-linked to one another by the actions of lysyl oxidase to form long fibrils. Collagen fibrils interact with small proteoglycans such as decorin or biglycan, as well as matricellular proteins such as thrombospondin 2. These interactions determine fibril size, packing, and organization so collagen fibrils are of uniform diameter and are packed together in a regular and highly organized pattern (Canty and associates, 2005). During cervical ripening, collagen fibrils are disorganized, and there is increased spacing between fibrils.

Matrix metalloproteases (MMPs) are proteases capable of degrading extracellular matrix proteins. Of these, collagenase members of the MMP family degrade collagen. Some studies support a role of MMPs in cervical ripening, whereas others suggest that the biomechanical changes are not consistent solely with collagenase activation and loss of collagen. For example, Buhimschi and colleagues (2004) performed tissue biomechanical studies in the rat and suggest that ripening correlates with changes in collagen's three-dimensional structure rather than its degradation by collagenases. Moreover, mouse and human studies document no changes in collagen content between nonpregnancy and term pregnancy (Myers and associates, 2008; Read and co-workers, 2007).

Collagen solubility—a marker of less mature collagen—is increased early in the cervical softening phase in mice and continues for the remainder of pregnancy (Read and colleagues, 2007). Increased solubility may result in part from a decline in expression of the cross-linking enzyme, lysyl oxidase, during pregnancy (Drewes and associates, 2007; Ozasa and co-workers,

1981). Although collagen solubility has not been determined during cervical softening in early human pregnancy, increased solubility of collagen during cervical ripening has been noted (Granström and colleagues, 1989; Myers and associates, 2008).

Thus, it is possible that dynamic changes in collagen structure rather than collagen content may regulate remodeling. Specifically, ultrastructure analysis by electron microscopy in the rat cervix suggests that collagen dispersion predominates rather than degradation during ripening (Yu and colleagues, 1995). Dispersion of collagen fibrils leads to a loss of tissue integrity and increased tissue compliance. In further support, polymorphisms or mutations in genes required for collagen assembly are associated with an increased incidence of cervical insufficiency (Anum, 2009; Paternoster, 1998; Rahman, 2003; Warren, 2007; and all their colleagues).

Glycosaminoglycans (GAGs). These are high-molecular-weight polysaccharides that contain amino sugars and can form complexes with proteins to form proteoglycans. One glycosaminoglycan is hyaluronan (HA), a carbohydrate polymer whose synthesis is carried out by hyaluronan synthase isoenzymes. In both women and mice, hyaluronan content and hyaluronan synthase 2 expression is increased in the cervix during ripening (Osmers and associates, 1993; Straach and co-workers, 2005).

Hyaluronans' functions are dependent on size, and the breakdown of large-molecular-weight HA to small-molecular-weight products is carried out by a family of enzymes termed hyaluronidases. Large-molecular-weight HA, which in the mouse cervix predominates during cervical ripening, has a dynamic role in creating and filling space to increase viscoelasticity and matrix disorganization. Low-molecular-weight HA has proinflammatory properties, and studies in mice reveal increases in low-molecular-weight HA during labor and the puerperium (Ruscheinsky and colleagues, 2008). The importance of regulated changes in HA size during cervical ripening and dilatation is supported by a study reporting administration of hyaluronidase to the cervix of term pregnant women. Administration resulted in a reduction in labor duration and a reduced incidence of cesarean delivery due to cervical malfunction (Spallacci and co-workers, 2007). Activation of intracellular signaling cascades and other biological functions requires interactions with cell-associated HA-binding proteins. There are several in the cervix and include the proteoglycan, *versican*, and the cell surface receptor, CD44 (Ruscheinsky and colleagues, 2008).

Proteoglycans. These glycoproteins are found in abundance in the cervix, and changes in proteoglycan composition within the cervical matrix also accompany cervical ripening. At least two small leucine-rich proteoglycans are expressed in the cervix—*decorin* and *biglycan*. Although mRNA content of these two does not change during cervical ripening, changes in proteoglycan content are reported during ripening in support of posttranslational regulation (Westergren-Thorsson and colleagues, 1998). Decorin and other family members interact with collagen and influence the packing and order of collagen fibrils (Ameye and co-workers, 2002). The net result of their decreased expression is a rearrangement of collagen such that collagen fibers are weakened, shortened, and disorganized. Mice deficient in decorin have loose, fragile skin due to the inability of collagen fibrils to form uniform, packed structures. (Danielson and associates, 1997).

Inflammatory Changes. The marked changes within the extracellular matrix during cervical ripening in Phase 2 are accompanied by stromal invasion with inflammatory cells. This has led to a model in which cervical ripening is considered an inflammatory process such that cervical chemoattractants attract inflammatory cells, which in turn release proteases that may aid degradation of collagen and other matrix components. In phase 3 or 4 of parturition, there is increased cervical expression of chemokines and collagenase/protease activity. It was assumed that processes regulating phases 3 and 4 of dilation and postpartum recovery of the cervix were similar to those in phase 2 of cervical ripening (Osman, 2003; Bokström, 1997; Sennström, 2000; Young, 2002, and all their colleagues). This, however, may not be the case. Recent observations from both human and animal studies have challenged the importance of inflammation in initiation of cervical ripening. For example, Sakamoto and associates (2004, 2005) found no correlation between the degree of clinical cervical ripening with cervical interleukin 8 tissue (IL-8) concentrations. Interleukin 8, a cytokine that chemoattracts neutrophils, however, is present in increased levels in cervical tissue collected after vaginal delivery—phases 3 and 4.

Word and colleagues (2005) described an animal model in which parturition fails due to a small rigid cervix despite uterine contractions. Although this model has a robust recruitment of inflammatory cells to the stromal matrix, cervical ripening does not develop. In mouse models, monocyte migration, but not activation, takes place prior to labor (Timmons and Mahendroo, 2006, 2007; Timmons and associates, 2009). Furthermore, tissue depletion of neutrophils before birth has no effect on the timing or success of parturition. Finally, activation of neutrophils, proinflammatory M1 macrophages, and alternatively, activated M2 macrophages is increased within 2 hours after birth, suggesting a role for inflammatory cells in postpartum cervical remodeling.

Induction and Prevention of Cervical Ripening. The exact mechanisms that lead to cervical ripening are still being defined, and therapies to prevent premature cervical ripening remain to be identified. Therapies to promote cervical ripening for labor induction include direct application of prostaglandins E_2 (PGE$_2$) and $F_{2\alpha}$ (PGF$_{2\alpha}$). These modify collagen and alter relative glycosaminoglycan concentrations. This property is useful clinically to aid labor induction (see Chap. 22, p. 502).

In some nonhuman species, the cascades of events that allow cervical ripening are induced by decreasing serum progesterone concentrations. And in humans, administration of progesterone antagonists causes cervical ripening. As discussed later, humans may have developed unique mechanisms to localize decreases in progesterone action in the cervix and myometrium.

Phase 3 of Parturition: Labor

Phase 3 is synonymous with active labor, that is, uterine contractions that bring about progressive cervical dilatation and delivery. Clinically, phase 3 is customarily divided into the three

stages of labor. These stages compose the commonly used labor graph shown in Figure 6-2. The clinical stages of labor may be summarized as follows:

1. The first stage begins when widely spaced uterine contractions of sufficient frequency, intensity, and duration are attained to bring about cervical thinning, termed *effacement*. This labor stage ends when the cervix is fully dilated—about 10 cm—to allow passage of the fetal head. The first stage of labor, therefore, is the *stage of cervical effacement and dilatation*
2. The second stage begins when cervical dilatation is complete, and ends with delivery. Thus, the second stage of labor is the *stage of fetal expulsion*
3. The third stage begins immediately after delivery of the fetus and ends with the delivery of the placenta. Thus, the third stage of labor is the *stage of placental separation and expulsion*.

First Stage of Labor: Clinical Onset of Labor

In some women, forceful uterine contractions that effect delivery begin suddenly. In others, the initiation of labor is heralded by spontaneous release of a small amount of blood-tinged mucus from the vagina. This extrusion of the mucus plug that had previously filled the cervical canal during pregnancy is referred to as "show" or "bloody show." There is very little blood with the mucous plug, and its passage indicates that labor is already in progress or likely will ensue in hours to days.

Uterine Labor Contractions. Unique among physiological muscular contractions, those of uterine smooth muscle during labor are painful. The pain's cause is not known definitely, but several possibilities have been suggested:

- Hypoxia of the contracted myometrium—such as that with angina pectoris
- Compression of nerve ganglia in the cervix and lower uterus by contracted interlocking muscle bundles
- Stretching of the cervix during dilatation
- Stretching of the peritoneum overlying the fundus.

Compression of nerve ganglia in the cervix and lower uterine segment by the contracting myometrium is an especially attractive hypothesis. Paracervical infiltration with a local anesthetic usually produces appreciable pain relief with contractions (see Chap. 19, p. 450). Uterine contractions are involuntary and for the most part, independent of extrauterine control. Neural blockade from epidural analgesia does not diminish their frequency or intensity. In other examples, myometrial contractions in paraplegic women and in women after bilateral lumbar sympathectomy are normal but painless.

Mechanical stretching of the cervix enhances uterine activity in several species, including humans. This phenomenon has been referred to as the *Ferguson reflex* (Ferguson, 1941). Its exact mechanism is not clear, and release of oxytocin has been suggested but not proven. Manipulation of the cervix and "stripping" the fetal membranes is associated with an increase in blood levels of prostaglandin $F_{2\alpha}$ metabolite (PGFM). As shown in Figure 6-4, this could also increase contractions (see also Chap. 22, p. 504).

The interval between contractions diminishes gradually from about 10 minutes at the onset of the first stage of labor to

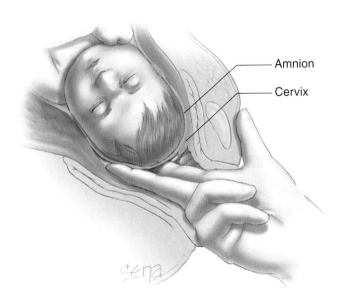

FIGURE 6-4 Clinically, membrane stripping may aid cervical ripening and in some cases, labor induction.

as little as 1 minute or less in the second stage. Periods of relaxation between contractions, however, are essential for fetal welfare. Unremitting contractions compromise uteroplacental blood flow sufficiently to cause fetal hypoxemia. In active-phase labor, the duration of each contraction ranges from 30 to 90 seconds, averaging about 1 minute. There is appreciable variability in contraction intensity during normal labor. Specifically, amnionic fluid pressures generated by contractions during spontaneous labor average approximately 40 mm Hg, but with variations from 20 to 60 mm Hg (see Chap. 18, p. 437).

Distinct Lower and Upper Uterine Segments. During active labor, the uterine divisions that were initiated in phase 2 of parturition become increasingly evident (**Figs. 6-5** and **6-6**). By abdominal palpation, even before rupture of the membranes, the two segments can sometimes be differentiated. The upper segment is firm during contractions, whereas the lower segment is softer, distended, and more passive. This mechanism is imperative because if the entire myometrium, including the lower uterine segment and cervix, were to contract simultaneously and with equal intensity, the net expulsive force would be decreased markedly. Thus, the upper segment contracts, retracts, and expels the fetus. In response to these contractions, the softened lower uterine segment and cervix dilate and thereby form a greatly expanded, thinned-out tube through which the fetus can pass.

The myometrium of the upper segment does not relax to its original length after contractions. Instead, it becomes relatively fixed at a shorter length. The upper active uterine segment contracts down on its diminishing contents, but myometrial tension remains constant. The net effect is to take up slack, thus maintaining the advantage gained in the expulsion of the fetus. Concurrently, the uterine musculature is kept in firm contact with the uterine contents. As the consequence of retraction, each successive contraction commences where its predecessor left off. Thus, the upper part of the uterine cavity becomes slightly smaller with each successive contraction. Because of the successive shortening of the muscular fibers, the upper active segment becomes progressively thickened throughout first- and second-stage labor (see Fig. 6-5). This process continues and results in a tremendously thickened upper uterine segment immediately after delivery.

Clinically, it is important to understand that the phenomenon of upper segment retraction is contingent upon a decrease in the volume of its contents. For this to happen, particularly early in labor when the entire uterus is virtually a closed sac with only minimal cervical dilatation, the musculature of the lower segment must stretch. This permits increasingly more of the uterine contents to occupy the lower segment. The upper segment retracts only to the extent that the lower segment distends and the cervix dilates.

Relaxation of the lower uterine segment mirrors the same gradual progression of retraction. Recall that after each contraction of the upper segment, the muscles do not return to the

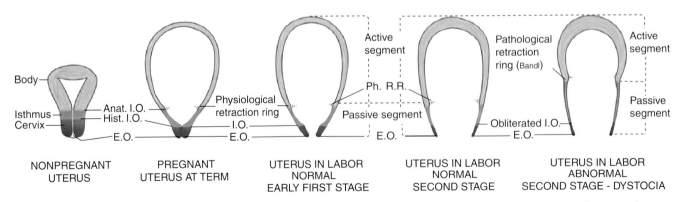

FIGURE 6-5 Sequence of development of the segments and rings in the uterus at term and in labor. Note comparison between the uterus of a nonpregnant woman, the uterus at term, and the uterus during labor. The passive lower uterine segment is derived from the isthmus, and the physiological retraction ring develops at the junction of the upper and lower uterine segments. The pathological retraction ring develops from the physiological ring. (Anat. I.O. = anatomical internal os; E.O. = external os; Hist. I.O. = histological internal os; Ph.R.R. = physiological retraction ring.)

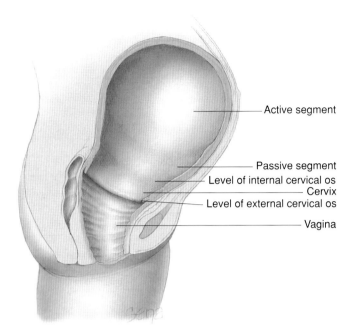

Active segment

Passive segment
Level of internal cervical os
Cervix
Level of external cervical os
Vagina

FIGURE 6-6 The uterus at the time of vaginal delivery. The active upper segment retracts around the presenting part as the fetus descends through the birth canal. In the passive lower segment, there is considerably less myometrial tone.

previous length, but tension remains essentially the same. By comparison, in the lower segment, successive lengthening of the fibers with labor is accompanied by thinning, normally to only a few millimeters in the thinnest part. As a result of the lower segment thinning and concomitant upper segment thickening, a boundary between the two is marked by a ridge on the inner uterine surface—the *physiological retraction ring.* When the thinning of the lower uterine segment is extreme, as in obstructed labor, the ring is prominent and forms a *pathological retraction ring* (see Fig. 6-5). This abnormal condition is also known as the *Bandl ring,* which is discussed further in Chapter 20 (p. 486).

Uterine Shape Changes During Labor. Each contraction produces an elongation of the ovoid uterine shape with a concomitant decrease in horizontal diameter. This change in shape has important effects on the process of labor. First, there is increased *fetal axis pressure.* The decreased horizontal diameter serves to straighten the fetal vertebral column. This presses the upper pole of the fetus firmly against the fundus, whereas the lower pole is thrust farther downward. The lengthening of the ovoid shape has been estimated at 5 and 10 cm. Second, with lengthening of the uterus, the longitudinal fibers are drawn taut. As a result, the lower segment and cervix are the only parts of the uterus that are flexible, and these are pulled upward and around the lower pole of the fetus.

Ancillary Forces in Labor. After the cervix is dilated fully, the most important force in fetal expulsion is that produced by maternal intra-abdominal pressure. Contraction of the abdom-

inal muscles simultaneously with forced respiratory efforts with the glottis closed is referred to as *pushing.* The nature of the force is similar to that with defecation, but the intensity usually is much greater. The importance of intra-abdominal pressure is attested to by prolonged descent during labor in paraplegic women. And although increased intra-abdominal pressure is necessary to complete second-stage labor, pushing accomplishes little in the first stage. It exhausts the mother, and its associated increased intrauterine pressures may be harmful to the fetus.

Cervical Changes During First-Stage Labor

As the result of contraction forces, two fundamental changes—effacement and dilatation—take place in the already-ripened cervix. For an average-sized fetal head to pass through the cervix, its canal must dilate to a diameter of approximately 10 cm. At this time, the cervix is said to be completely or fully dilated. Although there may be no fetal descent during cervical effacement, most commonly, the presenting fetal part descends somewhat as the cervix dilates. During second-stage labor in nulliparas, the presenting part typically descends slowly and steadily. In multiparas, however, particularly those of high parity, descent may be rapid.

Cervical effacement is "obliteration" or "taking up" of the cervix. It is manifest clinically by shortening of the cervical canal from a length of about 2 cm to a mere circular orifice with almost paper-thin edges. The muscular fibers at about the level of the internal cervical os are pulled upward, or "taken up," into the lower uterine segment. The condition of the external os remains temporarily unchanged (Fig. 6-7).

Effacement may be compared with a funneling process in which the whole length of a narrow cylinder is converted into a very obtuse, flaring funnel with a small circular opening. Because of increased myometrial activity during uterine preparedness for labor, appreciable effacement of a softened cervix sometimes is accomplished before active labor begins. Effacement causes expulsion of the mucous plug as the cervical canal is shortened.

Because the lower segment and cervix have lesser resistance during a contraction, a centrifugal pull is exerted on the cervix leading to distension, or *cervical dilatation* (Figs. 6-8). As uterine contractions cause pressure on the membranes, the hydrostatic action of the amnionic sac in turn dilates the cervical canal like a wedge. In the absence of intact membranes, the pressure of the presenting part against the cervix and lower uterine segment is similarly effective. Early rupture of the membranes does not retard cervical dilatation so long as the presenting fetal part is positioned to exert pressure against the cervix and lower segment. The process of cervical effacement and dilatation causes the formation of the *forebag* of amnionic fluid, which is the leading portion of the amnionic sac and fluid located in front of the presenting part.

Referring back to Figure 6-2, recall that cervical dilatation is divided into latent and active phases. The active phase is subdivided further into the acceleration phase, the phase of maximum slope, and the deceleration phase (Friedman, 1978). The duration of the latent phase is more variable and sensitive to changes by extraneous factors. For example, sedation may prolong the latent phase, and myometrial stimulation shortens it.

Multipara   Primigravida

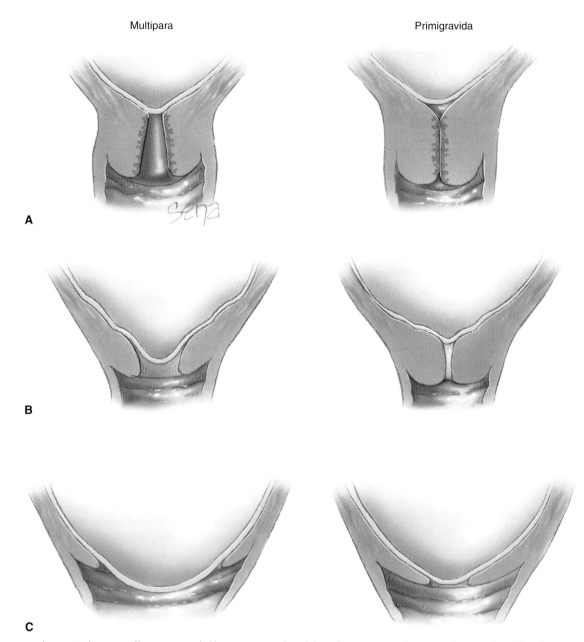

FIGURE 6-7 Schematic showing effacement and dilatation. **A.** Before labor, the primigravid cervix is long and undilated in contrast to that of the multipara, which has dilatation of the internal and external os. **B.** As effacement begins, the multiparous cervix shows dilatation and funneling of the internal os. This is less apparent in the primigravid cervix. **C.** As complete effacement is achieved in the primigravid cervix, dilation is minimal. The reverse is true in the multipara.

The latent phase duration has little bearing on the subsequent course of labor, whereas the characteristics of the accelerated phase are usually predictive of a particular labor outcome. Completion of cervical dilatation during the active phase is accomplished by cervical retraction about the presenting part. The first stage ends when cervical dilatation is complete. Once the second stage commences, only progressive descent of the presenting part will foretell further progress.

Second Stage of Labor: Fetal Descent

In many nulliparas, engagement of the head is accomplished before labor begins. That said, the head may not descend further until late in labor. In the descent pattern of normal labor, a typical

hyperbolic curve is formed when the station of the fetal head is plotted as a function of labor duration. *Station* describes descent of the fetal biparietal diameter in relation to a line drawn between maternal ischial spines (Chap. 17, p. 392). Active descent usually takes place after dilatation has progressed for some time (Fig. 6-9). In nulliparas, increased rates of descent are observed ordinarily during cervical dilatation phase of maximum slope. At this time, the speed of descent is also maximal and is maintained until the presenting part reaches the perineal floor (Friedman, 1978).

Pelvic Floor Changes During Labor

The birth canal is supported and is functionally closed by several layers of tissues that together form the pelvic floor. The

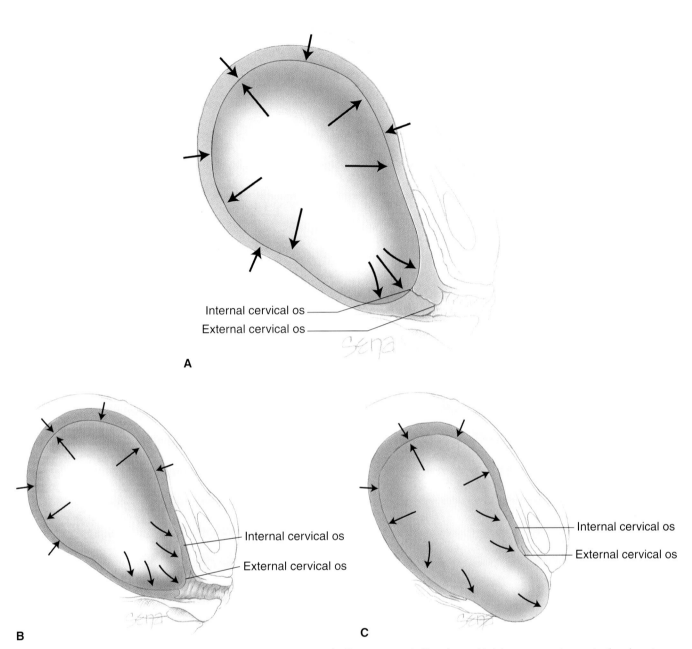

Internal cervical os
External cervical os

A

Internal cervical os
External cervical os

B

Internal cervical os
External cervical os

C

FIGURE 6-8 Hydrostatic action of membranes in effecting cervical effacement and dilatation. With labor progression, note the changing relations of the internal and external os in (A), (B), and (C). Although not shown in this diagram, with membrane rupture, the presenting part, applied to the cervix and the forming lower uterine segment, acts similarly.

most important structures are the levator ani muscle and the fibromuscular connective tissue covering its upper and lower surfaces. There are marked changes in the biomechanical properties of these structures and the vaginal wall during parturition resulting from changes in structure or composition of the extracellular matrix (Lowder and co-workers, 2007; Rahn and associates, 2008). The levator ani consists of the pubovisceral, puborectalis, and iliococcygeus muscles, which close the lower end of the pelvic cavity as a diaphragm. Thereby, a concave upper and a convex lower surface are presented (Chap. 2, p. 33). The posterior and lateral portions of the pelvic floor, which are not spanned by the levator ani, are occupied bilaterally by the piriformis and coccygeus muscles.

The levator ani muscle varies in thickness from 3 to 5 mm, although its margins encircling the rectum and vagina are somewhat thicker. During pregnancy, the levator ani usually undergoes hypertrophy, forming a thick band that extends backward from the pubis and encircles the vagina about 2 cm above the plane of the hymen. On contraction, the levator ani draws both the rectum and the vagina forward and upward in the direction of the symphysis pubis and thereby acts to close the vagina. The more superficial muscles of the perineum are too delicate to serve more than an accessory function.

In the first stage of labor, the membranes, when intact, and the fetal presenting part serve to dilate the upper vagina. The most marked change consists of the stretching of levator ani

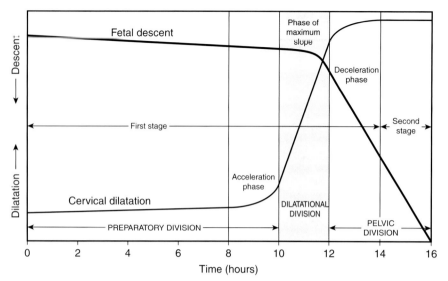

FIGURE 6-9 Labor course divided on the basis of expected evolution of the dilatation and descent curves into three functional divisions. The preparatory division includes the latent and acceleration phases. The dilatational division is the phase of maximum slope of dilatation. The pelvic division encompasses both the deceleration phase and the second stage, which is concurrent with the phase of maximum slope of fetal descent. (Redrawn from Friedman, 1978.)

muscle fibers. This is accompanied by thinning of the central portion of the perineum, which becomes transformed from a wedge-shaped, 5-cm-thick mass of tissue to a thin, almost transparent membranous structure less than 1 cm thick. When the perineum is distended maximally, the anus becomes markedly dilated and presents an opening that varies from 2 to 3 cm in diameter and through which the anterior wall of the rectum bulges. The extraordinary number and size of the blood vessels that supply the vagina and pelvic floor result in substantive blood loss if these tissues are torn.

Third Stage of Labor: Delivery of Placenta and Membranes

This stage begins immediately after delivery of the fetus and involves the separation and expulsion of the placenta and membranes. As the neonate is born, the uterus spontaneously contracts around its diminishing contents. Normally, by the time the infant is completely delivered, the uterine cavity is nearly obliterated. The organ consists of an almost solid mass of muscle, several centimeters thick, above the thinner lower segment. The uterine fundus now lies just below the level of the umbilicus.

This sudden diminution in uterine size is inevitably accompanied by a decrease in the area of the placental implantation site (Fig. 6-10). For the placenta to accommodate itself to this reduced area, it increases in thickness, but because of limited placental elasticity, it is forced to buckle. The resulting tension pulls the weakest layer of the decidua—the decidua spongiosa—from that site. Thus, placental separation follows disproportion created between the unchanged placental size and the reduced size of the implantation site. During cesarean delivery, this phenomenon may be directly observed when the placenta is implanted posteriorly.

Cleavage of the placenta is aided greatly by the loose structure of the spongy decidua, which may be likened to the row of perforations between postage stamps. As separation proceeds, a hematoma forms between the separating placenta and the decidua. The hematoma is usually the result, rather than the cause of the separation, because in some cases bleeding is negligible. The hematoma may, however, accelerate cleavage. Because placental separation is through its spongy layer, part of the decidua is cast off with the placenta, whereas the rest remains attached to the myometrium. The amount of decidual tissue retained at the placental site varies.

The placenta ordinarily separates within minutes after delivery. Occasionally, some degree of separation begins even before the third stage of labor. This probably accounts for certain cases of fetal heart rate decelerations that occur just before fetal expulsion.

Separation of Fetal Membranes

The great decrease in uterine cavity surface area simultaneously throws the fetal membranes—the amniochorion and the

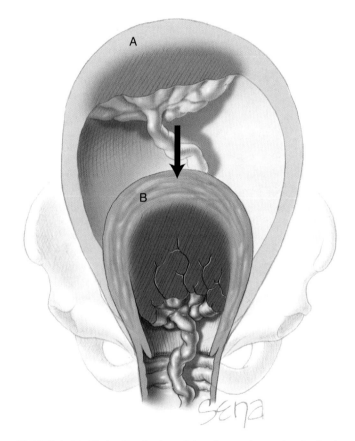

FIGURE 6-10 Diminution in size of the placental site after birth of the infant. **A.** Spatial relations before birth. **B.** Placental spatial relations after birth.

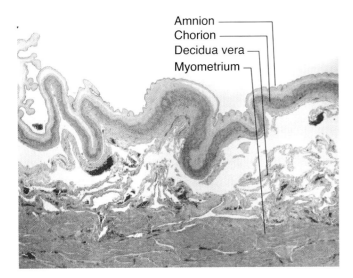

Amnion
Chorion
Decidua vera
Myometrium

FIGURE 6-11 Postpartum, membranes are thrown up into folds as the uterine cavity decreases in size (Used with permission from Dr. Kelley S. Carrick.).

parietal decidua—into innumerable folds (Fig. 6-11). Membranes usually remain in situ until placental separation is nearly completed. These are then peeled off the uterine wall, partly by further contraction of the myometrium and partly by traction that is exerted by the separated placenta, which lies in the lower segment or upper vagina. Following separation, the body of the uterus normally forms an almost solid mass of muscle, the anterior and posterior walls of which, each measuring 4 to 5 cm in thickness, lie in close apposition such that the uterine cavity is almost obliterated.

Placental Extrusion

After the placenta has separated and occupies the lower uterine segment or upper vagina, it may be expelled by increased abdominal pressure. Women in the recumbent position, however, frequently cannot expel the placenta spontaneously. Thus, completion of the third stage is accomplished usually by alternately compressing and elevating the fundus, while exerting minimal traction on the umbilical cord (Fig. 17-31, p. 398).

Most commonly during placental delivery, a retroplacental hematoma forms and pushes the center forward and causes it to separate toward the uterine cavity. Weighted by this hematoma, the placenta descends, drags the membranes, and peels them from their uterine attachment. Consequently, the glistening amnion, covering the placental surface, presents at the vulva. The retroplacental hematoma either follows the placenta or is found within the inverted sac. In this process, known as the *Schultze mechanism* of placental expulsion, blood from the placental site pours into the membrane sac and does not escape externally until after extrusion of the placenta. In the other method of placental extrusion, known as the *Duncan mechanism,* the placenta separates first at the periphery. As a result, blood collects between the membranes and the uterine wall and escapes from the vagina. In this circumstance, the placenta descends sideways, and the maternal surface appears first.

Phase 4 of Parturition: The Puerperium

Immediately and for about an hour or so after delivery, the myometrium remains in a state of rigid and persistent contraction and retraction. This directly compresses large uterine vessels and allows thrombosis of their lumens (Fig. 2-14, p. 25). For this reason, severe postpartum hemorrhage is prevented.

Concurrently during the early puerperium, a maternal-type behavior pattern develops and *maternal-neonatal bonding* begins. The onset of lactogenesis and milk let-down in mammary glands also is, in an evolutionary sense, crucial to the bringing forth of young. Both compression of uterine vessels and maternal-type behavior patterns are mediated by oxytocin (p. 159).

Uterine involution and cervical repair, both remodeling processes that restore these organs to the nonpregnant state, follow in a timely fashion. These protect the reproductive tract from invasion by commensal microorganisms and restore endometrial responsiveness to normal hormonal cyclicity. Reinstitution of ovulation signals preparation for the next pregnancy. This generally occurs within 4 to 6 weeks after birth, but it is dependent on the duration of breast feeding. Infertility usually persists as long as breast feeding is continued because of lactation-induced, prolactin-mediated anovulation and amenorrhea (Chap. 32, p. 694).

PHYSIOLOGICAL AND BIOCHEMICAL PROCESSES REGULATING PARTURITION

The physiological processes that result in the initiation of parturition and the onset of labor remain poorly defined. There are two general contemporaneous theorems concerning labor initiation. Viewed simplistically, these are the *loss of function of pregnancy maintenance factors* and the *synthesis of factors that induce parturition.* Selected tenets of these two postulates are incorporated into most theorems.

Some investigators also speculate that the mature fetus is the source of the initial signal for parturition commencement. Others suggest that one or more uterotonins, produced in increased amounts, or an increase in the population of its myometrial receptors is the proximate cause. Indeed, an obligatory role for one or more uterotonins is included in most parturition theories, as either a primary or a secondary phenomenon in the final events of childbirth. Both rely on careful regulation of smooth muscle contraction.

Anatomical and Physiological Considerations of the Myometrium

There are unique characteristics of smooth muscle, including myometrium, compared with those of skeletal muscle that may confer advantages for the myometrium in the efficiency of uterine contractions and delivery of the fetus. First, the degree of smooth-muscle cell shortening with contractions may be one order of magnitude greater than that attained in striated muscle cells. Second, forces can be exerted in smooth muscle cells in multiple directions, whereas the contraction force generated by skeletal muscle is always aligned with the axis of the muscle fibers. Third, smooth muscle is not organized in the same manner as skeletal muscle. In myometrium, the thick and thin filaments are found in long, random bundles throughout the cells. This plexiform arrangement aids greater shortening and force-generating capacity. Lastly, greater multidirectional force generation in the uterine fundus compared with that of the lower uterine segment permits versatility in expulsive force directionality. These forces thus can be brought to bear irrespective of the fetal lie or presentation.

Regulation of Myometrial Contraction and Relaxation

Myometrial contraction is controlled by the transcription of key genes, which produce proteins that repress or enhance cellular contractility. These proteins function to: (1) enhance the interactions between the actin and myosin proteins that cause muscle contraction; (2) increase excitability of individual myome-

trial cells; and (3) promote intracellular cross talk that allow development of synchronous contractions.

Actin-Myosin Interactions

The interaction of myosin and actin is essential to muscle contraction. This interaction requires that actin be converted from a globular to filamentous form. Moreover, actin must be attached to the cytoskeleton at focal points in the cell membrane to allow development of tension (Fig. 6-12). Actin must partner with myosin, which is comprised of multiple light and heavy chains. The interaction of myosin and actin causes activation of adenosine triphosphatase, adenosine triphosphate hydrolysis, and force generation. This interaction is effected by enzymatic phosphorylation of the 20-kDa light chain of myosin (Stull and colleagues, 1988, 1998). This phosphorylation reaction is catalyzed by the enzyme *myosin light-chain kinase*, which

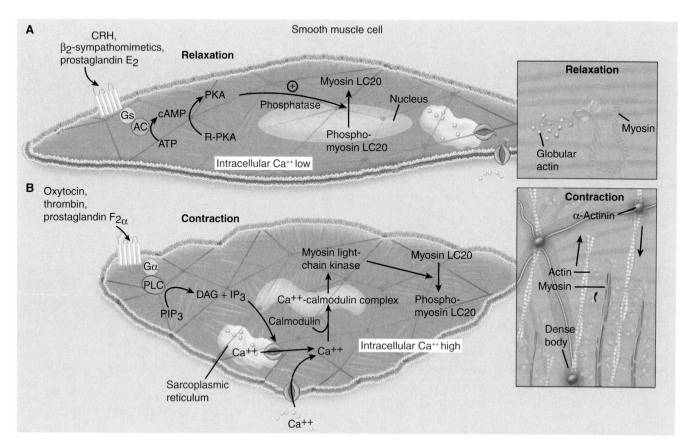

FIGURE 6-12 Uterine myocyte relaxation and contraction. **A.** Uterine relaxation is maintained by factors that increase myocyte cyclic adenosine monophosphate (cAMP). This activates protein kinase A (PKA) to promote phosphodiesterase activity with dephosphorylation of myosin light-chain kinase (MLCK). There are also processes that serve to maintain actin in a globular form, and thus to prevent fibril formation necessary for contractions. **B.** Uterine contractions result from reversal of these sequences. Actin now assumes a fibrillar form, and calcium enters the cell to combine with calmodulin to form complexes. These complexes activate MLCK to bring about phosphorylation of the myosin light chains. This generates ATPase activity to cause sliding of myosin over the actin fibrils, which is a uterine contractor. (AC = adenylyl cyclase; Ca^{++} = calcium; DAG = diacylglycerol; Gs and $G\alpha$ = G-receptor proteins; IP_3 = inositol triphosphate; LC20 = light chain 20; PIP_3 = phosphatidylinositol 3, 4, 5-triphosphate; PLC = phospholipase C; R-PKA = inactive protein kinase.) (Adapted from Smith R: Parturition. *N Engl J Med* 356(3):271–283, with permission. Copyright © 2007 Massachusetts Medical Society. All rights reserved.)

is activated by calcium. Calcium binds to calmodulin, a calcium-binding regulatory protein, which in turn binds to and activates myosin light-chain kinase.

Intracellular Calcium

Agents that promote contraction act on myometrial cells to increase intracellular cytosolic calcium concentration—$[Ca^{2+}]_i$—or allow an influx of extracellular calcium through ligand- or voltage-regulated calcium channels (see Fig. 6-12). For example, prostaglandin $F_{2\alpha}$ and oxytocin bind their receptors during labor, which opens ligand-activated calcium channels. Activation of these receptors also releases calcium from internal stores in the sarcoplasmic reticulum. This leads to a drop in electronegativity within the cell. Voltage-gated ion channels open, additional calcium ions move into the cell, and cellular depolarization follows. The increase in $[Ca^{2+}]_i$ is often transient, but contractions can be prolonged through the inhibition of myosin phosphatase activity (Woodcock and associates, 2004).

Conditions that decrease $[Ca^{2+}]_i$ and increase intracellular concentrations of cyclic adenosine monophosphate (cAMP) or cyclic guanosine monophosphate (cGMP) ordinarily promote uterine relaxation. Animal studies reveal the importance of small conductance calcium-activated K^+ isoform 3 (SK3) channels in maintenance of uterine relaxation. Expression of the SK3 channel declines at the end of pregnancy as contractility is increased (Pierce and colleagues, 2008). Agents such as corticotropin-releasing hormone (CRH) and prostaglandin E_2 increase intracellular cAMP. Another potential mechanism for maintenance of relaxation is the promotion of actin in a globular form rather than in fibrils, which is required for contraction (Macphee and Lye, 2000; Yu and López Bernal, 1998).

In addition to myocyte contractility, myocyte excitability is also regulated by changes in the electrochemical potential gradient across the plasma membrane. Prior to labor, myocytes maintain a relatively high interior electronegativity. This state is maintained by the combined actions of the ATPase-driven sodium-potassium pump and the large conductance, voltage- and Ca^{2+}-sensitive K channel—*maxi-K channels* (Parkington and Coleman, 2001). During uterine quiescence, the maxi-K channel is open and allows potassium to leave the cell to maintain interior electronegativity. At the time of labor, changes in electronegativity lead to depolarization and contraction (Brainard and colleagues, 2005; Chanrachakul and co-workers, 2003).

Another important facet of uterine contractility is the need for myocytes to work in synchrony to allow powerful waves of myometrial contraction. These contractions must be coordinated, be of sufficient amplitude, and be interspersed with periods of uterine relaxation to allow appropriate placental blood flow. As parturition progresses, there is increased synchronization of electrical uterine activity.

Myometrial Gap Junctions

As in other muscle cells, the cellular signals that control myometrial contraction and relaxation can be effectively transferred between cells through intercellular junctional channels. Communi-

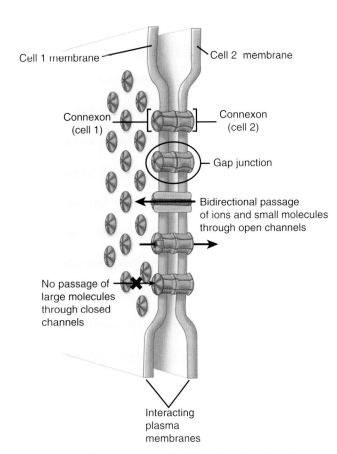

FIGURE 6-13 The protein subunits of gap junction channels are called connexins. Six connexins form a hemichannel (connexon), and two connexons (one from each cell) form a gap junction channel. Connexons and gap junction channels can be formed from one or more connexin proteins. The composition of the gap junction channel is important for their selectivity with regard to passage of molecules and communication between cells.

cation is established between myometrial cells by gap junctions, which aid the passage of electrical or ionic coupling currents as well as metabolite coupling. The transmembrane channels that make up the gap junctions consist of two protein "hemichannels" (Sáez and associates, 2005). These are termed *connexons*, and each is composed of six *connexin* subunit proteins (Fig. 6-13). These pairs of connexons establish a conduit between coupled cells for the exchange of small molecules that can be nutrients, waste products, metabolites, second messengers, or ions.

Optimal numbers of functional permeable gap junctions between myometrial cells are believed to be important for electrical myometrial synchrony. At least 21 human connexin genes have been identified. Four described in the uterus are connexins 26, 40, 43, and 45. Because connexin 43 junctions are scarce in the nonpregnant uterus, they are thought to be most important in gap junction formation during parturition. Most certainly, these increase in size and abundance during human parturition (Chow and Lye, 1994). Finally, mouse models deficient in connexin 43-enriched gap junctions exhibit delayed parturition, further supporting their role (Döring and colleagues, 2006; Tong, 2009).

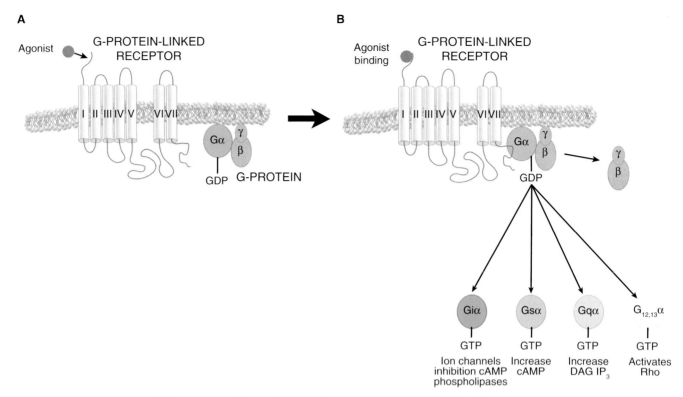

FIGURE 6-14 G-protein-coupled receptor signal transduction pathways. **A.** Receptors coupled to heterotrimeric guanosine-triphosphate (GTP)-binding proteins (G proteins) are integral transmembrane proteins that transduce extracellular signals to the cell interior. G-protein-coupled receptors exhibit a common structural motif consisting of seven membrane-spanning regions. **B.** Receptor occupation promotes interaction between the receptor and the G protein on the interior surface of the membrane. This induces an exchange of guanosine diphosphate (GDP) for GTP on the G protein α subunit and dissociation of the α subunit from the $\beta\gamma$ heterodimer. Depending on its isoform, the GTP-α subunit complex mediates intracellular signaling either indirectly by acting on effector molecules such as adenylyl cyclase (AC) or phospholipase C (PLC), or directly by regulating ion channel or kinase function. (cAMP = cyclic adenosine monophosphate; DAG = diacylglycerol; IP_3 = inositol triphosphate.)

Cell Surface Receptors

There are various cell surface receptors that can directly regulate myocyte contractile state. Three major classes are G-protein-linked, ion channel-linked, and enzyme-linked. Multiple examples of each have been identified in human myometrium. These further appear to be modified during the phases of parturition. Most G-protein-coupled receptors are associated with adenylyl cyclase activation—for example, CRHR1α and the LH receptors (Fig. 6-14). Other G-protein-coupled myometrial receptors, however, are associated with G-protein–mediated activation of phospholipase C.

Ligands for the G-protein-coupled receptors include neuropeptides, hormones, and autacoids. Many of these are available to the myometrium during pregnancy in high concentration by several routes. Modes include *endocrine*, via maternal blood; *paracrine*, via contiguous tissues or adjacent cells; or *autocrine*, by direct synthesis in the myocyte (Fig. 6-15). Importantly, myometrial response to a hormone can change during pregnancy. It therefore is conceivable that hormonal myometrial action is regulated by expression of the G-protein-coupled receptor, its associated G-proteins, and the effector plasma membrane proteins.

Cervical Dilatation During Labor

Cervical dilatation is characterized by a large influx of leukocytes into the cervical stroma (Sakamoto and co-workers, 2004, 2005). Cervical tissue levels of leukocyte chemoattractants such as IL-8 are increased just after delivery, as are IL-8 receptors. Identification of genes upregulated just after vaginal delivery further suggests that dilatation and early stages of postpartum repair are aided by inflammatory responses, apoptosis, and activation of proteases that degrade extracellular matrix components (Hassan and associates, 2006; Havelock and co-workers, 2005). The composition of glycosaminoglycans, proteoglycans, and poorly formed collagen fibrils that were necessary during ripening and dilatation must be rapidly removed to allow reorganization and recovery of cervical structure. In the days that follow completion of parturition, rapid recovery of cervical structure involves processes that resolve inflammation, promote tissue repair, and recreate dense cervical connective tissue and structural integrity.

Phase 1: Uterine Quiescence and Cervical Competence

The myometrial quiescence of parturition phase 1 is so remarkable and successful that it probably is induced by multiple

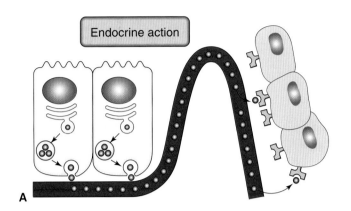

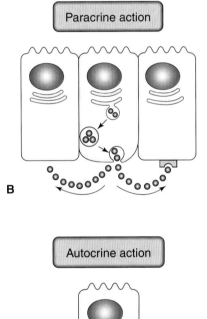

FIGURE 6-15 Different forms of cellular communication are depicted. **A.** Endocrine—chemical messenger travels through blood vessels to reach distant target cells. **B.** Paracrine—chemical messengers are released and diffuse to nearby target cells. **C.** Autocrine—chemical messengers are released by a cell whose membrane receptors then bind the messenger. (From Halvorson, 2008, with permission.)

independent and cooperative biomolecular processes. Individually, some of these processes may be redundant so that pregnancy may continue in the absence of one or more that normally contribute to pregnancy maintenance. It is likely that all manners of molecular systems—neural, endocrine, paracrine, and autocrine—are called on to implement and coordinate a state of relative uterine unresponsiveness. Moreover, a comple-

mentary system that protects the uterus against agents that could perturb the tranquil state of phase 1 also must be in place (Fig. 6-16).

Phase 1 of human parturition and its quiescent state are likely the result of many factors that include:

- Actions of estrogen and progesterone via intracellular receptors
- Myometrial cell plasma membrane receptor-mediated increases in cAMP
- The generation of cGMP
- Other systems, including modifications in myometrial cell ion channels.

Progesterone and Estrogen Contributions to Phase 1

In many species, the role of the sex steroid hormones is clear—progesterone inhibits and estrogen promotes the events leading to parturition. In humans, however, it seems most likely that both estrogen and progesterone are components of a broader-based molecular system that implements and maintains phase 1 of parturition. In many species, the removal of progesterone—or *progesterone withdrawal*—directly precedes the progression of phase 1 into phase 2 of parturition. In addition, providing progesterone to some species will delay parturition via a decrease in myometrial activity and continued maintenance of cervical competency (Challis and Lye, 1994). Studies in these species have led to a better understanding of why the progesterone-replete myometrium of phase 1 is relatively noncontractile.

Plasma levels of estrogen and progesterone in normal pregnancy are enormous and in great excess of the affinity constants for their receptors. For this reason, it is difficult to comprehend how relatively subtle changes in the ratio of their concentrations could modulate physiological processes during pregnancy. The teleological evidence, however, for an increased progesterone-to-estrogen ratio in the maintenance of pregnancy and a decline in the progesterone-to-estrogen ratio for parturition is overwhelming. In all species studied to date, including humans, administration of the progesterone-receptor antagonist mifepristone (RU486) or onapristone will promote some or all key features of parturition. These include cervical ripening, increased cervical distensibility, and increased uterine sensitivity to uterotonins (Bygdeman and co-workers, 1994; Chwalisz, 1994; Wolf and colleagues, 1993).

The exact role of estrogen in regulating human uterine activity and cervical competency is even less well understood. That said, it appears that estrogen can act to promote progesterone responsiveness, and in doing so, promote uterine quiescence. The estrogen receptor, acting via the estrogen-response element of the progesterone-receptor gene, induces progesterone-receptor synthesis, which allows increased progesterone-mediated function.

Steroid Hormone Regulation of Myometrial Cell-to-Cell Communication. Progesterone likely increases uterine quiescence by direct or indirect effects that cause decreased expression

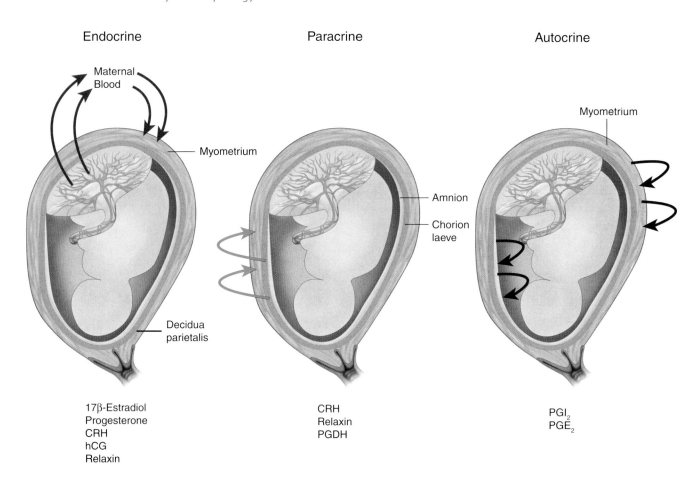

	Endocrine	Paracrine	Autocrine

17β-Estradiol
Progesterone
CRH
hCG
Relaxin

CRH
Relaxin
PGDH

PGI$_2$
PGE$_2$

FIGURE 6-16 Theoretical fail-safe system involving endocrine, paracrine, and autocrine mechanisms for the maintenance of phase 1 of parturition, uterine quiescence. (CRH = corticotropin-releasing hormone; hCG = human chorionic gonadotropin; PGE$_2$ = prostaglandin E$_2$; PGI$_2$ = prostaglandin I$_2$; PGDH = 15-hydroxy prostaglandin dehydrogenase.)

of the contraction-associated proteins (CAPs). Progesterone has been shown to inhibit expression of the gap junctional protein connexin 43 in several rodent models of labor, and progesterone administration prevents or delays labor (Fig. 6-17). Conversely, inhibition of progesterone activity at midgestation using the progesterone-receptor antagonist RU486 leads to a premature induction of myometrial connexin 43 protein production, and thus stimulates labor.

Estrogen treatment also promotes myometrial gap junction formation in some animals by increasing connexin 43 synthesis. The simultaneous administration of anti-estrogens prevents this (Burghardt and colleagues, 1984). Progesterone treatment, however, negates the stimulatory effect of estrogen on the development of gap junctions in some animals.

G-Protein–Coupled Receptors That Promote Myometrial Relaxation

A number of G-protein-coupled receptors that normally are associated with G$_{\alpha s}$-mediated activation of adenylyl cyclase and increased levels of cAMP are present in myometrium. These receptors together with appropriate ligands may act—in concert with sex steroid hormones—as part of a fail-safe system to maintain uterine quiescence (Price and associates, 2000; Sanborn and colleagues, 1998).

Beta-Adrenoreceptors. The β-adrenergic receptors have served as prototypes of cAMP signaling in causing myometrium relaxation. Most commonly, β-adrenergic receptors mediate G$_{\alpha s}$-stimulated increases in adenylyl cyclase, increased levels of cAMP, and myometrial cell relaxation. The rate-limiting factor in the β-receptor system is likely the number of receptors expressed and the level of adenylyl cyclase expression. The number of G-proteins in most systems far exceeds the number of receptors and effector molecules. These properties have led to development of β-mimetic agents that are used clinically to promote uterine quiescence and thereby forestall labor. Examples are ritodrine and terbutaline, which are discussed in Chapter 36 (p. 823).

Luteinizing Hormone (LH) and Human Chorionic Gonadotropin (hCG) Receptors. The G-protein-coupled receptor for LH-hCG has been demonstrated in myometrial smooth muscle and blood vessels (Lei and co-workers, 1992; Ziecik and colleagues, 1992). Levels of myometrial LH-hCG receptors during pregnancy are greater before than during labor (Zuo and colleagues, 1994). Chorionic gonadotropin acts to activate adenylyl cyclase by way of a plasma membrane receptor-G$_{\alpha s}$-linked system. This decreases contraction frequency and force and decreases the number of tissue-specific myometrial cell gap junctions (Ambrus and Rao, 1994; Eta and co-workers, 1994). Thus, high circulating levels of hCG may be one mechanism causing uterine quiescence.

Relaxin. This peptide hormone consists of an A and B chain and is structurally similar to the insulin family of proteins (Bogic and associates, 1995; Weiss, 1995). Relaxin mediates lengthening of the pubic ligament, cervical softening, vaginal relaxation, and inhibition of myometrial contractions. There are two separate human relaxin genes, designated H1 and H2. The H1 gene is primarily expressed in the decidua, trophoblast, and prostate, whereas the H2 gene is primarily expressed in the corpus luteum.

Relaxin in plasma of pregnant women is believed to originate exclusively by secretion from the corpus luteum. Plasma levels peak at about 1 ng/mL between 8 and 12 weeks and thereafter decline to lower levels that persist until term. The plasma membrane receptor for relaxin—*relaxin family peptide receptor 1 (RXFP1)*—mediates activation of adenylyl cyclase. Relaxin may promote myometrial relaxation. Although it inhibits contractions of nonpregnant myometrial strips, it does not inhibit those of uterine tissue taken from pregnant women.

Relaxin also effects cervical remodeling through cell proliferation and modulation of extracellular matrix components such as collagen and hyaluronan (Park and associates, 2005). Consistent with a role in cervical remodeling, mice deficient in relaxin or its RXFP1 receptor have difficult parturition and in some cases, are unable to deliver their young (Feng and co-workers, 2005).

Corticotropin-Releasing Hormone (CRH). This hormone is synthesized in the placenta and hypothalamus. As discussed later, CRH plasma levels increase dramatically during the final 6 to 8 weeks of normal pregnancy and have been implicated in the mechanisms controlling the timing of human parturition (Smith, 2007; Wadhwa and colleagues, 1998). Recent studies reveal a dual role of CRH during pregnancy and labor that is mediated by specific CRH-receptor variants and the signalling pathways they initiate (Zhang and co-workers, 2008). During phase 2, CRH binds the receptor CRH-R1, which acting through G5α protein and adenylate cyclase, leads to production of cAMP and subsequent inhibition of myometrial activity. In contrast, at term, CRH can activate the Gqα protein pathway, which favors myometrial contraction. Another aspect of CRH regulation is union of CRH to its binding protein, which can limit bioavailability. CRH-binding protein levels are high during pregnancy and are reported to decline at the time of labor.

Prostaglandins. The prostanoids interact with a family of eight different G-protein-coupled receptors, several of which are expressed in myometrium (Myatt and Lye, 2004).

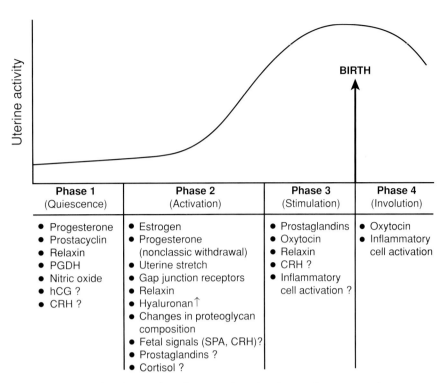

FIGURE 6-17 The key factors thought to regulate the phases of parturition. (CRH = corticotropin-releasing hormone; hCG = human chorionic gonadotropin; SPA = surfactant protein A.) (Adapted from JRG Challis, DM Sloboda, N Alfaidy, et al., 2002, *Reproduction*, Vol. 124, No. 1, p. 2, © Society for Reproduction and Fertility 2002, by permission.)

Prostaglandins most commonly have been considered as uterotonins. However, they have diverse effects, and some act as smooth muscle relaxants.

The major synthetic pathways involved in prostaglandin biosynthesis are shown in Figure 6-18. Prostaglandins are produced using plasma membrane–derived arachidonic acid, which usually is released by the action of the phospholipases A_2 or C on membrane phospholipids. Arachidonic acid can then act as substrate for both type 1 and type 2 prostaglandin H synthase—PGHS-1 and -2, also called cyclooxygenase-1 and -2—COX-1 and 2. Both PGHS isoforms convert arachidonic acid to the unstable endoperoxide prostaglandin G_2 and then to prostaglandin H_2. These enzymes are the target of many nonsteroidal anti-inflammatory drugs (NSAIDs). Indeed, ability of specific NSAIDs to work as tocolytics was considered promising until they were shown to have adverse effects on fetal physiology and development (see Chap. 14, p. 319) (Loudon and co-workers, 2003; Olson and colleagues, 2003, 2007). Through prostaglandin isomerases, prostaglandin H_2 is converted to active prostaglandins, including PGE_2, $PGF_{2\alpha}$, and PGI_2.

Prostaglandin isomerase expression is tissue-specific, thus controlling the relative production of various prostaglandins. Another important control point for prostaglandin activity is its metabolism, which most often is through the action of 15-hydroxyprostaglandin dehydrogenase (PGDH). Expression of this enzyme can be regulated in the uterus, which is important because of its ability to rapidly inactivate prostaglandins to their 15-keto metabolites.

The effect of prostaglandins on tissue targets is complicated in that there are a number of G-protein-coupled prostaglandin

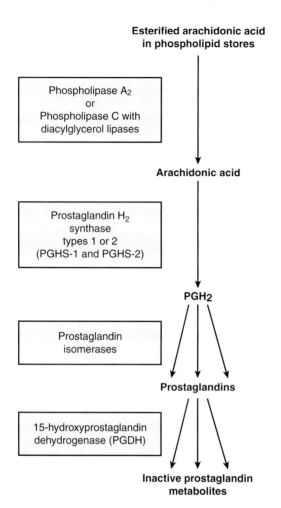

FIGURE 6-18 Overview of the prostaglandin biosynthetic pathway.

receptors (Coleman and associates, 1994). This family of receptors is classified according to the binding specificity of a given receptor to a particular prostaglandin. The receptors are TP—thromboxane A_2; DP—PGD_2; IP—prostacyclin or PGI_2; FP—$PGF_{2\alpha}$ receptor; and $EP_{1,2,3,and\,4}$-PGE_2 receptors. Both PGE_2 and PGI_2 could potentially act to maintain uterine quiescence by increasing cAMP signaling, yet PGE_2 can promote uterine contractility through binding to EP_1 and EP_3 receptors. And also, PGE_2, PGD_2, and PGI_2 have been shown to cause vascular smooth muscle relaxation and vasodilatation in many circumstances. Thus, either the generation of specific prostaglandins or the relative expression of the various prostaglandin receptors may determine myometrial responses to prostaglandins (Lyall, 2002; Olson, 2003, 2007; Smith, 2001; Smith, 1998, and all their colleagues).

In addition to gestational changes, other studies show that there may be regional changes in the upper and lower uterine segments. Expression of COX-2 was shown to be spatially regulated in myometrium and cervix in pregnancy and labor, and an increasing concentration gradient from the fundus to the cervix was noted (Havelock and associates, 2005). Thus, it is entirely possible that prostanoids contribute to myometrial relaxation at one stage of pregnancy and to regional—fundal—myometrial contractions—after initiation of parturition (Myatt and Lye,

2004). Animal studies suggest changes in relative levels of PGE_2 receptors in the term cervix (Schmitz and co-workers, 2006).

Atrial and Brain Natriuretic Peptides and Cyclic Guanosine Monophosphate (cGMP)

Activation of guanylyl cyclase increases intracellular cGMP levels, which also promotes smooth muscle relaxation (Word and colleagues, 1993). Guanylate cyclase activity and cGMP content is increased in pregnant myometrium before labor starts compared with after labor has begun (Telfer and colleagues, 2001). Intracellular cGMP levels can be stimulated by either atrial natriuretic peptide (ANP) and brain natriuretic peptide (BNP) receptors, which are both present in myometrium during pregnancy (Itoh and co-workers, 1994). BNP is secreted by amnion in large amounts, and ANP is expressed in placenta (Itoh and associates, 1993; Lim and Gude, 1995).

Soluble guanylyl cyclase is also activated by nitric oxide, which because of its hydrophobic nature, readily penetrates the plasma membrane to enter cells. Nitric oxide reacts with iron and stimulates it to produce cGMP and myometrial relaxation (Izumi and colleagues, 1993). Nitric oxide is synthesized in decidua, myometrial blood vessels, and nerves (Yallampalli and colleagues, 1994a, 1994b). Its role in possible uterine quiescence is not understood.

Accelerated Uterotonin Degradation and Phase 1 of Parturition

In addition to pregnancy-induced compounds that stimulate myometrial cell refractoriness, there are striking increases in the activities of enzymes that degrade or inactivate endogenously produced uterotonins. Some of these and their degradative enzymes include PGDH, which degrades prostaglandins; enkephalinase and endothelins; oxytocinase and oxytocin; diamine oxidase and histamine; catechol *O*-methyltransferase and catecholamines; angiotensinases and angiotensin-II; and platelet-activating factor (PAF) acetylhydrolase and PAF. Activities of several of these enzymes are increased by progesterone action and many decrease late in gestation (Bates, 1979; Casey, 1980; Germain, 1994, and all their colleagues).

Phase 2: Uterine Activation and Cervical Ripening

Classical Progesterone Withdrawal and Parturition

In species that exhibit progesterone withdrawal, progression of parturition to labor can be blocked by administering progesterone to the mother. In pregnant women, however, there are conflicting reports as to whether or not progesterone administration can delay the timely onset of parturition or prevent preterm labor. Some studies suggest that progesterone neither prevents preterm labor nor appears to extend labor, but others suggest the opposite (Mackenzie and associates, 2006). Clinically, any advantages to the use of progesterone or its metabolite, 17-hydroxyprogesterone, to decrease the incidence of preterm labor in high-risk populations seem minimal (Fonseca, 2007; Meis, 2003; Rouse, 2007, and all their colleagues). The 17-hydroxyprogesterone molecule binds and activates the progesterone receptor less so than progesterone. Further research may help explain its differential action and how it could be better used to prevent preterm labor.

Progesterone Receptor Antagonists and Human Parturition

When the steroidal antiprogestin, mifepristone or RU486, is administered during the latter phase of the ovarian cycle, it induces menstruation prematurely. It is also an effective abortifacient during early pregnancy (see Chap. 9, p. 232). Mifepristone is a classical steroid antagonist, acting at the level of the progesterone receptor. Although less effective in inducing abortion or labor in women later in pregnancy, mifepristone appears to have some effect on cervical ripening and increasing myometrial sensitivity to uterotonins (Chwalisz and Garfield, 1994; Chwalisz, 1994; Berkane and associates, 2005). These data suggest that humans have a mechanism for progesterone inactivation, whereby the myometrium and cervix becomes refractory to the blocking actions of progesterone.

Functional Progesterone Withdrawal in Human Parturition

As an alternative to classical progesterone withdrawal resulting from decreased secretion, research has focused on unique human mechanisms that have evolved to inhibit progesterone action. In theory, functional progesterone withdrawal or antagonism could be mediated through several mechanisms:

- Changes in the relative expression of the nuclear progesterone receptor (PR) protein isoforms, PR-A, PR-B, and PR-C
- Changes in the relative expression of membrane-bound progesterone receptors
- Posttranslational modifications of the progesterone receptor
- Alterations in progesterone receptor activity through changes in the expression of co-activators or co-repressors that directly influence receptor function
- Local inactivation of progesterone by steroid-metabolizing enzymes or synthesis of a natural antagonist.

Indeed, there is experimental evidence that lends support to each of these possibilities. Evidence now suggests that progesterone receptor activity is decreased late in gestation. As discussed in Chapter 3 (p. 41), there are numerous isoforms of the receptor—these include PR-A, PR-B, and PR-C. In vitro studies have led to the concept that PR-B is the principal mediator of progesterone actions, whereas PR-A and PR-C decrease progesterone responsiveness by repressing the transcriptional activation of the PR-B isoform. With respect to functional progesterone withdrawal, in a series of studies, it has been shown that there is a shift in the relative ratio of PR-A to PR-B within the myometrium late in gestation (Madsen, 2004; Mesiano, 2002; Pieber, 2001, and all their colleagues). Analysis of placental tissues for PR-A and PR-B suggests that the ratio is similarly modified in decidua and chorion, but that there is decreased overall progesterone receptor expression in the amnion (Haluska and co-workers, 2002). Similarly, studies of cervical stroma suggest changes in receptor isoforms (Stjernholm-Vladic

and associates, 2004). And Condon and associates (2006) reported that myometrial PR-C to PR-B ratio increased, but *only* in fundal—and not lower-segment—myometrium. PR coactivators have also been shown to decline in term myometrium, which may contribute to reduced progesterone action (Condon and associates, 2003).

In addition to the nuclear progesterone receptors described above, a number of membrane-associated progesterone receptors have been identified that include mPR_α, mPR_β, and mPR_γ. The first two couple to inhibitory G-proteins. Ligand binding to these receptors decreases cAMP levels and increases myosin phosphorylation, both of which promote uterine contractility. Although still not entirely clear, current evidence suggests that changes in expression of membrane PR isoforms may also promote the transition from myometrial quiescence to activation (Karteris and co-workers, 2006).

There is evidence in human and rodent models that local action of enzymes catabolize progesterone to metabolites that have a weak affinity for the progesterone receptor. One of these enzymes is steroid 5α-reductase type 1. In mice that cannot express this enzyme, the cervix does not ripen and parturition does not ensue (Mahendroo and colleagues, 1999). Similarly, mice deficient in the enzyme 20α-hydroxy-steroid dehydrogenase have delayed parturition (Piekorz and associates, 2005). A decline in 17β-hydroxysteroid dehydrogenase type 2 in the human cervix at term results in a net increase in estrogen and decline in progesterone (Andersson and co-workers, 2008).

And lastly, there is some support for antiprogestin-like activities of glucocorticoids on progesterone receptor activity (Karalis and co-workers, 1996). Because glucocorticoids play an important role in parturition initiation in several species, examining their potential role as an antiprogestin in humans warrants further study.

Taken together, all of these observations support the concept that multiple pathways exist for a functional progesterone withdrawal that includes changes in PR isoform and receptor coactivator levels and in local hormone metabolism to less active products.

Oxytocin Receptors

It is still controversial whether oxytocin plays a role in the early phases of uterine activation, or whether its sole function is in the expulsive phase of labor. Most studies of regulation of myometrial oxytocin receptor synthesis have been performed in the rat and mouse. Disruption of the oxytocin receptor gene in the mouse does not affect parturition. This suggests that, at least in this species, multiple systems likely ensure that parturition occurs. There is little doubt, however, that there is an increase in myometrial oxytocin receptors during phase 2 of parturition. Moreover, their activation results in increased phospholipase C activity and subsequent increases in cytosolic calcium and uterine contractility.

Progesterone and estradiol appear to be the primary regulators of oxytocin receptor expression. Estradiol treatment in vivo or in myometrial explants increases myometrial oxytocin receptors. This action, however, is prevented by simultaneous treatment with progesterone (Fuchs and colleagues, 1983). Progesterone also may act within the myometrial cell to increase oxytocin receptor degradation and inhibit oxytocin activation of its receptor at the cell surface (Bogacki and associates, 2002; Soloff and colleagues, 1983). These data indicate that one of the mechanisms whereby progesterone maintains uterine quiescence is through the inhibition of myometrial oxytocin response.

The increase in oxytocin receptors in nonhuman species appears to be mainly regulated either directly or indirectly by estradiol. Treatment of several species with estrogen leads to a uterine oxytocin receptors increase (Blanks and co-workers, 2003; Challis and Lye, 1994). The level of oxytocin receptor mRNA in human myometrium at term is greater than that found in preterm myometrium (Wathes and co-workers, 1999). Thus, increased receptors at term may be attributable to increased gene transcription. An estrogen response element, however, is not present in the oxytocin receptor gene, suggesting that the stimulatory effects of estrogen may be indirect.

Human studies suggest that inflammatory-related rapid-response genes may regulate oxytocin receptors (Bethin, 2003; Kimura, 1999; Massrieh, 2006, and all their colleagues). These receptors also are present in human endometrium and in decidua at term and stimulate prostaglandin production (Fuchs and associates, 1981). In addition, these receptors are found in the myometrium and at lower levels, in amniochorion–decidual tissues (Benedetto and associates, 1990; Wathes and co-workers, 1999).

Relaxin

Although relaxin may play a role in maintenance of uterine quiescence, it also has roles in phase 2 of parturition. These include remodeling of the extracellular matrix of the uterus, cervix, vagina, breast, and pubic symphysis as well as promoting cell proliferation and inhibiting apoptosis. Relaxin's actions on cell proliferation and apoptosis are mediated through the G-protein-coupled receptor, RXFP1, whereas some but not all actions of relaxin on matrix remodeling are mediated through RXFP1 (Samuel and co-workers, 2009; Yao and associates, 2008). Although the precise mechanisms for modulation of matrix turnover have not been fully elucidated, relaxin appears to mediate synthesis of glycosaminoglycans and proteoglycans and to degrade matrix macromolecules such as collagen by induction of matrix metalloproteases. Relaxin promotes growth of the cervix, vagina, and pubic symphysis and is necessary for breast remodeling for lactation. Consistent with its proposed roles, mice deficient in relaxin or the RXFP1 receptor have protracted labor, reduced growth of the cervix, vagina, and symphysis, and are unable to nurse because of incomplete nipple development (Feng, 2005; Park, 2005; Yao, 2008, and all their associates).

Fetal Contributions to Initiation of Parturition

It is intellectually intriguing to envision that the mature human fetus provides the signal to initiate parturition. Teleologically, this seems most logical because such a signal could be transmitted in several ways to suspend uterine quiescence. The fetus may provide a signal through a blood-borne agent that acts on the placenta. Research is ongoing to better understand the fetal sig-

nals that contribute to the initiation of parturition (Mendelson, 2009). Although signals may arise from the fetus, it is likely that the uterus and cervix first must be prepared for labor before a uterotonin produced by the fetus or elsewhere can be optimally effective (Casey and MacDonald, 1994).

Uterine Stretch and Parturition

There is now considerable evidence that fetal growth is an important component in uterine activation in phase 1 of parturition. In association with fetal growth, significant increases in myometrial tensile stress and amnionic fluid pressure follow (Fisk and co-workers, 1992). With uterine activation, stretch is required for induction of specific contraction-associated proteins (CAPs). Stretch increases expression of the gap junction protein—connexin 43, as well as oxytocin receptors. Others have hypothesized that stretch plays an integrated role with fetal–maternal endocrine cascades of uterine activation (Lyall and co-workers, 2002; Ou and colleagues, 1997, 1998).

Clinical support for a role of stretch comes from the observation that multifetal pregnancies are at a much greater risk for preterm labor than singletons (Gardner and co-workers, 1995). Preterm labor is also significantly more common in pregnancies complicated by hydramnios (Many and associates, 1996). Although the mechanisms causing preterm birth in these two examples are debated, a role for uterine stretch must be considered.

Cell signaling systems used by stretch to regulate the myometrial cell continue to be defined. This process—*mechanotransduction*—may include activation of cell-surface receptors or ion channels, transmission of signals through extracellular matrix, or release of autocrine molecules that act directly on myometrium (Shynlova and co-workers, 2009). For example, the extracellular matrix protein, fibronectin, and its cell surface receptor, alpha 5 integrin receptor, are induced in the rodent in response to stretch (Shynlova and colleagues, 2007). This interaction may aid force transduction during labor contraction by anchoring hypertrophied myocytes to the uterine extracellular matrix.

Fetal Endocrine Cascades Leading to Parturition

The ability of the fetus to provide endocrine signals that initiate parturition has been demonstrated in several species. More than 30 years ago, Liggins and associates (1967, 1973) demonstrated that the fetus provides the signal for the timely onset of parturition in sheep. This signal was shown to come from the fetal hypothalamic-pituitary-adrenal axis (Whittle and co-workers, 2001).

Defining the exact mechanisms regulating human parturition has proven more difficult, and all evidence suggests that it is not regulated in the exact manner seen in the sheep. Even so, activation of the human fetal hypothalamic–pituitary–adrenal placental axis is considered a critical component of normal parturition. Moreover, premature activation of this axis is considered to prompt many cases of preterm labor (Challis and co-workers, 2000, 2001). As in the sheep, steroid products of the human fetal adrenal gland are believed to have effects on the placenta and membranes that eventually transform myometrium from a quiescent to contractile state. A key component in the human may be the unique ability of the placenta to produce large amounts of corticotropin-releasing hormone (CRH).

Actions of Corticotropin-Releasing Hormone on the Fetal Adrenal Gland

The human fetal adrenal glands are morphologically, functionally, and physiologically remarkable organs. At term, the fetal adrenal glands weigh the same as those in the adult and are similar in size to the adjacent fetal kidney (Chap. 3, p. 69). The daily steroid production by the fetal adrenal glands near term is estimated to be 100 to 200 mg/day. This is higher than the 30 to 40 mg/day seen in adult glands at rest. Within the fetal adrenal gland, steroidogenic function and zonation differ from the adult. For example, significant amounts of cortisol are not produced in the fetal gland until the last trimester. As a result, fetal cortisol levels increase during the last weeks of gestation (Murphy, 1982). During this same period, levels of dehydroepiandrosterone sulfate (DHEA-S) production also are increasing significantly, leading to increases in maternal estrogens, particularly estriol.

These increases in fetal adrenal gland activity contrast with fetal pituitary adrenocorticotropic hormone (ACTH) levels, which do not increase until actual labor onset. Thus, substantial growth and increased steroid synthesis during latter gestation is at a time when fetal plasma ACTH levels are low (Winters and co-workers, 1974). It is presumed that alternate stimuli for growth and steroidogenesis are likely placentally derived. In support of this, the fetal zone of the adrenal gland undergoes rapid involution immediately after birth, when placenta-derived factors are no longer available.

Many favor CRH of placental origin to be a critical agent for fetal adrenal hypertrophy and increased steroidogenesis in late pregnancy. Some in vitro studies have shown that CRH stimulates fetal adrenal DHEA-S and cortisol biosynthesis (Parker and associates, 1999; Smith and co-workers, 1998). The ability of CRH to regulate the adrenal glands and of the adrenals to regulate placental CRH production supports the idea of a feed-forward endocrine cascade that initiates late in gestation (Fig. 6-19).

Placental Corticotropin-Releasing Hormone Production.

A CRH hormone identical to maternal and fetal hypothalamic CRH is synthesized by the placenta in relatively large amounts (Grino and associates, 1987; Saijonmaa and colleagues, 1988). One important difference is that, unlike hypothalamic CRH, which is under glucocorticoid negative feedback, cortisol has been shown to *stimulate* placental CRH production (Jones and co-workers, 1989; Marinoni and associates, 1998). This ability makes it possible to create a feed-forward endocrine cascade that does not end until separation of the fetus from the placenta at delivery.

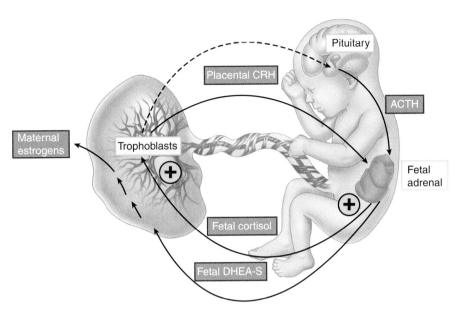

FIGURE 6-19 The placental–fetal adrenal endocrine cascade. In late gestation, placental corticotropin-releasing hormone (CRH) stimulates fetal adrenal production of dehydroepiandrosterone sulfate (DHEA-S) and cortisol. The latter stimulates production of placental CRH, which leads to a feed-forward cascade that enhances adrenal steroid hormone production. (ACTH = adrenocorticotropic hormone.)

Maternal plasma CRH levels are low in the first trimester and rise from midgestation to term. In the last 12 weeks, CRH plasma levels rise exponentially, peaking during labor and then falling precipitously after delivery (Frim and associates, 1988; Sasaki and colleagues, 1987). Amnionic fluid CRH levels similarly increase in late gestation. And although umbilical cord blood CRH levels are lower than those in maternal circulation, they are within the range of concentrations that are found to stimulate fetal adrenal steroidogenesis (Goland and co-workers, 1986, 1993; Perkins and associates, 1995).

Corticotropin-releasing hormone is the only trophic hormone–releasing factor to have a specific serum binding protein. During most of pregnancy, it appears that CRH-binding protein (CRH-BP) binds most maternal circulating CRH. Binding likely inactivates ACTH-stimulating activity of placental CRH (Lowry, 1993). During later pregnancy, however, CRH-BP levels in both maternal plasma and amnionic fluid decline at the same time CRH levels are strikingly increasing. This leads to markedly increased levels of bioavailable CRH (Perkins and co-workers, 1995; Petraglia and associates, 1997).

In pregnancies in which the fetus can be considered to be "stressed" from various complications, concentrations of CRH in fetal plasma, amnionic fluid, and maternal plasma are increased compared with those seen in normal gestation (Berkowitz, 1996; Goland, 1993; McGrath, 2002; Perkins, 1995, and all their co-workers). The placenta is likely the source for this increased CRH. For example, placental CRH content was fourfold higher in placentas from women with preeclampsia than in those from normal pregnancies (Perkins and co-workers, 1995). Moreover, the biological impact of increased CRH levels is likely to be amplified in such instances as a result of subnormal levels of CRH-BP (Petraglia and co-workers, 1996). Such increases in placental CRH production during normal gestation and the excessive secretion of placental CRH in complicated pregnancies may play a role in the normal gestational increases in fetal adrenal cortisol synthesis (Murphy, 1982). It also may result in the supranormal levels of umbilical cord blood cortisol noted in stressed neonates (Falkenberg and colleagues, 1999; Goland and co-workers, 1994).

Corticotropin-Releasing Hormones and Parturition Timing

Placental CRH has been proposed to play several roles in parturition regulation. Placental CRH may enhance fetal cortisol production to provide positive feedback so that the placenta produces more CRH. Resulting high levels of CRH may modulate myometrial contractility via interaction with the CRH receptor isoform, CRH-R1d. This isoform is known to enhance myometrial contractile response (Grammatopoulos, 1994, 1995, 1999; Hillhouse, 1993; Markovic, 2007, and all their colleagues). It has also been proposed that cortisol affects the myometrium indirectly by stimulating the fetal membranes to increase prostaglandin synthesis.

And finally, CRH has been shown to stimulate fetal adrenal C_{19}-steroid synthesis, thereby increasing substrate for placental aromatization. Increased production of estrogens would shift the estrogen-to-progesterone ratio and promote the expression of a series of contractile proteins in the myometrium, leading to a loss of myometrial quiescence.

Some have proposed that the rising level of CRH at the end of gestation reflects a *fetal-placental clock* (McLean and colleagues, 1995). CRH levels vary greatly among women, and it appears that the rate of increase in maternal CRH levels is a more accurate predictor of pregnancy outcome than is a single measurement (Leung and associates, 2001; McGrath and Smith, 2002). In this regard, the placenta and fetus, through endocrinological events, influence the timing of parturition at the end of normal gestation.

Fetal Lung Surfactant and Parturition

Surfactant protein A (SP-A) produced by the fetal lung is required for lung maturation. Its levels are increased in amnionic fluid at term in women and mice. Recent studies in the mouse suggest that the increasing SP-A concentrations in amnionic fluid activate fluid macrophages to migrate into the myometrium and induce a transcription factor—*nuclear factor-kB* (Condon and co-workers, 2004). This factor activates inflammatory response genes in the myometrium, which in turn promote uterine contractility. This model supports the supposition that fetal signals play a role in parturition initiation. The exact mechanisms by which SP-A activates myometrial contractility in women, however, remains to be clarified as studies in women suggest that fetal macrophages in the amnionic cavity do not enter the myometrium during labor (Kim and colleagues, 2006; Leong and associates, 2008). Pulmonary surfactant and components of surfactant such as platelet activating factor, when secreted into human amnionic fluid, have been reported to stimulate prostaglandin synthesis (PGE_2) and uterine contractility. This supports a function of SP-A in human parturition (Lopez and co-workers, 1988; Toyoshima and associates, 1995).

Fetal Anomalies and Delayed Parturition

There is fragmentary evidence that pregnancies with markedly diminished estrogen production may be associated with prolonged gestation. Some of these "natural experiments" include fetal anencephaly with adrenal hypoplasia and placental sulfatase deficiency. The broad range of gestational length seen with these disorders questions the exact role of estrogen in human parturition initiation.

Other fetal abnormalities that prevent or severely reduce the entry of fetal urine into amnionic fluid—renal agenesis, or into lung secretions—pulmonary hypoplasia, do not prolong human pregnancy. Thus, a fetal signal through the paracrine arm of the fetal–maternal communication system does not appear to be mandated for parturition initiation.

Some brain anomalies of the fetal calf, fetal lamb, and sometimes the human fetus delay the normal timing of parturition. More than a century ago, Rea (1898) observed an association between fetal anencephaly and prolonged human gestation. Malpas (1933) extended these observations and described a pregnancy with an anencephalic fetus that was prolonged to 374 days—53 weeks. He concluded that the association between anencephaly and prolonged gestation was attributable to anomalous fetal brain–pituitary–adrenal function. The adrenal glands of the anencephalic fetus are very small and at term, may be only 5 to 10 percent as large as those of a normal fetus. This is caused by developmental failure of the fetal zone that normally accounts for most of fetal adrenal mass and production of C_{19}-steroid hormones (see Chap. 3, p. 70). Such pregnancies are also associated with delayed labor (Anderson and Turnbull, 1973). These findings are suggestive that in humans, as in sheep, the fetal adrenal glands are important for the timely onset of parturition.

Systems to Ensure Success of Phase 3 of Parturition

Phase 3 of parturition is synonymous with uterine contractions that bring about progressive cervical dilatation and delivery. Current data favor the *uterotonins theory of labor initiation.* Increased uterotonin production would follow once phase 1 is suspended and uterine phase 2 processes are implemented. A number of uterotonins may be important to the success of phase 3, that is, active labor (see Fig. 6-17). Just as multiple processes likely contribute to myometrial unresponsiveness of phase 1 of parturition, other processes may contribute jointly to a system that ensures labor success.

Uterotonins that are candidates for labor induction include oxytocin, prostaglandins, serotonin, histamine, PAF, angiotensin II, and many others. All have been shown to stimulate smooth muscle contraction through G-protein coupling.

Oxytocin and Phase 3 of Parturition

Late in pregnancy, during phase 2 of parturition, there is a 50-fold or more increase in the number of myometrial oxytocin receptors (Fuchs and associates, 1982; Kimura and co-workers, 1996). This increase coincides with an increase in uterine contractile responsiveness to oxytocin (Soloff and co-workers, 1979). Moreover, prolonged gestation is associated with a delay in the increase of these receptors (Fuchs and colleagues, 1984).

Oxytocin—literally, *quick birth*—was the first uterotonin to be implicated in parturition initiation. This nanopeptide is synthesized in the magnocellular neurons of the supraoptic and paraventricular neurons (Fig. 6-20). The prohormone is transported with its carrier protein, *neurophysin*, along the axons to the neural lobe of the posterior pituitary gland in membrane-bound vesicles for storage and later release. The prohormone is converted enzymatically to oxytocin during transport (Gainer and colleagues, 1988; Leake, 1990). Although oxytocin does not appear to cause the initiation of parturition, it may be one of several participants to ensure labor effectiveness.

Role of Oxytocin in Phases 3 and 4 of Parturition. Because of successful labor induction with oxytocin, it was logically suspected in parturition initiation. First, in addition to its effectiveness in inducing labor at term, oxytocin is a potent uterotonin and occurs naturally in humans. Subsequent observations provide additional support for this theory:

- The number of oxytocin receptors strikingly increases in myometrial and decidual tissues near the end of gestation
- Oxytocin acts on decidual tissue to promote prostaglandin release
- Oxytocin is synthesized directly in decidual and extraembryonic fetal tissues and in the placenta (Chibbar and associates, 1993; Zingg and colleagues, 1995).

Although little evidence suggests a role for oxytocin in phase 2 of parturition, abundant data support its important role during second-stage labor and the puerperium—phase 4 of parturition. Specifically, there are increased maternal serum oxytocin levels: (1) during second-stage labor—the end of phase 3 of parturition, (2) in the early postpartum period, and (3) during breast feeding—phase 4 of parturition (Nissen and co-workers, 1995). Immediately after delivery of the fetus, placenta, and membranes—completion of parturition phase 3—firm and persistent uterine contraction and retraction are essential to prevent postpartum hemorrhage. Oxytocin likely causes persistent contractions.

Oxytocin infusion in women promotes increased levels of mRNAs in myometrial genes that encode proteins essential for uterine involution. These include interstitial collagenase, monocyte chemoattractant protein-1, interleukin-8, and urokinase plasminogen activator receptor. Therefore, oxytocin action at the end of labor and during phase 3 of parturition may be involved in uterine involution.

Prostaglandins and Phase 3 of Parturition

Although their role in phase 2—activation phase—of noncomplicated pregnancies is less well defined, a critical role for prostaglandins in phase 3 of parturition is clear (MacDonald and Casey, 1993). Evidence supportive of this theory includes:

- Levels of prostaglandins—or their metabolites, in amnionic fluid, maternal plasma, and maternal urine are increased during labor (Keirse, 1979)
- Treatment of pregnant women with prostaglandins, by any of several routes of administration, causes abortion or labor at all stages of gestation (Novy and Liggins, 1980)
- Administration of prostaglandin H synthase type 2 (PGHS-2) inhibitors to pregnant women will delay spontaneous labor onset and sometimes arrest preterm labor (Loudon and co-workers, 2003)

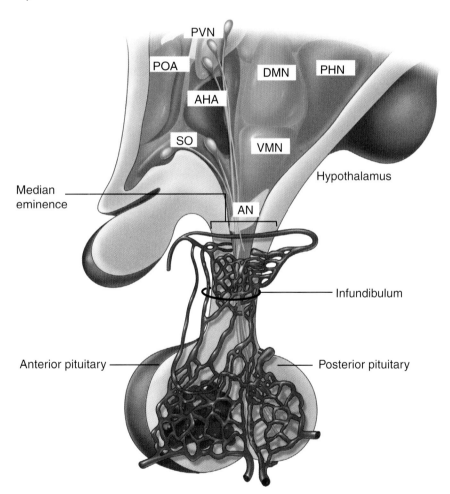

FIGURE 6-20 Hypothalamic-pituitary-adrenal (HPA) axis. Many reproductive functions are regulated by the HPA axis. During parturition, the magnocellular neurons in the maternal hypothalamus synthesize oxytocin, a uterotonin. Oxytocin in its prohormone form is transported to the posterior pituitary for storage and subsequent release. The fetal HPA axis begins to secrete hormones as early as 6-8 weeks of fetal life. During pregnancy and parturition, this axis plays important roles in regulating fetal DHEA-S production, which is the precursor for estrogen synthesis in the placenta, and in CRH production by the fetus and placenta. (AHA = anterior hypothalamic area; AN = arcuate nucleus; DMN = Dorsomedial nucleus; PHN = posterior hypothalamic nucleus; POA = preoptic area; PVN = paraventricular nucleus; SO = supraoptic nucleus; VMN = ventromedial nucleus.)

- Prostaglandin treatment of myometrial tissue in vitro sometimes causes contraction, dependent on the prostanoid tested and the physiological status of the tissue treated.

Uterine Events Regulating Prostaglandin Production.

During labor, the production of prostaglandins within the myometrium and decidua is an efficient mechanism of activating contractions. For example, PG synthesis is high and unchanging in the decidua during phase 2 and 3 of parturition, in support of a role of prostaglandins in activation and stimulation. The receptor for $PGF_{2\alpha}$ is increased in the decidua at term, and this increase most likely is the regulatory step in PG action in the uterus. The myometrium synthesizes PGHS-2 with the onset of labor, but most PG likely comes from the decidua.

The fetal membranes and placenta also produce prostaglandins. Prostaglandins, primarily PGE_2, but also $PGF_{2\alpha}$, are detected in amnionic fluid at all stages of gestation. As the fetus grows, prostaglandins levels in the amnionic fluid increase gradually. The major increases in amnionic fluid, however, are demonstrable after labor begins (Fig. 6-21). There are higher levels, which likely result as the cervix dilates and exposes decidual tissue (Fig. 6-22). These increased levels in the forebag as compared with the upper compartment are believed to be the result of an inflammatory response that signals the events leading to active labor. Together, the increases in cytokines and

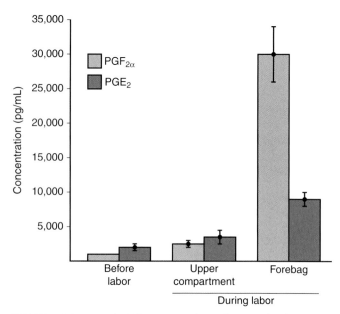

FIGURE 6-21 Mean (±SD) concentrations of prostaglandin $F_{2\alpha}$ ($PGF_{2\alpha}$) and prostaglandin E_2 (PGE_2) in amnionic fluid at term before labor and in the upper and forebag compartments during labor at all stages of cervical dilatation. (Data from MacDonald and Casey, 1993.)

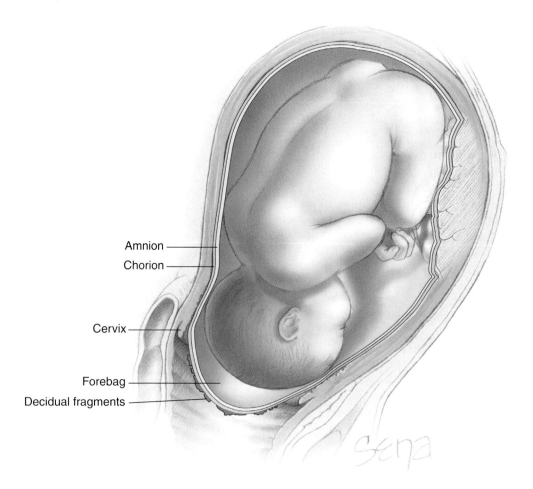

FIGURE 6-22 Sagittal view of the exposed forebag and attached decidual fragments after cervical dilatation during labor. (Redrawn from MacDonald and Casey, 1996.)

prostaglandins further degrade the extracellular matrix, thus weakening fetal membranes.

Findings of Kemp and co-workers (2002) and Kelly (2002) support a possibility that inflammatory mediators aid cervical dilatation and alterations to the lower uterine segment. It can be envisioned that they, along with the increased prostaglandins measured in vaginal fluid during labor, add to the relatively rapid cervical changes that are characteristic of parturition.

Platelet-Activating Factor (PAF)

There are a number of allergic and inflammatory responses in which PAF is involved. This mediator is produced in basophils, neutrophils, eosinophils, monocytes, and endothelial cells. The PAF receptor is a member of the G-protein–coupled receptor family of transmembrane receptors. Its stimulation by PAF increases myometrial cell calcium levels and promotes uterine contractions. Levels of PAF in amnionic fluid are increased during labor, and PAF treatment of myometrial tissue promotes contraction (Nishihara and associates, 1984; Zhu and colleagues, 1992). This factor is inactivated enzymatically by PAF-acetylhydrolase (PAF-AH), which is present in macrophages, which are found in large numbers in decidua (Prescott and associates, 1990). Thus, the myometrium may be protected from PAF action by PAF-AH during pregnancy.

Endothelin-1

The endothelins are a family of 21-amino acid peptides that powerfully induce myometrial contraction (Word and colleagues, 1990). The endothelin A receptor is preferentially expressed in smooth muscle and effects an increase in intracellular calcium. Endothelin-1 is produced in myometrium, and its potential contribution to phase 3 of parturition is not defined. Although endothelin-1 is also synthesized in amnion, it is unlikely that it is transported from the amnion or amnionic fluid to the myometrium without degradation (Eis and colleagues, 1992). Enkephalinase, which catalyzes the degradation of endothelin-1, is highly active in chorion laeve (Germain and associates, 1994).

Angiotensin II

There are two G-protein-linked angiotensin II receptors-expressed in the uterus—AT1 and AT2. In nonpregnant women, the AT2 receptor is predominant, but the AT1 receptor is preferentially expressed in pregnant women (Cox and associates, 1993). Angiotensin II binding to the plasma-membrane receptor evokes contraction. During pregnancy, the vascular smooth muscle that expresses the AT2 receptor is refractory to the pressor effects of infused angiotensin II (see Chap. 5, p. 120). In myometrium near term, however, angiotensin II may be another component of the uterotonin system of phase 3 of parturition. A potential mechanism for increased angiotensin II responsiveness in preeclampsia via increased levels of heterodimers between the vasopressor receptor AT1 and the vasodepressor receptor B2 also emphasizes a role of angiotensin II in the normal physiology of parturition (Quitterer and associates, 2004).

Corticotropin-Releasing Hormone (CRH)

Late in pregnancy—phase 2 or 3 of parturition—modification in the CRH receptor favors a switch from cAMP forma-

tion to increased myometrial cell calcium levels via protein kinase C activation. Oxytocin acts to attenuate CRH-stimulated accumulation of cAMP in myometrial tissue, and CRH augments the contraction-inducing potency of a given dose of oxytocin in human myometrial strips (Quartero and colleagues, 1991, 1992). Finally, CRH acts to increase myometrial contractile force in response to $PGF_{2\alpha}$ (Benedetto and associates, 1994).

Contribution of Intrauterine Tissues to Parturition

Although they have a potential role in parturition initiation, amnion, chorion laeve, and decidua parietalis more likely have an alternative role. The membranes and decidua comprise an important tissue shell around the fetus that serves as a physical, immunological, and metabolic shield that protects against the untimely initiation of parturition. Late in gestation, however, the fetal membranes may indeed act to prepare for labor.

Amnion. Virtually all of the membrane's tensile strength—resistance to tearing and rupture—is provided by the amnion (Chap. 3, p. 59). This avascular tissue is highly resistant to penetration by leukocytes, microorganisms, and neoplastic cells. It also constitutes a selective filter to prevent fetal particulate-bound lung and skin secretions from reaching the maternal compartment. In this manner, maternal tissues are protected from amnionic fluid constituents that could adversely affect decidual or myometrial function or adverse events such as amnionic fluid embolism (see Chap. 35, p. 788).

Several bioactive peptides and prostaglandins that cause myometrial relaxation or contraction are synthesized in amnion (Fig. 6-23). Late in pregnancy, amnionic prostaglandin biosynthesis is increased and phospholipase A_2 and PGHS-2 show increased activity (Johnson and colleagues, 2002). Accordingly, many hypothesize that prostaglandins regulate events leading to parturition. It is likely that amnion is the major source for amnionic fluid prostaglandins, and their role in activation of cascades that promote membrane rupture is clear. The influence of amnion-derived prostaglandins on uterine quiescence and activation, however, is less clear. This is because prostaglandin transport from the amnion through the chorion to access maternal tissues is limited by expression of the inactivating enzyme, prostaglandin dehydrogenase.

Chorion Laeve. This tissue layer also is primarily protective, and it provides immunological acceptance. The chorion laeve is also enriched with enzymes that inactivate uterotonins—for example, prostaglandin dehydrogenase (PGDH), oxytocinase, and enkephalinase (Cheung and co-workers, 1990; Germain and associates, 1994). As noted, PGDH inactivates amnion-derived prostaglandins. With chorionic rupture, this barrier would be lost, and prostaglandins could readily influence adjacent decidua and myometrium.

There is also evidence that PGDH levels found in the chorion decline during labor. This would allow increased prostaglandin-stimulated matrix metalloproteinase (MMP) activity associated with membrane rupture. It would further allow PG entry into the maternal compartment to promote myometrial contractility (Patel, 1999; Van Meir, 1996; Wu, 2000, and all their co-workers).

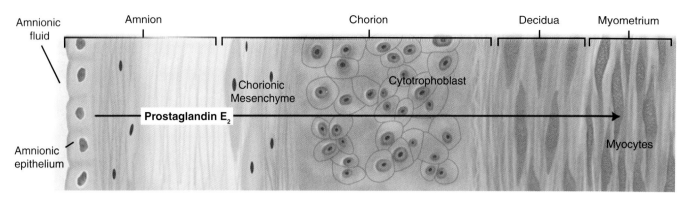

FIGURE 6-23 The amnion synthesizes prostaglandins, and late in pregnancy, synthesis is increased by increased phospholipase A_2 and prostaglandin H synthase, type 2 (PGHS-2) activity. During pregnancy, the transport of prostaglandins from the amnion to maternal tissues is limited by expression of the inactivating enzymes, prostaglandin dehydrogenase (PGDH), in the chorion. During labor, PGDH levels decline, and amnion-derived prostaglandins can influence membrane rupture and uterine contractility. The role of decidual activation in parturition is unclear but may involve local progesterone metabolism and increased prostaglandin receptor concentrations, thus enhancing uterine prostaglandin actions and cytokine production. (Adapted from Smith, 2007.)

It is likely that progesterone maintains chorion PGDH expression, whereas cortisol decreases its expression. Thus, PGDH levels would decrease late in gestation as fetal cortisol production increases and as part of progesterone withdrawal.

Decidua Parietalis. A metabolic contribution of decidua parietalis to parturition initiation is an appealing possibility for both anatomical and functional reasons. The generation of decidual uterotonins that act in a paracrine manner on contiguous myometrium is intuitive. In addition, decidua expresses steroid metabolizing enzymes such as $20_\alpha HSD$ and steroid $5_\alpha R1$ that may regulate local progesterone withdrawal. There is also evidence that decidual activation is an accompaniment of human parturition (Casey and MacDonald, 1988a, 1988b, 1990; MacDonald and colleagues, 1991). The central question is whether decidual activation precedes or follows labor onset.

Decidual activation appears to be localized to the exposed decidual fragments lining the forebag. Trauma, hypoxia, and exposure of forebag decidua to endotoxin lipopolysaccharide, microorganisms, and interleukin-1β (IL-1β) in the vaginal fluids provoke an inflammatory reaction—an inevitable and consistent sequela of labor. With this inflammation, cytokines are produced that can either increase uterotonin production—principally prostaglandins, or act directly on myometrium to cause contraction—for example, tumor necrosis factor-α (TNF-α) and interleukins 1, 6, 8, and 12. These molecules also can act as chemokines that recruit to the myometrium neutrophils and eosinophils, which further increase contractions and labor (Keelan and co-workers, 2003).

There is uncertainty whether PG concentration or output from the decidua increases with term labor onset. Olson and Ammann (2007) suggest that the major regulation of decidual PG action is not PG synthesis, but rather increased expression of the $PGF_{2\alpha}$ receptor.

Regulation of Phase 3 and 4 of Parturition: Summary

It is likely that multiple and possibly redundant processes contribute to the success of the three active labor phases once phase 1 of parturition is suspended and phase 2 is implemented. Phase 3 is highlighted by increased activation of G-protein-coupled receptors that inhibit cAMP formation, increase intracellular calcium stores, and promote interaction of actin and myosin and subsequent force generation. Simultaneously, cervical proteoglycan composition and collagen structure are altered to a form that promotes tissue distensibility and increased compliance. The net result is initiation of coordinated myometrial contractions of sufficient amplitude and frequency to dilate the prepared cervix and push the fetus through the birth canal. The source of regulatory ligands for these receptors varies from endocrine hormones such as oxytocin to locally produced prostaglandins.

In phase 4 of parturition, a complicated series of repair processes are initiated to resolve inflammatory responses and remove glycosaminoglycans, proteoglycans, and structurally compromised collagen. Simultaneously, matrix and cellular components required for complete uterine involution are synthesized, and the dense connective tissue and structural integrity of the cervix is reformed.

PHYSIOLOGY AND BIOCHEMISTRY OF PRETERM LABOR

Preterm birth has major human consequences—after congenital anomalies, it is the greatest cause of neonatal morbidity and mortality (Chap. 36, p. 804). Spontaneous preterm labor with intact fetal membranes is the most common cause of preterm delivery and accounts for about half of preterm births. In another quarter, preterm premature rupture of the membranes is almost always followed by preterm delivery. Many factors increase the likelihood of preterm delivery. Some of these are genetics, infection, nutrition, behavior, and the environment (Fig. 6-24).

Genetic Influence on Preterm Birth

Analogous to other complex disease processes, multiple coexistent genetic alterations and environment may lead to preterm birth (Esplin and Varner, 2005; Ward, 2008). There are polymorphisms

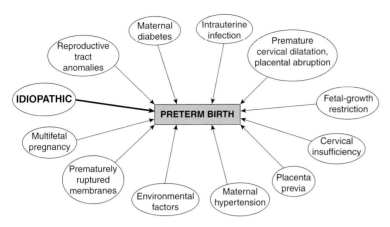

FIGURE 6-24 Risks for preterm birth. Approximately 50 percent of preterm births are idiopathic.

in genes associated with inflammation and infection and in those associated with collagen turnover (Velez and colleagues, 2008). Inherited mutations in genes regulating collagen assembly predispose individuals to cervical insufficiency or prematurely ruptured membranes (Anum, 2009; Wang, 2006; Warren, 2007, and all their associates).

Preterm Prematurely Ruptured Membranes (PPROM)

This term defines spontaneous rupture of the fetal membranes before 37 completed weeks and *before labor onset* (American College of Obstetricians and Gynecologists, 2007). Such rupture likely has a variety of causes, but many believe intrauterine infection to be a major predisposing event (Gomez and colleagues, 1997; Mercer, 2003).

Some studies suggest that the pathogenesis of preterm rupture relates to increased apoptosis of membranes' cellular components and to increased levels of specific proteases in membranes and amnionic fluid. Much of the membranes' tensile strength is provided by the extracellular matrix within the amnion. Interstitial amnionic collagens, primarily types I and III, are produced in mesenchymal cells and are the structural component most important for its strength (Casey and MacDonald, 1996). For that reason, collagen degradation has been a focus of research.

The matrix metalloproteinase (MMP) family is involved with normal tissue remodeling and particularly with collagen degradation. The MMP-2, MMP-3, and MMP-9 members of this family are found in higher concentrations in amnionic fluid from pregnancies with PPROM (Park and colleagues, 2003; Romero and associates, 2002). The activity of MMPs is in part regulated by tissue inhibitors of matrix metalloproteinases (TIMPs). Several of these inhibitors are found in lower concentrations in amnionic fluid from women with PPROM. Elevated MMP levels found at a time when protease inhibitor expression decreases supports further that their expression alters amnionic tensile strength. Studies of amniochorion explants have demonstrated that the expression of MMPs can be increased by treatment with IL-1, TNF-α, and IL-6 (Fortunato and colleagues, 1999a,b, 2002). Thus, MMP induction may be part of an in-

flammatory process. Proteins involved in the synthesis of mature cross-linked collagen or matrix proteins that bind collagen and promote tensile strength have also been found to be altered in PPROM (Wang and associates, 2006).

In pregnancies with PPROM, the amnion exhibits a higher degree of cell death than that in the term amnion (Arechavaleta-Velasco and colleagues, 2002; Fortunato and Menon, 2003). Markers of apoptosis with PPROM also show increased levels compared with those of term membranes. In vitro studies indicate that apoptosis is likely regulated by bacterial endotoxin IL-1β and TNF-α. Taken together, these observations suggest that many cases of PPROM result from activation of collagen degradation, alterations in collagen assembly, and cell death all leading to a weakened amnion.

A number of studies have been done to ascertain the incidence of infection-induced PPROM. Bacterial cultures of amnionic fluid support a role for infection in a significant proportion. A review of 18 studies comprised of almost 1500 women with PPROM found that in a third, bacteria were isolated from amnionic fluid (Goncalves and co-workers, 2002). Because of these findings, some have given prophylactic antimicrobial treatment to prevent PPROM. Although results are conflicting, there is evidence that early treatment of selected asymptomatic lower genital tract infections and active periodontal inflammation will reduce the incidence of PPROM and preterm birth (Chap. 36, p. 812).

Thus, there is compelling evidence that infection causes a significant proportion of PPROM cases. The inflammatory response that leads to membrane weakening is currently being defined. Research is focused on mediators of this process with a goal of identification of early markers for women at risk for PPROM.

Spontaneous Preterm Labor

Pregnancies with intact fetal membranes and spontaneous preterm labor—for clinical as well as research purposes—must be distinguished from those complicated by PPROM. Even so, pregnancies complicated by spontaneous preterm labor do not constitute a homogeneous group characterized singularly by early initiation of parturition. Among the more common associated findings are multifetal pregnancy, intrauterine infection, bleeding, placental infarction, premature cervical dilatation, cervical incompetence, uterine fundal abnormalities, and fetal anomalies. Severe maternal illness as a result of nonobstetrical infections, autoimmune diseases, and gestational hypertension also increases the risks for preterm labor. Taken together, these disorders cause about half of spontaneous preterm deliveries, and their relative contribution varies between populations.

Although there are unique aspects to each cause of preterm labor, recent studies have suggested that they share certain common denominators. Thus, fetal or maternal conditions provide important clues. It seems important to reemphasize that the actual process of preterm labor should be considered a final step—one that results from premature uterine activation that was initiated weeks before the onset of labor. Indeed, many forms of spontaneous preterm labor that result from premature initiation of phase 2 of parturition may be viewed in this light. Although the end result in preterm birth is the same as at term, namely cervical ripening and myometrial activation, recent studies question the idea that preterm birth is simply acceleration of the normal process. Identification of both common and uncommon factors has begun to explain the physiological processes of human parturition at term and preterm. Three major causes of spontaneous preterm labor include uterine distension, maternal–fetal stress, and infection.

Uterine Distension

There is no doubt that multifetal pregnancy and hydramnios lead to an increased risk of preterm birth (Chap. 39, p. 869). It is likely that early uterine distension acts to initiate expression of contraction-associated proteins (CAPs) in the myometrium. The CAP genes influenced by stretch include those coding for gap junction proteins such as connexin 43, for oxytocin receptors, and for prostaglandin synthase (Korita, 2002; Lyall, 2002; Sooranna, 2004, all their colleagues). Thus, excessive uterine stretch causes premature loss of myometrial quiescence.

Uterine stretch also leads to early activation of the placental-fetal endocrine cascade shown in Figure 6-17. The resulting early rise in maternal CRH and estrogen levels can further enhance the expression of myometrial CAP genes (Warren and co-workers, 1990; Wolfe and colleagues, 1988).

Finally, the influence of uterine stretch should be considered with regard to the cervix. For example, cervical length is an important risk factor for preterm birth in multifetal pregnancies (Goldenberg and co-workers, 1996). Prematurely increased stretch and endocrine activity may initiate events that shift the timing of uterine activation, including premature cervical ripening.

Maternal-Fetal Stress

The complexities of measuring "stress" lead to difficulty in defining its exact role (Lobel, 1994). That said, considerable evidence shows a correlation between some sort of maternal stress and preterm birth (Hedegaard, 1993; Hobel, 2003; Ruiz, 2003; Zambrana, 1999, and all their co-workers). Moreover, there is a correlation between maternal psychological stress and the placental–adrenal endocrine axis that provides a potential mechanism for stress-induced preterm birth (Lockwood, 1999; Wadhwa and associates, 2001).

As discussed earlier, the last trimester is marked by rising maternal serum levels of placental-derived CRH. This hormone works with ACTH to increase adult and fetal adrenal steroid hormone production, including the initiation of fetal cortisol biosynthesis. Rising levels of maternal and fetal cortisol further increase placental CRH secretion, which develops a feed-forward endocrine cascade that does not end until delivery (see Fig. 6-19). Rising levels of CRH further stimulate fetal adrenal DHEA-S biosynthesis, which acts as substrate to increase maternal plasma estrogens, particularly estriol.

It has been hypothesized that a premature rise in cortisol and estrogens results in an early loss of uterine quiescence. Supporting this hypothesis are numerous studies indicating that spontaneous preterm labor is associated with an early rise in maternal CRH levels (Holzman, 2001; McGrath, 2002; Moawad, 2002,

and all their co-workers). Levels of CRH in term and preterm women are similar. However, women destined for preterm labor exhibit a rise in CRH levels 2 to 6 weeks earlier (McLean and co-workers, 1995). This has been described as early as 18 weeks' gestation, leading some to suggest that CRH determination may provide a useful marker for preterm delivery. Because of large variations in CRH levels among pregnant women, however, a single CRH measurement has low sensitivity (Leung and colleagues, 2001; McGrath and associates, 2002). It may be that the *rate of increase* in maternal CRH levels may be a more accurate predictor of preterm birth. Confounding factors include CRH variability among ethnic groups. Another is that placental CRH enters the fetal circulation—albeit at lower levels than in the maternal circulation. In vitro studies have shown that CRH can directly stimulate fetal adrenal production of DHEA-S and cortisol (Parker and colleagues, 1999; Smith and co-workers, 1998).

If preterm delivery is associated with early activation of the fetal adrenal-placental endocrine cascade, maternal estrogen levels would likely be prematurely elevated. This is true, and an early rise of serum estriol concentrations is noted in women with subsequent preterm labor (Heine and co-workers, 2000; McGregor and associates, 1995). Physiologically, this premature rise in estrogens may alter myometrial quiescence.

Taken together, these observations suggest that preterm birth is associated, in many cases, with a maternal-fetal biological stress response. The nature and variety of the stressors that activate this cascade likely are broad. For example, CRH or estriol levels are prematurely elevated in preterm birth due to infection and multifetal pregnancies (Gravett and colleagues, 2000; Warren and co-workers, 1990). Thus, activation of this axis may be considered a common feature for initiation of phase 1 of parturition.

Infection and Preterm Labor

There is great interest in the role of infection as a primary cause of preterm labor in pregnancies with intact membranes. Many cases of preterm labor may result from intrauterine infection. This concept has been promoted because of widespread suspicion that subclinical infection is a common accompaniment and cause of preterm labor. The term "subclinical" has been used to describe infection that is accompanied by little or no clinical evidence of infection (Goncalves and co-workers, 2002; Iams and colleagues, 1987).

Certainly microorganisms are not recovered from the amnionic fluid in all women with preterm labor, In fact, the incidence of positive cultures varies from 10 to 40 percent and averages 15 percent (Goncalves and co-workers, 2002). Importantly, these women were more likely to develop clinical chorioamnionitis and preterm PROM than women with sterile cultures. Their neonates are also more likely to have complications (Hitti and co-workers, 2001). Although more severe when intra-amniotic infection is detected, intra-amniotic inflammation in the absence of detectable microorganisms is also a risk factor for the development of a fetal inflammatory response (Lee and associates, 2007, 2008). The earlier the onset of preterm labor, the greater is the likelihood of documented amnionic fluid infection (Goldenberg and associates, 2000; Watts and colleagues, 1992). At the same time, however, the incidence of culture-positive amnionic fluids collected by amniocentesis during spontaneous term labor is similar or even greater than it is during preterm labor (Gomez and colleagues, 1994; Romero and co-workers, 1993). It has been suggested that at term, amnionic fluid is infiltrated by bacteria as a consequence of labor, whereas in preterm pregnancies, bacteria represent an important cause of labor. Although plausible, this explanation questions the contribution of fetal infection as a major contributor to preterm birth.

Certainly, there are considerable data that associate chorioamnionitis with preterm labor (Goldenberg and associates, 2002; Üstün and colleagues, 2001). In such infections, the microbes may invade maternal tissue only and not amnionic fluid. Despite this, endotoxins can stimulate amnionic cells to secrete cytokines that enter amnionic fluid. This scenario may serve to explain the apparently contradictory observations concerning an association between amnionic fluid cytokines and preterm labor, in which microbes were not detectable in the amnionic fluid.

Sources for Intrauterine Infection. The patency of the female reproductive tract, although essential for achievement of

pregnancy and delivery, is theoretically problematic during phase 1 of parturition. It has been suggested that bacteria can gain access to intrauterine tissues through: (1) transplacental transfer of maternal systemic infection, (2) retrograde flow of infection into the peritoneal cavity via the fallopian tubes, or (3) ascending infection with bacteria from the vagina and cervix. The lower pole of the fetal membrane–decidual junction is contiguous with the orifice of the cervical canal, which in turn is patent to the vagina. This anatomical arrangement provides a passageway for microorganisms, and ascending infection is considered to be the most common. A thoughtful description of the potential degrees of intrauterine infection has been provided by Goncalves and co-workers (2002). They categorize intrauterine infection into four stages of microbial invasion that include bacterial vaginosis—stage I, decidual infection—stage II, amnionic infection—stage III, and finally, fetal systemic infection—stage IV. As expected, progression of these stages is thought to increase the effects on preterm birth and neonatal morbidity.

Based on these insights, it is straightforward to construct a theory for the pathogenesis of infection-induced preterm labor (Fig. 6-25). Ascending microorganisms colonize the decidua and possibly the membranes, where they then may enter

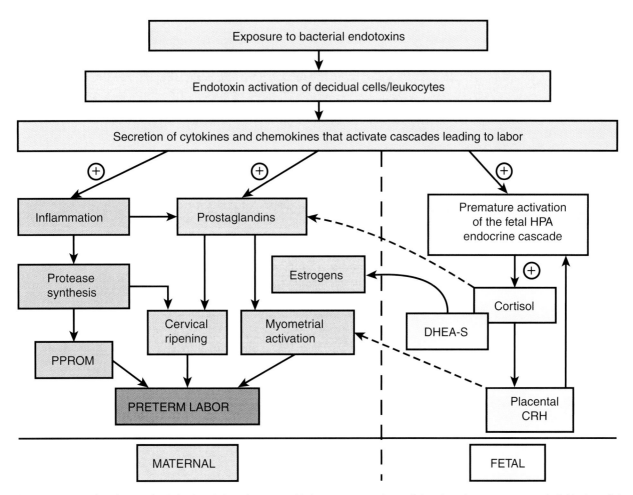

FIGURE 6-25 Potential pathways for infection-induced preterm birth. Exposure to bacterial endotoxins causes an early initiation of the normal processes associated with parturition, including cervical ripening, loss of uterine quiescence, and increased production of uterotonins. (CRH = corticotropin-releasing hormone; DHEA-S =dehydroepiandrosterone sulfate; HPA = hypothalamic–pituitary–adrenal; PPROM = preterm prematurely ruptured membranes.)

the amnionic sac. Lipopolysaccharide or other toxins elaborated by bacteria induce cytokine production in cells within the decidua, membranes, or fetus itself. Both lipopolysaccharide and cytokines then provoke prostaglandin release from the membranes, the decidua, or both. These influence both cervical ripening and loss of myometrial quiescence (Challis, 2002; Keelan, 2003; Loudon, 2003; Olson, 2003; and all their associates).

Microbes Associated with Preterm Birth. Some microorganisms—examples include *Gardnerella vaginalis, Fusobacterium, Mycoplasma hominis,* and *Ureaplasma urealyticum*—are detected more commonly than others in amnionic fluid of women with preterm labor (Gerber, 2003; Hillier, 1988; Romero, 1989; Yoon, 1998, and all their co-workers). This finding was interpreted by some as presumptive evidence that specific microorganisms are more commonly involved as pathogens in the induction of preterm labor. Another interpretation, however, is that given direct access to the membranes after cervical dilatation, selected microorganisms, such as fusobacteria, that are more capable of burrowing through these exposed tissues will do so. Fusobacteria are found in the vaginal fluid of only 9 percent of women but in 28 percent of positive amnionic fluid cultures from preterm labor pregnancies with intact membranes (Chaim and Mazor, 1992). Further studies are needed to better define these interactions.

Intrauterine Inflammatory Response to Infection. The initial inflammatory response elicited by bacterial toxins is mediated, in large measure, by specific receptors on mononuclear phagocytes, decidual cells, and trophoblasts. These *toll-like receptors* represent a family of receptors that has evolved to recognize pathogen-associated molecules (Janssens and Beyaert, 2003). Toll-like receptors are present in the placenta on trophoblast cells as well as on fixed and invading leukocytes (Chuang and Ulevitch, 2000; Gonzalez and colleagues, 2007; Holmlund and co-workers, 2002). Under the influence of ligands such as bacterial lipopolysaccharide, these receptors increase release of chemokines, cytokines, and prostaglandins as part of an inflammatory response. One example is IL-1β, which is produced rapidly after lipopolysaccharide stimulation (Dinarello, 2002). This cytokine in turn acts to promote a series of responses that include: (1) increased synthesis of others, that is, TNF-α, IL-6, and IL-8; (2) proliferation, activation, and migration of leukocytes; (3) modifications in extracellular matrix proteins; and (4) mitogenic and cytotoxic effects such as fever and acute phase response (El-Bastawissi and colleagues, 2000). Also, IL-1 promotes prostaglandin formation in many tissues, including myometrium, decidua, and amnion (Casey and co-workers, 1990). Thus, there appears to be a cascade of events once an inflammatory response is initiated that can result in preterm labor.

Origin of Cytokines in Intrauterine Infection. Cytokines within the normal term uterus are likely important for normal and preterm labor. The transfer of cytokines such as IL-1 from decidua across the membranes into amnionic fluid appears to be severely limited. Thus, it is likely that cytokines produced in maternal decidua and myometrium will have effects on that side, whereas cytokines produced in the membranes or in cells within the amnionic fluid will not be transferred to maternal tissues. In most cases of inflammation resulting from infection, resident and invading leukocytes produce the bulk of cytokines. Indeed, leukocytes—mainly neutrophils, macrophages, and T lymphocytes—infiltrate the cervix, lower uterine segment, and fundus at the time of labor. It was also shown that with preterm labor, leukocytes invade both membranes and cervix. Thus, invading leukocytes may be the major source of cytokines at the time of labor. Along with proinflammatory cytokines recent studies in women and animal models highlight the importance of the anti-inflammatory limb of the immune response in the parturition process (Gotsch and colleagues, 2008; Timmons and co-workers, 2009).

Immunohistochemical studies have shown in the term laboring uterus that both invading leukocytes and certain parenchymal cells produce cytokines. These leukocytes appear to be the primary source of myometrial cytokines, including IL-1, IL-6, IL-8, and TNF-α (Young and co-workers, 2002). By contrast, in the decidua, both stromal cells and leukocytes are likely to contribute because they have been shown to produce these same cytokines. In the cervix, glandular and surface epithelial cells appear to produce IL-6, IL-8, and TNF-α. Of these, IL-8 is considered a critical cytokine in cervical dilation, and it is produced in both cervical epithelial and stromal cells.

The presence of cytokines in amnionic fluid and their association with preterm labor has been well documented. But their exact cellular origin—with or without culturable microorganisms—has not been well defined. Although the rate of IL-1 secretion from forebag decidual tissue is great, Kent and colleagues (1994) found that there is negligible in vivo transfer of radiolabeled IL-1 across the membranes. Amnionic fluid IL-1 probably does not arise from amnion tissue, fetal urine, or fetal lung secretions. It most likely is secreted by mononuclear phagocytes or neutrophils activated and recruited into the amnionic fluid. Therefore, IL-1 in amnionic fluid likely is generated in situ from newly recruited cells. This scenario is supported by immunohistochemical studies (Young and co-workers, 2002). Thus, the amount of amnionic fluid IL-1 would be determined by the number of leukocytes recruited, their activational status, or the effect of amnionic fluid constituents on their rate of IL-1 secretion.

Leukocyte infiltration may be regulated by fetal membrane synthesis of specific chemokines. In term labor, there are increased amnionic fluid concentrations of the potent chemoattractant and monocyte-macrophage activator, *monocyte chemotactic protein-1 (MCP-1)*. As is true for prostaglandins and other cytokines, the levels of MCP-1 are much higher in the forebag compared with the upper compartment (Esplin and co-workers, 2003). Levels in preterm labor were significantly higher than those found in normal term amnionic fluid (Jacobsson and colleagues, 2003). It has been proposed that MCP-1 may be the factor that initiates fetal leukocyte infiltration of the placenta and membranes. In addition, the production of MCP-1 may act as a marker for intra-amnionic infection and inflammation.

Summary of Preterm Labor

Preterm labor is a pathological condition with multiple etiologies and has recently been termed the *preterm parturition syndrome* (Romero and associates, 2006). Most research in this field has been focused on the role of infection in mediating preterm birth. It is possible that intrauterine infection causes some cases currently categorized as idiopathic spontaneous preterm labor. There are a variety of sites for intrauterine infection—maternal, fetal, or both—and increasing evidence that the inflammatory response may have distinct and compartment-specific functions that differ between uterus, fetal membranes, and cervix in normal birth. Thus, determining the proportion of pregnancies that end prematurely because of infection is difficult. That said, it is clear that infection does not explain all causes of preterm birth.

In recent years, our understanding of other influences on the parturition process such as maternal nutrition before or during pregnancy, genetics, and dynamic regulation of changes in the extracellular matrix have led to new avenues of research and a broader understanding of this complicated and multifactorial process. The current and future application of genomic and bioinformatics as well as molecular and biochemical studies will shed light on pathways involved in term and preterm labor and identify processes critical to all phases of cervical remodeling and uterine function.

REFERENCES

American College of Obstetricians and Gynecologists: Premature rupture of membranes. Practice Bulletin No. 80, April 2007

Ameye L, Young MF: Mice deficient in small leucine-rich proteoglycans: Novel *in vivo* models for osteoporosis, osteoarthritis, Ehlers-Danlos syndrome, muscular dystrophy, and corneal diseases. Glycobiology 12:107R, 2002

Ambrus G, Rao Ch V: Novel regulation of pregnant human myometrial smooth muscle cell gap junctions by human chorionic gonadotropin. Endocrinology 135:2772, 1994

Anderson ABM, Turnbull AC: Comparative aspects of factors involved in the onset of labor in ovine and human pregnancy. In Klopper A, Gardner J (eds): Endocrine Factors in Labour. London, Cambridge University Press, 1973, p 141

Anderson J, Brown N, Mahendroo MS, et al: Utilization of different aquaporin water channels in the mouse cervix during pregnancy and parturition and in the models of preterm and delayed cervical ripening. Endocrinology 147:130, 2006

Andersson S, Minjarez D, Yost NP, et al: Estrogen and progesterone metabolism in the cervix during pregnancy and parturition. J Clin Endocrinol Metab 93(6):2366, 2008

Anum EA, Hill LD, Pandya A, et al: Connective tissue and related disorders and preterm birth: clues to genes contributing to prematurity. Placenta 30(3):207, 2009

Arechavaleta-Velasco F, Mayon-Gonzalez J, Gonzalez-Jimenez M, et al: Association of type II apoptosis and 92-kDa type IV collagenase expression in human amniochorion in prematurely ruptured membranes with tumor necrosis factor receptor-1 expression. J Soc Gynecol Investig 9:60, 2002

Bates GW, Edman CD, Porter JC, et al: Catechol-*O*-methyltransferase activity in erythrocytes of women taking oral contraceptive steroids. Am J Obstet Gynecol 133:691, 1979

Benedetto MT, DeCicco F, Rossiello F, et al: Oxytocin receptor in human fetal membranes at term and during delivery. J Steroid Biochem 35:205, 1990

Benedetto C, Petraglia F, Marozio L, et al: Corticotropin-releasing hormone increases prostaglandin-F$_{2\alpha}$ activity on human myometrium in vitro. Am J Obstet Gynecol 171:126, 1994

Berkane N, Verstraete L, Uzan S, et al: Use of mifepristone to ripen the cervix and induce labor in term pregnancies. Am J Obstet Gynecol 192:114, 2005

Berkowitz GS, Lapinski RH, Lockwood CJ, et al: Corticotropin-releasing factor and its binding protein: Maternal serum levels in term and preterm deliveries. Am J Obstet Gynecol 174:1477, 1996

Bethin KE, Nagai Y, Sladek R, et al: Microarray analysis of uterine gene expression in mouse and human pregnancy. Mol Endocrinol 17:1454, 2003

Blanks AM, Vatish M, Allen MJ, et al: Paracrine oxytocin and estradiol demonstrate a spatial increase in human intrauterine tissues with labor. J Clin Endocrinol Metab 88:3392, 2003

Bogacki M, Silvia WJ, Rekawiecki R, et al: Direct inhibitory effect of progesterone on oxytocin-induced secretion of prostaglandin F (2alpha) from bovine endometrial tissue. Biol Reprod 67:184, 2002

Bogic LV, Mandel M, Bryant-Greenwood GD: Relaxin gene expression in human reproductive tissues by in situ hybridization. J Clin Endocrinol Metab 80:130, 1995

Bokström H, Brännström M, Alexandersson M, et al: Leukocyte subpopulations in the human uterine cervical stroma at early and term pregnancy. Hum Reprod 12:586, 1997

Brainard AM, Miller AJ, Martens JR, et al: Maxi-K channels localize to caveolae in human myometrium: A role for an actin–channel–caveolin complex in the regulation of myometrial smooth muscle K$^+$ current. Am J Physiol Cell Physiol 289:C49, 2005

Buhimschi IA, Dussably L, Buhimschi CS, et al: Physical and biomechanical characteristics of rat cervical ripening are not consistent with increased collagenase activity. Am J Obstet Gynecol 191:1695, 2004

Burghardt RC, Mitchell PA, Kurten RC: Gap junction modulation in rat uterus, II. Effects of antiestrogens on myometrial and serosal cells. Biol Reprod 30:249, 1984

Bygdeman M, Swahn ML, Gemzell-Danielsson K, et al: The use of progesterone antagonists in combination with prostaglandin for termination of pregnancy. Hum Reprod 9:121, 1994

Canty EG, Kadler KE: Procollagen trafficking, processing and fibrillogenesis. Cell Sci 118:1341, 2005

Casey ML, MacDonald PC: Biomolecular processes in the initiation of parturition: Decidual activation. Clin Obstet Gynecol 31:533, 1988a

Casey ML, MacDonald PC: The role of a fetal–maternal paracrine system in the maintenance of pregnancy and the initiation of parturition. In Jones CT (ed): Fetal and Neonatal Development. Ithaca, NY, Perinatology, 1988b, p 521

Casey ML, MacDonald PC: Biomolecular mechanisms in human parturition: Activation of uterine decidua. In d'Arcangues C, Fraser IS, Newton JR, Odlind V (eds): Contraception and Mechanisms of Endometrial Bleeding. Cambridge, England, Cambridge University Press, 1990, p 501

Casey ML, MacDonald PC: Human parturition: Distinction between the initiation of parturition and the onset of labor. In Ducsay CA (ed): Seminars in Reproductive Endocrinology. New York, Thieme, 1993, p 272

Casey ML, MacDonald PC: Human parturition. In Bruner JP (ed): Infertility and Reproductive Medicine Clinics of North America. Philadelphia, Saunders, 1994, p 765

Casey ML, MacDonald PC: Transforming growth factor-beta inhibits progesterone-induced enkephalinase expression in human endometrial stromal cells. J Clin Endocrinol Metab 81:4022, 1996

Casey ML, MacDonald PC: The endocrinology of human parturition. Ann N Y Acad Sci 828:273, 1997

Casey ML, Cox SM, Word RA, et al: Cytokines and infection-induced preterm labour. Reprod Fertil Devel 2:499, 1990

Casey ML, Hemsell DL, MacDonald PC, et al: NAD$^+$-dependent 15-hydroxyprostaglandin dehydrogenase activity in human endometrium. Prostaglandins 19:115, 1980

Chaim W, Mazor M: Intraamniotic infection with fusobacteria. Arch Gynecol Obstet 251:1, 1992

Challis JR, Sloboda DM, Alfaidy N, et al: Prostaglandins and mechanisms of preterm birth. Reproduction 124:1, 2002

Challis JR, Smith SK: Fetal endocrine signals and preterm labor. Biol Neonate 79:163, 2001

Challis JRG, Lye SJ: Parturition. In Knobil E, Neill JD (eds): The Physiology of Reproduction, 2nd ed, Vol II. New York, Raven, 1994, p 985

Challis JRG, Matthews SG, Gibb W, et al: Endocrine and paracrine regulation of birth at term and preterm. Endocr Rev 21:514, 2000

Chanrachakul B, Matharoo-Ball B, Turner A, et al: Immunolocalization and protein expression of the alpha subunit of the large-conductance calcium-activated potassium channel in human myometrium. Reproduction 126:43, 2003

Cheung PY, Walton JC, Tai HH, et al: Immunocytochemical distribution and localization of 15-hydroxyprostaglandin dehydrogenase in human fetal membranes, decidua, and placenta. Am J Obstet Gynecol 163:1445, 1990

Chibbar R, Miller FD, Mitchell BF: Synthesis of oxytocin in amnion, chorion, and decidua may influence the timing of human parturition. J Clin Invest 91:185, 1993

Chow L, Lye SJ: Expression of the gap junction protein connexin-43 is increased in the human myometrium toward term and with the onset of labor. Am J Obstet Gynecol 170:788, 1994

Chuang TH, Ulevitch RJ: Cloning and characterization of a sub-family of human toll-like receptors: hTLR7, hTLR8, and hTLR9. Eur Cytokine Netw 11:372, 2000

Chwalisz K: The use of progesterone antagonists for cervical ripening and as an adjunct to labour and delivery. Hum Reprod Suppl 1:131, 1994

Chwalisz K, Garfield RE: Antiprogestins in the induction of labor. Ann N Y Acad Sci 734:387, 1994

Coleman RA, Smith WL, Narumiya S: Eighth International Union of Pharmacology. Classification of prostanoid receptors: Properties, distribution, and structure of the receptor and their subtypes. Pharmacol Rev 46:205, 1994

Condon JC, Hardy DB, Kovaric K, et al: Up-regulation of the progesterone receptor (PR)-C isoform in laboring myometrium by activation of nuclear factor-kappaB may contribute to the onset of labor through inhibition of PR function. Mol Endocrinol 20:764, 2006

Condon JC, Jeyasuria P, Faust JM, et al: Surfactant protein secreted by the maturing mouse fetal lung acts as a hormone that signals the initiation of parturition. Proc Natl Acad Sci U S A 101:4978, 2004

Condon JC, Jeyasuria P, Faust JM, et al: A decline in the levels of progesterone receptor coactivators in the pregnant uterus at term may antagonize progesterone receptor function and contribute to the initiation of parturition. Proc Natl Acad Sci U S A 100:9518, 2003

Cox BE, Ipson MA, Shaul PW, et al: Myometrial angiotensin II receptor subtypes change during ovine pregnancy. J Clin Invest 92:2240, 1993

Danforth DN, Veis A, Breen M, et al: The effect of pregnancy and labor on the human cervix: Changes in collagen, glycoproteins, and glycosaminoglycans. Am J Obstet Gynecol 120:641, 1974

Danielson KG, Baribault H, Holmes DF, et al: Targeted disruption of decorin leads to abnormal collagen fibril morphology and skin fragility. J Cell Biol 136(3):729, 1997

Dinarello CA: The IL-1 family and inflammatory diseases. Clin Exp Rheumatol 20:S1, 2002

Döring B, Shynlova O, Tsui P, et al: Ablation of connexin43 in uterine smooth muscle cells of the mouse causes delayed parturition. J Cell Sci 119:1715, 2006

Drewes PG, Yanagisawa H, Starcher B, et al: Pelvic organ prolapse in fibulin-5 knockout mice: Pregnancy-induced changes in elastic fiber homeostasis in mouse vagina. Am J Pathol 170:578, 2007

Eis AW, Mitchell MD, Myatt L: Endothelin transfer and endothelin effects on water transfer in human fetal membranes. Obstet Gynecol 79:411, 1992

El-Bastawissi AY, Williams MA, Riley DE, et al: Amniotic fluid interleukin-6 and preterm delivery: A review. Obstet Gynecol 95:1056, 2000

Esplin MS, Romero R, Chaiworapongsa T, et al: Amniotic fluid levels of immunoreactive monocyte chemotactic protein-1 increase during term parturition. J Matern Fetal Neonatal Med 14:51, 2003

Esplin MS, Varner MW: Genetic factors in preterm birth—the future. BJOG 112 Suppl 1:97, 2005

Eta E, Ambrus G, Rao CV: Direct regulation of human myometrial contractions by human chorionic gonadotropin. J Clin Endocrinol Metab 79:1582, 1994

Falkenberg ER, Davis RO, DuBard M, et al: Effects of maternal infections on fetal adrenal steroid production. Endocr Res 25:239, 1999

Feng S, Bogatcheva NV, Kamat AA, et al: Genetic targeting of relaxin and Ins13 signaling in mice. Ann N Y Acad Sci 1041:82, 2005

Ferguson JKW: A study of the motility of the intact uterus at term. Surg Gynecol Obstet 73:359, 1941

Fisk NM, Ronderos-Dumit D, Tannirandorn Y, et al: Normal amniotic pressure throughout gestation. Br J Obstet Gynaecol 99:18, 1992

Fonseca EB, Celik E, Para M, et al: Progesterone and the risk of preterm birth among women with a short cervix. N Engl J Med 357:462, 2007

Fortunato SJ, Menon R: IL-1 beta is a better inducer of apoptosis in human fetal membranes than IL-6. Placenta 24:922, 2003

Fortunato SJ, Menon R, Lombardi SJ: MMP/TIMP imbalance in amniotic fluid during PROM: An indirect support for endogenous pathway to membrane rupture. J Perinat Med 27:362, 1999a

Fortunato SJ, Menon R, Lombardi SJ: Stromelysins in placental membranes and amniotic fluid with premature rupture of membranes. Obstet Gynecol 94:435, 1999b

Fortunato SJ, Menon R, Lombardi SJ: Role of tumor necrosis factor-alpha in the premature rupture of membranes and preterm labor pathways. Am J Obstet Gynecol 187:1159, 2002

Friedman EA: Labor: Clinical Evaluation and Management, 2nd ed. New York, Appleton-Century-Crofts, 1978

Frim DM, Emanuel RL, Robinson BG, et al: J Clin Invest 82:287, 1988

Fuchs AR, Fuchs F, Husslein P, et al: Oxytocin receptors and human parturition. A dual role for oxytocin in the initiation of labor. Science 215:1396, 1982

Fuchs AR, Fuchs F, Husslein P, et al: Oxytocin receptors in the human uterus during pregnancy and parturition. Am J Obstet Gynecol 150:734, 1984

Fuchs AR, Husslein P, Fuchs F: Oxytocin and the initiation of human parturition, 2. Stimulation of prostaglandin production in human decidua by oxytocin. Am J Obstet Gynecol 141:694, 1981

Fuchs AR, Periyasamy S, Alexandrova M, et al: Correlation between oxytocin receptor concentration and responsiveness to oxytocin in pregnant rat myometrium: Effect of ovarian steroids. Endocrinology 113:742, 1983

Gainer H, Alstein M, Whitnall MH, et al: The biosynthesis and secretion of oxytocin and vasopressin. In Knobil E, Neill J (eds): The Physiology of Reproduction, Vol II. New York, Raven, 1988, p 2265

Gardner MO, Goldenberg RL, Cliver SP, et al: The origin and outcome of preterm twin pregnancies. Obstet Gynecol 85:553, 1995

Gerber S, Vial Y, Hohlfeld P, et al: Detection of Ureaplasma urealyticum in second-trimester amniotic fluid by polymerase chain reaction correlates with subsequent preterm labor and delivery. J Infect Dis 187:518, 2003

Germain A, Smith J, MacDonald PC, et al: Human fetal membrane contribution to the prevention of parturition: Uterotonin degradation. J Clin Endocrinol Metab 78:463, 1994

Goland RS, Jozak S, Conwell I: Placental corticotropin-releasing hormone and the hypercortisolism of pregnancy. Am J Obstet Gynecol 171:1287, 1994

Goland RS, Jozak S, Warren WB, et al: Elevated levels of umbilical cord plasma corticotropin-releasing hormone in growth-retarded fetuses. J Clin Endocrinol Metab 77:1174, 1993

Goland RS, Wardlaw SL, Stark RI, et al: High levels of corticotropin-releasing hormone immunoactivity in maternal and fetal plasma during pregnancy. J Clin Endocrinol Metab 63:1199, 1986

Goldenberg RL, Andrews WW, Hauth JC: Choriodecidual infection and preterm birth. Nutr Rev 60:S19, 2002

Goldenberg RL, Hauth JC, Andrews WW: Intrauterine infection and preterm delivery. N Engl J Med 342:1500, 2000

Goldenberg RL, Iams JD, Miodovnik M, et al: The preterm prediction study: Risk factors in twin gestations. National Institute of Child Health and Human Development Maternal-Fetal Medicine Units Network. Am J Obstet Gynecol 175:1047, 1996

Gomez R, Romero R, Edwin SS, et al: Pathogenesis of preterm labor and preterm premature rupture of membranes associated with intraamniotic infection. Infect Dis Clin North Am 11:135, 1997

Gomez R, Romero R, Glasasso M, et al: The value of amniotic fluid interleukin-6, white blood cell count, and gram stain in the diagnosis of microbial invasion of the amniotic cavity in patients at term. Am J Reprod Immunol 32:200, 1994

Goncalves LF, Chaiworapongsa T, Romero R: Intrauterine infection and prematurity. Ment Retard Dev Disabil Res Rev 8:3, 2002

Gonzalez JM, Xu H, Ofori E, et al: Toll-like receptors in the uterus, cervix, and placenta: Is pregnancy an immunosuppressed state? Am J Obstet Gynecol 197(3):296, 2007

Gotsch F, Romero R, Kusanovic JP, et al: The anti-inflammatory limb of the immune response in preterm labor, intra-amniotic infection/.inflammation, and spontaneous parturition at term: a role for interleukin-10. J Matern Fetal Neonatal Med 21(8):529, 2008

Grammatopoulos D, Milton NGN, Hillhouse EW: The human myometrial CRH receptor: G proteins and second messengers. Mol Cell Endocrinol 99:245, 1994

Grammatopoulos D, Thompson S, Hillhouse EW: The human myometrium expresses multiple isoforms of the corticotropin-releasing hormone receptor. J Clin Endocrinol Metab 80:2388, 1995

Grammatopoulos DK, Dai Y, Randeva HS, et al: A novel spliced variant of the type 1 corticotropin-releasing hormone receptor with a deletion in the seventh transmembrane domain present in the human pregnant term myometrium and fetal membranes. Mol Endocrinol 13:2189, 1999

Granström L, Ekman G, Ulmsten U, et al: Changes in the connective tissue of corpus uteri during ripening and labour in term pregnancy. Br J Obstet Gynaecol 96:1198, 1989

Gravett MG, Hitti J, Hess DL, et al: Intrauterine infection and preterm delivery: Evidence for activation of the fetal hypothalamic-pituitary-adrenal axis. Am J Obstet Gynecol 182:1404, 2000

Grino M, Chrousos GP, Margioris AN: The corticotropin releasing hormone gene is expressed in human placenta. Biochem Biophys Res Commun 148:1208, 1987

Haluska GJ, Wells TR, Hirst JJ, et al: Progesterone receptor localization and isoforms in myometrium, decidua, and fetal membranes from rhesus macaques: Evidence for functional progesterone withdrawal at parturition. J Soc Gynecol Invest 9:125, 2002

Halvorson LM: Reproductive Endocrinology. In Schorge JO, Schaffer JI, Halvorsen LM, et al (eds): Williams Gynecology, New York, McGraw-Hill, 2008

Hassan SS, Romero R, Haddad R, et al: The transcriptome of the uterine cervix before and after spontaneous term parturition. Am J Obstet Gynecol 195:778, 2006

Havelock J, Keller P, Muleba N, et al: Human myometrial gene expression before and during parturition. Biol Reprod 72:707, 2005

Hedegaard M, Henriksen TB, Sabroe S, et al: Psychological distress in pregnancy and preterm delivery. BMJ 307:234, 1993

Hegar A: Diagnose der frühesten Schwangersschaftsperiode. Deutsche Medizinische Wochenschrift 21:565, 1895

Heine RP, McGregor JA, Goodwin TM, et al: Serial salivary estriol to detect an increased risk of preterm birth. Obstet Gynecol 96:490, 2000

Hermanns-Lê T, Piérard G, Quatresooz P: Ehlers-Danlos-like dermal abnormalities in women with recurrent preterm premature rupture of fetal membranes. Am J Dermatopathol 27, 407, 2005

Hibbard JU, Tart M, Moawad AH: Cervical length at 16-22 weeks' gestation and risk for preterm delivery. Obstet Gynecol 96:972, 2000

Hillhouse EW, Grammatopoulos D, Milton NGN, et al: The identification of a human myometrial corticotropin-releasing hormone receptor that increases in affinity during pregnancy. J Clin Endocrinol Metab 76:736, 1993

Hillier SL, Martius J, Krohn M, et al: A case-control study of chorioamnionic infection and histologic chorioamnionitis in prematurity. N Engl J Med 319:972, 1988

Hitti J, Tarczy-Hornoch P, Murphy J, et al: Amniotic fluid infection, cytokines, and adverse outcome among infants at 34 weeks' gestation or less. Obstet Gynecol 98:1080, 2001

Hobel C, Culhane J: Role of psychosocial and nutritional stress on poor pregnancy outcome. J Nutr 133:1709S, 2003

Holmlund U, Cabers G, Dahlfors AR, et al: Expression and regulation of the pattern recognition receptors Toll-like receptor-2 and Toll-like receptor-4 in the human placenta. Immunology 107:145, 2002

Holzman C, Jetton J, Siler-Khodr T, et al: Second trimester corticotropin-releasing hormone levels in relation to preterm delivery and ethnicity. Obstet Gynecol 97:657, 2001

Iams JD, Clapp DH, Contox DA, et al: Does extraamniotic infection cause preterm labor? Gas-liquid chromatography studies of amniotic fluid in amnionitis, preterm labor, and normal controls. Obstet Gynecol 70:365, 1987

Iams JD, Goldenberg RL, Meis PJ, et al: The length of the cervix and the risk of spontaneous premature delivery. N Engl J Med 334:567, 1996

Itoh H, Sagawa N, Hasegawa M, et al: Brain natriuretic peptide is present in the human amniotic fluid and is secreted from amnion cells. J Clin Endocrinol Metab 76:907, 1993

Itoh H, Sagawa N, Hasegawa M, et al: Expression of biologically active receptors for natriuretic peptides in the human uterus during pregnancy. Biochem Biophys Res Commun 203:602, 1994

Izumi H, Yallampalli C, Garfield RE: Gestational changes in L-arginine-induced relaxation of pregnant rat and human myometrial smooth muscle. Am J Obstet Gynecol 169:1327, 1993

Jacobsson B, Holst RM, Wennerholm UR, et al: Monocyte chemotactic protein-1 in cervical and amniotic fluid: Relationship to microbial invasion of the amniotic cavity, intraamniotic inflammation, and preterm delivery. Am J Obstet Gynecol 189:1161, 2003

Janssens S, Beyaert R: Role of Toll-like receptors in pathogen recognition. Clin Microbiol Rev 16:637, 2003

Johnson RF, Mitchell CM, Giles WB, et al: The in vivo control of prostaglandin H synthase-2 messenger ribonucleic acid expression in the human amnion at parturition. J Clin Endocrinol Metab 87:2816, 2002

Jones SA, Brooks AN, Challis JR: Steroids modulate corticotropin-releasing hormone production in human fetal membranes and placenta. J Clin Endocrinol Metab 68:825, 1989

Karalis K, Goodwin G, Majzoub JA: Cortisol blockade of progesterone: A possible molecular mechanism involved in the initiation of human labor. Nat Med 2:556, 1996

Karteris E, Zervou S, Pang Y, et al: Progesterone signaling in human myometrium through two novel membrane G protein-coupled receptors: Potential role in functional progesterone withdrawal at term. Mol Endocrinol 20:1519, 2006

Keelan JA, Blumenstein M, Helliwell RJ, et al: Cytokines, prostaglandins and parturition—a review. Placenta 24:S33, 2003

Keirse MJNC: Prostaglandins in parturition. In Keirse M, Anderson A, Gravenhorst J (eds): Human Parturition. The Hague, Netherlands, Martinus Nijhoff, 1979, p 101

Kelly RW: Inflammatory mediators and cervical ripening. J Reprod Immunol 57:217, 2002

Kemp B, Menon R, Fortunato SJ, et al: Quantitation and localization of inflammatory cytokines interleukin-6 and interleukin-8 in the lower uterine segment during cervical dilatation. J Asst Reprod Genet 19:215, 2002

Kent AS, Sullivan MH, Elder MG: Transfer of cytokines through human fetal membranes. J Reprod Fertil 100:81, 1994

Kim CJ, Kim JS, Kim YM, et al: Fetal macrophages are not present in the myometrium of women with labor at term. Am J Obstet Gynecol 195:829, 2006

Kimura T, Ivell R, Rust W, et al: Molecular cloning of a human MafF homologue, which specifically binds to the oxytocin receptor gene in term myometrium. Biochem Biophys Res Commun 264:86, 1999

Kimura T, Takemura M, Nomura S, et al: Expression of oxytocin receptor in human pregnant myometrium. Endocrinology 137:780, 1996

Kokenyesi R, Armstrong LC, Agah A, et al: Thrombospondin 2 deficiency in pregnant mice results in premature softening of the uterine cervix. Biol Reprod 70:385, 2004

Korita D, Sagawa N, Itoh H, et al: Cyclic mechanical stretch augments prostacyclin production in cultured human uterine myometrial cells from pregnant women: Possible involvement of up-regulation of prostacyclin synthase expression. J Clin Endocrinol Metab 87:5209, 2002

Leake RD: Oxytocin in the initiation of labor. In Carsten ME, Miller JD (eds): Uterine Function. Molecular and Cellular Aspects. New York, Plenum, 1990, p 361

Lee SE, Romero R, Jung H: The intensity of the fetal inflammatory response in intraamniotic inflammation with and without microbial invasion of the amniotic cavity. Am J Obstet Gynecol 197(3):294, 2007

Lee SE, Romero R, Park CW: The frequency and significance of intraamniotic inflammation in patients with cervical insufficiency. Am J Obstet Gynecol 198(6):633, 2008

Lei ZM, Reshef E, Rao CV: The expression of human chorionic gonadotropin/luteinizing hormone receptors in human endometrial and myometrial blood vessels. J Clin Endocrinol Metab 75:651, 1992

Leong AS, Norman JE, Smith R: Vascular and myometrial changes in the human uterus at term. Reprod Sci 15:59, 2008

Leppert PC: Anatomy and physiology of cervical ripening. Clin Obstet Gynecol 38:267, 1995

Leung TN, Chung TK, Madsen G, et al: Rate of rise in maternal plasma corticotrophin-releasing hormone and its relation to gestational length. BJOG 108:527, 2001

Liggins GC: Ripening of the cervix. Semin Perinatol 2:261, 1978

Liggins GC, Fairclough RJ, Grieves SA, et al: The mechanism of initiation of parturition in the ewe. Recent Prog Horm Res 29:111, 1973

Liggins GC, Kennedy PC, Holm LW: Failure of initiation of parturition after electrocoagulation of the pituitary of the fetal lamb. Am J Obstet Gynecol 98:1080, 1967

Lim AT, Gude NM: Atrial natriuretic factor production by the human placenta. J Clin Endocrinol Metab 80:3091, 1995

Lobel M: Conceptualizations, measurement, and effects of prenatal maternal stress on birth outcomes. J Behav Med 17:225, 1994

Lockwood CJ: Stress-associated preterm delivery: The role of corticotropin-releasing hormone. Am J Obstet Gynecol 180:S264, 1999

Lopez BA, Newman GE, Phizackerley PJ, et al: Surfactant stimulates prostaglandin E production in human amnion. Br J Obstet Gynaecol 95:1013, 1988

Loudon JA, Groom KM, Bennett PR: Prostaglandin inhibitors in preterm labour. Best Pract Res Clin Obstet Gynaecol 17:731, 2003

Lowder JL, Debes KM, Moon DK, et al: Biomechanical adaptations of the rat vagina and supportive tissues in pregnancy to accommodate delivery. Obstet Gynecol 109:136, 2007

Lowry PJ: Corticotropin-releasing factor and its binding protein in human plasma. Ciba Found Symp 172:108, 1993

Lyall F, Lye S, Teoh T, et al: Expression of Gsalpha, connexin-43, connexin-26, and EP1, 3, and 4 receptors in myometrium of prelabor singleton versus multiple gestations and the effects of mechanical stretch and steroids on Gsalpha. J Soc Gynecol Investi 9:299, 2002

MacDonald PC, Casey ML: The accumulation of prostaglandins (PG) in amniotic fluid is an aftereffect of labor and not indicative of a role for PGE2 and PGE2 alpha in the initiation of human parturition. J Clin Endocrinol Metab 76:1332, 1993

MacDonald PC, Casey ML: Preterm birth. Sci Am 3:42, 1996

MacDonald PC, Koga S, Casey ML: Decidual activation in parturition: Examination of amniotic fluid for mediators of the inflammatory response. Ann N Y Acad Sci 622:315, 1991

Mackenzie R, Walker M, Armson A, et al: Progesterone for the prevention of preterm birth among women at increased risk: A systematic review and meta-analysis of randomized controlled trials. Am J Obstet Gynecol 194:1234, 2006

Macphee DJ, Lye SJ: Focal adhesion signaling in the rat myometrium is abruptly terminated with the onset of labor. Endocrinology 141:274, 2000

Madsen G, Zakar T, Ku CY, et al: Prostaglandins differentially modulate progesterone receptor-A and -B expression in human myometrial cells: Evidence for prostaglandin-induced functional progesterone withdrawal. J Clin Endocrinol Metab 89:1010, 2004

Mahendroo MS, Porter A, Russell DW, et al: The parturition defect in steroid 5alpha-reductase type 1 knockout mice is due to impaired cervical ripening. Mol Endocrinol 13:981, 1999

Malpas P: Postmaturity and malformation of the fetus. J Obstet Gynaecol Br Emp 40:1046, 1933

Many A, Lazebhnik N, Hill LM: The underlying cause of polyhydramnios determines prematurity. Prenat Diagn 16:55, 1996

Marinoni E, Korebrits C, Di Iorio R, et al: Effect of betamethasone in vivo on placental corticotropin-releasing hormone in human pregnancy. Am J Obstet Gynecol 178:770, 1998

Markovic D, Vatish M, Gu M, et al: The onset of labor alters corticotropin-releasing hormone type 1 receptor variant expression in human myometrium: Putative role of interleukin-1beta. Endocrinology 148:3205, 2007

Massrieh W, Derjuga A, Doualla-Bell F, et al: Regulation of the MAFF transcription factor by proinflammatory cytokines in mymetrial cells. Biol Reprod 74:699, 2006

McGrath S, McLean M, Smith D, et al: Maternal plasma corticotropin-releasing hormone trajectories vary depending on the cause of preterm delivery. Am J Obstet Gynecol 186:257, 2002

McGrath S, Smith R: Prediction of preterm delivery using plasma corticotrophin-releasing hormone and other biochemical variables. Ann Med 34:28, 2002

McGregor JA, Jackson GM, Lachelin GC, et al: Salivary estriol as risk assessment for preterm labor: A prospective trial. Am J Obstet Gynecol 173:1337, 1995

McLean M, Bisits A, Davies J, et al: A placental clock controlling the length of human pregnancy. Nat Med 1:460, 1995

Meis PJ, Klebanoff M, Thom E, et al: Prevention of recurrent preterm delivery by 17 alpha-hydroxyprogesterone caproate. N Engl J Med 348:2379, 2003

Mendelson CR: Minireview: Fetal-maternal hormonal signaling in pregnancy and labor. Mol Endocrinol 23(7):947, 2009

Mercer BM: Preterm premature rupture of the membranes. Obstet Gynecol 101:178, 2003

Mesiano S, Chan EC, Fitter JT, et al: Progesterone withdrawal and estrogen activation in human parturition are coordinated by progesterone receptor A expression in the myometrium. J Clin Endocrinol Metab 87:2924, 2002

Moawad AH, Goldenberg RL, Mercer B, et al: The Preterm Prediction Study: The value of serum alkaline phosphatase, alpha-fetoprotein, plasma corticotropin-releasing hormone, and other serum markers for the prediction of spontaneous preterm birth. Am J Obstet Gynecol 186:990, 2002

Murphy BE: Human fetal serum cortisol levels related to gestational age: Evidence of a midgestational fall and a steep late gestational rise independent of sex or mode of delivery. Am J Obstet Gynecol 144:276, 1982

Myatt L, Lye SJ: Expression, localization and function of prostaglandin receptors in myometrium. Prostaglandins Leukot Essent Fatty Acids 70:137, 2004

Myers KM, Paskaleva AP, House M, et al: Mechanical and biochemical properties of human cervical tissue. Acta Biomaterialia 4:104, 2008

Nishihira J, Ishibashi T, Mai Y, et al: Mass spectrometric evidence for the presence of platelet-activating factor (1-0-alkyl-2-sn-glycero-3-phosphocholine) in human amniotic fluid during labor. Lipids 19:907, 1984

Nissen E, Lilja G, Widstrom A-M, et al: Elevation of oxytocin levels early post partum in women. Acta Obstet Gynecol Scand 74:530, 1995

Novy MJ, Liggins GC: Role of prostaglandin, prostacyclin, and thromboxanes in the physiologic control of the uterus and in parturition. Semin Perinatol 4:45, 1980

Olson DM, Ammann C: Role of the prostaglandins in labour and prostaglandin receptor inhibitors in the prevention of preterm labour. Front Biosci 12:1329, 2007

Olson DM, Zaragoza DB, Shallow MC: Myometrial activation and preterm labour: Evidence supporting a role for the prostaglandin F receptor—a review. Placenta 24:S47, 2003

Osman I, Young A, Ledingham MA, et al: Leukocyte density and pro-inflammatory cytokine expression in human fetal membranes, decidua, cervix and myometrium before and during labour at term. Mol Hum Reprod 9:41, 2003

Osmers R, Rath W, Pflanz MA, et al: Glycosaminoglycans in cervical connective tissue during pregnancy and parturition. Obstet Gynecol 81:88, 1993

Ou CW, Chen ZQ, Qi S, et al: Increased expression of the rat myometrial oxytocin receptor messenger ribonucleic acid during labor requires both mechanical and hormonal signals. Biol Reprod 59:1055, 1998

Ou CW, Orsino A, Lye SJ: Expression of connexin-43 and connexin-26 in the rat myometrium during pregnancy and labor is differentially regulated by mechanical and hormonal signals. Endocrinology 138:5398, 1997

Ozasa H, Tominaga T, Nishimura T, et al: Lysyl oxidase activity in the mouse uterine cervix is physiologically regulated by estrogen. Endocrinology 109:618, 1981

Park J-I, Chang CL, Hsu SY: New insights into biological roles of relaxin and relaxin-related peptides. Rev Endocrine & Metabol Dis 6:291, 2005

Park KH, Chaiworapongsa T, Kim YM, et al: Matrix metalloproteinase 3 in parturition, premature rupture of the membranes, and microbial invasion of the amniotic cavity. J Perinat Med 31:12, 2003

Parker CR Jr, Stankovic AM, Goland RS: Corticotropin-releasing hormone stimulates steroidogenesis in cultured human adrenal cells. Mol Cell Endocrinol 155:19, 1999

Parkington HC, Coleman HA: Excitability in uterine smooth muscle. Front Horm Res 27:179, 2001

Patel FA, Clifton VL, Chwalisz K, et al: Steroid regulation of prostaglandin dehydrogenase activity and expression in human term placenta and chorio-decidua in relation to labor. J Clin Endocrinol Metab 84:291, 1999

Paternoster DM, Santarossa C, Vettore N, et al: Obstetric complications in Marfan's syndrome pregnancy. Minerva Ginecol 50:441, 1998

Perkins AV, Wolfe CD, Eben F, et al: Corticotrophin-releasing hormone-binding protein in human fetal plasma. J Endocrinol 146:395, 1995

Petraglia F, Florio P, Benedetto C, et al: High levels of corticotropin-releasing factor (CRF) are inversely correlated with low levels of maternal CRF-binding protein in pregnant women with pregnancy-induced hypertension. J Clin Endocrinol Metab 81:852, 1996

Petraglia F, Florio P, Simoncini T, et al: Cord plasma corticotropin-releasing factor-binding protein (CRF-BP) in term and preterm labour. Placenta 18:115, 1997

Pieber D, Allport VC, Hills F, et al: Interactions between progesterone receptor isoforms in myometrial cells in human labour. Mol Hum Reprod 7:875, 2001

Piekorz RP, Gingras S, Hoffmeyer A, et al: Regulation of progesterone levels during pregnancy and parturition by signal transducer and activator of transcription 5 and 20α-hydroxysteroid dehydrogenase. Molecul Endocrinol 19:431, 2005

Pierce SL, Kresowik JD, Lamping KG, et al: Overexpression of SK3 channels dampens uterine contractility to prevent preterm labor in mice. Biol Reprod 78:1058, 2008

Prescott SM, Zimmerman GA, McIntyre TM: Platelet activating factor. J Biol Chem 265:17381, 1990

Price SA, Pochun I, Phaneuf S, et al: Adenylyl cyclase isoforms in pregnant and nonpregnant human myometrium. J Endocrinol 164:21, 2000

Quartero HWP, Noort WA, Fry CH, et al: Role of prostaglandins and leukotrienes in the synergistic effect of oxytocin and corticotropin-releasing hormone (CRH) on the contraction force in human gestational myometrium. Prostaglandins 42:137, 1991

Quartero HWP, Strivatsa G, Gillham B: Role for cyclic adenosine monophosphate in the synergistic interaction between oxytocin and corticotrophin-releasing factor in isolated human gestational myometrium. Clin Endocrinol 36:141, 1992

Quitterer U, Lother H, Abdalla S: AT1 receptor heterodimers and angiotensin II responsiveness in preeclampsia. Semin Nephrol 24(2):115, 2004

Rahman J, Rahman FZ, Rahman W, et al: Obstetric and gynecologic complications in women with Marfan syndrome. J Reprod Med 48:723, 2003

Rahn DD, Ruff MD, Brown SA, et al: Biomechanical properties of the vaginal wall: Effect of pregnancy, elastic fiber deficiency, and pelvic organ prolapse. Am J Obstet Gynecol 198:590.e1, 2008

Rea C: Prolonged gestation, acrania, monstrosity and apparent placenta praevia in one obstetrical case. JAMA 30:1166, 1898

Read CP, Word RA, Ruscheinsky MA, et al: Cervical remodeling during pregnancy and parturition: Molecular characterization of the softening phase in mice. Reproduction 134:327, 2007

Romero R, Chaiworapongsa T, Espinoza J, et al: Fetal plasma MMP-9 concentrations are elevated in preterm premature rupture of the membranes. Am J Obstet Gynecol 187:1125, 2002

Romero R, Durum S, Dinarello CA, et al: Interleukin-1 stimulates prostaglandin biosynthesis by human amnion. Prostaglandins 37:13, 1989

Romero R, Espinoza J, Kusanovic JP, et al: The preterm parturition syndrome. BJOG 3:17, 2006

Romero R, Nores J, Mazor M, et al: Microbial invasion of the amniotic cavity during term labor. Prevalence and clinical significance. J Reprod Med 38:543, 1993

Rouse DJ, Caritis SN, Peaceman AM, et al: A trial of 17 alpha-hydroxyprogesterone caproate to prevent prematurity in twins. N Engl J Med 357:454, 2007

Ruiz RJ, Fullerton J, Dudley DJ: The interrelationship of maternal stress, endocrine factors and inflammation on gestational length. Obstet Gynecol Surv 58:415, 2003

Ruscheinsky M, De la Motte C, Mahendroo M: Hyaluronan and its binding proteins during cervical ripening and parturition: Dynamic changes in size, distribution and temporal sequence. Matrix Biol, March 17, 2008

Sáez JC, Retamal MA, Basilio D, et al: Connexin-based gap junction hemichannels: Gating mechanisms. Biochim Biophys Acta 1711:215, 2005

Saijonmaa O, Laatikainen T, Wahlstrom T: Corticotrophin-releasing factor in human placenta: Localization, concentration and release in vitro. Placenta 9:373, 1988

Sakamoto Y, Moran P, Bulmer JN, et al: Macrophages and not granulocytes are involved in cervical ripening. J Reprod Immunol 66(2):161, 2005

Sakamoto Y, Moran P, Searle RF, et al: Interleukin-8 is involved in cervical dilatation but not in prelabour cervical ripening. Clin Exp Immunol 138:151, 2004

Samuel CS, Royce SG, Chen B, et al: Relaxin family peptide receptor-1 protects against airway fibrosis during homeostasis but not against fibrosis associated with chronic allergic airways disease. Endocrinology 150(3):1495, 2009

Sanborn BM, Yue C, Wang W, et al: G-protein signaling pathways in myometrium: Affecting the balance between contraction and relaxation. Rev Reprod 3:196, 1998

Sasaki A, Shinkawa O, Margioris AN, et al: Immunoreactive corticotropin-releasing hormone in human plasma during pregnancy, labor, and delivery. J Clin Endocrinol Metab 64:224, 1987

Sennström MB, Ekman G, Westergren-Thorsson G, et al: Human cervical ripening, an inflammatory process mediated by cytokines. Mol Hum Reprod 6:375, 2000

Schmitz T, Levine BA, Nathanielsz PW: Localization and steroid regulation of prostaglandin E2 receptor protein expression in ovine cervix. Reproduction 131:743, 2006

Shynlova O, Tsui P, Jaffer S, et al: Integration of endocrine and mechanical signals in the regulation of myometrial functions during pregnancy and labour. Eur J Obstet Gynecol Reprod Biol 144(Suppl 1):S2, 2009

Shynlova O, Williams SJ, Draper H, et al: Uterine stretch regulates temporal and spatial expression of fibronectin protein and its alpha 5 integrin receptor in myometrium of unilaterally pregnant rates. Biol Reprod 77:880, 2007

Smith GC, Wu WX, Nathanielsz PW: Effects of gestational age and labor on expression of prostanoid receptor genes in baboon uterus. Biol Reprod 64:1131, 2001

Smith R: Parturition. N Engl J Med 356:271, 2007

Smith R, Mesiano S, Chan EC, et al: Corticotropin-releasing hormone directly and preferentially stimulates dehydroepiandrosterone sulfate secretion by human fetal adrenal cortical cells. J Clin Endocrinol Metab 83:2916, 1998

Soloff MS, Alexandrova M, Fernström MJ: Oxytocin receptors: Triggers for parturition and lactation? Science 204:1313, 1979

Soloff MS, Fernström MA, Periyasamy S, et al: Regulation of oxytocin receptor concentration in rat uterine explants by estrogen and progesterone. Can J Biochem Cell Biol 61:625, 1983

Sooranna SR, Lee Y, Kim LU, et al: Mechanical stretch activates type 2 cyclooxygenase via activator protein-1 transcription factor in human myometrial cells. Mol Hum Reprod 10:109, 2004

Spallicci MD, Chiea MA, Singer JM, et al: Use of hyaluronidase for cervical ripening: a randomized trial. Eur J Obstet Gynecol 130(1):46, 2007

Stjernholm-Vladic Y, Wang H, Stygar D, et al: Differential regulation of the progesterone receptor A and B in the human uterine cervix at parturition. Gynecol Endocrinol 18:41, 2004

Straach KJ, Shelton JM, Richardson JA, et al: Regulation of hyaluronan expression during cervical ripening. Glycobiology 15:55, 2005

Stull JT, Taylor DA, MacKenzie LW, et al: Biochemistry and physiology of smooth muscle contractility. In McNellis D, Challis JRG, MacDonald PC, et al (eds): Cellular and integrative mechanisms in the onset of labor. An NICHD workshop. Ithaca, NY, Perinatology, 1988, p 17

Stull JT, Lin PJ, Krueger JK, et al: Myosin light chain kinase: Functional domains and structural motifs. Acta Physiol Scand 164:471, 1998

Telfer JF, Itoh H, Thomson AJ, et al: Activity and expression of soluble and particulate guanylate cyclases in myometrium from nonpregnant and pregnant women: Down-regulation of soluble guanylate cyclase at term. J Clin Endocrinol Metab 86(12):5934, 2001

Timmons BC, Fairhurst AM, Mahendroo MS: Temporal changes in myeloid cells in the cervix during pregnancy and parturition. J Immunol 182(5):2700, 2009

Timmons BC, Mahendroo M: Processes regulating cervical ripening differ from cervical dilation and postpartum repair: Insights from gene expression studies. Reprod Sci 14:53, 2007

Timmons BC, Mahendroo MS: Timing of neutrophil activation and expression of proinflammatory markers to do not support a role for neutrophils in cervical ripening in the mouse. Biol Reprod 74:236, 2006

Tong D, Lu X, Wang HS, et al: A dominant loss-of-function GJA1(Cx43) mutant impairs parturition in the mouse, Biol Reprod 80(6):1099, 2009

Toyoshima K, Narahara H, Furukawa M, et al: Platelet-activating factor. Role of fetal lung development and relationship to normal and premature labor. Clin Perinatol 22(2):263 1995

Üstün C, Kocak I, Baris S, et al: Subclinical chorioamnionitis as an etiologic factor in preterm deliveries. Int J Obstet Gynecol 72:109, 2001

Van Meir CA, Sangha RK, Walton JC, et al: Immunoreactive 15-hydroxyprostaglandin dehydrogenase (PGDH) is reduced in fetal membranes from patients at preterm delivery in the presence of infection. Placenta 17:291, 1996

Velez DR, Fortunato SJ, Williams SM, et al: Interleukin-6 (IL-6) and receptor (IL6-R) gene haplotypes associate with amniotic fluid protein concentrations in preterm birth. Hum Mol Genet 17:1619, 2008

Wadhwa PD, Culhane JF, Rauh V, et al: Stress and preterm birth: Neuroendocrine, immune/inflammatory, and vascular mechanisms. Matern Child Health J 5:119, 2001

Wadhwa PD, Porto M, Garite TJ, et al: Maternal corticotropin-releasing hormone levels in the early third trimester predict length of gestation in human pregnancy. Am J Obstet Gynecol 179:1079, 1998

Wang H, Parry S, Macones G, et al: A functional SNP in the promoter of the SERPINH1 gene increases risk of preterm premature rupture of membranes in African Americans. PNAS 103:13463, 2006

Ward K: Genetic factors in common obstetric disorders. Clin Obstet Gynecol 51:74, 2008

Warren JE, Silver RM, Dalton J, et al: Collagen 1A1 and transforming growth factor-β polymorphisms in women with cervical insufficiency. Obstet Gynecol 110:619, 2007

Warren WB, Goland RS, Wardlaw SL, et al: Elevated maternal plasma corticotropin releasing hormone levels in twin gestation. J Perinat Med 18:39, 1990

Wathes DC, Borwick SC, Timmons PM, et al: Oxytocin receptor expression in human term and preterm gestational tissues prior to and following the onset of labour. J Endocrinol 161:143, 1999

Watts DH, Krohn MA, Hillier SL, et al: The association of occult amniotic fluid infection with gestational age and neonatal outcome among women in preterm labor. Obstet Gynecol 79:351, 1992

Weiss G: Relaxin used to produce the cervical ripening of labor. Clin Obstet Gynecol 38:293, 1995

Westergren-Thorsson G, Norman M, Björnsson S, et al: Differential expressions of mRNA for proteoglycans, collagens and transforming growth factor-beta in the human cervix during pregnancy and involution. Biochim Biophys Acta 1406:203, 1998

Whittle WL, Patel FA, Alfaidy N, et al: Glucocorticoid regulation of human and ovine parturition: The relationship between fetal hypothalamic-pituitary-adrenal axis activation and intrauterine prostaglandin production. Biol Reprod 64:1019, 2001

Winters AJ, Oliver C, Colston C, et al: Plasma ACTH levels in the human fetus and neonate as related to age and parturition. J Clin Endocrinol Metab 39:269, 1974

Wira CR, Grant-Tschudy KS, Crane-Godreau MA: Epithelial cells in the female reproductive tract: A central role as sentinels of immune protection. AJRI 53:65, 2005

Wolf JP, Simon J, Itskovitz J, et al: Progesterone antagonist RU 486 accommodates but does not induce labour and delivery in primates. Hum Reprod 8:759, 1993

Wolfe CD, Patel SP, Linton EA, et al: Plasma corticotrophin-releasing factor (CRF) in abnormal pregnancy. Br J Obstet Gynaecol 95:1003, 1988

Woodcock NA, Taylor CW, Thornton S: Effect of an oxytocin receptor antagonist and rho kinase inhibitor on the $[Ca^{++}]_i$ sensitivity of human myometrium. Am J Obstet Gynecol 190:222, 2004

Word RA, Kamm KE, Stull JT, et al: Endothelin increases cytoplasmic calcium and myosin phosphorylation in human myometrium. Am J Obstet Gynecol 162:1103, 1990

Word RA, Landrum CP, Timmons BC, et al: Transgene insertion on mouse chromosome 6 impairs function of the uterine cervix and causes failure of parturition. Biol Reprod 73:1046, 2005

Word RA, Li XH, Hnat M, et al: Dynamics of cervical remodeling during pregnancy and parturition: mechanisms and current concepts. Semin Reprod Med, 25(1):69, 2007

Word RA, Stull JT, Casey ML, et al: Contractile elements and myosin light chain phosphorylation in myometrial tissue from nonpregnant and pregnant women. J Clin Invest 92:29, 1993

Wu WX, Ma XH, Smith GC, et al: Prostaglandin dehydrogenase mRNA in baboon intrauterine tissues in late gestation and spontaneous labor. Am J Physiol Regul Integr Comp Physiol 279:R1082, 2000

Yallampalli C, Byam-Smith M, Nelson SO, et al: Steroid hormones modulate the production of nitric oxide and cGMP in the rat uterus. Endocrinology 134:1971, 1994a

Yallampalli C, Izumi H, Byam-Smith M, et al: An L-arginine-nitric oxide-cyclic guanosine monophosphate system exists in the uterus and inhibits contractility during pregnancy. Am J Obstet Gynecol 170:175, 1994b

Yao L, Agoulnik AI, Cooke S, et al: Relaxin acts on stromal cells to promote epithelial and stromal proliferation and inhibit apoptosis in the mouse cervix and vagina. Endocrinology 149(5):2072, 2008

Yoon BH, Romero R, Park JS, et al: Microbial invasion of the amniotic cavity with *Ureaplasma urealyticum* is associated with robust host response in fetal, amniotic, and maternal compartments. Am J Obstet Gynecol 179:1254, 1998

Young A, Thomson AJ, Ledingham M, et al: Immunolocalization of proinflammatory cytokines in myometrium, cervix, and fetal membranes during human parturition at term. Biol Reprod 66:445, 2002

Yu JT, López Bernal A: The cytoskeleton of human myometrial cells. J Reprod Fertil 112:185, 1998

Yu SY, Tozzi A, Babiarz J, et al: Collagen changes in rat cervix in pregnancy—Polarized light microscopic and electron microscopic studies. P.S.E.B.M. 209:360, 1995

Zambrana RE, Dunkel-Schetter C, Collins NL, et al: Mediators of ethnic-associated differences in infant birth weight. J Urban Health 76:102, 1999

Zhang LM, Want YK, Hui N, et al: Corticotropin-releasing hormone acts on CRH-R1 to inhibit the spontaneous contractility of non-labouring human myometrium at term. Life Sci 83(17-18):620, 2008

Zhu YP, Word RA, Johnston JM: The presence of PAF binding sites in human myometrium and its role in uterine contraction. Am J Obstet Gynecol 166:1222, 1992

Ziecik AJ, Derecka-Reszka K, Rzucidlo SJ: Extragonadal gonadotropin receptors, their distribution and function. J Physiol Pharmacol 43:33, 1992

Zingg HH, Rozen F, Chu K, et al: Oxytocin and oxytocin receptor gene expression in the uterus. Recent Prog Horm Res 50:255, 1995

Zuo J, Lei ZM, Rao CV: Human myometrial chorionic gonadotropin/luteinizing hormone receptors in preterm and term deliveries. J Clin Endocrinol Metab 79:907, 1994

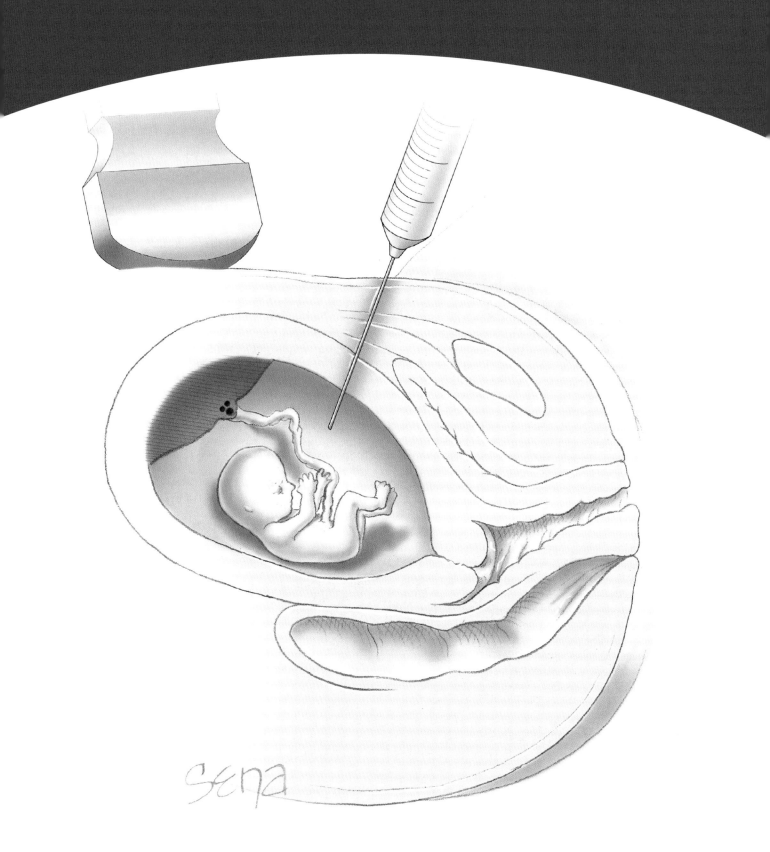

CHAPTER 7

Preconceptional Counseling

In 2006, the Centers for Disease Control and Prevention defined preconceptional care as "a set of interventions that aim to identify and modify biomedical, behavioral, and social risks to a woman's health or pregnancy outcome through prevention and management." In addition, it established the following goals for improving preconceptional care:

1. Improve knowledge, attitudes, and behaviors of men and women related to preconceptional health.
2. Assure that all women of childbearing age receive preconceptional care services—including evidence-based risk screening, health promotion, and interventions—that will enable them to enter pregnancy in optimal health.
3. Reduce risks indicated by a previous adverse pregnancy outcome through interconceptional interventions to prevent or minimize recurrent adverse outcomes.
4. Reduce the disparities in adverse pregnancy outcomes.

The American College of Obstetricians and Gynecologists (2005a) also has reinforced the importance of preconceptional and interpregnancy care. Moreover, recent data from the Centers for Disease Control and Prevention describe the health status of women who gave birth to live-born infants in the United States in 2004 (Table 7-1). This table demonstrates the high prevalence of many conditions that may be amenable to inter-vention during the preconceptional and interpregnancy periods (D'Angelo and associates, 2007).

BENEFITS OF PRECONCEPTIONAL COUNSELING

Randomized trials that evaluate preconceptional counseling efficacy are scarce, partly because withholding such counseling would be unethical. In addition, because maternal and perinatal outcomes are dependent on the interaction of various maternal, fetal, and environmental factors, it is often difficult to ascribe salutary outcomes to a specific intervention (Moos, 2004). That said, there are a few prospective and case-control studies that clearly demonstrate the successes of preconceptional counseling.

Unplanned Pregnancy

Counseling about potential pregnancy risks and preventative strategies must be provided before conception. By the time most women realize they are pregnant—1 to 2 weeks after the first missed period—the fetal spinal cord has already formed and the heart is beating. Thus, many prevention strategies, for example folic acid to prevent neural-tube defects, are ineffective if initiated at this time. It is estimated that up to half of all pregnancies are unplanned, and that these may be at greatest risk (American College of Obstetricians and Gynecologists, 2006; Finer and Henshaw, 2006). Women with unintended pregnancy are more likely to be young or single; have lower educational attainment; use tobacco, alcohol, or illicit drugs; and not supplement with folate (Cheng, 2009; Dott, 2009; Postlethwaite, 2009, and all their associates).

To assess the effectiveness of preconceptional counseling to reduce unintended pregnancies, Moos and colleagues (1996) studied the effects of a preconceptional care program instituted in a health department clinic. The 456 women given preconceptional counseling had a 50-percent greater likelihood of describing their subsequent pregnancies as intended compared

TABLE 7-1. Prevalence of Prepregnancy Maternal Behaviors, Experiences, Health Conditions, and Previous Poor Birth Outcomes in the United States in 2004

Factor	Prevalence (percent)
Tobacco use	23.2
Alcohol use	50.1
Multivitamin use	35.1
Contraceptive nonuse[a]	53.1
Dental visit	77.8
Health counseling	30.3
Physical abuse	3.6
Stress	18.5
Underweight	13.2
Overweight	13.1
Obesity	21.9
Diabetes	1.8
Asthma	6.9
Hypertension	2.2
Heart problem	1.2
Anemia	10.2
Prior low-birthweight infant	11.6
Prior preterm infant	11.9

[a]Among women who were not trying to become pregnant. Data from D'Angelo and associates (2007).

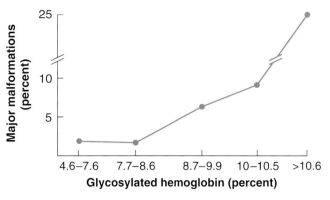

FIGURE 7-1. Relationship between first-trimester glycosylated hemoglobin values and risk for major congenital malformations in 320 women with insulin-dependent diabetes. (Data from Kitzmiller and associates, 1991.)

with 309 women with health care but no counseling, and a 65-percent greater likelihood compared with women with no healthcare prior to pregnancy. Family planning and contraception are discussed in Chapter 32.

CHRONIC MEDICAL DISORDERS

Diabetes Mellitus

Because maternal and fetal pathology associated with hyperglycemia is well known, diabetes is the prototype of a condition for which preconceptional counseling is beneficial. Diabetes-associated risks to both mother and fetus are discussed in detail in Chapter 52. Most important, many of these complications can be avoided if glucose control is optimized before conception. The American College of Obstetricians and Gynecologists (2005c) has concluded that preconceptional counseling for women with pregestational diabetes mellitus is both beneficial and cost-effective and should be encouraged.

Recommendations of the American Diabetes Association (2004) for the content of preconceptional care are listed in Table 7-2. Importantly, it advises that the preconceptional goal is to obtain the lowest hemoglobin A_{1c} level possible without undue risk of hypoglycemia in the mother. In addition to assessing diabetic control during the preceding 6 weeks, hemoglobin A_{1c} measurement can also be used to compute risks for major anomalies (Fig. 7-1). Although these data are from women with severe diabetes, the incidence of fetal anomalies in

women who have gestational diabetes and fasting hyperglycemia is increased fourfold compared with that in normal women (Sheffield and associates, 2002).

Efficacy of Counseling in Diabetic Women

Preconceptional counseling has been shown to decrease diabetes-related complications at all stages of pregnancy. For example, Leguizamón and colleagues (2007) identified 12 clinical studies comparing the incidence of major congenital anomalies in a combined total of 1618 women with insulin-dependent diabetes mellitus who received preconceptional care with a combined total of 1599 who did not. The rates of congenital anomalies in the two groups were 2.7 and 8.3 percent, respectively. Importantly, 10 of the 12 studies showed that preconceptional care is associated with significantly fewer malformations.

Dunne and co-workers (1999) reported that diabetic women who received counseling sought prenatal care earlier, had lower hemoglobin A_{1c} levels, and were less likely to smoke during pregnancy. Of the women who received counseling, none were delivered before 30 weeks compared with 17 percent in an uncounseled cohort. Finally, counseled women had fewer macrosomic infants—25 versus 40 percent; they had no growth-restricted infants compared with 8.5 percent; they had no neonatal deaths compared with 6 percent; and their infants had half as many admissions to the intensive care nursery—17 versus 34 percent. Similarly, Temple and associates (2006) found lower rates of adverse pregnancy outcome and preterm delivery in those receiving prepregnancy care.

It follows that preconceptional counseling reduces healthcare costs in diabetic women. Indeed, based upon their literature review, Reece and Homko (2007) found that for every dollar spent on a preconceptional care program for diabetic women between $1.86 and $5.19 was saved in direct medical costs averted. Surprisingly, despite such benefits, the proportion of diabetic women receiving preconceptional care remains low. In a study of approximately 300 women with diabetes enrolled in a managed-care plan, Kim and colleagues (2005) found that only about half reported receiving preconceptional counseling. Among the uninsured, the rates are undoubtedly even lower.

TABLE 7-2. American Diabetes Association Recommendations for the Preconceptional Care of Women with Diabetes

Medical and obstetrical history

- Duration and type of diabetes
- Acute complications, including history of infections, ketoacidosis, and hypoglycemia
- Chronic complications, including retinopathy, nephropathy, hypertension, atherosclerotic vascular disease, and neuropathy
- Diabetes management, including insulin regimen, use of glucose lowering agents, self-glucose monitoring regimens and results, nutrition, and physical activity
- Concomitant medical conditions
- Menstrual and pregnancy history, contraceptive use
- Support systems

Physical examination

- Blood pressure, including testing for orthostatic changes
- Retinal examination with pupillary dilatation
- Cardiovascular examination for evidence of cardiac or peripheral vascular disease—if present, screen for evidence of coronary artery disease
- Neurological examination

Laboratory evaluation

- Hemoglobin A_{1c}
- Serum creatinine
- Urine protein: protein excretion >190 mg/24 hours may increase the risk for hypertensive disorders during pregnancy (see Chap. 34, p. 719); protein excretion >400 mg/24 hours may increase the risk for fetal-growth restriction (see Chap. 38, p. 843).
- Thyroid function tests: 5- to 10-percent coincidence of type 1 diabetes and thyroid dysfunction (see Chap. 53, p. 1134).

Initial management plan

- Counseling
  - Risk and prevention of congenital anomalies
  - Fetal and neonatal complications of maternal diabetes (see Chap. 52, p. 1113)
  - Effects of pregnancy on maternal diabetic complications (see Chap. 52, p. 1116)
  - Risks of obstetrical complications that occur with increased frequency in diabetic pregnancies (see Chap. 52, p. 1113)
  - Need for effective contraception until glycemia is well controlled
- Insulin regimen selected to achieve the following goals:
  - Capillary plasma glucose before meals = 80–110 mg/dL
  - Capillary plasma glucose 2 hours after meals less than 155 mg/dL[a]
- Monitor hemoglobin A_{1c} levels at 1- to 2-month intervals until stable with the goal to achieve a concentration less than 1 percent above the normal range

[a] There are no data to suggest that postmeal glucose monitoring has a specific role in preconception diabetes care beyond what is needed to achieve the target hemoglobin A_{1c}. Thus, a focus on preprandial monitoring is recommended initially to assist patients in self-selection of insulin doses.
Copyright © 2004 American Diabetes Association. From Diabetes Care®, Vol. 27, 2004; S76-S78. Modified with permission from The American Diabetes Association.

Epilepsy

It is indisputable that women with epilepsy are two to three times more likely to have infants with structural anomalies than unaffected women (Wide and associates, 2004). Some reports indicate that epilepsy increases this risk, independent of the effects of antiseizure medication. This view is not held by all. Holmes and colleagues (2001) compared pregnancy outcomes in 509 epileptic women who took antiseizure medication with 606 who did not. They found that fetuses exposed to one drug had significantly fewer malformations than those exposed to two or more drugs—21 versus 28 percent. By contrast, the incidence of fetal defects of epileptic mothers who did not take medication was 8.5 percent—the same as in fetuses of women without seizure disorders.

Preconceptional counseling usually includes efforts to achieve control with monotherapy and with medications considered least teratogenic (Adab, 2004; Aguglia, 2009; Tomson, 2009, and all their associates). As shown in Table 7-3, some regimens used individually are less teratogenic than others. Results of a prospective registry, for example, indicate that the overall risk of major malformations associated with lamotrigine monotherapy is comparable with that of the general population. The risks of antiseizure medication are described in detail in Chapter 14 (p. 317). According to Jeha and Morris (2005), the American Academy of

TABLE 7-3. Antiepileptic Treatment Regimens and Their Association with Major Congenital Malformations

Regimen	Range of Major Congenital Malformations (percent)
Any antiepileptic drug	7.9
Lamotrigine monotherapy	2.1–2.9
Carbamazepine monotherapy	2.0–5.2
Phenobarbital monotherapy	4.7–6.5
Phenytoin monotherapy	3.4–10.5
Valproic acid monotherapy	8.6–16.7
Untreated	0.8–5.0
General population	1.6–2.2

Jeha LE and Morris HH. Optimizing outcomes in pregnant women with epilepsy. Cleve Clin J Med 2005; 72:938-945. Reprinted with permission. Copyright © 2005 Cleveland Clinic. All rights reserved.

Neurology recommends consideration for discontinuation of antiseizure medication in select women, including those who:

1. Have been seizure-free for 2 to 5 years
2. Have a single seizure type
3. Have a normal neurological examination and normal intelligence
4. Have an electroencephalogram that has normalized with treatment.

Epileptic women also are advised to take supplemental folic acid. Biale and Lewenthal (1984) performed a case-control study to evaluate effects of periconceptional folate supplementation in women taking anticonvulsants. Although 10 of 66 (15 percent) unsupplemented pregnancies resulted in offspring with congenital malformations, none of 33 neonates of supplemented women had anomalies. Similarly, in a case-control study using the Hungarian National Birth Registry, Kjær and colleagues (2008) concluded that risk of congenital abnormalities in fetuses exposed to carbamazepine, phenobarbital, phenytoin, and primidone is reduced—but not eliminated—by folic acid supplementation.

Vajda and colleagues (2008) recently reported results from the Australian Register of Antiepileptic Drugs in Pregnancy. They found that the risk of seizures during pregnancy was 50 to 70 percent less if the prepregnancy year was seizure free. Once one year without seizures had elapsed, there seemed to be relatively little further advantage in deferring pregnancy to avoid seizures during pregnancy.

Other Chronic Diseases

Cox and co-workers (1992) reviewed pregnancy outcomes of 1075 high-risk women who received preconceptional counseling. The 240 women with hypertension, renal disease, thyroid disease, asthma, or heart disease had significantly better outcomes than with their previous pregnancies. Indeed, 80 percent of those counseled were delivered of normal infants, compared with only 40 percent in the previous gestation which lacked prepregnancy counseling.

GENETIC DISEASES

The Centers for Disease Control and Prevention (2007) estimate that birth defects affect about one in every 33 babies born in the United States each year. Moreover, these defects are currently the leading cause of infant mortality and account for 20 percent of deaths. The benefits of preconceptional counseling usually are measured by comparing the incidence of new cases before and after initiation of a counseling program. Some examples of congenital conditions that clearly benefit from counseling include neural-tube defects, phenylketonuria, the thalassemias, Tay-Sachs, and other genetic diseases more common in individuals of Eastern European Jewish descent. Screening for heritable genetic diseases, including cystic fibrosis and fragile X syndrome, is further discussed in Chapter 13 (p. 297).

Neural-Tube Defects (NTDs)

The incidence of these defects is 1 to 2 per 1000 live births, and they are second only to cardiac anomalies as the most frequent structural fetal malformation (see Chap. 12, p. 281). Some NTDs, as well as congenital heart defects, are associated with a specific mutation in the methylene tetrahydrofolate reductase gene (677C → T). Adverse effects of this appear to be largely overcome by periconceptional folic acid supplementation (Ou and colleagues, 1996). Although its role is still controversial, low levels of vitamin B_{12} preconceptionally, similar to folate, may increase the risk of neural-tube defects (Molloy and co-workers, 2009; Thompson and colleagues, 2009).

The Medical Research Council on Vitamin Study Research Group (1991) conducted a randomized double-blind study of preconceptional folic acid therapy at 33 centers in seven European countries. Women with a previous affected child who took supplemental folic acid before conception and throughout the first trimester reduced their NTD recurrence risk by 72 percent. Perhaps more importantly, because 90 to 95 percent of infants with NTDs are born to women with no prior family history, Czeizel and Dudas (1992) showed that supplementation reduced the *a priori* risk of a *first* NTD occurrence.

Despite such benefit, in recent years, only 40 to 50 percent of women have taken folic acid supplementation during the periconceptional period (de Jong-van den Berg and co-workers, 2005; Goldberg and colleagues, 2006). The strongest predictor of use appears to be consultation with a health-care provider before conception. To improve supplementation, many countries fortify wheat and maize flour with folic acid to lower rates of NTDs (Bell and Oakley, 2008; Hamner and associates, 2009).

Phenylketonuria (PKU)

This inherited disorder of phenylalanine metabolism is an example of a disease in which the fetus is not at risk to inherit the disorder, but may be damaged by maternal disease. Specifically, individuals with PKU who eat an unrestricted diet have abnormally high blood phenylalanine levels. As discussed in Chapter 12 (p. 277), this amino acid readily crosses the placenta and can damage developing fetal organs, especially neural and cardiac tissues (Table 7-4). With appropriate preconceptional counseling and adherence to a phenylalanine-restricted diet before pregnancy,

TABLE 7-4. Frequency of Complications in the Offspring of Women with Untreated Phenylketonuria (Blood Phenylamine >1200 μmol/L)

Complication	Frequency in Affected Pregnancies (percent)
Spontaneous abortions	24
Mental retardation	92
Microcephaly	73
Congenital heart disease	12
Intrauterine growth restriction	40

Adapted with kind permission from Dr. François Maillot and Springer Science+Business Media: *Journal of Inherited Metabolic Disease*, A practical approach to maternal phenylketonuria management, Vol. 30, 2007, pp. 198–201, F Maillot, P Cook, M Lilburn, and PJ Lee, © SSIEM and Springer 2007.

the incidence of fetal malformations is dramatically reduced (Guttler, 1990; Hoeks, 2009; Koch, 1990, and all their associates).

The Maternal Phenylketonuria Collaborative Study confirmed the effectiveness of preconceptional care in almost 300 women with this disorder (Rouse and co-workers, 1997). Compared with infants whose mothers had poor dietary control, infants of those women with a low phenylalanine diet had a lower incidence of microcephaly—6 versus 15 percent, neurological abnormalities—4 versus 14 percent, and cardiac defects—none versus 16 percent. Similarly, Lee and colleagues (2005) found improved fetal birthweights, head circumferences, and intelligent quotient (IQ) scores in 110 newborns whose mothers began a phenylalanine-restricted diet before conception.

Thalassemias

These disorders of globin-chain synthesis are the most common single-gene disorders worldwide. As many as 200 million people carry a gene for one of these hemoglobinopathies, and hundreds of mutations are known to cause thalassemia syndromes (Chap. 51, p. 1090). In endemic areas such as Mediterranean and Southeast Asian countries, counseling and other prevention strategies have reduced the incidence of new cases by at least 80 percent (Angastiniotis and Modell, 1998). The American College of Obstetricians and Gynecologists (2007) recommends that individuals of such ancestry be offered carrier screening to allow them to make informed decisions regarding reproduction and prenatal diagnosis. Preimplantation genetic diagnosis of thalassemia is available for candidate patients (Chen and associates, 2008; Mohd Nasri and colleagues, 2009).

Experiences with a long-standing counseling program aimed at Montreal high school students at risk were summarized by Mitchell and colleagues (1996). During a 20-year period, 25,274 students of Mediterranean origin were counseled and tested for β-thalassemia. Within a few years of initiating the preconceptional program, all high-risk couples who requested prenatal diagnosis had already been counseled, and no affected children were born during those times.

Genetic Diseases More Prevalent in Individuals of Eastern European Jewish Descent

Most individuals of Jewish ancestry in North America are descended from Ashkenazi Jewish communities and are at an increased risk for having offspring with one of the autosomal recessive disorders listed in Table 7-5. The American College of Obstetricians and Gynecologists (2004) recommends preconceptional care for these women:

- The family history of individuals considering pregnancy—or who are already pregnant—should determine whether either member of the couple is of Eastern European (Ashkenazi) Jewish ancestry or has a relative with cystic fibrosis or a genetic condition listed in Table 7-5.
- Carrier screening for Tay-Sachs disease, Canavan disease, cystic fibrosis, and familial dysautonomia should be offered to Ashkenazi Jewish individuals before conception.
- Carrier screening is also available for mucolipidosis IV, Niemann-Pick disease type A, Fanconi anemia group C, Bloom syndrome, and Gaucher disease.
- When only one partner is of Ashkenazi Jewish descent, that individual should be screened first. If this individual is a carrier, the other partner is offered screening. The couple should be informed that the carrier frequency and detection rate in non-Jewish individuals is unknown for all of these disorders except Tay-Sachs disease and cystic fibrosis (see Table 7-5). Therefore, it is difficult to predict the couple's risk of having a child with the disorder.
- Individuals with a positive family history of one of these disorders should be offered carrier screening for the specific disorder and may benefit from genetic counseling (see Chap. 8, p. 200).
- When both partners are carriers of one of these disorders, they should be referred for genetic counseling and offered prenatal diagnosis.
- When an individual is found to be a carrier, he or she should be encouraged to inform relatives that they are at risk for carrying the same mutation.

Tay-Sachs Disease

The effectiveness of preconceptional counseling in reducing genetic disease has been most clearly demonstrated in Tay-Sachs disease. This disease is a severe, autosomal-recessive neurodegenerative disorder that leads to death in early childhood. In the early 1970s, there were approximately 60 new cases in the United States each year, primarily in individuals of Jewish heritage. An intensive worldwide campaign was initiated to counsel Jewish men and women of reproductive age to identify carriers through genetic testing, to provide prenatal testing for high-risk couples, and even to help heterozygote carriers choose unaffected mates. Within 8 years of the inception of this campaign, nearly 1 million young adults around the world had been tested and counseled. The incidence of new Tay-Sachs cases has plummeted to only approximately five new cases per year (Kaback and colleagues, 1993). Currently, most new cases are in the non-Jewish population.

TABLE 7-5. Clinical Features of Autosomal Recessive Genetic Diseases Frequent among Individuals of Eastern European Jewish Descent Amenable to Carrier Screening

Disorder	Disease Incidence	Carrier Frequency[a]	Detection Rate[a]	Description
Tay-Sachs disease	1/3000	1/30	Varies[b]	Caused by hexosaminidase A deficiency. Neurological motor and mental dysfunction with childhood death. No effective treatment
Canavan disease	1/6400	1/40	98%	Caused by aspartoacylase deficiency. Neurological disorder with developmental delay, hypotonia, large head, seizures, blindness, gastrointestinal reflux, and childhood death. No effective treatment
Cystic fibrosis	1/2500–3000	1/29	97%	See p. 178
Familial dysautonomia	1/3600	1/32	99%	Caused by mutations in IKBKAP gene. Neurological disorder with poor feeding, abnormal sweating, pain and temperature insensitivity, labile blood pressure, and scoliosis. No cure, but some treatments lengthen and improve quality of life
Fanconi anemia group C	1/32,000	1/89	99%	Usually caused by recessive mutation of any of several genes. Severe anemia, pancytopenia, developmental delay, failure to thrive, and later-childhood death. Congenital anomalies, microcephaly, and mental retardation may be present. Bone-marrow transplantation may be successful
Niemann-Pick disease type A	1/32,000	1/90	95%	Caused by sphingomyelinase deficiency. Neurodegenerative disorder with childhood death. No effective treatment
Mucolipidosis IV	1/62,500	1/127	95%	Neurodegenerative lysosomal storage disorder with growth failure, marked psychomotor retardation, and retinal degeneration. Life expectancy may be normal. There is no effective treatment
Bloom syndrome	1/40,000	1/100	95–97%	Increased chromosome breakage, susceptibility to infections and malignancies, growth deficiency, skin findings, and mental retardation. Death usually in 20s and related to cancer. No effective treatment
Gaucher disease (Type 1)	1/900	1/15	95%	Caused by β-glucosidase deficiency. Affects the spleen, liver, and bones. Develops at any age with a wide clinical spectrum including anemia, bruising and bleeding, hepatosplenomegaly, and osteoporosis. Enzyme therapy improves quality of life

[a]Non-Jewish carrier frequency and detection rates are unknown except for Tay-Sachs disease: 1 in 30 if French Canadian or Cajun ancestry and 1 in 300 for others, with a 98-percent carrier detection rate by Hex-A test.
[b]Detection is 98 percent by Hex-A test, 94 percent by DNA-based test.
Data from the American College of Obstetricians and Gynecologists (2004, 2005d) and the National Institute of Neurological Disorders and Stroke (2007a–d).

The American College of Obstetricians and Gynecologists (2005d) recommends the following regarding Tay-Sachs disease:

- Screening be offered before pregnancy if both members of a couple are of Ashkenazi Jewish, French-Canadian, or Cajun descent. Those with a family history consistent with Tay-Sachs disease should also be offered screening.

- When one member of a couple is at high risk as described above, but the other partner is not, the high-risk partner should be offered screening, especially if there is uncertainty about ancestry or if there is a consistent family history. If the high-risk partner is determined to be a carrier, the other partner also should be offered screening.

- Biochemical analysis by determining hexosaminidase A serum levels should be used for individuals in low-risk populations. Leukocyte testing must be used if the woman is already pregnant or taking oral contraceptives.
- Ambiguous or positive screening test results should be confirmed by biochemical and DNA analysis for the most common mutation. This will detect patients who carry genes associated with mild disease or pseudodeficiency states.
- If both partners are determined to be carriers of Tay-Sachs disease, genetic counseling and prenatal diagnosis should be offered.

PRECONCEPTIONAL COUNSELORS

Practitioners providing routine health maintenance have the best opportunity to provide preventive counseling. Gynecologists, internists, family practitioners, and pediatricians can do so at periodic health examinations. The occasion of a negative pregnancy test is an excellent time for counseling. Jack and associates (1995) administered a comprehensive preconceptional risk survey to 136 such women, and almost 95 percent reported at least one problem that could affect a future pregnancy. These included medical or reproductive problems—52 percent, family history of genetic diseases—50 percent, increased risk of human immunodeficiency virus (HIV)—30 percent, increased risk of hepatitis B and use of illegal substances—25 percent, alcohol use—17 percent, and nutritional risks—54 percent.

Basic advice regarding diet, alcohol and illicit drug use, smoking, vitamin intake, exercise, and other behaviors can be provided. Pertinent medical records should be reviewed. Counselors should be knowledgeable about relevant medical diseases, prior surgery, reproductive disorders, or genetic conditions, and must be able to interpret data and recommendations provided by other specialists. If the practitioner is uncomfortable providing counseling, the woman or couple should be referred to an appropriate counselor.

PRECONCEPTIONAL COUNSELING VISIT

Personal and Family History

A thorough review is taken of the medical, obstetrical, social, and family histories. Useful information is more likely to be obtained by asking specific questions about each history and about each family member than by asking general, open-ended questions. The interview may take 30 minutes to an hour. Some important information can be obtained by questionnaire, ideally at a routine prepregnancy visit. Prepared questionnaires are also available that address these topics. Answers are reviewed with the couple to ensure appropriate follow-up, including obtaining relevant medical records.

Medical History

Preconceptional counseling addresses all risk factors pertinent to mother and fetus. General points include how pregnancy will affect maternal health, and how a high-risk condition might affect the fetus. Finally, advice for improving outcome is provided. Almost any medical, obstetrical, or genetic condition warrants some consideration prior to pregnancy. These are discussed in

terms of general maternal and fetal risks, and suggestions for prepregnancy evaluation are offered. More detailed information on specific diseases is found in their relevant chapters.

Genetic Diseases

Women whose ethnic background, race, or personal or family history places them at increased risk to have a fetus with a genetic disease should receive appropriate counseling. This includes the possibility of prenatal diagnosis as discussed in Chapter 13. These women may require additional counseling visits to a trained genetic counselor. They also may benefit from consultation with other specialists, for example, anesthesiologists, cardiologists, or surgeons.

Reproductive History

Questions are asked regarding infertility; abnormal pregnancy outcomes, including miscarriage, ectopic pregnancy, and recurrent pregnancy loss; and obstetrical complications such as preeclampsia, placental abruption, and preterm delivery (Stubblefield and co-workers, 2008). Regarding this last complication, most studies to date have not disclosed significant benefits of proposed prophylactic regimens such as treatment of bacterial vaginosis or other interconceptional antimicrobial regimens to prevent spontaneous preterm birth (Andrews and colleagues, 2006; Allsworth and Peipert, 2007).

History of a prior stillborn infant is especially important. This was recently reviewed by Silver (2007).

When identified, specific complications can be managed as outlined in discussions of these topics, which are found in later chapters of this text.

Social History

Maternal Age

Women at both ends of the reproductive-age spectrum have unique outcomes that are considered.

Adolescent Pregnancy. According to the Centers for Disease Control and Prevention, 7.6 percent of births in 2002 in the United States were in women between the ages of 15 and 19 years. Although this represented a 9-percent decline since 2000, the adolescent pregnancy rate remains among the highest of all industrialized nations (Ventura and colleagues, 2006). Adolescents are more likely to be anemic, and they are at increased risk to have growth-restricted infants, preterm labor, and a higher infant mortality rate (Fraser and associates, 1995; Usta and co-workers, 2008). The incidence of sexually transmitted diseases—common in adolescents—is even higher during pregnancy (Niccolai and colleagues, 2003).

Because most of their pregnancies are unplanned, adolescents rarely seek preconceptional counseling. These young women usually are still growing and developing and thus have greater caloric requirements than older women. The normal or underweight adolescent should be advised to increase caloric intake by 400 kcal/day. Alternatively, as discussed in Chapter 43, the obese adolescent likely does not need additional calories. Nonjudgmental questioning may elicit a history of substance abuse.

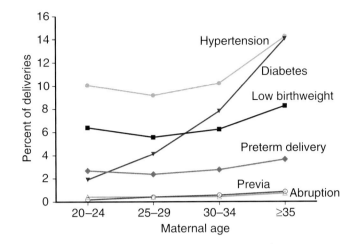

FIGURE 7-2. Incidence of selected pregnancy complications in relation to maternal age among 235,329 women delivered at Parkland Hospital, 1988–2007. (Used with permission from Dr. Donald McIntire.)

Pregnancy after Age 35. Currently, about 10 percent of pregnancies occur in women within this age group. The older woman is more likely to request preconceptional counseling, either because she has postponed pregnancy and now wishes to optimize her outcome, or because she plans to undergo infertility treatment. Some studies—including data from Parkland Hospital presented in Figure 7-2—indicate that after age 35, there is an increased risk for obstetrical complications as well as perinatal morbidity and mortality (Cunningham and Leveno, 1995; Huang and associates, 2008). The older woman who has a chronic illness or who is in poor physical condition usually has readily apparent risks. For the physically fit woman without medical problems, however, the risks are much lower than previously reported.

The maternal mortality rate is higher in women aged 35 and older. Compared with women in their 20s, women aged 35 to 39 are 2.5 times more likely and women aged 40 or more are 5.3 times more likely for pregnancy-related mortality (Geller and colleagues, 2006). According to Buehler and colleagues (1986), improved medical care may ameliorate these risks. They reviewed maternal deaths in the United States from 1974 through 1982. Through 1978, older women had a fivefold increased relative risk of maternal death compared with that of younger women. By 1982, however, the mortality rates for older women had decreased by 50 percent.

Maternal age-related fetal risks primarily stem from: (1) indicated preterm delivery for maternal complications such as hypertension and diabetes, (2) spontaneous preterm delivery, (3) fetal growth disorders related to chronic maternal disease or multifetal gestation, (4) fetal aneuploidy, and (5) pregnancies resulting from use of assisted reproductive technology.

Most researchers have found that fetal aneuploidy is the only congenital abnormality related to maternal age. A study of 577,000 births in British Columbia by Baird and co-workers (1991) and another of 574,000 live births in Sweden by Pradat (1992) found no association between nonaneuploid structural defects and maternal age. An exception was the study by Hollier and colleagues (2000) of nearly 103,000 pregnancies that included 3885 infants with congenital malformations delivered at Parkland Hospital. They reported that the incidence of nonaneuploid structural abnormalities increased significantly with maternal age. Some contend, however, that ascertainment bias was likely because older mothers commonly underwent targeted sonographic examination but not amniocentesis, and the study population was enriched with regional referrals for women with malformed fetuses.

Assisted Reproductive Techniques. Recall that older women have subfertility problems. And although the incidence of dizygotic twinning increases related to maternal age, the more important cause of multifetal gestation in older women follows the use of *assisted reproductive technology* and *ovulation induction*. Indeed, according to the Centers for Disease Control and Prevention, 40 percent of triplet and 17 percent of twin births in the United States in 2004 were the result of assisted reproductive technologies (Martin and associates, 2007). As discussed in Chapter 39 (p. 859), multifetal pregnancies account for much of the morbidity and mortality from preterm delivery (Schieve and colleagues, 2002; Strömberg and associates, 2002).

Over the past decade, experience has accrued that links assisted reproductive techniques to increased major congenital malformations. Hansen and co-workers (2002) reported that 9 percent of 837 infants conceived by in vitro fertilization and 8.6 percent of 301 infants conceived using intracytoplasmic sperm injection and had major birth defects—this compared with 4.2 percent in 4000 control women.

Paternal Age. Although there is an increased incidence of genetic diseases in offspring caused by new autosomal-dominant mutations in older men, the incidence is still low (see Chap. 12, p. 276). Accordingly, whether targeted sonographic examinations should be performed solely for advanced maternal or paternal age is controversial.

Recreational Drugs and Smoking

Fetal risks associated with alcohol, marijuana, cocaine, amphetamines, and heroin are discussed in Chapter 14 (see p. 326). The first step in preventing drug-related fetal risk is for the woman to honestly assess her usage. Questioning should be nonjudgmental. Alcoholism can be identified by asking the well-studied TACE questions, which correlate with *DSM-IV* criteria (Chang and associates, 1998). TACE is a series of four questions concerning <u>tolerance</u> to alcohol, being <u>annoyed</u> by comments about their drinking, attempts to <u>cut down</u>, and a history of drinking early in the morning—the <u>eye opener</u>.

In a Canadian study of more than 1000 postpartum patients, Tough and colleagues (2006) found that a high percentage of women reported alcohol use while trying to conceive. Specifically, nearly half of those planning for pregnancy reported a mean of 2.2 drinks daily during early gestation before they recognized that they were pregnant. Of note, Bailey and co-workers (2008) found that rates of binge drinking and marijuana use by men were unaffected by their partner's pregnancy. The frequency and pattern of such behaviors clearly underscore the opportunity for preconceptional counseling.

In 2005, approximately 10 percent of women giving birth in the United States smoked cigarettes, and this rate was roughly doubled in those mothers between ages 18 and 24 years as well as in those who did not graduate from high school (Martin and associates, 2007). Smoking affects fetal growth in a dose-dependent manner. It increases the risk of premature rupture of membranes, placenta previa, fetal-growth restriction, and low birthweight (American College of Obstetricians and Gynecologists, 2005e). Even passive exposure to environmental tobacco smoke appears to negatively affect birthweight (Hegaard and associates, 2006). Smoking has also been associated with sudden infant death syndrome (Pollack and co-workers, 2001). Lastly, smoking increases the risk of pregnancy complications related to vascular damage, such as uteroplacental insufficiency and placental abruption (see Chap. 35, p. 761).

After counseling, the woman should be provided with a prepregnancy program to reduce or eliminate smoking. A number of resources to assist with such a program are available from the American College of Obstetricians and Gynecologists (2005e).

Environmental Exposures

Everyone is exposed to environmental substances, but fortunately only a few agents have an impact on pregnancy outcome (Windham and Fenster, 2008). Exposures to infectious organisms and chemicals impart the greatest risk.

Methyl mercury is a recognized environmental contaminant for which all pregnant women are potentially at risk because certain kinds of large fish are contaminated (see Chap. 14, p. 323). Mercury is a neurotoxin that readily crosses the placenta and has adverse fetal effects (Jedrychowski and collaborators, 2006). Accordingly, the U.S. Food and Drug Administration (FDA) (2004) has recommended that pregnant women not eat shark, swordfish, king mackerel, or tilefish, and that they consume no more than 12 ounces of other kinds of shellfish or other fish per week. Albacore or "white" tuna has more mercury than other canned tuna. Oken and colleagues (2003) have provided data showing that since the original FDA advisory, there has been a decline of ingestion by pregnant women of suspect fish species.

Electromagnetic Energy. There is no evidence in humans or animals that exposure to various electromagnetic fields such as high-voltage power lines, electric blankets, microwave ovens, and cellular phones causes adverse fetal effects (O'Connor, 1999; Robert, 1999). Electrical shock is discussed further in Chapter 42 (p. 942).

Lifestyle and Work Habits

A number of personal and work habits as well as lifestyle issues may affect pregnancy outcome.

Diet

Pica for ice, laundry starch, clay, dirt, or other nonfood items should be discouraged (see Chap. 8, p. 211). In some cases, it may represent an unusual physiological response to iron deficiency (Federman and colleagues, 1997). Many vegetarian diets are protein deficient but can be corrected by increasing egg and cheese consumption. As discussed in Chapter 43, obesity is associated with a number of maternal complications such as hypertension, preeclampsia, gestational diabetes, labor abnormal-

ities, postterm pregnancy, cesarean delivery, and operative complications (American College of Obstetricians and Gynecologists, 2005b). It also appears to be associated with a range of structural anomalies (Stothard and colleagues, 2009). By comparing changes in prepregnancy body mass index (BMI), Villamor and Cnattingius (2006) found that modest increases in BMI before pregnancy could result in perinatal complications, even if a woman does not become overweight.

In addition to nutritional deficiencies, anorexia and bulimia increase the risk of associated maternal problems such as electrolyte disturbances, cardiac arrhythmias, and gastrointestinal pathology (Becker and associates, 1999). Pregnancy-related complications include greater risks of low birthweight, smaller head circumference, microcephaly, and small for gestational age (Kouba and co-workers, 2005).

Exercise

Conditioned pregnant women usually can continue to exercise throughout gestation (American College of Obstetricians and Gynecologists, 2002; Duncombe and associates, 2006). As discussed in Chapter 8 (p. 206), there are no data to suggest that exercise is deleterious during pregnancy. One caveat is that as pregnancy progresses, balance problems and joint relaxation may predispose to orthopedic injury. A woman should be advised not to exercise to exhaustion, and she should augment heat dissipation and fluid replacement. She should avoid supine positions, activities requiring good balance, and extreme weather conditions.

Domestic Abuse

Pregnancy can exacerbate interpersonal problems and is a time of increased risk from an abusive partner. According to the American College of Obstetricians and Gynecologists (2006), and as discussed in Chapter 42 (p. 936), from 1 to 20 percent of women are abused during pregnancy. Silverman and associates (2006) found that women reporting intimate partner violence during the year prior to pregnancy were at increased risk for a number of complications. These included hypertension, vaginal bleeding, hyperemesis, preterm delivery, and low-birthweight infants. Similarly, Rodrigues and colleagues (2008) found in a survey of more than 2600 consecutive postpartum women that 24 percent of mothers of preterm infants had experienced physical abuse during pregnancy compared with 8 percent of mothers of term newborns.

The interviewer should inquire about risk factors for domestic violence and should offer intervention as appropriate. Abuse is more likely in women whose partners abuse alcohol or drugs, are recently unemployed, have a poor education or low income, or have a history of arrest (Grisso and colleagues, 1999; Kyriacou and associates, 1999). In a survey of approximately 200 women who underwent violence screening during prenatal care, 97 percent reported that they were not embarrassed, angry, or offended when assessed (Renker and Tonkin, 2006).

Family History

The most thorough method for obtaining a family history is to construct a pedigree using the symbols shown in Figure 7-3. The health and reproductive status of each "blood relative" should be individually reviewed for medical illnesses, mental

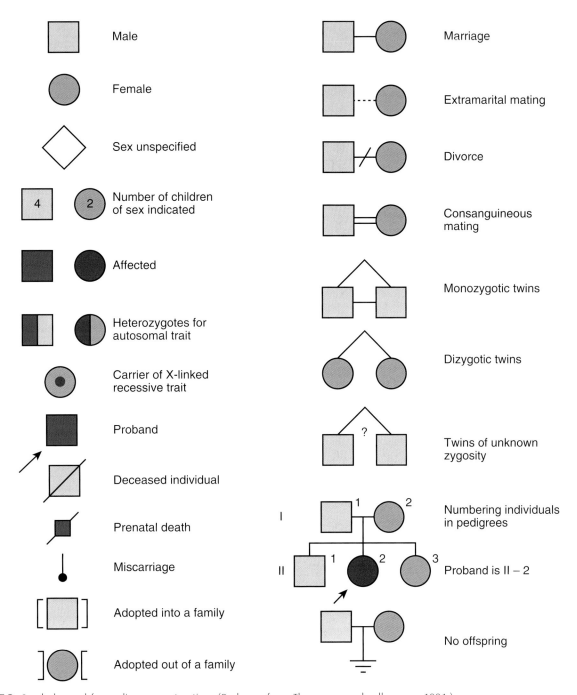

FIGURE 7-3. Symbols used for pedigree construction. (Redrawn from Thompson and colleagues, 1991.)

retardation, birth defects, infertility, and pregnancy loss. Certain racial, ethnic, or religious backgrounds may indicate increased risk for specific recessive disorders.

Although most women can provide some information regarding their history, their understanding may be limited. For example, several studies have shown that pregnant women often fail to report a birth defect in the family or report it incorrectly. It is thus important to verify the type of reported defect or genetic disease by reviewing pertinent medical records or by contacting affected relatives for additional information.

Immunizations

Preconceptional counseling includes assessment of immunity. Depending on health status, travel plans, and time of year, other

immunizations may be indicated as discussed in Chapter 8 (see Table 8-10, p. 208). Vaccines consist of toxoids—for example, tetanus; killed bacteria or viruses—such as influenza, pneumococcus, hepatitis B, meningococcus, and rabies; or attenuated live viruses—including varicella-zoster, measles, mumps, polio, rubella, chickenpox, and yellow fever. Immunization during pregnancy with toxoids or with killed bacteria or viruses has not been associated with adverse fetal outcomes. Alternatively, live-virus vaccines are not recommended during pregnancy and ideally should be given at least 1 month before attempts to conceive. Women inadvertently given measles, mumps, rubella, or varicella vaccines during pregnancy, however, are not necessarily advised to seek pregnancy termination. Most reports indicate that immunization to any of these agents poses only a theoretical risk to the fetus. Lastly, immunization to smallpox, anthrax, and other bioterrorist diseases should be discussed (see Chap. 58, p. 1230). Based upon their study of approximately 300 women who received smallpox vaccination near the time of conception, Ryan and co-workers (2008) found that rates of pregnancy loss, preterm birth, and birth defects were not higher than expected.

Screening Tests

Certain laboratory tests may be helpful in assessing the risk for and preventing some complications during pregnancy. These include basic tests that are usually performed during prenatal care and are discussed in Chapter 8. Some examples are that rubella, varicella, and hepatitis B immune status should be de-

termined so that vaccination can be carried out as part of preconceptional care. A hemogram will exclude most serious inherited anemias. Hemoglobin electrophoresis is performed in individuals at increased risk—for example, African-Americans for sickle syndromes and women of Mediterranean or Asian origin for thalassemias. As discussed on page 178, couples of Jewish ancestry are candidates for carrier testing for Tay-Sachs and Canavan disease, whereas Caucasians of northern European descent may elect screening for cystic fibrosis.

More specific tests may assist the evaluation of women with certain chronic medical diseases (Table 7-6). Examples of some, but certainly not all, chronic diseases that may be assessed by prenatal testing include kidney and cardiovascular diseases and diabetes.

TABLE 7-6.

Condition	Reference Chapter	Recommendations for Preconceptional Counseling
Abnormal weight	Chap. 43, p. 946	Calculate BMI yearly. (see Fig. 43-1, p. 947). *BMI ≥ 25 kg/m²*: Counsel on diet. Test for diabetes and metabolic syndrome if indicated. *BMI ≤ 18.5 kg/m²*: Assess for eating disorder
Cardiovascular disease	Chap. 44, p. 961 Chap. 14, p. 325	Counsel on cardiac risks during pregnancy. Optimize cardiac function, and offer effective contraception during this time and for those not desiring conception. Discuss warfarin, ACE inhibitor, and ARB teratogenicity and if possible, switch to less dangerous agent when conception planned. Offer genetic counseling to those with congenital cardiac anomalies (see Table 44-4, p. 961). Review situations for infective endocarditis
Chronic hypertension	Chap. 45, p. 985 Chap. 14, p. 319	Counsel on specific risks during pregnancy. Assess those with long-standing HTN for ventricular hypertrophy, retinopathy, and renal disease. Counsel women taking ACE inhibitors and ARBs on drug teratogenicity, on effective contraception during use, and on the need to switch agents prior to conception
Asthma	Chap. 46, p. 996	Counsel on asthma risks during pregnancy. Optimize pulmonary function and offer effective contraception during this time. Treat women with pharmacological step therapy for chronic asthma based on ACOG-ACAAI (2000) recommendations
Thrombophilia	Chap. 47, p. 1014	Question for personal or family history of thrombotic events or recurrent poor pregnancy outcomes. If found, counsel and screen those contemplating pregnancy. Offer genetic counseling to those with known thrombophilia. Discuss warfarin teratogenicity, offer effective contraception during use, and switch to a less teratogenic agent, if possible, prior to conception
Renal disease	Chap. 48, p. 1039 Chap. 14, p. 319	Counsel on specific risks during pregnancy. Optimize blood pressure control and offer effective contraception during this time. Counsel women taking ACE inhibitors and ARBs on their teratogenicity, on effective contraception during use, and on the need to switch agents prior to conception

TABLE 7-6. Continued

Condition	Reference Chapter	Recommendations for Preconceptional Counseling
Gastrointestinal disease	Chap. 49, p. 1054 Chap. 14, p. 320	*Inflammatory bowel disease:* Counsel affected women on subfertility risks and risks of adverse pregnancy outcomes. Discuss teratogenicity of methotrexate and the other immunomodulators, about which less is known, e.g., mycophenolate mofetil, etc. Offer effective contraception during their use and switch agents, if possible, prior to conception
Hepatobiliary disease	Chap. 50, p. 1067	*Hepatitis B*: Vaccinate all high-risk women prior to conception (Table 8-10, p. 208). Counsel chronic carriers on transmission prevention to partners and fetus *Hepatitis C*: Screen high-risk women. Counsel affected women on risks of disease and transmission. Refer for treatment, discuss ramifications of treatment during pregnancy, and offer effective contraception
Hematological disease	Chap. 51, p. 1085	*Sickle-cell disease:* Screen all black women. Counsel those with trait or disease. Test partner if desired *Thalassemias:* Screen women of southeast asian or mediterranean ancestry
Diabetes	Chap. 52, p. 1113	Advocate good glucose control, especially in periconceptional period to decrease known teratogenicity of overt diabetes. Evaluate for retinopathy, nephropathy, hypertension, etc. (See Table 7-2, p. 176)
Thyroid disease	Chap. 53, p. 1126	Screen those with thyroid disease symptoms. Ensure iodine-sufficient diet. Treat overt hyper- or hypothyroidism prior to conception. Counsel on risks to pregnancy outcome
Connective tissue disease	Chap. 54, p. 1146 Chap. 14, p. 320	*RA*: Counsel on flare risk after pregnancy. Discuss methotrexate and leflunomide teratogenicity, as well as possible effects of other immunomodulators. Offer effective contraception during their use and switch agents prior to conception. Halt NSAIDS by 27 weeks' gestation *SLE*: Counsel on risks during pregnancy. Optimize disease and offer effective contraception during this time and for those not desiring conception. Discuss mycophenolate mofetil and cyclophosphamide teratogenicity as well as possible effects of newer immunomodulators. Effective contraception during their use. If possible, switch agents prior to conception
Neurological and psychiatric disorders	Chap. 55, p. 1164 Chap. 14, p. 323	*Depression:* Screen for symptoms of depression. In those affected, counsel on risks of treatment and of untreated illness and high risk of exacerbation during pregnancy and the puerperium *Seizure disorder:* optimize seizure control using monotherapy if possible. (see p. 176 and Table 7-3)
Dermatological disease	Chap. 56, p. 1191 Chap. 14, p. 324	Discuss isotretinoin and etretinate teratogenicity, effective contraception during their use, and need to switch agents prior to conception
Cancer	Chap. 57, p. 1193 Chap. 14, p. 320	Counsel on fertility preservation options prior to cancer therapy and on decreased fertility following certain agents. Offer genetic counseling to those with mutation-linked cancers. Evaluate cardiac function in those given cardiotoxic agents, such as adriamycin. Obtain mammography for those given childhood chest radiotherapy. Discuss SERM teratogenicity, effective contraception during their use, and need to switch agents prior to conception. Review chemotherapy and discuss possible teratogenic effects if continued during pregnancy

(continued)

TABLE 7-6. Continued

Condition	Reference Chapter	Recommendations for Preconceptional Counseling
Infectious diseases	Chap. 58, p. 1210	*Asymptomatic bacteriuria:* No role for preconceptional screening *Bacterial Vaginosis:* No role for preconceptional screening *Influenza:* Vaccinate women who will be pregnant during flu season. Vaccinate high-risk women prior to flu season *Malaria:* Counsel to avoid travel to endemic areas during conception. If unable, offer effective contraception during travel or provide chemoprophylaxis for those planning pregnancy *Rubella:* Screen for rubella immunity. If nonimmune, vaccinate and counsel on the need for effective contraception during the subsequent 3 months *Tuberculosis:* Screen high-risk women and treat prior to conception *Tetanus:* Update vaccination, as needed, in all reproductive-aged women *Varicella:* Question regarding immunity. If nonimmune, vaccinate.
STDs	Chap. 59, p. 1235	*Gonorrhea, syphilis, chlamydial infection:* Screen high-risk women and treat as indicated *HIV:* Screen at-risk women. Counsel affected women on risks during pregnancy and on perinatal transmission. Discuss initiation of treatment prior to pregnancy to decrease transmission risk. Offer effective contraception to those not desiring conception *HPV:* Provide PAP smear screening. Vaccinate candidate patients *HSV:* Provide serological screening to asymptomatic women with affected partners. Counsel affected women on risks of perinatal transmission and of preventative measures during the third trimester and labor

ACAAI = American College of Allergy, Asthma, and Immunology; ACE = angiotensin-converting enzyme inhibitor; ARB = angiotensin-receptor blocker; ACOG = American College of Obstetricians and Gynecologists; BMI = body mass index; HIV = human immunodeficiency virus; HPV = human papillomavirus; HSV = herpes simplex virus; HTN = hypertension; NSAID = nonsteroidal anti-inflammatory drug; RA = rheumatoid arthritis; SERM = selective estrogen-receptor modulator; SLE = systemic lupus erythematosus; STD = sexually transmitted disease.
(Adapted from Jack and colleagues, 2008.)

REFERENCES

Adab N, Tudur SC, Vinten J, et al: Common antiepileptic drugs in pregnancy in women with epilepsy. Cochrane Database Syst Rev CD004848, 2004

Aguglia U, Barboni G, Battino D, et al: Italian Consensus Conference on Epilepsy and Pregnancy, Labor and Puerperium. Epilepsia 50:7, 2009

Allsworth JE, Peipert JF: Prevalence of bacterial vaginosis: 2001–2004 National Health and Nutrition Examination Survey Data. Obstet Gynecol 109:114, 2007

American Academy of Neurology: Practice parameter: Management issues for women with epilepsy (summary statement). Report of the Quality Standards Subcommittee of the American Academy of Neurology. Epilepsia 39:1226, 1998

American College of Obstetricians and Gynecologists: Exercise during pregnancy and the postpartum period. Committee Opinion No. 267, January 2002

American College of Obstetricians and Gynecologists: Prenatal and preconceptional carrier screening for genetic diseases in individuals of Eastern European Jewish descent. Committee Opinion No. 298, August 2004

American College of Obstetricians and Gynecologists: The importance of preconception care in the continuum of women's health care. Committee Opinion No. 313, September 2005a

American College of Obstetricians and Gynecologists: Obesity in pregnancy. Committee Opinion No. 315, September 2005b

American College of Obstetricians and Gynecologists: Pregestational diabetes mellitus. Practice Bulletin No. 60, March 2005c

American College of Obstetricians and Gynecologists: Screening for Tay-Sachs Disease. Committee Opinion No. 318, October 2005d

American College of Obstetricians and Gynecologists: Smoking cessation during pregnancy. Committee Opinion No. 316, October 2005e

American College of Obstetricians and Gynecologists: Psychosocial risk factors: Perinatal screening and intervention. Committee Opinion No. 343, August 2006

American College of Obstetricians and Gynecologists: Hemoglobinopathies in pregnancy. Practice Bulletin No. 78, January 2007

American College of Obstetricians and Gynecologists (ACOG) and American College of Allergy, Asthma and Immunology (ACAAI): The use of newer asthma and allergy medications during pregnancy. Ann Allergy Asthma Immunol 84(5):475, 2000

American Diabetes Association: Preconception care of women with diabetes. Diabetes Care 27:S76, 2004

Andrews WW, Goldenberg RL, Hauth JC, et al: Interconceptional antibiotics to prevent spontaneous preterm birth: A randomized clinical trial. Am J Obstet Gynecol 194:617, 2006

Angastiniotis M, Modell B: Global epidemiology of hemoglobin disorders. Ann NY Acad Sci 850:251, 1998

Bailey JA, Hill KG, Hawkins JD, et al: Men's and women's patterns of substance use around pregnancy. Birth 35:1, 2008

Baird PA, Saolovnick AD, Yee IM: Maternal age and birth defects: A population study. Lancet 338:527, 1991

Becker AE, Grinspoon SK, Klibanski A, et al: Eating disorders. N Engl J Med 340:14, 1999

Bell KN, Oakley Jr GP: Update on prevention of folic acid-preventable spina bifida and anencephaly. Birth Defects Res 85:102, 2009

Besculides M, Laraque F. Unintended pregnancy among the urban poor. J Urban Health 81: 340, 2004

Biale Y, Lewenthal H: Effect of folic acid supplementation on congenital malformations due to anticonvulsive drugs. Eur J Obstet Gynecol Reprod Biol 18:211, 1984

Buehler JW, Kaunitz AM, Hogue CJR, et al: Maternal mortality in women aged 35 years or older: United States. JAMA 255:53, 1986

Centers for Disease Control and Prevention: Birth defects. Available at: www.cdc.gov/node.do/id/0900f3ec8000dffe. Accessed January 12, 2007

Centers for Disease Control and Prevention: Recommendations to improve preconception health and health care—United States: A report of the CDC/ATSDR preconception care work group and the select panel on preconception care. MMWR 55:RR-6, 2006

Chang G, Wilkins-Haug L, Berman S, et al: Alcohol use and pregnancy: Improving identification. Obstet Gynecol 91:892, 1998

Chen SU, Su YN, Fang MY, et al: PGD of beta-thalassaemia and HLA haplotypes using OminiPlex whole genome amplification. Reprod Biomed Online 17:699, 2008

Cheng D, Schwarz EB, Douglas E, et al: Unintended pregnancy and associated maternal preconception, prenatal and postpartum behaviors. Contraception 79:194, 2009

Cox M, Whittle MJ, Byrne A, et al: Prepregnancy counseling: Experience from 1075 cases. Br J Obstet Gynaecol 99:873, 1992

Cunningham FG, Leveno KJ: Childbearing among older women—the message is cautiously optimistic. N Engl J Med 333:953, 1995

Czeizel AE, Dudas I: Prevention of the first occurrence of neural-tube defects by periconceptional vitamin supplementation. N Engl J Med 327:1832, 1992

D'Angelo D, Williams L, Morrow B, et al: Preconception and interconception health status of women who recently gave birth to a live-born infant – Pregnancy Risk Assessment Monitoring System (PRAMS), United States, 26 reporting areas, 2004. MMWR Surveillance Summaries 56(SS10):1-35, December 14, 2007

de Jong-van den Berg LTW, Hernandez-Diaz S, Werler MM, et al: Trends and predictors of folic acid awareness and periconceptional use in pregnant women. Am J Obstet Gynecol 192:121, 2005

Dott M, Rasmussen SA, Hogue CJ, et al: Association between pregnancy intention and reproductive-health related behaviors before and after pregnancy recognition, National Birth Defects Prevention Study, 1997–2002. Matern Child Health J [Epub ahead of print], 2009

Duncombe D, Skouteris H, Wertheim EH, et al: Vigorous exercise and birth outcomes in a sample of recreational exercisers: A prospective study across pregnancy. Aust NZ J Obstet Gynaecol 46:288, 2006

Dunne FP, Brydon P, Smith T, et al: Preconception diabetes care in insulin-dependent diabetes mellitus. QJM 92:175, 1999

Federman DG, Kirsner RS, Federman GS: Pica: Are you hungry for the facts? Conn Med 61:207, 1997

Finer LB, Henshaw SK: Disparities in the rates of unintended pregnancies in the United States, 1994 and 2001. Perspect Sex Reprod Health 38:90, 2006

Fraser AM, Brockert JE, Ward RH: Association of young maternal age with adverse reproductive outcomes. N Engl J Med 332:1113, 1995

Geller SE, Cox SM, Callaghan WM, et al: Morbidity and mortality in pregnancy: Laying the groundwork for safe motherhood. Womens Health Issues 16:176, 2006

Goldberg BB, Alvarado S, Chavez C, et al: Prevalence of periconceptional folic acid use and perceived barriers to the postgestation continuance of supplemental folic acid: Survey results from a Teratogen Information Service. Birth Defects Res Part A Clin Mol Teratol 76:193, 2006

Grisso JA, Schwarz DF, Hirschinger N, et al: Violent injuries among women in an urban area. N Engl J Med 341:1899, 1999

Guttler F, Lou H, Andresen J, et al: Cognitive development in offspring of untreated and preconceptionally treated maternal phenylketonuria. J Inherited Metab Dis 13:665, 1990

Hamner HC, Mulinare J, Cogswell ME, et al: Predicted contribution of folic acid fortification of corn masa flour to the usual folic acid intake for the US population: National Health and Nutrition Examination Survey 2001–2004. Am J Clin Nutr 89:305, 2009

Hansen M, Kurinczuk JJ, Bower C, et al: The risk of major birth defects after intracytoplasmic sperm injection and in vitro fertilization. N Engl J Med 346:725, 2002

Hegaard HK, Kjærgaard H, Møller LF, et al: The effect of environmental tobacco smoke during pregnancy on birth weight. Acta Obstet et Gynecol 85:675, 2006

Hoeks MP, den Heijer M, Janssen MC: Adult issues in phenylketonuria. J Med 67:2, 2009

Hollier LM, Leveno KJ, Kelly MA, et al: Maternal age and malformations in singleton births. Obstet Gynecol 96:701, 2000

Holmes LB, Harvey EA, Coull BA, et al: The teratogenicity of anticonvulsant drugs. N Engl J Med 344:1132, 2001

Huang L, Sauve R, Birkett N, et al: Maternal age and risk of stillbirth: A systematic review. CMAJ 178:165, 2008

Jack BW, Atrash H, Coonrod DV, et al: The clinical content of preconception care: an overview and preparation of this supplement. Am J Obstet Gynecol 199(6 Suppl 2):S266, 2008

Jack BW, Campanile C, McQuade W, et al: The negative pregnancy test. An opportunity for preconception care. Arch Fam Med 4:340, 1995

Jedrychowski W, Jankowski J, Flak E, et al: Effects of prenatal exposure of mercury on cognitive and psychomotor function in one-year-old infants: Epidemiologic cohort study in Poland. Ann Epidemiol 16:439, 2006

Jeha LE, Morris HH: Optimizing outcomes in pregnant women with epilepsy. Cleve Clin J Med 72:928, 2005

Kaback M, Lim-Steele J, Dabholkar D, et al: Tay Sachs disease: Carrier screening, prenatal diagnosis, and the molecular era. JAMA 270:2307, 1993

Kim C, Ferrara A, McEwen LN, et al: Preconception care in managed care: The translating research into action for diabetes study. Am J Obstet Gynecol 192:227, 2005

Kitzmiller JL, Gavin LA, Gin GD, et al: Preconception care of diabetics. JAMA 265:731, 1991

Kjær D, Horvath-Puhó E, Christensen J, et al: Antiepileptic drug use, folic acid supplementation, and congenital abnormalities: A population-based case-control study. BJOG 115:98, 2008

Koch R, Hanley W, Levy H, et al: A preliminary report of the collaborative study of maternal phenylketonuria in the United States and Canada. J Inherit Metab Dis 13:641, 1990

Kouba S, Hällström T, Lindholm C, et al: Pregnancy and neonatal outcomes in women with eating disorders. Obstet Gynecol 105:255, 2005

Kyriacou DN, Anglin D, Taliaferro E, et al: Risk factors for injury to women from domestic violence. N Engl J Med 341:1892, 1999

Lee PJ, Ridout D, Walter JH, et al: Maternal phenylketonuria: Report from the United Kingdom registry 1978-97. Arch Dis Child 90:143, 2005

Leguizamón G, Igarzabal ML, Reece EA: Periconceptional care of women with diabetes mellitus. Obstet Gynecol Clin N Am 34:225, 2007

Maillot F, Cook P, Lilburn M, et al: A practical approach to maternal phenylketonuria management. J Inherit Metab Dis 30:198, 2007

Martin JA, Hamilton BE, Sutton PD, et al: Births: Final data for 2005. Natl Vital Stat Rep, Vol. 56, No. 6. Hyattsville, MD: National Center for Health Statistics, 2007

Medical Research Council on Vitamin Study Research Group: Prevention of neural tube defects: Results of the Medical Research Council vitamin study. Lancet 338:131, 1991

Mitchell JJ, Capua A, Clow C, et al: Twenty-year outcome analysis of genetic screening programs for Tay-Sachs and beta-thalassemia disease carriers in high schools. Am J Hum Genet 59:793, 1996

Mohd Nasri NW, Jamal AR, Abdullah NC, et al: Preimplantation genetic diagnosis for β-thalassemia using single-cell DNA analysis for codons 17 and 26 of β-globin gene. Arch Med Res 40:1, 2009

Molloy AM, Kirke PN, Troendle JF, et al: Maternal vitamin B12 status and risk of neural tube defects in a population with high neural tube defect prevalence and no folic Acid fortification. Pediatrics 123(3):917, 2009

Moos MK: Preconceptional health promotion: Progress in changing a prevention paradigm. J Perinat Neonatal Nurs 18:2, 2004

Moos MK, Bangdiwala SI, Meibohm AR, et al: The impact of a preconceptional health promotion program on intendedness of pregnancy. Am J Perinatol 13:103, 1996

National Institute of Neurological Disorders and Stroke: NINDS Canavan disease information page. Available at: http://www.ninds.nih.gov/disorders/canavan/canavan.htm. Accessed March 11, 2007a

National Institute of Neurological Disorders and Stroke: NINDS Tay-Sachs disease information page. Available at: http://www.ninds.nih.gov/disorders/taysachs/taysachs.htm. Accessed March 11, 2007b

National Institute of Neurological Disorders and Stroke: NINDS Niemann-Pick disease information page. Available at: http://www.ninds.nih.gov/disorders/niemann/niemann.htm. Accessed March 11, 2007c

National Institute of Neurological Disorders and Stroke: NINDS Gaucher's disease information page. Available at: http://www.ninds.nih.gov/disorders/gauchers/gauchers.htm. Accessed March 11, 2007d

Niccolai LM, Ethier KA, Kershaw TS, et al: Pregnant adolescents at risk: Sexual behaviors and sexually transmitted disease prevalence. Am J Obstet Gynecol 188:63, 2003

O'Connor ME: Intrauterine effects in animals exposed to radiofrequency and microwave fields. Teratology 59:287, 1999

Oken E, Kleinman KP, Berland WE, et al: Decline in fish consumption among pregnant women after national mercury advisory. Obstet Gynecol 102:346, 2003

Ou CY, Stevenson RE, Brown VK, et al: 5, 10 Methylenetetrahydrofolate reductase genetic polymorphism as a risk factor for neural tube defects. Am J Med Genet 63:610, 1996

Pollack HA: Sudden infant death syndrome, maternal smoking during pregnancy, and the cost-effectiveness of smoking cessation intervention. Am J Public Health 91:432, 2001

Postlethwaite D, Armstrong MA, Hung Y-Y, et al: Pregnancy outcomes by pregnancy intention in a managed care setting. Matern Child Health J [Epub ahead of print], 2009

Pradat P. Epidemiology of major congenital heart defects in Sweden, 1981–1986. J Epidemiol Community Health 46:211, 1992

Reece EA, Homko CJ: Prepregnancy care and the prevention of fetal malformations in the pregnancy complicated by diabetes. Clin Obstet Gynecol 50:990: 2007

Renker PR, Tonkin P: Women's views of prenatal violence screening: Acceptability and confidentiality issues. Obstet Gynecol 107:348, 2006

Robert E: Intrauterine effects of electromagnetic fields (low frequency, mid-frequency RF, and microwave): Review of epidemiologic studies. Teratology 59:292, 1999

Rodrigues T, Rocha L, Barros H: Physical abuse during pregnancy and preterm delivery. Am J Obstet Gynecol 198:171.e1, 2008

Rouse B, Azen C, Koch R, et al: Maternal Phenylketonuria Collaborative Study (MPKUCS) offspring: Facial anomalies, malformations, and early neurological sequelae. Am J Med Genet 69:89, 1997

Ryan MA, Seward JF, for the Smallpox Vaccine in Pregnancy Registry Team: Pregnancy, birth, and infant health outcomes from the National Smallpox Vaccine in Pregnancy Registry, 2003–2006. Clin Infect Dis 46:S221, 2008

Schieve LA, Meikle SF, Ferre C, et al: Low and very low birth weight in infants conceived with use of assisted reproductive technology. N Engl J Med 346:731, 2002

Sheffield JS, Butler-Koster EL, Casey BM, et al: Maternal diabetes mellitus and infant malformations. Obstet Gynecol 100:925, 2002

Silver RM: Fetal death. Obstet Gynecol 109:153, 2007

Silverman JG, Decker MR, Reed E, et al: Intimate partner violence victimization prior to and during pregnancy among women residing in 26 U.S. states: Associations with maternal and neonatal health. Am J Obstet Gynecol 195:140, 2006

Stothard KJ, Tennant PW, Bell R, et al: Maternal overweight and obesity and the risk of congenital anomalies: A systematic review and meta-analysis. JAMA 301:636, 2009

Strömberg B, Dahlquist A, Ericson A, et al: Neurological sequelae in children born after in-vitro fertilisation: A population-based study. Lancet 359:461, 2002

Stubblefield PG, Coonrod DV, Reddy UM, et al: The clinical content of preconception care: Reproductive history. Am J Obstet Gynecol 199(6 Suppl 2):S373, 2008

Temple RC, Aldridge VJ, Murphy HR: Prepregnancy care and pregnancy outcomes in women with type 1 diabetes. Diabetes Care 29:1744, 2006

Thompson MD, Cole DE, Ray JG: Vitamin B-12 and neural tube defects: the Canadian experience. Am J Clin Nutr 89(2):697S, 2009

Thompson MW, McInnes RR, Huntington FW (eds): Genetics in Medicine, 5th ed. Philadelphia, Saunders, 1991

Tomson T, Battino D: Pregnancy and epilepsy: What should we tell our patients? J Neurol 256(6):856, 2009

Tough S, Tofflemire K, Clarke M, et al: Do women change their drinking behaviors while trying to conceive? An opportunity for preconception counseling. Clin Med Res 4:97, 2006

US Food and Drug Administration: What you need to know about mercury in fish and shellfish. 2004 EPA and FDA advice for: Women who might become pregnant, women who are pregnant, nursing mother, young children. EPA-823-R-04-005, March 2004. Available at: http://www.cfsan.fda.gov/. Accessed March 11, 2007

Usta IM, Zoorob D, Abu-Musa A, et al: Obstetric outcome of teenage pregnancies compared with adult pregnancies. Acta Obstet Gynecol 87:178, 2008

Vajda FJ, Hitchcock A, Graham J, et al: Seizure control in antiepileptic drug-treated pregnancy. Epilepsia 49:172, 2008

Ventura SJ, Abma JC, Mosher WD, et al: Recent trends in teenage pregnancy in the United States, 1990-2002. Health E-stats. Hyattsville, MD: National Center for Health Statistics. Released December 13, 2006

Villamor E, Cnattingius S: Interpregnancy weight change and risk of adverse pregnancy outcomes: A population-based study. Lancet 368:1164, 2006

Wide K, Winbladh B, Kallen B: Major malformations in infants exposed to antiepileptic drugs in utero, with emphasis on carbamazepine and valproic acid: A nation-wide population-based register study. 93:174, 2004

Windham G, Fenster L: Environmental contaminants and pregnancy outcomes. Fertil Steril 89:e111, 2008

CHAPTER 8

Prenatal Care

Organized prenatal care in the United States was introduced largely by social reformers and nurses. In 1901, Mrs. William Lowell Putnam of the Boston Infant Social Service Department began a program of nurse visits to women enrolled in the home delivery service of the Boston Lying-in Hospital (Merkatz and colleagues, 1990). It was so successful that a prenatal clinic was established in 1911. In 1915, J. Whitridge Williams reviewed 10,000 consecutive deliveries at Johns Hopkins Hospital and concluded that 40 percent of 705 perinatal deaths could have been prevented by prenatal care. In 1954, Nicholas J. Eastman credited organized prenatal care with having "done more to save mothers' lives in our time than any other single factor" (Speert, 1980). In the 1960s, Dr. Jack Pritchard established a network of university-operated prenatal clinics located in the most underserved communities in Dallas County. In large part because of increased accessibility, currently more than 95 percent of medically indigent women delivering at Parkland Hospital receive prenatal care. Importantly and related, the perinatal mortality rate of women in this system is less than that of the United States overall.

OVERVIEW OF PRENATAL CARE

Almost a century after its introduction, prenatal care has become one of the most frequently used health services in the United States. In 2006, more than 4.2 million births were registered in the United States (Martin and associates, 2009). In

2001, there were approximately 50 million prenatal visits—the median was 12.3 visits per pregnancy—and as shown in Figure 8-1, many women had 17 or more visits.

A new birth certificate form was introduced in 2003 and is now used by 19 states, with the remaining 31 states continuing to use the 1989 form. Unfortunately, data regarding the timing of prenatal care from these two systems are not comparable. For example, with the 1989 version that represents 2.2 million births, nearly 83 percent of women received first-trimester prenatal care in 2006. Conversely, those states using the 2003 version reported that only 69 percent of women received first-trimester care (Martin and associates, 2009). Although the difference is striking, it merely represents a change in reporting and is not a harbinger of diminished of prenatal care. Indeed, according to the Centers for Disease Control and Prevention (2008a), birth certificate data using the 1989 version show that more than 99 percent of women received some prenatal care in the third trimester.

Since the early 1990s, the largest gains in timely prenatal care have been among minority groups. As shown in Figure 8-2, however, disparity continues. In 2006, African American and Hispanic women were more than twice as likely as non-Hispanic white women to begin prenatal care after the first trimester (Martin and associates, 2009). Obstetrical and medical risk factors or complications identifiable during prenatal care are summarized in Table 8-1. Importantly, many of these complications are *treatable*.

Assessing Adequacy of Prenatal Care

A commonly employed system for measuring prenatal care adequacy is the index of Kessner and colleagues (1973). As shown in Table 8-2, this *Kessner Index* incorporates three items from the birth certificate: length of gestation, timing of the first prenatal visit, and number of visits. It does not, however, measure the quality of care, nor does it consider the relative risk of complications for the mother. Still, the index remains a useful measure of prenatal care adequacy. Using this index, the National Center for Health Statistics concluded that 12 percent of American

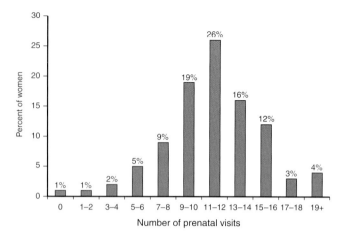

FIGURE 8-1 Frequency distribution of the number of prenatal visits for the United States in 2001. (Adapted from Martin and associates, 2002b.)

women who were delivered in 2000 received inadequate prenatal care (Martin and associates, 2002a).

The Centers for Disease Control and Prevention (2000) analyzed birth certificate data for the years 1989 to 1997 and found that half of women with delayed or no prenatal care wanted to begin care earlier. Reasons for inadequate prenatal care varied by social and ethnic group, age, and method of payment. The most common reason cited was late identification of pregnancy by the patient. The second most commonly cited barrier was lack of money or insurance for such care. The third was inability to obtain an appointment.

Effectiveness of Prenatal Care

Prenatal care designed during the early 1900s was focused on lowering the extremely high maternal mortality rates. Such care

undoubtedly contributed to the dramatic decline in maternal mortality rates from 690 per 100,000 births in 1920 to 50 per 100,000 by 1955 (Loudon, 1992). As discussed in Chapter 1 (p. 5), the current low maternal mortality rate of approximately 8 per 100,000 is likely associated with the high utilization of prenatal care. Indeed, in a population-based study from North Carolina, Harper and co-workers (2003) found that the risk of pregnancy-related maternal death was decreased fivefold among recipients of prenatal care.

There are other studies that attest to the efficacy of prenatal care. Herbst and associates (2003) found that no prenatal care was associated with more than a twofold increased risk of preterm birth. Schramm (1992) compared the costs and benefits of prenatal care in 1988 for more than 12,000 Medicaid patients in Missouri. For each $1 spent for prenatal care, there were estimated savings of $1.49 in newborn and postpartum costs. Vintzileos and colleagues (2002a) analyzed National Center for Health Statistics data for 1995 to 1997. They reported that women with prenatal care had an overall stillbirth rate of 2.7 per 1000 compared with 14.1 per 1000 for women without prenatal care—an adjusted relative risk of 3.3 for fetal death. Vintzileos and colleagues (2002b, 2003) later reported that prenatal care was associated with significantly lower rates of preterm births as well as neonatal death associated with several high-risk conditions that included placenta previa, fetal-growth restriction, and postterm pregnancy.

ORGANIZATION OF PRENATAL CARE

The essence of prenatal care is described by the American Academy of Pediatrics and the American College of Obstetricians and Gynecologists (2007) as: "A comprehensive antepartum care program involves a coordinated approach to medical care and psychosocial support that optimally begins before conception and extends throughout the antepartum period." This comprehensive program includes: (1) preconceptional care, (2) prompt diagnosis of pregnancy, (3) initial prenatal evaluation, and (4) follow-up prenatal visits.

Preconceptional Care

Because health during pregnancy depends on health before pregnancy, preconceptional care should logically be an integral prelude to prenatal care. As discussed in detail in Chapter 7, a comprehensive preconceptional care program has the potential to assist women by reducing risks, promoting healthy lifestyles, and improving readiness for pregnancy.

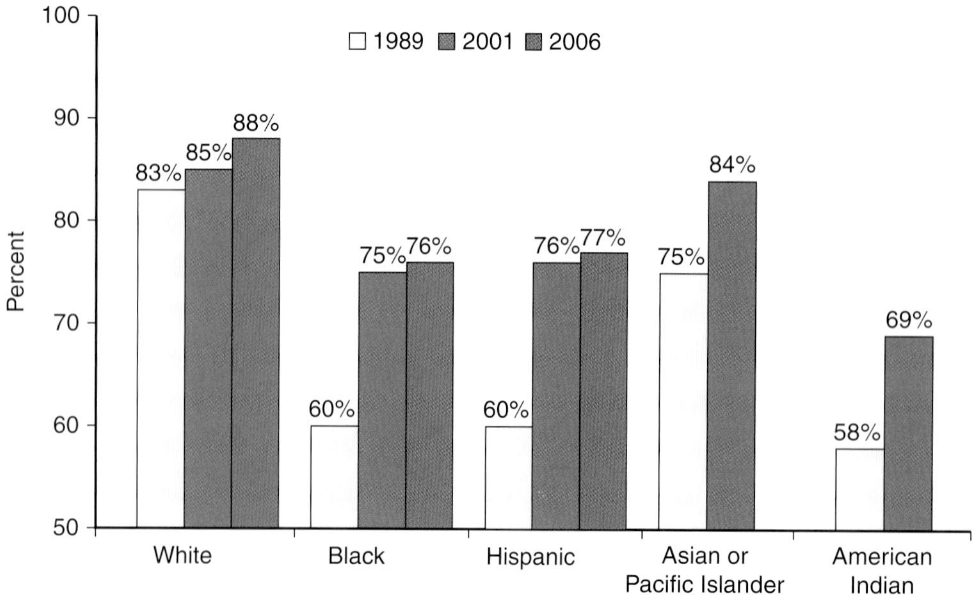

FIGURE 8-2 Percentage of women in the United States with prenatal care beginning in the first trimester by ethnicity in 1989, 2001, and 2006. (Adapted from Martin and associates, 2002b, 2009.)

TABLE 8-1. Obstetrical and Medical Risk Factors Detected During Prenatal Care in the United States in 2001

Risk Factor	Births	Percent
Total live births	4,025,933	100
Gestational hypertension	150,329	3.7
Diabetes	124,242	3.1
Anemia	99,558	2.5
Hydramnios/oligohydramnios	54,694	1.4
Lung disease	48,246	1.2
Genital herpes	33,560	0.8
Chronic hypertension	32,232	0.8
D (Rh) sensitization	26,933	0.7
Cardiac disease	20,698	0.5
Renal disease	12,045	0.3
Incompetent cervix	11,251	0.3
Hemoglobinopathy	3,141	0.1
Total	616,929	15.3

Data from Martin and associates (2002b).

TABLE 8-2. Kessner Index Criteria

Adequate Prenatal Care

Initial visit in first trimester and:

Weeks		Attended Prenatal Visits
17	and	2 or more
18–21	and	3 or more
22–25	and	4 or more
26–29	and	5 or more
30–31	and	6 or more
32–33	and	7 or more
34–35	and	8 or more
36 or more	and	9 or more

Inadequate Prenatal Care

Initial visit in third trimester or:

Weeks		Attended Prenatal Visits
17–21	and	None
22–29	and	1 or fewer
30–31	and	2 or fewer
32–33	and	3 or fewer
34 or more	and	4 or fewer

Intermediate Care

All other combinations

Reprinted with permission from *Contrasts in Health Status,* Vol. 1, © 1973 by the National Academy of Sciences, Courtesy of the National Academies Press, Washington, D.C.

Diagnosis of Pregnancy

The diagnosis of pregnancy usually begins when a woman presents with symptoms, and possibly a positive home urine pregnancy test result. Typically, such women receive confirmatory testing of urine or blood for human chorionic gonadotropin (hCG). There may be presumptive or diagnostic findings of pregnancy on examination. Sonography is often used, particularly in those cases in which there is question about pregnancy viability or location.

Signs and Symptoms

A number of clinical findings and symptoms may indicate an early pregnancy.

Cessation of Menses. The abrupt cessation of menstruation in a healthy reproductive-aged woman who previously has experienced spontaneous, cyclical, predictable menses is highly suggestive of pregnancy. As discussed in Chapter 3 (p. 44), there is appreciable variation in the length of the ovarian—and thus menstrual—cycle among women, and even in the same woman. Thus, amenorrhea is not a reliable indication of pregnancy until 10 days or more after expected menses onset. When a second menstrual period is missed, the probability of pregnancy is much greater.

Uterine bleeding somewhat suggestive of menstruation occurs occasionally after conception. One or two episodes of bloody discharge, somewhat reminiscent of and sometimes mistaken for menstruation, are not uncommon during the first month of pregnancy. Such episodes are interpreted to be physiological, and likely the consequence of blastocyst implantation.

Changes in Cervical Mucus. Dried cervical mucus examined microscopically has characteristic patterns dependent on the stage of the ovarian cycle and the presence or absence of pregnancy. Mucus crystallization necessary for the production of the fern pattern is dependent on an increased sodium chloride concentration. Cervical mucus is relatively rich in sodium chloride when estrogen, but not progesterone, is being produced. Thus, from approximately the 7th to the 18th day of the cycle, a fern-like pattern is seen (Fig. 8-3).

In contrast, progesterone secretion—even without a reduction in estrogen secretion—acts promptly to lower sodium chloride concentration to levels that prohibit ferning. During pregnancy, progesterone usually exerts a similar effect, even though the amount of estrogen produced is enormous. After approximately the 21st day, a different pattern forms that gives a beaded or cellular appearance (Fig. 8-4). This beaded pattern also is usually encountered during pregnancy. Thus, copious thin mucus with a fern pattern on drying makes early pregnancy unlikely.

Breast Changes. Anatomical changes in the breasts that accompany pregnancy are characteristic during a first pregnancy (see Chap. 5, p. 111). These are less obvious in multiparas, whose breasts may contain a small amount of milky material or colostrum for months or even years after the birth of their last child, especially if the child was breast fed.

Vaginal Mucosa. During pregnancy, the vaginal mucosa usually appears dark bluish- or purplish-red and congested—the

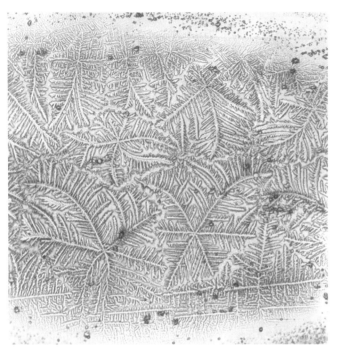

FIGURE 8-3 Photomicrograph of cervical mucus obtained on day 11 of the menstrual cycle. (Used with permission from Stephen W. Glenn on behalf of Dr. James C. Glenn.)

Chadwick sign, popularized by him in 1886. Although presumptive evidence of pregnancy, it is not conclusive.

Skin Changes. Increased pigmentation and changes in appearance of abdominal striae are common to, but not diagnostic of, pregnancy. They may be absent during pregnancy, and they may be seen in women taking estrogen-progestin contraceptives (see Chap. 5, p. 111 and Chap. 56, p. 1185).

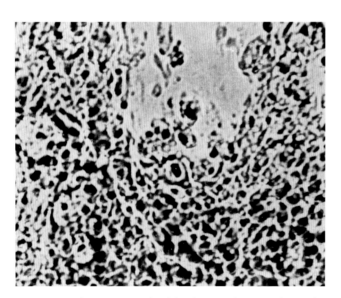

FIGURE 8-4 Photomicrograph of dried cervical mucus obtained from the cervical canal of a woman pregnant at 32 to 33 weeks. The beaded pattern is characteristic of progesterone action on the endocervical gland mucus composition. (Courtesy of Dr. J. C. Ullery.)

Changes in the Uterus. During the first few weeks of pregnancy, the increase in uterine size is limited principally to the anteroposterior diameter. By 12 weeks, the body of the uterus is almost globular with an average diameter of 8 cm. On bimanual examination, it feels doughy or elastic and sometimes becomes exceedingly soft. At 6 to 8 weeks' menstrual age, a firm cervix is felt which contrasts with the now softer fundus and compressible interposed softened isthmus—the *Hegar sign.* The softening at the isthmus may be so marked that the cervix and the body of the uterus seem to be separate organs.

When using a stethoscope for auscultation, the *uterine souffle* may be heard in the later months of pregnancy. This is a soft, blowing sound that is synchronous with the maternal pulse. It is produced by the passage of blood through the dilated uterine vessels and is heard most distinctly near the lower portion of the uterus. In contrast, the *funic souffle* is a sharp, whistling sound that is synchronous with the fetal pulse. It is caused by the rush of blood through the umbilical arteries and may not be heard consistently.

Cervical Changes. There is increased cervical softening as pregnancy advances. Other conditions, such as estrogen–progestin contraceptives, may also cause such softening. As pregnancy progresses, the external cervical os and cervical canal may become sufficiently patulous to admit the fingertip. However, the internal os should remain closed.

Perception of Fetal Movements. Maternal perception of fetal movement may depend on factors such as parity and habitus. In general, after a first successful pregnancy, a woman may first perceive fetal movements between 16 and 18 weeks. A primigravida may not appreciate fetal movements until approximately 2 weeks later (18 to 20 weeks). At approximately 20 weeks, depending on maternal habitus, an examiner can begin to detect fetal movements.

Pregnancy Tests

Detection of hCG in maternal blood and urine provides the basis for endocrine tests of pregnancy. This hormone is a glycoprotein with a high carbohydrate content. The molecule is a heterodimer composed of two dissimilar subunits, designated α and β, which are noncovalently linked (see Chap. 3, p. 63). The α-subunit is identical to those of luteinizing hormone (LH), follicle-stimulating hormone (FSH), and thyroid-stimulating hormone (TSH). HCG prevents involution of the corpus luteum, the principal site of progesterone formation during the first 6 weeks.

Trophoblast cells produce hCG in amounts that increase exponentially following implantation. With a sensitive test, the hormone can be detected in maternal plasma or urine by 8 to 9 days after ovulation. The doubling time of plasma hCG concentration is 1.4 to 2.0 days. As shown in Figure 8-5, serum hCG levels increase from the day of implantation and reach peak levels at 60 to 70 days. Thereafter, the concentration declines slowly until a nadir is reached at about 16 weeks.

Measurement of hCG. With the recognition that LH and hCG were composed of both an α- and a β-subunits, but that the β-subunits of each were structurally distinct, antibodies were

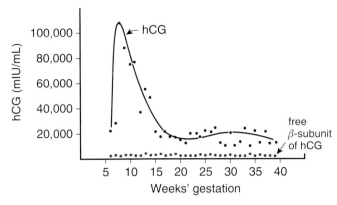

FIGURE 8-5 Mean concentration of human chorionic gonadotropin (hCG) in serum of women throughout normal pregnancy. The free β-subunit of hCG is in low concentration throughout pregnancy. (Data from Ashitaka and colleagues, 1980; Selenkow and co-workers, 1971.)

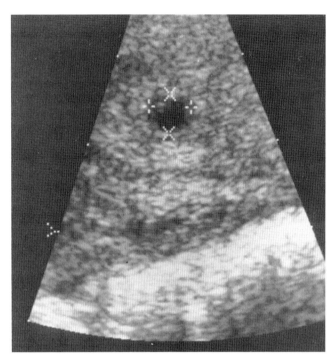

FIGURE 8-6 Abdominal sonogram demonstrating a gestational sac at 4 to 5 weeks' gestational (menstrual) age.

developed with high specificity for the β-subunit of hCG. This specificity is the basis for its detection, and numerous commercial immunoassays are available for measuring serum and urine levels of hCG. Although each immunoassay detects a slightly different mixture of hormone, its free subunits, or its metabolites, all are appropriate for pregnancy testing (Cole, 1998).

One commonly employed technique is the *sandwich-type immunoassay.* With this test, a monoclonal antibody against the β-subunit is bound to a solid-phase support. The attached antibody is then exposed to and binds hCG in the serum or urine specimen. A second antibody is then added to "sandwich" the bound hCG. In some assays, the second antibody is linked to an enzyme, such as alkaline phosphatase. When substrate for the enzyme is added, a color develops, the intensity of which is proportional to the amount of enzyme and thus to the amount of the second antibody bound. This, in turn, is a function of the amount of hCG in the test sample. The sensitivity for the laboratory detection of hCG in serum is as low as 1.0 mIU/mL using this technique. With extremely sensitive immunoradiometric assays, the detection limit is even lower (Wilcox and associates, 2001).

False-positive hCG test results are rare (Braunstein, 2002). A few women have circulating serum factors that may interact with the hCG antibody. The most common are heterophilic antibodies, which are human antibodies directed against animal-derived antigens used in immunoassays. Thus, women who have worked closely with animals are more likely to develop such antibodies and alternative laboratory techniques are available (American College of Obstetricians and Gynecologists, 2002a).

Home Pregnancy Tests. In 1999, approximately 19 million over-the-counter pregnancy test kits were sold in the United States with sales of almost $230 million (Wilcox and associates, 2001). Bastian and colleagues (1998) evaluated studies of home pregnancy test kits and found that testing done by volunteers achieved a mean 91-percent sensitivity. *Importantly, actual patients obtained only 75-percent sensitivity and a high false-negative result rate.*

Cole and colleagues (2004) also questioned the utility of home testing. They found that a detection limit of 12.5 mIU/ mL would be required to diagnose 95 percent of pregnancies at the time of

missed menses. In their study of the accuracy of 18 different home pregnancy tests, they also found that only one brand had this degree of sensitivity. Two other brands gave false-positive or invalid results. In fact, clearly positive results were given by only 44 percent of the brands at an hCG concentration of 100 mIU/mL. A test capable of detecting this level would be expected to identify only about 15 percent of pregnancies at the time of the missed menses.

Sonographic Recognition of Pregnancy

The use of transvaginal sonography has revolutionized imaging of early pregnancy and its growth and development. A gestational sac may be demonstrated by abdominal sonography after only 4 to 5 weeks' menstrual age (Fig. 8-6). By 35 days, a normal sac should be visible in all women, and after 6 weeks, heart motion should be seen. Up to 12 weeks, the crown-rump length is predictive of gestational age within 4 days (see Chap. 16, p. 350).

Initial Prenatal Evaluation

Prenatal care should be initiated as soon as there is a reasonable likelihood of pregnancy. The major goals are to:

1. Define the health status of the mother and fetus.
2. Estimate the gestational age.
3. Initiate a plan for continuing obstetrical care.

Typical components of the initial visit are summarized in Table 8-3. The initial plan for subsequent care may range from relatively infrequent routine visits to prompt hospitalization because of serious maternal or fetal disease.

Prenatal Record

Use of a standardized record within a perinatal healthcare system greatly aids antepartum and intrapartum management.

TABLE 8-3. Typical Components of Routine Prenatal Care

			Weeks		
	Text Referral	First Visit	15–20	24–28	29–41
History					
Complete	Chap. 8, p. 195	•			
Updated			•	•	•
Physical examination					
Complete	Chap. 8, p. 197	•			
Blood pressure	Chap. 34, p. 706	•	•	•	•
Maternal weight	Chap. 8, p. 200	•	•	•	•
Pelvic/cervical examination	Chap. 8, p. 197	•			
Fundal height	Chap. 8, p. 199	•	•	•	•
Fetal heart rate/position	Chap. 8, p. 200	•	•	•	•
Laboratory tests					
Hematocrit or hemoglobin	Chap. 51, p. 1079	•		•	
Blood type and Rh factor	Chap. 29, p. 618	•			
Antibody screen	Chap. 29, p. 618	•		A	
Pap smear screening	Chap. 57, p. 1201	•			
Glucose tolerance test	Chap. 52, p. 1105			•	
Fetal aneuploidy screening	Chap. 13, p. 292	B[a] and/or	B		
Neural-tube defect screening			B		
Cystic fibrosis screening	Chap. 13, p. 298	B or	B		
Urine protein assessment	Chap. 5, p. 124	•			
Urine culture	Chap. 48, p. 1034	•			
Rubella serology	Chap. 58, p. 1214	•			
Syphilis serology	Chap. 59, p. 1235	•			C
Gonococcal culture	Chap. 59, p. 1239	D			D
Chlamydial culture	Chap. 59, p. 1240	•			C
Hepatitis B serology	Chap. 59, p. 1067	•			
HIV serology	Chap. 59, p. 1246	B			
Group B streptococcus culture	Chap. 59, p. 1220				E

[a] First-trimester aneuploidy screening may be offered between 11 and 14 weeks.

HIV = human immunodeficiency virus.

A Performed at 28 weeks, if indicated.

B Test should be offered.

C High-risk women should be retested at the beginning of the third trimester.

D High-risk women should be screened at the first prenatal visit and again in the third trimester.

E Rectovaginal culture should be obtained between 35 and 37 weeks.

Standardizing documentation may allow communication and continuity of care between providers and enable objective measures of care quality to be evaluated over time and across different clinical settings (Gregory and associates, 2006). A prototype is provided by the American Academy of Pediatrics and the American College of Obstetricians and Gynecologists (2007).

Definitions. There are several definitions pertinent to establishment of an accurate prenatal record.

- *Nulligravida:* a woman who currently is not pregnant, nor has she ever been pregnant.
- *Gravida:* a woman who currently is pregnant or she has been in the past, irrespective of the pregnancy outcome. With the establishment of the first pregnancy, she becomes

a *primigravida,* and with successive pregnancies, a *multigravida.*

- *Nullipara:* a woman who has never completed a pregnancy beyond 20 weeks' gestation. She may or may not have been pregnant or may have had a spontaneous or elective abortion(s) or an ectopic pregnancy.
- *Primipara:* a woman who has been delivered only once of a fetus or fetuses born alive or dead with an estimated length of gestation of 20 or more weeks. In the past, a 500-g birthweight threshold was used to define parity. This threshold is no longer as pertinent because of the survival of infants with birthweights less than 500 g.
- *Multipara:* a woman who has completed two or more pregnancies to 20 weeks or more. Parity is determined by the

number of pregnancies reaching 20 weeks and not by the number of fetuses delivered. *Parity is the same (para 1) for a singleton or multifetal delivery or delivery of a live or stillborn infant.*

In some locales, the obstetrical history is summarized by a series of digits connected by dashes. These refer to the number of term infants, preterm infants, abortuses less than 20 weeks, and children currently alive. For example, a woman who is para 2–1–0–3 has had two term deliveries, one preterm delivery, and no abortuses, and has three living children. Because these are nonconventional, it is helpful to specify the outcome of any pregnancy that did not end normally.

Normal Pregnancy Duration. The mean duration of pregnancy calculated from the first day of the last normal menstrual period is very close to 280 days or 40 weeks. In a study of 427,581 singleton pregnancies from the Swedish Birth Registry, Bergsjø and colleagues (1990) found that the mean duration of pregnancy was 281 days with a standard deviation of 13 days.

It is customary to estimate the expected date of delivery by adding 7 days to the date of the first day of the last normal menstrual period and counting back 3 months—*Naegele's rule.* For example, if the last menstrual period began September 10, the expected date of delivery is June 17. A *gestational age* or *menstrual age* calculated in this way erroneously assumes pregnancy to have begun approximately 2 weeks before ovulation. Clinicians use this gestational age to mark temporal events during pregnancy. In contrast, embryologists and other reproductive biologists more often employ *ovulatory age* or *fertilization age,* both of which are typically 2 weeks shorter. Somewhat related, Bracken and Belanger (1989) tested the accuracy of various "pregnancy wheels" provided by three pharmaceutical companies and found that such devices predicted incorrect delivery dates in 40 to 60 percent of estimates, with a 5-day error being typical.

Trimesters. It has become customary to divide pregnancy into three equal epochs of approximately 3 calendar months. Historically, the first trimester extends through completion of 14 weeks, the second through 28 weeks, and the third includes the 29th through 42nd weeks of pregnancy. Thus, there are three periods of 14 weeks each. Certain major obstetrical problems tend to cluster in each of these time periods. For example, most spontaneous abortions take place during the first trimester, whereas most women with hypertensive disorders due to pregnancy are diagnosed during the third trimester.

In modern obstetrics, the clinical use of trimesters to describe a specific pregnancy is too imprecise. For example, it is inappropriate in cases of uterine hemorrhage to categorize the problem temporally as "third-trimester bleeding." Appropriate management for the mother and her fetus will vary remarkably, depending on whether bleeding begins early or late in the third trimester (see Chap. 35, p. 757). Because precise knowledge of fetal age is imperative for ideal obstetrical management, the clinically appropriate unit is *weeks of gestation completed.* And more recently, clinicians designate gestational age using completed weeks and days, for example, $33^{4/7}$ weeks or 33 + 4, for 33 completed weeks and 4 days.

History

For the most part, the same essentials go into appropriate history-taking from the pregnant woman as elsewhere in medicine. **Detailed information concerning past obstetrical history is crucial because many prior pregnancy complications tend to recur in subsequent pregnancies.**

The *menstrual history* is extremely important. The woman who spontaneously menstruates regularly every 28 days or so is most likely to ovulate at midcycle. Thus, gestational or menstrual age is the number of weeks since the onset of the last menstrual period. If her menstrual cycles were significantly longer than 28 to 30 days, ovulation more likely occurred well beyond 14 days. If the intervals were much longer and irregular, chronic anovulation is likely to have preceded some of the episodes identified as menses. *Without a history of regular, predictable, cyclic, spontaneous menses that suggest ovulatory cycles, accurate dating of pregnancy by history and physical examination is difficult.*

It is also important to ascertain whether or not *steroidal contraceptives* were used before the pregnancy. Because ovulation may not have resumed 2 weeks after the onset of the last withdrawal bleeding and instead may have occurred at an appreciably later and highly variable date, using the time of ovulation for predicting the time of conception in this circumstance may be erroneous. Use of sonography in early pregnancy will clarify gestational age in these situations.

Psychosocial Screening. The American College of Obstetricians and Gynecologists (2006) defines psychosocial risk factors as nonbiomedical factors that affect mental and physical well-being. The College advocates psychosocial screening at least once each trimester to increase the likelihood of identifying important issues and reducing adverse pregnancy outcomes. Screening for barriers to care includes lack of transportation, child care, or family support; unstable housing; unintended pregnancy; communication barriers; nutritional problems; cigarette smoking; substance abuse; depression; and safety concerns that include domestic violence. Such screening is performed regardless of social status, education level, or race and ethnicity. Shown in Table 8-4 is one recommended screening tool.

Cigarette Smoking. Smoking results in unequivocal adverse sequelae for pregnant women and their fetuses (United States Department of Health and Human Services, 2000). Maternal smoking data has been included on the birth certificate since 1989. The number of pregnant women who smoke continues to decline, and from 1990 to 2003, the reported rate decreased from 18 to 13 percent (American College of Obstetricians and Gynecologists, 2005b; Martin and associates, 2009). According to the Centers for Disease Control and Prevention (2007), 13 percent of women admitted to smoking during the last 3 months of pregnancy. Those most likely to smoke were younger and had less education.

Numerous adverse outcomes have been linked to smoking during pregnancy. Potential teratogenic effects are reviewed in Chapter 14 (p. 329). There is a twofold risk of placenta previa, placental abruption, and premature membrane rupture compared with nonsmokers. Further, babies born to women who

TABLE 8-4. Psychosocial Screening Tool

1. Yes   No   Do you have any problems (job, transportation, etc.) that prevent you from keeping your healthcare appointments?
2. Yes   No   Do you feel unsafe where you live?
3. Yes   No   In the past 2 months, have you used any form of tobacco?
4. Yes   No   In the past 2 months, have you used drugs or alcohol (including beer, wine, or mixed drinks)?
5. Yes   No   In the past year, have you been threatened, hit, slapped, or kicked by anyone you know?
6. Yes   No   Has anyone forced you to perform any sexual act that you did not want to do?
7. On a 1-to-5 scale, how do you rate your current stress level?

    1   2   3   4   5
    low   high

8. How many times have you moved in the past 12 months? _____
9. If you could change the timing of this pregnancy, would you want it: __ earlier; __ later; __ not at all; __ no change.

Reprinted, with permission, from Psychosocial risk factors: Perinatal screening intervention. ACOG Committee Opinion No. 343. American College of Obstetricians and Gynecologists. Obstet Gynecol 2006; 108:469.

smoke are approximately 30 percent more likely to be born preterm, weigh on average a half pound less, and are up to three times more likely to die of sudden infant death syndrome (SIDS) than infants born to nonsmokers (Centers for Disease Control and Prevention, 2007). In 2001, the incidence of low-birthweight infants born to American women who smoked during pregnancy was 11.9 percent compared with 7.3 percent born to nonsmokers (Martin and co-workers, 2002b). Finally, risks for spontaneous abortion, fetal death, and fetal digital anomalies are also increased (Man and Chang, 2006).

A number of pathophysiological mechanisms have been proposed to explain these adverse outcomes. They include fetal hypoxia from increased carboxyhemoglobin, reduced uteroplacental blood flow, and direct toxic effects of nicotine and other compounds in smoke (American College of Obstetricians and Gynecologists, 2005b; Jazayeri and colleagues, 1998). Nicotine transfer is so efficient that fetal nicotine exposure is greater than that of the mother (Luck and associates, 1985). Exposed fetuses have decreased heart rate variability, due to impaired autonomic regulation (Zeskind and colleagues, 2006). According to the American Academy of Pediatrics and the American College of Obstetricians and Gynecologists (2007), perinatal mortality rates would be reduced by 5 percent if maternal smoking was eliminated.

Smoking Cessation. The most successful efforts for smoking cessation during pregnancy involve interventions that emphasize how to stop. One example is a 5-step session lasting 15 minutes or less in which the provider: (1) *Asks* about smoking status; (2) *Advises* those who smoke to stop; (3) *Assesses* the willingness to quit within the next 30 days; (4) *Assists* interested patients by providing pregnancy-specific self-help materials; and (5) *Arranges* follow-up visits to track progress (American College of Obstetricians and Gynecologists, 2005b).

Nicotine replacement products have not been sufficiently evaluated to determine their effectiveness and safety in pregnancy. Interdiction is optimal—but not always pragmatic—before conception. Thus, the American College of Obstetricians

and Gynecologists (2005b) has concluded that it is reasonable to use nicotine medications during pregnancy if prior nonpharmacological attempts have failed. Wisborg and co-workers (2000) randomly assigned 250 women who smoked at least 10 cigarettes per day to receive a nicotine or a placebo patch beginning after the first trimester. Overall, 26 percent of these women stopped smoking, but there were no significant differences in smoking cessation, birthweight, or preterm delivery between the two groups. Importantly, no serious adverse effects from the patches were reported, but compliance with either treatment was low.

Alcohol Use During Pregnancy. Ethanol is a potent teratogen and can cause fetal alcohol syndrome characterized by growth restriction, facial abnormalities, and central nervous system dysfunction (see Chap. 14, p. 317). Women who are pregnant or considering pregnancy should abstain from using any alcoholic beverages. Such use is substantively underreported on the birth certificate—less than 1 percent of women reported any alcohol use during pregnancy in 2001 (Martin and colleagues, 2002b). But, according to the Centers for Disease Control and Prevention (2002a), approximately 13 percent of pregnant women used alcohol in 1999. Although this was down from 16 percent in 1995, it is unfortunate that rates of binge and frequent drinking during pregnancy have not declined.

Illicit Drug Use. It is estimated that 10 percent of fetuses are exposed to one or more illicit drugs (American Academy of Pediatrics and the American College of Obstetricians and Gynecologists, 2007). Agents may include heroin and other opiates, cocaine, amphetamines, barbiturates, and marijuana. Chronic use of large quantities is harmful to the fetus. Well-documented sequelae include fetal distress, low birthweight, and drug withdrawal soon after birth. Women who use such drugs frequently do not seek prenatal care or if they do, they may not admit to the use of such substances. El-Mohandes and associates (2003) reported that when women who use illicit drugs receive prenatal care, the risks for preterm birth and low birthweight are reduced.

The effects of several illicit drugs are considered in detail in Chapter 14 (p. 326). The American College of Obstetricians and Gynecologists (1999) has reviewed methods for screening women during pregnancy for use of illicit drugs and for alcohol abuse.

Domestic Violence Screening. The term *domestic violence* usually refers to violence against adolescent and adult females within the context of family or intimate relationships. Such violence has been increasingly recognized as a major public health problem (see Chap. 42, p. 936). Unfortunately, most abused women continue to be victimized during pregnancy. With the possible exception of preeclampsia, domestic violence is more prevalent than any major medical condition detectable through routine prenatal screening (American Academy of Pediatrics and the American College of Obstetricians and Gynecologists, 2007). The prevalence during pregnancy is estimated to be between 4 and 8 percent. As discussed in Chapter 42 (p. 936), intimate partner violence is associated with an increased risk of a number of adverse perinatal outcomes including preterm delivery, fetal-growth restriction, and perinatal death.

The American College of Obstetricians and Gynecologists (2006) has provided methods for screening for domestic violence and recommends their use at the first prenatal visit, then again at least once per trimester, and again at the postpartum visit. Webster and Holt (2004) found that a simple, six-question self-report survey is an effective alternative to direct questioning for identifying pregnant women who are experiencing partner violence. Physicians should be familiar with state laws that may require reporting of domestic violence—for example, child abuse is always reportable. Coordination with social services can be invaluable in such cases.

Physical Examination

A thorough, general physical examination should be completed at the initial prenatal encounter. Expected changes in physical examination findings resulting from normal pregnancy are addressed throughout Chapters 2 and 5.

Pelvic Examination. The cervix is visualized employing a speculum lubricated with warm water or water-based lubricant gel. Bluish-red passive hyperemia of the cervix is characteristic, but not of itself diagnostic, of pregnancy. Dilated, occluded cervical glands bulging beneath the ectocervical mucosa—*nabothian cysts*—may be prominent. The cervix is not normally dilated except at the external os. To identify cytological abnormalities, a Pap smear is performed, and specimens for identification of *Chlamydia trachomatis* and *Neisseria gonorrhoeae* are obtained.

Bimanual examination is completed by palpation, with special attention given to the consistency, length, and dilatation of the cervix; to uterine size and any adnexal masses; to the fetal presentation later in pregnancy; to the bony architecture of the pelvis; and to any anomalies of the vagina and perineum. All cervical, vaginal, and vulvar lesions are evaluated further by appropriate use of colposcopy, biopsy, culture, or dark-field examination. The perianal region should be visualized and digital rectal examination performed.

Laboratory Tests

Recommended routine tests at the first prenatal encounter are listed in Table 8-3 and normal ranges for pregnancy are found in the Appendix. The Institute of Medicine recommends universal human immunodeficiency virus (HIV) testing, with patient notification and right of refusal, as a routine part of prenatal care. The Centers for Disease Control and Prevention (2006b) as well as the American Academy of Pediatrics and the American College of Obstetricians and Gynecologists (2007) support this recommendation. If a woman declines testing, this should be recorded in the prenatal record. Pregnant women should also be screened for hepatitis B virus. Based on their prospective investigation of 1000 women, Murray and co-workers (2002) concluded that in the absence of hypertension, routine urinalysis beyond the initial prenatal visit was not necessary.

Chlamydial Infection. *Chlamydia trachomatis* is isolated from the cervix in 2 to 13 percent of pregnant women. The American Academy of Pediatrics and the American College of Obstetricians and Gynecologists (2007) recommend that all women be screened during the first prenatal visit, with additional third-trimester testing for those at increased risk. Risk factors include unmarried status, recent change in sexual partner or multiple concurrent partners, age under 25 years, inner-city residence, history or presence of other sexually transmitted diseases, and little or no prenatal care. Following treatment, repeat testing is recommended in 3 weeks (see Chap. 59, p. 1240). A negative prenatal test for chlamydia or gonorrhea should not preclude postpartum screening (Mahon and associates, 2002).

High-Risk Pregnancies

There are many risk factors that can be identified and given appropriate consideration in pregnancy management. Examples of common risk factors proposed by the American Academy of Pediatrics and the American College of Obstetricians and Gynecologists (2007) are shown in Table 8-5. In addition, Table 8-6 lists ongoing risk factors for which consultation may be indicated. Some conditions may require the involvement of a maternal-fetal medicine subspecialist, geneticist, pediatrician, anesthesiologist, or other medical specialist in the evaluation, counseling, and care of the woman and her fetus.

Subsequent Prenatal Visits

Subsequent prenatal visits have been traditionally scheduled at intervals of 4 weeks until 28 weeks, and then every 2 weeks until 36 weeks, and weekly thereafter. Women with complicated pregnancies often require return visits at 1- to 2-week intervals. For example, Luke and co-workers (2003) found that a specialized prenatal care program that emphasized nutrition and education and that required return visits every 2 weeks resulted in improved outcomes in twin pregnancies.

In 1986, the Department of Health and Human Services convened an expert panel to review the content of prenatal care. This report was subsequently re-evaluated and revised in 2005 (Gregory and associates, 2006). The panel recommended, among other things, early and continuing risk assessment that

TABLE 8-5. Recommended Consultation for Risk Factors Identified in Early Pregnancy[a]

Medical History and Conditions	
Asthma	
Symptomatic on medication	OBG
Severe (multiple hospitalizations)	MFM
Cardiac disease	
Cyanotic, prior myocardial infarction, aortic stenosis, pulmonary hypertension, Marfan syndrome, prosthetic valve, American Heart Association class II or greater (see Chap. 44, p. 959)	MFM
Other	OBG
Diabetes mellitus	
Class A–C	OBG
Class D or greater	MFM
Drug and alcohol use	OBG
Epilepsy (on medication)	OBG
Family history of genetic problems	
(Down syndrome, Tay-Sachs disease, phenylketonuria)	MFM
Hemoglobinopathy (SS, SC, S-thalassemia)	MFM
Hypertension	
Chronic, with renal or heart disease	MFM
Chronic, without renal or heart disease	OBG
Prior pulmonary embolus or deep vein thrombosis	OBG
Psychiatric illness	OBG
Pulmonary disease	
Severe obstructive or restrictive	MFM
Moderate	OBG
Renal disease	
Chronic, creatinine $\geq$ 3 mg/dL, $\pm$ hypertension	MFM
Chronic, other	OBG
Requirement for prolonged anticoagulation	MFM
Severe systemic disease	MFM
Obstetrical History and Conditions	
Age $\geq$35 years at delivery	OBG
Cesarean delivery, prior classical or vertical incision	OBG
Incompetent cervix	OBG
Prior fetal structural or chromosomal abnormality	MFM
Prior neonatal death	OBG
Prior fetal death	OBG
Prior preterm delivery or preterm ruptured membranes	OBG
Prior low birthweight (<2500 g)	OBG
Second-trimester pregnancy loss	OBG
Uterine leiomyomas or malformation	OBG
Initial Laboratory Tests	
Human immunodeficiency virus (HIV)	
Symptomatic or low CD4 count	MFM
Other	OBG
CDE (Rh) of other blood group isoimmunization (excluding ABO, Lewis)	MFM
Initial examination condylomata (extensive, covering vulva or vaginal opening)	OBG

[a] At the time of consultation, continued patient care should be determined by collaboration with the referring care provider or by transfer of care.

Used with permission of the American Academy of Pediatrics, American College of Obstetricians and Gynecologists. Guidelines for perinatal care. 6th ed. Elk Grove Village (IL): AAP; Washington, DC: ACOG; 2007. Copyright American Academy of Pediatrics and American College of Obstetricans and Gynecologists, 2007.

TABLE 8-6. Recommended Consultation for Ongoing Risk Factors Identified During Pregnancy[a]

Medical History and Conditions

Drugs/alcohol use	OBG
Proteinuria (≥2+ on catheterized sample, unexplained by urinary infection)	OBG
Pyelonephritis	OBG
Severe systemic disease that adversely affects pregnancy	OBG

Obstetrical History and Conditions

Blood pressure elevation (diastolic BP ≥90 mm Hg), no proteinuria	OBG
Fetal-growth restriction suspected	OBG
Fetal abnormality suspected by sonography	
Anencephaly	OBG
Other	MFM
Fetal demise	OBG
Gestational age 41 weeks	OBG
Herpes, active lesion at 36 weeks	OBG
Hydramnios or oligohydramnios by sonography	OBG
Hyperemesis, persistent, beyond first trimester	OBG
Multifetal gestation	OBG
Preterm labor, threatened	OBG
Premature rupture of membranes	OBG
Vaginal bleeding ≥14 weeks	OBG

Examination and Laboratory Findings

Abnormal MSAFP (high or low)	OBG
Abnormal Pap smear result	OBG
Anemia (hematocrit <28 percent, unresponsive to iron therapy)	OBG
Condylomata (extensive, covering labia and vaginal opening)	OBG
HIV	
Symptomatic or low CD4 count	MFM
Other	OBG
CDE (Rh) or other blood group isoimmunization (excluding ABO, Lewis)	MFM

[a] At the time of consultation, continued patient care should be determined by collaboration with the referring care provider or by transfer of care.
OBG = obstetrician-gynecologist; MFM = Maternal-fetal medicine specialist.
Used with permission of the American Academy of Pediatrics, American College of Obstetricians and Gynecologists. Guidelines for perinatal care. 6th ed. Elk Grove Village (IL): AAP; Washington, DC: ACOG; 2007. Copyright American Academy of Pediatrics and American College of Obstetricans and Gynecologists, 2007.

is patient specific, with flexibility of clinical visits; health promotion and education, including preconceptional care; medical and psychosocial interventions; standardized documentation; and expanded objectives of prenatal care—to include the health of the family up to 1 year after birth of the infant.

The World Health Organization conducted a multicenter randomized trial with almost 25,000 women comparing routine prenatal care with an experimental model designed to minimize visits (Villar and associates, 2001). In the new model, women were seen once in the first trimester and screened for certain risk factors. Those without any anticipated complications—80 percent of the women screened—were seen again at 26, 32, and 38 weeks. Compared with routine prenatal care, which required a median of eight visits, the new model required a median of only five visits. No disadvantages were found in women with fewer visits, and these findings were consistent with other randomized trials (Clement and co-workers, 1999; McDuffie and colleagues, 1996).

Prenatal Surveillance

At each return visit, steps are taken to determine the well-being of mother and fetus (see Table 8-3). Certain information is considered especially important—an example is assessment of gestational age and accurate measurement of blood pressure (Jones and associates, 2003). Evaluation typically includes:

Fetal
- Heart rate(s)
- Size—current and rate of change
- Amount of amnionic fluid
- Presenting part and station (late in pregnancy)
- Activity

Maternal
- Blood pressure—current and extent of change
- Weight—current and amount of change
- Symptoms—including headache, altered vision, abdominal pain, nausea and vomiting, bleeding, vaginal fluid leakage, and dysuria
- Height in centimeters of uterine fundus from symphysis
- Vaginal examination late in pregnancy often provides valuable information to include:
  1. Confirmation of the presenting part and its station (see Chap. 17, p. 374).
  2. Clinical estimation of pelvic capacity and its general configuration (see Chap. 2, p. 31).
  3. Consistency, effacement, and dilatation of the cervix.

Assessment of Gestational Age

This is one of the most important determinations at prenatal examinations. Precise knowledge of gestational age is important because a number of pregnancy complications may develop for which optimal treatment will depend on fetal age. Fortunately, it is possible to identify gestational age with considerable precision through an appropriately timed, carefully performed clinical examination, coupled with knowledge of the time of onset of the last menstrual period.

Fundal Height. Between 20 and 34 weeks, the height of the uterine fundus measured in centimeters correlates closely with gestational age in weeks (Calvert, 1982; Jimenez, 1983; Quaranta, 1981, and all their associates). The fundal height should be measured as the distance over the abdominal wall from the top of the symphysis pubis to the top of the fundus. *The bladder must be emptied before making the measurement.* For example, Worthen and Bustillo (1980) demonstrated that at 17 to 20 weeks, fundal height was 3 cm higher with a full bladder. Obesity may also distort this relationship. Unfortunately, using fundal height alone, fetal-growth restriction may be undiagnosed in up to a third of cases (American College of Obstetricians and Gynecologists, 2000).

Fetal Heart Sounds. The fetal heart can first be heard in most women between 16 and 19 weeks when carefully auscultated with a standard nonamplified stethoscope. The ability to hear unamplified fetal heart sounds will depend on factors such as patient size and hearing acuity of the examiner. Herbert and co-workers (1987) reported that the fetal heart was audible by 20 weeks in 80 percent of women. By 21 weeks, audible fetal heart sounds were present in 95 percent, and by 22 weeks they were heard in all. The fetal heart rate now ranges from 110 to 160 bpm and is heard as a double sound resembling the tick of a watch under a pillow. Because the fetus moves freely in amnionic fluid, the site on the maternal abdomen where fetal heart sounds can be heard best will vary.

Instruments incorporating Doppler ultrasound instruments are often used to easily detect fetal heart action, almost always by 10 weeks (see Chap. 18, p. 412). Using real-time sonography with a vaginal transducer, fetal cardiac activity can be seen as early as 5 menstrual weeks.

Sonography. In the United States, about two thirds of women have at least one prenatal sonographic examination (Martin and colleagues, 2005). And within the past decade, many women have an initial sonographic evaluation as part of first-trimester aneuploidy screening, followed by a standard examination in the second trimester to evaluate fetal anatomy. Indications for sonography are reviewed in Chapter 13 (p. 294). The American College of Obstetricians and Gynecologists (2009) has concluded that a physician is not obligated to perform sonography without a specific indication in a low-risk patient, but that if she requests sonography, it is reasonable to honor her request.

Subsequent Laboratory Tests

If initial results were normal, most tests need not be repeated (see Table 8-3). Fetal aneuploidy screening may be performed at 11 to 14 weeks and/or at 15 to 20 weeks, depending on the protocol selected (see Chap. 13, p. 292). Serum screening for neural-tube defects is offered at 15 to 20 weeks (see Chap. 13, p. 287). Hematocrit or hemoglobin determination, along with syphilis serology if it is prevalent in the population, should be repeated at 28 to 32 weeks (Hollier and co-workers, 2003; Kiss and colleagues, 2004). Women who are D (Rh) negative and are unsensitized should have an antibody screening test repeated at 28 to 29 weeks, with administration of anti-D immune globulin if they remain unsensitized.

Cystic fibrosis carrier screening should be offered to couples with a family history of cystic fibrosis and to Caucasian couples of European or Ashkenazi Jewish descent planning a pregnancy or seeking prenatal care. Ideally, screening is performed before conception or during the first or early second trimester. Information about cystic fibrosis screening also should be provided to patients in other racial and ethnic groups who are at lower risk (see Chap. 13, p. 298).

Group B Streptococcal (GBS) Infection. The American College of Obstetricians and Gynecologists (2002c) and the Cen-

ters for Disease Control and Prevention (2002b) recommend that vaginal and rectal GBS cultures be obtained in all women between 35 and 37 weeks. Intrapartum antimicrobial prophylaxis is given for those whose cultures are positive. Women with GBS bacteriuria or a previous infant with invasive disease are given empirical intrapartum prophylaxis. These infections are discussed in detail in Chapter 58 (p. 1220).

Gestational Diabetes. All pregnant women should be screened for gestational diabetes mellitus, whether by history, clinical factors, or routine laboratory testing. Although laboratory testing between 24 and 28 weeks is the most sensitive approach, there may be pregnant women at low risk who are less likely to benefit from testing (American Academy of Pediatrics and American College of Obstetricians and Gynecologists, 2007). Gestational diabetes is discussed in Chapter 52 (p. 1104).

Gonococcal Infection. Risk factors for gonorrhea are similar for those for *Chlamydia*. The American Academy of Pediatrics and the American College of Obstetricians and Gynecologists (2007) recommend that pregnant women with risk factors or symptoms be tested for *N. gonorrhoeae* at an early prenatal visit and again in the third trimester. Treatment is given for gonorrhea as well as possible coexisting chlamydial infection, as outlined in Chapter 59 (p. 1239).

Special Screening for Genetic Diseases. Selected screening should be offered to couples at increased risk based on family history or the ethnic or racial background (American College of Obstetricians and Gynecologists, 2004c, 2005c). These are discussed further in Chapters 12 (p. 275) and 13 (p. 296). Some examples include testing for Tay-Sachs disease for people of Eastern European Jewish or French Canadian ancestry; β-thalassemia for those of Mediterranean, Southeast Asian, Indian, Pakistani, or African ancestry; α-thalassemia for people of Southeast Asian or African ancestry; and sickle-cell anemia for people of African, Mediterranean, Middle Eastern, Caribbean, Latin American, or Indian descent.

NUTRITION

Recommendations for Weight Gain

For the first half of the 20th century, it was recommended that weight gain during pregnancy be limited to less than 20 lb or 9.1 kg. It was believed that such restriction would prevent gestational hypertension and fetal macrosomia. By the 1970s, however, women were encouraged to gain at least 25 lb or 11.4 kg to prevent preterm birth and fetal-growth restriction, a recommendation supported by subsequent research (Ehrenberg and associates, 2003). In 1990, the Institute of Medicine recommended a weight gain of 25 to 35 lb—11.5 to 16 kg—for women with a normal prepregnancy body mass index (BMI). This index is easily calculated using the chart shown in Figure 43-1 (p. 947). Weight gains recommended by the Institute of Medicine (1990) according to prepregnant BMI categories are shown in Table 8-7. The American Academy of Pediatrics and the American College of Obstetricians and Gynecologists (2007) have endorsed these guidelines. It is problematic,

TABLE 8-7. Recommended Ranges of Weight Gain During Singleton Gestations Stratified by Prepregnancy Body Mass Index[a]

Weight-for-Height Category		Recommended Total Weight Gain	
Category	BMI	kg	lb
Low	< 19.8	12.5–18	28–40
Normal	19.8–26	11.5–16	25–35
High	26–29	7–11.5	15–25
Obese	> 29	≥ 7	≥ 15

[a] The range for twin pregnancy is 35 to 45 lb (16 to 20 kg). Young adolescents (< 2 years after menarche) and African-American women should strive for gains at the upper end of the range. Shorter women (< 62 in. or < 157 cm) should strive for gains at the lower end of the range. BMI = body mass index.
From the Institute of Medicine (1990), with permission.

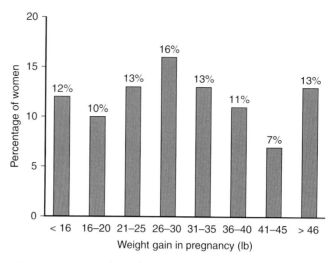

FIGURE 8-7 Maternal weight gains in the United States reported on the birth certificate in 2006. (From Martin and colleagues, 2009.)

however, that in 2003, 46 percent of women had weight gains above these guidelines (Catalano, 2007).

It has been recently emphasized by Catalano (2007) that when the Institute of Medicine guidelines were written, concern was focused on the low-birthweight infant, whereas currently the focus is on the obesity epidemic. This likely explains renewed interest in *lower* weight gains during pregnancy. As discussed in Chapter 43 (p. 949), obesity is associated with significantly increased risks for gestational hypertension, preeclampsia, gestational diabetes, macrosomia, and cesarean delivery. The risk appears "dose related" to prenatal weight gain. In a population-based cohort of more than 120,000 obese pregnant women, Kiel and associates (2007) found that those who gained *less than 15 pounds* had the lowest rates of preeclampsia, large-for-gestational age infants, and cesarean delivery. Among 100,000 women with normal prepregnancy body mass index, DeVader and colleagues (2007) found that those who gained less than 25 pounds during pregnancy had a lower risk for preeclampsia, failed induction, cephalopelvic disproportion, cesarean delivery, and large-for-gestational age infants. This cohort, however, had an increased risk for small-for-gestational age infants.

Overnutrition

There is irrefutable evidence that maternal weight gain during pregnancy influences birthweight. Martin and colleagues (2009) studied this using birth certificate data for 2006. As shown in Figure 8-7, 60 percent of pregnant women gained 26 lb or more. Maternal weight gain had a positive correlation with birthweight, and women with the greatest risk—14 percent—for delivering an infant weighing less than 2500 g were those with weight gains less than 16 lb. Nearly nineteen percent of births to women with such low weight gains were preterm. Cohen and associates (2001) studied more than 4000 pregnant women and concluded that ethnic differences in pregnancy outcomes were not explained by nutritional variations.

Severe Undernutrition

Meaningful studies of nutrition in human pregnancy are exceedingly difficult to design because experimental dietary deficiency is not ethical. In those instances in which severe nutritional deficiencies have been induced as a consequence of social, economic, or political disaster, coincidental events often have created many variables, the effects of which are not amenable to quantification. Some past experiences suggest, however, that in otherwise healthy women, a state of near starvation is required to establish clear differences in pregnancy outcome.

During the severe European winter of 1944–1945, nutritional deprivation of known intensity prevailed in a well-circumscribed area of The Netherlands occupied by the German military (Kyle and Pichard, 2006). At the lowest point during this *Dutch Hunger Winter,* rations reached 450 kcal/day, with generalized rather than selective malnutrition. Smith (1947) analyzed the outcomes of pregnancies that were in progress during this 6-month famine. Median infant birthweights decreased approximately 250 g and rose again after food became available. This indicated that birthweight can be influenced significantly by starvation during later pregnancy. The perinatal mortality rate, however, was not altered, nor was the incidence of malformations significantly increased. Interestingly, the frequency of pregnancy "toxemia" was found to decline.

Evidence of impaired brain development has been obtained in some animal fetuses whose mothers had been subjected to intense dietary deprivation. Subsequent intellectual development was studied by Stein and associates (1972) in young male adults whose mothers had been starved during pregnancy. The comprehensive study was made possible because all males at age 19 underwent compulsory examination for military service. It was concluded that severe dietary deprivation during pregnancy caused no detectable effects on subsequent mental performance.

A number of studies of the long-term consequences to this cohort of children born to nutritionally deprived women have been performed and were recently reviewed by Kyle and Pichard

(2006). Progeny exposed in mid to late pregnancy were lighter, shorter, and thinner at birth, and they had a higher incidence of subsequent diminished glucose tolerance, hypertension, reactive airway disease, dyslipidemia, and coronary artery disease. Early pregnancy exposure was associated with increased obesity in adult women but not men. Early exposure was also associated with increased central nervous system anomalies, schizophrenia, and schizophrenia-spectrum personality disorders.

These observations, as well as others, have led to the concept of *fetal programming* by which adult morbidity and mortality are related to fetal health. Known widely as the *Barker hypothesis*, as promulgated by Barker and colleagues (1989), this concept is discussed in Chapter 38 (p. 853).

Weight Retention after Pregnancy

Not all the weight gained during pregnancy is lost during and immediately after delivery (Hytten, 1991). Schauberger and co-workers (1992) studied prenatal and postpartum weights in 795 Wisconsin women. Their average weight gain was 28.6 lb or 4.8 kg. As shown in Figure 8-8, most maternal weight loss was at delivery—approximately 12 lb or 5.5 kg—and in the ensuing 2 weeks thereafter—approximately 9 lb or 4 kg. An additional 5.5 lb or 2.5 kg was lost between 2 weeks and 6 months postpartum. Thus, average total weight loss resulted in an average retained pregnancy weight of 3 lb or 1.4 kg. Overall, the more weight gained during pregnancy, the more that was lost postpartum. Interestingly, there is no relationship between prepregnancy BMI or prenatal weight gain and weight retention (American Academy of Pediatrics and American College of Obstetricians and Gynecologists, 2005a, 2007). Accruing weight with age—rather than parity—is considered the main factor affecting weight gain over time.

Recommended Dietary Allowances

Periodically, the Food and Nutrition Board of the Institute of Medicine (2008) publishes recommended dietary allowances,

including those for pregnant or lactating women. The latest recommendations are summarized in Table 8-8. Certain prenatal vitamin–mineral supplements may lead to intakes well in excess of the recommended allowances. Moreover, the use of excessive supplements, which often are self-prescribed, has led to concern about nutrient toxicities during pregnancy. Those with potentially toxic effects include iron, zinc, selenium, and vitamins A, B_6, C, and D. In particular, excessive vitamin A—more than 10,000 IU per day—may be teratogenic (see Chap. 14, p. 324). Vitamin and mineral intake more than twice the recommended daily dietary allowance shown in Table 8-8 should be avoided (American Academy of Pediatrics and American College of Obstetricians and Gynecologists, 2007).

Calories

As shown in Figure 8-9, pregnancy requires an additional 80,000 kcal—most are accumulated in the last 20 weeks. To meet this demand, a caloric increase of 100 to 300 kcal per day is recommended during pregnancy (American Academy of Pediatrics and American College of Obstetricians and Gynecologists, 2007). Calories are necessary for energy, and whenever caloric intake is inadequate, protein is metabolized rather than being spared for its vital role in fetal growth and development. Total physiological requirements during pregnancy are not necessarily the sum of ordinary nonpregnant requirements plus those specific to pregnancy. For example, the additional energy required during pregnancy may be compensated in whole or in part by reduced physical activity (Hytten, 1991).

Protein

To the basic protein needs of the nonpregnant woman are added the demands for growth and remodeling of the fetus, placenta, uterus, and breasts, as well as increased maternal blood volume (see Chap. 5, p. 113). During the second half of pregnancy, approximately 1000 g of protein are deposited, amounting to 5 to 6 g/day (Hytten and Leitch, 1971). The concentrations of most amino acids in maternal plasma fall markedly, including ornithine, glycine, taurine, and proline (Hytten, 1991). Exceptions during pregnancy are glutamic acid and alanine, which rise in concentration.

Preferably, most protein should be supplied from animal sources, such as meat, milk, eggs, cheese, poultry, and fish, because they furnish amino acids in optimal combinations. Milk and dairy products have long been considered nearly ideal sources of nutrients, especially protein and calcium, for pregnant or lactating women. Ingestion of specific fish and methylmercury toxicity are discussed on page 206.

Minerals

The intakes recommended by the Institute of Medicine (2008) for a variety of minerals are presented in Table 8-8. With the exception of iron, practically all diets that supply sufficient calories for appropriate weight gain will contain enough minerals to prevent deficiency if iodized foods are ingested.

Iron. The reasons for substantively increased iron requirements during pregnancy are discussed in Chapter 5 (p. 115). Of the approximately 300 mg of iron transferred to the fetus and

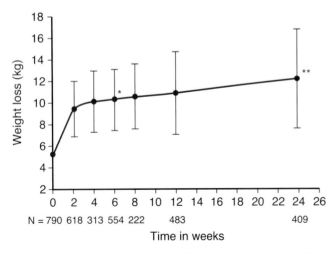

FIGURE 8-8 Cumulative weight loss from last antepartum visit to 6 months' postpartum. *Statistically different from 2-week weight loss, **Statistically different from 6-week weight loss. (From Schauberger and co-workers, 1992, with permission.)

TABLE 8-8. Recommended Daily Dietary Allowances for Adolescent and Adult Pregnant and Lactating Women

	Pregnant		Lactating	
Age (years)	14–18	19–50	14–18	19–50
Fat-soluble vitamins				
Vitamin A	750 μg	770 μg	1200 μg	1300 μg
Vitamin D[a]	5 μg	5 μg	5 μg	5 μg
Vitamin E	15 mg	15mg	19 mg	19 mg
Vitamin K[a]	75 μg	90 μg	75 μg	90 μg
Water-soluble vitamins				
Vitamin C	80 mg	85 mg	115 mg	120 mg
Thiamin	1.4 mg	1.4 mg	1.4 mg	1.4 mg
Riboflavin	1.4 mg	1.4 mg	1.6 mg	1.6 mg
Niacin	18 mg	18 mg	17 mg	17 mg
Vitamin B_6	1.9 mg	1.9 mg	2 mg	2 mg
Folate	600 μg	600 μg	500 μg	500 μg
Vitamin B_{12}	2.6 μg	2.6 μg	2.8 μg	2.8 μg
Minerals				
Calcium[a]	1300 mg	1000 mg	1300 mg	1000 mg
Sodium[a]	1.5 g	1.5 g	1.5 g	1.5 g
Potassium[a]	4.7 g	4.7 g	5.1 g	5.1 g
Iron	27 mg	27 mg	10 mg	9 mg
Zinc	12 mg	11 mg	13 mg	12 mg
Iodine	220 μg	220 μg	290 μg	290 μg
Selenium	60 μg	60 μg	70 μg	70 μg
Other				
Protein	71 g	71 g	71 g	71 g
Carbohydrate	175 g	175 g	210 g	210 g
Fiber[a]	28 g	28 g	29 g	29 g

[a]Recommendations measured as Adequate Intake (AI).
From the Food and Nutrition Board of the Institute of Medicine (2008).

placenta and the 500 mg incorporated into the expanding maternal hemoglobin mass, nearly all is used after midpregnancy. During that time, iron requirements imposed by pregnancy and maternal excretion total approximately 7 mg per day (Pritchard and Scott, 1970). Few women have sufficient

iron stores or dietary iron intake to supply this amount. Thus, the American Academy of Pediatrics and the American College of Obstetricians and Gynecologists (2007) endorse the recommendation by the National Academy of Sciences that at least 27 mg of ferrous iron supplement be given daily to pregnant women. This amount is contained in most prenatal vitamins.

Scott and co-workers (1970) established that as little as 30 mg of elemental iron, supplied as ferrous gluconate, sulfate, or fumarate and taken daily throughout the latter half of pregnancy, provides sufficient iron to meet the requirements of pregnancy and to protect preexisting iron stores. This amount will also provide for iron requirements for lactation. The pregnant woman may benefit from 60 to 100 mg of iron per day if she is large, has twin fetuses, begins supplementation late in pregnancy, takes iron irregularly, or has a somewhat depressed hemoglobin level. The woman who is overtly anemic from iron deficiency responds well to oral supplementation with iron salts (see Chap. 51, p. 1080).

Because iron requirements are slight during the first 4 months of pregnancy, it is *not necessary* to provide supplemental iron during this time. Withholding iron supplementation during the first trimester of pregnancy avoids the risk

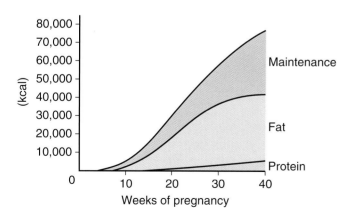

FIGURE 8-9 Cumulative kilocalories required for pregnancy. (From *Clinical Physiology in Obstetrics*, 3rd ed., G Chamberlain and F Broughton-Pipkin (eds). Copyright © 1998 Blackwell Science. Reproduced with permission of Blackwell Publishing Ltd.)

of aggravating nausea and vomiting (Gill and associates, 2009). Ingestion of iron at bedtime or on an empty stomach aids absorption and appears to minimize the possibility of an adverse gastrointestinal reaction.

Since 1997, the Food and Drug Administration (FDA) has required that iron preparations containing 30 mg or more of elemental iron per tablet be packaged as individual doses, such as in blister packages. This regulation is targeted at preventing accidental iron poisoning in children.

Calcium. As discussed in Chapter 5 (p. 114), the pregnant woman retains approximately 30 g of calcium, most of which is deposited in the fetus late in pregnancy (Pitkin, 1985). This amount of calcium represents only approximately 2.5 percent of total maternal calcium, most of which is in bone, and which can readily be mobilized for fetal growth. Moreover, Heaney and Skillman (1971) demonstrated increased calcium absorption by the intestine and progressive retention throughout pregnancy. Efforts to prevent preeclampsia using calcium supplementation have not proven efficacious, and it is not recommended for routine use during pregnancy (see Chap. 34, p. 727).

Zinc. Severe zinc deficiency may lead to poor appetite, suboptimal growth, and impaired wound healing. Profound zinc deficiency may cause dwarfism and hypogonadism. It may also lead to a specific skin disorder, *acrodermatitis enteropathica,* as the result of a rare, severe congenital zinc deficiency. Although the level of zinc supplementation that is safe for pregnant women has not been clearly established, recommended daily intake during pregnancy is approximately 12 mg.

Goldenberg and colleagues (1995) randomly assigned 580 indigent women to daily 25-mg zinc supplementation or placebo beginning at midpregnancy. Plasma zinc levels were significantly higher in women who received supplements. Infants born to zinc-supplemented women were slightly larger—mean increase 125 g—and had a slightly larger head circumference—mean 4 mm. Later, Osendarp and colleagues (2001) randomly assigned 420 women in Bangladesh to receive either daily 30-mg zinc supplementation or placebo from 12 to 16 weeks until delivery. Although supplementation did not improve birthweight, low-birthweight infants of mothers who received zinc had reduced risks of acute diarrhea, dysentery, and impetigo. In a follow-up study of these infants at 13 months, zinc supplementation was not found to confer any benefits on developmental outcome (Hamadani and co-workers, 2002).

Iodine. The use of iodized salt and bread products is recommended during pregnancy to offset the increased fetal requirements and maternal renal losses of iodine. Despite this, iodine intake has declined substantially in the past 15 years, and in some areas, it is probably inadequate (see Chap. 53, p. 1133). Interest in increasing dietary iodine was heightened by reports linking subclinical maternal hypothyroidism to adverse pregnancy outcomes and possible neurodevelopmental defects in children studied at age 7 years (Casey and associates, 2004; Haddow and colleagues, 1999). Severe maternal iodine deficiency predisposes offspring to endemic cretinism, characterized by multiple severe neurological defects. In parts of China and Africa where this condition is endemic, iodide supplementation very early in pregnancy prevents some cases of cretinism (Cao and colleagues, 1994).

Magnesium. Deficiency of magnesium as the consequence of pregnancy has not been recognized. Undoubtedly, during prolonged illness with no magnesium intake, the plasma level might become critically low, as it would in the absence of pregnancy. We have observed magnesium deficiency during pregnancy complicated by the consequences of previous intestinal bypass surgery.

Sibai and co-workers (1989) randomly assigned 400 normotensive primigravid women to 365 mg elemental magnesium supplementation or placebo tablets from 13 to 24 weeks. Supplementation did not improve any measures of pregnancy outcome.

Trace Metals. Copper, selenium, chromium, and manganese all have important roles in certain enzyme functions. In general, most are provided by an average diet. A severe geochemical selenium deficiency has been identified in a large area of China. Deficiency is manifested by a frequently fatal cardiomyopathy in young children and women of childbearing age. Conversely, selenium toxicity resulting from oversupplementation also has been observed. There is no reported need to supplement selenium in American women.

Potassium. The concentration of potassium in maternal plasma decreases by approximately 0.5 mEq/L by midpregnancy (Brown and colleagues, 1986). Potassium deficiency develops in the same circumstances as when a woman is not pregnant.

Fluoride. There is no evidence that supplemental fluoride during pregnancy is beneficial (Institute of Medicine, 1990). Maheshwari and co-workers (1983) found that fluoride metabolism is not altered appreciably during pregnancy. Horowitz and Heifetz (1967) concluded that there were no additional benefits from maternal ingestion of fluoridated water if the offspring ingested such water from birth.

Sa Roriz Fonteles and associates (2005) studied microdrill biopsies of deciduous teeth and concluded that prenatal fluoride provided no additional fluoride uptake compared with postnatal fluoride alone. Supplemental fluoride ingested by lactating women does not increase the fluoride concentration in breast milk (Ekstrand and colleagues, 1981).

Vitamins

The increased requirements for most vitamins during pregnancy shown in Table 8-8 usually are supplied by any general diet that provides adequate calories and protein. The exception is folic acid during times of unusual requirements, such as pregnancy complicated by protracted vomiting, hemolytic anemia, or multiple fetuses. That said, in impoverished countries, routine multivitamin supplementation reduced the incidence of low-birthweight and growth-restricted fetuses, but did not alter preterm delivery or perinatal mortality rates (Fawzi and colleagues, 2007).

Folic Acid. The Centers for Disease Control and Prevention (2004) estimated that the number of pregnancies affected by neural-tube defects has decreased from 4000 pregnancies per year to approximately 3000 per year since mandatory fortification of cereal products with folic acid in 1998. Perhaps more than half of all neural-tube defects can be prevented with daily intake of 400 μg of folic acid throughout the periconceptional period (Centers for Disease Control and Prevention, 1999). Putting 140 μg of folic acid into each 100 g of grain products may increase the folic acid intake of the average American woman of childbearing age by 100 μg per day. Because nutritional sources alone are insufficient, however, folic acid supplementation is still recommended (American College of Obstetricians and Gynecologists, 2003b). Using data from 15 international registries, Botto and associates (2006) demonstrated a significant reduction in neural-tube defects only in countries with folic acid *fortification* programs, but no decrease in areas with supplementation recommendations alone.

A woman with a prior child with a neural-tube defect can reduce the 2- to 5-percent recurrence risk by more than 70 percent with daily 4-mg folic acid supplements the month before conception and during the first trimester. As emphasized by the American Academy of Pediatrics and the American College of Obstetricians and Gynecologists (2007), this dose should be consumed as a separate supplement, that is, not as multivitamin tablets, to avoid excessive intake of fat-soluble vitamins. Unfortunately, surveys continue to suggest that many women, especially among minorities, remain unaware of the recommendations regarding folic acid supplementation (Perlow, 2001; Rinsky-Eng and Miller, 2002). This important relationship between folic acid deficiency and neural-tube defects is further discussed in Chapter 13 (p. 288).

Vitamin A. Dietary intake of vitamin A in the United States appears to be adequate, and routine supplementation during pregnancy is not recommended by the American College of Obstetricians and Gynecologists (1998b). Conversely, there is an association of birth defects with very high doses during pregnancy—10,000 to 50,000 IU daily. These malformations are similar to those produced by the vitamin A derivative isotretinoin—*Accutane*—which is a potent teratogen (see Chap. 14, p. 324). Beta-carotene, the precursor of vitamin A found in fruits and vegetables, has not been shown to produce vitamin A toxicity.

Vitamin A deficiency is an endemic nutrition problem in the developing world. West (2003) estimates that worldwide, 6 million pregnant women suffer from night blindness secondary to vitamin A deficiency. In 736 third-trimester Indian women, Radhika and colleagues (2002) found overt deficiency manifested as night blindness in 3 percent. Another 27 percent had subclinical vitamin A deficiency defined as a serum retinol concentration below 20 μg/dL. Vitamin A deficiency, whether overt or subclinical, was associated with an increased risk of anemia and spontaneous preterm birth.

Vitamin B$_{12}$. Maternal plasma vitamin B$_{12}$ levels decrease in normal pregnancy and result mostly from reduced plasma levels of carrier proteins—*transcobalamins* (see Chap. 51, p. 1082 and Appendix). Vitamin B$_{12}$ occurs naturally only in foods of animal origin, and strict vegetarians may give birth to infants whose B$_{12}$ stores are low. Likewise, because breast milk of a vegetarian mother contains little vitamin B$_{12}$, the deficiency may become profound in the breast-fed infant (Higginbottom and associates, 1978). Excessive ingestion of vitamin C also can lead to a functional deficiency of vitamin B$_{12}$. Although its role is still controversial, low levels of vitamin B$_{12}$ preconceptionally, similar to folate, may increase the risk of neural-tube defects (Molloy and co-workers, 2009; Thompson and colleagues, 2009).

Vitamin B$_6$—Pyridoxine. Limited clinical trials in pregnant women have failed to demonstrate any benefits of vitamin B$_6$ supplements (Thaver and associates, 2006). For women at high risk for inadequate nutrition—for example, substance abusers, adolescents, and those with multifetal gestations—a daily 2-mg supplement is recommended. Vitamin B$_6$, when combined with the antihistamine *doxylamine,* has been found helpful in many cases of nausea and vomiting of pregnancy (Boskovic and associates, 2003; Staroselsky and associates, 2007).

Vitamin C. The recommended dietary allowance for vitamin C during pregnancy is 80 to 85 mg/day—about 20 percent more than when nonpregnant (see Table 8-8). A reasonable diet should readily provide this amount. The maternal plasma level declines during pregnancy, whereas the cord level is higher, a phenomenon observed with most water-soluble vitamins.

Pragmatic Nutritional Surveillance

Although the science of nutrition continues in its perpetual struggle to identify the ideal amounts of protein, calories, vitamins, and minerals for the pregnant woman and her fetus, those directly responsible for their care may best discharge their duties as follows:

1. In general, advise the pregnant woman to eat what she wants in amounts she desires and salted to taste.
2. Ensure that there is ample food available in the case of socioeconomically deprived women.
3. Monitor weight gain, with a goal of approximately 25 to 35 lb in women with a normal BMI.
4. Periodically explore food intake by dietary recall to discover the occasional nutritionally absurd diet.
5. Give tablets of simple iron salts that provide at least 27 mg of iron daily. Give folate supplementation before and in the early weeks of pregnancy.
6. Recheck the hematocrit or hemoglobin concentration at 28 to 32 weeks to detect any significant decrease.

COMMON CONCERNS

Employment

More than half of the children in the United States are born to working mothers. Federal law prohibits employers from excluding women from job categories on the basis that they are or might become pregnant (Annas, 1991). The Family Medical Leave Act requires that covered employers must grant up to 12 workweeks of unpaid leave to an employee for the birth and care of a newborn child (United States Department of Labor, 2008). In the absence of complications, most women can continue to work until the onset of labor (American Academy of Pediatrics and American College of Obstetricians and Gynecologists, 2007).

Some types of work, however, may increase pregnancy complication risks. Mozurkewich and colleagues (2000) reviewed 29 studies that involved more than 160,000 pregnancies. With physically demanding work, women had a 20- to 60-percent increase in rates of preterm birth, fetal-growth restriction, or gestational hypertension. In a prospective study of more than 900 healthy nulliparas, Higgins and associates (2002) found that women who worked had a fivefold risk of preeclampsia. Newman and colleagues (2001) reported outcomes in 2929 women with singleton pregnancies studied by the Maternal–Fetal Medicine Units Network. Occupational fatigue—estimated by the number of hours standing, intensity of physical and mental demands, and environmental stressors—was associated with an increased risk of preterm membrane rupture. For women reporting the highest degrees of fatigue, the risk was 7.4 percent.

Thus, any occupation that subjects the pregnant woman to severe physical strain should be avoided. Ideally, no work or play should be continued to the extent that undue fatigue develops. Adequate periods of rest should be provided. It seems prudent to advise women with previous pregnancy complications that are at risk to recur—for example, preterm birth—to minimize physical work.

Exercise

In general, pregnant women do not need to limit exercise, provided they do not become excessively fatigued or risk injury. Clapp and associates (2000) randomly assigned 46 pregnant women who did not exercise regularly to either no exercise or to weight-bearing exercise beginning at 8 weeks. Exercise consisted of treadmill running, step aerobics, or stair stepper use for 20 minutes three to five times each week. They did this throughout pregnancy at an intensity between 55 and 60 percent of the preconceptional maximum aerobic capacity. Both placental size and birthweight were significantly greater in the exercise group. Duncombe and co-workers (2006) reported similar findings in 148 women. In contrast, Magann and colleagues (2002) prospectively analyzed exercise behavior in 750 healthy women and found that working women who exercised had smaller infants, more dysfunctional labors, and more frequent upper respiratory infections.

The American College of Obstetricians and Gynecologists (2002b) advises a thorough clinical evaluation be conducted before recommending an exercise program. In the absence of contraindications listed in Table 8-9, pregnant women should be encouraged to engage in regular, moderate-intensity physical activity 30 minutes or more a day. Each activity should be reviewed individually for its potential risk. Activities with a high risk of falling or abdominal trauma should be avoided. Similarly, scuba diving should be avoided because the fetus is at an increased risk for decompression sickness.

In the setting of certain pregnancy complications, it is wise to abstain from exercise and even limit physical activity. For example, some women with hypertensive disorders caused by pregnancy may benefit from being sedentary (see Chap. 34, p. 729), as may women with preterm labor, placenta previa, or multifetal gestation (see Chap. 39, p. 880); those suspected of having a growth-restricted fetus (see Chap. 38, p. 852); or those with severe cardiac or pulmonary disease (see Chap. 44, p. 958).

TABLE 8-9. Absolute and Relative Contraindications to Aerobic Exercise During Pregnancy

Absolute Contraindications
- Hemodynamically significant heart disease
- Restrictive lung disease
- Incompetent cervix/cerclage
- Multifetal gestation at risk for preterm labor
- Persistent second- or third-trimester bleeding
- Placenta previa after 26 weeks
- Preterm labor during the current pregnancy
- Ruptured membranes
- Preeclampsia/pregnancy-induced hypertension

Relative Contraindications
- Severe anemia
- Unevaluated maternal cardiac arrhythmia
- Chronic bronchitis
- Poorly controlled type 1 diabetes
- Extreme morbid obesity
- Extreme underweight (BMI <12)
- History of extremely sedentary lifestyle
- Fetal-growth restriction in current pregnancy
- Poorly controlled hypertension
- Orthopedic limitations
- Poorly controlled seizure disorder
- Poorly controlled hyperthyroidism
- Heavy smoker

Reprinted, with permission, from Exercise during pregnancy and the postpartum period. ACOG Committee Opinion No. 267. American College of Obstetricians and Gynecologists. *Obstet Gyn* 2002; 99:171-173.

Fish Consumption

Fish are an excellent source of protein, are low in saturated fats, and contain omega-3 fatty acids. Because nearly all fish and shellfish contain trace amounts of mercury, pregnant and lactating women are advised to avoid specific types of fish with potentially high methylmercury levels. These include shark, swordfish, king mackerel, and tile fish. It is further recommended that pregnant women ingest no more than 12 ounces or two servings of canned tuna per week and no more than 6 ounces of albacore or "white" tuna (U.S. Environmental Protection Agency, 2008). If the mercury content of locally caught fish is unknown, then overall fish consumption should be limited to 6 ounces per week. The recent ALSPAC study—Avon Longitudinal Study of Parents and Children, however, reported beneficial effects on pregnancy outcomes in women who consumed 340 g or more of seafood weekly (Hibbeln and co-workers, 2007).

Travel

Automobile Travel

The American College of Obstetricians and Gynecologists (1998a) has formulated guidelines for use of automobile passenger restraints during pregnancy (see Chap. 42, p. 937).

Women should be encouraged to wear properly positioned three-point restraints throughout pregnancy while riding in automobiles. The lap belt portion of the restraining belt should be placed under the abdomen and across her upper thighs. The belt should be comfortably snug. The shoulder belt also should be snugly positioned between the breasts. Available information suggests that airbags should not be disabled for the pregnant woman (American College of Obstetricians and Gynecologists, 1998a).

Air Travel

In general, air travel by the healthy woman has no harmful effect on pregnancy (Aerospace Medical Association, 2003). Travel in properly pressurized aircraft offers no unusual risk. Thus, in the absence of obstetrical or medical complications, the American Academy of Pediatrics and the American College of Obstetricians and Gynecologists (2004a, 2007) have concluded that pregnant women can safely fly up to 36 weeks. It is recommended that pregnant women observe the same precautions for air travel as the general population, including periodic movement of the lower extremities, ambulation at least hourly, and use of seatbelts while seated. A significant risk with travel, especially international travel, is acquisition of infectious diseases or developing a complication remote from adequate facilities (Ryan and associates, 2002).

Coitus

It is generally accepted that in healthy pregnant women, sexual intercourse usually is not harmful. Whenever abortion or preterm labor threatens, however, coitus should be avoided. Nearly 10,000 women enrolled in a prospective investigation by the Vaginal Infection and Prematurity Study Group were interviewed regarding sexual activity (Read and Klebanoff, 1993). They reported a decreased frequency of sexual intercourse with advancing gestation. By 36 weeks, 72 percent had intercourse less than once weekly. According to Bartellas and colleagues (2000), the decrease is attributed to decreased desire in 58 percent and fear of harm to the pregnancy in 48 percent.

Intercourse late in pregnancy specifically has not been found to be harmful. Grudzinskas and co-workers (1979) found no association between gestational age at delivery and the frequency of coitus during the last 4 weeks of pregnancy. Sayle and colleagues (2001) found no increased—and actually a decreased—risk of delivery within 2 weeks of intercourse. Tan and co-workers (2007) studied women scheduled for nonurgent labor induction and found that spontaneous labor ensued in half of each group who had and did not have intercourse.

Oral-vaginal intercourse is occasionally hazardous. Aronson and Nelson (1967) described a fatal air embolism late in pregnancy as a result of air blown into the vagina during cunnilingus. Other near-fatal cases have been described (Bernhardt and associates, 1988).

Dental Care

Examination of the teeth should be included in the prenatal examination, and good dental hygiene is encouraged. Periodontal disease has been linked to preterm labor (see Chap. 36, p. 812). Unfortunately, its treatment improves dental health but does not prevent preterm birth (Michalowicz and co-workers, 2006). Dental caries are not aggravated by pregnancy. Importantly, pregnancy is not a contraindication to dental treatment including dental radiographs (Giglio and associates, 2009).

Immunization

Current recommendations for immunizations during pregnancy are summarized in Table 8-10. Over the past decade, well-publicized concerns regarding childhood exposure to the thimerosal preservative in some vaccines led to parental prohibition. These results have proven groundless, but controversy continues (Sugarman, 2007; Thompson and co-workers, 2007; Tozzi and associates, 2009). Thus, they are recommended for use in pregnancy. The American College of Obstetricians and Gynecologists (2003a) stresses that current information on the safety of vaccines given during pregnancy is subject to change and can be verified from the Centers for Disease Control and Prevention website at http://www.cdc.gov/vaccines.

All women who will be pregnant during the influenza season should be offered vaccination, regardless of their stage of pregnancy. Those with underlying medical conditions that increase the risk for complications should be offered the vaccine before flu season starts (American Academy of Pediatrics and American College of Obstetricians and Gynecologists, 2007). Recently, Zaman and co-workers (2008) showed that prenatal maternal vaccination reduced influenza incidence in the first 6 months by 63 percent in infants born to these women. Moreover, it reduced all febrile respiratory illnesses in these children by a third.

Women who are susceptible to rubella during pregnancy should receive MMR—measles-mumps-rubella—vaccination postpartum. Although this vaccine is not recommended during pregnancy, congenital rubella syndrome has never resulted from its inadvertent use. There is no contraindication to MMR vaccination while breast feeding (American College of Obstetricians and Gynecologists, 2002d).

Biological Warfare and Vaccines

The tragic events of September 11, 2001, and the ongoing threat of bioterrorism require familiarity with smallpox and anthrax vaccines during pregnancy. The smallpox vaccine is made with live attenuated vaccinia virus related to smallpox and to cowpox viruses. Fetal vaccinia infection is rare, but it may result in abortion, stillbirth, or neonatal death. Thus, in nonemergency circumstances, vaccination is contraindicated during pregnancy and in women who might become pregnant within 28 days of vaccination (Centers for Disease Control and Prevention, 2006a). If, however, vaccination is inadvertently performed in early pregnancy, this is not grounds for termination (Suarez and Hankins, 2002). If the pregnant woman is at risk because of exposure to smallpox—either as a direct victim of a bioterrorist attack or as a close contact of an individual case—the risks from clinical smallpox substantially outweigh any potential risk from vaccination (Suarez and Hankins, 2002).

Anthrax vaccination has been limited principally to individuals who are occupationally exposed, such as special veterinarians, laboratory workers, and members of the armed forces. The vaccine contains no live virus and thus would not be

TABLE 8-10. Recommendations for Immunization During Pregnancy

Immunobiological Agent	Indications for Immunization During Pregnancy	Dose Schedule	Comments
Live Attenuated Virus Vaccines			
Measles	Contraindicated—see immune globulins	Single dose SC, preferably as MMR[a]	Vaccinate susceptible women postpartum. Breast feeding is not a contraindication
Mumps	Contraindicated	Single dose SC, preferably as MMR	Vaccinate susceptible women postpartum
Rubella	Contraindicated, but congenital rubella syndrome has never been described after vaccine	Single dose SC, preferably as MMR	Teratogenicity of vaccine is theoretical and not confirmed to date; vaccinate susceptible women postpartum
Poliomyelitis Oral = live attenuated; injection = enhanced-potency inactivated virus	Not routinely recommended for women in the United States, except women at increased risk of exposure[b]	Primary: Two doses of enhanced-potency inactivated virus SC at 4–8 week intervals and a 3rd dose 6–12 months after 2nd dose. Immediate protection: One dose oral polio vaccine (in outbreak setting)	Vaccine indicated for susceptible women traveling in endemic areas or in other high-risk situations
Yellow fever	Travel to high-risk areas	Single dose SC	Limited theoretical risk outweighed by risk of yellow fever
Varicella	Contraindicated, but no adverse outcomes reported in pregnancy	Two doses needed: 2nd dose given 4–8 weeks after 1st dose	Teratogenicity of vaccine is theoretical. Vaccination of susceptible women should be considered postpartum
Smallpox (vaccinia)	Contraindicated in pregnant women and in their household contacts	One dose SC, multiple pricks with lancet	Only vaccine known to cause fetal harm
Other			
Influenza	All pregnant women, regardless of trimester during flu season (Nov.-Mar.)	One dose IM every year	Inactivated virus vaccine
Rabies	Indications for prophylaxis not altered by pregnancy; each case considered individually	Public health authorities to be consulted for indications, dosage, and route of administration	Killed-virus vaccine
Hepatitis B	Pre-exposure and postexposure for women at risk of infection	Three-dose series IM at 0, 1, and 6 months	Used with hepatitis B immune globulin for some exposures. Exposed newborn needs birth-dose vaccination and immune globulin as soon as possible. All infants should receive birth dose of vaccine
Hepatitis A	Pre-exposure and postexposure if at risk (international travel)	Two-dose schedule IM, 6 months apart	Inactivated virus
Inactivated Bacterial Vaccines			
Pneumococcus	Indications not altered by pregnancy. Recommended for women with asplenia; metabolic, renal, cardiac, or pulmonary diseases; immunosuppression; or smokers	In adults, one dose only; consider repeat dose in 6 years for high-risk women	Polyvalent polysaccharide vaccine

(continued)

TABLE 8-10. Recommendations for Immunization During Pregnancy (*Continued*)

Immunobiological Agent	Indications for Immunization During Pregnancy	Dose Schedule	Comments
Inactivated Bacterial Vaccines			
Meningococcus	Indications not altered by pregnancy; vaccination recommended in unusual outbreaks	One dose; tetravalent vaccine	Antimicrobial prophylaxis if significant exposure
Typhoid	Not recommended routinely except for close, continued exposure or travel to endemic areas	Killed Primary: 2 injections IM 4 weeks apart Booster: One dose; schedule not yet determined	Killed, injectable vaccine or live attenuated oral vaccine. Oral vaccine preferred
Anthrax	See text	Six-dose primary vaccination, then annual booster vaccination	Preparation from cell-free filtrate of *B. anthracis*. No dead or live bacteria. Teratogenicity of vaccine theoretical
Toxoids			
Tetanus-diphtheria	Lack of primary series, or no booster within past 10 years	Primary: Two doses IM at 1–2 month interval with 3rd dose 6–12 months after the 2nd Booster: Single dose IM every 10 years after completion of primary series	Combined tetanus-diphtheria toxoids preferred: adult tetanus-diphtheria formulation. Updating immune status should be part of antepartum care
Specific Immune Globulins			
Hepatitis B	Postexposure prophylaxis	Depends on exposure (see Chap. 50, p. 1069)	Usually given with hepatitis B virus vaccine; exposed newborn needs immediate prophylaxis
Rabies	Postexposure prophylaxis	Half dose at injury site, half dose in deltoid	Used in conjunction with rabies killed-virus vaccine
Tetanus	Postexposure prophylaxis	One dose IM	Used in conjunction with tetanus toxoid
Varicella	Should be considered for exposed pregnant women to protect against maternal, not congenital, infection	One dose IM within 96 hours of exposure	Indicated also for newborns or women who developed varicella within 4 days before delivery or 2 days following delivery
Standard Immune Globulins			
Hepatitis A Hepatitis A virus vaccine should be used with hepatitis A immune globulin	Postexposure prophylaxis and high risk	0.02 mL/kg IM in one dose	Immune globulin should be given as soon as possible and within 2 weeks of exposure; infants born to women who are incubating the virus or are acutely ill at delivery should receive one dose of 0.5 mL as soon as possible after birth

[a] Two doses necessary for students entering institutions of higher education, newly hired medical personnel, and travel abroad.
[b] Inactivated polio vaccine recommended for nonimmunized adults at increased risk.
ID = intradermally; IM = intramuscularly; MMR = measles, mumps, rubella; PO = orally: and SC = subcutaneously.
Adapted from the Centers for Disease Control and Prevention, Recommendations of the Advisory Committee on Immunization Practices, 2003, 2005, 2006a, 2008b.

expected to pose significant risk to the fetus. Wiesen and Littell (2002) studied the reproductive outcomes of 385 women in the United States Army who became pregnant after vaccination and reported no adverse effects on fertility or pregnancy outcome.

Smallpox, anthrax, and other infections related to bioterrorism are discussed in Chapter 58 (p. 1230).

Caffeine

In 1980, the FDA advised pregnant women to limit caffeine intake. The Fourth International Caffeine Workshop concluded shortly thereafter that there was no evidence that caffeine had increased teratogenic or reproductive risks (Dews and colleagues, 1984). Caffeine is not a teratogen for small laboratory animals, but if given in massive doses it potentiates mutagenic effects of radiation and some chemicals. When infused intravenously into sheep, caffeine decreases uterine blood flow by 5 to 10 percent (Conover and colleagues, 1983).

Whether adverse outcomes may be related to caffeine consumption is somewhat controversial. In a case-control study, Klebanoff and co-workers (1999) measured paraxanthine, a biological serum marker of caffeine consumption, in 487 women with spontaneous abortions and in 2087 controls. Only extremely high levels, equivalent to more than 5 cups of coffee per day, were associated with abortion. Clausson and associates (2002) found no association of moderate caffeine consumption of less than 500 mg daily with low birthweight, fetal-growth restriction, or preterm delivery. Bech and associates (2007) randomly assigned more than 1200 pregnant women who drank at least three cups of coffee per day to caffeinated versus decaffeinated coffee. They found no difference in birthweight or gestational age at delivery between groups. However, the CARE study (2008) included 2635 low-risk pregnancies and found that the odds ratio for fetal-growth restriction was increased to approximately 1.4 among those whose daily caffeine consumption exceeded 200 mg throughout pregnancy compared with those who consumed less than 100 mg daily. The American Dietetic Association (2002) recommends that caffeine intake during pregnancy be limited to less than 300 mg daily, or approximately three, 5-oz cups of percolated coffee.

Nausea and Vomiting

These are common complaints during the first half of pregnancy. Nausea and vomiting of varying severity usually commence between the first and second missed menstrual period and continue until 14 to 16 weeks. Although nausea and vomiting tend to be worse in the morning—thus erroneously termed *morning sickness,* they frequently continue throughout the day. Lacroix and co-workers (2000) found that nausea and vomiting were reported by three fourths of pregnant women and lasted an average of 35 days. Half had relief by 14 weeks, and 90 percent by 22 weeks. In 80 percent of the women, nausea lasted all day. It was frequently described to have a character and intensity similar to that experienced by patients undergoing cancer chemotherapy.

Seldom is the treatment of nausea and vomiting of pregnancy so successful that the affected expectant mother is afforded complete relief. Fortunately, the unpleasantness and discomfort usually can be minimized. Eating small meals at more frequent intervals but stopping short of satiation is valuable. Borrelli and colleagues (2005) did a systematic literature search and reported that the herbal remedy, ginger, was likely effective. Mild symptoms usually respond to vitamin B_6 given along with doxylamine, but some women require phenothiazine or H_1-receptor blocker antiemetics (American College of Obstetricians and Gynecologists, 2004b). In some women, vomiting may be so severe that dehydration, electrolyte and acid–base disturbances, and starvation ketosis become serious problems. This is termed *hyperemesis gravidarum,* and its management is described in Chapter 49 (p. 1050).

Backache

Low back pain to some extent is reported in nearly 70 percent of pregnant women (Wang and colleagues, 2004). Minor degrees follow excessive strain or fatigue and excessive bending, lifting, or walking. Orvieto and associates (1994) studied 449 women and reported that back pain increased with duration of gestation. Prior low back pain and obesity were risk factors.

Back pain can be reduced by having women squat rather than bend over when reaching down, providing back support with a pillow when sitting down, and avoiding high-heeled shoes. Severe back pain should not be attributed simply to pregnancy until a thorough orthopedic examination has been conducted. Muscular spasm and tenderness, which often are classified clinically as acute strain or fibrositis, respond well to analgesics, heat, and rest. As discussed in Chapter 53, some women with severe back and hip pain may have *pregnancy-associated osteoporosis* (Dunne and colleagues, 1993). Severe pain also has other uncommon causes, such as disc disease, vertebral osteoarthritis, or septic arthritis (Smith and associates, 2008).

Norén and co-workers (2002) studied the long-term outcomes of 231 women who had some type of back pain during pregnancy. Residual pain 3 years after delivery was reported by approximately 20 percent. Women with combined lumbar back and posterior pelvic pain were at greatest risk for disability, which was attributed to impaired back extensor and hip abductor muscle functions (see Chap. 30, p. 656).

Varicosities

These enlarged veins generally result from congenital predisposition and are exaggerated by prolonged standing, pregnancy, and advancing age. Usually varicosities become more prominent as pregnancy advances, as weight increases, and as the length of time spent upright is prolonged. As discussed in Chapter 5 (p. 119), femoral venous pressure increases appreciably as pregnancy advances. The symptoms produced by varicosities vary from cosmetic blemishes and mild discomfort at the end of the day to severe discomfort that requires prolonged rest with elevated feet.

Treatment is generally limited to periodic rest with leg elevation, elastic stocking use, or both. Surgical correction during pregnancy generally is not advised, although occasionally the symptoms may be so severe that injection, ligation, or even stripping of the veins is necessary. Vulvar varicosities may be aided by application of a foam rubber pad suspended across the vulva by a belt. Rarely, large varicosities may rupture, resulting in profuse hemorrhage.

Hemorrhoids

Varicosities of the rectal veins may first appear during pregnancy because of increased venous pressure. More often, pregnancy causes an exacerbation or a recurrence of previous hemorrhoids. Pain and swelling usually are relieved by topically applied anesthetics, warm soaks, and stool-softening agents. Thrombosis of an external hemorrhoid can cause considerable pain, but the clot usually can be evacuated by incising the vein wall under topical anesthesia.

Heartburn

This symptom is one of the most common complaints of pregnant women and is caused by reflux of gastric contents into the lower esophagus. The increased frequency of regurgitation during pregnancy most likely results from the upward displacement and compression of the stomach by the uterus, combined with relaxation of the lower esophageal sphincter (see Chap. 5, p. 125). In most pregnant women, symptoms are mild and are relieved by a regimen of more frequent but smaller meals and avoidance of bending over or lying flat. Antacids may provide considerable relief. Aluminum hydroxide, magnesium trisilicate, or magnesium hydroxide alone or in combination are given. Management for symptoms that do not respond to these simple measures is discussed in Chapter 49 (p. 1052).

Pica

The cravings of pregnant women for strange foods are termed pica. At times, nonfoods such as ice—pagophagia, starch—amylophagia, or clay—geophagia may predominate. This desire has been considered by some to be triggered by severe iron deficiency. Although some women crave these items, and although the craving usually is ameliorated after correction of iron deficiency, not all pregnant women with pica are necessarily iron deficient. Indeed, if strange "foods" dominate the diet, iron deficiency will be aggravated or will develop eventually.

Patel and colleagues (2004) from the University of Alabama at Birmingham prospectively completed a dietary inventory on more than 3000 women during the second trimester. The prevalence of pica was 4 percent. The most common nonfood items ingested were starch in 64 percent, dirt in 14 percent, sourdough in 9 percent, and ice in 5 percent. The prevalence of anemia was 15 percent in women with pica compared with 6 percent in those without it. Interestingly, the rate of spontaneous preterm birth at less than 35 weeks was twice as high in women with pica.

Ptyalism

Women during pregnancy are occasionally distressed by profuse salivation. Although usually unexplained, the cause of such ptyalism sometimes appears to be stimulation of the salivary glands by the ingestion of starch.

Sleeping and Fatigue

Beginning early in pregnancy, many women experience fatigue and need increased amounts of sleep. This likely is due to the soporific effect of progesterone(s). Moreover, *sleep efficiency* is diminished because REM sleep is decreased and non-REM sleep prolonged (Pien and Schwab, 2004). Fatigue and nonrestful sleep may be exacerbated by morning sickness. By the late second trimester, total nocturnal sleep duration is decreased, and women usually begin to complain of sleep disturbances. Approximately half of women begin snoring (Izci and associates, 2005). By the third trimester, nearly all women have altered sleep. Although total nocturnal sleep time is similar to nonpregnancy, sleep efficiency is perturbed because REM sleep is decreased. Daytime naps and mild sedatives at bedtime such as diphenhydramine (Benadryl) are usually helpful.

Leukorrhea

Pregnant women commonly develop increased vaginal discharge, which in many instances is not pathological. Increased mucus secretion by cervical glands in response to hyperestrogenemia is undoubtedly a contributing factor. Occasionally, troublesome leukorrhea is the result of vulvovaginal infection. The majority of these in adult women are caused by bacterial vaginosis, candidiasis, or trichomoniasis (Eckert, 2006). These vulvovaginal infections are reviewed in Chapter 59 (p. 1246).

Cord Blood Banking

In the past 20 years, umbilical cord blood transplantation has been successfully performed more than 7000 times to treat hematopoietic cancers and a variety of genetic conditions in children and adults (Moise, 2005). There are two types of cord blood banks. Public banks promote allogenic donation, for use by a related or unrelated recipient, similar to blood product donation. Whereas private banks were initially developed to store stem cells for future autologous use, these banks charge fees for initial processing and annual storage. The American College of Obstetricians and Gynecologists (2008) has concluded that if a woman requests information on umbilical cord banking, information regarding advantages and disadvantages of public versus private banking should be disclosed. Some states have passed legislation that requires physicians to inform patients about cord blood banking options. Importantly, few transplants have been performed by using cord blood stored in the absence of a known indication in the recipient (Thornley and associates, 2009). The likelihood that cord blood would be used for the donor couple's child or family member is considered remote—at most, approximately 1 in 2700 individuals (American College of Obstetricians and Gynecologists, 2008). It is recommended that directed donation be considered when an immediate family member carries the diagnosis of a specific condition known to be treatable by hematopoietic transplantation.

REFERENCES

Aerospace Medical Association, Medical Guidelines Task Force: Medical guidelines for airline travel, 2nd ed. Aviat Space Environ Med 74:5, 2003

American Academy of Pediatrics and American College of Obstetricians and Gynecologists: Guidelines for perinatal care, 6th ed. 2007

American College of Obstetricians and Gynecologists: Obstetric aspects of trauma management. Educational Bulletin No. 251, September 1998a

American College of Obstetricians and Gynecologists: Vitamin A supplementation during pregnancy. Committee Opinion No. 196, January 1998b

American College of Obstetricians and Gynecologists: Psychosocial risk factors: Perinatal screening and intervention. Educational Bulletin No. 255, November 1999

American College of Obstetricians and Gynecologists: Intrauterine growth restriction. Practice Bulletin No. 12. Obstet Gynecol, January 2000

American College of Obstetricians and Gynecologists: Avoiding inappropriate clinical decisions based on false-positive human chorionic gonadotropin test results. Committee Opinion No. 278, November 2002a

American College of Obstetricians and Gynecologists: Exercise during pregnancy and the postpartum period. Committee Opinion No. 267, January 2002b

American College of Obstetricians and Gynecologists: Prevention of early-onset group B streptococcal disease in newborns. Committee Opinion No. 279, December 2002c

American College of Obstetricians and Gynecologists: Rubella vaccination. Committee Opinion No. 281, December 2002d

American College of Obstetricians and Gynecologists: Immunization during pregnancy. Committee Opinion No. 282, January 2003a

American College of Obstetricians and Gynecologists: Neural tube defects. Practice Bulletin No. 44, July 2003b

American College of Obstetricians and Gynecologists: Air travel during pregnancy. Committee Opinion No. 264, December 2001, Reaffirmed 2004a

American College of Obstetricians and Gynecologists: Nausea and vomiting of pregnancy. Practice Bulletin No. 52, April 2004b

American College of Obstetricians and Gynecologists: Prenatal and preconceptional carrier screening for genetic diseases in individuals of eastern European Jewish descent. Committee Opinion No. 298, August 2004c

American College of Obstetricians and Gynecologists: Ultrasonography in pregnancy. Practice Bulletin No. 58, December 2004d

American College of Obstetricians and Gynecologists: Obesity in pregnancy. Committee Opinion No. 315, September 2005a

American College of Obstetricians and Gynecologists: Smoking cessation during pregnancy. Committee Opinion No. 316, October 2005b

American College of Obstetricians and Gynecologists: Update on carrier screening for cystic fibrosis. Committee Opinion No. 325, December 2005c

American College of Obstetricians and Gynecologists: Psychosocial risk factors: Perinatal screening and intervention. Committee Opinion No. 343, August 2006

American College of Obstetricians and Gynecologists: Human immunodeficiency virus. Committee Opinion No. 389, December 2007

American College of Obstetricians and Gynecologists: Umbilical cord blood banking. Committee Opinion No. 399. Obstet Gynecol 111:475, 2008

American College of Obstetricians and Gynecologists: Ultrasonography in pregnancy. Practice Bulletin No. 101, December 2009

American Dietetic Association: Position of the American Dietetic Association: Nutrition and lifestyle for a healthy pregnancy outcome. J Am Diet Assoc 102:1479, 2002

Annas GJ: Fetal protection and employment discrimination—the Johnson Controls case. N Engl J Med 325:740, 1991

Aronson ME, Nelson PK: Fatal air embolism in pregnancy resulting from an unusual sex act. Obstet Gynecol 30:127, 1967

Ashitaka Y, Nishimura R, Takemori M, et al: Production and secretion of hCG and hCG subunits by trophoblastic tissue. In Segal S (ed): Chorionic Gonadotropins. New York, Plenum, 1980, p 151

Barker DJ, Osmond C, Law CM: The intrauterine and early postnatal origins of cardiovascular disease and chronic bronchitis. J Epidemiol Community Health 43:237,1989

Bartellas E, Crane JMG, Daley M, et al: Sexuality and sexual activity in pregnancy. Br J Obstet Gynaecol 107:964, 2000

Bastian LA, Nanda K, Hasselblad V, et al: Diagnostic efficiency of home pregnancy test kits. A meta-analysis. Arch Fam Med 7:465, 1998

Bech BH, Obel C, Henriksen TB, et al: Effect of reducing caffeine intake on birth weight and length of gestation: randomized controlled trial. BMJ 335:409, 2007

Bergsjø P, Denman DW III, Hoffman HJ, et al: Duration of human singleton pregnancy. A population-based study. Acta Obstet Gynecol Scand 69:197, 1990

Bernhardt TL, Goldmann RW, Thombs PA, et al: Hyperbaric oxygen treatment of cerebral air embolism from orogenital sex during pregnancy. Crit Care Med 16:729, 1988

Borrelli F, Capasso R, Aviello G, et al: Effectiveness and safety of ginger in the treatment of pregnancy-induced nausea and vomiting. Obstet Gynecol 105:849, 2005

Boskovic R, Einarson A, Maltepe C, et al: Dilectin therapy for nausea and vomiting of pregnancy: Effects of optimal dosing. J Obstet Gynaecol Can 25:830, 2003

Botto LD, Lisi A, Bower C, et al: Trends of selected malformations in relation to folic acid recommendations and fortification: An international assessment. Birth Defects Res A Clin Mol Teratol 76:693, 2006

Bracken MB, Belanger K: Calculation of delivery dates. N Engl J Med 321:1483, 1989

Braunstein GD: False-positive serum human chorionic gonadotropin results: Causes, characteristics, and recognition. Am J Obstet Gynecol 187:217, 2002

Brown MA, Sinosich MJ, Saunders DM, et al: Potassium regulation and progesterone-aldosterone interrelationships in human pregnancy: A prospective study. Am J Obstet Gynecol 155:349, 1986

Calvert JP, Crean EE, Newcombe RG, et al: Antenatal screening by measurement of symphysis–fundus height. BMJ 285:846, 1982

Cao XY, Jiang XM, Dou ZH, et al: Timing of vulnerability of the brain to iodine deficiency in endemic cretinism. N Engl J Med 331:1739, 1994

CARE study group: Maternal caffeine intake during pregnancy and risk of fetal growth restriction: A large prospective observational study. BMJ 337:a2332, 2008

Casey BM, Dashe JS, McIntire DD, et al: Subclinical hypothyroidism and pregnancy outcomes. Obstet Gynecol 105:239, 2005

Catalano PM: Increasing maternal obesity and weight gain during pregnancy: The obstetric problems of plentitude. Obstet Gynecol 110:743, 2007

Centers for Disease Control and Prevention: Knowledge and use of folic acid by women of childbearing age—United States 1995–1998. MMWR 48:16, 1999

Centers for Disease Control and Prevention: Entry into prenatal care—United States, 1989–1997. MMWR 49:393, 2000

Centers for Disease Control and Prevention: Alcohol use among women of childbearing age—United States, 1991–1999. MMWR 51:273, 2002a

Centers for Disease Control and Prevention: Prevention of perinatal group B streptococcal disease. MMWR 51:1, 2002b

Centers for Disease Control and Prevention: Recommendations of the Advisory Committee on Immunization Practices, 2003. Available at: http://www.cdc.gov/mmwr/preview/mmwrhtml/0002528. Accessed March 4, 2003

Centers for Disease Control and Prevention: Spina bifida and anencephaly before and after folic acid mandate—United States, 1995–1996 and 1999–2000. MMWR 53:362, 2004

Centers for Disease Control and Prevention: Prevention and control of meningococcal disease: Recommendations of the advisory committee on immunization practices (ACIP). MMWR 54:1, 2005

Centers for Disease Control and Prevention: General recommendations on immunization. Recommendations of the advisory committee on immunization practices (ACIP). MMWR 55:32, 2006a

Centers for Disease Control and Prevention: Revised recommendations for HIV testing of adults, adolescents, and pregnant women in health-care settings. MMWR 55:1, 2006b

Centers for Disease Control and Prevention: Tobacco use and pregnancy. Available at: http://www.cdc.gov/reproductivehealth/TobaccoUsePregnancy/index.htm. Accessed December 17, 2007

Centers for Disease Control and Prevention: National Vital Statistics System. Available at: http://www.cdc.gov.gov/nchs/nvss.htm. Accessed January 22, 2008a

Centers for Disease Control and Prevention: Prevention and control of influenza: Recommendations of the advisory committee on immunization practices (ACIP). MMWR 57:1, 2008b

Chadwick JR: Value of the bluish coloration of the vaginal entrance as a sign of pregnancy. Trans Am Gynecol Soc 11:399, 1886

Chamberlain G, Broughton-Pipkin F (eds): Clinical Physiology in Obstetrics, 3rd ed. Oxford, Blackwell Science, 1998

Clapp JF III, Kim H, Burciu B, et al: Beginning regular exercise in early pregnancy: Effect on fetoplacental growth. Am J Obstet Gynecol 183:1484, 2000

Clausson B, Granath F, Ekbom A, et al: Effect of caffeine exposure during pregnancy on birth weight and gestational age. Am J Epidemiol 155:429, 2002

Clement S, Candy B, Sikorski J, et al: Does reducing the frequency of routine antenatal visits have long term effects? Follow up of participants in a randomised controlled trial. Br J Obstet Gynaecol 106:367, 1999

Cohen GR, Curet LB, Levine RJ, et al: Ethnicity, nutrition, and birth outcomes in nulliparous women. Am J Obstet Gynecol 185:660, 2001

Cole LA: HCG, its free subunits and its metabolites: Roles in pregnancy and trophoblastic disease. J Reprod Med 43:3, 1998

Cole LA, Khanlian SA, Sutton JM, et al: Accuracy of home pregnancy tests at the time of missed menses. Am J Obstet Gynecol 190:100, 2004

Conover WB, Key TC, Resnik R: Maternal cardiovascular response to caffeine infusion in the pregnant ewe. Am J Obstet Gynecol 145:534, 1983

DeVader SR, Neeley HL, Myles TD, et al: Evaluation of gestational weight gain guidelines for women with normal prepregnancy body mass index. Obstet Gynecol 110:745, 2007

Dews P, Grice HC, Neims A, et al: Report of Fourth International Caffeine Workshop, Athens, 1982. Food Chem Toxicol 22:163, 1984

Duncombe D, Skouteris H, Wertheim EH, et al: Vigorous exercise and birth outcomes in a sample of recreational exercisers: a prospective study across pregnancy. Aust N Z J Obstet Gynaecol 46:288, 2006

Dunne F, Walters B, Marshall T, et al: Pregnancy associated osteoporosis. Clin Endocrinol 39:487, 1993

Eckert LO: Acute vulvovaginitis. N Engl J Med 355:1244, 2006

Ehrenberg HM, Dierker L, Milluzzi C, et al: Low maternal weight, failure to thrive in pregnancy, and adverse pregnancy outcomes. Am J Obstet Gynecol 189:1726, 2003

Ekstrand J, Boreus LO, de Chateau P: No evidence of transfer of fluoride from plasma to breast milk. Br Med J (Clin Res Ed) 283:761, 1981

El-Mohandes A, Herman AA, Kl-Khorazaty MN, et al: Prenatal care reduces the impact of illicit drug use on perinatal outcomes. J Perinatol 23:354, 2003

Fawzi WW, Msamanga GI, Urassa W, et al: Vitamins and perinatal outcomes among HIV-negative women in Tanzania. N Engl J Med 356:14, 2007

Food and Drug Administration: Food standards: Amendment of standards of identity for enriched grain products to require addition of folic acid. 61 Federal Register 8781, 1996

Food and Nutrition Board of the Institute of Medicine: Dietary Reference Intake. National Academy of Sciences, 2004. Available at: http://www.iom.edu/object.file/master/21/372/o.pdf. Accessed October 20, 2008

Giglio JA, Lanni SM, Laskin DM, et al: Oral health care for the pregnant patient. J Can Dent Assoc 75(1):43, 2009

Gill SK, Maltepe C, Koren G: The effectiveness of discontinuing iron-containing prenatal multivitamins on reducing the severity of nausea and vomiting of pregnancy. J Obstet Gynaecol 29(1):13, 2009

Goldenberg RL, Tamura T, Neggers Y, et al: The effect of zinc supplementation on pregnancy outcome. JAMA 274:463, 1995

Gregory KD, Johnson CT, Johnson TRB, et al: The content of prenatal care. Women's Health Issues 16:198, 2006

Grudzinskas JG, Watson C, Chard T: Does sexual intercourse cause fetal distress? Lancet 2:692, 1979

Haddow JE, Palomaki GE, Allan WC, et al: Maternal thyroid deficiency during pregnancy and subsequent neuropsychological development of the child. N Engl J Med 341:549, 1999

Hamadani JD, Fuchs GJ, Osendarp SJ, et al: Zinc supplementation during pregnancy and effects on mental development and behaviour of infants: A follow-up study. Lancet 360:290, 2002

Harper MA, Byington RP, Espeland MA, et al: Pregnancy-related death and health care services. Obstet Gynecol 102:273, 2003

Heaney RP, Skillman TG: Calcium metabolism in normal human pregnancy. J Clin Endocrinol Metab 33:661, 1971

Herbert WNP, Bruninghaus HM, Barefoot AB, et al: Clinical aspects of fetal heart auscultation. Obstet Gynecol 69:574, 1987

Herbst MA, Mercer BM, Beazley D, et al: Relationship of prenatal care and perinatal morbidity in low-birth-weight infants. Am J Obstet Gynecol 189:930, 2003

Hibbeln JR, Davis JM, Steer C, et al: Maternal seafood consumption in pregnancy and neurodevelopmental outcomes in childhood (ALSPAC study): An observation cohort study. Lancet 369:578, 2007

Higginbottom MC, Sweetman L, Nyhan WL: A syndrome of methylmalonic aciduria, homocystinuria, megaloblastic anemia and neurologic abnormalities in a vitamin B_{12}-deficient breast-fed infant of a strict vegetarian. N Engl J Med 299:317, 1978

Higgins JR, Walshe JJ, Conroy RM, et al: The relation between maternal work, ambulatory blood pressure, and pregnancy hypertension. J Epidemiol Community Health 56:389, 2002

Hollier LM, Hill J, Sheffield JS, et al: State laws regarding prenatal syphilis screening in the United States. Am J Obstet Gynecol 189:1178, 2003

Horowitz HS, Heifetz SB: Effects of prenatal exposure to fluoridation on dental caries. Public Health Rep 82:297, 1967

Hytten FE: Weight gain in pregnancy. In Hytten FE, Chamberlain G (eds): Clinical Physiology in Obstetrics, 2nd ed. Oxford, Blackwell, 1991, p 173

Hytten FE, Chamberlain G: Clinical Physiology in Obstetrics, 2nd ed. Oxford, Blackwell, 1991, p 152

Hytten FE, Leitch I: The Physiology of Human Pregnancy, 2nd ed. Oxford, Blackwell, 1971

Institute of Medicine: Nutrition During Pregnancy, 1. Weight Gain; 2. Nutrient Supplements. Washington, DC, National Academy Press, 1990

Institute of Medicine: Dietary reference intakes. Food and Nutrition Board, Institute of Medicine, National Academies 2004. Available at: www.iom.edu/cms/3788/21370.aspx. Accessed October 30, 2008

Izci B, Martin SE, Dundas KC, et al: Sleep complaints: snoring and daytime sleepiness in pregnant and pre-eclamptic women. Sleep Med 6:163, 2005

Jazayeri A, Tsibris JCM, Spellacy WN: Umbilical cord plasma erythropoietin levels in pregnancies complicated by maternal smoking. Am J Obstet Gynecol 178:433, 1998

Jimenez JM, Tyson JE, Reisch JS: Clinical measures of gestational age in normal pregnancies. Obstet Gynecol 61:438, 1983

Jones DW, Appel LJ, Sheps SG, et al: Measuring blood pressure accurately: New and persistent challenges. JAMA 289:1027, 2003

Kessner DM, Singer J, Kalk CE, et al: Infant death: An analysis by maternal risk and health care. In: Contrasts in Health Status, Vol 1. Washington, DC, Institute of Medicine, National Academy of Sciences, 1973, p 59

Kiel DW, Dodson EA, Artal R, et al: Gestational weight gain and pregnancy outcomes in obese women: How much is enough. Obstet Gynecol 110:752, 2007

Kiss H, Widham A, Geusau A, et al: Universal antenatal screening for syphilis: Is it still justified economically? A 10-year retrospective analysis. Eur J Obstet Gynecol Reprod Biol 112:24, 2004

Klebanoff MA, Levine RJ, DerSimonian R, et al: Maternal serum paraxanthine, a caffeine metabolite, and the risk of spontaneous abortion. N Engl J Med 341:1639, 1999

Kyle UG, Pichard C: The Dutch Famine of 1944–1945: A pathophysiological model of long-term consequences of wasting disease. Curr Opin Clin Nutr Metab Care 9:388, 2006

Lacroix R, Eason E, Melzack R: Nausea and vomiting during pregnancy: A prospective study of its frequency, intensity, and patterns of change. Am J Obstet Gynecol 182:931, 2000

Loudon I: Death in Childbirth. New York, Oxford University Press, 1992, p 577

Luck W, Nau H, Hansen R: Extent of nicotine and cotinine transfer to the human fetus, placenta and amniotic fluid of smoking mothers. Dev Pharmacol Ther 8:384, 1985

Luke B, Brown MB, Misiunas R, et al: Specialized prenatal care and maternal and infant outcomes in twin pregnancy. Am J Obstet Gynecol 934, 2003

Magann EF, Evans SF, Weitz B, et al: Antepartum, intrapartum, and neonatal significance of exercise on healthy low-risk pregnant working women. Obstet Gynecol 99:466, 2002

Maheshwari UR, King JC, Leybin L, et al: Fluoride balances during early and late pregnancy. J Occup Med 25:587, 1983

Mahon BE, Rosenman MB, Graham MF, et al: Postpartum *Chlamydia trachomatis* and *Neisseria gonorrhoeae* infections. Am J Obstet Gynecol 186:1320, 2002

Man LX, Chang B: Maternal cigarette smoking during pregnancy increases the risk of having a child with a congenital digital anomaly. Plast Reconstr Surg 117:301, 2006

Martin JA, Hamilton BE, Sutton PD, et al: Births: Final Data for 2003. Natl Vital Stat Rep 54:2, 2005

Martin JA, Hamilton BE, Sutton PD, et al: Births: Final Data for 2006. Natl Vital Stat Rep 57:7, 2009

Martin JA, Hamilton BE, Ventura SJ, et al: Births: Final Data for 2000. Natl Vital Stat Rep 50:1, February 12, 2002a

Martin JA, Hamilton BE, Ventura SJ, et al: Births: Final Data for 2001. Natl Vital Stat Rep 51:2, December 18, 2002b

Martin JA, Kung HC, Mathews TJ, et al: Annual summary of vital statistics: 2006. Pediatrics 121:788, 2008

McDuffie RS Jr, Beck A, Bischoff K, et al: Effect of frequency of prenatal care visits on perinatal outcome among low-risk women. A randomized controlled trial. JAMA 275:847, 1996

Merkatz IR, Thompson JE, Walsh LV: History of prenatal care. In Merkatz IR, Thompson JE (eds): New Perspectives on Prenatal Care. New York, Elsevier, 1990, p 14

Michalowicz BS, Hodges JS, DiAngelis AJ, et al: Treatment of periodontal disease and the risk of preterm birth. N Engl J Med 355;1885, 2006

Moise KJ: Umbilical cord stem cells. Obstet Gynecol 106:1393, 2005

Molloy AM, Kirke PN, Troendle JF, et al: Maternal vitamin B_{12} status and risk of neural tube defects in a population with high neural tube defect prevalence and no folic acid fortification. Pediatrics 123(3):917, 2009

Mozurkewich EL, Luke B, Avni M, et al: Working conditions and adverse pregnancy outcome: A meta-analysis. Obstet Gynecol 95:623, 2000

Murray N, Homer CS, Davis GK, et al: The clinical utility of routine urinalysis in pregnancy: A prospective study. Med J Aust 177:477, 2002

Newman RB, Goldenberg RL, Moawad AH, et al: Occupational fatigue and preterm premature rupture of membranes. Am J Obstet Gynecol 184:438, 2001

Norén L, Östgaard S, Johansson G, et al: Lumbar back and posterior pelvic pain during pregnancy: A 3-year follow-up. Eur Spine J 11:267, 2002

Orvieto R, Achiron A, Ben-Rafael Z, et al: Low-back pain of pregnancy. Acta Obstet Gynecol Scand 73:209, 1994

Osendarp SJ, van Raaij JM, Darmstadt GL, et al: Zinc supplementation during pregnancy and effects on growth and morbidity in low birthweight infants: A randomised placebo controlled trial. Lancet 357:1080, 2001

Patel MV, Nuthalapaty FS, Ramsey PS, et al: Pica: A neglected risk factor for preterm birth [abstract]. Obstet Gynecol 103:68S, 2004

Perlow JH: Comparative use and knowledge of preconceptional folic acid among Spanish- and English-speaking patient populations in Phoenix and Yuma, Arizona. Am J Obstet Gynecol 184:1263, 2001

Pien GW, Schwab RJ: Sleep disorders during pregnancy. Sleep 27:1405, 2004

Pitkin RM: Calcium metabolism in pregnancy and the perinatal period: A review. Am J Obstet Gynecol 151:99, 1985

Pivarnik JM, Mauer MB, Ayres NA, et al: Effects of chronic exercise on blood volume expansion and hematologic indices during pregnancy. Obstet Gynecol 83:265, 1994

Pritchard JA, Scott DE: Iron demands during pregnancy. In Hallberg L, Harwerth HG, Vannotti A (eds): Iron Deficiency: Pathogenesis, Clinical Aspects, Therapy. New York, Academic Press, 1970

Quaranta P, Currell R, Redman CWG, et al: Prediction of small-for-dates infants by measurement of symphysial-fundal height. Br J Obstet Gynaecol 88:115, 1981

Radhika MS, Bhaskaram P, Balakrishna N, et al: Effects of vitamin A deficiency during pregnancy on maternal and child health. Br J Obstet Gynaecol 109:689, 2002

Read JS, Klebanoff MA: Sexual intercourse during pregnancy and preterm delivery: Effects of vaginal microorganisms. Am J Obstet Gynecol 168:514, 1993

Rinsky-Eng J, Miller L: Knowledge, use, and education regarding folic acid supplementation: Continuation study of women in Colorado who had a pregnancy affected by a neural tube defect. Teratology 66:S29, 2002

Ryan ET, Wilson ME, Kain KC: Illness after international travel. N Engl J Med 347:505, 2002

Sa Roriz Fonteles C, Zero DT, Moss ME, et al: Fluoride concentrations in enamel and dentin of primary teeth after pre- and postnatal fluoride exposure. Caries Res 39:505, 2005

Sayle AE, Savitz DA, Thorp JM Jr, et al: Sexual activity during late pregnancy and risk of preterm delivery. Obstet Gynecol 97:283, 2001

Schauberger CW, Rooney BL, Brimer LM: Factors that influence weight loss in the puerperium. Obstet Gynecol 79:424, 1992

Schramm WF: Weighing costs and benefits of adequate prenatal care for 12,023 births in Missouri's Medicaid Program, 1988. Public Health Rep 107:647, November–December 1992

Scott DE, Pritchard JA, Saltin AS, et al: Iron deficiency during pregnancy. In Hallberg L, Harwerth HG, Vannotti A (eds): Iron Deficiency: Pathogenesis, Clinical Aspects, Therapy. New York, Academic Press, 1970

Selenkow HA, Varma K, Younger D, et al: Patterns of serum immunoreactive human placental lactogen (IR-HPL) and chorionic gonadotropin (IR-HCG) in diabetic pregnancy. Diabetes 20:696, 1971

Sibai BM, Villar MA, Bray E: Magnesium supplementation during pregnancy: A double-blind randomized controlled clinical trial. Am J Obstet Gynecol 161:115, 1989

Smith CA: Effects of maternal undernutrition upon the newborn infant in Holland (1944–1945). Am J Obstet Gynecol 30:229, 1947

Smith MW, Marcus PS, Wurtz LD: Orthopedic issues in pregnancy. Obstet Gynecol Surv 63:103, 2008

Speert H: Obstetrics and Gynecology in America: A History. Chicago, American College of Obstetricians and Gynecologists, 1980, p 142

Staroselsky A, Garcia-Bournissen F, Koren G: American Gastroenterological Association Institute medical position statement on the use of gastrointestinal medication in pregnancy. Gastroenterology 132:824, 2007

Stein Z, Susser M, Saenger G, et al: Nutrition and mental performance. Science 178:708, 1972

Suarez VR, Hankins GD: Smallpox and pregnancy: From eradicated disease to bioterrorist threat. Obstet Gynecol 100:87, 2002

Sugarman SD: Cases in vaccine court—legal battles over vaccines and autism. N Engl J Med 257:1275, 2007

Tan PC, Yow CM, Omar SZ: Effect of coital activity on onset of labor in women scheduled for labor induction. Obstet Gynecol 110:820, 2007

Thaver D, Saeed MA, Bhutta ZA: Pyridoxine (vitamin B_6) supplementation in pregnancy. Cochrane Database Syst Rev 2:CD000179, 2006

Thompson MD, Cole DE, Ray JG: Vitamin B_{12} and neural tube defects: the Canadian experience. Am J Clin Nutr 89(2):697S, 2009

Thompson WW, Price C, Goodson B, et al: Early thimerosal exposure and neuropsychological outcomes at 7 to 10 years. N Engl J Med 257:1281, 2007

Thornley I, Eapen M, Sung L, et al: Private cord blood banking: experiences and views of pediatric hematopoietic cell transplantation physicians. Pediatrics 123(3):1011, 2009

Tozzi AE, Bisiacchi P, Tarantino V, et al: Neuropsychological performance 10 years after immunization in infancy with thimerosal-containing vaccines. Pediatrics 123(2):475, 2009

United States Department of Health and Human Services: Reducing tobacco use: A report of the Surgeon General. Atlanta, GA, U.S. Department of Health and Human Services, Centers for Disease Control and Prevention, National Center for Chronic Disease Prevention and Health Promotion, Office on Smoking and Health, 2000

United States Department of Labor: Family and Medical Leave Act. Available at: www.dol.gov/esa/whd/fmla/. Accessed January 22, 2008

United States Environmental Protection Agency: What you need to know about mercury in fish and shellfish. Available at: www.epa.gov/waterscience/fish/advice/. Accessed March 13, 2008

Villar J, Báaqeel H, Piaggio G, et al: WHO antenatal care randomised trial for the evaluation of a new model of routine antenatal care. Lancet 357:1551, 2001

Vintzileos AM, Ananth CV, Smulian JC, et al: Prenatal care and black-white fetal death disparity in the United States: Heterogeneity by high-risk conditions. Obstet Gynecol 99:483, 2002a

Vintzileos AM, Ananth CV, Smulian JC, et al: The impact of prenatal care on neonatal deaths in the presence and absence of antenatal high-risk conditions. Am J Obstet Gynecol 186:1011, 2002b

Vintzileos AM, Ananth CV, Smulian JC, et al: The impact of prenatal care on preterm births among twin gestations in the United States, 1989–2000. Am J Obstet Gynecol 189:818, 2003

Wang SM, Dezinno P, Maranets I, et al: Low back pain during pregnancy: Prevalence, risk factors, and outcomes. Obstet Gynecol 104:65, 2004

Webster J, Holt V: Screening for partner violence: Direct questioning or self-report? Obstet Gynecol 103:299, 2004

West KP: Vitamin A deficiency disorders in children and women. Food Nutr Bull 24:S78, 2003

Wiesen AR, Littell CT: Relationship between prepregnancy anthrax vaccination and pregnancy and birth outcomes among U.S. Army women. JAMA 287:1556, 2002

Wilcox AJ, Baird DD, Dunson D, et al: Natural limits of pregnancy testing in relation to the expected menstrual period. JAMA 286:1759, 2001

Williams JW: The limitations and possibilities of prenatal care. JAMA 64:95, 1915

Wisborg K, Henriksen TB, Jespersen LB, et al: Nicotine patches for pregnant smokers: A randomized controlled study. Obstet Gynecol 96:967, 2000

Worthen N, Bustillo M: Effect of urinary bladder fullness on fundal height measurements. Am J Obstet Gynecol 138:759, 1980

Zaman K, Roy E, Arifeen SE, et al: Effectiveness of maternal influenza immunization in mothers and infants. N Engl J Med 359(15):1555, 2008

Zeskind PS, Gingras JL: Maternal cigarette-smoking during pregnancy disrupts rhythms in fetal heart rate. J Pediatr Psychology 31:5, 2006

CHAPTER 9

Abortion

The word *abortion* derives from the Latin *aboriri*—to miscarry. According to the New Shorter Oxford Dictionary (2002), abortion is premature birth before a live birth is possible, and in this sense it is synonymous with miscarriage. It also means an induced pregnancy termination to destroy the fetus. Although both terms are used interchangeably in a medical context, popular use of the word *abortion* by laypersons implies a deliberate pregnancy termination. Thus, many prefer *miscarriage* to refer to spontaneous fetal loss before viability. To add to confusion, widespread use of sonography and measurement of serum human chorionic gonadotropin levels allow identification of extremely early pregnancies along with terms to describe these. Some examples are *early pregnancy loss* or *early pregnancy failure*. Throughout this book, we employ all of these at one time or another.

The duration of pregnancy is also used to define and classify abortions for statistical and legal purposes (see Chap. 1, p. 3). For example, the National Center for Health Statistics, the Centers for Disease Control and Prevention, and the World Health Organization define *abortion* as pregnancy termination prior to 20 weeks' gestation or with a fetus born weighing less than 500 g. Despite this, definitions vary widely according to state laws.

SPONTANEOUS ABORTION

More than 80 percent of spontaneous abortions are in the first 12 weeks. As shown in Figure 9-1, at least half result from chromosomal anomalies. There also appears to be a 1.5 male:female gender ratio in early abortuses (Benirschke and Kaufmann, 2000). After the first trimester, both the abortion rate and the incidence of chromosomal anomalies decrease.

Hemorrhage into the decidua basalis, with adjacent tissue necrosis, usually accompanies early miscarriage. In these cases, the ovum detaches, and this stimulates uterine contractions that result in expulsion. When a gestational sac is opened, fluid is commonly found surrounding a small macerated fetus, or alternatively, there is no fetus—the so-called *blighted ovum*.

Incidence

The prevalence of spontaneous abortion varies according to diligence used in its identification. For example, Wilcox and colleagues (1988) studied 221 healthy women through 707 menstrual cycles. They found that 31 percent of pregnancies were lost after implantation. Importantly, using highly specific assays for minute concentrations of maternal serum β-human chorionic gonadotropin (β-hCG), two thirds of these early losses were designated as *clinically silent*.

A number of factors influence the spontaneous abortion rate, but it is not known at this time if those that are clinically silent are affected by some of these. For example, clinically apparent miscarriage increases with parity as well as with maternal and paternal age (Gracia, 2005; Warburton, 1964; Wilson, 1986, and all their colleagues). The frequency doubles from 12 percent in women younger than 20 years to 26 percent in those older than 40 years. For the same comparison of paternal ages, the frequency increases from 12 to 20 percent. But again, it is not known if clinically silent miscarriages are similarly affected by age and parity.

Although mechanisms responsible for abortion are not always apparent, during the first 3 months of pregnancy, death of the embryo or fetus nearly always precedes spontaneous expulsion. Thus, finding the cause of early abortion involves ascertaining the cause of fetal death. In later losses, the fetus usually

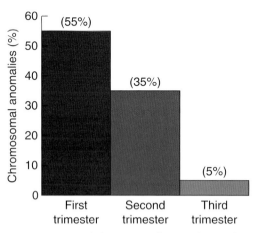

FIGURE 9-1 Frequency of chromosomal anomalies in abortuses and stillbirths during each trimester. Approximate percentages for each group are shown. (Data from Eiben, 1990; Fantel, 1980; Warburton, 1980, and all their colleagues.)

does not die before expulsion, and other explanations are sought.

Fetal Factors

Early spontaneous abortions commonly display a developmental abnormality of the zygote, embryo, fetus, or at times, the placenta. Of 1000 spontaneous abortions analyzed by Hertig and Sheldon (1943), half had a degenerated or absent embryo—the *blighted ovum* described previously. In 50 to 60 percent of spontaneously aborted embryos and early fetuses, abnormalities in chromosomal numbers account for most wastage (Table 9-1). Chromosomal errors become less common with advancing pregnancy and are found in approximately a third of second-trimester losses but in only 5 percent of third-trimester stillbirths (see Chap. 29, p. 630).

Aneuploid Abortion

Approximately 95 percent of chromosomal abnormalities are caused by maternal gametogenesis errors, whereas 5 percent are

due to paternal errors (Jacobs and Hassold, 1980). Those found most commonly in abortuses are listed in Table 9-1.

Autosomal trisomy is the most frequently identified chromosomal anomaly with first-trimester miscarriages. Although most trisomies result from *isolated nondisjunction*, balanced structural chromosomal rearrangements are present in one partner in 2 to 4 percent of couples with recurrent miscarriage (American College of Obstetricians and Gynecologists, 2001). Autosomal trisomies for all except chromosome number 1 have been identified in abortuses, and those with autosomes 13, 16, 18, 21, and 22 are most common. Bianco and colleagues (2006) recently described that a previous miscarriage increased the risk of a subsequent fetal aneuploidy from a baseline risk of 1.39 percent to 1.67 percent in almost 47,000 women. Two or three previous miscarriages increased this to 1.84 and 2.18 percent, respectively.

Monosomy X (45,X) is the single most common specific chromosomal abnormality. These cause Turner syndrome, which usually results in abortion and much less frequently in live-born females (Chap. 12, p. 270). Conversely, *autosomal monosomy* is rare and incompatible with life.

Triploidy is often associated with hydropic placental (molar) degeneration (Chap. 11, p. 258). Incomplete (partial) hydatidiform moles may be triploid or trisomic for only chromosome 16. Although these fetuses frequently abort early, the few carried longer are all grossly malformed. Advanced maternal and paternal age does not increase the incidence of triploidy.

Tetraploid abortuses are rarely live born and are most often aborted early in gestation.

Chromosomal structural abnormalities infrequently cause abortion. Some infants who are live born with a balanced translocation may appear normal as discussed on page 224.

Euploid Abortion

Chromosomally normal fetuses tend to abort later in gestation than those with aneuploidy. For example, although 75 percent of aneuploid abortions occurred before 8 weeks, euploid abortions peaked at approximately 13 weeks (Kajii, 1980). The incidence of euploid abortions increases dramatically after maternal age exceeds 35 years (Stein and co-workers, 1980).

TABLE 9-1. Chromosomal Findings in Abortuses

Chromosomal Studies	Incidence in Percent		
	Kajii et al. (1980)	Eiben et al. (1990)	Simpson (1980)
Normal (euploid)			
46,XY and 46,XX	46	51	54
Abnormal (aneuploid)			
Autosomal trisomy	31	31	22
Monosomy X (45,X)	10	5	9
Triploidy	7	6	8
Tetraploidy	2	4	3
Structural anomaly	2	2	2
Double or triple trisomy	2	0.9	0.7

Maternal Factors

The causes of euploid abortions are poorly understood, although a variety of medical disorders, environmental conditions, and developmental abnormalities have been implicated. The well-known influence of maternal age was discussed above.

Infections

According to the American College of Obstetricians and Gynecologists (2001), infections are an uncommon cause of early abortion. Even in their study of insulin-dependent diabetic women—presumably more susceptible to infection—Simpson and co-workers (1996) found no evidence of infection-induced miscarriage.

A number of specific infections have been studied. For example, although *Brucella abortus* and *Campylobacter fetus* cause abortion in cattle, they do not do so in humans (Sauerwein and associates, 1993). There is also no evidence that either *Listeria monocytogenes* or *Chlamydia trachomatis* stimulate abortions in humans (Feist, 1999; Osser, 1996; Paukku, 1999, and all their colleagues). In a prospective study, infection with herpes simplex virus in early pregnancy also did not increase the incidence (Brown and co-workers, 1997). Evidence that *Toxoplasma gondii* causes abortion in humans remains inconclusive.

Data concerning a link between some other infections and increased abortion are conflicting. For example, Quinn and co-workers (1983a, b) provided serological evidence that supports a role for *Mycoplasma hominis* and *Ureaplasma urealyticum.* Conversely, Temmerman and associates (1992) found no link between genital mycoplasma and spontaneous abortion. They did find abortion to be independently associated with serological evidence of syphilis and HIV-1 infection, and with vaginal colonization with group B streptococci. In contrast, van Benthem and associates (2000) reported that women had the same risk for spontaneous abortion before and after they had developed HIV infection. Oakeshott and associates (2002) reported an association between second, but not first-trimester miscarriage and *bacterial vaginosis* (see Chap. 59, p. 1246).

Chronic Debilitating Diseases

Early abortions are rarely secondary to chronic wasting diseases such as tuberculosis or carcinomatosis. Celiac sprue, however, has been reported to cause both male and female infertility and recurrent abortions (Sher and colleagues, 1994).

Endocrine Abnormalities

Hypothyroidism. Severe iodine deficiency may be associated with miscarriages (Castañeda and co-workers, 2002). Thyroid hormone deficiency is common in women, it is usually caused by an autoimmune disorder, but any effects of hypothyroidism on early pregnancy loss have not been adequately studied. Thyroid autoantibodies alone have been associated with an increased incidence of miscarriage (Abramson and Stagnaro-Green, 2001; Poppe and colleagues, 2008). As discussed on page 226, the data are less convincing that women with *recurrent miscarriage* have a greater incidence of antithyroid antibodies than normal controls.

Diabetes Mellitus

Spontaneous abortion and major congenital malformation rates are both increased in women with insulin-dependent diabetes. The risk appears related to the degree of metabolic control in early pregnancy. In a prospective study, Mills and associates (1988) reported that excellent glucose control within 21 days of conception resulted in a miscarriage rate similar to that in nondiabetic controls. Poor glucose control, however, resulted in a markedly increased abortion rate. Overt diabetes is a cause of recurrent pregnancy loss, and Craig and co-workers (2002) have reported a higher incidence of insulin resistance in these women. This is discussed further on page 226.

Nutrition

Dietary deficiency of any one nutrient or moderate deficiency of all nutrients does not appear to be an important cause of abortion. Even at the extreme, hyperemesis gravidarum with significant weight loss is rarely followed by miscarriage. In one study, Maconochie and associates (2007) found a reduced risk in women who ate fresh fruit and vegetables daily.

Drug Use and Environmental Factors

A variety of different agents have been reported to be associated with an increased incidence of abortion.

Tobacco. Smoking has been linked with an increased risk for euploid abortion (Kline and co-workers, 1980). Two studies suggested that the abortion risk increased in a linear fashion with cigarettes smoked per day (Armstrong and colleagues, 1992; Chatenoud and associates, 1998). Subsequent studies, however, failed to support this association (Maconochie, 2007; Rasch, 2003; Wisborg, 2003, and all their co-workers).

Alcohol. Both spontaneous abortion and fetal anomalies may result from frequent alcohol use during the first 8 weeks of pregnancy (Floyd and co-workers, 1999). The risk seems to be related to both frequency and dose (Armstrong and associates, 1992). A low level of alcohol consumption during pregnancy was not associated with a significant risk for abortion (Kesmodel and associates, 2002; Maconochie and co-workers, 2007).

Caffeine. Armstrong and associates (1992) reported that women who consumed at least five cups of coffee per day had a slightly increased abortion risk, and that above this threshold, the risk correlated linearly. Similarly, Cnattingius and colleagues (2000) observed a significantly increased abortion risk only in women who consumed at least 500 mg of caffeine daily—roughly equivalent to five cups of coffee. Klebanoff and associates (1999) reported that pregnant women in whom levels of the caffeine metabolite paraxanthine were extremely elevated had a twofold risk for miscarriage. They concluded that moderate caffeine consumption was unlikely to cause spontaneous abortion.

Radiation. In therapeutic doses given to treat malignancy, radiation is certainly an abortifacient (see Chap. 41, p. 915). Although lower doses are less toxic, the human dose to effect abortion is not precisely known. According to Brent (1999), exposure to less than five rads does not increase the risk for miscarriage.

Contraceptives. Oral contraceptives or spermicidal agents used in contraceptive creams and jellies are not associated with an increased miscarriage rate. When intrauterine devices fail to prevent pregnancy, however, the risk of abortion, and specifically septic abortion, increases substantively (see Chap. 32, p. 685).

Environmental Toxins. Accurately assessing the relationship between environmental exposures and miscarriage poses challenges. There may be difficulties in measuring the intensity and duration of exposure, and there is little information to conclusively indict or absolve any specific agent. Some studies include those by Barlow and Sullivan (1982), who found that arsenic, lead, formaldehyde, benzene, and ethylene oxide possibly cause miscarriages. Video display terminals and exposure to their accompanying electromagnetic fields do not adversely affect miscarriage rates (Schnorr and associates, 1991). Similarly, no effects were found with occupational exposure to ultrasound (Taskinen and colleagues, 1990). An increased risk of miscarriage has been described for dental assistants exposed to 3 or more hours of nitrous oxide per day in offices without gas-scavenging equipment (Rowland and co-workers, 1995). Before the use of such equipment, Boivin (1997) concluded that women occupationally exposed to anesthetic gases had an increased risk for miscarriage. In another meta-analysis, Dranitsaris and colleagues (2005) identified a small incremental risk for spontaneous abortion in female staff who worked with cytotoxic chemotherapeutic drugs.

Immunological Factors

A number of immune-mediated disorders are associated with early pregnancy loss. Many tend to be repetitive, and they are considered with recurrent miscarriage (p. 225).

Inherited Thrombophilias

Some genetic disorders of blood coagulation may increase the risk of both arterial and venous thrombosis. The better studied thrombophilias are caused by mutations of the genes for factor V Leiden, prothrombin, antithrombin, proteins C and S, and methylene tetrahydrofolate reductase (hyperhomocysteinemia). Because these are most commonly associated with recurrent miscarriage, they are considered on page 225.

Maternal Surgery

Uncomplicated abdominal or pelvic surgery performed during early pregnancy does not appear to increase the risk for abortion. Ovarian tumors are generally removed without interfering with pregnancy (see Chap. 40, p. 904). An important exception involves early removal of the corpus luteum or the ovary in which the corpus luteum resides. If performed prior to 10 weeks' gestation, supplemental progesterone is indicated. If between 8 and 10 weeks, then only one injection of intramuscular 17-hydroxyprogesterone caproate, 150 mg, is required immediately after surgery. If the corpus luteum is excised between 6 to 8 weeks, then two additional doses should be given one and two weeks after the first.

Trauma

Presumably, major abdominal trauma can precipitate abortion, however, this is unusual. Any effects of minor trauma are difficult to ascertain. In general, trauma contributes minimally to the incidence of abortion (see Chap. 42, p. 936).

Uterine Defects

Acquired Uterine Defects.
Large and multiple uterine leiomyomas are common, and they may cause miscarriage. In most instances, their location is more important than their size (see Chap. 40, p. 901). Uterine synechiae—*Asherman syndrome*—usually result from destruction of large areas of endometrium by curettage. A hysterosalpingogram may show characteristic multiple filling defects, but hysteroscopy is more accurate for diagnosis. With subsequent pregnancy, the amount of remaining endometrium may be insufficient to support the pregnancy, and abortion may ensue.

Developmental Uterine Defects.
Abnormal müllerian duct formation or fusion defects may develop spontaneously or may follow in utero exposure to diethylstilbestrol (DES) (see Chap. 40, p. 897). Although they can cause midpregnancy loss and other preterm birth and pregnancy complications, it is controversial whether uterine defects cause early miscarriage. As discussed on page 224, corrective procedures to prevent abortion, if done at all, should be performed as a last resort and with a full understanding that they may not be effective (American College of Obstetricians and Gynecologists, 2001).

Incompetent Cervix

This describes a discrete obstetrical entity characterized by painless cervical dilatation in the second trimester. It can be followed by prolapse and ballooning of membranes into the vagina, and ultimately, expulsion of an immature fetus. Unless effectively treated, this sequence may repeat in future pregnancies.

Unfortunately, women with pregnancies that abort in the second trimester often have histories and clinical findings that make it difficult to distinguish true cervical incompetence from other causes of midtrimester pregnancy loss. MacNaughton and colleagues (1993) studied almost 1300 women with nonclassical histories of cervical incompetence. In a randomized trial with the primary outcome of delivery before 33 weeks, cerclage was found to be beneficial, albeit marginally. Specifically, 13 percent of women in the cerclage group delivered prior to 33 weeks compared with 17 percent in the noncerclage group. Said another way, for every 25 cerclage procedures, one birth before 33 weeks was prevented.

Recently, interest has been focused on the use of transvaginal sonography to identify cervical incompetence. Some features—primarily cervical length—when measured at midpregnancy, may predict preterm delivery. Another is termed *funneling*—ballooning of the membranes into a dilated internal os, but with a closed external os (Owen and associates, 2003).

The clinical relevance of these cervical changes is not entirely clear. Three randomized cerclage trials that studied such women reported conflicting results. Rust and colleagues (2001) randomized 113 women with a cervical length of less than 25 mm or with substantive funneling to undergo either cerclage or expectant management. The incidence of preterm birth was 35 percent in the cerclage group and 36 percent in the control group. In a second study, To and colleagues (2004) randomly assigned 253 women to cerclage placement and reported that the risk of early preterm birth was not significantly reduced. The third study by Althuisius and colleagues (2001) randomized only 35 women, but results suggested that cerclage might be beneficial. At least at this time, the use of sonography to diagnose cervical incompetence is not recommended.

Etiology. Although the cause of cervical incompetence is obscure, previous trauma to the cervix such as dilatation and curettage, conization, cauterization, or amputation has been implicated. In a population-based Norwegian cohort study of more than 15,000 women who had undergone cervical conization, Albrechtsen and colleagues (2008) reported a fourfold risk of pregnancy loss before 24 weeks. Chasen and associates (2005) reported that neither prior dilatation and evacuation (D&E) nor dilatation and extraction (D&X) after 20 weeks increased the likelihood of an incompetent cervix. In other instances, abnormal cervical development, including that following exposure to DES in utero, may play a role (see Chap. 40, p. 897).

Evaluation and Treatment. Once confirmed, classical cervical incompetence is treated with cerclage, which surgically reinforces a weak cervix by some type of purse-string suturing. Bleeding, uterine contractions, or ruptured membranes are usually contraindications to cerclage. Sonography is performed to confirm a living fetus and to exclude major fetal anomalies. Cervical specimens are tested for gonorrhea and chlamydial infection, and these and other obvious cervical infections are treated. For at least a week before and after surgery, sexual intercourse is prohibited.

Cerclage ideally is performed prophylactically before cervical dilatation. In some cases, this is not possible, and *rescue cerclage* is performed emergently after the cervix is found to be dilated or effaced. Elective cerclage generally is performed between 12 and 16 weeks, but there is debate as to how late emergency cerclage should be performed. The conundrum is that the more advanced the pregnancy, the greater the risk that surgical intervention will stimulate preterm labor or membrane rupture. Although this is not evidence based, we usually do not perform cerclage after approximately 23 weeks, however, others recommend placement even later (Caruso and associates, 2000; Terkildsen and colleagues, 2003).

In a 10-year review of 75 women undergoing emergency cerclage procedures, Chasen and Silverman (1998) reported that 65 percent were delivered at 28 weeks or later, and half delivered after 36 weeks. Importantly, only 44 percent of those with bulging membranes at the time of cerclage reached 28 weeks. Caruso and associates (2000) reported their experience with emergency cerclage in 23 women from 17 to 27 weeks who had a dilated cervix and protruding membranes. Because only 11 live-born infants resulted, they concluded that success was unpredictable. Based on their 20-year experience with 116 women, Terkildsen and colleagues (2003) reported that nulli-

paras and those with bulging membranes were significantly more likely to be delivered before 28 weeks. Cerclage after 22 weeks, however, was associated with a better chance of delivery beyond 28 weeks.

If the clinical indication for cerclage is questionable, these women may be advised to decrease physical activity and abstain from intercourse. Most receive cervical examinations each week or every 2 weeks to assess effacement and dilatation. Unfortunately, rapid effacement and dilatation can develop despite such precautions (Witter, 1984).

Cerclage Procedures. Two types of vaginal operations are commonly used during pregnancy. The more simple procedure developed by McDonald (1963) is shown in Figure 9-2. The more complicated operation is a modification of the original procedure described by Shirodkar (1955) and shown in Figure 9-3. Compared with historical controls, women with classical histories of cervical incompetence have success rates approaching 85 to 90 percent when either technique is performed prophylactically (Caspi and associates, 1990; Kuhn and Pepperell, 1977). For these reasons, most practitioners reserve the modified Shirodkar procedure for women with a previous failure of the McDonald cerclage or those with structural cervical abnormalities.

During emergency cerclage, replacing the prolapsed amnionic sac back into the uterus will usually aid suture placement (Locatelli and associates, 1999). Tilting the operating table head down may be beneficial. And filling the bladder with 600 mL of saline through an indwelling Foley catheter usually will help to reduce prolapsing membranes. Unfortunately, this maneuver also can carry the cervix cephalad, away from the operating field. Some advocate placing a Foley catheter with a 30-mL balloon through the cervix and inflating the balloon to deflect the amnionic sac cephalad. The balloon is then deflated gradually as the cerclage suture is tightened.

Transabdominal cerclage with the suture placed at the uterine isthmus is used in some cases of severe anatomical defects of the cervix or cases of prior transvaginal cerclage failure (Cammarano and colleagues, 1995; Gibb and Salaria, 1995). In a review of 14 retrospective reports, Zaveri and associates (2002) concluded that when a prior transvaginal cerclage failed to prevent preterm delivery, the risk of perinatal death or delivery prior to 24 weeks following transabdominal cerclage (6 percent) was only slightly lower than the risk following repeat transvaginal cerclage (13 percent). Importantly, 3 percent of women who underwent transabdominal cerclage had serious operative complications, whereas there were none in women in the transvaginal group. Although transabdominal cerclage has been performed through the laparoscope, it generally requires laparotomy for initial suture placement and subsequent laparotomy for removal of the suture, for delivery of the fetus, or both.

Complications. Charles and Edward (1981) identified complications, especially infection, to be less frequent when elective cerclage was performed by 18 weeks. In the trial by MacNaughton and colleagues (1993), membrane rupture complicated only 1 of more than 600 procedures done before 19 weeks. Cerclage

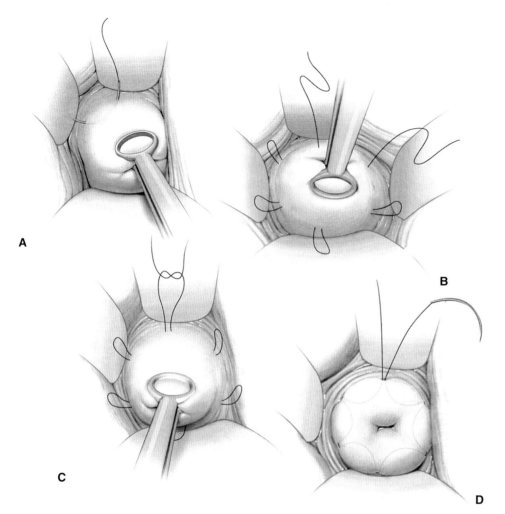

FIGURE 9-2 McDonald cerclage procedure for incompetent cervix. **A.** Start of the cerclage procedure with a number 2 monofilament suture being placed in the body of the cervix very near the level of the internal os. **B.** Continuation of suture placement in the body of the cervix so as to encircle the os. **C.** Completion of encirclement. **D.** The suture is tightened around the cervical canal sufficiently to reduce the diameter of the canal to 5 to 10 mm, and then the suture is tied. The effect of the suture placement on the cervical canal is apparent. A second suture placed somewhat higher may be of value if the first is not in close proximity to the internal os.

servation, or removal of the cerclage and labor induction (Barth, 1995). Insufficient data limit firm recommendations, and the optimal management remains controversial (O'Connor and associates, 1999).

Following the modified Shirodkar operation, the suture may be left in place, and cesarean delivery performed. Conversely, it may be removed, and vaginal delivery permitted.

Paternal Factors

Little is known about paternal factors in the genesis of miscarriage. Certainly, chromosomal abnormalities in sperm have been associated with abortion (Carrell and co-workers, 2003).

Clinical Classification of Spontaneous Abortion

Spontaneous abortion can be classified clinically a number of ways. Commonly used subgroups include threatened, inevitable, incomplete, and missed abortion. *Septic abortion* is the condition when the products of conception and uterus are infected. Finally, *recurrent miscarriage*—also termed *recurrent pregnancy loss*—describes consecutive early losses with implied similar etiology.

was associated with higher rates of subsequent hospitalization and tocolysis, as well as a doubling of the incidence of puerperal fever—6 percent versus 3 percent. Thomason and co-workers (1982) found that perioperative antimicrobial prophylaxis failed to prevent most infection, and tocolytics failed to arrest most labor. With clinical infection, the suture should be cut, and labor induced or augmented if necessary. Similarly, if signs of imminent abortion or delivery develop, the suture should be released at once. Failure to do so may enable vigorous uterine contractions to tear the uterus or cervix.

Membrane rupture during suture placement or within the first 48 hours following surgery is considered by some to be an indication for cerclage removal. Kuhn and Pepperell (1977) reported that rupture in the absence of labor increased the likelihood of serious fetal or maternal infection if the suture was left in situ and delivery was delayed. Still, the range of management options includes observation, removal of the cerclage and ob-

Threatened Abortion

The clinical diagnosis of *threatened abortion* is presumed when a bloody vaginal discharge or bleeding appears through a closed cervical os during the first half of pregnancy. These develop in 20 to 25 percent of women during early gestation and may persist for days or weeks. Approximately half of these pregnancies will abort, although the risk is substantially lower if fetal cardiac activity is visualized (Tongsong and colleagues, 1995).

Eddleman and associates (2006) designed an individualized risk assessment model for spontaneous pregnancy loss in more than 35,000 pregnancies. By far, bleeding during the current pregnancy was the most predictive risk factor for pregnancy loss. Even if abortion does not follow early bleeding, these fetuses are at increased risk for preterm delivery, low birthweight, and perinatal death (Johns and Jauniaux, 2006; Weiss and associates, 2002). Fortunately, the risk of a malformed surviving infant does not appear to be increased. Maternal risks include antepartum hemorrhage, manual removal of the placenta, and cesarean delivery (Wijesiriwardana and co-workers, 2006).

One physiological cause of bleeding occurs near the time of expected menses—*implantation bleeding.* Cervical lesions commonly bleed in early pregnancy, especially after intercourse. Cervical polyps and decidual reaction also tend to bleed in early gestation. Bleeding from these benign sources is not accompanied by lower abdominal pain and low backache.

With miscarriage, bleeding usually begins first, and cramping abdominal pain follows a few hours to several days later. The pain may present as anterior and clearly rhythmic cramps; as a persistent low backache, associated with a feeling of pelvic pressure; or as a dull, midline, suprapubic discomfort. Whichever form the pain takes, the combination of bleeding and pain predicts a poor prognosis for pregnancy continuation.

Because ectopic pregnancy, ovarian torsion, and the other types of abortion may mimic threatened abortion, women with early pregnancy bleeding and pain should be evaluated. With persistent or heavy bleeding, a hematocrit is performed, and if there is significant anemia or hypovolemia, then pregnancy evacuation is usually indicated.

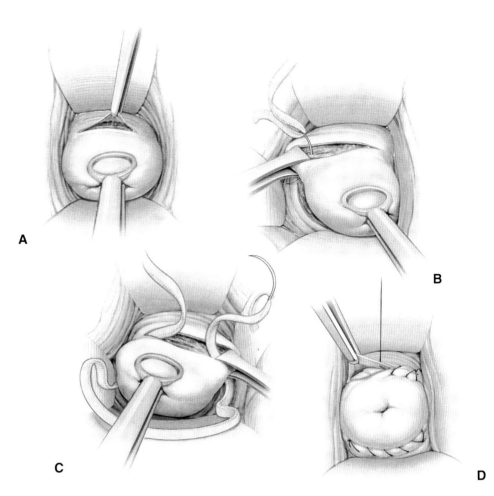

FIGURE 9-3 Modified Shirodkar cerclage for incompetent cervix. **A.** A transverse incision is made in the mucosa overlying the anterior cervix, and the bladder is pushed cephalad. **B.** A 5-mm Mersiline tape on a Mayo needle is passed anteriorly to posteriorly. **C.** The tape is then directed posteriorly to anteriorly on the other side of the cervix. Allis clamps placed so as to bunch the cervical tissue to diminish the distance the needle must travel submucosally facilitate placement of the tape. **D.** The tape is snugly tied anteriorly, after ensuring that all slack has been taken up. The cervical mucosa is then closed with continuous stitches of chromic suture to bury the anterior knot.

There are no effective therapies for threatened abortion. Bed rest, although often prescribed, does not alter its course. Acetaminophen-based analgesia may be given for discomfort. Typically, transvaginal sonography, serial serum quantitative human chorionic gonadotropin (hCG), and serum progesterone levels, used alone or in combination, are analyzed to ascertain if the fetus is alive and within the uterus. Because they are not 100-percent accurate to confirm fetal death, repeat evaluations may be necessary.

Ectopic pregnancy should always be considered in the differential diagnosis of threatened abortion. In one report, Condous and colleagues (2005) described 152 women with heavy bleeding who were diagnosed to have a completed miscarriage and an endometrial thickness < 15 mm. Almost 6 percent of these women were found to have an ectopic pregnancy on further evaluation.

It is imperative to recognize an early ectopic pregnancy before tubal rupture develops. Thus, for women with abnormal bleeding or pelvic pain who have low serum β-hCG levels, an

extrauterine pregnancy must be differentiated from a normal uterine pregnancy or an early miscarriage (Chap. 10, p. 243). Barnhart and colleagues (2004a) have provided data concerning composite serum β-hCG disappearance curves in women with early miscarriage (Fig. 9-4). They also provided similar data for symptomatic women with a normal early pregnancy (Barnhart and associates, 2004b).

Anti-D Immunoglobulin

The D-negative woman is given anti-D immunoglobulin following miscarriage because as many as 5 percent become isoimmunized without it. This practice is controversial with threatened abortion because it lacks evidence-based support (American College of Obstetricians and Gynecologists, 1999; Weissman and associates, 2002).

Inevitable Abortion

Gross rupture of the membranes, evidenced by leaking amnionic fluid in the presence of cervical dilatation, signals almost certain abortion. Commonly, either uterine contractions begin

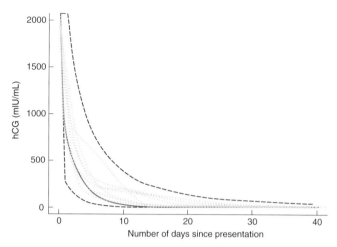

FIGURE 9-4 Composite curve describing decline in serial serum β-hCG values starting at a level of 2000 mIU/mL following early spontaneous miscarriage. The yellow dotted lines are individual patients. The solid blue line is the predicted curve based on the summary of all data, and the two red dashed lines represent the 95-percent confidence intervals. (From Barnhart, 2004a, with permission.)

promptly to cause miscarriage, or infection develops. Rarely, a gush of vaginal fluid during the first half of pregnancy is without serious consequence. If not emanating from the bladder, the fluid may have collected previously between the amnion and chorion. Because of this possibility, if a sudden discharge of fluid in early pregnancy occurs before pain, fever, or bleeding, then diminished activity with observation is reasonable. After 48 hours, if no additional amnionic fluid has escaped and if there is no bleeding, pain, or fever, then a woman may resume her usual activities except for any form of vaginal penetration. If, however, the gush of fluid is accompanied or followed by bleeding, pain, or fever, abortion should be considered inevitable, and the uterus emptied.

Incomplete Abortion

Bleeding ensues when the placenta, in whole or in part, detaches from the uterus. During *incomplete abortion*, the internal cervical os opens and allows passage of blood. The fetus and placenta may remain entirely in utero or may partially extrude through the dilated os. Before 10 weeks, the fetus and placenta are commonly expelled together, but later they are delivered separately. In some women, additional cervical dilatation is necessary before curettage is performed. In many cases, retained placental tissue simply lies loosely in the cervical canal, allowing easy extraction from an exposed external os with ring forceps. Suction curettage, as described later, effectively evacuates the uterus. In clinically stable women, expectant management of an incomplete abortion can also be a reasonable option (Blohm and colleagues, 2003).

Hemorrhage from incomplete abortion of a more advanced pregnancy is occasionally severe but rarely fatal. Therefore, in women with more advanced pregnancies or with heavy bleeding, evacuation is promptly performed. If there is fever, appropriate antibiotics are given before curettage.

Missed Abortion—Early Pregnancy Failure

The term *missed abortion* is contemporaneously imprecise because it was defined many decades before the advent of immunological pregnancy tests and sonography. It was used to describe dead products of conception that were retained for days, weeks, or even months in the uterus with a closed cervical os. Because spontaneous miscarriages are almost always preceded by embryofetal death, most were correctly referred to as "missed." In the typical instance, early pregnancy appears to be normal, with amenorrhea, nausea and vomiting, breast changes, and uterine growth. After embryonic death, there may or may not be vaginal bleeding or other symptoms of threatened abortion.

With sonography, confirmation of an anembryonic gestation or of fetal or embryonic death is possible (Fig. 9-5). Many women choose medical or surgical termination at the time of diagnosis. If the pregnancy is not terminated and if miscarriage does not follow for days or weeks, uterine size remains unchanged, and then gradually becomes smaller. Mammary changes usually regress, and women often lose a few pounds. Many women have no symptoms during this period except persistent amenorrhea. If the missed abortion terminates spontaneously, and most do, the process of expulsion is the same as in any abortion.

Septic Abortion

Maternal deaths associated with septic criminal abortions are rare in the United States. Occasionally, however, miscarriage and elective abortion may be complicated by severe infections (Barrett and co-workers, 2002; Fjerstad and associates, 2009). Endomyometritis is the most common manifestation of postabortal infection, but parametritis, peritonitis, septicemia, and even endocarditis occasionally develop (Vartian and Septimus, 1991). Treatment of infection includes prompt administration of intravenous broad-spectrum antibiotics followed by uterine evacuation. With severe sepsis syndrome, acute respiratory syndrome or disseminated intravascular coagulopathy may develop, and supportive care is essential (see Chap. 42, p. 932).

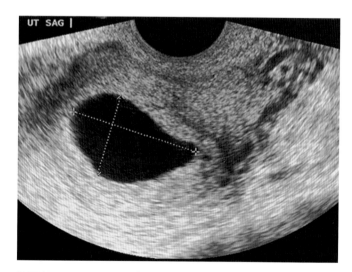

FIGURE 9-5 Transvaginal sonography displays an anembryonic gestation. (Used with permission from Dr. Elysia Moschos.)

TABLE 9-2. Some Randomized Controlled Studies for Management of Early Pregnancy Loss

Study	Type of Abortion	Treatment Arms	Outcomes
Blohm et al (2005)	"Signs of miscarriage" (n = 126)	1. Placebo 2. PGE$_1$, 400 μg vaginally	54% completed at 7 days 81% completed at 7 days; more pain, more analgesia
Trinder et al (2006)	Incomplete or missed SAB (n = 1200)	1. Expectant 2. PGE$_1$, 800 μg vaginally ± 200 mg mifepristone 3. Suction curettage	50% curettage 2% transfusions 38% curettage 1% transfusions 5% repeat curettage
Zhang et al (2005)	Pregnancy failure[a] (n = 652)	1. PGE$_1$, 800 μg vaginally 2. Vacuum aspiration	71% completed at 3 days; 84% by 8 days; 16% failure 97% successful
Weeks et al (2005)	Incomplete SAB (n = 312)	1. PGE$_1$, 600 μg vaginally 2. Vacuum aspiration	96% success, 1% complications 92% success, 10% complications
Dao et al (2007)	Incomplete SAB (n = 447)	1. PGE$_1$, 600 μg orally 2. Vacuum aspiration	95% completed 99% completed
Shwekerela et al (2007)	Incomplete SAB (n = 300)	1. PGE$_1$, 600 μg orally 2. Vacuum aspiration	99% completed 100% completed

[a]Includes anembryonic gestation, embryonic or fetal death, or incomplete or inevitable SAB.

PGE$_1$ = prostaglandin E$_1$; SAB = spontaneous abortion

In the past, criminal abortions and neglected incomplete abortions became infected by otherwise nonvirulent vaginal commensural bacteria such as *Clostridium perfringens*. These almost disappeared after abortion was legalized. However, in 2005, the Centers for Disease Control and Prevention reported four deaths associated with medical abortion from toxic shock syndrome caused by *Clostridium sordellii* infection. Fischer and colleagues (2005) detailed these infections and described clinical manifestations that began within 1 week after the medically induced abortion. The hallmark was severe endothelial injury with capillary leakage and hemoconcentration, hypotension, and profound leukocytosis. Since that time, Cohen and associates (2007) reported four other cases—two with *C. sordellii* and two with *C. perfringens*—that developed following spontaneous or induced abortions. Two were fatal. Daif and associates (2009) described a case of necrotizing fasciitis and toxic shock syndrome caused by group A streptococcal infection after elective medical abortion.

Management

With embryofetal death now easy to verify with current sonographic technology, management can be more individualized. Expectant, medical, and surgical management are all reasonable options unless there is serious bleeding or infection. Surgical treatment is definitive and predictable, but is invasive and not necessary for all women. Expectant and medical management may obviate curettage, but are associated with unpredictable bleeding, and some women will need unscheduled surgery. For example, in the observational study of Luise and colleagues (2002), 81 percent of almost 1100 women with suspected first-trimester miscarriage reported spontaneous resolution.

A number of randomized studies have been done to evaluate these methods. In many cases, however, the studies themselves are not comparable because different criteria were used for inclusion, and various protocols were employed. For example, emptying the uterus with medical therapy for early pregnancy failure has a higher success rate in those with vaginal bleeding compared with women with a more "intact" gestation (Creinin and colleagues, 2006). From the studies listed in Table 9-2, some generalizations can be made:

1. Success is dependent on the type of early pregnancy failure.
2. With spontaneous incomplete abortion, expectant management results in spontaneous completion in approximately half of cases.
3. For early pregnancy failure, otherwise not further defined, PGE$_1$ given orally or vaginally is effective in approximately 85 percent for completed abortion within 7 days.
4. Curettage is a quick resolution that is almost 100-percent successful in completing early pregnancy failures.

Thus, there are several management options that can be selected by the woman and her gynecologist. Of course, with dangerous hemorrhage or infection, prompt completion of abortion—either medically or surgically—is warranted.

RECURRENT MISCARRIAGE

This is also referred to as *recurrent spontaneous abortion* and *recurrent pregnancy loss*. It is classically defined as three or more consecutive pregnancy losses at 20 weeks or less or with fetal weights less than 500 grams. Most women with recurrent miscarriage have embryonic or early fetal loss, and the minority of losses are after 14 weeks. Although the definition includes three or more miscarriages, many agree that evaluation should at least be considered following two consecutive losses. This is because the risk of subsequent loss after two successive miscarriages is similar to that following three losses—approximately 30 percent (Harger and associates, 1983). Remarkably, the chance for successful pregnancy may approach 50 percent even after six losses (Poland and co-workers, 1977; Warburton and Fraser, 1964).

Recurrent miscarriage should be distinguished from sporadic pregnancy loss described in the previous section. Sporadic loss implies that intervening pregnancies have resulted in healthy infants. Others distinguish *primary recurrent miscarriage*—no successful pregnancies—from *secondary recurrent miscarriage*—one prior live birth—as the latter group does not reach a risk of subsequent loss of 32 percent until after three miscarriages. Thus, it is reasonable to delay evaluation of secondary recurrent loss until three consecutive losses (Poland and co-workers, 1977).

The causes of recurrent miscarriage parallel those of sporadic miscarriage, although the relative incidence differs between the two categories. For example, first-trimester losses with recurrent miscarriage have a significantly lower incidence of genetic anomalies (Sullivan and colleagues, 2004). In one series, normal karyotypes were identified in half of recurrent miscarriages but only a fourth of sporadic losses. The timing of the pregnancy losses may provide a clue to their cause. By way of another example, genetic factors most frequently result in early embryonic losses, whereas autoimmune or anatomical abnormalities are more likely to result in second-trimester losses (Schust and Hill, 2002).

Parental Chromosomal Abnormalities

Although these account for only 2 to 4 percent of recurrent losses, karyotypic evaluation of both parents remains a critical part of evaluation. Therapel and colleagues (1985) summarized data from 79 studies of couples with two or more miscarriages. These included 8208 women and 7834 men, and chromosomal abnormalities were detected in 2.9 percent—a fivefold greater incidence than for the general population. The ratio of female-to-male abnormalities was approximately 2:1. Balanced reciprocal translocations accounted for 50 percent of identified abnormalities; Robertsonian translocations for 24 percent; X chromosome mosaicism such as 47,XXY—*Klinefelter syndrome*—for 12 percent; and inversions and a variety of other anomalies comprised the remainder. Conversely, Hogge and associates (2007) reported that recurrent pregnancy loss is not associated with skewed X-inactivation—*transcriptional silencing*.

Inheritance of translocation syndromes is discussed in detail in Chapter 12 (p. 273). Briefly, if one parent carries a balanced translocation, the karyotype of a resultant pregnancy may be normal, the same balanced translocation, or an unbalanced translocation. Balanced translocations are likely to cause subsequent recurrent miscarriage in the offspring. An unbalanced translocation may produce a miscarriage, fetal anomaly, or stillbirth. Overall, however, the prognosis is good. Franssen and colleagues (2006) studied 247 couples with a balanced translocation and reported that almost 85 percent had at least one healthy infant. Thus, a history of second-trimester loss or fetal anomaly should raise the suspicion that an abnormal chromosome pattern is present in one parent. Couples with an abnormal karyotype should be offered preimplantation genetic counseling (Chap. 12, p. 301).

Routine karyotyping of products of conception is costly, may not accurately reflect the fetal karyotype, and we do not recommend it. That said, some recommend routine chromosomal analysis following a second consecutive miscarriage (Stephenson, 2006).

Anatomical Factors

A number of genital tract anatomical abnormalities have been implicated in recurrent miscarriage. According to Devi Wold and colleagues (2006), 15 percent of women with three or more consecutive miscarriages have a congenital or acquired uterine anomaly. These essentially are the same as those associated with all miscarriages and are discussed on page 218. They are also discussed in detail in Chapter 40 (p. 890). They include acquired uterine abnormalities such as intrauterine synechiae-*Asherman syndrome*, leiomyomas, and cervical incompetence. Developmental defects include septate, bicornuate, and unicornuate uterus as well as uterine didelphys. Also included are abnormalities associated with in utero exposure to DES.

The frequency of these anomalies in women with recurrent miscarriage varies widely depending on depth of evaluation and criteria set for abnormalcy. Salim and colleagues (2003) described nearly 2500 women who were screened for developmental uterine anomalies using three-dimensional sonography. Anomalies were identified in 24 percent of women with recurrent miscarriage, but in only 5 percent of normal controls. In other studies of women with recurrent miscarriage, the prevalence of uterine anomalies has been estimated to be only 7 to 15 percent (Ashton and co-workers, 1988; Makino and associates, 1992).

Treatment

As discussed on page 218, the evidence is not robust to link these anatomical anomalies with early pregnancy loss. It is therefore difficult to prove that their correction improves pregnancy outcome (American College of Obstetricians and Gynecologists, 2001). There are retrospective studies to support correction with some anomalies. Saygili-Yilmaz and colleagues (2003) reviewed pregnancy outcomes following hysteroscopic metroplasty in women who had a septate uterus and more than two prior miscarriages. In 59 such women, the incidence of miscarriage decreased from 96 to 10 percent following surgery, and term pregnancies increased from none to 70 percent (Saygili-Yilmaz and associates, 2002).

For uterine synechiae, hysteroscopic lysis is preferable to curettage. Katz and colleagues (1996) reported 90 women with synechiae who had at least two prior miscarriages or preterm perinatal deaths or both. With adhesiolysis, miscarriage rates decreased from 79 to 22 percent, and term pregnancies increased from 18 to 69 percent. Other studies have reported similar outcomes (Al-Inany, 2001; Goldenberg and associates, 1995).

As discussed in Chapter 40 (p. 903), it is controversial whether submucous myomas cause recurrent miscarriage more than infrequently. If symptomatic, most agree that submucosal and intracavitary fibroids should be excised. In studies of women undergoing in vitro fertilization, pregnancy outcomes were adversely affected by submucosal myomas, but not by those that were subserosal or intramural and less than 5 to 7 cm (Jun and co-workers, 2001; Ramzy and colleagues, 1998).

Immunological Factors

In their analysis of published studies, Yetman and Kutteh (1996) determined that 15 percent of more than 1000 women with recurrent miscarriage had recognized autoimmune factors. Two primary pathophysiological models are the *autoimmune theory*—immunity against self, and the *alloimmune theory*—immunity against another person.

Autoimmune Factors

Miscarriages are more common in women with systemic lupus erythematosus (Warren and Silver, 2004). Many of these women have antiphospholipid antibodies, which are a family of autoantibodies that bind to negatively charged phospholipids, phospholipids-binding proteins, or a combination of the two (Branch and Khamashta, 2003; Carp and colleagues, 2008). They also are found in women without lupus. Indeed, in up to 5 percent of normal pregnant women, lupus anticoagulant (LAC) and anticardiolipin antibody (ACA) have been linked with excessive pregnancy wastage. Instead of causing miscarriage, they more likely are found with fetal death after midpregnancy. Because of this, fetal death is one criterion for diagnosis of the *antiphospholipid syndrome* (American College of Obstetricians and Gynecologists, 2005a). These are discussed in Chapter 47 (p. 1017) and listed in Table 47-3 (p. 1018). This is the only autoimmune condition that can be correlated with adverse pregnancy outcome. Women with both a history of early fetal loss and high antibody levels may have a 70-percent miscarriage recurrence rate (Dudley and Branch, 1991). Antibodies to β_2-glycoprotein may be especially problematic, but not those to phosphatidyl serine (Alijotas-Reig and colleagues, 2008, 2009).

In a prospective study of 860 women screened for anticardiolipin antibody in the first trimester, Yasuda and colleagues (1995) reported that 7 percent tested positive. Miscarriage developed in 25 percent of the antibody-positive group, compared with only 10 percent of the negative group. In another study, however, Simpson and associates (1998) found no association between early pregnancy loss and the presence of either anticardiolipin antibody or lupus anticoagulant.

Treatment. There are treatment regimens for antiphospholipid syndrome that increase live birth rates. Kutteh (1996) randomized 50 affected women to receive either low-dose aspirin alone or low-dose aspirin plus heparin. Women who received both aspirin and heparin had a significantly greater percentage of viable infants—80 versus 44 percent, respectively. Rai and colleagues (1997) reported a 77-percent live-birth rate in women randomized to be given low-dose aspirin plus low-dose unfractionated heparin therapy—5000 units twice daily—

versus 42 percent with aspirin alone. In contrast, Farquharson and associates (2002) reported a 72-percent live-birth rate using low-dose aspirin alone, which was similar to a 78-percent rate in women given low-dose aspirin plus low-dose low-molecular weight heparin.

As emphasized by Branch and Khamashta (2003), the discrepant reports are confusing, and therapeutic guidelines are blurred. The American College of Obstetricians and Gynecologists (2005a) recommends low-dose aspirin—81 mg orally per day, along with unfractionated heparin—5000 units subcutaneously, twice daily. This therapy, begun when pregnancy is diagnosed, is continued until delivery. Although this treatment may improve overall pregnancy success, these women remain at high risk for preterm labor, prematurely ruptured membranes, fetal-growth restriction, preeclampsia, and placental abruption (Backos and colleagues, 1999; Rai and co-workers, 1997).

In addition to IgG and IgM anticardiolipin antibodies, there are antibody idiotypes directed to a large number of lipids (Bick and Baker, 2006). Their measurement is expensive, frequently poorly controlled, and of uncertain relevance in the diagnosis of recurrent miscarriage. Results are likewise inconclusive regarding testing for other antibodies including rheumatoid factor, antinuclear antibodies, and antithyroid antibodies.

Alloimmune Factors

It is suggested that normal pregnancy requires the formation of blocking factors that prevent maternal rejection of foreign fetal antigens that are paternally derived. A woman will not produce these serum blocking factors if she has human leukocyte antigens (HLAs) similar to those of her husband. Other alloimmune disorders have been posited to cause recurrent miscarriage, including altered natural killer (NK) cell activity and increased lymphocytotoxic antibodies. A variety of therapies to correct these disorders have been suggested, including the use of paternal-cell immunization, third-party donor leukocytes, trophoblast membrane infusion, and intravenous immunoglobulin. Most of these have not withstood rigorous scrutiny, some are potentially harmful, and thus we agree with Scott (2003) that immunotherapy cannot be recommended. One possible exception is intravenous immunoglobulin therapy for secondary recurrent miscarriage—women with recurrent early pregnancy losses following one previously successful birth (Hutton and associates, 2007).

Inherited Thrombophilias

These are genetically determined abnormal clotting factors that can cause pathological thrombosis from an imbalance between clotting and anticoagulation pathways. These are discussed in detail in Chapter 47, and their action is shown in Figure 47-1 (p. 1016). The most widely studied include resistance to activated protein C (aPC) caused by the *factor V Leiden mutation* or another; decreased or absent *antithrombin III* activity; the *prothrombin gene* mutation; and mutation in the gene for *methylene tetrahydrofolate reductase* that causes elevated serum levels of homocysteine—hyperhomocysteinemia.

Carp and associates (2002) and Adelberg and Kuller (2002) cast doubt on the importance of inherited thrombophilias in early miscarriage. As placental perfusion is minimal in very early pregnancy, thrombophilias may have greater clinical implications in later pregnancy. In a meta-analysis of 31 studies by Rey and colleagues (2003), recurrent miscarriage was most closely associated with the factor V Leiden and prothrombin gene mutation. The subject was recently reviewed by Kutteh and Triplett (2006) as well as Bick and Baker (2006). After their Cochrane Database review, Kaandorp and co-workers (2009) concluded that women with recurrent miscarriage and thrombophilia do not benefit from aspirin or heparin therapy.

Endocrinological Factors

Studies evaluating the relationship between various endocrinological abnormalities have been inconsistent and have generally been underpowered (American College of Obstetricians and Gynecologists, 2001). According to Arredondo and Noble (2006), 8 to 12 percent of recurrent miscarriages are the result of endocrine factors.

Progesterone Deficiency

Also termed *luteal phase defect*, insufficient progesterone secretion by the corpus luteum or placenta has been suggested to cause miscarriage. Deficient progesterone production, however, may be the consequence rather than the cause of early pregnancy failure (Salem and associates, 1984). Diagnostic criteria and efficacy of therapy for this proposed disorder require validation (American College of Obstetricians and Gynecologists, 2001). If the corpus luteum is removed surgically, such as for an ovarian tumor, progesterone replacement is indicated in pregnancies less than 8 to 10 weeks (p. 218).

Polycystic Ovarian Syndrome

Because of oligo- or anovulation, these women are subfertile. When pregnant, there also may be an increased risk for miscarriage, but this is controversial (Cocksedge and associates, 2008). Two possible mechanisms that have been suggested are elevations in luteinizing hormone (LH) and direct effects of hyperinsulinemia on ovarian function. If the elevated LH concentration causes miscarriage, then its inhibition during a gonadotropin ovulation induction cycle might decrease miscarriage rates. In the controlled trial by Clifford and co-workers (1996), however, this did not improve pregnancy outcome. The data implicating hyperinsulinemia in pregnancy loss are somewhat stronger. In two studies, miscarriage rates were decreased with metformin treatment before and during pregnancy (Glueck and associates, 2002; Jakubowicz and colleagues, 2002). Continuing metformin throughout pregnancy has been shown to also significantly reduce the incidence of insulin-requiring gestational diabetes as well as fetal-growth restriction.

Diabetes Mellitus

Spontaneous abortion and major congenital malformation rates are both increased in women with insulin-dependent diabetes (see Chap. 7, p. 175). This risk is also related to the degree of metabolic control in early pregnancy. Similar to women with polycystic ovary syndrome, some women with recurrent miscarriage have been reported to have increased insulin resistance (Craig and associates, 2002). Pregnancy loss from poorly controlled diabetes is substantively lowered with optimal metabolic control (see Chap. 52. p. 1114).

Hypothyroidism

Severe iodine deficiency is associated with excessive early pregnancy loss (p. 217). Thyroid hormone deficiency from an autoimmune cause is common in women, but any effects it has on miscarriage have not been adequately studied. And although thyroid autoantibodies are associated with an increased incidence of spontaneous abortion, their role in recurrent miscarriage is less convincing (Abramson and Stagnaro-Green, 2001; Lakasing and Williamson, 2005). In a study of 870 women with recurrent miscarriage, Rushworth and colleagues (2000) reported that those with antithyroid antibodies were just as likely to achieve a live birth as those without antibodies.

Because it is not clear that thyroid disease causes recurrent miscarriage, the American College of Obstetricians and Gynecologists (2001) concludes that there is no indication for screening asymptomatic women. Conversely, overt hypothyroidism may be difficult to detect clinically, testing is inexpensive, and treatment is highly effective. Thus, we recommend thyroid-stimulating hormone (TSH) screening for women with recurrent miscarriage.

Infections

Very few infections are firmly proven to cause early pregnancy loss (p. 217). Moreover, if any of those infections are associated with miscarriage, they are even less likely to cause recurrent miscarriage because maternal antibodies usually develop with the primary infection.

Evaluation and Management

The timing and extent of evaluation of women with recurrent miscarriage is based on maternal age, coexistent infertility, symptoms, and the level of anxiety. With otherwise normal findings, we perform a modicum of tests to include parental karyotyping, uterine cavity evaluation, and testing for antiphospholipid antibody syndrome. Approximately half of couples with recurrent miscarriage will have no explanatory findings. Nevertheless, their prognosis is reasonable. The meta-analysis by Jeng and colleagues (1995) of randomized, prospective studies of couples with unexplained recurrent miscarriage determined that 60 to 70 percent had a successful subsequent pregnancy with no treatment.

INDUCED ABORTION

An induced abortion is the medical or surgical termination of pregnancy before the time of fetal viability. In 2005, a total of 1.22 million legal abortions were reported to the Centers for Disease Control and Prevention (Gamble and colleagues, 2008). The total has decreased each year since 2002, but this at least partially results from clinics inconsistently reporting medically induced abortions (Strauss and colleagues, 2007). The *abortion ratio* was 238 abortions per 1000 live births, and the *abortion rate* was 16 per 1000 women aged 15 to 44 years. Half of these women were 24 years or younger, 80 percent were unmarried, and 53 percent were Caucasian. Approximately 60 percent of abortions were performed during the first 8 weeks, and 88 percent during the first 12 weeks of pregnancy.

Classification

Therapeutic Abortion

There are a number of diverse medical and surgical disorders that are indications for termination of pregnancy. Examples include persistent cardiac decompensation, especially with fixed pulmonary hypertension, advanced hypertensive vascular disease or diabetes, and malignancy. In cases of rape or incest, most consider termination reasonable. The most common indication currently is to prevent birth of a fetus with a significant anatomical, metabolic, or mental deformity. The seriousness of fetal deformities is wide ranging and frequently defies social, legal, or political classification.

Elective (Voluntary) Abortion

The interruption of pregnancy before viability at the request of the woman, but not for medical reasons, is usually termed *elective* or *voluntary abortion*. These procedures comprise most abortions done today, and according to the National Vital Statistics Reports, approximately one pregnancy is electively terminated for every four live births in the United States (Ventura and colleagues, 2008). The Executive Board of the American College of Obstetricians and Gynecologists (2004) supports the legal right of women to obtain an abortion prior to fetal viability and considers this a medical matter between a woman and her physician.

Abortion in the United States

In 1973, the United States Supreme Court legalized abortion. Until then, only therapeutic abortions could be performed legally in most states. The most common legal definition of therapeutic abortion until then was termination of pregnancy before fetal viability for the purpose of saving the life of the mother. A few states extended their laws to read "to prevent serious or permanent bodily injury to the mother" or "to preserve the life or health of the woman." Some states allowed abortion if a pregnancy was likely to result in the birth of an infant with grave malformations.

The legality of elective abortion was established by the Supreme Court in the case of *Roe v. Wade*. The Court defined the extent to which states might regulate abortion:

1. For the stage prior to approximately the end of the first trimester, the abortion decision and the procedure must be left to the medical judgment of the attending physician.
2. For the stage subsequent to approximately the end of the first trimester, the State, in promoting its interest in the health of the mother, may, if it chooses, regulate the abor-

tion procedures in ways that are reasonably related to maternal health.
3. For the stage subsequent to viability, the State, in promoting its interest in the potential of human life, may, if it chooses, regulate, and even proscribe abortion, except where necessary, in appropriate medical judgment, for the preservation of the life or health of the mother.

Since 1973, several other Supreme Court decisions merit citation. Borgmann and Jones (2000) have extensively reviewed these legal issues. These appellate cases originated with legislation, both state and national, that was introduced or enacted to regulate or dismantle the three provisions listed above. In general, these attempts were unsuccessful until 1989. At that time, the Supreme Court ruled in the case of *Webster v. Reproductive Health Services* that states could place restrictions interfering with provision of abortion services on such items as waiting periods, specific informed consent requirements, parental/spousal notification, and hospital requirements. Based upon this decision, there are now numerous individual state restrictions that limit choice and access to abortion services. In one example, the decision to enforce parental notification in Texas in 2000 was associated with decreased abortion rates but simultaneously increased unintended births among 17-year-olds (Joyce and associates, 2006).

Another recent choice-limiting decision is the federal law banning the poorly defined *partial birth abortion*. This law is under challenge on several fronts. The Supreme Court in 2007 voted 5 to 4 to uphold the Partial-Birth Abortion Ban Act of 2003 in its review of *Gonzales v. Carhart* from Nebraska. This was followed by editorials in the *New England Journal of Medicine* lamenting more governmental intrusion into medical practice as well as "chipping away at women's rights" described by Justice Ginsburg in her dissenting opinion (Charo, 2007; Greene, 2007). Their opinions are in line with that of the American College of Obstetricians and Gynecologists (2004) that states: *The intervention of legislative bodies into medical decision making is inappropriate, ill advised, and dangerous.*

Counseling before Elective Abortion

Three choices available to a woman considering an abortion include continued pregnancy with its risks and parental responsibilities; continued pregnancy with its risks and responsibilities of arranged adoption; or the choice of abortion with its risks. Knowledgeable and compassionate counselors should objectively describe and provide information about these choices so that a woman or couple can make an informed decision.

Techniques for Early Abortion

Abortion can be performed either medically or surgically by several techniques shown in Table 9-3. Distinctive clinical features of each technique are shown in Table 9-4. Paul and colleagues (1999) summarized in detail many abortion techniques. A first-trimester pregnancy may be removed surgically by uterine curettage or by a number of medical regimens.

TABLE 9-3. Abortion Techniques

Surgical Techniques
  Cervical dilatation followed by uterine evacuation
    Curettage
    Vacuum aspiration (suction curettage)
    Dilatation and evacuation (D&E)
    Dilatation and extraction (D&X)
  Menstrual aspiration
  Laparotomy
    Hysterotomy
    Hysterectomy
Medical Techniques
  Intravenous oxytocin
  Intra-amnionic hyperosmotic fluid
    20-percent saline
    30-percent urea
  Prostaglandins E_2, $F_{2\alpha}$, E_1, and analogues
    Intra-amnionic injection
    Extraovular injection
    Vaginal insertion
    Parenteral injection
    Oral ingestion
  Antiprogesterones—RU 486 (mifepristone) and
    epostane
  Methotrexate—intramuscular and oral
  Various combinations of the above

Residency Training in Abortion Techniques

Because of its inherent controversial aspects, abortion training for residents in obstetrics and gynecology has been both championed and assailed. The American College of Obstetricians and Gynecologists (2009) supports abortion training for residents. In some programs, such as the University of California at San Francisco, a special 6-week abortion-training elective for housestaff was implemented in 1980. From 1998 through 2003, 40 residents completed training and none opted out of the rotation (Steinauer and co-workers, 2005b). Other programs, such as ours at Parkland Memorial Hospital, teach residents the technical aspects of abortion by management of early missed abortions as well as pregnancy interruption for fetal

death, severe fetal anomalies, and maternal medical or surgical disorders. According to Eastwood and colleagues (2006), only 10 percent of programs provide no training in elective abortion.

Because of these differences, influenced by political and moral convictions, the American College of Obstetricians and Gynecologists (2004) respects the need and responsibility of healthcare providers to determine their individual positions based on personal beliefs. Certainly, physicians trained to care for women must be familiar with various abortion techniques so that complications can be managed or referrals made for suitable care (Steinauer and associates, 2005a).

Surgical Abortion

A pregnancy may be removed surgically through an appropriately dilated cervix or transabdominally by either hysterotomy or hysterectomy. In the absence of maternal systemic disease, abortion procedures do not require hospitalization. When abortion is performed outside a hospital setting, capabilities for cardiopulmonary resuscitation and for immediate transfer to a hospital must be available.

Dilatation and Curettage (D&C)

Transcervical approaches to surgical abortion require first dilating the cervix and then evacuating the pregnancy by mechanically scraping out the contents—sharp curettage, by suctioning out the contents—suction curettage, or both. Vacuum aspiration, the most common form of suction curettage, requires a rigid cannula attached to an electric-powered vacuum source (MacIsaac and Darney, 2000; Masch and Roman, 2005). Alternatively, manual vacuum aspiration uses a similar cannula that attaches to a handheld syringe for its vacuum source (Goldberg and associates, 2004). The likelihood of complications increases after the first trimester. These include uterine perforation, cervical laceration, hemorrhage, incomplete removal of the fetus and placenta, and infections. Accordingly, sharp or suction curettage should be performed before 14 to 15 weeks.

Evidence supports that antimicrobial prophylaxis should be provided to all women undergoing a transcervical surgical abortion. Based on their review of 11 randomized trials, Sawaya and associates (1996) concluded that antimicrobials decreased the risk of infection by approximately 40 percent. No one regimen

TABLE 9-4. Features of Medical and Surgical Abortion

Medical Abortion	Surgical Abortion
Usually avoids invasive procedure	Involves invasive procedure
Usually avoids anesthesia	Allows use of sedation if desired
Requires two or more visits	Usually requires one visit
Days to weeks to complete	Complete in a predictable period of time
Available during early pregnancy	Available during early pregnancy
High success rate (~95 percent)	High success rate (99 percent)
Bleeding moderate to heavy for short time	Bleeding commonly perceived as light
Requires follow-up to ensure completion of abortion	Does not require follow-up in all cases
Requires patient participation throughout a multistep process	Patient participation in a single-step process

Reprinted, with permission, from American College of Obstetricians and Gynecologists. Medical management of abortion. ACOG Practice Bulletin 67. Washington, DC: ACOG; 2005

appears superior. One convenient, inexpensive, and effective regimen is doxycycline, 100 mg orally twice daily for 7 days (Fjerstad and associates, 2009).

Dilatation and Evacuation (D&E)

Beginning at 16 weeks, fetal size and structure dictate use of this technique. Wide mechanical cervical dilatation, achieved with metal or hygroscopic dilators, precedes mechanical destruction and evacuation of fetal parts. With complete removal of the fetus, a large-bore vacuum curette is used to remove the placenta and remaining tissue.

Dilatation and Extraction (D&X)

This is similar to dilatation and evacuation except that suction evacuation of the intracranial contents after delivery of the fetal body through the dilated cervix aids extraction and minimizes uterine or cervical injury from instruments or fetal bones. In political parlance, this procedure has been termed *partial birth abortion,* discussed on page 227.

Hygroscopic Dilators. Trauma from mechanical dilatation can be minimized by using devices that slowly dilate the cervix (Fig. 9-6). These devices, called *hygroscopic dilators,* draw water from cervical tissues and expand, gradually dilating the cervix. One type of hygroscopic dilators originates from the stems of *Laminaria digitata* or *Laminaria japonica,* a brown seaweed. The stems are cut, peeled, shaped, dried, sterilized, and packaged according to size-small, 3 to 5 mm in diameter; medium, 6 to 8 mm; and large, 8 to 10 mm. The strongly hygroscopic laminaria presumably act by drawing water from proteoglycan complexes, causing the complexes to dissociate, and thereby allowing the cervix to soften and dilate.

Synthetic hygroscopic dilators, such as Lamicel and Dilapan-S, are also available. Lamicel is a slender, rod-shaped polyvinyl acetal sponge impregnated with anhydrous magnesium sulfate. Dilapan-S is an acrylic-based hydrogel rod. In 1995, Dilapan was removed from the U.S. market because of concerns over device fragmentation. It was reintroduced following Food and Drug Administration approval of a new device design (Food and Drug Administration, 2008).

To insert hygroscopic dilators, the cervix is cleansed with povidone-iodine solution and is grasped anteriorly with a tenaculum. A hygroscopic dilator of the appropriate size is then inserted using a uterine packing forceps so that the tip rests at the level of the internal os (see Fig. 9-6). After 4 to 6 hours, the laminaria will have swollen and dilated the cervix sufficiently to allow easier mechanical dilatation and curettage. Cramping frequently accompanies expansion of the laminaria.

An interesting dilemma is presented by the woman who has a hygroscopic dilator placed overnight in preparation for elective abortion, but who then changes her mind. Schneider and associates (1991) described this in first-trimester and 14 second-trimester pregnancies. Four patients returned to their original decision and aborted their pregnancies. Of the remaining 17, there were 14 term deliveries, two preterm deliveries, and one spontaneous abortion 2 weeks later. None of the women suffered infectious morbidity, including three untreated women whose cervical cultures were positive for chlamydia. In spite of this generally reassuring report, an attitude of irrevocability with regard to dilator placement and abortion seems prudent.

Prostaglandins. As an alternative to hygroscopic dilators, various prostaglandin preparations may be placed into the posterior vaginal fornix to aid subsequent dilatation. MacIsaac and colleagues (1999) randomized women to receive 400 μg of misoprostol placed vaginally 4 hours before first-trimester abortion versus laminaria placement. Misoprostol effected equal or greater dilatation, caused less pain on insertion, and produced similar side effects. It is important to emphasize that this 400-μg dose is far in excess of oral or vaginal dosing for labor induction (see Chap. 22, p. 503).

Technique for Dilatation and Curettage

After bimanual examination is performed to determine the size and orientation of the uterus, a speculum is inserted, and the cervix is swabbed with povidone-iodine or equivalent solution. The anterior cervical lip is grasped with a toothed tenaculum. The cervix, vagina, and uterus are richly supplied by nerves of Frankenhäuser plexus, which lies within connective tissue lateral to the

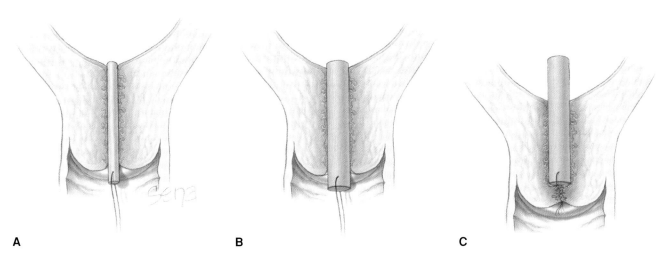

A   **B**   **C**

FIGURE 9-6 Insertion of laminaria prior to dilatation and curettage. **A.** Laminaria immediately after being appropriately placed with its upper end just through the internal os. **B.** Several hours later the laminaria is now swollen, and the cervix is dilated and softened. **C.** Laminaria inserted too far through the internal os; the laminaria may rupture the membranes.

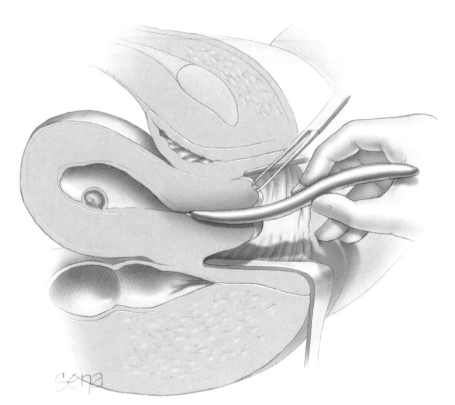

FIGURE 9-7 Dilatation of cervix with a Hegar dilator. Note that the fourth and fifth fingers rest against the perineum and buttocks, lateral to the vagina. This maneuver is an important safety measure because if the cervix relaxes abruptly, these fingers prevent a sudden and uncontrolled thrust of the dilator, a common cause of uterine perforation.

out with the thumb and forefinger only (Fig. 9-7). If beyond 16 weeks' gestation, the fetus is extracted, usually in parts, using Sopher forceps and other destructive instruments. Risks include uterine perforation, cervical laceration, and uterine bleeding due to the larger fetus and placenta and to the thinner uterine walls. Morbidity can be minimized if: (1) the cervix is adequately dilated before attempting to remove the products of conception, (2) instruments are introduced into the uterus and manipulated without force, and (3) all tissue is removed.

Complications. The incidence of uterine perforation associated with dilatation and curettage for elective abortion varies. Two important determinants are the skill of the clinician and the position of the uterus. The likelihood of perforation is greater if the uterus is retroverted. Accidental uterine perforation usually is recognized easily when the instrument passes without resistance deep into the pelvis. Observation may be sufficient if the uterine perforation is small, as when produced by a uterine sound or narrow dilator.

Although possible, Chen and colleagues (2008) reported no uterine scar separation in 78 women with prior cesarean delivery or myomectomy who then underwent medical or surgical abortion for early pregnancy failure.

Considerable intra-abdominal damage can be caused by instruments, especially suction and sharp curettes, passed through a uterine defect into the peritoneal cavity (Keegan and Forkowitz, 1982). In this circumstance, laparotomy to examine the abdominal contents is often the safest course of action. Depending on the circumstances, laparoscopy may be substituted. Unrecognized bowel injury can cause severe peritonitis and sepsis (Kambiss and associates, 2000).

Some women may develop cervical incompetence or uterine synechiae following dilatation and curettage. Rarely, abortion performed by curettage on more advanced pregnancies may induce sudden, severe consumptive coagulopathy, which can prove fatal. Those contemplating abortion should understand the potential for these rare but serious complications.

If prophylactic antimicrobials are given as described on page 228, pelvic sepsis is decreased by 40 to 90 percent, depending whether the procedure is surgical or medical. Most infections that develop respond readily to appropriate antimicrobial treatment (see Chap. 31, p. 662). Rarely, infections such as bacterial endocarditis will develop, but they can be fatal (Jeppson and associates, 2008).

uterosacral ligaments. Thus, paracervical injections are most effective if placed immediately lateral to the insertion of the uterosacral ligaments into the uterus. A local anesthetic, such as 5 mL of 1 or 2-percent lidocaine, may be injected at 4 and 8 o'clock at the cervical base. Mankowski and associates (2009) reported that an intracervical block with 5-mL aliquots of 1-percent lidocaine injected at 12, 3, 6, and 9 o'clock were equally as effective. Dilute vasopressin may be added to the local anesthetic to decrease blood loss (Keder, 2003).

If required, the cervix is further dilated with Hegar, Hank, or Pratt dilators until a suction cannula of the appropriate diameter can be inserted. Choosing the most appropriately sized cannula balances competing factors: small cannulas carry the risk of retained intrauterine tissue postoperatively, whereas large cannulas risk cervical injury and more discomfort. The fourth and fifth fingers of the hand introducing the dilator should rest on the perineum and buttocks as the dilator is pushed through the internal os (Fig. 9-7). This technique minimizes forceful dilatation and provides a safeguard against uterine perforation. Uterine sounding measures the depth and inclination of the uterine cavity prior to cannula insertion. The suction cannula is moved toward the fundus and then back toward the os and is turned circumferentially to cover the entire surface of the uterine cavity (Fig. 9-8). When no more tissue is aspirated, a gentle sharp curettage should follow to remove any remaining placental or fetal fragments (Fig. 9-9).

Because the uterus is characteristically perforated on the insertion of any instrument, manipulations should be carried

Menstrual Aspiration

Aspiration of the endometrial cavity can be completed using a flexible 5- or 6-mm Karman cannula that is attached to a syringe. When completed within 1 to 3 weeks after a missed menstrual period, this has been referred to as *menstrual extraction, menstrual induction, instant period, traumatic abortion, and mini-abortion.* At this early stage of gestation, pregnancy can be misdiagnosed, an implanted zygote can be missed by the curette, ectopic pregnancy can be unrecognized, or infrequently, a uterus can be perforated. Even so, Paul and associates (2002) reported a 98-percent success rate in more than 1000 women who underwent this procedure. A positive pregnancy test result will eliminate a needless procedure on a nonpregnant woman whose period has been delayed for other reasons.

To identify placenta in the aspirate, MacIsaac and Darney (2000) recommend that the syringe contents be rinsed in a strainer to remove blood, then placed in a clear plastic container with saline, and examined with back lighting. Placental tissue macroscopically appears soft, fluffy, and feathery. A magnifying lens, colposcope, or microscope also can improve visualization.

Manual Vacuum Aspiration

This office-based procedure is similar to menstrual aspiration but is used for early pregnancy failures as well as elective termination up to 12 weeks. Masch and Roman (2005) recommend that pregnancy terminations in the office with this method be limited to 10 weeks or less. Certainly, blood loss rises sharply between 10 and 12 weeks (Westfall and colleagues, 1998).

The procedure uses a hand-operated 60-mL syringe and cannula. A vacuum is created in the syringe and attached to the cannula, which is inserted transcervically into the uterus. The vacuum is activated and produces up to 60 mm Hg suction. Although complications are similar to other surgical methods, they are not increased (Goldberg and associates, 2004).

With pregnancies less than 8 weeks, no cervical preparation is required. After this time, some recommend either osmotic dilators placed the day before or misoprostol given 2 to 4 hours before the procedure. A paracervical block, with or without intravenous sedation, or conscious sedation is used for anesthesia.

Laparotomy

In a few circumstances, abdominal hysterotomy or hysterectomy for abortion is preferable to either curettage or medical

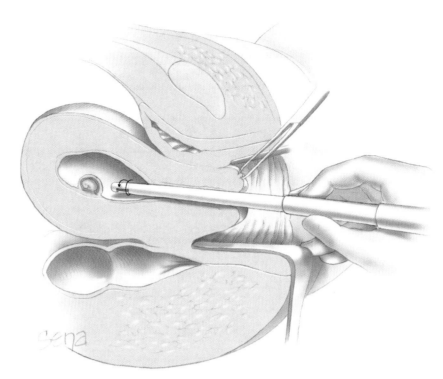

FIGURE 9-8 A suction curette is advanced to the uterine fundus and then back to the internal os. During its insertion and retraction, the curette is simultaneously rotated 360° several times to remove tissue circumferentially from the uterine walls.

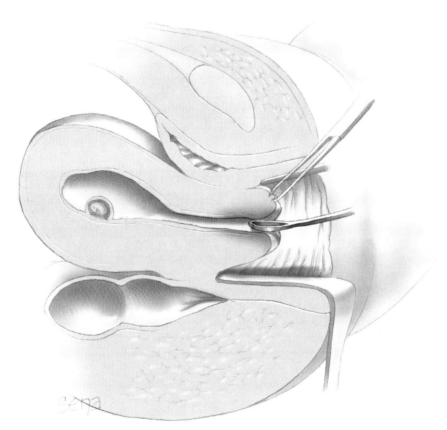

FIGURE 9-9 Introduction of a sharp curette. The instrument is held with the thumb and forefinger. In the upward movement of the curette, only the strength of these two fingers should be used.

induction. If significant uterine disease is present, hysterectomy may provide ideal treatment. Either hysterotomy with tubal ligation or on occasion, hysterectomy may be indicated for women who desire pregnancy termination and sterilization. At times, a failed medical induction during the second trimester may necessitate hysterotomy or hysterectomy.

Medical Abortion

Throughout history, many naturally occurring substances have been tried as abortifacients. In many cases, serious systemic illness or even death has resulted rather than abortion. Even today, only a few effective, safe abortifacient drugs are used.

According to the American College of Obstetricians and Gynecologists (2005b), outpatient medical abortion is an acceptable alternative to surgical abortion in appropriately selected women with pregnancies less than 49 days menstrual age. Beyond this point, the available data, although less robust, support surgical abortion as a preferable method of early abortion.

Three medications for early medical abortion have been widely studied and used: the antiprogestin *mifepristone*; the antimetabolite *methotrexate*; and the prostaglandin *misoprostol*. These agents cause abortion by increasing uterine contractility either by reversing the progesterone-induced inhibition of contractions—mifepristone and methotrexate or by stimulating the myometrium directly—misoprostol. In addition, mifepristone causes cervical collagen degradation, possibly because of increased expression of matrix metalloproteinase-2 (Clark and associates, 2006).

A variety of dosing schemes that have been proven effective are shown in Table 9-5. Mifepristone or methotrexate are administered initially, and followed after a specified time by misoprostol. Guest and associates (2007) randomized 450 women to be given 200 mg mifepristone orally followed by 800 μg misoprostol vaginally either 6 hours later or 36 to 48 hours later. When given at 36 to 48 hours, the success rate was 96 percent compared with 89 percent for the 6-hour group ($p < .05$). As discussed on page 223, at least for "pregnancy failures"—anembryonic gestation, embryonic or fetal death, and incomplete or inevitable abortion—800 μg misoprostol given vaginally as a sole agent was effective in causing complete expulsion by day 8 in 84-percent of women treated (Zhang and colleagues, 2005). Recently, Fjerstad and associates (2009) compared septic complications in more than 225,000 women undergoing a medical abortion. After changing the route of administration from vaginal to buccal misoprostol, along with providing 7-day postprocedure doxycycline prophylaxis, they documented a 93-percent decreased serious infection rate—from 0.93 per 1000 to 0.06 per 1000. Finally, both methotrexate and misoprostol are teratogens, and their use thus requires a commitment on the part of both a woman and her caregiver to complete the abortion.

Contraindications to medical abortion have evolved from the exclusion criteria of various medical abortion trials. In addition to specific allergies to the medicines, they have included an in situ intrauterine device, severe anemia, coagulopathy or anticoagulant use, and significant medical conditions such as active liver disease, cardiovascular disease, and uncontrolled seizure disorders. Additionally, because misoprostol can lower glucocorticoid activity, women with adrenal disease or with disorders requiring glucocorticoid therapy should be excluded (American

TABLE 9-5. Regimens for Medical Termination of Early Pregnancy

Mifepristone/Misoprostol
[a]Mifepristone, 100-600 mg orally followed by:
[b]Misoprostol, 200-600 μg orally or 800 μg vaginally in multiple doses over 6-72 hours.

Methotrexate/Misoprostol
[c]Methotrexate, 50 mg/m² intramuscularly or orally followed by:
[d]Misoprostol, 800 μg vaginally in 3-7 days. Repeat if needed 1 week after methotrexate initially given.

Misoprostol alone
800 μg vaginally, repeated for up to three doses.

[a]Doses of 200 versus 600 mg similarly effective.
[b]Oral route may be less effective and with more nausea and diarrhea. May be given sublingually, or buccally. Postprocedure pelvic infection significantly higher with vaginal versus oral route. Possibly more effective when given at 36-48 hours instead of at 6 hours.
[c]Efficacy similar for routes of administration.
[d]Similar efficacy when given on day 3 versus day 5.
Data from the American College of Obstetricians and Gynecologists (2005); Borgatta (2001); Bracken (2007); Chen (2008); Creinin (2001, 2007); Fjerstad (2009); Guest (2007); Hamoda (2005); Schaff (2000); Shannon (2006); von Hertzen (2007); Wiebe (1999, 2002); Winikoff (2008), and all their colleagues.

College of Obstetricians and Gynecologists, 2005b). A modified methotrexate dose should be given with caution—if at all—in women with renal insufficiency (Kelly and associates, 2006). Women contemplating medical abortion should receive thorough counseling of both medical and surgical approaches.

With the mifepristone regimen, according to the package labeling, misoprostol is to be provider administered. Afterwards the woman typically remains in the office for 4 hours, and if the pregnancy appears to have been expelled, she is examined to confirm expulsion. If during observation, the pregnancy does not appear to have been expelled, a pelvic examination is performed prior to discharge, and the woman is reappointed for 1 to 2 weeks. At this later appointment, if clinical examination or sonographic evaluation fails to confirm completed abortion, a suction procedure usually is done.

In regimens employing methotrexate, women are typically seen at least 24 hours after misoprostol, and approximately 7 days after methotrexate administration, at which time a sonographic examination is performed. If the pregnancy persists, another dose of misoprostol is given, and the woman is seen again in 1 week if fetal cardiac activity is present or in 4 weeks if there is no fetal cardiac activity. If by the second visit, abortion has not occurred, it is usually completed by suction curettage.

Bleeding and cramping with medical termination can be significantly worse than symptoms experienced with menses. Adequate pain medication, usually including a narcotic, should be provided. According to the American College of Obstetricians and Gynecologists (2005b), soaking two pads or more per hour for at least 2 hours is a threshold at which the woman should be instructed to contact her provider, who can determine whether she needs to be seen.

Early medical abortion is highly effective—90 to 98 percent of women will not require surgical intervention (Kahn and co-workers, 2000). According to Hausknecht (2003), there were only 139 complications reported to the manufacturer with mifepristone when given with misoprostol to 80,000 women for medical abortion.

Unnecessary surgical intervention in women undergoing medical abortion can be avoided if sonographic results are interpreted appropriately. Specifically, if no gestational sac is present, in the absence of heavy bleeding, intervention in most women is unnecessary. This is true even when, as is common, the uterus contains sonographically evident debris.

Second-Trimester Abortion

Invasive means of second-trimester medical abortion have long been available, and some are listed in Table 9-3. In the past 25 years, however, the ability to safely and effectively accomplish noninvasive second-trimester abortion has evolved considerably. Principal among these noninvasive methods are high-dose intravenous oxytocin and vaginal prostaglandin administration, including prostaglandin E_2 suppositories and prostaglandin E_1 (misoprostol) pills. Regardless of method, hygroscopic dilator placement as shown in Figure 9-6 will shorten the duration (Goldberg and colleagues, 2005).

Oxytocin

Given as a single agent in high doses, oxytocin will effect second-trimester abortion in 80 to 90 percent of cases. For more than 15 years, the regimen shown in Table 9-6 has been used with a high degree of safety and effectiveness at the University of Alabama. By mixing the oxytocin in an isotonic solution such as normal saline, and avoiding excessive administration of dilute intravenous solutions, we have not observed hyponatremia or water intoxication.

TABLE 9-6. Concentrated Oxytocin Protocol for Mid-trimester Abortion

50 units oxytocin in 500 mL of normal saline infused over 3 hr; 1-hr diuresis (no oxytocin)

100 units oxytocin in 500 mL of normal saline infused over 3 hr; 1-hr diuresis (no oxytocin)

150 units oxytocin in 500 mL of normal saline infused over 3 hr; 1-hr diuresis (no oxytocin)

200 units oxytocin in 500 mL of normal saline infused over 3 hr; 1-hr diuresis (no oxytocin)

250 units oxytocin in 500 mL of normal saline infused over 3 hr; 1-hr diuresis (no oxytocin)

300 units oxytocin in 500 mL of normal saline infused over 3 hr; 1-hr diuresis (no oxytocin)

Modified from Ramsey and Owen (2000), with permission

Prostaglandin E_2

Suppositories of 20 mg prostaglandin E_2 placed in the posterior vaginal fornix are a simple and effective means of effecting second-trimester abortion. This method is not more effective than high-dose oxytocin, and it causes more frequent side effects such as nausea, vomiting, fever, and diarrhea (Owen and associates, 1992). If prostaglandin E_2 is used, an antiemetic such as metoclopramide, an antipyretic such as acetaminophen, and an antidiarrheal such as diphenoxylate/atropine are given either to prevent or to treat symptoms.

Prostaglandin E_1

Misoprostol can be used easily and inexpensively as a single agent for second-trimester pregnancy termination. In their randomized trial, Ramsey and co-workers (2004) administered misoprostol, 600 μg vaginally followed by 400 μg every 4 hours. They reported that this effected abortion significantly faster than concentrated oxytocin given in combination with prostaglandin E_2—median time to abortion 12 versus 17 hours, respectively. Misoprostol achieved abortion within 24 hours in 95 percent of women compared with 85 percent in the other group. Importantly, only 2 percent of women in the misoprostol group required curettage for retained placenta compared with 15 percent in the oxytocin/prostaglandin E_2 group. Kapp and co-workers (2007) reported that mifepristone, 200 mg given 1 day before misoprostol, reduced median time to expulsion from 18 to 10 hours compared with a placebo group.

The outcome of medically induced second-trimester abortion after a previous cesarean delivery has been the subject of several reports. Although some early reports were discouraging, recent evidence is not so pessimistic. Systematic reviews by Berghella and colleagues (2009) as well as Goyal (2009) found that the risk of uterine rupture in these women given misoprostol was only about 0.3 to 0.4 percent

Consequences of Elective Abortion

Maternal Mortality

Legally induced abortion, performed by trained gynecologists, especially when performed during the first 2 months of pregnancy, has a mortality rate of less than 1 per 100,000 procedures (Grimes, 2006; Strauss and colleagues, 2007). Early abortions are safer, and the relative risk of dying as the consequence of abortion approximately doubles for each 2 weeks after 8 weeks' gestation. The Centers for Disease Control and Prevention recorded seven deaths related to legal abortion in 2004 (Gamble and associates, 2008). According to Horon (2005), such deaths are underreported.

Impact on Future Pregnancies

In a scholarly review of the impact of elective abortion on subsequent pregnancy outcome, Hogue (1986) summarized data from more than 200 publications. Data relating abortion to subsequent pregnancy outcome are observational and therefore subject to bias and uncontrolled confounding factors. All studies on this topic must be interpreted with these limitations in mind. That

TABLE 9-7. Outcomes in Next Pregnancy in 16,883 Women Who Had Either a Surgically or Medically Induced First-Trimester Abortion

Pregnancy Outcome	Incidence (Percent)[a]	
	Surgical	Medical
Ectopic pregnancy	2.3	2.4
Miscarriage	12.7	12.2
Preterm delivery	6.7	5.4
Birthweight <2500 g	5.1	4.0

[a]All comparisons $p > .05$.
Data from Virk and colleagues (2007).

said, fertility does not appear to be diminished by an elective abortion. Moreover, most studies indicate that vacuum aspiration does not increase the subsequent incidence of second-trimester spontaneous abortion or preterm delivery. The case-control French EPIPAGE study, however, found a 1.5-fold increased incidence of very preterm delivery—22 to 32 weeks—in women with a history of induced abortion (Moreau and colleagues, 2005). Subsequent ectopic pregnancies are not increased. Multiple sharp curettage abortion procedures may increase the subsequent risk of placenta previa, whereas vacuum aspiration procedures likely do not (Johnson and associates, 2003). In their recent meticulous systematic review, Swingle and co-workers (2009) found a significantly increased risk of preterm birth—OR 1.32—after either spontaneous or induced abortions.

The large population study from Denmark indicated that subsequent pregnancy outcomes are similar following medical and surgical methods of induced abortions. Using the Danish Abortion Registry of 30,349 procedures done from 1999 through 2004, Virk and colleagues (2007) provided data from 16,883 women who had a subsequent pregnancy through 2005. The results listed in Table 9-7 show very similar pregnancy outcomes.

CONTRACEPTION FOLLOWING MISCARRIAGE OR ABORTION

Ovulation may resume as early as 2 weeks after an early pregnancy is terminated, whether spontaneously or induced. Lahteenmaki and Luukkainen (1978) detected surges of luteinizing hormone (LH) 16 to 22 days after abortion in 15 of 18 women studied. Plasma progesterone levels, which had plummeted after the abortion, increased soon after LH surges. These hormonal events agree with histological changes observed in endometrial biopsies (Boyd and Holmstrom, 1972). **Therefore, if pregnancy is to be prevented, effective contraception should be initiated soon after abortion.** Reeves and associates (2007) have computed a lower unintended pregnancy rate in women who desire an intrauterine device if it is inserted at the time of pregnancy termination. Madden and Westhoff (2009) have shown similar benefits with depot medroxyprogesterone acetate (DMPA). Choices for contraception are discussed in Chapter 32.

REFERENCES

Abramson J, Stagnaro-Green A: Thyroid antibodies and fetal loss: An evolving story. Thyroid 11:57, 2001

Adelberg AM, Kuller JA: Thrombophilias and recurrent miscarriage. Obstet Gynecol Surv 57:703, 2002

Albrechtsen S, Rasmussen S, Thoresen S, et al: Pregnancy outcome in women before and after cervical conisation: Population based cohort study. BMJ 18:337, 2008

Alijotas-Reig J, Casellas-Caro M, Ferrer-Oliveras R, et al: Are anti-beta-glycoprotein-I antibodies markers for recurrent pregnancy loss in lupus anticoagulant/anticardiolipin seronegative women? Am J Reprod Immunol 60:229, 2008

Alijotas-Reig J, Ferrer-Oliveras R, Rodrigo-Anoro J, et al: Anti-β_2-glycoprotein-I and anti-phosphatidylserine antibodies in women with spontaneous pregnancy loss. Fertil Steril [Epub ahead of print], 2009

Al-Inany H: Intrauterine adhesions. An update. Acta Obstet Gynecol Scand 80:986, 2001

Althuisius SM, Dekker GA, Hummel P, et al: Final results of the cervical incompetence prevention randomized cerclage trial (CIPRACT): Therapeutic cerclage with bed rest versus bed rest alone. Am J Obstet Gynecol 185:1106, 2001

American College of Obstetricians and Gynecologists: Prevention of Rh D alloimmunization. Practice Bulletin No. 4, May 1999

American College of Obstetricians and Gynecologists: Management of recurrent early pregnancy loss. Practice Bulletin No. 24, February 2001

American College of Obstetricians and Gynecologists: Abortion policy. ACOG Statement of Policy issued by the ACOG Executive Board, July 2004

American College of Obstetricians and Gynecologists: Antiphospholipid syndrome. Practice Bulletin No. 68, November, 2005a

American College of Obstetricians and Gynecologists: Medical management of abortion. Practice Bulletin No. 67, October 2005b

American College of Obstetricians and Gynecologists: Abortion access and training. Committee Opinion No. 424, January 2009

Armstrong BG, McDonald AD, Sloan M: Cigarette, alcohol, and coffee consumption and spontaneous abortion. Am J Public Health 82:85, 1992

Arredondo F, Noble LS: Endocrinology of recurrent pregnancy loss. Semin Reprod Med 1:33, 2006

Ashton D, Amin HK, Richart RM, et al: The incidence of asymptomatic uterine anomalies in women undergoing transcervical tubal sterilization. Obstet Gynecol 72:28, 1988

Backos M, Rai R, Baxter N, et al: Pregnancy complications in women with recurrent miscarriage associated with antiphospholipid antibodies treated with low dose aspirin and heparin. Br J Obstet Gynecol 106:102, 1999

Barlow S, Sullivan FM: Reproductive Hazards of Industrial Chemicals: An Evaluation of Animal and Human Data. New York, Academic Press, 1982

Barnhart K, Sammel MD, Chung K, et al: Decline of serum human chorionic gonadotropin and spontaneous complete abortion: Defining the normal curve. Obstet Gynecol 104:975, 2004a

Barnhart KT, Sammel MD, Rinaudo PF: Symptomatic patients with an early viable intrauterine pregnancy: hCG curves redefined. Obstet Gynecol 104:50, 2004b

Barrett JP, Whiteside JL, Boardman LA: Fatal clostridial sepsis after spontaneous abortion. Obstet Gynecol 99:899, 2002

Barth WH: Operative procedures of the cervix. In Hankins GDV, Clark SL, Cunningham FG, et al (eds): Operative Obstetrics. Norwalk, CT, Appleton & Lange, 1995, p 753

Benirschke K, Kaufmann P: Pathology of the Human Placenta, 4th ed. New York, Springer-Verlag, 2000

Berghella V, Airoldi J, O'Neill AM, et al: Misoprostol for second trimester pregnancy termination in women with prior caesarean: a systematic review. BJOG 2009; DOI: 10.1111/j.1471-0528.2009.02190.x, 2009

Bianco K, Caughey AB, Shaffer BL, et al: History of miscarriage and increased incidence of fetal aneuploidy in subsequent pregnancy. Obstet Gynecol 107:1098, 2006

Bick RL, Baker WF Jr: Hereditary and acquired thrombophilia in pregnancy. In Bick RL (ed): Hematological Complications in Obstetrics, Pregnancy, and Gynecology. United Kingdom, Cambridge University Press, 2006, p 122

Blohm F, Fridén BE, Milsom I, et al: A randomized double blind trial comparing misoprostol or placebo in the management of early miscarriage. BJOG 112:1090, 2005

Blohm F, Fridén B, Platz-Christensen JJ, et al: Expectant management of first-trimester miscarriage in clinical practice. Acta Obstet Gynecol Scand 82:654, 2003

Boivin JF: Risk of spontaneous abortion in women occupationally exposed to anaesthetic gases: A meta-analysis. Occup Environ Med 54:541, 1997

Borgatta L, Burnhill MS, Tyson J, et al: Early medical abortion with methotrexate and misoprostol. Obstet Gynecol 97:11, 2001

Borgmann CE, Jones BS: Legal issues in the provision of medical abortion. Am J Obstet Gynecol 183:S84, 2000

Boulot P, Hoffet M, Bachelard B, et al: Late vaginal induced abortion after a previous cesarean birth: Potential for uterine rupture. Gynecol Obstet Invest 36:87, 1993

Boyd EF Jr, Holmstrom EG: Ovulation following therapeutic abortion. Am J Obstet Gynecol 113:469, 1972

Bracken H, Ngoc NTH, Schaff E, et al: Mifepristone followed in 24 hours to 48 hours by misoprostol for late first-trimester abortion. Obstet Gynecol 109:895, 2007

Branch DW, Khamashta MA: Antiphospholipid syndrome: Obstetric diagnosis, management, and controversies. Obstet Gynecol 101:1333, 2003

Brent RL: Utilization of developmental basic science principles in the evaluation of reproductive risks from pre- and postconception environmental radiation exposures. Teratology 59:182, 1999

Brown ZA, Selke S, Zeh J, et al: The acquisition of herpes simplex virus during pregnancy. N Engl J Med 337:509, 1997

Cammarano CL, Herron MA, Parer JT: Validity of indications for transabdominal cervicoisthmic cerclage for cervical incompetence. Am J Obstet Gynecol 172:1871, 1995

Carp H, Dolitzky M, Tur-Kaspa I, et al: Hereditary thrombophilias are not associated with a decreased live birth rate in women with recurrent miscarriage. Fertil Steril 78:58, 2002

Carp HJ, Meroni PL, Shoenfeld Y: Autoantibodies as predictors of pregnancy complications. Rheumatology (Oxford) 47:6, 2008

Carrell DT, Wilcox AL, Lowy L, et al: Male chromosomal factors of unexplained recurrent pregnancy loss. Obstet Gynecol 101:1229, 2003

Caruso A, Trivellini C, De Carolis S, et al: Emergency cerclage in the presence of protruding membranes: Is pregnancy outcome predictable? Acta Obstet Gynecol Scand 79:265, 2000

Caspi E, Schneider DF, Mor Z, et al: Cervical internal os cerclage: Description of a new technique and comparison with Shirodkar operation. Am J Perinatol 7:347, 1990

Castañeda R, Lechuga D, Ramos RI, et al: Endemic goiter in pregnant women: Utility of the simplified classification of thyroid size by palpation and urinary iodine as screening tests. BJOG 109:1366, 2002

Centers for Disease Control and Prevention: Abortion surveillance—United States, 2002. MMWR Surveill Summ 54:1, 2005

Chapman S, Crispens MA, Owen J, et al: Complications of midtrimester pregnancy terminations: The effect of prior cesarean delivery. Am J Obstet Gynecol 174:356, 1996

Charles D, Edward WR: Infectious complications of cervical cerclage. Am J Obstet Gynecol 141:1065, 1981

Charo RA: The partial death of abortion rights. N Engl J Med 356:1905, 2007

Chasen ST, Kalish RB, Gupta M, et al: Obstetric outcomes after surgical abortion at > or = 20 weeks' gestation. Am J Obstet Gynecol 193:1161, 2005

Chasen ST, Silverman NS: Mid-trimester emergent cerclage: A ten year single institution review. J Perinatol 18:338, 1998

Chatenoud L, Parazzini F, Di Cintio E, et al: Paternal and maternal smoking habits before conception and during the first trimester: Relation to spontaneous abortion. Ann Epidem 8:520, 1998

Chen BA, Reeves MF, Creinin MD, et al: Misoprostol for treatment of early pregnancy failure in women with previous uterine surgery. Am J Obstet Gynecol 198:626.e1, 2008

Clark K, Ji H, Feltovich H, et al: Mifepristone-induced cervical ripening: Structural, biomechanical, and molecular events. Am J Obstet Gynecol 194:1391, 2006

Clifford K, Rai R, Watson H, et al: Does suppressing luteinizing hormone secretion reduce the miscarriage rate? Results of a randomized controlled trial. BMJ 312:1508, 1996

Cnattingius S, Signorello LB, Anneren G, et al: Caffeine intake and the risk of first-trimester spontaneous abortion. N Engl J Med 343:1839, 2000

Cocksedge KA, Li TC, Saravelos SH, et al: A reappraisal of the role of polycystic ovary syndrome in recurrent miscarriage. Reprod Biomed Online 17:151, 2008

Cohen AL, Bhatnagar J, Reagan S, et al: Toxic shock associated with Clostridium sordellii and Clostridium perfringens after medical and spontaneous abortion. Obstet Gynecol 110:1027, 2007

Condous G, Okaro E, Khalid A, et al: Do we need to follow up complete miscarriages with serum human chorionic gonadotrophin levels? BJOG 112:827, 2005

Craig TB, Ke RW, Kutteh WH: Increase prevalence of insulin resistance in women with a history of recurrent pregnancy loss. Fertil Steril 78:487, 2002

Creinin MD, Huang X, Westhoff C: et al: Factors related to successful misoprostol treatment for early pregnancy failure. Obstet Gynecol 107:901, 2006

Creinin MD, Pymar HC, Schwartz JL: Mifepristone 100 mg in abortion regimens. Obstet Gynecol 98:434, 2001

Creinin MD, Schreiber CA, Bednarek P: Mifepristone and misoprostol administered simultaneously versus 24 hours apart for abortion. Obstet Gynecol 109:885, 2007

Daif JL, Levie M, Chudnoff S, et al: Group A streptococcus causing necrotizing fasciitis and toxic shock syndrome after medical termination of pregnancy. Obstet Gynecol 113:504, 2009

Dao B, Blum J, Thieba B, et al: Is misoprostol a safe, effective and acceptable alternative to manual vacuum aspiration for postabortion care? Results from a randomized trial in Burkina Faso, West Africa. BJOG 114:1368, 2007

Devi Wold AS, Pham N, Arici A: Anatomic factors in recurrent pregnancy loss. Semin Reprod Med 1:25, 2006

Dranitsaris G, Johnston M, Poirier S, et al: Are health care providers who work with cancer drugs at an increased risk for toxic events? A systematic review and meta-analysis of the literature. J Oncol Pharm Pract 2:69, 2005

Dudley DJ, Branch W: Antiphospholipid syndrome: A model for autoimmune pregnancy loss. Infert Reprod Med Clin North Am 2:149, 1991

Eastwood KL, Kacmar JE, Steinauer J, et al: Abortion training in United States obstetrics and gynecology residency programs. Obstet Gynecol 108:303, 2006

Eddleman K, Sullivan L, Stone J, et al: An individualized risk for spontaneous pregnancy loss: A risk function model. J Soc Gynecol Investig 13:197A, 2006

Eiben B, Bartels I, Bahr-Prosch S, et al: Cytogenetic analysis of 750 spontaneous abortions with the direct-preparation method of chorionic villi and its implications for studying genetic causes of pregnancy wastage. Am J Hum Genet 47:656, 1990

Fantel AG, Shepard TH, Vadheim-Roth C, et al: Embryonic and fetal phenotypes: Prevalence and other associated factors in a large study of spontaneous abortion. In Porter IH, Hook EM (eds): Human Embryonic and Fetal Death. New York, Academic Press, 1980, p 71

Farquharson RG, Quenby S, Greaves M: Antiphospholipid syndrome in pregnancy: A randomized, controlled trial of treatment. Obstet Gynecol 100:408, 2002

Feist A, Sydler T, Gebbers JJ, et al: No association of Chlamydia with abortion. J R Soc Med 92:237, 1999

Fischer M, Bhatnagar J, Guarner J, et al: Fatal toxic shock syndrome associated with Clostridium sordellii after medical abortion. N Engl J Med 353:2352, 2005

Fjerstad M, Trussell J, Sivin I, et al: Rates of serious infection after changes in regimens for medical abortion. N Engl J Med 361:145, 2009

Floyd RL, Decoufle P, Hungerford DW: Alcohol use prior to pregnancy recognition. Am J Prev Med 17:101, 1999

Food and Drug Administration, Center for Devices and Radiological Heath: PMA final decisions rendered for October 2002. Available at: http://www.fda.gov/cdrh/pma/pmaoct02.html. Accessed December 7, 2008

Franssen MT, Korevaar JC, van der Veen F, et al: Reproductive outcome after chromosome analysis in couples with two or more miscarriages: Case-control study. BMJ 332:759, 2006

Gamble SB, Strauss LT, Parker WY, et al: Abortion surveillance – United States, 2005. MMWR 57:SS-13, 2008

Gibb DM, Salaria DA: Transabdominal cervicoisthmic cerclage in the management of recurrent second trimester miscarriage and preterm delivery. Br J Obstet Gynaecol 102:802, 1995

Glueck CJ, Want P, Goldenberg N, et al: Pregnancy outcomes among women with polycystic ovary syndrome treated with metformin. Hum Reprod 17:2858, 2002

Goldberg AB, Dean G, Kang MS, et al: Manual versus electric vacuum aspiration for early first-trimester abortion: A controlled study of complication rates. Obstet Gynecol 103:101, 2004

Goldberg AB, Drey EA, Whitaker AK: Misoprostol compared with laminaria before early second-trimester surgical abortion: a randomized trial. Obstet Gynecol 106:234, 2005

Goldenberg M, Sivan E, Sharabi Z, et al: Reproductive outcome following hysteroscopic management of intrauterine septum and adhesions. Human Reprod 10:2663, 1995

Goyal V: Uterine rupture in second-trimester misoprostol-induced abortion of cesarean delivery. a systematic review. Obstet Gynecol 112:1117, 2009

Gracia CR, Sammel MD, Chittams J, et al: Risk factors for spontaneous abortion in early symptomatic first-trimester pregnancies. Obstet Gynecol 106:993, 2005

Greene MF: The intimidation of American physicians—Banning partial-birth abortion. N Engl J Med 356:2128, 2007

Grimes DA: Estimation of pregnancy-related mortality risk by pregnancy outcome, United States, 1991 to 1999. Am J Obstet Gynecol 194:92, 2006

Guest J, Chien PF, Thomson MA, et al: Randomised controlled trial comparing the efficacy of same-day administration of mifepristone and misoprostol for termination of pregnancy with the standard 36 to 48 hour protocol. BJOG 114:207, 2007

Hamoda H, Ashok PW, Flett GMM, et al: A randomised controlled trial of mifepristone in combination with misoprostol administered sublingually or vaginally for medical abortion up to 13 weeks of gestation. BJOG 112:1102, 2005

Harger JH, Archer DF, Marchese SG, et al: Etiology of recurrent pregnancy losses and outcome of subsequent pregnancies. Obstet Gynecol 62:574, 1983

Hausknecht R: Mifepristone and misoprostol for early medical abortion: 18 months experience in the United States. Contraception 67:463, 2003

Hertig AT, Sheldon WH: Minimal criteria required to prove prima facie case of traumatic abortion or miscarriage: An analysis of 1,000 spontaneous abortions. Ann Surg 117:596, 1943

Hogge WA, Prosen TL, Lanasa MC, et al: Recurrent spontaneous abortion and skewed X-inactivation: Is there an association? Am J Obstet Gynecol 196:384.e1, 2007

Hogue CJR: Impact of abortion on subsequent fecundity. Clin Obstet Gynaecol 13:95, 1986

Horon IL: Underreporting of maternal deaths on death certificates and the magnitude of the problem of maternal mortality. Am J Public Health 95:478, 2005

Hutton B, Sharma R, Fergusson D, et al: Use of intravenous immunoglobulin for treatment of recurrent miscarriage: A systematic review. BJOG 114:134, 2007

Jacobs PA, Hassold TJ: The origin of chromosomal abnormalities in spontaneous abortion. In Porter IH, Hook EB (eds): Human Embryonic and Fetal Death. New York, Academic Press, 1980, p 289

Jakubowicz DJ, Iuorno MJ, Jakubowicz S, et al: Effects of metformin on early pregnancy loss in the polycystic ovary syndrome. J Clin Endocrinol Metab 87:524, 2002

Jeng GT, Scott JR, Burmeister LF: A comparison of meta-analytic results using literature vs. individual patient data. Paternal cell immunization for recurrent miscarriage. JAMA 274:830, 1995

Jeppson PC, Park A, Chen CC: Multivalvular bacterial endocarditis after suction curettage abortion. Obstet Gynecol 112:452, 2008

Johns J, Jauniaux E: Threatened miscarriage as a predictor of obstetric outcome. Obstet Gynecol 107:845, 2006

Johnson LG, Mueller BA, Daling JR: The relationship of placenta previa and history of induced abortion. Int J Gynaecol Obstet 81:191, 2003

Joyce T, Kaestner R, Colman S: Changes in abortions and births and the Texas parental notification law. N Engl J Med 354:1031, 2006

Jun SH, Ginsburg ES, Racowsky C, et al: Uterine leiomyomas and their effect on in vitro fertilization outcome: A retrospective study. J Assist Reprod Genet 18:139, 2001

Kaandorp S, Di Nisio M, Goddijn M, et al: Aspiring or anticoagulants for treating recurrent miscarriage in women without antiphospholipid syndrome. Cochrane Database Syst Rev (1):CD004734, 2009

Kahn JG, Becker BJ, MacIsaac L, et al: The efficacy of medical abortion: A metaanalysis. Contraception 61:29, 2000

Kajii T, Ferrier A, Niikawa N, et al: Anatomic and chromosomal anomalies in 639 spontaneous abortions. Hum Genet 55:87, 1980

Kambiss SM, Hibbert ML, Macedonia C, et al: Uterine perforation resulting in bowel infarction: Sharp traumatic bowel and mesenteric injury at the time of pregnancy termination. Milit Med 165:81, 2000

Kapp N, Borgatta L, Stubblefield P, et al: Mifepristone in second-trimester medical abortion. Obstet Gynecol 110:1304, 2007

Katz A, Ben-Arie A, Lurie S, et al: Reproductive outcome following hysteroscopic adhesiolysis in Asherman's syndrome. Int J Fertil Menopausal Stud 41:462, 1996

Keder LM: Best practices in surgical abortion. Am J Obstet Gynecol 189:418, 2003

Keegan GT, Forkowitz MJ: A case report: Uretero-uterine fistula as a complication of elective abortion. J Urol 128:137, 1982

Kelly H, Harvey D, Moll S: A cautionary tale. Fatal outcome of methotrexate therapy given for management of ectopic pregnancy. Obstet Gynecol 107:439, 2006

Kesmodel U, Wisborg K, Olsen SF, et al: Moderate alcohol intake in pregnancy and the risk of spontaneous abortion. Alcohol 37:87, 2002

Klebanoff MA, Levine RJ, DerSimonian R, et al: Maternal serum paraxanthine, a caffeine metabolite, and the risk of spontaneous abortion. N Engl J Med 341:1639, 1999

Kline J, Stein ZA, Shrout P, et al: Drinking during pregnancy and spontaneous abortion. Lancet 2:176, 1980

Kuhn RPJ, Pepperell RJ: Cervical ligation: A review of 242 pregnancies. Aust NZ J Obstet Gynaecol 17:79, 1977

Kutteh WH: Antiphospholipid antibody-associated recurrent pregnancy loss: Treatment with heparin and low-dose aspirin is superior to low-dose aspirin alone. Am J Obstet Gynecol 174:1584, 1996

Kutteh WH, Triplett DA: Thrombophilias and recurrent pregnancy loss. Semin Reprod Med 1:54, 2006

Lahteenmaki P, Luukkainen T: Return of ovarian function after abortion. Clin Endocrinol 2:123, 1978

Lakasing L, Williamson C: Obstetric complications due to autoantibodies. Best Pract Res Clin Endocrinol Metab 19:149, 2005

Locatelli A, Vergani P, Bellini P, et al: Amnioreduction in emergency cerclage with prolapsed membranes: Comparison of two methods for reducing the membranes. Am J Perinatol 16:73, 1999

Luise C, Jermy K, May C, et al: Outcome of expectant management of spontaneous first trimester miscarriage: Observational study. BMJ 324:873, 2002

MacIsaac L, Darney P: Early surgical abortion: An alternative to and backup for medical abortion. Am J Obstet Gynecol 183:S76, 2000

MacIsaac L, Grossman D, Balistreri E, et al: A randomized controlled trial of laminaria, oral misoprostol, and vaginal misoprostol before abortion. Obstet Gynecol 93:766, 1999

MacNaughton MC, Chalmers IG, Dubowitz V, et al: Final report of the Medical Research Council/Royal College of Obstetricians and Gynaecologists Multicentre Randomized Trial of Cervical Cerclage. Br J Obster Gynaecol 100:516, 1993

Maconochie N, Doyle P, Prior S, et al: Risk factors for first trimester miscarriage—Results from a UK-population-based case-control study. BJOG 114:170, 2007

Madden T, Westhoff C: Rates of follow-up and repeat pregnancy in the 12 months after first-trimester induced abortion. Obstet Gynecol 113:663, 2009

Makino T, Hara T, Oka C, et al: Survey of 1120 Japanese women with a history of recurrent spontaneous abortions. Eur J Obstet Gynecol Reprod Biol 44:123, 1992

Mankowski JL, Kingston J, Moran T, et al: Paracervical compared with intracervical lidocaine for suction curettage. a randomized controlled trial. Obstet Gynecol 113:1052, 2009

Masch RJ, Roman AS: Uterine evacuation in the office. Contemp Obstet Gynecol 51:66, 2005

McDonald IA: Incompetent cervix as a cause of recurrent abortion. J Obstet Gynaecol Br Commonw 70:105, 1963

Mills JL, Simpson JL, Driscoll SG, et al: Incidence of spontaneous abortion among normal women and insulin-dependent diabetic women whose pregnancies were identified within 21 days of conception. N Engl J Med 319:1618, 1988

Moreau C, Kaminski M, Ancel PY, et al: Previous induced abortions and the risk of very preterm delivery: Results of the EPIPAGE study. BJOG 112:430, 2005

New Shorter Oxford English Dictionary, 5th ed. Trumble WR, Stevenson A (eds). New York, Oxford University Press, 2002, p 7

Ngoc NT, Blum J, Westheimer E, et al: Medical treatment of missed abortion using misoprostol. Int J Gynaec Obstet 87:138, 2004

Oakeshott P, Hay P, Hay S, et al: Association between bacterial vaginosis or chlamydial infection and miscarriage before 16 weeks' gestation: Prospective, community based cohort study. BMJ 325:1334, 2002

O'Connor S, Kuller JA, McMahon MJ: Management of cervical cerclage after preterm premature rupture of membranes. Obstet Gynecol Surv 54:391, 1999

Osser S, Persson K: Chlamydial antibodies in women who suffer miscarriage. Br J Obstet Gynaecol 103:137, 1996

Owen J, Hauth JC, Winkler CL, et al: Midtrimester pregnancy termination: A randomized trial of prostaglandin E2 versus concentrated oxytocin. Am J Obstet Gynecol 167:1112, 1992

Owen J, Iams JD, Hauth JC: Vaginal sonography and cervical incompetence. Am J Obstet Gynecol 188:586, 2003

Paukku M, Tulppala M, Puolakkainen M, et al: Lack of association between serum antibodies to *Chlamydia trachomatis* and a history of recurrent pregnancy loss. Fertil Steril 72:427, 1999

Paul M, Lichtenberg S, Borgatta L, et al (eds): A Clinician's Guide to Medical and Surgical Abortion. New York, Churchill Livingstone, 1999

Paul ME, Mitchell CM, Rogers AJ, et al: Early surgical abortion: Efficacy and safety. Am J Obstet Gynecol 187:407, 2002

Poland B, Miller J, Jones D, et al: Reproductive counseling in patients who have had a spontaneous abortion. Am J Obstet Gynecol 127:685, 1977

Poppe K, Velkeniers B, Glinoer D, et al: The role of thyroid autoimmunity in fertility and pregnancy. Nat Clin Pract Endocrinol Metab 4:394, 2008

Quinn PA, Shewchuck AB, Shuber J, et al: Efficacy of antibiotic therapy in preventing spontaneous pregnancy loss among couples colonized with genital mycoplasmas. Am J Obstet Gynecol 145:239, 1983a

Quinn PA, Shewchuck AB, Shuber J, et al: Serologic evidence of *Ureaplasma urealyticum* infection in women with spontaneous pregnancy loss. Am J Obstet Gynecol 145:245, 1983b

Rai R, Cohen H, Dave M, et al: Randomised controlled trial of aspirin and aspirin plus heparin in pregnant women with recurrent miscarriage associated with phospholipid antibodies (or antiphospholipid antibodies). BMJ 314:253, 1997

Ramsey PS, Owen J: Midtrimester cervical ripening and labor induction. Clin Obstet Gynecol 43(3):495, 2000

Ramsey PS, Savage K, Lincoln T, Owen J: Vaginal misoprostol versus concentrated oxytocin and vaginal PGE2 for second-trimester labor induction. Obstet Gynecol 104:138, 2004

Ramzy AM, Sattar M, Amin Y, et al: Uterine myomata and outcome of assisted reproduction. Hum Reprod 13:198, 1998

Rasch V: Cigarette, alcohol, and caffeine consumption: Risk factors for spontaneous abortion. Acta Obstet Gynecol Scand 82:182, 2003

Reeves MF, Smith KJ, Creinin MD: Contraceptive effectiveness of immediate compared with delayed insertion of intrauterine devices after abortion. Obstet Gynecol 109:1286, 2007

Rey E, Kahn SR, David M, et al: Thrombophilic disorders and fetal loss: A meta-analysis. Lancet 361:901, 2003

Rowland AS, Baird DD, Shore DL, et al: Nitrous oxide and spontaneous abortion in female dental assistants. Am J Epidemiol 141:531, 1995

Rushworth FH, Backos M, Rai R, et al: Prospective pregnancy outcome in untreated recurrent miscarriages with thyroid autoantibodies. Hum Reprod 15:1637, 2000

Rust OA, Atlas RO, Reed J, et al: Revisiting the short cervix detected by transvaginal ultrasound in the second trimester: Why cerclage may not help. Am J Obstet Gynecol 185·1098, 2001

Salem HT, Ghaneimah SA, Shaaban MM, et al: Prognostic value of biochemical tests in the assessment of fetal outcome in threatened abortion. Br J Obstet Gynaecol 91:382, 1984

Salim R, Regan L, Woelfer B, et al: A comparative study of the morphology of congenital uterine anomalies in women with and without a history of recurrent first trimester miscarriage. Hum Reprod 18:162, 2003

Sauerwein RW, Bisseling J, Horrevorts AM: Septic abortion associated with *Campylobacter fetus* subspecies *fetus* infection: Case report and review of the literature. Infection 21:33, 1993

Sawaya GF, Grady D, Kerlikowske K, et al: Antibiotics at the time of induced abortion: The case for universal prophylaxis based on a meta-analysis. Obstet Gynecol 87:884, 1996

Saygili-Yilmaz E, Yildiz S, Erman-Akar M, et al: Reproductive outcome of septate uterus after hysteroscopic metroplasty. Arch Gynecol Obstet 4:289, 2003

Saygili-Yilmaz ES, Erman-Akar M, Yildiz S, et al: A retrospective study on the reproductive outcome of the septate uterus corrected by hysteroscopic metroplasty. Int J Gynaecol Obstet 1:59, 2002

Schaff EA, Fielding SL, Westhoff C, et al: Vaginal misoprostol administered 1, 2, or 3 days after mifepristone for early medical abortion. A randomized trial. JAMA 284:1948, 2000

Schneider D, Golan A, Langer R, et al: Outcome of continued pregnancies after first and second trimester cervical dilatation by laminaria tents. Obstet Gynecol 78:1121, 1991

Schnorr TM, Grajewski BA, Hornung RW, et al: Video display terminals and the risk of spontaneous abortion. N Engl J Med 324:727, 1991

Schust D, Hill J: Recurrent pregnancy loss. In Berek J (eds): Novak's Gynecology, 13th ed. Philadelphia, Lippincott Williams & Wilkins, 2002

Scott JR. Immunotherapy for recurrent miscarriage. Cochrane Database Syst Rev (2):CD000112, 2003

Shannon C, Wiebe E, Jacot F: Regimens of misoprostol with mifepristone for early medical abortion: A randomized trial. BJOG 113:621, 2006

Sher KS, Jayanthi V, Probert CS, et al: Infertility, obstetric and gynaecological problems in coeliac sprue. Digest Dis 12:186, 1994

Shirodkar VN: A new method of operative treatment for habitual abortions in the second trimester of pregnancy. Antiseptic 52:299, 1955

Shwekerela B, Kalumuna R, Kipingili R, et al: Misoprostol for treatment of incomplete abortion at the regional hospital level: Results from Tanzania. BJOG 114:1363, 2007

Simpson JL: Genes, chromosomes, and reproductive failure. Fertil Steril 33:107, 1980

Simpson JL, Carson SA, Chesney C, et al: Lack of association between antiphospholipid antibodies and first-trimester spontaneous abortion: Prospective study of pregnancies detected within 21 days of conception. Fertil Steril 69:814, 1998

Simpson JL, Mills JL, Kim H, et al: Infectious processes: An infrequent cause of first trimester spontaneous abortions. Hum Reprod 11:668, 1996

Stein Z, Kline J, Susser E, et al: Maternal age and spontaneous abortion. In Porter IH, Hook EB (eds): Human Embryonic and Fetal Death. New York, Academic Press, 1980, p 107

Steinauer J, Darney P, Auerbach RD: Should all residents be trained to do abortions? Contemp Obstet Gynecol 51:56, 2005a

Steinauer J, Drey EA, Lewis R, et al: Obstetrics and gynecology resident satisfaction with an integrated, comprehensive abortion rotation. Obstet Gynecol 105:1335, 2005b

Stephenson MD: Management of recurrent early pregnancy loss. J Reprod Med 51:303, 2006

Strauss LT, Gamble SB, Parker WY, et al: Abortion surveillance—United States, 2004. MMWR Surveill Summ 56:1, 2007

Stubblefield PG, Naftolin F, Frigoletto F, Ryan KJ: Laminaria augmentation of intra-amniotic PGF midtrimester pregnancy termination. Prostaglandins 10:413, 1975

Sullivan AE, Silver RM, LaCoursiere DY, et al: Recurrent fetal aneuploidy and recurrent miscarriage. Obstet Gynecol 104:784, 2004

Supreme Court of the United States: Gonzales, Attorney General v. Carhart, et al. Certiorari to the United States Court of Appeals for the Eighth Circuit. Argued November 8, 2006—Decided April 18, 2007

Supreme Court of the United States: Jane Roe et al v Henry Wade, District Attorney of Dallas County. Opinion No. 70-18, January 22, 1973

Supreme Court of the United States: William Webster v Reproductive Health Services. Opinion No. 88-605, July 3, 1989

Swingle HM, Colaizy TT, Zimmerman MB, et al: Abortion and the risk of subsequent preterm birth. J Reprod Med 54:95, 2009

Taskinen H, Kyyrönen P, Hemminki K: Effects of ultrasound, shortwaves, and physical exertion on pregnancy outcome in physiotherapists. J Epidemiol Community Health 44:196, 1990

Temmerman M, Lopita MI, Sanghvi HC, et al: The role of maternal syphilis, gonorrhoea and HIV-1 infections in spontaneous abortion. Int J STD AIDS 3:418, 1992

Terkildsen MFC, Parilla BV, Kumar P, et al: Factors associated with success of emergent second-trimester cerclage. Obstet Gynecol 101:565, 2003

Therapel AT, Tharapel SA, Bannerman RM: Recurrent pregnancy losses and parental chromosome abnormalities: A review. Br J Obstet Gynecol 92:899, 1985

Thomason JL, Sampson MB, Beckman CR, et al: The incompetent cervix: A 1982 update. J Reprod Med 27:187, 1982

To MS, Alfirevic Z, Heath VCF, et al: Cervical cerclage for prevention of preterm delivery in women with short cervix: Randomised controlled trial. Lancet 363:1849, 2004

Tongsong T, Srisomboon J, Wanapirak C, et al: Pregnancy outcome of threatened abortion with demonstrable fetal cardiac activity: A cohort study. J Obstet Gynaecol 21:331, 1995

Trinder J, Brocklehurst P, Porter R, et al: Management of miscarriage: expectant, medical, or surgical? Results of randomised controlled trial (miscarriage treatment (MIST) trial). BMJ 332:1235, 2006

van Benthem BH, de Vincenzi I, Delmas MD, et al: Pregnancies before and after HIV diagnosis in a European cohort of HIV-infected women. European study on the natural history of HIV infection in women. AIDS 14:2171, 2000

Vartian CV, Septimus EJ: Tricuspid valve group B streptococcal endocarditis following elective abortion. Review Infect Dis 13:997, 1991

Ventura SJ, Abma JC, Mosher WD, et al: Estimated pregnancy rates by outcome for the United States, 1990–2004. Natl Vit Stat Rep Vol 56, No. 15, April 14, 2008

Virk J, Zhang J, Olsen J: Medical abortion and the risk of subsequent adverse pregnancy outcomes. N Engl J Med 357:648, 2007

von Hertzen H, Piaggio G, Huong NT, et al: Efficacy of two intervals and two routes of administration of misoprostol for termination of early pregnancy: A randomized controlled equivalence trial. Lancet 369:1938, 2007

Warburton D, Fraser FC: Spontaneous abortion risks in man: Data from reproductive histories collected in a medical genetics unit. Am J Hum Genet 16:1, 1964

Warburton D, Stein Z, Kline J, et al: Chromosome abnormalities in spontaneous abortion: Data from the New York City study. In Porter IH, Hook EB (eds): Human Embryonic and Fetal Death. New York, Academic Press, 1980, p 261

Warren JB, Silver RM: Autoimmune disease in pregnancy: Systemic lupus erythematosus and antiphospholipid syndrome. Obstet Gynecol Clin North Am 31:345, 2004

Weiss J, Malone F, Vidaver J, et al: Threatened abortion: A risk factor for poor pregnancy outcome—A population based screening study (The FASTER Trial). Am J Obstet Gynecol 187:S70, 2002

Weissman AM, Dawson JD, Rijhsinghani A, et al: Non-evidence-based use of Rho(D) immune globulin for threatened abortion by family practice and obstetric faculty physicians. J Reprod Med 47:909, 2002

Westfall JM, Sophocles A, Burggraf H, et al: Manual vacuum aspiration for first-trimester abortion. Arch Fam Med 7:559, 1998

Wiebe ER: Oral methotrexate compared with injected methotrexate when used with misoprostol for abortion. Am J Obstet Gynecol 181:149, 1999

Wiebe E, Dunn S, Guilbert E, et al: Comparison of abortions induced by methotrexate or mifepristone followed by misoprostol. Obstet Gynecol 99:813, 2002

Wijesiriwardana A, Bhattacharya S, Shetty A, et al: Obstetric outcome in women with threatened miscarriage in the first trimester. Obstet Gynecol 107:557, 2006

Wilcox AF, Weinberg CR, O'Connor JF, et al: Incidence of early loss of pregnancy. N Engl J Med 319:189, 1988

Wilson RD, Kendrick V, Wittmann BK, et al: Spontaneous abortion and pregnancy outcome after normal first-trimester ultrasound examination. Obstet Gynecol 67:352, 1986

Winikoff B, Dzuba IG, Creinin MD, et al: Two distinct oral routes of misoprostol in mefipristone medical abortion. a randomized controlled trial. Obstet Gynecol 112:1303, 2008

Wisborg K, Kesmodel U, Henriksen TB, et al: A prospective study of maternal smoking and spontaneous abortion. Acta Obstet Gynecol Scand 82:936, 2003

Witter FR: Negative sonographic findings followed by rapid cervical dilatation due to cervical incompetence. Obstet Gynecol 64:136, 1984

Yasuda M, Takakuwa K, Tokunaga A, et al: Prospective studies of the association between anticardiolipin antibody and outcome of pregnancy. Obstet Gynecol 86:555, 1995

Yetman DL, Kutteh WH: Antiphospholipid antibody panels and recurrent pregnancy loss: Prevalence of anticardiolipin antibodies compared with other antiphospholipid antibodies. Fertil Steril 66:540, 1996

Zaveri V, Aghajafari F, Amankwah K, et al: Abdominal versus vaginal cerclage after a failed transvaginal cerclage: A systematic review. Am J Obstet Gynecol 187:868, 2002

Zhang J, Gilles JM, Barnhart K, et al: A comparison of medical management with misoprostol and surgical management for early pregnancy failure. N Engl J Med 353:761, 2005

Ectopic Pregnancy

The blastocyst normally implants in the endometrial lining of the uterine cavity. Implantation anywhere else is considered an ectopic pregnancy. It is derived from the Greek *ektopos*—out of place. According to the American College of Obstetricians and Gynecologists (2008), 2 percent of all first-trimester pregnancies in the United States are ectopic, and these account for 6 percent of all pregnancy-related deaths. The risk of death from an extrauterine pregnancy is greater than that for pregnancy that either results in a live birth or is intentionally terminated. Moreover, the chance for a subsequent successful pregnancy is reduced after an ectopic pregnancy. With earlier diagnosis, however, both maternal survival and conservation of reproductive capacity are enhanced.

GENERAL CONSIDERATIONS

Classification

Nearly 95 percent of ectopic pregnancies are implanted in the various segments of the fallopian tubes (Fig. 10-1). Of these, most are ampullary implantations. The remaining 5 percent implant in the ovary, peritoneal cavity, or within the cervix. More recently,

cesarean scar pregnancies are reported to be more common than in the past. Occasionally, and usually with assisted reproductive technologies (ART), multifetal pregnancies implant simultaneously with either both ectopic, or one ectopic and the other intrauterine.

Risk Factors

Prior tubal damage, either from a previous ectopic pregnancy or from tubal surgery to relieve infertility or for sterilization, confers the highest risk for ectopic pregnancy (Table 10-1). After one previous ectopic pregnancy, the chance of another is approximately 10 percent (Ankum and colleagues, 1996; Skjeldestad and co-workers, 1998). Infertility, per se, as well as the use of ART to overcome it, is associated with substantively increased risks for ectopic pregnancy (Clayton and colleagues, 2006). The Society for Assisted Reproductive Technology and the American Society for Reproductive Medicine (2007) reported outcomes from more than 108,000 cycles performed in 2001. Ectopic pregnancy rates were 4.3 percent following zygote intrafallopian transfer (ZIFT) but only 1.8 percent with in vitro fertilization (IVF). And "atypical" implantations—cornual, abdominal, cervical, ovarian, and heterotopic pregnancy—are more common following ART procedures. Prior tubal infection or other sexually transmitted diseases are also common risk factors. And so is smoking, which may be a surrogate marker for these infections because of high-risk behavior (Saraiya and co-workers, 1998). Peritubal adhesions subsequent to salpingitis, postabortal or puerperal infection, appendicitis, or endometriosis may increase the risk for tubal pregnancy. One episode of salpingitis can be followed by a subsequent ectopic pregnancy in up to 9 percent of women (Centers for Disease Control and Prevention, 2007).

Failed Contraception

With any form of contraceptive, the *absolute* number of ectopic pregnancies is decreased because pregnancy occurs less often. In some contraceptive failures, however, the relative number of

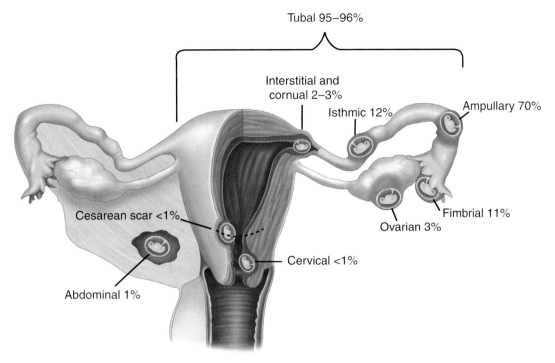

Tubal 95–96%

Interstitial and cornual 2–3%

Isthmic 12%

Ampullary 70%

Cesarean scar <1%

Fimbrial 11%

Ovarian 3%

Cervical <1%

Abdominal 1%

FIGURE 10-1 Sites of implantation of 1800 ectopic pregnancies from a 10-year population-based study. (Data from Callen, 2000; Bouyer and colleagues, 2003.)

ectopic pregnancies is increased. Examples include some forms of tubal sterilization, intrauterine devices, high-dose estrogen emergency contraception, and progestin-only minipills (Ory, 1981; Sivin, 1991).

Epidemiology

According to the Centers for Disease Control and Prevention (1995), the rate of ectopic pregnancies continued to increase in

the United States through the 1990s (Fig. 10-2). Thereafter, because of the increasing use of medical outpatient treatment, reliable data on the actual number of ectopic pregnancies are not available after 1990. That said, the 1.9-percent rate in 1992 is similar to that of 2.1 percent in more than 125,000 pregnancies reported from Kaiser Permanente of North California from 1997 to 2000 (Van Den Eeden and colleagues, 2005).

Increasing Ectopic Pregnancy Rates

A number of reasons at least partially explain the increased rate of ectopic pregnancies in the United States and many European countries. Some of these include:

1. Increasing prevalence of sexually transmitted infections, especially those caused by *Chlamydia trachomatis* (Centers for Disease Control and Prevention, 2007)
2. Identification through earlier diagnosis of some ectopic pregnancies otherwise destined to resorb spontaneously
3. Popularity of contraception that predisposes pregnancy failures to be ectopic
4. Tubal sterilization techniques that with contraceptive failure increase the likelihood of ectopic pregnancy
5. Assisted reproductive technology
6. Tubal surgery, including salpingotomy for tubal pregnancy and tuboplasty for infertility.

TABLE 10-1. Some Reported Risk Factors for Ectopic Pregnancy

Risk Factor	Relative Risk
Previous ectopic pregnancy	3–13
Tubal corrective surgery	4
Tubal sterilization	9
Intrauterine device	1–4.2
Documented tubal pathology	3.8–21
Infertility	2.5–3
Assisted reproductive technology	2–8
Previous genital infection	2–4
Chlamydia	2
Salpingitis	1.5–6.2
Smoking	1.7–4
Prior abortion	0.6–3
Multiple sexual partners	1.6–3.5
Prior cesarean delivery	1–2.1

Data from Bakken (2007a, b); Barnhart (2006); Bouyer (2003); Gala (2008); Karaer (2006); Virk (2007), and all their colleagues.

Mortality

According to the World Health Organization (2007), ectopic pregnancy is responsible for almost 5 percent of maternal deaths in developed countries. But deaths from ectopic pregnancy in the United States have become uncommon since the 1970s. As shown in Figure 10-2, the case-fatality rate from ectopic pregnancy

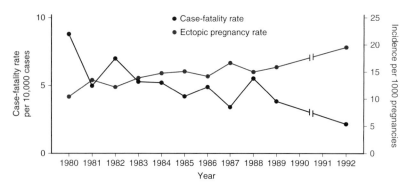

FIGURE 10-2 Case-fatality rate and incidence of ectopic pregnancy for the United States, 1980–1992. (From the Centers for Disease Control and Prevention, 1995.)

declined markedly from 1980 to 1992. This decrease is likely due to improved diagnosis and management. Still, according to Grimes (2006), from 1991 through 1999, estimated mortality rates for ectopic pregnancies were 32 per 100,000 deliveries compared with maternal death rates of 7 per 100,000 for liveborns. There remains a marked disparity between black and white women for both incidence and case-fatality rates. For example, Anderson and colleagues (2004) reported that the ectopic pregnancy-related mortality ratio in black women in Michigan was 18 times higher than for white women.

TUBAL PREGNANCY

The fertilized ovum may lodge in any portion of the oviduct, giving rise to ampullary, isthmic, and interstitial tubal pregnancies (see Fig. 10-1). In rare instances, the fertilized ovum may implant in the fimbriated extremity. The ampulla is the most frequent site, followed by the isthmus. Interstitial pregnancy accounts for only about 2 percent. From these primary types, secondary forms of tubo-abdominal, tubo-ovarian, and broad-ligament pregnancies occasionally develop.

Because the tube lacks a submucosal layer, the fertilized ovum promptly burrows through the epithelium, and the zygote comes to lie near or within the muscularis. The rapidly proliferating trophoblast may invade the subjacent muscularis, however, half of ampullary ectopic pregnancies stay within the tubal lumen with preservation of the muscularis layer in 85 percent (Senterman and associates, 1988). The embryo or fetus in an ectopic pregnancy is often absent or stunted.

Tubal Rupture

The invading, expanding products of conception may rupture the oviduct at any of several sites (Fig. 10-3). Before precise methods to measure human chorionic gonadotropin (hCG) were available, many cases of tubal pregnancy ended in rupture during the first trimester. As a rule, whenever there is tubal rupture in the first few weeks, the pregnancy is situated in the isthmic portion of the tube. When the fertilized ovum is implanted well within the interstitial portion, rupture usually occurs later (Fig. 10-4). Rupture is usually spontaneous, but it may follow coitus or bimanual examination. There are usually symptoms, and signs of hypovolemia are common.

Tubal Abortion

The frequency of tubal abortion depends in part on the implantation site. Abortion is common in ampullary pregnancies, whereas rupture is the usual outcome with isthmic pregnancies. With hemorrhage, there is further disruption of the connection between the placenta and membranes and the tubal wall. If placental separation is complete, all of the products of conception may be extruded through the fimbriated end into the peritoneal cavity. At this point, hemorrhage may cease and symptoms eventually disappear. Some bleeding usually persists as long as products remain in the oviduct. Blood slowly trickles from the tubal fimbria into the peritoneal cavity and typically pools in the rectouterine cul-de-sac. If the fimbriated extremity is occluded, the fallopian tube may gradually become distended by blood, forming a hematosalpinx.

Abdominal Pregnancy

With either tubal abortion or intraperitoneal rupture, the entire conceptus may be extruded from the tube, or if the rent is small, profuse hemorrhage may occur without extrusion. If an early conceptus is expelled essentially undamaged into the peritoneal cavity, its placental attachment may persist, or it may reimplant almost anywhere and grow as an abdominal pregnancy (Worley and colleagues, 2008). This is unusual, and most small conceptuses are resorbed. Occasionally, they may remain in the cul-de-sac for years as an encapsulated mass, or even become calcified to form a *lithopedion* (Berman and Katsiyiannis, 2001).

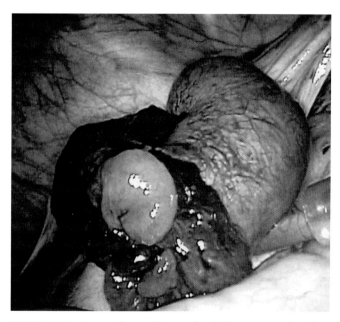

FIGURE 10-3 Ruptured ampullary early tubal pregnancy. (Used with permission from Dr. Togas Tulandi.)

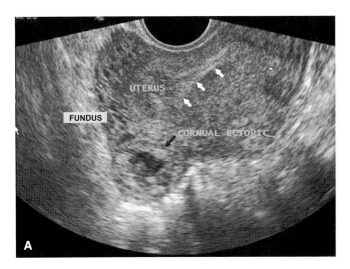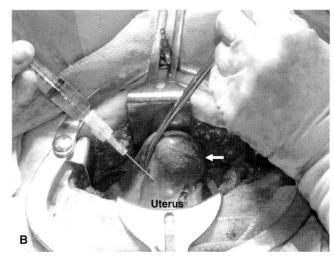

FIGURE 10-4 Cornual ectopic pregnancy. **A.** Transvaginal sonogram, parasagittal view shows an empty uterine cavity (*white arrows*) and a mass lateral to the uterine fundus (*red arrow*). (Courtesy of Dr. Elysia Moschos.) **B.** Intraoperative photograph during cornual resection of an ectopic pregnancy. A Pean clamp is placed across the round ligament, uteroovarian ligament, and fallopian tube distal to the cornual pregnancy (*white arrow*). The surgeon is injecting a dilute vasopressin solution at the cornual base prior to incision. (Used with permission from Dr. Marlene Corton.)

Broad Ligament Pregnancy

In zygotes implanted toward the mesosalpinx, rupture may occur at the portion of the tube not immediately covered by peritoneum. The gestational contents may be extruded into a space formed between the folds of the broad ligament and then become an intraligamentous or broad ligament pregnancy.

Interstitial and Cornual Pregnancy

Although used interchangeably, these are slightly different implantations. Cornual implantation describes those in the upper and lateral uterine cavity, whereas interstitial denotes those implanted within the proximal intramural portion of the tube (Malinowski and Bates, 2006). Together, they account for 2 to 3 percent of all tubal gestations (Fig. 10-1). In the past, rupture would not occur usually until 14 to 16 weeks, often with severe hemorrhage. Currently, interstitial and cornual pregnancy are usually diagnosed before rupture (Fig. 10-4). Both may be treated by cornual resection via laparotomy. Alternatively, several authors have described treatment with uterus-sparing laparoscopic surgery or methotrexate (Eun, 2009; Soriano, 2008; Tulandi, 2004, and all their associates).

Multifetal Ectopic Pregnancy

Heterotopic Ectopic Pregnancy

The word *heterotopic* pregnancy is used in place of the older term *combined* pregnancy. It defines a uterine pregnancy coexisting with a second pregnancy in an extrauterine location. Because, strictly speaking, heterotopic is synonymous with ectopic, the use of "heterotopic ectopic pregnancy" is tautological. Although most heterotopic pregnancies are tubal and uterine, they are also seen with ovarian, cervical, and other pregnancies.

The natural incidence of a tubal pregnancy accompanied by a coexisting uterine gestation is approximately 1 per 30,000

pregnancies. Because of ART, however, its incidence has increased to 1 in 7000 overall, and following ovulation induction, it may be as high as 0.5 to 1 percent (Mukul and Teal, 2007). A heterotopic pregnancy is more likely and should be considered with any of the following:

- Conception achieved by assisted reproductive techniques
- Persistent or rising hCG levels after dilatation and curettage for an induced or spontaneous abortion
- A uterine fundus larger than menstrual dates
- More than one corpus luteum
- Absent vaginal bleeding in the presence of signs and symptoms of an ectopic pregnancy
- Sonographic evidence of uterine and extrauterine pregnancy.

Multifetal Tubal Pregnancy

Twin tubal pregnancy with both embryos in the same tube as well as with one in each tube has been reported (Rolle and colleagues, 2004). Berkes and associates (2008) describe a rare case of three embryos implanting ectopically in one tube following IVF.

Clinical Manifestations

Women with a tubal pregnancy have diverse clinical manifestations that largely depend on whether there is rupture. Earlier patient presentation and more precise diagnostic technology have enabled identification before rupture in most cases. Typically, the woman does not suspect tubal pregnancy and assumes that she has a normal early pregnancy, or that she is having a miscarriage. **Symptoms and signs of ectopic pregnancy are often subtle or even absent.**

Without early diagnosis, the natural history of "classical" cases is characterized by variably delayed menstruation followed by slight vaginal bleeding or spotting. With rupture, there is usually severe lower abdominal and pelvic pain that is frequently described as sharp, stabbing, or tearing. Vasomotor disturbances develop, ranging from vertigo to syncope. There is tenderness during abdominal palpation, and bimanual pelvic examination, especially cervical motion, causes exquisite pain. The posterior vaginal fornix may bulge because of blood in the rectouterine cul-de-sac, or a tender, boggy mass may be felt to one side of the uterus. Symptoms of diaphragmatic irritation, characterized by pain in the neck or shoulder, especially on inspiration, develop in perhaps half of women with sizable intraperitoneal hemorrhage.

Symptoms and Signs

Most women present for care early in the course of a developing ectopic pregnancy. In some, the diagnosis is made even before the onset of symptoms. Common findings include the following:

1. *Pain.* Pelvic and abdominal pain are reported by 95 percent of women with tubal pregnancy. With more advanced gestation, Dorfman and associates (1984) reported that gastrointestinal symptoms (80 percent) and dizziness or light-headedness (58 percent) were common. With rupture, pain may be anywhere in the abdomen.
2. *Abnormal bleeding.* Amenorrhea with some degree of vaginal spotting or bleeding is reported by 60 to 80 percent of women with tubal pregnancy. Approximately one fourth mistake the bleeding for true menstruation. Although profuse vaginal bleeding is suggestive of an incomplete abortion, such bleeding occasionally is seen with tubal gestations.
3. *Abdominal and pelvic tenderness.* With early unruptured ectopic pregnancies, tenderness is uncommon. With rupture, however, exquisite tenderness during abdominal and vaginal examination, especially with cervical motion, is demonstrable in more than three fourths of women.
4. *Uterine changes.* Although minimal early, later the uterus may be pushed to one side by an ectopic mass. The uterus may also be enlarged due to hormonal stimulation. The degree to which the endometrium is converted to decidua is variable. The finding of uterine decidua without trophoblast *suggests* ectopic pregnancy, but absence of decidual tissue does not exclude it.
5. *Vital signs.* Although generally normal before rupture, responses to moderate hemorrhage include no change in vital signs, a slight rise in blood pressure, or a vasovagal response with bradycardia and hypotension. Birkhahn and colleagues (2003) noted that in 25 women with ruptured ectopic pregnancy, the majority on presentation had a heart rate of less than 100 beats per minute and a systolic blood pressure greater than 100 mm Hg. Blood pressure will fall and pulse will rise only if bleeding continues and hypovolemia becomes significant.

Diagnosis of Ectopic Pregnancy

Laboratory Tests

Human Chorionic Gonadotropin (β-hCG). Rapid and accurate determination of pregnancy is essential in evaluating women with complaints suggestive of ectopic pregnancy. Current serum and urine pregnancy tests that use enzyme-linked immunosorbent assays (ELISAs) for β-hCG are sensitive to levels of 10 to 20 mIU/mL and are positive in greater than 99 percent of ectopic pregnancies (Kalinski and Guss, 2002). However, rare cases of ectopic pregnancy with a negative serum β-hCG assay result have been reported (Grynberg and colleagues, 2009; Lee and Lamaro, 2009).

Serum Progesterone. A single progesterone measurement can be used to establish with high reliability that there is a normally developing pregnancy. A value exceeding 25 ng/mL excludes ectopic pregnancy with 92.5-percent sensitivity (Lipscomb and co-workers, 1999a; Pisarska and colleagues, 1998). Conversely, values below 5 ng/mL are found in only 0.3 percent of normal pregnancies (Mol and colleagues, 1998). Thus, values <5 ng/mL suggest either an intrauterine pregnancy with a dead fetus or an ectopic pregnancy. Because in most ectopic pregnancies, progesterone levels range between 10 and 25 ng/mL, the clinical utility is limited (American College of Obstetricians and Gynecologists, 2008).

Novel Serum Markers. A number of preliminary studies have been done to evaluate novel markers to detect ectopic pregnancy. These include vascular endothelial growth factor (VEGF), cancer antigen 125 (CA125), creatine kinase, fetal fibronectin, and mass spectrometry-based proteomics (Daniel, 1999; Ness, 1998; Predanic, 2000; Shankar, 2005, and all their co-workers). None of these are in current clinical use.

Hemogram. After hemorrhage, depleted blood volume is restored toward normal by hemodilution over the course of a day or longer. Even after substantive hemorrhage, hemoglobin or hematocrit readings may at first show only a slight reduction. Hence, after an acute hemorrhage, a decrease in hemoglobin or hematocrit level over several hours is a more valuable index of blood loss than is the initial level. In about half of women with a ruptured ectopic pregnancy, varying degrees of leukocytosis up to 30,000/μL may be documented.

Sonography

This imaging tool is indispensable to confirm the clinical diagnosis of suspected ectopic gestation. In many cases, its location and size are also ascertained by sonography.

Transvaginal Sonography (TVS). High-resolution transvaginal sonography has revolutionized the care of women with suspected ectopic pregnancy. It is an integral part of most algorithms directed at ectopic pregnancy identification and is discussed in that context on p. 243.

Transabdominal Sonography. Identification of tubal pregnancy products is difficult using transabdominal sonography. If a gestational sac is clearly identified within the uterine cavity, ectopic pregnancy is still a consideration if ART was used. Conversely, with sonographic absence of a uterine pregnancy, a positive assay for β-hCG, fluid in the cul-de-sac, and an abnormal pelvic mass, ectopic pregnancy is almost certain (Romero and associates, 1988). A uterine pregnancy usually is not recognized using abdominal sonography until 5 to 6 menstrual weeks or 28 days after timed ovulation (Batzer and co-workers, 1983).

Culdocentesis

This simple technique was used commonly in the past to identify hemoperitoneum. The cervix is pulled toward the symphysis with a tenaculum, and a long 16- or 18-gauge needle is inserted through the posterior vaginal fornix into the cul-de-sac. If present, fluid can be aspirated, however, failure to do so is interpreted only as unsatisfactory entry into the cul-de-sac and does not exclude an ectopic pregnancy, either ruptured or unruptured. Fluid containing fragments of old clots, or bloody fluid that does not clot, is compatible with the diagnosis of hemoperitoneum resulting from an ectopic pregnancy. If the blood subsequently clots, it may have been obtained from an adjacent blood vessel rather than from a bleeding ectopic pregnancy.

Multimodality Diagnosis

Ectopic pregnancies are identified with the combined use of clinical findings along with serum analyte testing and transvaginal sonography. A number of algorithms have been proposed, but most include five key components:

1. Transvaginal sonography
2. Serum β-hCG level—both the initial level and the pattern of subsequent rise or decline
3. Serum progesterone level
4. Uterine curettage
5. Laparoscopy and occasionally, laparotomy.

One algorithm for suspected ectopic pregnancy evaluation is shown in Figure 10-5. **The choice of diagnostic algorithm applies only to hemodynamically stable women—those with presumed rupture should undergo prompt surgical therapy.** For a suspected unruptured ectopic pregnancy, all diagnostic strategies involve trade-offs. Strategies that maximize detection of ectopic pregnancy may result in the interruption of one normal pregnancy for every 100 women evaluated. Conversely, those that reduce the potential for interruption of a normal pregnancy will delay diagnosis of more ectopic pregnancies. And some do not recommend diagnostic curettage as shown in the algorithm because it results in unnecessary medical or surgical therapy for ectopic pregnancy (Barnhart and colleagues, 2002).

Use of Transvaginal Sonography (TVS). In a woman in whom ectopic pregnancy is suspected, TVS is performed, and findings that indicate intrauterine or ectopic pregnancy are sought.

Endometrial Cavity. A trilaminar endometrial pattern is unique for diagnosis of ectopic pregnancy—its specificity is 94 percent, but with a sensitivity of only 38 percent (Hammoud and associates, 2005). Anechoic fluid collections, however, which would normally suggest an early intrauterine gestational sac, may also be seen with ectopic pregnancy. These include pseudogestational sac and decidual cyst:

1. All pregnancies induce an endometrial decidual reaction, and sloughing of the decidua can create an intracavitary fluid collection called a *pseudogestational sac*, or *pseudosac*. This one-layer sac characteristically lies in the midline within the endometrial cavity and can be seen contiguous with the endometrial stripe. In contrast, gestational sacs are usually eccentrically located (Dashefsky and colleagues, 1988). When a pseudosac is noted, the risk of ectopic pregnancy is increased (Nyberg and associates, 1987; Hill and co-workers, 1990).
2. A *decidual cyst* is identified as an anechoic area lying within the endometrium but remote from the canal and often at the endometrial-myometrial border. Ackerman and colleagues (1993) suggested this finding represents early decidual breakdown and precedes decidual cast formation. For these reasons, the American College of Obstetricians and Gynecologists (2004) advises caution in diagnosing an intrauterine pregnancy in the absence of a definite yolk sac or embryo. The yolk sac is typically seen within a gestational sac at 5.5 weeks' gestational age (Fig. 10-6).

Adnexa. When fallopian tubes and ovaries are visualized and an extrauterine yolk sac or embryo is identified, a tubal pregnancy is clearly confirmed (Fig. 10-6). But, such findings are present in only 15 to 30 percent of cases (Paul and co-workers, 2000).

In some cases, a *halo* or tubal ring surrounded by a thin hypoechoic area caused by subserosal edema can be seen. According to Burry and associates (1993), this has a positive-predictive value of 92 percent and a sensitivity of 95 percent. In their meta-analysis of 10 studies, Brown and Doubilet (1994) reported that the finding of any adnexal mass, other than a simple ovarian cyst, was the most accurate sonographic finding. It had a sensitivity of 84 percent, specificity of 99 percent, positive-predictive value of 96 percent, and negative-predictive value of 95 percent.

Differentiation of an ectopic pregnancy from a corpus luteum cyst can be challenging. With transvaginal color Doppler imaging, placental blood flow within the periphery of the complex adnexal mass—the *ring of fire*—can be seen (Fig. 10-7). This also may be seen with a corpus luteum of pregnancy. Swire and co-workers (2004) observed that the wall of the corpus luteum is less echogenic compared with both the tubal halo and the endometrium. They found that a spongiform, lace-like, or reticular pattern seen within the corpus luteum cyst is classical for hemorrhage.

Rectouterine Cul-De-Sac. Free peritoneal fluid suggests intra-abdominal bleeding. As little as 50 mL can be seen in the cul-de-sac using the transvaginal transducer, and transabdominal imaging helps to assess the extent of hemoperitoneum. Detection of peritoneal fluid in conjunction with an adnexal mass is highly predictive of ectopic pregnancy (Nyberg and associates, 1991).

At the current level of technology, the absence of suggestive sonographic findings does not exclude an ectopic pregnancy. That said, sonography has decreased the need for diagnostic laparoscopy and/or curettage to establish the diagnosis of ectopic pregnancy.

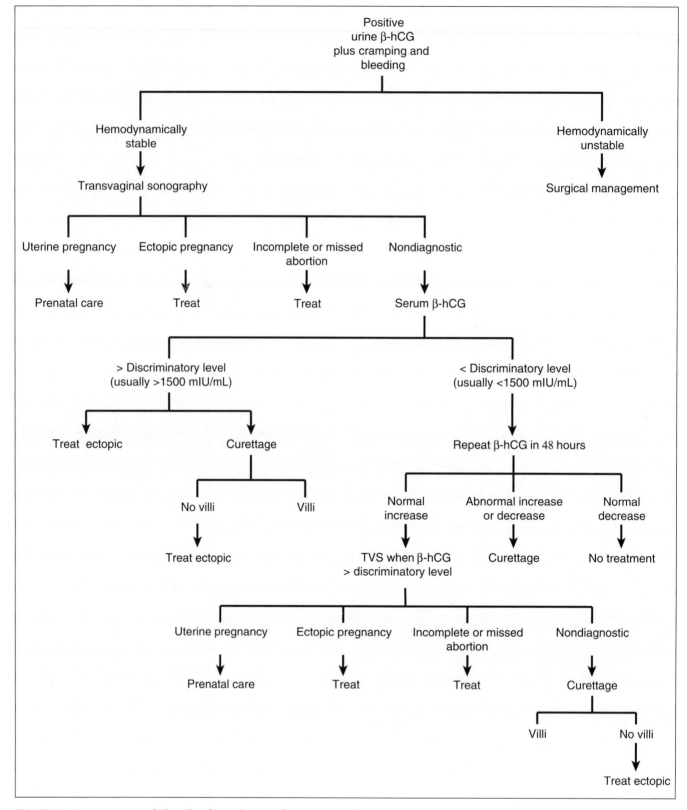

FIGURE 10-5 One suggested algorithm for evaluation of a woman with a suspected ectopic pregnancy. hCG = human chorionic gonadotropin; TVS = transvaginal sonography. (Modified from Gala, 2008.)

Nondiagnostic Transvaginal Sonography. In many cases, sonography is nondiagnostic and subsequent management is based on serial serum β-hCG values and repeated sonographic examinations. A number of investigators have described *discriminatory* β-hCG levels above which failure to visualize a uter-

ine pregnancy indicates with high reliability that the pregnancy either is not alive or is ectopic. Barnhart and colleagues (1994) reported that an empty uterus with a serum β-hCG concentration of ≥1500 mIU/mL was 100-percent accurate in excluding a live uterine pregnancy. Thus, if the initial β-hCG level exceeds

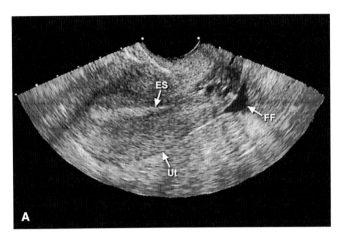
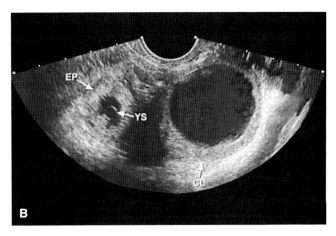

FIGURE 10-6 Vaginal sonogram of an ectopic pregnancy. **A.** The uterus (*Ut*) is seen with a normal endometrial stripe (*ES*). A small amount of free fluid (*FF*) is visible in the posterior cul-de-sac. **B.** The tubal ectopic pregnancy (*EP*) with its yolk sac (*YS*) is seen along with a corpus luteum (*CL*) cyst. (Used with permission from Dr. Michelle L. Robbin.)

the discriminatory level—1500 mIU/mL in this case, and no live intrauterine pregnancy is seen with TVS, then the diagnosis is narrowed to an intrauterine pregnancy with a dead fetus versus an ectopic pregnancy. Early multifetal gestation, of course, remains a possibility. Curettage will distinguish an ectopic from a nonliving uterine pregnancy. Conversely, if an intrauterine embryo, fetus, or placenta is identified by TVS, the diagnosis is apparent. When none of these is identified, tubal pregnancy is a probability.

If the initial β-hCG level is below the discriminatory value, early uterine pregnancy is a possibility, and serial assays of β-hCG, in conjunction with serial TVS evaluations, are usually done. Kadar and Romero (1987) reported that mean doubling time for serum β-hCG levels with early normal pregnancy was approximately 48 hours. The lowest normal value for this increase was 66 percent. Barnhart and co-workers (2004) reported a 53-percent 48-hour *minimum* rise with a 24-hour *minimum* rise of 24 percent (Table 10-2). Importantly, Silva and colleagues (2006) caution that a third of women with an ectopic pregnancy will have a 53-percent rise at 48 hours. They further reported that there is no single pattern to characterize ectopic

pregnancy and that approximately half have decreasing β-hCG levels, whereas the other half have increasing levels.

Failure to maintain this minimum rate of increased β-hCG production, along with an empty uterus, is suggestive of an ectopic pregnancy or completed abortion. Thus, appropriately selected women with a suspected ectopic pregnancy, but whose initial β-hCG level is below the discriminatory level, are seen at 2- to 3-day intervals for further evaluation. If the β-hCG level rises insufficiently, plateaus, or exceeds the discriminatory level without evidence of a uterine pregnancy by TVS, then a live intrauterine pregnancy can be excluded. Next, distinction between a nonliving intrauterine and an ectopic pregnancy is made by uterine curettage. Barnhart and associates (2003) reported that endometrial biopsy was less sensitive than curettage.

A single serum progesterone measurement may clarify the diagnosis in a few cases (American College of Obstetricians and Gynecologists, 2008; Stovall and associates, 1989, 1992). Most values, however, fall between customary normal values of 5 to 20 or 25 ng/mL. Buckley and colleagues (2000) reported progesterone levels to be conclusive in only a fourth of women. One caveat is that pregnancy achieved with ART may be associated with higher than usual progesterone levels (Perkins and associates, 2000). All drawbacks considered, serum levels of at least 25 ng/mL after spontaneous conception provide reassurance

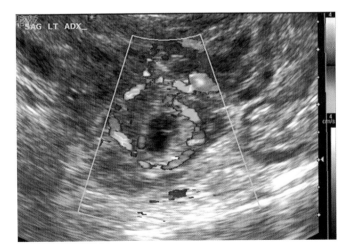

FIGURE 10-7 Color Doppler transvaginal sonogram of an ectopic pregnancy. The "ring of fire" reflects placental blood flow around the periphery of the pregnancy. This finding may also be seen with a corpus luteum cyst. (Used with permission from Dr. Elysia Moschos.)

TABLE 10-2. Lower Normal Limits for Percentage Increase of Serum β-hCG During Early Uterine Pregnancy

Sampling Interval (days)	Increase from Initial Value (percent)
1	24–29
2	53–66
3	114
4	175
5	255

Data from Barnhart (2004) and Kadar (1981) and their co-workers.

that an ectopic pregnancy is *unlikely*. Mol and colleagues (1998) performed a meta-analysis of 22 studies and reported that a serum progesterone level < 5 ng/mL predicted a dying pregnancy with almost 100-percent specificity but only 60-percent sensitivity. Values of > 20 ng/mL were 95-percent specific for a healthy normal pregnancy, but with only 40-percent sensitivity.

Laparoscopic Diagnosis

Direct visualization of the fallopian tubes and pelvis by laparoscopy offers a reliable diagnosis in most cases of suspected ectopic pregnancy. There is also a ready transition to definitive operative therapy, which is discussed subsequently.

Management

In many cases, early diagnosis allows definitive surgical or medical management of unruptured ectopic pregnancy—sometimes even before the onset of symptoms. In either case, treatment before rupture is associated with less morbidity and mortality and a better prognosis for fertility. D-negative women with an ectopic pregnancy who are not sensitized to D-antigen should be given anti-D immunoglobulin (see Chap. 29, p. 624).

Surgical Management

Laparoscopy is the preferred surgical treatment for ectopic pregnancy unless the woman is hemodynamically unstable. There have been only a few prospective studies in which laparotomy was compared with laparoscopic surgery. Hajenius and associates (2007) performed a Cochrane Database review, and their findings are summarized:

1. There were no significant differences in overall tubal patency following salpingostomy determined at second-look laparoscopy.

2. Each method was followed by a similar number of subsequent uterine pregnancies.
3. There were fewer subsequent ectopic pregnancies in women treated laparoscopically, although this was not statistically significant.
4. Laparoscopy resulted in shorter operative times, less blood loss, less analgesic requirements, and shorter hospital stays.
5. Laparoscopic surgery was slightly but significantly less successful in resolving tubal pregnancy.
6. The costs for laparoscopy were significantly less, although some argue that costs are similar when cases converted to laparotomy are considered.

As experience has accrued, cases previously managed by laparotomy—for example, ruptured tubal pregnancies or interstitial pregnancies—can safely be managed by laparoscopy (Sagiv and colleagues, 2001).

Tubal surgery is considered *conservative* when there is tubal salvage. Examples include salpingostomy, salpingotomy, and fimbrial expression of the ectopic pregnancy. *Radical surgery* is defined by salpingectomy. Conservative surgery may increase the rate of subsequent uterine pregnancy but is associated with higher rates of persistently functioning trophoblast (Bangsgaard and colleagues, 2003).

Salpingostomy. This procedure is used to remove a small pregnancy that is usually less than 2 cm in length and located in the distal third of the fallopian tube (**Fig. 10-8**). A 10- to 15-mm linear incision is made with unipolar needle cautery on the antimesenteric border over the pregnancy. The products usually will extrude from the incision and can be carefully removed or flushed out using high-pressure irrigation that more thoroughly removes the trophoblastic tissue (Al-Sunaidi and Tulandi, 2007). Small bleeding sites are controlled with needlepoint electrocoagulation or laser, and the incision is left unsutured to heal

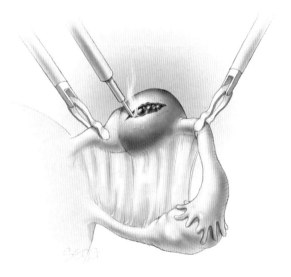 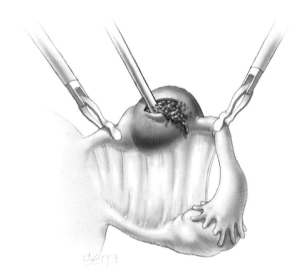

A   B

FIGURE 10-8 Linear salpingostomy for ectopic pregnancy. **A.** Linear incision for removal of a small tubal pregnancy is created on the antimesenteric border of the tube. **B.** Products of conception may be flushed from the tube using an irrigation probe. Alternatively, products may be removed with grasping forceps. Following evacuation of the tube, bleeding sites are treated with electrosurgical coagulation or laser, and the incision is not sutured. If the incision is closed, the procedure is termed a *salpingotomy*. (From Hoffman, 2008, with permission.)

by secondary intention. Natale and associates (2003) reported that serum β-hCG levels > 6000 mIU/mL are associated with a higher risk of implantation into the muscularis and thus with more tubal damage.

Salpingotomy. Seldom performed today, salpingotomy is essentially the same procedure as salpingostomy except that the incision is closed with delayed-absorbable suture. According to Tulandi and Saleh (1999), there is no difference in prognosis with or without suturing.

Salpingectomy. Tubal resection may be used for both ruptured and unruptured ectopic pregnancies. When removing the oviduct, it is advisable to excise a wedge of the outer third (or less) of the interstitial portion of the tube. This so-called *cornual resection* is done in an effort to minimize the rare recurrence of pregnancy in the tubal stump. Even with cornual resection, however, a subsequent interstitial pregnancy is not always prevented (Kalchman and Meltzer, 1966).

Persistent Trophoblast. Incomplete removal of trophoblast may result in persistent ectopic pregnancy. Because of this, Graczykowski and Mishell (1997) administered a "prophylactic" 1 mg/m^2 dose of methotrexate postoperatively. Persistent trophoblast complicates 5 to 20 percent of salpingostomies and can be identified by persistent or rising hCG levels. Usually β-hCG levels fall quickly and are at about 10 percent of preoperative values by day 12 (Hajenius and colleagues, 1995; Vermesh and associates, 1988). Also, if the postoperative day 1 serum β-hCG value is less than 50 percent of the preoperative value, then persistent trophoblast rarely is a problem (Spandorfer and co-workers, 1997).

According to Seifer (1997), factors that increase the risk of persistent ectopic pregnancy include:

1. Small pregnancies, that is, less than 2 cm
2. Early therapy, that is, before 42 menstrual days
3. Serum β-hCG levels exceeding 3000 mIU/mL
4. Implantation medial to the salpingostomy site.

In the face of persistent or increasing β-hCG, additional surgical or medical therapy is necessary.

Medical Management with Methotrexate

This folic acid antagonist is highly effective against rapidly proliferating trophoblast, and it has been used for more than 40 years to treat gestational trophoblastic disease (see Chap. 11, p. 263). It is also used for early pregnancy termination (see Chap. 9, p. 232). Tanaka and associates (1982) first used methotrexate to treat an interstitial pregnancy, and since then, it has been used successfully for all varieties of ectopic pregnancy. In the largest single-center series, Lipscomb and colleagues (1999a) reported a 91-percent success rate in 350 women given methotrexate therapy. Moreover, 80 percent of these women required only one dose.

Active intra-abdominal hemorrhage is a contraindication to chemotherapy. According to the Practice Committee of the American Society for Reproductive Medicine (2006), other absolute contraindications include intrauterine pregnancy; breast feeding; immunodeficiency, alcoholism; chronic hepatic, renal, or pulmonary disease; blood dyscrasias; and peptic ulcer disease.

Patient Selection. The best candidate for medical therapy is the woman who is asymptomatic, motivated, and compliant. With medical therapy, some classical predictors of success include:

1. *Initial serum β-hCG level.* This is the single best prognostic indicator of successful treatment with single-dose methotrexate. The prognostic value of the other two predictors is likely directly related to their relationship with β-hCG concentrations. Menon and co-workers (2007) performed a systematic review of studies totaling more than 500 women treated with single-dose methotrexate for ectopic pregnancy. They reported failure rates of 1.5 percent if the initial serum hCG concentration was <1000 mIU/mL; 5.6 percent with 1000-2000 mIU/mL; 3.8 percent with 2000-5000 mIU/mL; and 14.3 percent when levels were between 5000 and 10,000 mIU/mL.
2. *Ectopic pregnancy size.* Although these data are less precise, many early trials used "large size" as an exclusion criterion. Lipscomb and colleagues (1998) reported a 93-percent success rate with single-dose methotrexate when the ectopic mass was <3.5 cm, compared with success rates between 87 and 90 percent when the mass was >3.5 cm.
3. *Fetal cardiac activity.* Although this is a relative contraindication to medical therapy, the admonition is based on limited evidence. Most studies report increased failure rates if there is cardiac activity, Lipscomb and colleagues (1998) reported an 87-percent success rates in such cases.

Dose, Administration, and Toxicity. The three general schemes for methotrexate administration are shown in Table 10-3. These three are essentially those recommended by the American College of Obstetricians and Gynecologists (2008). In most studies, the intramuscular methotrexate dose was 50 mg/m^2. Although single-dose treatment is easier to administer and monitor than variable-dose therapy, it may have a higher failure rate (Hajenius and co-workers, 2007). And although methotrexate can be given orally, Lipscomb and co-workers (2002) reported it to be less effective than that given intramuscularly. Direct injection of methotrexate into the ectopic mass is seldom used with tubal ectopic pregnancy.

These regimens are associated with minimal laboratory changes and symptoms, although occasional toxicity may be severe. Kooi and Kock (1992) reviewed 16 studies and reported that adverse effects were resolved by 3 to 4 days after methotrexate was discontinued. The most common were liver involvement—12 percent, stomatitis—6 percent, and gastroenteritis—1 percent. One woman had bone marrow depression. Case reports also describe life-threatening neutropenia and fever, transient drug-induced pneumonitis, and alopecia, as well as death in a woman with renal failure (Buster and Pisarska, 1999; Kelly and colleagues, 2006). Importantly, nonsteroidal anti-inflammatory drugs may enhance methotrexate toxicity, whereas vitamins containing folic acid may lower its efficacy. Using anti-müllerian hormone assays, Oriol and co-workers (2008) concluded that ovarian reserve was not compromised by single-dose methotrexate therapy.

TABLE 10-3. Methotrexate Therapy for Primary Treatment of Ectopic Pregnancy

Regimen	Surveillance
Single dose[a] Methotrexate, 50 mg/m^2 IM	Measure β-hCG levels days 4 and 7: • If difference ≥ 15 percent, repeat weekly until undetectable • If difference < 15 percent between day 4 and 7 levels, repeat methotrexate dose and begin new day 1 • If fetal cardiac activity present day 7, repeat methotrexate dose, begin new day 1 • Surgical treatment if β-hCG levels not decreasing or fetal cardiac activity persists after three doses methotrexate
Two dose Methotrexate, 50 mg/m^2 IM, days 0, 4	Follow-up as for single-dose regimen
Variable dose (up to four doses): Methotrexate, 1 mg/kg IM, days 1, 3, 5, 7 Leucovorin, 0.1 mg/kg IM, days 2, 4, 6, 8	Measure β-hCG levels day 1, 3, 5, and 7. Continue alternate-day injections until β-hCG levels decrease ≥ 15 percent in 48 hours, or four doses of methotrexate given. Then, weekly β-hCG until undetectable

[a]Preferred by surgeons.
IM = intramuscular.
Regimens from Buster and Pisarska (1999), Kirk (2007), Lipscomb (2007), Pisarska (1998, 1999), and all their colleagues.

Monitoring Efficacy of Therapy. Serum β-hCG levels are used to monitor response to both medical and surgical therapy. Patterns of serum level decline described by Saraj and colleagues (1998) are shown in **Figure 10-9**. After linear salpingostomy, serum β-hCG levels *declined rapidly* over days and then more gradually, with a mean resolution time of about 20 days. In contrast, after single-dose methotrexate, mean serum β-hCG levels *increased* for the first 4 days, and then gradually declined with a mean resolution time of 27 days. Lipscomb and colleagues (1998) used single-dose methotrexate to successfully treat 287 women and reported that the average time to resolution—defined as serum hCG level < 15 mIU/mL, was 34 days. Importantly, the longest time was 109 days.

As shown in Table 10-3, monitoring single-dose therapy calls for serum β-hCG determinations at 4 and 7 days. About 15 to 20 percent of women require a second dose of methotrexate. Kirk and colleagues (2007) recently confirmed the efficacy of the "15 percent, day 4 and 7 rule." With variable-dose methotrexate, levels are measured at 48-hour intervals until they fall more than 15 percent. After successful treatment, weekly serum β-hCG determinations are measured until undetectable. Outpatient surveillance is preferred, but if there is any question of safety or compliance, the woman is hospitalized. Failure is judged when the β-hCG level plateaus or rises or tubal rupture occurs. Importantly, tubal rupture can occur in the face of declining β-hCG levels.

Separation Pain. An important observation is that 65 to 75 percent of women initially given methotrexate will have increasing pain beginning several days after therapy. This *separation pain* generally is mild and relieved by analgesics. In a series of 258 methotrexate-treated women by Lipscomb and colleagues (1999b), 20 percent had pain severe enough to require evaluation in the clinic or emergency room. Ultimately, 10 of these 53 underwent surgical exploration. Said another way, 20 percent of women given single-dose methotrexate will have significant pain, and 20 percent of these will require laparoscopy.

Persistent Ectopic Pregnancy. The failure rate is similar for either medical or surgical management (Table 10-4). In three randomized trials, 5 to 14 percent of women treated initially with methotrexate ultimately required surgery, whereas 4 to 20 percent of those undergoing laparoscopic resection eventually received methotrexate for persistent trophoblast (Fernandez, 1998; Hajenius, 1997, 2007; Saraj, 1998, and all their associates).

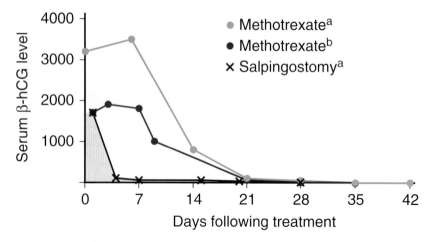

FIGURE 10-9 Schematic of comparative patterns of serum β-hCG level decline after single-dose methotrexate treatment or laparoscopic salpingostomy for unruptured ectopic pregnancy. Values are approximate. Yellow area is range *between* mean values reported by [a]Saraj and colleagues (1998) and those reported by [b]Dilbaz and associates (2006). Gray area represents area under the curve for mean values following salpingostomy reported by [a]Saraj and colleagues (1998).

TABLE 10-4. Representative Reproductive Performance in 3198 Women Following Primary Treatment for Ectopic Pregnancy

Management	Successful Treatment[a] (percent)	Tubal Patency[b] (percent)	Subsequent Pregnancy (percent)	
			Uterine	Ectopic
Salpingostomy	93	76	58	12
Methotrexate				
Single-dose	87	81	61	8
Variable-dose	93	75	52	8
Expectant	68	76	57	13

[a]Defined as resolution of ectopic pregnancy.
[b]Not all women were evaluated for patency.
Data from Buster and Krotz (2007).

Rupture of Persistent Ectopic Pregnancy. This is the worst form of primary therapy failure with a 5 to 10-percent occurrence in women treated medically. Lipscomb and associates (1998) described a 14-day mean time to rupture, but one woman had tubal rupture 32 days after single-dose methotrexate.

Expectant Management

In select cases, it is reasonable to observe very early tubal pregnancies that are associated with stable or falling serum β-hCG levels. As many as a third of such women will present with declining β-hCG levels (Shalev and colleagues, 1995). Stovall and Ling (1992) restrict expectant management to women with these criteria:

1. Tubal ectopic pregnancies only
2. Decreasing serial β-hCG levels
3. Diameter of the ectopic mass not >3.5 cm
4. No evidence of intra-abdominal bleeding or rupture by transvaginal sonography.

Trio and colleagues (1995) reported spontaneous resolution of ectopic pregnancy in 49 of 67, or 73 percent of selected women treated expectantly. Resolution without treatment was more likely if the initial serum β-hCG level was <1000 mIU/mL. In another 60 women managed expectantly, Shalev and associates (1995) reported spontaneous resolution in almost half.

With expectant management, subsequent rates of tubal patency and intrauterine pregnancy are comparable with surgery and medical management (see Table 10-4). **The potentially grave consequences of tubal rupture, coupled with the established safety of medical and surgical therapy, require that expectant therapy be undertaken only in appropriately selected and counseled women.** According to the American College of Obstetricians and Gynecologists (2008), 88 percent of ectopic pregnancies will resolve if the β-hCG is <200 mIU/mL.

ABDOMINAL PREGNANCY

Strictly defined, abdominal pregnancy is an implantation in the peritoneal cavity exclusive of tubal, ovarian, or intraligamentary implantations. Although a zygote can traverse the tube and implant primarily in the peritoneal cavity, most abdominal pregnancies are thought to follow early tubal rupture or abortion. In cases of advanced extrauterine pregnancy, it is not unusual that the placenta is still at least partially attached to the uterus or adnexa (Fig. 10-10). Worley and colleagues (2008) recently

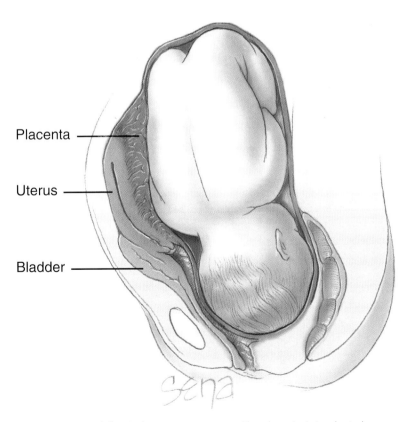

Placenta

Uterus

Bladder

FIGURE 10-10 Abdominal pregnancy at term. The placenta is implanted on the posterior surface of the uterus and broad ligament. The enlarged, flattened uterus is located just beneath the anterior abdominal wall. The cervix and vagina are dislodged anteriorly and superiorly by the large fetal head in the cul-de-sac.

described our experiences with 10 women with such pregnancies that were 18 to 43 weeks' gestational age—five of these were 26 weeks or greater. Although only three of 10 met strict criteria for abdominal pregnancy by the location of placental implantation, in all 10, the fetus was located intra-abdominally. The placenta was implanted in a massively dilated tube in three pregnancies at 18, 26, and 30 weeks; and two others were implanted in a rudimentary horn at 20 and 22 weeks. Naim and associates (2008) reported an advanced abdominal pregnancy from an earlier uterine rupture. These likely are to become more common because of cesarean scar pregnancy, discussed on page 253.

Because of these vicissitudes, the reported incidence of abdominal pregnancy will vary depending on definitions used. More than 20 years ago, the Centers for Disease Control and Prevention estimated its incidence to be 1 in 10,000 live births (Atrash and co-workers, 1987). In the report cited above from Parkland Hospital, advanced abdominal pregnancy had an incidence of about 1 in 25,000 births. Using the stricter criteria, however, the incidence was about 1 in 85,000.

Diagnosis

A high index of suspicion is warranted with advanced extrauterine gestations because they cause symptoms that are often vague and nonspecific. Presenting complaints may include abdominal pain, nausea and vomiting, bleeding or decreasing to absent fetal movements. Many women, however, are asymptomatic. Findings that might suggest the diagnosis include elevated levels of maternal serum alpha-fetoprotein (Costa and associates, 1991; Worley and co-workers, 2008). Although abnormal fetal positions can be palpated, the ease of palpating fetal parts is not a reliable sign. The cervix may be displaced, depending in part on the fetal position (Zeck and colleagues, 2007).

Sonography

Findings with an abdominal pregnancy using sonography most often do not provide an unequivocal diagnosis. Oligohydramnios is common but nonspecific. In some suspected cases, however, sonographic findings may be diagnostic. For example, the fetal head may be seen to lie immediately adjacent to the maternal bladder with no interposed uterine tissue (Kurtz and associates, 1982). Even with ideal conditions, however, a sonographic diagnosis of abdominal pregnancy is missed in half of cases (Costa and associates, 1991; Worley and colleagues, 2008).

Magnetic Resonance (MR) Imaging

This can be used to confirm a diagnosis of abdominal pregnancy following a suspicious sonographic examination (Fig. 10-11). Although described as accurate and specific by Harris and associates (1988) and Wagner and Burchardt (1995), our experiences are that it is not totally reliable. At our institutions, abdominal pregnancy has been incorrectly diagnosed as a placenta previa, and conversely, an intrauterine pregnancy with degenerating fibroids has been misdiagnosed as an abdominal pregnancy. Whenever an abdominal pregnancy is identified, MR imaging should be done to provide maximal information concerning placental implantation (Bertrand and colleagues, 2009).

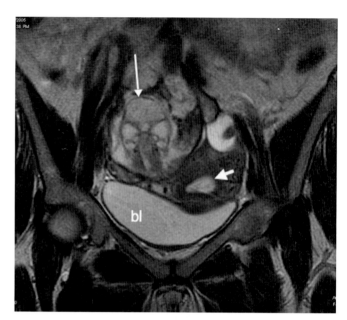

FIGURE 10-11 T2-weighted single-shot fast-spin echo (SSFSE) magnetic resonance coronal pelvic image of an 18-week abdominal pregnancy. The fetal head (*long arrow*) is not contained within the uterine cavity (*short arrow*). The maternal bladder (*bl*) is inferior to these structures. The high-signal-intensity area superior to the uterus is an ovarian cyst. (Reprinted from *American Journal of Obstetrics and Gynecology*, Vol. 198, No. 3, KC Worley, MD Hnat, and FG Cunningham, Advanced extrauterine pregnancy: Diagnostic and therapeutic challenges, pp. 297.e1–297.e7, Copyright 2008, with permission from Elsevier.)

Computed Tomography

Costa and associates (1991) maintain that computed tomography is superior to MR imaging, but its use is limited because of concerns for fetal radiation. In cases of certain abdominal pregnancy, and in the absence of MR imaging, knowledge of the placental implantation site would outweigh any fetal risks in our estimation.

Management

An abdominal pregnancy is life-threatening, and clinical management depends on the gestational age at diagnosis. Some recommend waiting until fetal viability with in-hospital observation if pregnancy is diagnosed after 24 weeks (Cartwright and associates, 1986; Hage and colleagues, 1988). Such management carries a risk for sudden and life-threatening hemorrhage, and we are of the opinion that termination generally is indicated when the diagnosis is made. Certainly, before 24 weeks, conservative treatment rarely is justified.

Once placental implantation has been assessed, several options are available. Preoperative angiographic embolization has been used successfully in some women with advanced abdominal pregnancy. Alternatively, catheters placed in the uterine arteries may be inflated to decrease intraoperative blood loss. In either case, vascularization of ectopic placental implantation may be difficult to occlude. Other preoperative considerations include insertion of ureteral catheters, bowel preparation, assurance of sufficient blood products, and availability of a multidisciplinary surgical team. Should such resources not be available, elective transfer of a woman with a known advanced extrauterine pregnancy to a tertiary care facility is recommended.

The principal surgical objectives with an abdominal pregnancy include delivery of the fetus and careful assessment of placental implantation without provoking hemorrhage. Anatomical derangements often complicate fetal delivery and increase the risk of intraoperative injury. After delivery, placental implantation is assessed carefully because the surrounding areas will be quite vascular even if there is no placental invasion.

Management of the Placenta

Placental removal may precipitate torrential hemorrhage because the normal hemostatic mechanism of myometrial contractions to constrict hypertrophied blood vessels is lacking. This can develop spontaneously or more likely, when the surgeon is attempting to locate the exact site of placental attachment. Therefore, it is best to avoid unnecessary exploration of surrounding organs. If it is obvious that the placenta can be safely removed or if there is already hemorrhage from its implantation site, then removal begins immediately. When possible, blood vessels supplying the placenta should be ligated first.

Leaving the Placenta in Situ. Some advocate leaving the placenta in place as the lesser of two evils. It decreases the chance of immediate life-threatening hemorrhage, but at the expense of long-term sequelae. Unfortunately, when left in the abdominal cavity, the placenta commonly becomes infected with subsequent formation of abscesses, adhesions, intestinal obstruction, and wound dehiscence (Bergstrom and colleagues, 1998; Martin and associates, 1988). Partial ureteral obstruction with reversible hydronephrosis has also been described (Weiss and Stone, 1994). In many of these cases, surgical removal becomes inevitable.

If the placenta is left, its involution may be monitored using sonography and serum β-hCG levels (France and Jackson, 1980; Martin and McCaul, 1990). Color Doppler sonography can be used to assess changes in blood flow. In some cases, and usually depending on its size, placental function rapidly declines, and the placenta is resorbed. In one case described by Belfar and associates (1986), placental resorption took more than 5 years. In the 10 women from Parkland Hospital described by Worley and colleagues (2008), the placenta was left implanted in two. Both developed disastrous complications with hemorrhage and infection.

Methotrexate use is controversial. It has been recommended to hasten involution and has been reported to cause accelerated placental destruction with accumulation of necrotic tissue and infection with abscess formation (Rahman and associates, 1982). It is difficult to envision a supporting role for the use of an antimetabolite for a senescent organ.

Maternal and Fetal Outcomes

The maternal mortality rate is increased substantively with advanced abdominal pregnancy. With appropriate preoperative planning, however, the mortality rate has been reduced from approximately 20 percent to less than 5 percent (Stevens, 1993). Fetal salvage in an abdominal pregnancy is gestational-

age dependent. In the cases from Parkland Hospital, all infants born after 26 weeks survived, albeit with numerous neonatal complications (Worley and associates, 2008). In an earlier review, Stevens (1993) found that survival of infants born after 30 weeks was 63 percent. He also reported fetal malformations and deformations in 20 percent. The most common deformations were facial or cranial asymmetry, or both, and various joint abnormalities. The most common malformations were limb deficiency and central nervous system anomalies.

OVARIAN PREGNANCY

Ectopic pregnancy implanted in the ovary is rare. Traditional risk factors for ovarian ectopic pregnancy are similar to those for tubal pregnancy, but use of an IUD seems to be disproportionately associated (Gray and Ruffolo, 1978; Pisarska and Carson, 1999). Although the ovary can accommodate more readily than the fallopian tube to the expanding pregnancy, rupture at an early stage is the usual consequence. This would seem more likely with a twin ovarian pregnancy (Garg and colleagues, 2009). Nonetheless, there are recorded cases in which ovarian pregnancies went to term, and a few infants survived (Williams and associates, 1982).

Diagnosis

Findings are likely to mimic those of a tubal pregnancy or a bleeding corpus luteum. Serious bleeding is seen in approximately one third of cases. At surgery, early ovarian pregnancies are likely to be considered corpus luteum cysts or a bleeding corpus luteum. Use of transvaginal sonography has resulted in a more frequent diagnosis of unruptured ovarian pregnancies (Marcus and Brinsden, 1993; Sidek and colleagues, 1994). Such early diagnosis may allow for a medical approach.

Management

The classical management for ovarian pregnancies has been surgical. Early bleeding for small lesions has been managed by ovarian wedge resection or cystectomy (Schwartz and colleagues, 1993). With larger lesions, ovariectomy is most often performed, and laparoscopy has been used to resect or to perform laser ablation (Goldenberg and associates, 1994; Herndon and colleagues, 2008). Finally, methotrexate has been used successfully to treat unruptured ovarian pregnancies (Chelmow and associates, 1994; Raziel and Golan, 1993; Shamma and Schwartz, 1992).

CERVICAL PREGNANCY

Implantation of the zygote in the cervix is uncommon, but the incidence is increasing as a result of ART (Ginsburg and co-workers, 1994; Peleg and associates, 1994). According to Jeng and colleagues (2007), 60 percent of women with a cervical pregnancy had previously undergone dilation and curettage. In a typical case, the endocervix is eroded by trophoblast, and the pregnancy proceeds to develop in the fibrous cervical wall. The higher the trophoblast is implanted in the cervical canal, the greater is its capacity to grow and hemorrhage. A heterotopic

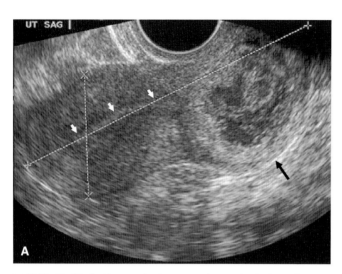
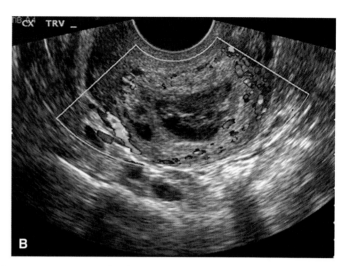

FIGURE 10-12 A. Transvaginal sonography, sagittal view of a cervical pregnancy. Sonographic findings with cervical pregnancy may include: (1) an hourglass uterine shape and ballooned cervical canal; (2) gestational tissue at the level of the cervix (*black arrow*); (3) absent intrauterine gestational tissue (*white arrows*); and (4) a portion of the endocervical canal seen interposed between the gestation and the endometrial canal. **B.** In a transverse view of the cervical pregnancy, Doppler color flow shows abundant vascularization. (Used with permission from Dr. Elysia Moschos.)

cervical pregnancy and a twin cervical pregnancy were recently reported by Shah (2009) and Trojano (2009) and their associates.

Painless vaginal bleeding is reported by 90 percent of women with a cervical pregnancy—a third of these have massive hemorrhage (Ushakov and colleagues, 1997). Only a fourth have abdominal pain with bleeding. As pregnancy progresses, a distended, thin-walled cervix with a partially dilated external os may be evident. Above the cervical mass, a slightly enlarged uterine fundus may be palpated. According to Jeng and colleagues (2007), a 14-week cervical pregnancy is the most advanced case reported. They described experiences with 38 referred cases at a mean of 8.8 weeks and whose serum β-hCG levels ranged from 2800 to 103,000 mIU/mL. Identification of cervical pregnancy is based on speculum examination, palpation, and transvaginal sonography. Findings include an empty uterus and a gestation filling the cervical canal as shown in Figure 10-12. Magnetic resonance imaging and three-dimensional sonography have been used to confirm the diagnosis (Bader-Armstrong and associates, 1989; Sherer and colleagues, 2008).

Management

In the past, hysterectomy was often necessary because of profuse hemorrhage that accompanied attempts at cervical pregnancy removal. With hysterectomy, the risk of urinary tract injury is increased because of the enlarged, barrel-shaped cervix. To avoid the morbidity of surgery and sterilization, other approaches have been developed.

Cerclage

Hemorrhage associated with cervical pregnancy can be managed successfully by placing a heavy silk ligature around the cervix (Bachus, 1990; Bernstein, 1981; Fruscalzo, 2008, and all their associates). This is similar to that with a McDonald cerclage discussed in Chapter 9 (p. 219). The suture effectively

ligates the bilateral descending cervical branches of the uterine artery at a level above the pregnancy to control bleeding. Mashiach and colleagues (2002) described the successful management and resolution of four cervical pregnancies using a Shirodkar cerclage. In one of these cases, a concurrent intrauterine pregnancy progressed to term, and a healthy infant was delivered vaginally.

Curettage and Tamponade

Nolan (1989) and Thomas (1991) and their associates recommend placement of hemostatic cervical sutures at 3 and 9 o'clock to ligate descending cervical branches of the uterine artery. Suction curettage is then performed, followed immediately by insertion of a Foley catheter into the cervical canal. The 30-mL catheter bulb is inflated, and the vagina is packed tightly with gauze to further tamponade bleeding. A suction catheter tip may be left above the vaginal packing to ensure adequate drainage and to monitor blood loss.

Arterial Embolization

Successful selective preoperative uterine artery embolization has been described by Nakao and colleagues (2008) as well as others. This technique, detailed in Chapter 35 (p. 797), also has been used successfully to control bleeding following medical therapy (Cosin and associates, 1997). Kung and colleagues (2004) employed a combination of laparoscopically assisted uterine artery ligation followed by hysteroscopic endocervical resection to successfully treat six cervical pregnancies.

Medical Management

Methotrexate and other medical treatments have been used successfully for cervical pregnancies. In many centers, including ours, methotrexate has become the first-line therapy in the stable woman. The general guidelines for methotrexate use for ectopic pregnancy are as described earlier (see Table 10-3). The drug has also been injected directly into the gestational sac with or without potassium chloride to induce fetal death (Kaplan, 1990; Marcovici, 1994; Timor-Tritsch, 1994, and all their colleagues).

Pregnancies of more than 6 weeks' duration generally require induction of fetal death with potassium chloride or prolonged methotrexate therapy. Kung and Chang (1999) reviewed 62 cases and reported that women in whom the fetus was alive had a higher failure rate with single-dose methotrexate. Verma and Goharkhay (2009) treated 24 cervical pregnancies with a single-dose intramuscular methotrexate protocol with doses between 50 and 75 mg/m². For women in whom fetal cardiac activity was detectable, sonographically guided fetal intracardiac injection of 2 mL (2 mEq/mL) potassium chloride (KCl) solution was added. If β-hCG levels did not decline more than 15 percent after 1 week, a second dose of methotrexate was given to some patients. Here again the experiences of Jeng and colleagues (2007) with 38 referred cases is instructive. Many of these were relatively far advanced—half were >9 weeks and 60 percent had fetal heart action. These women were treated with 50-mg methotrexate injected into the gestational sac with a 22-gauge *needle through the transducer.* If there was cardiac activity, then KCl was injected into the heart or thoracic cavity. Three women developed significant hemorrhage with membrane rupture. An intracervical Foley catheter was placed for tamponade for 3 days, and a second 50-mg methotrexate dose was given intramuscularly. Treatment was successful in all 38 women with a mean resolution of 38 days—range 21 to 68 days. Song and associates (2009) described management of 50 cases with similar results for regression in 30 given methotrexate. They observed that sonographic resolution lagged far behind serum β-hCG regression.

CESAREAN SCAR PREGNANCY (CSP)

Implantation of an otherwise normal pregnancy into a prior cesarean delivery uterine scar was reported more than 30 years ago by Larsen and Solomon (1978). These vary in size and in many ways are similar to a placenta increta with all of its proclivity to cause torrential hemorrhage (see Chap. 35, p. 778).

Incidence

From their reviews, Rotas (2006) and Ash (2007) and their colleagues cite an increasing incidence of cesarean scar pregnancies (CSP) of about 1:2000 pregnancies. This is likely to increase as does the cesarean delivery rate (see Chaps. 25 and 26). Indeed, these may comprise up to 5 percent of ectopic pregnancies in women with at least one prior cesarean delivery. It is not known if the incidence increases with multiple procedures or if it is affected by either one- or two-layer uterine incision closure. At least one case of recurrent scar pregnancy has been described (Holland and Bienstock, 2008).

Clinical Presentation

This varies depending on the gestational age, which ranges from 5 to 6 weeks up to midpregnancy. Pain and bleeding are most common, but up to 40 percent of women are asymptomatic, and the diagnosis is made during routine sonographic examination (Rotas and associates, 2006). In some cases, early rupture leads to an abdominal pregnancy (Teng and co-workers, 2007).

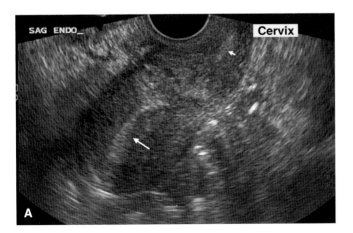

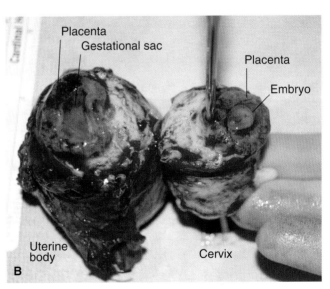

FIGURE 10-13 A. Transvaginal sonogram sagittal view shows a uterus with a cesarean scar pregnancy (CSP). The diagnosis is suggested by criteria that include an empty uterine cavity appearing as a bright hyperechoic endometrial stripe (*long, white arrow*); an empty cervical canal (*short, white arrow*); and an intracavitary mass seen in the anterior wall of the uterine isthmus (*red arrows*). (Courtesy of Dr. Elysia Moschos.) **B.** This hysterectomy specimen with a cesarean scar pregnancy is transversely sectioned at the level of the uterine isthmus and through the gestational sac. The uterine body lies to the left, and the cervix is on the right. A metal probe is placed through the endocervical canal to show the eccentric development of this gestation. Only a thin layer of myometrium overlies this pregnancy, which pushes anteriorly through the uterine wall. (Courtesy of Drs. Sunil Balgobin, Manisha Sharma, and Rebecca Stone.)

Diagnosis and Management

Presentation is too variable to have a concise recommendation for diagnosis. Suffice it to say, a high clinical index of suspicion is warranted in a woman with a prior cesarean delivery. Moschos and associates (2008) have described our experiences from Parkland Hospital with first-trimester sonographic diagnosis, and an example is shown in Figure 10-13. Management is gestational-age dependent and includes methotrexate treatment, curettage, hysteroscopic resection, uterine-preserving resection by laparotomy or laparoscopy, a combination of these, or hysterectomy (Ash, 2007; Demirel, 2009; Fylstra, 2003; Halperin, 2009; Rotas, 2006; Wang, 2006, and all their colleagues).

OTHER SITES OF ECTOPIC PREGNANCY

A number of intra-abdominal placental implantations have been cited in case reports. Most are variations on abdominal pregnancy as discussed on page 249. *Splenic pregnancy* has been reported by Mankodi and associates (1977) and Cormio and associates (2003). In their review, Shippey and colleagues (2007) found 14 cases of *hepatic pregnancy*. A few cases of *retroperitoneal pregnancy* have been reported (Goldberg and associates, 2007; Iwama and colleagues 2008). Khalil and associates (2006) found 16 cases of *omental pregnancy* reported since 1903. Although laparotomy is preferred by many for these ectopic abdominal pregnancies, Yi and colleagues (2008) described the laparoscopic excision of an omental pregnancy. Varma and co-workers (2003) described a live-born 35-week infant whose placenta implanted exclusively on the omentum. Fishman and co-workers (1998) described implantation of a 6-week *diaphragmatic pregnancy* in a woman with abdominal and shoulder pain, dyspnea, and a hemothorax.

REFERENCES

Ackerman TE, Levi CS, Lyons EA, et al: Decidual cyst: Endovaginal sonographic sign of ectopic pregnancy. Radiology 189(3):727, 1993

Al-Sunaidi M, Tulandi T: Surgical treatment of ectopic pregnancy. Semin Reprod Med 25(2):117, 2007

American College of Obstetricians and Gynecologists: Ultrasonography in pregnancy. Practice Bulletin No. 58, December 2004

American College of Obstetricians and Gynecologists: Medical management of ectopic pregnancy. Practice Bulletin No. 94, June 2008

Anderson FWJ, Hogan JG, Ansbacher R. Sudden death: Ectopic pregnancy mortality. Obstet Gynecol 103:1218, 2004

Ankum WM, Mol BWJ, Van der Veen F, et al: Risk factors for ectopic pregnancy: A meta-analysis. Fertil Steril 65:1093, 1996

Ash A, Smith A, Maxwell D: Caesarean scar pregnancy. BJOG 114:253, 2007

Atrash HK, Friede A, Hogue CJ: Abdominal pregnancy in the United States: Frequency and maternal mortality. Obstet Gynecol 69:333, 1987

Bachus KE, Stone D, Suh B, et al: Conservative management of cervical pregnancy with subsequent fertility. Am J Obstet Gynecol 162:450, 1990

Bader-Armstrong B, Shah Y, Rubens D: Use of ultrasound and magnetic resonance imaging in the diagnosis of cervical pregnancy. J Clin Ultrasound 17:283, 1989

Bakken IJ, Skjeldestad FE, Lydersen S, et al: Births and ectopic pregnancies in a large cohort of women tested for *Chlamydia trachomatis*. Sex Transm Dis 34:739, 2007a

Bakken IJ, Skjeldestad FE, Nordbo SA: *Chlamydia trachomatis* infections increase the risk for ectopic pregnancy: A population-based, nested case-control study. Sex Transm Dis 34:166, 2007b

Bangsgaard N, Lund CO, Ottesen B, et al: Improved fertility following conservative surgical treatment of ectopic pregnancy. Br J Obstet Gynaecol 110:765, 2003

Barnhart K, Mennuti MT, Benjamin I, et al: Prompt diagnosis of ectopic pregnancy in an emergency department setting. Obstet Gynecol 84:1010, 1994

Barnhart KT, Gracia CR, Reindl B, et al: Usefulness of Pipelle endometrial biopsy in the diagnosis of women at risk for ectopic pregnancy. Am J Obstet Gynecol 188:906, 2003

Barnhart KT, Katz I, Hummel A, et al: Presumed diagnosis of ectopic pregnancy. Obstet Gynecol 100:505, 2002

Barnhart KT, Sammel MD, Gracia CR, et al: Risk factors for ectopic pregnancy in women with symptomatic first-trimester pregnancies. Fertil Steril 86:36, 2006

Barnhart KT, Sammel MD, Rinaudo PF, et al: Symptomatic patients with an early viable intrauterine pregnancy: hCG curves redefined. Obstet Gynecol 104:50, 2004

Batzer FR, Weiner S, Corson SL, et al: Landmarks during the first forty-two days of gestation demonstrated by the beta-subunit of human chorionic gonadotropin and ultrasound. Am J Obstet Gynecol 146:973, 1983

Belfar HL, Kurtz AB, Wapner RJ: Long-term follow-up after removal of an abdominal pregnancy: Ultrasound evaluation of the involuting placenta. J Ultrasound Med 5:521, 1986

Bergstrom R, Mueller G, Yankowitz J: A case illustrating the continued dilemmas in treating abdominal pregnancy and a potential explanation for the high rate of postsurgical febrile morbidity. Gynecol Obstet Invest 46:268, 1998

Berkes E, Szendei G, Csabay L, et al: Unilateral triplet ectopic pregnancy after in vitro fertilization and embryo transfer. Fertil Steril 90(5):2003.e17, 2008

Berman BJ, Katsiyiannis WT: Images in clinical medicine. A medical mystery. N Engl J Med 345:1176, 2001

Bernstein D, Holzinger M, Ovadia J, et al: Conservative treatment of cervical pregnancy. Obstet Gynecol 58:741, 1981

Bertrand G, Le Ray C, Simard-Émond L, et al: Imaging in the management of abdominal pregnancy: A case report and review of the literature. J Obstet Gynaecol Can 31(1):57, 2009

Birkhahn RH, Gaieta TJ, Van Deusen SK, et al: The ability of traditional vital signs and shock index to identify ruptured ectopic pregnancy. Am J Obstet Gynecol 189:1293, 2003

Bouyer J, Coste J, Shojaei T, et al: Risk factors for ectopic pregnancy: A comprehensive analysis based on a large case-control, population-based study in France. Am J Epidemiol 157:185, 2003

Brown DL, Doubilet PM: Transvaginal sonography for diagnosing ectopic pregnancy: Positivity criteria and performance characteristics. J Ultrasound Med 13:259, 1994

Buckley RG, King KJ, Disney JD, et al: Serum progesterone testing to predict ectopic pregnancy in symptomatic first-trimester patients. Ann Emerg Med 36:95, 2000

Burry KA, Thurmond AS, Suby-Long TD, et al: Transvaginal ultrasonographic findings in surgically verified ectopic pregnancy. Am J Obstet Gynecol 168:1796, 1993

Buster JE, Krotz S: Reproductive performance after ectopic pregnancy. Sem Reprod Med 25:131, 2007

Buster JE, Pisarska MD: Medical management of ectopic pregnancy. Clin Obstet Gynecol 42:23, 1999

Callen PW (ed): Ultrasonography in Obstetrics and Gynecology, 4th ed., Philadelphia, WB Saunders, 2000, p 919

Cartwright PS, Brown JE, Davis RJ, et al: Advanced abdominal pregnancy associated with fetal pulmonary hypoplasia: Report of a case. Am J Obstet Gynecol 155:396, 1986

Centers for Disease Control and Prevention: Ectopic pregnancy—United States, 1990–1992. MMWR 1:46, 1995

Centers for Disease Control and Prevention: Sexually transmitted diseases. Surveillance 2006. Special focus profiles. Women and infants. cdc.gov/std/stats/womenandinf.htm. Modified November 13, 2007

Chelmow D, Gates E, Penzias AS: Laparoscopic diagnosis and methotrexate treatment of an ovarian pregnancy: A case report. Fertil Steril 62:879, 1994

Clayton HB, Schieve LA, Peterson HB, et al: Ectopic pregnancy risk with assisted reproductive technology procedures. Obstet Gynecol 107(3):595, 2006

Cormio G, Santamato S, Vimercati A, et al: Primary splenic pregnancy: A case report. J Reprod Med 48:479, 2003

Cosin JA, Bean M, Grow D, et al: The use of methotrexate and arterial embolization to avoid surgery in a case of cervical pregnancy. Fertil Steril 67:1169, 1997

Costa SD, Presley J, Bastert G: Advanced abdominal pregnancy. Obstet Gynecol Surv 46:515, 1991

Daniel Y, Geva E, Lerner-Geva L, et al: Levels of vascular endothelial growth factor are elevated in patients with ectopic pregnancy: Is this a novel marker? Fertil Steril 72:1013, 1999

Dashefsky SM, Lyons EA, Levi CS, et al: Suspected ectopic pregnancy: Endovaginal and transvesical US. Radiology 169:181, 1988

Demirel LC, Bodur H, Selam B, et al: Laparoscopic management of heterotopic cesarean scar pregnancy with preservation of intrauterine gestation and delivery at term: Case report. Fertil Steril 91(4):1293.e5, 2009

Dilbaz S, Caliskan E, Dilbaz B, et al: Predictors of methotrexate treatment failure in ectopic pregnancy. J Reprod Med 51:87, 2006

Dorfman SF, Grimes DA, Cates W Jr, et al: Ectopic pregnancy mortality, United States, 1979 to 1980: Clinical aspects. Obstet Gynecol 64:386, 1984

Eun DS, Choi YS, Choi J, et al: Laparoscopic cornuotomy using a temporary tourniquet suture and diluted vasopressin injection in interstitial pregnancy. Fertil Steril 91(5):1933, 2009

Fernandez H, Yves Vincent SCA, Pauthier S, et al: Randomized trial of conservative laparoscopic treatment and methotrexate administration in ectopic pregnancy and subsequent fertility. Hum Reprod 13:3239, 1998

Fishman DA, Padilla LA, Joob A, et al: Ectopic pregnancy causing hemothorax managed by thoracoscopy and actinomycin D. Obstet Gynecol 91:837, 1998

France JT, Jackson P: Maternal plasma and urinary hormone levels during and after a successful abdominal pregnancy. Br J Obstet Gynaecol 87:356, 1980

Fruscalzo A, Mai M, Löbbeke K, et al: A combined intrauterine and cervical pregnancy diagnosed in the 13th gestational week: Which type of management is more feasible and successful? Fertil Steril 89(2):456.e13 2008

Fylstra DL, Pound-Chang T, Miller MG, et al: Ectopic pregnancy within a cesarean delivery scar: A case report. Am J Obstet Gynecol 187:302, 2002

Gala RB: Ectopic pregnancy. In Schorge JO, Schaffer JI, Halvorson LM, et al (eds). Williams Gynecology. New York, McGraw-Hill, 2008, pp 160, 165, 170

Garg MK, Vyas S, Gulati A, et al: Primary twin ovarian pregnancy: Case report and review of the literature. J Clin Ultrasound 37(1):43, 2009

Ginsburg ES, Frates MC, Rein MS, et al: Early diagnosis and treatment of cervical pregnancy in an in vitro fertilization program. Fertil Steril 61:966, 1994

Goldberg J, Weinstein M, Kaulback K, et al: Massive retroperitoneal hematoma caused by retroperitoneal ectopic pregnancy. Female Patient 32(6):47, 2007

Goldenberg M, Bider D, Mashiach S, et al: Laparoscopic laser surgery of primary ovarian pregnancy. Hum Reprod 9:1337, 1994

Graczykowski JW, Mishell DR Jr: Methotrexate prophylaxis for persistent ectopic pregnancy after conservative treatment by salpingostomy. Obstet Gynecol 89:118, 1997

Gray CL, Ruffolo EH: Ovarian pregnancy associated with intrauterine contraceptive devices. Am J Obstet Gynecol 132:134, 1978

Grimes DA: Estimation of pregnancy-related mortality risk by pregnancy outcome, United States, 1991 to 1999. Am J Obstet Gynecol 194(1):92, 2006

Grynberg M, Teyssedre J, Andre C, et al: Rupture of ectopic pregnancy with negative serum beta-hCG leading to hemorrhagic shock. Obstet Gynecol 113:537, 2009

Hage ML, Wall LL, Killam A: Expectant management of abdominal pregnancy. A report of two cases. J Reprod Med 33:407, 1988

Hajenius PJ, Engelsbel S, Mol BW, et al: Randomised trial of systemic methotrexate versus laparoscopic salpingostomy in tubal pregnancy. Lancet 350:774, 1997

Hajenius PJ, Mol BWJ, Ankum WM, et al: Clearance curves of serum human chorionic gonadotropin for the diagnosis of persistent trophoblast. Hum Reprod 10:683, 1995

Hajenius PJ, Mol F, Mol BW, et al: Intervention for tubal ectopic pregnancy. Cochrane Database Syst Rev 24:CD000324, 2007

Halperin R, Schneider D, Mendlovic S, et al: Uterine-preserving emergency surgery for cesarean scar pregnancies: Another medical solution to an iatrogenic problem. Fertil Steril 91(6):2623, 2009

Hammoud AO, Hammoud I, Bujold E, et al: The role of sonographic endometrial patterns and endometrial thickness in the differential diagnosis of ectopic pregnancy. Am J Obstet Gynecol 192:1370, 2005

Harris MB, Angtuaco T, Frazier CN, et al: Diagnosis of a viable abdominal pregnancy by magnetic resonance imaging. Am J Obstet Gynecol 159:150, 1988

Herndon C, Garner EIO: Vaginal spotting was the only evidence of a crisis. Am J Obstet Gynecol 199:324.e1, 2008

Hill LM, Kislak S, Martin JG: Transvaginal sonographic detection of the pseudogestational sac associated with ectopic pregnancy. Obstet Gynecol 75(6):986, 1990

Hoffman BL: Surgeries for benign gynecologic conditions. In Schorge JO, Schaffer JI, Halvorsen LM, et al (eds), Williams Gynecology, New York, McGraw-Hill, 2008, p. 943

Holland MG, Bienstock JL: Recurrent ectopic pregnancy in a cesarean scar. Obstet Gynecol 111:541, 2008

Iwama H, Tsutsumi S, Igarashi H, et al: A case of retroperitoneal ectopic pregnancy following IVF-ET in a patient with previous bilateral salpingectomy. Am J Perinatol 25:33, 2008

Jeng CJ, Ko ML, Shen J: Transvaginal ultrasound-guided treatment of cervical pregnancy. Obstet Gynecol 109:1076, 2007

Kadar N, Romero R: Observations on the log human chorionic gonadotropin–time relationship in early pregnancy and its practical implications. Am J Obstet Gynecol 157:73, 1987

Kalchman GG, Meltzer RM: Interstitial pregnancy following homolateral salpingectomy: Report of 2 cases and a review of the literature. Am J Obstet Gynecol 96:1139, 1966

Kalinski MA, Guss DA: Hemorrhagic shock from a ruptured ectopic pregnancy in a patient with a negative urine pregnancy test result. Ann Emerg Med 40:102, 2002

Kaplan BR, Brandt T, Javaheri G, et al: Nonsurgical treatment of a viable cervical pregnancy with intra-amniotic methotrexate. Fertil Steril 53:941, 1990

Karaer A, Avsar FA, Batioglu S: Risk factors for ectopic pregnancy: A case-control study. Aust N Z J Obstet Gynaecol 46:521, 2006

Kelly H, Harvey D, Moll S: A cautionary tale: Fatal outcome of methotrexate therapy given for management of ectopic pregnancy. Obstet Gynecol 107:439, 2006

Khalil A, Aslam N, Haider H, et al: Laparoscopic management of a case of unexpected omental pregnancy. J Obstet Gynaecol 25:475, 2006

Kirk E, Condous G, Van Calster B, et al: A validation of the most commonly used protocol to predict the success of single-dose methotrexate in the treatment of ectopic pregnancy. Hum Reprod 22:858, 2007

Kooi S, Kock HC: A review of the literature on nonsurgical treatment in tubal pregnancy. Obstet Gynecol Surv 47:739, 1992

Kung FT, Chang SY: Efficacy of methotrexate treatment in viable and nonviable cervical pregnancies. Am J Obstet Gynecol 181:1438, 1999

Kung FT, Lin H, Hsu TY, et al: Differential diagnosis of suspected cervical pregnancy and conservative treatment with the combination of laparoscopy-assisted uterine artery ligation and hysteroscopic endocervical resection. Fertil Steril 81:1642, 2004

Kurtz AB, Dubbins PA, Wapner RJ, et al: Problem of abnormal fetal position. JAMA 247:3251, 1982

Larsen JV, Solomon MH: Pregnancy in a uterine scar sacculus—an unusual cause of postabortal haemorrhage. A case report. S Afr Med J 53(4):142, 1978

Lee JK, Lamaro VP: Ruptured tubal ectopic pregnancy with negative serum beta hCG–A case for ongoing vigilance? N Z Med J 122(1288):94, 2009

Lipscomb GH: Medical therapy for ectopic pregnancy. Semin Reprod Med 25:93, 2007

Lipscomb GH, Bran D, McCord ML, et al: Analysis of three hundred fifteen ectopic pregnancies treated with single-dose methotrexate. Am J Obstet Gynecol 178:1354, 1998

Lipscomb GH, McCord ML, Stovall TG, et al: Predictors of success of methotrexate treatment in women with tubal ectopic pregnancies. N Engl J Med 341:1974, 1999a

Lipscomb GH, Meyer NL, Flynn DE, et al: Oral methotrexate for treatment of ectopic pregnancy. Am J Obstet Gynecol 186:1192, 2002

Lipscomb GH, Puckett KJ, Bran D, et al: Management of separation pain after single-dose methotrexate therapy for ectopic pregnancy. Obstet Gynecol 93:590, 1999b

Malinowski A, Bates SK: Semantics and pitfalls in the diagnosis of cornual/interstitial pregnancy. Fertil Steril 86:1764.e11, 2006

Mankodi RC, Sankari K, Bhatt SM: Primary splenic pregnancy. Br J Obstet Gynaecol 84:634, 1977

Marcovici I, Rosenzweig BA, Brill AI, et al: Cervical pregnancy: Case reports and a current literature review. Obstet Gynecol Surv 49:49, 1994

Marcus SF, Brinsden PR: Primary ovarian pregnancy after in vitro fertilization and embryo transfer: Report of seven cases. Fertil Steril 60:167, 1993

Martin JN Jr, McCaul JF IV: Emergent management of abdominal pregnancy. Clin Obstet Gynecol 33:438, 1990

Martin JN Jr, Sessums JK, Martin RW, et al: Abdominal pregnancy: Current concepts of management. Obstet Gynecol 71:549, 1988

Mashiach S, Admon D, Oelsner G, et al: Cervical Shirodkar cerclage may be the treatment modality of choice for cervical pregnancy. Hum Reprod 17:493, 2002

Menon S, Colins J, Barnhart KT: Establishing a human chorionic gonadotropin cutoff to guide methotrexate treatment of ectopic pregnancy: A systematic review. Fertil Steril 87(3):481, 2007

Mol BWJ, Lijmer JG, Ankum WM, et al: The accuracy of single serum progesterone measurement in the diagnosis of ectopic pregnancy: A meta-analysis. Hum Reprod 13:3220, 1998

Moschos E, Sreenarasimhaiah S, Twickler DM: First-trimester diagnosis of cesarean scar ectopic pregnancy. J Clin Ultrasound 36(8):504, 2008

Mukul LV, Teal SB: Current management of ectopic pregnancy. Obstet Gynecol Clin North Am 34:403, 2007

Naim NM, Ahmad S, Siraj HH, et al: Advanced abdominal pregnancy resulting from late uterine rupture. Obstet Gynecol 111:502, 2008

Nakao Y, Yokoyama, Iwasaka T: Uterine artery embolization followed by dilation and curettage for cervical pregnancy. Obstet Gynecol 111:505, 2008

Natale AM, Candiani M, Merlo D, et al: Human chorionic gonadotropin level as a predictor of trophoblastic infiltration into the tubal wall in ectopic pregnancy: A blinded study. Fertil Steril 79:981, 2003

Ness RB, McLaughlin MT, Heine RP, et al: Fetal fibronectin as a marker to discriminate between ectopic and intrauterine pregnancies. Am J Obstet Gynecol 179:697, 1998

Nolan TE, Chandler PE, Hess LW, et al: Cervical pregnancy managed without hysterectomy. A case report. J Reprod Med 34:241, 1989

Nyberg DA, Hughes MP, Mack LA, et al: Extrauterine findings of ectopic pregnancy of transvaginal US: Importance of echogenic fluid. Radiology 178:823, 1991

Nyberg DA, Mack LA, Laing FC, et al: Distinguishing normal from abnormal gestational sac growth in early pregnancy. J Ultrasound Med 6(1):23, 1987

Oriol B, Barrio A, Pacheco A, et al: Systemic methotrexate to treat ectopic pregnancy does not affect ovarian reserve. Fertil Steril 90(5):1579, 2008

Ory HW: Ectopic pregnancy and intrauterine contraceptive devices: New perspectives. The woman's health study. Obstet Gynecol 57:137, 1981

Paul M, Schaff E, Nichols M: The roles of clinical assessment, human chorionic gonadotropin assays, and ultrasonography in medical abortion practice. Am J Obstet Gynecol 183:S34, 2000

Peleg D, Bar-Hava I, Neuman-Levin M, et al: Early diagnosis and successful nonsurgical treatment of viable combined intrauterine and cervical pregnancy. Fertil Steril 62:405, 1994

Perkins SL, Al-Ramahi M, Claman P: Comparison of serum progesterone as an indicator of pregnancy nonviability in spontaneously pregnant emergency room and infertility clinic patient populations. Fertil Steril 73:499, 2000

Pisarska MD, Carson SA: Incidence and risk factors for ectopic pregnancy. Clin Obstet Gynecol 42:2, 1999

Pisarska MD, Carson SA, Buster JE: Ectopic pregnancy. Lancet 351:1115, 1998

Practice Committee of the American Society for Reproductive Medicine: Medical treatment of ectopic pregnancy. 86:S96, 2006

Predanic M: Differentiating tubal abortion from viable ectopic pregnancy with serum CA-125 and beta-human chorionic gonadotropin determinations. Fertil Steril 73:522, 2000

Rahman MS, Al-Suleiman SA, Rahman J, et al: Advanced abdominal pregnancy—observations in 10 cases. Obstet Gynecol 59:366, 1982

Raziel A, Golan A: Primary ovarian pregnancy successfully treated with methotrexate. Am J Obstet Gynecol 169:1362, 1993

Rolle C, Wai C, Hoffman B: Unilateral twin ectopic pregnancy in a patient with multiple sexually transmitted infections. Infect Dis Obstet Gynecol 1:14, 2004

Romero R, Kadar N, Castro D, et al: The value of adnexal sonographic findings in the diagnosis of ectopic pregnancy. Am J Obstet Gynecol 158:52, 1988

Rotas MA, Haberman S, Levgur M: Cesarean scar ectopic pregnancies. Obstet Gynecol 107:1373, 2006

Sagiv R, Golan A, Arbel-Alon S, et al: Three conservative approaches to treatment of interstitial pregnancy. J Am Assoc Gynecol Laparosc 8:154, 2001

Saraiya M, Berg CJ, Kendrick JS, et al: Cigarette smoking as a risk factor for ectopic pregnancy. Am J Obstet Gynecol 178:493, 1998

Saraj AJ, Wilcox JG, Najmabadi S, et al: Resolution of hormonal markers of ectopic gestation: A randomized trial comparing single-dose intramuscular methotrexate with salpingostomy. Obstet Gynecol 92:989, 1998

Schwartz LB, Carcangiu ML, DeCherney AH: Primary ovarian pregnancy. A case report. J Reprod Med 38:155, 1993

Seifer DB: Persistent ectopic pregnancy: An argument for heightened vigilance and patient compliance. Fertil Steril 68:402, 1997

Senterman M, Jibodh R, Tualndi T: Histopathologic study of ampullary and isthmic tubal ectopic pregnancy. Am J Obstet Gynecol 159:939, 1988

Shah AA, Grotegut CA, Likes CE III, et al: Heterotopic cervical pregnancy treated with transvaginal ultrasound-guided aspiration resulting in cervical site varices within the myometrium. Fertil Steril 91:934.e19, 2009

Shalev E, Peleg D, Tsabari A, et al: Spontaneous resolution of ectopic tubal pregnancy: Natural history. Fertil Steril 63:15, 1995

Shamma FN, Schwartz LB: Primary peritoneal pregnancy successfully treated with methotrexate. Am J Obstet Gynecol 167:1307, 1992

Shankar R, Gude N, Cullinanae F, et al: An emerging role for comprehensive proteome analysis in human pregnancy research. Reproduction 129:685, 2005

Sherer DM, Gorelick C, Dalloul M, et al: Three-dimensional sonographic findings of a cervical pregnancy. J Ultrasound Med 27(1):155, 2008

Shippey SH, Bhoola SM, Royek AB, et al: Diagnosis and management of hepatic ectopic pregnancy. Obstet Gynecol 109:544, 2007

Sidek S, Lai SF, Lim-Tan SK: Primary ovarian pregnancy: Current diagnosis and management. Singapore Med J 35:71, 1994

Silva C, Sammel MD, Zhou L, et al: Human chorionic gonadotropin profile for women with ectopic pregnancy. Obstet Gynecol 107:605, 2006

Sivin I: Alternative estimates of ectopic pregnancy risks during contraception. Am J Obstet Gynecol 165:1900, 1991

Skjeldestad FE, Hadgu A, Eriksson N: Epidemiology of repeat ectopic pregnancy: a population-based prospective cohort study. Obstet Gynecol 91:129, 1998

Society for Assisted Reproductive Technology; American Society for Reproductive Medicine: Assisted reproductive technology in the United States: 2001 results generated from the American Society for Reproductive Medicine/Society for Assisted Reproductive Technology registry. Fertil Steril 87:1253, 2007

Song MJ, Moon MH, Kim JA, et al: Serial transvaginal sonographic findings of cervical ectopic pregnancy treated with high-dose methotrexate. J Ultrasound Med 28:55, 2009

Soriano D, Vicus D, Mashiach R, et al: Laparoscopic treatment of cornual pregnancy: A series of 20 consecutive cases. Fertil Steril 90(3):839, 2008

Spandorfer SD, Sawin SW, Benjamin I, et al: Postoperative day 1 serum human chorionic gonadotropin level as a predictor of persistent ectopic pregnancy after conservative surgical management. Fertil Steril 68:430, 1997

Stevens CA: Malformations and deformations in abdominal pregnancy. Am J Med Genet 47:1189, 1993

Stovall TG, Ling FW: Some new approaches to ectopic pregnancy management. Contemp Obstet Gynecol 37:35, 1992

Stovall TG, Ling FW, Carson SA, et al: Serum progesterone and uterine curettage in differential diagnosis of ectopic pregnancy. Fertil Steril 57:456, 1992

Stovall TG, Ling FW, Cope BJ, et al: Preventing ruptured ectopic pregnancy with a single serum progesterone. Am J Obstet Gynecol 160:1425, 1989

Swire MN, Castro-Aragon I, Levine D: Various sonographic appearances of the hemorrhagic corpus luteum cyst. Ultrasound Q 20:45, 2004

Tanaka T, Hayashi H, Kutsuzawa T, et al: Treatment of interstitial ectopic pregnancy with methotrexate: Report of a successful case. Fertil Steril 37:851, 1982

Teng HC, Kumar G, Ramli NM: A viable secondary intra-abdominal pregnancy resulting from rupture of uterine scar: Role of MRI. Br J Radiol 80:e134, 2007

Thomas RL, Gingold BR, Gallagher MW: Cervical pregnancy. A report of two cases. J Reprod Med 36:459, 1991

Timor-Tritsch IE, Monteagudo A, Mandeville EO, et al: Successful management of viable cervical pregnancy by local injection of methotrexate guided by transvaginal ultrasonography. Am J Obstet Gynecol 170:737, 1994

Trio D, Strobelt N, Picciolo C, et al: Prognostic factors for successful expectant management of ectopic pregnancy. Fertil Steril 63:469, 1995

Trojano G, Colafiglio G, Saliani N, et al: Successful management of a cervical twin pregnancy: neoadjuvant systematic methotrexate and prophylactic high cervical cerclage before curettage. Fertil Steril 91:935.e17, 2009

Tulandi T, A1-Jaroudi D: Interstitial pregnancy: Results generated from the Society of Reproductive Surgeons. Obstet Gynecol 103:47, 2004

Tulandi T, Saleh A: Surgical management of ectopic pregnancy. Clin Obstet Gynecol 42:31, 1999

Ushakov FB, Elchalal U, Aceman PJ, et al: Cervical pregnancy: Past and future. Obstet Gynecol Surv 52:45, 1997

Van Den Eeden SK, Shan J, Bruce C, et al: Ectopic pregnancy rate and treatment utilization in a large managed care organization. Obstet Gynecol 105:1052, 2005

Varma R, Mascarenhas L, James D. Successful outcome of advanced abdominal pregnancy with exclusive omental insertion. Ultrasound Obst Gyn 12:192, 2003

Verma U, Goharkhay N: Conservative management of cervical ectopic pregnancy. Fertil Steril 91(3):671, 2009

Vermesh M, Silva PD, Sauer MV, et al: Persistent tubal ectopic gestation: Patterns of circulating beta-human chorionic gonadotropin and progesterone and management options. Fertil Steril 50:584, 1988

Virk J, Zhang J, Olsen J: Medical abortion and the risk of subsequent adverse pregnancy outcomes. N Engl J Med 357:648, 2007

Wagner A, Burchardt AJ: MR imaging in advanced abdominal pregnancy. A case report of fetal death. Acta Radiol 36:193, 1995

Wang CJ, Chao AS, Yuen LT, et al: Endoscopic management of cesarean scar pregnancy. Fertil Steril 85:494, 2006

Weiss RE, Stone NN: Persistent maternal hydronephrosis after intra-abdominal pregnancy. J Urol 152:1196, 1994

Williams PC, Malvar TC, Kraft JR: Term ovarian pregnancy with delivery of a live female infant. Am J Obstet Gynecol 142:589, 1982

World Health Organization: Maternal mortality in 2005. Estimates developed by WHO, UNICEF, UNFPA and The World Bank. 2007

Worley KC, Hnat MD, Cunningham FG: Advanced extrauterine pregnancy: Diagnostic and therapeutic challenges. Am J Obstet Gynecol 198:297e1, 2008

Yi KW, Yeo MK, Shin JH, et al: Laparoscopic management of early omental pregnancy detected by magnetic resonance imaging. J Minim Invasive Gynecol 15:231, 2008

Zeck W, Kelters I, Winter R, et al: Lessons learned from four advanced abdominal pregnancies at an East African Health Center. J Perinat Med 35(4):278, 2007

CHAPTER 11

Gestational Trophoblastic Disease

The term *gestational trophoblastic disease* refers to a spectrum of pregnancy-related placental tumors. Gestational trophoblastic disease is divided into molar and nonmolar tumors. Nonmolar tumors are grouped as *gestational trophoblastic neoplasia*. The American College of Obstetricians and Gynecologists (2004) terms these as *malignant gestational trophoblastic disease*. Although these tumors are histologically distinct and have varying propensities to invade and metastasize, it became evident during the 1970s that histological confirmation was not necessary to provide effective treatment. Instead, a system was adopted based principally on clinical findings and serial serum measurements of human chorionic gonadotropin (β-hCG). A number of schemas have been used over the past 30 years to classify these tumors on the basis of malignant potential, and to direct clinical staging and optimal treatment. The International Federation of Gynecology and Obstetrics (FIGO) trophoblastic disease classification scheme is frequently used (Table 11-1). When these management algorithms are followed, most gestational tumors—both benign and malignant—are eminently curable (Berkowitz and Goldstein, 2009).

HYDATIDIFORM MOLE—MOLAR PREGNANCY

Molar pregnancy is characterized histologically by abnormalities of the chorionic villi that consist of trophoblastic proliferation and edema of villous stroma. Although moles usually occupy the uterine cavity, occasionally they develop as ectopic pregnancies (Abdul and co-workers, 2008; Chauhan and colleagues, 2004). The degree of tissue changes and absence or presence of a fetus

or embryonic elements is used to describe them as *complete* or *partial* (Table 11-2).

Complete Hydatidiform Mole

Features of a complete hydatidiform mole are shown in Table 11-2. Grossly, the chorionic villi appear as a mass of clear vesicles (Fig. 11-1). These vary in size from barely visible to a few centimeters and often hang in clusters from thin pedicles. Histologically, they typically show hydropic degeneration and villous edema; absence of villous blood vessels; varying degrees of proliferation of the trophoblastic epithelium; and absence of embryonic elements such as a fetus and amnion.

Ploidy

The chromosomal composition of complete moles is usually diploid and of paternal origin. About 85 percent are 46,XX with both sets of chromosomes paternal in origin (Wolf and Lage, 1995). Termed *androgenesis*, the ovum is fertilized by a haploid sperm, which duplicates its own chromosomes after meiosis. The chromosomes of the ovum are either absent or inactivated. In other complete moles, the chromosomal pattern may be 46,XY due to dispermic fertilization (Bagshawe and Lawler, 1982).

Lawler and colleagues (1991) described 200 molar pregnancies. Of the 151 complete moles, 128 or 85 percent were diploid, 3 were triploid, and 1 was haploid. Of the 49 partial moles, 86 percent were triploid. Niemann and co-workers (2006) approached this another way. They classified 162 moles as diploid and 105 as triploid without regard for other criteria for complete or partial moles. In this study, all persistent or malignant sequelae were in women with diploid moles.

Malignant Potential

Complete molar pregnancy has a higher incidence of malignant sequela compared with partial moles. In most studies, 15 to 20 percent of complete moles had evidence of persistent

TABLE 11-1. Classification of Gestational Trophoblastic Disease

Hydatidiform mole
  Complete
  Partial
Gestational trophoblastic neoplasia[a]
  Invasive mole
  Choriocarcinoma
  Placental site trophoblastic tumor
  Epithelioid trophoblastic tumor

[a]Also called malignant gestational trophoblastic disease. Modified from the International Federation of Gynecology and Obstetrics (FIGO Oncology Committee, 2002).

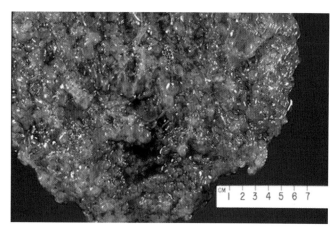

FIGURE 11-1 A complete or classical hydatidiform mole. (Courtesy of Dr. Michael G. O'Connor.)

trophoblastic disease (Kerkmeijer and colleagues, 2006; Soper, 2006). Interestingly, earlier molar evacuation does not lower this risk (Schorge and co-workers, 2000).

Partial Hydatidiform Mole

Features of a partial or incomplete molar pregnancy include some element of fetal tissue and hydatidiform changes that are focal and less advanced. There is slowly progressive swelling within the stroma of characteristically avascular chorionic villi, whereas vascular villi that have a functioning fetal-placental circulation are spared (Shapter and McLellan, 2001).

As shown in Table 11-2, the karyotype typically is triploid—69,XXX, 69,XXY, or much less commonly, 69,XYY. These are each composed of one maternal and two paternal haploid sets of chromosomes (Berkowitz and colleagues, 1986, 1991; Wolf and Lage, 1995). Only 3 of 270 molar pregnancies studied by Niemann and associates (2006) were tetraploid. The nonviable fetus associated with a triploid partial mole typically has multiple malformations (Philipp and co-workers, 2004). In the review by Jauniaux (1999), 82 percent of fetuses had symmetrical growth restriction.

The risk of persistent trophoblastic disease after a partial mole is substantially lower than that following a complete molar pregnancy (Table 11-2). Moreover, persistent disease seldom is choriocarcinoma. Seckl and associates (2000) documented only 3 of 3000 of partial moles to be complicated by choriocarcinoma. Growdon and co-workers (2006) found that higher postevacuation β-hCG levels correlated with increased risk for persistent disease. Specifically, levels ≥ 200 mIU/mL in the third through eighth week postevacuation were associated with at least a 35-percent risk of persistent disease.

Twin Molar Pregnancy

A twin gestation composed of a complete diploid molar pregnancy and a normal pregnancy is not rare (Fig. 11-2). Niemann and associates (2006) reported that 5 percent of diploid moles were part of a twin pregnancy with a fetus. Survival of the normal coexisting fetus is variable and depends on whether the diagnosis is made, and if so, whether problems from the molar component such as preeclampsia or hemorrhage develop. In their review, Vejerslev (1991) found that of 113 such pregnancies, 45 percent progressed to 28 weeks, and of these, 70 percent of neonates survived.

Compared with a partial mole, women with these types of twin pregnancies have a substantive risk of developing subsequent

TABLE 11-2. Features of Partial and Complete Hydatidiform Moles

Feature	Partial Mole	Complete Mole
Karyotype	Usually 69,XXX or 69,XXY	46,XX or 46,XY
Pathology		
Embryo fetus	Often present	Absent
Amnion, fetal red blood cells	Often present	Absent
Villous edema	Variable, focal	Diffuse
Trophoblastic proliferation	Variable, focal, slight to moderate	Variable, slight to severe
Clinical presentation		
Diagnosis	Missed abortion	Molar gestation
Uterine size	Small for dates	50% large for dates
Theca-lutein cysts	Rare	25–30%
Medical complications	Rare	Frequent
Persistent trophoblastic disease	1–5%	15–20%

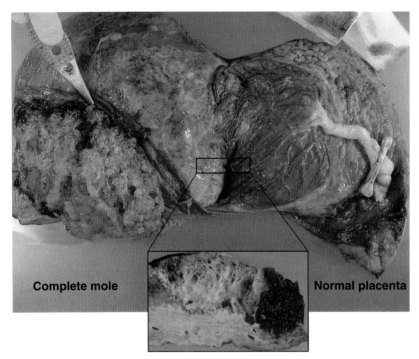

FIGURE 11-2 Photograph of placentas from a twin pregnancy with one normal twin and with a complete mole. The complete mole (*left*) shows the characteristic vesicular structure. The placenta on the *right* appears grossly normal. A transverse section through the border between these two is shown (*inset*). (Courtesy of Drs. April Bleich, Pamela Kothari, and Brian Levenson.)

gestational trophoblastic neoplasia. But this risk does not appear greater than following a singleton complete mole (Niemann and associates, 2007b). In their review of 77 pregnancies, Sebire and colleagues (2002b) reported that 21 percent of pregnancies not terminated subsequently required chemotherapy for persistent disease. This rate is not significantly different from the rate of 16 percent among women who terminate their pregnancies. In the series by Niemann and colleagues (2006), 25 percent of such twin pregnancies subsequently needed chemotherapy.

Histological Diagnosis of Hydatidiform Moles

Histological changes of complete and partial moles are listed in Table 11-2. Attempts to relate the histological structure of individual complete moles to their subsequent malignant potential have generally been disappointing (Fukunaga, 2005; Novak and Seah, 1954; Paradinas, 1997, and all their colleagues).

Cytometry

Moles evacuated early may have not yet developed the histological findings characteristic of their type. Thus, either *flow cytometry* or *automated image cytometry* can be used to determine cellular ploidy (Crisp and associates, 2003; Niemann and colleagues, 2006). Immunostaining techniques are also useful to highlight cells that are of pure paternal derivation from those of both maternal and paternal derivation (Genest and co-workers, 2002; Merchant and associates, 2005).

Theca-Lutein Cysts

In 25 to 60 percent of women with a complete mole, the ovaries contain multiple theca-lutein cysts. These may vary from microscopic to 10 cm or more in diameter. Their surfaces are smooth, often yellowish, and lined with lutein cells. They are thought to result from overstimulation of lutein elements by large amounts of hCG secreted by proliferating trophoblastic cells. Montz and colleagues (1988) reported that persistent gestational trophoblastic disease was more likely in women with theca-lutein cysts, especially if bilateral. This is logical because cysts are more likely with higher serum hCG levels, which may portend a worse prognosis (Niemann and co-workers, 2006). Such cysts are also seen with fetal hydrops, placental hypertrophy, and multifetal pregnancy (see Chap. 5, p. 110). Larger cysts may undergo torsion, infarction, and hemorrhage. Because they regress, oophorectomy is not performed unless the ovary is extensively infarcted.

Epidemiology and Risk Factors

The incidence of hydatidiform mole has been relatively constant in the United States and Europe at 1 to 2 per 1000 pregnancies (Drake and colleagues, 2006; Loukovarra and associates, 2005). It is more prevalent in Hispanics and American Indians (Smith and co-workers, 2006). Until recently, it was held to be much more frequent in some Asian countries however, these data were from hospital studies and thus misleading (Schorge and associates, 2000). In a Korean study, Kim and colleagues (2004) used current terminology and classification and reported a population-based incidence of 2 per 1000 deliveries.

Age

Maternal age at either extreme of the reproductive spectrum is a risk factor for molar pregnancy. Specifically, adolescents and women aged 36 to 40 years have a twofold risk and those over 40 years have an almost tenfold risk (Altman and associates, 2008; Sebire and colleagues, 2002a).

Prior Molar Pregnancy

There is a substantively increased risk for recurrent trophoblastic disease. In a review of 12 series totaling almost 5000 molar pregnancies, the frequency of recurrent moles was 1.3 percent (Loret de Mola and Goldfarb, 1995). The risk is 1.5 percent for a complete mole and 2.7 percent for a partial mole (Garrett and colleagues, 2008). With two prior molar pregnancies, Berkowitz and associates (1998) reported that 23 percent of women had a third mole! Repetitive hydatidiform moles in women with different partners suggest that an oocyte defect leads to molar development.

Other Risk Factors

Oral contraceptive use and its duration as well as previous miscarriage increase the chances for a molar pregnancy as much as twofold (Palmer and co-workers, 1999). Other studies implicate smoking, various vitamin deficiencies, and increased paternal age.

Clinical Course

The "typical" clinical presentation of women with a molar pregnancy has changed considerably over the past several decades because of earlier diagnosis. Most women present for pregnancy care early and undergo sonography, thus molar pregnancies are detected before they grow to larger sizes with more complications (Kerkmeijer and co-workers, 2009). In many ways, this changing presentation picture is analogous to that of ectopic pregnancy. In general, symptoms tend to be more pronounced with complete moles compared with partial moles (Drake and colleagues, 2006; Niemann and associates, 2007a).

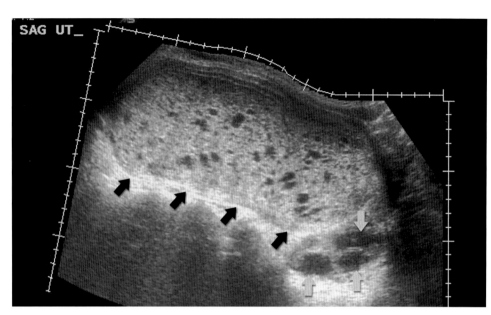

FIGURE 11-3 Sagittal sonogram image of a 20-week-sized uterus with a complete hydatidiform mole (*black arrows*) and associated ovarian theca-lutein cysts (*white arrows*).

Clinical Presentation

There is usually 1 to 2 months of *amenorrhea*. There may be significant *nausea and vomiting*. Eventually, *uterine bleeding* is almost universal and may vary from spotting to profuse hemorrhage. It may begin just before spontaneous molar abortion or more often, follow an intermittent course for weeks to months. In more advanced moles, there may be considerable concealed uterine hemorrhage with moderate iron-deficiency anemia.

In about half of cases, *uterine growth* is more rapid than expected. The uterus has a soft consistency. Large theca-lutein cysts may be difficult to distinguish from the enlarged uterus on bimanual examination. And although the uterus is enlarged, typically no fetal heart motion is detected.

As the consequence of the thyrotropin-like effect of hCG, plasma free thyroxine levels are often elevated and TSH levels are decreased. Despite this, clinically apparent *thyrotoxicosis* is unusual, but thyroid storm has been reported (Chiniwala and colleagues, 2008). In our experiences, the serum free-T_4 levels rapidly normalize after uterine evacuation. Occasionally, *early-onset preeclampsia* develops with a large mole. Because gestational hypertension is rarely seen before 24 weeks, preeclampsia that develops before this time should raise concerns for molar pregnancy. Interestingly, none of the 24 women with a complete mole described by Coukos and colleagues (1999) experienced hyperemesis, clinical thyrotoxicosis, or preeclampsia.

Trophoblastic Deportation or Embolization

Variable amounts of trophoblast escape into the pelvic venous system at the time of molar evacuation (Hankins and colleagues, 1987). In some women, this tissue subsequently invades the pulmonary parenchyma to cause persistent trophoblastic disease or overt metastases. Acutely, the volume of tissue may be sufficient to produce clinically apparent acute pulmonary embolism or edema. Although deportation of massive amounts of trophoblastic tissue is probably uncommon, fatalities have been described (Delmis and co-workers, 2000).

Diagnosis

Some women will present early with spontaneous passage of molar tissue. In most cases, however, there are varying durations of amenorrhea, usually followed by irregular bleeding. These almost always prompt pregnancy testing and sonography. If left untreated, spontaneous expulsion usually occurs around 16 weeks. The characteristic sonographic appearance of a complete mole includes a complex, echogenic uterine mass with numerous cystic spaces and no fetus or amnionic sac (Fig. 11-3). Sonographic features of a partial mole include a thickened, hydropic placenta with fetal tissue (Zhou and co-workers, 2005). Importantly, in early pregnancy, sonography will demonstrate the characteristic appearance in as few as a third of women with a partial mole (John and associates, 2005). Occasionally, molar pregnancy may be confused for a uterine leiomyoma or multifetal pregnancy.

Management

Current mortality rates from molar pregnancies have been practically reduced to zero by prompt diagnosis and appropriate therapy. There are two important basic tenets for management of all molar pregnancies. The first is evacuation of the mole, and the second is regular follow-up to detect persistent trophoblastic disease. Most clinicians obtain a preoperative chest radiograph, but unless there is evidence of extrauterine disease, computed tomography (CT) or magnetic resonance (MR) imaging to evaluate the liver or brain is not done routinely. Laboratory work includes a hemogram to assess anemia, blood type and antibody screen, serum hepatic transaminase levels to assess liver involvement, and a baseline serum β-hCG level (Soper, 2006). That said, Knowles and colleagues (2007) analyzed the effectiveness of preevacuation testing for suspected molar pregnancy. They concluded that hemogram and blood type with antibody screen alone were appropriate for most patients without suspicious signs or symptoms.

The unusual circumstance of twinning with a complete mole plus a fetus and placenta is problematic, especially if there are no apparent fetal anomalies found with sonography or karyotypic aberrations. Neither maternal risks nor the likelihood of a healthy offspring have been precisely established if pregnancy is continued (Vejerslev, 1991).

Prophylactic Chemotherapy

The long-term prognosis for women with a hydatidiform mole is not improved with prophylactic chemotherapy (Goldstein and Berkowitz, 1995). Because toxicity—including death—may be significant, it is not recommended routinely (American College of Obstetricians and Gynecologists, 2004).

Suction Curettage

Molar evacuation by suction curettage is usually the preferred treatment regardless of uterine size. For large moles, adequate anesthesia and blood-banking support is imperative. With a closed cervix, preoperative dilatation with an osmotic dilator may be helpful (see Chap. 9, p. 229). The cervix is then further dilated to allow insertion of a 10- to 12-mm suction curette. After most of the molar tissue has been removed, oxytocin is given. After the myometrium has contracted, *thorough but gentle curettage* with a large sharp curette usually is performed. We have found that intraoperative sonography helps to ensure that the uterine cavity has been emptied.

Other Methods of Termination

In the United States, only rarely are labor induction or hysterotomy used for molar evacuation. Both will likely increase blood loss and may increase the incidence of persistent trophoblastic disease (American College of Obstetricians and Gynecologists, 2004).

Hysterectomy

If no further pregnancies are desired, hysterectomy may be preferred to suction curettage. It is a logical procedure in women aged 40 and older, because at least a third of these women go on to develop persistent gestational trophoblastic neoplasia. Although hysterectomy does not eliminate this possibility, it markedly reduces its likelihood (Soper, 2006). Finally, hysterectomy is an important adjunct to treatment of chemoresistant tumors (Doumplis and colleagues, 2007; Lurain and associates, 2008).

Postevacuation Surveillance

Consistent follow-up is imperative for women in whom a molar pregnancy has been evacuated. The long-term goal is to ensure complete resolution of trophoblastic disease, with chemotherapy if necessary. The following steps are recommended:

1. Prevent pregnancy for a minimum of 6 months using hormonal contraception.
2. After a baseline serum β-hCG level is obtained within 48 hours *after* evacuation, levels are monitored every 1 to 2 weeks while still elevated. This is important to detect

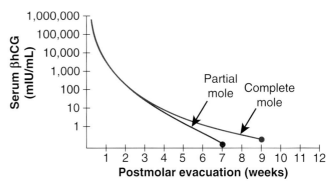

FIGURE 11-4 Schematic illustration of composite medians of β-subunit chorionic gonadotropin regression curves in women with a partial or complete hydatidiform mole. (Composite constructed using median data reported by Golfier (2007), Schlaerth (1981), Wolfberg (2004, 2005, 2006), and all their colleagues.)

persistent trophoblastic disease. Even small amounts of trophoblastic tissue can be detected by the assay. These levels should progressively fall to an undetectable level as shown in Figure 11-4.
3. Chemotherapy is not indicated as long as these serum levels continue to regress. A rise or persistent plateau demands evaluation for persistent gestational trophoblastic disease and usually treatment. An increase signifies trophoblastic proliferation that is most likely malignant unless the woman is again pregnant.
4. Once the β-hCG level falls to a normal level, serum β-hCG levels are determined monthly for another 6 months. If undetectable, surveillance can then be discontinued and pregnancy allowed.

Such intensive monitoring has a high noncompliance rate. Fortunately, recent observations indicate that verifying undetectable β-hCG levels for 6 months is likely unnecessary. A number of investigators have reported that no woman with a partial or complete mole whose serum β-hCG levels became undetectable subsequently developed persistent disease (Chan, 2006; Lavie, 2005; Wolfberg, 2004, 2006, and all their colleagues). As shown in Figure 11-4, the median times for this are 7 and 9 weeks, respectively. Although not a routine part of surveillance, postevacuation sonographic uterine examination may reveal myometrial nodules or hypervascularity, which may be associated predictors of subsequent gestational trophoblastic neoplasia (GTN) (Garavaglia and co-workers, 2009).

GESTATIONAL TROPHOBLASTIC NEOPLASIA

This group of placental tumors is characterized by their aggressive invasion into the myometrium and propensity to metastasize. Collectively, they are also termed *malignant gestational trophoblastic disease* by the American College of Obstetricians and Gynecologists (2004). Histologically these tumors include invasive mole, choriocarcinoma, placental site trophoblastic tumor, and epithelioid trophoblastic tumor. Because in most cases they are diagnosed by only persistently elevated serum β-hCG levels, there is no tissue available for pathological study. Criteria for diagnosis of postmolar gestational trophoblastic neoplasia are shown in Table 11-3.

TABLE 11-3. Criteria for Diagnosis of Gestational Trophoblastic Neoplasia or Postmolar Gestational Trophoblastic Disease

1. Plateau of serum β-hCG level (±10 percent) for four measurements during a period of 3 weeks or longer—days 1, 7, 14, 21.
2. Rise of serum β-hCG > 10 percent during three weekly consecutive measurements or longer, during a period of 2 weeks or more—days 1, 7, 14.
3. The serum β-hCG level remains detectable for 6 months or more.
4. Histological criteria for choriocarcinoma.

Criteria of the International Federation of Gynecology and Obstetrics (FIGO Oncology Committee, 2002).

Gestational trophoblastic neoplasia almost always develops with or follows some form of recognized pregnancy. Most follow a hydatidiform mole, but neoplasia may follow an abortion, normal pregnancy, or even an ectopic pregnancy (Cortés-Charry and co-workers, 2006; Nugent and associates, 2006).

Histopathological Classification

As discussed, the diagnosis of neoplasia is usually made by persistently elevated serum β-hCG levels without confirmation by pathological study. Importantly, management is not directed by histological findings.

Invasive Mole

This common manifestation of neoplasia is characterized by excessive trophoblastic overgrowth with extensive tissue invasion by trophoblastic cells and whole villi. There is penetration deep into the myometrium, sometimes with involvement of the peritoneum, adjacent parametrium, or vaginal vault. Such tumors almost always arise from partial or complete moles (Sebire and associates, 2005). They are locally invasive, but generally lack the pronounced tendency to widespread metastasis typical of choriocarcinoma.

Gestational Choriocarcinoma

This extremely malignant tumor may be considered a carcinoma of the chorionic epithelium. It has an incidence of about 1 in 30,000 pregnancies—two thirds develop after a normal delivery and a third follow molar gestations. It should be considered when persistent bleeding follows any pregnancy event (Soper, 2006).

The characteristic gross picture of these tumors is that of a rapidly growing mass invading both myometrium and blood vessels, causing hemorrhage and necrosis (Fig. 11-5). The tumor is dark red or purple and ragged or friable. If it involves the endometrium, then bleeding, sloughing, and infection of the surface usually occur early. Masses of tissue buried in the myometrium may extend outward, appearing on the uterus as dark, irregular nodules that eventually penetrate the peritoneum.

Although cytotrophoblastic and syncytial elements are involved, one or the other may predominate. Microscopically,

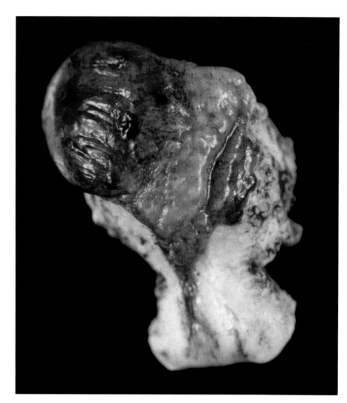

FIGURE 11-5 Choriocarcinoma is evident in the fundus of the hysterectomy specimen. (Courtesy of Dr. Ona Faye-Petersen.)

columns and sheets of these trophoblastic cells penetrate the muscle and blood vessels. They sometimes create a plexiform arrangement and at other times are completely disorganized, interspersed with clotted blood. And, in contrast to hydatidiform or invasive mole, there is not a villous pattern. Factors involved in malignant chorionic transformation are unknown, but its normal predisposition of invasive growth and erosion of blood vessels is greatly augmented.

Metastases often develop early and are generally blood-borne because of the affinity of trophoblastic cells for blood vessels. The most common sites are the lungs in more than 75 percent of cases, and the vagina in about 50 percent. Overall, Berry and colleagues (2008) reported vaginal metastases in 4.5 percent of 806 women with gestational trophoblastic neoplasia. The vulva, kidneys, liver, ovaries, brain, and bowel also may contain metastases (Fig. 11-6). Ovarian theca-lutein cysts are identified in over a third of cases.

Placental Site Trophoblastic Tumor

The rare variant of trophoblastic neoplasia arises from the placental implantation site following normal term pregnancy, spontaneous or induced abortion, or an ectopic or molar pregnancy (Feltmate and colleagues, 2001; Moore-Maxwell and Robboy, 2004). Histologically, there are intermediate trophoblastic cells, many of which are prolactin producing (Miller and associates, 1989). For this reason, serum β-hCG levels are relatively low compared with tumor mass. A high proportion of free β-hCG—over 30 percent—is accurate for diagnosis of this tumor (Cole and colleagues, 2008). Bleeding is the main presenting symptom. Locally invasive tumors are resistant to

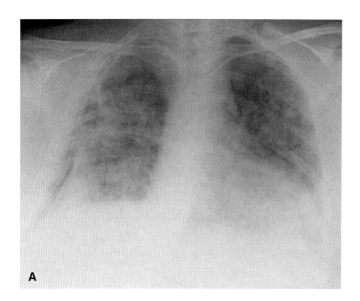

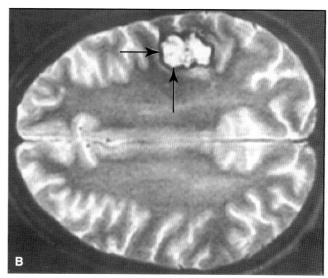

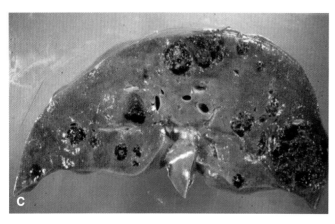

FIGURE 11-6 Metastatic choriocarcinoma. **A.** Chest radiograph demonstrates widespread metastatic lesions. (Courtesy of Dr. Michael G. O'Connor.) **B.** Cranial MRI scan shows a large metastasis on the left (*black arrows*). (Courtesy of Dr. Ilana Ariel.) **C.** Autopsy specimen shows multiple hemorrhagic hepatic metastasis. (Courtesy of Dr. Michael G. O'Connor.)

chemotherapy and hysterectomy is the best treatment (Baergen and associates, 2006). Cases managed without hysterectomy have been reported (Numnum and co-workers, 2006).

Epithelioid Trophoblastic Tumor

This rare trophoblastic tumor is distinct from gestational choriocarcinoma and placental site trophoblastic tumor (Macdonald and colleagues, 2008). In their recent review, Palmer and associates (2008) found only 52 reported cases. The preceding pregnancy event may be remote or, in some cases, cannot be confirmed. Epithelioid trophoblastic tumor develops from neoplastic transformation of chorionic-type intermediate trophoblast. Microscopically, it resembles placental site trophoblastic tumor, but the cells are smaller and display less nuclear pleomorphism (Allison and co-workers, 2006). Grossly, the tumor grows in a nodular fashion rather than the infiltrative pattern of placental site tumor. Hysterectomy is the primary method of treatment, but approximately a fourth of these women present with metastatic disease. There are too few reported cases to evaluate the efficacy of chemotherapy.

Clinical Course

The most common finding with gestational trophoblastic neoplasms is irregular bleeding associated with uterine subinvolu-

tion. The bleeding may be continuous or intermittent, with sudden and sometimes massive hemorrhage. Myometrial perforation from trophoblastic growth may cause intraperitoneal hemorrhage (Hancock and Tidy, 2002). Some women present with metastatic lesions to the vagina or vulva. In others, the uterine tumor has disappeared, leaving only distant metastases. If untreated, choriocarcinoma is invariably fatal.

Diagnosis

Consideration for the possibility of gestational trophoblastic neoplasia is the most important factor in diagnosis. Unusually persistent bleeding after pregnancy of any type should prompt measurement of serum β-hCG levels and consideration for diagnostic curettage. Persistent or rising serum β-hCG levels in the absence of pregnancy are indicative of trophoblastic neoplasia.

After thorough pelvic assessment, then hemogram, renal and liver function studies, and chest radiograph are obtained (Darby and associates, 2009). Solitary or multiple pulmonary nodules are suggestive of metastasis and should prompt further imaging of the brain, abdomen, and pelvis (Garner and colleagues, 2004). The threshold for additional imaging beyond chest radiograph should be low. Moodley and Moodley (2004) described three women with normal chest radiograph readings but who had lung metastases identified with CT-scanning. Positron emission computed tomography (PET/CT) scanning may also be useful (Niemann and co-workers, 2006).

Staging and Prognostic Scoring

Clinical staging is similar to that for ovarian cancer except that stage III allows pulmonary involvement. Risk assessment is done using the modified World Health Organization (WHO) Prognostic Scoring System (FIGO Oncology Committee, 2002). Scores of 0 to 4 are given for each category that includes age; type of antecedent pregnancy and interval from it; serum β-hCG concentration; size of tumor, its site, and the number of metastases; and previous chemotherapy. When summed, low-risk neoplasia generally includes cumulative scores of 0 to 6. Kohorn (2007) has proposed a dynamic scoring system that includes tumor response.

Treatment

In general, oncology referral is preferable. Single-agent chemotherapy is given for nonmetastatic or low-risk metastatic neoplasia (Horowitz and co-workers, 2009). Abrão and colleagues (2008) reviewed 108 low-risk cases and found methotrexate or actinomycin D alone equally effective compared with a combination of the two. Methotrexate is less toxic than actinomycin D, but both are usually curative (Chan and colleagues, 2006; Schorge and colleagues, 2008). There is no need for hospitalization to begin initial therapy (Carter and colleagues, 2008). Virtually all women with nonmetastatic tumors or low-risk gestational trophoblastic neoplasia are cured with these if treated early. In 150 women with low-risk GTN, Growden and co-workers (2009) found that metastatic disease, single-day methotrexate infusion, and complete mole histology were risk factors for additional chemotherapy beyond the first course.

Repeat curettage may cause perforation and is avoided unless there is bleeding or a substantial amount of retained molar tissue. On the other hand "debulking" by curettage hastens response (van Trommel and co-workers, 2005). For women who have completed childbearing, hysterectomy is an option. Carlini and colleagues (2006) reported a woman who responded to chemotherapy after selective uterine artery embolization for heavy vaginal bleeding.

Chemotherapy subsequent to the initial dose is guided by serial serum β-hCG levels. Of note, failure may be falsely assumed when *phantom hCG* caused by heterophilic antibodies interferes with the hCG assay (American College of Obstetricians and Gynecologists, 2004).

Women are classified as high risk when the modified WHO prognostic score is 7 or greater. In these women, combination chemotherapy—with its increased toxicity—has produced cure rates between 67 and 85 percent (Lurain and co-workers, 2006a; Soper, 2006). One is the *EMA-CO regimen—E*toposide, *M*ethotrexate, *A*ctinomycin D, *C*yclophosphamide, and *O*ncovin (vincristine). Surgery and radiotherapy are also frequently employed (Lurain and co-workers, 2006b).

Subsequent Pregnancy

Surveillance is, at a minimum, 6 months for molar pregnancy, 1 year for gestational trophoblastic neoplasia, and up to 2 years if there are metastases. Fertility is not impaired, and pregnancy outcomes are usually normal following successful treatment (Schorge and associates, 2000). The primary concern is the 2-percent risk for developing trophoblastic disease in a subsequent pregnancy (Garrett and colleagues, 2008).

REFERENCES

Abdul MA, Randawa AJ, Shehu SM: Ectopic (tubal) molar gestation: report of two cases. Niger J Clin Pract 11(4):392, 2008

Abrão RA, de Andrade JM, Tiezzi DG, et al: Treatment for low-risk gestational trophoblastic disease: Comparison of single-agent methotrexate, dactinomycin and combination regimens. Gynecol Oncol 108:149, 2008

Allison KH, Love JE, Garcia RL: Epithelioid trophoblastic tumor: Review of a rare neoplasm of the chorionic-type intermediate trophoblast. Arch Pathol Lab Med 130:1875, 2006

Altman AD, Bently B, Murray S, et al: Maternal age-related rate of gestational trophoblastic disease. Obstet Gynecol 112:244, 2008

American College of Obstetricians and Gynecologists: Bulletin #53. Diagnosis and treatment of gestational trophoblastic disease. Obstet Gynecol 103:1365, 2004

Baergen RN, Rutgers JL, Young RH, et al: Placental site trophoblastic tumor: A study of 55 cases and review of the literature emphasizing factors of prognostic significance. Gynecol Oncol 100:511, 2006

Bagshawe KD, Lawler SD: Commentary: Unmasking moles. Br J Obstet Gynaecol 89:255, 1982

Berkowitz RS, Goldstein DP: Current management of gestational trophoblastic diseases. Gynecol Oncol 112(3):654, 2009

Berkowitz RS, Goldstein DP, Bernstein MR: Advances in management of partial molar pregnancy. Contemp Obstet Gynecol 36:33, 1991

Berkowitz RS, Goldstein DP, Bernstein MR: Management of partial molar pregnancy. Contemp Obstet Gynecol 27:77, 1986

Berkowitz RS, Im SS, Bernstein MR, et al: Gestational trophoblastic disease. Subsequent pregnancy outcome, including repeat molar pregnancy. J Reprod Med 43:81, 1998

Berry E, Hagopian GS, Lurain JR: Vaginal metastases in gestational trophoblastic neoplasia. J Reprod Med 53:487, 2008

Carlini L, Villa A, Busci L, et al: Selective uterine artery embolization: A new therapeutic approach in a patient with low-risk gestational trophoblastic disease. Am J Obstet Gynecol 195:314, 2006

Carter LD, Hancock BW, Everard JE: Low-risk gestational trophoblastic neoplasia. Evaluating the need for initial inpatient treatment during low-dose methotrexate chemotherapy. J Reprod Med 53:525, 2008

Chan KK, Huang Y, Tam KF, et al: Single-dose methotrexate regiment in the treatment of low-risk gestational trophoblastic neoplasia. Am J Obstet Gynecol 195:1282, 2006

Chauhan S, Diamond MP, Johns DA: A case of molar ectopic pregnancy. Fertil Steril 81:1140, 2004

Chiniwala NU, Woolf PD, Bruno CP, et al: Thyroid storm caused by a partial hydatidiform mole. Thyroid 18:479, 2008

Cole LA, Khanlian SA, Muller CY: Blood test for placental site trophoblastic tumor and nontrophoblastic malignancy for evaluating patients with low positive human chorionic gonadotropin results. J Reprod Med 53:457, 2008

Cortés-Charry R, Figueira LM, García-Barriola V, et al: Gestational trophoblastic disease in ectopic pregnancy. A case series. J Reprod Med 51:760, 2006

Coukos G, Makrigiannakis A, Chung J, et al: Complete hydatidiform mole. A disease with a changing profile. J Reprod Med 44:698, 1999

Crisp H, Burton JL, Stewart R, et al: Refining the diagnosis of hydatidiform mole: Image ploidy analysis and p57KIP2 immunohistochemistry. Histopathology 43:363, 2003

Darby S, Jolley I, Pennington S, et al: Does chest CT matter in the staging of GTN? Gynecol Oncol 112:155, 2009

Delmis J, Pfeifer D, Ivanisecvic M, et al: Sudden death from trophoblastic embolism in pregnancy. Eur J Obstet Gynecol Reprod Biol 92:225, 2000

Doumplis D, Al-Khatib K, Sieunarine K, et al: A review of the management by hysterectomy of 25 cases of gestational trophoblastic tumors from March 1993 to January 2006. BJOG 114:1168, 2007

Drake RD, Rao GG, McIntire DD, et al: Gestational trophoblastic disease among Hispanic women: A 21-year hospital-based study. Gynecol Oncol 103:81, 2006

Feltmate CM, Genest DR, Wise L, et al: Placental site trophoblastic tumor: A 17-year experience at the New England Trophoblastic Disease Center. Gynecol Oncol 82:415, 2001

FIGO Oncology Committee: FIGO staging for gestational trophoblastic neoplasia 2000. Int J Gynecol Obstet 77:285, 2002

Fukunaga M, Katabuchi H, Nagasaka T, et al: Interobserver and intraobserver variability in the diagnosis of hydatidiform mole. Am J Surg Pathol 29:942, 2005

Garavaglia E, Gentile C, Cavoretto P, et al: Ultrasound imaging after evacuation as an adjunct to beta-hCG monitoring in posthydatidiform molar gestational trophoblastic neoplasia. Am J Obstet Gynecol 200(4):417.e1, 2009

Garner EI, Garrett A, Goldstein DP, et al: Significance of chest computed tomography findings in the evaluation and treatment of persistent gestational trophoblastic neoplasia. J Reprod Med 49:411, 2004

Garrett LA, Garner EIO, Feltmate CM, et al: Subsequent pregnancy outcomes in patients with molar pregnancy and persistent gestational trophoblastic neoplasia. J Reprod Med 53:481, 2008

Genest DR, Ruiz RE, Weremowicz S, et al: Do nontriploid partial hydatidiform moles exist? J Reprod Med 47:363, 2002

Goldstein DP, Berkowitz RS: Prophylactic chemotherapy of complete molar pregnancy. Semin Oncol 22:157, 1995

Golfier F, Raudrant D, Frappart L, et al: First epidemiologic data from the French Trophoblastic Disease Reference Center. Am J Obstet Gynecol 196:172.e1, 2007

Growdon WB, Wolfberg AJ, Feltmate CM, et al: Postevacuation hCG levels and risk of gestational trophoblastic neoplasia among women with partial molar pregnancies. J Reprod Med 51:871, 2006

Growdon WB, Wolfberg AJ, Goldstein DP, et al: Evaluating methotrexate treatment in patients with low-risk postmolar gestational trophoblastic neoplasia. Gynecol Oncol 112:353, 2009

Hancock BW, Tidy JA: Current management of molar pregnancy. J Reprod Med 47:347, 2002

Hankins GD, Wendel GD, Snyder RR, et al: Trophoblastic embolization during molar evacuation: Central hemodynamic observations. Obstet Gynecol 63:368, 1987

Horowitz NS, Goldstein DP, Berkowitz RS: Management of gestational trophoblastic neoplasia. Semin Oncol 36(2):181, 2009

Jauniaux E: Partial moles: From postnatal to prenatal diagnosis. Placenta 20:379, 1999

John J, Greenwold N, Buckley S, et al: A prospective study of ultrasound screening for molar pregnancies in missed miscarriages. Ultrasound Obstet Gynecol 25:493, 2005

Kerkmeijer LG, Massuger LF, Ten Kate-Booij MJ, et al: Earlier diagnosis and serum human chorionic gonadotropin regression in complete hydatidiform moles. Obstet Gynecol 113:326, 2009

Kerkmeijer L, Wielsma S, Bekkers R, et al: Guidelines following hydatidiform mole: A reappraisal. Obstet Gynaecol 46:112, 2006

Kim SJ, Lee C, Kwon SY, et al: Studying changes in the incidence, diagnosis and management of GTD: The South Korean model. J Reprod Med 49:643, 2004

Knowles LM, Drake RD, Ashfaq R, et al: Simplifying the preevacuation testing strategy for patients with molar pregnancy. J Reprod Med 52:685, 2007

Kohorn EI: Dynamic staging and risk factor scoring for gestational trophoblastic disease. Int J Gynecol Cancer 17:1124, 2007

Lavie I, Rao GG, Castrillon DH, et al: Duration of human chorionic gonadotropin surveillance for partial hydatidiform moles. Am J Obstet Gynecol 192:1362, 2005

Lawler SD, Fisher RA, Dent J: A prospective genetic study of complete and partial hydatidiform moles. Am J Obstet Gynecol 164:1270, 1991

Loret de Mola JR, Goldfarb JM: Reproductive performance of patients after gestational trophoblastic disease. Semin Oncol 22:193, 1995

Loukovaara M, Pukkala E, Lehtovirta P, et al: Epidemiology of hydatidiform mole in Finland, 1975 to 2001. Eur J Gynaecol Oncol 26:207, 2005

Lurain JR, Hoekstra AV, Schink J: Results of treatment of patients with gestational trophoblastic neoplasia referred to the Brewer Trophoblastic Disease Center after failure of treatment elsewhere (1979–2006). J Reprod Med 53:535, 2008

Lurain JR, Singh DK, Schink JC: Primary treatment of metastatic high-risk gestational trophoblastic neoplasia with EMA-CO chemotherapy. J Reprod Med 51: 767, 2006a

Lurain JR, Singh DK, Schink JC: Role of surgery in the management of high-risk gestational trophoblastic neoplasia. J Reprod 51:773, 2006b

Macdonald MC, Palmer JE, Hancock BW, et al: Diagnostic challenges in extrauterine epithelioid trophoblastic tumours: A report of two cases. Gynecol Oncol 108(2):452, 2008

Merchant SH, Amin MB, Viswanatha DS, et al: p57KIP2 immunohistochemistry in early molar pregnancies: Emphasis on its complementary role in the differential diagnosis of hydropic abortuses. Hum Pathol 36:180, 2005

Miller DS, Ballon SC, Teng NNH: Gestational trophoblastic diseases. In Brody SA, Ueland K (eds): Endocrine Disorders in Pregnancy. Norwalk, CT, Appleton and Lange, 1989, p 451

Montz FJ, Schlaerth JB, Morrow CP: The natural history of theca lutein cysts. Obstet Gynecol 72:247, 1988

Moodley M, Moodley J: Evaluation of chest x-ray findings to determine metastatic gestational trophoblastic disease according to the proposed new staging system: A case series. J Obstet Gynaecol 24:287, 2004

Moore-Maxwell CA, Robboy SJ: Placental site trophoblastic tumor arising from antecedent molar pregnancy. Gynecol Oncol 92:708, 2004

Niemann I, Petersen LK, Hansen ES, et al: Differences in current clinical features of diploid and triploid hydatidiform mole. BJOG 114:1273, 2007a

Niemann I, Petersen LK, Hansen ES, et al: Predictors of low risk of persistent trophoblastic disease in molar pregnancies. Obstet Gynecol 107:1006, 2006

Niemann I, Sunde L, Petersen LK: Evaluation of the risk of persistent trophoblastic disease after twin pregnancy with diploid hydatidiform mole and coexisting normal fetus. Am J Obstet Gynecol 197:45.e1, 2007b

Novak E, Seah CS: Choriocarcinoma of the uterus. Am J Obstet Gynecol 67:933, 1954

Nugent D, Hassadia A, Everard J, et al: Postpartum choriocarcinoma. Presentation, management and survival. J Reprod Med 51:819, 2006

Numnum MT, Kilgore LC, Conner MG, et al: Fertility sparing therapy in a patient with placental site trophoblastic tumor: A case report. Gynecol Oncol 103:1141, 2006

Palmer JE, Macdonald M, Wells M, et al: Epithelioid trophoblastic tumor. J Reprod Med 53:465, 2008

Palmer JR, Driscoll SG, Rosenberg L, et al: Oral contraceptive use and risk of gestational trophoblastic tumors. J Natl Cancer Inst 91:635, 1999

Paradinas FJ, Fisher RA, Browne P, et al: Diploid hydatidiform moles with fetal red blood cells in molar villi. 1—Pathology, incidence, and prognosis. J Pathol 181:183, 1997

Philipp T, Grillenberger K, Separovic ER, et al: Effects of triploidy on early human development. Prenat Diagn, 24:276, 2004

Schlaerth JB, Morrow CP, Kletzky OA, et al: Prognostic characteristics of serum human chorionic gonadotropin titer regression following molar pregnancy. Obstet Gynecol 58:478, 1981

Schorge JO: Gestational trophoblastic disease. In Schorge JO, Schaffer JI, Halvorson LM, et al (eds), Williams Gynecology. New York, McGraw-Hill, 2008, p 755

Schorge JO, Goldstein DP, Bernstein MR, et al: Recent advances in gestational trophoblastic disease. J Reprod Med 45:692, 2000

Sebire NJ, Foskett M, Fisher RA, et al: Risk of partial and complete hydatidiform molar pregnancy in relation to maternal age. Br J Obstet Gynaecol 109:99, 2002a

Sebire NJ, Foskett M, Fisher RA, et al: Persistent gestational trophoblastic disease is rarely, if ever, derived from non-molar first-trimester miscarriage. Med Hypotheses 64:689, 2005

Sebire NJ, Foskett M, Parainas FJ, et al: Outcome of twin pregnancies with complete hydatidiform mole and healthy co-twin. Lancet 359:2165, 2002b

Seckl MJ, Fisher RA, Salerno G, et al: Choriocarcinoma and partial hydatidiform moles. Lancet 356:36, 2000

Shapter AP, McLellan R: Gestational trophoblastic disease. Obstet Gynecol Clin North Am 28:805, 2001

Smith HO, Wiggins C, Verschraegen CF, et al: Changing trends in gestational trophoblastic disease. J Reprod Med 51:777, 2006

Soper JT: Gestational trophoblastic disease. Obstet Gynecol 108:176, 2006

van Trommel NE, Massuger LF, Verheijen RH, et al: The curative effect of a second curettage in persistent trophoblastic disease: A retrospective cohort survey. Gynecol Oncol 99:6, 2005

Vejerslev LO: Clinical management and diagnostic possibilities in hydatidiform mole with coexistent fetus. Obstet Gynecol Surv 46:577, 1991

Wolf NG, Lage JM: Genetic analysis of gestational trophoblastic disease: A review. Semin Oncol 22:113, 1995

Wolfberg AJ, Berkowitz RS, Goldstein DP, et al: Postevacuation hCG levels and risk of gestational trophoblastic neoplasia in women with complete molar pregnancy. Obstet Gynecol 106:548, 2005

Wolfberg AJ, Feltmate C, Goldstein DP, et al: Low risk of relapse after achieving undetectable hCG levels in women with complete molar pregnancy. Obstet Gynecol 104:551, 2004

Wolfberg AJ, Growdon WB, Feltmate CM, et al: Low risk of relapse after achieving undetectable hCG levels in women with partial molar pregnancy. Obstet Gynecol 108:393, 2006

Zhou Q, Lei XY, Xie Q, et al: Sonographic and Doppler imaging in the diagnosis and treatment of gestational trophoblastic disease: A 12-year experience. J Ultrasound Med 24:15, 2005

CHAPTER 12

Genetics

Genetics is the branch of science that deals with genes, heredity, and the variation of inherited characteristics. *Medical genetics* is the study of the etiology, pathogenesis, and natural history of human diseases that are at least partially genetic in origin. Diagnosis, management, and prevention of such diseases are also part of this field.

Genetic disease is common. Between 2 and 3 percent of newborns have a recognized structural defect, another 3 percent have a defect diagnosed by age 5, and by age 18, another 8 to 10 percent are discovered to have one or more functional or developmental abnormalities. Added to these is the susceptibility to many common diseases that have a genetic basis as well as most cancers, which develop as the result of cumulative mutations. All in all, an astounding two thirds of the population will experience a disease with a genetic component in their lifetimes. Tests available for the prenatal diagnosis of selected genetic diseases and the rationale accompanying their use are described throughout Chapter 13.

The *Human Genome Project,* supported principally by the National Human Genome Research Institute, accomplished complete sequencing of the human genome in 2003. Efforts have since focused on *genomics,* the study of functions and interactions of all genes, to better understand the biology of disease (Burke, 2003; McKusick and Ruddle, 2003). The *Online Mendelian Inheritance in Man—OMIM* was developed in 1985 by the National Library of Medicine in collaboration with Johns Hopkins University. In 1995, it was developed for the World Wide Web by the National Center for Biotechnology Informa-tion. It is an up-to-date compendium of human genes and phe-notypes. As of April 2009, the OMIM listed more than 12,700 unique genes with known sequence. Of these, greater than 12,000 are autosomal dominant or recessive, more than 600 are X- or Y-linked, and 37 are mitochondrial. OMIM has also cata-logued more than 2800 mendelian conditions that either have a known molecular basis or have an identified responsible gene that has been sequenced. And finally, the catalogue has more than 1500 conditions for which the molecular basis remains un-known. In the future, it is likely that consideration of individual genetic background and specific traits and susceptibilities will enhance routine medical care. From the foregoing, it is obvious that knowledge of genetic principles is essential for all clinicians.

CHROMOSOMAL ABNORMALITIES

The 22 pairs of autosomes and one pair of sex chromosomes can be affected by a wide range of numerical and structural ab-normalities that profoundly affect gene expression.

Standard Nomenclature

Karyotypes are reported using nomenclature agreed upon by the genetics community and codified as the International System for Human Cytogenetic Nomenclature (ISCN, 2009). Karyotypic abnormalities fall into two broad cate-gories—those of chromosome *number,* such as *trisomy,* and those of chromosome *structure,* such as a *translocation* or *dele-tion.* Each chromosome has a short arm—the "p" or *petit* arm and a long arm—the "q" arm—named for the next letter in the alphabet. The two arms are separated by the centromere. When reporting a karyotype, the total number of chromo-somes is listed first, corresponding to the number of cen-tromeres present. This is followed by the sex chromosomes—XX or XY, and then by a description of any structural variation or abnormality. Specific abnormalities are indicated

TABLE 12-1. Examples of Karyotype Designations Using the International System for Human Cytogenetic Nomenclature (2009)

Karyotype	Description
46,XY	Normal male chromosome constitution
47,XX,+21	Female with trisomy 21
47,XY,+21/46,XY	Male who is a mosaic of trisomy 21 cells and cells with normal constitution
46,XY,del(4)(p14)	Male with terminal deletion of the short arm of chromosome 4 at band p14
46,XX,dup(5)(p14p15.3)	Female with duplication of the short arm of chromosome 5 from band p14 to band p15.3
45,XY,der(13;14)(q10;q10)	Male with a "balanced" Robertsonian translocation of the long arms of chromosomes 13 and 14; the karyotype now has one normal 13, one normal 14, and the translocation chromosome, thereby reducing the chromosome number by 1 (to 45)
46,XY,t(11;22)(q23;q11.2)	Male with a balanced reciprocal translocation between chromosomes 11 and 22; breakpoints are at 11q23 and 22q11.2
46,XX,inv(3)(p21q13)	Inversion of chromosome 3 that extends from p21 to q13—because it includes the centromere, this is a pericentric inversion
46,X,r(X)(p22.1q27)	Female with one normal X chromosome and one ring X chromosome; the breakpoints indicate that the regions distal to p22.1 and q27 are deleted from the ring
46,X,i(X)(q10)	Female with one normal X chromosome and an isochromosome of the long arm of the X chromosome

Adapted from Jorde and colleagues (2006), courtesy of Dr. Fred Elder.

by standard abbreviations, such as *dup (duplication), del (deletion),* and *t (translocation).* The region or bands of the p or q arms affected are then specifically designated. Some examples of standard nomenclature for writing a karyotype are shown in Table 12-1.

Chromosomal abnormalities figure prominently in assessments of the impact of genetic disease, accounting for 50 percent of embryonic deaths, 5 to 7 percent of fetal losses, 6 to 11 percent of stillbirths and neonatal deaths, and 0.9 percent of live births (Hook, 1992; Jacobs and colleagues, 1992; Tolmie, 1995).

Abnormalities of Chromosome Number

The most easily recognized chromosomal abnormalities are numerical. *Aneuploidy* is inheritance of an extra chromosome—*trisomy,* or loss of a chromosome—*monosomy.* These differ from *polyploidy,* which is characterized by an abnormal number of an entire haploid chromosomal set—for example, triploidy, which is discussed below. The estimated incidence of aneuploidy and other chromosomal abnormalities is shown in Table 12-2.

Autosomal Trisomies

In most cases, trisomy results from meiotic *nondisjunction,* in which chromosomes: (1) fail to pair up, (2) pair up properly but

separate prematurely, or (3) fail to separate. The risk of autosomal trisomy increases with maternal age as shown in Figure 12-1. Oocytes are held suspended in midprophase of meiosis I from birth until ovulation—in some cases for 50 years. Aging is thought to break down chiasmata that keep paired chromosomes aligned. When meiosis is completed at the time of ovulation, nondisjunction causes one gamete to have two copies of the affected chromosome. And if fertilized, trisomy will result. The other gamete receives no copies and is monosomic if fertilized.

Male and female gametes are affected at different frequencies—3 to 4 percent of sperm and 10 to 20 percent of oocytes are aneuploid because of meiotic errors. Although each chromosome pair is equally likely to have a segregation error, only trisomies 21, 18, and 13 can result in a term pregnancy. And many fetuses with these common trisomies will be lost before term. Snijders and colleagues (1999) reported that with trisomy 21, the fetal death rate was 30 percent between 12 and 40 weeks and about 20 percent between 16 and 40 weeks. Other trisomies have severe abnormalities, resulting in even higher rates of pregnancy loss (Fig. 12-2). For example, trisomy 1 has never been reported. Trisomy 16 accounts for 16 percent of all first-trimester losses but is never seen later.

Trisomy 21. In 1866, J. L. H. Down described a group of mentally retarded children with distinctive physical features. Nearly

TABLE 12-2. Frequency and Distribution of Chromosomal Abnormalities

	Frequency (Percent)		
Abnormality	**Abortion**	**Stillborn**	**Liveborn**
Trisomy, all types	25	4	0.3
Sex chromosomal monosomy	8.7	0.1	0.05
Triploidy	6.4	0.2	—
Tetraploidy	2.4	—	—
Structural	2	0.8	0.5
Total	~50	~5	~0.9

Adapted from Hassold and Schwartz (2008), with permission.

100 years later, Lejeune and colleagues (1959) discovered that *Down syndrome* is caused by trisomy 21. The karyotype for trisomy 21, shown in Figure 12-3, occurs overall in 1 in 800 to 1000 newborns. Because it is the most common nonlethal trisomy, it is the focus of most genetic screening and testing protocols (see Chap. 13, p. 292). About 95 percent of Down syndrome cases result from maternal nondisjunction of chromosome 21 to 75 percent during meiosis I and 25 percent during meiosis II. The remaining 5 percent of Down syndrome cases result from mosaicism or a translocation, which is discussed below.

Some typical Down syndrome characteristics in newborns are shown in Figure 12-4. These infants have epicanthal folds with up-slanting palpebral fissures, a flat nasal bridge, a small head with flattened occiput, and marked hypotonia with tongue protrusion. There is frequently loose skin at the nape of the neck, as well as short fingers, a single palmar crease, hypoplasia of the middle phalanx of the fifth finger, and a prominent space or "sandal-toe-gap" between the first and second toes. Associated major abnormalities that may be visualized by sonographic examination include cardiac anomalies, particularly endocardial cushion defects, and gastrointestinal anomalies such as duodenal atresia (see Fig. 16-19, p. 359).

Children with Down syndrome have an increased incidence of leukemia and thyroid disease. Their intelligence quotient (IQ) ranges from 25 to 50, with a few individuals testing higher. Most affected children have social skills averaging 3 to 4 years ahead of their mental age.

Recurrence Risk. With a pregnancy complicated by trisomy 21 from nondisjunction, the woman has an approximate 1-percent risk for any trisomy in a subsequent pregnancy. This pertains until it is exceeded by her age-related risk, after which, her age-related risk predominates. Because of this risk, invasive prenatal diagnosis is offered as discussed in Chapter 13 (p. 299). Parental chromosomal studies are not necessary unless the trisomy was due to an unbalanced translocation. Females with Down syndrome are fertile, and approximately a third of their offspring will have Down syndrome (Scharrer and colleagues, 1975). Down syndrome males have markedly decreased spermatogenesis and are almost always sterile. That said, a few cases

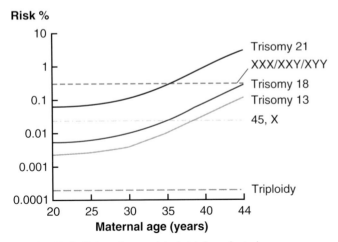

FIGURE 12-1 Maternal age-related risk for selected aneuploidies. (Redrawn from Nicolaides, 2004, with permission.)

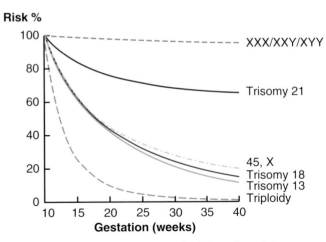

FIGURE 12-2 Gestational-age-related risk for selected chromosomal abnormalities, relative to the risk at 10 weeks' gestation. (Redrawn from Nicolaides, 2004, with permission.)

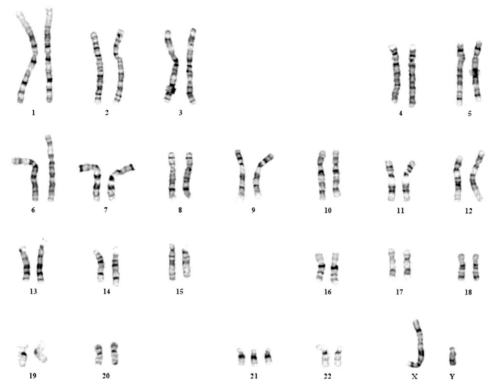

FIGURE 12-3 Abnormal male karyotype with trisomy 21, consistent with Down syndrome (47,XY, + 21). (Used with permission from Dr. Frederick Elder.)

of reproduction have been reported (Pradhan and co-workers, 2006; Zuhlke and co-workers, 1994).

Trisomy 18. Also known as *Edwards syndrome,* trisomy 18 has an overall frequency of 1 in 8000 newborns and is three to four times more common in females. As with other aneuploidies, its incidence is much higher in the first trimester, and 85 percent of fetuses die between 10 weeks and term (Fig. 12-2). Trisomy 18 fetuses usually are growth restricted, with a mean birthweight of 2340 g reported by Snijders and colleagues (1995).

Striking facial features include prominent occiput, rotated and malformed ears, short palpebral fissures, and a small mouth. The hands are often clenched, with the second and fifth fingers overlapping the third and fourth (Jones, 1997). Virtually every organ system can be affected by trisomy 18. Almost 95 percent have cardiac defects—most commonly ventricular or atrial septal defects or patent ductus arteriosus. Other anomalies include horseshoe kidney, radial bone aplasia, hemivertebrae, hernias, diastasis, and imperforate anus. These infants are usually frail and have frequent apneic spells. In a report from the National Center

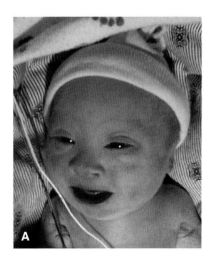
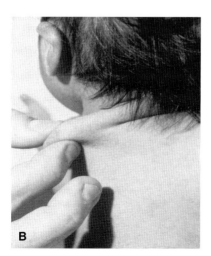
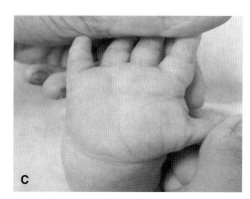

FIGURE 12-4 Trisomy 21—Down Syndrome. **A.** Characteristic facial appearance. **B.** Redundant nuchal tissue. **C.** Single transverse palmar crease. (Photographs courtesy of Dr. Charles P. Read and Dr. Lewis Weber.)

on Birth Defects and Developmental Disabilities, Rasmussen and associates (2003) described a median survival of 14 days. Up to 10 percent survived to 1 year, and rare reports describe profoundly retarded survivors older than 10 years.

If the pregnancy is continued, mode of delivery should be discussed in advance because these fetuses commonly have fetal heart rate abnormalities during labor. Indeed, in years past, more than half of undiagnosed cases were delivered by cesarean for "fetal distress" (Schneider and colleagues, 1981).

Trisomy 13. Known as *Patau syndrome,* trisomy 13 has an incidence of approximately 1 in 20,000 births. Common abnormalities include cardiac defects in 80 to 90 percent and holoprosencephaly in 70 percent. The latter may be accompanied by microcephaly, hypotelorism, and pronounced abnormalities of the orbits, nose, and palate. Affected fetuses also may have abnormal ears, an omphalocele, polycystic kidneys, radial bone aplasia, areas of skin aplasia, and polydactyly. In a review of 70 live-born infants with trisomy 13, Rasmussen and colleagues (2003) found a median survival of 7 days, and up to 10 percent survived to 1 year. Counseling regarding prenatal diagnosis and delivery is approached as described with trisomy 18.

Trisomy 13 is the only aneuploidy that has been associated with an increased risk for preeclampsia. Accompanied by hyperplacentosis, preeclampsia develops in up to half of pregnancies with trisomy 13 carried beyond the second trimester (Tuohy and James, 1992). Interestingly, chromosome 13 contains a gene for an angiogenic protein associated with preeclampsia—*soluble fms-like tyrosine kinase-1—sFlt-1* (see also Chap. 34, p. 714). Bdolah and colleagues (2006) found that mothers carrying trisomy 13 fetuses had increased levels of sFlt-1 early in pregnancy, which may be explained by the extra copy of chromosome 13. These investigators hypothesized that this may be the etiology of preeclampsia in such cases.

Other Trisomies. It is rare to see live-born neonates with other autosomal trisomies, although mosaicism involving a few other autosomal chromosomes has been reported.

Monosomy

Nondisjunction creates an equal number of nullisomic and disomic gametes. There is, however, no recognized association between maternal age and monosomy. This likely is because *autosomal monosomy* is almost universally incompatible with life, and thus monosomic conceptuses die before implantation (Garber and co-workers, 1996). As a rule, missing chromosomal material is more devastating than having extra chromosomal material. The one exception is *monosomy X—Turner syndrome,* which is discussed below.

Polyploidy

This is an abnormal number of complete haploid chromosomal sets. Polyploidy accounts for about 20 percent of abortions and is rarely seen in later pregnancies. Two thirds of *triploidy* cases result from fertilization of one egg by two sperm. The other third are caused by failure of one of the meiotic divisions, leading to a diploid chromosomal complement in either the egg or more frequently, the sperm. The origin of the extra set of chromosomes determines the phenotype. If the extra chromosomes are paternal—*diandric,* the result is usually a partial hydatidiform mole with abnormal fetal structures (see Chap. 11, p. 258). If the extra set of chromosomes is maternal—*digynic,* a fetus and placenta develop, but the fetus is severely growth restricted. Triploid fetuses of either kind are frequently dysmorphic.

If a woman has a triploid fetus that survived past the first trimester, the recurrence risk is 1 to 1.5 percent (Gardner and Sutherland, 1996). Thus, prenatal diagnosis is offered in subsequent pregnancies (see Chap. 13, p. 296).

Tetraploidy always results in 92,XXXX or 92,XXYY, suggesting a postzygotic failure to complete an early cleavage division (Nussbaum and colleagues, 2007). The conceptus invariably succumbs, and the recurrence risk for tetraploidy is minimal.

Sex Chromosome Abnormalities

45,X

Also called *Turner syndrome,* this is the only monosomy compatible with life. It is the most common aneuploidy in abortuses and accounts for 20 percent of first-trimester losses. Its prevalence is about 1 in 5000 liveborns (Sybert and McCauley, 2004).

There are three distinct phenotypes seen with 45,X. At least 98 percent of conceptuses are so abnormal that they abort early. The second phenotype is often identified by abnormal sonographic findings, which include cystic hygromas (see Fig. 16-12, p. 356). These frequently are accompanied by hydrops progressing to fetal demise. The third, and least common, phenotype is found in those born alive. Their features include short stature, broad chest with widely spaced nipples, congenital lymphedema with puffy fingers and toes, low hairline with webbed posterior neck, and minor bone and cartilage abnormalities. Between 30 and 50 percent have a major cardiac malformation, usually aortic coarctation or bicuspid aortic valve. Intelligence is generally in the normal range, although individuals frequently have visual-spatial organization deficits and difficulty with nonverbal problem solving and with interpretation of subtle social cues (Jones, 2006). Over 90 percent also have ovarian dysgenesis and require lifelong hormone replacement beginning just before adolescence.

The reason for the wide range in phenotypes is that approximately half of live-born infants with Turner syndrome have mosaicism. In such cases, there are two or more populations of cells—for example, 45,X/46,XX or 45,X/46,XY (Saenger, 1996; Sybert and McCauley, 2004). Sometimes mosaicism is detected in peripheral blood cells, and other times it is expressed only in tissues that are not routinely tested (Fernandez, 1996; Kim, 1999; Nazarenko, 1999, and all their colleagues). For reasons that are not clear, the missing X chromosome is paternally derived in 80 percent of cases (Cockwell and colleagues, 1991; Hassold and associates, 1991).

47,XXX

Approximately 1 in every 1000 female infants has an additional X chromosome—47,XXX. The extra X is maternally derived in more than 90 percent of cases (Milunsky and Milunsky, 2004). Fetuses with XXX do not have an increased incidence of anomalies, and infants do not have any unusual phenotypic features. There is variability in clinical presentation.

Tall stature is common, pubertal development is normal, and fertility is typically normal, although premature ovarian failure has been reported (Holland, 2001). Mental retardation is not a feature of XXX, but these children are at increased risk for a delay in language development and motor skills (Linden and Bender, 2002).

Females with four or five X chromosomes—48,XXXX or 49,XXXXX—are likely to have physical abnormalities apparent at birth. They exhibit varying degrees of mental retardation, and for both males and females, the IQ drops with each additional X chromosome.

47,XXY

Known as *Klinefelter syndrome*, 47,XXY is the most common sex chromosome abnormality. It occurs in approximately 1 per 600 male infants and results from addition of an extra X chromosome to a normal male karyotype. In approximately 50 percent of cases, the extra X chromosome is maternally derived, and in approximately 50 percent, it is paternal (Milunsky and Milunsky, 2004). There is a slight association with both advanced maternal or paternal age (Jacobs and Hassold, 1995; Lowe and colleagues, 2001).

As with XXX, fetuses with XXY do not have an increased incidence of anomalies, and infants do not have any unusual phenotypic features. Boys are typically tall, but although prepubertal development is normal, they do not virilize and thus require testosterone replacement. They have small testes, are infertile as a result of gonadal dysgenesis, and may develop gynecomastia. Mental retardation is not a feature of XXY. In general, IQ scores are within the normal range, although delays in speech, reading, and motor skills are not uncommon.

47,XYY

This aneuploidy occurs in about 1 in 1000 male infants. The extra Y chromosome is of course paternally derived, and there is no association with paternal age (Milunsky and Milunsky, 2004). The incidence of anomalies is not increased, and there are no unusual phenotypic features. Affected individuals tend to be tall, they have normal puberty, and fertility is unimpaired. Early reports indicating that XYY was associated with criminal or violent behavior suffered from ascertainment bias. Children are at increased risk for speech and neuromotor development problems but not for mental retardation. Linden and Bender (2002) followed a series of children prenatally diagnosed with XYY and found their mean IQ scores to be above average.

Males with more than two Y chromosomes—48,XYYY—or with both additional X and Y chromosomes—48,XXYY or 49,XXXYY—have obvious physical abnormalities and significant mental retardation.

Abnormalities of Chromosome Structure

Structural chromosome abnormalities include deletions, duplications, and microdeletions/microduplications; Robertsonian and reciprocal translocations; isochromosomes; paracentric and pericentric inversions; ring chromosomes; and mosaicism. Each is described using the terminology shown in Table 12-1. In general, identification of a fetus with a structural chromosomal abnormality raises two questions:

1. What phenotypic abnormalities or later developmental abnormalities are associated with this finding?
2. Is parental karyotyping indicated—specifically, are the parents at increased risk to carry this abnormality? If so, what is their risk to have future affected offspring?

Deletions and Duplications

A deletion simply means that a portion of a chromosome is missing. A duplication means that a portion of a chromosome has been included twice. These errors are described by the location of the two break points within the chromosome. Some deletions involve segments of DNA large enough to be seen with standard cytogenetic karyotyping. Common deletions are often referred to by eponyms—one example is *del 5p*, which also is called *cri du chat syndrome*.

Most deletions and duplications occur during meiosis and result from malalignment or mismatching during pairing of homologous chromosomes. If the two chromosomes are not aligned properly, the malaligned segment may be deleted as shown in Figure 12-5. If the mismatch remains and the two chromosomes recombine, the result may be a deletion in one and a duplication in the other. If a deletion or duplication is identified in a fetus or child, the parents should be tested to

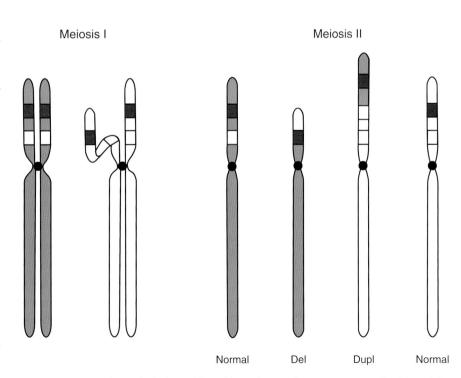

FIGURE 12-5 A mismatch during pairing of homologous chromosomes may lead to a deletion in one chromosome and a duplication in the other. (del = deletion; dup = duplication.)

Meiosis I   Meiosis II

Normal   Del   Dupl   Normal

TABLE 12-3. Some Microdeletion Syndromes Detectable by Fluorescence in-Situ Hybridization

Syndrome	Features	Location
Alagille	Dysmorphic facies, cholestatic jaundice, pulmonic stenosis, butterfly vertebrae, absent deep tendon reflexes, poor school performance	20p11.23–20p12.2
Angelman	Dysmorphic facies—"happy puppet" appearance, mental retardation, ataxia, hypotonia, seizures	15q11.2-q13 (maternal genes)
Cri du chat	Growth restriction, hypotonia, severe mental retardation, abnormal laryngeal development with "cat-like" cry	5p15.2–15.3
Kallmann 1	Hypogonadotropic hypogonadism and anosmia	Xp22.3
Miller-Dieker	Severe neuronal migration abnormalities with lissencephaly, microcephaly, failure to thrive, dysmorphic facies	17p13.3
Prader-Willi	Obesity, hypotonia, mental retardation, short stature, hypogonadotropic hypogonadism, small hands and feet	15q11.2-q13 (paternal genes)
Saethre-Chotzen	Acrocephaly, asymmetry of the skull and face, partial syndactyly of fingers and toes	7p21.1
Smith-Magenis	Dysmorphic facies, speech delay, hearing loss, sleep disturbances, self-destructive behaviors	17p11.2
Velocardiofacial/ DiGeorge	May include conotruncal cardiac defects, cleft palate, velopharyngeal incompetence, thymic and parathyroid abnormalities, learning disability, characteristic facial appearance	22q11.2
Williams-Beuren	Aortic stenosis, peripheral pulmonary arterial stenoses, elfin facies, mental retardation, short stature, infantile hypercalcemia	7q11.23
Wolf-Hirschhorn	Dysmorphic facies, severe mental retardation, polydactyly, cutis aplasia, seizures	4p16.3

Adapted from Online Mendelian Inheritance in Man (2009).

determine if either carries a balanced translocation, as this would significantly increase the recurrence risk.

Microdeletion Syndromes. Some deletions are not large enough to be recognized by traditional karyotyping and thus, molecular cytogenetic techniques are required. *Fluorescence in-situ hybridization (FISH)* may be used to detect microdeletions associated with *contiguous gene syndromes*—deletion of a stretch of DNA that contains multiple genes. These deletions cause clinically recognizable syndromes that may include serious but unrelated phenotypic abnormalities. Deletions can occur in any region, however, several are found more frequently than expected by chance alone. This is thought to result from a greater propensity for certain regions to break. Some microdeletion syndromes detectable by FISH are listed in Table 12-3, and FISH technique is discussed on page 283.

DiGeorge and Shprintzen Phenotypes. Both of these phenotypes result from the same 22q11.2 microdeletion (Driscoll and colleagues, 1993). In a population-based study, Botto and colleagues (2003) reported its prevalence to be about 1 in 6000 among whites, blacks, and Asians, and 1 in 3800 among Hispanics. More than 80 percent of patients had heart defects, and

a third had major extracardiac anomalies. The deletion accounted for about 1 in 70 cases of major heart defects within the general birth population (Botto and colleagues, 2003).

Shprintzen phenotype is also called *velocardiofacial syndrome.* Affected individuals may have cleft palate, velopharyngeal incompetence, prominent nose, a long face with recessed mandible, cardiac defects, learning difficulties, and short stature. By contrast, the DiGeorge phenotype is characterized by thymic hypo- or aplasia, parathyroid hypo- or aplasia, and conotruncal cardiac malformations. Typical facies includes short palpebral fissures, micrognathia with a short philtrum, and ear anomalies. Mental development is usually normal. The 22q11.2 microdeletion also accounts for a large proportion of conotruncal heart defects in individuals who do not have extracardiac features of either DiGeorge or Shprintzen syndromes (Botto and associates, 2003).

How two so obviously disparate phenotypes can be caused by the same microdeletion has intrigued geneticists since their discovery. One hypothesis is that DiGeorge and Shprintzen phenotypes represent two extremes of a spectrum of abnormalities caused by identical deletions. Another possibility is that each syndrome is caused by a different contiguous gene deletion at the 22q11.2 location. If so, then current cytogenetic methods cannot distinguish differences between the two.

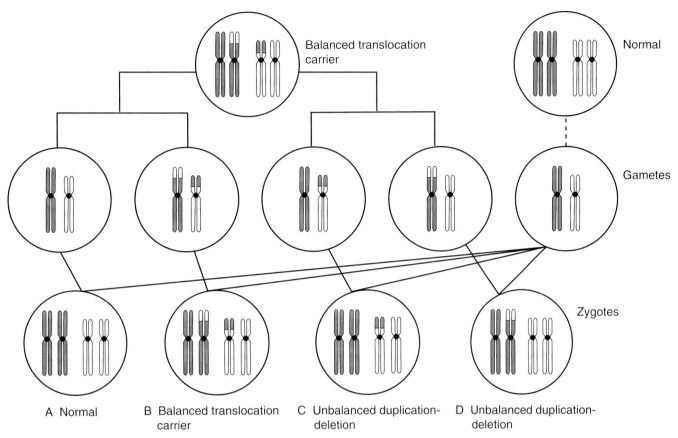

A Normal   B Balanced translocation   C Unbalanced duplication-   D Unbalanced duplication-
carrier   deletion   deletion

FIGURE 12-6 A carrier of a balanced translocation may produce offspring who are also carriers of the balanced rearrangement **(B)**, offspring with unbalanced translocations **(C, D)**, or offspring with normal chromosomal complements **(A)**.

Microduplication Syndromes. Recently, attention has been focused on genomic syndromes that are characterized by duplication of the very DNA regions that are deleted in recognized microdeletion syndromes. For example, Hassed and colleagues (2004) described four family members with features of the velocardiofacial syndrome, each of whom was found to have an *interstitial microduplication* of 22q11.2—the region *deleted* in this syndrome. Microduplications of the deleted regions in both the *Smith-Magenis syndrome* and the *Williams-Beuren syndrome* also produce clinical syndromes very similar to their respective microdeletion counterparts (Potocki and colleagues, 2000; Somerville and associates, 2005).

Chromosomal Translocations

These are DNA rearrangements in which a segment of DNA breaks away from one chromosome and attaches to another chromosome. The rearranged chromosomes are called *derivative (der) chromosomes*. There are two types of translocations— *reciprocal* and *Robertsonian*.

Reciprocal Translocations. Also termed a double-segment translocation, reciprocal translocation is a rearrangement of chromosomal material in which there are breaks in two different chromosomes, and the fragments are exchanged before the breaks are repaired. If no chromosomal material is gained or lost in this process, it is a *balanced translocation*. Although the transposition of chromosomal segments can cause abnormalities due to repositioning of specific genes, in most cases gene function is

not affected and the balanced carrier is phenotypically normal. And offspring who inherit either the two normal chromosomes or the two translocated chromosomes usually have a normal phenotype. Fryns and associates (1992) reported a 6.4-percent incidence of a major anomaly with a balanced translocation— including the 3-percent background risk.

Carriers of a balanced translocation can produce *unbalanced* gametes that result in abnormal offspring. As shown in Figure 12-6, if one of the translocated chromosomes and one of the normal co-chromosomes are included in the oocyte or sperm, the result following fertilization will be monosomy for part of one chromosome and trisomy for part of another. The observed risk of many specific translocations can be estimated by a genetic counselor. In general, translocation carriers identified after the birth of an abnormal child have a 5- to 30-percent risk of having liveborn offspring with unbalanced chromosomes. Carriers identified for other reasons, for example, during an infertility evaluation, have only a 5-percent risk, probably because their gametes are so abnormal that conceptions are nonviable.

Robertsonian Translocations. These result when the long arms of two individual acrocentric chromosomes—for example, chromosomes 13 and 14—fuse at the centromere to form one derivative chromosome. Translocations may involve any of the acrocentric chromosomes—chromosomes 13, 14, 15, 21, and 22. That said, almost all Robertsonian translocations involve chromosome 14 (Levitan, 1988). Fusion at the centromeres results in the loss of one centromere and the *satellite regions* which comprise the short arms of each chromosome. These regions contain only genes coding for ribosomal RNA, which also are present in multiple copies on other acrocentric chromosomes. As long as the fused q arms are intact, the translocation carrier is usually phenotypically normal. Because the number of centromeres determines the chromosome count, the typical carrier of a Robertsonian translocation will have only 45 chromosomes.

Robertsonian carriers have reproductive difficulties. If the fused chromosomes are homologous—from the same chromosome pair—the carrier makes only unbalanced gametes. Each egg or sperm contains either both copies of the translocated chromosome, which would result in trisomy if fertilized, or no copy, which would result in monosomy. If the fused chromosomes are nonhomologous, four of the six possible gametes would be abnormal. Some are nonviable, and the actual observed incidence of abnormal offspring is only 15 percent if the translocation is carried by the mother, and 2 percent if carried by the father.

Robertsonian translocations are common. Their incidence overall is about 1 in 1000 newborns—equal to all other translocations combined. These translocations, however, are not a major cause of miscarriage. They are found in less than 5 percent of couples with recurrent pregnancy loss (Smith and Gaha, 1990). Still, identification of a Robertsonian translocation has tremendous impact on reproductive plans and may have implications for other family members. When a fetus or child is found to have a translocation trisomy, chromosomal studies of both parents should be performed. If neither parent is a carrier and the translocation occurred spontaneously, the recurrence risk is extremely low.

Isochromosomes

These abnormal chromosomes are composed of either two q arms or two p arms of one chromosome fused together. Isochromosomes are thought to arise when the centromere breaks transversely instead of longitudinally during meiosis II or mitosis. They also may result from a meiotic error in a chromosome with a Robertsonian translocation. An isochromosome made of the q arms of an acrocentric chromosome behaves like a homologous Robertsonian translocation because no important genetic material is lost. Conversely, such a carrier could produce only abnormal unbalanced gametes. When an isochromosome involves nonacrocentric chromosomes that have p arms containing functional genetic material, the fusion and abnormal centromere break results in two isochromosomes—one composed of both p arms and one composed of both q arms. It is likely that one of these isochromosomes would be lost during cell division, resulting in the deletion of all the genes located on the lost arm. Thus, a carrier is usually phenotypically abnormal, and produces abnormal gametes. An example is isochromosome X, which causes the full Turner syndrome phenotype.

Chromosomal Inversion

These occur when there are two breaks in the same chromosome, and the intervening genetic material is inverted before the breaks are repaired. Although no genetic material is lost or duplicated, the rearrangement may alter gene function. There are two types—*pericentric* and *paracentric*.

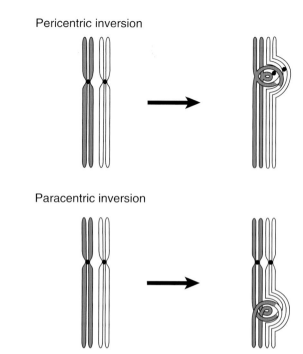

FIGURE 12-7 Mechanism of meiosis in the setting of either **(A)** pericentric inversion (one involving the centromere) or **(B)** paracentric inversion (not involving the centromere). Individuals with pericentric inversions are at increased risk to produce offspring with a duplication/deletion. Those with paracentric inversions are at increased risk for early pregnancy loss.

Pericentric Inversion. This results when the breaks are in each arm of the chromosome so that the inverted chromosome material includes the centromere (Fig. 12-7). Because such inversions cause problems in chromosomal alignment during meiosis, the carrier is at high risk to produce abnormal gametes and thus, abnormal offspring. The risk can be calculated for each specific inversion, but in general, the observed risk is 5 to 10 percent if ascertainment was prompted after the birth of an abnormal child, and 1 to 3 percent if ascertainment was prompted by another reason (Gardner and Sutherland, 1996).

Paracentric Inversion. With a paracentric inversion, the inverted material is from only one arm, and the centromere is not within the inverted segment (Fig. 12-7). The carrier makes either normal balanced gametes or gametes that are so abnormal as to preclude fertilization. Thus, although infertility may be a problem, the risk of abnormal offspring is extremely low.

Ring Chromosome

When there are deletions from both ends of a chromosome, the ends may unite, forming a ring chromosome. If the deletions are substantial, the carrier is phenotypically abnormal. One example is *ring X chromosome,* which may result in the Turner syndrome phenotype.

Telomeres are the physical ends of linear chromosomes. They are specialized nucleoprotein complexes that have important functions in the protection, replication, and stabilization of the chromosomal ends. If only the telomeres are lost, all important genetic material is retained, and the carrier is essentially balanced. The

TABLE 12-4. Mosaicism Encountered in Amnionic Fluid Culture

Type	Prevalence	Description and Significance
Level I	2–3 percent	Single cell with an abnormal karyotype in a single culture—confined to one of several flasks or to one of several colonies on a coverslip. This is usually a cell-culture artifact (pseudomosaicism).
Level II	1 percent	Multiple cells with an abnormal karyotype in a single culture—confined to one of several flasks or to one of several colonies on a coverslip. This is also usually a cell-culture artifact (pseudomosaicism).
Level III	0.1–0.3 percent	Multiple cells in multiple cultures with an abnormal karyotype. Further testing warranted, as a second cell line may be present in the fetus in 60–70 percent of cases (true mosaicism).

ring, however, prevents normal chromosome alignment during meiosis and thus produces abnormal gametes. It also disrupts cell division, which may cause abnormal growth of many tissues and lead to small stature, borderline to moderate mental deficiency, and minor dysmorphisms (Gardner and Sutherland, 1996).

A ring chromosome may form de novo or may be inherited from a carrier parent. In cases of parent-to-child transmission, the mother is the carrier, possibly because a ring chromosome compromises spermatogenesis.

Chromosomal Mosaicism

An individual with mosaicism has two or more cytogenetically distinct cell lines derived from a single zygote. The phenotypic expression of mosaicism depends on many factors, including whether the cytogenetically abnormal cells involve the placenta, the fetus, part of the fetus, or some combination. Mosaicism encountered in cultured amnionic fluid may or may not reflect the actual fetal chromosome complement. Different levels of mosaicism and their clinical significance are presented in Table 12-4. When the abnormal cells involve only a single flask of amnionic fluid, the result is more likely *pseudomosaicism* and explained by cell-culture artifact (Bui and colleagues, 1984; Hsu and Perlis, 1984). When abnormal cells involve multiple cultures, however, true mosaicism is more likely, and further testing of fetal blood or even skin fibroblasts may be warranted. In these cases, a second cell line may be present in 60 to 70 percent of fetuses (Hsu and Perlis, 1984; Worton and Stern, 1984). Consultation with a geneticist may be helpful in evaluating the degree of risk posed by amnionic fluid mosaicism or pseudomosaicism for selected chromosomes, as well as to determine the need for additional testing.

Confined Placental Mosaicism

Studies of chorionic villus sampling have shown that 2 percent of placentas are mosaic, even though the associated fetus is usually normal (Henderson and associates, 1996). Such *confined placental mosaicism* seems to be chromosome specific. Mosaicism involving chromosomes 2, 7, 8, 10, and 12 is usually caused by a mitotic error, whereas that involving chromosomes 9, 16, and 22 is more likely to result from partial correction of a meiotic error (Robinson and colleagues, 1997).

Confined placental mosaicism may have either positive or negative effects. It may play a role in the survival of some cytogenetically abnormal fetuses. For example, trisomy 13 and 18 fetuses who survive to term may do so only because of early "trisomic correction" in some cells that become trophoblasts (Kalousek and co-workers, 1989). Growth restriction may be influenced by *which* chromosome is lost during the trisomic correction. If the fetus retains two normal copies of the chromosome, but both copies are from the same parent, growth may be impaired. This event is referred to as *uniparental disomy* and is discussed later. Conversely, some cytogenetically normal fetuses may have severe growth restriction because the placenta contains a population of aneuploid cells that impair its function (Kalousek and Dill, 1983).

Gonadal mosaicism is confined to the gonads. It likely arises as the result of a mitotic error in cells destined to become the gonad, resulting in a population of abnormal germ cells. Because spermatogonia and oogonia divide throughout fetal life, and spermatogonia continue to divide throughout adulthood, gonadal mosaicism may also be the result of a meiotic error in previously normal dividing germ cells. Gonadal mosaicism may explain de novo autosomal dominant mutations in the offspring of normal parents. This may cause such diseases as achondroplasia or osteogenesis imperfecta as well as X-linked diseases such as Duchenne muscular dystrophy. It also explains the recurrence of such diseases in more than one child in a previously unaffected family. It is because of the potential for gonadal mosaicism that the recurrence risk after the birth of a child with a disease caused by a "new" mutation is approximately 6 percent.

MODES OF INHERITANCE

Monogenic (Mendelian) Inheritance

A monogenic disorder is caused by a mutation or alteration in a single locus or gene in one or both members of a gene pair. Monogenic disorders are also called mendelian to signify that their transmission follows the laws of inheritance proposed by Gregor Mendel. Traditional modes of mendelian inheritance include autosomal dominant, autosomal recessive, X-linked, and Y-linked. Other monogenic patterns of inheritance include mitochondrial inheritance, uniparental disomy, imprinting, and trinucleotide repeat expansion, that is, *anticipation* (Guttmacher and Collins, 2002).

By age 25, about 0.4 percent of the population exhibits an abnormality attributed to a monogenic disorder, and 2 percent will have at least one such disorder during their lifetime.

It is important to emphasize that it is the *phenotype* that is dominant or recessive, not the genes. In some dominant diseases, for example, the normal gene may still be directing the production of normal protein, but the phenotype is determined by protein produced by the abnormal gene. Likewise, the heterozygous carrier of some recessive diseases may produce detectable levels of the abnormal gene product, but he or she does not display features of the disease because the phenotype is directed by the product of the normal co-gene. For example, erythrocytes from carriers of sickle-cell anemia contain about 30 percent hemoglobin S, however, because the remaining hemoglobin is A, these cells do not sickle under normal oxygen conditions.

Although transmission patterns of these diseases are consistent with mendelian inheritance, their phenotypes are strongly influenced by modifying genes and environmental factors. Some common single-gene disorders affecting adults are listed in Table 12-5.

Autosomal Dominant Inheritance

If only one member of a gene pair determines the phenotype, that gene is considered to be dominant. An individual carrying a gene that causes an autosomal dominant disease has a 50-percent chance of passing on the affected gene with each conception. A gene with a dominant mutation generally specifies the phenotype in preference to the normal gene. That said, not all individuals will necessarily manifest an autosomal dominant condition the same way. Factors that affect the phenotype of an autosomal dominant condition include *penetrance, expressivity,* and occasionally, presence of *co-dominant genes.*

Penetrance. This term describes whether or not an autosomal dominant gene is expressed at all. A gene with some kind of recognizable phenotypic expression in all individuals has 100-percent penetrance. If some carriers express the gene but some do not, then penetrance is *incomplete.* This is quantitatively expressed by the ratio of those individuals with any phenotypic characteristics of the gene to the total number of gene carriers. For example, a gene that is expressed in some way in 80 percent of individuals who have that gene is 80-percent penetrant. Incomplete penetrance may explain why some autosomal dominant diseases appear to "skip" generations.

Expressivity. This term refers to the degree to which the phenotypic features are expressed. If all individuals carrying the affected gene do not have identical phenotypes, the gene has *variable expressivity.* Expressivity of a gene can range from complete or severe manifestations to only mild features of the disease. An example of a disease with variable expressivity is neurofibromatosis.

Co-dominant Genes. If alleles in a gene pair are different from each other, but both are expressed in the phenotype, they are considered to be co-dominant. A common example is the human major blood groups—because their genes are co-dominant, both A and B red-cell antigens can be expressed simultaneously in one individual. Another example is the several genes responsible for hemoglobinopathies. The individual with one gene directing pro-

TABLE 12-5. Some Common Single-Gene Disorders

Autosomal Dominant
Achondroplasia
Acute intermittent porphyria
Adult polycystic kidney disease
Antithrombin III deficiency
BRCA1 and BRCA2 breast cancer
Ehlers-Danlos syndrome
Familial adenomatous polyposis
Familial hypercholesterolemia
Hereditary hemorrhagic telangiectasia
Hereditary spherocytosis
Huntington disease
Hypertrophic obstructive cardiomyopathy
Long QT syndrome
Marfan syndrome
Myotonic dystrophy
Neurofibromatosis type 1 and 2
Tuberous sclerosis
von Willebrand disease

Autosomal Recessive
α_1-Antitrypsin deficiency
Congenital adrenal hyperplasia
Cystic fibrosis
Gaucher disease
Hemochromatosis
Homocystinuria
Phenylketonuria
Sickle cell anemia
Tay-Sachs disease
Thalassemia syndromes
Wilson disease

X Linked
Androgen insensitivity syndrome
Chronic granulomatous disease
Color blindness
Fabry disease
Fragile X syndrome
Glucose-6-phosphate deficiency
Hemophilia A and B
Hypophosphatemic rickets
Muscular dystrophy—Duchenne and Becker
Ocular albinism type 1 and 2

duction of sickle hemoglobin and the other directing production of hemoglobin C produces both S and C hemoglobins.

Advanced Paternal Age. Increasing paternal age significantly increases the risk of spontaneous new mutations. These may result in offspring with autosomal dominant disorders, such as neurofibromatosis or achondroplasia (Friedman, 1981). Such new mutations may also result in offspring carrying X-linked conditions, and they may be a factor in early pregnancy loss. The incidence of new autosomal dominant mutations among newborns whose fathers are 40 years old is at least 0.3 percent. There is some evidence that paternal age also may affect the incidence of isolated structural abnormalities (McIntosh and colleagues, 1995).

Advanced paternal age is *not* associated with an increased risk for aneuploidy, probably because aneuploid sperm cannot fertilize an egg.

Autosomal Recessive Inheritance

A trait that is recessive is expressed only when both copies of the gene function identically. Thus, autosomal recessive diseases develop only when both gene copies are abnormal. Phenotypic alterations in gene carriers—that is, *heterozygotes*—usually are undetectable clinically but may be recognized at the biochemical or cellular level. For example, many enzyme deficiency diseases are autosomal recessive. The enzyme level in a carrier will be about half of normal, but because enzymes are made in great excess, this reduction usually does not cause disease. It does, however, represent a phenotypic alteration and can be used for screening purposes. Other recessive conditions do not produce any phenotypic changes in the carrier and can be identified only by molecular methods.

Unless they are screened for a specific disease, such as cystic fibrosis, carriers usually are recognized only after the birth of an affected child or the diagnosis of an affected family member (see Chap. 13, p. 297). A couple whose child has an autosomal recessive disease has a 25-percent recurrence risk with each conception. The likelihood that a normal sibling of an affected child is a carrier of the gene is two out of three. Thus, 1/4 of offspring will be homozygous normal, 2/4 will be heterozygote carriers, and 1/4 will be homozygous abnormal. Another way to look at this is that three of four children will be phenotypically normal, and two of these three will be carriers.

The carrier child will not have affected children, unless his or her partner is also a heterozygous carrier or is homozygous and has the disease. Because genes leading to rare autosomal recessive conditions have a low prevalence in the general population, the chance that a partner will be a gene carrier is low unless the couple is either related or is a member of an at-risk population (American College of Obstetricians and Gynecologists, 2004).

Inborn Errors of Metabolism. Most of these autosomal recessive diseases result from the absence of a crucial enzyme leading to incomplete metabolism of proteins, sugars, or fats. The metabolic intermediates that build up are toxic to a variety of tissues, resulting in mental retardation or other abnormalities.

Phenylketonuria (PKU). This classic example of an autosomal recessive defect results from diminished or absent *phenylalanine hydroxylase* activity. Homozygotes are unable to metabolize phenylalanine to tyrosine. If the diet is unrestricted, incomplete protein metabolism leads to abnormally high phenylalanine levels that cause neurological damage and mental retardation. There also is hypopigmented hair, eyes, and skin because phenylalanine competitively inhibits tyrosine hydrolase, which is essential for melanin production. The disease affects 1 in 10,000 to 15,000 white newborns. There is tremendous geographical and ethnic variation, with incidences ranging from 5 to 190 cases per million.

PKU is notable for two reasons. First, it is one of the few metabolic disorders for which treatment exists. Homozygotes who ingest a phenylalanine-restricted diet can avoid many of the clinical consequences of the disease. Early diagnosis and limitation of dietary phenylalanine beginning in infancy are essential to prevent neurological damage. Accordingly, all states and many countries now mandate newborn screening for PKU, and about 100 cases per million births are identified worldwide. The special diet should be continued indefinitely, as patients who abandon the phenylalanine-restricted diet are reported to have a significantly lower IQ (Koch and co-workers, 2000).

The second reason is that women with PKU are at risk to have otherwise normal heterozygous offspring who sustain damage in utero as a result of being exposed to high phenylalanine concentrations during pregnancy. Phenylalanine readily crosses the placenta, and hyperphenylalaninemia has significant risk for miscarriage and for offspring with mental retardation, microcephaly, low birth weight, and congenital heart defects. For this reason, women with PKU should adhere to the phenylalanine-restricted diet if they are contemplating pregnancy, and then throughout pregnancy (Clarke, 2003). In the Maternal Phenylketonuria Collaborative Study, 572 pregnancies were followed over 18 years. Findings showed that maintenance of serum phenylalanine levels in the 160 to 360 μmol/L—2 to 6 mg/dL—range significantly reduced the risk of fetal abnormalities (Koch and colleagues, 2003; Platt and co-workers, 2000). The study further demonstrated that women who established optimal phenylalanine levels of 120 to 360 μmol/L between 0 and 10 weeks had children with mean IQ in the normal range at age 6 to 7 years (Koch and colleagues, 2003).

Consanguinity. Two individuals are considered consanguineous if they have at least one ancestor in common. First-degree relatives share half of their genes, second-degree relatives share a fourth, and third-degree relatives—cousins—share one eighth. Because of the potential for shared deleterious genes, consanguineous unions are at increased risk to produce children with otherwise rare autosomal recessive diseases. They are also at increased risk to have offspring with multifactorial conditions that are subsequently discussed.

First-cousin marriages, the most frequent consanguineous mating, carry a twofold increased risk over background of abnormal offspring—4 to 6 percent if there is no family history of genetic disease. If one of the partners has a sibling with an autosomal recessive disease, the risk of affected offspring is many times higher than if he or she had chosen an unrelated partner.

Incest is defined as a sexual relationship between first-degree relatives such as parent and child or brother and sister and is universally illegal. Progeny of such unions carry the highest risk of abnormal outcome, and up to 40 percent of offspring are abnormal as a result of both recessive and multifactorial disorders (Friere-Maia, 1984; Nadiri, 1979).

X-Linked and Y-linked Inheritance

Most X-linked diseases are recessive. Some of the best known examples are color blindness, hemophilia A, and Duchenne muscular dystrophy. When a woman carries a gene causing an

X-linked recessive condition, each son has a 50-percent risk of being affected, and each daughter has a 50-percent chance of being a carrier.

Males carrying an X-linked recessive gene are usually affected because they lack a second X chromosome to express the normal dominant gene. When a male has an X-linked disease, none of his sons will be affected because they cannot receive the abnormal X-linked gene from him. Women carrying an X-linked recessive gene are generally unaffected by the disease it causes. In some cases, however, because of skewed *lyonization*—inactivation of one X chromosome in each cell—female carriers may have features of the condition. An example is a woman who has the gene for hemophilia A and who herself has bleeding tendencies (Plug and colleagues, 2006). Similarly, some female carriers of Duchenne muscular dystrophy may develop cardiomyopathy and conduction defects (Politano and colleagues, 1996). Identification of such symptoms may be valuable in caring for the pregnant woman and providing accurate prenatal diagnosis.

X-linked dominant disorders mainly affect females because they tend to be lethal in male offspring. Examples include focal dermal hypoplasia, vitamin D-resistant rickets, and incontinentia pigmenti.

The Y chromosome carries genes important for sex determination and a variety of cellular functions such as spermatogenesis and bone development. Deletion of genes on the long arm results in severe spermatogenic defects, whereas genes at the tip of the short arm are critical for chromosomal pairing during meiosis and for fertility.

Mitochondrial Inheritance

Each human cell contains hundreds of mitochondria, each containing its own genome and associated replication system. In this sense, they behave autonomously. Mitochondria are inherited exclusively from the mother. Human oocytes contain approximately 100,000 mitochondria, but sperm contain only 100 and these are destroyed after fertilization. Each mitochondrion has multiple copies of a 16.5-kb circular DNA molecule that contains 37 unique genes. Mitochondrial DNA encodes peptides required for oxidative phosphorylation, as well as ribosomal and transfer RNAs.

Because mitochondria contain genetic information, their inheritance allows the transmission of genes from mother to offspring without the possibility of recombination. If a mitochondrial mutation occurs, it may segregate into a daughter cell during cell division and thus be propagated. If an oocyte containing largely mutated mitochondrial DNA is fertilized, the offspring may have a mitochondrial disease. Mitochondrial diseases have a characteristic transmission pattern—individuals of both sexes can be affected, but transmission is only through females.

As of April 2009, 26 mitochondrial diseases or conditions with known molecular basis were described in the OMIM website. Examples include myoclonic epilepsy with ragged red fibers (MERRF), Leber optic atrophy, Kearns-Sayre syndrome, Leigh syndrome, and interestingly, susceptibility to both aminoglycoside-induced deafness and chloramphenicol toxicity.

TABLE 12-6. Some Disorders Caused by DNA Triplet Repeat Expansion

Dentatorubral pallidoluysian atrophy
Fragile X syndrome
Friedreich ataxia
Huntington disease
Kennedy disease—spinal bulbar muscular atrophy
Myotonic dystrophy
Spinocerebellar ataxias

DNA Triplet Repeat Expansion—Anticipation

Mendel's first law states that genes are passed unchanged from parent to progeny. Barring the new mutations, this law still applies to many genes or traits. Certain genes, however, are unstable, and their size, and consequently their function, may be altered as they are transmitted from parent to child. This is manifested clinically by *anticipation*, a phenomenon in which disease symptoms seem to be more severe and to appear at an earlier age in each successive generation. Examples include fragile X syndrome and myotonic dystrophy, both of which are caused by expansion of a repeated trinucleotide segment of DNA. Examples of other DNA triplet (trinucleotide) repeat diseases are shown in Table 12-6.

Fragile X Syndrome. This is the most common form of *familial* mental retardation and affects about 1 in 4000 males and 1 in 8000 females (American College of Obstetricians and Gynecologists, 2006). It is an X-linked disorder characterized by mental retardation that is borderline to severe. Males have an average IQ score of 35 to 45, whereas the IQ in females is generally higher (Nelson, 1995). Affected individuals also may have autistic behavior, attention-deficit/hyperactivity disorder—ADHD, as well as speech and language problems. The physical phenotype includes a narrow face with large jaw, long prominent ears, and macroorchidism in postpubertal males.

Fragile X is caused by expansion of a repeated trinucleotide DNA segment—CGG, that is, cytosine-guanine-guanine—at chromosome Xq27. When the CGG number reaches a critical size, the *fragile X mental retardation 1 (FMR1)* gene becomes methylated and thereby inactivated, and thus, *FMR1 protein* is not produced (Migeon, 1993). The number of repeats and the degree of methylation determines whether or not an individual is affected by the syndrome, as well as its severity (Cutillo, 1994). Clinically, four groups have been described:

1. Full mutation—more than 200 repeats
2. Premutation—61 to 200 repeats
3. Intermediate—41 to 60 repeats
4. Unaffected—fewer than 40 repeats

Males who have the full mutation typically have methylation of the FMR1 gene and full expression of the syndrome. In females, expression is variable, due to X-inactivation of the affected X chromosome.

Although individuals with premutations were initially considered to be normal, more recent research has been focused on three

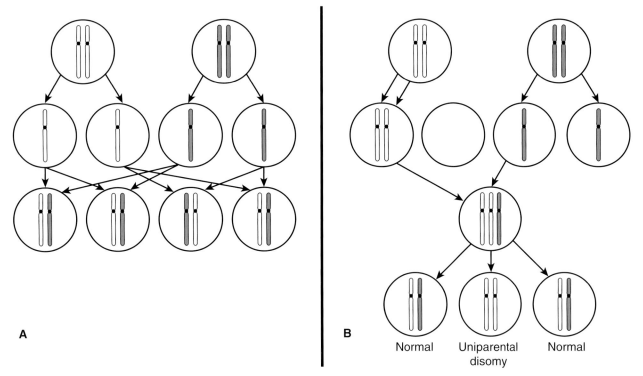

Normal   Uniparental   Normal
                disomy

FIGURE 12-8 *Mechanism of uniparental disomy arising from trisomic "rescue."* **A.** In normal meiosis, one member of each pair of homologous chromosomes is inherited from each parent. **B.** If nondisjunction results in a trisomic conceptus, one homologue is sometimes lost. In a third of cases, loss of one homologue leads to uniparental disomy.

conditions that may manifest: late-onset neurodegenerative disorder with tremor and ataxia, particularly in males; premature ovarian failure in 20 to 30 percent of females; and autism or autistic-like behavior among children (Hagerman and Hagerman, 2004).

Whether a fetus will inherit the full mutation for fragile X syndrome depends on the gender of the transmitting parent and the number of CGG repeats in that parental gene. When transmitted by a male, the number of repeats usually remains stable—the premutation is transmitted without expanding to a full mutation. When transmitted by a female with a premutation, the FMR1 gene can expand during meiosis, particularly if the CGG repeat number exceeds 90. If a woman carries a premutation that increases in size as she transmits it to her offspring, then her child is at risk to have the full fragile X syndrome (Cutillo, 1994). If she carries an intermediate repeat number—41 to 60 repeats—expansion to a full mutation is unlikely.

Prenatal diagnosis of fragile X may be accomplished using Southern blot analysis and polymerase chain reaction to determine the CGG repeat number and the gene methylation status. These tests are discussed subsequently. Amniocentesis is preferred, because gene methylation status may not be reliably assessed from chorionic villi. It is reasonable to refer individuals with a history of mental retardation, developmental delay of unknown etiology, or autism for genetic evaluation because 2 to 6 percent will be determined to have fragile X (Curry and colleagues, 1997; Wenstrom and associates, 1999).

Uniparental Disomy

In this situation, both members of one pair of chromosomes are inherited from the *same* parent, instead of one member being

inherited from *each* parent. Often, uniparental disomy does not have clinical consequences. Some exceptions are when it involves chromosomes 6, 7, 11, 14, or 15. These offspring are at increased risk for an abnormality that results from parent-of-origin differences in gene expression (Shaffer and colleagues, 2001). Although several genetic mechanisms may cause uniparental disomy, the most common is "trisomic rescue" as shown in Figure 12-8. After a nondisjunction event produces a trisomic conceptus, one of the three homologues may be lost. This will result in uniparental disomy for that chromosome in a third of cases.

Isodisomy is the unique situation in which an individual receives two identical copies of one chromosome in a pair from one parent. This mechanism explains some cases of cystic fibrosis, in which only one parent is a carrier but the fetus inherits two copies of the same abnormal chromosome from that parent (Spence and co-workers, 1988; Spotila and colleagues, 1992). It also has been implicated in abnormal growth related to placental mosaicism (Robinson and colleagues, 1997).

Imprinting

This term describes the process by which certain genes are inherited in an inactivated or *transcriptionally silent* state at one of the parental loci in the offspring (Hall, 1990). This type of gene inactivation is determined by the gender of the transmitting parent and may be reversed in the next generation. Imprinting affects gene expression by *epigenetic control*; that is, it changes the phenotype by altering gene expression and not by permanently altering the genotype. When a gene is inherited in an imprinted state, gene function is directed by the co-gene inherited

TABLE 12-7. Some Disorders That Can Involve Imprinting

Disorder	Chromosomal Region	Parental Origin
Angelman	15q11-q13	Maternal
Beckwith-Wiedemann	11p15.5	Paternal
Myoclonic-dystonia	7q21	Maternal
Prader-Willi	15q11-q13	Paternal
Pseudohypoparathyroidism	20q13.2	Depends on type
Russell-Silver syndrome	7p11.2	Maternal

Adapted from Online Mendelian Inheritance in Man (2009).

from the other parent, so imprinting exerts an effect by control-ling the "dosage" of specific genes.

Selected diseases that can involve imprinting are shown in Table 12-7. A useful example includes two very different diseases that may be caused by microdeletion, uniparental disomy, or imprinting for the 15q11-q13 region of DNA:

1. *Prader–Willi syndrome* is characterized by obesity and hyperphagia; short stature; small hands, feet, and external genitalia; and mild mental retardation. In over 70 percent of cases, Prader-Willi is caused by microdeletion or disrup-tion for the *paternal* 15q11-q13. The remainder of cases are due to *maternal* uniparental disomy or due to imprinting—with the *paternal* genes inactive (Online Mendelian Inheri-tance in Man, 2008).

2. *Angelman syndrome* includes normal stature and weight; se-vere mental retardation; absent speech; seizure disorder; ataxia and jerky arm movements; and paroxysms of inappro-priate laughter. In approximately 70 percent of cases, Angel-man syndrome is caused by microdeletion or disruption for the *maternal* 15q11-q13. In 2 percent, the syndrome is caused by *paternal* uniparental disomy, and another 2 to 3 percent are due to imprinting—with the *maternal* genes in-activated (Online Mendelian Inheritance in Man, 2008).

There are a number of other examples of imprinting important to obstetricians. A *complete hydatidiform mole,* which has a pater-nally derived diploid chromosomal complement, is characterized by the abundant growth of placental tissue with no fetal structures (see Chap. 11, p. 257). Conversely, an *ovarian teratoma,* which has a maternally derived diploid chromosomal complement, is charac-terized by the growth of various fetal tissues but no placental struc-tures (Porter and Gilks, 1993). It thus appears that paternal genes are vital for placental development, and maternal genes are essen-tial for fetal development, but both must be present in every cell for normal fetal growth and development.

Multifactorial and Polygenic Inheritance

Polygenic traits are determined by the combined effects of more than one gene, and *multifactorial traits* are determined by multi-ple genes and environmental factors. Most inherited traits are multifactorial or polygenic. Birth defects caused by such inheri-tance are recognized by their tendency to recur in families, but not according to a mendelian inheritance pattern. The empirical

recurrence risk for first-degree relatives usually is quoted as 3 to 5 percent. Multifactorial traits can be classified in several ways, but the most logical is to categorize them as continuously vari-able traits, threshold traits, or complex disorders of adult life.

Continuously Variable Traits

A trait is continuously variable if it has a normal distribution in the general population, such as height or head size. Abnormalcy for a trait is defined as a measurement greater than two standard deviations above or below the population mean. Continuously variable traits are believed to result from the individually small effects of many genes combined with environmental factors. They tend to be less extreme in the offspring of affected individ-uals, because of the statistical principle of regression to the mean.

Threshold Traits

These traits do not appear until a certain threshold is exceeded. Factors that create liability or propensity for the trait are nor-mally distributed, and only individuals at the extreme of this distribution exceed the threshold and have the trait or defect. The phenotypic abnormality is thus an all-or-none phenome-non. Individuals in high-risk families have enough abnormal genes or environmental influences that their liability is close to the threshold, and in certain family members, the threshold is crossed. Cleft lip and palate and pyloric stenosis are examples of threshold traits.

Certain threshold traits have a predilection for one gender, indicating that males and females have a different liability threshold (Fig. 12-9). An example is pyloric stenosis, which is more common in males. If a female has pyloric stenosis, it is likely that she inherited even more abnormal genes or predis-posing factors than are usually necessary to produce pyloric stenosis in males. The recurrence risk for her children or siblings is thus higher than the expected 3 to 5 percent. Her male sib-lings or offspring would have the highest liability, because they not only will inherit more than the usual number of predispos-ing genes but also are the more susceptible sex.

Finally, the recurrence risk of threshold traits is also higher if the defect is severe, again suggesting the presence of more ab-normal genes or influences. For example, the recurrence risk af-ter the birth of a child with bilateral cleft lip and palate is 8 per-cent, compared with only 4 percent for unilateral cleft lip without cleft palate (Melnick and associates, 1980).

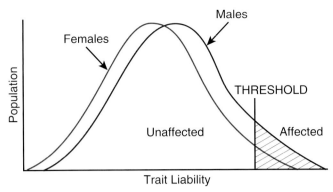

FIGURE 12-9 Schematic example of a threshold trait such as pyloric stenosis that has a predilection for males. Each gender is normally distributed, but at the same threshold, more males than females will develop the condition.

Complex Disorders of Adult Life

These are traits in which many genes determine the susceptibility to environmental factors, with disease resulting from the most unfavorable combination of both. Examples include common disorders such as heart disease or hypertension. These are usually familial and behave as threshold traits, but with environmental influence as an important cofactor. In recent years, many specific gene mutations have been characterized that may cause these common conditions. For example, as of April 2009, the OMIM website listed more than 700 specific entries for "Diabetes." In some diseases, the identity of the associated gene provides a clue to pathogenesis, whereas in others the related gene may simply serve as a disease marker.

Examples of Multifactorial or Polygenic Defects

Various birth defects and common diseases exhibit multifactorial or polygenic inheritance. These diseases have certain inherent characteristics that help to distinguish them from disorders with other modes of inheritance (Table 12-8). When assessing

---

TABLE 12-8. Characteristics of Multifactorial Diseases

There is a genetic contribution
- No mendelian pattern of inheritance
- No evidence of single-gene disorder

Nongenetic factors are also involved in disease causation
- Lack of penetrance despite predisposing genotype
- Monozygotic twins may be discordant

Familial aggregation may be present
- Relatives are more likely to have disease-predisposing alleles

Expression more common among close relatives
- Becomes less common in less closely related relatives, fewer predisposing alleles
- Greater concordance in monozygotic than dizygotic twins

Adapted from Nussbaum and colleagues (2007).

---

risks for a familial multifactorial trait, it is important to consider the degree of relatedness of the affected relative to the fetus, not the parents. An affected first-degree relative—parents or siblings of the fetus—results in a substantial risk increase, but risk declines exponentially with successively more distant relationships. Two examples are cardiac defects and neural-tube defects.

Cardiac Defects. Structural heart anomalies are the most common birth defects worldwide, with an incidence of 8 per 1000 births. More than 100 genes believed to be involved in cardiovascular morphogenesis have been identified, including those directing production of various transcription factors, secreted proteins, extracellular proteins, and protein receptors (Olson, 2006; Weismann and Gelb, 2007). These gene products are likely involved in the development of specific cardiac tissues and structures. For example, folic acid and the methylene tetrahydrofolate reductase (MTHFR) mutation influence the development of cardiac defects (Wenstrom and co-workers, 2001). Importantly, periconceptional folic acid-containing multivitamin supplementation may reduce their incidence (Czeizel, 1998).

Observed recurrence risks for common congenital heart defects are shown in Table 12-9. If the exact nature of the defect is known, the most specific risk should be quoted when counseling. Otherwise, couples can be informed of the empirical risk of having a child with a cardiac defect. This is 5 to 6 percent if the mother has the defect and 2 to 3 percent if the father has the defect (Burn and associates, 1998). Specific defects, which may have recurrence risks four- to sixfold higher, include hypoplastic left heart, bicuspid aortic valve, and aortic coarctation (Lin and Garver, 1988; Nora and Nora, 1988).

Neural-Tube Defects. Isolated, that is, nonsyndromic, neural-tube defects are the second most common congenital structural abnormalities after cardiac defects. Their prenatal diagnosis and sonographic features are described in Chapters 13 (p. 287) and 16 (p. 354), respectively.

Neural-tube defects are classic examples of multifactorial inheritance. Their development is influenced by environment, diet, physiological abnormalities such as hyperthermia or hyperglycemia, teratogen exposure, family history, ethnic origin, fetal gender, amnionic fluid nutrients, and various genes. Neural-tube defects associated with type 1 diabetes mellitus are more likely to be cranial or cervical-thoracic; with valproic acid exposure, lumbosacral defects; and with hyperthermia, anencephaly (Becerra and colleagues, 1990; Hunter, 1984; Lindhout and associates, 1992).

Hibbard and Smithells (1965) postulated more than 40 years ago that abnormal folate metabolism was responsible for many neural-tube malformations. Decades later, a thermolabile variant of the enzyme 5,10-methylene tetrahydrofolate reductase (MTHFR), which plays a key role in folate metabolism, was shown to be associated with neural-tube defects. This enzyme transfers a methyl group from folic acid to convert homocysteine to methionine. One abnormal form of MTHFR carries a mutation at position 677 of its gene and has reduced enzymatic activity. Folic acid supplementation likely works by overcoming this relative enzyme deficiency. Because some defects develop in fetuses with normal 677 C→T alleles, and because

TABLE 12-9. Recurrence Risk (percent) for Congenital Heart Defects If Siblings or Parents Are Affected

	Father	Mother	1 Sibling	2 Siblings
Ventricular septal defects	2	6–10	3	10
Atrial septal defects	1.5	4–4.5	2.5	8
Fallot tetralogy	1.5	2.5	2.5	8
Pulmonary stenosis	2	4–6.5	2	6
Aortic stenosis	3	13–18	2	6
Coarctation	2	4	2	6

Adapted from Nora and Nora (1988), with permission.

folic acid supplementation does not prevent all cases, other unknown genes or factors are presumed to be involved.

Without folic acid supplementation, the empirical recurrence risk after one affected child is 3 to 4 percent, and after two affected children it is 10 percent. With supplementation, the risk after one affected child decreases by 70 percent to less than 1 percent (Czeizel and Dudas, 1992; MRC Vitamin Study Research Group, 1991).

Importantly, prenatal folic acid supplementation in all women may also significantly decrease the incidence of first occurrences of neural-tube defects. Since 1998, the Food and Drug Administration has required fortification of cereal grain products calculated so that the average woman ingests daily an extra 200 μg of folic acid. In the United States, the incidence of neural-tube defects has decreased by a fourth following folic acid fortification (Centers for Disease Control and Prevention, 2004; De Wals and associates, 2003).

GENETIC TESTS

Cytogenetic Analysis

Any tissue containing dividing cells or cells that can be stimulated to divide is suitable for cytogenetic analysis. The dividing cells are arrested in metaphase, and the chromosomes are stained to reveal light and dark bands. The most commonly used technique is Giemsa staining, which yields the G-bands shown in Figure 12-3. The unique banding pattern of each chromosome aids its identification as well as detection of deleted, duplicated, or rearranged segments. The accuracy of cytogenetic analysis increases with the number of bands produced. High-resolution metaphase banding routinely yields 450 to 550 visible bands per haploid chromosome set. Banding of prophase chromosomes generally yields 850 bands.

Because only dividing cells can be evaluated, the rapidity with which results are obtained correlates with the rapidity of cell growth in culture. Fetal blood cells often produce results in 36 to 48 hours. Amnionic fluid, which contains epithelial cells, gastrointestinal mucosal cells, and amniocytes usually yields results in 5 to 14 days. If fetal skin fibroblasts are evaluated postmortem, stimulation of cell growth can be more difficult, and cytogenetic analysis may take 2 to 3 weeks.

Fluorescence In Situ Hybridization (FISH)

This procedure provides a rapid method for determining numerical changes of selected chromosomes and confirming the presence or absence of a specific gene or DNA sequence. FISH is particularly useful for the rapid identification of a specific aneuploidy that may alter clinical management—for example, detection of trisomy 18 or verification of suspected microdeletion or duplication syndromes.

The cells are fixed onto a glass slide, and fluorescently labeled chromosome or gene probes are allowed to hybridize to the fixed chromosomes as shown in Figures 12-10 and 12-11. Each probe is a DNA sequence that is complementary to a unique region of the chromosome or gene being investigated, thus preventing cross reaction with other chromosomes. If the DNA sequence of interest is present, hybridization is detected as a bright signal visible by microscopy. The number of signals indicates the number of chromosomes or genes of that type in the cell being analyzed. FISH does not provide information about the entire chromosomal complement, merely the specific chromosomal region or gene of interest.

The most common prenatal application of FISH involves probing interphase chromosomes with DNA sequences specific to chromosomes 21, 18, 13, X, and Y. Probes are also available to aid identification of a number of microdeletion syndromes. Shown in Figure 12-11 is an example of interphase FISH using α-satellite probes for chromosomes 18, X, and Y, in this case demonstrating three signals for chromosome 18—trisomy 18. In a review by Tepperberg and colleagues (2001) of more than 45,000 cases, the concordance between FISH analysis for these chromosomes and a standard cytogenetic karyotype was 99.8 percent. Whenever a FISH analysis is performed, confirmation with standard cytogenetic evaluation is recommended by the American College of Medical Genetics (2000).

Southern Blotting

Named for its inventor, Edward Southern, this technique allows identification of one or several DNA fragments of interest

Probe creation

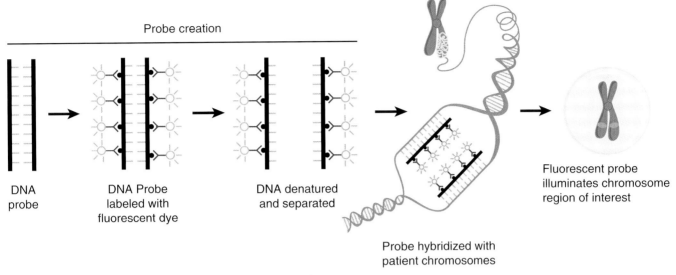

FIGURE 12-10 Steps in fluorescence in situ hybridization (FISH).

from among the million or so typically obtained by enzyme digestion of the entire human genome. As illustrated in Figure 12-12, DNA is digested with a restriction endonuclease enzyme, the resulting fragments are separated from each other using agarose gel electrophoresis, and then the fragments are transferred to a nitrocellulose membrane that binds DNA. Probes homologous for the DNA segment of interest are then hybridized to the DNA already bound to the membrane, with a marker that permits their identification. Basic principles of the Southern blot technique also can be applied to RNA, in

which case it is called *Northern blotting,* and to proteins—*Western blotting.*

Polymerase Chain Reaction (PCR)

PCR enables the rapid synthesis of large amounts of a specific DNA sequence or gene. For this, the entire gene sequence or the sequences at the beginning and end of the gene must be known. PCR involves three steps that are repeated many times. First, double-stranded DNA is denatured by heating. Then, oligonucleotide primers corresponding to the target sequence on each separated DNA strand are added and anneal to either end of the target sequence. Finally, a mixture of nucleotides and heat-stable DNA polymerase is added to elongate the primer sequence, and new complementary strands of DNA are synthesized. The procedure is repeated over and over with exponential amplification of the DNA segment.

Linkage Analysis

If a specific disease-causing gene has not been identified, linkage analysis may be helpful. In such cases, the likelihood that an individual, for example, a fetus, has inherited the abnormal trait can be estimated. Linkage analysis allows the location of different genes to be determined, along with their approximate distances from each other. Limitations of this technique are that it is imprecise, that it depends on family size and availability of family members for testing, and that it relies on the presence of informative markers near the gene.

Specific scattered markers are selected for study, based on the suspected location of the gene responsible for the condition. DNA from each family member is next analyzed to determine whether any of the selected markers are transmitted along with the disease gene. If individuals with the disease have the marker and individuals without the disease do not, the gene causing the disease is said to be linked to the marker, suggesting that they are close to each other on the same chromosome.

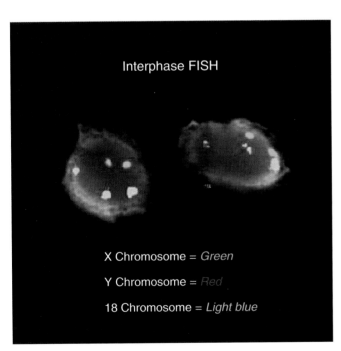

Interphase FISH

X Chromosome = *Green*

Y Chromosome = *Red*

18 Chromosome = *Light blue*

FIGURE 12-11 Interphase fluorescence in situ hybridization (FISH) using α-satellite probes for chromosomes 18, X, and Y. In this case, the three light blue signals, two green signals, and absence of red signals indicates that this is a female fetus with trisomy 18. (Used with permission from Dr. Frederick Elder.)

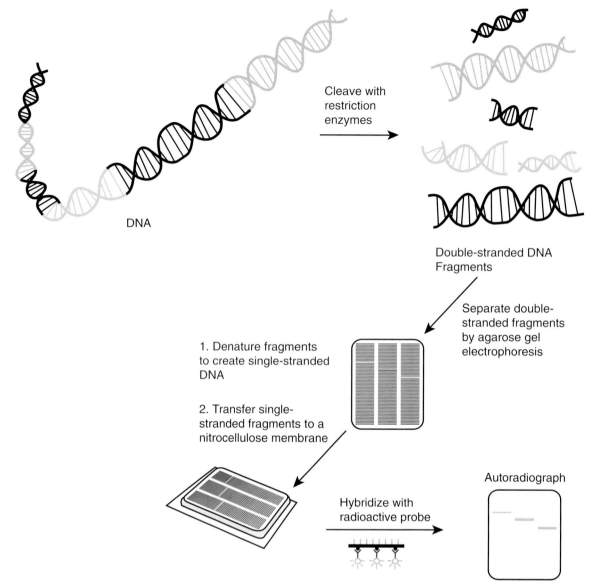

Cleave with restriction enzymes

DNA

Double-stranded DNA Fragments

Separate double-stranded fragments by agarose gel electrophoresis

1. Denature fragments to create single-stranded DNA

2. Transfer single-stranded fragments to a nitrocellulose membrane

Hybridize with radioactive probe

Autoradiograph

FIGURE 12-12 Southern blotting analysis. Genomic DNA is isolated from leukocytes or amniocytes and digested with a restriction enzyme. This procedure yields a series of reproducible fragments that are separated by agarose gel electrophoresis. The separated DNA fragments are then transferred ("blotted") to a nitrocellulose membrane that binds DNA. The membrane is treated with a solution containing a radioactive single-stranded nucleic acid probe, which forms a double-stranded nucleic acid complex at membrane sites when homologous DNA is present. These regions are then detected by autoradiography.

Comparative Genomic Hybridization (CGH) Arrays

CGH arrays take advantage of the principles of PCR and nucleic acid hybridization to screen DNA for many genes or mutations simultaneously. A microarray platform contains DNA fragments of known sequence. DNA from the tested individual is labeled with a fluorescent dye and exposed to the DNA fragments fixed on the chip. Normal control DNA is labeled with a different fluorescent probe. The intensity of fluorescent probe signals is then read by a laser scanner.

There are important limitations of this technology in its present form. It cannot detect balanced structural chromosomal rearrangements such as balanced translocations or inversions. Genetic polymorphisms identified with it may or may not be clinically significant. Although the use of CGH arrays is currently investigational, it is anticipated that this technology will one day revolutionize genetic screening for prenatal diagnosis.

REFERENCES

American College of Medical Genetics: Technical and clinical assessment of fluorescence in situ hybridization: An ACMG/ASHG position statement. I. Technical Considerations. Genet Med 2(6):356, 2000

American College of Obstetricians and Gynecologists: Prenatal and preconceptional carrier screening for genetic diseases in individuals of Eastern European Jewish descent. Committee Opinion No. 298, August 2004

American College of Obstetricians and Gynecologists: Screening for fragile X syndrome. Committee Opinion No. 338, June 2006

Bdolah Y, Palomaki GE, Yaron Y, et al: Circulating angiogenic proteins in trisomy 13. Am J Obstet Gynecol 194:239, 2006

Becerra JE, Khoury MJ, Cordero JF, et al: Diabetes mellitus during pregnancy and the risks for specific birth defects: A population-based case-control study. Pediatrics 85:1, 1990

Botto LD, May K, Fernhoff PM, et al: Population-based study of 22q11.2 deletion: Phenotype, incidence, and contribution to major birth defects in the population. Pediatrics 112:101, 2003

Bui TH, Iselius L, Lindsten J: European collaborative study on prenatal diagnosis: Mosaicism, pseudomosaicism and single abnormal cells in amniotic fluid cultures. Prenat Diagn Spring; 4 Spec No:145, 1984

Burke W: Genomics as a probe for disease biology. N Engl J Med 349:969, 2003

Burn J, Brennan P, Little J, et al: Recurrence risks in offspring of adults with major heart defects: Results from first cohort of British collaborative study. Lancet 351:311, 1998

Centers for Disease Control and Prevention: Spina bifida and anencephaly before and after folic acid mandate—United States, 1995–1996 and 1999–2000. MMWR 53:362, 2004

Clarke JTR: The Maternal Phenylketonuria Project: A summary of progress and challenges for the future. Pediatrics 112:1584, 2003

Cockwell A, MacKenzie M, Youings S, et al: A cytogenetic and molecular study of a series of 45 X fetuses and their parents. J Med Genet 28:151, 1991

Curry CJ, Stevenson RE, Aughton D, et al: Evaluation of mental retardation: Recommendations of a consensus conference. Am J Med Genet 72:468, 1997

Cutillo DM: Fragile X syndrome. Genet Teratol 2:1, 1994

Czeizel AE: Periconceptional folic acid containing multivitamin supplementation. Eur J Obstet Gynecol Reprod Biol 78:151, 1998

Czeizel AE, Dudas I: Prevention of the first occurrence of neural-tube defects by periconceptional vitamin supplementation. N Engl J Med 327:1832, 1992

De Wals P, Rusen ID, Lee NS, et al: Trend in prevalence of neural tube defects in Quebec. Birth Defects Res Part A 67:919, 2003

Driscoll DA, Salvin J, Sellinger B, et al: Prevalence of 22q11 microdeletions in DiGeorge and velocardiofacial syndromes: Implications for genetic counselling and prenatal diagnosis. J Med Genet 30:813, 1993

Fernandez R, Mendez J, Pasaro E: Turner syndrome: A study of chromosomal mosaicism. Hum Genet 98:29, 1996

Friedman HM: Genetic disease in the offspring of older fathers. Obstet Gynecol 57:745, 1981

Friere-Maia N: Effects of consanguineous marriages on morbidity and precocious mortality: Genetic counseling. Am J Med Genet 18:401, 1984

Fryns JP, Kleczkowski A, Kubien E, et al: On the excess of mental retardation and/or congenital malformations in apparently balanced reciprocal translocations. A critical review of the Leuven data. Genet Counsel 2:185, 1992

Garber AP, Schreck R, Carlson DE: Fetal loss. In Rimoin DL, Connor JM, Pyeritz RE (eds): Emery and Rimoin's Principles and Practice of Medical Genetics, 3rd ed. New York, Churchill Livingstone, 1996

Gardner RJM, Sutherland GR: Chromosome Abnormalities and Genetic Counseling, 2nd ed. Oxford Monographs on Medical Genetics No. 29. Oxford, Oxford University Press, 1996

Guttmacher AE, Collins FS: Genomic medicine—A primer (review article). New Engl J Med, 347:1512, 2002

Hagerman PJ, Hagerman RJ: The fragile-X premutation: A maturing perspective. Am J Hum Genet 74:805, 2004

Hall JG: Genomic imprinting: Review and relevance to human diseases. Am J Hum Genet 46:857, 1990

Hassed SH, Hopcus-Niccum D, Zhang L, et al: A new genomic duplication syndrome complementary to the velocardiofacial (22q11 deletion) syndrome. Clin Genet 65:400, 2004

Hassold T, Arnovitz K, Jacobs PA, et al: The parental origin of the missing or additional chromosome in 45,X and 47,XXX females. Birth Defects Orig Artic Ser 26:297, 1991

Hassold TJ, Schwartz S: Chromosome disorders. In Fauci AS, Braunwald E, Kasper DL, et al (eds): Harrison's Internal Medicine, 17th ed. New York, McGraw-Hill, 2008

Henderson KG, Shaw TE, Barrett IJ, et al: Distribution of mosaicism in human placentae. Hum Genet 97:650, 1996

Hibbard ED, Smithells RW: Folic acid metabolism and human embryopathy. Lancet 1:1254, 1965

Holland CM: 47,XXX in an adolescent with premature ovarian failure and autoimmune disease. J Pediatr Adolesc Gynecol 14:77, 2001

Hook EB: Prevalence, risks, and recurrence. In Brock DJH, Rodeck CH, Ferguson-Smith MA (eds): Prenatal Diagnosis and Screening. Edinburgh, Churchill Livingstone, 1992, p 351

Hsu LY, Perlis TE: United States survey on chromosome mosaicism and pseudomosaicism in prenatal diagnosis. Prenat Diagn 4:97, 1984

Hunter AGW: Neural tube defects in Eastern Ontario and Western Quebec: Demography and family data. Am J Med Genet 19:45, 1984

International System for Human Cytogenetic Nomenclature (ISCN): Recommendations for the International Standing Committee on Human Cytogenetics Nomenclature. Shaffer LG, Slovak ML, Campbell LJ (eds). Karger Publishers, 2009

Jacobs PA, Browne C, Gregson N, et al: Estimates of the frequency of chromosome abnormalities detectable in unselected newborns using moderate levels of banding. J Med Genet 29:103, 1992

Jacobs PA, Hassold TJ: The origin of numerical chromosomal abnormalities. Adv Genet 33:101, 1995

Jones KL: Smith's recognizable patterns of human malformation, 6th ed. Philadelphia, Elsevier Saunders, 2006

Jorde LB, Carey JC, Bamshad MJ, et al: Medical Genetics, 3rd edition, Philadelphia, Elsevier-Mosby-Saunders, 2006

Kalousek DK, Barrett IJ, McGillivray BC: Placental mosaicism and intrauterine survival of trisomies 13 and 18. Am J Hum Genet 44:338, 1989

Kalousek DK, Dill FJ: Chromosomal mosaicism confined to the placenta in human conceptions. Science 221:665, 1983

Kim SS, Jung SC, Kim JH, et al: Chromosome abnormalities in a referred population for suspected chromosomal aberrations: A report of 4117 cases. J Korean Med Sci 14:373, 1999

Koch R, Hanley W, Levy H, et al: Maternal phenylketonuria: An international study. Mol Genet Metab 71:233, 2000

Koch R, Hanley W, Levy H, et al: The Maternal Phenylketonuria International Study: 1984-2002. Pediatrics 112:1523, 2003

Lejeune J, Turpin R, Gautier M: Chromosomic diagnosis of mongolism. Arch Fr Pediatr 16:962, 1959

Levitan M: Textbook of Human Genetics, 3rd ed. New York, Oxford University Press, 1988

Lin AE, Garver KL: Genetic counseling for congenital heart defects. J Pediatr 113:1105, 1988

Linden MG, Bender BG: Fifty-one prenatally diagnosed children and adolescents with sex chromosome abnormalities. Am J Med Genet 110:11, 2002

Lindhout D, Omtzigt JGC, Cornel MC: Spectrum of neural tube defects in 34 infants prenatally exposed to antiepileptic drugs. Neurology 42(suppl 5):111, 1992

Lowe X, Eskenazi B, Nelson DO, et al: Frequency of XY sperm increases with age in fathers of boys with Klinefelter syndrome. Am J Hum Genet 69:1046, 2001

McIntosh GC, Olshan AF, Baird PA: Paternal age and the rise of birth defects in offspring. Epidemiology 6:282, 1995

McKusick VA, Ruddle FH: A new discipline, a new name, a new journal. Genomics 1:1, 2003

Melnick M, Bixler D, Fogh-Andersen P: Cleft lip +/- cleft palate: An overview of the literature and an analysis of Danish cases born between 1941 and 1968. Am J Med Genet 6:83, 1980

Migeon BR: Role of DNA methylation in X-inactivation and the fragile X syndrome. Am J Med Genet 47:685, 1993

Milunsky A, Milunsky JM: Genetic counseling: Preconception, prenatal, and perinatal. In Milunsky A (ed), Genetic Disorders of the Fetus: Diagnosis, Prevention, and Treatment, 5th ed. Baltimore and London, Johns Hopkins University Press, 2004

MRC Vitamin Study Research Group: Prevention of neural tube defects: Results of the Medical Research Council Vitamin Study. Lancet 338:131, 1991

Nadiri S: Congenital abnormalities in newborns of consanguineous and nonconsanguineous parents. Obstet Gynecol 53:195, 1979

Nazarenko SA, Timoshevsky VA, Sukhanova NN: High frequency of tissue-specific mosaicism in Turner syndrome patients. Clin Genet 56:59, 1999

Nelson DL: The fragile X syndromes. Sem Cell Biol 6:5, 1995

Nicolaides KH: The 11 to 13+6 Weeks Scan. Fetal Medicine Foundation, London, 2004

Nora JJ, Nora AH: Updates on counseling the family with a first-degree relative with a congenital heart defect. Am J Med Genet 29:137, 1988

Nussbaum RL, McInnes RR, Willard HF: Thompson and Thompson—Genetics in Medicine, 7th ed. Philadelphia, Saunders-Elsevier, 2007

Olson EN: Gene regulatory networks in the evolution and development of the heart. Science 313:1922, 2006

Online Mendelian Inheritance in Man (OMIM). McKusick-Nathans Institute for Genetic Medicine, Johns Hopkins University (Baltimore, MD) and National Center for Biotechnology Information, National Library of Medicine (Bethesda, MD). Available at: http://www.ncbi.nlm.nih.gov/omim/. Accessed April 6, 2009

Platt LD, Koch R, Hanley WB, et al: The international study of pregnancy outcome in women with maternal phenylketonuria: Report of a 12-year study. Am J Obstet Gynecol 182:326, 2000

Plug I, Mauser-Bunschoten EP, Brocker-Vriends AH, et al: Bleeding in carriers of hemophilia. Blood 108:52, 2006

Politano L, Nigro V, Nigro G, et al: Development of cardiomyopathy in female carriers of Duchenne and Becker muscular dystrophy carriers. JAMA 275:1335, 1996

Porter S, Gilks CB: Genomic imprinting: A proposed explanation for the different behaviors of testicular and ovarian germ cell tumors. Med Hypotheses 41:37, 1993

Potocki L, Shaw CJ, Stankiewicz P, et al: Variability in clinical phenotype despite common chromosomal deletion in Smith-Magenis syndrome [del (17)(p11.2p11.2)]. Genet Med 5(6):430, 2003

Potocki L, Chen KS, Park SS, et al: Molecular mechanism for duplication 17p11.2-the homologous recombination reciprocal of the Smith-Magenis microdeletion. Nat Genet 24(1):84, 2000

Pradhan M, Dalal A, Khan F, Agrawal S: Fertility in men with Down syndrome: A case report. Fertil Steril 86:1765, 2006

Rasmussen SA, Wong L-Y, Yang Q, et al: Population-based analyses of mortality in trisomy 13 and trisomy 18. Pediatrics 111:777, 2003

Robinson WP, Barrett IJ, Bernard L, et al: Meiotic origin of trisomy in confined placental mosaicism is correlated with presence of fetal uniparental disomy, high levels of trisomy in trophoblast, and increased risk of fetal intrauterine growth restriction. Am J Hum Genet 60:917, 1997

Saenger P: Turner's syndrome. N Engl J Med 335:1749, 1996

Scharrer S, Stengel-Rutkowski S, Rodewald-Rudescu A, et al: Reproduction in a female patient with Down's syndrome. Case report of a 46,XY child showing slight phenotypical anomalies born to a 47,XX, +21 mother. Humangenetik 26:207, 1975

Schneider AS, Mennuti MT, Zackai EH: High cesarean section rate in trisomy 18 births: A potential indication for late prenatal diagnosis. Am J Obstet Gynecol 140:367, 1981

Shaffer LG, Agan N, Goldberg JD, et al: American College of Medical Genetics Statement on Diagnostic Testing for Uniparental Disomy. Genet Med 3:206, 2001

Smith A, Gaha TJ: Data on families of chromosome translocation carriers ascertained because of habitual spontaneous abortion. Aust N Z J Obstet Gynaecol 30:57, 1990

Snijders RJM, Sebire NJ, Nicolaides KH: Maternal age and gestational age-specific risk for chromosomal defects. Fetal Diagn Ther 10:356, 1995

Snijders RJM, Sundberg K, Holzgreve W, et al: Maternal age- and gestation-specific risk for trisomy 21. Ultrasound Obstet Gynecol 13:167, 1999

Somerville MJ, Mervis CB, Young EJ, et al: Severe expressive-language delay related to duplication of the Williams-Beuren locus. N Engl J Med 353:1694, 2005

Spence JE, Perciaccante RG, Greig FM, et al: Uniparental disomy as a mechanism for human genetic disease. Am J Hum Genet 42:217, 1988

Spotila LD, Sereda L, Prockop DJ: Partial isodisomy for maternal chromosome 7 and short stature in an individual with a mutation at the COLIA2 locus. Am J Hum Genet 51:1396, 1992

Sybert VP, McCauley E: Turner's syndrome. N Engl J Med 351:1227, 2004

Tepperberg J, Pettenati MJ, Rao PN, et al: Prenatal diagnosis using interphase fluorescence in situ hybridization (FISH): 2-year multi-center retrospective study and review of the literature. Prenat Diagn 21(4):293, 2001

Tolmie JL: Chromosome disorders. In Whittle MJ, Connor JM (eds): Prenatal Diagnosis in Obstetric Practice. Oxford, Blackwell Scientific, 1995, p 34

Tuohy JF, James DK: Pre-eclampsia and trisomy 13. Br J Obstet Gynaecol 99:891, 1992

Weismann CG, Gelb BD: The genetics of congenital heart disease: A review of recent developments. Curr Opin Cardiol 22:200, 2007

Wenstrom KD, Descartes M, Franklin J, et al: A five year experience with fragile X screening of high risk gravidas. Am J Obstet Gynecol 181:789, 1999

Wenstrom KD, Johanning GL, Johnston KE, et al: Association of the C677T methylenetetrahydrofolate reductase mutation and elevated homocysteine levels with congenital cardiac malformations. Am J Obstet Gynecol 184:806, 2001

Worton RG, Stern R: A Canadian collaborative study of mosaicism in amniotic fluid cell cultures. Prenat Diagn 4:131, 1984;

Zuhlke C, Thies U, Braulke I, et al: Down syndrome and male fertility: PCR-derived fingerprinting, serological and andrological investigations. Clin Genet 46:324, 1994

CHAPTER 13

Prenatal Diagnosis and Fetal Therapy

The incidence of major abnormalities apparent at birth is 2 to 3 percent. These anomalies cause a significant portion of neonatal deaths, and more than a fourth of all pediatric hospital admissions result from genetic disorders (Lee and colleagues, 2001). *Prenatal diagnosis* is the science of identifying structural or functional abnormalities—birth defects—in the fetus. With this information, clinicians hope to provide appropriate counseling and optimize outcome. In some cases, fetal therapy can be used to improve the intrauterine environment. Therapy may include blood product transfusion, administration of medication transplacentally or via the fetal circulation, laser or radiofrequency ablation of vascular anastomoses, amnioreduction, shunt placement, or more extensive fetal surgery.

ETIOLOGY OF BIRTH DEFECTS

Birth defects can arise in at least three ways. The most common type of structural fetal abnormality is a *malformation*—an intrinsic abnormality "programmed" in development, regardless of whether a precise genetic etiology is known. An example is spina bifida. The second type is a *deformation* caused when a genetically normal fetus develops abnormally because of mechanical forces imposed by the uterine environment. An example is an otherwise normal limb that develops contractures because of prolonged oligohydramnios. The third type is a *disruption*, which is a more severe change in form or function that occurs when genetically normal tissue is modified as the result of a specific insult. An example is damage from an amnionic band causing a cephalocele or limb-reduction abnormality.

Sometimes multiple structural or developmental abnormalities occur together in one individual. A cluster of several anomalies or defects can be a *syndrome*, meaning that all the abnormalities have the same cause—for example, trisomy 18 (see Chap. 12, p. 269). Anomalies also may comprise a *sequence*, meaning that all developed sequentially as result of one initial insult—for example, oligohydramnios leading to pulmonary hypoplasia, limb contractures, and facial deformities. Finally, a group of anomalies may be considered an *association*, in which particular anomalies occur together frequently but do not seem to be linked etiologically—for example, *VATER*, association of vertebral defects, anal atresia, tracheoesophageal fistula with esophageal atresia, and radial dysplasia. It is readily apparent that classification of fetal anomalies can be challenging, and reclassification may be required.

PRENATAL DIAGNOSIS OF NEURAL-TUBE DEFECTS

Neural-Tube Defects (NTDs)

The open neural-tube defects include *anencephaly*, *spina bifida*, *cephalocele*, and other rare spinal fusion (*schisis*) abnormalities. Features of these anomalies are reviewed in Chapter 16 (p. 354). As a class, these defects of neurulation occur in 1.4 to 2 per 1000 pregnancies and are the second most common class of birth defect after cardiac anomalies (American College of Obstetricians and Gynecologists, 2003). In the 1970s, Brock and associates (1972, 1973) observed that pregnancies complicated by a NTD had higher levels of alpha-fetoprotein (AFP) in maternal serum and amnionic fluid. This formed the basis for the first maternal serum screening test for a birth defect.

The results of a landmark trial were reported by Wald and associates (1977), who described the United Kingdom Collaborative Study on Alpha-Fetoprotein in Relation to Neural-Tube Defects. This study demonstrated the efficacy of maternal serum AFP screening for NTDs. Maternal serum AFP concentration at 16 to 18 weeks was found to exceed 2.5 multiples of the median (MoM) in 88 percent of women carrying fetuses with anencephaly and in 79 percent with spina bifida (Wald and co-workers, 1977). These benefits were subsequently confirmed by others and adopted in the United States and Europe by the mid-1980s (Burton, 1983; Haddow, 1983; Milunsky, 1980, and all their co-workers).

Risk Factors for Neural-Tube Defects

Almost 95 percent of NTDs occur in the absence of recognized risk factor or family history—hence the need for routine screening. There are, however, specific risk factors, some of which are listed in Table 13-1. Genetic causes are the largest category, and NTDs are multifactorial disorders (Chap. 12, p. 281). The recurrence risk is approximately 4 percent if a couple has previously had a child with either anencephaly or spina bifida, 5 percent if either parent was born with a NTD, and as high as 10 percent if a couple has two affected children. One etiology for this in some populations is a common mutation in the methylene tetrahydrofolate reductase (MTHFR) gene—677C→T—which leads to impaired homocysteine and folate metabolism and increases the risk for NTDs and probably cardiac malformations (Dalal, 2007; Grandone, 2006; Munoz, 2007, and all their colleagues). NTDs are also a component of more than 80 genetic syndromes, many of which include other fetal anomalies amenable to prenatal diagnosis (Milunsky and Canick, 2004).

Other risk factors for NTD include environmental exposures, such as hyperthermia; certain medications, especially those that disturb folic acid metabolism; and hyperglycemia from insulin-dependent diabetes. Although the exact mechanism by which diabetes causes a NTD is unknown, research in rodents has focused on the role of embryonic hyperglycemia causing increased oxidative metabolism (Loeken, 2005; Zhao and Reece, 2005). In mice, oxidative stress leads to decreased expression of one or more genes involved in neuroepithelial and neural crest development, effectively arresting the process of neural-tube closure.

There are also certain racial/ethnic groups, as well as populations living in high-risk geographical regions, that have an increased incidence of NTDs. For example, the United Kingdom has the highest frequency of NTDs—1 percent, whereas the overall incidence in the United States is only 0.2 percent. Within the U.S., Mexican-born women have an unexplained twofold increased risk (Velie and colleagues, 2006). The frequency of defects in high-risk populations is probably related to both ethnic-genetic background and environmental influences such as diet (see Chap. 12, p. 281).

Many women at increased risk for NTD benefit from taking 4 mg of folic acid daily before conception and through the first trimester (see also Chap. 7, p. 177). These include individuals with one or more prior affected children or if either the pregnant woman or her partner *has* a NTD. Although data are limited,

TABLE 13-1. Some Risk Factors for Neural-Tube Defects

Genetic cause
- Family history—multifactorial inheritance
- MTHFR mutation—677C→T
- Syndromes with autosomal recessive inheritance
  Meckel-Gruber
  Roberts
  Joubert
  Jarcho-Levin
  HARDE—hydrocephalus–agyria–retinal dysplasia–
    encephalocele
- Aneuploidy
  Trisomy 13
  Trisomy 18
  Triploidy

Exposure to certain environmental agents
- Diabetes—hyperglycemia
- Hyperthermia
  Hot tub or sauna
  Fever (controversial)
- Medications
  Valproic acid
  Carbamazepine
  Coumadin
  Aminopterin
  Thalidomide
  Efavirenz

Geographical region—ethnicity, diet, other factor
- United Kingdom
- India
- China
- Egypt
- Mexico
- Southern Appalachian United States

MTHFR = methylene tetrahydrofolate reductase.

folic acid supplementation may not decrease the NTD risk in women with valproic acid exposure, high temperature in the first trimester or hot tub exposure, or diabetes (American College of Obstetricians and Gynecologists, 2003). The role of lower doses of folic acid supplementation to reduce the first occurrence of NTDs in low-risk women is reviewed in Chapter 8, p. 204).

Alpha-Fetoprotein (AFP)

This glycoprotein is synthesized early in gestation by the fetal yolk sac and later by the fetal gastrointestinal tract and liver (see Chap. 4, p. 79). It is the major serum protein in the embryo-fetus and is analogous to albumin. As shown in Figure 13-1, its concentration increases steadily in both fetal serum and amnionic fluid until 13 weeks, after which, levels rapidly decrease. Conversely, AFP is found in steadily increasing quantities in maternal serum after 12 weeks. The normal concentration

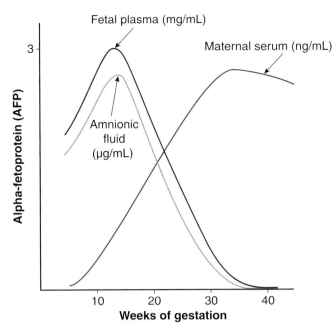

FIGURE 13-1 Diagram of alpha-fetoprotein (AFP) concentration across gestational age in fetal plasma, amnionic fluid, and maternal serum. The scale refers to the fetal plasma level, which is approximately 150 times greater than the amnionic fluid concentration and 50,000 times greater than the maternal serum concentration.

gradient between fetal plasma and maternal serum is on the order of 50,000:1. Fetal body wall defects uncovered by integument, such as NTDs and ventral wall defects, permit AFP to leak into the amnionic fluid, resulting in maternal serum AFP levels that may be dramatically increased.

Maternal Serum AFP Screening

The American College of Obstetricians and Gynecologists (2003) recommends that all women be offered second-trimester AFP screening. This is a component of multiple marker serum screening and is generally offered between 15 and 20 weeks. It should be performed within a protocol that includes quality control, counseling, and follow-up. Maternal serum AFP is measured in nanograms/milliter (ng/mL) and reported as a multiple of the median (MoM) of the unaffected population. Converting the results to MoM normalizes the distribution of AFP levels and permits comparison of results from different laboratories and populations. Using a maternal serum AFP level of 2.0 or 2.5 MoM as the upper limit of normal, most laboratories report a sensitivity—detection rate—of at least 90 percent for anencephaly and 80 percent for spina bifida, at a screen-positive rate of 3 to 5 percent (Milunsky and Canick, 2004). The positive-predictive value, those with AFP elevation who have an affected fetus, is only 2 to 6 percent. Thus, an abnormal screening test

should be followed by counseling and consideration for a diagnostic test. The reason that the detection rate is not higher is explained by the overlap in AFP distributions in affected and unaffected pregnancies as shown in Figure 13-2.

Several factors influence the maternal serum AFP level and are taken into consideration when calculating the AFP MoM:

1. Maternal weight—Because AFP is a fetal product measured in the maternal circulation, accurate maternal weight reflects the volume of distribution
2. Gestational age—Maternal serum AFP concentration increases by approximately 15 percent per week during the second trimester, thus accurate gestational age is essential (Knight and Palomaki, 1992)
3. Race or ethnicity—African-American women have at least 10-percent higher serum AFP concentrations despite having a lower NTD risk (Benn and colleagues, 1997)
4. Diabetes—Women with overt diabetes have a three- to fourfold increased risk for an NTD, but their serum AFP levels may be as much as 20 percent lower than those of nondiabetics (Greene and colleagues, 1988). Although most laboratories continue to adjust for diabetes, it is unclear at this time if this is necessary for those with tight glycemic control (Sancken and Bartels, 2001)
5. Multifetal gestation—A higher screening threshold value is used in twin pregnancies, and the detection rate as well as false-positive rate will depend on the threshold selected (Cuckle and colleagues, 1990). For example, at Parkland Hospital, AFP is considered elevated in a twin pregnancy if greater than 3.5 MoM, but other laboratories use 4.0 or even 5.0 MoM.

One algorithm for evaluating maternal serum AFP is shown in Figure 13-3. With an elevated value, if not already performed, evaluation begins with a standard sonographic examination, which can reliably exclude three common causes of AFP elevation: underestimation of gestational age, multifetal gestation, and fetal demise. Most cases of neural-tube defects may be detected or suspected during this initial examination (Dashe and colleagues, 2006). Once the screening test is confirmed to be abnormal, the patient is offered diagnostic evaluation as subsequently discussed.

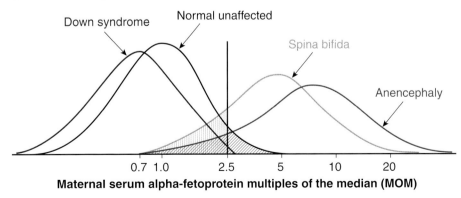

FIGURE 13-2 Maternal serum alpha-fetoprotein distribution for singleton pregnancies at 15 to 20 weeks. The screen cut-off value of 2.5 multiples of the median is expected to result in a false-positive rate of up to 5 percent (*black hatched area*) and false-negative rates of up to 20 percent for spina bifida (*tan hatched area*) and 10 percent for anencephaly (*red hatched area*).

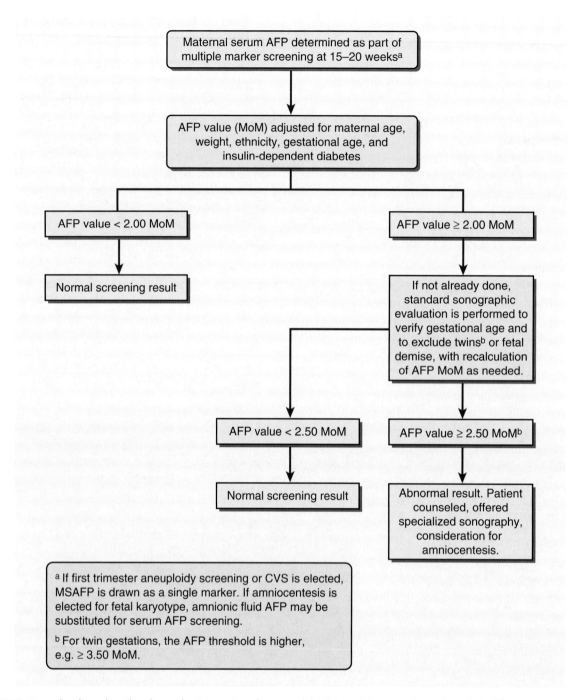

FIGURE 13-3 Example of an algorithm for evaluating maternal serum alpha-fetoprotein screening values (MSAFP).

In addition to NTDs, many other types of birth defects and placental abnormalities are associated with AFP elevation (Table 13-2). The likelihood that a pregnancy is affected by a fetal or placental abnormality increases in proportion to the AFP level. Greater than 40 percent of pregnancies are abnormal if the AFP level is greater than 7 MoM (Reichler and co-workers, 1994).

Evaluation of Maternal Serum AFP Elevation

Women with abnormally elevated serum AFP levels should be referred for genetic counseling and offered a diagnostic test, such as specialized sonographic evaluation and amniocentesis. Those with certain risk factors and normal AFP levels are also offered diagnostic testing. Risk factors include a personal history of NTD, a first-degree relative with NTD, insulin-dependent diabetes, and first-trimester exposure to medication associated with increased NTD risk.

Specialized Sonography. More than two decades ago, Nicolaides and associates (1986) described frontal bone scalloping—the "lemon sign"—shown in Figure 13-4, and bowing of the cerebellum with effacement of the cisterna magna—the "banana sign" shown in Figure 13-5—in second-trimester fetuses with open spina bifida. These investigators also noted that small biparietal diameter and ventriculomegaly frequently were present in such cases. In their review, Watson and associates

TABLE 13-2. Some Conditions Associated with Abnormal Maternal Serum Alpha-Fetoprotein Concentrations

Elevated Levels
Underestimated gestational age
Multifetal gestation
Fetal death
Neural-tube defects
Gastroschisis
Omphalocele
Low maternal weight
Pilonidal cysts
Esophageal or intestinal obstruction
Liver necrosis
Cystic hygroma
Sacrococcygeal teratoma
Urinary obstruction
Renal anomalies—polycystic kidneys, renal agenesis
Congenital nephrosis
Osteogenesis imperfecta
Congenital skin defects
Cloacal exstrophy
Chorioangioma of placenta
Placental abruption
Oligohydramnios
Preeclampsia
Low birthweight
Maternal hepatoma or teratoma

Low Levels
Obesity[a]
Diabetes[a]
Chromosomal trisomies
Gestational trophoblastic disease
Fetal death
Overestimated gestational age

[a]Adjustments in formula used to calculate risk.

(1991) reported that 99 percent of fetuses with open spina bifida had one or more of these findings.

Transverse and sagittal images of the spine are increasingly used to characterize the size and location of spinal defects (see Fig. 16-9, p. 355). Indeed, experienced investigators have described nearly 100-percent detection of open NTDs (Nadel, 1990; Norem, 2005; Sepulveda, 1995, and all their colleagues). Overall NTD risk may be reduced by at least 95 percent when no spine or cranial abnormalities is observed (Hogge, 1989; Morrow, 1991; Van den Hof, 1990, and all their associates).

Many centers now use specialized sonography as the primary method of evaluating an elevated serum AFP. And although amniocentesis is offered, many women no longer opt for it. Importantly, as recommended by the American College of Obstetricians and Gynecologists (2003), women should be counseled regarding risks and benefits of both diagnostic tests, the risk associated with their degree of AFP elevation or with other risk

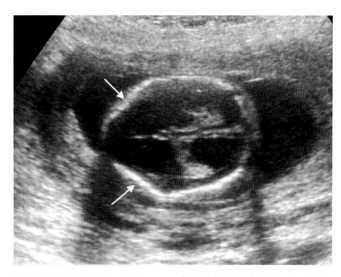

FIGURE 13-4 In this axial image of the fetal head at the level of the lateral ventricles, inward bowing or scalloping of the frontal bones (*arrows*) in the setting of spina bifida produces the "lemon sign." The image also depicts ventriculomegaly.

factors, and the quality and findings of the sonographic examination before making a decision.

Amniocentesis. Until relatively recently, an elevated maternal serum AFP level prompted amniocentesis to determine the amnionic fluid AFP level. If this was also elevated, an assay for acetylcholinesterase was performed, and if positive, it was considered diagnostic of a NTD. The overall sensitivity is about 98 percent for open NTDs, with a false-positive rate of 0.4 percent (Milunsky and Carick, 2004). In one series of nearly 10,000 pregnancies, amniocentesis for AFP and acetylcholinesterase detected 100 percent of anencephaly and open spina bifida cases, with a false-positive rate of only 0.2 percent (Loft and colleagues, 1993). However, other fetal abnormalities may be

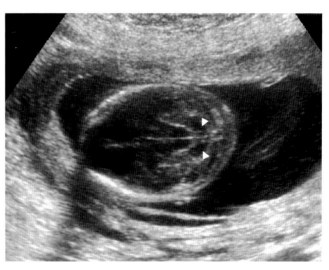

FIGURE 13-5 In this image of the fetal head at the level of the posterior fossa, downward herniation of the cerebellum (*white arrows*), with effacement of the cisterna magna, produces the "banana sign."

associated with both elevated amnionic fluid AFP and positive assay for acetylcholinesterase, including ventral wall defects, esophageal atresia, fetal teratoma, cloacal exstrophy, and skin abnormalities such as epidermolysis bullosa. And although amniocentesis was once considered the "gold standard" for diagnosis of open NTDs, in many centers it has been replaced by, or used in conjunction with, specialized sonography.

If amniocentesis is elected, it is somewhat controversial whether concurrent fetal karyotyping should be offered. If the maternal serum AFP level is elevated, but with *normal* amnionic fluid AFP level and no sonographically detectable fetal anomaly, Thiagarajah and colleagues (1995) found no increased risk for an abnormal karyotype in more than 600 pregnancies. Conversely, Feuchtbaum and associates (1995) reported a 1.1-percent rate of chromosomal anomalies in 8097 pregnancies—twice the expected prevalence. Gonzalez and associates (1996) reported that in women with an elevated serum and an elevated amnionic fluid AFP level but no visible fetal anomaly, the risk for chromosomal abnormalities was fivefold above background risk. The risk for chromosomal defects is higher whenever a NTD is *diagnosed*. In a review of more than 17,000 prenatal diagnosis cases, Hume and associates (1996) observed a aneuploidy rate in the 106 fetuses with an isolated NTD. At Parkland Hospital, amniocentesis for fetal karyotype is offered following sonographic diagnosis of NTD.

Unexplained Maternal Serum AFP Elevation

When no fetal or placental abnormality is detected after a specialized sonographic evaluation, with or without amniocentesis, the AFP elevation is considered *unexplained*. These pregnancies are at increased risk for a variety of subsequent adverse pregnancy outcomes (see Table 13-2). Some include a fetal anomaly not detectable prenatally, fetal-growth restriction, oligohydramnios, placental abruption, preterm membrane rupture, preterm birth, and even fetal death (Katz, 1990; Simpson, 1991; Waller, 1991, and all their associates). Many of these complications are assumed to result from placental damage or dysfunction. However, often neither the etiology nor optimal management is clear. No specific program of maternal or fetal surveillance has been found to favorably affect pregnancy outcomes (Cunningham and Gilstrap, 1991). At Parkland Hospital, prenatal care for these women is not altered unless a specific complication arises. Despite the extensive list of *possible* adverse outcomes, most women with unexplained AFP elevation have normal outcomes.

Management of the Fetus with a Neural-Tube Defect

The optimal timing and method of delivery for an affected fetus are controversial. Reports are retrospective and suffer from various biases. That said, an equal number of reports support cesarean versus vaginal delivery (Bensen and co-workers, 1988; Luthy and colleagues, 1991; Sakala and Andree, 1990). Cesarean delivery might reduce the risk of mechanical trauma and fetal spinal infection. Moreover, delivery can be scheduled to allow precise timing so that the appropriate management team can be assembled. It is best that the delivery time and method

be determined on a case-by-case basis. Fetal surgical repair of meningomyelocele is being studied in a multicenter trial as described on page 306.

PRENATAL DIAGNOSIS OF DOWN SYNDROME AND OTHER ANEUPLOIDIES

Aneuploidy Screening Protocols

As discussed in Chapter 12, the risk of fetal trisomy increases considerably with maternal age and rises most rapidly beginning at age 35 (see Fig. 12-1, p. 268). Traditionally, age 35 has been selected as the threshold for "advanced maternal age." Thus, until the mid-1980s, prenatal diagnostic testing for fetal aneuploidy was offered only to women who would be 35 or older at delivery. After Merkatz and colleagues (1984) reported that pregnancies with fetal Down syndrome were characterized by low maternal serum AFP levels at 15 to 20 weeks, screening for Down syndrome became available to younger women. If the serum screening test identified a younger woman as having the same or greater risk for fetal trisomy 21 as a woman 35 years of age at delivery—about 1 in 375—the result was considered abnormal, and amniocentesis was offered.

During the past two decades, the field of prenatal diagnosis has undergone major advances. The addition of other serum analytes to second-trimester screening has improved trisomy 21 detection by three- to fourfold, and as high as 80 percent with the quadruple marker test (Malone and colleagues, 2005). Perhaps more impressive, comparable results can be achieved at 11 to 14 weeks by using a combination of the fetal nuchal translucency measurement and serum markers (American College of Obstetricians and Gynecologists, 2007b). These screening tests have even greater detection rates in older women because the prevalence of aneuploidy is higher.

Because of these improved detection rates with screening technology, the American College of Obstetricians and Gynecologists (2007b) recommends that *all* women who present for prenatal care before 20 weeks be offered screening. Thus, regardless of age, all women are counseled regarding the differences between screening and diagnostic tests, and they are given the option of invasive diagnostic testing.

There are a number of approaches to fetal aneuploidy screening as shown in Table 13-3. Sonography and maternal serum markers can be used in the first trimester, second trimester, or as a combination of first- and second-trimester tests. Of the screening options currently available, each has its own advantages (Reddy and Mennuti, 2006). The College thus recommends that, depending on available tests, physicians should determine which strategies best meet the needs of their patients. Screening tests such as those presented in Table 13-3 typically have false-positive rates of approximately 5 percent.

Second-Trimester Screening

As discussed above, it was discovered in the 1980s that multiple maternal serum markers could reliably differentiate pregnancies affected by trisomy 18 and 21 from unaffected pregnancies. At 15 to 20 weeks, Down syndrome pregnancies are characterized by an AFP value of approximately 0.7 MoM, human chorionic

TABLE 13-3. Selected Down Syndrome Screening Strategies

Strategy	Analytes	Detection Rate[a] (Percent)
First-trimester screen	NT, PAPP-A, hCG or free β-hCG	79–87
NT (First trimester)	NT	64–70
Triple test	MSAFP, hCG or free β-hCG, uE3	60–69
Quadruple (Quad) test	MSAFP, hCG or free β-hCG, uE3, inh	67–81
Integrated screen	First-trimester screen & Quad test—results withheld until Quad test completed	94–96
Stepwise sequential screen	First-trimester screen & Quad test — 1% offered diagnostic test after first trimester screen — 99% proceed to Quad test, results withheld until Quad test completed	90–95
Contingent sequential screen	First-trimester screen & Quad test — 1% offered diagnostic test after first-trimester screen — 15% proceed to Quad test, results withheld until Quad test completed — 84% have no additional test after first-trimester screen	88–94

[a]Based on a 5-percent positive screen rate.

Free β-hCG = free β-subunit hCG; hCG = human chorionic gonadotropin; inh = dimeric inhibin α; MSAFP = maternal serum alpha-fetoprotein; NT = nuchal translucency; PAPP-A = pregnancy-associated plasma protein-A; uE3 = unconjugated estriol.

Data from Cuckle (2005), Malone (2005), Wapner (2003), and all their colleagues.

gonadotropin (hCG) level of approximately 2.0 MoM, and unconjugated estriol concentration of approximately 0.8 MoM (Bogart, 1987; Merkatz, 1984; Wald, 1988a, b, and all their coworkers). This "triple test" can detect as many as 65 to 70 percent of trisomy 21 cases. The test is also used to screen for trisomy 18, in which all three serum markers are decreased. A fourth marker, dimeric inhibin alpha, was subsequently added to make the quadruple or "quad" test. Values of about 1.8 MoM are reported in Down syndrome pregnancies (Spencer and colleagues, 1996).

Accurate gestational age is essential for expected detection rates when multiple markers are used. For example, Wald and colleagues (1996) found that for a 5-percent false-positive rate, the quad test could detect 70 percent of Down syndrome fetuses in pregnancies dated by last menstrual period alone compared with 77 percent in pregnancies dated by second-trimester sonography. In a large study of pregnancies dated by first-trimester sonography, the sensitivity of the quad test exceeded 80 percent (Malone and colleagues, 2005).

Multiple-marker screening tests are based on a composite likelihood ratio determined by levels of all analytes. The maternal age-related risk is then multiplied by this ratio. A positive screening test indicates *increased risk*, but it is not diagnostic of Down syndrome or another aneuploidy. Conversely, a negative screening test indicates that the *risk* is not increased, but it does not guarantee a normal fetus. After gestational age is confirmed by sonography,

women with a positive screening test result should be offered amniocentesis or fetal blood sampling for fetal karyotyping (American College of Obstetricians and Gynecologists, 2007b).

First-Trimester Screening

This is performed between 11 and 14 weeks. Protocols in current use include maternal serum analyte screening, sonographic evaluation, or a combination of both. Two maternal serum analytes are tested, hCG (or free βhCG) and pregnancy-associated plasma protein A (PAPP-A) (Haddow and associates, 1998). In the first trimester, serum hCG levels are higher, approximately 2.0 MoM, and PAPP-A levels are lower, approximately 0.4 MoM, with a Down syndrome fetus.

The most commonly used first-trimester screening protocol combines these two serum markers with the sonographic *nuchal translucency*, which is discussed below. Using this protocol, Down syndrome detection in large prospective trials ranges from 79 to 87 percent with a false-positive rate of 5 percent (see Table 13-3). These results are comparable to second-trimester quad screening (American College of Obstetricians and Gynecologists, 2007b). All screening tests for fetal aneuploidy are less sensitive in younger women because of lower prevalence rates. Gestational age also affects the accuracy of Down syndrome detection. Testing sensitivity is approximately 5 percent lower if performed at 13 instead of 11 weeks (Malone and colleagues, 2005).

In addition to trisomy 21, other abnormalities are also identified by first-trimester screening. For example, Nicolaides (2004) reported approximately 90-percent sensitivity for trisomies 18 and 13 with a 1-percent false-positive rate. Moreover, results may be abnormal in the setting of a number of structural fetal anomalies (Souka and colleagues 2001). There is also strong association between increasing nuchal translucency, which is detailed subsequently, and fetal cardiac anomalies (Atzei and colleagues, 2005; Simpson and colleagues, 2007). Because of this, the American College of Obstetricians and Gynecologists (2007b) recommends that when the nuchal translucency measurement is 3.5 mm or greater with a normal fetal karyotype, then targeted sonographic examination, fetal echocardiography, or both should be considered.

There are several logistical concerns with first-trimester screening. One is that because fewer than 10 percent of maternal-fetal medicine specialists perform chorionic villus sampling (CVS), the advantage of early diagnosis may be lost. A second is that women still require serum AFP testing in the second trimester. Another is that second-trimester screening will need to be provided for the one third of women who present for prenatal care after the first trimester.

Combined First- and Second-Trimester Screening

As first-trimester screening has become incorporated into practice, research efforts have focused on whether screening efficacy may be even further improved by combining the currently available first- and second-trimester screening technologies. A number of strategies have been developed (see Table 13-3):

1. *Integrated screening* combines results of both the first- and second-trimester screening tests into a single risk. Integrated screening has the highest Down syndrome detection rate—90 to 96 percent. The disadvantage, however, is that results are not available until the second-trimester screening test has been completed. A form of integrated screening, *serum integrated screening,* incorporates the serum markers of the first-trimester screening test with second-trimester quadruple marker testing. It may be offered if nuchal translucency measurement is not available, but it is significantly less effective than when nuchal translucency is included (American College of Obstetricians and Gynecologists, 2007b).

2. *Sequential screening* discloses results of first-trimester screening to women at highest risk, thus allowing them the option of earlier invasive testing. There are two testing strategies in this category:

   a. *Stepwise sequential screening* is for women with first-trimester screen results indicating particular risk for trisomy 21—for example, the top 1 percent, which may include 70 percent of trisomy 21 fetuses. These women are informed and offered invasive testing (Cuckle and associates, 2005). The remainder—about 99 percent—of women undergo second-trimester screening

   b. *Contingent sequential screening* is similar to stepwise screening, except that women are divided into three groups: high, moderate, and low risk. Those at highest

risk—the top 1 percent—are counseled and offered invasive testing. Those at lowest risk—perhaps 80 to 85 percent—have no further testing. Only women at moderate risk—about 15 to 20 percent—go on to second-trimester screening (Cuckle and associates, 2005). This option is the most cost-effective for population screening because second-trimester screening is obviated in up to 85 percent of prenatal patients.

Integrated and sequential screening strategies require coordination between the practitioner and the laboratory to ensure that the second sample is obtained during the appropriate gestational window, sent to the same laboratory, and appropriately linked to first-trimester results. Not all laboratories are currently capable of integrating first- and second-trimester results because of laboratory inexperience or patent issues. Finally, the need for repeated visits at precise times may create special challenges for clinics serving indigent patients.

Sonographic Screening for Aneuploidy

Major Structural Defects

Because 2 to 3 percent of infants are found to have major birth defects, it is not uncommon for a major structural anomaly to be discovered during a routine sonographic examination. An isolated malformation may be multifactorial—for example, a cardiac defect or a NTD, or it may be part of a genetic syndrome. With a syndrome, the fetus may have other abnormalities that are undetectable by sonography but that affect the prognosis—for example, mental retardation. Aneuploidy is often associated with both major anatomical malformations and minor markers, which are discussed below. With few exceptions, the specific aneuploidy risk associated with most major anomalies is high enough to merit offering invasive fetal testing (Table 13-4).

Although the finding of a major anomaly often increases the aneuploidy risk, it should not be assumed that aneuploid fetuses will have a sonographically detectable major malformation. For example, only 25 to 30 percent of second-trimester fetuses with Down syndrome will have a major malformation that can be identified sonographically (Vintzileos and Egan, 1995). Most fetuses with trisomy 18, trisomy 13, and triploidy—aneuploidies much more likely to be lethal in utero—will have major sonographic abnormalities.

Second-Trimester Sonographic Markers—"Soft Signs"

For more than two decades, investigators have recognized that the sonographic detection of aneuploidy, particularly Down syndrome, may be increased by the addition of minor sonographic markers that are collectively referred to as "soft signs." In the absence of aneuploidy or an associated major malformation, these minor abnormalities usually do not significantly affect the fetal prognosis. A host of features seen sonographically in some Down fetuses are listed in Table 13-5. Six of these have been the focus of "genetic sonogram" studies, in which likelihood ratios have been calculated and are shown in Table 13-6. The aneuploidy risk increases with the number of markers identified.

TABLE 13-4. Aneuploidy Risk Associated with Selected Major Fetal Anomalies

Abnormality	Approximate Population Incidence	Aneuploidy Risk (Percent)	Common Aneuploidies[a]
Cystic hygroma	1/300 EU;1/2000 B	50	45X,21,18,13, triploidy
Nonimmune hydrops	1/1500–4000 B	10–20	21,18,13,45X triploidy
Ventriculomegaly	1/700–3000 B	5–25	13,18,21, triploidy
Holoprosencephaly	1/16,000 B	40–60	13,18,22, triploidy
Dandy Walker complex	1/30,000 B	30–50	18,13,21, triploidy
Cleft lip/palate	1/500–3000 B	5–15	18,13
Cardiac defects	5–8/1000 B	10–30	21,18,13,45X, 22q microdeletion
Diaphragmatic hernia	1/2500–10,000 B	5–15	18,13,21
Esophageal atresia	1/2000–4000 B	10–40	18,21
Duodenal atresia	1/5000 B	30–40	21
Jejunal/ileal atresia	1/3000 B	Minimal	None
Gastroschisis	1/2000–5000 B	Minimal	None
Omphalocele	1/4000 B	30–50	18,13,21, triploidy
Clubfoot	1/1000 B	5–20	18,13

[a]Numbers indicate autosomal trisomies except where indicated, for example, 45 X indicates monosomy X.
B = birth; EU = early ultrasound.
Data from Callen (2000); Malone (2005); Nyberg (2003); Santiago-Munoz (2007), and all their colleagues.

The incorporation of minor markers into second-trimester screening protocols has been studied largely in high-risk populations, with reported detection of Down syndrome of 50 to 75 percent (American College of Obstetricians and Gynecologists, 2007b). Unfortunately, at least 10 percent of unaffected pregnancies will have one of these markers, significantly limiting their utility for general population screening (Bromley and colleagues, 2002; Nyberg and Souter, 2003). Their use is also hampered by lack of standard measurement criteria and clear definition of what constitutes an abnormal finding. There are new markers, such as fetal nasal bone hypoplasia, which may hold promise (Gianferrari and colleagues, 2007). Currently the American College of Obstetricians and Gynecologists (2007b) recommends that risk adjustment based on second-trimester sonographic markers be limited to specialized centers and those conducting research in this area.

First-Trimester Nuchal Translucency

The increased sonolucent area at the back of the fetal neck is termed the nuchal translucency, or NT (see Fig. 16-1, p. 351). During the 1990s, it became apparent that this sign was associated with Down syndrome and other aneuploidies, genetic syndromes, and birth defects (Souka and co-workers 1998). Specifically, if the NT measurement is abnormally increased, approximately a third of such fetuses will have a chromosome abnormality, and half of these are Down syndrome (Snijders and colleagues, 1998). Increased NT itself is not a fetal abnormality, but rather a marker or soft sign that confers increased risk. When expressed as a multiple of the median, the NT measurement can be combined with serum analytes to calculate an accurate composite risk.

The major drawbacks are that NT measurement requires specific training, standardization, use of appropriate ultrasound equipment, and ongoing quality assessment. For these reasons, the American College of Obstetricians and Gynecologists (2007b) recommends that this procedure be limited to centers and individuals who can meet these criteria. Used alone, and as shown in Table 13-3, NT measurement will identify 64 to 70 percent of cases of Down syndrome (Malone and colleagues, 2005). When combined with serum markers, and again shown

TABLE 13-5. Second-Trimester Markers or "Soft Signs" Associated with Some Down Syndrome Fetuses

Sonographic Marker

Nuchal fold thickening
Nasal bone absence or hypoplasia
Shortened frontal lobe or brachycephaly
Short ear length
Echogenic intracardiac focus
Echogenic bowel
Mild renal pelvis dilation
Widened iliac angle
Widened gap between first and second toes—"sandal gap"
Clinodactyly, hypoplastic mid-phalanx of fifth digit
Single transverse palmar crease
Short femur
Short humerus

TABLE 13-6. Likelihood Ratios and False-Positive Rates for Isolated Second-Trimester Markers Used in Down Syndrome Screening Protocols

Sonographic Marker	Likelihood Ratio	Prevalence in Unaffected Fetuses (Percent)
Nuchal fold thickening	11–17	0.5
Mild renal pelvis dilation	1.5–1.9	2.0–2.2
Echogenic intracardiac focus	1.4–2.8	3.8–3.9[a]
Echogenic bowel	6.1–6.7	0.5–0.7
Short femur	1.2–2.7	3.7–3.9
Short humerus	5.1–7.5	0.4
Any 1 marker	1.9–2.0	10.0–11.3
2 markers	6.2–9.7	1.6–2.0
3 or more markers	80–115	0.1–0.3

[a]Higher in Asian individuals
Data from Bromley (2002), Nyberg (2001), Smith-Bindman (2001), and all their co-workers.

in Table 13-3, NT measurement detects 79 to 87 percent of Down fetuses. For this reason, the use of NT alone is recommended only in selected circumstances—for example, multifetal gestation (American College of Obstetricians and Gynecologists, 2007b).

Absent Nasal Bone

This first-trimester marker is also much more common in fetuses with Down syndrome. Cicero and colleagues (2001) examined 701 women at high risk for a Down fetus at 11 to 14 weeks. They were studied prior to amniocentesis for advanced maternal age or an abnormal fetal NT measurement. The investigators reported the nasal bone to be absent in 73 percent of Down syndrome fetuses, but in only 0.5 percent of karyotypically normal fetuses. In the FASTER—First and Second Trimester Evaluation of Risk—trial of more than 6300 women of average risk, Malone and colleagues (2005) found *no* case of Down syndrome detected by nasal bone assessment. They concluded that nasal bone sonography is more difficult to accomplish than nuchal translucency. They further concluded that nasal bone assessment is a poor screening tool in the general population.

The Maternal Fetal Medicine Nuchal Translucency Oversight Committee recently recommended that nasal bone assessment should be used only as a secondary or contingency marker in screening protocols (Rosen and associates, 2007). The Committee emphasized that further evaluation in a low-risk population is needed. Further, it recommended that educational and credentialing procedures be established.

FETUSES AT INCREASED RISK FOR GENETIC DISORDERS

Fetal Aneuploidy

At least 8 percent of conceptuses are aneuploid, and these account for 50 percent of first-trimester abortions and 5 to 7 percent of all stillbirths and neonatal deaths. Some factors that

increase the fetal aneuploidy risk are listed in Table 13-7. Individuals with these risk factors may be candidates for genetic counseling. Although maternal age of 35 years or older is no longer used as a threshold to determine who is offered prenatal diagnosis (American College of Obstetricians and Gynecologists, 2007b), it is the most common risk factor for fetal aneuploidy. Risks for Down syndrome and any aneuploidy according to maternal age are presented for singletons in Table 13-8 and for dizygotic twins in Table 13-9. As discussed, many women 35 or older now elect prenatal aneuploidy screening in the first or second trimester, and this modifies their age-related risk. Aneuploidy risks associated with numerical chromosomal abnormalities and chromosomal rearrangements are discussed in Chapter 12 (p. 267).

TABLE 13-7. Women with Increased Risk of Fetal Aneuploidy

Singleton pregnancy and maternal age older than 35 at delivery[a]
Dizygotic twin pregnancy and maternal age older than 31 at delivery
Previous autosomal trisomy birth
Previous 47,XXX or 47,XXY birth
Patient or partner is carrier of chromosome translocation
Patient or partner is carrier of chromosomal inversion
History of triploidy
Some cases of repetitive early pregnancy losses
Patient or partner has aneuploidy
Major fetal structural defect by sonography

[a]All women, regardless of age, should have the option of invasive testing (American College of Obstetricians and Gynecologists, 2007a).

TABLE 13-8. Singleton Gestation—Maternal Age-Related Risk for Down Syndrome and Any Aneuploidy at Midtrimester and at Term

Maternal Age	Down Syndrome		Any Aneuploidy	
	Midtrimester	Term	Midtrimester	Term
35	1/250	1/384	1/132	1/204
36	1/192	1/303	1/105	1/167
37	1/149	1/227	1/83	1/130
38	1/115	1/175	1/65	1/103
39	1/89	1/137	1/53	1/81
40	1/69	1/106	1/40	1/63
41	1/53	1/81	1/31	1/50
42	1/41	1/64	1/25	1/39
43	1/31	1/50	1/19	1/30
44	1/25	1/38	1/15	1/24
45	1/19	1/30	1/12	1/19

From Hook and co-workers (1983), with permission.

Familial Genetic Disease

Couples with a personal or family history of a heritable genetic disorder should be offered genetic counseling and provided with a calculated or estimated risk of having an affected fetus. Specific molecular tests for a variety of common genetic diseases are available. The risk of a disease for which the responsible gene has not been identified can sometimes be estimated by comparing fetal DNA with that of affected and unaffected family members using *restriction fragment length polymorphism analysis.* For some diseases, no laboratory tests may be available. In some cases, risk may be refined by sonographic examination if there are associated fetal structural abnormalities or by determination of fetal gender if the disease is X-linked.

A major issue that remains unresolved for many genetic disorders is phenotype prediction. For example, the disease may have variable penetrance and expressivity, and the phenotype may be modified by pre- and postnatal environmental influences. For these reasons, identification of a specific disease gene often is not sufficient to allow prediction of the phenotype of an affected fetus, even when there have been other affected siblings or family members. The phenotype of cystic fibrosis, for example, can vary widely within a family as discussed subsequently. Phenotype prediction is especially difficult when there are no living affected family members, or when the disease gene is identified as the result of population screening (see Chap. 12, p. 276).

Ethnic Groups at High Risk

Some otherwise rare recessive genes are found with increased frequency in certain racial or ethnic groups—examples are

TABLE 13-9. Dizygotic Twin Pregnancy—Maternal Age-Related Risk for Down Syndrome and Any Aneuploidy at Midtrimester and at Term[a]

Maternal Age	Down Syndrome		Any Aneuploidy	
	Midtrimester	Term	Midtrimester	Term
32	1/256	1/409	1/149	1/171
33	1/206	1/319	1/116	1/151
34	1/160	1/257	1/91	1/126
35	1/125	1/199	1/71	1/101
36	1/98	1/153	1/56	1/82
37	1/77	1/118	1/44	1/67
38	1/60	1/92	1/35	1/54
39	1/47	1/72	1/27	1/44
40	1/37	1/56	1/21	1/35
41	1/29	1/44	1/17	1/28
42	1/23	1/33	1/13	1/22

From Meyers and colleagues (1997), with permission.
[a]Risk applies to one or both fetuses.

TABLE 13-10. Autosomal Recessive Diseases Found with Increased Frequency in Certain Ethnic Groups

Disease	Heritage of Groups at Increased Risk
Hemoglobinopathies	African, Mediterranean, Caribbean, Latin American, Middle Eastern, Southeast Asian
Thalassemia	Mediterranean, Asian
Inborn errors of metabolism: Tay-Sachs disease, Canavan disease, familial dysautonomia, Fanconi anemia group C, Niemann-Pick disease type A, mucolipidosis IV, Bloom syndrome, Gaucher disease	Ashkenazi Jewish
Cystic fibrosis	Caucasians of North European descent, Ashkenazi Jewish, Native American (Zuni, Pueblo)
Tyrosinemia, Morquio syndrome	French Canadian

given in Table 13-10. This increased frequency results from generations who procreate only within their own groups because of religious or ethnic prohibitions or geographical isolation. A phenomenon called the *founder effect* occurs when an otherwise rare gene that is found with increased frequency within a certain population can be traced back to a single family member or small group of ancestors. Some autosomal recessive conditions for which it is recommended that carrier screening be offered to individuals at increased risk are discussed below.

Cystic Fibrosis (CF)

This autosomal recessive disorder is caused by a mutation in a gene on the long arm of chromosome 7 that encodes a protein termed the *cystic fibrosis conductance transmembrane regulator (CFTR)*. More than 1500 mutations in this large gene had been described by the Cystic Fibrosis Consortium (2008) in their database. As shown in Table 13-11, the CF carrier frequency is about 1 in 25 in Caucasian and Native Americans and those of Ashkenazi Jewish (Eastern European) descent, 1 in 46 Hispanic Americans, 1 in 65 African Americans, and 1 in 94 Asian Americans. Some individuals have mild disease or only a single affected organ—for example, chronic pancreatitis (see Chap. 46, p. 1007).

This tremendous range of clinical expression likely reflects both the degree to which protein function is changed by the mutation and the variation in exposure and susceptibility to environmental factors.

Carrier Screening. The American College of Obstetricians and Gynecologists (2007c) recommends that information about CF screening be made available to all couples. The current screening panel contains 23 pan-ethnic CF gene mutations. The panel can detect 88 percent of CF carriers who are Caucasian and 94 percent who are Ashkenazi Jewish. However, the test detects only 72 percent in Hispanic Americans and 65 percent in African Americans. Although a negative screening test result does not preclude the possibility of carrying a less-common mutation, it does reduce the risk substantively from the background rate (see Table 13-11). When both partners are from higher-risk groups, including Caucasian, European, or Ashkenazi Jewish ethnicity, carrier screening should be offered before conception or early in pregnancy. For individuals with a family history of CF, it is helpful to obtain records of the CFTR mutation. If the mutation has not been identified, screening with an expanded mutation panel or even complete CFTR gene sequencing may be necessary.

TABLE 13-11. Cystic Fibrosis Detection and Carrier Rates Before and After Testing

Racial or Ethnic Group	Detection Rate (Percent)	Carrier Rate Before Test	Carrier Risk After Negative Test
Ashkenazi Jewish	94	1/24	~1 in 400
Non-Hispanic Caucasian	88	1/25	~1 in 208
Hispanic American	72	1/46	~1 in 164
African American	65	1/65	~1 in 186
Asian American	49	1/94	~1 in 184

Reprinted, with permission, from Update on carrier screening for cystic fibrosis. ACOG Committee Opinion No. 325. American College of Obstetricians and Gynecologists. Obstet Gynecol 2005; 106:1465–8.

Fetal Testing. If both parents are carriers, the fetus can be tested using chorionic villus sampling or amniocentesis to determine whether it inherited either or both parental mutations. Phenotype prediction is fairly accurate if the mutations are ΔF508 or W1282X. Other mutations are less closely associated with disease symptoms, and thus phenotype prediction and pregnancy management are difficult. Prognosis is determined primarily by pulmonary status, and there is poor genotype–phenotype correlation between these other mutations and the severity of pulmonary disease.

Autosomal Recessive Diseases in Individuals of Ashkenazi Jewish Descent

The carrier rate among individuals of Ashkenazi Jewish heritage is approximately 1 in 30 for Tay-Sachs disease, 1 in 40 for Canavan disease, and 1 in 32 for familial dysautonomia. Fortunately, the detection rate of screening tests for each is at least 98 percent in this population. Because of their relatively high prevalence and consistently severe and predictable phenotype, the American College of Obstetricians and Gynecologists (2008) recommends that carrier screening for these three conditions be offered to Ashkenazi Jewish individuals, either before conception or during early pregnancy (see Chap. 7, p. 178). There are a number of other autosomal recessive diseases that are also more common in Ashkenazi Jews and are amenable to carrier screening, with detection rates of at least 95 percent (American College of Obstetricians and Gynecologists, 2008). These include Fanconi anemia group C, Niemann-Pick disease type A, mucolipidosis IV, Bloom syndrome, and Gaucher disease. Patient education materials can be made available so that those who are interested can request additional information or carrier screening if desired.

DIAGNOSTIC TECHNIQUES

Second-Trimester Amniocentesis

Amniocentesis for genetic diagnosis usually is performed between 15 and 20 weeks. In the United States, it is the procedure most commonly used to diagnose fetal aneuploidy and other genetic disorders. The safety of amniocentesis has been confirmed in several multicenter studies (Canadian Early and Mid-Trimester Amniocentesis Trial Group, 1998; NICHD National Registry for Amniocentesis Study Group, 1976). As shown in Figure 13-6, sonographic guidance is used to pass a 20- to 22-gauge spinal needle into the amnionic sac while avoiding the placenta, umbilical cord, and fetus. Because the initial 1 or 2 mL of fluid aspirate may be contaminated with maternal cells, it is either discarded or used for amnionic fluid AFP testing. Another approximately 20 mL of fluid is then collected for fetal karyotyping, and the needle is removed. Sonographically the uterine puncture site is observed for bleeding, and fetal cardiac motion is documented at the end of the procedure.

Complications are infrequent and include transient vaginal spotting or amnionic fluid leakage in 1 to 2 percent and chorioamnionitis in less than 0.1 percent. Needle injuries to the

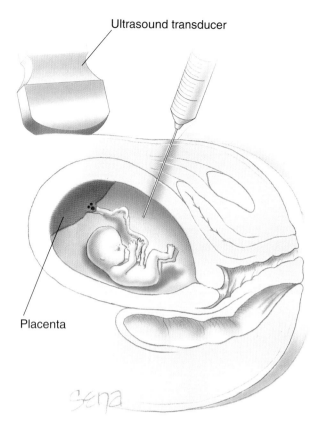

FIGURE 13-6 Amniocentesis.

fetus are rare. Fetal cells obtained during amniocentesis rarely fail to grow in culture. However, this is more likely if the fetus is abnormal (Persutte and Lenke, 1995). Digital PCR of uncultured amniocytes and chorionic villous tissue provides rapid detection of aneuploidy and may prove promising for expanded clinical use (Fan and associates, 2009).

Although early studies reported a fetal loss of about 0.5 percent, a large trial involving 35,003 women cited the procedure-related fetal loss rate to be 0.06 percent (Eddleman and colleagues, 2006). Based on recent studies, the American College of Obstetricians and Gynecologists (2007a) concluded that the procedure-related loss is approximately 1 in 300 to 500. Some losses are unrelated to amniocentesis but instead due to preexisting abnormalities such as placental abruption, abnormal placental implantation, fetal anomalies, uterine anomalies, and infection. Wenstrom and colleagues (1996) analyzed 66 fetal deaths following nearly 12,000 second-trimester amniocenteses and found that 12 percent were caused by preexisting intrauterine infection. A number of other postprocedural deaths have no apparent etiology.

Early Amniocentesis

These procedures are performed between 11 and 14 weeks. For a number of reasons, early amniocentesis is less satisfactory than standard second-trimester amniocentesis. The technique is the same as for traditional amniocentesis, although puncture of the sac may be more challenging due to lack of membrane fusion to the uterine wall. Less fluid is typically withdrawn, approximately 1 mL for each week of gestation (Nicolaides, 1994; Shulman, 1994; Sundberg, 1997, and all their associates).

Early amniocentesis has higher rates of postprocedural complications. One fetal complication that stands out is talipes equinovarus—*clubfoot*. Data from the Canadian Early and Mid-Trimester Amniocentesis Trial (1998) that involved nearly 4400 women undergoing early amniocentesis showed that rates of amnionic fluid leakage, fetal loss, and talipes equinovarus were all significantly higher following early compared with traditional amniocentesis. A trial involving 3775 women found that early amniocentesis was associated with a fourfold increased rate of talipes equinovarus compared with chorionic villus sampling (Philip and colleagues, 2004). Another problem with early amniocentesis is that there are more cell culture failures, thus necessitating a second procedure. For all these reasons, the American College of Obstetricians and Gynecologists (2007a) recommends against the use of early amniocentesis.

Chorionic Villus Sampling (CVS)

Biopsy of chorionic villi is generally performed at 10 to 13 weeks. Samples may be obtained transcervically or transabdominally, depending on which route allows easiest access to the placenta (**Fig. 13-7**). Relative contraindications include vaginal bleeding or spotting, active genital tract infection, extreme uterine ante- or retroflexion, or body habitus precluding easy uterine access or clear sonographic visualization of its contents.

The indications for CVS are essentially the same as for amniocentesis, except for a few analyses that specifically require either amnionic fluid or placental tissue. The primary advantage of villous biopsy is that results are available earlier in pregnancy, which lessens parental anxiety when results are normal. It also allows earlier and safer methods of pregnancy termination when results are abnormal.

Complications of CVS are similar to those for amniocentesis. The incidence of amnionic fluid leakage or infection is less than 0.5 percent (American College of Obstetricians and Gynecologists, 2007a). In a randomized trial involving nearly 4000 women, Jackson and colleagues (1992) compared transcervical CVS with transabdominal CVS and found no significant difference in fetal safety. The American College of Obstetricians and Gynecologists (2007a) has concluded that the fetal loss rate is the same after either types of CVS.

Early reports of an association between CVS and limb-reduction defects and oromandibular limb hypogenesis caused a great deal of concern (Burton, 1992; Firth, 1991, 1994; Hsieh, 1995, and all their colleagues). Subsequently, it was shown that limb-reduction defects were associated with CVS performed earlier in gestation—typically around 7 weeks. Thus, when CVS is performed by an experienced operator after 10 weeks, the incidence of limb-reduction defects is the same as background (Evans and Wapner, 2005; Kuliev and co-workers, 1996).

Laboratory Results

Midtrimester amniocentesis is associated with the lowest incidence of uninformative results—up to 0.8 percent. This compares with 0.8 to 1.5 percent for transcervical CVS and 0.7 to 1.9 percent for transabdominal CVS (Canadian Collaborative CVS–Amniocentesis Clinical Trial Group, 1989; Philip and co-workers, 2004; Rhoads and colleagues, 1989). Uninformative data usually are the result of an inadequate sample or the detection of mosaicism—more than one distinct cell line in a single chorionic villous sample. In these circumstances, such findings rarely represent true fetal mosaicism, but instead usually indicate *confined placental mosaicism*, or *pseudomosaicism* (see Chap. 12, p. 275).

Fetal Blood Sampling

Also called percutaneous umbilical blood sampling (PUBS) or cordocentesis, this procedure was first described by Daffos and colleagues (1983). It is performed primarily for assessment and treatment of confirmed red cell or platelet alloimmunization and in the evaluation of nonimmune hydrops (see Chap. 29, p. 623). Often, when severe fetal anemia is suspected, Doppler evaluation of the fetal middle cerebral artery peak systolic velocity is first performed. This is a noninvasive method of detecting severe fetal anemia, used prior to proceeding with fetal blood sampling and/or intrauterine transfusion. Fetal blood sampling also can be used to obtain cells for genetic analysis when CVS or amniocentesis results are confusing or when rapid diagnosis is necessary. Karyotyping of fetal blood usually can be accomplished within 24 to 48 hours. Blood can also be analyzed for metabolic and hematological studies, acid–base analysis, viral and bacterial cultures, polymerase chain reaction and other genetic techniques, and immunological studies.

Technique

Under direct sonographic guidance, the operator uses a 22-gauge spinal needle to puncture the umbilical vein, usually at or near its placental origin, and blood is withdrawn. This is shown in **Figure 13-8**. A free loop of cord also can be accessed for

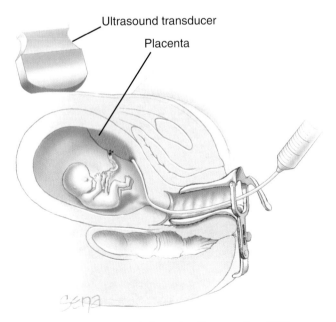

FIGURE 13-7 Transcervical chorionic villus sampling (CVS).

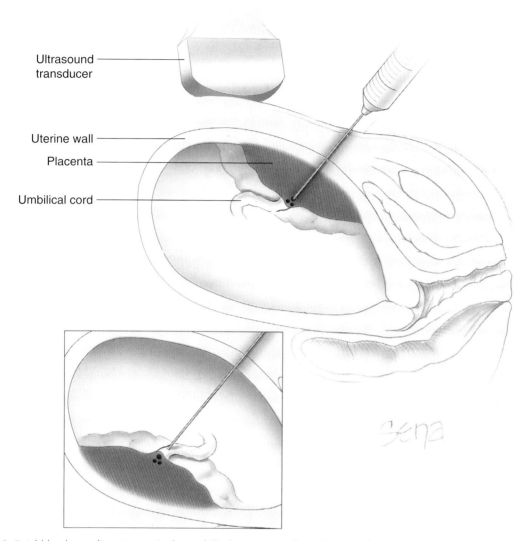

Ultrasound transducer

Uterine wall

Placenta

Umbilical cord

FIGURE 13-8 Fetal blood sampling. Access to the umbilical vein varies depending on placental location and cord position. With an anterior placenta, the needle may traverse the placenta. **Inset:** With posterior placentation, the needle passes through amnionic fluid before penetrating the umbilical vein. Alternately, a free loop of cord may be accessed.

venipuncture. Arterial puncture should be avoided because it may result in vasospasm and fetal bradycardia.

Complications

These may include cord vessel bleeding—50 percent, cord hematoma—17 percent, fetal-maternal hemorrhage—66 percent with an anterior placenta and 17 percent with a posterior placenta, and fetal bradycardia—3 to 12 percent (Ghidini and associates, 1993). Most complications are transitory with complete fetal recovery, but some result in fetal death. The procedure-related fetal death rate is cited to be 1.4 percent, but varies according to the indication as well as fetal status (Ghidini and colleagues, 1993; Maxwell and associates, 1991).

Fetal Tissue Biopsy

There are many genetic conditions for which there is no specific molecular test. Sometimes, prenatal diagnosis can only be accomplished by direct analysis of fetal tissue obtained by sonographically guided biopsy. Linkage analysis has been used for the diagnosis of familial disorders, but it is possible only if there are living, informative, affected family members (see Chap. 12, p. 283). The technique has been used for muscle biopsy to diagnose muscular dystrophy or mitochondrial myopathy (Evans and colleagues, 1994). And skin biopsy has been used to diagnose epidermolysis bullosa (Elias and co-workers, 1994).

Preimplantation Genetic Diagnosis

With the use of assisted reproductive technologies, zygotes affected with a severe genetic disorder can be identified so that they are not used for in vitro fertilization. As a result, only unaffected embryos are selected for implantation. The technique has been performed to diagnose nearly 200 different single-gene disorders such as cystic fibrosis, sickle-cell disease, or β-thalassemia;

to determine gender in X-linked diseases; and although controversial, to match for human leukocyte antigens for potential umbilical cord stem cell transplant for an affected sibling (de Wert, 2007; Flake, 2003; Fragouli, 2007; Grewal, 2004; Jiao, 2003; Rund and Rachmilewitz, 2005; Xu, 2004, and all their colleagues).

Several techniques have been reported. *Polar body analysis* is attractive because the first and second polar bodies normally are expelled, and their removal should not affect fetal development. Because most biopsied polar bodies are in metaphase, the chromosomes in these cells also are suitable for fluorescence in situ hybridization (FISH) analysis, which is discussed in Chapter 12 (p. 282) (Munne, 2001). A second technique is *blastomere biopsy* of the 3-day-old embryo at the 6- to 10-cell stage. One cell is removed through a hole made in the zona pellucida. Loss of one totipotent cell at this stage supposedly has little or no effect on the developing embryo. Even so, in a report by El-Toukhy and co-workers (2003), there was a lower implantation rate when previously biopsied frozen embryos were thawed and transferred. This technique is complex and still under development. New techniques such as whole-genome multiple displacement amplification from single cells may allow even more broad diagnoses (Spits and colleagues, 2006).

The American College of Obstetricians and Gynecologists (2009) recently reviewed the topic of preimplantaton genetic *screening* for aneuploidy using FISH. The College concluded that current data does not support use of this technology solely for advanced maternal age, that it does not improve in vitro fertilization success, and that it may be detrimental.

Fetal Cells in the Maternal Circulation

More than 50 years ago, various types of fetal cells were identified in the maternal circulation (Douglas and colleagues, 1959). It is now known that fetal cells likely are present in all pregnant women, although the concentration is very low—only 2 to 6 cells per mL of maternal blood (Bianchi and Hanson, 2006). Isolation of these cells for prenatal analysis might obviate the need for invasive procedures (Ober-Berman and associates, 2009). Most research in this area focuses on cell sorting techniques, which take advantage of unique cell surface proteins and other characteristics that distinguish fetal from maternal cells. These techniques include density gradient or protein separation, fluorescence-activated cell sorting, and magnetic-activated cell sorting (Bianchi and Hanson, 2006).

Nucleated red blood cells are most easily isolated. Fetal cells obtained this way have been evaluated for genetic diseases such as β-thalassemia as well as for fetal red cell D-antigen typing (Geifman-Holtzman and colleagues, 1996; Rund and Rachmilewitz, 2005). Karyotyping using FISH techniques may also be possible in some cases (Poon and co-workers, 2000). In a National Institutes of Health (NIH)-sponsored trial of fetal cell isolation, 1292 pregnant women with male fetuses were evaluated. In 41 percent, at least one XY male cell was detected using FISH (Bianchi and colleagues, 2002). The sensitivity was higher if a chromosomal abnormality was present—at least one aneuploid cell was detected by FISH in 74 percent of aneuploid fetuses.

The study of fetal cells in the maternal circulation is fascinating from the perspective of autoimmune disease as well. Fetal cells may persist in the maternal circulation for decades following delivery. There is evidence that persistent fetal cells play a role in the development of maternal autoimmune diseases, such as scleroderma and thyroiditis, possibly through a graft-versus-host phenomenon (see Chap. 53, p. 1127, and Chap. 54, p. 1146). Remarkably, there is even some evidence that fetal cells acquired during pregnancy might have a therapeutic role (Bianchi, 2004).

Several problems have hampered clinical implementation of this technology. There has been no universal fetal cell surface or cytoplasmic marker that identifies cells as being from the fetus. However, the maspin gene, a tumor suppressor gene that is hypomethylated in the placenta, has shown promise (Chim and colleagues, 2005). It still remains difficult to isolate a quantity of fetal cells sufficient for analysis or to isolate a pure sample devoid of maternal cells. And because some fetal cells appear to be immortal in the maternal circulation, it may not be possible to determine whether isolated cells are from the current or a past pregnancy. A recent NIH workshop concluded that there is need for standardization of techniques used for cell-free fetal DNA analysis (Bianchi and Hanson, 2006). The panel also noted that direct-to-consumer early fetal gender detection has become widely available, but that the accuracy is controversial. Noninvasive Rh CDE genotyping is now clinically available in several European countries and will likely soon be available in the United States.

FETAL THERAPY

Although prenatal treatment is currently not feasible for most fetal abnormalities, interventions have been developed during the past two decades that have dramatically altered the course of selected fetal anomalies and conditions. The 2004 NIH-sponsored multidisciplinary workshop on fetal treatment was designed to develop a plan for evaluation of such in-utero therapy (Chescheir and Socol, 2005).

Even when treatment is not available, there may be significant benefit from prenatal diagnosis of an anomaly or aneuploidy. For example, diagnosis may allow psychological preparation, and findings may alter delivery plans. Some neonates will benefit from delivery at a specialized center with immediate access to pediatric surgery or other subspecialists. In other cases, knowledge of a severe or lethal anomaly may allow for an informed decision about pregnancy termination or a decision not to perform cesarean delivery for fetal indications. Along with a maternal-fetal medicine or genetics referral, consultation with pediatric subspecialist(s) is often helpful.

Fetal Transfusion

The intrauterine transfusion of red blood cells has radically altered the natural history of fetal anemia due to alloimmunization and other causes. In many cases, a morbid and even lethal condition now is almost always treatable. Transfusions have also been used to treat fetal thrombocytopenia.

Fetal Anemia

There are many causes of fetal anemia, including alloimmunization, infection, genetic diseases such as thalassemia, and fetal-to-maternal hemorrhage. Anemia may be identified by fetal blood sampling as discussed, or in many cases, by Doppler evaluation of the fetal middle cerebral artery peak systolic velocity (see Chap. 16, p. 364). In the past, maternal *CDE alloimmunization* was the most common cause of hemolytic disease affecting the fetus (see Chap. 29, p. 619). Anti-D immunoglobulin given antepartum and at delivery has significantly diminished its incidence, but many other red cell antigens can also produce hemolytic anemia. The natural history of severe anemia usually is development of heart failure, hydrops, and ultimately death. The advent of fetal transfusion therapy has resulted in survival rates that exceed 90 percent with severe anemia without hydrops, and 70 percent if hydrops has developed (Schumacher and Moise, 1996).

Fetuses with *parvovirus B19 infection*, especially those infected before 20 weeks, may develop severe anemia from red cell hypoplasia. Although the fetus may spontaneously recover, most recommend transfusion if severe anemia is detected (see Chap. 58, p. 1215). Unfortunately, some fetuses develop viral myocarditis in addition to anemia and may not respond to transfusion therapy. Moreover, others may have sequelae of infection despite timely treatment. Surveillance of 24 fetuses given transfusions for anemia from parvovirus infection was provided by Nagel and colleagues (2007). Of 16 survivors aged 6 months to 8 years, neurodevelopmental status was abnormal in a third. These investigators found that neurological disability was not related to the severity of anemia or acidemia and proposed an infection-related cause.

Other causes of fetal anemia may be amenable to therapy. *Fetal-to-maternal hemorrhage* may be treated with fetal transfusion if the hemorrhage is significant but not ongoing. Unfortunately, it is not possible to determine whether irreversible neurological injury from cerebral hypoperfusion has already occurred (see Chap. 29, p. 617). Transfusions have also been used to treat fetal anemia from *hemoglobin Bart disease* (see Chap. 51, p. 1090).

Platelet transfusions for fetal *alloimmune thrombocytopenia* has been well described. Unfortunately, there is significant morbidity associated with the frequent transfusions required, and procedure-related fetal loss rates average approximately 5 percent per pregnancy (Berkowitz and co-workers, 2006). For this reason, most reserve platelet transfusions for cases refractory to medical therapy with high-dose immunoglobulin G, with or without corticosteroids (see Chap. 29, p. 629).

Technique. Using sonographic guidance, intravascular transfusion into the umbilical vein is generally considered the preferred method of fetal transfusion, although some employ intraperitoneal transfusion. In the setting of hydrops, peritoneal absorption is impaired, and intravascular transfusion is considered the optimal method (Moise, 2002). The red cells are generally type O, D-negative, cytomegalovirus negative, packed to a hematocrit of about 80 percent, irradiated, and leukocyte-poor. The fetal-placental volume allows a relatively rapid infusion of a relatively large quantity of blood. Prior to blood infusion, a paralytic agent such as vecuronium may be given to the fetus to minimize movements and potential trauma. The target hematocrit is approximately 40 to 50 percent in the nonhydropic fetus. The volume transfused may be estimated by multiplying the estimated fetal weight by 0.02 for each 10 percent increase in hematocrit needed (Giannina and colleagues, 1998). In the severely anemic fetus, less blood is transfused initially, and the next transfusion is planned 2 days later. Subsequent transfusions usually take place every 2 to 4 weeks, depending on the hematocrit.

Fetal Medical Therapy

There are several fetal conditions that have been shown to be amenable to maternal-fetal therapy. In such cases, medication administered to the mother is transported transplacentally and exerts beneficial effects on the fetus.

Thyrotoxicosis

Some euthyroid women with Graves thyrotoxicosis who have undergone radioiodine thyroid ablation will continue to produce IgG thyroid-stimulating antibodies that cross the placenta to cause fetal thyrotoxicosis (see Chap. 53, p. 1127). Fetal thyroid status can be assessed by cordocentesis for thyroid hormones. If hyperthyroidism is confirmed, propylthiouracil administered to the mother is carried transplacentally to suppress the fetal thyroid (Wenstrom and associates, 1990).

Congenital Adrenal Hyperplasia

Several autosomal recessive enzyme deficiencies cause congenital adrenal hyperplasia (CAH) characterized by impaired synthesis of cortisol from cholesterol by the adrenal cortex (see Chap. 4, p. 102). The 21-hydroxylase deficiency accounts for more than 90 percent of cases. The classic form has a population incidence of approximately 1:15,000. In selected populations, however, it is higher—for example, 1:300 in Yupik Alaskan Eskimos and 1:5000 in Saudi Arabians (New and Nimkarn, 2007). Due to excessive fetal adrenal androgen production, the condition can cause female virilization (see Chap. 4, p. 102). These newborns may be at risk for salt-wasting adrenal crises, and all states require newborn testing.

Treatment to prevent virilization must begin early, ideally prior to 9 weeks, *before it is known whether the fetus will be affected or even its gender*. One regimen is dexamethasone, given orally to the mother at a dosage of 20 μg/kg/d in three divided doses. Typically, treatment is begun and prenatal diagnosis with either CVS or amniocentesis is performed later. If testing shows that the fetus has a male karyotype, dexamethasone is stopped. If molecular genetic testing demonstrates that a female fetus is affected or if testing is indeterminate, treatment is continued until term. In affected families, clinically available molecular genetic testing can identify 80 to 98 percent of cases (New and Nimkarn, 2007).

Arrhythmias

As many as 1 percent of pregnancies are complicated by a fetal arrhythmia (Copel and associates, 2000). Fetal M-mode sonography is used to clarify the relationship between atrial and ventricular beats and thereby diagnose the type of rhythm disturbance. Most are benign atrial extrasystoles (premature atrial contractions), which usually resolve before delivery with maturity of the conduction system.

Sustained tachyarrhythmias—most commonly from supraventricular tachycardia or atrial flutter—can lead to cardiac decompensation and hydrops if untreated. Maternal administration of antiarrhythmic drugs that cross the placenta is used to convert to a normal rhythm or to lower the baseline heart rate and thereby forestall failure. A variety of medications have been used, most commonly digoxin, sotalol, flecainide and procainamide. Their selection depends on the type of tachyarrhythmia as well as provider familiarity and experience with the drug, but digoxin is usually the first-line agent. Amiodarone therapy has been associated with neonatal hypothyroidism, which may be severe (Niinikoski and co-workers, 2007; Simpson, 2006).

Antiarrhythmic medications may have significant maternal and fetal risks, particularly because therapy may require dosages at the upper end of the therapeutic range for adults. A maternal electrocardiogram should be performed before and during therapy. If the fetus has become hydropic, the drug may need to be administered directly via the umbilical vein (Mangione and co-workers, 1999; Simpson, 2006).

Congenital Infections

A number of infectious agents cross the placenta and cause fetal infection with serious consequences. Prompt maternal treatment—and thus fetal treatment—may prevent or mitigate associated fetal morbidity. One dramatic example is timely treatment of maternal syphilis. Many causes of treatment "failures" are due to recognition *after* fetal infection is too advanced to respond. Diagnosis and treatment of sexually transmitted and other infectious diseases that may infect and affect the fetus are discussed throughout Chapters 58 and 59.

Metabolic Disorders

A number of inherited metabolic disorders have been treated in utero with impressive outcomes. Fetal *methylmalonic acidemia* has been treated with maternal oral and intramuscular vitamin B_{12} therapy, which is continued after birth and is associated with normal development into adulthood (Ampola and co-workers, 1975; O'Brien and Bianchi, 2005). Fetal umbilical vein and intraperitoneal transfusions of fresh-frozen plasma have been used to treat *Smith-Lemli-Opitz syndrome* (Irons and colleagues, 1999). And maternal oral L-serine supplementation has been used to treat fetal *3-phosphoglycerate-dehydrogenase deficiency* (de Koning and colleagues, 2004.)

Fetal Stem Cell Transplantation

In theory, stem cell transplantation could be used to treat a variety of hematological, metabolic, and immunological diseases and could serve as a delivery vehicle for gene transfer to treat other genetic conditions. The fetal period is ideal for this because in the first and early second trimesters, the fetus does not have an adaptive immune response to foreign antigens and has therefore been described as *preimmune* (Tiblad and Westgren,

2008). Other advantages are that pretreatment chemotherapy or radiation is not necessary prior to transplantation and that there is less risk for graft-versus-host disease.

Animal models have been developed to study fetal bone marrow transplantation. Studies have focused on identifying the optimal gestation age for transplantation, as well as the best source of hemopoietic stem cells such as fetal blood or liver, cord blood, parental bone marrow or circulating hemopoietic progenitor cells, or mesenchymal stem cells (Le Blanc and associates, 2005).

To date, human fetal stem cell transplantation has been most successful in the treatment of immunodeficiency syndromes, which suggests that even the early fetus has some degree of immunocompetence. Engraftment has been achieved in fetuses with severe combined immunodeficiency and bare lymphocyte syndrome and had a benign clinical course (Tiblad and Westgren, 2008). Treatment of other immunodeficiencies, including chronic granulomatous disease and Chediak-Higashi syndrome, and treatment of some storage diseases have not been successful. Stem cell transplantation has been used to treat some hemoglobinopathies. Fetuses with sickle-cell anemia have not achieved engraftment. In some with α- and β-thalassemia, despite achieving engraftment, children have remained transfusion dependent (Tiblad and Westgren, 2008; Westgren and colleagues, 1996). A fetus with osteogenesis imperfecta type II who was transplanted with fetal mesenchymal stem cells developed both engraftment and chimerism (Le Blanc and colleagues, 2005). Although long-term outcome of such cases remains uncertain, the technology holds a great deal of promise.

Fetal Gene Therapy

With advances in genetic technologies and progress in the identification of genes responsible for inherited disease, efforts have focused on therapeutic gene transfer. This has been attempted only in animal models, with limited success and significant challenges (David and Peebles, 2008). Certain inherited metabolic conditions in which tissue damage begins shortly after or even before birth would be ideal for early therapy by gene transfer. In Tay-Sachs disease, for example, central nervous system cells exhibit the characteristic pathology as early as 9 weeks after conception (Grabowski and colleagues, 1984). Early gene therapy also has the potential of requiring only one treatment, which would be definitive and would span a lifetime.

A number of criteria—not yet met—are considered requisite for the development of therapeutic gene transfer:

1. The normal gene can be inserted into the target cells and remain there long enough to have the desired effect. Potential types of vectors include nonviral agents, such as cationic polymers and cationic liposomes, and viruses—adenovirus, retrovirus, and lentiviruses (David and Peebles, 2008)

2. The level of expression of the new gene will be appropriate after a single application

3. The new gene will not harm the cell or the individual (Anderson, 1984). For example, two children who received gene therapy for severe combined immunodeficiency disease developed T-cell leukemia. Leukemia was a

consequence of the gene vector inserting near an oncogene, thereby activating the oncogene and increasing leukemia susceptibility (Berns, 2004).

Other unresolved issues include the timing of the procedure, that is, preconceptional, at the time of fertilization, prior to implantation, or during embryogenesis or fetal development. Which are the ideal recipient or target cells? Finally, which are the safest methods? Efficient techniques for in vivo gene targeting have yet to be developed, and the possibility of ex vivo gene transfer raises ethical considerations.

Fetal Surgery

The prospect of treating severe fetal anomalies in utero has been a topic of intense interest for more than two decades. Pioneering work in animals led to the development of *open fetal surgery*, in which maternal hysterotomy and partial exteriorization of the fetus are performed to permit surgery for selected life-threatening anomalies. Currently, such expertise is available at only a few centers in the United States and for only a few fetal conditions. Because it entails substantive fetal and maternal risks, these procedures are considered only when they might reasonably be expected to improve fetal outcome and when withholding them would undoubtedly be catastrophic.

Although the indications for open fetal surgery are limited, the number of conditions amenable to less invasive therapy has expanded, particularly during the past decade. These procedures are not without risk, but maternal morbidity and fetal preterm delivery may be reduced. A number of fetal abnormalities treatable antepartum or intrapartum are shown in Table 13-12. For any fetal therapy, it is important that appropriate selection criteria be established and verified, that each procedure be perfected and tested successfully in experimental animals, and that its efficacy in human pregnancy be rigorously evaluated prior to widespread implementation (Harrison and colleagues, 1980; Moise and associates, 1995). Chescheir (2009) further recommends that we must understand how fetal therapy is altered after a maternal-fetal intervention.

Open Fetal Surgery

These procedures require a highly skilled team from different disciplines, as well as extensive case management with education and counseling. To gain fetal access, the mother must undergo general endotracheal anesthesia to suppress both uterine contractions and fetal responses. Using sonographic guidance to avoid the placental edge, a hysterotomy incision is made with a stapling device that seals the edges to permit hemostasis. Warmed fluid is continuously infused into the uterus thorough a rapid infusion device. The fetus is gently manipulated to permit pulse oximetry monitoring and venous access in case fluids or blood are emergently needed (Fig. 13-9). At this point, fetal surgery is performed. The hysterotomy is then closed and tocolysis begun. Later in the pregnancy, delivery is completed by cesarean.

In a review of 87 open fetal surgery procedures from the Fetal Treatment Center of the University of California, San Francisco, Golombeck and colleagues (2006) reported the following morbidities: maternal pulmonary edema—28 percent, maternal blood transfusion—13 percent, preterm labor and delivery—33

TABLE 13-12. Some Abnormalities Amenable to Fetal Surgery

Open Fetal Surgery
- Cystic adenomatoid malformation
- Extralobar pulmonary sequestration
- Sacrococcygeal teratoma
- Spina bifida

Fetoscopic Surgery
- Twin-twin transfusion: laser of placental anastamoses
- Diaphragmatic hernia: fetal endoscopic tracheal occlusion (FETO)
- Posterior urethral valves: cystoscopic laser
- Congenital high airway obstruction: vocal cord laser
- Amnionic band release

Percutaneous Procedures
- Shunt therapy
    - Posterior-urethral valves/bladder outlet obstruction
    - Pleural effusion: chylothorax or sequestration
    - Dominant cyst in congenital cystic adenomatoid malformation (CCAM)
- Radiofrequency ablation
    - Twin-reversed arterial perfusion (TRAP) sequence
    - Monochorionic twins with severe anomaly(ies) of 1 twin
    - Chorioangioma
- Fetal intracardiac catheter procedures
    - Aortic or pulmonic valvuloplasty for stenosis
    - Atrial septostomy for hypoplastic left heart with restrictive atrial septum

Ex-utero-intrapartum-treatment(EXIT) procedures
- Congenital diaphragmatic hernia after FETO
- Congenital high airway obstruction sequence (CHAOS)
- Severe micrognathia
- EXIT-to-resection
    - Resection of fetal thoracic or mediastinal mass
    - Tumors involving airway/neck
- EXIT-to-extracorporeal membrane oxygenation (ECMO)
    - Congenital diaphragmatic hernia (if no fetal surgery)

---

percent, prematurely ruptured membranes—52 percent, chorion-amnion separation—20 percent, chorioamnionitis—9 percent, and placental abruption—9 percent. Other potential risks include later uterine rupture, maternal sepsis, and fetal death during or following the procedure.

Some conditions for which open fetal surgery is offered include thoracic masses with hydrops, such as *congenital cystic adenomatoid malformation* (CCAM) and *extralobar pulmonary sequestration; spina bifida; and sacrococcygeal teratoma* (SCT) with evidence of high-output cardiac failure (see Fig. 13-9). For fetuses with CCAM, Adzick and colleagues (1998) found that once hydrops had developed, none of 25 fetuses survived without treatment, whereas eight of 13 survived with fetal lobectomy. For 30 fetuses with a sacrococcygeal teratoma, Hendrick

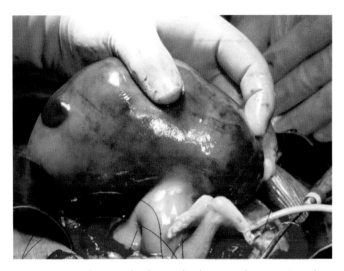

FIGURE 13-9 Photograph of open fetal surgery for resection of a sacrococcygeal teratoma. Hysterotomy has been completed, and the caudal portion of the fetus has been delivered onto the surgical field. The tumor is held by the surgeon's hand. (Used with permission from Dr. Timothy M. Crombleholme of the Fetal Care Center of Cincinnati.)

and colleagues (2004) reported that only four were amenable to tumor debulking—three survived following delivery at mean gestational age of 29 weeks.

Unlike open fetal surgery for other abnormalities, surgery for *spina bifida* is controversial, because the condition itself is not lethal. However, isolated open spinal defects usually result in permanent neurological damage, and in-utero repair can potentially limit the damage from chronic exposure to amnionic fluid (Heffez and associates, 1990). Proponents report that early experience suggests a decreased need for ventriculoperitoneal shunting and resolution of hindbrain herniation (Johnson and colleagues, 2003). As of 2009, prenatal surgical closure of fetal spine defects is available as part of an NIH-sponsored multicenter research trial

entitled *Management of Myelomeningocele Study—MOMS* (moms@biostat.bsc.gwu.edu).

In the past, open fetal surgery was also attempted for cases of isolated *congenital diaphragmatic hernia*. The goal was to replace the liver within the abdominal cavity and repair the defect. Unfortunately, umbilical vein occlusion led to intraoperative fetal deaths, and overall survival was not improved. Efforts have since focused on fetoscopic tracheal occlusion for this anomaly, which is discussed subsequently.

Fetoscopic Surgery

Fetoscopy compares to open fetal surgery as laparoscopy does to laparotomy. To perform surgery using fiberoptic endoscopes only 1 to 2 mm in diameter and instruments such as lasers that fit through 3 to 5 mm cannulae has revolutionized treatments available for selected fetal conditions. These state-of-the-art procedures are performed almost exclusively at highly specialized centers, and most are considered investigational.

Risks are lower than with open fetal surgery but can still be formidable. For endoscopic procedures that entail minimally invasive laparotomy for access, Golombeck and colleagues (2006) reported complications of maternal pulmonary edema—25 percent, preterm delivery—27 percent, prematurely ruptured membranes—44 percent, chorion-amnion separation—65 percent, and placental abruption—6 percent. Other risks include maternal infection or injury and fetal death.

Examples of conditions treated by fetoscopy include twin-twin transfusion syndrome (TTTS), congenital diaphragmatic hernia—fetal tracheal occlusion, cystoscopic laser treatment of posterior urethral valves, laser therapy of vocal cord occlusion in congenital high-airway obstruction sequence, and release of amnionic bands.

Twin-Twin Transfusion Syndrome (TTTS). Laser therapy for TTTS has been the most commonly used example of fetoscopic surgery (Fig. 13-10). With this procedure, laser energy ablates

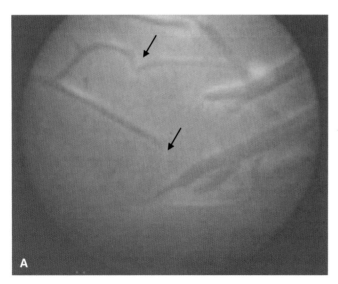
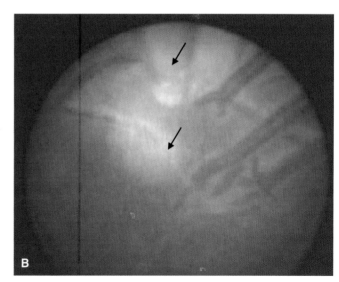

FIGURE 13-10 Laser therapy for twin-twin transfusion syndrome (TTTS). Fetoscopic photograph of the placental fetal surface. **A.** Vascular anastomoses (*arrows*) are shown before selective laser ablation. **B.** Sites of ablation are seen as blanched yellow-white areas (*arrows*). (Used with permission from Dr. Timothy M. Crombleholme of the Fetal Care Center of Cincinnati.)

pathological vascular anastomoses within a monochorionic twin placenta (see Chap. 39, p. 872). Even with such therapy, evaluation and management of TTTS remains challenging (Norton, 2007). For example, the relationship between placental angioarchitecture and pregnancy outcome is not fully understood, and neurological complications and preterm birth remain common. Treatment is even less likely to be successful in pregnancy after 26 weeks (Crombleholme and colleagues, 2007). Finally, fetal cardiovascular compromise plays a significant role in perinatal outcome (Rychik and associates, 2007; Van Mieghem and co-workers, 2009).

Fetal Endoscopic Tracheal Occlusion (FETO) for Congenital Diaphragmatic Hernia (CDH).

Fetoscopic therapy has been rigorously evaluated in infants with this condition. With an isolated diaphragmatic hernia and with specialized care and postnatal surgery, mortality rates approximate 30 percent (Reickert and colleagues, 1998). The major prenatal findings used to identify candidates for fetal therapy—those at risk for lethal pulmonary hypoplasia—include a significant amount of liver within the thorax and a low lung-to-head ratio—the cross-sectional area of the right lung divided by the head circumference. The rationale for FETO is that by placing a silicone balloon between the fetal carina and vocal cords, the normal egress of lung fluid is halted, and the lungs will expand despite the presence of abdominal organs in the chest. The balloon is removed at delivery via the ex-utero-intrapartum-treatment (EXIT) procedure, which is discussed subsequently.

Although initial results were promising, FETO is currently controversial. Harrison and co-workers (2003) from the University of California Fetal Treatment Center conducted a randomized trial of FETO in 24 fetuses with a diaphragmatic hernia who had predicted survival of less than 40 percent with conventional neonatal surgical correction. Because there was approximately 75-percent survival in both groups at 90 days, the trial was discontinued. In other countries—particularly in Europe—FETO continues to be performed in fetuses with otherwise poor prognoses (Deprest and colleagues, 2006).

Percutaneous Procedures

Sonographic guidance can be used to permit therapy with a shunt, radiofrequency ablation needle, or angioplasty catheter. Although risks are lower than with open fetal surgery, risks include maternal infection, preterm labor or prematurely ruptured membranes, and fetal injury or loss. Fetal thoracic and urinary shunts have become increasingly available however, treatment with radiofrequency ablation and especially angioplasty remain investigational and largely confined to highly specialized centers.

Fetal Shunt Therapy. Percutaneous shunts have been used to drain fluid in cases of selected urinary and thoracic abnormalities. *Urinary shunts* are primarily used in cases of fetal *bladder-outlet obstruction*—for example, *posterior urethral valves*—that would otherwise be lethal. The rationale is that allowing urine to drain from the bladder into the amnionic cavity might preserve renal function and protect against pulmonary hypoplasia

TABLE 13-13. Optimal Fetal Urinary Electrolyte and Protein Values in Cases of Bladder Outlet Obstruction

Analyte	Threshold value
Sodium	<100 mmol/L
Chloride	<90 mmol/L
Calcium	<8 mg/dL
Osmolality	<200 mmol/L
β_2-microglobulin	<6 mg/L
Total protein	<20 mg/dL

Fetal renal status is assessed by 3 percutaneous bladder drainages at 48- to 72-hour intervals.
If all values are below the thresholds listed, good prognosis.
If 1 or 2 values exceed the thresholds, prognosis is borderline.
If 3 or more values exceed the thresholds, poor prognosis.

Adapted from Biard and colleagues (2005).

from oligohydramnios. Potential candidates are fetuses without other severe anomalies or aneuploidy and who have no sonographic features that confer poor prognosis, for example, renal cortical cysts. Only male fetuses are treated because in females the type of anomaly tends to be even more severe. Serial bladder drainage or vesicocentesis is performed to determine the urine electrolyte and protein content to classify the renal prognosis as good, borderline, or poor (Table 13-13). The procedure is performed by inserting a small trocar and cannula into the fetal bladder under sonographic guidance. This is followed by placement of a double-pigtail catheter (Freedman and colleagues, 2000). In their review of long-term outcomes of children treated with vesicoamnionic shunts, Biard and colleagues (2005) reported overall 1-year survival to be 90 percent. One third of surviving children required dialysis or renal transplantation.

Thoracic shunts from the fetal pleural cavity into the amnionic cavity are performed to drain large pleural effusions. These may accrue with a *chylothorax,* or they may accompany *pulmonary sequestration.* Shunts have also been used to drain a dominant cyst in fetuses with *congenital cystic adenomatoid malformation.* These shunts are associated with fetal loss rates of 5 percent (Wilson and Johnson, 2003). In their review of controlled observational studies of these pulmonary drainage procedures in more than 600 fetuses, Knox and colleagues (2006) found that perinatal survival was significantly improved if there was fetal hydrops, but not in milder cases.

Radiofrequency Ablation Procedure (RFA). With this procedure, high-frequency alternating current is used to coagulate and desiccate tissue. Recently this has become a favored modality for the treatment of *twin-reversed arterial perfusion (TRAP) sequence* or *acardiac twin* (see Chap. 39, p. 872). It is

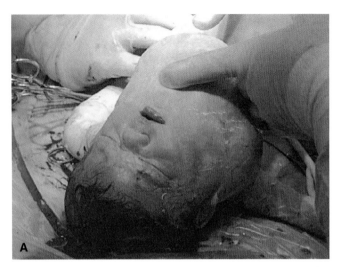
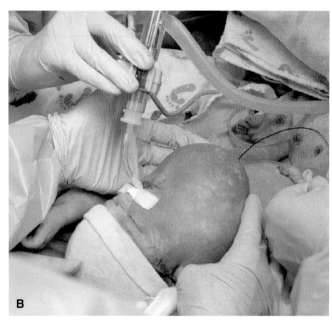

FIGURE 13-11 A. Ex-utero intrapartum treatment—EXIT—procedure. This fetus was diagnosed prenatally with large lymphatic abnormality of the neck, lower face, and mediastinum. The EXIT procedure was planned because of concern for tracheal compression and possibly deviation. Upon delivery of the head, with the placental circulation maintained, the surgeon evaluates the airway and prepares to attempt intubation. **B.** Infant following a controlled intubation, oxygenating well, and supported by the neonatal intensive care unit team. (Courtesy of Drs. Michael Zaretsky and Julie Y. Lo.)

also used for selective termination for other monochorionic twin complications. Without treatment, the mortality rate for the normal or pump twin in TRAP sequence exceeds 50 percent, and it is even higher with larger acardiac twins. Under sonographic guidance, a 17- or 19-gauge RFA needle is placed into the base of the umbilical cord of the acardiac twin, within the abdomen. After a 2-cm area of coagulation is achieved, color Doppler sonography is used to verify that there is no longer flow into the acardiac twin. Lee (2007) and Livingston (2007) and their colleagues performed this procedure in more than 20 pregnancies and reported nearly 90-percent survival of the normal twin. Recently, Lee and co-workers (2009) reported the largest series—83 patients—treated with RFA of the acardiac mass in TRAP sequence and confirmed the effectiveness of this technique.

Fetal Intracardiac Catheter Procedures. Selected fetal cardiac lesions are concerning because of their progression during gestation. For example, severe fetal aortic stenosis detected in the early second trimester may progress to a hypoplastic left heart by the third trimester (Simpson and Sharland, 1997). In 22 fetuses with critical aortic stenosis, Wilkins-Haug and associates (2006) performed aortic valvuloplasty by inserting a 19-gauge cannula into the left ventricle and passing a 0.014-inch guide wire with a coronary artery angioplasty catheter through the aortic valve orifice. Although initially attempted using sonographic guidance alone, maternal laparotomy was required in two thirds of cases to achieve optimal positioning. Of 18 live births, only three had biventricular circulation and did not require a Norword procedure to treat hypoplastic left heart (Wilkins-Haug and colleagues, 2006). This technique has also been used for pulmonic valvuloplasty and atrial septostomy. It remains investigational.

Ex Utero Intrapartum Treatment (EXIT)

This procedure is designed to allow the fetus/infant to remain perfused by the placental circulation after being partially delivered so that life-saving treatment can be performed prior to complete delivery. EXIT procedures have been performed for more than 15 years. As reviewed by Hirose and colleagues (2004), EXIT was initially used to treat airway obstruction after fetal surgery—FETO, as previously discussed. The technique has also been used to treat airway obstruction caused by neck masses and laryngeal or tracheal atresia or stenosis (Fig. 13-11) (Steigman and associates, 2009). More recently, Kunisaki and co-workers (2007) used the EXIT procedure as a bridge to extracorporeal membrane oxygenation (ECMO). This is used so that infants with large thoracic masses can undergo immediate resection. These investigators have also used EXIT-to-ECMO for managing infants with severe congenital diaphragmatic hernia (Morris and co-workers, 2009).

REFERENCES

Adzick NS, Harrison MR, Crombleholme TM, et al: Fetal lung lesions: Management and outcome. Am J Obstet Gynecol 179:884, 1998

American College of Obstetricians and Gynecologists: Neural tube defects. Practice Bulletin No. 44, July 2003

American College of Obstetricians and Gynecologists: Invasive prenatal testing for aneuploidy. Practice Bulletin No. 88, December, 2007a

American College of Obstetricians and Gynecologists: Screening for fetal chromosomal abnormalities. Practice Bulletin No. 77, January, 2007b

American College of Obstetricians and Gynecologists: Update on carrier screening for cystic fibrosis. Obstet Gynecol 106:1465, 2005, reaffirmed 2007c

American College of Obstetricians and Gynecologists: Prenatal and preconceptional carrier screening for genetic diseases in individuals of Eastern European Jewish descent. Committee Opinion No. 298, August 2004, reaffirmed 2008

American College of Obstetricians and Gynecologists: Preimplantation genetic screening for aneuploidy. Committee opinion No. 430, March 2009

Ampola M, Mahoney MJ, Nakamura E, et al: Prenatal therapy of a patient with vitamin B$_{12}$-responsive methylmalonic acidemia. N Engl J Med 293:313, 1975

Anderson WF: Prospects for human gene therapy. Science 226:401, 1984

Atzei A, Gajewska K, Huggon IC, et al: Relationship between nuchal translucency thickness and prevalence of major cardiac defects in fetuses with normal karyotype. Ultrasound Obstet Gynecol 26:154, 2005

Benn PA, Clive JM, Collins R: Medians for second-trimester maternal serum α-fetoprotein, human chorionic gonadotropin, and unconjugated estriol: Differences between races or ethnic groups. Clin Chem 43:333, 1997

Bensen JT, Dillard RG, Burton BK: Open spina bifida: Does cesarean section delivery improve prognosis? Obstet Gynecol 71:532, 1988

Berkowitz RL, Bussel JB, McFarland JG: Alloimmune thrombocytopenia: State of the art 2006. Review article. Am J Obstet Gynecol 195:907, 2006

Berns A: Good news for gene therapy. N Engl J Med 350:1679, 2004

Bianchi DW: Fetomaternal cell traffic, pregnancy-associated progenitor cells, and autoimmune disease. Best Pract Res Clin Obstet Gynaecol 18:959, 2004

Bianchi DW, Hanson J: Sharpening the tools: A summary of a National Institutes of Health workshop on new technologies for detection of fetal cells in maternal blood for early prenatal diagnosis. J Matern Fetal Neonatal Med 19:199, 2006

Bianchi DW, Simpson JL, Jackson LG, et al: Fetal gender and aneuploidy detection using fetal cells in maternal blood: Analysis of NIFTY I data. National Institute of Child Health and Development Fetal Cell Isolation Study. Prenat Diagn 22:609, 2002

Biard JM, Johnson MP, Carr MC, et al: Long-term outcomes in children treated by prenatal vesicoamniotic shunting for lower urinary tract obstruction. Obstet Gynecol 106:503, 2005

Bogart MH, Pandian MR, Jones OW: Abnormal maternal serum chorionic gonadotropin levels in pregnancies with fetal chromosome abnormalities. Prenat Diagn 7:623, 1987

Brock DJ, Bolton AE, Monaghan JM: Prenatal diagnosis of anencephaly through maternal serum-alpha-fetoprotein measurement. Lancet 2:923, 1973

Brock DJ, Sutcliffe RG: Alpha-fetoprotein in the antenatal diagnosis of anencephaly and spina bifida. Lancet 2:197, 1972

Bromley B, Lieberman E, Shipp TD, et al: The genetic sonogram, a method for risk assessment for Down syndrome in the mid trimester. J Ultrasound Med 21:1087, 2002

Burton BK, Schulz CJ, Burd LI: Limb anomalies associated with chorionic villus sampling. Obstet Gynecol 79:726, 1992

Burton BK, Sowers SG, Nelson LH: Maternal serum α-fetoprotein screening in North Carolina: Experience with more than twelve thousand pregnancies. Am J Obstet Gynecol 146:439, 1983

Callen PW: Ultrasonography in Obstetrics and Gynecology, 4th ed. Philadelphia, WB Sanders, 2000

Canadian Collaborative CVS–Amniocentesis Clinical Trial Group: Multicentre randomised clinical trial of chorion villus sampling and amniocentesis. Lancet 7:1, 1989

Canadian Early and Mid-Trimester Amniocentesis Trial (CEMAT) Group: Randomised trial to assess safety and fetal outcome of early and midtrimester amniocentesis. Lancet 351:242, 1998

Chescheir NC: Maternal-fetal surgery: Where are we and how did we get here? Clinical expert series, Obstet Gynecol 113:717, 2009

Chescheir NC, Socol M: The National Institutes of Health Workshop on fetal treatment: Needs assessment and future directions. Current Commentary. Obstet Gynecol 106:828, 2005

Chim SS, Tong YK, Chiu RW, et al: Detection of the placental epigenetic signature of the maspin gene in maternal plasma. Proc Natl Acad Sci USA 102:753, 2005

Cicero S, Curcio P, Papageorghiou A, et al: Absence of nasal bone in fetuses with trisomy 21 at 11–14 weeks of gestation: An observational study. Lancet 358:1665, 2001

Copel JA, Liang RI, Demasio K, et al: The clinical significance of the irregular fetal heart rhythm. Am J Obstet Gynecol 182:813, 2000

Crombleholme TM, Shera D, Lee H, et al: A prospective, randomized, multicenter trial of amnioreduction vs selective fetoscopic laser photocoagulation for the treatment of twin-twin transfusion syndrome. Am J Obstet Gynecol 197:396, 2007

Cuckle H, Benn P, Wright D: Down syndrome screening in the first and/or second trimester: Model predicted performance using meta-analysis parameters. Semin Perinatol 29:252, 2005

Cuckle H, Wald N, Stevenson JD, et al: Maternal serum alpha-fetoprotein screening for open neural tube defects in twin pregnancies. Prenat Diagn 10:71, 1990

Cunningham FG, Gilstrap LC: Maternal serum alpha-fetoprotein screening. N Engl J Med 325:55, 1991

Cystic Fibrosis Consortium: Cystic Fibrosis Mutation Database: Available at http://www.genet.sickkids.on.ca/cftr/app. Accessed May 20, 2008

Daffos F, Capella-Pavlovsky M, Forestier F: A new procedure for fetal blood sampling in utero: Preliminary results of fifty-three cases. Am J Obstet Gynecol 146:985, 1983

Dalal A, Pradhan M, Tiwari D, et al: MTHFR 677C-T and 1298 A-T polymorphisms: Evaluation of maternal genotypic risk and association with level of neural tube defect. Gynecol Obstet Invest 63:146, 2007

Dashe JS, Twickler DM, Santos-Ramos R, et al: Alpha-fetoprotein detection of neural tube defects and the impact of standard ultrasound. Am J Obstet Gynecol 195:1623, 2006

David AL, Peebles D: Gene therapy for the fetus: Is there a future? Best Pract Res Clin Obstet Gynaecol 22:203, 2008

Deprest J, Jani J, Van Schoubroeck D, et al: Current consequences of prenatal diagnosis of congenital diaphragmatic hernia. J Pediatr Surg 41:423, 2006

de Koning TJ, Klomp LW, van Oppen AC, et al: Prenatal and early postnatal treatment in 3-phosphoglycerate-dehydrogenase deficiency. Lancet 364:2221, 2004

de Wert G, Liebaers I, Van De Velde H: The future (r)evolution of preimplantation genetic diagnosis/human leukocyte antigen testing: Ethical reflections. Stem Cells 25(9):2167, 2007

Douglas GW, Thomas L, Carr M, et al: Trophoblasts in the circulating blood during pregnancy. Am J Obstet Gynecol 58:960, 1959

Eddleman KA, Malone FD, Sullivan L, et al: Pregnancy loss rates after midtrimester amniocentesis. Obstet Gynecol 108:1067, 2006

El-Toukhy T, Khalaf Y, Al-Darazi K, et al: Effect of blastomere loss on the outcome of frozen embryo replacement cycles. Fertil Steril 79:1106, 2003

Elias S, Emerson DS, Simpson JL, et al: Ultrasound-guided fetal skin sampling for prenatal diagnosis of genodermatoses. Obstet Gynecol 83:337, 1994

Evans MI, Hoffman EP, Cadrin C, et al: Fetal muscle biopsy: Collaborative experience with varied indications. Obstet Gynecol 84:913, 1994

Evans MI, Wapner RJ: Invasive prenatal diagnostic procedures. Semin Perinatol 29:215, 2005

Fan C, Blumenfeld Y, Chueh J, et al: Digital PCR enables rapid prenatal diagnosis of fetal aneuploidy. Abstract No 65. Presented at the 29th Annual Meeting of the Society for Maternal-Fetal Medicine. 26-31 January 2009

Feuchtbaum LB, Cunningham G, Waller DK, et al: Fetal karyotyping for chromosome abnormalities after an unexplained elevated maternal serum alpha-fetoprotein screening. Obstet Gynecol 86:248, 1995

Firth HV, Boyd PA, Chamberlain PF, et al: Analysis of limb reduction defects in babies exposed to chorionic villus sampling. Lancet 343:1069, 1994

Firth HV, Boyd PA, Chamberlain P, et al: Severe limb abnormalities after chorion villus sampling at 56–66 days' gestation. Lancet 337:762, 1991

Flake AW: Stem cell and genetic therapies for the fetus. Semin Pediatr Surg 12:202, 2003

Fragouli E: Preimplantation genetic diagnosis: Present and future. J Assist Reprod Genet 24:201, 2007

Freedman AL, Johnson MP, Gonzalez R: Fetal therapy for obstructive uropathy: Past, present . . . future? Pediatr Nephrol 14:167, 2000

Geifman-Holtzman O, Bernstein IM, Berry SM, et al: Fetal RhD genotyping in fetal cells flow sorted from maternal blood. Am J Obstet Gynecol 174:818, 1996

Ghidini A, Sepulveda W, Lockwood CJ, et al: Complications of fetal blood sampling. Am J Obstet Gynecol 168:1339, 1993

Gianferrari EA, Benn PA, Dries L, et al: Absent or shortened nasal bone length and the detection of Down syndrome in second-trimester fetuses. Obstet Gynecol 109:371, 2007

Giannina G, Moise KJ Jr, Dorman K: A simple method to estimate the volume for fetal intravascular transfusion. Fetal Diagn Ther 13:94, 1998

Golombeck K, Ball RH, Lee H, et al: Maternal morbidity after maternal-fetal surgery. Am J Obstet Gynecol 194:834, 2006

Gonzalez D, Barret T, Apuzzio J: Utility of routine fetal karyotyping for patients undergoing amniocentesis for elevated maternal serum alpha-fetoprotein. Am J Obstet Gynecol 174:436, 1996

Grabowski GA, Kruse JR, Goldberg JD, et al: First-trimester prenatal diagnosis of Tay-Sachs disease. Am J Hum Genet 36:1369, 1984

Grandone E, Corrao AM, Colaizzo D, et al: Homocysteine metabolism in families from southern Italy with neural tube defects: Role of genetic and nutritional determinants. Prenat Diagn 26:1, 2006

Greene MF, Haddow JE, Palomaki GE, et al: Maternal serum alpha-fetoprotein levels in diabetic pregnancies. Lancet 2:345, 1988

Grewal SS, Kahn JP, MacMillan ML, et al: Successful hematopoietic stem cell transplantation for Fanconi anemia from an unaffected HLA-genotype-identical sibling selected using preimplantation genetic diagnosis. Blood 103:1147, 2004

Haddow JE, Kloza EM, Smith DE, et al: Data from an alpha-fetoprotein pilot screening program in Maine. Obstet Gynecol 62:556, 1983

Haddow JE, Palomaki G, Knight GJ, et al: Screening of maternal serum for fetal Down's syndrome in the first trimester. N Engl J Med 338:955, 1998

Harrison MR, Jester JA, Ross NA: Correction of congenital diaphragmatic hernia in utero. I. The model: Intrathoracic balloon produces fatal pulmonary hypoplasia. Surgery 88:174, 1980

Harrison MR, Keller RL, Hawgood SB, et al: A randomized trial of fetal endoscopic tracheal occlusion for severe fetal congenital diaphragmatic hernia. N Engl J Med 349:1916, 2003

Heffez DS, Aryanpur J, Hutchins GM, et al: The paralysis associated with myelomeningocele: Clinical and experimental data implicating a preventable spinal cord injury. Neurosurgery 26:987, 1990

Hendrick HL, Flake AW, Crombleholme TM, et al: Sacrococcygeal teratoma: Prenatal assessment, fetal intervention, and outcome. J Pediatr Surg 39:430, 2004

Hirose S, Farmer DL, Lee H, et al: The ex utero intrapartum treatment procedure: Looking back at EXIT. J Pediatr Surg 39:375, 2004

Hogge WA, Thiagarajah S, Ferguson JE, et al: The role of ultrasonography and amniocentesis in the evaluation of pregnancies at risk for neural tube defects. Am J Obstet Gynecol 161:520, 1989

Hook EB, Cross PK, Schreinemachers DM: Chromosomal abnormality rates at amniocentesis and in live-born infants. JAMA 249:2034, 1983

Hsieh FJ, Shyu MK, Sheu BC, et al: Limb defects after chorionic villus sampling. Obstet Gynecol 85:84, 1995

Hume RF Jr, Drugan A, Reichler A, et al: Aneuploidy among prenatally detected neural tube defects. Am J Med Genet 61:171, 1996

Irons MB, Nores J, Stewart TL, et al: Antenatal therapy of Smith-Lemli-Opitz syndrome. Fetal Diagn Ther 14:133, 1999

Jackson LG, Zachary JM, Fowler SE, et al: A randomized comparison of transcervical and transabdominal chorionic-villus sampling. The U.S. National Institute of Child Health and Human Development Chorionic-Villus Sampling and Amniocentesis Study Group. N Engl J Med 327:636, 1992

Jiao Z, Zhou C, Li J, et al: Birth of healthy children after preimplantation diagnosis of beta-thalassemia by whole-genome amplification. Prenat Diagn 23:646, 2003

Johnson MP, Sutton LN, Rintoul N, et al: Fetal myelomeningocele repair: Short-term clinical outcomes. Am J Obstet Gynecol 189:482, 2003

Katz VL, Chescheir NC, Cefalo RC: Unexplained elevations of maternal serum alpha-fetoprotein. Obstet Gynecol Surv 45:719, 1990

Knight GK, Palomaki GE: Maternal serum alpha-fetoprotein and the detection of open neural tube defects. In: Elias S, Simpson JL, eds., Maternal Serum Screening. New York: Churchill Livingstone, p 41, 1992

Knox EM, Kilby MD, Martin WL, et al: In-utero pulmonary drainage in the management of primary hydrothorax and congenital cystic lung lesion: A systematic review. Ultrasound Obstet Gynecol 28:726, 2006

Kuliev A, Jackson L, Froster U, et al: Chorionic villus sampling safety. Report of World Health Organization/EURO meeting in association with the Seventh International Conference on Early Prenatal Diagnosis of Genetic Diseases, Tel Aviv, Israel, May 21, 1994. Am J Obstet Gynecol 174:807, 1996

Kunisaki SM, Fauza DO, Barnewolt CE, et al: Ex utero intrapartum treatment with placement on extracorporeal membrane oxygenation for fetal thoracic masses. J Pediatr Surg 42:420, 2007

Le Blanc K, Götherström C, Ringdén O, et al: Fetal mesenchymal stem-cell engraftment in bone after in utero transplantation in a patient with severe osteogenesis imperfecta. Transplantation 79:1607, 2005

Lee H, Crombleholme T, Wilson D: Radiofrequency ablation for twin-reversed arterial perfusion: The North American Fetal Treatment Network (NAFNET) experience. Abstract No 7. Presented at the 29th Annual Meeting of the Society for Maternal-Fetal Medicine. 26–31 January 2009

Lee H, Wagner AJ, Sy E, et al: Efficacy of radiofrequency ablation for twin-reversed arterial perfusion sequence. Am J Obstet Gynecol 196:459, 2007

Lee K, Khoshnood B, Chen L, et al: Infant mortality from congenital malformations in the United States, 1970–1997. Obstet Gynecol 98:620, 2001

Livingston JC, Lim FY, Polzin W, et al: Intrafetal radiofrequency ablation for twin reversed arterial perfusion (TRAP): A single-center experience. Am J Obstet Gynecol 197:399, 2007

Loeken M: Current perspectives on the causes of neural tube defects resulting from diabetic pregnancy. Am J Med Genet Part C (Semin Med Genet) 135C:77, 2005

Loft AG, Hogdall E, Larsen SO, et al: A comparison of amniotic fluid alpha-fetoprotein and acetylcholinesterase in the prenatal diagnosis of open neural tube defects and anterior abdominal wall defects. Prenatal Diagn 13:93, 1993

Luthy DA, Wardinsky T, Shurtleff DB, et al: Cesarean section before the onset of labor and subsequent motor function in infants with meningomyelocele diagnosed antenatally. N Engl J Med 324:662, 1991

Malone FD, Ball RH, Nyberg DA, et al: First-trimester nasal bone evaluation for aneuploidy in the general population. Obstet Gynecol 105:901, 2005

Malone FD, Canick JA, Ball RH, et al: First-trimester or second-trimester screening, or both, for Down's syndrome. N Engl J Med 353:2001, 2005

Mangione R, Guyon F, Vergnaud A, et al: Successful treatment of refractory supraventricular tachycardia by repeat intravascular injection of amiodarone in a fetus with hydrops. Eur J Obstet Gynecol Reprod Biol 86:105, 1999

Maxwell DJ, Johnson P, Hurley P, et al: Fetal blood sampling and pregnancy loss in relation to indication. Br J Obstet Gynaecol 98:892, 1991

Merkatz IR, Nitowsky HM, Macri JN, et al: An association between low maternal serum α-fetoprotein and fetal chromosomal abnormalities. Am J Obstet Gynecol 148:886, 1984

Meyers C, Adam R, Dungan J, et al: Aneuploidy in twin gestations: When is maternal age advanced? Obstet Gynecol 89:248, 1997

Milunsky A, Alpert E, Neff RK, et al: Prenatal diagnosis of neural tube defects. IV. Maternal serum alpha-fetoprotein screening. Obstet Gynecol 55:60, 1980

Milunsky A, Canick JA: Maternal serum screening for neural tube and other defects. In Milunsky A (ed): Genetic Disorders and the Fetus. Diagnosis, Prevention, and Treatment, 5th ed. Baltimore and London the Johns Hopkins University Press, 2004, p 719

Moise KJ: Management of rhesus alloimmunization in pregnancy. Obstet Gynecol 100:600, 2002

Moise KJ Jr, Belfort M, Saade G: Iatrogenic gastroschisis in the treatment of diaphragmatic hernia. Am J Obstet Gynecol 172:715, 1995

Morris LM, Lim FY, Crombleholme TM: Ex utero intrapartum treatment procedure: a peripartum management strategy in particularly challenging cases. J Pediatr 154(1):126, 2009

Morrow RJ, McNay MB, Whittle MJ: Ultrasound detection of neural tube defects in patients with elevated maternal serum alpha-fetoprotein. Obstet Gynecol 78:1055, 1991

Munne S: Preimplantation genetic diagnosis of structural abnormalities. Mol Cell Endocrinol 183:S55, 2001

Munoz JB, Lacasana M, Cavazos RG, et al: Methylenetetrahydrofolate reductase gene polymorphisms and risk of anencephaly in Mexico. Mol Hum Reprod 13:419, 2007

Nadel AS, Green JK, Holmes LB, et al: Absence of need for amniocentesis in patients with elevated levels of maternal serum alpha-fetoprotein and normal ultrasonographic examinations. N Engl J Med 323:557, 1990

Nagel HT, DeHaan TR, Vandenbussche FP, et al: Long-term outcome after fetal transfusion for hydrops associated with parvovirus B19 infection. Obstet Gynecol 109:42, 2007.

New MI, Nimkarn S: 21-hydroxylase-deficient urogenital adrenal hyperplasia. Gene Review www.genetests.org Updated 7 September 2007

NICHD National Registry for Amniocentesis Study Group: Midtrimester amniocentesis for prenatal diagnosis. JAMA 236:1471, 1976

Nicolaides KH, Campbell S, Gabbe SG, et al: Ultrasound screening for spina bifida: Cranial and cerebellar signs. Lancet 12:72, 1986

Nicolaides K, Brizot M de L, Patel F, et al: Comparison of chorionic villus sampling and amniocentesis for fetal karyotyping at 10–13 weeks' gestation. Lancet 344:435, 1994

Nicolaides KH: Nuchal translucency and other first-trimester sonographic markers of chromosomal abnormalities. Review article. Am J Obstet Gynecol 191:45, 2004

Niinikoski H, Mamalainen Am, Ekblad H, et al: Neonatal hypothyroidism after amiodarone therapy. Acta Paediatrica 96:773, 2007

Norem CT, Schoen EJ, Walton DL, et al: Routine ultrasonography compared with maternal serum alpha-fetoprotein for neural tube defect screening. Obstet Gynecol 106:747, 2005

Norton ME: Evaluation and management of twin-twin transfusion syndrome: Still a challenge. Am J Obstet Gynecol 196:606, 2007

Nyberg DA, Souter VL: Use of genetic sonography for adjusting the risk for fetal Down syndrome. Semin Perinatol 27:130, 2003

Nyberg DA, Souter VL, El-Bastawissi A, et al: Isolated sonographic markers for detection of fetal Down syndrome in the second trimester of pregnancy. J Ultrasound Med 20:1053, 2001

Ober-Berman J, Xiong Y, Wagner C, et al: Accuracy of noninvasive prenatal diagnosis of fetal single gene disorders from maternal blood. Abstract No 618. Presented at the 29th Annual Meeting of the Society for Maternal-Fetal Medicine. 26–31 January 2009

O'Brien B, Bianchi DW: Fetal therapy for single gene disorders. Clin Obstet Gynecol 48:885, 2005

Persutte WH, Lenke RR: Failure of amniotic-fluid-cell growth: Is it related to fetal aneuploidy? Lancet 345:96, 1995

Philip J, Silver RK, Wilson RD, et al: Late first-trimester invasive prenatal diagnosis: Results of an international randomized trial. Obstet Gynecol 103:1164, 2004

Poon LL, Leung TN, Lau TK, et al: Prenatal detection of fetal Down's syndrome from maternal plasma. Lancet 356:1819, 2000

Reddy UM, Mennuti MT: Incorporating first-trimester Down syndrome studies in to prenatal screening. Obstet Gynecol 107:167, 2006

Reichler A, Hume RF Jr, Drugan A, et al: Risk of anomalies as a function of level of elevated maternal serum α-fetoprotein. Am J Obstet Gynecol 171:1052, 1994

Reickert CA, Hirschl RB, Atkinson JB, et al: Congenital diaphragmatic hernia survival and use of extracorporeal life support at selected level III nurseries with multimodality support. Surgery 123:305, 1998

Rhoads GG, Jackson LG, Schlesselman SE, et al: The safety and efficacy of chorionic villus sampling for early prenatal diagnosis of cytogenetic abnormalities. N Engl J Med 320:609, 1989

Rosen T, D'Alton ME, Platt LD, et al: First-trimester ultrasound assessment of the nasal bone to screen for aneuploidy. Obstet Gynecol 110:339, 2007

Rund D, Rachmilewitz E: β-Thalassemia. N Engl J Med 353:1135, 2005

Rychik J, Tian Z, Bebbington M, et al: The twin-twin transfusion syndrome: Spectrum of cardiovascular abnormality and development of a cardiovascular score to assess severity of disease. Am J Obstet Gynecol 197:392, 2007

Sakala EP, Andree I: Optimal route of delivery for meningomyelocele. Obstet Gynecol Surv 45:209, 1990

Sancken U, Bartels I: Biochemical screening for chromosomal disorders and neural tube defects (NTD): Is adjustment of maternal alpha-fetoprotein (AFP) still appropriate in insulin-dependent diabetes mellitus (IDDM)? Prenat Diagn 21:383, 2001

Santiago-Munoz PC, McIntire DD, Barber RG, et al: Outcomes of pregnancies with fetal gastroschisis. Obstet Gynecol 110:663, 2007

Schumacher B, Moise KJ Jr: Fetal transfusion for red blood cell alloimmunization in pregnancy. Obstet Gynecol 88:137, 1996

Sepulveda W, Donaldson A, Johnson RD, et al: Are routine alpha-fetoprotein and acetylcholinesterase determinations still necessary at second-trimester amniocentesis? Impact of high-resolution ultrasonography. Obstet Gynecol 85:107, 1995

Shulman LP, Elias S, Phillips OP, et al: Amniocentesis performed at 14 weeks' gestation or earlier: Comparison with first-trimester transabdominal chorionic villus sampling. Obstet Gynecol 83:543, 1994

Simpson JL: Fetal arrhythmias. Ultrasound Obstet Gynecol 27:599, 2006

Simpson JL, Elias S, Morgan CD, et al: Does unexplained second trimester (15 to 20 weeks' gestation) maternal serum alpha-fetoprotein elevation presage adverse perinatal outcome? Pitfalls and preliminary studies with late second- and third-trimester maternal serum alpha-fetoprotein. Am J Obstet Gynecol 164:829, 1991

Simpson JM, Sharland GK: Natural history and outcome of aortic stenosis diagnosed prenatally. Heart 77:205, 1997

Simpson LL, Malone FD, Bianchi DW, et al: Nuchal translucency and the risk of congenital heart disease. Obstet Gynecol 109:376, 2007

Smith-Bindman R, Hosmer W, Feldstein VA, et al: Second-trimester ultrasound to detect fetuses with Down syndrome. A meta-analysis. JAMA 285:1044, 2001

Snijders RJ, Noble P, Sebire N, et al: UK multicentre project on assessment of risk of trisomy 21 by maternal age and fetal nuchal-translucency thickness at 10–14 weeks of gestation. Fetal Medicine Foundation First Trimester Screening Group. Lancet 352:337, 1998

Souka AP, Krampl E, Bakalis S, et al: Outcome of pregnancy in chromosomally normal fetuses with increased nuchal translucency in the first trimester. Ultrasound Obstet Gynecol 18:9, 2001

Souka AP, Snijders RJ, Novakov A, et al: Defects and syndromes in chromosomally normal fetuses with increased nuchal translucency thickness at 10-14 weeks of gestation. Ultrasound Obstet Gynecol 11:388, 1998

Spencer K, Wallace EM, Ritoe S: Second-trimester dimeric inhibin-A in Down's syndrome screening. Prenat Diagn 15:1101, 1996

Spits C, LeCaignec C, DeRycke M, et al: Whole-genome multiple displacement amplification from single cells. Nat Protocols 1:1965, 2006

Steigman SA, Nemes L, Barnewolt CE, et al: Differential risk for neonatal surgical airway intervention in prenatally diagnosed neck masses. J Pediatr Surg 44(1):76, 2009

Sundberg K, Bang J, Smidt-Jensen S, et al: Randomised study of risk of fetal loss related to early amniocentesis versus chorionic villus sampling. Lancet 350:697, 1997

Thiagarajah S, Stroud CB, Vavelidis F, et al: Elevated maternal serum α-fetoprotein levels: What is the risk of fetal aneuploidy? Am J Obstet Gynecol 173:388, 1995

Tiblad E, Westgren M: Fetal stem-cell transplantation. Best Pract Res Clin Obstet Gynaecol 22:189, 2008

Van den Hof MC, Nicolaides KH, Campbell J, et al: Evaluation of the lemon and banana signs in one hundred thirty fetuses with open spina bifida. Am J Obstet Gynecol 162:322, 1990

Van Mieghem T, Klaritsch P, Doné E, et al: Assessment of fetal cardiac function before and after therapy for twin-to-twin transfusion syndrome. Am J Obstet Gynecol 200(4):400.e1, 2009

Velie EM, Shaw GM, Malcoe LH, et al: Understanding the increased risk of neural tube defect-affected pregnancies among Mexico-born women in California: Immigration and anthropomorphic factors. Paediatr Perinat Epidemiol 20:219, 2006

Vintzileos AJ, Egan JF: Adjusting the risk for trisomy 21 on the basis of second-trimester ultrasonography. Am J Obstet Gynecol 172:837, 1995

Wald NJ, Cuckle H, Brock JH, et al: Maternal serum-alpha-fetoprotein measurement in antenatal screening for anencephaly and spina bifida in early pregnancy. Report of UK Collaborative Study on Alpha-Fetoprotein in Relation to Neural-tube Defects. Lancet 1:1323, 1977

Wald NJ, Cuckle HS, Densem JW, et al: Maternal serum unconjugated oestriol as an antenatal screening test for Down's syndrome. Br J Obstet Gynaecol 95:334, 1988a

Wald NJ, Cuckle HS, Densem JW, et al: Maternal serum screening for Down's syndrome in early pregnancy. BMJ 297:1029, 1988b

Wald NJ, Densem JW, Muttukrishna S, et al: Prenatal screening for Down's syndrome using inhibin-A as a serum marker. Prenat Diagn 16:143, 1996

Waller DK, Lustig LS, Cunningham GC, et al: Second-trimester maternal serum alpha-fetoprotein levels and the risk of subsequent fetal death. N Engl J Med 325:6, 1991

Wapner R, Thom E, Simpson JL, et al: First-trimester screening for trisomies 21 and 18. N Engl J Med 349:1471, 2003

Watson WJ, Chescheir NC, Katz VL, et al: The role of ultrasound in evaluation of patients with elevated maternal serum alpha-fetoprotein: A review. Obstet Gynecol 78:123, 1991

Wenstrom KD, Andrews WW, Tamura T, et al: Elevated amniotic fluid interleukin-6 levels at genetic amniocentesis predict subsequent pregnancy loss. Am J Obstet Gynecol 174:830, 1996

Wenstrom KD, Weiner CP, Williamson RA, et al: Prenatal diagnosis of fetal hyperthyroidism using funipuncture. Obstet Gynecol 76:513, 1990

Westgren M, Ringden O, Eik-Nes S, et al: Lack of evidence of permanent engraftment after in utero fetal stem cell transplantation in congenital hemoglobinopathies. Transplantation 61:1176, 1996

Wilkins-Haug LE, Tworetzky W, Benson CB, et al: Factors affecting technical success of fetal aortic valve dilatation. Ultrasound Obstet Gynecol 28:47, 2006

Wilson RD, Johnson MP: Prenatal ultrasound guided percutaneous shunts for obstructive uropathy and thoracic disease. Semin Pediatr Surg 12:182, 2003

Xu K, Rosenwaks Z, Beaverson K, et al: Preimplantation genetic diagnosis for retinoblastoma: The first reported liveborn. Am J Ophthalmol 137:18, 2004

Zhao Z, Reece EA: Experimental mechanisms of diabetic embryopathy and strategies for developing therapeutic interventions. J Soc Gynecol Invest 12:449, 2005

CHAPTER 14

Teratology and Medications That Affect the Fetus

In the United States, approximately 3 percent of infants have a major structural malformation that is detectable at birth. By age 5, another 3 percent have been diagnosed with a malformation, and another 8 to 10 percent are discovered to have one or more functional or developmental abnormalities by age 18. For most birth defects—approximately 65 percent, the etiology is unknown (Schardein, 2000). Importantly, chemically induced birth defects, which include those caused by medications, are believed to account for less than 1 percent of all birth defects (Center for Drug Evaluation and Research, 2005). Selected examples of confirmed teratogens are listed in Table 14-1.

Medications are commonly prescribed for pregnant women, and in France, Lacroix and colleagues (2000) found this to average 13.6 medications. Nearly all drugs in pregnancy are used off-label because of the paucity of research and clinical trials. The study of medication use in pregnancy is hampered at least in part by the difficulty of studying this special population given the vulnerability of the developing fetus. In addition, there are numerous physiological changes in pregnancy such as alterations in blood volume, plasma proteins, and gastric emptying and transit time that affect dosing and distribution of drugs.

TERATOLOGY

A *teratogen* is any agent—chemicals, viruses, environmental agents, physical factors, and drugs—that acts during embryonic or fetal development to produce a permanent alteration of form or function. The word *teratogen* is derived from the Greek *teratos,* meaning monster. A *hadegen*—after Hades, the god who possessed a helmet conferring invisibility—is an agent that interferes with normal maturation and function of an organ. A *trophogen* is an agent that alters growth. Hadegens and trophogens generally affect processes occurring after organogenesis or even after birth. Chemical or physical exposures that act as hadegens or trophogens are much harder to document. For simplification, most authors use the word *teratogen* to refer to all three types of agents.

Evaluation of Potential Teratogens

A birth defect in a newborn exposed prenatally to a certain drug, chemical, or environmental agent arouses concern that the agent is a teratogen. The two approaches used currently to identify teratogenicity after a drug is released for clinical use include follow-up studies and case-control surveillance (Mitchell, 2003). Before such culpability is established, specific criteria that follow the tenets in Table 14-2 must be considered:

- *The defect must be completely characterized.* This is preferably done by a geneticist or dysmorphologist. Many genetic and environmental factors produce similar anomalies. For example, although cleft lip and palate are associated with antenatal hydantoin exposure, there are also more than 200 known genetic causes (Murray, 1995). Identical defects with different etiologies are called *phenocopies.* It is easiest to prove causation when a rare exposure produces a rare defect, when at least three cases with the same exposure have been identified, and when the defect is severe.

TABLE 14-1. Selected Drugs or Substances Suspected or Proven to Be Human Teratogens

Alcohol	Methimazole
Angiotensin-converting enzyme inhibitors and angiotensin-receptor blockers	Methyl mercury
	Methotrexate
Aminopterin	Misoprostol
Androgens	Mycophenolate
Bexarotene	Paroxetine
Bosentan	Penicillamine
Carbamazepine	Phenobarbital
Chloramphenicol	Phenytoin
Chlorbiphenyls	Radioactive iodine
Cocaine	Ribavirin
Corticosteroids	Streptomycin
Cyclophosphamide	Tamoxifen
Danazol	Tetracycline
Diethylstilbestrol (DES)	Thalidomide
Efavirenz	Tobacco
Etretinate	Toluene
Isotretinoin	Tretinoin
Leflunomide	Valproate
Lithium	Warfarin

- *The agent must cross the placenta.* Although with few exceptions, all drugs cross the placenta, the drug must do so in sufficient *quantity* to directly influence fetal development or alter maternal or placental metabolism to exert an indirect fetal effect. Placental transfer depends on maternal metabolism; on specific characteristics of the drug, such as

TABLE 14-2. Criteria for Proof of Human Teratogenicity

1. Careful delineation of clinical cases
2. Rare environmental exposure associated with rare defect, with at least three reported cases—easiest if defect is severe
3. Proof that the agent acts on the embryo or fetus, directly or indirectly
4. Proven exposure to agent at critical time(s) in prenatal development
5. The association must be biologically plausible
6. Consistent findings by two or more epidemiological studies of high quality:
   (a) Control of confounding factors
   (b) Sufficient numbers
   (c) Exclusion of positive and negative bias factors
   (d) Prospective studies, if possible
   (e) Relative risk of three or more
7. Teratogenicity in experimental animals, especially primates

Modified from Czeizel and Rockenbauer (1997), Shepard (2001), and Yaffe and Briggs (2003).

protein binding and storage, molecular size, electrical charge, and lipid solubility; and on placental metabolism, such as with cytochrome P_{450} enzyme systems. In early pregnancy, the placenta also has a relatively thick membrane that slows diffusion (Leppik and Rask, 1988).

- *Exposure must occur during a critical developmental period.* Syndromes resulting from teratogen exposure are named according to the time of exposure. Those within the first 8 weeks result in an *embryopathy,* and after 8 weeks, a *fetopathy.*
  1. The *preimplantation period* is the 2 weeks from fertilization to implantation and has traditionally been called the "all or none" period. The zygote undergoes cleavage, and an insult damaging a large number of cells usually causes death of the embryo. If only a few cells are injured, compensation is usually possible with continued normal development (Clayton-Smith and Donnai, 1996). Animal studies have shown that some insults—those that appreciably diminish the number of cells in the inner cell mass—can produce a dose-dependent diminution in body length or size (Iahnaccone and co-workers, 1987).
  2. The *embryonic period* is from the second through the eighth week. It encompasses organogenesis and is thus the most crucial with regard to structural malformations. The critical developmental period for each organ system is shown in Figure 14-1.
  3. Maturation and functional development continue after 8 weeks, and during this *fetal period,* certain organs remain vulnerable. For example, the brain remains susceptible throughout pregnancy to environmental influences such as alcohol exposure. Alteration in cardiac blood flow during the fetal period can result in deformations such as hypoplastic left heart or aortic coarctation (Clark, 1984).

- *There must be a biologically plausible association.* Because both birth defects and drug or environmental exposures are common, it is always possible that an exposure and a defect are temporally but not causally related. For example, pregnant women frequently express concern about ingesting food or drinks containing aspartame. This compound, however, is metabolized to aspartic acid, which does not cross the placenta; to phenylalanine, which is metabolized; and to methanol, which is produced from aspartame in quantities lower than those released from an equal amount of metabolized fruit juice. Thus, it is not biologically plausible that aspartame is a teratogen.

- *Epidemiological findings must be consistent.* The initial evaluation of teratogen exposure is usually retrospective and may be hampered by recall bias, inadequate reporting, and incomplete assessment of the exposed population. The investigation is often confounded by a variety of dosages, concomitant drug therapy, and maternal disease(s). Familial and environmental factors can also influence development of birth defects. Thus, an important criterion for proving teratogenicity is that two or more high-quality epidemiological studies should report similar findings. These studies should control for confounding factors, exclude positive and negative biases, include a sufficient number of cases, and be conducted prospectively. Additionally, a relative risk greater than 3 is generally

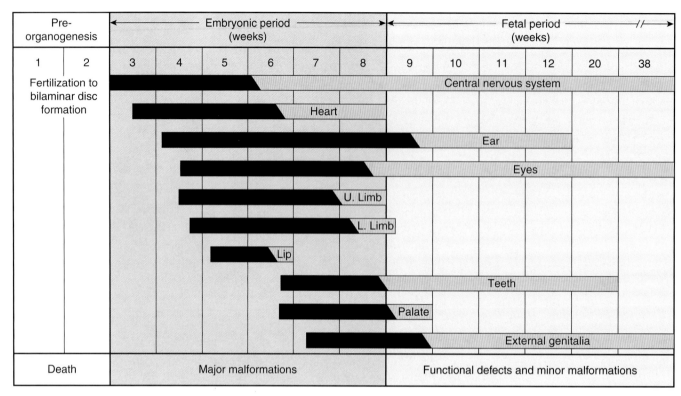

FIGURE 14-1 Timing of organogenesis during the embryonic period. (From Sadler, 1990, with permission.)

necessary to support the hypothesis, and a lesser risk should be interpreted with caution (Khouri and colleagues, 1992).

An illustration of the advantages of prospective evaluation is the Canadian multicenter study of lithium exposure (Jacobson and colleagues, 1992). Multiple case reports had associated lithium use with the rare *Ebstein anomaly* of the heart. When 148 exposed women were carefully evaluated prospectively, there was only one case of Ebstein anomaly, leading to the conclusion that lithium is not an important human teratogen, but that targeted sonography and fetal echocardiography are indicated following exposure. Suspected teratogens rarely are evaluated epidemiologically, and as a result, drug safety information frequently is derived from case reports and small series. Nonscientific and biased reporting has contributed to assertions—subsequently proven false—about the safety of widely used drugs. In many cases these assertions prompted litigation and cessation of manufacture of some very useful drugs. An example is *Bendectin,* a drug that was safe and effective for the treatment of nausea and vomiting in early pregnancy. More than 30 million women used this drug worldwide, and the 3-percent congenital anomaly rate among exposed fetuses was not different from the background rate (McKeigue and associates, 1994). Despite evidence that Bendectin was not teratogenic, it was the subject of numerous lawsuits, and the financial burden of defending these suits forced its withdrawal. Thereafter, hospitalizations for hyperemesis doubled (Koren and co-workers, 1998).

• *The suspected teratogen causes a defect in an animal.* If a drug or environmental exposure causes birth defects in experimental animals, it may be harmful to the human fetus

(Brent, 2004a, 2004b). Human teratogenicity is more likely if the agent produces an adverse effect in many different species, especially subhuman primates.

The problems associated with reliance on animal data are illustrated by thalidomide. Although one of the most potent human teratogens was known, its teratogenicity was not recognized until thousands of infants had been born with thalidomide embryopathy because it produced no defects in several animal species studied.

Food and Drug Administration Classifications

To provide therapeutic guidance, a system for rating drug safety in pregnancy was developed in 1979 by the Food and Drug Administration (FDA). The system was designed to assist physicians by simplifying risk-benefit information with categories represented by letters that are listed in the classification shown in Table 14-3. The general consensus is that this system is not ideal. Many drug ratings are based on animal data, case reports, and limited or no human data, with information rarely updated. Because the manufacturer rates the product, discrepancies are common. This may be one reason why Lacroix and associates (2000) found that more than half of pregnant women in France were prescribed a medication from category D. Rather than simplifying counseling, this system places the onus on the clinician to interpret category information according to timing of exposure, dose, route, other medications used, and underlying medical condition(s).

The FDA acknowledges important limitations of the system. One is that drugs in categories D and X, and to a certain extent those in category C, may pose similar risks but are categorized

TABLE 14-3. Food and Drug Administration Categories for Drugs and Medications

Category A: Studies in pregnant women have not shown an increased risk for fetal abnormalities if administered during the first (second, third, or all) trimester(s) of pregnancy, and the possibility of fetal harm appears remote.

Fewer than 1 percent of all medications are in this category. Examples include levothyroxine, potassium supplementation, and prenatal vitamins, when taken at recommended doses.

Category B: Animal reproduction studies have been performed and have revealed no evidence of impaired fertility or harm to the fetus. Prescribing information should specify kind of animal and how dose compares with human dose.

or

Animal studies have shown an adverse effect, but adequate and well-controlled studies in pregnant women have failed to demonstrate a risk to the fetus during the first trimester of pregnancy, and there is no evidence of a risk in later trimesters.

Examples include many antibiotics, such as penicillins, macrolides, and most cephalosporins.

Category C: Animal reproduction studies have shown that this medication is teratogenic (or embryocidal or has other adverse effect), and there are no adequate and well-controlled studies in pregnant women. Prescribing information should specify kind of animal and how dose compares with human dose.

or

There are no animal reproduction studies and no adequate and well-controlled studies in humans.

Approximately two thirds of all medications are in this category. It contains medications commonly used to treat potentially life-threatening medical conditions, such as albuterol for asthma, zidovudine and lamivudine for human immunodeficiency viral infection, and many antihypertensives, including β-blockers and calcium-channel blockers.

Category D: This medication can cause fetal harm when administered to a pregnant woman. If this drug is used during pregnancy or if a woman becomes pregnant while taking this medication, she should be apprised of the potential hazard to the fetus.

This category also contains medications used to treat potentially life-threatening medical conditions, for example: systemic corticosteroids, azathioprine, phenytoin, carbamazepine, valproic acid, and lithium.

Category X: This medication is contraindicated in women who are or may become pregnant. It may cause fetal harm. If this drug is used during pregnancy or if a woman becomes pregnant while taking this medication, she should be apprised of the potential hazard to the fetus.

There are a few medications in this category that have never been shown to cause fetal harm but should be avoided nonetheless such as the rubella vaccine.

---

differently based on different risk-benefit considerations. Another drawback is that merely having categories creates the impression that drugs within a category pose similar risks, which is not the case. Concern has also been raised that reliance on the drug categories to make complex decisions about therapy for pregnant women may often be inappropriate.

Because of these problems, the FDA has proposed new rules for labeling drugs for use by pregnant women. Specifically, the Center for Drug Evaluation and Research (Food and Drug Administration, 2008) would remove the A-X categories and replace them with a narrative *fetal risk summary, clinical considerations,* and *inadvertent exposure* including registries available. This evidence-based rating system is currently under development. Meanwhile, the most current and accurate information can be obtained through online reproductive toxicity services such as *Reprotox* and *TERIS.*

GENETIC AND PHYSIOLOGICAL MECHANISMS OF TERATOGENICITY

Teratogens likely act by disturbing specific physiological processes, which leads to cell death, altered tissue growth, or abnormal cellular differentiation. Because abnormal physiological processes may be induced in many different cells or tissues, teratogenic exposure commonly results in multiple effects. Drugs

may produce similar phenotypes if they disturb similar pathophysiological processes. The *fetal hydantoin syndrome,* subsequently discussed, illustrates this concept. Exposure may cause any combination of growth impairment, developmental delay, craniofacial abnormalities, hypoplasia of the distal phalanges, and widely spaced nipples. This phenotype shares features with that associated with prenatal exposure to carbamazepine and is similar to fetal alcohol syndrome (Vorhees and associates, 1988).

Disruption of Folic Acid Metabolism

Several congenital anomalies, including neural-tube defects, cardiac defects, cleft lip and palate, and even Down syndrome, are thought to arise, at least in part, from disturbance of folic acid metabolic pathways. Folic acid is essential for the production of methionine, which is required for methylation reactions and thus production of proteins, lipids, and myelin. Hydantoin, carbamazepine, valproic acid, and phenobarbital impair folate absorption or act as antagonists. They can lead to decreased periconceptional folate levels in women with epilepsy and to fetal malformations (Dansky and colleagues, 1987; Hiilesmaa and co-workers, 1983).

A study by Hernandez-Diaz and colleagues (2000) that included 5832 infants with birth defects and 8387 control infants is instructive. They showed that fetuses who were exposed during embryogenesis to anticonvulsant medications that act as folic acid antagonists had a two- to threefold increased risk for oral clefts, cardiac defects, and urinary tract abnormalities. Although periconceptional folate supplementation lowers the malformation rate, women with epilepsy should be given the fewest number of drugs possible during pregnancy as well as folic acid supplementation (Lewis and co-workers, 1998; Zhu and Zhou, 1989).

Fetal Genetic Composition

It is believed that many multifactorial anomalies are caused by the interaction of environment and certain altered genes. One well-known example is mutation of the gene for *methylene tetrahydrofolate reductase—MTHFR 677C → T*. This mutation is associated with neural-tube defects and other malformations, but only when the mother has inadequate folic acid intake.

Another example is that fetuses exposed to hydantoin are most likely to develop anomalies if they are homozygous for a gene mutation resulting in abnormally low levels of *epoxide hydrolase* (Buehler and associates, 1990). Hydantoin, carbamazepine, and phenobarbital are metabolized by microsomes to arene oxides or epoxides. These oxidative intermediates normally are detoxified by cytoplasmic *epoxide hydrolase,* but because fetal epoxide hydrolase activity is weak, oxidative intermediates accumulate in fetal tissue (Horning and colleagues, 1974). These free oxide radicals have carcinogenic, mutagenic, and other toxic effects that are dose related and increase with multidrug therapy (Buehler and associates, 1990; Lindhout and co-workers, 1984).

There is also a reported association between cigarette smoking and isolated cleft palate, but only in individuals with an uncommon polymorphism in the gene for *transforming growth factor-1—TGF-1*. The risk of clefts in individuals with this allele is increased two- to sevenfold (Hwang and colleagues, 1995; Shaw and co-workers, 1996).

Homeobox Genes

These are highly conserved genes that share a region of homology. They are regulatory and encode nuclear proteins that act as transcription factors to control the expression of other developmentally important genes (Boncinelli, 1997). They are essential for establishing positional identity of various structures along the body axis from the branchial area to the coccyx. The arrangement of the genes along the chromosome corresponds to the arrangement of the body areas they control and the order in which they are activated (Faiella and collaborators, 1994).

An example of homeobox gene teratogenicity is retinoic acid. During embryogenesis, retinoids such as vitamin A activate genes essential for normal growth and tissue differentiation. Retinoic acid is a potent teratogen that can activate these genes prematurely, resulting in chaotic gene expression at sensitive stages of development (Soprano and Soprano, 1995). This mechanism has been linked to abnormalities in the hindbrain and limb buds. Another example is valproic acid, which is believed to preferentially alter the expression of the homeobox *Hox genes.* Disregulation of Hox-gene expression by valproic acid may prevent normal closure of the posterior neuropore (Faiella and colleagues, 1994). Interestingly, the affected Hox genes, *Hox d8, d10,* and *d11*, all control posterior structures.

This corresponds with clinical observations that most neural-tube defects caused by valproic acid are in the lumbosacral area.

Paternal Exposures

In some cases, paternal exposures to drugs or environmental influences may increase the risk of adverse fetal outcome (Robaire and Hales, 1993). Several mechanisms are postulated. One is the induction of a gene mutation or chromosomal abnormality in sperm. Because the process by which germ cells mature into functional spermatogonia takes 64 days, drug exposure at any time during the 2 months prior to conception could result in a mutation. A second possibility is that during intercourse a drug in seminal fluid could directly contact the fetus. And a third is that paternal germ cell exposure to drugs or environmental agents may alter gene expression (Trasler and Doerksen, 1999).

Some studies support these hypotheses. For example, ethyl alcohol, cyclophosphamide, lead, and certain opiates have been associated with an increased risk of behavioral defects in the offspring of exposed male rodents (Nelson and colleagues, 1996). In humans, paternal environmental exposure to mercury, lead, solvents, pesticides, anesthetic gases, or hydrocarbons may be associated with early pregnancy loss (Savitz and associates, 1994). Offspring of men employed in the art or textile industries have been reported to be at increased risk for stillbirth, preterm delivery, and growth restriction. Others who may have an increased risk of having anomalous offspring include janitors, woodworkers, firemen, printers, and painters (Olshan and co-workers, 1991; Schnitzer and associates, 1995).

COUNSELING FOR TERATOGEN EXPOSURE

Questions regarding medication and illicit drug use should be part of routine preconceptional and prenatal care. Often women who request genetic counseling for prenatal drug exposure have misinformation regarding risk. Koren and colleagues (1989) reported that a fourth of women exposed to nonteratogenic drugs thought they had a 25-percent risk of fetal anomalies—that is, a risk equivalent to thalidomide exposure. Women also may underestimate the background risk of birth defects in the general population. Such misleading information can be amplified by the referral source, who may exaggerate risk—and even offer pregnancy termination—or by inaccurate reports in the lay press.

Counseling should include possible fetal risks from drug exposure, as well as possible teratogenic risks or genetic implications of the condition for which the drug was prescribed. Importantly, the manner in which information is presented affects the perception of risk. Jasper and colleagues (2001) showed that women given *negative information*—such as a 1- to 3-percent chance of having a malformed newborn—are more likely to perceive an exaggerated risk than women given *positive information*, that is, the 97- to 99-percent chance of having a child without a malformation. Ideally, women should be counseled preconceptionally as discussed throughout Chapter 7. In reality, however, patients often do not seek care or report possible adverse exposures until *after* conception.

With a few notable exceptions, most commonly prescribed drugs and medications can be used with relative safety during pregnancy.

For the few drugs believed to be teratogenic, counseling should emphasize *relative risk*. All women have an approximate 3-percent chance of having a neonate with a birth defect. Although exposure to a confirmed teratogen may increase this risk, it is usually increased by only 1 or 2 percent, or at most, doubled or tripled. The concept of *risk versus benefit* also should be introduced. Some untreated diseases pose a more serious threat to both mother and fetus than any theoretical risks from medication exposure.

EXAMPLES OF KNOWN AND SUSPECTED TERATOGENS

Fortunately, the number of drugs or medications strongly suspected or proven to be human teratogens is small (see Table 14-1). In addition, in nearly every clinical situation potentially requiring therapy with a known teratogen, there are several alternate drugs that can be given with relative safety. In general, because there are no adequate and well-controlled studies in pregnant women for most medications, and because animal reproduction studies are not always predictive of human response, the use of any medication in pregnancy must be carefully considered and only used if clearly needed.

Alcohol

Ethyl alcohol is one of the most potent teratogens known. As many as 70 percent of Americans drink alcohol socially, and its use during pregnancy varies by population. Ethen and associates (2009) published data from the National Birth Defects Prevention Study that 30 percent of women report drinking alcohol during pregnancy. This rate is approximately threefold higher than that found in a 2002 survey by the Centers for Disease Control and Prevention (2004).

The fetal effects of alcohol abuse have been recognized at least since the 1800s. Lemoine and associates (1968) categorized the wide spectrum of alcohol-related fetal defects, in what is now known as the *fetal alcohol syndrome* (Table 14-4). The Institute of Medicine (1996) has estimated that the prevalence of the syndrome ranges from 0.6 to 3 per 1000 births, and the prevalence of alcohol-related birth defects and neurobehavioral disorders is 9 per 1000 births. Thus, alcohol is one of the most frequent nongenetic causes of mental retardation as well as the leading cause of preventable birth defects in the United States.

Clinical Characteristics

Fetal alcohol syndrome has specific criteria, which are enumerated in Table 14-4. These were updated by a national task force of the Centers for Disease Control and Prevention and include dysmorphic facial features, pre- or postnatal growth impairment, and central nervous system abnormalities that may be structural, neurological, or functional (Bertrand and colleagues, 2005). The distinctive facial features are shown in Figure 14-2. Affected individuals may have other alcohol-related major and minor birth defects, including cardiac and renal anomalies, orthopedic problems, and abnormalities of the eyes and ears. *Fetal alcohol spectrum disorder* is an umbrella term that includes the full range of prenatal alcohol damage that may not meet the criteria for fetal alcohol syndrome and is esti-

TABLE 14-4. Fetal Alcohol Syndrome and Alcohol-Related Birth Defects

Fetal Alcohol Syndrome Diagnostic Criteria—all required
I. Dysmorphic facial features
   a. Small palpebral fissures
   b. Thin vermilion border
   c. Smooth philtrum
II. Prenatal and/or postnatal growth impairment
III. Central nervous system abnormalities
   a. Structural: Head size < 10th percentile, significant brain abnormality on imaging
   b. Neurological
   c. Functional: Global cognitive or intellectual deficits, functional deficits in at least three domains

Alcohol-Related Birth Defects
I. Cardiac: atrial or ventricular septal defect, aberrant great vessels, conotruncal heart defects
II. Skeletal: radioulnar synostosis, vertebral segmentation defects, joint contractures, scoliosis
III. Renal: aplastic or hypoplastic kidneys, dysplastic kidneys, horseshoe kidney, ureteral duplication
IV. Eyes: strabismus, ptosis, retinal vascular abnormalities, optic nerve hypoplasia
V. Ears: conductive or neurosensory hearing loss
VI. Minor: hypoplastic nails, clinodactyly, pectus carinatum or excavatum, camptodactyly, "hockey stick" palmar creases, refractive errors, "railroad track" ears

Modified from Bertrand and co-workers (2005) and Hoyme and colleagues (2005).

mated to occur in up to 1 in 100 children born in the United States (Burd, 2003; Guerri, 2009; Sampson, 1997, and all their associates).

Dose Effect

Binge drinking has been linked to an increased risk of stillbirth (Strandberg-Larsen and co-workers, 2008). However, the minimum amount of alcohol required to produce adverse fetal consequences is unknown (Henderson and colleagues, 2007). Fetal vulnerability varies due to genetic factors, nutritional status, environmental factors, coexisting disease, and maternal age (Abel, 1995). Wass and colleagues (2001) monitored fetal brain growth sonographically in 167 pregnant women. They found that of the fetuses whose mothers drank an average of 8 ounces of alcohol per day, 23 percent had a frontal cortex measurement below the 10th percentile compared with only 4 percent of nonexposed fetuses. Unfortunately, fetal alcohol syndrome cannot be reliably diagnosed prenatally, although in some cases, major abnormalities or growth restriction may suggest it.

Anticonvulsant Medications

Women with epilepsy have an increased risk of fetal malformations that is usually estimated to be two to three times the

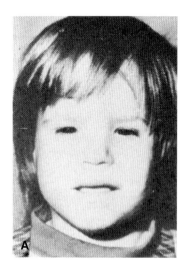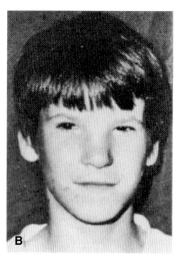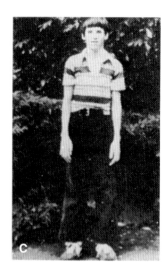

FIGURE 14-2 Fetal alcohol syndrome. **A.** At 2½ years. **B, C.** At 12 years. Note persistence of short palpebral fissures, epicanthal folds, flat midface, hypoplastic philtrum, and thin upper vermilion border. This individual also has the short, lean prepubertal stature characteristic of young males with fetal alcohol syndrome. (Reprinted from *The Lancet,* Vol. 326, AP Streissguth, SK Clarren, and KL Jones, Natural history of the fetal alcohol syndrome: A 10-year-follow-up of eleven patients, pp. 85–91, Copyright 1985, with permission from Elsevier.)

background rate. There has been controversy as to whether the increased risk is due to the underlying seizure disorder or the medication(s) used to treat it (Holmes and colleagues, 2001). Recent data suggest that the risks are not as great as once thought. For example, a meta-analysis by Fried and associates (2004) from the Toronto Motherisk Program showed that women with untreated epilepsy had a similar risk for major fetal malformations as did nonepileptic control women. And in the United Kingdom Epilepsy and Pregnancy Registry of 3400 women, the major fetal malformation rate was 3 percent with untreated epilepsy and 3 percent with epilepsy treated with monotherapy (Morrow and colleagues, 2006). In fact, only women who were treated with valproate had a significantly increased risk for malformations—the risk was 9 percent if valproate was part of polytherapy.

Malformations of all types are more prevalent with high serum anticonvulsant concentrations. Moreover, the need for drug therapy, for high serum levels, and for multiple medications also reflects severity of epilepsy. Thus, it is also possible that at least part of the increased risk is related to epilepsy itself or some other aspects of the maternal condition. The most frequently reported defects—whether or not the mother takes medication—are orofacial clefts, cardiac malformations, and neural-tube defects. For example, clefts develop almost 10 times more frequently than in the general population.

The most commonly used potentially teratogenic anticonvulsants and their fetal effects are listed in Table 14-5. Several of these produce a similar constellation of malformations, typified by the *fetal hydantoin syndrome* shown in

TABLE 14-5. Teratogenic Effects of Common Anticonvulsant Medications

Drug	Abnormalities Described	Affected	Pregnancy Category
Valproate	Neural-tube defects, clefts, skeletal abnormalities, developmental delay	1–2% with monotherapy, 9–12% with polytherapy	D
Phenytoin	Fetal hydantoin syndrome: craniofacial anomalies, fingernail hypoplasia, growth deficiency, developmental delay, cardiac defects, clefts	5–11%	D
Carbamazepine	Fetal hydantoin syndrome, spina bifida	1–2%	D
Phenobarbital	Clefts, cardiac anomalies, urinary tract malformations	10–20%	D
Lamotrigine	Inhibits dihydrofolate reductase, lowering fetal folate levels. Registry data suggest increased risk for clefts	4-fold with monotherapy, 10-fold with polytherapy	C
Topiramate	Registry data suggest increased risk for clefts	2%	C
Levetiracetam	Theoretical—skeletal abnormalities and impaired growth in animals at doses similar to or greater than human therapeutic doses	Too few cases reported to assess risk	C

From Cunningham (2005), Holmes (2008), Hunt (2006, 2008), Morrow (2006), UCB, Inc. (2008), and all their associates.

Figure 14-3. Other medications, such as *phenobarbital,* act by lowering fetal folate levels and may thereby cause defects associated with impaired folic acid metabolism, such as neural-tube defects, oral clefts, cardiac anomalies, and urinary tract malformations (see Chap. 12, p. 281).

There are limited data available for the newer anticonvulsants—*levetiracetam, lamotrigine,* and *topiramate.* Cases reported thus far through registries suggest that the risk for oral clefts may be increased with either lamotrigine or topiramate (Holmes and associates, 2008; Hunt and co-workers, 2008) (Table 14-5). But because most birth defects are so infrequent, even a severalfold increase would not necessarily be apparent with the relatively small number of cases reported. Given limitations of the available data, many obstetricians and neurologists choose to maintain the woman on whichever medication(s) had best stabilized her seizures prior to pregnancy.

Angiotensin-Converting Enzyme (ACE) Inhibitors and Angiotensin-Receptor Blockers

It has been known for 20 years that ACE inhibitors are fetotoxic, and more recently they have also been associated with embryotoxicity. The most frequently associated agent is *enalapril,* although *captopril* and *lisinopril* have also been implicated. Because angiotensin-receptor blockers exert their effects through a similar mechanism, concerns about toxicity have been generalized to include this entire category of medications. These drugs disrupt the fetal renin-angiotensin system, which is essential for normal renal development (Guron and Friberg, 2000). In addition, they may provoke prolonged fetal hypotension and hypoperfusion, thus initiating a sequence of events leading to renal ischemia, renal tubular dysgenesis, and anuria (Pryde and colleagues, 1993; Schubiger and associates, 1988). The resulting oligohydramnios may prevent normal lung development and lead to limb contractures. Reduced perfusion also causes growth restriction, relative limb shortening, and maldevelopment of the calvarium (Barr and Cohen, 1991). Because these changes occur after organogenesis, and thus during the fetal period, they are termed *ACE inhibitor fetopathy* (see p. 313).

Cooper and colleagues (2006) recently described 209 children whose mothers were prescribed ACE inhibitors in the first trimester. They reported that 8 percent had major congenital anomalies—predominantly cardiovascular and central nervous system malformations—a rate 2.7 times higher than that observed in more than 29,000 control infants. Given the many therapeutic options for treating hypertension during pregnancy, it is recommended that ACE inhibitors and angiotensin-receptor blocking agents be avoided.

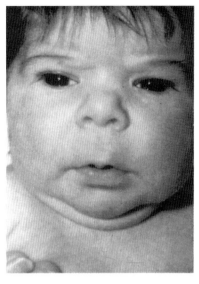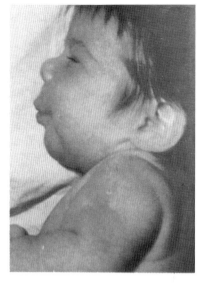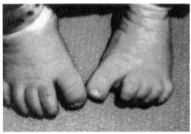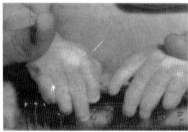

FIGURE 14-3 Fetal hydantoin syndrome. Upper: facial features including upturned nose, mild midfacial hypoplasia, and long upper lip with thin vermilion border. Lower: distal digital hypoplasia. (From Buehler BA, Delimont D, van Waes M, et al: Prenatal prediction of risk of the fetal hydantoin syndrome. *N Engl J Med* 322:1567, with permission. Copyright © 1990 Massachusetts Medical Society. All rights reserved.)

Antifungals

Fluconazole and Itraconazole

There have been several reports of congenital malformations associated with fluconazole. Exposed newborns had skull abnormalities, cleft palate, humeral-radial fusion, and other arm abnormalities (Aleck and Bartley, 1997). There have also been reports associating itraconazole with limb defects and other adverse outcomes. Despite this, large cohort studies suggest that neither drug is teratogenic (Bar-Oz, 2000; Carter, 2008; Sorenson, 1999, and all their colleagues).

Anti-inflammatory Agents

Nonsteroidal Anti-Inflammatory Drugs (NSAIDs)

These are not considered to be teratogenic, but they can have adverse fetal effects when used in the third trimester (Parilla, 2004; Rebordosa and colleagues, 2008). *Indomethacin* in particular is reported to cause constriction of the fetal ductus arteriosus with subsequent pulmonary hypertension (Marpeau and associates, 1994; Rasanen and Jouppila, 1995). It may also decrease fetal urine output and thereby reduce amnionic fluid volume, presumably by increasing vasopressin levels and responsiveness to it (van der Heijden and colleagues, 1994; Walker and associates, 1994). These complications appear to be more likely when the drug is taken for longer than 72 hours. In one series of more than 60 pregnancies, ductal constriction developed in 50 percent, with a significantly increased incidence after 30 weeks (Vermillion and colleagues, 1997). Fortunately, ductal flow velocity returned to normal following discontinuation of therapy in all cases. There also are associations of indomethacin with intraventricular hemorrhage, bronchopulmonary dysplasia, and necrotizing enterocolitis. Some reports indicate that low-birthweight neonates who are delivered preterm within 48 hours of indomethacin exposure are at highest risk (Major and associates, 1994; Norton and co-workers, 1993). Studies conducted after neonatal surfactant treatment became available have not confirmed this association (Gardner and colleagues, 1996).

Leflunomide

This is a pyrimidine-synthesis inhibitor used to treat rheumatoid arthritis (see Chap. 54, p. 1157). It currently is considered contraindicated in pregnancy. This is because in animal studies with multiple species, hydrocephalus, eye anomalies, skeletal abnormalities, and embryo death have been reported with amounts given at or below human-equivalent exposure (Sanofi-aventis Pharmaceuticals, 2007). It can take 2 years after discontinuation for the active metabolite of leflunomide to return to nondetectable plasma levels. The manufacturer has developed a cholestyramine treatment/washout plan in the event of unintended pregnancy. There are also guidelines and a cholestyramine treatment plan available for men taking this medication who are contemplating fathering a child (Brent, 2001).

Antimalarials

Chloroquine is valuable as a first-line antimalarial treatment and for chemoprophylaxis. In high doses, it is also effective against rheumatoid arthritis and systemic lupus erythematosus (Ruiz-Irastorza and associates, 2009; Vroom and co-workers, 2006). *Quinine* and *quinidine* are reserved for severely ill women with chloroquine-resistant malaria. There has been no increased rate of congenital anomalies in the offspring of mothers given any of these antimalarial drugs during pregnancy (McGready and co-workers, 2001, 2002). Daily use of chloroquine for lupus and other connective-tissue diseases has been shown to cause maternal retinopathy but no adverse fetal effects (Araiza-Casillas and colleagues, 2004; Costedoat-Chalumeau and co-workers, 2003). Second- or third-trimester use of *mefloquine* for asymptomatic malaria treatment has been associated with a fivefold increased risk of stillbirth (Nosten and colleagues, 1999). According to Briggs and colleagues (2005), however, accumulated evidence supports its safety.

Antimicrobials

Aminoglycosides

Maternal administration can result in toxic fetal blood levels, but this can be avoided by using lower divided doses (Regev and colleagues, 2000). Although both nephrotoxicity and ototoxicity have been reported in preterm newborns and adults treated with *gentamicin* or *streptomycin*, congenital defects resulting from prenatal exposure have not been confirmed.

Chloramphenicol

This readily crosses the placenta and results in significant fetal blood levels. The incidence of congenital anomalies does not appear to be increased in exposed fetuses. When given to the preterm neonate, the *gray baby syndrome* may develop. This is manifested by cyanosis, vascular collapse, and death. It seems unlikely that fetal serum levels obtained from maternal administration would cause this syndrome.

Sulfonamides

Although these agents readily cross the placenta, fetal blood levels are lower than maternal levels. Sulfonamides do not appear to pose any significant teratogenic risk (Briggs and colleagues, 2005). They displace bilirubin from protein binding sites, raising theoretical concerns about hyperbilirubinemia in the preterm neonate if used near delivery (see Chap. 29, p. 625).

Tetracyclines

Tetracycline may cause yellow-brown discoloration of deciduous teeth or be deposited in fetal long bones when used after 25 weeks (Kutscher and associates, 1966). The risk of dental caries, however, is not increased in exposed children (Billing and associates, 2004). One acceptable use is treatment of maternal syphilis in penicillin-allergic women for whom desensitization is not feasible (see Chap. 59, p. 1238).

Antineoplastic Agents

Cyclophosphamide

In the first trimester, this alkylating agent inflicts a chemical insult on developing fetal tissues, resulting in cell death and heritable DNA alterations in surviving cells. The most common fetal anomalies are missing and hypoplastic digits, believed to be caused by necrosis of limb buds and DNA damage in surviving cells (Manson and associates, 1982). Other defects include cleft palate, single coronary artery, imperforate anus, and fetal-growth restriction with microcephaly (Kirshon and colleagues, 1988). Nurses who administer cyclophosphamide may be at increased risk for fetal loss, but there are no adequate epidemiological studies (Glantz, 1994).

Methotrexate and Aminopterin

These drugs alter folic acid metabolism, which is essential for normal cell replication (Sutton and co-workers, 1998). Methotrexate commonly is prescribed in gynecology for ectopic pregnancy or as an abortifacient (see Chap. 9, p. 232 and Chap. 10, p. 247). It is also used for psoriasis and some connective-tissue diseases (see Chap. 54, p. 1150 and Chap. 56, p. 1191). Principal features of fetal methotrexate-aminopterin syndrome are growth restriction, failure of calvarial ossification, craniosynostosis, hypoplastic supraorbital ridges, small posteriorly rotated ears, micrognathia, and severe limb abnormalities (Del Campo and associates, 1999). The critical period for their development is 8 to 10 menstrual weeks. After a review of 20 first-trimester exposures, Feldcamp and Carey (1993) calculated that a dosage of 10 mg/week is necessary to produce abnormalities. The standard 50 mg/m^2 dose for ectopic pregnancy or elective abortion easily exceeds this, and ongoing pregnancies after methotrexate treatment—especially if used in conjunction with misoprostol—raise concerns for fetal malformations (Creinin and Vittinghoff, 1994).

Tamoxifen

This nonsteroidal selective estrogen-receptor modulator (SERM) is used as an adjuvant to treat breast cancer (see Chap. 57, p. 1195). Although not found to be teratogenic for all animals, it is *fetotoxic* in rats and marmosets, in which it produces deaths and impaired growth, and is *carcinogenic* in rats and mice. In rodents, tamoxifen causes changes similar to those seen following maternal diethylstilbestrol (DES) exposure as subsequently discussed. There are limited human data available. Tamoxifen is pregnancy category D, and it is recommended that exposed offspring be followed for up to 20 years to assess the risk of carcinogenicity (Briggs and colleagues, 2005).

Antivirals

Amantadine is used in pregnancy to prevent, modify, or treat influenza infections (see Chap. 46, p. 1003). This drug is embryotoxic and teratogenic in animals at high doses, but data regarding its safety in pregnancy are limited (Centers for Disease Control and Prevention, 2003). Several case reports and case series in which amantadine was given during the first trimester suggest a possible association with cardiac defects, but the information provided is too limited to allow risk assessment (Pandit and colleagues, 1994; Rosa, 1994).

Ribavirin is given by aerosol inhalation to treat respiratory syncytial virus infections in infants and young children. Pregnant women may be exposed to the drug while working in intensive care nurseries. The drug is highly teratogenic in all animal species studied and consistently produces skull, palate, eye, jaw, limb, skeleton, and gastrointestinal abnormalities in rodent models (Briggs and colleagues, 2005). Although human exposures are rare, the manufacturers consider it Category X and contraindicated for use in pregnancy.

As discussed in Chapter 59 (p. 1250), the use of antiviral medications for human immunodeficiency virus (HIV) infections during pregnancy is growing. These agents inhibit host intracellular viral replication through their action on RNA or DNA substrates. A registry chronicling their maternal and fetal effects has been established by several manufacturers, and it can be accessed for current information at http://www.apregistry.com/. Watts and associates (2004) reported that nearly 1400 first-trimester exposed pregnancies have been followed through this registry thus far, and no significant increase in birth defects has been noted following exposure to lamivudine, nelfinavir, nevirapine, stavudine, or zidovudine.

Another drug used to treat HIV infection is *efavirenz,* a nonnucleoside reverse transcriptase inhibitor. Three of 20 cynomolgus monkeys treated with doses of efavirenz comparable with human doses had birth defects—anencephaly, cleft palate, and microphthalmia (Bristol-Meyers Squibb, 2008). It is reassuring, however, that the Antiretroviral Pregnancy Registry Steering Committee (2004) reported 159 human pregnancies with first-trimester exposure and found neither an increased risk for birth defects nor a particular pattern of defects. At this time, data are limited and options for treating pregnant women are best individualized.

Bosentan

This is an endothelin-receptor antagonist used to treat pulmonary hypertension (see Chap. 44, p. 970). Bosentan is teratogenic in rats, causing abnormalities of the head, face, and large blood vessels, and it is also carcinogenic in rats and mice (Actelion Pharmaceuticals, 2005). No human data are available, but based on these concerning animal data, the manufacturer has rated bosentan category X (Briggs and associates, 2005). Moreover, the package insert recommends pregnancy be excluded before starting treatment and prevented with two concurrent forms of birth control thereafter. As any hormonal contraceptives—oral, injectable, or implantable—may not be completely effective in women on bosentan, it is recommended that they not be the sole means of contraception.

Hormones

The primordial structures that will become the external genitalia are bipotential for the first 9 weeks (see Chap. 4, p. 98). Between 9 and 14 weeks, the testis secretes androgen and the male fetus develops a male perineal phenotype. Because the ovaries do not secrete androgens, the female fetus continues to develop a female phenotype, which is completed by 20 weeks. Exposure to exogenous sex hormones before 7 completed weeks generally has no effect on external structures. Between 7 and 12 weeks, however, female genital tissue is responsive to exogenous androgens and exposure can result in full masculinization. The tissue continues to exhibit some response until 20 weeks, with exposure causing partial masculinization or genital ambiguity.

Those areas of the brain with high concentrations of estrogen and androgen receptors are also influenced by hormonal exposure. Hormones program the central nervous system for gender identity, sexual behavior, levels of aggression, and gender-specific play behaviors. The critical period for hormonal influence on behavior is much later than that for the external genitalia, with the degree of behavioral alteration proportional to dose and length of exposure.

Androgens

One example of the fetal effects from early exposure to androgens is autosomal recessive *congenital adrenal hyperplasia* (see Chap. 4, p. 102). Exposure to exogenous androgens can induce similar fetal effects, but masculinization from exogenous androgens does not progress after birth (Stevenson, 1993b).

Testosterone and Anabolic Steroids. Androgen exposure in reproductive-aged women occurs primarily as the result of anabolic steroids used to increase lean body mass and muscular strength. Synthetic testosterones are the most effective and are taken in doses 10 to 40 times higher than physiological doses. In adult women, these compounds cause extreme and irreversible virilization, liver dysfunction, and mood and libido disorders. Exposure of a female fetus results in varying degrees of virilization, including labioscrotal fusion after first-trimester exposure and phallic enlargement from later fetal exposure (Grumbach and Ducharme, 1960; Schardein, 1985). An example is shown in Figure 4-19 (p. 102). Normal female maturation usually occurs at puberty, although surgery may be necessary to give a more feminine appearance to the virilized genitalia.

Androgenic Progestins. These testosterone derivatives currently are used as contraceptives. In studies of rats and nonhuman primates, antenatal exposure to *medroxyprogesterone acetate* given as an intramuscular depot contraceptive has been associated with virilization of female fetuses and feminization of male fetuses. Fortunately, no association between this agent and any congenital defects in humans has been established (see Chap. 32, p. 682). *Norethindrone,* a progesterone-only contraceptive, is estimated to cause female fetus masculinization in 1 percent of exposures (Schardein, 1985).

Danazol. This ethinyl testosterone derivative has weak androgenic activity. It is prescribed primarily for endometriosis but also is used to treat immune thrombocytopenic purpura, migraine headaches, premenstrual syndrome, and some breast diseases. In a review of its inadvertent use during early pregnancy, Brunskill (1992) reported that 40 percent of 57 exposed female fetuses were virilized. There was a dose-related pattern of clitoromegaly, fused labia, and urogenital sinus malformation, most of which required surgical correction.

Estrogens

Most of the many available estrogen compounds do not affect fetal development. *Oral contraceptives,* as discussed in Chapter 32 (p. 675), have not been associated with congenital anomalies (Raman-Wilms and colleagues, 1995). *Tamoxifen* is a selective estrogen-receptor modulator and is discussed with other antineoplastic agents on page 321.

Diethylstilbestrol (DES). From 1940 to 1971, between 2 million and 10 million pregnant women took this synthetic estrogen to "support" high-risk pregnancies (Giusti and co-workers, 1995). The drug later was shown to have no beneficial effects, and its use for this purpose was abandoned. Herbst and colleagues (1971) reported a series of eight prenatally exposed women who developed vaginal clear-cell adenocarcinoma. Subsequent studies showed that the absolute cancer risk in prenatally exposed women is approximately 1 per 1000. A registry established by the National Institutes of Health reported that half of 384 cancer patients were exposed before 12 weeks and 70 percent before 17 weeks (Melnick and colleagues, 1987). Malignancy was not dose related, and there was no relationship between location of the tumor and timing of exposure. For these reasons and because its absolute risk is low, some authors categorize DES as an *incomplete carcinogen.*

The drug also produces both structural and functional abnormalities (Salle and colleagues, 1996). By 18 weeks, the müllerian-derived cuboidal-columnar epithelium lining the vagina should be replaced by squamous epithelium originating from the urogenital sinus. DES interrupts this transition in up to half of exposed female fetuses, resulting in excess cervical eversion—*ectropion*, and ectopic vaginal glandular epithelium—*adenosis*. These lesions have malignant potential, and DES-exposed women have a twofold increase in vaginal and cervical intraepithelial neoplasia (Vessey, 1989). Approximately a fourth of exposed females have structural abnormalities of the cervix or vagina (Robboy and associates, 1984). The most commonly reported abnormalities include a hypoplastic, T-shaped uterine

cavity; cervical collars, hoods, septa, and coxcombs; and "withered" fallopian tubes (Goldberg and Falcone, 1999). As discussed in Chapter 40 (p. 897), these women are at increased risk for poor pregnancy outcomes related to uterine malformations, decreased endometrial thickness, and reduced uterine perfusion (Kaufman and colleagues, 2000). Exposed men have normal sexual function and fertility but are at increased risk for epididymal cysts, microphallus, cryptorchidism, and testicular hypoplasia (Stillman, 1982). Klip and associates (2002) reported that sons of women exposed in utero had an increased risk of hypospadias.

Immunosuppressants

Corticosteroids

Hydrocortisone, prednisone, and other corticosteroids are commonly used to treat serious medical conditions such as asthma and autoimmune disease. In animal studies, they have been associated with cleft palate. In a 10-year prospective cohort study by the Motherisk Program and the University of Toronto, corticosteroid exposure was not associated with an increased risk for major malformations (Park-Wyllie and colleagues, 2000). A meta-analysis by the same investigators, however, did demonstrate an increased incidence of facial clefts. The odds ratio for clefts in case-control series was increased approximately threefold—an absolute risk of 3 per 1000 (Park-Wyllie and colleagues, 2000). Based on these findings, systemic corticosteroids are category D if used in the first trimester, however, they are not considered to represent a major teratogenic risk.

Mycophenolate Mofetil

This inosine monophosphate dehydrogenase inhibitor, and a related agent, *mycophenolic acid,* are used to prevent rejection in recipients of kidney, liver, or heart transplantation. They have also been used in the treatment of autoimmune disease. In 2007, the FDA revised the prescribing information for these medications to pregnancy category D, based on reports of increased risks of spontaneous abortion and selected anomalies in exposed pregnancies (Food and Drug Administration, 2008). Of 33 pregnancies in the National Transplantation Pregnancy Registry exposed to *mycophenolate mofetil,* 45 percent experienced a spontaneous loss, and 22 percent of surviving infants had malformations. The majority of reported malformations have involved the ear and include bilateral microtia, anotia, and/or atresia of the external auditory canals. In addition, oral clefts have been described. Importantly, inosine monophosphate dehydrogenase inhibitors may decrease the efficacy of oral contraceptives. Because of these risks, the manufacturer states that women must use two different types of effective birth control for 1 month before starting use of these immunosuppressants, during their use, and for 6 weeks after stopping their use (Roche Laboratories, 2008).

Iodine Preparations

Radioactive iodine-131 is used to treat thyroid malignancies and hyperthyroidism, and it is used diagnostically for thyroid scanning. It is contraindicated during pregnancy because it readily crosses the placenta and is avidly concentrated in the fetal thyroid by the end of the first trimester. High doses of radiation may ablate the fetal thyroid as well as increase the future risk for childhood thyroid cancer. Although fetal thyroid hormone production is believed to begin at approximately 10 weeks, it would seem prudent to avoid radioiodide at any gestational age (see also Chap. 41, p. 921 and Chap. 53, p. 1128).

Methyl Mercury

Although not a drug, methyl mercury is a known teratogen. Reports from Minimata, Japan, and from rural Iraq, the sites of two major methyl mercury industrial spills, indicate that the developing nervous system is particularly susceptible to the effects of mercury. Prenatal exposure causes disturbances in neuronal cell division and migration, resulting in a range of defects from developmental delay and mild neurological abnormalities to microcephaly and severe brain damage (Choi and colleagues, 1978).

Although there have been no recent episodes of large-scale methyl mercury contamination in the United States, pregnant women worldwide are currently at risk of exposure. Mercury enters the ecosystem through industrial pollution, which joins surface water and eventually reaches the ocean. Several varieties of older large fish, notably tuna, shark, king mackerel, and tilefish, absorb and retain mercury from the water or ingest it when they eat smaller fish and aquatic organisms. Women who eat these fish ingest mercury, which is metabolized to inorganic mercury by intestinal microflora and eliminated by demethylation and fecal excretion. The process is slow, with an elimination half-time of 45 to 70 days (Clarkson, 2002). Because large quantities of contaminated fish ingested during pregnancy may expose a fetus to unsafe mercury levels, the Environmental Protection Agency and the Food and Drug Administration (2008) currently recommend that pregnant women not eat shark, swordfish, king mackerel, or tilefish. Regarding other fish, a pregnant woman should eat each week no more than 6 ounces of albacore tuna or 12 ounces of fish or shellfish thought to be low in mercury (see Chap. 8, p. 206).

Psychiatric Medications

Lithium

This drug is used for manic-depressive illness (see Chap. 55, p. 1179). As discussed on page 314, it has been associated with the rare *Ebstein anomaly*, which is characterized by a downward or apical displacement of the tricuspid valve that leads to atrialization of the right ventricle. In the Lithium Baby Register, by 1977, there were five cases of Ebstein anomaly among 183 reported exposed pregnancies (Weinstein, 1977). Subsequently, in a prospective multicenter study of 148 exposed pregnancies, there was only one such case, leading to the conclusion that lithium may not be an important teratogen (Jacobson and colleagues, 1992). Currently, targeted sonography with fetal echocardiography is recommended for women who take lithium in the first trimester.

Lithium also may cause transient neonatal toxicity. Effects have included hypothyroidism, diabetes insipidus, cardiomegaly, bradycardia, electrocardiogram abnormalities, cyanosis, and hypotonia (Briggs and associates, 2005).

Selective Serotonin-Reuptake Inhibitors (SSRIs)

In a study of seven health plans including nearly 119,000 pregnant women, Andrade and co-workers (2008) reported that 8 percent were prescribed antidepressants. As a class, these are the most commonly used antidepressants in pregnancy (see Chap. 55, p. 1177). Included are citalopram, escitalopram, fluoxetine, fluvoxamine, paroxetine, and sertraline.

Teratogenicity. In 2005, data from a Swedish national registry and a U.S. insurance claims database raised concerns that the rate of congenital cardiac malformations was increased 1.5- to 2-fold following first-trimester paroxetine exposure (GlaxoSmithKline, 2008). The two studies included more than 12,000 pregnant women prescribed antidepressants, including approximately 1600 women who used paroxetine in the first trimester. The overall rate of infants with cardiovascular malformations among women who took paroxetine was increased approximately 0.5 to 1.0 percentage points above the rate for infants with other antidepressant exposure in utero. Most of these defects were atrial and ventricular septal defects, which are the most common congenital cardiac anomalies and are also among the most difficult to reliably detect with prenatal sonography. Based on these findings, the manufacturer changed the pregnancy category of paroxetine, but not other SSRIs, from C to D. Also, the American College of Obstetricians and Gynecologists (2007) recommended that paroxetine use be avoided in women who are either pregnant or planning pregnancy and that fetal echocardiography should be considered for women with early pregnancy paroxetine exposure.

Subsequent to these events, two large case-control studies from multisite surveillance programs have reported potential teratogenicity of paroxetine and other SSRI medications. From the National Birth Defects Prevention Study, Alwan and associates (2007) did not find an increased risk of cardiovascular anomalies but did identify a two- to threefold increased risk for omphalocele, craniosynostosis, and anencephaly. This risk—approximately 2 per 1000 infants—was primarily with paroxetine exposure. In the other study, Louik and colleagues (2007) from the Sloane Epidemiology Center did not identify a risk for any of these birth defects. They did, however, report an association with paroxetine and cardiac right outflow tract abnormalities as well as with sertraline and cardiac septal defects and omphalocele. Because of the large number of outcomes analyzed, the American College of Obstetricians and Gynecologists (2007) concluded that the absolute risk of any birth defect is very small and that SSRIs are not major teratogens.

Neonatal Effects. There are two types of neonatal effects that have been described following maternal SSRI use in pregnancy. A neonatal behavioral syndrome has been observed in up to a fourth of fetuses exposed in the last trimester (Chambers and associates, 2006; Costei and colleagues, 2002). In a review of 13 case reports and nine cohort studies that included 990 pregnancies with such exposure, Moses-Kolko and co-workers (2005) calculated a significant overall risk ratio of 3.0 for this syndrome. Most reported cases followed paroxetine or fluoxetine exposure. Common features are jitteriness or shivering, increased muscle tone, feeding or digestive disturbances, irritability or agitation, and respiratory distress.

Generally, the syndrome is considered to be mild and self-limited, lasting usually approximately 2 days. Management typically consists of supportive care. Jordan and colleagues (2008) found that affected infants were not more likely to be transferred to a special care nursery or to require longer hospitalization than infants of mothers whose depression was not treated with medication. Rarely, there may be a severe form of this syndrome—reported in only 0.3 percent of infants—manifested by seizures, hyperpyrexia, excessive weight loss, and need for intubation. These findings are similar to those in adults from SSRI toxicity or from drug discontinuation (Levin, 2004).

The second neonatal syndrome is rare and manifested by persistent pulmonary hypertension in the newborn (PPHN). It is characterized by high pulmonary vascular resistance, right-to-left shunting, and profound hypoxemia. Mortality rates are as high as 20 percent, and many survivors have long-term morbidity (Jankov and McNamara, 2005). In a case-control study, Chambers and colleagues (2006) compared 377 women whose infants had pulmonary hypertension with 836 women with unaffected infants. Fetuses exposed to maternal SSRIs after 20 weeks had a sixfold increased risk for pulmonary hypertension. The absolute risk among exposed infants was 6 to 12 per 1000—approximately 1 percent.

The American College of Obstetricians and Gynecologists (2007) has stressed that the potential risks of SSRI use in pregnancy must be considered in the context of the risk of depression relapse if their administration is discontinued. Thus, treatment with these medications during pregnancy should be individualized.

Retinoids

These compounds, especially vitamin A, are essential for normal growth, tissue differentiation, reproduction, and vision (Gudas, 1994). As discussed earlier, retinoids are believed to activate clusters of homeobox genes during embryogenesis (Soprano and Soprano, 1995).

Vitamin A

There are two natural forms of vitamin A. *Beta-carotene* is a precursor of provitamin A. It is found in fruits and vegetables and has never been shown to cause birth defects (Oakley and Erickson, 1995). *Retinol* is preformed vitamin A. Many foods contain vitamin A, but animal liver contains the most. Several reports of prenatal supplementation have associated high doses of vitamin A with congenital anomalies. However, they were clouded by small numbers, unknown daily dose, and absence of any recognizable pattern of observed defects. Two cohort studies have also been inconclusive (Conway, 1958; Rothman and coworkers, 1995). The only prospective study included 423 women who contacted European Teratology Services to report exposure (Mastroiacovo and associates, 1999). These women had ingested from 10,000 to 300,000 IU of vitamin A daily during the first 9 weeks of pregnancy. Only three exposed newborns had birth defects, and there was no relationship between vitamin dose and outcome. It seems reasonable to avoid doses higher than the recommended daily allowance of 5000 IU (American College of Obstetricians and Gynecologists, 1995).

Nohynek and colleagues (2006) found that human topical exposure to retinol- or retinyl ester-containing cosmetic creams at 30,000 IU/day did not affect plasma levels of retinol, retinyl esters, or retinoic acids.

Bexarotene

This is a member of a subclass of retinoids used to treat refractory T-cell lymphoma. When given to rats in amounts comparable to human doses, eye and ear abnormalities, cleft palate, and incomplete ossification resulted (Eisai, 2007). This medication is considered contraindicated during pregnancy. Moreover, male patients who have partners who could become pregnant are advised to use condoms during sexual intercourse if they are taking bexarotene and for one month after discontinuing therapy.

Isotretinoin

Some isomers of vitamin A are used primarily for dermatological disorders because they stimulate epithelial cell differentiation (see Chap. 56, p. 1191). *Isotretinoin,* which is 13-*cis*-retinoic acid, is effective for treatment of cystic acne. **Isotretinoin is considered one of the most potent teratogens in common use.** First-trimester exposure is associated with a high rate of fetal loss, and the 26-fold increased malformation rate in survivors is similar to that for thalidomide (Lammer and coworkers, 1985). Abnormalities have been described only with first-trimester use. Because it is rapidly cleared—the mean serum half-life is 12 hours—anomalies are not increased in women who discontinue therapy before conception (Dai and colleagues, 1989).

Malformations typically involve the cranium and face, heart, central nervous system, and thymus. The craniofacial malformation most strongly associated with isotretinoin—microtia or anotia—is bilateral, but often asymmetrical. These defects frequently appear in conjunction with agenesis or stenoses of the external ear canal (Fig. 14-4). Other defects include cleft palate and maldevelopment of the facial bones and cranium. The most frequent cardiac anomalies are conotruncal or outflow tract defects, and hydrocephalus is the most common central nervous system defect. Thymic abnormalities include aplasia, hypoplasia, or malposition.

Dai and colleagues (1992) summarized 433 exposed pregnancies and did not find any safe first-trimester exposure period or dose. Despite the well-publicized hazards associated with prenatal isotretinoin use, as well as efforts by the manufacturer to highlight these reproductive risks, exposures continue to be reported. The FDA-mandated web-based pregnancy risk management system—the iPLEDGE program—requires that all patients, physicians, and pharmacies participate in an attempt to eliminate fetal exposure (www.ipledgeprogram.com).

Etretinate

This orally administered retinoid is used to treat psoriasis. **Etretinate is associated with severe anomalies similar to those with isotretinoin**. One important difference is that anomalies are observed even when conception occurs *after* discontinuation of etretinate. The drug is lipophilic, has a half-life of 120 days, and has been detected in serum almost 3 years after therapy

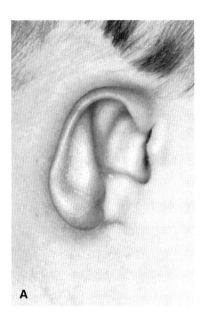

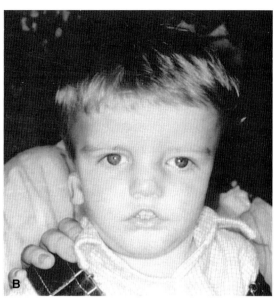

FIGURE 14-4 Isotretinoin embryopathy. **A**. Bilateral microtia or anotia with stenosis of external ear canal. **B**. Flat, depressed nasal bridge and ocular hypertelorism. (Photograph courtesy of Dr. Edward Lammer.)

(DiGiovanna and colleagues, 1984; Thomson and Cordero, 1989). It is unknown how long the teratogenic effects persist, but Lammer (1988) reported malformations up to 51 weeks after discontinuation! If possible, women who plan future childbearing should not use this drug. If etretinate is used, Geiger and associates (1994) suggest that women wait at least 2 years after concluding treatment before conceiving.

Tretinoin

This is all-*trans*-retinoic acid, and it most often is used as a gel preparation for topical treatment of acne vulgaris. When the gel is used, the skin metabolizes most of the drug with minimal apparent absorption. In two studies totaling 221 neonates born to women who used topical tretinoin during early pregnancy, there were no observed increases in rates of congenital anomalies (Jick and colleagues, 1993; Loureiro and colleagues, 2005). Four cases have been reported in which first-trimester topical use resulted in fetal defects similar to those associated with isotretinoin (Reprotox, 2008b). In all, however, the doses were unknown, and in one case, another medication was concurrently used.

Tretinoin is also available in an oral form for use as antineoplastic therapy for acute promyelocytic leukemia at doses 9000 to 14,000 times greater than those used topically. Like other retinoids, this form is likely to be highly teratogenic, although no affected fetuses have been reported to date (Briggs and colleagues, 2005).

Thalidomide

This anxiolytic and sedative drug is likely the most notorious human teratogen. It produces malformations in approximately 20 percent of fetuses exposed during the specific time window from 34 to 50 days menstrual age. Defects primarily are limited to structures derived from the mesodermal layer, such as limbs, ears, cardiovascular system, and bowel musculature. A wide variety of limb-reduction defects have been associated with thalidomide, with upper limbs usually more severely affected.

Bone defects range from abnormal shape or size to total absence of a bone or limb segment—*phocomelia*. Limb-reduction defects may be the result of dysmorphogenesis—seen also with warfarin and phenytoin—or of vascular disruption of a normally formed limb—seen also with misoprostol, chorionic villus sampling, and phenytoin (Holmes, 2002).

Thalidomide was available from 1956 to 1960 before its teratogenicity was discovered. The ensuing disaster was instructive of a number of important teratological principles. First, the placenta had been believed to be a perfect barrier that was impervious to toxic substances unless given in maternally lethal doses (Dally, 1998). Second, the extreme variability in species susceptibility to drugs and chemicals had not yet been appreciated. Thus, because thalidomide produced no defects in experimental mice and rats, it was assumed to be safe for humans. Third, thalidomide demonstrated the close relationship between the timing of exposure and the type of defect (Knapp and co-workers, 1962). For example, upper limb phocomelia developed only after exposure during days 27 to 30—coincidental with appearance of the upper limb buds at day 27. Lower limb phocomelia was associated with exposure during days 30 to 33, gallbladder aplasia at 42 to 43 days, duodenal atresia at 40 to 47 days—and so on for a number of malformations.

Thalidomide was removed from the drug market, but in the past decade a number of immunomodulating uses were discovered (Franks and associates, 2004). It was approved in the United States in 1999 for the treatment of erythema nodosum leprosum (Ances, 2002). It also has been shown effective for the treatment of cutaneous lupus erythematosus, chronic graft-versus-host disease, prurigo nodularis, and certain malignancies (Maurer and co-workers, 2004; Pro and associates, 2004). For obvious reasons, it is recommended that reproductive-aged women taking thalidomide use two highly effective forms of birth control. However, despite ample warnings, thalidomide-affected children continue to be born in countries where the drug is available (Castilla and co-workers, 1996).

Warfarin (Coumadin Derivatives)

These anticoagulants, which include warfarin and dicumarol, are low molecular weight, readily cross the placenta, and can cause significant adverse teratogenic and fetal effects. Ginsberg and Hirsh (1989) reviewed 186 studies involving 1325 exposed pregnancies and reported that 9 percent of exposed fetuses suffered permanent deformity or disability, and 17 percent of these fetuses died. Schaefer and colleagues (2006) compared 666 women exposed to vitamin K antagonists—63 were exposed to

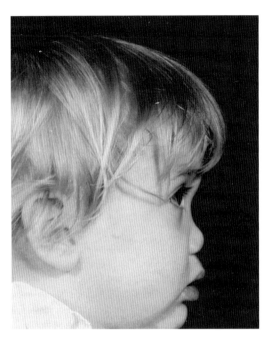

FIGURE 14-5 Warfarin embryopathy or fetal warfarin syndrome: nasal hypoplasia and depressed nasal bridge. (Courtesy of Dr. Mary Jo Harrod.)

warfarin—with 1094 nonexposed controls and found more structural defects and other adverse pregnancy outcomes. The rate of embryopathies, however, was less than 1 percent.

It was concluded that two distinct types of defects result from exposure during two different developmental periods. If exposed between the sixth and ninth weeks, the fetus is at risk for *warfarin embryopathy*. This is characterized by nasal and midface hypoplasia, such as shown in **Figure 14-5**, and stippled vertebral and femoral epiphyses. Importantly, vitamin K-dependent clotting factors are not demonstrable in the embryo, and it is thought that warfarin derivatives exert their teratogenic effect by inhibiting posttranslational carboxylation of coagulation proteins (Hall and associates, 1980). The syndrome is a phenocopy of *chondrodysplasia punctata*, a group of genetic diseases thought to be caused by inherited defects in osteocalcin. There are data that suggest that the risk of warfarin embryopathy is dose dependent. In a study of 43 women with mechanical heart valves treated with warfarin during 58 pregnancies, Vitale and colleagues (1999) found that warfarin embryopathy and fetal wastage developed only when a dose exceeding 5 mg daily was taken throughout the first trimester. In these women, the incidence of embryopathy was 8 percent, and that of spontaneous abortion was 72 percent.

During the second and third trimesters, the defects associated with fetal exposure to warfarin likely result from hemorrhage leading to disharmonic growth and deformation from scarring in any of several organs (Warkany, 1976). Defects may be regionally extensive and include dorsal midline central nervous system dysplasia, such as agenesis of the corpus callosum, Dandy-Walker malformation, and midline cerebellar atrophy; ventral midline dysplasia such as microphthalmia, optic atrophy, and blindness; and developmental delay and mental retardation (Hall and colleagues, 1980).

Herbal Remedies

It is difficult to estimate the risk or safety of various herbal remedies because they are not regulated by the FDA. Thus, the identity and quantity of all ingredients are frequently unknown. Few human or animal studies of their teratogenic potential have been reported, and knowledge of complications has essentially been limited to reports of acute toxicity (Hepner and co-workers, 2002; Sheehan, 1998). In general, because it is not possible to assess the effects of herbal remedies on the developing fetus, pregnant women should be counseled to avoid these substances.

A number of herbal preparations with possible adverse physiological or pharmacological effects are listed in Table 14-6. In addition, *Echinacea* causes fragmentation of hamster sperm (Ondrizek and associates, 1999). *Black cohosh*, used to speed labor and treat premenstrual symptoms, contains a chemical that acts similarly to estrogen. *Gingko*, touted as an aid to memory and mental clarity, can interfere with the effects of monoamine oxidase-inhibiting drugs and has anticoagulant properties. Real *licorice* contains *glycyrrhizin*, which has hypertensive and potassium-wasting effects. *Soy* products contain phytoestrogen.

Certain herbal remedies may act as abortifacients. For example, *blue* and *black cohosh* appear to directly stimulate uterine musculature. *Pennyroyal* appears to work by irritating the bladder and uterus and causing strong uterine contractions. The drug also can cause liver damage, renal failure, and disseminated intravascular coagulation and has been associated with several maternal deaths (Black, 1985).

Recreational Drugs

It is estimated that at least 10 percent of fetuses are exposed to one or more illicit drugs (American Academy of Pediatrics and the American College of Obstetricians and Gynecologists, 2007). As discussed on page 317, alcohol is a known significant teratogen, and because it is legally obtained and ubiquitous, its use confounds that of illicit drugs. Other confounding factors include poor maternal health, malnutrition, infectious diseases, and polydrug abuse. Several different drugs may be used at the same time, and the combination may cause a worse outcome than expected with drugs used alone. Furthermore, many illegal substances contain contaminants such as lead, cyanide, cellulose, herbicides, and pesticides. And, substances commonly added as diluents include fine glass beads, powdered sugar, finely ground sawdust, strychnine, arsenic, antihistamines, and even coumadin. Some of these diluents and impurities may independently have serious adverse perinatal effects.

Amphetamines

These sympathomimetic agents can be used as central nervous system stimulants, as anorectics, or as treatment of narcolepsy. Various amphetamines are teratogenic at very high doses in mice (Reprotox, 2008a). But in four cohort studies of 818 women who took amphetamines during early pregnancy, the frequencies of major and minor congenital anomalies were no greater than those for controls (Heinonen and colleagues, 1983; Little and associates, 1988; Milkovich and van den Berg, 1977). *Methamphetamines* are used to treat obesity and narcolepsy in adults and

TABLE 14-6. Possible Adverse Effects of Some Herbal Medicines

Herb and Common Name	Relevant Pharmacological Effects	Perioperative Concerns
Echinacea: *purple coneflower root*	Activation of cell-mediated immunity	Allergic reactions; decreased effectiveness of immunosuppressants; potential for immunosuppression with long-term use
Ephedra: *ma huang*	Tachycardia and hypertension through direct and indirect sympathomimetic effects	Hypertension, arrhythmias with myocardial ischemia and stroke; long-term use depletes endogenous catecholamines; life-threatening interaction with monoamine oxidase inhibitors
Garlic: *ajo*	Inhibition of platelet aggregation; increased fibrinolysis; equivocal antihypertensive activity	Increased risk of bleeding, especially when combined with other medications that inhibit platelet aggregation
Ginger	COX inhibitor	Increased risk of bleeding
Ginseng	Lowers blood glucose; inhibition of platelet aggregation; increased PT and aPTT in animals	Hypoglycemia; increased risk of bleeding; decreased anticoagulation effect of warfarin
Glucosamine and chondroitin		Worsening of diabetes
Kava: *awa, intoxicating pepper, kawa*	Sedation, anxiolysis	Increased sedative effect of anesthetics; effects of tolerance and withdrawal unknown
St. John wort: *amber, goat weed, hardhay, hypericum, klamatheweed*	Inhibition of neurotransmitter reuptake, monoamine oxidase inhibition unlikely	Induction of cytochrome P_{450} affecting cyclosporine, warfarin, steroids, protease inhibitors, and possibly benzodiazepines, calcium-channel blockers, and many other drugs
Valerian: *all heal, garden heliotrope, vandal root*	Sedation	Increased sedative effect of anesthetics; liver damage; benzodiazepine-like acute withdrawal; potential to increase anesthetic requirements with long-term use
Yohimbe		Hypertension, arrhythmias

aPTT = activated partial thromboplastin times; COX = cyclooxygenase; PT = prothrombin time.
From Ang-Lee and colleagues (2001), Briggs and associates (2005), and Consumer Reports on Health (2003).

hyperkinetic children. These drugs often are used to dilute other illicit drugs. Methamphetamine use has been associated with symmetrical fetal-growth restriction but does not appear to increase the frequency of congenital anomalies (Little and colleagues, 1988; Ramin and associates, 1992). Methylamphetamine, known as *speed, ice, crank,* and *crystal meth,* produces defects in mice, rats, and rabbits, but has not been associated with defects in humans. Methylenedioxymethamphetamine (MDMA)—known as *ecstasy*—is in the amphetamine family. In animal studies, it is not teratogenic, and limited data suggest no increased risk of human teratogenicity or fetal toxicity (Briggs and colleagues, 2005).

Cocaine

This alkaloid is derived from the leaves of the South American tree *Erythroxylon coca.* It is a highly effective topical anesthetic and local vasoconstrictor. It is also a central nervous system

stimulant through sympathomimetic action via dopamine. It is one of the most widely abused drugs, and the National Survey on Drug Use and Health (2007) reported that it accounted for more than 10 percent of illicit drug use in the United States.

Most of the adverse outcomes associated with cocaine result from its vasoconstrictive and hypertensive effects. The risk of vascular disruption within the embryo, fetus, or placenta is highest *after* the first trimester and likely accounts for the increased incidence of stillbirth with this drug (Hoyme and associates, 1990). A number of cocaine-related congenital anomalies resulting from vascular disruption have been described. These include skull defects, cutis aplasia, porencephaly, subependymal and periventricular cysts, ileal atresia, cardiac anomalies, and visceral infarcts (Cohen and associates, 1994; Little and colleagues, 1989; Stevenson, 1993a). Results from the population-based Atlanta Birth Defects Case-Control Study showed that cocaine use increased the risk fourfold for urinary tract defects (Chavez and colleagues, 1988). Prune-belly anomaly also has been reported (Bingol and co-workers, 1986; Chasnoff and colleagues, 1985, 1988).

Cocaine has been associated with microcephaly and behavioral abnormalities (Rivkin and associates, 2008). There are, however, few prospective studies of its effect on psychomotor development. Singer and colleagues (2002) reported a prospective study of 218 cocaine-exposed infants and 197 unexposed controls. At age 2 years, compared with control infants, the cocaine-exposed infants had significantly more cognitive defects and twice the rate of developmental delay. Cognitive impairments persisted at age 4 years (Singer and associates, 2004).

Not all studies, however, support the concept of cocaine as a major teratogen. Reports of cocaine-induced limb-reduction defects have been disputed (Hume and co-workers, 1997). One prospective longitudinal cohort study of 272 offspring of crack-cocaine users found no increase in the number or pattern of birth defects (Behnke and co-workers, 2001). Because few reports address dosage or total fetal exposure during pregnancy, it is difficult to estimate the ultimate fetal risk associated with antenatal cocaine use.

Opiates (Narcotics)

Heroin. In most studies, the frequency of congenital anomalies is not higher with heroin use (Little and associates, 1990b). In one cohort study of 830 exposed neonates, the frequency of anomalies was 2.4 percent, similar to the background risk (Ostrea and Chavez, 1979). Other types of morbidity, such as fetal-growth restriction, perinatal death, and several perinatal complications, are common in the offspring of narcotic-addicted mothers (Lifschitz and colleagues, 1983; Little and co-workers, 1990b). It is not clear whether these complications are due to fetal heroin exposure or to generally poor maternal health. Postnatal growth of these children appears to be normal in most cases, although the average head circumference is smaller than that of unexposed children. There also may be mild developmental delay or behavioral disturbances (Chasnoff and colleagues, 1986; Lifschitz and co-workers, 1983).

Withdrawal symptoms such as tremors, irritability, sneezing, vomiting, fever, diarrhea, and occasionally seizures are observed in 40 to 80 percent of newborns born to heroin-addicted women (Alroomi and colleagues, 1988). Although these symptoms may be prolonged, they usually persist for fewer than 10 days. Logically, higher doses of maternal methadone are associated with longer required lengths of neonatal abstinence syndrome treatment (Lim and co-workers, 2009). Abnormal respiratory function during sleep often persists and may be a factor in the increased incidence of sudden infant death syndrome in exposed newborns (Kandall and associates, 1993).

Methadone. This *synthetic* opioid narcotic structurally resembles propoxyphene and is used primarily as maintenance therapy for narcotic addiction. Although large doses are teratogenic in rodents, congenital anomalies were not increased above background in cohort studies and clinical series of neonates born to women on methadone maintenance therapy (Stimmel and Adamsons, 1976). Withdrawal symptoms, however, are fre-

quent, and birthweights are often lower than expected (Briggs and colleagues, 2005). Chasnoff and co-workers (1987) compared 52 cocaine-using pregnant women with 73 former heroin addicts maintained on methadone. They found a significantly higher rate of preterm labor, rapid labor, placental abruption, and meconium staining among cocaine users. Withdrawal from methadone is more severe than from heroin and more protracted—up to 3 weeks—due to the much longer half-life of methadone. That said, the best maintenance agonist for pregnant women has not been found (Minozzi and associates, 2008).

Marijuana

Also known as *hashish*, in earlier studies, marijuana was used by nearly 15 percent of pregnant women (Abel and Sokol, 1988; Chasnoff and colleagues, 1990). The active ingredient is *delta-9-tetrahydrocannabinol (THC)*, which in high doses is teratogenic for animals. There is no evidence, however, that marijuana is associated with human anomalies. The birthweight of exposed fetuses has been reported to be lower in some studies but not others (Greenland, 1983; Linn, 1983; Shiono, 1995, and all their colleagues).

Miscellaneous Drugs

Phencyclidine (PCP), known as *angel dust,* is not associated with congenital anomalies. Neonatal withdrawal, characterized by tremors, jitteriness, and irritability, is observed in more than half of exposed newborns. Golden and colleagues (1987) reported that the incidence of structural malformations was not increased in 94 phencyclidine-exposed infants, but confirmed an increased incidence of newborn behavioral and developmental abnormalities. *"T's and blues"* is a street mixture of the narcotic analgesic *pentazocine (Talwin)* and the over-the-counter antihistamine *tripelennamine (Pyribenzamine).* It has not been associated with an increased incidence of congenital anomalies (Little and co-workers, 1990a; von Almen and Miller, 1984).

Classically known as *lysergic acid diethylamide (LSD),* these are amine alkaloids obtained only through chemical synthesis. There is no evidence that this drug is a human teratogen. Some investigators have found increased frequencies of chromosomal breakage in somatic cells of mothers who used lysergic acid as well as in their prenatally exposed newborns. However, such breakage does not appear to correlate with an increased risk for congenital anomalies.

Toluene is present in paints and glue and when intentionally inhaled, can produce lightheadedness, dizziness, and loss of consciousness. Prenatal abuse is associated with *toluene embryopathy.* The phenotype has been compared with fetal alcohol syndrome and includes pre- and postnatal growth deficiency, microcephaly, and characteristic facial and hand findings—midface hypoplasia, short palpebral fissures, wide nasal bridge, and abnormal palmar creases (Pearson and colleagues, 1994). Developmental delays have been reported in approximately 40 percent of exposed children (Arnold and colleagues, 1994). Fortunately, the maximum occupational exposure is estimated to be only a fraction of that experienced by abusers and is not expected to cause significant fetal risk (Wilkins-Haug, 1997).

Tobacco

Cigarette smoke contains a complex mixture of substances including nicotine, cotinine, cyanide, thiocyanate, carbon monoxide, cadmium, lead, and various hydrocarbons (Stillerman and colleagues, 2008). In addition to being fetotoxic, many of these substances have vasoactive effects or reduce oxygen levels. The best-documented reproductive outcome related to smoking is a direct dose-response reduction in fetal growth. Newborns of mothers who smoke weigh an average of 200 g less than those of nonsmokers, and heavy smoking results in more severe weight reduction (D'Souza and associates, 1981). Smoking doubles the risk of low birthweight and increases the risk of fetal-growth restriction two- to threefold (Werler, 1997). Mercer and colleagues (2008) have shown that this disparity can be detected sonographically between 10 and 20 weeks. Women who stop smoking early in pregnancy generally have neonates with normal birthweights (Cliver and co-workers, 1995). Smoking also may cause a slightly increased incidence of subfertility, spontaneous abortion, placenta previa and abruption, and preterm delivery. These effects are discussed in more detail in Chapters 35 (p. 761), 36 (p. 811), and 38 (p. 848).

It is plausible that the vasoactive properties of tobacco smoke could produce congenital defects related to vascular disturbances. Martinez-Frias and colleagues (1999) observed in smokers a twofold risk of *Poland sequence*, which is caused by an interruption in the vascular supply to one side of the fetal chest and ipsilateral arm. Smoking was found associated with an increased risk for congenital heart disease in a dose-related manner (Malik and co-workers, 2008). Smoking at least 20 cigarettes a day combined with the use of vasoconstrictive drugs such as amphetamines and decongestants also appears to result in a fourfold risk of gastroschisis and small intestinal atresia (Werler and associates, 2003).

Smoking has been associated with cleft lip and palate in individuals heterozygous or homozygous for an uncommon polymorphism in the transforming growth factor gene (Shaw and colleagues, 1996). When exposed prenatally to cigarette smoke, these individuals have twice the risk of combined cleft lip and palate, and four to seven times the risk for cleft palate alone (Hwang and associates, 1995; Shaw and co-workers, 1996). A study that used the National Vital Statistics System natality data from more than 6 million live births in the United States found an association between maternal smoking and hydrocephaly, microcephaly, omphalocele, gastroschisis, cleft lip and palate, and hand abnormalities (Honein and colleagues, 2001).

REFERENCES

Abel EL, Hannigan, JH: Maternal risk factors in fetal alcohol syndrome: Provocative and permissive influences. Neurotoxicol Teratol 17(4):445, 1995
Abel EL, Sokol RJ: Marijuana and cocaine use during pregnancy. In Niebyl J (ed): Drug Use in Pregnancy, 2nd ed. Philadelphia, Lea and Febiger, 1988, p 223
Actelion Pharmaceuticals: Tracleer (bosentan) full prescribing information, 2005. Available at: http://www.tracleer.com/pdf/PI_4pg_TR2454_032707_FINAL.pdf. Accessed August 7, 2008
Aleck KA, Bartley DL: Multiple malformation syndrome following fluconazole use in pregnancy: Report of an additional patient. Am J Med Genet 72:253, 1997
Alroomi LG, Davidson J, Evans TJ, et al: Maternal narcotic abuse and the newborn. Arch Dis Child 63:81, 1988
Alwan S, Reefhuis J, Rasmussen SA, et al: Use of selective serotonin-reuptake inhibitors in pregnancy and the risk of birth defects. National Birth Defects Prevention Study. N Engl J Med 356:2684, 2007
American Academy of Pediatrics and American College of Obstetricians and Gynecologists: Guidelines for Perinatal Care, 6th ed. 2007
American College of Obstetricians and Gynecologists: Vitamin A supplementation during pregnancy. Committee Opinion No. 157, September 1995
American College of Obstetricians and Gynecologists: Use of psychiatric medications during pregnancy and lactation. Practice Bulletin No. 87, November 2007
Ances BM: New concerns about thalidomide. Obstet Gynecol 99:125, 2002
Andrade SE, Raebel MA, Brown J, et al: Use of antidepressant medications during pregnancy: A multisite study. Am J Obstet Gynecol 198(2):194, 2008
Ang-Lee MK, Moss J, Yuan CS: Herbal medicines and perioperative care. JAMA 286:208, 2001
Antiretroviral Pregnancy Registry Steering Committee: Antiretroviral pregnancy international interim report for 1 January 1989 through 31 January 2004. Wilmington, NC, Registry Coordinating Center, 2004
Araiza-Casillas R, Cardenas F, Morales Y, et al: Factors associated with chloroquine-induced retinopathy in rheumatic diseases. Lupus 13:119, 2004
Arnold GL, Kirby RS, Langendoerfer S, et al: Toluene embryopathy: Clinical delineation and developmental follow-up. Pediatrics 93:216, 1994
Bar-Oz B, Moretti ME, Bishai R, et al: Pregnancy outcome after in utero exposure to itraconazole: A prospective cohort study. Am J Obstet Gynecol 183:617, 2000
Barr M, Cohen MM: ACE inhibitor fetopathy and hypocalvaria: The kidney-skull connection. Teratology 44:485, 1991
Behnke M, Eyler FD, Garvan CW, et al: The search for congenital malformations in newborns with fetal cocaine exposure. Pediatrics 107:E74, 2001
Bertrand J, Floyd RL, Weber MK: Fetal Alcohol Syndrome Prevention Team, Division of Birth Defects and Developmental Disabilities, National Center on Birth Defects and Developmental Disabilities, Centers for Disease Control and Prevention (CDC). Guidelines for identifying and referring persons with fetal alcohol syndrome. MMWR 54:1, 2005
Billings RJ, Berkowitz RI, Watson G: Teeth. Pediatrics 113(4):1120, 2004
Bingol N, Fuchs M, Holipas N, et al: Prune belly syndrome associated with maternal cocaine abuse. Am J Hum Genet 39:A51, 1986
Black DR: Pregnancy unaffected by pennyroyal usage. J Am Osteopath Assoc 85:282, 1985
Boncinelli E: Homeobox genes and disease. Curr Opin Genet Dev 7:331, 1997
Brent RL: Environmental causes of human congenital malformations: The pediatrician's role in dealing with these complex clinical problems caused by a multiplicity of environmental and genetic factors. Pediatrics 113:957, 2004a
Brent RL: Teratogen update: Reproductive risks of leflunomide (Arava), a pyrimidine synthesis inhibitor: Counseling women taking leflunomide before or during pregnancy and men taking leflunomide who are contemplating fathering a child. Teratology 63(2):106, 2001
Brent RL: Utilization of animal studies to determine the effects and human risks of environmental toxicants (drugs, chemicals, and physical agents). Pediatrics 113:984, 2004b
Briggs GG, Freeman RK, Yaffe SJ: Drugs in Pregnancy and Lactation, 7th ed. Philadelphia, Lippincott Williams & Wilkins, 2005
Bristol-Myers Squibb: Sustiva product information, 2000. Available at: http://packageinserts.bms.com/pi/pi_sustiva.pdf. Accessed August 7, 2008
Brunskill PJ: The effects of fetal exposure to danazol. Br J Obstet Gynaecol 99:212, 1992
Buehler BA, Delimont D, van Waes M, et al: Prenatal prediction of risk of the fetal hydantoin syndrome. N Engl J Med 322:1567, 1990
Burd L, Cotsonas-Hassler TM, Martsolf JT, et al: Recognition and management of fetal alcohol syndrome. Neurotoxicol Teratol 25:681, 2003
Carter TC, Druschell CM, Romitti PA, et al: Antifungal drugs and the risk of selected birth defects. Am J Obstet Gynecol 198(20):191, 2008
Castilla EE, Ashton-Prolla O, Barreda-Mejia E, et al: Thalidomide, a current teratogen in South America. Teratology 54:273, 1996
Center for Drug Evaluation and Research: Reviewer guidance. Evaluating the risks of drug exposure in human pregnancies. Food and Drug Administration, April 2005. Available at: www.fda/gov/cder/guidance/index.htm. Accessed March 12, 2008
Centers for Disease Control and Prevention: Alcohol consumption among women who are pregnant or who might become pregnant. United States, 2002. MMWR 53: 1178, 2004
Centers for Disease Control and Prevention: Antiviral agents for influenza: Background information for clinicians. CDC Fact Sheet, December 16, 2003
Chambers CD, Hernandez-Diaz S, Van Marter LJ, et al: Selective serotonin-reuptake inhibitors and risk of persistent pulmonary hypertension of the newborn. N Engl J Med 354(6):579, 2006

Chasnoff IJ, Burns KA, Burns WJ: Cocaine use in pregnancy: Perinatal morbidity and mortality. Neurotoxicol Teratol 9:291, 1987

Chasnoff IJ, Burns KA, Burns WJ, et al: Prenatal drug exposure: Effects on neonatal and infant growth development. Neurotoxicol Teratol 8:357, 1986

Chasnoff IJ, Burns WJ, Schnoll SH, et al: Cocaine use in pregnancy. N Engl J Med 313:666, 1985

Chasnoff IJ, Chisum GM, Kaplan WE: Maternal cocaine use and genitourinary tract malformations. Teratology 37:201, 1988

Chasnoff IJ, Landress HJ, Barrett ME: The prevalence of illicit drug or alcohol use during pregnancy and the discrepancies in mandatory reporting in Pinellas County, Florida. N Engl J Med 322:1202, 1990

Chavez GF, Mulinare J, Cordero JF: Maternal cocaine use and the risk for genitourinary tract defects: An epidemiologic approach. Am J Hum Genet 43:A43, 1988

Choi BH, Lapham LW, Amin-Zaki L, et al: Abnormal neuronal migration, deranged cerebellar cortical organization, and diffuse white matter astrocytosis of human fetal brain. A major effect of methyl mercury poisoning in utero. J Neuropathol Neurol 37:719, 1978

Clark EB: Neck web and congenital heart defects: A pathogenic association in 45 X-O Turner syndrome? Teratology 29:355, 1984

Clarkson TW: The three modern faces of mercury. Environ Health Perspect 110:11, 2002

Clayton-Smith J, Donnai D: Human malformations. In Rimoin DL, Connor JM, Pyeritz RE (eds): Emery and Rimoin's Principles and Practice of Medical Genetics, 3rd ed. New York, Churchill Livingstone, 1996, p 383

Cliver SP, Goldenberg RL, Lutter R, et al: The effect of cigarette smoking on neonatal anthropometric measurements. Obstet Gynecol 85:625, 1995

Cohen HL, Sloves JH, Laungani S, et al: Neurosonographic findings in full-term infants born to maternal cocaine abusers: Visualization of subependymal and periventricular cysts. J Clin Ultrasound 22:327, 1994

Consumer Reports on Health: When good drugs do bad things. Consumer Reports on Health, July 2003, p 8

Conway H: Effect of supplemental vitamin therapy on the limitation of incidence of cleft lip and cleft palate in humans. Plast Reconstr Surg 22:450, 1958

Cooper WO, Hernandez-Diaz S, Arbogast PG, et al: Major congenital malformation after first-trimester exposure to ACE inhibitors. N Engl J Med 354:2443, 2006

Costedoat-Chalumeau N, Amoura Z, Duhaut P, et al: Safety of hydroxychloroquine in pregnant patients with connective tissue diseases: A study of one hundred thirty-three cases compared with a control group. Arthritis Rheum 48:3207, 2003

Costei AM, Kozer E, Ho T, et al: Perinatal outcome following third trimester exposure to paroxetine. Arch Pediatr Adolesc Med 156:1129, 2002

Creinin MD, Vittinghoff E: Methotrexate and misoprostol vs misoprostol alone for early abortion: A randomized controlled trial. JAMA 272:1190, 1994

Cunningham M, Tennis P, and the International Lamotrigine Pregnancy Registry Scientific Advisory Committee: Lamotrigine and the risk of malformations in pregnancy. Neurology 64:955, 2005

Czeizel AE, Rockenbauer M: Population-based case-control study of teratogenic potential of corticosteroids. Teratology 56:335, 1997

D'Souza SW, Black P, Richards B: Smoking in pregnancy: Associations with skinfold thickness, maternal weight gain, and fetal size at birth. BMJ 282:1661, 1981

Dai WS, Hsu MA, Itri LM: Safety of pregnancy after discontinuation of isotretinoin. Arch Dermatol 125:362, 1989

Dai WS, LaBraico JM, Stern RS: Epidemiology of isotretinoin exposure during pregnancy. J Am Acad Dermatol 26:599, 1992

Dally A: Thalidomide: Was the tragedy preventable? Lancet 351:1197, 1998

Dansky LV, Andermann E, Rosenblatt D, et al: Anticonvulsants, folate levels, and pregnancy outcome: A prospective study. Ann Neurol 21:176, 1987

Del Campo M, Kosaki K, Bennett FC, et al: Developmental delay in fetal aminopterin/methotrexate syndrome. Teratology 60:10, 1999

DiGiovanna JJ, Zezh LA, Ruddel ME, et al: Etretinate: Persistent serum levels of a potent teratogen. Clin Res 32:579A, 1984

Eisai Inc.: Targretin product information, 2007. Available at: http://www.eisai.com/pdf_files/TargretinGelM%20PI%20rev-1%20ver-1%20jan07.pdf. Accessed August 7, 2008

Environmental Protection Agency and Food and Drug Administration: What you need to know about mercury in fish and shellfish. 2004. Advice for women who might become pregnant, women who are pregnant, nursing mothers, young children. EPA-823-F-04-009. Updated August 2008

Ethen MK, Ramadhani TA, Scheurele AE, et al: National Birth Defects Prevention Study. Alcohol consumption by women before and during pregnancy. Matern Child Health J 13(2):274, 2009

Faiella A, Zappavigna V, Mavilio F, et al: Inhibition of retinoic acid-induced activation of 3' human HOXB genes by antisense oligonucleotides affects sequential activation of genes located upstream in the four HOX clusters. Proc Natl Acad Sci USA 7:5335, 1994

Feldcamp M, Carey JC: Clinical teratology counseling and consultation case report: Low dose methotrexate exposure in the early weeks of pregnancy. Teratology 47:533, 1993

Food and Drug Administration: Information for healthcare professionals mycophenolate mofetil (marketed as Cellcept) and mycophenolic acid (marketed as Myfortic). 5-16-2008. Available at: http://www.fda.gov/cder/drug/InfoSheets/HCP/mycophelolateHCP.htm. Accessed April 12, 2009

Food and Drug Administration: Pregnancy categories for prescription drugs. FDA Bulletin, September 1979

Food and Drug Administration: Summary of proposed rules on pregnancy and lactation labeling. 2008. Available at: http://www.fda.gov/cber/rules/frpreglac.pdf. Accessed November 15, 2008

Franks ME, Macpherson GR, Figg WD: Thalidomide. Lancet 363:1802, 2004

Fried S, Kozer E, Nulman I, et al: Malformation rates in children with untreated epilepsy: A meta-analysis. Drug Saf 27(3):197, 2004

Gardner MO, Owen J, Skelly S, et al: Preterm delivery after indomethacin. A risk factor for neonatal complications? J Reprod Med 41:903, 1996

Geiger JM, Baudin M, Saurat JH: Teratogenic risk with etretinate and acitretin treatment. Dermatology 189:109, 1994

Ginsberg JS, Hirsh J: Anticoagulants during pregnancy. Annu Rev Med 40:79, 1989

Giusti RM, Iwamoto K, Hatch EE: Diethylstilbestrol revisited: A review of the long-term health effects. Ann Intern Med 122:778, 1995

Glantz JC: Reproductive toxicology of alkylating agents. Obstet Gynecol Surv 49:709, 1994

GlaxoSmithKline: Paxil (paroxetine hydrochloride) prescribing information, January 2008. Available at: http://us.gsk.com/products/assets/us_paxil.pdf. Accessed August 7, 2008

Goldberg JM, Falcone T: Effect of diethylstilbestrol on reproductive functions. Fertil Steril 72:1, 1999

Golden NL, Kuhnert BR, Sokol RJ, et al: Neonatal manifestations of maternal phencyclidine exposure. J Perinat Med 15:185, 1987

Greenland S, Richwald GA, Honda GD: The effects of marijuana use during pregnancy, 2. A study in a low-risk home delivery population. Drug Alcohol Depend 11:359, 1983

Grumbach MM, Ducharme JR: The effects of androgens on fetal sexual development. Androgen-induced female pseudohermaphrodism. Fertil Steril 11:157, 1960

Gudas LJ: Retinoids and vertebrate development. J Biol Chem 269:15399, 1994

Guerri C, Bazinet A, Riley EP: Foetal alcohol spectrum disorders and alterations in brain and behaviour. Alcohol Alcohol 44(2):108, 2009

Guron G, Friberg P: An intact renin-angiotensin system is a prerequisite for normal renal development. J Hypertension 18:123, 2000

Hall JG, Pauli RM, Wilson K: Maternal and fetal sequelae of anticoagulation during pregnancy. Am J Med 68:122, 1980

Heinonen OP, Slone D, Shapiro S: Birth Defects and Drugs in Pregnancy. Littleton. MA, John Wright Publishing Sciences Group, 1983

Henderson J, Gray R, Brocklehurst P. Systematic review of effects of low-moderate prenatal alcohol exposure on pregnancy outcome. BJOG 114:243, 2007

Hepner DL, Harnett M, Segal S, et al: Herbal medicine use in parturients. Anesth Analg 94:690, 2002

Herbst AL, Ulfelder H, Poskanzer DC: Adenocarcinoma of the vagina. Association of maternal stilbestrol therapy. N Engl J Med 284:878, 1971

Hernandez-Diaz S, Werler MM, Walker AM, et al: Folic acid antagonists during pregnancy and the risk of birth defects. N Engl J Med 343:1608, 2000

Hiilesmaa VK, Teramo K, Granstrom ML, et al: Serum folate concentrations in women with epilepsy. BMJ 287:577, 1983

Holmes LB: Teratogen-induced limb defects. Am J Med Genet 112:297, 2002

Holmes LB, Baldwin EJ, Smith CR, et al: Increased frequency of isolated cleft palate in infants exposed to lamotrigine during pregnancy. Neurology 70 (22 Pt 2):2152, 2008

Holmes LB, Harvey EA, Coull BA, et al: The teratogenicity of anticonvulsant drugs. N Engl J Med 344:1132, 2001

Honein MA, Paulozzi LJ, Watkins ML: Maternal smoking and birth defects: Validity of birth certificate data for effect estimation. Public Health Rep 116:327, 2001

Horning MG, Stratton C, Wilson A, et al: Detection of 5-(3,4)-diphenylhydantoin in the newborn human. Anal Lett 4:537, 1974

Hoyme HE, Jones KL, Dixon SD, et al: Prenatal cocaine exposure and fetal vascular disruption. Pediatrics 85:743, 1990

Hoyme HE, May PA, Kalberg WO, et al: A practical clinical approach to diagnosis of fetal alcohol spectrum disorders: Clarification of the 1996 Institute of Medicine criteria. Pediatrics 115(1):39, 2005

Hume RF Jr, Martin LS, Bottoms SF, et al: Vascular disruption birth defects and history of prenatal cocaine exposure: A case control study. Fetal Diagn Ther 12:292, 1997

Hunt S, Craig J, Russell A, et al: Levetiracetam in pregnancy: Preliminary experience from the UK Epilepsy and Pregnancy Register. Neurology 67:1876, 2006

Hunt S, Russell WH, Smithson L, et al: Topriamate in pregnancy: preliminary experience from the UK epilepsy and pregnancy register. Neurology 71:272, 2008

Hwang SJ, Beaty TH, Panny SR, et al: Association study of transforming growth factor alpha (TGFα) Tag 1 polymorphism and oral clefts. Am J Epidemiol 14:629, 1995

Iahnaccone PM, Bossert NL, Connelly CS: Disruption of embryonic and fetal development due to preimplantation chemical insults: A critical review. Am J Obstet Gynecol 157:476, 1987

Institute of Medicine, National Academy of Sciences. Fetal Alcohol Syndrome: Diagnosis, Epidemiology, Prevention and Treatment. Washington, DC, National Academies Press, 1996

iPLEDGE program announcement – FDA. Available at http://www.fda.gov/cder/drug/advisory/isotretinoin2005.htm. Accessed April 5, 2007

Jacobson SJ, Jones K, Johnson K, et al: Prospective multicentre study of pregnancy outcome after lithium exposure during first trimester. Lancet 339:530, 1992

Jankov RP, McNamara PJ. Inhaled nitric oxide therapy for persistent pulmonary hypertension of the newborn: When is it enough? J Crit Care 20:294, 2005

Jasper JD, Goel R, Einarson A, et al: Effects of framing on teratogenic risk perception in pregnant women. Lancet 358:1237, 2001

Jick SS, Terris BZ, Jick H: First trimester topical tretinoin and congenital disorders. Lancet 341:1664, 1993

Jordan AE, Jackson GL, Deardorff D, et al: Serotonin reuptake inhibitor use in pregnancy and the neonatal behavioral syndrome. J Matern Fetal Neonatal Med 21(10):745, 2008

Kandall SR, Gaines J, Habel L, et al: Relationship of maternal substance abuse to subsequent sudden infant death syndrome in offspring. J Pediatr 123:120, 1993

Kaufman RH, Adam E, Hatch EE, et al: Continued follow-up of pregnancy outcomes in diethylstilbestrol-exposed offspring. Obstet Gynecol 96:483, 2000

Khouri MI, James IM, Flanders WD, et al: Interpretation of recurring weak association obtained from epidemiologic studies of suspected human teratogens. Teratology 46:69, 1992

Kirshon B, Wasserstrum N, Willis R, et al: Teratogenic effects of first trimester cyclophosphamide therapy. Obstet Gynecol 72:462, 1988

Klip H, Verloop J, van Gool JD, et al: Hypospadias in sons of women exposed to diethylstilbestrol in utero: A cohort study. Lancet 359:1102, 2002

Knapp K, Lenz W, Nowack E: Multiple congenital abnormalities. Lancet 2:725, 1962

Koren G, Bologa M, Long D, et al: Perception of teratogenic risk by pregnant women exposed to drugs and chemicals during the first trimester. Am J Obstet Gynecol 160:1190, 1989

Koren G, Pastuszak A, Ito S: Drugs in pregnancy. Review. N Engl J Med 338:112, 1998

Kutscher AH, Zegarelli EV, Tovell HM, et al: Discoloration of deciduous teeth induced by administration of tetracycline antepartum. Am J Obstet Gynecol 96:291, 1966

Lacroix I, Damase-Michel C, Lapeyre-Mestre M, et al: Prescription of drugs during pregnancy in France. Lancet 356:1735, 2000

Lammer EJ: Embryopathy in infant conceived one year after termination of maternal etretinate. Lancet 2:1080, 1988

Lammer EJ, Chen DT, Hoar RM, et al: Retinoic acid embryopathy. N Engl J Med 313:837, 1985

Lemoine P: Les enfants de parents alcooliques. Ovest Med 21:476, 1968

Leppik IE, Rask CA: Pharmacokinetics of antiepileptic drugs during pregnancy. Semin Neurol 8:240, 1988

Lewis DP, Van Dyke DC, Stumbo PJ, et al: Drug and environmental factors associated with adverse pregnancy outcomes. Part I: Antiepileptic drugs, contraceptives, smoking, and folate. Ann Pharm 32:802, 1998

Levin R: Neonatal adverse events associated with in utero SSRI/SNRI exposure. U.S. Food and Drug Administration. Available at: www.fda.gov/ohrms/-dockets/ac/04/slides/2004-4050S1_11_Levin.ppt. Accessed March 26, 2008

Lifschitz MH, Wilson GS, Smith EO, et al: Fetal and postnatal growth of children born to narcotic-dependent women. J Pediatr 102:686, 1983

Lim S, Prasad MR, Samuels P, et al: High-dose methadone in pregnant women and its effect on duration of neonatal abstinence syndrome. Am J Obstet Gynecol 200(1):70.e1, 2009

Lindhout D, Rene JE, Hoppener A, et al: Teratogenicity of antiepileptic drug combinations with special emphasis on epoxidation of carbamazepine. Epilepsia 25:77, 1984

Linn S, Schoenbaum SC, Monson RR, et al: The association of marijuana use with outcome of pregnancy. Am J Public Health 73:1161, 1983

Little BB, Snell LM, Gilstrap LC, et al: Effects of Ts and blues abuse during pregnancy on maternal and infant health status. Am J Perinatol 7:359, 1990a

Little BB, Snell LM, Gilstrap LC: Methamphetamine abuse during pregnancy: Outcome and fetal effects. Obstet Gynecol 72:541, 1988

Little BB, Snell LM, Klein VR, et al: Cocaine abuse during pregnancy: Maternal and fetal implications. Obstet Gynecol 73:157, 1989

Little BB, Snell LM, Klein VR, et al: Maternal and fetal effects of heroin addiction during pregnancy. J Reprod Med 35:159, 1990b

Louik C, Lin AE, Werler MM, et al: First-trimester use of selective serotonin-reuptake inhibitors and the risk of birth defects. N Engl J Med 356:2675, 2007

Loureiro KD, Kao KK, Jones KL, et al: Minor malformations characteristic of the retinoic acid embryopathy and other birth outcomes in children of women exposed to topical tretinoin during early pregnancy. Am J Med Genetics Part A 136A(2):117, 2005

Major CA, Lewis DF, Harding JA, et al: Tocolysis with indomethacin increases the incidence of necrotizing enterocolitis in the low-birth-weight neonate. Am J Obstet Gynecol 170:102, 1994

Malik S, Cleves MA, Honein MA, et al: Maternal smoking and congenital heart defects. Pediatrics 121(4):e810, 2008

Manson JM, Papa L, Miller ML, et al: Studies of DNA damage and cell death in embryonic limb buds induced by teratogenic exposure to cyclophosphamide. Teratog Carcinog Mutagen 2:47, 1982

Marpeau L, Bouillie J, Barrat J, et al: Obstetrical advantages and perinatal risks of indomethacin: A report of 818 cases. Fetal Diagn Ther 9:110, 1994

Martinez-Frias ML, Czeizel AE, Rodriguez-Pinilla E, et al: Smoking during pregnancy and Poland sequence: Results of a population-based registry and a case-control registry. Teratology 59:35, 1999

Mastroiacovo P, Mazzone T, Addis A, et al: High vitamin A intake in early pregnancy and major malformations: A multicenter prospective controlled study. Teratology 59:7, 1999

Maurer T, Poncelet A, Berger T: Thalidomide treatment for prurigo nodularis in human immunodeficiency virus-infected subjects: Efficacy and risk of neuropathy. Arch Dermatol 140:845, 2004

McGready R, Cho T, Keo NK, et al: Artemisinin antimalarials in pregnancy: A prospective treatment study of 539 episodes of multidrug-resistant *Plasmodium falciparum.* Clin Infect Dis 33:2009, 2001

McGready R, Thwai KL, Cho T, et al: The effects of quinine and chloroquine antimalaria treatments in the first trimester of pregnancy. Trans R Soc Trop Med Hyg 96:180, 2002

McKeigue PM, Lamm SH, Linn S, et al: Bendectin and birth defects: I. A meta-analysis of the epidemiologic studies. Teratology 50:27, 1994

Melnick S, Cole P, Anderson D, et al: Rates and risks of diethylstilbestrol-related clear-cell adenocarcinoma of the vagina and cervix. N Engl J Med 316:514, 1987

Mercer BM, Merlino AA, Milluzzi CJ, et al: Small fetal size before 20 weeks' gestation: Associations with maternal tobacco use, early preterm birth, and low birthweight. Am J Obstet Gynecol 198(6):673, 2008

Milkovich L, van den Berg BJ: Effects of antenatal exposure to anorectic drugs. Am J Obstet Gynecol 129:637, 1977

Minozzi S, Amato L, Vecchi S: Maintenance agonist treatments for opiate dependent pregnant women. Cochrane Database Syst Rev April 16;(2):CD006318, 2008

Mitchell AA: Systematic identification of drugs that cause birth defects—a new opportunity. N Engl J Med 349:26, 2003

Morrow JI, Russell A, Guthrie E, et al: Malformation risks of antiepileptic drugs in pregnancy: A prospective study from the UK Epilepsy and Pregnancy Register. J Neurol Neurosurg Psych 77:193, 2006

Moses-Kolko EI, Bogen D, Perel J, et al: Neonatal signs after late in utero exposure to serotonin reuptake inhibitors. Literature review and implications for clinical applications. JAMA 293:2372, 2005

Murray JC: Face facts: Genes, environment, and clefts. Am J Hum Genet 57:3227, 1995

National Survey on Drug Use and Health: National findings. Substance Abuse and Mental Health Services Administration, Office of Applied Studies. Department of Health and Human Services. Available at: http://www.oas.samhsa.gov/-nsduh/2k7nsduh/2k7results.pdf. Accessed November 11, 2008

Nelson BK, Moorman WJ, Schrader SM: Review of experimental male-mediated behavioral and neurochemical disorders. Neurotoxicology 18:611, 1996

Nohynek GJ, Meuling WJA, Vaes WHJ, et al: Repeated topical treatment, in contrast to single oral doses, with vitamin A containing preparations does not affect plasma concentrations of retinol, retinyl esters or retinoic acids in female subjects of child-bearing age. Toxicol Lett 163:65, 2006

Norton ME, Merrill J, Cooper BA, et al: Neonatal complications after the administration of indomethacin for preterm labor. N Engl J Med 329(22), 1993

Nosten F, Vincenti M, Simpson J, et al: The effects of mefloquine treatment in pregnancy. Clin Infect Dis 28:808, 1999

Oakley GP, Erickson JD: Vitamin A and birth defects. N Engl J Med 333:1414, 1995

Olshan AF, Teschke K, Baird PA: Paternal occupation and congenital anomalies. Am J Ind Med 20:447, 1991

Ondrizek RR, Chan PJ, Patton WC, et al: An alternative medicine study of herbal effects on the penetration of zonafree hamster oocytes and the integrity of sperm deoxyribonucleic acid. Fertil Steril 71:517, 1999

Ostrea EM, Chavez CJ: Perinatal problems (excluding neonatal withdrawal) in maternal drug addiction: A study of 830 cases. J Pediatr 94:292, 1979

Pandit PB, Chitayat D, Jefferies AL, et al: Tibial hemimelia and tetralogy of Fallot associated with first trimester exposure to amantadine. Reprod Toxicol 8:89, 1994

Parilla BV: Using indomethacin as a tocolytic. Contemp Ob/Gyn 49:90, 2004

Park-Wyllie L, Mazzota P, Pastuszak A, et al: Birth defects after maternal exposure to corticosteroids: Prospective cohort study and meta-analysis of epidemiological studies. Teratology 62(6):385, 2000

Pearson MA, Hoyme HE, Seaver LH, et al: Toluene embryopathy: Delineation of the phenotype and comparison with fetal alcohol syndrome. Pediatrics 93:211, 1994

Pro B, Younes A, Albitar M, et al: Thalidomide for patients with recurrent lymphoma. Cancer 100:1186, 2004

Pryde PG, Sedman AB, Nugent CE, et al: Angiotensin converting enzyme inhibitor fetopathy. J Am Soc Nephrol 3:1575, 1993

Raman-Wilms L, Tseng AL, Wighardt S, et al: Fetal genital effects of first-trimester sex hormone exposure: A meta-analysis. Obstet Gynecol 85:141, 1995

Ramin SM, Little BB, Trimmer KJ, et al: Methamphetamine use during pregnancy. Am J Obstet Gynecol 166:353, 1992

Rasanen J, Jouppila P: Fetal cardiac function and ductus arteriosus during indomethacin and sulindac therapy for threatened preterm labor: A randomized study. Am J Obstet Gynecol 173:20, 1995

Rebordosa C, Kogevinas M, Horváth-Puhó E, et al: Acetaminophen use during pregnancy: Effects on risk for congenital abnormalities. Am J Obstet Gynecol 198(2):178, 2008

Regev RH, Litmanowitz I, Arnon S, et al: Gentamicin serum concentrations in neonates born to gentamicin-treated mothers. Pediat Infect Dis J 19:890, 2000

Reprotox: Reproductive Toxicology Center: Amphetamines. Available at: http://reprotox.org/data. Accessed November 11, 2008a

Reprotox: Reproductive Toxicology Center: Tretinoin. Available at: http://reprotox.org/data/1428.html. Accessed November 11, 2008b

Rivkin MJ, Davis PE, Lemaster JL, et al: Volumetric MRI study of brain in children with intrauterine exposure to cocaine, alcohol, tobacco, and marijuana. Pediatrics 121(4):741, 2008

Robaire B, Hales BF: Paternal exposure to chemicals before conception. BMJ 307:341, 1993

Robboy SJ, Noller KL, O'Brien P, et al: Increased incidence of cervical and vaginal dysplasia in 3,980 diethylstilbestrol- exposed young women. Experience of the National Collaborative Diethylstilbestrol Adenosis Project. JAMA 252:2979, 1984

Roche Laboratories Inc.: CellCept package insert, December 2008. Available at: http://www.rocheusa.com/products/cellcept/pi.pdf. Accessed April 12, 2009

Rosa F: Amantadine pregnancy experience. Reprod Toxicol 8:531, 1994

Rothman KJ, Moore LL, Singer MR, et al: Teratogenicity of high vitamin A intake. N Engl J Med 333:1369, 1995

Ruiz-Irastorza G, Ramos-Casals M, Brito-Zeron P: Clinical efficacy and side effects of antimalarials in systemic lupus erythematosus: a systematic review. Ann Rheum Dis [Epub ahead of print], 2009

Sadler TW: Langman's Medical Embryology, 6th ed. Baltimore, Williams & Wilkins, 1990, p 130

Salle B, Sergeant P, Awada A, et al: Transvaginal ultrasound studies of vascular and morphological changes in uteri exposed to diethylstilbestrol in utero. Hum Reprod 11:2531, 1996

Sampson PD, Streissguth AP, Bookstein FL, et al: Incidence of fetal alcohol syndrome and prevalence of alcohol-related neurodevelopmental disorder. Teratology 56(5):317 1997

Sanofi-aventis Pharmaceuticals: Arava product information, 2007. Available at: http://products.sanofi-aventis.us/arava/arava.pdf. Accessed August 7, 2008

Savitz DA, Sonnenfeld N, Olshan AF: Review of epidemiological studies of paternal occupational exposure and spontaneous abortion. Am J Ind Med 25:361, 1994

Schaefer C, Hannemann D, Meister R, et al: Vitamin K antagonists and pregnancy outcome—A multicenter prospective study. Thromb Haemost 95(6):949, 2006

Schardein JL: Chemically Induced Birth Defects, 3rd ed. New York, Marcel Dekker, 2000

Schardein JL: Congenital abnormalities and hormones during pregnancy: A clinical review. Teratology 22:251, 1985

Schnitzer PG, Olshan AF, Erickson JD: Paternal occupation and risk of birth defects in the offspring. Epidemiology 6:577, 1995

Schubiger G, Flury G, Nussberger J: Enalapril for pregnancy induced hypertension: Acute renal failure in the neonate. Ann Intern Med 108:215, 1988

Shaw GM, Velie EM, Schaffer D: Risk of neural tube defect affected pregnancies among obese women. JAMA 275:1093, 1996

Sheehan DM: Herbal medicines, phytoestrogens and toxicity: Risk:benefit considerations. Proc Soc Exp Biol Med 217:379, 1998

Shepard TH: Catalog of Teratogenic Agents, 10th ed. Baltimore, The Johns Hopkins University Press, 2001

Shiono PH, Klebanoff MA, Nugent RP, et al: The impact of cocaine and marijuana use on low birth weight and preterm birth: A multicenter study. Am J Obstet Gynecol 172:19, 1995

Singer LT, Arendt R, Minnes S, et al: Cognitive and motor outcomes of cocaine-exposed infants. JAMA 287:1952, 2002

Singer LT, Minnes S, Short E, et al: Cognitive outcomes of preschool children with prenatal cocaine exposure. JAMA 292:1021, 2004

Soprano DR, Soprano KJ: Retinoids as teratogens. Annu Rev Nutr 15:111, 1995

Sorenson HT, Nelsen GL, Olesen C, et al: Risk of malformations and other outcomes in children exposed to fluconazole in utero. Br J Clin Pharmacol 48:234, 1999

Stevenson RE: Causes of human anomalies: An overview and historical perspective. Human malformations and related anomalies. In Stevenson RE, Hall JG, Goodman RM (eds): Human Malformations and Related Anomalies. New York, Oxford University Press, 1993a, p 3

Stevenson RE: The environmental basis of human anomalies. In Stevenson RE, Hall JG, Goodman RM (eds): Human Malformations and Related Anomalies. New York, Oxford University Press, 1993b, p 137

Stillerman KP, Mattison DR, Giudice LC, et al: Environmental exposures and adverse pregnancy outcomes: A review of the science. Reprod Sci 15(7):631, 2008

Stillman RJ: In utero exposure to diethylstilbestrol: Adverse effects on the reproductive tract and reproductive performance in male and female offspring. Am J Obstet Gynecol 142:905, 1982

Stimmel B, Adamsons K: Narcotic dependency in pregnancy. Methadone maintenance compared to use of street drugs. JAMA 235:1121, 1976

Strandberg-Larsen K, Nielsen NR, Grønbaek M, et al: Binge drinking in pregnancy and risk of fetal death. Obstet Gynecol 111(3):602, 2008

Streissguth AP, Clarren SK, Jones KL: Natural history of fetal alcohol syndrome: A 10-year follow-up of eleven patients. Lancet 2:85, 1985

Sutton C, McIvor RS, Vagt M, et al: Methotrexate-resistant form of dihydroreductase protects transgenic murine embryos from teratogenic effects of methotrexate. Pediatr Dev Pathol 1:503, 1998

Thomson EJ, Cordero JF: The new teratogens: Accutane and other vitamin-A analogs. MCN Am J Matern Child Nurs 14:244, 1989

Trasler JM, Doerksen T: Teratogen update: Paternal exposures—reproductive risks. Teratology 60:161, 1999

UCB, Inc: Keppra prescribing information, 2008. Available at: http://www.keppraxr.com/hcp/includes/pdf/Keppra_XR_Prescribing_Information.pdf. Accessed April 12, 2009

van der Heijden BJ, Carlus C, Narcy F, et al: Persistent anuria, neonatal death, and renal microcystic lesions after prenatal exposure to indomethacin. Am J Obstet Gynecol 171:617, 1994

Vermillion ST, Scardo JA, Lashus AG, et al: The effect of indomethacin tocolysis on fetal ductus arteriosus constriction with advancing gestational age. Am J Obstet Gynecol 177:256, 1997

Vessey MP: Epidemiological studies of the effects of diethylstilbestrol. IARC Sci Publ 335, 1989

Vitale N, DeFeo M, De Santo LS, et al: Dose-dependent fetal complications of warfarin in pregnant women with mechanical heart valves. J Am Coll Cardiol 33:1637, 1999

von Almen WF, Miller JM: Ts and blues in pregnancy. J Reprod Med 31:236, 1984

Vorhees CV, Minck Dr, Berry HK: Anticonvulsants and brain development. Prog Brain Res 73:229, 1988

Vroom F, de Walle HE, van de Laar MA, et al: Disease-modifying antirheumatic drugs in pregnancy: current status and implications for the future. Drug Saf 29(10):845, 2006

Walker MPR, Moore TR, Brace RA: Indomethacin and arginine vasopressin interaction in the fetal kidney. A mechanism of oliguria. Am J Obstet Gynecol 171:1234, 1994

Warkany J: Warfarin embryopathy. Teratology 14:205, 1976

Wass TS, Persutte WH, Hobbins JC: The impact of prenatal alcohol exposure on frontal cortex development in utero. Am J Obstet Gynecol 185:737, 2001

Watts DH, Covington DL, Beckerman K, et al: Assessing the risk of birth defects associated with antiretroviral exposure during pregnancy. Am J Obstet Gynecol 191(3):985, 2004

Weinstein MR: Recent advances in clinical psychopharmacology. I. Lithium carbonate. Hosp Form 12:759, 1977

Werler MM: Teratogen update: Smoking and reproductive outcomes. Teratology 55:382, 1997

Werler MM, Sheehan JE, Mitchell AA: Association of vasoconstrictive exposures with risks of gastroschisis and small intestinal atresia. Epidemiology 14:349, 2003

Wilkins-Haug L: Teratogen Update: Toluene. Teratology 55:145, 1997

Yaffe SJ, Briggs GG: Is this drug going to harm my baby? Contemp Ob/Gyn 48:57, 2003

Zhu M, Zhou S: Reduction of the teratogenic effects of phenytoin by folic acid and a mixture of folic acid, vitamins, amino acids: A preliminary trial. Epilepsia 30:246, 1989

CHAPTER 15

Antepartum Assessment

According to the American College of Obstetricians and Gynecologists and the American Academy of Pediatrics (2007), the goals of antepartum fetal surveillance include prevention of fetal death and avoidance of unnecessary interventions. Current techniques employed to forecast fetal well-being focus on fetal physical activities, including heart rate, movement, breathing, and amnionic fluid production. In most cases, a negative, that is, normal test result is highly reassuring, because fetal deaths within 1 week of a normal test are rare. Indeed, negative-predictive values—a true negative test—for most of the tests described are 99.8 percent or higher. In contrast, estimates of the positive-predictive values—a true positive test—for abnormal test results are low and range between 10 and 40 percent. Importantly, the widespread use of antepartum fetal surveillance is primarily based on circumstantial evidence because there have been no definitive randomized clinical trials.

FETAL MOVEMENTS

Passive unstimulated fetal activity commences as early as 7 weeks and becomes more sophisticated and coordinated by the end of pregnancy (Vindla and James, 1995). Indeed, beyond 8 menstrual weeks, fetal body movements are never absent for periods exceeding 13 minutes (DeVries and co-workers, 1985). Between 20 and 30 weeks, general body movements become organized, and the fetus starts to show rest-activity cycles (Sorokin and co-workers, 1982). In the third trimester, fetal movement maturation continues until approximately 36 weeks, when behavioral states are established in most normal fetuses. Nijhuis and colleagues (1982) studied fetal heart rate patterns, general body movements, and eye movements and described four fetal behavioral states:

- **State 1F** is a quiescent state—quiet sleep—with a narrow oscillatory bandwidth of the fetal heart rate
- **State 2F** includes frequent gross body movements, continuous eye movements, and wider oscillation of the fetal heart rate. This state is analogous to rapid eye movement (REM) or active sleep in the neonate
- **State 3F** includes continuous eye movements in the absence of body movements and no heart rate accelerations. The existence of this state is disputed (Pillai and James, 1990a)
- **State 4F** is one of vigorous body movement with continuous eye movements and heart rate accelerations. This state corresponds to the awake state in infants.

Fetuses spend most of their time in states 1F and 2F. For example, at 38 weeks, 75 percent of time is spent in these two states (Nijhuis and colleagues, 1982).

These behavioral states—particularly 1F and 2F, which correspond to quiet sleep and active sleep—have been used to develop an increasingly sophisticated understanding of fetal behavior. Oosterhof and co-workers (1993) studied fetal urine

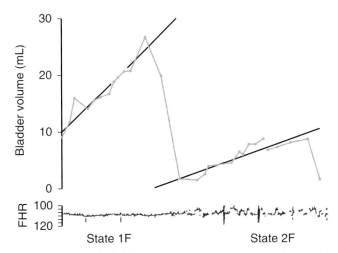

FIGURE 15-1 Fetal bladder volume measurements together with fetal heart rate variation record in relation to 1F or 2F behavior states. State 1F fetal heart rate has a narrow bandwidth consistent with quiet sleep. State 2F heart rate shows wide oscillation of the baseline consistent with active sleep. (Modified from Oosterhof and co-workers, 1993, with permission.)

tric sensors. Weak, strong, and rolling movements were described, and their relative contributions to total weekly movements throughout the last half of pregnancy were quantified. As pregnancy advances, weak movements decrease and are superseded by more vigorous movements, which increase for several weeks and then subside at term. Presumably, declining amnionic fluid and space account for diminishing activity at term. Figure 15-2 shows fetal movements during the last half of gestation in 127 pregnancies with normal outcomes. The mean number of weekly movements calculated from 12-hour daily recording periods increased from approximately 200 at 20 weeks to a maximum of 575 movements at 32 weeks. Fetal movements then declined to an average of 282 at 40 weeks. Normal weekly maternal counts of fetal movements ranged between 50 and 950, with large daily variations that included counts as low as 4 to 10 per 12-hour period in normal pregnancies.

Clinical Application

In 1973, Sadovsky and Yaffe described seven case reports of pregnancies with decreased fetal activity that preceded fetal death. Since then, various methods have been described to quantify fetal movement as a way of prognosticating well-being. Methods include use of a tocodynamometer, visualization with sonography, and maternal subjective perceptions. Most investigators have reported excellent correlation between maternally perceived fetal motion and movements documented by instrumentation. For example, Rayburn (1980) found that 80 percent of all movements observed during sonographic monitoring were perceived by the mother. In contrast, Johnson and colleagues (1992) reported that beyond 36 weeks, mothers perceived only 16 percent of fetal body movements recorded by a Doppler device. Fetal motions lasting more than 20 seconds were identified more accurately by the mother than shorter episodes.

Although several fetal movement counting protocols have been used, neither the optimal number of movements nor the

production in normal pregnancies in states 1F or 2F. As shown in Figure 15-1, bladder volumes increased during state 1F quiet sleep. During state 2F, the fetal heart rate baseline bandwidth increased appreciably, and bladder volume was significantly diminished. The latter was due to fetal voiding as well as decreased urine production. These phenomena were interpreted to represent reduced renal blood flow during active sleep.

An important determinant of fetal activity appears to be sleep-awake cycles, which are independent of the maternal sleep-awake state. *Sleep cyclicity* has been described as varying from about 20 minutes to as much as 75 minutes. Timor-Tritsch and associates (1978) reported that the mean length of the quiet or inactive state for term fetuses was 23 minutes. Patrick and associates (1982) measured gross fetal body movements with real-time sonography for 24-hour periods in 31 normal pregnancies and found the longest period of inactivity to be 75 minutes. Amnionic fluid volume is another important determinant of fetal activity. Sherer and colleagues (1996) assessed the number of fetal movements in 465 pregnancies during biophysical profile testing in relation to amnionic fluid volume estimated using sonography. They observed decreased fetal activity with diminished amnionic volumes and suggested that a restricted uterine space might physically limit fetal movements.

Sadovsky and colleagues (1979b) studied fetal movements in 120 normal pregnancies and classified the movements into three categories according to both maternal perceptions and independent recordings using piezoelec-

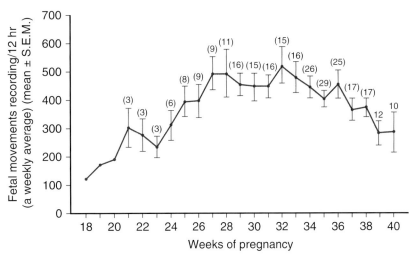

FIGURE 15-2 Graph depicts averages of fetal movements counted during 12-hour periods (mean ± SEM). (From Sadovsky and associates, 1979a, with permission.)

ideal duration for counting them has been defined. For example, in one method, perception of 10 fetal movements in up to 2 hours is considered normal (Moore and Piaquadio, 1989). In another, women are instructed to count fetal movements for 1 hour a day, and the count is accepted as reassuring if it equals or exceeds a previously established baseline count (Neldam, 1983). The American College of Obstetricians and Gynecologists (2002) suggests that one approach to assessing fetal movement is to have the woman count distinct fetal movements on a daily basis after 28 weeks' gestation. The perception of 10 distinct movements in up to 2 hours is considered reassuring. The counting can be discontinued for that day after 10 movements.

Commonly, women may present in the third trimester complaining of subjectively reduced fetal movement. Harrington and colleagues (1998) reported that 7 percent of 6793 women delivered at a London hospital presented with a complaint of decreased fetal movement. Fetal heart rate monitoring tests were employed if sonographic scans for fetal growth or Doppler velocimetry were abnormal. The pregnancy outcomes for women who complained of decreased fetal movement were not significantly different from those for women without this complaint. Nonetheless, the authors recommended evaluation to reassure the mother.

Grant and co-workers (1989) performed an unparalleled investigation of maternally perceived fetal movements and pregnancy outcome. More than 68,000 pregnancies were randomly assigned between 28 and 32 weeks. Women in the fetal movement arm of the study were instructed by specially employed midwives to record the time needed to feel 10 movements each day. This required an average of 2.7 hours each day. Women in the control group were informally asked about movements during prenatal visits. Reports of decreased fetal motion were evaluated with tests of fetal well-being. Antepartum death rates for normally formed singletons were similar in the two study groups regardless of prior risk status. Despite the counting policy, most stillborn fetuses were dead by the time the mothers reported for medical attention. Importantly, these investigators did not conclude that maternal perceptions of fetal activity were meaningless. Conversely, they concluded that informal maternal perceptions were as valuable as formally counted and recorded fetal movement.

FETAL BREATHING

After decades of uncertainty as to whether the fetus normally breathes, Dawes and co-workers (1972) showed small inward and outward flows of tracheal fluid, indicating fetal thoracic movement in sheep. These chest wall movements differed from those following birth in that they were discontinuous. Another interesting feature of fetal respiration was *paradoxical chest wall movement.* As shown in **Figure 15-3**, during inspiration the chest wall paradoxically collapses and the abdomen protrudes (Johnson and co-workers, 1988). In the newborn or adult, the opposite occurs. One interpretation of the paradoxical respiratory motion might be coughing to clear amnionic fluid debris. Although the physiological basis for the breathing reflex is not completely understood, such exchange of amnionic fluid appears to be essential for normal lung development.

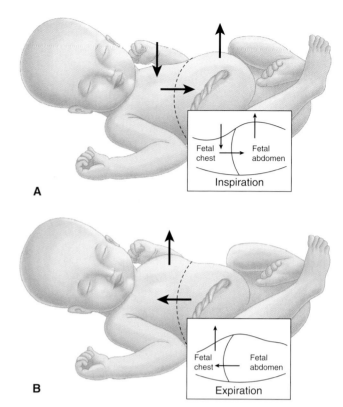

FIGURE 15-3 Paradoxical chest movement with fetal respiration. (Adapted from Johnson and co-workers, 1988.)

Dawes (1974) identified two types of respiratory movements. The first are *gasps or sighs,* which occurred at a frequency of 1 to 4 per minute. The second, *irregular bursts of breathing,* occurred at rates up to 240 cycles per minute. These latter rapid respiratory movements were associated with REM. Badalian and co-workers (1993) studied the maturation of normal fetal breathing using color flow and spectral Doppler analysis of nasal fluid flow as an index of lung function. They suggested that fetal respiratory rate decreased in conjunction with increased respiratory volume at 33 to 36 weeks and coincidental with lung maturation.

Many investigators have examined fetal breathing movements, using sonography to determine whether monitoring chest wall movements might be of benefit to evaluate fetal health. Several variables in addition to hypoxia were found to affect fetal respiratory movements. These included labor—during which it is normal for respiration to cease—hypoglycemia, sound stimuli, cigarette smoking, amniocentesis, impending preterm labor, gestational age, and the fetal heart rate itself.

Because fetal breathing movements are episodic, interpretation of fetal health when respirations are absent may be tenuous. Patrick and associates (1980) performed continuous 24-hour observation periods using sonography in an effort to characterize fetal breathing patterns during the last 10 weeks of pregnancy. A total of 1224 hours of fetal observation was completed in 51 pregnancies. Figure 15-4 shows the percentage of time spent breathing near term. Clearly, there is diurnal variation, because breathing substantively diminishes during the night. In addition, breathing activity increases somewhat following maternal meals. Total absence of breathing was observed

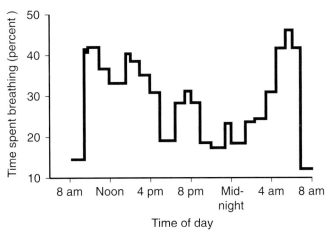

FIGURE 15-4 The percentage of time spent breathing by 11 fetuses at 38 to 39 weeks demonstrated a significant increase in fetal breathing activity after breakfast. Breathing activity diminished during the day and reached its minimum between 8 pm and midnight hours. There was a significant increase in the percentage of time spent breathing between 4 and 7 am, when mothers were asleep. (Adapted from Patrick and co-workers, 1980.)

TABLE 15-1. Criteria for Interpretation of the Contraction Stress Test

- Negative: no late or significant variable decelerations
- Positive: late decelerations following 50% or more of contractions (even if the contraction frequency is fewer than three in 10 minutes)
- Equivocal-suspicious: intermittent late decelerations or significant variable decelerations
- Equivocal-hyperstimulatory: fetal heart rate decelerations that occur in the presence of contractions more frequent than every 2 minutes or lasting longer than 90 seconds
- Unsatisfactory: fewer than three contractions in 10 minutes or an uninterpretable tracing

Reprinted, with permission, from the American College of Obstetricians and Gynecologists. Antepartum fetal surveillance. ACOG Practice Bulletin 9. Washington, DC: ACOG; 2007.

in some of these normal fetuses for up to 122 minutes, indicating that fetal evaluation to diagnose absent respiratory motion may require long periods of observation.

The potential for breathing activity to be an important marker of fetal health is unfulfilled because of the multiplicity of factors that normally affect breathing. Most clinical applications have included assessment of other fetal biophysical indices, such as heart rate. As will be discussed, fetal breathing has become a component of the *biophysical profile.*

CONTRACTION STRESS TESTING

As amnionic fluid pressure increases with uterine contractions, myometrial pressure exceeds collapsing pressure for vessels coursing through uterine muscle, ultimately decreasing blood flow to the intervillous space. Brief periods of impaired oxygen exchange result, and if uteroplacental pathology is present, these elicit late fetal heart rate decelerations (see Chap. 18, p. 421). Contractions also may produce a pattern of variable decelerations as a result of cord compression, suggesting oligohydramnios, which is often a concomitant of placental insufficiency.

Ray and colleagues (1972) used this concept in 66 complicated pregnancies and developed what they termed the *oxytocin challenge test* and later called the *contraction stress test.* Contractions were induced using intravenous oxytocin, and the fetal heart rate response was recorded using standard monitoring. The criterion for a positive (abnormal) test was uniform repetitive late fetal heart rate decelerations. These reflected the uterine contraction waveform and had an onset at or beyond the acme of a contraction. Such late decelerations could be the result of uteroplacental insufficiency. The tests were generally repeated on a weekly basis, and the investigators concluded that negative (normal) contraction stress tests forecast fetal health. One disadvantage cited was that the average contraction stress test required 90 minutes to complete.

Fetal heart rate and uterine contractions are recorded simultaneously with an external monitor. If at least three spontaneous contractions of 40 seconds or longer are present in 10 minutes, no uterine stimulation is necessary (American College of Obstetricians and Gynecologists, 2007). Contractions are induced with either oxytocin or nipple stimulation if there are fewer than three in 10 minutes. If oxytocin is preferred, a dilute intravenous infusion is initiated at a rate of 0.5 mU/min and doubled every 20 minutes until a satisfactory contraction pattern is established (Freeman, 1975). The results of the contraction stress test are interpreted according to the criteria shown in Table 15-1.

Nipple stimulation to induce uterine contractions is usually successful for contraction stress testing (Huddleston and associates, 1984). One method recommended by the American College of Obstetricians and Gynecologists (2007) involves a woman rubbing one nipple through her clothing for 2 minutes or until a contraction begins. She is instructed to restart after 5 minutes if the first nipple stimulation did not induce three contractions in 10 minutes. Advantages include reduced cost and shortened testing times. Although Schellpfeffer and associates (1985) reported unpredictable uterine hyperstimulation and fetal distress, others did not find excessive activity to be harmful (Frager and Miyazaki, 1987).

NONSTRESS TESTS

Freeman (1975) and Lee and colleagues (1975) introduced the *nonstress test* to describe fetal heart rate acceleration in response to fetal movement as a sign of fetal health. This test involved the use of Doppler-detected fetal heart rate acceleration coincident with fetal movements perceived by the mother. By the end of the 1970s, the nonstress test had become the primary method of testing fetal health. The nonstress test was easier to perform, and normal results were used to further discriminate false-positive contraction stress tests. Simplistically, the nonstress test is primarily a test of *fetal condition,* and it differs from the contraction stress test, which is a test of *uteroplacental function.* Currently, nonstress testing is the most widely used primary testing method for assessment of fetal well-being and has also been incorporated into the biophysical profile testing system subsequently discussed.

Fetal Heart Rate Acceleration

The fetal heart rate normally is increased or decreased by autonomic influences mediated by sympathetic or parasympathetic impulses from brainstem centers. Beat-to-beat variability is also under the control of the autonomic nervous system (Matsuura and colleagues, 1996). Consequently, pathological loss of acceleration may be seen in conjunction with significantly decreased beat-to-beat variability of the fetal heart rate (see Chap. 18, p. 414). Loss of such reactivity, however, is most commonly associated with sleep cycles, discussed earlier. It also may be caused by central depression from medications or maternal cigarette smoking (Jansson and co-workers, 2005; Oncken and colleagues, 2002).

The nonstress test is based on the hypothesis that the heart rate of a fetus who is not acidotic as a result of hypoxia or neurological depression will temporarily accelerate in response to fetal movement (Fig. 15-5). Fetal movements during testing are identified by maternal perception and recorded. Similarly, Smith and colleagues (1988) observed a decrease in the number of accelerations in preterm fetuses subsequently found to have lower umbilical artery blood PO_2 values.

Gestational age influences acceleration or reactivity of fetal heart rate. Pillai and James (1990b) studied the development of fetal heart rate acceleration patterns during normal pregnancy. The percentage of body movements accompanied by acceleration and the amplitude of these accelerations increased with gestational age (Fig. 15-6). Guinn and colleagues (1998) studied nonstress test results between 25 and 28 weeks in 188 pregnancies that ultimately had normal outcomes. Only 70 percent of these normal fetuses demonstrated the required 15 beats per minute (bpm) or more of heart rate acceleration. Lesser degrees of acceleration, that is, 10 bpm, occurred in 90 percent of the fetuses.

The National Institute of Child Health and Human Development Fetal Monitoring Workshop (1997) has defined normal acceleration based on gestational age. The acme of acceleration is 15 bpm or more above the baseline rate, and the acceleration lasts 15 seconds or longer but less than 2 minutes in fetuses at or beyond 32 weeks. Before 32 weeks, accelerations are defined as having an acme 10 bpm or more above baseline for 10 seconds or longer.

Normal Nonstress Tests

There have been many different definitions of normal nonstress test results. They vary as to the number, amplitude, and duration of acceleration, as well as the test duration. The definition currently recommended by the American College of Obstetricians and Gynecologists and the American Academy of Pediatrics (2007) is two or more accelerations that peak at 15 bpm or more above baseline, each lasting 15 seconds or more, and all occurring within 20 minutes of beginning the test (Fig. 15-7). It was also recommended that accelerations with or without fetal movements be accepted, and that a 40-minute or longer tracing—to account for fetal sleep cycles—should be performed before concluding that there was insufficient fetal reactivity. Miller and colleagues (1996b) reviewed outcomes in fetuses with nonstress tests considered as nonreactive because there was only one acceleration. They concluded that one acceleration was just as reliable as two in predicting healthy fetal status.

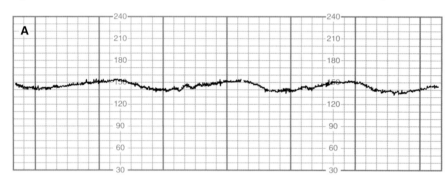
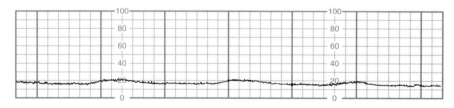
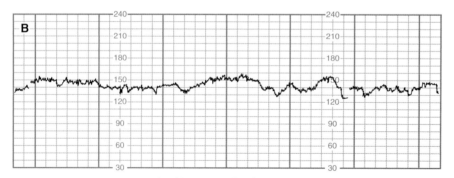

FIGURE 15-5 Two antepartum fetal heart rate (FHR) tracings in a 28-week pregnant woman with diabetic ketoacidosis. **A.** FHR tracing (*upper panel*) and accompanying contraction tracing (*second panel*). Tracing, obtained during maternal and fetal acidemia shows absence of accelerations, diminished variability, and late decelerations with weak spontaneous contractions. **B.** FHR tracing shows return of normal accelerations and variability of the fetal heart rate following correction of maternal acidemia.

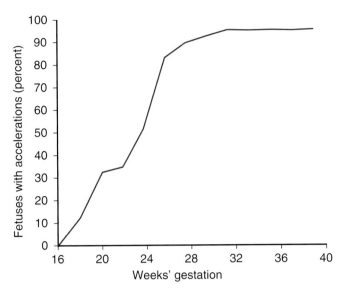

FIGURE 15-6 Percentage of fetuses with at least one acceleration of 15 beats/min sustained for 15 sec concurrent with fetal movement. (Adapted from Pillai and James, 1990b.)

tests, blinded to specific patient clinical data, to a national sample of obstetricians for their interpretations. He concluded that although nonstress testing is popular, the reliability of test interpretation needs improvement. Such problems with subjective interpretation have prompted efforts to computerize analysis of nonstress tests. Pardey and colleagues (2002) have developed such a system—*Sonicaid Fetal Care.* Turan and colleagues (2007) evaluated the *Oxford Sonicaid 8002 cCTG* system in 58 growth-restricted fetuses and compared findings with those obtained by multiple other tests. They concluded that the computerized system performed best when used with umbilical venous Doppler findings or as a substitute for the traditional nonstress test in the biophysical profile score.

Abnormal Nonstress Tests

There are abnormal nonstress test patterns that reliably forecast severe fetal jeopardy. Hammacher and co-workers (1968) described tracings with what they termed a *silent oscillatory pattern.* This pattern consisted of a fetal heart rate baseline that oscillated less than 5 bpm and presumably indicated absent acceleration and beat-to-beat variability. Hammacher considered this pattern ominous.

Visser and associates (1980) described a "terminal cardiotocogram," which included: (1) baseline oscillation of less than 5 bpm, (2) absent accelerations, and (3) late decelerations with spontaneous uterine contractions. These results were similar to experiences from Parkland Hospital in which absence of accelerations during an 80-minute recording period in 27 fetuses was associated consistently with evidence of uteroplacental pathology (Leveno and associates, 1983). The latter included fetal-growth restriction in 75 percent, oligohydramnios in 80 percent, fetal acidosis in 40 percent, meconium in 30 percent, and placental infarction in 93 percent. Thus, the lack of fetal heart rate acceleration, when not due to maternal sedation, is an ominous finding (Fig. 15-8). Similarly, Devoe and co-workers (1985) concluded that nonstress tests that were nonreactive for 90 minutes were almost invariably—93 percent—associated with significant perinatal pathology.

Although a normal number and amplitude of accelerations seems to reflect fetal well-being, "insufficient acceleration" does not invariably predict fetal compromise. Indeed, some investigators have reported 90-percent or higher false-positive rates (Devoe and associates, 1986). Because healthy fetuses may not move for periods of up to 75 minutes, Brown and Patrick (1981) considered that a longer duration of nonstress testing might increase the positive-predictive value of an abnormal, that is, nonreactive, test. They concluded that either the test became reactive during a period up to 80 minutes or the test remained nonreactive for 120 minutes, indicating that the fetus was very ill.

Not only are there many different definitions of normal nonstress test results, but the reproducibility of interpretations is problematic. For example, Hage (1985) mailed five nonstress

Interval between Testing

The interval between tests, originally rather arbitrarily set at 7 days, appears to have been shortened as experience evolved with nonstress testing. According to the American College of Obstetricians and Gynecologists (2007), more frequent testing is advocated by some investigators for women with postterm pregnancy, multifetal gestation, type 1 diabetes mellitus, fetal-growth restriction, or gestational hypertension (Devoe, 2008; Freeman, 2008; Graves, 2007; Kennelly and Sturgiss, 2007). In these circumstances, some investigators perform twice-weekly tests, with additional testing performed

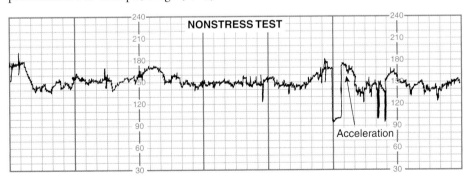

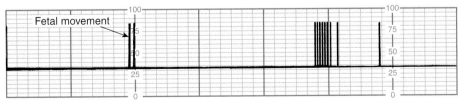

FIGURE 15-7 Reactive nonstress test. In the upper panel, notice increase of fetal heart rate to more than 15 beats/min for longer than 15 sec following fetal movements, indicated by the vertical marks (*lower panel*).

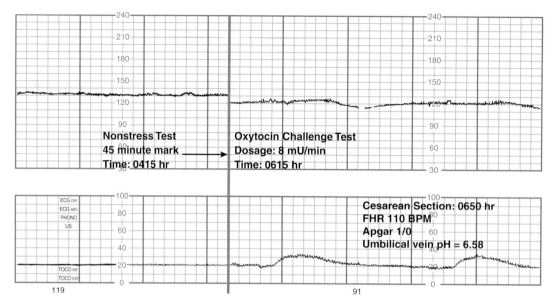

FIGURE 15-8 Nonreactive nonstress test (*left side of tracing*) followed by contraction stress test showing mild, late decelerations (*right side of tracing*). Cesarean delivery was performed, and the severely acidemic fetus could not be resuscitated.

for maternal or fetal deterioration regardless of the time elapsed since the last test. Others perform nonstress tests daily or even more frequently, for example, with severe preeclampsia remote from term (see Chap. 34, p. 728).

Decelerations During Nonstress Testing

Fetal movements commonly produce heart rate decelerations. Timor-Tritsch and associates (1978) reported this during non-stress testing in half to two thirds of tracings, depending on the vigor of the fetal motion. This high incidence of decelerations inevitably makes interpretation of their significance problematic. Indeed, Meis and co-workers (1986) reported that variable fetal heart rate decelerations during nonstress tests were not a sign of fetal compromise. The American College of Obstetricians and Gynecologists (2007) has concluded that variable decelerations, if nonrepetitive and brief—less than 30 seconds—do not indicate fetal compromise or the need for obstetrical intervention. In contrast, repetitive variable decelerations—at least three in 20 minutes—even if mild, have been associated with an increased risk of cesarean delivery for fetal distress. Decelerations lasting 1 minute or longer have been reported to have an even worse prognosis (Bourgeois, 1984; Druzin, 1981; Pazos, 1982, and all their co-workers).

Hoskins and associates (1991) attempted to refine interpretation of testing that shows variable decelerations by adding sonographic estimation of amnionic fluid volume. The incidence of cesarean delivery for intrapartum fetal distress progressively increased concurrently with the severity of variable decelerations and decline of amnionic fluid volume. Severe variable decelerations during a nonstress test plus an amnionic fluid index of ≤ 5 cm resulted in a 75-percent cesarean delivery rate. Fetal distress in labor, however, also frequently developed in those pregnancies with variable decelerations but with normal amounts of amnionic fluid. Similar results were reported by Grubb and Paul (1992).

False-Normal Nonstress Tests

Smith and associates (1987) performed a detailed analysis of the causes of fetal death within 7 days of normal nonstress tests. The most common indication for testing was postterm pregnancy. The mean interval between testing and death was 4 days, with a range of 1 to 7 days. The single most common autopsy finding was meconium aspiration, often associated with some type of umbilical cord abnormality. They concluded that an acute asphyxial insult had provoked fetal gasping. They also concluded that nonstress testing was inadequate to preclude such an acute asphyxial event and that other biophysical characteristics might be beneficial. For example, assessment of amnionic fluid volume was considered valuable. Other ascribed frequent causes of fetal death included intrauterine infection, abnormal cord position, malformations, and placental abruption.

ACOUSTIC STIMULATION TESTS

Loud external sounds have been used to startle the fetus and thereby provoke heart rate acceleration—an *acoustic stimulation nonstress test*. A commercially available acoustic stimulator is positioned on the maternal abdomen, and a stimulus of 1 to 2 seconds is applied (Eller and associates, 1995). This may be repeated up to three times for up to 3 seconds (American College of Obstetricians and Gynecologists, 2007). A positive response is defined as the rapid appearance of a qualifying acceleration following stimulation (Devoe, 2008). Perez-Delboy and colleagues (2002) randomized 113 women to nonstress testing with and without vibroacoustic stimulation. Such stimulation shortened the average time for nonstress testing from 24 to 15 minutes.

TABLE 15-2. Components and Their Scores for the Biophysical Profile

Component	Score 2	Score 0
Nonstress test[a]	≥2 accelerations of ≥15 beats/min for ≥15 sec within 20–40 min	0 or 1 acceleration within 20–40 min
Fetal breathing	≥1 episode of rhythmic breathing lasting ≥30 sec within 30 min	<30 sec of breathing within 30 min
Fetal movement	≥3 discrete body or limb movements within 30 min	<3 discrete movements
Fetal tone	≥1 episode of extremity extension and subsequent return to flexion	0 extension/flexion events
Amnionic fluid volume[b]	A pocket of amnionic fluid that measures at least 2 cm in two planes perpendicular to each other (2 × 2 cm pocket)	Largest single vertical pocket ≤2 cm

[a] May be omitted if all four sonographic components are normal.
[b] Further evaluation warranted, regardless of biophysical composite score, if largest vertical amnionic fluid pocket ≤2 cm.

BIOPHYSICAL PROFILE

Manning and colleagues (1980) proposed the combined use of five fetal biophysical variables as a more accurate means of assessing fetal health than a single element. Required equipment includes a sonography machine and Doppler ultrasound to record fetal heart rate. Typically, these tests require 30 to 60 minutes of examiner time. Shown in Table 15-2 are the five biophysical components assessed, which include: (1) fetal heart rate acceleration, (2) fetal breathing, (3) fetal movements, (4) fetal tone, and (5) amnionic fluid volume. Normal variables were assigned a score of 2 each and abnormal variables, a score of 0. Thus, the highest score possible for a normal fetus is 10. Kopecky and associates (2000) observed that 10 to 15 mg of morphine sulfate administered to a mother caused a significant decrease in the biophysical score by suppressing fetal breathing and heart rate acceleration.

Manning and colleagues (1987) tested more than 19,000 pregnancies using the biophysical profile interpretation and management shown in Table 15-3. They reported a false-normal test rate, defined as an antepartum death of a structurally normal fetus, of approximately 1 per 1000. More than 97 percent of the pregnancies tested had normal test results. The most common identifiable causes of fetal death after a normal biophysical profile include fetomaternal hemorrhage, umbilical cord accidents, and placental abruption (Dayal and associates, 1999).

Manning and co-workers (1993) published a remarkable description of 493 fetuses in which biophysical scores were performed immediately before measurement of umbilical venous blood pH values obtained via cordocentesis. Approximately 20 percent of tested fetuses had growth restriction, and the remainder had alloimmune hemolytic anemia. As shown in Figure 15-9, a biophysical score of 0 was invariably associated with

significant fetal acidemia, whereas normal score of 8 or 10 was associated with normal pH. An equivocal test result—a score of 6—was a poor predictor of abnormal outcome. A decrease from an abnormal result—a score of 2 or 4—to a very abnormal score (0) was a progressively more accurate predictor of abnormal outcome.

Salvesen and colleagues (1993) correlated the biophysical profile with umbilical venous blood pH obtained at cordocentesis in 41 pregnancies complicated by diabetes. They also found that abnormal pH was significantly associated with abnormal biophysical profile scores. They concluded, however, that the biophysical profile was of limited value in the prediction of fetal pH, because nine mildly acidemic fetuses had normal antepartum tests. Weiner and colleagues (1996) assessed the meaning of antepartum fetal tests in 135 overtly growth-restricted fetuses and came to a similar conclusion. They found that morbidity and mortality in severe fetal-growth restriction were determined primarily by gestational age and birthweight and not by abnormal fetal tests. Lalor and associates (2008) recently updated the Cochrane review and concluded that there is insufficient evidence at this time to support the use of the biophysical profile as a test of fetal well-being in high-risk pregnancies. Kaur and associates (2008) performed daily biophysical profiles to ascertain the optimal delivery time in 48 growth-restricted preterm fetuses who weighed < 1000 g. Despite scores of 8 in 27 fetuses and 6 in 13, there were six deaths and 21 acidotic fetuses. They conclude that a high incidence of false-positive and –negative results is seen in very preterm fetuses.

Modified Biophysical Profile

Because the biophysical profile is labor intensive and requires a person trained in sonography, Clark and co-workers (1989) used

TABLE 15-3. Biophysical Profile Score, Interpretation, and Pregnancy Management

Biophysical Profile Score	Interpretation	Recommended Management
10	Normal, nonasphyxiated fetus	No fetal indication for intervention; repeat test weekly except in diabetic patients and postterm pregnancy (twice weekly)
8/10 (Normal AFV) 8/8 (NST not done)	Normal, nonasphyxiated fetus	No fetal indication for intervention; repeat testing per protocol
8/10 (Decreased AFV)	Chronic fetal asphyxia suspected	Deliver
6	Possible fetal asphyxia	If amnionic fluid volume abnormal, deliver If normal fluid at >36 weeks with favorable cervix, deliver If repeat test ≤6, deliver If repeat test >6, observe and repeat per protocol
4	Probable fetal asphyxia	Repeat testing same day; if biophysical profile score ≤6, deliver
0 to 2	Almost certain fetal asphyxia	Deliver

AFV = amnionic fluid volume; NST = nonstress test.
From Manning and colleagues (1987), with permission.

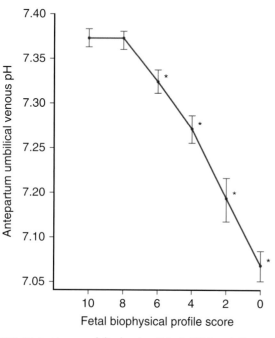

FIGURE 15-9 Mean umbilical vein pH (±2 SD) in relation to fetal biophysical profile score category. (This figure was published in *American Journal of Obstetrics & Gynecology*, Vol. 169, No. 4, FA Manning, R Snijders, CR Harman, et al., Fetal biophysical profile score. VI. Correlation with antepartum umbilical venous fetal pH, pp. 755–763, Copyright Elsevier 1993.)

an abbreviated biophysical profile as their first-line antepartum screening test in 2628 singleton pregnancies. Specifically, a vibroacoustic nonstress test was performed twice weekly and combined with amnionic fluid index determination (see Chap. 21, p. 490). An amnionic fluid index of <5 cm was considered abnormal. This abbreviated biophysical profile required approximately 10 minutes to perform, and they concluded that it was a superb method of antepartum surveillance because there were no unexpected fetal deaths.

Nageotte and colleagues (1994) also combined biweekly nonstress tests with the amnionic fluid index and considered ≤5 cm to be abnormal. They performed 17,429 modified biophysical profiles in 2774 women and concluded that such testing was an excellent method of fetal surveillance. Miller and associates (1996a) reported results with more than 54,000 modified biophysical profiles performed in 15,400 high-risk pregnancies. They described a false-negative rate of 0.8 per 1000 and a false-positive rate of 1.5 percent.

The American College of Obstetricians and Gynecologists and the American Academy of Pediatrics (2007) have concluded that the modified biophysical profile test is as predictive of fetal well-being as other approaches to biophysical fetal surveillance.

AMNIONIC FLUID VOLUME

Amnionic fluid volume is commonly evaluated in women with complaints of decreased fetal movement (Frøen and colleagues, 2008). Moreover, amnionic fluid has become an integral component in the antepartum assessment of pregnancies at risk for fetal death. This is based on the rationale that decreased utero-placental perfusion may lead to diminished fetal renal blood flow, decreased urine production, and ultimately, oligohydramnios. As discussed in Chapter 21 (p. 490), the amnionic fluid index, the deepest vertical pocket, and the 2 × 2-cm pocket used in the biophysical profile are some sonographic techniques used to estimate amnionic fluid volume (Chamberlain, 1984; Manning, 1984; Nabhan, 2008; Rutherford, 1987, and all their colleagues).

In their review of 42 reports on the amnionic fluid index published between 1987 and 1997, Chauhan and co-workers (1999) concluded that an index of ≤ 5.0 cm significantly increased the risk of either cesarean delivery for fetal distress or a low 5-minute Apgar score. Similarly, in a retrospective analysis of 6423 pregnancies managed at Parkland Hospital, Casey and colleagues (2000) found that an amnionic fluid index of ≤ 5 cm was associated with significantly increased perinatal morbidity and mortality rates. Locatelli and associates (2004) reported an increased risk of low-birthweight infants if there was oligohydramnios so defined.

Not all investigators agree with the concept that an index of ≤ 5 cm portends adverse outcomes. Magann and colleagues (1999, 2004) concluded that the index was a poor diagnostic test and that it better predicted normal than abnormal volumes. Driggers and co-workers (2004) and Zhang and associates (2004) did not find a correlation with poor outcomes in pregnancies in which the index was below 5 cm. In the only randomized trial reported to date, Conway and colleagues (2000) concluded that nonintervention to permit spontaneous onset of labor was as effective as induction in term pregnancies with amnionic fluid index values ≤5 cm.

DOPPLER VELOCIMETRY

Doppler ultrasound is a noninvasive technique to assess blood flow by characterizing downstream impedance (see Chap. 16, p. 362). Three fetal vascular circuits, which include the umbilical artery, middle cerebral artery, and ductus venosus, are currently being assessed using Doppler technology to determine fetal health and help time delivery for growth-restricted fetuses. Maternal uterine artery Doppler velocimetry has also been evaluated in efforts to predict placental dysfunction. The goal of such testing is to optimize the time of delivery—late enough to avoid complications of preterm delivery and early enough to avoid stillbirth (Ghidini, 2007).

Doppler Blood Flow Velocity

Wave forms were first studied systematically in the umbilical arteries late in pregnancy, and abnormal wave forms correlated with hypovascularity of the umbilical placental villous structure such as shown in Figure 15-10 (Trudinger, 2007). It was shown that 60 to 70 percent of the small placental arterial channels would need to be obliterated before the umbilical artery Doppler waveform became abnormal. Such extensive placental vascular pathology has a major effect on the fetal circulation. According to Trudinger (2007), because more than 40 percent of the combined fetal ventricular output is directed to the placenta, obliteration of vascular channels in the placental-umbilical circulation increases afterload and leads to fetal hypoxemia.

This in turn leads to dilatation and redistribution of middle cerebral artery blood flow. Ultimately, pressure rises in the ductus venosus due to afterload in the right side of the fetal heart. Thus, it is postulated that such placental vascular dysfunction results in increased umbilical artery blood flow resistance, which progresses to decreased middle cerebral artery impedance followed ultimately by abnormal flow in the ductus venosus (Baschat, 2004). In this scenario, abnormal Doppler waveforms in the ductus venosus are a late finding in the progression of fetal deterioration due to chronic hypoxemia.

Umbilical Artery Velocimetry

The use of Doppler ultrasound to measure blood flow in pregnancy was described at the end of the 1970s (Trudinger, 2007). The umbilical artery systolic-diastolic (S/D) ratio is considered abnormal if it is above the 95th percentile for gestational age or

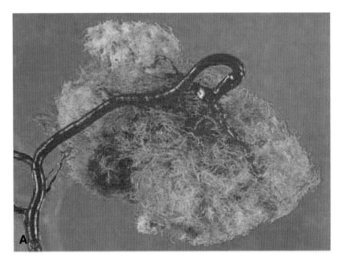

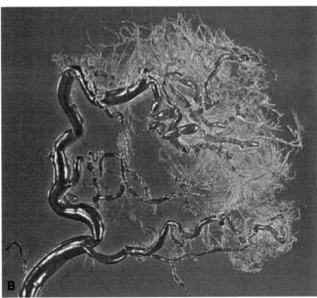

FIGURE 15-10 Acrylic casts of the umbilical arterial vascular tree within a placental lobule. They were prepared by injection of the umbilical artery at the site of cord insertion and later acid digestion of the tissue. **A.** Normal placenta. **B.** Placenta from a pregnancy with absent end diastolic flow in the umbilical artery recorded before delivery. (From Trudinger, 2007, with permission.)

if diastolic flow is either absent or reversed (see Chap. 16, p. 363). Absent or reversed end-diastolic flow as shown in Figure 15-11 signifies increased impedance to umbilical artery blood flow (see also Fig. 16-27, p. 364). It is reported to result from poorly vascularized placental villi and is seen in extreme cases of fetal-growth restriction (Todros and co-workers, 1999). Zelop and colleagues (1996) found that the perinatal mortality rate for absent end-diastolic flow was approximately 10 percent, and for reversed end-diastolic flow, it approximated 33 percent. Spinillo and associates (2005) studied neurodevelopmental outcome at 2 years of age in 266 growth-restricted fetuses delivered between 24 and 35 weeks' gestation following umbilical artery Doppler testing. Of infants with absent or reversed flow in the umbilical artery, 8 percent had evidence of cerebral palsy, compared with 1 percent of those in whom Doppler flow was either normal or was above the 95th percentile but without reversed flow.

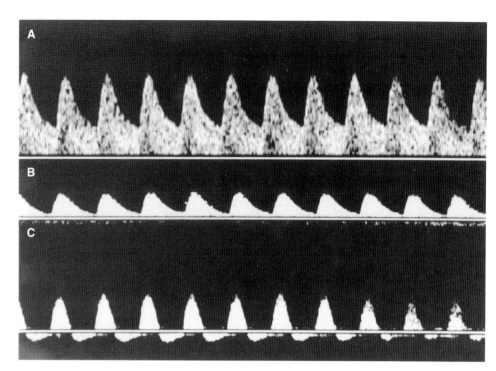

FIGURE 15-11 Three studies of fetal umbilical artery velocimetry. The peaks represent systolic velocity, and the troughs show the diastolic velocity. **A.** Normal velocimetry pattern. **B.** Velocity is zero during diastole (trough reaches the horizontal line). **C.** Arterial velocity is reversed during diastole (trough is below horizontal line).

Doppler ultrasound of the umbilical artery has been subjected to more extensive assessment with randomized controlled trials than has any previous test of fetal health. Williams and colleagues (2003) randomized 1360 high-risk women to either nonstress testing or Doppler velocimetry. They found a significantly increased incidence of cesarean delivery for fetal distress in the nonstress test group compared with that for those tested with Doppler velocimetry—8.7 versus 4.6 percent, respectively. One interpretation of this finding is that the nonstress test more frequently identified fetuses in jeopardy. Conversely, Gonzalez and associates (2007) found that abnormal umbilical artery Doppler findings in a cohort of growth-restricted fetuses were the best predictors of perinatal outcomes.

The utility of umbilical artery Doppler velocimetry was reviewed by the American College of Obstetricians and Gynecologists (2000, 2004). It was concluded that no benefit has been demonstrated other than in pregnancies with suspected fetal-growth restriction. Specifically, no benefits have been demonstrated for velocimetry for other conditions such as postterm pregnancy, diabetes, systemic lupus erythematosus, or antiphospholipid antibody syndrome. Similarly, velocimetry has not proved of value as a screening test for detecting fetal compromise in the general obstetrical population.

Middle Cerebral Artery

Doppler velocimetry interrogation of the middle cerebral artery (MCA) has received particular attention because of observa-

tions that the hypoxic fetus attempts *brain sparing* by reducing cerebrovascular impedance and thus increasing blood flow. Such brain sparing in growth-restricted fetuses has been documented by Konje and colleagues (2001) to undergo reversal. They reported that 8 of 17 fetuses with this reversal died. Ott and co-workers (1998) randomized 665 women undergoing modified biophysical profiles to either the profile alone or combined with middle cerebral to umbilical artery velocity flow assessment. There were no significant differences in pregnancy outcomes between these two study groups.

In a different application, Oepkes and colleagues (2006) used MCA Doppler velocimetry to detect severe fetal anemia in 165 fetuses with D alloimmunization. They prospectively compared serial amniocentesis for measurement of bilirubin levels with Doppler measurement of peak systolic velocity in the middle cerebral artery. These investigators concluded that Doppler could safely replace amniocentesis in the management of isoimmunized pregnancies. Indeed, Doppler velocimetry of the MCA is useful for detection and management of fetal anemia of any cause (Moise, 2008). The American College of Obstetricians and Gynecologists (2006) also concluded that such use of Doppler is appropriate in centers with personnel trained in the procedure (see Chap. 16, p. 364).

Ductus Venosus

The use of Doppler ultrasound to assess the fetal venous circulation is the most recent application of this technology. Bilardo and colleagues (2004) prospectively studied umbilical artery and ductus venosus Doppler results in 70 growth-restricted fetuses at 26 to 33 weeks' gestation. They concluded that ductus venosus Doppler velocimetry was the best predictor of perinatal outcome. Importantly, however, negative or reversed flow in the ductus venous was a late finding because these fetuses had already sustained irreversible multiorgan damage due to hypoxemia. Also, gestational age at delivery was a major determinant of perinatal outcome independent of ductus venous flow. Specifically, 36 percent of growth-restricted fetuses delivered between 26 and 29 weeks succumbed compared with 5 percent delivered from 30 to 33 weeks.

Baschat and co-workers (2007) systemically studied 604 growth-restricted fetuses using umbilical artery, middle cerebral artery, and ductus venosus Doppler velocimetry and reached conclusions similar to those of Bilardo and colleagues (2004). Specifically, absent or reversed flow in the ductus venosus was associated with profound generalized fetal metabolic collapse. They too reported that gestational age was a powerful cofactor in ultimate perinatal outcome for growth-restricted fetuses delivered before 30 weeks. Put another way, by the time severely abnormal flow is seen in the ductus venosus, it is too late because the fetus is already near death. However, earlier delivery puts the fetus at risk for death due to preterm delivery. Ghidini (2007) concluded that these reports do not support routine use of ductus venous Doppler in the monitoring of growth-restricted fetuses and recommended further study.

Uterine Artery

Vascular resistance in the uterine circulation normally decreases in the first half of pregnancy due to invasion of maternal uterine vessels by trophoblastic tissue (see Chap. 3, p. 54). This process can be detected using Doppler flow velocimetry of the uterine arteries. Uterine artery Doppler may be most helpful in assessing pregnancies at high risk of complications related to uteroplacental insufficiency (Abramowicz and Sheiner, 2008). Persistence or development of high-resistance patterns have been linked to a variety of pregnancy complications (Lees and co-workers, 2001; Yu and associates, 2005). In a study of 30,519 unselected British women, Smith and colleagues (2007) assessed uterine artery velocimetry at 22 to 24 weeks. The risk of fetal death before 32 weeks when associated with abruption, preeclampsia, or fetal-growth restriction was significantly linked to high-resistance flow. They and others suggest continued research on the role of uterine artery Doppler velocimetry as a screening tool to detect pregnancies at risk for stillbirth (Reddy and associates, 2008).

CURRENT ANTENATAL TESTING RECOMMENDATIONS

According to the American College of Obstetricians and Gynecologists (2007), there is no "best test" to evaluate fetal well-being. Three testing systems—contraction stress test, nonstress test, and biophysical profile—have different end points to consider depending on the clinical situation. The American College of Obstetricians and Gynecologists (2002) patient education pamphlet describes these tests of fetal well-being and summarizes as follows: "Monitoring helps you and your doctor during your pregnancy by telling more about the well-being of the baby. If a test result suggests that there may be a problem, this does not always mean that the baby is in trouble. It simply may mean that you need special care or more tests. Discuss any questions you have about monitoring with your doctor."

The most important consideration in deciding when to begin antepartum testing is the prognosis for neonatal survival. The severity of maternal disease is another important consideration. In general, with the majority of high-risk pregnancies, most authorities recommend that testing begin by 32 to 34 weeks. Pregnancies with severe complications might require testing as early as 26 to 28 weeks. The frequency for repeating tests has been arbitrarily set at 7 days, but more frequent testing is often done.

Significance of Fetal Testing

Does antenatal fetal testing really improve fetal outcome? Platt and co-workers (1987) reviewed its impact between 1971 and 1985 at Los Angeles County Hospital. During this 15-year period, more than 200,000 pregnancies were managed, and nearly 17,000 of these women underwent antepartum testing of various types. Fetal surveillance increased from less than 1 percent of pregnancies in the early 1970s to 15 percent in the mid-1980s. These authors concluded that such testing was clearly beneficial because the fetal death rate was significantly less in the tested high-risk pregnancies compared with the rate in those not tested.

A contrasting opinion on the benefits of antenatal fetal testing was offered by Thacker and Berkelman (1986). It was their view that efficacy is best evaluated in randomized controlled trials. After reviewing 600 reports, they found only four such trials, all performed with the nonstress test, and none with the contraction stress test. The numbers in these four trials were considered too small to detect important benefits and did not support the use of either test. Enkin and colleagues (2000) reviewed evidence in the Cochrane Library from controlled trials of antepartum fetal surveillance. They concluded that "despite their widespread use, most tests of fetal well-being should be considered of experimental value only rather than validated clinical tools."

Another important and unanswered question is whether antepartum fetal surveillance identifies fetal asphyxia early enough to prevent brain damage. Todd and co-workers (1992) attempted to correlate cognitive development in infants up to age 2 years following either abnormal umbilical artery velocimetry or nonstress test results. Only abnormal nonstress tests were associated with marginally poorer cognitive outcomes. These investigators concluded that by the time fetal compromise is diagnosed with antenatal testing, fetal damage has already been sustained. Low and colleagues (2003) reached a similar conclusion in their study of 36 preterm infants delivered based on antepartum test results. Manning and co-workers (1998) studied the incidence of cerebral palsy in 26,290 high-risk pregnancies managed with serial biophysical profile testing. They compared these outcomes with those of 58,657 low-risk pregnancies in which antepartum testing was not performed. The rate of cerebral palsy was 1.3 per 1000 in tested pregnancies compared with 4.7 per 1000 in untested women.

Antenatal forecasts of fetal health have clearly been the focus of intense interest for more than two decades. When such testing is reviewed, several themes emerge:

1. Methods of fetal forecasting have evolved continually, a phenomenon that at least suggests dissatisfaction with the precision or efficacy of any given method

2. The fetal biophysical performance is characterized by wide ranges of normal biological variation, resulting in difficulty determining when such performance should be considered abnormal. *How many movements, respirations, or accelerations? In what time period?* Unable to easily quantify normal fetal biophysical performance, most investigators have resorted to somewhat arbitrary answers to such questions

3. Despite the invention of increasingly complex testing methods, abnormal results are seldom reliable, prompting many clinicians to use antenatal testing to forecast fetal *wellness* rather than *illness.*

REFERENCES

Abramowicz JS, Sheiner E: Ultrasound of the placenta: A systemic approach. Part II: Function assessment (Doppler). Placenta 29(11):921, 2008

American College of Obstetricians and Gynecologists: Intrauterine growth restriction. Practice Bulletin No. 12, January 2000

American College of Obstetricians and Gynecologists: Special tests for monitoring fetal health. Patient Education Pamphlet, January 2002

American College of Obstetricians and Gynecologists: Ultrasonography in pregnancy. Practice Bulletin No. 50, December 2004

American College of Obstetricians and Gynecologists: Management of alloimmunization during pregnancy. Practice Bulletin No. 75, August 2006

American College of Obstetricians and Gynecologists: Antepartum fetal surveillance. Practice Bulletin No. 9, October 1999, Reaffirmed 2007

American College of Obstetricians and Gynecologists and the American Academy of Pediatrics. Guidelines for Perinatal Care, 6th ed. October 2007

Badalian SS, Chao CR, Fox HE, et al: Fetal breathing-related nasal fluid flow velocity in uncomplicated pregnancies. Am J Obstet Gynecol 169:563, 1993

Baschat AA: Opinion and Review: Doppler application in the delivery timing in the preterm growth-restricted fetus: Another step in the right direction. Ultrasound Obstet Gynecol 23:118, 2004

Baschat AA, Cosmi E, Bilardo C, et al: Predictors of neonatal outcome in early-onset placental dysfunction. Obstet Gynecol 109:253, 2007

Bilardo CM, Wolf H, Stigter RH, et al: Relationship between monitoring parameters and perinatal outcome in severe, early intrauterine growth restriction. Ultrasound Obstet Gynecol 23:199, 2004

Bourgeois FJ, Thiagarajah S, Harbert GN Jr: The significance of fetal heart rate decelerations during nonstress testing. Am J Obstet Gynecol 150:213, 1984

Brown R, Patrick J: The nonstress test: How long is enough? Am J Obstet Gynecol 141:646, 1981

Casey BM, McIntire DD, Bloom SL, et al: Pregnancy outcomes after antepartum diagnosis of oligohydramnios at or beyond 34 weeks' gestation. Am J Obstet Gynecol 182:909, 2000

Chamberlain PF, Manning FA, Morrison I, et al: Ultrasound evaluation of amniotic fluid volume. II. The relationship of increased amniotic fluid volume to perinatal outcome. Am J Obstet Gynecol 150:250, 1984

Chauhan SP, Sanderson M, Hendrix NW, et al: Perinatal outcomes and amniotic fluid index in the antepartum and intrapartum periods: A meta-analysis. Am J Obstet Gynecol 181:1473, 1999

Clark SL, Sabey P, Jolley K: Nonstress testing with acoustic stimulation and amnionic fluid volume assessment: 5973 tests without unexpected fetal death. Am J Obstet Gynecol 160:694, 1989

Conway DL, Groth S, Adkins WB, et al: Management of isolated oligohydramnios in the term pregnancy: A randomized clinical trial. Am J Obstet Gynecol 182:S21, 2000

Dawes GS: Breathing before birth in animals and man. An essay in medicine. Physiol Med 290:557, 1974

Dawes GS, Fox HE, Leduc BM, et al: Respiratory movements and rapid eye movement sleep in the foetal lamb. J Physiol 220:119, 1972

Dayal AK, Manning FA, Berck DJ, et al: Fetal death after normal biophysical profile score: An eighteen year experience. Am J Obstet Gynecol 181:1231, 1999

Devoe LD: Antenatal fetal assessment: Multifetal gestation—an overview. Semin Perinatol 32:281, 2008

Devoe LD, Castillo RA, Sherline DM: The nonstress test as a diagnostic test: A critical reappraisal. Am J Obstet Gynecol 152:1047, 1986

Devoe LD, McKenzie J, Searle NS, et al: Clinical sequelae of the extended nonstress test. Am J Obstet Gynecol 151:1074, 1985

DeVries JIP, Visser GHA, Prechtl NFR: The emergence of fetal behavior. II. Quantitative aspects. Early Hum Dev 12:99, 1985

Driggers RW, Holcroft CJ, Blakemore KJ, et al: An amniotic fluid index ≤ 5 cm within 7 days of delivery in the third trimester is not associated with decreasing umbilical arterial pH and base excess. J Perinatol 24:72, 2004

Druzin ML, Gratacos J, Keegan KA, et al: Antepartum fetal heart rate testing, 7. The significance of fetal bradycardia. Am J Obstet Gynecol 139:194, 1981

Eller DP, Scardo JA, Dillon AE, et al: Distance from an intrauterine hydrophone as a factor affecting intrauterine sound pressure levels produced by the vibroacoustic stimulation test. Am J Obstet Gynecol 173:523, 1995

Enkin M, Keirse MJNC, Renfrew M, et al: A Guide to Effective Care in Pregnancy and Childbirth, 3rd ed. New York, Oxford University Press, 2000, p 225

Frager NB, Miyazaki FS: Intrauterine monitoring of contractions during breast stimulation. Obstet Gynecol 69:767, 1987

Freeman RK: Antepartum testing in patients with hypertensive disorders in pregnancy. Semin Perinatol 32:271, 2008

Freeman RK: The use of the oxytocin challenge test for antepartum clinical evaluation of uteroplacental respiratory function. Am J Obstet Gynecol 121:481, 1975

Frøen JF, Tviet JV, Saastad E, et al: Management of decreased fetal movements. Semin Perinatol 32(4):307, 2008

Ghidini A: Doppler of the ductus venosus in severe preterm fetal growth restriction. A test in search of a purpose? Obstet Gynecol 109:250, 2007

Gonzalez JM, Stamilio DM, Ural S, et al: Relationship between abnormal fetal testing and adverse perinatal outcomes in intrauterine growth restriction. Am J Obstet Gynecol 196:e48, 2007

Grant A, Elbourne D, Valentin L, et al: Routine formal fetal movement counting and risk of antepartum late death in normally formed singletons. Lancet 2:345, 1989

Graves CR: Antepartum fetal surveillance and timing of delivery in the pregnancy complicated by diabetes mellitus. Clin Obstet Gynecol 50:1007, 2007

Grubb DK, Paul RH: Amnionic fluid index and prolonged antepartum fetal heart rate decelerations. Obstet Gynecol 79:558, 1992

Guinn DA, Kimberlin KF, Wigton TR, et al: Fetal heart rate characteristics at 25 to 28 weeks gestation. Am J Perinatol 15:507, 1998

Hage ML: Interpretation of nonstress tests. Am J Obstet Gynecol 153:490, 1985

Hammacher K, Hüter KA, Bokelmann J, et al: Foetal heart frequency and perinatal condition of the foetus and newborn. Gynaecologia 166:349, 1968

Harrington K, Thompson O, Jorden L, et al: Obstetric outcomes in women who present with a reduction in fetal movements in the third trimester of pregnancy. J Perinat Med 26:77, 1998

Hoskins IA, Frieden FJ, Young BK: Variable decelerations in reactive nonstress tests with decreased amnionic fluid index predict fetal compromise. Am J Obstet Gynecol 165:1094, 1991

Huddleston JF, Sutliff JG, Robinson D: Contraction stress test by intermittent nipple stimulation. Obstet Gynecol 63:669, 1984

Jansson LM, DiPietro J, Elko PA-C: Fetal response to maternal methadone administration. Am J Obstet Gynecol 193:611, 2005

Johnson MJ, Paine LL, Mulder HH, et al: Population differences of fetal biophysical and behavioral characteristics. Am J Obstet Gynecol 166:138, 1992

Johnson T, Besinger R, Thomas R: New clues to fetal behavior and well-being. Contemp Ob/Gyn, May 1988

Kaur S, Picconi JL, Chadha R, et al: Biophysical profile in the treatment of intrauterine growth-restricted fetuses who weigh <1000 g. Am J Obstet Gynecol 199:264.e1, 2008

Kennelly MM, Sturgiss SN: Management of small-for-gestational-age twins with absent/reversed end diastolic flow in the umbilical artery: Outcome of a policy of daily biophysical profile (BPP). Prenat Diagn 27:77, 2007

Konje JC, Bell SC, Taylor DT: Abnormal Doppler velocimetry and blood flow volume in the middle cerebral artery in very severe intrauterine growth restriction: Is the occurrence of reversal of compensatory flow too late? Br J Obstet Gynaecol 108:973, 2001

Kopecky EA, Ryan ML, Barrett JFR, et al: Fetal response to maternally administered morphine. Am J Obstet Gynecol 183:424, 2000

Lalor JG, Fawole B, Alfirevic Z, et al: Biophysical profile for fetal assessment in high risk pregnancies. Cochrane Database Syst Rev CD000038, January 23, 2008

Lee CY, DiLoreto PC, O'Lane JM: A study of fetal heart rate acceleration patterns. Obstet Gynecol 45:142, 1975

Lees C, Parra M, Missfelder-Lobos H, et al: Individualized risk assessment for adverse pregnancy outcome by uterine artery Doppler at 23 weeks. Obstet Gynecol 98:369, 2001

Leveno KJ, Williams ML, DePalma RT, et al: Perinatal outcome in the absence of antepartum fetal heart rate acceleration. Obstet Gynecol 61:347, 1983

Locatelli A, Vergani P, Toso L, et al: Perinatal outcome associated with oligohydramnios in uncomplicated term pregnancies. Arch Gynecol Obstet 269:130, 2004

Low JA, Killen H, Derrick EJ: Antepartum fetal complexia in the preterm pregnancy. Am J Obstet Gynecol 188:461, 2003

Magann EF, Chauhan SP, Kinsella MJ, et al: Antenatal testing among 1001 patients at high risk: The role of ultrasonographic estimates of amniotic fluid volume. Am J Obstet Gynecol 180:1330, 1999

Magann EF, Doherty DA, Chauhan SP, et al: How well do the amniotic fluid index and single deepest pocket indices (below the 3rd and 5th and above the 95th and 97th percentiles) predict oligohydramnios and hydramnios? Am J Obstet Gynecol 190:164, 2004

Manning FA, Bondaji N, Harman CR, et al: Fetal assessment based on fetal biophysical profile scoring VIII: The incidence of cerebral palsy in tested and untested perinates. Am J Obstet Gynecol 178:696, 1998

Manning FA, Harman CR, Morrison I, et al: Fetal assessment based on fetal biophysical profile scoring, IV. An analysis of perinatal morbidity and mortality. Am J Obstet Gynecol 150:245, 1984

Manning FA, Morrison I, Harman CR, et al: Fetal assessment based on fetal biophysical profile scoring: Experience in 19,221 referred high-risk pregnancies, 2. An analysis of false-negative fetal deaths. Am J Obstet Gynecol 157:880, 1987

Manning FA, Platt LD, Sipos L: Antepartum fetal evaluation: Development of a fetal biophysical profile. Am J Obstet Gynecol 136:787, 1980

Manning FA, Snijders R, Harman CR, et al: Fetal biophysical profile score, VI. Correlation with antepartum umbilical venous fetal pH. Am J Obstet Gynecol 169:755, 1993

Matsuura M, Murata Y, Hirano T, et al: The effects of developing autonomous nervous system on FHR variabilities determined by the power spectral analysis. Am J Obstet Gynecol 174:380, 1996

Meis PJ, Ureda JR, Swain M, et al: Variable decelerations during nonstress tests are not a sign of fetal compromise. Am J Obstet Gynecol 154:586, 1986

Miller DA, Rabello YA, Paul RH: The modified biophysical profile: Antepartum testing in the 1990s. Am J Obstet Gynecol 174:812, 1996a

Miller F, Miller D, Paul R, et al: Is one fetal heart rate acceleration during a nonstress test as reliable as two in predicting fetal status? Am J Obstet Gynecol 174:337, 1996b

Moise KJ Jr: The usefulness of middle cerebral artery Doppler assessment in the treatment of the fetus at risk for anemia. Am J Obstet Gynecol 198:161. e1, 2008

Moore TR, Piaquadio K: A prospective evaluation of fetal movement screening to reduce the incidence of antepartum fetal death. Am J Obstet Gynecol 160:1075, 1989

Nabhan AF, Abdelmoula YA: Amniotic fluid index versus single deepest vertical pocket as a screening test for preventing adverse pregnancy outcome. Cochrane Database Syst Rev 3:CD006593, 2008

Nageotte MP, Towers CV, Asrat T, et al: Perinatal outcome with the modified biophysical profile. Am J Obstet Gynecol 170:1672, 1994

National Institute of Child Health and Human Development Research Planning Workshop. Electronic fetal heart rate monitoring: Research guidelines for interpretation. Am J Obstet Gynecol 177:1385, 1997

Neldam S: Fetal movements as an indicator of fetal well being. Dan Med Bull 30:274, 1983

Nijhuis JG, Prechtl HFR, Martin CB Jr, et al: Are there behavioural states in the human fetus? Early Hum Dev 6:177, 1982

Oepkes D, Seaward G, Vandenbussche FPHA, et al: Doppler ultrasonography versus amniocentesis to predict fetal anemia. N Engl J Med 355:156, 2006

Oncken C, Kranzler H, O'Malley P, et al: The effect of cigarette smoking on fetal heart rate characteristics. Obstet Gynecol 99:751, 2002

Oosterhof H, vd Stege JG, Lander M, et al: Urine production rate is related to behavioural states in the near term human fetus. Br J Obstet Gynaecol 100:920, 1993

Ott WJ, Mora G, Arias F, et al: Comparison of the modified biophysical profile to a "new" biophysical profile incorporating the middle cerebral artery to umbilical artery velocity flow systolic/diastolic ratio. Am J Obstet Gynecol 178:1346, 1998

Pardey J, Moulden M, Redmon CWG: A computer system for numerical analysis of nonstress tests. Am J Obstet Gynecol 186:1095, 2002

Patrick J, Campbell K, Carmichael L, et al: Patterns of gross fetal body movements over 24-hour observation intervals during the last 10 weeks of pregnancy. Am J Obstet Gynecol 142:363, 1982

Patrick J, Campbell K, Carmichael L, et al: Patterns of human fetal breathing during the last 10 weeks of pregnancy. Obstet Gynecol 56:24, 1980

Pazos R, Vuolo K, Aladjem S, et al: Association of spontaneous fetal heart rate decelerations during antepartum nonstress testing and intrauterine growth retardation. Am J Obstet Gynecol 144:574, 1982

Perez-Delboy A, Weiss J, Michels A, et al: A randomized trial of vibroacoustic stimulation for antenatal fetal testing. Am J Obstet Gynecol 187:S146, 2002

Pillai M, James D: Behavioural states in normal mature human fetuses. Arch Dis Child 65:39, 1990a

Pillai M, James D: The development of fetal heart rate patterns during normal pregnancy. Obstet Gynecol 76:812, 1990b

Platt LD, Paul RH, Phelan J, et al: Fifteen years of experience with antepartum fetal testing. Am J Obstet Gynecol 156:1509, 1987

Ray M, Freeman R, Pine S, et al: Clinical experience with the oxytocin challenge test. Am J Obstet Gynecol 114:1, 1972

Rayburn WF: Clinical significance of perceptible fetal motion. Am J Obstet Gynecol 138:210, 1980

Reddy UM, Filly RA, Copel JA, et al: Prenatal imaging: Ultrasonography and magnetic resonance imaging. Obstet Gynecol 112(1):145, 2008

Rutherford SE, Phelan JP, Smith CV, et al: The four-quadrant assessment of amniotic fluid volume: An adjunct to antepartum fetal heart rate testing. Obstet Gynecol 70:353, 1987

Sadovsky E, Evron S, Weinstein D: Daily fetal movement recording in normal pregnancy. Riv Obstet Ginecol Practica Med Perinatal 59:395, 1979a

Sadovsky E, Laufer N, Allen JW: The incidence of different types of fetal movement during pregnancy. Br J Obstet Gynaecol 86:10, 1979b

Sadovsky E, Yaffe H: Daily fetal movement recording and fetal prognosis. Obstet Gynecol 41:845, 1973

Salvesen DR, Freeman J, Brudenell JM, et al: Prediction of fetal acidemia in pregnancies complicated by maternal diabetes by biophysical scoring and fetal heart rate monitoring. Br J Obstet Gynaecol 100:227, 1993

Schellpfeffer MA, Hoyle D, Johnson JWC: Antepartum uterine hypercontractility secondary to nipple stimulation. Obstet Gynecol 65:588, 1985

Sherer DM, Spong CY, Ghidini A, et al: In preterm fetuses decreased amniotic fluid volume is associated with decreased fetal movements. Am J Obstet Gynecol 174:344, 1996

Smith CV, Nguyen HN, Kovacs B, et al: Fetal death following antepartum fetal heart rate testing: A review of 65 cases. Obstet Gynecol 70:18, 1987

Smith GCS, Yu CKH, Papageorghiou AT, et al: Maternal uterine artery Doppler flow velocimetry and the risk of stillbirth. Obstet Gynecol 109:144, 2007

Smith JH, Anand KJ, Cotes PM, et al: Antenatal fetal heart rate variation in relation to the respiratory and metabolic status of the compromised human fetus. Br J Obstet Gynaecol 95:980, 1988

Sorokin Y, Bottoms SF, Dierker CJ, et al: The clustering of fetal heart rate changes and fetal movements in pregnancies between 20 and 30 weeks gestation. Am J Obstet Gynecol 143:952, 1982

Spinillo A, Montanari L, Bergante C, et al: Prognostic value of umbilical artery Doppler studies in unselected preterm deliveries. Obstet Gynecol 105:613, 2005

Thacker SB, Berkelman RL: Assessing the diagnostic accuracy and efficacy of selected antepartum fetal surveillance techniques. Obstet Gynecol Surv 41:121, 1986

Timor-Tritsch IE, Dierker LJ, Hertz RH, et al: Studies of antepartum behavioral state in the human fetus at term. Am J Obstet Gynecol 132:524, 1978

Todd AL, Tridinger BJ, Cole MJ, et al: Antenatal tests of fetal welfare and development at age 2 years. Am J Obstet Gynecol 167:66, 1992

Todros T, Sciarrone A, Piccoli E, et al: Umbilical Doppler waveforms and placental villous angiogenesis in pregnancies complicated by fetal growth restriction. Obstet Gynecol 93:499, 1999

Trudinger B: Doppler: More or less? Editorial in Ultrasound Obstet Gynecol 29:243, 2007

Turan S, Turan OM, Berg C, et al: Computerized fetal heart rate analysis, Doppler ultrasound and biophysical profile score in the prediction of acid-base status of growth-restricted fetuses. Ultrasound Obstet Gynecol 30:750, 2007

Vindla S, James D: Fetal behavior as a test of fetal well-being. Br J Obstet Gynaecol 102:597, 1995

Visser GHA, Redman CWG, Huisjes HJ, et al: Nonstressed antepartum heart rate monitoring: Implications of decelerations after spontaneous contractions. Am J Obstet Gynecol 138:429, 1980

Weiner Z, Divon MY, Katz N, et al: Multi-variant analysis of antepartum fetal test in predicting neonatal outcome of growth retarded fetuses. Am J Obstet Gynecol 174:338, 1996

Williams KP, Farquharson DF, Bebbington M, et al: Screening for fetal well-being in a high-risk pregnant population comparing the nonstress test with umbilical artery Doppler velocimetry: A randomized controlled clinical trial. Am J Obstet Gynecol 188:1366, 2003

Yu CK, Smith GC, Papageorghiou AT, et al: Fetal Medicine Foundation Second Trimester Screening Group An integrated model for the prediction of preeclampsia using maternal factors and uterine artery Doppler velocimetry in unselected low-risk women. Am J Obstet Gynecol 193:429, 2005

Zelop CM, Richardson DK, Heffner LJ: Outcomes of severely abnormal umbilical artery Doppler velocimetry in structurally normal singleton fetuses. Obstet Gynecol 87:434, 1996

Zhang J, Troendle J, Meikle S, et al: Isolated oligohydramnios is not associated with adverse perinatal outcomes. Br J Obstet Gynaecol 111:220, 2004

Fetal Imaging

Recent advances in fetal imaging have been the result of technological achievements in sonography and magnetic resonance imaging, with dramatic improvements in resolution and image display. Both 3- and 4-dimensional ultrasound imagings have continued to evolve, and Doppler applications have expanded. Magnetic resonance imaging has added immensely to the already profound impact of sonography on obstetrics. A sonographic examination performed with the exacting recommended standards of the American Institute of Ultrasound in Medicine (2007) offers vital information about fetal anatomy, physiology, growth, and well-being.

SONOGRAPHY IN OBSTETRICS

Since the first obstetrical application of sonographic imaging by Donald and co-workers (1958), this technique has become indispensable for fetal evaluation.

Technology

The real-time image on the ultrasound screen is produced by sound waves reflected back from organs, fluids, and tissue interfaces of the fetus within the uterus. Transducers made of piezo-

electric crystals convert electrical energy into sound waves that are emitted in synchronized pulses, then "listen" for the returning echoes. Because air is a poor transmitter of high-frequency sound waves, soluble gel is applied to the skin to act as a coupling agent. Sound waves pass through layers of tissue, encounter an interface between tissues of different densities, and are reflected back to the transducer. Dense tissue such as bone produces high-velocity reflected waves, which are displayed brightly on the screen. Conversely, fluid generates few reflected waves and appears dark or anechoic on the screen. The electrical pulses created by the echoes are converted into digital representations, the most common of which is the 2-dimensional real-time image. Depending on settings, these digital images can be generated at 50 to greater than 100 frames/second. Postprocessing techniques then smooth the combined images and yield the appearance of real-time imaging.

Higher-frequency transducers yield better image resolution, whereas lower frequencies penetrate tissue more effectively. Current transducers offer wide-bandwidth technology, which allows them to perform over a range of frequencies. In the second trimester, a 4- to 6-megahertz-bandwidth transducer is often in close enough proximity to the fetus to provide precise images. However, by the third trimester, a lower frequency 2- to 5-megahertz-bandwidth transducer may be needed for penetration, but can lead to compromised resolution. This explains why resolution is often poor when imaging obese patients and why low-frequency transducers are needed to *reach* the fetus through the maternal tissues (Dashe and colleagues, 2009). In early pregnancy, 4- to 9-megahertz-bandwidth vaginal transducers provide excellent resolution because the small embryo is close to the transducer.

Safety

Sonography should be performed only with a valid medical indication and with the lowest possible exposure setting to gain necessary information—the ALARA principle—As Low As Reasonably

Achievable (American Institute of Ultrasound in Medicine, 2007, 2008). As discussed in Chapter 41 (p. 921), recent studies have suggested that prolonged exposure to ultrasound affects the migration of brain cells in fetal mice (Rakic, 2006). These findings have not altered the use of sonography in pregnant women because clinical application is unlikely to harm the human fetus. Duplex Doppler coupled with real-time imaging requires monitoring of the *thermal index*, which is displayed during its use. Microbubble ultrasound contrast agents are not used in pregnancy because they might raise the *mechanical index* (see Chap. 41, p. 921).

The American Institute of Ultrasound in Medicine (2003) recommends that fetal sonography be performed only by professionals who have been trained to recognize medically important conditions such as fetal anomalies, artifacts that may mimic pathology, and techniques to avoid ultrasound exposure beyond what is considered safe for the fetus. Importantly, the use of sonography for "keepsake fetal imaging" is not condoned by either the American Institute of Ultrasound in Medicine (2007) or the Food and Drug Administration (Rados, 2004).

Clinical Applications

Accurate assessment of gestational age, fetal growth, and the detection of fetal and placental abnormalities are major benefits of sonography. The American Institute of Ultrasound in Medicine (2007), in conjunction with the American College of Obstetrics and Gynecology (2009) and the American College of Radiology (2007), has updated guidelines for obstetrical sonographic studies. The sensitivity of sonography for detecting fetal anomalies varies according to factors such as gestational age, maternal habitus, position of the fetus, features of the equipment, skill of the sonographer, and the specific abnormality in question. All women undergoing sonographic examination should be counseled about its limitations. Although it will never be possible to detect all structural abnormalities, significant advances have been made.

TABLE 16-1. Some Indications for First-Trimester Ultrasound Examination

1. Confirm an intrauterine pregnancy
2. Evaluate a suspected ectopic pregnancy
3. Define the cause of vaginal bleeding
4. Evaluate pelvic pain
5. Estimate gestational age
6. Diagnose or evaluate multifetal gestations
7. Confirm cardiac activity
8. Assist chorionic villus sampling, embryo transfer, and localization and removal of an intrauterine device
9. Assess for certain fetal anomalies, such as anencephaly, in high-risk patients
10. Evaluate maternal pelvic masses and/or uterine abnormalities
11. Measure nuchal translucency when part of a screening program for fetal aneuploidy
12. Evaluate suspected gestational trophoblastic disease

From the American Institute of Ultrasound in Medicine (2007), with permission.

First-Trimester Evaluation

Indications for performing sonography in the first 14 weeks are listed in Table 16-1. Early pregnancy can be evaluated using transabdominal or transvaginal sonography, or both. The components listed in Table 16-2 should be assessed. With transvaginal scanning, the gestational sac is reliably seen in the uterus by 5 weeks, and fetal echoes and cardiac activity by 6 weeks. The crown-rump length is the most accurate biometric predictor of gestational age. This image should be obtained in a sagittal plane and include neither the yolk sac nor a limb bud. If carefully performed, it has a variation of only 3 to 5 days.

TABLE 16-2. Components of Standard Ultrasound Examination by Trimester

First Trimester	Second and Third Trimester
1. Gestational sac location	1. Fetal number; multifetal gestations: amnionicity, chorionicity, fetal sizes, amnionic fluid volume, and fetal genitalia, if visualized
2. Embryo and/or yolk sac identification	2. Presentation
3. Crown-rump length	3. Fetal cardiac activity
4. Cardiac activity	4. Placental location and its relationship to the internal cervical os
5. Fetal number, including amnionicity and chorionicity of multiples when possible	5. Amnionic fluid volume
6. Assessment of embryonic/fetal anatomy appropriate for the first trimester	6. Gestational age
7. Evaluation of the uterus, adnexa, and cul-de-sac	7. Fetal weight
8. Assessment of the fetal nuchal region if possible	8. Evaluation of the uterus, adnexa, and cervix
	9. Fetal anatomical survey, including documentation of technical limitations

Modified from the American Institute of Ultrasound in Medicine (2007), with permission.

With first-trimester sonography, anembryonic gestation, embryonic demise, and molar and ectopic pregnancies can all be reliably diagnosed (see Chaps. 9, 10, and 11). Using transvaginal examination, cardiac motion is typically observed when the embryo has reached 5 mm in length. Multifetal gestation can be identified early, and this is the optimal time to determine chorionicity (see Chap. 39, p. 865). The first trimester is the ideal time to evaluate certain maternal pelvic structures, including the uterus, adnexa, and cul-de-sac, however, cervical length is best evaluated in the second trimester.

Fetal Abnormalities

Assessment for certain fetal anomalies, such as *anencephaly* in patients at increased risk, is considered an acceptable indication for first-trimester sonographic examination (Table 16-1). Research has also focused on the potential detection of fetal anomalies and syndromes in the late first trimester (Bahado-Singh and Cheng, 2004). Dane and colleagues (2007) reported that 17 of 24 fetal defects discovered by transvaginal sonography in 1290 women were seen in the first trimester. These included central nervous system, neck, neural tube, and cardiac malformations. Similarly, Souka and associates (2006) reported a detection rate of 50 percent for anomalies with sonography during this time.

Nuchal Translucency. This is the maximum thickness of the subcutaneous translucent area between the skin and soft tissue overlying the fetal spine at the back of the neck (Fig. 16-1). It is measured in the sagittal plane between 11 and 14 weeks using precise criteria (Table 16-3). When increased, there is a higher risk for fetal aneuploidy and a variety of structural anomalies. As discussed in Chapter 13 (p. 295), nuchal translucency measurement, combined with maternal serum chorionic gonadotropin and pregnancy-associated plasma protein A assess-

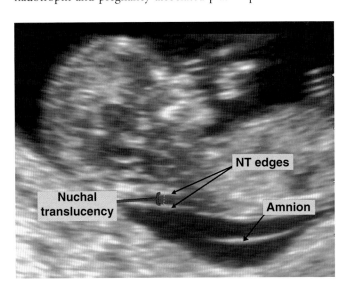

FIGURE 16-1 The nuchal translucency (*NT*) measurement is the maximum thickness of the subcutaneous translucent area between the skin and soft tissue overlying the fetal spine at the back of the neck. Calipers are placed on the inner borders of the nuchal space, at its widest portion, perpendicular to the long axis of the fetus. In this normal fetus at 12 weeks' gestation, the measurement is 2.0 mm. (Used with permission from Dr. Robyn Horsager.)

TABLE 16-3. Guidelines for Nuchal Translucency (NT) Measurement

1. The margins of NT edges must be clear enough for proper caliper placement
2. The fetus must be in the midsagittal plane
3. The image must be magnified so that it is filled by the fetal head, neck, and upper thorax
4. The fetal neck must be in a neutral position, not flexed and not hyperextended
5. The amnion must be seen as separate from the NT line
6. Electronic calipers must be used to perform the measurement
7. Calipers must be placed on the inner borders of the nuchal space with none of the horizontal crossbar itself protruding into the space
8. The calipers must be placed perpendicular to the long axis of the fetus
9. The measurement must be obtained at the widest space of the NT

From the American Institute of Ultrasound in Medicine (2007), with permission.

ment, has gained widespread use for first-trimester aneuploidy screening.

Second- and Third-Trimester Evaluations

The many indications for second- and third-trimester sonographic examinations are listed in Table 16-4. There are three types of sonographic evaluations: *standard, specialized,* and *limited.*

1. The *standard*—also termed *basic*—obstetrical sonographic examination is most commonly performed. Its components are listed in Table 16-2, including a survey of fetal anatomy, which is listed in Table 16-5. When multifetal gestations are studied, documentation includes the number(s) of chorions and amnions, comparison of fetal sizes, estimation of amnionic fluid volume in each sac, and description of fetal genitalia if visualized. Fetal anatomy may be adequately assessed after approximately 18 weeks. If a complete survey of fetal anatomy cannot be obtained—for example, due to oligohydramnios, fetal position, or maternal obesity—the limitation should be noted in the report (American College of Obstetricians and Gynecologists, 2009; American Institute of Ultrasound in Medicine, 2007).

2. There are several types of *specialized* examinations. The *targeted* examination is a detailed anatomical survey performed when an anomaly is suspected on the basis of history, maternal serum screening test abnormalities, or abnormal findings from a standard examination. Other *specialized* examinations include fetal echocardiography, Doppler evaluation, biophysical profile, or additional biometric studies. Specialized studies are performed and interpreted by an experienced operator who determines the examination components on a

TABLE 16-4. Some Indications for Second- or Third-Trimester Ultrasound Examination

Estimation of gestational age
Evaluation of fetal growth
Vaginal bleeding
Abdominal/pelvic pain
Cervical insufficiency
Determination of fetal presentation
Suspected multifetal gestation
Adjunct to amniocentesis or other procedure
Significant uterine size/clinical date discrepancy
Pelvic mass
Suspected molar pregnancy
Adjunct to cervical cerclage
Suspected ectopic pregnancy
Suspected fetal death
Suspected uterine abnormality
Evaluation of fetal well-being
Suspected hydramnios or oligohydramnios
Suspected placental abruption
Adjunct to external cephalic version
Preterm prematurely ruptured membranes and/or preterm labor
Abnormal biochemical markers
Follow-up evaluation of a fetal anomaly
Follow-up evaluation of placental location for suspected placenta previa
History of congenital anomaly in prior pregnancy
Evaluation of fetal condition in late registrants for prenatal care
Findings that may increase the risk for aneuploidy
Screening for fetal anomalies

Adapted from the National Institutes of Health (1984) by the American Institute of Ultrasound in Medicine (2007).

TABLE 16-5. Minimal Elements of a Standard Examination of Fetal Anatomy

Head, face, and neck
  Cerebellum
  Choroid plexus
  Cisterna magna
  Lateral cerebral ventricles
  Midline falx
  Cavum septum pellucidum
  Upper lip
  Consideration of nuchal fold measurement
Chest
  Four-chamber view of heart
  Evaluation of both outflow tracts if technically feasible
Abdomen
  Stomach—presence, size, and situs
  Kidneys
  Bladder
  Umbilical cord insertion into fetal abdomen
  Umbilical cord vessel number
Spine
  Cervical, thoracic, lumbar, and sacral spine
Extremities
  Legs and arms—presence or absence
Gender
  Indicated in low-risk pregnancies only for evaluation of multifetal gestations

From the American Institute of Ultrasound in Medicine (2007), with permission.

case-by-case basis (American College of Obstetricians and Gynecologists, 2009).

3. The *limited* examination is performed when a specific question requires investigation. Examples include amnionic fluid assessment, placental location, or evaluation of fetal presentation or viability. In most cases, limited examinations are appropriate only when a prior complete examination is on record (American Institute of Ultrasound in Medicine, 2007).

Fetal Biometry

Various formulas and nomograms allow accurate assessment of gestational age and describe normal growth of fetal structures. Equipment software computes the estimated gestational age from the crown-rump length. It also estimates gestational age and fetal weight using measurements of the biparietal diameter, head and abdominal circumference, and femur length. Estimates are typically most accurate when multiple parameters are used with nomograms derived from fetuses of similar ethnic or racial background living at similar altitude. Even the best models may over- or underestimate fetal weight by as much as 15 percent (American Institute of Ultrasound in Medicine, 2007). Nomograms for individual structures such as the fetal cerebellum, ears, interocular and binocular orbital distances, thoracic circumference, kidneys, long bones, and feet may be used to address specific questions about organ system abnormalities or syndromes.

Gestational Age

Crown-rump length is most accurate in the first trimester. Biparietal diameter (BPD) is most accurate from 14 to 26 weeks, with a variation of 7 to 10 days. The BPD is measured from the outer edge of the proximal skull to the inner edge of the distal skull, at the level of the thalami and cavum septum pellucidum (Fig. 16-2). The head circumference (HC) also is measured. If the head shape is flattened—*dolichocephaly*, or rounded—*brachycephaly*, the HC is more reliable than the BPD. The femur length (FL) correlates well with both BPD and gestational age. It is measured with the beam perpendicular to the long axis of the shaft, excluding the epiphysis, and has a variation of 7 to 11 days in the second trimester (Fig. 16-3). The abdominal circumference (AC) has the widest variation, up to 2 to 3 weeks, because it involves soft tissue. This circumference is most affected by fetal

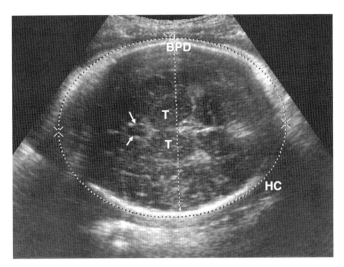

FIGURE 16-2 The transthalamic view is a transverse (axial) image obtained at the level of the thalami (*T*) and cavum septum pellucidum (*bounded by arrows*). The biparietal diameter (*BPD*) and head circumference (*HC*) are measured in this view.

growth. The AC is measured at the skin line in a transverse view of the fetus at the level of the fetal stomach and umbilical vein (Fig. 16-4).

The variability of gestational age estimation increases with advancing pregnancy. Individual measurements are least accurate in the third trimester, and estimates are improved by averaging the four parameters. If one parameter differs significantly from the others, it may be excluded from the calculation. The outlier could result from poor visibility, but it could also indicate a fetal abnormality or growth problem. Sonography performed to evaluate fetal growth should typically be performed at least 2 to 4 weeks apart (American College of Obstetricians and Gynecologists, 2009; American Institute of Ultrasound in Medicine, 2007).

Amnionic Fluid

Determination of amnionic fluid volume is an important method of fetal assessment and is discussed in Chapter 21 (p. 490). Subjectively, oligohydramnios is obvious crowding of the fetus and absence of significant fluid pockets. Conversely, hydramnios is apparent fluid excess.

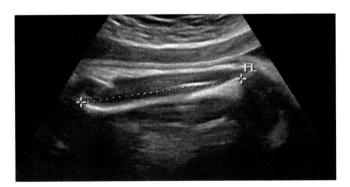

FIGURE 16-3 Example of the femur length (*FL*), obtained perpendicular to the femoral shaft.

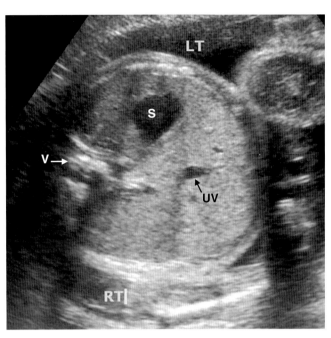

FIGURE 16-4 The abdominal circumference is measured in the transverse plane, at the level of the stomach (*S*) and the confluence of the umbilical vein (*UV*) with the portal sinus. The fetal vertebral body (*V*) aids in orienting anteroposterior anatomy of the image slice.

Several objective measurements have been used to evaluate amnionic fluid volume. The most widely used is the *amnionic fluid index (AFI)*, which is calculated by adding the depth in centimeters of the largest vertical pocket in each of four equal uterine quadrants (Phelan and colleagues, 1987). Reference ranges have been established from 16 weeks onward, and in most normal pregnancies, the AFI ranges between 8 and 24 cm (see Fig. 21-1, p. 491). Another method measures the largest vertical pocket of amnionic fluid. The normal range is 2 to 8 cm. Values < 2 cm signify oligohydramnios, whereas those > 8 cm define hydramnios. This latter method is commonly used for twin pregnancies (Fig. 16-5).

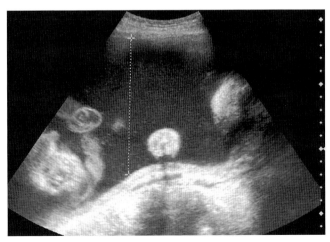

FIGURE 16-5 The largest vertical pocket of amnionic fluid is increased (11 cm) in this twin pregnancy complicated by twin-twin transfusion syndrome.

NORMAL AND ABNORMAL FETAL ANATOMY

An important goal of sonographic evaluation is to categorize fetal components as anatomically normal or abnormal. Deviations from normal typically prompt specialized examination. In the discussion that follows, only a few of literally hundreds of fetal anomalies are described.

Central Nervous System

Anomalies of the fetal brain are among the most common, and sonography is extremely useful to detect and characterize them. Three transverse (axial) views are imaged: (1) the *transthalamic view* is used to measure BPD and HC and includes the thalami and cavum septum pellucidum (see Fig. 16-2); (2) the *transventricular view* includes the atria of the lateral ventricles, which contain the echogenic choroid plexus (Fig. 16-6); (3) the *transcerebellar view* is obtained by angling the view back through the posterior fossa (Fig. 16-7). Here, the cerebellum and cisterna magna are typically measured. Between 15 and 22 weeks, the cerebellar diameter in millimeters is roughly equivalent to the gestational age in weeks (Goldstein and associates, 1987).

Abnormalities detected in any of these three views suggest a possible fetal brain anomaly. Specialized evaluation may permit accurate diagnosis of abnormalities such as neural-tube defects, ventriculomegaly, holoprosencephaly, hydranencephaly, Dandy-Walker malformation, agenesis of the corpus callosum, porencephaly, or intracranial tumor.

Neural-Tube Defects

These malformations are the second most common class of congenital anomalies—cardiac anomalies are the most common. Neural-tube defects are found in approximately 1.6 per 1000 live births in the United States, and their incidence is as high as 8 per 1000 in the United Kingdom. Defects result from incomplete closure of the neural tube by the embryonic age of

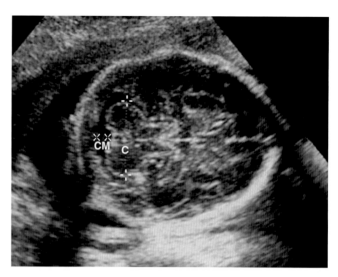

FIGURE 16-7 Transcerebellar view of the posterior fossa, demonstrating measurement of the cerebellum (*C*) and cisterna magna (*CM*).

26 to 28 days. Prenatal diagnosis with maternal serum alpha-fetoprotein screening and sonography are discussed in detail in Chapter 13 (p. 287).

Anencephaly is a lethal defect characterized by absence of the brain and cranium above the base of the skull and orbits (Fig. 16-8). It can be diagnosed in the late first trimester, and with adequate visualization, virtually all cases may be diagnosed in the second trimester. Inability to obtain a view of the biparietal diameter should raise suspicion. Hydramnios from impaired fetal swallowing is common in the third trimester.

Cephalocele—also termed encephalocele—is a herniation of meninges and brain tissue through a cranial defect, typically an occipital midline defect. Associated hydrocephalus and microcephaly are common, and there is a high incidence of mental impairment among surviving infants. Cephalocele is an important

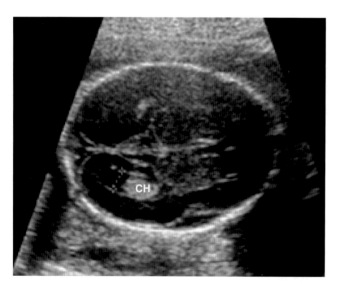

FIGURE 16-6 Transventricular view of the atrium of the lateral ventricle, which is marked by calipers and contains the echogenic choroid plexus (*CH*).

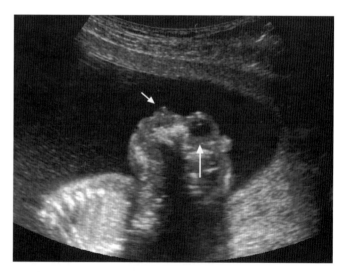

FIGURE 16-8 Anencephaly. This sagittal image shows the absence of forebrain and cranium above the skull base and orbit. The long white arrow points to the fetal orbit, and the short white arrow indicates the nose.

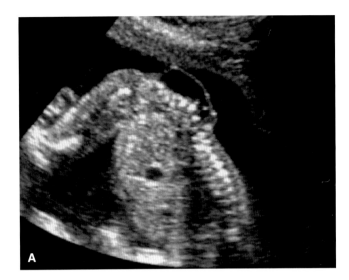

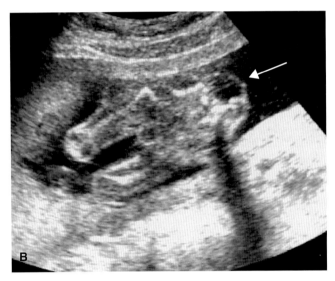

FIGURE 16-9 Sagittal (**A**) and transverse (**B**) views of the spine in a fetus with a large lumbosacral meningomyelocele (*arrow*).

feature of the autosomal recessive *Meckel-Gruber syndrome.* A cephalocele that is not in the occipital midline may be caused by the *amnionic band sequence.*

Spina bifida is an opening in the vertebrae through which a meningeal sac may protrude. In 90 percent of cases, the sac contains neural elements, and the anomaly is termed a *meningomyelocele.* When a meningeal sac alone protrudes through the defect, it is a *meningocele.* Spinal defects usually can be imaged in multiple planes (Fig. 16-9). Transverse images provide the best visualization of the extent of the defect and overlying soft tissue. Movement of the lower extremities does not predict normal function after birth. The *Arnold-Chiari II* malformation associated with spina bifida occurs when downward displacement of the spinal cord pulls a portion of the cerebellum through the foramen magnum into the upper cervical canal. Classically, fetuses with spina bifida have one or more of the following sonographic cranial findings: scalloping of the frontal bones—the so-called "lemon sign" (see Fig. 13-4, p. 291), bowing of the cerebellum with effacement of the cisterna magna—the "banana sign" (see Fig. 13-5), small biparietal diameter, and ventriculomegaly (Campbell and colleagues, 1987).

Ventriculomegaly

Enlargement of the cerebral ventricles is a nonspecific marker of abnormal brain development (Pilu, 2008; Wyldes and Watkinson, 2004). The lateral ventricle is commonly measured at its *atrium,* which is the confluence of the temporal and occipital horns (see Fig. 16-6). The atrial measurement is normally between 5 and 10 mm from 15 weeks until term. Mild ventriculomegaly is diagnosed when the atrial width measures 10 to 15 mm, and overt or severe ventriculomegaly when it exceeds 15 mm (Fig. 16-10). A *dangling choroid plexus* characteristically is found in severe cases (Cardoza and associates, 1988a, 1988b; Mahony and colleagues, 1988).

Ventriculomegaly may be caused by a wide variety of genetic and environmental insults, and prognosis is determined by both etiology and rate of progression. Generally, the larger the atrium, the greater the likelihood of abnormal outcome (Gaglioti and co-workers, 2009; Joó and associates, 2008). Initial evaluation of ventricular enlargement includes a thorough examination of fetal anatomy, fetal karyotyping, and testing for congenital infections such as cytomegalovirus and toxoplasmosis (Chap. 58, p. 1210). That said, even when ventriculomegaly is mild and appears isolated, counseling may be a challenge, because the prognosis is variable. Bloom and colleagues (1997) found that a third of infants prenatally diagnosed with isolated and mild ventriculomegaly were developmentally delayed.

Holoprosencephaly

With this abnormality, the prosencephalon fails to divide completely into two separate cerebral hemispheres and underlying diencephalic structures. As a result, in the most severe form— *alobar holoprosencephaly*—a single monoventricle, with or without a covering mantle of cortex, surrounds the fused central thalami (Fig. 16-11). Differentiation into two cerebral hemispheres is induced by prechordal mesenchyme, which is also responsible for differentiation of the midline face. Thus, there may be associated anomalies of the eyes or orbits—hypotelorism or cyclopia;

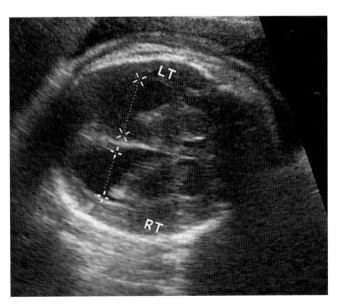

FIGURE 16-10 The atria appear unusually prominent in this fetus with ventriculomegaly (caliper measurements 20 mm).

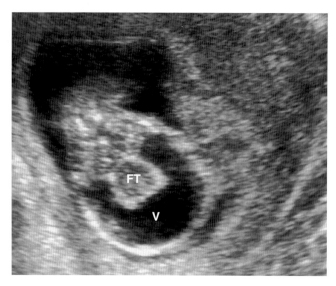

FIGURE 16-11 In this 14-week fetus with a lobar holoprosencephaly, the thalami are fused (*FT*) and surrounded by a monoventricle (*V*).

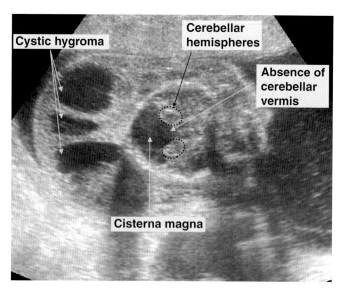

FIGURE 16-12 This 17-week fetus has a Dandy-Walker malformation of the posterior fossa, as well as large, septated cystic hygromas. The cerebellar hemispheres are visibly separated, with absence of the cerebellar vermis, such that the fourth ventricle communicates with the cisterna magna. The cystic hygromas are the fluid-filled sacs that extend from the posterior aspect of the neck.

nose—arhinia or proboscis; and lips—median cleft. The birth prevalence is 1 in 10,000 to 15,000, although it is much more common in abortuses. Approximately half of all cases have a chromosomal abnormality, particularly trisomy 13, although other aneuploidies and at least nine separate gene mutations have also been reported (Shiota and colleagues, 2007). Fetal karyotyping should be offered when this anomaly is identified.

Dandy-Walker Malformation

Originally described by Dandy and Blackfan (1914), this abnormality of the posterior fossa is characterized by agenesis of the cerebellar vermis, enlargement of the posterior fossa, and elevation of the tentorium. The birth prevalence is approximately 1 per 12,000 (Long and colleagues, 2006). Sonographically, fluid in the enlarged cisterna magna visibly communicates with the fourth ventricle through the defect in the cerebellar vermis, with visible separation of the cerebellar hemispheres (Fig. 16-12). Ventriculomegaly is common.

The Dandy-Walker malformation is associated with a large number of genetic and sporadic syndromes, aneuploidies, congenital viral infections, and some teratogens, all of which greatly affect the prognosis. Thus, the initial evaluation mirrors that for ventriculomegaly (p. 355). Even when vermian agenesis appears to be partial and relatively subtle, there is a high incidence of associated anomalies, and the prognosis is typically poor (Ecker and colleagues, 2000; Long and associates, 2006). Figure 16-2 depicts a fetus with Dandy-Walker malformation and septated cystic hygromas in the setting of aneuploidy.

Cystic Hygroma

This is a malformation of the lymphatic system in which fluid-filled sacs extend from the posterior neck (Fig. 16–12). Cystic hygromas are often large and multiseptated. They typically develop as part of a lymphatic obstruction sequence, in which lymph from the head fails to drain into the jugular vein and accumulates instead in jugular lymphatic sacs. The enlarged thoracic duct can impinge on the developing heart. Cystic hygromas are associated with an increased risk for cardiac malformations. In some cases, these are flow-related anomalies such as a hypoplastic left heart or coarctation of the aorta.

Approximately 60 to 70 percent of cystic hygromas cases are associated with aneuploidy. Of fetuses with cystic hygromas diagnosed in the second trimester, approximately 75 percent of aneuploid cases are 45,X— *Turner syndrome* (Johnson and colleagues, 1993; Shulman and associates, 1992). When cystic hygromas are diagnosed in the first trimester, the most common aneuploidy is *trisomy 21*, as reported in Malone and co-workers (2005). In this prospective series, first-trimester fetuses with cystic hygromas were five times more likely to be aneuploid than the fetuses with an increased nuchal translucency. Cystic hygromas also may be an isolated finding or part of a genetic syndrome such as *Noonan syndrome* (Lee and associates, 2009).

Large cystic hygromas are usually found in the setting of hydrops fetalis, rarely resolve, and carry a poor prognosis. Small hygromas may undergo spontaneous resolution, and provided that the fetal karyotype and echocardiography are normal, the prognosis *may* be good (Shulman and co-workers, 1992; Trauffer and associates, 1994).

Thorax

The lungs are best visualized after 20 to 25 weeks and appear as homogeneous structures surrounding the heart. In the four-chamber view of the chest, they comprise approximately two thirds of the area. A variety of thoracic malformations including cystic adenomatoid malformation, extralobar pulmonary sequestration, and bronchogenic cysts may be seen sonographically as cystic or solid space-occupying lesions. Fetal therapy for such lesions is discussed in Chapter 13 (p. 305).

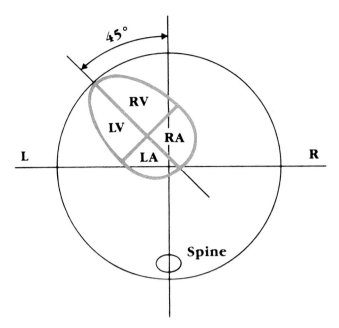

FIGURE 16-13 Diagram demonstrating measurement of the cardiac axis from the four-chamber view of the fetal heart. (L = left; LA = left atrium; LV = left ventricle; R = right; RA = right atrium; RV = right ventricle.) (Redrawn from Comstock CH: Normal fetal heart axis and position, *Obstetrics & Gynecology*, 1987, vol. 70, no. 2, pp. 255–259, with permission.)

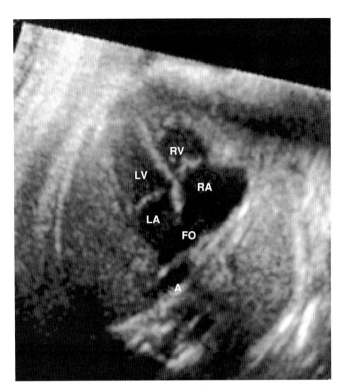

FIGURE 16-14 Four-chamber view of the fetal heart, showing the location of the left and right atria (*LA, RA*), left and right ventricles (*LV, RV*), foramen ovale (*FO*), and descending thoracic aorta (*A*).

Diaphragmatic Hernia

The incidence of congenital diaphragmatic hernia is approximately 1 per 3700 births (Wenstrom and colleagues, 1991). They are left-sided and posterior in 90 percent, and the most common sonographic finding is repositioning of the heart to the middle or right side of the thorax by the stomach and bowel. With improved technology, visualization of the liver within the thorax is increasingly common. Associated findings include absence of the stomach bubble within the abdomen, small abdominal circumference, and bowel peristalsis seen in the fetal chest. Almost half of cases are associated with other major anomalies or aneuploidy. Thus, a thorough evaluation of all fetal structures should be performed, and amniocentesis for fetal karyotyping should be offered. Fetal therapy for diaphragmatic hernia is discussed in Chapter 13 (p. 307).

Heart

As a group, cardiac malformations are the most common congenital anomalies with an incidence of approximately 8 per 1000 live births (see Chap. 12, p. 281). Almost 90 percent of cardiac defects are multifactorial or polygenic, another 1 to 2 percent are the result of a single-gene disorder or a gene-deletion syndrome, and 1 to 2 percent result from exposure to a teratogen such as isotretinoin, hydantoin, or diabetic hyperglycemia. *Up to 30 to 40 percent of cardiac defects diagnosed prenatally are associated with chromosomal abnormalities* (Moore and co-workers, 2004; Paladini and colleagues, 2002). Thus, their recognition should prompt fetal karyotyping. Fortunately, up to 50 to 70 percent of aneuploid fetuses have extracardiac anomalies that are identifiable sonographically. The most frequently encountered aneuploidies are Down syndrome, trisomies 18 and 13, and Turner syndrome (45,X).

Components of the Examination

The standard cardiac assessment includes a four-chamber view, evaluation of rate and rhythm, and, if possible, evaluation of the cardiac outflow tracts.

The four-chamber view is a transverse plane through the fetal thorax at a level immediately above the diaphragm (Figs. 16-13 and 16-14). It allows evaluation of heart size, its position in the chest, cardiac axis, atria and ventricles, foramen ovale, atrial septum primum, interventricular septum, and atrioventricular valves. The two atria and ventricles should be similar in size, respectively, and the apex of the heart should form a 45-degree angle with the left anterior chest wall (Fig. 16–13). Abnormalities of cardiac axis are frequently encountered in the setting of structural cardiac anomalies. Smith and colleagues (1995) found that 75 percent of fetuses with congenital heart anomalies had an axis angle that exceeded 75 degrees. Similarly, Shipp and co-workers (1995) found that 45 percent of those with abnormal hearts had left axis deviation.

The American Institute of Ultrasound in Medicine (2007) recommends that if technically feasible, each standard examination should attempt to evaluate both left and right ventricular outflow tracts (Fig. 16-15). Evaluation of the cardiac outflow tracts may aid detection of abnormalities not initially appreciated in the four-chamber view, such as transposition of the great vessels, Fallot tetralogy, or truncus arteriosus.

A specialized examination with fetal echocardiography is typically performed if there are any of the following: abnormality noted in the four-chamber or outflow tract views, arrhythmia, presence of extracardiac anomaly that confers increased risk, known genetic syndrome that may include a cardiac defect,

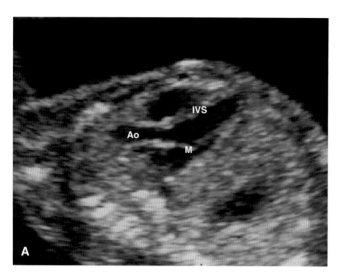
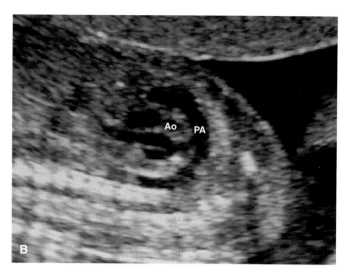

FIGURE 16-15 Views of the left and right ventricular outflow tracts. **A.** The left ventricular outflow tract demonstrates the continuity of the interventricular septum (*IVS*) and mitral valve (*M*) with the walls of the aorta (*Ao*). **B.** The right ventricular outflow tract shows the normal orientation of the aorta (*Ao*) and pulmonary artery (*PA*).

increased nuchal translucency in the first trimester in a fetus with a normal karyotype, insulin-treated diabetes prior to pregnancy, family history of congenital heart defect (see Chap. 12, p. 281), or exposure to a medication associated with increased risk for cardiac malformations.

Abdominal Wall

The integrity of the abdominal wall at the level of the cord insertion is assessed during the standard examination (Fig. 16-16). *Gastroschisis* and *omphalocele*, collectively termed *ventral wall defects,* are relatively common fetal anomalies. As discussed in Chapter 13 (p. 290), they are often detected because of elevated maternal serum alpha-fetoprotein screening.

Gastroschisis

This is a full-thickness abdominal wall defect typically located to the right of the umbilical cord insertion, and bowel herniates through the defect into the amnionic cavity (Fig. 16-17). Its inci-

dence is 1 per 2000 to 5000 pregnancies, and it is the one major anomaly more common in infants of younger mothers. Santiago-Munoz and colleagues (2007) reported an average maternal age of approximately 20 years in 60 pregnancies complicated by gastroschisis. Associated bowel abnormalities such as *jejunal atresia* are found in 15 to 30 percent of cases and are believed to be a result of vascular damage or mechanical trauma. The anomaly is not associated with an increased risk for aneuploidy and usually has a survival rate of approximately 90 percent (Kitchanan, 2000; Nembhard, 2001; Santiago-Munoz, 2007, and all their colleagues).

Fetuses with gastroschisis are at increased risk for growth restriction, affecting 15 to nearly 40 percent (Puligandla and associates, 2004; Santiago-Munoz and co-workers, 2007). Infants with growth restriction, however, did not have increased mortality rates or longer hospitalization compared with affected infants who were normally grown. Ergün and colleagues (2005) reported that in 75 infants with gastroschisis, the only risk factor associated with longer hospitalization was delivery before 36 weeks.

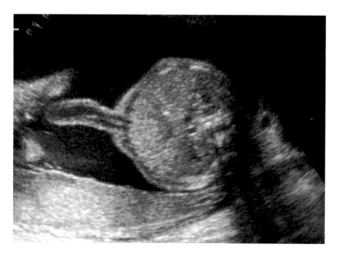

FIGURE 16-16 Transverse sonogram of a second-trimester fetus with an intact anterior abdominal wall and normal cord insertion.

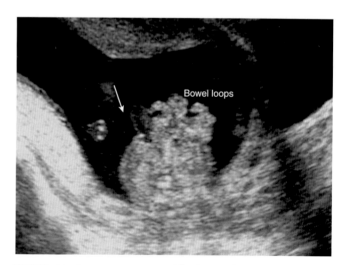

FIGURE 16-17 Transverse view of fetal abdomen. In this fetus with gastroschisis, extruded bowel loops are floating in the amnionic fluid to the right of the normal umbilical cord insertion site (*arrow*).

Omphalocele

This anomaly complicates approximately 1 per 5000 pregnancies. It forms when the lateral ectomesodermal folds fail to meet in the midline, leaving the abdominal contents covered only by a two-layered sac of amnion and peritoneum. The umbilical cord inserts into the apex of the sac (Fig. 16-18). In over half of cases, an omphalocele is associated with other major anomalies or aneuploidy. It also is a component of syndromes such as *Beckwith–Wiedemann, cloacal exstrophy,* and *pentalogy of Cantrell.* The smaller the defect, the greater the risk for aneuploidy (De Veciana and associates, 1994). The prognosis is determined by the size of the omphalocele and also by accompanying genetic or structural abnormalities (Heider and co-workers, 2004). Like other major anomalies, identification of an omphalocele mandates a complete fetal evaluation, and karyotyping is recommended.

Gastrointestinal Tract

The stomach is visible in nearly all fetuses after 14 weeks, and the liver, spleen, gallbladder, and bowel can be identified in many second- and third-trimester fetuses. Nonvisualization of the stomach within the abdomen is associated with a number of abnormalities. These include esophageal atresia, diaphragmatic hernia, abdominal wall defects, and neurological abnormalities that inhibit fetal swallowing. If the stomach is not seen on initial examination, the examination should be repeated. Millener and co-workers (1993), however, found that even with subsequent visualization of the stomach, a third of fetuses had an abnormal outcome.

The appearance of the bowel changes with fetal maturation. Occasionally it may appear bright, or echogenic, particularly if a higher frequency transducer is used (Vincoff and associates, 1999). Echogenic bowel is most commonly a normal variant or indicative of swallowed intra-amnionic blood. However, when the bowel appears as bright as fetal bone, there is a slightly increased risk for underlying gastrointestinal malformation, congenital infection such as cytomegalovirus, cystic fibrosis, and trisomy 21 (see Chap. 13, p. 296).

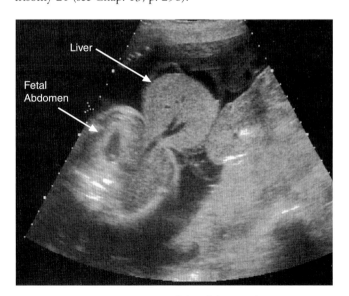

FIGURE 16-18 Transverse view of the abdomen showing an omphalocele as a large abdominal wall defect with exteriorized liver covered by a thin membrane.

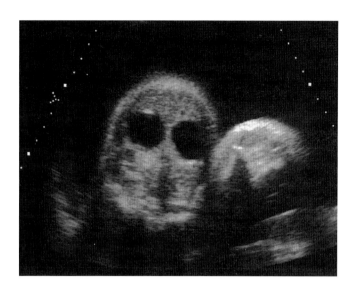

FIGURE 16-19 Double-bubble sign of duodenal atresia is seen on this axial abdominal image of the fetus.

Gastrointestinal Atresia

Most atresias are characterized by obstruction with proximal bowel dilatation. In general, the more proximal the obstruction, the more likely it is to be associated with hydramnios.

Esophageal atresia may be suspected when the stomach cannot be visualized and hydramnios is present. That said, in up to 90 percent of cases, a concomitant *tracheoesophageal fistula* allows fluid to enter the stomach, and thus prenatal detection is problematic (Pretorius and colleagues, 1987a). Approximately half of fetuses with esophageal atresia have associated anomalies, including aneuploidy in 20 percent and growth restriction in 40 percent. Cardiac malformations are especially common.

Duodenal atresia occurs in approximately 1 in 10,000 live births (Robertson and colleagues, 1994). It is associated with the sonographic *double-bubble sign,* which represents distension of the stomach and the first part of the duodenum (Fig. 16-19). This finding is usually not present prior to 24 weeks. Demonstrating continuity between the stomach and proximal duodenum will differentiate duodenal atresia from other causes of abdominal cystic structures. Approximately 30 percent of fetuses with duodenal atresia diagnosed antenatally have trisomy 21, and more than half have other anomalies. Obstructions in the more distal small bowel usually result in multiple dilated loops that may have increased peristaltic activity.

Large bowel obstructions and *anal atresia* are less readily diagnosed by sonography because hydramnios is not a typical feature, and the bowel may not be significantly dilated. The transverse view through the pelvis may reveal the enlarged rectum as a fluid-filled structure between the bladder and the sacrum.

Kidneys and Urinary Tract

Fetal kidneys are easily visible adjacent to the fetal spine, frequently as early as 14 weeks, and routinely by 18 weeks. Reference tables are available to provide normal kidney dimensions throughout pregnancy. The placenta and membranes are the major source of amnionic fluid early in pregnancy, but after 18 weeks, most of the fluid is produced by the kidneys. Fetal urine production increases from 5 mL/hr at 20 weeks to approximately 50 mL/hr at term (Rabinowitz and co-workers, 1989). Unexplained oligohydramnios suggests a urinary tract abnormality, whereas normal amnionic fluid volume in the second half of pregnancy suggests urinary tract patency with at least one functioning kidney.

Renal Agenesis

One or both kidneys are congenitally absent in 1 in 4000 births. The kidney is not visible, and the adrenal gland typically enlarges to fill the renal fossa. Hoffman and colleagues (1992) have aptly termed this the *lying down adrenal sign.* If renal agenesis is bilateral, no urine is produced, and the resulting anhydramnios leads to pulmonary hypoplasia, limb contractures, a distinctive compressed face, and death from cord compression or pulmonary hypoplasia. When this combination of abnormalities results from renal agenesis, it is called *Potter syndrome,* after Dr. Edith Potter, who described it in 1946. When these abnormalities result from scant amnionic fluid of some other etiology, it is called *Potter sequence.*

Polycystic Kidney Disease

Of the hereditary polycystic diseases, only the infantile form of autosomal recessive polycystic kidney disease may be reliably diagnosed antenatally. As discussed in Chapter 48 (p. 1042), the autosomal dominant condition usually does not manifest until adulthood, although prenatal diagnosis has been described (Pretorius and associates, 1987b). Infantile polycystic kidney disease is characterized by abnormally large kidneys that fill the fetal abdomen and appear to have a solid, ground-glass texture (Fig. 16-20). The abdominal circumference is enlarged, and there is

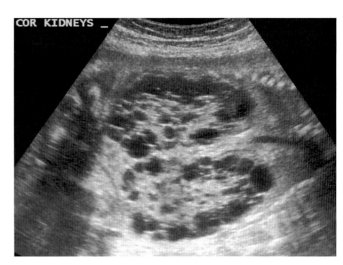

FIGURE 16-21 Coronal view of the fetal abdomen and lower thorax displays multiple cysts of varying sizes, which do not communicate in the retroperitoneal region of this fetus with multicystic dysplastic kidneys.

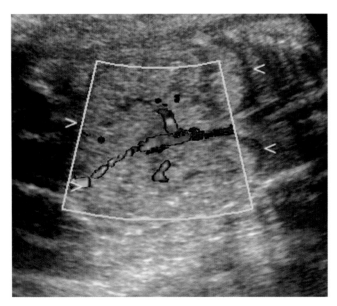

FIGURE 16-20 Coronal view of fetal abdomen and lower thorax displays the classic appearance of bilaterally enlarged echogenic kidneys in this fetus with autosomal recessive infantile polycystic kidneys. Arrows mark the upper and lower poles of each kidney. The renal arteries and aorta are seen with color Doppler mapping.

severe oligohydramnios. The cystic changes can only be identified microscopically.

Multicystic Dysplastic Kidney Disease

These renal changes arise from complete obstruction or atresia at the level of the renal pelvis or proximal ureter prior to 10 weeks. The diagnosis usually can be made antenatally by identifying abnormally dense renal parenchyma with multiple peripheral cysts of varying size that do not communicate with each other or with the renal pelvis (Fig. 16-21). This finding should be distinguished from obstructive pyelectasis, in which the fluid-filled areas can be seen to connect. The prognosis for fetuses with multicystic dysplastic kidney disease is generally good if findings are unilateral and amnionic fluid volume is normal. If bilateral, as in Figure 16-21, the prognosis is poor.

Ureteropelvic Junction Obstruction

This condition is the most common cause of neonatal hydronephrosis and affects males at least twice as often as females. The actual obstruction is generally functional rather than anatomical, and it is bilateral in a third of cases (Fig. 16-22). It is characterized by dilatation of the renal pelvis—*pyelectasis.* Various measurements taken at all gestational ages are used to predict fetuses that will require postnatal evaluation (Corteville, 1991; Mandell, 1991; Wilson, 1997, and all their colleagues). A commonly used upper limit for the normal renal pelvis diameter is 4 mm before 20 weeks. If this limit is exceeded, sonography is performed again at 34 weeks. If the pelvis is then greater than 7 mm, evaluation in the neonatal period should be considered.

Adra and co-workers (1995) found that two thirds of fetuses with pyelectasis > 8 mm had an abnormality at birth. Similarly, Ismaili and associates (2003) reported that a diameter of at least 7 mm in a third-trimester fetus had a 70-percent positive-predictive value for a renal abnormality. Yamamura and colleagues

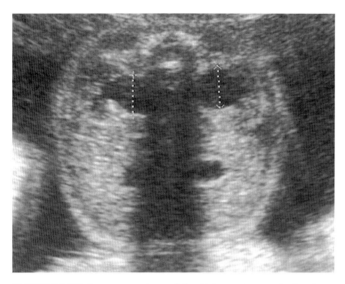

FIGURE 16-22 Transverse view of the kidneys demonstrating hydronephrosis (*calipers*) in a fetus with ureteropelvic junction obstruction.

(2007) recently evaluated mild fetal pyelectasis and found that a single third-trimester follow-up evaluation was a safe and cost-effective management. Specifically, none of the 244 fetuses in their series required antenatal interventions or progressed to severe pyelectasis to justify more intensive follow-up evaluations.

Collecting System Duplication

This is the most common genitourinary anomaly and is found in up to 4 percent of the population. The characteristic obstruction of the upper pole is evident as pyelectasis, often associated with a dilated ureter that may be mistaken for a loop of bowel, as well as with an ectopic ureterocele within the bladder. Reflux of the lower pole moiety is common. In the neonatal period, additional testing such as voiding cystourethrography will determine whether antimicrobial treatment is needed to minimize urinary infections and will assist with planning follow-up or surgical intervention.

Bladder Outlet Obstruction

This distal obstruction of the urinary tract is more common in male fetuses, and the most common etiology is *posterior urethral valves*. Characteristically, there is dilatation of the bladder and proximal urethra. As a result, the urethra resembles a keyhole, and the bladder wall is thickened. Oligohydramnios portends a poor prognosis because of pulmonary hypoplasia. Unfortunately, the outcome is not uniformly good even with a normal amount of fluid. As with other obstructive uropathies, prenatal diagnosis allows some affected fetuses to benefit from early intervention postnatally or even consideration of in utero therapy (see Chap. 13, p. 307).

3- AND 4-DIMENSIONAL SONOGRAPHY

The goal of 3-D imaging is to obtain a volume and then to render that volume to enhance real-time 2-dimensional findings. Special transducers are used to obtain volumes as still images—

3D—and as a function of time—4D. By sophisticated postprocessing, a variety of different displays can be produced. Because of the obvious appeal of a 3-D portrait of the fetal face, surface rendering is the most popular technique and is well known to the lay public (Fig. 16-23). And for selected anomalies, such as those of the face and skeleton, 3-D may provide additional useful information (Goncalves and associates, 2005). However, comparisons of 3-D with conventional 2-D sonography for the diagnosis of most congenital anomalies have *not* demonstrated an improvement in overall detection (Goncalves and co-workers, 2006; Reddy and colleagues, 2008). The American College of Obstetricians and Gynecologists (2009) recently affirmed that proof of a clinical advantage of 3D sonography in general is lacking. Thus, the precise utility of this exciting technology has yet to be fully determined.

One potential advantage of 3-D volume acquisition is the ability to reformat images in any plane. For example, if the image is obtained in the typical axial plane, volume acquisition can allow the image can be reformatted in sagittal, coronal, or even oblique planes. Sequential "slices" can be generated, similar to computed tomographic (CT) or magnetic resonance (MR) imaging. Applications of this technique include evaluation of intracranial anatomy in the sagittal plane—for example, the corpus callosum, and evaluation of the palate and skeletal system (Benacerraf, 2006; Pilu, 2008; Timor-Tritsch, 2000, and all their colleagues).

Recently, 4-D imaging has also been used to improve visualization of cardiac anatomy. Postprocessing algorithms and techniques have taken advantage of real-time image volumes—with and without color Doppler mapping. An example is *spatiotemporal image correlation—STIC*. They are used to evaluate the

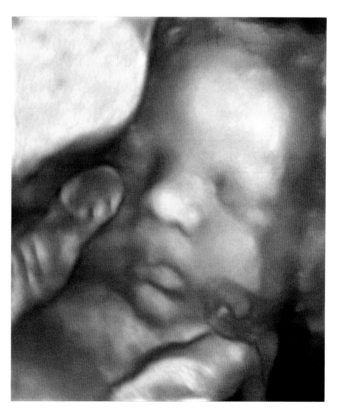

FIGURE 16-23 Surface rendered 3-dimensional image of the fetal face at 33 weeks' gestation.

complex cardiac anatomy and function (DeVore and associates, 2003; Espinoza and colleagues, 2008). Addition of an inversion-mode algorithm may aid imaging of blood flow within the heart and great vessels and may even allow measurement of ventricular blood volume (Goncalves and co-workers, 2004). Systematic approaches or protocols for using these new techniques to evaluate cardiac anatomy and physiology are under development (Espinoza and associates, 2007).

Limitations

There are several limitations to 3-D sonography. To adequately image a fetal surface structure in 3-D, it must be surrounded by amnionic fluid, because crowding by adjacent structures obscures the captured image. Image processing with 3-D sonography lengthens time to completion of the study, although Benacerraf and colleagues (2006) have demonstrated that this can be shortened with experience. Further, there are limitations on image resolution, data storage, and manipulation (Michailidis and co-workers, 2001; Pretorius and colleagues, 2001). The American Institute of Ultrasound in Medicine (2005) and the American College of Obstetricians and Gynecologists (2009) currently recommend that 3-D ultrasound be used only as an adjunct to conventional sonography.

DOPPLER

The use of Doppler in obstetrics has been primarily in the areas of duplex velocimetry and color mapping. The Doppler shift is a phenomenon that occurs when a source of light or sound waves is moving relative to an observer and is detected by the observer as a shift in the wave frequency. When sound waves strike a moving target, the frequency of the sound waves reflected back is shifted proportionate to the velocity and direction of the moving target. Because the magnitude and direction of the frequency shift depend on the relative motion of the moving target, the velocity and direction of the target can be determined.

Important to obstetrics, Doppler may be used to determine the volume and rate of blood flow through maternal and fetal vessels. In this situation, the sound source is the ultrasound transducer, the moving target is the column of red blood cells flowing through the circulation, and the reflected sound waves are observed by the ultrasound transducer. Two types of Doppler are used in medicine:

1. *Continuous wave Doppler* equipment has two separate types of crystals—one transmits high-frequency sound waves, and another continuously receives signals. It cannot be used for imaging of the blood vessel(s). In M-mode echocardiography, continuous wave Doppler is used to evaluate motion through time.
2. *Pulse wave Doppler* uses only one crystal, which transmits the signal and then waits until the returning signal is received before transmitting another one. It allows precise targeting and visualization of the vessel of interest. Pulse wave Doppler also can be configured to allow color-flow mapping with software that displays blood flowing away from the transducer as blue and blood flowing toward the transducer as red. Various combinations of pulse wave Doppler, color-flow Doppler, and real-time sonography are commercially available and are loosely referred to as *duplex Doppler.*

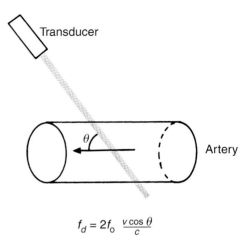

$$f_d = 2f_o \frac{v\cos\theta}{c}$$

FIGURE 16-24 Doppler equation: Ultrasound emanating from the transducer with initial frequency f_o strikes blood moving at velocity v. Reflected frequency f_d is dependent on angle τ; between beam of sound and vessel. (From Copel and associates, 1988.)

Clinical Applications

The Doppler equation shown in **Figure 16-24** contains the variables that affect the Doppler shift. An important source of error when calculating flow or velocity is the angle between sound waves from the transducer and flow within the vessel—termed the *angle of insonation* and abbreviated as theta—θ. Because cosine θ is a component of the equation, measurement error becomes large when the angle of insonation is not close to zero, in other words, when blood flow is not coming *directly* toward or away from the transducer. Thus, ratios are used to compare different waveform components, allowing cosine θ to cancel out of the equation. **Figure 16-25** is a schematic of the Doppler waveform and describes the three ratios commonly

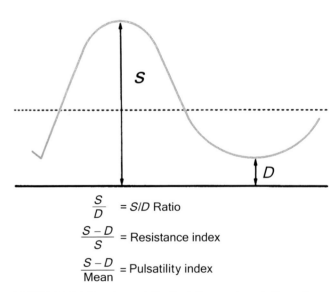

$$\frac{S}{D} = S/D \text{ Ratio}$$

$$\frac{S-D}{S} = \text{Resistance index}$$

$$\frac{S-D}{\text{Mean}} = \text{Pulsatility index}$$

FIGURE 16-25 Doppler systolic–diastolic waveform indices of blood flow velocity. The mean is calculated from computer-digitized waveforms. (D = diastole; S = systole.) (This figure was published in *American Journal of Obstetrics & Gynecology*, Vol. 164, No. 4, JA Low, The current status of maternal and fetal blood flow velocimetry, pp. 1049–1063, Copyright Elsevier 1991.)

used. The simplest is the *systolic-diastolic ratio (S/D ratio)*, which compares maximum (peak) systolic flow with end-diastolic flow, thereby evaluating downstream impedance to flow.

Flow in numerous maternal and fetal vessels have been studied to better understand antenatal pathophysiology. Figure 16-26 illustrates several vessels and their corresponding waveforms. The following discussion is limited to selected obstetrical applications.

Umbilical Artery

This vessel normally has forward flow throughout the cardiac cycle, and the amount of flow during diastole increases as gestation advances. Thus, the *S/D* ratio *decreases,* from about 4.0 at 20 weeks to 2.0 at term. The *S/D* ratio is generally less than 3.0 after 30 weeks. As discussed in Chapter 15 (p. 343), umbilical artery Doppler has been subjected to more rigorous assessment than has any previous test of fetal health (Alfirevic and Neilson, 1995). This measurement is considered to be a useful adjunct in the management of pregnancies complicated by fetal-growth restriction (American College of Obstetricians and Gynecologists, 2008). It is not recommended for screening of low-risk pregnancies or for complications other than growth restriction.

Umbilical artery Doppler is considered abnormal if the *S/D* ratio is above the 95th percentile for gestational age. In extreme cases of growth restriction, end-diastolic flow may become absent or even reversed (Fig. 16-27). These should prompt a complete fetal evaluation—almost half of cases are associated with fetal aneuploidy or a major anomaly (Wenstrom and associates, 1991). In the absence of a reversible maternal complication or a fetal anomaly, *reversed* end-diastolic flow suggests severe fetal circulatory compromise and usually prompts immediate delivery. Sezik and colleagues (2004) reported that fetuses of preeclamptic women who had absent or reversed end-diastolic flow were more likely to have hypoglycemia and polycythemia.

Ductus Arteriosus

Doppler evaluation of the ductus arteriosus has been used primarily to monitor fetuses exposed to indomethacin and other nonsteroidal anti-inflammatory agents—NSAIDs. Indomethacin, which is used for tocolysis, may cause ductal constriction or closure (Huhta and colleagues, 1987). The resulting increased

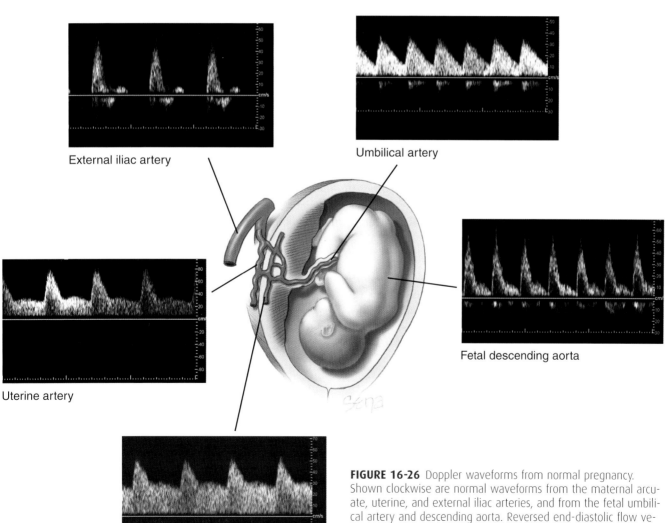

External iliac artery

Umbilical artery

Uterine artery

Fetal descending aorta

Arcuate artery

FIGURE 16-26 Doppler waveforms from normal pregnancy. Shown clockwise are normal waveforms from the maternal arcuate, uterine, and external iliac arteries, and from the fetal umbilical artery and descending aorta. Reversed end-diastolic flow velocity is apparent in the external iliac artery, whereas continuous diastolic flow characterizes the uterine and arcuate vessels. Finally, note the greatly diminished end-diastolic flow in the fetal descending aorta.

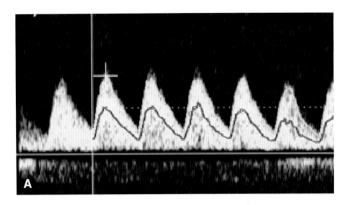

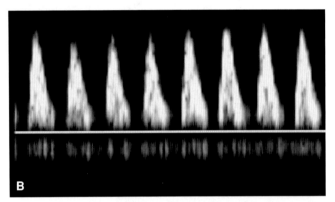

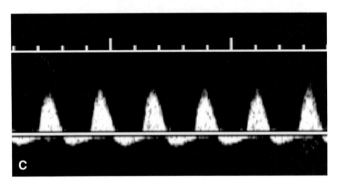

FIGURE 16-27 Umbilical artery Doppler waveforms. **A.** Normal diastolic flow. **B.** Absence of end-diastolic flow. **C.** Reversed end-diastolic flow.

pulmonary flow may cause reactive hypertrophy of the pulmonary arterioles and eventual development of pulmonary hypertension (see Chap. 36, p. 825). Ductal constriction can be reversed, and its persistence may be directly related to increasing dosage and duration of NSAID administration. In a review of 12 randomized controlled trials involving more than 200 exposed pregnancies, Koren and colleagues (2006) reported that NSAIDs increased the odds of ductal constriction by 15-fold. They also concluded that this was a low estimate because most of the pregnancies were exposed for 72 hours or less. In general, ductal constriction is a potentially serious complication that should be avoided. Thus, drug administration duration is typically limited to < 72 hours, and those on NSAIDs are closely monitored so that these can be discontinued if constriction is identified.

Uterine Artery

Uterine blood flow is estimated to increase from 50 mL/min early in gestation to 500 to 750 mL/min by term (see Chap. 5,

p. 108). The uterine artery Doppler waveform is unique and characterized by high diastolic flow velocities similar to those in systole (Fig. 16-26). There is also highly turbulent flow, which displays a spectrum of many different velocities. Increased resistance to flow and development of a diastolic notch have been associated with pregnancy-induced hypertension (Arduini, 1987; Fleischer, 1986; Harrington, 1996; North, 1994, and all their colleagues). More recently, Zeeman and co-workers (2003) confirmed that increased impedance of uterine artery velocimetry at 16 to 20 weeks was predictive of superimposed preeclampsia developing in women with chronic hypertension. In a report from the recent workshop on prenatal imaging held by the National Institute of Child Health and Human Development, Reddy and associates (2008) concluded that perinatal benefits of uterine artery Doppler screening have not yet been demonstrated.

Middle Cerebral Artery (MCA)

Doppler measurement of middle cerebral artery velocimetry has been studied and employed clinically for detection of fetal anemia and in the assessment of growth restriction. Although accurate measurement of velocity in other vessels may be limited by high insonating angles, MCA measurements are an exception. Anatomically, the path of this artery is such that flow velocity approaches the transducer "head-on," and the fontanel allows easy insonation (Fig. 16-28).

With fetal anemia, the peak systolic velocity is increased due to increased cardiac output and decreased blood viscosity (Segata and Mari, 2004). This has permitted the reliable, noninvasive detection of fetal anemia in cases of bloodgroup alloimmunization. More than a decade ago, Mari and colleagues (1995) performed MCA velocity studies in 135 normal fetuses and 39 with alloimmunization. They showed that anemic fetuses had a peak systolic velocity above the normal mean. In a subsequent collaborative study of 376 pregnancies, Mari and colleagues (2000) used a threshold of 1.50 multiple of the median (MoM) for peak systolic velocity to correctly identify all fetuses with moderate or severe anemia. The false-positive rate was 12 percent. Others have since reported similar findings (Bahado-Singh and colleagues, 2000; Cosmi and associates, 2002). In many centers, MCA peak systolic velocity has replaced invasive testing with amniocentesis for the detection of fetal anemia (see Chap. 29, p. 622).

MCA Doppler has also been studied as an adjunct to the evaluation of fetal-growth restriction. It is believed that there is a progression of Doppler findings in severely affected fetuses such that increased impedance of flow in the umbilical artery may be detected first. This is followed by redistribution of flow to the brain, with decreasing resistance that has been termed *brain sparing*, and eventually by abnormalities in venous flow (Mari, 2007; Reddy, 2008; Turan, 2008, and all their colleagues). Unfortunately, this brain-sparing effect has not been shown to be protective for the fetus—in fact, it is more likely the opposite. At this time, MCA Doppler has *not* been adopted as standard practice in the management of growth restriction, and its utility in the timing of delivery of such fetuses is uncertain.

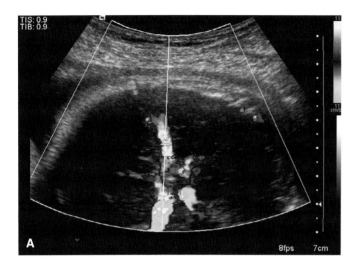

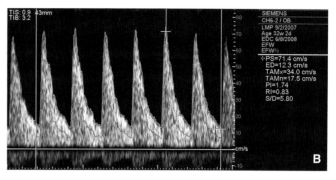

FIGURE 16-28 Middle cerebral artery color Doppler (**A**) and waveform (**B**) in a 32-week fetus with elevated peak systolic velocity secondary to fetal anemia from Rh alloimmunization.

Ductus Venosus

In the setting of severe fetal-growth restriction, cardiac dysfunction may lead to venous flow abnormalities, including pulsatile flow in the umbilical vein and abnormal ductus venosus waveforms (Reddy and associates, 2008). Ductus venosus abnormalities may identify preterm growth-restricted fetuses that are at greatest risk for adverse outcomes (Baschat, 2003, 2004; Bilardo and co-workers, 2004; Figueras and associates, 2009). Trudinger (2007) has proposed that understanding and treatment of the underlying placental vasculopathy are likely to be more important for improving outcomes than for focusing on early delivery. In the workshop on prenatal imaging held by the National Institute of Child Health and Human Development, Reddy and colleagues (2008) concluded that use of venous Doppler for the management of fetal-growth restriction requires demonstration of perinatal benefit before adoption.

Newer applications of color mapping onto the M-mode tracing permit exquisite evaluation of wall motion and blood velocity and categorization of complex arrhythmias (Fig. 16-29). Importantly, some of these, for example, supraventricular tachycardias, can be treated to prevent or reverse heart failure. Others, such as premature atrial contractions, resolve spontaneously without intervention. Antenatal treatment is discussed in Chapter 13 (p. 303).

MAGNETIC RESONANCE (MR) IMAGING

The fetus was first studied with MR imagining in the mid-1980s when image acquisition was slow and motion artifact was problematic. Since then, technological advances allowing fast-acquisition MR protocols have been developed. These include SSFSE—Single Shot Fast Spin Echo sequence; HASTE—Half-

M-MODE ECHOCARDIOGRAPHY

Motion-mode, or M-mode sonography is a linear display of the events of the cardiac cycle, with time on the x-axis and motion on the y-axis. It is used commonly to measure the fetal heart rate, and deviations from the normal rate and rhythm are readily apparent. If there is an abnormality, an evaluation of cardiac anatomy is performed. M-mode echocardiography may allow precise characterization of an arrhythmia, including separate evaluation of atrial and ventricular waveforms. It can be used to assess ventricular function and atrial and ventricular outputs, as well as the timing of these events.

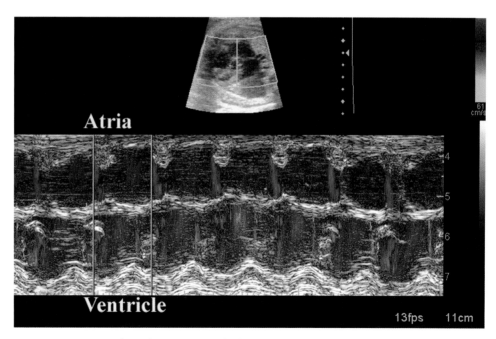

FIGURE 16-29 M-mode with superimposed color Doppler demonstrates the normal concordance between the atrial and ventricular contractions.

Fourier Acquisition Single shot Turbo spin Echo sequence; RARE—Rapid Acquisition with Relaxation Enhancement sequence; and echo-planar imaging. Images are acquired within 1 second or less, eliminating the need for sedation because motion artifact is significantly reduced.

Technologically speaking, MR imaging is superior to sonography because it is hindered only minimally by bony interfaces, maternal obesity, oligohydramnios, or an engaged fetal head. Pragmatically, however, MR imaging is not portable, and it can be time-consuming. Thus, it currently is used as an adjunct to fetal sonography, especially for complex abnormalities of the central nervous system, thorax, and gastrointestinal and genitourinary systems (Farhataziz, 2005; Hawkins, 2008; Matsuoka, 2003; Twickler, 2003, and all their associates).

Safety

MR imaging uses no ionizing radiation however, theoretical concerns include the effects of fluctuating electromagnetic fields and high sound-intensity levels. The strength of the magnetic field is measured in *tesla (T)*. A number of animal and tissue studies have been conducted that address the biological effects of electromagnetic fields. In one, Wiskirchen and colleagues (1999) studied long-term effects of repetitive exposure of human lung fibroblasts to a static 1.5 T magnetic field. They found that exposed and control cells had similar proliferation.

Human studies, although relatively few in number, support the safety of fetal MR imaging. Kanal (1994) reported a large epidemiological retrospective study of nurses and technologists working with MR imaging in which rates of pregnancy loss, infertility, low birth weight, and preterm birth were compared before and after employment. There was no increased incidence of adverse outcome in the MR-exposed group. Two follow-up studies from Nottingham, England, described children exposed to echo-planar MR in utero. In one, Baker and colleagues (1994b) did a three-year follow-up of 20 children and found no increased incidence of disease or disability. In the second, Clements and associates (2000) prospectively followed 20 infants exposed in utero to echo-planar MR imaging and found that pediatric assessments at age 9 months were normal.

Glover and colleagues (1995) attempted to mimic the sound level experienced by the fetal ear during an MR procedure. An adult volunteer swallowed a microphone connected to a thin lead, and the stomach was filled with a liter of fluid to represent the amnionic sac. There was at least a 30-dB attenuation in intensity from the body surface to the fluid-filled stomach. This reduced the acoustic sound pressure down from the dangerous threshold of 120 dB to an acceptable level < 90 dB. This is considerably less than the 135 dB experienced when vibroacoustic stimulation is used (see Chap. 18, p. 427). Arulkuman and associates (1991) reported no evidence of hearing loss in 450 babies exposed to vibroacoustic stimulation. Finally, fetal heart rate patterns and movements during MR procedures demonstrated no change (Vadeyar, 2000).

Studies in pregnancy reported to date have been performed with a magnet strength of 1.5 T or less. It is recommended that informed consent be obtained when fetal MR is performed. In more than 1600 MR procedures performed during pregnancy at the University of Texas Southwestern Medical Center over the past 8 years, there have been no patient safety issues. Maternal anxiety from claustrophobia or fear of the equipment was encountered in less than 1 percent. To reduce maternal anxiety in this small group, a one-time oral dose of diazepam, 5 to 10 mg, or lorazepam, 1 to 2 mg, is given. For some equipment, the maternal weight limit is 350 pounds—thus some obese women will not be candidates (Zaretsky and Twickler, 2003d).

Fetal Anatomic Survey

Although there is experience with normal fetal anatomy imaged with MR imaging, there have been no comparisons with contemporaneous sonography. Zaretsky and colleagues (2003b) applied the American College of Obstetrics and Gynecology ultrasound criteria to an axial sequence and reported that 85 percent of the anatomical targets were adequately visualized. Using axial, coronal, and sagittal MR acquisitions, this same group found that 99 percent of targeted anatomy—excluding the heart—was visualized (Zaretsky and associates, 2003a). In both studies, nonfetal components that included the placenta, amnionic fluid, and maternal pelvis were visualized adequately. These studies and others indicate that MR imaging is more informative beyond 20 weeks.

Central Nervous System

Although sonography is the preferred method of imaging fetal intracranial abnormalities, MR images are superior in many ways because of the improved resolution. Thus, MR imaging is a valuable adjunct in the antenatal diagnosis of some suspected cranial anomalies. Very fast T2 weighted images produce excellent tissue contrast, and cerebrospinal-fluid-containing structures are hyperintense or bright. This allows exquisite detail of the posterior fossa, midline structures, and cerebral cortex. Near-field attenuation caused by the fetal skull on sonography is not a problem with MR imaging, and this feature allows accurate determination of lesion bilaterality. Another major advantage is acquisition of images in the axial, coronal, and sagittal planes in reference to the fetus or the maternal pelvis. Sagittal fetal images are very helpful, for example, in evaluating the corpus callosum when there is mild ventriculomegaly. T1-weighted images are occasionally used to differentiate between fat and hemorrhage.

Routine MR biometry includes BPD, occipitofrontal diameter (OFD), cerebellar width, and cisterna magna and bilateral atrial measurements. Twickler and associates (2002) measured ventricle and cisterna magna values in 60 fetuses from 14 weeks to term. They reported that although atrial measurements are slightly smaller with MR compared with sonography, cisterna magna measurements were similar. Tables have been established for measurements of multiple components of normal brain biometry, including corpus callosum length and cerebellar vermis (Garel, 2004; Tilea and colleagues, 2009).

Fetal Brain Development

Levine and Barnes (1999a) reported that cortical maturation evaluated with MR imaging accurately portrayed cerebral gyration and sulcation patterns of embryological development. This is important because fetuses with a cerebral abnormality may have a significant lag time in cortical development. And although sonography is limited to evaluate subtle early migrational abnormalities, MR imaging is more accurate, and even more so later in gestation.

Second Opinion MR Imaging Evaluation

At least three large studies have assessed second-opinion MR examination for a cerebral abnormality detected by sonography and its ability to confirm or change a diagnosis and possibly alter clinical management. Levine and co-workers (1999b) evaluated 66 fetuses with such abnormalities and found that MR imaging provided additional information in nearly 60 percent and changed the diagnosis in 40 percent. Importantly, management was clearly changed in 15 percent. Simon and colleagues (2000) studied 73 fetuses with brain anomalies and reported that MR imaging findings changed management in almost half. Twickler and co-workers (2003) reported that MR imaging provided valuable additional information in 65 percent of 72 fetuses. Moreover, in half of these 46 cases, the diagnosis was changed, and this altered clinical management in a third. Evaluation with MR imaging was more likely to confirm sonographic findings prior to 24 weeks, but beyond that 24 weeks, a change of diagnosis or additional information was more frequently found.

The most common reason for fetal MR evaluation is isolated ventriculomegaly. Commonly associated abnormalities may not be well visualized with sonography. For example, in the study by Twickler and associates (2003), the diagnosis of marked ventriculomegaly was narrowed to a more precise diagnosis such as aqueductal stenosis or hydranencephaly (Fig. 16-30). Another

was from mild ventriculomegaly to more specific diagnoses such as corpus callosum agenesis and migrational abnormalities. These findings were recently confirmed by Benacerraf and colleagues (2007). These more precise diagnoses impact patient counseling and, to a lesser degree, clinical management.

Cerebral Lesions with Multifetal Gestation

Hu and Twickler (2006) recently reviewed MR findings with complicated multifetal gestations. MR imaging has been used to evaluate monochorionic twin gestations for the possibility of hemorrhage or periventricular leukomalacia in the setting of twin-twin transfusion syndrome or with demise of one twin. Documentation of these problems is particularly important when placental ablation of the vascular anastomoses is considered (see Chap. 13, p. 306, and Chap. 39, p. 874).

Thorax

MR imaging is used to further evaluate thoracic masses and abnormalities to delineate their location and size and to quantify the volume of remaining lung tissue. The tissue contrast between normal lung tissue and thoracic lesions is excellent in most cases. Thoracic abnormalities that are studied further with MR imaging include congenital cystic adenomatoid malformations (CCAM), bronchopulmonary sequestrations (BPS), congenital diaphragmatic hernias (CDH), and chylothoraces (Fig. 16-31). It is also helpful with abnormalities that cause pulmonary hypoplasia such as renal and skeletal dysplasias.

MR imaging is an excellent adjunct to sonography to evaluate fetuses with a congenital diaphragmatic hernia. It aids determination of liver position and identification of abdominal

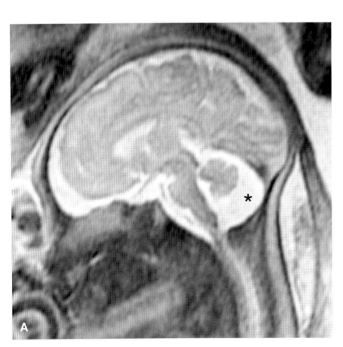
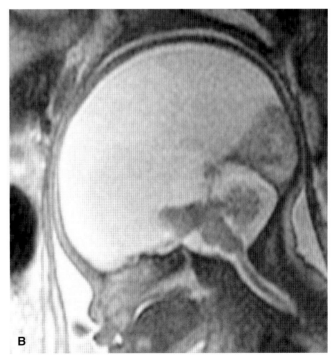

FIGURE 16-30 Magnetic resonance imaging of the fetal brain. **A.** Midline sagittal image of a 37-week fetal brain with a prominent cisterna magna (*asterisk*) and normal vermis. **B.** Midline sagittal image of a 35-week fetal brain with hydranencephaly.

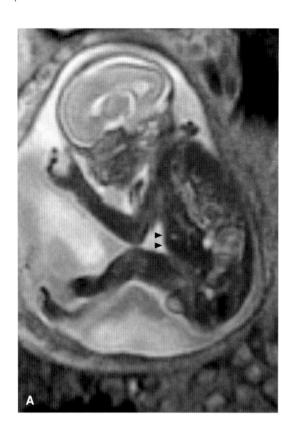

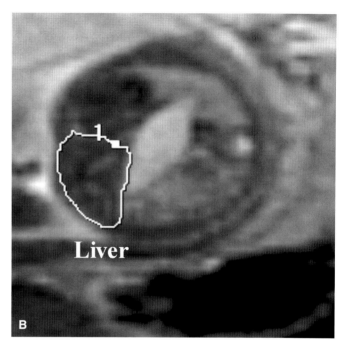

FIGURE 16-31 Magnetic resonance image of a 26-week fetus with congenital diaphragmatic hernia involving the liver. **A.** On this sagittal image, black arrowheads point to the liver in the chest. **B.** The liver is outlined in the axial plane.

contents within the chest (Fig. 16-31) (Hedrick, 2007; Walsh, 2000; Worley, 2009, and all their associates). Findings have been especially helpful in right-sided diaphragmatic hernias.

In some of these cases, prognosis can be estimated by the amount of normal lung tissue that remains or by the percentage of thorax occupied by the fetal liver (Kilian and co-workers, 2009; Worley and colleagues, 2009). However, the lung volume/gestational age ratio as a predictor of lethality with diaphragmatic hernia has shown little utility. In contrast, with renal disorders, this ratio was significantly different between groups with lethal and nonlethal malformations (Zaretsky and colleagues, 2005a).

Abdomen

In many cases, sonography accurately diagnoses genitourinary abnormalities and is the preferred modality. With oligohydramnios or maternal obesity, however, MR imaging is useful to evaluate complex anomalies. Poutamo and co-workers (2000) evaluated 24 fetuses with either oligohydramnios or a suspected urinary tract abnormality. MR evaluation alone led to the diagnosis in eight cases. It added information in 5 of 12 cases complicated by oligohydramnios and in three of 10 cases with normal amnionic fluid volumes. Caire and colleagues (2003) also found MR imaging to be an excellent technique for studying complex anatomical genitourinary malformations.

Determining the origin of a fetal cystic abdominal mass is difficult, especially in the third trimester. In some cases, MR imaging can help differentiate between genitourinary and gastrointestinal abnormalities. The signal intensity of meconium in the colon and urine in the bladder were evaluated in 80 fe-

tuses by Farhataziz and colleagues (2005). They reported that characteristic MR signals of each were most helpful after 24 weeks. In over half of suspected gastrointestinal or genitourinary abnormalities, T1-weighted images added additional information.

Placenta

The clinical importance of identifying women with placenta accreta is discussed in Chapter 35 (p. 776). These women are at risk for severe hemorrhage and hysterectomy, and MR imaging findings may help in surgical planning and patient counseling. Sonography is used to identify myometrial invasion, and MR evaluation can be used as an adjunct in indeterminate cases.

Levine and co-workers (1997) compared the accuracy of MR imaging with that of transabdominal and transvaginal grayscale sonography with color and power Doppler. Transvaginal sonography was adequate to diagnose six of seven cases of accreta. The remaining case was a posterior placenta accreta that was diagnosed accurately using MR imaging. These investigators reported MR imaging to be helpful only in cases in which the placenta lay outside the range for both transabdominal and transvaginal sonography. Conversely, Warshak and associates (2006) compared MR imaging with sonography and found MR imaging to be superior to evaluate myometrial invasion. Our experience is that sonography is excellent to determine myometrial involvement (Fig. 16-32). If sonography with Doppler color flow mapping demonstrates large intraplacental lakes and myometrial thickness < 1 mm, the sensitivity for myometrial invasion is 100 percent (Twickler and colleagues,

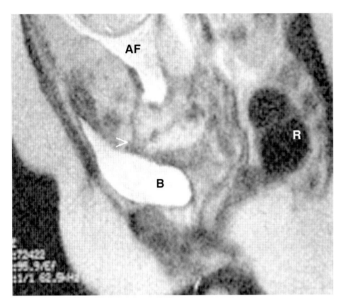

FIGURE 16-32 Magnetic resonance image of placenta increta at 35 weeks. A bridging vessel (*arrowhead*) between the retroplacental vessels and bladder serosal interface. AF = amnionic fluid; B = bladder; R = rectum.

2000). Identification of placenta percreta with bladder wall invasion is less accurate even when both sonography and MR imaging are used.

Fetal and Uterine Volumetry

MR imaging has been used to determine specific organ volumes, and it is potentially useful to reconstruct a 3-D image. Garden and co-workers (1996) used serial MR imaging and reported volume determinations of the fetus and the fetal liver, lungs, and brain. Baker and associates (1994a) calculated fetal weight determined by volume and reported that it compared favorably with sonographic estimated weight. Zaretsky and colleagues (2003c) studied the accuracy of MR imaging versus sonography for fetal weight estimation in 80 women and found good correlations using the Baker equation.

Pelvimetry

A number of studies have used MR pelvimetry to assess pelvic capacity and predict vaginal delivery (see Chap. 20, p. 472). None has been found clinically valuable (Zaretsky and colleagues, 2005b).

REFERENCES

Adra AM, Mejides AA, Dennaoui MS. et al: Fetal pyelectasis: Is it always "physiologic"? Am J Obstet Gynecol 173:1263, 1995
Alfirevic Z, Neilson JP: Doppler ultrasonography in high-risk pregnancies: Systematic review with meta-analysis. Am J Obstet Gynecol 172:1379, 1995
American College of Obstetricians and Gynecologists: Guidelines for diagnostic imaging during pregnancy. Committee Opinion No. 299, September 2004
American College of Obstetricians and Gynecologists: Screening for fetal chromosomal abnormalities. Practice Bulletin No. 77, January 2007
American College of Obstetricians and Gynecologists: Ultrasonography in pregnancy. Practice Bulletin No. 101, February 2009

American College of Radiology: Reporting obstetrical ultrasound codes. ACR Bulletin 62:24, 2007
American Institute of Ultrasound in Medicine (AIUM): American Institute of Ultrasound in Medicine Consensus Report on Potential Bioeffects of Diagnostic Ultrasound. J Ultrasound Med 27:503, 2008
American Institute of Ultrasound in Medicine (AIUM): Practice guideline for the performance of obstetric ultrasound examinations, pp. 2–7. October 2007
Arduini D, Rizzo G, Romanini C, et al: Utero-placental blood flow velocity waveforms as predictors of pregnancy-induced hypertension. Eur J Obstet Gynecol Reprod Biol 26:335, 1987
Arulkuman S, Skurr B, Tong H, et al: No evidence of hearing loss due to fetal acoustic stimulation test. Obstet Gynecol 78:283, 1991
Bahado-Singh RO, Cheng CS: First trimester prenatal diagnosis. Curr Opin Obstet Gynecol 16:177, 2004
Bahado-Singh RO, Oz AU, Hsu C, et al: Middle cerebral artery Doppler velocimetric deceleration angle as a predictor of fetal anemia in Rh-alloimmunized fetuses without hydrops. Am J Obstet Gynecol 183:746, 2000
Baker PN, Johnson IR, Gowland PA, et al: Fetal weight estimation by echo-planar magnetic resonance imaging. Lancet 343:644, 1994a
Baker PN, Johnson IR, Harvey PR, et al: A three-year follow-up of children imaged in utero with echo-planar magnetic resonance. Am J Obstet Gynecol 170:32, 1994b
Baschat AA: Doppler application in the delivery timing of the preterm growth-restricted fetus: Another step in the right direction. Ultrasound Obstet Gynecol 23:111, 2004
Baschat AA: Relationship between placental blood flow resistance and precordial venous Doppler indices. Ultrasound Obstet Gynecol 22:561, 2003
Benacerraf BR, Benson CB, Abuhamad AZ, et al: Three- and 4-dimensional ultrasound in obstetrics and gynecology: Proceedings of the American Institute of Ultrasound in Medicine Consensus Conference. Ultrasound Med 24:1587, 2005
Benacerraf BR, Shipp TD, Bromley B, et al: Three-dimensional US of the fetus: Volume imaging. Radiology 238:988, 2006
Benacerraf BR, Shipp TD, Bromley B, et al: What does magnetic resonance imaging add to the prenatal sonographic diagnosis of ventriculomegaly? J Ultrasound Med 26:1513, 2007
Bilardo CM, Wolf H, Stigter RH, et al: Relationship between monitoring parameters and perinatal outcome in severe, early intrauterine growth restriction. Ultrasound Obstet Gynecol 23:119, 2004
Bloom SL, Bloom DD, DellaNebbia C, et al: The developmental outcome of children with antenatal mild isolated ventriculomegaly. Obstet Gynecol 90:93, 1997
Caire JT, Ramus RM, Magee KP, et al: MRI of fetal genitourinary anomalies. AJR Am J Roentgenol 181:1381, 2003
Campbell J, Gilbert WM, Nicolaides, et al: Ultrasound screening for spina bifida: Cranial and cerebellar signs in a high-risk population. Obstet Gynecol 70(2):247, 1987
Cardoza JD, Filly RA, Podrasky AE: The dangling choroid plexus: A sonographic observation of value in excluding ventriculomegaly. AJR Am J Roentgenol 151:767, 1988a
Cardoza JD, Goldstein RB, Filly RA: Exclusion of fetal ventriculomegaly with a single measurement: The width of the lateral ventricular atrium. Radiology 169:711, 1988b
Clements H, Duncan KE, Fielding K, et al: Infants exposed to MRI in utero have a normal paediatric assessment of 9 months of age. Br J Radiol 73:190, 2000
Copel JA, Grannum PA, Hobbins JC, et al: Doppler Ultrasound in Obstetrics. Williams Obstetrics, 17th ed. (Suppl 16), Norwalk, CT, Appleton and Lange, 1988
Corteville J, Gray D, Crane J: Congenital hydronephrosis: Correlation of fetal ultrasonographic finding with infant outcome. Am J Obstet Gynecol 165:384, 1991
Cosmi E, Mari G, Delle CL, et al: Noninvasive diagnosis by Doppler ultrasonography of fetal anemia resulting from parvovirus infection. Am J Obstet Gynecol 187:1290, 2002
Dandy WE, Blackfan KD: Internal hydrocephalus: An experimental, clinical, and pathological study. Am J Dis Child 8:406, 1914
Dane B, Dane C, Sivri D, et al: Ultrasound screening for fetal major abnormalities at 11-14 weeks. Acta Obstet Gynecol Scand 86:666, 2007
Dashe JS, McIntire DD, Twickler DM: Effect of maternal obesity on the ultrasound detection of anomalous fetuses. 113:1, 2009
De Veciana M, Major CA, Porto M: Prediction of an abnormal karyotype in fetuses with omphalocele. Prenat Diagn 14:487, 1994
DeVore GR, Falkensammer P, Sklansky MS, et al: Spatio-temporal image correlation (STIC): New technology for evaluation of the fetal heart. Ultrasound Obstet Gynecol 22:380, 2003

Donald I, MacVicar J, Brown TG: Investigation of abdominal masses by pulsed ultrasound. Lancet 7032:1188, 1958

Ecker JL, Shipp TD, Bromley B, et al: The sonographic diagnosis of Dandy-Walker and Dandy-Walker variant: Associated findings and outcomes. Prenat Diagn 20:328, 2000

Ergün O, Barksdale E, Ergün FS, et al: The timing of delivery of infants with gastroschisis influences outcome. J Pediatr Surg 40:424, 2005

Espinoza J, Gotsch F, Kusanovic JP, et al: Changes in fetal cardiac geometry with gestation: Implications for 3- and 4-dimensional fetal echocardiography. J Ultrasound Med 26:437, 2007

Espinoza J, Romero R, Kusanovic JP, Gotsch F, et al: Standardized views of the fetal heart using four-dimensional sonographic and tomographic imaging. Ultrasound Obstet Gynecol 31:233, 2008

Farhataziz N, Engels JE, Ramus RM, et al: Fetal MRI of urine and meconium by gestational age for the diagnosis of genitourinary and gastrointestinal abnormalities. AJR Am J Roentgenol 184:1891, 2005

Figueras F, Benavides A, Del Rio M, et al: Monitoring of fetuses with intrauterine growth restriction: longitudinal changes in ductus venosus and aortic isthmus flow. Ultrasound Obstet Gynecol 33(1):39, 2009

Fleischer A, Schulman H, Farmakides G, et al: Uterine artery Doppler velocimetry in pregnant women with hypertension. Am J Obstet Gynecol 154:806, 1986

Gaglioti P, Oberto M, Todros T: The significance of fetal ventriculomegaly: Etiology, short-and long-term outcomes. Prenat Diagn 29(4):381, 2009

Garden AS, Roberts N: Fetal and fetal organ volume estimations with magnetic resonance imaging. Am J Obstet Gynecol 175:442, 1996

Garel C: Development of the fetal brain. In MRI of the Fetal Brain: Normal Development and Cerebral Pathologies. New York, Springer, 2004

Glover P, Hykin J, Gowland P, et al: An assessment of the intrauterine sound intensity level during obstetric echo-planar magnetic resonance imaging. Br J Radiol 68:1090, 1995

Goldstein I, Reece EA, Pilu G, et al: Cerebellar measurements with ultrasonography in the evaluation of fetal growth and development. Am J Obstet Gynecol 156:1065, 1987

Goncalves LF, Lee W, Espinoza J, et al: Three- and 4-dimensional ultrasound in obstetric practice: Does it help? J Ultrasound Med 24:1599, 2005

Goncalves LF, Nien JK, Espinoza J, et al: What does 2-dimensional imaging add to 3- and 4-dimensional obstetric ultrasonography? J Ultrasound Med 25:691, 2006

Goncalves LF, Espinoza J, Lee W, et al: Three- and four-dimensional reconstruction of the aortic and ductal arches using inversion mode: A new rendering algorithm for visualization of fluid-filled anatomical structures. Ultrasound Obstet Gynecol 24:696, 2004

Harrington K, Cooper D, Lees C, et al: Doppler ultrasound of the uterine arteries: The importance of bilateral notching in the prediction of pre-eclampsia, placental abruption or delivery of a small-for-gestational-age baby. Ultrasound Obstet Gynecol 7:182, 1996

Hawkins JS, Dashe JS, Twickler DM: Magnetic resonance imaging diagnosis of severe fetal renal anomalies. Am J Obstet Gynecol 198:328.e1, 2008

Hedrick HL, Danzer E, Merchant A, et al: Liver position and lung-to-head ratio for prediction of extracorporeal membrane oxygenation and survival in isolated left congenital diaphragmatic hernia. Am J Obstet Gynecol 197:422.e1, 2007

Heider AL, Strauss RA, Kuller JA: Omphalocele: Clinical outcomes in cases with normal karyotypes. Am J Obstet Gynecol 190:135, 2004

Hoffman CK, Filly RA, Callen PW: The "lying down" adrenal sign: A sonographic indicator of renal agenesis or ectopia in fetuses and neonates. J Ultrasound Med 11:533, 1992

Hu LS, Caire J, Twickler DM: MR findings of complicated multifetal gestations. Obstet Gynecol 36(1): 76, 2006

Huhta JC, Moise KJ, Fisher DJ, et al: Detection and quantitation of construction of the fetal ductus arteriosus by Doppler echocardiography. Circulation 75:406, 1987

Ismaili K, Hall M, Donner C, et al: Results of systematic screening for minor degrees of fetal renal pelvis dilatation in an unselected population. Am J Obstet Gynecol 188:242, 2003

Johnson MP, Johnson A, Holzgreve W, et al: First-trimester simple hygroma: Cause and outcome. Am J Obstet Gynecol 168:156, 1993

Joó JG, Tóth Z, Beke A, et al: Etiology, prenatal diagnoses and outcome of ventriculomegaly in 230 cases. Fetal Diagn Ther 24(3):254, 2008

Kanal E: Pregnancy and the safety of magnetic resonance imaging. MRI Clin N Am 2:309, 1994

Kilian AK, Schaible T, Hofmann V, et al: Congenital diaphragmatic hernia: predictive value of MRI relative lung-to-head ratio compared with MRI fetal lung volume and sonographic lung-to-head ratio. AJR 192(1):153, 2009

Kitchanan S, Patole SK, Muller R, et al: Neonatal outcome of gastroschisis and exomphalos: A 10-year review. J Paediatric Child Health 36:428, 2000

Koren G, Florescu A, Costei AM, et al: Nonsteroidal antiinflammatory drugs during third trimester and the risk of premature closure of the ductus arteriosus: A meta-analysis. Ann Pharmacother 40(5):824, 2006

Lee KA, Williams B, Roza K, et al: PTPN11 analysis for the prenatal diagnosis of Noonan syndrome in fetuses with abnormal ultrasound findings. Clin Genet 75(2):190, 2009

Levine D, Barnes PD: Cortical maturation in normal and abnormal fetuses as assessed with prenatal MR imaging. Radiology 210:751, 1999a

Levine D, Barnes PD, Madsen JR, et al: Central nervous system abnormalities assessed with prenatal magnetic resonance imaging. Obstet Gynecol 94:1011, 1999b

Levine D, Hulka CA, Ludmir J, et al: Placenta accreta: Evaluation with color Doppler US, power Doppler US, and MR imaging. Radiology 205:773, 1997

Long A, Moran P, Robson S: Outcome of fetal cerebral posterior fossa anomalies. Prenat Diagn 26:707, 2006

Low JA: The current status of maternal and fetal blood flow velocimetry. Am J Obstet Gynecol 164:1049, 1991

Mahony BS, Nyberg DA, Hirsch JH, et al: Mild idiopathic lateral cerebral ventricular dilatation in utero: Sonographic evaluation. Radiology 169:715, 1988

Malone FD, Ball RH, Nyberg DA, et al: First-trimester septated cystic hygroma: Prevalence, natural history, and pediatric outcome. Obstet Gynecol 106:288, 2005

Mandell J, Blythe B, Peters C, et al: Structural genitourinary defects detected in utero. Radiology 178:193, 1991

Mari G, Abuhamad AZ, Uerpairojkit B, et al: Blood flow velocity waveforms of the abdominal arteries in appropriate- and small-for-gestational-age fetuses. Ultrasound Obstet Gynecol 6:15, 1995

Mari G, Deter RL, Carpenter RL, et al: Noninvasive diagnosis by Doppler ultrasonography of fetal anemia due to maternal red-cell alloimmunization. Collaborative group for Doppler assessment of the blood velocity in anemic fetuses. N Engl J Med 342:9, 2000

Mari G, Hanif F, Drennan K, et al: Staging of intrauterine growth-restricted fetuses. J Ultrasound Med 26:1469, 2007

Matsuoka S, Takeuchi K, Yamanaka Y, et al: Comparison of magnetic resonance imaging and ultrasonography in the prenatal diagnosis of congenital thoracic abnormalities. Fetal Diagn Ther 18:447, 2003

Michailidis GD, Economides DL, Schild RL: The role of three-dimensional ultrasound in obstetrics. Curr Opin Obstet Gynecol 13:207, 2001

Millener PB, Anderson NG, Chisholm RJ: Prognostic significance of nonvisualization of the fetal stomach by sonography. AJR Am J Roentgenol 160:827, 1993

Moore JW, Binder CA, Berry R: Prenatal diagnosis of aneuploidy and deletion 22q11.2 in fetuses with ultrasound detection of cardiac defects. Am J Obstet Gynecol 191(6):2068, 2004

National Institutes of Health: Diagnostic ultrasound imaging in pregnancy: Report of a consensus. NIH Publication 84-667, 1984

Nembhard WN, Waller DK, Sever LE, et al: Patterns of first-year survival among infants with selected congenital anomalies in Texas, 1995-1997. Teratology 64:267, 2001

North RA, Ferrier C, Long D, et al: Uterine artery Doppler flow velocity waveforms in the second trimester for the prediction of preeclampsia and fetal growth retardation. Obstet Gynecol 83:378, 1994

Paladini D, Russo M, Teodoro A, et al: Prenatal diagnosis of congenital heart disease in the Naples area during the years 1994–1999 – the experience of a joint fetal-pediatric cardiology unit. Prenatal Diagn 22(7):545, 2002

Phelan JP, Ahn MO, Smith CV, et al: Amnionic fluid index measurements during pregnancy. J Reprod Med 32:601, 1987

Pilu G: Ultrasound evaluation of the fetal neural axis. In Callen PW (ed), Ultrasonography in Obstetrics and Gynecology. Saunders Elsevier, 2008, p 366

Potter EL: Bilateral renal agenesis. J Pediatr 29:68, 1946

Poutamo J, Vanninen R, Partanen K, et al: Diagnosing fetal urinary tract abnormalities: Benefits of MRI compared to ultrasonography. Acta Obstet Gynecol Scand 79:63, 2000

Pretorius DH, Borok NN, Coffler MS, et al: Three-dimensional ultrasound in obstetrics and gynecology. Radiol Clin North Am 39:499, 2001

Pretorius DH, Drose JA, Dennis MA, et al: Tracheoesophageal fistula in utero: Twenty-two cases. J Ultrasound Med 6:509, 1987a

Pretorius DH, Lee ME, Manco-Johnson ML, et al: Diagnosis of autosomal dominant polycystic kidney disease in utero and in the young infant. J Ultrasound Med 6:249, 1987b

Puligandla PS, Janvier A, Flageole H, et al: The significance of intrauterine growth restriction is different from prematurity for the outcome of infants with gastroschisis. J Pediatr Surg 39:1200, 2004

Rabinowitz R, Peters MT, Vyas S, et al: Measurement of fetal urine production in normal pregnancy by real-time ultrasonography. Am J Obstet Gynecol 161:1264, 1989

Rados C: FDA cautions against ultrasound "keepsake" images. FDA Consumer Magazine 38(1):9, 2004

Rakic P: Ultrasound effects on fetal brains questioned. RSNA News 16(11):8, 2006

Reddy UM, Filly RA, Copel JA: Prenatal imaging: Ultrasonography and magnetic resonance imaging (current commentary). Obstet Gynecol 112:145, 2008

Robertson FM, Crombleholme TM, Paidas M, et al: Prenatal diagnosis and management of gastrointestinal disorders. Semin Perinatol 18:182, 1994

Santiago-Munoz PC, McIntire DD, Barber RG, et al: Outcomes of pregnancies with fetal gastroschisis. Obstet Gynecol 110:663, 2007

Segata M, Mari G: Fetal anemia: New technologies. Curr Opin Obstet Gynecol 16:153, 2004

Sezik M, Tuncay G, Yapar EG: Prediction of adverse neonatal outcomes in preeclampsia by absent or reversed end-diastolic flow velocity in the umbilical artery. Gynecol Obstet Invest 57:109, 2004

Shiota K, Yamada S, Komada M, et al: Research review: Embryogenesis of holoprosencephaly. Am J Med Genet 143A:3079, 2007

Shipp TD, Bromley B, Hornberger LK, et al: Levorotation of the fetal cardiac axis: A clue for the presence of congenital heart disease. Obstet Gynecol 85:97, 1995

Shulman LP, Emerson DS, Felker RE, et al: High frequency of cytogenetic abnormalities in fetuses with cystic hygroma diagnosed in the first trimester. Obstet Gynecol 80:80, 1992

Simon EM, Goldstein RB, Coakley FV, et al: Fast MR imaging of fetal CNS anomalies in utero. Am J Neuroradiol 21:1688, 2000

Smith RS, Comstock CH, Kirk JS, et al: Ultrasonographic left cardiac axis deviation: A marker for fetal anomalies. Obstet Gynecol 85:187, 1995

Souka AP, Pilalis A, Kavalakis I, et al: Screening for major structural abnormalities at the 11- to 14-week ultrasound scan. Am J Obstet Gynecol 194:393, 2006

Tilea B, Alberti C, Adamsbaum C, et al: Cerebral biometry in fetal magnetic resonance imaging: New reference data. Ultrasound Obstet Gynecol 33(2):173, 2009

Timor-Tritsch IE, Monteagudo A, Mayberry P: Three-dimensional ultrasound evaluation of the fetal brain: The three horn view. Ultrasound Obstet Gynecol 16:302, 2000

Trauffer PML, Anderson CE, Johnson A, et al: The natural history of euploid pregnancies with first-trimester cystic hygromas. Am J Obstet Gynecol 170:1279, 1994

Trudinger B: Editorial. Doppler: More or less? Ultrasound Obstet Gynecol 29:243, 2007

Turan OM, Turan S, Gungor S, et al: Progression of Doppler abnormalities in intrauterine growth restriction. Ultrasound Obstet Gynecol 32:160, 2008

Twickler DM, Lucas MJ, Balis AB, et al: Color flow mapping for myometrial invasion in women with a prior cesarean delivery. J Matern Fetal Med 9:330, 2000

Twickler DM, Magee KP, Caire J, et al: Second-opinion magnetic resonance imaging for suspected fetal central nervous system abnormalities. Am J Obstet Gynecol 188:492, 2003

Twickler DM, Reichel T, McIntire DD, et al: Fetal central nervous system ventricle and cisterna magna measurements by magnetic resonance imaging. Am J Obstet Gynecol 187:927, 2002

Vadeyar SH, Moore RJ, Strachan BK, et al: Effect of fetal magnetic resonance imaging on fetal heart rate patterns. Am J Obstet Gynecol 182:666, 2000

Vincoff NS, Callen PW, Smith-Bindman R, et al: Effect of ultrasound transducer frequency on the appearance of the fetal bowel. J Ultrasound Med 18:799, 1999

Walsh DS, Hubbard AM, Olutoye OO, et al: Assessment of fetal lung volumes and liver herniation with magnetic resonance imaging in congenital diaphragmatic hernia. Am J Obstet Gynecol 183:1067, 2000

Warshak CR, Eskander R, Hull AD, et al: Accuracy of ultrasonography and magnetic resonance imaging in the diagnosis of placenta accreta. Obstet Gynecol 108:573, 2006

Wenstrom KD, Weiner CP, Williamson RA: Diverse maternal and fetal pathology associated with absent diastolic flow in the umbilical artery of high-risk fetuses. Obstet Gynecol 77:374, 1991

Wilson R, Lynch S, Lessoway V: Fetal pyelectasis: Comparison of postnatal renal pathology with unilateral and bilateral pyelectasis. Prenat Diagn 17:451, 1997

Wiskirchen J, Groenewaeller EF, Kehlbach R, et al: Long-term effects of repetitive exposure to a static magnetic field 1.5 T on proliferation of human fetal lung fibroblasts. Magn Reson Med 41:464, 1999

Worley KC, Dashe JS, Oliver Q, et al: Magnetic resonance imaging as a predictor of outcome in fetuses with isolated congenital diaphragmatic hernia. Am J Obstet Gynecol 200:318.e1, 2009

Wyldes M, Watkinson M: Isolated mild fetal ventriculomegaly. Arch Dis Child Fetal Neonatal Ed 89:F9, 2004

Yamamura Y, Swartout JP, Anderson EA, et al: Management of mild fetal pyelectasis: A comparative analysis. J Ultrasound Med 26:1539, 2007

Zaretsky M, Ramus R, McIntire D, et al: MRI calculation of lung volumes to predict outcome in fetuses with genitourinary abnormalities. AJR Am J Roentgenol 185:1328, 2005a

Zaretsky MV, Alexander JM, McIntire DD, et al: Magnetic resonance imaging pelvimetry and the prediction of labor dystocia. Obstet Gynecol 106:919, 2005b

Zaretsky MV, McIntire DD, Twickler DM: Feasibility of the fetal anatomic and maternal pelvic survey by magnetic resonance imaging at term. Am J Obstet Gynecol 189:997, 2003a

Zaretsky MV, Ramus RM, Twickler DM: Single uterine fast acquisition magnetic resonance fetal surgery: Is it feasible? J Matern Fetal Neonatal Med 14:107, 2003b

Zaretsky M, Reichel TF, McIntire D, et al: Comparison of magnetic resonance imaging to ultrasound in the estimation of birth weight at term. Am J Obstet Gynecol 189:1017, 2003c

Zaretsky MV, Twickler DM: Magnetic imaging in obstetrics. Clin Obstet Gynecol 46:868, 2003d

Zeeman GG, McIntire DD, Twickler DM: Maternal and fetal artery Doppler findings in women with chronic hypertension who subsequently develop superimposed pre-eclampsia. J Matern Fetal Neonatal Med 14:318, 2003

LABOR AND DELIVERY

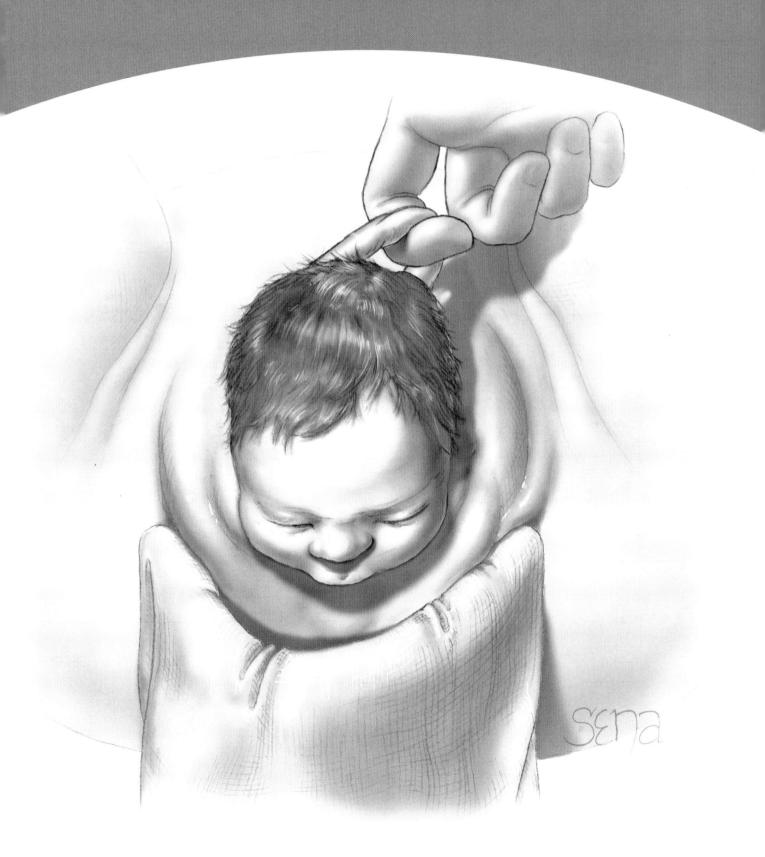

CHAPTER 17

Normal Labor and Delivery

Childbirth is the period from the onset of regular uterine contractions until expulsion of the placenta. The process by which this normally occurs is called *labor*—a term that in the obstetrical context takes on several connotations from the English language. According to the *New Shorter Oxford English Dictionary* (1993), toil, trouble, suffering, bodily exertion, especially when painful, and an outcome of work are all characteristics of *labor* and thus implicated in the process of childbirth. Such connotations all seem appropriate to us and emphasize the need for all attendants to be supportive of the laboring woman's needs, particularly in regard to effective pain relief.

At Parkland Hospital in 2007, only 50 percent of 13,991 women with singleton cephalic presentations at term had a spontaneous labor and delivery. The remainder had ineffective labor requiring augmentation, had other medical and obstetrical complications requiring induction of labor, or underwent cesarean delivery. It seems excessive to consider 50 percent of parturients as "abnormal" because they did not spontaneously labor and deliver. Hence, the distinction between normal and abnormal is often subjective. This high prevalence of labor abnormalities, however, can be used to underscore the importance of labor events in the successful outcome of pregnancy.

MECHANISMS OF LABOR

At the onset of labor, the position of the fetus with respect to the birth canal is critical to the route of delivery. Thus, fetal position

within the uterine cavity should be determined at the onset of labor.

Fetal Lie, Presentation, Attitude, and Position

Fetal orientation relative to the maternal pelvis is described in terms of fetal lie, presentation, attitude, and position.

Fetal Lie

The relation of the fetal long axis to that of the mother is termed *fetal lie* and is either *longitudinal* or *transverse*. Occasionally, the fetal and the maternal axes may cross at a 45-degree angle, forming an *oblique lie*, which is unstable and always becomes longitudinal or transverse during labor. A longitudinal lie is present in greater than 99 percent of labors at term. Predisposing factors for transverse lies include multiparity, placenta previa, hydramnios, and uterine anomalies (see Chap. 20, p. 476).

Fetal Presentation

The *presenting part* is that portion of the fetal body that is either foremost within the birth canal or in closest proximity to it. It can be felt through the cervix on vaginal examination. Accordingly, in longitudinal lies, the presenting part is either the fetal head or breech, creating *cephalic* and *breech presentations*, respectively. When the fetus lies with the long axis transversely, the *shoulder* is the presenting part and is felt through the cervix on vaginal examination. Table 17-1 describes the incidences of the various fetal presentations.

Cephalic Presentation. Such presentations are classified according to the relationship between the head and body of the fetus (Fig. 17-1). Ordinarily, the head is flexed sharply so that the chin is in contact with the thorax. The occipital fontanel is the presenting part, and this presentation is referred to as a *vertex* or *occiput presentation*. Much less commonly, the fetal neck may be sharply extended so that the occiput and back come in contact,

TABLE 17-1. Fetal Presentation in 68,097 Singleton Pregnancies at Parkland Hospital

Presentation	Percent	Incidence
Cephalic	96.8	—
Breech	2.7	1:36
Transverse lie	0.3	1:335
Compound	0.1	1:1000
Face	0.5	1:2000
Brow	0.01	1:10,000

and the face is foremost in the birth canal—*face presentation* (see Fig. 20-6, p. 474). The fetal head may assume a position between these extremes, partially flexed in some cases, with the anterior (large) fontanel, or bregma, presenting—*sinciput presentation*—or partially extended in other cases, to have a *brow presentation* (see Fig. 20-8, p. 476). These latter two presentations are usually transient. As labor progresses, sinciput and brow presentations almost always convert into vertex or face presentations by neck flexion or extension, respectively. Failure to do so can lead to dystocia, as discussed in Chapter 20 (p. 476).

The term fetus usually presents with the vertex, most logically because the uterus is piriform or pear shaped. Although the fetal head at term is slightly larger than the breech, the entire *podalic pole* of the fetus—that is, the breech and its flexed extremities—is bulkier and more mobile than the cephalic pole. The *cephalic pole* is composed of the fetal head only. Until approximately 32 weeks, the amnionic cavity is large compared with the fetal mass, and there is no crowding of the fetus by the uterine walls. Subsequently, however, the ratio of amnionic fluid volume decreases relative to the increasing fetal mass. As a result, the uterine walls are apposed more closely to the fetal parts.

If presenting by the breech, the fetus often changes polarity to make use of the roomier fundus for its bulkier and more mobile podalic pole. As discussed in Chapter 24 (p. 527 and Fig. 24-1), the incidence of breech presentation decreases with gestational age. It is approximately 25 percent at 28 weeks, 17 percent at 30 weeks, 11 percent at 32 weeks, and then decreases to approximately 3 percent at term. The high incidence of breech presentation in hydrocephalic fetuses is in accord with this theory, because in this circumstance, the fetal cephalic pole is larger than its podalic pole.

Breech Presentation. When the fetus presents as a breech, the three general configurations are *frank, complete,* and *footling presentations* and are described in Chapter 24 (p. 527). Breech presentation may result from circumstances that prevent normal version from taking place,

for example, a septum that protrudes into the uterine cavity (see Chap. 40, p. 897). A peculiarity of fetal attitude, particularly extension of the vertebral column as seen in frank breeches, also may prevent the fetus from turning. If the placenta is implanted in the lower uterine segment, it may distort normal intrauterine anatomy and result in a breech presentation.

Fetal Attitude or Posture

In the later months of pregnancy the fetus assumes a characteristic posture described as attitude or habitus (see Fig. 17-1). As a rule, the fetus forms an ovoid mass that corresponds roughly to the shape of the uterine cavity. The fetus becomes folded or bent upon itself in such a manner that the back becomes markedly convex; the head is sharply flexed so that the chin is almost in contact with the chest; the thighs are flexed over the abdomen; and the legs are bent at the knees. In all cephalic presentations, the arms are usually crossed over the thorax or become parallel to the sides. The umbilical cord lies in the space between them and the lower extremities. This characteristic posture results from the mode of fetal growth and its accommodation to the uterine cavity.

Abnormal exceptions to this attitude occur as the fetal head becomes progressively more extended from the vertex to the face presentation (see Fig. 17-1). This results in a progressive change in fetal attitude from a convex (flexed) to a concave (extended) contour of the vertebral column.

Fetal Position

Position refers to the relationship of an arbitrarily chosen portion of the fetal presenting part to the right or left side of the birth canal. Accordingly, with each presentation there may be two positions—right or left. The fetal occiput, chin (mentum), and sacrum are the determining points in vertex, face, and breech presentations, respectively (Figs. 17-2 to 17-6). Because the presenting part may be in either the left or right position, there are left and right occipital, left and right mental, and left and right sacral presentations, abbreviated as LO and RO, LM and RM, and LS and RS, respectively.

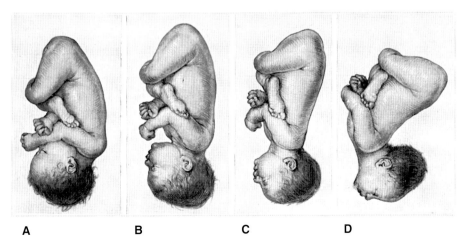

A   **B**   **C**   **D**

FIGURE 17-1 Longitudinal lie. Cephalic presentation. Differences in attitude of the fetal body in **(A)** vertex, **(B)** sinciput, **(C)** brow, and **(D)** face presentations. Note changes in fetal attitude in relation to fetal vertex as the fetal head becomes less flexed.

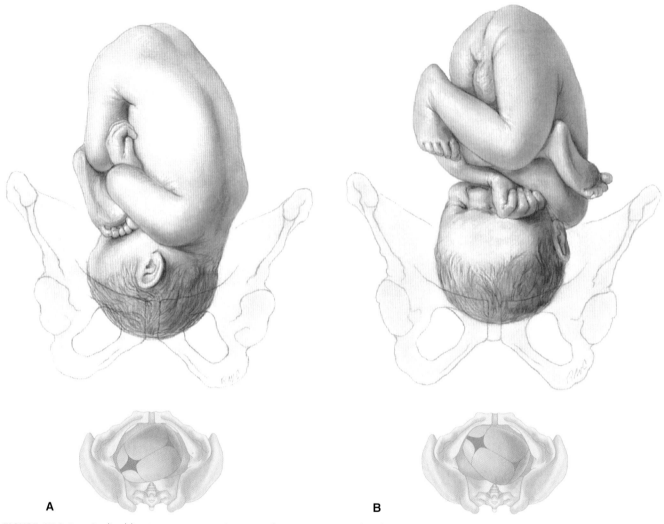

FIGURE 17-2 Longitudinal lie. Vertex presentation. **A.** Left occiput anterior (LOA). **B.** Left occiput posterior (LOP).

Varieties of Presentations and Positions

For still more accurate orientation, the relationship of a given portion of the presenting part to the anterior, transverse, or posterior portion of the maternal pelvis is considered. Because the presenting part in right or left positions may be directed anteriorly (A), transversely (T), or posteriorly (P), there are six varieties of each of the three presentations (see Figs. 17-2 to 17-6). Thus, in an occiput presentation, the presentation, position, and variety may be abbreviated in clockwise fashion as:

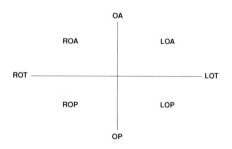

Approximately two thirds of all vertex presentations are in the left occiput position, and one third in the right.

In shoulder presentations, the acromion (scapula) is the portion of the fetus arbitrarily chosen for orientation with the maternal pelvis. One example of the terminology sometimes employed for this purpose is illustrated in Figure 17-7. The acromion or back of the fetus may be directed either posteriorly or anteriorly and superiorly or inferiorly (see Chap. 20, p. 476). Because it is impossible to differentiate exactly the several varieties of shoulder presentation by clinical examination and because such differentiation serves no practical purpose, it is customary to refer to all transverse lies simply as *shoulder presentations.* Another term used is *transverse lie,* with *back up* or *back down.*

Diagnosis of Fetal Presentation and Position

Several methods can be used to diagnose fetal presentation and position. These include abdominal palpation, vaginal examination, auscultation, and, in certain doubtful cases, sonography. Occasionally plain radiographs, computed tomography, or magnetic resonance imaging may be used.

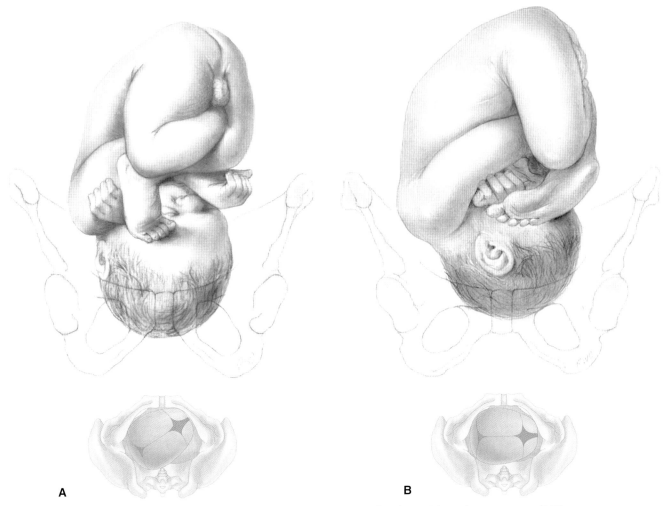

FIGURE 17-3 Longitudinal lie. Vertex presentation. **A**. Right occiput posterior (ROP). **B**. Right occiput transverse (ROT).

Abdominal Palpation—Leopold Maneuvers

Abdominal examination can be conducted systematically employing the four maneuvers described by Leopold in 1894 and shown in Figure 17-8. The mother lies supine and comfortably positioned with her abdomen bared. These maneuvers may be difficult if not impossible to perform and interpret if the patient is obese, if there is excessive amnionic fluid, or if the placenta is anteriorly implanted.

1. The first maneuver permits identification of which fetal pole—that is, cephalic or podalic—occupies the uterine fundus. The breech gives the sensation of a large, nodular mass, whereas the head feels hard and round and is more mobile and ballottable
2. Performed after determination of fetal lie, the second maneuver is accomplished as the palms are placed on either side of the maternal abdomen, and gentle but deep pressure is exerted. On one side, a hard, resistant structure is felt—the back. On the other, numerous small, irregular, mobile parts are felt—the fetal extremities. By noting whether the back is directed anteriorly, transversely, or posteriorly, the orientation of the fetus can be determined

3. The third maneuver is performed by grasping with the thumb and fingers of one hand the lower portion of the maternal abdomen just above the symphysis pubis. If the presenting part is not engaged, a movable mass will be felt, usually the head. The differentiation between head and breech is made as in the first maneuver. If the presenting part is deeply engaged, however, the findings from this maneuver are simply indicative that the lower fetal pole is in the pelvis, and details are then defined by the fourth maneuver
4. To perform the fourth maneuver, the examiner faces the mother's feet and, with the tips of the first three fingers of each hand, exerts deep pressure in the direction of the axis of the pelvic inlet. In many instances, when the head has descended into the pelvis, the anterior shoulder may be differentiated readily by the third maneuver.

Abdominal palpation can be performed throughout the latter months of pregnancy and during and between the contractions of labor. With experience, it is possible to estimate the size of the fetus. According to Lydon-Rochelle and colleagues (1993), experienced clinicians accurately identify fetal malpresentation using Leopold maneuvers with a high sensitivity—88

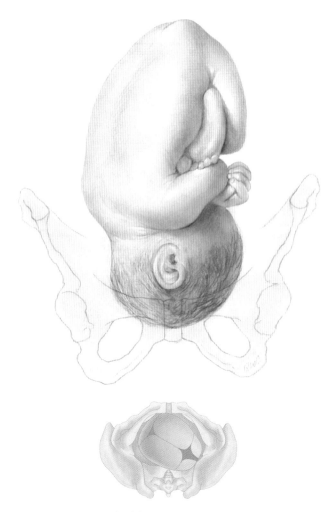

FIGURE 17-4 Longitudinal lie. Vertex presentation. Right occiput anterior (ROA).

percent, specificity—94 percent, positive-predictive value—74 percent, and negative-predictive value—97 percent.

Vaginal Examination

Before labor, the diagnosis of fetal presentation and position by vaginal examination is often inconclusive because the presenting part must be palpated through a closed cervix and lower uterine segment. With the onset of labor and after cervical dilatation, vertex presentations and their positions are recognized by palpation of the various fetal sutures and fontanels. Face and breech presentations are identified by palpation of the facial features and the fetal sacrum, respectively.

In attempting to determine presentation and position by vaginal examination, it is advisable to pursue a definite routine, comprising four movements:

1. The examiner inserts two fingers into the vagina and the presenting part is found. Differentiation of vertex, face, and breech is then accomplished readily
2. If the vertex is presenting, the fingers are directed posteriorly and then swept forward over the fetal head toward the maternal symphysis (**Fig. 17-9**). During this

movement, the fingers necessarily cross the sagittal suture and its course is delineated
3. The positions of the two fontanels then are ascertained. The fingers are passed to the most anterior extension of the sagittal suture, and the fontanel encountered there is examined and identified. Then, with a sweeping motion, the fingers pass along the suture to the other end of the head until the other fontanel is felt and differentiated (**Fig. 17-10**)
4. The station, or extent to which the presenting part has descended into the pelvis, can also be established at this time (see p. 392). Using these maneuvers, the various sutures and fontanels are located readily (see Fig. 4-9, p. 84).

Sonography and Radiography

Sonographic techniques can aid identification of fetal position, especially in obese women or in women with rigid abdominal walls. In some clinical situations, information obtained radiographically justifies the minimal risk from a single x-ray exposure (see Chap. 41, p. 915). Zahalka and colleagues (2005) compared digital examinations with transvaginal and transabdominal sonography for determination of fetal head position during second-stage labor and reported that transvaginal sonography was superior.

Mechanisms of Labor with Occiput Anterior Presentation

In most cases, the vertex enters the pelvis with the sagittal suture lying in the transverse pelvic diameter. The fetus enters the pelvis in the *left occiput transverse (LOT)* position in 40 percent of labors and in the *right occiput transverse (ROT)* position in 20 percent (Caldwell and associates, 1934). In *occiput anterior positions—LOA or ROA*—the head either enters the pelvis with the occiput rotated 45 degrees anteriorly from the transverse position, or subsequently does so. The mechanism of labor in all these presentations is usually similar.

The positional changes in the presenting part required to navigate the pelvic canal constitute the *mechanisms of labor*. The *cardinal movements of labor* are engagement, descent, flexion, internal rotation, extension, external rotation, and expulsion (**Fig. 17-11**). During labor, these movements not only are sequential but also show great temporal overlap. For example, as part of engagement, there is both flexion and descent of the head. It is impossible for the movements to be completed unless the presenting part descends simultaneously. Concomitantly, uterine contractions effect important modifications in fetal attitude, or habitus, especially after the head has descended into the pelvis. These changes consist principally of fetal straightening, with loss of dorsal convexity and closer application of the extremities to the body. As a result, the fetal ovoid is transformed into a cylinder, with the smallest possible cross section typically passing through the birth canal.

Engagement

The mechanism by which the biparietal diameter—the greatest transverse diameter in an occiput presentation—passes through the pelvic inlet is designated *engagement*. The fetal head may

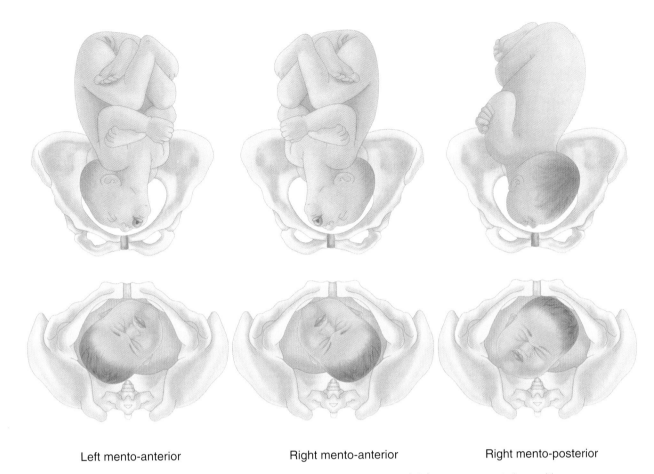

Left mento-anterior   Right mento-anterior   Right mento-posterior

FIGURE 17-5 Longitudinal lie. Face presentation. Left and right mentum anterior and right mentum posterior positions.

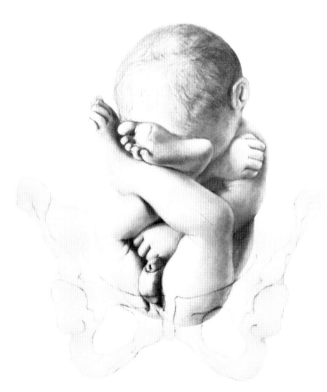

FIGURE 17-6 Longitudinal lie. Breech presentation. Left sacrum posterior (LSP).

engage during the last few weeks of pregnancy or not until after labor commencement. In many multiparous and some nulliparous women, the fetal head is freely movable above the pelvic inlet at labor onset. In this circumstance, the head is sometimes referred to as "floating." A normal-sized head usually does not engage with its sagittal suture directed anteroposteriorly. Instead, the fetal head usually enters the pelvic inlet either transversely or obliquely.

Asynclitism. Although the fetal head tends to accommodate to the transverse axis of the pelvic inlet, the sagittal suture, while remaining parallel to that axis, may not lie exactly midway between the symphysis and the sacral promontory. The sagittal suture frequently is deflected either posteriorly toward the promontory or anteriorly toward the symphysis (Fig. 17-12). Such lateral deflection to a more anterior or posterior position in the pelvis is called *asynclitism*. If the sagittal suture approaches the sacral promontory, more of the anterior parietal bone presents itself to the examining fingers, and the condition is called *anterior asynclitism*. If, however, the sagittal suture lies close to the symphysis, more of the posterior parietal bone will present, and the condition is called *posterior asynclitism*. With extreme posterior asynclitism, the posterior ear may be easily palpated.

Moderate degrees of asynclitism are the rule in normal labor. However, if severe, the condition is a common reason for cephalopelvic disproportion even with an otherwise normal-sized

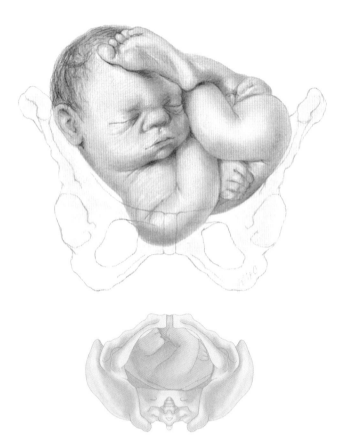

FIGURE 17-7 Transverse lie. Right acromiodorsoposterior (RADP). The shoulder of the fetus is to the mother's right, and the back is posterior.

pelvis. Successive shifting from posterior to anterior asynclitism aids descent.

Descent

This movement is the first requisite for birth of the newborn. In nulliparas, engagement may take place before the onset of labor, and further descent may not follow until the onset of the second stage. In multiparous women, descent usually begins with engagement. Descent is brought about by one or more of four forces: (1) pressure of the amnionic fluid, (2) direct pressure of the fundus upon the breech with contractions, (3) bearing-down efforts of maternal abdominal muscles, and (4) extension and straightening of the fetal body.

Flexion

As soon as the descending head meets resistance, whether from the cervix, walls of the pelvis, or pelvic floor, then flexion of the head normally results. In this movement, the chin is brought into more intimate contact with the fetal thorax, and the appreciably shorter suboccipitobregmatic diameter is substituted for the longer occipitofrontal diameter (Figs. 17-13 and 17-14).

Internal Rotation

This movement consists of a turning of the head in such a manner that the occiput gradually moves toward the symphysis

pubis anteriorly from its original position or less commonly, posteriorly toward the hollow of the sacrum (Figs. 17-15, 17-16, and 17-17). Internal rotation is essential for the completion of labor, except when the fetus is unusually small.

Calkins (1939) studied more than 5000 women in labor to the time of internal rotation. He concluded that in approximately two thirds, internal rotation is completed by the time the head reaches the pelvic floor; in about another fourth, internal rotation is completed very shortly after the head reaches the pelvic floor; and in the remaining 5 percent, anterior rotation does not take place. When the head fails to turn until reaching the pelvic floor, it typically rotates during the next one or two contractions in multiparas. In nulliparas, rotation usually occurs during the next three to five contractions.

Extension

After internal rotation, the sharply flexed head reaches the vulva and undergoes extension. If the sharply flexed head, on reaching the pelvic floor, did not extend but was driven farther downward, it would impinge on the posterior portion of the perineum and would eventually be forced through the tissues of the perineum. When the head presses upon the pelvic floor, however, two forces come into play. The first force, exerted by the uterus, acts more posteriorly, and the second, supplied by the resistant pelvic floor and the symphysis, acts more anteriorly. The resultant vector is in the direction of the vulvar opening, thereby causing head extension. This brings the base of the occiput into direct contact with the inferior margin of the symphysis pubis (see Fig. 17-16).

With progressive distension of the perineum and vaginal opening, an increasingly larger portion of the occiput gradually appears. The head is born as the occiput, bregma, forehead, nose, mouth, and finally the chin pass successively over the anterior margin of the perineum (see Fig. 17-17). Immediately after its delivery, the head drops downward so that the chin lies over the maternal anus.

External Rotation

The delivered head next undergoes *restitution* (see Fig. 17-11). If the occiput was originally directed toward the left, it rotates toward the left ischial tuberosity. If it was originally directed toward the right, the occiput rotates to the right. Restitution of the head to the oblique position is followed by completion of external rotation to the transverse position. This movement corresponds to rotation of the fetal body and serves to bring its bisacromial diameter into relation with the anteroposterior diameter of the pelvic outlet. Thus, one shoulder is anterior behind the symphysis and the other is posterior. This movement apparently is brought about by the same pelvic factors that produced internal rotation of the head.

Expulsion

Almost immediately after external rotation, the anterior shoulder appears under the symphysis pubis, and the perineum soon becomes distended by the posterior shoulder. After delivery of the shoulders, the rest of the body quickly passes.

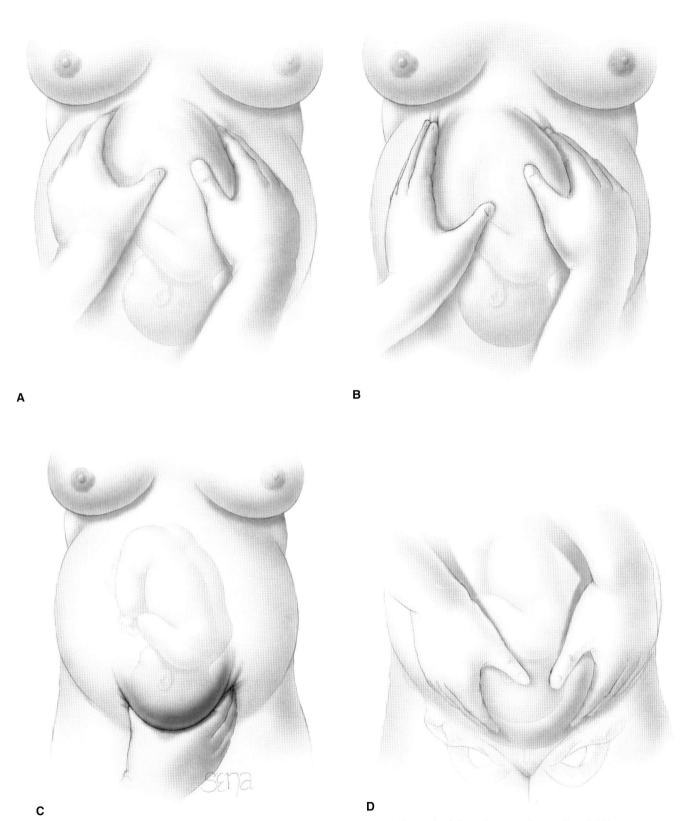

A

B

C

D

FIGURE 17-8 Leopold maneuvers (**A-D**) performed in fetus with a longitudinal lie in the left occiput anterior position (LOA).

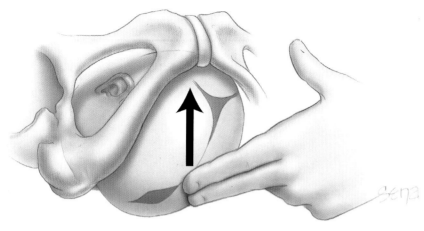

FIGURE 17-9 Locating the sagittal suture by vaginal examination.

immediately over the cervical os becomes edematous (see Fig. 29-12, p. 635). This swelling known as the *caput succedaneum* (Figs. 17-18 and 17-19). It usually attains a thickness of only a few millimeters, but in prolonged labors it may be sufficiently extensive to prevent the differentiation of the various sutures and fontanels. More commonly, the caput is formed when the head is in the lower portion of the birth canal and frequently only after the resistance of a rigid vaginal outlet is encountered. Because it develops over the most dependent area of the head, one may deduce the original fetal head position by noting the location of the caput succedaneum.

Mechanisms of Labor with Occiput Posterior Presentation

In approximately 20 percent of labors, the fetus enters the pelvis in an *occiput posterior (OP)* position. The right occiput posterior (ROP) is slightly more common than the left (LOP) (Caldwell and associates, 1934). It appears likely from radiographic evidence that posterior positions are more often associated with a narrow forepelvis. They also are more commonly seen in association with anterior placentation (Gardberg and Tuppurainen, 1994a).

In most occiput posterior presentations, the mechanism of labor is identical to that observed in the transverse and anterior varieties, except that the occiput has to internally rotate to the symphysis pubis through 135 degrees, instead of 90 and 45 degrees, respectively (see Fig. 17-17).

With effective contractions, adequate flexion of the head, and a fetus of average size, most posteriorly positioned occiputs rotate promptly as soon as they reach the pelvic floor, and labor is not lengthened appreciably. In perhaps 5 to 10 percent of cases, however, rotation may be incomplete or may not take place at all, especially if the fetus is large (Gardberg and Tuppurainen, 1994b). Poor contractions, faulty flexion of the head, or epidural analgesia, which diminishes abdominal muscular pushing and relaxes the muscles of the pelvic floor, may predispose to incomplete rotation. If rotation is incomplete, transverse arrest may result. If no rotation toward the symphysis takes place, the occiput may remain in the direct occiput posterior position, a condition known as *persistent occiput posterior*. Both persistent occiput posterior and transverse arrest represent deviations from the normal mechanisms of labor and are considered further in Chapter 20.

Changes in Shape of the Fetal Head

Caput Succedaneum

In vertex presentations, the fetal head changes shape as the result of labor forces. In prolonged labors before complete cervical dilatation, the portion of the fetal scalp

Molding

The change in fetal head shape from external compressive forces is referred to as *molding*. Possibly related to Braxton Hicks contractions, some molding develops before labor. Most studies indicate that there is seldom overlapping of the parietal bones. A "locking" mechanism at the coronal and lambdoidal connections actually prevents such overlapping (Carlan and colleagues, 1991). Molding results in a shortened suboccipitobregmatic diameter and a lengthened mentovertical diameter. These changes are of greatest importance in women with contracted pelves or asynclitic presentations. In these circumstances, the degree to which the head is capable of molding may make the difference between spontaneous vaginal delivery and an operative delivery. Some older literature cited severe head molding as a cause for possible cerebral trauma. Because of the multitude of associated factors, for example, prolonged labor with fetal sepsis and acidosis, it is impossible to link molding to any alleged fetal or neonatal neurological sequelae. Most cases of molding resolve within the week following delivery, although persistent cases have been described (Graham and Kumar, 2006).

CHARACTERISTICS OF NORMAL LABOR

The greatest impediment to understanding normal labor is recognizing its start. The strict definition of labor—*uterine contractions that bring about demonstrable effacement and dilatation*

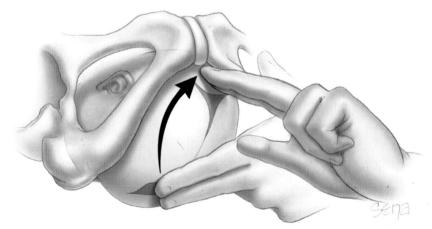

FIGURE 17-10 Differentiating the fontanels by vaginal examination.

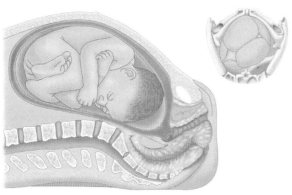

1. Head floating, before engagement

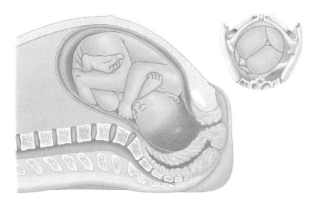

2. Engagement, descent, flexion

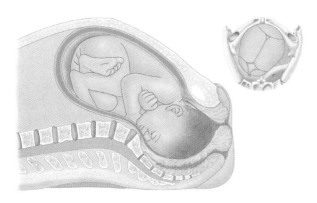

3. Further descent, internal rotation

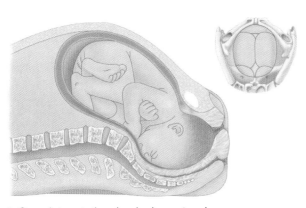

4. Complete rotation, beginning extension

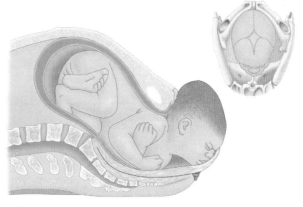

5. Complete extension

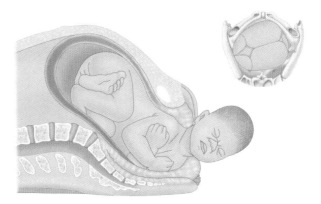

6. Restitution (external rotation)

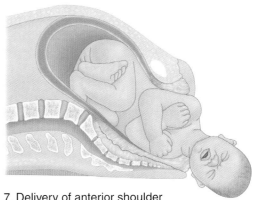

7. Delivery of anterior shoulder

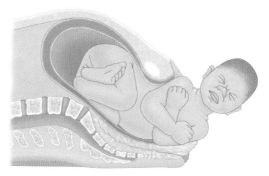

8. Delivery of posterior shoulder

FIGURE 17-11 Cardinal movements of labor and delivery from a left occiput anterior position.

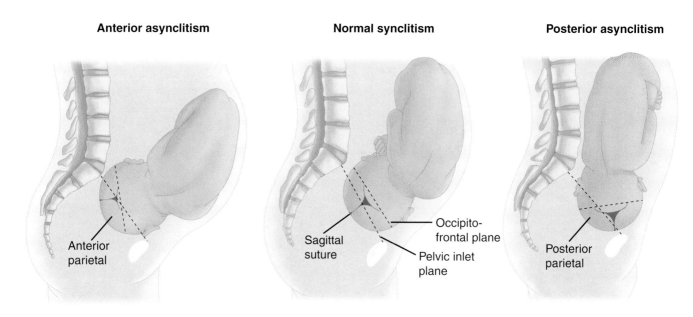

Anterior asynclitism   **Normal synclitism**   **Posterior asynclitism**

Anterior parietal — Sagittal suture — Occipito-frontal plane — Pelvic inlet plane — Posterior parietal

FIGURE 17-12 Synclitism and asynclitism.

of the cervix—does not easily aid the clinician in determining when labor has actually begun, because this diagnosis is confirmed only retrospectively. Several methods may be used to define its start. One defines onset as the clock time when painful contractions become regular. Unfortunately, uterine activity that causes discomfort, but that does not represent true labor, may develop at any time during pregnancy. False labor often stops spontaneously, or it may proceed rapidly into effective contractions.

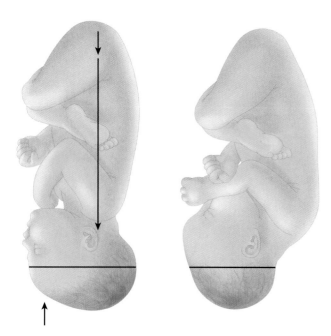

FIGURE 17-13 Lever action produces flexion of the head. Conversion from occipitofrontal to suboccipitobregmatic diameter typically reduces the anteroposterior diameter from nearly 12 to 9.5 cm.

A second method defines the onset of labor as beginning at the time of admission to the labor unit. At the National Maternity Hospital in Dublin, efforts have been made to codify admission criteria (O'Driscoll and colleagues, 1984). These criteria at term require painful uterine contractions accompanied by any one of the following: (1) ruptured membranes, (2) bloody "show," or (3) complete cervical effacement.

In the United States, admission for labor is frequently based on the extent of dilatation accompanied by painful contractions. When a woman presents with intact membranes, a cervical dilatation of 3 to 4 cm or greater is presumed to be a reasonably reliable threshold for the diagnosis of labor. In this case, labor onset commences with the time of admission. This presumptive method obviates many of the uncertainties in diagnosing labor during earlier stages of cervical dilatation.

First Stage of Labor

Assuming that the diagnosis has been confirmed, then what are the expectations for the progress of normal labor? A scientific approach was begun by Friedman (1954), who described a characteristic sigmoid pattern for labor by graphing cervical dilatation against time. This graphic approach, based on statistical observations, changed labor management. Friedman developed the concept of three functional divisions of labor to describe the physiological objectives of each division as shown in Figure 17-20:

1. During the *preparatory division,* although the cervix dilates little, its connective tissue components change considerably (see Chap. 6, p. 138). Sedation and conduction analgesia are capable of arresting this division of labor.
2. The *dilatational division,* during which dilatation proceeds at its most rapid rate, is unaffected by sedation or conduction analgesia.
3. The *pelvic division* commences with the deceleration phase of cervical dilatation. The classic mechanisms of labor that

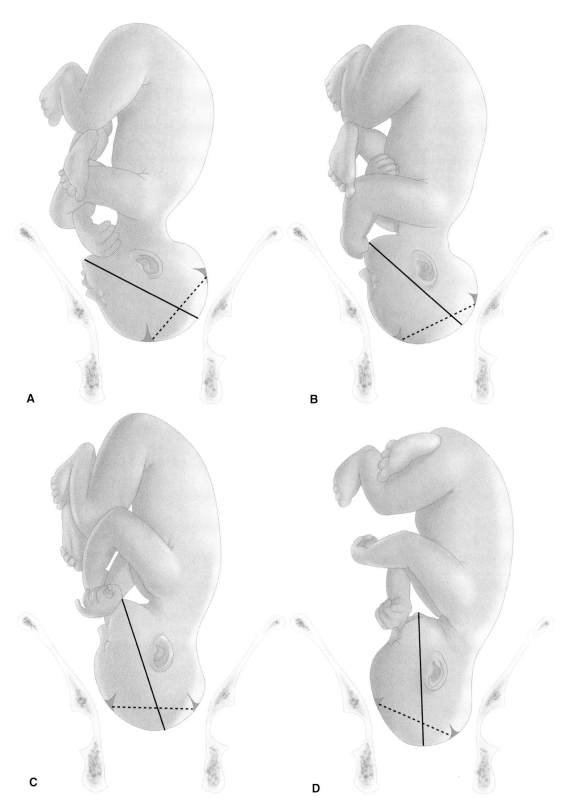

FIGURE 17-14 Four degrees of head flexion. The solid line represents the occipitomental diameter, whereas the broken line connects the center of the anterior fontanel with the posterior fontanel. **A.** Flexion poor. **B.** Flexion moderate. **C.** Flexion advanced. **D.** Flexion complete. Note that with complete flexion, the chin is on the chest. The suboccipitobregmatic diameter, the shortest anteroposterior diameter of the fetal head, is passing through the pelvic inlet.

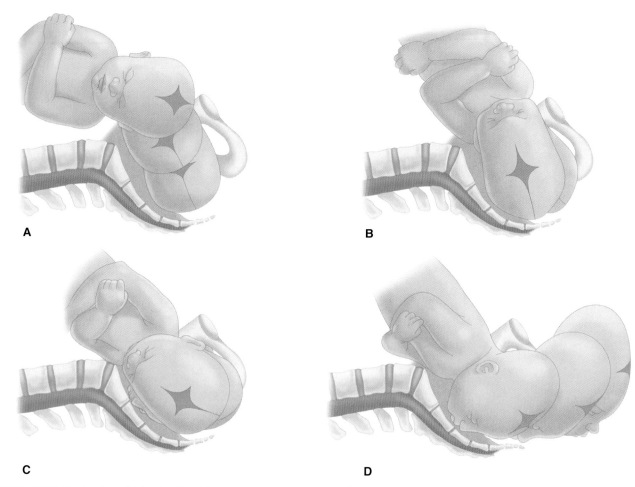

FIGURE 17-15 Mechanism of labor for the left occiput transverse position, lateral view. **A.** Engagement. **B.** Posterior asynclitism at the pelvic brim followed by lateral flexion. **C.** After engagement, further descent. **D.** Rotation and extension.

involve the cardinal fetal movements of the cephalic presentation—engagement, flexion, descent, internal rotation, extension, and external rotation—take place principally during the pelvic division. In actual practice, however, the onset of the pelvic division is seldom clearly identifiable.

As shown in Figure 17-20, the pattern of cervical dilatation during the preparatory and dilatational divisions of normal labor is a sigmoid curve. Two phases of cervical dilatation are defined. The *latent phase* corresponds to the preparatory division, and the *active phase,* to the dilatational division. Friedman subdivided the active phase into the *acceleration phase,* the *phase of maximum slope,* and the *deceleration phase* (Fig. 17-21).

Latent Phase

The onset of latent labor, as defined by Friedman (1972), is the point at which the mother perceives regular contractions. The latent phase for most women ends at between 3 and 5 cm of dilatation. This threshold may be clinically useful, for it defines cervical dilatation limits beyond which active labor can be expected.

This concept of a latent phase has great significance in understanding normal human labor because labor is considerably longer when a latent phase is included. To better illustrate this,

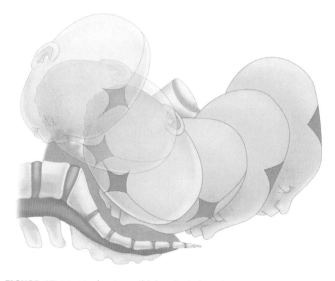

FIGURE 17-16 Mechanism of labor for left occiput anterior position.

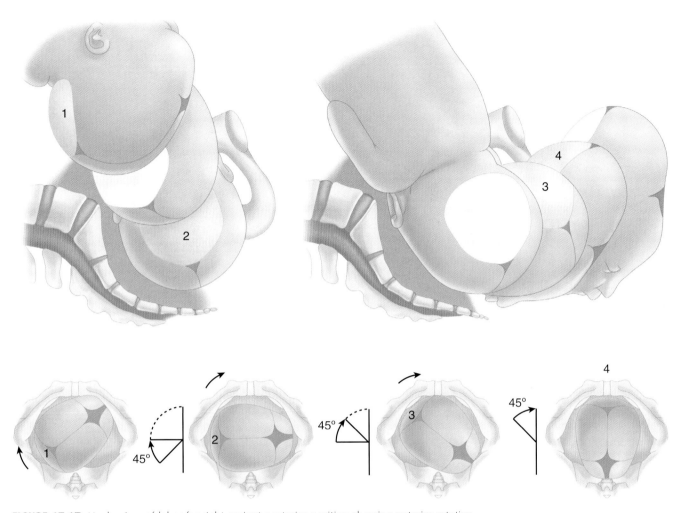

FIGURE 17-17 Mechanism of labor for right occiput posterior position showing anterior rotation.

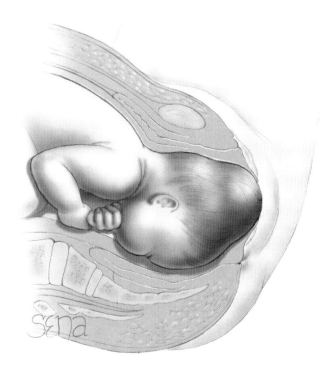

FIGURE 17-18 Formation of caput succedaneum.

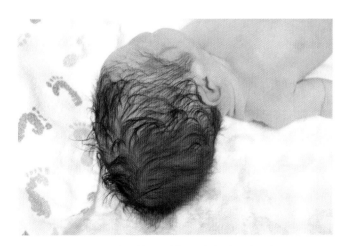

FIGURE 17-19 Considerable molding of the head and caput succedaneum formation in a recently delivered newborn.

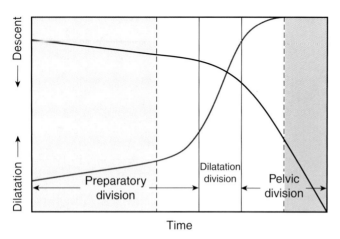

FIGURE 17-20 Labor course divided functionally on the basis of dilatation and descent curves into: (1) a preparatory division, including latent and acceleration phases; (2) a dilatational division, occupying the phase of maximum slope; and (3) a pelvic division, encompassing both deceleration phase and second stage concurrent with the phase of maximum slope of descent. (Courtesy of Dr. L. Casey; redrawn from Friedman, 1978.)

Figure 17-22 shows eight labor curves from nulliparas in whom labor was diagnosed beginning with their admission, rather than with the onset of regular contractions. When labor is defined similarly, there is remarkable similarity of individual labor curves.

Prolonged Latent Phase. Friedman and Sachtleben (1963) defined this by a latent phase exceeding 20 hours in the nullipara and 14 hours in the multipara. These times corresponded to the 95th percentiles. Factors that affected duration of the latent phase included excessive sedation or epidural analgesia;

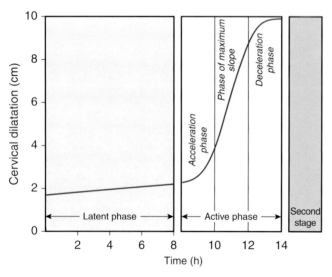

FIGURE 17-21 Composite of the average dilatation curve for nulliparous labor. The first stage is divided into a relatively flat latent phase and a rapidly progressive active phase. In the active phase, there are three identifiable component parts that include an acceleration phase, a phase of maximum slope, and a deceleration phase. (Courtesy of Dr. L. Casey; redrawn from Friedman, 1978.)

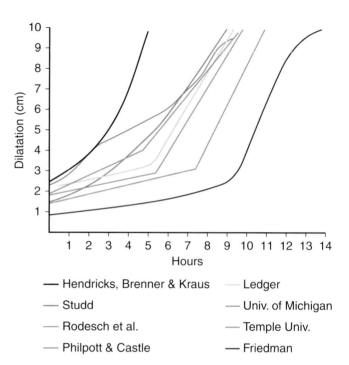

— Hendricks, Brenner & Kraus	⋯ Ledger
— Studd	— Univ. of Michigan
— Rodesch et al.	— Temple Univ.
— Philpott & Castle	— Friedman

FIGURE 17-22 Progress of labor in primigravid women from the time of admission. When the starting point on the abscissa begins with admission to the hospital, a latent phase is not observed.

unfavorable cervical condition, that is, thick, uneffaced, or undilated; and false labor. Following heavy sedation, 85 percent of women progressed to active labor. In another 10 percent, uterine contractions ceased, suggesting that they had false labor. The remaining 5 percent experienced persistence of an abnormal latent phase and required oxytocin stimulation. Amniotomy was discouraged because of the 10-percent incidence of false labor. Sokol and colleagues (1977) reported a 3- to 4-percent incidence of prolonged latent phase, regardless of parity. Friedman (1972) reported that prolongation of the latent phase did not adversely influence fetal or maternal morbidity or mortality rates, but Chelmow and co-workers (1993) disputed the long-held belief that prolongation of the latent phase is benign.

Active Labor

As shown in Figure 17-22, the progress of labor in nulliparous women has particular significance because these curves all reveal a rapid change in the slope of cervical dilatation rates between 3 and 5 cm. *Thus, cervical dilatation of 3 to 5 cm or more, in the presence of uterine contractions, can be taken to reliably represent the threshold for active labor.* Similarly, these curves provide useful guideposts for labor management.

Turning again to Friedman (1955), the mean duration of active-phase labor in nulliparas was 4.9 hours. But the standard deviation of 3.4 hours is large; hence, the active phase was reported to have a statistical maximum of 11.7 hours. Indeed, rates of cervical dilatation ranged from a minimum of 1.2 up to 6.8 cm/hr. Friedman (1972) also found that multiparas progress somewhat faster in active-phase labor, with a *minimum* normal rate of 1.5 cm/hr. His analysis of active-phase labor concomitantly describes rates of fetal descent and cervical dilatation (see Fig. 17-20). Descent begins in the later stage of active dilatation, commencing at 7 to 8 cm in nulliparas and becoming most rapid after 8 cm.

Active-Phase Abnormalities. Abnormalities in this labor phase are common. Sokol and co-workers (1977) reported that 25 percent of nulliparous and 15 percent of multiparous labors were complicated by an active-phase abnormality. Friedman (1972) subdivided active-phase problems into *protraction* and *arrest disorders*. He defined protraction as a *slow rate* of cervical dilatation or descent, which for nulliparas was less than 1.2 cm dilatation per hour or less than 1 cm descent per hour. For multiparas, protraction was defined as less than 1.5 cm dilatation per hour or less than 2 cm descent per hour. He defined arrest as a *complete cessation* of dilatation or descent. *Arrest of dilatation* was defined as 2 hours with no cervical change, and *arrest of descent* as 1 hour without fetal descent.

The prognosis for protraction and arrest disorders differed considerably. Friedman found that approximately 30 percent of women with protraction disorders had cephalopelvic disproportion, compared with 45 percent of women in whom an arrest disorder developed. Abnormal labor patterns, diagnostic criteria, and treatment methods according to Cohen and Friedman (1983) are summarized in Chapter 20 (see p. 465 and Table 20-2).

Factors contributing to both protraction and arrest disorders were excessive sedation, epidural analgesia, and fetal malposition. In both protraction and arrest disorders, Friedman recommended fetopelvic evaluation to identify cephalopelvic disproportion. Recommended therapy for protraction disorders was expectant management, whereas oxytocin was advised for arrest disorders in the absence of cephalopelvic disproportion. During those times, x-ray pelvimetry was frequently used to identify cephalopelvic disproportion—a method now known to be notoriously inaccurate (see Chap. 20, p. 472). Still, it is remarkable that of the 500 women studied, only 2 percent had a cesarean delivery. By way of comparison, Henry and colleagues (2008) recently described a 67-percent cesarean delivery rate for 1014 women with active-phase arrest. These differences must be kept in mind when considering the significance of various labor abnormalities described by Friedman.

Hendricks and co-workers (1970) challenged Friedman's conclusions about the course of normal human labor. Their principal differences included: (1) absence of a latent phase, (2) no deceleration phase, (3) brevity of labor, and (4) dilatation at similar rates for nulliparas and multiparas after 4 cm. They disputed the concept of a latent phase because they observed that the cervix dilated and effaced slowly during the 4 weeks preceding labor. They contended that the *latent phase* actually progressed over several weeks. They also reported that labor was relatively rapid. Specifically, the average time from admission to complete dilatation was 4.8 hours for nulliparas and 3.2 hours for multiparas.

There have been other reports in which investigators have reassessed the Friedman labor curves. Zhang and colleagues (2002) plotted detailed data on 1329 nulliparous women in spontaneous labor at term and found that the average curve differed markedly from the Friedman curve. Specifically, the cervix dilated more slowly in the active phase, and it took 5.5 hours to progress from 4 cm to 10 cm compared with only 2.5 hours in the Friedman curve. Alexander and colleagues (2002), in a study performed at Parkland Hospital, found that epidural analgesia lengthened the active phase of the Friedman labor curve by 1 hour. This increase was the result of a slightly slower, but significant rate of cervical dilatation—1.4 cm/hr in women given epidural analgesia compared with 1.6 cm/hr in those without such analgesia. Gurewitsch and colleagues (2002, 2003) studied the labor and descent curves of women with greater and lesser parity. They concluded that poor progress from 4 to 6 cm should not be considered abnormal and that women with high parity should not be expected to progress faster than those with lower parity. Greenberg and colleagues (2006) studied ethnic differences in the labor length in 27,521 women and concluded that the Friedman curves should be modified to account for ethnic differences.

Second Stage of Labor

This stage begins when cervical dilatation is complete and ends with fetal delivery. The median duration is approximately 50 minutes for nulliparas and about 20 minutes for multiparas, but it is highly variable (Kilpatrick and Laros, 1989). In a woman of higher parity with a previously dilated vagina and perineum, two or three expulsive efforts after full cervical dilatation may suffice to complete delivery. Conversely, in a woman with a contracted pelvis, a large fetus, or with impaired expulsive efforts from conduction analgesia or sedation, the second stage may become abnormally long. Abnormalities of the second stage of labor are described in Chapter 20 (see p. 468).

Duration of Labor

Our understanding of the normal duration of labor may be clouded by the many clinical variables that affect conduct of labor in modern obstetrical units. Kilpatrick and Laros (1989) reported that the mean length of first- and second-stage labor was approximately 9 hours in nulliparous women without regional analgesia, and that the 95th percentile upper limit was 18.5 hours. Corresponding times for multiparous women were a mean of 6 hours with a 95th percentile maximum of 13.5 hours. These authors defined labor onset as the time when a woman recalled regular, painful contractions every 3 to 5 minutes that led to cervical change.

Spontaneous labor was analyzed in nearly 25,000 women delivered at term at Parkland Hospital in the early 1990s. Almost 80 percent of women were admitted with a cervical dilatation of 5 cm or less. Parity—nulliparous versus multiparous—and cervical dilatation at admission were significant determinants of the length of spontaneous labor. The median time from admission to spontaneous delivery for all parturients was 3.5 hours, and 95 percent of all women delivered within 10.1 hours. These results suggest that normal human labor is relatively short. Zhang and associates (2009a, b) described similar findings in their study of 126,887 deliveries from 12 institutions over the United States.

Summary of Normal Labor

Labor is characterized by brevity and considerable biological variation. Active labor can be reliably diagnosed when cervical dilatation is 3 cm or more in the presence of uterine contractions. Once this cervical dilatation threshold is reached, normal progression to delivery can be expected, depending on parity, in the ensuing 4 to 6 hours. Anticipated progress during a 1- to 2-hour second stage is monitored to ensure fetal safety. Finally, most women in spontaneous labor, regardless of parity, if left unaided, will deliver within approximately 10 hours after admission for spontaneous labor. Insufficient uterine activity is a common and correctable cause of abnormal labor progress. *Therefore, when time breaches in normal labor boundaries are the only pregnancy complications, interventions other than cesarean delivery must be considered before resorting to this method of delivery for failure to progress.*

MANAGEMENT OF NORMAL LABOR AND DELIVERY

The ideal management of labor and delivery requires two potentially opposing viewpoints on the part of clinicians. First, birthing should be recognized as a normal physiological process that most women experience without complications. Second, intrapartum complications, often arising quickly and unexpectedly, should be anticipated. Thus, clinicians must simultaneously make every woman and her supporters feel comfortable, yet ensure safety for the mother and newborn should complications suddenly develop. The American Academy of Pediatrics and the American College of Obstetricians and Gynecologists (2007) have collaborated in the development of *Guidelines for Perinatal Care.* These provide detailed information on the appropriate content of intrapartum care, including both personnel and facility requirements. Shown in Table 17-2 are the recommended nurse-to-patient ratios recommended for labor and delivery. Shown in Table 17-3 are the recommended room dimensions for these functions.

TABLE 17-2. Recommended Nurse/Patient Ratios for Labor and Delivery

Nurse/Patient Ratio	Clinical Setting
1:2	Patients in labor
1:1	Patients in second-stage labor
1:1	Patients with medical or obstetrical complications
1:2	Oxytocin induction or augmentation of labor
1:1	Coverage initiation of epidural analgesia
1:1	Circulation for cesarean delivery

Used with permission of the American Academy of Pediatrics, American College of Obstetricians and Gynecologists. Guidelines for perinatal care. 6th ed. Elk Grove Village (IL): AAP; Washington, DC: ACOG; 2007. Copyright American Academy of Pediatrics and American College of Obstetricans and Gynecologists, 2007.

TABLE 17-3. Recommended Minimum Room Dimensions for Labor and Delivery

Function	Net Floor Space (square feet)
Labor	100–160 per bed
LDR—labor, delivery, and recovery	256
LDRP—LDR plus postpartum	
Vaginal delivery	350
Cesarean delivery	400

Used with permission of the American Academy of Pediatrics, American College of Obstetricians and Gynecologists. Guidelines for perinatal care. 6th ed. Elk Grove Village (IL): AAP; Washington, DC: ACOG; 2007. Copyright American Academy of Pediatrics and American College of Obstetricans and Gynecologists, 2007.

Admission Procedures

Pregnant women should be urged to report early in labor rather than to procrastinate until delivery is imminent for fear that they might be experiencing false labor. Early admittance to the labor and delivery unit is important, especially if during antepartum care the woman, her fetus, or both have been identified as being at risk.

Identification of Labor

Although the differentiation between false and true labor is difficult at times, the diagnosis usually can be clarified by contraction frequency and intensity and by cervical dilatation as shown in Table 17-4. Use of an algorithm to help diagnose active labor was associated with more home discharges after initial prelabor assessment (Cheyne and colleagues, 2008). Another study showed that a formalized approach to labor assessment improved patient satisfaction with little effect on pregnancy outcomes (Hodnett and co-workers, 2008). In those instances when a diagnosis of labor cannot be established with certainty, observation for a longer period of time is often wise.

Pates and colleagues (2007) studied the commonly used recommendations given to pregnant women that, in the absence of ruptured membranes or bleeding, uterine contractions 5 minutes apart for 1 hour—that is, ≥ 12 contractions in 1 hour—may signify labor onset. Among 768 women studied at Parkland Hospital, active labor defined as cervical dilatation ≥ 4 cm

TABLE 17-4. Characteristics of True versus False Labor

Characteristic	True Labor	False Labor
Contractions		
Rhythm	Regular	Irregular
Intervals	Gradually shorten	Unchanged
Intensity	Gradually increases	Unchanged
Discomfort		
Location	Back and abdomen	Lower abdomen
Sedation	No effect	Usually relieved
Cervical dilatation	Yes	No

was diagnosed within 24 hours in three fourths of women with 12 or more contractions per hour. Bailit and colleagues (2005) compared labor outcomes of 6121 women who presented in active labor defined as uterine contractions plus cervical dilatation ≥ 4 cm with those of 2697 women who presented in the latent phase. Women admitted during latent-phase labor had more active-phase arrest, need for oxytocin labor stimulation, and chorioamnionitis. It was concluded that physician interventions in women presenting in the latent phase may have been the cause of subsequent labor abnormalities.

Emergency Medical Treatment and Labor Act (EMTALA)

Congress enacted EMTALA in 1986 to ensure public access to emergency services regardless of the ability to pay. All Medicare-participating hospitals with emergency services must provide an appropriate screening examination for any pregnant woman experiencing contractions who comes to the emergency department for evaluation. The most recent iteration of these regulations went into effect on November 10, 2003 (Federal Register, 2003).

The definition of an emergency condition makes specific reference to a pregnant woman who is having contractions. Labor is defined as "the process of childbirth beginning with the latent phase of labor continuing through delivery of the placenta. A woman experiencing contractions is in true labor unless a physician certifies that after a reasonable time of observation the woman is in false labor." A woman in true labor is considered "unstable" for interhospital transfer purposes until the newborn and placenta are delivered. An unstable woman may, however, be transferred at the direction of the patient or by a physician who certifies that the benefits of treatment at another facility outweigh the risks of transfer. Physicians and hospitals violating these federal requirements are subject to civil penalties of up to $50,000 and termination from the Medicare program.

Preadmission and Admission Electronic Fetal Heart Rate Monitoring

As discussed in Chapter 18 (p. 410), electronic fetal heart rate monitoring is routinely used for high-risk pregnancies commencing at admission. Some investigators recommend monitoring women with low-risk pregnancies upon admission as a test of fetal well-being—the so-called *fetal admission test*. If no fetal rate abnormalities are detected, continuous electronic monitoring is replaced by intermittent assessment for the remainder of labor. We are of the view that electronic fetal heart rate monitoring is reasonable in the preadmission evaluation of women, including those who subsequently are discharged. At Parkland Hospital, external electronic monitoring is performed for at least 1 hour before discharging the woman who was ascertained to have false labor.

Home Births

A major emphasis of obstetrical care during the 20th century was the movement to birthing in hospitals rather than in homes. In 2006, 99 percent of births in the United States took place in hospitals (Martin and colleagues, 2009). Of the other

1 percent, 65 percent were in homes and 28 percent in birthing centers. The results of studies comparing neonatal and perinatal mortality rates associated with intended home deliveries with those of hospital deliveries have been conflicting. Most suggest an increased risk with home delivery. In their recent evidence-based systematic review, Berghella and colleagues (2008) found good-quality data to favor hospital birth.

Vital Signs and Review of Pregnancy Record

Maternal blood pressure, temperature, pulse, and respiratory rate are recorded. The pregnancy record is promptly reviewed to identify complications. Problems identified or anticipated during prenatal care should be displayed prominently in the pregnancy record.

Vaginal Examination

Most often, *unless there has been bleeding in excess of bloody show,* a vaginal examination is performed. The gloved index and second fingers are then introduced into the vagina while avoiding the anal region (Fig. 17-23). The number of vaginal examinations correlates with infection-related morbidity, especially in cases of early membrane rupture.

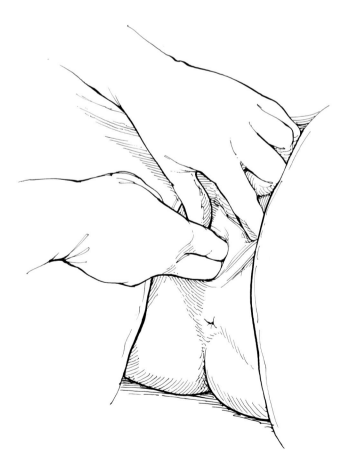

FIGURE 17-23 To perform vaginal examination, the labia have been separated with one hand, and the first and second fingers of the other hand are carefully inserted into the introitus.

Detection of Ruptured Membranes

The woman should be instructed during the antepartum period to be aware of fluid leakage from the vagina and to report such an event promptly. Rupture of the membranes is significant for three reasons. First, if the presenting part is not fixed in the pelvis, the possibility of umbilical cord prolapse and compression is greatly increased. Second, labor is likely to begin soon if the pregnancy is at or near term. Third, if delivery is delayed after membrane rupture, intrauterine infection is more likely as the time interval increases (Herbst and Källén, 2007).

Upon sterile speculum examination, ruptured membranes are diagnosed when amnionic fluid is seen pooling in the posterior fornix or clear fluid is flowing from the cervical canal. Although several diagnostic tests for the detection of ruptured membranes have been recommended, none is completely reliable. If the diagnosis remains uncertain, another method involves pH determination of vaginal fluid. The pH of vaginal secretions normally ranges from 4.5 to 5.5, whereas that of amnionic fluid is usually 7.0 to 7.5. The use of the indicator *nitrazine* to identify ruptured membranes is a simple and fairly reliable method. Test papers are impregnated with the dye, and the color of the reaction between these paper strips and vaginal fluids is interpreted by comparison with a standard color chart. A pH above 6.5 is consistent with ruptured membranes. False-positive test results may occur with coexistent blood, semen, or bacterial vaginosis, whereas false-negative tests may result with scant fluid (American Academy of Pediatrics and American College of Obstetricians and Gynecologists, 2007).

Other tests include arborization or ferning of vaginal fluid, which suggests amnionic rather than cervical fluid. Amnionic fluid crystallizes to form a fernlike pattern due to its relative concentrations of sodium chloride, proteins, and carbohydrates (see Fig. 8-3, p. 192). Detection of alpha-fetoprotein in the vaginal vault has been used to identify amnionic fluid (Yamada and colleagues, 1998). Identification may also follow injection of indigo carmine into the amnionic sac via abdominal amniocentesis.

Cervical Examination

The degree of *cervical effacement* usually is expressed in terms of the length of the cervical canal compared with that of an uneffaced cervix. When the length of the cervix is reduced by one half, it is 50-percent effaced. When the cervix becomes as thin as the adjacent lower uterine segment, it is completely, or 100-percent, effaced.

Cervical dilatation is determined by estimating the average diameter of the cervical opening by sweeping the examining finger from the margin of the cervical opening on one side to that on the opposite side. The diameter traversed is estimated in centimeters. The cervix is said to be dilated fully when the diameter measures 10 cm, because the presenting part of a term-size newborn usually can pass through a cervix this widely dilated.

The *position* of the cervix is determined by the relationship of the cervical os to the fetal head and is categorized as posterior, midposition, or anterior. Along with position, the *consistency* of cervix is determined to be soft, firm, or intermediate between these two.

The level—or *station*—of the presenting fetal part in the birth canal is described in relationship to the ischial spines, which are halfway between the pelvic inlet and the pelvic outlet. When the lowermost portion of the presenting fetal part is at the level of the spines, it is designated as being at zero (0) station. In the past, the long axis of the birth canal above and below the ischial spines was arbitrarily divided into thirds by some and into fifths (approximately 1 cm) by other groups. In 1989, the American College of Obstetricians and Gynecologists adopted the classification of station that divides the pelvis above and below the spines into fifths. Each fifth represents a centimeter above or below the spines. Thus, as the presenting fetal part descends from the inlet *toward* the ischial spines, the designation is −5, −4, −3, −2, −1, then 0 station. Below the spines, as the presenting fetal part descends, it passes +1, +2, +3, +4, and +5 stations to delivery. Station +5 cm corresponds to the fetal head being visible at the introitus.

If the leading part of the fetal head is at 0 station or below, most often the fetal head has engaged—thus, the biparietal plane has passed through the pelvic inlet. *If the head is unusually molded or if there is an extensive caput formation or both, engagement might not have taken place although the head appears to be at 0 station.*

In a study done at five teaching centers in Denver, residents, nurses, and faculty were surveyed to determine what definitions were being used to describe fetal station (Carollo and colleagues, 2004). Four different definitions were in use. Disturbingly, these investigators found that few caregivers were aware that others were using different definitions of station! Dupuis and colleagues (2005) tested the reliability of clinical estimations of station using the position of the leading part in centimeters above or below the spines as recommended by the American Academy of Pediatrics and the American college of Obstetricians and Gynecologists (2007). A birth simulator was used in which station could be precisely measured and compared with the vaginal examination done by clinicians. They reported that the clinical examiners were incorrect a third of the time.

These five characteristics: cervical dilatation, effacement, consistency, position, and fetal station are assessed when tabulating the Bishop score. This score is commonly used to predict labor induction outcome and is discussed in Chapter 22 (p. 501).

Laboratory Studies

When the woman is admitted in labor, most often the hematocrit or hemoglobin concentration should be rechecked. The hematocrit can be measured easily and quickly. At Parkland Hospital, blood is collected in a standard collection tube with anticoagulant. From this, a heparinized capillary tube is filled to spin in a microhematocrit centrifuge in the labor and delivery unit. This provides a hematocrit value within 3 minutes. The initial collection tube is also sent to the hematology laboratory for evaluation. Another labeled tube of blood is allowed to clot and is kept available for blood type and screen, if needed. A final sample is collected for routine serology. We obtain a urine specimen for protein determination in hypertensive women only (see Chap. 34, p. 707). In some labor units, however, a clean-catch voided specimen is examined in all women for protein and glucose.

Women who have had no prenatal care should be considered to be at risk for syphilis, hepatitis B, and human immunodeficiency virus (HIV) (see Chap. 59, p. 1235). In patients with no prior prenatal care, these laboratory studies, as well as a blood type and antibody screen, should be performed (Amcrican Academy of Pediatrics and American College of Obstetricians and Gynecologists, 2002). Some states, for example, Texas, require routine testing for syphilis, hepatitis B, and HIV in all women admitted to labor and delivery units even if these were done during prenatal care.

Management of the First Stage of Labor

As soon as possible after admittance, the remainder of the general examination is completed. A clinician can best reach a conclusion about the normalcy of the pregnancy when all examinations, including record and laboratory review, are completed. A rational plan for monitoring labor then can be established based on the needs of the fetus and the mother. Because there are marked individual variations in lengths of labor, precise statements as to its anticipated duration are unwise.

Monitoring Fetal Well-Being During Labor

This is discussed in detail in Chapter 18. Briefly, the American Academy of Pediatrics and American College of Obstetricians and Gynecologists (2007) recommend that during the first stage of labor, in the absence of any abnormalities, the fetal heart rate should be checked immediately after a contraction at least every 30 minutes and then every 15 minutes during the second stage. If continuous electronic monitoring is used, the tracing is evaluated at least every 30 minutes during the first stage and at least every 15 minutes during second-stage labor. For women with pregnancies at risk, fetal heart auscultation is performed at least every 15 minutes during the first stage of labor and every 5 minutes during the second stage. Continuous electronic monitoring may be used with evaluation of the tracing every 15 minutes during the first stage of labor, and every 5 minutes during the second stage.

Uterine Contractions

Although usually assessed by electronic monitoring as also discussed in Chapter 18, contractions can be both quantitatively and qualitatively evaluated manually. With the palm of the hand resting lightly on the uterus, the time of contraction onset is determined. Its intensity is gauged from the degree of firmness the uterus achieves. At the acme of effective contractions, the finger or thumb cannot readily indent the uterus during a "firm" contraction. The time at which the contraction disappears is noted next. This sequence is repeated to evaluate the frequency, duration, and intensity of uterine contractions.

Maternal Vital Signs

Temperature, pulse, and blood pressure are evaluated at least every 4 hours. If membranes have been ruptured for many hours before labor onset or if there is a borderline temperature elevation, the temperature is checked hourly. Moreover, with prolonged membrane rupture, defined as greater than 18 hours, antimicrobial administration for prevention of group B streptococcal infections is recommended. This is discussed in Chapter 58 (see p. 1220).

Subsequent Vaginal Examinations

During the first stage of labor, the need for subsequent vaginal examinations to monitor cervical change and presenting part position will vary considerably. When the membranes rupture, an examination should be performed expeditiously if the fetal head was not definitely engaged at the previous vaginal examination. This excludes umbilical cord prolapse. The fetal heart rate should also be checked immediately and during the next uterine contraction to help detect occult umbilical cord compression. At Parkland Hospital, periodic pelvic examinations are typically performed at 2- to 3-hour intervals to evaluate labor progress (see p. 405).

Oral Intake

Food should be withheld during active labor and delivery. Gastric emptying time is remarkably prolonged once labor is established and analgesics are administered. As a consequence, ingested food and most medications remain in the stomach and are not absorbed. Instead, they may be vomited and aspirated (see Chap. 19, p. 460). According to the American Academy of Pediatrics and the American College of Obstetricians and Gynecologists (2007), sips of clear liquids, occasional ice chips, and lip moisturizers are permitted.

Intravenous Fluids

Although it has become customary in many hospitals to establish an intravenous infusion system routinely early in labor, there is seldom any real need for such in the normal pregnant woman at least until analgesia is administered. An intravenous infusion system is advantageous during the immediate puerperium to administer oxytocin prophylactically and at times therapeutically when uterine atony persists. Moreover, with longer labors, the administration of glucose, sodium, and water to the otherwise fasting woman at the rate of 60 to 120 mL/hr prevents dehydration and acidosis. Shrivastava and associates (2009) noted shorter labors in nulliparas delivering vaginal who were provided an intravenous normal saline (NS) with dextrose solution compared with those given NS solution only. Garite and colleagues (2000) randomly assigned 195 women in labor to receive either 125 or 250 mL/hr of lactated Ringer or isotonic sodium chloride solution. The mean volume of total intravenous fluid was 2008 mL in the 125 mL/hr group and 2487 mL in the 250 mL/hr group. Labor lasted more than 12 hours in significantly more (26 versus 13 percent) of the women given a 125 mL/hr infusion compared with those given 250 mL/hr—26 versus 13 percent, respectively.

Maternal Position

The normal laboring woman need not be confined to bed early in labor. A comfortable chair may be beneficial psychologically and perhaps physiologically. In bed, the laboring woman should be allowed to assume the position she finds most comfortable—this will be lateral recumbency most of the time. She must not be restricted to lying supine because of resultant aortocaval compression and its potential to lower uterine perfusion (see Chap. 5, p. 120). Bloom and colleagues (1998) conducted a randomized trial of walking during labor in more than 1000 women with low-risk pregnancies. They found that walking neither enhanced nor impaired active labor and that it was not harmful. Lawrence and associates (2009) reached similar findings in their Cochrane database review.

Analgesia

This is discussed in detail in Chapter 19. In general, pain relief should depend on the needs and desires of the woman. The American College of Obstetricians and Gynecologists (2009) has specified optimal goals for anesthesia care in obstetrics.

Amniotomy

If the membranes are intact, there is a great temptation, even during normal labor, to perform amniotomy. The presumed benefits are more rapid labor, earlier detection of meconium-stained amnionic fluid, and the opportunity to apply an electrode to the fetus or insert a pressure catheter into the uterine cavity for monitoring. The advantages and disadvantages of amniotomy are discussed in Chapter 22 (p. 508). Importantly, the fetal head must be well applied to the cervix and not be dislodged from the pelvis during the procedure to avert umbilical cord prolapse.

Urinary Bladder Function

Bladder distension should be avoided because it can hinder descent of the fetal presenting part and lead to subsequent bladder hypotonia and infection. During each abdominal examination, the suprapubic region should be inspected and palpated to detect distension. If the bladder is readily seen or palpated above the symphysis, the woman should be encouraged to void. At times, she can ambulate with assistance to a toilet and successfully void, even though she cannot void on a bedpan. If the bladder is distended and she cannot void, catheterization is indicated. Carley and colleagues (2002) found that 51 of 11,332 vaginal deliveries (1 in 200) were complicated by urinary retention. Most women resumed normal voiding before discharge from the hospital. Musselwhite and associates (2007) reported retention in 4.7 percent of women who had labor epidural analgesia. Risk factors that increased likelihood of retention were primiparity, oxytocin-induced or -augmented labor, perineal lacerations, instrumented delivery, catheterization during labor, and labor with duration more than 10 hours.

Management of the Second Stage of Labor

With full cervical dilatation, which signifies the onset of the second stage, a woman typically begins to bear down. With descent of the presenting part, she develops the urge to defecate. Uterine contractions and the accompanying expulsive forces may now last 1½ minutes and recur at an interval no longer than 1 minute. As discussed on page 389, the median duration of the second stage is 50 minutes in nulliparas and 20 minutes in multiparas, although the interval can be highly variable. Monitoring of the fetal heart rate is discussed on page 393, and interpretation of second-stage electronic fetal heart rate patterns is discussed in Chapter 18 (p. 425).

Expulsive Efforts

In most cases, bearing down is reflexive and spontaneous during second-stage labor. Occasionally, a woman may not employ her expulsive forces to good advantage and coaching is desirable. Her legs should be half-flexed so that she can push with them against the mattress. When the next uterine contraction begins, she is instructed to exert downward pressure as though she were straining at stool. In a randomized study from Istanbul, Yildirim and Beji (2008) reported that open-glottis pushing while breathing out was superior to the closed-glottis breath-held Valsalva-type pushing. The former method resulted in a shorter second stage and better cord acid-base values. A woman is not encouraged to push beyond the completion of each contraction. Instead, she and her fetus should be allowed to rest and recover. During this period of actively bearing down, the fetal heart rate auscultated immediately after the contraction is likely to be slow but should recover to normal range before the next expulsive effort.

A number of positions during the second stage have been recommended to augment pushing efforts. Eason and colleagues (2000) performed an extensive review of various positions and their effect on the incidence of perineal trauma. They found that the supported upright position had no advantages over the recumbent one. Upright positions include sitting, kneeling, squatting, or resting with the back at a 30-degree elevation. Conversely, in their systematic review, Berghella and colleagues (2008) reported good-quality data that supported the upright position. Fetal and obstetrical outcomes appear to be unaffected whether pushing is coached or uncoached during second-stage labor (Bloom and co-workers, 2006; Hansen and associates, 2002). The maternal effects of coached pushing were reported by Schaffer and colleagues (2005), who performed urodynamic testing in primiparas 3 months following delivery. Those coached to push during second-stage labor had decreased bladder capacity and decreased first urge to void compared with women encouraged to push or rest as desired. The long-term effects of this practice are yet to be defined.

As the head descends through the pelvis, feces frequently are expelled by the woman. With further descent, the perineum begins to bulge and the overlying skin becomes stretched. Now the scalp of the fetus may be visible through the vulvar opening. At this time, the woman and her fetus are prepared for delivery.

Preparation for Delivery

Delivery can be accomplished with the mother in a variety of positions. The most widely used and often the most satisfactory one is the dorsal lithotomy position. At Parkland Hospital, the lithotomy position is not mandated for normal deliveries. In many birthing rooms, delivery is accomplished with the woman lying flat on the bed.

For better exposure, leg holders or stirrups are used. In placing the legs in holders, care should be taken not to separate the legs too widely or place one leg higher than the other. This may exert pulling forces on the perineum that might easily result in extension of a spontaneous tear or of an episiotomy into a fourth-degree laceration. The popliteal region should rest comfortably in the proximal portion and the heel in the distal portion of the leg holder. The legs are not strapped into the stirrups, thereby allowing quick flexion of the thighs backward onto the abdomen should shoulder dystocia develop (see Chapter 20, p. 481). The legs may cramp during the second stage, in part, because of pressure by the fetal head on nerves in the pelvis. They may be relieved by changing the position of the leg or by brief massage, but leg cramps should never be ignored.

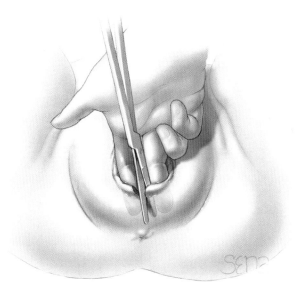

FIGURE 17-24 Midline episiotomy being made. Two fingers are insinuated between the perineum and fetal head, and the episiotomy is then cut vertically downward.

Preparation for delivery should include vulvar and perineal cleansing. If desired, sterile drapes may be placed in such a way that only the immediate area around the vulva is exposed. In the past, the major reason for care in scrubbing, gowning, and gloving was to protect the laboring woman from the introduction of infectious agents. Although these considerations remain valid, infectious disease exposure concerns today must also be extended to healthcare providers.

Spontaneous Delivery

Delivery of the Head

With each contraction, the perineum bulges increasingly. The vulvovaginal opening is dilated by the fetal head (Fig. 17-24), gradually forming an ovoid and, finally, an almost circular open-

ing (Fig. 17-25). This encirclement of the largest head diameter by the vulvar ring is known as *crowning*. Unless an episiotomy has been made as described later, the perineum thins and especially in nulliparous women, may undergo spontaneous laceration. Slow delivery of the head while instructing the mother not to push may decrease lacerations according to Laine and co-workers (2008). The anus becomes greatly stretched and protuberant, and the anterior wall of the rectum may be easily seen through it.

There once was considerable controversy concerning whether an episiotomy should be cut routinely. It is now clear that an episiotomy will increase the risk of a tear into the external anal sphincter or the rectum or both. Conversely, anterior tears involving the urethra and labia are more common in women in whom an episiotomy is not cut. Most, including us, advocate individualization and do not routinely perform episiotomy. This issue is discussed in detail on page 401.

Ritgen Maneuver. When the head distends the vulva and perineum enough to open the vaginal introitus to a diameter of 5 cm or more, a towel-draped, gloved hand may be used to exert forward pressure on the chin of the fetus through the perineum just in front of the coccyx. Concurrently, the other hand exerts pressure superiorly against the occiput (Fig. 17-26). This maneuver is simpler than that originally described by Ritgen (1855), and it is customarily designated the *modified Ritgen maneuver* (Cunningham, 2008).

This maneuver allows controlled delivery of the head (Fig. 17-27). It also favors neck extension so that the head is delivered with its smallest diameters passing through the introitus and over the perineum. Mayerhofer and colleagues (2002) have challenged the use of the Ritgen maneuver because it was associated with more third-degree lacerations and more frequent use of episiotomy. They preferred the "hands-poised" method, in

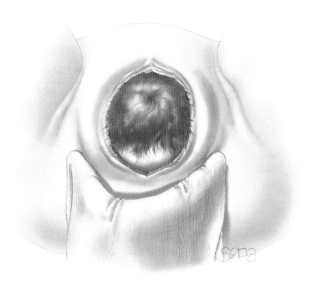

FIGURE 17-25 Delivery of the head. The occiput is being kept close to the symphysis by moderate pressure to the fetal chin at the tip of the maternal coccyx.

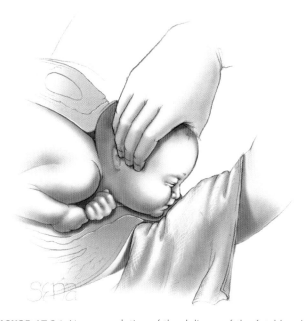

FIGURE 17-26 Near completion of the delivery of the fetal head by the modified Ritgen maneuver. Moderate upward pressure is applied to the fetal chin by the posterior hand covered with a sterile towel, while the suboccipital region of the fetal head is held against the symphysis.

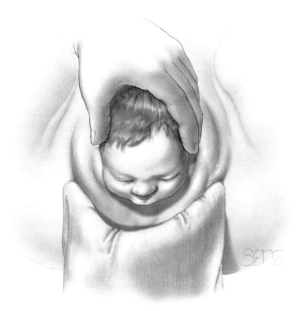

FIGURE 17-27 Delivery of the head. The mouth appears over the perineum.

which the attendant did not touch the perineum during delivery of the head. This method had similar associated laceration rates as the modified Ritgen maneuver, but with a lower incidence of third-degree tears. Recently, Jönsson and associates (2008) reported results of their trial of 1623 women. They found a similar incidence of third- and fourth-degree tears—5.5 versus 4.4 percent—in women assigned to the Ritgen maneuver versus simple perineal support.

Delivery of the Shoulders

After its delivery, the fetal head falls posteriorly, bringing the face almost into contact with the maternal anus. As described on page 380, the occiput promptly turns toward one of the maternal thighs, and the head assumes a transverse position (Fig. 17-28). This movement of restitution—external

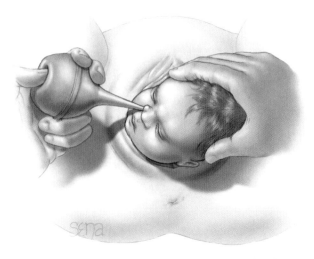

FIGURE 17-28 Aspirating the nose and mouth immediately after delivery of the head.

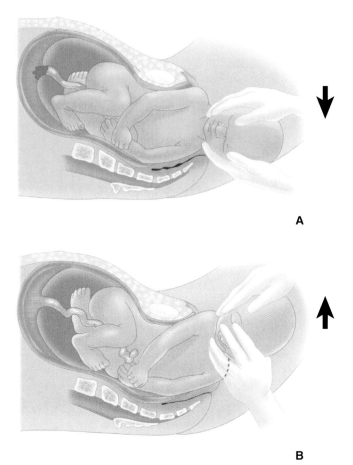

FIGURE 17-29 A. Gentle downward traction to effect descent of the anterior shoulder. **B.** Delivery of the anterior shoulder completed. Gentle upward traction to deliver the posterior shoulder.

rotation—indicates that the bisacromial diameter, which is the transverse diameter of the thorax, has rotated into the anteroposterior diameter of the pelvis.

Most often, the shoulders appear at the vulva just after external rotation and are born spontaneously. If delayed, immediate extraction may appear advisable. The sides of the head are grasped with two hands, and gentle downward traction is applied until the anterior shoulder appears under the pubic arch (Fig. 17-29). Some prefer to deliver the anterior shoulder prior to suctioning the nasopharynx or checking for a nuchal cord to avoid shoulder dystocia. Next, by an upward movement, the posterior shoulder is delivered (see Fig. 17-29).

The rest of the body almost always follows the shoulders without difficulty. With prolonged delay, however, its birth may be hastened by moderate traction on the head and moderate pressure on the uterine fundus. Hooking the fingers in the axillae should be avoided. This may injure the nerves of the upper extremity and produce a transient or possibly permanent paralysis. Traction, furthermore, should be exerted only in the direction of the long axis of the neonate. If applied obliquely, it causes bending of the neck and excessive stretching of the brachial plexus (see Chap. 29, p. 636).

Immediately after delivery of the newborn, there is usually a gush of amnionic fluid, often blood-tinged but not grossly bloody.

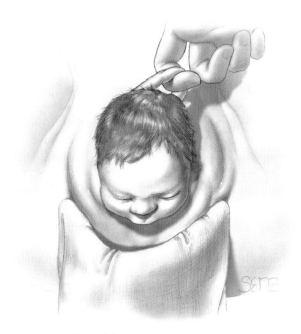

FIGURE 17-30 The umbilical cord is identified around the neck and is readily slipped over the head.

Clearing the Nasopharynx

Once the thorax is delivered and the newborn can inspire, the face is quickly wiped and the nares and mouth are aspirated, as demonstrated in Figure 17-28. This minimizes fetal aspiration of amnionic fluid, particulate matter, and blood.

Nuchal Cord

Following delivery of the anterior shoulder, a finger should be passed to the fetal neck to determine whether it is encircled by one or more coils of the umbilical cord (Fig. 17-30). A nuchal cord is found in approximately 25 percent of deliveries and ordinarily causes no harm. If a coil of umbilical cord is felt, it should be slipped over the head if loose enough. If applied too tightly, the loop should be cut between two clamps and the neonate promptly delivered.

Clamping the Cord

The umbilical cord is cut between two clamps placed 4 to 5 cm from the fetal abdomen, and later an umbilical cord clamp is applied 2 to 3 cm from the fetal abdomen. A plastic clamp that is safe, efficient, and fairly inexpensive, such as the Double Grip Umbilical Clamp (Hollister), is used at Parkland Hospital.

Timing of Cord Clamping. If after delivery the newborn is placed at or below the level of the vaginal introitus for 3 minutes and the fetoplacental circulation is not immediately occluded by cord clamping, an average of 80 mL of blood may be shifted from the placenta to the neonate (Yao and Lind, 1974). This provides approximately 50 mg of iron, which reduces the frequency of iron-deficiency anemia later in infancy. At the same time, however, increased bilirubin from the added erythrocytes contributes further to hyperbilirubinemia (see

Chap. 29, p. 625). In their recent Cochrane Database review of randomized trials, McDonald and Middleton (2008) reported that delaying cord clamping until 1 minute after birth increased the newborn hemoglobin concentration 2.2 g/dL compared with clamping within the first 60 seconds. At the same time, early clamping reduced the risk of phototherapy by 40 percent.

Our policy is to clamp the cord after first thoroughly clearing the airway, all of which usually requires approximately 30 seconds. The newborn is not elevated above the introitus at vaginal delivery or much above the maternal abdominal wall at the time of cesarean delivery.

Management of the Third Stage of Labor

Immediately after delivery of the newborn, the size of the uterine fundus and its consistency are examined. If the uterus remains firm and there is no unusual bleeding, watchful waiting until the placenta separates is the usual practice. Massage is not employed, but the fundus is frequently palpated to make certain that it does not become atonic and filled with blood from placental separation.

Signs of Placental Separation

Because attempts to express the placenta prior to its separation are futile and possibly dangerous, the clinician should be alert to the following signs of placental separation:

1. The uterus becomes globular and as a rule, firmer
2. There is often a sudden gush of blood
3. The uterus rises in the abdomen because the placenta, having separated, passes down into the lower uterine segment and vagina. Here, its bulk pushes the uterus upward
4. The umbilical cord protrudes farther out of the vagina, indicating that the placenta has descended.

These signs sometimes appear within 1 minute after delivery of the newborn and usually within 5 minutes. When the placenta has separated, it should be determined that the uterus is firmly contracted. The mother may be asked to bear down, and the intra-abdominal pressure may be adequate to expel the placenta. If these efforts fail or if spontaneous expulsion is not possible because of anesthesia, then after ensuring that the uterus is contracted firmly, pressure is exerted with the hand on the fundus to propel the detached placenta into the vagina, as depicted and described in Figure 17-31. This approach has been termed *physiological management* as later contrasted with *active management* of the third stage (Thilaganathan and colleagues, 1993).

Delivery of the Placenta

Expression of the placenta should never be forced before placental separation lest the uterus becomes inverted. **Traction on the umbilical cord must not be used to pull the placenta out of the uterus.** Uterine inversion is one of the grave complications associated with delivery, and it constitutes an emergency requiring immediate attention (see Chap. 35, p. 780). As downward pressure toward the vagina is applied to the body of the uterus, the umbilical cord is kept slightly taut (see Fig. 17-31). The uterus is then lifted cephalad with the abdominal hand.

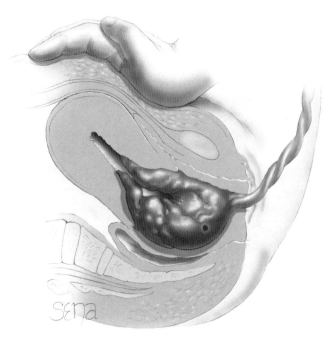

FIGURE 17-31 Expression of placenta. Note that the hand is *not* trying to push the fundus of the uterus through the birth canal! As the placenta leaves the uterus and enters the vagina, the uterus is elevated by the hand on the abdomen while the cord is held in position. The mother can aid in the delivery of the placenta by bearing down. As the placenta reaches the perineum, the cord is lifted, which in turn lifts the placenta out of the vagina.

This maneuver is repeated until the placenta reaches the introitus (Prendiville and associates, 1988b). As the placenta passes through the introitus, pressure on the uterus is stopped. The placenta is then gently lifted away from the introitus (Fig. 17-32). Care is taken to prevent the membranes from being torn off and left behind. If the membranes start to tear, they are

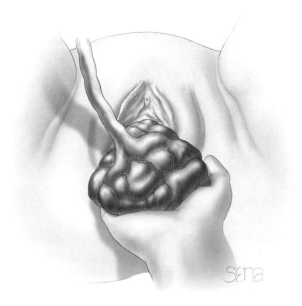

FIGURE 17-32 The placenta is removed from the vagina by lifting the cord.

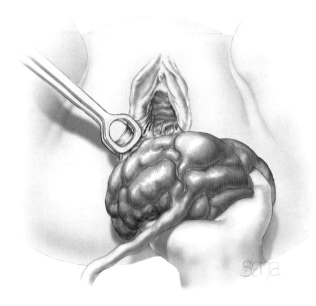

FIGURE 17-33 Membranes that were somewhat adherent to the uterine lining are separated by gentle traction with a ring forceps.

grasped with a clamp and removed by gentle teasing (Fig. 17-33). The maternal surface of the placenta should be examined carefully to ensure that no placental fragments are left in the uterus.

Manual Removal of Placenta

Occasionally, the placenta will not separate promptly. This is especially common in cases of preterm delivery (Dombrowski and colleagues, 1995). If there is brisk bleeding and the placenta cannot be delivered by the above technique, manual removal of the placenta is indicated, using the safeguards described in Chapter 35 (p. 774). It is unclear as to the length of time that should elapse in the absence of bleeding before the placenta is manually removed (Deneux-Tharaux and co-workers, 2009). If induction analgesia is still intact, some obstetricians practice routine manual removal of any placenta that has not separated spontaneously by the time they have completed delivery of the newborn and care of the cord. Proof of the benefits of this practice, however, has not been established, and most obstetricians await spontaneous placental separation unless bleeding is excessive. The American College of Obstetricians and Gynecologists (2003b) has concluded that there are no data to either support or refute the use of prophylactic antimicrobials when manual removal is performed.

Management of the Third Stage

Uterine massage following placental delivery is recommended by many to prevent postpartum hemorrhage. We support this but note that evidence for this practice is lacking (Hofmeyr and associates, 2008). Oxytocin, ergonovine, and methylergonovine are all employed widely in the normal third stage of labor, but the timing of their administration differs in various institutions. Oxytocin, and especially ergonovine, given before delivery of the placenta will decrease blood loss (Prendiville and associates, 1988a). If they are given before delivery of the placenta, however, they may entrap an undiagnosed, undelivered second twin. However, Jackson and colleagues (2001) randomly assigned 1486 women to infusions of 20 units of oxytocin diluted in 500 mL normal saline begun before or after placental delivery and found no differences in outcomes.

If an intravenous infusion is in place, our standard practice has been to add 20 units (2 mL) of oxytocin per liter of infusate. This solution is administered after delivery of the placenta at a rate of 10 mL/min (200 mU/min) for a few minutes until the uterus remains firmly contracted and bleeding is controlled. The infusion rate then is reduced to 1 to 2 mL/min until the mother is ready for transfer from the recovery suite to the postpartum unit. The infusion is usually then discontinued.

Oxytocin

The synthetic form of the octapeptide oxytocin is commercially available in the United States as Syntocinon and Pitocin. Each milliliter of injectable oxytocin, which is not effective by mouth, contains 10 USP units. The half-life of intravenously infused oxytocin is approximately 3 minutes. Before delivery, the spontaneously laboring uterus is typically exquisitely sensitive to oxytocin and dosing is carefully titrated to achieve adequate contractions (see Chap. 22, p. 506). After delivery of the fetus, however, these dangers no longer exist and fixed dosing, as described earlier, may be used.

Cardiovascular Effects

More than 30 years ago, Secher and co-workers (1978) reported that, even in healthy women, an intravenous bolus of 10 units of oxytocin caused a marked transient fall in blood pressure with an abrupt increase in cardiac output. More recently, Svanström and associates (2008) confirmed those findings in 10 otherwise healthy women following cesarean delivery. Mean pulse rate increased 28 bpm, mean arterial pressure decreased 33 mm Hg, and electrocardiogram changes of myocardial ischemia as well as chest pain and subjective discomfort were noted. These hemodynamic changes could be dangerous for women hypovolemic from hemorrhage or those with cardiac disease. **Thus, oxytocin should not be given intravenously as a large bolus.** Rather, it should be given as a dilute solution by continuous intravenous infusion or as an intramuscular injection in a dose of 10 USP units. In cases of postpartum hemorrhage, direct injection into the uterus, either transvaginally or transabdominally, following a vaginal birth or cesarean delivery has proven effective.

The use of nipple stimulation in the third stage of labor also has been shown to increase uterine pressures and to decrease third-stage duration and blood loss (Irons and associates, 1994). Indeed, results were similar to those achieved using the combination of oxytocin (5 units) and ergometrine (0.5 mg).

Water Intoxication. The considerable antidiuretic action of oxytocin can cause water intoxication. With high-dose oxytocin, it is possible to produce water intoxication if the oxytocin is administered in a large volume of electrolyte-free aqueous dextrose solution (Whalley and Pritchard, 1963). For example, Schwartz and Jones (1978) described convulsions in both the mother and her newborn following administration of 6.5 liters of 5-percent dextrose solution and 36 units of oxytocin predelivery. The sodium concentration in cord plasma was 114 mEq/L.

In general, if oxytocin is to be administered in high doses for a considerable period of time, its concentration should be increased rather than increasing the flow rate of a more dilute solution (see Chap. 22, p. 507). Consideration also should be given to use of either normal saline or lactated Ringer solution in these circumstances.

Ergonovine and Methylergonovine

These are ergot alkaloids with similar activity levels in myometrium. Methylergonovine is also called ergometrine and ergostetrine. Whether given intravenously, intramuscularly, or orally, both these agents are powerful stimulants of myometrial contraction, exerting an effect that may persist for hours. In pregnant women, an intravenous dose of as little as 0.1 mg or an oral dose of only 0.25 mg results in a tetanic uterine contraction. Effects develop almost immediately after intravenous injection of the drug and within a few minutes after intramuscular or oral administration. Moreover, the response is sustained with little tendency toward relaxation. For this reason, they are dangerous for the fetus and mother prior to delivery.

Parenteral administration of ergot alkaloids, especially by the intravenous route, sometimes initiates transient hypertension. This is more likely to be severe in the woman with gestational hypertension or who is prone to develop hypertension. Browning (1974) described serious side effects attributable to 0.5 mg of ergonovine administered intramuscularly to four postpartum women. Two of these promptly became severely hypertensive, the third became hypertensive and convulsed, and the fourth suffered cardiac arrest. We have seen an instance of such profound vasoconstriction from these compounds when given intravenously that all peripheral pulses were lost, and sodium nitroprusside was required to restore perfusion. Unfortunately, the mother sustained cerebral hypoxic ischemic injury.

Studies of Oxytocin and Ergot Alkaloids. Choy and co-workers (2002) randomly assigned 991 women to receive intravenous oxytocin or intramuscular syntometrine for prevention of third-stage blood loss. Syntometrine is a combined oxytocin and ergonovine agent. They reported oxytocin to be preferable because syntometrine induced hypertension in 3 percent of women. In a similar study of 600 women, Orji and associates (2008) also reported no differences except for increased nausea, vomiting, and hypertension in the syntometrine group.

Munn and co-workers (2001) compared two oxytocin dosage regimens for prevention of uterine atony at cesarean delivery. Either 10 units or 80 units of oxytocin in 500 mL of lactated Ringer solution were infused during the 30 minutes following delivery of the newborn. The rate of uterine atony was significantly lower in the high-dose regimen group compared with that of the lower-dose group—19 versus 39 percent, respectively.

Prostaglandins

Analogs of prostaglandins are not used routinely for management of third-stage labor. Villar and colleagues (2002) reviewed prophylactic use of misoprostol to prevent postpartum hemorrhage and concluded that oxytocin or oxytocin-ergot preparations are more effective. Other prostaglandins such as 15-methyl prostaglandin $F_{2\alpha}$ are reserved for treatment of uterine atony with hemorrhage (see Chap. 35, p. 774).

"Fourth Stage" of Labor

The placenta, membranes, and umbilical cord should be examined for completeness and for anomalies, as described in Chapter 27. The hour immediately following delivery is critical, and it has been designated by some as the *fourth stage of labor*. Although oxytocics are administered, postpartum hemorrhage as the result of uterine atony is more likely at this time. Consequently, the uterus and perineum should be frequently evaluated. The American Academy of Pediatrics and the American College of Obstetricians and Gynecologists (2007) recommend

that maternal blood pressure and pulse be recorded immediately after delivery and every 15 minutes for the first hour.

Lacerations of the Birth Canal

Lacerations of the vagina and perineum are classified as first- through fourth-degree lacerations or perineal tears. *First-degree* lacerations involve the fourchette, perineal skin, and vaginal mucous membrane but not the underlying fascia and muscle (Fig. 17-34). These included periurethral lacerations, which may bleed profusely. *Second-degree* lacerations involve, in addition, the fascia and muscles of the perineal body but not the anal sphincter. These tears usually extend upward on one or both sides of the vagina, forming an irregular triangular injury.

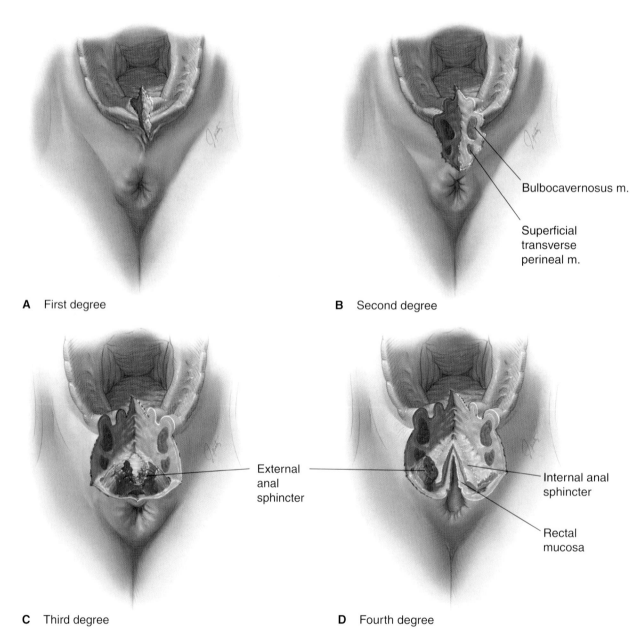

A First degree

B Second degree

Bulbocavernosus m.

Superficial transverse perineal m.

C Third degree

External anal sphincter

D Fourth degree

Internal anal sphincter

Rectal mucosa

FIGURE 17-34 Classification of perineal lacerations. **A.** First-degree laceration is a superficial tear that involves the vaginal mucosa and/or perineal skin. **B.** A second-degree laceration extends into the fascia and muscles that surround the vagina. **C.** A third-degree laceration extends into or through the external anal sphincter muscle. **D.** A fourth-degree laceration extends into the anorectal lumen and thus involves disruption of both the external and internal anal sphincters. (Courtesy of Drs. Marlene Corton and Shayzreen Roshanravan.)

Third-degree lacerations extend farther to involve the anal sphincter. A *fourth-degree* laceration extends through the rectum's mucosa to expose its lumen.

Laceration Risks and Morbidity

Perineal tears may follow any vaginal delivery, but Combs and associates (1990) identified factors associated with an increased risk of third- and fourth-degree lacerations. These include midline episiotomy, nulliparity, second-stage arrest of labor, persistent occiput posterior position, mid or low forceps, use of local anesthetics, and Asian race.

Morbidity rates rise as laceration severity increases. Venkatesh and colleagues (1989) reported a 5-percent incidence of third- and fourth-degree perineal tears in 20,500 vaginal deliveries. Approximately 10 percent of these 1040 primary repairs had a postoperative wound disruption and two thirds required surgical correction. Williams and Chames (2006) found that mediolateral episiotomy was the most powerful predictor of wound disruption. Goldaber and associates (1993) found that 21 of 390 or 5.4 percent of women with fourth-degree lacerations experienced significant morbidity. There were 1.8 percent dehiscences, 2.8 percent infections with dehiscences, and 0.8 percent with isolated infections. Although administration of a perioperative 2-g intravenous dose of cefazolin reduced rates of this morbidity, it was not totally eliminated.

Because repair of perineal lacerations is virtually the same as that of episiotomy incisions, albeit sometimes less satisfactory because of tear irregularities, the technique of laceration repair is discussed with episiotomy repair.

Episiotomy

In a strict sense, episiotomy is incision of the pudenda. Perineotomy is incision of the perineum. In common parlance, however, the term *episiotomy* often is used synonymously with *perineotomy,* a practice that we follow here. The incision may be made in the midline, creating a *median* or *midline episiotomy.* It may also begin in the midline but be directed laterally and downward away from the rectum, termed a *mediolateral episiotomy.*

Purposes of Episiotomy

Although still a common obstetrical procedure, the use of episiotomy has decreased remarkably over the past 25 years. Weber and Meyn (2002) used the National Hospital Discharge Survey to analyze use of episiotomy between 1979 and 1997 in the United States. Approximately 65 percent of women delivered vaginally in 1979 had an episiotomy compared with 39 percent by 1997. By 2003, the rate had decreased to approximately 18 percent (Martin and colleagues, 2005). Through the 1970s, it was common practice to cut an episiotomy for almost all women having their first delivery. The reasons for its popularity included substitution of a straight surgical incision, which was easier to repair, for the ragged laceration that otherwise might result. The long-held beliefs that postoperative pain is less and healing improved with an episiotomy compared with a tear,

however, appeared to be incorrect (Larsson and colleagues, 1991).

Another commonly cited but unproven benefit of routine episiotomy was that it prevented pelvic floor complications—that is, vaginal wall support defects and incontinence. A number of observational studies and randomized trials, however, showed that routine episiotomy is associated with an *increased* incidence of anal sphincter and rectal tears (Angioli, 2000; Eason, 2000; Nager and Helliwell, 2001; Rodriguez, 2008, and all their colleagues).

Carroli and Mignini (2009) reviewed the Cochrane Pregnancy and Childbirth Group trials registry. There were lower rates of posterior perineal trauma, surgical repair, and healing complications in the restricted-use group. Alternatively, the incidence of anterior perineal trauma was lower in the routine-use group.

With these findings came the realization that episiotomy did not protect the perineal body and contributed to anal sphincter incontinence by increasing the risk of third- and fourth-degree tears. Signorello and associates (2000) reported that fecal and flatus incontinence were increased four- to sixfold in women with an episiotomy compared with a group of women delivered with an intact perineum. Even compared with spontaneous lacerations, episiotomy tripled the risk of fecal incontinence and doubled it for flatus incontinence. Episiotomy without extension did not lower this risk. Despite repair of a third-degree extension, 30 to 40 percent of women have long-term anal incontinence (Gjessing and co-workers, 1998; Poen and colleagues, 1998). Finally, Alperin and associates (2008) recently reported that episiotomy performed for the first delivery conferred a five-fold risk for second-degree or worse lacerations with the second delivery.

For all of these reasons, the American College of Obstetricians and Gynecologists (2006) has concluded that restricted use of episiotomy is preferred to routine use. We are of the view that the procedure should be applied selectively for appropriate indications. These include fetal indications such as shoulder dystocia and breech delivery, forceps or vacuum extractor deliveries, occiput posterior positions, and instances in which failure to perform an episiotomy will result in perineal rupture. *The final rule is that there is no substitute for surgical judgment and common sense.*

Timing of Episiotomy

If performed unnecessarily early, bleeding from the episiotomy may be considerable during the interim between incision and delivery. If it is performed too late, lacerations will not be prevented. Typically, episiotomy is completed when the head is visible during a contraction to a diameter of 3 to 4 cm (see Fig. 17-24). When used in conjunction with forceps delivery, most perform an episiotomy after application of the blades (see Chap. 23, p. 514).

Midline versus Mediolateral Episiotomy

Differences between the two types of episiotomies are summarized in Table 17-5. Except for the important issue of third- and fourth-degree extensions, midline episiotomy is superior. Anthony

TABLE 17-5. Midline Versus Mediolateral Episiotomy

	Type of Episiotomy	
Characteristic	Midline	Mediolateral
Surgical repair	Easy	More difficult
Faulty healing	Rare	More common
Postoperative pain	Minimal	Common
Anatomical results	Excellent	Occasionally faulty
Blood loss	Less	More
Dyspareunia	Rare	Occasional
Extensions	Common	Uncommon

and colleagues (1994) presented data from the Dutch National Obstetric Database of more than 43,000 deliveries. They found a more than fourfold decrease in severe perineal lacerations following mediolateral episiotomy compared with rates after midline incision. Proper selection of cases can minimize this one disadvantage. For example, Kudish and co-workers (2006) advised against midline episiotomy with operative vaginal delivery because of an increased incidence of anal sphincter tears.

Episiotomy Repair

Typically, episiotomy repair is deferred until the placenta has been delivered. This policy permits undivided attention to the signs of placental separation and delivery. A further advantage is

that episiotomy repair is not interrupted or disrupted by the obvious necessity of delivering the placenta, especially if manual removal must be performed. The major disadvantage is continuing blood loss until the repair is completed.

Technique. There are many ways to close an episiotomy incision, but *hemostasis and anatomical restoration without excessive suturing are essential* for success with any method. Adequate analgesia is imperative, and Sanders and co-workers (2002) emphasized that women without regional analgesia can experience high levels of pain during perineal suturing. A technique that commonly is employed is shown in Figure 17-35. Mornar and Perlow (2008) have shown that blunt needles are suitable and likely decrease the incidence of needlestick injuries. The suture material commonly used is 2-0 chromic catgut. Sutures made of polyglycolic acid derivatives are also commonly used. A decrease in postsurgical pain is cited as the major advantage of synthetic materials. However, closures with these materials occasionally require suture removal from the repair site because of pain or dyspareunia. Kettle and co-workers (2002) randomly assigned 1542 women with perineal lacerations or episiotomies to undergo continuous versus interrupted repair with rapidly absorbed polyglactin 910 (Vicryl Rapids, Ethicon) or standard polyglactin 910 sutures. The former typically is absorbed by 42 days and the latter not for approximately 90 days. The continuous method was associated with less perineal pain. The rapidly absorbed material was associated with lower rates of suture removal compared with standard polyglactin—3 versus 13 percent. In another randomized study comparing continuous

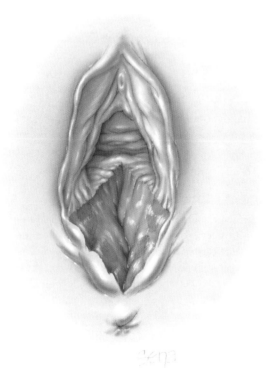

A

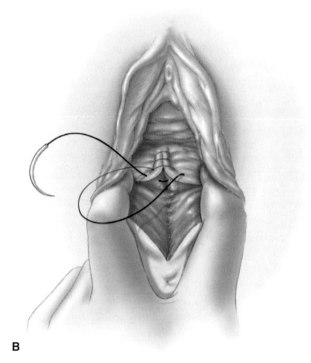

B

FIGURE 17-35 Repair of midline episiotomy. **A.** Disruption of the hymenal ring and bulbocavernosus and superficial transverse perineal muscle are seen within the diamond-shaped incision following episiotomy. **B.** Absorbable 2-0 or 3-0 suture is used for continuous closure of the vaginal mucosa and submucosa. (*Continued*)

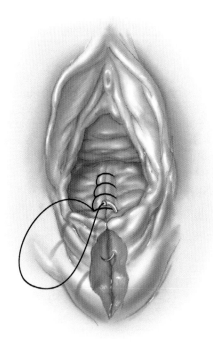

C

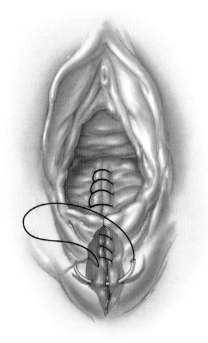

D

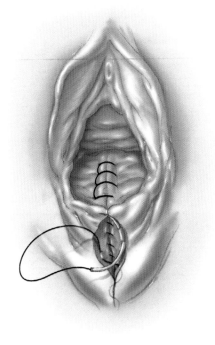

E

FIGURE 17-35 *Continued* **C.** After closing the vaginal incision and reapproximating the cut margins of the hymenal ring, the needle and suture are positioned to close the perineal incision. **D.** A continuous closure with absorbable 2-0 or 3-0 suture is used to close the fascia and muscles of the incised perineum. **E.** The continuous suture is then carried upward as a subcuticular stitch. The final knot it, tied proximally to the hymenal ring.

versus interrupted closure, Valenzuela (2009) and Kindberg (2008) and their associates found no differences in the techniques.

Repair of Fourth-Degree Laceration. The end-to-end technique of repairing a fourth-degree laceration is shown in Figure 17-36. Other techniques have been described, but in all, it is

essential to approximate the torn edges of the rectal mucosa with sutures placed in the rectal muscularis approximately 0.5 cm apart. This muscular layer then is covered with a layer of fascia. Finally, the cut ends of the anal sphincter are isolated, approximated, and sutured together with three or four interrupted stitches. The remainder of the repair is the same as for an episiotomy.

The overlapping technique is an alternative method to approximate the external anal sphincter. Despite promising initial results with this technique, more recent data based on a randomized controlled trial do not support that this method yields superior anatomical or functional results compared with those of the traditional end-to-end technique (Fitzpatrick and colleagues, 2000; Sultan and co-workers, 1999). Thus, more emphasis should be placed on prevention of anal sphincter lacerations (Cunningham, 2008). Postrepair, stool softeners should be prescribed for a week, and enemas should be avoided. Prophylactic antimicrobials should be considered, as described by Goldaber and associates (1993). Unfortunately, normal function is not always ensured even with correct and complete surgical repair. Some women may experience continuing fecal incontinence caused by injury to the innervation of the pelvic floor musculature (Roberts and co-workers, 1990).

Pain after Episiotomy

Pudendal block analgesia will help to relieve perineal pain postoperatively (Aissaoui and associates, 2008). Application of ice packs helps to reduce swelling and allay discomfort. In one randomized trial, Minassian and colleagues (2002) reported that topical application of 5-percent lidocaine ointment was not effective in relieving episiotomy or perineal laceration discomfort. Analgesics such as codeine give considerable relief. **Because pain may be a signal of a large vulvar, paravaginal, or ischiorectal hematoma or perineal cellulitis, it is essential to examine these sites carefully if pain is severe or persistent.** Management of these complications is discussed in Chapter 35 (p. 783).

Signorello and co-workers (2001) surveyed 615 women 6 months postpartum and reported that those delivered with an intact perineum reported better sexual function compared with

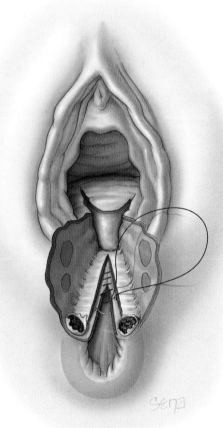

A

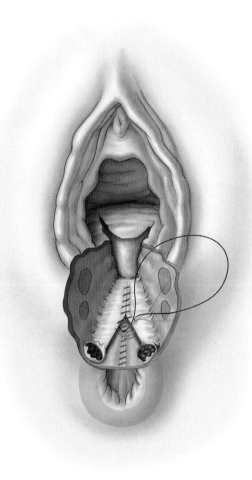

B

FIGURE 17-36 Layered repair of a fourth-degree perineal laceration. **A.** Approximation of the anorectal mucosa and submucosa in a running or interrupted fashion using fine absorbable suture such as 3-0 or 4-0 chromic or Vicryl. During this suturing, the superior extent of the anterior anal laceration is identified, and the sutures are placed through the submucosa of the anorectum approximately 0.5 cm apart down to the anal verge. **B.** A second layer is placed through the rectal muscularis using 3-0 Vicryl suture in a running or interrupted fashion. This "reinforcing layer" should incorporate the torn ends of the internal anal sphincter, which is identified as the thickening of the circular smooth muscle layer at the distal 2 to 3 cm of the anal canal. It can be identified as the glistening white fibrous structure lying between the anal canal submucosa and the fibers of the external anal sphincter (EAS). In many cases, the internal sphincter retracts laterally and must be sought and retrieved for repair. (*Continued*)

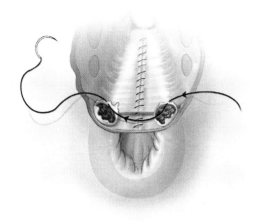

C

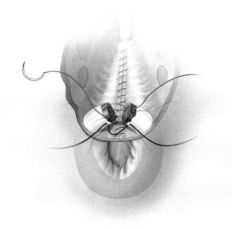

D

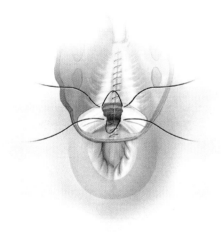

E

FIGURE 17-36 *Continued.* In overview, with traditional end-to-end approximation of the EAS, a suture is placed through the EAS muscle, and four to six simple interrupted 2-0 or 3-0 Vicryl sutures are placed at the 3, 6, 9, and 12 o'clock positions through the EAS muscle's connective tissue capsule. The sutures through the inferior and posterior portions of the sphincter should be placed first and tied last to aid this part of the repair. Initially with closure, the disrupted ends of the striated (EAS) muscle and capsule are identified and grasped with Allis clamps.**C.** Suture through the posterior wall of the external anal sphincter (EAS) capsule. **D.** Sutures through the EAS (*blue suture*) and inferior capsule wall. **E.** Sutures to reapproximate the anterior and superior walls of the EAS capsule. The remainder of the repair is similar to that described for a midline episiotomy in FIGURE 17-35.

those who had perineal trauma. In another follow-up of 2490 women, Rådestad and associates (2008) reported delayed intercourse at 3 and 6 months, but not at 1 year in women with and without perineal trauma. Finally, Brubaker and colleagues (2008) reported that women with anal sphincter lacerations at delivery had decreased sexual activity at 6 months.

LABOR MANAGEMENT PROTOCOLS

An orderly and systematic approach to labor management results in reproducible maternal and perinatal outcomes. This was recently proven by Althabe and co-workers (2008), who randomized implementation of evidence-based care in 19 hospitals in Argentina and Uruguay. Several labor management protocols are subsequently presented. These include those from the

National Maternity Hospital in Dublin, the World Health Organization, and from Parkland Hospital.

Active Management of Labor

More than 30 years ago, O'Driscoll and colleagues (1984) at the National Maternity Hospital in Dublin pioneered the concept that a disciplined, standardized labor management protocol reduced the number of cesarean deliveries for dystocia. Their overall cesarean delivery rate was 5 percent in the 1970s and 1980s with such management. The approach is now referred to as *active management of labor.* Two of its components—amniotomy and oxytocin—have been widely used, especially in English-speaking countries outside the United States (Thornton and Lilford, 1994). With this protocol, labor is diagnosed when painful contractions are accompanied by complete cervical effacement, bloody "show," or ruptured membranes. Women with such findings are committed to delivery within 12 hours. Pelvic examination is performed each hour for the next 3 hours, and thereafter at 2-hour intervals. When dilatation has not increased by at least 1 cm/hr, amniotomy is performed. Progress is again assessed at 2 hours and high-dose oxytocin infusion, described in Chapter 22 (p. 506), is started unless dilatation of at least 1 cm/hr is documented. Women are constantly attended by midwives.

If membranes rupture prior to admission, oxytocin is begun for no progress at the 1-hour mark. No special equipment is used, either to dispense oxytocin or to monitor its effects, and electronic uterine contraction monitoring is not used. Oxytocin is dispensed by gravity and regulated by a personal nurse. The solution contains 10 units of oxytocin in 1 L of dextrose and water. The total dose may not exceed 10 units, and the infusion rate may not exceed 30 to 40 mU/min. In the Dublin protocol, scalp blood sampling is used as the definitive test for fetal distress.

López-Zeno and colleagues (1992) prospectively compared such active management with their "traditional" approach to labor management at Northwestern Memorial Hospital in Chicago. They randomly assigned 705 nulliparas with uncomplicated pregnancies in spontaneous labor at term. The cesarean delivery rate was statistically lower with active versus traditional management—10.5 versus 14.1 percent, respectively. Subsequent studies did not show this. Wei and associates (2009) in a Cochrane database review found a modest reduction in cesarean delivery rates when active management of labor was compared with standard care. Frigoletto and co-workers (1995) reported another randomized trial with 1934 nulliparous women at Brigham and Women's Hospital in Boston. Although they found that such management somewhat shortened labor, it did not affect the cesarean delivery rate. These observations have since been reported by many others (Impey, 2000; Nicholson, 2008; Rogers, 1997; Sadler, 2000, and all their associates). The American College of Obstetricians and Gynecologists (2003a) concluded that active management of labor may shorten labor, although it has not consistently been shown to reduce rates of cesarean delivery. In a recent Cochrane Database systematic analysis, Brown and colleagues (2008) reached similar conclusions.

World Health Organization Partogram

A *partogram* was designed by the World Health Organization (WHO) for use in developing countries (Dujardin and co-workers, 1992). According to Orji (2008), the partograph is similar for nulliparas and multiparas. Labor is divided into a latent phase, which should last no longer than 8 hours, and an active phase. The active phase starts at 3 cm dilatation, and progress should be no slower than 1 cm/hr. A 4-hour wait is recommended before intervention when the active phase is slow. Labor is graphed, and analysis includes use of alert and action lines. Lavender and colleagues (2006) randomized 3000 nulliparous women to labor interventions at 2 hours versus 4 hours as recommended by WHO. Their cesarean delivery rate was unaffected, and they concluded that interventions

such as amniotomy and oxytocin were needlessly increased using the 2-hour time interval. After their recent Cochrane Database systematic review, Lavender and associates (2008) do not recommend use of the partograph for standard labor management.

Parkland Hospital Labor Management Protocol

During the 1980s, the obstetrical volume at Parkland Hospital doubled to approximately 15,000 births per year. In response, a second delivery unit for women with uncomplicated term pregnancies was designed. This provided a unique opportunity to implement and evaluate a standardized protocol for labor management. Its design was based on the approach that had evolved at our hospital up to that time. This emphasized the implementation of specific, sequential interventions when abnormal labor was suspected. This approach currently is used in both complicated and uncomplicated pregnancies.

Women are admitted if active labor—defined as cervical dilatation of 3 to 4 cm or more in the presence of uterine contractions—is diagnosed or if ruptured membranes are confirmed. Management guidelines summarized in **Figure 17-37** stipulate that a pelvic examination be performed approximately every 2 hours. Ineffective labor is suspected when the cervix does not dilate within approximately 2 hours of admission. Amniotomy is then performed, and labor progress determined at the next 2-hour evaluation. In women whose labors do not progress, an intrauterine pressure catheter is placed to assess uterine function. Hypotonic contractions and no cervical dilatation after an additional 2 to 3 hours result in stimulation of labor using the high-dose oxytocin regimen described in Chapter 22 (p. 506). The goal is uterine activity of 200 to 250 Montevideo units for 2 to 4 hours before dystocia can be diagnosed.

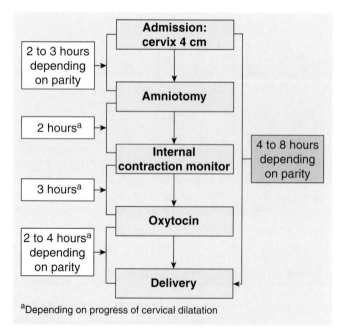

FIGURE 17-37 Schematic of labor management protocol in use at Parkland hospital. The total admission-to-delivery times are shorter than the potential sum of the intervention intervals because not every woman requires every intervention.

Dilatation rates of 1 to 2 cm/hr are accepted as evidence of progress after satisfactory uterine activity has been established with oxytocin. As shown in Figure 17-37, this can require up to 8 hours or more before cesarean delivery is performed for dystocia. The cumulative time required to effect this stepwise management approach permits many women to establish effective labor. This management protocol has been evaluated in more than 20,000 women with uncomplicated pregnancies. Cesarean delivery rates in nulliparous and parous women were 8.7 and 1.5 percent, respectively. Importantly, these labor interventions and the relatively infrequent use of cesarean delivery did not jeopardize the fetus-newborn.

REFERENCES

Aissaoui Y, Bruyère R, Mustapha H, et al: A randomized controlled trial of pudendal nerve block for pain relief after episiotomy. Anesth Analg 107:625, 2008

Alexander JM, Sharma SK, McIntire DD, et al: Epidural analgesia lengthens the Friedman active phase of labor. Obstet Gynecol 100:46, 2002

Alperin M, Krohn MA, Parviainen K: Episiotomy and increase in the risk of obstetric laceration in a subsequent vaginal delivery. Obstet Gynecol 111:1274, 2008

Althabe F, Buekens P, Bergel E, et al: A behavioral intervention to improve obstetrical care. N Engl J Med 358:1929, 2008

American Academy of Pediatrics and the American College of Obstetricians and Gynecologists: Guidelines for Perinatal Care, 5th ed. Washington, DC, AAP and ACOG, 2002

American Academy of Pediatrics and the American College of Obstetricians and Gynecologists: Guidelines for Perinatal Care, 6th ed. Washington, DC, AAP and ACOG, 2007

American College of Obstetricians and Gynecologists: Obstetric forceps. Committee Opinion 71, 1989

American College of Obstetricians and Gynecologists: Dystocia and augmentation of labor. Practice Bulletin No. 49, December 2003a

American College of Obstetricians and Gynecologists: Prophylactic antibiotics in labor and delivery. Practice Bulletin No. 47, October 2003b

American College of Obstetricians and Gynecologists: Episiotomy. Practice Bulletin No. 71, April 2006

American College of Obstetricians and Gynecologists: Optimal goals for anesthesia care in obstetrics. Committee Opinion No. 433, May 2009

Angioli R, Gomez-Marin O, Cantuaria G, et al: Severe perineal lacerations during vaginal delivery: The University of Miami experience. Am J Obstet Gynecol 182:1083, 2000

Anthony S, Buitendijk SE, Zondervan KT, et al: Episiotomies and the occurrence of severe perineal lacerations. Br J Obstet Gynaecol 101:1064, 1994

Bailit JL, Dierker L, Blanchard MH, et al: Outcomes of women presenting in active versus latent phase of spontaneous labor. Obstet Gynecol 105:77, 2005

Berghella V, Baxter JK, Chauhan SP: Evidence-based labor and delivery management. Am J Obstet Gynecol 199:445, 2008

Bloom SL, Casey BM, Schaffer JI, et al: A randomized trial of coached versus uncoached maternal pushing during the second stage of labor. Am J Obstet Gynecol 194:10, 2006

Bloom SL, McIntire DD, Kelly MA, et al: Lack of effect of walking on labor and delivery. N Engl J Med 339:76, 1998

Brown HC, Paranjothy S, Dowswell T, et al: Package of care for active management in labour for reducing caesarean section rates in low-risk women. Cochrane Database Syst Rev 8:CD004907, 2008

Browning DJ: Serious side effects of ergometrine and its use in routine obstetric practice. Med J Aust 1:957, 1974

Brubaker L, Handa VL, Bradley CS, et al: Sexual function 6 months after first delivery. Obstet Gynecol 111:1040, 2008

Caldwell WE, Moloy HC, D'Esopo DA: A roentgenologic study of the mechanism of engagement of the fetal head. Am J Obstet Gynecol 28:824, 1934

Calkins LA: The etiology of occiput presentations. Am J Obstet Gynecol 37:618, 1939

Carlan SJ, Wyble L, Lense J, et al: Fetal head molding: Diagnosis by ultrasound and a review of the literature. J Perinatol 11:105, 1991

Carley ME, Carley JM, Vasdev G, et al: Factors that are associated with clinically overt postpartum urinary retention after vaginal delivery. Am J Obstet Gynecol 187:430, 2002

Carollo TC, Reuter JM, Galan HL, et al: Defining fetal station. Am J Obstet Gynecol 191:1793, 2004

Carroli G, Mignini L: Episiotomy for vaginal birth. Cochrane Database Syst Rev 1:CD000081, 2009

Chelmow D, Kilpatrick SJ, Laros RK Jr: Maternal and neonatal outcomes after prolonged latent phase. Obstet Gynecol 81:486, 1993

Cheyne H, Hundley V, Dowding D, et al: Effects of algorithm for diagnosis of active labour: Cluster randomized trial. BMJ 337:a2396, 2008

Choy CMY, Lau WC, Tam WH, et al: A randomized controlled trial of intramuscular syntometrine and intravenous oxytocin in the management of the third stage of labor. Br J Obstet Gynaecol 109:173, 2002

Cohen W, Friedman EA (eds): Management of Labor. Baltimore, University Park Press, 1983

Combs CA, Robertson PA, Laros RK: Risk factors for third-degree and fourth-degree perineal lacerations in forceps and vacuum deliveries. Am J Obstet Gynecol 163:100, 1990

Cunningham FG: The Ritgen maneuver: Another sacred cow questioned. Obstet Gynecol 112:210, 2008

Deneux-Tharaux C, Macfarlane A, Winter C, et al: Policies for manual removal of placenta at vaginal delivery: variations in timing within Europe. BJOG 116(1):119, 2009

Dombrowski MP, Bottoms SF, Saleh AAA, et al: Third stage of labor: Analysis of duration and clinical practice. Am J Obstet Gynecol 172:1279, 1995

Dujardin B, De Schampheleire I, Sene H, et al: Value of the alert and action lines on the partogram. Lancet 339:1336, 1992

Dupuis O, Silveira R, Zentner A, et al: Birth simulator: Reliability of transvaginal assessment of fetal head station as defined by the American College of Obstetricians and Gynecologists classification. Am J Obstet Gynecol 192:868, 2005.

Eason E, Feldman P: Much ado about a little cut: Is episiotomy worthwhile? Obstet Gynecol 95:616, 2000

Eason E, Labrecque M, Wells G, et al: Preventing perineal trauma during childbirth: A systematic review. Obstet Gynecol 95:464, 2000

Federal Register, Vol 68, No. 174, p 53222, September 9, 2003

Fitzpatrick M, Behan M, O'Connell PR, et al: A randomized clinical trial comparing primary overlap with approximation repair of third-degree obstetric tears. Am J Obstet Gynecol 183:1220, 2000

Friedman E: The graphic analysis of labor. Am J Obstet Gynecol 68:1568, 1954

Friedman EA: An objective approach to the diagnosis and management of abnormal labor. Bull NY Acad Med 48:842, 1972

Friedman EA: Labor: Clinical Evaluation and Management, 2nd ed. New York, Appleton-Century-Crofts, 1978

Friedman EA: Primigravid labor: A graphicostatistical analysis. Obstet Gynecol 6:567, 1955

Friedman EA, Sachtleben MR: Amniotomy and the course of labor. Obstet Gynecol 22:755, 1963

Frigoletto FD Jr, Lieberman E, Lang JM, et al: A clinical trial of active management of labor. N Engl J Med 333:745, 1995

Gardberg M, Tuppurainen M: Anterior placental location predisposes for occiput posterior presentation near term. Acta Obstet Gynecol Scand 73:151, 1994a

Gardberg M, Tuppurainen M: Persistent occiput posterior presentation—a clinical problem. Acta Obstet Gynecol Scand 73:45, 1994b

Garite TJ, Weeks J, Peters-Phair K, et al: A randomized controlled trial of the effect of increased intravenous hydration on the course of labor in nulliparous women. Am J Obstet Gynecol 183:1544, 2000

Gjessing H, Backe B, Sahlin Y: Third degree obstetric tears; outcome after primary repair. Acta Obstet Gynecol Scand 77:736, 1998

Goldaber KG, Wendel PJ, McIntire DD, et al: Postpartum perineal morbidity after fourth-degree perineal repair. Am J Obstet Gynecol 168:489, 1993

Graham JM Jr, Kumar A: Diagnosis and management of extensive vertex birth molding. Clin Pediatr (Phila) 45(7):672, 2006

Greenberg MB, Cheng YW, Hopkins LM, et al: Are there ethnic differences in the length of labor? Am J Obstet Gynecol 195:743, 2006

Gurewitsch ED, Diament P, Fong J, et al: The labor curve of the grand multipara: Does progress of labor continue to improve with additional childbearing? Am J Obstet Gynecol 186:1331, 2002

Gurewitsch ED, Johnson E, Allen RH, et al: The descent curve of the grand multiparous woman. Am J Obstet Gynecol 189:1036, 2003

Hansen SL, Clark SL, Foster JC: Active pushing versus passive fetal descent in the second stage of labor: A randomized controlled trial. Obstet Gynecol 99:29, 2002

Hendricks CH, Brenner WE: Cardiovascular effects of oxytocic drugs used postpartum. Am J Obstet Gynecol 108:751, 1970

Henry DE, Cheng YW, Shaffer BL, et al: Perinatal outcomes in the setting of active phase arrest of labor. Obstet Gynecol 112:1109, 2008

Herbst A, Källén K: Time between membrane rupture and delivery and septicemia in term neonates. Obstet Gynecol 110:612, 2007

Hodnett ED, Stremler R, Willan AR, et al: Effect on birth outcomes of a formalized approach to care in hospital labour assessment units: International, randomized controlled trial. BMJ 337:a1021, 2008

Hofmeyr GJ, Abdel-Aleem H, Abdel-Aleem MA: Uterine massage for preventing postpartum haemorrhage. Cochrane Database Syst Rev 16:CD006431, 2008

Impey L, Hobson J, O'Herlihy C: Graphic analysis of actively managed labor: Prospective computation of labor progress in 500 consecutive nulliparous women in spontaneous labor at term. Am J Obstet Gynecol 183:438, 2000

Irons DW, Sriskandabalan P, Bullough CH: A simple alternative to parental oxytocics for the third stage of labor. Int J Gynaecol Obstet 46:15, 1994

Jackson KW, Allbert JR, Schemmer GK, et al: A randomized controlled trial comparing oxytocin administration before and after placental delivery in the prevention of postpartum hemorrhage. Am J Obstet Gynecol 185:873, 2001

Jönsson ER, Elfaghi I, Rydhström, et al: Modified Ritgen's maneuver for anal sphincter injury at delivery: A randomized controlled trial. Obstet Gynecol 112:212, 2008

Kettle C, Hills RK, Jones P, et al: Continuous versus interrupted perineal repair with standard or rapidly absorbed sutures after spontaneous vaginal birth: A randomized controlled trial. Lancet 359:2217, 2002

Kilpatrick SJ, Laros RK Jr: Characteristics of normal labor. Obstet Gynecol 74:85, 1989

Kindberg S, Stehouwer M, Hvidman L, et al: Postpartum perineal repair performed by midwives: A randomized trial comparing two suture techniques leaving the skin unsutured. BJOG 115:472, 2008

Kudish B, Blackwell S, Mcneeley G, et al: Operative vaginal delivery and midline episiotomy: A bad combination for the perineum. Am J Obstet Gynecol 195:749, 2006

Laine K, Pirhonen T, Rolland R, et al: Decreasing the incidence of anal sphincter tears during delivery. Obstet Gynecol 111:1053, 2008

Larsson P, Platz-Christensen J, Bergman B, et al: Advantage or disadvantage of episiotomy compared with spontaneous perineal laceration. Gynecol Obstet Invest 31:213, 1991

Lavender T, Alfirevic A, Walkinshaw S: Effect of different partogram action lines on birth outcomes. Obstet Gynecol 108:295, 2006

Lavender T, Hart A, Smyth RM: Effect of partogram use on outcomes for women in spontaneous labour at term. Cochrane Database Syst Rev 8:CD005461, 2008

Lawrence A, Lewis L, Hofmeyr GJ, et al: Maternal positions and mobility during first stage labour. Cochrane Database Syst Rev 2:CD003934, 2009

Leopold J: Conduct of normal births through external examination alone. Arch Gynaekol 45:337, 1894

López-Zeno JA, Peaceman AM, Adashek JA, et al: A controlled trial of a program for the active management of labor. N Engl J Med 326:450, 1992

Lydon-Rochelle M, Albers L, Gorwoda J, et al: Accuracy of Leopold maneuvers in screening for malpresentation: A prospective study. Birth 20:132, 1993

Martin JA, Hamilton BE, Sutton PD, et al: Births: Final data for 2002. National Vital Statistics Reports, Vol 52, No 10. Hyattsville, MD, National Center for Health Statistics, 2003

Martin JA, Hamilton BE, Sutton PD, et al: Births: Final data for 2003. National Vital Statistics Reports, Vol 54, No 2. Hyattsville, MD, National Center for Health Statistics, 2005

Martin JA, Hamilton BE, Sutton PD, et al: Births: Final data for 2006. National Vital Statistics Reports, Vol 57, No 7. Hyattsville, MD, National Center for Health Statistics, 2009

Mayerhofer K, Bodner-Adler B, Bodner K, et al: Traditional care of the perineum during birth: A prospective, randomized, multicenter study of 1,076 women. J Reprod Med 47:477, 2002

McDonald SJ, Middleton P: Effect of timing of umbilical cord clamping of term infants on maternal and neonatal outcomes. Cochrane Database Syst Rev 16:CD004074, 2008

Minassian VA, Jazayeri A, Prien SD, et al: Randomized trial of lidocaine ointment versus placebo for the treatment of postpartum perineal pain. Obstet Gynecol 100:1239, 2002

Mornar SJ, Perlow JH: Blunt suture needle use in laceration and episiotomy repair at vaginal delivery. Am J Obstet Gynecol 198:e14, 2008

Munn MB, Owen J, Vincent J, et al: Comparison of two oxytocin regimens to prevent uterine atony at cesarean delivery: A randomized controlled trial. Obstet Gynecol 98:386, 2001

Musselwhite KL, Faris P, Moore K, et al: Use of epidural anesthesia and the risk of acute postpartum urinary retention. Am J Obstet Gynecol 196:472, 2007

Nager CW, Helliwell JP: Episiotomy increases perineal laceration length in primiparous women. Am J Obstet Gynecol 185:444, 2001

New Shorter Oxford English Dictionary. New York, Oxford University Press, 1993

Nicholson JM, Parry S, Caughey AB, et al: The impact of the active management of risk in pregnancy at term on birth outcomes: A randomized clinical trial. Am J Obstet Gynecol 198:511.e1, 2008

O'Driscoll K, Foley M, MacDonald D: Active management of labor as an alternative to cesarean section for dystocia. Obstet Gynecol 63:485, 1984

Orji E: Evaluating progress of labor in nulliparas and multiparas using the modified WHO partograph. Int J Gynaecol Obstet 102:249, 2008

Orji E, Agwu F, Loto O, et al: A randomized comparative study of prophylactic oxytocin versus ergometrine in the third stage of labor. Int J Gynaecol Obstet 101:129, 2008

Pates JA, McIntire DD, Leveno KJ: Uterine contractions preceding labor. Obstet Gynecol 110:566, 2007

Poen AC, Felt-Bersma RJ, Strijers RL, et al: Third-degree obstetric perineal tear: Long-term clinical and functional results after primary repair. Br J Surg 85:1433, 1998

Prendiville W, Elbourne D, Chalmers I: The effects of routine oxytocic administration in the management of the third stage of labour: An overview of the evidence from controlled trials. Br J Obstet Gynaecol 95:3, 1988a

Prendiville WJ, Harding JE, Elbourne DR, et al: The Bristol third stage trial: Active versus physiological management of third stage of labour. Br Med J 297:1295, 1988b

Rådestad I, Olsson A, Nissen E, et al: Tears in the vagina, perineum, sphincter ani, and rectum and first sexual intercourse after childbirth: A nationwide follow-up. Birth 35:98, 2008

Ritgen G: Concerning his method for protection of the perineum. Monatschrift für Geburtskunde 6:21, 1855. See English translation, Wynn RM: Am J Obstet Gynecol 93:421, 1965

Roberts PL, Coller JA, Schoetz DJ, et al: Manometric assessment of patients with obstetric injuries and fecal incontinence. Dis Colon Rectum 33:16, 1990

Rodriguez A, Arenas EA, Osorio AL, et al: Selective vs routine midline episiotomy for the prevention of third- or fourth-degree lacerations in nulliparous women. Am J Obstet Gynecol 198:285.e1, 2008

Rogers R, Gelson GJ, Miller AC, et al: Active management of labor: Does it make a difference? Am J Obstet Gynecol 177:599, 1997

Sadler LC, Davison T, McCowan LME: A randomized controlled trial and meta-analysis of active management of labour. Br J Obstet Gynaecol 107:909, 2000

Sanders J, Campbell R, Peters TJ: Effectiveness of pain relief during perineal suturing. Br J Obstet Gynaecol 109:1066, 2002

Schaffer JI, Bloom SL, Casey BM, et al: A randomized trial of the effects of coached vs uncoached maternal pushing during the second stage of labor on postpartum pelvic floor structure and function. Am J Obstet Gynecol 192:1692, 2005

Schwartz RH, Jones RWA: Transplacental hyponatremia due to oxytocin. Br Med J 1:152, 1978

Secher NJ, Arnso P, Wallin L: Haemodynamic effects of oxytocin (Syntocinon) and methylergometrine (Methergin) on the systemic and pulmonary circulations of pregnant anaesthetized women. Acta Obstet Gynecol Scand 57:97, 1978

Shrivastava VK, Garite TJ, Jenkins SM, et al: A randomized, double-blinded, controlled trial comparing parenteral normal saline with and without dextrose on the course of labor in nulliparas. Am J Obstet Gynecol 200(4):379.e1, 2009

Signorello LB, Harlow BL, Chekos AK, et al: Midline episiotomy and anal incontinence: Retrospective cohort study. Br Med J 320:86, 2000

Signorello LB, Harlow BL, Chekos AK, et al: Postpartum sexual functioning and its relationship to perineal trauma: A retrospective cohort study of primiparous women. Am J Obstet Gynecol 184:881, 2001

Sokol RJ, Stojkov J, Chik L, et al: Normal and abnormal labor progress: I. A quantitative assessment and survey of the literature. J Reprod Med 18:47, 1977

Sultan AH, Monga AK, Kumar D, et al: Primary repair of obstetric anal sphincter rupture using the overlap technique. Br J Obstet Gynaecol 106:318, 1999

Svanström MC, Biber B, Hanes M, et al: Signs of myocardial ischaemia after injection of oxytocin: A randomized double-blind comparison of oxytocin and methylergometrine during caesarean section. Br J Anaesth 100:683, 2008

Thilaganathan B, Cutner A, Latimer J, et al: Management of the third-stage of labour in women at low risk of postpartum haemorrhage. Eur J Obstet Gynecol Reprod Biol 48:19, 1993

Thornton JG, Lilford RJ: Active management of labour: Current knowledge and research issues. Br Med J 309:366, 1994

Valenzuela P, Saiz Puente MS, Valero JL, et al: Continuous versus interrupted sutures for repair of episiotomy or second-degree perineal tears: a randomised controlled trial. BJOG 116(3):436, 2009

Venkatesh KS, Ramanujam PS, Larson DM, et al: Anorectal complications of vaginal delivery. Dis Colon Rectum 32:1039, 1989

Villar J, Gülmezoglu AM, Hofmeyr GJ, et al: Systematic review of randomized controlled trials of misoprostol to prevent postpartum hemorrhage. Obstet Gynecol 100:1301, 2001

Weber AM, Meyn L: Episiotomy use in the United States, 1979–1997. Obstet Gynecol 100:1177, 2002

Wei S, Wo BL, Xu H, et al: Early amniotomy and early oxytocin for prevention of, or therapy for, delay in first stage spontaneous labour compared with routine care. Cochrane Database Syst Rev 2:CD006794, 2009

Whalley PJ, Pritchard JA: Oxytocin and water intoxication. JAMA 186:601, 1963

Williams MK, Chames MC: Risk factors for the breakdown of perineal laceration repair after vaginal delivery. Am J Obstet Gynecol 195:755, 2006

Yamada H, Kishida T, Negishi H, et al: Silent premature rupture of membranes, detected and monitored serially by an AFP kit. J Obstet Gynaecol Res 24:103, 1998

Yao AC, Lind J: Placental transfusion. Am J Dis Child 127:128, 1974

Yildirim G, Beji NK: Effects of pushing techniques in birth on mother and fetus: A randomized study. Birth 35:25, 2008

Zahalka N, Sadan O, Malinger G, et al: Comparison of transvaginal sonography with digital examination and transabdominal sonography for the determination of fetal head position in the second stage of labor. Am J Obstet Gynecol 193:381, 2005

Zhang J, Troendle J, Mikolajczyk R, et al: Natural history of labor progression [Abstract 134]. Presented at the 29th Annual Meeting of the Society for Maternal-Fetal Medicine in San Diego, CA, January 26–31, 2009a

Zhang J, Troendle JF, Yancey MK: Reassessing the labor curve in nulliparous women. Am J Obstet Gynecol 187:824, 2002

Zhang J, Vanveldhuisen P, Troendle J, et al: Normal labor patterns in U.S. women [Abstract 80]. Presented at the 29th Annual Meeting of the Society for Maternal–Fetal Medicine in San Diego, CA, January 26–31, 2009b

Intrapartum Assessment

Following earlier work by Hon (1958), continuous electronic fetal monitoring (EFM) was introduced into obstetrical practice in the late 1960s. No longer were intrapartum fetal surveillance and the suspicion of fetal distress based upon periodic auscultation with a fetoscope. Instead, the continuous graph-paper portrayal of the fetal heart rate was potentially diagnostic in assessing pathophysiological events affecting the fetus. Indeed, there were great expectations that:

- Electronic fetal heart rate monitoring provided accurate information
- The information was of value in diagnosing fetal distress
- It would be possible to intervene to prevent fetal death or morbidity
- Continuous electronic fetal heart rate monitoring was superior to intermittent methods.

When first introduced, electronic fetal heart rate monitoring was used primarily in complicated pregnancies, but gradually became used in most pregnancies. By 1978, it was estimated that nearly two thirds of American women were being monitored electronically during labor (Banta and Thacker, 1979). In 2002, approximately 3.4 million American women, comprising 85 percent of all live births, underwent electronic fetal monitoring (Martin and colleagues, 2003). Indeed, fetal monitoring has become the most prevalent obstetrical procedure in the United States (American College of Obstetricians and Gynecologists, 2005).

ELECTRONIC FETAL MONITORING

Internal Electronic Monitoring

The fetal heart rate may be measured by attaching a bipolar spiral electrode directly to the fetus (Fig. 18-1). The wire electrode penetrates the fetal scalp, and the second pole is a metal wing on the electrode. Vaginal body fluids create a saline electrical bridge that completes the circuit and permits measurement of the voltage differences between the two poles. The two wires of the bipolar electrode are attached to a reference electrode on the maternal thigh to eliminate electrical interference. The electrical fetal cardiac signal—P wave, QRS complex, and T wave—is amplified and fed into a cardiotachometer for heart rate calculation. The peak R-wave voltage is the portion of the fetal electrocardiogram most reliably detected.

An example of the method of fetal heart rate processing employed when a scalp electrode is used is shown in Figure 18-2. Time (t) in milliseconds between fetal R waves is fed into a cardiotachometer, where a new fetal heart rate is set with the arrival of each new R wave. As also shown in Figure 18-2, a premature atrial contraction is computed as a heart rate acceleration because the interval (t_2) is shorter than the preceding one (t_1). The phenomenon of continuous R-to-R wave fetal heart rate computation is known as *beat-to-beat variability*. The physiological event being counted, however, is not a mechanical event corresponding to a heartbeat but rather an electrical event.

Electrical cardiac complexes detected by the electrode include those generated by the mother. Although the maternal electrocardiogram (ECG) signal is approximately five times stronger than the fetal ECG, its amplitude is diminished when it is recorded through the fetal scalp electrode. In a live fetus, this low maternal ECG signal is detected but masked by the fetal ECG. If the fetus is dead, the weaker maternal signal will be

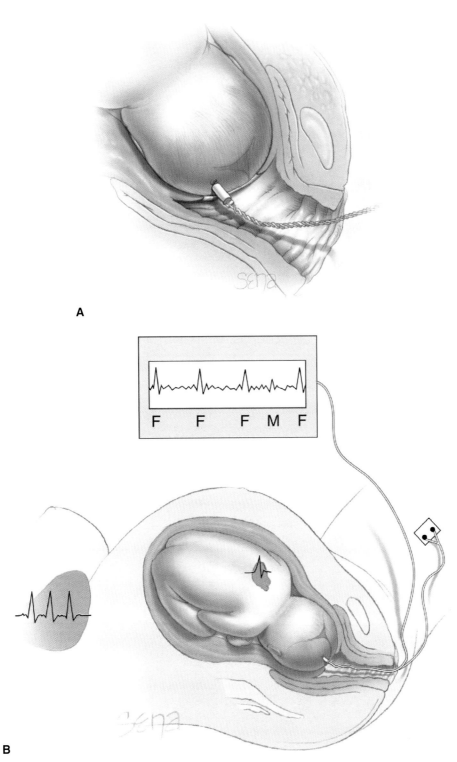

A

F   F   F M F

B

FIGURE 18-1 Internal electronic fetal monitoring. **A.** Scalp electrode penetrates the fetal scalp by means of a coiled electrode. **B.** Schematic representation of a bipolar electrode attached to the fetal scalp for detection of fetal QRS complexes (F). Also shown is the maternal heart and corresponding electrical complex (M) that is detected.

amplified and displayed as the "fetal" heart rate (Freeman and co-workers, 2003). Shown in Figure 18-3 are simultaneous recordings of maternal chest wall ECG signals and fetal scalp electrode ECG signals. This fetus is experiencing premature atrial contractions, which cause the cardiotachometer to rapidly and erratically seek new heart rates, resulting in the "spiking" shown in the standard fetal monitor tracing. Importantly, when the fetus is dead, the maternal R waves are still detected by the scalp electrode as the next best signal and are counted by the cardiotachometer (Fig. 18-4).

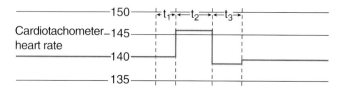

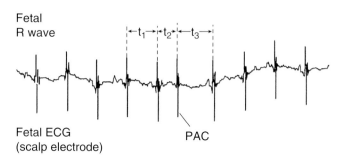

FIGURE 18-2 Schematic representation of fetal electrocardiographic signals used to compute continuing beat-to-beat heart rate with scalp electrodes. Time intervals (t_1, t_2, t_3) in milliseconds between successive fetal R waves are used by cardiotachometer to compute instantaneous fetal heart rate. (ECG = electrocardiogram; PAC = premature atrial contraction.)

External (Indirect) Electronic Monitoring

The necessity for membrane rupture and uterine invasion may be avoided by use of external detectors to monitor fetal heart action and uterine activity. External monitoring, however, does not provide the precision of fetal heart rate measurement or the quantification of uterine pressure afforded by internal monitoring.

The fetal heart rate is detected through the maternal abdominal wall using the *ultrasound Doppler principle* (Fig. 18-5). Ultrasound waves undergo a shift in frequency as they are reflected from moving fetal heart valves and from pulsatile blood ejected during systole (see Chap. 16, p. 362).

The unit consists of a transducer that emits ultrasound and a sensor to detect a shift in frequency of the reflected sound. The transducer is placed on the maternal abdomen at a site where fetal heart action is best detected. A coupling gel must be applied because air conducts ultrasound poorly. The device is held in position by a belt. Care should be taken that maternal arterial pulsations are not confused with fetal cardiac motion (Neilson and associates, 2008).

Ultrasound Doppler signals are edited electronically before fetal heart rate data are printed onto the bedside monitor tracing paper. Reflected ultrasound signals from moving fetal heart valves are analyzed through a microprocessor that compares incoming signals with the most recent previous signal. This process, called *autocorrelation*, is based on the premise that the fetal heart rate has regularity whereas "noise" is random and without regularity. Several fetal heart motions must be deemed electronically acceptable by the microprocessor before the fetal heart rate is printed. Such electronic editing has greatly improved the tracing quality of the externally recorded fetal heart rate.

Fetal Heart Rate Patterns

It is now generally accepted that interpretation of fetal heart rate patterns can be problematic because of the lack of agreement on definitions and nomenclature (American College of Obstetricians and Gynecologists, 2005). The National Institute of Child Health and Human Development (NICHD) Research Planning Workshop (1997) brought together investigators with expertise in the field to propose standardized, unambiguous definitions for interpretation of fetal heart rate patterns during labor. The definitions proposed as a result of this workshop will be used in this chapter (Table 18-1). First, it is important to recognize that interpretation of electronic fetal heart rate data is based on the visual pattern of the heart rate as portrayed on chart recorder graph paper. Thus, the choice of vertical and horizontal scaling greatly affects the appearance of the fetal heart rate. Scaling factors recommended by the workshop are 30 beats per minute (beats/min or bpm) per vertical cm (range, 30 to 240 beats/min) and 3 cm/min chart recorder paper speed. Fetal heart rate variation is falsely displayed at the slower 1 cm/min paper speed compared with that of the smoother baseline recorded at 3 cm/min (Fig. 18-6). Thus, pattern recognition can be considerably distorted depending on the scaling factors used.

Baseline Fetal Heart Activity

Baseline fetal heart activity refers to the modal characteristics that prevail apart from periodic accelerations or decelerations associated with uterine contractions. Descriptive characteristics of baseline fetal heart activity include *rate, beat-to-beat variability, fetal arrhythmia*, and distinct patterns such as *sinusoidal* or *saltatory* fetal heart rates.

Rate

With increasing fetal maturation, the heart rate decreases. This continues postnatally such that the average rate is 90 beats/min by age 8 (Behrman, 1992). Pillai and James (1990) longitudinally studied fetal heart rate characteristics in 43 normal pregnancies. The baseline fetal heart rate decreased an average of 24 beats/min between 16 weeks and term, or approximately 1 beat/min per week. It is postulated that this normal gradual slowing of the fetal heart rate corresponds to maturation of parasympathetic (vagal) heart control (Renou and co-workers, 1969).

The baseline fetal heart rate is the approximate mean rate rounded to increments of 5 beats/min during a 10-minute tracing segment. In any 10-minute window, the minimum interpretable baseline duration must be at least 2 minutes. If the baseline fetal heart rate is less than 110 beats/min, it is termed *bradycardia*. If the baseline rate is greater than 160 beats/min, it is termed *tachycardia*. The average fetal heart rate is considered the result of tonic balance between *accelerator* and *decelerator* influences on pacemaker cells. In this concept, the sympathetic system is the accelerator influence, and the parasympathetic system is the decelerator factor mediated via vagal slowing of heart rate (Dawes, 1985). Heart rate also is under the control of

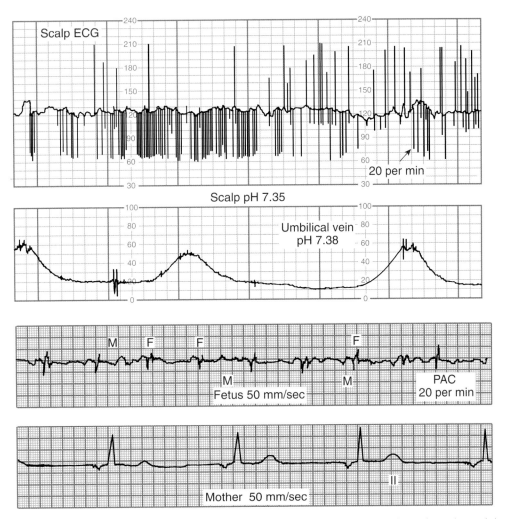

FIGURE 18-3 The top tracing shows standard fetal monitor tracing of heart rate using fetal scalp electrode. Spiking of the fetal rate in the monitor tracing is due to premature atrial contractions. The second panel displays accompanying contractions. The bottom two tracings represent cardiac electrical complexes detected from fetal scalp and maternal chest wall electrodes. (ECG = electrocardiogram; F = fetus; M = mother; PAC = fetal premature atrial contraction.)

arterial chemoreceptors such that both hypoxia and hypercapnia can modulate rate. More severe and prolonged hypoxia, with a rising blood lactate level and severe metabolic acidemia, induces a prolonged fall in heart rate (Thakor and Giussani, 2009).

Bradycardia. During the third trimester, the normal mean baseline fetal heart rate has generally been accepted to be between 120 and 160 beats/min. The lower normal limit is disputed internationally, with some investigators recommending 110 beats/min (Manassiev, 1996). Pragmatically, a rate between 100 and 119 beats/min, in the absence of other changes, usually is not considered to represent fetal compromise. Such low but potentially normal baseline heart rates also have been attributed to head compression from occiput posterior or transverse positions, particularly during second-stage labor (Young and Weinstein, 1976). Such mild bradycardias were observed in 2 percent of monitored pregnancies and averaged approximately 50 minutes in duration. Freeman and colleagues (2003) have concluded that bradycardia within the range of 80 to 120

beats/min with good variability is reassuring. Interpretation of rates less than 80 beats/min is problematic, and such rates generally are considered nonreassuring.

Some causes of fetal bradycardia include congenital heart block and serious fetal compromise (Jaeggi, 2008, Kodama, 2009, Larma, 2007, and all their associates). Figure 18-7 shows bradycardia in a fetus dying from placental abruption. Maternal hypothermia under general anesthesia for repair of a cerebral aneurysm or during maternal cardiopulmonary bypass for open-heart surgery also can cause fetal bradycardia. Sustained fetal bradycardia in the setting of severe pyelonephritis and maternal hypothermia also has been reported (Hankins and coworkers, 1997). These infants apparently are not harmed by several hours of such bradycardia.

Tachycardia. Fetal tachycardia is defined as a baseline heart rate in excess of 160 beats/min. The most common explanation for fetal tachycardia is maternal fever from chorioamnionitis, although fever from any source can increase baseline fetal heart rate. Such infections also have been observed to

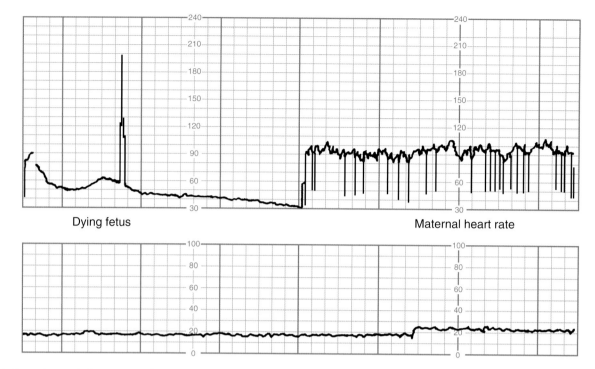

Dying fetus

Maternal heart rate

FIGURE 18-4 Placental abruption. In the upper panel, the fetal scalp electrode first detected the heart rate of the dying fetus. After fetal death, the maternal electrocardiogram complex is detected and recorded. The second panel displays an absence of uterine contractions.

induce fetal tachycardia before overt maternal fever is diagnosed (Gilstrap and associates, 1987). Fetal tachycardia caused by maternal infection typically is not associated with fetal compromise unless there are associated periodic heart rate changes or fetal sepsis.

Other causes of fetal tachycardia include fetal compromise, cardiac arrhythmias, and maternal administration of parasympathetic (atropine) or sympathomimetic (terbutaline) drugs. The key feature to distinguish fetal compromise in association with tachycardia seems to be concomitant heart rate decelerations. Prompt relief of the compromising event, such as correction of maternal hypotension caused by epidural analgesia, can result in fetal recovery.

Wandering Baseline. This baseline rate is unsteady and "wanders" between 120 and 160 beats/min (Freeman and colleagues, 2003). This rare finding is suggestive of a neurologically abnormal fetus and may occur as a preterminal event.

Beat-to-Beat Variability

Baseline variability is an important index of cardiovascular function and appears to be regulated largely by the autonomic nervous system (Kozuma and colleagues, 1997). That is, a sympathetic and parasympathetic "push and pull" mediated via the sinoatrial node produces moment-to-moment or beat-to-beat oscillation of the baseline heart rate. Such change of the heart rate is defined as baseline variability. Variability is further divided into short term and long term.

Short-term variability reflects the instantaneous change in fetal heart rate from one beat—or R wave—to the next. This variability is a measure of the time interval between cardiac systoles (Fig. 18-8). Short-term variability can most reliably be determined to be normally present only when electrocardiac cycles are measured directly with a scalp electrode. *Long-term variability* is used to describe the oscillatory changes that occur during the course of 1 minute and result in the waviness of the baseline (Fig. 18-9). The normal frequency of such waves is three to five cycles per minute (Freeman and associates, 2003).

It should be recognized that precise quantitative analysis of both short- and long-term variability presents a number of

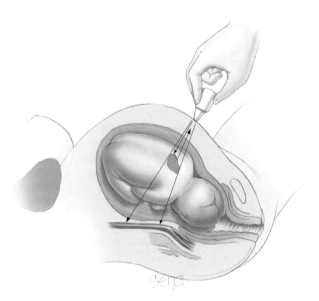

FIGURE 18-5 Ultrasound Doppler principle used externally to measure fetal heart motions. Pulsations of the maternal aorta also may be detected and erroneously counted. (Adapted from Klavan and co-workers, 1977, with permission.)

TABLE 18-1. The National Institute of Child Health and Human Development Research Planning Workshop Definitions of Fetal Heart Rate Patterns

Pattern	Workshop Interpretations
Baseline	• The mean FHR rounded to increments of 5 bpm during a 10-min segment, excluding: — Periodic or episodic changes — Periods of marked FHR variability — Segments of baseline that differ > 25 bpm
Baseline variability	• The baseline must be for a minimum of 2 min in any 10-min segment • Fluctuations in the FHR of two cycles per min or greater • Variability is visually quantified as the amplitude of peak-to-trough in bpm — Absent—amplitude range undetectable — Minimal—amplitude range detectable but ≤ 5 bpm — Moderate (normal)—amplitude range 6–25 bpm — Marked—amplitude range > 25 bpm
Acceleration	• A visually apparent increase—onset to peak in less than 30 sec—in the FHR from the most recently calculated baseline • The duration of an acceleration is defined as the time from the initial change in FHR from the baseline to the return of the FHR to the baseline • At 32 weeks and beyond, an acceleration has an acme of ≥ 15 bpm above baseline, with a duration of ≥ 15 sec but < 2 min • Before 32 weeks, an acceleration has an acme ≥ 10 bpm above baseline, with a duration of ≥ 10 sec but < 2 min • Prolonged acceleration lasts ≥ 2 min, but < 10 min • If an acceleration lasts ≥ 10 min, it is baseline change
Bradycardia	• Baseline FHR < 110 bpm
Early deceleration	• In association with a uterine contraction, a visually apparent, usually symmetrical, gradual—onset to nadir ≥ 30 sec—decrease in FHR with return to baseline • Nadir of the deceleration occurs at the same time as the peak of the contraction
Late deceleration	• In association with a uterine contraction, a visually apparent, gradual—onset to nadir ≥ 30 sec decrease in FHR with return to baseline • Onset, nadir, and recovery of the deceleration occur after the beginning, peak, and end of the contraction, respectively
Tachycardia	• Baseline FHR > 160 bpm
Variable deceleration	• An abrupt onset to nadir < 30 sec, visually apparent decrease in the FHR below the baseline • The decrease in FHR is ≥ 15 bpm, with a duration of ≥ 15 sec but < 2 min
Prolonged deceleration	• Visually apparent decrease in the FHR below the baseline • Deceleration is ≥ 15 bpm, lasting ≥ 2 min but < 10 min from onset to return to baseline

BPM = beats per minute; FHR = fetal heart rate.
Reprinted from *American Journal of Obstetrics & Gynecology*, Vol. 177, No. 6, National Institute of Child Health and Human Development Research Planning Workshop, Electronic fetal heart rate monitoring: Research guidelines for interpretation, pp. 1385–1390, Copyright 1997, with permission from Elsevier.

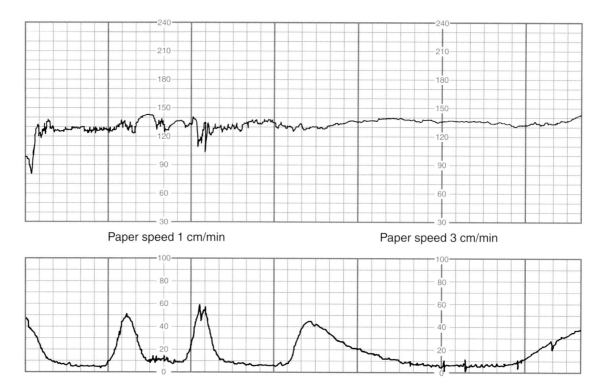

Paper speed 1 cm/min   Paper speed 3 cm/min

FIGURE 18-6 Fetal heart rate obtained by scalp electrode (*upper panel*) and recorded at 1 cm/min compared with that at 3 cm/min chart recorder paper speed. Concurrent uterine contractions are shown in the (*lower panel*).

frustrating problems due to technical and scaling factors. For example, Parer and co-workers (1985) evaluated 22 mathematical formulas designed to quantify heart rate variability and found most to be unsatisfactory. Consequently, most clinical interpretation is based on visual analysis with subjective judgment of the smoothness or flatness of the baseline. According to Freeman and

colleagues (2003), there is no current evidence that the distinction between short- and long-term variability has any clinical relevance. Similarly, the NICHD Workshop (1997) did not recommend differentiating short- and long-term variability because in actual practice they are visually determined as a unit. The workshop panel defined baseline variability as those baseline fluctuations of two cycles per minute or greater. They recommended the criteria shown in **Figure 18-10** for quantification of variability. Normal beat-to-beat variability was accepted to be 6 to 25 beats/min.

Increased Variability. Several physiological and pathological processes can affect or interfere with beat-to-beat variability. Dawes and co-workers (1981) described increased variability during *fetal breathing*. In healthy infants, short-term variability is attributable to respiratory sinus arrhythmia (Divon and associates, 1986). *Fetal body movements* also affect variability (Van Geijn and colleagues, 1980). Pillai and James (1990) reported increased baseline variability with *advancing gestation*. Up to 30 weeks, baseline characteristics were similar during both fetal rest and activity. After 30 weeks, fetal inactivity was

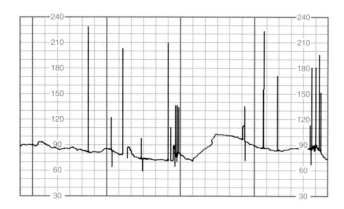

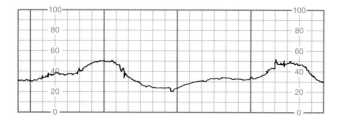

FIGURE 18-7 Fetal bradycardia measured with a scalp electrode (*upper panel*) in a pregnancy complicated by placental abruption and subsequent fetal death. Concurrent uterine contractions are shown in the (*lower panel*).

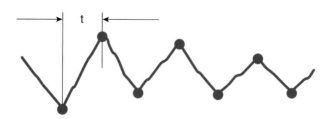

FIGURE 18-8 Schematic representation of short-term beat-to-beat variability measured by a fetal scalp electrode. (t = time interval between successive fetal R waves.) (Adapted from Klavan and co-workers, 1977.)

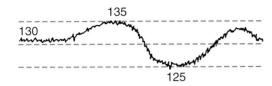

FIGURE 18-9 Schematic representation of long-term beat-to-beat variability of the fetal heart rate ranging between 125 and 135 beats/min. (Adapted from Klavan and associates, 1977.)

associated with diminished baseline variability and conversely, variability was increased during fetal activity. Fetal gender does not affect heart rate variability (Ogueh and Steer, 1998).

The baseline fetal heart rate becomes more physiologically fixed (less variable) as the rate increases. Conversely, there is more instability or variability of the baseline at lower heart rates. This phenomenon presumably reflects less cardiovascular physiological wandering as beat-to-beat intervals shorten due to increasing heart rate.

Decreased Variability. Diminished beat-to-beat variability can be an ominous sign indicating a seriously compromised fetus. Paul and co-workers (1975) reported that loss of variability in combination with decelerations was associated with *fetal acidemia*. They analyzed variability in the 20 minutes preceding delivery in 194 pregnancies. Decreased variability was defined as 5 or fewer beats/min excursion of the baseline (see Fig. 18-10), whereas acceptable variability exceeded this range. Fetal scalp pH was measured 1119 times in these pregnancies, and mean values were found to be increasingly more acidemic when decreased variability was added to progressively intense heart rate decelerations. For example, mean fetal scalp pH of approximately 7.10 was found when severe decelerations were combined with 5 beats/min or less variability, compared with a pH approximately 7.20 when greater variability was associated with similarly severe decelerations. Severe *maternal acidemia* also can cause decreased fetal beat-to-beat variability, as shown in Figure 18-11 in a mother with diabetic ketoacidosis.

The precise pathological mechanisms by which fetal hypoxemia results in diminished beat-to-beat variability are not totally understood. Interestingly, mild degrees of fetal hypoxemia have been reported actually to *increase* variability, at least at the outset of the hypoxic episode (Murotsuki and co-workers, 1997). According to Dawes (1985), it seems probable that the loss of variability is a result of metabolic acidemia that causes depression of the fetal brainstem or the heart itself. Thus, diminished beat-to-beat variability, when it reflects fetal compromise, likely reflects acidemia rather than hypoxia.

A common cause of diminished beat-to-beat variability is *analgesic drugs* given during labor (see Chap. 19, p. 446). A large variety of central nervous system depressant drugs can cause transient diminished beat-to-beat variability. Included are narcotics, barbiturates, phenothiazines, tranquilizers, and general anesthetics. Diminished variability occurs regularly within 5 to 10 minutes following intravenous meperidine administration, and the effects may last up to 60 minutes or longer depending on the dosage given (Petrie, 1993). Butorphanol given intravenously diminishes fetal heart rate reactivity (Schucker and associates, 1996). Hill and colleagues (2003), in a study performed at Parkland Hospital, found that 5 beats/min or less variability occurred in 30 percent of

women given continuous intravenous meperidine compared with 7 percent in those given continuous labor epidural analgesia using 0.0625-percent bupivacaine and 2 μg/mL of fentanyl.

Magnesium sulfate, widely used in the United States for tocolysis as well as management of hypertensive women, has been arguably associated with diminished beat-to-beat variability. Hallak and colleagues (1999) randomly assigned 34 normal, nonlaboring women to standard magnesium sulfate infusion versus isotonic saline. Magnesium sulfate was associated with statistically decreased variability only in the third hour of the infusion. However, the average decrease in variability was deemed clinically insignificant because the mean variability was 2.7 beats/min in the third hour of magnesium infusion compared with 2.8 beats/min at baseline. Magnesium sulfate also blunted the frequency of accelerations.

It is generally believed that reduced baseline heart rate variability is the single most reliable sign of fetal compromise. For example, Smith and co-workers (1988) performed a computerized analysis of beat-to-beat variability in growth-restricted fetuses *before* labor. They observed that diminished variability (4.2 beats/min or less) that was maintained for 1 hour was diagnostic of developing acidemia and imminent fetal death. By contrast, Samueloff and associates (1994) evaluated variability as a predictor of fetal outcome during labor in 2200 consecutive deliveries. They concluded that variability by itself could not be used as the only indicator of fetal well-being. Conversely, they also concluded that good variability should not be interpreted as necessarily reassuring.

In summary, beat-to-beat variability is affected by a variety of pathological and physiological mechanisms. Variability has considerably different meaning depending on the clinical setting. The development of decreased variability in the absence of decelerations is unlikely to be due to fetal hypoxia (Davidson and co-workers, 1992). A persistently flat fetal heart rate baseline—absent variability—within the normal baseline rate range and without decelerations may reflect a previous insult to the fetus that has resulted in neurological damage (Freeman and colleagues, 2003).

Cardiac Arrhythmia

When fetal cardiac arrhythmias are first suspected using electronic monitoring, findings can include baseline bradycardia, tachycardia, or most commonly in our experience, *abrupt baseline spiking* (Fig. 18-12). Intermittent baseline bradycardia is frequently due to congenital heart block. As discussed in Chapter 54 (p. 1150), conduction defects, most commonly complete atrioventricular (AV) block, usually are found in association with maternal connective-tissue diseases. Documentation of an arrhythmia can only be accomplished, practically speaking, when scalp electrodes are used. Some fetal monitors can be adapted to output the scalp electrode signals into an electrocardiographic recorder. Because only a single lead is obtained, analysis and interpretation of rhythm and rate disturbances are severely limited.

Southall and associates (1980) studied antepartum fetal cardiac rate and rhythm disturbances in 934 normal pregnancies between 30 and 40 weeks. Arrhythmias, episodes of bradycardia less than 100 beats/min, or tachycardia greater than 180 beats/min were encountered in 3 percent. Most supraventricular arrhythmias are of little significance during labor unless there is coexistent heart failure as evidenced by fetal hydrops.

SECTION 4

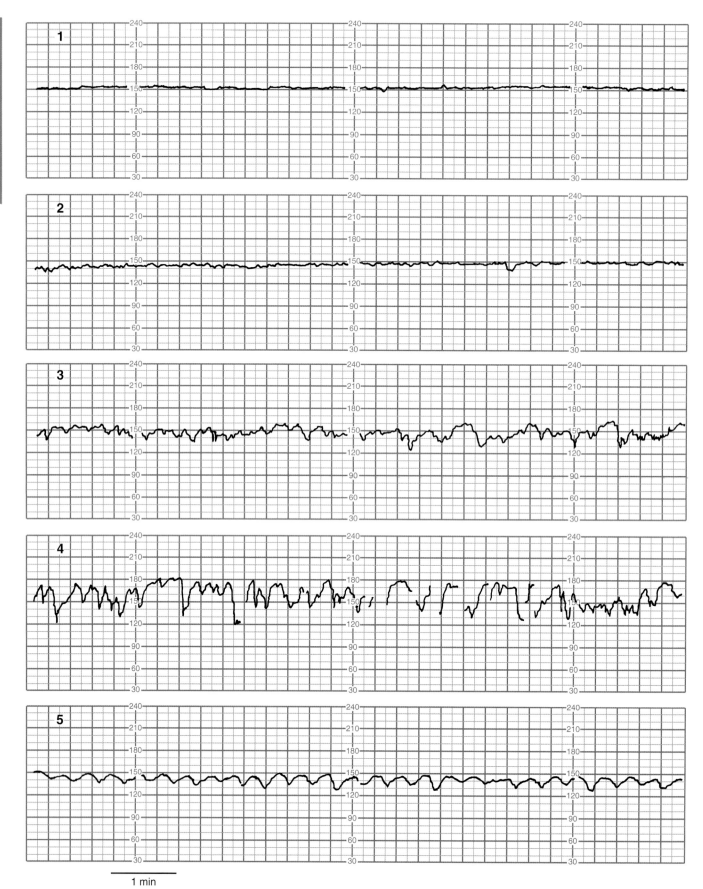

1 min

FIGURE 18-10 Panels 1–4: Grades of baseline fetal heart rate variability—irregular fluctuations in the baseline of 2 cycles per minute or greater. **1.** Undetectable, absent variability. **2.** Minimal variability, ≤5 beats/min. **3.** Moderate (normal) variability, 6 to 25 beats/min. **4.** Marked variability, >25 beats/min. **Panel 5:** Sinusoidal pattern. The sinusoidal pattern differs from variability in that it has a smooth, sinelike pattern of regular fluctuation and is excluded in the definition of fetal heart rate variability. (Adapted from National Institute of Child Health and Human Development Research Planning Workshop, 1997.)

TABLE 17-5. Midline Versus Mediolateral Episiotomy

Characteristic	Type of Episiotomy	
	Midline	Mediolateral
Surgical repair	Easy	More difficult
Faulty healing	Rare	More common
Postoperative pain	Minimal	Common
Anatomical results	Excellent	Occasionally faulty
Blood loss	Less	More
Dyspareunia	Rare	Occasional
Extensions	Common	Uncommon

and colleagues (1994) presented data from the Dutch National Obstetric Database of more than 43,000 deliveries. They found a more than fourfold decrease in severe perineal lacerations following mediolateral episiotomy compared with rates after midline incision. Proper selection of cases can minimize this one disadvantage. For example, Kudish and co-workers (2006) advised against midline episiotomy with operative vaginal delivery because of an increased incidence of anal sphincter tears.

Episiotomy Repair

Typically, episiotomy repair is deferred until the placenta has been delivered. This policy permits undivided attention to the signs of placental separation and delivery. A further advantage is

that episiotomy repair is not interrupted or disrupted by the obvious necessity of delivering the placenta, especially if manual removal must be performed. The major disadvantage is continuing blood loss until the repair is completed.

Technique. There are many ways to close an episiotomy incision, but *hemostasis and anatomical restoration without excessive suturing are essential* for success with any method. Adequate analgesia is imperative, and Sanders and co-workers (2002) emphasized that women without regional analgesia can experience high levels of pain during perineal suturing. A technique that commonly is employed is shown in Figure 17-35. Mornar and Perlow (2008) have shown that blunt needles are suitable and likely decrease the incidence of needlestick injuries. The suture material commonly used is 2-0 chromic catgut. Sutures made of polyglycolic acid derivatives are also commonly used. A decrease in postsurgical pain is cited as the major advantage of synthetic materials. However, closures with these materials occasionally require suture removal from the repair site because of pain or dyspareunia. Kettle and co-workers (2002) randomly assigned 1542 women with perineal lacerations or episiotomies to undergo continuous versus interrupted repair with rapidly absorbed polyglactin 910 (Vicryl Rapids, Ethicon) or standard polyglactin 910 sutures. The former typically is absorbed by 42 days and the latter not for approximately 90 days. The continuous method was associated with less perineal pain. The rapidly absorbed material was associated with lower rates of suture removal compared with standard polyglactin—3 versus 13 percent. In another randomized study comparing continuous

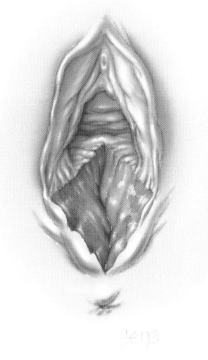

A

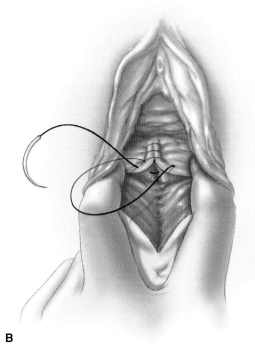

B

FIGURE 17-35 Repair of midline episiotomy. **A.** Disruption of the hymenal ring and bulbocavernosus and superficial transverse perineal muscle are seen within the diamond-shaped incision following episiotomy. **B.** Absorbable 2-0 or 3-0 suture is used for continuous closure of the vaginal mucosa and submucosa. (*Continued*)

Third-degree lacerations extend farther to involve the anal sphincter. A *fourth-degree* laceration extends through the rectum's mucosa to expose its lumen.

Laceration Risks and Morbidity

Perineal tears may follow any vaginal delivery, but Combs and associates (1990) identified factors associated with an increased risk of third- and fourth-degree lacerations. These include midline episiotomy, nulliparity, second-stage arrest of labor, persistent occiput posterior position, mid or low forceps, use of local anesthetics, and Asian race.

Morbidity rates rise as laceration severity increases. Venkatesh and colleagues (1989) reported a 5-percent incidence of third- and fourth-degree perineal tears in 20,500 vaginal deliveries. Approximately 10 percent of these 1040 primary repairs had a postoperative wound disruption and two thirds required surgical correction. Williams and Chames (2006) found that mediolateral episiotomy was the most powerful predictor of wound disruption. Goldaber and associates (1993) found that 21 of 390 or 5.4 percent of women with fourth-degree lacerations experienced significant morbidity. There were 1.8 percent dehiscences, 2.8 percent infections with dehiscences, and 0.8 percent with isolated infections. Although administration of a perioperative 2-g intravenous dose of cefazolin reduced rates of this morbidity, it was not totally eliminated.

Because repair of perineal lacerations is virtually the same as that of episiotomy incisions, albeit sometimes less satisfactory because of tear irregularities, the technique of laceration repair is discussed with episiotomy repair.

Episiotomy

In a strict sense, episiotomy is incision of the pudenda. Perineotomy is incision of the perineum. In common parlance, however, the term *episiotomy* often is used synonymously with *perineotomy*, a practice that we follow here. The incision may be made in the midline, creating a *median* or *midline episiotomy*. It may also begin in the midline but be directed laterally and downward away from the rectum, termed a *mediolateral episiotomy*.

Purposes of Episiotomy

Although still a common obstetrical procedure, the use of episiotomy has decreased remarkably over the past 25 years. Weber and Meyn (2002) used the National Hospital Discharge Survey to analyze use of episiotomy between 1979 and 1997 in the United States. Approximately 65 percent of women delivered vaginally in 1979 had an episiotomy compared with 39 percent by 1997. By 2003, the rate had decreased to approximately 18 percent (Martin and colleagues, 2005). Through the 1970s, it was common practice to cut an episiotomy for almost all women having their first delivery. The reasons for its popularity included substitution of a straight surgical incision, which was easier to repair, for the ragged laceration that otherwise might result. The long-held beliefs that postoperative pain is less and healing improved with an episiotomy compared with a tear,

however, appeared to be incorrect (Larsson and colleagues, 1991).

Another commonly cited but unproven benefit of routine episiotomy was that it prevented pelvic floor complications—that is, vaginal wall support defects and incontinence. A number of observational studies and randomized trials, however, showed that routine episiotomy is associated with an *increased* incidence of anal sphincter and rectal tears (Angioli, 2000; Eason, 2000; Nager and Helliwell, 2001; Rodriguez, 2008, and all their colleagues).

Carroli and Mignini (2009) reviewed the Cochrane Pregnancy and Childbirth Group trials registry. There were lower rates of posterior perineal trauma, surgical repair, and healing complications in the restricted-use group. Alternatively, the incidence of anterior perineal trauma was lower in the routine-use group.

With these findings came the realization that episiotomy did not protect the perineal body and contributed to anal sphincter incontinence by increasing the risk of third- and fourth-degree tears. Signorello and associates (2000) reported that fecal and flatus incontinence were increased four- to sixfold in women with an episiotomy compared with a group of women delivered with an intact perineum. Even compared with spontaneous lacerations, episiotomy tripled the risk of fecal incontinence and doubled it for flatus incontinence. Episiotomy without extension did not lower this risk. Despite repair of a third-degree extension, 30 to 40 percent of women have long-term anal incontinence (Gjessing and co-workers, 1998; Poen and colleagues, 1998). Finally, Alperin and associates (2008) recently reported that episiotomy performed for the first delivery conferred a fivefold risk for second-degree or worse lacerations with the second delivery.

For all of these reasons, the American College of Obstetricians and Gynecologists (2006) has concluded that restricted use of episiotomy is preferred to routine use. We are of the view that the procedure should be applied selectively for appropriate indications. These include fetal indications such as shoulder dystocia and breech delivery, forceps or vacuum extractor deliveries, occiput posterior positions, and instances in which failure to perform an episiotomy will result in perineal rupture. *The final rule is that there is no substitute for surgical judgment and common sense.*

Timing of Episiotomy

If performed unnecessarily early, bleeding from the episiotomy may be considerable during the interim between incision and delivery. If it is performed too late, lacerations will not be prevented. Typically, episiotomy is completed when the head is visible during a contraction to a diameter of 3 to 4 cm (see Fig. 17-24). When used in conjunction with forceps delivery, most perform an episiotomy after application of the blades (see Chap. 23, p. 514).

Midline versus Mediolateral Episiotomy

Differences between the two types of episiotomies are summarized in Table 17-5. Except for the important issue of third- and fourth-degree extensions, midline episiotomy is superior. Anthony

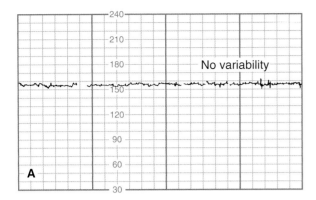

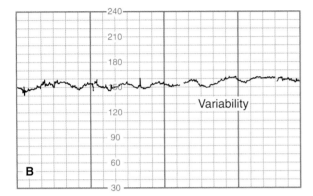

FIGURE 18-11 A. External fetal heart recording showing lack of long-term variability at 31 weeks during maternal diabetic ketoacidosis (pH 7.09). **B.** Recovery of fetal long-term variability after correction of maternal acidemia.

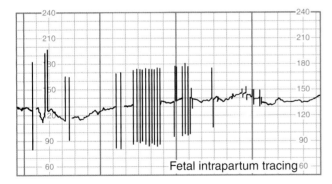

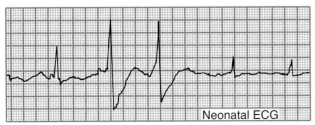

FIGURE 18-12 Internal fetal monitoring at term demonstrated occasional abrupt beat-to-beat fetal heart rate spiking due to erratic extrasystoles shown in the superimposed fetal electrocardiogram. The normal infant was delivered spontaneously and had a normal cardiac rhythm in the nursery.

Many supraventricular arrhythmias disappear in the immediate neonatal period, although some are associated with structural cardiac defects (Api and Carvalho, 2009). Copel and co-workers (2000) used echocardiography to evaluate 614 fetuses referred for auscultated irregular heart rate without hydrops. Only 10 fetuses (2 percent) were found to have significant arrhythmias, and all but one of these infant survived.

Boldt and colleagues (2003) followed 292 consecutive fetuses diagnosed with a cardiac arrhythmia through birth and into childhood. Atrial extrasystoles comprised the most common arrhythmia (68 percent), followed by atrial tachycardias (12 percent), atrioventricular block (12 percent), sinus bradycardia (5 percent), and ventricular extrasystoles (2.5 percent). Chromosomal anomalies were found in 1.7 percent of the fetuses. Fetal hydrops developed in 11 percent, and 2 percent had intrauterine death. Fetal hydrops was a bad prognostic finding. Overall, 93 percent of the study population was alive at a median follow-up period of 5 years, and 3 percent—7 infants, had neurological handicaps. Ninety-seven percent of the infants with atrial extrasystoles lived, and none suffered neurological injury. Only 6 percent required postnatal cardiac medications. Lopriore and associates (2009) found low rates of death and long-term neurological impairment in fetuses with supraventricular tachycardia or atrial flutter. In contrast, higher mortality rates were noted in those with atrioventricular block.

Although most fetal arrhythmias are of little consequence during labor when there is no evidence of fetal hydrops, such arrhythmias impair interpretation of intrapartum heart rate tracings. Sonographic evaluation of fetal anatomy as well as echocardiography may be useful. Some clinicians use fetal scalp sampling as an adjunct. Generally, in the absence of fetal hydrops, neonatal outcome is not measurably improved by pregnancy intervention. At Parkland Hospital, intrapartum fetal cardiac arrhythmias, especially in the presence of clear amnionic fluid, are managed conservatively. Freeman and colleagues (2003) have extensively reviewed interpretation of the fetal electrocardiogram during labor.

Sinusoidal Heart Rate

A true sinusoidal pattern such as that shown in panel 5 of Figure 18-10 may be observed with severe fetal anemia from Rh isoimmunization, feto-maternal hemorrhage, twin-twin transfusion syndrome, or vasa previa with bleeding; with fetal intracranial hemorrhage; and with severe fetal asphyxia (Modanlou and Murata, 2004). Insignificant sinusoidal patterns have been reported following administration of meperidine, morphine, alphaprodine, and butorphanol (Angel, 1984; Egley, 1991; Epstein, 1982, and all their associates). Shown in Figure 18-13 is a sinusoidal pattern seen with maternal meperidine administration. An important characteristic of this pattern when due to narcotics is the sine frequency of 6 cycles per minute. A sinusoidal pattern also has been described with chorioamnionitis, fetal distress, and umbilical cord occlusion (Murphy and associates, 1991). Young and co-workers (1980a) and Johnson and colleagues (1981) concluded that intrapartum sinusoidal fetal heart patterns were not generally associated with fetal compromise.

Modanlou and Freeman (1982), based on their extensive review, proposed adoption of a strict definition:

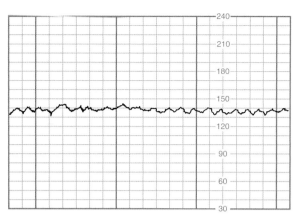

FIGURE 18-13 Sinusoidal fetal heart rate pattern associated with maternal intravenous meperidine administration. Sine waves are occurring at a rate of 6 cycles per minute.

1. Stable baseline heart rate of 120 to 160 beats/min with regular oscillations
2. Amplitude of 5 to 15 beats/min (rarely greater)
3. Long-term variability frequency of 2 to 5 cycles per minute.
4. Fixed or flat short-term variability
5. Oscillation of the sinusoidal waveform above or below a baseline
6. Absence of accelerations.

Although these criteria were selected to define a sinusoidal pattern that is most likely ominous, they observed that the pattern associated with alphaprodine is indistinguishable. Other investigators have proposed a classification of sinusoidal heart rate patterns into mild (amplitude 5 to 15 beats/min), intermediate (16 to 24 beats/min), and major (25 or more beats/min) to quantify fetal risk (Murphy and associates, 1991; Neesham and co-workers, 1993).

Some investigators have defined intrapartum sine wave–like baseline variation with periods of acceleration as *pseudosinusoidal.* Murphy and co-workers (1991) reported that pseudosinusoidal patterns were seen in 15 percent of monitored labors. Mild pseudosinusoidal patterns were associated with use of meperidine and epidural analgesia. Intermediate pseudosinusoidal patterns were linked to fetal sucking or transient episodes of fetal hypoxia caused by umbilical cord compression. Egley and colleagues (1991) reported that 4 percent of fetuses demonstrated sinusoidal patterns transiently during normal labor. These authors observed patterns for up to 90 minutes in some cases and also in association with oxytocin or alphaprodine usage, or both.

The pathophysiology of sinusoidal patterns is unclear, in part due to various definitions. There seems to be general agreement that *antepartum* sine wave baseline undulation portends severe fetal anemia. However, few D-isoimmunized fetuses develop this pattern (Nicolaides and associates, 1989). The sinusoidal pattern has been reported to develop or disappear after fetal transfusion (Del Valle and associates, 1992; Lowe and co-workers, 1984). Ikeda and colleagues (1999) have proposed, based on studies in fetal lambs, that the sinusoidal fetal heart rate pattern is related to waves of arterial blood pressure, reflecting oscillations in the baroreceptor–chemoreceptor feedback mechanism for control of the circulation.

Periodic Fetal Heart Rate Changes

The periodic fetal heart rate refers to deviations from baseline that are related to uterine contractions. *Acceleration* refers to an increase in fetal heart rate above baseline and *deceleration* to a decrease below the baseline rate. The nomenclature most commonly used in the United States is based upon the *timing* of the deceleration in relation to contractions—thus, *early, late,* or *variable* in onset related to the corresponding uterine contraction. The waveform of these decelerations is also significant for pattern recognition. In early and late decelerations, the slope of fetal heart rate change is gradual, resulting in a curvilinear and uniform or symmetrical waveform. With variable decelerations, the slope of fetal heart rate change is abrupt and erratic, giving the waveform a jagged appearance. It has been proposed that decelerations be defined as *recurrent* if they occur with 50 percent or more of contractions in any 20-minute period (NICHD Research Planning Workshop, 1997).

Another system now used less often to describe decelerations is based on the pathophysiological events considered most likely to cause the pattern. In this system, early decelerations are termed *head compression,* late decelerations are termed *uteroplacental insufficiency,* and variable decelerations become *cord compression patterns.* The nomenclature of type I (early), type II (late), and type III (variable) "dips" proposed by Caldeyro-Barcia and co-workers (1973) is not used in the United States.

Accelerations. An acceleration is a visually apparent abrupt increase—defined as onset of acceleration to a peak in less than 30 seconds—in the fetal heart rate baseline (NICHD Research Planning Workshop, 1997). According to Freeman and co-workers (2003), accelerations most often occur antepartum, in early labor, and in association with variable decelerations. Proposed mechanisms for intrapartum accelerations include fetal movement, stimulation by uterine contractions, umbilical cord occlusion, and fetal stimulation during pelvic examination. Fetal scalp blood sampling and acoustic stimulation also incite fetal heart rate acceleration (Clark and associates, 1982). Finally, acceleration can occur during labor without any apparent stimulus. Indeed, accelerations are common in labor and are nearly always associated with fetal movement. These accelerations are virtually always reassuring and almost always confirm that the fetus is not acidemic at that time.

Accelerations seem to have the same physiological explanations as beat-to-beat variability in that they represent intact neurohormonal cardiovascular control mechanisms linked to fetal behavioral states. Krebs and co-workers (1982) analyzed electronic heart rate tracings in nearly 2000 fetuses and found sporadic accelerations during labor in 99.8 percent. The presence of fetal heart accelerations during the first or last 30 minutes, or both, was a favorable sign for fetal well-being. The absence of such accelerations during labor, however, is not necessarily an unfavorable sign unless coincidental with other nonreassuring changes. There is about a 50-percent chance of acidemia in the fetus who fails to respond to stimulation in the presence of an otherwise nonreassuring pattern (Clark and colleagues, 1984; Smith and associates, 1986).

Early Deceleration. Early deceleration of the fetal heart rate consists of a gradual decrease and return to baseline associated with a contraction (Fig. 18-14). Such early deceleration was first

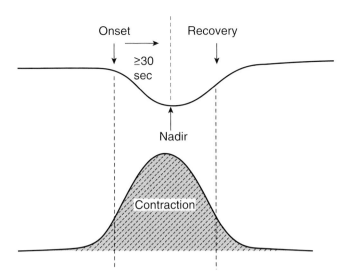

FIGURE 18-14 Features of early fetal heart rate deceleration. Characteristics include gradual decrease in the heart rate with both onset and recovery coincident with the onset and recovery of the contraction. The nadir of the deceleration is 30 seconds or more after the onset of the deceleration.

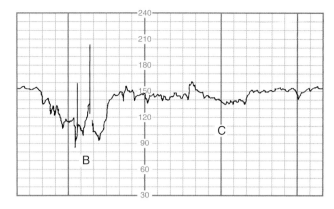

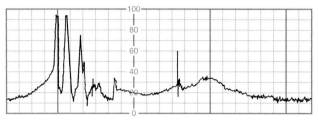

FIGURE 18-15 Two different fetal heart rate patterns during second-stage labor that are likely both due to head compression *(upper panel)*. Maternal pushing efforts *(lower panel)* correspond to the spikes with uterine contractions. Fetal heart rate deceleration **(C)**, is consistent with the pattern of head compression shown in Figure 18-14. Deceleration **(B)**, however, is "variable" in appearance because of its jagged configuration and may alternatively represent cord occlusion.

described by Hon (1958). He observed that there was a drop in heart rate with uterine contractions and that this was related to cervical dilatation. He considered these findings to be physiological.

Freeman and co-workers (2003) defined early decelerations as those generally seen in active labor between 4 and 7 cm dilatation. In their definition, the degree of deceleration is generally proportional to the contraction strength and rarely falls below 100 to 110 beats/min or 20 to 30 beats/min below baseline. Such decelerations are common during active labor and are not associated with tachycardia, loss of variability, or other fetal heart rate changes. Importantly, early decelerations are not associated with fetal hypoxia, acidemia, or low Apgar scores.

Head compression probably causes vagal nerve activation as a result of dural stimulation, and that mediates the heart rate deceleration (Paul and colleagues, 1964). Ball and Parer (1992) concluded that fetal head compression is a likely cause not only of the deceleration shown in Figure 18-14 but also of those shown in Figure 18-15, which typically occur during second-stage labor. Indeed, they observed that head compression is the likely cause of many variable decelerations classically attributed to cord compression.

Late Deceleration. The fetal heart rate response to uterine contractions can be an index of either uterine perfusion or placental function. A late deceleration is a smooth, gradual, symmetrical decrease in fetal heart rate beginning at or after the peak of the contraction and returning to baseline only after the contraction has ended (American College of Obstetricians and Gynecologists, 1995). In most cases, the onset, nadir, and recovery of the deceleration occur after the beginning, peak, and ending of the contraction, respectively (Fig. 18-16). The magnitude of late decelerations is rarely more than 30 to 40 beats/min below baseline and typically not more than 10 to 20 beats/min. Late decelerations usually are not accompanied by accelerations.

Myers and associates (1973) studied monkeys in which they compromised uteroplacental perfusion by lowering maternal aortic blood pressure. The interval or lag from the contraction onset until the late deceleration onset was directly related to basal fetal oxygenation. They demonstrated that the length of the lag phase was predictive of the fetal PO_2 but not fetal pH. The lower the fetal PO_2 prior to contractions, the shorter the lag phase to onset of late decelerations. This lag period reflected the time necessary

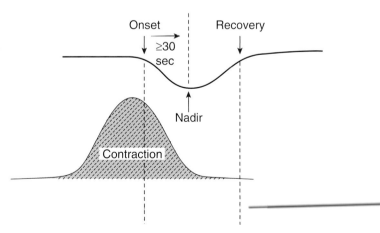

FIGURE 18-16 Features of late fetal heart rate deceleration. Characteristics include gradual decrease in the heart rate with the nadir and recovery occurring after the end of the contraction. The nadir of the deceleration occurs 30 seconds or more after the onset of the deceleration.

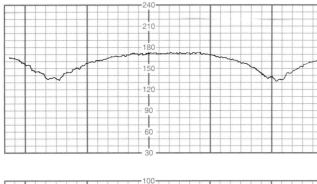

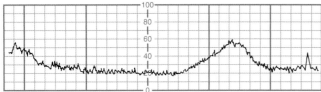

FIGURE 18-17 Late decelerations due to uteroplacental insufficiency resulting from placental abruption. Immediate cesarean delivery was performed. Umbilical artery pH was 7.05 and the P_{O_2} was 11 mm Hg.

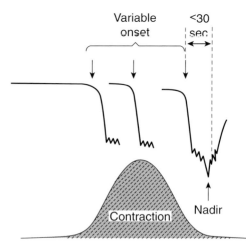

FIGURE 18-18 Features of variable fetal heart rate decelerations. Characteristics include an abrupt decrease in the heart rate and onset that commonly varies with successive contractions. The decelerations measure ≤ 15 beats/min for 15 seconds or longer and have an onset-to-nadir phase of less than 30 seconds. Total duration is less than 2 minutes.

for the fetal P_{O_2} to fall below a critical level necessary to stimulate arterial chemoreceptors, which mediated decelerations.

Murata and co-workers (1982) also showed that a late deceleration was the first fetal heart rate consequence of uteroplacental-induced hypoxia. During the course of progressive hypoxia that led to death over 2 to 13 days, monkey fetuses invariably exhibited late decelerations before development of acidemia. Variability of the baseline heart rate disappeared as acidemia developed.

A large number of clinical circumstances can result in late decelerations. Generally, any process that causes maternal hypotension, excessive uterine activity, or placental dysfunction can induce late decelerations. The two most common causes are hypotension from epidural analgesia and uterine hyperactivity caused by oxytocin stimulation. Maternal diseases such as hypertension, diabetes, and collagen-vascular disorders can cause chronic placental dysfunction. Placental abruption can cause acute late decelerations (Fig. 18-17).

Variable Decelerations. The most common deceleration patterns encountered during labor are variable decelerations attributed to umbilical cord occlusion. Melchior and Bernard (1985) identified variable decelerations in 40 percent of more than 7000 monitor tracings when labor had progressed to 5 cm dilatation and in 83 percent by the end of the first labor stage. Variable deceleration of the fetal heart rate is defined as a visually apparent *abrupt* decrease in rate. The onset of deceleration commonly varies with successive contractions (Fig. 18-18). The duration is less than 2 minutes.

Very early in the development of electronic monitoring, Hon (1959) tested the effects of umbilical cord compression on fetal heart rate (Fig. 18-19). Similar complete occlusion of the

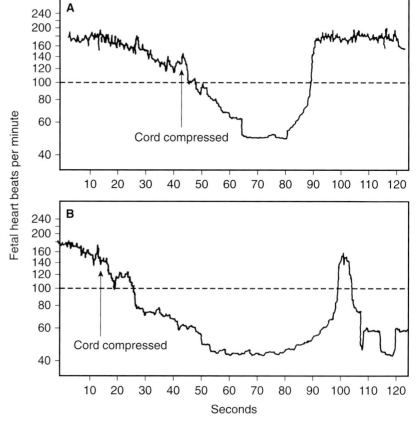

FIGURE 18-19 Fetal heart rate effects of cord compression. Panel **(A)** shows the effects of 25-second compression compared with those of 40 seconds in panel **(B)**. (This figure was redrawn from *American Journal of Obstetrics & Gynecology*, Vol. 78, No. 1, EH Hon, The fetal heart rate patterns preceding death in utero, pp. 47–56, Copyright Elsevier 1959.)

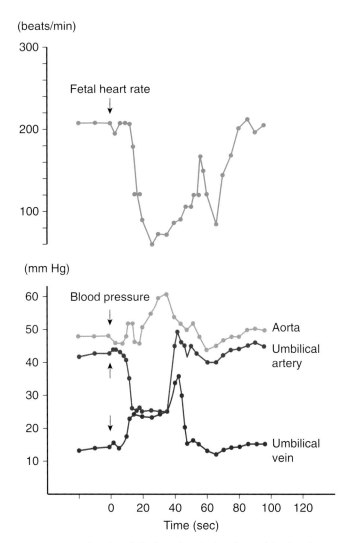

FIGURE 18-20 Total umbilical cord occlusion (*arrow*) in the sheep fetus is accompanied by an increase in fetal aortic blood pressure. Blood pressure changes in the umbilical vessels are also shown. (Adapted from Kunzel, 1985, with permission.)

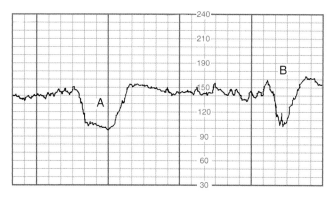

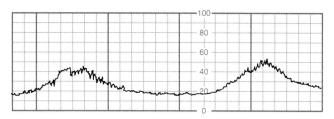

FIGURE 18-21 Varying (variable) fetal heart rate decelerations. Deceleration **(B)** exhibits "shoulders" of acceleration compared with deceleration **(A)**. (Adapted from Kunzel, 1985, with permission.)

umbilical cord in experimental animals produces abrupt, jagged-appearing deceleration of the fetal heart rate (Fig. 18-20). Concomitantly, fetal aortic pressure increases. Itskovitz and co-workers (1983) observed that variable decelerations in fetal lambs occurred only after umbilical blood flow was reduced by at least 50 percent.

Two types of variable decelerations are shown in Figure 18-21. The deceleration denoted by A is very much like that seen with complete umbilical cord occlusion in experimental animals (see Fig. 18-20). Deceleration B, however, has a different configuration because of the "shoulders" of acceleration before and after the deceleration component. Lee and co-workers (1975) proposed that this variation of variable deceleration was caused by differing degrees of partial cord occlusion. In this physiological scheme, occlusion of only the vein reduces fetal blood return, thereby triggering a baroreceptor-mediated acceleration. Subsequent complete occlusion results in fetal systemic hypertension due to obstruction of umbilical artery flow. This stimulates a baroreceptor-mediated deceleration. Presumably, the aftercoming shoulder of acceleration represents the same events occurring in reverse (Fig. 18-22).

Ball and Parer (1992) concluded that variable decelerations are mediated vagally and that the vagal response may be due to chemoreceptor or baroreceptor activity or both. Partial or complete cord occlusion produces an increase in afterload (baroreceptor) and a decrease in fetal arterial oxygen content (chemoreceptor). These both result in vagal activity leading to deceleration. In fetal monkeys, the baroreceptor reflexes appear to operate during the first 15 to 20 seconds of umbilical cord occlusion followed by decline in PO_2 at approximately 30 seconds, which then serves as a chemoreceptor stimulus (Mueller-Heubach and Battelli, 1982).

Thus, variable decelerations represent fetal heart rate reflexes that reflect either blood pressure changes due to interruption of umbilical flow or changes in oxygenation. It is likely that most fetuses have experienced brief but recurrent periods of hypoxia due to umbilical cord compression during gestation. The frequency and inevitability of cord occlusion undoubtedly have provided the fetus with these physiological mechanisms as a means of coping. The great dilemma for the obstetrician in managing variable fetal heart rate decelerations is determining when variable decelerations are pathological. The American College of Obstetricians and Gynecologists (1995) has defined *significant* variable decelerations as those decreasing to less than 70 beats/min and lasting more than 60 seconds.

Other fetal heart rate patterns have been associated with umbilical cord compression. *Saltatory* baseline heart rate (Fig. 18-23) was first described by Hammacher and colleagues (1968) and linked to umbilical cord complications during labor. The pattern consists of rapidly recurring couplets of acceleration and deceleration causing relatively large oscillations of the baseline fetal heart rate. We also observed a relationship between cord occlusion and the saltatory pattern (Leveno and associates, 1984). In the absence of other fetal heart rate findings,

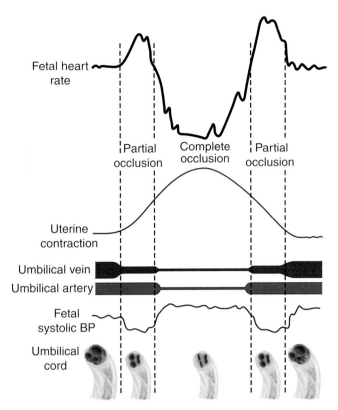

FIGURE 18-22 Schematic representation of the fetal heart rate effects with partial and complete umbilical cord occlusion. Uterine pressures generated early in a contraction cause cord compression predominantly of the thin-walled umbilical vein. The resulting decrease in fetal cardiac output leads to an initial compensatory rise in fetal heart rate. As cord compression intensifies, umbilical arteries are then also compressed. The resulting rise in fetal systolic blood pressure leads to a vagal-mediated fetal heart rate deceleration. As the contraction abates and compression is relieved first on the umbilical arteries, elevated fetal systolic blood pressures drop and the deceleration resolves. A final increase in fetal heart rate is seen as a result of persistent umbilical vein occlusion. With completion of the uterine contraction and cord compression, the fetal heart rate returns to baseline. (BP = blood pressure). (Adapted from Lee and colleagues, 1975.)

these do not signal fetal compromise. *Lambda* is a pattern involving an acceleration followed by a variable deceleration with no acceleration at the end of the deceleration. This pattern typically is seen in early labor and is not ominous (Freeman and colleagues, 2003). This lambda pattern may result from mild cord compression or stretch. *Overshoot* is a variable deceleration followed by acceleration. The clinical significance of this pattern is controversial (Westgate and associates, 2001).

Prolonged Deceleration

This pattern, which is shown in Figure 18-24, is defined as an isolated deceleration lasting 2 minutes or longer but less than 10 minutes from onset to return to baseline (NICHD Research Planning Workshop, 1997). Prolonged decelerations are difficult to interpret because they are seen in many different clinical situations. Some of the more common causes include cervical examination, uterine hyperactivity, cord entanglement, and maternal supine hypotension.

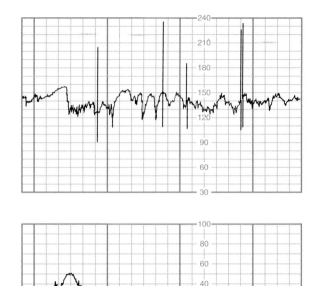

FIGURE 18-23 Saltatory baseline fetal heart rate showing rapidly recurring couplets of acceleration combined with deceleration.

Epidural, spinal, or paracervical analgesia may induce prolonged deceleration of the fetal heart rate. For example, Eberle and colleagues (1998) reported that prolonged decelerations occurred in 4 percent of normal parturients given either epidural or intrathecal labor analgesia. Hill and associates (2003) observed prolonged deceleration in 1 percent of women given epidural analgesia during labor at Parkland Hospital. Other causes of prolonged deceleration include maternal hypoperfusion or hypoxia from any cause, placental abruption, umbilical cord knots or prolapse, maternal seizures including eclampsia

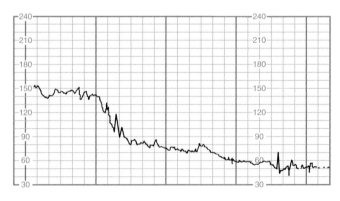

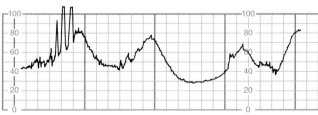

FIGURE 18-24 Prolonged fetal heart rate deceleration due to uterine hyperactivity. Approximately 3 minutes of the tracing are shown, but the fetal heart rate returned to normal after uterine hypertonus resolved. Vaginal delivery later ensued.

and epilepsy, application of a fetal scalp electrode, impending birth, or even maternal Valsalva maneuver.

The placenta is very effective in resuscitating the fetus if the original insult does not recur immediately. Occasionally, such self-limited prolonged decelerations are followed by loss of beat-to-beat variability, baseline tachycardia, and even a period of late decelerations, all of which resolve as the fetus recovers. Freeman and co-workers (2003) emphasize rightfully that the fetus may die during prolonged decelerations. Thus, management of prolonged decelerations can be extremely tenuous. Management of isolated prolonged decelerations is based upon bedside clinical judgment, which inevitably will sometimes be imperfect given the unpredictability of these decelerations.

Fetal Heart Rate Patterns During Second-Stage Labor

Decelerations are virtually ubiquitous during the second stage. In fact, Melchior and Bernard (1985) reported that only 1.4 percent of more than 7000 deliveries did not have decelerations during second-stage labor. Both cord compression and fetal head compression have been implicated as causes of decelerations and baseline bradycardia during second-stage labor. The high incidence of such patterns minimized their potential significance during the early development and interpretation of electronic monitoring. For example, Boehm (1975) described profound, prolonged fetal heart rate deceleration in 10 minutes preceding vaginal delivery of 18 healthy infants. Subsequently, Herbert and Boehm (1981) reported another 18 pregnancies with similar prolonged decelerations during second-stage labor. There was one stillbirth and one neonatal death. These experiences attest to the unpredictability of the fetal heart rate during second-stage labor.

Spong and colleagues (1998) analyzed the characteristics of second-stage variable fetal heart rate decelerations in 250 deliveries and found that as the total number of decelerations to less than 70 beats/min increased, the 5-minute Apgar score decreased. Put another way, the longer a fetus was exposed to variable decelerations, the lower the Apgar score at 5 minutes.

Picquard and co-workers (1988) analyzed heart rate patterns during second-stage labor in 234 women in an attempt to identify specific patterns to diagnose fetal compromise. Loss of beat-to-beat variability and baseline fetal heart rate less than 90 beats/min were predictive of fetal acidemia. Krebs and associates (1981) also found that persistent or progressive baseline bradycardia and baseline tachycardia were associated with low Apgar scores. Gull and colleagues (1996) observed that abrupt fetal heart rate deceleration to less than 100 beats/min, and associated with loss of beat-to-beat variability for 4 minutes or longer, was predictive of fetal acidemia. Thus, abnormal baseline heart rate—either bradycardia or tachycardia, absent beat-to-beat variability, or both—in the presence of second-stage decelerations, is associated with increased but not inevitable fetal compromise (Fig. 18-25).

Admission Fetal Monitoring in Low-Risk Pregnancies

In this application of electronic fetal monitoring, women with low-risk pregnancies are monitored for a short time on admission for labor, and continuous monitoring is used only if abnormalities of the fetal heart rate are subsequently identified. Mires and colleagues (2001) randomly assigned 3752 low-risk women in spontaneous labor at the time of admission to either auscultation of the fetal heart rate using Doppler during and immediately after at least one contraction or to 20 minutes of

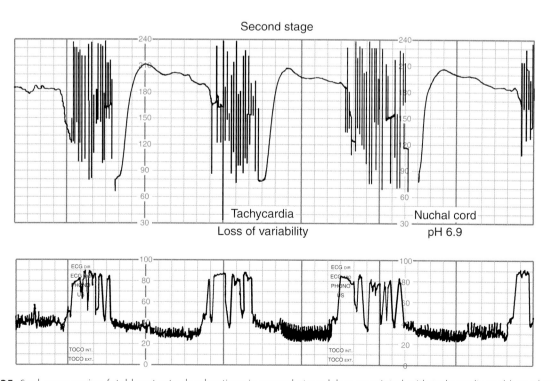

FIGURE 18-25 Cord compression fetal heart rate decelerations in second-stage labor associated with tachycardia and loss of variability. The umbilical cord arterial pH was 6.9.

electronic fetal monitoring. Use of admission electronic fetal monitoring did not improve infant outcome. Moreover, its use resulted in increased interventions, including operative delivery. Impey and associates (2003) performed a similar study in 8588 low-risk women and also found no improvement in infant outcome. More than half of the women enrolled in these studies, whether they received admission electronic monitoring or auscultation, eventually required continuous monitoring for diagnosed abnormalities in the fetal heart rate.

Complications of Electronic Fetal Monitoring

Injury to the fetal scalp or breech by the electrode is rarely a major problem, although application at some other site—such as the eye in case of a face presentation—can prove serious. Rarely, a fetal vessel in the placenta may be ruptured by catheter placement (Trudinger and Pryse-Davies, 1978). Severe cord compression has been described from entanglement with the catheter. Penetration of the placenta, causing hemorrhage and possibly uterine perforation during catheter insertion, has led to serious morbidity, as well as spurious recordings that resulted in inappropriate management.

Both the fetus and the mother may be at increased risk of *infection* as the consequence of internal monitoring. Scalp wounds from the electrode may become infected, and subsequent cranial osteomyelitis has been reported (Brook, 2005; Eggink and co-workers, 2004; McGregor and McFarren, 1989). Puerperal infection increased from 12 percent in externally monitored women to 18 percent in those in whom an internal apparatus was used (Faro and associates, 1990). The American Academy of Pediatrics and the American College of Obstetricians and Gynecologists (2007) have recommended that certain maternal infections, including human immunodeficiency virus (HIV), herpes simplex virus, hepatitis B virus, and hepatitis C virus, are relative contraindications to internal fetal heart rate monitoring.

OTHER INTRAPARTUM ASSESSMENT TECHNIQUES

Fetal Scalp Blood Sampling

According to the American College of Obstetricians and Gynecologists (1995), measurements of the pH in capillary scalp blood may help to identify the fetus in serious distress. However, that said, it also emphasized that neither normal nor abnormal scalp pH results have been shown to be predictive of infant outcome. The College also indicated that the procedure is now used uncommonly.

Technique

An illuminated endoscope is inserted through the dilated cervix after membrane rupture so as to press firmly against the fetal scalp (Fig. 18-26). The skin is wiped clean with a cotton swab and coated with a silicone gel to cause the blood to accumulate as discrete globules. An incision is made through the skin to a

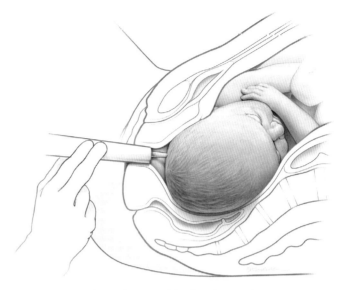

FIGURE 18-26 The technique of fetal scalp sampling using an amnioscope. The end of the endoscope is displaced from the fetal vertex approximately 2 cm to show the disposable blade against the fetal scalp before incision. (Adapted from Hamilton and McKeown, 1974.)

depth of 2 mm with a special blade on a long handle. As a drop of blood forms on the surface, it is immediately collected into a heparinized glass capillary tube. The pH of the blood is measured promptly.

Interpretation

The pH of fetal capillary scalp blood is usually lower than that of umbilical venous blood and approaches that of umbilical arterial blood. Zalar and Quilligan (1979) recommended the following protocol to try to confirm fetal distress. If the pH is greater than 7.25, labor is observed. If the pH is between 7.20 and 7.25, the pH measurement is repeated within 30 minutes. If the pH is less than 7.20, another scalp blood sample is collected immediately, and the mother is taken to an operating room and prepared for surgery. Delivery is performed promptly if the low pH is confirmed. Otherwise, labor is allowed to continue, and scalp blood samples are repeated periodically.

The only benefits reported for scalp pH testing are fewer cesarean deliveries for fetal distress (Young and co-workers, 1980b). Goodwin and associates (1994), however, in a study of 112,000 deliveries, showed a decrease in the scalp pH sampling rate from approximately 1.8 percent in the mid-1980s to 0.03 percent by 1992 with no increased delivery rate for fetal distress. They concluded that scalp pH sampling was unnecessary. Kruger and colleagues (1999) have advocated the use of fetal scalp blood lactate concentration as an adjunct to pH. Wiberg-Itzel and colleagues (2008) randomized 1496 fetuses to scalp blood pH analysis and 1496 to scalp blood lactate analysis. They found either to be equivalent in predicting fetal acidemia. The advantage of lactate measurement was that a smaller amount of blood was needed, which led to a lower procedure failure rate compared with scalp sampling for pH.

Scalp Stimulation

Clark and associates (1984) have suggested that scalp stimulation is an alternative to scalp blood sampling. This proposal was based on the observation that acceleration of the heart rate in response to pinching of the scalp with an Allis clamp just prior to obtaining blood was invariably associated with a normal pH. Conversely, failure to provoke acceleration was not uniformly predictive of fetal acidemia. Later, Elimian and associates (1997) reported that of 58 cases in which the fetal heart rate accelerated 10 beats/min or more after 15 seconds of gentle digital stroking of the scalp, 100 percent had a scalp pH of 7.20 or greater. Without an acceleration, however, only 30 percent had a scalp pH less than 7.20.

Vibroacoustic Stimulation

Fetal heart rate acceleration in response to vibroacoustic stimulation has been recommended as a substitute for scalp sampling (Edersheim and colleagues, 1987). The technique uses an electronic artificial larynx placed approximately 1 centimeter from or directly onto the maternal abdomen (see Chap. 15, p. 340). Response to vibroacoustic stimulation is considered normal if a fetal heart rate acceleration of at least 15 beats/min for at least 15 seconds occurs within 15 seconds after the stimulation and with prolonged fetal movements (Sherer, 1994). Lin and colleagues (2001) prospectively studied vibroacoustic stimulation in 113 women in labor with either moderate to severe variable or late fetal heart rate decelerations. They concluded that this technique is an effective predictor of fetal acidosis in the setting of variable decelerations. However, the predictability for fetal acidosis in the setting of late decelerations is limited. Other investigators have reported that although vibroacoustic stimulation in second-stage labor is associated with fetal heart rate reactivity, the quality of the response did not predict neonatal outcome or enhance labor management (Anyaegbunam and associates, 1994).

Skupski and co-workers (2002) performed a meta-analysis of reports on intrapartum fetal stimulation tests published between 1966 and 2000. Four types of fetal stimulation were analyzed and included scalp puncture for pH testing, Allis clamp pinching of the fetal scalp, vibroacoustic stimulation, and digital stroking of the scalp. Results were similar for all four methods. These investigators concluded that intrapartum stimulation tests were useful to exclude fetal acidemia. However, they cautioned that these tests are "less than perfect."

Fetal Pulse Oximetry

Using technology similar to that of adult pulse oximetry, instrumentation has been developed that may allow assessment of fetal oxyhemoglobin saturation once membranes are ruptured. A unique padlike sensor such as shown in Figure 18-27 is inserted through the cervix and positioned against the fetal face, where it is held in place by the uterine wall. Vintzileos and associates (2005) described the use of a transabdominal fetal pulse oximeter in a preliminary study of six women. As reviewed by Yam and co-workers (2000), the transcervical de-

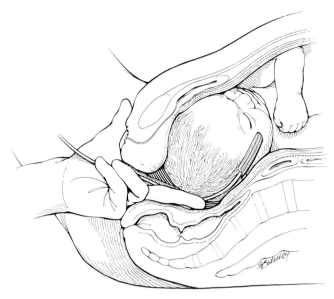

FIGURE 18-27 Schematic diagram of fetal pulse oximeter sensor placement.

vice has been used extensively by many investigators and has been reported to reliably register fetal oxygen saturation in 70 to 95 percent of women throughout 50 to 88 percent of their labors. The lower limit for normal fetal oxygen saturation is generally considered to be 30 percent by most investigators (Gorenberg and colleagues, 2003; Stiller and associates, 2002). As shown in Figure 18-28, however, fetal oxygen saturation normally varies greatly when measured in umbilical artery blood (Arikan and colleagues, 2000). Bloom and associates (1999) reported that brief, transient fetal oxygen saturations below 30 percent were common during labor because such values were observed in 53 percent of fetuses with normal outcomes. Saturation values below 30 percent, however, when persistent for 2 minutes or longer, were associated with an increased risk of potential fetal compromise.

Garite and colleagues (2000) randomly assigned 1010 women with term pregnancies and in whom predefined abnormal fetal heart rate patterns developed to either conventional fetal monitoring alone or fetal monitoring plus continuous fetal pulse oximetry. Cesarean delivery for fetal distress was performed when pulse oximetry values remained less than 30 percent for the entire interval between two contractions or when the fetal heart rate patterns met predefined guidelines. The use of fetal pulse oximetry significantly reduced the rate of cesarean delivery for nonreassuring fetal status from 10.2 to 4.5 percent. Alternatively, the cesarean delivery rate for dystocia increased significantly from 9 to 19 percent when pulse oximetry was used. There were no neonatal benefits or adverse effects associated with fetal pulse oximetry. Based on these observations, the Obstetrics and Gynecology Devices Panel of the Medical Devices Advisory Committee of the Food and Drug Administration (FDA) in 2000 approved marketing of the Nellcor N-400 Fetal Oxygen Monitoring System. Since then, another three randomized trials of fetal pulse oximetry have been reported:

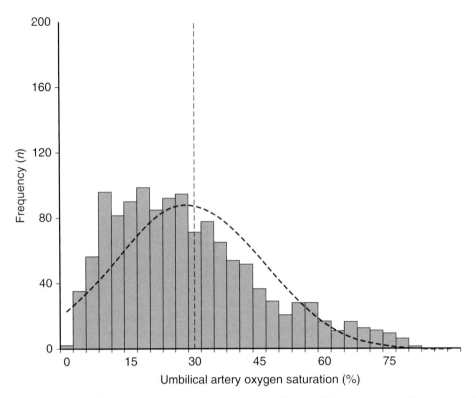

FIGURE 18-28 Frequency distribution of umbilical artery oxygen saturation values in 1281 vigorous newborn infants. Dotted line indicates normal distribution. (Reproduced from *BJOG*, Vol. 107, Issue 8, GM Arikan, HS Scholz, E Petru, MCH Haeusler, J Haas, and PAM Weiss, Cord blood oxygen saturation in vigorous infants at birth: What is normal? 987–994, 2000, with the permission of the Royal College of Obstetricians and Gynaecologists.)

1. Klauser and colleagues (2005) randomly assigned 360 women with nonreassuring fetal heart rate patterns to standard fetal monitoring plus fetal pulse oximetry or to standard monitoring alone and found no benefits for oximetry

2. East and associates (2006) from Australia randomized 600 women with nonreassuring fetal heart rate patterns to standard monitoring either alone or with added fetal pulse oximetry. These investigators reported that addition of oximetry significantly reduced cesarean deliveries for a nonreassuring fetal heart rate pattern. They further reported, however, that neonatal outcomes were not different between the study groups

3. Bloom and co-workers (2006) reported the largest trial, performed by the Maternal-Fetal Units Network. A total of 5341 women in labor at term underwent placement of the fetal oximetry sensor, but the information was randomly withheld from care providers. Unlike the earlier studies, participants were not required to have nonreassuring fetal heart rate patterns. Sensor application was generally successful and fetal oxygen saturation values were registered 75 percent of the time. Knowledge of fetal oxygen saturation did not change the rates of cesarean delivery in the overall population or in the subgroup of 2168 women who had nonreassuring fetal heart rate patterns. Moreover, neonatal outcomes were not improved by knowledge of fetal oxygen saturation status.

Because of these findings, in 2005, the manufacturer discontinued sale of the fetal oximeter system in the United States.

Fetal Electrocardiography

Because as fetal hypoxia worsens, there are changes in the T-wave and in the ST segment of the fetal ECG, several investigators have assessed the value of analyzing these parameters as an adjunct to conventional fetal monitoring. The technique requires internal monitoring of the fetal heart rate and special equipment to process the fetal ECG. The rationale behind this technology is based on the observation that the mature fetus exposed to hypoxemia develops an elevated ST segment with a progressive rise in T-wave height that can be expressed as a T:QRS ratio (Fig. 18-29). It is postulated that increasing T:QRS ratios reflect fetal cardiac ability to adapt to hypoxia and appears before neurological damage. Progression of hypoxia results in an increasingly negative ST-segment deflection such that it appears as a biphasic waveform (Fig. 18-30). In 2005, the manufacturer—Neoventa Medical—received FDA approval for their ST analysis system, named STAN system (Food and Drug Administration, 2009). Westgate and co-workers (1993) studied the benefits of monitoring ST-segment changes in a randomized trial of 2400 pregnancies. Infant outcomes were not improved compared with those in whom conventional fetal monitoring alone was used. However, there was a reduction in the cesarean delivery rate for fetal distress.

In another randomized trial of 4966 Swedish women, Amer-Wåhlin and colleagues (2001, 2007) found that the addition of ST analysis to conventional fetal monitoring significantly reduced cesarean delivery rates for fetal distress as well as metabolic

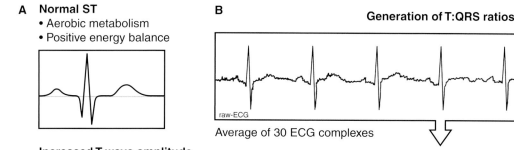

A. Normal ST
- Aerobic metabolism
- Positive energy balance

Increased T-wave amplitude
- Hypoxia/anaerobic metabolism
- Adrenaline surge

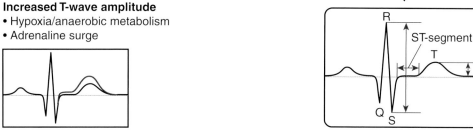

B. Generation of T:QRS ratios

raw-ECG
Average of 30 ECG complexes

R
ST-segment
T
$\frac{T}{QRS}$ ratio
Q
S

FIGURE 18-29 A. ST segment changes in normal and hypoxic conditions. **B.** Generation of T:QRS ratios. (Redrawn with permission from *Contemporary OB/GYN(Technology),* September 15, 2006, pp. 6–10. *Contemporary OB/GYN (Technology)* is a copyrighted publication of Advanstar Communications Inc. All rights reserved.)

acidemia in umbilical artery blood. Subsequently, experience was reported with clinical application of STAN monitoring at a London hospital (Doria and associates, 2007). Introduction of STAN as a clinical practice did not change the incidence of operative delivery or neonatal encephalopathy. In another study, ST data were collected from all fetuses (Norén and co-workers, 2003). There were 29 infants with adverse outcomes that included death in 3, neonatal encephalopathy in 7, or metabolic acidemia in 19. Of these, 22 had abnormal ST waveforms. A serious confounding factor in interpretation of this study is the long intervals of abnormal fetal heart rate patterns before intervention. For example, the median interval before delivery—during which time the fetal heart rate pattern was significantly abnormal—was almost 3 hours in the infants with encephalopathy. When American obstetricians were shown these very same fetal monitoring tracings, they more often would have intervened compared with their European counterparts (Ross and colleagues, 2004). It must be considered that ST abnormalities might occur late in the course of fetal compromise. Neilson (2006) reviewed the Cochrane Database to assess fetal ECG analysis during labor. There were 8872 women in which such monitoring was performed. He concluded that fetal ST segment waveform analysis was perhaps useful in

preventing fetal acidosis and neonatal encephalopathy when standard fetal heart rate (FHR) monitoring suggested abnormal patterns. Although no randomized trials have yet been performed in the United States, the Maternal-Fetal Medicine Units Network has one under development.

Intrapartum Doppler Velocimetry

Doppler analysis of the umbilical artery has been studied as another potential adjunct to conventional fetal monitoring. Further described in Chapter 16 (p. 363), abnormal Doppler waveforms may signify pathological umbilical-placental vessel resistance. From their review, Farrell and co-workers (1999) concluded that this technique was a poor predictor of adverse perinatal outcomes. They concluded that Doppler velocimetry had little, if any, role in fetal surveillance during labor.

FETAL DISTRESS

The terms *fetal distress* and *birth asphyxia* are too broad and vague to be applied with any precision to clinical situations (American College of Obstetricians and Gynecologists, 2004). Uncertainty about the diagnosis based on interpretation of fetal heart rate patterns has given rise to descriptions such as *reassuring* or *nonreassuring*. The term "reassuring" suggests a restoration of confidence by a particular pattern, whereas "nonreassuring" suggests inability to remove doubt. These patterns during labor are dynamic such that they can rapidly change from reassuring to nonreassuring and vice versa. In this situation, obstetricians experience surges of both confidence and doubt. Put another way, most diagnoses of fetal distress using heart rate patterns occur when obstetricians lose confidence or cannot assuage doubts about fetal condition. *These assessments are subjective clinical judgments inevitably subject to imperfection and must be recognized as such.*

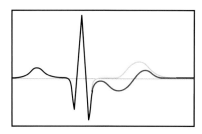

FIGURE 18-30 Biphasic ST-segment waveform with progressive fetal hypoxia. (Adapted from Devoe, 2006, courtesy of Neoventa Medical.)

Pathophysiology

Why is the diagnosis of fetal distress based on heart rate patterns so tenuous? One explanation is that these patterns are more a reflection of fetal physiology than of pathology. Physiological control of heart rate includes a variety of interconnected mechanisms that depend on blood flow as well as oxygenation. Moreover, the activity of these control mechanisms is influenced by the preexisting state of fetal oxygenation, for example, as seen with chronic placental insufficiency. Importantly, the fetus is tethered by an umbilical cord, whereby blood flow is constantly in jeopardy. Moreover, normal labor is a process of increasing acidemia (Rogers and colleagues, 1998). Thus, normal labor is a process of repeated fetal hypoxic events resulting inevitably in acidemia. Put another way, and assuming that "asphyxia" can be defined as hypoxia leading to acidemia, normal parturition is an asphyxiating event for the fetus.

Diagnosis

Because of the above uncertainties, it follows that identification of "fetal distress" based upon fetal heart rate patterns is imprecise and controversial. It is well known that experts in interpretation of these patterns often disagree with each other. In fact, Parer (1997), a strong advocate of electronic fetal heart rate monitoring and an organizer of the 1997 NICHD fetal monitoring workshop, lightheartedly compared the experts in attendance with marine iguanas of the Galapagos Islands, to wit: "all on the same beach but facing different directions and spitting at one another constantly!"

Ayres-de-Campos and colleagues (1999) investigated interobserver agreement of interpretation of fetal heart rate patterns and found that agreement—or conversely, disagreement—was related to whether the pattern was normal, suspicious, or pathological. Specifically, experts agreed on 62 percent of normal patterns, 42 percent of suspicious patterns, and only 25 percent of pathological patterns. Keith and co-workers (1995) asked each of 17 experts to review 50 tracings on two occasions, at least 1 month apart. About 20 percent changed their own interpretations, and approximately 25 percent did not agree with the interpretations of their colleagues. And although Murphy and colleagues (2003) concluded that at least part of the interpretation problem is due to a lack of formalized education in American training programs, this is obviously only a small modifier. Put another way, how can the teacher enlighten the student if the teacher is uncertain?

Evaluation of Classification Systems

Research efforts have been designed to test the utility of well-defined fetal heart rate classification systems. Berkus and associates (1999) retrospectively analyzed fetal heart rate patterns during the last 30 minutes of labor in 1859 term pregnancies. The study was designed to determine if specific patterns or combinations of patterns predicted neonatal outcome. Indisputably normal fetal heart rate patterns were recorded within 30 minutes of delivery in only 26 percent of cases. Prolonged bradycardia or tachycardia or fetal heart rate patterns that combined the absence of accelerations with severe variable or late decelerations were associated with an increased incidence of adverse infant outcome. Low and colleagues (1999) analyzed fetal

heart rate patterns of term infants born with significant metabolic acidemia—defined as an umbilical artery base deficit > 16 mmol/L. Only 71 of 23,000 fetuses had acidemia this severe, and although patterns with absent baseline variability were the most specific, they were identified in only 17 percent of the 71 acidemic fetuses.

Dellinger and co-workers (2000) analyzed intrapartum fetal heart rate patterns in 898 pregnancies using a classification system of their own design. Fetal heart rate patterns during the hour before delivery were classified as "normal," "stress," or "distress." Fetal "distress" was diagnosed in 1 percent of tracings, 70 percent were classified as "normal," and a third were "intermediate" patterns. The fetal "distress" group contained patterns with zero variability *plus* late or moderate-to-severe variable decelerations or with baseline rates < 110 beats/min for 5 minutes or longer. Outcomes such as cesarean delivery, fetal acidemia, and admission to the intensive care nursery were significantly related to the fetal heart rate pattern. These investigators concluded that their classification system accurately predicted normal outcomes for fetuses as well as discriminating true fetal distress. Others have used computer programs in an effort to improve interpretation of fetal heart rate patterns, but with variable results (Agrawal, 2003; Bellver, 2004; Devoe, 2000; Reddy, 2009, and all their colleagues). Most recently, Parer and Ikeda (2007) have developed a framework for standardized management of intrapartum fetal heart rate patterns. They identified 134 patterns and color-coded each pattern. Those with no threat of fetal acidemia were coded green, and no intervention was required. Those with a severe threat of acidemia were coded red, and rapid delivery was recommended. The authors emphasized that their proposed framework required clinical testing before it could be concluded to be effective.

National Institutes of Health Workshops on Definitions and Interpretations

The National Institute of Child Health and Human Development (1997) held a succession of workshops in 1995 and 1996 to develop standardized and unambiguous definitions of FHR tracings and published recommendations for interpreting FHR patterns. As described by Spong (2008), the goal of these definitions was to allow FHR patterns to be more precisely interpreted, and these definitions were adopted by the American College of Obstetricians and Gynecologists (2005) as shown in Table 18-1. In 2008, the NICHD reconvened a second workshop to reevaluate the 1997 recommendations and to clarify terminology (Macones and co-workers, 2008). The major changes included categorizations of FHR interpretations into a three-tier system shown in Table 18-2. The new terminology for defining uterine contractions is described subsequently in the section on surveillance of uterine activity (p. 437).

Status of Fetal Heart Rate Pattern Interpretation

After almost 40 years of experience with interpretation of fetal heart rate patterns, evidence is finally emerging that some combinations of fetal heart rate characteristics can be meaningfully used to identify normal and severely abnormal fetuses. As

TABLE 18-2. Three-Tier Fetal Heart Interpretation System Recommended by the 2008 NICHD Workshop on Electronic Fetal Monitoring

Category I—Normal
Include all of the following:
- Baseline rate: 110–160 bpm
- Baseline FHR variability: moderate
- Late or variable decelerations: absent
- Early decelerations: present or absent
- Accelerations: present or absent

Category II—Indeterminate
Include all FHR tracings not categorized as Category I or III. Category II tracings may represent an appreciable fraction of those encountered in clinical care. Examples include any of the following:

Baseline rate
- Bradycardia not accompanied by absent baseline variability
- Tachycardia

Baseline FHR variability
- Minimal baseline variability
- Absent baseline variability not accompanied by recurrent decelerations
- Marked baseline variability

Accelerations
- Absence of induced accelerations after fetal stimulation

Periodic or episodic decelerations
- Recurrent variable decelerations accompanied by minimal or moderate baseline variability
- Prolonged deceleration ≥ 2 minutes but < 10 minutes
- Recurrent late decelerations with moderate baseline variability
- Variable decelerations with other characteristics, such as slow return to baseline, "overshoots," or "shoulders"

Category III—Abnormal
Include either:
- Absent baseline FHR variability and any of the following:
  Recurrent late decelerations
  Recurrent variable decelerations
  Bradycardia
- Sinusoidal pattern

bpm = beats per minute; FHR = fetal heart rate; NICHD = National Institute of Child Health and Human Development. From Macones and colleagues (2008), with permission.

shown in Tables 18-1 and 18-2, true fetal distress patterns appear to be those in which beat-to-beat variability is zero in conjunction with severe decelerations or persistent baseline rate changes, or both. Fortunately, such fetal distress is rare. One ex-

planation for the persistent failure to scientifically establish the benefits of fetal heart rate monitoring is the rarity of such fetal distress, effectively precluding statistically significant results from clinical trials (Hornbuckle and colleagues, 2000).

Meconium in the Amnionic Fluid

Obstetrical teaching throughout the past century has included the concept that meconium passage is a potential warning of fetal asphyxia. In 1903, J. Whitridge Williams observed and attributed meconium passage to "relaxation of the sphincter ani muscle induced by faulty aeration of the (fetal) blood." Obstetricians, however, have also long realized that the detection of meconium during labor is problematic in the prediction of fetal distress or asphyxia. In their review, Katz and Bowes (1992) emphasized the prognostic uncertainty of meconium by referring to the topic as a "murky subject." Indeed, although 12 to 22 percent of labors are complicated by meconium, only a few are linked to infant mortality. In an investigation from Parkland Hospital, meconium was found to be a "low-risk" obstetrical hazard because the perinatal mortality rate attributable to meconium was 1 death per 1000 live births (Nathan and co-workers, 1994).

Three theories have been suggested to explain fetal passage of meconium and, in part, may explain the tenuous connection between its detection and infant mortality. The pathological explanation proposes that fetuses pass meconium in response to hypoxia and that meconium therefore signals fetal compromise (Walker, 1953). Alternatively, in utero passage of meconium may represent normal gastrointestinal tract maturation under neural control (Mathews and Warshaw, 1979). Third, meconium passage could follow vagal stimulation from common but transient umbilical cord entrapment and resultant increased peristalsis (Hon and colleagues, 1961). Thus, meconium release also could represent physiological processes.

Ramin and associates (1996) studied almost 8000 pregnancies with meconium-stained amnionic fluid delivered at Parkland Hospital. Meconium aspiration syndrome was significantly associated with fetal acidemia at birth. Other significant correlates of aspiration included cesarean delivery, forceps to expedite delivery, intrapartum heart rate abnormalities, depressed Apgar scores, and need for assisted ventilation at delivery. Analysis of the type of fetal acidemia based on umbilical blood gases suggested that the fetal compromise associated with meconium aspiration syndrome was an acute event, because most acidemic fetuses had abnormally increased PCO_2 values rather than a pure metabolic acidemia.

Dawes and co-workers (1972) observed that such hypercarbia in fetal lambs induces gasping and resultant increased amnionic fluid inhalation. Jovanovic and Nguyen (1989) observed that meconium gasped into the fetal lungs caused aspiration syndrome only in asphyxiated animals. Ramin and co-workers (1996) hypothesized that the pathophysiology of meconium aspiration syndrome includes, but is not limited to, fetal hypercarbia, which stimulates fetal respiration leading to aspiration of meconium into the alveoli. Lung parenchymal injury is secondary to acidemia-induced alveolar cell damage. In this pathophysiological scenario, meconium in amnionic fluid is a fetal environmental hazard rather than a marker of preexistent compromise. This proposed pathophysiological sequence is not all-inclusive, because it does not account for approximately half of the cases of meconium aspiration syndrome in which the fetus was not acidemic at birth.

From the foregoing, it was concluded that the high incidence of meconium observed in the amnionic fluid during labor often represents fetal passage of gastrointestinal contents in conjunction with normal physiological processes. Although normal, such meconium becomes an environmental hazard when fetal acidemia supervenes. Importantly, such acidemia occurs acutely, and therefore meconium aspiration is unpredictable and likely unpreventable. Moreover, Greenwood and colleagues (2003) showed that clear amnionic fluid was also a poor predictor. In a prospective study of 8394 women with clear amnionic fluid, they found that clear fluid was an unreliable sign of fetal well-being.

There is accumulating evidence that many infants with meconium aspiration syndrome have suffered chronic hypoxia before birth (Ghidini and Spong, 2001). For example, Blackwell and associates (2001) found that 60 percent of infants diagnosed as having meconium aspiration syndrome had umbilical artery blood pH ≥ 7.20, suggesting that the syndrome was unrelated to the neonatal condition at delivery. Similarly, markers of chronic hypoxia, such as fetal erythropoietin levels and nucleated red blood cell counts in newborn infants, suggest that chronic hypoxia is involved in many cases of meconium aspiration syndrome (Dollberg and colleagues, 2001; Jazayeri and colleagues, 2000).

Routine obstetrical management of a newborn with meconium-stained amnionic fluid has generally included intrapartum suctioning of the oropharynx and nasopharynx on the perineum after delivery of the head, but before delivery of the shoulder. The new guidelines from the American College of Obstetricians and Gynecologists (2007), however, recommend that such infants no longer routinely receive intrapartum suctioning because it does not prevent meconium aspiration syndrome (Chap. 28, p. 628). If the infant is depressed, the trachea is intubated, and meconium suctioned from beneath the glottis. If the newborn is vigorous, defined as having strong respiratory efforts, good muscle tone, and a heart rate > 100 bpm, then tracheal suction is not necessary and may injure the vocal cords.

Management Options

The principal management options for significantly variable fetal heart rate patterns consist of correcting any fetal insult, if possible. Measures suggested by the American College of Obstetricians and Gynecologists (2005) are listed in Table 18-3. Moving the mother to the lateral position, correcting maternal hypotension caused by regional analgesia, and discontinuing oxytocin serve to improve uteroplacental perfusion. Examination is done to exclude prolapsed cord or impending delivery. Simpson and James (2005) assessed benefits of three maneuvers in 52 women with fetal O_2 saturation sensors already in place. They used intravenous hydration—500 to 1000 mL of lactated Ringers solutions given over 20 minutes; lateral versus supine position; and using a nonrebreather mask administered supplemental oxygen at 10 L/min. Each of these maneu-

TABLE 18-3. Initial Evaluation and Treatment of Nonreassuring Fetal Heart Rate Patterns

- Discontinuation of any labor stimulating agent Cervical examination to assess for umbilical cord prolapse or rapid cervical dilation or descent of the fetal head
- Changing maternal position to left or right lateral recumbent position, reducing compression of the vena cava and improving uteroplacental blood flow
- Monitoring maternal blood pressure level for evidence of hypotension, especially in those with regional anesthesia—if present, treatment with ephedrine or phenylephrine may be warranted
- Assessment of patient for uterine hyperstimulation by evaluating uterine contraction frequency and duration

From American College of Obstetricians and Gynecologists, *Intrapartum Fetal Heart Rate Monitoring*, ACOG Practice Bulletin 70, Washington, DC: ACOG, 2005, with permission.

vers significantly increased fetal oxygen saturation levels, although the increments were small.

Tocolysis

A single intravenous or subcutaneous injection of 0.25 mg of terbutaline sulfate given to relax the uterus has been described as a temporizing maneuver in the management of nonreassuring fetal heart rate patterns during labor. The rationale is that inhibition of uterine contractions might improve fetal oxygenation, thus achieving in utero resuscitation. Cook and Spinnato (1994) described their experience with terbutaline tocolysis for fetal resuscitation in 368 pregnancies over a 10-year period. Such resuscitation improved fetal scalp blood pH values, although all fetuses underwent cesarean delivery. These investigators concluded that although the studies were small and rarely randomized, most reported favorable results with terbutaline tocolysis for nonreassuring patterns. Small intravenous doses of nitroglycerin—60 to 180 µg—also have been reported to be beneficial (Mercier and colleagues, 1997).

Amnioinfusion

Gabbe and co-workers (1976) showed in monkeys that removal of amnionic fluid produced variable decelerations and that replenishment of fluid with saline relieved the decelerations. Miyazaki and Taylor (1983) infused saline through an intrauterine pressure catheter in laboring women who had either variable decelerations or prolonged decelerations attributed to cord entrapment. Such therapy improved the heart rate pattern in half of the women studied. Later, Miyazaki and Nevarez (1985) randomly assigned 96 nulliparous women in labor with cord compression patterns and found that those who were treated with amnioinfusion required cesarean delivery for fetal distress less often.

Based on many of these early reports, transvaginal amnioinfusion has been extended into three clinical areas:

1. Treatment of variable or prolonged decelerations
2. Prophylaxis for women with oligohydramnios, as with prolonged ruptured membranes
3. Attempts to dilute or wash out thick meconium (see Chap. 21, p. 497).

Many different amnioinfusion protocols have been reported, but most include a 500- to 800-mL bolus of warmed normal saline followed by a continuous infusion of approximately 3 mL per minute (Owen and co-workers, 1990; Pressman and Blakemore, 1996). In another study, Rinehart and colleagues (2000) randomly gave either 500-mL boluses of normal saline at room temperature alone or 500-mL boluses plus continuous infusion of 3 mL per minute. Their study included 65 women with variable decelerations, and the investigators found neither method to be superior. Wenstrom and associates (1995) surveyed use of amnioinfusion in teaching hospitals in the United States. The procedure was used in 96 percent of the 186 centers surveyed, and it was estimated that 3 to 4 percent of all women delivered at these centers received such infusion. Potential complications of amnioinfusion are summarized in Table 18-4.

Prophylactic Amnioinfusion for Variable Decelerations.
Hofmeyr (1998) used the Cochrane Database to specifically analyze the effects of amnioinfusion in the management of fetal heart rate patterns associated with umbilical cord compression. There were 14 suitable studies identified, most with fewer than 200 participants. It was concluded that amnioinfusion appeared to be useful in reducing the occurrence of variable decelerations, improving neonatal outcome, and reducing cesarean delivery rates for "fetal distress." Based largely on this review, the American College of Obstetricians and Gynecologists (2005) recommends consideration of amnioinfusion with persistent variable decelerations.

TABLE 18-4. Complications Associated with Amnioinfusion from a Survey of 186 Obstetrical Centers

Complication	Centers Reporting No. (%)
Uterine hypertonus	27 (14)
Abnormal fetal heart rate tracing	17 (9)
Chorioamnionitis	7 (4)
Cord prolapse	5 (2)
Uterine rupture	4 (2)
Maternal cardiac or respiratory compromise	3 (2)
Placental abruption	2 (1)
Maternal death	2 (1)

Adapted from Wenstrom and colleagues (1995), with permission.

Prophylactic Amnioinfusion for Oligohydramnios.
Amnioinfusion in women with oligohydramnios has been used prophylactically in an effort to avoid intrapartum fetal heart rate patterns from cord occlusion. Nageotte and co-workers (1991) found that such amnioinfusion resulted in significantly decreased frequency and severity of variable decelerations in labor. There was no improvement, however, in the cesarean delivery rate or condition of term infants. In a randomized investigation, Macri and colleagues (1992) studied prophylactic amnioinfusion in 170 term and postterm pregnancies complicated by both thick meconium and oligohydramnios. Amnioinfusion significantly reduced cesarean delivery rates for fetal distress as well as meconium aspiration syndrome. In contrast, Ogundipe and associates (1994) randomly assigned 116 term pregnancies with an amnionic fluid index of < 5 cm to receive prophylactic amnioinfusion or standard obstetrical care. There were no significant differences in overall cesarean delivery rates, delivery rates for fetal distress, or umbilical gas studies.

Amnioinfusion for Meconium-Stained Amnionic Fluid.
Pierce and associates (2000) summarized the results of 13 prospective trials of intrapartum amnioinfusion in 1924 women with moderate to thick meconium-stained fluid. Infants born to women treated by amnioinfusion were significantly less likely to have meconium below the vocal cords and were less likely to develop meconium aspiration syndrome than infants born to women not undergoing amnioinfusion. The cesarean delivery rate was also lower in the amnioinfusion group. Similar results were reported by Rathore and colleagues (2002). In contrast, a number of investigators were not supportive of amnioinfusion for meconium staining. For example, Usta and associates (1995) reported that amnioinfusion was not feasible in half of women with moderate or thick meconium who were randomized to this treatment. These investigators were unable to demonstrate any improvement in neonatal outcomes. Spong and co-workers (1994) also concluded that although prophylactic amnioinfusion did dilute meconium, it did not improve perinatal outcome. Lastly, Fraser and colleagues (2005) randomized amnioinfusion in 1998 women with thick meconium staining of the amnionic fluid in labor and found no benefits. Because of these findings, the American College of Obstetricians and Gynecologists (2006a) does not recommend amnioinfusion to dilute meconium-stained amnionic fluid.

Xu and co-workers (2007) recently performed a systematic review of randomized controlled trials done to evaluate benefits of amnioinfusion for women in labor complicated by meconium-stained amnionic fluid. They separated the reporting centers based on availability or nonavailability of continuous electronic fetal monitoring—standard versus limited intrapartum surveillance, respectively (Table 18-5). Importantly, amnioinfusion did not decrease the incidence of meconium-aspiration syndrome in the standard surveillance group. It did, however, in the group with limited surveillance—2.4 versus 10 percent for amnioinfusion versus controls—RR = 0.25 (0.13–0.47). These reviewers concluded that amnioinfusion in areas with limited resources may be used to lower the incidence of meconium-aspiration syndrome.

TABLE 18-5. Results of Randomized Controlled Trials of Amnioinfusion versus Standard Intrapartum Surveillance of Women in Labor with Meconium-Stained Amnionic Fluid

Outcome	Treatment Group		RR (95% CI)
	Amnioinfusion No. (%)	Control No. (%)	
Meconium-aspiration syndrome	55/1576 (3.5)	64/1062 (6.0)	0.59 (0.28–1.25)
Meconium beneath cords	83/1538 (5.4)	210/1564[a] (13.4)	0.29 (0.14–0.57)
5-minute Apgar < 7	36/1425 (2.5)	46/1443 (3.2)	0.9 (0.58–1.41)
Neonatal pH < 7.2	188/903 (20.8)	226/885[a] (25.5)	0.62 (0.40–0.96)
Cesarean delivery	471/1586 (29.7)	474/1598 (29.7)	0.89 (0.73–1.10)

[a]Comparison between treatment groups is significant ($p < .05$).
Data from Xu and associates (2007).

Fetal Heart Rate Patterns and Brain Damage

Attempts to correlate fetal heart rate patterns with brain damage have been based primarily on studies of infants identified as a result of medicolegal actions. For example, Rosen and Dickinson (1992) analyzed intrapartum fetal heart rate patterns in 55 such cases and found no specific pattern that correlated with neurological injury. Phelan and Ahn (1994) reported that among 48 fetuses later found to be neurologically impaired, a persistent nonreactive fetal heart rate tracing was already present at the time of admission in 70 percent. They concluded that fetal neurological injury occurred predominately prior to arrival to the hospital. When they looked retrospectively at heart rate patterns in 209 brain-damaged infants, they concluded that there was not a single unique pattern associated with fetal neurological injury (Ahn and co-workers, 1996). Identical results were reported by Williams and Galerneau (2004), who also found that neonatal seizures due to hypoxic ischemic encephalopathy were related to nonspecific abnormal fetal heart rate patterns only when the patterns had been present for an average of 72 minutes. Most recently, Graham and associates (2006) reviewed the world literature published between 1966 and 2006 on the effect of fetal heart rate monitoring to prevent perinatal brain injury and found no benefit.

Experimental Evidence

Fetal heart rate patterns necessary for perinatal brain damage have been studied in experimental animals. Myers (1972) described the effects of complete and partial asphyxia in rhesus monkeys in studies of brain damage due to perinatal asphyxia. Complete asphyxia was produced by total occlusion of umbilical blood flow that led to prolonged deceleration (Fig. 18-31). Fetal arterial pH did not reach 7.0 until about 8 minutes after complete cessation of oxygenation and umbilical flow. At least 10 minutes of such prolonged deceleration was required before there was evidence of brain damage in surviving fetuses.

Myers (1972) also produced partial asphyxia in rhesus monkeys by impeding maternal aortic blood flow. This resulted in late decelerations due to uterine and placental hypoperfusion. He observed that several hours of these late decelerations did not damage the fetal brain unless the pH fell below 7.0. Indeed, Adamsons and Myers (1977) reported subsequently that late

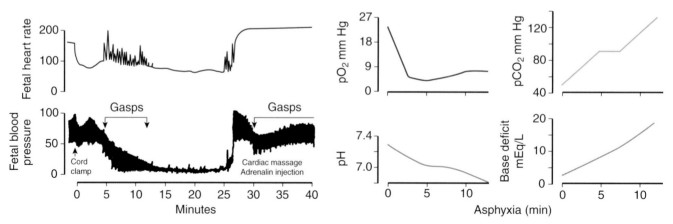

FIGURE 18-31 Prolonged deceleration in a rhesus monkey shown with blood pressure and biochemical changes during total occlusion of umbilical cord blood flow. (Adapted from Myers, 1972.)

decelerations were a marker of partial asphyxia long before brain damage occurred.

The most common fetal heart rate pattern during labor—due to umbilical cord occlusion—requires considerable time to significantly affect the fetus in experimental animals. Clapp and colleagues (1988) partially occluded the umbilical cord for 1 minute every 3 minutes in fetal sheep. Rocha and colleagues (2004) totally occluded the umbilical cord for 90 seconds every 30 minutes for 3 to 5 hours a day for 4 days without producing necrotic brain cell injury. The results from experiments such as these suggest that the effects of umbilical cord entrapment depend on the degree of occlusion—partial versus total, the duration of individual occlusions, and the frequency of such occlusions.

Human Evidence. The contribution of intrapartum events to subsequent neurological handicaps has been greatly overestimated as discussed in further detail in Chapter 29 (p. 612). Nelson and Grether (1998) performed a population-based study of children with disabling spastic cerebral palsy in which they compared intrapartum records of these children with matched controls. Intrapartum fetal heart rate abnormalities did not distinguish between children with cerebral palsy and normal controls. Badawi and colleagues (1998) performed a case-control population-based study of infants with cerebral palsy in Western Australia. Only 5 percent of the brain-damaged infants had intrapartum factors. This fact led them to conclude that most cerebral palsy is unrelated to labor events. Shown in Table 18-6 are some of the other pathologies associated with cerebral palsy.

Low and co-workers (1989) divided perinatal brain damage found following an asphyxial event into three categories based on microscopic findings:

1. From 18 to 48 hours—neuronal necrosis with pyknosis or lysis of the nucleus in shriveled eosinophilic cells
2. From 48 to 72 hours—more intense neuronal necrosis with macrophage response

---

TABLE 18-6. Some Major, Nonintrapartum Pathologies Associated with Cerebral Palsy

- Preterm delivery
- Placental hemorrhage—previa, abruption
- Multifetal pregnancy
- Genetic disorders and anomalies
- Fetal infection—e.g., cytomegalovirus, toxoplasmosis, funisitis, villitis
- Fetal-growth restriction
- Maternal disease—e.g., diabetes, hypertension, viral illness
- Placental infarction, thrombosis
- Tight nuchal cord
- Childhood causes
- Fetal anemia—e.g., hemorrhage, anti-D isoimmunization

Adapted from Strijbis and colleagues (2006).

3. More than 3 days—all the preceding plus astrocytic response with gliosis and in some, early cavitation.

Abnormal brain histopathology was not observed with acute, lethal asphyxia. Moreover, 43 percent of brain damage episodes occurred prior to labor, and 25 percent were in the neonatal period. In another investigation, Low and associates (1984) estimated that more than 1 hour of fetal hypoxia associated with profound metabolic acidemia—pH less than 7.0—was required before neurological abnormalities could be diagnosed at age 6 to 12 months. Low and co-workers (1988) identified 37 term infants with profound metabolic acidemia at birth, followed them for 1 year, and found major neurological deficits in 13 percent. Minor deficits were diagnosed in 10 infants, and the remaining 60 percent were normal. These investigators further observed that intrapartum fetal asphyxia with metabolic acidemia at delivery in both the term and preterm fetus was marked by severe complications not only of the central nervous system, but also of the respiratory and renal systems (Low and colleagues, 1994, 1995).

Clearly, for brain damage to occur, the fetus must be exposed to much more than a brief period of hypoxia. Moreover, the hypoxia must cause profound, just barely sublethal metabolic acidemia. The American College of Obstetricians and Gynecologists (2006b) specifies that such hypoxic-ischemic encephalopathy will show other signs of damage to include: (1) metabolic acidosis in umbilical cord artery blood—pH < 7 and base deficit $\geq$ 12 mmol/L; (2) Apgar scores 0–3 beyond 5 minutes, and (3) neurological sequelae—seizures, coma, hypotonia, and one or more of cardiovascular, gastrointestinal, hematological, pulmonary, hepatic, or renal system dysfunction. Accordingly, the American College of Obstetricians and Gynecologists (2006b) recommends umbilical cord gases be obtained whenever there is cesarean delivery for fetal compromise, a low 5-minute Apgar score, severe fetal-growth restriction, an abnormal fetal heart rate tracing, maternal thyroid disease, or multifetal gestation. Fetal heart rate patterns consistent with these sublethal conditions are fortunately rare.

These observations strengthen the position of the American College of Obstetricians and Gynecologists (2006b) on the criteria necessary to consider birth asphyxia as a cause of cerebral palsy as discussed in detail in Chapter 29 (p. 612). These include cord blood evidence of metabolic acidosis and early onset of severe or moderate encephalopathy. Importantly, spastic quadriplegia and, less commonly, dyskinetic cerebral palsy are the only types of cerebral palsy associated with acute hypoxic intrapartum events. Unilateral brain lesions—hemiplegia or diplegia—are not a result of intrapartum hypoxia.

Benefits of Electronic Fetal Heart Rate Monitoring

There are several fallacious assumptions behind expectations of improved perinatal outcome with electronic monitoring. One assumption is that fetal distress is a slowly developing phenomenon and that electronic monitoring makes possible early detection of the compromised fetus. This assumption is illogical; that is, how can all fetuses die slowly? Another presumption is that all fetal damage develops in the hospital. Within the past 20 years, attention has been focused on the reality that most damaged fetuses suffered insults before arrival at labor units. The very term *fetal monitor* implies that this inanimate technology in some fashion "monitors." The assumption is made that if a dead or damaged infant is delivered, the tracing strip must provide some clue, because this device was monitoring fetal condition. All of these assumptions led to great expectations and fostered the belief that all dead or damaged neonates were preventable. Parer and King (2000) reviewed reasons why fetal heart rate monitoring did not live up to its expectations. These unwarranted expectations have greatly fueled litigation in obstetrics. Indeed, Symonds (1994) reported that 70 percent of all liability claims related to fetal brain damage are based on reputed abnormalities seen in the electronic fetal monitor tracing.

By the end of the 1970s, questions about the efficacy, safety, and costs of electronic monitoring were being voiced from the Office of Technology Assessment, the United States Congress, and the Centers for Disease Control and Prevention. Banta and Thacker (2002) reviewed 25 years of the controversy on the benefits, or lack thereof, of electronic fetal monitoring. Parer (2003) points out that the controversy continues and that ". . . to justify our continued use of EFM, we need to clean up our house. We must come to some agreement on a national level about interpretation and management."

Parkland Hospital Experience: Selective versus Universal Monitoring

In July 1982, an investigation began at Parkland Hospital to ascertain whether all women in labor should undergo electronic monitoring (Leveno and co-workers, 1986). In alternating months, universal electronic monitoring was rotated with selective heart rate monitoring, which was the prevailing practice.

During the 3-year investigation, 17,410 labors were managed using universal electronic monitoring. No significant differences were found in any perinatal outcomes. There was a significantly small increase in the cesarean delivery rate for fetal distress associated with universal monitoring. Thus, increased application of electronic monitoring at Parkland Hospital did not improve perinatal results, but it increased the frequency of cesarean delivery for fetal distress.

Summary of Randomized Studies. Thacker and associates (1995) identified 12 randomized clinical trials of electronic fetal monitoring from 1966 to 1994. There were 58,624 total pregnancies included in these studies. These authors concluded that the benefits once claimed for electronic monitoring are clearly more modest than were believed and appear to be primarily in the prevention of neonatal seizures. Long-term implications of this outcome, however, appear less serious than once believed. Abnormal neurological consequences were not consistently higher among children monitored by auscultation compared with electronic methods. The authors concurred with the position of the American College of Obstetricians and Gynecologists (1995) on intrapartum fetal surveillance.

Current Recommendations

The methods most commonly used for intrapartum fetal heart rate monitoring include auscultation with a fetal stethoscope or a Doppler ultrasound device, or continuous electronic monitoring of the heart rate and uterine contractions. No scientific evidence has identified the most effective method, including the frequency or duration of fetal surveillance that ensures optimum results. Summarized in Table 18-7 are the current recommendations of the American Academy of Pediatrics and the American College of Obstetricians and Gynecologists (2007). Intermittent auscultation or continuous electronic monitoring is considered an acceptable method of intrapartum surveillance

TABLE 18-7. Guidelines for Methods of Intrapartum Fetal Heart Rate Monitoring

Surveillance	Low-Risk Pregnancies	High-Risk Pregnancies
Acceptable methods		
Intermittent auscultation	Yes	Yes[a]
Continuous electronic monitoring (internal or external)	Yes	Yes[b]
Evaluation intervals		
First-stage labor (active)	30 min	15 min[a,b]
Second-stage labor	15 min	5 min[a,c]

[a]Preferably before, during, and after a uterine contraction.
[b]Includes tracing evaluation and charting at least every 15 minutes.
[c]Tracing should be evaluated at least every 5 minutes.
From the American Academy of Pediatrics and the American College of Obstetricians and Gynecologists (2007).

in both low- and high-risk pregnancies. The recommended interval between checking the heart rate, however, is longer in the uncomplicated pregnancy. When auscultation is used, it is recommended that it be performed after a contraction and for 60 seconds. It also is recommended that a 1-to-1 nurse–patient ratio be used if auscultation is employed.

INTRAPARTUM SURVEILLANCE OF UTERINE ACTIVITY

Analysis of electronically measured uterine activity permits some generalities concerning the relationship of certain contraction patterns to labor outcome. There is considerable normal variation, however, and caution must be exercised before judging true labor or its absence solely from study of a monitor tracing. Uterine muscle efficiency to effect delivery varies greatly. To use an analogy, 100-meter sprinters all have the same muscle groups yet cross the finish line at different times.

Internal Uterine Pressure Monitoring

Amnionic fluid pressure is measured between and during contractions by a fluid-filled plastic catheter with its distal tip located above the presenting part (Fig. 18-32). The catheter is connected to a strain-gauge pressure sensor adjusted to the same level as the catheter tip in the uterus. The amplified electrical signal produced in the strain gauge by variation in pressure within the fluid system is recorded on a calibrated moving paper strip simultaneously with the fetal heart rate recording. Intrauterine pressure catheters are now available that have the pressure sensor in the catheter tip, which obviates the need for the fluid column.

External Monitoring

Uterine contractions can be measured by a displacement transducer in which the transducer button, or "plunger," is held against the abdominal wall. As the uterus contracts, the button moves in proportion to the strength of the contraction. This movement is converted into a measurable electrical signal that indicates the *relative* intensity of the contraction—it does not give an accurate measure of intensity. However, external monitoring can give a good indication of the onset, peak, and end of the contraction.

Patterns of Uterine Activity

Caldeyro-Barcia and Poseiro (1960), from Montevideo, Uruguay, were pioneers who have done much to elucidate the patterns of spontaneous uterine activity throughout pregnancy. Contractile waves of uterine activity were usually measured using intra-amnionic pressure catheters. But early in their studies, as many as four simultaneous intramyometrial microballoons were also used to record uterine pressure. These investigators also introduced the concept of *Montevideo units* to define uterine activity (see Chap. 20, p. 467). By this definition, uterine performance is the product of the intensity—increased uterine pressure above baseline tone—of a contraction in mm Hg mul-

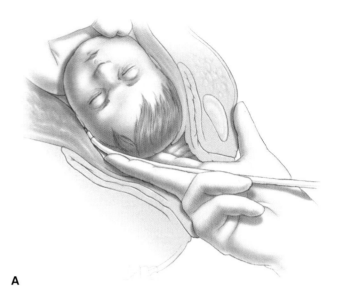

A

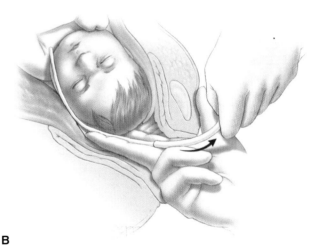

B

FIGURE 18-32 Placement of an intrauterine pressure catheter to monitor contractions and their pressures. **A.** The white catheter, contained within the blue introducer, is inserted into the birth canal and placed along one side of the fetal head. **B.** The catheter is then gently advanced into the uterus, and the introducer is withdrawn.

tiplied by contraction frequency per 10 minutes. For example, three contractions in 10 minutes, each of 50 mm Hg intensity, would equal 150 Montevideo units.

During the first 30 weeks, uterine activity is comparatively quiescent. Contractions are seldom greater than 20 mm Hg, and these have been equated with those first described in 1872 by John Braxton Hicks. Uterine activity increases gradually after 30 weeks, and it is noteworthy that these *Braxton Hicks contractions* also increase in intensity and frequency. Further increases in uterine activity are typical of the last weeks of pregnancy, termed *prelabor*. During this phase, the cervix ripens (see Chap. 6, p. 138).

According to Caldeyro-Barcia and Poseiro (1960), clinical labor usually commences when uterine activity reaches values between 80 and 120 Montevideo units. This translates into approximately three contractions of 40 mm Hg every 10 minutes.

Importantly, there is no clear-cut division between prelabor and labor, but rather a gradual and progressive transition.

During first-stage labor, uterine contractions increase progressively in intensity from approximately 25 mm Hg at commencement of labor to 50 mm Hg at the end. At the same time, frequency increases from three to five contractions per 10 minutes, and uterine baseline tone from 8 to 12 mm Hg. Uterine activity further increases during second-stage labor, aided by maternal pushing. Indeed, contractions of 80 to 100 mm Hg are typical and occur as frequently as five to six per 10 minutes. Interestingly, the duration of uterine contractions—60 to 80 seconds—does not increase appreciably from early active labor through the second stage (Bakker and associates, 2007; Pontonnier and colleagues, 1975). Presumably, this duration constancy serves fetal respiratory gas exchange. During a uterine contraction, the intervillous space, where respiratory gas exchange occurs, becomes isolated. This leads to functional fetal "breath holding," which has a 60- to 80-second limit that remains relatively constant.

Caldeyro-Barcia and Poseiro (1960) also observed empirically that uterine contractions are clinically palpable only after their intensity exceeds 10 mm Hg. Moreover, until the intensity

of contractions reaches 40 mm Hg, the uterine wall can readily be depressed by the finger. At greater intensity, the uterine wall then becomes so hard that it resists easy depression. Uterine contractions usually are not associated with pain until their intensity exceeds 15 mm Hg, presumably because this is the minimum pressure required for distending the lower uterine segment and cervix. It follows that Braxton Hicks contractions exceeding 15 mm Hg may be perceived as uncomfortable because distension of the uterus, cervix, and birth canal is generally thought to elicit discomfort.

Hendricks (1968) observed that "the clinician makes great demands upon the uterus." The uterus is expected to remain well relaxed during pregnancy, to contract effectively but intermittently during labor, and then to remain in a state of almost constant contraction for several hours postpartum. Figure 18-33 demonstrates an example of normal uterine activity during labor. Uterine activity progressively and gradually increases from prelabor through late labor. Interestingly, as shown in Figure 18-33, uterine contractions after birth are identical to those resulting in delivery of the infant. It is therefore not surprising that the uterus that performs poorly before delivery is also prone to atony and puerperal hemorrhage.

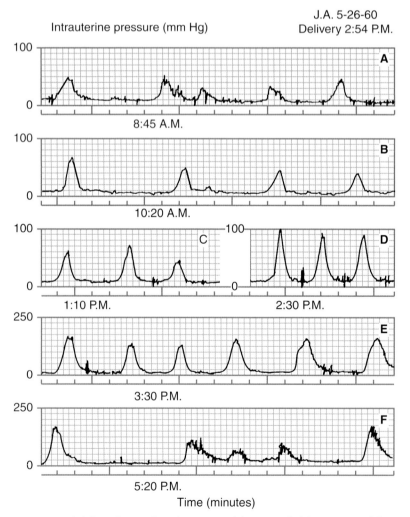

FIGURE 18-33 Intrauterine pressure recorded through a single catheter. **A.** Prelabor. **B.** Early labor. **C.** Active labor. **D.** Late labor. **E.** Spontaneous activity ½ hour postpartum. **F.** Spontaneous activity 2½ hours postpartum. (Adapted from Hendricks, 1968, with permission.)

Origin and Propagation of Contractions

The uterus has not been studied extensively in terms of its non-hormonal physiological mechanisms of function. The normal contractile wave of labor originates near the uterine end of one of the fallopian tubes. Thus, these areas act as "pacemakers" (Fig. 18-34). The right pacemaker usually predominates over the left and starts most contractile waves. Contractions spread from the pacemaker area throughout the uterus at 2 cm/sec, depolarizing the whole organ within 15 seconds. This depolarization wave propagates downward toward the cervix. Intensity is greatest in the fundus, and it diminishes in the lower uterus. This phenomenon is thought to reflect reductions in myometrial thickness from the fundus to the cervix. Presumably, this descending gradient of pressure serves to direct fetal descent toward the cervix as well as to efface the cervix. Importantly, all parts of the uterus are synchronized and reach their peak pressure almost simultaneously, giving rise to the curvilinear waveform shown in Figure 18-34. Young and Zhang (2004) have shown that the initiation of each contraction is triggered by a tissue-level bioelectric event.

The pacemaker theory also serves to explain the varying intensity of adjacent coupled contractions shown in panels A and B of Figure 18-33. Such coupling was termed *incoordination* by Caldeyro-Barcia and Poseiro (1960). A contractile wave begins in one cornual-region pacemaker, but does not synchronously depolarize the entire uterus. As a result, another contraction begins in the contralateral pacemaker and produces the second contractile wave of the couplet. These small contractions alternating with larger ones appear to be typical of early labor. Indeed, labor may progress with such uterine activity, albeit at a slower pace. These authors also observed that labor would progress slowly if regular contractions were hypotonic—that is, contractions with intensity less than 25 mm Hg or frequency less than 2 per 10 minutes. Similar observations were made by Seitchik (1981) in a computer-aided analysis comparing women in active labor with those in arrested labor. Normal labor was characterized by a minimum of three contractions that averaged greater than 25 mm Hg and less than 4-minute intervals between contractions. A lesser amount of uterine activity was associated with arrest of active labor. Prospective diagnosis of hypotonic labor cannot be reliably based simply on a few uterine pressures.

Hauth and co-workers (1986) quantified uterine contraction pressures in 109 women at term who received oxytocin for

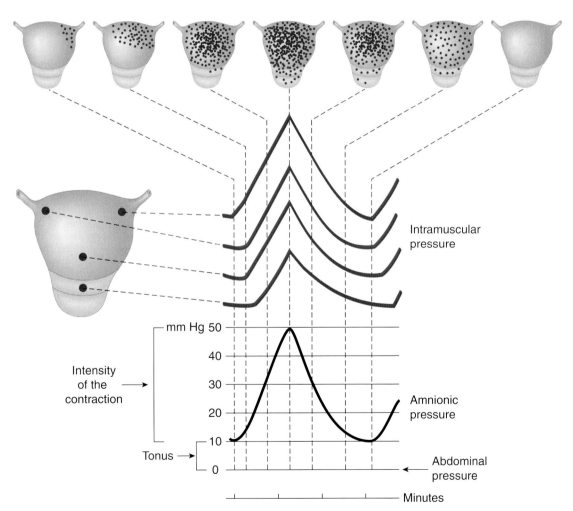

FIGURE 18-34 Schematic representation of the normal contractile wave of labor. Large uterus on the left shows the four points at which intramyometrial pressure was recorded with microballoons. Four corresponding pressure tracings are shown in relation to each other by shading on the small uteri at top. (Adapted from Caldeyro-Barcia and Poseiro, 1960.)

labor induction or augmentation. Most of these women achieved 200 to 225 Montevideo units, and 40 percent had up to 300 units to effect delivery. The authors suggested that these levels of uterine activity should be sought before consideration of cesarean delivery for presumed dystocia.

REFERENCES

Adamsons K, Myers RE: Late decelerations and brain tolerance of the fetal monkey to intrapartum asphyxia. Am J Obstet Gynecol 128:893, 1977

Agrawal SK, Doucette F, Gratton R, et al: Intrapartum computerized fetal heart rate parameters and metabolic acidosis at birth. Obstet Gynecol 102:731, 2003

Ahn MO, Korst L, Phelan JP: Intrapartum fetal heart rate patterns in 209 brain damaged infants. Am J Obstet Gynecol 174:492, 1996

Amer-Wåhlin I, Arulkumaran S, Hagberg H, et al: Fetal electrocardiogram: ST waveform analysis in intrapartum surveillance. BJOG 114:1191, 2007

Amer-Wåhlin I, Hellsten C, Norén H, et al: Cardiotocography only versus cardiotocography plus ST analysis of fetal electrocardiogram for intrapartum fetal monitoring: A Swedish randomized controlled trial. Lancet 358:534, 2001

American Academy of Pediatrics and the American College of Obstetricians and Gynecologists: Intrapartum and postpartum care of the mother. In Guidelines for Perinatal Care, 6th ed. Washington, DC, 2007, p 146

American College of Obstetricians and Gynecologists: Fetal heart rate patterns: Monitoring, interpretation, and management. Technical Bulletin No. 207, July 1995

American College of Obstetricians and Gynecologists: Inappropriate use of the terms fetal distress and birth asphyxia. Committee Opinion No. 303, October 2004

American College of Obstetricians and Gynecologists: Intrapartum fetal heart rate monitoring. Practice Bulletin No. 70, December 2005

American College of Obstetricians and Gynecologists: Amnioinfusion does not prevent meconium aspiration syndrome. Committee Opinion No. 346, October 2006a

American College of Obstetricians and Gynecologists: Umbilical cord blood gas and acid-base analysis. Committee Opinion No. 348, November 2006b

American College of Obstetricians and Gynecologists: Management of delivery of a newborn with meconium stained amniotic fluid. Committee Opinion No. 379, September 2007

Angel J, Knuppel R, Lake M: Sinusoidal fetal heart rate patterns associated with intravenous butorphanol administration. Am J Obstet Gynecol 149:465, 1984

Anyaegbunam AM, Ditchik A, Stoessel R, et al: Vibroacoustic stimulation of the fetus entering the second stage of labor. Obstet Gynecol 83:963, 1994

Api O, Carvalho JS: Fetal dysrhythmias. Best Pract Res Clin Obstet Gynaecol 22(1):31, 2008

Arikan GM, Scholz HS, Petru E, et al: Cord blood oxygen saturation in vigorous infants at birth: What is normal? Br J Obstet Gynaecol 107:987, 2000

Ayres-de-Campos D, Bernardes J, Costa-Pereira A, et al: Inconsistencies in classification by experts of cardiotocograms and subsequent clinical decision. Br J Obstet Gynaecol 106:1307, 1999

Badawi N, Kurinczuk J, Keogh JM, et al: Intrapartum risk factors for newborn encephalopathy: The Western Australia case-control study. BMJ 317:1554, 1998

Bakker PC, Kurver PH, Duik DJ, et al: Elevated uterine activity increases the risk of fetal acidosis at birth. Am J Obstet Gynecol 196:313, 2007

Ball RH, Parer JT: The physiologic mechanisms of variable decelerations. Am J Obstet Gynecol 166:1683, 1992

Banta HD, Thacker SB: Assessing the costs and benefits of electronic fetal monitoring. Obstet Gynecol Surv 34:627, 1979

Banta HD, Thacker SB: Electronic fetal monitoring: Lessons from a formative case of health technology assessment. Int J Technol Assess Health Care 18:762, 2002

Behrman RE: The cardiovascular system. In Behrman RE, Kliegman RM, Nelson WE, et al (eds): Nelson Textbook of Pediatrics, 14th ed. Philadelphia, Saunders, 1992, p 1127

Bellver J, Perales A, Maiques V, et al: Can antepartum computerized cardiotocography predict the evolution of intrapartum acid-base status in normal fetuses? Acta Obstet Gynecol Scand 83:267, 2004

Berkus MD, Langer O, Samueloff A, et al: Electronic fetal monitoring: What's reassuring? Acta Obstet Gynecol Scand 78:15, 1999

Blackwell SC, Moldenhauer J, Hassan SS, et al: Meconium aspiration syndrome in term neonates with normal acid-base status at delivery: Is it different? Am J Obstet Gynecol 184:1422, 2001

Bloom SL, Spong CY, Thom E, et al: Fetal pulse oximetry and cesarean delivery. N Engl J Med 335:21, 2006

Bloom SL, Swindle RG, McIntire DD, et al: Fetal pulse oximetry: Duration of desaturation and intrapartum outcome. Obstet Gynecol 93:1036, 1999

Boehm FH: Prolonged end stage fetal heart rate deceleration. Obstet Gynecol 45:579, 1975

Boldt T, Eronen M, Andersson S: Long-term outcome in fetuses with cardiac arrhythmias. Obstet Gynecol 102:1372, 2003

Brook I: Infected neonatal cephalohematomas caused by anaerobic bacteria. J Perinat Med 33(3):255, 2005

Caldeyro-Barcia R, Mendez-Bauer C, Poseiro JJ, et al: Fetal monitoring in labor. In Walloch HJ, Gold EM, Lis EF (eds): Maternal and Child Health Practices. Springfield, IL, Thomas, 1973, p 332

Caldeyro-Barcia R, Poseiro JJ: Physiology of the uterine contraction. Clin Obstet Gynecol 3:386, 1960

Clapp JF, Peress NS, Wesley M, et al: Brain damage after intermittent partial cord occlusion in the chronically instrumented fetal lamb. Am J Obstet Gynecol 159:504, 1988

Clark SL, Gimovsky ML, Miller FC: Fetal heart rate response to scalp blood sampling. Am J Obstet Gynecol 14:706, 1982

Clark SL, Gimovsky ML, Miller FC: The scalp stimulation test: A clinical alternative to fetal scalp blood sampling. Am J Obstet Gynecol 148:274, 1984

Cook VD, Spinnato JA: Terbutaline tocolysis prior to cesarean section for fetal distress. J Matern Fetal Med 3:219, 1994

Copel JA, Liang RI, Demasio K, et al: The clinical significance of the irregular fetal heart rhythm. Am J Obstet Gynecol 182:813, 2000

Davidson SR, Rankin JH, Martin CB Jr, et al: Fetal heart rate variability and behavioral state: Analysis by power spectrum. Am J Obstet Gynecol 167:717, 1992

Dawes GS: The control of fetal heart rate and its variability in counts. In Kunzel W (ed): Fetal Heart Rate Monitoring. Berlin, Springer-Verlag, 1985, p 188

Dawes GS, Fox HE, Leduc BM, et al: Respiratory movements and rapid eye movement sleep in the foetal lamb. J Physiol 220:119, 1972

Dawes GS, Visser GHA, Goodman JDS, et al: Numerical analysis of the human fetal heart rate: Modulation by breathing and movement. Am J Obstet Gynecol 140:535, 1981

Del Valle GO, Joffe GM, Izquierdo LA, et al: Acute posttraumatic fetal anemia treated with fetal intravascular transfusion. Am J Obstet Gynecol 166:127, 1992

Dellinger EH, Boehm FH, Crane MM: Electronic fetal heart rate monitoring: Early neonatal outcomes associated with normal rate, fetal stress, and fetal distress. Am J Obstet Gynecol 182:214, 2000

Devoe L: ECG analysis: The next generation in electronic fetal monitoring? Contemporary Ob/Gyn, September 15, 2006, p 6

Devoe L, Golde S, Kilman Y, et al: A comparison of visual analyses of intrapartum fetal heart rate tracings according to the new National Institute of Child Health and Human Development guidelines with computer analyses by an automated fetal heart rate monitoring system. Am J Obstet Gynecol 183:361, 2000

Divon MY, Winkler H, Yeh SY, et al: Diminished respiratory sinus arrhythmia in asphyxiated term infants. Am J Obstet Gynecol 155:1263, 1986

Dollberg S, Livny S, Mordecheyev N, et al: Nucleated red blood cells in meconium aspiration syndrome. Obstet Gynecol 97:593, 2001

Doria V, Papageorghiou AT, Gustafsson A, et al: Review of the first 1502 cases of ECG-ST waveform analysis during labour in a teaching hospital. BJOG 114:1202, 2007

East CE, Brennecke SP, King JF, et al: The effect of intrapartum fetal pulse oximetry, in the presence of a nonreassuring fetal heart rate pattern, on operative delivery rates: A multicenter, randomized, controlled trial (the FOREMOST trial). Am J Obstet Gynecol 194:606, 2006

Eberle RL, Norris MC, Eberle AM, et al: The effect of maternal position on fetal heart rate during epidural or intrathecal labor analgesia. Am J Obstet Gynecol 179:150, 1998

Edersheim TG, Hutson JM, Druzin ML, et al: Fetal heart rate response to vibratory acoustic stimulation predicts fetal pH in labor. Am J Obstet Gynecol 157:1557, 1987

Eggink BH, Richardson CJ, Rowen JL: Gardnerella vaginalis–infected scalp hematoma associated with electronic fetal monitoring. Pediatr Infect Dis J 23:276, 2004

Egley CC, Bowes WA, Wagner D: Sinusoidal fetal heart rate pattern during labor. Am J Perinatol 8:197, 1991

Elimian A, Figueroa R, Tejani N: Intrapartum assessment of fetal well-being: A comparison of scalp stimulation with scalp pH sampling. Obstet Gynecol 89:373, 1997

Epstein H, Waxman A, Gleicher N, et al: Meperidine induced sinusoidal fetal heart rate pattern and reversal with naloxone. Obstet Gynecol 59:225, 1982

Faro S, Martens MG, Hammill HA, et al: Antibiotic prophylaxis: Is there a difference? Am J Obstet Gynecol 162:900, 1990

Farrell T, Chien PFW, Gordon A: Intrapartum umbilical artery Doppler velocimetry as a predictor of adverse perinatal outcome: a systematic review. Br J Obstet Gynaecol 106:783, 1999

Food and Drug Administration: OxiFirst Fetal Oxygen Saturation Monitoring System. New device approval. Available at: www.fda.gov/cdrh/mda/docs/p990053.pdf. Accessed January 5, 2009

Food and Drug Administration: STAN S31 Fetal Heart Monitor – P020001. New device approval. Available at: http://www.fda.gov/cdrh/mda/docs/p020001.html Accessed May 7, 2009

Fraser WD, Hofmeyer J, Lede R, et al: Amnioinfusion for the prevention of the meconium aspiration syndrome. N Engl J Med 353:9, 2005

Freeman RK, Garite TH, Nageotte MP: Fetal Heart Rate Monitoring, 3rd ed. Philadelphia, Lippincott Williams & Wilkins, 2003

Gabbe SG, Ettinger BB, Freeman RK, et al: Umbilical cord compression associated with amniotomy: Laboratory observations. Am J Obstet Gynecol 126:353, 1976

Garite TJ, Dildy GA, McNamara H, et al: A multicenter controlled trial of fetal pulse oximetry in the intrapartum management of nonreassuring fetal heart rate patterns. Am J Obstet Gynecol 183:1049, 2000

Ghidini A, Spong CY: Severe meconium aspiration syndrome is not caused by aspiration of meconium. Am J Obstet Gynecol 185:931, 2001

Gilstrap LC III, Hauth JC, Hankins GDV, et al: Second stage fetal heart rate abnormalities and type of neonatal acidemia. Obstet Gynecol 70:191, 1987

Goodwin TM, Milner-Masterson L, Paul RH: Elimination of fetal scalp blood sampling on a large clinical service. Obstet Gynecol 83:971, 1994

Gorenberg DM, Pattillo C, Hendi P, et al: Fetal pulse oximetry: Correlation between oxygen desaturation, duration, and frequency and neonatal outcomes. Am J Obstet Gynecol 189:136, 2003

Graham EM, Petersen SM, Christo DK, et al: Intrapartum electronic fetal heart rate monitoring and the prevention of perinatal brain injury. Obstet Gynecol 108:656, 2006

Greenwood C, Lalchandani S, MacQuillan K, et al: Meconium passed in labor: How reassuring is clear amniotic fluid? Obstet Gynecol 102:89, 2003

Gull I, Jaffa AJ, Oren M, et al: Acid accumulation during end-stage bradycardia in term fetuses: How long is too long? Br J Obstet Gynaecol 103:1096, 1996

Hallak M, Martinez-Poyer J, Kruger ML, et al: The effect of magnesium sulfate on fetal heart rate parameters: A randomized, placebo-controlled trial. Am J Obstet Gynecol 181:1122, 1999

Hamilton LA Jr, McKeown MJ: Biochemical and electronic monitoring of the fetus. In Wynn RM (ed): Obstetrics and Gynecology Annual, 1973. New York, Appleton-Century-Crofts, 1974

Hammacher K, Huter K, Bokelmann J, et al: Foetal heart frequency and perinatal conditions of the fetus and newborn. Gynaecologia 166:349, 1968

Hankins GDV, Leicht TL, Van Houk JW: Prolonged fetal bradycardia secondary to maternal hypothermia in response to urosepsis. Am J Perinatol 14:217, 1997

Hauth JC, Hankins GV, Gilstrap LC, et al: Uterine contraction pressures with oxytocin induction/augmentation. Obstet Gynecol 68:305, 1986

Hendricks CH: Uterine contractility changes in the early puerperium. In Anderson GV, Quilligan EJ (eds): Clinical Obstetrics and Gynecology, Thromboembolic Disorders, Physiology of Labor. New York, Harper & Row, 1968, p 125

Herbert CM, Boehm FH: Prolonged end-stage fetal heart deceleration: A re-analysis. Obstet Gynecol 57:589, 1981

Hicks JB: On the contractions of the uterus throughout pregnancy. Trans Obstet Soc Lond 13, 1872

Hill JB, Alexander JM, Sharma SK, et al: A comparison of the effects of epidural and meperidine analgesia during labor on fetal heart rate. Obstet Gynecol 102:333, 2003

Hofmeyr GJ: Amnioinfusion for umbilical cord compression in labour. Cochrane Database Syst Rev 1:CD000013, 1998

Hon EH: The electronic evaluation of the fetal heart rate. Am J Obstet Gynecol 75:1215, 1958

Hon EH: The fetal heart rate patterns preceding death in utero. Am J Obstet Gynecol 78:47, 1959

Hon EH, Bradfield AM, Hess OW: The electronic evaluation of the fetal heart rate. Am J Obstet Gynecol 82:291, 1961

Hornbuckle J, Vail A, Abrams KR, et al: Bayesian interpretation of trials: The example of intrapartum electronic fetal heart rate monitoring. Br J Obstet Gynaecol 107:3, 2000

Ikeda T, Murata Y, Quilligan EJ, et al: Two sinusoidal heart rate patterns in fetal lambs undergoing extracorporeal membrane oxygenation. Am J Obstet Gynecol 180:462, 1999

Impey L, Raymonds M, MacQuillan K, et al: Admission cardiotocography: A randomised controlled trial. Lancet 361:465, 2003

Itskovitz J, LaGamma EF, Rudoloph AM: Heart rate and blood pressure response to umbilical cord compression in fetal lambs with special reference to the mechanisms of variable deceleration. Am J Obstet Gynecol 147:451, 1983

Jaeggi ET, Friedberg MK: Diagnosis and management of fetal bradyarrhythmias. Pacing Clin Electrophysiol 31 Suppl 1:S50, 2008

Jazayeri A, Politz L, Tsibris JCM, et al: Fetal erythropoietin levels in pregnancies complicated by meconium passage: Does meconium suggest fetal hypoxia? Am J Obstet Gynecol 183:188, 2000

Johnson TR Jr, Compton AA, Rotmeusch J, et al: Significance of the sinusoidal fetal heart rate pattern. Am J Obstet Gynecol 139:446, 1981

Jovanovic R, Nguyen HT: Experimental meconium aspiration in guinea pigs. Obstet Gynecol 73:652, 1989

Katz VL, Bowes WA: Meconium aspiration syndrome: Reflections on a murky subject. Am J Obstet Gynecol 166:171, 1992

Keith RDF, Beckley S, Garibaldi JM, et al: A multicentre comparative study of 17 experts and an intelligent computer system for managing labour using the cardiotocogram. Br J Obstet Gynaecol 102:688, 1995

Klauser CK, Christensen EE, Chauhan SP, et al: Use of fetal pulse oximetry among high-risk women in labor: A randomized clinical trial. Am J Obstet Gynecol 192:1810, 2005

Klavan M, Laver AT, Boscola MA: Clinical concepts of fetal heart rate monitoring. Waltham, MA, Hewlett-Packard, 1977

Kozuma S, Watanabe T, Bennet L, et al: The effect of carotid sinus denervation on fetal heart rate variation in normoxia, hypoxia and post-hypoxia in fetal sleep. Br J Obstet Gynaecol 104:460, 1997

Krebs HB, Petres RE, Dunn LJ: Intrapartum fetal heart rate monitoring, 5. Fetal heart rate patterns in the second stage of labor. Am J Obstet Gynecol 140:435, 1981

Krebs HB, Petres RE, Dunn LJ, et al: Intrapartum fetal heart rate monitoring, 6. Prognostic significance of accelerations. Am J Obstet Gynecol 142:297, 1982

Kruger K, Hallberg B, Blennow M, et al: Predictive value of fetal scalp blood lactate concentration and pH as markers of neurologic disability. Am J Obstet Gynecol 181:1072, 1999

Künzel W: Fetal heart rate alterations in partial and total cord occlusion. In Kunzel W (ed): Fetal Heart Rate Monitoring: Clinical Practice and Pathophysiology. Berlin, Springer-Verlag, 1985, p 114

Larma JD, Silva AM, Holcroft CJ, et al: Intrapartum electronic fetal heart rate monitoring and the identification of metabolic acidosis and hypoxic-ischemic encephalopathy. Am J Obstet Gynecol 197(3):301.e1, 2007

Lee CV, DiLaretto PC, Lane JM: A study of fetal heart rate acceleration patterns. Obstet Gynecol 45:142, 1975

Leveno KJ, Cunningham FG, Nelson S: Prospective comparison of selective and universal electronic fetal monitoring in 34,995 pregnancies. N Engl J Med 315:615, 1986

Leveno KJ, Quirk JG, Cunningham FG, et al: Prolonged pregnancy: Observations concerning the causes of fetal distress. Am J Obstet Gynecol 150:465, 1984

Lin CC, Vassallo B, Mittendorf R: Is intrapartum vibroacoustic stimulation an effective predictor of fetal acidosis? J Perinat Med 29:506, 2001

Lopriore E, Aziz MI, Nagel HT, et al: Long-term neurodevelopmental outcome after fetal arrhythmia. Am J Obstet Gynecol [Epub ahead of print] Apr 2, 2009

Low JA, Galbraith RS, Muir DW, et al: Factors associated with motor and cognitive deficits in children after intrapartum fetal hypoxia. Am J Obstet Gynecol 148:533, 1984

Low JA, Galbraith RS, Muir DW, et al: Motor and cognitive deficits after intrapartum asphyxia in the mature fetus. Am J Obstet Gynecol 158:356, 1988

Low JA, Panagiotopoulos C, Derrick EJ: Newborn complications after intrapartum asphyxia with metabolic acidosis in the term fetus. Am J Obstet Gynecol 170:1081, 1994

Low JA, Panagiotopoulos C, Derrick EJ: Newborn complications after intrapartum asphyxia with metabolic acidosis in the preterm fetus. Am J Obstet Gynecol 172:805, 1995

Low JA, Robertson DR, Simpson LL: Temporal relationships of neuropathologic conditions caused by perinatal asphyxia. Am J Obstet Gynecol 160:608, 1989

Low JA, Victory R, Derrick J: Predictive value of electronic fetal monitoring for intrapartum fetal asphyxia with metabolic acidosis. Obstet Gynecol 93:285, 1999

Lowe TW, Leveno KJ, Quirk JG, et al: Sinusoidal fetal heart rate patterns after intrauterine transfusion. Obstet Gynecol 64:215, 1984

Macones GA, Hankins GD, Spong CY, et al: The 2008 National Institute of Child Health and Human Development Workshop report on electronic fetal monitoring. Update on definitions, interpretations, research guidelines. Obstet Gynecol 112:661, 2008

Macri CJ, Schrimmer DB, Leung A, et al: Prophylactic amnioinfusion improves outcome of pregnancy complicated by thick meconium and oligohydramnios. Am J Obstet Gynecol 167:117, 1992

Manassiev N: What is the normal heart rate of a term fetus? Br J Obstet Gynaecol 103:1272, 1996

Martin JA, Hamilton BE, Sutton PD, et al: Births: Final data for 2002. National Vital Statistics Report, Vol. 52, No. 1. Hyattsville, MD, National Center for Health Statistics, 2003

Mathews TG, Warshaw JB: Relevance of the gestational age distribution of meconium passage in utero. Pediatrics 64:30, 1979

McGregor JA, McFarren T: Neonatal cranial osteomyelitis: A complication of fetal monitoring. Obstet Gynecol 73(2):490, 1989

Melchior J, Bernard N: Incidence and pattern of fetal heart rate alterations during labor. In Kunzel W (ed): Fetal Heart Rate Monitoring: Clinical Practice and Pathophysiology. Berlin, Springer-Verlag, 1985, p 73

Mercier FJ, Dounas M, Bouaziz H, et al: Intravenous nitroglycerin to relieve intrapartum fetal distress related to uterine hyperactivity: A prospective observation study. Anesth Analg 84:1117, 1997

Mires G, Williams F, Howie P: Randomised controlled trial of cardiotocography versus Doppler auscultation of fetal heart at admission in labour in low risk obstetric population. BMJ 322:1457, 2001

Miyazaki FS, Nevarez F: Saline amnioinfusion for relief of repetitive variable decelerations: A prospective randomized study. Am J Obstet Gynecol 153:301, 1985

Miyazaki FS, Taylor NA: Saline amnioinfusion for relief of variable or prolonged decelerations. Am J Obstet Gynecol 146:670, 1983

Modanlou H, Freeman RK: Sinusoidal fetal heart rate pattern: Its definition and clinical significance. Am J Obstet Gynecol 142:1033, 1982

Modanlou HD, Murata Y: Sinusoidal heart rate pattern: Reappraisal of its definition and clinical significance. J Obstet Gynaecol Res 30(3):169, 2004

Mueller-Heubach E, Battelli AF: Variable heart rate decelerations and transcutaneous P_{O_2} (tc P_{O_2}) during umbilical cord occlusion in the fetal monkey. Am J Obstet Gynecol 144:796, 1982

Murata Y, Martin CB, Ikenoue T, et al: Fetal heart rate accelerations and late decelerations during the course of intrauterine death in chronically catheterized rhesus monkeys. Am J Obstet Gynecol 144:218, 1982

Murotsuki J, Bocking AD, Gagnon R: Fetal heart rate patterns in growth-restricted fetal sleep induced by chronic fetal placental embolization. Am J Obstet Gynecol 176:282, 1997

Murphy AA, Halamek LP, Lyell DJ, et al: Training and competency assessment in electronic fetal monitoring: A national survey. Obstet Gynecol 101:1243, 2003

Murphy KW, Russell V, Collins A, et al: The prevalence, aetiology and clinical significance of pseudo-sinusoidal fetal heart rate patterns in labour. Br J Obstet Gynaecol 98:1093, 1991

Myers RE: Two patterns of perinatal brain damage and their conditions of occurrence. Am J Obstet Gynecol 112:246, 1972

Myers RE, Mueller-Heubach E, Adamsons K: Predictability of the state of fetal oxygenation from a quantitative analysis of the components of late deceleration. Am J Obstet Gynecol 115:1083, 1973

Nageotte MP, Bertucci L, Towers CV, et al: Prophylactic amnioinfusion in pregnancies complicated by oligohydramnios: A prospective study. Obstet Gynecol 77:677, 1991

Nathan L, Leveno KJ, Carmody TJ, et al: Meconium: A 1990s perspective on an old obstetric hazard. Obstet Gynecol 83:328, 1994

National Institute of Child Health and Human Development Research Planning Workshop: Electronic fetal heart rate monitoring: Research guidelines for integration. Am J Obstet Gynecol 177:1385, 1997

Neesham DE, Umstad MP, Cincotta RB, et al: Pseudo-sinusoidal fetal heart rate pattern and fetal anemia: Case report and review. Aust NZ J Obstet Gynaecol 33:386, 1993

Neilson DR Jr, Freeman RK, Mangan S: Signal ambiguity resulting in unexpected outcome with external fetal heart rate monitoring. Am J Obstet Gynecol 198:717, 2008

Neilson JP: Fetal electrocardiogram (ECG) for fetal monitoring during labour. Cochrane Database System Rev 3:CD000116, 2006

Nelson KB, Grether JK: Potentially asphyxiating conditions and cerebral palsy in infants of normal birth weight. Am J Obstet Gynecol 179:567, 1998

Nicolaides KH, Sadovsky G, Cetin E: Fetal heart rate patterns in red blood cell isoimmunized pregnancies. Am J Obstet Gynecol 161:351, 1989

Norén H, Amer-Wåhlin I, Hagberg H, et al: Fetal electrocardiography in labor and neonatal outcome: Data from the Swedish randomized controlled trial on intrapartum fetal monitoring. Am J Obstet Gynecol 188:183, 2003

Ogueh O, Steer P: Gender does not affect fetal heart rate variation. Br J Obstet Gynaecol 105:1312, 1998

Ogundipe OA, Spong CY, Ross MG: Prophylactic amnioinfusion for oligohydramnios: A re-evaluation. Obstet Gynecol 84:544, 1994

Owen J, Henson BV, Hauth JC: A prospective randomized study of saline solution amnioinfusion. Am J Obstet Gynecol 162:1146, 1990

Parer J: NIH sets the terms for fetal heart rate pattern interpretation. OB/Gyn News, September 1, 1997

Parer JT: Electronic fetal heart rate monitoring: A story of survival. Obstet Gynecol Surv 58:561, 2003

Parer JT, Ikeda T: A framework for standardized management of intrapartum fetal heart rate pattern. Am J Obstet Gynecol 197:26, 2007

Parer JT, King T: Fetal heart rate monitoring: Is it salvageable? Am J Obstet Gynecol 182:982, 2000

Parer WJ, Parer JT, Holbrook RH, et al: Validity of mathematical models of quantitating fetal heart rate variability. Am J Obstet Gynecol 153:402, 1985

Paul RH, Snidon AK, Yeh SY: Clinical fetal monitoring, 7. The evaluation and significance of intrapartum baseline FHR variability. Am J Obstet Gynecol 123:206, 1975

Paul WM, Quilligan EJ, MacLachlan T: Cardiovascular phenomena associated with fetal head compression. Am J Obstet Gynecol 90:824, 1964

Petrie RH: Dose/response effects of intravenous meperidine in fetal heart rate variability. J Matern Fetal Med 2:215, 1993

Phelan JP, Ahn MO: Perinatal observations in forty-eight neurologically impaired term infants. Am J Obstet Gynecol 171:424, 1994

Picquard F, Hsiung R, Mattauer M, et al: The validity of fetal heart rate monitoring during the second stage of labor. Obstet Gynecol 72:746, 1988

Pierce J, Gaudier FL, Sanchez-Ramos L: Intrapartum amnioinfusion for meconium-stained fluid: Meta-analysis of prospective clinical trials. Obstet Gynecol 95:1051, 2000

Pillai M, James D: The development of fetal heart rate patterns during normal pregnancy. Obstet Gynecol 76:812, 1990

Pontonnier G, Puech F, Grandjean H, et al: Some physical and biochemical parameters during normal labour. Fetal and maternal study. Biol Neonate 26:159, 1975

Pressman EK, Blakemore KJ: A prospective randomized trial of two solutions for intrapartum amnioinfusion: Effects on fetal electrolytes, osmolality, and acid-base status. Am J Obstet Gynecol 175:945, 1996

Ramin KD, Leveno KJ, Kelly MS, et al: Amnionic fluid meconium: A fetal environmental hazard. Obstet Gynecol 87:181, 1996

Rathore AM, Singh R, Ramji S, et al: Randomised trial of amnioinfusion during labour with meconium stained amniotic fluid. Br J Obstet Gynaecol 109:17, 2002

Reddy A, Moulden M, Redman CW: Antepartum high-frequency fetal heart rate sinusoidal rhythm: computerized detection and fetal anemia. Am J Obstet Gynecol 200(4):407.e1, 2009

Renou P, Warwick N, Wood C: Autonomic control of fetal heart rate. Am J Obstet Gynecol 105:949, 1969

Rinehart BK, Terrone DA, Barrow JH, et al: Randomized trial of intermittent or continuous amnioinfusion for variable decelerations. Obstet Gynecol 96:571, 2000

Rocha E, Hammond R, Richardson B: Necrotic cell injury in the preterm and near-term ovine fetal brain after intermittent umbilical cord occlusion. Am J Obstet Gynecol 191:488, 2004

Rogers MS, Mongelli M, Tsang KH, et al: Lipid peroxidation in cord blood at birth: The effect of labour. Br J Obstet Gynaecol 105:739, 1998

Rosen MG, Dickinson JC: The incidence of cerebral palsy. Am J Obstet Gynecol 167:417, 1992

Ross M, Devoe L, Rosen K: Improved intrapartum fetal assessment with addition of ST-segment analysis of fetal heart rate (FHR) tracings: Trial among U.S. clinicians. Am J Obstet Gynecol 189:S183, 2004

Samueloff A, Langer O, Berkus M, et al: Is fetal heart rate variability a good predictor of fetal outcome? Acta Obstet Gynecol Scand 73:39, 1994

Schucker JL, Sarno AP, Egerman RS, et al: The effect of butorphanol on the fetal heart rate reactivity during labor. Am J Obstet Gynecol 174:491, 1996

Seitchik J: Quantitating uterine contractility in a clinical context. Obstet Gynecol 57:453, 1981

Sherer DM: Blunted fetal response to vibroacoustic stimulation associated with maternal intravenous magnesium sulfate therapy. Am J Perinatol 11:401, 1994

Simpson KR, James DC: Efficacy of intrauterine resuscitation techniques in improving fetal oxygen status during labor. Obstet Gynecol 105:1362, 2005

Skupski DW, Rosenberg CR, Eglinton GS: Intrapartum fetal stimulation tests: A meta-analysis. Obstet Gynecol 99:129, 2002

Smith CV, Nguyen HN, Phelan JP, et al: Intrapartum assessment of fetal well-being: A comparison of fetal acoustic stimulation with acid–base determinations. Am J Obstet Gynecol 155:726, 1986

Smith JH, Anand KJ, Cotes PM, et al: Antenatal fetal heart rate variation in relation to the respiratory and metabolic status of the compromised human fetus. Br J Obstet Gynaecol 95:980, 1988

Southall DP, Richards J, Hardwick RA, et al: Prospective study of fetal heart rate and rhythm patterns. Arch Dis Child 55:506, 1980

Spong CY: Electronic fetal heart rate monitoring: Another look. Obstet Gynecol 112:506, 2008

Spong CY, Ogundipe OA, Ross MG: Prophylactic amnioinfusion for meconium-stained amniotic fluid. Am J Obstet Gynecol 171:931, 1994

Spong CY, Rasul C, Collea JV, et al: Characterization and prognostic significance of variable decelerations in the second stage of labor. Am J Perinatol 15:369, 1998

Stiller R, von Mering R, König V, et al: How well does reflectance pulse oximetry reflect intrapartum fetal acidosis? Am J Obstet Gynecol 186:1351, 2002

Strijbis EM, Oudman I, van Essen P, et al: Cerebral palsy and the application of the international criteria for acute intrapartum hypoxia. Obstet Gynecol 107(6):1357, 2006

Symonds EM: Fetal monitoring: Medical and legal implications for the practitioner. Curr Opin Obstet Gynecol 6:430, 1994

Thacker SB, Stroup DF, Peterson HB: Efficacy and safety of intrapartum electronic fetal monitoring: An update. Obstet Gynecol 86:613, 1995

Thakor AS, Giussani DA: Effects of acute acidemia on the fetal cardiovascular defense to acute hypoxemia. Am J Physiol Regul Integr Comp Physiol 296(1):R90, 2009

Trudinger BJ, Pryse-Davies J: Fetal hazards of the intrauterine pressure catheter: Five case reports. Br J Obstet Gynaecol 85:567, 1978

Usta IM, Mercer BM, Aswad NK, et al: The impact of a policy of amnioinfusion for meconium-stained amniotic fluid. Obstet Gynecol 85:237, 1995

Van Geijn HP, Jongsma HN, deHaan J, et al: Heart rate as an indicator of the behavioral state. Am J Obstet Gynecol 136:1061, 1980

Vintzileos AM, Nioka S, Lake M, et al: Transabdominal fetal pulse oximetry with near-infrared spectroscopy. Am J Obstet Gynecol 192(1):129, 2005

Walker J: Foetal anoxia. J Obstet Gynaecol Br Commonw 61:162, 1953

Wenstrom K, Andrews WW, Maher JE: Amnioinfusion survey: Prevalence protocols and complications. Obstet Gynecol 86:572, 1995

Westgate J, Harris M, Curnow JSH, et al: Plymouth randomized trial of cardiotocogram only versus ST waveform plus cardiotocogram for intrapartum monitoring in 2400 cases. Am J Obstet Gynecol 169:1151, 1993

Westgate JA, Bennet L, De Haan HH, et al: Fetal heart rate overshoot during repeated umbilical cord occlusion in sheep. Obstet Gynecol 97:454, 2001

Wiberg-Itzel E, Lipponer C, Norman M, et al: Determination of pH or lactate in fetal scalp blood in management of intrapartum fetal distress: Randomised controlled multicenter trial. BMJ 336:1284, 2008

Williams JW: Williams Obstetrics, 1st ed. New York, Appleton, 1903

Williams K, Galerneau F: Comparison of intrapartum fetal heart rate tracings in patients with neonatal seizures vs no seizures, what are the differences? J Perinat Med 32:422, 2004

Xu H, Hofmeyr J, Roy C, et al: Intrapartum amnioinfusion for meconium-stained amniotic fluid: A systematic review of randomised controlled trials. BJOG 114:383, 2007

Yam J, Chua S, Arulkumaran S: Intrapartum fetal pulse oximetry. Part I: Principles and technical issues. Obstet Gynecol Surv 55:163, 2000

Young BK, Katz M, Wilson SJ: Sinusoidal fetal heart rate, 1. Clinical significance. Am J Obstet Gynecol 136:587, 1980a

Young BK, Weinstein HM: Moderate fetal bradycardia. Am J Obstet Gynecol 126:271, 1976

Young DC, Gray JH, Luther ER, et al: Fetal scalp blood pH sampling: Its value in an active obstetric unit. Am J Obstet Gynecol 136:276, 1980b

Young RC, Zhang P: Functional separation of deep cytoplasmic calcium from subplasmalemmal space calcium in cultured human uterine smooth muscle cells. Cell Calcium 36(1):11, 2004

Zalar RW, Quilligan EJ: The influence of scalp sampling on the cesarean section rate for fetal distress. Am J Obstet Gynecol 135:239, 1979

Obstetrical Anesthesia

Obstetrical anesthesia presents unique challenges. Labor begins without warning, and anesthesia may be required within minutes of a full meal. Vomiting with aspiration of gastric contents is a constant threat. The usual physiological adaptations of pregnancy require special consideration, especially with disorders such as preeclampsia, placental abruption, or sepsis syndrome.

Of all anesthesia-related deaths in the U.S. from 1995 to 2005, 3.6 percent were in pregnant women (Li and co-workers, 2009). Anesthesia complications caused 1.6 percent of pregnancy-related maternal deaths in the United States from 1991 through 1997 (Berg and co-workers, 2003). Of the 855 pregnancy-associated deaths described by Mhyre and colleagues (2007), anesthesia was related to 2.3 percent. Data from the Pregnancy Mortality Surveillance Program of the Centers for Disease Control and Prevention indicate that anesthesia-related maternal mortality rates have declined significantly (Chang and colleagues, 2003). Supportive of this, Deneux-Tharaux and colleagues (2005) reported that there were no maternal deaths from anesthetic complications in Massachusetts and North Carolina during 1999 and 2000. Finally, Kuklina and co-workers

(2009) reviewed obstetrical morbidity in the U.S. and reported a decrease in severe anesthesia complications—2 per 1000 in 1999 compared with 1.1 per 1000 in 2005.

Several factors have contributed to improved safety of obstetrical anesthesia. Hawkins and colleagues (1997b) and D'Angelo (2007) concluded that the most significant factor is the increased use of regional analgesia. Increased availability of in-house anesthesia coverage almost certainly is another important reason (Hawkins and associates, 1997a, b; Nagaya and associates, 2000).

GENERAL PRINCIPLES

Obstetrical Anesthesia Services

The American College of Obstetricians and Gynecologists (2002) reaffirmed its joint position with the American Society of Anesthesiologists that a woman's request for labor pain relief is sufficient medical indication for its provision. The American Academy of Pediatrics and the American College of Obstetricians and Gynecologists (2007) have specified that it is the responsibility of the obstetrician or certified nurse-midwife, in consultation with an anesthesiologist, if appropriate, to formulate a suitable plan for pain relief. Identification of any of the risk factors shown in Table 19-1 should prompt consultation with anesthesia personnel to permit a joint management plan. This plan should include strategies to minimize the need for emergency anesthesia in women for whom such anesthesia would be especially hazardous. To help guide these decisions, the American Society of Anesthesiologists Task Force on Obstetrical Anesthesia (2007) has recently updated its Practice Guidelines.

Goals for optimizing obstetrical anesthesia services have been jointly established by the American College of Obstetricians and Gynecologists and the American Society of Anesthesiologists (2004, 2009):

TABLE 19-1. Maternal Risk Factors That Should Prompt Anesthesia Consultation

- Marked obesity
- Severe edema or anatomical abnormalities of the face, neck, or spine, including trauma or surgery
- Abnormal dentition, small mandible, or difficulty opening the mouth
- Extremely short stature, short neck, or arthritis of the neck
- Goiter
- Serious maternal medical problems, such as cardiac, pulmonary, or neurological disease
- Bleeding disorders
- Severe preeclampsia
- Previous history of anesthetic complications
- Obstetrical complications likely to lead to operative delivery—examples include placenta previa or higher-order multifetal gestation

From the American Academy of Pediatrics and the American College of Obstetricians and Gynecologists, 2007, with permission.

1. Availability of a licensed practitioner who is credentialed to administer an appropriate anesthetic whenever necessary and to maintain support of vital functions in an obstetrical emergency.
2. Availability of anesthesia personnel to permit the start of a cesarean delivery within 30 minutes of the decision to perform the procedure.
3. Anesthesia personnel immediately available to perform an emergency cesarean delivery during the active labor of a woman attempting vaginal birth after cesarean (see Chap. 26, p. 571).
4. Appointment of a qualified anesthesiologist to be responsible for all anesthetics administered.
5. Availability of a qualified physician with obstetrical privileges to perform operative vaginal or cesarean delivery during administration of anesthesia.
6. Availability of equipment, facilities, and support personnel equal to that provided in the surgical suite.
7. Immediate availability of personnel, other than the surgical team, to assume responsibility for resuscitation of a depressed newborn (see Chap. 28, p. 591).

To meet these goals, 24-hour in-house anesthesia coverage is usually necessary. Providing such services in smaller facilities is more challenging—a problem underscored by the fact that approximately one third of all hospitals providing obstetrical care have fewer than 500 deliveries per year (American College of Obstetricians and Gynecologists, 2009).

Bell and colleagues (2000) calculated the financial burden that may be incurred when trying to provide "24/7" obstetrical anesthesia coverage. Given the average indemnity and Medicaid reimbursement for labor epidural analgesia, they concluded that such coverage could not operate profitably at their tertiary referral institution. Compounding this burden, some third-party payers have denied reimbursement for epidural analgesia in the absence of a specific medical indication—an approach repudiated by the American College of Obstetricians and Gynecologists and the American Society of Anesthesiologists (2004).

Role of an Obstetrician

Every obstetrician should be proficient in local and pudendal analgesia that may be administered in appropriately selected circumstances. In general, however, it is preferable for an anesthesiologist or anesthetist to provide pain relief so that the obstetrician can focus attention on the laboring woman and her fetus. **General anesthesia should be administered only by those with special training.**

Principles of Pain Relief

In a scholarly review, Lowe (2002) emphasized that the experience of labor pain is a highly individual reflection of variable stimuli that are uniquely received and interpreted by each woman. These stimuli are modified by emotional, motivational, cognitive, social, and cultural circumstances. The complexity and individuality of the experience suggest that a woman and her caregivers may have a limited ability to anticipate her pain experience prior to labor. Thus, choice among a variety of methods of pain relief is desirable.

NONPHARMACOLOGICAL METHODS OF PAIN CONTROL

Fear and the unknown potentiate pain. A woman who is free from fear, and who has confidence in the obstetrical staff that cares for her, usually requires smaller amounts of analgesia. Read (1944) emphasized that the intensity of pain during labor is related in large measure to emotional tension. He urged that women be well informed about the physiology of parturition and the various hospital procedures they may experience during labor and delivery. Lamaze (1970) subsequently described his psychoprophylactic method, which emphasized childbirth as a natural physiological process. Pain often can be lessened by teaching pregnant women relaxed breathing and their labor partners psychological support techniques. These concepts have considerably reduced the use of potent analgesic, sedative, and amnestic drugs during labor and delivery.

When motivated women have been prepared for childbirth, pain and anxiety during labor have been found to be diminished significantly, and labors are even shorter (Melzack, 1984; Saisto and associates, 2001). In addition, the presence of a supportive spouse or other family member, of conscientious labor attendants, and of a considerate obstetrician who instills confidence have all been found to be of considerable benefit. In one study, Kennell and associates (1991) randomly assigned 412 nulliparous women in labor either to continuous emotional support from an experienced companion or to monitoring by an inconspicuous observer who did not interact with the laboring woman. The cesarean delivery rate was significantly lower in the continuous support group compared with that of the hands-off monitored group—8 versus 13 percent—as was the frequency of epidural analgesia for vaginal delivery—8 versus 23 percent.

TABLE 19-2. Parenteral Agents for Labor Pain

Agent	Usual Dose	Frequency	Onset	Neonatal Half-Life
Meperidine	25–50 mg (IV) 50–100 mg (IM)	Q 2–4 hr Q 1–2 hr	5 min (IV) 30–45 min (IM)	13–22.4 hr 63 hr for active metabolites
Fentanyl	50–100 μg (IV)	Q 1 hr	1 min	5.3 hr
Nalbuphine	10 mg (IV or IM)	Q 3 hr	2–3 min (IV) 15 min (IM)	4.1 hr
Butorphanol	1–2 mg (IV or IM)	Q 4 hr	1–2 (IV) 10–30 min (IM)	Not known Similar to nalbuphine in adults
Morphine	2–5 mg (IV) 10 mg (IM)	Q 4 hr	5 min (IV) 30–40 min (IM)	7.1 hr

IV = intravenously; IM = intramuscularly; Q = every.
Reprinted, with permission, from American College of Obstetricians and Gynecologists. Obstetric analgesia and anesthesia. ACOG Practice Bulletin 36. Washington, DC: ACOG; 2002.

ANALGESIA AND SEDATION DURING LABOR

When uterine contractions and cervical dilatation cause discomfort, pain relief with a narcotic such as meperidine, plus one of the tranquilizer drugs such as promethazine, is usually appropriate. With a successful program of analgesia and sedation, the mother should rest quietly between contractions. In this circumstance, discomfort usually is felt at the acme of an effective uterine contraction, but the pain is generally not unbearable. Appropriate drug selection and administration of the medications shown in Table 19-2 should safely accomplish these objectives for the great majority of women in labor.

Parenteral Agents

Meperidine and Promethazine

Meperidine, 50 to 100 mg, with promethazine, 25 mg, may be administered intramuscularly at intervals of 2 to 4 hours. A more rapid effect is achieved by giving meperidine intravenously in doses of 25 to 50 mg every 1 to 2 hours. Whereas analgesia is maximal 30 to 45 minutes after an intramuscular injection, it develops almost immediately following intravenous administration. Meperidine readily crosses the placenta, and its half-life in the newborn is approximately 13 hours or longer (American College of Obstetricians and Gynecologists, 2002). Its depressant effect in the fetus follows closely behind the peak maternal analgesic effect.

According to Bricker and Lavender (2002), meperidine is the most common opioid used worldwide for pain relief from labor. Tsui and associates (2004) found meperidine to be superior to placebo for pain relief in the first stage of labor. In a randomized investigation of epidural analgesia conducted at Parkland Hospital, patient-controlled intravenous analgesia with meperidine was found to be an inexpensive and reasonably effective method for labor analgesia (Sharma and colleagues, 1997). Women randomized to self-administered analgesia were given 50-mg meperidine with 25-mg promethazine intravenously as an initial bolus. Thereafter, an infusion pump was set to deliver 15 mg of meperidine every 10 minutes as needed until delivery. Neonatal

sedation, as measured by need for naloxone treatment in the delivery room, was identified in 3 percent of newborns.

Butorphanol (Stadol)

This synthetic narcotic, given in 1- to 2-mg doses, compares favorably with 40 to 60 mg of meperidine (Quilligan and colleagues, 1980). The major side effects are somnolence, dizziness, and dysphoria. Neonatal respiratory depression is reported to be less than with meperidine, but care must be taken that the two drugs are not given contiguously because butorphanol antagonizes the narcotic effects of meperidine. Angel and colleagues (1984) and Hatjis and Meis (1986) described a sinusoidal fetal heart rate pattern following butorphanol administration (see Chap. 18, p. 419).

Fentanyl

This short-acting and potent synthetic opioid may be given in doses of 50 to 100 μg intravenously every hour. Its main disadvantage is a short duration of action, which requires frequent dosing or the use of a patient-controlled intravenous pump. Moreover, Atkinson and associates (1994) reported that butorphanol provided better initial analgesia than fentanyl and was associated with fewer requests for more medication or for epidural analgesia.

Efficacy and Safety of Parenteral Agents

Parenteral sedation is not without risks. Hawkins and colleagues (1997b) reported that 4 of 129 maternal anesthetic-related deaths were from such sedation—one from aspiration, two from inadequate ventilation, and one from overdosage. As discussed, narcotics used during labor may cause newborn respiratory depression.

Narcotic Antagonists

Naloxone is a narcotic antagonist capable of reversing respiratory depression induced by opioid narcotics. It acts by displacing the narcotic from specific receptors in the central nervous system. Withdrawal symptoms may be precipitated in recipients who are physically dependent on narcotics. For this reason, naloxone is contraindicated in a newborn of a narcotic-addicted mother (American Academy of Pediatrics and American College of Obstetricians and Gynecologists, 2007). After adequate ventilation has been established, naloxone may be given to reverse respiratory depression in a newborn infant whose mother received narcotics (see Chap. 28, p. 593).

Nitrous Oxide

A self-administered mixture of 50-percent nitrous oxide (N_2O) and oxygen provides satisfactory analgesia during labor for many women (Rosen, 2002a). Some preparations are premixed in a single cylinder (*Entonox*), and in others, a blender mixes the two gases from separate tanks (*Nitronox*). The gases are connected to a breathing circuit through a valve that opens only when the patient inspires. The use of intermittent nitrous oxide for labor pain has been reviewed by Rosen (2002a) and the following technique suggested:

1. Instruct the woman to take slow deep breaths and to begin inhaling 30 seconds before the next anticipated contraction and to cease when the contraction starts to recede
2. Remove the mask between contractions and encourage her to breathe normally. No one but the patient or knowledgeable personnel should hold the mask
3. Instruct a caregiver to remain in verbal contact with the patient
4. Provide the expectation that the pain will likely not be eliminated, but that the gas should provide some relief

5. Ensure intravenous access, pulse oximetry, and adequate scavenging of exhaled gases
6. Use with additional caution after previous opioid administration because the combination can more easily render a woman unconscious and unable to protect her airway.

REGIONAL ANALGESIA

Various nerve blocks have been developed over the years to provide pain relief during labor and delivery. They are correctly referred to as *regional analgesics.*

Sensory Innervation of the Genital Tract

Uterine Innervation

Pain during the first stage of labor is generated largely from the uterus. Visceral sensory fibers from the uterus, cervix, and upper vagina traverse through the Frankenhäuser ganglion, which lies just lateral to the cervix, and enter into the pelvic plexus and then into the middle and superior internal iliac plexuses (Fig. 19-1). From there, the fibers travel in the lumbar and lower thoracic sympathetic chains to enter the spinal cord through the white rami communicantes associated with the T10 through T12 and L1 nerves. Early in labor, the pain of uterine contractions is transmitted predominantly through the T11 and T12 nerves.

The motor pathways to the uterus leave the spinal cord at the level of T7 and T8 vertebrae. Theoretically, any method of sensory block that does not also block motor pathways to the uterus can be used for analgesia during labor.

Lower Genital Tract Innervation

Pain with vaginal delivery arises from stimuli from the lower genital tract. These are transmitted primarily through the pudendal nerve, the peripheral branches of which provide sensory innervation to the perineum, anus, and the more medial and inferior parts of the vulva and clitoris. The pudendal nerve passes beneath the posterior surface of the sacrospinous ligament just as the ligament attaches to the ischial spine. As discussed in Chapter 2 (p. 19), sensory nerve fibers of the pudendal nerve are derived from ventral branches of the S2 through S4 nerves.

Anesthetic Agents

Some of the more commonly used local anesthetics, along with their usual concentrations, doses, and durations of action, are summarized in Table 19-3. The dose of

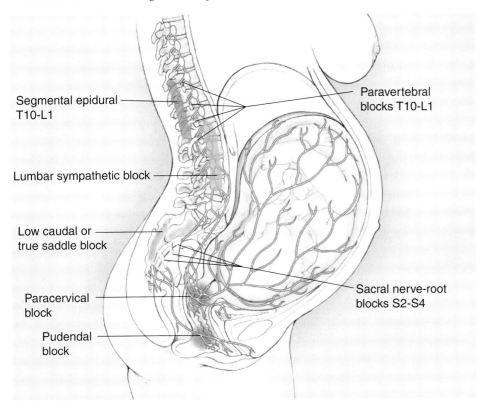

FIGURE 19-1 Pathways of labor pain. Pain stimuli from the cervix and uterus travel through the paracervical region and the pelvic and hypogastric plexus to enter the lumbar sympathetic chain. Through the white rami communicantes of the T10, T11, T12, and L1 spinal nerves, they enter the dorsal horn of the spinal cord. Blockade at different levels along this path can alleviate the visceral component of labor pain. (Adapted from Eltzschig HK, Lieberman ES, and Camann WR: Medical progress: Regional anesthesia and analgesia for labor and delivery. *N Engl J Med* 348:319, with permission. Copyright © 2003 Massachusetts Medical Society. All rights reserved.)

TABLE 19-3. Some Local Anesthetic Agents Used in Obstetrics

Plain Solutions

Anesthetic Agent	Usual Concentration (percent)	Usual Volume (mL)	Usual Dose (mg)	Onset	Average Duration (min)	Clinical Use
Amino-esters						
2-Chloroprocaine	1–2	20–30	400–600	Rapid	15–30	Local or pudendal block
	2–3	15–25	300–750		30–60	Epidural (not subarachnoid) for cesarean delivery
Tetracaine	0.2	—	4	Slow	75–150	Low spinal block/6% glucose[a]
	0.5	—	7–10		75–150	Spinal for cesarean delivery/5% glucose[a]
Amino-amides						
Lidocaine	1	20–30	200–300	Rapid	30–60	Local or pudendal block
	2	15–30	300–450		60–90	Epidural for cesarean delivery
	5	1–1.5	50–75		45–60	Spinal for cesarean or puerperal tubal ligation/7.5% glucose[a]
	5	0.5–1	25–50		30–60	Spinal for vaginal delivery/7.5% glucose[a]
Bupivacaine	0.5	15–20	50–100	Slow	90–150	Epidural for cesarean delivery
	0.25	8–10	20–25		60–90	Epidural for labor
	0.75	1–1.5	7.5–11		60–120	Spinal for cesarean delivery/ 8.25% glucose[a]
Ropivacaine	0.5	15–20	75–100	Slow	90–150	Epidural for cesarean delivery
	0.25	8–10	20–25		60–90	Epidural for labor

[a]Addition of glucose to local anesthetics creates a hyperbaric solution, which is heavier and denser than cerebrospinal fluid. (Courtesy of Dr. Shiv Sharma and Dr. Donald Wallace.)

each agent varies widely and is dependent on the particular nerve block and physical status of the woman. The onset, duration, and quality of analgesia can be enhanced by increasing the dose. This can be done safely only by incrementally administering small-volume boluses of the agent and by carefully monitoring early warning signs of toxicity. Administration of these agents must be followed by appropriate monitoring for adverse reactions. Equipment and personnel to manage these reactions must be immediately available.

Most often, serious toxicity follows inadvertent intravenous injection. For this reason, when epidural analgesia is initiated, dilute epinephrine is sometimes added and given as a test dose. A sudden significant rise in the maternal heart rate or blood pressure immediately after administration suggests intravenous catheter placement. Personnel using these agents must be cognizant that these agents are manufactured in more than one concentration and ampule size, which increases the potential for dosing errors. Systemic toxicity from local anesthetics typically manifests in the central nervous and cardiovascular systems.

Central Nervous System Toxicity

Early symptoms are those of *stimulation* but, as serum levels increase, *depression* follows. Symptoms may include light-headedness, dizziness, tinnitus, metallic taste, and numbness of the tongue and mouth. Patients may show bizarre behavior, slurred speech, muscle fasciculation and excitation, and ultimately, generalized convulsions, followed by loss of consciousness. The convulsions should be controlled, an airway established, and oxygen delivered. Succinylcholine abolishes the peripheral manifestations of the convulsions and allows tracheal intubation. Thiopental or diazepam act centrally to inhibit convulsions. Magnesium sulfate, administered according to the regimen for eclampsia, also controls convulsions (see Chap. 34, p. 737). Abnormal fetal heart rate patterns such as late decelerations or persistent bradycardia may develop from maternal hypoxia and lactic acidosis induced by convulsions. With arrest of convulsions, administration of oxygen, and application of other supportive measures, the fetus usually recovers more quickly in utero than following immediate cesarean delivery. Moreover, the mother is better served if delivery is forestalled until the intensity of hypoxia and metabolic acidosis has diminished.

Cardiovascular Toxicity

These manifestations generally develop later than those from cerebral toxicity, but may not develop at all because they are induced by higher serum drug levels. The notable exception is bupivacaine, which is associated with the development of neurotoxicity and cardiotoxicity at virtually identical levels (Mulroy, 2002). Because of this risk of systemic toxicity, use of 0.75-percent solution of bupivacaine for epidural injection was proscribed by the Food and Drug Administration in 1984. Similar to neurotoxicity, cardiovascular toxicity is characterized first by stimulation and then by depression. Accordingly, there is hypertension and tachycardia, which soon is followed by hypotension, cardiac arrhythmias, and impaired uteroplacental perfusion.

Hypotension is managed initially by turning the woman onto either side to avoid aortocaval compression. A crystalloid solution is infused rapidly along with intravenously administered ephedrine. Emergency cesarean delivery should be considered if maternal vital signs have not been restored within 5 minutes of cardiac arrest (see Chap. 42, p. 942). As with convulsions, however, the fetus is likely to recover more quickly in utero once maternal cardiac output is reestablished.

Pudendal Block

This block is a relatively safe and simple method of providing analgesia for spontaneous delivery. As shown in Figure 19-2, a tubular introducer that allows 1.0 to 1.5 cm of a 15-cm 22-gauge needle to protrude beyond its tip is used to guide the needle into position over the pudendal nerve. The end of the introducer is placed against the vaginal mucosa just beneath the tip of the ischial spine. The needle is pushed beyond the tip of the director into the mucosa and a mucosal wheal is made with 1 mL of 1-percent lidocaine solution or an equivalent dose of another local anesthetic (Table 19-3). To guard against intravascular infusion, aspiration is attempted before this and all subsequent injections. The needle is then advanced until it touches the sacrospinous ligament, which is infiltrated with 3 mL of lidocaine. The needle is advanced farther through the ligament, and as it pierces the loose areolar tissue behind the ligament, the resistance of the plunger decreases. Another 3 mL of solution is injected into this region. Next, the needle is withdrawn into the introducer, which is moved to just above the ischial spine. The needle is inserted through the mucosa and 3 more mL is deposited. The procedure is then repeated on the other side.

Within 3 to 4 minutes of injection, the successful pudendal block will allow pinching of the lower vagina and posterior vulva bilaterally without pain. If delivery occurs before the pudendal block becomes effective and an episiotomy is indicated, then the fourchette, perineum, and adjacent vagina can be infiltrated with 5 to 10 mL of 1-percent lidocaine solution directly at the site where the episiotomy is to be made. By the time of the repair, the pudendal block usually has become effective.

Pudendal block usually does not provide adequate analgesia when delivery requires extensive obstetrical manipulation. Moreover, such analgesia is usually inadequate for women in whom complete visualization of the cervix and upper vagina or manual exploration of the uterine cavity is indicated.

Complications

As previously described, intravascular injection of a local anesthetic agent may cause serious systemic toxicity. Hematoma formation from perforation of a blood vessel is most likely when there is a coagulopathy (Lee and colleagues, 2004). Rarely, severe infection may originate at the injection site. The infection may spread posterior to the hip joint, into the gluteal musculature, or into the retropsoas space (Svancarek and associates, 1977).

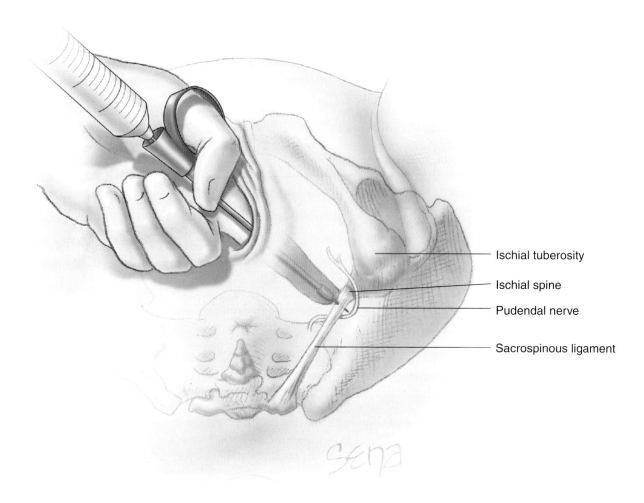

FIGURE 19-2 Local infiltration of the pudendal nerve. Transvaginal technique showing the needle extended beyond the needle guard and passing through the sacrospinous ligament to reach the pudendal nerve.

Ischial tuberosity

Ischial spine

Pudendal nerve

Sacrospinous ligament

Paracervical Block

This block usually provides satisfactory pain relief during the first stage of labor. We do not use it routinely in our institutions. Because the pudendal nerves are not blocked, however, additional analgesia is required for delivery. For paracervical blockade, usually lidocaine or chloroprocaine, 5 to 10 mL of a 1-percent solution, is injected into the cervix laterally at 3 and 9 o'clock. Bupivacaine is contraindicated because of an increased risk of cardiotoxicity (American Academy of Pediatrics and American College of Obstetricians and Gynecologists, 2007; Rosen, 2002b). Because these anesthetics are relatively short acting, paracervical block may have to be repeated during labor.

Complications

Fetal bradycardia is a worrisome complication that occurs in approximately 15 percent of paracervical blocks (Rosen, 2002b). Bradycardia usually develops within 10 minutes and may last up to 30 minutes. Doppler studies have shown an increase in the pulsatility index of the uterine arteries following paracervical blockade (see Chap. 16, p. 364). These observations support the hypothesis of drug-induced arterial vasospasm as a cause of fetal bradycardia (Manninen and co-workers, 2000). For these reasons, paracervical block should not be used in situations of potential fetal compromise.

Spinal (Subarachnoid) Block

Introduction of a local anesthetic into the subarachnoid space to effect analgesia has long been used for delivery. Advantages include a short procedure time, rapid onset of blockade, and high success rate. Because of the smaller subarachnoid space during pregnancy, likely the consequence of engorgement of the internal vertebral venous plexus, the same amount of anesthetic agent in the same volume of solution produces a much higher blockade in parturients than in nonpregnant women.

Vaginal Delivery

Low spinal block can be used for forceps or vacuum delivery. The level of analgesia should extend to the T10 dermatome, which corresponds to the level of the umbilicus. Blockade to this level provides excellent relief from the pain of uterine contractions (see Fig. 19-1).

Several local anesthetic agents have been used for spinal analgesia. Addition of glucose to any of these agents creates a hyperbaric solution, which is heavier and denser than cerebrospinal fluid. A sitting position causes a hyperbaric solution to settle caudally, whereas a lateral position will have a greater effect on the dependent side. Lidocaine given in a hyperbaric solution produces excellent analgesia and has the advantage of a rapid onset and relatively short duration. Bupivacaine in an 8.25-percent dextrose solution provides satisfactory anesthesia to the lower vagina and the perineum for more than 1 hour. Neither is administered until the cervix is fully dilated and all other criteria for safe forceps delivery have been fulfilled (see Chap. 23, p. 513). Preanalgesic intravenous hydration with 1 L of crystalloid solution will prevent or minimize hypotension in many cases.

Cesarean Delivery

A level of sensory blockade extending to the T4 dermatome is desired for cesarean delivery (see Fig. 19-3). Depending on maternal size, 10 to 12 mg of bupivacaine in a hyperbaric solution or 50 to 75 mg of lidocaine hyperbaric solution are administered. The addition of 20 to 25 mg of fentanyl increases the rapidity of blockade onset and reduces shivering. The addition of 0.2 mg of morphine improves pain control during delivery and postoperatively.

Complications of Regional Analgesia

Shown in Table 19-4 are some of the more common complications associated with regional analgesia. The estimated incidences were derived from 19 studies published between 1987 and 2000, as well as data from the Maternal-Fetal Medicine Units (MFMU) Network, which included more than 37,000 women undergoing cesarean delivery (Bloom and colleagues, 2005). Importantly, obese women have significantly impaired ventilation and thus close clinical monitoring is imperative (von Ungern-Sternberg and associates, 2004).

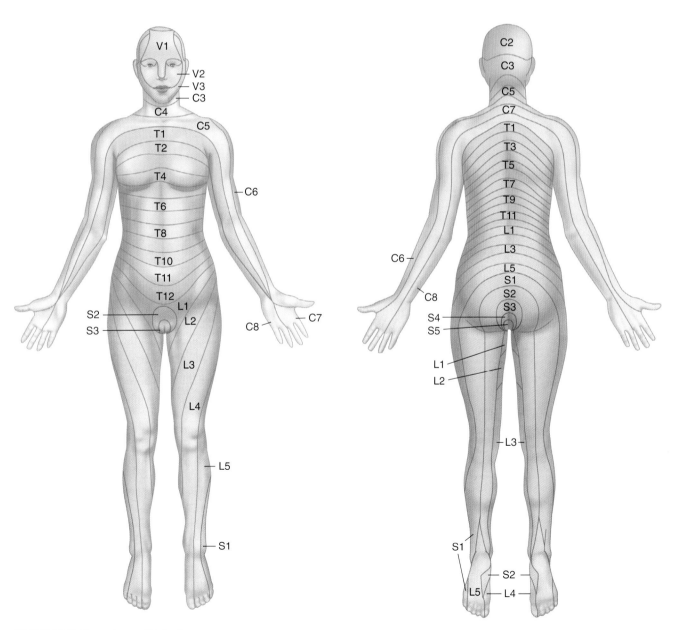

FIGURE 19-3 Dermatome distribution.

TABLE 19-4. Complications of Regional Analgesia Techniques

Complication	Incidence (percent) from ACOG[a]			Incidence (percent) from MFMU[b]		
	Spinal (n = N/A)	Epidural (n = N/A)	Combined[c] (n = N/A)	Spinal (n = 14,797)	Epidural (n = 15,443)	Combined[c] (n = 4375)
Hypotension[d]	25–67	28–31	—	—	—	—
Postdural puncture headache	1.5–3	2	1–2.8	0.5	0.3	0.5
Pruritus	41–85	1.3–26	41–85	—	—	—
Failed regional blockade (need for GETA)	—	—	—	2.1	4.3	1.7
High spinal blockade	—	—	—	0.06	0.07	0.07
Chemical meningitis or epidural abscess or hematoma	—	—	—	0	0	0

[a]ACOG = American College of Obstetricians and Gynecologists. Incidence based upon 19 reports published between 1987–2000.
[b]MFMU = Maternal-Fetal Medicine Units Network of the National Institute of Child Health and Human Development.
[c]Combined = combined spinal-epidural analgesia technique.
[d]Women were given intravenous prehydration before analgesia injected.
GETA = general endotracheal anesthesia; N/A = data not available.
Data from the American College of Obstetricians and Gynecologists (2002) and Bloom and colleagues (2005).

Hypotension

This common complication may develop soon after injection of the local anesthetic agent. It is the consequence of vasodilatation from sympathetic blockade and is compounded by obstructed venous return due to uterine compression of the great vessels. **In the supine position, even in the absence of maternal hypotension measured in the brachial artery, placental blood flow may still be significantly reduced.** Treatment includes uterine displacement by left lateral positioning of the patient, intravenous hydration, and intravenous bolus injections of ephedrine or phenylephrine.

Ephedrine is a sympathomimetic drug that binds to alpha- and beta-receptors but also indirectly enhances norepinephrine release. It raises blood pressure by increasing heart rate and cardiac output and by variably elevating peripheral vascular resistance. In animal studies, ephedrine preserves uteroplacental blood flow during pregnancy compared with alpha$_1$-receptor agonists. For this reason, it is a preferred vasopressor for obstetric use. Phenylephrine is a pure alpha agonist and raises blood pressure solely through vasoconstriction. A meta-analysis of seven randomized trials by Lee and colleagues (2002b) suggests that the safety profiles of ephedrine and phenylephrine are comparable.

In a randomized trial at Parkland Hospital, Morgan and colleagues (2000) found that from the standpoint of umbilical artery pH at birth, epinephrine used as needed to maintain blood pressure during spinal injection was superior to prophylactic ephedrine. Mean pH in the former group was 7.26 and in the latter 7.12. Following their systematic review of 14 reports, Lee and colleagues (2002a) question whether routine prophylactic ephedrine is needed for elective cesarean delivery. Ngan Kee and associates (2004) have used prophylactic phenylephrine infusion without the fetal acidemia reported with prophylactic ephedrine use.

High Spinal Blockade

Most often, complete spinal blockade follows administration of an excessive dose of local anesthetic agent. This is certainly not always the case, because accidental total spinal block has even occurred following an epidural test dose (Palkar and associates, 1992). With complete spinal block, hypotension and apnea promptly develop and must be immediately treated to prevent cardiac arrest. In the undelivered woman: (1) the uterus is immediately displaced laterally to minimize aortocaval compression, (2) effective ventilation is established, preferably with tracheal intubation, and (3) intravenous fluids and ephedrine are given to correct hypotension.

Spinal (Postdural Puncture) Headache

Leakage of cerebrospinal fluid from the site of puncture of the meninges can lead to spinal headache. Presumably, when the woman sits or stands, the diminished volume of cerebrospinal fluid creates traction on pain-sensitive central nervous system structures. Rates of this complication can be reduced by using a small-gauge spinal needle and avoiding multiple punctures. In a prospective, randomized study of five different spinal needles, Vallejo and colleagues (2000) concluded that Sprotte and Whitacre needles had the lowest risks of postdural puncture headaches. In a recent study by Sprigge and Harper (2008), the incidence of postdural puncture headache was 1 percent in more than 5000 women undergoing spinal analgesia.

There is no good evidence that placing a woman absolutely flat on her back for several hours is effective in preventing headache. Vigorous hydration may be of value, but compelling evidence to support its use is also lacking. The administration of *caffeine,* a cerebral vasoconstrictor, has been shown in randomized studies to afford temporary relief (Sechzer and Abel, 1978; Camann and colleagues, 1990).

With severe headache, an *epidural blood patch* is most effective. A few milliliters of autologous blood are obtained aseptically by venipuncture into a tube *without anticoagulant.* This blood is injected into the epidural space at the site of the dural puncture. Relief is immediate and complications uncommon. In a randomized trial of 64 women, Scavone and colleagues (2004) found that prophylactic blood patch did not decrease either the incidence of postdural puncture headache or the need for a subsequent therapeutic blood patch.

If a headache does not have the pathognomonic postural characteristics or persists despite treatment with a blood patch, other diagnoses should be considered. For example, Chisholm and Campbell (2001) described a case of superior sagittal sinus thrombosis that manifested as a postural headache. Chan and Paech (2004) have described persistent cerebrospinal fluid leak in three women. Smarkusky and colleagues (2006) described pneumocephalus, which caused immediate cephalgia. Finally, Dawley and Hendrix (2009) reported an intracranial subdural hematoma after spinal anesthesia.

Convulsions. In rare instances, postdural puncture cephalgia is associated with temporary blindness and convulsions. Shearer and colleagues (1995) described eight such cases associated with 19,000 regional analgesic procedures. It is presumed that these too are caused by cerebrospinal fluid hypotension. Immediate treatment of seizures and blood patch was effective in all cases.

Bladder Dysfunction

With spinal analgesia, bladder sensation is likely to be obtunded and bladder emptying impaired for several hours after delivery. As a consequence, bladder distension is a frequent postpartum complication, especially if appreciable volumes of intravenous fluid are given.

Oxytocics and Hypertension

Paradoxically, hypertension from ergonovine or methylergonovine injections following delivery is more common in women who have received a spinal or epidural block.

Arachnoiditis and Meningitis

Local anesthetics are no longer preserved in alcohol, formalin, or other toxic solutes, and disposable equipment is used by most. These practices, coupled with aseptic technique, have made meningitis and arachnoiditis rare but have not eliminated them (Harding, 1994; Newton, 1994; Sandkovsky, 2009, and all their associates).

Contraindications to Spinal Analgesia

Shown in Table 19-5 are the absolute contraindications to regional analgesia according to the American College of Obstetricians and Gynecologists (2002). Obstetrical complications that are associated with maternal hypovolemia and hypotension—for example, severe hemorrhage—are contraindications to the use of spinal blockade. The additive cardiovascular effects of spinal

TABLE 19-5. Absolute Contraindications to Regional Analgesia

- Refractory maternal hypotension
- Maternal coagulopathy
- Maternal use of once-daily dose of low-molecular-weight heparin within 12 hours
- Untreated maternal bacteremia
- Skin infection over site of needle placement
- Increased intracranial pressure caused by a mass lesion

Reprinted, with permission, from American College of Obstetricians and Gynecologists. Obstetric analgesia and anesthesia. ACOG Practice Bulletin 36. Washington, DC: ACOG; 2002.

blockade in the presence of acute blood loss in nonpregnant patients were documented by Kennedy and co-workers (1968).

Disorders of coagulation and defective hemostasis also preclude the use of spinal analgesia (see Chap. 47, p. 1022). Although there are no randomized studies to guide the management of anticoagulation at the time of delivery, consensus opinion suggests that women given subcutaneous unfractionated heparin or low-molecular-weight heparin should be instructed to stop therapy when labor begins (Krivak and Zorn, 2007). Subarachnoid puncture is also contraindicated if there is cellulitis at the site of needle entry. Neurological disorders are considered by many to be a contraindication, if for no other reason than that exacerbation of the neurological disease might be attributed without cause to the anesthetic agent. Other maternal conditions, such as significant aortic stenosis or pulmonary hypertension, are also relative contraindications to the use of spinal analgesia (see Chap. 44, p. 958).

Preeclampsia

As with significant hemorrhage, severe preeclampsia is another complication in which markedly decreased blood pressure can be predicted when spinal analgesia is used. Gambling and Writer (1999) concluded that with severe preeclampsia, epidural analgesia is preferable to spinal blockade and especially preferable to a general anesthetic. Dyer and associates (2007), however, also concluded that single-dose spinal analgesia for cesarean delivery is safe.

As subsequently discussed, hypotension is also a risk with epidural analgesia and severe preeclampsia. Wallace and colleagues (1995) randomly assigned 80 women with severe preeclampsia undergoing cesarean delivery to receive general anesthesia or either epidural or combined spinal-epidural analgesia. There were no differences in maternal or neonatal outcomes. However, 30 percent of women given epidural analgesia and 22 percent of those given spinal-epidural blockade developed hypotension—the average reduction in mean arterial pressure was between 15 and 25 percent. In another randomized study of 100 women with severe preeclampsia, Visalyaputra and co-workers (2005) reported similar maternal and neonatal

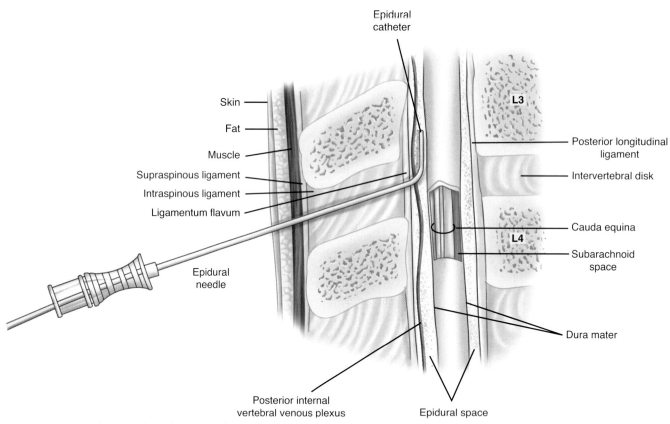

Epidural
catheter

Skin

Fat

Muscle

Supraspinous ligament

Intraspinous ligament

Ligamentum flavum

Epidural
needle

L3

Posterior longitudinal
ligament

Intervertebral disk

Cauda equina

L4

Subarachnoid
space

Dura mater

Posterior internal
vertebral venous plexus

Epidural space

FIGURE 19-4 Introduction of a catheter into the epidural space through a Tuohy needle.

outcomes with spinal versus epidural analgesia given for cesarean delivery.

Epidural Analgesia

Relief of labor and childbirth pain, including cesarean delivery, can be accomplished by injection of a local anesthetic agent into the epidural or peridural space (Fig. 19-4). This potential space contains areolar tissue, fat, lymphatics, and the internal venous plexus. This plexus becomes engorged during pregnancy such that the volume of the epidural space is appreciably reduced. Entry for obstetrical analgesia is usually through a lumbar intervertebral space. Although only one injection may be given, usually an indwelling catheter is placed for repeat injections or continuous infusion using a volumetric pump.

Continuous Lumbar Epidural Block

Complete analgesia for the pain of labor and vaginal delivery necessitates a block from the T10 to the S5 dermatomes (Figs. 19-1 and 19-3). For cesarean delivery, a block extending from the T4 to the S1 dermatomes is desired. The spread of the anesthetic depends upon the location of the catheter tip; the dose, concentration, and volume of anesthetic agent used (see Table 19-3); and whether the mother is head-down, horizontal, or head-up (Setayesh and colleagues, 2001). Individual variations in anatomy or presence of synechiae may preclude a completely satisfactory block. Finally, the catheter tip may migrate from its original location during the course of labor.

Technique. One example of the sequential steps and techniques for performance of epidural analgesia is detailed in Table 19-6. Before injection of the local anesthetic agent's therapeutic dose, a test dose is given. The woman is observed for features of toxicity from intravascular injection and for signs of spinal blockade from subarachnoid injection. If these are absent, only then is a full dose given. Analgesia is maintained by intermittent boluses of similar volume, or small volumes of the drug are delivered continuously by infusion pump (Halpern and Carvalho, 2009). The addition of small doses of a short-acting narcotic—fentanyl or sufentanil—has been shown to improve analgesic efficacy while avoiding motor blockade (Chestnut and colleagues, 1988). **Appropriate resuscitation equipment and drugs must be available during administration of epidural analgesia.**

Complications

Epidural analgesia usually provides unparalleled relief from the pain of labor and delivery. That said, as shown in Table 19-4, there are certain problems inherent in its use. As with spinal blockade, it is imperative that close monitoring, including the level of analgesia, be performed by trained personnel.

Total Spinal Blockade. Dural puncture with inadvertent subarachnoid injection may cause total spinal blockade. Sprigge and Harper (2008) cited an incidence of 0.91 percent recognized accidental dural punctures at the time of epidural analgesia in more than 18,000 women. Personnel and facilities must

TABLE 19-6. Technique for Labor Epidural Analgesia

1. Informed consent is obtained, and the obstetrician consulted.
2. Monitoring includes the following:
   - Blood pressure every 1 to 2 minutes for 15 minutes after giving a bolus of local anesthetic.
   - Continuous maternal heart rate monitoring during analgesia induction.
   - Continuous fetal heart rate monitoring.
   - Continual verbal communication.
3. Hydration with 500 to 1000 mL of lactated Ringer solution.
4. The woman assumes a lateral decubitus or sitting position.
5. The epidural space is identified with a loss-of-resistance technique.
6. The epidural catheter is threaded 3 to 5 cm into the epidural space.
7. A test dose of 3 mL of 1.5% lidocaine with 1:200,000 epinephrine or 3 mL of 0.25% bupivacaine with 1:200,000 epinephrine is injected after careful aspiration to avert intravascular injection and after a uterine contraction. This minimizes the chance of confusing tachycardia that results from labor pain with that of tachycardia from intravenous injection of the test dose.
8. If the test dose is negative, one or two 5-mL doses of 0.25% bupivacaine are injected to achieve a sensory T10 level.
9. After 15 to 20 minutes, the block is assessed using loss of sensation to cold or pinprick. If no block is evident, the catheter is replaced. If the block is asymmetrical, the epidural catheter is withdrawn 0.5 to 1.0 cm and an additional 3 to 5 mL of 0.25% bupivacaine is injected. If the block remains inadequate, the catheter is replaced.
10. The woman is positioned in the lateral or semilateral position to avoid aortocaval compression.
11. Subsequently, maternal blood pressure is recorded every 5 to 15 minutes. The fetal heart rate is monitored continuously.
12. The level of analgesia and intensity of motor blockade are assessed at least hourly.

This table was published in Local anesthetic techniques, by B Glosten, in *Obstetric Anesthesia: Principles and Practice*, 2nd ed., DH Chestnut (ed), p. 363, Copyright Elsevier 1999.

be immediately available to manage this complication as described on page 452.

Ineffective Analgesia. Using currently popular continuous epidural infusion regimens such as 0.125-percent bupivacaine with 2-mg/mL fentanyl, 90 percent of women rate their pain relief as good to excellent (Sharma and colleagues, 1997). Alternatively, a few women find epidural analgesia to be inadequate for labor. In a study of almost 2000 parturients, Hess and associates (2001) found that approximately 12 percent complained of three or more episodes of pain or pressure. Risk factors for such breakthrough pain included nulliparity, heavier fetal weights, and epidural catheter placement at an earlier cervical dilatation. Dresner and colleagues (2006) reported that epidural analgesia was more likely to fail as body mass index increased. If the epidural analgesia is allowed to dissipate before another injection of anesthetic drug, subsequent pain relief may be delayed, incomplete, or both.

In some women, epidural analgesia is not sufficient for cesarean delivery. For example, in the MFMU Network study cited earlier, 4 percent of women initially given epidural analgesia required a general anesthetic for cesarean delivery (Bloom and colleagues, 2005). Also, at times, perineal analgesia for delivery is difficult to obtain, especially with the lumbar epidural technique. When this situation is encountered, pudendal block or systemic analgesia or rarely general anesthesia may be added.

Hypotension. Sympathetic blockade from epidurally injected analgesic agents may cause hypotension and decreased cardiac output. In normal pregnant women, hypotension induced by epidural analgesia usually can be prevented by rapid infusion of 500 to 1000 mL of crystalloid solution as described for spinal analgesia. Danilenko-Dixon and associates (1996) showed that maintaining a lateral position minimized hypotension compared with the supine position. Despite these precautions, hypotension is the most common side effect and is severe enough to require treatment in a third of women (Sharma and colleagues, 1997).

Central Nervous Stimulation. Convulsions are an uncommon but serious complication, the immediate management of which was described previously. Also cited was the case described by Smarkusky and co-workers (2006) of acute onset of intrapartum headache due to a postdural pneumocephalus.

Maternal Fever. Since the observation by Fusi and associates (1989) that the mean temperature increased in laboring women given epidural analgesia, a number of randomized and retrospective cohort studies have confirmed that some women develop intrapartum fever following this procedure. Many studies are limited by inability to control for other risk factors, such as length of labor, duration of ruptured membranes, and number of vaginal examinations (Yancey and co-workers, 2001a). With this in mind, the frequency of intrapartum fever associated with epidural analgesia was found by Lieberman and O'Donoghue (2002) to be 10 to 15 percent above the baseline rate.

The two general theories concerning the etiology of maternal hyperthermia are *maternal-fetal infection* or *dysregulation of body temperature*. Dashe and co-workers (1999) studied placental histopathology in laboring women given epidural analgesia and identified intrapartum fever only when there was placental inflammation. This suggests that fever is due to infection. The other

TABLE 19-7. Selected Labor Events in 2703 Nulliparous Women Randomized to Epidural Analgesia or Intravenous Meperidine Analgesia

Event[a]	Epidural Analgesia (n = 1339)	Intravenous Meperidine (n = 1364)	p Value
Labor outcomes			
First-stage duration (hr)[b]	8.1 ± 5	7.5 ± 5	0.011
Second-stage duration (min)	60 ± 56	47 ± 57	<0.001
Oxytocin after analgesia	641 (48)	546 (40)	<0.001
Type of delivery			
Spontaneous vaginal	1027 (77)	1122 (82)	<0.001
Forceps	172 (13)	101 (7)	<0.001
Cesarean	140 (10.5)	141 (10.3)	0.92

[a]Data are presented as n(%) or mean ± SD.
[b]First stage = initiation of analgesia to complete cervical dilatation.
Adapted from Sharma and colleagues, 2004, with permission.

proposed mechanisms include alteration of the hypothalamic thermoregulatory set point, impairment of peripheral thermoreceptor input to the central nervous system with selective blockage of warm stimuli, or imbalance between heat production and heat loss (Yancey and co-workers, 2001a). To support this theory, Goetzl and colleagues (2007) reported that hyperthermia is seen in a minority of women and that it develops soon after epidural injection. Whatever the mechanism, women with persistent fever are usually treated with antimicrobials for presumed chorioamnionitis.

Back Pain. An association between epidural analgesia and back pain has been reported by some, but not all (Breen, 1994; Howell, 2001; MacArthur, 1997, and all their colleagues). In a prospective cohort study, Butler and Fuller (1998) reported that back pain after delivery was common with epidural analgesia, however, persistent pain was uncommon. Based on their systematic review, Lieberman and O'Donoghue (2002) concluded that available data do not support an association between epidural analgesia and development of de novo, long-term backache.

Miscellaneous Complications. A spinal or epidural hematoma rarely complicates placement of an epidural catheter (Grant, 2007). Epidural abscesses are equally rare (Darouiche, 2006). Uncommonly, the plastic epidural catheter is sheared off (Noblett and co-workers, 2007).

Effect on Labor

Most studies, including the combined five randomized trials from Parkland Hospital shown in Table 19-7, report that epidural analgesia prolongs labor and increases the use of oxytocin stimulation. Alexander and associates (2002) examined the effects of epidural analgesia on the Friedman (1955) labor curve described in Chapter 17 (p. 389). There were 459 nulliparas randomly assigned to patient-controlled epidural analgesia or patient-controlled intravenous meperidine. Compared with Friedman's original criteria, epidural analgesia prolonged the active phase of labor by 1 hour. As shown in Table 19-7, epidural analgesia also increases the need for operative vaginal instrumented delivery because of prolonged second-stage labor, but importantly, without adverse neonatal effects (Chestnut, 1999; Thorp and Breedlove, 1996). A more contemporaneous concern is perineal trauma associated with instrumented delivery. This relationship is discussed in detail in Chapter 17 (p. 401) and Chapter 23 (p. 519).

Fetal Heart Rate

Hill and colleagues (2003) examined the effects of epidural analgesia with 0.25-percent bupivacaine on fetal heart rate patterns. Compared with intravenous meperidine, no deleterious effects were identified. In fact, reduced beat-to-beat variability and fewer accelerations were more common in fetuses whose mothers received meperidine (see Chap. 18, p. 417). Based on their systematic review of eight studies, Reynolds and co-workers (2002) reported that epidural analgesia was associated with improved neonatal acid-base status compared with meperidine.

Cesarean Delivery

A more contentious issue in the past was whether epidural analgesia increased the risk for cesarean delivery. Evidence that it did was from the era when dense blocks of local anesthetic agents were used that impaired motor function and therefore likely contributed to increased rates of cesarean delivery. As techniques were refined, many investigators were of the opinion that epidural administration of *dilute* anesthetic solutions did not increase cesarean delivery rates (Chestnut, 1997; Thompson and colleagues, 1998). Several studies conducted at Parkland Hospital were designed to answer this and related questions. From 1995 to 2002, a total of 2703 nulliparous women at term and in spontaneous labor were enrolled in five trials to evaluate epidural analgesia techniques compared with methods for administration of intravenous meperidine. The results from these are summarized in Figure 19-5 and show that epidural analgesia does not significantly increase cesarean delivery rates.

Yancey and co-workers (1999) described the effects of an on-demand labor epidural analgesia service at Tripler Army Hospital in Hawaii. This followed a policy change in military medical centers. As a result, the incidence of labor epidural analgesia

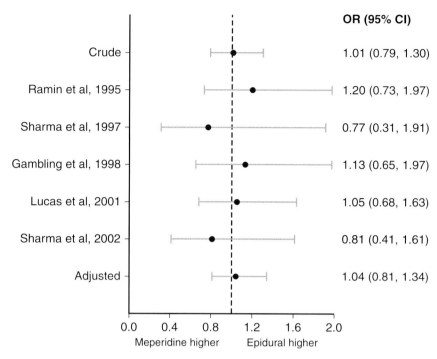

FIGURE 19-5 Results of five studies comparing the incidence of cesarean delivery in women given either epidural analgesia or intravenous meperidine. The individual odds ratios (ORs) with 95-percent confidence intervals (CIs) for each randomized study, as well as overall crude and adjusted ORs with 95-percent CIs, are shown. An OR of less than 1.0 favored epidural over meperidine analgesia. (From Sharma and associates, 2004, with permission.)

increased from 1 percent before the policy to 60 percent within 2 years. The primary cesarean delivery rate was 13.4 percent before and 13.2 percent after this dramatic change. In a follow-up study, Yancey and co-workers (2001b) reported that fetal malpresentations at vaginal delivery were not more common after epidural usage increased. The only significant difference that they found was an increased duration of second-stage labor of approximately 25 minutes (Zhang and co-workers, 2001).

Based on these randomized studies and a meta-analysis of 14 such trials, Sharma and Leveno (2003) and Leighton and Halpern (2002) concluded that epidural analgesia is not associated with an increased rate of cesarean deliveries.

Timing of Epidural Placement

In several retrospective studies, epidural placement in early labor was linked to an increased risk of cesarean delivery (Lieberman, 1996; Rogers, 1999; Seyb, 1999, and all their co-workers). These observations prompted at least five randomized trials, which showed that timing of epidural placement has no effect on the risk of cesarean birth, forceps delivery, or fetal malposition (Chestnut, 1994a, b; Luxman, 1998; Ohel, 2006; Wong, 2005, 2009, and all their associates). Thus, withholding epidural placement until some arbitrary cervical dilation has been reached is unsupportable and serves only to deny women maximal labor pain relief.

Safety

The relative safety of epidural analgesia is attested to by the extraordinary experiences reported by Crawford (1985) from the

Birmingham Maternity Hospital in England. From 1968 through 1985, more than 26,000 women were given epidural analgesia for labor, and there were no maternal deaths. The nine potentially life-threatening complications followed either inadvertent intravenous or intrathecal injection of lidocaine, bupivacaine, or both. Similarly, according to the Confidential Enquiries into Maternal Deaths in the United Kingdom between 2003 and 2005, there were only a few anesthesia-related deaths associated with epidural use (Lewis, 2007).

There were no anesthesia-related maternal deaths among nearly 20,000 women who received epidural analgesia in the MFMU Network study cited earlier (Bloom and colleagues, 2005). And finally, Ruppen and associates (2006) reviewed data from 27 studies involving 1.4 million pregnant women who received epidural analgesia. They calculated risks of 1:145,000 for deep epidural infection, 1:168,000 for epidural hematoma, and 1:240,000 for persistent neurological injury.

Contraindications

As with spinal analgesia, contraindications to epidural analgesia include actual or anticipated serious maternal hemorrhage, infection at or near the sites for puncture, and suspicion of neurological disease (see Table 19-5).

Thrombocytopenia. Although low platelet counts are intuitively worrisome, the level at which epidural bleeding *might* develop is unknown according to the American Society of Anesthesiologists Task Force on Obstetrical Anesthesia (2007). Epidural hematomas are extremely rare, and incidence of nerve damage from a hematoma is estimated to be 1 in 150,000 (Grant, 2007). The American College of Obstetricians and Gynecologists (2002) has concluded that women with a platelet count of 50,000 to 100,000/μL may be candidates for regional analgesia.

Anticoagulation. Women receiving anticoagulation therapy who are given regional analgesia are at increased risk for spinal cord hematoma and compression (see Chap. 47, p. 1022). The American College of Obstetricians and Gynecologists (2002) has concluded the following:

1. Women receiving unfractionated heparin therapy should be able to receive regional analgesia if they have a normal activated partial thromboplastin time (aPTT)
2. Women receiving prophylactic doses of unfractionated heparin or low-dose aspirin are not at increased risk and can be offered regional analgesia
3. For women receiving once-daily low-dose low-molecular-weight heparin, regional analgesia should not be placed until 12 hours after the last injection

4. Low-molecular-weight heparin should be withheld for at least 2 hours after the removal of an epidural catheter

5. The safety of regional analgesia in women receiving twice-daily low-molecular-weight heparin has not been studied sufficiently. It is not known whether delaying regional analgesia for 24 hours after the last injection is adequate.

Severe Preeclampsia-Eclampsia. Potential concerns with epidural analgesia in those with severe preeclampsia include hypotension as well as hypertension from pressor agents given to correct hypotension. Additionally, there is the potential for pulmonary edema following infusion of large volumes of crystalloid. These are outweighed by disadvantages of general anesthesia. Tracheal intubation may be difficult because of upper airway edema. Moreover, general anesthesia can lead to severe, sudden hypertension that can cause pulmonary or cerebral edema or intracranial hemorrhage.

With improved techniques for infusion of dilute local anesthetics into the epidural space, most obstetricians and obstetrical anesthesiologists have come to favor epidural blockade for labor and delivery in women with severe preeclampsia (Cheek and Samuels, 1991; Gambling and Writer, 1999; Gutsche, 1986). There seems to be no argument that epidural analgesia for women with severe preeclampsia-eclampsia can be safely used when specially trained anesthesiologists and obstetricians are responsible for the woman and her fetus (American College of Obstetricians and Gynecologists, 2002; Cunningham and Leveno, 1995). In a study from Parkland Hospital, Lucas and colleagues (2001) randomly assigned 738 women with hypertension to epidural analgesia or patient-controlled intravenous analgesia during labor. A standardized protocol for prehydration, incremental epidural administration, and ephedrine use was employed. They concluded that labor epidural analgesia was safe in women with hypertensive disorders. In a similar study from the University of Alabama at Birmingham, Head and colleagues (2002) randomly assigned 116 women with severe preeclampsia to receive either intrapartum epidural or patient-controlled intravenous opioid analgesia. Epidural analgesia provided superior pain relief without a significant increase in maternal or neonatal complications.

Intravenous Fluid Preload. Women with severe preeclampsia have remarkably diminished intravascular volume compared with normal pregnancy (Zeeman and colleagues, 2009). Conversely, total body water is increased because of the capillary leak caused by endothelial cell activation (see Chap. 34, p. 712). This imbalance is manifested as pathological peripheral edema, proteinuria, ascites, and total lung water. For all of these reasons, aggressive volume replacement increases the risk for pulmonary edema, especially in the first 72 hours postpartum (Clark and colleagues, 1985; Cotton and associates, 1986). In one study, Hogg and associates (1999) reported that 3.5 percent of women with severe preeclampsia developed pulmonary edema when preloaded without a protocol limitation to volume. Importantly, this risk can be reduced or obviated with judicious prehydration—usually with 500 to 1000 mL of crystalloid solution. Specifically, in the study by Lucas and colleagues (2001) cited earlier, there were no instances of pulmonary edema among the women in whom crystalloid preload was limited to 500 mL. Moreover, vasodilation produced by epidural blockade is less abrupt if the analgesia level is achieved slowly with dilute solutions of local anesthetic agents. This allows maintenance of blood pressure while simultaneously avoiding infusion of large volumes of crystalloid.

With vigorous intravenous crystalloid therapy, there is also concern about development of cerebral edema (see Chap. 34, p. 724). Moreover, Heller and co-workers (1983) demonstrated that most cases of *pharyngolaryngeal edema* were related to aggressive volume therapy.

Epidural Opiate Analgesia

Injection of opiates into the epidural space to relieve pain from labor has become popular. Their mechanism of action derives from interaction with specific receptors in the dorsal horn and dorsal roots. Opiates alone usually will not provide adequate analgesia, and they most often are given with a local anesthetic agent such as bupivacaine. The major advantages of using such a combination are the rapid onset of pain relief, a decrease in shivering, and less dense motor blockade (Meister and colleagues, 2000). Side effects are common and include pruritus and urinary retention. Immediate or delayed respiratory depression is worrisome (Ackerman and colleagues, 1992). Naloxone, given intravenously, will abolish these symptoms without affecting the analgesic action.

COMBINED SPINAL–EPIDURAL TECHNIQUES

The combination of spinal and epidural techniques has increased in popularity and may provide rapid and effective analgesia for labor as well as for cesarean delivery. An introducer needle is first placed in the epidural space. A small-gauge spinal needle is then introduced through the epidural needle into the subarachnoid space—this is called the *needle-through-needle technique*. A single bolus of an opioid, sometimes in combination with a local anesthetic, is injected into the subarachnoid space. The spinal needle is withdrawn, and an epidural catheter is then placed through the introducer needle. The use of a subarachnoid opioid bolus results in the rapid onset of profound pain relief with virtually no motor blockade. The epidural catheter permits repeated dosing of analgesia. However, in a randomized comparison, Abrão and associates (2009) reported that combined spinal-epidural analgesia was associated with a greater incidence of fetal heart rate abnormalities related to uterine hypertonus than was epidural analgesia alone.

LOCAL INFILTRATION FOR CESAREAN DELIVERY

A local block is occasionally useful to augment an inadequate or "patchy" regional block that was given in an emergency. On more rare occasions, local infiltration may be used to perform an emergency cesarean delivery to save the life of a fetus in the absence of any anesthesia support.

Technique

In one technique, the skin is infiltrated in the line of the proposed incision, and the subcutaneous, muscle, and rectus sheath layers are injected as the abdomen is opened. A dilute solution of lidocaine—30 mL of 2-percent with 1:200,000 epinephrine diluted with 60 mL of normal saline—is prepared, and a total of

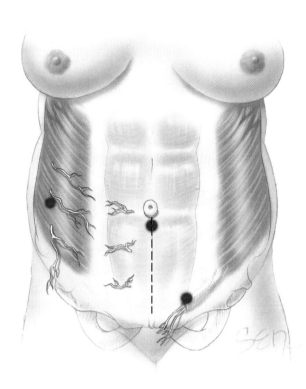

FIGURE 19-6 Local anesthetic block for cesarean delivery. The first injection site is halfway between the costal margin and iliac crest in the midaxillary line to block the 10th, 11th, and 12th intercostal nerves. A second injection at the external inguinal ring blocks branches of the genitofemoral and ilioinguinal nerves. These sites are infiltrated bilaterally. A final site is along the line of proposed skin incision.

100 to 120 mL is infiltrated. Injection of large volumes into the fatty layers, which are relatively devoid of nerve supply, is avoided to limit the total dose of local anesthetic needed.

A second technique involves a field block of the major branches supplying the abdominal wall, to include the 10th, 11th, and 12th intercostal nerves and the ilioinguinal and genitofemoral nerves (Busby, 1963). As shown in Figure 19-6, the former group of nerves is located at a point midway between the costal margin and iliac crest in the midaxillary line. The latter group is found at the level of the external inguinal ring. Only one skin puncture is made at each of the four sites (right and left sides). At the intercostal block site, the needle is directed medially and injection is carried down to the transversalis fascia, avoiding injection of the subcutaneous fat. Approximately 5 to 8 mL of 0.5-percent lidocaine is injected. The procedure is repeated at a 45-degree angle cephalad and caudad to this line. The other side is then injected. At the ilioinguinal and genitofemoral sites, the injection is started at a site 2 to 3 cm lateral from the pubic tubercle at a 45-degree angle. Finally, the skin overlying the planned incision is injected.

GENERAL ANESTHESIA

The increased safety of regional analgesia has increased the relative risk of general anesthesia. The case-fatality rate of general anesthesia for cesarean delivery is estimated to be approximately 32 per million live births compared with 1.9 per million for re-

gional analgesia (Hawkins and associates, 1997b). In the Michigan Mortality Surveillance report by Mhyre and colleagues (2007), 4 of 8 anesthesia-related maternal deaths were associated with the use of general anesthesia.

One common cause of death cited for general anesthesia is failed intubation. This occurs in approximately 1 of every 250 general anesthetics administered to pregnant women—a tenfold higher rate than in nonpregnant patients (Barnardo and Jenkins, 2000). The American College of Obstetricians and Gynecologists (2002) has concluded that this relative increase in morbidity and mortality rates suggests that regional analgesia is the preferred method of pain control and should be used unless contraindicated (see Table 19-5). Indeed, in the MFMU Network study that has been cited, 93 percent of more than 37,000 cesarean deliveries were attempted with regional analgesia (Bloom and colleagues, 2005). Trained personnel and specialized equipment—including fiberoptic intubation—are mandatory for the safe use of general anesthesia.

Patient Preparation

Prior to anesthesia induction, several steps should be taken to help minimize the risk of complications for the mother and fetus. These include the use of antacids, lateral uterine displacement, and preoxygenation.

Antacids

The practice of administering antacids shortly before induction of anesthesia has probably done more to decrease mortality rates from general anesthesia than any other single practice (Gibbs and Banner, 1984). The American Society of Anesthesiologists Task Force on Obstetrical Anesthesia (2007) recommends timely administration of a nonparticulate antacid, an H_2-receptor antagonist, or metoclopramide. For many years, we have recommended administration of 30 mL of Bicitra—sodium citrate with citric acid—within a few minutes of the anticipated time of anesthesia induction, by either general or major regional block. If more than 1 hour has passed between when a first dose was given and when anesthesia is induced, then a second dose is given.

Uterine Displacement

As discussed in Chapter 5 (p. 120), the uterus may compress the inferior vena cava and aorta when the mother is supine. With lateral uterine displacement, the duration of general anesthesia has less effect on neonatal condition than when the woman remains supine (Crawford and colleagues, 1972).

Preoxygenation

Because functional reserve lung capacity is reduced, pregnant women become hypoxemic more rapidly during periods of apnea than do nonpregnant patients. Obesity exacerbates this tendency (McClelland and associates, 2009). To minimize hypoxia between the time of muscle relaxant injection and intubation, it is important first to replace nitrogen in the lungs with oxygen. This is accomplished by administering 100-percent oxygen via face mask for 2 to 3 minutes prior to anesthesia induction. In an emergency, four vital capacity breaths of 100-percent oxygen via a tight breathing circuit will provide similar benefit (Norris and Dewan, 1985).

Induction of Anesthesia

Thiopental

This thiobarbiturate given intravenously is widely used and offers easy and rapid induction, prompt recovery, and minimal risk of vomiting. Thiopental and similar compounds are poor analgesic agents, and administration of sufficient drug given alone to maintain anesthesia may cause appreciable newborn depression.

Ketamine

This agent also may be used to render a patient unconscious. Doses of 1 mg/kg induce general anesthesia. Alternatively, given intravenously in low doses of 0.2 to 0.3 mg/kg, ketamine may be used to produce analgesia and sedation just prior to vaginal delivery. Ketamine may also prove useful in women with acute hemorrhage because, unlike thiopental, it is not associated with hypotension. Conversely, it usually causes a rise in blood pressure, and thus it generally should be avoided in women who are already hypertensive. Unpleasant delirium and hallucinations are commonly induced by this agent.

Intubation

Immediately after a patient is rendered unconscious, a muscle relaxant is given to aid intubation. *Succinylcholine,* a rapid-onset and short-acting agent, commonly is used. Cricoid pressure—the *Sellick maneuver*—is used by a trained assistant to occlude the esophagus from the onset of induction until intubation is completed. Before the operation begins, proper placement of the endotracheal tube must be confirmed.

Failed Intubation

Although uncommon, failed intubation is a major cause of anesthesia-related maternal mortality (Wallace and Sidawi, 1997). In their review of 67 maternal deaths associated with general anesthesia, Hawkins and colleagues (1997b) reported that 22 percent were secondary to induction or intubation problems. A history of previous difficulties with intubation as well as a careful assessment of anatomical features of the neck and of maxillofacial, pharyngeal, and laryngeal structures may help predict a difficult intubation. Even in cases in which the initial airway assessment was unremarkable, edema may develop intrapartum and present considerable difficulties (Farcon and associates, 1994). Morbid obesity is also a major risk factor for failed or difficult intubation. The American Society of Anesthesiologists Task Force on Obstetrical Anesthesia (2007) stresses the importance of appropriate preoperative preparation to include the immediate availability of specialized equipment. These include a variety of different shaped laryngoscopes, laryngeal mask airways, a fiber-optic bronchoscope, and a transtracheal ventilation set, as well as liberal use of awake oral intubation techniques.

Management. An important principle is to start the operative procedure only after it has been ascertained that tracheal intubation has been successful and that adequate ventilation can be accomplished. Even with an abnormal fetal heart rate pattern, initiation of cesarean delivery will only serve to complicate matters if there is difficult or failed intubation. Frequently, the woman must be allowed to awaken and a different technique used, such as an awake intubation or regional analgesia.

Following failed intubation, the woman is ventilated by mask and cricoid pressure is applied to reduce the chance of aspiration (Cooper and colleagues, 1994). Surgery may proceed with mask ventilation, or the woman may be allowed to awaken. In those cases in which the woman has been paralyzed and in which ventilation cannot be reestablished by insertion of an oral airway, laryngeal mask airway, or use of a fiberoptic laryngoscope to intubate the trachea, a life-threatening emergency exists. To restore ventilation, percutaneous or even open cricothyrotomy is performed, and jet ventilation begun (Reisner and colleagues, 1999). Failed intubation drills have been recommended to optimize response to such an emergency (Lewis, 2007; Nair and Alderson, 2006).

Gas Anesthetics

Once the endotracheal tube is secured, a 50:50 mixture of nitrous oxide and oxygen is administered to provide analgesia. Usually, a volatile halogenated agent is added to provide amnesia and additional analgesia. The mechanisms of action of inhaled anesthetics have been reviewed by Campagna and colleagues (2003).

Volatile Anesthetics

The most commonly used volatile anesthetics in the United States include *isoflurane* and two of its derivatives, *desflurane* and *sevoflurane.* They are usually added in low concentrations to the nitrous oxide-oxygen mixture to provide amnesia. They are potent, nonexplosive agents that produce remarkable uterine relaxation when given in high concentrations. These are used when relaxation is a requisite such as for internal podalic version of the second twin (see Chap. 39, p. 883), breech decomposition (see Chap. 24, p. 535), and replacement of the acutely inverted uterus (see Chap. 35, p. 780).

Extubation

The tracheal tube may be safely removed only if the woman is conscious to a degree that enables her to follow commands and is capable of maintaining oxygen saturation with spontaneous respiration. Consideration should be given to emptying the stomach via a nasogastric tube prior to extubation. As induction has become safer, extubation may now be more perilous. Of 15 anesthesia-related deaths of pregnant women from 1985 to 2003 in Michigan, none occurred during induction, whereas five resulted from hypoventilation or airway obstruction during emergence, extubation, or recovery (Mhyre and colleagues, 2007).

Aspiration

Massive gastric acidic inhalation causing pulmonary insufficiency from aspiration pneumonitis was first described by the obstetrician Mendelson, and the syndrome bears his name (Marik, 2001). Such pneumonitis has in the past been the most common cause of anesthetic deaths in obstetrics and therefore deserves special attention. In a survey of maternal deaths between 1979 and 1990, the Centers for Disease Control and Prevention identified that inhalation of gastric contents was associated with 23 percent of the 129 anesthesia-related deaths (Hawkins and colleagues, 1997b). To minimize the occurrence of this complication, antacids should be given routinely, intubation should be accompanied by cricoid pressure, and regional analgesia should be employed when possible.

Fasting

According to the American Society of Anesthesiologists Task Force on Obstetrical Anesthesia (2007), there is insufficient data regarding fasting times for clear liquids and the risk of pulmonary aspiration during labor. Recommendations are that modest amounts of clear liquids such as water, clear tea, black coffee, carbonated beverages, and pulp-free fruit juices be allowed in uncomplicated laboring women. Obvious solid foods should be avoided. The Task Force also recommended a fasting period of 6 to 8 hours, depending on the type of food ingested, for uncomplicated parturients undergoing elective cesarean delivery or puerperal tubal ligation.

Pathophysiology

In 1952, Teabeaut demonstrated experimentally that if the pH of aspirated fluid was below 2.5, severe chemical pneumonitis developed. It was later demonstrated that the pH of gastric juice of nearly half of women tested intrapartum was below 2.5 (Taylor and Pryse-Davies, 1966). The right mainstem bronchus usually offers the simplest pathway for aspirated material to reach the lung parenchyma, and therefore the right lower lobe is most often involved. In severe cases, there is bilateral widespread involvement.

The woman who aspirates may develop evidence of respiratory distress immediately or as long as several hours after aspiration, depending in part on the material aspirated and the severity of the response. Aspiration of a large amount of solid material causes obvious signs of airway obstruction. Smaller particles without acidic liquid may lead to patchy atelectasis and later to bronchopneumonia.

When highly acidic liquid is inspired, decreased oxygen saturation along with tachypnea, bronchospasm, rhonchi, rales, atelectasis, cyanosis, tachycardia, and hypotension are likely to develop. At the sites of injury, there is pulmonary capillary leakage and exudation of protein-rich fluid containing numerous erythrocytes into the lung interstitium and alveoli. This causes decreased pulmonary compliance, shunting of blood, and severe hypoxemia. Radiographic changes may not appear immediately, and they may be variable, although the right lung most often is affected. Therefore, chest radiographs alone should not be used to exclude aspiration.

Treatment

The methods recommended for treatment of aspiration have changed appreciably in recent years, indicating that previous therapy was not very successful. Suspicion of aspiration of gastric contents demands close monitoring for evidence of pulmonary damage. Respiratory rate and oxygen saturation as measured by pulse oximetry are the most sensitive and earliest indicators of injury.

As much of the inhaled fluid as possible should be immediately wiped out of the mouth and removed from the pharynx and trachea by suction. Saline lavage may further disseminate the acid throughout the lung and is not recommended. If large particulate matter is inspired, bronchoscopy may be indicated to relieve airway obstruction. There is no convincing clinical or experimental evidence that corticosteroid therapy or prophylac-

tic antimicrobial administration is beneficial (Marik, 2001). If clinical evidence of infection develops, however, then vigorous treatment is given. If acute respiratory distress syndrome develops, mechanical ventilation with positive end-expiratory pressure may prove lifesaving (see Chap. 42, p. 930).

REFERENCES

Abrão KC, Francisco RP, Miyadahira S, et al: Elevation of uterine basal tone and fetal heart rate abnormalities after labor analgesia: A randomized controlled trial. Obstet Gynecol 113(10):41, 2009

Ackerman WE III, Juneja M, Spinnato JA: Epidural opioids' OB advantages. Contemp Obstet Gynecol 37:68, 1992

Alexander JM, Sharma SK, McIntire DD, et al: Epidural analgesia lengthens the Friedman active phase of labor. Obstet Gynecol 100:46, 2002

American Academy of Pediatrics and American College of Obstetricians and Gynecologists: Guidelines for Perinatal Care, 6th ed. Washington, DC, 2007

American College of Obstetricians and Gynecologists: Obstetric analgesia and anesthesia. Practice Bulletin 36, July 2002

American College of Obstetricians and Gynecologists: Optimal goals for anesthesia care in obstetrics. Committee Opinion No. 433, May 2009

American College of Obstetricians and Gynecologists and the American Society of Anesthesiologists: Pain relief during labor. Committee Opinion No. 297, July 2004

American Society of Anesthesiologists Task Force on Obstetrical Anesthesia: Practice guidelines for obstetrical anesthesia. Anesthesiology 106:843, 2007

Angel JL, Knuppel RA, Lake M: Sinusoidal fetal heart rate pattern associated with intravenous butorphanol administration: A case report. Am J Obstet Gynecol 149:465, 1984

Atkinson BD, Truitt LJ, Rayburn WF, et al: Double-blind comparison of intravenous butorphanol (Stadol) and fentanyl (Sublimaze) for analgesia during labor. Am J Obstet Gynecol 171:993, 1994

Barnardo PD, Jenkins JG: Failed tracheal intubation in obstetrics: A 6-year review in the UK region. Anaesthesia 55:690, 2000

Bell ED, Penning DH, Cousineau EF, et al: How much labor is in a labor epidural? Manpower cost and reimbursement for an obstetric analgesia service in a teaching institution. Anesthesiology 92:851, 2000

Berg CJ, Chang J, Callaghan WM, et al: Pregnancy-related mortality in the United States, 1991–1997. Obstet Gynecol 101:289, 2003

Bloom SL, Spong CY, Weiner SJ, et al: Complications of anesthesia for cesarean delivery. Obstet Gynecol 106:281, 2005

Breen TW, Ransil BJ, Groves PA, et al: Factors associated with back pain after childbirth. Anesthesiology 81:29, 1994

Bricker L, Lavender T: Parenteral opioids for labor pain relief: A systematic review. Am J Obstet Gynecol 186:S94, 2002

Busby T: Local anesthesia for cesarean section. Am J Obstet Gynecol 87:399, 1963

Butler R, Fuller J: Back pain following epidural anaesthesia in labour. Can J Anaesth 45:724, 1998

Camann WR, Murray RS, Mushlin PS, et al: Effects of oral caffeine on postdural puncture headache: A double-blinded, placebo-controlled trial. Anesth Analg 70:181, 1990

Campagna JA, Miller KW, Forman SA: Mechanisms of actions of inhaled anesthetics. N Engl J Med 348:2110, 2003

Chan BO, Paech MJ: Persistent cerebrospinal fluid leak: A complication of the combined spinal-epidural technique. Anesth Analg 98:828, 2004

Chang J, Elam-Evans LD, Berg CJ, et al: Pregnancy-related mortality surveillance—United States, 1991–1999. MMWR 52:1, 2003

Cheek TG, Samuels P: Pregnancy induced hypertension. In Datta S (ed): Anesthesia and Management of High-Risk Pregnancy. St Louis, Mosby-Year Book, 1991

Chestnut DH: Effect on the progress of labor and method of delivery. In Chestnut DH (ed): Obstetric Anesthesia: Principles and Practice, 2nd ed. St Louis: Mosby-Year Book, 1999, p 408

Chestnut DH: Epidural analgesia and the incidence of cesarean section: Time for another close look. Anesthesiology 87:472, 1997

Chestnut DH, McGrath JM, Vincent RD Jr, et al: Does early administration of epidural analgesia affect obstetric outcome in nulliparous women who are in spontaneous labor? Anesthesiology 80:1201, 1994a

Chestnut DH, Owen CL, Bates JN, et al: Continuous infusion epidural analgesia during labor: A randomized, double-blind comparison of 0.625% bupivacaine/0.0002% fentanyl versus 0.125% bupivacaine. Anesthesiology 68:754, 1988

Chestnut DH, Vincent RD Jr, McGrather JM, et al: Does early administration of epidural analgesia affect obstetric outcome in nulliparous women who are receiving intravenous oxytocin? Anesthesiology 80:1193, 1994b

Chisholm ME, Campbell DC: Postpartum postural headache due to superior sagittal sinus thrombosis mistaken for spontaneous intracranial hypotension. Can J Anaesth 48:302, 2001

Clark SL, Divon MY, Phelan JP: Preeclampsia/eclampsia: Hemodynamic and neurologic correlations. Obstet Gynecol 66:337, 1985

Cooper SD, Benumof JL, Ozaki GT: Evaluation of the Bullard laryngoscope using the new intubating stylet: Comparison with conventional laryngoscopy. Anesth Analg 79:965, 1994

Cotton DB, Longmire S, Jones MM, et al: Cardiovascular alterations in severe pregnancy-induced hypertension: Effects of intravenous nitroglycerin coupled with blood volume expansion. Am J Obstet Gynecol 154:1053, 1986

Crawford JS: Some maternal complications of epidural analgesia for labour. Anaesthesia 40:1219, 1985

Crawford JS, Burton M, Davies P: Time and lateral tilt at caesarean section. Br J Anaesth 44:477, 1972

Cunningham FG, Leveno KJ: Obstetrical concerns for anesthetic management of severe preeclampsia. Williams Obstetrics, 19th ed (Suppl 10). Norwalk, Conn, Appleton and Lange, December 1994/January 1995

D'Angelo R: Anesthesia-related maternal mortality: A pat on the back or a call to arms? Anesthesiology 106(6):1082, 2007

Danilenko-Dixon DR, Tefft L, Haydon B, et al: The effect of maternal position on cardiac output with epidural analgesia in labor [Abstract]. Am J Obstet Gynecol 174:332, 1996

Darouiche RO: Spinal epidural abscess. N Engl J Med 355:2012, 2006

Dashe JS, Rogers BB, McIntire DD, et al: Epidural analgesia and intrapartum fever: Placental findings. Obstet Gynecol 93:341, 1999

Dawley B, Hendrix A: Intracranial subdural hematoma after spinal anesthesia in a parturient. Obstet Gynecol 113(2):570, 2009

Deneux-Tharaux C, Berg C, Bouvier-Colle M-H, Gissler M, et al: Underreporting of pregnancy-related mortality in the United States and Europe. Obstet Gynecol 106:684, 2005

Dresner M, Brocklesby J, Bamber J: Audit of the influence of body mass index on the performance of epidural analgesia in labour and the subsequent mode of delivery. Br J Obstet Gynaecol 113:1178, 2006

Dyer RA, Piercy JL, Reed AR: The role of the anaesthetist in the management of the pre-eclamptic patient. Curr Opin Anaesthesiol 20(3):168, 2007

Eltzschig HK, Lieberman ES, Camann WR: Regional anesthesia and analgesia for labor and delivery. N Engl J Med 348:319, 2003

Farcon EL, Kim MH, Marx GF: Changing Mallampati score during labour. Can J Anaesth 41:50, 1994

Friedman EA: Primigravid labor: A graphicostatistical analysis. Obstet Gynecol 6:567, 1955

Fusi L, Steer PJ, Maresh MJA, et al: Maternal pyrexia associated with the use of epidural analgesia in labour. Lancet 1:1250, 1989

Gambling DR, Writer D: Hypertensive disorders. In Chestnut DH (ed): Obstetric Anesthesia: Principles and Practice, 2nd ed. St Louis, Mosby-Year Book, 1999, p 875

Gibbs CP, Banner TC: Effectiveness of Bicitra as a preoperative antacid. Anesthesiology 61:97, 1984

Glosten B: Local anesthetic techniques. In Chestnut DH (ed): Obstetric Anesthesia: Principles and Practice, 2nd ed. St Louis, Mosby-Year Book, 1999, p 363

Goetzl L, Rivers J, Zighelboim I, et al: Intrapartum epidural analgesia and maternal temperature regulation. Obstet Gynecol 109:687, 2007

Grant GJ: Safely giving regional anesthesia to gravidas with clotting disorders. Contemp OB Gyn August, 2007

Gutsche BB: The experts opine: The role of epidural anesthesia in preeclampsia. Surv Anesthesiol 30:304, 1986

Halpern SH, Carvalho B: Patient-controlled epidural analgesia for labor. Anesth Analg 108(3):921, 2009

Harding SA, Collis RE, Morgan BM: Meningitis after combined spinal–extradural anaesthesia in obstetrics. Br J Anaesth 73:545, 1994

Hatjis CG, Meis PJ: Sinusoidal fetal heart rate pattern associated with butorphanol administration. Obstet Gynecol 67:377, 1986

Hawkins JL, Gibbs CP, Orleans M, et al: Obstetric anesthesia work force survey, 1981 versus 1992. Anesthesiology 87:135, 1997a

Hawkins JL, Koonin LM, Palmer SK, et al: Anesthesia-related deaths during obstetric delivery in the United States, 1979–1990. Anesthesiology 86:277, 1997b

Head BB, Owen J, Vincent RD, et al: A randomized trial of intrapartum analgesia in women with severe preeclampsia. Obstet Gynecol 99:452, 2002

Heller PJ, Scheider EP, Marx GF: Pharyngolaryngeal edema as a presenting symptom in preeclampsia. Obstet Gynecol 62:523, 1983

Hess PE, Pratt SD, Lucas TP, et al: Predictors of breakthrough pain during labor epidural analgesia. Anesth Analg 93:414, 2001

Hill JB, Alexander JM, Sharma SK, et al: A comparison of the effects of epidural and meperidine analgesia during labor on fetal heart rate. Obstet Gynecol 102:333, 2003.

Hogg B, Hauth JC, Caritis SN, et al: Safety of labor epidural anesthesia for women with severe hypertensive disease. Am J Obstet Gynecol 181:1096, 1999

Howell CJ, Kidd C, Roberts W, et al: A randomized controlled trial of epidural compared with non-epidural analgesia in labour. Br J Obstet Gynaecol 108:27, 2001

Kennedy WF Jr, Bonica JJ, Akamatsu TJ, et al: Cardiovascular and respiratory effects of subarachnoid block in the presence of acute blood loss. Anesthesiology 29:29, 1968

Kennell J, Klaus M, McGrath S, et al: Continuous emotional support during labor in a U.S. hospital: A randomized controlled trial. JAMA 265:2197, 1991

Krivak TC, Zorn KK: Venous thromboembolism in obstetrics and gynecology. Obstet Gynecol 109(3):761, 2007

Kuklina EV, Meikle SF, Jamieson DJ, et al: Severe obstetric morbidity in the United States: 1998–2005. Obstet Gynecol 113:293, 2009

Lamaze F: Painless Childbirth: Psychoprophylactic Method. Chicago, Henry Regnery, 1970

Lee A, Ngan Kee WD, Gin T: Prophylactic ephedrine prevents hypotension during spinal anesthesia for cesarean delivery but does not improve neonatal outcome: A quantitative systematic review. Can J Anaesth 49:588, 2002a

Lee A, Ngan Kee WD, Gin T: A quantitative, systematic review of randomized controlled trials of ephedrine versus phenylephrine for the management of hypotension during spinal anesthesia for cesarean delivery. Anesth Analg 94:920, 2002b

Lee LA, Posner KL, Domino KB, et al: Injuries associated with regional anesthesia in the 1980s and 1990s: A closed claims analysis. Anesthesiology 101:143, 2004

Leighton BL, Halpern SH: The effects of epidural analgesia on labor, maternal, and neonatal outcomes: A systematic review. Am J Obstet Gynecol 186:569, 2002

Lewis G (ed): The Confidential Enquiry into Maternal and Child Health (CEMACH). Saving Mothers' Lives. London, CEMACH, 2007

Li G, Warner M, Lang BH et al: Epidemiology of anesthesia-related mortality in the United States, 1999–2005. Anesthesiology 110(4):759, 2009

Lieberman E, Lang JM, Cohen A, et al: Association of epidural analgesia with cesarean delivery in nulliparas. Obstet Gynecol 88:993, 1996

Lieberman E, O'Donoghue C: Unintended effects of epidural analgesia during labor: A systematic review. Am J Obstet Gynecol 186:531, 2002

Lowe NK: The nature of labor pain. Am J Obstet Gynecol 106:S16, 2002

Lucas MJ, Sharma SK, McIntire DD, et al: A randomized trial of labor analgesia in women with pregnancy-induced hypertension. Am J Obstet Gynecol 185:970, 2001

Luxman D, Wholman I, Groutz A, et al: The effect of early epidural block administration on the progression and outcome of labor. Int J Obstet Anesth 7:161, 1998

MacArthur AJ, MacArthur C, Weeks SK: Is epidural anesthesia in labor associated with chronic low back pain? A prospective cohort study. Anesth Analg 85:1066, 1997

Manninen T, Aantaa R, Salonen M, et al: A comparison of the hemodynamic effects of paracervical block and epidural anesthesia for labor analgesia. Acta Anaesthesiol Scand 44:441, 2000

Marik PE: Aspiration pneumonitis and aspiration pneumonia. N Engl J Med 344:665, 2001

McClelland SH, Bogod DG, Hardman JG: Pre-oxygenation and apnoea in pregnancy: Changes during labour and with obstetric morbidity in a computational simulation. Anaesthesia 64(4):371, 2009

Meister GC, D'Angelo R, Owen M, et al: A comparison of epidural analgesia with 0.125% ropivacaine with fentanyl versus 0.125% bupivacaine with fentanyl during labor. Anesth Analg 90:632, 2000

Melzack R: The myth of painless childbirth. Pain 19:321, 1984

Mhyre JM, Riesner MN, Polley LS, et al: A series of anesthesia-related maternal deaths in Michigan, 1985–2003. Anesthesiology 106:1096, 2007

Morgan D, Philip J, Sharma S, et al: A neonatal outcome with ephedrine infusions with or without preloading during spinal anesthesia for cesarean section. Society of Anesthesiologists and Perinatologists, Montreal, Quebec, Canada. Anesthesiology (supplement):A5, 2000

Mulroy MF: Systemic toxicity and cardiotoxicity from local anesthetics: Incidence and preventive measures. Reg Anesth Pain Med 27:556, 2002

Ngan Kee WD, Khaw KS, Ng FF, et al: Prophylactic phenylephrine infusion for preventing hypotension during spinal anesthesia for cesarean delivery. Anesth Analg 98:815, 2004

Nair A, Alderson JD: Failed intubation drill in obstetrics. Int J Obstet Anes 15(2):172, 2006

Nagaya K, Fetters MD, Ishikawa M, et al: Causes of maternal mortality in Japan. JAMA 283:2661, 2000

Newton JA Jr, Lesnik IK, Kennedy CA: *Streptococcus salivarius* meningitis following spinal anesthesia. Clin Infect Dis 18:840, 1994

Noblett K, McKinney A, Kim R: Sheared epidural catheter during an elective procedure. Obstet Gynecol 109:566, 2007

Norris MC, Dewan DM: Preoxygenation for cesarean section: A comparison of two techniques. Anesthesiology 62:827, 1985

Ohel G, Gonen R, Vaida S, et al: Early versus late initiation of epidural analgesia in labor: Does it increase the risk of cesarean section? A randomized trial. Am J Obstet Gynecol 194:600, 2006

Palkar NV, Boudreaux RC, Mankad AV: Accidental total spinal block: A complication of an epidural test dose. Can J Anaesth 39:1058, 1992

Quilligan EJ, Keegan KA, Donahue MJ: Double-blind comparison of intravenously injected butorphanol and meperidine in parturients. Int J Gynaecol Obstet 18:363, 1980

Read GD: Childbirth without Fear. New York, Harper, 1944, p 192

Reisner LS, Benumof JL, Cooper SD: The difficult airway: Risk, prophylaxis, and management. In Chestnut DH (ed): Obstetric Anesthesia: Principles and Practice, 2nd ed. St Louis, Mosby-Year Book, 1999, p 611

Reynolds F, Sharma SK, Seed PT: Analgesia in labour and fetal acid-base balance: A meta-analysis comparing epidural with systemic opioid analgesia. Br J Obstet Gynaecol 109:1344, 2002

Rogers R, Gilson G, Kammerer-Doak D: Epidural analgesia and active management of labor: Effects on length of labor and mode of delivery. Obstet Gynecol 93:995, 1999

Rosen MA: Nitrous oxide for relief of labor pain: A systematic review. Am J Obstet Gynecol 186:S110, 2002a

Rosen MA: Paracervical block for labor analgesia: A brief historic review. Am J Obstet Gynecol 186:S127, 2002b

Ruppen W, Derry S, McQuay H, et al: Incidence of epidural hematoma, infection, and neurologic injury in obstetric patients with epidural analgesia/anesthesia. Anesthesiology 105:394, 2006

Saisto T, Salmela-Aro K, Nurmi JE, et al: A randomized controlled trial of intervention in fear of childbirth. Obstet Gynecol 98:820, 2001

Sandkovsky U, Mihu MR, Adeyeye A, et al: Iatrogenic meningitis in an obstetric patient after combined spinal-epidural analgesia: Case report and review of the literature. South Med J 102(3):287, 2009

Scavone BM, Wong CA, Sullivan JT, et al: Efficacy of a prophylactic epidural blood patch in preventing post dural puncture headache in parturients after inadvertent dural puncture. Anesthesiology 101:1422, 2004

Sechzer PH, Abel L: Post-spinal anesthesia headache treated with caffeine. Evaluation with demand method. Part I. Curr Therap Res 24:307, 1978

Setayesh AR, Kholdebarin AR, Moghadam MS, et al: The Trendelenburg position increases the spread and accelerates the onset of epidural anesthesia for cesarean section. Can J Anaesth 48:890, 2001

Seyb ST, Berka RJ, Socol ML, et al: Risk of cesarean delivery with elective induction of labor at term in nulliparous women. Obstet Gynecol 94:600, 1999

Sharma SK, Leveno KJ: Regional analgesia and progress of labor. Clin Obstet Gynecol 46:633, 2003

Sharma SK, McIntire DD, Wiley J, et al: Labor analgesia and cesarean delivery. An individual patient meta-analysis of nulliparous women. Anesthesiology 100:142, 2004

Sharma SK, Sidawi JE, Ramin SM, et al: Cesarean delivery: A randomized trial of epidural versus patient-controlled meperidine analgesia during labor. Anesthesiology 87:487, 1997

Shearer VE, Jhaveri HS, Cunningham FG: Puerperal seizures after post-dural puncture headache. Obstet Gynecol 85:255, 1995

Smarkusky L, DeCarvalho H, Bermudez A, et al: Acute onset headache complicating labor epidural caused by intrapartum pneumocephalus. Obstet Gynecol 108:795, 2006

Sprigge JS, Harper SJ: Accidental dural puncture and post dural puncture headache in obstetric anaesthesia: Presentation and management: A 23-year survey in a district general hospital. Anaesthesia 63:36, 2008

Svancarek W, Chirino O, Schaefer G Jr, et al: Retropsoas and subgluteal abscesses following paracervical and pudendal anesthesia. JAMA 237:892, 1977

Taylor G, Pryse-Davies J: The prophylactic use of antacids in the prevention of the acid pulmonary aspiration syndrome (Mendelson's syndrome). Lancet 1:288, 1966

Teabeaut JR II: Aspiration of gastric contents: An experimental study. Am J Pathol 28:51, 1952

Thompson TT, Thorp JM, Mayer D, et al: Does epidural analgesia cause dystocia? J Clin Anesth 10:58, 1998

Thorp JA, Breedlove G: Epidural analgesia in labor: An evaluation of risks and benefits. Birth 23:63, 1996

Tsui MHY, Kee WDN, Ng FF, et al: A double blinded randomized placebo-controlled study of intramuscular pethidine for pain relief in the first stage of labour. Br J Obstet Gynaecol 111:648, 2004

Vallejo MC, Mandell GL, Sabo DP, et al: Postdural puncture headache: A randomized comparison of five spinal needles in obstetric patients. Anesth Analg 91:916, 2000

Visalyaputra S, Rodanant O, Somboonviboon W, et al: Spinal versus epidural anesthesia for cesarean delivery in severe preeclampsia: A prospective randomized, multicenter study. Anesth Analg 101:862, 2005

von Ungern-Sternberg BS, Regli A, Bucher E, et al: Impact of spinal anaesthesia and obesity on maternal respiratory function during elective Caesarean section. Anaesthesia 59:743, 2004

Wallace DH, Leveno KJ, Cunningham FG, et al: Randomized comparison of general and regional anesthesia for cesarean delivery in pregnancies complicated by severe preeclampsia. Obstet Gynecol 86:193, 1995

Wallace DH, Sidawi JE: Complications of obstetrical anesthesia. Williams Obstetrics, 20th ed (Suppl 3). Norwalk, Conn, Appleton & Lange, June/July, 1997

Wong CA, McCarthy RJ, Sullivan JT, et al: Early compared with late neuraxial analgesia in nulliparous labor induction. Obstet Gynecol 113(5):1066, 2009

Wong CA, Scavone BM, Peaceman AM, et al: The risk of cesarean delivery with neuraxial analgesia given early versus late in labor. N Engl J Med 352:655, 2005

Yancey MK, Pierce B, Schweitzer D, et al: Observations on labor epidural analgesia and operative delivery rates. Am J Obstet Gynecol 180:353, 1999

Yancey MK, Zhang J, Schwarz J, et al: Labor epidural analgesia and intrapartum maternal hyperthermia. Obstet Gynecol 98:763, 2001a

Yancey MK, Zhang J, Schweitzer DL, et al: Epidural analgesia and fetal head malposition at vaginal delivery. Obstet Gynecol 97:608, 2001b

Zeeman GG, Cunningham FG, Pritchard JA: The magnitude of hemoconcentration with eclampsia. Hypertens Preg 28(2):127, 2009

Zhang J, Yancey MK, Klebanoff MA, et al: Does epidural analgesia prolong labor and increase risk of cesarean delivery? A natural experiment. Am J Obstet Gynecol 185:128, 2001

Abnormal Labor

In 2007, the cesarean delivery rate was 31.8 percent—the highest level ever reported for the United States (Hamilton and co-workers, 2009). According to the American College of Obstetricians and Gynecologists (2003), approximately 60 percent of primary cesarean deliveries in the United States are attributable to the diagnosis of dystocia. Roy (2003) has proposed that this high frequency results from environmental changes that are developing more rapidly than Darwinian natural selection. Humans are poorly adapted to the affluence of the modern diet, and one result is dystocia. Evidence in support of this comes from Barau and associates (2006), who analyzed prepregnancy body mass index (BMI) and the risk of cesarean delivery. They studied 16,592 singleton births and reported a linear association between BMI and cesarean delivery. This has been similarly shown by others (Leung, 2008; Nuthalapaty, 2004; Roman, 2008; Treacy, 2006; Wilkes, 2003, and all their colleagues). As further discussed in Chapter 43, Getahun and co-workers (2007) reported that obesity is associated with an increased cesarean delivery rate. Interestingly, these researchers found that a decrease in weight from obese to normal eliminates this risk.

OVERVIEW OF DYSTOCIA

Dystocia literally means *difficult labor* and is characterized by abnormally slow labor progress. It arises from four distinct abnormalities that may exist singly or in combination:

1. Abnormalities of the expulsive forces. Uterine contractions may be insufficiently strong or inappropriately coordinated to efface and dilate the cervix—uterine dysfunction. Also, there may be inadequate voluntary maternal muscle effort during second-stage labor.
2. Abnormalities of presentation, position, or development of the fetus.
3. Abnormalities of the maternal bony pelvis—that is, pelvic contraction.
4. Abnormalities of soft tissues of the reproductive tract that form an obstacle to fetal descent (see Chap. 40, p. 890).

More simply, these abnormalities can be mechanistically simplified into three categories that include abnormalities of: the *powers*—uterine contractility and maternal expulsive effort; the *passenger*—the fetus; and the *passage*—the pelvis. Common clinical findings in women with these labor abnormalities are summarized in Table 20-1.

Dystocia Definitions

Combinations of the abnormalities shown in Table 20-1 often interact to produce dysfunctional labor. Today, expressions such as *cephalopelvic disproportion* and *failure to progress* often are used to describe ineffective labors:

1. The expression *cephalopelvic disproportion* came into use prior to the 20th century to describe obstructed labor resulting from disparity between the size of the fetal head and maternal pelvis. But the term originated at a time when the main indication for cesarean delivery was overt pelvic

Abnormal Labor **465**

CHAPTER 20

TABLE 20-1. Common Clinical Findings in Women with Ineffective Labor

Inadequate cervical dilation or fetal descent:
  Protracted labor—slow progress
  Arrested labor—no progress
  Inadequate expulsive effort—ineffective pushing

Fetopelvic disproportion:
  Excessive fetal size
  Inadequate pelvic capacity
  Malpresentation or position of the fetus

Ruptured membranes without labor

contracture due to rickets (Olah and Neilson, 1994). Such absolute disproportion is now rare, and most cases result from malposition of the fetal head within the pelvis (asynclitism) or from ineffective uterine contractions. True disproportion is a tenuous diagnosis because two thirds or more of women undergoing cesarean delivery for this reason subsequently deliver even larger newborns vaginally (see Chap. 26, p. 565).

2. *Failure to progress* in either spontaneous or stimulated labor has become an increasingly popular description of ineffectual labor. This term is used to include lack of progressive cervical dilatation or lack of fetal descent. Most precisely, however, the specific terms and their definitions should be used to describe abnormal labor (Table 20-2).

Overdiagnosis of Dystocia

As discussed, dystocia is the most common current indication for primary cesarean delivery. Gifford and colleagues (2000) reported that lack of progress in labor was the reason for 68 percent of unplanned cesarean deliveries for cephalic-presenting fetuses.

It is generally agreed that dystocia leading to cesarean delivery is overdiagnosed in the United States and elsewhere. The reasons for this, however, are controversial. Those implicated have included incorrect diagnosis, epidural analgesia, fear of litigation, and even clinician convenience (Lieberman and coworkers, 1996; Savage and Francome, 1994; Thorp and colleagues, 1993a).

It appears that variability of criteria for diagnosis is a major determinant of this increase. For example, Gifford and associates (2000) found that almost 25 percent of the cesarean deliveries performed annually in the United States for lack of progress were in women with cervical dilatation of only 0 to 3 cm (Fig. 20-1). This practice is contrary to recommendations of the American College of Obstetricians and Gynecologists (1995a) that the cervix be dilated to 4 cm or more before dystocia is diagnosed. Thus, the diagnosis often is made before active labor, and therefore before an adequate trial of labor. Another factor implicated is insufficient oxytocin stimulation of labor in women with slow labor (Rouse and Owen, 1999b). King (1993) found that cesarean deliveries for dystocia in private patients in the United Kingdom were related to office hours and surgery schedules whereas the timing of procedures for fetal distress were evenly distributed throughout the day.

TABLE 20-2. Abnormal Labor Patterns, Diagnostic Criteria, and Methods of Treatment

	Diagnostic Criteria			
Labor Pattern	**Nulliparas**	**Multiparas**	**Preferred Treatment**	**Exceptional Treatment**
Prolongation Disorder				
Prolonged latent phase	> 20 hr	> 14 hr	Bed rest	Oxytocin or cesarean delivery for urgent problems
Protraction Disorders				
Protracted active-phase dilatation	< 1.2 cm/hr	< 1.5 cm/hr	Expectant and support	Cesarean delivery for CPD
Protracted descent	< 1 cm/hr	< 2 cm/hr		
Arrest Disorders				
Prolonged deceleration phase	> 3 hr	> 1 hr	Evaluate for CPD: CPD: cesarean delivery No CPD: oxytocin	Rest if exhausted Cesarean delivery
Secondary arrest of dilatation	> 2 hr	> 2 hr		
Arrest of descent	> 1 hr	> 1 hr		
Failure of descent	No descent in deceleration phase or second stage			

CPD = cephalopelvic disproportion.
Modified from Cohen and Friedman (1983).

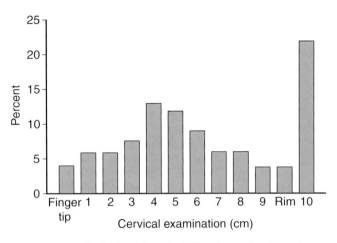

FIGURE 20-1 Distribution of cervical dilatation at the time of cesarean delivery for dystocia. (Adapted from Gifford and colleagues, 2000, with permission.)

Mechanisms of Dystocia

Dystocia described by Williams (1903) in the first edition of this text is still true today. Figure 20-2 is from that edition, and it demonstrates the mechanical process of labor and the potential obstacles. The cervix and lower uterus are shown at the end of pregnancy and at the end of labor. At the end of pregnancy, the fetal head, to traverse the birth canal, must encounter a relatively thicker lower uterine segment and undilated cervix. The uterine fundus muscle is less developed and presumably less powerful. Uterine contractions, cervical resistance, and the forward pressure exerted by the leading fetal part are the factors influencing the progress of first-stage labor (see Chap. 6, p. 141).

After complete cervical dilatation (see Fig. 20-2), however, the mechanical relationship between the fetal head size and position and the pelvic capacity, namely *fetopelvic proportion*, becomes clearer as the fetus descends. Accordingly, abnormalities in fetopelvic proportions become more apparent once the second stage is reached.

Uterine muscle malfunction can result from uterine overdistension or obstructed labor or both. Thus, ineffective labor is generally accepted as a possible warning sign of fetopelvic disproportion.

Artificial separation of labor abnormalities into pure *uterine dysfunction* and *fetopelvic disproportion* simplifies classification, but is an incomplete characterization because these two abnormalities are so closely interlinked. Indeed, according to the American College of Obstetricians and Gynecologists (1995a), the bony pelvis rarely limits vaginal delivery.

In the absence of objective means of precisely distinguishing these two causes of labor failure, clinicians must rely on a *trial of labor* to determine if labor can be successful in effecting vaginal delivery. In our opinion, defining the adequacy of a trial of labor is a priority in moderating the primary cesarean delivery rate for dystocia.

ABNORMALITIES OF THE EXPULSIVE FORCES

Cervical dilatation and propulsion and expulsion of the fetus are brought about by contractions of the uterus, reinforced during the second stage by voluntary or involuntary muscular action of the abdominal wall—"pushing." The diagnosis of uterine dysfunction in the latent phase is difficult and sometimes can be made only in retrospect (see Chap. 17, p. 389). Women who are not yet in active labor commonly are erroneously treated for uterine dysfunction.

During the past 50 to 60 years, there have been at least three significant advances in the treatment of uterine dysfunction:

1. Realization that undue prolongation of labor may contribute to maternal and perinatal morbidity and mortality rates.
2. Use of dilute intravenous infusion of oxytocin in the treatment of certain types of uterine dysfunction.
3. More frequent use of cesarean delivery rather than difficult midforceps delivery when oxytocin fails or its use is inappropriate.

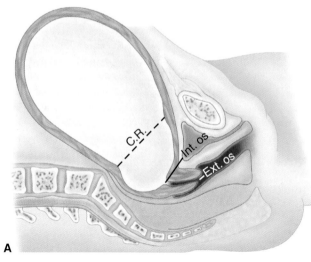
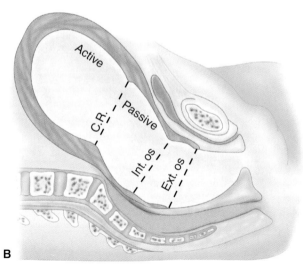

FIGURE 20-2 Diagrams of the birth canal **(A)** at the end of pregnancy and **(B)** during the second stage of labor, showing formation of the birth canal. (C.R. = contraction ring; Int. = internal; Ext = external.) (Adapted from from Williams, 1903.)

Types of Uterine Dysfunction

Reynolds and co-workers (1948) emphasized that uterine contractions of normal labor are characterized by a gradient of myometrial activity. These forces are greatest and last longest at the fundus—considered fundal dominance—and they diminish toward the cervix. Caldeyro-Barcia and colleagues (1950) from Montevideo, Uruguay, inserted small balloons into the myometrium at various levels (see Chap. 18, p. 437). They reported that in addition to a gradient of activity, there was a time differential in the onset of the contractions in the fundus, midzone, and lower uterine segments. Larks (1960) described the stimulus as starting in one cornu and then several milliseconds later in the other. The excitation waves then join and sweep over the fundus and down the uterus. The Montevideo group also ascertained that the lower limit of contraction pressure required to dilate the cervix is 15 mm Hg. This figure is in agreement with the findings of Hendricks and co-workers (1959), who reported that normal spontaneous contractions often exert pressures of approximately 60 mm Hg.

From these observations, it is possible to define two types of uterine dysfunction. In the more common *hypotonic uterine dysfunction,* there is no basal hypertonus and uterine contractions have a normal gradient pattern (synchronous), but pressure during a contraction is insufficient to dilate the cervix. In the second type, *hypertonic uterine dysfunction* or *incoordinate uterine dysfunction,* either basal tone is elevated appreciably or the pressure gradient is distorted. Gradient distortion may result from contraction of the uterine midsegment with more force than the fundus or from complete asynchronism of the impulses originating in each cornu or a combination of these two.

Active-Phase Disorders

Labor abnormalities are clinically divided into either slower-than-normal progress—*protraction disorder*—or complete cessation of progress—*arrest disorder.* A woman must be in the active phase of labor with cervical dilatation to at least 3 to 4 cm to be diagnosed with either of these. Handa and Laros (1993) diagnosed active-phase arrest, defined as no dilatation for 2 hours or more, in 5 percent of term nulliparas. This incidence has not changed since the 1950s (Friedman, 1978). Inadequate uterine contractions, defined as less than 180 Montevideo units, calculated as shown in Figure 20-3, were diagnosed in 80 percent of women with active-phase arrest.

Protraction disorders are less well described, and the time necessary before diagnosing slow progress is undefined. The World Health Organization (1994) has proposed a labor management *partograph* in which protraction is defined as less than 1 cm/hr cervical dilatation for a minimum of 4 hours. Criteria for the diagnosis of protraction and arrest disorders have been recommended by the American College of Obstetricians and Gynecologists (1995a). These criteria were adapted from those of Cohen and Friedman (1983), shown in Table 20-2.

Hauth and co-workers (1986, 1991) reported that when labor is effectively induced or augmented with oxytocin, 90 percent of women achieve 200 to 225 Montevideo units, and 40 percent achieve at least 300 Montevideo units. These results suggest that there are certain minimums of uterine activity that should be achieved before performing cesarean delivery for dystocia. Accordingly, the American College of Obstetricians and Gynecologists (1989) has suggested that before the diagnosis of arrest during first-stage labor is made, both of these criteria should be met:

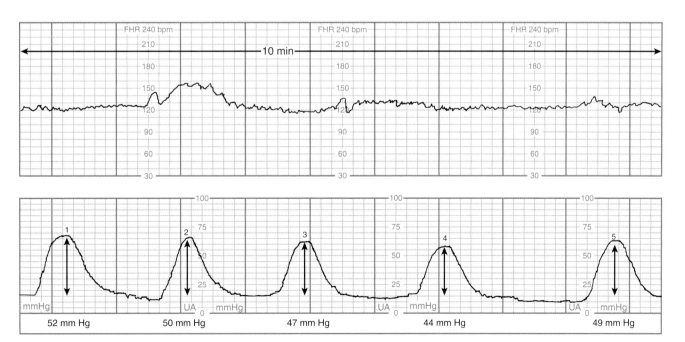

FIGURE 20-3 Montevideo units are calculated by subtracting the baseline uterine pressure from the peak contraction pressure for each contraction in a 10-minute window and adding the pressures generated by each contraction. In the example shown, there were five contractions, producing pressure changes of 52, 50, 47, 44, and 49 mm Hg, respectively. The sum of these five contractions is 242 Montevideo units.

1. The latent phase has been completed, and the cervix is dilated 4 cm or more.
2. A uterine contraction pattern of 200 Montevideo units or more in a 10-minute period has been present for 2 hours without cervical change.

Rouse and Owen (1999b) have challenged the "2-hour rule" on the grounds that a longer time, that is, at least 4 hours, is necessary before concluding that the active phase of labor has failed. We agree.

Second-Stage Disorders

As discussed in Chapter 17 (see p. 389 and Fig. 17-20), fetal descent largely follows complete dilatation. Moreover, the second stage incorporates many of the cardinal movements necessary for the fetus to negotiate the birth canal. Accordingly, disproportion of the fetus and pelvis frequently becomes apparent during second-stage labor.

Until recently, there have been unquestioned second-stage rules that limited its duration. These rules were established in American obstetrics by the beginning of the 20th century. They stemmed from concerns about maternal and fetal health, likely regarding infection and led to difficult forceps operations. The second stage in nulliparas was limited to 2 hours and extended to 3 hours when regional analgesia was used. For multiparas, 1 hour was the limit, extended to 2 hours with regional analgesia. At Parkland Hospital during 1999, only 6 percent of second-stage labors in nulliparas at term exceeded 2 hours.

Cohen (1977) investigated the fetal effects of second-stage labor length at Beth Israel Hospital. He included 4403 term nulliparas in whom electronic fetal heart rate monitoring was performed. The neonatal mortality rate was not increased in women whose second-stage labor exceeded 2 hours. Epidural analgesia was used commonly, and this likely accounted for the large number of pregnancies with a prolonged second stage. These data influenced decisions to permit an additional hour for the second stage when regional analgesia was used.

Menticoglou and colleagues (1995a, b) challenged the prevailing dictums on the duration of the second stage. These arose because of grave neonatal injuries associated with forceps rotations to shorten second-stage labor. As a result, they

allowed a longer second stage to decrease the vaginal operative delivery rate. Between 1988 and 1992, second-stage labor exceeded 2 hours in a fourth of 6041 nulliparas at term. Labor epidural analgesia was used in 55 percent. The length of the second stage, even in those lasting up to 6 hours or more, was not related to neonatal outcome. These results were attributed to careful use of electronic monitoring and scalp pH measurements. These investigators concluded that there is no compelling reason to intervene with a possibly difficult forceps or vacuum extraction because a certain number of hours have elapsed. They observed, however, that after 3 hours in the second stage, delivery by cesarean or other operative method increased progressively. By 5 hours, the prospects for spontaneous delivery in the subsequent hour are only 10 to 15 percent.

Myles and Santolaya (2003) analyzed both the maternal and neonatal consequences of prolonged second-stage labor in 7818 women in Chicago between 1996 and 1999. Maternal outcomes in relation to the duration of second-stage labor are shown in Table 20-3. Neonatal mortality and morbidity rates were not related to the length of the second stage.

Maternal Pushing Efforts. With full cervical dilatation, most women cannot resist the urge to "bear down" or "push" each time the uterus contracts (see Chap. 17, p. 394). The combined force created by contractions of the uterus and abdominal musculature propels the fetus downward. Bloom and colleagues (2006) studied effects of actively coaching expulsive efforts. They reported that although the second stage was slightly shorter in the coached women, there were no other maternal or neonatal advantages.

At times, force created by abdominal musculature is compromised sufficiently to slow or even prevent spontaneous vaginal delivery. Heavy sedation or regional analgesia may reduce the reflex urge to push and may impair the ability to contract abdominal muscles sufficiently. In other instances, the inherent urge to push is overridden by the intense pain created by bearing down. Two approaches to second-stage pushing in women with epidural analgesia have yielded contradictory results. The first advocates pushing forcefully with contractions after complete dilation, regardless of the urge to push. With the second, analgesia infusion is stopped and

TABLE 20-3. Clinical Outcomes in Relation to the Duration of Second-Stage Labor

	Duration of Second Stage		
Clinical Outcome	< 2 hr n = 6259 (%)	2-4 hr n = 384 (%)	> 4 hr n = 148 (%)
Cesarean delivery	1.2	9.2	34.5
Instrumented delivery	3.4	16.0	35.1
Perineal trauma	3.6	13.4	26.7
Postpartum hemorrhage	2.3	5.0	9.1
Chorioamnionitis	2.3	8.9	14.2

Adapted from Myles and Santolaya (2003).

pushing begun only after the woman regains the sensory urge to bear down. Fraser and co-workers (2000) found that delayed pushing reduced difficult operative deliveries, whereas Manyonda and associates (1990) reported the opposite. Hansen and colleagues (2002) randomly assigned 252 women with epidural analgesia to one of the two approaches. There were no adverse maternal or neonatal outcomes linked to delayed pushing despite significantly prolonging second-stage labor. Plunkett and co-workers (2003), in a similar study, confirmed these findings.

Fetal Station at Onset of Active Labor

Descent of the leading edge of the presenting part to the level of the ischial spines (0 station) is defined as engagement. Friedman and Sachtleben (1965, 1976) reported a significant association between higher station at the onset of labor and subsequent dystocia. Handa and Laros (1993) found that fetal station at the time of arrested labor was also a risk factor for dystocia. Roshanfekr and associates (1999) analyzed fetal station in 803 nulliparous women at term in active labor. At admission, approximately 30 percent with the fetal head at or below 0 station had a 5-percent cesarean delivery rate. This is compared with a 14-percent rate for those with higher stations. The prognosis for dystocia, however, was not related to incrementally higher fetal head stations above the pelvic midplane (0 station). Importantly, 86 percent of nulliparous women without fetal head engagement at diagnosis of active labor delivered vaginally. These observations apply especially for parous women because the head typically descends later in labor.

Reported Causes of Uterine Dysfunction

Various labor factors have been implicated as causes of uterine dysfunction.

Epidural Analgesia

It is important to emphasize that epidural analgesia can slow labor (Sharma and Leveno, 2000). As shown in Table 20-4, epidural analgesia has been associated with lengthening of both first- and second-stage labor and with slowing of the rate of fetal descent. This is documented further in Chapter 19 (p. 456).

Chorioamnionitis

Because of the association of prolonged labor with maternal intrapartum infection, some clinicians have suggested that infection itself contributes to abnormal uterine activity. Satin and co-workers (1992) studied the effects of chorioamnionitis on oxytocin stimulation in 266 pregnancies. Infection diagnosed late in labor was found to be a marker of cesarean delivery for dystocia, whereas this was not observed in women diagnosed as having chorioamnionitis early in labor. Specifically, 40 percent of women developing chorioamnionitis after requiring oxytocin for dysfunctional labor later required cesarean delivery for dystocia. It is likely that uterine infection in this clinical setting is a consequence of dysfunctional, prolonged labor rather than a cause of dystocia.

Maternal Position During Labor

Advocacy for recumbency or ambulation during labor has vacillated. Proponents of walking report it to shorten labor, decrease rates of oxytocin augmentation, decrease the need for analgesia, and lower the frequency of operative vaginal delivery (Flynn and co-workers, 1978; Read and colleagues, 1981).

According to Miller (1983), the uterus contracts more frequently but with less intensity with the mother lying on her back rather than on her side. Conversely, contraction frequency and intensity have been reported to increase with sitting or standing. Lupe and Gross (1986) concluded, however, that there is no conclusive evidence that upright maternal posture or ambulation improves labor. They reported that women preferred to lie on their side or sit in bed. Few chose to walk, fewer to squat, and none wanted the knee-chest position. They tended to assume fetal positions in later labor. Most women enthusiastic about ambulation returned to bed when active labor began (Carlson and associates, 1986; Williams and co-workers, 1980).

Bloom and colleagues (1998) conducted a randomized trial to study the effects of walking during first-stage labor. In 1067 women with uncomplicated term pregnancies delivered at Parkland Hospital, these investigators reported that ambulation did not affect labor duration. Ambulation did not reduce the need for analgesia nor was it harmful to the fetus-neonate. Because of these observations, we give women without complications the option of electing either recumbency or supervised ambulation during labor. This policy is in agreement with the American

TABLE 20-4. Effect of Epidural Analgesia on the Progress of Labor in 199 Nulliparous Women Delivered Spontaneously at Parkland Hospital

Labor Characteristics[a]	Epidural Analgesia	Meperidine Analgesia	*p* value
Cervical dilatation at analgesia	4.1 cm	4.2 cm	NS
Active phase	7.9 hr	6.3 hr	.005
Second stage	60 min	48 min	.03
Fetal descent	4.2 cm/hr	7.9 cm/hr	.003

[a]Mean values are listed.
NS = not stated.
Reprinted from *American Journal of Obstetrics & Gynecology*, Vol. 178, No. 3, JM Alexander, MJ Lucas, SM Ramin, et al., The course of labor with and without epidural analgesia, pp. 516–520, Copyright 1998, with permission from Elsevier.

College of Obstetricians and Gynecologists (2003), which has concluded that ambulation in labor is not harmful, and mobility may result in greater comfort.

Birthing Position in Second-Stage Labor

Considerable interest has been shown in alternative second-stage labor birth positions and their effect on labor. Gupta and Hofmeyr (2004) in their Cochrane database review compared upright positions with supine or lithotomy positions. Upright positions included sitting in a "birthing chair," kneeling, squatting, or resting with the back at a 30-degree elevation. With these positions, they found a 4-minute shorter interval to delivery, less pain, and lower incidences of nonreassuring fetal heart rate patterns and of operative vaginal delivery. They did report increased rates of blood loss exceeding 500 mL. Berghella and colleagues (2008) hypothesized that parity, less intense aortocaval compression, improved fetal alignment, and larger pelvic outlet diameters might explain these findings. In an earlier study, Russell (1969) described a 20- to 30-percent increase in the area of the pelvic outlet with squatting compared with that in the supine position. Finally, Babayer and associates (1998) cautioned that prolonged sitting or squatting during the second stage may cause peroneal neuropathy.

Water Immersion

A birthing tub or bath has been advocated as a means of relaxation that may contribute to more efficient labor. Cluett and colleagues (2004) randomly assigned 99 laboring women at term in first-stage labor identified to have dystocia to immersion in a birthing pool or to oxytocin augmentation. Water immersion lowered the rate of epidural analgesia use but did not alter the rate of operative delivery. More infants of women in the immersion group were admitted to the neonatal intensive care unit (NICU). These findings were similar to their Cochrane database review except that NICU admissions were not increased in their review (Cluett and Burns, 2009).

Robertson and associates (1998) reported that immersion was not associated with chorioamnionitis or endometritis. Moreover, Kwee and co-workers (2000) studied the effects of immersion in 20 women and reported that blood pressure decreased, whereas fetal heart rate was unaffected. Neonatal complications unique to underwater birth that have been described include drowning, hyponatremia, waterborne infection, cord rupture, and polycythemia (Austin and colleagues, 1997; Pinette and associates, 2004).

RUPTURED MEMBRANES WITHOUT LABOR

Membrane rupture at term without spontaneous uterine contractions complicates approximately 8 percent of pregnancies. Until recently, management generally included labor stimulation if contractions did not begin after 6 to 12 hours. This intervention evolved approximately 40 years ago because of maternal and fetal complications due to chorioamnionitis (Calkins, 1952). Such routine intervention was the accepted practice until challenged by Kappy and co-workers (1979), who reported excessive cesarean delivery in term pregnancies with

ruptured membranes managed with labor stimulation compared with those expectantly managed.

Hannah (1996) and Peleg (1999) and their associates enrolled a total of 5042 pregnancies with ruptured membranes in a randomized investigation. They measured the effects of induction versus expectant management and also compared induction using intravenous oxytocin with that using prostaglandin E_2 gel. There were approximately 1200 pregnancies in each of the four study arms. They concluded that labor induction with intravenous oxytocin was the preferred management. This determination was based on significantly fewer intrapartum and postpartum infections in women whose labor was induced. There were no significant differences in cesarean delivery rates. Subsequent analysis by Hannah and colleagues (2000) indicated increased adverse outcomes when expectant management at home was compared with in-hospital observation. Mozurkewich and associates (2009) reported lower rates of chorioamnionitis, metritis, and NICU admissions for women with term ruptured membranes whose labors were induced compared with those managed expectantly. At Parkland Hospital, labor is induced soon after admission when ruptured membranes are confirmed at term.

PRECIPITOUS LABOR AND DELIVERY

Not only can labor be too slow, but it also can be abnormally rapid. *Precipitous labor* is extremely rapid labor and delivery. It may result from an abnormally low resistance of the soft parts of the birth canal, from abnormally strong uterine and abdominal contractions, or *rarely* from the absence of painful sensations and thus a lack of awareness of vigorous labor.

Definition and Incidence

According to Hughes (1972), precipitous labor terminates in expulsion of the fetus in less than 3 hours. Using this definition, 89,047 live births—2 percent—were complicated by precipitous labor in the United States during 2006 (Martin and co-workers, 2009). Despite this incidence, there is little published information concerning adverse effects.

Maternal Effects

Precipitous labor and delivery seldom are accompanied by serious maternal complications if the cervix is effaced appreciably and compliant, if the vagina has been stretched previously, and if the perineum is relaxed. Conversely, vigorous uterine contractions combined with a long, firm cervix and a noncompliant birth canal may lead to uterine rupture or extensive lacerations of the cervix, vagina, vulva, or perineum. It is in these latter circumstances that the rare condition of *amnionic fluid embolism* most likely develops (see Chap. 35, p. 788). **The uterus that contracts with unusual vigor before delivery is likely to be hypotonic after delivery, with hemorrhage from the placental implantation site as the consequence.** Postpartum hemorrhage from uterine atony is discussed in Chapter 35 (p. 774).

Mahon and colleagues (1994) described 99 pregnancies delivered within 3 hours of labor onset. *Short labors* were defined as a rate of cervical dilatation of 5 cm/hr or faster for nulliparas and 10 cm/hr for multiparas. Such short labors were more common in multiparas who typically had contractions at intervals less than 2 minutes and were associated with placental abruption, meconium, postpartum hemorrhage, cocaine abuse, and low Apgar scores.

Fetal and Neonatal Effects

Adverse perinatal outcomes from precipitous labor may be increased considerably for several reasons. The tumultuous uterine contractions, often with negligible intervals of relaxation, prevent appropriate uterine blood flow and fetal oxygenation. Resistance of the birth canal may rarely cause intracranial trauma. Acker and colleagues (1988) reported that Erb or Duchenne brachial palsy was associated with such labors in a third of cases (see Chap. 29, p. 636). Finally, during an unattended birth, the newborn may fall to the floor and be injured, or it may need resuscitation that is not immediately available.

Treatment

Unusually forceful spontaneous uterine contractions are not likely to be modified to a significant degree by analgesia. The use of tocolytic agents such as magnesium sulfate is unproven in these circumstances. Use of general anesthesia with agents that impair uterine contractibility, such as isoflurane, is often excessively heroic. Certainly, any oxytocin agents being administered should be stopped immediately.

FETOPELVIC DISPROPORTION

Fetopelvic disproportion arises from diminished pelvic capacity, excessive fetal size, or more usually, a combination of both.

Pelvic Capacity

Any contraction of the pelvic diameters that diminishes its capacity can create dystocia during labor. There may be contractions of the pelvic inlet, the midpelvis, or the pelvic outlet, or a generally contracted pelvis may be caused by combinations of these. Normal pelvic dimension are additionally discussed in Chapter 2 (p. 31).

Contracted Inlet

The pelvic inlet usually is considered to be contracted if its shortest anteroposterior diameter is less than 10 cm or if the greatest transverse diameter is less than 12 cm. The anteroposterior diameter of the inlet is commonly approximated by manually measuring the diagonal conjugate, which is approximately 1.5 cm greater (see Chap. 2, p. 31). Therefore, inlet contraction usually is defined as a diagonal conjugate of less than 11.5 cm.

Using clinical and at times, imaging pelvimetry, it is important to identify the shortest anteroposterior diameter through which the fetal head must pass. Occasionally, the body of the first sacral vertebra is displaced forward so that the shortest distance may actually be between this abnormal sacral promontory and the symphysis pubis.

Prior to labor, the fetal biparietal diameter has been shown to *average* from 9.5 to as much as 9.8 cm. Therefore, it might prove difficult or even impossible for some fetuses to pass through an inlet that has an anteroposterior diameter of less than 10 cm. Mengert (1948) and Kaltreider (1952), employing x-ray pelvimetry, demonstrated that the incidence of difficult deliveries is increased to a similar degree when either the anteroposterior diameter of the inlet is less than 10 cm or the transverse diameter is less than 12 cm. As expected, when both diameters are contracted, dystocia is much greater than when only one is contracted.

A small woman is likely to have a small pelvis, but she is also likely to have a small neonate. Thoms (1937) studied 362 nulliparas and found the mean birthweight of their offspring was significantly lower—280 g—in women with a small pelvis than in those with a medium or large pelvis. In veterinary obstetrics, in most species, maternal size rather than paternal size is the important determinant of fetal size.

Normally, cervical dilatation is aided by hydrostatic action of the unruptured membranes or after their rupture, by direct application of the presenting part against the cervix (see Fig. 6-8, p. 145). In contracted pelves, however, because the head is arrested in the pelvic inlet, the entire force exerted by the uterus acts directly on the portion of membranes that contact the dilating cervix. Consequently, early spontaneous rupture of the membranes is more likely.

After membrane rupture, absent pressure by the head against the cervix and lower uterine segment predisposes to less effective contractions. Hence, further dilatation may proceed very slowly or not at all. Cibils and Hendricks (1965) reported that the mechanical adaptation of the fetal passenger to the bony passage plays an important part in determining the efficiency of contractions. The better the adaptation, the more efficient are the contractions. Thus, cervical response to labor provides a prognostic view of labor outcome in women with inlet contraction.

A contracted inlet plays an important part in the production of abnormal presentations. In normal nulliparas, the presenting part at term commonly descends into the pelvic cavity before the onset of labor. When the inlet is contracted considerably, however, descent usually does not take place until after labor onset, if at all. Cephalic presentations still predominate, but the head floats freely over the pelvic inlet or rests more laterally in one of the iliac fossae. Accordingly, very slight influences may cause the fetus to assume other presentations. *In women with contracted pelves, face and shoulder presentations are encountered three times more frequently, and the cord prolapses four to six times more often.*

Contracted Midpelvis

This finding is more common than inlet contraction. It frequently causes transverse arrest of the fetal head, which potentially can lead to a difficult midforceps operation or to cesarean delivery.

The obstetrical plane of the midpelvis extends from the inferior margin of the symphysis pubis through the ischial spines and touches the sacrum near the junction of the fourth and fifth vertebrae (see Chap. 2, p. 32). A transverse line theoretically connecting the ischial spines divides the midpelvis into anterior and posterior portions. The former is bounded anteriorly by the lower border of the symphysis pubis and laterally by the ischiopubic rami. The posterior portion is bounded dorsally by the sacrum and laterally by the sacrospinous ligaments, forming the lower limits of the sacrosciatic notch.

Average midpelvis measurements are as follows: *transverse,* or interischial spinous, 10.5 cm; *anteroposterior,* from the lower border of the symphysis pubis to the junction of S4-S5, 11.5 cm; and *posterior sagittal,* from the midpoint of the interspinous line to the same point on the sacrum, 5 cm. The definition of midpelvic contractions has not been established with the same precision possible for inlet contractions. Even so, the midpelvis is likely contracted when the sum of the interspinous and posterior sagittal diameters of the midpelvis—normal, 10.5 plus 5 cm, or 15.5 cm—falls to 13.5 cm or less. This concept was emphasized by Chen and Huang (1982) in evaluating possible midpelvic contraction. There is reason to suspect midpelvic contraction whenever the interspinous diameter is less than 10 cm. When it measures less than 8 cm, the midpelvis is contracted.

Although there is no precise manual method of measuring midpelvic dimensions, a suggestion of contraction sometimes can be inferred if the spines are prominent, the pelvic sidewalls converge, or the sacrosciatic notch is narrow. Moreover, Eller and Mengert (1948) noted that the relationship between the intertuberous and interspinous diameters of the ischium is sufficiently constant that narrowing of the interspinous diameter can be anticipated when the intertuberous diameter is narrow. A normal intertuberous diameter, however, does not always exclude a narrow interspinous diameter.

Contracted Outlet

This finding usually is defined as an interischial tuberous diameter of 8 cm or less. The pelvic outlet may be roughly likened to two triangles, with the interischial tuberous diameter constituting the base of both. The sides of the anterior triangle are the pubic rami, and its apex is the inferoposterior surface of the symphysis pubis. The posterior triangle has no bony sides but is limited at its apex by the tip of the last sacral vertebra—not the tip of the coccyx. Diminution of the intertuberous diameter with consequent narrowing of the anterior triangle must inevitably force the fetal head posteriorly. Floberg and associates (1987) reported that outlet contractions were found in almost 1 percent of more than 1400 unselected nulliparas with term pregnancies. A contracted outlet may cause dystocia not so much by itself as through the often-associated midpelvic contraction. *Outlet contraction without concomitant midplane contraction is rare.*

Although the disproportion between the fetal head and the pelvic outlet is not sufficiently great to give rise to severe dystocia, it may play an important part in the production of perineal tears. With increasing narrowing of the pubic arch, the occiput cannot emerge directly beneath the symphysis pubis but is forced increasingly farther down upon the ischiopubic rami. The perineum, consequently, becomes increasingly distended and thus exposed to greater danger of laceration.

Pelvic Fractures

Speer and Peltier (1972) reviewed experiences with pelvic fractures and pregnancy. Trauma from automobile collisions was the most common cause of pelvic fractures. With bilateral fractures of the pubic rami, compromise of the birth canal capacity by callus formation or malunion was common. A history of pelvic fracture warrants careful review of previous radiographs and possibly computed tomographic pelvimetry later in pregnancy.

Estimation of Pelvic Capacity

The techniques for clinical evaluation using digital examination of the bony pelvis during labor are described in detail in Chapter 2 (p. 31). Briefly, the examiner attempts to judge the anteroposterior diameter of the inlet—the diagonal conjugate, the interspinous diameter of the midpelvis, and the intertuberous distances of the pelvic outlet. A narrow pelvic arch of less than 90 degrees can signify a narrow pelvis. An unengaged fetal head can indicate either excessive fetal head size or reduced pelvic inlet capacity.

X-Ray Pelvimetry. Even when widely used, the prognosis for successful vaginal delivery in any given pregnancy cannot be established using x-ray pelvimetry alone (Mengert, 1948). Thus, x-ray pelvimetry is considered to be of limited value in the management of labor with a cephalic presentation (American College of Obstetricians and Gynecologists, 1995b).

Computed Tomographic (CT) Scanning. Advantages of CT pelvimetry, such as that shown in Figure 20-4, compared with those of conventional x-ray pelvimetry include reduced radiation exposure, greater accuracy, and easier performance. With either method, costs are comparable and x-ray exposure is small (see Chap. 41, p. 918). With conventional x-ray pelvimetry, the mean gonadal exposure is estimated by the Committee on Radiological Hazards to Patients to be 885 mrad (Osborn, 1963). Depending on the machine and technique employed, fetal doses with computed tomography may range from 250 to 1500 mrad (Moore and Shearer, 1989).

Magnetic Resonance (MR) Imaging. The advantages of MR pelvimetry include lack of ionizing radiation, accurate measurements, complete fetal imaging, and the potential for evaluating soft tissue dystocia (McCarthy, 1986; Stark and coworkers, 1985). Zaretsky and colleagues (2005) used MR imaging to measure pelvic and fetal head volume in an effort to identify those women at greatest risk of undergoing cesarean delivery for dystocia. Although significant associations were found with some of the measures and cesarean delivery for dystocia, they could not with accuracy predict which woman would require cesarean delivery. Others have reported similar findings (Sporri and co-workers, 1997).

Fetal Dimensions in Fetopelvic Disproportion

Fetal size alone is seldom a suitable explanation for failed labor. Even with the evolution of current technology, a fetal size threshold to predict fetopelvic disproportion is still elusive. Most cases of disproportion arise in fetuses whose weight is well within the range of the general obstetrical population. As shown

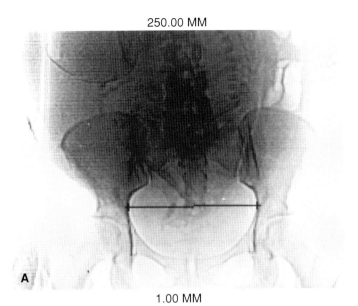

A

1.00 MM

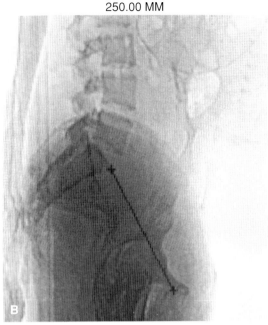

B

1.00 MM

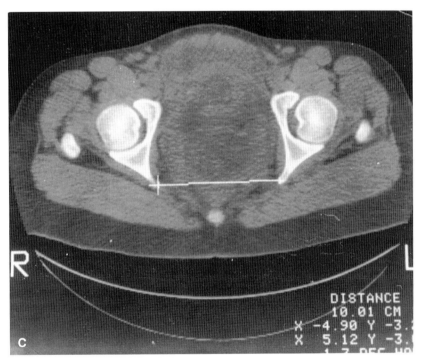

C

DISTANCE
10.01 CM
X -4.90 Y -3.
X 5.12 Y -3.

FIGURE 20-4 A. Anteroposterior view of a digital radiograph. Illustrated is the measurement of the transverse diameter of the pelvic inlet using an electronic cursor. The fetal body is clearly outlined. **B.** Lateral view of a digital radiograph. Illustrated are measurements of the anteroposterior diameters of the inlet using the electronic cursor. **C.** An axial computed tomographic section through the midpelvis. The level of the fovea of the femoral heads was ascertained from the anteroposterior digital radiograph because it corresponds to the level of the ischial spines. The interspinous diameter is measured using the electronic cursor. The total fetal radiation dose using the three exposures shown in parts **(A-C)** is approximately 250 mrad.

in Figure 20-5, two thirds of neonates who required cesarean delivery after failed forceps delivery weighed less than 3700 g. Thus, other factors, such as malposition of the head, obstruct fetal passage through the birth canal. These include asynclitism, occiput posterior position, and face and brow presentations.

Estimation of Fetal Head Size

Efforts to clinically and radiographically predict fetopelvic disproportion based on fetal head size have proved disappointing. Müller (1880) and Hillis (1930) described a clinical maneuver to predict disproportion. The fetal brow and the suboccipital

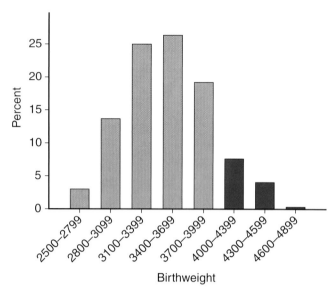

FIGURE 20-5 Birthweight distribution of 362 newborns delivered by cesarean at Parkland Hospital (1989–1999) after a failed attempt to effect vaginal delivery with forceps. Only 12 percent (n = 44) of the newborns weighed > 4000 g (*dark bars*).

region are grasped through the abdominal wall with the fingers, and firm pressure is directed downward in the axis of the inlet. If no disproportion exists, the head readily enters the pelvis, and vaginal delivery can be predicted. Thorp and colleagues (1993b) performed a prospective evaluation of the *Mueller-Hillis maneuver* and concluded that there was no relationship between dystocia and failed descent during the maneuver.

Measurements of fetal head diameters using plain radiographic techniques are not used because of parallax distortions. The biparietal diameter and head circumference can be measured sonographically, and there have been attempts to use this information in the management of dystocia. Thurnau and co-workers (1991) used the *fetal-pelvic index* to identify labor complications. Unfortunately, the sensitivity of such measurements to predict cephalopelvic disproportion is poor (Ferguson and associates, 1998). We are of the view that there is no currently satisfactory method for accurate prediction of fetopelvic disproportion based on head size.

Face Presentation

With this presentation, the head is hyperextended so that the occiput is in contact with the fetal back, and the chin (mentum) is presenting **(Fig. 20-6)**. The fetal face may present with the chin (mentum) anteriorly or posteriorly, relative to the maternal symphysis pubis (see Chap. 17, p. 379). Although many may persist, many mentum posterior presentations convert spontaneously to anterior even in late labor (Duff, 1981). If not, the fetal brow (bregma) is pressed against the maternal symphysis pubis. This position precludes flexion of the fetal head necessary to negotiate the birth canal.

Cruikshank and White (1973) reported an incidence of 1 in 600, or 0.17 percent. As shown in Table 17-1 (p. 375), among more than 70,000 singleton newborns delivered at Parkland, approximately 1 in 2000 had a face presentation at delivery.

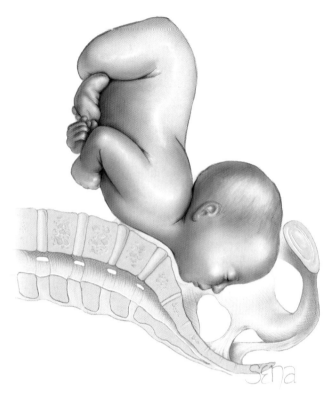

FIGURE 20-6 Face presentation. The occiput is the longer end of the head lever. The chin is directly posterior. Vaginal delivery is impossible unless the chin rotates anteriorly.

Etiology. Causes of face presentations are numerous and include conditions that favor extension or prevent head flexion. Preterm infants, with their smaller head dimensions, can engage prior to conversion to vertex position (Shaffer and associates, 2006b). In exceptional instances, marked enlargement of the neck or coils of cord around the neck may cause extension. Bashiri and colleagues (2008) reported that fetal malformations and hydramnios were risk factors for face or brow presentations. Anencephalic fetuses naturally present by the face.

Extended positions develop more frequently when the pelvis is contracted or the fetus is very large. In a series of 141 face presentations studied by Hellman and co-workers (1950), the incidence of inlet contraction was 40 percent. This high incidence of pelvic contraction should be kept in mind when considering management.

High parity is a predisposing factor to face presentation (Fuchs and colleagues, 1985). In these cases, a pendulous abdomen permits the back of the fetus to sag forward or laterally, often in the same direction in which the occiput points. This promotes extension of the cervical and thoracic spine.

Diagnosis. Face presentation is diagnosed by vaginal examination and palpation of facial features. As discussed in Chapter 24 (p. 528), it is possible to mistake a breech for a face presentation because the anus may be mistaken for the mouth and the ischial tuberosities for the malar prominences. The radiographic demonstration of the hyperextended head with the facial bones at or below the pelvic inlet is characteristic.

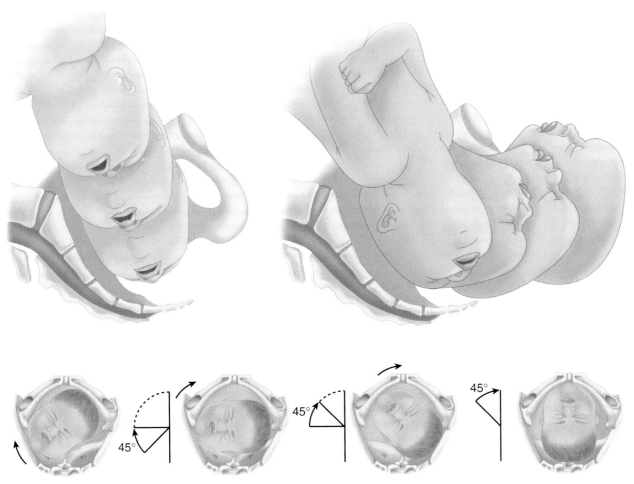

FIGURE 20-7 Mechanism of labor for right mentoposterior position with subsequent rotation of the mentum anteriorly and delivery.

Mechanism of Labor. Face presentations rarely are observed above the pelvic inlet. Instead, the brow generally presents early and is usually converted to present the face after further extension of the head during descent. The mechanism of labor in these cases consists of the cardinal movements of descent, internal rotation, and flexion, and the accessory movements of extension and external rotation (Fig. 20-7). Descent is brought about by the same factors as in cephalic presentations. Extension results from the relation of the fetal body to the deflected head, which is converted into a two-armed lever, the longer arm of which extends from the occipital condyles to the occiput. When resistance is encountered, the occiput must be pushed toward the back of the fetus while the chin descends.

The objective of internal rotation of the face is to bring the chin under the symphysis pubis. Only in this way can the neck traverse the posterior surface of the symphysis pubis. If the chin rotates directly posteriorly, the relatively short neck cannot span the anterior surface of the sacrum, which measures about 12 cm in length. Moreover, the fetal brow (bregma) is pressed against the maternal symphysis pubis. This position precludes flexion necessary to negotiate the birth canal. Hence, birth of the head from a mentum posterior position is impossible unless the shoulders enter the pelvis at the same time, an event that is

impossible except when the fetus is extremely small or macerated. Internal rotation results from the same factors as in vertex presentations.

After anterior rotation and descent, the chin and mouth appear at the vulva, the undersurface of the chin presses against the symphysis, and the head is delivered by flexion (see Fig. 20-8). The nose, eyes, brow (bregma), and occiput then appear in succession over the anterior margin of the perineum. After birth of the head, the occiput sags backward toward the anus. Next, the chin rotates externally to the side toward which it was originally directed, and the shoulders are born as in cephalic presentations.

Edema may sometimes significantly distort the face. At the same time, the skull undergoes considerable molding, manifested by an increase in length of the occipitomental diameter of the head.

Management. In the absence of a contracted pelvis, and with effective labor, successful vaginal delivery usually will follow. Fetal heart rate monitoring is probably better done with external devices to avoid damage to the face and eyes. Because face presentations among term-size fetuses are more common when there is some degree of pelvic inlet contraction, cesarean delivery

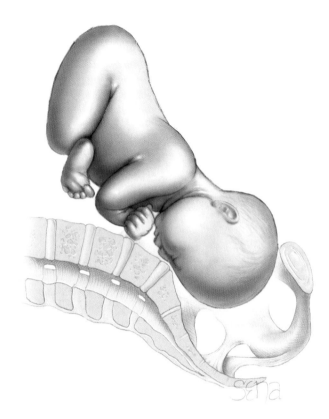

FIGURE 20-8 Brow posterior presentation.

frequently is indicated. Attempts to convert a face presentation manually into a vertex presentation, manual or forceps rotation of a persistently posterior chin to a mentum anterior position, and internal podalic version and extraction are dangerous and not attempted.

Brow Presentation

This rare presentation is diagnosed when that portion of the fetal head between the orbital ridge and the anterior fontanel presents at the pelvic inlet. As shown in **Figure 20-8**, the fetal head thus occupies a position midway between full flexion (occiput) and extension (face). Except when the fetal head is small or the pelvis is unusually large, engagement of the fetal head and subsequent delivery cannot take place as long as the brow presentation persists.

Etiology and Diagnosis. The causes of persistent brow presentation are the same as those for face presentation. A brow presentation is commonly unstable and often converts to a face or an occiput presentation (Cruikshank and White, 1973). The presentation may be recognized by abdominal palpation when both the occiput and chin can be palpated easily, but vaginal examination is usually necessary. The frontal sutures, large anterior fontanel, orbital ridges, eyes, and root of the nose are felt on vaginal examination, but neither the mouth nor the chin is palpable.

Mechanism of Labor. With a very small fetus and a large pelvis, labor is generally easy, but with a larger fetus, it is usually difficult. This is because engagement is impossible until there is

marked molding that shortens the occipitomental diameter or more commonly, until there is either flexion to an occiput presentation or extension to a face presentation. The considerable molding essential for vaginal delivery of a persistent brow characteristically deforms the head. The caput succedaneum is over the forehead, and it may be so extensive that identification of the brow by palpation is impossible. In these instances, the forehead is prominent and squared, and the occipitomental diameter is diminished.

In transient brow presentations, the prognosis depends on the ultimate presentation. If the brow persists, prognosis is poor for vaginal delivery unless the fetus is small or the birth canal is large. Principles of management are the same as those for a face presentation.

Transverse Lie

In this position, the long axis of the fetus is approximately perpendicular to that of the mother. When the long axis forms an acute angle, an *oblique lie* results. The latter is usually only transitory, because either a longitudinal or transverse lie commonly results when labor supervenes. For this reason, the oblique lie is called an *unstable lie* in Great Britain.

In a transverse lie, the shoulder is usually positioned over the pelvic inlet. The head occupies one iliac fossa, and the breech the other. This creates a *shoulder presentation* in which the side of the mother on which the acromion rests determines the designation of the lie as right or left acromial. And because in either position the back may be directed anteriorly or posteriorly, superiorly or inferiorly, it is customary to distinguish varieties as dorsoanterior and dorsoposterior (**Fig. 20-9**).

Transverse lie was found once in 322 singleton deliveries (0.3 percent) at both the Mayo Clinic and the University of Iowa Hospital (Cruikshank and White, 1973; Johnson, 1964). This is remarkably similar to the incidence at Parkland Hospital of approximately 1 in 335 singleton fetuses.

Etiology. Some of the more common causes of transverse lie include: (1) abdominal wall relaxation from high parity, (2) preterm fetus, (3) placenta previa, (4) abnormal uterine anatomy, (5) hydramnios, and (6) contracted pelvis.

Women with four or more deliveries have a 10-fold incidence of transverse lie compared with nulliparas. A relaxed and pendulous abdomen allows the uterus to fall forward, deflecting the long axis of the fetus away from the axis of the birth canal and into an oblique or transverse position. Placenta previa and pelvic contraction act similarly. A transverse or oblique lie occasionally develops in labor from an initial longitudinal position.

Diagnosis. A transverse lie is usually recognized easily, often by inspection alone. The abdomen is unusually wide, whereas the uterine fundus extends to only slightly above the umbilicus. No fetal pole is detected in the fundus, and the ballottable head is found in one iliac fossa and the breech in the other. The position of the back is readily identifiable. When the back is anterior (see Fig. 20-9), a hard resistance plane extends across the front of the abdomen. When it is posterior, irregular nodulations representing fetal small parts are felt through the abdominal wall.

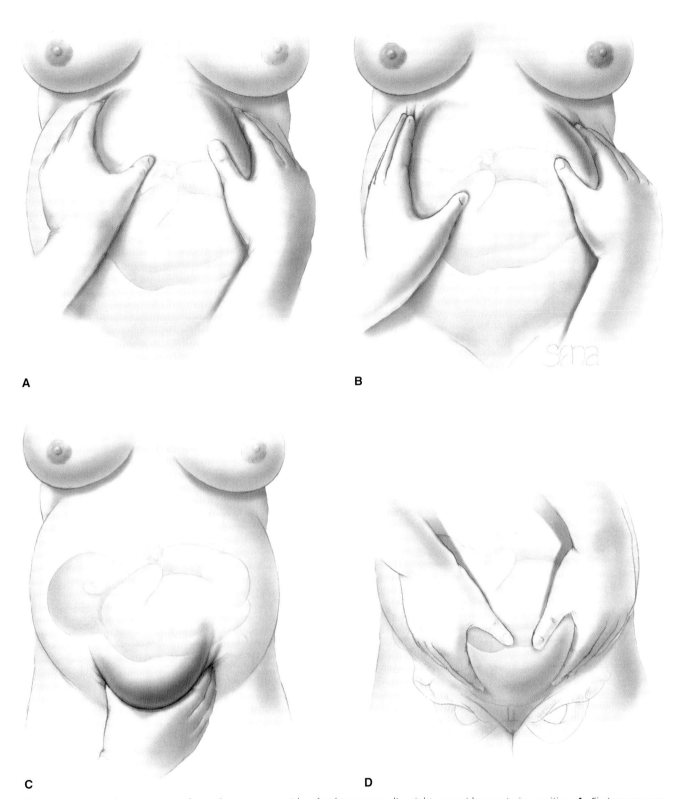

A

B

C

D

FIGURE 20-9 Leopold maneuver performed on women with a fetal transverse lie, right acromidorsoanterior position. **A.** First maneuver. **B.** Second maneuver. **C.** Third maneuver. **D.** Fourth maneuver.

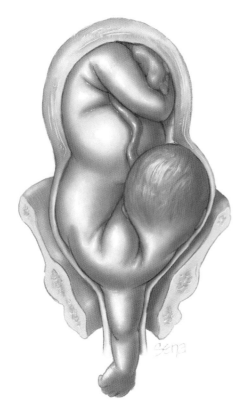

FIGURE 20-10 Neglected shoulder presentation. A thick muscular band forming a pathological retraction ring has developed just above the thin lower uterine segment. The force generated during a uterine contraction is directed centripetally at and above the level of the pathological retraction ring. This serves to stretch further and possibly to rupture the thin lower segment below the retraction ring.

On vaginal examination, in the early stages of labor, if the side of the thorax can be reached, it may be recognized by the "gridiron" feel of the ribs. With further dilatation, the scapula and the clavicle are distinguished on opposite sides of the thorax. The position of the axilla indicates the side of the mother toward which the shoulder is directed.

Mechanism of Labor. Spontaneous delivery of a fully developed newborn is impossible with a persistent transverse lie. After rupture of the membranes, if labor continues, the fetal shoulder is forced into the pelvis, and the corresponding arm frequently prolapses (Fig. 20-10). After some descent, the shoulder is arrested by the margins of the pelvic inlet, with the head in one iliac fossa and the breech in the other. As labor continues, the shoulder is impacted firmly in the upper part of the pelvis. The uterus then contracts vigorously in an unsuccessful attempt to overcome the obstacle. With time, a retraction ring rises increasingly higher and becomes more marked. With this *neglected transverse lie,* the uterus will eventually rupture. Even without this complication, morbidity is increased because of the frequent association with placenta previa, the increased likelihood of cord prolapse, and the necessity for major operative efforts.

If the fetus is small—usually less than 800 g—and the pelvis is large, spontaneous delivery is possible despite persistence of

the abnormal lie. The fetus is compressed with the head forced against its abdomen. A portion of the thoracic wall below the shoulder thus becomes the most dependent part, appearing at the vulva. The head and thorax then pass through the pelvic cavity at the same time. The fetus, which is doubled upon itself and thus sometimes referred to as *conduplicato corpore,* is expelled.

Management. Active labor in a woman with a transverse lie is usually an indication for cesarean delivery. Before labor or early in labor, with the membranes intact, attempts at external version are worthwhile in the absence of other complications. If the fetal head can be maneuvered by abdominal manipulation into the pelvis, it should be held there during the next several contractions in an attempt to fix the head in the pelvis.

With cesarean delivery, because neither the feet nor the head of the fetus occupies the lower uterine segment, a low transverse incision into the uterus may lead to difficult fetal extraction. This is especially true of dorsoanterior presentations. Therefore, a vertical incision is typically indicated (see Chap. 25, p. 555).

Compound Presentation

In a compound presentation, an extremity prolapses alongside the presenting part, and both present simultaneously in the pelvis (Fig. 20-11).

Incidence and Etiology. Goplerud and Eastman (1953) identified a hand or arm prolapsed alongside the head once in every 700 deliveries. Much less common was prolapse of one or both lower extremities alongside a cephalic presentation or a hand

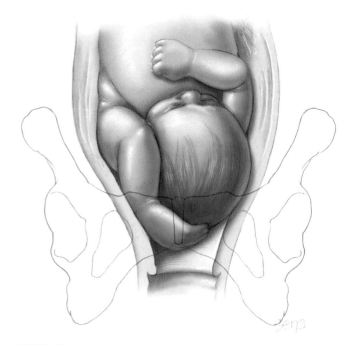

FIGURE 20-11 Compound presentation. The left hand is lying in front of the vertex. With further labor, the hand and arm may retract from the birth canal, and the head may then descend normally.

alongside a breech. At Parkland Hospital, compound presentations were identified in only 68 of more than 70,000 singleton fetuses—an incidence of approximately 1 in 1000. Causes of compound presentations are conditions that prevent complete occlusion of the pelvic inlet by the fetal head, including preterm labor (Goplerud and Eastman, 1953).

Management and Prognosis. In most cases, the prolapsed part should be left alone, because most often it will not interfere with labor. If the arm is prolapsed alongside the head, the condition should be observed closely to ascertain whether the arm retracts out of the way with descent of the presenting part. If it fails to retract and if it appears to prevent descent of the head, the prolapsed arm should be pushed gently upward and the head simultaneously downward by fundal pressure. Tebes and co-workers (1999) described a tragic outcome in a newborn delivered spontaneously with the hand alongside the head. The infant developed ischemic necrosis of the presenting forearm, which required amputation. In general, rates of perinatal mortality and morbidity are increased as a result of concomitant preterm delivery, prolapsed cord, and traumatic obstetrical procedures.

Persistent Occiput Posterior Position

Most occiput posterior positions undergo spontaneous anterior rotation followed by uncomplicated delivery. Although the precise reasons for failure of spontaneous rotation are not known, transverse narrowing of the midpelvis is undoubtedly a contributing factor. Gardberg and associates (1998) used sonography to record the position of the fetal head in 408 term pregnancies at entry into labor (Fig. 20-12). Early in labor, approximately 15 percent of fetuses were occiput posterior, and 5 percent were in this position at delivery. Importantly, two thirds of occiput posterior deliveries occurred with fetuses who were occiput anterior at the beginning of labor. Thus, most occiput posterior presentations at delivery are the result of malrotation of occiput anterior position during labor, and almost 90 percent of occiput posterior presentations at the outset of labor spontaneously rotate anteriorly.

Labor and delivery need not differ remarkably from that with the occiput anterior. Progress may be determined by assessing cervical dilatation and descent of the head. In most instances, delivery usually can be accomplished without great difficulty once the head reaches the perineum. The possibilities for vaginal delivery are: (1) spontaneous delivery, (2) forceps delivery with the occiput posterior, (3) manual rotation to the occiput anterior followed by spontaneous or forceps delivery, and (4) forceps rotation to occiput anterior and delivery.

Spontaneous Delivery. If the pelvic outlet is roomy and the vaginal outlet and perineum are somewhat relaxed from previous deliveries, rapid spontaneous delivery often will take place. If the vaginal outlet is resistant to stretch and the perineum is firm, late first-stage or second-stage labor or both may be appreciably prolonged. During each expulsive effort, the head is driven against the perineum to a much greater degree than when anterior. Therefore, forceps delivery often is indicated. A generous episiotomy usually is needed.

Forceps Delivery as an Occiput Posterior. The need for more traction can be minimized if perineal resistance is lowered by creating a larger episiotomy. The use of forceps and a large episiotomy warrant more complete analgesia than may be achieved with pudendal block and local perineal infiltration. The forceps are applied bilaterally along the occipitomental diameter, as described in Chapter 23 (p. 516).

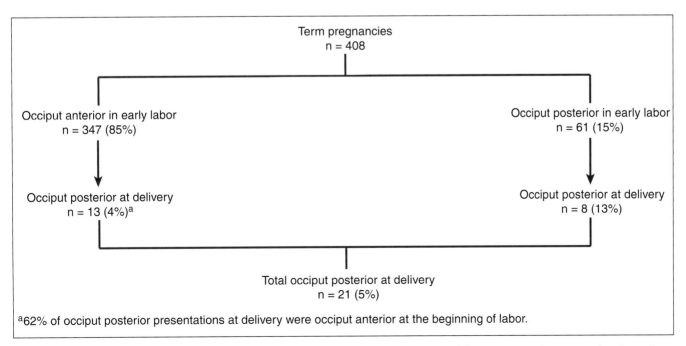

FIGURE 20-12 Occiput posterior presentation in early labor compared with presentation at delivery. Sonography was used to determine position of the fetal head in early labor. (From Gardberg and associates, 1998.)

Infrequently, protrusion of fetal scalp through the introitus is the consequence of marked elongation of the fetal head from molding combined with formation of a large caput succedaneum. In some cases, the head may not even be engaged—that is, the biparietal diameter may not have passed through the pelvic inlet. In these, labor is characteristically long and descent of the head is slow. Careful palpation above the symphysis may disclose the fetal head to be above the pelvic inlet. Prompt cesarean delivery is appropriate.

Manual Rotation. The requirements for forceps rotation must be met before performing a manual rotation. When the hand is introduced to locate the posterior ear and thus confirm the posterior position, the occiput often spontaneously rotates toward the anterior position. If not, the head may be grasped with the fingers over one ear and the thumb over the other and rotation of the occiput to the anterior position attempted (see Chap. 23, p. 516). Shaffer and associates (2006a) performed manual rotation in 742 women with fetuses in occiput posterior or occiput transverse positions. Of those successfully rotated, only 2 percent required cesarean delivery.

Forceps Rotation. If the head is engaged, the cervix fully dilated, and the pelvis adequate, forceps rotation may be attempted. These circumstances most likely prevail when expulsive efforts of the mother during the second stage are ineffective. Rotation with forceps is described in Chapter 23 p. 517).

Menticoglou and co-workers (1995b) reviewed the obstetrical features of 15 newborns with birth-related high-cervical spinal cord injuries in 13 Canadian hospitals between 1982 and 1994. All of these neonates underwent cephalic delivery with forceps rotation of 90 degrees or more from occipitoposterior or occipitotransverse positions. Investigators could not determine whether these serious, albeit rare, fetal injuries resulted from mismanagement or from an intrinsic risk of properly performed forceps rotation. They estimated that this complication developed in less than 1 per 1000 forceps rotations.

Outcome. There are notable differences when persistent occiput posterior position is compared with the occiput anterior. Cheng and colleagues (2006) compared outcomes of 2591 women with persistent occiput position to those of 28,801 women with occiput anterior presentations. Virtually every possible delivery complication was found more frequently with a persistent occiput posterior. Only 46 percent of these women delivered spontaneously, and they accounted for 9 percent of cesarean deliveries performed. In addition, occiput posterior position at delivery was associated with increased adverse short-term neonatal outcomes. Similar results were reported by Ponkey (2003) and Fitzpatrick (2001) and their associates.

At Parkland Hospital, spontaneous delivery is preferred. Either manual rotation to the anterior position followed by forceps delivery or forceps delivery from the occiput posterior position is used for the others. If neither can be completed with relative ease, cesarean delivery is performed.

Persistent Occiput Transverse Position

In the absence of a pelvic architecture abnormality or asynclitism, the occiput transverse position is usually transitory. Thus, unless contractions are hypotonic, spontaneous anterior rotation usually is completed rapidly.

Delivery. If rotation ceases because of poor expulsive forces and pelvic contractures are absent, vaginal delivery usually can be accomplished readily in a number of ways. The easiest is that the occiput may be manually rotated anteriorly or posteriorly. If successful, Le Ray and co-workers (2007) reported a 4-percent cesarean delivery rate compared with nearly 60-percent in women who failed manual rotation. Alternatively, some clinicians apply Kielland forceps to the occiput transverse position as described in Chapter 23 (p. 517). These forceps are used to rotate the occiput to the anterior position. The head is delivered either with the same forceps or with Simpson or Tucker–McLane forceps. If spontaneous rotation fails because of hypotonic uterine contractions *without cephalopelvic disproportion,* oxytocin may be infused and closely monitored.

The genesis of the occiput transverse position is not always so simple or the treatment so benign. With the platypelloid (anteroposteriorly flattened) and the android (heart-shaped) pelves, there may not be adequate room for rotation of the occiput to either the anterior or the posterior position (see Fig. 2-24, p. 33). With the android pelvis, the head may not even be engaged, yet the scalp may be visible through the vaginal introitus as the consequence of considerable molding and caput formation. Consequently, if forceps delivery is attempted, undue force should be avoided.

Dystocia from Hydrocephalus

Macrocephaly from excessive accumulation of cerebrospinal fluid may prohibit vaginal delivery. Normal fetal head circumference at term ranges between 32 and 38 cm. With hydrocephalus, the circumference often exceeds 50 cm and may reach 80 cm. Fluid volume is usually between 500 and 1500 mL but as much as 5 L may accumulate. For a number of reasons, discussed in Chapter 13 (p. 287), it is uncommon with births at term. Associated defects are frequent, especially neural-tube defects. Breech presentation is found in at least a third of fetuses and may present problems in undiagnosed cases (**Fig. 20-13**).

Management. If the biparietal diameter (BPD) is < 10 cm or if the head circumference is < 36 cm, vaginal delivery may be permitted (Anteby and Yagel, 2003). In many cases, however, the macrocephalic head must be reduced in size to deliver it. Even with cesarean delivery, it may be desirable to remove cerebrospinal fluid just before incising the uterus to circumvent extensions of a low transverse or vertical incision or to avoid deliberately creating a long vertical uterine incision. Removal of fluid by *cephalocentesis* was a mainstay in the historical intrapartum management of hydrocephalus, but it has come under considerable scrutiny in recent years. Chervenak and colleagues (1985) described results of cephalocentesis in 11 fetuses for whom the procedure was used to permit vaginal or cesarean delivery. Ten of these fetuses died either in utero or within 3 hours of delivery. Seven had intracranial bleeding at autopsy. Chervenak

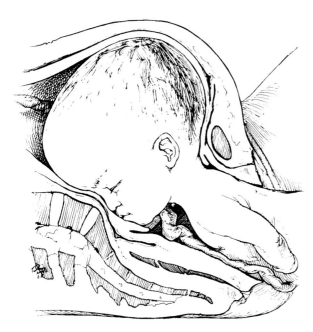

FIGURE 20-13 Severe dystocia from hydrocephalus and breech presentation. Note the distension of the lower uterine segment.

and McCullough (1986) and Chasen and associates (2001) advocate that cephalocentesis use be limited to fetuses with severe associated abnormalities. They recommended that all others be delivered abdominally. Such management requires precise knowledge of the extent of fetal malformations, which is not always possible.

Fetal Abdominal Distension

Enlargement of the fetal abdomen sufficient to cause dystocia is usually the result of a *greatly distended bladder, ascites,* or *enlargement of the kidneys or liver.* Occasionally, the edematous fetal abdomen may attain such proportions that spontaneous delivery is impossible (Fig. 20-14). These abnormalities are frequently diagnosed sonographically before delivery, and the decision must be made whether or not to perform cesarean delivery (Clark and co-workers, 1985). In general, fetal prognosis is poor, regardless of the delivery method.

SHOULDER DYSTOCIA

The incidence of shoulder dystocia varies greatly depending on the criteria used for diagnosis. For example, Gross and co-workers (1987) reported that 0.9 percent of almost 11,000 vaginal deliveries were coded for shoulder dystocia at the Toronto General Hospital. True shoulder dystocia, however, diagnosed as such when maneuvers were required to deliver the shoulders in addition to downward traction and episiotomy, was identified in only 0.2 percent. Current reports cite an incidence of shoulder dystocia that varies between 0.6 percent and 1.4 percent (American College of Obstetricians and Gynecologists, 2002; Gottlieb and Galan, 2007).

There is evidence that the incidence of shoulder dystocia has increased in recent decades, likely due to increasing birthweight (Hopwood, 1982; MacKenzie and colleagues, 2007). The increased incidence may be due to more attention to its appropriate documentation (Nocon and co-workers, 1993). As discussed in Chapter 38 (p. 853), gross fetal birthweight—*macrosomia*—is important, but distribution of excessive tissue with *large-for-gestational age* infants is also important in its etiology.

The use of maneuvers to define shoulder dystocia has been appropriately questioned (Beall and associates, 1998; Spong and colleagues, 1995). In deliveries in which shoulder dystocia is anticipated, one or more maneuvers may be used prophylactically, and the diagnosis not recorded. In other cases, one or two maneuvers may be used with rapid resolution of dystocia and with an excellent

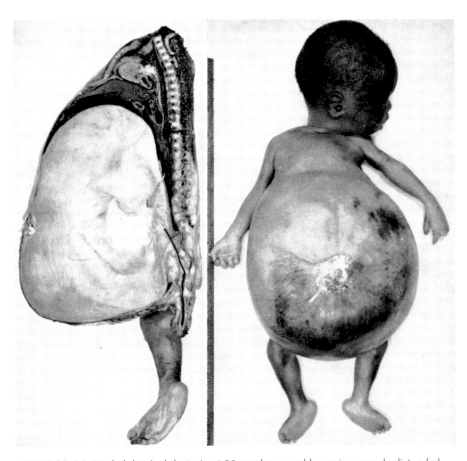

FIGURE 20-14 Fetal abdominal dystocia at 28 weeks caused by an immensely distended bladder. Delivery was made possible by expression of fluid through a bladder perforation at the level of the fetal umbilicus. Section shows the interior of the bladder and compression of organs of abdominal and thoracic cavities. A black thread has been laid in the urethra. (This figure was published in *American Journal of Obstetrics & Gynecology*, Vol. 29, JE Savage, Dystocia due to dilation of the fetal urinary bladder, p. 267, Copyright Elsevier 1935.)

outcome, and the diagnosis also is not recorded. Spong and colleagues (1995) attempted to more objectively define shoulder dystocia by witnessing 250 unselected deliveries and timing the intervals from delivery of the head, to delivery of the shoulders, and to completion of the birth. The incidence of 11 percent, defined by the use of obstetrical maneuvers, was much higher than previously reported. Only half were recorded as such by the clinicians. The mean head-to-body delivery time in normal births was 24 seconds compared with 79 seconds in those with shoulder dystocia. These investigators proposed that a head-to-body delivery time exceeding 60 seconds be used to define shoulder dystocia.

Maternal Consequences

Postpartum hemorrhage, usually from uterine atony, but also from vaginal and cervical lacerations, is the major maternal risk from shoulder dystocia (Benedetti and Gabbe, 1978; Parks and Ziel, 1978).

Fetal Consequences

Shoulder dystocia may be associated with significant fetal morbidity and even mortality. Gherman and co-workers (1998) reviewed 285 cases of shoulder dystocia and found that 25 percent were associated with fetal injuries. Transient Erb or Duchenne brachial plexopathy accounted for two thirds of injuries. In this same cohort of 285 infants, 38 percent had a clavicular fracture, and 17 percent sustained a humeral fracture. There was one neonatal death, and four newborns had persistent brachial plexopathy injuries. Mehta and associates (2007) found a similar number of injuries in a study of 205 shoulder dystocia cases in which 36 or 17.5 percent had injury—again, most involved the brachial plexus.

Brachial Plexopathy

Nerve injury to the brachial plexus may be localized to the upper or lower part of the plexus (see Chap. 29, p. 636). It usually results from stretch on the plexus during passage of the fetus through the birth canal and subsequent delivery. Downward traction on the brachial plexus during delivery of the anterior shoulder is thought to present a particular risk for such stretch.

Importantly, this is likely not the only factor that can result in brachial plexus injury. Using computer modeling, Gonik and colleagues (2003) demonstrated that stretching of the brachial plexus is greater from endogenous forces, which include maternal push-

ing and uterine contractions, than from iatrogenic applied force. Moreover, Jennett and associates (2001, 2002) have presented evidence that brachial plexus injuries may precede delivery itself and may occur even prior to labor. Consistent with this evidence, Alexander and co-workers (2008) reported four cases of brachial plexus in women undergoing cesarean delivery without labor.

Erb palsy and Klumpke paralysis may result from injury to the brachial plexus. These are fully described in Chapter 29 (p. 636). Chauhan and colleagues (2005) reported the incidence and outcome of brachial plexus injury during a 22-year period from 1980 to 2002. There were 89 injuries identified in 89,978 deliveries. Of the 85 delivering vaginally, only half were associated with shoulder dystocia. Importantly, 88 percent of the injuries resolved by 1 year of life.

Clavicular Fracture

These fractures are relatively common and have been diagnosed in 0.4 percent of newborns delivered vaginally at Parkland Hospital (Roberts and co-workers, 1995). Although at times associated with shoulder dystocia, the clavicle often fractures without any suspect clinical events. Investigators have concluded that isolated clavicular fractures are unavoidable, unpredictable, and have no clinical consequences (Lam and colleagues, 2002).

Prediction and Prevention of Shoulder Dystocia

There has been considerable evolution in obstetrical thinking about the preventability of shoulder dystocia. Although there are clearly several risk factors associated with shoulder dystocia, identification of individual instances before the fact has proven to be impossible.

Risk Factors

Various maternal, intrapartum, and fetal characteristics have been implicated in the development of shoulder dystocia. Several, including obesity, multiparity, and diabetes, all exert their effects because of associated increased birthweight. For example, Keller and co-workers (1991) identified shoulder dystocia in 7 percent of pregnancies complicated by gestational diabetes. Similarly, the association of postterm pregnancy with shoulder dystocia is likely because many fetuses continue to grow after 42 weeks (see Chap. 37, p. 837). Table 20-5 shows the incidence of shoulder dystocia related to birthweight groupings at Parkland

TABLE 20-5. Incidence of Shoulder Dystocia According to Birthweight Grouping in Singleton Neonates Delivered Vaginally in 1994 at Parkland Hospital

Birthweight Group	Births No.	Shoulder Dystocia No. (%)
≤ 3000 g	2953	0
3001–3500 g	4309	14 (0.3)
3501–4000 g	2839	28 (1.0)
4001–4500 g	704	38 (5.4)
> 4500 g	91	17 (19.0)
All weights	10,896	97 (0.9)

Hospital during 1994. Clearly, shoulder dystocia rates increase with greater birthweight, but almost half of the newborns with shoulder dystocia weighed less than 4000 g.

Despite this, some advocate identification of macrosomia with sonography and liberal use of cesarean delivery to avoid shoulder dystocia (O'Leary, 1992). Others have disputed the concept that cesarean delivery is indicated for large fetuses, even those estimated to weigh 4500 g. Rouse and Owen (1999a) concluded that a prophylactic cesarean delivery policy for macrosomic newborns would require more than 1000 cesarean deliveries and millions of dollars to avert a single permanent brachial plexus injury. The American College of Obstetricians and Gynecologists (2002) has concluded that performing cesarean deliveries for all women suspected of carrying a macrosomic fetus is not appropriate, except possibly for an estimated fetal weight > 5000 g in nondiabetic women and > 4500 g in those with diabetes.

Intrapartum complications associated with development of shoulder dystocia include midforceps delivery and prolonged first- and second-stage labor (Baskett and Allen, 1995; Nocon and associates, 1993). Conversely, McFarland and co-workers (1995) found that abnormalities of first- and second-stage labor were not useful predictors. Beall and colleagues (2003) randomly assigned 128 women with a fetus estimated to weigh > 3800 g to delivery with or without prophylactic McRoberts maneuvers. They found that such use of this maneuver was not beneficial.

Prior Shoulder Dystocia. Most have reported an increased risk of recurrent shoulder dystocia with a range from 13 to 25 percent (Ginsberg and Moisidis, 2001; Moore and associates, 2008; Usta and co-workers, 2008). In contrast, Baskett and Allen (1995) found the recurrence risk to be only 1 to 2 percent. Gurewitsch and colleagues (2007) have suggested that shoulder dystocia prevention in the general population is neither feasible nor cost-effective, but that intervention in women with a prior history of shoulder dystocia may minimize recurrence and the associated morbidities. The American College of Obstetricians and Gynecologists (2002) recommends that estimated fetal weight, gestational age, maternal glucose intolerance, and severity of prior neonatal injury should be evaluated and risks and benefits of cesarean delivery discussed with any woman with a history of shoulder dystocia.

Summary

The American College of Obstetricians and Gynecologists (2002) reviewed studies and concluded that:

1. Most cases of shoulder dystocia cannot be accurately predicted or prevented.
2. Elective induction of labor or elective cesarean delivery for all women suspected of having a macrosomic fetus is not appropriate.
3. Planned cesarean delivery may be considered for the nondiabetic woman with a fetus whose estimated fetal weight is > 5000 g or for the diabetic woman whose fetus is estimated to weigh > 4500 g.

Management

Because shoulder dystocia cannot be accurately predicted, clinicians should be well versed in its management principles. Fol-

lowing delivery of the head, the umbilical cord is compressed within the vagina, and fetal oxygenation declines. Thus, reduction in the time from delivery of the head to delivery of the body is of great importance for survival. An initial gentle attempt at traction, assisted by maternal expulsive efforts, is recommended. Some clinicians have advocated performing a large episiotomy, and adequate analgesia is certainly ideal. Moreover, a variety of techniques can be used to free the anterior shoulder from its impacted position behind the symphysis pubis:

Moderate *suprapubic pressure* can be applied by an assistant while downward traction is applied to the fetal head.

The *McRoberts maneuver* was described by Gonik and associates (1983) and named for William A. McRoberts, Jr., who popularized its use at the University of Texas at Houston. The maneuver consists of removing the legs from the stirrups and sharply flexing them up onto the abdomen (Fig. 20-15). Gherman and colleagues (2000) analyzed the McRoberts maneuver using x-ray pelvimetry. They found that the procedure caused straightening of the sacrum relative to the lumbar vertebrae, rotation of the symphysis pubis toward the maternal head, and a decrease in the angle of pelvic inclination. Although this does not increase pelvic dimensions, pelvic rotation cephalad tends to free the impacted anterior shoulder. Gonik and co-workers (1989) tested the McRoberts position objectively with laboratory models and found that the maneuver reduced the forces needed to free the fetal shoulder.

Woods (1943) reported that by progressively rotating the posterior shoulder 180 degrees in a corkscrew fashion, the impacted anterior shoulder could be released. This is frequently referred to as the *Woods corkscrew maneuver* (Fig. 20-16).

Delivery of the posterior shoulder consists of carefully sweeping the posterior arm of the fetus across the chest, followed by delivery of the arm. The shoulder girdle is then rotated into one of the oblique diameters of the pelvis with subsequent delivery of the anterior shoulder (Fig. 20-17).

Rubin (1964) recommended two maneuvers. First, the fetal shoulders are rocked from side to side by applying force to the maternal abdomen. If this is not successful, the pelvic hand reaches the most easily accessible fetal shoulder, which is then pushed toward the anterior surface of the chest. This maneuver most often results in abduction of both shoulders, which in turn produces a smaller shoulder-to-shoulder diameter. This permits displacement of the anterior shoulder from behind the symphysis pubis (Fig. 20-18).

Deliberate *fracture of the clavicle* by pressing the anterior clavicle against the pubic ramus can be performed to free the shoulder impaction. In practice, however, it is difficult to deliberately fracture the clavicle of a large neonate. If successful, the fracture will heal rapidly and is usually trivial compared with brachial nerve injury, asphyxia, or death.

Hibbard (1982) recommended that pressure be applied to the fetal jaw and neck in the direction of the maternal rectum, with strong fundal pressure applied by an assistant as the anterior shoulder is freed. Strong fundal pressure, however, applied at the wrong time may result in even further impaction of the anterior shoulder. Gross and associates (1987) reported that fundal pressure in the absence of other maneuvers "resulted in a 77-percent complication rate and was strongly associated with (fetal) orthopedic and neurologic damage."

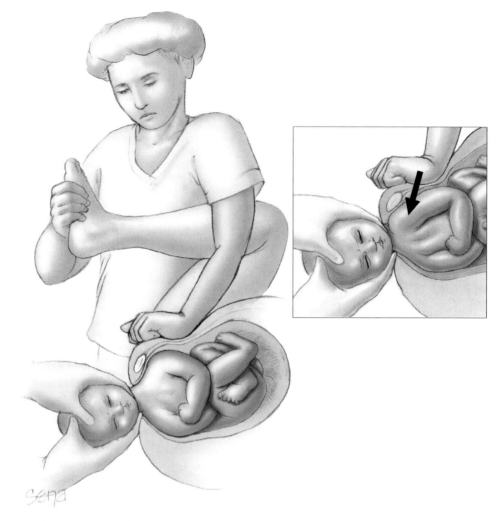

FIGURE 20-15 The McRoberts maneuver. The maneuver consists of removing the legs from the stirrups and sharply flexing the thighs up onto the abdomen. The assistant is also providing suprapubic pressure simultaneously (*arrow*).

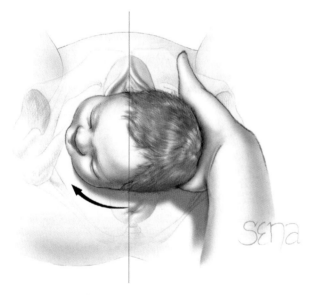

FIGURE 20-16 Woods maneuver. The hand is placed behind the posterior shoulder of the fetus. The shoulder is then rotated progressively 180 degrees in a corkscrew manner so that the impacted anterior shoulder is released.

Sandberg (1985) reported the *Zavanelli maneuver* for cephalic replacement into the pelvis followed by cesarean delivery. The first part of the maneuver consists of returning the head to the occiput anterior or posterior position. The operator flexes the head and slowly pushes it back into the vagina, following which cesarean delivery is performed. Terbutaline, 0.25 mg, is given subcutaneously to produce uterine relaxation.

Sandberg (1999) has subsequently reviewed 103 reported cases in which the Zavanelli maneuver was used. This maneuver was successful in 91 percent of cephalic cases and in all cases of breech head entrapments. Despite successful replacement, fetal injuries were still common in the desperate circumstances under which the Zavanelli maneuver was used. They reported six stillbirths, eight neonatal deaths, and 10 neonates who suffered brain damage. Uterine rupture also was reported. Ross and Beall (2006) report a case of dislocation of the cervical spine and associated stillbirth in an attempt to deliver a macrosomic infant from an impacted shoulder with this maneuver.

Cleidotomy consists of cutting the clavicle with scissors or other sharp instruments and is usually used for a dead fetus (Schramm, 1983). *Symphysiotomy* also has been applied successfully, as

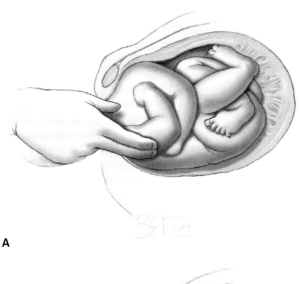

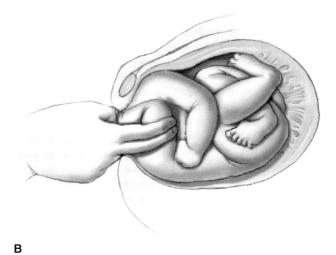

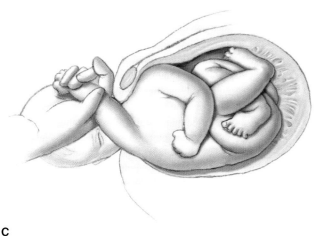

FIGURE 20-17 Shoulder dystocia with impacted anterior shoulder of the fetus. **A.** The operator's hand is introduced into the vagina along the fetal posterior humerus. **B.** The arm is splinted and swept across the chest, keeping the arm flexed at the elbow. **C.** The fetal hand is grasped and the arm extended along the side of the face. The posterior arm is delivered from the vagina.

described by Hartfield (1986). Goodwin and colleagues (1997) reported three cases in which symphysiotomy was performed after the Zavanelli maneuver had failed. All three neonates died, and maternal morbidity was significant due to urinary tract injury.

Hernandez and Wendel (1990) suggested use of a *shoulder dystocia drill* to better organize emergency management of an impacted shoulder:

1. Call for help—mobilize assistants, an anesthesiologist, and a pediatrician. Initially, a gentle attempt at traction is made. Drain the bladder if it is distended.
2. A generous episiotomy—consider mediolateral or episioproctotomy—may afford room posteriorly.
3. Suprapubic pressure is used initially by most practitioners because it has the advantage of simplicity. Only one assistant is needed to provide suprapubic pressure while normal downward traction is applied to the fetal head.
4. The McRoberts maneuver requires two assistants. Each assistant grasps a leg and sharply flexes the maternal thigh against the abdomen.

These maneuvers will resolve most cases of shoulder dystocia. If they fail, however, the following steps may be attempted:

1. The Woods screw maneuver.

2. Delivery of the posterior arm is attempted, but with a fully extended arm, this is usually difficult to accomplish.

Other techniques generally should be reserved for cases in which all other maneuvers have failed. These include intentional fracture of the anterior clavicle or humerus and the Zavanelli maneuver. Crofts (2006, 2007), Goffman (2008), Draycott (2008) and their colleagues have shown benefit from shoulder dystocia training using simulation-based education. The American College of Obstetricians and Gynecologists (2002) has concluded that there is no evidence that any one maneuver is superior to another in releasing an impacted shoulder or reducing the chance of injury. Performance of the McRoberts maneuver, however, was deemed a reasonable initial approach.

MATERNAL AND FETAL COMPLICATIONS WITH DYSTOCIA

Dystocia, especially if labor is prolonged, is associated with an increased incidence of several common obstetrical and neonatal complications. Although maternal and fetal effects resulting from dystocia are divided arbitrarily in the following discussion, dystocia may result in serious consequences to either or both simultaneously. Many are discussed in detail in other chapters.

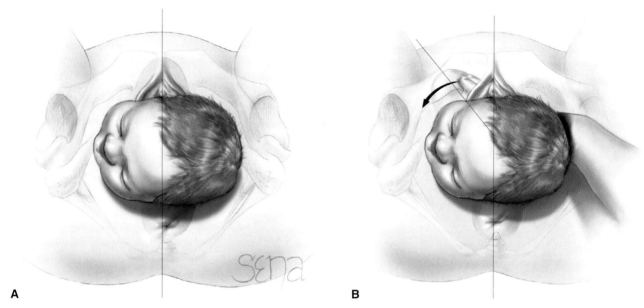

FIGURE 20-18 The second Rubin maneuver. **A.** The shoulder-to-shoulder diameter is aligned vertically. **B.** The more easily accessible fetal shoulder (the anterior is shown here) is pushed toward the anterior chest wall of the fetus (*arrow*). Most often, this results in abduction of both shoulders, reducing the shoulder-to-shoulder diameter and freeing the impacted anterior shoulder.

Maternal Complications

Intrapartum chorioamnionitis and postpartum pelvic infection are more common with desultory and prolonged labors (see Chap. 31, p. 661). Postpartum hemorrhage from atony is increased with prolonged and augmented labors and is discussed in Chapter 35 (p. 774). Hemorrhage from cesarean delivery is contributory, and there is a higher incidence of uterine tears with hysterotomy if the fetal head is impacted in the pelvis.

Uterine Rupture

Abnormal thinning of the lower uterine segment creates a serious danger during prolonged labor, particularly in women of high parity and in those with a prior cesarean delivery (see Chap. 35, p. 784). When disproportion is so pronounced that there is no engagement or descent, the lower uterine segment becomes increasingly stretched, and rupture may follow. In such cases, there is usually an exaggeration of the normal *contraction ring* shown in Figure 20-2 and also described in Chapter 6 (p. 143 and Fig. 6-3).

Pathological Retraction Ring. Localized rings or constrictions of the uterus develop in association with prolonged obstructed labors that are seldom encountered today. The *pathological retraction ring of Bandl* is associated with marked stretching and thinning of the lower uterine segment. The ring may be seen clearly as a uterine indentation and signifies impending rupture of the lower uterine segment.

Following birth of a first twin, a pathological ring may still develop occasionally as hourglass constrictions of the uterus. The ring can sometimes be relaxed and delivery effected with appropriate general anesthesia, but occasionally prompt ce-

sarean delivery offers a better prognosis for the second twin (see Chap. 39, p. 882).

Fistula Formation

With dystocia, the presenting part is firmly wedged into the pelvic inlet and does not advance for a considerable time. Tissues of the birth canal lying between the leading part and the pelvic wall may be subjected to excessive pressure. Because of impaired circulation, necrosis may result and become evident several days after delivery as vesicovaginal, vesicocervical, or rectovaginal fistulas. Most often, pressure necrosis follows a very prolonged second stage. They are rarely seen today except in undeveloped countries.

Pelvic Floor Injury

Injury to the pelvic floor muscles, nerve supply, or interconnecting fascia is a common consequence of vaginal delivery, particularly if the delivery is difficult (Branham, 2007; Kearney, 2006; Weidner, 2006, and all their associates). During childbirth, the pelvic floor is exposed to direct compression from the fetal head and to downward pressure from maternal expulsive efforts. These forces stretch and distend the pelvic floor, resulting in functional and anatomical alterations in the muscles, nerves, and connective tissues (see Fig. 2-26, p. 34). There is accumulating concern that such effects on the pelvic floor during childbirth lead to urinary and anal incontinence and to pelvic organ prolapse (Delancey, 2008; Dietz, 2005; Nichols, 2005, and all their colleagues). As discussed in Chapter 17 (p. 400), the anal sphincter is torn in 3 to 6 percent of deliveries, and approximately half of these women report subsequent fecal or gas incontinence (Zetterstrom and co-workers, 1999).

At Parkland Hospital, Casey and colleagues (2005) found that the incidence of pelvic floor dysfunction symptoms were increased with forceps delivery, birthweight > 4000 g, and episiotomy. In an earlier poll of English female obstetricians, 30 percent expressed preference for an elective cesarean delivery rather than vaginal delivery and cited avoidance of pelvic floor injury as the explanation for their choice (Wagner, 2000). Many of these long-term sequelae have contributed to the current trend of *cesarean delivery for maternal request* discussed in Chapter 25 (p. 548).

Childbirth has also been increasingly recognized as one of many factors leading to pelvic floor prolapse (American College of Obstetricians and Gynecologists, 2007; Schaffer and Hughes, 2008). And according to Nygaard (2006), de novo postpartum incontinence, although uncommon, is likely caused by childbirth and should be the focus of preventative measures. Clearly, there is uncertainty regarding the long-term impact of childbirth-associated pelvic floor injury, and several groups are studying this.

Postpartum Lower Extremity Nerve Injury

Wong and colleagues (2003) reviewed neurological injury involving the lower extremities in association with labor and delivery. The most common mechanism is external compression of the peroneal nerve, usually caused by inappropriate leg positioning in stirrups, especially during a prolonged second-stage labor. These and other injuries are discussed in Chapter 30 (p. 656). Fortunately, symptoms resolve within 6 months of delivery in most women.

Perinatal Complications

Similar to the mother, the incidence of peripartum fetal sepsis is increased with longer labors. Mechanical injuries are more common because there are more operative as well as traumatic injuries. *Caput succedaneum* may be impressive and *molding*, is shown in Figure 17-19 (p. 387), and is commonly seen with dystocia (Buchmann and Libhaber, 2008). It must be distinguished from a *cephalohematoma*. These other injuries are discussed in Chapter 29 (p. 633).

REFERENCES

Acker DB, Gregory KD, Sachs BP, et al: Risk factors for Erb-Duchenne palsy. Obstet Gynecol 71:389, 1988
Alexander JM, Leveno KJ, Hauth J, et al: Fetal injury associated with cesarean delivery. Obstet Gynecol 108:885, 2008
Alexander JM, Lucas MJ, Ramin SM, et al: The course of labor with and without epidural analgesia. Am J Obstet Gynecol 178:516, 1998
American College of Obstetricians and Gynecologists: Dystocia. Technical Bulletin No. 137, December 1989
American College of Obstetricians and Gynecologists: Dystocia and the augmentation of labor. Technical Bulletin No. 218, December 1995a
American College of Obstetricians and Gynecologists: Guidelines for diagnostic imaging during pregnancy. Committee Opinion No. 158, September 1995b
American College of Obstetricians and Gynecologists: Shoulder dystocia. Practice Bulletin No. 40, November 2002
American College of Obstetricians and Gynecologists: Dystocia and augmentation of labor. Practice Bulletin No. 49, December 2003
American College of Obstetricians and Gynecologists: Pelvic organ prolapse. Practice Bulletin No. 79, February 2007

Anteby EY, Yagel S: Route of delivery of fetuses with structural abnormalities. Eur J Obstet Gynecol Reprod Biol 106(1):5, 2003
Austin T, Bridges N, Markiewicz M, et al: Severe neonatal polycythaemia after third stage of labour underwater. Lancet 350 (9089):1445, 1997
Babayer M, Bodack MP, Creatura C: Common peroneal neuropathy secondary to squatting during childbirth. Obstet Gynecol 91:830, 1998
Barau G, Robillazrd PY, Hulsey TC, et al: Linear association between maternal pre-pregnancy body mass index and risk of cesarean section in term deliveries. BJOG 113:1173, 2006
Bashiri A, Burstein E, Bar-David J, et al: Face and brow presentation: Independent risk factors. J Matern Fetal Neonatal Med 21(6):357, 2008
Baskett TF, Allen AC: Perinatal implications of shoulder dystocia. Obstet Gynecol 86:15, 1995
Beall MH, Spong C, McKay J, et al: Objective definition of shoulder dystocia: A prospective evaluation. Am J Obstet Gynecol 179:934, 1998
Beall MH, Spong CY, Ross MG: A randomized controlled trial of prophylactic maneuvers to reduce head-to-body delivery time in patients at risk for shoulder dystocia. Obstet Gynecol 102:31, 2003
Benedetti TJ, Gabbe SG: Shoulder dystocia. A complication of fetal macrosomia and prolonged second stage of labor with mid-pelvic delivery. Obstet Gynecol 52:526, 1978
Berghella V, Baxter JK, Chauhan SP: Evidence-based labor and delivery management. Am J Obstet Gynecol 199(5):445, 2008
Bloom SL, Casey BM, Schaffer JI, et al: A randomized trial of coached versus uncoached maternal pushing during the second stage of labor. Am J Obstet Gynecol 194; 10, 2006
Bloom SL, McIntire DD, Kelly MA, et al: Lack of effect of walking on labor and delivery. N Engl J Med 339:76, 1998
Branham V, Thomas J, Jaffe T, et al: Levator ani abnormality 6 weeks after delivery persists at 6 months. Am J Obstet Gynecol 197(1):65.e1, 2007
Buchmann EJ, Libhaber E: Sagittal suture overlap in cephalopelvic disproportion: Blinded and non-participant assessment. Acta Obstet Gynecol Scand 87(7):731, 2008
Caldeyro-Barcia R, Alvarez H, Reynolds SRM: A better understanding of uterine contractility through simultaneous recording with an internal and a seven channel external method. Surg Obstet Gynecol 91:641, 1950
Calkins LA: Premature spontaneous rupture of the membranes. Am J Obstet Gynecol 64:871, 1952
Carlson JM, Diehl JA, Murray MS, et al: Maternal position during parturition in normal labor. Obstet Gynecol 68:443, 1986
Casey BM, Schaffer JI, Bloom SL: Obstetric antecedents for postpartum pelvic floor dysfunction. Am J Obstet Gynecol 192:1655, 2005
Chasen ST, Chervenak FA, McCullough LB: The role of cephalocentesis in modern obstetrics. Am J Obstet Gynecol 185:734, 2001
Chauhan SP, Rose CH, Gherman RB, et al: Brachial plexus injury: A 23-year experience from a tertiary center. Am J Obstet Gynecol 192:1795, 2005
Chen HY, Huang SC: Evaluation of midpelvic contraction. Int Surg 67:516, 1982
Cheng YW, Shaffer BL, Caughey AB: The association between persistent occiput posterior position and neonatal outcomes. Obstet Gynecol 107:837, 2006
Chervenak FA, Berkowitz RL, Tortona M, et al: The management of fetal hydrocephalus. Am J Obstet Gynecol 151:933, 1985
Chervenak FA, McCullough LB: Ethical analysis of the intrapartum management of pregnancy complicated by fetal hydrocephalus with macrocephaly. Obstet Gynecol 68:720, 1986
Cibils LA, Hendricks CH: Normal labor in vertex presentation. Am J Obstet Gynecol 91:385, 1965
Clark S, DeVore GR, Platt LD: The role of ultrasound in the aggressive management of obstructed labor secondary to fetal malformations. Am J Obstet Gynecol 152:1042, 1985
Cluett ER, Burns E: Immersion in water in labour and birth. Cochrane Database Syst Rev 2:CD000111, 2009
Cluett ER, Pickering RM, Getliffe K, et al: Randomised controlled trial of labouring in water compared with standard augmentation for management of dystocia in first stage of labour. BMJ 328:314, 2004
Cohen W: Influence of the duration of second stage labor on perinatal outcome and puerperal morbidity. Obstet Gynecol 49:266, 1977
Cohen W, Friedman EA (eds): Management of Labor. Baltimore, University Park Press, 1983
Crofts JF, Bartlett C, Ellis D, et al: Training for shoulder dystocia: A trial of simulation using low-fidelity and high-fidelity mannequins. Obstet Gynecol 108:1477, 2006
Crofts JF, Bartlett C, Ellis D, et al: Management of shoulder dystocia: Skill retention 6 and 12 months after training. Obstet Gynecol 110:1069, 2007

Cruikshank DP, White CA: Obstetric malpresentations: Twenty years' experience. Am J Obstet Gynecol 116:1097, 1973

Delancey JO, Kane LL, Miller JM, et al: Graphic integration of causal factors of pelvic floor disorders: An integrated life span model. Am J Obstet Gynecol 199(6):610.e1, 2008

Dietz HP, Lanzarone V: Levator trauma after vaginal delivery. Obstet Gynecol 106(4):707, 2005

Draycott TJ, Crofts JF, Ash JP, et al: Improving neonatal outcome through practical shoulder dystocia training. Obstet Gynecol 112:12, 2008

Duff P: Diagnosis and management of face presentation. Obstet Gynecol 57:105, 1981

Eller WC, Mengert WF: Recognition of mid-pelvic contraction. Am J Obstet Gynecol 53:252, 1947

Ferguson JE, Newberry YG, DeAngelis GA, et al: The fetal-pelvic index has minimal utility in predicting fetal-pelvic disproportion. Am J Obstet Gynecol 179:1186, 1998

Fitzpatrick M, McQuillan K, O'Herlihy C: Influence of persistent occiput posterior position on delivery outcome. Obstet Gynecol 98:1027, 2001

Floberg J, Belfrage P, Ohlsén H: Influence of pelvic outlet capacity on labor: A prospective pelvimetry study of 1429 unselected primi-paras. Acta Obstet Gynecol Scand 66:121, 1987

Flynn AM, Kelly J, Hollins G, et al: Ambulation in labour. BMJ 2:591, 1978

Fraser WD, Marcoux S, Krauss I, et al: Multicenter, randomized, controlled trial of delayed pushing for nulliparous women in the second stage of labor with continuous epidural analgesia. Am J Obstet Gynecol 182:1165, 2000

Friedman EA: Labor. Clinical Evaluation and Management, 2nd ed. New York, Appleton-Century-Crofts, 1978

Friedman EA, Sachtleben MR: Station of the fetal presenting part II: Effect on the course of labor. Am J Obstet Gynecol 93:530, 1965

Friedman EA, Sachtleben MR: Station of the fetal presenting part IV: Arrest of descent in nulliparas. Obstet Gynecol 47:129, 1976

Fuchs K, Peretz BA, Marcovici R, et al: The grand multipara—is it a problem? Int J Gynaecol Obstet 73:321, 1985

Gardberg M, Laakkonen E, Salevaara M: Intrapartum sonography and persistent occiput posterior position: A study of 408 deliveries. Obstet Gynecol 91:746, 1998

Getahun D, Kaminsky LM, Elsasser DA, et al: Changes in prepregnancy body mass index between pregnancies and risk of primary cesarean delivery. Am J Obstet Gynecol 197:376, 2007

Gherman RB, Ouzounian JG, Goodwin TM: Obstetric maneuvers for shoulder dystocia and associated fetal morbidity. Am J Obstet Gynecol 178:1126, 1998

Gherman RB, Tramont J, Muffley P, et al: Analysis of McRoberts' maneuver by x-ray pelvimetry. Obstet Gynecol 95:43, 2000

Gifford DS, Morton SC, Fiske M, et al: Lack of progress in labor as a reason for cesarean. Obstet Gynecol 95:589, 2000

Ginsberg NA, Moisidis C: How to predict recurrent shoulder dystocia. Am J Obstet Gynecol 184:1427, 2001

Goffman D, Heo H, Pardanani S, et al: Improving shoulder dystocia management among resident and attending physicians using simulations. Am J Obstet Gynecol 199:294, 2008

Gonik B, Allen R, Sorab J: Objective evaluation of the shoulder dystocia phenomenon: Effect of maternal pelvic orientation on force reduction. Obstet Gynecol 74:44, 1989

Gonik B, Stringer CA, Held B: An alternate maneuver for management of shoulder dystocia. Am J Obstet Gynecol 145:882, 1983

Gonik B, Zhang N, Grimm MJ: Defining forces that are associated with shoulder dystocia: The use of a mathematic dynamic computer model. Am J Obstet Gynecol 188:1068, 2003

Goodwin TM, Banks E, Millar LK, et al: Catastrophic shoulder dystocia and emergency symphysiotomy. Am J Obstet Gynecol 177:463, 1997

Goplerud J, Eastman NJ: Compound presentation: Survey of 65 cases. Obstet Gynecol 1:59, 1953

Gottlieb AG, Galan HL: Shoulder dystocia: An update. Obstet Gynecol Clin N Am 34:501, 2007

Gross SJ, Shime J, Farine D: Shoulder dystocia: Predictors and outcome: A five-year review. Am J Obstet Gynecol 156:334, 1987

Gupta JK, Hofmeyr GJ: Position for women during second stage of labour. Cochrane Database Syst Rev (1):CD002006, 2004

Gurewitsch ED, Johnson TL, Allen RH: After shoulder dystocia: managing the subsequent pregnancy and delivery. Semin Perinatol 31(3):185, 2007

Hamilton BE, Martin JA, Ventura SJ: Births: Preliminary data for 2007. National Vital Statistics Reports Vol 57, No 12. Hyattsville, MD, National Center for Health Statistics, 2009

Handa VL, Laros RK: Active-phase arrest in labor: Predictors of cesarean delivery in a nulliparous population. Obstet Gynecol 81:758, 1993

Hannah ME, Hodnett ED, Willan A, et al: Prelabor rupture of the membranes at term: Expectant management at home or in hospital? Obstet Gynecol 96:533, 2000

Hannah M, Ohlsson A, Farine D, et al: International Term PROM Trial: A RCT of induction of labor for prelabor rupture of membranes at term. Am J Obstet Gynecol 174:303, 1996

Hansen SL, Clark SL, Foster JC: Active pushing versus passive fetal descent in the second stage of labor: A randomized controlled trial. Obstet Gynecol 99:29, 2002

Hartfield VJ: Symphysiotomy for shoulder dystocia. Am J Obstet Gynecol 155:228, 1986

Hauth JC, Hankins GD, Gilstrap LC III: Uterine contraction pressures achieved in parturients with active phase arrest. Obstet Gynecol 78:344, 1991

Hauth JC, Hankins GD, Gilstrap LC III, et al: Uterine contraction pressures with oxytocin induction/augmentation. Obstet Gynecol 68:305, 1986

Hellman LM, Epperson JWW, Connally F: Face and brow presentation: The experience of the Johns Hopkins Hospital, 1896 to 1948. Am J Obstet Gynecol 59:831, 1950

Hendricks CH, Quilligan EJ, Tyler AB, et al: Pressure relationships between intervillous space and amniotic fluid in human term pregnancy. Am J Obstet Gynecol 77:1028, 1959

Hernandez C, Wendel GD: Shoulder dystocia. In Pitkin RM (ed): Clinical Obstetrics and Gynecology, Vol XXXIII. Hagerstown, Pa, Lippincott, 1990, p 526

Hibbard LT: Coping with shoulder dystocia. Contemp Ob/Gyn 20:229, 1982

Hillis DS: Diagnosis of contracted pelvis by the impression method. Surg Gynecol Obstet 51:857, 1930

Hopwood HG: Shoulder dystocia: Fifteen years' experience in a community hospital. Am J Obstet Gynecol 144:162, 1982

Hughes EC: Obstetric-Gynecologic Terminology. Philadelphia, Davis, 1972, p 390

Jennett RJ, Tarby TJ: Disuse osteoporosis as evidence of brachial plexus palsy due to intrauterine fetal maladaptation. Am J Obstet Gynecol 185:236, 2001

Jennett RJ, Tarby TJ, Krauss RL: Erb's palsy contrast with Klumpke's and total palsy: Different mechanisms are involved. Am J Obstet Gynecol 186:1216, 2002

Johnson CE: Transverse presentation of the fetus. JAMA 187:642, 1964

Kaltreider DF: Criteria of midplane contraction. Am J Obstet Gynecol 63:392, 1952

Kappy KA, Cetrulo C, Knuppel RA: Premature rupture of membranes: Conservative approach. Am J Obstet Gynecol 134:655, 1979

Kearney R, Miller JM, Ashton-Miller JA, et al: Obstetric factors associated with levator ani muscle injury after vaginal birth. Obstet Gynecol 107(1):144, 2006

Keller JD, Lopez-Zeno JA, Dooley SL, et al: Shoulder dystocia and birth trauma in gestational diabetes: A five year experience. Am J Obstet Gynecol 165:928, 1991

King JF: Obstetric intervention and the economic imperative. Br J Obstet Gynaecol 100:1063, 1993

Kwee A, Graziosi GCM, van Leeuwen JHS, et al: The effect of immersion on haemodynamic and fetal measures in uncomplicated pregnancies of nulliparous women. Br J Obstet Gynaecol 107:663, 2000

Lam MH, Wong GY, Lao TT: Reappraisal of neonatal clavicular fracture: Relationship between infant size and neonatal morbidity. Obstet Gynecol 100:115, 2002

Larks SD: Electrohysterography. Springfield, Ill, Thomas, 1960

Le Ray C, Serres P, Schmitz T, et al: Manual rotation in occiput posterior or transverse positions: Risk factors and consequences on the cesarean delivery rate. Obstet Gynecol 110(4):873, 2007

Leung TY, Leung TN, Sahota DS, et al: Trends in maternal obesity and associated risks of adverse pregnancy outcomes in a population of Chinese women. BJOG 115:1529, 2008

Lieberman E, Lang JM, Cohen A, et al: Association of epidural analgesia with cesarean delivery in nulliparas. Obstet Gynecol 88:993, 1996

Lupe PJ, Gross TL: Maternal upright posture and mobility in labor: A review. Obstet Gynecol 67:727, 1986

MacKenzie IZ, Shah M, Lean K, et al: Management of shoulder dystocia: Trends in incidence and maternal and neonatal morbidity. Obstet Gynecol 110:1059, 2007

Mahon TR, Chazotte C, Cohen WR: Short labor: Characteristics and outcome. Obstet Gynecol 84:47, 1994

Manyonda IT, Shaw DE, Drife JO: The effect of delayed pushing in the second stage of labor with continuous lumbar epidural analgesia. Acta Obstet Gynecol Scand 69:291, 1990

Martin JA, Hamilton BE, Sutton PD, et al: Births: Final Data for 2006. National Vital Statistics Reports, Vol 57, No 7. Hyattsville, Md, National Center for Health Statistics, 2009

McCarthy S: Magnetic resonance imaging in obstetrics and gynecology. Magn Reson Imaging 4:59, 1986

McFarland M, Hod M, Piper JM, et al: Are labor abnormalities more common in shoulder dystocia? Am J Obstet Gynecol 173:1211, 1995

Mehta SH, Blackwell SC, Chadha R, et al: Shoulder dystocia and the next delivery: Outcomes and management. J Matern Fetal Med 20;729, 2007

Mengert WF: Estimation of pelvic capacity. JAMA 138:169, 1948

Menticoglou SM, Manning F, Harman C, et al: Perinatal outcomes in relation to second-stage duration. Am J Obstet Gynecol 173:906, 1995a

Menticoglou SM, Perlman M, Manning FA: High cervical spinal cord injury in neonates delivered with forceps: Report of 15 cases. Obstet Gynecol 86:589, 1995b

Miller FC: Uterine motility in spontaneous labor. Clin Obstet Gynecol 26:78, 1983

Moore HM, Reed SD, Batra M, et al: Risk factors for recurrent shoulder dystocia, Washington state, 1987–2004. Am J Obstet Gynecol 198:e16, 2008

Moore MM, Shearer DR: Fetal dose estimates for CT pelvimetry. Radiology 171:265, 1989

Mozurkewich E, Chilimigras J, Koepke E, et al: Indications for induction of labour: A best-evidence review. BJOG 116(5):626, 2009

Müller: On the frequency and etiology of general pelvic contraction. Arch Gynaek 16:155, 1880

Myles TD, Santolaya J: Maternal and neonatal outcomes in patients with a prolonged second stage of labor. Obstet Gynecol 102(1):52, 2003

Nichols CM, Ramakrishnan V, Gill EJ, et al: Anal incontinence in women with and those without pelvic floor disorders. Obstet Gynecol 106(6):1266, 2005

Nocon JJ, McKenzie DK, Thomas LJ, et al: Shoulder dystocia: An analysis of risks and obstetric maneuvers. Am J Obstet Gynecol 168:1732, 1993

Nuthalapaty FS, Rouse DJ, Owen J: The association of maternal weight with cesarean risk, labor duration, and cervical dilation rate during labor induction. Obstet Gynecol 103:452, 2004

Nygaard I: Urogynecology: The importance of long-term follow-up. Obstet Gynecol 108:244, 2006

Olah KSJ, Neilson J: Failure to progress in the management of labour. Br J Obstet Gynaecol 101:1, 1994

O'Leary JA: Shoulder Dystocia and Birth Injury. New York, McGraw-Hill, 1992, p 75

Osborn SB: The implications of the Committee on Radiological Hazards to Patients (Adrian Committee), 1. Variations in the radiation dose received by the patient in diagnostic radiology. Br J Radiol 36:230, 1963

Parks DG, Ziel HK: Macrosomia: A proposed indication for primary cesarean section. Obstet Gynecol 52:407, 1978

Peleg D, Hannah ME, Hodnett ED, et al: Predictors of cesarean delivery after prelabor rupture of membranes at term. Obstet Gynecol 93:1031, 1999

Pinette MG, Wax J, Wilson E: The risks of underwater birth. Am J Obstet Gynecol 190(5):1211, 2004

Plunkett BA, Lin A, Wong CA, et al: Management of the second stage of labor in nulliparas with continuous epidural analgesia. Obstet Gynecol 102:109, 2003

Ponkey SE, Cohen AP, Heffner LJ, et al: Persistent fetal occiput posterior position: Obstetric outcomes. Obstet Gynecol 101:915, 2003

Read JA, Miller FC, Paul RH: Randomized trial of ambulation versus oxytocin for labor enhancement: A preliminary report. Am J Obstet Gynecol 139:669, 1981

Reynolds SRM, Heard OO, Bruns P, et al: A multichannel strain-gauge tocodynamometer: An instrument for studying patterns of uterine contractions in pregnant women. Bull Johns Hopkins Hosp 82:446, 1948

Roberts SW, Hernandez C, Maberry MC, et al: Obstetric clavicular fracture: The enigma of normal birth. Obstet Gynecol 86:978, 1995

Robertson PA, Huang LJ, Croughan-Minihane MS, et al: Is there an association between water baths during labor and the development of chorioamnionitis or endometritis? Am J Obstet Gynecol 178:1215, 1998

Roman H, Goffinet F, Hulsey TF, et al: Maternal body mass index at delivery and risk of cesarean due to dystocia in low risk pregnancies. Acta Obstet Gynecol Scand 87(2):163, 2008

Roshanfekr D, Blakemore KJ, Lee J, et al: Station at onset of active labor in nulliparous patients and risk of cesarean delivery. Obstet Gynecol 93:329, 1999

Ross MG, Beall MH: Cervical neck dislocation associated with Zavanelli maneuver. Obstet Gynecol 108(2):737, 2006

Rouse DJ, Owen J: Prophylactic cesarean delivery for fetal macrosomia diagnosed by means of ultrasonography—a Faustian bargain? Am J Obstet Gynecol 181:332, 1999a

Rouse DJ, Owen J, Hauth JC: Active-phase labor arrest: Oxytocin augmentation for at least 4 hours. Obstet Gynecol 93:323, 1999b

Roy RP: A Darwinian view of obstructed labor. Obstet Gynecol 101:397, 2003

Rubin A: Management of shoulder dystocia. JAMA 189:835, 1964

Russell JG: Moulding of the pelvic outlet. J Obstet Gynaecol Br Commonw 76:817, 1969

Sandberg EC: The Zavanelli maneuver: A potentially revolutionary method for the resolution of shoulder dystocia. Am J Obstet Gynecol 152:479, 1985

Sandberg EC: The Zavanelli maneuver: 12 years of recorded experience. Obstet Gynecol 93:312, 1999

Satin AJ, Maberry MC, Leveno KJ, et al: Chorioamnionitis: A harbinger of dystocia. Obstet Gynecol 79:913, 1992

Savage JE: Dystocia due to dilation of the fetal urinary bladder. Am J Obstet Gynecol 29:267, 1935

Savage W, Francome C: British cesarean section rates: Have we reached a plateau? Br J Obstet Gynaecol 101:645, 1994

Schaffer JI, Hughes D: Pelvic organ prolapse. In Schorge JO, Schaffer JI, Halvorsen LM, et al (eds): Williams Gynecology, New York, McGraw-Hill, 2008

Schramm M: Impacted shoulders—a personal experience. Aust NZ J Obstet Gynaecol 23:28, 1983

Shaffer BL, Cheng YW, Vargas JE, et al: Manual rotation of the fetal occiput: Predictors of success and delivery. Am J Obstet Gynecol 194(5):e7-9, 2006a

Shaffer BL, Cheng YW, Vargas JE, et al: Face presentation: Predictors and delivery route. Am J Obstet Gynecol 194(5):e10, 2006b

Sharma SK, Leveno KJ: Update: Epidural analgesia during labor does not increase cesarean births. Curr Anesth Rep 2:18, 2000

Speer DP, Peltier LF: Pelvic fractures and pregnancy. J Trauma 12:474, 1972

Spong CY, Beall M, Rodrigues D, et al: An objective definition of shoulder dystocia: Prolonged head-to-body delivery intervals and/or the use of ancillary obstetric maneuvers. Obstet Gynecol 86:433, 1995

Sporri S, Hanggi W, Brahetti A, et al: Pelvimetry by magnetic resonance imaging as a diagnostic tool to evaluate dystocia. Obstet Gynecol 89:902, 1997

Stark DD, McCarthy SM, Filly RA, et al: Pelvimetry by magnetic resonance imaging. Am J Radiol 144:947, 1985

Tebes CC, Mehta P, Calhoun DA, et al: Congenital ischemic forearm necrosis associated with a compound presentation. J Matern Fetal Med 8:281, 1999

Thoms H: The obstetrical significance of pelvic variations: A study of 450 primiparous women. BMJ 2:210, 1937

Thorp JA, Hu DH, Albin RM, et al: The effect of intrapartum epidural analgesia on nulliparous labor: A randomized, controlled, prospective trial. Am J Obstet Gynecol 169:851, 1993a

Thorp JM Jr, Pahel-Short L, Bowes WA Jr: The Mueller-Hillis maneuver: Can it be used to predict dystocia? Obstet Gynecol 82:519, 1993b

Thurnau GR, Scates DH, Morgan MA: The fetal-pelvic index: A method of identifying fetal-pelvic disproportion in women attempting vaginal birth after previous cesarean delivery. Am J Obstet Gynecol 165:353, 1991

Treacy A, Robson M, O'Herlihy C: Dystocia increases with advancing maternal age. Am J Obstet Gynecol 195:760, 2006

Usta HM, Hayek S, Yahya F, et al: Shoulder dystocia: What is the risk of recurrence. Acta Obstet Gynecol 87:992, 2008

Ventura SJ, Martin JA, Curtin SC, et al: Births: Final data for 1998. National Vital Statistics Reports, Vol 48, No 3. Hyattsville, Md, National Center for Health Statistics, 2000

Wagner M: Choosing caesarean section. Lancet 356:1677, 2000

Weidner AC, Jamison MG, Branham V, et al: Neuropathic injury to the levator ani occurs in 1 in 4 primiparous women. Am J Obstet Gynecol 195(6):1851, 2006

Wilkes PT, Wolf DM, Kronbach DW, et al: Risk factors for cesarean delivery at presentation of nulliparous patients in labor. Obstet Gynecol 102:1352, 2003

Williams JW: Obstetrics: A Textbook for the Use of Students and Practitioners, 1st ed. New York, Appleton, 1903, p 282

Williams RM, Thom MH, Studd JW: A study of the benefits and acceptability of ambulation in spontaneous labor. Br J Obstet Gynaecol 87:122, 1980

Wong CA, Scavone BM, Dugan S, et al: Incidence of postpartum lumbosacral spine and lower extremity nerve injuries. Obstet Gynecol 101:279, 2003

Woods CE: A principle of physics is applicable to shoulder delivery. Am J Obstet Gynecol 45:796, 1943

World Health Organization: Partographic management of labour. Lancet 343:1399, 1994

Zaretsky MV, Alexander JM, McIntire DD, et al: Magnetic resonance imaging pelvimetry and the prediction of labor dystocia. Obstet Gynecol 106:919, 2005

Zetterstrom J, Lopez A, Auzen B, et al: Anal sphincter tears at vaginal delivery: Risk factors and clinical outcome of primary repair. Obstet Gynecol 94:21, 1999

CHAPTER 21

Disorders of Amnionic Fluid Volume

Amnionic fluid serves several roles during pregnancy. It creates a physical space for the fetal skeleton to shape normally, promotes normal fetal lung development, and helps to avert compression of the umbilical cord. The most common intrinsic abnormalities that are encountered clinically are either too much or too little amnionic fluid.

NORMAL AMNIONIC FLUID VOLUME

Normally, amnionic fluid volume reaches 1 L by 36 weeks and decreases thereafter to less than 200 mL at 42 weeks (Table 21-1). Diminished fluid is termed *oligohydramnios*. Somewhat arbitrarily, more than 2 L of amnionic fluid is considered excessive and is termed *hydramnios* or *polyhydramnios*. In rare instances, the uterus may contain an enormous quantity of fluid, with reports of as much as 15 L. In most instances, chronic hydramnios develops, which is the gradual increase of excessive fluid. In acute hydramnios, the uterus may become markedly distended within a few days.

Measurement of Amnionic Fluid

Over the past decades, a number of sonographic methods have been used to measure the amount of amnionic fluid. Phelan and colleagues (1987) described quantification using the *amnionic fluid index—AFI*. This is calculated by adding the vertical depths of the largest pocket in each of four equal uterine quadrants. According to their calculations, significant hydramnios is

defined by an index greater than 24 cm. Magann and colleagues (2000) performed a cross-sectional study of longitudinal changes in the amnionic fluid index in normal pregnancies (Fig. 21-1). Their curve and the ones of Hinh and Ladinsky (2005) and Machado and colleagues (2007) show a peak AFI at approximately 32 weeks followed by a steady decline until 42 weeks. Normal values for multifetal pregnancy have been provided by Porter and associates (1996) and Hill and co-workers (2000) and are discussed further in Chapter 39 (p. 879).

The group from the University of Mississippi has performed several investigations to assess the sonographic accuracy of AFI evaluation. Magann and associates (1992) compared AFI values with measurements obtained by dye dilution. They used this technique to measure amnionic fluid in 40 women undergoing amniocentesis in late pregnancy. They found that the AFI was reasonably reliable in determining normal or increased amnionic fluid but was inaccurate in diagnosing oligohydramnios. In comparison with other tools of amnionic fluid measurement, this group showed poor correlation among the AFI, the two-diameter fluid pocket, and the single deepest-pocket methods (Chauhan, 1997; Johnson, 2007; Magann, 2003a, b, 2004, and all their associates). In addition, Morris and colleagues (2003) studied 1584 women at term and found that the AFI was superior to the single deepest pocket. Magann and colleagues (2001) evaluated the addition of color Doppler imaging and concluded that its concurrent use with AFI measurements leads to overdiagnosis of oligohydramnios. Peedicayil and colleagues (1994) emphasized that borderline values should be repeated before interventions are undertaken.

Several factors may modulate the AFI. For example, Yancey and Richards (1994) reported that high altitude—6000 ft—was associated with an increased index. Most, but not all, have reported that maternal hydration increased the index (Bush, 1996; Deka, 2001; Kerr, 1996; Kilpatrick, 1993; Magann, 2003c, and all their associates). This effect dissipates by 24 hours and has not been proven to improve outcome (Malhotra and Deka, 2004).

TABLE 21-1. Typical Amnionic Fluid Volume

Weeks' Gestation	Fetus (g)	Placenta (g)	Amnionic Fluid (mL)	Percent Fluid
16	100	100	200	50
28	1000	200	1000	45
36	2500	400	900	24
40	3300	500	800	17

From Queenan (1991), with permission.

Conversely, fluid restriction or dehydration may lower the AFI. In postterm pregnancy, Oz and colleagues (2002) investigated the etiology of oligohydramnios. They found a reduction in renal artery end-diastolic velocity, suggesting that increased arterial impedance is an important etiological factor. Ross and colleagues (1996) administered 1-deamino-[8-D-arginine] vasopressin (DDAVP) to women with oligohydramnios. This resulted in maternal serum hypoosmolality—285 to 265 mOsm/kg—that was associated with an increase in the AFI from 4 to 8 cm within 8 hours.

HYDRAMNIOS

Incidence

Excessive amnionic fluid is identified in approximately 1 percent of pregnancies. The diagnosis usually is suspected clinically and confirmed by sonographic examination. An extreme example is shown in Figure 21-2. Most investigators define hydramnios as an AFI of greater than 24 to 25 cm—corresponding to greater than the 95th or 97.5th percentiles. Using an index of 25 cm or greater, Biggio and colleagues (1999) reported a 1-percent incidence in more than 36,000 women examined at the University of Alabama. These observations confirmed the findings of Hill and associates (1987). These findings, summarized in Figure 21-3, included 80 percent with mild hydramnios—defined as pockets measuring 8 to 11 cm in vertical dimension. Moderate hydramnios—defined as a pocket containing only small parts and measuring 12 to 15 cm deep—was found in 15 percent. Only 5 percent had severe hydramnios, defined by a free-floating fetus found in pockets of fluid of 16 cm or greater. Golan and co-workers (1993) reported remarkably similar findings in nearly 14,000 women.

Causes of Hydramnios

The degree of hydramnios, as well as its prognosis, is often related to

the cause. Many reports are biased because they consist of observations from women referred for targeted sonographic evaluation. Others are population based but still may not reflect an accurate incidence unless universal sonographic screening is performed. In either case, obvious pathological hydramnios frequently is associated with fetal malformations, especially of the central nervous system or gastrointestinal tract. For example, hydramnios accompanies approximately half of cases of anencephaly and esophageal atresia. In the study by Hill and associates (1987), the cause of mild hydramnios was identified in only 15 percent of cases. Conversely, with moderate or severe hydramnios, the etiology was identified in more than 90 percent, and fetal anomalies were present in half of these cases. The opposite is not true, however, and in the Spanish Collaborative Study of Congenital Malformations with more than 27,000 anomalous fetuses, only 3.7 percent had hydramnios, whereas another 3 percent had oligohydramnios (Martinez-Frias and colleagues, 1999).

Damato and colleagues (1993) reported findings from 105 women referred for evaluation of excessive fluid, of whom

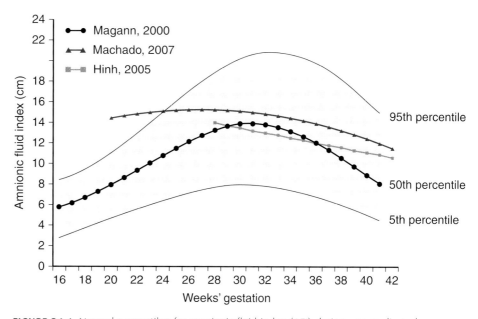

FIGURE 21-1 Normal percentiles for amnionic fluid index (AFI) during uncomplicated pregnancy. Black curves represent the 5th, 50th, and 95th percentile values from Magann and co-workers (2000). Red and tan curves represent 50th percentile values from Machado and colleagues (2007) and from Hinh and Ladinsky (2005), respectively.

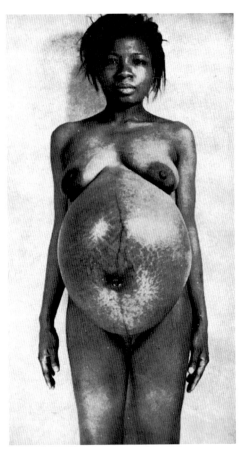

FIGURE 21-2 Advanced degree of hydramnios—5500 mL of amnionic fluid was measured at delivery.

almost 65 percent had an abnormal outcome. There were 47 singletons with one or more abnormalities that included gastrointestinal anomalies (15), nonimmune hydrops (12), chromosomal abnormalities (7), and central nervous system (12), thoracic (9), skeletal (8), and cardiac malformations (4). Among 19 twin pregnancies, 12 involved twin-twin transfusion syndrome, and only two of the 19 were normal.

Other less common causes of hydramnios include fetal pseudohypoaldosteronism, fetal Bartter or hyperprostaglandin E syndrome, fetal nephrogenic diabetes insipidus, placental chorioangioma, fetal sacrococcygeal teratoma, and maternal substance abuse (Narchi and colleagues, 2000; Panting-Kemp and associates, 2002).

Idiopathic hydramnios is excess amnionic fluid not associated with congenital anomalies, malformations, maternal diabetes, isoimmunization, infection, tumors or multifetal gestation. It occurs in approximately half of all hydramnios cases. However, even when sonography and radiography show an apparently normal fetus, the prognosis is still guarded, because fetal malformations and chromosomal abnormalities are common. For example, Brady and colleagues (1992) identified 125 cases of unexplained or idiopathic hydramnios in 5000 population-based pregnancies. Of these, two fetuses had trisomy 18 and two had trisomy 21.

Pathogenesis

Early in pregnancy, the amnionic cavity is filled with fluid very similar in composition to extracellular fluid. During the first

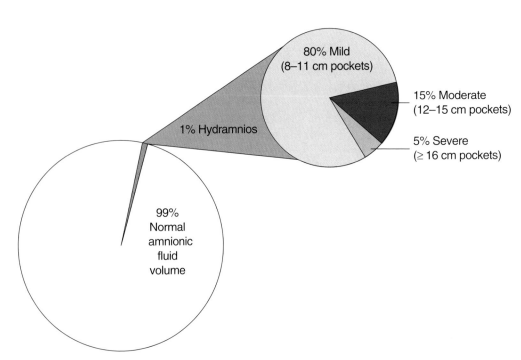

FIGURE 21-3 Amnionic fluid indexes in 36,796 pregnancies studied sonographically at 20 weeks or greater. (Data from Biggio and associates, 1999.)

half of pregnancy, transfer of water and other small molecules takes place not only across the amnion but also through fetal skin. During the second trimester, the fetus begins to urinate, swallow, and inspire amnionic fluid (Abramovich and colleagues, 1979; Duenhoelter and Pritchard, 1976). These processes have a modulating role in the control of fluid volume. Although the major source of amnionic fluid in hydramnios has most often been assumed to be the amnionic epithelium, no histological changes in amnion or chemical changes in amnionic fluid have been found.

The role of aquaporins—cell membrane water-channel proteins—has received attention recently. Some of these transmembrane proteins are expressed in fetal membranes and possibly ensure amnionic fluid homeostasis (Liu and associates, 2008; Wang and colleagues, 2007). Water-channel aquaporin 1 (AQP1) expression was found to be increased in membranes—especially reflected amnion—of pregnancies complicated by idiopathic hydramnios (Mann and associates, 2006). Additionally, aquaporin-1 knockout mice produce a greater volume of dilute amnionic fluid than do normal controls (Mann and coworkers, 2005).

Because the fetus normally swallows amnionic fluid, it has been assumed that this mechanism is one of the ways by which the volume is controlled. The theory gains validity by the nearly constant presence of hydramnios when fetal swallowing is inhibited, as in cases of esophageal atresia. But swallowing is not the only mechanism for preventing hydramnios. Specifically, Pritchard (1966) and Abramovich (1970) found in some instances of gross hydramnios that appreciable volumes of fluid were swallowed.

In cases of anencephaly and spina bifida, increased transudation of fluid from the exposed meninges into the amnionic cavity may result in hydramnios. Another possible explanation in anencephaly, which is not associated with abnormal swallowing, is excessive urination caused either by stimulation of cerebrospinal centers deprived of their protective coverings or by lack of antidiuretic effect because of impaired arginine vasopressin secretion.

In hydramnios associated with twin-twin transfusion syndrome (TTTS) in monozygotic twin pregnancy, the hypothesis has been advanced that one fetus usurps the greater part of the circulation common to both twins and develops cardiac hypertrophy, which in turn results in increased urine output (see Chap. 39, p. 874). Naeye and Blanc (1972) identified dilated renal tubules, an enlarged bladder, and increased urinary output in the recipient twin in the early neonatal period. This suggests that increased fetal urine production is responsible for hydramnios. Conversely, donor members of twin-twin transfusion syndrome pairs had dystrophic renal tubules and oligohydramnios. Several investigators have implicated the renin-angiotensin system in the fluid volume discordancy seen with TTTS (Galea and coworkers, 2008; Mahieu-Caputo and associates, 2000, 2005).

The hydramnios that commonly develops with maternal diabetes during the third trimester remains unexplained. One theory is that maternal hyperglycemia causes fetal hyperglycemia, resulting in osmotic diuresis. Bar-Hava and associates (1994) reported that increases in third-trimester amnionic fluid volume in women with gestational diabetes correlated with hyper-

glycemia the day prior to fluid measurement. Nordin and colleagues (2006) reported an association between the level of hypoglycemia and the diagnosis of hydramnios. Women requiring insulin had a fivefold increased risk of hydramnios compared with pregnant women with normal glucose control.

Clinical Manifestations

Major maternal symptoms accompanying hydramnios arise primarily from pressure exerted within the overdistended uterus and upon adjacent organs. When distension is excessive, the mother may suffer from severe dyspnea, and in extreme cases, she may be able to breathe only when upright (see Fig. 21-2). Edema, the consequence of major venous system compression by the enlarged uterus, is common. Swelling tends to be especially severe in the lower extremities, the vulva, and the abdominal wall. Rarely, oliguria may result from ureteral obstruction by the enlarged uterus (see Chap. 48, p. 1046). Hydramnios associated with fetal hydrops may cause the *mirror syndrome*, whereby the maternal condition mimics the fetus in that she develops edema and proteinuria, and frequently, preeclampsia (Carbillon and colleagues, 1997). This was originally described by Ballantyne in 1892, and it is discussed further in Chapter 29 (p. 627).

With chronic hydramnios, the accumulation of fluid takes place gradually, and a woman may tolerate excessive abdominal distension with relatively little discomfort. In acute hydramnios, however, distension may lead to disturbances sufficiently serious to be threatening. Acute hydramnios tends to develop earlier in pregnancy than does the chronic form—often as early as 16 to 20 weeks—and it may rapidly expand the uterus. As a rule, acute hydramnios leads to labor before 28 weeks, or the symptoms become so severe that intervention is mandatory.

Diagnosis

The primary clinical finding with hydramnios is uterine enlargement in association with difficulty in palpating fetal small parts and in hearing fetal heart tones. In severe cases, the uterine wall may be so tense that it is impossible to palpate any fetal parts (see Fig. 21-2). The differentiation among hydramnios, ascites, or a large ovarian cyst usually can be made by sonographic evaluation.

Pregnancy Outcome

The most frequent maternal complications associated with hydramnios are placental abruption, uterine dysfunction, and postpartum hemorrhage. The placenta may prematurely separate extensively after a rapid decrease in uterine surface area following uterine decompression due to amnionic fluid escape (see Chap. 35, p. 761). Uterine dysfunction and postpartum hemorrhage result from uterine atony consequent to overdistension. Abnormal fetal presentations and operative intervention are also common.

In general, the more severe the degree of hydramnios, the higher the perinatal mortality rate. The population-based study from the University of Alabama at Birmingham included more than 40,000 women (Biggio and co-workers, 1999). These investigators compared 370 women identified as having hydramnios with more than 36,000 women with normal fluid

TABLE 21-2. Outcomes in Women Identified to Have Hydramnios after 20 Weeks Compared with 36,426 Control Women with a Normal Amnionic Fluid Index

	Amnionic Fluid Index (AFI)			Hydramnios (n = 370)		
Factor	Hydramnios (n = 370)	Normal AFI (n = 36,426)	*p*	Diabetic (n = 71)	Nondiabetic (n = 299)	*p*
Perinatal outcomes						
Anomalies	8.4%	0.3%	<.001	0	10.4%	.005
Growth restriction	3.8%	6.7%	0.3	0	4.7%	NS
Aneuploidy	1/370	1/3643	.10	0/71	1/299	NS
Mortality	49/1000	14/1000	<.001	0/1000	60/1000	.03
Maternal outcomes						
Cesarean delivery	47%	16.4%	<.001	70%	42%	<.001
Diabetes	19.5%	3.2%	<.001			

NS = not significant.
Data from Biggio and colleagues (1999).

volume studied at 20 weeks' gestation or later. As shown in Table 21-2, hydramnios was found to portend a significantly increased risk for adverse outcomes. Most of these were in non-diabetic women with hydramnios. Magann and colleagues (2007) found that idiopathic hydramnios is associated with fetal macrosomia, a higher risk of adverse pregnancy outcomes, and a two- to fivefold increase in perinatal mortality rates. A 12-month follow-up of infants from 24 pregnancies complicated by unexplained hydramnios found that 80 percent had normal outcomes. Of abnormal outcomes, there were two perinatal deaths, and three neonates with either West syndrome, polyuric syndrome, or pulmonary stenosis, respectively (Touboul and colleagues, 2007). Conversely, Panting-Kemp and co-workers (1999) found that idiopathic hydramnios was not associated with increased adverse outcomes except for cesarean delivery.

Furman and co-workers (2000) described substantively increased adverse perinatal outcomes if fetal-growth restriction accompanies hydramnios. Perinatal mortality rates are increased further by preterm delivery, and fetal death complicates up to 40 percent of pregnancies with hydramnios and an anomalous fetus. Other associated conditions adding to poor outcomes are erythroblastosis, maternal diabetes, and umbilical cord prolapse.

Midtrimester Hydramnios

The prognosis of midtrimester hydramnios depends on the severity. As with other cases, mild hydramnios has a reasonably good outcome. Glantz and co-workers (1994) studied 47 consecutive singleton pregnancies with a single deepest pocket of 6 to 10 cm that was identified at 14 to 27 weeks. Excessive fluid resolved spontaneously in three fourths of these pregnancies, and perinatal outcomes were similar to matched controls without hydramnios. In the group in which hydramnios persisted, two of 10 had fetal aneuploidy.

Management

Minor degrees of hydramnios rarely require treatment. Even moderate degrees with some discomfort usually can be managed without intervention until labor ensues or until the membranes rupture spontaneously. If dyspnea or abdominal pain is present or if ambulation is difficult, hospitalization becomes necessary. Bed rest, diuretics, and water and salt restriction are ineffective. More recently, indomethacin therapy has been used for symptomatic hydramnios.

Amniocentesis

The principal purpose of amniocentesis is to relieve maternal distress, and to that end, it is transiently successful. Amnionic fluid also can be tested to predict fetal lung maturity as described in Chapter 29 (p. 606). Elliott and associates (1994) reported results from 200 therapeutic amniocenteses in 94 women with hydramnios. Common causes included twin-twin transfusion syndrome—38 percent, idiopathic—26 percent, fetal or chromosomal anomalies—17 percent, and diabetes—12 percent. They removed a mean of 1650 mL of fluid at each procedure and gained an average duration-to-delivery of 7 weeks. Only three procedures were complicated—one woman had ruptured membranes, one developed chorioamnionitis, and another suffered placental abruption after 10 L of fluid were removed. Leung and co-workers (2004) cited a 3-percent incidence of complications in 134 rapid aminodrainage procedures.

Technique. To remove amnionic fluid, a clinician inserts a commercially available plastic catheter that tightly covers an 18-gauge needle through the locally anesthetized abdominal wall into the amnionic sac. The needle is withdrawn, and an intravenous infusion set is connected to the catheter hub. The opposite end of the tubing is dropped into a graduated cylinder placed at floor level. The flow of amnionic fluid is controlled with the tubing screw clamp so that approximately 500 mL/hr is withdrawn. After 1500 to 2000 mL have been collected, the uterus usually has decreased in size sufficiently that the catheter may be withdrawn from the amnionic sac. At the same time, maternal relief is dramatic, and the danger of placental separation from decompression is slight. Using strict aseptic technique, this procedure can be repeated as necessary to provide patient comfort. Elliott and colleagues (1994) used wall suction and removed 1000 mL over 20 minutes (50 mL/min). However, we prefer more gradual removal.

Amniotomy

The disadvantage inherent with amniotomy during labor in women with excessive fluid is the possibility of cord prolapse and especially of placental abruption. Slow removal of fluid by amniocentesis helps to obviate these dangers.

Indomethacin Therapy

In their review of several studies, Kramer and colleagues (1994) concluded that indomethacin impairs fetal lung liquid production or enhances absorption, decreases fetal urine production, and increases fluid movement across fetal membranes. Maternal doses employed by most investigators range from 1.5 to 3 mg/kg per day. Cabrol and associates (1987) used indomethacin therapy for 2 to 11 weeks in eight women with idiopathic hydramnios from 24 to 35 weeks. Hydramnios, defined by at least one 8-cm fluid pocket, improved in all cases. There were no serious adverse effects, and the outcomes were good. Mamopoulos and colleagues (1990) treated 15 women—11 were diabetic—who had hydramnios at 25 to 32 weeks. Amnionic fluid volume decreased in all women after indomethacin was begun. The fluid in the maximum pocket decreased from a mean of 10.7 cm at 27 weeks to 5.9 cm after therapy. The outcome was good in all 15 newborns. Kriplani and colleagues (2001) successfully treated a patient with indomethacin who had hydramnios from a placental chorioangioma.

A major concern for the use of indomethacin is the potential for closure of the fetal ductus arteriosus (see Chap. 14, p. 319). Moise and colleagues (1988) reported that seven of 14 fetuses whose mothers received indomethacin had ductal constriction detected by Doppler study. Persistent constriction was not demonstrated in the reports described earlier in this section nor has it been described in studies in which indomethacin was given for tocolysis (Kramer and colleagues, 1994).

OLIGOHYDRAMNIOS

In rare instances, the volume of amnionic fluid may fall far below the normal limits and occasionally be reduced to only a few milliliters. In general, oligohydramnios developing early in pregnancy is less common and frequently has a poor prognosis. By contrast, in pregnancies that continue beyond term, diminished fluid volume may be found often. Marks and Divon (1992) found oligohydramnios—defined as an AFI of 5 cm or less—in 12 percent of 511 pregnancies of 41 weeks or greater. In 121 women studied longitudinally, there was a mean decrease of 25 percent per week in the AFI beyond 41 weeks. Gagnon and colleagues (2002) found that chronic severe

TABLE 21-3. Conditions Associated with Oligohydramnios

Fetal
　Chromosomal abnormalities
　Congenital anomalies
　Growth restriction
　Demise
　Postterm pregnancy
　Ruptured membranes

Placenta
　Abruption
　Twin-twin transfusion

Maternal
　Uteroplacental insufficiency
　Hypertension
　Preeclampsia
　Diabetes

Drugs
　Prostaglandin synthase inhibitors
　Angiotensin-converting enzyme inhibitors

Idiopathic

From Peipert and Donnenfeld (1991), with permission.

placental insufficiency caused a reduction in amnionic fluid volume not attributable to reduced fetal urine production. The risk of cord compression, and in turn fetal distress, is increased with diminished fluid in all labors, but especially in posterm pregnancy (Grubb and Paul, 1992; Leveno and colleagues, 1984).

Early-Onset Oligohydramnios

A number of varied conditions have been associated with diminished amnionic fluid, and some are listed in Table 21-3. Oligohydramnios almost always is evident when there is either obstruction of the fetal urinary tract or renal agenesis. Therefore, anuria almost certainly has an etiological role in such cases. A chronic leak from a defect in the fetal membranes may reduce the volume of fluid appreciably, but most often labor soon ensues. Exposure to angiotensin-converting enzyme inhibitors has been associated with oligohydramnios (see Chap. 14, p. 319).

From 15 to 25 percent of cases of oligohydramnios are associated with the fetal anomalies shown in Table 21-4. Diminished fluid decreases the accuracy of sonographic imaging. For example, Pryde and co-workers (2000) were able to visualize fetal structures in only half of women referred for midtrimester oligohydramnios. After amnioinfusion, they were able to visualize 77 percent of routinely imaged structures. Identification of associated anomalies increased from 12 to 31 percent of fetuses.

Prognosis

Fetal outcome is generally poor with early-onset oligohydramnios. Shenker and colleagues (1991) described 80 pregnancies in which only half of the fetuses survived. Mercer and Brown (1986) described 34 midtrimester pregnancies complicated by

TABLE 21-4. Congenital Anomalies Associated with Oligohydramnios

Amnionic band syndrome
Cardiac: Fallot tetralogy, septal defects
Central nervous system: holoprosencephaly,
   meningocoele, encephalocoele, microcephaly
Chromosomal abnormalities: triploidy, trisomy 18,
   Turner syndrome
Cloacal dysgenesis
Cystic hygroma
Diaphragmatic hernia
Genitourinary: renal agenesis, renal dysplasia, urethral
   obstruction, bladder exstrophy, Meckel-Gruber
   syndrome, ureteropelvic junction obstruction,
   prune-belly syndrome
Hypothyroidism
Skeletal: sirenomelia, sacral agenesis, absent radius,
   facial clefting
TRAP (twin reverse arterial perfusion) sequence
Twin-twin transfusion
VACTERL (vertebral, anal, cardiac, tracheo-esophageal,
   renal, limb) association

Adapted from McCurdy and Seeds (1993) and Peipert and Donnenfeld (1991).

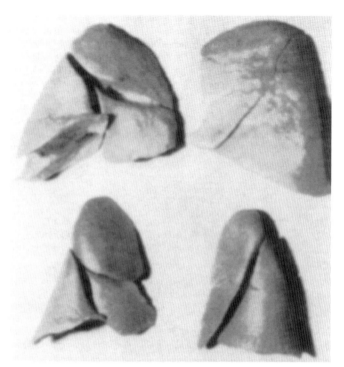

FIGURE 21-4 Normal-sized lungs (*top*) are shown in comparison with hypoplastic lungs (*bottom*) of fetuses at the same gestational age. (Reproduced from *BJOG*, Vol. 101, Issue X, MJ Newbould, M Lendon, and AJ Barson, Oligohydramnios sequence: The spectrum of renal malformations, 598, 1994, with the permission of the Royal College of Obstetricians and Gynaecologists.)

oligohydramnios defined by the absence of amnionic fluid pockets greater than 1 cm. Nine fetuses—a fourth— had anomalies, and 10 of the 25 who were phenotypically normal either aborted spontaneously or were stillborn because of severe maternal hypertension, restricted fetal growth, or placental abruption. Of the 14 liveborn infants, 8 were preterm and 7 died. The six infants who were delivered at term did well. Garmel and co-workers (1997) observed that appropriately grown fetuses associated with oligohydramnios prior to 37 weeks had a threefold increase in preterm birth but not of later growth restriction or fetal death.

Newbould and colleagues (1994) described autopsy findings in 89 infants with the Potter sequence or Potter syndrome (see Chap. 16, p. 360). Only 3 percent had a normal renal tract; 34 percent had bilateral renal agenesis; 34 percent had bilateral cystic dysplasia; 9 percent had unilateral agenesis with dysplasia; and 10 percent had minor urinary abnormalities.

Otherwise normal infants may suffer the consequences of early-onset severely diminished amnionic fluid. Adhesions between the amnion may entrap fetal parts and cause serious deformities, including amputation. Moreover, because the fetus is subjected to pressure from all sides, musculoskeletal deformities such as clubfoot are observed frequently.

Pulmonary Hypoplasia

The presence of oligohydramnios markedly increases the fetal risk for pulmonary hyperplasia such as shown in Figure 21-4. Its incidence at birth approximates 1 per 1000 infants, but when amnionic fluid is scant, pulmonary hypoplasia is com-

mon (Moessinger and colleagues, 1989). Winn and associates (2000) performed a prospective cohort study in 163 cases of oligohydramnios that followed prematurely ruptured membranes at 15 to 28 weeks. Almost 13 percent of fetuses developed pulmonary hypoplasia. When rupture occurred at earlier gestational ages, hypoplasia was more common. Kilbride and co-workers (1996) studied 115 women with prematurely ruptured membranes before 29 weeks. There ultimately were seven stillbirths and 40 neonatal deaths and a calculated perinatal mortality rate of 409 per 1000. The risk of lethal pulmonary hypoplasia was 20 percent. Adverse outcomes were more likely with earlier rupture as well as duration exceeding 14 days.

According to Fox and Badalian (1994) and Lauria and colleagues (1995), there are three possibilities that account for pulmonary hypoplasia. First, thoracic compression may prevent chest wall excursion and lung expansion. Second, lack of fetal breathing movements decreases lung inflow. The third and the most widely accepted model involves a failure to retain intrapulmonary amnionic fluid or an increased outflow with impaired lung growth and development. Albuquerque and colleagues (2002) found a relationship between oligohydramnios and spinal flexion in the human fetus that also may contribute to fetal pulmonary hypoplasia.

Oligohydramnios in Late Pregnancy

Using an amnionic fluid index of less that 5 cm, Casey and co-workers (2000) cited an incidence of oligohydramnios of

TABLE 21-5. Pregnancy Outcomes (in percent) in 147 Women with Oligohydramnios at 34 Weeks

Factor	Oligohydramnios[a] (n = 147)	Normal AFI (n = 6276)	p
Labor induction	42	18	<.001
Nonreassuring FHR	48	39	<.03
Cesarean for FHR	5	3	.18
Stillbirth	14/1000	3/1000	<.03
Neonatal ICU	7	2	<.001
Meconium aspiration	1	0.1	<.001
Neonatal death	5	0.3	<.001
Fetal-growth restriction	24	9	<.001
Fetal malformation	10	2.5	<.001

[a]AFI ≤ 5.0 cm.
AFI = amnionic fluid index; FHR = fetal heart rate pattern; ICU = intensive care unit.
Data from Casey and co-workers (2000).

2.3 percent in more than 6400 pregnancies undergoing sonography after 34 weeks at Parkland Hospital. They confirmed previous observations that this finding is associated with an increased risk of adverse perinatal outcomes (Table 21-5).

Management of oligohydramnios in late pregnancy depends on the clinical situation. Initially, an evaluation for fetal anomalies and growth is critical. In a pregnancy complicated by oligohydramnios and fetal-growth restriction, close fetal surveillance is important because of associated morbidity. In many cases, evidence for fetal or maternal compromise will override potential complications from preterm delivery. However, oligohydramnios detected before 36 weeks in the presence of normal fetal anatomy and growth may be managed expectantly in conjunction with increased fetal surveillance (see Chap. 15, p. 334).

The outcomes of pregnancies with intrapartum oligohydramnios are conflicting. Chauhan and associates (1999) performed meta-analysis of 18 studies comprising more than 10,500 pregnancies in which the intrapartum AFI was less than 5 cm. Compared with controls whose index was greater than 5 cm, women with oligohydramnios had a significantly increased 2.2-fold risk for cesarean delivery for fetal distress and a 5.2-fold increased risk for a 5-minute Apgar score of less than 7. Cord compression during labor is common with oligohydramnios. Baron and colleagues (1995) reported a 50-percent increase in variable decelerations during labor and a sevenfold increased cesarean delivery rate in these women. Divon and associates (1995) studied 638 women with a postterm pregnancy in labor and observed that only those whose amnionic fluid index was 5 cm or less had fetal heart rate decelerations and meconium. Interestingly, Chauhan and colleagues (1995) showed that diminished amnionic fluid index increased the cesarean delivery rate only in women whose labor attendants were made aware of the findings!

Conversely, using the RADIUS trial database, Zhang and colleagues (2004) reported that oligohydramnios of this degree was not associated with adverse perinatal outcomes. Similarly, Magann and co-workers (1999) did not find that associated oligohydramnios increased risks for intrapartum complications. Casey and co-workers (2000) showed a 25-percent increase in nonreassuring fetal heart rate patterns when women with oligohydramnios were compared with normal controls. Despite this, the cesarean delivery rate for pregnancies with this finding increased only from 3 to 5 percent (see Table 21-5).

Amnioinfusion

Numerous studies have evaluated whether intrapartum amnioinfusion may prevent fetal morbidity from meconium-stained fluid—often associated with oligohydramnios. Pierce and colleagues (2000) performed meta-analysis of 13 such studies of more than 1900 women. They found that amnioinfusion resulted in significantly decreased adverse outcomes that included meconium beneath the cords (OR 0.18), meconium aspiration syndrome (OR 0.30), neonatal acidemia (OR 0.42), and cesarean delivery rate (0.74). Conversely, Spong and associates (1994) found no benefits when they compared therapeutic with prophylactic amnioinfusion for meconium. Indeed, meconium aspiration syndrome occurred only in the group undergoing therapeutic amnioinfusion. Surprisingly, only 16 percent of the group randomized to expectant therapy ultimately required amnioinfusion for variable fetal heart rate decelerations. These findings are in agreement with reviews of outcomes before and after amnioinfusion protocols were implemented (De Meeus, 1997; Rogers, 1996; Usta, 1995, and all their colleagues).

Fraser and associates (2005) reported results from a 56-center, 13-country international trial of amnioinfusion in 1998 women at term in labor and with thick meconium. They found that amnioinfusion did not reduce the risk of meconium aspiration syndrome, cesarean delivery, or other major indicators of maternal or neonatal morbidity. The incidence of perinatal death or meconium aspiration syndrome was not significantly different—4.5 versus 3.4 percent in the amnioinfused women compared with controls. Finally, Xu and colleagues (2007) recently performed a meta-analysis of 12 trials that included more than 4000 women randomly assigned to amnioinfusion versus no treatment. When outcomes in 1999 women undergoing amnioinfusion were compared with those in 2031 control women, there was no evidence that amnioinfusion reduced the risk of meconium aspiration syndrome (RR 0.59, 95% CI 0.28–1.25), 5-minute Apgar score <7 (RR 0.9, 95% CI 0.58–1.41), or cesarean delivery (RR 0.89, 95% CI 0.73–1.1).

Finally, a number of maternal deaths have been associated with amnioinfusion in pregnancies complicated by thick meconium-stained fluid (Dibble and Elliot, 1992; Maher and colleagues, 1994). In at least seven of these cases, rapid labor was thought to play a major role (Dorairajan and Soundararaghavan, 2005).

Taken together, these results suggest that routine prophylactic amnioinfusion for labors complicated by meconium-stained amnionic fluid is not warranted. Indeed, the American College of Obstetricians and Gynecologists (2006) concluded that routine prophylactic amnioinfusion for this reason is not recommended. The College, however, concluded that amnioinfusion is a reasonable approach in the treatment of repetitive variable decelerations, regardless of amnionic fluid meconium status. Amnioinfusion is discussed in greater detail in Chapter 29 (p. 628), and the technique is described in Chapter 18 (p. 433).

REFERENCES

Abramovich DR: Fetal factors influencing the volume and composition of liquor amnii. J Obstet Gynaecol Br Commonw 77:865, 1970

Abramovich DR, Garden A, Jandial L, et al: Fetal swallowing and voiding in relation to hydramnios. Obstet Gynecol 54:15, 1979

Albuquerque CA, Smith KR, Saywers TE, et al: Relations between oligohydramnios and spinal flexion in the human fetus. Early Hum Dev 68:119, 2002

American College of Obstetricians and Gynecologists: Amnioinfusion does not prevent meconium aspiration syndrome. Obstet Gynecol 108:1053, 2006

Ballantyne JW: The Diseases and Deformities of the Foetus. Edinburgh, Scotland, Oliver and Boyd, 1892

Bar-Hava I, Scarpelli SA, Barnhard Y, et al: Amniotic fluid volume reflects recent glycemic status in gestational diabetes mellitus. Am J Obstet Gynecol 171:952, 1994

Baron C, Morgan MA, Garite TJ: The impact of amniotic fluid volume assessed intrapartum on perinatal outcome. Am J Obstet Gynecol 173:167, 1995

Biggio JR Jr, Wenstrom KD, Dubard MB, et al: Hydramnios prediction of adverse perinatal outcome. Obstet Gynecol 94:773, 1999

Brady K, Polzin WJ, Kopelman JN, et al: Risk of chromosomal abnormalities in patients with idiopathic polyhydramnios. Obstet Gynecol 79:234, 1992

Bush J, Minkoff H, McCalla S, et al: The effect of intravenous fluid load on amniotic fluid index in patients with oligohydramnios. Am J Obstet Gynecol 174:379, 1996

Cabrol D, Landesman R, Muller J, et al: Treatment of polyhydramnios with prostaglandin synthetase inhibitor (indomethacin). Am J Obstet Gynecol 157:422, 1987

Carbillon L, Oury JF, Guerin JM, et al: Clinical biological features of Ballantyne syndrome and the role of placental hydrops. Obstet Gynecol Surv 52:310, 1997

Casey BM, McIntire DD, Bloom SL, et al: Pregnancy outcomes after antepartum diagnosis of oligohydramnios at or beyond 34 weeks' gestation. Am J Obstet Gynecol 182:909, 2000

Chauhan SP, Magann EF, Morrison JC, et al: Ultrasonographic assessment of amniotic fluid does not reflect actual amniotic fluid volume. Am J Obstet Gynecol 177:291, 1997

Chauhan SP, Sanderson M, Hendrix NW, et al: Perinatal outcome and amniotic fluid index in the antepartum and intrapartum periods: A meta-analysis. Am J Obstet Gynecol 181:1473, 1999

Chauhan SP, Washburne JF, Magann EF, et al: A randomized study to assess the efficacy of the amniotic fluid index as a fetal admission test. Obstet Gynecol 86:9, 1995

Damato N, Filly RA, Goldstein RB, et al: Frequency of fetal anomalies in sonographically detected polyhydramnios. J Ultrasound Med 12:11, 1993

Deka D, Malhotra B: Role of maternal oral hydration in increasing amniotic fluid volume in pregnant women with oligohydramnios. Int J Gynaecol Obstet 73:155, 2001

De Meeus JB, D'Halluin G, Bascou V, et al: Prophylactic intrapartum amnioinfusion: A controlled retrospective study of 135 cases. Eur J Obstet Gynecol Reprod Biol 72:141, 1997

Dibble LA, Elliot JP: Possible amniotic fluid embolism associated with amnioinfusion. J Matern Fetal Med 1:263, 1992

Divon MY, Marks AD, Henderson CE: Longitudinal measurement of amniotic fluid index in postterm pregnancies and its association with fetal outcome. Am J Obstet Gynecol 172:142, 1995

Dorairajan G, Soundararaghavan S: Maternal death after intrapartum saline amnioinfusion—report of two cases. BJOG 112:1331, 2005

Duenhoelter JH, Pritchard JA: Fetal respiration: quantitative measurements of amnionic fluid inspired near term by human and rhesus fetuses. Am J Obstet Gynecol 125(3):306, 1976

Elliott JP, Sawyer AT, Radin TG, et al: Large-volume therapeutic amniocentesis in the treatment of hydramnios. Obstet Gynecol 84:1025, 1994

Fox HE, Badalian SS: Ultrasound prediction of fetal pulmonary hypoplasia in pregnancies complicated by oligohydramnios and in cases of congenital diaphragmatic hernia: A review. Am J Perinatol 11:104, 1994

Fraser WD, Hofmeyr J, Lede R, et al: Amnioinfusion for the prevention of the meconium aspiration syndrome. Amnioinfusion Trial Group. N Engl J Med 353:909, 2005

Furman B, Erez O, Senior L, et al: Hydramnios and small for gestational age: Prevalence and clinical significance. Acta Obstet Gynecol Scand 79:31, 2000

Gagnon R, Harding R, Brace RA: Amniotic fluid and fetal urinary responses to severe placental insufficiency in sheep. Am J Obstet Gynecol 186:1076, 2002

Galea P, Barigye O, Wee L, et al: The placenta contributes to activation of the renin angiotensin system in twin-twin transfusion syndrome. Placenta 29(8):734, 2008

Garmel SH, Chelmow D, Sha SJ, et al: Oligohydramnios and the appropriately grown fetus. Am J Perinatol 14:359, 1997

Glantz JC, Abramowicz JS, Sherer DM: Significance of idiopathic midtrimester polyhydramnios. Am J Perinatol 11:305, 1994

Golan A, Wolman I, Saller Y, et al: Hydramnios in singleton pregnancy: Sonographic prevalence and etiology. Gynecol Obstet Invest 35:91, 1993

Grubb DK, Paul RH: Amniotic fluid index and prolonged antepartum fetal heart rate decelerations. Obstet Gynecol 79:558, 1992

Hill LM, Breckle R, Thomas ML, et al: Polyhydramnios: Ultrasonically detected prevalence and neonatal outcome. Obstet Gynecol 69:21, 1987

Hill LM, Krohn M, Lazebnik N, et al: The amniotic fluid index in normal twin pregnancies. Am J Obstet Gynecol 182:950, 2000

Hinh ND, Ladinsky JL: Amniotic fluid index measurements in normal pregnancy after 28 gestational weeks. Int J Gynaecol Obstet 91:132, 2005

Johnson JM, Chauhan SP, Ennen CS, et al: A comparison of 3 criteria of oligohydramnios in identifying peripartum complications: A secondary analysis. Am J Obstet Gynecol 197:207.e1, 2007

Kerr J, Borgida AF, Hardardottir H, et al: Maternal hydration and its effect on the amniotic fluid index. Am J Obstet Gynecol 174:416, 1996

Kilbride HW, Yeast J, Thibeault DW: Defining limits of survival: Lethal pulmonary hypoplasia after midtrimester premature rupture of membranes. Am J Obstet Gynecol 175:675, 1996

Kilpatrick SJ, Safford KL: Maternal hydration increases amniotic fluid index in women with normal amniotic fluid. Obstet Gynecol 81:49, 1993

Kramer WB, Van den Veyver IB, Kirshon B: Treatment of polyhydramnios with indomethacin. Clin Perinatol 21:615, 1994

Kriplani A, Abbi M, Banerjee N, et al: Indomethacin therapy in the treatment of polyhydramnios due to placental chorioangioma. J Obstet Gynaecol Res 27:245, 2001

Lauria MR, Gonik B, Romero R: Pulmonary hypoplasia: Pathogenesis, diagnosis, and antenatal prediction. Obstet Gynecol 86:466, 1995

Leung WC, Jouannic JM, Hyett J, et al: Procedure-related complications of rapid amniodrainage in the treatment of polyhydramnios. Ultrasound Obstet Gynecol 23:154, 2004

Leveno KJ, Quirk JG Jr, Cunningham FG, et al: Prolonged pregnancy, 1. Observations concerning the causes of fetal distress. Am J Obstet Gynecol 150:465, 1984

Liu H, Zheng Z, Wintour EM: Aquaporins and fetal fluid balance. Placenta 29:840, 2008

Machado MR, Cecatti JG, Krupa F, et al: Curve of amniotic fluid index measurements in low risk pregnancy. Acta Obstet Gynecol Scand 86:37, 2007

Magann EF, Chauhan SP, Bofill JA, et al: Comparability of the amniotic fluid index and single deepest pocket measurements in clinical practice. Aust NZ J Obstet Gynaecol 43:75, 2003a

Magann EF, Chauhan SP, Doherty DA, et al: A review of idiopathic hydramnios and pregnancy outcomes. Obstet Gynecol Surv 62:795, 2007

Magann EF, Chauhan SP, Martin JN: Is amniotic fluid volume status predictive of fetal acidosis at delivery? Aust NZ J Obstet Gynaecol 43:129, 2003b

Magann EF, Doherty DA, Chauhan SP, et al: Effect of maternal hydration on amniotic fluid volume. Obstet Gynecol 101:1261, 2003c

Magann EF, Doherty DA, Chauhan SP, et al: How well do the amniotic fluid index and single deepest pocket indices (below the 3rd and 5th and above the 95th and 97th percentiles) predict oligohydramnios and hydramnios? Am J Obstet Gynecol 190:164, 2004

Magann EF, Chauhan SP, Barrilleaux PS, et al: Ultrasound estimate of amniotic fluid volume: Color Doppler overdiagnosis of oligohydramnios. Obstet Gynecol 98:71, 2001

Magann EF, Kinsella MJ, Chauhan SP, et al: Does an amniotic fluid index of </ = 5 cm necessitate delivery in high-risk pregnancies? A case-control study. Am J Obstet Gynecol 180:1354, 1999

Magann EF, Nolan TE, Hess LW, et al: Measurement of amniotic fluid volume: Accuracy of ultrasonography techniques. Am J Obstet Gynecol 167:1533, 1992

Magann EF, Sanderson M, Martin JN, et al: The amniotic fluid index, single deepest pocket, and two-diameter pocket in normal human pregnancy. Am J Obstet Gynecol 182:1581, 2000

Maher JE, Wenstrom KD, Hauth JC, et al: Amniotic fluid embolism after saline amnioinfusion: Two cases and review of the literature. Obstet Gynecol 83:851, 1994

Mahieu-Caputo D, Dommergues M, Delezoide AL, et al: Twin-to-twin transfusion syndrome. Role of the fetal renin-angiotensin system. Am J Pathol 156(2):629, 2000

Mahieu-Caputo D, Meulemans A, Martinovic J, et al: Paradoxic activation of the renin-angiotensin system in twin-twin transfusion syndrome: an explanation for cardiovascular disturbances in the recipient. Pediatr Res 58(4):685, 2005

Malhotra B, Deka D: Duration of the increase in amniotic fluid index (AFI) after acute maternal hydration. Arch Gynecol Obstet 269:173, 2004

Mamopoulos M, Assimakopoulos E, Reece EA, et al: Maternal indomethacin therapy in the treatment of polyhydramnios. Am J Obstet Gynecol 162:1225, 1990

Mann S, Dvorak N, Gilbert H, et al: Steady-state levels of aquaporin 1 mRNA expression are increased in idiopathic polyhydramnios. Am J Obstet Gynecol 194:884, 2006

Mann SE, Ricke EA, Torres EA, et al: A novel model of polyhydramnios: Amniotic fluid volume is increased in aquaporin 1 knockout mice. Am J Obstet Gynecol 192:2041, 2005

Marks AD, Divon MY: Longitudinal study of the amniotic fluid index in postdates pregnancy. Obstet Gynecol 79:229, 1992

Martinez-Frias ML, Bermejo E, Rodriguez-Pinilla E, et al: Maternal and fetal factors related to abnormal amniotic fluid. J Perinatol 19:514, 1999

McCurdy CM Jr, Seeds JW: Oligohydramnios: Problems and treatment. Semin Perinatol 17:183, 1993

Mercer LJ, Brown LG: Fetal outcome with oligohydramnios in the second trimester. Obstet Gynecol 67:840, 1986

Moessinger AC, Santiago A, Paneth NS, et al: Time-trends in necropsy prevalence and birth prevalence of lung hypoplasia. Paediatr Perinat Epidemiol 3:421, 1989

Moise KJ Jr, Huhta JC, Sharif DS, et al: Indomethacin in the treatment of premature labor: Effects on the fetal ductus arteriosus. N Engl J Med 319:327, 1988

Morris JM, Thompson K, Smithey J, et al: The usefulness of ultrasound assessment of amniotic fluid in predicting adverse outcome in prolonged pregnancy: A prospective blinded observational study. BJOG 110:989, 2003

Naeye RL, Blanc WA: Fetal renal structure and the genesis of amniotic fluid disorders. Am J Pathol 67:95, 1972

Narchi H, Santos M, Kulayat N: Polyhydramnios as a sign of fetal pseudohypoaldosteronism. Int J Gynaecol Obstet 69:53, 2000

Newbould MJ, Lendon M, Barson AJ: Oligohydramnios sequence: The spectrum of renal malformations. Br J Obstet Gynaecol 101:598, 1994

Nordin NM, Wei JW, Naing NN, et al: Comparison of maternal-fetal outcomes in gestational diabetes and lesser degrees of glucose intolerance. J Obstet Gynaecol Res 32(1):107, 2006

Oz AU, Holub B, Mendilcioglu I, et al: Renal artery Doppler investigation of the etiology of oligohydramnios in postterm pregnancy. Obstet Gynecol 100:715, 2002

Panting-Kemp A, Nguyen T, Castro L: Substance abuse and polyhydramnios. Am J Obstet Gynecol 187:602, 2002

Panting-Kemp A, Nguyen T, Chang E, et al: Idiopathic polyhydramnios and perinatal outcome. Am J Obstet Gynecol 181:1079, 1999

Peedicayil A, Mathai M, Regi A, et al: Inter- and intra-observer variation in the amniotic fluid index. Obstet Gynecol 84:848, 1994

Peipert JF, Donnenfeld AE: Oligohydramnios: A review. Obstet Gynecol Surv 46:325, 1991

Phelan JP, Smith CV, Broussard P, et al: Amniotic fluid volume assessment with the four-quadrant technique at 36–42 weeks' gestation. J Reprod Med 32:540, 1987

Pierce J, Gaudier FL, Sanchez-Ramos L: Intrapartum amnioinfusion for meconium-stained fluid: Meta-analysis of prospective clinical trials. Obstet Gynecol 95:1051, 2000

Porter TF, Dildy GA, Blanchard JR, et al: Normal values for amniotic fluid index during uncomplicated twin pregnancy. Obstet Gynecol 87:699, 1996

Pritchard JA: Fetal swallowing and amniotic fluid volume. Obstet Gynecol 28:606, 1966

Pryde PG, Hallak M, Lauria MR, et al: Severe oligohydramnios with intact membranes: An indication for diagnostic amnioinfusion. Fetal Diagn Ther 15:46, 2000

Queenan JT: Polyhydramnios and oligohydramnios. Contemp Obstet Gynecol 36:60, 1991

Rogers MS, Lau TK, Wang CC, et al: Amnioinfusion for the prevention of meconium aspiration during labour. Aust NZ J Obstet Gynaecol 36:407, 1996

Ross MG, Cedars L, Nijland MJ, et al: Treatment of oligohydramnios with maternal 1-deamino-[8-D-arginine] vasopressin–induced plasma hypoosmolality. Am J Obstet Gynecol 174:1608, 1996

Shenker L, Reed KL, Anderson CF, et al: Significance of oligohydramnios complicating pregnancy. Am J Obstet Gynecol 164:1597, 1991

Spong CY, Ogundipe OA, Ross MG: Prophylactic amnioinfusion for meconium-stained amniotic fluid. Am J Obstet Gynecol 171:931, 1994

Touboul C, Boileau P, Picone O, et al: Outcome of children born out of pregnancies complicated by unexplained polyhydramnios. BJOG 114:489, 2007

Usta IM, Mercer BM, Aswad NK, et al: The impact of a policy of amnioinfusion for meconium-stained amniotic fluid. Obstet Gynecol 85:237, 1995

Wang S, Amidi F, Yin S, et al: Cyclic adenosine monophosphate regulation of aquaporin gene expression in human amnion epithelia. Reprod Sci 14:234, 2007

Winn HN, Chen M, Amon E, et al: Neonatal pulmonary hypoplasia and perinatal mortality in patients with midtrimester rupture of amniotic membranes—a critical analysis. Am J Obstet Gynecol 182:1638, 2000

Xu H, Hofmeyr J, Roy C, et al: Intrapartum amnioinfusion for meconium-stained amniotic fluid: A systematic review of randomised controlled trials. BJOG 114:383, 2007

Yancey MK, Richards DS: Effect of altitude on the amniotic fluid index. J Reprod Med 39:101, 1994

Zhang J, Troendle J, Meikle S, et al: Isolated oligohydramnios is not associated with adverse perinatal outcomes. BJOG 111:220, 2004

CHAPTER 22

Labor Induction

Induction implies stimulation of contractions before the spontaneous onset of labor, with or without ruptured membranes. *Augmentation* refers to stimulation of spontaneous contractions that are considered inadequate because of failed cervical dilation and fetal descent. According to the National Center for Health Statistics, the incidence of labor induction in the United States more than doubled from 9.5 percent in 1991 to 22.5 percent in 2006 (Martin and associates, 2009). The incidence is variable between practices. For example, at Parkland Hospital approximately 35 percent of labors are induced or augmented. By comparison, at the University of Alabama at Birmingham Hospital, labor is induced in about 20 percent of women, and another 35 percent are given oxytocin for augmentation—a total of 55 percent. This chapter includes an overview of indications for labor induction and augmentation, as well as a description of various techniques to effect pre-induction cervical ripening.

LABOR INDUCTION

Indications

Induction is indicated when the benefits to either mother or fetus outweigh those of continuing the pregnancy. Indications include immediate conditions such as ruptured membranes with chorioamnionitis or severe preeclampsia. The more common indications include membrane rupture without labor, gestational hypertension, nonreassuring fetal status, postterm pregnancy, and various maternal medical conditions such as chronic hypertension and diabetes (American College of Obstetricians and Gynecologists, 1999a).

There are a number of techniques available to induce or augment labor, and these are discussed separately. Importantly, and as recommended in *Guidelines for Perinatal Care*, each obstetrical department should have its own written protocols that describe administration of oxytocin and other uterotonics (American Academy of Pediatrics and American College of Obstetricians and Gynecologists, 2007).

Contraindications

Contraindications to induction are similar to those that preclude spontaneous labor or delivery. Fetal factors include appreciable macrosomia, multifetal gestation, severe hydrocephalus, malpresentation, or nonreassuring fetal status. The few maternal contraindications are related to prior uterine incision type, contracted or distorted pelvic anatomy, abnormal placentation, and conditions such as active genital herpes infection or cervical cancer.

Risks

Maternal complication rates that are increased in association with labor induction include cesarean delivery, chorioamnionitis, and uterine atony.

Cesarean Delivery Rate

This is especially increased in nulliparas undergoing induction (Luthy and colleagues, 2004; Yeast and associates, 1999). A number of investigators have reported two- to threefold risks (Hoffman and Sciscione, 2003; Maslow and Sweeny, 2000; Smith and colleagues, 2003). Moreover, these rates are inversely related with favorability of the cervix at induction, that is, the Bishop score (Vahratian and colleagues, 2005; Vroucnraets and associates, 2005).

However, pre-induction cervical ripening may not lower the cesarean delivery rate in a nullipara with an unfavorable cervix (Mercer, 2005). In a retrospective cohort study, Hamar and associates (2001) found that the rate of cesarean delivery following elective induction was significantly increased in women without antepartum complications and with a Bishop score of 7 or greater compared with those with spontaneous labor.

In nulliparas more than 41 weeks with an unengaged vertex, the risk of cesarean delivery increases 12-fold compared with that of those with an engaged vertex (Shin and associates, 2004). There is no increased risk if the engaged fetal head is occiput posterior at the time of induction (Peregrine and colleagues, 2007).

Chorioamnionitis

Women whose labor is induced have an increased incidence of chorioamnionitis compared with those in spontaneous labor (American College of Obstetricians and Gynecologists, 1999a).

Uterine Atony

Postpartum atony and hemorrhage are more common in women undergoing induction or augmentation. Intractable atony was the indication for a third of all cesarean hysterectomies. This indication was more prevalent in women with induced or augmented labor or in those with chorioamnionitis. Shellhaas and associates (2001) reported data from nearly 137,000 deliveries in the Maternal-Fetal Units Network. There were 146 emergent postpartum hysterectomies done—about 1 per 1000 vaginal deliveries versus 1 per 200 cesarean deliveries. Importantly, 41 percent of all hysterectomies followed primary cesarean delivery. Kastner and colleagues (2002) reported similar findings.

Elective Labor Induction

There can be no doubt that elective induction for convenience of the practitioner or the woman and her family has become more prevalent. Glantz (2003) estimated that a fourth of all labor inductions were elective. Despite this, the American College of Obstetricians and Gynecologists (1999a) does not support this practice, except for logistical reasons such as a risk of rapid labor, a woman who lives a long distance from the hospital, or psychosocial indications. We are also of the opinion that routine elective induction at term is not justified, because of the increased risk for severe, albeit infrequent, adverse maternal outcomes. Tita (2009) and Clark (2009) and their colleagues have reported also significant and appreciable adverse neonatal morbidity with elective delivery prior to 39 completed weeks and without consideration or documentation of the American College of Obstetricians and Gynecologists criteria (2007, 2008) detailed in Chapters 26 (p. 571) and 29 (p. 606). If elective induction is considered at term, these risks must be discussed and informed consent obtained.

Oshiro and associates (2009) implemented guidelines to discourage deliveries prior to 39 completed weeks. Fisch and co-workers (2009) also developed and enforced similar guidelines at their institution. Both groups of investigators reported significant decreases in rates of elective deliveries following initiation of guidelines.

Expectations of Labor Induction

Several factors increase the success of labor induction and include multiparity, body mass index (BMI) <30, favorable cervix, and birthweight <3500 g (Peregrine and associates, 2006; Pevzner and co-workers, 2009). In many cases, it seems that the uterus is simply poorly prepared for labor. One example is an "unripe cervix." It is also likely that the increase in cesarean deliveries associated with induction is strongly influenced by the duration of the induction attempt, especially in the circumstance of an unfavorable cervix. Rouse and colleagues (2000) reported characteristics of failed labor induction in a prospective management protocol for 509 women, of whom 360 were nulliparas. The cesarean delivery rate was 9 percent in parous women but 25 percent in nulliparas. The authors concluded that by requiring a minimum of 12 hours of uterine stimulation with oxytocin after membrane rupture, many nulliparas who remained in the latent phase of labor at 6 and 9 hours eventually entered active labor and had a safe vaginal delivery. Simon and Grobman (2005) reported that only 2 percent of nulliparas never achieved active phase labor before cesarean delivery. They concluded that a latent phase as long as 18 hours during induction allowed most of these women to achieve a vaginal delivery without a significantly increased risk of maternal or neonatal morbidity.

The duration for either labor induction or augmentation and successful delivery has received too little attention. More precise data are needed to understand the wide range of individual management. For example, Garcia and associates (2001), after adjustment for case mix, reported that the cesarean delivery rate was about 30 percent lower at academic medical centers compared with that at community hospitals. Doyle and colleagues (2002) reported that cesarean deliveries in a community hospital were twice that of a county hospital.

PREINDUCTION CERVICAL RIPENING

The condition of the cervix—or "favorability"—is important to successful labor induction.

Cervical "Favorability"

One quantifiable method used to predict outcomes of labor induction is the score described by Bishop (1964) and presented in Table 22-1. A *Bishop score* of 9 conveys a high likelihood for a successful induction. Most practitioners would consider that a woman whose cervix is 2 cm dilated, 80 percent effaced, soft, and midposition and a fetal occiput at −1 station would have a successful labor induction. For research purposes, a Bishop score of 4 or less identifies an unfavorable cervix and may be an indication for cervical ripening.

As an alternate to the Bishop score, Hatfield and associates (2007) performed a meta-analysis of 20 trials in which cervical length was assessed by transvaginal sonography and used to

TABLE 22-1. Bishop Scoring System Used for Assessment of Inducibility

	Factor				
Score	Dilatation (cm)	Effacement (Percent)	Station (−3 to +2)	Cervical Consistency	Cervical Position
0	Closed	0–30	−3	Firm	Posterior
1	1–2	40–50	−2	Medium	Midposition
2	3–4	60–70	−1	Soft	Anterior
3	≥5	≥80	+1, +2	—	—

predict successful induction. Because of the heterogeneity of study criteria—including the definition of "successful induction"—the authors concluded that the question was still unanswered. They, as did Crane (2006), found that cervical length determination by sonography was not superior to use of the Bishop score.

Unfortunately, women too frequently have an indication for induction but with an unfavorable cervix. As favorability or Bishop score decreases, there is an increasingly unsuccessful induction rate. Thus, considerable research has been directed toward various techniques to "ripen" the cervix prior to stimulation of uterine contractions. In many cases, the techniques used to improve cervical favorability also stimulate contractions. Thus, they may be used to induce labor. Methods used for cervical ripening include pharmacological preparations and various forms of mechanical cervical distension.

Pharmacological Techniques

Prostaglandin E_2

Local application of prostaglandin E_2—dinoprostone—is commonly used for cervical ripening (American College of Obstetricians and Gynecologists, 1999a, b). Its gel form—Prepidil—is available in a 2.5-mL syringe for an intracervical application of 0.5 mg of dinoprostone. With the woman supine, the tip of a pre-filled syringe is placed intracervically, and the gel is deposited just below the internal cervical os. After application she remains reclined for at least 30 minutes. Doses may be repeated every 6 hours, with a maximum of three doses recommended in 24 hours.

Owen and colleagues (1991) did a meta-analysis of 18 studies with 1811 women. They found that prostaglandin E_2 improved Bishop scores and when coupled with oxytocin, lowered induction-to-delivery times compared with those of women treated with oxytocin alone. Unfortunately, they found no benefit in lowering the cesarean delivery rate.

A 10-mg dinoprostone vaginal insert—Cervidil—is also approved for cervical ripening. This is a thin, flat, rectangular polymeric wafer held within a small, white mesh polyester sac (Fig. 22-1). The sac has a long attached tail to allow easy removal from the vagina. The insert provides slower release of medication—0.3 mg/hr—than the gel form. Combined with oxytocin, these inserts have been reported to shorten the induction-to-delivery interval (Bolnick and associates, 2004). Cervidil is used as a single dose placed transversely in the posterior vaginal fornix. Lubricant should be used sparingly, if at all, with insertion. Excessive lubricant can coat and hinder the release of dinoprostone. Following insertion, a woman should remain recumbent for at least 2 hours. The insert is removed after 12 hours or with labor onset.

Administration. Prostaglandin preparations should only be administered in or near the delivery suite, and uterine activity and fetal heart rate monitoring should be performed (American College of Obstetricians and Gynecologists, 1995b). These guidelines stem from the risk that prostaglandin preparations may cause uterine tachysystole. When contractions begin, they are usually apparent in the first hour and show peak activity in the first 4 hours (Bernstein, 1991; Miller and colleagues, 1991). When Perry and Leaphart (2004) compared intracervical gel with the intravaginal insert, they found that intravaginal placement resulted in quicker delivery—11.7 versus 16.2 hours. However, when more than two sequential doses of a prostaglandin E_2 insert were used, Chan and associates (2004) reported that 59 percent of women required emergency cesarean delivery. According to manufacturer guidelines, oxytocin induction that follows prostaglandin use for cervical ripening should be delayed for 6 to 12 hours following prostaglandin E_2 administration.

Side Effects. Uterine tachysystole has been reported to follow vaginally administered prostaglandin E_2 in 1 to 5 percent of women (Brindley and Sokol, 1988; Rayburn, 1989). Although

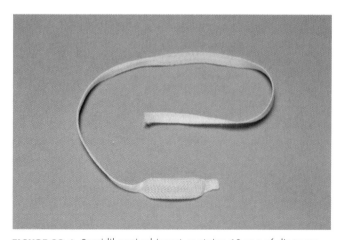

FIGURE 22-1 Cervidil vaginal insert contains 10 mg of dinoprostone designed to release approximately 0.3 mg/hr over a 10-hour period. (Used with permission of Forest Laboratories, Inc., New York, New York).

definitions may vary among studies, most use the terms defined by the American College of Obstetricians and Gynecologists (1999a) to describe increased uterine activity as follows:

1. *Uterine tachysystole* is defined as ≥6 contractions in a 10-minute period.
2. *Uterine hypertonus* is described as a single contraction lasting longer than 2 minutes.
3. *Uterine hyperstimulation* is when either condition leads to a nonreassuring fetal heart rate pattern.

Because hyperstimulation that can cause fetal compromise may develop when prostaglandins are used with preexisting spontaneous labor, such use is not recommended. If hyperstimulation occurs with the 10-mg insert, its removal by pulling on the tail of the surrounding net sac will usually reverse this effect. Irrigation to remove the gel preparation has not been helpful.

Contraindications to prostaglandin agents in general include asthma, glaucoma, or increased intraocular pressure. Moreover, manufacturer recommendations caution against its use in women with ruptured membranes.

Prostaglandin E₁

Misoprostol—Cytotec—is a synthetic prostaglandin E_1, approved as a 100- or 200-μg tablet for prevention of peptic ulcers. It has been used "off label" for preinduction cervical ripening and may be administered orally or vaginally. The tablets are stable at room temperature.

Although it has become widespread, the off-label use of misoprostol is controversial (Wagner, 2005; Weeks and associates, 2005). In 2000, G. D. Searle & Company notified physicians that misoprostol is not approved for labor induction or abortion. Despite this, the American College of Obstetricians and Gynecologists (2000) quickly reaffirmed its recommendation for use of the drug because of proven safety and efficacy. It currently is the prostaglandin of choice for these purposes at both Parkland Hospital and the University of Alabama at Birmingham Hospital.

Vaginal Administration. Several investigators have reported that misoprostol tablets placed into the vagina were either of equivalent or superior efficacy compared with intracervical prostaglandin E_2 gel (von Gemund and associates, 2004; Wing and co-workers, 1995a, b). The American College of Obstetricians and Gynecologists (1999b) reviewed 19 randomized trials in which more than 1900 women were given intravaginal misoprostol in doses ranging from 25 to 200 μg. They recommended the 25-μg dose—a fourth of a 100-μg tablet. The drug is evenly distributed among these quartered tablets.

Misoprostol use may decrease the need for oxytocin induction and reduce induction-to-delivery intervals (Sanchez-Ramos and colleagues, 1997). Hofmeyr and associates (2003) reviewed the Cochrane database and support these recommendations, but caution that rates of uterine hyperstimulation with adverse fetal heart rate changes are increased with their use. A 50-μg misoprostol intravaginal dose has been associated with significantly increased uterine tachysystole, meconium passage, and meconium aspiration compared with prostaglandin E_2 gel (Wing and co-workers, 1995a, b). A 25-μg intravaginal dose was

found comparable to dinoprostone regarding adverse neonatal outcome (von Gemund and associates, 2004).

Uterine rupture has been reported by Wing and colleagues (1998) with prostaglandin E_1 use in women with a prior cesarean delivery. Indeed, Plaut and associates (1999) reported uterine rupture in 5 of 89—6 percent—of women who had a prior cesarean incision and who were induced with misoprostol. This is compared with only 1 of 423 such women not given misoprostol. Currently, the consensus is that prior uterine surgery, including cesarean delivery, precludes the use of misoprostol (American College of Obstetricians and Gynecologists, 2004).

Oral Administration. Prostaglandin E_1 tablets are also effective when given orally. Windrim and associates (1997) reported oral misoprostol administration to be of similar efficacy as intravaginal administration for cervical ripening. Wing (2000) and Hall (2002) and their associates reported that a 100-μg oral dose was as effective as a 25-μg intravaginal dose.

Labor Induction with Prostaglandin E₁. Both vaginal and oral misoprostol may be used for either cervical ripening or labor induction. Hofmeyer and Gulmezoglu (2007) performed a Cochrane systematic review and found vaginal misoprostol, followed by oxytocin if needed, to be superior to oxytocin alone for labor induction. Rates of cesarean delivery section were variable. Some studies showed decreased rates with misoprostol, whereas others found no difference in rates.

It appears that 100 μg of oral or 25 μg of vaginal misoprostol is similar in efficacy to intravenous oxytocin for labor induction in women at or near term with either prematurely ruptured membranes or a favorable cervix (Lin and co-workers, 2005; Lo and associates, 2003). Misoprostol may be associated with an increased rate of hyperstimulation. In addition, induction with PGE_1 may prove ineffective and require subsequent augmentation with oxytocin. Thus, there are trade-offs regarding the risks, costs, and ease of administration of the two drugs, but either is suitable for labor induction. For *labor augmentation*, results of a pilot study showed oral misoprostol, 75 μg given at 4-hour intervals for a maximum of two doses, to be safe and effective (Villano and colleagues, 2010).

Nitric Oxide Donors

Several findings have led to a search for agents that stimulate nitric oxide (NO) production locally to be used for clinical purposes (Chanrachakul and co-workers, 2000). First, nitric oxide is likely a mediator of cervical ripening (see Chap. 3, p. 138). Also, cervical NO metabolites are increased at the beginning of uterine contractions. Lastly, cervical NO production is very low in postterm pregnancy (Väisänen-Tommiska and colleagues, 2003, 2004).

Bullarbo and colleagues (2007) recently reviewed rationale and use of the NO donors *isosorbide mononitrate* and *glyceryl trinitrate*. Isosorbide mononitrate induces cervical cyclo-oxygenase 2 (Ekerhovd and colleagues, 2002). It also induces cervical ultrastructure rearrangement similar to that seen with spontaneous cervical ripening (Thomson and associates, 1997; Ekerhovd and colleagues, 2003).

Clinical trials have not shown NO donors to be as effective as prostaglandin E_2 to effect cervical ripening (Chanrachakul and associates, 2001; Osman and colleagues, 2006). And the addition of isosorbide mononitrate to either dinoprostone or misoprostol did not enhance cervical ripening either in early pregnancy or at term and did not shorten time to vaginal delivery (Collingham, 2009; Ledingham, 2001; Wölfler, 2006, and all their co-workers).

Mechanical Techniques

Transcervical Catheter

A Foley catheter may be placed through the internal cervical os. Downward tension that is created by taping the catheter to the thigh can lead to cervical ripening. A modification of this, termed *extra-amnionic saline infusion (EASI),* consists of a constant saline infusion through the catheter into the space between the internal cervical os and placental membranes (Fig. 22-2). Catheter placement, with or without continuous saline infusion, results in improved cervical favorability and frequently stimulates contractions (Guinn and associates, 2004). Sherman and colleagues (1996) summarized the results of 13 trials with balloon-tipped catheters to effect cervical dilatation. They concluded that, with or without saline infusion, the method led to rapid improvement in Bishop scores and shorter labors. Karjane and co-workers (2006) reported that chorioamnionitis was less frequent when infusion was done compared with no infusion—6 versus 16 percent.

Labor Induction. Especially with saline infusion, the transcervical catheter technique is also effective for initiating labor, and several comparative studies have been done. Chung and colleagues (2003) randomized 135 women to labor induction with vaginal

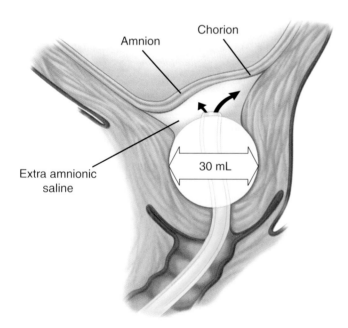

FIGURE 22-2 Extra-amnionic saline infusion (EASI) through 26F Foley catheter is placed through the cervix. The 30-mL balloon is inflated with saline and pulled snugly against the internal os, and the catheter taped to the thigh. Room-temperature normal saline is infused through the catheter port of the Foley at 30 or 40 mL/hour by intravenous infusion pump.

misoprostol, extra-amnionic Foley catheter with bulb inflation to 30 mL, or both therapies. Outcomes were similar in all three groups, and there was no apparent benefit of combining these two techniques. Conversely, Culver and colleagues (2004) compared oxytocin plus an intracervical Foley catheter with 25-μg vaginal misoprostol every 4 hours in women with a Bishop score less than 6. The mean induction-to-delivery time was significantly shorter in the catheter-plus-oxytocin group—16 versus 22 hours. Levy and associates (2004) reported that the use of an 80-mL Foley transcervical catheter balloon compared with that of a 30-mL for cervical ripening was significantly more effective.

Extra-amnionic Saline Infusion (EASI)

This technique has been reported to significantly improve the Bishop score and decrease induction-to-delivery times compared with: (1) 50-μg intravaginal misoprostol tablets, (2) 0.5 mg of intracervical prostaglandin E_2, (3) 50-μg oral misoprostol (Goldman and Wigton, 1999; Vengalil and colleagues, 1998). In another study, Guinn and colleagues (2000) randomized women to intracervical prostaglandin E_2, laminaria plus intravenous oxytocin, or EASI plus oxytocin. The cesarean delivery rate was similar with all three interventions. The mean induction-to-delivery time of 18 hours with catheter infusion was significantly less than the 21 hours with laminaria plus oxytocin or the 25 hours with prostaglandin E_2 gel.

In one follow-up study, Sciscione and co-workers (2004) concluded that cervical ripening with a Foley catheter did not increase the risk of preterm birth in a subsequent pregnancy.

Hygroscopic Cervical Dilators

Cervical dilatation can be accomplished using hygroscopic osmotic cervical dilators, as described for early pregnancy termination (see Chap. 9, p. 229). These mechanical dilators have long been successfully used when inserted prior to pregnancy termination (Hale and Pion, 1972). More recently, they have also been used for cervical ripening before labor induction. Intuitive concerns of ascending infection have not been verified. Thus, their use appears to be safe, although anaphylaxis has followed laminaria insertion (Cole and Bruck, 2000; Nguyen and Hoffman, 1995). Dilators are attractive because of their low cost and easy placement and removal.

Gilson and associates (1996) reported a rapid improvement of cervical favorability in women randomized to hygroscopic dilators prior to oxytocin induction. There was, however, no beneficial effect on the vaginal delivery rate or induction-to-delivery times compared with those of women given oxytocin only. In the randomized study cited earlier, Guinn and co-workers (2000) reported a longer induction-to-delivery time with cervical dilators plus oxytocin compared with that of EASI plus oxytocin.

Membrane Stripping for Labor Induction

Induction of labor by membrane "stripping" is a common practice (see Fig. 6-4, p. 142). McColgin and colleagues (1990) reported that stripping was safe and decreased the incidence of postterm gestation. They documented significantly increased serum levels of endogenous prostaglandins with stripping (McColgin and associates, 1993). Allott and Palmer (1993) randomized 195 women with normal pregnancies beyond 40 weeks to digital cervical examination either with or without membrane stripping. The women were examined as outpatients. Two thirds of those who underwent stripping entered spontaneous labor within 72 hours compared with one third of the other group. The incidence of ruptured membranes, infection, and bleeding was not increased. Importantly, subsequent induction for postterm pregnancy at 42 weeks was significantly decreased with stripping.

Summary of Preinduction Cervical Ripening

These techniques are widely used when labor induction is indicated for a woman with an "unripe cervix." Some of the preinduction techniques described may have benefits when compared with oxytocin induction alone (Table 22-2). Some are quite successful for induction. That said, there are few data to support the premise that any of these techniques results in a reduction in cesarean delivery rates or in lower maternal or neonatal morbidity compared with those of women in whom such techniques are not used.

LABOR INDUCTION AND AUGMENTATION WITH OXYTOCIN

In most instances, pre-induction cervical ripening and labor induction are simply a continuum. Often, as described above, "ripening" will also stimulate labor. If not, however, induction or augmentation may be continued with diluted intravenous solutions of oxytocin given by infusion pump.

TABLE 22-2. Some Commonly Used Regimens for Pre-induction Cervical Ripening and/or Labor Induction

Techniques	Agent	Route/Dose	Comments
Pharmacological			
Prostaglandin E$_2$	Dinoprostone gel, 0.5 mg (Prepidil)	Cervical 0.5 mg; repeat in 6 hr; permit 3 doses total	1. Shorter I-D times with oxytocin infusion than oxytocin alone
	Dinoprostone insert, 10 mg (Cervidil)	Posterior fornix, 10 mg	2. Insert has shorter I-D times than gel
			3. 6–12 hr interval from last insert to oxytocin infusion
Prostaglandin E$_1$[a]	Misoprostol tablet, 100–200 μg (Cytotec)	Vaginal, 25 μg; repeat 3–6 hr prn	1. Contractions within 30–60 min
		Oral, 50–100 μg; repeat 3–6 hr prn	2. Comparable success with oxytocin for ruptured membranes at term and/or favorable cervix
			3. Tachysystole common with doses >25 μg dosed vaginally
Mechanical			
Transcervical 36F Foley catheter	30-mL balloon		1. Improves Bishop scores rapidly
			2. 80-mL balloon more effective
			3. Combined with oxytocin infusion is superior to PGE$_1$ vaginally
			4. Results improved with EASI
Hygroscopic dilators		Laminaria, magnesium sulfate	1. Rapidly improves Bishop score
			2. May not shorten I-D times with oxytocin

[a]Off-label use.
EASI = extra-amnionic saline infusion at 30–40 mL/hr; I-D = induction-to-delivery.

Synthetic oxytocin is one of the most commonly used medications in the United States. It was the first polypeptide hormone synthesized, an achievement for which the 1955 Nobel Prize in chemistry was awarded (du Vigneaud and co-workers, 1953). Regarding labor, it may be used for induction or for augmentation of labor.

With oxytocin use, the American College of Obstetricians and Gynecologists (1999a) recommends fetal heart rate and contraction monitoring similar to that for any high-risk pregnancy. Contractions can be monitored either by palpation or by electronic means of recording uterine activity (see Chap. 18, p. 437). One caveat with palpation is that contraction pressures cannot be accurately quantified (Arrabal and Nagey, 1996).

Techniques

Intravenous Oxytocin Administration

The goal of induction or augmentation is to effect uterine activity sufficient to produce cervical change and fetal descent, while avoiding development of a nonreassuring fetal status. In general, oxytocin should be discontinued if the number of contractions persists with a frequency greater than five in a 10-minute period or seven in a 15-minute period or with a persistent nonreassuring fetal heart rate pattern. Discontinuation of oxytocin nearly always rapidly decreases the frequency of contractions. When oxytocin is stopped, its concentration in plasma rapidly falls because the mean half-life is approximately 5 minutes. Seitchik and co-workers (1984) found that the uterus contracts within 3 to 5 minutes of beginning an oxytocin infusion and that a plasma steady-state is reached in 40 minutes. Response is highly variable and depends on preexisting uterine activity, cervical status, pregnancy duration, and individual biological differences. Caldeyro-Barcia and Poseiro (1960) reported that the uterine response to oxytocin increases from 20 to 30 weeks and increases rapidly at term (see Chap. 18, p. 437).

Oxytocin Dosage. A 1-mL ampule containing 10 units usually is diluted into 1000 mL of a crystalloid solution and administered by infusion pump. A typical infusate consists of 10 or 20 units—or 10,000 to 20,000 mU—mixed into 1000 mL of lactated Ringer solution. This mixture results in an oxytocin concentration of 10 or 20 mU/mL, respectively. To avoid bolus administration, the infusion should be inserted into the main intravenous line close to the venipuncture site.

A number of oxytocin regimens for labor stimulation are recommended by the American College of Obstetricians and Gynecologists (1999a). These and others are shown in Table 22-3. Initially, only variations of low-dose protocols were used in the United States. In 1984, O'Driscoll and colleagues (1984) from Dublin described a protocol for the active management of labor that called for oxytocin at a starting dosage of 6 mU/min and advanced in 6-mU/min increments. Subsequent comparative trials during the 1990s were done to compare high-dose—4 to 6 mU/min—versus conventional low-dose—0.5 to 1.5 mU/min—regimens both for labor induction and for augmentation.

From Parkland Hospital, Satin and colleagues (1992) evaluated an oxytocin regimen using an initial and incremental dosage of 6 mU/min compared with one using 1 mU/min. Increases at 20-minute intervals were provided as needed. Among 1112 women undergoing induction, the 6-mU/min regimen resulted in a shorter mean admission-to-delivery time, fewer failed inductions, and no cases of neonatal sepsis. Among 1676 women who had labor augmentation, those who received the 6-mU/min regimen had a shorter duration-to-delivery time, fewer forceps deliveries, fewer cesarean deliveries for dystocia, and decreased intrapartum chorioamnionitis or neonatal sepsis. With this protocol, uterine hyperstimulation is managed by oxytocin discontinuation followed by resumption when indicated and at half the stopping dosage. Thereafter, the dosage is increased at 3 mU/min when appropriate instead of the usual 6-mU/min increase for women without hyperstimulation. No adverse neonatal effects were observed.

Xenakis and colleagues (1995) reported benefits using an incremental oxytocin regimen starting at 4 mU/min. In a comparative study of 1307 women by Merrill and Zlatnik (1999), 816 were randomized for labor induction and 816 for augmentation with incremental oxytocin given at either 1.5 or 4.5 mU/min. Women randomized to the 4.5 mU/min dosage had significantly decreased mean durations of induction-to-second-stage labor and induction-to-delivery. Nulliparas randomized to the 4.5 mU/min dosage had a significantly lower

TABLE 22-3. Various Low- and High-Dose Oxytocin Regimens Used for Labor Induction

Regimen	Starting Dose (mU/min)	Incremental Increase (mU/min)	Interval (min)
Low-Dose	0.5–1.5	1	15–40
	2	4, 8, 12, 16, 20 25, 30	15
High-Dose	4	4	15
	4.5	4.5	15–30
	6	6[a]	20–40[b]

[a]With hyperstimulation and after oxytocin infusion is discontinued, it is restarted at ½ the previous dose and increased at 3 mU/min incremental doses.
[b]Hyperstimulation is more common with shorter intervals.
Data from Merrill and Zlatnik (1999), Satin and associates (1992, 1994), and Xenakis and colleagues (1995).

cesarean delivery rate for dystocia compared with those given 1.5 mU/min dosage—5.9 versus 11.9 percent.

Thus, benefits favor higher-dose regimens of 4.5 to 6 mU/min compared with lower dosages of 0.5 to 1.5 mU/min. In 1990, routine use of the 6-mU/min oxytocin beginning and incremental dosage was incorporated at Parkland Hospital and continues through today. At the University of Alabama at Birmingham, a 2-mU/min beginning and incremental oxytocin regimen is administered. In both cases, these dosages are employed for either labor induction or augmentation.

Interval between Incremental Dosing

Intervals to increase oxytocin doses vary from 15 to 40 minutes (see Table 22-2). Satin and colleagues (1994) addressed this aspect with a 6-mU/min regimen providing increases at either 20- or 40-minute intervals. Women assigned to the 20-minute interval regimen for labor augmentation had a significant reduction in the rate of cesarean delivery for dystocia compared with that for the 40-minute interval regimen—8 versus 12 percent. As perhaps expected, uterine hyperstimulation was significantly more frequent with the 20-minute regimen.

Other investigators report even more frequent incremental increases. Frigoletto and associates (1995) and Xenakis and co-workers (1995) began oxytocin at 4 mU/min with increases as needed every 15 minutes. Merrill and Zlatnik (1999) started with 4.5 mU/min with increases every 30 minutes. López-Zeno and colleagues (1992) began at 6 mU/min with increases every 15 minutes. Thus, there are a number of acceptable oxytocin protocols that at least appear dissimilar. But a comparison of protocols from two of our institutions indicates that this is not so:

1. The Parkland Hospital protocol calls for a starting dose of oxytocin at 6 mU/min, with 6-mU/min increases every 40 minutes, but employs flexible dosing based on hyperstimulation.
2. The University of Alabama at Birmingham Hospital protocol begins oxytocin at 2 mU/min and increases it as needed every 15 minutes to 4, 8, 12, 16, 20, 25, and 30 mU/min.

Thus, although the regimens at first appear disparate, if there is no uterine activity, either regimen is delivering 12 mU/min by 45 minutes into the infusion.

Maximal Dosage

The *maximal* effective dose of oxytocin to achieve adequate contractions in all women is different. Wen and colleagues (2001) studied 1151 consecutive nulliparas and found that the likelihood of progression to a vaginal delivery decreased at and beyond an oxytocin dosage of 36 mU/min. At a dosage of 72 mU/min, however, half of the nulliparas were delivered vaginally. Thus, if contractions are not adequate—less than 200 Montevideo units—and if the fetal status is reassuring and labor has arrested, an oxytocin infusion dose greater than 48 mU/min has no apparent risks.

Risks versus Benefits

Unless the uterus is scarred, uterine rupture associated with oxytocin infusion is rare, even in parous women (see Chap. 35, p. 784). Flannelly and associates (1993) reported no uterine ruptures, with or without oxytocin, in 27,829 *nulliparas*. There were eight instances of overt uterine rupture during labor in 48,718 *parous* women— but only one of these was associated with oxytocin use.

Oxytocin has amino-acid homology similar to arginine vasopressin. Thus, not surprisingly, it has significant antidiuretic action, and when infused at dosages of 20 mU/min or more, renal free water clearance decreases markedly. If aqueous fluids are infused in appreciable amounts along with oxytocin, *water intoxication* can lead to convulsions, coma, and even death. In general, if oxytocin is to be administered in high doses for a considerable period of time, its concentration should be increased rather than increasing the flow rate of a more dilute solution. Consideration also should be given to use of either normal saline or lactated Ringer solution in these circumstances.

Uterine Contraction Pressures

Contraction forces in spontaneously laboring women range from 90 to 390 Montevideo units. As discussed in Chapter 20 (p. 467), the latter are calculated by subtracting the baseline uterine pressure from the peak contraction pressure for each contraction in a 10-minute window. The pressures generated by each contraction are then summed. Caldeyro-Barcia and associates (1950) and Seitchik and colleagues (1984) found that the mean or median spontaneous uterine contraction pattern resulting in a progression to a vaginal delivery was between 140 and 150 Montevideo units.

In the management of active-phase arrest, and with no contraindication to intravenous oxytocin, decisions must be made with knowledge of the safe upper range of uterine activity. Hauth and co-workers (1986) described an effective and safe protocol for oxytocin augmentation for active-phase arrest with which greater than 90 percent of women achieved an average of at least 200 to 225 Montevideo units. Hauth and associates (1991) later reported that nearly all women in whom active-phase arrest persisted, despite oxytocin, generated more than 200 Montevideo units. Importantly, despite no labor progression, there were no adverse maternal or perinatal effects in those undergoing cesarean delivery. There are no data regarding safety and efficacy of contraction patterns in women with a prior cesarean delivery, with twins, or with an overdistended uterus.

Duration of Oxytocin Administration—Active Phase Arrest

First-stage arrest of labor is defined by the American College of Obstetricians and Gynecologists (1989, 1995a) as a completed latent phase along with contractions exceeding 200 Montevideo units for more than 2 hours without cervical change. Some investigators have attempted to define a more accurate duration for active-phase arrest. Arulkumaran and associates (1987) extended the 2-hour limit to 4 hours and reported a 1.3-percent cesarean delivery rate in women who continued to have adequate contractions and progressive cervical dilatation of at least 1 cm/hr. In women without progressive cervical dilatation who were allowed another 4 hours of labor, half required cesarean delivery.

Rouse and colleagues (1999) prospectively managed 542 women at term with active-phase arrest and no other complications. Their protocol was to achieve a sustained pattern of at least 200 Montevideo units for a *minimum* of 4 hours. This time frame was extended to 6 hours if activity of 200 Montevideo units or greater could not be sustained. Almost 92 percent of these women were delivered vaginally. As discussed in Chapter 20 (p. 467), these and other studies support the practice to allow an active-phase arrest of 4 hours (Rouse and associates, 2001). Solheim and colleagues (2009) also support the quality and cost effectiveness of allowing an active-phase arrest of 4 hours.

Zhang and co-workers (2002) analyzed labor duration from 4 cm to complete dilatation in 1329 nulliparas at term. They found that before dilatation of 7 cm was reached, lack of progress for more than 2 hours was not uncommon in those who delivered vaginally. Alexander and colleagues (2002) reported that epidural analgesia prolonged active labor by 1 hour compared with duration of the active phase as defined by Friedman (1955). Consideration of these changes in the management of labor, especially in nulliparas, may safely reduce the cesarean delivery rate.

Amniotomy

A common indication for artificial rupture of the membranes—*surgical amniotomy*—includes the need for direct monitoring of the fetal heart rate or uterine contractions, or both. During amniotomy, to minimize the risk of cord prolapse, care should be taken to avoid dislodging the fetal head. Fundal or suprapubic pressure or both may reduce the risk of cord prolapse. Some clinicians prefer to rupture membranes during a contraction. If the vertex is not well applied to the lower uterine segment, a gradual egress of amnionic fluid can sometimes be accomplished by several membrane punctures with a 26-gauge needle held with a ring forceps and with direct visualization using a vaginal speculum. In many of these, however, membranes tear and fluid is lost rapidly. The fetal heart rate should be assessed before and immediately after amniotomy.

Elective Amniotomy

Membrane rupture with the intention of accelerating labor is commonly performed. In the investigations presented in Table 22-4, amniotomy at about 5 cm dilation accelerated spontaneous labor by 1 to 2 hours. Importantly, neither the need for oxytocin stimulation nor the overall cesarean delivery rate was increased. Although mild and moderate cord compression patterns were increased following amniotomy, cesarean delivery for fetal distress was not increased. Most importantly, there were no adverse perinatal effects.

Amniotomy Induction

Artificial rupture of the membranes—sometimes called surgical induction—can be used to induce labor, and it always implies a commitment to delivery. The main disadvantage of amniotomy used alone for labor induction is the unpredictable and occasionally long interval to labor onset. That said, in a randomized trial, Bakos and Bäckström (1987) found that amniotomy alone or combined with oxytocin was superior to oxytocin alone. Mercer and colleagues (1995) randomized 209 women undergoing oxytocin induction to either early amniotomy at 1 to 2 cm, or late amniotomy at 5 cm. Early amniotomy was associated with significant 4-hour shorter labor. With early amniotomy, however, there was an increased incidence of chorioamnionitis.

Amniotomy Augmentation

It is common practice to perform amniotomy when labor is abnormally slow. Rouse and co-workers (1994) found that amniotomy with oxytocin augmentation for arrested active-phase labor shortened the time to delivery by 44 minutes compared with that of oxytocin alone. Although amniotomy did not affect the route of delivery, one drawback was that it significantly increased the incidence of chorioamnionitis.

ACTIVE MANAGEMENT OF LABOR

This term describes a codified approach to the management of labor, which is discussed in detail in Chapter 17 (p. 405).

TABLE 22-4. Randomized Clinical Trials of Elective Amniotomy in Early Spontaneous Labor at Term

Study	Number	Effects of Amniotomy					
		Mean Dilatation at Amniotomy	Mean Shortening of Labor	Need for Oxytocin	Cesarean Delivery Rate	Abnormal Tracing	Neonatal Effects
Fraser and co workers (1993)	925	<5 cm	125 min	None	None[a]	None	None
Garite and associates (1993)	459	5.5 cm	81 min	Decreased	None	Increased[b]	None
UK Amniotomy Group (1994)	1463	5.1 cm	60 min	None	None	NA	None

[a]No effect on overall rate; cesarean delivery for fetal distress significantly increased.
[b]Increased mild and moderate umbilical cord compression patterns.
NA = not assessed.

REFERENCES

Alexander JM, Sharma SK, McIntire D, et al: Epidural analgesia lengthens the Friedman active phase of labor. Obstet Gynecol 100:46, 2002

Allott HA, Palmer CR: Sweeping the membranes: A valid procedure in stimulating the onset of labour? Br J Obstet Gynaecol 100:898, 1993

American Academy of Pediatrics and American College of Obstetricians and Gynecologists: Guidelines for Perinatal Care, 6th ed. 2007, p 148

American College of Obstetricians and Gynecologists: Dystocia. Technical Bulletin No. 137, December 1989

American College of Obstetricians and Gynecologists: Dystocia and the augmentation of labor. Technical Bulletin No. 218, December 1995a

American College of Obstetricians and Gynecologists: Induction of labor. Technical Bulletin No. 217, December 1995b

American College of Obstetricians and Gynecologists: Induction of labor. Practice Bulletin No. 10, November 1999a

American College of Obstetricians and Gynecologists: Induction of labor with misoprostol. Committee Opinion No. 228, November 1999b

American College of Obstetricians and Gynecologists: Response to Searle's drug warning on misoprostol. Committee Opinion No. 248, December 2000

American College of Obstetricians and Gynecologists: Vaginal birth after cesarean delivery. Practice Bulletin No. 54, July 2004

American College of Obstetricians and Gynecologists: Fetal lung maturity. Practice Bulletin No. 97, September 2008

Arrabal PP, Nagey DA: Is manual palpation of uterine contractions accurate? Am J Obstet Gynecol 174:217, 1996

Arulkumaran S, Koh CH, Ingemarsson I, et al: Augmentation of labour—mode of delivery related to cervimetric progress. Aust NZ J Obstet Gynaecol 27:304, 1987

Bakos O, Bäckström T: Induction of labor: A prospective, randomized study into amniotomy and oxytocin as induction methods in a total unselected population. Acta Obstet Gynecol Scand 66:537, 1987

Bernstein P: Prostaglandin E$_2$ gel for cervical ripening and labour induction: A multi-centre placebo-controlled trial. Can Med Assoc J 145:1249, 1991

Bishop EH: Pelvic scoring for elective induction. Obstet Gynecol 24:266, 1964

Bolnick JM, Velazquez MD, Gonzalez JL, et al: Randomized trial between two active labor management protocols in the presence of an unfavorable cervix. Am J Obstet Gynecol 190:124, 2004

Brindley BA, Sokol RJ: Induction and augmentation of labor. Basis and methods for current practice. Obstet Gynecol Surv 43:730, 1988

Bullarbo M, Orrskog ME, Andersch B, et al: Outpatient vaginal administration of the nitric oxide donor isosorbide mononitrate for cervical ripening and labor induction postterm: A randomized controlled study. Am J Obstet Gynecol 196:50.e1, 2007

Caldeyro-Barcia R, Alvarez H, Reynolds SRM: A better understanding of uterine contractility through simultaneous recording with an internal and a seven channel external method. Surg Obstet Gynecol 91:641, 1950

Caldeyro-Barcia R, Poseiro JJ: Physiology of the uterine contraction. Clin Obstet Gynecol 3:386, 1960

Chan LY, Fu L, Leung TN, et al: Obstetrical outcomes after cervical ripening by multiple doses of vaginal prostaglandin E$_2$. Acta Obstet Gynecol Scand 83:70, 2004

Chanrachakul B, Herabutya Y, Punyavachira P: Potential efficacy of nitric oxide for cervical ripening in pregnancy at term. Int J Gynaecol Obstet 71(3):217, 2000

Chanrachakul B, Herabutya Y, Punyavachira P: Randomized comparison of glyceryl trinitrate and prostaglandin E$_2$ for cervical ripening at term. Obstet Gynecol 96:549, 2000

Chung JH, Huang WH, Rumney P, et al: A prospective, randomized controlled trial comparing misoprostol, Foley catheter, and combination misoprostol-Foley for labor induction. Am J Obstet Gynecol 189:1031, 2003

Clark SL, Miller DD, Belfort MA, et al: Neonatal and maternal outcomes associated with elective term delivery. Am J Obstet Gynecol 200(2):156.e1, 2009

Cole DS, Bruck LR: Anaphylaxis after laminaria insertion. Obstet Gynecol 95:1025, 2000

Collingham J, Fuh K, Caughey A, et al: Randomized clinical trial of cervical ripening and labor induction using oral misoprostol with or without intravaginal isosorbide mononitrate. Abstract No 145. Presented at the 29th Annual Meeting of the Society for Maternal-Fetal Medicine. 26–31 January 2009

Crane JMG: Transvaginal ultrasound cervical length and successful labor induction [Abstract]. Obstet Gynecol 107:60S, 2006

Culver J, Strauss RA, Brody S, et al: A randomized trial comparing vaginal misoprostol versus Foley catheter with concurrent oxytocin for labor induction in nulliparous women. Am J Perinatol 21:139, 2004

Doyle N, Ramin Su, Yeomans E, et al: Cesarean section: Community versus county hospital. Am J Obstet Gynecol 187:S110, 2002

du Vigneaud V, Ressler C, Swan JM, et al: The synthesis of oxytocin. J Am Chem Soc 75:4879, 1953

Ekerhovd E, Bullarbo M, Andersch B, et al: Vaginal administration of the nitric oxide donor isosorbide mononitrate for cervical ripening at term: A randomized controlled study. Am J Obstet Gynecol 189:1692, 2003

Ekerhovd E, Weijdegård B, Brännström I, et al: Nitric oxide induced cervical ripening in the human: Involvement of cyclic guanosine monophosphate, prostaglandin F$_{2\alpha}$, and prostaglandin E$_2$. Am J Obstet Gynecol 186:745, 2002

Fisch JM, English D, Pedaline S, et al: Labor induction process improvement: A patient quality-of-care initiative. Obstet Gynecol 113(4):797, 2009

Flannelly GM, Turner MJ, Rassmussen MJ, et al: Rupture of the uterus in Dublin: An update. J Obstet Gynecol 13:440, 1993

Fraser W, Marcoux S, Moutquin JM, et al: Effect of early amniotomy on the risk of dystocia in nulliparous women. N Engl J Med 328:1145, 1993

Friedman EA: Primigravid labor: A graphicostatistical analysis. Obstet Gynecol 6:567, 1955

Frigoletto FD, Lieberman E, Lang JM, et al: A clinical trial of active management of labor. N Engl J Med 333:745, 1995

Garcia FAR, Miller HB, Huggins GR, et al: Effect of academic affiliation and obstetric volume on clinical outcome and cost of childbirth. Obstet Gynecol 97:567, 2001

Garite TJ, Porto M, Carlson NJ, et al: The influence of elective amniotomy on fetal heart rate patterns and the course of labor in term patients: A randomized study. Am J Obstet Gynecol 168:1827, 1993

Glantz JC: Labor induction rate variation in upstate New York: What is the difference? Birth 30:68, 2003

Gilson GJ, Russell DJ, Izquierdo LA, et al: A prospective randomized evaluation of a hygroscopic cervical dilator, Dilapan, in the preinduction ripening of patients undergoing induction of labor. Am J Obstet Gynecol 175:145, 1996

Goldman JB, Wigton TR: A randomized comparison of extraamniotic saline infusion and intracervical dinoprostone gel for cervical ripening. Obstet Gynecol 93:271, 1999

Guinn DA, Davies JK, Jones RO, et al: Labor induction in women with an unfavorable Bishop score: Randomized controlled trial of intrauterine Foley catheter with concurrent oxytocin infusion versus Foley catheter with extra-amniotic saline infusion with concurrent oxytocin infusion. Am J Obstet 191:225, 2004

Guinn DA, Goepfert AR, Christine M, et al: Extra-amniotic saline infusion, laminaria, or prostaglandin E$_2$ gel for labor induction with unfavorable cervix: A randomized trial. Obstet Gynecol 96:106, 2000

Hale RW, Pion RJ: Laminaria: An underutilized clinical adjunct. Clin Obstet Gynecol 15:829, 1972

Hall R, Duarte-Gardea M, Harlass F: Oral versus vaginal misoprostol for labor induction. Obstet Gynecol 99:1044, 2002

Hamar B, Mann S, Greenberg P, et al: Low-risk inductions of labor and cesarean delivery for nulliparous and parous women at term. Am J Obstet Gynecol 185:S215, 2001

Hatfield AS, Sanchez-Ramos L, Kaunitz AM: Sonographic cervical assessment to predict the success of labor induction: A systematic review with meta-analysis. Am J Obstet Gynecol 197:186, 2007

Hauth JC, Hankins GD, Gilstrap LC III: Uterine contraction pressures with oxytocin induction/augmentation. Obstet Gynecol 68:305, 1986

Hauth JC, Hankins GD, Gilstrap LC III: Uterine contraction pressures achieved in parturients with active phase arrest. Obstet Gynecol 78:344, 1991

Hoffman MK, Sciscione AC: Elective induction with cervical ripening increases the risk of cesarean delivery in multiparous women. Obstet Gynecol 101:7S, 2003

Hofmeyr GJ, Gülmezoglu AM: Vaginal misoprostol for cervical ripening and induction of labour. Cochrane Database Syst Rev 1: CD000941, 2003

Karjane NW, Brock EL, Walsh SW: Induction of labor using a Foley balloon, with and without extra-amniotic saline infusion. Obstet Gynecol 107:234, 2006

Kastner ES, Figueroa R, Garry D, et al: Emergency peripartum hysterectomy: Experience at a community teaching hospital. Obstet Gynecol 99:971, 2002

Ledingham MA, Thomson AJ, Lunan CB, et al: A comparison of isosorbide mononitrate, misoprostol and combination therapy for first trimester preoperative cervical ripening: A randomised controlled trial. Br J Obstet Gynecol 108:276, 2001

Levy R, Kanengiser B, Furman B, et al: A randomized trial comparing a 30-mL and an 80-mL Foley catheter balloon for preinduction cervical ripening. Am J Obstet Gynecol 191:1632, 2004

Lin MG, Nuthalapaty FS, Carver AR, et al: Misoprostol for labor induction in women with term premature rupture of membranes: A meta-analysis. Obstet Gynecol 106:593, 2005

Lo JY, Alexander JM, McIntire DD, et al: Ruptured membranes at term: Randomized, double-blind trial of oral misoprostol for labor induction. Obstet Gynecol 101:685, 2003

López-Zeno JA, Peaceman AM, Adashek JA, et al: A controlled trial of a program for the active management of labor. N Engl J Med 326:450, 1992

Luthy DA, Malmgren JA, Zingheim RW: Cesarean delivery after elective induction in nulliparous women: The physician effect. Am J Obstet Gynecol 191:1511, 2004

Martin JA, Hamilton BE, Sutton PD, et al: Births: final data for 2006. National Vital Statistics Reports, Vol 57, No 7. Hyattsville, MD, National Center for Health Statistics, 2009

Maslow AS, Sweeny AL: Elective induction of labor as a risk factor for cesarean delivery among low-risk women at term. Obstet Gynecol 95:917, 2000

McColgin SW, Bennett WA, Roach H, et al: Parturitional factors associated with membrane stripping. Am J Obstet Gynecol 169:71, 1993

McColgin SW, Hampton HL, McCaul JF, et al: Stripping of membranes at term: Can it safely reduce the incidence of post-term pregnancy? Obstet Gynecol 76:678, 1990

Mercer BM: Induction of labor in the nulliparous gravida with an unfavorable cervix. Obstet Gynecol 105:688, 2005

Mercer BM, McNanley T, O'Brien JM, et al: Early versus late amniotomy for labor induction: A randomized trial. Am J Obstet Gynecol 173:1371, 1995

Merrill DC, Zlatnik FJ: Randomized, double-masked comparison of oxytocin dosage in induction and augmentation of labor. Obstet Gynecol 94:455, 1999

Miller AM, Rayburn WF, Smith CV: Patterns of uterine activity after intravaginal prostaglandin E$_2$ during preinduction cervical ripening. Am J Obstet Gynecol 165:1006, 1991

National Institutes of Health: NIH Conference Statement: National Institutes of Health state-of-the-science conference statement: Cesarean delivery on maternal request, March 27-29, 2006. Obstet Gynecol 107:1386, 2006

Nguyen MT, Hoffman DR: Anaphylaxis to laminaria. J Allergy Clin Immunol 95:138, 1995

O'Driscoll K, Foley M, MacDonald D: Active management of labor as an alternative to cesarean section for dystocia. Obstet Gynecol 63:485, 1984

Oshiro BT, Henry E, Wilson J, et al: Decreasing elective deliveries before 39 weeks of gestation in an integrated health care system. Obstet Gynecol 113(4):804, 2009

Osman I, MacKenzie F, Norrie J, et al: The "PRIM" study: A randomized comparison of prostaglandin E$_2$ gel with the nitric oxide donor isosorbide mononitrate for cervical ripening before the induction of labor at term. Am J Obstet Gynecol 194:1012, 2006

Owen J, Winkler CL, Harris BA, et al: A randomized, double-blind trial of prostaglandin E2 gel for cervical ripening and meta-analysis. Am J Obstet Gynecol 165:991, 1991

Peregrine E, O'Brien P, Jauniaux E: Impact on delivery outcome of ultrasonographic fetal head position prior to induction of labor. Obstet Gynecol 109:618, 2007

Peregrine E, O'Brien P, Omar R, et al: Clinical and ultrasound parameters to predict the risk of cesarean delivery after induction of labor. Obstet Gynecol 107(2 Pt 1):227, 2006

Perry MY, Leaphart WL: Randomized trial of intracervical versus posterior fornix dinoprostone for induction of labor. Obstet Gynecol 103:13, 2004

Pevzner L, Rumney P, Petersen R, et al: Predicting a successful induction of labor: A secondary analysis of misoprostol vaginal insert trial. Abstract No 218. Presented at the 29th Annual Meeting of the Society for Maternal-Fetal Medicine. 26–31 January 2009

Plaut MM, Schwartz ML, Lubarsky SL: Uterine rupture associated with the use of misoprostol in the gravid patient with a previous cesarean section. Am J Obstet Gynecol 180:1535, 1999

Rayburn WF: Prostaglandin E$_2$ gel for cervical ripening and induction of labor: A critical analysis. Am J Obstet Gynecol 160:529, 1989

Rouse DJ, McCullough C, Wren AL, et al: Active-phase labor arrest: A randomized trial of chorioamnion management. Obstet Gynecol 83:937, 1994

Rouse DJ, Owen J, Hauth JC: Active-phase labor arrest: Oxytocin augmentation for at least 4 hours. Obstet Gynecol 93:323, 1999

Rouse D, Owen J, Hauth JC: Criteria for failed labor induction: Prospective evaluation of a standardized protocol. Obstet Gynecol 96:671, 2000

Rouse DJ, Owen J, Savage KG, et al: Active phase labor arrest: Revisiting the 2-hour minimum Obstet Gynecol 98:550, 2001

Sanchez-Ramos L, Kaunitz AM, Wears RL, et al: Misoprostol for cervical ripening and labor induction: A meta-analysis. Obstet Gynecol 89:633, 1997

Satin AJ, Leveno KJ, Sherman ML, et al: High- versus low-dose oxytocin for labor stimulation. Obstet Gynecol 80:111, 1992

Satin AJ, Leveno KJ, Sherman ML, et al: High-dose oxytocin: 20- versus 40-minute dosage interval. Obstet Gynecol 83:234, 1994

Sciscione A, Larkin M, O'Shea A, et al: Preinduction cervical ripening with the Foley catheter and the risk of subsequent preterm birth. Am J Obstet Gynecol 190:751, 2004

Seitchik J, Amico J, Robinson AG, et al: Oxytocin augmentation of dysfunctional labor, 4. Oxytocin pharmacokinetics. Am J Obstet Gynecol 150:225, 1984

Shellhaas C for the NICHD MFMU Network: The MFMU cesarean registry: Cesarean hysterectomy—its indications, morbidities, and mortality. Am J Obstet Gynecol 185:S123, 2001

Sherman DJ, Frenkel E, Tovbin J, et al: Ripening of the unfavorable cervix with extraamniotic catheter balloon: Clinical experience and review. Obstet Gynecol Surv 51:621, 1996

Shin KS, Brubaker KL, Ackerson LM: Risk of cesarean delivery in nulliparous women at greater than 41 weeks' gestational age with an unengaged vertex. Am J Obstet Gynecol 190:129, 2004

Simon CE, Grobman WA: When has an induction failed? Obstet Gynecol 105: 705, 2005

Smith KM, Hoffman MK, Sciscione A: Elective induction of labor in nulliparous women increases the risk of cesarean delivery. Obstet Gynecol 101:45S, 2003

Solheim K, Myers D, Sparks T, et al: Continuing a tral of labor after 2 hours of active-phase labor arrest: A cost-effectiveness analysis. Abstract No 205. Presented at the 29th Annual Meeting of the Society for Maternal-Fetal Medicine. 26–31 January 2009

Thomson AJ, Lunan CB, Cameron AD, et al: Nitric oxide donors induce ripening of the human uterine cervix: a randomised controlled trial. Br J Obstet Gynecol 104:1054, 1997

Tita AT, Landon MB, Spong CY, et al: Timing of elective repeat cesarean delivery at term and neonatal outcomes. N Engl J Med 360(2):111, 2009

UK Amniotomy Group: A multicentre randomised trial of amniotomy in spontaneous first labour at term. Br J Obstet Gynaecol 101:307, 1994

Vahratian A, Zhang J, Troendle JF, et al: Labor progression and risk of cesarean delivery in electively induced nulliparas. Obstet Gynecol 105: 698, 2005

Väisänen-Tommiska M, Nuutila M, Aittomäki K, et al: Nitric oxide metabolites in cervical fluid during pregnancy: Further evidence for the role of cervical nitric oxide in cervical ripening. Am J Obstet Gynecol 188:779, 2003

Väisänen-Tommiska M, Nuutila M, Ylikorkala O: Cervical nitric oxide release in women postterm. Obstet Gynecol 103:657, 2004

Vengalil SR, Guinn DA, Olabi NF, et al: A randomized trial of misoprostol and extra-amniotic saline infusion for cervical ripening and labor induction. Obstet Gynecol 91:774, 1998

Villano KS, Lo JY, Alexander JM: A dose-finding study of oral misoprostol for labor augmentation. Am J Obstet Gynecol [In press], 2010

von Gemund N, Scherjon S, LeCessie S, et al: A randomized trial comparing low dose vaginal misoprostol and dinoprostone for labour induction. Br J Obstet Gynaecol 111:42, 2004

Vrouenraets FPJM, Roumen FJME, Dehing CJG, et al: Bishop score and risk of cesarean delivery after induction of labor in nulliparous women. Am J Obstet Gynecol 105: 690, 2005

Wagner M: Off-label use of misoprostol in obstetrics: A cautionary tale. BJOG 112: 266, 2005

Weeks AD, Fiala C, Safar P: Misoprostol and the debate over off-label drug use. BJOG 112: 269, 2005

Wen T, Beceir A, Xenakis E, et al: Is there a maximum effective dose of Pitocin? Am J Obstet Gynecol 185:S212, 2001

Windrim R, Bennett K, Mundle W, et al: Oral administration of misoprostol for labor induction: A randomized controlled trial. Obstet Gynecol 89:392, 1997

Wing DA, Jones MM, Rahall A, et al: A comparison of misoprostol and prostaglandin E$_2$ gel for preinduction cervical ripening and labor induction. Am J Obstet Gynecol 172:1804, 1995a

Wing DA, Lovett K, Paul RH: Disruption of prior uterine incision following misoprostol for labor induction in women with previous cesarean delivery. Obstet Gynecol 91:828, 1998

Wing DA, Park MR, Paul RH: A randomized comparison of oral and intravaginal misoprostol for labor induction. Obstet Gynecol 95:905, 2000

Wing DA, Rahall A, Jones MM, et al: Misoprostol: An effective agent for cervical ripening and labor induction. Am J Obstet Gynecol 172:1811, 1995b

Wölfler MM, Facchinetti F, Venturini P, et al: Induction of labor at term using isosorbide mononitrate simultaneously with dinoprostone compared to dinoprostone treatment alone: A randomized, controlled trial. Am J Obstet Gynecol 195:1617, 2006

Xenakis EMJ, Langer O, Piper JM, et al: Low-dose versus high-dose oxytocin augmentation of labor—a randomized trial. Am J Obstet Gynecol 173: 1874, 1995

Yeast JD, Jones A, Poskin M: Induction of labor and the relationship to cesarean delivery: A review of 7001 consecutive inductions. Am J Obstet Gynecol 180:628, 1999

Zhang J, Troendle JF, Yancey MK: Reassessing the labor curve in nulliparous women. Am J Obstet Gynecol 187:824, 2002

CHAPTER 23

Forceps Delivery and Vacuum Extraction

The precise incidence of operative vaginal delivery in the United States is unknown. According to the National Vital Statistics Report, forceps or vacuum delivery was coded on the birth certificate as the method of delivery for 4.5 percent of vaginal births in the United States in 2006 (Martin and colleagues, 2009).

FORCEPS DELIVERY

True forceps were first devised in the late 16th or beginning of the 17th century. The reader is referred to the 19th and earlier editions of *Williams Obstetrics* regarding their history.

Forceps Designs

These instruments basically consist of two crossing branches. Each branch has four components: blade, shank, lock, and handle. Each blade has two curves: The *cephalic curve* conforms to the shape of the fetal head, and the *pelvic curve* corresponds more or less to the axis of the birth canal (Fig. 23-1). Some varieties are *fenestrated* or *pseudofenestrated* to permit a firmer grasp of the fetal head.

The blades are connected to the handles by the *shanks*. The common method of articulation, the *English lock,* consists of a socket located on the shank at the junction with the handle, into which fits a socket similarly located on the opposite shank

(Figs. 23-1 and 23-2). A *sliding lock* is used in some forceps, such as Kielland forceps (Fig. 23-3).

Classification of Forceps Deliveries

The current classification of the American College of Obstetricians and Gynecologists (2000, 2002) for forceps and vacuum operations is summarized in Table 23-1. It emphasizes the two most important discriminators of risk for both mother and infant: *station* and *rotation.* Station is measured in centimeters, -5 to 0 to $+5$. Deliveries are categorized as outlet, low, and midpelvic procedures. *High forceps* in which instruments are applied above 0 station have no place in contemporary obstetrics.

Incidence of Forceps Delivery

Over the past decade, as the cesarean delivery rate has risen, the rate of operative vaginal delivery has fallen. The latter was 9.8 percent in 1994, and fell to 4.5 percent of all births in the United States in 2006 (Martin and colleagues, 2009). In a study from the United States National Hospital Discharge Survey, Kozak and Weeks (2002) reported that forceps deliveries decreased 17.7 to 4.0 per 100 vaginal deliveries from 1980 to 2000. During this same 20-year period, the vacuum delivery rate increased from 0.7 to 8.4 per 100 vaginal deliveries.

Effects of Regional Analgesia

Epidural analgesia may be associated with failure of spontaneous rotation to an occiput anterior position. It also may slow second-stage labor and decrease maternal expulsive efforts. Both of these may predispose to instrumented delivery. Sharma and colleagues (2004) analyzed the outcomes of 2703 nulliparas who were enrolled in one of five randomized trials performed at Parkland Hospital to ascertain the effects of labor analgesia. Women given epidural analgesia had a twofold increased rate of forceps delivery compared with those given intravenous

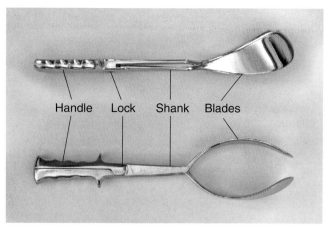

FIGURE 23-1 Tucker–McLane forceps. The blade is solid and the shank is narrow.

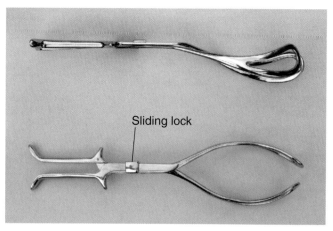

FIGURE 23-3 Kielland forceps. The characteristic features are the sliding lock, minimal pelvic curvature, and light weight.

analgesia—13 versus 7 percent. Similarly, in their meta-analysis of epidural versus opioid analgesia, Halpern and colleagues (1998) reported that women receiving epidural analgesia were twice as likely to have an instrumented delivery. Both studies are consistent with a comprehensive systematic review performed by Lieberman and O'Donoghue (2002).

Training

As the rate of operative vaginal delivery has declined, so have opportunities for training. In 1999, Hankins and colleagues reported that fewer than half of the residency directors expected proficiency with midforceps delivery, and today, far fewer would. From a training standpoint, in many programs even low and outlet forceps procedures have reached critically low levels. Thus, traditional hands-on training will likely evolve. For example, Dupuis and colleagues (2006, 2009) have developed a sophisticated forceps simulation system that utilizes spatial location sensors to track the trajectories of forceps blades. Leslie and associates (2005) used an isometric strength testing unit with real-time visual feedback to optimize traction force exerted

by residents during simulated forceps deliveries. Cheong and co-workers (2004) reported lowered rates of maternal and neonatal morbidity associated with instrumented delivery in their hospital after the implementation of a formal instrumented delivery education program that included a manikin and pelvic model.

Function of Forceps

Although the most important function of forceps is *traction*, forceps may be invaluable for *rotation*, particularly for occiput transverse and posterior positions. In general, Simpson forceps are used to deliver the fetus with a molded head, as is common in nulliparous women. The Tucker-McLane instrument is often used for the fetus with a rounded head, which more characteristically is seen in multiparas. In most situations, however, either instrument is appropriate.

Forces Exerted by the Forceps

The force produced by the forceps on the fetal skull is a complex function of both traction and compression by the forceps, as well as friction produced by maternal tissues. It is impossible to ascertain the amount of force exerted by forceps for an individual patient.

Indications for Forceps

When it is technically feasible and can be safely accomplished, termination of second-stage labor by forceps or vacuum extraction delivery is indicated in any condition threatening the mother or fetus that is likely to be relieved by delivery. Some *maternal indications* include heart disease, pulmonary injury or compromise, intrapartum infection, certain neurological conditions, exhaustion, or prolonged second-stage labor. For nulliparas, the latter is defined by the American College of Obstetricians and Gynecologists (2002) as more than 3 hours with, and more than 2 hours without, regional analgesia. In the parous woman, a prolonged second stage is defined as more than 2 hours with, and more than 1 hour without, regional analgesia. Shortening of second-stage labor for maternal reasons should generally be performed from either a low or outlet station.

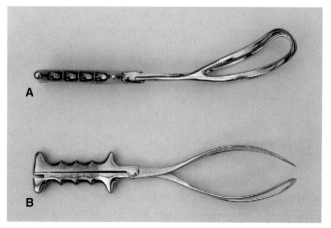

FIGURE 23-2 Simpson forceps. **A.** Note the ample pelvic curve in the blades. **B.** The cephalic curve is evident in the articulated blades. The fenestrated blade and the wide shank in front of English-style lock characterize the Simpson forceps.

TABLE 23-1. Classification of Forceps Delivery according to Station and Rotation[a]

Procedure	Criteria
Outlet forceps	1. Scalp is visible at the introitus without separating the labia 2. Fetal skull has reached pelvic floor 3. Sagittal suture is in anteroposterior diameter or right or left occiput anterior or posterior position 4. Fetal head is at or on perineum, and 5. Rotation does not exceed 45 degrees
Low forceps	Leading point of fetal skull is at station $\geq$ +2 cm, and not on the pelvic floor, and: • Rotation is 45 degrees or less, *or* • Rotation is greater than 45 degrees.
Midforceps	Station is between 0 and +2 cm.
High	Not included in classification.

[a]Classification for the vacuum delivery system is the same as for forceps except that vacuum is used for traction but not rotation.
Used with permission of the American Academy of Pediatrics, American College of Obstetricians and Gynecologists. Guidelines for perinatal care. 6th ed. Elk Grove Village (IL): AAP; Washington, DC: ACOG; 2007. Copyright American Academy of Pediatrics and American College of Obstetricans and Gynecologists, 2007.

Presuming that all prerequisites for instrumented delivery are met, some *fetal indications* for operative vaginal delivery include prolapse of the umbilical cord, premature separation of the placenta, or a nonreassuring fetal heart rate pattern.

Elective and Outlet Forceps

Forceps generally should not be used electively until the criteria for outlet forceps have been met. The fetal head must be on the perineal floor with the sagittal suture no more than 45 degrees from the anteroposterior diameter. In these circumstances, forceps delivery is a simple and safe operation (Hagadorn-Freathy and associates, 1991). That said, however, there is no evidence that use of prophylactic forceps is *beneficial* in the otherwise normal term labor and delivery.

Prophylactic Outlet Forceps for Low-Birthweight Fetuses

In the past, it was taught that forceps delivery was somewhat protective of the fragile head of the preterm infant. Fairweather (1981) reported no significant differences in outcomes in neonates who weighed 500 to 1500 g between those delivered spontaneously and those by outlet forceps. Schwartz and colleagues (1983) reported similar findings. Thus, it appears that there is no obvious advantage to routine outlet forceps delivery of a small fetus.

Prerequisites for Forceps Application

There are at least six prerequisites for successful application of forceps:

1. The cervix must be completely dilated.
2. The membranes must be ruptured.
3. The head must be engaged. Extensive caput succedaneum formation and molding sometimes make determination of

the station difficult. With difficulties of station assignment, it is important to realize that what is assumed to be a low-forceps procedure may actually be a more difficult midforceps operation.
4. The fetus must present a vertex, or present a face with the chin anterior.
5. The position of the fetal head must be precisely known.
6. There should be no suspected cephalopelvic disproportion.

Preparation for Forceps Delivery

Although pudendal block analgesia may prove adequate for outlet forceps operations, regional analgesia or general anesthesia is preferable for low-forceps or midpelvic procedures. The bladder should be emptied.

The exact position of the fetal head must be known for a proper cephalic application. With the head low in the pelvis, position is determined by examination of the sagittal suture and the fontanels. When the head is at a higher station, an absolute determination can be made by locating the posterior ear.

Outlet Forceps Delivery

Forceps Application

Delivery by outlet forceps of the occiput anterior fetal head is illustrated in Figures 23-4 through 23-7. In such circumstances, the small (posterior) fontanel is directed toward the symphysis pubis. The forceps, if applied to the sides of the pelvis, grasp the head ideally. The forceps are applied as follows: Two or more fingers of the right hand are introduced inside the left posterior portion of the vulva and into the vagina beside the fetal head. The handle of the left branch is then grasped between the thumb and two fingers of the left hand. The tip of the blade is then gently

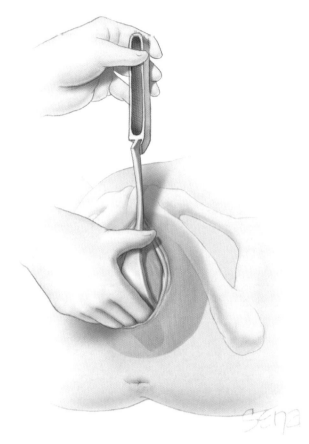

FIGURE 23-4 The left handle of the forceps is held in the left hand. The blade is introduced into the left side of the pelvis between the fetal head and fingers of the operator's right hand.

passed into the vagina between the fetal head and the palmar surface of the fingers of the right hand (see Fig. 23-4). For application of the right blade, two or more fingers of the left hand are introduced into the right, posterior portion of the vagina to serve as a guide for the right blade. This blade is held in the right hand and introduced into the vagina as described for the left blade. After positioning, the branches are articulated (see Fig. 23-7).

The blades are constructed so that their cephalic curve is closely adapted to the sides of the fetal head. The biparietal diameter of the fetal head corresponds to the greatest distance between the appropriately applied blades. Consequently, the head of the fetus is perfectly grasped only when the long axis of the blades corresponds to the occipitomental diameter. Thus, the major portion of the blade is lying over the face. If the fetus is in an occiput anterior position, then the concave margins of the blades are directed toward the sagittal suture. If the fetus is in an occiput posterior position, then the concave margins are directed toward the fetal face.

Applied as such, the forceps should not slip, and traction may be applied most advantageously. With most forceps, if one blade is applied over the brow and the other over the occiput, the instrument cannot be locked, or if locked, the blades will slip off when traction is applied (Fig. 23-8). For these reasons, the forceps must be applied directly to the sides of the fetal head along the occipitomental diameter.

Appropriateness of Application

For the occiput anterior position, appropriately applied blades are equidistant from the sagittal suture. In the occiput posterior position, the blades are equidistant from the midline of the face and brow.

Traction

If necessary, rotation to occiput anterior is performed before traction is applied (Fig. 23-9). When it is certain that the blades are placed satisfactorily, then gentle, intermittent, horizontal traction is exerted until the perineum begins to bulge (Fig. 23-10). With traction, as the vulva is distended by the occiput, an episiotomy may be performed if indicated (Fig. 23-11).

Additional horizontal traction is applied, and the handles are gradually elevated, eventually pointing almost directly upward as the parietal bones emerge (Figs. 23-12 and 23-13). As the handles are raised, the head is extended. During the birth of the head, spontaneous delivery should be simulated as closely as possible. Traction should therefore be intermittent, and the

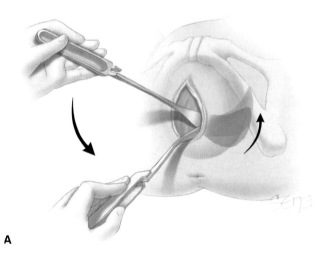

A

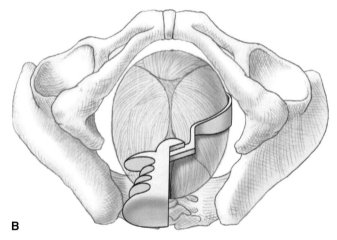

B

FIGURE 23-5 A. Continued insertion of the left blade. Note the arc of the handles as they rotate to be applied to the mother's left. **B.** First blade in place.

the forceps in place to control the advance of the head. However, the thickness of the blades adds to the distension of the vulva, thus increasing the likelihood of laceration or necessitating a large episiotomy. To prevent this, the forceps may be removed and delivery completed by the modified Ritgen maneuver (Fig. 23-14). If the forceps are removed prematurely, the modified Ritgen maneuver may prove to be ineffective or unduly difficult.

Low- and Midforceps Operations

When the head lies above the perineum, the sagittal suture usually occupies an oblique or transverse diameter of the pelvis. In such cases, the forceps should always be applied to the sides of the head.

Left Occiput Anterior Position

The right hand, introduced into the left posterior segment of the vagina, should identify the posteriorly located left ear. At the same time, the right hand serves as a guide for introduction of the left branch of the forceps, which is held in the left hand and applied over the left ear. Two fingers of the left hand are then introduced into the right posterior portion of the pelvis.

The right branch of the forceps, held in the right hand, is then introduced along the left hand as a guide. It must then be applied over the anterior ear of the fetus by gently sweeping the blade anteriorly until it lies directly opposite the blade that was introduced first.

Right Occiput Anterior Position

The blades are introduced similarly as above, but in the opposite directions off the vertical. After the blades have been applied to the sides of the head, the left handle and shank lie above the right. Consequently, the forceps do not immediately articulate. Locking of the branches is easily effected, however, by rotating the left around the right to bring the lock into proper position.

Occiput Transverse Positions

The forceps are introduced similarly, as described, but with the first blade applied over the posterior ear and the second rotated anteriorly to a position opposite the first. In this case, one blade lies in front of the sacrum and the other behind the symphysis. Simpson or Tucker-McLane forceps or one of their modifications is generally used. In some cases the specialized Kielland forceps may be used.

Rotation from Anterior and Transverse Positions

When the occiput is obliquely anterior, it gradually rotates spontaneously to the symphysis pubis as traction is exerted.

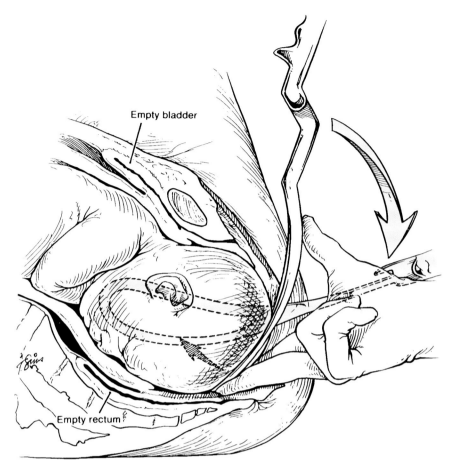

FIGURE 23-6 Sagittal view of first-blade application. The fetus is presenting as vertex with occiput anterior crowning. The application of the left blade of the Simpson forceps is shown. Next, the right blade is applied and the blades are articulated.

head should be allowed to recede in intervals, as in spontaneous labor. Except when urgently indicated, as in severe fetal bradycardia, delivery should be sufficiently slow, deliberate, and gentle to prevent undue head compression. It is preferable to apply traction only with each uterine contraction.

After the vulva has been well distended by the head, the delivery may be completed in several ways. Some clinicians keep

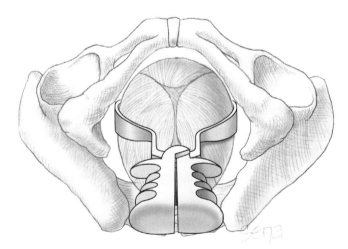

FIGURE 23-7 The vertex is now occiput anterior, and the forceps are symmetrically placed and articulated.

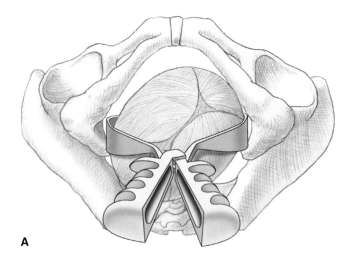

A

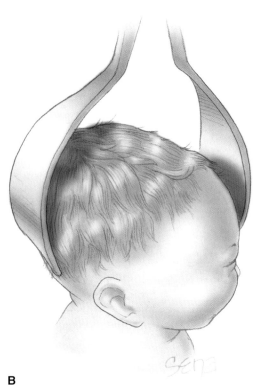

B

FIGURE 23-8 Incorrect application of forceps. **A.** One blade over the occiput and the other over the brow. Forceps cannot be locked. **B.** With incorrect placement, blades tend to slip off with traction.

When it is directly transverse, however, a rotary motion of the forceps is required. Rotation counterclockwise from the left side toward the midline is required when the occiput is directed toward the left, and in the reverse direction when it is directed toward the right side of the pelvis. Infrequently, when forceps are used in transverse positions in anteroposteriorly flattened—platypelloid—pelves, rotation should not be attempted until the fetal head has reached or approached the pelvic floor. Regardless of the original position of the head, delivery eventually is accomplished by exerting traction downward until the occiput appears at the vulva. After this, the rest of the operation is completed as previously described.

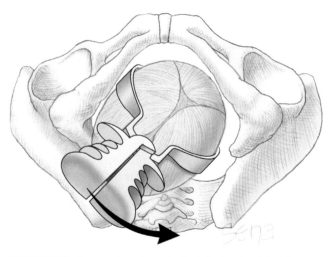

FIGURE 23-9 Forceps have been locked. Vertex is rotated from left occiput anterior to occiput anterior (*arrow*).

Occiput Posterior Positions

Prompt delivery may at times become necessary when the small occipital fontanel is directed toward one of the sacroiliac synchondroses, that is, in right occiput posterior or left occiput posterior positions. When delivery is required in either instance, the head is often imperfectly flexed. In some cases, when the hand is introduced into the vagina to locate the posterior ear, the occiput rotates spontaneously toward the anterior, indicating that manual rotation of the fetal head might easily be accomplished.

Manual Rotation

A hand with the palm upward is inserted into the vagina and the fingers are brought in contact with the side of the fetal head that is to be rotated toward the anterior position, while the thumb is placed over the opposite side of the head. With the occiput in a right posterior position, the left hand is used to rotate the occiput anteriorly in a clockwise direction. The right hand is used for the left occiput posterior position. The head must not be disengaged during rotation. After the occiput has reached the anterior position, labor may be allowed to continue, or forceps can be used. Le Ray and colleagues (2007) reported a success rate of greater than 90 percent, and two thirds required only one attempt.

Forceps Delivery of Occiput Posterior

If manual rotation cannot be easily accomplished, application of the blades to the head in the posterior position and delivery from the occiput posterior position may be the safest procedure (Fig. 23-15). In many cases, the cause of the persistent occiput posterior position and of the difficulty in accomplishing

group. Within the occiput posterior group, operative delivery was associated with a higher incidence of severe perineal lacerations—35 versus 16 percent; vaginal lacerations—18 versus 7 percent; and episiotomy—95 versus 74 percent, than was spontaneous delivery. Damron and Capeless (2004) reported a third- or fourth-degree perineal laceration in 72 percent of 118 women with occiput posterior forceps deliveries. From The Netherlands, de Leeuw and collaborators (2008) studied more than 28,500 operative vaginal deliveries and reported similar findings. Consequences of these perineal tears are discussed in Chapter 17 (p. 400). Infants delivered from the occiput posterior position had a higher incidence of Erb

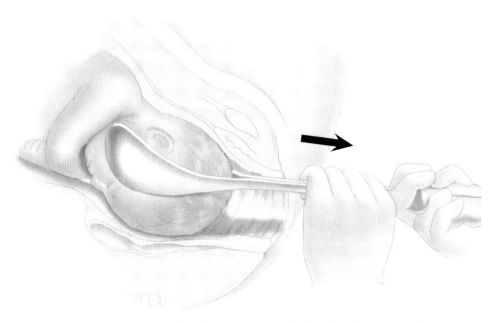

FIGURE 23-10 Occiput anterior. Delivery by low forceps. The direction of gentle traction for delivery of the head is indicated.

rotation is an anthropoid pelvis, the architecture of which opposes rotation and predisposes to posterior delivery. When the occiput is directly posterior, horizontal traction should be applied until the base of the nose is under the symphysis. The handles should then be slowly elevated until the occiput gradually emerges over the anterior margin of the perineum. Then, the forceps are directed in a downward motion, and the nose, face, and chin successively emerge from the vulva.

Occiput posterior delivery causes greater distension of the vulva, and a large episiotomy may be needed. Pearl and associates (1993) reviewed 564 occiput posterior deliveries and compared them with 1068 controls. The occiput posterior group had a higher incidence of severe perineal lacerations and extensive episiotomy compared with that of the occiput anterior

and facial nerve palsies, 1 and 2 percent, respectively, than did those delivered from the occiput anterior position.

Forceps Rotations of Occiput Oblique Posterior

For rotations, either Tucker-McLane, Simpson, or Kielland forceps may be used. The oblique occiput may be rotated 45 degrees to the posterior position, or 135 degrees to the anterior position (Fig. 23-16). If rotation is performed with Tucker-McLane or Simpson forceps, the head must be flexed, but this is not necessary with Kielland forceps because they have a less pronounced pelvic curve. In rotating the occiput anteriorly with Tucker-McLane or Simpson forceps, the pelvic curvature, originally directed upward, is, at the completion of rotation, inverted and directed posteriorly. Attempted delivery with the instrument in that position is likely to cause vaginal sulcus tears and sidewall lacerations. To avoid such trauma, it is essential to remove and reapply the instrument as described below.

Occiput Transverse Rotation

Specialized skill and training are essential when performing this technically difficult operative vaginal procedure. Either standard forceps, such as pseudofenestrated Simpson, or specialized forceps, such as Kielland, are employed. The latter have a sliding lock and almost no pelvic curve (see Fig. 23-3). On each handle is a small knob that indicates the direction of the occiput. The station of the fetal head must be accurately ascertained to be at, or preferably below, the level of the ischial spines, especially in the presence of extreme molding.

Kielland described two methods of applying the anterior blade:

1. With the *wandering* or *gliding* method, the anterior blade is introduced at the side of the pelvis over the brow or face. The blade is then arched around the brow or face to an anterior position, with the handle of the blade held close to

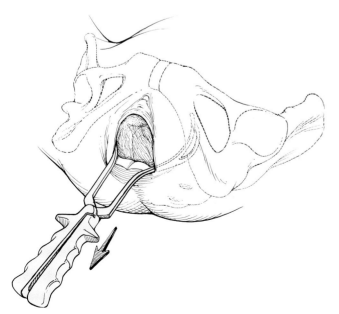

FIGURE 23-11 Horizontal traction.

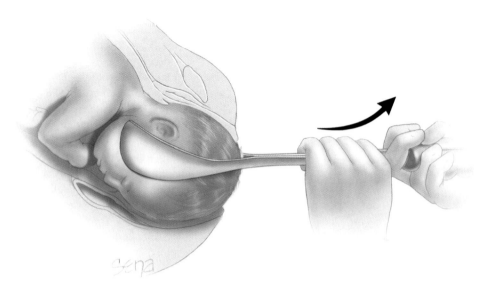

FIGURE 23-12 Upward arching traction (*arrow*) is used as the head is delivered.

the opposite maternal buttock throughout the maneuver. The second blade is introduced posteriorly and the branches are locked.

2. With the *direct* or *classical* application, the anterior blade is introduced first with its cephalic curve directed upward, curving under the symphysis. After it has been advanced far enough into the lower uterine cavity, it is turned on its axis through 180 degrees to adapt the cephalic curvature to the head. For a more detailed description Kielland forceps procedures, see the second edition of *Operative Obstetrics* (Gilstrap, 2002).

Face Presentation Forceps Delivery

With a mentum anterior face presentation, forceps can be used to effect vaginal delivery. The blades are applied to the sides of

the head along the occipitomental diameter, with the pelvic curve directed toward the neck. Downward traction is exerted until the chin appears under the symphysis. Then, by an upward movement, the face is slowly extracted, with the nose, eyes, brow, and occiput appearing in succession over the anterior margin of the perineum (Fig. 23-17). Forceps should not be applied to the mentum posterior presentation because vaginal delivery is impossible.

Morbidity from Forceps Operations

Maternal Morbidity

The relationship of maternal morbidity to forceps deliveries should be considered on two levels. First, and overall, the maternal morbidity from indicated forceps delivery is most properly compared with the morbidity from cesarean delivery, and not to that from spontaneous vaginal delivery. This is because

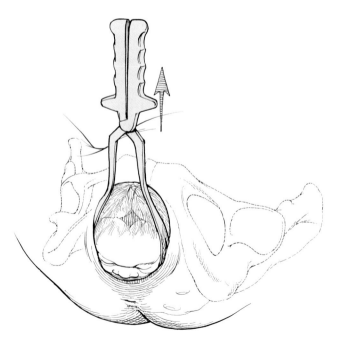

FIGURE 23-13 Upward traction (*arrow*) is continued as the head is delivered.

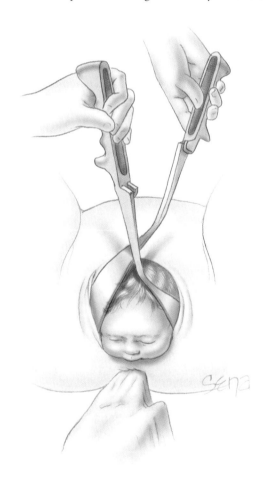

FIGURE 23-14 Forceps may be disarticulated as the head is delivered. Modified Ritgen maneuver may be used to complete delivery of the head.

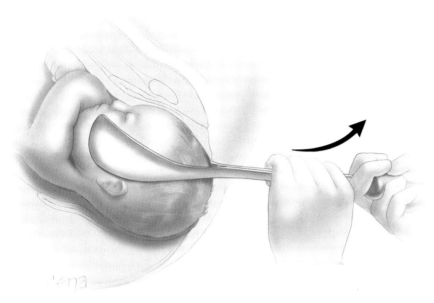

FIGURE 23-15 Outlet forceps delivery from an occiput posterior position. The head should be flexed after the bregma passes under the symphysis.

the alternative to indicated forceps delivery is cesarean delivery. Second, among women undergoing forceps delivery, the higher the station, and/or the greater the degree of rotation, the more likely it is that morbidity in the form of lacerations and blood loss will occur.

Lacerations and Episiotomy. As documented by a number of studies, the very conditions that lead to indications for operative vaginal delivery also increase the need for episiotomy and the likelihood of lacerations (de Leeuw and colleagues, 2008). Moreover, station and degree of instrumented rotation correlate with morbidity. Hagadorn-Freathy and co-workers (1991) reported a 13-percent rate of third- and fourth-degree episiotomy extensions and vaginal lacerations for outlet forceps, 22 percent for low forceps with less than 45 degrees rotation, 44 percent for low forceps with more than 45 degrees rotation, and 37 percent for midforceps deliveries. Bofill and colleagues (1996a, b) found

a significant association of moderate and severe perineal injuries with indicated operative deliveries, use of forceps versus vacuum extractor, the need for episiotomy, and delivery from other than outlet station. These findings are consistent with the recent report of FitzGerald and associates (2007).

Coincidental with overall efforts to reduce routine episiotomy use, Ecker and colleagues (1997) reported a significant decrease in the episiotomy rate with both forceps—96 to 30 percent—as well as vacuum—89 to 39 percent—deliveries from 1984 to 1994. During this time, there was a decrease in fourth-degree but no change in third-degree lacerations. In a review of more than 34,000 vaginal births by Goldberg and colleagues (2002), episiotomy rates decreased from 70 percent in 1983 to 19 percent in 2000. Forceps deliveries, however, were associated with higher episiotomy rates as well as third- and fourth-degree lacerations compared with those of spontaneous delivery.

Urinary and Fecal Incontinence. *Short-term effects* of forceps and vacuum deliveries, especially midcavity deliveries, include postpartum urinary retention and bladder dysfunction (Carley and co-workers, 2002). Arya and colleagues (2001) reported that urinary incontinence after forceps delivery was more likely to persist than incontinence associated with vacuum or spontaneous delivery.

Regarding *long-term effects*, there are a now a number of studies indicating that even spontaneous vaginal delivery will, in some women, be followed by urinary and fecal incontinence. Incontinence is temporary and improves with time in some of these. In others, however, it persists and may worsen over years. Extensive episiotomies or lacerations, especially of the anal sphincter, are more likely to cause problems with incontinence than spontaneous vaginal delivery alone (Pollack and associates, 2004; Pregazzi and colleagues, 2002). Because forceps deliveries are associated with an increased incidence of episiotomy and extension or laceration, it is not surprising that forceps use has been associated in some reports with higher rates of anal and urinary incontinence (Baydock and co-workers, 2009; Fitzpatrick and colleagues, 2003; Viktrup and Lose, 2001). Thus, the anterior compartment—responsible for bladder function, or the posterior

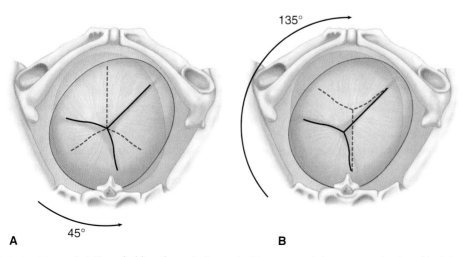

FIGURE 23-16 Rotation of obliquely posterior occiput to sacrum **(A)** or to symphysis pubis **(B)**.

135°

45°

A

B

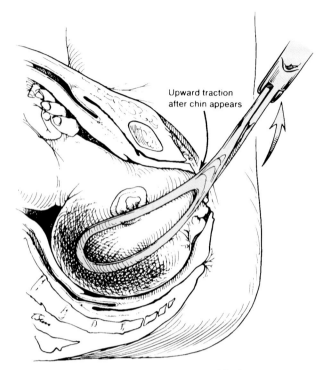

Upward traction
after chin appears

FIGURE 23-17 Face presentation, mentum (chin) anterior. Delivery with outlet forceps (Simpson).

compartment—responsible for anal function, or both may be involved.

Anal sphincter dysfunction, although associated with spontaneous delivery, is increased with instrumental vaginal delivery, episiotomy extensions, and deep lacerations. Eason and colleagues (2000, 2002) evaluated 949 Canadian women 3 months after delivery. Three percent had fecal incontinence, and more than a fourth had flatus incontinence. Both were more common in women who had had anal sphincter injuries and forceps delivery. Sultan and colleagues (1993) reported defecatory symptoms in 38 percent of women after forceps delivery, 12 percent following vacuum delivery, and 4 percent after spontaneous delivery with either a mediolateral episiotomy or second-degree lacerations. Pretlove and associates (2008) performed a systematic Cochrane Library review that included more than 12,000 deliveries. Within the year following delivery, women delivered by forceps had a twofold increased incidence of anal incontinence. Muscle injury is responsible for most anal dysfunction, however, pudendal nerve damage also plays a role (Tetzschner and colleagues, 1998).

Although the short-term effects on anorectal function associated with operative vaginal delivery are of concern, studies of long-term morbidity are conflicting. For example, in a 34-year follow-up after forceps delivery, Bollard and colleagues (2003) reported that significant fecal and urinary incontinence was no more likely after forceps delivery than after vaginal delivery. In a 30-year follow-up study, Nygaard and co-workers (1997) documented incontinence of flatus in 31, 43, and 36 percent of women who had experienced a disrupted sphincter, an episiotomy, or cesarean delivery, respectively. Conversely, in a 6-year follow-up of 3813 women, MacArthur and associates (2005) found an overall 3.6-percent prevalence of anal inconti-

nence. First delivery by forceps was associated with a doubled risk of anal incontinence relative to spontaneous vaginal delivery. They also reported that cesarean delivery was not protective.

Febrile Morbidity. Postpartum uterine infection and pelvic cellulitis are more frequent, and often more severe, in women following cesarean delivery compared with that following operative vaginal delivery (Robertson and colleagues, 1990).

Perinatal Morbidity

Direct morbidity to the fetus caused by forceps is usually from trauma. Facial nerve palsy was reported by Falco and Eriksson (1990) in 0.9 percent of 8415 infants delivered by forceps compared with 0.02 percent among 35,877 delivered spontaneously or by cesarean. The former included infants delivered by high and midforceps. Importantly, almost 90 percent of these facial palsies underwent complete spontaneous resolution. Brachial plexus injury was reported by Gilbert and co-workers (1999) to be more frequent among infants delivered with forceps or vacuum than those delivered spontaneously. They analyzed data from more than 1 million deliveries in California and described rates of injury of 5, 4, and 1.5 per thousand with forceps, vacuum, and spontaneous delivery, respectively.

Forceps and vacuum deliveries were associated with intracranial hemorrhage more commonly than spontaneous delivery in a study by Towner and colleagues (1999). They reviewed 583,340 term nulliparous women delivered in California between 1992 and 1994. A third of these underwent cesarean, forceps, or vacuum delivery, and they were compared with those delivered spontaneously. As shown in Table 23-2, the incidence of intracranial hemorrhage was highest in infants delivered by forceps, vacuum, or cesarean after labor had started, and comparable across these groups. Combined attempts with vacuum and forceps had the highest rate. These investigators concluded that abnormal labor, and not the method of delivery per se, was the common risk factor.

Morbidity from Midforceps Deliveries

Numerous reports have described the association of neonatal morbidity and midforceps operations. Several factors must be considered when interpreting these studies. First and foremost, most were conducted prior to the redefined classification of

TABLE 23-2. Effect of Method of Delivery on Incidence of Neonatal Intracranial Hemorrhage (ICH)

Delivery	ICH
Vacuum and forceps	1:280
Forceps	1:664
Vacuum	1:860
Cesarean with labor	1:907
Spontaneous	1:1900
Cesarean without labor	1:2750

Data from Towner and colleagues (1999).

forceps in 1988 by the American College of Obstetricians and Gynecologists (2000). Thus, in these earlier studies, midforceps were not defined clearly and included deliveries from relatively high stations (0 to +1), as well as those with difficult forceps rotations. Second, spontaneous vaginal deliveries are not appropriate controls for midforceps. Supportive of this is the study of Towner and colleagues (1999) in which infants delivered by cesarean after commencement of labor had the same risk of intracranial hemorrhage as those delivered by forceps. Finally, there is no uniformity in the criteria used to define immediate fetal morbidity.

There are only a few studies done applying the updated 1988 classification. In one, Robertson and associates (1990) reported significantly higher neonatal morbidity in the midforceps group compared with infants born by cesarean delivery.

The study cited earlier by Hagadorn-Freathy and colleagues (1991) was a prospective investigation designed to test the validity of the 1988 classification for fetal risk discrimination. They classified 357 forceps deliveries using both the pre-1988 and 1988 classifications and compared outcomes. Facial nerve palsy developed in 1.3 percent of infants delivered by outlet forceps and 3.2 percent of those delivered by midforceps using the pre-1988 classification. This compared with rates of 0.9 percent for outlet forceps, 1.7 percent for low forceps, and 9.2 percent for midforceps using the 1988 classification. Thus, the 1988 classification seems to usefully discriminate among the risks associated with outlet, low-, and midpelvic forceps deliveries. Because of increased maternal and neonatal morbidity rates compared with those for low-forceps operations, midforceps deliveries are seldom performed now.

Long-Term Infant Morbidity

For many decades, controversy has attended forceps vis-à-vis their relationship to long-term neurodevelopmental outcomes. Particularly controversial has been the possible association between forceps delivery and decreased measures of intelligence. Some of the early studies used data from the Collaborative Perinatal Project. In one, Broman and co-workers (1975) controlled for socioeconomic status, race, and gender. They reported that infants delivered by midforceps had slightly higher intelligence scores at age 4 years compared with those of children delivered spontaneously. Using the same database, Friedman and associates (1977, 1984) analyzed intelligence assessments at or after age 7 years. They concluded that children delivered by midforceps had lower mean intelligence quotients (IQs) compared with children delivered by outlet forceps. In yet another report from this same database, Dierker and colleagues (1986) compared long-term outcomes of children delivered by midforceps with those of children delivered by cesarean after dystocia. The strength of this study is the appropriateness of the control group. These investigators reported that delivery by midforceps was not associated with neurodevelopmental disability.

In another study of long-term morbidity of midforceps deliveries, Nilsen (1984) evaluated 18-year-old men when they were drafted into the Norwegian Army. The study found that those delivered by Kielland forceps had higher intelligence scores than those delivered spontaneously, by vacuum extraction, or by cesarean. Similar data reported by Seidman and colleagues (1991) from more than 32,000 Israeli Defense Forces draftees are shown in Table 23-3. Likewise, Wesley and colleagues (1992) assessed 1746 children and found no significant differences in intelligence test scores at age 5 years in spontaneous, forceps, or vacuum deliveries. Murphy and co-workers (2004) found no association between forceps delivery and epilepsy in a cohort of 21,441 adults, 9 percent of whom had been delivered by forceps. Finally, Bahl and associates (2007) performed a prospective cohort study of the children of 264 women who underwent operative delivery. Their incidence of adverse outcomes was similar whether delivered by successful forceps delivery, failed forceps with cesarean delivery, or immediate cesarean delivery.

TABLE 23-3. Intelligence Test Scores at Age 17 for Subjects Born in Jerusalem between 1964 and 1970

	Mean Intelligence Score ($\pm$SE)	
Type of Delivery	**Unadjusted**	**Adjusted[a]**
Spontaneous (n = 29,136)	105.4 (0.1)	105.7 (0.1)
Forceps (n = 567)	108.2 (0.7)	104.6 (0.4)
Vacuum extraction (n = 1207)	109.6 (0.5)	105.9 (0.4)
Cesarean delivery (n = 1335)	105.4 (0.4)	103.7 (0.1)

SE = standard error.
[a]Adjusted by multiple regression for confounding effects of sex, birthweight, ethnic origin, birth order, maternal age, and paternal and maternal education and social class.
Reprinted from *The Lancet*, Vol. 337, DS Seidman, A Laor, R Gale, DK Stevenson, S Mashiach, and YL Danon, Long-term effects of vacuum and forceps deliveries, pp. 1583–1585, Copyright 1991, with permission from Elsevier.

Conclusions Regarding Morbidity From Forceps

Although it is clear that midforceps operations are associated with the most significant maternal and neonatal risks, the bulk of studies in which morbid events were reported are from an era when cesarean delivery rates were around 5 percent. Thus, they undoubtedly included many difficult and even ill-advised forceps deliveries that would, in all likelihood, never be attempted today.

Also relevant to contemporary instrumented delivery is the widespread use of epidural analgesia (Lieberman and O'Donoghue, 2002). The need for forceps or vacuum delivery in women using this form of labor pain relief often results from inadequate maternal expulsive forces against a relaxed pelvic sling. Because of this, such deliveries are not usually associated with either relative or absolute cephalopelvic disproportion. Although it is prudent in these cases to allow a longer second-stage labor, in some circumstances, delivery is indicated sooner. Forceps deliveries for epidural-associated labor abnormalities are likely to be safer than the same operation performed in women with prolonged labor or midpelvic arrest unassociated with conduction analgesia.

It seems reasonable to conclude that outlet and low-forceps operations, as classified by the scheme proposed by the American College of Obstetricians and Gynecologists (2000), can be performed safely for both mother and fetus if the basic guidelines set forth in this chapter are carefully observed.

Trial of Forceps and Failed Forceps

If an attempt at operative vaginal delivery is anticipated to be difficult, the attempt should be considered a trial. With an operating room both equipped and staffed for immediate cesarean delivery, the trial may proceed. If a satisfactory application of the forceps cannot be achieved, then the procedure is abandoned and delivery accomplished by use of either vacuum extraction or cesarean. Once application has been achieved and in conjunction with contractions and maternal expulsive efforts, gentle downward pulls are made on the forceps. If there is no descent, the procedure should be abandoned and cesarean delivery performed.

In a study of 122 women who had a trial of midcavity forceps or vacuum extraction in a setting with full preparations to proceed to cesarean section, Lowe (1987) found no significant difference in immediate neonatal or maternal morbidity compared with that of 42 women delivered for similar indications by cesarean but without such a trial of instrumentation. Conversely, neonatal morbidity was higher in 61 women who had "unexpected" forceps or vacuum failure in which there was no prior preparation for immediate cesarean delivery. Ben-Haroush and colleagues (2007) reported a 1.3-percent failed forceps rate in 821 attempts. This compares with a 10-percent failed vacuum rate during 4299 attempts. Factors associated with failure were persistent occiput posterior position, absence of regional or general anesthesia, and birthweight greater than 4000 g.

To avoid morbidity with failed forceps or vacuum delivery, the American College of Obstetricians and Gynecologists (2000) cautions that these trials should be attempted only if the clinical assessment is highly suggestive of a successful outcome. We also emphasize proper training.

VACUUM EXTRACTION

In the United States, the device is referred to as the vacuum extractor, whereas in Europe it is commonly referred to as a *ventouse*—from French, literally, *soft cup* (Fig. 23-18A). Theoretical advantages of the vacuum extractor compared with forceps include: (1) avoidance of insertion of space-occupying steel blades within the vagina, (2) no requirement for precise positioning over the fetal head, (3) less maternal trauma, and (4) less intracranial pressure during traction. All previously described instruments were unsuccessful until Malmström (1954) applied a new principle, that is, traction on a metal cap designed so that the suction creates an artificial caput—chignon—within the cup that holds firmly and allows adequate traction.

As with forceps choice, the decision to use a metal or a soft cup appears regional. In the United States, the metal cup generally has been replaced by newer soft-cup vacuum extractors. As emphasized by Duchon and associates (1998), however, high-pressure vacuum generates large amounts of force regardless of the cup used. A wide variety of soft-cup extractors and vacuum devices are available. The former differ in their shape, size, rigidity, and reusability. The main difference among the latter is whether the device is handheld and actuated by the operator, or whether an assistant holds and operates the pump. Shown in Figure 23-18A is the system currently used at the University of Alabama at Birmingham Hospital.

A number of investigators have studied outcome in rigid and soft cups. Loghis and colleagues (1992) compared results of 200 women delivered using a metal cup with those of 200 women in whom a pliable cup was used. No differences were found in the rate of birth canal trauma—11 versus 13 percent; major neonatal scalp trauma—6.5 versus 5.5 percent; neonatal jaundice—15.5 versus 13.5 percent; or Apgar scores. Kuit and co-workers (1993) found that the only advantage of the soft cups was a lower incidence of scalp injury. They reported a 14-percent episiotomy extension rate with both rigid and pliable cups. Associated perineal lacerations developed with 16 percent of rigid cup extractions and 10 percent with the pliable cup. Johanson and Menon (2000a) analyzed results from nine randomized trials. They found that soft cups had an almost twofold failure rate but half the number of scalp injuries compared with rigid cups. In a similar review, Vacca (2002) concluded that there were fewer scalp lacerations with the soft cup, but that the rate of cephalohematomas and subgaleal hemorrhage was similar between soft and rigid cups.

Indications and Prerequisites for Vacuum Delivery

Generally, vacuum extraction is reserved for fetuses who have attained a gestational age of at least 34 weeks. Otherwise, the indications and prerequisites for its use are the same as for forceps delivery (American College of Obstetricians and Gynecologists, 2000). From their review of vacuum extraction, Koscica and Gimovsky (2002) concluded that contraindications include

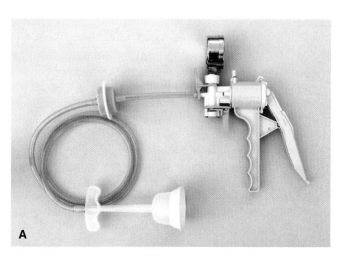

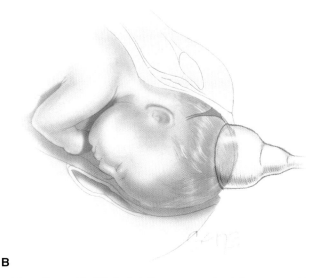

FIGURE 23-18 A. Vacuum delivery system: The Mityvac pump is attached to a disposable MitySoft Bell vacuum-assist delivery cup with tubing and filter. **B.** Cup in place.

operator inexperience, inability to assess fetal position, high station, and suspicion of cephalopelvic disproportion. Contraindications for delivery using vacuum extraction include face or other nonvertex presentations, or fetal coagulopathy. Recent scalp blood sampling is a relative contraindication, however, this sampling is infrequently used.

Technique

Proper cup placement is the most important determinant of success in vacuum extraction. The center of the cup should be over the sagittal suture and about 3 cm in front of the posterior fontanel toward the face (Fig. 23-18B). Anterior placement on the fetal cranium—near the anterior fontanel rather than over the occiput—will result in cervical spine extension unless the fetus is small. Similarly, asymmetrical placement relative to the sagittal suture may worsen asynclitism. Cup placement for elective use in occiput anterior positions is seldom difficult. In contrast, when the indication for delivery is failure to descend caused by occipital malposition, with or without asynclitism or deflexion, cup placement can be difficult.

Entrapment of maternal soft tissue predisposes the mother to lacerations and hemorrhage and virtually ensures cup dislodgement. The full circumference of the cup should be palpated both before and after the vacuum has been created as well as prior to traction to ensure that such entrapment has not occurred. When using rigid cups, it is recommended that the vacuum be created gradually by increasing the suction by 0.2 kg/cm^2 every 2 minutes until a negative pressure of 0.8 kg/cm^2 is reached. With soft cups, negative pressure can be increased to 0.8 kg/cm^2 over as little as 1 minute (Hankins and associates, 1995; Kuit and colleagues, 1993). Some authors suggest that 0.6 kg/cm^2 is the optimal peak pressure (Lucas, 1994). Listed in Table 23-4 are conversions of various units of pressures used by different instruments.

Traction should be intermittent and coordinated with maternal expulsive efforts. Traction may be initiated by using a two-handed technique, that is, the fingers of one hand are

placed against the suction cup, while the other hand grasps the handle of the instrument. Manual torque to the cup should be avoided as it may cause cephalohematomas and with metal cups, "cookie-cutter"–type scalp lacerations. Vacuum extraction should be considered a trial, and without early and clear evidence of descent toward delivery, an alternate delivery approach should be considered. As a general guideline, progressive descent should accompany each traction attempt. Neither data nor consensus are available regarding the number of pulls required to effect delivery, the maximum number of cup pop-offs that can be tolerated, or optimal total duration of the procedure. Cup dislodgement due to technical failure or less than optimal placement should not be equated with dislodgement under ideal conditions of exact cup placement and optimal vacuum maintenance. The former may merit either additional attempts at placement and delivery or alternatively, a trial of forceps (Ezenagu and colleagues, 1999; Williams and co-workers, 1991). As with forceps procedures, there should be a willingness to abandon attempts at vacuum extraction if satisfactory progress is not made (American College of Obstetricians and Gynecologists, 2000).

TABLE 23-4. Table of Vacuum Pressure Conversions

mm Hg	in Hg	lb/in^2	kg/cm^2
100	3.9	1.9	0.13
200	7.9	3.9	0.27
300	11.8	5.8	0.41
400	15.7	7.7	0.54
500	19.7	9.7	0.68
600	23.6	11.6	0.82

Reprinted from MJ Lucas, The role of vacuum extraction in modern obstetrics [Review], *Clinical Obstetrics & Gynecology*, Vol. 37, No. 4, pp. 794–805, 1994, with permission.

524   Labor and Delivery

SECTION 4

Complications

Complications of the vacuum extractor include scalp lacerations and bruising, subgaleal hematomas, cephalohematomas, intracranial hemorrhage, neonatal jaundice, subconjunctival hemorrhage, clavicular fracture, shoulder dystocia, injury of sixth and seventh cranial nerves, Erb palsy, retinal hemorrhage, and fetal death (Broekhuizen and associates, 1987; Galbraith, 1994; Govaert and colleagues, 1992). That said, Berkus and associates (1985) found no increase in rates of serious neonatal morbidity, including retinal hemorrhage, for the Silastic vacuum extractor compared with that associated with spontaneous delivery.

The Food and Drug Administration (FDA) issued a Public Health Advisory in 1998 regarding the possible association of vacuum-assisted delivery with serious fetal complications, including death. During a 4-year period, the FDA received reports of nine serious fetal injuries and 12 newborn deaths, which was a significant increase over the preceding 11 years. In a response to this advisory, the American College of Obstetricians and Gynecologists (1998) issued a Committee Opinion recommending the continued use of vacuum-assisted delivery devices when appropriate. They estimated that there is approximately one adverse event per 45,455 vacuum extractions per year.

Subsequently, Ross and colleagues (2000) reviewed the FDA Manufacturer and User Facility Device Experience (MAUDE) Database for the six months after the FDA advisory. These investigators concluded that adverse events due to the vacuum may in fact occur at a substantially higher rate than previously reported. Simonson and co-workers (2007) employed systematic radiographic and sonographic screening in 913 successful term vacuum-assisted deliveries and reported a fairly high reservoir of complications, including a 5-percent rate of skull fracture, and a 1-percent rate of intracranial hemorrhage. Complications were more frequent among nulliparas, midcavity deliveries, after more than three traction attempts, and after cup dislodgement. Reassuringly, all infants with skull fracture were asymptomatic, as were seven of the eight infants with intracranial hemorrhage. There were no cases of subgaleal hemorrhage.

Recommendations Regarding Vacuum Delivery

Considering the 1998 FDA Public Health Advisory, the following recommendations seem reasonable:

1. The classification of vacuum deliveries should be the same as that used for forceps deliveries (including station).
2. The same indications and contraindications used for forceps deliveries should be applied to vacuum-assisted deliveries.
3. The vacuum should not be applied to an unengaged vertex, that is, above 0 station.
4. The individual performing or supervising the procedure should be an experienced operator.
5. The operator should be willing to abandon the procedure if it does not proceed easily or if the cup dislodges more than three times.

COMPARISON OF VACUUM EXTRACTION WITH FORCEPS

There have been numerous studies comparing vacuum extraction with forceps deliveries. Vacca and associates (1983) conducted a randomized, prospective study comparing metal cup vacuum extraction with forceps delivery. They reported a higher frequency of maternal trauma and blood loss in the forceps group, but an increase in the incidence of neonatal jaundice in the vacuum group. Macleod and co-workers (2008) found lower episiotomy rates with vacuum delivery compared with forceps delivery. Bofill and colleagues (1996b) randomized 637 women to forceps versus vacuum extraction with the Mityvac M-cup. There were significantly more third- and fourth-degree lacerations—29 versus 12 percent—in the forceps-delivered group. Conversely, the incidence of both shoulder dystocia and cephalohematoma was approximately doubled in the vacuum group—15 versus 6 percent, and 37 versus 19 percent, respectively. Caughey and associates (2005) reported lower overall rates of shoulder dystocia, but the same relative relationship between the vacuum and forceps—3.5 percent versus 1.5 percent. Fitzpatrick and colleagues (2003) randomized 130 women to vacuum or forceps delivery. At 3 months, symptoms of fecal incontinence were more common in women delivered with forceps than with vacuum—59 versus 33 percent.

Although retinal hemorrhage occasionally is seen with vacuum usage, it has no apparent long-term effects. Johanson and Menon (2000b) analyzed 10 randomized trials and confirmed that vacuum extraction was associated with less maternal but more fetal trauma, for example, cephalohematoma and retinal hemorrhage.

The data are sparse regarding long-term neurological outcome in newborns delivered by vacuum extraction. In the report of an 18-year follow-up by Nilsen (1984), the mean intelligence score of 38 male infants delivered by vacuum was not different from the national average. Seidman and associates (1991) reported in their adjusted analysis that mean IQ score at age 17 in those delivered by vacuum or forceps was virtually the same as those delivered spontaneously (see Table 23-3). Johanson and colleagues (1999) performed a 5-year follow-up of a randomized trial of forceps versus vacuum delivery in more than 600 women and reported that there were no significant differences in child development in the two groups.

REFERENCES

American Academy of Pediatrics and the American College of Obstetricians and Gynecologists. Guidelines for Perinatal Care, 6th ed. Washington, DC, AAP and ACOG, 2007, p 158

American College of Obstetricians and Gynecologists: Delivery by vacuum extraction. Committee on Obstetric Practice, No. 208, 1998

American College of Obstetricians and Gynecologists: Operative vaginal delivery. Practice Bulletin No. 17, June 2000

Arya LA, Jackson ND, Myers DL, et al: Risk of new-onset urinary incontinence after forceps and vacuum delivery in primiparous women. Am J Obstet Gynecol 185:1318, 2001

Bahl R, Patel RR, Swingler R, et al: Neurodevelopmental outcome at 5 years after operative delivery in the second stage of labor: A cohort study. Am J Obstet Gynecol 197:147, 2007

Baydock SA, Flood C, Schulz JA, et al: Prevalence and risk factors for urinary and fecal incontinence four months after vaginal delivery. J Obstet Gynaecol Can 31(1):36, 2009

Ben-Haroush A, Melamed N, Kaplan B, et al: Predictors of failed operative vaginal delivery: A single-center experience. Am J Obstet Gynecol 197:308.e1, 2007

Berkus MD, Ramamurthy RS, O'Connor PS, et al: Cohort study of silastic obstetric vacuum cup deliveries, 1. Safety of the instrument. Obstet Gynecol 66:503, 1985

Bofill JA, Rust OA, Devidas M, et al: Prognostic factors for moderate and severe maternal genital tract laceration with operative vaginal delivery. Am J Obstet Gynecol 174:353, 1996a

Bofill JA, Rust OA, Schorr SJ, et al: A randomized prospective trial of the obstetric forceps versus the M-cup. Am J Obstet Gynecol 174:354, 1996b

Bollard RC, Gardiner A, Duthie GS, et al: Anal sphincter injury, fecal and urinary incontinence: A 34-year follow-up after forceps delivery. Dis Colon Rectum 46:1083, 2003

Broekhuizen FF, Washington JM, Johnson F, et al: Vacuum extraction versus forceps delivery: Indications and complications, 1979 to 1984. Obstet Gynecol 69:338, 1987

Broman SH, Nichols PL, Kennedy WA: Preschool IQ: Prenatal and Early Developmental Correlates. Hillside, NJ, Erlbaum, 1975

Carley ME, Carley JM, Vasdev G, et al: Factors that are associated with clinically overt postpartum urinary retention after vaginal delivery. Am J Obstet Gynecol 187:430, 2002

Caughey AB, Sandberg PL, Zlatnik MG, et al: Forceps compared with vacuum. Rates of neonatal and maternal morbidity. Obstet Gynecol 106:908, 2005

Cheong YC, Abdullahi H, Lashen H, et al: Can formal education and training improve the outcome of instrumental delivery? Eur J Obstet Gynecol 113:139, 2004

Damron DP, Capeless EL: Operative vaginal delivery: A comparison of forceps and vacuum for success rate and risk of rectal sphincter injury. Am J Obstet Gynecol 191:907, 2004

de Leeuw JW, de Wit C, Kuijken JP, et al: Mediolateral episiotomy reduces the risk for anal sphincter injury during operative vaginal delivery. BJOG 115:104, 2008

Dierker LJ, Rosen MG, Thompson K, et al: Midforceps deliveries: Long-term outcome of infants. Am J Obstet Gynecol 154:764, 1986

Duchon MA, DeMund MA, Brown RH: Laboratory comparison of modern vacuum extractors. Obstet Gynecol 72:155, 1998

Dupuis O, Moreau R, Pham MT: Assessment of forceps blade orientations during their placement using an instrumented childbirth simulator. BJOG 116(2):327, 2009

Dupuis O, Moreau R, Silveira R, et al: A new obstetric forceps for the training of junior doctors: A comparison of the spatial dispersion of forceps blade trajectories between junior and senior obstetricians. Am J Obstet Gynecol 194:1524, 2006

Eason E, Labrecque M, Marcoux S, et al: Anal incontinence after childbirth. CMAJ 166:326, 2002

Eason E, Labrecque M, Wells G, et al: Preventing perineal trauma during childbirth: A systematic review. Obstet Gynecol 95:464, 2000

Ecker JL, Tan WM, Bansal RK, et al: Is there a benefit to episiotomy at operative vaginal delivery? Observations over ten years in a stable population. Am J Obstet Gynecol 176:411, 1997

Ezenagu LC, Kakaria R, Bofill JA: Sequential use of instruments at operative vaginal delivery: Is it safe? Am J Obstet Gynecol 180:1446, 1999

Fairweather D: Obstetric management and follow-up of the very low-birthweight infant. J Reprod Med 26:387, 1981

Falco NA, Eriksson E: Facial nerve palsy in the newborn: Incidence and outcome. Plast Reconstr Surg 85:1, 1990

FDA Public Health Advisory: Need for CAUTION When Using Vacuum Assisted Delivery Devices. May 21, 1998

FitzGerald MP, Weber AM, Howden N, et al: Risk factors for anal sphincter tear during vaginal delivery. Obstet Gynecol 109:29, 2007

Fitzpatrick M, Behan M, O'Connell PR, et al: Randomised clinical trial to assess anal sphincter function following forceps or vacuum assisted vaginal delivery. Br J Obstet Gynaecol 110:424, 2003

Friedman EA, Sachtleben MR, Bresky PA: Dysfunctional labor, 12. Long-term effects on the fetus. Am J Obstet Gynecol 127:779, 1977

Friedman EA, Sachtleben-Murray MR, Dahrouge D, et al: Long-term effects of labor and delivery on offspring: A matched-pair analysis. Am J Obstet Gynecol 150:941, 1984

Galbraith RS: Incidence of neonatal sixth nerve palsy in relation to mode of delivery. Am J Obstet Gynecol 170:1158, 1994

Gilbert WM, Nesbitt TS, Danielsen B: Associated factors in 1611 cases of brachial plexus injury. Obstet Gynecol 93:536, 1999

Gilstrap LC III: Forceps delivery. In Gilstrap LC III, Cunningham FG, VanDorsten JP (eds): Operative Obstetrics, 2nd ed. New York, McGraw-Hill, 2002

Goldberg J, Holtz D, Hyslop T, et al: Has the use of routine episiotomy decreased? Examination of episiotomy rates from 1983 to 2000. Obstet Gynecol 99:395, 2002

Govaert P, Vanhaesebrouck P, de Praeter C: Traumatic neonatal intracranial bleeding and stroke. Arch Dis Child 67:840, 1992

Hagadorn-Freathy AS, Yeomans ER, Hankins GDV: Validation of the 1988 ACOG forceps classification system. Obstet Gynecol 77:356, 1991

Halpern SH, Leighton BL, Ohisson A, et al: Effect of epidural vs parenteral opioid analgesia on the progress of labor. JAMA 280:2105, 1998

Hankins GDV, Clark SL, Cunningham FG, et al: Vacuum delivery. In: Operative Obstetrics. Norwalk, Conn, Appleton & Lange, 1995

Hankins GD, Uckan E, Rowe TF, et al: Forceps and vacuum delivery: Expectations of residency and fellowship training program directors. Am J Perinatol 16:23, 1999

Johanson R, Menon V: Soft versus rigid vacuum extractor cups for assisted vaginal delivery. Cochrane Database Syst Rev 2:CD000446, 2000a

Johanson RB, Heycock E, Carter J, et al: Maternal and child health after assisted vaginal delivery: Five-year follow up of a randomised controlled study comparing forceps and ventouse. Br J Obstet Gynaecol 106:544, 1999

Johanson RB, Menon BK: Vacuum extraction forceps for assisted vaginal delivery. Cochrane Database Syst Rev 2:CD000224, 2000b

Koscica KL, Gimovsky ML: Vacuum extraction. Optimizing outcomes. Reducing legal risk. OBG Management April 2002, p 89

Kozak LJ, Weeks JD: U.S. trends in obstetric procedures, 1990–2000. Birth 29:157, 2002

Kuit JA, Eppinga HG, Wallenburg HCS, et al: A randomized comparison of vacuum extraction delivery with a rigid and a pliable cup. Obstet Gynecol 82:280, 1993

Le Ray C, Serres P, Schmitz T, et al: Manual rotation in occiput posterior or transverse positions. Obstet Gynecol 110:873, 2007

Leslie KK, Dipasquale-Lehnerz P, Smith M: Obstetric forceps training using visual feedback and the isometric strength testing unit. Obstet Gynecol 105:377, 2005

Lieberman E, O'Donoghue C: Unintended effects of epidural analgesia during labor: A systematic review. Am J Obstet Gynecol 186:S31, 2002

Loghis C, Pyrgiotis E, Panayotopoulos N, et al: Comparison between metal cup and silicon rubber cup vacuum extractor. Eur J Obstet Gynecol Reprod Biol 45:173, 1992

Lowe B: Fear of failure: A place for the trial of instrumental delivery. Br J Obstet Gynaecol 94:60, 1987

Lucas MJ: The role of vacuum extraction in modern obstetrics (review). Clin Obstet Gynecol 37:794, 1994

MacArthur C, Glazener C, Lancashire R, et al: Faecal incontinence and mode of first and subsequent delivery: A six-year longitudinal study. Br J Obstet Gynaecol 112:1075, 2005

Macleod M, Strachan B, Bahl R, et al: A prospective cohort study of maternal and neonatal morbidity in relation to use of episiotomy at operative vaginal delivery. BJOG 115(13):1688, 2008

Malmström T: The vacuum extractor, an obstetrical instrument. Acta Obstet Gynecol Scand Suppl 4:33, 1954

Martin JA, Hamilton BE, Sutton PD, et al: Births: Final Data for 2006. National Vital Statistics Reports, Vol 57, No 7. Hyattsville, Md, National Center for Health Statistics, 2009

Murphy DJ, Libby G, Chien P, et al: Cohort study of forceps delivery and the risk of epilepsy in adulthood. Am J Obstet Gynecol 191:392, 2004

Nilsen ST: Boys born by forceps and vacuum extraction examined at 18 years of age. Acta Obstet Gynecol Scand 63:549, 1984

Nygaard IE, Rao SS, Dawson JD: Anal incontinence after anal sphincter disruption: A 30 year retrospective cohort study. Obstet Gynecol 89:896, 1997

Pearl ML, Roberts JM, Laros RK, et al: Vaginal delivery from the persistent occiput posterior position: Influence on maternal and neonatal morbidity. J Reprod Med 38:955, 1993

Pollack J, Nordenstram J, Brismar S, et al: Anal incontinence after vaginal delivery: A five-year prospective cohort study. Obstet Gynecol 104:1397, 2004

Pregazzi R, Sartore A, Troiano L, et al: Postpartum urinary symptoms: Prevalence and risk factors. Eur J Obstet Gynecol Reprod Biol 103:179, 2002

Pretlove SJ, Thompson PJ, Toozs-Hobson PM, et al: Does the mode of delivery predispose women to anal incontinence in the first year postpartum? A comparative systematic review. BJOG 115:421, 2008

Robertson PA, Laros RK, Zhao RL: Neonatal and maternal outcome in low-pelvic and mid-pelvic operative deliveries. Am J Obstet Gynecol 162:1436, 1990

Ross MG, Fresquez M, El-Haddad MA: Impact of FDA advisory on reported vacuum-assisted delivery and morbidity. J Matern Fetal Med 9:321, 2000

Schwartz DB, Miodovnik M, Lavin JP Jr: Neonatal outcome among low birth weight infants delivered spontaneously or by low forceps. Obstet Gynecol 62:283, 1983

Seidman DS, Laor A, Gale R, et al: Long-term effects of vacuum and forceps deliveries. Lancet 337:1583, 1991

Sharma SK, McIntire DD, Wiley J, et al: Labor analgesia and cesarean delivery: An individual patient meta-analysis of nulliparous women. Anesthesiology 100:142, 2004

Simonson C, Barlow P, Dehennin N, et al: Neonatal complications of vacuum-assisted delivery. Obstet Gynecol 109:626, 2007

Sultan AH, Kamm MA, Bartram CI, et al: Anal sphincter trauma during instrumental delivery. Int J Gynaecol Obstet 43:263, 1993

Tetzschner T, Sorensen M, Lose G, et al: Anal and urinary incontinence after obstetric and sphincter rupture. Ugeskr Laeger 160:3218, 1998

Towner D, Castro MA, Eby-Wilkens E, et al: Effect of mode of delivery in nulliparous women on neonatal intracranial injury. N Engl J Med 341:1709, 1999

Vacca A: Vacuum-assisted delivery. Best Pract Res Clin Obstet Gynaecol 16:17, 2002

Vacca A, Grant A, Wyatt G, et al: Portsmouth operative delivery trial: A comparison of vacuum extraction and forceps delivery. Br J Obstet Gynaecol 90:1107, 1983

Viktrup L, Lose G: The risk of stress incontinence 5 years after first delivery. Am J Obstet Gynecol 185:82, 2001

Wesley B, Van den Berg B, Reece EA: The effect of operative vaginal delivery on cognitive development. Am J Obstet Gynecol 166:288, 1992

Williams MC, Knuppel RA, O'Brien WF, et al: A randomized comparison of assisted vaginal delivery by obstetric forceps and polyethylene vacuum cup. Obstet Gynecol 78:789, 1991

CHAPTER 24

Breech Presentation and Delivery

When the buttocks of the fetus enter the pelvis before the head, the presentation is *breech*. The term probably derives from the same word as *britches,* which described a cloth covering the loins and thighs. Breech presentation is more common remote from term because the bulk of each fetal pole is more similar. Most often, however, as term approaches, the fetus turns spontaneously to a cephalic presentation because the increasing bulk of the buttocks seeks the more spacious fundus. But, breech presentation persists in 3 to 4 percent of singleton deliveries at term (Fig. 24-1). For example, the annual rate of breech presentation at delivery in nearly 270,000 singleton newborns at Parkland Hospital has varied from only 3.3 to 3.9 percent during the past 20 years.

ASSOCIATED FACTORS

As term approaches, the uterine cavity usually accommodates the fetus in a longitudinal lie with the vertex presenting. Factors other than gestational age that predispose to breech presentation include hydramnios, high parity with uterine relaxation, multiple fetuses, oligohydramnios, hydrocephaly, anencephaly, previous breech delivery, uterine anomalies, placenta previa, fundal placental implantation, and pelvic tumors. Vendittelli and colleagues (2008) recently described a twofold incidence of breech presentation and prior cesarean delivery.

DIAGNOSIS

Definitions

The varying relations between the lower extremities and buttocks of breech presentations form the categories of frank, complete, and incomplete breech presentations. With a *frank breech* presentation, the lower extremities are flexed at the hips and extended at the knees, and thus the feet lie in close proximity to the head (Fig. 24-2). A *complete breech* presentation differs in that one or both knees are flexed (Fig. 24-3). With *incomplete breech* presentation, one or both hips are not flexed, and one or both feet or knees lie below the breech, such that a foot or knee is lowermost in the birth canal (Fig. 24-4). *Footling breech* is an incomplete breech with one or both feet below the breech.

In perhaps 5 percent of term breech presentations, the fetal head may be in extreme hyperextension. These presentations have been referred to as the *stargazer fetus,* and in Britain as the *flying foetus.* With such hyperextension, vaginal delivery may result in injury to the cervical spinal cord. Thus, if present after labor has begun, this is an indication for cesarean delivery (Svenningsen and associates, 1985).

Abdominal Examination

Use of the *Leopold maneuvers* to ascertain fetal presentation is discussed in Chapter 17 (p. 377). The accuracy of palpation varies (Lydon-Rochelle, 1993; Nassar, 2006, and all their coworkers; Thorp, 1991). Thus, with suspected breech presentation—or any presentation other than cephalic—sonographic evaluation is indicated.

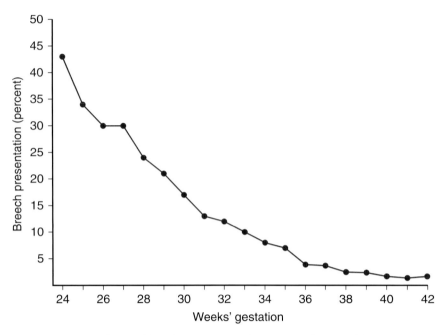

FIGURE 24-1 Prevalence of breech presentation by gestational age at delivery in 58,842 singleton pregnancies at the University of Alabama at Birmingham Hospitals, 1991 to 2006. (Used with permission from the Center for Women's Reproductive Health, University of Alabama at Birmingham.)

With the first Leopold maneuver, the hard, round, readily ballottable fetal head may be found to occupy the fundus. The second maneuver indicates the back to be on one side of the abdomen and the small parts on the other. With the third maneuver, if not engaged, the breech is movable above the pelvic inlet. After engagement, the fourth maneuver shows the firm breech to be beneath the symphysis.

Vaginal Examination

With the frank breech presentation, both ischial tuberosities, the sacrum, and the anus usually are palpable, and after further fetal descent, the external genitalia may be distinguished. Especially when labor is prolonged, the buttocks may become markedly swollen, rendering differentiation of a face and breech difficult. In some cases, the anus may be mistaken for the mouth and the ischial tuberosities for the malar eminences. With careful examination, however, the finger encounters muscular resistance with the anus, whereas the firmer, less yielding jaws are felt through the mouth. The finger, upon removal from the anus, may be stained with meconium. The mouth and malar eminences form a triangular shape, whereas the ischial tuberosities and anus lie in a straight line.

The sacrum and its spinous processes are palpated to establish the position and presentation. As with cephalic presentations and as described in Chapter 17 (p. 375), fetal positions are designated as left sacrum anterior (LSA), right sacrum anterior (RSA), left sacrum posterior (LSP), right sacrum posterior (RSP), or sacrum transverse (ST) to reflect the relationship of the fetal sacrum to the maternal pelvis.

Regarding presentation, with a complete breech, the feet may be felt alongside the buttocks. In footling presentations, one or both feet are inferior to the buttocks. When the breech has descended farther into the pelvic cavity, the genitalia may be felt.

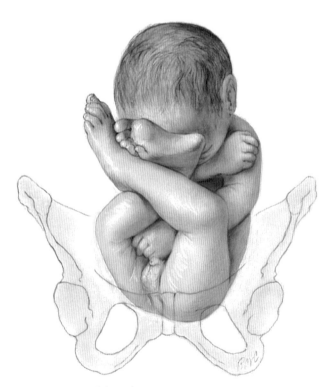

FIGURE 24-2 Frank breech presentation.

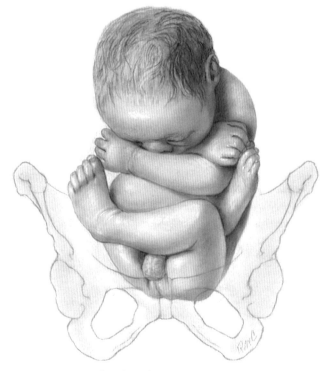

FIGURE 24-3 Complete breech presentation.

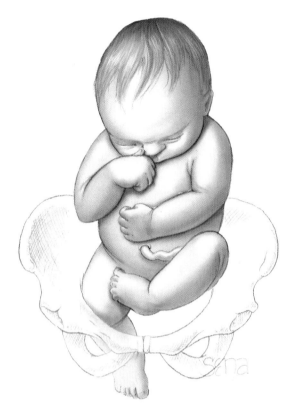

FIGURE 24-4 Incomplete breech presentation.

Imaging Techniques

Because most are preterm, in many fetuses, the breech is smaller than the aftercoming head. Moreover, unlike cephalic presentations, the head of a breech-presenting fetus is not permitted to undergo molding during labor. Thus to avoid trapping of the head following delivery of the breech, pelvic dimensions should be assessed prior to vaginal delivery. In addition, the type of breech and degree of neck flexion or extension should be identified. To evaluate these, there are several imaging techniques.

Sonography

The best confirmation of a suspected breech presentation is with sonography. It also can provide information regarding the breech type and neck angle (Fontenot and associates, 1997; Rojansky and colleagues, 1994).

Other Methods

Computed tomographic (CT) scanning also can be used and will also provide pelvic measurements and configuration with lower doses of radiation than standard radiographs (see Chap. 20, p. 472). *Magnetic resonance (MR) imaging* provides reliable information about pelvic capacity and architecture without ionizing radiation, but it is not always readily available (van Loon and colleagues, 1997).

Pelvimetry. The role of radiographic pelvimetry to help determine the mode of delivery for breech presentation is controversial. Cheng and Hannah (1993) reviewed 15 studies of term-presenting breeches in which either radiographic or CT pelvimetry was used. They concluded that the utility of pelvimetry was difficult to assess because "permissible" pelvic dimensions varied

among studies. Also, in most of these studies, there was no correlation between pelvic measurements and labor outcome. At Parkland Hospital, we use CT pelvimetry when possible to assess the *critical dimensions* of the pelvis (see Chap. 2, p. 31).

COMPLICATIONS

In the persistent breech presentation, an increased frequency of the following complications can be anticipated:

- Prolapsed cord
- Placenta previa
- Congenital anomalies
- Uterine anomalies and tumors
- Difficult delivery
- Increased maternal and perinatal morbidity

PROGNOSIS

Adverse pregnancy outcomes may be increased for both mother and fetus.

Maternal Morbidity

Because of the greater frequency of operative delivery, there is a higher rate of maternal morbidity for pregnancies complicated by persistent breech presentation. The most worrisome are genital tract lacerations. Intrauterine maneuvers, especially with a thinned lower uterine segment, or delivery of the aftercoming head through an incompletely dilated cervix, may cause rupture of the uterus, lacerations of the cervix and vaginal walls, or both. Such manipulations also may lead to extensions of the episiotomy and deep perineal tears. Anesthesia sufficient to induce appreciable uterine relaxation may cause uterine atony and in turn, postpartum hemorrhage. Finally, manual manipulations within the birth canal increase the risk of infection.

The maternal mortality rate may even be increased. Schutte and colleagues (2007) reported the deaths of four women in the Netherlands from 2000 to 2002 as a result of elective cesarean delivery for breech presentation—a case fatality rate of 0.47 maternal deaths per 1000 births.

Perinatal Morbidity and Mortality

The major contributors to perinatal loss are preterm delivery, congenital anomalies, and birth trauma. In their study reported more than 30 years ago, Brenner and associates (1974) found that at every stage of gestation, neonatal deaths were significantly greater among breeches. One reason was that congenital abnormalities were identified in 6.3 percent of breech-presenting fetuses compared with 2.4 percent of those who were not breech. However, in an analysis of 57,819 pregnancies in the Netherlands, corrected for gestational age, congenital defects, and birthweight, Schutte and colleagues (1985) reported that the perinatal mortality rate was higher in breech—compared with cephalic—presenting newborns. These investigators concluded that breech presentation may not be coincidental, but rather is a consequence of poor fetal quality.

More contemporaneous outcomes are improved because of careful assessment before attempted vaginal delivery and because of increased cesarean delivery rates, which generally exceed 60 percent. For example, Albrechtsen and colleagues (1997) reported that the perinatal mortality rate in 45,579 breech deliveries decreased from 9 percent in the period from 1967 through 1976 to 3 percent from 1987 through 1994. Herbst (2005) analyzed 22,549 term breech deliveries from 1991 to 2001 and reported a remarkably low combined perinatal and infant mortality rate of 0.63 percent.

Fetal Injuries

Several specific injuries are associated with vaginal breech deliveries. Fracture of the humerus and clavicle cannot always be avoided, and fracture of the femur may be sustained during difficult breech extractions. Such fractures are associated with both vaginal and cesarean deliveries (Awwad and colleagues, 1993; Vasa and Kim, 1990). Neonatal perineal tears have been reported as a complication of spinal electrode use (Freud and associates, 1993). Hematomas of the sternocleidomastoid muscles occasionally develop after delivery, although they usually disappear spontaneously. More serious problems, however, may follow separation of the epiphyses of the scapula, humerus, or femur. There is no evidence that the incidence of congenital hip dislocations is increased (Clausen and Nielsen, 1988).

Upper extremity paralysis may follow pressure on the brachial plexus by the fingers in exerting traction, but more frequently it is caused by overstretching the neck while freeing the arms. Geutjens and colleagues (1996) described 36 newborns with brachial plexus injury following vaginal breech delivery. In 80 percent, there was avulsion of the upper cervical spine roots. This injury cannot be treated adequately by microsurgical nerve grafting and carries a poor prognosis for shoulder function. When the fetus is extracted forcibly through a contracted pelvis, spoon-shaped depressions or actual fractures of the skull may result. Occasionally, even the fetal neck may be broken when great force is employed. Testicular injury, in some cases severe enough to result in anorchia, may follow vaginal breech delivery (Tiwary, 1989).

Term Breech Fetus

Cheng and Hannah (1993) conducted a comprehensive review of 24 studies encompassing 11,721 women. Studies were selected that compared *planned* vaginal with *planned* cesarean delivery for the term, singleton breech fetus. The corrected perinatal mortality rate ranged from 0 to 48 per 1000 births. All but two of the 77 perinatal deaths were in women allowed to deliver vaginally. The main causes of death were head entrapment, cerebral injury and intracranial hemorrhage, cord prolapse, and intrapartum asphyxia. The overall neonatal mortality and morbidity rates resulting from trauma were increased almost fourfold in the planned vaginal delivery groups. Similarly, Gifford and co-workers (1995) performed a meta-analysis of outcomes after term breech delivery, and they too reported that a trial of labor was associated with an increased risk of perinatal injury or death. Their analysis included only two randomized trials. Although these two trials concluded that vaginal breech delivery was relatively safe, only 110 women were actually allowed a trial of labor. This small number does not provide sufficient power to demonstrate differences in outcomes such as perinatal death and birth injury (Eller and Van Dorsten, 1995).

Preterm Breech Fetus

There are no randomized studies regarding delivery of the preterm breech fetus. A number of older retrospective studies yielded conflicting results. Studies published since 1990, however, generally report no excessive risks (Gravenhorst and co-workers, 1993; Wolf and colleagues, 1999). In a multicenter study, Malloy and co-workers (1991) described findings from the National Institute of Child Health and Human Development-sponsored Neonatal Research Network of 437 very-low-birthweight breech newborns. After adjusting for several variables, the risk of intraventricular hemorrhage and death was not significantly affected by the mode of delivery for fetuses weighing less than 1500 g. In a similar report from France, Kayem and co-workers (2008) described neonatal outcomes in 169 breech deliveries from 26 to 30 weeks. The neonatal death risk—11 versus 7 percent—was similar in infants undergoing planned vaginal versus planned cesarean delivery.

Current Status of Vaginal Breech Delivery

There are a number of events during the past decade that have had a marked influence on the mode of delivery for the breech-presenting fetus. Some of these changes are now summarized.

The Randomised Multicentre Trial

The multinational study performed by the Term Breech Trial Collaborative Group reported by Hannah and colleagues (2000) had a significant impact on obstetrical management. The trial included 1041 women randomly assigned to planned cesarean and 1042 to planned vaginal delivery. In the planned vaginal delivery group, 57 percent were actually delivered vaginally. Overall, planned cesarean delivery was associated with a lower risk of perinatal mortality compared with planned vaginal delivery—3 per 1000 versus 13 per 1000. Planned cesarean delivery was also associated with a lower risk of "serious" neonatal morbidity—1.4 versus 3.8 percent. Maternal complications were similar between the groups.

As subsequently discussed, the almost immediate effect of these results was an abrupt and almost complete decline in the rate of attempted vaginal breech deliveries. For example, in the Netherlands, the cesarean delivery rate for term breeches increased from 50 percent in the 33 months preceding the publication of the trial to 80 percent in the 25 months after its publication (Rietberg and associates, 2005).

United States, 2000–2005

In 2001, the American College of Obstetricians and Gynecologists published Committee Opinion No. 265, which concluded that except in cases of "advanced labor" and "imminent delivery"—not otherwise defined—women with persistent singleton breech presentation at term should undergo a planned cesarean delivery. These opinions arose from the previously discussed study by Hannah and colleagues (2000). Since that time, the number of vaginal breech deliveries has diminished. For example, in 2004, 87 percent of breech fetuses in the United States were born by cesarean delivery. As a result, the number of skilled operators with the ability to safely select and vaginally deliver breech fetuses continues to dwindle. Obvious medicolegal concerns make it difficult to train new physicians to perform such deliveries.

For a number of reasons, we took issue with Committee Opinion No. 265 (Hauth and Cunningham, 2002). Our objections primarily centered on reliance on the Randomized Multicentre Trial. More recently, Glezerman (2006) again codified some of these criticisms:

1. Among the 1025 women enrolled from countries with low perinatal mortality rates, perinatal deaths were infrequent and did not differ significantly between groups—none in 514 women in the planned cesarean compared with 3 of 511 in the planned vaginal delivery group.
2. Most outcomes included in the "serious" neonatal morbidity composite do not actually portend long-term disability.
3. Fewer than 10 percent of women in the trial underwent pelvimetry using plain radiography, CT scanning, or MR imaging.
4. In more than 30 percent of women, the attitude of the fetal head was determined only by clinical methods.

As it happens, these criticisms subsequently were proven valid. Whyte and colleagues (2004) reported the 2-year outcomes for children born during the original multicenter trial. They found that planned cesarean delivery was not associated with a reduction in the rate of death or developmental delay. Specifically in the planned cesarean delivery group, the rate was 3.1 percent compared with 2.8 percent in the vaginal delivery group. Similar results were reported from Norway by Eide and associates (2005), who analyzed findings from more than 390,000 men who had intelligence testing at mandatory military registration. More than 8000 of these men—2 percent—were delivered from the breech position. The investigators concluded that presentation at birth did not affect intellectual performance. They also found that cesarean delivery of breech-presenting fetuses was not associated with *improved* intelligence-testing performance.

There are also a number of contemporaneous single-center studies that support a trial of vaginal delivery for selected breech-presenting term fetuses. Irion and associates (1998) reported significantly fewer maternal complications, but no difference in corrected neonatal morbidity or mortality rates between 385 *attempted* vaginal breech deliveries—70 percent of whom were delivered vaginally—and 320 planned cesarean deliveries. Giuliani and associates (2002) reported that in their institution, vaginal breech delivery was performed in half of 699 consecutive, term, breech-presenting fetuses. There were no short- or long-term differences in outcomes for fetuses delivered by either route. Alarab and associates (2004) reported no serious adverse neonatal outcomes in the fourth of 146 term breech fetuses delivered vaginally over a 3½-year period. Excellent outcomes for singleton breech fetuses after planned vaginal birth have also been reported by Uotila (2005), Krupitz (2005), Pradhan (2005), and their colleagues.

Results from a large prospective European study were reported by Goffinet and co-workers (2006). They analyzed outcomes of 8105 term singleton breech-presenting fetuses from 174 French and Belgium hospitals. The decision on mode of delivery and the management of those who labored followed fairly stringent guidelines put forth by the French College of Obstetricians and Gynecologists and which are consistent with those outlined below. Vaginal delivery was planned in about a third—2526—of these women, and it was successful in 1796 of these—71 percent. The perinatal mortality or serious neonatal morbidity rates were low. Importantly, they did not differ between the planned vaginal and planned cesarean group—1.6 versus 1.5 percent, respectively. The single neonatal death was a nonmalformed newborn who was in the planned cesarean group.

United States, after 2005

In response to the 2-year outcomes from the Multicentre International Trial, as well as some of the other reports cited above, the American College of Obstetricians and Gynecologists (2006) modified its stance concerning breech delivery. Specifically, Committee Opinion No. 340 states that "the decision regarding the mode of delivery should depend on the experience of the health care provider" and that "planned vaginal delivery of a term singleton breech fetus may be reasonable under hospital-specific protocol guidelines."

These newer guidelines seem more reasonable to define state-of-the-art practices. The problem of a continuing source of experienced operators is real (Chinnock and Robson, 2007). Some institutions have responded to diminished training opportunities in innovative ways. For example, Deering and colleagues (2006) utilized a birth simulator to improve resident competence in vaginal breech delivery. Finally, as aptly stated by Gimovsky and associates (2007), the "understandable but elusive desire to be 100-percent correct complicates the issue"!

Recommendations for Delivery

A diligent search for any other complications, actual or anticipated, that might justify cesarean delivery has become a feature of most philosophies for managing singleton breech delivery. Cesarean delivery is commonly, but not exclusively, used in the following circumstances:

1. A large fetus
2. Any degree of contraction or unfavorable shape of the pelvis determined clinically or with CT pelvimetry
3. A hyperextended head
4. When delivery is indicated in the absence of spontaneous labor
5. Uterine dysfunction—some would use oxytocin augmentation
6. Incomplete or footling breech presentation
7. An apparently healthy and viable preterm fetus with the mother in either active labor or in whom delivery is indicated
8. Severe fetal-growth restriction
9. Previous perinatal death or children suffering from birth trauma
10. A request for sterilization
11. Lack of an experienced operator.

For a favorable outcome with any breech delivery, at the very minimum, the birth canal must be sufficiently large to allow passage of the fetus without trauma. The cervix must be fully dilated, and if not, then a cesarean delivery nearly always is the more appropriate method of delivery when suspected fetal compromise develops.

TECHNIQUES FOR BREECH DELIVERY

Labor and Spontaneous Delivery

There are important fundamental differences between labor and delivery in cephalic and breech presentations. With a cephalic presentation, once the head is delivered, the rest of the body typically follows without difficulty. With a breech, however, successively larger and very much less compressible parts are born. Spontaneous complete expulsion of the fetus that presents as a breech, as subsequently described, is seldom accomplished successfully. Therefore, as a rule, vaginal delivery requires skilled participation for a favorable outcome.

Methods of Vaginal Delivery

There are three general methods of breech delivery through the vagina:

1. *Spontaneous breech delivery.* The fetus is expelled entirely spontaneously without any traction or manipulation other than support of the newborn.
2. *Partial breech extraction.* The fetus is delivered spontaneously as far as the umbilicus, but the remainder of the body is extracted or delivered with operator traction and assisted maneuvers, with or without maternal expulsive efforts.
3. *Total breech extraction.* The entire body of the fetus is extracted by the obstetrician.

Labor Induction and Augmentation

Induction or augmentation of labor in women with a breech presentation is controversial. Many years ago, Brenner and associates (1974) found similar perinatal outcomes in newborns with induced versus spontaneous labor. In oxytocin-augmented labor, however, infant mortality rates were higher and Apgar scores were lower. Fait and colleagues (1998) reported that 12 of 23 women with an unripe cervix who underwent induction had a successful breech vaginal delivery with no neonatal complications. Su and colleagues (2003) reported that avoiding labor augmentation and having an experienced obstetrician present at birth significantly reduces the risk of adverse perinatal outcomes.

At Parkland Hospital, cesarean delivery is preferred to oxytocin induction or augmentation with a viable fetus. Amniotomy induction is suitable. At the University of Alabama at Birmingham, oxytocin is employed if clinical factors are favorable for vaginal delivery and if CT pelvimetry confirms an adequate pelvis.

Management of Labor

On arrival, rapid assessment should be made to establish the status of the membranes, labor, and fetal condition. Surveillance of fetal heart rate and uterine contractions is begun at admission. Immediate recruitment of necessary staff should include:

1. An obstetrician skilled in the art of breech extraction
2. An associate to assist with the delivery

3. Anesthesia personnel who can ensure adequate analgesia or anesthesia when needed
4. An individual trained newborn resuscitation.

In addition, the nursery is notified. For the mother, an intravenous catheter is inserted, and an infusion begun. Emergency induction of anesthesia or maternal resuscitation following hemorrhage from lacerations or from uterine atony are but two of many reasons that may require immediate intravenous access.

Stage of Labor

Assessment of cervical dilatation and effacement and the station of the presenting part is essential for planning the route of delivery. If labor is too far advanced, there may not be sufficient time to obtain pelvimetry. This alone, however, should not force the decision for cesarean delivery. Biswas and Johnstone (1993) found that among 267 term breech presentations, satisfactory progress in labor was the best indicator of pelvic adequacy. Nwosu and colleagues (1993) reported similar findings.

Fetal Condition

In many cases, sonographic fetal evaluation was done as part of prenatal care. If not, the presence of gross fetal abnormalities, such as hydrocephaly or anencephaly, can be rapidly ascertained with the use of sonography. This will help to ensure that a cesarean delivery is not performed under emergency conditions for an anomalous fetus with no chance of survival. For vaginal delivery, the fetal head should not be extended. As discussed, it is usually possible to ascertain head flexion and to exclude extension with sonography (Fontenot and colleagues, 1997; Rojansky and co-workers, 1994). If not possible, then simple two-view radiography of the abdomen can be used.

Fetal Monitoring

Additional help is required for managing labor and delivery of a breech presentation. One-on-one nursing is ideal during labor because of the risk of cord prolapse or occlusion, and physicians must be readily available should there be an emergency. Guidelines for monitoring the high-risk fetus are applied as discussed in Chapter 17 (p. 393). During the first stage of labor, the fetal heart rate is recorded at least every 15 minutes. Most clinicians prefer continuous electronic monitoring.

When membranes are ruptured, either spontaneously or artificially, the risk of cord prolapse is appreciably increased. The frequency of cord prolapse is increased when the fetus is small or when the breech is not frank (Barrett, 1991; Collea and colleagues, 1978. Therefore, a vaginal examination should be performed following rupture to check for cord prolapse. To detect occult cord prolapse, special attention should be directed to the fetal heart rate for the first 5 to 10 minutes following membrane rupture.

Soernes and Bakke (1986) confirmed earlier observations that umbilical cord length is significantly shorter in breech presentations. Moreover, multiple coils of cord entangling the fetus are more common with breech presentations (Spellacy and associates, 1966). These umbilical cord abnormalities likely play a role both in the development of breech presentation and in the relatively high incidence of nonreassuring fetal heart rate patterns in labor.

Route of Delivery

The choice of abdominal or vaginal delivery is based on factors discussed on page 531. As outlined by the American College of Obstetricians and Gynecologists (2006), risks versus benefits are discussed with the woman. If possible, this is done before admission.

Cardinal Movements with Breech Delivery

Engagement and descent of the breech usually take place with the bitrochanteric diameter in one of the oblique pelvic diameters. The anterior hip usually descends more rapidly than the posterior hip, and when the resistance of the pelvic floor is met, internal rotation of 45 degrees usually follows, bringing the anterior hip toward the pubic arch and allowing the bitrochanteric diameter to occupy the anteroposterior diameter of the pelvic outlet. If the posterior extremity is prolapsed, however, it, rather than the anterior hip, rotates to the symphysis pubis.

After rotation, descent continues until the perineum is distended by the advancing breech, and the anterior hip appears at the vulva. By lateral flexion of the fetal body, the posterior hip then is forced over the perineum, which retracts over the buttocks, thus allowing the infant to straighten out when the anterior hip is born. The legs and feet follow the breech and may be born spontaneously or require aid.

After the birth of the breech, there is slight external rotation, with the back turning anteriorly as the shoulders are brought into relation with one of the oblique diameters of the pelvis. The shoulders then descend rapidly and undergo internal rotation, with the bisacromial diameter occupying the anteroposterior plane. Immediately following the shoulders, the head, which is normally sharply flexed upon the thorax, enters the pelvis in one of the oblique diameters and then rotates in such a manner as to bring the posterior portion of the neck under the symphysis pubis. The head is then born in flexion.

The breech may engage in the transverse diameter of the pelvis, with the sacrum directed anteriorly or posteriorly. The mechanism of labor in the transverse position differs only in that internal rotation is through an arc of 90 rather than 45 degrees. Infrequently, rotation occurs in such a manner that the back of the fetus is directed posteriorly instead of anteriorly. Such rotation should be prevented if possible. Although the head may be delivered by allowing the chin and face to pass beneath the symphysis, the slightest traction on the body may cause extension of the head, which increases the diameter of the head that must pass through the pelvis.

Partial Breech Extraction

Delivery is easier, and in turn, morbidity and mortality rates are probably lower, when the breech is allowed to deliver spontaneously to the umbilicus. Delivery of the breech draws the umbilicus and attached cord into the pelvis, which compresses the cord. Therefore, once the breech has passed beyond the vaginal introitus, the abdomen, thorax, arms, and head must be deliv-

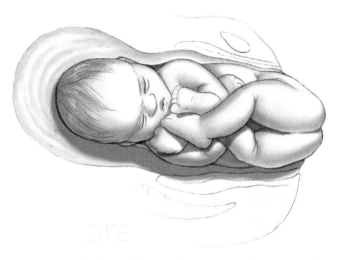

FIGURE 24-5 The hips of the frank breech are delivering over the perineum.

ered promptly. If a nonreassuring fetal heart rate pattern develops before this time, however, a decision must be made whether to perform manual extraction or cesarean delivery.

With all breech deliveries, unless there is considerable relaxation of the perineum, an episiotomy should be made. The episiotomy is an important adjunct to any type of breech delivery. The posterior hip will deliver, usually from the 6 o'clock position, and often with sufficient pressure to evoke passage of thick meconium at this point (Fig. 24-5). The anterior hip then delivers, followed by external rotation to a sacrum anterior position. The mother should be encouraged to continue to push, as the cord is now drawn well down into the birth canal and likely is being compressed or stretched causing fetal bradycardia. As the fetus continues to descend, the legs are sequentially delivered by splinting the medial aspect of each femur with the operator's fingers positioned parallel to each femur, and by exerting pressure laterally to sweep each leg away from the midline.

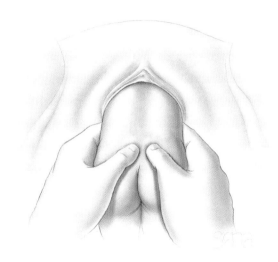

FIGURE 24-6 Delivery of the body. The hands are applied, but not above the pelvic girdle. Gentle downward rotational traction is accomplished until the scapulas are clearly visible.

Following delivery of the legs, the fetal bony pelvis is grasped with both hands, using a cloth towel moistened with warm water. The fingers should rest on the anterior superior iliac crests and the thumbs on the sacrum, minimizing the chance of fetal abdominal soft tissue injury (Fig. 24-6). Maternal expulsive efforts are used in conjunction with continued gentle downward operator rotational traction to effect delivery. Gentle downward traction is combined with an initial 90-degree rotation of the fetal pelvis through one arc and then a 180-degree rotation to the other, to effect delivery of the scapulas and arms (Figs. 24-7 and 24-8).

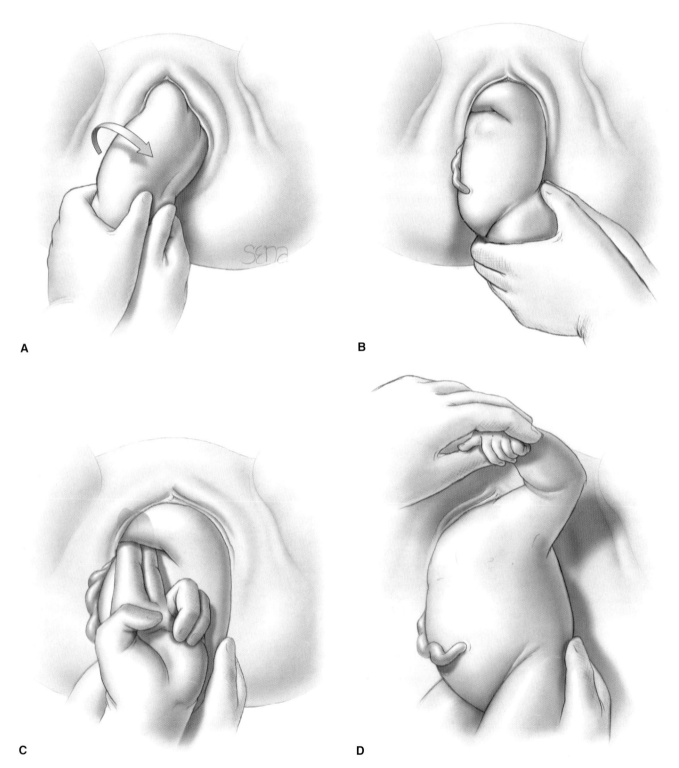

A

B

C

D

FIGURE 24-7 Clockwise rotation of the fetal pelvis 90 degrees brings the sacrum from anterior to left sacrum transverse. Simultaneously, the application of gentle downward traction effects delivery of the scapula **(A)** and arm **(B–D)**.

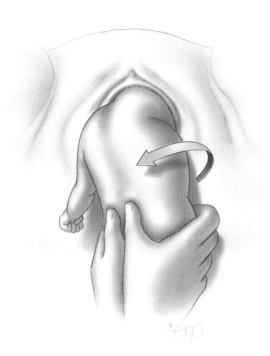

FIGURE 24-8 Counterclockwise rotation from sacrum anterior to right sacrum transverse along with gentle downward traction effects delivery of the right scapula.

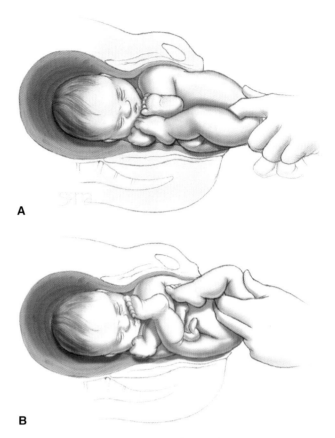

A

B

FIGURE 24-9 A. Extraction of frank breech using fingers in groins. **B.** Once the hips are delivered, each hip and knee is flexed to deliver them from the vagina.

These rotational and downward traction maneuvers will decrease the persistence of nuchal arms, which can prevent further descent and may result in a traumatic delivery. These maneuvers are frequently most easily effected with the operator at the level of the maternal pelvis and with one knee on the floor. When the scapulas are clearly visible, delivery is then completed as subsequently described for the complete or incomplete breech (p. 536).

Total Breech Extraction

Frank Breech Extraction

At times, extraction of a frank breech may be required and can be accomplished by moderate traction exerted by a finger in each groin and aided by a generous episiotomy (Fig. 24-9). If moderate traction does not affect delivery, then vaginal delivery can be accomplished only by breech decomposition. This procedure involves manipulation within the birth canal to convert the frank breech into a footling breech. It is accomplished more readily if the membranes have ruptured recently, and it becomes extremely difficult if there is minimal amnionic fluid. In such cases, the uterus may have become tightly contracted around the fetus. Pharmacological relaxation by general anesthesia, intravenous magnesium sulfate, or a beta-mimetic such as terbutaline, 250 µg subcutaneously, may be required.

Breech decomposition is accomplished by the maneuver attributed to Pinard (1889). It aids in bringing the fetal feet within reach of the operator. As shown in Figure 24-10, two fingers are carried up along one extremity to the knee to push

it away from the midline. Spontaneous flexion usually follows, and the foot of the fetus is felt to impinge on the back of the hand. The fetal foot then may be grasped and brought down.

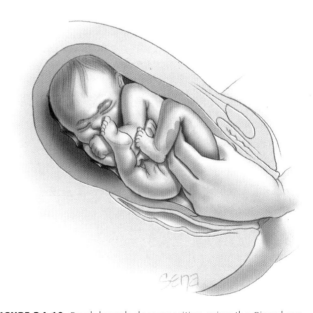

FIGURE 24-10 Frank breech decomposition using the Pinard maneuver. Two fingers are inserted along one extremity to the knee, which is then pushed away from the midline after spontaneous flexion. Traction is used to deliver a foot into the vagina.

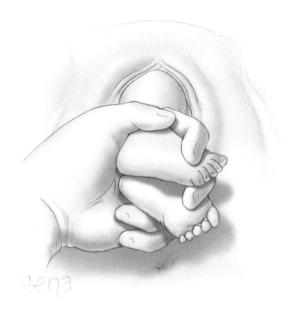

FIGURE 24-11 Complete breech extraction begins with traction on the feet and ankles.

Complete or Incomplete Breech Extraction

During total extraction of a complete or incomplete breech, the hand is introduced through the vagina and both feet of the fetus are grasped. The ankles are held with the second finger lying between them and with gentle traction, the feet are brought through the vulva. If difficulty is experienced in grasping both feet, first one foot should be drawn into the vagina but not through the introitus, and then the other foot is advanced in a similar fashion. Now both feet are grasped and pulled through the vulva simultaneously (Fig. 24-11).

As the legs begin to emerge through the vulva, downward gentle traction is then continued. As the legs emerge, successively higher portions are grasped, first the calves and then the thighs. When the breech appears at the vaginal outlet, gentle traction is applied until the hips are delivered. As the buttocks emerge, the back of the fetus usually rotates to the anterior. The thumbs are then placed over the sacrum and the fingers over the hips, and assisted breech delivery is completed, as described previously (see Fig. 24-6). As the scapulas become visible, the back of the fetus tends to turn spontaneously toward the side of the mother to which it was originally directed.

A cardinal rule in successful breech extraction is to employ steady, gentle, downward rotational traction until the lower halves of the scapulas are delivered, making no attempt at delivery of the shoulders and arms until one axilla becomes visible. The appearance of one axilla indicates that the time has arrived for delivery of the shoulders. It makes little difference which shoulder is delivered first, and there are two methods for delivery of the shoulders:

1. In the first method, with the scapulas visible, the trunk is rotated in such a way that the anterior shoulder and arm appear at the vulva and can easily be released and delivered first (see Fig. 24-7). The body of the fetus is then rotated in the reverse direction to deliver the other shoulder and arm (see Fig. 24-8).

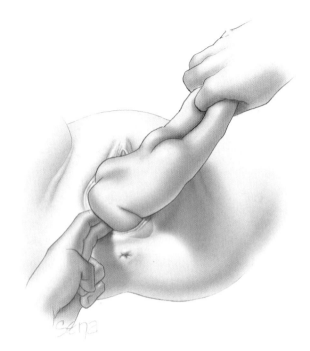

FIGURE 24-12 As breech extraction continues, upward traction is employed, effecting delivery of the posterior shoulder. This is followed by delivery of the posterior arm.

2. The second method is employed if trunk rotation is unsuccessful. With this maneuver, the posterior shoulder is delivered first. The feet are grasped in one hand and drawn upward over the inner thigh of the mother toward which the ventral surface of the fetus is directed (Fig. 24-12). In this manner, leverage is exerted on the posterior shoulder, which slides out over the perineal margin, usually followed by the arm and hand. Then, by depressing the body of the fetus, the anterior shoulder emerges beneath the pubic arch, and the arm and hand usually follow spontaneously. Thereafter, the back tends to rotate spontaneously in the direction of the symphysis. If upward rotation fails to occur, it is completed by manual rotation of the body. Delivery of the head may then be accomplished.

Unfortunately, the process is not always so simple, and it is sometimes necessary first to free and deliver the arms. These maneuvers are less likely to be required if rotational traction is employed and attempts to deliver the shoulders until an axilla becomes visible are avoided. **Attempts to free the arms immediately after the costal margins emerge should be avoided.** There is more space available in the posterior and lateral segments of the normal pelvis than elsewhere. Therefore, in difficult cases, the posterior arm should be freed first. Because the corresponding axilla is already visible, upward traction on the feet is continued, and two fingers of the other hand are passed along the humerus until the elbow is reached (see Fig. 24-12). The fingers are placed parallel to the humerus and used to splint the arm, which is swept downward and delivered through the vulva.

To deliver the anterior arm, depression of the body of the fetus is sometimes all that is required to allow the anterior arm to slip out spontaneously. In other instances, the anterior arm can be swept down over the thorax using two fingers as a splint.

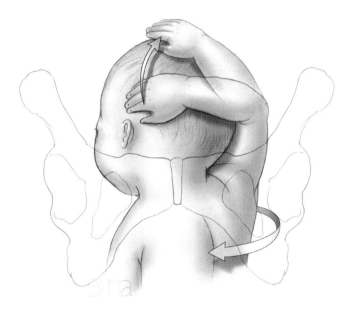

FIGURE 24-13 Reduction of nuchal arm being accomplished by rotating the fetus through half a circle counterclockwise so that the friction exerted by the birth canal will draw the elbow toward the face.

In some cases, the body must be held with the thumbs over the scapulas and rotated to bring the undelivered shoulder near the closest sacrosciatic notch. The legs then are carried upward to bring the ventral surface of the fetus to the opposite inner thigh of the mother. Subsequently, the arm can be delivered as described previously. If the arms have become extended over the head, their delivery, although more difficult, usually can be accomplished by the maneuvers just described. In so doing, particular care must be taken by the operator to carry the fingers up

to the elbow and to use them as a splint to prevent fracture of the humerus.

Nuchal Arm. As discussed earlier, one or both fetal arms occasionally may be found around the back of the neck—the nuchal arm—and impacted at the pelvic inlet. In this situation, delivery is more difficult. If the nuchal arm cannot be freed in the manner described, extraction may be aided, especially with a single nuchal arm, by rotating the fetus through half a circle in such a direction that the friction exerted by the birth canal will serve to draw the elbow toward the face (Fig. 24-13). Should rotation of the fetus fail to free the nuchal arm(s), it may be necessary to push the fetus upward in an attempt to release it. If the rotation is still unsuccessful, the nuchal arm often is extracted by hooking a finger(s) over it and forcing the arm over the shoulder, and down the ventral surface for delivery of the arm. In this event, fracture of the humerus or clavicle is very common.

Delivery of the Aftercoming Head

The fetal head may be extracted with forceps or by one of the following maneuvers.

Mauriceau Maneuver

The index and middle finger of one hand are applied over the maxilla, to flex the head, while the fetal body rests on the palm of the hand and forearm (Fig. 24-14). The forearm is straddled by the fetal legs. Two fingers of the other hand then are hooked over the fetal neck, and grasping the shoulders, downward traction is applied until the suboccipital region appears under the symphysis. Gentle suprapubic pressure simultaneously applied by an assistant helps keep the head flexed. The body then is elevated toward the maternal abdomen, and the mouth, nose, brow, and eventually the occiput emerge successively over the perineum. **With this maneuver, the operator uses both hands simultaneously and in tandem to exert continuous downward gentle traction simultaneously on the fetal neck and on the maxilla.** At the same time, appropriate suprapubic pressure applied by an assistant is helpful in delivery of the head (see Fig. 24-14).

Modified Prague Maneuver

Rarely, the back of the fetus fails to rotate to the anterior. When this occurs, rotation of the back to the anterior may be achieved by using stronger traction on the fetal legs or bony pelvis. If the back still remains oriented

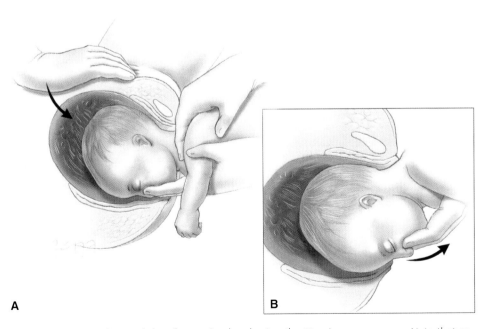

FIGURE 24-14 A. Delivery of the aftercoming head using the Mauriceau maneuver. Note that as the fetal head is being delivered, flexion of the head is maintained by suprapubic pressure provided by an assistant. **B.** Pressure on the maxilla is applied simultaneously by the operator as upward and outward traction is exerted.

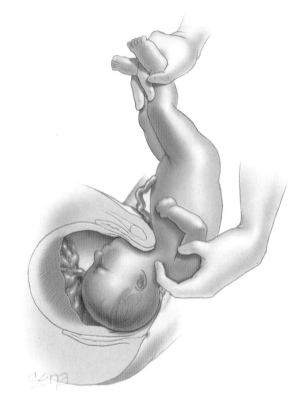

FIGURE 24-15 Delivery of the aftercoming head using the modified Prague maneuver necessitated by failure of the fetal trunk to rotate anteriorly.

posteriorly, extraction may be accomplished using the Mauriceau maneuver and delivering the fetus back down. If this is impossible, the fetus still may be delivered using the modified Prague maneuver, which, as practiced today, consists of two fingers of one hand grasping the shoulders of the back-down fetus from below while the other hand draws the feet up over the maternal abdomen (Fig. 24-15).

Forceps to Aftercoming Head

Specialized forceps can be used to deliver the aftercoming head. *Piper forceps,* shown in Figure 24-16, or divergent *Laufe forceps* may be applied electively or when the Mauriceau maneuver cannot be accomplished easily. The blades of the forceps should not be applied to the aftercoming head until it has been brought into the pelvis by gentle traction, combined with suprapubic pressure, and is engaged. Suspension of the body of the fetus in a towel effectively holds the fetus and helps keep the arms out of the way.

Entrapment of the Aftercoming Head

Occasionally—especially with a small preterm fetus—the incompletely dilated cervix will constrict around the neck and impede delivery of the aftercoming head. At this point, it must be assumed that there is significant and even total cord compression, and thus time is of the essence. With gentle traction on the fetal body, the cervix, at times, may be manually slipped over the occiput. If this is not successful, then

Dührssen incisions as shown in Figure 24-17 may be necessary. Other alternatives include intravenous nitroglycerin—typically 100 μg—to provide cervical relaxation for relief of head entrapment (Dufour and colleagues, 1997; Wessen and associates, 1995). There is, however, no compelling evidence of its efficacy for this purpose. General anesthesia is another option.

As a last resort, replacement of the fetus higher into the vagina and uterus, followed by cesarean delivery, can be used to rescue an entrapped breech fetus that cannot be delivered vaginally. Steyn and Pieper (1994) described use of the *Zavanelli maneuver*—cesarean delivery after replacement of the fetus back into the uterus—to deliver a healthy 2590-g newborn with head entrapment. Sandberg (1999) reviewed 11 breech deliveries in which this maneuver was used.

In some countries, *symphysiotomy* is used to widen the anterior pelvis. Sunday-Adeoye and colleagues (2004) reported that at the Mater Misericordiae Hospital, in Nigeria, 3.7 percent of 27,477 deliveries from 1982 to 1989 were accomplished with symphysiotomy! In his review, Menticoglou (1990) reported that its use has been associated with good infant outcomes in 80 percent of reported cases. Lack of operator training and the potential to cause serious maternal injury explain its rare use in this country (Goodwin and colleagues, 1997).

ANALGESIA AND ANESTHESIA

Continuous epidural analgesia, as described in Chapter 19 (p. 454), is advocated by some as ideal for women in labor with a breech presentation. Confino and colleagues (1985) reviewed the outcomes of 371 singleton breech fetuses delivered vaginally. About 25 percent of these women had been given continuous epidural analgesia, and oxytocin augmentation was necessary to effect delivery in half of them. Although first-stage labor was not longer than in a control group not given epidural analgesia, the second stage was prolonged significantly in women whose fetuses weighed more than 2500 g. It was doubled if the fetus weighed more than 3500 g. Chadha and associates (1992) reported similar findings. These potential disadvantages must be weighed against the advantages of better pain relief and importantly, increased pelvic relaxation should extensive manipulation be required to complete delivery.

Analgesia for episiotomy and intravaginal manipulations that are needed for breech extraction usually can be accomplished with pudendal block and local infiltration of the perineum. Nitrous oxide plus oxygen inhalation provides further relief from pain. If general anesthesia is required, it can be induced quickly with thiopental plus a muscle relaxant and maintained with nitrous oxide.

Anesthesia for breech decomposition and extraction must provide sufficient relaxation to allow intrauterine manipulations. Although successful decomposition has been accomplished using epidural or spinal analgesia, increased uterine tone may render the operation more difficult. Under such conditions, general anesthesia with a halogenated agent may be required to relax the uterus as well as to provide analgesia.

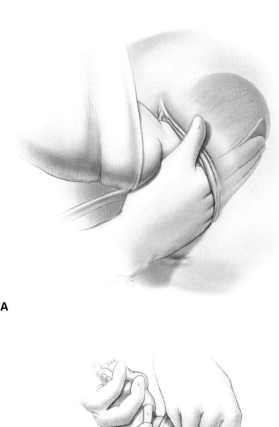

A

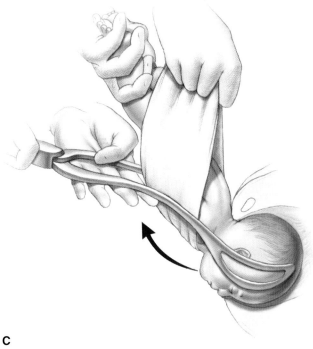

C

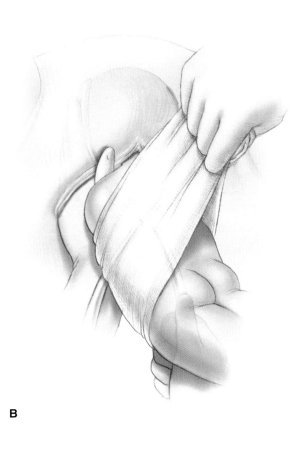

B

FIGURE 24-16 Piper forceps for delivery of the aftercoming head. **A.** The fetal body is held elevated using a warm towel and the left blade of forceps applied to the aftercoming head. **B.** The right blade is applied with the body still elevated. **C.** Forceps delivery of aftercoming head. Note the direction of movement shown by the arrow.

VERSION

Version is a procedure in which the fetal presentation is altered by physical manipulation, either substituting one pole of a longitudinal presentation for the other, or converting an oblique or transverse lie into a longitudinal presentation. According to whether the head or breech is made the presenting part, the operation is designated *cephalic* or *podalic version,* respectively. In *external version,* the manipulations are performed exclusively through the abdominal wall. In *internal version,* they are accomplished inside the uterine cavity.

External Cephalic Version

In the United States, Van Dorsten and co-workers (1981) rekindled interest in this procedure, and the American College of Obstetricians and Gynecologists (2006) recommends that version should be offered and attempted whenever possible. The

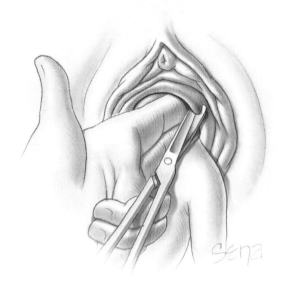

FIGURE 24-17 Dührssen incision being cut at 2 o'clock, which is followed by a second incision at 10 o'clock. Infrequently, an additional incision is required at 6 o'clock. The incisions are so placed as to minimize bleeding from the laterally located cervical branches of the uterine cavity. After delivery, the incisions are repaired as described in Chapter 35 (p. 783).

success rate for external version ranges from 35 to 86 percent, with an average of 58 percent (American College of Obstetricians and Gynecologists, 2000). In their review of 25 reports through 1991, Zhang and co-workers (1993) reported an average success rate of 65 percent. Moreover, they observed that after successful version, almost all fetuses remain cephalic.

Interestingly, several reports suggest that even after successful version, the risk of cesarean delivery does not completely revert to the institutional baseline for vertex presentations, and that dystocia, malpresentation, and nonreassuring fetal heart patterns may be more common after successful version (Chan and colleagues, 2004; Vézina and associates, 2004). Also, failure is not always absolute. Ben-Meir and colleagues (2007) reported a spontaneous version rate of 7 percent among 226 failed versions—2 percent among nulliparas and 13 percent among parous women.

Indications

In general, when a breech presentation is recognized prior to labor in a woman who has reached 36 weeks' gestation, external cephalic version should be considered. Before this time, there is a relatively high incidence of recurrence. After 36 weeks, however, the likelihood of spontaneous version is low (Hickok and colleagues, 1992; Westgren and co-workers, 1985). Moreover, if version results in the need for immediate delivery, complications of iatrogenic preterm delivery generally are not severe.

Version is contraindicated if vaginal delivery is not an option. Examples include placenta previa or nonreassuring fetal status. A prior uterine incision is a relative contraindication, although in small studies external version was not associated with uterine rupture in women who had previously undergone

TABLE 24-1. Factors That May Modify the Success of External Cephalic Version

Increase Success
Increasing parity
Ample amnionic fluid
Unengaged fetus
Tocolysis

Decrease Success
Engaged fetus
Tense uterus
Inability to palpate head
Obesity
Anterior placenta
Fetal spine anterior or posterior
Labor

cesarean delivery (Abenhaim, 2009; Flamm, 1991; Sela, 2009, and all their associates). At the University of Alabama at Birmingham, decisions about version in women with a prior cesarean incision are individualized. At Parkland Hospital, external version is not attempted in these women. Obviously, larger studies are needed to better characterize risks versus benefits.

Factors Associated with Successful Version

A number of associated factors can improve or lessen the chances of a successful version attempt (Table 24-1). Increasing parity and increasing amnionic fluid index are consistent factors associated with success (Boucher, 2003; Hutton, 2008; Kok, 2008; Zhang, 1993, and all their co-workers). Kok and colleagues (2009) reported improved success also in those with a posterior placenta and complete breech position.

A number of factors are predictive of *failed version*. Lau and associates (1997) identified three: (1) an engaged presenting part, (2) difficult palpation of the fetal head, and (3) a uterus tense to palpation. When all three were present, there were no successes; with two, success was less than 20 percent; and if none was present, the success rate was 94 percent. In a secondary analysis of a randomized trial that included 178 women undergoing attempted version, Hutton and colleagues (2008) reported that an unengaged presenting part improved the success rate. They recommended consideration for attempted version before engagement, that is, earlier in pregnancy. Other reported determinants of failed version include maternal obesity, anterior placenta, cervical dilatation, and anterior or posterior positioning of the fetal spine (Fortunato and associates, 1988; Newman and colleagues, 1993).

Transverse Lie

Women with a transverse lie usually are excluded from analyses of breech version because the overall success rate approaches 90 percent (Newman and colleagues, 1993).

Technique

External cephalic version should be carried out in an area that has ready access to a facility equipped to perform emergency cesarean deliveries (American College of Obstetricians and

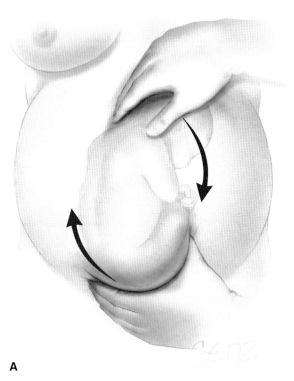
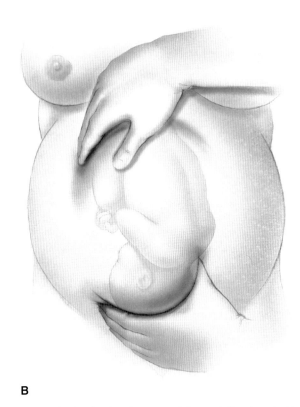

A   B

FIGURE 24-18 External cephalic version. **A.** Clockwise pressure is exerted against the fetal poles. **B.** Successful completion is noted by feeling the head above the symphysis during Leopold examination.

Gynecologists, 2000). Sonographic examination is performed to confirm nonvertex presentation and adequacy of amnionic fluid volume, to exclude obvious fetal anomalies if not done previously, and to identify placental location. External monitoring is performed to assess fetal heart rate reactivity. Anti-D immune globulin is given if indicated.

A *forward roll* of the fetus usually is attempted first. As shown in Figure 24-18, each hand grasps one of the fetal poles, and the buttocks are elevated from the maternal pelvis and displaced laterally. The buttocks are then gently guided toward the fundus, while the head is directed toward the pelvis. If the forward roll is unsuccessful, then a *backward flip* is attempted. Version attempts are discontinued for excessive discomfort, persistently abnormal fetal heart rate, or after multiple failed attempts. The nonstress test is repeated after version until a normal test result is obtained.

Tocolysis

Although many clinicians recommend uterine relaxation with a tocolytic agent, their impact on success is controversial. For example, Robertson and associates (1987) used ritodrine, Tan and colleagues (1989) used salbutamol, and Yanny and associates (2000) used glyceryl trinitrate, but none observed apparent benefits. Indeed, Bujold and colleagues (2003) conducted a placebo-controlled trial of 99 women and reported that sublingual nitroglycerin was associated with a *lower* version success rate than placebo—48 versus 63 percent. In another randomized trial, however, Fernandez and co-workers (1996) reported that the success rate with subcutaneous terbutaline-52 percent-was significantly higher

than without—27 percent. Our policies at the University of Alabama at Birmingham and at Parkland Hospital are to administer 250 μg of terbutaline subcutaneously to most women prior to attempted version. When maternal tachycardia—a known side effect of terbutaline—is noted, then the version attempt is begun.

Conduction Analgesia

Epidural analgesia has been reported to increase the success of version. In a randomized trial, Schorr and co-workers (1997) found that epidural analgesia given with terbutaline tocolysis resulted in a 60-percent success rate compared with 30 percent of women given only terbutaline. In another randomized trial of 108 women, Mancuso and associates (2000) reported a success rate of 59 percent with epidural analgesia versus 33 percent without.

Spinal analgesia has also been used for external version. Weiniger and associates (2007) reported in a small trial of 70 women that spinal analgesia increased the success rate of version. In the trials of Dugoff (2001) and Delisle (2001) and their colleagues, it was not of benefit. According to the American College of Obstetricians and Gynecologists (2000), there is not enough consistent evidence to recommend conduction analgesia routinely for external version.

Other Methods

There are some unconventional interventions that have been used to help effect version. Cardini and Weixen (1998) performed a randomized trial to evaluate *moxibustion*. This involves burning the herbal preparation *moxa* to generate heat to stimulate acupuncture point BL67—to promote spontaneous breech version. Women in the intervention group experienced significantly increased fetal movements and more often had a cephalic presentation at delivery. These astounding results were not replicated in a follow-up study by Cardini and co-workers (2005). Mehl (1994) found *hypnosis* with suggestions for relaxation to be effective. Finally, Crawford (2005) described a case report of successful use of an old folk remedy—application of ice to the abdomen—to cause version.

Complications

Risks of external version include placental abruption, uterine rupture, fetomaternal hemorrhage, isoimmunization, preterm labor, fetal compromise, and even death. Most worrisome is the report by Stine and co-workers (1985) of a maternal death due to amnionic fluid embolism. That said, fetal deaths are rare (Zhang and colleagues, 1993).

With the exception of rare severe complications, based on a comprehensive review, Collaris and Oei (2004) concluded that external cephalic version is safe. One caveat was that complications were more common when conduction analgesia was used. Use of nitrous oxide or conduction analgesia was associated with twice as many abnormal fetal heart rate tracings. Moreover, vaginal bleeding and procedure-related emergency cesarean deliveries were increased tenfold. These reviewers concluded that diminished pain in these women likely encouraged overzealous application of force during the version attempts, which led to complications. More recently, Collins and associates (2007) report very low complication rates and an emergency cesarean rate of only 0.5 percent in 805 consecutive external cephalic version attempts at the John Radcliffe Hospital in Oxford, England.

Internal Podalic Version

This maneuver is used only for delivery of a second twin. It consists of the insertion of a hand into the uterine cavity to turn the fetus manually. The operator seizes one or both feet and draws them through the fully dilated cervix while using the other hand transabdominally to push the upper portion of the fetal body in the opposite direction as shown in Chapter 39 (p. 883). This is followed by breech extraction.

REFERENCES

Abenhaim HA, Varin J, Boucher M: External cephalic version among women with a previous cesarean delivery: Report on 36 cases and review of the literature. J Perinat Med 37(2):156, 2009

Alarab M, Regan C, O'Connell MP, et al: Singleton vaginal breech delivery at term: Still a safe option. Obstet Gynecol 103:407, 2004

Albrechtsen S, Rasmussen S, Reigstad H, et al: Evaluation of a protocol for selecting fetuses in breech presentation for vaginal delivery or cesarean section. Am J Obstet Gynecol 177:586, 1997

American College of Obstetricians and Gynecologists: External cephalic version. Practice Bulletin No. 13, February 2000

American College of Obstetricians and Gynecologists: Mode of term singleton breech delivery. Committee Opinion No. 265, December 2001

American College of Obstetricians and Gynecologists: Mode of term in singleton breech delivery. Committee Opinion No. 340, July 2006

Awwad JT, Nahhas DE, Karam KS: Femur fracture during cesarean breech delivery. Int J Gynaecol Obstet 43:324, 1993

Barrett JM: Funic reduction for the management of umbilical cord prolapse. Am J Obstet Gynecol 165:654, 1991

Ben-Meir A, Elram T, Tsafrir A, et al: The incidence of spontaneous version after failed external cephalic version. Am J Obstet Gynecol 196(2):157, 2007

Biswas A, Johnstone MJ: Term breech delivery: Does x-ray pelvimetry help? Aust NZ J Obstet Gynaecol 33:150, 1993

Boucher M, Bujold E, Marquette GP, et al: The relationship between amniotic fluid index and successful external cephalic version: A 14-year experience. Am J Obstet Gynecol 189:751, 2003

Brenner WE, Bruce RD, Hendricks CH: The characteristics and perils of breech presentation. Am J Obstet Gynecol 118:700, 1974

Bujold E, Boucher M, Rinfret D, et al: Sublingual nitroglycerin versus placebo as a tocolytic for external cephalic version: A randomized controlled trial in parous women. Am J Obstet Gynecol 189:1070, 2003

Cardini F, Weixin H: Moxibustion for correction of breech presentation: A randomized controlled trial. JAMA 280:1580, 1998

Cardini F, Lombardo P, Regalia AL, et al: A randomized controlled trial of moxibustion for breech presentation. Br J Obstet Gynaecol 112(6):743, 2005

Chadha YC, Mahmood TA, Dick MJ, et al: Breech delivery and epidural analgesia. Br J Obstet Gynaecol 99:96, 1992

Chan LY, Tang JL, Tsoi KF, et al: Intrapartum cesarean delivery after successful external cephalic version: A meta-analysis. Obstet Gynecol 104:155, 2004

Cheng M, Hannah M: Breech delivery at term: A critical review of the literature. Obstet Gynecol 82:605, 1993

Chinnock M, Robson S: Obstetric trainees' experience in vaginal breech delivery. Obstet Gynecol 110:900, 2007

Clausen I, Nielsen KT: Breech position, delivery route and congenital hip dislocation. Acta Obstet Gynecol Scand 67:595, 1988

Collaris RJ, Oei SG: External cephalic version: A safe procedure? A systematic review of version-related risks. Acta Obstet Gynecol Scand 83:511, 2004

Collea JV, Rabin SC, Weghorst GR, et al: The randomized management of term frank breech presentation: Vaginal delivery vs cesarean section. Am J Obstet Gynecol 131:186, 1978

Collins S, Ellaway P, Harrington D, et al: The complications of external cephalic version: Results from 805 consecutive attempts. Br J Obstet Gynaecol 114(5):636, 2007

Confino E, Ismajovich B, Rudick V, et al: Extradural analgesia in the management of singleton breech delivery. Br J Anaesth 57:892, 1985

Crawford MP: Use of external abdominal ice to complete external cephalic version in term breech pregnancy. J Am Board Fam Pract 18(4):312, 2005

Deering S, Brown J, Hodor J, et al: Simulation training and resident performance of singleton vaginal breech delivery. Obstet Gynecol 107(1): 86, 2006

de Meeus JB, Ellia F, Magnin G: External cephalic version after previous cesarean section: A series of 38 cases. Eur J Obstet Gynecol Reprod Biol 81:65, 1998

Delisle MF, Kamani AA, Douglas MJ, et al: Antepartum external cephalic version under spinal anesthesia: A randomized controlled study [Abstract]. J Obstet Gynaecol Can 25:S13, 2003

Dufour PH, Vinatier D, Orazi G, et al: The use of intravenous nitroglycerin for emergency cervico-uterine relaxation. Acta Obstet Gynecol Scand 76:287, 1997

Dugoff L, Stamm CA, Jones OW III, et al: The effect of spinal anesthesia on the success rate of external cephalic version: A randomized trial. Obstet Gynecol 93:345, 1999

Eide MG, Øyen N, Skjaerven R, et al: Breech delivery and intelligence: A population-based study of 8,738 breech infants. Obstet Gynecol 105(1):4, 2005

Eller DP, Van Dorsten JP: Route of delivery for the breech presentation: A conundrum. Am J Obstet Gynecol 173: 393, 1995

Fait G, Daniel Y, Lessing JB, et al: Can labor with breech presentation be induced? Gynecol Obstet Investig 469:181, 1998

Fernandez CO, Bloom S, Wendel G: A prospective, randomized, blinded comparison of terbutaline versus placebo for singleton, term external cephalic version. Am J Obstet Gynecol 174:326, 1996

Flamm BL, Fried MW, Lonky NM, et al: External cephalic version after previous cesarean section. Am J Obstet Gynecol 165:370, 1991

Fontenot T, Campbell B, Mitchell-Tutt E, et al: Radiographic evaluation of breech presentation: Is it necessary? Ultrasound Obstet 10:338, 1997

Fortunato SJ, Mercer LJ, Guzick DS: External cephalic version with tocolysis: Factors associated with success. Obstet Gynecol 72:59, 1988

Freud E, Orvieto R, Merlob P: Neonatal labioperineal tear from fetal scalp electrode insertion, a case report. J Reprod Med 38:647, 1993

Geutjens G, Gilbert A, Helsen K: Obstetric brachial plexus palsy associated with breech delivery. A different pattern of injury. J Bone Joint Surg [Br] 78:303, 1996

Gifford DS, Morton SC, Fiske M, et al: A meta-analysis of infant outcomes after breech delivery. Obstet Gynecol 85:1047, 1995

Gimovsky ML, Rosa E, Bronshtein E: Update on breech. Contemp ObGyn September 2007

Gimovsky ML, Wallace RL, Schifrin BS, et al: Randomized management of the nonfrank breech presentation at term: A preliminary report. Am J Obstet Gynecol 146:34, 1983

Giuliani A, Scholl WMJ, Basver A, et al: Mode of delivery and outcome of 699 term singleton breech deliveries at a single center. Am J Obstet Gynecol 187:1694, 2002

Glezerman M: Five years to the term breech trial: The rise and fall of a randomized controlled trial. Am J Obstet Gynecol 194(1):20, 2006

Goffinet F, Carayol M, Foidart JM, et al: Is planned vaginal delivery for breech presentation at term still an option? Results of an observational prospective survey in France and Belgium. Am J Obstet Gynecol 194(4):1002, 2006

Goodwin TM, Banks E, Millar LK, et al: Catastrophic shoulder dystocia and emergency symphysiotomy. Am J Obstet Gynecol 177:463, 1997

Gravenhorst JB, Schreuder AM, Veen S, et al: Breech delivery in very preterm and very-low-birthweight infants in the Netherlands. Br J Obstet Gynaecol 100:411, 1993

Hannah ME, Hannah WJ, Hewson SA, et al: Planned caesarean section versus planned vaginal birth for breech presentation at term: A randomised multicentre trial. Lancet 356:1375,2000

Hauth JC, Cunningham FG: Vaginal breech delivery is still justified. Obstet Gynecol 99:1115, 2002

Herbst A: Term breech delivery in Sweden: Mortality relative to fetal presentation and planned mode of delivery. Acta Obstet Gynecol Scand 84(6):593, 2005

Hickok DE, Gordon DC, Milberg JA, et al: The frequency of breech presentation by gestational age at birth: A large population-based study. Am J Obstet Gynecol 166:851, 1992

Hutton EK, Saunders CA, Tu M, et al: Factors associated with a successful external cephalic version in the early ECV trial. J Obstet Gynaecol Can 30(1):23, 2008

Irion O, Hirsbrunner Almagbaly PH, Morabia A: Planned vaginal delivery versus elective caesarean section: A study of 705 singleton term breech presentations. Br J Obstet Gynaecol 105:710, 1998

Kayem G, Baumann R, Goffinet F, et al: Early preterm breech delivery: Is a policy of planned vaginal delivery associated with increased risk of neonatal death? Am J Obstet Gynecol 198(3):289.e1, 2008

Kok M, Cnossen J, Gravendeel L, et al: Clinical factors to predict the outcome of external cephalic version: A metaanalysis. Am J Obstet Gynecol 199(6):630.e1, 2008

Kok M, Cnossen J, Gravendeel L, et al: Ultrasound factors to predict the outcome of external cephalic version: A meta-analysis. Ultrasound Obstet Gynecol 33(1):76, 2009

Krupitz H, Arzt W, Ebner T, et al: Assisted vaginal delivery versus caesarean section in breech presentation. Acta Obstet Gynecol Scand 84(6):588, 2005

Lau TK, Lo KWK, Wan D, et al: Predictors of successful external cephalic version at term: A prospective study. Br J Obstet Gynaecol 104:798, 1997

Lydon-Rochelle M, Albers L, Gorwoda J, et al: Accuracy of Leopold maneuvers in screening for malpresentation: A prospective study. Birth 20:132, 1993

Malloy MH, Onstad L, Wright E: National Institute of Child Health and Human Development Neonatal Research Network: The effect of cesarean delivery on birth outcome in very-low-birthweight infants. Obstet Gynecol 77:498, 1991

Mancuso KM, Yancey MK, Murphy JA, et al: Epidural analgesia for cephalic version: A randomized trial. Obstet Gynecol 95:648, 2000

Mehl LE: Hypnosis and conversion of the breech to the vertex presentation. Arch Fam Med 3:881, 1994

Menticoglou SM: Symphysiotomy for the trapped aftercoming parts of the breech: A review of the literature and a plea for its use. Aust NZ J Obstet Gynaecol 30:1, 1990

Nassar N, Roberts CL, Cameron CA, et al: Diagnostic accuracy of clinical examination for detection of non-cephalic presentation in late pregnancy: Cross sectional analytic study. Br Med J 333:578, 2006

Newman RB, Peacock BS, Van Dorsten JP: Predicting success of external cephalic version. Am J Obstet Gynecol 169:245, 1993

Nwosu EC, Walkinshaw S, Chia P: Undiagnosed breech. Br J Obstet Gynaecol 100:531, 1993

Pinard A: On version by external maneuvers. In: Traite de Palper Abdominal. Paris, 1889

Pradhan P, Mohajer M, Deshpande S: Outcome of term breech births: 10-year experience at a district general hospital. Br J Obstet Gynaecol 112(2):218, 2005

Rietberg CC, Elferink-Stinkens PM, Visser GH: The effect of the Term Breech Trial on medical intervention behaviour and neonatal outcome in The Netherlands: An analysis of 35,453 term breech infants. Br J Obstet Gynaecol 112(2):205, 2005

Robertson AW, Kopelman JN, Read JA, et al: External cephalic version at term: Is a tocolytic necessary? Obstet Gynecol 70:896, 1987

Rojansky N, Tanos V, Lewin A, et al: Sonographic evaluation of fetal head extension and maternal pelvis in cases of breech presentation. Acta Obstet Gynecol Scand 73:607, 1994

Sandberg EC: The Zavanelli maneuver: 12 years of recorded experience. Obstet Gynecol 93:312, 1999

Schorr SJ, Speights SE, Ross EL, et al: A randomized trial of epidural anesthesia to improve external cephalic version success. Am J Obstet Gynecol 177:1133, 1997

Schutte JM, Steegers EA, Santema JG, et al: Maternal deaths after elective cesarean section for breech presentation in the Netherlands. Acta Obstet Gynecol Scand 86(2):240, 2007

Schutte MF, van Hemel OJS, van de Berg C, et al: Perinatal mortality in breech presentations as compared to vertex presentations in singleton pregnancies: An analysis based upon 57,819 computer-registered pregnancies in the Netherlands. Eur J Obstet Gynecol Reprod Biol 19:391, 1985

Sela HY, Fiegenberg T, Ben-Meir A, et al: Safety and efficacy of external cephalic version for women with a previous cesarean delivery. Eur J Obstet Gynecol Reprod Biol 142(2):111, 2009

Soernes T, Bakke T: The length of the human umbilical cord in vertex and breech presentations. Am J Obstet Gynecol 154:1086, 1986

Spellacy WN, Gravem H, Fisch RO: The umbilical cord complications of true knots, nuchal cords, and cord around the body. Am J Obstet Gynecol 94:1136, 1966

Steyn W, Pieper C: Favorable neonatal outcome after fetal entrapment and partially successful Zavanelli maneuver in a case of breech presentation. Am J Perinatol 11:348, 1994

Stine LE, Phelan JP, Wallace R, et al: Update on external cephalic version performed at term. Obstet Gynecol 65:642, 1985

Su M, McLeod L, Ross S, et al: Factors associated with adverse perinatal outcome in the Term Breech Trial. Am J Obstet Gynecol 189:740, 2003

Sunday-Adeoye IM, Okonta P, Twomey D: Symphysiotomy at the Mater Misericordiae Hospital Afikpo, Ebonyi State of Nigeria (1982-1999): A review of 1013 cases. J Obstet Gynecol 24(5):525, 2004

Svenningsen NW, Westgren M, Ingemarsson I: Modern strategy for the term breech delivery—A study with a 4-year follow-up of the infants. J Perinat Med 13:117, 1985

Tan GW, Jen SW, Tan SL: A prospective randomised controlled trial of external cephalic version comparing two methods of uterine tocolysis with a non-tocolysis group. Singapore Med J 30:155, 1989

Thorp JM Jr, Jenkins T, Watson W: Utility of Leopold maneuvers in screening for malpresentation. Obstet Gynecol 78:394, 1991

Tiwary CM: Testicular injury in breech delivery: Possible implications. Urology 34:210, 1989

Uotila J, Tuimala R, Kirkinen P: Good perinatal outcome in selective vaginal breech delivery at term. Acta Obstet Gynecol Scand 84(6):578, 2005

Van Dorsten JP, Schifrin BS, Wallace RL: Randomized control trial of external cephalic version with tocolysis in late pregnancy. Am J Obstet Gynecol 141:417, 1981

van Loon AJ, Mantingh A, Serlier EK, et al: Randomised controlled trial of magnetic resonance pelvimetry in breech presentation at term. Lancet 350:1799, 1997

Vasa R, Kim MR: Fracture of the femur at cesarean section: Case report and review of literature. Am J Perinatol 7:46, 1990

Vendittelli F, Rivière O, Creen-Hébert C, et al: Is a breech presentation at term more frequent in women with a history of cesarean delivery? Am J Obstet Gynecol 198(5):521.e1, 2008

Vézina Y, Bujold E, Varin J, et al: Cesarean delivery after successful external cephalic version of breech presentation at term: A comparative study. Am J Obstet Gynecol 190:763, 2004

Weiniger CF, Ginosar Y, Elchalal U, et al: External cephalic version for breech presentation with or without spinal analgesia in nulliparous women at term. Obstet Gynecol 110:1343, 2007

Wessen A, Elowsson P, Axemo P, et al: The use of intravenous nitroglycerin for emergency cervico-uterine relaxation. Acta Anaesthesiol Scand 39:847, 1995

Westgren M, Edvall H, Nordstrom L, et al: Spontaneous cephalic version of breech presentation in the last trimester. Br J Obstet Gynaecol 92:19, 1985

Whyte H, Hannah ME, Saigal S, et al: Outcomes of children at 2 years after planned cesarean birth versus planned vaginal birth for breech presentation at term: The International Randomized Term Breech Trial. Am J Obstet Gynecol 191(3):864, 2004

Wolf H, Schaap AHP, Bruinse HW, et al: Vaginal delivery compared with caesarean section in early preterm breech delivery: A comparison of long term outcome. Br J Obstet Gynaecol 106:486, 1999

Yanny H, Johanson R, Baldwin KJ, et al: Double-blind randomised controlled trial of glyceryl trinitrate spray for external cephalic version. Br J Obstet Gynaecol 107:562, 2000

Zhang J, Bowes WA, Fortney JA: Efficacy of external cephalic version, including safety, cost-benefit analysis, and impact on the cesarean delivery rate. Obstet Gynecol 82:306, 1993

CHAPTER 24

Cesarean Delivery and Peripartum Hysterectomy

Cesarean delivery is defined as the birth of a fetus through incisions in the abdominal wall (laparotomy) and the uterine wall (hysterotomy). This definition does not include removal of the fetus from the abdominal cavity in the case of rupture of the uterus or in the case of an abdominal pregnancy. In some cases, and most often because of emergent complications such as intractable hemorrhage, abdominal hysterectomy is indicated following delivery. When performed at the time of cesarean delivery, the operation is termed *cesarean hysterectomy.* If done within a short time after vaginal delivery, it is termed *postpartum hysterectomy.*

HISTORICAL BACKGROUND

The origin of the term *cesarean* is obscure, and three principal explanations have been suggested.

In the first, according to legend, Julius Caesar was born in this manner, with the result that the procedure became known as the Caesarean operation. Several circumstances weaken this explanation. First, the mother of Julius Caesar lived for many years after his birth in 100 BC, and as late as the 17th century, the operation was almost invariably fatal. Second, the operation, whether performed on the living or the dead, is not mentioned by any medical writer before the Middle Ages. Historical details of the origin of the family name Caesar are found in the monograph by Pickrell (1935).

The second explanation is that the name of the operation is derived from a Roman law, supposedly created in the 8th century BC by Numa Pompilius, ordering that the procedure be performed upon women dying in the last few weeks of pregnancy in the hope of saving the child. This *lex regia*—king's rule or law—later became the *lex caesarea* under the emperors, and the operation itself became known as the caesarean operation. The German term *Kaiserschnitt*—Kaiser cut—reflects this derivation.

The third explanation is that the word *caesarean* was derived sometime in the Middle Ages from the Latin verb *caedere, to cut.* This explanation seems most logical, but exactly when it was first applied to the operation is uncertain. Because *section* is derived from the Latin verb *seco*, which also means *cut*, the term *caesarean section* seems tautological—thus *cesarean delivery* is used. In the United States, the *ae* in the first syllable of *caesarean* is replaced with the letter *e*. In the United Kingdom, Australia, and most commonwealth nations, the *ae* is retained.

A more extensive review of the history of cesarean delivery can be found in the 22nd edition of *Williams Obstetrics* (Cunningham and colleagues, 2005), as well as in works by Boley (1991) and Sewell (1993).

CONTEMPORARY STATUS OF CESAREAN DELIVERY

Frequency

From 1970 to 2007, the cesarean delivery rate in the United States rose from 4.5 percent of all deliveries to 31.8 percent (Hamilton and colleagues, 2009; MacDorman and associates, 2008). This increase has been steady with the exception of the years between 1989 and 1996 when the annual rate of cesarean delivery actually decreased (Fig. 25-1). This decrease was largely due to a significantly increased rate of vaginal birth after cesarean (VBAC) and to a closely mirrored decrease in the primary rate

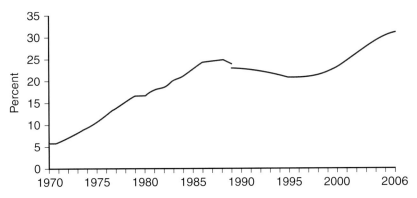

FIGURE 25-1 Total cesarean delivery rate: United States, 1970–2006. (Reprinted from *Clinics in Perinatology*, Vol. 35, No. 2, MF MacDorman, F Menacker, E Declercq, Cesarean birth in the United States: Epidemiology, trends, and outcomes, pp. 293–307, Copyright 2008, with permission from Elsevier.)

(Fig. 25-2). These trends were short lived, and in 2007, the primary cesarean delivery rate was above 30 percent, whereas VBAC rates dropped to 8.5 percent (Hamilton and associates, 2009).

In response to the increased use of cesarean delivery, the American College of Obstetricians and Gynecologists Task Force on Cesarean Delivery Rates (2000) recommended two benchmarks for the United States for the year 2010. Goals included a cesarean rate of 15.5 percent for nulliparous women at 37 weeks or more with a singleton cephalic presentation and secondly, a vaginal birth rate after a prior cesarean of 37 percent in women at 37 weeks or more with a singleton cephalic presentation who had a prior low transverse cesarean delivery. These goals are consistent with the 15-percent cesarean rate established by the U.S. Department of Health and Human Services *Healthy People 2010* program for primiparous, low-risk women. The department's mid-decade review of the program (2006), however, showed no progress on this goal.

The reasons for the continued increase in the cesarean rates are not completely understood, but some explanations include the following:

1. Women are having fewer children, thus, a greater percentage of births are among *nulliparas,* who are at increased risk for cesarean delivery.

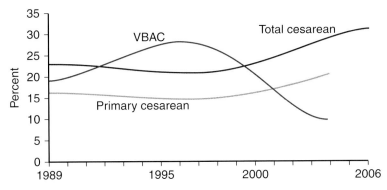

FIGURE 25-2 Total cesarean delivery rate, United States, 1989–2006, and primary cesarean and vaginal birth after cesarean (VBAC) rates, 1989–2004. (Reprinted from *Clinics in Perinatology*, Vol. 35, No. 2, MF MacDorman, F Menacker, E Declercq, Cesarean birth in the United States: Epidemiology, trends, and outcomes, pp. 293–307, Copyright 2008, with permission from Elsevier.)

2. The average *maternal age* is rising, and older women, especially nulliparas, are at increased risk of cesarean delivery (Fig. 25-3).

3. The use of *electronic fetal monitoring* is widespread. This technique is associated with an increased cesarean delivery rate compared with intermittent fetal heart rate auscultation (see Chap. 18, p. 436). Although cesarean delivery performed primarily for "fetal distress" comprises only a minority of all such procedures, in many more cases, concern for an abnormal or "nonreassuring" fetal heart rate tracing lowers the threshold for cesarean deliveries performed for abnormal progress of labor.

4. Most fetuses presenting as *breech* are now delivered by cesarean (see Chap. 24, p. 531).

5. The incidence of *forceps and vacuum deliveries* has decreased (see Chap. 23, p. 511).

6. Rates of *labor induction* continue to rise, and induced labor, especially among nulliparas, increases the risk of cesarean delivery (see Chap. 22, p. 500).

7. The prevalence of *obesity* has risen dramatically, and obesity increases the risk of cesarean delivery (see Chap. 43, p. 950).

8. Rates of cesarean delivery for women with preeclampsia have increased, whereas rates of labor induction in these patients has declined. In Norway, for example, cesarean delivery increased from 16.4 percent for nulliparous preeclamptics during 1967–1978, to 35.4 percent during 1979–1990, and to 37 percent during 1991–2003 (Basso and colleagues, 2006).

9. *Vaginal birth after cesarean—VBAC—*has decreased from a high of 26 percent in 1996 to a rate of 8.5 percent in 2007 (see Chap. 26, p. 565) (Hamilton and associates, 2009).

10. Elective cesarean deliveries are increasingly being performed for a variety of indications including concern for *pelvic floor injury* associated with vaginal birth, medically indicated *preterm birth*, to reduce the risk of *fetal injury*, and for *patient request* (Ananth and co-workers, 2005; Nygaard and Cruikshank, 2003).

11. *Malpractice litigation* continues to contribute significantly to the present cesarean rate. In a compilation of medical malpractice claim data for the years 1985 through 2003, obstetrics accounted for the largest number of claims paid (Texas Medical Liability Trust, 2004). A brain-damaged infant was one of the most prevalent patient conditions, and overall, the average indemnity paid on obstetrical claims was 28 percent greater than for the other 24 specialties included in the report. This data is especially troubling in view of the well-documented lack of association between cesarean delivery and any reduction in childhood neurological problems. According to Foley and colleagues (2002), the incidence of neither neonatal seizures nor cerebral palsy diminished as the rate of cesarean delivery increased (see Chap. 29, p. 611).

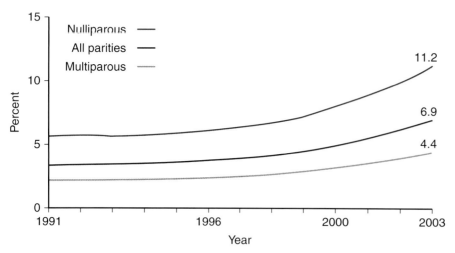

FIGURE 25-3 Primary cesarean delivery rates by parity for women with no indicated risk factors in the United States from 1991 to 2003. Women with term vertex singletons, with birthweight <4000 grams, and no reported medical risk factors or complications of labor or delivery. (Reprinted from *Seminars in Perinatology,* Vol. 30, No. 5, F Menacker, E Declercq, MF MacDorman, Cesarean delivery: Background, trends, and epidemiology, pp. 235–241, Copyright 2006, with permission from Elsevier.)

Indications

As shown in Table 25-1, repeat cesarean deliveries and those performed for dystocia have been the leading indications in both the United States and other western industrialized countries. Although it is not possible to catalog comprehensively all appropriate indications for cesarean delivery, more than 85 percent are performed because of prior cesarean delivery, dystocia, fetal distress, or breech presentation.

For women in whom scheduled cesarean delivery is selected, the risk of adverse neonatal respiratory outcome increases in those delivered before 39 weeks (Clark, 2009; Oshiro, 2009; Tita, 2009, and all their colleagues). The American College of Obste-

tricians and Gynecologists (2008) recommends that fetal pulmonary maturity should be confirmed before scheduled delivery at less than 39 weeks of gestation unless fetal maturity can be determined from historical criteria (see Table 26-4. p. 571).

Dystocia

Some form of dystocia is the most frequent indication for cesarean delivery in the United States. An analysis of dystocia as a contributing factor to the cesarean rate is difficult, however, because of the heterogeneity inherent in the condition (see Chap. 20, p. 464). Indeed, there are 28 different World Health Organization (2007) ICD-10 codes applicable to cesarean delivery performed for a labor abnormality! Descriptive terms vary from more precise definitions promulgated by Friedman (1978)—*secondary arrest of dilatation, arrest of descent*—to more ambiguous and commonly used terms such as *cephalopelvic disproportion* and *failure to progress.*

Fetal Distress

Electronic fetal monitoring was employed in 85 percent of labors in the United States in 2003 (Martin and colleagues, 2005). Its use increases the cesarean delivery rate, perhaps by as much as 40 percent (Thacker and associates, 2001). Unfortunately, despite initial optimism, it has become well established that management based on electronic monitoring is no better in reducing the risk of cerebral palsy or perinatal death than that based on intermittent heart rate auscultation. Indeed, the performance of cesarean delivery per se may have no bearing on the neurodevelopmental prognosis of the infant. Scheller and Nelson (1994), in a report from the National Institutes of Health, and Lien and associates (1995) presented data specifically refuting any association between cesarean delivery and either cerebral palsy or seizures.

Pertinent to the diagnosis of fetal distress are the recommendations of the American Academy of Pediatrics and the American College of Obstetricians and Gynecologists (2007) that facilities giving obstetrical care have the capability of initiating a cesarean delivery within 30 minutes of the decision to operate. Misinterpretations of this guideline are common. Specifically, this recommendation addresses facilities and does not govern clinical decision-making. There is no nationally recognized standard of care that codifies an acceptable time interval for performance of cesarean delivery. In most instances, operative delivery is not necessary within this 30-minute time frame. Bloom and co-workers (2001) reported for Maternal-Fetal Medicine Units (MFMU) Network that 69 percent of 7450 cesareans performed in labor commenced more than 30 minutes after the decision to operate. In a second study, Bloom and colleagues (2006) evaluated cesarean deliveries performed for emergency indications. They reported that failure

TABLE 25-1. Indication for Cesarean Delivery from the Maternal-Fetal Medicine Units Network

	Cesarean Deliveries (%)[a]
Primary	**21,798**
Dystocia	8122 (37)
Nonreassuring fetal heart rate	5404 (25)
Abnormal presentation	4321 (20)
Other	3323 (15)
Unsuccessful trial of forceps or vacuum	628 (3)
Repeat	**15,312**
No VBAC attempt	12,565 (82)
Failed VBAC	2687 (17)
Unsuccessful trial of forceps or vacuum	60 (0.4)

[a]Data are shown as number (%).
VBAC = vaginal birth after cesarean.
Adapted from Alexander and co-workers (2006).

TABLE 25-2. Selected Complications Associated with Emergency Cesarean Delivery According to Decision-to-Incision Interval from the Maternal-Fetal Medicine Units Network

	30 Minutes or Less (n = 1814)	31 Minutes or More (n = 994)	p
Maternal Outcome[a]			
Endometritis	212 (11.7)	129 (13.0)	.32
Wound complication	23 (1.3)	9 (0.9)	.39
Operative injury	5 (0.3)	5 (0.5)	
Neonatal Outcome[a]			
5-minute Apgar score ≤3	18 (1.0)	9 (0.9)	.82
Umbilical artery pH <7.0[b]	52 (4.8)	9 (1.6)	.001
Hypoxic ischemic encephalopathy	12 (0.7)	5 (0.5)	.61
Fetal death in labor	3 (0.2)	0 (0.0)	.31
Neonatal death			
With no malformations	7 (0.4)	1 (0.1)	.27
With malformations	8 (0.4)	3 (0.3)	.76

[a]Data are shown as number (%).
[b]Umbilical artery pH was missing for 41 percent of the infants.
Modified from Bloom and colleagues (2006).

to achieve a cesarean delivery decision-to-incision time of less than 30 minutes was not associated with a negative impact on neonatal outcome (Table 25-2). On the other hand, when faced with an acute, catastrophic deterioration in fetal condition, cesarean delivery usually is indicated as rapidly as possible, and purposeful delays of any time would be inappropriate.

Breech Presentation

Management of the breech-presenting fetus is discussed in Chapter 24. Concern for fetal injury, as well as the infrequency with which a breech presentation meets criteria for a trial of labor, make it likely that its contribution to the overall cesarean delivery rate will remain relatively static.

Prior Cesarean Delivery

Management of the woman with a prior cesarean delivery is discussed in Chapter 26.

Methods to Decrease Cesarean Delivery Rates

Several investigators have documented the feasibility of achieving significant reductions in institutional cesarean delivery rates without increased perinatal morbidity or mortality rates (DeMott, 1990; DeMuylder, 1990; Porreco, 1990; Pridijian, 1991; Sanchez-Ramos, 1990, and all their co-workers). Programs aimed at reducing the number of cesarean deliveries generally are focused on educating physicians, peer reviewing, encouraging a trial of labor after prior transverse cesarean delivery, and restricting cesarean deliveries for dystocia only to women who meet strictly defined criteria. In a randomized study from 34 Latin American hospitals, Althabe and colleagues (2004) reported that a mandatory second opinion was associated with a small, but significant, reduction in the cesarean delivery rate without an adverse effect on maternal or perinatal morbidity.

Maternal Mortality and Morbidity

In the United States, maternal death attributable solely to cesarean delivery is rare. Even so, large data sets attest to the mortality risks. Clark and colleagues (2008), in a review of nearly 1.5 million pregnancies, found maternal mortality rates of 2.2 per 100,000 cesarean deliveries. In another study, Hall and Bewley (1999) compiled data from more than 2 million births in the United Kingdom from 1994 through 1996. They showed that whereas emergency cesarean delivery was associated with an almost ninefold risk of maternal death compared with that of vaginal delivery, even elective cesarean delivery was associated with an almost threefold risk.

Rates of severe obstetrical complications increased in the U.S. from 1998–1999 to 2004–2005. Many of these increases were associated with the rising cesarean delivery rate (Kuklina and co-workers, 2009). The maternal morbidity rate is increased twofold with cesarean delivery compared with vaginal delivery (Villar and associates, 2007). Principal sources are puerperal infection, hemorrhage, and thromboembolism (Burrows and associates, 2004). Others are listed in Table 25-3, and not all morbidity is immediate. Declerq and colleagues (2007) reported that rehospitalization in the 30 days following cesarean delivery was more than twice as common as after vaginal delivery—75 versus 19 hospitalizations per 1000 deliveries. Rajasekar and Hall (1997) reported that the incidence of bladder laceration with cesarean operation was 1.4 per 1000 procedures, and the incidence of ureteral injury was 0.3 per 1000. Although bladder injury was immediately identified, the diagnosis of ureteral

TABLE 25-3. Complications Associated with Low-Risk Planned Cesarean Delivery[a] Compared with Planned Vaginal Delivery among Healthy Women in Canada, 1991–2005

Complication	Type of Planned Delivery[b]	
	Cesarean (n = 46,766)	Vaginal (n = 2,292,420)
Overall morbidity	1279 (2.73)	20,639 (0.9)
Hysterectomy	39 (0.09)	254 (0.01)
Transfusion	11 (0.02)	1500 (0.07)
Anesthetic complications	247 (0.53)	4793 (0.21)
Hypovolemic shock	3 (0.01)	435 (0.02)[c]
Cardiac arrest	89 (0.19)	887 (0.04)
Venous thromboembolism	28 (0.06)	623 (0.03)
Puerperal infection	281 (0.60)	4833 (0.21)
Wound disruption	41 (0.09)	1151 (0.05)
Wound hematoma	607 (1.3)	6263 (0.27)
In-hospital deaths	0	41 (0.002)

[a] Healthy women with a singleton gestation and no previous cesarean deliveries who underwent cesarean delivery for breech presentation were used as a surrogate for a low-risk planned cesarean delivery group.
[b] Data are shown as number (%).
[c] Nonsignificant comparison. For all other comparisons $p < .05$.
Modified from Liu and co-workers (2007).

injury often was delayed. Uterine infection is relatively common after cesarean delivery. The diagnosis and management of pelvic and wound infections following cesarean delivery are discussed in Chapter 31. Women with prior cesarean delivery have increased rates of uterine rupture in subsequent pregnancy compared with those with only prior vaginal deliveries. Fortunately, however, the risk of rupture is low, and the overall risk was found by Spong and colleagues (2007) to approximate 0.3 percent. As discussed in Chapter 43 (see p. 950), morbidity associated with cesarean delivery is increased dramatically in obese women. All of these morbidities, as well as the increased recovery time, result in a twofold increase in costs for cesarean versus vaginal delivery (Henderson and associates, 2001).

Patient Choice in Cesarean Delivery

As cesarean delivery has become safer and more commonly performed, and women have taken a more active role in their obstetrical care, it has been argued that women should be able to choose to undergo elective cesarean delivery (Harer, 2000). This has become one of the most important and controversial issues currently facing our specialty. Although the rate is difficult to determine with precision, elective cesarean delivery is on the rise and by one estimate, has increased 50 percent in the past decade (Meikle and colleagues, 2005). Gossman and associates (2005) estimated that 2.5 percent of all births in the United States in 2003 were defined as *cesarean delivery on maternal request (CDMR)*. Reasons for mothers to request cesarean delivery include avoidance of pelvic floor injury during vaginal birth, reduced risk of fetal injury, avoidance of the uncertainty and pain of labor, and convenience. Importantly,

Worley and colleagues (2009) found that approximately one third of the pregnant women who delivered at their institution entered spontaneous labor at term, and 96 percent of these delivered vaginally without adverse neonatal outcomes. Thus, the debate surrounding CDMR includes its medical rationale from both a maternal and fetal-neonatal standpoint, the concept of informed free choice by the woman, and the autonomy of the physicians in offering this choice.

To address this, the National Institute of Health held a State-of-the-Science Conference on Cesarean Delivery on Maternal Request. A panel of experts critically reviewed available literature to form recommendations based on risks and benefits identified. It is noteworthy that most of the maternal and neonatal outcomes examined had insufficient data to permit such recommendations. Indeed, one of the main conclusions of the conference was that more high-quality research is needed to fully evaluate the issues. This was also the conclusion of the American College of Obstetricians and Gynecologists (2007a).

The panel was able to draw some conclusions from the existing data. Cesarean delivery on maternal request should not be performed prior to 39 weeks' gestation unless there is evidence of fetal lung maturity. It should be avoided in women desiring several children because of the risk of placenta accreta (see Chap. 35, p. 776). Finally, it should not be motivated by the unavailability of effective pain management.

Ethics

Cesarean delivery on maternal request has numerous ethical concepts that have been debated. Bewley and Cockburn (2002a, b) argue that the concept of elective cesarean delivery lacks both ethical and medical merit. Others have concluded that currently available evidence does not support *routine* elective cesarean delivery. However, it does ethically support an obstetrical decision to accede to an *informed* patient's request for such a delivery (Kalish and associates, 2008; Minkoff, 2006; Minkoff and Chervenak, 2003). Clearly, and usually only with the benefit of hindsight, it can be said that some women and infants who have undergone difficult vaginal birth may have been better served by cesarean delivery. In most cases, however, clinically robust means of prospectively identifying otherwise uncomplicated pregnancies in which the woman or her fetus-infant would benefit from elective cesarean delivery are lacking. At this time, we conclude that it is difficult to justify a *laissez faire* approach to this major operation.

TECHNIQUE FOR CESAREAN DELIVERY

With minor variations, surgical performance of cesarean delivery is comparable worldwide. Most steps are founded on evidence-based data, and these have been reviewed by Berghella and associates (2005).

Abdominal Incision

Usually either a midline vertical or a suprapubic transverse incision is used. Only in special circumstances would a paramedian or midtransverse incision be employed.

Vertical Incision

An infraumbilical midline vertical incision is quickest to create. The incision should be of sufficient length to allow delivery of the infant without difficulty. Therefore, its length should correspond with the estimated fetal size. Sharp dissection is performed to the level of the anterior rectus sheath, which is freed of subcutaneous fat to expose a 2-cm-wide strip of fascia in the midline. Some surgeons prefer to incise the rectus sheath with the scalpel throughout the length of the fascial incision. Others prefer to make a small opening and then incise the fascial layer with scissors. The rectus and the pyramidalis muscles are separated in the midline by sharp and blunt dissection to expose transversalis fascia and peritoneum.

The transversalis fascia and preperitoneal fat are dissected carefully to reach the underlying peritoneum. The peritoneum near the upper end of the incision is opened carefully, either bluntly, or by elevating it with two hemostats placed about 2 cm apart. The tented fold of peritoneum between the clamps is then examined and palpated to be sure that omentum, bowel, or bladder is not adjacent. In women who have had previous intra-abdominal surgery, including cesarean delivery, omentum or bowel may be adherent to the undersurface of the peritoneum. *In women with obstructed labor, the bladder may be pushed cephalad almost to the level of the umbilicus* (see Chap. 20, p. 486). The peritoneum is incised superiorly to the upper pole of the incision and downward to just above the peritoneal reflection over the bladder.

Transverse Incisions

With the modified *Pfannenstiel incision,* the skin and subcutaneous tissue are incised using a lower, transverse, slightly curvilinear inci-

sion. The incision is made at the level of the pubic hairline and is extended somewhat beyond the lateral borders of the rectus muscles. Sharp dissection is continued through the subcutaneous layer to the level of the fascia. The superficial epigastric vessels can usually be identified halfway between the skin and fascia, several centimeters from the midline. If lacerated, these may be suture ligated or coagulated with an electrosurgical blade. After the subcutaneous tissue has been separated from the underlying fascia for 1 cm or so on each side, the fascia is incised. At this level, the anterior abdominal fascia is typically composed of two visible layers, the aponeuroses from the external oblique muscle and a fused layer containing aponeuroses of the internal oblique and transverse abdominis muscles. Ideally, the two layers are individually incised during lateral extension of the fascial incision. The inferior epigastric vessels typically lie outside the lateral border of the rectus abdominis muscle and beneath the fused aponeuroses of the internal oblique and transverse abdominis muscles. Thus, extension of the fascial incision further laterally may cut these vessels. Therefore, if lateral extension is required, these vessels should be identified and cauterized or ligated to prevent bleeding and vessel retraction if lacerated.

Sequentially, first the superior and then the inferior edge of the fascia is grasped with suitable clamps and elevated by the assistant as the operator separates the fascial sheath from the underlying rectus muscles either bluntly or sharply. Blood vessels coursing between the muscles and fascia are clamped, cut, and ligated, or they are fulgurated with electrocautery. Meticulous hemostasis is imperative to lower rates of infection and bleeding. The fascial separation is carried near enough to the umbilicus to permit an adequate midline longitudinal incision of the peritoneum. The rectus muscles are then separated in the midline to expose the underlying peritoneum. The peritoneum is opened as discussed earlier.

The Pfannenstiel incision follows Langer lines of skin tension, and thus, excellent cosmetic results can be achieved. It also offers decreased rates of postoperative pain, of fascial wound dehiscence, and of incisional hernia. Whether it is stronger and less likely to undergo dehiscence is debated (Hendrix and coworkers, 2000). The Pfannenstiel incision is often discouraged for cases in which a large operating space is essential or in which access to the upper abdomen may be required. With repeat cesarean delivery, reentry through a Pfannenstiel incision usually is more time consuming and difficult because of scarring.

When a transverse incision is desired and more room is needed, the *Maylard incision* provides a safe option (Ayers and Morley, 1987; Giacalone and colleagues, 2002). In this incision, the rectus muscles are divided sharply or with electrocautery. The incision also may be especially useful in women with significant scarring from previous transverse incisions.

Uterine Incisions

Most often, the lower uterine segment is incised transversely as described by Kerr in 1921. Occasionally, a low-segment vertical incision as described by Krönig in 1912 may be used. The so-called *classical incision* is a vertical incision into the body of the uterus above the lower uterine segment and reaches the uterine fundus. This incision is seldom used today, and indications are discussed on page 555. For most cesarean deliveries, the transverse incision is preferred. Compared with a

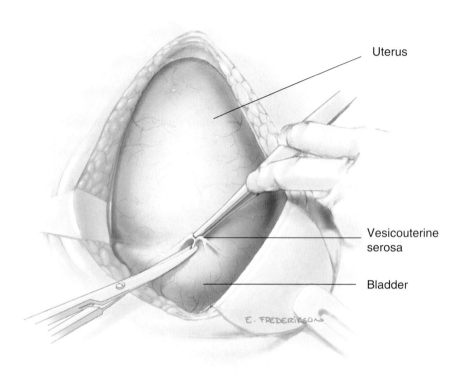

FIGURE 25-4 The loose vesicouterine serosa is grasped with forceps and incised with Metzenbaum scissors.

classical incision, it is easier to repair, is located at a site least likely to rupture during a subsequent pregnancy, and does not promote adherence of bowel or omentum to the incisional line.

Technique for Transverse Cesarean Incision

Commonly, the uterus is found to be dextrorotated so that the left round ligament is more anterior and closer to the midline than the right. With thick meconium or infected amnionic fluid, some surgeons prefer to put a moistened laparotomy pack in each lateral peritoneal gutter to absorb fluid and blood that escape from the opened uterus. The reflection of peritoneum above the upper margin of the bladder and overlying the anterior lower uterine segment—the *bladder flap*—is grasped in the midline with forceps and incised transversely with scissors (Fig. 25-4). Scissors are inserted between the vesicouterine serosa and myometrium of the lower uterine segment. The scissors are pushed laterally from the midline, and then withdrawn while partially opening the blades intermittently. This separates a 2-cm–wide strip of serosa, which is then incised. As the lateral margin on each side is approached, the scissors are directed somewhat more cephalad (Fig. 25-5). The lower flap of peritoneum is elevated, and the bladder is gently separated by blunt or sharp dissection from the underlying myometrium (Fig. 25-6). In general, the separation of bladder should not exceed 5 cm in depth and usually should be less. It is possible, especially with an effaced, dilated cervix, to dissect downward so deeply as inadvertently to expose and then enter the underlying vagina rather than the lower uterine segment.

The uterus is entered through the lower uterine segment approximately 1 cm below the upper margin of the peritoneal

reflection. It is important to place the uterine incision relatively higher in women with advanced or complete cervical dilatation to minimize both lateral extension of the incision into the uterine arteries and unintended entry into the vagina. This is done by using the vesicouterine serosal reflection as a guide.

The uterus can be incised by a variety of techniques. Each is initiated by using a scalpel to transversely incise the exposed lower uterine segment for 1 to 2 cm in the midline (Fig. 25-7). This must be done carefully to avoid injury to the fetus. Skin laceration was the most common fetal injury seen with 37,110 cesarean deliveries in the Maternal Fetal Medicine Units Network study reported by Alexander and colleagues (2006). Careful blunt entry using hemostats or fingertip to split the muscle may be helpful. Once the uterus is opened, the incision can be extended by cutting laterally and then slightly upward with bandage scissors. Alternatively, when the lower uterine segment is thin, the incision can be extended by simply spreading the incision, using lateral and upward pressure applied with each index finger (Fig. 25-8). Although Rodriguez and associates (1994) reported that blunt and sharp extensions of the initial uterine incision are equivalent in terms of safety and postoperative complications, Magann and colleagues (2002) reported that sharp extension increased blood loss and the need for transfusion.

The uterine incision should be made large enough to allow delivery of the head and trunk of the fetus without either tearing into or having to cut into the uterine vessels

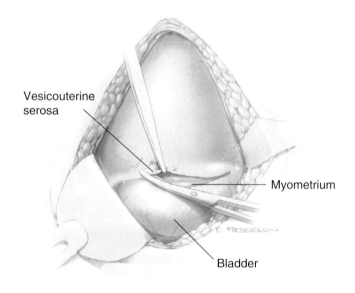

FIGURE 25-5 The loose serosa above the upper margin of the bladder is elevated and incised laterally.

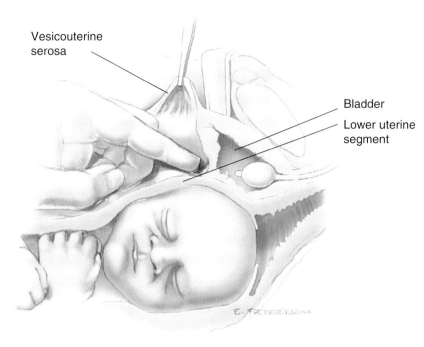

FIGURE 25-6 Cross section shows blunt dissection of the bladder off the uterus to expose the lower uterine segment.

that course through the lateral margins of the uterus. If the placenta is encountered in the line of incision, it must be either detached or incised. When the placenta is incised, fetal hemorrhage may be severe. Thus, delivery and cord clamping should be performed as soon as possible in such cases.

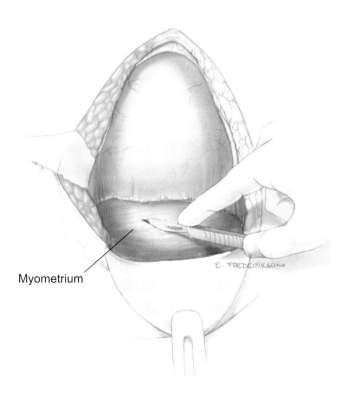

FIGURE 25-7 The myometrium is carefully incised to avoid cutting the fetal head.

Although the Pfannenstiel-Kerr technique for abdominal and uterine entry has been used for decades, newer methods have been suggested. The Joel-Cohen and Misgav-Ladach methods use an abdominal incision placed higher than the Pfannenstiel and use blunt dissection of all encountered layers following sharp skin incision (Joel-Cohen, 1977; Stark, 1995). These have been associated with lower rates of intraoperative blood loss, puerperal fever, and postoperative pain and with shorter operative times. Long-term outcomes with these techniques, such as subsequent rupture of the uterus, are unknown (Hofmeyr and co-workers, 2008).

Delivery of the Infant

In a cephalic presentation, a hand is slipped into the uterine cavity between the symphysis and fetal head. The head is elevated gently with the fingers and palm through the incision, aided by modest transabdominal fundal pressure (Fig. 25-9). After a long labor with cephalopelvic disproportion, the fetal head may be tightly wedged in the birth canal. Upward pressure exerted by a hand in the vagina by an assistant will help to dislodge the head and allow its delivery above the symphysis. Alternatively, in women without labor, the fetal head may be unmolded, and without a leading cephalic point, the round head may be difficult to lift through the uterine incision. In such instances, either forceps or a vacuum device may be used to deliver the fetal head (Fig. 25-10). The shoulders then are delivered using gentle traction plus fundal pressure (Fig. 25-11). The rest of the body readily follows. To minimize fetal aspiration of amnionic fluid, exposed nares and mouth are aspirated with a bulb syringe.

After the shoulders are delivered, an intravenous infusion containing two ampules or 20 units of oxytocin per liter of crystalloid is infused at 10 mL/min until the uterus contracts satisfactorily. After this, the rate can be reduced. Bolus doses of 5 to 10 units are avoided because of associated hypotension. Munn and colleagues (2001) studied a much higher initial concentration using a solution of 80 units of oxytocin in 500 mL of crystalloid, which was infused at about 17 mL/min. They reported that this approach significantly reduced the need for additional uterotonic agents.

The umbilical cord is clamped, and the newborn is given to the team member who will conduct resuscitative efforts as needed (see Chap. 28, p. 591). The uterine incision is observed for any vigorously bleeding sites. These should be promptly clamped with Pennington or ring forceps or similar instruments. The placenta is then delivered unless it has already done so spontaneously. Many surgeons prefer manual removal, but spontaneous delivery, as shown in Fig. 25-12, along with some cord traction has been shown to reduce the risk of operative blood loss and infection (Anorlu, 2008; Atkinson, 1996; Baksu, 2005, and all their colleagues). Fundal massage, begun as soon as the fetus is delivered, reduces bleeding and hastens placental delivery.

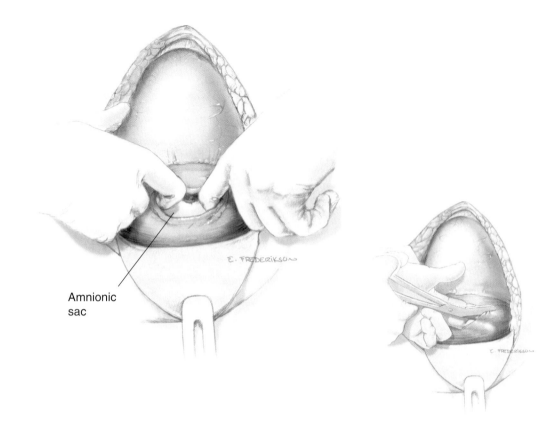

Amnionic
sac

FIGURE 25-8 After entering the uterine cavity, the incision is extended laterally with fingers or with bandage scissors (*inset*).

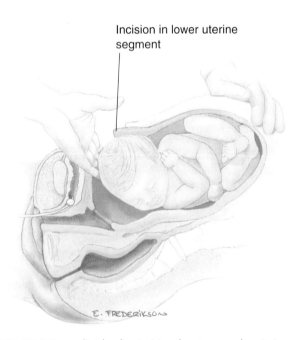

Incision in lower uterine
segment

FIGURE 25-9 Immediately after incising the uterus and rupturing the fetal membranes, the fingers are insinuated between the symphysis pubis and the fetal head until the posterior surface of the head is reached. The head is lifted carefully anteriorly and as necessary, superiorly to bring it from beneath the symphysis forward through the uterine and abdominal incisions. As the fetal head is lifted through the incision, pressure usually is applied to the uterine fundus through the abdominal wall to help expel the fetus.

The American Academy of Pediatrics and the American College of Obstetricians and Gynecologists (2007) recommend that "a qualified person who is skilled in neonatal resuscitation should be in the operative delivery room, with all equipment needed for neonatal resuscitation, to care for the neonate." Jacob and Phenninger (1997) compared 834 cesarean deliveries with 834 low-risk vaginal deliveries. They found that, with regional analgesia, there is rarely a need for infant resuscitation after elective repeat cesarean delivery or cesarean delivery for dystocia without fetal heart rate abnormalities, and that a pediatrician may not be necessary at such deliveries. At Parkland Hospital, pediatric nurse practitioners attend uncomplicated, scheduled cesarean deliveries.

Uterine Repair

After delivery of the placenta, the uterus may be lifted through the incision onto the draped abdominal wall, and the fundus covered with a moistened laparotomy pack. Although some clinicians prefer to avoid it, uterine exteriorization often has advantages that outweigh its disadvantages. For example, the relaxed, atonic uterus can be recognized quickly and massage applied. The incision and bleeding points are more easily visualized and repaired, especially if there have been extensions laterally. Adnexal exposure is superior, and thus, tubal sterilization is easier. The principal disadvantage is from discomfort and vomiting caused by traction in cesarean deliveries performed

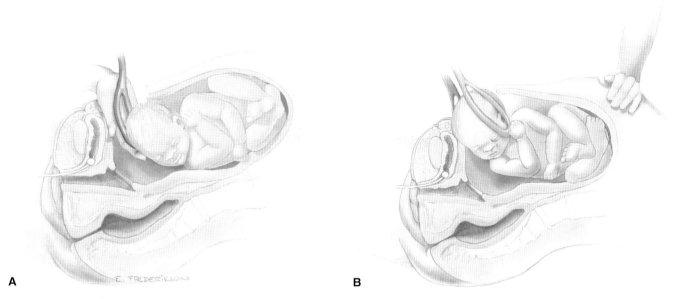

A   **B**

FIGURE 25-10 A. The first C-section forcep blade is placed. **B.** Slight upward and outward traction is used to lift the head through the incision.

under regional analgesia. Neither febrile morbidity nor blood loss appears to be increased with uterine exteriorization prior to repair (Coutinho and co-workers, 2008; Walsh and Walsh, 2009).

Immediately after delivery and examination of the placenta, the uterine cavity is inspected and either suctioned or wiped out with a gauze pack to remove avulsed membranes, vernix, clots, and other debris. The upper and lower cut edges and each lateral angle of the uterine incision are examined carefully for bleeding. Individually clamped large vessels are best ligated with a suture. Concern has been expressed by some clinicians that sutures through the decidua may lead to endometriosis in the hysterotomy scar, but this is rare.

The uterine incision is then closed with one or two layers of continuous 0- or #1 absorbable suture. Chromic suture is used by many, but some prefer synthetic delayed-absorbable sutures.

Hauth and colleagues (1992) randomized 906 women to either one- or two-layer closure using 1-0 chromic gut. A continuous locking one-layer closure required less operative time and fewer additional hemostatic sutures. In a follow-up report of 164 women delivered subsequently, the type of uterine closure did not significantly affect several maternal and fetal complications in the next pregnancy (Chapman and associates, 1997). Similarly, Durnwald and Mercer (2003) reported no uterine ruptures in 182 women who underwent a trial of labor after single-layer closure compared with four ruptures in 340 women (1.2 percent) after double-layer closure. By contrast, Bujold and associates (2002) reported that single-layer closure was associated with a fourfold increased risk of uterine rupture during a subsequent trial of labor. Further study is needed to resolve this issue (see Chap. 26, p. 569).

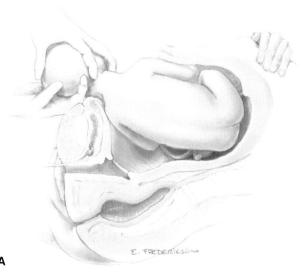
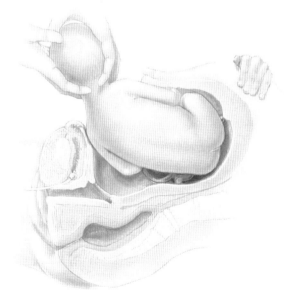

A   **B**

FIGURE 25-11 The anterior **(A)** and then the posterior shoulder **(B)** are delivered.

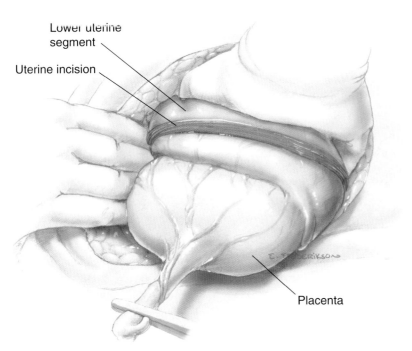

Lower uterine segment

Uterine incision

Placenta

FIGURE 25-12 Placenta bulging through the uterine incision as the uterus contracts. A hand gently massages the fundus to help aid placental separation.

At both Parkland and the University of Alabama at Birmingham Hospitals, we favor the one-layer uterine closure. The initial suture is placed just beyond one angle of the uterine incision. A running-lock suture, which creates a more hemostatic closure, is then performed with each suture penetrating the full thickness of

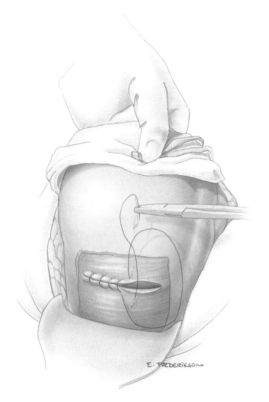

FIGURE 25-13 The cut edges of the uterine incision are approximated with a running-lock suture.

the myometrium (Fig. 25-13). It is important to carefully select the site of each stitch and to avoid withdrawing the needle once it penetrates the myometrium. This minimizes the perforation of unligated vessels and subsequent bleeding. The running-lock suture is continued just beyond the opposite incision angle. Especially when the lower segment is thin, satisfactory approximation of the cut edges usually can be obtained with one layer of suture. If approximation is not satisfactory after a single-layer continuous closure, or if bleeding sites persist, then more sutures are required. Either another layer of sutures may be placed to achieve approximation and hemostasis, or individual bleeding sites can be secured with figure-of-eight or mattress sutures.

Traditionally, serosal edges overlying the uterus and bladder have been approximated with a continuous 2-0 chromic catgut suture. Multiple randomized trials suggest that omission of this step causes no postoperative complications (Grundsell, 1998; Hull and Varner, 1991; Irion, 1996; Nagele, 1996; Pietrantoni, 1991, and all their associates). Specifically, not approximating the bladder flap is unlikely to increase adhesion formation or long-term morbidity (Roset and colleagues, 2003; Tulandi and Al-Jaroudi, 2003). Data are conflicting as to whether nonclosure of parietal peritoneum decreases postoperative discomfort and adhesions and need for analgesia (Chanrachakul, 2002; Lyell, 2005; Rafique, 2002; and all their colleagues).

If tubal sterilization is to be performed, it is now done as described in Chapter 33 (see p. 698).

Abdominal Closure

All packs are removed, and the paracolic gutters and cul-de-sac are emptied of blood and amnionic fluid using gentle suction. Some surgeons irrigate the gutters and cul-de-sac, especially in the presence of infection or meconium. A small randomized trial by Harrigill and colleagues (2003) supports that this step is not necessary in low-risk women who undergo cesarean delivery in the absence of amnionitis. After the sponge and instrument counts are found to be correct, the abdominal incision is closed in layers. As previously discussed, many surgeons omit the parietal peritoneal closure because it serves little purpose. If there is distended bowel in the incision site, however, we find that peritoneal closure may help to protect the bowel when fascial sutures are placed. As each layer is closed, bleeding sites are located, clamped, and ligated or coagulated with an electrosurgical blade. The rectus muscles are allowed to fall into place, and the subfascial space is meticulously checked for hemostasis. With significant diastasis, the rectus muscles may be approximated with one or two figure-of-eight sutures of 0 or #1 chromic gut suture. The overlying rectus fascia is closed either with interrupted 0-gauge delayed-absorbable sutures that are placed lateral to the fascial edges and no more than 1 cm apart, or by a continuous, nonlocking technique with a delay-absorbable suture.

The subcutaneous tissue usually need not be closed if it is less than 2 cm thick, and the skin is closed with vertical mattress sutures of 3-0 or 4-0 silk or equivalent suture; with a running 4-0 subcuticular stitch using delayed-absorbable suture; or with skin clips. If the subcutaneous tissue is at least 2 cm thick, it should be closed. In a randomized prospective study of more than 1400 women undergoing cesarean delivery, Bohman and colleagues (1992) reported a significantly decreased frequency of superficial wound disruption when the subcutaneous layer was approximated. Based on their systematic review of six studies, Chelmow and colleagues (2004) concluded that suturing the subcutaneous tissue at cesarean delivery decreases the risk of wound disruption by 34 percent in women with fat thickness greater than 2 cm. Addition of a subcutaneous drain with closure, however, does not prevent significant wound complications (Hellums and colleagues, 2007; Ramsey and associates, 2005).

Technique for Classical Cesarean Incision

Occasionally it is necessary to use a classical incision for delivery. Some indications stem from difficulty in exposing or safely entering the lower uterine segment. For example, a *densely adhered bladder* from previous surgery is encountered; a *leiomyoma* occupies the lower uterine segment; the cervix has been *invaded by cancer*; *massive maternal obesity* precludes safe access to the lower uterine segment; and some cases of *placenta previa with anterior implantation*, especially in the case where the placenta has grown through a prior uterine incision—*placenta increta or percreta*.

In other instances, fetal indications dictate the need. *Transverse lie of a large fetus*, especially if the membranes are ruptured and the shoulder is impacted in the birth canal, usually necessitates a classical incision. A fetus presenting as a back-down transverse lie may be particularly difficult to deliver through a transverse uterine incision. Sometimes when the fetus is very small, especially if breech, and the lower uterine segment is not thinned out, a classical incision is the best choice. Finally, if there are multiple fetuses, a classical incision may be preferable.

Uterine Incision

A vertical uterine incision is initiated with a scalpel beginning as low as possible, depending on how well the lower segment is thinned out. If adhesions, insufficient exposure, a tumor, or placenta percreta preclude development of a bladder flap, then the incision is made above the level of the bladder. Once the uterus is entered with a scalpel, the incision is extended cephalad with bandage scissors until it is sufficiently long to permit delivery of the fetus. Numerous large vessels that bleed profusely are commonly encountered within the myometrium.

Uterine Repair

One method employs a layer of continuous 0- or #1 chromic catgut to approximate the deeper halves of the incision. The outer half of the uterine incision is then closed with similar suture, using either a continuous stitch or figure-of-eight sutures. No unnecessary needle tracts should be made lest myometrial vessels be perforated leading to subsequent hemorrhage or hematoma. To achieve good approximation and to prevent the

suture from tearing through the myometrium, it is helpful to have an assistant compress the uterus on each side of the wound toward the midline as each suture is placed and tied. The edges of the uterine serosa, if not already so, are approximated with continuous 2-0 chromic catgut. The operation is then completed as described earlier.

Postmortem Cesarean Delivery

At times, cesarean delivery is performed in a woman who has just died, or who is expected to do so momentarily (Capobianco and colleagues, 2008). The issue of cesarean delivery to aid in cardiopulmonary resuscitation of the mother is further discussed in Chapter 42 (see p. 942).

PERIPARTUM HYSTERECTOMY

Hysterectomy performed at or following delivery may be lifesaving if there is severe obstetrical hemorrhage. It can be carried out in conjunction with cesarean delivery or following vaginal delivery. In a study of almost 29,000 cesarean deliveries, Shellhaas and colleagues (2001) reported that hysterectomy was performed in 1 in every 200 cesarean deliveries. If all deliveries are considered, the rate ranges from 0.4 to 0.8 percent (Briery, 2007; Forna, 2004; Glaze, 2008; Knight, 2008, and all their associates).

Indications

Most procedures are performed to arrest hemorrhage from intractable uterine atony, lower-segment bleeding associated with the uterine incision or placental implantation, uterine rupture, or uterine vessel laceration (Flood, 2009; Knight, 2008; Muench, 2008; Silver, 2006, and all their co-workers). These conditions are discussed in Chapter 35. Large leiomyomas may preclude satisfactory hysterotomy closure and thus necessitate hysterectomy. Elective indications for peripartum hysterectomy include large or symptomatic leiomyomas and severe cervical dysplasia or carcinoma in situ.

Major complications of peripartum hysterectomy compared with cesarean delivery are increased blood loss and greater risk of urinary tract damage. An important factor affecting the complication rate is whether the operation is performed electively or emergently. As shown in Table 25-4, the morbidity rate associated with emergency hysterectomy is substantively increased. Seago and associates (1999) reported that the rate of intraoperative and postoperative complications among 100 women who underwent planned cesarean hysterectomy was not increased compared with that of a control group of 37 women who underwent cesarean delivery followed by hysterectomy performed within the subsequent 6 months.

Although pelvic vessels are appreciably hypertrophied, hysterectomy usually is aided by the ease of tissue plane development in pregnant women. Blood loss is usually appreciable because hysterectomy performed for hemorrhage almost always is associated with torrential bleeding. Indeed, as shown in Table 25-4, 83 percent of women undergoing emergency peripartum hysterectomy required transfusions compared with only 28 percent of those undergoing a planned hysterectomy. Preoperative preparation such as intravascular balloon placement in cases of

TABLE 25-4. Comparison of Morbidity Rates with Elective Versus Emergency Peripartum Hysterectomy

Complication	Complications in Percent[a]	
	Elective (n = 345)	Emergency (n = 644)
Transfusions	28	83
Urinary tract injury	1.8	5.6
Surgical infection	21	25
Death	0	1.4

[a]All complications not reported by all studies. Averages calculated from reported data. Data from Briery (2007), Castaneda (2000), Glaze (2008), Kastner (2002), Kwee (2006), Plauche (1995), Sakse (2008), Zelop (1993), Zorlu (1998), and all their colleagues.

placenta percreta as described by Shrivastava and colleagues (2007) is discussed in Chapter 35 (p. 776).

Technique for Peripartum Hysterectomy

Supracervical or total hysterectomy is performed using standard operative techniques. Initially, placement of a self-retaining retractor such as a Balfour is not necessary. Satisfactory exposure is best obtained with cephalad traction on the uterus by an assistant, along with handheld retractors such as a Richardson or Deaver. The bladder flap is deflected downward to the level of the cervix if possible. After cesarean delivery and placental removal, if the hysterotomy incision is bleeding appreciably, either it can be sutured, or Pennington or sponge-forceps can be applied for hemostasis. If bleeding is minimal, neither maneuver is necessary.

The round ligaments close to the uterus are divided between Heaney or Kocher clamps and doubly ligated (Fig. 25-14). Either 0- or #1 suture can be used. The incision in the vesicouterine serosa that was made to mobilize the bladder is extended laterally and upward through the anterior leaf of the broad ligament to reach the incised round ligaments. The posterior leaf of the broad ligament adjacent to the uterus is perforated just beneath the fallopian tubes, utero-ovarian ligaments, and ovarian vessels (Fig. 25-15). These vessels then are doubly clamped close to the uterus and divided, and the lateral pedicle is doubly ligated (Fig. 25-16). The posterior leaf of the broad ligament is divided inferiorly toward the uterosacral ligaments (Fig. 25-17). Next, the bladder and attached peritoneal flap are again deflected and dissected from the lower uterine segment and retracted out of the operative field. If the bladder flap is unusually adherent, as it may be after previous hysterotomy incisions, careful sharp dissection may be necessary (Fig. 25-18).

Special care is required from this point on to avoid injury to the ureters, which pass beneath the uterine arteries. To help accomplish this, an assistant places constant traction on the uterus in the direction away from the side on which the uterine vessels are being ligated. The ascending uterine artery and veins on either side are identified near their origin. These pedicles are then doubly clamped immediately adjacent to the uterus, divided,

and doubly suture ligated. As shown in Figure 25-19, we prefer to use three heavy clamps, incise the tissue between the most medial and two lateral clamps, and then ligate the two pedicles in the clamps lateral to the uterus.

In cases of profuse hemorrhage, it may be more advantageous to rapidly double clamp and divide all of the vascular pedicles between clamps to gain hemostasis and then return to suture ligate all of the pedicles.

Supracervical Hysterectomy

To perform a subtotal hysterectomy, it is necessary only to amputate the body of the uterus immediately below the level of

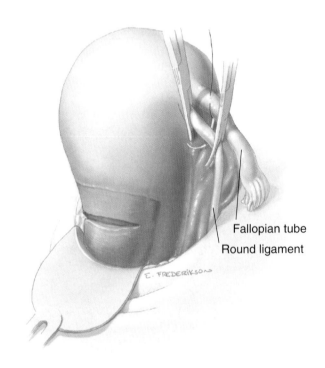

Fallopian tube
Round ligament

E. FREDERIKSON

FIGURE 25-14 The round ligaments are clamped, ligated, and transected bilaterally.

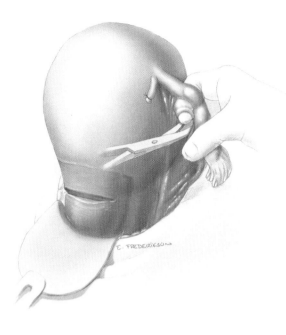

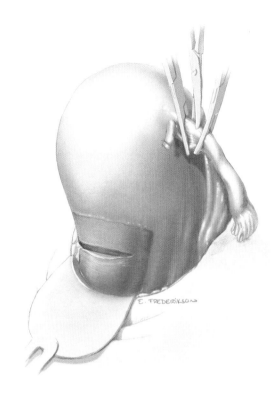

FIGURE 25-15 The posterior leaf of the broad ligament adjacent to the uterus is perforated just beneath the fallopian tube, utero-ovarian ligaments, and ovarian vessels.

FIGURE 25-16 The utero-ovarian ligament and fallopian tube are clamped and cut bilaterally.

uterine artery ligation. The cervical stump may be closed with continuous or interrupted chromic catgut sutures. Subtotal hysterectomy is often all that is necessary to stop hemorrhage and may be the more prudent operation for selected women (Jones, 1999; Kastner, 2002; Learman, 2003; Munro, 1997, and all their associates).

Total Hysterectomy

Even if total hysterectomy is planned, we find it in many cases technically easier to finish the operation after amputating the uterine fundus and placing Ochsner or Kocher clamps on the stump for traction and hemostasis. Self-retaining retractors also may be placed at this time. To remove the cervix, it is necessary to extensively mobilize the bladder. This will help carry the ureters caudad as the bladder is retracted beneath the symphysis and will prevent laceration or suturing of the bladder during cervical excision and vaginal cuff closure. If the cervix is effaced and dilated appreciably, the cervicovaginal junction after delivery may be identified through a vertical uterine incision made anteriorly in the midline, either through the open hysterotomy incision or through an incision created at the level of the ligated uterine vessels. A finger is directed inferiorly through the incision to identify the free margin of the dilated, effaced cervix and the anterior vaginal fornix. The contaminated glove is replaced. Another useful method to identify the cervical margins is to transvaginally place four metal skin clips or brightly colored sutures at 12, 3, 6, and 9 o'clock positions on the cervical edges prior to hysterectomy.

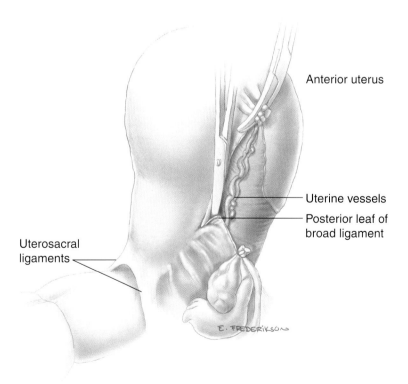

Anterior uterus

Uterine vessels

Posterior leaf of broad ligament

Uterosacral ligaments

FIGURE 25-17 The posterior leaf of the broad ligament is divided inferiorly toward the uterosacral ligament.

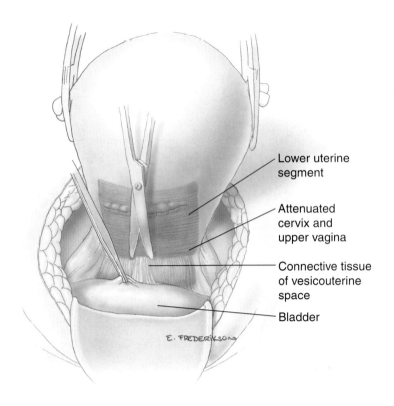

Lower uterine segment

Attenuated cervix and upper vagina

Connective tissue of vesicouterine space

Bladder

FIGURE 25-18 The bladder is dissected sharply from the lower uterine segment.

The cardinal ligaments, the uterosacral ligaments, and the many large vessels these ligaments contain are clamped systematically with Heaney-type curved clamps, Ochsner-type straight clamps, or similar instruments (Fig. 25-20). The clamps are placed as close to the cervix as possible, taking care not to include excessive tissue in each clamp. The tissue between the pair of clamps is incised and the distal pedicle suture ligated. These steps are repeated until the level of the lateral vaginal fornix is reached. In this way, the descending branches of the uterine vessels are clamped, cut, and ligated as the cervix is dissected from the cardinal ligaments.

Immediately below the level of the cervix, a curved clamp is placed across the lateral vaginal fornix, and the tissue is incised medially to the clamp (Fig. 25-21). The excised lateral vaginal fornix can be simultaneously doubly ligated and sutured to the stump of the cardinal ligament. The cervix is inspected to ensure that it has been completely removed, and the vagina is then repaired. Each of the angles of the lateral vaginal fornix is secured to the cardinal and uterosacral ligaments (Fig. 25-22). Following this step, some surgeons prefer to close the vagina using figure-of-eight chromic catgut sutures. Others achieve hemostasis by

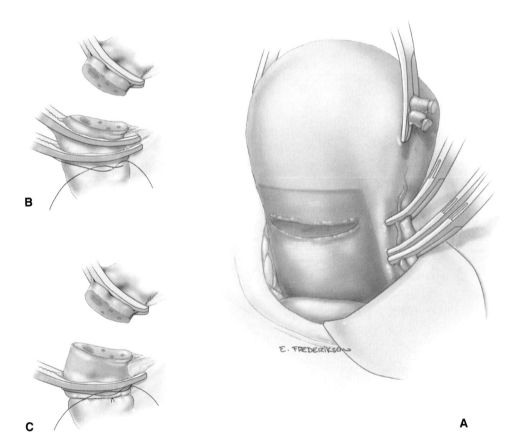

FIGURE 25-19 A. The uterine artery and veins on either side are doubly clamped immediately adjacent to the uterus and divided. **B, C.** The vascular pedicle is doubly suture ligated.

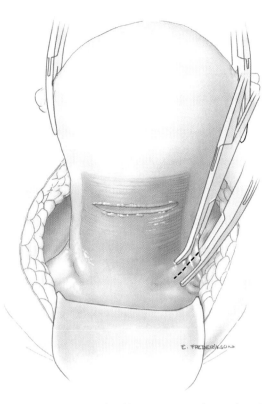

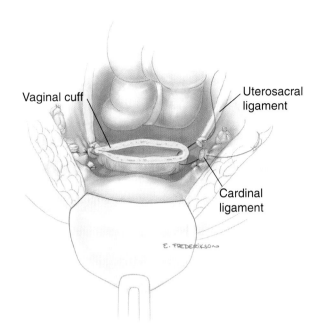

FIGURE 25-22 The lateral angles of the vaginal cuff are secured to the cardinal and uterosacral ligaments.

FIGURE 25-20 The cardinal ligaments are clamped, incised, and ligated.

using a running-lock stitch of chromic catgut suture placed through the mucosa and adjacent endopelvic fascia around the circumference of the vaginal cuff (Fig. 25-23).

If a self-retaining retractor has not already been placed, some clinicians choose to insert the instrument at this point. The

bowel is then packed out of the field, and all sites are examined carefully for bleeding. One technique is to perform a systematic bilateral survey from the fallopian tube and ovarian ligament pedicles to the vaginal vault and bladder flap. Bleeding sites are ligated with care to avoid the ureters. The abdominal wall normally is closed in layers, as previously described (p. 554).

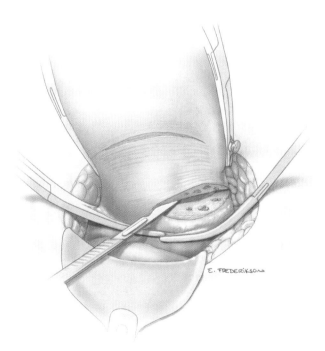

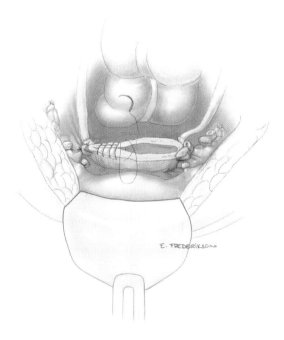

FIGURE 25-21 A curved clamp is placed across the lateral vaginal fornix below the level of the cervix, and the tissue incised medially to the point of the clamp.

FIGURE 25-23 A running-lock suture approximates the vaginal wall edges.

Oophorectomy

Most studies indicate that in 5 percent of postpartum hysterectomies, one adnexum will have to be removed to stop bleeding (Plauche, 1995). In the recent report by Briery and colleagues (2007), a fourth of women had unilateral or bilateral oophorectomy. That said, during any hysterectomy, a decision as to the fate of the ovaries must be made. For women who are approaching menopause, the decision is not difficult, but few women who undergo cesarean hysterectomy are of this age.

Cystotomy

Rarely and usually in women who have had a previous cesarean delivery, injury to the bladder may occur, usually in the form of an incidental cystotomy. This complication is more common in women undergoing cesarean hysterectomy.

Bladder injury is typically identified at the time of surgery, and initially, a gush of clear fluid into the operating field may be seen. If laceration is suspected, it may be confirmed with instillation of sterile infant formula through a Foley catheter into the bladder. Leakage of opaque milk aids in identifying a laceration and delineating its borders. Additionally, cystoscopy may be indicated to further define bladder injury. Repair at the primary surgery is preferred and lowers the risk of postoperative vesicovaginal fistula formation. Once ureteral patency is confirmed, the bladder may be closed with a two- or three-layer running closure using a 3-0 absorbable or delayed-absorbable suture (**Fig. 25-24**). The first layer inverts the mucosa into the bladder, and subsequent layers reapproximate

bladder muscularis. Postoperative care requires continuous bladder drainage for 7 to 10 days.

PERIPARTUM MANAGEMENT

Preoperative Care

If cesarean delivery is planned, a sedative may be given at bedtime the night before the operation. In general, no other sedatives, narcotics, or tranquilizers are administered until after the infant is born. Oral intake is stopped at least 8 hours before surgery. The woman scheduled for repeat cesarean delivery typically is admitted the day of surgery and evaluated by the obstetrician and the anesthesiologist. The hematocrit is rechecked, as is the indirect Coombs test. If the latter is positive, then availability of compatible blood must be ensured. An antacid, such as Bicitra, 30 mL, is given orally shortly before conduction analgesia or induction with general anesthesia to minimize the risk of lung injury from gastric acid aspiration (see Chap. 19, p. 460). An indwelling bladder catheter is placed. If hair obscures the operative field it should be removed the day of surgery by clipping or shaving. If shaving is performed the night before surgery, the risk of wound infection is increased. According to the American College of Obstetricians and Gynecologists (2007b), there are insufficient data to determine the value of fetal monitoring prior to *scheduled* cesarean delivery in women without risk factors. That said, fetal heart tones should be documented prior to surgery.

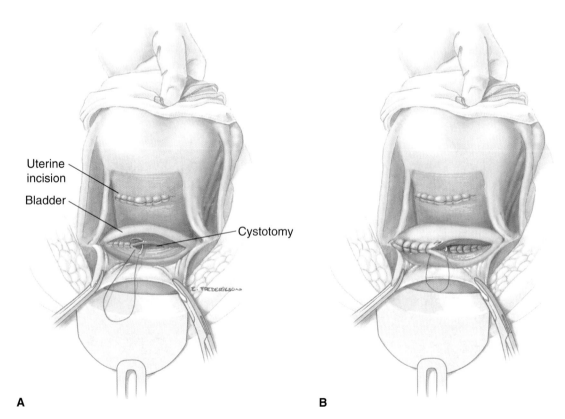

Uterine incision

Bladder

Cystotomy

E. FREDERIKSON

A   **B**

FIGURE 25-24 Cystotomy repair. **A.** The primary layer inverts the bladder mucosa with running or interrupted sutures of 3-0 delayed-absorbable or absorbable suture. **B.** Second and possibly a third layer approximate the bladder muscularis to reinforce the incision closure.

Intravenous Fluids

Requirements for intravenous fluids, including blood, during and after cesarean delivery can vary considerably. Intravenously administered fluids consist of either lactated Ringer solution or a similar crystalloid solution with 5-percent dextrose. Typically, at least 2 to 3 L are infused during surgery. Blood loss with uncomplicated cesarean delivery approximates 1000 mL. The woman of average size with a hematocrit of 30 percent or more and a normally expanded blood and extracellular fluid volume most often will tolerate blood loss up to 2000 mL without difficulty. Unappreciated bleeding through the vagina during the procedure, bleeding concealed in the uterus after its closure, or both commonly lead to underestimation.

Although blood loss averages about 1500 mL with elective cesarean hysterectomy, it is variable (Pritchard, 1965). Thus, throughout the procedure and subsequently, while in the recovery area, blood pressure and urine flow are monitored closely.

Prevention of Postoperative Infection

Febrile morbidity is frequent after cesarean delivery. A large number of randomized trials have demonstrated that a single dose of an antimicrobial agent given at the time of cesarean delivery will serve to decrease infectious morbidity significantly. This is true of high-risk laboring patients as well as those undergoing elective cesarean delivery (American College of Obstetricians and Gynecologists, 2003). For women in labor or with ruptured membranes, most clinicians recommend a single 2-g dose of a β-lactam drug—either a cephalosporin or extended-spectrum penicillin—after delivery of the newborn. The delay of prophylactic antibiotic administration after the delivery of the infant has been due to concerns surrounding neonatal exposure to antibiotics and the potential effect on neonatal sepsis evaluation. Some authors have found no effect on maternal infection rates whether prophylaxis is administered at the time of the skin incision or at cord clamping (Thigpen and co-workers, 2005). Others, however, reported decreased rates if given at the earlier time (Sullivan and associates, 2007; Tita and colleagues, 2009). Currently, the original concerns regarding effect on neonatal infections have not been adequately dispelled.

Postoperative pelvic infection is the most frequent cause of febrile morbidity and develops in up to 20 percent of these women despite peripartum prophylactic antimicrobials (Goepfert and associates, 2001). The addition of azithromycin to a standard first- or second-generation cephalosporin prophylactic dose was found to decrease the risk of postoperative endometritis compared with cephalosporin alone (Tita and colleagues, 2008, 2009). Treatment of uterine infection and its complications are discussed in Chapter 31 (p. 661).

Recovery Suite

Postoperatively, the amount of bleeding from the vagina must be monitored closely, and the uterine fundus must be identified frequently by palpation to ensure that the uterus is remaining firmly contracted. Unfortunately, as conduction analgesia fades or the woman awakens from general anesthesia, palpation of the abdomen is likely to produce considerable discomfort. This can be made tolerable by giving an effective analgesic intravenously, such as meperidine, 75 to 100 mg, or morphine, 10 to 15 mg. A thick dressing with an abundance of adhesive tape over the abdomen interferes with fundal palpation and massage and later causes discomfort as the tape is removed. Deep breathing and coughing are encouraged. Once the mother is fully awake, bleeding is minimal, blood pressure is satisfactory, and urine flow is at least 30 mL/hr, she may be transferred to her room.

Subsequent Care

Analgesia

For the woman of average size, meperidine, 50 to 75 mg, is given intramuscularly as often as every 3 hours as needed for discomfort (Table 25-5). Alternatively, morphine sulfate, 10 to 15 mg, is similarly administered. An antiemetic, such as promethazine, 25 mg, usually is given along with the narcotic. Intravenous meperidine or morphine via a patient-controlled pump is an even more effective alternative to bolus therapy in the immediate postoperative period (Table 25-5). The pump typically is programmed to deliver a continuous infusion of drug. The woman can supplement with intermittent boluses, the frequency of which are determined by the "lock-out" interval. In a trial at Parkland Hospital, morphine provided superior pain relief to meperidine and was associated with significantly

---

TABLE 25-5. Typical Settings for Administration of Intravenous Opioids via a Patient-Controlled Analgesia Pump

Recovery room:
   IV meperidine, 25 mg every 5 min up to 100 mg
   or
   IV morphine, 2 mg every 5 min up to 10 mg

Postpartum ward (first 24 h after surgery):[a]
   IM meperidine, 50–75 mg every 3–4 h as needed
   or
   PCA intravenous meperidine, 10 mg with a 6 min lockout interval and maximum dose of 200 mg in 4 h as needed. An additional 25-mg booster dose was permitted for a maximum of 2 doses
   or
   IM morphine, 10–15 mg every 3–4 h as needed
   or
   PCA intravenous morphine, 1 mg with a 6-min lockout interval and maximum dose of 30 mg in 4 h as needed. An additional 2-mg booster dose was permitted for a maximum of 2 doses

[a]Each postpartum ward regimen also included promethazine, 25 mg intravenously every 6 h as needed for nausea.
IM = intramuscular; IV = intravenous; PCA = patient-controlled analgesia.
Reprinted from *American Journal of Obstetrics & Gynecology*, Vol. 190, No. 5, NP Yost, SL Bloom, MK Sibley, et al., A hospital-sponsored quality improvement study of pain management after cesarean delivery, pp. 1341–1346, Copyright 2004, with permission from Elsevier.

higher rates of breast-feeding continuation and infant rooming-in (Yost and colleagues, 2004).

Vital Signs

After transfer to her room, the woman is assessed at least hourly for 4 hours and thereafter, at intervals of 4 hours. Blood pressure, pulse, temperature, uterine tone, urine output, and amount of bleeding are evaluated.

Fluid Therapy and Diet

The puerperium is characterized by excretion of fluid that was retained during pregnancy. Moreover, with the typical cesarean delivery, significant extracellular fluid sequestration in bowel wall and lumen does not occur, unless it was necessary to pack the bowel away from the operative field or peritonitis develops. Thus, the woman who undergoes cesarean delivery rarely develops fluid sequestration in the so-called third space. On the contrary, she normally begins surgery with a physiologically enlarged extravascular volume acquired during pregnancy that she mobilizes and excretes after delivery. Therefore, large volumes of intravenous fluids during and subsequent to surgery are not needed to replace sequestered extracellular fluid. As a generalization, 3 L of fluid should prove adequate during the first 24 hours after surgery. If urine output falls below 30 mL/hr, however, the woman should be reevaluated promptly. The cause of the oliguria may range from unrecognized blood loss to an antidiuretic effect from infused oxytocin.

Exception to this typical pattern of fluid mobilization include pathological constriction of the extracellular fluid compartment from severe preeclampsia, vomiting, fever, prolonged labor without adequate fluid intake, significant blood loss, or sepsis.

Bladder and Bowel Function

The bladder catheter most often can be removed by 12 hours postoperatively or more conveniently, the morning after surgery. The prevalence of urinary retention following cesarean delivery approximates 3 percent, and a failure to progress in labor following surgery is an identified risk (Chai and associates, 2008). Thus, surveillance for bladder overdistension should be implemented as with vaginal delivery.

In uncomplicated cases, solid food may be offered within 8 hours of surgery (Bar, 2008; Kramer, 1996; Orji, 2009, and all their co-workers). Although some degree of adynamic ileus follows virtually every abdominal operation, in most cases of cesarean delivery it is negligible. Symptoms include abdominal distension and gas pains, and an inability to pass flatus or stool. The pathophysiology of postoperative ileus is complex and involves hormonal, neural, and local factors that are incompletely understood (Livingston and Passaro, 1990). If associated with otherwise unexplained fever, an unrecognized bowel injury may be responsible. Treatment for ileus has changed little during the past several decades and involves intravenous fluid and electrolyte supplementation. If severe, nasogastric decompression is necessary. Frequently, a 10-mg bisacodyl rectal suppository provides appreciable relief.

Ambulation

Women undergoing cesarean have a two- to 20-fold increased of risk of pulmonary embolism compared with those delivering vaginally. Risks include age > 35; BMI > 30; parity >3; emergency cesarean; cesarean hysterectomy; concurrent infection, major illness, preeclampsia, or gross varicosities; recent immobility; and prior deep-venous thrombosis or thrombophilia (Marik and Plante, 2008). Early ambulation lowers the risk of venous thrombosis and pulmonary embolism (see Chap. 47, p. 1013).

In most instances, by the day after surgery, a woman should get briefly out of bed with assistance at least twice to walk. Ambulation can be timed so that a recently administered analgesic will minimize the discomfort. By the second day, she may walk without assistance.

Wound Care

The incision is inspected each day, and the skin sutures or clips often can be removed on the fourth day after surgery. However, if there is concern for superficial wound separation, as in the obese patient, the suture or clips should remain in place for 7 to 10 days. By the third postpartum day, showering is not harmful to the incision.

Laboratory

The hematocrit is routinely measured the morning after surgery. It is checked sooner if there was unusual blood loss or if there is oliguria or other evidence to suggest hypovolemia. If the hematocrit is decreased significantly from the preoperative level, the measurement is repeated and a search is instituted to identify the cause of the decline. If the hematocrit stabilizes, the mother can be allowed to ambulate, and if there is little likelihood of further blood loss, iron therapy is preferred to transfusion.

Breast Care

Breast feeding can be initiated the day of surgery. If the mother elects not to breast feed, a binder that supports the breasts without marked compression usually will minimize discomfort (see Chap. 30, p. 651).

Hospital Discharge

Unless there are complications during the puerperium, the mother generally is discharged on the third or fourth postpartum day (see Chap. 30, p. 657). Strong and associates (1993) have presented data suggesting that discharge on day 2 may be appropriate for properly selected and motivated women. Activities during the first week should be restricted to self-care and care of her baby with assistance. Brooten and colleagues (1994) successfully combined early discharge with nurse-specialist transitional home care.

REFERENCES

Alexander JM, Leveno KJ, Hauth J, et al: Fetal injury associated with cesarean delivery. Obstet Gynecol 108(4):885, 2006

Althabe F, Belizn JM, Villar J, et al: Mandatory second opinion to reduce rates of unnecessary caesarean sections in Latin America: A cluster randomised controlled trial. Lancet.12;363:1934, 2004

American Academy of Pediatrics and American College of Obstetricians and Gynecologists: Guidelines for Perinatal Care, 6th ed. Elk Grove, Ill, American Academy of Pediatrics, 2007

American College of Obstetricians and Gynecologists, Task Force on Cesarean Delivery Rates: Evaluation of cesarean delivery. June 2000

American College of Obstetricians and Gynecologists: Prophylactic antibiotics in labor and delivery. Practice Bulletin No. 47, October 2003

American College of Obstetricians and Gynecologists: Cesarean delivery on maternal request. Committee Opinion No. 394, December 2007a

American College of Obstetricians and Gynecologists: Fetal monitoring prior to scheduled Cesarean delivery. Committee Opinion No. 382. Obstet Gynecol 110(4):961, 2007b

American College of Obstetricians and Gynecologists: Fetal lung maturity. Practice Bulletin No. 97, September 2008

Ananth CV, Joseph KS, Oyelese Y, et al: Trends in preterm birth and perinatal mortality among singletons: United States, 1989 through 2000. Obstet Gynecol105:1084, 2005

Anorlu RI, Maholwana B, Hofmeyr GJ: Methods of delivering the placenta at caesarean section. Cochrane Database Syst Rev Jul 16;(3):CD004737, 2008

Atkinson MW, Owen J, Wren A, et al: The effect of manual removal of the placenta on post-cesarean endometritis. Obstet Gynecol 87:99, 1996

Ayers JWT, Morley GW: Surgical incision for cesarean section. Obstet Gynecol 70:706, 1987

Baksu A, Kalan A, Ozkan A, et al: The effect of placental removal method and site of uterine repair on postcesarean endometritis and operative blood loss. Acta Obstet Gynecol Scand 84(3):266, 2005

Bar G, Scheiner E, Lezerovitz A, et al: Early maternal feeding following caesarean delivery: A prospective randomized study. Acta Obstet Gynecol Scand 87(1):68, 2008

Basso O, Rasmussen S, Weinberg C, et al: Trends in fetal and infant survival following preeclampsia. JAMA 296:11, 2006

Berghella V, Baxter JK, Chauhan SP: Evidence-based surgery for cesarean delivery. Am J Obstet Gynecol 193(5):1607, 2005

Bewley S, Cockburn J: The unethics of "request" caesarean section [Commentary]. Br J Obstet Gynaecol 109:593, 2002a

Bewley S, Cockburn J: The unfacts of "request" caesarean section [Commentary]. Br J Obstet Gynaecol 109:597, 2002b

Bloom SL, for the National Institute of Child Health and Human Development Maternal–Fetal Medicine Units Cesarean Registry: Decision to incision times and infant outcome. Am J Obstet Gynecol 185:S121, 2001

Bloom SL, Leveno KJ, Spong CY, et al: Decision-to-incision times and maternal and fetal outcomes. Obstet Gynecol 108(1):6, 2006

Bohman VR, Gilstrap L, Leveno K, et al: Subcutaneous tissue: To close or not to close at cesarean section. Am J Obstet Gynecol 166:407, 1992

Boley JP: The history of cesarean section. Can Med Assoc J 145:319, 1991

Briery CM, Rose CH, Hudson WT, et al: Planned vs emergent cesarean hysterectomy. Am J Obstet Gynecol, 197(2):154.e1, 2007

Brooten D, Roncoli M, Finkler S, et al: A randomized trial of early hospital discharge and home follow-up of women having cesarean birth. Obstet Gynecol 84:832, 1994

Bujold E, Bujold C, Hamilton EF, et al: The impact of a single-layer or double-layer closure on uterine rupture. Am J Obstet Gynecol 186:1326, 2002

Burrows LJ, Meyn LA, Weber AM: Maternal morbidity associated with vaginal versus cesarean delivery. Obstet Gynecol. 103:907, 2004

Capobianco G, Balata A, Mannazzu MC, et al: Perimortem cesarean delivery 30 minutes after a laboring patient jumped from a fourth-floor window: Baby survives and is normal at age 4 years. Am J Obstet Gynecol 198(1):15, 2008

Castaneda S, Karrison T, Cibils LA: Peripartum hysterectomy. J Perinat Med 28(6):472, 2000

Chai AH, Wong T, Mak HL, et al: Prevalence and associated risk factors of retention of urine after caesarean section. Int Urogynecol J Pelvic Floor Dysfunct 194(4):537, 2008

Chanrachakul B, Hamontri S, Herabutya Y: A randomized comparison of postcesarean pain between closure and nonclosure of peritoneum. Eur J Obstet Gynecol Reprod Biol 101:31, 2002

Chapman SJ, Owen J, Hauth JC: One versus two-layer closure of a low transverse cesarean: The next pregnancy. Obstet Gynecol 89:16, 1997

Chelmow D, Rodriguez EJ, Sabatini MM: Suture closure of subcutaneous fat and wound disruption after cesarean delivery: A meta-analysis. Obstet Gynecol. 103:974, 2004

Clark SL, Belfort MA, Dildy GA, et al: Maternal death in the 21st century: Causes, prevention, and relationship to cesarean delivery. Am J Obstet Gynecol 199(1):36.e1, 2008

Clark SL, Miller DD, Belfort MA, et al: Neonatal and maternal outcomes associated with elective term delivery. Am J Obstet Gynecol 200(2):156.e1, 2009

Coutinho IC, Ramos de Morim MM, Katz L, et al: Uterine exteriorization compared with in situ repair at cesarean delivery. Obstet Gynecol 111:639, 2008

Cunningham FG, Leveno KL, Bloom SL, et al: Cesarean delivery and peripartum hysterectomy. In: Williams Obstetrics, 22nd ed. New York, McGraw-Hill, 2005, p 588

Declercq E, Barger M, Cabra JH, et al: Maternal outcomes associated with planned primary cesarean births compared with planned vaginal births. Obstet Gynecol 109(3):669, 2007

DeMott RK, Sandmire HF: The Green Bay cesarean section study, 1. The physician factor as a determinant of cesarean birth rates. Am J Obstet Gynecol 162:1593, 1990

DeMuylder X, Thiery M: The cesarean delivery rate can be safely reduced in a developing country. Obstet Gynecol 75:60, 1990

Durnwald C, Mercer B: Uterine rupture, perioperative and perinatal morbidity after single-layer and double-layer closure at cesarean delivery. Am J Obstet Gynecol 189:925, 2003

Flood KM, Said S, Geary M, et al: Changing trends in peripartum hysterectomy over the last 4 decades. Am J Obstet Gynecol 200(6):632.e1, 2009

Foley M, Alarab M, O'Herlighy C: Neonatal seizures and peripartum deaths: Lack of correlation with cesarean rate [Abstract]. Am J Obstet Gynecol 187:S102, 2002

Forna F, Miles AM, Jamieson DJ: Emergency peripartum hysterectomy: A comparison of cesarean and postpartum hysterectomy. Am J Obstet Gynecol 190:1440, 2004

Friedman EA: Labor, Clinical Evaluation and Management. New York, Appleton, 1978

Giacalone PL, Daures JP, Vignal J, et al: Pfannenstiel versus Maylard incision for cesarean delivery: A randomized controlled trial. Obstet Gynecol 99:745, 2002

Glaze S, Ekwalanga P, Roberts G, et al: Peripartum hysterectomy: 1999 to 2006. Obstet Gynecol 111(3):732, 2008

Goepfert A, for the National Institute of Child Health and Human Development Maternal–Fetal Medicine Units Network: The MFMU Cesarean Registry: Infectious morbidity following primary cesarean section. Am J Obstet Gynecol 185:S192, 2001

Gossman GL, Joesch JM, Tanfer K: Trends in maternal request cesarean delivery from 1991 to 2004. Obstet Gynecol 108: 1506, 2006

Grundsell HS, Rizk DE, Kumar RM: Randomized study of non-closure of peritoneum in lower segment cesarean section. Acta Obstet Gynecol Scand 77:110, 1998

Hall MH, Bewley S: Maternal mortality and mode of delivery. Lancet 354:776, 1999

Hamilton BE, Martin JA, Sutton PD, et al: Births: Final data for 2004. National Vital Statistics Reports, Vol 55, No.1. Hyattsville, Md, National Center for Health Statistics, 2006

Hamilton BE, Martin JA, Ventura SJ: Births: Preliminary Data for 2007. National Vital Statistics Reports, Vol 57, No 12. Hyattsville, Md, National Center for Health Statistics, 2009

Harer W: Patient choice caesarean. Am Coll Obstet Gynecol Clin Rev 5:2, 2000

Harrigill KM, Miller HS, Haynes DE: The effect of intraabdominal irrigation at cesarean delivery on maternal morbidity: A randomized trial. Obstet Gynecol 101:80, 2003

Hauth JC, Owen J, Davis RO, et al: Transverse uterine incision closure: One versus two layers. Am J Obstet Gynecol 167:1108, 1992

Hellums EK, Lin MG, Ramsey PS: Prophylactic subcutaneous drainage for prevention of wound complications after cesarean delivery—a metaanalysis. Am J Obstet Gynecol 197(3):229, 2007

Henderson J, McCandlish R, Kumiega L, et al: Systematic review of economic aspects of alternative modes of delivery. Br J Obstet Gynaecol 108:149, 2001

Hendrix SL, Schimp V, Martin J, et al: The legendary superior strength of the Pfannenstiel incision: A myth? Am J Obstet Gynecol 182:1446, 2000

Hofmeyr GJ, Mathai M, Shah A, et al: Techniques for caesarean section. Cochrane Database Syst Rev 1:CD004662, 2008

Hull DB, Varner MW: A randomized study of closure of the peritoneum at cesarean delivery. Obstet Gynecol 77:818, 1991

Irion O, Luzuy F, Beguin F: Nonclosure of the visceral and parietal peritoneum at caesarean section: A randomised controlled trial. Br J Obstet Gynaecol 103:690, 1996

Jacob J, Phenninger J: Cesarean deliveries: When is a pediatrician necessary? Obstet Gynecol 89:217, 1997

Joel-Cohen S: Abdominal and Vaginal Hysterectomy: New Techniques Based on Time and Motion Studies. London, William Heinemann Medical Books, 1977

Jones DE, Shackelford DP, Brame RG: Supracervical hysterectomy: Back to the future? Am J Obstet Gynecol 180:513, 1999

Kalish RB, McCullough LB, Chervenak FA: Patient choice cesarean delivery: Ethical issues. Curr Opin Obstet Gynecol 20:116, 2008

Kastner ES, Figueroa R, Garry D, et al: Emergency peripartum hysterectomy: Experience at a community teaching hospital. Obstet Gynecol 99:971, 2002

Kerr JMM: The lower uterine segment incision in conservative caesarean section. J Obstet Gynaecol Br Emp 28:475, 1921

Knight M, Kurinczuk JJ, Spark P, et al: Cesarean delivery and peripartum hysterectomy. Obstet Gynecol 111(1):97, 2008

Kramer R, Van Someren J, Qualls C, et al: Postoperative management of cesarean section patients: The effect of immediate feeding on the incidence of ileus. Obstet Gynecol 88:29, 1996

Krönig B: Transperitonealer cervikaler Kaiserschnitt. In: Doderlein A, Krönig B (eds): Operative Gynakologie. 1912, p 879

Kuklina EV, Meikle SF, Jamieson DJ, et al: Severe obstetric morbidity in the United States: 1998–2005. Obstet Gynecol 113(2 Pt 1):293, 2009

Kwee A, Bots ML, Visser GH, et al: Emergency peripartum hysterectomy: A prospective study in The Netherlands. Eur J Obstet Gynecol Reprod Biol 124(2).187-92, 2006.

Learman LA, Summitt RL, Varner RE, et al: A randomized comparison of total or supracervical hysterectomy: Surgical complications and clinical outcomes. Obstet Gynecol 102:453, 2003

Lien JM, Towers CV, Quilligan EJ, et al: Term early-onset neonatal seizures: Obstetric characteristics, etiologic classifications, and perinatal care. Obstet Gynecol 85:163, 1995

Liu SL, Liston RM, Joseph KS, et al: Maternal mortality and severe morbidity associated with low-risk planned cesarean delivery versus planned vaginal delivery at term. CMAJ 176(4):455, 2007

Livingston EH, Passaro EP: Postoperative ileus. Dig Dis Sci 35:21, 1990

Lyell DJ, Caughey AB, Hu E, et al: Peritoneal closure at primary cesarean delivery and adhesions. Obstet Gynecol 106(2):275, 2005

MacDorman MF, Menacker F, Declercq E: Cesarean birth in the United States: Epidemiology, trends, and outcomes. Clin Perinatol 35(2):293, 2008

Magann EF, Chauhan SP, Bufkin L, et al: Intra-operative haemorrhage by blunt versus sharp expansion of the uterine incision at caesarean delivery: A randomised clinical trial. Br J Obstet Gynaecol 109:448, 2002

Marik PE, Plante LA: Venous thromboembolic disease and pregnancy. N Engl J Med 359(19):2025, 2008

Martin JA, Hamilton BE, Sutton PD, et al: Births: Final data for 2002. Natl Vital Stat Rep 52(10):1, 2003

Martin JA, Hamilton BE, Sutton PD, et al: Births: Final Data for 2003. National Vital Statistics Reports, Vol 54, No 2. Hyattsville, Md, National Center for Health Statistics, 2005

Martin JA, Hamilton BE, Sutton PD, et al: Births: Final data for 2004. Natl Vital Stat Rep 55(1):1, 2006

Meikle SF, Steiner CA, Zhang, J, Lawrence WL: A national estimate of the elective primary cesarean delivery rate. Obstet Gynecol 105:751, 2005

Menacker F, Declercq E, Macdorman MF: Cesarean delivery: background, trends, and epidemiology. Semin Perinatol 30(5):235, 2006

Minkoff H: The ethics of cesarean section by choice. Semin Perinatol 30(5):309, 2006

Minkoff H, Chervenak FA: Elective primary cesarean delivery. N Engl J Med 348:946, 2003

Muench MV, Baschatt AA, Oyelese Y, et al: Gravid hysterectomy: A decade of experience at an academic referral center. J Reprod Med 53(4):271, 2008

Munn MB, Owen J, Vincent R, et al: Comparison of two oxytocin regimens to prevent uterine atony at cesarean delivery: A randomized controlled trial. Obstet Gynecol 98:386, 2001

Munro MG: Supracervical hysterectomy: A time for reappraisal. Obstet Gynecol 89:133, 1997

Nagele F, Karas H, Spitzer D, et al: Closure or nonclosure of the visceral peritoneum at cesarean delivery. Am J Obstet Gynecol 174:1366, 1996

National Institutes of Health State-of-the-Science Conference Statement: Cesarean delivery on maternal request. March 27-29, 2006. 107:6, 2006

Nygaard I, Cruikshank DP: Should all women be offered elective cesarean delivery? Obstet Gynecol 102:217, 2003

Orji EO, Olabode TO, Kuti O, et al: A randomised controlled trial of early initiation of oral feeding after cesarean section. J Matern Fetal Neonatal Med 22(1):65, 2009

Oshiro BT, Henry E, Wilson J, et al: Decreasing elective deliveries before 39 weeks of gestation in an integrated health care system. Obstet Gynecol 113(4):804, 2009

Pickrell K: An inquiry into the history of cesarean section. Bull Soc Med Hist (Chicago) 4:414, 1935

Pietrantoni M, Parsons MT, O'Brien WF, et al: Peritoneal closure or nonclosure at cesarean. Obstet Gynecol 77:293, 1991

Plauche WC: Obstetric hysterectomy. In Hankins GDV, Clark SL, Cunningham FG, et al (eds): Operative Obstetrics. Norwalk, Conn, Appleton & Lange, 1995, p 333

Porreco RP: Meeting the challenge of the rising cesarean birth rate. Obstet Gynecol 75:133, 1990

Pridijian G, Hibbard JU, Moawad AH: Cesarean: Changing the trends. Obstet Gynecol 77:195, 1991

Pritchard JA: Changes in the blood volume during pregnancy and delivery. Anesthesiology 26:393, 1965

Rafique Z, Shibli KU, Russell IF, et al: A randomised controlled trial of the closure or non-closure of peritoneum at caesarean section: Effect on postoperative pain. Br J Obstet Gynaecol 109:694, 2002

Rajasekar D, Hall M: Urinary tract injuries during obstetric intervention. Br J Obstet Gynaecol 104:731, 1997

Ramsey PS, White AM, Guinn DA, et al: Subcutaneous tissue reapproximation, alone or in combination with drain, in obese women undergoing cesarean delivery. Obstet Gynecol 105(5 Pt 1):967, 2005

Rodriguez AI, Porter KB, O'Brien WF: Blunt versus sharp expansion of the uterine incision in low-segment transverse cesarean section. Am J Obstet Gynecol 171:1022, 1994

Roset E, Boulvain M, Irion O: Nonclosure of the peritoneum during cesarean section: Long-term follow-up of a randomized controlled trial. Eur J Obstet Gynecol Reprod Biol 108:40, 2003

Sakse A, Weber T, Nickelsen C, et al: Peripartum hysterectomy in Denmark 1995-2004. Acta Obstet Gynecol Scand 86(12):1472, 2007

Sanchez-Ramos L, Kaunitz AM, Peterson HB, et al: Reducing cesarean sections at a teaching hospital. Am J Obstet Gynecol 163:1081, 1990

Scheller JM, Nelson KB: Does cesarean delivery prevent cerebral palsy or other neurologic problems of childhood? Obstet Gynecol 83:624, 1994

Seago DP, Roberts WE, Johnson VK, et al: Planned cesarean hysterectomy: A preferred alternative to separate operations. Am J Obstet Gynecol 180:1385, 1999

Sewell JE: Cesarean Section—A Brief History. Washington, DC, American College of Obstetricians and Gynecologists, 1993

Shellhaas C for the National Institute of Child Health and Human Development Maternal–Fetal Medicine Units Network: The MFMU Cesarean Registry: Cesarean hysterectomy—its indications, morbidities, and mortality. Am J Obstet Gynecol 185:S123, 2001

Shrivastava V, Nageotte M, Major C, et al: Case-control comparison of cesarean hysterectomy with and without prophylactic placement of intravascular balloon catheters for placenta accreta. Am J Obstet Gynecol 197(4):402.e1, 2007

Silver RM, Landon MB, Rouse DJ, et al: Maternal morbidity associated with multiple repeat cesarean deliveries. Obstet Gynecol 107:1226, 2006

Spong CY, Landon MB, Gilbert S, et al: Risk of uterine rupture and adverse perinatal outcome at term after cesarean delivery. Obstet Gynecol 110(4):801, 2007

Stark M, Chavkin Y, Kupfersztain C, et al: Evaluation of combinations of procedures in cesarean section. Int J Gynecol Obstet 48(3):273, 1995

Strong TH, Brown WL Jr, Brown WL, et al: Experience with early postcesarean hospital dismissal. Am J Obstet Gynecol 169:116, 1993

Sullivan SA, Smith T, Chang E, et al: Administration of cefazolin prior to skin incision is superior to cefazolin at cord clamping in preventing postcesarean infectious morbidity: A randomized controlled trial. Am J Obstet Gynecol 196:455, 2007

Texas Medical Liability Trust: PIAA releases national closed claim data. The Reporter, November-December 2004

Thigpen BD, Hood WA, Chauhan S, et al: Timing of prophylactic antibiotic administration in the uninfected laboring gravida: A randomized clinical trial. Am J Obstet Gynecol 192:1864, 2005

Thacker SB, Stroup D, Chang M: Continuous electronic heart rate monitoring for fetal assessment during labor. Cochrane Database Syst Rev 2:CD000063, 2001

Tita AT, Hauth JC, Grimes A, et al: Decreasing incidence of postcesarean endometritis with extended–spectrum antibiotic prophylaxis. Obstet Gynecol 111(1):51, 2008

Tita AT, Landon MB, Spong CY, et al: Timing of elective repeat cesarean delivery at term and neonatal outcomes. N Engl J Med 360(2):111, 2009

Tita AT, Rouse DJ, Blackwell S, et al: Emerging concepts in antibiotic prophylaxis for cesarean delivery: A systematic review. Obstet Gynecol 113(3):675, 2009

Tulandi T, Al-Jaroudi D: Nonclosure of peritoneum: A reappraisal. Am J Obstet Gynecol 189:609, 2003

U.S. Department of Health and Human Services: Healthy People 2010 Midcourse Review. 2006 Available at: http://www.healthypeople.gov/data/midcourse/pdf/ExecutiveSummary.pdf Accessed July 27, 2008

U.S. Department of Health and Human Services: Healthy People 2010, 2nd ed. With Understanding and Improving Health and Objectives for Improving Health. 2 vols. Washington, DC, U.S. Government Printing Office, November 2000

Villar J, Carroli G, Zavaleta N, et al: Maternal and neonatal individual risks and benefits associated with caesarean delivery: Multicentre prospective study. BJM 335:1025, 2007

Walsh CA, Walsh SR: Extraabdominal vs intraabdominal uterine repair at cesarean delivery: A metaanalysis. Am J Obstet Gynecol 200(6):625.e1, 2009

World Health Organization: International statistical classification of diseases and related health problems, 10th revision, version for 2007. Available at: http://www.who.int/classifications/apps/icd/icd10online/. Accessed July 27, 2008

Worley KC, McIntire DD, Leveno KJ: The prognosis for spontaneous labor in women with uncomplicated term pregnancies: Implications for cesarean delivery on maternal request. Obstet Gynecol 113(4):812, 2009

Yost NP, Bloom SL, Sibley MK, et al: A hospital-sponsored quality improvement study of pain management after cesarean delivery. Am J Obstet Gynecol 190:1341, 2004

Zelop CM, Harlow BL, Frigoletto FD Jr, et al: Emergency peripartum hysterectomy. Am J Obstet Gynecol 168:1443, 1993

Zorlu CG, Turan C, Isik AZ, et al: Emergency hysterectomy in modern obstetric practice. Changing clinical perspective in time. Acta Obstet Gynecol Scand 77(2):186, 1998

CHAPTER 26

Prior Cesarean Delivery

Few issues in modern obstetrics have been as controversial as the management of the woman who has had a prior cesarean delivery. For many decades, a scarred uterus was believed by most to contraindicate labor out of fear of uterine rupture. In 1916 Cragin made his famous, oft-quoted, and now seemingly excessive pronouncement, "Once a cesarean, always a cesarean." Recall that when this statement was made, the classical vertical uterine incision was used almost universally. Even so, some of his contemporaries did not totally agree with his pronouncement. For example, J. Whitridge Williams (1917) termed the statement "an exaggeration" in the fourth edition of *Williams Obstetrics.*

In the 1920s the technique of low-transverse uterine incision was introduced by Kerr (1921). Leading obstetrical institutions subsequently reported that although catastrophic uterine rupture developed in at least 4 percent of prior classical incisions, only about 0.5 percent of transverse incisions ruptured. And while caution reigned, beginning in the 1950s comfort with the low-transverse incisions resulted in a number of reports that described the de facto policy of a trial of labor in some women without recurring indications for cesarean delivery. And even with repeat cesarean delivery being the stated norm, Hellman and Pritchard

(1971) wrote in the 14th edition of *Williams Obstetrics* that "many reliable institutions, however, report a 30-to 40-percent rate of vaginal deliveries following cesarean section without difficulty." In 1978, Merrill and Gibbs reported that subsequent vaginal delivery was safely accomplished at the University of Texas at San Antonio in 83 percent of women with a prior cesarean delivery.

Thus, interest was rekindled in vaginal birth especially as the rates of primary cesarean delivery were increasing at an unprecedented pace. Between 1980 and 1988, for example, the cesarean rate jumped from 17 to 25 percent. Meanwhile, more evidence had accrued that uterine rupture was infrequent and rarely catastrophic. In an effort to address the rising cesarean delivery rate, the American College of Obstetricians and Gynecologists (1988) recommended that most women with one previous low-transverse cesarean delivery should be counseled to attempt labor in a subsequent pregnancy. Accordingly, the frequency of vaginal birth after cesarean—commonly referred to as *VBAC*—increased significantly. And as shown in Figure 26-1, by 1996 almost a third of women with a prior cesarean were being delivered vaginally. Pitkin (1991), who was editor of *Obstetrics & Gynecology* at that time, wrote that "without question, the most remarkable change in obstetric practice over the last decade was management of the woman with prior cesarean delivery."

TRIAL OF LABOR VERSUS REPEAT CESAREAN DELIVERY

Associated Risks

Beginning in 1989, as the number of women attempting vaginal delivery increased, there were a growing number of reports that described increased rates of uterine rupture and perinatal morbidity and mortality leading some to suggest that VBAC might be riskier than anticipated (Flamm, 1997; Leveno, 1999; Scott, 1991). In 1998 and 1999, the American College of Obstetricians and Gynecologists issued updated Practice Bulletins supporting VBAC, but also urging a more cautious approach. Subsequently,

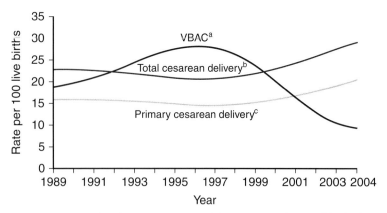

FIGURE 26-1 Total and primary cesarean delivery rates and vaginal birth after previous cesarean (VBAC) rate: United States, 1989–2004. [a]VBAC = number of vaginal births after previous cesarean delivery per 100 births. [b]Percentage of all live births by cesarean delivery. [c]Number of primary cesarean deliveries per 100 live births to women without a prior cesarean delivery. From National Institutes of Health State-of-the-Science Conference Statement, 2006.

fewer women attempted VBAC, and there was a corresponding increase in the overall cesarean delivery rate (see Fig. 26-1). In 2007, VBAC rates in the U.S. decreased to a rate of 8.5 percent (Hamilton and associates, 2009).

Fetal Risk

Uterine rupture and its associated complications clearly are increased with a trial of labor. But some have argued that these factors should weigh only minimally in the decision to attempt

VBAC because their absolute risk is low. One of the largest and most comprehensive studies designed to examine risks associated with VBAC was conducted by the Maternal-Fetal Medicine Units (MFMU) Network and reported by Landon and colleagues (2004). In this prospective study conducted at 19 academic medical centers, the outcomes of nearly 18,000 women who attempted a trial of labor were compared with those of more than 15,000 women who underwent elective repeat cesarean delivery. As shown in Table 26-1, although the risk of uterine rupture was higher among women undergoing a trial of labor, the absolute risk was small—only 7 per 1000. To the contrary, however, there were no uterine ruptures in the elective cesarean delivery group. Of note, rates of stillbirth and hypoxic ischemic encephalopathy were significantly greater in the trial of labor arm. Others have reported similar results (Chauhan and colleagues, 2003; Mozurkewich and Hutton, 2000).

In another study, Smith and associates (2002) analyzed outcomes associated with a trial of labor compared with those of planned repeat cesarean delivery in nearly 25,000 women with a prior cesarean delivery. The risk of delivery-related perinatal death was 1.3 per 1000 among the 15,515 women who attempted VBAC. Although the absolute risk was again small, this rate was *11 times greater* than the risk of perinatal death in 9014 women who planned repeat cesarean delivery.

Collectively, these data suggest that the absolute risk of uterine rupture attributable to a trial of labor resulting in death or

TABLE 26-1. Complications in Women with a Prior Cesarean Delivery Enrolled in the NICHD Maternal-Fetal Medicine Units Network, 1999–2002

Complication	Trial of Labor Group n = 17,898 (%)	Elective Repeat Cesarean Group n = 15,801 (%)	Odds Ratio (95% Confidence Interval)	p-value
Uterine rupture	124 (0.7)	0	N/A	<.001
Uterine dehiscence	119 (0.7)	76 (0.5)	1.38 (1.04–1.85)	.03
Hysterectomy	41 (0.2)	47 (0.3)	0.77 (0.51–1.17)	.22
Thromboembolic disease	7 (0.04)	10 (0.1)	0.62 (0.24–1.62)	.32
Transfusion	304 (1.7)	158 (1.0)	1.71 (1.41–2.08)	<.001
Uterine infection	517 (2.9)	285 (1.8)	1.62 (1.40–1.87)	<.001
Maternal death	3 (0.02)	7 (0.04)	0.38 (0.10–1.46)	.21
Antepartum stillbirth[a]				
37–38 weeks	18 (0.4)	8 (0.1)	2.93 (1.27–6.75)	.008
39 weeks or more	16 (0.2)	5 (0.1)	2.70 (0.99–7.38)	.07
Intrapartum stillbirth[a]				
37–38 weeks	1	0	N/A	.43
39 weeks or more	1	0	N/A	1.00
Term HIE[a]	12 (0.08)	0	N/A	<.001
Term neonatal death[a]	13 (0.08)	7 (0.05)	1.82 (0.73–4.57)	.19

[a]Denominator is 15,338 for the trial of labor group and 15,014 for the elective repeat cesarean delivery group.
HIE = hypoxic ischemic encephalopathy; N/A = not applicable; NICHD = National Institute of Child Health and Human Development.
Adapted from Landon MB, Hauth JC, Leveno KJ, et al: Maternal and perinatal outcomes associated with a trial of labor after prior cesarean delivery. *N Engl J Med* 351:2581, with permission. Copyright © 2004 Massachusetts Medical Society. All rights reserved.

injury to the fetus is approximately 1 per 1000. Thus, the major controversy surrounding the management of women with a prior cesarean delivery stems from the question: *Is a 1 per 1000 risk of having an otherwise healthy fetus die or be damaged as a result of a trial of labor acceptable?*

Maternal Risk

Another potential argument in support of VBAC has been that a trial of labor is associated with reduced risks for the mother compared with those of a repeat cesarean delivery. Most studies suggest that the maternal *mortality* rate does not differ significantly between women undergoing a trial of labor compared with those undergoing an elective repeat cesarean (Landon and collaborators, 2004; Mozurkewich and Hutton, 2000). In a retrospective cohort study of more than 300,000 Canadian women with a prior cesarean delivery, Wen and associates (2005) found an increased—albeit statistically nonsignificant—maternal mortality rate with elective repeat cesarean delivery. Specifically, the maternal death rate for women undergoing an elective repeat cesarean delivery was 5.6 per 100,000 compared with 1.6 per 100,000 for those having a trial of labor.

Estimates of maternal *morbidity* have produced conflicting results. In the meta-analysis by Mozurkewich and Hutton (2000), women undergoing a trial of labor were approximately half as likely to require a blood transfusion or hysterectomy compared with those undergoing repeat cesarean delivery. Conversely, in the MFMU Network study cited earlier, Landon and co-workers (2004) observed that the risks of transfusion and infection were significantly greater for women attempting a trial of labor (see Table 26-1). Rossi and D'Addario (2008) reported similar findings in their meta-analysis. McMahon and associates (1996), in a population-based study of 6138 women, found that major complications—hysterectomy, uterine rupture, or operative injury—were almost twice as common in women undergoing a trial of labor compared with those undergoing an elective second cesarean delivery. Moreover, compared with a successful trial of labor, the risk of these major complications was fivefold greater in women whose attempt at a vaginal delivery failed. Similarly, El-Sayed and associates (2007) found a fivefold higher rate of chorioamnionitis and a twofold higher rate of hemorrhage among women with a failed trial of labor compared with those having a successful attempt. Finally, after their meta-analysis, Rossi and D'Addario (2008) also reported an increased incidence of overall maternal complications when women with a failed VBAC were compared with those undergoing successful VBAC—17 versus 3 percent, respectively.

Patient Preference

As described in Chapter 25 (p. 547), compared with vaginal delivery, cesarean birth is associated with increased risks. Some of these are anesthesia complications, hemorrhage, damage to the bladder and other organs, pelvic infection, and adhesion formation. Moreover, many of these risks escalate progressively with increasing numbers of cesarean deliveries (Silver and associates, 2006).

Despite these potential concerns, an elective repeat cesarean delivery is considered by many women to be preferable to a trial of labor. Frequent reasons include the convenience of a scheduled delivery and the fear of a prolonged and potentially dangerous labor. Abitbol and associates (1993) found that these preferences persisted despite extensive antepartum counseling. They interviewed women at discharge and of those who selected repeat cesarean delivery, 93 percent reported satisfaction. This compared with only 53 percent of women overall who elected a trial of labor and 80 percent of those who had an uncomplicated trial of labor.

CANDIDATES FOR A TRIAL OF LABOR

Selection of women best suited for a trial of labor is particularly challenging. Indeed, reviews by Hashima (2004) and Guise (2004) and their associates led them to conclude that there are few high-quality data available to guide this clinical decision. Clearly, however, the fewer the number of complicating risk factors, the greater is the likelihood of success (Gregory and co-workers, 2008).

In a recent secondary analysis of the MFMU Network study cited earlier, Grobman and colleagues (2007b) developed a nomogram to help predict a successful trial of labor (Fig. 26-2). These investigators also used this tool to predict risk of associated maternal morbidity with VBAC (Grobman and colleagues, 2009). The model is applicable only to women with one prior cesarean delivery who are at term. In a comparable effort, Srinivas and associates (2007) concluded that the use of only six variables—maternal age and race, gestational age, type of labor, prior cesarean indication, and history of vaginal delivery—could not be reliably used to predict successful VBAC. And in a third study, Macones and associates (2006) attempted to develop a clinical model to predict uterine rupture. They incorporated many antepartum and intrapartum factors and concluded that rupture was not predictable with either individual or multiple clinical characteristics. The investigators from the MFMU Network reached a similar conclusion (Grobman and colleagues, 2008).

Despite these limitations for precision, a number of points are pertinent to the evaluation of women for a trial of labor. Current recommendations of the American College of Obstetricians and Gynecologists (2004) for selecting appropriate candidates are listed in Table 26-2.

TABLE 26-2. Some Factors for Consideration in Selection of Candidates for Vaginal Birth after Cesarean Delivery (VBAC)

- One previous prior low-transverse cesarean delivery
- Clinically adequate pelvis
- No other uterine scars or previous rupture
- Physician immediately available throughout active labor capable of monitoring labor and performing an emergency cesarean delivery
- Availability of anesthesia and personnel for emergency cesarean delivery

Reprinted, with permission, from American College of Obstetricians and Gynecologists. Vaginal birth after previous cesarean delivery. ACOG Practice Bulletin 54. Washington, DC: ACOG; 2004.

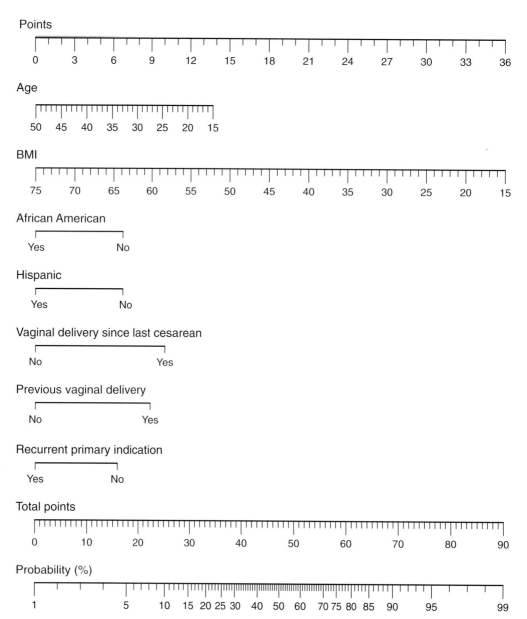

FIGURE 26-2 Predictive nomogram for probability of vaginal birth after cesarean delivery (VBAC). This nomogram is used by locating each patient characteristic and finding the number of points on the uppermost scale to which that characteristic corresponds. For example, a maternal age of 26 years corresponds to approximately 10 points. The sum of points generated from each of these characteristics is compared with the "total points" scale, and the predicted probability of VBAC is determined from the corresponding point on the lowermost scale. As an example, the woman with 60 total points has a 75- to 80-percent chance of a successful VBAC. (Reproduced from Grobman and colleagues, 2007b, with permission.)

Type of Prior Uterine Incision

Women with a transverse scar confined to the lower uterine segment have the lowest risk of symptomatic scar separation during a subsequent pregnancy (Table 26-3). The highest risks are with prior vertical incisions extending into the fundus such as the classical incision shown in Figure 26-3. Importantly, in some women, the classical scar will rupture before the onset of labor, and this can happen several weeks before term. In a review of 157 women with a prior classical cesarean delivery, Chauhan and colleagues (2002) reported that one woman had a complete uterine rupture prior to the onset of labor, whereas 9 percent had a uterine dehiscence.

The risk of uterine rupture in women with a prior vertical incision that did not extend into the fundus is unclear. Martin (1997) and Shipp (1999) and their co-workers reported that these low vertical uterine incisions did not have an increased risk for rupture compared with that of low transverse incisions. The American College of Obstetricians and Gynecologists (2004) concluded that, although there is limited evidence, women with a prior vertical incision in the lower uterine segment without fundal extension may be candidates for VBAC. This is in contrast to prior classical or T-shaped uterine incisions, which are considered contraindications to labor.

TABLE 26-3. Types of Prior Uterine Incisions and Estimated Risks for Uterine Rupture

Prior Incision	Estimated Rupture Rate (Percent)
Classical	4–9
T-shaped	4–9
Low-vertical[a]	1–7
Low-transverse	0.2–1.5
Prior uterine rupture	
Lower segment	6
Upper uterus	32

[a]See text for definition.
Data from the American College of Obstetricians and Gynecologists (1999, 2004), Chauhan (2002), Martin (1997), Reyes-Ceja (1969), Ritchie (1971), Shipp (1999), and all their colleagues.

Nowadays, there are very few indications for a primary vertical incision, and in those instances—for example, preterm breech fetus with an undeveloped lower segment—the "low vertical" incision almost invariably extends into the active segment. It is not known, however, how far upward the incision has to extend before risks become those of a true classical incision. It is helpful in the operative report to document its exact extent.

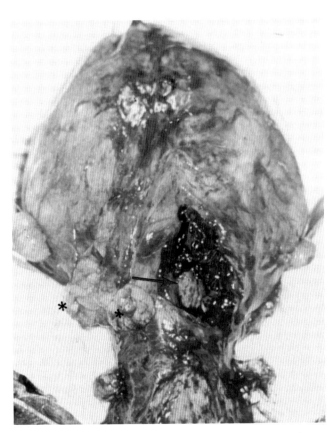

FIGURE 26-3 Ruptured vertical cesarean section scar (*arrow*) identified at time of repeat cesarean delivery early in labor. The asterisk to the left indicates some of the sites of densely adherent omentum.

And although the type of prior incision was not known, Sciscione and associates (2008) reported that women who had a prior preterm cesarean delivery were approximately twice as likely to suffer a uterine rupture compared with those with a prior term cesarean delivery. This may be in part explained by the increased likelihood of extension of the uterine incision into the contractile portion. Harper and co-workers (2009), however, did not find a significantly increased rate of rupture during subsequent VBAC in those with a prior cesarean delivery performed at ≤ 34 weeks.

There are special considerations for women with uterine malformations who have undergone cesarean delivery. Earlier reports suggested that the risks for uterine rupture in a subsequent pregnancy may be as high as with a classical incision. Specifically, Ravasia and associates (1999) in a study of 25 women with müllerian duct anomalies and a prior low transverse cesarean delivery reported that subsequent uterine rupture occurred in 2 women— 8 percent. Importantly, and as discussed later (see p. 572), both of these women had labor induced with prostaglandin E_2 gel. In a more recent study, Erez and co-workers (2007) described the outcomes of 165 women with müllerian duct anomalies who had one prior cesarean delivery. In this retrospective study, 103 of the women attempted a trial of labor, and 61 percent of these delivered vaginally. There were no cases of uterine rupture—and in only 10 women was labor induced—and maternal morbidity rates were comparable with similar women without müllerian anomalies (Chap. 40, p. 891).

Given the wide range of risk for uterine rupture associated with various types of prior uterine incisions, it is not surprising that most fellows of the American College of Obstetricians and Gynecologists consider the type of prior incision to be the most important factor when considering a trial of labor (Coleman and co-workers, 2005).

Prior Uterine Rupture

Women who have previously sustained a uterine rupture are at increased risk for recurrence during a subsequent attempted VBAC. As shown in Table 26-3, those with a previous low-segment rupture have a 6-percent recurrence risk, whereas prior upper uterine rupture confers a 32-percent risk (Reyes-Ceja and associates, 1969; Ritchie, 1971). We believe that women with prior uterine ruptures or classical or T-shaped incisions ideally should undergo repeat cesarean delivery when fetal pulmonary maturity is assured, and preferably prior to the onset of labor. They should also be counseled regarding the hazards of unattended labor and signs of possible uterine rupture.

Closure of Prior Incision

As discussed in Chapter 25 (see p. 552), the low-transverse uterine incision can be sutured in either one or two layers. Whether the risk of subsequent uterine rupture is affected by these is unclear. Chapman (1997) and Tucker (1993) and their associates found no relationship between a one- and two-layer closure and the risk of subsequent uterine rupture. And although Durnwald and Mercer (2003) also found no increased risk of rupture, they reported that uterine dehiscence was more common after single-layer closure. In contrast, Bujold and co-workers (2002) found that a single-layer closure was associated with nearly a fourfold increased risk of rupture compared with a double-layer closure. In response, Vidaeff and Lucas (2003) argued that experimental models of wound healing have not demonstrated advantages of a double-layer closure. Because of potentially confounding variables inherent in this type of retrospective study, they concluded that the evidence is insufficient to routinely recommend a double-layer closure. At our institutions we routinely suture the low-segment incision with one running locking suture (see Chap. 25, p. 552).

Interdelivery Interval

It seems logical to assume that the risk of uterine rupture would be increased if a hysterotomy scar did not have sufficient time to heal. Magnetic resonance imaging studies of myometrial healing suggest that complete uterine involution and restoration of anatomy may require at least 6 months (Dicle and colleagues, 1997). To explore this issue further, Shipp and associates (2001) examined the relationship between interdelivery interval and uterine rupture in 2409 women who had one prior cesarean delivery. Uterine rupture developed in 29 women—1.4 percent. Interdelivery intervals of 18 months or less were associated with a threefold increased risk of symptomatic rupture during a subsequent trial of labor compared with intervals greater than 18 months. Similarly, Stamilio and co-workers (2007) noted a threefold increased risk of uterine rupture in women with an interpregnancy interval of less than 6 months compared with one of 6 months or longer. However, interpregnancy intervals of 6 to 18 months did not significantly increase the risk of uterine rupture or maternal morbidity.

Number of Prior Cesarean Incisions

It also seems logical that the risk of uterine rupture would increase with the number of previous cesarean deliveries. Miller and colleagues (1994) studied 12,707 such women undergoing a trial of labor. They reported rupture rates of 0.6 percent following one cesarean delivery and 1.8 percent for women with two prior cesarean deliveries. Similarly, Macones and associates (2005a) reported a twofold increase in the rate of uterine rupture among women attempting trial of labor after two prior cesarean deliveries—1.8 percent—compared with those with one—0.9 percent. In contrast, analysis of the MFMU Network database by Landon and co-workers (2006) did not confirm this. Instead, they reported an insignificant difference in the uterine rupture rate in 975 women with multiple prior cesarean deliveries compared with 16,915 women with a single prior operation—0.9 versus 0.7 percent, respectively.

Prior Vaginal Delivery

Any previous vaginal delivery, either before or following a cesarean birth, significantly improves the prognosis for a subsequent vaginal delivery with either spontaneous or induced labor (Grinstead and Grobman, 2004; Hendler and co-workers, 2004; Mercer and colleagues, 2008). Prior vaginal delivery also lowers the risk of subsequent uterine rupture and other mor-

bidities (Cahill and co-workers, 2006; Zelop and associates, 2000). Indeed, the most favorable prognostic factor is prior vaginal delivery. The American College of Obstetricians and Gynecologists (2004) has taken the position that for women with two prior low transverse cesarean deliveries, only those with a prior vaginal delivery should be considered candidates for a spontaneous trial of labor.

Indication for Prior Cesarean Delivery

The success rate for a trial of labor depends to some extent on the indication for the previous cesarean delivery. Generally, 60 to 80 percent of labor trials after prior cesarean birth result in vaginal delivery (American College of Obstetricians and Gynecologists, 2004). In a large series reported by Wing and Paul (1999), 91 percent of women whose first cesarean delivery was for breech presentation subsequently delivered vaginally. If fetal distress was the original indication, the success rate was 84 percent. Importantly, only 38 percent delivered vaginally if the fetus born during a trial of labor birth had a birthweight exceeding the initial pregnancy birthweight by more than 500 g.

Prior dystocia is an important predictor of vaginal delivery after prior cesarean. In more than 1900 women, Peaceman and associates (2006) found that those with dystocia as the original indication had a significantly lower success rate compared with those with other indications—54 versus 67 percent, respectively. Bujold and Gauthier (2001) reported a 75-percent vaginal delivery rate in women whose prior cesarean delivery was for second-stage dystocia.

Fetal Size

It has not been conclusively proven that increasing fetal size increases the risk for uterine rupture with VBAC. Zelop and associates (2001) compared the outcomes of almost 2750 women undergoing a trial of labor of whom 1.1 percent had a uterine rupture. The rate increased—albeit not significantly—with increasing fetal weight—1.0 percent for <4000 g, 1.6 percent for >4000 g, and 2.4 percent for >4250 g. Similarly, Elkousy and colleagues (2003) reported that for women attempting VBAC who had no previous vaginal deliveries, the relative risk of rupture doubled if birthweight was >4000 g. Finally, women who attempt a trial of labor with a preterm fetus have lower rupture rates with successful vaginal delivery rates that are the same or higher as for other conditions discussed (Durnwald and associates, 2006; Quiñones and colleagues, 2005).

Multifetal Gestation

Perhaps surprisingly, twin pregnancy does not appear to increase the risk of uterine rupture with VBAC. Ford and associates (2006) analyzed the outcomes of 1850 such women with a prior cesarean delivery who attempted a trial of labor. The uterine rupture rate was 0.9 percent, and the rate of successful vaginal delivery was 45 percent. Similar studies by Cahill (2005) and Varner (2007) and their colleagues reported rupture rates of 0.7 to 1.1 percent and vaginal delivery rates of 75 to 85 percent.

TABLE 26-4. Timing of Elective Repeat Cesarean Delivery at Term and Neonatal Outcomes

Outcome	Wk 37 (n = 834) (%)	Wk 38 (n = 3909) (%)	Wk 39 (n = 6512) (%)	Wk 40 (n = 1385) (%)	p for trend[a]
Any adverse outcome or death	15.3	11.0	8.0	7.3	<0.001
Admission to the NICU	12.8	8.1	5.9	4.8	<0.001
Adverse respiratory outcome					
RDS	3.7	1.9	0.9	0.9	<0.001
RDS or TTN	8.2	5.5	3.4	3.0	<0.001
Ventilation in 1st 24 hr	1.9	0.9	0.4	0.4	<0.001
Newborn sepsis[b]	7.0	4.0	2.5	2.7	<0.001
Proven case	0.4	0.1	0.1	0.1	0.260
Treated hypoglycemia	2.4	0.9	0.7	0.8	<0.001
Hospitalization ≥ 5 days	9.1	5.7	3.6	4.1	<0.001

[a]The p value was calculated by the Cochran-Armitage test for trend for the period from 37 to 39 weeks only.
[b]Newborn sepsis includes both suspected and proven infections.
NICU = neonatal intensive care unit; RDS = respiratory distress syndrome; TTN = transient tachypnea of the newborn.
Used with permission of the American Academy of Pediatrics, American College of Obstetricians and Gynecologists. Guidelines for perinatal care. 6th ed. Elk Grove Village (IL): AAP; Washington, DC: ACOG; 2007. Copyright American Academy of Pediatrics and American College of Obstetricans and Gynecologists, 2007.

Maternal Obesity

Obesity decreases the success of VBAC. Hibbard and colleagues (2006) reported the following vaginal delivery rates: 85 percent with a normal body mass index (BMI), 78 percent with a BMI between 25 and 30, 70 percent with a BMI between 30 and 40, and 61 percent with a BMI of 40 or more. Similar findings were reported by Juhasz and associates (2005).

LABOR AND DELIVERY CONSIDERATIONS

If elective repeat cesarean delivery is planned, it is essential that the fetus be mature. Significant and appreciable adverse neonatal morbidity has been reported with elective delivery prior to 39 completed weeks (Table 26-4) (Clark and colleagues, 2009; Tita and co-workers, 2009). The American Academy of Pediatrics and the American College of Obstetricians and Gynecologists (2007) have established guidelines shown in Table 26-5 for timing an elective operation. If none of the four is met, then fetal pulmonary maturity should be documented by amnionic fluid analysis before elective repeat cesarean delivery. Techniques for amnionic fluid assessment are outlined by the American College of Obstetricians and Gynecologists (2008) and described in Chapter 29 (p. 606). Alternatively, spontaneous labor is awaited.

Informed Consent

No woman with a prior uterine incision should be forced to undergo a trial of labor. Instead, the risks and benefits of a trial of labor versus a repeat cesarean delivery should be discussed. The ultimate decision to attempt VBAC should be made by the informed woman in conjunction with her physician. The American Academy of Pediatrics and the American College of Obstetricians and Gynecologists (2007) recommend that the issues listed in Table 26-6 be addressed in arriving at that decision.

Intrapartum Care

The guidelines listed in Table 26-2 are used in the care of women who have chosen a trial of labor. Lavin and co-workers (2002) surveyed all hospitals in Ohio to determine the number that actually

TABLE 26-5. Criteria for Establishment of Fetal Maturity

Fetal maturity may be assumed if one of the following criteria is met:
1. Fetal heart sounds have been documented for 20 weeks by nonelectronic fetoscope or for 30 weeks by Doppler ultrasound.
2. It has been 36 weeks since a positive serum or urine hCG pregnancy test was performed by a reliable laboratory.
3. A sonographic measurement of the crown-rump length, obtained at 6 to 11 weeks, supports a current gestational age of 39 weeks or more.
4. Clinical history and physical and sonographic examination performed at 12 to 20 weeks support current gestational age of 39 weeks or more.

Used with permission of the American Academy of Pediatrics, American College of Obstetricians and Gynecologists. Guidelines for perinatal care. 6th ed. Elk Grove Village (IL): AAP; Washington, DC: ACOG; 2007. Copyright American Academy of Pediatrics and American College of Obstetricans and Gynecologists, 2007.

TABLE 26-6. Recommended Counseling Points for Women With a Prior Cesarean Delivery

- Advantages of a successful vaginal delivery, for example, shorter postpartum hospital stay; less painful, more rapid recovery; and others.
- Contraindications to a trial of labor, for example, prior classical cesarean, previous uterine rupture, lack of resources to perform emergency cesarean delivery during labor, and others.
- Relative contraindications, for example, two prior uterine surgeries with no previous vaginal delivery.
- Risk of uterine rupture—generally less than 1 percent.
- Increased risk of uterine rupture with multiple uterine surgeries, uterine tachysystole, attempts at cervical ripening or labor induction with oxytocin.
- Uterine rupture has been associated with fetal death as well as severe neonatal neurological injury and may occur no matter what resources are available to manage it.

From the American College of Obstetricians and Gynecologists and American Academy of Pediatrics (2007), with permission.

had an obstetrician, anesthesia personnel, and a surgical team immediately available—present in the hospital—when a woman attempted a VBAC. A complete complement was available in 15 percent of Level I, 63 percent of Level II, and 100 percent of Level III institutions. Because VBAC attempts were equally distributed among the institutions, it is obvious that many women are undergoing a trial of labor under less than optimal conditions.

Similar concerns were raised by Bucklin and associates (2005) after their 2001 obstetrical anesthesia workforce survey. They reported that hospital by-laws require an anesthesiologist to be in-hospital for women attempting a VBAC without epidural analgesia in 86 percent of hospitals that have at least 1500 annual deliveries, 45 percent of hospitals with 500 to 1499 deliveries, and 33 percent of those with 100 to 500 deliveries.

Cervical Ripening and Labor Stimulation

Most evidence suggests that any attempt to stimulate cervical ripening or to induce or augment labor increases the uterine rupture risk in women undergoing a trial of labor.

Oxytocin

Induction or augmentation of labor with oxytocin has been implicated in increased rates of uterine rupture in women attempting VBAC. In the MFMU Network study reported by Landon and colleagues (2004), uterine rupture was more frequent in those women induced with oxytocin alone—1.1 percent—compared with those in spontaneous labor—0.4 percent. Among women in this trial who had never had a prior vaginal delivery, the uterine rupture risk associated with an oxytocin induction was 1.8 percent—a fourfold increased risk compared with spontaneous labor (Grobman and co-workers,

2007a). These observations are similar to those of Zelop and associates (1999), who reported a 2.3 percent uterine rupture rate with labor induction compared with 1 percent of women whose labor was augmented or 0.4 percent with spontaneous labor.

Cahill and colleagues (2008) found that as the infusion dose of oxytocin increased, so did the risk of uterine rupture. At their maximum infusion dose of 21 to 30 mU/min, the risk of uterine rupture was fourfold greater than that in women not given oxytocin. Goetzl and associates (2001) described similar findings. They concluded that differences in the dose or patterns of oxytocin use associated with uterine rupture were not substantive enough to develop safer induction protocols.

Experiences at Parkland Hospital. Our experiences with uterine ruptures led us to discontinue oxytocin use for labor induction or augmentation in women with a prior cesarean delivery. Specifically, between 1986 and 1990, a trial of labor was undertaken by 2044 of 7049 women—29 percent—with a prior cesarean. Of these, 1482 or 73 percent delivered vaginally. In women who labored spontaneously, uterine rupture with part of the fetus extruded outside of the uterus was identified in three women—a rate of 1.5 per 1000. But in another 307 women who were given oxytocin during their trial of labor, there were three uterine ruptures—a significantly increased rate of 10 per 1000. Because of this sixfold increase with oxytocin use, we adopted the conservative approach.

Prostaglandins

A number of prostaglandin preparations that are commonly employed for cervical ripening or labor induction are discussed in Chapter 22 (p. 502). Their use in women with a prior cesarean delivery is less clear. The studies that have been published, however, urge caution with prostaglandin use in these women.

Wing and colleagues (1998) described a comparative study of prostaglandin E_1—*misoprostol*—versus oxytocin for labor induction in women with a prior cesarean delivery. They terminated their trial after two of the first 17 women assigned to misoprostol developed a uterine rupture. There are several studies that evaluated other prostaglandins for labor induction. In general, they also demonstrated an increased risk of uterine rupture, albeit with variable rates. Ravasia and colleagues (2000) compared uterine rupture in 172 women given prostaglandin E_2 gel with 1544 women in spontaneous labor. The rate of rupture was significantly greater in women treated with prostaglandin E_2 gel—2.9 percent—compared with 0.9 percent in those with spontaneous labor. Lydon-Rochelle and associates (2001) performed a retrospective population-based study. They found that induction of labor with prostaglandins for VBAC increased the uterine rupture risk more than 15-fold compared with elective repeat cesarean delivery. Based in large part on the results of this latter study, the American College of Obstetricians and Gynecologists (2002, 2004) discouraged the use of prostaglandin analogs for cervical ripening or labor induction in women attempting a VBAC.

It is important to note, however, that subsequent studies repeated over the intervening years have been less ominous. For example, in the MFMU Network study cited previously, Landon and colleagues (2004) reported a uterine rupture rate of 1.4 percent when any prostaglandin was used in combination with oxytocin.

But in the subgroup of 227 women in whom labor was induced with a prostaglandin only, there were no ruptures. Macones and co-workers (2005b) reported similar findings. They found that intravaginal prostaglandins alone, *excluding misoprostol*, were not associated with an increased risk of uterine rupture. Importantly, they found that sequential use of a prostaglandin followed by oxytocin was associated with a threefold-increased risk of rupture compared with spontaneous labor. Kayani and Alfirevic (2005) reported two ruptures in 52 women with such sequential use.

In an interesting report, Buhimschi and colleagues (2005) found that women given prostaglandins were more likely to rupture at the site of their old scar. In contrast, women given oxytocin were more likely to rupture at a site *remote* from the old scar. They hypothesized that prostaglandins might induce biochemical modifications in the lower uterine segment scar that predispose it to rupture during labor.

After again reviewing contemporaneous reports, the American College of Obstetricians and Gynecologists (2006) concluded that labor induction in women who attempt a VBAC is a reasonable option. The College advises that potentially increased risk of uterine rupture associated with any induction should be discussed with the woman and documented. Finally, selection of women most likely to have a successful VBAC, as well as avoiding misoprostol and sequential use of prostaglandins and oxytocin, appear to offer the lowest risk of uterine rupture.

Epidural Analgesia

Concerns that epidural analgesia for labor might mask the pain of uterine rupture have not been verified (Farmer and colleagues, 1991; Flamm and associates, 1994). Less than 10 percent of women with scar separation experience pain and bleeding, and fetal heart rate decelerations are the most likely sign of rupture (Flamm and associates, 1990; Kieser and Baskett, 2002). Successful VBAC rates are similar, and in some cases higher, among women with labor epidural analgesia compared with those using other forms of analgesia (Landon and co-workers, 2005; Stovall and colleagues, 1987). The American Academy of Pediatrics and the American College of Obstetricians and Gynecologists (2007) have concluded that epidural analgesia may safely be used during a trial of labor. Importantly, they also recommend that the anesthesia service be available whenever a woman with a prior cesarean delivery is admitted in active labor.

Uterine Scar Exploration

Most clinicians routinely document the integrity of a prior scar by palpation following successful vaginal delivery. Alternatively, uterine exploration is considered by others to be unnecessary. Currently, the benefits of scar evaluation in the asymptomatic women are unclear. There is general agreement, however, that surgical correction of a scar dehiscence is necessary only if significant bleeding is encountered. Asymptomatic separations do not generally require exploratory laparotomy and repair. Our practice is to routinely examine these prior incision sites. Any decision for laparotomy and repair takes into consideration the extent of the tear as well as whether the peritoneal cavity is entered.

External Cephalic Version

Limited data suggest that external cephalic version for breech presentation may be as successful in women with a prior cesarean delivery who are contemplating a trial of labor (American College of Obstetricians and Gynecologists, 2004). This procedure is addressed in Chapter 24 (p. 539).

UTERINE RUPTURE

Classification

Uterine rupture typically is classified as either: (1) *complete* when all layers of the uterine wall are separated, or (2) *incomplete* when the uterine muscle is separated but the visceral peritoneum is intact. Incomplete rupture is also commonly referred to as *uterine dehiscence*. As expected, morbidity and mortality rates are appreciably greater when rupture is complete. The greatest risk factor for either form of rupture is prior cesarean delivery (see Fig. 26-3). In a review of all cases of uterine rupture in Nova Scotia between 1988 and 1997, Kieser and Baskett (2002) reported that 92 percent were in women with a prior cesarean birth. Other causes of uterine rupture are discussed in Chapter 35 (see p. 784).

Diagnosis

Prior to developing hypovolemic shock, symptoms and physical findings in women with uterine rupture may appear bizarre unless the possibility is kept in mind. For example, hemoperitoneum from a ruptured uterus may result in diaphragmatic irritation with pain referred to the chest—directing one to a diagnosis of pulmonary or amnionic fluid embolism instead of uterine rupture. The most common sign of uterine rupture is a nonreassuring fetal heart rate pattern with variable heart rate decelerations that may evolve into late decelerations, bradycardia, and death (American Academy of Pediatrics and American College of Obstetricians and Gynecologists, 2007). Contrary to older teachings, few women experience cessation of contractions following uterine rupture, and the use of intrauterine pressure catheters has not been shown to assist reliably in the diagnosis (Rodriguez and associates, 1989).

In some women, the appearance of uterine rupture is identical to that of placental abruption. In most, however, there is remarkably little appreciable pain or tenderness. Also, because most women in labor are treated for discomfort with either narcotics or epidural analgesia, pain and tenderness may not be readily apparent. The condition usually becomes evident because of signs of fetal distress and occasionally because of maternal hypovolemia from concealed hemorrhage.

If the fetal presenting part has entered the pelvis with labor, loss of station may be detected by pelvic examination. If the fetus is partly or totally extruded from the site of uterine rupture, abdominal palpation or vaginal examination may be helpful to identify the presenting part, which will have moved away from the pelvic inlet. A firm contracted uterus may at times be felt alongside the fetus.

Prognosis

With rupture and expulsion of the fetus into the peritoneal cavity, the chances for intact fetal survival are dismal, and reported mortality rates range from 50 to 75 percent. Fetal condition depends on the degree to which the placental implantation remains intact, although this can change within minutes. With rupture, the only chance of fetal survival is afforded by immediate delivery, most often by laparotomy. Otherwise, hypoxia from both placental separation and maternal hypovolemia is inevitable. If rupture is followed by immediate total placental separation, then very few intact fetuses will be salvaged. For example, in the August 2008 issue of *acog Today*, the emergency team at Sharp Mary Birch Hospital for Women is described. After training, the "decision-to-incision" time was decreased to 14 ± 5.6 minutes. Thus, even in the best of circumstances, fetal salvage will be impaired.

In a study using the Swedish Birth Registry, Kaczmarczyk and colleagues (2007) found that the risk of neonatal death following uterine rupture was 5 percent—a 60-fold increase in the risk compared with pregnancies not complicated by uterine rupture. In the MFMU Network study, 7 of the 114 uterine ruptures—6 percent—associated with a trial of labor were complicated by the development of hypoxic ischemic encephalopathy (Spong and associates, 2007).

Maternal deaths from rupture are uncommon. For example, of 2.5 million women who gave birth in Canada between 1991 and 2001, there were 1898 cases of uterine rupture, and four of these—0.2 percent—resulted in maternal death (Wen and associates, 2005). In other regions of the world, however, maternal mortality rates associated with uterine rupture are much higher. In a report from rural India, for example, the maternal mortality rate associated with uterine rupture was 30 percent (Chatterjee and Bhaduri, 2007).

Hysterectomy versus Repair

With complete rupture during a trial of labor, hysterectomy may be required. In the reports by McMahon (1996) and Miller (1997) and their colleagues, 10 to 20 percent of such women required hysterectomy for hemostasis. In selected cases, however, suture repair with uterine preservation may be performed. Sheth (1968) described outcomes from a series of 66 women in whom repair of a uterine rupture was elected rather than hysterectomy. In 25 instances, the repair was accompanied by tubal sterilization. Thirteen of the 41 mothers who did not have tubal sterilization had a total of 21 subsequent pregnancies, and uterine rupture recurred in four of these—approximately 25 percent. More recently, Usta and associates (2007) identified 37 women with a prior complete uterine rupture delivered over a 25-year period in Lebanon. Hysterectomy was performed in 11, and in the remaining 26 women, the rupture was repaired. Twelve of these women had 24 subsequent pregnancies, of which one third were complicated by recurrent uterine rupture. Hysterectomy is described in Chapter 25 (see p. 556), and management of obstetrical hemorrhage is detailed in Chapter 35 (p. 791).

COMPLICATIONS WITH MULTIPLE REPEAT CESAREAN DELIVERIES

Because of the concerns with attempting a trial of labor—even in the woman with excellent criteria that forecast successful

VBAC—most women in the United States chose elective repeat cesarean delivery (see Fig. 26-1). This choice is not without a number of significant maternal complications that increase in women who have multiple repeat operations. The incidences of some common complications for women with one prior transverse cesarean delivery who undergo an elective repeat cesarean delivery were shown in Table 26-1.

The MFMU Network addressed issues of increased morbidity in a cohort of 30,132 women who had from one to six repeat cesarean deliveries (Silver and associates, 2006). This report addressed a list of morbidities, most of which increased as a trend with increasing number of repeat operations. The rates of some of the more common or serious complications are depicted in Figure 26-4. In addition to ones shown, injuries to the bowel or bladder, admissions to an intensive care unit or ventilator therapy, operative time and hospitalization, and maternal mortality showed significantly increasing trends. Similar results have been reported by Nisenblat (2006) and Usta (2005) and their colleagues.

One particular complication that is especially worrisome is the significantly increased risks for placenta previa with growth into the prior cesarean delivery scar. In some cases a percreta may invade the bladder or other adjacent structures. Difficult resection carries an inordinately high risk of hysterectomy, massive hemorrhage with transfusions, and maternal mortality. Management is described in detail in Chapter 35 (p. 776).

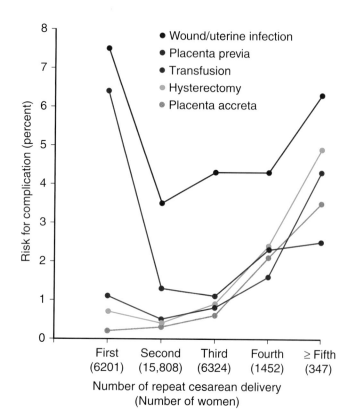

FIGURE 26-4 Maternal-Fetal Medicine Units Network: Rates of some complications with increasing number of repeat cesarean deliveries. (Data from Silver and colleagues, 2006.)

STATE OF VBAC IN 2009

In the United States, VBAC rates have ebbed and flowed from virtually none, to a significant increase, and then to a current decreasing trend. Reasons for this pendulum swing are multifaceted. The most prominent driving force in the repeat cesarean delivery rate is the slow but steady increase in the primary cesarean delivery rate shown in Figure 26-1. Also shown is the effect that decreasing VBAC rates have on the total cesarean delivery rate. The risks versus benefits, along with the pros and cons of a woman electing a trial of labor for VBAC versus elective repeat cesarean delivery, can be complex. The "best answer" for a given woman with a prior cesarean delivery is unknown. Thus, she and her partner are encouraged to actively participate with her healthcare provider in the final decision after appropriate counseling. To minimize some of the confusion in arriving at the decision, the National Institutes of Health is planning a Consensus Development Conference to elucidate the current knowledge on VBAC and its various scenarios. At this time, these deliberations are scheduled to be presented in the spring of 2010.

REFERENCES

Abitbol MM, Castillo I, Taylor UB, et al: Vaginal birth after cesarean section: The patient's point of view. Am Fam Physician 47:129, 1993

acog Today: OB Team Stat improves emergency response. August 2008, p 11

American Academy of Pediatrics and the American College of Obstetricians and Gynecologists: Guidelines for Perinatal Care, 6th ed., 2007

American College of Obstetricians and Gynecologists: Guidelines for vaginal delivery after a previous cesarean birth. Committee Opinion No. 64, October 1988

American College of Obstetricians and Gynecologists: Vaginal birth after previous cesarean delivery. Practice Bulletin No. 2, October 1998

American College of Obstetricians and Gynecologists: Vaginal birth after previous cesarean delivery. Practice Bulletin No. 5, July 1999

American College of Obstetricians and Gynecologists: Induction of labor for vaginal birth after cesarean delivery. Committee Opinion No. 271, April 2002

American College of Obstetricians and Gynecologists: Vaginal birth after previous cesarean delivery. Practice Bulletin No. 54, July 2004

American College of Obstetricians and Gynecologists Committee on Obstetric Practice: Induction of labor for vaginal birth after cesarean delivery. ACOG Committee Opinion No. 342, 2006

American College of Obstetricians and Gynecologists: Fetal lung maturity. Practice Bulletin No. 97, September 2008

Bucklin BA, Hawkins JL, Anderson JR, et al: Obstetric anesthesia workforce survey: Twenty-year update. Anesthesiology 103:645, 2005

Buhimschi CS, Buhimschi IA, Patel S, et al: Rupture of the uterine scar during term labour: Contractility or biochemistry? BJOG 112:38, 2005

Bujold E, Bujold C, Hamilton EF, et al: The impact of a single-layer or double-layer closure on uterine rupture. Am J Obstet Gynecol 186:1326, 2002

Bujold E, Gauthier RJ: Should we allow a trial of labor after a previous cesarean for dystocia in the second stage of labor? Obstet Gynecol 98:652, 2001

Cahill A, Stamilio DM, Paré E, et al: Vaginal birth after cesarean (VBAC) attempt in twin pregnancies: Is it safe? Am J Obstet Gynecol 193:1050, 2005

Cahill AG, Stamilio DM, Odibo A, et al: Is vaginal birth after cesarean (VBAC) or elective repeat cesarean safer in women with a prior vaginal delivery? Am J Obstet Gynecol 195:1143, 2006

Cahill AG, Waterman BM, Stamilio DM, et al: Higher maximum doses of oxytocin are associated with an unacceptably high risk for uterine rupture in patients attempting vaginal birth after cesarean delivery. Am J Obstet Gynecol 199:32.e1, 2008

Chapman SJ, Owen J, Hauth JC: One- versus two-layer closure of a low transverse cesarean: The next pregnancy. Obstet Gynecol 89:16, 1997

Chatterjee SR, Bhaduri S: Clinical analysis of 40 cases of uterine rupture at Durgapur Subdivisional Hospital: An observational study. J Indian Med Assoc 105:510, 2007

Chauhan SP, Magann EF, Wiggs CD, et al: Pregnancy after classic cesarean delivery. Obstet Gynecol 100:946, 2002

Chauhan SP, Martin JN Jr, Henrichs CE, et al: Maternal and perinatal complications with uterine rupture in 142,075 patients who attempted vaginal birth after cesarean delivery: A review of the literature. Am J Obstet Gynecol 189:408, 2003

Clark SL, Miller DD, Belfort MA, et al: Neonatal and maternal outcomes associated with elective term delivery. Am J Obstet Gynecol 200(2):156.e1, 2009

Coleman VH, Erickson K, Schulkin J, et al: Vaginal birth after cesarean delivery. J Reprod Med 50:261, 2005

Cragin E: Conservatism in obstetrics. NY Med J 104:1, 1916

Dicle O, Kücükler C, Pirnar T: Magnetic resonance imaging evaluation of incision healing after cesarean sections. Eur Radiol 7:31, 1997

Durnwald C, Mercer B: Uterine rupture, perioperative and perinatal morbidity after single-layer and double-layer closure at cesarean delivery. Am J Obstet Gynecol 189:925, 2003

Durnwald CP, Rouse DJ, Leveno KJ, et al: The Maternal-Fetal Medicine Units Cesarean Registry: Safety and efficacy of a trial of labor in preterm pregnancy after a prior cesarean delivery. Am J Obstet Gynecol 195:1119, 2006

Elkousy MA, Sammel M, Stevens E, et al: The effect of birth weight on vaginal birth after cesarean delivery success rates. Am J Obstet Gynecol 188:824, 2003

El-Sayed YY, Watkins MM, Fix M, et al: Perinatal outcomes after successful and failed trials of labor after cesarean delivery. Am J Obstet Gynecol 196:583.e1, 2007

Erez O, Dulder D, Novack L, et al: Trial of labor and vaginal birth after cesarean section in patients with uterine Müllerian anomalies: A population-based study. Am J Obstet Gynecol 196:537.e1, 2007

Farmer RM, Kirschbaum T, Potter D, et al: Uterine rupture during trial of labor after previous cesarean section. Am J Obstet Gynecol 165:996, 1991

Flamm BL: Once a cesarean, always a controversy. Obstet Gynecol 90:312, 1997

Flamm BL, Goings JR, Liu Y, et al: Elective repeat cesarean delivery versus trial of labor: A prospective multicenter study. Obstet Gynecol 83:927, 1994

Flamm BL, Newman LA, Thomas SJ, et al: Vaginal birth after cesarean delivery: Results of a 5-year multicenter collaborative study. Obstet Gynecol 76:750, 1990

Ford AA, Bateman BT, Simpson LL: Vaginal birth after cesarean delivery in twin gestations: A large, nationwide sample of deliveries. Am J Obstet Gynecol 195:1138, 2006

Goetzl L, Shipp TD, Cohen A, et al: Oxytocin dose and the risk of uterine rupture in trial of labor after cesarean. Obstet Gynecol 97:381, 2001

Gregory KD, Korst LM, Fridman M, et al: Vaginal birth after cesarean: Clinical risk factors associated with adverse outcome. Am J Obstet Gynecol 198:452.e1, 2008

Grinstead J, Grobman WA: Induction of labor after one prior cesarean: Predictors of vaginal delivery. Obstet Gynecol 103:534, 2004

Grobman WA, Gilbert S, Landon MB, et al: Outcomes of induction of labor after one prior cesarean. Obstet Gynecol 109:262, 2007a

Grobman WA, Lai Y, Landon MB, et al: Can a prediction model for vaginal birth after cesarean also predict the probability of morbidity related to a trial of labor? Am J Obstet Gynecol 200(1):56.e1, 2009

Grobman WA, Lai Y, Landon MB, et al: Development of a nomogram for prediction of vaginal birth after cesarean delivery. Obstet Gynecol 109:806, 2007b

Grobman WA, Lai Y, Landon MB, et al: Prediction of uterine rupture associated with attempted vaginal birth after cesarean delivery. Am J Obstet Gynecol 199:30.e1, 2008

Guise J-M, Berlin M, McDonagh M, et al: Safety of vaginal birth after cesarean: A systematic review. Obstet Gynecol 103:420, 2004

Hamilton BE, Martin JA, Ventura SJ: Births: Preliminary Data for 2007. National Vital Statistics Reports, Vol 57, No 12. Hyattsville, Md, National Center for Health Statistics, 2009

Harper LM, Cahill AG, Stamilio DM, et al: Effect of gestational age at the prior cesarean delivery on maternal morbidity in subsequent VBAC attempt. Am J Obstet Gynecol 200(3):276.e1, 2009

Hashima JN, Eden KB, Osterweil P, et al: Predicting vaginal birth after cesarean delivery: A review of prognostic factors and screening tools. Am J Obstet Gynecol 190:547, 2004

Hellman LM, Pritchard JA: Williams Obstetrics, 14th ed. Meredith Corporation, 1971, p 941

Hendler I, Gauthier RJ, Bujold E: The effects of prior vaginal delivery compared to prior VBAC on the outcomes of current trial of VBAC [Abstract 384]. J Soc Gynecol Investig 11:202A, 2004

Hibbard JU, Gilbert S, Landon MB, et al: Trial of labor or repeat cesarean delivery in women with morbid obesity and previous cesarean delivery. Obstet Gynecol 108:125, 2006

Juhasz G, Gyamfi C, Gyamfi P, et al: Effect of body mass index and excessive weight gain on success of vaginal birth after cesarean delivery. Obstet Gynecol 106:741, 2005

Kaczmarczyk M, Sparén P, Terry P, et al: Risk factors for uterine rupture and neonatal consequences of uterine rupture: A population-based study of successive pregnancies in Sweden. BJOG 114:1208, 2007

Kayani SI, Alfirevic Z: Uterine rupture after induction of labour in women with previous caesarean section. BJOG 112:451, 2005

Kerr JN: The lower uterine segment incision in conservative cesarean section. J Obstet Gynaecol Br Emp 28:475, 1921

Kieser KE, Baskett TF: A 10-year population-based study of uterine rupture. Obstet Gynecol 100:749, 2002

Landon MB, Hauth JC, Leveno KJ, et al: Maternal and perinatal outcomes associated with a trial of labor after prior cesarean delivery. N Engl J Med 351:2581, 2004

Landon MB, Leindecker S, Spong CY, et al: The MFMU Cesarean Registry: Factors affecting the success of trial of labor after previous cesarean delivery. Am J Obstet Gynecol 193:1016, 2005

Landon MB, Spong CY, Thom E, et al: Risk of uterine rupture with a trial of labor in women with multiple and single prior cesarean delivery. Obstet Gynecol 108:12, 2006

Lavin JP, DiPasquale L, Crane S, et al: A state-wide assessment of the obstetric, anesthesia, and operative team personnel who are available to manage the labors and deliveries and to treat the complications of women who attempt vaginal birth after cesarean delivery. Am J Obstet Gynecol 187:611, 2002

Leveno KJ: Controversies in OB-Gyn: Should we rethink the criteria for VBAC? Contemp Ob/Gyn, January 1999

Lydon-Rochelle M, Holt VL, Easterling TR, et al: Risk of uterine rupture during labor among women with a prior cesarean delivery. N Engl J Med 345:3, 2001

Macones GA, Cahill A, Pare E, et al: Obstetric outcomes in women with two prior cesarean deliveries: Is vaginal birth after cesarean delivery a viable option? Am J Obstet Gynecol 192:1223, 2005a

Macones GA, Cahill AG, Stamilio DM, et al: Can uterine rupture in patients attempting vaginal birth after cesarean delivery be predicted? Am J Obstet Gynecol 195:1148, 2006

Macones GA, Peipert J, Nelson DB, et al: Maternal complications with vaginal birth after cesarean delivery: A multicenter study. Am J Obstet Gynecol 193:1656, 2005b

Martin JN, Perry KG, Roberts WE, et al: The care for trial of labor in the patients with a prior low-segment vertical cesarean incision. Am J Obstet Gynecol 177:144, 1997

McMahon MJ, Luther ER, Bowes WA Jr, et al: Comparison of a trial of labor with an elective second cesarean section. N Engl J Med 335:689, 1996

Mercer BM, Gilbert S, Landon MB, et al: Labor outcomes with increasing number of prior vaginal births after cesarean delivery. Obstet Gynecol 111:285, 2008

Merrill BS, Gibbs CE: Planned vaginal delivery following cesarean section. Obstet Gynecol 52:50, 1978

Miller DA, Diaz FG, Paul RH: Vaginal birth after cesarean: A 10-year experience. Obstet Gynecol 84:255, 1994

Miller DA, Goodwin TM, Gherman RB, et al: Intrapartum rupture of the unscarred uterus. Obstet Gynecol 89:671, 1997

Mozurkewich EL, Hutton EK: Elective repeat cesarean delivery versus trial of labor: A meta-analysis of the literature from 1989 to 1999. Am J Obstet Gynecol 183:1187, 2000

National Institutes of Health State-of-the-Science Conference Statement: Cesarean delivery on maternal request. NIH Consens Sci Statements 23:5, 2006

Nisenblat V, Barak S, Griness OB, et al: Maternal complications associated with multiple cesarean deliveries. Obstet Gynecol 108:21, 2006

Peaceman AM, Gersnoviez R, Landon MB, et al: The MFMU cesarean registry: Impact of fetal size on trial of labor success for patients with previous cesarean for dystocia. Am J Obstet Gynecol 195:1127, 2006

Pitkin RM: Once a cesarean? Obstet Gynecol 77:939, 1991

Quiñones JN, Stamilio DM, Paré E, et al: The effect of prematurity on vaginal birth after cesarean delivery: Success and maternal morbidity. Obstet Gynecol 105:519, 2005

Ravasia DJ, Brain PH, Pollard JK: Incidence of uterine rupture among women with müllerian duct anomalies who attempt vaginal birth after cesarean delivery. Am J Obstet Gynecol 181:877, 1999

Ravasia DJ, Wood SL, Pollard JK: Uterine rupture during induced trial of labor among women with previous cesarean delivery. Am J Obstet Gynecol 183:1176, 2000

Reyes-Ceja L, Cabrera R, Insfran E, et al: Pregnancy following previous uterine rupture: Study of 19 patients. Obstet Gynecol 34:387, 1969

Ritchie EH: Pregnancy after rupture of the pregnant uterus: A report of 36 pregnancies and a study of cases reported since 1932. J Obstet Gynaecol Br Commonw 78:642, 1971

Rodriguez MH, Masaki DI, Phelan JP, et al: Uterine rupture: Are intrauterine pressure catheters useful in the diagnosis? Am J Obstet Gynecol 161:666, 1989

Rossi AC, D'Addario V: Maternal morbidity following a trial of labor after cesarean section vs elective repeat cesarean delivery: A systematic review with metaanalysis. Am J Obstet Gynecol 199(3):224, 2008

Sciscione AC, Landon MB, Leveno KJ, et al: Previous preterm cesarean delivery and risk of subsequent uterine rupture. Obstet Gynecol 111:648, 2008

Scott JR: Mandatory trial of labor after cesarean delivery: An alternative viewpoint. Obstet Gynecol 77:811, 1991

Sheth SS: Results of treatment of rupture of the uterus by suturing. J Obstet Gynaecol Br Commonw 75:55, 1968

Shipp TD, Zelop CM, Repke JT, et al: Interdelivery interval and risk of symptomatic uterine rupture. Obstet Gynecol 97:175, 2001

Shipp TD, Zelop CM, Repke JT, et al: Intrapartum uterine rupture and dehiscence in patients with prior lower uterine segment vertical and transverse incisions. Obstet Gynecol 94:735, 1999

Silver RM, Landon MB, Rouse DJ, et al: Maternal morbidity associated with multiple repeat cesarean deliveries. Obstet Gynecol 207:1226, 2006

Smith GC, Pell JP, Cameron AD, et al: Risk of perinatal death associated with labor after previous cesarean delivery in uncomplicated term pregnancies. JAMA 287:2684, 2002

Spong CY, Landon MB, Gilbert S, et al: Risk of uterine rupture and adverse perinatal outcome at term after cesarean delivery. Obstet Gynecol 110:801, 2007

Srinivas SK, Stamilio DM, Stevens EJ, et al: Predicting failure of a vaginal birth attempt after cesarean delivery. Obstet Gynecol 109:800, 2007

Stamilio DM, DeFranco E, Paré E, et al: Short interpregnancy interval. Risk of uterine rupture and complications of vaginal birth after cesarean delivery. Obstet Gynecol 110, 1075, 2007

Stovall TG, Shaver DC, Soloman SK, et al: Trial of labor in previous cesarean section patients, excluding classical cesarean sections. Obstet Gynecol 70:713, 1987

Tita AT, Landon MB, Spong CY, et al: Timing of elective repeat cesarean delivery at term and neonatal outcomes. N Engl J Med 360(2):111, 2009

Tucker JM, Hauth JC, Hodgkins P, et al: Trial of labor after a one- or two-layer closure of a low transverse uterine incision. Am J Obstet Gynecol 168:545, 1993

Usta IM, Hamdi MA, Abu Musa AA, et al: Pregnancy outcome in patients with previous uterine rupture. Acta Obstet Gynecol 86:172, 2007

Usta IM, Hobeika EM, Abu-Musa AA, et al: Placenta previa-accreta: Risk factors and complications. Am J Obstet Gynecol 193:1045, 2005

Varner MW, Thom E, Spong CY, et al: Trial of labor after one previous cesarean delivery for multifetal gestation. Obstet Gynecol 110:814, 2007

Vidaeff AC, Lucas MJ: Impact of single- or double-layer closure on uterine rupture [Letter]. Am J Obstet Gynecol 188:602, 2003

Wen SW, Huang L, Liston R, et al: Severe maternal morbidity in Canada, 1991-2001. CMAJ 173:759, 2005

Williams JW: Obstetrics: A Text-book for the Use of Students and Practitioners, 4th ed. New York, Appleton, 1917

Williams Obstetrics, 14th ed. Williams JW, Hellman LM, Pritchard JA (eds). New York, Appleton-Century-Crofts, 1971, p 941

Wing DA, Lovett K, Paul RH: Disruption of prior uterine incision following misoprostol for labor induction in women with previous cesarean delivery. Obstet Gynecol 91:828, 1998

Wing DA, Paul RH: Vaginal birth after cesarean section: Selection and management. Clin Obstet Gynecol 42:836, 1999

Zelop CM, Shipp TD, Repke JT, et al: Uterine rupture during induced or augmented labor in gravid women with one prior cesarean delivery. Am J Obstet Gynecol 181:882, 1999

Zelop CM, Shipp TD, Repke JT, et al: Effect of previous vaginal delivery on the risk of uterine rupture during a subsequent trial of labor. Am J Obstet Gynecol 183:1184, 2000

Zelop CM, Shipp TD, Repke JT, et al: Outcomes of trial of labor following previous cesarean delivery among women with fetuses weighing >4000 g. Am J Obstet Gynecol 185:903, 2001

CHAPTER 27

Abnormalities of the Placenta, Umbilical Cord, and Membranes

With basic knowledge of placental implantation, development, and anatomy presented in Chapter 3, clinicians can more easily understand the genesis of abnormal placental types. Much of the ever-growing knowledge of placental pathology was stimulated by a nucleus of placental pathologists that includes, among others, Benirschke, Driscoll, Fox, Naeye, Salafia, and Faye-Petersen. For a detailed account of these disorders, the reader is referred to the 5th edition of *Pathology of the Human Placenta* by Benirschke and colleagues (2006) and the 2nd edition of the *Handbook of Placental Pathology* by Faye-Petersen and associates (2006).

ABNORMALITIES OF THE PLACENTA

Abnormal Shape or Implantation

Most placentas are either round or oval, but variations are common. As discussed in this chapter, many of these have clinical importance.

Multiple Placentas with a Single Fetus

Uncommonly, the placenta forms as separate, near equally sized disks. The cord inserts between the two placental lobes—either into a connecting chorionic bridge or into intervening membranes. This condition is termed *bilobate placenta,* but is also known as *bipartite placenta* or *placenta duplex* (Fig. 27-1). Fox and Sebire (2007) reported its incidence to be approximately 1

in 350 deliveries. A placenta containing three or more lobes is rare and termed *multilobate.*

Succenturiate Lobe

These placentas are a smaller version of the bilobate placenta. One or more small accessory lobes develop in the membranes at a distance from the main placenta, to which they usually have vascular connections of fetal origin. Although its incidence has been cited by Benirschke and associates (2006) to be as high as 5 percent, we have encountered these much less frequently. Suzuki and co-workers (2009) noted a twofold higher incidence of succenturiate lobes in twin placentas. The accessory lobe may sometimes be retained in the uterus after delivery and may cause serious hemorrhage. In some cases, an accompanying vasa previa may cause dangerous fetal hemorrhage at delivery.

Placenta Membranacea

Rarely, all or a large part of the fetal membranes are covered by functioning villi. Placenta membranacea may occasionally give rise to serious hemorrhage because of associated placenta previa or accreta (Greenberg and colleagues, 1991).

Ring-Shaped Placenta

In fewer than 1 in 6000 deliveries, the placenta is annular in shape, and sometimes a complete ring of placental tissue is present. This development may be a variant of placenta membranacea. Because of tissue atrophy in a portion of the ring, a horseshoe shape is more common. These abnormalities appear to be associated with a greater likelihood of antepartum and postpartum bleeding and fetal-growth restriction (Faye-Petersen and colleagues, 2006).

Placenta Fenestrata

In this rare anomaly, the central portion of a discoidal placenta is missing. In some instances, there is an actual hole in the placenta, but more often, the defect involves only villous tissue,

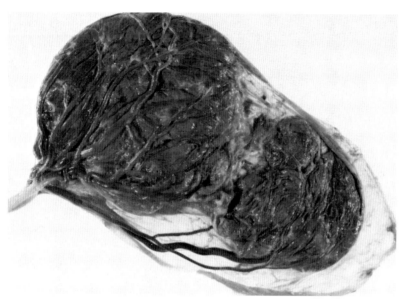

FIGURE 27-1 Bilobate placenta with marginal insertion of the umbilical cord. There also is partial velamentous insertion of the cord with the fetal vessels traversing the membranes to reach the smaller lobe on the right.

and the chorionic plate remains intact. Clinically, it may erroneously prompt a search for a retained placental lobule.

Extrachorial Placentation

When the chorionic plate, which is on the fetal side of the placenta, is smaller than the placental basal plate, which is located on the maternal side, the periphery is uncovered, and the term *extrachorial placenta* is used (Fig. 27-2). If the fetal surface of such a placenta presents a central depression surrounded by a thickened, gray-white ring, it is called a *circumvallate placenta*. The ring is composed of a double fold of chorion and amnion, with degenerated decidua and fibrin in between. Within the ring, the fetal surface presents the usual appearance, except that the large vessels terminate abruptly at the ring edge. When the ring does not have the central depression, the placenta is described as *circummarginate* (see Fig. 27-2).

With circumvallate placentas, there is an increased risk of antepartum hemorrhage—from both placental abruption and fetal hemorrhage—as well as of preterm delivery, perinatal mortality, and congenital malformations (Lademacher and co-workers, 1981; Suzuki, 2008). Adverse clinical outcomes with circummarginate placentas are less well defined.

Placenta Accreta, Increta, and Percreta

These abnormalities are serious variations in which trophoblastic tissues invade the myometrium to varying depths. They are much more likely with placenta previa or with implantation over a prior uterine incision or perforation. Torrential hemorrhage is a frequent complication (see Chap. 35, p. 776).

Circulatory Disturbances

Conceptually, placental perfusion disorders may be grouped into: (1) those that disrupted maternal blood flow to or within the placenta and (2) those that disturb fetal blood flow through

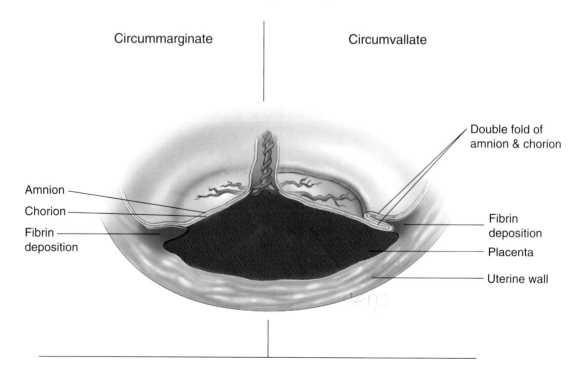

Circummarginate | Circumvallate

Amnion
Chorion
Fibrin deposition

Double fold of amnion & chorion
Fibrin deposition
Placenta
Uterine wall

FIGURE 27-2 Circumvallate *(right)* and circummarginate *(left)* varieties of extrachorial placentas. With circumvallate placenta, the double fold of amnion and chorion creates the broad white ring seen on the fetal surface of these placentas. Circummarginate placentas lack this double fold and white ring.

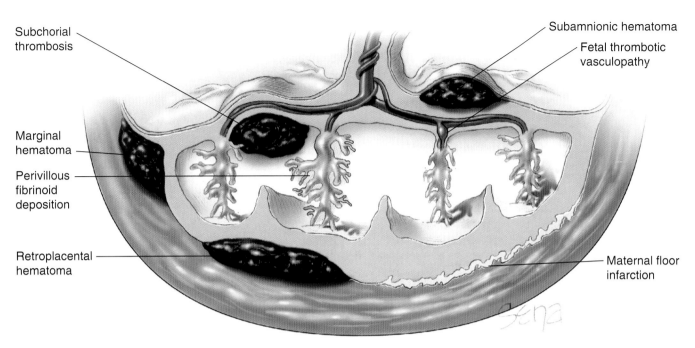

FIGURE 27-3 Potential sites of placental circulatory disturbances. (Adapted from Faye-Peterson and colleagues, 2006.)

the villi. Many of these lesions are common and are found in normal mature placentas. Although they limit maximal placental blood flow, the placenta's functional reserve is great. Some estimate that the placenta can lose up to 30 percent of its villi without untoward fetal effect (Fox and Sebire, 2007). If lesions are extensive, however, they have the potential to profoundly limit fetal growth.

Maternal Blood Flow Disruption

A number of lesions can restrict or abate intervillous blood flow.

Maternal Floor Infarction. Erroneously termed *infarction*, this condition deposits a dense fibrinoid layer on the placental basal plate (Fig. 27-3). This thick, white, firm, corrugated surface acts as a blockade to normal maternal blood flow. These infarctions are associated with fetal growth restriction, abortion, preterm delivery, and stillbirths (Andres and co-workers, 1990; Mandsager and colleagues, 1994). It occasionally recurs in subsequent pregnancies. Their etiopathogenesis is not well defined, although it may be associated with maternal thrombophilia (Gogia and Machin, 2008; Katz and associates, 2002; Sebire and colleagues, 2002, 2003). These lesions are considered in further detail in Chapter 47 p. 1014).

Perivillous Fibrinoid Deposition. These small yellow-white nodules within the placenta are considered a normal part of placental aging. They form when normal maternal blood flow currents around an individual villus are slowed, which leads to blood stasis and fibrin deposition. This layer of fibrin diminishes oxygenation to the villus and results in syncytiotrophoblast necrosis (Faye-Petersen and colleagues, 2006). When extreme, this lesion can cause fetal growth restriction or fetal demise.

Hematoma. Placental hematomas are described in a number of ways depicted in Figure 27-3. These include: (1) *retroplacental hematoma*—between the placenta and its adjacent decidua; (2) *marginal hematoma*—between the chorion and decidua and also clinically called subchorionic hemorrhage; (3) *subchorial thrombosis*, also known as *Breus mole*—along the roof of the intervillous space and beneath the chorionic plate; and (4) *subamnionic hematoma*—between the placenta and amnion.

Large retroplacental, marginal, and subchorial collections have been associated with higher rates of miscarriage, abruption, fetal-growth restriction, preterm delivery, and adherent placenta (Ball, 1996; Madu, 2006; Nagy, 2003; Nyberg, 1987, and all their colleagues). Subamnionic hematomas are of fetal vessel origin and discussed later.

Infarction. Chorionic villi receive oxygen solely from maternal circulation through the uteroplacental vessels, which jet blood into the intervillous space. Uteroplacental diseases that diminish or obstruct this connection can lead to villous infarction. Although these are common lesions in mature placentas, if they are numerous, placental insufficiency may develop. When they are thick, centrally located, and randomly distributed, they may be associated with preeclampsia or lupus anticoagulant.

Fetal Blood Flow Disruption

There are a number of lesions that may restrict fetoplacental blood flow.

Fetal Thrombotic Vasculopathy. Fetal blood flows from the two umbilical arteries into the placenta. These arteries divide and send branches out across the placental surface. Eventually, these supply individual stem villi, which may thrombose and obstruct fetal blood flow (see Fig. 27-3). Distal to the point of obstruction, affected portions of the villus are rendered nonfunctional. Thrombi are normally found in mature placentas but may become clinically significant if a large portion of villi is lost.

Hematoma. As indicated, subamnionic hematomas lie between the placenta and amnion (see Fig. 27-3). These hematomas most often are acute events during third-stage labor when cord traction ruptures a vessel near the cord insertion. With chronic lesions, fetomaternal hemorrhage or fetal-growth restriction have been reported (Deans and Jauniaux, 1998). In addition, these may be confused with other potentially dangerous placental masses such as chorioangioma, which is discussed subsequently (Sepulveda, 2000; Van Den Bosch, 2000; Volpe, 2008, and all their associates).

Placental Calcification

Calcium salts may be deposited throughout the placenta, but are most common on maternal surface in the basal plate. Calcification is associated with nulliparity, higher socioeconomic status, and greater maternal serum calcium levels (Fox and Sebire, 2007). Calcifications can be seen with sonography, however, criteria to grade its degree have not been found useful to predict neonatal outcome (Hill, 1983; McKenna, 2005; Montan, 1986; Sau, 2004 and all their colleagues).

Hypertrophic Villous Lesions

Striking enlargement of the chorionic villi is commonly seen in association with severe erythroblastosis and fetal hydrops. It also has been described in maternal diabetes, fetal congestive heart failure, and maternal-fetal syphilis (Sheffield and colleagues, 2002). Many of these conditions are discussed in Chapter 29.

Placental Tumors

Gestational Trophoblastic Disease

These pregnancy-related trophoblastic proliferative abnormalities are discussed in Chapter 11.

Chorioangioma

Because of the resemblance of their components to the blood vessels and stroma of the chorionic villus, the term *chorioangioma*—or *chorangioma*—is considered the most appropriate designation. These are the only benign tumors of the placenta and have an incidence of approximately 1 percent (Guschmann and associates, 2003).

Levels of maternal serum alpha-fetoprotein (MSAFP) may be elevated with these and may prompt sonographic evaluation (see Chap. 13, p. 290). A well-circumscribed, rounded, predominantly hypoechoic lesion near the chorionic surface and protruding into the amnionic cavity is a common characteristic (Fig. 27-4). Documenting increased blood flow by color Doppler can assist in distinguishing these lesions from other placental masses (Prapas, 2000).

Small growths are usually asymptomatic. Large tumors, typically those measuring greater than 5 cm, however, may be

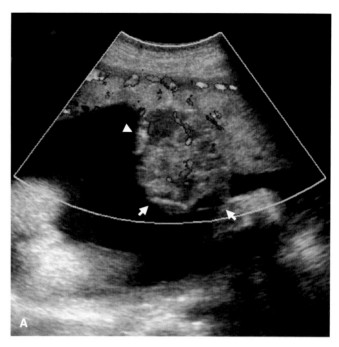

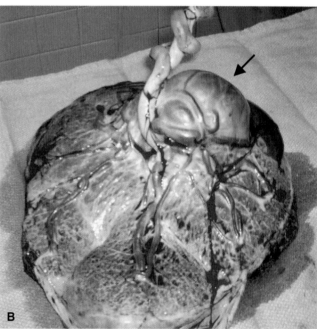

FIGURE 27-4 Placental chorioangioma. **A.** Color Doppler imaging displays blood flow through a large chorioangioma. The tumor border is outlined by white arrows. **B.** After delivery, the chorioangioma is seen as a round, well-circumcised mass (*black arrow*) protruding from the fetal surface.

associated with significant arteriovenous shunting within the placenta, leading to fetal anemia and hydrops (see Chap. 29, p. 626). Antepartum hemorrhage, preterm delivery, amnionic fluid abnormalities, and fetal growth restriction may also complicate large tumors (Sepulveda and associates, 2003a; Zalel and co-workers, 2002). Because of severe fetal sequelae with large tumors, treatment may include an attempt to reduce blood flow to the tumor by means of vessel occlusion or ablation (Lau, 2003; Nicolini, 1999; Quintero, 1996; Sepulveda, 2009, and all their colleagues).

Tumors Metastatic to the Placenta

Malignant tumors rarely metastasize to the placenta. Of those that do, melanomas, leukemias and lymphomas, and breast cancer are the most common (Al-Adnani and co-workers, 2007). Tumor cells usually are confined within the intervillous space. As a result, metastasis to the fetus is uncommon, but is most often seen with melanoma (Alexander and colleagues, 2003; Altman and associates, 2003).

ABNORMALITIES OF THE MEMBRANES

Meconium Staining

The presence of meconium in amnionic fluid is relatively common, and incidences range from 12 to 20 percent (Ghidini and Spong, 2001; Oyelese and co-workers, 2006; Tran and associates, 2004). Staining of the amnion can be obvious within 1 to 3 hours after meconium passage (Miller and colleagues, 1985). More-prolonged exposure results in staining of the chorion, umbilical cord, and decidua. According to Benirschke and colleagues (2006), meconium passage cannot be timed or dated accurately.

Meconium may be passed in a variety of clinical settings. First, in most fetuses, meconium passage is prevented by tonic anal sphincter contraction and by lack of intestinal peristalsis. Thus, preterm fetuses, with immature gastrointestinal mechanisms, infrequently pass meconium. In contrast, for postterm fetuses, whose intestinal tracts are mature, meconium passage may be normal, and stained fluid is seen in approximately 30 percent of these deliveries (Katz and Bowes, 1992; Tybulewicz and co-workers, 2004; Walsh and Fanaroff, 2007). Secondly, vagal stimulation produced by cord or head compression may be associated with meconium passage in the absence of fetal distress. Lastly, meconium passage is also associated with fetal acidosis, nonreassuring fetal heart rate patterns, and low Apgar scores (Krebs and co-workers, 1980; Nathan and colleagues, 1994). In these cases, theories suggest that fetal hypoxia produces relaxation of the anal sphincter and gasping of the fetus with subsequent in utero aspiration of meconium. If aspirated by the fetus before or during birth, meconium can obstruct the airways, leading to severe hypoxia, inflammation, and infection—*meconium aspiration syndrome.*

Neonatal effects of meconium aspiration syndrome are found in Chapter 29 (p. 628). One serious maternal risk is that meconium-laden amnionic fluid embolism greatly increases maternal mortality rates from cardiorespiratory failure and consumptive coagulopathy (see Chap. 35, p. 788). In addition, the risk of puerperal metritis with meconium-stained amnionic fluid is increased two- to fourfold (Jazayeri and colleagues, 2002; Tran and co-workers, 2004).

Chorioamnionitis

A variety of organisms may infect the membranes, umbilical cord, and eventually the fetus. Routes of infection include ascending infection from the lower genital tract, hematogenous spread from maternal blood, direct spread from the endometrium or fallopian tube, and iatrogenic contamination during invasive procedures (see Fig. 36-10, p. 813). Of these, ascending infection is most common and frequently is associated with prolonged membrane rupture and long labor.

In general, vaginal bacteria are excluded from the upper reproductive tract by a closed internal cervical os and intracervical mucus plug. Entry of organisms can create initial infection of the chorion and adjacent decidua in the area overlying the internal os. Subsequently, progression leads to full-thickness involvement of the membranes—*chorioamnionitis.* Organisms may then spread along the chorioamnionic surface and infect the amnionic fluid. There can be subsequent inflammation of the chorionic plate and of the umbilical cord—*funisitis* (Al-Adnani and Sebire, 2007; Goldenberg and co-workers, 2000; Redline, 2006). Fetal infection may result from hematogenous routes, aspiration, swallowing, or other direct contact with infected amnionic fluid and is discussed in Chapter 36 (p. 812).

Grossly, infection is characterized by clouding of the membranes. There also may be a foul odor, depending on bacterial species and concentration. Occult chorioamnionitis, caused by a wide variety of microorganisms, frequently is cited as a possible explanation for many otherwise unexplained cases of ruptured membranes, preterm labor, or both (see Chap. 6, p. 163).

Other Abnormalities

Amnion nodosum is a placental lesion consisting of numerous small, light-tan nodules on the amnion that overlies the placenta. It is considered a hallmark of prolonged and severe oligohydramnios (Adeniran and Stanek, 2007). *Amnionic bands* are caused when disruption of the amnion leads to formation of bands or strings that entrap the fetus and impair growth and development of the involved structure (see Chap. 29, p. 637).

ABNORMALITIES OF THE UMBILICAL CORD

The cord develops in close association with the amnion, as described in Chapter 3 (p. 61). It serves a vital function, but it unfortunately is susceptible to entanglement, compression, and occlusion.

Cord Measurements

Length

Most cords are 50 to 60 cm long, and very few are abnormally short or long. Short cords may be associated with adverse perinatal outcomes such as fetal-growth restriction, congenital malformations, intrapartum distress, and a twofold risk of death (Berg and Rayburn, 1995; Krakowiak and associates, 2004). Excessively long cords are more likely to be associated with cord prolapse or entanglement and with fetal anomalies, distress, and demise.

Cord length is influenced positively by both the volume of amnionic fluid and fetal mobility. Miller and associates (1981) identified higher rates of appreciably shortened cords if there was chronic fetal constraint from oligohydramnios or decreased fetal movement, such as that seen with Down syndrome or limb dysfunction.

Diameter

Antenatal determination of cord length has technical limitations. For this reason, investigators have evaluated cord diameter as a predictive fetal marker. Although lean umbilical cords have been associated with poor fetal growth and large-diameter cords with macrosomia, the clinical utility of this parameter is still unclear (Barbieri, 2008; Cromi, 2007; Raio 1999b, 2003, and all their colleagues).

Cord Coiling

In most cases, the umbilical vessels spiral through the cord, and a predictable number of coils per unit length can be determined. This *umbilical coiling index (UCI)* is defined as the number of complete coils divided by the length of the cord in centimeters (Strong and colleagues, 1994). Antenatally, coiling can be determined sonographically, although with lower sensitivity than measurement postpartum (Predanic and associates, 2005a). Clinically, hypocoiling has been linked with fetal demise, whereas hypercoiling is related to fetal-growth restriction and intrapartum fetal acidosis and asphyxia. Both have been linked to trisomies and single umbilical artery (de Laat and co-workers, 2005, 2006, 2007; Predanic and colleagues, 2005c).

Vessel Number

Single Umbilical Artery

In a review of nearly 350,000 deliveries, Heifetz (1984) found an incidence of a single artery to be 0.63 percent in liveborns, 1.92 percent in perinatal deaths, and 3 percent in twins. The incidence is increased considerably in women with diabetes, epilepsy, preeclampsia, antepartum hemorrhage, oligohydramnios or hydramnios, and chromosomal abnormalities (Byrne and Blanc, 1985; Leung and Robson, 1989). Although several theories exist, secondary atrophy of a previously normal umbilical artery is most commonly accepted as the etiology.

In many cases, a single umbilical artery is detected by routine sonographic screening. Hill and co-workers (2001) reported that the number of cord vessels could be quantified sonographically in almost 98 percent of cases studied between 17 and 36 weeks.

For most fetuses, a two-vessel cord is an isolated finding and not associated with other anomalies. But up to a third of all infants with only one umbilical artery have associated anomalies (Gornall, 2003; Pierce, 2001; Prucka, 2004, and all their colleagues) Perinatal prognosis is better if a two-vessel umbilical cord is an *isolated sonographic finding.* Moreover, many investigators have found no increased risk of aneuploidy if no other structural abnormalities accompany a two-vessel cord (Budorick and co-workers 2001; Lubusky and associates, 2007). Conversely, Catanzarite (1995) described 46 fetuses with this isolated sonographic finding, and two had lethal chromosomal abnormalities and a third had a tracheoesophageal fistula. Data from studies evaluating the risk of growth restriction in otherwise normal fetuses with a single umbilical artery are contradictory (Goldkrand, 2001; Predanic, 2005b; Wiegand, 2008, and all their colleagues).

If a two-vessel cord is a *nonisolated finding,* the risk of aneuploidy is increased (Granese and associates, 2007). There are a number of associated anomalies, and Martinez-Frias (2008) reported associated increased frequency of renal agenesis, imperforate anus, and vertebral defects.

Hyrtl Anastomosis. This connection between the two umbilical arteries is found within approximately 3 cm of the placental insertion of the cord. Found in most placentas, this anastomosis acts as a pressure-equalizing system between umbilical arteries (Gordon and associates, 2007). As a result, redistribution of pressure gradients and blood flow improves placental perfusion, especially during uterine contractions or during compression of one umbilical artery. Fetuses with a single umbilical artery, lack this safety valve. This may partially explain the increased rate of otherwise unexplained fetal demise in late pregnancy or during labor in these fetuses (Raio and co-workers, 1999a, 2001).

Four-Vessel Cord

Careful inspection may disclose a venous remnant. These are uncommon, and their association with an increased risk of congenital anomalies is unclear (Meyer and colleagues, 1969; Jeanty, 1990).

Fused Umbilical Artery

During embryological development, the umbilical artery rarely may fail to split, and as a result, creates a fused shared lumen. This may extend through the entire cord, but if partial, it is typically found toward the cord's placental insertion (Yamada and colleagues, 2005). Fujikura (2003) noted higher rates of marginal or velamentous cord insertion, but not congenital fetal anomalies.

Cord Insertion

Marginal Insertion

The cord usually is inserted at or near the center of the fetal surface of the placenta. Cord insertion at the placental margin is sometimes referred to as a *Battledore placenta* (Fig. 27-5). It is

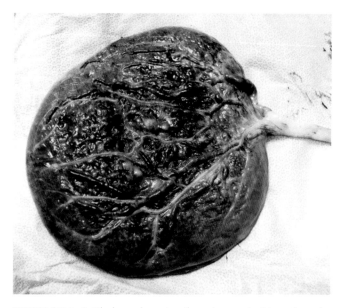

FIGURE 27-5 Battledore placenta—there is marginal insertion of the cord.

found in about 7 percent of term placentas (Benirschke and associates, 2006). With the exception of the cord being pulled off during delivery of the placenta, it is of little clinical significance (Liu and co-workers, 2002).

Furcate Insertion

In this uncommon anomaly, the insertion site is normal, but umbilical vessels lose their protective Wharton jelly shortly before insertion. As a result, they are covered only by amnion and prone to compression, twisting, and thrombosis.

Velamentous Insertion

This type of insertion is of considerable clinical importance. The umbilical vessels spread within the membranes at a distance from the placental margin, which they reach surrounded only by a fold of amnion (Fig. 27-6). As a result, vessels are vulnerable to compression, which may lead to fetal anoxia. Although their incidence is approximately 1 percent, velamentous insertion develops in more commonly with placenta previa and multifetal gestations (Feldman and associates, 2002; Fox and Sebire, 2007; Papinniemi and co-workers, 2007).

Vasa Previa. In some cases of velamentous insertion, placental vessels overlie the cervix, lie between the cervix and the presenting fetal part, and are supported only by membranes. As a result, vessels are vulnerable not only to compression, which may lead to fetal anoxia, but also to laceration, which can lead to fetal exsanguination. Fortunately, vasa previa is uncommon, and Lee and co-workers (2000) identified it in 1 in 5200 pregnancies. Risk factors include bilobate or succenturiate placentas and second-trimester placenta previa, with or without later migration (Baulies and associates, 2007; Suzuki and Igarashi, 2008). It is also increased in pregnancies

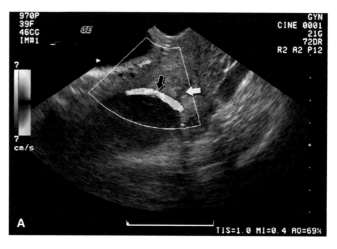

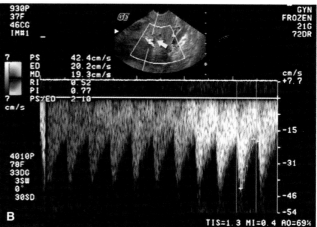

FIGURE 27-7 Vasa previa. **A.** Transvaginal sonogram with color mapping shows the large vessel (*black arrow*) covering the internal os of the cervix (*yellow arrow*). **B.** Doppler waveform of the vessel shows the typical appearance of the umbilical artery with a rate of 150 beats per minute.

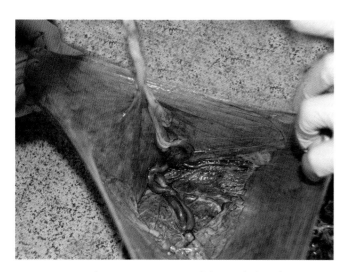

FIGURE 27-6 Velamentous insertion of the cord. The placenta and membranes have been inverted to expose the amnion. Part of the fetal surface of the placenta appears at the bottom of the photograph. The large fetal vessels extend from the cord insertion and within the membranes. From the proximity of the vessels to the site of membrane rupture, it can be seen how a vessel could easily be torn by digital manipulation or descent of the fetal head during labor.

conceived by in vitro fertilization (IVF), and this is believed to stem from greater rates of abnormal cord insertion with pregnancies so conceived (Schachter and associates, 2003).

Antepartum diagnosis results in improved rates of fetal survival compared with intrapartum diagnosis (Oyelese and associates, 2004). Thus, vasa previa would ideally be identified early, and scheduled cesarean delivery planned. Clinically, an examiner is occasionally able to palpate or directly see a tubular fetal vessel in the membranes overlying the presenting part. With endovaginal sonography, a vessel may be identified as echogenic, parallel or circular line near the cervix (Fig. 27-7). Because of a low sensitivity for imaging vasa previa with sonography, color Doppler examination is recommended when vasa previa is suspected. Canterino and colleagues (2005) have also described use of 3D-sonography with power Doppler angiography.

Whenever there is hemorrhage antepartum or intrapartum, the possibility of vasa previa and a ruptured fetal vessel should be considered. Determination of bleeding as fetal or maternal is possible, and a variety of tests may be used. Each relies on the increased resistance of fetal hemoglobin compared with maternal to denaturing by alkaline reagents (Lindqvist and Gren,

2007; Oyelese and co-workers, 1999). Unfortunately, the amount of fetal blood that can be shed without killing the fetus is relatively small. Thus, in many cases, fetal death is virtually instantaneous.

Cord Abnormalities Capable of Impeding Blood Flow

Several mechanical and vascular abnormalities of the umbilical cord are capable of impairing fetal–placental blood flow.

Knots

False knots appear as knobs protruding from the cord surface and are focal redundancies of a vessel or Wharton jelly, with no clinical significance. With *true knots,* active fetal movements create cord knotting. The incidence of true knots is approximately 1 percent, and these are more common in monoamnionic twins. The risk of stillbirth is increased five- to tenfold in those with true knots (Airas and Heinonen, 2002; Sørnes, 2000). In live fetuses, although heart rate abnormalities are increased during labor with this complication, cord blood acid-base values are usually normal (Airas and Heinonen, 2002; Maher and Conti, 1996).

Loops

The cord frequently becomes coiled around portions of the fetus, and this is more likely with longer cords. Those looped around the neck are termed a *nuchal cord,* and several large studies have reported one loop of nuchal cord in 20 to 34 percent of deliveries; two loops in 2.5 to 5 percent; and three loops in 0.2 to 0.5 percent (Kan and Eastman, 1957; Sørnes, 1995; Spellacy and associates, 1966). As labor progresses, contractions may compress the cord vessels and create fetal heart rate decelerations that persist until the contraction ceases. In labor, 20 percent of fetuses with a nuchal cord have moderate or severe variable heart rate decelerations, and they are also more likely to have a lower umbilical artery pH (Hankins and colleagues, 1987). Fortunately, coiling of the cord around the neck is an uncommon cause of adverse perinatal outcome (Mastrobattista and co-workers; 2005; Sheiner and associates, 2006).

Funic Presentation

Uncommonly, the umbilical cord may be the presenting part in labor and most often is associated with fetal malpresentation. Cord prolapse or fetal heart rate abnormalities is an associated labor finding, although funic presentation may be identified antenatally with sonography and with color flow Doppler (Ezra and co-workers, 2003; Raga and associates, 1996). If present during labor, cesarean delivery is typically indicated.

Umbilical Cord Stricture

This is a focal narrowing of the cord diameter that typically develops in the area of fetal umbilical insertion (Peng and co-workers, 2006). Absence of Wharton jelly and stenosis or obliteration of cord vessels at the narrow segment are characteristic pathological features (Sun and associates, 1995). Most fetuses are stillborn (French and colleagues, 2005).

Hematoma

These accumulations of blood are associated with short cords, trauma, and entanglement. They may result from a varix rupture, usually of the umbilical vein, with effusion of blood into the cord. Hematomas also may be caused by umbilical vessel venipuncture.

Cysts

Cord cysts occasionally may be found along the course of the cord and are designated true cysts or pseudocysts, according to their origin. *True cysts* are epithelium-lined remnants of the allantois and may co-exist with a persistently patent urachus. In contrast, the more common *pseudocysts* form from local degeneration of Wharton jelly. Both have a similar sonographic appearance.

Single umbilical cord cysts found in the first trimester tend to resolve completely, whereas multiple cysts may portend miscarriage or aneuploidy (Ghezzi and co-workers, 2003; Sepulveda and colleagues, 1999b). Moreover, pseudocysts persisting beyond this can be associated with structural and chromosomal anomalies defects, especially trisomy 18 and 13 (Sepulveda and associates, 1999a; Smith and colleagues, 1996).

Thrombosis

Intrauterine thrombosis of umbilical cord vessels is a rare event (Fig. 27-8). Approximately 70 percent are venous, 20 percent are venous and arterial, and 10 percent are arterial thromboses (Heifetz, 1988). Venous thromboses have lower perinatal morbidity and mortality rates than those in the artery. The latter is associated with fetal-growth restriction and fetal demise (Klaritsch and associates, 2008; Sato and Benirschke, 2006; Singh and co-workers, 2003).

Vessel Dilatation

An *umbilical vein varix* is a marked focal dilatation that may develop within the intra-amnionic part of the umbilical vein or within its fetal intra-abdominal portion. Those found intra-abdominally have increased rates of fetal demise, structural anomalies, and aneuploidy (Fung and co-workers, 2005). The most common complications are varix rupture, varix thrombosis, compression of the umbilical artery, and fetal cardiac failure due to increased preload (Mulch and associates, 2006).

An *umbilical artery aneurysm* is a rare congenital thinning of the vessel wall with diminished support from Wharton jelly. Indeed, most form at or near the cord insertion into the placenta, where this support is absent. There is an association with single umbilical artery, trisomy 18, fetal-growth restriction, and stillbirth (Sepulveda and colleagues, 2003b; Weber and associates, 2007). It has been suggested that these aneurysms lead to fetal hypoxia and death by umbilical vein compression.

PATHOLOGICAL EXAMINATION

Most authorities agree that routine placental examination by a pathologist is not indicated, although there still is debate as to which placentas should be submitted. The College of American

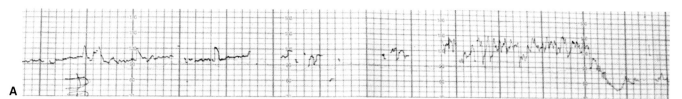

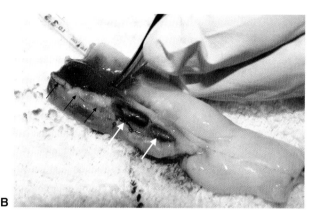

FIGURE 27-8 A. Fetal heart rate tracing shows an initially reassuring and reactive pattern. The fetal heart rate becomes erratic and is followed by persistent fetal bradycardia, which prompts emergent cesarean delivery. **B.** A segment of the umbilical cord following delivery. A neonatal endotracheal tube is seen in the umbilical vein, which is held by forceps. One of the umbilical arteries has been dissected from the surrounding Wharton jelly *(black arrows)*. Two distinct thrombi are seen within this vessel *(white arrows)*. (Used with permission from Dr. J. Seth Hawkins.)

Pathologists recommends routine examination for an extensive list of indications (Langston and colleagues, 1997). Using these guidelines, Curtin and co-workers (2007) computed that 37 percent of all placentas would be submitted. The American College of Obstetricians and Gynecologists (1993) concluded that there are insufficient data to support all of these recommendations.

TABLE 27-1. Some Indications for Placental Examination by a Pathologist

Maternal fever
Chorioamnionitis
Placental abruption
Hypertension
Thyroid disease
Autoimmune disease, thrombosis, or other disorder associated with vasculitis
Meconium
Cord abnormalities
Gross placental abnormalities
Stillbirth/early neonatal death
Neonatal neurological problems
Multifetal gestation
Fetal-growth restriction
Acidotic newborn
Low Apgar scores
Very-low-birthweight infant
Unexpectedly "flat" term or near-term infant[a]

[a]An infant in whom the obstetrical surveillance has been reassuring but who has low Apgar scores or other evidence of poor performance in the delivery room. Infection is a classic cause.
From Gibbs and colleagues (2004), with permission.

Certainly, all agree that the placenta and cord should be examined in the delivery room. The decision to request pathological examination will depend on clinical and placental findings. At this time, some correlation of specific placental findings with both short- and long-term neonatal outcomes is possible. Gibbs and co-workers (2004), based largely on conclusions reached in the 2003 American College of Obstetricians and Gynecologists/American Academy of Pediatrics publication, *Neonatal Encephalopathy and Cerebral Palsy*, provide the indications shown in Table 27-1.

REFERENCES

Adeniran AJ, Stanek J: Amnion nodosum revisited: Clinicopathologic and placental correlations. Arch Pathol Lab Med 131:1829, 2007

Airas U, Heinonen S: Clinical significance of true umbilical knots: A population-based analysis. Am J Perinatol 19:127, 2002

Al-Adnani M, Kiho L, Scheimberg I: Maternal pancreatic carcinoma metastatic to the placenta: A case report and literature review. Pediatr Dev Pathol 10:61, 2007

Al-Adnani M, Sebire NJ: The role of perinatal pathological examination in subclinical infection in obstetrics. Best Pract Res Clin Obstet Gynaecol 21:505, 2007

Alexander A, Samlowski WE, Grossman D, et al: Metastatic melanoma in pregnancy: Risk of transplacental metastases in the infant. J Clin Oncol 21:2179, 2003

Altman JF, Lowe L, Redman B, et al: Placental metastasis of maternal melanoma. J Am Acad Dermatol 49:1150, 2003

American College of Obstetricians and Gynecologists, American Academy of Pediatrics: Neonatal Encephalopathy and Cerebral Palsy: Defining the Pathogenesis and Pathophysiology. Washington, DC, ACOG; 2003.

American College of Obstetricians and Gynecologists: Committee on Obstetrics: Maternal-Fetal Medicine. Placental Pathology No. 125, July 1993

Andres RL, Kuyper W, Resnik R, et al: The association of maternal floor infarction of the placenta with adverse perinatal outcome. Am J Obstet Gynecol 163:935, 1990

Ball RH, Ade CM, Schoenborn JA, et al: The clinical significance of ultrasonographically detected subchorionic hemorrhages. Am J Obstet Gynecol 174:996, 1996

Barbieri C, Cecatti JG, Krupa F, et al: Validation study of the capacity of the reference curves of ultrasonographic measurements of the umbilical cord to identify deviations in estimated fetal weight. Acta Obstet Gynecol Scand 87:286, 2008

Baulies S, Maiz N, Muñoz A, et al: Prenatal ultrasound diagnosis of vasa praevia and analysis of risk factors. Prenat Diagn 27:595, 2007

Benirschke K, Kaufmann P, Baergen R: Pathology of the Human Placenta, 5th ed. New York, Springer, 2006, pp 353, 401, 455

Berg TG, Rayburn WF: Umbilical cord length and acid-base balance at delivery. J Reprod Med 40:9, 1995

Budorick NE, Kelly TF, Dunn JA, et al: The single umbilical artery in a high-risk patient population: What should be offered? J Ultrasound Med 20:619, 2001

Byrne J, Blanc WA: Malformations and chromosome anomalies in spontaneously aborted fetuses with single umbilical artery. Am J Obstet Gynecol 151:340, 1985

Canterino JC, Modestin-Sorrentino M, Muench MV, et al: Vasa previa: Prenatal diagnosis and evaluation with 3-dimensional sonography and power angiography. J Ultrasound Med 24:721, 2005

Catanzarite VA, Hendricks SK, Maida C, et al: Prenatal diagnosis of the two-vessel cord: Implications for patient counseling and obstetric management. Ultrasound Obstet Gynecol 5:75, 1995

Cromi A, Ghezzi F, Di Naro E, et al: Large cross-sectional area of the umbilical cord as a predictor of fetal macrosomia. Ultrasound Obstet Gynecol 30:804, 2007

Curtin WM, Krauss S, Metlay LA, et al: Pathologic examination of the placenta and observed practice. Obstet Gynecol 109:35, 2007

de Laat MW, Franx A, Bots ML, et al: Umbilical coiling index in normal and complicated pregnancies. Obstet Gynecol 107:1049, 2006

de Laat MW, Franx A, van Alderen ED, et al: The umbilical coiling index, a review of the literature. J Matern Fetal Neonatal Med 17:93, 2005

de Laat MW, van Alderen ED, Franx A, et al: The umbilical coiling index in complicated pregnancy. Eur J Obstet Gynecol Reprod Biol 130:66, 2007

Deans A, Jauniaux E: Prenatal diagnosis and outcome of subamniotic hematomas. Ultrasound Obstet Gynecol 11:319, 1998

Ezra Y, Strasberg SR, Farine D: Does cord presentation on ultrasound predict cord prolapse? Gynecol Obstet Invest 56:6, 2003

Faye-Petersen OM, Heller DS, Joshi VV: Handbook of Placental Pathology, 2nd ed. London, Taylor & Francis, 2006, pp 27, 29, 39, 83

Feldman DM, Borgida AF, Trymbulak WP, et al: Clinical implications of velamentous cord insertion in triplet gestations. Am J Obstet Gynecol 186:809, 2002

Fox H, Sebire NJ: Pathology of the Placenta, 3rd ed. Philadelphia, Saunders, 2007, pp 79, 99, 133, 484

French AE, Gregg VH, Newberry Y, et al: Umbilical cord stricture: A cause of recurrent fetal death. Obstet Gynecol 105:1235, 2005

Fujikura T: Fused umbilical arteries near placental cord insertion. Am J Obstet Gynecol 188:765, 2003

Fujikura T, Klionsky B: The significance of meconium staining. Am J Obstet Gynecol 121:45, 1975

Fung TY, Leung TN, Leung TY, et al: Fetal intra-abdominal umbilical vein varix: What is the clinical significance? Ultrasound Obstet Gynecol 25:149, 2005

Ghezzi F, Raio L, Di Naro E, et al: Single and multiple umbilical cord cysts in early gestation: Two different entities. Ultrasound Obstet Gynecol 21:213, 2003

Ghidini A, Spong CY: Severe meconium aspiration syndrome is not caused by aspiration of meconium. Am J Obstet Gynecol 185:931, 2001

Gibbs RS, Rosenberg AR, Warren CJ, et al: Suggestions for practice to accompany neonatal encephalopathy and cerebral palsy. Obstet Gynecol 103:778, 2004

Gogia N, Machin GA: Maternal thrombophilias are associated with specific placental lesions. Pediatr Dev Pathol 11(6):424, 2008

Goldenberg RL, Hauth JC, Andrews WW: Intrauterine infection and preterm delivery. N Engl J Med 342:1500, 2000

Goldkrand JW, Pettigrew C, Lentz SU, et al: Volumetric umbilical artery blood flow: Comparison of the normal versus the single umbilical artery cord. J Matern Fetal Med 10:116, 2001

Gordon Z, Eytan O, Jaffa AJ, et al: Hemodynamic analysis of Hyrtl anastomosis in human placenta. Am J Physiol Regul Integra Comp Physiol 292:R977, 2007

Gornall AS, Kurinczuk JJ, Konje JC: Antenatal detection of a single umbilical artery: Does it matter? Prenat Diagn 23:117, 2003

Granese R, Coco C, Jeanty P: The value of single umbilical artery in the prediction of fetal aneuploidy: Findings in 12,672 pregnant women. Ultrasound Q 23:117, 2007

Greenberg JA, Sorem KA, Shifren JL, et al: Placenta membranacea with placenta increta: A case report and literature review. Obstet Gynecol 78:512, 1991

Guschmann M, Henrich W, Entezami M, et al: Chorioangioma—new insights into a well-known problem. I. Results of a clinical and morphological study of 136 cases. J Perinatal Med 31:163, 2003

Hankins GD, Snyder RR, Hauth JC, et al: Nuchal cords and neonatal outcome. Obstet Gynecol 70:687, 1987

Heifetz SA: Single umbilical artery: A statistical analysis of 237 autopsy cases and a review of the literature. Perspect Pediatr Pathol 8:345, 1984

Heifetz SA: Thrombosis of the umbilical cord: Analysis of 52 cases and literature review. Pediatr Pathol 8:37, 1988

Hill LM, Breckle R, Ragozzino MW, et al: Grade 3 placentation: Incidence and neonatal outcome. Obstet Gynecol 61:728, 1983

Hill LM, Wibner D, Gonzales P, et al: Validity of transabdominal sonography in the detection of a two-vessel umbilical cord. Obstet Gynecol 98:837, 2001

Jazayeri A, Jazayeri MK, Sahinler M, et al: Is meconium passage a risk factor for maternal infection in term pregnancy? Obstet Gynecol 99:548, 2002

Jeanty P: Persistent right umbilical vein: An ominous prenatal finding? Radiology 177:735, 1990

Kan PS, Eastman NJ: Coiling of the umbilical cord around the foetal neck. Br J Obstet Gynaecol 64:227, 1957

Katz VL, Bowes WA Jr: Meconium aspiration syndrome: Reflections on a murky subject. Am J Obstet Gynecol 166:171, 1992

Katz VL, DiTomasso J, Farmer R, et al: Activated protein C resistance associated with maternal floor infarction treated with low-molecular-weight heparin. Am J Perinatol 19:273, 2002

Klaritsch P, Haeusler M, Karpf E, et al: Spontaneous intrauterine umbilical artery thrombosis leading to severe fetal growth restriction. Placenta 29:374, 2008

Krakowiak P, Smith EN, de Bruyn G, et al: Risk factors and outcomes associated with a short umbilical cord. Obstet Gynecol 103:119, 2004

Krebs HB, Petres RE, Dunn LJ: Intrapartum fetal heart rate monitoring. III. Association of meconium with abnormal fetal heart rate patterns. Am J Obstet Gynecol 137:936, 1980

Lademacher DS, Vermeulen RCW, Harten JJVD, et al: Circumvallate placenta and congenital malformation. Lancet 1:732, 1981

Langston C, Kaplan C, Macpherson T, et al: Practice guideline for examination of the placenta. Arch Pathol Lab Med 121:449, 1997

Lau TK, Leung TY, Yu SC, et al: Prenatal treatment of chorioangioma by microcoil embolisation. BJOG 110:70, 2003

Lee W, Lee VL, Kirk JS, et al: Vasa previa: Prenatal diagnosis, natural evolution and clinical outcome. Obstet Gynecol 95:572, 2000

Leung AK, Robson WL: Single umbilical artery: A report of 159 cases. Am J Dis Child 143:108, 1989

Lindqvist PG, Gren P: An easy-to-use method for detecting fetal hemoglobin—a test to identify bleeding from vasa previa. Eur J Obstet Gynecol Reprod Biol 131:151, 2007

Liu CC, Pretorius DH, Scioscia AL, et al: Sonographic prenatal diagnosis of marginal placental cord insertion: Clinical importance. Ultrasound Med 21:627, 2002

Lubusky M, Dhaifalah I, Prochazka M, et al: Single umbilical artery and its siding in the second trimester of pregnancy: Relation to chromosomal defects. Prenat Diagn 27:327, 2007

Madu AE: Breus' mole in pregnancy. J Obstet Gynaecol 26:815, 2006

Maher JT, Conti JA: A comparison of umbilical cord blood gas values between newborns with and without true knots. Obstet Gynecol 88:863, 1996

Mandsager NT, Bendon R, Mostello D, et al: Maternal floor infarction of the placenta: Prenatal diagnosis and clinical significance. Obstet Gynecol 83:750, 1994

Martinez-Frias ML, Bermejo E, Rodriguez-Pinilla E, et al: Does single umbilical artery (SUA) predict any type of congenital defect? Clinical-epidemiological analysis of a large consecutive series of malformed infants. Am J Med Genet A 146:15, 2008

Mastrobattista JM, Hollier LM, Yeomans ER, et al: Effects of nuchal cord on birthweight and immediate neonatal outcomes. Am J Perinatol 22:83, 2005

McKenna D, Tharmaratnam S, Mahsud S, et al: Ultrasonic evidence of placental calcification at 36 weeks' gestation: Maternal and fetal outcomes. Acta Obstet Gynecol Scand 84:7, 2005

Meyer WW, Lind J, Moinian M: An accessory fourth vessel of the umbilical cord: A preliminary study. Am J Obstet Gynecol 105:1063, 1969

Miller PW, Coen RW, Benirschke K: Dating the time interval from meconium passage to birth. Obstet Gynecol 66:459, 1985

Miller ME, Higginbottom M, Smith DW: Short umbilical cord: Its origin and relevance. Pediatrics 67:618, 1981

Montan S, Jörgensen C, Svalenius E, et al: Placental grading with ultrasound in hypertensive and normotensive pregnancies: A prospective, consecutive study. Acta Obstet Gynecol Scand 65:477, 1986

Mulch AD, Stallings SP, Salafia CM: Elevated maternal serum alpha-fetoprotein, umbilical vein varix, and mesenchymal dysplasia: Are they related? Prenat Diagn 26:659, 2006

Nagy S, Bush M, Stone J, et al: Clinical significance of subchorionic and retroplacental hematomas detected in the first trimester of pregnancy. Obstet Gynecol 102:94, 2003

Nathan L, Leveno KJ, Carmody TJ III, et al: Meconium: A 1990s perspective on an old obstetric hazard. Obstet Gynecol 83:329, 1994

Nicolini U, Zuliani G, Caravelli E, et al: Alcohol injection: A new method of treating placental chorioangiomas. Lancet 353(9165):1674, 1999

Nyberg DA, Cyr DR, Mack LA, et al: Sonographic spectrum of placental abruption. AJR Am J Roentgenol 148:161, 1987

Oyelese Y, Catanzarite V, Prefumo F, et al: Vasa previa: The impact of prenatal diagnosis on outcomes. Obstet Gynecol 103:937, 2004

Oyelese Y, Culin A, Ananth CV, et al: Meconium-stained amniotic fluid across gestation and neonatal acid-base status. Obstet Gynecol 108:345, 2006

Oyelese KO, Turner M, Lees C, et al: Vasa previa: An avoidable obstetric tragedy. Obstet Gynecol Surv 54:138, 1999

Papinniemi M, Keski-Nisula L, Heinonen S: Placental ratio and risk of velamentous umbilical cord insertion are increased in women with placenta previa. Am J Perinatol 24:353, 2007

Peng HQ, Levitin-Smith M, Rochelson B, et al: Umbilical cord stricture and overcoiling are common causes of fetal demise. Pediatr Dev Pathol 9:14, 2006

Pierce BT, Dance VD, Wagner RK, et al: Perinatal outcome following fetal single umbilical artery diagnosis. J Matern Fetal Med 10:59, 2001

Prapas N, Liang RI, Hunter D, et al: Color Doppler imaging of placental masses: Differential diagnosis and fetal outcome. Ultrasound Obstet Gynecol 16:559, 2000

Predanic M, Perni SC, Chasen ST, et al: Assessment of umbilical cord coiling during the routine fetal sonographic anatomic survey in the second trimester. J Ultrasound Med 24:185, 2005a

Predanic M, Perni SC, Friedman A, et al: Fetal growth assessment and neonatal birth weight in fetuses with an isolated single umbilical artery. Obstet Gynecol 105:1093 2005b

Predanic M, Perni SC, Chasen ST, et al: Ultrasound evaluation of abnormal umbilical cord coiling in second trimester of gestation in association with adverse pregnancy outcome. Am J Obstet Gynecol 193:387, 2005c

Prucka S, Clemens M, Craven C, et al: Single umbilical artery: What does it mean for the fetus? A case-control analysis of pathologically ascertained cases. Genet Med 6:54, 2004

Quintero RA, Reich H, Romero R, et al: In utero endoscopic devascularization of a large chorioangioma. Ultrasound Obstet Gynecol 8:48, 1996

Raga F, Osborne N, Ballester MJ, et al: Color flow Doppler: A useful instrument in the diagnosis of funic presentation. J Natl Med Assoc 88:94, 1996

Raio L, Ghezzi F, Di Naro E, et al: Prenatal assessment of the Hyrtl anastomosis and evaluation of its function: Case report. Hum Reprod 14:1890, 1999a

Raio L, Ghezzi F, Di Naro E, et al: Sonographic measurement of the umbilical cord and fetal anthropometric parameters. Eur J Obstet Gynecol Reprod Biol 83:131, 1999b

Raio L, Ghezzi F, Di Naro E, et al: In-utero characterization of the blood flow in the Hyrtl anastomosis. Placenta 22:597, 2001

Raio L, Ghezzi F, Di Naro E, et al: Umbilical cord morphologic characteristics and umbilical artery Doppler parameters in intrauterine growth-restricted fetuses. J Ultrasound Med 22:1341, 2003

Redline RW: Inflammatory responses in the placenta and umbilical cord. Semin Fetal Neonatal Med 11:296, 2006

Sato Y, Benirschke K: Umbilical arterial thrombosis with vascular wall necrosis: Clinicopathologic findings of 11 cases. Placenta 27:715, 2006

Sau A, Seed P, Langford K: Intraobserver and interobserver variation in the sonographic grading of placental maturity. Ultrasound Obstet Gynecol 23:374, 2004

Schachter M, Tovbin Y, Arieli S, et al: In vitro fertilization is a risk factor for vasa previa. Fertil Steril 79:1254, 2003

Sebire NJ, Backos M, El Gaddal S, et al: Placental pathology, antiphospholipid antibodies, and pregnancy outcome in recurrent miscarriage patients. Obstet Gynecol 101:258, 2003

Sebire NJ, Backos M, Goldin RD, et al: Placental massive perivillous fibrin deposition associated with antiphospholipid antibody syndrome. Br J Obstet Gynaecol 109:570, 2002

Sepulveda W, Alcalde JL, Schnapp C: Perinatal outcome after prenatal diagnosis of placental chorioangioma. Obstet Gynecol 102:1028, 2003a

Sepulveda W, Aviles G, Carstens E, et al: Prenatal diagnosis of solid placental masses: The value of color flow imaging. Ultrasound Obstet Gynecol 16:554, 2000

Sepulveda W, Corral E, Kottmann C, et al: Umbilical artery aneurysm: Prenatal identification in three fetuses with trisomy 18. Ultrasound Obstet Gynecol 21:213, 2003b

Sepulveda W, Gutierrez J, Sanchez, et al: Pseudocyst of the umbilical cord: Prenatal sonographic appearance and clinical significance. Obstet Gynecol 93:377, 1999a

Sepulveda W, Leible S, Ulloa A, et al: Clinical significance of first trimester umbilical cord cysts. J Ultrasound Med 18(2):95, 1999b

Sepulveda W, Wong AE, Herrera L, et al: Endoscopic laser coagulation of feeding vessels in large placental chorioangiomas: Report of three cases and review of invasive treatment options. Prenat Diagn 29(3):201, 2009

Sheffield JS, Sánchez PJ, Wendel GD Jr, et al: Placental histopathology of congenital syphilis. Obstet Gynecol 100:126, 2002

Sheiner E, Abramowicz JS, Levy A, et al: Nuchal cord is not associated with adverse perinatal outcome. Arch Gynecol Obstet 274:81, 2006

Singh V, Khanum S, Singh M: Umbilical cord lesions in early intrauterine fetal demise. Arch Pathol Lab Med 127:850, 2003

Smith GN, Walker M, Johnston S: The sonographic finding of persistent umbilical cord cystic masses is associated with lethal aneuploidy and/or congenital anomalies. Prenat Diagn 16:1141, 1996

Sørnes T: Umbilical cord encirclements and fetal growth restriction. Obstet Gynecol 86:725, 1995

Sørnes T: Umbilical cord knots. Acta Obstet Gynecol Scand 79:157, 2000

Spellacy WN, Gravem H, Fisch RO: The umbilical cord complications of true knots, nuchal coils and cords around the body. Report from the collaborative study of cerebral palsy. Am J Obstet Gynecol 94:1136, 1966

Strong TH Jr, Jarles DL, Vega JS, et al: The umbilical coiling index. Am J Obstet Gynecol 170(1 Pt 1):29, 1994

Sun Y, Arbuckle S, Hocking G, et al: Umbilical cord stricture and intrauterine fetal death. Pediatr Pathol Lab Med 15:723, 1995

Suzuki S: Clinical significance of pregnancies with circumvallate placenta. J Obstet Gynaecol Res 34:51, 2008

Suzuki S, Igarashi M: Clinical significance of pregnancies with succenturiate lobes of placenta. Arch Gynecol Obstet 277:299, 2008

Suzuki S, Igarashi M, Inde Y, et al: Abnormally shaped placentae in twin pregnancy. Arch Gynecol Obstet [Epub ahead of print], 2009

Tran SH, Caughey AB, Musei TJ: Meconium-stained amniotic fluid is associated with puerperal infections. Am J Obstet Gynecol 191:2175, 2004

Tybulewicz AT, Clegg SK, Fonfé GJ, et al: Preterm meconium staining of the amniotic fluid: Associated findings and risk of adverse clinical outcome. Arch Dis Child Fetal Neonatal Ed 89:F328, 2004

Van Den Bosch T, Van Schoubroeck D, Cornelis A, et al: Prenatal diagnosis of a subamniotic hematoma. Fetal Diagn Ther 15:32, 2000

Volpe G, Volpe N, Fucci L, et al: Subamniotic hematoma: 3D and color Doppler imaging in the differential diagnosis of placental masses and fetal outcome. Minerva Ginecol 60:255, 2008

Walsh MC, Fanaroff JM: Meconium stained fluid: Approach to the mother and the baby. Clin Perinatol 34:653, 2007

Wanapirak C, Tongsong T, Sirichotiyakul S, et al: Alcholization: The choice of intrautcrine treatment for chorioangioma. J Obstet Gynaecol Res 28:71, 2002

Weber MA, Sau A, Maxwell DJ, et al: Third trimester intrauterine fetal death caused by arterial aneurysm of the umbilical cord. Pediatr Deve Pathol 10:305, 2007

Wiegand S, McKenna DS, Croom C, et al: Serial sonographic growth assessment in pregnancies complicated by an isolated single umbilical artery. Am J Perinatol 25:149, 2008

Yamada S, Hamanishi J, Tanada S, et al: Embryogenesis of fused umbilical arteries in human embryos. Am J Obstet Gynecol 193:1709, 2005

Zalel Y, Weisz B, Gamzu R, et al: Chorioangiomas of the placenta: Sonographic and Doppler flow characteristics. Ultrasound Med 21:909, 2002

FETUS AND NEWBORN

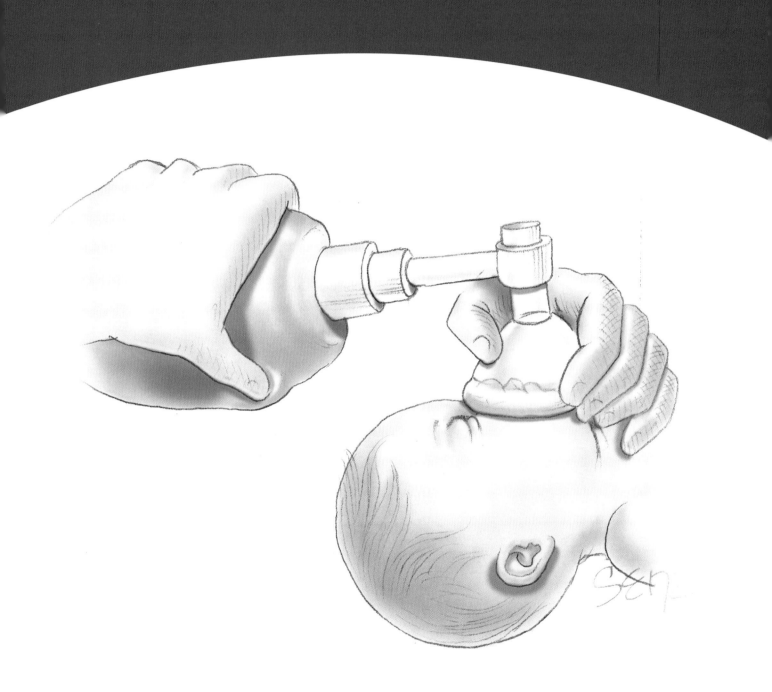

CHAPTER 28

The Newborn Infant

Immediately following birth, infant survival depends on a prompt and orderly conversion to air breathing. Fluid-filled alveoli expand with air, perfusion must be established, and oxygen and carbon dioxide exchanged.

INITIATION OF AIR BREATHING

Stimuli to Breathe Air

The newborn begins to breathe and cry almost immediately after birth, indicating the establishment of active respiration. Factors that appear to influence the first breath of air include:

1. Physical *stimulation,* such as handling the neonate during delivery
2. *Deprivation of oxygen and accumulation of carbon dioxide,* which serve to increase the frequency and magnitude of breathing movements both before and after birth (Dawes, 1974)
3. *Compression of the thorax,* which during pelvic descent and vaginal birth forces an amount of fluid from the respiratory tract equivalent to about a fourth of the ultimate functional residual capacity (Saunders and Milner, 1978).

Aeration of the newborn lung does not involve the inflation of a collapsed structure, but instead, the rapid replacement of bronchial and alveolar fluid by air. After delivery, the residual alveolar fluid is cleared through the pulmonary circulation and to a lesser degree, through the pulmonary lymphatics (Chernick, 1978). Delay in removal of fluid from the alveoli probably contributes to the syndrome of *transient tachypnea of the newborn (TTN)* (Guglani and co-workers, 2008). As fluid is replaced by air, the compression of the pulmonary vasculature is reduced considerably and in turn, resistance to blood flow is lowered. With the fall in pulmonary arterial blood pressure, the ductus arteriosus normally closes (see Fig. 4-12, p. 90).

High negative intrathoracic pressures are required to bring about the initial entry of air into the fluid-filled alveoli. Normally, from the first breath after birth, progressively more residual air accumulates in the lung, and with each successive breath, lower pulmonary opening pressure is required. In the normal mature newborn, by approximately the fifth breath, pressure-volume changes achieved with each respiration are very similar to those of the adult. Thus, the breathing pattern shifts from the shallow episodic inspirations characteristic of the fetus to regular, deeper inhalations (see Chap. 15, p. 336). Surfactant—synthesized by type II pneumocytes and already present—lowers alveolar surface tension and thereby prevents collapse of the lung with each expiration. Lack of sufficient surfactant, common in preterm infants, leads to the prompt development of *respiratory distress syndrome* (see Chap. 29, p. 605).

MANAGEMENT OF DELIVERY

Immediate Care

Before and during delivery, careful consideration must be given to several determinants of neonatal well-being including: (1) health status of the mother; (2) prenatal complications, including any suspected fetal malformations; (3) gestational age; (4) labor complications; (5) duration of labor and ruptured membranes; (6) type and duration of anesthesia; (7) difficulty with delivery; and (8) medications given during labor and their amounts, times given, and routes of administration.

The American Academy of Pediatrics and the American College of Obstetricians and Gynecologists (2007) recommend attendance at delivery of at least one person whose primary responsibility is the neonate and who is capable of initiating resuscitation. Either that person or someone else who is immediately available should have the skills required to perform complete resuscitation.

Newborn Resuscitation

Approximately 10 percent of newborns require some degree of active resuscitation to stimulate breathing, and 1 percent require extensive resuscitation (International Liaison Committee on Resuscitation, 2006). It is perhaps not coincidental that the risk of death for newborns delivered at home in Washington State between 1989 and 1996 was nearly twice that of those delivered in hospitals (Pang and co-workers, 2002). When deprived of oxygen, either before or after birth, neonates demonstrate a well-defined sequence of events leading to apnea. As shown in Figure 28-1, oxygen deprivation results initially in a transient period of rapid breathing. If such deprivation persists, however, breathing stops and the infant enters a stage of *primary apnea*. This stage is accompanied by a fall in heart rate and loss of neuromuscular tone. Simple stimulation and exposure to oxygen will usually reverse primary apnea. If oxygen deprivation and asphyxia persist, however, the newborn will develop deep gasping respirations, followed by *secondary apnea*. This latter stage is associated with a further decline in heart rate, falling blood pressure, and loss of neuromuscular tone. Neonates in secondary apnea will not respond to stimulation and will not spontaneously resume respiratory efforts. Unless ventilation is assisted, death follows. Clinically, primary and secondary apnea are indistinguishable. Thus, secondary apnea must be assumed and resuscitation of the apneic newborn must be started immediately.

Resuscitation Protocol

The following is a summary of the guidelines for neonatal resuscitation recommended by the International Liaison Committee on Resuscitation (2006).

Basic Steps. As shown in Figure 28-2, the newborn is first placed in a warm environment to minimize heat loss. Next, the airway is cleared as necessary. If the delivery is complicated by meconium and the infant is not vigorous, tracheal intubation is recommended as subsequently discussed to allow suctioning before further resuscitative efforts are performed. The infant is then dried and stimulated after which respiratory effort, heart rate, and color are assessed. In most instances, the newborn will take a breath within a few seconds of birth and cry within half a minute. If the infant is breathing, the heart rate is greater than 100 bpm, and the skin of the central portion of the body and mucous membranes are pink, then routine supportive care is provided.

Ventilation. Apnea, gasping respirations, or bradycardia beyond 30 seconds after delivery should prompt administration of *positive-pressure ventilation* (Fig. 28-3). Assisted ventilation rates of 30 to 60 breaths per minute are commonly employed. Adequate ventilation is indicated by bilateral rise of the chest, ability to auscultate breath sounds, and improvement of heart rate and color. If ventilation is inadequate, the head position should be checked as shown in Figure 28-3, secretions cleared, and if necessary, inflation pressure increased.

Failure by the newborn to establish effective respirations may result from a variety of complications, including the following:

- Hypoxemia or acidosis from any cause
- Drugs administered to the mother prior to delivery
- Immaturity
- Upper airway obstruction
- Pneumothorax
- Lung abnormalities, either intrinsic—for example, hypoplasia, or extrinsic—for example, diaphragmatic hernia
- Aspiration of meconium-laden amnionic fluid
- Central nervous system developmental abnormality
- Septicemia.

Endotracheal Intubation. If bag-and-mask ventilation is ineffective or prolonged, tracheal intubation should be performed. Other indications include the need for chest compressions or tracheal administration of medications, or special circumstances such as extremely low birthweight or congenital diaphragmatic hernia. A laryngoscope with a straight blade—size 0 for a preterm infant and size 1 for a term neonate—is introduced at the side of the mouth and then directed posteriorly toward the oropharynx (Fig. 28-4). The laryngoscope is next moved gently into the space, termed the vallecula, between the base of the

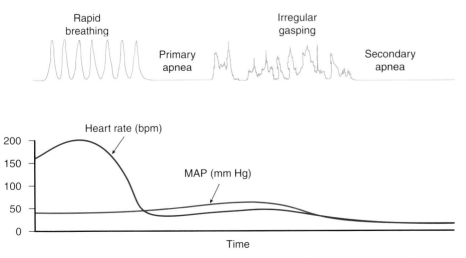

FIGURE 28-1 Physiological changes associated with primary and secondary apnea in the newborn. (Adapted from Kattwinkel, 2000.)

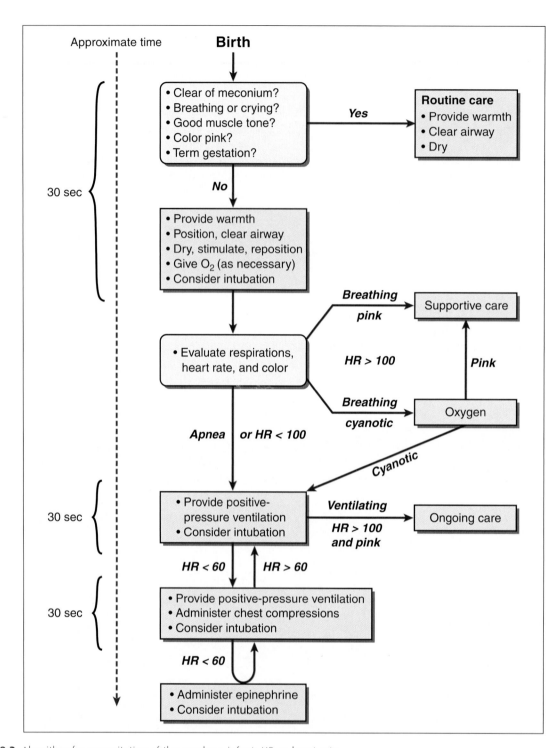

FIGURE 28-2 Algorithm for resuscitation of the newborn infant. HR = heart rate.

tongue and the epiglottis. Gentle elevation of the tip of the laryngoscope will raise the epiglottis and expose the glottis and the vocal cords. The tube is then introduced through the vocal cords. Gentle cricoid pressure may be useful. Suggested tube sizes and depth of insertion are shown in Table 28-1.

Several steps are taken to ensure that the tube is positioned in the trachea and not the esophagus: observation for symmetrical chest wall motion; auscultation for equal breath sounds, especially in the axillae; and auscultation for the absence of breath sounds or gur-

gling over the stomach. Given that meconium, blood, mucus, and particulate debris in amnionic fluid or in the birth canal may have been inhaled prior to delivery, any foreign material encountered in the tracheal tube is suctioned immediately. During suctioning a negative pressure of 80 to 100 mm Hg is applied as the cannula is slowly withdrawn. The endotracheal tube is then replaced. Kaiser and colleagues (2008) caution that suctioning in very-low-birth-weight infants causes potentially deleterious increases of up to 30 percent in cerebral blood flow velocity.

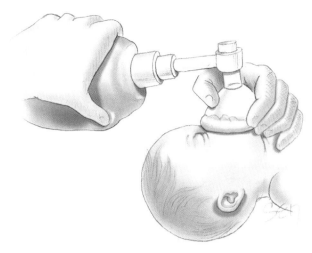

FIGURE 28-3 Correct use of bag-and-mask ventilation. The head should be in a sniffing position with the tip of the nose pointing to the ceiling, and care should be taken to avoid hyperextension of the neck.

Using an appropriate ventilation bag attached to the tracheal tube, puffs of air are delivered into the tube at 1- to 2-second intervals with a force adequate to gently lift the chest wall. Pressures of 25 to 35 cm H_2O typically will expand the alveoli without causing pneumothorax, pneumomediastinum, or other barotrauma. If ventilatory pressure is not being monitored, an increase in heart rate should be used to indicate adequate inflation pressure. If there is central cyanosis, the air should be oxygen-enriched.

Chest Compressions. If the heart rate remains below 60 bpm despite adequate ventilation with 100-percent oxygen for 30 seconds, chest compressions are initiated. Compressions are delivered on the lower third of the sternum at a depth sufficient to generate a palpable pulse. A 3:1 ratio of compressions to ventilations is recommended, with 90 compressions and 30 breaths to achieve approximately 120 events each minute. The heart rate is reassessed every 30 seconds, and chest compressions are continued until the spontaneous heart rate is at least 60 bpm.

Medications and Volume Expansion. Epinephrine is indicated when the heart rate remains below 60 bpm after a mini-

mum of 30 seconds of adequate ventilation and chest compressions. Epinephrine is particularly indicated if there is asystole. The recommended intravenous dose is 0.01 to 0.03 mg/kg, that is, 0.1 to 0.3 mL/kg of a 1:10,000 solution. If given through the tracheal tube, higher doses are employed, up to 0.1 mg/kg, that is, 1 mL/kg. Epinephrine is repeated every 3 to 5 minutes as indicated.

Volume expansion should be considered when blood loss is suspected, the infant appears to be in shock, or the response to resuscitative measures is inadequate. An isotonic crystalloid solution, such as normal saline or Ringer lactate, is recommended. Symptomatic anemia may require transfusion of red blood cells. The initial dose of either type of volume expander is 10 mL/kg given by slow intravenous push over 5 to 10 minutes. This is delivered via a catheter placed into the umbilical vein.

Routine use of *sodium bicarbonate* during neonatal resuscitation is controversial and usually not done. The hyperosmolarity and CO_2-generating properties of bicarbonate may be detrimental to myocardial and cerebral function (Kette and associates, 1991). If sodium bicarbonate is used during prolonged arrests unresponsive to other therapy, it should be administered only after establishment of adequate ventilation and circulation.

Naloxone is a narcotic antagonist indicated for reversal of respiratory depression in a newborn whose mother received narcotics within 4 hours of delivery. It is not recommended as part of initial resuscitation, and heart rate and color should be restored by adequate ventilation prior to naloxone administration. The standard dose of naloxone is 0.1 mg/kg, although this has been poorly studied. Because the narcotic duration of action may exceed that of naloxone, continued monitoring of respiratory function is essential, and repeated doses may be necessary. Based on their systematic review of nine studies, McGuire and Fowlie (2003) concluded that *prophylactic* naloxone administration has not been shown to have any clinical benefits. Gill and Colvin (2007) question its use at all.

Discontinuation of Resuscitation. As expected, newborns with cardiopulmonary arrest who do not respond promptly to resuscitation are at great risk for mortality and if they survive, severe morbidity. Haddad and associates (2000) described 33 infants born without cardiac or respiratory effort that persisted for at least the first 5 minutes of life, and in whom resuscitation was attempted. Of 11 survivors, five had clinical or radiological signs of neurological injury, four were lost to follow-up, and the

TABLE 28-1. Suggested Endotracheal Tube Size and Depth of Insertion

Weight (g)	Gestational Age (wk)	Tube Size (mm) (Inside diameter)	Depth of Insertion from Upper Lip (cm)
<1000	<28	2.5	6–7
1000–2000	28–34	3.0	7–8
2000–3000	34–38	3.5	8–9
>3000	>38	3.5–4.0	>9

Compiled from Kattwinkel (2006) used with permission of the American Academy of Pediatrics, *Textbook of Neonatal Resuscitation*, 5th ed., Copyright American Academy of Pediatrics and American Heart Association, 2006.

other two had normal neurological development. The International Liaison Committee on Resuscitation (2006) concluded that discontinuation of resuscitative efforts may be appropriate if there are no signs of life after 10 minutes of continuous and adequate resuscitative efforts. This is because continued resuscitation is associated with a very high mortality rate or severe neurodevelopmental disability.

METHODS USED TO EVALUATE NEWBORN CONDITION

Apgar Score

This scoring system is a useful clinical tool to identify those neonates who require resuscitation as well as to assess the effectiveness of any resuscitative measures (Apgar, 1953). As shown in Table 28-2, each of the five easily identifiable characteristics—heart rate, respiratory effort, muscle tone, reflex irritability, and color—is assessed and assigned a value of 0 to 2. The total score, based on the sum of the five components, is determined 1 and 5 minutes after delivery.

The 1-minute Apgar score reflects the need for immediate resuscitation. The 5-minute score, and particularly the change in score between 1 and 5 minutes, is a useful index of the effectiveness of resuscitative efforts. The 5-minute Apgar score also has prognostic significance for neonatal survival, because survival is related closely to the condition of the neonate in the delivery room (Apgar and associates, 1958). In an analysis of more than 150,000 infants delivered at Parkland Hospital, Casey and associates (2001b) assessed

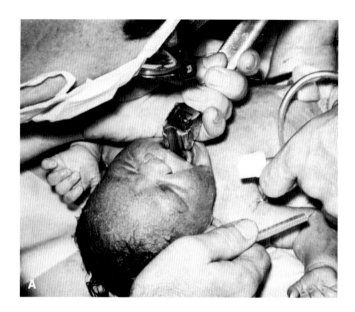

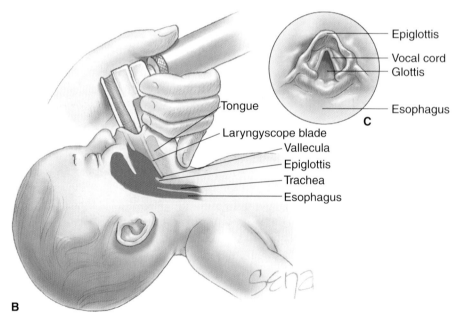

FIGURE 28-4 A. Use of laryngoscope to insert a tracheal tube under direct vision. **B.** Sagittal view during intubation. The laryngoscope blade is inserted between the tongue base and epiglottis. Upward tilting of the tongue also lifts the epiglottis. **C.** The endotracheal tube is then threaded below the epiglottis and between the vocal cords to enter the trachea.

TABLE 28-2. Apgar Scoring System

Sign	0 Points	1 Point	2 Points
Heart rate	Absent	<100 bpm	≥100 bpm
Respiratory effort	Absent	Slow, irregular	Good, crying
Muscle tone	Flaccid	Some flexion of extremities	Active motion
Reflex irritability	No response	Grimace	Vigorous cry
Color	Blue, pale	Body pink, extremities blue	Completely pink

Data from Apgar (1953).

the contemporaneous significance of the 5-minute score for predicting survival during the first 28 days of life. They found that in term neonates, the risk of neonatal death was approximately 1 in 5000 for those with Apgar scores of 7 to 10. This risk compares with a mortality rate of 1 in 4 for term infants with scores of 3 or less. Low 5-minute scores were comparably predictive of neonatal death in preterm infants. These investigators concluded that the Apgar scoring system is as relevant for the prediction of neonatal survival today as it was almost 50 years ago.

There have been attempts to use Apgar scores to define asphyxial injury and to predict subsequent neurological outcome—uses for which the Apgar score was never intended. Such associations are difficult to measure with reliability given that both asphyxial injury and low Apgar scores are infrequent outcomes. For example, according to United States birth certificate records for 2006, only 1.6 percent of newborns had a 5-minute score below 7 (Martin and co-workers, 2009). Similarly, in a population-based study of more than 1 million term infants born in Sweden between 1988 and 1997, the incidence of 5-minute Apgar scores of 3 or less was approximately 2 per 1000 (Thorngren-Jerneck and Herbst, 2001).

Despite the methodological challenges, erroneous definitions of asphyxia by many groups were established solely based upon low Apgar scores. These prompted the American College of Obstetricians and Gynecologists and the American Academy of Pediatrics to issue a joint statement in 1986 concerning "Use and Abuse of the Apgar Score." The statement was updated in 1996 and has been reaffirmed several times, the most recent in 2006. Important caveats regarding Apgar score interpretation addressed in this statement include the following:

1. Because certain elements of the Apgar score are partially dependent on the physiological maturity of the newborn, a healthy preterm infant may receive a low score only because of immaturity (Amon and associates, 1987; Catlin and co-workers, 1986).
2. Given that Apgar scores may be influenced by a variety of factors including, but not limited to, fetal malformations, maternal medications, and infection, to equate the presence of a low Apgar score solely with asphyxia or hypoxia represents a misuse of the score.
3. Correlation of the Apgar score with adverse future neurological outcome increases when the score remains 3 or less at 10, 15, and 20 minutes, but still does not indicate the cause of future disability (Freeman and Nelson, 1988; Nelson and Ellenberg, 1981).
4. The Apgar score alone cannot establish hypoxia as the cause of cerebral palsy (Chap. 29, p. 613). A neonate who has had an asphyxial insult proximate to delivery that is severe enough to result in acute neurological injury should demonstrate all of the following: (1) profound acidemia with cord artery blood pH < 7 and acid-base deficit ≥ 12mmol/L; (2) Apgar score of 0–3 persisting for 10 minutes or longer; (3) neurological manifestations such as seizures, coma, or hypotonia; and (4) multisystem organ dysfunction—cardiovascular, gastrointestinal, hematological, pulmonary, or renal.

Umbilical Cord Blood Acid–Base Studies

Blood taken from umbilical vessels may be used for acid-base studies to assess the metabolic status of the neonate. Blood collection is performed following delivery by immediately isolating a 10- to 20-cm segment of cord with two clamps near the neonate and two clamps nearer the placenta. The importance of clamping the cord is underscored by the fact that delays of 20 to 30 seconds can alter both the PCO_2 and pH (Lievaart and de-Jong, 1984). The cord is then cut between the two proximal and two distal clamps.

Arterial blood is drawn from the isolated segment of cord into a 1- to 2-ml commercially prepared plastic syringe containing lyophilized heparin or a similar syringe that has been flushed with a heparin solution containing 1000 U/mL. The needle is capped and the syringe transported, on ice, to the laboratory. Although efforts should be made for prompt transport, neither the pH nor PCO_2 change significantly in blood kept at room temperature for up to 60 minutes (Duerbeck and associates, 1992). In fact, Chauhan and colleagues (1994) developed mathematical models allowing reasonable prediction of birth acid–base status in properly collected cord blood samples analyzed as late as 60 hours after delivery.

Fetal Acid-Base Physiology

The fetus produces both carbonic and organic acids. Carbonic acid (H_2CO_3) is formed by oxidative metabolism of CO_2. The fetus usually rapidly clears CO_2 through the placental circulation, which limits the buildup of carbonic acid. When H_2CO_3 accumulates in fetal blood and there is no concurrent increase in organic acids—as occurs in impaired placental exchange—the result is termed *respiratory acidemia.*

Organic acids primarily include lactic and β-hydroxybutyric acids. Increased levels of these acids follow persistent placental exchange impairment and result from anaerobic glycolysis. These organic acids are cleared slowly from fetal blood, and when they accumulate without a concurrent increase in H_2CO_3, the result is termed *metabolic acidemia.* With the development of metabolic acidemia, bicarbonate (HCO_3^-) decreases because it is used to buffer the organic acid. An increase in H_2CO_3 accompanied by an increase in organic acid reflected by decreased HCO_3^- causes *mixed respiratory-metabolic acidemia.*

In the fetus, respiratory and metabolic acidemia, and ultimately tissue acidosis, are most likely part of a progressively worsening continuum. This is different from the adult pathophysiology, in which distinct conditions result in either respiratory (pulmonary disease) or metabolic (diabetes) acidemia. In the fetus, the placenta serves as both the lungs and to a certain degree, the kidneys. One principal cause of developing fetal acidemia is a decrease in uteroplacental perfusion. This results in the retention of CO_2 (respiratory acidemia), and if protracted and severe enough, a mixed or metabolic acidemia.

Assuming that maternal pH and blood gases are normal, the actual pH of fetal blood is dependent on the proportion of carbonic and organic acids as well as the amount of bicarbonate, which is the major buffer in blood. This can best be illustrated by the Henderson–Hasselbalch equation:

$$pH = pK + \log \frac{[base]}{[acid]} \quad or, \quad pH = pK + \log \frac{HCO_3^-}{H_2CO_3}$$

For clinical purposes, HCO_3^- represents the metabolic component and is reported in mEq/L. The H_2CO_3 concentration represents the respiratory component and is reported as the P_{CO_2} in mm Hg. Thus:

$$pH = pK + \log \frac{metabolic \ (HCO_3^- \ mEq/L)}{respiratory \ (PCO_2 \ mmHg)}$$

The result of this equation is a pH value. However, pH is a logarithmic term and does not give a linear measure of acid accumulation. For example, a change in hydrogen ion concentration associated with a fall in pH from 7.0 to 6.9 is almost twice that which is associated with a fall in pH from 7.3 to 7.2. For this reason, the *delta base* offers a more linear measure of the degree of accumulation of metabolic acid (Armstrong and Stenson, 2007). The change in base, or delta base, is a calculated number used as a measure of the change in buffering capacity of bicarbonate (HCO_3^-). For example, HCO_3^- concentration will be decreased with a metabolic acidemia as it is consumed to maintain a normal pH. A *base deficit* occurs when HCO_3^- concentration decreases to below normal levels, and a *base excess* occurs when HCO_3^- values are above normal. Importantly, a mixed respiratory–metabolic acidemia with a large base deficit and a low HCO_3^-—less than 12 mmol/L—is more often associated with a depressed neonate than is a mixed acidemia with a minimal base deficit and a more nearly normal HCO_3^-. A nomogram for calculating the delta base has been published by Siggaard-Anderson (1963).

Clinical Significance of Acidemia

Fetal oxygenation and pH generally decline during the course of normal labor (Dildy and co-workers, 1994). Normal umbilical cord blood pH and blood gas values at delivery in term newborns are summarized in Table 28-3. Similar values have been measured in preterm infants (Dickinson and co-workers, 1992; Ramin and associates, 1989; Riley and Johnson, 1993). Using data from more than 19,000 deliveries, the lower limits of normal pH in the newborn have been found to range from 7.04 to 7.10 (Boylan and Parisi, 1994). Thus, these values should be considered to define neonatal acidemia. Most fetuses will tolerate intrapartum acidemia with a pH as low as 7.00 without incurring neurological impairment (Freeman and Nelson, 1988; Gilstrap and associates, 1989). Supportive of this threshold, Goldaber and associates (1991) found that there were significantly more neonatal deaths and infants with neurological dysfunction below a pH of 7.00 (Table 28-4).

Another important prognostic consideration is the direction of pH change from birth to the immediate neonatal period. Casey and co-workers (2001a) found that the risk of seizures during the first 24 hours of life was reduced fivefold if an umbilical artery cord pH below 7.2 normalized within 2 hours after delivery.

In the fetus, *metabolic acidemia* develops when oxygen deprivation is of sufficient duration and magnitude to require anaerobic metabolism for fetal cellular energy needs. Low and associates (1997) defined fetal acidosis as a base deficit of greater than 12 mmol/L and severe fetal acidosis as a base deficit greater than 16 mmol/L. In the study of more than 150,000 newborns cited earlier, Casey and associates (2001b) defined metabolic acidemia using umbilical cord blood gas cutoffs that were 2 standard deviations below the mean, that is, an umbilical artery blood pH less than 7.00 accompanied by a P_{CO_2} of no more than 76.3 mm Hg

---

TABLE 28-3. Umbilical Cord Blood pH and Blood Gas Values in Normal Term Newborns

	Study		
Values	Ramin et al, 1989[a] (n = 1292)[c]	Riley and Johnson, 1993[b] (n = 3522)[c]	Arikan et al, 2000[a] (n = 1281)[d]
Arterial Blood			
pH	7.28 (0.07)	7.27 (0.069)	7.25 (7.08)[b]
Pco$_2$ (mm Hg)	49.9 (14.2)	50.3 (11.1)	50.0 (75)[d]
HCO$_3^-$ (mEq/L)	23.1 (2.8)	22.0 (3.6)	—
Base excess (mEq/L)	–3.6 (2.8)	–2.7 (2.8)	–4.3 (–11.1)[d]
Venous Blood			
pH	—	7.34 (0.063)	—
Pco$_2$ (mm Hg)	—	40.7 (7.9)	—
HCO$_3^-$ (mEq/L)	—	21.4 (2.5)	—
Base excess (mEq/L)	—	–2.4 (2)	—

[a]Infants of selected women with uncomplicated vaginal deliveries.
[b]Infants of unselected women with vaginal deliveries.
[c]Shown as mean (SD).
[d]Shown as median and 2.5 or 97.5 centile.

TABLE 28-4. Umbilical Arterial Blood pH Related to Neonatal Morbidity, Mortality, and Apgar Scores in Term Infants

	Umbilical Artery pH			
Complication	<7.00 (n = 87) No. (%)	7.00–7.04 (n = 95) No. (%)	7.05–7.09 (n = 290) No. (%)	7.10–7.14 (n = 798) No. (%)
Seizure	11 (13)	4 (4.2)	0	2 (0.3)
Neonatal deaths	7 (8)	1 (1.1)	0	3 (0.4)
Intensive care nursery	34 (39)	12 (13)	17 (5.9)	22 (2.8)
Intubated	12 (14)	6 (6.3)	5 (1.7)	5 (0.6)
Apgar scores ≤ 3				
1 minute	24 (27.6)	8 (8.4)	12 (4.1)	19 (2.4)
5 minutes	9 (10.3)	1 (1.1)	1 (0.3)	0

From Goldaber and associates (1991), with permission.

(higher values indicate a respiratory component), HCO_3^- concentration of no more than 17.7 mmol/L, and base deficit of at least 10.3 mEq/L. From the standpoint of *possible* cerebral palsy causation, the American Academy of Pediatrics and the American College of Obstetricians and Gynecologists (2003), in their widely endorsed monograph, defined metabolic acidosis as umbilical arterial pH <7.0 and a base deficit of at least 12 mmol/L.

Metabolic acidemia is associated with a high rate of multiorgan dysfunction. In rare cases, such hypoxia-induced metabolic acidemia may be so severe as to cause subsequent neurological impairment. In fact, a fetus without such acidemia cannot by definition have suffered recent hypoxic-induced injury. Even severe metabolic acidosis, however, is poorly predictive of subsequent neurological impairment in the term neonate. Although metabolic acidosis was associated with an increase in immediate neonatal complications in a group of infants with depressed 5-minute Apgar scores, Socol and colleagues (1994) found no difference in umbilical artery blood gas measurements among infants who subsequently developed cerebral palsy and those with normal long-term neurological outcome. In very-low-birthweight infants—those less than 1000 g—newborn acid-base status may be more closely linked to long-term neurological outcome (Gaudier and co-workers, 1994; Low and associates, 1995). In the study cited above, Casey and associates (2001b) measured the association between metabolic acidemia, low Apgar scores, and neonatal death in term and preterm infants. As shown in Figure 28-5, relative to newborns with a 5-minute Apgar score of at least 7, the risk of neonatal death was more than 3200-fold greater in term infants with metabolic acidemia and 5-minute scores of 3 or less.

Respiratory acidemia generally develops as a result of an acute interruption in placental gas exchange with subsequent CO_2 retention. Transient umbilical cord compression is the most common antecedent factor. In general, respiratory acidemia is not harmful to the fetus. Low and co-workers (1994) found no increase in newborn complications after respiratory acidosis. The degree to which pH is affected by P_{CO_2}, the respiratory component of the acidosis, can be calculated. First, the upper normal neonatal P_{CO_2} (49 mm Hg) is subtracted from the cord blood gas P_{CO_2} value. Each 10 additional mm Hg P_{CO_2} will

lower the pH by 0.08 units (Eisenberg and colleagues, 1987). Thus, in a mixed respiratory–metabolic acidemia, the benign respiratory component can be calculated as in the following example: During labor, an acute cord prolapse occurred and the fetus was delivered by cesarean 20 minutes later. The umbilical artery blood gas pH was 6.95, with a P_{CO_2} of 89 mm Hg. To calculate the degree to which the cord compression and subsequent impairment of CO_2 exchange affected the pH, the relationship given earlier is applied: 89 mm Hg minus 49 mm Hg = 40 mm Hg (excess CO_2). To correct pH: (40 ÷ 10) × 0.08 = 0.32; 6.95 + 0.32 = 7.27. Therefore, the pH prior to cord prolapse was approximately 7.27, well within normal limits. Thus, the entire pH resulted from respiratory acidosis.

Recommendations for Cord Blood Gas Determinations

A cost-effectiveness analysis for universal cord blood gas measurements has not been conducted. In some centers, cord gas analysis is performed in all neonates at birth. The American

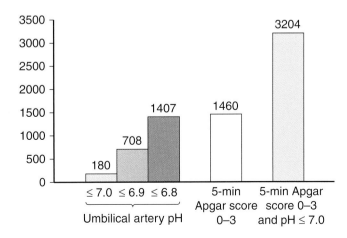

FIGURE 28-5 Relative risk for neonatal death in term infants with low Apgar score or umbilical artery acidemia—or both. Actual number of infants are cited above each bar.

College of Obstetricians and Gynecologists (2006) recommends that cord blood gas and pH analyses be obtained in the following circumstances:

1. Cesarean delivery for fetal compromise
2. Low 5-minute Apgar score
3. Severe growth restriction
4. Abnormal fetal heart rate tracing
5. Maternal thyroid disease
6. Intrapartum fever
7. Multifetal gestation.

Although umbilical cord acid-base blood determinations are poorly predictive of either immediate or long-term adverse neurological outcome, they provide the most objective evidence of the fetal metabolic status at birth.

PREVENTIVE CARE

Eye Infection Prophylaxis

Gonococcal Infection

In the past, blindness was common in children who developed *gonococcal ophthalmia neonatorum* contracted from passage through the infected birth canal (Schneider, 1984). In 1884, Credé, a German obstetrician, introduced a 1-percent ophthalmic solution of silver nitrate that largely eliminated blindness due to *Neisseria gonorrhoeae.* A variety of other antimicrobials have also proven to be effective, and gonococcal ophthalmia neonatorum prophylaxis is now mandatory for all neonates (American Academy of Pediatrics and American College of Obstetricians and Gynecologists, 2007). The Centers for Disease Control and Prevention (2006) recommendations for gonococcal eye prophylaxis include a single application of either 0.5-percent erythromycin ophthalmic ointment or 1-percent tetracycline ophthalmic ointment soon after delivery. Treatment of presumptive gonococcal ophthalmia—conjunctivitis in a neonate born to a mother with untreated gonorrhea—is given with single-dose ceftriaxone, 25 to 50 mg/kg, either intramuscularly or intravenously, not to exceed 125 mg. Culture for both gonorrhea and chlamydia (an approved non-culture based method may be substituted) should be obtained prior to treatment.

Chlamydial Infection

Adequate neonatal prophylaxis against *chlamydial conjunctivitis* is complex. From 12 to 25 percent of neonates delivered vaginally of mothers with an active chlamydial infection will develop conjunctivitis (Teoh and Reynolds, 2003). Although it is reasonable to expect that tetracycline and erythromycin ophthalmic ointments applied at birth as described above would reduce the incidence of chlamydial conjunctivitis, this is not the case. In a study from Kenya, Isenberg and colleagues (1995) showed that 2.5-percent povidone-iodine solution was superior to either 1-percent silver nitrate solution or 0.5-percent erythromycin ointment in preventing chlamydial conjunctivitis. In another study from Iran, povidone-iodine eye drops were twice as effective in preventing clinical conjunctivitis as erythromycin drops—9 versus 18 percent failure rate, respectively (Ali and associates, 2007). Accord-

ing to the Centers for Disease Control and Prevention (2006), the effectiveness of topical prophylaxis is unclear, and any case of conjunctivitis in a newborn less than 1 month old should prompt consideration for chlamydial infection.

Hepatitis B Immunization

Routine immunization of all newborns against hepatitis B prior to hospital discharge has been recommended since 1991. The Centers for Disease Control and Prevention (2005) recommends thimerosal-free vaccine. This vaccine does not appear to increase the number of febrile episodes, sepsis evaluations, or adverse neurological sequelae (Lewis and associates, 2001). If the mother is seropositive for hepatitis B surface-antigen, the neonate should also be passively immunized with hepatitis B immune globulin (see Chap. 50, p. 1070).

Vitamin K

This injection is provided to prevent vitamin K-dependent hemorrhagic disease of the newborn, which is discussed in Chapter 29 (p. 629). A 0.5- to 1-mg single-dose intramuscular administration of vitamin K within 1 hour of birth is recommended by the American Academy of Pediatrics and American College of Obstetricians and Gynecologists (2007).

Universal Newborn Screening

Newborn screening programs began in the early 1960s when a test for phenylketonuria (PKU) could be carried out on blood samples collected on filter paper (Guthrie and Susi, 1963). Subsequently, screening for a number of other disorders has been mandated by various state laws (American College of Obstetricians and Gynecologists, 2007b).

Technical advances have made a large number of relatively simply performed mass screening tests available for newborn conditions. In response to calls for a uniform national policy, the Maternal and Child Health Bureau (2005) appointed a committee of the American College of Medical Genetics to develop such panels. A *core panel* of 29 congenital conditions in five categories is shown in Table 28-5. Most of these are done using *tandem spectroscopy.* Neonatal screening for hearing loss was shown in a Dutch study to diagnose problems a mean of 6 months earlier and improve outcomes (Durieux-Smith and colleagues, 2008).

Most states require that the core panel be performed. Supplemental conditions—*secondary targets*—are also listed on the Maternal and Child Health Bureau web site. Some states require some of these 24 in addition to their mandated core panel. Each practitioner needs to be familiar with their individual state's requirements, available at http://genes-r-us.uthscsa.edu.

ROUTINE NEWBORN CARE

Estimation of Gestational Age

An estimate of newborn gestational age may be made very soon after delivery (Fig. 28-6). The relationship between gestational age and birthweight should be used to identify neonates at risk

TABLE 28-5. Newborn Screening Core Panel

Acylcarnitine Disorders[a]				
Organic Acid Metabolism	Fatty Acid Metabolism	Amino Acid Metabolism[a]	Hemoglobin Disorders	Others
Isovaleric	Medium-chain acyl-CoA dehydrogenase	Phenylketonuria	SS disease	Congenital hypothyroidism
Glutaric type I	Very long-chain acyl-CoA dehydrogenase	Maple syrup (urine)	S-β-thalassemia	Biotinidase
3-hydroxy-3-methyl glutaric	Long-chain 3-OH acyl-CoA dehydrogenase	Homocystinuria	SC disease	Congenital adrenal hyperplasia
Multiple carboxylase	Trifunctional protein	Citrullinemia		Galactosemia
Methylmalonic mutase	Carnitine uptake	Arginosuccinic		Hearing loss
3-methylcrotonyl-CoA carboxylase		Tyrosinemia I		Cystic fibrosis
Methylmalonic acid (cobalamine A, B)				
Propionic				
3-ketothiolase				

[a]Determined by tandem mass spectrometry.
From Maternal and Child Health Bureau (2005).

for complications (McIntire and colleagues, 1999). For example, neonates who are either small- or large-for-gestational-age are at increased risk for hypoglycemia and polycythemia, and measurements of blood glucose and hematocrit are indicated (American Academy of Pediatrics and American College of Obstetricians and Gynecologists, 2007).

Skin Care

Following delivery, excess vernix, blood, and meconium should be gently wiped off. Any remaining vernix is readily absorbed and disappears entirely within 24 hours. The first bath should be postponed until the temperature of the neonate has stabilized.

Umbilical Cord

Loss of water from the Wharton jelly leads to mummification of the umbilical cord shortly after birth. Within 24 hours, the cord stump loses its characteristic bluish-white, moist appearance and soon becomes dry and black. Within several days to weeks, the stump sloughs and leaves a small, granulating wound, which after healing forms the umbilicus. Separation usually takes place within the first 2 weeks, with a range of 3 to 45 days (Novack and colleagues, 1988). The umbilical cord dries more quickly and separates more readily when exposed to air. Thus, a dressing is not recommended.

Serious umbilical infections sometimes are encountered. The most likely offending organisms are *Staphylococcus aureus, Escherichia coli,* and group B streptococcus. Because the umbilical stump in such cases may present no outward sign of infection, the diagnosis may be elusive. Strict aseptic precautions should be observed in the immediate care of the cord. In a randomized study of 766 newborns, Janssen and co-workers (2003) showed that triple-dye applied to the cord was superior to soap

and water care in preventing colonization and exudate formation. Mullany and colleagues (2006), in a randomized trial of over 15,000 Nepalese newborns, found that cleansing the cord stump with 4-percent chlorhexidine reduced severe omphalitis by 75 percent compared with cleansing with soap and water.

Feeding

According to the American College of Obstetricians and Gynecologists (2007a), exclusive breast feeding is preferred until 6 months. In many hospitals, infants begin breast feeding in the delivery room. Most term newborns thrive best when fed at intervals of every 2 to 4 hours. Preterm or growth-restricted newborns require feedings at shorter intervals. In most instances, a 3-hour interval is satisfactory. The proper length of each feeding depends on several factors, such as the quantity of breast milk, the readiness with which it can be obtained from the breast, and the avidity with which the infant nurses. It is generally advisable for the infant to nurse for 5 minutes at each breast for the first 4 days, or until the mother has a supply of milk. After the fourth day, the newborn nurses up to 10 minutes on each breast.

A goal established by the U.S. Public Health Service for *Healthy People 2010* is to increase the proportion of mothers who breast feed their infants (U.S. Department of Health and Human Services, 2000). Substantial progress toward this goal has been made. In 2008, 74 percent of infants were breast fed at least once, and 31 percent were breast fed exclusively for at least 3 months (Centers for Disease Control and Prevention, 2009). Breast feeding is discussed further in Chapter 30 (p. 651).

Initial Weight Loss

Because most neonates actually receive little nutriment for the first 3 or 4 days of life, they progressively lose weight until the flow of maternal milk has been established or other feeding is

Neuromuscular Maturity

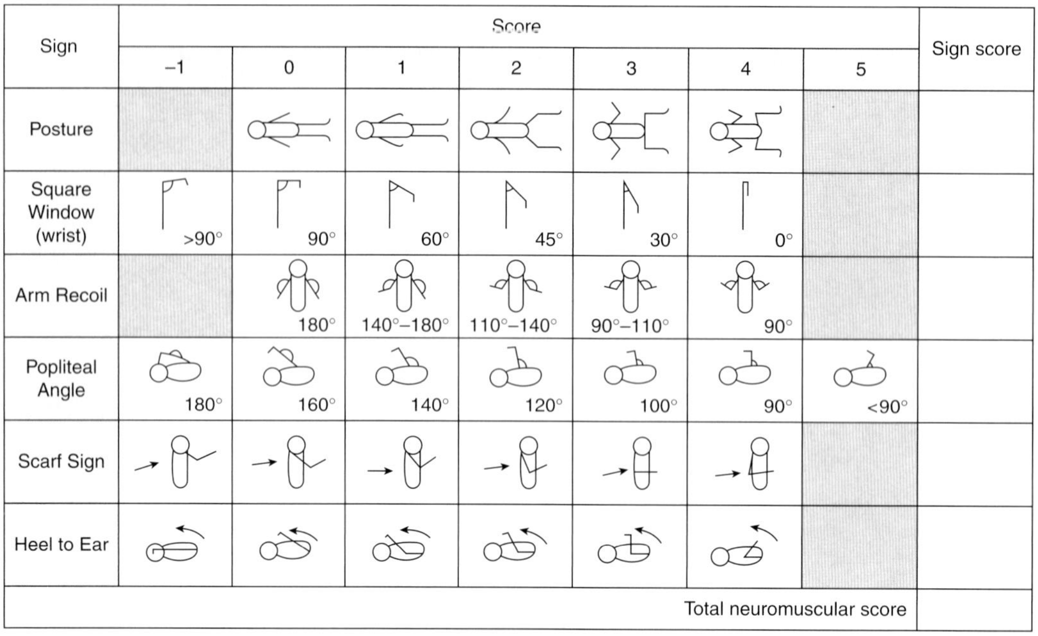

Sign	Score							Sign score
	−1	0	1	2	3	4	5	
Posture								
Square Window (wrist)	>90°	90°	60°	45°	30°	0°		
Arm Recoil		180°	140°–180°	110°–140°	90°–110°	90°		
Popliteal Angle	180°	160°	140°	120°	100°	90°	<90°	
Scarf Sign								
Heel to Ear								
						Total neuromuscular score		

Physical Maturity

Sign	Score							Sign score
Skin	Sticky friable transparent	gelatinous red, translucent	smooth pink, visible veins	superficial peeling &/or rash, few veins	cracking pale areas rare veins	parchment deep cracking no vessels	leathery cracked wrinkled	
Lanugo	none	sparse	abundant	thinning	bald areas	mostly bald		
Plantar Surface	heel–toe 40–50 mm:−1 <40 mm:−2	>50 mm no crease	faint red marks	anterior transverse crease only	creases ant. 2/3	creases over entire sole		
Breast	imperceptible	barely perceptible	flat areola no bud	stippled areola 1–2 mm bud	raised areola 3–4 mm bud	full areola 5–10 mm bud		
Eye/Ear	lids fused loosely:−1 tightly:−2	lids open pinna flat stays folded	sl. curved pinna; soft; slow recoil	well–curved pinna; soft but ready recoil	formed & firm instant recoil	thick cartilage ear stiff		
Genitals male	scrotum flat, smooth	scrotum empty faint rugae	testes in upper canal rare rugae	testes descending few rugae	testes down good rugae	testes pendulous deep rugae		
Genitals female	clitoris prominent labia flat	prominent clitoris small labia minora	prominent clitoris enlarging minora	majora & minora equally prominent	majora large minora small	majora cover clitoris & minora		
						Total physical maturity score		

Maturity Rating

score	weeks
−10	20
5	22
0	24
5	26
10	28
15	30
20	32
25	34
30	36
35	38
40	40
45	42
50	44

FIGURE 28-6 Ballard score for estimating gestational age. (Reprinted from *The Journal of Pediatrics,* Vol. 119, No. 3, JL Ballard, JC Khoury, K Wedig, et al., New Ballard Score, expanded to include extremely premature infants, pp. 417–423, Copyright 1991, with permission from Elsevier.)

instituted. Preterm infants lose relatively more weight and regain their birthweight more slowly than term newborns. Infants who are small-for-gestational-age but otherwise healthy regain their initial weight more quickly when fed than those born preterm.

If the normal newborn is nourished properly, birthweight usually is regained by the end of the 10th day. Thereafter, the weight typically increases steadily at the rate of about 25 g/day

for the first few months. Birthweight doubles by 5 months of age and triples by the end of the first year.

Stools and Urine

For the first 2 or 3 days after birth, the contents of the colon are composed of soft, brownish-green *meconium*. This consists of desquamated epithelial cells from the intestinal tract, mucus, epidermal cells, and lanugo (fetal hair) that have been swallowed along with amnionic fluid. The characteristic color results from bile pigments. During fetal life and for a few hours after birth, the intestinal contents are sterile, but bacteria quickly colonize the bowel.

Meconium stooling is seen in 90 percent of newborns within the first 24 hours, and most of the rest within 36 hours. Newborns first void usually shortly after birth, but may not until the second day. The passage of meconium and urine indicates patency of the gastrointestinal and urinary tracts. Failure of the newborn to stool or urinate after these times suggests a congenital defect, such as imperforate anus or a urethral valve. After the third or fourth day, as the consequence of ingesting milk, meconium is replaced by light-yellow homogenous feces with a consistency similar to peanut butter.

Icterus Neonatorum

Between the second and fifth day of life approximately one third of all neonates develop so-called *physiological jaundice of the newborn.* Serum bilirubin levels at birth are normally 1.8 to 2.8 mg/dL. These levels increase during the next few days but with wide individual variation. Between the third and fourth day, the bilirubin in term newborns commonly exceeds 5 mg/dL, the concentration at which jaundice is usually noticeable. Most of the bilirubin is free, that is, unconjugated. In the liver, bilirubin is bound or conjugated to glucuronic acid and excreted into bile. With hepatic immaturity, less bilirubin is conjugated with glucuronic acid and leads to reduced excretion in bile (see Chap. 29, p. 625). By an alternate method, reabsorption of free bilirubin may result from the enzymatic splitting of bilirubin glucuronide by intestinal conjugase activity in the newborn intestine. This effect also appears to contribute significantly to transient hyperbilirubinemia. In preterm neonates, jaundice is more common and usually more severe and prolonged than in term newborns, because of even lower hepatic conjugation rates. Increased erythrocyte destruction from any cause also contributes to hyperbilirubinemia.

The standard and noninvasive treatment of an affected newborn is phototherapy. With this, the neonate is exposed to a specific light wavelength that is absorbed by the bilirubin molecule. As a result, unconjugated bilirubin in the skin is converted to a water-soluble stereoisomer, which is then excreted in bile.

Circumcision

This subject has been controversial for the past 20 years. For centuries, newborn male circumcision has been performed as a religious ritual. That said, current scientific evidence suggests that several medical benefits accrue from circumcision. A review by the American Academy of Pediatrics Task Force on Circumcision (1989) reported that the procedure prevented phimosis, paraphimosis, and balanoposthitis, and it decreased the incidence of penile cancer. The Task Force also cited an increased incidence of cervical cancer among sexual partners of uncircumcised men infected with human papillomavirus (HPV). The associations between circumcision and reduced risks of penile human papillomavirus infection and cervical cancer in sexual partners have been corroborated by Castellsagué and associates (2002).

Ten years later, however, the American Academy of Pediatrics (1999) concluded that existing evidence is insufficient to recommend *routine* neonatal circumcision—a position that is endorsed by the American College of Obstetricians and Gynecologists (American Academy of Pediatrics and the American College of Obstetricians and Gynecologists, 2007). Others have argued that the existing data support a recommendation for routine circumcision (Schoen and associates, 2000). In two large randomized trials from regions of Africa with a high prevalence of human immunodeficiency virus (HIV), adult male circumcision was found to lower the risk of HIV acquisition by half (Bailey and co-workers, 2007; Gray and colleagues, 2007). Tobian and associates (2009) found adult male circumcision also decreased incidences of HIV, HPV, and herpesvirus-2 infections.

It is currently recommended that parents should make an informed choice after being given accurate and unbiased information. Nelson and associates (2005) estimated that from 1997 to 2000, 61 percent of newborn males in the United States were circumcised. Another problem is who should provide these services—obstetricians, pediatricians, urologists, or midlevel providers (Johnson and colleagues, 2007).

Surgical Technique

Newborn circumcision should be performed only on a healthy neonate. Other contraindications include any genital abnormalities such as hypospadias and a family history of a bleeding disorder unless excluded in the infant. The most commonly used instruments are shown in Figure 28-7 and include Gomco and Mogen clamps and the Plastibell device. Compared with the

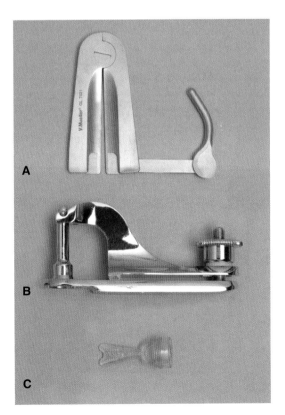

FIGURE 28-7 A. Mogen clamp. The arms of the clamp open to 3 mm maximum width. **B.** Gomco clamp, assembled. **C.** Plastibell clamp.

Gomco procedure, Kaufman and colleagues (2002) reported that the Mogen technique required less time to perform and was associated with less apparent discomfort for the newborn. Regardless of the method used, the goal is to remove enough shaft skin and inner preputial epithelium so that the glans is exposed sufficiently to prevent phimosis. In all techniques: (1) the amount of external skin to be removed must be accurately estimated, (2) the preputial orifice must be dilated to visualize the glans and ensure that it is normal, (3) the inner preputial epithelium must be freed from the glans epithelium, and (4) the circumcision device must be left in place long enough to produce hemostasis before amputating the prepuce (Lerman and Liao, 2001). For a detailed description of surgical techniques see the second edition of *Operative Obstetrics* (Gilstrap and colleagues, 2002).

Anesthesia for Circumcision. The American Academy of Pediatrics (1999) recommends that if circumcision is performed, procedural analgesia should be provided. A variety of techniques for pain relief have been described, including lidocaine-prilocaine topical cream, local analgesia infiltration, and dorsal penile nerve block and ring block. Stang and colleagues (1988) reported that dorsal penile nerve block reduced behavioral distress and modified the adrenocortical stress response in neonates undergoing circumcision. This observation was confirmed in subsequent clinical studies (Arnett and co-workers, 1990; Fontaine and Toffler, 1991). The results of these studies favor the dorsal penile nerve block or the ring block techniques compared with topical analgesia (Hardwick-Smith, 1998; Lander, 1997; Taddio, 1997, and their colleagues). The use of a pacifier dipped in sucrose also appears beneficial (Kaufman and colleagues, 2002).

After appropriate penile cleansing, the *ring block technique* consists of placing a wheal of 1-percent lidocaine at the base of the penis and advancing the needle in a 180-degree arc around the base of the penis first to one side and then the other to achieve a circumferential ring of analgesia. The maximum dose of lidocaine is 1.0 mL. The addition of a buffering agent does not appear to offer a benefit (Newton and co-workers, 1999). **No vasoactive compounds such as epinephrine should ever be added to the local analgesic agent.**

Complications of Circumcision. As with any surgical procedure, there is a risk of bleeding, infection, and hematoma formation. These risks, however, are low (Christakis and colleagues, 2000). Unusual complications reported as isolated cases include amputation of the distal glans (Neulander and colleagues, 1996), infection with human immunodeficiency virus-1 (HIV-1) and other sexually transmitted diseases (Nicoll, 1997), meatal stenosis (Upadhyay and associates, 1998), penile denudation (Orozco-Sanchez and Neri-Vela, 1991), penile destruction with electrosurgical coagulation (Gearhart and Rock, 1989), subsequent epidermal inclusion cyst and urethrocutaneous fistula (Amukele and associates, 2003), and ischemia following the inappropriate use of lidocaine with epinephrine (Berens and Pontus, 1990).

Rooming-In

This model of maternity care place newborns in their mothers' rooms instead of central nurseries. Termed *rooming-in*,

this approach first appeared in hospitals in the United States in the early 1940s (Temkin, 2002). In part, rooming-in stems from a trend to make all phases of childbearing as natural as possible and to foster mother-child relationships at an early date. By 24 hours, the mother is generally fully ambulatory. Thereafter, with rooming-in, she can usually provide routine care for herself and her newborn. An obvious advantage is her increased ability to assume full care of the infant when she arrives home.

Hospital Discharge

Traditionally, the newborn is discharged with its mother, and in most cases, maternal stay has determined that of the neonate. From 1970 to the mid-1990s, average maternal postpartum length of stay declined steadily, and many mothers were discharged in under 48 hours. Although it is clear that most newborns can be safely discharged within 48 hours, this is not uniformly true. For example, using data from the Canadian Institute for Health Information, Liu and colleagues (2000) examined readmission rates in more than 2.1 million neonatal discharges. As the length of hospital stay decreased from 4.2 days in 1990 to 2.7 days in 1997, the readmission rate increased from 27 to 38 per 1000 births. Dehydration and jaundice accounted for most of these readmissions. Using Washington state neonatal discharge data, Malkin and co-workers (2000) found that the 28-day mortality rate was increased fourfold and the 1-year mortality rate increased twofold in newborns discharged within 30 hours of birth.

Because of the increased scrutiny regarding short hospital stays, federal legislation—*The Newborns' and Mothers' Health Protection Act of 1996*—was enacted to prohibit insurers from restricting hospital stays for mothers and newborns to less than 2 days for vaginal delivery or 4 days for cesarean delivery. As a result, the average length of hospital stay for childbirth increased from 2.1 days in 1995 to 2.5 days in 2000. This increase reflected the reduced number of very short hospital stays following childbirth (Hall and Owings, 2002). Although Mosen and associates (2002) found that implementation of the new legislation was associated with a 6-percent increase in cost, readmission rates within 7 days of discharge decreased by nearly half. In their analysis of over 662,000 births in California, Datar and Sood (2006) found decreased rates of readmission of 9, 12, and 20 percent, respectively, at 1, 2, and 3 years after the legislation was implemented.

REFERENCES

Ali A, Khadije D, Elahe A, et al: Prophylaxis of ophthalmia neonatorum comparison of Betadine, erythromycin and no prophylaxis. J Trop Pediatr 53(6):388, 2007

American Academy of Pediatrics, Committee on Fetus and Newborn: Use and abuse of the Apgar score. Pediatrics 78:1148, 1986

American Academy of Pediatrics, Task Force on Circumcision: Report of the Task Force on Circumcision. Pediatrics 84:388, 1989

American Academy of Pediatrics, Task Force on Circumcision: Circumcision Policy Statement. Pediatrics 103:686, 1999

American Academy of Pediatrics and the American College of Obstetricians and Gynecologists: Care of the neonate. In: Guidelines for Perinatal Care, 5th ed. Washington, DC, AAP and ACOG, 2007

American College of Obstetricians and Gynecologists and the American Academy of Pediatrics: Neonatal encephalopathy and cerebral palsy: Defining the pathogenesis and pathophysiology. January 2003

American College of Obstetricians and Gynecologists and the American Academy of Pediatrics: The Apgar score. Committee Opinion No. 333, May 2006

American College of Obstetricians and Gynecologists: Umbilical cord blood gas and acid–base analysis. Committee Opinion No. 348, November 2006

American College of Obstetricians and Gynecologists: Breastfeeding: Maternal and infant aspects. Committee Opinion No. 361, February 2007a

American College of Obstetricians and Gynecologists: Newborn screening. Committee Opinion No. 393, December 2007b

Amon E, Sibai BM, Anderson GD, et al: Obstetric variables predicting survival of the immature newborn ($\leq$1000 gm): A five-year experience in a single perinatal center. Am J Obstet Gynecol 156:1380, 1987

Amukele SA, Lee GW, Stock JA, et al: 20-year experience with iatrogenic penile injury. J Urol 170:1691, 2003

Apgar V: A proposal for a new method of evaluation of the newborn infant. Curr Res Anesth Analg 32:260, 1953

Apgar V, Holaday DA, James LS, et al: Evaluation of the newborn infant— second report. JAMA 168:1985, 1958

Arikan GM, Scholz HS, Petru E, et al: Cord blood oxygen saturation in vigorous infants at birth: What is normal? Br J Obstet Gynaecol 107:987, 2000

Armstrong L, Stenson BJ: Use of umbilical cord blood gas analysis in the assessment of the newborn. Arch Dis Child Fetal Neonatal Ed 92:430, 2007

Arnett RM, Jones JS, Horger EO III: Effectiveness of 1% lidocaine dorsal penile nerve block in infant circumcision. Am J Obstet Gynecol 163:1074, 1990

Bailey RC, Moses S, Parker CB, et al: Male circumcision for HIV prevention in young men in Kismu, Kenya: A randomized controlled trial. Lancet 369:643, 2007

Ballard JL, Khoury JC, Wedig K, et al: New Ballard score, expanded to include extremely premature infants. J Pediatr 119:417, 1991

Berens R, Pontus SP Jr: A complication associated with dorsal penile nerve block. Reg Anesth 15:309, 1990

Boylan PC, Parisi VM: Fetal acid–base balance. In Creasy RK, Resnik R (eds): Maternal–Fetal Medicine, 3rd ed. Philadelphia, Saunders, 1994

Casey BM, Goldaber KG, McIntire DD, et al: Outcomes among term infants when two-hour postnatal pH is compared with pH at delivery. Am J Obstet Gynecol 184:447, 2001a

Casey BM, McIntire DD, Leveno KJ: The continuing value of the Apgar score for the assessment of newborn infants. N Engl J Med 344:467, 2001b

Castellsagué X, Bosch FX, Muñoz N, et al: Male circumcision, penile human papillomavirus infection, and cervical cancer in female partners. N Engl J Med 346:1105, 2002

Catlin EA, Carpenter MW, Brann BS, et al: The Apgar score revisited: Influence of gestational age. J Pediatr 109:865, 1986

Centers for Disease Control and Prevention: Breastfeeding Report Card — United States, 2008. Available at: http://www.cdc.gov/breastfeeding/pdf/ 2008%20Breastfeeding%20Report%20Card.pdf. Accessed May 18, 2009

Centers for Disease Control and Prevention: A comprehensive immunization strategy to eliminate transmission of hepatitis B virus infection in the United States. MMWR 54(RR16):1, 2005

Centers for Disease Control and Prevention: Sexually transmitted diseases treatment guidelines, 2006. MMWR 55(RR11):1, 2006

Chauhan SP, Cowan BD, Meydrech EF, et al: Determination of fetal acidemia at birth from a remote umbilical arterial blood gas analysis. Am J Obstet Gynecol 170:1705, 1994

Chernick V: Fetal breathing movements and the onset of breathing at birth. Clin Perinatol 5:257, 1978

Christakis DA, Harvey E, Zerr DM, et al: A trade-off analysis of routine newborn circumcision. Pediatrics 105:246, 2000

Credé CSF: Die Verhütung der Augenenzündung der Neugeborenen. Berlin, Hirschwald, 1884

Datar A, Sood N: Impact of postpartum hospital-stay legislation on newborn length of stay, readmission, and mortality in California. Pediatrics 118:63, 2006

Dawes GS: Breathing before birth in animals or man. N Engl J Med 290:557, 1974

Dickinson JE, Eriksen NL, Meyer BA, et al: The effect of preterm birth on umbilical cord blood gases. Obstet Gynecol 79:575, 1992

Dildy GA, van den Berg PP, Katz M, et al: Intrapartum fetal pulse oximetry: Fetal oxygen saturation trends during labor and relation to delivery outcome. Am J Obstet Gynecol 171:679, 1994

Duerbeck NB, Chaffin DG, Seeds JW: A practical approach to umbilical artery pH and blood gas determinations. Obstet Gynecol 79:959, 1992

Durieux-Smith A, Fitzpatrick E, Whittingham J: Universal newborn hearing screening: A question of evidence. Int J Audiol 47(1):12, 2008

Eisenberg MS, Cummins RO, Ho MT: Code Blue: Cardiac Arrest and Resuscitation. Philadelphia, Saunders, 1987, p 146

Fontaine P, Toffler WL: Dorsal penile nerve block for newborn circumcision. Am Fam Physician 43:1327, 1991

Freeman JM, Nelson KB: Intrapartum asphyxia and cerebral palsy. Pediatrics 82:240, 1988

Gaudier FL, Goldenberg RL, Nelson KG, et al: Acid–base status at birth and subsequent neurosensory impairment in surviving 500 to 1000 gm infants. Am J Obstet Gynecol 170:48, 1994

Gearhart JP, Rock JA: Total ablation of the penis after circumcision with electrocautery: A method of management and long-term follow-up. J Urol 142:799, 1989

Gill AW, Colvin J: Use of naloxone during neonatal circumcision in Australia: Compliance with published guidelines. J Paediatr Child Health 43:795, 2007

Gilstrap LC, Cunningham FG, VanDorsten JP (eds): Operative Obstetrics, 2nd ed. New York, McGraw-Hill, 2002, p 657

Gilstrap LC III, Leveno KJ, Burris J, et al: Diagnosis of birth asphyxia on the basis of fetal pH, Apgar score, and newborn cerebral dysfunction. Am J Obstet Gynecol 161:825, 1989

Goldaber KG, Gilstrap LC III, Leveno KJ, et al: Pathologic fetal acidemia. Obstet Gynecol 78:1103, 1991

Gray RH, Kigozi G, Serwadda D, et al: Male circumcision for HIV prevention in Rakai, Uganda: A randomized trial. Lancet 369:657, 2007

Guglani L, Lakshminrusimha S, Ryan RM: Transient tachypnea of the newborn. Pediatr Rev 29(11):e59, 2008

Guthrie R, Susi A: A simple phenylalanine method for detecting phenylketonuria in large populations of newborn infants. Pediatrics 32:338, 1963

Haddad B, Mercer BM, Livingston JC, et al: Outcome after successful resuscitation of babies born with Apgar scores of 0 at both 1 and 5 minutes. Am J Obstet Gynecol 182:1210, 2000

Hall MJ, Owings MF: 2000 National hospital discharge survey. Advance Data from Vital and Health Statistics, No 329. Hyattsville, Md: National Center for Health Statistics, 2002

Hardwick-Smith S, Mastrobattista JM, Wallace PA, et al: Ring block for neonatal circumcision. Obstet Gynecol 91:930, 1998

International Liaison Committee on Resuscitation (ILCOR) Consensus on Science with Treatment Recommendations for Pediatric and Neonatal Patients: Neonatal resuscitation. Pediatrics 117:978, 2006

Isenberg SJ, Apt L, Wood M: A controlled trial of povidone-iodine as prophylaxis against ophthalmia neonatorum. N Engl J Med 332:562, 1995

Janssen PA, Selwood BL, Dobson SR, et al: To dye or not to dye: A randomized clinical trial of a triple dye/alcohol regime versus dry cord care. Pediatrics 111:15, 2003

Johnson TRB, Pituch K, Brackbill EL, et al: Why and how a Department of Obstetrics and Gynecology stopped doing routine newborn male circumcision. Obstet Gynecol 109(3):750, 2007

Kaiser JR, Gauss CH, Williams DK: Tracheal suctioning is associated with prolonged disturbances of cerebral hemodynamics in very low birth weight infants. J Perinatol 28(1):34, 2008

Kattwinkel J: Textbook of Neonatal Resuscitation, 5th ed. American Academy of Pediatrics and American Heart Association, 2006

Kaufman GE, Cimo S, Miller LW, et al: An evaluation of the effects of sucrose on neonatal pain with 2 commonly used circumcision methods. Am J Obstet Gynecol 186:564, 2002

Kette F, Weil MH, Gazmuri RJ: Buffer solutions may compromise cardiac resuscitation by reducing coronary perfusion pressure. JAMA 266:2121, 1991

Lander J, Brady-Fryer B, Metcalfe JB, et al: Comparison of ring block, dorsal penile nerve block, and topical anesthesia for neonatal circumcision: A randomized controlled trial. JAMA 278:2157, 1997

Lerman SE, Liao JC: Neonatal circumcision. Pediatr Clin North Am 48:1539, 2001

Lewis E, Shinefield HR, Woodruff BA, et al: Safety of neonatal hepatitis B vaccine administration. Pediatr Infect Dis J 20:1049, 2001

Lievaart M, deJong PA: Acid–base equilibrium in umbilical cord blood and time of cord clamping. Obstet Gynecol 63:44, 1984

Liu S, Wen SW, McMillan D, et al: Increased neonatal readmission rate associated with decreased length of hospital stay at birth in Canada. Can J Public Health 91:46, 2000

Low JA, Lindsay BG, Derrick EJ: Threshold of metabolic acidosis associated with newborn complications. Am J Obstet Gynecol 177:1391, 1997

Low JA, Panagiotopoulos C, Derrick EJ: Newborn complications after intrapartum asphyxia with metabolic acidosis in the preterm fetus. Am J Obstet Gynecol 172:805, 1995

Low JA, Panagiotopoulos C, Derrick EJ: Newborn complications after intrapartum asphyxia with metabolic acidosis in the term fetus. Am J Obstet Gynecol 170:1081, 1994

Malkin JD, Garber S, Broder MS, et al: Infant mortality and early postpartum discharge. Obstet Gynecol 96:183, 2000

Martin JA, Hamilton BE, Sutton PD, et al. Births: Final data for 2004. National Vital Statistics Reports, vol 55, no 1. Hyattsville, MD: National Center for Health Statistics. 2006

Martin JA, Hamilton BE, Sutton PD, et al: Births: Final Data for 2006. National Vital Statistics Reports, Vol 57, No 7. Hyattsville, Md, National Center for Health Statistics, 2009

Maternal and Child Health Bureau: Newborn screening: Towards a uniform screening panel and system. Executive Summary. Rockville, MD: MCHB, 2005 http://mchb.hrsa.gov/screening/summary.htm, accessed April 27, 2008

McGuire W, Fowlie PW: Naloxone for narcotic exposed newborn infants: Systematic review. Arch Dis Child Fetal Neonatal Ed 88:F308, 2003

McIntire DD, Bloom SL, Casey BM, Leveno KJ: Birth weight in relation to morbidity and mortality among newborn infants. N Engl J Med 340:1234, 1999

Mosen DM, Clark SL, Mundorff MB, et al: The medical and economic impact of the Newborns' and Mothers' Health Protection Act. Obstet Gynecol 99:116, 2002

Mullany LC, Darmstadt GL, Khatry SK, et al: Topical applications of chlorhexidine to the umbilical cord for prevention of omphalitis and neonatal mortality in southern Nepal: A community-based, cluster randomized trial. Lancet 367:910, 2006

Nelson CP, Dunn R, Wan J, et al: The increasing incidence of newborn circumcision: Data from the nationwide inpatient sample. J Urol 173:978, 2005

Nelson KB, Ellenberg JH: Apgar scores as predictors of chronic neurologic disability. Pediatrics 68:36, 1981

Neulander E, Walfisch S, Kaneti J: Amputation of distal penile glans during neonatal ritual circumcision—a rare complication. Br J Urol 77:924, 1996

Newton CW, Mulnix N, Baer L, et al: Plain and buffered lidocaine for neonatal circumcision. Obstet Gynecol 93:350, 1999

Nicoll A: Routine male neonatal circumcision and risk of infection with HIV-1 and other sexually transmitted diseases. Arch Dis Child 77:194, 1997

Novack AH, Mueller B, Ochs H: Umbilical cord separation in the normal newborn. Am J Dis Child 142:220, 1988

Orozco-Sanchez J, Neri-Vela R: Total denudation of the penis in circumcision. Description of a plastic technique for repair of the penis. Bol Med Hosp Infant Mex 48:565, 1991

Pang JWY, Heffelfinger JD, Huang GJ, et al: Outcomes of planned home births in Washington state: 1989–1996. Obstet Gynecol 100:253, 2002

Ramin SM, Gilstrap LC, Leveno KJ, et al: Umbilical artery acid–base status in the preterm infant. Obstet Gynecol 74:256, 1989

Riley RJ, Johnson JWC: Collecting and analyzing cord blood gases. Clin Obstet Gynecol 36:13, 1993

Saunders RA, Milner AD: Pulmonary pressure/volume relationships during the last phase of delivery and the first postnatal breaths in human subjects. J Pediatr 93:667, 1978

Schneider G: Silver nitrate prophylaxis. Can Med Assoc J 131:193, 1984

Schoen EJ, Wiswell TE, Moses S: New policy on circumcision—cause for concern. Pediatrics 105:620, 2000

Siggaard-Anderson O: Blood acid–base alignment nomogram. Scand J Clin Laborat Invest 15:211, 1963

Socol ML, Garcia PM, Riter S: Depressed Apgar scores, acid–base status, and neurologic outcome. Am J Obstet Gynecol 170:991, 1994

Stang HJ, Gunnar MR, Snellman L, et al: Local anesthesia for neonatal circumcision: Effects on distress and cortisol response. JAMA 259:1507, 1988

Taddio A, Stevens B, Craig K, et al: Efficacy and safety of lidocaine-prilocaine cream for pain during circumcision. N Engl J Med 336:1197, 1997

Temkin E: Rooming-in: Redesigning hospitals and motherhood in Cold War America. Bull Hist Med 76:271, 2002

Teoh D, Reynolds S: Diagnosis and management of pediatric conjunctivitis. Pediatr Emerg Care 19:48, 2003

Thorngren-Jerneck K, Herbst A: Low 5-minute Apgar score: A population-based register study of 1 million term births. Obstet Gynecol 98:65, 2001

Tobian AA, Serwadda D, Quinn TC, et al: Male circumcision for the prevention of HSV-2 and HPV infections and syphilis. N Engl J Med 360(13):1298, 2009

Upadhyay V, Hammodat HM, Pease PWB: Post circumcision meatal stenosis: 12 years' experience. NZ Med J 111:57, 1998

U.S. Department of Health and Human Services: Healthy People 2010, Vol II. Washington, DC, USDHHS, Objective 16–19, 2000

CHAPTER 29

Diseases and Injuries of the Fetus and Newborn

The fetus and newborn infant are susceptible to a large number of diseases. Because many disorders have a different presentation and course in term as compared with preterm infants, they are considered separately (see Chap. 36, p. 804). Disorders that are the direct consequence of maternal disease are discussed in chapters pertinent to specific maternal conditions. Because most perinatal infections arise as a result of maternal infection or colonization, they are considered in Chapters 58 and 59.

DISEASES COMMON IN THE PRETERM FETUS AND NEWBORN

Respiratory Distress Syndrome

To provide blood gas exchange immediately following delivery, the lungs must rapidly fill with air while being cleared of fluid. Concurrently, pulmonary arterial blood flow must increase remarkably. Some of the fluid is expressed as the chest is compressed during vaginal delivery, and the remainder is absorbed through the pulmonary lymphatics. Sufficient surfactant, synthesized by type II pneumocytes, is essential to stabilize the air-expanded alveoli. It lowers surface tension and thereby prevents lung collapse during expiration (see Chap. 4, p. 95). If surfactant is inadequate, hyaline membranes form in the distal bronchioles and alveoli, and respiratory distress develops.

Although *respiratory distress syndrome (RDS)* is generally a disease of preterm neonates, it does develop in term newborns, especially in the setting of sepsis or meconium aspiration. In recent years, mortality rates from RDS have decreased because of antenatal corticosteroid and newborn surfactant therapy (Jobe, 2004; Martin, 2004). Male infants are more likely to develop RDS than females, and white infants are more frequently and severely affected than black infants.

Clinical Course

In typical RDS, tachypnea develops, the chest wall retracts, and expiration is accompanied by *grunting* and *nostril flaring.* Shunting of blood through nonventilated lung contributes to hypoxemia and metabolic and respiratory acidosis. Poor peripheral circulation and systemic hypotension may be evident. The chest radiograph shows a diffuse reticulogranular infiltrate and an air-filled tracheobronchial tree—*air bronchogram.*

Respiratory insufficiency also can be caused by sepsis, pneumonia, meconium aspiration, pneumothorax, persistent fetal circulation, heart failure, and malformations involving thoracic structures, such as diaphragmatic hernia. Evidence is also accruing that there may be common mutations in surfactant protein production that cause RDS (Garmany and colleagues, 2008; Shulenin and associates, 2004).

Pathology

With inadequate surfactant, alveoli are unstable, and low pressures cause collapse at end expiration. Pneumocyte nutrition is compromised by hypoxia and systemic hypotension. There may be partial persistence of the fetal circulation that leads to pulmonary hypertension and a relative right-to-left shunt. Eventually, there is ischemic necrosis of alveolar cells. When oxygen therapy is initiated, the pulmonary vascular bed dilates, and the shunt reverses. Protein-filled fluid leaks into the alveolar ducts, and the cells lining the ducts slough. Hyaline membranes composed of fibrin-rich protein and cellular debris line the dilated alveoli and terminal bronchioles. The epithelium underlying the membrane becomes necrotic. Following hematoxylin-eosin staining, these membranes appear amorphous and eosinophilic, like hyaline cartilage. Because of this, respiratory distress in the newborn is also termed *hyaline membrane disease.*

Treatment

The most important factor influencing survival is neonatal intensive care. Although hypoxemia is indicative of the need for oxygen, excess oxygen can damage the pulmonary epithelium and the retina. Advances in mechanical ventilation technology have improved neonatal survival. For example, *continuous positive airway pressure (CPAP)* prevents the collapse of unstable alveoli and allows high inspired-oxygen concentrations to be reduced, thereby minimizing toxicity. Disadvantages include disturbance of the endothelium and epithelium—caused by overstretching, which results in barotrauma and impaired venous return (Verbrugge and Lachmann, 1999). *High-frequency oscillatory ventilation* may reduce the risk of barotrauma by using a constant, low-distending pressure and small variations or oscillations to promote alveolar patency. This technique allows optimal lung volume to be maintained and carbon dioxide to be cleared without damaging alveoli. Although mechanical ventilation has undoubtedly improved survival, it is also an important factor in the genesis of chronic lung disease—*bronchopulmonary dysplasia.*

Treatment of the ventilator-dependent neonate with *glucocorticoids* was used for many years to prevent chronic lung disease. The American Academy of Pediatrics (2002) now recommends against their use because of limited benefits and increased adverse neuropsychological effects. Yeh and colleagues (2004) described significantly impaired motor and cognitive function and school performance in exposed neonates. The results of a Cochrane Review by Halliday and co-workers (2009) support late postnatal corticosteroid treatment only for infants who could not be weaned from mechanical ventilation.

In some studies, *inhaled nitric oxide* was shown to be associated with improved outcomes for infants undergoing mechanical ventilation (Ballard, 2006; Kinsella, 2006; Mestan, 2005; Schreiber, 2003, and all their colleagues). Another study done by van Meurs and associates (2005) showed no benefits. Currently, such treatment is considered investigational (Chock and co-workers, 2009; Stark, 2006).

Surfactant Prophylaxis

Exogenous surfactant products can prevent hyaline membrane disease. They contain biological or animal surfactants such as bovine—*Survanta,* calf—*Infasurf,* porcine—*Curosurf,* or synthetic—*Exosurf.* In a Cochrane Review, Pfister and associates (2007) found that animal-derived and synthetic surfactant were comparable. Lucinactant—*Surfaxin R*—is a synthetic form that contains sinulpeptide KL4 to diminish lung inflammation (Zhu and co-workers, 2008).

Surfactant therapy has been credited for the largest drop in infant mortality rates observed in 25 years (Jobe, 1993). It has been used for *prophylaxis* of preterm at-risk infants and for *rescue* of those with established disease. Antenatal corticosteroids and surfactant given together result in an even greater reduction in the overall death rate. In a Cochrane Review, Seger and Soll (2009) found that infants who receive prophylactic surfactant had a decreased risk of pneumothorax, pulmonary interstitial emphysema, bronchopulmonary dysplasia, and mortality.

Complications

Persistent hyperoxia injures the lung, especially the alveoli and capillaries. High oxygen concentrations given at high pressures can cause *bronchopulmonary dysplasia.* With this, alveolar and bronchiolar epithelial damage leads to hypoxia, hypercarbia, and chronic oxygen dependence from peribronchial and interstitial fibrosis. According to Baraldi and Filippone (2007), most cases are now seen in infants born before 30 weeks and represent a developmental disorder secondary to alveolarization injury. Severe disease and death rates are decreasing, however, long-term pulmonary dysfunction is later encountered. *Pulmonary hypertension* is another frequent complication. If hyperoxemia is sustained, the infant also is at risk of developing *retinopathy of prematurity,* formerly called *retrolental fibroplasia* (see p. 607). When any of these develop, the likelihood of subsequent neurosensory impairment is substantively increased (Schmidt and colleagues, 2003).

Prevention

With the possible exception of progesterone therapy to prevent recurrent preterm birth, there are no methods to prevent or treat preterm labor (see Chap. 36, p. 816). The National Institutes of Health (1994, 2000) concluded that a single course of antenatal corticosteroid therapy reduced respiratory distress and intraventricular hemorrhage in preterm infants born between 24 and 34 weeks (see p. 609). The American College of Obstetricians and Gynecologists and American Academy of Pediatrics (2003) considers all women at risk for preterm birth in this gestational age range to be potential candidates for therapy. This is discussed further is Chapter 36 (p. 821). After 34 weeks, approximately 4 percent of infants develop respiratory distress syndrome (Fuchs and colleagues, 2009).

Amniocentesis for Fetal Lung Maturity

Delivery for fetal indications is necessary when the risks to the fetus from a hostile intrauterine environment are greater than the risk of severe neonatal problems, including respiratory distress, even if the fetus is preterm. If this degree of risk is not present and the criteria for elective delivery at term are not met, then amniocentesis and amnionic fluid analysis are used to confirm fetal lung maturity. To accomplish this, several methods can be used to determine the relative concentration of surfactant-active phospholipids in this amnionic fluid. Fluid acquisition is similar to that described for second-trimester amniocentesis (see Chap. 13, p. 299). Complications requiring urgent delivery arise in up to 1 percent of procedures (American College of Obstetricians and Gynecologists, 2008a). Following analysis, the probability of respiratory distress developing in a given infant depends on the test used and fetal gestational age. Importantly, administration of corticosteroids to induce pulmonary maturation has variable effects on some of these tests.

Lecithin–Sphingomyelin (L/S) Ratio. Although not used nearly as much as in the past, the labor-intensive *L/S ratio* for

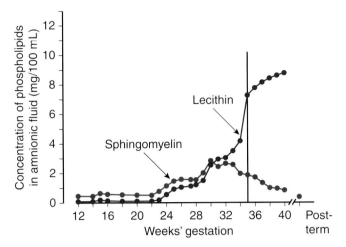

FIGURE 29-1 Changes in mean concentrations of lecithin and sphingomyelin in amnionic fluid during gestation in normal pregnancy. (This figure was published in *American Journal of Obstetrics & Gynecology,* Vol. 115, No. 4, L Gluck and MV Kulovich, Lecithin-sphingomyelin ratios in amniotic fluid in normal and abnormal pregnancy, pp. 539–546, Copyright Elsevier 1973.)

many years was the gold-standard test. Dipalmitoylphosphatidylcholine—DPPC, that is, lecithin—along with phosphatidylinositol and especially phosphatidylglycerol is an important component of the surface-active layer that prevents alveolar collapse (see Chap. 4, p. 96). Before 34 weeks, lecithin and sphingomyelin are present in amnionic fluid in similar concentrations. At 32 to 34 weeks, the concentration of lecithin relative to sphingomyelin begins to rise (Fig. 29-1).

Gluck and co-workers (1971) reported that the risk of neonatal respiratory distress is slight whenever the concentration of lecithin is at least twice that of sphingomyelin (L/S ratio). Conversely, there is increased risk of respiratory distress when this ratio is below 2 (Table 29-1). Because lecithin and sphingomyelin are found in blood and meconium, contamination with these substances may lower a mature L/S ratio (Buhi and Spellacy, 1975).

Phosphatidylglycerol (PG). It was held for many years that respiratory distress may develop despite an L/S ratio greater than 2 in infants of women with diabetes. Some recommend that phosphatidylglycerol be documented in amnionic fluid of these women. At this time, it is unclear if either diabetes, per se, or its level of control causes false-positive phospholipid test results for lung maturity (American College of Obstetricians and Gynecologists, 2008a).

Fluorescence Polarization. This automated assay measures the surfactant-to-albumin ratio in uncentrifuged amnionic fluid and gives results in approximately 30 minutes. When a ratio of 50 or greater was obtained with the commercially available *TDx-FLM* test, Steinfeld and colleagues (1992) predicted fetal lung maturity in 100 percent of cases. Subsequent investigators found the TDx-FLM to be equal or superior to the L/S ratio, foam stability index, or phosphatidylglycerol assessment, including in diabetic pregnancies (Eriksen and associates, 1996; Karcher and co-workers, 2005). The recently modified *TDx-FLM II* is used by many hospitals as their first-line test of pulmonary maturity with a threshold value of 55 mg/g ratio (see Table 29-1).

Other Tests. The *foam stability* or *shake test* depends on the ability of surfactant in amnionic fluid, when mixed appropriately with ethanol, to generate stable foam at the air–liquid interface (Clements and associates, 1972). Problems include errors caused by slight contamination and frequent false-negative test results. Alternatively, the *Lumadex-FSI test, fluorescent polarization (microviscometry),* and *amnionic fluid absorbance at 650-nm wavelength* have all been used with variable success. The *lamellar body count* is a rapid, simple, and accurate method of assessing fetal lung maturity and is comparable to TDx-FLM and L/S ratio (Karcher and colleagues, 2005).

Retinopathy of Prematurity

Formerly known as *retrolental fibroplasia,* by 1950, retinopathy of prematurity had become the largest single cause of blindness in this country. After the discovery that the disease resulted from hyperoxemia, its frequency decreased remarkably. The fetal retina vascularizes centrifugally from the optic nerve starting at approximately the fourth month and continues until shortly after birth. During vascularization, excessive oxygen induces severe retinal vasoconstriction with endothelial damage and vessel obliteration, especially in the temporal portion. Neovascularization results, and the new vessels penetrate the retina and extend into the vitreous. Here, they are prone to leak proteins or burst with subsequent hemorrhage. Adhesions then form, which detach the retina.

Precise levels of hyperoxemia that can be sustained without causing retinopathy are not known. Preterm birth results in a "relative" hyperoxia compared with in utero oxygen content even in infants not exposed to higher FiO_2.

Intraventricular Hemorrhage

There are four major categories of intracranial hemorrhage in the neonate (Volpe, 1995). *Subdural hemorrhage* is usually the result of trauma. *Subarachnoid hemorrhage* and *intracerebellar hemorrhage* usually result from trauma in term infants and hypoxia in preterm infants. *Periventricular-intraventricular hemorrhage* results from either trauma or asphyxia in half of term infants and has no discernible cause in a fourth. In preterm neonates, the pathogenesis of periventricular hemorrhage is multifactorial and includes hypoxic-ischemic events, anatomical factors, coagulopathy, and many others. The prognosis after hemorrhage depends on its location and extent. For example, subdural and subarachnoid hemorrhage often result in minimal, if any, neurological abnormalities. Bleeding into the parenchyma, however, can cause serious permanent damage.

Periventricular–Intraventricular Hemorrhage

When the fragile capillaries in the germinal matrix rupture, there is bleeding into surrounding tissues that may extend into the ventricular system and brain parenchyma. This type of hemorrhage is common in preterm neonates, especially those born before 32 weeks, but it can also develop at later gestational ages and even in term neonates.

Most hemorrhages develop within 72 hours of birth, but they have been observed as late as 24 days (Perlman and Volpe, 1986). Because intraventricular hemorrhage usually is recognized

TABLE 29-1. Commonly Used Direct Tests of Fetal Lung Maturity

Test[a]	Technique	Time and Ease of Testing[b]	Threshold	Mature Negative-Predictive Value	Immature Positive-Predictive Value[c]	Blood Contamination Affects Results	Meconium Contamination Affects Results	Vaginal Pool Sample
Lecithin/sphingomyelin ratio	Thin-layer chromatography	4+	2–3.5	95–100	33–50	Yes	Yes	No
Phosphatidylglycerol	Thin-layer chromatography	4+	Present (usually greater than 3% of total phospholipids)	95–100	23–53	No	No	Yes
	Antisera with AminoStat-FLM	1+	0.5 = low positive; 2 = high positive	95–100	23–53	No	No	Yes
Fluorescence polarization	Fluorescence polarization with TDx-FLM II	1+	≥ 55 mg/g of albumin[d]	96–100	47–61	Yes	Yes	Yes
Foam-stability index	Ethanol added to amnionic fluid, solution shaken, presence of stable bubbles at meniscus noted	2+	≥ 47	95	51	Yes	Yes	No
Optical density at 650 nm	Spectrophotometric reading	1+	Optical density ≥ 0.15	98	13	NA	NA	NA
Lamellar body counts	Counts using counter commercial hematology	2+	30,000–40,000 (investigational)	97–98	29–35	Yes	No	NA

Typical Predictive Value (Percent) spans the Mature Negative-Predictive Value and Immature Positive-Predictive Value columns.

[a]Commercial versions are available for all tests except optical density and lamellar body counts.

[b]Range in complexity: 1+ indicates procedure is simple, procedure is available all the time, procedure time is short, and personnel effort is not intensive; 4+ indicates procedure is complex or difficult, time consuming, and therefore, frequently not available at all times.

[c]Positive-predictive value is the probability of neonatal respiratory distress syndrome when the fetal lung maturity test result is immature.

[d]The manufacturer has reformulated the product and revised the testing procedure. Currently, the threshold for maturity is 55; with the original assay, it was 70.

NA = not available.

Reprinted, with permission, from American College of Obstetricians and Gynecologists. Fetal lung maturity. ACOG Practice Bulletin 97. Washington, DC: ACOG; 2008.

within 3 days of delivery, its genesis is often erroneously attributed to birth events. It is important to realize that *prelabor* intraventricular hemorrhage also can occur (Achiron and associates, 1993; Nores and co-workers, 1996).

Almost half of hemorrhages are clinically silent, and most small germinal matrix hemorrhages and those confined to the cerebral ventricles resolve without impairment (Weindling, 1995). Large lesions can result in hydrocephalus or in degenerated cystic areas termed *periventricular leukomalacia* (p. 610). Importantly, the extent of periventricular leukomalacia correlates with the risk of cerebral palsy.

Pathology

There is damage to the germinal matrix capillary network, which predisposes to subsequent extravasation of blood into the surrounding tissue. In preterm infants, this capillary network is especially fragile for several reasons. First, the subependymal germinal matrix provides poor support for the vessels coursing through it. Secondly, venous anatomy in this region causes stasis and congestion, which makes vessels susceptible to bursting with increased intravascular pressure. Thirdly, vascular autoregulation is impaired before 32 weeks (Matsuda and colleagues, 2006; Volpe and Hill, 1987).

Even if extensive hemorrhage or other complications of preterm birth do not cause death, survivors can have major neurodevelopmental handicaps. DeVries and co-workers (1985) attribute most long-term sequelae of intraventricular-periventricular hemorrhage to *periventricular leukomalacia.* These degenerated cystic areas develop *most* commonly as a result of ischemia and *least* commonly in direct response to hemorrhage.

Incidence and Severity

The incidence of ventricular hemorrhage depends on gestational age at birth. Approximately half of all neonates born before 34 weeks but only 4 percent of those born at term will have some evidence of hemorrhage (Hayden and associates, 1985). Very-low-birthweight infants have the earliest onset of hemorrhage, the greatest likelihood of parenchymal tissue involvement, and thus the highest mortality rate (Perlman and Volpe, 1986). Preterm black infants are at disparate risk for intraventricular hemorrhage (Reddick and associates, 2008).

The severity of intraventricular hemorrhage can be assessed by neuroimaging studies. Papile and colleagues (1978) devised the most widely used grading scheme to quantify the extent of a lesion and estimate prognosis.

Grade I—hemorrhage limited to the germinal matrix
Grade II—intraventricular hemorrhage
Grade III—hemorrhage with ventricular dilatation
Grade IV—parenchymal extension of hemorrhage

Jakobi and colleagues (1992) showed that infants with grade I or II intraventricular hemorrhage had a greater than 90-percent survival rate and a 3-percent rate of handicap—similar to control infants of the same age. The survival rate for infants with grade III or IV hemorrhage, however, was only 50 percent. Extremely-low-birthweight infants with grade I or II hemorrhage have poorer neurodevelopmental outcomes at 20 months than

controls (Patra and associates, 2006). The most recent data from the Neonatal Research Network indicate that 30 percent of infants born weighing 501 to 1500 g develop intracranial hemorrhage, and 12 percent are grade III or IV (Fanaroff and colleagues, 2007).

Contributing Factors. Events that predispose to germinal matrix hemorrhage and subsequent periventricular leukomalacia are multifactorial and complex. As discussed, the preterm fetus has fragile intracranial blood vessels that make it particularly susceptible. Moreover, preterm birth is frequently associated with infection, which further predisposes to endothelial activation, platelet adherence, and thrombi (Redline and associates, 2008). Luthy and co-workers (1987) reported a threefold increased risk for grade III or IV hemorrhage in neonates with a cord arterial pH < 7.2. Respiratory distress syndrome and mechanical ventilation are commonly associated factors (Sarkar and co-workers, 2009). Lesko and colleagues (1986) reported that heparin, often used to maintain vascular catheter patency in intensive care units, was associated with a fourfold increased risk of geminal matrix hemorrhage.

Prevention with Antenatal Corticosteroids

Administration of corticosteroids at least 24 hours before delivery appears to prevent or reduce the incidence and severity of intraventricular hemorrhage. A Consensus Development Conference of the National Institutes of Health (1994) concluded that such therapy reduced rates of mortality, respiratory distress, and intraventricular hemorrhage in preterm infants born between 24 and 32 weeks and that the benefits were additive with those from surfactant therapy. The consensus panel also concluded that benefits of antenatal steroid therapy probably extend to women with preterm premature membrane rupture. A second consensus statement by the National Institutes of Health (2000) recommended that repeated courses of corticosteroids should not be given because there were insufficient data to prove benefit or to document the safety of multiple courses (see Chap. 36, p. 821).

Subsequently, the Maternal Fetal Medicine Units Network reported that repeated corticosteroid courses were associated with some improved preterm neonatal outcomes, but also with reduced birthweight and increased risk for fetal-growth restriction (Wapner and colleagues, 2006). Surveillance of this cohort through age 2 to 3 years found that children exposed to repeated—versus single-dose steroid courses—did not differ significantly in physical or neurocognitive measures (Wapner and colleagues, 2007). It was worrisome, however, that there was a nonsignificant 5.7-fold relative risk of cerebral palsy in infants exposed to multiple steroid courses. At the same time, the 2-year follow-up of the Australasian Collaborative Trial was reported by Crowther and associates (2007). In more than 1100 infants, the incidence of cerebral palsy was almost identical—4.2 versus 4.8 percent—in those given repeated versus single-course steroids, respectively.

Another possibility is "rescue-dose corticosteroid" therapy. Garite and co-workers (2009) evaluated short-term outcomes in 437 women who completed the initial steroid course before 30 weeks, but at least 14 days had elapsed. These women were randomized to receive a single additional "rescue dose" of corticosteroid versus placebo. For those delivered < 34 weeks, the steroid group had significantly less respiratory distress syndrome, ventilator support, and surfactant use.

Studies with follow-up of more than 30 years are now being reported from the New Zealand cohort of adults exposed to single-dose antenatal steroids. Treatment was not associated with neuropsychological or cardiovascular dysfunction, but there was a slightly increased rate of insulin resistance compared with that of the placebo group (Dalziel and co-workers, 2005a, b).

As discussed in Chapter 36 (p. 821), at this time, we follow recommendations for single-course therapy by the American College of Obstetricians and Gynecologists (2008b).

Other Preventative Methods. The efficacy of *phenobarbital*, *vitamin K*, *vitamin E*, or *indomethacin* in diminishing the frequency and severity of intracranial hemorrhage, when administered either to the neonate or to the mother during labor, remains controversial (Chiswick, 1991; Hanigan, 1988; Thorp, 1995, and all their colleagues). Data from a variety of sources suggest that *magnesium sulfate* may prevent the sequelae of periventricular hemorrhage, as discussed on page 614.

It is generally agreed that avoiding significant hypoxia both before and after preterm delivery is of paramount importance (Low and co-workers, 1995). There is presently no convincing evidence, however, that routine cesarean delivery for the preterm fetus presenting cephalic will decrease the incidence of periventricular hemorrhage. Anderson and associates (1992) found no significant difference in the overall *frequency* of hemorrhage in infants whose birthweights were below 1750 g and who were delivered without labor compared with those delivered during latent or active labor. Infants delivered of mothers in active labor, however, tended to have more grade III or IV hemorrhages.

Periventricular Leukomalacia

This pathological description refers to cystic areas deep in brain white matter that develop after hemorrhagic *or* ischemic infarction. Tissue ischemia leads to regional necrosis, and because brain tissue does not regenerate, these irreversibly damaged areas appear as echolucent cysts on neuroimaging studies. They generally require at least 2 weeks to develop but have been reported to develop as long as 4 months after the initial insult. Thus, their presence at birth may help to determine the timing of a hemorrhagic event.

Association with Cerebral Palsy

Allan and co-workers (1997) found that the highest rates of cerebral palsy in 505 infants weighing between 600 and 1250 g were associated with periventricular leukomalacia (37 percent) and ventriculomegaly (30 percent). DeVries and colleagues (1993) followed 504 infants born at 34 weeks or less. At least two thirds had localized cystic periventricular leukomalacia, and 100 percent of those with extensive cystic areas developed cerebral palsy. Conversely, only 11 percent of those with transient cysts developed cerebral palsy. Hsu and co-workers (1996) showed that the size of the cyst(s) correlates directly with the risk for cerebral palsy. Fujimoto and colleagues (1994) demonstrated that symmetrical cystic lesions convey the highest risk.

Intraventricular Hemorrhage as a Cause

A variety of clinical and pathological data link severe intraventricular hemorrhage—grade III or IV—and resulting periventricular leukomalacia to cerebral palsy (p. 612). As described earlier, grade I or II hemorrhages usually resolve without extensive tissue injury. Luthy and associates (1987) reported a 16-fold increased risk of cerebral palsy for low-birthweight infants who had grade III or IV hemorrhage compared with the risk in infants who had either none or grade I or II hemorrhage.

Ischemia as a Cause

Consideration of brain development explains why very preterm infants are most susceptible to ischemia and periventricular leukomalacia. Before 32 weeks, the vascular anatomy of the brain is composed of two systems. One penetrates into the cortex—the *ventriculopedal system*. The other reaches down to the ventricles, but then curves to flow outward—the *ventriculofugal system* (Weindling, 1995). There are no vascular anastomoses connecting these two systems. As a result, the area between these systems, through which the pyramidal tracts pass near the lateral cerebral ventricles, is a watershed area vulnerable to ischemia. Vascular insufficiency before 32 weeks leading to ischemia would affect this watershed area first. Resulting damage of the pyramidal tracts would cause spastic diplegia. After 32 weeks, vascular flow shifts toward the cortex. Thus, hypoxic injury after this time primarily damages the cortical region.

Perinatal Infection as a Cause

Periventricular leukomalacia is more strongly linked to infection and inflammation than to intraventricular hemorrhage. Zupan and associates (1996) studied 753 infants born between 24 and 32 weeks, 9 percent of whom developed periventricular leukomalacia. Those born before 28 weeks or who had inflammatory events during the last days to weeks before delivery or who had both were at highest risk. Perlman and co-workers (1996) found that periventricular leukomalacia was strongly associated with prolonged membrane rupture, chorioamnionitis, and neonatal hypotension. Bailis and associates (2009) reported that chronic—and not acute—placental inflammation was associated with leukomalacia.

Fetal infection may be the key element in the pathway between preterm birth, intracranial hemorrhage, periventricular leukomalacia, and cerebral palsy (Dammann and Leviton, 1997; Yoon and colleagues, 1997a, 2000, 2001). In the pathway proposed in **Figure 29-2**, antenatal reproductive tract infection evokes the production of cytokines such as tumor necrosis factor and interleukins-1, -6, and -8. These in turn stimulate prostaglandin production and preterm labor (see Chap. 36, p. 812). Preterm intracranial blood vessels are susceptible to rupture and damage, and the cytokines that stimulate preterm labor also have direct toxic effects on oligodendrocytes and myelin. Vessel rupture, tissue hypoxia, and cytokine-mediated damage result in massive neuronal cell death. Glutamate is released, stimulating membrane receptors to allow excess calcium to enter the neurons. High intracellular calcium levels are toxic to white matter, and glutamate may be directly toxic to oligodendrocytes (Oka and associates, 1993).

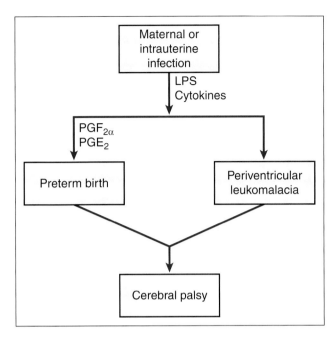

FIGURE 29-2 Schematic representation of the hypothesized pathway between maternal or intrauterine infection and preterm birth or periventricular leukomalacia. Both potentially lead to cerebral palsy. LPS = lipopolysaccharide; PG = prostaglandin.

Many studies have shown that infection and cytokines can directly damage the immature brain. Inoculation of rabbit embryos with *Escherichia coli* causes histological damage in white matter (Yoon and colleagues, 1997a). Moreover, tumor necrosis factor and interleukin-6 were more frequently found in the brains of infants who died with periventricular leukomalacia (Yoon and co-workers, 1997b). Cytokines are strongly linked to white matter lesions even when organisms cannot be demonstrated (Yoon and associates, 2000).

Infection appears to be important even when separated from preterm birth. Verma and colleagues (1997) studied outcomes in 285 infants born after preterm labor and 279 infants born after preterm prematurely ruptured membranes. These researchers compared these outcomes with those of 149 infants who were delivered preterm for other reasons. The incidence and severity of intraventricular hemorrhage and periventricular leukomalacia were highest in those infants with spontaneous labor or membrane rupture and were increased even more with chorioamnionitis. Grether and Nelson (1997) studied children whose birthweight was greater than 2500 g and found a ninefold increased risk of cerebral palsy with either intrapartum maternal fever or chorioamnionitis. They noted a 19-fold risk if there was neonatal infection. Wu and co-workers (2003) studied more than 231,500 singletons born at ≥ 36 weeks and reported a fourfold increased risk of cerebral palsy with clinical chorioamnionitis. Finally, Stoll and colleagues (2004) studied 6093 extremely-low-birthweight infants and found neonatal infections to be associated with a 50-percent rate of neurodevelopmental impairment.

Andrews and co-workers (2008) recently provided data that raise questions regarding an increased incidence of adverse neurodevelopmental outcomes related to chorioamnionitis. In a co-

hort of infants born between 23 and 32 weeks, they studied a number of surrogate indicators and direct markers of in utero inflammation that included clinical findings, cytokine levels, histological findings, and microbial culture results. Infants undergoing comprehensive psychoneurological testing had similar incidences of IQ < 70, cerebral palsy, or both, regardless of these markers. They interpreted their findings to support current practices that employ efforts to delay delivery with preterm pregnancies in the absence of overt intrauterine infection. This does not apply to preterm pregnancies in which *clinical chorioamnionitis* is diagnosed as illustrated by the Canadian Neonatal Network study reported by Soraisham and co-workers (2009). Of 3094 singletons born < 33 weeks, 15 percent had evidence of clinical chorioamnionitis—foul-smelling amnionic fluid, maternal fever, uterine tenderness, fetal tachycardia, and maternal leukocytosis. Compared with noninfected infants, those in the latter group had significantly increased rates of early-onset sepsis—4.8 versus 0.9 percent—and some intraventricular hemorrhage—22 versus 12 percent.

Brain Disorders

Few events evoke more fear and apprehension in parents and obstetricians than the specter of "brain damage." This term immediately conjures visions of disabling cerebral palsy and hopeless mental retardation. Although most brain disorders or injuries are less horrific, they nevertheless are a major source of psychological and economical damage.

The persistence for so many years of the presumed birth-injury etiology for cerebral damage was a major reason for the escalating rate of cesarean delivery through the 1970s and 1980s. Because in most cases, the injury for cerebral palsy does not occur peripartum, increases in cesarean delivery rates did not result in a significant decline in cerebral palsy rates.

Brain disorders or damage, including cerebral palsy, are a complex and multifactorial process caused by a combination of genetic, physiological, environmental, and obstetrical factors. For years, the term *birth asphyxia*—indicating a neurological injury during birth—was inappropriately applied to many infants. Fortunately, objective definitions have subsequently evolved. To clarify the potential role of intrapartum events in causing permanent neurological injury, the American College of Obstetricians and Gynecologists (1998, 2004) developed a precise definition of birth asphyxia that includes all of these three:

1. Profound metabolic or mixed acidemia (pH < 7.0) determined on an umbilical cord arterial blood sample
2. Persistent Apgar score of 0 to 3 for longer than 5 minutes
3. Evidence of neonatal neurological sequelae such as seizures, coma, or hypotonia or of dysfunction of one or more of the following systems: cardiovascular, gastrointestinal, hematological, pulmonary, or renal.

When these three factors are associated with brain injury, they suggest that perinatal *hypoxic ischemic encephalopathy* developed. More importantly, their absence helped to forge the crucial link between *antepartum* events that cause most cases of cerebral palsy.

Neonatal Encephalopathy

The American College of Obstetricians and Gynecologists and the American Academy of Pediatrics (2003) convened the Task Force on Neonatal Encephalopathy and Cerebral Palsy to review scientific data on these topics. It defined encephalopathy as some combination of abnormal consciousness, tone, reflexes, feeding, respiration, or seizures in the term or near-term infant. The Task Force concluded that there were many different causes, which may or may not result in permanent sequelae—cerebral palsy being but one. Moreover, cerebral palsy can be attributed to an intrapartum event only if the affected child develops *hypoxic ischemic encephalopathy*. Further, of the several forms of cerebral palsy, only the spastic quadriplegic type can result from an acute interruption of blood supply prior to delivery. Hemiparetic or hemiplegic cerebral palsy, spastic diplegia, and ataxia are unlikely to result from an intrapartum event. Purely dyskinetic or ataxic cerebral palsy, especially when accompanied by a learning disorder, usually has a genetic origin (Nelson and Grether, 1998).

Although there is no doubt that some cases of cerebral palsy arise from intrapartum hypoxic–ischemic events, accumulated data indicate that at least 70 percent of all cases of neonatal encephalopathy result from an event *prior* to the onset of labor. To address this, the Task Force developed four essential criteria that, if all are present, define an acute intrapartum event sufficient to cause cerebral palsy:

1. Evidence of metabolic acidosis in fetal umbilical arterial blood obtained at delivery: pH < 7.0 *and* base deficit of ≥ 12 mmol/L
2. Early onset of severe or moderate neonatal encephalopathy in infants born at 34 or more weeks
3. Cerebral palsy of spastic quadriplegic or dyskinetic type
4. Exclusion of other possible etiologies such as trauma, coagulation disorders, infections, or genetic disorders.

The Task Force also developed five criteria that, if occurring together, suggest that the supposed insult occurred within 0 to 48 hours of delivery:

1. A sentinel hypoxic event occurring immediately before or during labor
2. Sudden and sustained fetal bradycardia or the absence of fetal heart rate variability in the presence of persistent, late, or variable decelerations, usually after a hypoxic sentinel event when the fetal heart rate pattern was previously normal
3. Apgar scores of 0 to 3 beyond 5 minutes
4. Onset of multisystem dysfunction within 72 hours of birth
5. Early imaging study showing evidence of acute, nonfocal cerebral abnormality.

Strijbis and associates (2006) applied these criteria to 213 children with cerebral palsy and found them useful to audit causation and to exclude primary intrapartum hypoxia.

Prophylactic Hypothermia. Recent trials have demonstrated the efficacy of hypothermia for hypoxic ischemic encephalopathy to prevent death and moderate-to-severe disability in term infants (Gluckman and colleagues, 2005; Shankaran and associates, 2005). Total body cooling therapy to 33.5°C is based on extensive animal literature, which shows that a reduction in brain temperature immediately after a hypoxic-ischemic insult improves outcome. Its use is currently investigational pending outcomes from ongoing randomized trials (Blackmon and Stark, 2006).

Cerebral Palsy

This term refers to a group of conditions that are characterized by chronic movement or posture abnormalities that are cerebral in origin, arise early in life, and are nonprogressive (Nelson, 2003). Epilepsy and mental retardation frequently accompany cerebral palsy but seldom are associated with perinatal asphyxia in the absence of cerebral palsy.

Cerebral palsy is commonly classified by the type of neurological dysfunction—spastic, dyskinetic, or ataxic—as well as the number and distribution of limbs involved—quadriplegia, diplegia, hemiplegia, or monoplegia. The major types and their frequencies are:

- *Spastic quadriplegia,* which has a strong association with mental retardation and seizure disorders—20 percent
- *Diplegia,* which is common in preterm or low-birthweight infants—30 percent
- *Hemiplegia*—30 percent
- *Choreoathetoid types*—15 percent
- *Mixed varieties* (Freeman and Nelson, 1988; Rosen and Dickinson, 1992).

Significant mental retardation, defined as an intelligence quotient (IQ) of less than 50, is associated with 25 percent of cerebral palsy cases.

Incidence and Epidemiological Correlates. According to the Centers for Disease Control and Prevention, the prevalence of cerebral palsy in the United States was 3.1 per 1000 children in 2000 (Bhasin and co-workers, 2006). Importantly, this rate either has remained essentially unchanged or has increased since the 1950s (Torfs and colleagues, 1990; Winter and associates, 2002). In some countries, the incidence has risen because advances in the care of very preterm infants have improved their survival, but not their neurological prognosis. For example, Moster and co-workers (2008) presented long-term follow-up studies of more than 900,000 births in Norway entered into the compulsory national registry. Of nonanomalous term infants, the rate of cerebral palsy was 0.1 percent compared with 9.1 percent in those born at 23 to 27 weeks. The figures for mental retardation for infants born in these epochs were 0.4 versus 4.4 percent, respectively.

Nelson and Ellenberg (1984, 1985, 1986a, b) have made seminal observations to our understanding of cerebral palsy. Their studies included data from the Collaborative Perinatal Project, which followed offspring of almost 54,000 pregnancies until age 7. They found that the important antecedents and most commonly associated risk factors for cerebral palsy were: (1) evidence of genetic abnormalities, such as maternal mental retardation, fetal microcephaly, and fetal congenital malformations; (2) birthweight less than 2000 g; (3) gestational age at birth less than 32 weeks; and (4) infection. Obstetrical complications were not strongly predictive of cerebral palsy. Indeed, only approximately

TABLE 29-2. Prenatal and Perinatal Risk Factors in Children with Cerebral Palsy

Risk Factors	Risk Ratio	95% CI
Long menstrual cycle (>36 days)[a]	9.0	2.2–37.1
Hydramnios[a]	6.9	1.0–49.3
Premature placental separation[a]	7.6	2.7–21.1
Intervals between pregnancies < 3 months or > 3 years	3.7	1.0–4.4
Birthweight < 2000 g[a]	4.2	1.8–10.2
Spontaneous preterm labor	3.4	1.7–6.7
Preterm delivery at 23–27 weeks	78.9	56.5–110
Breech, face, or transverse lie[a]	3.8	1.6–9.1
Severe birth defect[a]	5.6	8.1–30.0
Nonsevere birth defect	6.1	3.1–11.8
Time to cry > 5 minutes[a]	9.0	4.3–18.8
Low placental weight[a]	3.6	1.5–8.4

[a]Also associated with cerebral palsy in the Collaborative Perinatal Project.
From Livinec (2005), Moster (2008), Nelson and Ellenberg (1985, 1986a, b), Torfs (1990), and all their colleagues.

20 percent of affected children had markers of perinatal asphyxia. By contrast, more than half had associated congenital malformations, low birthweight, microcephaly, or another explanation for the brain disorder. They concluded that the causes of most cerebral palsy cases were unknown and that no foreseeable single intervention would likely prevent a large proportion of cases.

Torfs and associates (1990) reported similar findings in 55 children with cerebral palsy from more than 19,000 enrolled in the California Child Health and Development Studies. The strongest predictors of cerebral palsy included a congenital anomaly, low birthweight, low placental weight, or abnormal fetal position. These factors were similar to those identified in the Collaborative Perinatal Project (Table 29-2). Interestingly, cesarean delivery or low-, mid-, and even high-forceps delivery did not correlate with cerebral palsy (see Chap. 25, p. 545). Similarly, the Maternal Fetal Medicine Units Network studied nearly 800 infants with birthweights less than 1000 g and showed that only low birthweight and early gestational age correlated with neonatal neurological morbidity (Goepfert and associates, 1996). From Sweden, Thorngren-Jerneck and Herbst (2006) studied 2306 infants with cerebral palsy and found that preterm birth was a factor in a third. Other risk factors included fetal-growth disorders, placental abruption, type 1 diabetes, preeclampsia, and maternal age older than 40 years (Wu and associates, 2006). A high incidence of microcephaly in neonates with isolated congenital heart lesions was reported by Barbu and co-workers (2009). This finding led them to speculate that brain injury was due to chronic fetal hypoxemia.

Redline (2005, 2008) has made important observations concerning correlation of placental lesions with neurodevelopmental abnormalities (see Chap. 27, p. 585). Perhaps related, Gibson and associates (2005) found that some inherited fetal thrombophilias were associated with cerebral palsy.

Intrapartum Events. The Task Force on Neonatal Encephalopathy and Cerebral Palsy determined that only 1.6 cases of cerebral palsy per 10,000 deliveries are attributable solely to intrapartum hypoxia. This finding is supported by many studies. For example, Stanley and Blair (1991) performed a case-control study of all cases of cerebral palsy in Western Australia from 1975 to 1980. They reported that intrapartum injury as the cause of cerebral palsy was unlikely in 92 percent of cases; in 3.3 percent, it was possible; and in only 4.9 percent was it likely. Phelan and associates (1996) reviewed fetal monitor tracings from 209 infants with neonatal neurological impairment and classified 75 percent as nonpreventable. Strijbis and associates (2006) could attribute only 2 percent of 213 cases of cerebral palsy to intrapartum hypoxia.

Consistent with this, data from a variety of sources indicate that continuous electronic fetal monitoring in labor neither predicts nor reduces the risk of cerebral palsy compared with intermittent auscultation (Clark and Hankins, 2003; Grant, 1989; MacDonald, 1985; Thacker, 1995, and all their associates). These and other studies led the American College of Obstetricians and Gynecologists (2005) to conclude that electronic fetal monitoring does not reduce the incidence of long-term neurological impairment.

Importantly, there does not appear to be any specific fetal heart rate pattern that predicts cerebral palsy, and a number of studies have found no relationship between the clinical response to abnormal fetal heart rate patterns and neurological outcome (Melone, 1991; Nelson, 1996; Niswander, 1984, and all their colleagues). In fact, an abnormal heart rate pattern in fetuses who ultimately develop cerebral palsy may reflect preexisting neurological abnormality and not ongoing, remedial injury (Phelan and Ahn, 1994).

Apgar Scores. A variety of data show that Apgar scores alone are generally poor predictors of neurological impairment. Nelson and Ellenberg (1984) reported that in the absence of obstetrical complications, low Apgar scores alone were not associated with a high level of risk. In infants who had 5-minute

Apgar scores of 3 or less combined with a complicated birth, however, the incidence of cerebral palsy was increased appreciably. Dijxhoorn and colleagues (1986) reported similar findings. The American College of Obstetricians and Gynecologists (1996) concluded that low Apgar scores at 1 and 5 minutes identify infants who need resuscitation, but that alone these are not evidence for hypoxia sufficient to result in neurological damage (see Chap. 28, p. 594). Exceptions are survivors with Apgar scores of zero at 10 minutes. Harrington and colleagues (2007) reviewed 94 such infants admitted alive to the neonatal intensive care unit—78 died, and all survivors who were assessed had long-term disabilities.

Umbilical Cord Blood Gas Studies. An important part of the definition of neonatal asphyxia is metabolic acidosis (see Chap. 28, p. 595). In its absence, significant intrapartum hypoxia or asphyxia generally is excluded. When used alone, however, umbilical cord acid-base determinations have proven no more helpful than the 1- and 5-minute Apgar scores in predicting long-term neurological sequelae. Dijxhoorn and associates (1986) studied 805 term newborns delivered vaginally. They reported that the largest number of neurologically abnormal infants had low Apgar scores but a normal cord arterial pH. This indicated that intrapartum hypoxia was not the major cause of neurological morbidity.

Data from several studies demonstrate that a pH < 7.0 is the threshold for clinically significant acidemia (Gilstrap and associates, 1989; Goldaber and colleagues, 1991). In a later study of more than 150,000 infants, Casey and co-workers (2001) used umbilical artery pH to assess the predictability of neonatal death within 28 days. As the pH fell to 7.0 or less, the likelihood of neonatal death escalated and increased 1400-fold with a cord pH of 6.8 or lower in term newborns. When the cord pH was 7.0 or less and the 5-minute Apgar score was 0 to 3, the relative risk of neonatal death was increased by 3204!

Newborn complications increase coincident with the severity of acidemia at birth. According to the American College of Obstetricians and Gynecologists (2006c), encephalopathy develops in 10 percent of newborns whose umbilical arterial base deficit is 12 to 16 mmol/L, and in 40 percent whose deficit is > 16 mmol/L.

Nucleated Red Blood Cells. These immature red cells enter the circulation in response to hypoxia or hemorrhage. Their quantification has been proposed as a measure of hypoxia. And because increased production of nucleated red cells takes place over time, it has been suggested that these counts can be used to measure the duration of hypoxia (Naeye and Localio, 1995). Most studies do not support this, and others have not been able to reproduce these findings (Hankins and co-workers, 2002; Silva and colleagues, 2006). As summarized by the Task Force on Neonatal Encephalopathy and Cerebral Palsy, the significance of both nucleated erythrocytes and lymphocytes as markers for hypoxic injury is currently imprecise and unclear.

Prevention

In preterm infants, corticosteroid therapy may reduce the incidence of intraventricular hemorrhage as discussed on page 609.

In addition, prophylaxis or aggressive treatment of infection may protect against neurological injury.

Because epidemiological evidence suggested that maternal magnesium sulfate therapy had a fetal neuroprotective effect, three large randomized trials have been performed to investigate this hypothesis. An Australian randomized trial by Crowther and colleagues (2003) included 1063 women at imminent risk of delivery before 30 weeks. A multicenter French trial reported by Marret and associates (2008) included 573 pregnancies at < 33 weeks. The most convincing evidence for magnesium neuroprotection is from the National Institute of Child Health and Human Development (NICHD) Maternal-Fetal Medicine Units Network study reported by Rouse and colleagues (2008). The *Beneficial Effects of Antenatal Magnesium Sulfate— BEAM—Study* randomized more than 2220 women at 24 to 31 weeks, most with either preterm labor or preterm prematurely ruptured membranes. Mortality rates were not affected, but rates of *moderate or severe cerebral palsy* were significantly lower in the magnesium-exposed children whose mothers were enrolled between 24 and 27 weeks. Doyle and co-workers (2009) performed a Cochrane database meta-analysis of these and two other studies, totaling 6145 women at risk for preterm birth. They reported significantly decreased rates of cerebral palsy— RR 0.68 (0.54 to 0.87) as well as gross motor dysfunction—RR 0.61 (0.44 to 0.85) in infants exposed to magnesium compared with those in nonexposed infants. These results are discussed in detail in Chapter 36 (p. 824).

Neuroimaging Studies

The use of sonography, computed-tomography, and magnetic-resonance imaging studies has greatly added to the understanding of the etiology and evolution of perinatal brain lesions, including hypoxic-ischemic encephalopathy. According to the Task Force, imaging studies are generally normal if performed on the day of birth in an infant with perinatal asphyxia (American College of Obstetricians and Gynecologists, 2003). Magnetic resonance (MR) with diffusion-weighted imaging (DWI) will show evidence of injury by approximately 24 hours. Abnormal diffusion peaks at approximately 5 days and disappears within 2 weeks. Computed tomography (CT) scans show decreased density in the thalami or basal ganglia after 24 hours, and these persist for 5 to 7 days. On sonography, there is increasing echogenicity in the thalami and basal ganglia, which progresses over 2 to 3 days and persists for 5 to 7 days. The Task Force concluded that imaging studies are helpful in timing an injury, but provide only a window in time without absolute precision.

MR imaging is the best diagnostic method to identify and characterize neonatal strokes (Nelson and Lynch, 2004; Raju and colleagues, 2007). Woodward and associates (2006) studied 167 infants born before 30 weeks. In 21 percent, moderate-to-severe abnormalities of white matter were identified by MR imaging done at term-equivalent weeks of age. These abnormalities were associated with three- to 10-fold increases in cognitive and motor delay, cerebral palsy, and neurosensory impairment. Wu and co-workers (2006) studied 273 infants born after 36 weeks who were later diagnosed with cerebral palsy. Of these, 227 were studied by MR imaging and 46 by CT

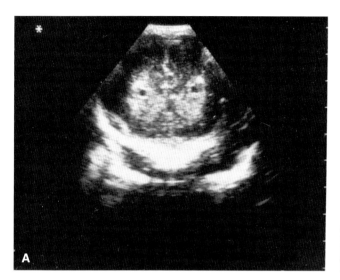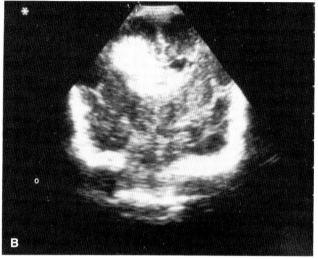

FIGURE 29-3 Preterm infant delivered at 27 weeks because of placental abruption. **A.** Sonogram of the head performed on the first postnatal day shows small bilateral cysts in the periventricular white matter and bilateral germinal-matrix hemorrhages. These findings indicate a much older lesion than one caused by perinatal asphyxia. **B.** A second sonographic evaluation on day 3 of life showed bilateral intraventricular hemorrhage and a large right-sided intraparenchymal echodensity. (Used with from Dr. Jeffrey M. Perlman.)

scanning. A third of all of these studies were normal; focal arterial infarction was seen in 22 percent; brain malformations in 14 percent; and periventricular white-matter injuries in 12 percent. Bax and co-workers (2006) used MR imaging to study 351 children who had cerebral palsy. Almost 88 percent of MR scans were abnormal. The most common finding was white-matter damage including periventricular leukomalacia—43 percent, basal ganglia lesions—13 percent, cortical and subcortical lesions—9 percent, malformations—9 percent, and focal infarcts—7 percent.

Cranial sonography also provides useful information. For example, Locatelli and colleagues (2009) found a significantly increased incidence of neurological damage in the 20 percent of 225 preterm infants who had intraventricular hemorrhage, periventricular leukomalacia, or both. The development of periventricular leukomalacia is shown in Figure 29-3. In this case, because cysts take days to weeks to develop, a sonographic examination performed on day 1 was critical in diagnosing *antenatal* brain injury. Intraventricular hemorrhage was found to be a secondary insult that developed in the nursery. In some infants, sonography provides findings different but complementary to those of CT scanning. In Figure 29-4, grade III intraventricular hemorrhage was seen at birth by CT scanning, but sonographic examination done the same day also identified periventricular leukomalacia from an injury well before birth.

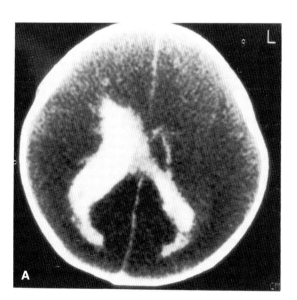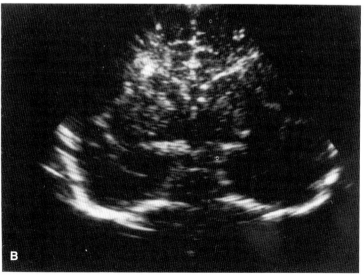

FIGURE 29-4 This term infant was born depressed. **A.** The computed tomographic (CT) scan done on day 1 demonstrates a grade III intraventricular hemorrhage. **B.** Sonogram confirmed intraventricular hemorrhage, however, bilateral cystic periventricular leukomalacia was also seen, which was not observed on the CT scan. These findings documented a severe antenatal brain insult of 4 to 5 weeks' duration. (From Perlman and Cunningham, 1993.)

Computed tomographic and MR imaging have also been used in older children to define the timing of cerebral injury. Some children were born preterm, but others were at term. For example, Wiklund and colleagues (1991a, b) studied children between 5 and 16 years of age with hemiplegic cerebral palsy—28 of these had been born preterm, whereas 83 were born at term. Almost 75 percent of all 111 children had abnormal CT findings. In more than half of term infants, CT findings suggested a *prenatal* injury. In contrast, as many as 70 percent of those delivered preterm had findings that confirmed an insult in early *postnatal* life. Cortical and subcortical injury suggestive of a perinatal injury was found in 19 percent.

Neonatal Encephalopathy in Term Infants

Mature infants also can suffer neurological insults, resulting in permanent compromise. Recall that neonatal encephalopathy is a defined syndrome of disturbed neurological function consisting of difficulty in initiating and maintaining respiration, depressed tone and reflexes, subnormal level of consciousness, and frequently, seizures. It generally is believed to be the consequence of a hypoxic-ischemic insult, although the timing of the insult is not always known. *Mild encephalopathy* is generally defined as hyperalertness, irritability, jitteriness, and hypertonia and hypotonia. *Moderate encephalopathy* includes lethargy, severe hypertonia, and occasional seizures, whereas *severe encephalopathy* is defined by coma, multiple seizures, and recurrent apnea.

Severe encephalopathy is a more important predictor of cerebral palsy and future cognitive defects than either mild or moderate types (Robertson and Finer, 1985). Poor postnatal brain growth is an early sign of neurological compromise. In one study, Cordes and colleagues (1994) performed serial head circumference measurements of 54 term infants with hypoxic-ischemic encephalopathy. They found that a 3.1-percent difference in the expected/observed head circumference in the first 4 months of life was predictive of microcephaly. Permanent impairment was predictable with 90-percent specificity.

Mental Retardation

Severe mental retardation has a prevalence of 3 per 1000 children. Etiological factors are shown in Table 29-3. Some genetic causes are discussed throughout Chapter 12. Preterm birth is a common association (Moster and colleagues, 2008). Isolated mental retardation—without epilepsy or cerebral palsy—is seldom associated with perinatal hypoxia (Nelson and Ellenberg, 1984, 1985, 1986a, b).

Seizure Disorders

The incidence of seizure disorders in infants < 1000 g was reported to be 9 percent in an Italian study (Falchi and colleagues, 2009). Although these may accompany cerebral palsy, isolated seizure disorders or epilepsy usually are not caused by perinatal hypoxia. Nelson and Ellenberg (1986b) determined that the major predictors of seizure disorders were fetal malformations—cerebral and noncerebral; family history of seizures; and neonatal seizures.

TABLE 29-3. Some Etiological Factors for Severe Mental Retardation

Factor	Percent
Prenatal	**73**
Chromosomal	36
Mutant genes	7
Multiple congenital anomalies	20
Acquired—infections, diabetes, growth restriction	10
Perinatal	**10**
Asphyxia or hypoxia	5
Unidentified causes	5
Postnatal	**11**
Unknown	**6**

Modified from Rosen and Hobel (1986), with permission.

Necrotizing Enterocolitis

This newborn bowel disorder has clinical findings of abdominal distention, ileus, and bloody stools. There is usually radiological evidence of *pneumatosis intestinalis*—bowel wall gas derived from invading bacteria. Bowel perforation may prompt resection.

The disease is seen primarily in low-birthweight infants but occasionally is encountered in mature neonates. Various hypothesized causes include perinatal hypotension, hypoxia, sepsis, umbilical catheterization, exchange transfusions, and the feeding of cow milk and hypertonic solutions (Kliegman and Fanaroff, 1984). All of these can ultimately lead to intestinal ischemia, and reperfusion injury also likely has a role (Czyrko and associates, 1991). The unifying hypothesis for these pathological processes is the uncontrolled inflammatory response to bacterial colonization of the preterm intestine (Grave and coworkers, 2007).

Treatment for necrotizing enterocolitis is controversial. A randomized trial of laparotomy versus peritoneal drainage found no difference in survival in preterm infants (Moss and associates, 2006). In an observational study, however, Blakely and colleagues (2006) found that laparotomy had a more favorable outcome than drainage for death rates and neurodevelopmental outcomes assessed at 18 to 22 months.

Infant Outcomes in Extreme Preterm Birth

All of the concerns previously described are amplified in infants born at 22 to 25 weeks. Currently, depending on many factors, this gestational age range is considered the threshold of viability. This is discussed in detail in Chapter 36 (p. 807). Also discussed there are perinatal outcomes of these very- and extremely low-birthweight infants.

The Neonatal Research Network reviewed 4446 infants born at 22 to 25 weeks' gestation (Tyson and associates, 2008). They reported that the likelihood of a favorable outcome with intensive care can be estimated by consideration of gestational age, sex, exposure to antenatal corticosteroids, singleton versus multifetal birth, and birthweight. Based on this, a tool is available for clinicians to utilize these factors (www.nichd.nih.gov/neonatal_estimates).

Anemia

After 35 weeks, the mean cord hemoglobin concentration is approximately 17 g/dL and values below 14 g/dL are abnormal. The neonatal hemoglobin value may rise as much as 20 percent if blood is transfused from the placenta. McDonald and Middleton (2008) performed a systematic review of 11 trials with nearly 3000 deliveries and compared early with late cord clamping. Late clamping was associated with a mean increase in hemoglobin concentration of 2.2 g/dL, however, it almost doubled the incidence of hyperbilirubinemia requiring phototherapy. Alternatively, if the placenta is cut or torn, if a fetal vessel is perforated or lacerated, or if the infant is held well above the level of the placenta for some time before cord clamping, the hemoglobin concentration may fall.

Fetal-to-Maternal Hemorrhage

Fetal red cells in the maternal circulation can be identified by use of the acid elution principle first described by Kleihauer, Brown, and Betke, or by any of several modifications. Fetal erythrocytes contain hemoglobin F, which is more resistant to acid elution than hemoglobin A. After exposure to acid, only fetal hemoglobin remains. Fetal red cells can then be identified by uptake of a special stain and quantified on a peripheral smear (Fig. 29-5). This test is accurate unless the maternal red cells carry excess fetal hemoglobin as the result of a hemoglobinopathy.

During all pregnancies, very small volumes of blood cells escape from the fetal compartment into the maternal intervillous space. This is important for several reasons. It is the cause of maternal red cell isoimmunization, as discussed on page 618. Second, routine fetal-to-maternal cell transfer may someday serve as the basis for a screening test for fetal aneuploidy using mater-

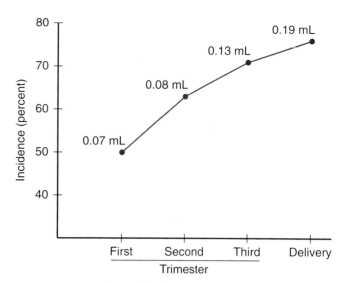

FIGURE 29-6 Incidence of fetal-to-maternal hemorrhage during pregnancy. The numbers at each data point represent total volume of fetal blood estimated to have been transferred into the maternal circulation. (Data from Choavaratana and colleagues, 1997.)

nal peripheral blood (see Chap. 13, p. 302). Lastly, it is now known that fetal stem cells or lymphocytes persist in certain maternal tissues. Such maternal-fetal *hybridization* or *microchimerism* can incite an immune response that may be the instigating factor in certain autoimmune diseases such as thyroiditis, scleroderma, and lupus erythematosus (see Chap. 54, p. 1146).

Choavaratana and colleagues (1997) performed serial Kleihauer–Betke tests in 2000 pregnant women and found that, although the *incidence* of fetal-maternal hemorrhage in each trimester was high, the *volume transfused* was very small (Fig. 29-6). How often fetomaternal hemorrhage exceeds 30 mL is controversial. Bowman (1985) reported that only 21 of 9000 women had fetal hemorrhage of this magnitude. Salim and associates (2005) studied fetomaternal hemorrhage of this magnitude in more than 800 women. Their original estimates were calculated erroneously because of an error in the 21st edition of *Williams Obstetrics*. When calculated using the correct formula, almost 4 percent of women had fetomaternal hemorrhages of 30 mL or greater whether delivered vaginally or by cesarean (Salim and Shalev, 2006). Other events that may cause sufficient hemorrhage to incite isoimmunization are shown in Table 29-4.

D-positive fetal red blood cells in D-negative maternal blood can also be detected, albeit nonquantitatively, by the *rosette test*. Maternal red cells are mixed with anti-D antibodies, which coat any D-positive fetal cells present in the sample. Indicator red cells bearing the D-antigen are then added, and rosettes form around the fetal cells as the indicator cells attach to them by the antibodies. Rosettes indicate that fetal D-positive cells are present.

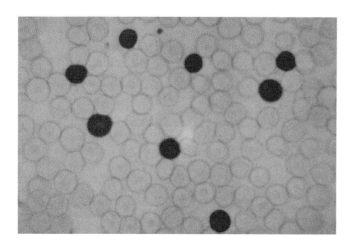

FIGURE 29-5 Massive fetal-to-maternal hemorrhage. After acid-elution treatment, fetal red cells rich in hemoglobin F stain darkly, whereas maternal red cells with only very small amounts of hemoglobin F stain lightly.

Sequelae

If the fetus becomes severely anemic, a sinusoidal heart rate pattern may develop (see Chap. 18, p. 419). Although not

TABLE 29-4. Causes of Fetomaternal Hemorrhage That May Incite Red Cell Antigen Isoimmunization

Early pregnancy loss
Miscarriage
Missed abortion
Elective abortion
Ectopic pregnancy

Procedures
Chorionic villus sampling
Amniocentesis
Fetal blood sampling

Other
Idiopathic
Maternal trauma
Manual placental removal
External version

pathognomonic of fetal anemia, it should prompt immediate evaluation. In general, anemia occurring gradually or chronically, as in isoimmunization, is better tolerated by the fetus than anemia that develops acutely. Chronic anemia may not produce fetal heart rate abnormalities until the fetus is moribund. In contrast, significant acute hemorrhage is poorly tolerated by the fetus and often causes profound neurological fetal impairment, usually from hypotension and cerebral hypoperfusion, ischemia, and infarction.

Because such pathophysiological organ damage occurs acutely, subsequent obstetrical management usually will not change the outcome. De Alemida and Bowman (1994) described 27 cases of fetal-maternal hemorrhage exceeding 80 mL. Despite appropriate management, almost half of these infants died or developed spastic diplegia. Indeed, in the study by Samadi and colleagues (1996), severe fetal-to-maternal hemorrhage caused 5 percent of all stillbirths. This likely is an underestimate because in some cases—about 20 percent—ABO incompatibilities would cause maternal isoagglutinins to rapidly destroy ABO-incompatible fetal erythrocytes. In most cases, the etiology of such hemorrhage is undetermined. For example, placental abruption seldom is the cause. Trauma, however, such as with vehicular accidents can cause placental tearing or "fracture" with significant fetal hemorrhage (see Chap. 42, p. 936). The fetal effects of acute hemorrhage also are illustrated by monochorionic twinning complicated by *twin-twin transfusion syndrome* (see Chap. 39, p. 874). Arterial and venous anastomoses are found in virtually all monochorionic twins. If there is an acute transfer of blood from the donor to the recipient twin, hypotension with hypoperfusion and cerebral infarction, as well as death, can occur.

Management

Once fetal-maternal hemorrhage is recognized, the volume of fetal blood loss can be quantified. The volume may influence obstetrical management and is essential to determining the appropriate dose of D-immunoglobulin when the woman is

D-negative. Using basic physiological principles, the amount of fetal hemorrhage may be calculated from the results of a Kleihauer–Betke (KB) stain using the formula:

$$\text{Fetal blood volume} = \frac{\text{MBV} \times \text{maternal Hct} \times \% \text{ fetal cells in KB}}{\text{newborn Hct}}$$

where MBV = maternal blood volume (approximately 5000 mL in normal-sized normotensive women at term) and Hct = hematocrit. Thus, for 1.7-percent positive KB-stained cells in a woman of average size with a hematocrit of 35 percent giving birth to a term infant weighing 3000 g and whose hematocrit is 0.5:

$$\text{Fetal blood volume} = \frac{5000 \times 0.35 \times 0.017}{0.5} = 60 \text{ mL}$$

The fetal-placental blood volume at term is 125 mL/kg, which is 375 mL for this 3000-g fetus. Thus, this fetus has lost 30 mL of red cells over time into the maternal circulation. This is equivalent to 60 mL of whole blood, because the hematocrit is 50 percent in a term fetus. This amount represents approximately 15 percent (60 ÷ 375 mL) of the fetal-placental volume. This loss should be well tolerated hemodynamically, but would require two 300-μg doses of anti-D immunoglobulin to prevent isoimmunization.

Isoimmunization

Pathophysiology

There are currently 29 blood groups and more than 600 red cell antigens that are recognized by the International Society of Blood Transfusing (Hosoi, 2008). Although some of them are immunologically and genetically important, many are so rare as to be of little clinical significance. Any individual who lacks a specific red cell antigen may produce an antibody when exposed to that antigen. Such antibodies can prove harmful to that individual if she receives a blood transfusion, or they may be harmful to her fetus during that pregnancy. Accordingly, blood banks routinely screen for erythrocyte antigens.

Most persons carry at least one red cell antigen inherited from their father but lacking in their mother. Thus, the mother could be sensitized if enough fetal erythrocytes reached her circulation to elicit an immune response. Even so, isoimmunization is actually rare for the following reasons: (1) low prevalence of incompatible red cell antigens; (2) insufficient transplacental passage of fetal antigens or maternal antibodies; (3) maternal-fetal ABO incompatibility, which leads to rapid clearance of fetal cells before they elicit an immune response; (4) variable antigenicity; and (5) variable maternal immune response to the antigen, with some antigens provoking only minimal response. Considering all these factors, it is not surprising that for all pregnant women there is only a 1-percent chance of D-isoimmunization by 6 months postpartum and that isoimmunization does not always lead to erythroblastosis fetalis.

The incidence of sensitization to red cell antigens at each stage of pregnancy has been studied most extensively in D-negative women. A D-negative woman delivered of a D-positive, ABO-compatible infant has a likelihood of isoimmunization of 16 percent. Two percent will be immunized by the time of delivery, 7 percent will have anti-D antibody by 6 months postpartum, and the remaining 7 percent will be "sensibilized" (Bowman, 1985). In sensibilized women, anti-D antibodies are produced at such a low level that they are not detected during or after the index pregnancy. Instead, they are identified early in a subsequent pregnancy when rechallenged by another D-positive fetus.

ABO Blood Group System

Although incompatibility for the major blood group antigens A and B is the most common cause of hemolytic disease in the newborn, the resulting anemia is usually mild. Approximately 20 percent of all infants have an ABO maternal blood group incompatibility, but only 5 percent are clinically affected. ABO incompatibility is different from CDE incompatibility for several reasons:

- ABO disease frequently is seen in firstborn infants. This is because most group O women have anti-A and anti-B isoagglutinins antedating pregnancy. These are attributed to exposure to bacteria displaying similar antigens

- Most species of anti-A and anti-B antibodies are immunoglobulin M (IgM), which cannot cross the placenta and therefore cannot reach fetal erythrocytes. In addition, fetal red cells have fewer A and B antigenic sites than adult cells and are thus less immunogenic. Thus, there is no need to monitor for fetal hemolysis, and there is no justification for early delivery

- The disease is invariably milder than D-isoimmunization and rarely results in significant anemia. Affected infants typically do not have erythroblastosis fetalis, but rather have neonatal anemia and jaundice, which can be treated with phototherapy

- ABO isoimmunization can affect future pregnancies, but unlike CDE disease, it rarely becomes progressively more severe. Katz and co-workers (1982) identified a recurrence in 87 percent. Of these, 62 percent required treatment, most often limited to neonatal phototherapy.

Because of these reasons, ABO isoimmunization is a disease of pediatric rather than obstetrical concern. Although there is no need for antenatal monitoring, careful neonatal observation is essential because hyperbilirubinemia may require treatment. Treatment usually consists of phototherapy or simple or exchange transfusion with O-negative blood (see p. 625).

CDE (Rhesus) Blood Group System

This system includes five red cell proteins or antigens: C, c, D, E, and e. No "d" antigen has been identified, and Rh- or D-negativity is defined as the absence of the D-antigen. There are, however, D-antigen variants that cause hemolytic disease (Bush and associates, 2003; Cannon and colleagues, 2003). Some of these include weak D, D^u, and partial D (Prasad and co-workers, 2006).

The CDE antigens are of considerable clinical importance because many D-negative individuals become isoimmunized after a single exposure. The two responsible genes—D and CE—

are located on the short arm of chromosome 1 and are inherited together, independent of other blood group genes. Like many genes, their incidence varies according to racial origin. Native Americans, Inuits, and Chinese and other Asiatic peoples have 99-percent D positivity. Approximately 93 percent of African-Americans are D-positive, but only 87 percent of Caucasians are. Of all racial and ethnic groups studied thus far, the Basques show the highest incidence of D-negativity at 34 percent.

The C-, c-, E-, and e-antigens have lower immunogenicity than the D-antigen, but they too can cause erythroblastosis fetalis. **All pregnant women should be tested routinely for D-antigen erythrocytes and for irregular antibodies in their serum.** Barss and colleagues (1988) demonstrated that this need be done only once during each pregnancy in D-positive women, and this is currently recommended by the American Association of Blood Banks.

Other Blood Group Incompatibilities

Because routine administration of anti-D immunoglobulin prevents most cases of anti-D-isoimmunization, proportionately more cases of significant antenatal hemolytic disease are now caused by the less common red cell antigens. Such sensitization is suggested by a positive indirect Coombs test performed to screen for abnormal antibodies in maternal serum (Table 29-5).

Several large studies indicate that anti-red cell antibodies are found in 1 percent of pregnancies (Bowell and colleagues, 1986; Howard and associates, 1998). From 40 to 60 percent of these are directed against the CDE antibodies. Anti-D is the most common, followed by anti-E, anti-c, and anti-C. A third of fetuses with either anti-C or anti-Ce alloimmunization described by Bowman and colleagues (1992b) had hemolysis but none had severe disease. In contrast, Hackney and co-workers (2004) reported that 12 of 46 anti-c isoimmunized fetuses had serious hemolysis, and eight of these 12 required transfusions.

Anti-Kell antibodies are also frequent. A fourth of all antibodies found are from the *Lewis system*. These do not cause hemolysis because Lewis antigens do not develop on fetal erythrocytes and are not expressed until a few weeks after birth.

Kell Antigen. Approximately 90 percent of Caucasians are Kell negative. Kell type is not routinely determined, and 90 percent of cases of anti-Kell sensitization result from transfusion with Kell-positive blood. As with CDE antigens, Kell sensitization also can develop as the result of maternal–fetal incompatibility. Kell sensitization may be clinically more severe than D-sensitization because anti-Kell antibodies also attach to fetal bone marrow erythrocyte precursors, thus preventing a hemopoietic response to anemia. Thus, there usually is a more rapid and severe anemia than with anti-D sensitization (Weiner and Widness, 1996).

Because fewer erythrocytes are produced, there is less hemolysis and less amnionic fluid bilirubin. As a result, severe anemia may not be predicted by either the maternal anti-Kell titer or the level of amnionic fluid bilirubin. Caine and Mueller-Heubach (1986) described 13 Kell-sensitized pregnancies with a Kell-positive fetus. Five of these resulted in hydrops or perinatal death despite favorable amnionic fluid studies 1 week before

TABLE 29-5. Atypical Antibodies and Their Relationship to Fetal Hemolytic Disease

Blood Group System	Antigens Related to Hemolytic Disease	Hemolytic Disease Severity	Proposed Management
Lewis	*		
I	*		
Kell	K	Mild to severe[†]	Fetal assessment
	k, Ko, Kp[a] Kp[b], Js[a], Js[b]	Mild	Routine obstetric care
Rh (non-D)	E, C, c	Mild to severe[†]	Fetal assessment
Duffy	Fy[a]	Mild to severe[†]	Fetal assessment
	Fy[b]	[‡]	Routine obstetric care
	By[3]	Mild	Routine obstetric care
Kidd	Jk[a]	Mild to severe	Fetal assessment
	Jk[b], Jk[3]	Mild	Routine obstetric care
MNSs	M, S, s, U	Mild to severe	Fetal assessment
	N	Mild	Routine obstetric care
	Mi[a]	Moderate	Fetal assessment
MSSSs	Mt[a]	Moderate	Fetal assessment
	Vw, Mur, Hil, Hut	Mild	Routine obstetric care
Lutheran	Lu[a], Lu[b]	Mild	Routine obstetric care
Diego	D1[a], Di[b]	Mild to severe	Fetal assessment
Xg	Xg[a]	Mild	Routine obstetric care
P	PP$_{1pk}$(Tj[a])	Mild to severe	Fetal assessment
Public antigens	Yt[a]	Moderate to severe	Fetal assessment
	Yt[b], Lan, Ge, Jr[a], CO[1-b-]	Mild	Routine obstetric care
	En[a]	Moderate	Fetal assessment
	Co[a]	Severe	Fetal assessment
Private antigens	Batty, Becker, Berrens, Evans, Gonzales, Hunt, Jobbins, Rm, Ven,Wright[b]	Mild	Routine obstetric care
	Biles, Heibel, Radin, Zd	Moderate	Fetal assessment
	Good, Wright[a]	Severe	Fetal assessment

*Not a proven cause of hemolytic disease of the newborn.
[†]With hydrops fetalis.
[‡]Not a cause of hemolytic disease of the newborn.
Reprinted, with permission, from American College of Obstetricians and Gynecologists. Management of alloimmunization during pregnancy. ACOG Practice Bulletin 75. Washington, DC: ACOG; 2006.

delivery. Bowman and colleagues (1992a) reviewed 20 Kell-sensitized pregnancies, in which exchange transfusions were required in four, and four fetuses died. Because of this disparate severity of Kell sensitization, some investigators recommend evaluation when the maternal anti-Kell titer is 1:8 or greater. In addition, Weiner and Widness (1996) suggest that the initial evaluation be accomplished by cordocentesis instead of amniocentesis, because fetal anemia from Kell sensitization is usually more severe than indicated by the amnionic fluid bilirubin level. Determination of fetal middle cerebral artery (MCA) velocity by Doppler obviates this, as discussed subsequently. Van Wamelen and associates (2007) studied 41 women and concluded that for timely detection of severe fetal anemia, pregnancies in women with anti-Kell titers ≥ 1:2 should be closely monitored by peak MCA systolic velocity beginning at 16 to 17 weeks.

Other Antigens. Kidd (Jk[a]), Duffy (Fy[a]), c-, E-, and to a lesser extent C-antigens can all cause erythroblastosis as severe

as that associated with sensitization to D-antigen (see Table 29-5). Two Duffy antigens have been identified, Fy[a] and Fy[b], and some African-Americans lack both. Fy[a] is the most immunogenic. The Kidd system also has two antigens, Jk[a] and Jk[b], with the population distribution as follows: Jk (a+b−), 26 percent; Jk (a−b+), 24 percent; and Jk (a+b+), 50 percent (Alper, 1977). In their report of 20 cases of Jk[a] isoimmunization, Franco and colleagues (2009) reported that all but one were mild.

If an IgG red cell antibody is detected and there is any doubt as to its significance, the clinician should err on the side of caution, and the pregnancy should be evaluated. As shown in Table 29-5, many rare or *private antigens* have been associated with severe isoimmunization (Rouse and Weiner, 1990).

Immune Hydrops

The abnormal collection of fluid in more than one area of the fetal body, such as ascites and pleural effusion, is termed *hydrops fetalis*. Its causes usually are categorized as immune and nonim-

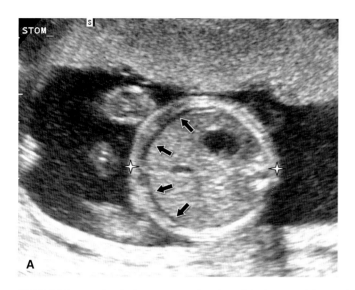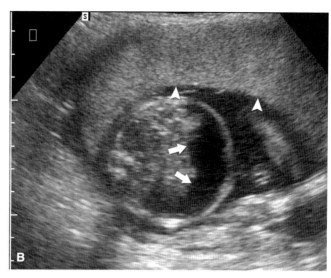

FIGURE 29-7 Hydropic fetus. **A.** Fetal ascites (*black arrows*) beneath the anasarca of the fetal abdominal wall (*white cursors*). **B.** Placental thickening (*arrowheads*) and marked pelvic ascites (*arrows*) are also seen in another image of the same fetus.

mune. In immune hydrops such as that with D-isoimmunization, excessive and prolonged hemolysis causes anemia, which in turn stimulates marked marrow erythroid hyperplasia. It also stimulates extramedullary hematopoiesis in the spleen and liver with eventual hepatic dysfunction. There may be cardiac enlargement and pulmonary hemorrhage. Fluid collects in the fetal thorax, abdominal cavity, or skin. The placenta is markedly edematous, enlarged, and boggy. It contains large, prominent cotyledons and edematous villi. Pleural effusions may be so severe as to restrict lung development, which causes pulmonary compromise after birth. Ascites, hepatomegaly, and splenomegaly may lead to severe labor dystocia. Severe hydropic changes are easily seen with sonography (Fig. 29-7).

The precise pathophysiology of hydrops remains unknown. Theories include heart failure from profound anemia and hypoxia, portal hypertension due to hepatic parenchymal disruption caused by extramedullary hemopoiesis, and decreased colloid oncotic pressure resulting from liver dysfunction and hypoproteinemia. The data from several studies indicate that in most cases, the degree and duration of anemia is the major factor causing and influencing the severity of ascites (Pasman and associates, 2006). Secondary factors include hypoproteinemia caused by liver dysfunction and capillary endothelial leakage resulting from tissue hypoxia. Both of these lead to protein loss and decreased colloid oncotic pressure, which worsen hydrops. For example, Nicolaides and colleagues (1985) performed percutaneous umbilical artery blood sampling in 17 severely D-isoimmunized fetuses at 18 to 25 weeks. All fetuses with hydrops had hemoglobin values less than 3.8 g/dL, plasma protein concentrations less than 2 standard deviations below the normal mean,

and substantive protein concentrations in ascitic fluid. Conversely, none of the fetuses with hemoglobin values exceeding 4 g/dL were hydropic, even though six of 10 also had hypoproteinemia of the same magnitude as the hydropic fetuses.

Weiner and co-workers (1989) evaluated umbilical venous pressure during 20 antenatal transfusions in isoimmunized pregnancies. Significantly elevated pressures found in hydropic fetuses normalized within 24 hours of transfusion. Because portal hypertension cannot resolve so rapidly, this suggests that the elevated pressure was actually due to hypoxic myocardial dysfunction, which was reversed by transfusions.

Fetuses with hydrops may die in utero from profound anemia and circulatory failure (Fig. 29-8). One sign of severe anemia and impending death is the sinusoidal fetal heart rate pattern (see Chap. 18 p. 419). In addition, hydropic placental changes

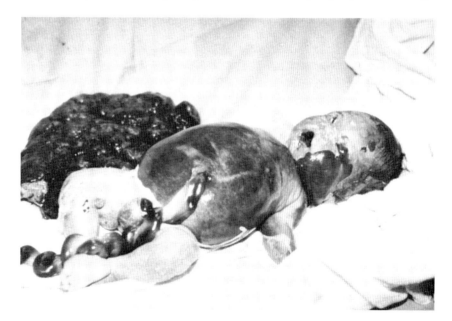

FIGURE 29-8 Severe erythroblastosis fetalis. Hydropic, macerated stillborn infant and characteristically large placenta.

leading to placentomegaly can cause preeclampsia. Ironically, the preeclamptic mother may develop severe edema mimicking that of the fetus—this is referred to as the *mirror syndrome* (see p. 627).

The liveborn hydropic infant appears pale, edematous, and limp at birth and usually requires resuscitation. The spleen and liver are enlarged, and there may be widespread ecchymosis or scattered petechiae. Dyspnea and circulatory collapse are common. Hyperbilirubinemia is discussed subsequently on page 625.

Perinatal Mortality

Perinatal deaths from hemolytic disease caused by D-isoimmunization have decreased dramatically since adoption of the policy of routine preventative administration of D-immunoglobulin to all D-negative women during or immediately after pregnancy. Survival also has been increased by antenatal transfusions or preterm delivery of affected fetuses if necessary (Bowman and colleagues, 1977; Fretts and co-workers, 1992). The advent of fetal transfusion therapy has resulted in survival rates exceeding 90 percent for severe anemia alone, and 70 percent if hydrops has developed (Moise, 2008).

Identification of the Isoimmunized Pregnancy

It is routine practice to perform blood typing and antibody screen at the first prenatal visit, and unbound antibodies in maternal serum are detected by the *indirect Coombs test*. If positive, specific antibodies are identified, and their immunoglobulin subtype is determined as either IgG or IgM. Only IgG antibodies are concerning because IgM antibodies cannot cross the placenta. If the IgG antibodies are known to cause fetal hemolytic anemia as shown in Table 29-5, the titer is quantified. The *critical titer* is the level for a particular antibody that requires further evaluation. This may be different for each antibody and is determined individually by each laboratory. For example, the critical titer for anti-D antibodies is usually 1:16. Thus, a titer of $\geq$ 1:16 indicates the possibility of severe hemolytic disease. The critical titers for other antibodies are often assumed to be 1:16 as well, although most laboratories have insufficient data to support this assumption. An important exception is Kell sensitization. The critical titer for anti-Kell antibody is 1:8 or even less as discussed on page 619.

Determining Fetal Genotype.

The presence of maternal anti-D antibodies does not necessarily mean that the fetus will be affected or is even D-positive. This may be for several reasons. For example, in a previously sensitized or sensibilized woman, the antibody titer may rise to high levels during a subsequent pregnancy even when the fetus is D-negative—the *amnestic response*. Additionally, half of all fetuses with antigen-positive Caucasian fathers are D-antigen negative, because half of D-positive Caucasian males are D-antigen heterozygous (Race and Sanger, 1975). Moreover, many women sensitized to non-D red cell antigens become immunized after a blood transfusion, and the antigen may not be present on paternal erythrocytes. Examples include other CE group and Kell antigens.

Determining zygosity of the father for the D-antigen is helpful, and DNA-based analysis will establish this. **But before paternal testing is pursued, it is imperative that any possibility of nonpaternity be disclosed.** If the father is homozygous for D, then there is a 100-percent chance of a D-positive fetus, and fetal genotyping is not necessary. Paternal heterozygosity can be estimated by co-inheritance of CcEe phenotypes, but this is inexact (Moise, 2008).

If the father is heterozygous or if paternal DNA-based testing cannot be performed, fetal genotyping is performed on samples of chorionic villous amniocytes or fetal blood. Reference laboratories are also able to analyze amniocytes for E, c, Kell, Kidd, M, and Duffy antigens. Likely, others will also soon be available. Noninvasive fetal D genotyping by using *cell-free fetal DNA* in maternal plasma is currently used in some European countries (Gautier and colleagues, 2005; Hahn and Chitty, 2008). Fetal DNA from maternal plasma or fetal cells is 85- to 95-percent accurate for D-antigen determination (Arntfield, 2009; Bianchi, 2005; Geifman-Holtzman, 2006, and all their co-workers). Currently, there are no such FDA-approved testing strategies available in the United States (see also Chap. 13, p. 302).

Management of Isoimmunization

Management is individualized and consists of maternal antibody titer surveillance, sonographic monitoring of the fetal middle cerebral artery peak systolic velocity, amnionic fluid bilirubin studies, or fetal blood sampling. Accurate pregnancy dating is critical. The gestational age at which fetal anemia developed in the last pregnancy is important because anemia tends to occur earlier and be sequentially more severe. In the first sensitized pregnancy, a positive antibody screen with a titer below the critical level should be followed with repeated titers at timely intervals, usually monthly. Once the critical titer has been met or exceeded, subsequent titers are not helpful, and further evaluation is required. If this is not the first sensitized pregnancy, then the pregnancy is considered to be at risk, and maternal antibody titers are unreliable.

Middle Cerebral Artery (MCA) Peak Systolic Velocity.

In most specialized centers, serial measurement of the peak systolic velocity of the fetal middle cerebral artery has replaced amniocentesis for detection of fetal anemia (American College of Obstetrics and Gynecology, 2006b). The technique is discussed in Chapter 16 (p. 364). The anemic fetus shunts blood preferentially to the brain to maintain adequate oxygenation. The peak MCA systolic velocity increases because of increased cardiac output and decreased blood viscosity (Moise, 2008). In a collaborative study, Mari and colleagues (2000) measured this velocity serially in 111 fetuses at risk for anemia and in 265 normal fetuses. A threshold of > 1.5 MoM correctly identified all fetuses with moderate or severe anemia. The sensitivity was 100 percent, and false-positive rate was 12 percent. A Doppler waveform illustrating this is shown in Chapter 16 (Fig. 16-28, p. 365). More recently, Oepkes and co-workers (2006) compared Doppler velocimetry to amnionic-fluid bilirubin studies. They reported that Doppler studies had an 88-percent sensitivity and 85-percent accuracy, whereas bilirubin studies had a 76 percent sensitivity, 77-percent specificity, and 76-percent accuracy. As discussed on page 624, velocimetry is less sensitive to predict anemia following fetal transfusions. Doppler results are shown in Figure 29-9. From a retrospective analysis, Sau and

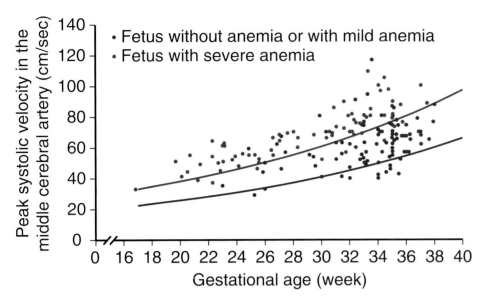

FIGURE 29-9 Doppler measurements of the peak systolic velocity in the middle cerebral artery in 165 fetuses at risk for severe anemia. The blue line indicates the median peak systolic velocity in normal pregnancies, and the red line shows 1.5 multiples of the median. (Reprinted from Oepkes D, Seaward PG, Vandenbussche FP, et al: Doppler ultrasonography versus amniocentesis to predict fetal anemia. *N Engl J Med* 355(2):156–164, with permission. Copyright © 2006 Massachusetts Medical Society. All rights reserved.)

colleagues (2009) also suggested that the noninvasive method was preferred.

If the MCA peak systolic velocity exceeds 1.5 MoM, the fetus is likely to be anemic. Further evaluation by fetal blood sampling is then necessary to determine the need for transfusions.

Amnionic Fluid Spectral Analysis

Almost 50 years ago, Liley (1961) demonstrated the utility of amnionic fluid spectral analysis to measure the bilirubin concentration to estimate the severity of hemolysis, and thus to indirectly assess anemia. It is less widely used now, but Moise (2008) recommends its parallel use initially with MCA Doppler flow studies to verify accuracy as centers gain experience with velocimetry. It is also used when Doppler velocimetry is not readily available.

Because amnionic fluid bilirubin levels are low, the concentration is measured by a spectrophotometer and is demonstrable as a change in absorbance at 450 nm—this difference is referred to as ΔOD_{450}. The likelihood of fetal anemia is determined by plotting the ΔOD_{450} value on a graph that is divided into several zones. The original Liley graph is valid from 27 to 42 weeks and contains three zones. Zone 1 generally indicates a D-negative fetus or one with only mild disease. Zone 2 indicates that anemia is present. In lower zone 2, the anticipated hemoglobin level is 11.0 to 13.9 g/dL, whereas in upper zone 2, hemoglobin values range from 8.0 to 10.9 g/dL. Zone 3 indicates severe anemia with hemoglobin values below 8.0 g/dL (Liley, 1961). Recently, Pasman and colleagues (2008) have observed a closer correlation of severe fetal anemia with a bilirubin/albumin ratio compared with the Liley or Queenan graphs.

Use of the "Liley curve" allowed decisions regarding management. At that time, the options were fetal intraperitoneal transfusions or preterm delivery. The Liley graph was subsequently modified by Queenan and associates (1993). These investigators

studied 845 amnionic fluid samples from 75 D-immunized and 520 unaffected pregnancies and constructed a Liley-type curve that begins at 14 weeks (Fig. 29-10). As can be seen, the naturally high amnionic fluid bilirubin level at midpregnancy results in a large *indeterminate zone*. Importantly, bilirubin concentrations in this zone do not accurately predict fetal hemoglobin concentration. For this reason, when evaluation indicates that severe fetal anemia or hydrops before 25 weeks is likely, many forego amniocentesis and instead perform fetal blood sampling.

Fetal Blood Transfusions. With evidence of fetal anemia, hepatomegaly, or hydrops or with non-reassuring fetal testing, management is determined by gestational age. The near-mature fetus should be delivered. The preterm fetus can be evaluated using fetal blood sampling, and transfusions are given as necessary as described in Chapter 13 (p. 301). Fetal hemoglobin, hematocrit, reticulocyte count, and indirect Coombs titer are determined to predict the onset of anemia if the fetus is not yet affected (Weiner and associates, 1991a).

Nicolaides and co-workers (1988) recommend that transfusions be commenced when the hemoglobin level is at least 2 g/dL below the mean for normal fetuses of corresponding gestational age (see Chap. 4, p. 91). Others recommend transfusions when the fetal hematocrit is below 30 percent—2 standard deviations below the mean at all gestational ages (Weiner and associates, 1991b). Fetal

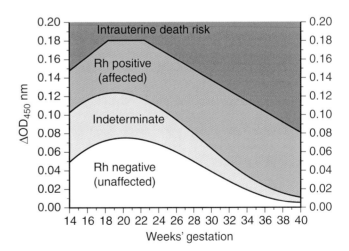

FIGURE 29-10 Proposed amnionic fluid ΔOD_{450} management zones in pregnancies from 14 to 40 weeks. (This figure was published in *American Journal of Obstetrics & Gynecology*, Vol. 168, No. 5, JT Queenan, PT Thomas, TP Tomai, et al., Deviation of amniotic fluid optical density at a wavelength of 450 nm in Rh isoimmunized pregnancies from 14 to 40 weeks' gestation: A proposal for clinical management, pp. 1370–1376, Copyright Elsevier 1993.)

intraperitoneal and intraumbilical blood transfusions are discussed in detail in Chapter 13 (p. 302). With severe early-onset hemolytic disease, intraperitoneal transfusions are done because it is technically difficult to gain vascular access in the cord (Howe and Michaitidis, 2007). With an older and larger fetus, most prefer intravascular transfusions.

Over the past decade or so, perinatal outcomes have been reasonably good. From the Netherlands, van Kamp and colleagues (2005) reported outcomes of 254 fetuses treated with intravascular transfusions. Overall survival was 89 percent, and 12 of 19 perinatal deaths were procedure related. Of 740 transfusions, 15 percent were performed before 24 weeks. Howe and Michaitidis (2007) performed intraperitoneal transfusions in five severely affected fetuses with D-isoimmunization beginning at 15 to 16 weeks. Each fetus received four or five transfusions before umbilical cord size allowed access. All five were delivered at 34 to 35 weeks and survived. Scheier (2006) and Klumper (2009) and their associates reported that MCA peak velocity is less accurate in predicting anemia after one transfusion, and even less so after two or more. As a rule, to predict the next transfusion, the fetal hematocrit decreases 1 volume percent per day.

Treatments that have not been effective include plasmapheresis, administration of promethazine or D-positive erythrocyte membranes in enteric capsules, and immunosuppression with corticosteroids.

Delivery. The goal of management is delivery of a reasonably mature healthy fetus. When management includes serial amnionic fluid ΔOD_{450} measurement or fetal transfusions, fetal well-being should be closely monitored with techniques discussed in Chapter 15. According to the American College of Obstetricians and Gynecologists (2006b), with appropriate management, extremely preterm delivery usually can be avoided.

Neonatal Care and Outcome. Some advocate that the last transfusion for the severely affected fetus be given at 30 to 32 weeks with antenatal corticosteroid administration and delivery at 32 to 34 weeks. Others continue transfusion until 36 weeks. In either case, cord blood is obtained at delivery for hemoglobin concentration and direct Coombs testing. If the infant is overtly anemic, it is often best to complete the initial exchange transfusion promptly with recently collected type-O, D-negative red cells. For infants who are not overtly anemic, the need for exchange transfusion is determined by the rate of increase in bilirubin concentration, the maturity of the infant, and the presence of other complications.

Most fetal transfusion survivors develop normally. In one long-term follow-up study, Grab and colleagues (1999) reported outcomes of 35 fetuses who had severe isoimmunization or immune hydrops and who were given antenatal intravascular transfusions. At age 1, only one had mild psychomotor disabilities, and another had delayed speech development. At up to age 6 years, however, none of the survivors, including those with hydrops, had either moderate or severe neurological impairment. Harper and associates (2006) provided a mean 10-year follow-up of 18 hydropic fetuses who underwent intravascular transfusions. Two fetuses died, two of the 16 survivors had

major neurological handicaps, but the remainder had neuropsychological findings similar to those of their siblings.

Anti-D Immunoglobulin

D-isoimmunization is prevented by administration of high-titer anti-D antibodies extracted by cold alcohol plasma fractionation and ultrafiltration. A standard intramuscular dose provides 300 μg of D-antibody as determined by radioimmunoassay. It is given to the D-negative nonsensitized mother to prevent sensitization after pregnancy-related events that could result in fetal-maternal hemorrhage as discussed on page 617 and listed in Table 29-4. Although sensitization can follow spontaneous miscarriage as well as early elective pregnancy termination, the precise incidence is not known (Hannafin and colleagues, 2006). Still, most recommend that D-negative women receive anti-D immunoglobulin (American College of Obstetricians and Gynecologists, 1999b). A 50-μg "mini dose" is available for these early pregnancy indications.

Routine Antepartum Administration. One dose of anti-D immunoglobulin is given prophylactically to all D-negative women at approximately 28 weeks, and a second dose is given after delivery if the infant is D-positive (American College of Obstetricians and Gynecologists, 1999b). Without such prophylaxis, Bowman and Pollock (1978) showed that 1.8 percent of D-negative women will become isoimmunized by silent fetal-maternal hemorrhage. When such prophylaxis is given, only 0.07 percent of susceptible women are sensitized. Despite a policy for antepartum immunoglobin administration, MacKenzie and associates (2006a) reported that the "real world" sensitization rate was 0.4 percent.

Regardless of antepartum administration at 28 weeks, a second dose is required after delivery because the half-life of immunoglobulin is only 24 days and protective levels predictably persist for only 6 weeks or so. In addition, fetal-maternal hemorrhage is more likely at delivery (see Fig. 29-6). Each 300-μg dose will protect the average-sized mother from a fetal hemorrhage of up to 15 mL of D-positive red cells or 30 mL of fetal whole blood. The initial 300-μg dose will produce a weakly positive—1:1 to 1:4—indirect Coombs titer in the mother. As the body mass index increases above 27 to 40 kg/m^2, serum antibody levels decrease by 30 to 60 percent (MacKenzie and associates, 2006b; Woelfer and co-workers, 2004). Rarely, a small amount of antibody crosses the placenta and results in a weakly positive direct Coombs test in cord and infant blood. This small amount causes negligible fetal hemolysis.

D-negative women who receive blood products are also at risk of becoming sensitized. Although they should be given only D-negative red cells, platelet transfusions and plasmapheresis can provide sufficient D-antigen to cause sensitization. This can be prevented by an injection of D-immunoglobulin. And most recommend routine administration when there is blunt maternal trauma, although its necessity has not been proven (Thorp, 2008). In many cases, anticipated fetomaternal hemorrhage is mild and likely protected by the 28-week dose of immunoglobulin. For example, Boucher and colleagues (2008) demonstrated this in more than 1300 trials of external cephalic version. **Still, when there is doubt about**

whether to give anti–D immunoglobulin, it should be given. Even if not needed, it will cause no harm, but failing to give it when needed can have severe consequences.

Large Fetal-to-Maternal Hemorrhage. With more severe fetal-maternal hemorrhage, one 300-μg dose of D-immunoglobulin may not be sufficient. Ness and colleagues (1987) studied 800 D-negative mothers and reported that the incidence of fetal-maternal transfusion exceeding 30 mL of whole blood, the quantity neutralized by one dose of immunoglobulin, was 1 percent. Another 5.6 percent of these pregnancies had fetal-maternal hemorrhage of between 11 and 30 mL. Adeniji and colleagues (2008) recently reported similar findings. Thus, at least 1 percent, and perhaps more, of susceptible mothers would have been given insufficient immunoglobulin if not tested. Importantly, these investigators determined that if extra D-immunoglobulin is considered only for women with risk factors such as abdominal trauma, placental abruption, placenta previa, intrauterine manipulation, multifetal gestation, or manual removal of the placenta, half of women requiring more than the 300-μg dose would be missed. Stedman and co-workers (1986) used the erythrocyte rosette test and reported similar results.

Because of the above observations, the American Association of Blood Banks recommends that all D-negative women be tested at delivery with the Kleihauer-Betke or rosette test (Snyder, 1998). The dosage of anti-D immunoglobulin is calculated from the estimated volume of the fetal-to-maternal hemorrhage described on page 618. One 300-μg ampule is given for each 30 mL of fetal whole blood to be neutralized. To determine if the dose was adequate after it is given, the indirect Coombs test is performed. A positive result indicates that there is excess anti–D-immunoglobulin in maternal serum, thus demonstrating that the dose was sufficient.

D^u-Antigen. Identification of the D^u-antigen may cause confusion or result in designation of the blood type as "weak D-positive." The D^u-antigen is actually a variant of the D-antigen, and women confirmed to be D^u-positive are therefore D-positive and do not need immunoglobulin (American College of Obstetricians and Gynecologists, 1999b). If a D-negative woman delivers a D^u-positive infant, she should be given D-immunoglobulin. As before, if there is any doubt about D-antigen status, then immunoglobin should be given.

Maternal-to-Fetal Hemorrhage

It is now recognized that in virtually all pregnancies, small amounts of maternal blood enter the fetal circulation. Unlike *fetal-to-maternal* bleeding, physiologically significant *maternal-to-fetal* hemorrhage is uncommon. Rarely, the D-negative fetus is exposed to maternal D-antigen and becomes sensitized. When such a female fetus reaches adulthood, she will produce anti-D antibodies even before or early in her first pregnancy. This mechanism of isoimmunization is called the *grandmother theory* because the fetus in the current pregnancy is jeopardized by antibodies initially provoked by its grandmother's erythrocytes. Major blood group (ABO) incompatibility offers appre-

ciable protection against D-sensitization of the fetus. D-negative infants born to D-positive mothers are not routinely given D-immunoglobulin prophylaxis.

Hyperbilirubinemia

Unconjugated or free bilirubin is readily transferred across the placenta from mother to fetus, if the maternal plasma level is high. Although conjugated bilirubin glucuronide is water soluble and normally is excreted into bile and urine when the plasma level is elevated, unconjugated bilirubin is not excreted this way.

Kernicterus

This condition may result from unconjugated hyperbilirubinemia in the newborn—especially if preterm. Bilirubin deposition and staining in the basal ganglia and hippocampus results in profound neuronal degeneration in these regions. Surviving infants show spasticity, muscular incoordination, and varying degrees of mental retardation. There is a positive correlation between unconjugated bilirubin levels above 18 to 20 mg/dL and kernicterus. Despite this, kernicterus may develop at much lower concentrations, especially in very preterm infants. In a follow-up study from the Collaborative Perinatal Project, levels of total serum bilirubin ≥25 mg/dL correlated with kernicterus only in those infants with a positive Coombs test (Kezniewicz and Newman, 2009).

Physiological Jaundice

By far the most common form of unconjugated nonhemolytic jaundice is so-called *physiological jaundice*. In the mature infant, serum bilirubin usually increases for 3 to 4 days to levels up to 10 mg/dL, and then concentrations fall rapidly. Perhaps 15 percent of infants are diagnosed with jaundice (Burke and associates, 2009). In one large study, 1 to 2 percent of infants 35 weeks or older had a serum bilirubin level > 20 mg/dL (Eggert and colleagues, 2006). In preterm infants, the rise is greater and more prolonged.

Treatment

Phototherapy is now widely used to treat hyperbilirubinemia because light increases oxidation of bilirubin. This enhances renal clearance and lowers serum bilirubin levels. Light that penetrates the skin also increases peripheral blood flow, which further enhances photo-oxidation. The randomized trial of 1974 extremely low-birthweight infants treated by the Neonatal Research Network showed that aggressive phototherapy reduced rates of neurodevelopmental impairment even further (Norris and colleagues, 2008).

Rarely, exchange transfusion is required. Newman and associates (2006) showed that when serum bilirubin levels in near-term or term infants exceed 25 mg/dL, therapy will prevent adverse neurodevelopmental outcomes. According to Burke and colleagues (2009), hospitalizations for kernicterus in term infants decreased from 5.1 per 100,000 in 1988 to 1.5 per 100,000 in 1994 and has remained at this level since then. Maisels and McDonagh (2008) recently provided a scholarly treatise on bilirubin metabolism and phototherapy.

Nonimmune Hydrops Fetalis

As defined on page 620, hydrops is characterized by excess fluid in two or more body areas such as the thorax, abdomen, or skin. It is often associated with hydramnios and a hydropic, thickened placenta. Because obstetrical sonographic examination has become routine, hydrops is frequently identified prenatally, and in many cases, the etiology can be determined. The reported incidence varies. Santolaya and colleagues (1992) identified hydrops in 0.6 percent of 12,572 pregnancies undergoing sonographic evaluation and were able to determine the etiology in 77 percent. Nonimmune causes were by far the most common—87 percent—and two thirds were due to intrinsic fetal or placental abnormalities. Heinonen and colleagues (2000) reported a much lower incidence of 1 per 1700 pregnancies, and they were able to determine etiology in 95 percent. In some cases, fetal ascites develops without other features of hydrops, and the overall prognosis is better (Favre and co-workers, 2004).

Bellini and co-workers (2009) recently performed a systematic review of 51 relevant publications describing 5437 pregnancies complicated by nonimmune hydrops. They classified these into 14 categories that are shown in Table 29-6. Cardiovascular disorders comprised almost 22 percent and included structural and functional abnormalities. Although chromosomal anomalies—13 percent—were varied, hematological causes— 10 percent—usually had a final common pathophysiological pathway with anemia and heart failure. Other causes are shown in Table 29-6.

Etiology

There is an ever-lengthening list of specific disorders that can lead to nonimmune hydrops (Table 29-7). *Cystic hygromas* are one of the most common associations, especially when hydrops is identified in the first or early second trimester (see Table 29-6). As discussed in Chapter 16 (p. 356), most of these are the result of aneuploidy. *Cardiac anomalies* have been implicated in 20 to 45 percent of nonimmune hydrops cases (Allan, 1986; Castillo, 1986; Gough, 1986; Santolaya, 1992,

TABLE 29-6. Categories of Disorders Causing Nonimmune Hydrops Fetalis in 5437 Pregnancies

Category	Percent
Cardiovascular	21.7
Chromosomal	13.4
Hematological	10.4
Infections	6.7
Thoracic	6.0
Lymphatic	5.7
Twin-twin transfusion	5.6
Syndromic	4.4
Urinary tract	2.3
Others	6.0
Idiopathic	17.8

Data from Bellini and colleagues, 2009

and all their co-workers). Fetal heart failure also can result from arrhythmias, arterial-venous malformations or immune- or infection-related myocarditis.

Perhaps another one third of fetal hydrops results from *multiple malformations* or *chromosomal anomalies*. Shulman and colleagues (2000) reported that more than 80 percent of cases of dramatic and extensive subcutaneous edema—*space-suit hydrops*—recognized in the first trimester are associated with chromosomal abnormalities.

In multifetal pregnancies, hydrops of one twin is usually from the *twin-twin transfusion syndrome* (see Chap. 39, p. 874). Hydrops can be due to heart failure either from volume overload and hypertensive cardiomyopathy in the recipient twin or from myocardial dysfunction secondary to severe anemia in the donor twin.

Other causes of severe anemia that can lead to hydrops include parvovirus infection, chorioangioma, acute fetal-maternal hemorrhage, and α_4-thalassemia (American College of Obstetricians and Gynecologists, 1999a; Duff and associates, 2009). In San Francisco, which has a large Asian population, 10 percent of hydrops was caused by α_4-thalassemia (Holzgreve and associates, 1984). *Inborn errors of metabolism* such as Gaucher disease, GM 1 gangliosidosis, and sialidosis can cause recurrent hydrops (Lefebvre and colleagues, 1999). Rarely, a *lymphatic anomaly* can result in isolated chylothorax or chylous ascites. Although these fluid collections alone do not qualify as hydrops, chylothorax can ultimately result in a treatable cause of hydrops.

Prognosis

Overall, the outcome for fetal hydrops of any cause is generally poor, however, the later it develops, the better the prognosis. In a study of 82 hydropic fetuses, McCoy and colleagues (1995) observed that if hydrops was evident before 24 weeks, the fetal mortality rate was 95 percent. Conversely, euploid fetuses with hydrops who survived to at least 24 weeks and who had structurally normal hearts had a survival rate of 20 percent.

Diagnosis

In some cases, targeted sonographic and laboratory evaluations will identify the cause of fetal hydrops—for example, those caused by a congenital anomaly, arrhythmia, or twin complication. Depending on the circumstances, helpful maternal blood tests might include hemoglobin electrophoresis, Kleihauer-Betke stain, indirect Coombs test, and serological tests for syphilis, toxoplasmosis, cytomegalovirus, rubella, and parvovirus B19. Amniocentesis is considered for karyotyping and for evidence of infection. Middle cerebral artery peak systolic velocity may suggest fetal anemia, which may prompt fetal blood sampling.

Management

In only a few instances is fetal hydrops amenable to treatment. For example, some tachyarrhythmias can be treated pharmacologically (see Chap. 13, p. 303). Severe anemia can be treated with blood transfusions. In addition, hydrops of one fetus in twin-twin transfusion syndrome may resolve with laser ablation of abnormal vascular anastomoses (see Chap. 13, p. 306

TABLE 29-7. Some Causes of Nonimmune Hydrops Fetalis

Fetal causes

Anomalies

Cardiac	Atrial or ventricular septal defect, hypoplastic left heart, pulmonary valve insufficiency, Ebstein subaortic stenosis, dilated heart, A-V canal defect, single ventricle, Fallot tetralogy, premature closure of foramen ovale, subendocardial fibroelastosis
Thoracic	Diaphragmatic hernia, cystic adenomatous malformation, pulmonary hypoplasia, lung hamartoma, mediastinal teratoma, chylothorax
Gastrointestinal	Jejunal atresia, midgut volvulus, intestinal malrotation or duplication, meconium peritonitis
Urological	Urethral stenosis or atresia, posterior bladder neck obstruction, bladder perforation, prune belly, neurogenic bladder, ureterocele
Syndromes	Thanatophoric dwarfism, arthrogryposis multiplex congenita, asphyxiating thoracic dystrophy, hypophosphatasia, osteogenesis imperfecta, achondroplasia, achondrogenesis, recessive cystic hygroma, and Neu-Laxova, Saldino-Noonan, and Pena-Shokeir type I syndromes
Conduction defects	Supraventricular tachycardias, heart block (including with maternal lupus erythematosus)
Miscellaneous	Cystic hygroma, congenital lymphedema, polysplenia syndrome, neuroblastoma, tuberous sclerosis, sacrococcygeal teratoma
Aneuploidies	Trisomy 21 and other trisomies, Turner syndrome, triploidy
Vascular	A-V shunts, large vessel thromboses (cava, portal, or femoral vein), Kasabach-Merritt syndrome
Infections	Cytomegalovirus, toxoplasmosis, syphilis, listeriosis, hepatitis, rubella, parvovirus, leptospirosis, Chagas disease
Multifetal pregnancy	Twin-twin transfusion syndrome, twin reverse-arterial perfusion (TRAP) syndrome
Miscellaneous	α_4-thalassemia (Bart hemoglobin), twisted ovarian cyst, fetal trauma, anemia, Gaucher disease, gangliosidosis, sialidosis

Placental causes — Chorioangioma, fetomaternal hemorrhage, A-V shunts, placenta trauma with fetal hemorrhage, twin-twin transfusion syndrome

Maternal causes

Medications	Indomethacin

and Chap. 39, p. 872). In most cases, however, hydrops cannot be treated and ultimately proves fatal for the fetus or newborn. In general, if nonimmune hydrops persists and cardiac abnormalities and aneuploidy have been excluded and if the fetus is mature enough that survival is likely, delivery should be accomplished. Very preterm fetuses usually are managed expectantly. Although hydrops usually persists or worsens with time, it occasionally resolves spontaneously (Mueller-Heubach and Mazer, 1983).

Maternal Complications

Preterm labor is common because of associated hydramnios. Placental abruption or uterine atony sometimes follows sudden decompression of an overdistended uterus, and retained placenta is common. Fetal hydrops was associated with a significant 2.3-fold increased risk for preeclampsia (Wu and colleagues, 2009). In one variant—the maternal *mirror syndrome*—the mother develops preeclampsia along with severe edema that is similar to that of the fetus. This unique complication of hydrops is believed to be caused by vascular changes in the swollen, hydropic placenta (Midgley and Hardrug, 2000). The observations of Kusanovic and co-workers (2008) show that this likely is related to antiangiogenic factors produced by hyperplacentosis (see Chap. 34, p. 714). Duthie and Walkinshaw

(1995) and Goeden and Worthington (2005) each describe a woman with parvovirus-associated fetal hydrops and severe preeclampsia at midpregnancy that resolved a few weeks after fetal anemia and hydrops had resolved.

Fetal Cardiac Arrhythmias

Abnormal fetal heart rhythms are now recognized frequently because of extensive use of real-time sonography and Doppler technology. Most arrhythmias are transient and benign, but some tachyarrhythmias, if sustained, can result in heart failure and fetal death. Fetal arrhythmias and their treatment are discussed in Chapter 13 (p. 303).

Congenital Heart Block

Brucato and co-workers (2003) reviewed 1825 cases of congenital heart block from 38 studies. They reported that antenatal diagnosis is associated with a much poorer prognosis and a higher risk of late-onset dilated cardiomyopathy than a diagnosis made in childhood. The recurrence risk of congenital heart block in subsequent pregnancy is high because this defect is associated with anticardiac antibodies. Many of these women have, or subsequently develop, systemic lupus erythematosus or another connective-tissue disease. Conversely, of all the women who produce anti–SS-A, only 1 in 20 have fetuses with cardiac disease (see Chap. 54, p. 1150).

Approximately half of cases of congenital heart block are caused by maternal anti-SS-A (anti-Ro) antibody that binds to tissue in the conduction tracts (Taylor and colleagues, 1986). Conduction tissue inflammation provoked by these antibodies can lead to permanent damage, and symptomatic survivors frequently require a pacemaker at birth. Not all affected fetuses have heart block, and anti-SS-A antibodies can affix to other cardiac tissues as well. If there is extensive myocarditis, the prognosis is poor. Cuneo and associates (2009) showed that if these antibodies are associated with effusions, bradyarrhythmias, or endocardial fibroelastosis, then progressive worsening may occur after birth. There are intriguing data from Stevens and associates (2003) that provide evidence that these affected myocytes may arise from maternal cell engraftment. Such *microchimerism* is discussed in Chapter 54 (p. 1146).

Fetal Treatment. Robinson and co-workers (2001) used terbutaline to transiently increase the heart rate of seven fetuses with a ventricular rate below 60. Fetal pacemaker placement may be an option. Saleeb and colleagues (1999) reviewed the treatment of 50 fetuses with heart block caused by maternal SS-A and SS-B antibodies. They concluded that fluorinated steroids significantly improved outcome and resulted in the resolution of pleural effusions, ascites, or hydrops in 13 of 18 treated cases. Currently, there are no completed controlled trials from which to draw conclusions.

DISEASES OF THE TERM FETUS AND NEONATE

Respiratory Distress Syndrome

Term infants can have respiratory complications, although these are much less frequent than in those born preterm. Common causes in term infants include sepsis, especially from group B streptococcal disease and intrauterine-acquired pneumonia; persistent pulmonary hypertension of the newborn; meconium aspiration syndrome; and pulmonary hemorrhage.

Advances in neonatal care have improved survival with these conditions. High-frequency oscillatory and jet ventilation improves oxygenation without high ventilatory pressures. Moreover, nitric oxide is a specific pulmonary vasodilator. Finer and Barrington (2000) reported a meta-analysis of 11 trials of therapy in infants 34 weeks or older with respiratory failure. They found that nitric oxide significantly improved oxygenation, reduced mortality rates, and decreased the need for extracorporeal membrane oxygenation (p. 606).

Meconium Aspiration Syndrome

This disorder results from peripartum inhalation of meconium-stained amnionic fluid. Inhalation leads to chemical pneumonitis with inflammation of pulmonary tissues, mechanical airway obstruction, and hypoxia. Singh and colleagues (2009) reported its incidence to be 1.8 percent in more than 162,000 term neonates. In severe cases, it progresses to persistent pulmonary hypertension, other morbidity, and death. Even with prompt and appropriate therapy, seriously affected infants frequently die or suffer long-term neurological sequelae.

Risk Factors

In up to 20 percent of pregnancies at term, amnionic fluid is contaminated by meconium. Its passage into a normal amnionic fluid volume results in light meconium staining, and its aspiration before labor is relatively common. In healthy, well-oxygenated fetuses, this diluted meconium is readily cleared from the lungs by normal physiological mechanisms. In some, however, the inhaled meconium is not cleared, and meconium aspiration syndrome results. It can occur after normal labor, but is more likely when the meconium is thick, the pregnancy is postterm, or the fetus is growth-restricted. Putting these together, pregnancies at highest risk are those with diminished amnionic fluid volume and with cord compression or uteroplacental insufficiency that may cause meconium passage (Leveno and colleagues, 1984). In these cases, the meconium remains thick and undiluted, and the compromised fetus cannot clear it.

Prevention

Unfortunately, pathological meconium aspiration cannot be predicted by the fetal heart rate tracing (Chap. 18, p. 431) (Dooley and colleagues, 1985). Early studies reported that the incidence of meconium aspiration syndrome could be reduced by *oropharyngeal suctioning* following delivery of the fetal head, but before delivery of the chest. Accordingly, this became the standard of care. Subsequently, however, several reports showed that strict adherence to this protocol did not reduce the incidence of meconium aspiration syndrome (Davis and colleagues, 1985; Wiswell and co-workers, 1990). Moreover, it was noted that associated pulmonary hypertension is characterized by abnormal arterial muscularization that begins well before birth. Because of such findings, Katz and Bowes (1992) concluded that only chronically asphyxiated fetuses develop meconium aspiration syndrome. They postulated that chronic antepartum asphyxia leads to pulmonary vascular damage, pulmonary hypertension, and persistent fetal circulation. Similarly, Richey (1995) and Bloom (1996) and their associates found no correlation between markers of *acute* asphyxia, such as umbilical artery acidosis, and meconium aspiration.

To settle this issue, an 11-center randomized trial of intrapartum suctioning versus no suctioning with meconium-stained amnionic fluid was done. Results reported by Vain and colleagues (2004) showed an identical 4-percent incidence of meconium aspiration syndrome in both groups. This led to a recommendation against routine intrapartum oropharyngeal and nasopharyngeal suctioning in the presence of meconium-stained fluid by the American Heart Association and American Academy of Pediatrics (2006) as well as the American College of Obstetricians and Gynecologists (2007). Instead, depressed newborns should be intubated and suctioned to remove meconium or other aspirated material from beneath the glottis. This is also discussed in Chapter 28 (p. 591).

Amnioinfusion

Saline infused into the amnionic cavity may be beneficial when meconium staining is thick and there are recurrent variable decelerations (Spong and associates, 1994). The technique is described in Chapters 18 (p. 433) and 21 (p. 497). Amnioinfusion probably poses little or no increased risk (Wenstrom and co-workers, 1995). Unfortunately, it does not benefit fetuses in whom meconium aspiration syndrome has already developed before labor (Byrne and Gau, 1987). A multicenter randomized trial of almost 2000 women who were laboring at 36 weeks or later and who had thick meconium-stained fluid was designed to evaluate amnioinfusion. Pregnancies were stratified by presence or absence of variable decelerations (Fraser and colleagues, 2005). Amnioinfusion did not reduce the perinatal death rate—0.5 percent in both groups. There was no difference in the rate of moderate or severe meconium aspiration—4.4 versus 3.1 percent, with and without amnioinfusion, respectively. Finally, there was not a significant reduction in cesarean delivery—32 versus 29 percent, respectively. For these reasons, the American College of Obstetrics and Gynecologists (2006a) does not recommend amnioinfusion to reduce meconium aspiration syndrome.

Hemorrhagic Disease of the Newborn

This disorder is characterized by spontaneous internal or external bleeding beginning any time after birth. Most hemorrhagic disease results from abnormally low levels of the vitamin K–dependent clotting factors—V, VII, IX, X, prothrombin, and proteins C and S (Zipursky, 1999). Early bleeding may begin within 48 hours after birth in infants whose mothers took anticonvulsants during pregnancy. In these cases, the depressed factor levels result from their decreased maternal hepatic synthesis and from the generally poor transplacental passage of vitamin K. Classic hemorrhagic disease, which becomes apparent from 2 to 5 days after birth, develops in infants not treated with vitamin K at birth. Late hemorrhage occurs at 2 to 12 weeks in infants who are exclusively breast fed, because breast milk contains very low levels of vitamin K. Other causes include hemophilia, congenital syphilis, sepsis, thrombocytopenia purpura, erythroblastosis, and intracranial hemorrhage.

Prophylaxis

Hemorrhagic disease can be avoided by the intramuscular injection of 1 mg of vitamin K_1 (phytonadione) at delivery. Oral administration is not effective, and maternal administration of vitamin K prior to delivery results in very little transport to the fetus. For treatment of active bleeding, vitamin K is injected intravenously. Reports of an association between the administration of vitamin K to newborns and subsequent development of childhood leukemia have been disproved (Zipursky, 1999).

Thrombocytopenia

There are a number of causes of neonatal thrombocytopenia, and these include immune disorders, infections, some drugs, and congenital syndromes. For example, parvovirus-related hydrops, discussed on page 626, is associated with severe thrombocytopenia in a third of cases (Segata and co-workers, 2007). Thrombocytopenia affects a third of all infants admitted to neonatal intensive care units (Sola-Visner and associates, 2009).

It is more common in those with respiratory distress complicated by hypoxia or sepsis.

Immune Thrombocytopenia

Rarely, antiplatelet IgG is transferred from the mother, causing thrombocytopenia in the fetus-neonate. In these cases, fetal thrombocytopenia is usually mild and is found in association with maternal autoimmune disease, especially immune thrombocytopenia. Importantly, neonatal platelet levels often fall rapidly after birth, reaching a nadir at 48 to 72 hours of life. Although corticosteroid therapy usually increases maternal platelet levels, it generally does not affect fetal platelets. Despite this, fetal platelet counts are usually adequate to allow vaginal delivery without an increased risk of intrapartum hemorrhage and without the need for fetal platelet sampling (see Chap. 51, p. 1094).

Alloimmune Thrombocytopenia

This condition is also referred to as *AIT* or *NAIT—neonatal AIT*—and it differs from immune thrombocytopenia in several important ways. It is caused by maternal isoimmunization to fetal platelet antigens in a manner similar to D-antigen isoimmunization discussed on page 618. Thus, the maternal platelet count is normal and isoimmunization is not suspected until after the birth of an affected child. In some cases, antepartum fetal intracranial hemorrhage is diagnosed. Of note, isoimmune thrombocytopenia, even in the first affected infant, is frequently severe and commonly develops before the third trimester. Fetal intracranial hemorrhage develops in up to 20 percent of severely affected fetuses, even as early as 20 weeks. Chronic villitis has been described in untreated cases (Althaus and colleagues, 2005).

Maternal isoimmunization is most often against the platelet antigen HPA-1a—formerly called PL A1—which is found in 98 percent of the population. The susceptible mother lacks this common antigen and becomes immunized when exposed to the fetal platelet antigen. Recall that some degree of fetal-maternal hemorrhage occurs in most pregnancies (see p. 617). Based on the incidence of HPA-1a negativity, 1 in 50 pregnancies is at risk. Yet the incidence of isoimmune thrombocytopenia is only 1 in 1000 to 1 in 5000 pregnancies (Berkowitz and associates, 2006a; Bussel and Primiani, 2008). The paucity of expected cases is explicable because fetal-maternal hemorrhage sufficient to provoke an immune response occurs in only 5 to 10 percent of pregnancies.

Antibodies other than anti-HPA-1a are responsible for 20 percent of cases. These include HPA-1b, HPA-3a, and HPA-5b (Davoren and associates, 2004). An extensive list of these was provided by Berkowitz and co-workers (2006a).

Diagnosis and Management. Progress in identification and treatment of affected fetuses was reviewed by Berkowitz and colleagues (2006b). The diagnosis is usually made after the first pregnancy in a woman with a normal platelet count. There is no evidence of immunological disorder, and her infant has unexplained severe thrombocytopenia. Fetal alloimmune thrombocytopenia recurs in 70 to 90 percent of subsequent pregnancies, is often severe, and usually develops earlier with each successive pregnancy. Indeed, half of such fetuses who undergo cordocentesis blood sampling will have a platelet count $< 20,000/\mu L$.

Because of severe thrombocytopenia in fetuses in subsequent pregnancies, invasive therapy such as platelet transfusions is problematic. Fortunately, weekly maternal intravenous infusions of immunoglobulin (IVIG), 1 g/kg/week, usually result in fetal platelet levels high enough to prevent spontaneous hemorrhage. For non-responders, maternal prednisone therapy is given also. Although Berkowitz and colleagues (2006b) recommend cesarean delivery in most cases, van den Akker and associates (2006) reported vaginal delivery to be safe in women given weekly immunoglobulin infusions and whose previous infant did not have intracranial hemorrhage. According to the Medical Letter, in 2006, such therapy cost $40 to $55 per gram. Despite this, Thung and Grobman (2005) calculated that it is cost effective.

Preeclampsia and Eclampsia

Fetal thrombocytopenia is not caused by preeclampsia–eclampsia. Pritchard and colleagues (1987) at Parkland Hospital studied a large number of mother-infant pairs in pregnancies complicated by hypertension and identified no cases in which neonatal thrombocytopenia correlated with maternal thrombocytopenia (see Chap. 34, p. 717).

Polycythemia and Hyperviscosity

Neonatal polycythemia and blood hyperviscosity develop as the result of chronic hypoxia in utero, from acute transfusion from the placenta or a twin at delivery, or more rarely, from maternal-fetal hemorrhage. As the hematocrit rises above 65, blood viscosity markedly increases. Signs and symptoms include plethora, cyanosis, and neurological aberrations. Laboratory findings include hyperbilirubinemia, thrombocytopenia, fragmented erythrocytes, and hypoglycemia. Treatment consists of partial exchange transfusion with plasma to lower the hematocrit.

FETAL DEATH

From the foregoing sections, it is apparent that a number of maternal and fetal conditions can result in fetal demise. With advances in obstetrics, clinical genetics, maternal-fetal and neonatal medicine, and perinatal pathology, a number of stillbirths that previously would have been categorized as "unexplained" can now be attributed to specific causes. In many cases, this information makes management of subsequent pregnancies easier. Sonography allows rapid confirmation of fetal death, which frequently prompts labor induction (see Chap. 22, p. 500).

Definition of Fetal Mortality

Statistics on perinatal outcome compiled by the Centers for Disease Control and Prevention and the Vital Statistics Reports include only those dead fetuses and neonates born at after 19 weeks, or if gestational age is not available, weighing 350 g or more (MacDorman and Kirmeyer, 2009). As shown in Figure 29-11, stillbirths are more common with decreasing gestational age. The fetal mortality rate for the United States has steadily declined since 1985 from 7.8 to 6.2 per 1000 live births. Before this, an even more impressive decline was likely because deaths of infants with anomalies were "prevented" by early pregnancy

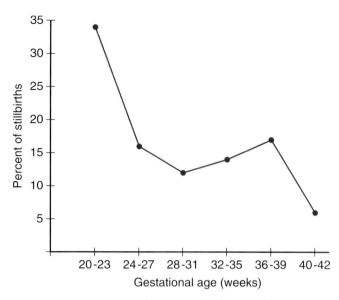

FIGURE 29-11 Proportion of 25,653 stillbirths according to gestational-age epochs in the United States in 2003—National Vital Statistics Reports. (Data from MacDorman and colleagues, 2007.)

terminations (Fretts and associates, 1992). There are a number of risk factors for stillbirth that were recently reviewed by Reddy (2007) and Silver (2007). These include black race, increasing maternal age, obesity, smoking, prior stillbirth, fetal-growth restriction, and maternal diseases. And Bukowski and associates (2009) linked excessive rates of stillbirth infants with fetal macrosomia defined as growth potential > 90th percentile. In some of these—for example, advancing maternal age, multiple factors are likely interactive (Huang and colleagues, 2008). Finally, the fetal death rate is increased fourfold in multifetal pregnancies (American College of Obstetricians and Gynecologists, 2009).

Causes of Fetal Death

The three general categories of fetal death shown in Table 29-8 are fetal, placental, and maternal. Autopsy performed by a pathologist with expertise in fetal and placental disorders, assisted by a team including maternal-fetal medicine, genetic, and pediatric specialists, often can determine the cause of death. Faye-Petersen (1999), Horn (2004), and their associates reviewed autopsies performed by such teams and found that the cause of death was identified in as many as 94 percent of cases. Determining the cause of preterm deaths is more difficult (Yudkin and colleagues, 1987).

Fetal Causes

Some type of fetal abnormality accounts for 25 to 40 percent of all stillbirths (see Table 29-8). The reported incidence of *major congenital malformations* in stillborns is highly variable because of ascertainment bias. It depends on whether autopsy was performed and if so, the experience, interest, and training of the pathologist (Cartlidge and co-workers, 1995a). For example, most stillbirths attributed to fetal causes in Wisconsin had a major structural malformation identified at autopsy (Pauli and

TABLE 29-8. Categories and Causes of Fetal Death

Fetal—25 to 40 percent
  Chromosomal anomalies
  Nonchromosomal birth defects
  Nonimmune hydrops
  Infections—viruses, bacteria, protozoa
Placental—25 to 35 percent
  Prematurely ruptured membranes
  Abruption
  Fetomaternal hemorrhage
  Cord accident
  Placental insufficiency
  Intrapartum asphyxia
  Previa
  Twin-twin transfusion
  Chorioamnionitis
Maternal—5 to 10 percent
  Diabetes
  Hypertensive disorders
  Obesity
  Age > 35 years
  Thyroid disease
  Renal disease
  Antiphospholipid antibodies
  Thrombophilias
  Smoking
  Illicit drugs and alcohol
  Infections and sepsis
  Preterm labor
  Abnormal labor
  Uterine rupture
  Postterm pregnancy
Unexplained—15 to 35 percent

From Cunningham and Hollier (1997), Eller and colleagues (2006), Reddy (2007), and Silver (2007).

Reiser, 1994). Conversely, in a study of 403 stillbirths reported by Copper and colleagues (1994), malformations were identified prenatally in only 5.6 percent. Faye-Petersen and associates (1999) found that a third of fetal deaths were caused by structural anomalies. Neural-tube defects, hydrops, isolated hydrocephalus, and complex congenital heart disease were the most common. Major structural anomalies, hydrops, and aneuploidy are particularly amenable to antenatal diagnosis.

Stillbirths caused by fetal infection are also common, especially when ascending bacterial infections of amnionic fluid and placental sources are considered. In indigent and inner-city women, congenital syphilis can be a common cause of fetal death (see Chap. 59, p. 761). Other potentially lethal infections include those caused by cytomegalovirus and parvovirus B19, as well as rubella, varicella, listeriosis, borreliosis, toxoplasmosis, and many more (Duff and colleagues, 2009; McClure and Goldenberg, 2009).

Placental Causes

Many fetal deaths due to placental abnormalities could also be categorized as having maternal or fetal causes. For example, placental abruption is associated with hypertension in approximately half of cases and could thus be considered a "maternal" cause. Placental insufficiency from aneuploidy could be considered a "fetal" cause. With these caveats in mind, perhaps 15 to 25 percent of fetal deaths are attributed to problems of the placenta, membranes, or cord (Fretts and Usher, 1997).

Placental abruption is the most common single identifiable cause of fetal death (see Chap. 35, p. 761). Fretts and Usher (1997) determined abruption to be the cause of death in 14 percent of stillborns. At Parkland Hospital, approximately 10 percent of third-trimester stillbirths are from abruption.

Significant *placental* and *membrane infection* is usually associated with fetal infection. Exceptions include tuberculosis and malaria. In some cases, microscopic examination of the placenta and membranes may help to identify an infectious cause (Duff and associates, 2009). Chorioamnionitis is characterized by mononuclear and polymorphonuclear leukocytes infiltrating the chorion (see Chap. 27, p. 581). Preterm stillbirths are more likely to be associated with these infections that include aerobic and anaerobic bacterial species as well as mycoplasma and ureaplasma (Goldenberg and associates, 2008; Onderdonk and co-workers, 2008).

Placental infarcts appear as areas of fibrinoid trophoblastic degeneration, calcification, and ischemic infarction from spiral artery occlusion. Marginal and subchorionic infarcts are common and usually of no import. These lesions and their clinical significance are discussed further in Chapter 27 (p. 579).

Fetal-maternal hemorrhage sufficient to cause fetal death was reported in 4.7 percent of 319 fetal deaths at Los Angeles County Women's Hospital in which Kleihauer-Betke stains of maternal blood had been performed (Samadi and associates, 1996). Although usually spontaneous, such hemorrhage is common with severe maternal trauma (see Chap. 42, p. 936).

Twin-twin transfusion syndrome is a common cause of fetal death in monochorionic multifetal pregnancy (see Chap. 39, p. 874).

Maternal Causes

Although they appear to make only a small contribution to fetal deaths, maternal factors may be underestimated. Some pathologies with a strong maternal component—for example, placental abruption or isoimmunization—often are attributed to placental or fetal causes. *Hypertensive disorders* and *diabetes* are the two most commonly cited maternal diseases and are associated with 5 to 8 percent of stillbirths (Alessandri and colleagues, 1992; Fretts and Usher, 1997). As discussed in Chapter 45 (p. 988), chronic hypertension is especially associated with increased fetal death (Aagaard-Tillery and co-workers, 2006; August and Lindheimer, 2009). Perhaps related, overweight and obese women have an increased risk of stillbirth (Chu and associates, 2007; Getahun and co-workers, 2007). Extremes of reproductive age—even when adjusted for known associations such as anomalies and maternal medical disorders—are complicated by a higher fetal death rate (Bateman and Simpson, 2006;

Reddy and associates, 2006; Wyatt and colleagues, 2005). The concept of severe maternal morbidity is discussed in Chapter 1 (p. 6). In developing countries, and intuitively so in developed nations, the stillbirth rate may be increased manyfold with severe maternal morbidities (Cham and associates, 2009).

Lupus anticoagulant and *anticardiolipin antibodies* are associated with decidual vasculopathy, placental infarction, fetal-growth restriction, recurrent abortion, and fetal death (see Chap. 54, p. 1151). Although women with these autoantibodies and other *thrombophilias* clearly are at increased risk for adverse pregnancy outcomes, very few otherwise unexplained stillbirths can be attributed solely to such antibodies (Reddy, 2007). These disorders are discussed in detail in Chapter 47 (p. 1014) and Chapter 54 (p. 1154).

Evaluation of the Stillborn

Determining the cause of fetal death aids the psychological adaptation to a significant loss, helps to assuage the guilt that is part of grieving, makes counseling regarding recurrence more accurate, and may prompt therapy or intervention to prevent a similar outcome in the next pregnancy (American College of Obstetricians and Gynecologists, 2009). Identification of inherited syndromes also provides useful information for other family members.

Clinical Examination

A thorough examination of the fetus, placenta, and membranes should be performed at delivery and recorded in the chart. The details of relevant prenatal events should be provided. Photographs should be taken for the record whenever possible, and a full radiograph of the fetus—a "fetogram"—may be performed. MR imaging and sonography may also be considered (American College of Obstetricians and Gynecologists, 2009). These are especially important in providing anatomical information if parents decline a full autopsy. The checklist used at Parkland Hospital to format the stillbirth note is outlined in Table 29-9.

Laboratory Evaluation

If autopsy and chromosomal studies are performed, up to 35 percent of stillborns are discovered to have major structural anomalies (Faye-Petersen and associates, 1999). Approximately 20 percent have dysmorphic features or skeletal abnormalities, and 8 percent have chromosomal abnormalities (Pauli and Reiser, 1994; Saller and colleagues, 1995). The American College of Obstetricians and Gynecologists (2009) recommends ideally karyotyping all stillborns. In the absence of morphological anomalies, up to 5 percent of stillborns will have a chromosomal abnormality (Korteweg and associates, 2008).

Appropriate consent must be obtained to take fetal tissue samples, including fluid obtained postmortem by needle aspiration. A total of 3 mL of fetal blood, obtained from the umbilical cord (preferably) or by cardiac puncture, is placed into a sterile, heparinized tube for cytogenetic studies. If blood cannot be obtained, the American College of Obstetricians and Gynecologists (2009) recommends at least one of the following samples: (1) a placental block about 1×1 cm taken below the

cord insertion site in the unfixed specimen; (2) umbilical cord segment about 1.5 cm long; or (3) internal fetal tissue specimen such as costochondral junction or patella (skin is no longer recommended). Tissue is washed with sterile saline prior to placement in lactated Ringer solution or sterile cytogenetic medium. Placement in formalin or alcohol kills remaining viable cells and prevents cytogenetic analysis.

A full karyotype may not be possible in cases with prolonged fetal death. Still, Korteweg and co-workers (2008) reported that in a third of macerated fetuses, they successfully performed cytogenetic analysis. Fluorescence in situ hybridization might be used to exclude numerical abnormalities or to look for certain common deletions such as that causing DiGeorge syndrome. Maternal blood should be obtained for Kleihauer-Betke staining, for antiphospholipid antibodies and lupus anticoagulant testing if indicated, and for serum glucose measurement to exclude overt diabetes.

Autopsy

Patients should be offered and encouraged to allow a full autopsy, but valuable information also can be obtained from limited studies. A gross external examination, combined with photography, radiography, MR imaging, bacterial cultures, and selective use of chromosomal and histopathological studies often can aid in determining the cause of death (Reddy, 2007; Silver, 2007).

TABLE 29-9. Protocol for Examination of Stillborns

Infant Description
  Malformations
  Skin staining
  Degree of maceration
  Color—pale, plethoric
Umbilical Cord
  Prolapse
  Entanglement—neck, arms, legs
  Hematomas or strictures
  Number of vessels
  Length
  Wharton jelly—normal, absent
Amnionic Fluid
  Color—meconium, blood
  Consistency
  Volume
Placenta
  Weight
  Staining—meconium
  Adherent clots
  Structural abnormalities—circumvallate or accessory lobes, velamentous insertion
  Edema—hydropic changes
Membranes
  Stained—meconium, cloudy
  Thickening

From Cunningham and Hollier (1997).

A complete autopsy is much more likely to yield valuable information. An analysis of 400 consecutive fetal deaths in Wales found that autopsy altered the presumed cause of death in 13 percent and provided new information in another 26 percent (Cartlidge and Stewart, 1995b). Studies show that autopsy results changed the recurrence risk estimates and parental counseling in 25 to 50 percent of cases (Faye-Petersen and colleagues, 1999; Silver, 2007).

In many centers, maternal records and autopsy findings are reviewed on a monthly basis by a stillbirth committee composed of maternal-fetal medicine specialists, neonatologists, clinical geneticists, and perinatal pathologists. If possible, the cause of death is assigned based on available evidence. Most importantly, parents should then be contacted and offered counseling regarding the cause of death, the recurrence risk if any, and strategies to avoid recurrence in future pregnancies.

Psychological Aspects

Fetal death is psychologically traumatic for the woman and her family. Further stress results from an interval of more than 24 hours between the diagnosis of fetal death and the induction of labor, not seeing her infant for as long as she desires, and having no tokens of remembrance (Radestad and colleagues, 1996). The woman experiencing a stillbirth or even an early miscarriage is at increased risk for postpartum depression and should be closely monitored (see Chap. 55, p. 1176).

Pregnancy After Previous Stillbirth

In a population-based Missouri study, Sharma and associates (2006) reported a stillbirth rate of 22.7 per 1000 in women with a prior fetal death. That said, there are very few conditions associated with recurrent stillbirth. According to Silver (2007), losses associated with placental insufficiency and preterm labor are more likely to recur, whereas those due to infection and multifetal pregnancy are less likely to do so. In fact, Surkan and co-workers (2004) found that delivery of a growth-restricted *liveborn* term infant was associated with a twofold increased risk of a subsequent stillbirth. With a growth-restricted preterm *liveborn*, this risk was increased fivefold. According to the American College of Obstetricians and Gynecologists (2009) the low-risk woman who has had an unexplained stillborn has a pregnancy-risk increased about tenfold. Because most occur earlier in gestation, the risk of a stillborn after 37 weeks is only 1.8 per 1000.

Other than hereditary disorders, only maternal conditions such as diabetes, chronic hypertension, or some thrombophilias increase the risk of recurrence. Losses that occur early in pregnancy are associated with a higher risk. Goldenberg and colleagues (1993) studied 95 women with a pregnancy loss at 13 to 24 weeks and found that in their next pregnancy, almost 40 percent delivered preterm, 5 percent had a stillbirth, and 6 percent had a neonatal death.

Prenatal Evaluation

Knowledge of the cause of fetal death results in a more precise calculation of individual recurrence risk and in many cases, allows a management plan to be made. For example, a cord accident would not be expected to recur. In contrast, aneuploidy generally has a 1-percent recurrence risk, and familial DiGeorge syndrome has a 50-percent recurrence. The latter two could be detected in subsequent pregnancies by chorionic villous sampling or amniocentesis. As discussed, infectious causes are unlikely to recur.

Maternal medical disorders associated with prior stillbirth are often easily identified. In some cases, intervention either preconceptionally or early in pregnancy improves outcome in subsequent pregnancies (see Chap. 7, p. 174). One example is tight preconceptional glucose control in diabetic women. Placental abruption, which has a 10-percent recurrence, often is associated with chronic hypertension that could possibly be reduced with more stringent blood pressure control or early delivery (Pritchard and colleagues, 1991). Finally, there is some evidence that recurrent fetal loss due to antiphospholipid antibodies can be decreased with treatment (see Chap. 54, p. 1151). This is more likely if fetal death was associated with placental insufficiency, growth restriction, or placental infarction (Reddy and colleagues, 2007).

Management of Subsequent Pregnancy

Few studies address management of the woman who has suffered a prior fetal death. The few modifiable risk factors such as hypertension and diabetes control are addressed. Some first- and second-trimester screening schemes may be enlightening. According to Reddy (2007), because almost half of fetal deaths are associated with growth restriction, fetal sonographic anatomical assessment at midpregnancy is followed by serial growth studies beginning at 28 weeks.

Weeks and colleagues (1995) evaluated fetal biophysical testing in 300 women whose only indication was prior stillbirth. There was only one recurrent stillbirth, and only three fetuses had abnormal testing results before 32 weeks. There was no relationship between the gestational age of the previous stillborn and the incidence or timing of abnormal test results or fetal jeopardy in the subsequent pregnancy. They concluded that antepartum surveillance should begin at 32 weeks or later in the otherwise healthy woman with a history of stillbirth. This recommendation is supported by the American College of Obstetricians and Gynecologists (2009) with the caveat that it increases the iatrogenic preterm delivery rate.

INJURIES OF THE FETUS AND NEWBORN

There are a number of birth injuries that can potentially complicate all types of deliveries. Some are more likely associated with "traumatic" delivery by forceps or vacuum, and others follow otherwise uncomplicated spontaneous delivery. Many are now discussed, and the remainder are described elsewhere in connection with specific obstetrical complications that lead to or contribute to the injury.

Incidence and Types of Injuries

There are few population studies available. In one from Nova Scotia from 1988 through 2001 that included 119,432 singleton, nonanomalous, vertex-presenting fetuses, the overall risk of trauma was 2 percent (Baskett and associates, 2007). But only

TABLE 29-10. Incidence of Major and Minor Trauma at Delivery—Nova Scotia, 1988–2001

Type of Delivery (Rate of Trauma)	Number	Trauma at Delivery	
		Major[a]	Minor[b]
Spontaneous (14 per 1000)	88,324	1:835	1:77
Assisted			
Vacuum (71 per 1000)	3175	1:265	1:15
Forceps (58 per 1000)	10,478	1:194	1:19
Failed assisted			
Vacuum (105 per 1000)	609	1:120	1:10
Forceps (56 per 1000)	714	1:143	1:20
Cesarean (8.6 per 1000)	16,132	1:3226	1:120
Labor (12 per 1000)	10,731	1:2682	1:84
No labor (1.2 per 1000)	5401	1:5401	1:900
All (19.5 per 1000)	119,432	1:639 (1.6 per 1000)	1:56 (18 per 1000)

[a]Major trauma = depressed skull fracture, intracranial hemorrhage, brachial plexopathy, or combination.
[b]Minor trauma = linear skull fracture, other fractures, facial palsy, cephalohematoma, or combination.
Data from Baskett and co-workers (2007).

0.16 percent of this was major trauma. As shown in Table 29-10, major trauma was most frequently associated with failed instrumented delivery, and the lowest incidence was with cesarean delivery without labor. Minor traumatic injuries followed a comparable pattern. Simonson and co-workers (2007) provided similar observations for 913 vacuum-assisted deliveries. Alexander and colleagues (2006), in the NICHD Maternal-Fetal Medicine Units Network study of 37,110 cesarean deliveries, reported 400 injuries for a 1.1-percent fetal injury rate. Most of these—260 or 0.7 percent—were skin lacerations, and there also were 88 cephalohematomas, 11 clavicular fractures, 11 facial nerve palsies, nine brachial plexopathies, and six skull fractures.

Head Injury

The fetus or infant can sustain a number of traumatic head injuries during labor or at delivery. They can be external and obvious or intracranial and even covert. Some are spontaneous, whereas others are associated with instrumented deliveries. These were reviewed recently by Doumouchtsis and Arulkumaran (2008).

Spontaneous Intracranial Hemorrhage

Fetal or neonatal intracranial hemorrhage can occur at any of several sites (Table 29-11). Isolated intraventricular hemorrhage into the germinal matrix, without associated subarach-

TABLE 29-11. Major Types of Intracranial Hemorrhage in the Newborn

Type	Gestational Age	Incidence and Severity	Cause(s) and Pathogenesis
Subdural	Term > preterm	Uncommon, Serious	Venous tears, Trauma common
Subarachnoid	Preterm > term	Common, Benign	Trauma—term, "Hypoxia"—preterm
Intracerebellar	Preterm > term	Uncommon, Serious	Multifactorial
Intraventricular	Preterm	Common, Serious	Germinal matrix, Multifactorial
Miscellaneous	Term > preterm	Uncommon, Variable	Trauma, hemorrhagic infarction, coagulopathy, vascular defect, ECMO

ECMO = extracorporeal membrane oxygenation.
Data from Volpe (1995).

noid or subdural bleeding, is the most common type of intracranial hemorrhage. As discussed on page 607, it usually occurs spontaneously as the result of immaturity and generally does not result from traumatic delivery or obstetrical factors (Hayden and colleagues, 1985). Infants weighing less than 1500 g are most susceptible.

Spontaneous intracranial hemorrhage also has been documented in healthy term neonates (Huang and Robertson, 2004). In a prospective study, Whitby and associates (2004) used MR imaging in such infants and found that 6 percent of those delivered spontaneously and 28 percent of those delivered by forceps had a subdural hemorrhage. None of these infants had clinical findings, and hematomas resolved in all by 4 weeks.

The fetal head has considerable plasticity and may undergo appreciable molding during passage through the birth canal. The dimensions of the head actually change during the second stage, with lengthening of the occipitofrontal diameter of the skull. Rarely, severe molding can result in tearing of the bridging veins from the cerebral cortex to the sagittal sinus or in rupture of the internal cerebral veins, of the vein of Galen at its junctions with the straight sinus, or of the tentorium itself. Compression of the skull can stretch the tentorium cerebelli and can tear the vein of Galen or its tributaries. As a result, intracranial hemorrhage and/or subdural subarachnoid hemorrhage may occur even after an apparently uneventful vaginal delivery. With vacuum-assisted deliveries, Simonson and colleagues (2007) reported an incidence of 0.87 percent of asymptomatic intracranial hemorrhage. Subgaleal hemorrhages associated with instrumented delivery can have a poor prognosis (Chang and co-workers, 2007).

Traumatic Intraventricular Hemorrhage

Birth trauma is not a common cause of intracranial hemorrhage. The elimination of difficult forceps operations and appropriate management of breech delivery have contributed significantly to a reduction in the incidence of all birth injuries. For example, in more than 190,000 singleton infants greater than 2500 g born in the United Kingdom in 1994 and 1995,

O'Mahony and colleagues (2005) reported an incidence of death from mechanical birth injury to be 3.1 per 100,000 births. As detailed in Chapter 23 (p. 520), appropriate use of forceps or vacuum delivery does not lead to increased intracranial hemorrhage or other neonatal injury (American College of Obstetricians and Gynecologists, 2000).

Infants suffering intracranial hemorrhage from mechanical injury, such as subdural hemorrhage from tentorial tears or massive infratentorial hemorrhage, have neurological abnormalities from the time of birth (Volpe, 1995). Severely affected infants have stupor or coma, nuchal rigidity, and opisthotonus that worsen over minutes to hours. Some infants who are born depressed appear to improve until approximately 12 hours of age, but then drowsiness, apathy, feeble cry, pallor, failure to nurse, dyspnea, cyanosis, vomiting, and convulsions become evident.

Subarachnoid hemorrhage is usually minor with no symptoms, but seizures with an interictal period may manifest. In some infants, there is catastrophic deterioration. Sonography, CT, or MR imaging of the head are useful for diagnosis and also have contributed appreciably to an understanding of the etiology and frequency of some forms of intracranial hemorrhage (Perlman and Cunningham, 1993).

Cephalohematoma

In the study from Nova Scotia, cephalohematomas were identified in 1.6 percent of all births (Baskett and co-workers, 2007). They are usually caused by injury to the periosteum of the skull during labor and delivery and rarely develop in the absence of birth trauma. For example, Simonson and colleagues (2007) reported an 11-percent incidence in 913 term infants successfully delivered by vacuum extraction. In the network study cited above of cesarean delivery outcomes, Alexander and associates (2006) found a 0.3-percent incidence of cephalohematoma. The hemorrhage may develop over one or both parietal bones, and palpable edges can be appreciated as the blood reaches the limits of the periosteum (Fig. 29-12).

A cephalohematoma may not be apparent until hours after delivery, when bleeding sufficient to raise the periosteum has occurred. It often grows larger, disappearing only after weeks or

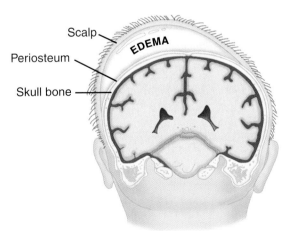
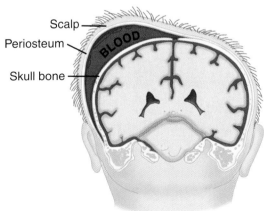

FIGURE 29-12 Difference between a large caput succedaneum (*left*) and cephalohematoma (*right*). In a caput succedaneum, the effusion overlies the periosteum and consists of edema fluid. In a cephalohematoma, it lies under the periosteum and consists of blood.

even months. The infant may become anemic. In contrast, caput succedaneum, also shown in Figure 29-12, consists of a focal swelling of the scalp from edema that overlies the periosteum. Swelling from caput succedaneum is maximal at birth, rapidly grows smaller, and usually disappears within hours or a few days. Occasionally, it becomes infected and an abscess may form (Kersten and co-workers, 2008).

Nerve Injuries

Spinal Injury

Overstretching of the spinal cord and associated hemorrhage may follow excessive traction during delivery, and there may be actual fracture or dislocation of the vertebrae. Menticoglou and associates (1995) described 15 neonates with this type of high cervical spinal cord injury and found that all of the injuries were associated with forceps rotations during delivery. Spinal cord injury also can occur during breech delivery.

Brachial Plexopathy

These injuries are relatively common and are identified between 1 in 500 to 1 in 1000 term births (Baskett and associates, 2007; Joyner and colleagues, 2006). Three types of brachial plexus damage have been described. Damage to the upper plexus is called *Erb* or *Duchenne paralysis* and involves C5 and C6 and occasionally C7. Injury leads to paralysis of the deltoid and infraspinatus muscles and the flexor muscles of the forearm. The affected arm is held straight and internally rotated, the elbow is extended, and the wrist and fingers flexed. Function of the fingers usually is retained. Because lateral head traction is frequently employed to effect delivery of the shoulders in normal vertex presentations, Erb paralysis can follow even deliveries that do not appear difficult.

Damage to the lower plexus—C8 and T1—results in *Klumpke paralysis*, in which the hand is flaccid. Total involvement of all brachial plexus nerve roots results in flaccidity of both arm and hand. With this kind of severe damage, there may also be *Horner syndrome* on the affected side—ptosis and pupillary meiosis resulting from interruption of nerve fibers in the cervical sympathetic chain.

With brachial plexus injury, increasing birthweight and breech delivery are significant risk factors. In a study of 130 infants with brachial plexus injuries, Ubachs and colleagues (1995) found that cases involving C5 to C6 nerve roots were frequently associated with breech delivery. More extensive damage involving C5 to C7 or C5 to T1 often followed difficult cephalic deliveries. Unfortunately, and as discussed in Chapter 20 (p. 481), shoulder dystocia cannot be predicted reliably. Thus, it is fortunate that most nerve injuries resolve with conservative therapy. Surgical repair is reserved for persistent cases due to nerve root avulsion (Malessy and Pondaag, 2009).

Facial Paralysis

Pressure on the facial nerve as it emerges from the stylomastoid foramen can cause damage resulting in facial paralysis. The incidence ranges from less than 1 to 7.5 per 1000 term births and is likely influenced by the vigor with which the diagnosis is sought (Levine and colleagues, 1984; White and associates, 1996). Facial paralysis may be apparent at delivery or may develop shortly after birth (Fig. 29-13). It most commonly is associated with normal spontaneous or cesarean delivery (Levine and co-workers, 1984). Only approximately 20 percent are associated with forceps deliveries (White and associates, 1996). In these deliveries, facial nerve damage can be caused by pressure exerted by the posterior blade when forceps have been placed obliquely on the fetal head. In these cases, forceps marks

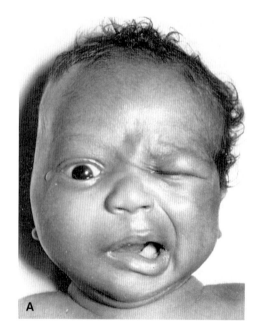
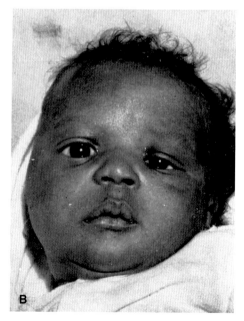

FIGURE 29-13 A. Paralysis of the right side of the face 15 minutes after forceps delivery. The grimace is limited to the left face because the right side is flaccid. **B.** Same infant 24 hours later. Recovery was complete in another 24 hours.

indicate the cause of injury. Spontaneous recovery within a few days is the rule. Injuries to the sixth cranial nerve, with resultant lateral rectus ocular muscle paralysis, following operative vaginal delivery have also been reported (Galbraith, 1994).

Skeletal and Muscle Injuries

Fractures

Clavicular fractures are common, unpredictable, and unavoidable complications of normal birth. Their incidence is 3 to 18 per 1000 live births (Roberts and associates, 1995; Turpenny and Nimmo, 1993). In a cohort of newborns with such fractures, Chez and colleagues (1994) were unable to identify a specific factor that could be changed to avoid these fractures.

Humeral fractures are not common. Difficulty encountered in the delivery of the shoulders in cephalic deliveries and of extended arms in breech deliveries often produces such fractures. Up to 70 percent of cases, however, follow uneventful delivery (Turpenny and Nimmo, 1993). Humeral fractures are often of the greenstick type, although complete fracture with overriding bones may occur. Palpation of the clavicles and long bones should be performed on all newborns when a fracture is suspected. Crepitation or unusual irregularity should prompt radiographic examination.

Femoral fractures are relatively rare and usually associated with breech delivery.

Mandibular fractures have been reported and were recently reviewed by Vasconcelos and associates (2009). *Skull fracture* was identified in 3.7 per 100,000 births in nearly 2 million deliveries in two areas of France between 1990 and 2000 (Dupuis and co-workers, 2005). Almost 75 percent were associated with instrumented deliveries, and the others with spontaneous or cesarean delivery. In the radiograph shown in Figure 29-14, a focal but markedly depressed skull fracture is apparent. Labor was characterized by vigorous contractions, full dilatation of the cervix, and arrest of descent of the head, which was tightly wedged in the pelvis. The fracture likely resulted from compression of the skull against the sacral promontory, from lifting hand pressure by the surgeon, or from upward hand pressure by an assistant who helped to push the head out of the birth canal at cesarean delivery. Surgical decompression of the fracture was successful.

Muscular Injuries

The sternocleidomastoid muscle may be injured, particularly during breech delivery. There may be a tear of the muscle or the fascial sheath, leading to a hematoma and gradual cicatricial contraction. As the neck lengthens in the process of normal growth, the head is gradually turned toward the side of the injury—a condition known as *torticollis*. The damaged muscle is less elastic and does not elongate at the same rate as its normal contralateral counterpart. Roemer (1954) reported that 27 of 44 infants showing this deformity had been delivered by breech or internal podalic version. He postulated that lateral hyperextension sufficient to rupture the sternocleidomastoid may occur as the aftercoming head passes over the sacral promontory.

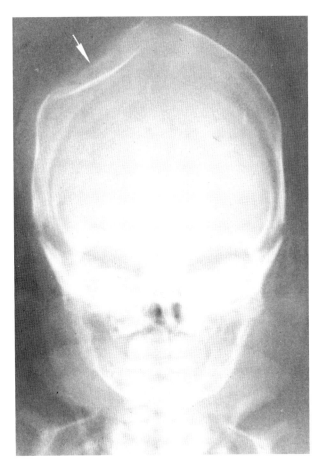

FIGURE 29-14 Depressed skull fracture (*arrow*) evident immediately after cesarean delivery. Labor had progressed, and the head was deep in the pelvis. Dislodgment of the head from the birth canal was performed by an assistant using manual pressure upward through the vagina.

Congenital Injuries

Amnionic Band Syndrome

A free strip of amnion can form a focal ring around an extremity or digit, eventually producing enough constriction to cause damage or even amputation of the encircled structure. Occasionally, the amputated part may be found within the uterus. The genesis of such bands is debated. Streeter (1930) and others proposed that a localized failure of germ plasm or an inherent developmental abnormality of the involved structures is responsible for the abnormalities. Torpin (1968) and others contend that the lesions are the consequence of early rupture of the amnion. Soldado and colleagues (2006) have developed an animal model to study this further. These lesions must be differentiated from limb-reduction defects associated with chorionic villus sampling done before 9 weeks as discussed in Chapter 13 (p. 300).

Congenital Postural Deformities

An otherwise normal fetal structure may be deformed by mechanical factors arising from chronically low volumes of amnionic fluid, by restriction of movement imposed by the small size and inappropriate shape of an abnormal uterine cavity, or by the presence of additional fetuses. Such mechanical deformations include talipes equinovarus, that is, clubfoot; scoliosis; and hip dislocation (Miller and co-workers, 1981). Talipes equinovarus and other positional foot abnormalities are associated with membrane rupture from early amniocentesis between 11 and 13 weeks (see Chap. 13, p. 299). Finally, hypoplastic lungs also can result from oligohydramnios (see Chap. 21, p. 496).

REFERENCES

Aagaard-Tillery KM, Holmgren C, Lacoursiere DY, et al: Factors associated with nonanomalous stillbirths: The Utah Stillbirth Database 1992-2002. Am J Obstet Gynecol 194:849, 2006

Achiron R, Pinchas OH, Reichman B, et al: Fetal intracranial haemorrhage: Clinical significance of in-utero ultrasonic diagnosis. Br J Obstet Gynaecol 100:995, 1993

Adeniji AO, Mabayoje VO, Raji AA, et al: Feto-maternal haemorrhage in parturients: Incidence and its determinants. J Obstet Gynaecol 28:60, 2008

Alessandri LM, Stanley FJ, Garner JB, et al: A case-control study of unexplained antepartum stillbirths. Br J Obstet Gynaecol 99:711, 1992

Alexander JM, Leveno KJ, Hauth J, et al: Fetal injury associated with cesarean delivery. Obstet Gynecol 108:885, 2006

Allan LD, Crawford DC, Sheridan R, et al: Aetiology of non-immune hydrops: The value of echocardiography. Br J Obstet Gynaecol 93:223, 1986

Allan WC, Vohr B, Makuch RW, et al: Antecedents of cerebral palsy in a multicenter trial on indomethacin for intraventricular hemorrhage. Arch Pediatr Adolesc Med 151:580, 1997

Alper CA: Blood groups I. Physiology. In Beck WS (ed): Hematology. Cambridge, Mass, MIT Press, 1977, p 299

Althaus J, Weir EG, Askin F, et al: Chronic villitis in untreated neonatal alloimmune thrombocytopenia: An etiology for severe early intrauterine growth restriction and the effect of intravenous immunoglobulin therapy. Am J Obstet Gynecol 193:1100, 2005

American Academy of Pediatrics. Postnatal corticosteroids to treat or prevent chronic lung disease in preterm infants. Pediatrics 109:330, 2002

American Academy of Pediatrics and American College of Obstetricians and Gynecologists: Guidelines for Perinatal Care, 6th Edition. 2007, p 210

American College of Obstetricians and Gynecologists: Fetal heart rate patterns: Monitoring, interpretation, and management. Technical Bulletin No. 207, July 1995

American College of Obstetricians and Gynecologists: Genetic evaluation of stillbirths and neonatal deaths. Committee Opinion No. 178, November 1996

American College of Obstetricians and Gynecologists: Inappropriate use of the terms fetal distress and birth asphyxia. Committee Opinion No. 197, February 1998

American College of Obstetricians and Gynecologists: Antepartum fetal surveillance. Practice Bulletin No. 9, October 1999a

American College of Obstetricians and Gynecologists: Prevention of RhD alloimmunization. Clinical Management Guidelines No. 4, May 1999b

American College of Obstetricians and Gynecologists: Operative vaginal delivery. Practice Bulletin No. 17, June 2000

American College of Obstetricians and Gynecologists: Inappropriate use of the terms fetal distress and birth asphyxia. Committee Opinion No. 303, October 2004

American College of Obstetricians and Gynecologists: Intrapartum fetal heart rate monitoring. Practice Bulletin No. 70, December 2005

American College of Obstetricians and Gynecologists: Amnioinfusion does not prevent meconium aspiration syndrome. Committee Opinion No. 346, 2006a

American College of Obstetricians and Gynecologists: Management of alloimmunization. Practice Bulletin No. 75, August 2006b

American College of Obstetricians and Gynecologists: Umbilical cord blood gas and acid-base analysis. Committee Opinion No. 348, November 2006c

American College of Obstetricians and Gynecologists: Management of delivery of a newborn with meconium-stained amnionic fluid. Committee Opinion No. 379, September 2007

American College of Obstetricians and Gynecologists: Fetal lung maturity. Practice Bulletin No. 97, September 2008a

American College of Obstetricians and Gynecologists: Antenatal corticosteroid therapy for fetal maturation. Committee Opinion No. 402, March 2008b

American College of Obstetricians and Gynecologists: Management of stillbirth. Practice Bulletin No.102, March 2009

American College of Obstetricians and Gynecologists and American Academy of Pediatrics: Neonatal encephalopathy and cerebral palsy. Defining the pathogenesis and pathophysiology. January 2003

American Heart Association and American Academy of Pediatrics. 2005 American Heart Association Guidelines for Cardiopulmonary Resuscitation and Emergency Cardiovascular Care of Pediatric and Neonatal Patients: Neonatal Resuscitation guidelines. Pediatrics 117:e1029, 2006

Anderson GD, Bada HS, Shaver DC, et al: The effect of cesarean section on intraventricular hemorrhage in the preterm infant. Am J Obstet Gynecol 166:1091, 1992

Andrews WW, Cliver SP, Biasini F, et al: Early preterm birth: Association between in utero exposure to acute inflammation and severe neurodevelopmental disability at 6 years of age. Am J Obstet Gynecol 198:466, 2008

Arntfield S, Ainsworth P, Mackay J, et al: Prenatal diagnosis of fetal RHD type using free fetal DNA (FFDNA) in maternal plasma: A pilot study. Am J Obstet Gynecol 201:43.e1, 2009

August P, Lindheimer MD: Chronic hypertension and pregnancy. In Lindheimer MD, Roberts JM, Cunningham FG (eds): Chesley's Hypertensive Disorders in Pregnancy. Elsevier, Inc., New York, In press, 2009

Bailis A, Maleki Z, Askin F, et al: Histopathological placental features associated with development of periventricular leukomalacia in preterm infants. Am J Obstet Gynecol, In press, 2009

Ballard RA, Truog WE, Cnaan A, et al: Inhaled nitric oxide in preterm infants undergoing mechanical ventilation. N Engl J Med 355:343, 2006

Baraldi E, Filippone M: Chronic lung disease after premature birth. N Engl J Med 357:1946, 2007

Barbu D, Mert I, Kruger M, et al: Evidence of fetal central nervous system injury in isolated congenital heart defects: microcephaly at birth. Am J Obstet Gynecol 201:43.e1, 2009

Barss VA, Frigoletto FD, Konugres A: The cost of irregular antibody screening. Am J Obstet Gynecol 159:428, 1988

Baskett TF, Allen VM, O'Connell CM, et al: Fetal trauma in term pregnancy. Am J Obstet Gynecol 197:499.e1, 2007

Bateman BT, Simpson LL: Higher rate of stillbirth at the extremes of reproductive age: A large nationwide sample of deliveries in the United States. Am J Obstet Gynecol 194:840, 2006

Bax M, Tydeman C, Flodmark O: Clinical and MRI correlates of cerebral palsy: The European cerebral palsy study. JAMA 296:1602, 2006

Bellini C, Hennekam RC, Fulcheri E, et al: Etiology of nonimmune hydrops fetalis: A systematic review. Am J Med Genet A 149A(5):844, 2009

Berkowitz RL, Bussel JB, McFarland JG: Alloimmune thrombocytopenia: State of the art 2006. Am J Obstet Gynecol 195:907, 2006a

Berkowitz RL, Kolb EA, McFarland JG, et al: Parallel randomized trials of risk-based therapy for fetal alloimmune thrombocytopenia. Obstet Gynecol 107:91, 2006b

Bhasin TK, Brocksen S, Avchen RN, et al: Prevalence of four developmental disabilities among children aged 8 years—Metropolitan Atlanta developmental disabilities surveillance program, 1996 and 2000. MMWR 55:22, 2006

Bianchi DW, Avent ND, Costa JM, et al: Noninvasive prenatal diagnosis of fetal rhesus D. Obstet Gynecol 106:841, 2005

Blackmon LR, Stark AR: American Academy of Pediatrics Committee on Fetus and Newborn. Hypothermia: A neuroprotective therapy for neonatal hypoxic-ischemic encephalopathy. Pediatrics 117:942, 2006

Blakely ML, Tyson JE, Lally KP, et al: Laparotomy versus peritoneal drainage for necrotizing enterocolitis or isolated intestinal perforation in extremely low birth weight infants: Outcomes through 18 months adjusted age. Pediatrics 117:e680, 2006

Bloom S, Ramin S, Neyman S, et al: Meconium stained amniotic fluid: Is it associated with elevated erythropoietin levels? Am J Obstet Gynecol 174:360, 1996

Boucher M, Marquette GP, Varin J, et al: Fetomaternal hemorrhage during external cephalic version. Obstet Gynecol 112:79, 2008

Bowell PJ, Allen DL, Entwistle CC: Blood group antibody screening tests during pregnancy. Br J Obstet Gynaecol 93:1038, 1986

Bowman JM: Controversies in Rh prophylaxis: Who needs Rh immune globulin and when should it be given? Am J Obstet Gynecol 151:289, 1985

Bowman JM, Chown B, Lewis M, et al: Rh isoimmunization, Manitoba, 1963–1975. Can Med Assoc J 116:282, 1977

Bowman JM, Pollock JM: Antenatal Rh prophylaxis: 28 week gestation service program. Can Med Assoc J 118:622, 1978

Bowman JM, Pollock JM, Manning FA, et al: Maternal Kell blood group alloimmunization. Obstet Gynecol 79:239, 1992a

Bowman JM, Pollock JM, Manning FA, et al: Severe anti-C hemolytic disease of the newborn. Am J Obstet Gynecol 166:1239, 1992b

Brucato A, Jonzon A, Friedman D, et al: Proposal for a new definition of a congenital complete atrioventricular block. Lupus 12:427, 2003

Buhi WC, Spellacy WN: Effects of blood or meconium on the determination of the amniotic fluid lecithin/sphingomyelin ratio. Am J Obstet Gynecol 121:321, 1975

Bukowski R, Malone FD, Porter TF, et al: Fetal macrosomia increases risk of stillbirth. Am J Obstet Gynecol, In press, 2009

Burke BL, Robbins JM, Bird TM, et al: Trends in hospitalizations for neonatal jaundice and kernicterus in the United States, 1988–2005. Pediatrics 123(2):524, 2009

Bush MC, Gaddipati S, Berkowitz R: Noninvasive management of Rh partial null (D–) to supplement traditional management of Rh isoimmunization. Obstet Gynaecol 102:1145, 2003

Bussel JB, Primiani A: Fetal and neonatal alloimmune thrombocytopenia: Progress and ongoing debates. Blood Rev 22:33, 2008

Byrne DL, Gau G: In utero meconium aspiration: An unpreventable cause of neonatal death. Br J Obstet Gynecol 94:813, 1987

Caine ME, Mueller-Heubach E: Kell sensitization in pregnancy. Am J Obstet Gynecol 154:85, 1986

Cannon M, Pierce R, Taber EB, et al: Fatal hydrops fetalis caused by anti-D in a mother with partial D. Obstet Gynecol 102:1143, 2003

Cartlidge PHT, Dawson AT, Stewart JH, et al: Value and quality of perinatal and infant postmortem examination: Cohort analysis of 400 consecutive deaths. BMJ 310:155, 1995a

Cartlidge PHT, Stewart JH: Effect of changing the stillbirth definition on evaluation of perinatal mortality rates. Lancet 346:486, 1995b

Casey BM, McIntire DD, Leveno KJ: The continuing value of the Apgar score for the assessment of newborn infants. N Engl J Med 344:467, 2001

Castillo RA, Devoe LD, Hadi HA, et al: Nonimmune hydrops fetalis: Clinical experience and factors related to a poor outcome. Am J Obstet Gynecol 155:812, 1986

Cham M, Sundby J, Vangen S: Fetal outcome in severe maternal morbidity: Too many stillbirths. Acta Obstet Gynecol Scand 88(3):343, 2009

Chang HY, Peng CC, Kao HA, et al: Neonatal subgaleal hemorrhage: Clinical presentation, treatment, and predictors of poor prognosis. Pediatr Int 49:903, 2007

Chez RA, Carlan S, Greenberg SL, et al: Fractured clavicle is an unavoidable event. Am J Obstet Gynecol 174:797, 1994

Chiswick M, Gladman G, Sinha S, et al: Vitamin E supplementation and periventricular hemorrhage in the newborn. Am J Clin Nutr 53:370S, 1991

Choavaratana R, Uer-Areewong S, Makanantakocol S: Fetomaternal transfusion in normal pregnancy and during delivery. J Med Assoc Thai 80:96, 1997

Chock VY, Van Meurs KP, Hintz SR, et al: Inhaled nitric oxide for preterm premature rupture of membranes, oligohydramnios, and pulmonary hypoplasia. Am J Perinatol 26(4):317, 2009

Chu SY, Kim SY, Lau J, et al: Maternal obesity and risk of stillbirth: A meta-analysis. Am J Obstet Gynecol 197(3):223, 2007

Clark SL, Hankins GD: Temporal and demographic trends in cerebral palsy—fact and fiction. Am J Obstet Gynecol 188:628, 2003

Clements JA, Platzker ACG, Tierney DF, et al: Assessment of the risk of respiratory distress syndrome by a rapid test for surfactant in amniotic fluid. N Engl J Med 286:1077, 1972

Copper RL, Goldenberg RL, DuBard MB, et al: Risk factors for fetal death in white, black, and Hispanic women. Obstet Gynecol 94:490, 1994

Cordes I, Roland EH, Lupton BA, et al: Early prediction of the development of microcephaly after hypoxic ischemic encephalopathy in the full-term newborn. Pediatrics 93:703, 1994

Crowther CA, Doyle LW, Haslam RR, et al: Outcomes at 2 years of age after repeat doses of antenatal corticosteroids. N Engl J Med 357:1179, 2007

Crowther CA, Hiller JE, Doyle LW, et al: Effect of magnesium sulfate given for neuroprotection before preterm birth. A randomized controlled trial. JAMA 290:2669, 2003

Cuneo B, Strasburger J, Imran N, et al: SSA/SSB antibody mediated fetal cardiac disease with normal AV conduction. Am J Obstet Gynecol, In press, 2009

Cunningham FG, Hollier LM: Fetal death. In: Williams Obstetrics, 20th ed (Suppl 4). Norwalk, Conn, Appleton & Lange, August/September 1997

Czyrko C, Steigman C, Turley DL, et al: The role of reperfusion injury in occlusive intestinal ischemia of the neonate: Malonaldehyde-derived fluorescent products and correlation of histology. J Surg Res 51:1, 1991

Dalziel SR, Lim VK, Lambert A, et al: Antenatal exposure to betamethasone: Psychological functioning and health related quality of life 31 years after inclusion in randomized controlled trial. BMJ 331(7518): 665, 2005a

Dalziel SR, Walker NK, Parag V, et al: Cardiovascular risk factors after antenatal exposure to betamethasone: 30-year follow-up of a randomized controlled trial. Lancet 365:1856, 2005b

Dammann O, Leviton A: Maternal intrauterine infection, cytokines, and brain damage in the preterm newborn. Pediatr Res 42:1, 1997

Davis RO, Phillips JB III, Harris BA Jr, et al: Fatal meconium aspiration syndrome occurring despite airway management considered appropriate. Am J Obstet Gynecol 141:731, 1985

Davoren A, Curtis BR, Aster RH, et al: Human platelet antigen-specific alloantibodies implicated in 1162 cases of neonatal alloimmune thrombocytopenia. Transfusion 44:1220, 2004

de Almida V, Bowman JM: Massive fetomaternal hemorrhage: Manitoba experience. Obstet Gynecol 83:323, 1994

DeVries LS, Dubowitz V, Lary S, et al: Predictive value of cranial ultrasound in the newborn baby: A reappraisal. Lancet 2:137, 1985

DeVries LS, Eken P, Groenendaal F, et al: Correlation between the degree of periventricular leukomalacia diagnosed using cranial ultrasound and MRI later in infancy in children with cerebral palsy. Neuropediatrics 24:263, 1993

Dijxhoorn MJ, Visser GHA, Fidler VJ, et al: Apgar score, meconium and acidemia at birth in relation to neonatal neurological morbidity in term infants. Br J Obstet Gynaecol 86:217, 1986

Dooley SL, Pesavento DJ, Depp R, et al: Meconium below the vocal cords at delivery: Correlation with intrapartum events. Am J Obstet Gynecol 153:767, 1985

Doumouchtsis SK, Arulkumaran S: Head trauma after instrumental births. Clin Perinatol 35:69, 2008

Doyle LW, Crowther CA, Middleton P, et al: Magnesium sulphate for women at risk of preterm birth for neuroprotection of the fetus. Cochrane Database Syst Rev 1:CD004661, 2009

Duff P, Barth WH, Post MD: Case 4-2009: A 39-year-old pregnant woman with fever after a trip to Africa. N Engl J Med 360:508, 2009

Dupuis O, Silveira R, Dupont C, et al: Comparison of "instrument-associated" and "spontaneous" obstetric depressed skull fractures in a cohort of 68 neonates. Am J Obstet Gynecol 192:165, 2005

Duthie SJ, Walkinshaw SA: Parvovirus associated fetal hydrops: Reversal of pregnancy induced proteinuric hypertension by in utero fetal transfusion. Br J Obstet Gynaecol 102:1011, 1995

Eggert LD, Wiedmeier SE, Wilson J, et al: The effect of instituting a prehospital-discharge newborn bilirubin screening program in an 18-hospital health system. Pediatrics 117:e855, 2006

Eller AG, Branch DW, Byrne JL: Stillbirth at term. Obstet Gynecol 108(2):442, 2006

Eriksen N, Tey A, Prieto J, et al: Fetal lung maturity in diabetic patients using the TDx FLM assay. Am J Obstet Gynecol 174:348, 1996

Falchi M, Palmas G, Pisano T, et al: Incidence of epilepsy in extremely low-birthweight infants (<1,000 g): A population study of central and southern Sardinia. Epilepsia 1:37, 2009

Fanaroff AA, Stoll BJ, Wright LL, et al: Trends in neonatal morbidity and mortality for very low birthweight infants. Am J Obstet Gynecol 196:147.e1, 2007

Favre R, Dreux S, Dommergues M, et al: Nonimmune fetal ascites: A series of 79 cases. Am J Obstet Gynecol 190:407, 2004

Faye-Petersen OM, Guinn DA, Wenstrom KD: Value of perinatal autopsy. Obstet Gynecol 94:915, 1999

Finer NN, Barrington KJ: Nitric oxide therapy for the newborn. Semin Perinatol 24:59, 2000

Franco A, Rossi K, Drugh D, et al: Management of anti-Jka alloimmunization. J Reprod Med 54:121, 2009

Fraser WD, Hofmeyr J, Lede R, et al: Amnioinfusion for the prevention of the meconium aspiration syndrome. Amnioinfusion Trial Group. N Engl J Med 353:909, 2005

Freeman JM, Nelson KB: Intrapartum asphyxia and cerebral palsy. Pediatrics 82:240, 1988

Fretts RC, Boyd ME, Usher RH, et al: The changing pattern of fetal death, 1961–1988. Obstet Gynecol 79:35, 1992

Fretts RC, Usher RH: Causes of fetal death in women of advanced maternal age. Obstet Gynecol 89:40, 1997

Fuchs K, Albright C, Scott K, et al: Obstetric factors affecting respiratory morbidity among late preterm infants. Am J Obstet Gynecol, In press, 2009

Fujimoto S, Yamaguchi N, Togari H, et al: Cerebral palsy of the cystic periventricular leukomalacia in low-birth-weight infants. Acta Paediatr 83:397, 1994

Galbraith RS: Incidence of sixth nerve palsy in relation to mode of delivery. Am J Obstet Gynecol 170:1158, 1994

Garite TJ, Kurtzman J, Maurel K, et al: Impact of a "rescue course" of antenatal corticosteroids: A multicenter randomized placebo-controlled trial. Am J Obstet Gynecol 200(3):248.e1, 2009

Garmany TH, Wambach JA, Heins HB, et al: Population and disease-based prevalence of the common mutations associated with surfactant deficiency. Pediatr Res 63(6):645, 2008

Gautier E, Benachi A, Giovangrandi Y, et al: Fetal RhD genotyping by maternal serum analysis: A two-year experience. Am J Obstet Gynecol 192:666, 2005

Geifman-Holtzman O, Grotegut CA, Gaughan JP: Diagnostic accuracy of non-invasive fetal Rh genotyping from maternal blood—A meta-analysis. Am J Obstet Gynecol 195:1163, 2006

Getahun D, Ananth CV, Kinzler WL: Risk factors for antepartum and intrapartum stillbirth: A population-based study. Am J Obstet Gynecol 196(6):530, 2007

Gibson CS, MacLennan AH, Hague WM, et al: Associations between inherited thrombophilias, gestational age, and cerebral palsy. Am J Obstet Gynecol 193:1437, 2005

Gilstrap LC III, Leveno KJ, Burris J, et al: Diagnosis of asphyxia on the basis of fetal pH, Apgar score, and newborn cerebral dysfunction. Am J Obstet Gynecol 161:825, 1989

Gluck L, Kulovich MV: Lecithin-sphingomyelin ratios in amniotic fluid in normal and abnormal pregnancy. Am J Obstet Gynecol 115:539, 1973

Gluck L, Kulovich MV, Borer RC Jr, et al: Diagnosis of the respiratory distress syndrome by amniocentesis. Am J Obstet Gynecol 109:440, 1971

Gluckman PD, Wyatt JS, Azzopardi D, et al: Selective head cooling with mild systemic hypothermia after neonatal encephalopathy: Multicentre randomised trial. Lancet 365:663, 2005

Goeden AM, Worthington D: Spontaneous resolution of mirror syndrome. Obstet Gynecol 106:1183, 2005

Goepfert AR, Goldenberg RL, Hauth JC, et al: Obstetrical determinants of neonatal neurological morbidity. Am J Obstet Gynecol 174:470, 1996

Goldaber KG, Gilstrap LC 3rd, Leveno KJ, et al: Pathologic fetal acidemia. Obstet Gynecol 78:1103, 1991

Goldenberg RL, Andrews WW, Goepfert AR, et al: The Alabama Preterm Birth Study: Umbilical cord blood *Ureaplasma urealyticum* and *Mycoplasma hominis* cultures in very preterm newborn infants. Am J Obstet Gynecol 198:43.e1, 2008

Goldenberg RL, Mayberry SK, Cooper RL, et al: Pregnancy outcome following a second-trimester loss. Obstet Gynecol 81:444, 1993

Gough JD, Keeling JW, Castle B, et al: The obstetric management of non-immunological hydrops. Br J Obstet Gynaecol 93:226, 1986

Grab D, Paulus WE, Bommer A, et al: Treatment of fetal erythroblastosis by intravascular transfusions: Outcome at 6 years. Obstet Gynecol 93:165, 1999

Grant A, O'Brien N, Joy MT, et al: Cerebral palsy among children born during the Dublin randomized trial of intrapartum monitoring. Lancet 2:1233, 1989

Grave G, Nelson SA, Walker A, et al: New therapies and preventive approaches for necrotizing enterocolitis: Report of a research planning workshop. Ped Res 62:1, 2007

Grether JK, Nelson KB: Maternal infection and cerebral palsy in infants of normal birth weight. JAMA 278:207, 1997

Hackney DN, Knudtson EJ, Rossi KQ, et al: Management of pregnancies complicated by anti-c isoimmunization. Obstet Gynecol 103:24, 2004

Hahn S, Chitty LS: Noninvasive prenatal diagnosis: Current practice and future perspectives. Curr Opin Obstet Gynec 10:146, 2008

Halliday HL, Ehrenkranz RA, Doyle LW: Late(>7 days) postnatal corticosteroids for chronic lung disease in preterm infants. Cochrane Database Syst Rev 1:CD001145, 2009

Hanigan WC, Kennedy G, Roemisch F, et al: Administration of indomethacin for the prevention of periventricular–intraventricular hemorrhage in high-risk neonates. J Pediatr 112:941, 1988

Hankins GD, Koen S, Gei AF, et al: Neonatal organ system injury in acute birth asphyxia sufficient to result in neonatal encephalopathy. Obstet Gynecol 99:688, 2002

Hannafin B, Lovecchio F, Blackburn P: Do Rh-negative women with first trimester spontaneous abortions need Rh immune globulin? Am J Emerg Med 24:487, 2006

Harper DC, Wsingle HM, Weiner CP, et al: Long-term neurodevelopmental outcome and brain volume after treatment for hydrops fetalis by in utero intravascular transfusions. Am J Obstet Gynecol 195:192, 2006

Harrington DJ, Redman CW, Moulden M, et al: Long-term outcome in surviving infants with Apgar at 10 minutes: A systematic review of the literature and hospital-based cohort. Am J Obstet Gynecol 196:463, 2007

Hayden CK, Shattuck KE, Richardson CJ, et al: Subependymal germinal matrix hemorrhage in full-term neonates. Pediatrics 75:714, 1985

Heinonen S, Ruynamen M, Kirkinen P: Etiology and outcome of second trimester nonimmunological fetal hydrops. Scand J Obstet Gynecol 79:15, 2000

Holzgreve W, Curry CJR, Golbus MS, et al: Investigation of nonimmune hydrops fetalis. Am J Obstet Gynecol 150:805, 1984

Horn LC, Langner A, Stiehl P, et al: Identification of the causes of intrauterine death during 310 consecutive autopsies. Eur J Obstet Gynecol Reprod Biol 113:134, 2004

Hosoi E: Biological and clinical aspects of ABO blood group system. J Med Invest 55:174, 2008

Howard H, Martlew V, McFadyen I, et al: Consequences for fetus and neonate of maternal red cell allo-immunization. Arch Dis Child Fetal Neonat Ed 78:F62, 1998

Howe DT, Michaitidis GD: Intraperitoneal transfusion in severe, early-onset Rh isoimmunization. Obstet Gynecol 110:880, 2007

Hsu N, Hung KL, Tsai ML, et al: The association of periventricular echodensity of cerebral palsy in preterm infants. Zhonghua Min Guo Xiao Er Ke Yi Xue Hui Za Zhi 37:433, 1996

Huang AH, Robertson RL: Spontaneous superficial parenchymal and leptomeningeal hemorrhage in term neonates. Am J Neuroradiol 25:469, 2004

Huang L, Sauve R, Birkett N, et al: Maternal age and risk of stillbirth: A systematic review. CMAJ 178:165, 2008

Jakobi P, Weissman A, Zimmer EZ, et al: Survival and long-term morbidity in preterm infants with and without a clinical diagnosis of periventricular, intraventricular hemorrhage. Eur J Obstet Gynecol Reprod Biol 46:73, 1992

Jobe AH: Pulmonary surfactant therapy. N Engl J Med 328:861, 1993

Jobe AH: Postnatal corticosteroids for preterm infants—do what we say, not what we do. N Engl J Med 350:1349, 2004

Joyner B, Soto MA, Adam HM: Brachial Plexus Injury. Pediatr Rev 27:238, 2006

Karcher R, Sykes E, Batton D, et al: Gestational age-specific predicted risk of neonatal respiratory distress syndrome using lamellar body count and surfactant-to-albumin ratio in amniotic fluid. Am J Obstet Gynecol 193:1680, 2005

Katz LV, Bowes WA: Meconium aspiration syndrome: Reflections on a murky subject. Am J Obstet Gynecol 166:171, 1992

Katz MA, Kanto WP Jr, Korotkein JH: Recurrence rate of ABO hemolytic disease of the newborn. Obstet Gynecol 59:611, 1982

Kersten CM, Moellering CM, Mato S: Spontaneous drainage of neonatal cephalohematoma: A delayed complication of scalp abscess. Clin Pediatr 47:183, 2008

Kinsella JP, Cutter GR, Walsh WF, et al: Early inhaled nitric oxide therapy in premature newborns with respiratory failure. N Engl J Med 355:354, 2006

Kliegman RM, Fanaroff AA: Necrotizing enterocolitis. N Engl J Med 310:1093, 1984

Klumper F, Pasman S, Van Kamp I, et al: MCA Doppler assessment to time serial intrauterine transfusions in red cell alloimmunized pregnancies? Am J Obstet Gynecol, In press, 2009

Korteweg FJ, Bouman K, Erwich JJ, et al: Cytogenetic analysis after evaluation of 750 fetal deaths. Obstet Gynecol 111:865, 2008

Kusanovic JP, Romero R, Espinoza J, et al: Twin-to-twin transfusion syndrome: An antiangiogenic state? Am J Obstet Gynecol 198:382.e1, 2008

Kuzniewicz M, Newman TB: Interaction of hemolysis and hyperbilirubinemia on neurodevelopmental outcomes in the collaborative perinatal project. Pediatrics 123(3): 1045, 2009

Lefebvre G, Wehbe G, Heron D, et al: Recurrent nonimmune hydrops fetalis: A prepresentation of sciatic acid storage disease. Genet Couns 10:277, 1999

Lesko SM, Mitchell AA, Epstein MF, et al: Heparin use as a risk factor for intraventricular hemorrhage in low-birth-weight infants. N Engl J Med 314:1156, 1986

Leveno KJ, Quirk JG Jr, Cunningham FG, et al: Prolonged pregnancy. I. Observations concerning the causes of fetal distress. Am J Obstet Gynecol 150:465, 1984

Levine MG, Holroyde J, Woods JR, et al: Birth trauma: Incidence and predisposing factors. Obstet Gynecol 63:792, 1984

Liley AW: Liquor amnii analysis in management of pregnancy complicated by rhesus sensitization. Am J Obstet Gynecol 82:1359, 1961

Livinec F, Ancel PY, Marret S, et al: Prenatal risk factors for cerebral palsy in very preterm singletons and twins. Obstet Gynecol 105:1341, 2005

Locatelli A, Andreani M, Pizzardi A, et al: Neonatal ultrasonographic (US) predictors of infant neurologic damage (ND) among babies with birth weight <1500 grams. Am J Obstet Gynecol, In press, 2009

Low JA, Panagiotopoulos C, Derrick EJ: Newborn complications after intrapartum asphyxia with metabolic acidosis in the preterm fetus. Am J Obstet Gynecol 172:805, 1995

Luthy DA, Shy KK, Strickland D, et al: Status of infants at birth and risk for adverse neonatal events and long-term sequelae: A study in low birthweight infants. Am J Obstet Gynecol 157:676, 1987

MacDonald D, Grant A, Sheridan-Pereira M, et al: The Dublin randomized controlled trial of intrapartum fetal heart rate monitoring. Am J Obstet Gynecol 152:524, 1985

MacDorman MF, Kirmeyer S: Fetal and perinatal mortality, United States, 2005. Natl Vital Stat Rep 57(8):1, 2009

MacDorman MF, Hoyert DL, Martin JA, et al: Fetal and perinatal mortality, United States, 2003. National Vital Statistics Reports Vol. 55, No. 6, Hyattsville, MD; National Center for Health Statistics, 2007

MacKenzie IZ, Findlay J, Thompson K, et al: Compliance with routine antenatal rhesus D prophylaxis and the impact on sensitizations: Observations over 14 years. BJOG 113:839, 2006a

MacKenzie IZ, Roseman F, Findlay J, et al: The kinetics of routine antenatal prophylactic intramuscular injections of polyclonal anti-D immunoglobulin. BJOG 113:97, 2006b

Maisels MJ, McDonagh AF: Phototherapy for neonatal jaundice. N Engl J Med 358:920, 2008

Malessy MJ, Pondaag W: Obstetric brachial plexus injuries. Neurosurg Clin N Am 20(1):1, 2009

Mari G, Deter RL, Carpenter RL, et al: Noninvasive diagnosis by Doppler ultrasonography of fetal anemia due to maternal red-cell alloimmunization. N Engl J Med 342:9, 2000

Marret S, Marpeau L, Follet-Bouhamed C, et al: Effect of magnesium sulphate on mortality and neurologic morbidity of the very-preterm newborn (of less than 33 weeks) with two-year neurological outcome: Results of the prospective PREMAG trial. Gynecol Obstet Fertil 36:278, 2008

Martin RJ: Nitric oxide for preemies—not so fast. N Engl J Med 349:2157, 2004

Matsuda T, Okuyama K, Cho K, et al: Cerebral hemodynamics during the induction of antenatal periventricular leukomalacia by hemorrhagic hypotension in chronically instrumented fetal sheep. Am J Obstet Gynecol 194:1057, 2006

McClure EM, Goldenberg RL: Infection and stillbirth. Semin Fetal Neonatal Med 14(4):182, 2009

McCoy MC, Katz VL, Could N, et al: Non-immune hydrops after 20 weeks' gestation: Review of 10 years' experience with suggestions for management. Obstet Gynecol 85:578, 1995

McDonald SJ, Middleton P: Effect of timing of umbilical cord clamping of term infants on maternal and neonatal outcomes. Cochrane Database Syst Rev 16(2):CD004074, 2008

Medical Letter: Intravenous immunoglobin (IVIG). Volume 48, Issue 1245, October 9, 2006

Melone PJ, Ernest JM, O'Shea MD Jr, et al: Appropriateness of intrapartum fetal heart rate management and risk of cerebral palsy. Am J Obstet Gynecol 165:272, 1991

Menticoglou SM, Perlman M, Manning FA: High cervical spinal cord injury in neonates delivered with forceps: Report of 15 cases. Obstet Gynecol 86:589, 1995

Mestan KK, Marks JD, Hecox K, et al: Neurodevelopmental outcomes of premature infants treated with inhaled nitric oxide. N Engl J Med 353:23, 2005

Midgley DY, Hardrug K: The mirror syndrome. Eur J Obstet Gynecol Reprod Biol 8:201, 2000

Miller ME, Graham JM Jr, Higginbotton MC, et al: Compression-related defects from early amnion rupture: Evidence for mechanical teratogenesis. J Pediatr 98:292, 1981

Moise KJ Jr: Management of rhesus alloimmunization in pregnancy. Obstet Gynecol 112:164, 2008

Morris BH, Oh W, Tyson JE, et al: Aggressive vs. conservative phototherapy for infants with extremely low birth weight. N Engl J Med 359(18):1885, 2008

Moss RL, Dimmitt RA, Barnhart DC, et al: Laparotomy versus peritoneal drainage for necrotizing enterocolitis and perforation. N Engl J Med 354:2225, 2006

Moster D, Lie RT, Markestad T: Long-term medical and social consequences of preterm birth. N Engl J Med 359:262, 2008

Mueller-Heubach E, Mazer J: Sonographically documented disappearance of fetal ascites. Obstet Gynecol 61:253, 1983

Naeye RL, Localio AR: Determining the time before birth when ischemia and hypoxemia initiated cerebral palsy. Obstet Gynecol 86:713, 1995

National Institutes of Health: Antenatal corticosteroids revisited: Repeat courses. NIH Consensus Statement Online 17:1, August 17–18, 2000

National Institutes of Health: Consensus Development Conference on the effects of corticosteroids for fetal maturation on perinatal outcomes. Consensus Development Conference statement. Bethesda, MD, NIH, 1994

Nelson KB: Can we prevent cerebral palsy? N Engl J Med 349:1765, 2003

Nelson KB, Dambrosia JM, Ting TY, et al: Uncertain value of electronic fetal monitoring in predicting cerebral palsy. N Engl J Med 334:613, 1996

Nelson KB, Ellenberg JH: Obstetric complications as risk factors for cerebral palsy or seizure disorders. JAMA 251:1843, 1984

Nelson KB, Ellenberg JH: Antecedents of cerebral palsy: Univariate analysis of risks. Am J Dis Child 139:1031, 1985

Nelson KB, Ellenberg JH: Antecedents of cerebral palsy: Multivariate analysis of risk. N Engl J Med 315:81, 1986a

Nelson KB, Ellenberg JH: Antecedents of seizure disorders in early childhood. Am J Dis Child 140:1053, 1986b

Nelson KB, Grether JK: Potentially asphyxiating conditions and spastic cerebral palsy in infants of normal birth weight. Am J Obstet Gynecol 179:507, 1998

Nelson KB, Lynch JK: Stroke in newborn infants. Lancet Neurol 3:150, 2004

Ness PM, Baldwin ML, Niebyl JR: Clinical high-risk designation does not predict excess fetal–maternal hemorrhage. Am J Obstet Gynecol 156:154, 1987

Newman TB, Liljestrand P, Jeremy RJ, et al: Outcomes among newborns with total serum bilirubin levels of 25 mg per deciliter or more. N Engl J Med 354:1889, 2006

Nicolaides KH, Clewell WH, Mibashan RS, et al: Fetal haemoglobin measurement in the assessment of red cell isoimmunization. Lancet 1:1073, 1988

Nicolaides KH, Warenski JC, Rodeck CH: The relationship of fetal plasma protein concentration and hemoglobin level to the development of hydrops in rhesus isoimmunization. Am J Obstet Gynecol 152:341, 1985

Niswander K, Henson G, Elbourne D, et al: Adverse outcome of pregnancy and the quality of obstetric care. Lancet 2:827, 1984

Nores J, Roberts A, Carr S: Prenatal diagnosis and management of fetuses with intracranial hemorrhage. Am J Obstet Gynecol 174:424, 1996

Oepkes D, Seaward PG, Vandenbussche FP, et al: Doppler ultrasonography versus amniocentesis to predict fetal anemia. N Engl J Med 355:156, 2006

Oka A, Belliveau MJ, Rosenberg PA, et al: Vulnerability of oligodendroglia to glutamate: Pharmacology, mechanisms, and prevention. J Neurosc 13:1441, 1993

O'Mahony F, Settatree R, Platt C, et al: Review of singleton fetal and neonatal deaths associated with cranial trauma and cephalic delivery during a national intrapartum-related confidential enquiry. BJOG 112:619, 2005

Onderdonk AB, Delaney ML, DuBois AM: Detection of bacteria in placental tissues obtained from extremely low gestational age neonates. Am J Obstet Gynecol 198:110.e1, 2008

Papile LA, Burstein J, Burstein R, et al: Incidence and evolution of subependymal and intraventricular hemorrhage: A study of infants with birth weights less than 1500 gm. J Pediatr 92:529, 1978

Pasman SA, Meerman RH, Vandenbussche FP, et al: Hypoalbuminemia: A cause of fetal hydrops? Am J Obstet Gynecol 194:972, 2006

Pasman SA, Sikkel E, Le Cessie S, et al: Bilirubin/albumin ratios in fetal blood and amniotic fluid in rhesus immunization. Obstet Gynecol 111:1083, 2008

Patra K, Wilson-Costello D, Taylor HG, et al: Grades I-II intraventricular hemorrhage in extremely low birth weight infants: Effects on neurodevelopment. J Pediatr 149:169, 2006

Pauli RM, Reiser CA: Wisconsin Stillbirth Service Program: II. Analysis of diagnoses and diagnostic categories in the first 1,000 referrals. Am J Med Genet 50:135, 1994

Perlman JM, Cunningham FG: Fetal and neonatal hypoxic ischemic cerebral injury. In: Williams Obstetrics, 18th ed (Suppl 21). Norwalk, Conn, Appleton & Lange, December/January 1993

Perlman JM, Risser R, Broyles RS: Bilateral cystic periventricular leukomalacia in the premature infant: Associated risk factors. Pediatrics 97:822, 1996

Perlman JM, Volpe JJ: Intraventricular hemorrhage in extremely small premature infants. Am J Dis Child 140:1122, 1986

Pfister RH, Soll RF, Wiswell T: Protein containing synthetic surfactant versus animal derived surfactant extract for the prevention and treatment of respiratory distress syndrome. Cochrane Database Syst Rev 4:CD006069, 2007

Phelan JP, Ahn MO: Perinatal observations in forty-eight neurologically impaired term infants. Am J Obstet Gynecol 171:424, 1994

Phelan JP, Ahn MO, Korst L, et al: Is intrapartum fetal brain injury in the term fetus preventable? Am J Obstet Gynecol 174:318, 1996

Prasad MR, Krugh D, Rossi KQ, et al: Anti-D in Rh positive pregnancies. Am J Obstet Gynecol 195:1158, 2006

Pritchard JA, Cunningham FG, Pritchard SA, et al: How often does maternal preeclampsia–eclampsia incite thrombocytopenia in the fetus? Obstet Gynecol 69:292, 1987

Pritchard JA, Cunningham FG, Pritchard SA, et al: On reducing the frequency of severe abruptio placentae. Am J Obstet Gynecol 165:1345, 1991

Queenan JT, Thomas PT, Tomai TP, et al: Deviation in amniotic fluid optical density at a wavelength of 450 nm in Rh isoimmunized pregnancies from 14 to 40 weeks' gestation: A proposal for clinical management. Am J Obstet Gynecol 168:1370, 1993

Race RR, Sanger R: Blood Groups in Man, 6th ed. Oxford, England, Blackwell, 1975

Radestad I, Steineck G, Nordin C, et al: Psychological complications after stillbirth—influence of memories and immediate management: Population based study. BMJ 312:1505, 1996

Raju TNK, Nelson KB, Ferriero D, et al: Ischemic perinatal stroke: Summary of a workshop sponsored by the NICHD and NINDS. Pediatrics 120:1, 2007

Reddick K, Canzoneri B, Roeder H, et al: Racial disparities and neonatal outcomes in preterm infants with intraventricular hemorrhage. Am J Obstet Gynecol, 199(6):S71, 2008

Reddy UM: Prediction and prevention of recurrent stillbirth. Obstet Gynecol 110:1151, 2007

Reddy UM, Ko C-W, Willinger M: Maternal age and the risk of stillbirth throughout pregnancy in the United States. Am J Obstet Gynecol 195:764, 2006

Redline RW: Severe fetal placental vascular lesions in term infants with neurologic impairment. Am J Obstet Gynecol 192:452, 2005

Redline RW: Placental pathology: A systematic approach with clinical correlations. Placenta 22:S86, 2008

Redline RW, Sagar P, King ME, et al: Case 12-2008: A newborn infant with intermittent apnea and seizures. N Engl J Med 358:1713, 2008

Richey S, Ramin SM, Bawdon RE, et al: Markers of acute and chronic asphyxia in infants with meconium-stained amniotic fluid. Am J Obstet Gynecol 172:1212, 1995

Roberts SW, Hernandez C, Maberry MC, et al: Obstetric clavicular fracture: The enigma of normal birth. Obstet Gynecol 86:978, 1995

Robertson C, Finer N: Term infants with hypoxic-ischemic encephalopathy: Outcome at 3.5 years. Dev Med Child Neurol 27:473, 1985

Robinson BV, Ettedgui JA, Sherman FS: Use of terbutaline in the treatment of complete heart block in the fetus. Cardiol Young 11:683, 2001

Roemer RJ: Relation of torticollis to breech delivery. Am J Obstet Gynecol 67:1146, 1954

Rosen MG, Dickinson JC: The incidence of cerebral palsy. Am J Obstet Gynecol 167:417, 1992

Rosen MG, Hobel CJ: Prenatal and perinatal factors associated with brain disorders. Obstet Gynecol 68:416, 1986

Rouse DJ, Hirtz DG, Thom E, et al: A randomized controlled trial of magnesium sulfate for the prevention of cerebral palsy. N Engl J Med 359(9):895, 2008

Rouse D, Weiner C: Ongoing fetomaternal hemorrhage treated by serial fetal intravascular transfusions. Obstet Gynecol 76:974, 1990

Saleeb S, Copel J, Friedman D, et al: Comparison of treatment with fluorinated glucocorticoids to the natural history of autoantibody–associated congenital heart block: Retrospective review of the research registry for neonatal lupus. Arthritis Rheum 42:2335, 1999

Salim R, BenShlomo I, Nachum Z, et al: The incidence of large fetomaternal hemorrhage and the Kleihauer-Betke test. Obstet Gynecol 105:1039, 2005

Salim R, Shalev E: The incidence of large fetomaternal hemorrhage and the Kleihauer-Betke test (Reply). Obstet Gynecol 107:207, 2006

Saller DN Jr, Lesser KB, Harrel U, et al: The clinical utility of the perinatal autopsy. JAMA 273:663, 1995

Samadi R, Miller D, Settlage R, et al: Massive fetomaternal hemorrhage and fetal death: Is it predictable? Am J Obstet Gynecol 174:391, 1996

Santolaya J, Alley D, Jaffe R, et al: Antenatal classification of hydrops fetalis. Obstet Gynecol 79:256, 1992

Sarkar S, Bhagat I, Dechert R, et al: Severe intraventricular hemorrhage in preterm infants: Comparison of risk factors and short-term neonatal morbidities between grade 3 and grade 4 intraventricular hemorrhage. Am J Perinatol 26:419, 2009

Sau A, El-Matary A, Newton L, et al: Management of red cell alloimmunized pregnancies using conventional methods compared with that of middle cerebral artery peak systolic velocity. Acta Obstet Gynecol Scand 88(4), 2009

Scheier M, Hernandez-Andrade E, Fonseca EB, et al: Prediction of severe fetal anemia in red blood cell alloimmunization after previous intrauterine transfusions. Am J Obstet Gynecol 195:1550, 2006

Schmidt B, Asztalos EV, Roberts RS, et al: Impact of bronchopulmonary dysplasia, brain injury, and severe retinopathy on the outcome of extremely low-birth-weight infants at 18 months. JAMA 289:1124, 2003

Schreiber MD, Gin-Mestan K, Marks JD, et al: Inhaled nitric oxide in premature infants with the respiratory distress syndrome. N Engl J Med 349:2099, 2003

Seger N, Soll R: Animal derived surfactant extract for treatment of respiratory distress syndrome. Cochrane Database Syst Rev 2:CD007836, 2009

Segata M, Chaoui R, Khalek N, et al: Fetal thrombocytopenia secondary to parvovirus infection. Am J Obstet Gynecol 196:61.e1, 2007

Shankaran S, Laptook AR, Ehrenkranz RA, et al: Whole-body hypothermia for neonates with hypoxic-ischemic encephalopathy. N Engl J Med 353:1574, 2005

Sharma PP, Salihu HM, Oyelese Y, et al: Is race a determinant of stillbirth recurrence? Obstet Gynecol 107:391, 2006

Shulenin S, Nogee LM, Annilo T, et al: ABCA3 gene mutations in newborns with fatal surfactant deficiency. N Engl J Med 350:1296, 2004

Shulman LP, Phillips OP, Emerson DS, et al: Fetal "space-suit" hydrops in the first trimester: Differentiating risk for chromosome abnormalities by delineating characteristics of nuchal translucency. Prenat Diagn 20:30, 2000

Silva AM, Smith RN, Lehmann CU, et al: Neonatal nucleated red blood cells and the prediction of cerebral white matter injury in preterm infants. Obstet Gynecol 107:550, 2006

Silver RM: Fetal death. Obstet Gynecol 109:153, 2007

Simonson C, Barlow P, Dehennin N, et al: Neonatal complications of vacuum-assisted delivery. Obstet Gynecol 110:189, 2007

Singh BS, Clark RH, Powers RJ, et al: Meconium aspiration syndrome remains a significant problem in the NICU: Outcomes and treatment patterns in term neonates admitted for intensive care during a ten-year period. J Perinatol 29(7):497, 2009

Snyder EL: Prevention of hemolytic disease of the newborn due to anti-D. Prenatal/perinatal testing and Rh immune globulin administration. Am Assoc Blood Banks Assoc Bull 98:1 (Level III), 1998

Sola-Visner M, Sallmon H, Brown R: New insights into the mechanisms of nonimmune thrombocytopenia in neonates. Semin Perinatol 33(1):43, 2009

Soldado F, Peiro JL, Aguirre M, et al: Extremity amniotic band syndrome in fetal lamb. I: An experimental model of limb amputation. Am J Obstet Gynecol 195:1607, 2006

Soll RF, Morley CJ: Prophylactic versus selective use of surfactant in preventing morbidity and mortality in preterm infants. Cochrane Database Syst Rev 2:CD000510, 2001

Soraisham AS, Singhal Nalini, McMillan DD, et al: A multicenter study on the clinical outcome of chorioamnionitis in preterm infants. Am J Obstet Gynecol 200:372.e1, 2009

Spong CY, Ogundipe OA, Ross MG: Prophylactic amnioinfusion for meconium stained amniotic fluid. Am J Obstet Gynecol 171:931, 1994

Stanley FJ, Blair E: Why have we failed to reduce the frequency of cerebral palsy? Med J Aust 154:623, 1991

Stark AR: Inhaled NO for preterm infants—getting to yes? N Engl J Med 355:404, 2006

Stedman CM, Baudin JC, White CA, et al: Use of the erythrocyte rosette test to screen for excessive fetomaternal hemorrhage in Rh-negative women. Am J Obstet Gynecol 154:1363, 1986

Steinfeld JD, Samuels P, Bulley MA, et al: The utility of the TDx test in the assessment of fetal lung maturity. Obstet Gynecol 79:460, 1992

Stevens AM, Hermes HM, Rutledge JC, et al: Myocardial-tissue-specific phenotype of maternal microchimerism in neonatal lupus congenital heart block. Lancet 362:1617, 2003

Stoll BJ, Hansen NI, Adams-Chapman I, et al: Neurodevelopmental and growth impairment among extremely low-birth-weight infants with neonatal infection. JAMA 292:2357, 2004

Streeter GL: Focal deficiencies in fetal tissues and their relation to intrauterine amputations. Contrib Embryol 22:1, 1930

Strijbis EM, Oudman I, van Essen P, et al: Cerebral palsy and the application of the international criteria for acute intrapartum hypoxia. Obstet Gynecol 107:1357, 2006

Surkan PJ, Stephansson O, Dickman PW, et al: Previous preterm and small-for-gestational-age births and the subsequent risk of stillbirth. N Engl J Med 350:754, 2004

Taylor PV, Scott JS, Gerlis LM, et al: Maternal antibodies against fetal cardiac antigens in congenital complete heart block. N Engl J Med 315:667, 1986

Thacker SB, Stroup DF, Peterson HB: Efficacy and safety of intrapartum electronic fetal monitoring: An update. Obstet Gynecol 86:613, 1995

Thorngren-Jerneck K, Herbst A: Perinatal factors associated with cerebral palsy in children born in Sweden. Obstet Gynecol 108:1499, 2006

Thorp JA, Ferette-Smith D, Gaston L, et al: Antenatal vitamin K and phenobarbital for preventing intracranial hemorrhage in the premature newborn: A randomized double-blind placebo-controlled trial. Am J Obstet Gynecol 172:253, 1995

Thorp JM: Utilization of anti-RhD in the emergency department after blunt trauma. Obstet Gynecol Surv 63:112, 2008

Thung SF, Grobman WA: The cost effectiveness of empiric intravenous immunoglobulin for the antepartum treatment of fetal and neonatal alloimmune thrombocytopenia. Am J Obstet Gynecol 193:1094, 2005

Torfs CP, van den Berg B, Oechsli FW, et al: Prenatal and perinatal factors in the etiology of cerebral palsy. J Pediatr 116:615, 1990

Torpin R: Fetal malformations caused by amnion rupture during gestation. Springfield, Ill, Thomas, 1968

Turpenny PD, Nimmo A: Fractured clavicle of the newborn in a population with a high prevalence of grand-multiparity: Analysis of 78 consecutive cases. Br J Obstet Gynaecol 100:338, 1993

Tyson JE, Parikh NA, Langer J, et al: Intensive care for extreme prematurity—moving beyond gestational age. N Engl J Med 358:1672, 2008

Ubachs JMH, Slooff ACJ, Peeters LLH: Obstetric antecedents of surgically treated obstetric brachial plexus injuries. Br J Obstet Gynaecol 102:813, 1995

Vain NE, Szyld EG, Prudent LM, et al: Oropharyngeal and nasopharyngeal suctioning of meconium-stained neonates before delivery of their shoulders: Multicentre, randomized controlled trial. Lancet 364:597, 2004

van den Akker ES, Oepkes D, Brand A, et al: Vaginal delivery for fetuses at risk of alloimmune thrombocytopenia? BJOG 113:781, 2006

van Kamp IL, Klumper FJ, Oepkes D, et al: Complications of intrauterine intravascular transfusion for fetal anemia due to maternal red-cell alloimmunization. Am J Obstet Gynecol 192:171, 2005

van Meurs KP, Wright LL, Ehrenkranz RA, et al: Inhaled nitric oxide for premature infants with severe respiratory failure. N Engl J Med 353:13, 2005 van Wamelen DJ, Klumper FJ, de Haas M, et al: Obstetric history and antibody titer in estimating severity of Kell alloimmunization in pregnancy. Obstet Gynecol 109:1093, 2007

Vasconcelos BC, Lago CA, Nogueira RV, et al: Mandibular fracture in a premature infant: A case report and review of the literature. J Oral Maxillofac Surg 67(1):218, 2009

Verbrugge SJ, Lachmann B: Mechanisms of ventilation-induced lung injury: Physiological rationale to prevent it. Monaldi Arch Chest Dis 54:22, 1999

Verma U, Tejani N, Klein S, et al: Obstetric antecedents of intraventricular hemorrhage and periventricular leukomalacia in the low-birth-weight neonate. Am J Obstet Gynecol 176:275, 1997

Volpe JJ: Neurology of the Newborn, 3rd ed. Philadelphia, Saunders, 1995, p 373

Volpe JJ, Hill A: Neurologic disorders. In Avery GB (ed): Neonatology, 3rd ed. Philadelphia, JB Lippincott, 1987, p 1073

Wapner RJ, Sorokin Y, Mele L, et al: Long-term outcomes after repeated doses of antenatal corticosteroids. N Engl J Med 357:1190, 2007

Wapner RJ, Sorokin Y, Thom EA, et al: Single versus weekly courses of antenatal corticosteroids: Evaluation of safety and efficacy Am J Obstet Gynecol 195:633, 2006

Weeks JW, Asrat T, Morgan MA, et al: Antepartum surveillance for a history of stillbirth: When to begin? Am J Obstet Gynecol 172:486, 1995

Weindling M: Periventricular haemorrhage and periventricular leukomalacia. Br J Obstet Gynaecol 102:278, 1995

Weiner CP, Pelzer GD, Heilskov J, et al: The effect of intravascular transfusion on umbilical venous pressure in anemic fetuses with and without hydrops. Am J Obstet Gynecol 161:1498, 1989

Weiner CP, Wenstrom KD, Sipes SL, et al: Risk factors for cordocentesis and fetal intravascular transfusion. Am J Obstet Gynecol 165:1020, 1991a

Weiner CP, Widness JA: Decreased fetal erythropoiesis and hemolysis in Kell hemolytic anemia. Am J Obstet Gynecol 174:547, 1996

Weiner CP, Williamson RA, Wenstrom KD, et al: Management of fetal hemolytic disease by cordocentesis: I. Prediction of fetal anemia. Am J Obstet Gynecol 165:546, 1991b

Wenstrom KD, Andrews WW, Maher JE: Amnioinfusion survey: Prevalence, protocols, and complications. Obstet Gynecol 86:572, 1995

Whitby EH, Griffiths PD, Rutter S, et al: Frequency and natural history of subdural haemorrhages in babies and relation to obstetrical factors. Lancet 363:846, 2004

White DA, Pressman EK, Hanna GV, et al: Facial nerve palsy—frequencies associated with spontaneous, forceps and cesarean deliveries. Am J Obstet Gynecol 174:353, 1996

Wiklund LM, Uvebrant P, Flodmark O: Computed tomography as an adjunct in etiological analysis of hemiplegic cerebral palsy, 1. Children born preterm. Neuropediatrics 22:50, 1991a

Wiklund LM, Uvebrant P, Flodmark O: Computed tomography as an adjunct in etiological analysis of hemiplegic cerebral palsy, 2. Children born at term. Neuropediatrics 22:121, 1991b

Winter S, Autry A, Boyle C, et al: Trends in the prevalence of cerebral palsy in a population-based study. Pediatrics 110:1220, 2002

Wiswell TE, Tuggle JM, Turner BS: Meconium aspiration syndrome: Have we made a difference? Pediatrics 85:715, 1990

Woelfer B, Schuchter K, Janisiw M, et al: Postdelivery levels of anti-D IgG prophylaxis in mothers depend on maternal body weight. Transfusion 44:512, 2004

Woodward LJ, Anderson PJ, Austin NC, et al: Neonatal MRI to predict neurodevelopmental outcomes in preterm infants. N Engl J Med 355:685, 2006

Wu DW, Cheng YW, Rand L, et al: Hydrops and preeclampsia: Another look into mirror syndrome. Am J Obstet Gynecol, In press, 2009

Wu YW, Croen LA, Shah SJ, et al: Cerebral palsy in a term population: Risk factors and neuroimaging findings. Pediatrics 118:691, 2006

Wu YW, Escobar GJ, Grether JK, et al: Chorioamnionitis and cerebral palsy in term and near-term infants. JAMA 290:2677, 2003

Wyatt PR, Owolabi T, Meier C, et al: Age-specific risk of fetal loss observed in a second trimester serum screening population. Am J Obstet Gynecol 192:240, 2005

Yeh TF, Lin YJ, Lin HC, et al: Outcomes at school age after postnatal dexamethasone therapy for lung disease of prematurity. N Engl J Med 350:1304, 2004

Yoon BH, Kim CJ, Romero R, et al: Experimentally induced intrauterine infection causes fetal brain white matter lesions in rabbits. Am J Obstet Gynecol 177:797, 1997a

Yoon BH, Romero R, Kim CJ, et al: High expression of tumor necrosis factor-alpha and interleukin-6 in periventricular leukomalacia. Am J Obstet Gynecol 177:406, 1997b

Yoon BH, Romero R, Moon JB, et al: Clinical significance of intra-amniotic inflammation in patients with preterm labor and intact membranes. Am J Obstet Gynecol 185:1130, 2001

Yoon BH, Romero R, Park JS, et al: Fetal exposure to an intra-amniotic inflammation and the development of cerebral palsy at the age of three years. Am J Obstet Gynecol 182:675, 2000

Yudkin PL, Wood L, Redman CWG: Risk of unexplained stillbirth at different gestational ages. Lancet 1:1192, 1987

Zhu Y, Miller TL, Chidekel A, et al: KL4-surfactant (lucinactant) protects human airway epithelium from hyperoxia. Pediatr Res 64(2):154, 2008

Zipursky A: Prevention of vitamin K deficiency bleeding in newborns [Review]. Br J Haematol 104:430, 1999

Zupan V, Gonzalez P, Lacaze-Masmonteil T, et al: Periventricular leukomalacia: Risk factors revisited. Dev Med Child Neurol 38:1061, 1996

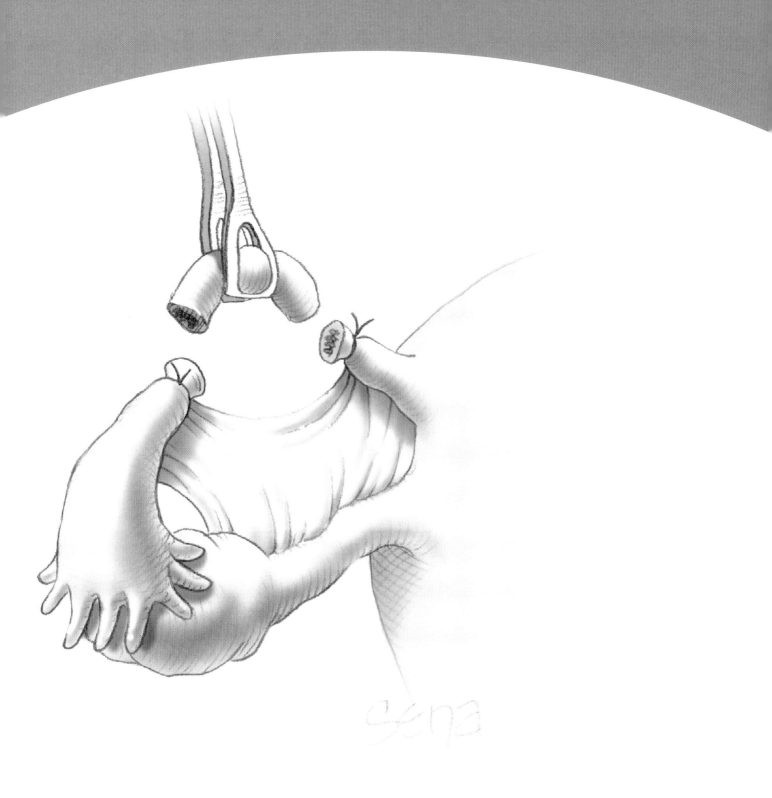

CHAPTER 30

The Puerperium

The puerperium is the period of time encompassing the first few weeks following birth. The duration of this "period" is understandably inexact, and it is considered by most to be between 4 and 6 weeks. Although a relatively uncomplex time compared with pregnancy, the puerperium is characterized by many physiological changes. Some of these changes may be simply bothersome for the new mother, although serious complications can also arise.

Some mothers have feelings of abandonment following delivery because of a newly aimed focus upon the infant. Thus, the puerperium may be a time of intense anxiety for many women. To illustrate this, data gathered by the Pregnancy Risk Assessment Monitoring System—*PRAMS*—is informative. This ongoing population based surveillance system was initiated in 1987 by the Centers for Disease Control and Prevention (2007a) to better understand why infant mortality rates had plateaued. The system collects data concerning maternal attitudes and experiences before, during, and shortly after pregnancy. Kanotra and colleagues (2007) analyzed data in a 10-state area in 2000 to assess challenges that women faced from 2 to 9 months following delivery. Their main findings are listed in Table 30-1.

ANATOMICAL, PHYSIOLOGICAL, AND CLINICAL ASPECTS

Vagina and Vaginal Outlet

Early in the puerperium, the vagina and its outlet form a capacious, smooth-walled passage that gradually diminishes in size but rarely returns to nulliparous dimensions. Rugae begin to reappear by the third week but are not as prominent as before. The hymen is represented by several small tags of tissue, which scar to form the *myrtiform caruncles.* Vaginal epithelium begins to proliferate by 4 to 6 weeks, usually coincidental with resumed ovarian estrogen production. Lacerations or stretching of the perineum during delivery may result in relaxation of the vaginal outlet. Some damage to the pelvic floor may be inevitable, and parturition predisposes to uterine prolapse as well as urinary and anal incontinence. This is a matter of great contemporaneous concern and is discussed in detail in Chapter 17 (p. 401).

Uterus

Vessels

The massively increased uterine blood flow necessary to maintain pregnancy is made possible by significant hypertrophy and remodeling of all pelvic vessels. After delivery, their caliber diminishes to approximately the size of the prepregnant state. Within the puerperal uterus, larger blood vessels become obliterated by hyaline changes, gradually resorbed, and replaced by smaller ones. Minor vestiges of the larger vessels, however, may persist for years.

Cervix and Lower Uterine Segment

During labor, the outer cervical margin, which corresponds to the external os, is usually lacerated, especially laterally. The cervical opening contracts slowly and for a few days immediately after labor readily admits two fingers. By the end of the first week, this opening narrows, the cervix thickens, and the endocervical canal reforms. The external os does not completely resume its pregravid appearance. It remains somewhat wider, and typically, bilateral depressions at the site of lacerations become permanent. These changes are characteristic of a parous cervix. The markedly thinned-out lower uterine segment contracts and retracts, but not as forcefully as the uterine corpus. During the next few weeks, the lower segment is converted from a clearly distinct substructure large enough to accommodate the fetal

TABLE 30-1. Pregnancy Risk Assessment Surveillance System—PRAMS[a]. Concerns Raised by Women in the First 2–9 Months Postpartum

Concerns	Percent
1. Need for social support	32
2. Breast feeding issues	24
3. Inadequate education about newborn care	21
4. Help with postpartum depression	10
5. Perceived need for extended hospital stay	8
6. Need for maternal insurance coverage postpartum	6

[a]Centers for Disease Control and Prevention (2007a). Data from Kanotra and associates (2007).

head, to a barely discernible uterine isthmus located between the corpus and internal os.

Cervical epithelium also undergoes considerable remodeling, and this actually may be salutary. For example, Ahdoot and colleagues (1998) found that about half of women showed regression of high-grade dysplasia following vaginal delivery.

Uterine Involution

Immediately after placental expulsion, the fundus of the contracted uterus lies slightly below the umbilicus. It consists mostly of myometrium covered by serosa and lined by basal decidua. The anterior and posterior walls, in close apposition, each measure 4 to 5 cm thick (Buhimschi and colleagues, 2003). Immediately postpartum, the uterus weighs approximately 1000 g. Because the blood vessels are compressed by the contracted myometrium, the uterus on section appears ischemic compared with the reddish-purple hyperemic pregnant organ.

During the puerperium, a truly remarkable *tour de force* of destruction or deconstruction begins. Two days after delivery, the uterus begins to involute, as shown in Figure 30-1, and at 1 week, it weighs about 500 g. By 2 weeks, it weighs about 300 g and has descended into the true pelvis. Around 4 weeks after delivery, it regains its previous nonpregnant size of 100 g or less. The total number of muscle cells probably does not decrease appreciably. Instead, the individual cells decrease markedly in size—from 500-800 μm by 5 to 10 μm at term to 50-90 μm by 2.5-5 μm postpartum. Involution of the connective tissue framework occurs equally rapidly.

Because separation of the placenta and membranes involves the spongy layer, the decidua basalis is not sloughed. The decidua that remains has striking variations in thickness, has an irregular jagged appearance, and is infiltrated with blood, especially at the placental site (see Fig. 30-1).

Sonographic Findings. It takes up to 5 weeks for the uterine cavity to regress to its nonpregnant state of a potential space. Tekay and Jouppila (1993) studied 42 normal women postpartum and identified fluid in the endometrial cavity in 78 percent at 2 weeks, 52 percent at 3 weeks, 30 percent at 4 weeks, and 10 percent at 5 weeks. Wachsberg and Kurtz (1992) followed 72 women and identified gas in the endometrial cavity in 19 percent within 3 days after delivery. In 7 percent, it was seen at 3 weeks. Finally, using Doppler ultrasound, Sohn and colleagues (1988) described continuously increasing uterine artery vascular resistance during the first 5 postpartum days.

Afterpains

In primiparas, the uterus tends to remain tonically contracted following delivery. However, in multiparas, it often contracts vigorously at intervals and gives rise to *afterpains*, which are similar to but milder than the pain of labor contractions. They are

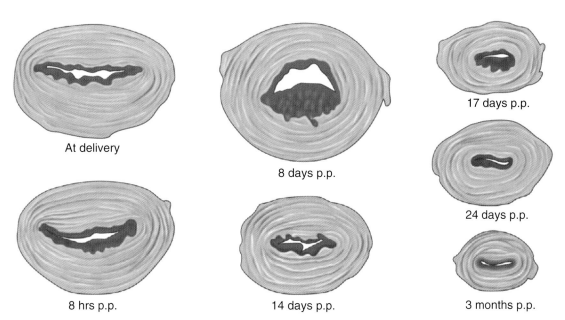

At delivery

8 days p.p.

17 days p.p.

8 hrs p.p.

14 days p.p.

24 days p.p.

3 months p.p.

FIGURE 30-1 Cross sections of uteri made at the level of the involuting placental site at varying times after delivery. p.p. = postpartum. (Redrawn from Williams, 1931.)

more pronounced as parity increases and worsen when the infant suckles, likely because of oxytocin release (Holdcroft and colleagues, 2003). Usually, afterpains decrease in intensity and become mild by the third day.

Lochia

Early in the puerperium, sloughing of decidual tissue results in a vaginal discharge of variable quantity. The discharge is termed *lochia* and consists of erythrocytes, shredded decidua, epithelial cells, and bacteria. For the first few days after delivery, there is blood sufficient to color it red—*lochia rubra*. After 3 or 4 days, lochia becomes progressively pale in color—*lochia serosa*. After about the 10th day, because of an admixture of leukocytes and reduced fluid content, lochia assumes a white or yellowish-white color—*lochia alba*. Lochia persists for up to 4 to 8 weeks after delivery (Visness and co-workers, 1997).

Endometrial Regeneration

Within 2 or 3 days after delivery, the remaining decidua becomes differentiated into two layers. The superficial layer becomes necrotic and is sloughed in the lochia. The basal layer adjacent to the myometrium remains intact and is the source of new endometrium. The endometrium arises from proliferation of the endometrial glandular remnants and the stroma of the interglandular connective tissue.

Endometrial regeneration is rapid, except at the placental site. Within a week or so, the free surface becomes covered by epithelium, and Sharman (1953) identified fully restored endometrium in all biopsy specimens obtained from the 16th day onward. Histological endometritis is part of the normal reparative process. Moreover, microscopic inflammatory changes characteristic of acute salpingitis are seen in almost half of postpartum women between 5 and 15 days. However, these do not reflect infection (Andrews, 1951).

Subinvolution

This term describes an arrest or a retardation of involution. It is accompanied by prolongation of lochial discharge and irregular or excessive uterine bleeding, which sometimes may be profuse. On bimanual examination, the uterus is larger and softer than would be expected. Both retention of placental fragments and pelvic infection may cause subinvolution. Ergonovine or methylergonovine (Methergine), 0.2 mg every 3 to 4 hours for 24 to 48 hours, is recommended by some for subinvolution, but its efficacy is questionable. On the other hand, bacterial metritis responds to oral antimicrobial therapy. Wager and colleagues (1980) reported that almost a third of cases of late postpartum uterine infection are caused by *Chlamydia trachomatis*. Thus, azithromycin or doxycycline therapy is appropriate empirical therapy.

Andrew and colleagues (1989) described 25 cases of hemorrhage between 7 and 40 days postpartum associated with non-involuted uteroplacental arteries. These abnormal arteries were filled with thrombi and lacked an endothelial lining. Perivascular trophoblasts were also identified in the vessel walls. They postulated that subinvolution, at least with regard to placental vessels, may represent an aberrant interaction between uterine cells and trophoblast.

Placental Site Involution

Complete extrusion of the placental site takes up to 6 weeks (Williams, 1931). When this process is defective, late-onset puerperal hemorrhage may ensue. Immediately after delivery, the placental site is approximately the size of the palm, but it rapidly decreases thereafter. Within hours of delivery, the placental site normally consists of many thrombosed vessels that ultimately undergo organization (see Fig. 30-1). By the end of the second week, it is 3 to 4 cm in diameter.

Williams (1931) described placental site involution as a process of exfoliation, which is in great part brought about by the undermining of the implantation site by growth of endometrial tissue. Thus, involution is not simply absorption in situ. Exfoliation consists of both extension and "downgrowth" of endometrium from the margins of the placental site, as well as development of endometrial tissue from the glands and stroma left deep in the decidua basalis after placental separation. Anderson and Davis (1968) concluded that placental site exfoliation results from sloughing of infarcted and necrotic superficial tissues followed by a remodeling process.

Late Postpartum Hemorrhage

The American College of Obstetricians and Gynecologists (2006) defines *secondary postpartum hemorrhage* as bleeding 24 hours to 12 weeks after delivery. Clinically worrisome uterine hemorrhage develops within 1 to 2 weeks in perhaps 1 percent of women. Such bleeding most often is the result of abnormal involution of the placental site. It occasionally is caused by retention of a placental fragment. Usually the retained piece undergoes necrosis with deposition of fibrin and may eventually form a so-called *placental polyp*. As the eschar of the polyp detaches from the myometrium, hemorrhage may be brisk. Demers (2005) and Salman (2008) and their associates have described delayed postpartum hemorrhage caused by von Willebrand disease (see Chap. 51, p. 1097).

Management. Because few women with delayed hemorrhage have retained placental fragments, we do not routinely perform curettage. Lee and associates (1981) studied 27 women with significant bleeding after the first postpartum day. In 20, sonographic evaluation revealed an empty uterus, and only one woman of the 27 had retained placental tissue. Importantly, in some with delayed hemorrhage, curettage will worsen bleeding by avulsing part of the implantation site. Thus, in a stable patient, if sonographic examination shows an empty cavity, then oxytocin, ergonovine, methylergonovine, or a prostaglandin analog is given. Antimicrobials are added if uterine infection is suspected. If large clots are seen in the uterine cavity with sonography, then *gentle* suction curettage is considered. Otherwise curettage is carried out only if appreciable bleeding persists or recurs after medical management.

Urinary Tract

Bladder trauma is associated most closely with the length of labor and thus to some degree is a normal accompaniment of vaginal delivery. Funnell and associates (1954) used cystoscopy immediately postpartum and described varying degrees of submucosal hemorrhage and edema. Postpartum, the bladder has an increased capacity and a relative insensitivity to intravesical pressure. Thus, overdistension, incomplete emptying, and excessive residual urine are common. Their management is discussed on page 655.

The dilated ureters and renal pelves return to their prepregnant state over the course of 2 to 8 weeks after delivery (see Chap. 5, p. 123). Urinary tract infection is of concern because residual urine and bacteriuria in a traumatized bladder, coupled with a dilated collecting system, are conducive to infection.

Incontinence

Urinary incontinence in the first few days postpartum is uncommon. That said, there is increasing attention to the potential for the development of urinary incontinence subsequent to pregnancy. Recent and ongoing evaluations have focused on the effect of delivery on urinary and anal incontinence as well as pelvic organ prolapse. These long-term effects are complex in origin and are related to numerous factors that may cause neuromuscular damage. For example, MacArthur and colleagues (2006) found that 14 percent of parous women who had delivered exclusively by cesarean reported incontinence when monitored long-term. Risks of incontinence from vaginal, perineal, and anal sphincter lacerations and from episiotomy are considered in detail in Chapter 17 (p. 401). Importantly, the debate concerning avoidance of such injuries by *elective primary cesarean delivery* was addressed in detail by a National Institutes of Health (NIH) sponsored State-of-the-Science Conference in March 2006 (see Chap. 25, p. 548). Chiarelli and Cockburn (2002) reported on a randomized trial to reduce the prevalence and severity of urinary incontinence. They found that multifaceted intervention that included pelvic floor exercises was effective.

Peritoneum and Abdominal Wall

The broad and round ligaments require considerable time to recover from the stretching and loosening that occur during pregnancy. As a result of ruptured elastic fibers in the skin and prolonged distension caused by the pregnant uterus, the abdominal wall remains soft and flaccid. Several weeks are required for these structures to return to normal. Recovery is aided by exercise. Except for silvery striae, the abdominal wall usually resumes its prepregnancy appearance. When muscles remain atonic, however, the abdominal wall also remains lax. Marked separation of the rectus muscles—*diastasis recti*—may result.

Blood and Fluid Changes

Marked leukocytosis and thrombocytosis may occur during and after labor. The white blood cell count sometimes reaches 30,000/μL, with the increase predominantly due to granulocytes. There is a relative lymphopenia and an absolute eosinopenia. Normally, during the first few postpartum days, hemoglobin concentration and hematocrit fluctuate moderately. If they fall much below the levels present just prior to labor, a considerable amount of blood has been lost (see Chap. 35, p. 761).

Although not extensively studied, in most women, blood volume has nearly returned to its nonpregnant level by 1 week after delivery. Cardiac output usually remains elevated for 24 to 48 hours postpartum and declines to nonpregnant values by 10 days

(Robson and colleagues, 1987). Heart rate changes follow this pattern. Systemic vascular resistance follows inversely. It remains in the lower range characteristic of pregnancy for 2 days postpartum and then begins to steadily increase to normal nonpregnant values.

Pregnancy-induced changes in blood coagulation factors persist for variable periods during the puerperium. Elevation of plasma fibrinogen is maintained at least through the first week, and hence, so is the sedimentation rate.

Normal pregnancy is associated with an appreciable increase in extracellular water, and postpartum diuresis is a physiological reversal of this process. This regularly occurs between the second and fifth days and corresponds with loss of residual pregnancy hypervolemia. In preeclampsia, both retention of fluid antepartum and diuresis postpartum may be greatly increased (see Chap. 34, p. 718).

Weight Loss

In addition to the loss of 5 to 6 kg due to uterine evacuation and normal blood loss, there is usually a further decrease of 2 to 3 kg through diuresis. Chesley and co-workers (1959) demonstrated a decrease in sodium space of about 2 L during the first week postpartum. According to Schauberger and co-investigators (1992), women approach their self-reported prepregnancy weight 6 months after delivery but still retain an average surplus of 1.4 kg (3 lb). Indigent women are more likely to retain weight gained during pregnancy (Olson and associates, 2003).

BREASTS AND LACTATION

Anatomically, each mature mammary gland or breast is composed of 15 to 25 lobes. They are arranged radially and are separated from one another by varying amounts of fat. Each lobe consists of several lobules, which in turn are composed of large numbers of alveoli. Each alveolus is provided with a small duct that joins others to form a single larger duct for each lobe as shown in Figure 30-2. These *lactiferous ducts* open separately on the nipple, where they may be distinguished as minute but distinct orifices. The alveolar secretory epithelium synthesizes the various milk constituents.

Colostrum

After delivery, the breasts begin to secrete colostrum, which is a deep lemon-yellow liquid. It usually can be expressed from the nipples by the second postpartum day. Compared with mature milk, colostrum contains more minerals and amino acids (Chuang and associates, 2005). It also has more protein, much of which is globulin, but less sugar and fat. Secretion persists for approximately 5 days, with gradual conversion to mature milk during the ensuing 4 weeks. Colostrum contains antibodies, and its content of immunoglobulin A (IgA) offers the newborn protection against enteric pathogens. Other host resistance factors found in colostrum and milk include complement, macrophages, lymphocytes, lactoferrin, lactoperoxidase, and lysozymes.

Milk

Human milk is a suspension of fat and protein in a carbohydrate-mineral solution. A nursing mother easily produces 600 mL of

Whey is milk serum and has been shown to contain large amounts of interleukin-6 (Saito and co-workers, 1991). It is associated closely with local IgA production by the breast. *Prolactin* appears to be actively secreted into breast milk (Yuen, 1988). *Epidermal growth factor (EGF)* has been identified in human milk, and because it is not destroyed by gastric proteolytic enzymes, it may be absorbed to promote growth and maturation of newborn intestinal mucosa (McCleary, 1991).

Endocrinology of Lactation

The precise humoral and neural mechanisms involved in lactation are complex. Progesterone, estrogen, and placental lactogen, as well as prolactin, cortisol, and insulin, appear to act in concert to stimulate the growth and development of the milk-secreting apparatus (Porter, 1974). With delivery, there is an abrupt and profound decrease in the levels of progesterone and estrogen. This decrease removes the inhibitory influence of progesterone on α-lactalbumin production by the rough endoplasmic reticulum. Increased α-lactalbumin stimulates lactose synthase to increase milk lactose. Progesterone withdrawal also allows prolactin to act unopposed in its stimulation of α-lactalbumin production.

The intensity and duration of subsequent lactation are controlled, in large part, by the repetitive stimulus of nursing. Prolactin is essential for lactation, and women with extensive pituitary necrosis—*Sheehan syndrome*—do not lactate (see Chap. 53, p. 1140). Although plasma prolactin levels fall after delivery to levels lower than during

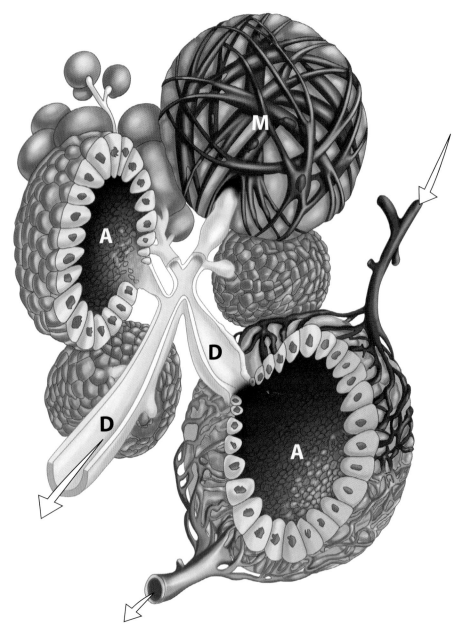

FIGURE 30-2 Graphic demonstration of the alveolar and ductal system. Note the myoepithelial fibers (*M*) that surround the outside of the uppermost alveolus. The secretions from the glandular elements are extruded into the lumen of the alveoli (*A*) and ejected by the myoepithelial cells into the ductal system (*D*), which empties through the nipple. Arterial blood supply to the alveolus is identified by the upper right arrow and venous drainage by the arrow beneath. (Redrawn from Dr. John C. Porter.)

milk daily, and maternal gestational weight gain has little impact on its quantity or quality (Institute of Medicine, 1990). Milk is isotonic with plasma, and lactose accounts for half of the osmotic pressure. Essential amino acids are derived from blood, and nonessential amino acids are derived in part from blood or synthesized in the mammary gland. Most milk proteins are unique and include α-lactalbumin, β-lactoglobulin, and casein. Fatty acids are synthesized in the alveoli from glucose and are secreted by an apocrine-like process. All vitamins except K are found in human milk, but in variable amounts. Vitamin D content is low—22 IU/mL, and newborn supplementation is recommended by the American Academy of Pediatrics (Wagner and colleagues, 2008).

pregnancy, each act of suckling triggers a rise in levels (McNeilly and associates, 1983). Presumably a stimulus from the breast curtails the release of dopamine (prolactin-inhibiting factor) from the hypothalamus, and this in turn transiently induces increased prolactin secretion.

The neurohypophysis secretes oxytocin in pulsatile fashion. This stimulates milk expression from a lactating breast by causing contraction of myoepithelial cells in the alveoli and small milk ducts (see Fig. 30-2). Milk ejection, or *letting down*, is a reflex initiated especially by suckling, which stimulates the neurohypophysis to liberate oxytocin. The reflex may even be provoked by an infant cry and can be inhibited by maternal fright or stress.

TABLE 30-2. Established and Potential Protective Effects on Infants of Human Milk and Breast Feeding

Decreased Incidence/Severity	Possible Protective Effects
Diarrhea	Sudden infant death syndrome
Lower respiratory infection	Type 1 diabetes
Otitis media	Inflammatory bowel disease
Bacteremia	Lymphoma
Bacterial meningitis	Allergies
Botulism	Chronic digestive diseases
Necrotizing enterocolitis	
Urinary infections	

From the American Academy of Pediatrics (1997).

Immunological Consequences of Breast Feeding

Antibodies in human colostrum and milk are poorly absorbed by infants. This does not lessen their importance because the predominant immunoglobulin is secretory IgA. This macromolecule is secreted across mucous membranes and has important antimicrobial functions. Milk contains secretory IgA antibodies against *Escherichia coli,* and breast-fed infants are less prone to enteric infections than bottle-fed infants (Cravioto and associates, 1991). Human milk also provides protection against rotavirus infections, which cause up to half of cases of infant gastroenteritis in this country (Newburg and associates, 1998). Breast feeding also likely reduces the risk of atopic dermatitis and wheezing illnesses in early childhood (Friedman and Zeiger, 2005).

Much attention has been directed to the role of maternal breast-milk lymphocytes in the immunological processes of the newborn. Milk contains both T and B lymphocytes, but the T lymphocytes appear to differ from those found in blood. Specifically, milk T lymphocytes are almost exclusively composed of cells that exhibit specific membrane antigens, including the LFA-1 high-memory T-cell phenotype. These memory T cells appear to be another avenue for the neonate to benefit from the maternal immunological experience (Bertotto and associates, 1990). Lymphocytes in colostrum undergo blastoid transformation in vitro following exposure to specific antigens.

Nursing

Human milk is ideal food for neonates. It provides age-specific nutrients as well as immunological factors and antibacterial substances (American College of Obstetricians and Gynecologists, 2007). Milk also contains factors that act as biological signals for promoting cellular growth and differentiation. The American Academy of Pediatrics (1997) has provided a list of benefits of nursing as outlined in Table 30-2. For both mother and infant, the benefits of breast feeding are likely long-term. For example, women who breast feed have a lower risk of breast cancer, and their children have increased adult intelligence independent of a wide range of possible confounding factors (Collaborative Group on Hormonal Factors in Breast Cancer, 2002; Kramer and associates, 2008). Breast feeding is associated with decreased postpartum weight retention (Baker and co-workers,

2008). Moreover, women in the Nurses' Health Study who reported breast feeding for at least two cumulative years had a 23-percent lower risk of coronary heart disease (Stuebe and colleagues, 2009).

Because of associated health benefits, one of the goals of the United States Public Health Service for year 2010 is to increase breast-feeding rates (Centers for Disease Control and Prevention, 2007b). Educational initiatives to include the father and peer counseling may improve these rates (Bonuck, 2005; Merewood, 2005; Pisacane, 2005; Wolfberg, 2004, and all their colleagues). Moreover, The Baby Friendly Hospital Initiative is an international program developed to increase rates of exclusive breast feeding and to extend its duration. It is based on the World Health Organization (1998) *Ten Steps to Successful Breast-feeding,* which are shown in Table 30-3. Worldwide, almost

TABLE 30-3. Ten Steps to Successful Breast Feeding

1. Have a written breast feeding policy that is regularly communicated to all healthcare staff
2. Train all staff in skills necessary to implement this policy
3. Inform all pregnant women about the benefits and management of breast feeding
4. Help mothers initiate breast feeding within an hour of birth
5. Show mothers how to breast feed and how to sustain lactation, even if they should be separated from their infants
6. Feed newborn infants nothing but breast milk, unless medically indicated, and under no circumstances provide breast milk substitutes, feeding bottles, or pacifiers free of charge or at low cost
7. Practice rooming-in, which allows mothers and infants to remain together 24 hours a day
8. Encourage breast feeding on demand
9. Give no artificial pacifiers to breast feeding infants
10. Help start breast feeding support groups and refer mothers to them

Adapted from the World Health Organization (1998).

20,000 hospitals are designated as "baby-friendly." There are also a variety of individual resources available for breast-feeding mothers that include online information from the American Academy of Pediatrics (http://www.aap.org) and La Leche League International (http://www.lalecheleague.org).

Breast Engorgement

Women who do not breast feed may experience engorgement, milk leakage, and breast pain, which peaks at 3 to 5 days after delivery (Spitz and associates, 1998). As many as half require analgesia for breast-pain relief. Up to 10 percent of women report severe pain up to 14 days.

Breasts should be supported with a well-fitting brassiere. Pharmacological or hormonal agents are not recommended to suppress lactation. Instead, ice packs and oral analgesics for 12 to 24 hours can be used to relieve discomfort. A breast binder is used at Parkland Hospital for these women, and a "sports bra" is used at the University of Alabama Hospital.

Milk Fever

Puerperal fever from breast engorgement is common. Before breast feeding was commonplace, Almeida and Kitay (1986) reported that 13 percent of postpartum women had fever that ranged from 37.8 to 39°C from engorgement. Fever seldom persisted for longer than 4 to 16 hours. The incidence and severity of engorgement, and fever associated with it, are much lower if women breast feed. Other causes of fever, especially those due to infection, must be excluded.

Contraception for Breast-Feeding Women

Ovulation may resume as early as 3 weeks after delivery, even in lactating women. Its timing depends on individual biological variation as well as the intensity of breast feeding. Progestin-only contraceptives—"mini-pills," depot medroxyprogesterone, or progestin implants—do not affect the quality or quantity of milk. Estrogen-progestin contraceptives likely reduce the quantity of breast milk, but under the proper circumstances, they too can be used by breast-feeding women. These hormonal methods are summarized in Table 30-4 and are discussed in Chapter 32 (p. 673).

Contraindications to Breast Feeding

Nursing is contraindicated in women who take street drugs or do not control their alcohol use; have an infant with galactosemia; have human immunodeficiency virus (HIV) infection; have active, untreated tuberculosis; take certain medications; or are undergoing treatment for breast cancer (American College of Obstetricians and Gynecologists, 2007). Breast feeding has been recognized for some time as a mode of HIV transmission. Nduati and colleagues (2000) randomly assigned 401 HIV-seropositive mother–infant pairs in Kenya to formula or breast feeding. At age 2 years, the rate of viral infection in breast-fed children was 37 percent—compared with 21 percent in formula-fed children.

Other viral infections do not contraindicate breast feeding. For example, with maternal cytomegalovirus infection, both

TABLE 30-4. Recommendations for Hormonal Contraception If Used by Breast-Feeding Women

- Progestin-only oral contraceptives prescribed or dispensed at discharge from the hospital to be started 2–3 weeks postpartum—for example, the first Sunday after the newborn is 2 weeks old
- Depot medroxyprogesterone acetate initiated at 6 weeks postpartum[a]
- Hormonal implants inserted at 6 weeks postpartum
- The levonorgestrel intrauterine system can be inserted at 6 weeks postpartum
- Combined estrogen-progestin contraceptives, if prescribed, should not be started before 6 weeks postpartum, and only when lactation is well established and the infant's nutritional status appropriate.

[a]There are certain clinical situations in which earlier initiation might be considered.
Reprinted, with permission, from American College of Obstetricians and Gynecologists. Breastfeeding: Maternal and infant aspects. ACOG Clin Rev 2007; 12 (1 suppl): 1-16.

virus and antibodies are present in breast milk. And although hepatitis B virus is excreted in milk, breast feeding is not contraindicated if hepatitis B immune globulin is given to these infants (American College of Obstetricians and Gynecologists, 2007). Maternal hepatitis C infection is not a contraindication because the 4-percent risk of infant transmission is the same for breast- and bottle-fed infants (Centers for Disease Control and Prevention, 1998). Women with active herpes simplex virus may suckle their infants if there are no breast lesions and if particular care is directed to hand washing before nursing.

Care of Breasts

The nipples require little attention other than cleanliness and attention to skin fissures. Fissured nipples render nursing painful, and they may have a deleterious influence on milk production. These cracks also provide a portal of entry for pyogenic bacteria. Because dried milk is likely to accumulate and irritate the nipples, washing the areola with water and mild soap is helpful before and after nursing. When the nipples are irritated or fissured, it may be necessary to use topical lanolin and a nipple shield for 24 hours or longer. If fissuring is severe, the infant should not be permitted to nurse on the affected side. Instead, the breast should be emptied regularly with a pump until the lesions are healed.

Proper technique for positioning the mother and infant during nursing has been reviewed by the American College of Obstetricians and Gynecologists (2007). This includes proper techniques for *latch-on* of the infant during suckling.

Drugs Secreted in Milk

Most drugs given to the mother are secreted in breast milk. However, the amount of drug ingested by the infant typically is small. Many factors influence drug excretion, including plasma

TABLE 30-5. Drugs That Have Been Associated with Significant Effects on Some Nursing Infants

Drug	Reported Effect[a]
Acebutolol	Hypotension, bradycardia, tachypnea
5-Aminosalicylic acid	Diarrhea (one case)
Atenolol	Cyanosis, bradycardia
Bromocriptine	Suppresses lactation, may be hazardous to the mother
Aspirin (salicylates)	Metabolic acidosis (one case)
Clemastine	Drowsiness, irritability, refusal to feed, high-pitched cry, neck stiffness (one case)
Ergotamine	Vomiting, diarrhea, convulsions—doses used in migraine medications
Lithium	A third to half therapeutic blood concentration in infants
Phenindione	Anticoagulant—increased prothrombin and partial thromboplastin time in one infant—not used in United States
Phenobarbital	Sedation; infantile spasms after weaning from milk containing phenobarbital; methemoglobinemia (one case)
Primidone	Sedation, feeding problems
Sulfasalazine	Bloody diarrhea (one case)

[a]Blood concentration in the infant may be of clinical importance.
Used with permission of the American Academy of Pediatrics, American College of Obstetricians and Gynecologists. Guidelines for perinatal care. 6th ed. Elk Grove Village (IL): AAP; Washington, DC: ACOG; 2007. Copyright American Academy of Pediatrics and American College of Obstetricans and Gynecologists, 2007.

concentration, degree of protein binding, plasma and milk pH, degree of ionization, lipid solubility, and molecular weight. The ratio of drug concentrations in breast milk to those in maternal plasma is the *milk-to-plasma drug-concentration ratio*. Most drugs have a milk-to-plasma ratio of 1 or less, about 25 percent have a ratio of more than 1, and about 15 percent have a ratio greater than 2 (Ito, 2000). Ideally, to minimize infant exposure, medication selection for the mother should favor drugs with a shorter half-life, poorer oral absorption, and lower lipid solubility. If multiple, daily drug doses are required, then each is taken by the mother *after* the closest feed. Single daily-dosed drugs may be taken just prior to the longest infant sleep interval—usually at bedtime (Spencer and co-workers, 2002).

There are only a few drugs that need to be avoided while breast feeding (Table 30-5). Cytotoxic drugs may interfere with cellular metabolism and potentially cause immune suppression or neutropenia, affect growth, or at least theoretically, increase the risk of childhood cancer. Examples include cyclophosphamide, cyclosporine, doxorubicin, and methotrexate. If a medication presents a concern, then the importance of therapy should be ascertained, as well as whether a safer alternative is available and whether neonatal exposure can be minimized if the medication dose is taken immediately after each breast feeding (American Academy of Pediatrics and the American College of Obstetricians and Gynecologists, 2007).

Radioactive isotopes of copper, gallium, indium, iodine, sodium, and technetium rapidly appear in breast milk. Consultation with a nuclear medicine specialist is recommended before performing a diagnostic study with these isotopes. The goal is to use a radionuclide with the shortest excretion time in breast milk. The

mother should pump her breasts before the study and store enough milk in a freezer for feeding the infant. After the study, she should pump her breasts to maintain milk production but discard all milk produced during the time that radioactivity is present. This ranges from 15 hours up to 2 weeks, depending on the isotope used.

Mastitis

Parenchymatous infection of the mammary glands is a rare complication antepartum but is estimated to develop in up to a third of breast-feeding women (Barbosa-Cesnik and associates, 2003). In our experiences, its incidence is much lower and probably less than 1 percent. Symptoms of suppurative mastitis seldom appear before the end of the first week postpartum and as a rule, not until the third or fourth week. Infection almost invariably is unilateral, and marked engorgement usually precedes inflammation. Symptoms include chills or actual rigor, which are soon followed by fever and tachycardia. The breast becomes hard and reddened, and there is severe pain. About 10 percent of women with mastitis develop an abscess. Detection of fluctuation may be difficult, and sonography may be helpful to detect an abscess.

Etiology

In earlier studies, *Staphylococcus aureus* was the most commonly isolated organism. Matheson and colleagues (1988) reported it in 40 percent of women with mastitis. Other commonly isolated organisms are coagulase-negative staphylococci and viridans streptococci. The immediate source of organisms that cause mastitis is almost always the infant's nose and throat. Bacteria enter the breast through the nipple at the site of a fissure or small abrasion.

The infecting organism can usually be cultured from milk. Toxic shock syndrome from mastitis caused by *S. aureus* has been reported (Demey and associates, 1989; Fujiwara and Endo, 2001).

At times, suppurative mastitis reaches epidemic levels among nursing mothers. Such outbreaks most often coincide with the appearance of a new strain of antibiotic-resistant staphylococcus. A contemporaneous example is community-acquired methicillin-resistant *S. aureus* (CA-MRSA), which has rapidly become the most commonly isolated staphylococcal species in some areas (Klevens and co-workers, 2007; Pallin and colleagues, 2008). At Parkland Hospital from 2000 to 2004, Laibl and associates (2005) reported that a fourth of CA-MRSA isolates were from women with puerperal mastitis. Hospital-acquired MRSA may cause mastitis when the infant becomes colonized after hand contact with nursery personnel who are colonized. In turn, these infants may spread CA-MRSA (Centers for Disease Control and Prevention, 2006). Stafford and colleagues (2008) noted a higher incidence of subsequent abscess in those with CA-MRSA-associated mastitis.

Treatment

Provided that appropriate therapy for mastitis is started before suppuration begins, the infection usually resolves within 48 hours. Abscess formation is more common with *S. aureus* infection (Matheson and associates, 1988). Most recommend that milk be expressed from the affected breast onto a swab and cultured before beginning therapy. Bacterial identification and antimicrobial sensitivities provide information mandatory for a successful surveillance program of nosocomial infections.

The initial antimicrobial choice is influenced by the current experience with staphylococcal infections at the institution. Although most are community-acquired organisms, as discussed above, these frequently include CA-MRSA. Dicloxacillin, 500 mg orally four times daily, may be started empirically. Erythromycin is given to women who are penicillin sensitive. If the infection is caused by resistant, penicillinase-producing staphylococci, or if resistant organisms are suspected while awaiting the results of culture, then vancomycin or another anti-MRSA antimicrobial should be given. Even though clinical response may be prompt, treatment should be continued for 10 to 14 days.

Marshall and colleagues (1975) demonstrated the importance of continued breast feeding. They reported that the only three abscesses that developed in 65 women with mastitis were in 15 women who quit breast feeding. Thomsen and co-workers (1984) observed that vigorous milk expression was sufficient treatment alone. Sometimes the infant will not nurse on the inflamed breast. This probably is not related to any changes in the milk taste but is secondary to engorgement and edema, which can make the areola harder to grip. Pumping can alleviate this. When nursing bilaterally, it is best to begin suckling on the uninvolved breast. This allows let-down to commence before moving to the tender breast.

Breast Abscess

In a population-based study of nearly 1.5 million Swedish women, the incidence of breast abscess was 0.1 percent (Kvist and Rydhstroem, 2005). An abscess should be suspected when defervescence does not follow within 48 to 72 hours of mastitis treatment, or when a mass is palpable. Traditional therapy is surgical drainage, which usually requires general anesthesia. The incision should be made corresponding to Langer skin lines for a cosmetic result (Stehman, 1990). In early cases, a single incision over the most dependent portion of fluctuation is usually sufficient, but multiple abscesses require several incisions and disruption of loculations. The resulting cavity is loosely packed with gauze, which should be replaced at the end of 24 hours by a smaller pack. A less invasive alternative is sonographic-guided needle aspiration using local anesthesia, which has success rates of 80 to 90 percent (O'Hara and colleagues, 1996; Schwarz and Shrestha, 2001).

Galactocele

Occasionally a milk duct becomes obstructed by inspissated secretions, and milk may accumulate in one or more mammary lobes. The amount is ordinarily limited, but an excess may form a fluctuant mass—a galactocele—that may cause pressure symptoms and have the appearance of an abscess. It may resolve spontaneously or require aspiration.

Accessory Breast Tissue

Extra breasts—*polymastia*, or extra nipples—*polythelia*, may develop along the former embryonic mammary ridge. Also termed the *milk line*, this line extends from the axilla to the groin bilaterally. The incidence of accessory breast tissue ranges from 0.22 to 6 percent in the general population (Loukas and colleagues, 2007). Breasts may be so small as to be mistaken for pigmented moles, or when without a nipple, for lymphadenopathy or a lipoma. Polymastia has no obstetrical significance, although occasionally their enlargement during pregnancy or engorgement postpartum may result in discomfort and anxiety.

Nipples

Occasionally lactiferous ducts open directly into a depression at the center of the areola. With these depressed nipples, nursing is difficult. If the depression is not deep, milk sometimes can be made available by use of a breast pump. If instead the nipple is greatly inverted, daily attempts should be made during the last few months of pregnancy to draw the nipple out with the fingers.

Abnormalities of Secretion

There are marked individual variations in the amount of milk secreted. Many of these are dependent not on general maternal health but on breast glandular development. Rarely, there is complete lack of mammary secretion—*agalactia*. Occasionally, mammary secretion is excessive—*polygalactia*.

CARE OF THE MOTHER DURING THE PUERPERIUM

Hospital Care

For the first hour after delivery, blood pressure and pulse should be taken every 15 minutes, or more frequently if indicated. The amount of vaginal bleeding is monitored, and the fundus palpated to ensure that it is well contracted. If relaxation is detected, the uterus should be massaged through the abdominal wall until it remains contracted. The addition of uterotonins is sometimes required. Blood may accumulate within the uterus without external bleeding. This may be detected early by detecting uterine enlargement during fundal palpation in the first postdelivery hours. Because the likelihood of significant hemorrhage is greatest immediately postpartum, even in normal cases, the uterus is closely monitored for at least 1 hour after delivery. Postpartum hemorrhage is discussed in Chapter 35 (p. 773).

If regional analgesia or general anesthesia is used for labor or delivery, the mother should be observed in an appropriately equipped and staffed recovery area.

Early Ambulation

Women are out of bed within a few hours after delivery. An attendant should be present for at least the first time, in case the woman becomes syncopal. The many confirmed advantages of early ambulation include fewer bladder complications and less frequent constipation. Early ambulation has reduced the frequency of puerperal venous thrombosis and pulmonary embolism (see Chap. 47, p. 1019).

Perineal Care

The woman is instructed to cleanse the vulva from anterior to posterior—the vulva toward the anus. An ice bag applied to the perineum may help reduce edema and discomfort during the first several hours if there is a laceration or an episiotomy. Most women also appear to obtain a measure of relief from the periodic application of a local anesthetic spray. Severe discomfort usually indicates a problem, such as a hematoma within the first day or so, and infection after the third or fourth day (see Chap. 35, p. 783). **Severe perineal, vaginal, or rectal pain always warrants careful inspection and palpation.** Beginning approximately 24 hours after delivery, moist heat as provided with warm sitz baths can be used to reduce local discomfort. Tub bathing after uncomplicated delivery is allowed. The episiotomy incision normally is firmly healed and nearly asymptomatic by the third week.

Bladder Function

Bladder filling after delivery may be variable. In most units, intravenous fluids are infused during labor and for an hour after delivery. Oxytocin, in doses that have an antidiuretic effect, is commonly infused postpartum, and rapid bladder filling is common. Moreover, both bladder sensation and capability to empty spontaneously may be diminished by local or conduction analgesia, by episiotomy or lacerations, and by instrumented delivery. Thus, urinary retention with bladder overdistension is common in the early puerperium. Ching-Chung and colleagues (2002) reported retention in 4 percent of women delivered vaginally. Musselwhite and associates (2007) reported retention in 4.7 percent of women who had labor epidural analgesia. Risk factors that increased likelihood of retention were primiparity, oxytocin-induced or -augmented labor, perineal lacerations, instrumented delivery, catheterization during labor, and labor with duration over 10 hours.

Prevention of bladder overdistension demands observation after delivery to ensure that the bladder does not overfill and that with each voiding, it empties adequately. The enlarged bladder can be palpated suprapubically, or it is evident abdominally indirectly as it elevates the fundus above the umbilicus. Van Os and Van der Linden (2006) have investigated the use of an automated sonography system to detect high bladder volumes and thus postpartum urinary retention.

Management

If a woman has not voided within 4 hours after delivery, it is likely that she cannot. If she has trouble voiding initially, she also is likely to have further trouble. An examination for perineal and genital-tract hematomas is made. With an overdistended bladder, an indwelling catheter should be left in place until the factors causing retention have abated. Even without a demonstrable cause, it usually is best to leave the catheter in place for at least 24 hours. This prevents recurrence and allows recovery of normal bladder tone and sensation.

When the catheter is removed, it is necessary subsequently to demonstrate ability to void appropriately. If a woman cannot void after 4 hours, she should be catheterized and the urine volume measured. If more than 200 mL, the bladder is not functioning appropriately, and the catheter is left for another day. If less than 200 mL of urine is obtained, the catheter can be removed and the bladder rechecked subsequently as described. Harris and colleagues (1977) reported that 40 percent of such women develop bacteriuria, and thus, a single-dose or short course of antimicrobial therapy is reasonable after the catheter is removed.

Subsequent Discomfort

Discomfort and its causes following cesarean delivery are considered in Chapter 25 (p. 561). During the first few days after vaginal delivery, the mother may be uncomfortable for a variety of reasons, including afterpains, episiotomy and lacerations, breast engorgement, and at times, postdural puncture headache. Mild analgesics containing codeine, aspirin, or acetaminophen, preferably in combinations, are given as frequently as every 3 hours during the first few days.

Depression

It is fairly common for a mother to exhibit some degree of depressed mood a few days after delivery. Termed *postpartum blues,* this likely is the consequence of a number of factors that include emotional letdown that follows the excitement and fears experienced during pregnancy and delivery, discomforts of the early puerperium, fatigue from sleep deprivation, anxiety over the ability to provide appropriate infant care, and body image concerns.

In most women, effective treatment includes anticipation, recognition, and reassurance. This disorder is usually mild and self-limited to 2 to 3 days, although it sometimes lasts for up to 10 days. Should these moods persist or worsen, evaluation is done for symptoms of major depression. Gavin and associates (2005) in a systematic review found depression in almost 20 percent of postpartum women. A recent analysis of the PRAMS database reported its prevalence to range from 12 to 20 percent in 17 states (Centers for Disease Control and Prevention, 2008). In a state-wide study from New Jersey, low-income women with pregestational or gestational diabetes had a twofold risk of perinatal or postpartum depression (Kozhimannil and colleagues,

2009). In women with preexisting psychiatric disorders, the first month after childbirth is associated with increased risk of psychiatric readmission (Munk-Olsen and co-workers, 2009). Further evaluation and management is discussed in Chapter 55 (p. 1176). Suicidal or infanticidal ideation is dealt with emergently. Because major postpartum depression recurs in at least a fourth of women in subsequent pregnancies, some recommend pharmacological prophylaxis beginning in late pregnancy or immediately postpartum (Wisner and co-workers, 2004).

Abdominal Wall Relaxation

If the abdomen is unusually flabby or pendulous, an ordinary girdle is often satisfactory. An abdominal binder is at best a temporary measure. Exercises to restore abdominal wall tone may be started anytime after vaginal delivery and as soon as abdominal soreness diminishes after cesarean delivery.

Diet

There are no dietary restrictions for women who have been delivered vaginally. Two hours after a normal vaginal delivery, if there are no complications, a woman should be allowed to eat. With breast feeding, the number of calories and protein consumed during pregnancy should be increased slightly as recommended by the Food and Nutrition Board of the National Research Council (see Chap. 8, p. 202). If the mother does not breast feed, dietary requirements are the same as for a nonpregnant woman.

It is standard practice in our hospitals to continue iron supplementation for at least 3 months after delivery and to check the hematocrit at the first postpartum visit.

Thromboembolic Disease

The frequency of deep-venous thrombosis and pulmonary embolism complicating pregnancy and the puerperium has decreased in recent years (see Chap. 47, p. 1019). Almost half of thromboembolic events associated with pregnancy develop in the puerperium. Jacobsen and colleagues (2008) recently reported that pulmonary embolism is most common in the first 6 weeks postpartum.

Neuromuscular and Joint Problems

Pain in the pelvic girdle, hips, or lower extremities may be due to stretching or tearing injuries sustained at normal or difficult delivery.

Obstetrical Neuropathies

Pressure on branches of the lumbosacral nerve plexus during labor may be manifest by complaints of intense neuralgia or cramplike pains extending down one or both legs as soon as the head descends into the pelvis. If the nerve is injured, pain may continue after delivery, and there also may be variable degrees of sensory loss or muscle paralysis. In some cases, there is footdrop, which can be secondary to injury at the level of the lumbosacral root, lumbosacral plexus, sciatic nerve, or common fibular (peroneal) nerve. Components of the lumbosacral plexus cross the pelvic brim and can be compressed by the fetal head or by forceps. The common fibular nerves may be externally compressed when the legs are positioned in stirrups, especially during a prolonged second stage of labor.

The incidence of obstetrical neuropathy is relatively common. Wong and colleagues (2003) evaluated more than 6000 consecutively delivered women at Northwestern University and found that approximately 1 percent had a confirmed nerve injury. Lateral femoral cutaneous neuropathies were the most common (24), followed by femoral neuropathies (14). A motor deficit accompanied a third of injuries. Nulliparity, prolonged second-stage labor, and pushing for a long duration in the semi-Fowler position were risk factors. The median duration of symptoms was 2 months, and the range was 2 weeks to 18 months.

Muscle Injuries

Pelvic or hip muscles and tendons can be stretched, torn, or separated during even normal labor. If nerve injury is excluded, we have found that magnetic resonance (MR) imaging is informative. An example is shown in Figure 30-3. Most of these resolve with antiinflammatory agents and physical therapy. Rarely, there may be septic pyomyositis as described by Sokolov and colleagues (2007).

Pelvic Bone and Joint Problems

Separation of the symphysis pubis or one of the sacroiliac synchondroses during labor may be followed by pain and marked

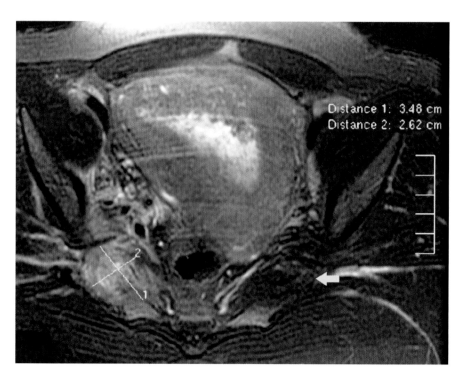

FIGURE 30-3 Magnetic resonance image of a piriformis hematoma. A large inhomogeneous mass of the right piriformis muscle consistent with a hematoma (*yellow cursor measurements*) is compared with the normal appearing left piriformis muscle (*yellow arrow*).

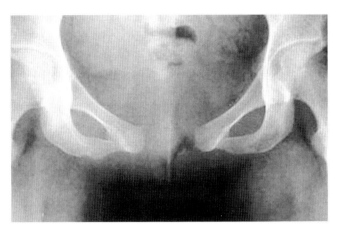

FIGURE 30-4 Radiograph demonstrating a 5-cm pubic diastasis immediately after vaginal delivery. Pain diminished over several weeks. Six months later, a repeat radiograph showed a 1-cm symphyseal gap. (Reprinted from Chang D and Markman BS: Spontaneous resolution of a pubic-symphysis diastasis. *N Engl J Med* 346:39, with permission. Copyright © 2002 Massachusetts Medical Society. All rights reserved.)

interference with locomotion (Fig. 30-4). Estimates of their frequency vary widely from 1 in 600 to 1 in 30,000 deliveries (Reis and colleagues, 1932; Taylor and Sonson, 1986). In our experiences, symptomatic separations are uncommon. When they are symptomatic, the onset of pain is often acute during delivery, but symptoms may manifest either antepartum or up to 48 hours postpartum (Snow and Neubert, 1997). Treatment is generally conservative, with rest in a lateral decubitus position and an appropriately fitted pelvic binder. Surgery is occasionally necessary in some symphyseal separations of more than 4 cm (Kharrazi and colleagues, 1997). Recurrence is more than 50 percent in subsequent pregnancy, and Culligan and associates (2002) recommend consideration of cesarean delivery. In some cases, fractures of the sacrum or pubic ramus are caused by even uncomplicated deliveries (Alonso-Burgos and colleagues, 2007). The latter are more likely with osteoporosis associated with heparin or corticosteroid therapy (Cunningham, 2005). This is discussed further in Chapter 53.

Immunizations

The D-negative woman who is not isoimmunized and whose infant is D-positive is given 300 μg of anti-D immune globulin shortly after delivery (see Chap. 29, p. 624). Women who are not already immune to rubella or rubeola measles are excellent candidates for combined measles-mumps-rubella vaccination before discharge (see Chap. 8, p. 208). Unless contraindicated, a diphtheria-tetanus toxoid booster injection is also given to postpartum women prior to discharge at Parkland Hospital.

Time of Discharge

Following uncomplicated vaginal delivery, hospitalization is seldom warranted for more than 48 hours. A woman should receive instructions concerning anticipated normal physiological changes of the puerperium, including lochia patterns, weight loss from diuresis, and milk let-down. She also should receive instructions concerning fever, excessive vaginal bleeding, or leg pain, swelling, or tenderness. Shortness of breath or chest pain warrants immediate concern.

Early Discharge

The length of hospital stays following labor and delivery is now regulated by federal law. Currently, the norms are hospital stays of up to 48 hours following uncomplicated vaginal delivery and up to 96 hours following uncomplicated cesarean delivery (American Academy of Pediatrics and the American College of Obstetricians and Gynecologists, 2007). Earlier hospital discharge is acceptable for appropriately selected women if they desire it.

Contraception

During the hospital stay, a concerted effort should be made to provide family planning education. Steroidal contraception and its effects on lactation are discussed in Chapter 32 (p. 694). Other forms of contraception are discussed throughout Chapter 32 and sterilization procedures in Chapter 33.

If a woman is not breast feeding, menses usually return within 6 to 8 weeks. At times, however, it is difficult clinically to assign a specific date to the first menstrual period after delivery. Only about 20 percent of women ovulate preceding the first menses (Hytten, 1995). A minority of women bleed small to moderate amounts intermittently, starting soon after delivery. Ovulation occurs at a mean of 7 weeks, but ranges from 5 to 11 weeks (Perez and associates, 1972). That said, ovulation before 28 days has been described (Hytten, 1995). Thus, conception is possible during the artificially defined 6-week puerperium. **Women who become sexually active during the puerperium, and who do not desire to conceive should initiate contraception.** This message is not universally delivered to women, nor is it always heeded. For example, Kelly and associates (2005) reported that by the third month postpartum, 58 percent of adolescents had resumed sexual intercourse, but only 80 percent of these were using contraception.

Breast Feeding and Ovulation

Women who breast feed ovulate much less frequently compared with those who do not, and there are great variations. Lactating women may first menstruate as early as the second or as late as the 18th month after delivery. Campbell and Gray (1993) analyzed daily urine specimens to determine the time of ovulation in 92 women. As shown in Figure 30-5, breast feeding in general delays resumption of ovulation, although as already emphasized, it does not invariably forestall it. Other findings in their study included the following:

1. Resumption of ovulation was frequently marked by return of normal menstrual bleeding
2. Breast-feeding episodes lasting 15 minutes seven times each day delayed resumption of ovulation
3. Ovulation can occur without bleeding
4. Bleeding can be anovulatory
5. The risk of pregnancy in breast-feeding women was approximately 4 percent per year

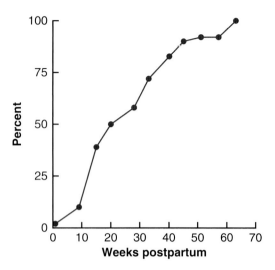

FIGURE 30-5 Cumulative proportion of breast-feeding women who ovulated during the first 70 weeks following delivery. (Data from Campbell and Gray, 1993.)

HOME CARE

Coitus

There are no evidence-based rules concerning resumption of coitus after delivery. It seems best to use common sense. After 2 weeks, coitus may be resumed *based on desire and comfort.* Barrett and colleagues (2000) reported that almost 90 percent of 484 primiparous women resumed sexual activity by 6 months. And although 65 percent of these reported problems, only 15 percent discussed them with a healthcare provider.

Intercourse *too soon* may be unpleasant, if not frankly painful, due to incomplete healing of the episiotomy or lacera-

tions. Moreover, the vaginal epithelium is thin and very little lubrication follows sexual stimulation. This likely is due to the hypoestrogenic state following delivery and lasting until ovulation resumes. It may be particularly problematic in breast-feeding women who are hypoestrogenic for many months postpartum (Palmer and Likis, 2003; Wisniewski and Wilkinson, 1991). For treatment, small amounts of topical estrogen cream can be applied daily for several weeks to vaginal and vulvar tissues. Additionally, vaginal lubricants may be used with coitus.

Late Maternal Morbidity

Taken together, major and minor maternal morbidity are surprisingly common in the months following childbirth (MacArthur and colleagues, 1991). In a survey of 1249 British mothers followed for up to 18 months, 3 percent required hospital readmission within 8 weeks (Glazener and co-workers, 1995). Milder health problems during the first 8 weeks were reported by 87 percent. And as shown in Table 30-6, almost three fourths continued to have a variety of problems for up to 18 months. Thus, although reported problems declined with time, they did so more slowly than generally assumed. Further reports by Lydon-Rochelle (2001), McGovern (2006), Thompson (2002), and all their colleagues described similar findings. From the foregoing, maternal morbidity following delivery is common, and at least historically, it was underappreciated. These studies called for a greater awareness of the needs of women as they convalesce from birthing.

Postpartum Follow-Up Care

By discharge, women who had an uncomplicated course can resume most activities, including bathing, driving, and household functions. Jimenez and Newton (1979) tabulated cross-cultural

TABLE 30-6. Puerperal Morbidity in Percent Reported by Women after Hospital Discharge

Morbidity	By 8 Weeks Postpartum	2 to 18 Months Postpartum
Feeling tired	59	54
Breast problems	36	20
Anemia	25	7
Backache	24	20
Hemorrhoids	23	15
Headache	22	15
Tearfulness/depression	21	17
Constipation	20	7
Suture breakdown	16	—
Vaginal discharge	15	8
Others[a]	2–7	1–8
At least one of the above	87	76

[a]Includes abnormal bleeding, urinary incontinence or infection, difficulty voiding, and hypertension.
Reproduced from *BJOG*, Vol. 102, Issue 4, CMA Glazener, M Abdalla, P Stroud, A Templeton, IT Russell, and S Naji, Postnatal maternal morbidity: Extent, causes, prevention and treatment, 282–287, 1995, with the permission of the Royal College of Obstetricians and Gynaecologists.

information on 202 societies from different international geographic regions. Following childbirth, most societies did not restrict work activity, and approximately half expected a return to full duties within 2 weeks. Tulman and Fawcett (1988) later reported that only half of mothers regained their usual level of energy by 6 weeks postpartum. Women who delivered vaginally were twice as likely to have normal energy levels at this time compared with those with a cesarean delivery. Ideally, the care and nurturing of the infant should be provided by the mother with ample help from the father.

The American Academy of Pediatrics and the American College of Obstetricians and Gynecologists (2007) recommend a postpartum visit between 4 and 6 weeks. This has proven quite satisfactory to identify abnormalities beyond the immediate puerperium as well as to initiate contraceptive practices. The Centers for Disease Control and Prevention (2007c) recently reported follow-up data from the Pregnancy Risk Assessment Monitoring System (PRAMS) database. Although overall compliance with postpartum visits was 90 percent, it ranged from 65 to 80 percent in adolescents, poorly educated or indigent women, and those with no prenatal care.

REFERENCES

Ahdoot D, Van Nostrand KM, Nguyen NJ, et al: The effect of route of delivery on regression of abnormal cervical cytologic findings in the postpartum period. Am J Obstet Gynecol 178:1116, 1998

Almeida OD Jr, Kitay DZ: Lactation suppression and puerperal fever. Am J Obstet Gynecol 154:940, 1986

Alonso-Burgos A, Royo P, Diaz L, et al: Labor-related sacral and pubic fractures. J Bone Joint Surg 89:396, 2007

American Academy of Pediatrics, American College of Obstetricians and Gynecologists: Guidelines for Perinatal Care, 6th ed. American Academy of Pediatrics, Elk Grove Village, IL; American College of Obstetricians and Gynecologists, Washington, DC, 2007, pp 171, 242

American Academy of Pediatrics, Work Group on Breastfeeding. Breastfeeding and the use of human milk. Pediatrics 100:1035, 1997

American College of Obstetricians and Gynecologists: Postpartum hemorrhage. Practice Bulletin 76, October 2006

American College of Obstetricians and Gynecologists Clinical Review. Special Report from ACOG. Breastfeeding: Maternal and infant aspects. 2007

Anderson WR, Davis J: Placental site involution. Am J Obstet Gynecol 102:23, 1968

Andrew AC, Bulmer JN, Wells M, et al: Subinvolution of the uteroplacental arteries in the human placental bed. Histopathology 15:395, 1989

Andrews MC: Epithelial changes in the puerperal fallopian tube. Am J Obstet Gynecol 62:28, 1951

Baker JL, Gamborg M, Heitmann BL, et al: Breastfeeding reduces postpartum weight retention. Am J Clin Nutr 88(6):1543, 2008

Barbosa-Cesnik C, Schwartz K, Foxman B: Lactation mastitis. JAMA 289:1609, 2003

Barrett G, Pendry E, Peacock J, et al: Women's sexual health after childbirth. BJOG 107:186, 2000

Bertotto A, Gerli R, Fabietti G, et al: Human breast milk T lymphocytes display the phenotype and functional characteristics of memory T cells. Eur J Immunol 20:1877, 1990

Bonuck KA, Trombley M, Freeman K, et al: Randomized, controlled trial of a prenatal and postnatal lactation consultant intervention on duration and intensity of breastfeeding up to 12 months. Pediatrics 116:1413, 2005

Buhimschi CS, Buhimschi IA, Manlinow AM, et al: Myometrial thickness during human labor and immediately post partum. Am J Obstet Gynecol 188:553, 2003

Campbell OMR, Gray RH: Characteristics and determinants of postpartum ovarian function in women in the United States. Am J Obstet Gynecol 169:55, 1993

Centers for Disease Control and Prevention: Recommendations for prevention and control of hepatitis C virus (HCV) infection and HCV-related chronic disease. MMWR 47:1, 1998

Centers for Disease Control and Prevention: Community-associated methicillin-resistant *Staphylococcus aureus* infection among healthy newborns—Chicago and Los Angeles County, 2004. MMWR 55:329, 2006

Centers for Disease Control and Prevention: Pregnancy risk assessment monitoring system (PRAMS). http://www.cdc.gov/prams/ Modified June 2007a

Centers for Disease Control and Prevention: Breastfeeding trends and updated national health objectives for exclusive breastfeeding—United States, birth years 2000—2004. MMWR 56:760, 2007b

Centers for Disease Control and Prevention: Postpartum care visits—11 states and New York City, 2004. MMWR 56:1312, 2007c

Centers for Disease Control and Prevention: Prevalence of self-reported postpartum depressive symptoms—17 states, 2004-2005. MMWR 57:361, 2008

Chang D, Markman BS: Spontaneous resolution of a pubic-symphysis diastasis. N Engl J Med 346:39, 2002

Chesley LC, Valenti C, Uichano L: Alterations in body fluid compartments and exchangeable sodium in early puerperium. Am J Obstet Gynecol 77:1054, 1959

Chiarelli P, Cockburn J: Promoting urinary continence in women after delivery: Randomised controlled trial. BMJ 324:1241, 2002

Ching-Chung L, Shuenn-Dhy C, Ling-Hong T, et al: Postpartum urinary retention: Assessment of contributing factors and long-term clinical impact. Aust N Z J Obstet Gynaecol 42:365, 2002

Chuang CK, Lin SP, Lee HC, et al: Free amino acids in full-term and preterm human milk and infant formula. J Pediatr Gastroenterol Nutr 40:496, 2005

Collaborative Group on Hormonal Factors in Breast Cancer: Breast cancer and breastfeeding: Collaborative reanalysis of individual data from 47 epidemiological studies in 30 countries, including 50,302 women with breast cancer and 96,973 women without the disease. Lancet 360:187, 2002

Cravioto A, Tello A, Villafan H, et al: Inhibition of localized adhesion of enteropathogenic *Escherichia coli* to HEp-2 cells by immunoglobulin and oligosaccharide fractions of human colostrum and breast milk. J Infect Dis 163:1247, 1991

Culligan P, Hill S, Heit M: Rupture of the symphysis pubis during vaginal delivery followed by two subsequent uneventful pregnancies. Obstet Gynecol 100:1114, 2002

Cunningham FG: Screening for osteoporosis. N Engl J Med 353(18):1975, 2005

Demers C, Derzko C, David M, et al: Gynaecological and obstetric management of women with inherited bleeding disorders. J Obstet Gynaecol Can 27:707, 2005

Demey HE, Hautekeete MI, Buytaert P, et al: Mastitis and toxic shock syndrome. A case report. Acta Obstet Gynecol Scand 68:87, 1989

Friedman NJ and Zeiger RS: The role of breast-feeding in the development of allergies and asthma. J Allerg Clin Immunol 115:1238, 2005

Fujiwara Y, Endo S: A case of toxic shock syndrome secondary to mastitis caused by methicillin-resistant *Staphylococcus aureus*. Kansenshogaku Zasshi 75:898, 2001

Funnell JW, Klawans AH, Cottrell TLC: The postpartum bladder. Am J Obstet Gynecol 67:1249, 1954

Gavin NI, Gaynes BN, Lohr KN, et al: Perinatal depression. A systematic review of prevalence and incidence. Obstet Gynecol 106:1071, 2005

Glazener CM, Abdalla M, Stroud P, et al: Postnatal maternal morbidity: Extent, causes, prevention and treatment. Br J Obstet Gynaecol 102:282, 1995

Harris RE, Thomas VL, Hui GW: Postpartum surveillance for urinary tract infection: Patients at risk of developing pyelonephritis after catheterization. South Med J 70:1273, 1977

Holdcroft A, Snidvongs S, Cason A, et al: Pain and uterine contractions during breast feeding in the immediate post-partum period increase with parity. Pain 104:589, 2003

Hytten F: The Clinical Physiology of the Puerperium. London, Farrand Press, 1995

Institute of Medicine: Nutrition During Pregnancy. Washington, DC, National Academy of Science, 1990, p 202

Ito S: Drug therapy for breast-feeding women. N Engl J Med 343:118, 2000

Jacobsen AF, Skjeldestad FE, Sandset PM: Incidence and risk patterns of venous thromboembolism in pregnancy and puerperium—a register-based case-control study. Am J Obstet Gynecol 198:233, 2008

Jimenez MH, Newton N: Activity and work during pregnancy and the postpartum period: A cross-cultural study of 202 societies. Am J Obstet Gynecol 135:171, 1979

Kanotra S, D'Angelo D, Phares TM, et al: Challenges faced by new mothers in the early postpartum period: An analysis of comment data from the 2000 pregnancy risk assessment monitoring system (PRAMS) survey. Matern Child Health J 11(6):549, 2007

Kelly LS, Sheeder J, Stevens-Simon C: Why lightning strikes twice: Postpartum resumption of sexual activity during adolescence. J Pediatr Adolesc Gynecol 18:327, 2005

Kharrazi FD, Rodgers WB, Kennedy JG, et al: Parturition-induced pelvic dislocation: A report of four cases. J Orthop Trauma 11:277, 1997

Klevens RM, Morrison MA, Nadle J, et al: Invasive methicillin-resistant *Staphylococcus aureus* infections in the United States. JAMA 298:1763, 2007

Kozhimannil KB, Pereira MA, Harlow BL: Association between diabetes and perinatal depression among low-income mothers. JAMA 301(8):842, 2009

Kramer MS, Aboud F, Mironova E, et al: Breastfeeding and child cognitive development: New evidence from a large randomized trial. Arch Gen Psychiatry 65(5):578, 2008

Kvist LJ, Rydhstroem H: Factors related to breast abscess after delivery: A population-based study. BJOG 112:1070, 2005

Laibl VR, Sheffield JS, Roberts S, et al: Clinical presentation of community-acquired methicillin-resistant *Staphylococcus aureus* in pregnancy. Obstet Gynecol 106:461, 2005

Lee CY, Madrazo B, Drukker BH: Ultrasonic evaluation of the postpartum uterus in the management of postpartum bleeding. Obstet Gynecol 58:227, 1981

Loukas M, Clarke P, Tubbs RS: Accessory breasts: A historical and current perspective. Am Surg 73(5):525, 2007

Lydon-Rochelle MT, Holt VL, Martin DP: Delivery method and self-reported postpartum general health status among primiparous women. Paediatr Perinat Epidemiol 15:232, 2001

MacArthur C, Glazener C, Wilson PD, et al: Persistent urinary incontinence and delivery mode history: A six-year longitudinal study. Br J Obstet Gynaecol 113:218, 2006

MacArthur C, Lewis M, Knox EG: Health after childbirth. Br J Obstet Gynaecol 98:1193, 1991

Marshall BR, Hepper JK, Zirbel CC: Sporadic puerperal mastitis—an infection that need not interrupt lactation. JAMA 344:1377, 1975

Matheson I, Aursnes I, Horgen M, et al: Bacteriological findings and clinical symptoms in relation to clinical outcome in puerperal mastitis. Acta Obstet Gynecol Scand 67:723, 1988

McCleary MJ: Epidermal growth factor: An important constituent of human milk. J Hum Lact 7:123, 1991

McGovern P, Dowd B, Gjerdingen D, et al: Postpartum health of employed mothers 5 weeks after childbirth. Ann Fam Med 4:159, 2006

McNeilly AS, Robinson ICA, Houston MJ, et al: Release of oxytocin and prolactin in response to suckling. BMJ (Clin Res Ed) 286:257, 1983

Merewood A, Mehta SD, Chamberlain LB, et al: Breastfeeding rates in U.S. baby-friendly hospitals: Results of a national survey. Pediatrics 116:628, 2005

Munk-Olsen T, Laursen TM, Mendelson T, et al: Risks and predictors of readmission for a mental disorder during the postpartum period. Arch Gen Psychiatry 66(2):189, 2009

Musselwhite KL, Faris P, Moore K, et al: Use of epidural anesthesia and the risk of acute postpartum urinary retention. Am J Obstet Gynecol 196:472, 2007

Nduati R, John G, Mbori-Ngacha D, et al: Effect of breastfeeding and formula feeding on transmission of HIV-1: A randomized clinical trial. JAMA 283:1167, 2000

Newburg DS, Peterson JA, Ruiz-Palacias GM, et al: Role of human-milk lactadherin in protection against symptomatic rotavirus infection. Lancet 351:1160, 1998

O'Hara RJ, Dexter SPL, Fox JN: Conservative management of infective mastitis and breast abscesses after ultrasonographic assessment. Br J Surg 83:1413, 1996

Olson CM, Strawderman MS, Hinton PS, et al: Gestational weight gain and postpartum behavior associated with weight change from early pregnancy to 1 y postpartum. Int J Obes Relat Metab Disord 27:117, 2003

Pallin DJ, Egan DJ, Pelletier AJ, et al: Increased U.S. emergency department visits for skin and soft tissue infections, and changes in antibiotic choices, during the emergence of community-associated methicillin-resistant *Staphylococcus aureus*. Ann Emerg Med 51:291, 2008

Palmer AR, Likis FE: Lactational atrophic vaginitis. J Midwifery Womens Health 48:282, 2003

Perez A, Vela P, Masnick GS, et al: First ovulation after childbirth: The effect of breastfeeding. Am J Obstet Gynecol 114:1041, 1972

Pisacane A, Continisio GI, Aldinucci M, et al: A controlled trial of the father's role in breastfeeding promotion. Pediatrics 116:e494, 2005

Porter JC: Proceedings: Hormonal regulation of breast development and activity. J Invest Dermatol 63:85, 1974

Reis RA, Baer JL, Arens RA, et al: Traumatic separation of the symphysis pubis during spontaneous labor: With a clinical and x-ray study of the normal symphysis pubis during pregnancy and the puerperium. Surg Gynecol Obstet 55:336, 1932

Robson SC, Dunlop W, Hunter S: Haemodynamic changes during the early puerperium. BMJ (Clin Res Ed) 294:1065, 1987

Saito S, Maruyama M, Kato Y, et al: Detection of IL-6 in human milk and its involvement in IgA production. J Reprod Immunol 20:267, 1991

Salman MC, Cil B, Esin S, et al: Late postpartum hemorrhage due to von Willebrand disease managed with uterine artery embolization. Obstet Gynecol 111:573, 2008

Schauberger CW, Rooney BL, Brimer LM: Factors that influence weight loss in the puerperium. Obstet Gynecol 79:424, 1992

Schwarz RJ, Shrestha R: Needle aspiration of breast abscesses. Am J Surg 182:117, 2001

Sharman A: Postpartum regeneration of the human endometrium. J Anat 87:1, 1953

Snow RE, Neubert AG: Peripartum pubic symphysis separation: A case series and review of the literature. Obstet Gynecol Surv 52:438, 1997

Sohn C, Fendel H, Kesternich P: Involution-induced changes in arterial uterine blood flow. Z Geburtshilfe Perinatol 192:203, 1988

Sokolov KM, Krey E, Miller LG, et al: Postpartum iliopsoas pyomyositis due to community-acquired methicillin-resistant *Staphylococcus aureus*. Obstet Gynecol 110:535, 2007

Spencer JP, Gonzalez LS III, Barnhart DJ: Medications in the breast-feeding mother. Am Fam Physician 65(2):170, 2002

Spitz AM, Lee NC, Peterson HB: Treatment for lactation suppression: Little progress in one hundred years. Am J Obstet Gynecol 179:1485, 1998

Stafford I, Hernandez J, Laibl V, et al: Community-acquired methicillin-resistant Staphylococcus aureus among patients with puerperal mastitis requiring hospitalization. Obstet Gynecol 112(3):533, 2008

Stehman FB: Infections and inflammations of the breast. In Hindle WH (ed): Breast Disease for Gynecologists. Norwalk, CT, Appleton & Lange, 1990, p 151

Stuebe AM, Michels KB, Willett WC, et al: Duration of lactation and incidence of myocardial infarction in middle to late adulthood. Am J Obstet Gynecol 200(2):138.e1, 2009

Taylor RN, Sonson RD: Separation of the pubic symphysis. An underrecognized peripartum complication. J Reprod Med 31:203, 1986

Tekay A, Jouppila P: A longitudinal Doppler ultrasonographic assessment of the alterations in peripheral vascular resistance of uterine arteries and ultrasonographic findings of the involuting uterus during the puerperium. Am J Obstet Gynecol 168(1 Pt 1):190, 1993

Thompson JF, Roberts CL, Currie M, et al: Prevalence and persistence of health problems after childbirth: Associations with parity and method of birth. Birth 29:83, 2002

Thomsen AC, Espersen T, Maigaard S: Course and treatment of milk stasis, noninfectious inflammation of the breast, and infectious mastitis in nursing women. Am J Obstet Gynecol 149:492, 1984

Tulman L, Fawcett J: Return of functional ability after childbirth. Nurs Res 37:77, 1988

Van Os AFM and Van der Linden PJQ: Reliability of an automatic ultrasound system in the post partum period in measuring urinary retention. Acta Obstet Gynecol Scand 85:604, 2006

Visness CM, Kennedy KI, Ramos R: The duration and character of postpartum bleeding among breast-feeding women. Obstet Gynecol 89:159, 1997

Wachsberg RH, Kurtz AB: Gas within the endometrial cavity at postpartum US: A normal finding after spontaneous vaginal delivery. Radiology 183:431, 1992

Wager GP, Martin DH, Koutsky L, et al: Puerperal infectious morbidity: Relationship to route of delivery and to antepartum *Chlamydia trachomatis* infection. Am J Obstet Gynecol 138:1028, 1980

Wagner CL, Greer FR, American Academy of Pediatrics Section on Breastfeeding, American Academy of Pediatrics Committee on Nutrition: Prevention of rickets and vitamin D deficiency in infants, children, and adolescents. Pediatrics 122(5):1142, 2008

Williams JW: Regeneration of the uterine mucosa after delivery with especial reference to the placental site. Am J Obstet Gynecol 22:664, 1931

Wisner KL, Perel JM, Peindl KS, et al: Prevention of postpartum depression: A pilot randomized clinical trial. Am J Psychiatry 161:1290, 2004

Wisniewski PM, Wilkinson EJ: Postpartum vaginal atrophy. Am J Obstet Gynecol 165(4 Pt 2):1249, 1991

Wolfberg AJ, Michels KB, Shields W, et al: Dads as breastfeeding advocates: Results from a randomized controlled trial of an educational intervention. Am J Obstet Gynecol 191:708, 2004

Wong CA, Scavone BM, Dugan S, et al: Incidence of postpartum lumbosacral spine and lower extremity nerve injuries. Obstet Gynecol 101:279, 2003

World Health Organization. Ten steps to successful breastfeeding. Geneva: WHO, 1998

Yuen BH: Prolactin in human milk: The influence of nursing and the duration of postpartum lactation. Am J Obstet Gynecol 158:583, 1988

CHAPTER 31

Puerperal Infection

Puerperal infection is a general term used to describe any bacterial infection of the genital tract after delivery. The earliest reference to puerperal infection is found in the works of Hippocrates from the 5th century BC, *De Mulierum Morbis*. He attributed the condition to retention of bowel contents. The history of puerperal infection is discussed in greater detail in previous editions of *Williams Obstetrics*.

Along with preeclampsia and obstetrical hemorrhage, puerperal infection formed the lethal triad of causes of maternal deaths for many decades of the 20th century. Fortunately, because of effective antimicrobials, maternal deaths from infection have become uncommon. Berg and associates (2003) reported results from the Pregnancy Mortality Surveillance System, which contained 3201 maternal deaths in the United States from 1991 through 1997. Infection caused 13 percent of pregnancy-related deaths and was the fifth leading cause of death. In a similar analysis of the North Carolina population from 1991 through 1999, Berg and colleagues (2005) reported that 40 percent of infection-related maternal deaths were preventable.

PUERPERAL FEVER

A number of factors can cause fever—a temperature of 38.0°C (100.4°F) or higher—in the puerperium. **Most persistent fevers after childbirth are caused by genital tract infection.**

Filker and Monif (1979) reported that only about 20 percent of women febrile within the first 24 hours after giving birth vaginally were subsequently diagnosed with pelvic infection. This was in contrast to 70 percent of those undergoing cesarean delivery. It must be emphasized that spiking fevers of 39°C or higher that develop within the first 24 hours postpartum may be associated with virulent pelvic infection caused by group A streptococcus. Other common causes of puerperal fever are breast engorgement and pyelonephritis or occasionally respiratory complications after cesarean delivery (Maharaj, 2007).

About 15 percent of women who do not breast feed develop postpartum fever from breast engorgement. This figure is lower in breast-feeding women (see Chap. 30, p. 652). Attributable fever rarely exceeds 39°C in the first few postpartum days and usually lasts less than 24 hours. Acute pyelonephritis has a variable clinical picture, and postpartum, the first sign of renal infection may be fever, followed later by costovertebral angle tenderness, nausea, and vomiting. Atelectasis is caused by hypoventilation and is best prevented by coughing and deep breathing on a fixed schedule following surgery. Fever associated with atelectasis is thought to follow infection by normal flora that proliferate distal to obstructing mucous plugs. Minor temperature elevations in the puerperium may also occasionally be caused by superficial or deep-venous thrombosis of the legs.

UTERINE INFECTION

Postpartum uterine infection has been called variously *endometritis, endomyometritis,* and *endoparametritis.* Because infection involves not only the decidua but also the myometrium and parametrial tissues, we prefer the inclusive term *metritis with pelvic cellulitis.*

Predisposing Factors

The route of delivery is the single most significant risk factor for the development of uterine infection (Burrows and associates,

2004; Koroukian, 2004). In the French Confidential Enquiry on Maternal Deaths, Deneux-Tharaux and colleagues (2006) cited a nearly 25-fold increased infection-related mortality rate with cesarean versus vaginal delivery. Rehospitalization rates for wound complications and endometritis were increased significantly in women undergoing a planned primary cesarean delivery compared with those having a planned vaginal birth (Declercq, 2007).

Vaginal Delivery

Compared with cesarean delivery, metritis following vaginal delivery is relatively uncommon. Women delivered vaginally at Parkland Hospital have a 1- to 2-percent incidence of metritis. Women at high risk for infection because of membrane rupture, prolonged labor, and multiple cervical examinations have a 5- to 6-percent incidence of metritis after vaginal delivery. If there is intrapartum chorioamnionitis, the risk of persistent uterine infection increases to 13 percent (Maberry and colleagues, 1991). Finally, manual removal of the placenta, discussed in Chapter 35 (p. 774), increased the puerperal metritis rate three-fold in the study by Baksu and associates (2005).

Cesarean Delivery

Single-dose perioperative antimicrobial prophylaxis is given almost universally at cesarean delivery. The American College of Obstetricians and Gynecologists (2003) recommends such prophylaxis for women at high risk for postpartum infection (see Chap. 25, p. 561). Such single-dose antimicrobial prophylaxis has done more to decrease the incidence and severity of postcesarean delivery infections than any other practice in the past 30 years.

The magnitude of the risk is exemplified from reports that predate antimicrobial prophylaxis. In 1973, Sweet and Ledger reported an overall incidence of uterine infection of 13 percent among affluent women who underwent cesarean delivery compared with 27 percent of indigent women. Cunningham and associates (1978) described an overall incidence of 50 percent in women who had cesarean delivery at Parkland Hospital. Important risk factors for infection following surgery included prolonged labor, membrane rupture, multiple cervical examinations, and internal fetal monitoring. Women with all of these factors who were not given perioperative prophylaxis had a 90-percent serious pelvic infection rate (DePalma and colleagues, 1982).

Other Risk Factors

It is generally accepted that pelvic infection is more common in women of lower socioeconomic status compared with those more advantaged (Maharaj, 2007). Except in extreme cases usually not seen in this country, it is unlikely that anemia or poor nutrition predispose to infection. *Bacterial colonization* of the lower genital tract with certain microorganisms—for example, group B streptococcus, *Chlamydia trachomatis, Mycoplasma hominis, Ureaplasma urealyticum,* and *Gardnerella vaginalis*—has been associated with an increased risk of postpartum infection (Andrews, 1995; Jacobsson, 2002; Watts, 1990, and all their colleagues). Other factors associated with an increased risk of infection include cesarean delivery for *multifetal gestation, young maternal age and nulliparity, prolonged labor induction, obesity,* and *meconium-stained amnionic fluid* (Jazayeri, 2002; Kabiru and Raynor, 2004; Myles, 2002, and all their colleagues).

Bacteriology

Most female pelvic infections are caused by bacteria indigenous to the female genital tract. Over the past decade, there have been reports of group A β-hemolytic streptococcus causing toxic shock-like syndrome and life-threatening infection (Aronoff and Mulla, 2008; Castagnola, 2008; Nathan and Leveno, 1994; Palep-Singh, 2007, and all their colleagues). Prematurely ruptured membranes is a prominent risk factor (Anteby and associates, 1999). In two reviews by Crum (2002) and Udagawa (1999) and their colleagues, women in whom group A streptococcal infection was manifested before, during, or within 12 hours of delivery had a maternal mortality rate of almost 90 percent and fetal mortality rate of greater than 50 percent. In the past 5 years, skin and soft-tissue infections due to community-acquired methicillin-resistant *Staphylococcus aureus*—CA-MRSA—have become common (see Chap. 58, p. 1223). As of 2009, these strains are not a common agent of puerperal metritis, but they are causative in incisional wound infections (Anderson and co-workers, 2007; Patel and colleagues, 2007). And Rotas and associates (2007) reported a woman with episiotomy cellulitis with CA-MRSA and hematogenously spread necrotizing pneumonia.

Common Pathogens

Bacteria commonly responsible for female genital tract infections are listed in Table 31-1. Generally, infections are polymicrobial, which promotes bacterial synergy. Other factors that promote virulence are hematomas and devitalized tissue. Although the cervix and vagina routinely harbor such bacteria, the uterine cavity is usually sterile before rupture of the amnionic sac. As the consequence of labor and delivery and associated manipulations, the amnionic fluid and uterus commonly become contaminated with anaerobic and aerobic bacteria (Fig. 31-1). In studies done before the use of antimicrobial prophylaxis, Gilstrap and Cunningham

---

TABLE 31-1. Bacteria Commonly Responsible for Female Genital Infections

Aerobes
Gram-positive cocci—group A, B, and D streptococci, enterococcus, *Staphylococcus aureus, Staphylococcus epidermidis*
Gram-negative bacteria—*Escherichia coli, Klebsiella, Proteus* species
Gram-variable—*Gardnerella vaginalis*

Others
Mycoplasma and *Chlamydia* species, *Neisseria gonorrhoeae*

Anaerobes
Cocci—*Peptostreptococcus* and *Peptococcus* species
Others—*Clostridium* and *Fusobacterium* species *Mobiluncus* species

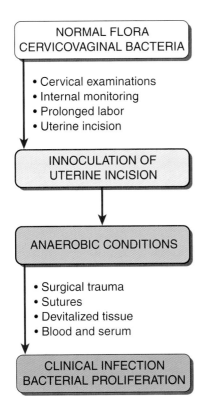

```
NORMAL FLORA
CERVICOVAGINAL BACTERIA
```

- Cervical examinations
- Internal monitoring
- Prolonged labor
- Uterine incision

```
INNOCULATION OF
UTERINE INCISION
```

```
ANAEROBIC CONDITIONS
```

- Surgical trauma
- Sutures
- Devitalized tissue
- Blood and serum

```
CLINICAL INFECTION
BACTERIAL PROLIFERATION
```

FIGURE 31-1 Pathogenesis of metritis following cesarean delivery. (Adapted from Gilstrap and Cunningham, 1979.)

(1979) cultured amnionic fluid obtained at cesarean delivery in women in labor with membranes ruptured more than 6 hours. All had bacterial growth and an average of 2.5 organisms was identified from each specimen. Anaerobic and aerobic organisms were identified in 63 percent, anaerobes alone in 30 percent, and aerobes alone in only 7 percent. Anaerobes included *Peptostreptococcus* and *Peptococcus* species in 45 percent, *Bacteroides* species in 9 percent, and *Clostridium* species in 3 percent. Aerobes included *Enterococcus* in 14 percent, group B streptococcus in 8 percent, and *Escherichia coli* in 9 percent of isolates. Sherman and co-workers (1999) later showed that bacterial isolates at cesarean delivery correlated with those taken at 3 days postpartum in those with metritis.

The role of other organisms in the etiology of these infections is unclear. Chlamydial infections have been implicated in late-onset, indolent metritis (Ismail and associates, 1985). Observations of Chaim and colleagues (2003) suggest that when cervical colonization of *U. urealyticum* is heavy, it may contribute to the development of metritis. Finally, Jacobsson and colleagues (2002) reported a threefold risk of puerperal infection in a group of Swedish women in whom bacterial vaginosis was identified in early pregnancy.

Bacterial Cultures

Routine pretreatment genital tract cultures are of little clinical use and add significant costs. Similarly, routine blood cultures seldom modify care. In two earlier studies done before perioperative prophylaxis was used, blood cultures were positive in 13 percent of women with postcesarean metritis at Parkland

Hospital and 24 percent in those at Los Angeles County Hospital (Cunningham and colleagues, 1978; DiZerega and co-workers, 1979). In a more recent Finnish study, Kankuri and associates (2003) confirmed bacteremia in only 5 percent of almost 800 women with puerperal sepsis.

PATHOGENESIS

Puerperal infection following vaginal delivery primarily involves the placental implantation site, decidua and adjacent myometrium, or cervicovaginal lacerations. The pathogenesis of uterine infection following cesarean delivery is that of an infected surgical incision (see Fig. 31-1). Bacteria that colonize the cervix and vagina gain access to amnionic fluid during labor, and postpartum, they invade devitalized uterine tissue. Parametrial cellulitis next follows with infection of the pelvic retroperitoneal fibroareolar connective tissue. With early treatment, infection is contained within the paravaginal tissue but may extend deeply into the pelvis.

CLINICAL COURSE

Fever is the most important criterion for the diagnosis of postpartum metritis. Intuitively, the degree of fever is believed proportional to the extent of infection and sepsis syndrome (see Chap. 42, p. 932). Temperatures commonly are 38 to 39°C. Chills that accompany fever suggest bacteremia. Women usually complain of abdominal pain, and parametrial tenderness is elicited on abdominal and bimanual examination. Although an offensive odor may develop, many women have foul-smelling lochia without evidence for infection. Other infections, notably those due to group A β-hemolytic streptococci, are frequently associated with scanty, odorless lochia. Leukocytosis may range from 15,000 to 30,000 cells/μL, but recall that cesarean delivery itself increases the leukocyte count (Hartmann and co-workers, 2000).

Treatment

If mild metritis develops after a woman has been discharged following vaginal delivery, outpatient treatment with an oral antimicrobial agent is usually sufficient. For moderate to severe infections, however, intravenous therapy with a broad-spectrum antimicrobial regimen is indicated. Improvement follows in 48 to 72 hours in nearly 90 percent of women treated with one of several regimens. Persistent fever after this interval mandates a careful search for causes of refractory pelvic infection. These include a parametrial phlegmon—an area of intense cellulitis; an abdominal incisional or pelvic abscess or infected hematoma; and septic pelvic thrombophlebitis. In our experience, persistent fever is seldom due to antimicrobial-resistant bacteria or due to drug side effects. The woman may be discharged home after she has been afebrile for at least 24 hours. Further oral antimicrobial therapy is not needed (Dinsmoor and colleagues, 1991; French and Smaill, 2002).

Choice of Antimicrobials

Although therapy is empirical, initial treatment following cesarean delivery is directed against most of the mixed flora shown

TABLE 31-2. Antimicrobial Regimens for Pelvic Infection Following Cesarean Delivery

Regimen	Comments
Clindamycin 900 mg + gentamicin 1.5 mg/kg, q8h intravenously	"Gold standard," 90–97% efficacy, once-daily gentamicin dosing acceptable + Ampicillin added to regimen with sepsis syndrome or suspected enterococcal infection
Clindamycin + aztreonam	Gentamicin substitute with renal insufficiency
Extended-spectrum penicillins	Piperacillin, ampicillin/sulbactam
Extended-spectrum cephalosporins	Cefotetan, cefoxitin, cefotaxime
Imipenem + cilastatin	Reserved for special indications

in Table 31-1, which typically cause puerperal infections. Such broad-spectrum antimicrobial coverage is often not necessary to treat infection following vaginal delivery, and as many as 90 percent of these infections respond to regimens such as ampicillin plus gentamicin. In contrast, anaerobic coverage is included for infections following cesarean delivery (Table 31-2).

In 1979, DiZerega and colleagues compared the effectiveness of clindamycin plus gentamicin with that of penicillin G plus gentamicin for treatment of pelvic infections following cesarean delivery. Women given the *clindamycin-gentamicin* regimen had a 95-percent response rate, and this regimen is still considered by most to be the standard by which others are measured (French and Smaill, 2002). Because enterococcal infections may persist despite this standard therapy, many add ampicillin to the clindamycin-gentamicin regimen, either initially or if there is no response by 48 to 72 hours (Brumfield and associates, 2000).

Many authorities recommend that serum gentamicin levels be periodically monitored, although at the University of Alabama and Parkland Hospitals, we do not routinely do so if the woman has normal renal function. Liu and associates (1999) compared multiple-dosing versus once-daily dosing with gentamicin and found that both provided adequate serum levels. Once-daily dosing has a cure rate similar to 8-hour dosing (Livingston and colleagues, 2003).

Because of potential nephrotoxicity and ototoxicity with gentamicin in the event of diminished glomerular filtration, some have recommended a combination of clindamycin and a second-generation cephalosporin to treat such women. Others recommend a combination of clindamycin and aztreonam, a monobactam compound with activity similar to the aminoglycosides.

The spectra of β-*lactam antimicrobials* include activity against many anaerobic pathogens. Some examples include cephalosporins such as cefoxitin, cefotetan, and cefotaxime, as well as extended-spectrum penicillins such as piperacillin, ticarcillin, and mezlocillin. β Lactam antimicrobials are inherently safe and except for allergic reactions, are free of major toxicity. The β-*lactamase inhibitors*, clavulanic acid, sulbactam, and tazobactam, have been combined with ampicillin, amoxicillin, ticarcillin, and piperacillin to extend their spectra. *Metronidazole* has superior in vitro activity against most anaerobes. This agent given with ampicillin and an aminoglycoside provides coverage against most organisms encountered in serious pelvic infections.

Imipenem is a carbapenem that has broad-spectrum coverage against most organisms associated with metritis. It is used in combination with *cilastatin*, which inhibits renal metabolism of imipenem. Although this combination is effective in most cases of metritis, it seems reasonable from both a medical and an economic standpoint to reserve it for more serious infections.

Prevention of Infection

Over the years, a number of strategies have been tested to prevent or at least mitigate the severity of postpartum infections.

Perioperative Antimicrobial Prophylaxis. As noted, administration of antimicrobial prophylaxis at the time of cesarean delivery has remarkably reduced the rate of postoperative pelvic and wound infections. Numerous studies have shown that prophylactic antimicrobials reduce the rate of pelvic infection by 70 to 80 percent (Chelmow and colleagues, 2001; Smaill and Hofmeyr, 2002). The observed benefit applies to both elective and nonelective cesarean delivery and also includes a reduction in abdominal incisional infections.

Single-dose prophylaxis with ampicillin or a first-generation cephalosporin is ideal, and both are as effective as broad-spectrum agents or a multiple-dose regimen (American College of Obstetricians and Gynecologists, 2003). A recent report of extended-spectrum prophylaxis with azithromycin added to standard single-dose prophylaxis showed a significant reduction in postcesarean metritis (Tita and colleagues, 2008). These findings need to be verified. Women known to be colonized with methicillin-resistant *Staphylococcus aureus*—MRSA—are given vancomycin in addition to a cephalosporin (see Chap. 58, p. 1223). Finally, the infection rate is lowered more if the selected antimicrobial is given before the skin incision compared with cord clamping (Constantine, 2008; Kaimal, 2008; Sullivan, 2007, and all their co-workers).

A number of locally applied antimicrobials have been evaluated to prevent puerperal infection. At best, the results of these studies are mixed. Intrapartum vaginal irrigation with *chlorhexidine* did not reduce the incidence of postpartum infection in trials conducted by Rouse and colleagues (1997, 2003). Likewise, Reid and associates (2001) reported that *povidone-iodine* vaginal irrigation before cesarean delivery had no effect on the incidence of fever, metritis, or abdominal incisional infection. Conversely, Starr and colleagues (2005) reported that women who underwent preoperative vaginal cleansing with povidone-iodine had a significantly lower infection rate following cesarean delivery—7 versus 14 percent. In a placebo-controlled trial, Pitt and colleagues (2001) applied 5 grams of *metronidazole gel* preoperatively as an adjunct to perioperative antimicrobial prophylaxis. They reported reduction in the rate of metritis from 17 to 7 percent with the gel but no significant effect on febrile morbidity or wound infections.

Treatment of Vaginitis. Prenatal treatment of asymptomatic vaginal infections has not been shown to prevent postpartum pelvic infections. Carey and associates (2000) reported no beneficial effects for women treated for asymptomatic bacterial vaginosis. Similarly, Klebanoff and colleagues (2001) reported a similar postpartum infection rate in women treated for second-trimester asymptomatic *Trichomonas vaginalis* infection compared with that of placebo-treated women.

Operative Technique. A number of technical maneuvers to alter the rate of postpartum infections in women undergoing cesarean delivery have been studied. For example, allowing the placenta to separate spontaneously compared with removing it manually lowers the risk of infection, but changing gloves by the surgical team after placental delivery does not (Atkinson and associates, 1996). Exteriorizing the uterus to close the hysterotomy may decrease febrile morbidity (Jacobs-Jokhan and Hofmeyr, 2004). No differences were found in postoperative infection rates when single- versus two-layer uterine closure was compared (Hauth and colleagues, 1992). Similarly, infection rates are not appreciably affected by closure versus nonclosure of the peritoneum (Bamigboye and Hofmer, 2003; Tulandi and Al-Jaroudi, 2003). Importantly, although closure of subcutaneous tissue in obese women does not lower the rate of wound infection, it does decrease the incidence of wound separation (Chelmow, 2004; Magann, 2002; Naumann, 1995, and all their colleagues).

Complications of Pelvic Infections

In more than 90 percent of women, metritis responds to treatment within 48 to 72 hours. In the remainder, any of several complications may arise. As with other aspects of puerperal infections, the incidence and severity of complications are remarkably decreased by perioperative antimicrobial prophylaxis.

Wound Infections

When prophylactic antimicrobials are given as described above, the incidence of abdominal incisional infections following cesarean delivery is less than 2 percent (Andrews and colleagues, 2003). The incidence in some cases averaged 6 percent and ranged from 3 to 15 percent (Chaim and associates, 2000; Owen and Andrews, 1994). Wound infection is a common cause of persistent fever in women treated for metritis. Other risk factors for wound infections include obesity, diabetes, corticosteroid therapy, immunosuppression, anemia, hypertension, and inadequate hemostasis with hematoma formation.

Incisional abscesses that develop following cesarean delivery usually cause fever or are responsible for its persistence beginning about the fourth day. In many cases, antimicrobials had been given for uterine infection, and thus, fever is persistent. Wound erythema and drainage usually accompany it. Although organisms that cause wound infections are generally the same as those isolated from amnionic fluid at cesarean delivery, hospital-acquired pathogens occasionally are causative (Emmons and colleagues, 1988; Owen and Andrews, 1994). Treatment includes antimicrobials and surgical drainage, with careful inspection to ensure that the fascia is intact.

With local wound care given two to three times daily, secondary en bloc closure at 4 to 6 days of tissue involved in superficial wound infection can usually be accomplished (Wechter and associates, 2005). With this closure, a polypropylene or nylon suture of appropriate gauge enters 3 cm from one wound edge. It crosses the wound to incorporate the full wound thickness and emerges 3 cm from the other wound edge. These are placed in series to close the opening. In most cases, sutures may be removed on postprocedural day 10.

Wound Dehiscence. Disruption or dehiscence refers to separation of the fascial layer. This is a serious complication and requires secondary closure of the incision in the operating room. McNeeley and colleagues (1998) reported fascial dehiscence in about 1 of 300 operations in almost 9000 women undergoing cesarean delivery. Most disruptions manifested on about the fifth postoperative day and were accompanied by a serosanguineous discharge. Two thirds of 27 fascial dehiscences identified in this study were associated with concurrent fascial infection and tissue necrosis.

Necrotizing Fasciitis. This uncommon, severe wound infection is associated with high mortality. In obstetrics, necrotizing fasciitis may involve abdominal incisions, or it may complicate episiotomy or other perineal lacerations. As the name implies, there is significant tissue necrosis. Of the risk factors for fasciitis summarized by Owen and Andrews (1994), three of these—*diabetes*, *obesity*, and *hypertension*—are relatively common in pregnant women. Like pelvic infections, these usually are polymicrobial and are caused by organisms that comprise normal vaginal flora. In some cases, however, infection is caused by a single virulent bacterial species such as group A β-hemolytic streptococcus. Occasionally, necrotizing infections are caused by rarely encountered pathogens (Swartz, 2004).

Goepfert and colleagues (1997) reviewed their experiences at the University of Alabama Birmingham Hospital from 1987 through 1994. Nine cases of necrotizing fasciitis complicated over 5000 cesarean deliveries—1.8 per 1000. In two women, the infection was fatal. In a report from Brigham and Womens and Massachusetts General Hospitals, Schorge and colleagues (1998) described five women with fasciitis following cesarean delivery. None of these women had predisposing risk factors, and none died.

Treatment consists of broad-spectrum antibiotics along with prompt wide fascial debridement until healthy bleeding tissue is encountered. With extensive resection, synthetic mesh may be required to close the fascial incision (Gallup and Meguiar, 2004; McNeeley and associates, 1998).

Peritonitis

It is unusual for peritonitis to develop following cesarean delivery. It is almost invariably preceded by metritis and uterine incisional necrosis and dehiscence. Other cases may be due to inadvertent bowel injury at cesarean delivery. Yet another cause is peritonitis following rupture of a parametrial or adnexal abscess. Finally, it may rarely be encountered after vaginal delivery.

In postpartum women, there is an important caveat to remember: **Abdominal rigidity may not be prominent with puerperal peritonitis because of abdominal wall laxity from pregnancy.** Pain may be severe, but frequently, the first symptoms of peritonitis are those of *adynamic ileus.* Marked bowel distension may develop, and these findings are unusual after uncomplicated cesarean delivery. If the infection begins in an intact uterus and extends into the peritoneum, antimicrobial treatment alone usually suffices. Conversely, peritonitis caused by uterine incisional necrosis or bowel perforation must be treated surgically.

Adnexal Infections

An *ovarian abscess* rarely develops in the puerperium. These are presumably caused by bacterial invasion through a rent in the ovarian capsule (Wetchler and Dunn, 1985). The abscess is usually unilateral, and women typically present 1 to 2 weeks after delivery. Rupture is common and peritonitis may be severe.

Parametrial Phlegmon

In some women in whom metritis develops following cesarean delivery, parametrial cellulitis is intensive and forms an area of induration, or *phlegmon,* within the leaves of the broad ligament (Fig. 31-2). These infections should be considered when fever persists longer than 72 hours despite intravenous antimicrobial therapy (DePalma and colleagues, 1982).

Phlegmons are usually unilateral, and they frequently are limited to the parametrial area at the base of the broad ligament. If the inflammatory reaction is more intense, cellulitis extends along natural lines of cleavage. The most common form of extension is laterally along the broad ligament, with a tendency to extend to the pelvic sidewall. Occasionally, posterior extension may involve the rectovaginal septum, producing a firm mass posterior to the cervix.

Severe cellulitis of the uterine incision may lead to necrosis and separation. Extrusion of purulent material commonly leads to peritonitis. Because puerperal metritis with cellulitis is typically a retroperitoneal infection, evidence of peritonitis suggests the possibility of uterine incisional necrosis, or less commonly, a bowel injury or other lesion as described above.

In most women with a phlegmon, clinical improvement follows continued treatment with a broad-spectrum antimicrobial regimen. Typically, fever resolves in 5 to 7 days, but in some cases, it is longer. Absorption of the induration may require several days to weeks. Surgery is reserved for women in whom uterine incisional necrosis is suspected. In rare cases, uterine debridement and resuturing of the incision are feasible (Rivlin and colleagues, 2004). For most, hysterectomy and surgical debridement are needed and are predictably difficult. There is often appreciable blood loss. Frequently, the cervix and lower uterine segment are involved with an intensive inflammatory process that extends to the pelvic sidewall to encompass one or both ureters. The adnexa are seldom involved, and one or both ovaries usually can be conserved.

Imaging Studies. Persistent puerperal infections can be evaluated using computed tomography (CT) or magnetic resonance (MR) imaging. Brown and colleagues (1991) used CT imaging in 74 women in whom pelvic infection was refractory to antimicrobial therapy. They found at least one abnormal radiological finding in 75 percent of these women. Maldjian and associates (1999) used MR imaging in 50 women with persistent fever and found a bladder flap hematoma in two thirds. In three women, parametrial edema was seen, and another two had a pelvic hematoma.

Uterine incisional dehiscence is sometimes suspected by CT scanning images (Figs. 31-3 and 31-4). These must be interpreted within the clinical context because apparent uterine incisional defects thought to represent edema can be seen even on images after uncomplicated cesarean delivery (Twickler and colleagues, 1991).

Pelvic Abscess

Rarely, a parametrial phlegmon suppurates, forming a fluctuant broad ligament mass that may point above the inguinal ligament. These abscesses may dissect anteriorly as shown in Figure 31-4 and be amenable to CT-directed needle drainage. Occasionally they dissect posteriorly to the rectovaginal septum, where surgical drainage is easily effected by colpotomy incision.

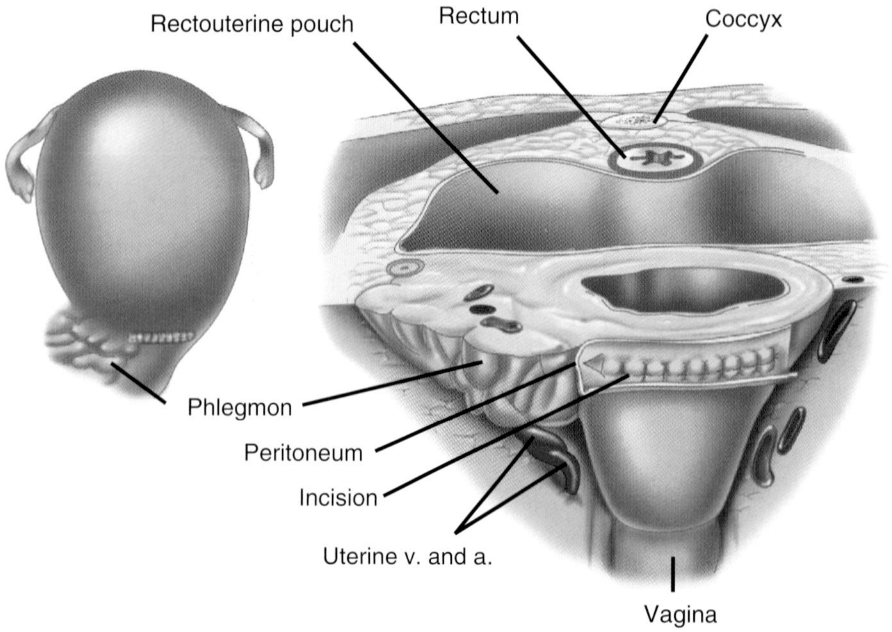

FIGURE 31-2 Parametrial phlegmon. Cellulitis causes induration in the right parametrium adjacent to the uterine cesarean incision. Induration extends to the pelvic sidewall. On bimanual pelvic examination, a phlegmon is palpable as a firm, three-dimensional mass.

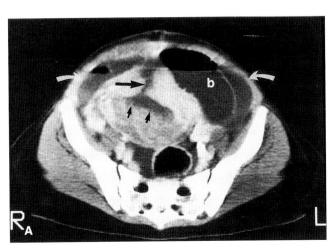
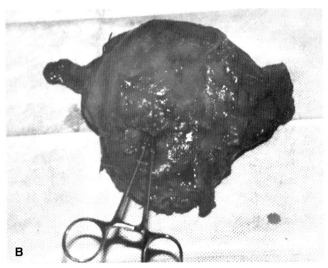

FIGURE 31-3 A. Pelvic computed tomography scan of dehiscence caused by infection of a vertical cesarean incision. Endometrial fluid (*small black arrows*) communicates with parametrial fluid (*curved white arrows*) through the uterine defect (*large black arrow*). A dilated bowel loop (*b*) is adjacent to the uterus on the left. **B.** Supracervical hysterectomy specimen with instrument through uterine dehiscence.

A *psoas abscess* is rare, and despite antimicrobial therapy, percutaneous drainage may be required (Shahabi and colleagues, 2002; Swanson and co-workers, 2008).

Septic Pelvic Thrombophlebitis

This was a common complication in the preantibotic era. Collins and colleagues (1951) described suppurative thrombophlebitis in 70 women cared for from 1937 through 1946 at Charity Hospital in New Orleans. Septic embolization was common and caused a third of maternal deaths during that period. With the advent of antimicrobial therapy, the mortality rate and need for surgical therapy for these infections diminished.

Pathogenesis. Puerperal infection may extend along venous routes and cause thrombosis as shown in Figure 31-5. Lym-

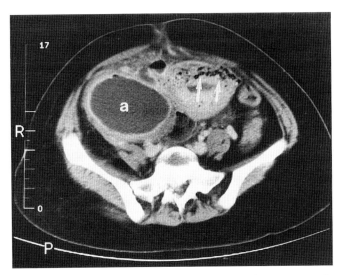

FIGURE 31-4 Pelvic computed tomography scan showing necrosis of the uterine incision with gas in the myometrium (*arrows*). There is also a large right-sided parametrial abscess (*a*).

phangitis often coexists. The ovarian veins may then become involved because they drain the upper uterus and therefore, the placental implantation site. The experiences of Witlin and Sibai (1995) and Brown and colleagues (1999) suggest that puerperal septic thrombophlebitis is likely to involve one or both ovarian venous plexuses (Fig. 31-6). In a fourth of women, the clot extends into the inferior vena cava and occasionally to the renal vein.

Incidence. During a five-year survey of 45,000 women who were delivered at Parkland Hospital, Brown and associates (1999) found an incidence of septic pelvic thrombophlebitis of 1:9000 following vaginal delivery and 1:800 with cesarean delivery. The overall incidence of 1:3000 deliveries was similar to the 1:2000 reported by Dunnihoo and colleagues (1991). In a cohort of 16,650 women undergoing primary cesarean delivery, Rouse and associates (2004) reported an incidence of 1:400 with cesarean delivery—it was about 1:175 if there was antecedent chorioamnionitis, and 1:500 if there was no intrapartum infection.

Management. Women with septic thrombophlebitis usually have clinical improvement of pelvic infection with antimicrobial treatment, however, they continue to have fever. Although there occasionally is pain in one or both lower quadrants, patients are usually asymptomatic except for chills. Diagnosis can be confirmed by either pelvic CT or MR imaging (Klima and Snyder, 2008; Sheffield and Cunningham, 2001). Using both, Brown and co-workers (1999) found that 20 percent of 69 women with metritis who had fever despite 5 days of appropriate therapy had septic pelvic thrombophlebitis. Before imaging methods were available, the *heparin challenge test* was advocated. Supposedly after intravenous heparin was given, if fever abated, this was considered diagnostic of pelvic phlebitis (Josey and Staggers, 1974). This was subsequently disproved by Brown and colleagues (1986) as well as by Witlin and Sibai (1995). Although Garcia and colleagues (2006) and Klima and Snyder (2008) advocate heparin administration, we do not use or recommend anticoagulation. In a randomized study of 14 women by Brown and

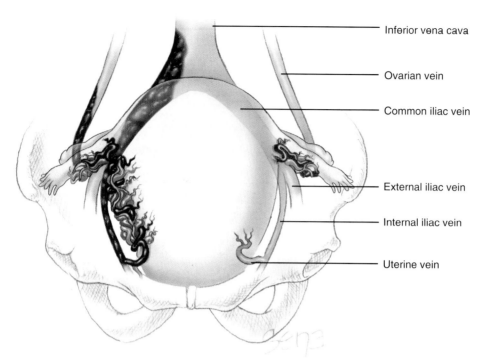

FIGURE 31-5 Routes of extension of septic pelvic thrombophlebitis. Any pelvic vessel and the inferior vena cava may be involved as shown on the left. The clot in the right common iliac vein extends from the uterine and internal iliac veins and into the inferior vena cava.

associates (1999), the addition of heparin to antimicrobial therapy for septic pelvic thrombophlebitis did not hasten recovery or improve outcome. Certainly, there is no evidence for long-term anticoagulation as given for "bland" venous thromboembolism.

Infections of the Perineum, Vagina, and Cervix

Episiotomy infections are not common because the operation is performed much less frequently now than in the past (American

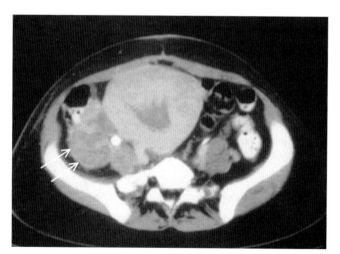

FIGURE 31-6 Pelvic computed tomography scan with contrast shows enlargement of the right ovarian venous plexus with low density of the lumens. The clotted vessels were easily palpable in this thin woman who had delivered vaginally 3 days earlier.

College of Obstetricians and Gynecologists, 2006). Reasons for this are discussed further in Chapter 17 (p. 401). Even more than 25 years ago, Owen and Hauth (1990) described only 10 episiotomy infections in 20,000 women delivered at the University of Alabama at Birmingham. With infection, dehiscence is a concern. Ramin and colleagues (1992) reported that 0.5 percent of episiotomy wounds dehisced at Parkland Hospital, and 80 percent of these were due to infection. More recently, Uygur and colleagues (2004) reported a 1-percent dehiscence rate and attributed two thirds to infection. There are no data to suggest that dehiscence is related to faulty repair.

Infection of a fourth-degree laceration is likely to be more serious. Goldaber and colleagues (1993) described 390 such women of whom 5.4 percent had morbidity—2.8 percent had infection and dehiscence, 1.8 percent had only dehiscence, and 0.8 percent only infection. Although life-threatening septic shock is rare, it may still occur as a result of an infected episiotomy (Soltesz and colleagues, 1999).

Pathogenesis and Clinical Course

Episiotomy dehiscence is most commonly associated with infection as discussed above. Other factors include coagulation disorders, smoking, and human papillomavirus infection (Ramin and Gilstrap, 1994). Local pain and dysuria, with or without urinary retention, are common symptoms. Ramin and colleagues (1992), evaluating a series of 34 women with episiotomy dehiscence, reported that the most common findings were pain in 65 percent, purulent discharge in 65 percent, and fever in 44 percent. In extreme cases, the entire vulva may become edematous, ulcerated, and covered with exudate.

Vaginal lacerations may become infected directly or by extension from the perineum. The mucosa becomes red and swollen and may then become necrotic and slough. Parametrial extension may result in lymphangitis.

Cervical lacerations are common but seldom are noticeably infected and may manifest as metritis. Deep lacerations which extend directly into the tissue at the base of the broad ligament may become infected and cause lymphangitis, parametritis, and bacteremia.

Treatment

Infected episiotomies are managed like other infected surgical wounds. Drainage is established, and in most cases, sutures are removed and the infected wound debrided. In some women with obvious cellulitis but no purulence, broad-spectrum

TABLE 31-3. Preoperative Protocol for Early Repair of Episiotomy Dehiscence

Open wound, remove sutures, begin intravenous antimicrobials

Wound care
  Sitz bath several times daily or hydrotherapy
  Adequate analgesia or anesthesia—regional analgesia or general anesthesia may be necessary for the first few debridements
  Scrub wound twice daily with a povidone-iodine solution
  Debride necrotic tissue

Closure when afebrile and with pink, healthy granulation tissue

Bowel preparation for fourth-degree repairs

antimicrobial therapy with close observation may be appropriate. With dehiscence, local wound care is continued along with intravenous antimicrobials. Hauth and colleagues (1986) were the first to advocate early repair after infection subsided, and other studies have confirmed the efficacy of this approach. Hankins and co-workers (1990) described early repair of episiotomy dehiscence in 31 women with an average duration of 6 days from dehiscence to episiotomy repair. All but two had a successful repair. Each of the two women with failures developed a pinpoint rectovaginal fistula that was treated successfully with a small rectal flap. Ramin and colleagues (1992) reported successful early repair of episiotomy dehiscence associated with infection in 32 of 34 women (94 percent), and Uygur and colleagues (2004) noted a similarly high percentage. Rarely, intestinal diversion may be required to allow healing (Rose and associates, 2005).

Technique for Early Repair. Before performing early repair, diligent preparation is essential as outlined in Table 31-3. **Most important is that the surgical wound must be properly cleaned and free of infection.** As shown in Figure 31-7, once the surface of the episiotomy wound is free of infection and exudate and covered by pink granulation tissue, secondary repair can be accomplished. The tissue must be adequately mobilized, with special attention to identify and mobilize the anal sphincter muscle. Secondary closure of the episiotomy is accomplished in layers, as described for primary episiotomy closure (see Chap. 17, p. 402). Postoperative care includes local wound care, low-residue diet, stool softeners, and nothing per vagina or rectum until healed.

Necrotizing Fasciitis

A rare but frequently fatal complication of perineal and vaginal wound infections is deep soft-tissue infection involving muscle and fascia. Although women with diabetes or women who are immunocompromised are more vulnerable, these serious infections may develop

in otherwise healthy women. Their microbiology appears to be similar to those of other pelvic infections, as well as necrotizing fasciitis of the abdominal wall incision described on page 662. Although uncommon today, Shy and Eschenbach (1979) reported that during the 1970s necrotizing fasciitis of the episiotomy was responsible for three of 15 maternal deaths in King County, Washington.

Necrotizing fasciitis of the episiotomy site may involve any of the several superficial or deep perineal fascial layers, and thus may extend to the thighs, buttocks, and abdominal wall (Fig. 31-8). Although some virulent infections, for example, from group A β-hemolytic streptococci, develop early postpartum, these infections typically do not cause symptoms until 3 to 5 days after delivery. Clinical findings vary, and it is frequently difficult to differentiate more innocuous superficial perineal infections from an ominous deep fascial one. A high index of suspicion, with surgical exploration if the diagnosis is uncertain, may be lifesaving. We aggressively pursue early exploration. Certainly, if myofasciitis progresses, the woman may become ill from septicemia. Profound hemoconcentration from capillary leakage with circulatory failure commonly occurs, and death may soon follow as described in Chapter 42 (p. 933).

Early diagnosis, surgical debridement, antimicrobials, and intensive care are of paramount importance in the successful treatment of necrotizing soft-tissue infections (Gallup and Meguiar, 2004; Urschel, 1999). Surgery includes extensive debridement of all infected tissue, leaving wide margins of healthy tissue. This may include extensive vulvar debridement with unroofing and excision of abdominal, thigh, or buttock fascia (see Fig. 31-8). Mortality is virtually universal without surgical treatment, and rates approach 50 percent even if extensive debridement is performed.

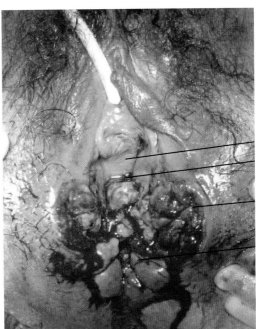

Anterior vaginal wall
Vaginal opening
Disrupted perineum
Rectal mucosa

FIGURE 31-7 Dehiscence of fourth-degree episiotomy. Secondary repair is done when the wound surface is free of exudate and covered by pink granulation tissue. (Courtesy of Dr. Scott Roberts.)

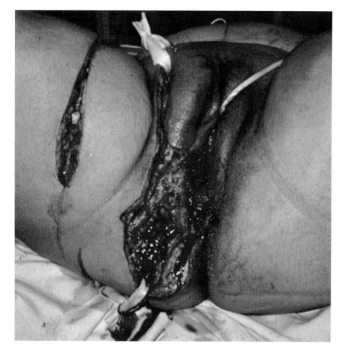

FIGURE 31-8 Necrotizing fasciitis complicating an episiotomy infection. Postpartum day 3, this woman had severe perineal pain and edema of the episiotomy site. Prompt extensive debridement and fasciotomy on her right inner thigh was completed. Cultures grew *Escherichia coli, Streptococcus viridans,* group D streptococcus, *Corynebacterium* species, *Bacteroides fragilis,* and *Clostridium* species. Blood cultures were positive for *Bacteroides fragilis.* She survived.

TOXIC SHOCK SYNDROME

This acute febrile illness with severe multisystem derangement has a case-fatality rate of 10 to 15 percent. There is usually fever, headache, mental confusion, diffuse macular erythematous rash, subcutaneous edema, nausea, vomiting, watery diarrhea, and marked hemoconcentration. Renal failure followed by hepatic failure, disseminated intravascular coagulation, and circulatory collapse may follow in rapid sequence. During recovery, the rash-covered areas undergo desquamation. *Staphylococcus aureus* has been recovered from almost all afflicted persons. Specifically, a staphylococcal exotoxin, termed *toxic shock syndrome toxin-1—* TSST-1—causes the clinical manifestations by provoking profound endothelial injury. A very small amount of TSST-1 has been shown to activate 5 to 30 percent of T cells to create a "cytokine storm" as described by Que (2005) and Heying (2007) and their colleagues. Treatment is discussed in Chapter 42 (p. 932).

In some cases, infection is not apparent, and colonization of a mucosal surface is the presumed source. From 10 to 20 percent of pregnant women have vaginal colonization with *S. aureus,* and thus it is not surprising that the disease develops in postpartum women (Chen and colleagues, 2006; Guerinot and co-workers, 1982). Almost identical findings of toxic shock were reported by Robbie and associates (2000) in women with infection complicated by *Clostridium sordellii* colonization.

During the 1990s, sporadic reports of virulent group A β-hemolytic streptococcal infection began to appear as discussed on page 662. Infection is complicated in some cases by *streptococcal toxic shock syndrome* produced when pyrogenic exotoxin is elaborated. Serotypes M1 and M3 are particularly virulent (Beres and associates, 2004; Okumura and colleagues, 2004).

Delayed diagnosis and treatment may be associated with fetal or maternal mortality (Crum and colleagues 2002; Schummer and Schummer 2002). Principal therapy for toxic shock is supportive, while allowing reversal of capillary endothelial injury (see Chap. 42, p. 934). Antimicrobial therapy to include staphylococcal and streptococcal coverage is given. With evidence of pelvic infection, antimicrobial therapy must also include agents used for polymicrobial infections. Women with these infections often require extensive wound debridement and possibly hysterectomy. Because the toxin is so potent, the mortality rate is correspondingly high (Hotchkiss and Karl, 2003).

REFERENCES

American College of Obstetricians and Gynecologists: Prophylactic antibiotics in labor and delivery. Practice Bulletin No. 47, October 2003
American College of Obstetricians and Gynecologists: Episiotomy. Practice Bulletin No. 71, April 2006
Anderson DJ, Sexton DJ, Kanafani ZA, et al: Severe surgical site infection in community hospitals: Epidemiology, key procedures, and the changing prevalence of methicillin-resistant *Staphylococcus aureus.* Infect Control Hosp Epidemiol 28 (9):1047, 2007
Andrews WW, Hauth JC, Cliver SP, et al: Randomized clinical trial of extended spectrum antibiotic prophylaxis with coverage for *Ureaplasma urealyticum* to reduce post-cesarean delivery endometritis. Obstet Gynecol 101:1183, 2003
Andrews WW, Shah SR, Goldenberg RL, et al: Association of post-cesarean delivery endometritis with colonization of the chorioamnion by *Ureaplasma urealyticum.* Obstet Gynecol 85:509, 1995
Anteby EY, Yagel S, Hanoch J, et al: Puerperal and intrapartum group A streptococcal infection. Infect Dis Obstet Gynecol 7:276, 1999
Aronoff DM, Mulla ZD: Postpartum invasive group A streptococcal disease in the modern era. Infect Dis Obstet Gynecol 796892, 2008
Atkinson MW, Owen J, Wren A, et al: The effect of manual removal of the placenta on post-cesarean endometritis. Obstet Gynecol 87:99, 1996
Baksu A, Kalan A, Ozkan A, et al: The effect of placental removal method and site of uterine repair on postcesarean endometritis and operative blood loss. Acta Obstet Gynecol Scand 84(3):266, 2005
Bamigboye AA, Hofmeyr GJ: Closure versus non-closure of the peritoneum at caesarean section. Cochrane Database Syst Rev 4:CD000163, 2003
Beres SB, Sylva GL, Sturdevant DE, et al: Genome-wide molecular dissection of serotype M3 group A *Streptococcus* strains causing two epidemics of invasive infections. Proc Natl Acad Sci USA 101:11833, 2004
Berg CJ, Chang J, Callaghan WM, et al: Pregnancy-related mortality in the United States, 1991–1997. Obstet Gynecol 101:289, 2003
Berg CJ, Harper MA, Atkinson SM, et al: Preventability of pregnancy-related deaths: Results of a state-wide review. Obstet Gynecol 106:1228, 2005
Brown CEL, Dunn DH, Harrell R, et al: Computed tomography for evaluation of puerperal infection. Surg Gynecol Obstet 172:2, 1991
Brown CEL, Lowe TW, Cunningham FG, et al: Puerperal pelvic thrombophlebitis: Impact on diagnosis and treatment using x-ray computed tomography and magnetic resonance imaging. Obstet Gynecol 68:789, 1986
Brown CEL, Stettler RW, Twickler D, et al: Puerperal septic pelvic thrombophlebitis: Incidence and response to heparin therapy. Am J Obstet Gynecol 181:143, 1999
Brumfield, CG, Hauth JC, Andrews WW: Puerperal infection after cesarean delivery: Evaluation of a standardized protocol. Am J Obstet Gynecol 182:1147, 2000
Burrows LJ, Meyn LA, Weber AM: Maternal morbidity associated with vaginal versus cesarean delivery. Obstet Gynecol 103:907, 2004
Carey JC, Klebanoff MA, Hauth JC, et al: Metronidazole to prevent preterm delivery in pregnant women with asymptomatic bacterial vaginosis. N Engl J Med 342:534, 2000
Castagnola DE, Hoffman MK, Carlson J, et al: Necrotizing cervical and uterine infection in the postpartum period caused by Group A *Streptococcus.* Obstet Gynecol 111:533, 2008
Chaim W, Bashiri A, Bar-David J, et al: Prevalence and clinical significance of postpartum endometritis and wound infection. Infect Dis Obstet Gynecol 8:77, 2000

Chaim W, Horowitz S, David JB, et al: Ureaplasma urealyticum in the development of postpartum endometritis. Eur J Obstet Reprod Biol 15:145, 2003

Chelmow D, Rodriguez EJ, Sabatini MM: Suture closure of subcutaneous fat and wound disruption after cesarean delivery: A meta-analysis. Obstet Gynecol 103:974, 2004

Chelmow D, Ruehli MS, Huang E: Prophylactic use of antibiotics for non-laboring patients undergoing cesarean delivery with intact membranes: A meta-analysis. Am J Obstet Gynecol 184:656, 2001

Chen KT, Huard RC, Della-Latta P, et al: Prevalence of methicillin-sensitive and methicillin-resistant *Staphylococcus aureus* in pregnant women. 108:482, 2006

Collins CG, McCallum EA, Nelson EW, et al: Suppurative pelvic thrombophlebitis: 1. Incidence, pathology, etiology; 2. Symptomatology and diagnosis; 3. Surgical techniques: A study of 70 patients treated by ligation of the inferior vena cava and ovarian veins. Surgery 30:298, 1951

Costantine MM, Rahman M, Ghulmiyah L, et al: Timing of perioperative antibiotics for cesarean delivery: A metaanalysis. Am J Obstet Gynecol 199(3):301.e1, 2008

Crum NF, Chun HM, Gaylord TG, et al: Group A streptococcal toxic shock syndrome developing in the third trimester of pregnancy. Infect Dis Obstet Gynecol 10:209, 2002

Cunningham FG, Hauth JC, Strong JD, et al: Infectious morbidity following cesarean: Comparison of two treatment regimens. Obstet Gynecol 52:656, 1978

Declercq E, Barger M, Cabral HJ, et al: Maternal outcomes associated with planned primary cesarean births compared with planned vaginal births. Obstet Gynecol 109:669, 2007

Deneux-Tharaux C, Carmona E, Bouvier-Colle MH, et al: Postpartum maternal mortality and cesarean delivery. Obstet Gynecol 108:541, 2006

DePalma RT, Cunningham FG, Leveno KJ, et al: Continuing investigation of women at high risk for infection following cesarean delivery. Obstet Gynecol 60:53, 1982

Dinsmoor MJ, Newton ER, Gibbs RS: A randomized, double-blind placebo-controlled trial of oral antibiotic therapy following intravenous antibiotic therapy for postpartum endometritis. Obstet Gynecol 77:60, 1991

DiZerega G, Yonekura L, Roy S, et al: A comparison of clindamycin-gentamicin and penicillin gentamicin in the treatment of post-cesarean section endomyometritis. Am J Obstet Gynecol 134:238, 1979

Dunnihoo DR, Gallaspy JW, Wise RB, et al: Postpartum ovarian vein thrombophlebitis: A review. Obstet Gynecol Surv 46:415, 1991

Emmons SL, Krohn M, Jackson M, et al: Development of wound infections among women undergoing cesarean section. Obstet Gynecol 72:559, 1988

Filker RS, Monif GRG: Postpartum septicemia due to group G streptococci. Obstet Gynecol 53;28S, 1979

French LM, Smaill FM: Antibiotic regimens for endometritis after delivery. In: Cochrane Library, Chichester, Wiley Issue 1, 2002

Gallup DG, Meguiar RV: Coping with necrotizing fasciitis. Contemp Ob/Gyn 49:38, 2004

Garcia J, Aboujaoude R, Apuzzio J, et al: Septic pelvic thrombophlebitis: Diagnosis and management. Infect Dis Obstet Gynecol 2006(15614):1, 2006

Gilstrap LC III, Cunningham FG: The bacterial pathogenesis of infection following cesarean section. Obstet Gynecol 53:545, 1979

Goepfert AR, Guinn DA, Andrews WW, et al: Necrotizing fasciitis after cesarean section. Obstet Gynecol 89:409, 1997

Goldaber KG, Wendel PJ, McIntire DD, et al: Postpartum perineal morbidity after fourth degree perineal repair. Am J Obstet Gynecol 168:489, 1993

Guerinot GT, Gitomer SD, Sanko SR: Postpartum patient with toxic shock syndrome. Obstet Gynecol 59:43S, 1982

Hankins GDV, Hauth JC, Gilstrap LC, et al: Early repair of episiotomy dehiscence. Obstet Gynecol 75:48, 1990

Hartmann KE, Barrett KE, Reid VC, et al: Clinical usefulness of white blood cell count after cesarean delivery. Obstet Gynecol 96:295, 2000

Hauth JC, Gilstrap LC III, Ward SC, et al: Early repair of an external sphincter ani muscle and rectal mucosal dehiscence. Obstet Gynecol 67:806, 1986

Hauth JC, Owen J, Davis RO: Transverse uterine incision closure: One versus two layers. Am J Obstet Gynecol 167:1108, 1992

Heying R, van de Gevel J, Que YA, et al: Fibronectin-binding proteins and clumping factor A in *Staphylococcus aureus* experimental endocarditis: FnBPA is sufficient to activate human endothelial cells. Thromb Haemost 97:617, 2007

Hotchkiss RS, Karl IE: The pathophysiology and treatment of sepsis. N Engl J Med 348:2, 2003

Ismail MA, Chandler AE, Beem ME: Chlamydial colonization of the cervix in pregnant adolescents. J Reprod Med 30:549, 1985

Jacobs-Jokhan D, Hofmeyr G: Extra-abdominal versus intra-abdominal repair of the uterine incision at caesarean section. Cochrane Database Syst Rev 4:CD000085, 2004

Jacobsson B, Pernevi P, Chidekel L, et al: Bacterial vaginosis in early pregnancy may predispose for preterm birth and postpartum endometritis. Acta Obstet Gynecol Scand 81:1006, 2002

Jazayeri A, Jazayeri MK, Sahinler M, et al: Is meconium passage a risk factor for maternal infection in term pregnancies? Obstet Gynecol 99:548, 2002

Josey WE, Staggers SR Jr: Heparin therapy in septic pelvic thrombophlebitis: A study of 46 cases. Am J Obstet Gynecol 120:228, 1974

Kabiru W, Raynor BD: Obstetric outcomes associated with increase in BMI category during pregnancy. Am J Obstet Gynecol 191:928, 2004

Kaimal AJ, Zlatnik MG, Cheng YW, et al: Effect of a change in policy regarding the timing of prophylactic antibiotics on the rate of postcesarean delivery surgical-site infections. Am J Obstet Gynecol 199(3):310.e1, 2008

Kankuri E, Kurki T, Carlson P, et al: Incidence, treatment and outcome of peripartum sepsis. Acta Obstet Gynecol Scand 82:730, 2003

Klebanoff MA, Carey JC, Hauth JC, et al: Failure of metronidazole to prevent preterm delivery among pregnant women with asymptomatic *Trichomonas vaginalis* infection. N Engl J Med 345:487, 2001

Klima, DA, Snyder TE: Postpartum ovarian vein thrombosis. Obstet Gynecol 111:431, 2008

Koroukian SM: Relative risk of postpartum complications in the Ohio Medicaid population: Vaginal versus cesarean delivery. Med Care Res Rev 61:203, 2004

Livingston JC, Llata E, Rinehart E, et al: Gentamicin and clindamycin therapy in postpartum endometritis: The efficacy of daily dosing versus dosing every 8 hours. Am J Obstet Gynecol 188:149, 2003

Liu C, Abate B, Reyes M, et al: Single daily dosing of gentamicin: Pharmacokinetic comparison of two dosing methodologies for postpartum endometritis. Infect Dis Obstet Gynecol 7:133, 1999

Maberry MC, Gilstrap LC, Bawdon RE, et al: Anaerobic coverage for intra-amnionic infection: Maternal and perinatal impact. Am J Perinatol 8:338, 1991

Magann EF, Chauhan SP, Rodts-Palenik S, et al: Subcutaneous stitch closure versus subcutaneous drain to prevent wound disruption after cesarean delivery: A randomized clinical trial. Am J Obstet Gynecol 186:1119, 2002

Maharaj D: Puerperal pyrexia: A review. Part II: Obstet Gynecol Surv 62:400, 2007

Maldjian C, Adam R, Maldjian J, et al: MRI appearance of the pelvis in the post cesarean-section patient. Magn Reson Imaging 17:223, 1999

McNeeley SG Jr, Hendrix SL, Bennett SM, et al: Synthetic graft placement in the treatment of fascial dehiscence with necrosis and infection. Am J Obstet Gynecol 179:1430, 1998

Myles TD, Gooch J, Santolaya J: Obesity as an independent risk factor for infectious morbidity in patients who undergo cesarean delivery. Obstet Gynecol 100:959, 2002

Nathan L, Leveno KJ: Group A streptococcal puerperal sepsis: Historical review and 1990s resurgence. Infect Dis Obstet Gynecol 1:252, 1994

Naumann RW, Hauth JC, Owen J, et al: Subcutaneous tissue approximation in relation to wound disruption after cesarean delivery in obese women. Obstet Gynecol 85:412, 1995

Okumura K, Schroff R, Campbell R, et al: Group A streptococcal puerperal sepsis with retroperitoneal involvement developing in a late postpartum woman: Case report. Am Surg 70:730, 2004

Owen J, Andrews WW: Wound complications after cesarean section. Clin Obstet Gynecol 27:842, 1994

Owen J, Hauth JC: Episiotomy infection and dehiscence. In Gilstrap LC III, Faro S (eds): Infections in Pregnancy. New York, Liss, P 61, 1990

Palep-Singh M, Jayaprakasan J, Hopkisson JF: Peripartum group A streptococcal sepsis: A case report. J Reprod Med 52 (10):977, 2007

Patel M, Kumar RA, Stamm AM, et al: USA300 genotype community-associated methicillin-resistant *Staphylococcus aureus* as a cause of surgical site infection. J Clin Microbiol 45 (10):3431, 2007

Pitt C, Sanchez-Ramos L, Kaunitz AM: Adjunctive intravaginal metronidazole for the prevention of postcesarean endometritis: A randomized controlled trial. Obstet Gynecol 98:745, 2001

Que YA, Haefliger JA, Piroth L, et al: Fibrinogen and fibronectin binding cooperative for valve infection and invasion in *Staphylococcus aureus* experimental endocarditis. J Exp Med 201:1627, 2005

Ramin SM, Gilstrap LC: Episiotomy and early repair of dehiscence. Clin Obstet Gynecol 37:816, 1994

Ramin SM, Ramus R, Little B, et al: Early repair of episiotomy dehiscence associated with infection. Am J Obstet Gynecol 167:1104, 1992

Reid VC, Hartmann KE, McMahon M, et al: Vaginal preparation with povidone iodine and postcesarean infections morbidity: A randomized controlled trial. Obstet Gynecol 97:147, 2001

Rivlin ME, Carroll CS, Morrison JC: Conservative surgery for uterine incisional necrosis complicating cesarean delivery. Obstet Gynecol 103:1105, 2004

Robbie LA, Dummer S, Booth NA, et al: Plasminogen activator inhibitor 2 and urokinase-type plasminogen activator in plasma and leucocytes in patients with severe sepsis. Br J Haematol 109:342, 2000

Rose CH, Blessitt KL, Araghizadeh F: Episiotomy dehiscence that required intestinal diversion. Am J Obstet Gynecol 193:1759, 2005

Rotas M, McCalla S, Liu C, et al: Methicillin-resistant *Staphylococcus aureus* necrotizing pneumonia arising from an infected episiotomy site. Obstet Gynecol 109:533, 2007

Rouse DJ, Cliver S, Lincoln TL, et al: Clinical trial of chlorhexidine vaginal irrigation to prevent peripartal infection in nulliparous women. Am J Obstet Gynecol 189:166, 2003

Rouse DJ, Hauth JC, Andrews WW, et al: Chlorhexidine vaginal irrigation for the prevention of peripartal infection: A placebo-controlled randomized clinical trial. Am J Obstet Gynecol 176: 617, 1997

Rouse DJ, Landon M, Leveno KJ, et al: The maternal-fetal medicine units cesarean registry: Chorioamnionitis at term and its duration-relationship to outcomes. Am J Obstet Gynecol 191:211, 2004

Saleem S, Reza T, McClure EM, et al: Chlorhexidine vaginal and neonatal wipes in home births in Pakistan: A randomized controlled trial. Obstet Gynecol 110:977

Schorge JO, Granter SR, Lerner LH, et al: Postpartum and vulvar necrotizing fasciitis: Early clinical diagnosis and histopathologic correlation. J Reprod Med 43:586, 1998

Schummer W, Schummer C: Two cases of delayed diagnosis of postpartal streptococcal toxic shock syndrome. Infect Dis Obstet Gynecol 10:217, 2002

Shahabi S, Klein JP, Rinaudo PF: Primary psoas abscess complicating a normal vaginal delivery. Obstet Gynecol 99:906, 2002

Sheffield JS, Cunningham FG: Detecting and treating septic pelvic thrombophlebitis. Contemp Ob/Gyn 3:15, 2001

Sherman D, Lurie S, Betzer M, et al: Uterine flora at cesarean and its relationship to postpartum endometritis. Obstet Gynecol 94:787, 1999

Shy KK, Eschenbach DA: Fatal perineal cellulitis from an episiotomy site. Obstet Gynecol 52:293, 1979

Smaill F, Hofmeyr GJ: Antibiotic prophylaxis for cesarean section. Cochrane Database Syst Rev 2:CD000933, 2002

Soltesz S, Biedler A, Ohlmann P, et al: Puerperal sepsis due to infected episiotomy wound. Zentralbl Gynakol 121:441, 1999

Starr RV, Zurawski J, Ismail M: Preoperative vaginal preparation with povidone-iodine and the risk of postcesarean endometritis. Obstet Gynecol 105:1024, 2005

Sullivan SA, Smith T, Change E, et al: Administration of cefazolin prior to skin incision is superior to cefazolin at cord clamping in preventing postcesarean infectious morbidity: A randomized, controlled trial. Am J Obstet Gynecol 196:455.e1, 2007

Swanson A, Lau KK, Kornman T, et al: Primary psoas muscle abscess in pregnancy. Aust NZ J Obstet Gynaecol 48(6):607, 2008

Swartz MN: Cellulitis. N Engl J Med 350:904, 2004

Sweet RL, Ledger WJ: Puerperal infectious morbidity. A two year review. Am J Obstet Gynecol 117:1093, 1973

Tita ATN, Hauth JC, Grimes A, et al: Decreasing incidence of postcesarean endometritis with extended-spectrum antibiotic prophylaxis. Obstet Gynecol 111:51, 2008

Tulandi T, Al-Jaroudi D: Nonclosure of peritoneum: A reappraisal. Am J Obstet Gynecol 189:609, 2003

Twickler DM, Setiawan AT, Harrell RS, et al: CT appearance of the pelvis after cesarean section. Am J Roentgenol 156:523, 1991

Udagawa H, Oshio Y, Shimizu Y: Serious group A streptococcal infection around delivery. Obstet Gynecol 94:153, 1999

Urschel JD: Necrotizing soft tissue infections. Postgrad Med J 75:645, 1999

Uygur D, Yesildaglar N, Kis S, et al: Early repair of episiotomy dehiscence. Aust N Z J Obstet Gynaecol 44:244, 2004

Watts DH, Krohn MA, Hillier SL, et al: Bacterial vaginosis as a risk factor for post-cesarean endometritis. Obstet Gynecol 75:52, 1990

Wechter ME, Pearlman MD, Hartmann KE: Reclosure of the disrupted laparotomy wound. A systematic review. Obstet Gynecol 106:376, 2005

Wetchler SJ, Dunn LJ: Ovarian abscess. Report of a case and a review of the literature. Obstet Gynecol Surv 40:476, 1985

Witlin AG, Sibai BM: Postpartum ovarian vein thrombosis after vaginal delivery: A report of 11 cases. Obstet Gynecol 85:775, 1995

Contraception

For sexually active fertile women who do not use contraception, pregnancy rates approach 90 percent at 1 year. For those who do not desire pregnancy, fertility regulation is now possible, and a variety of effective contraceptive methods are shown in Table 32-1. None is completely without side effects or categorically without danger. **One tenet emphasized throughout this chapter is that contraception usually poses less risk than does pregnancy.**

Nationally representative data concerning contraceptive use are shown in Figure 32-1. With use during the first year, wide variations can be seen between estimated failure rates of perfect and typical use (Table 32-2). Many of these rates can be appreciably reduced with effective motivation and education (Gilliam and co-workers, 2004). The World Health Organization has crafted four evidence-based guides for family planning, which encompass topics of contraceptive selection, patient counseling, and method use. These are available at the World Health Organization website: http://www.who.int/reproductive-health/publications/family_planning.html.

HORMONAL CONTRACEPTIVES

These are currently available in oral, injectable, transdermal-patch, and transvaginal-ring forms. Oral contraceptive pills are a combination of estrogen and progestin—"the pill"—are or progestin only. Other forms contain progestins alone or a combination of estrogen and progestin. Male hormonal contraceptive options have been evaluated in human trials and may be an option in the future (Blithe, 2008; Gu and associates, 2009; Mommers and co-workers, 2008).

Estrogen Plus Progestin Contraceptives

Combination oral contraceptives (COCs) are the most frequently used method of hormonal contraception, and an almost bewildering variety that are marketed are listed in Table 32-3. Most are also available as generics, and the U.S. Food and Drug Administration (FDA) (2008) confirms the bioequivalence of COC generics. Moreover, the American College of Obstetricians and Gynecologists (2007a) supports the use of either branded or generic COCs.

Mechanisms of Action

The contraceptive actions of COCs are multiple, but the most important effect is to prevent ovulation by suppression of hypothalamic gonadotropin-releasing factors. This in turn prevents pituitary secretion of follicle-stimulating hormone (FSH) and luteinizing hormone (LH). Progestins prevent ovulation by suppressing LH and also thicken cervical mucus, thereby retarding sperm passage. In addition, they render the endometrium unfavorable for implantation. Estrogen prevents ovulation by suppressing FSH release. It also stabilizes the endometrium, which prevents intermenstrual bleeding—also known as *breakthrough bleeding.*

The net effect is extremely effective ovulation suppression, inhibition of sperm migration through cervical mucus, and creation of an unfavorable endometrium for implantation. Thus, they provide virtually absolute protection against conception if taken as directed.

Pharmacology

In the United States, the *estrogens* used for contraception are *ethinyl estradiol* and much less commonly, its 3-methyl ether,

TABLE 32-1. Contraceptive Methods Currently Used in the United States

Combination estrogen and progestin contraceptives
  Pills
  Transdermal patch
  Vaginal ring
Progestin-only
  Pills
  Injectable (intramuscular, subcutaneous)
  Subdermal implant
  Intrauterine device
Copper intrauterine device
Physical, chemical, or barrier techniques
Preejaculatory withdrawal
Sexual abstinence around the time of ovulation
Breast feeding
Permanent sterilization

mestranol. Almost all currently available *progestins* are 19-nortestosterone derivatives, but one is an aldosterone derivative. Although individual progestins are initially chosen because of their progestational potencies, they are often compared and prescribed based on their presumed progestational, estrogenic, and especially their androgenic effects. A scientific basis for such selective prescribing, however, is lacking (Wallach and Grimes, 2000).

Dosage

Over time, the estrogen and progestin contents of COCs have been reduced remarkably to minimize hormone-related adverse effects. Currently, the lowest acceptable dose is limited by their ability to prevent pregnancy and unacceptable breakthrough bleeding. Although daily estrogen content varies from 20 to 50 μg of ethinyl estradiol, most contain 35 μg or less (see Table 32-3). The amount of progestin varies in two ways. In some formulations, the progestin dose remains constant during the cycle—*monophasic.* In others, the progestin and in some, the estrogen dose varies during the cycle—*biphasic* and *triphasic.*

Phasic pills were developed to reduce the amount of total progestin per cycle without sacrificing contraceptive efficacy or cycle control. The reduction is achieved by beginning with a low dose of progestin and increasing it later in the contraceptive cycle. Despite the theoretic advantage of lower total progesterone dose per cycle, this has not been borne out clinically (Moreau and colleagues, 2007; van Vliet and associates, 2006).

Administration

With the exception of one preparation, COCs are taken daily for a specified time (21 to 81 days) and then omitted for a specified time (4 to 7 days) called the "pill-free interval." During these

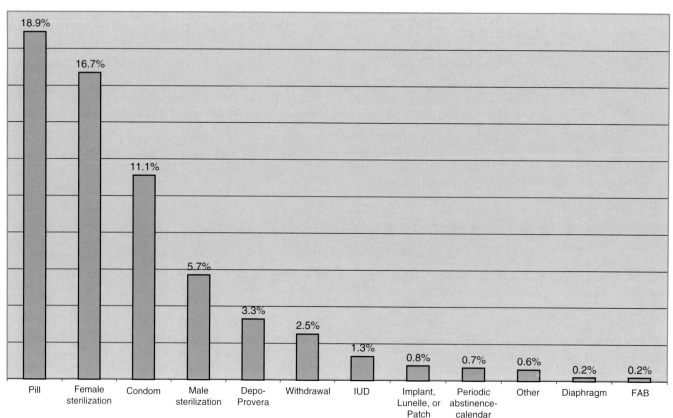

Method Use Among all Contraceptors

FIGURE 32-1 Contraceptive use in the United States, 2002, for users aged 15 to 44. DMPA = depot medroxyprogesterone acetate; FAB = fertility awareness-based method; IUD = intrauterine device. (Data from Chandra and co-workers, 2005.)

TABLE 32-2. Contraceptive Failure Rates During the First Year of Use

Method	Percent of Women with Pregnancy	
	Perfect Use	Typical Use
None	85	85
Combination pill	0.3	8
Progestin-only pill ("mini-pill")	0.5	8
Intrauterine devices:		
Mirena levonorgestrel device	0.1	0.1
ParaGard T 380A	0.6	0.8
Patch	0.3	8
Depot medroxyprogesterone	0.3	3.1
Combined injectable	0.5	3
Levonorgestrel implants	0.05	0.05
NuvaRing vaginal ring	8	0.3
Female sterilization	0.5	0.5
Male sterilization	0.1	0.15
Spermicides	18	29
Periodic abstinence		
Calendar	9	20
Ovulation method	3	
Symptothermal	2	
Postovulation	1	
Withdrawal	4	27
Cervical cap		
Parous women	26	32
Nulliparous women	9	16
Sponge		
Parous women	20	32
Nulliparous women	9	16
Diaphragm and spermicides	6	16
Condom		
Male	2	15
Female	5	21
Emergency contraception	>75% reduction	

Modified from Speroff and Darney, 2001, and Trussell, 2004.

pill-free days, withdrawal bleeding is expected. One trend of pills with lower estrogen doses is to shorten the pill-free interval, which seems to reduce the occurrence of intermenstrual bleeding (Nakajima and colleagues, 2007). For example, *Loestrin 24 Fe* and *Yaz* provide hormones for 24 days followed by 4 pill-free days. Alternatively, longer durations of active hormone, designed to minimize the number of withdrawal episodes, have been implemented (Edelman and co-workers, 2006). These extended-cycle products, such as *Seasonale* and *Seasonique*, produce a 13-week cycle, that is, 12 weeks of hormone use, followed by a week for withdrawal menses. More recently, in 2007, the FDA approved the first continuous COC, *Lybrel*, which is taken 365 days of each year.

Pill Usage

Ideally, women should begin COCs on the first day of a menstrual cycle, in which case a back-up contraceptive method is unnecessary. With the more traditional "Sunday start," women begin pills on the first Sunday that follows menses onset, and a back-up method is needed for 1 week to prevent conception. With the "Quick Start" method, COCs are started on any day, commonly the day prescribed, regardless of cycle timing. A back-up method is used during the first week. This latter approach improves short-term compliance (Westhoff and co-workers, 2002, 2007b). If the woman is already pregnant during Quick Start initiation, COCs are not teratogenic (see Chap. 14, p. 322) (Lammer and Cordero, 1986). Similarly, same-day initiation can be implemented with the contraceptive vaginal ring or patch (Murthy and co-workers, 2005; Schafer and associates, 2006).

For maximum efficiency, pills should be taken at the same time each day. If one dose is missed, contraception is likely not diminished with higher-dose monophasic COCs. Doubling the next dose will minimize breakthrough bleeding and maintain the pill schedule. If several doses are missed or lower-dose pills are used, the pill may be stopped, and an effective barrier

TABLE 32-3. Combination Oral Contraceptives Available in the United States

Product Name[a]	Estrogen	μg (days)[b]	Progestin	mg (days)	
Monophasic Preparations					
20 μg estrogen					
Yaz	EE	20 (24)	Drospirenone	3.00	
Alesse, Aviane, Lutera; Levlite, Lessina, Sronyx	EE	20	Levonorgestrel	0.10	
Loestrin 1/20, Junel 1/20, Microgestin 1/20	EE	20	Norethindrone acetate	1.00	
Loestrin 24 Fe	EE	20 (24)	Norethindrone acetate	1.00	(24)
30–35 μg estrogen					
Desogen, Ortho-Cept, Apri, Reclipsen, Solia	EE	30	Desogestrel	0.15	
Yasmin	EE	30	Drospirenone	3.00	
Demulen 1/35, Kelnor, Zovia 1/35	EE	35	Ethynodiol diacetate	1.00	
Levlen, Nordette, Levora, Portia	EE	30	Levonorgestrel	0.15	
Lo/Ovral, Cryselle, Low-Ogestrel	EE	30	Norgestrel	0.30	
Ovcon-35, Balziva, Zenchent	EE	35	Norethindrone	0.40	
Femcon Fe	EE	35	Norethindrone	0.40	
Brevicon; Modicon, Necon 0.5/35, Nortrel 0.5/35; Nelova 0.5/35E	EE	35	Norethindrone	0.50	
Ortho-Novum 1/35, Necon 1/35, Nortrel 1/35, Nelova 1/35E; Norinyl 1+35	EE	35	Norethindrone	1.00	
Loestrin 1.5/30, Junel 1.5/30, Microgestin 1.5/30	EE	30	Norethindrone acetate	1.50	
Ortho-Cyclen, Sprintec, Mononessa	EE	35	Norgestimate	0.25	
50 μg estrogen					
Ovral, Ogestrel	EE	50	Norgestrel	0.50	
Demulen 1/50, Zovia 1/50	EE	50	Ethynodiol diacetate	1.00	
Nelova 1/50M	Mes	50	Norethindrone	1.00	
Norinyl 1+50; Ortho-Novum 1/50, Necon 1/50	Mes	50	Norethindrone	1.00	
Ovcon 50	EE	50	Norethindrone	1.00	
Multiphasic Preparations					
20 μg estrogen					
Mircette, Kariva	EE	20 (21) 0 (2) 10 (5)	Desogestrel	0.15	
25 μg estrogen					
Ortho Tri-Cyclen Lo	EE	25	Norgestimate	0.18	(7)
				0.215	(7)
				0.25	(7)
Cyclessa, Velivet	EE	25	Desogestrel	0.1	(7)
				0.125	(7)
				0.15	(7)
30–35 μg estrogen					
Ortho Tri-Cyclen, Tri-Sprintec, Trinessa, Tri-Previfem	EE	35	Norgestimate	0.18	(7)
				0.215	(7)
				0.25	(7)
Tri-Levlen, Triphasil, Trivora, Enpresse	EE	30 (6) 40 (5) 30 (10)	Levonorgestrel	0.05 (6) 0.075 (5) 0.125 (10)	
Estrostep	EE	20 (5) 30 (7) 35 (9)	Norethindrone acetate	1.00	
Estrostep Fe, Tri-Legest Fe, Tilia Fe	EE	20 (5) 30 (7) 35 (9)	Norethindrone acetate	1.00	
Jenest	EE	35	Norethindrone	0.50 (7) 1.00 (14)	
Ortho-Novum 10/11, Necon 10/11, Nelova 10/11	EE	35	Norethindrone	0.50 (10) 1.00 (11)	

TABLE 32-3. Combination Oral Contraceptives Available in the United States (Continued)

Product Name[a]	Estrogen	μg (days)[b]	Progestin	mg (days)	
Ortho-Novum 7/7/7, Necon 7/7/7, Nortrel 7/7/7	EE	35	Norethindrone	0.50	(7)
				0.75	(7)
				1.00	(7)
Tri-Norinyl, Aranelle, Leena	EE	35	Norethindrone	0.50	(7)
				1.00	(9)
				0.50	(5)
Progestin-Only Preparations					
Ovrette	None		Norgestrel	0.075	(c)
Micronor, Errin; Nor-QD, Camila, Nor-BE, Jolivette	None		Norethindrone	0.35	(c)
Extended-Cycle Preparations					
Seasonale[c], Quasense[c], Jolessa[c]	EE	30 (84)	Levonorgestrel	0.15	(84)
Seasonique[d]	EE	30 (84)	Levonorgestrel	0.15	(84)
	EE	10 (7)			
Continuous Preparation					
Lybrel[e]	EE	20 (28)	Levonorgestrel	0.09	

EE = ethinyl estradiol; Mes = mestranol.
Numbers in parentheses = number of days at a particular dosage.
(c) = continuous use.
[a]Purple ink denotes original name brand. Black ink denotes subsequent generics.
[b]Administered for 21 days, variations listed in parentheses.
[c]12 weeks of active pills, 1 week of inert pills.
[d]12 weeks of active pills, 1 week of ethinyl estradiol only.
[e]One pill every day, 365 days each year.
Compiled from U.S. Food and Drug Administration, 2008a.

technique used until menses. The pill may then be restarted after this withdrawal bleeding. Alternatively, a new pack can be started immediately following identification of missed pills, and a barrier method used as a back-up method for 1 week. If there is no withdrawal bleeding, the woman should continue her pills but seek attention to exclude pregnancy.

Drug Interactions

Combination oral contraceptives interfere with the actions of some drugs (Table 32-4). Conversely, some drugs decrease the effectiveness of COCs (Table 32-5).

Beneficial Effects

When used reliably, COCs offer effective rapidly reversible methods of pregnancy prevention. In addition, there are a number of noncontraceptive benefits (European Society of Human Reproduction and Embryology, 2005). Some are listed in Table 32-6.

Possible Adverse Effects

A number of metabolic changes, often qualitatively similar to those of pregnancy, have been identified in women taking oral contraceptives. For example, total plasma thyroxine (T_4) and thyroid-binding proteins are elevated. Plasma cortisol concentration increases with a nearly comparable increase in transcortin. Therefore, these pregnancy-like effects should be

considered when evaluating laboratory tests in women using COCs.

Lipoproteins and Lipids. In general, COCs increase serum levels of triglycerides and total cholesterol. Estrogen decreases the concentration of low-density lipoprotein (LDL) cholesterol and increases high-density lipoprotein (HDL) cholesterol. Some progestins cause the reverse. Despite this, the clinical consequences of these perturbations have almost certainly been overstated. Oral contraceptives are not atherogenic, and their impact on lipids is inconsequential for most women (Wallach and Grimes, 2000). But in women with dyslipidemias, the American College of Obstetricians and Gynecologists (2006b) recommends assessment of lipid levels following initiation of COCs. In women with LDL cholesterol levels >160 mg/dL, or if there are multiple additional risk factors for cardiovascular disease, alternative contraceptive methods are recommended.

Carbohydrate Metabolism. There are limited effects on carbohydrate metabolism with current low-dose formulations in women who do not have diabetes. In addition, the risk of developing diabetes is not increased (Lopez and colleagues, 2007; Kim and associates, 2002). Moreover, COCs may be used in nonsmoking, diabetic women younger than 35 years who have no associated vascular disease (American College of Obstetricians and Gynecologists, 2006b).

TABLE 32-4. Drugs Whose Effectiveness Is Influenced by Combination Oral Contraceptives

Interacting Drug	Documentation	Management
Analgesics		
Acetaminophen	Adequate	Larger doses of analgesic may be required
Aspirin	Probable	Larger doses of analgesic may be required
Meperidine	Suspected	Smaller doses of analgesic may be required
Morphine	Probable	Larger doses of analgesic may be required
Anticoagulants		
Dicumarol, warfarin	Controversial	
Antidepressants		
Imipramine	Suspected	Decrease dosage about a third
Tranquilizers		
Diazepam	Suspected	Decrease dose
Alprazolam		
Temazepam	Possible	May need to increase dose
Other benzodiazepines	Suspected	Observe for increased effect
Anti-inflammatories		
Corticosteroids	Adequate	Watch for potentiation of effects, decrease dose accordingly
Bronchodilators		
Aminophylline	Adequate	Reduce starting dose by a third
Theophylline		
Caffeine		
Antihypertensives		
Cyclopenthiazide	Adequate	Increase dose
Metoprolol	Suspected	May need to lower dose
Antibiotics		
Troleandomycin	Suspected liver damage	Avoid
Cyclosporine	Possible	May use smaller dose
Antiretrovirals	Variable	See the manufacturer or other[a]

[a]UCSF: HIV INSite, 2005. UCSF = University of California at San Francisco.
Modified from Wallach, 2000, with permission.

TABLE 32-5. Drugs That May Reduce Combined Hormonal Contraceptive Efficacy

Interacting Drug	Documentation
Antituberculous	
Rifampin	Established—reduced efficacy <50 μg EE
Antifungals	
Griseofulvin	Strongly suspected
Anticonvulsants and Sedatives	
Phenytoin, mephenytoin, phenobarbital, primidone, carbamazepine, ethosuximide	Strongly suspected—reduced efficacy <50-μg EE, trials lacking
Antibiotics	
Tetracycline, doxycycline	Two small studies find no association
Penicillins	No association documented
Ciprofloxacin	No effect on efficacy of 30-μg EE + desogestrel
Ofloxacin	No effect on efficacy of a 30-μg EE + levonorgestrel
Antiretrovirals	Variable effects—see the manufacturer or other[a]

[a]UCSF: HIV Insite, 2005. UCSF = University of California at San Francisco.
Modified after Wallach, 2000, with permission.

TABLE 32-6. Some Benefits of Combined Estrogen Plus Progestin Oral Contraceptives

Increased bone density
Reduced menstrual blood loss and anemia
Decreased risk of ectopic pregnancy
Improved dysmenorrhea from endometriosis
Fewer premenstrual complaints
Decreased risk of endometrial and ovarian cancer
Reduction in various benign breast diseases
Inhibition of hirsutism progression
Improvement of acne
Prevention of atherogenesis
Decreased incidence and severity of acute salpingitis
Decreased activity of rheumatoid arthritis

Protein Metabolism. Estrogens increase hepatic production of a variety of globulins. One is sex-hormone binding globulin (SHBG), which leads to decreased bioavailable testosterone concentrations and its consequent effects. Angiotensinogen production is also augmented by COCs, and its conversion by renin to angiotensin I may be associated with "pill-induced hypertension" discussed subsequently. Fibrinogen, and likely factors II, VII, IX, X, XII, and XIII, are all increased in direct proportion to estrogen dose (Comp, 1996; Kaunitz, 1999). Associated risks for venous and arterial thrombosis are also discussed subsequently.

Hepatic Effects. Cholestasis and cholestatic jaundice are uncommon, but they resolve when COCs are discontinued. There are conflicting reports regarding the risk for cholelithiasis and cholecystectomy with COC use. If the risk exists, it appears small (Stuart and colleagues, 2007). Although active hepatitis is a contraindication to COC use, there is no reason to withhold oral contraceptives from women who have recovered.

Neoplasia. A stimulatory effect on some cancers is always a concern with female sex steroids. Fortunately, most studies indicate that overall, COCs are not associated with an increased risk of cancer (Hannaford and associates, 2007). In fact, a protective effect against ovarian and endometrial cancer has been shown (Collaborative Group on Epidemiological Studies of Ovarian Cancer, 2008; Cancer and Steroid Hormone Study, 1987). Protection from these cancers decreases, however, as time from pill use increases (Tworoger and co-workers, 2007). Rates of colorectal cancer appear to be reduced in ever users (Kabat and co-workers, 2008).

Although COC use in the past was linked to development of *hepatic focal nodular hyperplasia* and *benign hepatic adenoma,* large studies do not support this (Heinemann and colleagues, 1998). There is also no evidence for increased risk of *hepatocellular cancer* (Maheshwari and colleagues, 2007).

Because a third of cases of malignant melanoma in women develop during childbearing years, an association with hormonal and reproductive factors has been sought. To date, however, no association between COCs and melanoma has been identified (Lens and associates, 2008).

The relative risk of *cervical dysplasia* and *cervical cancer* is increased in current COC users, but this declines after use is discontinued. Following 10 or more years, risk returns to that of never users (International Collaboration of Epidemiological Studies of Cervical Cancer, 2007). Furthermore, after cervical dysplasia treatment, rates of recurrence are not increased by COC use (Frega and colleagues, 2008).

It is unclear whether COCs contribute to the development of *breast cancer.* The Collaborative Group on Hormonal Factors in Breast Cancer (1996) analyzed data from 54 studies that included more than 53,000 women with and more than 100,000 without breast cancer. There was a small but significantly increased relative risk for breast cancer of 1.24 for current users, 1.16 for those 1 to 4 years after stopping, and 1.07 for those 5 to 9 years after stopping. In this study, tumors associated with COC use tended to be less aggressive and to be detected at an earlier stage—a finding consistent with the possibility that the increased risk of breast cancer was due to greater surveillance among users. In women who are carriers of the BRCA1 or BRCA2 mutation, risks for breast cancer are not increased by COC use (Brohet and associates, 2007). With regard to *benign breast disease,* COCs appear to lower rates (Vessey and Yeates, 2007).

Nutrition. Aberrations in the levels of several *nutrients,* similar to changes induced by normal pregnancy, have been described for women who use oral contraceptives. Lower plasma levels have been described for ascorbic acid, folic acid, vitamin B_6 (pyridoxine), vitamin B_{12}, niacin, riboflavin, and zinc. An adequate diet, however, is sufficient for any detrimental deficiency (Mooij and co-workers, 1991). Although it is widely held that COCs lead to weight gain, studies have not verified this (Gallo and associates, 2008).

Cardiovascular Effects. A number of infrequent but significant cardiovascular risks are associated with COC use. These include thromboembolic disease, myocardial infarction, and stroke. For women with prior history of these events, COCs should not be considered (Table 32-7). And because these complications are increased in women older than 35 years and who smoke, COCs are not recommended for this population.

It has long been known that the risk of *deep-venous thrombosis and pulmonary embolism* is increased in women who use COCs (Stadel, 1981). These clearly are estrogen-dose related, and rates have been substantively decreased with lower-dose formulations containing 20 to 35 μg of ethinyl estradiol (Westhoff, 1998). Even with increased risk, the incidence with COCs use is only 3 to 4 per 10,000 woman-years (Mishell, 2000). Moreover, the risk is lower than the incidence of 5 to 6 per 10,000 woman-years estimated for pregnancy (see Chap. 47, p. 1013). The enhanced risk of thromboembolism appears to decrease rapidly once COCs are stopped.

Those most at risk for venous thrombosis and embolism include women with protein C or S deficiencies (Comp, 1996). Other clinical factors that increase the risk of venous thrombosis and embolism with COC use are hypertension, obesity, diabetes, smoking, and a sedentary lifestyle (Pomp and co-workers, 2007, 2008). Contraceptive use during the month before a major operative procedure appears to double the risk for postoperative

TABLE 32-7. Typical Package Insert Listing Contraindications and a Warning about the Use of Combination Oral Contraceptives

CONTRAINDICATIONS: Combination contraceptives should not be used in women with:

Thrombophlebitis or thromboembolic disorders
History of deep-vein thrombophlebitis or thrombotic disorders
Cerebrovascular or coronary-artery disease
Thrombogenic cardiac valvulopathies
Thrombogenic heart arrhythmias
Diabetes with vascular involvement
Severe hypertension
Known or suspected breast carcinoma
Carcinoma of the endometrium or other known or suspected estrogen-dependent neoplasia
Undiagnosed abnormal genital bleeding
Cholestatic jaundice of pregnancy or jaundice with pill use
Hepatic adenomas or carcinomas, or active liver disease with abnormal liver function
Known or suspected pregnancy
Major surgery with prolonged immobilization

WARNINGS
Cigarette smoking increases the risk of serious cardiovascular side effects from oral-contraceptive use. This risk increases with age and with the extent of smoking (in epidemiological studies, 15 or more cigarettes per day was associated with a significantly increased risk) and is quite marked in women over 35 years of age. Women who use oral contraceptives should be strongly advised not to smoke.

From Physicians Desk Reference, 2009.

thromboembolism (Robinson and co-workers, 1991). The American College of Obstetricians and Gynecologists (2007c) recommends balancing the risks of thromboembolism with those of unintended pregnancy during the 4 to 6 weeks required to reverse the thrombogenic effects of COCs prior to surgery.

According to the World Health Organization Collaborative Study (1998), the increase of *ischemic and hemorrhagic strokes* in nonsmoking women younger than 35 years is about 10 and 25 events per 1 million woman years, respectively. Several studies have concluded that the use of COCs by healthy, nonsmoking women is not associated with an increased risk of either type strokes (World Health Organization Collaborative Study, 1996). Conversely, women who have hypertension, smoke, or have migraine headaches with visual aura *and* use oral contraceptives have an increased risk of strokes (MacClellan and associates, 2007). Because the absolute risk of stroke is low, however, the American College of Obstetricians and Gynecologists (2006b) has concluded that COCs may be considered for women with migraines that lack focal neurological signs if they are otherwise healthy, normotensive nonsmokers younger than 35 years.

Oral contraceptives containing low-dose estrogen and low-androgenic progestins are not associated with an increased risk of *myocardial infarction* in nonsmokers (Margolis and associates, 2007; World Health Organization Collaborative Study, 1997). Smoking is an independent risk factor for myocardial infarction, and oral contraceptives act synergistically to increase this risk, especially after age 35 (Craft and Hannaford, 1989).

The estrogen component of COCs increases plasma angiotensinogen (renin substrate) to levels near those found in normal pregnancy. And although most women demonstrate these changes, low-dose COCs formulations rarely, if ever, cause clinically significant hypertension (Chasan-Taber and colleagues, 1996). A history of gestational hypertension does not preclude subsequent COC use. Because the absolute risk of stroke is low in hypertensive women using COCs, those with well-controlled uncomplicated hypertension who are nonsmokers, otherwise healthy, and younger than 35 may be considered for their use (American College of Obstetricians and Gynecologists, 2006b).

Effects on Reproduction. At least 90 percent of women who previously ovulated regularly begin to do so within 3 months after discontinuance of oral contraceptives. There is no evidence that COCs are teratogenic (Rothman and Louik, 1978; Savolainen and associates, 1981).

Lactation. Very small quantities of the hormones are excreted in breast milk, but no adverse effects on infants have been reported (World Health Organization, 1988). There is concern that these agents reduce the volume of breast milk, although data are limited (Truitt and colleagues, 2003). Alternatively, progestin-only oral contraceptives have little effect on lactation, provide excellent contraception, and thus may be preferred in women who are exclusively breast feeding their infants as subsequently discussed (p. 694).

Mood Changes. Low-dose estrogen formulations are not associated with depression or premenstrual mood changes, and indeed, may improve the latter (Joffe and associates, 2007). This is especially true with the drospirenone-containing COCs, *Yaz* and *Yasmin* (Bayer HealthCare, Wayne, NJ). Several studies have shown improvement in symptoms for women with premenstrual dysphoric disorder (PMDD) who use these (Lopez, 2009; Pearlstein, 2005; Yonkers, 2005, and all their associates, 2005). In fact, the FDA has approved indications to include treatment of premenstrual syndrome and moderate acne vulgaris for women requesting oral contraception.

Drospirenone is an analog of the aldosterone antagonist, spironolactone, and the dose of drospirenone in COCs currently marketed has properties similar to 25 mg of this diuretic (Seeger and co-workers, 2007). It displays antiandrogenic activity, and its antimineralocorticoid properties may, in theory, cause potassium retention, leading to hyperkalemia (Krattenmacher, 2000). Thus, drospirenone should not be prescribed for those with renal or adrenal insufficiency or with hepatic dysfunction. Moreover, monitoring of serum potassium levels is recommended in the first month for patients chronically treated concomitantly with any drug associated with potassium retention. These include nonsteroidal anti-inflammatory drugs

(NSAIDs), angiotensin-converting enzyme (ACE) inhibitors, angiotensin II antagonists, heparin, aldosterone antagonists, and potassium-sparing diuretics (Bayer HealthCare Pharmaceuticals, 2007b). All of this is recommended in the face of evidence that oral drospirenone in doses used in current COCs has no significant effect on serum potassium levels in patients with mild or moderate renal insufficiency (Schürmann and co-workers, 2006).

Infection. There are conflicting data concerning a role for COCs and episodic vulvovaginal candidiasis, although lower rates of bacterial vaginosis have been reported (Geiger and Foxman, 1996; Riggs and colleagues, 2007). Most but not all studies show increased rates of *Chlamydia trachomatis* infection in COC users, but not of *Neisseria gonorrhoeae* (Baeten and co-workers, 2001; Stuart and colleagues, 2003). Ness and co-workers (2001) found that COCs did not decrease the incidence of pelvic inflammatory disease but did modify its clinical severity. Some but not all studies suggest that COCs increase susceptibility to human immunodeficiency virus (HIV) infection and its progression (Baeten and associates, 2007a, b; Morrison and co-workers, 2007).

Other Effects. The progestin component of COCs reduces serum free testosterone levels and inhibits 5α-reductase to limit conversion of testosterone to its active metabolite, dihydrotestosterone. The estrogen component increases sex-hormone binding globulin (SHBG) production and also lowers circulating androgen levels. The expected results of these actions are to improve androgen-related conditions such as acne and hirsutism.

Hyperpigmentation of the face and forehead—chloasma—is more likely in women who demonstrated such a change during pregnancy. This is seen less commonly with the low-dose estrogen formulations. *Cervical mucorrhea,* likely due to cervical ectopy, is common in response to the estrogen component of COCs (Critchlow and colleagues, 1995). COCs may decrease formation of uterine *leiomyomas* in some women (Parazzini and co-workers, 1992). Although previously used for treating functional ovarian cysts, low-dose COCs have no effects (Grimes and colleagues, 2006b).

Transdermal Administration

The *Ortho Evra patch* (Ortho-McNeil Pharmaceutical, Raritan, NJ) has an inner layer containing an adhesive and hormone matrix, and a water-resistant outer layer. As a result, women can wear the patch in bathtubs, showers, swimming pools, saunas, and whirlpools without decreased efficacy. The patch may be applied to buttocks, upper outer arm, lower abdomen, or upper torso, but the breasts are avoided (Fig. 32-2). Because the hormones are combined with the adhesive, improper skin adherence will lower hormone absorption and efficacy. Therefore, if a patch is so poorly adhered that it requires reinforcement with tape, it should be replaced.

Initiation of the patch is the same as for COCs, and a new patch is applied weekly for 3 weeks, followed by a patch-free week to allow withdrawal bleeding. Although a patch is ideally worn no longer than 7 days, hormone levels remain in an effective range for up to 9 days, and this affords a 2-day window for patch change delays (Abrams and co-workers, 2001).

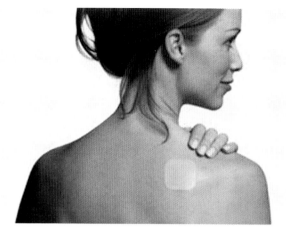

FIGURE 32-2 OrthoEvra transdermal contraceptive patch. (Courtesy of Ortho-McNeil Pharmaceuticals.)

Audet and co-workers (2001) found that the patch was slightly more effective than a low-dose oral contraceptive, with respective pregnancy rates 1.2 versus 2.2 pregnancies per 100 woman-years. Moreover, compliance appears to be improved compared with oral regimens (Dittrich and associates, 2002). In general, the patch shows a comparable side effect profile with COC pills. However, application-site reaction and breast tenderness are more frequent during initial cycles in patch wearers (Urdl and co-workers, 2005).

Obesity—90 kg or greater—may be associated with an increased risk for patch contraceptive failure (Zieman and associates, 2002). There is conflicting data that the patch has higher rates of venous thromboembolism (VTE) than COCs, and the package insert reflects these concerns. Specifically, studies by Jick and co-workers (2006a, b, 2007) have shown no increased rates of thromboembolism, ischemic stroke, or myocardial infarction. Conversely, Cole and associates (2007) reported a twofold increased rate of these three.

Summary for the Patch

For women who prefer weekly application rather than daily dosing, the patch provides an effective alternative hormonal contraceptive method. Candidates should weigh less than 90 kg and have no risk factors for cardiovascular disease and thromboembolism. Its other metabolic and physiological effects are substantively the same as for low-dose oral contraceptives, although the accumulated experience with the patch is small compared with that of COCs.

Transvaginal Administration

The *NuvaRing* (Organon USA, Roseland, NJ) is a flexible intravaginal hormonal contraceptive ring. Constructed of ethinyl vinyl acetate, the ring measures 54 mm in diameter and 4 mm in cross-section (Fig. 32-3). Its core contains ethinyl estradiol and the progestin, etonogestrel. These are released at rates of 15 μg and 120 μg per day, respectively and absorbed across the vaginal epithelium. Although this release results in systemic hormone levels lower than that from low-dose oral and patch

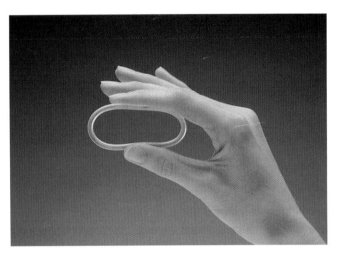

FIGURE 32-3 NuvaRing: estrogen-progestin-releasing vaginal contraceptive ring. (Courtesy of Organon, USA.)

contraceptive formulations, ovulation inhibition is complete (van den Heuvel and associates, 2005).

Before dispensing, the rings are refrigerated, and once dispensed, their shelf life is 4 months. The ring is placed within 5 days of menses onset and after 3 weeks of use, is removed for 1 week to allow withdrawal bleeding. Contraception will still be afforded if a ring is left in place for a fourth week. For rings left in place longer than 4 weeks, however, pregnancy should be excluded, a new ring placed, and alternative method used for 7 days (Organon USA, 2005).

Both usage compliance and contraceptive efficacy are comparable with that of COCs (Ahrendt and co-workers, 2006). Breakthrough bleeding is uncommon and appears less frequently than with pill use (Bjarnadóttir and colleagues, 2002). Patient satisfaction is high with this method, although vaginitis, ring-related events, and leukorrhea are more common (Oddsson and associates, 2005). Despite this, no deleterious affect on vaginal flora or on lower reproductive-tract or endometrial epithelia have been found (Bulten, 2005; Fraser, 2000; Veres, 2004, and their co-workers). Approximately 70 percent of partners report being able to feel the ring during intercourse (Dieben and colleagues, 2002). If this is bothersome, the ring may be removed for intercourse but should be replaced within 3 hours.

Intramuscular Administration

Lunelle is a contraceptive injection containing 25 mg of medroxyprogesterone acetate and 5 mg of estradiol cypionate. In 2002, prefilled Lunelle syringes were recalled by the manufacturer due to lack of assurance of full contraceptive potency. Although still FDA-approved, this method is no longer available in the United States.

Progestational Contraceptives

Oral Progestins

So-called *mini-pills* are progestin-only contraceptives that are taken daily. Unlike COCs, they do not reliably inhibit ovulation. Rather, their effectiveness depends more on alterations in cervical mucus and effects on the endometrium. Because mucus changes are not sustained longer than 24 hours, mini-pills should be taken at the same time every day to be maximally effective. These contraceptives have not achieved widespread popularity because of a much higher incidence of irregular bleeding and a somewhat higher pregnancy rate than COCs.

Benefits. Progestin-only pills have minimal if any effect on carbohydrate metabolism or coagulation, and they do not cause or exacerbate hypertension. They may be ideal for some women who are at increased risk of cardiovascular complications. Moreover, the mini-pill is often an excellent choice for lactating women. In combination with breast feeding, it is virtually 100-percent effective for up to 6 months and does not impair milk production.

Disadvantages. These contraceptives must be taken at about the same or nearly the same time each day. **If a progestin-only pill is taken even 4 hours late, a back-up form of contraception must be used for the next 48 hours.** And their effectiveness is decreased by the medications shown in Table 32-5. As with other hormonal contraceptive failures and pregnancy, there is a relative increase in the proportion of ectopic pregnancies (Sivin, 1991). Functional ovarian cysts develop with a greater frequency in women using these agents, although they do not usually necessitate intervention. Irregular uterine bleeding is another distinct disadvantage and may manifest as amenorrhea, metrorrhagia, or menorrhagia.

Contraindications. Progestin-only pills are contraindicated in women with unexplained uterine bleeding, known breast cancer, benign or malignant liver tumors, pregnancy, or acute liver disease (Ortho-McNeil Pharmaceutical, 2007).

Injectable Progestin Contraceptives

Both intramuscular depot medroxyprogesterone acetate (Depo-Provera), 150 mg every 3 months, and norethisterone enanthate (Norigest), 200 mg every 2 months, are injectable progestin contraceptives that have been effectively used worldwide for years. Depot medroxyprogesterone (DMPA) is injected into the deltoid or gluteus muscle without massage to ensure that the drug is released slowly. Alternatively, a subcutaneous version, *depo-SubQ provera 104,* is available and is injected into the subcutaneous tissue of the anterior thigh or abdomen every 3 months. This subcutaneous preparation contains 104 mg of DMPA, which is absorbed more slowly than the intramuscular formulation. Thus, even with a third less medication per dose, it maintains serum progestin levels sufficient to suppress ovulation for 3 months (Jain and associates, 2004). Currently, DMPA contraceptions are used in the United States by about 5 percent of women aged 18 to 44 who use contraception, and this method is particularly popular with adolescents (Mosher and co-workers, 2004).

The mechanisms of action are multiple and include ovulation inhibition, increased cervical mucus viscosity, and creation of an endometrium unfavorable for ovum implantation. Initial injection should begin within the first 5 days following menses onset. Therapeutic serum MPA levels sufficient to exert a consistent contraceptive effect are observed by 24 hours. Thus, no back-up contraceptive method is required if initiated within 5 days of menses onset (Haider and Darney, 2007). DMPA is an effective method with perfect-use pregnancy rates of 0.3 percent (Said and co-workers, 1986). Typical-use failure rates, however, approximate 7 percent at 12 months (Kost and associates, 2008).

Benefits. Injected progestins offer the convenience of a 3-month dosing schedule, contraceptive effectiveness comparable with or better than COCs, and minimal to no lactation impairment (American College of Obstetricians and Gynecologists, 2000). Iron-deficiency anemia is less likely in long-term users because of amenorrhea, which develops after 5 years in 80 percent of women (Gardner and Mishell, 1970).

Disadvantages. The principal disadvantages of depot progestins include irregular menstrual bleeding and prolonged anovulation after discontinuation, which results in delayed fertility resumption. Cromer and associates (1994) reported that a fourth of women discontinued its use in the first year because of irregular bleeding. After injections are stopped, a fourth do not resume regular menses for up to 1 year (Gardner and Mishell, 1970).

Although DMPA use does not affect overall breast cancer risk, there is a small increased risk in recent or current users (Skegg and co-workers, 1995). Cervical and hepatic malignancy do not appear to be increased, and the risk of ovarian and endometrial cancers is decreased (Kaunitz, 1996; World Health Organization, 1991).

Weight gain is generally attributed to DMPA, although not all studies have found this effect (Bahamondes and co-workers, 2001; Moore and associates, 1995). Weight gain is comparable between the two depot forms (Westhoff and co-workers, 2007c). Breast tenderness is reported by some users, as is depression, although a causal link for the latter has not been demonstrated.

In long-term users, loss of bone mineral density (BMD) is a potential problem (Scholes and colleagues, 1999). In 2004, the FDA added a black box warning to DMPA labeling which notes that this concern is probably most relevant for adolescents, who are building bone mass, and perimenopausal women, who will soon have increased bone loss during menopause. It is the opinion of the World Health Organization (1998) and American College of Obstetricians and Gynecologists (2008) that DMPA should not be restricted in those high-risk groups. However, the overall risks and benefits for continuing use should be reevaluated over time (d'Arcangues, 2006). It is somewhat reassuring that bone loss appears to be reversible after discontinuation of therapy but is still not complete after 18 to 24 months (Clark and colleagues, 2006; Scholes and co-workers, 2002).

DMPA use has not been shown to increase the risk for thromboembolism, stroke, or cardiovascular disease. Still, prior thromboembolism is considered a contraindication to its use. Other contraindications to DMPA include pregnancy, undiagnosed vaginal bleeding, breast cancer, cerebrovascular disease, or significant liver disease (Pfizer, 2006, 2007).

Progestin Implants

Levonorgestrel Implants

The *Norplant System* (Wyeth-Ayerst) provides levonorgestrel in six silastic rods that are implanted subdermally. Despite the

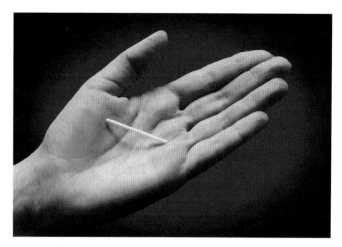

FIGURE 32-4 Implanon insert. (Courtesy of Organon, USA.)

effectiveness, safety, and patient satisfaction with this contraceptive, its use waned dramatically in the United States after a flurry of litigation. The manufacturer stopped distributing the system in July 2002.

Jadelle (Bayer Schering Pharma Oy, Turku, Finland), originally named Norplant-2, is a two-rod system similar to *Norplant*. It provides similar contraception for 3 years, but its two rods significantly shorten implant removal time (Sivin and co-workers, 2001). *Jadelle* has been approved for use, although it has not been marketed or distributed in the United States (Population Council, 2008).

Etonogestrel Implant

Approved by the FDA in 2006, *Implanon* (Organon, Roseland, NJ) is a single-rod subdermal implant with 68 mg of the progestin etonogestrel (ENG), and an ethylene vinyl acetate copolymer cover (Fig. 32-4). The implant is placed in the medial surface of the upper arm 6 to 8 cm from the elbow in the biceps groove within 5 days of onset of menses. It may be used as contraception for 3 years and then replaced at the same site or opposite arm.

Progestin is released continuously to suppress ovulation as the primary contraceptive action, although cervical mucus thickening and an atrophic endometrium add to its efficacy. Return of ovulation after implant removal is rapid. It is a highly effective method, and Croxatto and Mäkäräinen (1998) reported no pregnancies with its use during 53,530 cycles.

Implanon is not radiopaque, and a misplaced implant may be identified with sonography using a 10- to 15-MHz linear array transducer (Shulman and Gabriel, 2006). In some cases, magnetic resonance imaging may be required (Merki-Feld and associates, 2001).

Weight gain is neither a prominent side effect nor a common reason for implant discontinuation (Funk and co-workers, 2005). The ENG implant does not significantly affect bone mineral density, lipid profile, or liver enzymes (Beerthuizen and associates, 2000; Biswas and co-workers, 2003, 2004). The most frequently reported adverse event leading to removal was prolonged and frequent bleeding (Bitzer and colleagues, 2004). Contraindications for ENG implant use are those for DMPA.

INTRAUTERINE DEVICE (IUD)

In the United States, many are of the opinion that the intrauterine device (IUD) is an underused contraceptive. Although only about 1 percent of reproductive-aged women in the United States use this method, IUDs are the most commonly used method of reversible contraception worldwide (Chandra and colleagues, 2005; d'Arcanques, 2007).

Types of Intrauterine Devices

Devices that are *chemically inert* are composed of a nonabsorbable material, most often polyethylene, and impregnated with barium sulfate for radiopacity. Those that are *chemically active* have continuous elution of copper or a progestin. Currently, only chemically active IUDs are available in the United States. Most IUDs are described as *framed*, that is, formed as a rigid structure. *Frameless* IUDs have higher expulsion rates and are not used in the United States. They contain bracelets of copper that are crimped onto a string and affixed to the fundal myometrium (O'Brien and Marfleet, 2005).

The two chemically active IUDs currently approved for use in the United States include a progestin-releasing device (*Mirena*, Bayer HealthCare Pharmaceuticals, Wayne, NJ). It releases levonorgestrel into the uterus at a relatively constant rate of 20 μg/day, which reduces systemic effects. It has a T-shaped radiopaque frame, whose stem is wrapped with a cylinder reservoir, composed of a polydimethylsiloxane-levonorgestrel mixture. There are two trailing brown strings attached to the stem.

The second device is the T 380A IUD (*ParaGard*, Duramed Pharmaceuticals, Pomona, NY). It is a polyethylene and barium sulfate, T-shaped frame wound with copper. Specifically, 314 mm^2 of fine copper wire wrap the stem, and the arms each have 33-mm^2 copper bracelets, thus totaling 380 mm^2 of copper. Two strings extend from the base of the stem. Originally blue, the strings are now white.

Changing IUD Perceptions

With new information on safety, the IUD is once again gaining in popularity for several reasons:

1. IUDs are "use and forget" effective reversible contraceptive methods that do not have to be replaced for 10 years with the *ParaGard* and for 5 years with the *Mirena*
2. It is now better established that the major actions of IUDs are contraceptive, not abortifacient
3. The risk of pelvic infections is markedly reduced with the currently used monofilament string and with techniques to ensure safer insertion
4. The risk of an associated ectopic pregnancy has been clarified. Specifically, the contraceptive effect decreases the absolute number of ectopic pregnancies by approximately 50 percent compared with that of women not using contraception (World Health Organization, 1985, 1987). With failure, however, pregnancy is more likely to be ectopic (Furlong, 2002)
5. Legal liability appears to be less because the FDA currently classifies IUDs as drugs (Mishell and Sulak, 1997). As such,

the manufacturers must provide product information to be read by women prior to insertion (Bayer HealthCare Pharmaceuticals, 2007a; Duramed Pharmaceuticals, 2006). Signed consent forms that include a list of risks and benefits are also required.

Efficacy

These two types of IUDs are effective contraceptives, and their ability to prevent pregnancy is similar overall to that of tubal sterilization (American College of Obstetricians and Gynecologists, 2003). Importantly, pregnancy rates decrease progressively after the first year of use (Vessey and associates, 1983). For example, the levonorgestrel intrauterine system (LNG-IUS) has a typical-user failure rate of 0.1 percent after 1 year of use, and a <0.5-percent cumulative pregnancy rate by 5 years. This is lower than that of the copper-containing ParaGard with a 1-year rate of 0.8 percent and 5-year rates of 0.3 to 0.6 percent (Thonneau and Almont, 2008; Trussell, 2004). Finally, IUDs have 1-year continuation rates of 80 percent, which is slightly greater than that of 70 percent for oral contraceptives.

Contraceptive Action

These mechanisms have not been precisely defined and are a subject of ongoing debate. At one time, interference with successful implantation of the fertilized ovum was believed to be the main mode of IUD action but now is considered less important than its prevention of fertilization (Stanford and Mikolajczyk, 2002).

Within the uterus, an intense local endometrial inflammatory response is induced, especially by copper-containing devices. Cellular and humoral components of this inflammation are expressed in endometrial tissue and in fluid filling the uterine cavity and fallopian tubes. These lead to decreased sperm and egg viability (Ortiz and Croxatto, 2007). In the unlikely event that fertilization does occur, the same inflammatory actions are directed against the blastocyst, and the endometrium is transformed into a hostile site for implantation. With copper IUD, copper levels increase in the mucus of users and lower sperm motility and viability (Jecht and Bernstein, 1973).

With the LNG-IUS, in addition to an inflammatory reaction, progestin release in long-time users causes glandular atrophy and stromal decidualization. Moreover, progestins create scant viscous cervical mucus that hinders sperm motility. The LNG-IUS may also inconsistently release sufficient progestin to inhibit ovulation.

Other Beneficial Effects

Despite higher up-front costs of IUDs, their extended use makes their long-term cost-effectiveness competitive with or superior to other contraceptives (Trussell and co-workers, 2009). Many women with contraindications to COCs can often use these devices. These are quickly reversible method of contraception, and fertility is not impaired (Hov and associates, 2007). There is no increased risk of genital tract or breast neoplasia, and both IUDs are associated with a decreased risk of endometrial cancer (Curtis, 2007; Backman, 2005; Beining, 2008, and all their colleagues). Lastly, the LNG-IUS produces lower systemic progestin levels compared with DMPA, and thus, bone mineral density losses and weight gain are avoided (Bahamondes and colleagues, 2006; Yela and co-workers, 2006).

Adverse Effects

Adverse effects from IUDs include abnormal uterine bleeding, dysmenorrhea, expulsion, or uterine perforation. With extended use and advancing user age, however, pregnancy, expulsion, and bleeding complications decrease in frequency. Functional ovarian cysts are more frequent in the early months of LNG-IUS use but typically resolve spontaneously (Inki and associates, 2002).

Uterine Perforation

Clinically apparent or silent *uterine perforation* may occur while inserting a uterine sound or during IUD insertion. Rates approximate 1 per 1000 insertions (Harrison-Woolrych and associates, 2003). Although devices may migrate spontaneously into and through the uterine wall, most perforations occur, or at least begin, at the time of insertion. Some have found that IUD perforation, rotation, or embedding may cause excessive bleeding (Faundes and colleagues, 1997; Pizarro and associates, 1989). Evaluation of perforation is discussed subsequently. Another adverse effect is *abortion of an unsuspected pregnancy* following insertion, but a urine pregnancy test prior to insertion will obviate this. The frequency of both complications depends on operator skill and the precautions taken to detect pregnancy.

Expulsion

Loss of an IUD from the uterus is most common during the first month. Thus, these women should be examined about 1 month following insertion, usually after menses, to identify the tail trailing from the cervix. Barrier contraception may be desirable during this first month, especially if a device has been expelled previously. Following this, a woman should be instructed to palpate the strings protruding from the cervix each month after menses.

Lost Device

When the tail of an IUD cannot be visualized, the device may have been expelled, or it may have perforated the uterus. In either event, pregnancy is possible. Conversely, the IUD tail simply may be in the uterine cavity along with a normally positioned device. After excluding pregnancy, the uterine cavity is probed gently with a Randall stone clamp or with a specialized rod with a terminal hook to retrieve the string. **Never assume that the device has been expelled unless it was seen.**

When the tail is not visible, and the device is not felt by gentle probing of the uterine cavity, sonography can be used to ascertain if the device is within the uterus. If inconclusive or if no device is seen, then a plain radiograph of the abdomen and pelvis is taken with a sound inserted into the uterine cavity. Computed tomography (CT) scanning, MR imaging, and hysteroscopy are yet other alternatives (Peri and colleagues, 2007). It is safe to perform MR imaging at 1.5 tesla (T) with an IUD in place (Pasquale and associates, 1997). Moreover, at 3 T, it also appears to be safe with copper IUDs (Zieman and Kanal, 2007).

A device may penetrate the muscular uterine wall to varying degrees. Part of the device may extend into the peritoneal cavity, or part may remain firmly fixed in the myometrium, usually running parallel to the long axis of the uterus. It may penetrate into the cervix and actually protrude into the vagina. If located outside the uterus, a device of inert material, such as the Lippes Loop, may or may not cause harm. Chemically inert devices usually are removed easily from the peritoneal cavity by laparoscopy or colpotomy. An extrauterine copper-bearing device induces an intense local inflammatory reaction and adhesions. Thus, copper-bearing devices are more firmly adhered, and laparotomy may be necessary. Perforations of large and small bowel and bowel fistulas, with attendant morbidity, have been reported remote from insertion.

Cramping and Bleeding

Discomfort with insertion may stem from difficult uterine sounding or cervical stenosis, especially in nulliparas. If problematic, cervical softening typically follows use of misoprostol, 400 μg sublingually 1 to 3 hours prior to insertion (Sääv and associates, 2007). *Cramping* and some *bleeding* are common soon after insertion. Cramping is minimized by administering an NSAID an hour prior to insertion.

Menorrhagia

The amount of menstrual bleeding is commonly increased with use of the copper IUD. As this may cause iron-deficiency anemia, iron supplementation is given, and hemoglobin concentration or hematocrit is measured annually. Menorrhagia can be troubling, and up to 15 percent of women have the copper device removed because of this (Hatcher and associates, 1998). NSAIDs reduce bleeding and are considered first-line therapy for this (Grimes and associates, 2006a). In contrast, the LNG-IUS is associated with progressive amenorrhea, which is reported by a third of users after 2 years and by 60 percent after 12 years (Ronnerdag and Odlind, 1999).

Infection

The device-related risk of infection is increased only during the first 20 days following insertion (Farley and associates, 1992). Antimicrobial prophylaxis confers little benefit and is not recommended with insertion (Grimes and Schulz, 2001a; Walsh and colleagues, 1998). Moreover, the American Heart Association does not recommend infective endocarditis prophylaxis with insertion (Wilson and co-workers, 2007).

Fortunately, infection risk is not increased with long-term IUD use. Correspondingly, IUDs appear to cause little, if any, increase in the risk of infertility from infection among women at low risk for sexually transmitted infections (Hubacher and colleagues, 2001). For these reasons, the American College of Obstetricians and Gynecologists (2005b, 2007b) recommends that women who are at low risk for sexually transmitted diseases, including adolescents, are good candidates for IUDs.

Pelvic infection that does develop in a woman with an IUD may be of several forms. *Septic abortion* mandates immediate curettage. *Tubo-ovarian abscesses*—sometimes unilateral—have been reported and are treated aggressively. With suspected infection, the IUD should be removed.

Actinomyces Infection

Actinomyces israelii is a gram-positive, slow-growing, anaerobic bacterium that rarely leads to infection and abscess. It is found to be part of the indigenous genital flora of healthy women (Persson and Holmberg, 1984). Some have found it more frequently in the vaginal flora of IUD users, and rates of colonization increase with duration of IUD use (Curtis and Pine, 1981). *Actinomyces* is also identified in Papanicolaou smears, and Fiorino (1996) cited a 7-percent incidence in IUD users compared with less than 1 percent in nonusers.

In the absence of symptoms, the incidental finding of *Actinomyces* on cytology is problematic. First, infection is rare, even in those identified to harbor the bacteria. Reviews by Lippes (1999) and Westhoff (2007a) suggest that asymptomatic women may retain their IUD and do not require antibiotic treatment. The American College of Obstetricians and Gynecologists (2005b) lists four management options for asymptomatic women:

1. Expectant management
2. Extended oral antibiotic treatment with the IUD in place
3. IUD removal
4. IUD removal followed by antibiotic treatment.

Importantly, if signs or symptoms of infection develop in women who harbor *Actinomyces*, the device should be removed and antimicrobial therapy instituted. Early findings include fever, weight loss, abdominal pain, and abnormal vaginal bleeding or discharge. *Actinomyces* is sensitive to antimicrobials with gram-positive coverage, notably the penicillins.

Pregnancy with an IUD

It is important to identify women who become pregnant while using an IUD. Until about 14 weeks, the tail may be visible through the cervix, and if seen, it should be removed. This action reduces subsequent complications such as late abortion, sepsis, and preterm birth (Alvior, 1973). Tatum and co-workers (1976) reported an abortion rate of 54 percent with the device left in place compared with a rate of 25 percent if it was promptly removed.

If the tail is not visible, attempts to locate and remove the device may result in abortion. However, some practitioners have successfully used sonography to assist in the removal of devices without visible strings (Schiesser and co-workers, 2004). After fetal viability is reached, it is unclear whether it is better to remove an IUD whose string is visible and accessible or leave it in place. There is no evidence that fetal malformations are increased with a device in place (Tatum and associates, 1976).

Second-trimester abortion with an IUD in place is more likely to be infected (Vessey and associates, 1974). *Sepsis may be fulminant and fatal.* Pregnant women with a device in utero who demonstrate any evidence of pelvic infection are treated with intensive antimicrobial therapy and prompt uterine evacuation. Because of these risks, a woman should be given the option of early pregnancy termination if the device cannot be removed. In women who give birth with a device in place, appropriate steps should be taken at delivery to identify the IUD and to remove it.

TABLE 32-8. Contraindications to Use of an Intrauterine Device (IUD)

General:

1. Pregnancy or suspicion of pregnancy
2. Abnormalities of the uterus resulting in distortion of the uterine cavity
3. Acute pelvic inflammatory disease or a history of pelvic inflammatory disease unless there has been a subsequent uterine pregnancy
4. Postpartum endometritis or infected abortion in the past 3 months
5. Known or suspected uterine or cervical neoplasia, or unresolved abnormal cytological smear
6. Genital bleeding of unknown etiology
7. Untreated acute cervicitis or vaginitis, including bacterial vaginosis, until infection is controlled
8. Woman or her partner has multiple sexual partners
9. Conditions associated with increased susceptibility to infections with microorganisms—these include but are not limited to leukemia, acquired immune deficiency syndrome (AIDS), and intravenous drug abuse
10. History of ectopic pregnancy or condition that would predispose to ectopic pregnancy
11. Genital actinomycosis
12. A previously inserted IUD that has not been removed

Additionally, the ParaGard T 380A® (because of its copper content) should not be inserted when one or more of the following conditions exist:

1. Wilson disease
2. Copper allergy

Additionally, Mirena® insertion is contraindicated when one or more of the following conditions exist:

1. Hypersensitivity to any component of this product
2. Known or suspected carcinoma of the breast
3. Acute liver disease or tumor

Modified from Physicians Desk Reference, 2009.

Contraindications

Shown in Table 32-8 are manufacturers' contraindications to IUD use. Because levonorgestrel released by the LNG-IUS may inhibit tubal mobility, a previous ectopic pregnancy or other predisposing risk factors are additional contraindications. The IUD is safe and effective in HIV-infected women and may be used in other selected immunosuppressed women such as those with systemic lupus erythematosus (American College of Obstetricians and Gynecologists, 2006; Stringer and co-workers, 2007).

Insertion

Timing of insertion influences the ease of placement as well as pregnancy and expulsion rates. Insertion near the end of normal menstruation, when the cervix is usually softer and somewhat more dilated, may be easier, and at the same time may exclude early pregnancy. But insertion is not limited to this time. For the woman who is sure she is not pregnant and does not want to be pregnant, insertion is done at any time.

Immediate postpartum insertion is practiced in some areas. Grimes and colleagues (2001b) concluded that it is safe to do so, however, the expulsion rate and possibly pregnancy rates are higher than with later insertion. The recommendation has been made, therefore, to wait for at least 6 to 8 weeks after delivery to reduce expulsion rates and to minimize the risk of perforation. Women delivered at Parkland Hospital are seen 3 weeks' postpartum, and IUDs are inserted 6 weeks' postpartum or sooner if involution is complete. After early miscarriage or abortion, the device may be inserted immediately.

Before insertion, several procedural steps are carried out. Any contraindications are identified, and if none, then the woman is counseled and written consent obtained. An oral NSAID, with or without codeine, can be used to allay cramps. Misoprostol, 400 µg sublingually, may soften a rigid or stenotic cervix. Bimanual pelvic examination is performed to identify the position and size of the uterus. Abnormalities are evaluated as they may contraindicate insertion. Mucopurulent cervicitis or significant vaginitis should be appropriately treated and resolved before insertion.

The cervical surface is cleansed with an antiseptic solution, and sterile instruments and a sterile device should be used. A tenaculum is placed on the cervical lip, and the canal and uterine cavity are straightened by applying gentle traction. The uterus is then sounded to identify the direction and depth of the uterine cavity. Specific steps of ParaGard and Mirena insertion are shown in Figures 32-5 and 32-6 and outlined in their respective package inserts, available at: http://www.paragard.com/custom_images/ppi_eng.pdf and http://berlex.bayerhealthcare.com/html/products/pi/Mirena_PI.pdf?C = &c.

Following insertion, only the threads should be visible trailing from the cervix. These are trimmed to allow 3 to 4 cm to protrude into the vagina and their length is recorded. If there is suspicion that the device is not in the correct position, then placement should be confirmed, using sonography if necessary. If the IUD is not positioned completely within the uterus, it is removed and replaced with a new device. An expelled or partially expelled device should not be reinserted.

BARRIER METHODS

For many years, condoms, vaginal spermicidal agents, and vaginal diaphragms have been used for contraception with variable success (see Table 32-2).

Male Condom

These long-available products provide effective contraception, and their failure rate with strongly motivated couples has been as low as 3 or 4 per 100 couple-years of exposure (Vessey and co-workers, 1982). Generally, and during the first year of use especially, the failure rate is much higher. The contraceptive effectiveness of the male condom is enhanced appreciably by a reservoir tip and probably by the addition of spermicidal lubri-

cant. The contraceptive effectiveness is further improved by use of an intravaginal spermicidal agent. Such agents, as well as those used for lubrication, should be water-based. Oil-based products destroy latex condoms and diaphragms.

Speroff and Darney (2001) emphasize the following key steps to ensure maximal condom effectiveness:

1. A condom must be used with every coital act
2. It should be in place before contact of the penis with the vagina
3. Withdrawal must occur with the penis still erect
4. The base of the condom must be held during withdrawal
5. Either an intravaginal spermicide or a condom lubricated with spermicide should be employed.

Infection Prevention

When used properly, condoms provide considerable but not absolute protection against a broad range of sexually transmitted diseases. These include HIV, gonorrhea, syphilis, herpes, chlamydia, and trichomoniasis. There is also decreased risk for bacterial vaginosis (Hutchinson and co-workers, 2007). Condoms also may prevent and ameliorate premalignant cervical changes, presumably by blocking transmission of human papillomavirus (Manhart and Koutsky, 2002; Winer and colleagues, 2006).

Latex Sensitivity

For individuals sensitive to latex, condoms made from lamb intestines are effective, but they do not provide protection against infection. Fortunately, nonallergenic condoms have been developed and are comprised of polyurethane or of synthetic elastomers. Polyurethane condoms are effective against sexually transmitted diseases but have a higher breakage and slippage rate than latex condoms (Gallo and co-workers, 2006). In a randomized trial of 901 couples, Steiner and colleagues (2003) documented breakage and slippage at 8.4 percent with polyurethane condoms compared with 3.2 percent with latex condoms. Respective 6-month typical pregnancy probabilities were 9.0 compared with 5.4 percent.

Female Condom (Vaginal Pouch)

The only female condom available is marketed as the *FC Female Condom* (The Female Health Company, Chicago, IL). It is a polyurethane sheath with one flexible polyurethane ring at each end. The open ring remains outside the vagina, and the closed internal ring is fitted under the symphysis like a diaphragm (Fig. 32-7). The female condom can be used with both water-based and oil-based lubricants. Male condoms should not be used concurrently because simultaneous use may cause friction that leads to condom slipping, tearing, and displacement. Following use, the female condom outer ring should be twisted to seal the condom so that no semen spills out.

The female condom has an acceptability rate of about 60 percent for women and 80 percent for men. However, the pregnancy rate is higher than with the male condom (see Table 32-2). The female condom has a 0.6-percent breakage rate. The slippage and displacement rate is about 3 percent compared with 3 to 8 percent for male condoms. In vitro tests have shown the condom to be impermeable to HIV, cytomegalovirus, and hepatitis B virus.

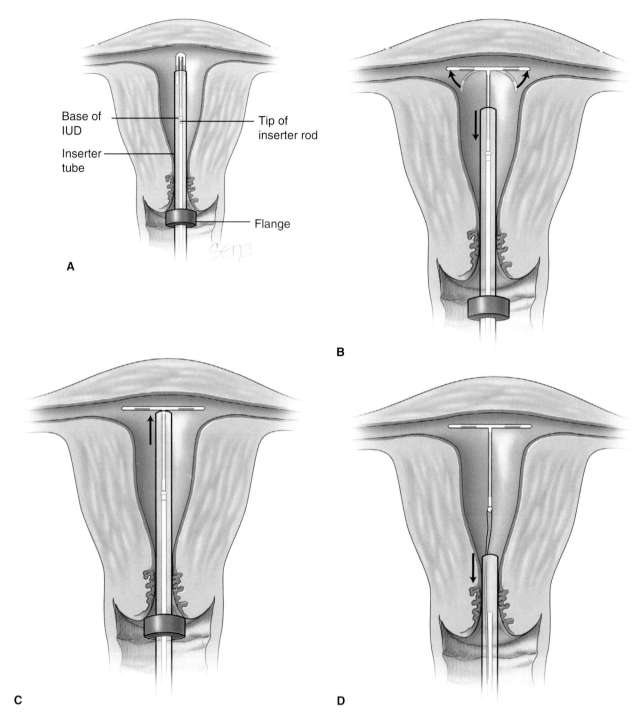

Base of IUD

Tip of inserter rod

Inserter tube

Flange

A

B

C

D

FIGURE 32-5 Insertion of ParaGard T 380A. The uterus is sounded, and the IUD is loaded into its inserter tube not more than 5 minutes before insertion. A blue plastic flange on the outside of the inserter tube is positioned from the IUD tip to reflect this depth. The IUD arms should lie in the same plane as the flat portion of the blue flange. **A.** The inserter tube, with the IUD loaded, is passed into the endometrial cavity. A long, solid, white inserter rod abuts the base of the IUD. When the blue flange contacts the cervix, insertion stops. **B.** To release the IUD arms, the solid white rod within the inserter tube is held steady, while the inserter tube is withdrawn no more than 1 cm. **C.** The inserter tube, not the inserter rod, is then carefully moved upward toward the top of the uterus until slight resistance is felt. At no time during insertion is the inserter rod advanced forward. **D.** First, the solid white rod and then the inserter tube are withdrawn individually. At completion, only the threads should be visible protruding from the cervix. These are trimmed to allow 3 to 4 cm to extend into the vagina.

Spermicides

These contraceptives are marketed variously as creams, jellies, suppositories, films, and aerosol foam. They are used widely in the United States, especially by women who find other methods unacceptable. They are useful especially for women who need temporary protection, for example, during the first week after starting oral contraceptives or while nursing. Most agents can be purchased without a prescription.

Typically, spermicides function by providing a physical barrier to sperm penetration as well as a chemical spermicidal action. The active ingredient is nonoxynol-9 or octoxynol-9.

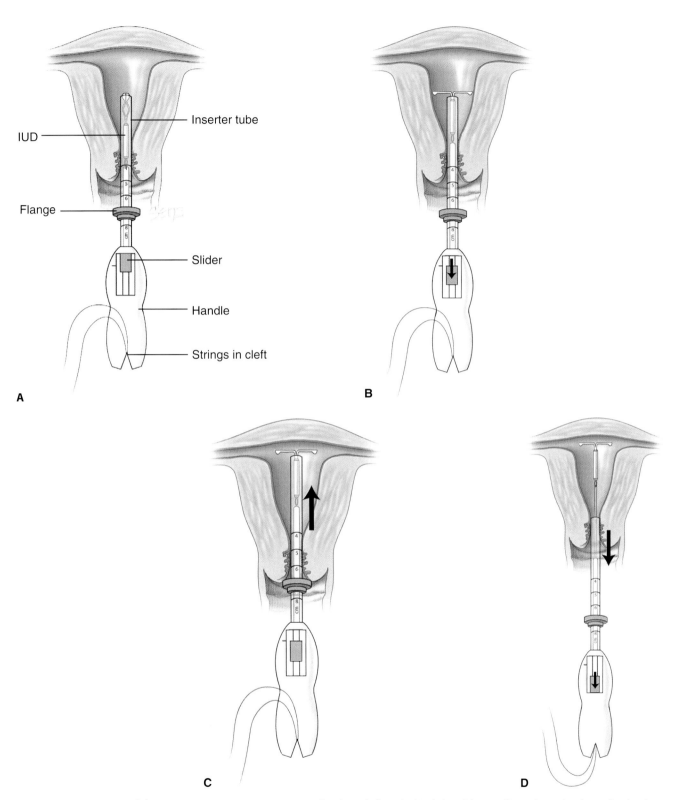

FIGURE 32-6 Insertion of the Mirena intrauterine system. Initially, threads from behind the slider are first released to hang freely. The slider found on the handle should be positioned at the top of the handle nearest the device. The IUD arms are oriented horizontally. A flange on the outside of the inserter tube is positioned from the IUD tip to reflect the depth found with uterine sounding. **A.** As both free threads are pulled, the Mirena IUD is drawn into the inserter tube. The threads are then tightly fixed from below into the handle's cleft. In these depictions, the inserter tube has been foreshortened. The inserter tube is gently inserted into the uterus until the flange lies 1.5 to 2 cm from the external cervical os to allow the arms to open. **B.** While holding the inserter steady, the IUD arms are released by pulling the slider back to reach the raised horizontal mark on the handle but no further. **C.** The inserter is then gently guided into the uterine cavity until its flange touches the cervix. **D.** The device is released by holding the inserter firmly in position, and pulling the slider down all the way. The threads will be released automatically from the cleft. The inserter may then be removed and IUD strings trimmed.

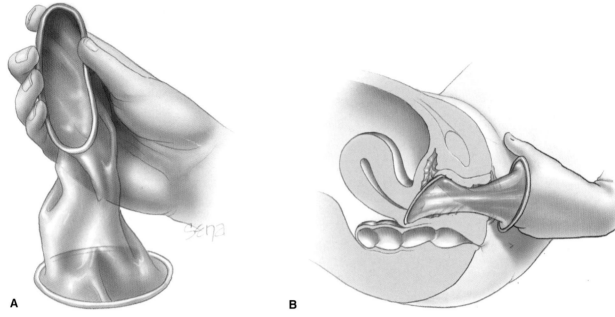

FIGURE 32-7 FC female condom insertion and positioning. **A.** The inner ring is squeezed for insertion. The sheath is inserted similarly to a diaphragm. **B.** The inner ring is pushed inward with an index finger.

Spermicides must be deposited high in the vagina in contact with the cervix shortly before intercourse. Their duration of maximal effectiveness is usually no more than 1 hour. Thereafter, they must be reinserted before repeat intercourse. Douching should be avoided for at least 6 hours after intercourse. High pregnancy rates are primarily attributable to inconsistent use rather than to method failure. Even if inserted regularly and correctly, however, foam preparations probably result in 5 to 12 pregnancies per 100 woman-years of use. They are not teratogenic (Briggs and colleagues, 2005).

Nonoxynol-9 does not provide protection against sexually transmitted infections. There is currently much interest in combination spermicides/microbicides, which are female-controlled contraceptives that can also protect against sexually transmitted diseases, including HIV infection (D'Cruz and Ucken, 2004; Palliser and colleagues, 2006).

Diaphragm Plus Spermicide

The diaphragm consists of a circular latex dome of various diameters supported by a circumferential latex-covered metal spring. It is effective when used in combination with spermicidal jelly or cream. The spermicide is applied into the dome cup and along the rim. The device is then positioned so that the cup faces the cervix and that the cervix, vaginal fornices, and anterior vaginal wall are partitioned effectively from the remainder of the vagina and the penis. In this fashion, the centrally placed spermicidal agent is held against the cervix. When appropriately positioned, one rim is lodged deep in the posterior vaginal fornix, and the opposite rim fits behind the inner surface of the symphysis and immediately below the urethra (Fig. 32-8). If a diaphragm is too small, it will not remain

in place. If it is too large, it is uncomfortable when forced into position. A cystocele or uterine prolapse typically leads to instability and expulsion. Because size and spring flexibility must be individualized, the diaphragm is available only by prescription.

With use, the diaphragm and spermicidal agent can be inserted hours before intercourse, but if more than 6 hours elapse, additional spermicide should be placed in the upper vagina for

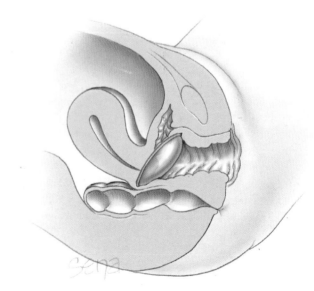

FIGURE 32-8 A diaphragm in place creates a physical barrier between the vagina and cervix.

maximum protection and be reapplied before each coital episode. The diaphragm should not be removed for at least 6 hours after intercourse. Because *toxic shock syndrome* has been described following its use, it may be worthwhile to remove the diaphragm at 6 hours, or at least the next morning, to minimize this uncommon event (see Chap. 31, p. 670). Diaphragm use results in a lower incidence of sexually transmitted diseases compared with condom use (Rosenberg and colleagues, 1992). Conversely, diaphragm use is associated with a slight increase in the rate of urinary infections, presumably from urethral irritation by the ring under the symphysis.

The diaphragm requires a high level of motivation for proper use. Vessey and colleagues (1982) reported a pregnancy rate of only 1.9 to 2.4 per 100 woman-years for motivated users. The unintended pregnancy rate is lower in women older than 35 years than that in those younger than 30.

Contraceptive Sponge

The Today contraceptive sponge (Synova Healthcare, Media, PA) was removed from the market in 1995 because of production modification cost increases. Since 2005, it is again available, from a new manufacturer, as an over-the-counter, one-size-fits-all device. The nonoxynol-9–impregnated polyurethane disc is 2.5 cm thick and 5.5 cm wide, and it has a dimple on one side and satin loop on the other (Fig. 32-9). The sponge is moistened with tap water and gently squeezed to create light suds. It is then positioned with the dimple placed directly against the cervix. The sponge can be inserted for up to 24 hours prior to intercourse, and while in place, it provides contraception regardless of coital frequency. It should remain in place for 6 hours after intercourse. Pregnancy is prevented primarily by the spermicide nonoxynol-9 and to a lesser extent, by covering the cervix and absorbing semen.

Although the sponge is possibly more convenient than the diaphragm or condom, it is less effective than either, as seen in Table 32-2 (Kuyoh and co-workers, 2003). Most common causes for method discontinuance are pregnancy, irritation, dis-

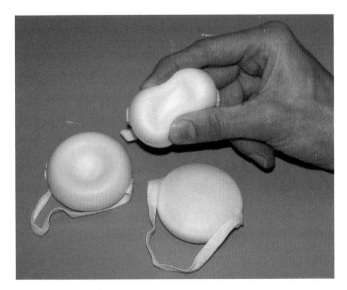

FIGURE 32-9 Today sponge.

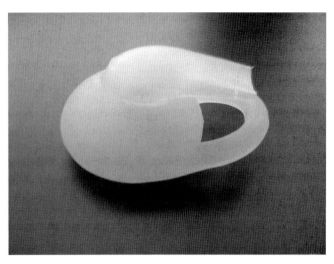

FIGURE 32-10 Lea's Shield. (Used with permission from the Cervical Barrier Advancement Society and Ibis Reproductive Health.)

comfort, or vaginitis (Beckman and associates, 1989). As discussed in Chapter 31 (p. 670), toxic shock syndrome (TSS) has been reported with the contraceptive sponge. The risk of toxic shock is rare, and there is evidence that the sponge may limit production of the responsible staphylococcal exotoxin (Remington and associates, 1987). Still, it is recommended that the sponge not be used during menses or the puerperium.

Cervical Cap

The *Prentif* cavity-rim cervical cap was approved for use by the FDA in 1988. The flexible, cup-like device is made of natural rubber and is fitted around the base of the cervix. It can be self-inserted and allowed to remain in place for up to 48 hours. It should be used with a spermicide applied once at insertion. If properly fitted and used correctly, the cap is comparable in effectiveness to the diaphragm (Richwald and colleagues, 1989). The cervical cap is relatively costly, and overall, incorrect fitting and/or improper placement make it less effective than the diaphragm plus spermicide (see Table 32-2).

Lea's Shield

Lea's Shield (Yama, Inc., Union, NJ) is a reusable, washable barrier made of silicone, which is placed against the cervix (Fig. 32-10). The device comes in one size, which simplifies the fitting process. It may be inserted any time prior to intercourse and must be left in place for at least 8 hours afterwards. When used with spermicide, and adjusted for age, the reported 6-month life-table pregnancy rate was 5.6 per 100 users (Mauck and associates, 1996).

FERTILITY AWARENESS-BASED METHODS

This form of contraception includes all family planning methods that attempt to identify fertile time each cycle and then modify sexual behavior. When fertility awareness-based (FAB) methods involve sexual abstinence during the fertile time, this technique is called *natural family planning—NFP*. When these methods involve occasionally using a barrier method during the fertile time, the method is called *fertility awareness-combined methods—FACM* (Jennings and colleagues, 2004).

Because the ovum is probably susceptible to successful fertilization for only 12 to 24 hours after ovulation, periodic abstinence has intuitive appeal as a means of birth control. Pregnancy rates, however, with various methods of periodic abstinence have been estimated from 5 to 40 per 100 woman-years (Population Reports, 1981). In other words, the unwanted pregnancy rate during the first year of use is approximately 20 percent (see Table 32-2).

Standard Days Method

This method was developed by the Institute for Reproductive Health at Georgetown University. Its users avoid unprotected intercourse during cycle days 8 through 19. For successful use, women must have regular monthly cycles of 26 to 32 days. Those who use the *standard days method* can use *Cycle-Beads* (Cycle Technologies, Washington, DC) to keep track of their days.

Calendar Rhythm Method

This method requires counting the number of days in the shortest and longest menstrual cycle during a 6- to 12-month span. From the shortest cycle, 18 days are subtracted to calculate the first fertile day. From the longest cycle, 11 days are subtracted to identify the last fertile day. This is problematic because ovulation most often occurs 14 days before the onset of the next menses. Because this is not necessarily 14 days *after* the onset of the last menses, the *calendar rhythm method* is not reliable.

Temperature Rhythm Method

This method relies on *slight* changes—sustained 0.4 degree Fahrenheit increases—in the basal body temperature that usually occur just before ovulation. This method is much more likely to be successful if, during each menstrual cycle, intercourse is avoided until well after the ovulatory temperature rise. For this method to be most effective, the woman must abstain from intercourse from the first day of menses through the third day after the increase in temperature. For obvious reasons, this is not a popular method! With excellent compliance, however, the unwanted pregnancy is approximately 2 percent the first year.

Cervical Mucus Rhythm Method

This so-called *Billings method* depends on awareness of vaginal "dryness" and "wetness." These are the consequences of changes in the amount and quality of cervical mucus at different times in the menstrual cycle. Abstinence is required from the beginning of menses until 4 days after slippery mucus is identified. Although this method has not achieved popularity, when it is used accurately, the first-year failure rate is approximately 3 percent.

Symptothermal Method

This method combines the use of changes in cervical mucus— onset of fertile period, changes in basal body temperature—end

of fertile period, and calculations to estimate the time of ovulation. Although this method is more complex to learn and apply, it does not appreciably improve reliability. The use of home kits to detect LH increases in the urine on the day prior to ovulation may improve the accuracy of periodic abstinence methods (Hatcher and associates, 2007).

EMERGENCY CONTRACEPTION

Many women present for contraceptive care following consensual but unprotected sexual intercourse, or in some cases, following sexual assault. In these situations, a number of methods substantially decrease the likelihood of an unwanted pregnancy when used correctly. Current methods of emergency contraception include COCs, progestin-only products, copper-containing IUDs, and mifepristone. Patients can obtain information regarding emergency contraception by calling 1-888-NOT-2-LATE (888-668-2528) or accessing The Emergency Contraception Website: http://ec.princeton.edu/.

History

For many decades it was known that pharmacological doses of estrogens would prevent pregnancy when given for recent unprotected intercourse. A study by Demers (1971) published in the *New England Journal of Medicine* was entitled "The Morning-After Pill," which referred to diethylstilbestrol (DES) used successfully as a postcoital contraceptive. It was never approved for this purpose, and in fact, the FDA discouraged the practice. Nevertheless, DES was widely prescribed off-label to prevent pregnancy. For example, beginning in the 1960s, it was routinely offered to women who were "at risk" for pregnancy following sexual assault and who were cared for at the Parkland Hospital Ob-Gyn Emergency Room. DES production by Eli Lilly, the last U.S. manufacturer, ceased in 1997.

In 1974, Yuzpe and colleagues published their pilot study of the use of combined hormone—100 μg ethinyl estradiol plus 1.0 mg dL-norgestrel—for postcoital contraception, and subsequently the *Yuzpe method* was found effective. In 1997, the FDA declared the Yuzpe method to be safe and effective for this off-label use and in 1998, approved the Yuzpe-method *Preven Emergency Contraceptive Kit* for prescriptive use. This kit was discontinued by the manufacturer in 2004.

In 1999, the FDA approved *Plan B*, which was the first progestin-only emergency contraceptive for prescriptive use. Because of its efficacy and safety, and especially its intent in preventing unwanted adolescent pregnancy, a number of organizations, including the American College of Obstetricians and Gynecologists and the American Academy of Pediatrics, recommended over-the-counter (OTC) availability (Drazen and colleagues, 2004). In 2009, the FDA allowed the manufacturer to market Plan B without a prescription to women 17 years and older.

Hormonal Emergency Contraception

Estrogen-Progestin Combinations

For reasons discussed above, this is also known as the *Yuzpe method*. A minimum of 100 μg of ethinyl estradiol and 0.5 mg of levonorgestrel is given as shown in Table 32-9. The only FDA-approved dedicated estrogen- and progesterone-containing product was the *Preven Emergency Contraceptive Kit*, which was for emergency contraception. These COC regimens are more effective the sooner they are taken after unprotected intercourse. The first dose is taken ideally within 72 hours of intercourse but may be given up to 120 hours. The initial dose is followed 12 hours later by a second dose. Emergency hormonal contraceptive regimens are highly effective and decrease the risk of pregnancy by up to 94 percent (American College of Obstetricians and Gynecologists, 2005a).

Nausea and vomiting are major problems due to high-dose estrogen in these regimens. For this reason, an oral antiemetic may be prescribed at least 1 hour before each dose. Oral pretreatment with 50-mg meclizine or with 10 mg of metoclopramide effectively decreases nausea (Ragan and associates, 2003; Raymond and colleagues, 2000). If a woman vomits within 2 hours of a dose, the dose must be repeated.

Progestin-Only Preparations

This progestin-only product provides two tablets, each containing 0.75 mg levonorgestrel. Optimally, the first dose is taken within 72 hours of unprotected coitus but may be given up to 120 hours. The second dose follows 12 hours later, although Ngai and colleagues (2005) showed that a 24-hour interval between the doses was also effective. Alternatively, a single, one-time 1.5-mg dose of levonorgestrel may be used.

The pregnancy rate with Plan B of 1.1 percent compares favorably with that of 3.2 percent in a similar group of women treated with the Yuzpe regimen. The major mechanism with all of these is inhibition or delay of ovulation. Other mechanisms include alteration of the endometrium, sperm penetration, and tubal motility. **Established pregnancies are not harmed.**

Copper-Containing Intrauterine Devices

Fasoli and co-workers (1989) summarized nine studies that included results from 879 women who accepted some type of copper-containing IUD as a sole method of postcoital contraception. The only reported pregnancy aborted spontaneously. Trussell and Stewart (1998) reported that when the IUD was inserted up to 5 days after unprotected intercourse, the failure rate was 1 percent. A secondary advantage is that this method also puts in place an effective 10-year method of contraception.

TABLE 32-9. Prescriptive Equivalents of Dedicated Products and Common Oral Contraceptives for Use as Emergency Contraception

Trade Name	Formulation	Pills per Dose[a]
Dedicated Products		
Plan B	0.75 mg levonorgestrel	1
Oral Contraceptives[b]		
Ogestrel, Ovral	0.05 mg EE 0.5 mg norgestrel	2
Cryselle, Low-Ogestrel, Lo/Ovral,	0.03 mg EE 0.3 mg norgestrel	4
Jolessa, Levlen, Levora, Nordette, Portia Quasense, Seasonale, Seasonique (blue-green)	0.03 mg EE 0.15 mg levonorgestrel	4
TriLevlen (yellow), Triphasil (yellow), Trivora (pink), Enpresse (orange)	0.03 mg EE 0.125 mg levonorgestrel	4
Alesse, Levlite, Aviane, Lutera, Lessina, Sryonx	0.02 mg EE 0.1 mg levonorgestrel	5

[a]Treatment consists of two doses taken 12 hours apart. Use of an antiemetic agent before each dose will lessen the risk of nausea, which is a common side effect.
[b]For these multiphasic formulations, the color in parentheses indicates which pills to use for emergency contraception.
EE = ethinyl estradiol.

Mifepristone (RU 486)

This medication is discussed in Chapter 9 (p. 232) and relies on its antiprogesterone effects to delay or inhibit ovulation as its means of postcoital contraception. A single 10-mg dose provides pregnancy prevention comparable with that of *Plan B* (Task Force on Postovulatory Methods of Fertility Regulation, 1999; von Hertzen and associates, 2002). There are few side effects with mifepristone, and compared with the Yuzpe method it is better tolerated and more effective (Ashok and colleagues, 2002, 2004). In the United States, mifepristone is not used for emergency contraception because of its high cost and because it is not manufactured or marketed in an appropriate dose. Another progesterone-receptor modulator—CDB-2914—was reported by Creinin and colleagues (2006) to be as effective as levonorgestrel in preliminary studies.

LACTATION

For mothers who are nursing exclusively, ovulation during the first 10 weeks after delivery is unlikely. Nursing, however, is not a reliable method of family planning for women whose infants are on a daytime-only feeding schedule. **Waiting for first menses involves a risk of pregnancy, because ovulation usually antedates menstruation.** Certainly, after the first menses, contraception is essential unless the woman desires pregnancy. Estrogen-progestin contraceptives may reduce both the rate and the duration of milk production. The benefits from prevention of pregnancy by the use of combined oral contraceptives would appear to outweigh the risks in selected patients. According to the American College of Obstetricians and Gynecologists (2000), progestin-only contraceptives are the preferred choice in most cases. In addition, IUDs have been recommended for the lactating sexually active woman following uterine involution.

REFERENCES

Abrams LS, Skee DM, Wong FA, et al: Pharmacokinetics of norelgestromin and ethinyl estradiol from two consecutive contraceptive patches. J Clin Pharmacol 41:1232, 2001

Ahrendt HJ, Nisand I, Bastianelli C, et al: Efficacy, acceptability and tolerability of the combined contraceptive ring, NuvaRing, compared with an oral contraceptive containing 30 microg of ethinyl estradiol and 3 mg of drospirenone. Contraception 74:451, 2006

Alvior Jr GT: Pregnancy outcome with removal of intrauterine device. Obstet Gynecol 41(6):894, 1973

American College of Obstetricians and Gynecologists: Breastfeeding: Maternal and infant aspects. Educational Bulletin No. 258, July 2000

American College of Obstetricians and Gynecologists: Benefits and risks of sterilization. Practice Bulletin No. 46, September 2003

American College of Obstetricians and Gynecologists. Emergency contraception. Practice Bulletin No. 69, December 2005a

American College of Obstetricians and Gynecologists: Intrauterine device. Practice Bulletin No. 59, January 2005b

American College of Obstetricians and Gynecologists: Use of hormonal contraception in women with coexisting medical conditions. Practice Bulletin No. 73, Obstet Gynecol 107:1453, 2006

American College of Obstetricians and Gynecologists: Brand versus generic oral contraceptives. Committee Opinion No. 375, Obstet Gynecol 110:447, 2007a

American College of Obstetricians and Gynecologists: Intrauterine device and adolescents. Committee Opinion No. 392, December 2007b

American College of Obstetricians and Gynecologists: Prevention of deep vein thrombosis and pulmonary embolism. Practice Bulletin No. 84, Obstet Gynecol 110:429, 2007c

American College of Obstetricians and Gynecologists: Depot medroxyprogesterone acetate and bone effects. Practice Bulletin No. 415, September 2008

Ashok PW, Hamoda H, Flett GM et al: Mifepristone versus the Yuzpe regimens (PC4) for emergency contraception. Int J Gynaecol Obstet 87:188, 2004

Ashok PW, Stalder C, Wagaarachchi PT, et al: A randomized study comparing a low dose of mifepristone and the Yuzpe regimen for emergency contraception. Br J Obstet Gynaecol 109:553, 2002

Audet MC, Moreau M, Koltun WD, et al: Evaluation of contraceptive efficacy and cycle control of a transdermal contraceptive patch vs an oral contraceptive: A randomized controlled trial. JAMA 285:2347, 2001

Backman T, Rauramo I, Jaakkola K, et al: Use of the levonorgestrel-releasing intrauterine system and breast cancer. Obstet Gynecol 106:813, 2005

Baeten JM, Benki S, Chohan V, et al: Hormonal contraceptive use, herpes simplex virus infection, and risk of HIV-1 acquisition among Kenyan women. AIDS, 21:1771, 2007a

Baeten JM, Lavreys L, Overbaugh J: The influence of hormonal contraceptive use on HIV-1 transmission and disease progression. Clin Infect Dis 45:360, 2007b

Baeten JM, Nyange PM, Richardson BA, et al: Hormonal contraception and risk of sexually transmitted disease acquisition: Results from a prospective study. Am J Obstet Gynecol 185:380, 2001

Bahamondes L, Del Castillo S, Tabares G: Comparison of weight increase in users of depot medroxyprogesterone acetate and copper IUD up to 5 years. Contraception 64(4):223, 2001

Bahamondes L, Espejo-Arce X, Hidalgo MM, et al: A cross-sectional study of the forearm bone density of long-term users of levonorgestrel-releasing intrauterine system. Hum Reprod 21:1316, 2006

Bayer HealthCare Pharmaceuticals: Mirena (levonorgestrel-releasing intrauterine system). Patient information, 2007a. Available at: http://berlex.bayer-healthcare.com/html/products/pi/mirena_patient_insert.pdf?C = &c. Accessed February 16, 2008

Bayer HealthCare Pharmaceuticals: Yasmin, drospirenone and ethinyl estradiol tablets, Physician labeling, 2007b. Available at: http://berlex.bayerhealth-care.com/html/products/pi/fhc/Yasmin_PI.pdf. Accessed February 22, 2008

Beckman LJ, Murray J, Harvey SM: The contraceptive sponge: Factors in initiation and discontinuation of use. Contraception 40:481, 1989

Beining RM, Dennis LK, Smith EM, et al: Meta-analysis of intrauterine device use and risk of endometrial cancer. Ann Epidemiol 18 (6):492, 2008

Beerthuizen R, van Beek A, Massai R, et al: Hum Reprod 15:118, 2000

Biswas A, Biswas S, Viegas OA: Effect of etonogestrel subdermal contraceptive implant (Implanon) on liver function tests—a randomized comparative study with Norplant implants. Contraception 70:379, 2004

Biswas A, Viegas OA, Roy AC: Effect of Implanon and Norplant subdermal contraceptive implants on serum lipids—a randomized comparative study. Contraception 68:189, 2003

Bitzer J, Tschudin S, Alder J, et al: Acceptability and side-effects of Implanon in Switzerland: A retrospective study by the Implanon Swiss Study Group. Eur J Contracept Reprod Health Care 9:278, 2004

Bjarnadóttir RI, Tuppurainen M, Killick SR: Comparison of cycle control with a combined contraceptive vaginal ring and oral levonorgestrel/ethinyl estradiol. Am J Obstet Gynecol 186:389, 2002

Briggs GG, Freeman RK, Yaffe SJ: Drugs in Pregnancy and Lactation, 7th ed. Baltimore, Williams & Wilkins, 2005

Brohet RM, Goldgar DE, Easton DF, et al: Oral contraceptives and breast cancer risk in the international BRCA 1/2 carrier cohort study: A report from EMBRACE, GENEPSO, GEO-HEBON, and the IBCCS Collaborating Group. J Clin Oncol 25:5327, 2007

Bulten J, Grefte J, Siebers B, et al: The combined contraceptive vaginal ring (NuvaRing) and endometrial histology. Contraception 72:362, 2005

Cancer and Steroid Hormone Study of the Centers for Disease Control and the National Institute of Child Health and Development: Combination oral contraceptive use and the risk of endometrial cancer. JAMA 257:796, 1987

Chandra A, Martinez GM, Mosher WD, et al: Fertility, family planning, and reproductive health of U.S. women: Data from the 2002 National Survey of Family Growth. National Center for Health Statistics. Vital Health Stat 23:1, 2005

Chasan-Taber L, Willett WC, Manson JE, et al: Prospective study of oral contraceptives and hypertension among women in the United States. Circulation 94:483, 1996

Clark MK, Sowers M, Levy B, et al: Bone mineral density loss and recovery during 48 months in first-time users of depot medroxyprogesterone acetate. Fertil Steril 86:1466, 2006

Cole JA, Norman H, Doherty M, et al: Venous thromboembolism, myocardial infarction, and stroke among transdermal contraceptive system users. Obstet Gynecol 109:339, 2007

Collaborative Group on Epidemiological Studies of Ovarian Cancer, Beral V, Doll R, Hermon C, Peto R, Reeves G. Ovarian cancer and oral contraceptives: Collaborative reanalysis of data of 45 epidemiological studies including 23,257 women with ovarian cancer and 87,303 controls. Lancet 371:303, 2008

Collaborative Group on Hormonal Factors in Breast Cancer: Breast cancer and hormonal contraceptives: Collaborative reanalysis of individual data on

53,297 women with breast cancer and 100,239 women without cancer from 54 epidemiological studies. Lancet 347:1713, 1996

Comp PC: Coagulation and thrombosis with OC use: Physiology and clinical relevance. Dialogues Contracept 5:1, 1996

Craft P, Hannaford PC: Risk factors for acute myocardial infarction in women: Evidence from the Royal College of General Practitioners' Oral Contraceptive Study. BMJ 298:165, 1989

Creinin MD, Schlaff W, Archer DF, et al: Progesterone receptor modulator for emergency contraception. Obstet Gynecol 108:1089, 2006

Critchlow CW, Wölner-Hanssen P, Eschenback DA, et al: Determinants of cervical ectopia and of cervicitis: Age, oral contraception, specific cervical infection, smoking, and douching. Am J Obstet Gynecol 173:534, 1995

Cromer BA, Smith RD, Blair JM, et al: A prospective study of adolescents who choose among levonorgestrel implant (Norplant), medroxyprogesterone acetate (Depo-Provera), or the combined oral contraceptive pill as contraception. Pediatrics 94:687, 1994

Croxatto HB, Mäkäräinen L: The pharmacodynamics and efficacy of Implanon. An overview of the data. Contraception 58:91S, 1998

Curtis EM, Pine L: *Actinomyces* in the vaginas of women with and without intrauterine contraceptive devices. Am J Obstet Gynecol 140:880, 1981

Curtis KM, Marchbanks PA, Peterson HG: Neoplasia with use of intrauterine devices. Contraception 75:S60, 2007

d'Arcangues C: WHO statement on hormonal contraception and bone health. Contraception 73:443, 2006

d'Arcangues C: Worldwide use of intrauterine devices for contraception. Contraception 75:S2, 2007

D'Cruz OJ, Uckun FM: Clinical development of microbicides for the prevention of HIV infection. Curr Pharm Des 10:315, 2004

Demers, LM: The morning-after pill. N Engl J Med 284:1034, 1971

Dieben TO, Roumen FJ, Apter D: Efficacy, cycle control, and user acceptability of a novel combined contraceptive vagina ring. Obstet Gynecol 100:585, 2002

Dittrich R, Parker L, Rosen JB, et al: Transdermal contraception: Evaluation of three transdermal norelgestromin/ethinyl estradiol doses in a randomized, multicenter, dose-response study. Am J Obstet Gynecol 186:15, 2002

Drazen JM, Greene MF, Wood AJJ: The FDA, politics, and Plan B. N Engl J Med 350:15, 2004

Duramed Pharmaceuticals: ParaGard intrauterine copper contraceptive. Patient information package insert, 2006. Available at: http://www.paragard.com/custom_images/ppi_eng.pdf. Accessed February 16, 2008

Edelman A, Gallo MF, Nichols MD, et al: Continuous versus cyclic use of combined oral contraceptives for contraception: Systematic Cochrane review of randomized controlled trials. Hum Reprod 21:573, 2006

European Society of Human Reproduction and Embryology. ESHRE Capri Workshop Group: Noncontraceptive health benefits of combined oral contraception. Hum Reprod Update 11:513, 2005

Farley TMM, Rosenberg MJ, Rowe PJ, et al: Intrauterine devices and pelvic inflammatory disease: An international perspective. Lancet 339:785, 1992

Fasoli M, Parazzini F, Cecchetti G, et al: Post-coital contraception: An overview of published studies. Contraception 39:459, 1989

Faundes D, Bahamondes L, Faundes A, et al: No relationship between the IUD position evaluated by ultrasound and complaints of bleeding and pain. Contraception 56:43, 1997

Fiorino AS: Intrauterine contraceptive device–associated actinomycotic abscess and *Actinomyces* detection on cervical smear. Obstet Gynecol 87:142, 1996

Fraser IS, Lacarra M, Mishell DR, et al: Vaginal epithelial surface appearances in women using vaginal rings for contraception. Contraception 61:131, 2000

Frega A, Scardamaglia P, Piazze J, et al: Oral contraceptives and clinical recurrence of human papillomavirus lesions and cervical intraepithelial neoplasia following treatment. Int J Gynaecol Obstet 100:175, 2008

Funk S, Miller MM, Mishell Jr DR, Archer DF, et al: Safety and efficacy of Implanon, a single-rod implantable contraceptive containing etonogestrel. Contraception 71:319, 2005

Furlong LA: Ectopic pregnancy risk when contraception fails. J Reprod Med 47:881, 2002

Gallo MF, Grimes DA, Lopez LM, et al: Non-latex versus latex male condoms for contraception. Cochrane Database Syst Rev (1):CD003550, 2006

Gallo MF, Lopez LM, Grimes DA, et al: Combination contraceptives: Effects on weight. Cochrane Database Syst Rev 4: CD003987, 2008

Gardner JM, Mishell DR Jr: Analysis of bleeding patterns and resumption of fertility following discontinuation of a long-acting injectable contraceptive. Fertil Steril 21:286, 1970

Geiger AM, Foxman B: Risk factors for vulvovaginal candidiasis: A case-control study among university students. Epidemiology 7:182, 1996

Gilliam M, Knight S, McCarthy M Jr: Success with oral contraceptives: A pilot study. Contraception 69:413, 2004

Grimes DA, Hubacher D, Lopez LM, Schulz KF. Non-steroidal anti-inflammatory drugs for heavy bleeding or pain associated with intrauterine-device use. Cochrane Database Syst Rev 4:CD006034, 2006a

Grimes DA, Jones LB, Lopez LM, et al: Oral contraceptives for functional ovarian cysts. Cochrane Database Syst Rev 4:CD006134, 2006b

Grimes DA, Schulz KF: Antibiotic prophylaxis for intrauterine contraceptive device insertion. Cochrane Database Syst Rev (2):CD001327, 2001a

Grimes DA, Schulz KF, Van Vliet H, et al: Immediate post-partum insertion of intrauterine devices. Cochrane Database Syst Rev 2:CD003036, 2001b

Gu Y, Liang X, Wu W: Multicenter contraceptive efficacy trial of injectable testosterone undecanoate in Chinese men. J Clin Endocrinol Metab 94(6):1910, 2009

Haider S, Darney PD: Injectable contraception. Clin Obstet Gynecol 50:898, 2007

Hannaford PC, Selvaraj S, Elliott AM, et al: Cancer risk among users of oral contraceptives: Cohort data from the Royal College of General Practitioners' oral contraception study. BMJ 335:651, 2007

Harrison-Woolrych M, Ashton J, Coulter D: Uterine perforation on intrauterine device insertion: Is the incidence higher than previously reported? Contraception 67:53, 2003

Hatcher RA, Trussell J, Stewart F, et al: Contraceptive Technology, 17th ed. New York, Ardent Media, 1998

Hatcher RA, Trussell J, Nelson AL, et al: Contraceptive Technology, 19th ed. New York, Ardent Media, 2007

Heinemann LA, Weimann A, Gerken G, et al: Modern oral contraceptive use and benign liver tumors: The German Benign Liver Tumor Case-Control Study. Eur J Contracept Reprod Health Care 3:194, 1998

Hov GG, Skjeldestad FE, Hilstad T: Use of IUD and subsequent fertility—follow-up after participation in a randomized clinical trial. Contraception 75:88, 2007

Hubacher D, Lara-Ricalde R, Taylor DJ, et al: Use of copper intrauterine devices and the risk of tubal infertility among nulligravid women. N Engl J Med 345:561, 2001

Hutchinson KB, Kip KE, Ness RB: Condom use and its association with bacterial vaginosis and bacterial vaginosis-associated vaginal microflora. Epidemiology 18:702, 2007

Inki P, Hurskainin R, Palo P, et al: Comparison of ovarian cyst formation in women using the levonorgestrel-releasing intrauterine system vs. hysterectomy. Ultrasound Obstet Gynecol 20:381, 2002

International Collaboration of Epidemiological Studies of Cervical Cancer: Cervical cancer and hormonal contraceptives: Collaborative reanalysis of individual data for 16573 women with cervical cancer and 35,509 women without cervical cancer from 24 epidemiological studies. Lancet 370:1609, 2007

Jain J, Jakimiuk AJ, Bode FR, et al: Contraceptive efficacy and safety of DMPA-SC. Contraception 70:269, 2004

Jecht EW, Bernstein GS: The influence of copper on the motility of human spermatozoa. Contraception 7:381, 1973

Jennings VH, Arevalo M, Kowal D: Fertility awareness-based methods. In Hatch RA, Trussell J, Stewart F, et al (eds): Contraceptive Technology, 18th ed. New York, Ardent Media, 2004, p 317

Jick SS, Jick H: Cerebral venous sinus thrombosis in users of four hormonal contraceptives: Levonorgestrel-containing oral contraceptives, norgestimate-containing oral contraceptives, desogestrel-containing oral contraceptives and the contraceptive patch. Contraception 74:290, 2006a

Jick SS, Kaye JA, Russmann S, et al: Risk of nonfatal venous thromboembolism in women using a contraceptive transdermal patch and oral contraceptives containing norgestimate and 35 microg of ethinyl estradiol. Contraception 73:223, 2006b

Jick S, Kaye JA, Lin L, et al: Further results on the risk of nonfatal venous thromboembolism in users of the contraceptive transdermal patch compared to users of oral contraceptives containing norgestimate and 35 μg of ethinyl estradiol. Contraception 76:4, 2007

Joffe J, Petrillo LF, Viguera AC, et al: Treatment of premenstrual worsening depression with adjunctive oral contraceptive pills: A preliminary report. J Clin Psychiatry 68:1954, 2007

Kabat GC, Miller AB, Rohan TE: Oral contraceptive use, hormone replacement therapy, reproductive history and risk of colorectal cancer in women. Int J Cancer 122:643, 2008

Kamischke A, Nieschlag E: Progress towards hormonal male contraception. Trends Pharmacol Sci 25:49, 2004

Kaunitz AM: Depot medroxyprogesterone acetate contraception and the risk of breast and gynecologic cancer. J Reprod Med 45:419, 1996

Kim C, Siscovick DS, Sidney S, et al: Oral contraceptive use and association with glucose, insulin, and diabetes in young adult women: The CARDIA Study. Coronary Artery Risk Development in Young Adults. Diabetes Care 25:1027, 2002

Kost K, Singh S, Vaughan B, et al: Estimates of contraceptive failure from the 2002 National Survey of Family Growth. Contraception 77:10, 2008

Krattenmacher R: Drospirenone: Pharmacology and pharmacokinetics of a unique progestogen. Contraception 62:29, 2000

Kuyoh MA, Toroitich-Ruto C, Grimes DA, et al: Sponge versus diaphragm for contraception: A Cochrane review. Contraception 67:15, 2003

Lammer EJ, Cordero JF: Exogenous sex hormone exposure and the risk for major malformations. JAMA 255:3128, 1986

Lens M, Bataille V: Melanoma in relation to reproductive and hormonal factors in women: Current review on controversial issues. Cancer Causes Control 19:437, 2008

Lippes J: Pelvic actinomycosis: A review and preliminary look at prevalence. Am J Obstet Gynecol 180:265, 1999

Lopez LM, Grimes DA, Schulz KF: Steroidal contraceptives: Effect on carbohydrate metabolism in women without diabetes mellitus. Cochrane Database Syst Apr 18 (2):CD006133, 2007

Lopez LM, Kaptein AA, Helmerhorst FM: Oral contraceptives containing drospirenone for premenstrual syndrome. Cochrane Database Syst Rev 2:CD006586, 2009

MacClellan LR, Giles W, Cole J, et al: Probable migraine with visual aura and risk of ischemic stroke: The Stroke Prevention in Young Women Study. Stroke 38:2438, 2007

Maheshwari S, Sarraj A, Kramer J, et al: Oral contraception and the risk of hepatocellular carcinoma. J Hepatol 47:506, 2007

Manhart LE, Koutsky LA: Do condoms prevent genital HPV infection, external genital warts, or cervical neoplasia? A meta-analysis. Sex Transm Dis 29:725, 2002

Margolis KL, Adami HO, Luo J, et al: A prospective study of oral contraceptive use and risk of myocardial infarction among Swedish women. Fertil Steril 88:310, 2007

Mauck C, Glover LH, Miller E, et al: Lea's Shield: A study of the safety and efficacy of a new vaginal barrier contraceptive used with and without spermicide. Contraception 53:329, 1996

Merki-Feld GS, Brekenfeld C, Migge, et al: Nonpalpable ultrasonographically not detectable Implanon rods can be localized by magnetic resonance imaging. Contraception 63:325, 2001

Mishell DR Jr: Oral contraceptives and cardiovascular events: Summary and application of data. Int J Fertil 45:121, 2000

Mishell DR Jr, Sulak PJ: The IUD: Dispelling the myths and assessing the potential. Dialogues Contracept 5:1, 1997

Mommers E, Kersemaekers WM, Elliesen J, et al: Male hormonal contraception: a double-blind, placebo-controlled study. J Clin Endocrinol Metab 93(7):2572, 2008

Mooij PN, Thomas CMG, Doesburg WH, et al: Multivitamin supplementation in oral contraceptive users. Contraception 44:277, 1991

Moore LL, Valuck R, McDougall C, et al: A comparative study of one-year weight gain among users of medroxyprogesterone acetate, levonorgestrel implants, and oral contraceptives. Contraception 52:215, 1995

Morrison CS, Richardson BA, Mmiro F, et al: Hormonal contraception and the risk of HIV acquisition. AIDS 21:85, 2007

Moreau C, Trussell J, Gilbert F, et al: Oral contraceptive tolerance: Does the type of pill matter? Obstet Gynecol 109:1277, 2007

Mosher WD, Martinez GM, Chandra A, et al: Use of contraception and use of family planning services in the United States: 1982–2002. Adv Data 10:1, 2004

Murthy AS, Creinin MD, Harwood B, et al: Same-day initiation of the transdermal hormonal delivery system (contraceptive patch) versus traditional initiation methods. Contraception 72(5):333, 2005

Nakajima ST, Archer DF, Ellman H: Efficacy and safety of a new 24-day oral contraceptive regimen of norethindrone acetate 1 mg/ethinyl estradiol 20 micro g (Loestrin 24 Fe). Contraception 75:16, 2007

Ness RB, Soper DE, Holley RL, et al: Hormonal and barrier contraception and risk of upper genital tract disease in the PID evaluation and Clinical Health (PEACH) study. Am J Obstet Gynecol 185:121, 2001

Ngai SW, Fan S, Li S, et al: A randomized trial to compare 24 h versus 12 h double dose regimen of levonorgestrel for emergency contraception. Hum Reprod 20:307, 2005

O'Brien PA, Marfleet C: Frameless versus classical intrauterine device for contraception. Cochrane Database Syst Rev Jan 25 (1):CD003282, 2005

Oddsson K, Leifels-Fischer B, Wiel-Masson D, et al: Superior cycle control with a contraceptive vaginal ring compared with an oral contraceptive containing 30 microg ethinylestradiol and 150 microg levonorgestrel: A randomized trial. Hum Reprod 20:557, 2005

Organon USA: NuvaRing package insert. 2005 Available at: http://www.nuvaring.com/Authfiles/Images/309_76063.pdf. Accessed February 3, 2008

Ortho-McNeil Pharmaceutical: Micronor Prescribing Information, Revised 2007. Available at: http://www.ortho-mcneilpharmaceutical.com/ortho-mcneilpharmaceutical/shared/pi/micro.pdf#zoom = 100. Accessed March 1, 2008

Ortiz ME, Croxatto HB: Copper-T intrauterine device and levonorgestrel intrauterine system: Biological bases of their mechanism of action. Contraception 75:S16, 2007

Palliser D, Chowdbury D, Wang QY, et al: An siRNA-based microbicide protects mice from lethal herpes simplex virus 2 infection. Nature 439:89, 2006

Parazzini F, Negri E, La Vecchia C, et al: Oral contraceptive use and risk of uterine fibroids. Obstet Gynecol 79:430, 1992

Pasquale SA, Russer TJ, Foldes R, et al: Lack of interaction between magnetic resonance imaging and the copper-T380A IUD. Contraception. 55(3):169, 1997

Pearlstein TB, Bachmann GA, Zacur HA, et al: Treatment of premenstrual dysphoric disorder with a new drospirenone-containing oral contraceptive formulation. Contraception 72:414, 2005

Peri N, Graham D, Levine D: Imaging of intrauterine contraceptive devices. J Ultrasound Med 26:1389, 2007

Persson E, Holmberg K: A longitudinal study of *Actinomyces israelii* in the female genital tract. Acta Obstet Gynecol Scand 63:207, 1984

Pfizer: Depo-Provera, Contraceptive Injection, medroxyprogesterone acetate injectable suspension, USP, Physician Information, 2006. Available at: http://www.pfizer.com/files/products/uspi_depo_provera_contraceptive.pdf. Accessed February 19, 2008

Pfizer: Depo-subQ provera 104, medroxyprogesterone acetate injectable suspension, Physician Information, 2007. Available at: http://www.pfizer.com/files/products/uspi_depo_subq_provera.pdf. Accessed February 19, 2008

Pizarro E, Schoenstedt G, Mehech G, et al: Uterine cavity and the location of IUDs following administration of meclofenamic acid to menorrhagic women. A pilot study. Contraception 40:413, 1989

Pomp ER, le Cessie S, Rosendaal FR, et al: Risk of venous thrombosis: Obesity and its joint effect with oral contraceptive use and prothrombotic mutations. Br J Haematol 139(2):289, 2007

Pomp ER, Rosendaal FR, Doggen CJ: Smoking increases the risk of venous thrombosis and acts synergistically with oral contraceptive use. Am J Hematol 83:97, 2008

Population Council: Jadelle® Implants: Research and Development. Available at: http://www.popcouncil.org/biomed/jadellefaqresearch.html. Accessed February 17, 2008

Population Reports: Periodic abstinence: How well do new approaches work? Series L, No. 3, September 1981, p 33

Ragan RE, Rock RW, Buck HW: Metoclopramide pretreatment attenuates emergency contraceptive-associated nausea. Am J Obstet Gynecol 188:330, 2003

Raymond EG, Creinin MD, Barnhart KT, et al: Meclizine for prevention of nausea associated with use of emergency contraceptive pills: A randomized study. Obstet Gynecol 95:271, 2000

Remington KM, Buller RS, Kelly JR: Effect of the Today contraceptive sponge on growth and toxic shock syndrome toxin-1 production by *Staphylococcus aureus*. Obstet Gynecol 69:563, 1987

Richwald GA, Greenland S, Gerber MM, et al: Effectiveness of the cavity-rim cervical cap: Results of a large clinical study. Obstet Gynecol 74:143, 1989

Riggs M, Klevanoff M, Nansel T, et al: Longitudinal association between hormonal contraceptives and bacterial vaginosis in women of reproductive age. Sex Transm Dis 34:954, 2007

Robinson GE, Burren T, Mackie IJ, et al: Changes in haemostasis after stopping the combined contraceptive pill: Implications for major surgery. BMJ 302:269, 1991

Ronnerdag M, Odlind V: Health effects of long-term use of the intrauterine levonorgestrel-releasing system. Acta Obstet Gynecol Scand 78:716, 1999

Rosenberg MJ, Davidson AJ, Chen JH, et al: Barrier contraceptives and sexually transmitted diseases in women: A comparison of female-dependent methods and condoms. Am J Public Health 82:669, 1992

Rothman KJ, Louik C: Oral contraceptives and birth defects. N Engl J Med 299:522, 1978

Sääv I, Aronsson A, Marions L, et al: Cervical priming with sublingual misoprostol prior to insertion of an intrauterine device in nulliparous women: A randomized controlled trial. Hum Reprod 22:2647, 2007

Said S, Omar K, Koetsawang S, et al: A multicentred phase III comparative clinical trial of depot-medroxyprogesterone acetate given three-monthly at doses of 100 mg or 150 mg: 1. Contraceptive efficacy and side effects. Contraception 34:223, 1986

Savolainen E, Saksela E, Saxen L: Teratogenic hazards of oral contraceptives analyzed in a national malformation register. Am J Obstet Gynecol 140:521, 1981

Schafer JE, Osborne LM, Davis AR, et al: Acceptability and satisfaction using Quick Start with the contraceptive vaginal ring versus an oral contraceptive. Contraception 73(5):488, 2006

Schiesser M, Lapaire O, Tercanli S, et al: Lost intrauterine devices during pregnancy: Maternal and fetal outcome after ultrasound-guided extraction. An analysis of 82 cases. Ultrasound Obstet Gynecol 23:486, 2004

Schlaff WD, Carson SA, Luciano A, et al: Subcutaneous injection of depot medroxyprogesterone acetate compared with leuprolide acetate in the treatment of endometriosis-associated pain. Fertil Steril 85.314, 2006

Scholes D, LaCroix AS, Ichikawa LE, et al: Injectable hormone contraception and bone density: Results from a prospective study. Epidemiology 13:581, 2002

Scholes D, LaCroix AS, Ott SM, et al: Bone mineral density in women using depot medroxyprogesterone acetate for contraception. Obstet Gynecol 93:233, 1999

Schürmann R, Blode H, Benda N, et al: Effect of drospirenone on serum potassium and drospirenone pharmacokinetics in women with normal or impaired renal function. J Clin Pharmacol 46:867, 2006

Seeger JD, Loughlin J, Eng PM, et al: Risk of thromboembolism in women taking ethinylestradiol/drospirenone and other oral contraceptives. Obstet Gynecol 110:587, 2007

Shulman LP, Gabriel H: Management and localization strategies for the nonpalpable Implanon rod. Contraception 73:325, 2006

Sivin I: Alternative estimates of ectopic pregnancy risks during contraception. Am J Obstet Gynecol 165:1900, 1991

Sivin I, Wan L, Ranta S, et al: Levonorgestrel concentrations during 7 years of continuous use of Jadelle contraceptive implants. Contraception 64:43, 2001

Skegg DCG, Noonan EA, Paul C, et al: Depot medroxyprogesterone acetate and breast cancer. JAMA 273:799, 1995

Speroff L, Darney PD: A Clinical Guide for Contraception, 3rd ed. Philadelphia, Lippincott Williams & Wilkins, 2001, pp 66, 99, 240, 284

Stadel BV: Oral contraceptives and cardiovascular disease. N Engl J Med 305:612, 1981

Stanford JB, Mikolajczyk RT: Mechanisms of action of intrauterine devices: Update and estimation of postfertilization effects. Obstet Gynecol 187:1699, 2002

Steiner MJ, Dominik R, Rountree W, et al: Contraceptive effectiveness of a polyurethane condom and a latex condom: A randomized controlled trial. Obstet Gynecol 101:539, 2003

Stringer EM, Kaseba C, Levy J, et al: A randomized trial of the intrauterine contraceptive device vs hormonal contraception in women who are infected with the human immunodeficiency virus. Am J Obstet Gynecol 197:144, 2007

Stuart GS, Castaño PM: Sexually transmitted infections and contraceptives: Selective issues. Obstet Gynecol Clin North Am 30:795, 2003

Stuart GS, Tang JH, Heartwell SF, et al: A high cholecystectomy rate in a cohort of Mexican American women who are postpartum at the time of oral contraceptive pill initiation. Contraception 76:357, 2007

Task Force on Postovulatory Methods of Fertility Regulation: Comparison of three single doses of mifepristone as emergency contraception: A randomized trial. Lancet 353:697, 1999

Tatum HJ, Schmidt FH, Jain AK: Management and outcome of pregnancies associated with Copper-T intrauterine contraceptive device. Am J Obstet Gynecol 126:869, 1976

Thonneau PF, Almont TE: Contraceptive efficacy of intrauterine devices. Am J Obstet Gynecol 198:248, 2008

Truitt ST, Fraser AB, Grimes DA, et al: Hormonal contraception during lactation: Systematic review of randomized controlled trials. Contraception 68:233, 2003

Trussell J: Contraceptive failure in the United States. Contraception 70:89, 2004

Trussell J, Lalla AM, Doan QV, et al: Cost effectiveness of contraceptives in the United States. Contraception 79(1):5, 2009

Trussell J, Stewart F: An update on emergency contraception. Dialogues Contracept 5:1, 1998

Tworoger SS, Fairfield KM, Colditz GA, et al: Association of oral contraceptive use, other contraceptive methods, and infertility with ovarian cancer risk. Am J Epidemiol 166(8):894, 2007

Urdl W, Apter D, Alperstein A, et al: Contraceptive efficacy, compliance and beyond: Factors related to satisfaction with once-weekly transdermal compared with oral contraception. Eur J Obstet Gynecol Reprod Biol 121:202, 2005

U.S. Food and Drug Administration: Approved drug products with therapeutic equivalence evaluations, 28th ed. Rockville, 2008. Available at: http://www.fda.gov/cder/ob. Accessed February 27, 2008a

U.S. Food and Drug Administration: Black box warning added concerning long-term use of Depo-Provera Contraceptive Injection. FDA Talk Paper, November 17, 2004. Available at: http://www.fda.gov/bbs/topics/ANSWERS/2004/ANS01325.html. Accessed February 17, 2008

U.S. Food and Drug Administration: Plan B (0.75mg levonorgestrel) Tablets Information. Available at: http://www.fda.gov/cder/drug/infopage/planB/default.htm Accessed May 19, 2009

van den Heuvel MW, van Bragt AJ, Alnabawu AK, et al: Comparison of ethinylestradiol pharmacokinetics in three hormonal contraceptive formulations: The vaginal ring, the transdermal patch and an oral contraceptive. Contraception 72:168, 2005

van Vliet HA, Grimes DA, Lopez LM: Triphasic versus monophasic oral contraceptives for contraception. Cochrane Database Sys Rev (3):CD003553, 2006

Veres S, Miller L, Burington B: A comparison between the vaginal ring and oral contraceptives. Obstet Gynecol 104:555, 2004

Vessey M, Yeates D: Oral contraceptives and benign breast disease: An update of findings in a large cohort study. Contraception 76:418, 2007

Vessey MP, Johnson B, Doll R, et al: Outcome of pregnancy in women using intrauterine devices. Lancet 1:495, 1974

Vessey MP, Lawless M, McPherson K, et al: Fertility after stopping use of intrauterine contraceptive device. BMJ 286:106, 1983

Vessey MP, Lawless M, Yeates D: Efficacy of different contraceptive methods. Lancet 1:841, 1982

von Hertzen H, Piaggio G, Ding J et al: Low dose mifepristone and two regimens of levonorgestrel for emergency contraception: A WHO multicentre randomized trial. Lancet 360:1803, 2002

Wallach M, Grimes DA (eds): Modern Oral Contraception. Updates from The Contraception Report. Totowa, NJ, Emron, 2000, pp 26, 90, 194–195

Walsh T, Grimes D, Frezieres R, et al: Randomised controlled trial of prophylactic antibiotics before insertion of intrauterine devices. IUD study group. Lancet 351:1005, 1998

Westhoff C: IUDs and colonization or infection with *Actinomyces*. Contraception 75:S48, 2007a

Westhoff C, Heartwell S, Edwards S, et al: Initiation of oral contraceptive using a quick start compared with a conventional start: A randomized controlled trial. Obstet Gynecol 109:1270, 2007b

Westhoff C, Jain JK, Milson, et al: Changes in weight with depot medroxyprogesterone acetate subcutaneous injection 104 mg/0.65 mL. Contraception 75:261, 2007c

Westhoff C, Kerns J, Morroni C, et al: Quick start: Novel oral contraceptive initiation method. Contraception 66:141, 2002

Westhoff CL: Oral contraceptives and thrombosis: An overview of study methods and recent results. Am J Obstet Gynecol 179:S38, 1998

Wilson W, Taubert KA, Gewitz M, et al: Prevention of infective endocarditis: Guidelines from the American Heart Association: A guideline from the American Heart Association Rheumatic Fever, Endocarditis, and Kawasaki Disease Committee, Council on Cardiovascular Surgery and Anesthesia, and the Quality of Care and Outcomes Research Interdisciplinary Working Group. Circulation 116:1736, 2007

Winer RL, Hughes JP, Feng Q, et al: Condom use and the risk of genital human papillomavirus infection in young women. N Engl J Med 354:2645, 2006

World Health Organization: A multinational case-control study of ectopic pregnancy. Clin Reprod Fertil 3:131, 1985

World Health Organization: Mechanism of action, safety and efficacy of intrauterine devices. Technical Report No. 753, Geneva, Switzerland, WHO, 1987

World Health Organization: Effects of hormonal contraceptives on breast milk composition and infant growth. Stud Fam Plann 19/361, 1988

World Health Organization: Depot-medroxyprogesterone acetate (DMPA) and risk of endometrial cancer. Int J Cancer 49:186, 1991

World Health Organization: Ischaemic stroke and combined oral contraceptives: Results of an international, multi-center case-control study. Lancet 348:498, 1996

World Health Organization: Acute myocardial infarction and combined oral contraceptives: Results of an international multi-center case-control study. Lancet 349:1202, 1997

World Health Organization: Cardiovascular disease and use of oral and injectable progestogen-only contraceptives and combined injectable contraceptives. Results of an international, multicenter, case-control study. Contraception 57:315, 1998

Yela DA, Monteiro IM, Bahamondes LG, et al: Weight variation in users of the levonorgestrel-releasing intrauterine system, of the copper IUD and of medroxyprogesterone acetate in Brazil. [Article in Portuguese] Rev Assoc Med Bras 52:32, 2006

Yonkers KA, Brown C, Pearlstein TB, et al: Efficacy of a new low-dose oral contraceptive with drospirenone in premenstrual dysphoric disorder. Obstet Gynecol 106:492, 2005

Yuzpe AA, Thurlow HJ, Ramzy I, et al: Post coital contraception—a pilot study. J Reprod Med 13:53, 1974

Zieman M, Guillebaud J, Weisberg E, et al: Contraceptive efficacy and cycle control with the Ortho Evra/Evra transdermal system: The analysis of pooled data. Fertil Steril 77:S13, 2002

Zieman M, Kanal E: Copper T 380A IUD and magnetic resonance imaging. Contraception 75:93, 2007

CHAPTER 33

Sterilization

Sterilization has become a popular choice of contraceptive for millions of men and women in the United States as well as in many countries worldwide. This procedure is indicated in those requesting sterilization and who clearly understand its permanence and its difficult and often unsuccessful reversal. A woman should be counseled regarding alternative contraceptive choices (American College of Obstetricians and Gynecologists, 2007).

FEMALE STERILIZATION

Female sterilization is the contraceptive method selected by 28 percent of couples in the United States (American College of Obstetricians and Gynecologists, 2003). And for women aged 35 to 44 years, surgical sterilization was their most commonly reported form of contraception (Bensyl and associates, 2005; Huber and Huber, 2009).

Sterilization is usually accomplished by occlusion or division of the fallopian tubes. This can be performed at any time, but at least half are performed in conjunction with cesarean or vaginal delivery and are termed *puerperal* (MacKay and associates, 2001). *Nonpuerperal* surgical tubal sterilization is usually accomplished via laparoscopy in an outpatient surgical center. Hysteroscopic or minilaparotomy approaches to occlusion are also available.

Puerperal Tubal Sterilization

For several days after delivery, the fallopian tubes are accessible at the umbilicus directly beneath the abdominal wall. Wall laxity allows easy repositioning of the abdominal incision over each uterine cornu. Thus, puerperal sterilization is technically simple, and hospitalization need not be prolonged. Some prefer to perform sterilization immediately following delivery, although others wait for 12 to 24 hours (Bucklin and Smith, 1999). At Parkland and the University of Alabama Hospitals, puerperal tubal ligation is performed in the obstetrical surgical suite the morning after delivery. This minimizes hospital stays but allows the likelihood of postpartum hemorrhage to diminish. In addition, the status of the newborn can be better ascertained.

Various techniques are now used to disrupt tubal patency. In general, a midtubal segment of fallopian tube is excised, and the severed ends seal by fibrosis and reperitonealization. Commonly used methods of interval sterilization include the Parkland, Pomeroy, and modified Pomeroy techniques (American College of Obstetricians and Gynecologists, 2003). Irving and Uchida techniques or Kroener fimbriectomy are rarely used because they involve increased dissection, operative time, and chance of mesosalpingeal injury. With fimbriectomy, unfavorably high failure rates stem from recanalization of the proximal tubal portion (Pati and Cullins, 2000).

Surgical Technique

A small infraumbilical incision is made. The fallopian tube is identified by grasping its midportion with a Babcock clamp, and the distal fimbria is identified. This prevents confusing the round ligament with the midportion of the tube. A common reason for sterilization failure is ligation of the wrong structure, typically the round ligament. Therefore, identification and isolation of the distal tube prior to ligation is required. **Whenever the tube is inadvertently dropped, it is mandatory to repeat this identification procedure.** Surgical steps are outlined for each method in Figures 33-1 and 33-2.

Failure Rates

Puerperal sterilization fails for two major reasons. First, surgical errors include transection of the round ligament or only partial transection of the tube. Thus, both tubal segments are submitted

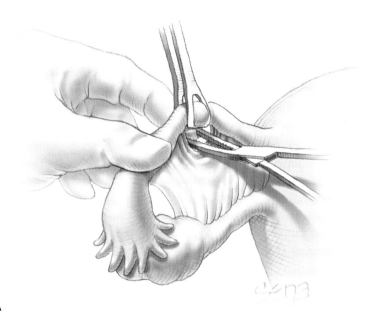

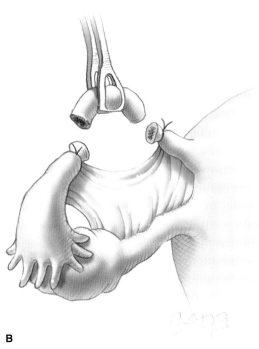

FIGURE 33-1 Parkland method. **A.** An avascular site in the mesosalpinx adjacent to the fallopian tube is perforated with a small hemostat. The jaws are opened to separate the fallopian tube from the adjacent mesosalpinx for approximately 2.5 cm. **B.** The freed fallopian tube is ligated proximally and distally with 0-chromic suture. The intervening segment of approximately 2 cm is excised, and the excision site is inspected for hemostasis. This method was designed to avoid the initial intimate proximity of the cut ends of the fallopian tube inherent with the Pomeroy procedure. (From Hoffman, 2008, with permission.)

for pathological confirmation. Secondly, a fistulous tract or spontaneous reanastomosis forms between the severed tubal stumps.

In their first report, investigators from the Collaborative Review of Sterilization (CREST) study described follow-up of 10,863 women who had undergone tubal sterilization from 1978 through 1986 (Peterson and colleagues, 1996). The failure rates for various procedures are summarized in Figure 33-3. Specifically, with the Parkland method, during four decades, the failure rate has been less than 1 in 400 procedures. It is readily

apparent that puerperal sterilization is highly effective, with a short- and long-term failure rate that is better than those of most interval procedures.

Nonpuerperal (Interval) Surgical Tubal Sterilization

Techniques for surgical nonpuerperal tubal sterilization, including modifications, basically consist of:

1. ligation and resection at laparotomy, as described earlier for puerperal sterilization
2. application of a variety of permanent rings, clips, or inserts to the fallopian tubes, by laparoscopy or hysteroscopy
3. electrocoagulation of a tubal segment, again usually through a laparoscope.

Surgical Approaches

In the United States, laparoscopic tubal ligation is the leading method of interval female sterilization (American College of Obstetricians and Gynecologists, 2003). The procedure is frequently performed in an ambulatory surgical setting under general anesthesia. In almost all cases, the woman can be discharged within several hours.

Minilaparotomy using a 3-cm suprapubic incision is also popular, especially in resource-poor countries (Kulier and colleagues, 2002). Although not commonly used, the peritoneal cavity can be entered through the posterior vaginal fornix—*colpotomy* or *culdotomy*—to perform tubal interruption.

Major morbidity is rare with either minilaparotomy or laparoscopy. In the study by Kulier and associates (2002), minor morbidity was twice as common with a minilaparotomy.

Laparoscopic Methods of Tubal Interruption

A number of techniques or devices can be used to accomplish tubal sterilization via laparoscopy. Details of these have been provided by a number of reviews (Hoffman, 2008; Pati and Cullins, 2000; Peterson, 2008).

Electrocoagulation is used for destruction of a segment of tube with either unipolar or bipolar electrical current. Although unipolar electrocoagulation has the lowest long-term failure rate, it also has the highest serious complication rate (see Fig. 33-3). For this reason, bipolar coagulation is usually chosen (American College of Obstetricians and Gynecologists, 2003). Because electrosurgical coagulation destroys a large segment of tube, surgical reversal is difficult if not impossible.

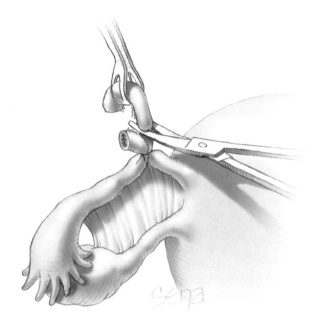

FIGURE 33-2 Surgical sterilization: Pomeroy method. Plain catgut is used to ligate a knuckle of tube to ensure prompt absorption of the ligature and subsequent separation of the severed tubal ends. (From Hoffman, 2008, with permission.)

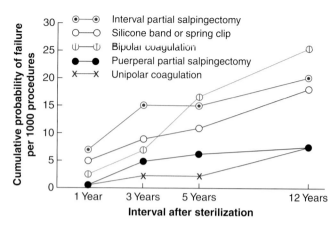

FIGURE 33-3 Data from the U.S. Collaborative Review of Sterilization (CREST) shows the cumulative probability of pregnancy per 1000 procedures by five methods of tubal sterilization. (Data from Peterson and co-workers, 1996.)

Mechanical methods of occlusion can be accomplished with a silastic rubber band such as the Falope Ring and the Tubal Ring; the spring-loaded Hulka-Clemens Clip—also known as the Wolf Clip; or the silicone-lined titanium Filshie Clip (Fig. 33-4). As shown in Figure 33-3, all these methods have favorable long-term success rates.

Failure Rates

The reasons for failure of surgical interval tubal sterilization are not always apparent, but some are:

1. Surgical errors likely account for 30 to 50 percent of cases
2. An occlusion method failure may result from fistula formation, especially with electrosurgical procedures. Faulty clips may not be sufficiently occlusive, or the fallopian tube may spontaneously reanastomose
3. Equipment failure, such as a defective current for electrosurgery, may be causative
4. The woman was already pregnant at the time of surgery—a so-called *luteal phase pregnancy.* To limit this possibility, surgery may ideally be performed during the follicular phase, and an effective contraceptive method used prior to surgery
5. In some cases, proper placement of clips is documented, and no reason is found (Belot and colleagues, 2008)

Some sterilization methods have lower failure rates than others. Even with the same procedure, there are variations in failure rates. For example, when fewer than three tubal sites are coagulated, the 5-year cumulative probability of pregnancy is about 12 per 1000 procedures. This compares with only 3 per 1000 if three or more sites are coagulated (Peterson and associates, 1999). Importantly, Soderstrom (1985) found that most sterilization failures were not preventable. The American College of Obstetricians and Gynecologists (1996) concluded that "pregnancies after sterilization may occur without any technical errors."

Long-Term Complications

In addition to the 15-year cumulative pregnancy rates shown in Figure 33-3, there are other long-term effects.

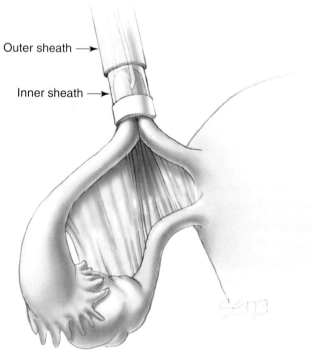

FIGURE 33-4 Silastic band (Falope Ring) placement. Applicator tongs draw a portion of tube up into an inner sheath. An outer sheath then pushes a silastic band off the inner sheath and onto the base of the tubal loop. (From Hoffman, 2008, with permission.)

Ectopic Pregnancy. Approximately half of pregnancies that follow a failed electrocoagulation procedure are ectopic, compared with only 10 percent following failure of a ring, clip, or tubal resection method (Hatcher and colleagues, 1990; Hendrix and associates, 1999). **Any symptoms of pregnancy in a woman after tubal sterilization must be investigated, and an ectopic pregnancy should be excluded.** Diagnosis and management are discussed in detail in Chapter 10.

Other Effects. Following sterilization *ovarian* and *breast cancer* risks are either decreased or unaffected (Eliassen, 2006; Iversen, 2007; Tworoger, 2007; Westhoff 2000, and all their co-workers). Moreover, Levgur and Duvivier (2000) reported that women who had undergone tubal sterilization were highly unlikely to subsequently have *salpingitis*. Holt and colleagues (2003) noted that an almost twofold increased incidence of *functional ovarian cysts* follows tubal sterilization.

Less objective but important psychological sequelae of sterilization have also been evaluated. In the CREST study, Costello and colleagues (2002) found that tubal ligation did not change *sexual interest or pleasure* in 80 percent of women. In most of the 20 percent of women who did report a change, *positive effects* were 10 to 15 times more likely.

Invariably, a number of women express *regrets about sterilization* (Curtis and colleagues, 2006; Kelekçi and co-workers, 2005). In the CREST study, Jamieson and co-workers (2002) reported that by 5 years, 7 percent of women who had undergone tubal ligation had regrets. This is not limited to their own sterilization, because 6.1 percent of women whose husbands had undergone vasectomy had similar regrets.

Posttubal Ligation Syndrome.
Menorrhagia and intermenstrual bleeding following sterilization has been termed the *posttubal ligation syndrome*. Observations from the CREST study have questioned such an association. Peterson and colleagues (2000) compared long-term outcomes of 9514 women who had undergone tubal sterilization with a cohort of 573 women whose partners had undergone vasectomy. They found that both groups had similar risks for menorrhagia, intermenstrual bleeding, and dysmenorrhea. In fact, they found that women who had undergone sterilization had *decreased* duration and volume of menstrual flow as well as *less* dysmenorrhea. There was, however, an increased incidence of cycle irregularity in the sterilized women.

The cause of these findings remains enigmatic. Several investigators have reported no significant change in serum levels of sex steroid

hormones or their releasing factors (Gentile and associates, 2006; Harlow and co-workers, 2002). Timonen and co-workers (2002) reported a transient increase in follicular phase serum estradiol levels that normalized by 12 months.

Reversal of Tubal Sterilization

No woman should undergo tubal sterilization believing that subsequent fertility is guaranteed by either surgery or in vitro fertilization. Both approaches are technically difficult, expensive, and not always successful. Success rates vary greatly depending on the age of the woman, the amount of tube remaining, and the technology used (Boeckxstaens and colleagues, 2007). With surgical reversals, pregnancy rates varied from 45 to 85 percent (Trussell and associates, 2003; Van Voorhis, 2000). **Almost 10 percent of women who undergo reversal of tubal sterilization have an ectopic pregnancy.**

Hysterectomy

In the absence of uterine or other pelvic disease, hysterectomy solely for sterilization at the time of cesarean delivery, early in the puerperium, or even remote from pregnancy is difficult to justify. It carries significantly increased surgical morbidity compared with tubal sterilization (Jamieson and co-workers, 2000; Johnson and colleagues, 2005).

Transcervical Sterilization

Sterilization has been performed using hysteroscopy to visualize the tubal ostia and obliterate them with a variety of compounds or devices.

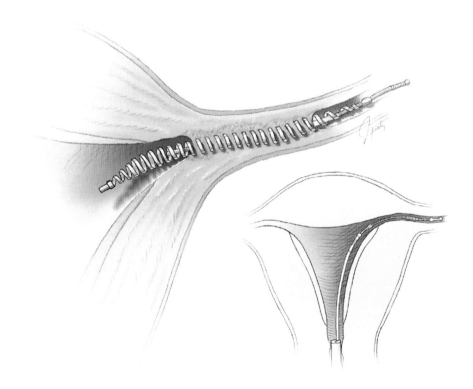

FIGURE 33-5 Essure microinsert placement hysteroscopically and ingrowth of tissue. (From Hoffman, 2008, with permission.)

Intratubal Devices

Tubes can be occluded by hysteroscopic insertion of some type of mechanical device into the proximal tube (Fig. 33-5). One of these, *Essure*, was approved by the Food and Drug Administration in 2002. This device is a microinsert that has a fine stainless steel inner coil enclosed in polyester fibers and an expandable outer coil of *Nitinol*—a nickel and titanium alloy. The outer coil expands after placement allowing the inner fibers also to expand. Over time, these synthetic fibers incite a chronic inflammatory response and prompt local tissue ingrowth from the surrounding tube (Valle and colleagues, 2001). This ingrowth leads to complete tubal lumen occlusion. This procedure requires hysterosalpingography 3 months following surgery to confirm occlusion (Wittmer and associates, 2006a, b). Some have evaluated the effectiveness of sonography to confirm occlusion or alternatively, dislodgement (Booker, 2008; Veersema, 2005; Weston, 2005, and all their colleagues).

Sedation, paracervical block, or both may be used for hysteroscopic placement of Essure microinserts. Bilateral placement is achieved in 88 to 96 percent of cases (Kerin, 2003; Levie, 2006; Miño, 2007; Ubeda, 2004, and all their colleagues). Thus, these devices cannot be placed in all women, and some do not tolerate the procedure awake (Duffy and colleagues, 2005). Postprocedure, a few women cannot tolerate the device because of intractable pelvic pain (Beckwith, 2008).

Preliminary results with this device have been encouraging (Association of Reproductive Health Professionals, 2002; Magos, 2004). Cooper and associates (2003) reported proper insertion in 464 of 507 women, and there were no pregnancies in more than 9600 woman-months.

Causes for pregnancy following Essure placement include conception prior to insertion, insert migration, uterine perforation, and noncompliance with hysterosalpingography or its misinterpretation (Levy, 2007; Moses, 2007; Ory, 2008, and all their colleagues).

Two additional inserts, *Ovion* and *Adiana*, similarly rely on tissue ingrowth for tubal occlusion. These currently are not available (Abbott, 2007; Vancaillie and associates, 2009; Zurawin and Ayensu-Coker, 2007).

Intratubal Chemical Methods

Several compounds may be used in tubal sterilization to sclerose or obstruct the tubal ostia, but none is currently available for use in the United States (Ogburn and Espey, 2007). Liquid silicone may be injected transcervically into the tubes, where it hardens, forming *silicone plugs* (Reed and Erb, 1983). Alternatively, tubal injections with the adhesive *methylcyanoacrylate* cause inflammation, necrosis, and fibrosis (Brundin, 1991). Tubal insertion of *quinacrine pellets* has been done in hundreds of thousands of women in other countries to achieve tubal occlusion. Because of concerns about carcinogenesis, the World Health Organization at one time recommended halting quinacrine use (Lippes, 2002). Since then, long-term follow-up studies from Vietnam have not shown an increased risk of cancer. However, investigators report high 1-, 5-, and 10-year cumulative pregnancy rates of 3, 10, and 12 percent, respectively (Sokal and colleagues, 2008a, b). Alternatively, *erythromycin* placed tubally to incite inflammation has been investigated, but it has an unacceptably high one-year failure rate of 36 percent (Bairagy and Mullick, 2004). Other mechanical inserts are less commonly used and are described by Abbott (2005, 2007) in his reviews.

MALE STERILIZATION

Availability of male contraceptives has traditionally been limited to condoms and vasectomy. According to their review, Page and associates (2008) cite 90- to 95-percent efficacy rates for experimental hormonal-based male contraceptives. They also cite promising nonhormonal methods of targeting sperm motility. But these are currently unavailable.

At this time, up to a half million men in the United States undergo vasectomy each year (Barone and co-workers, 2006; Magnani and colleagues, 1999). Through a small incision or alternatively through a puncture in the scrotum, the lumen of the vas deferens is disrupted to block the passage of sperm from the testes (Fig. 33-6). There are fewer minor surgical complications with the no-scalpel method than with the traditional incision technique, but each is equally effective (Cook and co-workers, 2007). In addition to surgical transection, obstruction with vas deferens plugs or clips is under investigation (Rowlands, 2009).

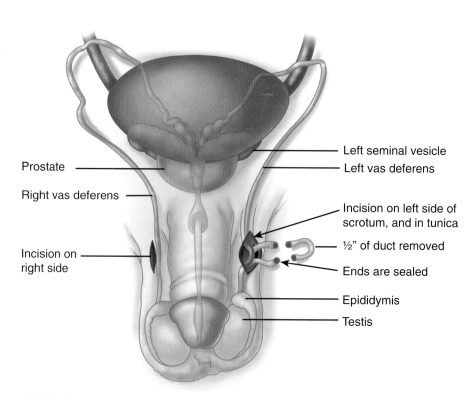

Prostate

Right vas deferens

Incision on right side

Left seminal vesicle

Left vas deferens

Incision on left side of scrotum, and in tunica

½" of duct removed

Ends are sealed

Epididymis

Testis

FIGURE 33-6 Anatomy of male reproductive system, showing procedure for vasectomy.

There is no doubt that vasectomy is safer than tubal sterilization because it is less invasive and is performed with local analgesia (American College of Obstetricians and Gynecologists, 2003). In their review, Hendrix and colleagues (1999) found that, compared with vasectomy, female tubal sterilization has a 20-fold increased complication rate, a 10- to 37-fold failure rate, and costs three times as much. Teachey (2008) described a rare death from a massive pulmonary embolism in a healthy 35-year-old man thought to be induced by limited mobilization following vasectomy.

Disadvantageously, sterilization following vasectomy is not immediate. Complete expulsion of sperm stored in the reproductive tract beyond the interrupted vas deferens takes about 3 months or 20 ejaculations (American College of Obstetricians and Gynecologists, 1996). Although most protocols dictate that semen should be analyzed until two consecutive sperm counts are zero, many investigators suggest that collection of only one azoospermic semen analysis is sufficient evidence of sterility (Bodiwala, 2007; Bradshaw, 2001; Griffin, 2005, and all their associates). During the period before azoospermia is documented, another form of contraception should be used.

The failure rate for vasectomy during the first year is 9.4 per 1000 procedures but only 11.4 per 1000 at 2, 3, and 5 years (Jamieson and colleagues, 2004). Failures result from unprotected intercourse too soon after ligation, incomplete occlusion of the vas deferens, or recanalization (Awsare, 2005; Deneux-Tharaux, 2004; Jamieson, 2004, and all their associates).

Restoration of Fertility

Success after vasectomy reversal depends on several factors, and fibrosis increases with time (Raleigh and colleagues, 2004). With reversal, results typically are superior using microsurgical techniques (American Society of Reproductive Medicine Practice Committee, 2006). Bolduc and associates (2007) reported that success was more likely with shorter obstructive intervals, same female partner, use of surgical clips when vasectomy was done, and presence of a sperm granuloma.

Long-Term Effects

Other than regrets, long-term consequences are rare (Amundsen and Ramakrishnan, 2004). Although formerly items of concern, increased atherogenesis or immune-complex mediated disease are no longer linked to vasectomy (Giovannucci, 1992; Goldacre, 1983; Massey, 1984, and all their associates). Moreover, there is no convincing evidence of an increased incidence of *testicular cancer* following vasectomy (Møller and co-workers, 1994). Earlier studies found evidence to associate development of *prostatic carcinoma* after vasectomy (Giovannucci and associates, 1993a, b; Hayes and co-workers, 1993). However, most reviewers have found no strong causal association between the two (Bernal-Delgado and colleagues, 1998; Holt and associates, 2008; Schwingl and Guess, 2000). A weak association may be explicable by greater scrutiny of men who have undergone vasectomy (Grönberg, 2003). Indeed, the long-term effects of vasectomy are few, although troublesome chronic scrotal pain may develop in up to 15 percent of men (Choe, 1996; Leslie, 2007; Manikandan, 2004; McMahon, 1992, and all their co-workers).

REFERENCES

Abbott J: Transcervical sterilization. Best Pract Res Clin Obstet Gynaecol 19:743, 2005
Abbott J: Transcervical sterilization. Curr Opin Obstet Gynecol 19:325, 2007
American College of Obstetricians and Gynecologists: Sterilization. ACOG Technical Bulletin No. 222, April 1996
American College of Obstetricians and Gynecologists: Benefits and risks of sterilization. Practice Bulletin No. 46, September 2003
American College of Obstetricians and Gynecologists Committee on Ethics: ACOG Committee Opinion No. 371, July 2007. Sterilization of women, including those with mental disabilities. Obstet Gynecol 110:217, 2007
American Society for Reproductive Medicine Practice Committee: Vasectomy reversal. Fertil Steril 86:S268, 2006
Amundsen GA, Ramakrishnan K: Vasectomy: A "seminal" analysis. South Med J 97:54, 2004
Association of Reproductive Health Professionals: Clinical Proceedings. Clinical Update on Transcervical Sterilization. Washington, DC, 2002
Awsare N, Krishnan J, Goustead GB, et al: Complications of vasectomy. Ann R Coll Surg Engl 87:406, 2005
Bairagy NR, Mullick BC: Use of erythromycin for nonsurgical female sterilization in West Bengal, India: A study of 790 cases. Contraception 69:47, 2004
Barone MA, Hutchison PL, Johnson CH, et al: Vasectomy in the Unites States, 2002. J Urol 176:232, 2006
Beckwith AW: Persistent pain after hysteroscopic sterilization with microinserts. Obstet Gynecol 111:511, 2008
Belot F, Louboutin A, Fauconnier A: Failure of sterilization after clip placement. Obstet Gynecol 111:515, 2008
Bensyl DM, Iuliano DA, Carter M, et al: Contraceptive use—United States and territories, Behavioral Risk Factor Surveillance System, 2002. MMWR Surveill Summ 54:1, 2005
Bernal-Delgado E, Latour-Pérez J, Pradas-Arnal F, et al: The association between vasectomy and prostate cancer: A systematic review of the literature. Fertil Steril 70:201, 1998
Bodiwala D, Jeyarajah S, Terry TR, et al: The first semen analysis after vasectomy: Timing and definition of success. BJU Int 99:727, 2007
Boeckxstaens A, Devroey P, Collins J: Getting pregnant after tubal sterilization: Surgical reversal or IVF? Hum Reprod 22:2660, 2007
Bolduc S, Fischer MA, Deceuninck G, et al: Factors predicting overall success: A review of 747 microsurgical vasovasostomies. Can Urol Assoc J 1(4):388, 2007
Booker CJ, Yarwood JL, Dodson WC: Dislodged Essure microinsert. Fertil Steril 89:964, 2008
Bradshaw HD, Rosario DJ, James MJ, et al: Review of current practice to establish success after vasectomy. Br J Surg 88:290, 2001
Brundin J: Transcervical sterilization in the human female by hysteroscopic application of hydrogelic occlusive devices into the intramural parts of the fallopian tubes: 10 years experience of the P-block. Eur J Obstet Gynecol Reprod Biol 39:41, 1991
Bucklin BA, Smith CV: Postpartum tubal ligation: Safety, timing and other implications for anesthesia. Anesth Analg 89:1269, 1999
Choe JM, Kirkemo AK: Questionnaire-based outcomes study of nononcological post-vasectomy complications. J Urol 155:1284, 1996
Cook LA, Pun A, van Vliet H, et al: Scalpel versus no-scalpel incision for vasectomy. Cochrane Database Syst Rev 18:CD004112, 2007
Cooper JM, Carignan CS, Cher D, et al: Microinsert nonincisional hysteroscopic sterilization. Obstet Gynecol 102:59, 2003
Costello C, Hillis S, Marchbanks P, et al: The effect of interval tubal sterilization on sexual interest and pleasure. Obstet Gynecol 100:3, 2002
Curtis KM, Mohllajee AP, Peterson HB: Regret following female sterilization at a young age: a systematic review. Contraception 73:205, 2006
Deneux-Tharaux C, Kahn E, Nazarali H, et al: Pregnancy rates after vasectomy: A survey of U.S. urologists. Contraception 69:401, 2004
Duffy S, Marsh F, Rogerson L, et al: Female sterilization: A cohort controlled comparative study of ESSURE *versus* laparoscopic sterilization. BJOG 112:1522, 2005
Eliassen AH, Colditz GA, Rosner B, et al: Tubal sterilization in relation to breast cancer risk. Int J Cancer 118:2026, 2006
Famuyide AO, Hopkins MR, El-Nashar SA, et al: Hysteroscopic sterilization in women with severe cardiac disease: Experience at a tertiary center. Mayo Clin Proc 83:431, 2008
Gentile GP, Helbig DW, Zacur H, et al: Hormone levels before and after tubal sterilization. Contraception 73:507, 2006
Giovannucci E, Ascherio A, Rimm EB, et al: A prospective study of vasectomy and prostate cancer in U.S. men. JAMA 269:876, 1993a
Giovannucci E, Tosteson TD, Speizer FE, et al: A retrospective cohort study of vasectomy and prostate cancer in U.S. men. JAMA 269:878, 1993b

Giovannucci E, Tosteson TD, Speizer FE, et al: A long-term study of mortality in men who have undergone vasectomy. N Engl J Med 326:1392, 1992

Goldacre JM, Holford TR, Vessey MP: Cardiovascular disease and vasectomy. N Engl J Med 308:805, 1983

Griffin T, Tooher R, Nowakowski K, et al: How little is enough? The evidence for post-vasectomy testing. J Urol 174:29, 2005

Grönberg H: Prostate cancer epidemiology. Lancet 361:859, 2003

Harlow BL, Missmer S, Cramer D, et al: Does tubal sterilization influence the subsequent risk of menorrhagia or dysmenorrhea? Fertil Steril 77:4, 2002

Hatcher RA, Stewart F, Trussell J, et al: Contraceptive Technology, 15th ed. New York, Irvington, 1990, pp 391, 403, 416

Hayes RB, Pottern CM, Greenberg R, et al: Vasectomy and prostate cancer in U.S. blacks and whites. Am J Epidemiol 137:263, 1993

Hendrix NW, Chauhan SP, Morrison JC: Sterilization and its consequences. Obstet Gynecol Surv 54:766, 1999

Hoffman BL: Surgeries for benign gynecologic conditions. In Schorge JO, Schaffer JI, Halvorsen LM, et al (eds): Williams Gynecology. New York, McGraw-Hill, 2008, p 937

Holt SK, Salinas CA, Stanford JL: Vasectomy and the risk of prostate cancer. J Urol 180(6):2565, 2008

Holt VL, Cushing-Haugen KL, Daling JR: Oral contraceptives, tubal sterilization, and functional ovarian cyst risk. Obstet Gynecol 102:252, 2003

Huber LR, Huber KR: Contraceptive choices of women 35-44 year of age: Findings from the Behavioral Risk Factor Surveillance System. Ann Epidemiol (Epub ahead of print) 2009

Iversen L, Hannaford PC, Elliott AM: Tubal sterilization, all-cause death, and cancer among women in the United Kingdom: Evidence from the Royal College of General Practitioners' Oral Contraception Study. Am J Obstet Gynecol 196:447.e1-447.e8, 2007

Jamieson DJ, Costello C, Trussell J, et al: The risk of pregnancy after vasectomy. Obstet Gynecol 103:848, 2004

Jamieson DJ, Hillis SD, Duerr A, et al: Complications of interval laparoscopic tubal sterilization: Findings from the United States Collaborative Review of Sterilization. Obstet Gynecol 96:997, 2000

Jamieson DJ, Kaufman SC, Costello C, et al: A comparison of women's regret after vasectomy versus tubal sterilization. Obstet Gynecol 99:1073, 2002

Johnson N, Barlow D, Lethaby A, et al: Surgical approach to hysterectomy for benign gynaecological disease. Cochrane Database Syst Rev 1:CD003677, 2005

Kelekçi S, Erdemoglu E, Kutluk S, et al: Risk factors for tubal ligation: Regret and psychological effects. Impact of Beck Depression Inventory. Contraception 71:417, 2005

Kerin JF, Cooper JM, Price T, et al: Hysteroscopic sterilization using a micro-insert device: Results of a multicentre Phase II study. Hum Reprod 18:1223, 2003

Kulier R, Boulvain M, Walker D, et al: Minilaparotomy and endoscopic techniques for tubal sterilization. Cochrane Database Syst Rev 2002(3): CD001328

Leslie TA, Illing RO, Cranston DW, et al: The incidence of chronic scrotal pain after vasectomy: A prospective audit. BJU Int 100:1330, 2007

Levgur M, Duvivier R: Pelvic inflammatory disease after tubal sterilization: A review. Obstet Gynecol Surv 55:41, 2000

Levie MD, Chudnoff SG: Prospective analysis of office-base hysteroscopic sterilization. J Minim Invasive Gynecol 13:98, 2006

Levy B, Levie MD, Childers ME: A summary of reported pregnancies after hysteroscopic sterilization. J Minim Invasive Gynecol 14:271, 2007

Lippes J: Quinacrine sterilization: The imperative need for clinical trials. Fertil Steril 77:1106, 2002

MacKay AP, Kieke BA, Koonin LM, et al: Tubal sterilization in the United States, 1994–1996. Fam Plann Perspect 33:161, 2001

Magnani RJ, Haws JM, Morgan GT, et al: Vasectomy in the United States, 1991 and 1995. Am J Public Health 89:92, 1999

Magos A, Chapman L: Hysteroscopic tubal sterilization. Obstet Gynecol Clin North Am 31:705, 2004

Manikandan R, Srirangam SJ, Pearson E, et al: Early and late morbidity after vasectomy: A comparison of chronic scrotal pain at 1 and 10 years. BJU Int 93:571, 2004

Massey FJ Jr, Bertstein GS, O'Fallon WM, et al: Vasectomy and health. Results from a large cohort study. JAMA 252:1023, 1984

McMahon AJ, Buckley J, Taylor A, et al: Chronic testicular pain following vasectomy. B J Urol 69:188, 1992

Miño M, Arjona JE, Cordón J, et al: Success rate and patient satisfaction with the Essure™ sterilization in an outpatient setting: A prospective study of 857 women. BJOG 114:763, 2007

Møller H, Knudsen LB, Lynge E: Risk of testicular cancer after vasectomy: Cohort study of over 73,000 men. BMJ 309:295, 1994

Moses AW, Burgis JT, Bacon JL, et al: Pregnancy after Essure® placement: Report of two cases. Fertil Steril 89:724.e9-11, 2008

Ogburn T, Espey E: Transcervical sterilization: Past, present and future. Obstet Gynecol Clin N Am 34:57, 2007

Ory EM, Hines RS, Cleland WH, et al: Pregnancy after microinsert sterilization with tubal occlusion confirmed by hysterosalpingogram. Obstet Gynecol 111:508, 2008

Page ST, Amory JK, Bremner WJ: Advances in male contraception. Endocr Rev 29:465, 2008

Pati S, Cullins V: Female sterilization: Evidence. Obstet Gynecol Clin North Am 27:859, 2000

Peterson HB: Sterilization. Obstet Gynecol 111:189, 2008

Peterson HB, Jeng G, Folger SG, et al: The risk of menstrual abnormalities after tubal sterilization. N Engl J Med 343:1681, 2000

Peterson HB, Xia Z, Hughes JM, et al: The risk of pregnancy after tubal sterilization: Findings from the U.S. Collaborative Review of Sterilization. Am J Obstet Gynecol 174:1161, 1996

Peterson HB, Xia Z, Wilcox LS, et al: Pregnancy after tubal sterilization with bipolar electrocoagulation. U.S. Collaborative Review of Sterilization Working Group. Obstet Gynecol 94:163, 1999

Peterson HB, Xia Z, Wilcox LS, et al: Pregnancy after tubal sterilization with silicone rubber band and spring clip application. Obstet Gynecol 97:205, 2001

Podolsky ML, Desai NA, Wagers TP, et al: Hysteroscopic tubal occlusion: Sterilization after failed laparoscopic or abdominal approaches. Obstet Gynecol 111:513, 2008

Raleigh D, O'Donnell L, Southwick GJ, et al: Stereological analysis of the human testis after vasectomy indicates impairment of spermatogenic efficiency with increasing obstructive interval. Fertil Steril 81:1595, 2004

Reed III TP, Erb R: Hysteroscopic tubal occlusion with silicone rubber. Obstet Gynecol 61:388, 1983

Rowlands S: New technologies in contraception. BJOG 116:230, 2009

Schwingl PJ, Guess HA: Safety and effectiveness of vasectomy. Fertil Steril 73:923, 2000

Soderstrom RM: Sterilization failures and their causes. Am J Obstet Gynecol 152:395, 1985

Sokal DC, Hieu do T, Loan ND, et al: Contraceptive effectiveness of two insertions of quinacrine: Results from 10-year follow-up in Vietnam. Contraception 78:61, 2008a

Sokal DC, Hieu do T, Loan ND, et al: Safety of quinacrine contraceptive pellets: Results from 10-year follow-up in Vietnam. Contraception 78:66, 2008b

Teachey DT: Saddle pulmonary embolism as a complication of vasectomy. Urology 71:351.e5, 2008

Timonen S, Tuominin J, Irjala K, et al: Ovarian function and regulation of the hypothalamic-pituitary-ovarian axis after tubal sterilization. J Reprod Med 47:131, 2002

Trussell J, Guilbert E, Hedley A: Sterilization failure, sterilization reversal, and pregnancy after sterilization reversal of Quebec. Obstet Gynecol 101:677, 2003

Tworoger SS, Fairfield KM, Colditz GA, et al: Association of oral contraceptive use, other contraceptive methods, and infertility with ovarian cancer risk. Am J Epidemiol 166:894, 2007

Ubeda A, Labastida R, Dexeus S: Essure: A new device for hysteroscopic tubal sterilization in an outpatient setting. Fertil Steril 82:196, 2004

Valle RF, Carignan CS, Wright TC, et al: Tissue response to the STOP microcoil transcervical permanent contraceptive device: Results from a prehysterectomy study. Fertil Steril 76:974, 2001

Vancaillie TG, Anderson TL, Johns DA: A 12-month prospective evaluation of transcervical sterilization using implantable polymer matrices. Obstet Gynecol 112(6):1270, 2008

Van Voorhis BJ: Comparison of tubal ligation reversal procedures. Clin Obstet Gynecol 43:641, 2000

Veersema S, Vleugels MPH, Timmermans A, et al: Follow-up of successful bilateral placement of Essure® microinserts with ultrasound. Fertil Steril 84:1733, 2005

Westhoff C, Davis A: Tubal sterilization: Focus on the U.S. experience. Fertil Steril 73:913, 2000

Weston G, Bowditch J: Office ultrasound should be the first-line investigation for confirmation of correct ESSURE placement. Aust NZ J Obstet Gynaecol 45:312, 2005

Wittmer MH, Brown DL, Hartman RP, et al: Sonography, CT, and MRI appearance of the Essure microinsert permanent birth control device. AJR 187:959, 2006a

Wittmer MH, Famuyde AO, Creedon DJ, et al: Hysterosalpingography for assessing efficacy of Essure microinsert permanent birth control device. AJR 187:955, 2006b

Zurawin RK, Ayensu-Coker L: Innovations in contraception: A review. Clin Obstet Gynecol 50:425, 2007

OBSTETRICAL COMPLICATIONS

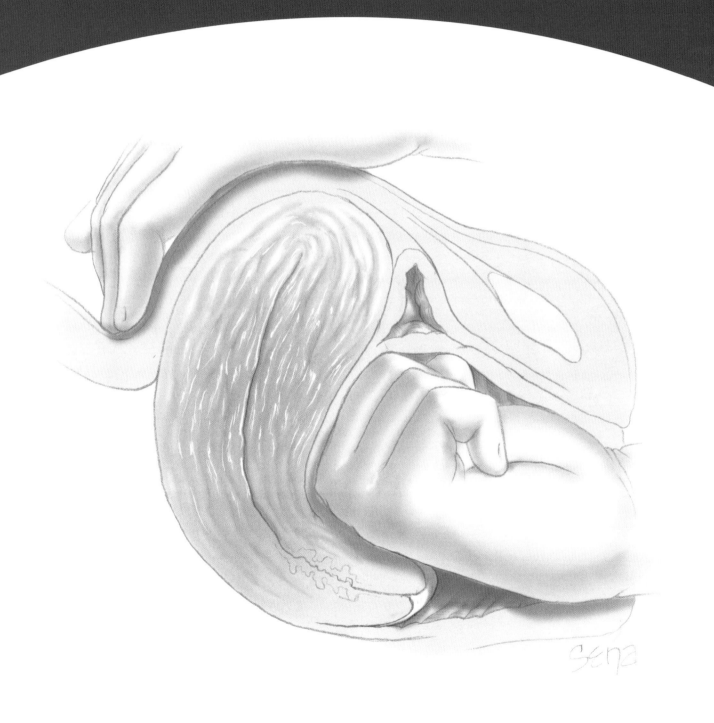

CHAPTER 34

Pregnancy Hypertension

Hypertensive disorders complicate 5 to 10 percent of all pregnancies, and together they form one member of the deadly triad, along with hemorrhage and infection, that contribute greatly to maternal morbidity and mortality rates. With hypertension, the *preeclampsia syndrome*, either alone or superimposed on chronic hypertension, is the most dangerous. As subsequently discussed, new-onset nonproteinuric hypertension during pregnancy—termed *gestational hypertension*—is followed by signs and symptoms of preeclampsia almost half the time, and preeclampsia is identified in 3.9 percent of all pregnancies (Martin and colleagues, 2009). The World Health Organization systematically reviews maternal mortality worldwide (Khan and colleagues, 2006). In developed countries, 16 percent of maternal deaths were due to hypertensive disorders. This percentage is greater than three other leading causes: hemorrhage—13 percent, abortion—8 percent, and sepsis—2 percent. In the United States from 1991 to 1997, Berg and colleagues (2003) reported that almost 16 percent of 3201 maternal deaths were from complications of pregnancy-related hypertension. Importantly, Berg and co-workers (2005) later re-

ported that over half of these hypertension-related deaths were preventable.

How pregnancy incites or aggravates hypertension remains unsolved despite decades of intensive research. Indeed, hypertensive disorders remain among the most significant and intriguing unsolved problems in obstetrics.

TERMINOLOGY AND CLASSIFICATION

The term gestational hypertension as used in previous editions of this book was chosen by Dr. Jack Pritchard to describe any new-onset uncomplicated hypertension during pregnancy when no evidence of the preeclampsia syndrome was apparent. Unfortunately, confusion arose by some using the term for both gestational hypertension and preeclampsia. We have thus adopted the schema of the Working Group of the NHBPEP—National High Blood Pressure Education Program (2000).

The Working Group classification of hypertensive disorders complicating pregnancy as shown in Table 34-1 describes four types of hypertensive disease:

1. Gestational hypertension—formerly termed pregnancy-induced hypertension. If preeclampsia syndrome does not develop and hypertension resolves by 12 weeks postpartum, it is redesignated as transient hypertension
2. Preeclampsia and eclampsia syndrome
3. Preeclampsia syndrome superimposed on chronic hypertension
4. Chronic hypertension.

An important feature of this classification is differentiating preeclampsia and eclampsia from other hypertensive disorders because the former two are potentially more ominous. This concept is also important to interpret and appreciate studies that address the etiology, pathogenesis, and clinical management of pregnancy-related hypertensive disorders.

TABLE 34-1. Diagnosis of Hypertensive Disorders Complicating Pregnancy

Gestational Hypertension:
- Systolic BP ≥140 or diastolic BP ≥90 mm Hg for first time during pregnancy
- No proteinuria
- BP returns to normal before 12 weeks postpartum
- Final diagnosis made only postpartum
- May have other signs or symptoms of preeclampsia, for example, epigastric discomfort or thrombocytopenia

Preeclampsia:
Minimum criteria:
- BP ≥ 140/90 mm Hg after 20 weeks' gestation
- Proteinuria ≥ 300 mg/24 hours or ≥ 1+ dipstick

Increased certainty of preeclampsia:
- BP ≥ 160/110 mm Hg
- Proteinuria 2.0 g/24 hours or ≥ 2+ dipstick
- Serum creatinine >1.2 mg/dL unless known to be previously elevated
- Platelets < 100,000/μL
- Microangiopathic hemolysis—increased LDH
- Elevated serum transaminase levels—ALT or AST
- Persistent headache or other cerebral or visual disturbance
- Persistent epigastric pain

Eclampsia:
- Seizures that cannot be attributed to other causes in a woman with preeclampsia

Superimposed Preeclampsia On Chronic Hypertension:
- New-onset proteinuria ≥ 300 mg/24 hours in hypertensive women but no proteinuria before 20 weeks' gestation
- A sudden increase in proteinuria or blood pressure or platelet count < 100,000/μL in women with hypertension and proteinuria before 20 weeks' gestation

Chronic Hypertension:
- BP ≥ 140/90 mm Hg before pregnancy or diagnosed before 20 weeks' gestation not attributable to gestational trophoblastic disease

or

- Hypertension first diagnosed after 20 weeks' gestation and persistent after 12 weeks postpartum

ALT = alanine aminotransferase; AST = aspartate aminotransferase; BP = blood pressure; LDH = lactate dehydrogenase.
National High Blood Pressure Education Program Working Group Report on High Blood Pressure in Pregnancy (2000).

DIAGNOSIS

Hypertension is diagnosed empirically when appropriately taken blood pressure exceeds 140 mm Hg systolic or 90 mm Hg diastolic. Korotkoff phase V is used to define diastolic pressure. In the past, it had been recommended that an incremental increase from midpregnancy values by 30 mm Hg systolic or 15 mm Hg diastolic pressure be used as diagnostic criteria, even when absolute values were below 140/90 mm Hg. These criteria are no longer recommended because evidence shows that such women are not likely to experience increased adverse pregnancy outcomes (Levine and co-workers, 2000; North and colleagues, 1999). That said, women who have a rise in pressure of 30 mm Hg systolic or 15 mm Hg diastolic should be seen more frequently. There is no doubt that

eclamptic seizures develop in some women whose blood pressures have been below 140/90 mm Hg (Alexander and associates, 2006). Edema is also no longer used as a diagnostic criterion because it is too common in normal pregnancy to be discriminant.

Gestational Hypertension

The diagnosis of gestational hypertension is made in women whose blood pressure reaches 140/90 mm Hg or greater for the first time after midpregnancy, but in whom *proteinuria is not identified* (see Table 34-1). Almost half of these women subsequently develop preeclampsia syndrome, which includes signs such as proteinuria and thrombocytopenia or symptoms such as headaches or epigastric pain. Gestational hypertension is reclassified as *transient hypertension* if evidence for preeclampsia does not develop, and the blood pressure returns to normal by 12 weeks postpartum.

Proteinuria is the surrogate objective marker that defines the system wide endothelial leak, which characterizes the preeclampsia syndrome. Even so, when blood pressure increases appreciably, it is dangerous to both mother and fetus to ignore this rise because proteinuria has not yet developed. As Chesley (1985) emphasized, 10 percent of eclamptic seizures develop before overt proteinuria is identified.

Preeclampsia

As shown throughout this chapter, preeclampsia is best described as a *pregnancy-specific syndrome that can affect virtually every organ system*. As discussed, although preeclampsia is much more than simply gestational hypertension with proteinuria, appearance of proteinuria remains an important objective diagnostic criterion. Proteinuria is defined by 24-hour urinary protein excretion exceeding 300 mg, a urine protein:creatinine ratio of ≥ 0.3, or persistent 30 mg/dL (1+ dipstick) protein in random urine samples (Lindheimer and colleagues, 2008a). None of these values are sacrosanct. Urine concentrations vary widely during the day, and so too will dipstick readings. Thus, assessment may even show a 1+ to 2+ value from concentrated urine specimens from women who excrete < 300 mg/day. As discussed on page 719, it is likely that determination of a spot urine:creatinine ratio will be a suitable replacement for a 24-hour measurement.

As emphasized in Table 34-1, the more severe the hypertension or proteinuria, the more certain is the diagnosis of preeclampsia as well as its adverse outcomes. Similarly, abnormal laboratory findings in tests of renal, hepatic, and hematological function increase the certainty of preeclampsia. Persistent premonitory symptoms of eclampsia, such as headache and epigastric pain, also increase the certainty. That said, some women may have *atypical preeclampsia* with all aspects of the syndrome, but without hypertension or proteinuria, or both (Sibai and Stella, 2009).

Indicators of Severity of Preeclampsia

The markers listed in Table 34-1 are also used to classify the severity of the preeclampsia syndrome. Many use the American College of Obstetricians and Gynecologists dichotomous "mild" and "severe." Thus, in many classifications, criteria are given for the diagnosis of "severe" preeclampsia, and the alternate classification is either implied or specifically termed "mild," "less severe," or "nonsevere" (Alexander and associates, 2003; Lindheimer and co-workers, 2008b). These are used because there are no generally agreed-upon criteria for "moderate" preeclampsia—an elusive third category. Criteria listed in Table 34-2 are categorized as "severe" versus "nonsevere." Parenthetically, the latter includes "moderate" and "mild," although they are not specifically defined.

Headaches or *visual disturbances* such as *scotomata* can be premonitory symptoms of eclampsia. *Epigastric or right upper quadrant pain* frequently accompanies hepatocellular necrosis, ischemia, and edema that stretch Glisson capsule. This characteristic pain is frequently accompanied by elevated serum hepatic transaminase levels. *Thrombocytopenia* is also characteristic of worsening preeclampsia. It probably is caused by platelet activation and aggregation as well as microangiopathic hemolysis induced by severe vasospasm. Other factors indicative of severe preeclampsia include renal or cardiac involvement as well as obvious fetal-growth restriction, which attest to its duration.

The more profound these signs and symptoms, the less likely it is that they can be temporized, and the more likely it is that delivery will be indicated. **The differentiation between nonsevere and severe gestational hypertension or preeclampsia can be misleading because what might be apparently mild disease may progress rapidly to severe disease.**

Eclampsia

The onset of convulsions in a woman with preeclampsia that cannot be attributed to other causes is termed *eclampsia*. The seizures are generalized and may appear before, during, or after

TABLE 34-2. Indicators of Severity of Gestational Hypertensive Disorders[a]

Abnormality	Nonsevere	Severe
Diastolic blood pressure	<110 mm Hg	≥110 mm Hg
Systolic blood pressure	<160 mm Hg	≥160 mm Hg
Proteinuria	≤2+	≥3+
Headache	Absent	Present
Visual disturbances	Absent	Present
Upper abdominal pain	Absent	Present
Oliguria	Absent	Present
Convulsion (eclampsia)	Absent	Present
Serum creatinine	Normal	Elevated
Thrombocytopenia	Absent	Present
Serum transaminase elevation	Minimal	Marked
Fetal-growth restriction	Absent	Obvious
Pulmonary edema	Absent	Present

[a]Compare with criteria in Table 34-1.

labor. In older reports, up to 10 percent of eclamptic women, especially nulliparas, did not develop seizures until after 48 hours postpartum (Sibai, 2005). Others have reported that up to a fourth of eclamptic seizures developed beyond 48 hours postpartum (Chames and co-workers, 2002). Our experiences from Parkland Hospital are that delayed postpartum eclampsia continues to occur in less than 10 percent of cases as we first reported more than 20 years ago (Alexander and co-workers, 2006; Brown and colleagues, 1987). These also are the observations from 222 women with eclampsia during a recent 2-year period in The Netherlands (Zwart and associates, 2008).

Preeclampsia Superimposed on Chronic Hypertension

All *chronic hypertensive disorders*, regardless of their cause, predispose to development of superimposed preeclampsia and eclampsia. The diagnosis of chronic underlying hypertension is based on findings listed in Table 34-1. These disorders can create difficult problems with diagnosis and management in women who are not seen until after midpregnancy. This is because blood pressure normally decreases during the second and early third trimesters in both normotensive and chronically hypertensive women (see Chap. 45, p. 984). Thus, a woman with previously undiagnosed chronic vascular disease, who is seen for the first time at 20 weeks, frequently has blood pressure within the normal range. During the third trimester, however, as blood pressure returns to its originally hypertensive level, it may be difficult to determine whether hypertension is chronic or induced by pregnancy. Even a careful search for evidence of preexisting end-organ damage may be futile as many of these women have mild disease. Thus, there may be no evidence of ventricular hypertrophy, chronic retinal vascular changes, or mild renal dysfunction.

In some women with chronic hypertension, blood pressure increases to obviously abnormal levels, and this is typically after 24 weeks. If accompanied by proteinuria, then superimposed preeclampsia is diagnosed. Superimposed preeclampsia commonly may develop earlier in pregnancy than "pure" preeclampsia. Superimposed disease tends to be more severe and often is accompanied by fetal-growth restriction. The same criteria shown in Table 34-2 are also used to further characterize severity of superimposed preeclampsia.

INCIDENCE AND RISK FACTORS

Preeclampsia often affects young and nulliparous women, whereas older women are at greater risk for chronic hypertension with superimposed preeclampsia. Also, the incidence is markedly influenced by race and ethnicity—and thus by genetic predisposition. Other factors include environmental, socioeconomic, and even seasonal influences (Lawlor, 2005; Palmer, 1999; Spencer, 2009, and all their co-workers).

With consideration for these vicissitudes, in a number of worldwide studies reviewed by Sibai and Cunningham (2009), the incidence of preeclampsia in nulliparous populations ranges from 3 to 10 percent. The incidence of preeclampsia in multiparas is also variable but is less than that for nulliparas. However, Ananth and Basso (2009) reported that the risk for stillbirths was more likely in hypertensive multiparas compared with nulliparas.

Other risk factors associated with preeclampsia include obesity, multifetal gestation, maternal age older than 35 years, and African-American ethnicity (Conde-Agudelo and Belizan, 2000; Sibai and colleagues, 1997; Walker, 2000). The relationship between maternal weight and the risk of preeclampsia is progressive. It increases from 4.3 percent for women with a body mass index (BMI) < 20 kg/m^2 to 13.3 percent in those with a BMI > 35 kg/m^2. In women with a twin gestation compared with those with singletons, the incidence of gestational hypertension—13 versus 6 percent, and the incidence of preeclampsia—13 versus 5 percent, are both significantly increased (Sibai and co-workers, 2000). The incidence is unrelated to zygosity (Maxwell and associates, 2001).

Although smoking during pregnancy causes a variety of adverse pregnancy outcomes, ironically, it has consistently been associated with a *reduced risk* of hypertension during pregnancy (Bainbridge and associates, 2005; Zhang and colleagues, 1999). Placenta previa has also been reported to reduce the risk of hypertensive disorders in pregnancy (Ananth and colleagues, 1997).

In the woman who was normotensive during her first pregnancy, the incidence of preeclampsia in a subsequent pregnancy is lower than cited above. In a population-based retrospective cohort analysis, Getahun and colleagues (2007) studied almost 137,000 second pregnancies in such women. The incidence for preeclampsia in white women was 1.8 percent compared with 3 percent in African-American women. Again, obesity was a major risk factor.

Eclampsia Incidence

Because it is somewhat preventable by adequate prenatal care, the incidence of eclampsia has decreased over the years. In developed countries, its incidence probably averages 1 in 2000 deliveries. In the National Vital Statistics Report, Ventura and colleagues (2000) estimated that the incidence in the United States in 1998 was approximately 1 in 3250. According to the Royal College of Obstetricians and Gynaecologists (2006), in the United Kingdom, it approximates 1 in 2000. And Akkawi and co-workers (2009) reported it to be 1 in 2500 in Dublin, Andersgaard and associates (2006) as 1 per 2000 for Scandinavia, and Zwart and co-workers (2008) as 1 per 1600 for The Netherlands.

ETIOPATHOGENESIS

Any satisfactory theory concerning the etiology and pathogenesis of preeclampsia must account for the observation that gestational hypertensive disorders are more likely to develop in women who:

- Are exposed to chorionic villi for the first time
- Are exposed to a superabundance of chorionic villi, as with twins or hydatidiform mole
- Have preexisting renal or cardiovascular disease
- Are genetically predisposed to hypertension developing during pregnancy.

A fetus is not a requisite for preeclampsia. And although chorionic villi are essential, they need not be located within the uterus. For example, Worley and associates (2008) reported a 30-percent incidence in women with an extrauterine pregnancy exceeding 18 weeks' gestation. Regardless of precipitating etiology, the cascade of events that leads to the preeclampsia syndrome is characterized by a host of abnormalities that result in vascular endothelial damage and subsequent vasospasm, transudation of plasma, and ischemic and thrombotic sequelae.

Preeclampsia as a Two-Stage Disorder

Observations that abnormal interfaces between maternal, paternal, and fetal tissues may cause preeclampsia have led to hypotheses that the syndrome is a two-stage disorder. In this scenario, there is a spectrum to include "maternal and placental preeclampsia" (Ness and Roberts, 1996). According to Redman and colleagues (2009), stage 1 is caused by faulty endovascular trophoblastic remodeling that downstream causes the stage 2 clinical syndrome (Fig. 34-1). There certainly is evidence that *some* cases of preeclampsia fit this theory. Importantly, stage 2 is susceptible to modification by preexisting maternal conditions that include cardiac or renal disease, diabetes, obesity, or hereditary influences. Such compartmentalization seems artificial, and it seems logical that there likely is a continuous process.

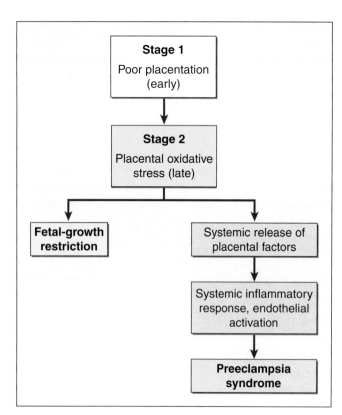

FIGURE 34-1 Schematic outlines the theory that the preeclampsia syndrome is a "two-stage disorder." Stage 1 is preclinical and characterized by faulty trophoblastic vascular remodeling of uterine arteries that causes placental hypoxia. Stage 2 is caused by release of placental factors into the maternal circulation causing systemic inflammatory response and endothelial activation. (Adapted from Borzychowski, 2006, and Redman, 2009, and their colleagues.)

Thus, although perhaps helpful to classify the syndrome for research purposes, preeclampsia is clinically more realistically a continuum of worsening disease. Moreover, evidence is accruing that many "isoforms" exist as discussed below.

Etiology

Writings describing eclampsia have been traced as far back as 2200 BC (Lindheimer and colleagues, 2009). And an imposing number of mechanisms have been proposed to explain its cause. Instead of being simply "one disease," preeclampsia appears to be a culmination of factors that likely involve a number of maternal, placental, and fetal factors. Those currently considered important include:

1. Placental implantation with abnormal trophoblastic invasion of uterine vessels
2. Immunological maladaptive tolerance between maternal, paternal (placental), and fetal tissues
3. Maternal maladaptation to cardiovascular or inflammatory changes of normal pregnancy
4. Genetic factors including inherited predisposing genes as well as epigenetic influences.

Abnormal Trophoblastic Invasion

In normal implantation, shown schematically in Figure 34-2, the uterine spiral arterioles undergo extensive remodeling as they are invaded by endovascular trophoblasts (see also Chap. 3, p. 54). These cells replace the vascular endothelial and muscular linings to enlarge the vessel diameter. The veins are invaded only superficially. In preeclampsia, however, there may be *incomplete trophoblastic invasion*. With such shallow invasion, decidual vessels, but not myometrial vessels, become lined with endovascular trophoblasts. The deeper myometrial arterioles do not lose their endothelial lining and musculoelastic tissue, and their mean external diameter is only half that of vessels in normal placentas (Fisher and colleagues, 2009). Madazli and associates (2000) showed that the magnitude of defective trophoblastic invasion of the spiral arteries correlates with the severity of the hypertensive disorder.

Using electron microscopy, De Wolf and co-workers (1980) examined arteries taken from the implantation site. They reported that early preeclamptic changes included endothelial damage, insudation of plasma constituents into vessel walls, proliferation of myointimal cells, and medial necrosis. Lipid accumulated first in myointimal cells and then within macrophages. Such lipid-laden cells and associated findings, as shown in Figure 34-3, were referred to as *atherosis* by Hertig (1945). Typically, the vessels affected by atherosis develop aneurysmal dilatation (Khong, 1991).

Thus, it is likely that the abnormally narrow spiral arteriolar lumen impairs placental blood flow. Diminished perfusion and a hypoxic environment eventually lead to release of *placental debris* that incites a systemic inflammatory response as described by Redman and Sargent (2008) and subsequently discussed. Fisher and colleagues (2009) have recently provided an elegant review of the molecular mechanisms involved in these interactions.

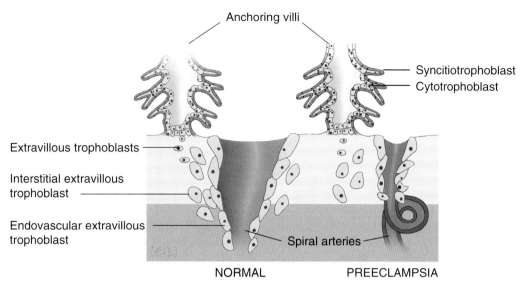

FIGURE 34-2 A. Normal third-trimester placental implantation shows proliferation of extravillous trophoblasts from an anchoring villus. These trophoblasts invade the decidua and extend into the walls of the spiral arteriole to replace the endothelium and muscular wall. This remodeling creates a dilated low-resistance vessel. **B.** Placenta in preeclamptic or fetal-growth restricted pregnancy shows defective implantation. This is characterized by incomplete invasion of the spiral arteriolar wall by extravillous trophoblasts and results in a small-caliber vessel with high resistance.

Immunological Factors

Maternal immune tolerance to paternally derived placental and fetal antigens is discussed in Chapter 3 (p. 58). Loss of this tolerance, or perhaps its *dysregulation*, is another theory cited to account for preeclampsia syndrome. Certainly the histological changes at the maternal-placental interface are suggestive of acute graft rejection (Labarrere, 1988). Some of these factors are shown in Table 34-3.

There are also inferential data that suggest an immune-mediated disorder. For example, the risk of preeclampsia is appreciably enhanced in circumstances in which formation of blocking antibodies to placental antigenic sites *might* be impaired. In this scenario, the first pregnancy would carry a higher risk. Tol-

erance dysregulation might also explain an increased risk when the paternal antigenic load is increased, that is, with two sets of paternal chromosomes—a "double dose." For example, women with molar pregnancies have a high incidence of early-onset preeclampsia. Also, women with a trisomy 13 fetus have a 30- to 40-percent incidence of preeclampsia. Bdolah and associates (2006) showed that these women also have elevated serum levels of antiangiogenic factors. The gene for one of these factors, sFLT-1, is on chromosome 13. Conversely, women previously exposed to paternal antigens, such as a prior pregnancy—with the same, but not different partner—are "immunized" against preeclampsia. This phenomenon is not as apparent in women with a prior abortion. Strickland and

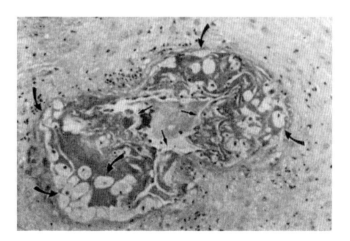

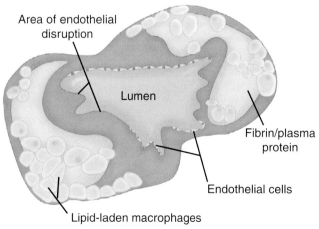

FIGURE 34-3 Atherosis is demonstrated in this blood vessel from a placental bed (*left*, photomicrograph; *right*, schematic diagram of the photomicrograph). Disruption of the endothelium results in a narrowed lumen because of accumulation of plasma proteins and foamy macrophages beneath the endothelium. In the left photograph, some of the foamy macrophages are shown by *curved arrows*, and *straight arrows* highlight areas of endothelial disruption. (Modified from BB Rogers, SL Bloom, and KJ Leveno, Atherosis revisited: Current concepts on the pathophysiology of implantation site, *Obstetrical & Gynecological Survey*, Vol. 54, No. 3, pp. 189–195, 1999, with permission.)

Obstetrical Complications

TABLE 34-3. Some Examples of Inherited Immunogenetic Factors That May Modify Genotype and Phenotype Expression in Preeclampsia

"Immunization" from a prior gestation
Inherited haplotypes for HLA-A, -B, -D, -Ia, -II
Inherited haplotypes for NK-cell receptors—also called killer-immunoglobulin-like receptors—KIR
Possibly shared susceptibility genes with diabetes and chronic hypertension

HLA = human leukocyte antigen; NK = natural killer.
From Ward and Lindheimer (2009).

associates (1986) studied more than 29,000 pregnancies at Parkland Hospital and reported that hypertensive disorders were significantly decreased, but not by much—22 versus 25 percent—in women who previously had miscarried compared with nulligravidas. Other studies have shown that multiparous women impregnated by a new consort have an increased risk of preeclampsia (Mostello and co-workers, 2002).

Redman and colleagues (2009) recently reviewed the possible role of *immune maladaptation* in the pathophysiology of preeclampsia. Early in a pregnancy destined to be preeclamptic, extravillous trophoblast express reduced amounts of immunosuppressive human leukocyte antigen G (HLA-G). This may contribute to defective placental vascularization in stage 1. Recall that as discussed in Chapter 3 (p. 59), during normal pregnancy, T-helper (Th) lymphocytes are produced so that type 2 activity is increased in relation to type 1—termed *type 2 bias* (Redman and Sargent, 2008). Th$_2$ cells promote humoral immunity, whereas Th$_1$ cells stimulate inflammatory cytokine secretion. Beginning in the early second trimester in women who develop preeclampsia, Th$_1$ action is increased and the Th$_1$/Th$_2$ ratio changes. Contributors to an enhanced immunologically mediated inflammatory reaction are stimulated by placental *microparticles*, as well as by adipocytes (Redman and Sargent, 2008).

Endothelial Cell Activation

In many ways, inflammatory changes are thought to be a continuation of the stage 1 changes caused by defective placentation discussed above. In response to placental factors released by ischemic changes or by any other inciting cause, a cascade of events is set in motion (Taylor and colleagues, 2009). Thus, antiangiogenic and metabolic factors and other inflammatory mediators are thought to provoke endothelial cell injury.

It has been proposed that endothelial cell dysfunction is due to an extreme activated state of leukocytes in the maternal circulation (Faas, 2000; Gervasi, 2001; Redman, 1999, and all their colleagues). Briefly, cytokines such as tumor necrosis factor-α (TNF-α) and the interleukins (IL) may contribute to the oxidative stress associated with preeclampsia. This is characterized by reactive oxygen species and free radicals that lead to formation of self-propagating lipid peroxides (Manten and associ-

ates, 2005). These in turn generate highly toxic radicals that injure endothelial cells, modify their nitric oxide production, and interfere with prostaglandin balance. Other consequences of oxidative stress include production of the lipid-laden macrophage foam cells seen in atherosis and shown in Figure 34-2; activation of microvascular coagulation manifest by thrombocytopenia; and increased capillary permeability manifest by edema and proteinuria.

These observations on the effects of oxidative stress in preeclampsia have given rise to increased interest in the potential benefit of antioxidants to prevent preeclampsia. Antioxidants are from a diverse family of compounds that function to prevent overproduction of and damage caused by noxious free radicals. Examples of antioxidants include vitamin E (α-tocopherol), vitamin C (ascorbic acid), and β-carotene. Dietary supplementation with these antioxidants to prevent preeclampsia has thus far proven unsuccessful and is discussed further on page 727.

Nutritional Factors

John and co-workers (2002) showed that in the general population a diet high in fruits and vegetables that have antioxidant activity is associated with decreased blood pressure. Zhang and associates (2002) reported that the incidence of preeclampsia was doubled in women whose daily intake of ascorbic acid was less than 85 mg. These studies were followed by randomized trials to study dietary supplementation. Villar and associates (2006) showed that calcium supplementation in populations with a *low dietary calcium intake* had a small effect to lower perinatal mortality rates, but no effect on the incidence of preeclampsia (see p. 727). In a number of trials, supplementation with the antioxidant vitamins C and E showed no beneficial effects.

Genetic Factors

Preeclampsia is a multifactorial, polygenic disorder. In their comprehensive review, Ward and Lindheimer (2009) cite an incident risk for preeclampsia of 20 to 40 percent for daughters of preeclamptic mothers; 11 to 37 percent for sisters of preeclamptic women; and 22 to 47 percent in twin studies. In a study by Nilsson and co-workers (2004) that included almost 1.2 million Swedish births, they reported a genetic component for gestational hypertension as well as preeclampsia. They also reported 60-percent concordance in monozygotic female twin pairs.

This hereditary predisposition likely is the result of interactions of literally hundreds of inherited genes—both maternal and paternal—that control myriad enzymatic and metabolic functions throughout every organ system. Thus, the clinical manifestation in any given woman with the preeclampsia syndrome will occupy a spectrum as discussed under the two-stage concept on page 710. In this regard, phenotypic expression will differ among similar genotypes depending on interactions with environmental factors.

Candidate Genes. From their recent review, Ward and Lindheimer (2009) found that more than 70 genes have been studied for their possible association with preeclampsia. Seven of

TABLE 34-4. Genes Frequently Studied for Their Association with Preeclampsia Syndrome

Gene (Polymorphism)	Function Affected	Chromosome	Biological Association
MTHFR (C677T)	Methylene tetrahydrofolate reductase	1p36.3	Vascular diseases
F5 (Leiden)	Factor V$_{Leiden}$	1q23	Thrombophilia—may coexist with other thrombophilic genes
AGT (M235T)	Angiotensinogen	1q42-q43	Blood pressure regulation, linked to essential hypertension
HLA (Various)	Human leukocyte antigens	6p21.3	Immunity
NOS3 (Glu 298 Asp)	Endothelial nitric oxide	7q36	Vascular endothelial function
F2 (G20210A)	Prothrombin (factor II)	11p11-q12	Coagulation—weakly associated, studied with other thrombophilic genes
ACE (I/D^{at}Intron 16)	Angiotensin-converting enzyme	17q23	Blood pressure regulation

Adapted from Ward and Lindheimer, 2009.

these that have been investigated widely are listed in Table 34-4. More than 100 studies of these seven genes were considered, and fewer than half reported a positive significant association with the gene(s) analyzed. Polymorphisms of the genes for Fas, hypoxia-inducible factor-1α protein (HIF-1α), IL-1β, lymphotoxin-α, transforming growth factor beta 3 (TGF-β3), and TNF have also been studied with varying results (Borowski, 2009; Hefler, 2001; Lachmeijer, 2001; Livingston, 2001; Wilson, 2009, and all their colleagues).

Because of the heterogeneity of the preeclampsia syndrome, and especially the other genetic and environmental factors that interact with its complex phenotypic expression, it is doubtful that any *one* candidate gene will be found responsible.

Other Genetic Variables. There is an extensive list of other variables that affect genotypic and phenotypic expression of the preeclampsia syndrome. Some include:

1. Multiple genotypes: maternal and paternal (fetal and placental)
2. Subgroups: associated disorders such as diabetes and characteristics such as parity
3. Genomic ethnicity: frequency of polymorphisms, genetic drift, founder effect, and selection
4. Gene-gene interaction: specific alleles or products of two or more genes affect one another and thus the phenotype
5. Epigenetic phenomena: variations in expression of a functional stable gene, for example, monozygotic twin differences
6. Gene-environmental interactions—these are infinite.

Pathogenesis

Vasospasm

The concept of vasospasm was advanced by Volhard (1918) based on his direct observations of small blood vessels in the nail beds, ocular fundi, and bulbar conjunctivae. It was also surmised from histological changes seen in various affected organs (Hinselmann, 1924; Landesman and co-workers, 1954). Vascular constriction causes increased resistance and subsequent hypertension. At the same time, endothelial cell damage causes interstitial leakage through which blood constituents, including platelets and fibrinogen, are deposited subendothelially. Wang and colleagues (2002) have also demonstrated disruption of endothelial junctional proteins. Suzuki and co-workers (2003) described ultrastructural changes in the subendothelial region of resistance arteries in preeclamptic women. With diminished blood flow because of maldistribution, ischemia of the surrounding tissues would lead to necrosis, hemorrhage, and other end-organ disturbances characteristic of the syndrome.

Endothelial Cell Activation

During the past two decades, endothelial cell activation has become the centerpiece in the contemporary understanding of the pathogenesis of preeclampsia. In this scheme, unknown factor(s)—likely placental in origin—are secreted into the maternal circulation and provoke activation and dysfunction of the vascular endothelium. The clinical syndrome of preeclampsia is thought to result from these widespread endothelial cell changes. In addition to microparticles, Grundmann and associates (2008) have reported that *circulating endothelial cell—CEC*—levels are significantly elevated fourfold in the peripheral blood of preeclamptic women.

Intact endothelium has anticoagulant properties, and endothelial cells blunt the response of vascular smooth muscle to agonists by releasing nitric oxide. Damaged or activated endothelial cells may produce less nitric oxide and secrete substances that promote coagulation and increase sensitivity to vasopressors (Gant and co-workers, 1974). Further evidence of endothelial activation includes the characteristic changes in glomerular capillary endothelial morphology, increased capillary permeability, and elevated blood concentrations of substances associated with endothelial activation. These latter substances are transferable, and serum from women with preeclampsia stimulates some of these substances in greater amounts. It seems likely that multiple factors in plasma of preeclamptic women combine to have these vasoactive effects (Myers and associates, 2007; Walsh, 2009).

Increased Pressor Responses. As discussed in Chapter 5 (p. 120), pregnant women normally develop refractoriness to infused vasopressors (Abdul-Karim and Assali, 1961). Women with early preeclampsia, however, have increased vascular reactivity to infused norepinephrine and angiotensin II (Raab and co-workers, 1956; Talledo and associates, 1968). Moreover, increased sensitivity to angiotensin II clearly precedes the onset of gestational hypertension. Gant and colleagues (1974) showed that normotensive nulliparas remained refractory to infused angiotensin II, but those who subsequently became hypertensive lost this refractoriness several weeks before the onset of hypertension.

Prostaglandins. A number of prostanoids are thought to be central to the pathophysiology of the preeclampsia syndrome. Specifically, the blunted pressor response seen in normal pregnancy is at least partially due to decreased vascular responsiveness mediated by endothelial prostaglandin synthesis. For example, compared with normal pregnancy, endothelial prostacyclin (PGI_2) production is decreased in preeclampsia. This action appears to be mediated by phospholipase A_2 (Taylor and Roberts, 1999). At the same time, thromboxane A_2 secretion by platelets is increased, and the prostacyclin:thromboxane A_2 ratio decreases. The net result favors increased sensitivity to infused angiotensin II, and ultimately, vasoconstriction (Spitz and colleagues, 1988). Chavarria and co-workers (2003) have provided evidence that these changes are apparent as early as 22 weeks in women who later develop preeclampsia.

Nitric Oxide. This potent vasodilator is synthesized from L-arginine by endothelial cells. Withdrawal of nitric oxide results in a clinical picture similar to preeclampsia in a pregnant animal model (Conrad and Vernier, 1989). Inhibition of nitric oxide synthesis increases mean arterial pressure, decreases heart rate, and reverses the pregnancy-induced refractoriness to vasopressors. In humans, nitric oxide likely is the compound that maintains the normal low-pressure vasodilated state characteristic of fetoplacental perfusion (Myatt and co-workers, 1992; Weiner and associates, 1992). It also is produced by fetal endothelium and is increased in response to preeclampsia, diabetes, and infection (Parra and associates, 2001; von Mandach and co-workers, 2003).

The effects of nitric oxide production in preeclampsia are unclear (Taylor and associates, 2009). It appears that the syndrome is associated with decreased endothelial nitric oxide synthase expression, thus increasing nitric oxide inactivation. These responses may be race-related, with African-American women producing more nitric oxide (Wallace and co-workers, 2009).

Endothelins

These 21-amino acid peptides are potent vasoconstrictors, and endothelin-1 (ET-1) is the primary isoform produced by human endothelium (Mastrogiannis and co-workers, 1991). Plasma ET-1 levels are increased in normotensive pregnant women, but women with preeclampsia have even higher levels (Ajne, 2003; Clark, 1992; Nova, 1991, and all their associates). According to Taylor and Roberts (1999), the placenta is not the source of increased ET-1 concentrations, and they likely arise from systemic endothelial activation. Interestingly, treatment of preeclamptic women with magnesium sulfate lowers ET-1 concentrations (Sagsoz and Kucukozkan, 2003).

Angiogenic and Antiangiogenic Proteins

Placental vasculogenesis is evident by 21 days after conception. There is an ever-expanding list of pro- and antiangiogenic substances involved in placental vascular development. The families of vascular endothelial growth factor (VEGF) and angiopoietins (Ang) gene products are most extensively studied. *Angiogenic imbalance* is used to describe excessive amounts of antiangiogenic factors that are hypothesized to be stimulated by worsening hypoxia at the uteroplacental interface. Trophoblastic tissue of women destined to develop preeclampsia overproduces at least two antiangiogenic peptides that enter the maternal circulation (Karumanchi and colleagues, 2009):

1. *Soluble Fms-like tyrosine kinase 1 (sFlt-1)* is a variant of the Flt-1 receptor for placental growth factor (PlGF) and vascular endothelial growth factor (VEGF). Increased maternal sFlt-1 levels inactivate and decrease circulating free PlGF and VEGF concentrations leading to endothelial dysfunction (Maynard and associates, 2003). As shown in **Figure 34-4A**, sFlt-1 levels begin to increase in maternal serum months before preeclampsia is evident.
2. *Soluble endoglin (sEng)* is a placenta-derived 65-kDa molecule that blocks endoglin—also called CD105—which is a co-receptor for the TGF-β family. This soluble form of endoglin inhibits various TGF-β isotopes from binding to endothelial receptors and results in decreased endothelial nitric oxide-dependent vasodilatation (Levine and co-workers, 2006; Venkatesha and associates, 2006). As shown in **Figure 34-4B**, sEng serum levels also begin to increase months before clinical preeclampsia develops.

The cause of placental overproduction of antiangiogenic proteins remains an enigma. The soluble forms are not increased in the fetal circulation or amnionic fluid, and their levels in maternal blood dissipate after delivery (Staff and co-workers, 2007). Research currently is focused on immunological mechanisms, oxidative stress, mitochondrial pathology, and hypoxia genes (Karumanchi and colleagues, 2009). Clinical research is directed at use of antiangiogenic proteins in the prediction and diagnosis of preeclampsia. In a systematic review, Widmer and associates (2007) concluded that retrospective studies show that third-trimester elevation of Sflt-1 levels and decreased PlGF concentrations correlate with preeclampsia development after 25 weeks. These results require verification in prospective studies.

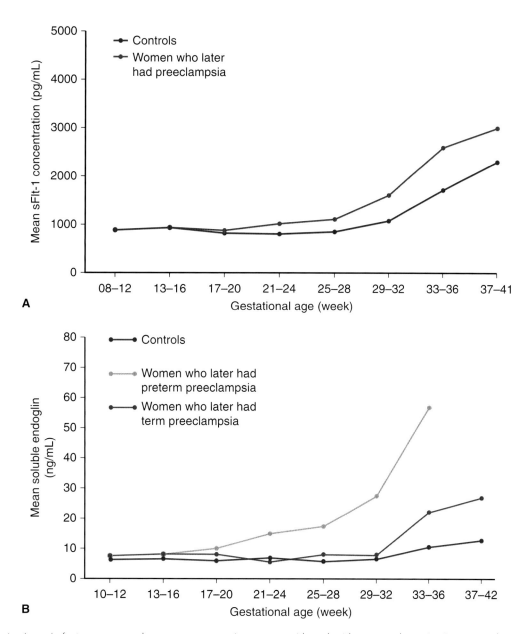

FIGURE 34-4 Angiogenic factors measured across pregnancy in women with and without preeclampsia. **A.** Mean sFlt-1 serum concentrations after logarithmic transformation show divergence of values before and after preeclampsia developed. **B.** Mean serum concentrations of soluble endoglin after logarithmic transformation also show divergence before and after preeclampsia developed. (Adapted from Levine and co-workers, 2006.)

PATHOPHYSIOLOGY

Although the cause of preeclampsia still remains unknown, evidence for its manifestation begins early in pregnancy with covert pathophysiological changes that gain momentum across gestation and eventually become clinically apparent. Unless delivery supervenes, these changes ultimately result in multi-organ involvement with a clinical spectrum ranging from barely noticeable to one of cataclysmic pathophysiological deterioration that can be life threatening for both mother and fetus. As discussed, these are thought to be a consequence of vasospasm, endothelial dysfunction, and ischemia. Although the myriad of maternal consequences of the preeclampsia syndrome are usu-

ally described in terms of individual organ systems, they frequently are multiple and they clinically overlap.

Cardiovascular System

Severe disturbances of normal cardiovascular function are common with preeclampsia or eclampsia. These are related to: (1) increased cardiac afterload caused by hypertension; (2) cardiac preload, which is substantively affected by pathologically diminished hypervolemia of pregnancy or is iatrogenically increased by intravenous crystalloid or oncotic solutions; and (3) endothelial activation with extravasation of intravascular fluid into the extracellular space, and importantly, into the lungs

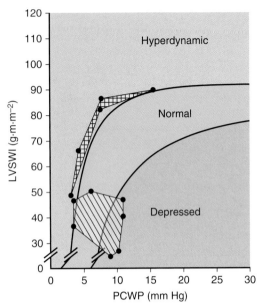

FIGURE 34-5 Ventricular function in normally pregnant women (*striped area*) and in women with eclampsia (*boxed area*) is plotted on a Braunwald ventricular function curve. Normal values are from Clark and colleagues (1989) and those for eclampsia are from Hankins and associates (1984).

(see Chap. 42, p. 929). As discussed in Chapter 5 (p. 118), during normal pregnancy, left ventricular mass increases, but there is no convincing evidence that additional structural changes are induced by preeclampsia (Hibbard and colleagues, 2009).

Hemodynamic Changes

The cardiovascular aberrations of pregnancy-related hypertensive disorders vary depending on a number of factors. These aberrations center around increased afterload and include severity of hypertension, presence of underlying chronic disease, presence of preeclampsia, and stage of the clinical course in which they are studied. There are claims that in some women these changes may even precede the onset of hypertension (Bosio, 1999; De Paco, 2008; Easterling, 1990; Hibbard, 2009, and all their colleagues). Nevertheless, with the clinical onset of preeclampsia, there is reduction in cardiac output likely due to increased peripheral resistance.

There are a number of studies in which data were obtained using invasive hemodynamic methods. Importantly, both nonhypertensive pregnant women and those with severe preeclampsia have normal or hyperdynamic ventricular function, as shown in Figure 34-5. In both of these groups, cardiac output is appropriate for left-sided filling pressures. Data from preeclamptic women obtained by invasive hemodynamic studies are confounded because of the heterogeneity of populations and interventions that also may significantly alter these measurements, such as substantive crystalloid infusions, antihypertensive agents, and magnesium sulfate. Ventricular function studies of preeclamptic women from a number of investigations are shown in Figure 34-6. Although cardiac function was hyperdynamic in all women, filling pressures were dependent on intravenous fluid infusions. Specifically, aggressive hydration resulted in hyperdynamic ventricular function in most women. Importantly, this is also accompanied by elevated pulmonary capillary wedge pressures. In some of these women, pulmonary edema may develop despite normal ventricular function because of an alveolar endothelial-epithelial leak that is compounded by decreased oncotic pressure from a low serum albumin concentration (American College of Obstetricians and Gynecologists, 2002a). Similar values of cardiac function were reported earlier by Lang and co-workers (1991) and more recently by Tihtonen and colleagues (2006), who used noninvasive impedance cardiography.

Thus, hyperdynamic ventricular function was largely a result of low wedge pressures and not a result of augmented myocardial contractility measured as left ventricular stroke work index. By comparison, women given appreciably larger volumes of fluid commonly had filling pressures that exceeded normal, but their ventricular function remained hyperdynamic because of increased cardiac output.

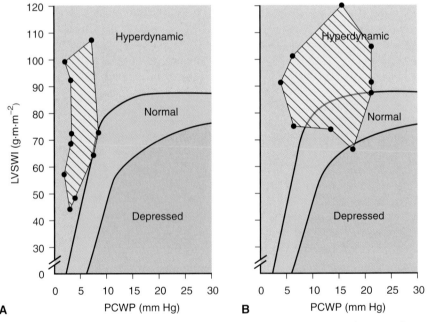

FIGURE 34-6 Ventricular function in women with severe preeclampsia–eclampsia plotted on the Braunwald ventricular function curve. The pulmonary capillary wedge pressures (PCWP) are lower in those managed with restricted fluid administration (*striped area in* **A**) compared with women managed with aggressive fluid therapy (*striped area in* **B**). In those managed with aggressive fluid infusions, eight developed pulmonary edema despite normal to hyperdynamic ventricular function in all but one. Data for **A** are from Benedetti (1980) and Hankins (1984) and colleagues and for **B** from Rafferty and Berkowitz (1980) and Phelan and Yurth (1982).

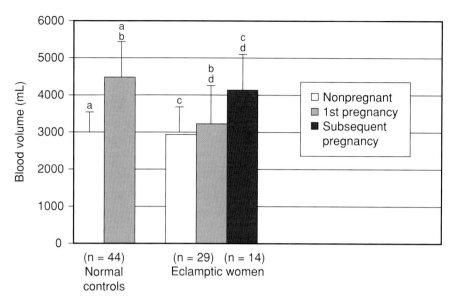

FIGURE 34-7 Bar graph comparing nonpregnant mean blood volumes with those obtained at the time of delivery in a group of women with normal pregnancy, eclampsia in their first pregnancy, and subsequent normal pregnancy in some of the women who had eclampsia. Extensions above bars represent one standard deviation. Comparison between values with identical lowercase letters, that is, a-a, b-b, c-c, d-d, are significant *p* < .001. (Data from Zeeman and Cunningham, 2009, with permission.)

cyte destruction as subsequently described. Vasospasm and endothelial leakage of plasma may persist for a variable amount of time after delivery as the endothelium undergoes repair. As this takes place, vasoconstriction reverses, and as the blood volume increases, the hematocrit usually falls. Thus, women with eclampsia:

- Are unduly sensitive to vigorous fluid therapy administered in an attempt to expand the contracted blood volume to normal pregnancy levels.
- Are sensitive to amounts of blood loss at delivery that are considered normal for a normotensive woman.

Blood and Coagulation

Hematological abnormalities develop in some women with preeclampsia. Among those commonly identified is thrombocytopenia, which at times may become so severe as to be life threatening. In addition, the levels of some plasma clotting factors may be decreased, and erythrocytes may display bizarre shapes and undergo rapid hemolysis.

Thrombocytopenia

Thrombocytopenia with eclampsia has been described at least since 1922 by Stancke. Because it is common, the platelet count is routinely measured in women with any form of gestational hypertension. The frequency and intensity of thrombocytopenia vary and are dependent on the severity and duration of the preeclampsia syndrome as well as the frequency with which platelet counts are performed (Heilmann and colleagues, 2007; Hupuczi and coworkers, 2007). Overt thrombocytopenia—defined by a platelet count < 100,000/μL—indicates severe disease (see Table 34-2). In general, the lower the platelet count, the higher the rates of maternal and fetal morbidity and mortality (Leduc and co-workers, 1992). In most cases, delivery is advisable because thrombocytopenia usually continues to worsen. After delivery, the platelet count may continue to decrease for the first day or so. It then usually increases progressively to reach a normal level usually within 3 to 5 days. In some instances, for example, with HELLP syndrome, the platelet count continues to fall after delivery. In some women whose platelet counts do not nadir until 48 to 72 hours, preeclampsia syndrome may be incorrectly attributed to one of the thrombotic microangiopathies (see Chap. 51, p. 1095).

Other Platelet Abnormalities. In addition to thrombocytopenia, there are myriad other platelet alterations described with the preeclampsia syndrome. These were recently reviewed by Kenny and associates (2009) and include platelet activation with increased degranulation, thromboxane A₂ release, and decreased lifespan. Paradoxically, in most studies, in vitro platelet aggregation is decreased compared with the normal increase characteristic of pregnancy (Kenny and associates, 2009). This

Blood Volume

It has been known for nearly 100 years that *hemoconcentration* is a hallmark of eclampsia. Zeeman and colleagues (2009a) expanded the previous observations of Pritchard and co-workers (1984). They found that in *eclamptic* women, the normally expected hypervolemia is severely curtailed and in some women, even absent (Fig. 34-7). Women of average size should have a blood volume of nearly 5000 mL during the last several weeks of a normal pregnancy, compared with approximately 3500 mL when not pregnant. With eclampsia, however, much or all of the anticipated normal excess 1500 mL is lost. Such hemoconcentration results from generalized vasoconstriction that follows endothelial activation and leakage of plasma into the interstitial space because of increased permeability. In women with *preeclampsia*, and depending on its severity, hemoconcentration is usually not as marked. Women with gestational hypertension, but without preeclampsia, usually have a normal blood volume (Silver and colleagues, 1998).

For women with severe hemoconcentration, it was once taught that an acute fall in hematocrit suggested resolution of preeclampsia. In this scenario, hemodilution follows endothelial healing with return of interstitial fluid into the intravascular space. **While this is somewhat correct, it is important to recognize that a substantive cause of this fall in hematocrit is usually the consequence of blood loss at delivery.** It may also be partially the result of increased erythro-

likely is due to platelet "exhaustion" following in vivo activation. Although the cause is unknown, immunological processes or simply platelet deposition at sites of endothelial damage may be implicated. Platelet-bound and circulating platelet-bindable immunoglobulins are increased, which suggest platelet surface alterations (Samuels and colleagues, 1987).

Neonatal Thrombocytopenia. In a large clinical study, Pritchard and colleagues (1987) showed that severe thrombocytopenia did not develop in the fetus or infant in preeclamptic women. In fact, these investigators found no cases of fetal thrombocytopenia despite severe maternal thrombocytopenia. *Maternal thrombocytopenia in hypertensive women is not a fetal indication for cesarean delivery.*

Hemolysis

Severe preeclampsia is frequently accompanied by evidence of hemolysis, which is semiquantified by elevated serum lactate dehydrogenase levels. Other evidence comes from schizocytosis, spherocytosis, and reticulocytosis in peripheral blood (Cunningham and associates, 1985; Pritchard and colleagues, 1954, 1976). These derangements result in part from microangiopathic hemolysis caused by endothelial disruption with platelet adherence and fibrin deposition. Sanchez-Ramos and colleagues (1994) described increased erythrocyte membrane fluidity with HELLP syndrome, and Cunningham and co-workers (1995) postulated that these changes were due to serum lipid alterations. Erythrocytic membrane changes, increased adhesiveness, and aggregation may also facilitate a hypercoagulable state (Gamzu and co-workers, 2001; Grisaru and associates, 1997).

HELLP Syndrome. In addition to hemolysis and thrombocytopenia, it also became appreciated that elevated serum liver transaminase levels were commonly found with severe preeclampsia and were indicative of hepatocellular necrosis (Chesley, 1978). Weinstein (1982) referred to this combination of events as the *HELLP syndrome*—and this moniker now is used worldwide. As shown in Table 34-2, facets of the HELLP syndrome are included in criteria that differentiate severe from nonsevere preeclampsia. It is discussed in further detail on page 720.

Coagulation

Subtle changes consistent with intravascular coagulation, and less often erythrocyte destruction, commonly are found with preeclampsia and especially eclampsia (Kenny and colleagues, 2009). Some of these changes include increased factor VIII consumption, increased levels of fibrinopeptides A and B and of fibrin degradation products, and decreased levels of regulatory proteins—antithrombin III and protein C and S. That said, there is little evidence that these abnormalities are clinically significant (Chesley, 1978; Pritchard and associates, 1984). Except for thrombocytopenia discussed above, coagulation aberrations generally are mild. Unless there is associated placental abruption, plasma fibrinogen levels do not differ remarkably from levels found in normal pregnancy, and fibrin degradation products are elevated only occasionally. Barron and colleagues (1999)

found that routine laboratory assessment of coagulation, including prothrombin time, activated partial thromboplastin time, and plasma fibrinogen level, to be unnecessary in the management of pregnancy-associated hypertensive disorders.

Other Clotting Factors. The *thrombophilias* are clotting factor deficiencies that lead to hypercoagulability. They may be associated with early-onset preeclampsia (see Table 47-3, p. 1018). *Fibronectin*, a glycoprotein associated with vascular endothelial cell basement membrane, is elevated in women with preeclampsia (Brubaker and colleagues, 1992). This observation is consistent with the view that preeclampsia causes vascular endothelial injury with subsequent hematological aberrations.

Volume Homeostasis

Endocrine Changes

Plasma levels of *renin, angiotensin II, angiotensin 1-7, and aldosterone* are substantively increased during normal pregnancy. With preeclampsia, and despite decreased blood volume, these values decrease substantively, but still remain above nonpregnant values (Luft and colleagues, 2009).

Deoxycorticosterone (DOC) is a potent mineralocorticoid that is increased remarkably in normal pregnancy (see Chap. 5, p. 129). This results from conversion of plasma progesterone to DOC rather than increased maternal adrenal secretion. Because of this, DOC secretion is not reduced by sodium retention or hypertension, and it may explain why women with preeclampsia retain sodium (Winkel and co-workers, 1980).

Vasopressin levels are similar in nonpregnant, normally pregnant, and preeclamptic women even though the latter two have substantively decreased plasma osmolality (Dürr and Lindheimer, 1999). It is yet unclear whether serum concentrations of *atrial natriuretic peptide* remain unchanged, or whether they are increased during normal pregnancy despite the increased plasma volume (Luft and colleagues, 2009). This peptide is released on atrial wall stretching from blood volume expansion, and it responds to cardiac contractility. Secretion of atrial natriuretic peptide is increased in women with preeclampsia (Borghi and associates, 2000; Luft and colleagues, 2009).

Fluid and Electrolyte Changes

In women with severe preeclampsia, the volume of *extracellular fluid,* manifest as edema, is usually much greater than that of normal pregnant women. The mechanism responsible for pathological fluid retention is thought to be endothelial injury. In addition to generalized edema and proteinuria, these women have reduced plasma oncotic pressure. This reduction creates a filtration imbalance and further displaces intravascular fluid into the surrounding interstitium.

Electrolyte concentrations do not differ appreciably in women with preeclampsia compared with those of normal pregnant women. This may not be the case if there has been vigorous diuretic therapy, sodium restriction, or administration of free water with sufficient oxytocin to produce antidiuresis.

Following an eclamptic convulsion, the serum pH and *bicarbonate* concentration are lowered due to lactic acidosis and compensatory respiratory loss of carbon dioxide. The intensity of acidosis relates to the amount of lactic acid produced and the rate at which carbon dioxide is exhaled.

Kidney

During normal pregnancy, renal blood flow and glomerular filtration rate are increased appreciably (see Chap. 5, p. 123 and Appendix). With development of preeclampsia, there may be a number of reversible anatomical and pathophysiological changes. Of clinical importance, renal perfusion and glomerular filtration are reduced. Levels that are much less than normal nonpregnant values are infrequent and are the consequence of severe disease.

Mildly diminished glomerular filtration may result from a reduced plasma volume. Most of the decrement is probably from increased renal afferent arteriolar resistance that may be elevated up to fivefold (Conrad and co-workers, 2009). There are also morphological changes characterized by glomerular endotheliosis blocking the filtration barrier. Diminished filtration causes serum creatinine values to rise to values seen in nonpregnant individuals, that is, 1 mg/mL, but sometimes even higher (Lindheimer and colleagues, 2008a).

In most preeclamptic women, urine sodium concentration is elevated. Urine osmolality, urine:plasma creatinine ratio, and fractional excretion of sodium are also indicative that a prerenal mechanism is involved. Kirshon and co-workers (1988) infused dopamine intravenously into oliguric women with preeclampsia, and this renal vasodilator stimulated increased urine output, fractional sodium excretion, and free water clearance. As was shown in Figure 34-6, crystalloid infusion increases left ventricular filling pressure, and although oliguria temporarily improves, rapid infusions may cause clinically apparent pulmonary edema. *Intensive intravenous fluid therapy is not indicated for these women with oliguria, unless diminished urine output is caused by hemorrhage.*

Plasma uric acid concentration is typically elevated in preeclampsia. The elevation exceeds the reduction in glomerular filtration rate and likely is also due to enhanced tubular reabsorption (Chesley and Williams, 1945). At the same time, preeclampsia is associated with diminished urinary excretion of calcium perhaps because of increased tubular reabsorption (Taufield and associates, 1987). Another possibility is from increased placental urate production compensatory to increased oxidative stress.

Proteinuria

At least some degree of proteinuria will establish the diagnosis of preeclampsia-eclampsia. Proteinuria may develop late, and some women may be delivered—or have an eclamptic convulsion—before it appears. For example, Sibai (2004) reported that 10 to 15 percent of women with HELLP syndrome did not have proteinuria at presentation. Zwart and associates (2008) reported that 17 percent of eclamptic women did not have proteinuria by the time of seizures.

Another problem is that the optimal method of establishing either abnormal levels of urine protein or albumin remains to be defined. Chen and co-workers (2008) have shown that clean-catch and catheterized urine specimens correlate well. But dipstick qualitative determinations depend on urinary concentration and are notorious for false-positive and negative results. For a 24-hour quantitative specimen, the standard "consensus" threshold value used is > 300 mg/24 h—or its extrapolated equivalent in shorter collections. Importantly, this has not been irrefutably established.

Determination of urinary protein: or albumin:creatinine ratio may supplant the cumbersome 24-hour quantification (Kyle and colleagues, 2008). In a recent systematic review, Papanna and associates (2008) concluded that random urine protein: creatinine ratios that are below 130 to 150 mg/g—0.13 to 0.15—indicate that the likelihood of proteinuria exceeding 300 mg/day is low. Midrange ratios, that is, 300 mg/g—0.3—have poor sensitivity and specificity. These investigators recommend that with midrange values, a 24-hour specimen be measured for accuracy.

There are several methods used to measure proteinuria, and none detect all of the various proteins normally excreted. A more accurate method involves measurement of albumin excretion. Albumin filtration exceeds that of larger globulins, and with glomerular disease such as preeclampsia, much of the protein in urine is albumin. Newly available test kits permit rapid measurement of urinary albumin:creatinine ratios in an outpatient setting (Kyle and co-workers, 2008).

Finally, although worsening or nephrotic-range proteinuria has been considered by most to be a sign of severe disease, this may not be the case (Airoldi and Weinstein, 2007). Thus, the quantity of protein excretion alone as an indicator of preeclampsia severity is currently being investigated.

Anatomical Changes

Changes identifiable by light and electron microscopy were commonly found in the kidney of eclamptic women at autopsy by Sheehan and Lynch (1973). Glomeruli are enlarged by approximately 20 percent, they are "bloodless," and capillary loops variably are dilated and contracted. Endothelial cells are swollen, and this was termed *glomerular capillary endotheliosis* by Spargo and associates (1959). Endothelial cells are often so swollen that they block or partially block the capillary lumens (Fig. 34-8). Homogeneous subendothelial deposits of proteins and fibrin-like material are seen.

There is evidence that endothelial swelling results from angiogenic factor "withdrawal" that is caused by the free protein complexing with the circulating antiangiogenic protein receptor discussed on page 714 (Eremina and associates, 2007; Karumanchi and colleagues, 2009). The angiogenic protein is crucial for podocyte health, and its inactivation by the antiangiogenic receptors leads to podocyte dysfunction and endothelial swelling. Consistent with this, Garovic and co-workers (2007) have shown increased excretion of urinary podocyte cells with eclampsia, a phenomenon shared by other proteinuric disorders. Of interest, podocytes are epithelial cells, and thus renal pathology is both endothelial and epithelial (see Fig. 34-8).

Acute Renal Failure (Acute Kidney Injury)

Rarely is *acute tubular necrosis* caused by preeclampsia alone. Although mild degrees are encountered in neglected cases, clinically apparent renal failure is invariably induced by coexistent hemorrhagic hypotension. This is usually caused by severe obstetrical hemorrhage for which adequate blood replacement was not given (see Chap. 48, p. 1045). Drakeley and co-workers (2002) described 72 women with preeclampsia and renal failure. Half had HELLP syndrome and a third had placental abruption. As discussed on page 721, Haddad and colleagues (2000) reported that 5 percent of 183 women with HELLP syndrome developed acute renal failure. Half of these also had a placental abruption, and most had postpartum hemorrhage. Rarely, irreversible *renal cortical necrosis* develops.

Liver

Hepatic changes in women with fatal eclampsia were described in 1856 by Virchow. The characteristic lesions commonly found were regions of periportal hemorrhage in the liver periphery. In their elegant autopsy studies, Sheehan and Lynch (1973) described that some degree of hepatic infarction accompanied hemorrhage in almost half of women who died with eclampsia. These corresponded with reports that had appeared during the 1960s describing elevated serum hepatic transaminase levels. Along with the earlier observations by Pritchard and colleagues (1954), who described hemolysis and thrombocytopenia with eclampsia, this constellation of hemolysis, hepatocellular necrosis, and thrombocytopenia was later termed *HELLP syndrome* by Weinstein (1985) to call attention to its seriousness (see p. 718).

Extensive anatomical lesions such as shown in Figure 34-9 are seldom identified with liver biopsy in nonfatal cases (Barton

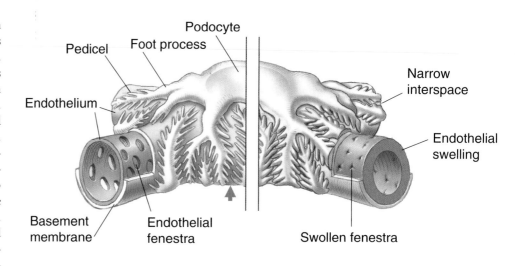

FIGURE 34-8 Schematic showing glomerular capillary endotheliosis. The capillary of the normal glomerulus shown on the left has wide endothelial fenestrations, and the pedicels emanating from the podocytes are widely spaced (*arrow*). The illustration on the right is of a glomerulus with changes induced by the preeclampsia syndrome. The endothelial cells are swollen and their fenestrae narrowed, as are the pedicels that now abut each other.

and colleagues, 1992). From a pragmatic point, liver involvement with preeclampsia may be clinically significant in the following circumstances:

1. Symptomatic involvement, typically manifest by moderate to severe right-upper or midepigastric pain and tenderness, is usually only seen with severe disease. In many cases, such women also have elevated serum aminotransferase levels—aspartate transferase (AST) or alanine transferase (ALT). In some cases, however, the amount of hepatic tissue involved with infarction may be surprisingly extensive, yet still clinically insignificant. In our experiences, infarction may be worsened by hypotension from obstetrical hemorrhage, and it may result in hepatic failure (Alexander and colleagues, 2009).

2. Asymptomatic elevations of serum hepatic transaminase levels—AST and ALT—are considered markers for severe preeclampsia. Values seldom exceed 500 U/L, but have been reported to exceed 2000 U/L in some women (see also Chap. 50, p. 1064). In general, serum levels inversely follow platelet levels, and they both usually normalize within 3 days following delivery.

3. Hepatic hemorrhage from areas of infarction may extend to form a hepatic hematoma. These in turn may extend to form a subcapsular hematoma that may rupture. They can be identified using computed tomography (CT) scanning or magnetic resonance (MR) imaging as shown in Figure 34-10. Unruptured hematomas are probably more common than clinically suspected, and are more likely with HELLP syndrome (Carlson and Bader, 2004; Rosen and colleagues, 2003). Although once considered a surgical condition, contemporaneous management usually consists of observation and conservative treatment of hematomas unless hemorrhage is ongoing (Barton and Sibai, 1999). In

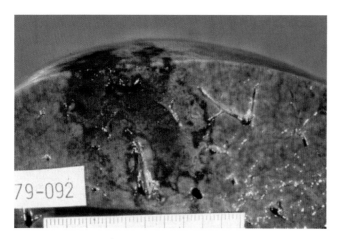

FIGURE 34-9 Gross liver specimen from a woman with preeclampsia who died from severe acidosis and liver failure. Periportal hemorrhagic necrosis was seen microscopically. (From Cunningham, 1993.)

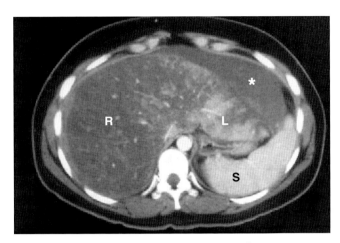

FIGURE 34-10 Abdominal CT-imaging performed postpartum in a woman with severe HELLP syndrome. A large subcapsular hematoma (*asterisk*) extends over the left lobe (*L*). The right lobe (*R*) has a heterogenous, hypodense appearance that represents widespread necrosis but with "sparing" of the left lobe—compare perfusion with normal spleen (*S*). (From Hay JE, Liver disease in pregnancy, *Hepatology*, vol. 47, no. 3, pp. 1067–1076. Copyright © 2008 American Association for the Study of Liver Diseases. Reproduced with permission of John Wiley & Sons, Inc.)

some cases, however, prompt surgical intervention may be lifesaving. Rinehart and co-workers (1999) reviewed 121 cases associated with preeclampsia, and the mortality rate was 30 percent. Rarely, liver transplant becomes necessary (Hunter and associates, 1995; Wicke and colleagues, 2004).

4. Acute fatty liver of pregnancy is sometimes confused with preeclampsia (Sibai, 2007). It too has an onset in late pregnancy, and often there is accompanying hypertension, elevated serum transaminase and creatinine levels, and thrombocytopenia (see Chap. 50, p. 1065).

Because there is no universally accepted definition of HELLP syndrome, its incidence varies by investigator, but when it is identified, the likelihood of hepatic hematoma and rupture is substantively increased. In a multicenter study, Haddad and colleagues (2000) described 183 women with HELLP syndrome of whom 40 percent had adverse outcomes including two maternal deaths. The incidence of subcapsular liver hematoma was 1.6 percent. Other complications included eclampsia—6 percent, placental abruption—10 percent, acute kidney injury—5 percent, and pulmonary edema—10 percent. Other serious complications included stroke, coagulopathy, acute respiratory distress syndrome, and sepsis.

There seems to be little doubt that women with preeclampsia complicated by the HELLP syndrome have worse outcomes than those without these findings. In their review of 693 women with HELLP syndrome, Keiser and co-workers (2009) reported that 10 percent had concurrent eclampsia. Sep and colleagues (2009) also described a significantly increased risk for complications in women with HELLP syndrome compared with those with "isolated preeclampsia." These included eclampsia—15 vs 4 percent, preterm birth—93 vs 78 percent, and perinatal mortality rate—9 vs 4 percent, respectively. They postulate that because of these marked clinical differences that the two disorders

likely have distinct pathogenesis. Given all of the variables contributing to the incidence and pathophysiology of preeclampsia as discussed on page 709, this is a reasonable conclusion. Sibai and Stella (2009) recently discussed some of these aspects under the rubric of "atypical preeclampsia-eclampsia."

Brain

Headaches and visual symptoms are common with severe preeclampsia, and associated convulsions define eclampsia. The earliest anatomical descriptions of brain involvement came from autopsy specimens, but CT- and MR-imaging and Doppler studies have added much new and important insight into cerebrovascular involvement.

Neuroanatomical Lesions

Most descriptions of the brain in eclamptic women are taken from eras when mortality rates were high. One consistent finding was that brain pathology accounted for only about a third of fatal cases such as the one shown in Figure 34-11. Most deaths were from pulmonary edema, and brain lesions were coincidental. Thus, although gross intracerebral hemorrhage was seen in up to 60 percent of eclamptic women, it was fatal in only half of these (Melrose, 1984; Richards and colleagues, 1988; Sheehan and Lynch, 1973). As shown in Figure 34-12, other principal lesions found at autopsy of eclamptic women were cortical and subcortical petechial hemorrhages. Other frequently described major lesions include subcortical edema, multiple nonhemorrhagic areas of "softening" throughout the brain, hemorrhagic areas in the white matter, and hemorrhage in the basal ganglia or pons, often with rupture into the ventricles. The classical microscopic vascular lesions consist of fibrinoid necrosis of the arterial wall and perivascular microinfarcts and hemorrhages.

Cerebrovascular Pathophysiology

Within the past several decades, clinical, pathological, and neuroimaging findings have led to two general theories to explain cerebral abnormalities associated with eclampsia. Importantly,

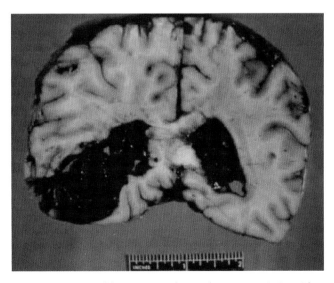

FIGURE 34-11 Fatal hypertensive hemorrhage in a primigravid woman with eclampsia.

endothelial cell dysfunction that characterizes the preeclampsia syndrome likely plays a key role in both:

1. The first theory suggests that in response to acute and severe hypertension, cerebrovascular overregulation leads to vasospasm (Trommer and associates, 1988). This presumption is based on the angiographic appearance of diffuse or multifocal segmental narrowings suggestive of vasospasm (Ito and co-workers, 1995). In this scheme, diminished cerebral blood flow is hypothesized to result in ischemia, cytotoxic edema, and eventually, tissue infarction. There is little objective evidence to support this.

2. The second theory is that sudden elevations in systemic blood pressure exceed the normal cerebrovascular autoregulatory capacity (Hauser and associates, 1988; Schwartz and co-workers, 2000). Regions of forced vasodilation and vasoconstriction develop, especially in arterial boundary zones. At the capillary level, disruption of the end-capillary pressure causes increased hydrostatic pressure, hyperperfusion, and extravasation of plasma and red cells through endothelial tight-junction openings leading to the accumulation of vasogenic edema. This theory is incomplete also because few eclamptic women have mean arterial pressures that exceed limits of autoregulation—approximately 160 mm Hg.

It seems reasonable to conclude that the most likely mechanism is a combination of the two. Thus, the preeclampsia syndrome has endothelial activation that is associated with an interendothelial cell leak that develops at blood pressure levels much lower than those causing vasogenic edema and has a loss of upper-limit autoregulation (Zeeman and colleagues, 2009b). This was described as the *reversible posterior leukoencephalopathy syndrome* by Hinchey and colleagues (1996). More recently, it is usually referred to as the *posterior reversible encephalopathy syndrome—PRES* (Narbone and associates, 2006).

Seizures consist of excessive release of excitatory neurotransmitters—especially glutamate; massive depolarization of network neurons; and bursts of action potentials (Meldrum, 2002). Clinical and experimental evidence suggest that extended seizures can cause significant brain injury and later brain dysfunction.

Cerebral Blood Flow

Autoregulation is the mechanism by which cerebral blood flow remains relatively constant despite alterations in cerebral perfusion pressure. In nonpregnant individuals, this mechanism protects the brain from hyperperfusion during mean arterial pressures up to 160 mm Hg. These are pressures far greater than those seen in all but a few women with eclampsia. Thus, to explain eclamptic seizures, it was theorized that autoregulation must be altered by pregnancy. And although species differences must be considered, studies by Cipolla and colleagues (2007,

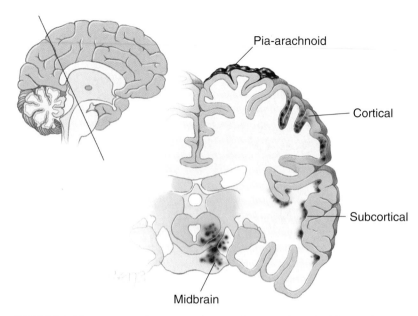

FIGURE 34-12 Composite illustration showing location of cerebral hemorrhages and petechiae in women with eclampsia. Insert shows the level of the brain from which the main image was constructed. (Data from Sheehan and Lynch, 1973.)

2009) have convincingly shown that autoregulation is unchanged across pregnancy in rats.

Using exacting MR imaging techniques, Zeeman and colleagues (2003) showed that cerebral blood flow across pregnancy is similar to nonpregnant values until it decreases significantly by 20 percent during the last trimester. Zeeman and co-workers (2004b) also documented significantly increased cerebral blood flow in women with severe preeclampsia compared with that of normotensive pregnant controls. Taken together, these findings suggest that eclampsia occurs when cerebral hyperperfusion forces capillary fluid interstitially because of endothelial activation and leads to perivascular edema seen with the preeclampsia syndrome. In this regard, eclampsia has similarities to PRES.

Clinical Manifestations

There are several neurological manifestations of the preeclampsia syndrome. Each signifies severe involvement and requires immediate attention:

1. *Headache and scotomata* are thought to arise from cerebrovascular hyperperfusion that has a predilection for the occipital lobes. According to Sibai (2005) and Zwart and associates (2008), 50 to 75 percent of women have headaches and 20 to 30 percent have visual changes preceding eclamptic convulsions. The headaches may be mild to severe and intermittent to constant. In our experiences, they are unique in that they usually improve after magnesium sulfate infusion is initiated.

2. Convulsions are diagnostic for eclampsia.

3. *Blindness* is rare with preeclampsia alone, but it complicates eclamptic convulsions in up to 15 percent of women (Cunningham and colleagues, 1995). Blindness has been reported to develop up to a week or more following

delivery (Chambers and Cain, 2004). There are at least two types of blindness as discussed subsequently.

4. *Generalized cerebral edema* may develop and is usually manifest by mental status changes that vary from confusion to coma. This situation is particularly dangerous because fatal supratentorial herniation may result.

Neuroimaging Studies. With CT imaging, localized hypodense lesions at the gray-white matter junction, primarily in the parieto-occipital lobes, are typically found in eclampsia. Such lesions may also be seen in the frontal and inferior temporal lobes, the basal ganglia, and thalamus (Brown and colleagues, 1988). The spectrum of brain involvement is wide, and increasing involvement can be identified with CT imaging. Involvement of the occipital lobes or diffuse cerebral edema may create symptoms such as blindness, lethargy, and confusion (Cunningham and Twickler, 2000). In the latter cases, widespread edema shows as a marked compression or even obliteration of the cerebral ventricles. Such women may develop signs of impending life-threatening transtentorial herniation.

A number of MR imaging acquisitions are used to study eclamptic women. Common findings are hyperintense T2 lesions in the subcortical and cortical regions of the parietal and occipital lobes, with occasional involvement of basal ganglia and/or the brainstem (Zeeman and associates, 2004a). An example demonstrating involvement of the occipital lobes is shown in Figure 34-13. Although these PRES lesions are almost universal in women with eclampsia, their incidence in women with preeclampsia is less frequent. They are more likely to be found in women who have severe disease and who have neurological symptoms (Schwartz and co-workers, 2000). And although usually reversible, a fourth of these hyperintense lesions represent cerebral infarctions that have persistent findings (Loureiro and associates, 2003; Zeeman and co-workers, 2004a).

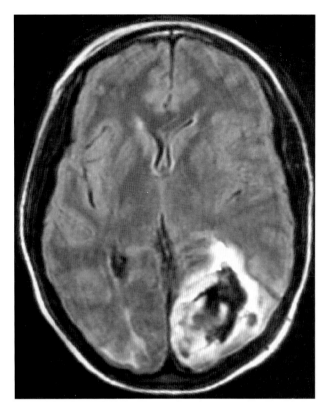

FIGURE 34-14 Cranial magnetic resonance imaging performed 3 days postpartum in a woman with eclampsia and HELLP syndrome. Neurovisual defects persisted at 1 year causing job disability. (From Murphy and Ayazifar, 2005, with permission.)

Visual Changes and Blindness

Scotomata, blurred vision, or diplopia are common with severe preeclampsia and eclampsia. These usually abate with magnesium sulfate therapy and/or lowered blood pressure. Blindness is less common, is usually reversible, and may arise from three potential areas. These are the visual cortex of the occipital lobe, the lateral geniculate nuclei, and retina. In the retina, lesions may include ischemia, infarction, and detachment.

Occipital blindness is also called *amaurosis*—from the Greek *dimming*. Affected women usually have evidence of extensive occipital lobe vasogenic edema on imaging studies. Of 15 women cared for at Parkland Hospital, blindness lasted from 4 hours to 8 days, but it resolved completely in all cases (Cunningham and associates, 1995). Rarely, extensive cerebral infarctions may result in total or partial visual defects (Fig. 34-14).

Blindness from retinal lesions caused by either retinal ischemia or infarction is also called *Purtscher retinopathy* (Fig. 34-15). Moseman and Shelton (2002) described a woman with permanent blindness due to a combination of infarctions in the retina as well as in the lateral geniculate nucleus bilaterally. In many cases of eclampsia-associated blindness, visual acuity improves, but if caused by retinal artery occlusion, vision may be permanently impaired (Blodi and associates, 1990; Lara-Torre and colleagues, 2002).

Finally, *retinal detachment* may also cause altered vision, although it is usually unilateral and seldom causes total visual loss. Occasionally, it coexists with cortical edema and accompanying visual defects. Asymptomatic serous retinal detachment is

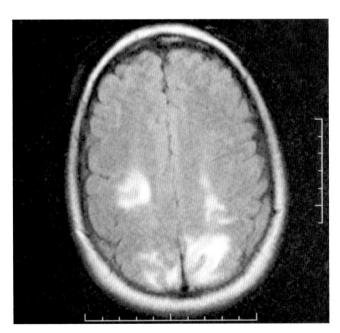

FIGURE 34-13 Magnetic resonance imaging in a nulliparous woman with eclampsia. Multilobe T2-flair high-signal lesions are apparent. (Courtesy of Dr. Gerda Zeeman.)

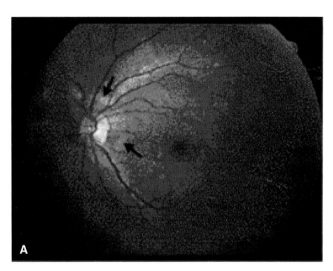
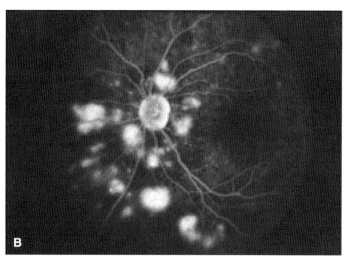

FIGURE 34-15 Purtscher retinopathy caused by choroidal ischemia in preeclampsia syndrome. **A.** Ophthalmoscopy shows scattered yellowish, opaque lesions of the retina (*arrows*). **B.** The late phase of fluorescein angiography shows areas of intense hyperfluorescence representing pooling of extravasated dye. (From Lam and Chan, 2001, with permission.)

relatively common and is obvious by examination (Saito and Tano, 1998). Surgical treatment is seldom indicated, the prognosis generally is good, and vision usually returns to normal within a week.

Cerebral Edema

Clinical manifestations suggesting widespread cerebral edema are worrisome. During a 13-year period, 10 of 175 women with eclampsia at Parkland Hospital were diagnosed with symptomatic cerebral edema (Cunningham and Twickler, 2000). Symptoms ranged from lethargy, confusion, and blurred vision to obtundation and coma. In some cases, symptoms waxed and waned. Mental status changes generally correlated with the degree of involvement seen with CT and MR imaging studies. Three women with generalized edema were comatose and had imaging findings of impending transtentorial herniation. One of these died from herniation.

Clinically, we have observed that these women are very susceptible to sudden and severe blood pressure elevations, which acutely worsen the widespread vasogenic edema. Thus, careful blood pressure control is essential. Consideration is given for treatment with mannitol or dexamethasone.

Long-Term Neurocognitive Sequelae

Women with eclampsia have been shown to suffer excessive cognitive decline when studied 5 to 10 years following an eclamptic pregnancy. This is discussed further on page 749.

Uteroplacental Perfusion

Defects in trophoblastic invasion and placentation germane to development of the preeclampsia syndrome and fetal-growth restriction were discussed on page 710. And of immense clinical importance, compromised uteroplacental perfusion from vasospasm is almost certainly a major culprit in the genesis of increased perinatal morbidity and mortality rates. Thus, measurement of uterine, intervillous, and placental blood flow would

likely be informative. Attempts to assess these in humans have been hampered by several obstacles that include inaccessibility of the placenta, the complexity of its venous effluent, and the need for radioisotopes or invasive techniques that are unsuitable for human research.

Measurement of uterine artery blood flow velocity has been used to estimate resistance to uteroplacental blood flow (see Chap. 16, p. 364). Vascular resistance is estimated by comparing arterial systolic and diastolic velocity waveforms. By the completion of placentation, impedance to uterine artery blood flow is markedly decreased. However, with abnormal placentation, abnormally high resistance persists (Ghidini and Locatelli, 2008). Earlier studies were done to assess this by measuring peak systolic:diastolic velocity ratios from uterine and umbilical arteries in preeclamptic pregnancies. The results were interpreted as showing that in some cases, but certainly not all, there was increased resistance (Fleischer and colleagues, 1986; Trudinger and Cook, 1990). Another Doppler waveform—uterine artery "notching"—has been reported to be associated with subsequent increased risks for preeclampsia or growth-restricted infants (Groom and co-workers, 2009).

Matijevic and Johnson (1999) measured resistance in *uterine spiral arteries*. Impedance was higher in peripheral than in central vessels. This has been termed a "ring-like" distribution. Mean resistance was higher in all women with preeclampsia compared with that in normotensive controls. Ong and colleagues (2003) used magnetic resonance imaging and other techniques to assess placental perfusion ex vivo in myometrial arteries removed from women with preeclampsia or fetal-growth restriction. They confirmed that in both conditions myometrial arteries exhibited endothelium-dependent vasodilatory response. Moreover, other pregnancy conditions such as fetal-growth restriction are also associated with increased resistance (Urban and co-workers, 2007).

Despite the above findings, evidence for compromised uteroplacental circulation is found in only a minority of women who go on to develop preeclampsia. Indeed, when preeclampsia develops during the third trimester, only a third of women with severe disease have abnormal uterine artery velocimetry (Li and colleagues, 2005). And in a study of 50 women with HELLP syndrome, only a third had abnormal uterine artery waveforms (Bush and associates, 2001). In general, the extent of abnormal waveforms correlates with severity of fetal involvement (Ghidini and Locatelli, 2008; Groom and colleagues, 2009).

PREDICTION AND PREVENTION

Prediction

Measurement in early pregnancy—or across pregnancy—of a variety of biological, biochemical, and biophysical markers implicated in the pathophysiology of preeclampsia has been proposed to predict its development. Attempts have been made to identify early markers of faulty placentation, impaired placental perfusion, endothelial cell activation and dysfunction, and activation of coagulation. For the most, these have resulted in testing strategies with poor sensitivity and with poor positive-predictive value for preeclampsia (Conde-Agudelo and colleagues, 2009; Lindheimer and associates, 2008b; Sibai, 2003). Currently there are no screening tests that are reliable, valid, and economical. There are, however, combinations of tests, some yet to be adequately evaluated, that may be promising (Levine and Lindheimer, 2009; Poon and co-workers, 2009). A major goal of the Maternal-Fetal Medicine Units Network (MFMU) is to identify such techniques.

The list of predictive factors evaluated during the last three decades is legion. Some are listed in Table 34-5, which is by no means all inclusive. Conde-Agudelo and associates (2009) have recently provided a thorough review of many of these testing strategies.

Placental Perfusion/Vascular Resistance-Related Tests

Most of these are cumbersome and time consuming.

Provocative Pressor Tests. There are three tests extensively evaluated to assess blood pressure increase in response to a stimulus. The "roll-over test" measures the hypertensive response in women at 28 to 32 weeks who are resting in the left lateral decubitus position and then "roll over" to assume a supine position. The *isometric exercise test* employs the same principle by squeezing a handball. The *angiotensin II infusion test* is performed by giving incrementally increasing doses intravenously, and the hypertensive response is quantified. In their updated meta-analysis, Conde-Agudelo and associates (2009) found sensitivities of all three tests to range from 55 to 70 percent with specificities of approximately 85 percent.

Uterine Artery Doppler Velocimetry. Faulty trophoblastic invasion of the spiral arteries, which is depicted in Figure 34-2, results in diminished placental perfusion and upstream increased uterine artery resistance. Increased uterine artery velocimetry determined by Doppler ultrasound—in the first or middle trimester—should provide indirect evidence of this process and thus serve as a predictive test for preeclampsia (Gebb and associates, 2009a, b; Groom and co-workers, 2009). As described on page 724 and in Chapter 16 (p. 364), increased flow resistance results in an abnormal waveform represented by an increased diastolic notch. A number of flow velocity waveforms—alone or in combination—have been investigated for preeclampsia prediction. At this time, none is suitable for clinical use (Conde-Agudelo and associates, 2009).

Pulse Wave Analysis. Like the uterine artery, finger arterial pulse "stiffness" is an indicator of cardiovascular risk. Investigators have evaluated its usefulness in preeclampsia prediction (Vollebregt and colleagues, 2009).

TABLE 34-5. Predictive Tests for Development of the Preeclampsia Syndrome

Testing Related To:	Examples
Placental perfusion/ vascular resistance	Roll-over test, isometric handgrip or cold pressor test, angiotensin-II infusion, midtrimester mean arterial pressure, platelet angiotensin-II binding, renin, 24-hour ambulatory blood pressure monitoring, uterine artery or fetal transcranial Doppler velocimetry
Fetal-placental unit endocrine dysfunction	Human chorionic gonadotropin (hCG), alpha-fetoprotein (AFP), estriol, pregnancy-associated protein A (PAPP A), inhibin A, activin A, placental protein 13, corticotropin-releasing hormone
Renal dysfunction	Serum uric acid, microalbuminuria, urinary calcium or kallikrein, microtransferrinuria, N-acetyl-β-glucosaminidase
Endothelial dysfunction/ oxidant stress	Platelet count and activation, fibronectin, endothelial adhesion molecules, prostaglandin, thromboxane, C-reactive protein, cytokines, endothelin, neurokinin B, homocysteine, lipids, antiphospholipid antibodies, plasminogen activator-inhibitor (PAI), leptin, p-selectin, angiogenic factors to include placental growth factor (PlGF), vascular endothelial growth factor (VEGF), fms-like tyrosine kinase receptor-1 (sFlt-1), endoglin
Others/miscellaneous	Antithrombin-III(AT-3), atrial natriuretic peptide (ANP), β₂-microglobulin, genetic markers, free fetal DNA, serum proteonomic markers

Adapted from Conde-Agudelo and associates (2009).

Fetal-Placental Unit Endocrine Dysfunction

A number of serum analytes that have been proposed to help predict preeclampsia are shown in Table 34-5. Newer ones are continuously added (Jeyabalan, 2009; Kanasaki, 2008; Kenny, 2009, and all their associates). Many of these gained widespread use in the 1980s to identify fetal malformations and were also found to be associated with other pregnancy abnormalities such as neural-tube defects and aneuploidy (see Chap. 13, p. 292). Although touted as such, in general, none of these tests has been shown to be clinically beneficial for hypertension prediction.

Renal Dysfunction-Related Tests

Some of the earliest studies to find predictive tests were related to preeclampsia-induced renal dysfunction.

Serum Uric Acid. One of the earliest laboratory manifestations of preeclampsia is hyperuricemia (Powers and associates, 2006). It likely results from reduced uric acid clearance from diminished glomerular filtration, increased tubular reabsorption, and decreased secretion (Lindheimer and colleagues, 2008a). It is used by some to define preeclampsia, but Cnossen and associates (2006) reported that its sensitivity ranged from 0 to 55 percent and specificity from 77 to 95 percent.

Microalbuminuria. A number of investigators have evaluated the potential value of microalbuminuria as a predictive test for preeclampsia. As reviewed by Conde-Agudelo and associates (2009), sensitivities ranging from 7 to 90 percent and specificities between 29 and 97 percent indicate a poor clinical predictive value. A recent study by Poon and colleagues (2008) likewise found unacceptable sensitivity and specificity for urine albumin:creatinine ratios.

Endothelial Dysfunction and Oxidant Stress-Related Tests

As discussed on page 713, overwhelming evidence indicates that endothelial activation is a major participant in the pathophysiology of the preeclampsia syndrome. As a result, compounds such as those listed in Table 34-5 are found in circulating blood of affected women, and some have been assessed for their predictive value.

Fibronectins. These high-molecular-weight glycoproteins serve a variety of cellular functions that include adhesion and morphology, migration, phagocytosis, and hemostasis (Chavarria and co-workers, 2002). Fibronectins are released from endothelial cells and extracellular matrix following endothelial injury. More than 20 years ago, Stubbs and colleagues (1984) reported that plasma concentrations were elevated in women with preeclampsia. Following their recent systematic review, Leeflang and associates (2007) concluded that neither cellular nor total fibronectin was clinically useful to predict preeclampsia.

Coagulation Activation. Thrombocytopenia and platelet dysfunction are integral features of preeclampsia as discussed on page 717. Platelet activation causes increased destruction and decreased concentrations. Mean platelet volume increases because of young platelet age (Kenny and colleagues, 2009). Although markers of coagulation activation are increased, the substantive overlap with levels in normotensive pregnant women prevents their predictive use.

Oxidative Stress. Increased levels of lipid peroxides coupled with decreased antioxidant activity have raised the possibility that markers of oxidative stress might predict preeclampsia (Walsh, 1994). For example, malondialdehyde is a marker of lipid peroxidation. Other markers are a variety of pro-oxidants or potentiators of pro-oxidants, including iron, transferrin, and ferritin; blood lipids, including triglycerides, free fatty acids, and lipoproteins; and antioxidants, including ascorbic acid and vitamin E (Bainbridge, 2005; Hubel, 1996; Powers, 2000, and all their colleagues). They are not predictive, but treatment to prevent preeclampsia with some of these has been studied as discussed on page 727.

Hyperhomocysteinemia causes oxidative stress and endothelial cell dysfunction and is found in preeclampsia. Although women with elevated serum homocysteine levels at midpregnancy had a three- to fourfold risk of preeclampsia, these tests have not shown to be clinically useful predictors (D'Anna, 2004; Mignini, 2005; Zeeman, 2003, and all their colleagues).

Angiogenic Factors. As discussed on page 714, evidence has accrued that an imbalance between proangiogenic and antiangiogenic factors is related to the pathogenesis of preeclampsia. Serum levels of proangiogenic factors, such as vascular endothelial growth factor (VEGF) and placental growth factor (PlGF), begin to decrease before clinical preeclampsia develops. And, recall as shown in Figure 34-4 that at the same time, levels of some antiangiogenic factors such as soluble fms-like tyrosine kinase 1 (sFlt-1) and soluble endoglin (sEng) are increased (Maynard and colleagues, 2008). Because of these findings, measurement of their plasma levels may serve as predictive tests for preeclampsia.

Conde-Agudelo and associates (2009) recently reviewed the predictive accuracy of some of these factors for severe preeclampsia. Sensitivities for all cases of preeclampsia ranged from 59 to 100 percent and specificity from 43 to 100 percent. The predictive accuracy was higher for early-onset preeclampsia.

These preliminary results suggest a clinical role for preeclampsia prediction. However, until better substantiated, their clinical usefulness is not recommended (Widmer and colleagues, 2007). Automated assays are being evaluated (Sunderji and associates, 2009). The World Health Organization began a multicenter trial in 2008 to evaluate these factors with plans to enroll 12,000 women.

Free Fetal DNA

Using polymerase chain reaction, free fetal DNA can be detected in maternal plasma (Lo and colleagues, 1997). Holzgreve and associates (1998) reported that fetal-maternal cell trafficking is increased in pregnancies complicated by preeclampsia. It is hypothesized that free DNA is released by accelerated apoptosis of cytotrophoblasts (DiFederico and colleagues, 1999). From their review, Conde-Agudelo and associates (2009) concluded that free fetal DNA quantification is not useful for prediction purposes.

TABLE 34-6. Some Methods to Prevent Preeclampsia That Have Been Evaluated in Randomized Trials

Dietary manipulation—low-salt diet, calcium supplementation, fish oil supplementation

Cardiovascular drugs—diuretics, antihypertensive drugs

Antioxidants—ascorbic acid (vitamin C), α-tocopherol (vitamin E)

Antithrombotic drugs—low-dose aspirin, aspirin/dipyridamole, aspirin + heparin, aspirin + ketanserin

Modified from Sibai and Cunningham (2009).

Prevention

A variety of strategies used to prevent or modify the severity of preeclampsia have been evaluated. Some are listed in Table 34-6. In general, none of these has been found to be clinically efficacious.

Dietary Manipulation

A favorite of many theorists and faddists for centuries, dietary "treatment" for preeclampsia has produced some interesting abuses as chronicled by Chesley (1978).

Low-Salt Diet. One of the earliest research efforts to prevent preeclampsia was salt restriction (De Snoo, 1937). This interdiction was followed by years of inappropriate diuretic therapy, after which these practices were discarded. Ironically, it was not until relatively recently that the first randomized trial was done by Knuist and colleagues (1998), who showed that a sodium-restricted diet was ineffective in preventing preeclampsia in 361 women.

Calcium Supplementation. Studies performed in the 1980s outside the United States showed that women with low dietary calcium intake were at significantly increased risk for gestational hypertension (Belizan and Villar, 1980; López-Jaramillo and associates, 1989; Marya and colleagues, 1987). An impressive number of trials have since been performed including one by the National Institute of Child Health and Human Development that included more than 4500 nulliparous women (Levine and colleagues, 1997). In aggregate, these trials have shown that unless women are calcium deficient, supplementation has no salutary effects (Sibai and Cunningham, 2009).

Fish Oil Supplementation. Cardioprotective fatty acids found in some fatty fishes are plentiful in diets of Scandinavians and American Eskimos. The most common dietary sources are EPA—eicosapentaenoic acid—and ALA—alpha-linoleic acid. With proclamations that supplementation with these fatty acids would prevent inflammatory-mediated atherogenesis, it was not a quantum leap to posit that they might prevent preeclampsia syndrome. Unfortunately, randomized trials conducted thus far have shown no such benefits (Makrides, 2006; Olafsdottir, 2006; Olsen, 2000, and all their colleagues).

Antihypertensive Drugs

Because of the putative effects of sodium restriction, it was not surprising that diuretic therapy became popular with the introduction of chlorothiazide in 1957 (Finnerty and colleagues, 1958; Flowers and co-workers, 1962). In their recent meta-analysis, Churchill and colleagues (2007) summarized nine randomized trials that included more than 7000 pregnant women. They found that women given diuretics had a decreased incidence of edema and hypertension, but not of preeclampsia.

Because women with chronic hypertension are at high risk for preeclampsia, several randomized trials—only a few placebo-controlled—have been done to evaluate various antihypertensive drugs to reduce the incidence of superimposed preeclampsia. A critical analysis of these trials failed to demonstrate such a reduction (Sibai and Cunningham, 2009).

Antioxidants

There are inferential data that an imbalance between oxidant and antioxidant activity may have an important role in the pathogenesis of preeclampsia (see p. 726). Two naturally occurring antioxidants—vitamins C and E—may decrease such oxidation. Moreover, women who developed preeclampsia were found to have reduced plasma levels of these two vitamins (Raijmakers and associates, 2004). Thus, dietary supplementation was proposed as a method to improve the oxidative capability of women at risk for preeclampsia.

There have now been a number of quality randomized studies to evaluate this possibility in women at high risk for preeclampsia (Poston, 2006; Rumbold, 2006; Villar, 2007, and all their co-workers). Most recently, Roberts (2009) reported the Maternal-Fetal Medicine Units Network trial that included almost 10,000 low-risk nulliparas. None of these studies showed reduction of preeclampsia in women given antioxidant vitamins compared with those given placebo.

Antithrombotic Agents

There are ample theoretical reasons that antithrombotic agents might reduce the incidence of preeclampsia. As discussed on page 713, the syndrome is characterized by vasospasm, endothelial cell dysfunction, and activation of platelets and the coagulation-hemostasis system. Moreover, prostaglandin imbalance(s) may be operative, and other sequelae of preeclampsia include placental infarction and spiral artery thrombosis.

Low-Dose Aspirin. In oral doses of 50 to 150 mg daily, aspirin effectively inhibits platelet thromboxane A2 biosynthesis with minimal effects on vascular prostacyclin production (Wallenburg and associates, 1986). But results from clinical trials have shown limited benefits. For example, results shown in Table 34-7 are from the Maternal-Fetal Medicine Units Network, and none of the outcomes was significantly improved. The Paris Collaborative Group performed a meta-analysis of the efficacy and safety of antiplatelet agents—predominantly aspirin—to

TABLE 34-7. Maternal-Fetal Medicine Units Network Trial of Low-Dose Aspirin in Women at High Risk for Preeclampsia

		Preeclampsia (Percent)[a]	
Risk Factors	No.	Aspirin	Placebo
Normotensive, no proteinuria	1613	14.5	17.7
Proteinuria plus hypertension	119	31.7	22.0
Proteinuria only	48	25.0	33.3
Hypertension only	723	24.8	25.0
Insulin-dependent diabetes	462	18.3	21.6
Chronic hypertension	763	26.0	24.6
Multifetal gestation	678	11.5	15.9
Previous preeclampsia	600	16.7	19.0

[a]No statistical difference for any comparison between groups.
Data from Caritis and associates (1998).

prevent preeclampsia (Askie and colleagues, 2007). They included 31 randomized trials involving 32,217 women. For women assigned to receive antiplatelet agents, the relative risk of preeclampsia was decreased significantly by 10 percent for development of preeclampsia, superimposed preeclampsia, preterm delivery, or any pregnancy with an adverse outcome. The number-needed-to-treat (NNT), however, was high. Because of these marginal benefits, it seems reasonable to individualize use of low-dose aspirin to prevent recurrent preeclampsia (Sibai and Cunningham, 2009).

Low-Dose Aspirin plus Heparin. Because of the high prevalence of placental thrombotic lesions found with severe preeclampsia, there have been several observational trials to evaluate heparin treatment for affected women. Sergis and associates (2006) reviewed effects of prophylaxis with low-molecular-weight heparin plus low-dose aspirin on pregnancy outcomes in women with a history of severe early-onset preeclampsia and low-birthweight infants. They reported better pregnancy outcomes in women given low-molecular-weight heparin plus low-dose aspirin compared with those given low-dose aspirin alone. At this time, it is not possible to make recommendations from these observational data.

MANAGEMENT

Pregnancy complicated by gestational hypertension is managed according to severity, gestational age, and presence of preeclampsia. Tenets of management, as emphasized earlier, also take into consideration endothelial cell injury and multi-organ dysfunction caused by the preeclampsia syndrome.

Preeclampsia cannot always be diagnosed definitively. Thus, given the explosive nature of the disorder, both the American College of Obstetricians and Gynecologists (2002a) and the National High Blood Pressure Education Program (NHBPEP) Working Group (2000) recommend more frequent prenatal visits, even if preeclampsia is only "suspected." *Increases in systolic and diastolic blood pressure can be either normal physiological*

changes or signs of developing pathology. Increased surveillance permits more prompt recognition of ominous changes in blood pressure, critical laboratory findings, and development of clinical signs and symptoms.

The basic management objectives for any pregnancy complicated by preeclampsia are:

1. Termination of pregnancy with the least possible trauma to mother and fetus
2. Birth of an infant who subsequently thrives
3. Complete restoration of health to the mother.

In many women with preeclampsia, especially those at or near term, all three objectives are served equally well by induction of labor. *One of the most important clinical questions for successful management is precise knowledge of fetal age.*

Early Diagnosis of Preeclampsia

Traditionally, the frequency of prenatal visits is increased during the third trimester, and this aids early detection of preeclampsia. Women without overt hypertension, but in whom early developing preeclampsia is suspected during routine prenatal visits, are seen more frequently. The protocol used successfully for many years at Parkland Hospital for women with new-onset diastolic blood pressures > 80 mm Hg but < 90 mm Hg or with sudden abnormal weight gain of more than 2 pounds per week includes return visits minimally at 7-day intervals, and preferably at 3- to 4-day intervals. Outpatient surveillance is continued unless overt hypertension, proteinuria, headache, visual disturbances, or epigastric discomfort supervene. Women with overt new-onset hypertension—either diastolic pressures 90 mm Hg or greater or systolic pressures 140 mm Hg or greater—are admitted for 2 to 3 days to determine if the increase is due to preeclampsia and if so, to evaluate its severity. Women with persistent severe disease are observed closely, and many are delivered. Conversely, women with apparently mild disease can often be managed as outpatients, although we have a low threshold for continued hospitalization in the nullipara.

Evaluation

Hospitalization is considered at least initially for women with new-onset hypertension, especially if there is persistent or worsening hypertension or development of proteinuria. A systematic evaluation is instituted to include the following:

- Detailed examination followed by daily scrutiny for clinical findings such as headache, visual disturbances, epigastric pain, and rapid weight gain
- Weight determined daily
- Analysis for proteinuria on admittance and at least every 2 days thereafter
- Blood pressure readings in the sitting position with an appropriate-size cuff every 4 hours, except between 2400 and 0600 unless previous readings had become elevated
- Measurements of plasma or serum creatinine and liver transaminase levels, and hemogram to include platelet quantification. The frequency of testing is determined by the severity of hypertension. Some recommend measurement of serum uric acid and lactic acid dehydrogenase levels as well as coagulation studies, but studies have called into question the value of these tests (Conde-Agudelo, 2009; Cnossen, 2006; Thangaratinam, 2006, and all their colleagues).
- Evaluation of fetal size and well-being and amnionic fluid volume either clinically or using sonography.

Goals of such management include early identification of worsening preeclampsia and development of a management scheme that includes a plan for timely delivery. If any of these observations lead to a diagnosis of severe preeclampsia as previously defined by the criteria in Table 34-2, further management is subsequently described.

Reduced physical activity throughout much of the day is likely beneficial. Absolute bed rest is not necessary. Ample protein and calories should be included in the diet, and sodium and fluid intake should not be limited or forced. Further management depends on: (1) severity of preeclampsia, (2) gestational age, and (3) condition of the cervix.

Fortunately, many cases are sufficiently mild and near enough to term that they can be managed conservatively until labor commences spontaneously or until the cervix becomes favorable for labor induction. Complete abatement of all signs and symptoms, however, is uncommon until after delivery. *Almost certainly, the underlying disease persists until after delivery!*

Consideration for Delivery

Termination of pregnancy is the only cure for preeclampsia. Headache, visual disturbances, or epigastric pain is indicative that convulsions may be imminent, and oliguria is another ominous sign. Severe preeclampsia demands anticonvulsant and usually antihypertensive therapy followed by delivery. Treatment is identical to that described subsequently for eclampsia. The prime objectives are to forestall convulsions, to prevent intracranial hemorrhage and serious damage to other vital organs, and to deliver a healthy infant.

When the fetus is preterm, the tendency is to temporize in the hope that a few more weeks in utero will reduce the risk of neonatal death or serious morbidity from prematurity. As dis-

cussed, such a policy certainly is justified in milder cases. Assessments of fetal well-being and placental function are performed, especially when the fetus is immature. Most recommend frequent performance of various tests to assess fetal well-being as described by the American College of Obstetricians and Gynecologists (1999). These include the *nonstress test* or the *biophysical profile* (see Chap. 15, pp. 337 and 341). Measurement of the lecithin-sphingomyelin (L/S) ratio in amnionic fluid may provide evidence of lung maturity (see Chap. 29, p. 606).

With moderate or severe preeclampsia that does not improve after hospitalization, delivery is usually advisable for the welfare of both mother and fetus. Labor induction is carried out, usually with preinduction cervical ripening with a prostaglandin or osmotic dilator (see Chap. 22, p. 501). Whenever it appears that induction almost certainly will not succeed, or attempts have failed, cesarean delivery is indicated for more severe cases.

For a woman near term, with a soft, partially effaced cervix, even milder degrees of preeclampsia probably carry more risk to the mother and her fetus-infant than does induction of labor. However, Barton and colleagues (2009) have recently quantified excessive neonatal morbidity in women delivered before 38 weeks despite having stable mild nonproteinuric gestational hypertension.

Elective Cesarean Delivery

Once severe preeclampsia is diagnosed, labor induction and vaginal delivery have traditionally been considered ideal. Temporization with an immature fetus is considered subsequently. Several concerns, including an unfavorable cervix, a perceived sense of urgency because of the severity of preeclampsia, and the need to coordinate neonatal intensive care, have led some to advocate cesarean delivery. Alexander and colleagues (1999) reviewed 278 singleton liveborns weighing 750 to 1500 g delivered of women with severe preeclampsia at Parkland Hospital. In half of the women, labor was induced, and the remainder underwent cesarean delivery without labor. Induction was successful in accomplishing vaginal delivery in a third, and it was not harmful to the very-low-birthweight infants. Alanis and associates (2008) reported similar observations. In their recent systematic review, Le Ray and co-workers (2009) confirmed these conclusions.

Hospitalization versus Outpatient Management

For women with mild to moderate stable hypertension—whether or not preeclampsia has been confirmed—continued surveillance in the hospital, at home for some reliable patients, or through a day-care unit is carried out. At least intuitively, reduced physical activity throughout much of the day seems beneficial. A number of observational studies and randomized trials have addressed the benefits of inpatient care and outpatient management.

Somewhat related, Abenhaim and colleagues (2008) reported a retrospective cohort study of 677 women hospitalized for bed rest because of threatened preterm delivery. When outcomes of these women were compared with those of the general obstetrical population, bed rest was associated with a significantly reduced risk of developing preeclampsia—RR 0.27 (CI 0.16–0.48). In a review of two small randomized trials totaling 106 women at high risk for preeclampsia, prophylactic bed rest 4 to 6 hours daily at home was successful in significantly lowering the incidence of preeclampsia but not gestational hypertension (Meher and Duely, 2006).

These and other observations support the claim that restricted activity alters the underlying pathophysiology of the preeclampsia syndrome. As for "complete bed rest," this is likely unachievable because of the severe restrictions it places on the otherwise well woman, and it also predisposes to thromboembolism (Knight and co-workers, 2007).

High-Risk Pregnancy Unit

An inpatient antepartum unit was established in 1973 at Parkland Hospital by Dr. Peggy Whalley in large part to provide care for women with hypertensive disorders. Initial results from this unit were reported by Hauth (1976) and Gilstrap (1978) and their colleagues. Most women hospitalized have a beneficial response characterized by disappearance or improvement of hypertension. *These women are not "cured," and nearly 90 percent have recurrent hypertension before or during labor.* By the end of 2006, more than 9000 nulliparous women with mild to moderate early-onset hypertension during pregnancy had been managed successfully in this unit. Provider costs—*not* charges—for this relatively simple physical facility, modest nursing care, no drugs other than iron and folate supplements, and few essential laboratory tests are minimal compared with the cost of neonatal intensive care for a preterm infant.

Home Healthcare

Many clinicians believe that further hospitalization is not warranted if hypertension abates within a few days, and this has legitimized third-party payers to deny hospital reimbursement. Consequently, most women with mild to moderate hypertension are managed at home. Outpatient management may continue as long as the disease does not worsen and if fetal jeopardy is not suspected. Sedentary activity throughout the greater part of the day is recommended. These women are instructed in detail to report symptoms. Home blood pressure and urine protein monitoring or frequent evaluations by a visiting nurse may prove beneficial. Lo and co-workers (2002) cautioned about the use of certain automated home blood pressure monitors that may fail to detect severe hypertension.

In an observational study by Barton and colleagues (2002), 1182 nulliparous women with mild gestational hypertension—20 percent had proteinuria—were managed with home health care. Their mean gestational ages were 32 to 33 weeks at enrollment and 36 to 37 weeks at the time of delivery. Severe preeclampsia developed in approximately 20 percent, about 3 percent developed HELLP syndrome, and two women had eclampsia. Perinatal outcomes were generally good. In approximately 20 percent, there was fetal-growth restriction, and the perinatal mortality rate was 4.2 per 1000.

Several prospective studies have been designed to compare continued hospitalization with either home healthcare or a day-

care unit. In a pilot study from Parkland Hospital, Horsager and associates (1995) randomly assigned 72 nulliparas with new-onset hypertension from 27 to 37 weeks either to continued hospitalization or to outpatient care. In all of these women, proteinuria had receded to less than 500 mg per day when randomized. Outpatient management included daily blood pressure monitoring by the patient or her family. Weight and spot urine protein determinations were evaluated three times weekly. A home health nurse visited twice weekly, and the women were seen weekly in the clinic. Perinatal outcomes were similar in each group. The only significant difference was that women in the home care group developed severe preeclampsia significantly more frequently than hospitalized women—42 versus 25 percent.

A larger randomized trial reported by Crowther and co-workers (1992) included 218 women with mild gestational nonproteinuric hypertension. After evaluation, half remained hospitalized, whereas the other half was managed as outpatients. As shown in Table 34-8, the mean duration of hospitalization was 22.2 days for women with inpatient management compared with only 6.5 days in the home care group. Preterm delivery before 34 and before 37 weeks was increased twofold in the outpatient group, but maternal and infant outcomes otherwise were similar.

Day-Care Unit

Another approach, now common in European countries, is day care. This approach has been evaluated by several investigators. In the study by Tuffnell and associates (1992), 54 women with hypertension after 26 weeks were assigned to either day care or routine management (Table 34-8). Hospitalizations, progression to overt preeclampsia, and labor inductions were significantly increased in the routine management group. Turnbull and co-workers (2004) enrolled 395 women who were randomly assigned to either day care or inpatient management (Table 34-8). Almost 95 percent had mild to moderate hypertension—288 without proteinuria and 86 with ≥ 1+ proteinuria. Fetal outcomes overall were good, there were no neonatal deaths, and none of the women developed eclampsia or HELLP syndrome. Surprisingly, costs for either scheme were not significantly different. Perhaps not surprisingly, general satisfaction favored day care.

Antepartum Hospitalization versus Outpatient Care

From the above, it can be seen that either inpatient or close outpatient management is appropriate for the woman with mild de novo hypertension, with or without nonsevere preeclampsia. Most of these studies were carried out in academic centers with dedicated management teams. That said, the key to success is close follow-up and a conscientious patient.

Antihypertensive Therapy for Mild to Moderate Hypertension

The use of antihypertensive drugs in attempts to prolong pregnancy or modify perinatal outcomes in pregnancies complicated by various types and severities of hypertensive disorders

TABLE 34-8. Randomized Clinical Trials Comparing Hospitalization versus Routine Care for Women with Mild Gestational Hypertension or Preeclampsia

Study Groups	N	Para$_0$ (%)	Chronic Htn (%)	EGA (wks)	Prot (%)	EGA (wks)	<37 wks (%)	<34 wks (%)	Mean Hosp (d)	Mean BW (g)	SGA (%)	PMR (%)
Crowther et al (1992)	218[a]											
Hospitalization	110	13	14	35.3	0	38.3	12	1.8	22.2	3080	14	0
Outpatient	108	13	17	34.6	0	38.2	22	3.7	6.5	3060	14	0
Tuffnell et al (1992)	54											
Day Unit	24	57	23	36	0	39.8	—	—	1.1	3320	—	0
Usual Care	30	54	21	36.5	21	39	—	—	5.1	3340	—	0
Turnbull et al (2004)	374[b]											
Hospitalization	125	63	0	35.9	22	39	—	—	8.5	3330	3.8	0
Day Unit	249	62	0	36.2	22	39.7	—	—	7.2	3300	2.3	0

Definitions: BW = birthweight; EGA = estimated gestational age; Htn = hypertension; PMR = perinatal mortality rate; Prot = proteinuria; SGA = small-for-gestational-age.
[a]Excluded women with proteinuria at entry.
[b]Included women with ≤ 1+ proteinuria.

has been of considerable interest. Treatment for women with chronic hypertension complicating pregnancy is discussed in detail in Chapter 45 (p. 988).

Drug treatment for early mild preeclampsia has been disappointing as shown in representative randomized trials listed in Table 34-9. Sibai and colleagues (1987a) evaluated the effectiveness of labetalol and hospitalization compared with hospitalization alone in 200 nulliparous women with gestational hypertension from 26 to 35 weeks. Although women given labetalol had significantly lower mean blood pressures, there

TABLE 34-9. Randomized Placebo-Controlled Trials of Antihypertensive Therapy for Early Mild Gestational Hypertension

Study	Study Drug (number)	Prolongation Pregnancy (days)	Severe Hypertension[a] (%)	Cesarean Delivery (%)	Placental Abruption (%)	Mean Birthweight (g)	Growth Restriction (%)	Neonatal Deaths
Sibai et al (1987a)[a]	Labetalol (100)	21.3	5	36	2	2205	19[c]	1
200 inpatients	Placebo (100)	20.1	15[c]	32	0	2260	9	0
Sibai et al (1992)[b]	Nifedipine 100)	22.3	9	43	3	2405	8	0
200 outpatients	Placebo (100)	22.5	18[c]	35	2	2510	4	0
Pickles et al (1992)	Labetalol (70)	26.6	9	24	NS	NS	NS	NS
144 outpatients	Placebo (74)	23.1	10	26	NS	NS	NS	NS
Wide-Swensson et al (1995)	Isradipine (54)	23.1	22	26	NS	NS	NS	0
111 outpatients	Placebo (57)	29.8	29	19	NS	NS	NS	0

[a]All women had preeclampsia.
[b]Includes postpartum hypertension.
[c]$p < .05$ when study drug compared with placebo.
NS = not stated.

were no differences between the groups in terms of mean pregnancy prolongation, gestational age at delivery, or birthweight. The cesarean delivery rates were similar, as were the number of infants admitted to special-care nurseries. *Growth-restricted infants were significantly twice as frequent in women given labetalol—19 versus 9 percent.*

The three other studies listed in Table 34-9 were performed to compare labetalol or the calcium-channel blockers, nifedipine and isradipine, with placebo. In none of these studies were any benefits of antihypertensive treatment shown. Von Dadelszen and Magee (2002) updated their previous meta-analysis and again concluded that treatment-induced decreases in maternal blood pressure may adversely affect fetal growth.

Abalos and colleagues (2007) reviewed randomized trials of active antihypertensive therapy compared with either no treatment or placebo given to women with mild to moderate gestational hypertension. These reviewers included 46 trials enrolling 4282 women and reported that, except for a halving of the risk for developing severe hypertension, active antihypertensive therapy had no beneficial effects. In contrast to the findings by von Dadelszen and Magee (2002) cited above, they reported that fetal-growth restriction *was not increased* in treated women. Similarly, it is controversial whether β-blocking agents cause fetal-growth restriction if given across pregnancy for chronic hypertension (August and Lindheimer, 2009; Umans and colleagues, 2009). Thus, any salutary or adverse effects of antihypertensive therapy seem minimal at most.

Delayed Delivery

Delayed Delivery with Early-Onset Severe Preeclampsia

For many years, it was the practice that all women with severe preeclampsia were delivered without delay. During the past 20 years, however, another approach for women with severe preeclampsia remote from term has been advocated by several investigators worldwide. This calls for "conservative" or "expectant" management with the aim of improving neonatal outcome without compromising maternal safety. Aspects of such management always include careful daily—and usually more frequent—inpatient monitoring of the woman and fetus, with or without antihypertensive drugs.

Theoretically, antihypertensive therapy has potential application when severe preeclampsia develops before neonatal survival is likely. Such management is controversial, and it may be dangerous. In one of the first studies, Sibai and the Memphis group (1985) attempted to prolong pregnancy because of fetal immaturity in 60 women with severe preeclampsia between 18 and 27 weeks. The results were disastrous. *The perinatal mortality rate was 87 percent. Although no mothers died, 13 suffered placental abruption, 10 had eclampsia, 3 developed renal failure, 2 had hypertensive encephalopathy, and one each had an intracerebral hemorrhage and a ruptured hepatic hematoma.*

Because of these catastrophic outcomes, the Memphis group redefined their study criteria and performed a randomized trial of expectant versus aggressive management of 95 women who had severe preeclampsia but with more advanced gestations of

28 to 32 weeks (Sibai and associates, 1994). *Women with HELLP syndrome were excluded from this trial.* Aggressive management included glucocorticoid administration for fetal lung maturation followed by delivery in 48 hours. Expectantly managed women were observed at bed rest and given either labetalol or nifedipine orally to control severe hypertension. In this study, pregnancy was prolonged for a mean of 15.4 days in the expectant management group. An overall improvement in neonatal outcomes was also reported.

Following these experiences, expectant management became more commonly practiced, but with the caveat that women with HELLP syndrome or growth-restricted fetuses were usually excluded. But in a subsequent follow-up observational study, the Memphis group compared outcomes in 133 preeclamptic women with and 136 without HELLP syndrome who presented between 24 and 36 weeks (Abramovici and co-workers, 1999). Women were subdivided into three study groups: The first group included those with hemolysis, elevated liver enzymes, *and* low platelets—*complete HELLP syndrome*. The second group included women with *partial HELLP syndrome*—defined as either one or two but not three of these laboratory findings. The third group included women who had severe preeclampsia without HELLP syndrome laboratory findings. Perinatal outcomes were similar in each group, and importantly, outcomes were not improved with procrastination. Despite this, the investigators concluded that women with partial HELLP syndrome, as well as those with severe preeclampsia alone, could be managed expectantly.

Sibai and Barton (2007) recently reviewed most reports since the early 1990s of expectant management of severe preeclampsia. Outcomes reported from seven studies published since 2000 are shown in Table 34-10. A total of more than 1200 women were included, and although the average time gained ranged from 5 to 10 days, their morbidity rates were formidable. As shown, serious complications included placental abruption, HELLP syndrome, pulmonary edema, renal failure, and eclampsia. Moreover, perinatal mortality rates averaged from 39 to 133 per 1000. Fetal-growth restriction was common, and in the study from The Netherlands by Ganzevoort and associates (2005a, b), it was an astounding 94 percent. It has been shown that perinatal mortality rates are disproportionately high in these growth-restricted infants, but maternal outcomes were not appreciably different from pregnancies in women without growth-restricted fetuses (Haddad and co-workers, 2007; Shear and colleagues, 2005).

Barber and associates (2009) conducted a 10-year review of 3408 women with severe preeclampsia from 24 to 32 weeks who had been entered into the California vital statistics database. They found that increasing lengths of antepartum hospital stays were associated with slight but significantly increased rates of maternal and neonatal morbidity.

Expectant Management of Midtrimester Severe Preeclampsia

A number of small studies have focused on expectant management of severe preeclampsia syndrome *before 28 weeks*. In their recent review, Bombrys and colleagues (2008) found eight such studies that included nearly 200 women with severe preeclampsia with an onset from less than 24 and up to 26 completed

TABLE 34-10. Maternal and Perinatal Outcomes with Expectant Management of Severe Preeclampsia from 24 to 34 Weeks

Study	EGA at Enrollment Wks (Range)	No.	Days Gained	Maternal Outcomes (percent)					Perinatal Outcomes (percent)	
				Placental Abruption	HELLP Syndrome	Pulmonary Edema	ARF	Eclampsia	SGA	PMR
Hall (2001)	26–34	340	11	20	5.2	2.1	1.7	1.2	36	9.0
Vigil-DeGracia (2003)	24–34	129	8.5	8.5	8.5	2.3	1.6	0	22	7.0
Haddad (2004)	24–34	239	5	8.7	14	3.8	0	0	24	5.4
Oettle (2005)	24–34	131[a]	11.6	23	4.6	0.8	2.3	2.3	NS	13.8
Shear (2005)	24–34	155	5.3	5.8	27	3.9	NS	1.9	62	3.9
Ganzevoort (2005a, b)	24–34	216	11	1.8	18	3.6	NS	1.8	94	18
Bombrys (2009)	27–34	66	5	11	8	9	3	0	27	1.5
Weighted averages	24–34	1276	8.7	11	13.3	3.1	1.4	1.0	43	9

[a]Includes one maternal death.
ARF = acute renal failure; EGA = estimated gestational age; HELLP = hemolysis, elevated liver enzymes, low platelet count; NS = not stated; PMR = perinatal mortality rate; SGA = small-for-gestational age.

weeks. Maternal complications were common, and there were no infant survivors in those presenting before 23 weeks. Thus, the authors recommended pregnancy termination for these women. For those at 23 weeks, the perinatal survival rate was 18 percent, but long-term perinatal morbidity is yet unknown. For women with pregnancies at 24 to 26 weeks, perinatal survival approached 60 percent, and it averaged almost 90 percent for those at 26 weeks.

Results from five studies published since 2000 of women with severe midtrimester preeclampsia who were managed expectantly are shown in Table 34-11. As can be seen, there are extraordinarily high maternal and perinatal morbidity and mortality rates in these extremely preterm pregnancies. Because of these results, at this time, there are inadequate contemporane-

ous comparative studies attesting to the perinatal benefits of such expectant treatment versus early delivery in the face of serious maternal complications that approach 50 percent.

Glucocorticoids for Lung Maturation

In attempts to enhance fetal lung maturation, glucocorticoids have been administered to women with severe hypertension who are remote from term. Treatment does not seem to worsen maternal hypertension, and a decrease in the incidence of respiratory distress and improved fetal survival has been cited. That said, there is only one randomized trial of corticosteroids given to hypertensive women for fetal lung maturation (Amorim and associates, 1999). This trial included 218 women with severe preeclampsia between 26 and 34 weeks who were randomly

TABLE 34-11. Maternal and Perinatal Outcomes (Percent) with Expectant Management in Women with Midtrimester Severe Preeclampsia

Study	No.	Maternal Complications	Perinatal Mortality
Hall et al (2001)	8	36	88
Gaugler-Senden et al (2006)	26	65[a]	82
Budden et al (2006)	31	71	71
Bombrys et al (2008)	46	38–64	43
Jenkins et al (2002)	39	54	90
Weighted average	140	60	65

[a]One maternal death.

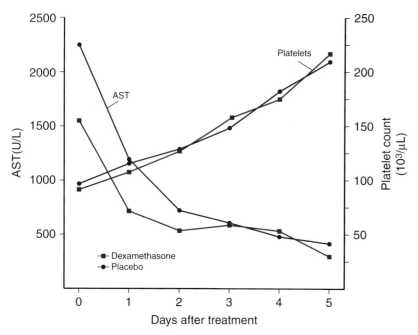

FIGURE 34-16 Recovery times for platelet counts and serum aspartate transferase (AST) levels in women with HELLP syndrome assigned to receive treatment with dexamethasone or placebo. (Data from Katz and colleagues, 2008.)

assigned to betamethasone or placebo administration. Neonatal complications, including respiratory distress, intraventricular hemorrhage, and death, were decreased significantly when betamethasone was given compared with placebo. However, there were two maternal deaths and 18 stillbirths. We add these findings to buttress our unenthusiastic acceptance of attempts to prolong gestation in many of these women (Bloom and Leveno, 2003; Leveno and Cunningham, 2009).

Corticosteroids to Ameliorate HELLP Syndrome

More than 25 years ago, Thiagarajah and colleagues (1984) suggested that glucocorticoids might also play a role in treatment of the laboratory abnormalities associated with the HELLP syndrome. Subsequently, Tompkins (1999) and O'Brien (2002) and their associates reported less than salutary effects. Martin and coworkers (2003) reviewed outcomes of almost 500 such women at their institution. From 1994 to 2000, 90 percent of women with HELLP syndrome were treated. Their outcomes were more favorable than the retrospective cohort from 1985 to 1991, during which time only 16 percent were treated with corticosteroids. Their randomized trial, although comparing two corticosteroids, did not include a nontreated group (Isler and co-workers, 2001).

Since these observational studies, there have been at least two prospective randomized trials designed to address this question. Fonseca and colleagues (2005) randomized 132 women with HELLP syndrome to either dexamethasone or placebo administration. Outcomes assessed included duration of hospitalization, recovery time of abnormal laboratory test results, recovery of clinical parameters, and complications that included acute renal failure, pulmonary edema, eclampsia, and death. None of these was significantly different between the two groups. In a similar blinded study, Katz and co-workers (2008) randomized 105 postpartum women with HELLP syndrome to

treatment with dexamethasone or placebo. They analyzed outcomes similar to the Fonseca study and found no advantage to dexamethasone. Shown in Figure 34-16 are recovery times for platelet counts and serum aspartate transferase (AST) levels. These recoveries are almost identical in the two groups. For these reasons, we do not recommend corticosteroid treatment for thrombocytopenia.

Risks versus Benefits of Delayed Delivery

Taken in toto, these studies require comment about repeated claims that expectant management of severe preeclampsia is beneficial. Undoubtedly, the overriding reason to terminate pregnancies with severe preeclampsia is maternal safety. There are no data to suggest that expectant management is beneficial for the mother. Indeed, it seems obvious that a delay to prolong gestation in women with severe preeclampsia may have serious maternal consequences such as those shown in Table 34-10. Notably, placental abruption develops in approximately 20 percent and pulmonary edema in about 4 percent. Moreover, there are substantive risks for eclampsia, cerebrovascular hemorrhage, and maternal death. These observations are especially pertinent when considered along with the absence of convincing evidence that perinatal outcomes are markedly improved by the average prolongation of pregnancy of about 1 week. If undertaken, shown in Table 34-12 are some criteria

---

TABLE 34-12. Some Indications for Delivery with Early-Onset Severe Preeclampsia

Maternal

Persistent severe headache or visual changes; eclampsia

Shortness of breath; chest tightness with rales and/or $S_aO_2 < 94$ percent breathing room air; pulmonary edema

Uncontrolled severe hypertension despite treatment

Oliguria < 500 mL/24 hr or serum creatinine $\geq$ 1.5 mg/dL

Persistent platelet counts < 100,000/μL

Suspected abruption, progressive labor, and/or ruptured membranes

Fetal

Severe growth restriction—< 5th percentile for EGA

Persistent severe oligohydramnios—AFI < 5 cm

Biophysical profile $\leq$ 4 done 6 hr apart

Reversed end-diastolic umbilical artery flow

Fetal death

AFI = amnionic fluid index; EGA = estimated gestational age; S_aO_2 = oxygen saturation.
From Sibai and Barton (2007).

recommended by Sibai and Barton (2007) that should promote consideration for delivery.

Eclampsia

Preeclampsia complicated by generalized tonic-clonic convulsions increases appreciably the risk to both mother and fetus. In an earlier study, Mattar and Sibai (2000) described outcomes in 399 consecutive women with eclampsia from 1977 through 1998. Major maternal complications included placental abruption—10 percent, neurological deficits—7 percent, aspiration pneumonia—7 percent, pulmonary edema—5 percent, cardiopulmonary arrest—4 percent, and acute renal failure—4 percent. Moreover, 1 percent of these women died.

European maternity units also report excessive maternal and perinatal morbidity and mortality rates with eclampsia. In a report from Scandinavia encompassing a 2-year period ending in 2000, Andersgaard and associates (2006) described 232 women with eclampsia. Although there was but a single maternal death, a third of the women experienced major complications that included HELLP syndrome, renal failure, pulmonary edema, pulmonary embolism, and stroke. The United Kingdom Obstetric Surveillance System (UKOSS) updated audit by Knight (2007) described maternal outcomes in 214 eclamptic women. There were no maternal deaths, and although outcomes were improved since the previous audit, five women experienced cerebral hemorrhage. In The Netherlands during 2 years ending in 2006, there were three maternal deaths among 222 eclamptic women (Zwart and colleagues, 2008). From Dublin, Akkawi and co-workers (2009) reported four maternal deaths among 247 eclamptic women. Thus, in developed countries, the maternal mortality rate is about 1 percent in women with eclampsia—in perspective, this is 1000-fold increased over the national maternal death rates for these countries.

Almost without exception, preeclampsia precedes the onset of eclamptic convulsions. Depending on whether convulsions appear before, during, or after labor, eclampsia is designated as antepartum, intrapartum, or postpartum. Eclampsia is most common in the last trimester and becomes increasingly more frequent as term approaches. In more recent years, there has been an increasing shift in the incidence of eclampsia toward the postpartum period. This is presumably related to improved access to prenatal care, earlier detection of preeclampsia, and prophylactic use of magnesium sulfate (Chames and colleagues, 2002). Importantly, other diagnoses should be considered in women with the onset of convulsions more than 48 hours postpartum or in women with focal neurological deficits, prolonged coma, or atypical eclampsia (Sibai, 2005).

Immediate Management of Seizure

Eclamptic seizures may be violent. During seizures, the woman must be protected, especially her airway. So forceful are the muscular movements that the woman may throw herself out of her bed, and if not protected, her tongue is bitten by the violent action of the jaws (Fig. 34-17). This phase, in which the muscles alternately contract and relax, may last approximately a minute. Gradually, the muscular movements become smaller

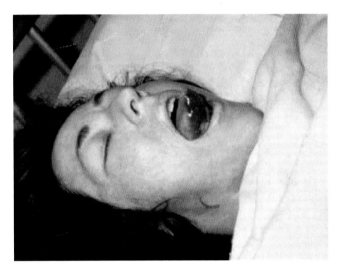

FIGURE 34-17 Hematoma of tongue from laceration during an eclamptic convulsion. Thrombocytopenia may have contributed to the bleeding.

and less frequent, and finally the woman lies motionless. After a seizure, the woman is postictal, but in some, a coma of variable duration ensues. When the convulsions are infrequent, the woman usually recovers some degree of consciousness after each attack. As the woman arouses, a semiconscious combative state may ensue. In severe cases, coma persists from one convulsion to another, and death may result. In rare instances, a single convulsion may be followed by coma from which the woman may never emerge. However, as a rule, death does not occur until after frequent convulsions. Finally and also rarely, convulsions continue unabated—*status epilepticus*—and require deep sedation and even general anesthesia.

Respirations after an eclamptic convulsion are usually increased in rate and may reach 50 or more per minute in response to hypercarbia, lactic acidemia, and transient hypoxia. Cyanosis may be observed in severe cases. High fever is a grave sign because it probably results from cerebrovascular hemorrhage.

Proteinuria is usually present and frequently pronounced. Urine output may be diminished appreciably, and occasionally anuria develops. There may be hemoglobinuria, but hemoglobinemia is observed rarely. Often, as shown in Figure 34-18, peripheral and facial edema is pronounced—at times, massive—but it may also be absent.

As with severe preeclampsia, after delivery, an increase in urinary output is usually an early sign of improvement. If there is renal dysfunction, serum creatinine levels should be monitored. Proteinuria and edema ordinarily disappear within a week postpartum (see Fig. 34-18). In most cases, blood pressure returns to normal within a few days to 2 weeks after delivery. As subsequently discussed, the longer hypertension persists postpartum, and the more severe it is, the more likely the patient also has chronic vascular disease.

In antepartum eclampsia, labor may begin spontaneously shortly after convulsions ensue and may progress rapidly. If the convulsion occurs during labor, contractions may increase in frequency and intensity, and the duration of labor may be

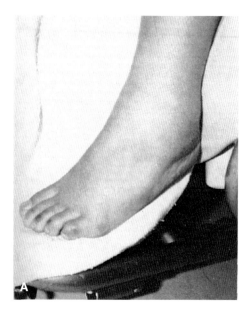
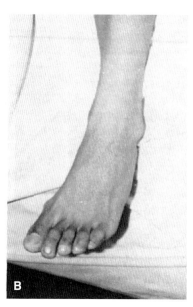

FIGURE 34-18 A. Severe edema in a young nulliparous woman with antepartum eclampsia. **B.** The same woman 3 days after delivery. The remarkable clearance of pedal edema, accompanied by diuresis and a 28-pound weight loss, was spontaneous and unprovoked by diuretic therapy.(From Cunningham and Pritchard, 1984, with permission.)

shortened. Because of maternal hypoxemia and lactic acidemia caused by convulsions, it is not unusual for fetal bradycardia to follow a seizure (Fig. 34-19). Bradycardia usually recovers within 3 to 5 minutes. However, if it persists more than approximately 10 minutes, then another cause such as placental abruption or imminent delivery must be considered.

Pulmonary edema may follow eclamptic convulsions. This usually is caused by aspiration pneumonitis from gastric content inhalation during vomiting that frequently accompanies convulsions. In some women, pulmonary edema may be caused by ventricular failure from increased afterload that may result from severe hypertension and vigorous intravenous fluid administration. Such pulmonary edema from ventricular failure is more common in morbidly obese women and in those with previously unappreciated chronic hypertension.

Occasionally, sudden death occurs synchronously with an eclamptic convulsion, or it follows shortly thereafter. Most often in these cases, death results from a massive cerebral hemorrhage (see Fig. 34-11). Hemiplegia may result from sublethal hemorrhage. Cerebral hemorrhages are more likely in older women with underlying chronic hypertension as discussed on page 721. Rarely, they may be due to a ruptured cerebral berry aneurysm or arteriovenous malformation (Witlin and co-workers, 1997a).

In approximately 10 percent of women, some degree of blindness follows a seizure. Blindness seldom develops spontaneously with preeclampsia. Two causes of blindness or impaired vision are varying degrees of retinal detachment or occipital lobe ischemia and edema (see p. 723). In both instances, the prognosis for return to normal function is good and is usually complete within a week postpartum (Cunningham and associates, 1995). Approximately 5 percent of women have substantively altered consciousness, including persistent coma, following a seizure. This is due to extensive cerebral edema, and transtentorial herniation may cause death as discussed on page 724 (Cunningham and Twickler, 2000).

Rarely, eclampsia is followed by psychosis, and the woman becomes violent. This usually lasts for several days to 2 weeks, but the prognosis for return to normal function is good, provided there was no preexisting mental illness. It is presumed to be similar to postpartum psychosis discussed in detail in Chapter 55 (p. 1179). Antipsychotic medications in carefully titrated doses have proved effective in the few cases of posteclampsia psychosis treated at Parkland Hospital.

Differential Diagnosis

Generally, eclampsia is more likely to be diagnosed too frequently rather than overlooked. Epilepsy, encephalitis, meningitis, cerebral tumor, cysticercosis, and ruptured cerebral aneurysm during late pregnancy and the puerperium may simulate eclampsia. **Until other such causes are excluded, however, all pregnant women with convulsions should be considered to have eclampsia.**

Management of Eclampsia

As reviewed by Chesley (1978), it has been long recognized in American obstetrics that magnesium sulfate is highly effective in preventing convulsions in

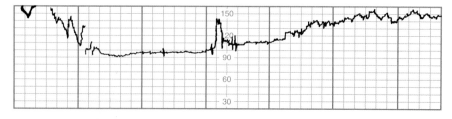
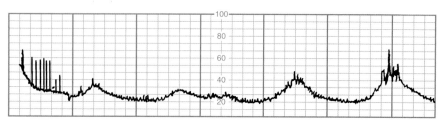

FIGURE 34-19 Fetal bradycardia following an intrapartum eclamptic convulsion. Bradycardia resolved and beat-to-beat variability returned approximately 5 minutes following the seizure.

women with preeclampsia and in stopping them in those with eclampsia. He cited observational data by Pritchard and colleagues (1955, 1975) from Parkland Hospital and from his own institution, Kings County Hospital in Brooklyn. At that time, most eclampsia regimens used in the United States adhered to a similar philosophy still in use today, and the tenets of which include the following:

1. Control of convulsions using an intravenously administered loading dose of magnesium sulfate. This is followed by a continuous infusion of magnesium sulfate
2. Intermittent administration of an antihypertensive medication to lower blood pressure whenever it is considered dangerously high
3. Avoidance of diuretics unless there is obvious pulmonary edema, limitation of intravenous fluid administration unless fluid loss is excessive, and avoidance of hyperosmotic agents
4. Delivery of the fetus to achieve a "cure."

Magnesium Sulfate to Control Convulsions

In more severe cases of preeclampsia, as well as in eclampsia, magnesium sulfate administered parenterally is an effective anticonvulsant that avoids producing central nervous system depression in either the mother or the infant. It may be given intravenously by continuous infusion or intramuscularly by intermittent injection (Table 34-13). The dosages for severe preeclampsia are the same as for eclampsia. Because labor and delivery is a more likely time for convulsions to develop, women with preeclampsia-eclampsia usually are given magnesium sulfate during labor and for 24 hours postpartum.

Magnesium sulfate is almost universally administered intravenously, and in most units, the intramuscular route has been abandoned. Of concern, magnesium sulfate solutions, although inexpensive to prepare, are not readily available in all parts of the developing world. And even when the solutions are available, the technology to infuse them may not be. Therefore, it should not be forgotten that the drug can be administered intramuscularly and that this route is as effective as intravenous administration. In a recent report from India, Chowdhury and colleagues (2009) showed that the two regimens were equivalent in preventing recurrent convulsions and maternal deaths in 630 women with eclampsia.

Magnesium sulfate is not given to treat hypertension. Based on a number of studies cited subsequently, as well as extensive clinical observations, magnesium most likely exerts a specific anticonvulsant action on the cerebral cortex. Typically, the mother stops convulsing after the initial 4-g loading dose. By an hour or two, she regains consciousness sufficiently to be oriented to place and time.

The magnesium sulfate dosages presented in Table 34-13 usually result in plasma magnesium levels illustrated in Figure 34-20. When magnesium sulfate is given to arrest eclamptic seizures, 10 to 15 percent of women have a subsequent convulsion. If so, an additional 2-g dose of magnesium sulfate in a 20-percent solution is slowly administered intravenously. In a small woman, this additional 2-g dose may be used once, but it can be given twice if needed in a larger woman. In only five of 245 women with eclampsia at Parkland Hospital was it necessary to use supplementary medication to control convulsions (Pritchard and associates, 1984). An intravenous barbiturate such as amobarbital or thiopental is given slowly. Midazolam or lorazepam may be given in a small single dose because

---

TABLE 34-13. Magnesium Sulfate Dosage Schedule Dosage Schedule for Severe Preeclampsia and Eclampsia

Continuous Intravenous Infusion
1. Give 4- to 6-g loading dose of magnesium sulfate diluted in 100 mL of IV fluid administered over 15–20 min
2. Begin 2 g/hr in 100 mL of IV maintenance infusion. Some recommend 1 g/hr
3. Monitor for magnesium toxicity:
   a. Assess deep tendon reflexes periodically
   b. Some measure serum magnesium level at 4–6 hr and adjust infusion to maintain levels between 4 and 7 meq/L (4.8 to 8.4 mg/dL)
   c. Measure serum magnesium levels if serum creatinine ≥ 1.0 mg/dL
4. Magnesium sulfate is discontinued 24 hr after delivery

Intermittent Intramuscular Injections
1. Give 4 g of magnesium sulfate ($MgSO_4 \cdot 7H_2O$ USP) as a 20% solution intravenously at a rate not to exceed 1 g/min
2. Follow promptly with 10 g of 50% magnesium sulfate solution, one-half (5 g) injected deeply in the upper outer quadrant of both buttocks through a 3-inch-long 20-gauge needle. (Addition of 1.0 mL of 2% lidocaine minimizes discomfort.) If convulsions persist after 15 min, give up to 2 g more intravenously as a 20% solution at a rate not to exceed 1 g/min. If the woman is large, up to 4 g may be given slowly
3. Every 4 hr thereafter give 5 g of a 50% solution of magnesium sulfate injected deeply in the upper outer quadrant of alternate buttocks, but only after ensuring that:
   a. The patellar reflex is present,
   b. Respirations are not depressed, and
   c. Urine output the previous 4 hr exceeded 100 mL
4. Magnesium sulfate is discontinued 24 hr after delivery

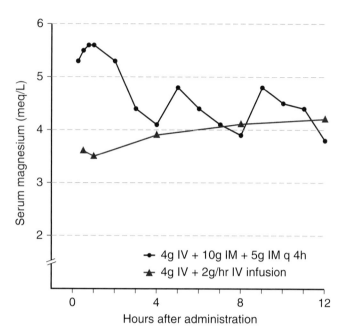

FIGURE 34-20 Comparison of serum magnesium levels in meq/L following a 4-g intravenous loading dose of magnesium sulfate and then maintained by either an intramuscular or continuing infusion. Multiply by 1.2 to convert meq/L to mg/dL. (Data from Sibai and colleagues, 1984.)

prolonged use is associated with a higher mortality rate (Royal College of Obstetricians and Gynaecologists, 2006).

Maintenance magnesium sulfate therapy is continued for 24 hours after delivery. For eclampsia that develops postpartum, magnesium sulfate is administered for 24 hours after the onset of convulsions. Ehrenberg and Mercer (2006) studied abbreviated postpartum magnesium administration in 200 women with *mild* preeclampsia. Of 101 women randomized to 12-hour treatment, seven had worsening preeclampsia, and treatment was extended to 24 hours. None of these 101 women and none of the other cohort of 95 given the 24-hour magnesium infusion developed eclampsia. This abbreviated regimen needs further study before being routinely administered for severe preeclampsia or eclampsia.

Pharmacology and Toxicology. Magnesium sulfate USP is $MgSO_4 \cdot 7H_2O$ and not simple $MgSO_4$. Parenterally administered magnesium is cleared almost totally by renal excretion, and magnesium intoxication is unusual when the glomerular filtration rate is maintained or only slightly decreased. Adequate urine output usually correlates with preserved glomerular filtration rates. That said, magnesium excretion is not urine flow dependent, and urinary volume per unit time does not, per se, predict renal function. Thus, serum creatinine levels must be measured to detect signs of declining glomerular filtration rate.

Eclamptic convulsions are almost always prevented or arrested by plasma magnesium levels maintained at 4 to 7 meq/L, 4.8 to 8.4 mg/dL, or 2.0 to 3.5 mmol/L. Although laboratories typically report *total* magnesium levels, free or *ionized* magnesium is the active moiety for suppressing neuronal excitability. Taber and associates (2002) found that there is a poor correlation between total and ionized levels. Further studies are neces-

sary to determine if either measurement provides a superior method for surveillance. As shown in Figure 34-20, after a 4-g intravenous loading dose, magnesium levels observed with the intramuscular regimen and those observed with the maintenance infusion of 2 g per hour are similar. In our experience with the infusion, a number of women require 3 g/hr to maintain effective plasma levels of magnesium. That said, most do not recommend routine magnesium level measurements (American College of Obstetricians and Gynecologists, 2002a; Royal College of Obstetricians and Gynaecologists, 2006).

Patellar reflexes disappear when the plasma magnesium level reaches 10 meq/L—about 12 mg/dL—presumably because of a curariform action. This sign serves to warn of impending magnesium toxicity. When plasma levels rise above 10 meq/L, breathing becomes weakened, and at 12 meq/L or more, respiratory paralysis and respiratory arrest follow. Somjen and colleagues (1966) induced marked hypermagnesemia in themselves by intravenous infusion and achieved plasma levels up to 15 meq/L. Predictably, at such high plasma levels, respiratory depression developed that necessitated mechanical ventilation, but depression of the sensorium was not dramatic as long as hypoxia was prevented.

Treatment with calcium gluconate or calcium chloride, 1 g intravenously, along with withholding further magnesium sulfate, usually reverses mild to moderate respiratory depression. One of these agents should be readily available. Unfortunately, the effects of intravenously administered calcium may be short-lived if there is a steady-state toxic level. For severe respiratory depression and arrest, prompt tracheal intubation and mechanical ventilation are lifesaving. Direct toxic effects on the myocardium from high levels of magnesium are uncommon. It appears that the cardiac dysfunction associated with magnesium is due to respiratory arrest and hypoxia. With appropriate ventilation, cardiac action is satisfactory even when plasma levels are exceedingly high (McCubbin and co-workers, 1981).

Because magnesium is cleared almost exclusively by renal excretion, the dosages described will become excessive if glomerular filtration is decreased substantively. The initial 4-g loading dose of magnesium sulfate can be safely administered regardless of renal function. It is important to administer the standard loading dose and not to reduce it under the mistaken conception that diminished renal function requires it. This is because after distribution, a loading dose achieves the desired therapeutic level, and the infusion maintains the steady-state level. *Thus, only the maintenance infusion rate should be altered with diminished glomerular filtration rate.* Renal function is estimated by measuring plasma creatinine. Whenever plasma creatinine levels are > 1.0 mg/mL, serum magnesium levels are used to adjust the infusion rate.

Acute cardiovascular effects of parenteral magnesium in women with severe preeclampsia have been studied using data obtained by pulmonary and radial artery catheterization. After a 4-g intravenous dose administered over 15 minutes, mean arterial blood pressure fell slightly, accompanied by a 13-percent increase in cardiac index (Cotton and colleagues, 1986b). Thus, magnesium decreased systemic vascular resistance and mean arterial pressure, and at the same time increased cardiac output without evidence of myocardial depression. These findings were coincidental with transient nausea and flushing, and the cardiovascular effects persisted for only 15 minutes despite continued magnesium infusion.

Thurnau and associates (1987) showed that there was a small but highly significant increase in total magnesium concentration in the cerebrospinal fluid with magnesium therapy. The magnitude of the increase was directly proportional to the corresponding serum concentration.

Magnesium is anticonvulsant and neuroprotective in a number of animal models. Some proposed mechanisms of action include: (1) reduced presynaptic release of the neurotransmitter glutamate, (2) blockade of glutamatergic N-methyl-D-aspartate (NMDA) receptors, (3) potentiation of adenosine action, (4) improved mitochondrial calcium buffering, and (5) blockage of calcium entry via voltage-gated channels (Arango and Mejia-Mantilla, 2006). Because hippocampal seizures can be blocked by magnesium, this implicates the NMDA receptor in eclamptic convulsions (Hallak and associates, 1998). These studies also confirm that magnesium has a central anticonvulsant effect.

Uterine Effects. Relatively high serum magnesium concentrations depress myometrial contractility both in vivo and in vitro. With the regimen described and the plasma levels that result, no evidence of myometrial depression has been observed beyond a transient decrease in activity during and immediately after the initial intravenous loading dose. Leveno and colleagues (1998) compared outcomes in 480 nulliparous women given phenytoin for preeclampsia with outcomes in 425 preeclamptic women given magnesium sulfate. Magnesium did not significantly alter the need for oxytocin stimulation of labor, admission-to-delivery intervals, or route of delivery. Similar results have been reported by others (Atkinson, 1995; Szal, 1999; Witlin, 1997b, and all their colleagues).

The mechanisms by which magnesium might inhibit uterine contractility are not established. However, these mechanisms are generally assumed to depend on its effects on intracellular calcium as discussed in detail in Chapter 6 (p. 148). Inhibition of uterine contractility is magnesium dose dependent, and serum levels of at least 8 to 10 meq/L are necessary to inhibit uterine contractions (Watt-Morse and colleagues, 1995). This likely explains why there are few if any uterine effects seen clinically when magnesium sulfate is given for preeclampsia. And as discussed in Chapter 36 (p. 824), magnesium is also not considered by many to be an effective tocolytic agent.

Fetal Effects. Maternal magnesium administered parenterally promptly crosses the placenta to achieve equilibrium in fetal serum and less so in amnionic fluid (Hallak and co-workers, 1993). Levels in amnionic fluid increase with duration of maternal infusion (Gortzak-Uzen and associates, 2005). Neonatal depression occurs only if there is *severe* hypermagnesemia at delivery. Neonatal compromise after therapy with magnesium sulfate is usually not problematic (Cunningham and Pritchard, 1984; Hallak and associates, 1999a). Whether magnesium sulfate affects the fetal heart rate pattern—specifically beat-to-beat variability—is controversial. In a randomized investigation, Hallak and colleagues (1999b) compared an infusion of magnesium sulfate with saline and reported that magnesium was associated with a small and clinically insignificant decrease in heart rate variability.

Observational studies have suggested a protective effect of magnesium against the development of cerebral palsy in very-low-birthweight infants (Nelson and Grether, 1995; Schendel and colleagues, 1996). At least five randomized trials have also assessed neuroprotective fetal effects. Moreover, Doyle and associates (2009) conducted a meta-analysis of five randomized trials that enrolled a total of 6145 infants born to women who were likely to give birth before 37 weeks. These women were randomly allocated to receive treatment with magnesium sulfate or placebo to prevent preeclampsia or preterm labor or to provide neuroprotection. Rates of substantive gross motor dysfunction were significantly decreased in infants exposed to therapeutic magnesium—0.61(CI 0.44–0.85). These findings are discussed in detail in Chapters 29 (p. 614) and 36 (p. 824).

Clinical Efficacy of Magnesium Sulfate Therapy. The multinational Eclampsia Trial Collaborative Group study (1995) involved 1687 women with eclampsia who were randomly allocated to different anticonvulsant regimens. In one cohort, 453 women were randomly assigned to be given magnesium sulfate and compared with 452 given diazepam. In a second cohort, 388 eclamptic women were randomly assigned to be given magnesium sulfate and compared with 387 women given phenytoin. The results of these and other comparative studies that each enrolled at least 50 women are summarized in Table 34-14. In aggregate, magnesium sulfate therapy was associated with a significantly lower incidence of recurrent seizures compared with women given an alternative anticonvulsant—9.7 versus 23 percent. Importantly, the maternal death rate of 3.1 percent with magnesium sulfate was significantly lower than that of 4.9 percent for the other regimens.

Management of Severe Hypertension

Dangerous hypertension can cause cerebrovascular hemorrhage, hypertensive encephalopathy and can trigger eclamptic convulsions in women with preeclampsia. Other complications include hypertensive afterload congestive heart failure and placental abruption.

Accordingly, the National High Blood Pressure Education Program Working Group (2000) specifically recommended that treatment include lowering systolic pressures to ≤ 160 mm Hg. Moreover, Martin and associates (2005) provided provocative observations that highlight the importance of treating systolic hypertension. They described 28 selected women with severe preeclampsia who suffered an associated stroke. Most of these were hemorrhagic—93 percent—and all women had systolic pressures > 160 mm Hg before suffering their stroke. By contrast, only 20 percent of these same women had diastolic pressures > 110 mm Hg. It seems likely that at least half of serious hemorrhagic strokes associated with preeclampsia are in women with chronic hypertension (Cunningham, 2005). Chronic hypertension results in development of *Charcot-Bouchard aneurysms* in the deeply penetrating arteries of the lenticulostriate branch of the middle cerebral artery. These supply the basal ganglia, putamen, thalamus, and adjacent deep white matter, as well as the pons and deep cerebellum. These aneurysmal

TABLE 34-14. Randomized Comparative Trials of Magnesium Sulfate with Another Anticonvulsant to Prevent Recurrent Eclamptic Convulsions

Study	Comparison Drug	Recurrent Seizures			Maternal Deaths		
		MgSO$_4$(%)	Other Drug (%)	RR (95% CI)	MgSO$_4$ (%)	Other Drug (%)	RR (95% CI)
Crowther et al (1990)	Diazepam	5/24	7/27	0.80 (0.29–2.2)	1/24	0/27	
Bhalla et al (1994)	Lytic cocktail	1/45	11/45	0.09 (0.1–0.68)	0/45	2/45	
Eclampsia Trial Collaborative Group (1995)	Phenytoin	60/453	126/452	0.48 (0.36–0.63)	10/388	20/387	0.5 (0.24–1.00)
	Diazepam	22/388	66/387	0.33 (0.21–0.53)	17/453	24/452	0.74 (0.40–1.36)
Totals		88/910 (9.7)	210/911 (23)	0.41 (0.32–0.51)	28/910 (3.1)	45/911 (4.9)	0.62 (0.39–0.99)

Data adapted from Leveno and Cunningham (2009) and Sibai and Cunningham (2009).

weakenings predispose these small arteries to rupture with sudden hypertension.

Because of these observations, our policy has been to treat women whose systolic blood pressures reach ≥ 160 mm Hg or whose diastolic pressures reach ≥ 110 mm Hg.

Antihypertensive Agents. There are several drugs available for rapid lowering of dangerously elevated blood pressure in women with the gestational hypertensive disorders. The three most commonly employed in North America and Europe are hydralazine, labetalol, and nifedipine. For years, parenteral hydralazine was the only one of the three available. However, when parenteral labetalol was later introduced, it was considered by most to be equally effective for obstetrical use. Orally administered nifedipine then became available, and this has gained popularity as first-line treatment for severe gestational hypertension.

Hydralazine. This is still a commonly used antihypertensive agent in the United States for treatment of women with severe gestational hypertension. Hydralazine is administered intravenously with a 5-mg initial dose, and this is followed by 5- to 10-mg doses at 15- to 20-minute intervals until a satisfactory response is achieved (American College of Obstetricians and Gynecologists, 2002a). Some limit the total dose to 30 mg per treatment cycle (Sibai, 2003). The target response antepartum or intrapartum is a decrease in diastolic blood pressure to 90 to 100 mm Hg, but not lower, lest placental perfusion be compromised. Hydralazine so administered has proven remarkably effective in the prevention of cerebral hemorrhage. Its onset of action can be as rapid as 10 minutes. Although repeated administration every 15 to 20 minutes may theoretically lead to undesirable hypotension, this has not been our experience.

At both Parkland Hospital and the University of Alabama at Birmingham Hospital, between 5 and 10 percent of all pregnant women with intrapartum hypertensive disorders are given a parenteral antihypertensive agent. Most often, we use hydralazine as

described. We do not limit the total dose, and seldom has a second antihypertensive agent been needed. We estimate that at least 5000 women have been so treated at Parkland during the past 40 years. Although less popular in Europe, hydralazine is used in some centers according to the Royal College of Obstetricians and Gynaecologists (2006). A dissenting opinion for first-line intrapartum use of hydralazine was voiced by the Vancouver group after their first meta-analysis (Magee and colleagues, 2003). They reached a similar conclusion after a more recent systematic review (Magee and co-workers, 2009). At the same time, however, Umans and associates (2009) concluded that objective outcomes data did not support the use of one drug over another.

As with any antihypertensive agent, the tendency to give a larger initial dose of hydralazine when the blood pressure is higher must be avoided. The response to even 5- to 10-mg doses cannot be predicted by the level of hypertension. Thus, our protocol is to always administer 5 mg as the initial dose. An adverse response to exceeding this initial dose is shown in **Figure 34-21**. This woman had chronic hypertension complicated by severe superimposed preeclampsia, and hydralazine was injected more frequently than recommended. Her blood pressure decreased in less than 1 hour from 240–270/130–150 mm Hg to 110/80 mm Hg. Fetal heart rate decelerations characteristic of uteroplacental insufficiency were evident when the pressure fell to 110/80 mm Hg. These decelerations persisted until her blood pressure was increased with rapid crystalloid infusion. In some cases, this fetal response to diminished uterine perfusion may be confused with placental abruption and may result in unnecessary emergent cesarean delivery.

Labetalol. Another effective antihypertensive agent commonly used in the United States is intravenous labetalol—an α_1- and nonselective β-blocker. Some prefer its use over hydralazine because of fewer side effects (Sibai, 2003). At Parkland Hospital, we give 10 mg intravenously initially. If the blood pressure has not decreased to the desirable level in 10 minutes, then 20 mg is given. The next 10-minute incremental dose is 40 mg and is

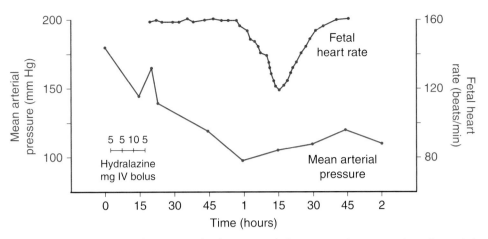

FIGURE 34-21 Effects of acute blood pressure decrease on fetal status. Hydralazine was given at 5-minute intervals instead of 15-minute intervals. The mean arterial pressure decreased from 180 to 90 mm Hg within 1 hour and was associated with fetal bradycardia. Rapid crystalloid infusion raised the mean pressure to 115 mm Hg and the fetus recovered.

followed by another 40 mg if needed. If a salutary response is not achieved, then an 80-mg dose is given. Sibai (2003) recommends 20 to 40 mg every 10 to 15 minutes as needed for a maximum dose of 220 mg per treatment cycle. The NHBPEP Working Group (2000) and the American College of Obstetricians and Gynecologists (2002a) recommend starting with a 20-mg intravenous bolus. If not effective within 10 minutes, this is followed by 40 mg, then 80 mg every 10 minutes but not to exceed a 220-mg total dose per episode treated.

Hydralazine versus Labetalol. Comparative studies of these two antihypertensive agents show equivalent results. In one, Mabie and colleagues (1987) compared intravenous hydralazine with labetalol for blood pressure control in 60 peripartum women. Labetalol lowered blood pressure more rapidly, and associated tachycardia was minimal, but hydralazine lowered mean arterial pressures to safe levels more effectively. In another trial, Vigil-De Gracia and associates (2007) randomized 200 severely hypertensive intrapartum women to be given either: (1) intravenous hydralazine—5 mg, which could be given every 20 minutes and repeated to a maximum of five doses, or (2) intravenous labetalol—20 mg initially, followed by 40 mg in 20 minutes and then 80 mg every 20 minutes if needed up to a maximum 300-mg dose. Maternal and neonatal outcomes were similar. Hydralazine caused significantly more maternal tachycardia and palpitations, whereas labetalol more frequently caused maternal hypotension and bradycardia. Other than maternal tachycardia with hydralazine and occasional maternal bradycardia with labetalol, we have not encountered arrhythmias with either drug.

Nifedipine. This calcium-channel blocking agent has become popular because of its efficacy for control of acute pregnancy-related hypertension. The NHBPEP Working Group (2000) and the Royal College of Obstetricians and Gynaecologists (2006) recommend a 10-mg initial oral dose to be repeated in 30 minutes if necessary. Nifedipine given sublingually is no longer recommended. Randomized trials that compared nifedipine with labetalol found neither drug definitively superior to the other (Scardo and associates, 1999; Vermillion and co-workers, 1999).

Other Antihypertensive Agents. A few other generally available antihypertensive agents have been tested in clinical trials but are not widely used. Belfort and associates (1990) administered the calcium antagonist, *verapamil*, by intravenous infusion at 5 to 10 mg per hour. Mean arterial pressure was lowered by 20 percent. Belfort and co-workers (1996, 2003) reported that *nimodipine* given either by continuous infusion or orally was effective to lower blood pressure in women with severe preeclampsia. Bolte and colleagues (1998, 2001) reported good results in preeclamptic women given intravenous *ketanserin*, a selective serotonergic ($5HT_{2A}$) receptor blocker. *Nitroprusside* or *nitroglycerine* is recommended by some if there is not optimal response to first-line agents (National High Blood Pressure Education Program Working Group, 2000). With these latter two agents, fetal cyanide toxicity may develop after 4 hours. We have not had the need for either due to our consistent success with first-line treatment using hydralazine, labetalol, or a combination of the two given in succession, but never simultaneously.

There are experimental antihypertensive drugs that may become useful for preeclampsia treatment. Two of these are *calcitonin gene related peptide (CGRP)*, which is a 37-amino acid potent vasodilator, and *endogenous digitalis-like factors*, also called *cardiotonic steroids* (Bagrov and Shapiro, 2008; Márquez-Rodas and colleagues, 2006).

Diuretics. Potent diuresis can further compromise placental perfusion. Immediate effects include depletion of intravascular volume, which most often is already reduced compared with that of normal pregnancy (see p. 717). Therefore, before delivery, diuretics are not used to lower blood pressure (Zeeman and co-workers, 2009a; Zondervan and associates, 1988). We limit antepartum use of furosemide or similar drugs solely to treatment of pulmonary edema.

Fluid Therapy

Lactated Ringer solution is administered routinely at the rate of 60 mL to no more than 125 mL per hour unless there is unusual fluid loss from vomiting, diarrhea, or diaphoresis, or more likely, there is excessive blood loss with delivery. Oliguria is common with severe preeclampsia. Thus, coupled with the knowledge that maternal blood volume is likely constricted compared with that of normal pregnancy, it is tempting to administer intravenous fluids more vigorously. However, controlled, conservative fluid administration is preferred for the typical woman with eclampsia who already has excessive extracellular fluid that is inappropriately distributed between intravascular and extravascular spaces. As discussed on page 716, infusion of large fluid volumes enhances the maldistribution of extravascular fluid and thereby appreciably increases the risk of pulmonary and cerebral edema (Sciscione, 2003; Sibai, 1987b; Zinaman, 1985, and all their co-workers).

Pulmonary Edema. Women with severe preeclampsia-eclampsia who develop pulmonary edema most often do so postpartum (Cunningham and colleagues, 1986; Zinaman and associates, 1985). First, aspiration of gastric contents, which may be the result of convulsions, anesthesia, or oversedation, should be excluded. As discussed in Chapter 42 (p. 929), there are three common causes of pulmonary edema in women with severe preeclampsia syndrome—pulmonary capillary permeability edema, cardiogenic edema, or a combination of the two.

Most women with severe preeclampsia will have some mild pulmonary congestion from permeability edema. This is caused by normal pregnancy changes magnified by the preeclampsia syndrome as discussed in Chapter 5 (p. 121). Importantly, plasma oncotic pressure decreases appreciably in normal term pregnancy because of decreased serum albumin concentration, and oncotic pressure falls even more with preeclampsia (Zinaman and associates, 1985). And both increased extravascular fluid oncotic pressure and increased capillary permeability have been described in women with preeclampsia (Brown and colleagues, 1989; Øian and associates, 1986).

Invasive Hemodynamic Monitoring. Knowledge concerning cardiovascular and hemodynamic pathophysiological alterations associated with severe preeclampsia-eclampsia has accrued from studies done using invasive monitoring and a flow-directed pulmonary artery catheter (see Figs. 34-5 and 34-6). A few reviews have addressed such monitoring in obstetrics (Clark and Cotton, 1988; Nolan and colleagues, 1992). Two conditions frequently cited as indications are preeclampsia associated with either oliguria or pulmonary edema. Somewhat ironically, it is usually vigorous treatment of the former that results in most cases of the latter. The American College of Obstetricians and Gynecologists (2002a) recommends such monitoring be reserved for severely preeclamptic women with accompanying severe cardiac disease, renal disease, or both or in cases of refractory hypertension, oliguria, and pulmonary edema.

Plasma Volume Expansion

Because the preeclampsia syndrome is associated with hemoconcentration directly proportional to syndrome severity, attempts to expand blood volume seem reasonable, at least intuitively (Ganzevoort and associates, 2004). This reasoning has led some to infuse various fluids, starch polymers, albumin con-

centrates, or combinations thereof in attempts to expand blood volume.

There are, however, observational studies that describe serious complications—especially pulmonary edema—with volume expansion. For example, López-Llera and colleagues (1982) reported that vigorous volume expansion in more than 700 eclamptic women was associated with a high incidence of pulmonary edema. Benedetti and associates (1985) described pulmonary edema in 7 of 10 women with severe preeclampsia who were given colloid therapy. Moreover, Sibai and co-workers (1987b) cited excessive colloid and crystalloid infusions as causing most of their reported 37 cases of pulmonary edema associated with severe preeclampsia-eclampsia. In general, these studies were not controlled or even comparative (Habek and colleagues, 2006).

The Amsterdam randomized study reported by Ganzevoort and co-workers (2005a, b) was a well-designed investigation done to evaluate volume expansion. A total of 216 women with severe preeclampsia were enrolled between 24 and 34 weeks' gestation. They also included women whose preeclampsia was complicated by HELLP syndrome, eclampsia, or fetal-growth restriction. All women were given magnesium sulfate to prevent eclampsia, betamethasone to promote pulmonary maturity, ketanserine to control dangerous hypertension, and normal saline infusions restricted to only deliver medications. In the group randomly assigned to volume expansion, each woman was given 250 mL of 6-percent hydroxyethyl starch infused over 4 hours twice daily. Their maternal and perinatal outcomes were compared with a control group and are shown in Table 34-15. None of these outcomes was significantly different between the two groups. Importantly, serious maternal morbidity and a substantive perinatal mortality rate accompanied their "expectant" management (see Table 34-10).

Prevention of Eclampsia

There have been a number of randomized trials designed to test the efficacy of seizure prophylaxis for women with gestational hypertension, with or without proteinuria, and thus preeclampsia. In most of these, magnesium sulfate was compared with either another anticonvulsant or with a placebo. *In all studies, magnesium sulfate was reported to be superior to the comparator agent to prevent eclampsia.* Four of the larger studies are summarized in Table 34-16. Lucas and colleagues (1995) reported that magnesium sulfate therapy was superior to phenytoin to prevent eclamptic seizures in women with gestational hypertension including those with all severities of preeclampsia. Belfort and associates (2003) compared magnesium sulfate and nimodipine— a calcium-channel blocker with specific cerebral vasodilator activity—for eclampsia prevention. In this unblinded randomized trial involving 1650 women with severe preeclampsia, the rate of eclampsia was more than threefold higher for women allocated to the nimodipine group—2.6 versus 0.8 percent compared with the group given magnesium sulfate.

The largest comparative study was the *MAGnesium Sulfate for Prevention of Eclampsia* (MAGPIE Trial Collaboration Group, 2002). More than 10,000 women with severe preeclampsia from 33 countries were randomly allocated to treatment

TABLE 34-15. Maternal and Perinatal Outcomes in a Randomized Trial of Plasma Volume Expansion versus Saline Infusion in 216 Women with Severe Preeclampsia between 24 and 34 Weeks

Outcomes	Control Group[a] (n = 105)	Treatment Group[a] (n = 111)
Maternal Outcomes (percent)		
Eclampsia (after enrollment)	1.9	1.8
HELLP (after enrollment)	19.0	17.0
Pulmonary edema	2.9	4.5
Placental abruption	3.8	1.0
Hepatic hematoma	1.0	0.0
Encephalopathy	2.9	1.8
Perinatal Outcomes		
Fetal deaths (percent)	7	12
Prolongation pregnancy (mean)	11.6 days	6.7 days
EGA at death (mean)	26.7 weeks	26.3 weeks
Birthweight (mean)	625 g	640 g
Live births (percent)	93	88
Prolongation pregnancy (mean)	10.5 days	7.4 days
EGA at delivery (mean)	31.6 weeks	31.4 weeks
Assisted ventilation (percent)	40	45
RDS (percent)	30	35
Chronic lung disease (percent)	7.6	8.1
Neonatal death (percent)	7.6	8.1
Perinatal mortality rate	142/1000	207/1000

[a]All comparisons $p > 0.05$.
EGA = estimated gestational age; HELLP = hemolysis, elevated liver enzymes, low platelet count; RDS = respiratory distress syndrome.
Data from Ganzevoort and colleagues (2005a, b).

TABLE 34-16. Randomized Comparative Trials of Prophylaxis with Magnesium Sulfate and Placebo or Another Anticonvulsant in Women with Gestational Hypertension

	Women with Seizures/Total Number Treated		
Study Inclusions	Magnesium Sulfate No. (%)	Control Treatment No. (%)	Comparison*
Lucas et al (1995) Gestational hypertension[a]	0/1049 (0)	Phenytoin 10/1089 (0.9)	$p < 0.001$
Coetzee et al (1998) Severe preeclampsia	1/345 (0.3)	Placebo 11/340 (3.2)	RR = 0.09 (0.1–0.69)
Magpie Trial (2002)[b] Severe preeclampsia	40/5055 (0.8)	Placebo 96/5055 (1.9)	RR = 0.42 (0.26–0.60)
Belfort et al (2003) Severe preeclampsia	7/831 (0.8)	Nimodipine 21/819 (2.6)	RR = 0.33 (0.14–0.77)

*All comparisons significant $p < 0.05$.
[a]Included women with and without proteinuria and those with all severities of preeclampsia.
[b]Magpie Trial Collaboration Group (2002).

with magnesium sulfate or placebo. Women given magnesium had a 58-percent significantly lower risk of eclampsia than those given placebo. Women given placebo and who developed eclampsia were treated with magnesium sulfate. Smyth and colleagues (2009) provided follow-up data of infants born to these mothers given magnesium sulfate. At about 18 months, child behavior did not differ in those exposed to versus those not exposed to magnesium sulfate.

Who Should Be Given Magnesium Sulfate?

Magnesium will prevent more seizures in women with correspondingly worse disease. Severity is difficult to quantify, and thus it is difficult to decide which individual woman might benefit most from prophylaxis. *In the United States, the consensus is that women judged to have severe preeclampsia should be given magnesium sulfate prophylaxis.* This is also the recommendation of the American College of Obstetricians and Gynecologists (2002a). As discussed, criteria that establish "severity" are not totally uniform, and many use those promulgated by the NHBPEP Working Group (2000), which are listed in Table 34-1. For women with "nonsevere" disease—again variably defined—the guidelines are even less clear-cut.

In many other countries, and principally following dissemination of the Magpie Trial Collaboration Group (2002) study results, magnesium sulfate is now recommended for women with severe preeclampsia. In some, however, debate continues concerning whether therapy should be reserved for women who have an eclamptic seizure. We are of the opinion that eclamptic seizures are dangerous for reasons discussed on page 735. Maternal mortality rates of up to 5 percent have been reported even in recent studies (Andersgaard, 2006; Benhamou, 2009; Schutte, 2008; Zwart, 2008, and all their colleagues). Moreover, there are substantively increased perinatal mortality rates in both industrialized countries as well as underdeveloped ones (Basso, 2006; Chowdhury, 2009; Knight, 2007; Schutte, 2008; Zwart, 2008, and all their associates). Finally, the possibility of adverse long-term neuropsychological sequelae of eclampsia described by Aukes (2007, 2009) and Postma (2009) and their colleagues, which is discussed on page 749, have raised additional concerns that eclamptic seizures perhaps are not "benign."

Parkland Hospital Study of Selective versus Universal Magnesium Sulfate Prophylaxis

Debate in the United States currently centers around which women with nonsevere gestational hypertension should be given magnesium sulfate prophylaxis. An opportunity to address these questions was afforded by a change in magnesium sulfate prophylaxis protocol for women delivering at Parkland Hospital beginning in 2000. Prior to this time, Lucas and colleagues (1995) had found the risk of eclampsia without magnesium prophylaxis to be 1 in 100 or less in women with *mild preeclampsia.* Up until 2000, all women with gestational hypertension were given maintenance magnesium prophylaxis intramuscularly as first described by Pritchard in 1955. After 2000, we instituted a standardized protocol for intravenously administered magnesium sulfate. At the same time, we also changed our practice of universal seizure prophylaxis for all

TABLE 34-17. Selective versus Universal Magnesium Sulfate Prophylaxis: Parkland Hospital Criteria to Define Severity of Gestational Hypertension

In a woman with new-onset proteinuric hypertension, at least one of the following criteria is required:
- Systolic BP ≥ 160 or diastolic BP ≥ 110 mm Hg
- Proteinuria ≥ 2+ as measured by dipstick in a catheterized urine specimen
- Serum creatinine > 1.2 mg/dL
- Platelet count < 100,000/μL
- Aspartate transaminase (AST) elevated two times above upper limit of normal range
- Persistent headache or scotomata
- Persistent midepigastric or right-upper quadrant pain

BP = blood pressure.
Criteria based on those from National High Blood Pressure Education Program Working Group (2000) and American College of Obstetricians and Gynecologists (2002a) and cited by Alexander and associates (2006).

women with gestational hypertension to one of selective prophylaxis given only to women who met our criteria for severe gestational hypertension. These criteria shown in Table 34-17 included women with ≥ 2+ proteinuria measured by dipstick in a catheterized urine specimen.

Following this protocol change, 60 percent of 6431 women with gestational hypertension during a 4½-year period were given magnesium sulfate prophylaxis. Of the 40 percent with nonsevere hypertension who were not treated, 27 women developed eclamptic seizures—1 in 92. The seizure rate was only 1 in 358 for 3935 women with criteria for severe disease who were given magnesium sulfate and thus were treatment failures. To assess morbidity, outcomes in 87 eclamptic women were compared with those in all 6431 noneclamptic hypertensive women. Although most maternal outcomes were similar, as shown in Table 34-18, almost a fourth of women with eclampsia who underwent emergent cesarean delivery required general anesthesia. This is of great concern because eclamptic women have laryngotracheal edema and are at a higher risk for failed intubation, gastric acid aspiration, and death (American College of Obstetricians and Gynecologists, 2002b). Neonatal outcomes were also of concern because the composite morbidity defined in Table 34-18 was significantly increased tenfold in eclamptic compared with noneclamptic women—12 versus 1 percent, respectively.

Thus, if one uses the Parkland criteria for nonsevere gestational hypertension, about 1 of 100 such women who are not given magnesium sulfate prophylaxis can be expected to have an eclamptic seizure. A fourth of these women likely will require emergent cesarean delivery with attendant maternal and perinatal morbidity and mortality from general anesthesia. From this, it appears that the major question regarding management of nonsevere gestational hypertension remains: Is it acceptable to avoid unnecessary treatment of 99 women to risk eclampsia in one?

TABLE 34-18. Selected Pregnancy Outcomes in 6518 Women with Gestational Hypertension According to Whether They Developed Eclampsia

Pregnancy Outcomes	Eclampsia No. (%)	Gestational Hypertension[a] No. (%)	p value
Number	87	6431	
Maternal			
Cesarean delivery	32 (37)	2423 (38)	0.86
Placental abruption	1 (1)	72 (1)	0.98
General anesthesia[b]	20 (23)	270 (4)	< 0.001
Neonatal			
Composite morbidity[c]	10 (12)	240 (1)	0.04

[a]Includes women who had preeclampsia.
[b]Emergent cesarean delivery.
[c]One or more: cord artery pH < 7.0; 5-minute Apgar score < 4; perinatal death; or unanticipated admission of term infant to an intensive care nursery.
Data from Alexander and colleagues (2006).

Delivery

To avoid maternal risks from cesarean delivery, steps to effect vaginal delivery are used initially in women with eclampsia. Following a seizure, labor often ensues spontaneously or can be induced successfully even in women remote from term (Alanis and associates, 2008). An immediate cure does not promptly follow delivery by any route, but serious morbidity is less common during the puerperium in women delivered vaginally.

Blood Loss at Delivery

Hemoconcentration or lack of normal pregnancy-induced hypervolemia is an almost predictable feature of severe preeclampsia-eclampsia as quantified by Zeeman and associates (2009) and shown in Figure 34-6. **These women, who consequently lack normal pregnancy hypervolemia, are much less tolerant of even normal blood loss than are normotensive pregnant women.** It is of great importance to recognize that an appreciable fall in blood pressure soon after delivery most often means excessive blood loss and not sudden resolution of vasospasm and endothelial damage. When oliguria follows delivery, the hematocrit should be evaluated frequently to help detect excessive blood loss. If identified, hemorrhage should be treated appropriately by careful blood transfusion.

Analgesia and Anesthesia

During the past 20 years, the use of conduction analgesia for women with preeclampsia syndrome has proven ideal. Initial problems with this method included hypotension and diminished uterine perfusion caused by sympathetic blockade in these women with attenuated hypervolemia. Development of techniques that used slow induction of epidural analgesia with dilute solutions of anesthetic agents were reported to counter the need for rapid infusion of large volumes of crystalloid or colloid to correct maternal hypotension and usually averts pulmonary edema (Hogg and colleagues, 1999; Wallace and co-workers, 1995). Moreover, epidural blockade avoids stimulation caused by tracheal intubation, which can cause sudden severe hypertension. Such blood pressure increases, in turn, can cause pulmonary edema, cerebral edema, or intracranial hemorrhage (Lavies and co-workers, 1989). Finally, tracheal intubation may be particularly difficult and thus hazardous in women with airway edema due to preeclampsia (American College of Obstetricians and Gynecologists, 2002b).

At least two randomized studies have been performed to evaluate these methods of analgesia and anesthesia. Wallace and colleagues (1995) studied 80 women with severe preeclampsia at a mean gestational age of 34.8 weeks who were to undergo cesarean delivery. They had not been given labor epidural analgesia and were randomized to receive general anesthesia, epidural analgesia, or combined spinal-epidural analgesia. Their mean preoperative blood pressure approximated 170/110 mm Hg, and all had proteinuria. Anesthetic and obstetrical management included antihypertensive drug therapy and limited intravenous fluids. Perinatal outcomes in each group were similar. Maternal hypotension resulting from regional analgesia was managed with judicious intravenous fluid administration. Similarly, maternal blood pressure was managed to avert severe hypertension in women undergoing general anesthesia (Fig. 34-22). There were no serious maternal or fetal complications attributable to any of the three anesthetic methods. It was concluded that all three are acceptable for use in women with pregnancies complicated by severe preeclampsia if steps are taken to ensure a careful approach to either method. A similar conclusion was reached by Dyer and colleagues (2003) following their randomized study of spinal analgesia versus general anesthesia in 70 women with preeclampsia and a nonreassuring fetal heart rate tracing. Dyer and associates (2008) later showed that decreased vascular resistance and mean arterial blood pressure induced by

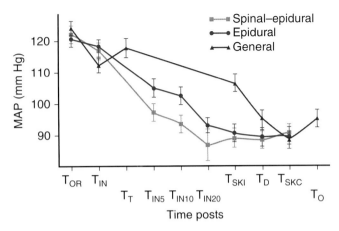

FIGURE 34-22 Blood pressure effects of general anesthesia versus epidural or spinal–epidural analgesia for cesarean delivery in 80 women with severe preeclampsia. MAP = mean arterial pressure. Time posts (T): OR = operating room; IN = induction of anesthesia; T = tracheal intubation; IN5 = induction + 5 min; IN10 = induction + 10 min; IN20 = induction + 20 min; SKI = skin incision; D = delivery; SKC = skin closure; O = extubation. (From Wallace and associates, 1995, with permission.)

epidural blockade were effectively counteracted by phenylephrine infusion to maintain cardiac output.

In a study from the University of Alabama at Birmingham, Head and co-workers (2002) randomly assigned 116 women with severe preeclampsia to receive either epidural or patient-controlled intravenous meperidine analgesia during labor. A standardized protocol limited intravenous fluids to 100 mL/hour. More women—9 percent—from the group assigned to epidural analgesia required ephedrine for hypotension. As expected, pain relief was superior in the epidural group but otherwise, maternal and neonatal complications were similar between groups. One woman in each group developed pulmonary edema.

In the past, some believed that epidural analgesia was an important factor in the intrapartum *treatment* of women with preeclampsia (Gutsche and Cheek, 1993). Lucas and associates (2001) studied 738 laboring women at Parkland Hospital who were 36 weeks or more and who had gestational hypertension of varying severity. Patients were randomly assigned to receive either epidural analgesia or patient-controlled intravenous

meperidine analgesia. Maternal and infant outcomes were similar in the two study groups. As shown in Table 34-19, although epidural analgesia resulted in a greater decrement of mean maternal arterial pressure compared with meperidine, it was not superior in preventing recurrent severe hypertension later in labor. Thus, labor epidural analgesia should not be misconstrued to be a therapy for hypertension.

For these reasons, judicious fluid administration in severely preeclamptic women who receive regional analgesia is key in their management. Newsome and associates (1986) showed that epidural blockade in women with severe preeclampsia caused elevation of pulmonary capillary wedge pressures. It is clear that aggressive volume replacement in these women increases their risk for pulmonary edema, especially in the first 72 hours postpartum (Clark and colleagues, 1985; Cotton and co-workers, 1986a). When pulmonary edema develops, there is also concern for development of cerebral edema. Finally, Heller and associates (1983) demonstrated that most cases of pharyngolaryngeal edema were related to aggressive volume therapy.

Persistent Severe Postpartum Hypertension

The potential problem of antihypertensive agents causing serious compromise of uteroplacental perfusion and thus of fetal well-being is obviated by delivery. Postpartum, if difficulty arises in controlling severe hypertension or if intravenous hydralazine or labetalol are being used repeatedly, then oral regimens can be given. Examples include labetalol or another β-blocker, nifedipine or another calcium-channel blocker, and possible addition of a thiazide diuretic. Persistent or refractory hypertension is likely due to mobilization of interstitial edema fluid and redistribution into the intravenous compartment, underlying chronic hypertension, or usually both (Tan and deSwiet, 2002). In women with chronic hypertension and left-ventricular hypertrophy, severe postpartum hypertension can cause pulmonary edema from cardiac failure (Cunningham and colleagues, 1986; Sibai and co-workers, 1987a).

Furosemide

Because persistence of severe hypertension corresponds to the onset and length of diuresis and extracellular fluid mobilization,

TABLE 34-19. Comparison of Cardiovascular Effects of Epidural versus Patient-Controlled Meperidine Analgesia During Labor in Women with Gestational Hypertension

	Labor Analgesia		
Hemodynamic Change	Epidural (n = 372)	Meperidine (n = 366)	p value
Mean arterial pressure change (mean)	−25 mm Hg	−15 mm Hg	< 0.001
Ephedrine for hypotension	11%	0	< 0.001
Severe hypertension after analgesia (BP ≥ 160/110 mm Hg)	< 1%	1%	NS

NS = not significant.
Data from Lucas and associates (2001).

it seems logical that furosemide-augmented diuresis might serve to hasten blood pressure control. To study this, Ascarelli and associates (2005) designed a randomized trial that included 264 postpartum preeclamptic women. After onset of spontaneous diuresis, patients were randomly assigned to 20-mg oral furosemide given daily versus no therapy. Compared with women with mild disease, those with severe preeclampsia had a lower mean systolic blood pressure at 2 days—142 versus 153 mm Hg—and less often required antihypertensive therapy during the remainder of hospitalization—14 versus 26 percent, respectively.

We have used a simple method to estimate excessive extracellular/interstitial fluid. The *postpartum weight* is compared with the last recorded recent *prenatal weight*, either from the last clinic visit or upon admission for delivery. On average, soon after delivery, maternal weight should be reduced by at least 10 to 15 pounds depending on birthweight, amnionic fluid volume, placental weight, and blood loss. Because of various interventions, especially intravenous crystalloid infusions given during operative vaginal or cesarean delivery, women with severe preeclampsia often have a postpartum weight *in excess of their last prenatal weight*. If this weight increase is associated with severe persistent postpartum hypertension, diuresis with intravenous furosemide is usually helpful.

Plasma Exchange

Martin and colleagues (1995) have described an atypical syndrome in which severe preeclampsia-eclampsia persists despite delivery. These investigators described 18 such women who they encountered over a 10-year period. They advocate single or multiple plasma exchange for these women. In some cases, 3 L of plasma was exchanged three times—a 36- to 45-donor unit exposure for each patient—before a response was forthcoming. Others have described plasma exchange performed in postpartum women with HELLP syndrome (Förster and associates, 2002; Obeidat and colleagues, 2002). In all of these cases, however, the distinction between HELLP syndrome and thrombotic thrombocytopenic purpura or hemolytic uremic syndrome was not clear. As further discussed in Chapter 51 (p. 1095), in our experiences with more than 50,000 women with gestational hypertension among nearly 400,000 pregnancies cared for at Parkland Hospital through 2009, we have encountered very few women with persistent postpartum hypertension, thrombocytopenia, and renal dysfunction who were diagnosed as having a thrombotic microangiopathy (Dashe and co-workers, 1998). As concluded by Martin and colleagues (2008) after their review of 166 pregnancies complicated by thrombotic thrombocytopenic purpura, a rapid diagnostic test such as that for ADAMTS-13 enzyme activity might be helpful to differentiate most of these.

Postpartum Angiopathy. Another cause of persistent hypertension, seizures, and central nervous system findings is termed postpartum angiopathy. Also known as the *reversible cerebral vasoconstriction syndrome*, it is more common in women, and is associated with a myriad of different precipitating events, with pregnancy and the puerperium being just one of these (Singhal and co-workers, 2009). In some cases, vasoconstriction may be

so severe as to cause cerebral ischemia and areas of infarction. The appropriate management is not known at this time.

LONG-TERM CONSEQUENCES

Women with hypertension identified during pregnancy should be evaluated during the first several months postpartum. They are counseled about long-term risks. As discussed earlier, the longer hypertension identified during pregnancy persists postpartum, the greater the likelihood that the woman has chronic hypertension. The Working Group concluded that hypertension attributable to pregnancy should resolve within 12 weeks of delivery (National High Blood Pressure Education Program, 2000). Persistence beyond this time is considered to be chronic hypertension (see Chap. 45, p. 983). The Magpie Trial Follow-Up Collaborative Group (2007) reported that 20 percent of 3375 preeclamptic women seen at a median of 26 months postpartum had hypertension. But even if hypertension does not persist in the short term, there is now convincing evidence that the risk for long-term cardiovascular morbidity is significantly increased in preeclamptic women as subsequently discussed.

Counseling for Future Pregnancies

Women who have had either gestational hypertension or preeclampsia are at higher risk to develop hypertensive and metabolic complications in future pregnancies. Generally, the earlier preeclampsia is diagnosed during the index pregnancy, the greater the likelihood of recurrence. For example, Sibai and colleagues (1986, 1991) found that nulliparous women diagnosed with preeclampsia before 30 weeks have a recurrence risk as high as 40 percent during a subsequent pregnancy.

In a study of 511 Icelandic women with gestational hypertension during their first pregnancy, Hjartardottir and co-workers (2006) reported an astonishing 70-percent recurrence risk for hypertension in the second pregnancy. Although most of these women had recurrent gestational hypertension, 5 percent had preeclampsia and 16 percent had chronic hypertension. The 151 women with preeclampsia in the first pregnancy had an overall 58-percent recurrence rate—over half had gestational hypertension and about a fourth each had either preeclampsia or chronic hypertensive disease. In a much larger study from the Denmark Birth Registry, Lykke and co-workers (2009b) analyzed singleton births in more than 535,000 women who had a first and second delivery from 1978 to 2007. Women whose first pregnancy was complicated by preeclampsia between 32 and 36 weeks had a significant twofold increased incidence of preeclampsia in their second pregnancy 25 versus 14 percent—compared with women who were normotensive during the first pregnancy. They also found that preterm delivery and fetal-growth restriction in the first pregnancy slightly, albeit significantly, increased the risk for preeclampsia in the second pregnancy.

Women with HELLP syndrome have a substantive risk for recurrence in subsequent pregnancies. In an earlier study, Sibai and colleagues (1995) found this to be approximately 5 percent, but this same group later described a 26-percent recurrence risk (Habli and co-workers, 2009). The true recurrence risk likely lies between these two extremes. Even if HELLP syndrome does not recur with subsequent recurrent preeclampsia, there is a high incidence of preterm delivery, fetal-growth restriction, placental abruption, and cesarean delivery (Habli and associates, 2009; Hnat and colleagues, 2002).

Some women with early-onset severe preeclampsia are found to have underlying thrombophilias (see p. 718). These disorders may also complicate subsequent pregnancies. For example, Facchinetti and associates (2009) reported a twofold increased risk for recurrent preeclampsia in women with a thrombophilia and preeclampsia compared with preeclamptic women without thrombophilia identified. In addition, these inherited disorders also affect overall long-term health (see Chap. 47, p. 1014).

Long-Term Sequelae

Cardiovascular and Neurovascular Morbidity

With the advent of national databases, several long-term studies confirm that any hypertension during pregnancy is a marker for increased rates of later cardiovascular-related morbidity and mortality. In a case-control study from Iceland, Arnadottir and colleagues (2005) analyzed outcomes for 325 women who had hypertension complicating pregnancy and who were delivered from 1931 through 1947. At a median follow-up of 50 years, 60 percent of hypertensive women compared with only 53 percent of controls had died. Compared with 629 normotensive pregnant controls, the prevalences of *ischemic heart*

disease—24 versus 15 percent, and *stroke*—9.5 versus 6.5 percent, were significantly increased in the women who had had hypertension during pregnancy. In a Swedish population study of more than 400,000 nulliparous women delivered between 1973 and 1982, Wikström and co-workers (2005) also found an increased incidence of ischemic heart disease in women with prior pregnancy-associated hypertension.

Lykke and associates (2009a) cited findings from a Danish registry of more than 780,000 nulliparous women having a singleton delivery from 1978 to 2007. After a mean follow-up of almost 15 years, the incidence of *chronic hypertension* was significantly increased 5.2-fold in those who had gestational hypertension, 3.5-fold after mild preeclampsia, and 6.4-fold after severe preeclampsia. After two hypertensive pregnancies, there was a 5.9-fold increase in the incidence of chronic hypertension. Importantly, these investigators also reported a significant 3.5-fold increased risk for *type 2 diabetes*.

Bellamy and co-workers (2007) recently performed a systematic review and meta-analysis of long-term risks for cardiovascular disease in women with preeclampsia. As shown in Figure 34-23, the risks in later life were increased for hypertension, ischemic heart disease, stroke, venous thromboembolism, as well as all-cause mortality. As emphasized by Harskamp and associates (2007), a number of cofactors or comorbidities are related to acquisition of these long-term adverse outcomes associated with pregnancy hypertension. These include but are not limited to the metabolic syndrome, diabetes, obesity, dyslipidemia, and atherosclerosis. These conclusions are underscored by the

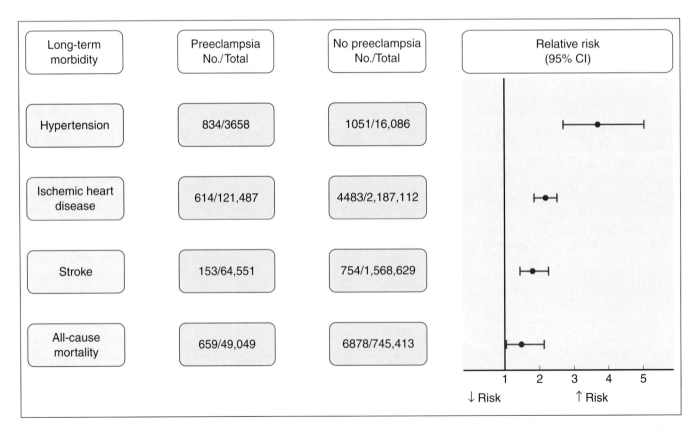

FIGURE 34-23 Long-term cardiovascular consequences of preeclampsia. All differences $p \leq .001$ except p = 0.03 for all-cause mortality. (Data from Bellamy and colleagues, 2007.)

findings of Berends and colleagues (2008), who confirmed shared constitutional risks for long-term vascular related risks in preeclamptic women as well as in their parents. Similar preliminary observations were recently reported by Smith and associates (2009) in an ongoing investigation.

Renal Sequelae

In a 40-year study of Norwegian birth and end-stage renal disease linked registries, Vikse and associates (2008) found that although the absolute risk of renal failure was small, preeclampsia was associated with a fourfold increased risk. Women with recurrent preeclampsia had an even greater risk. These data need to be considered in light of the findings that 15 to 20 percent of women with preeclampsia who undergo renal biopsy have evidence of chronic renal disease (Chesley, 1978). In another long-term follow-up study, Spaan and co-workers (2009) compared formerly preeclamptic women with a cohort of women who were normotensive at delivery. At 20 years following delivery, preeclamptic women were significantly more likely to be chronically hypertensive—55 versus 7 percent—compared with control women. They also had higher peripheral vascular and renal vascular resistance and decreased renal blood flow. These data do not permit conclusions of cause versus effect.

Neurological Sequelae

Until recently, it was commonly held that eclamptic seizures have no significant long-term sequelae. Findings have now accrued, however, that this is not always the case. Recall that almost all eclamptic women have multifocal areas of perivascular edema, as discussed on page 722. Approximately one fourth also have areas of cerebral infarctions. Recent preliminary data are compatible with long-term persistence of brain white matter lesions incurred at the time of eclamptic convulsions (Aukes and colleagues, 2009). When studied with MR imaging at a mean of 7.1 years, 40 percent of formerly eclamptic women had more and larger aggregate white matter lesions compared with only 17 percent of normotensive control women. The clinical relevance of these observations is not yet known. In studies designed to assess this, Aukes and colleagues (2007) reported that formerly eclamptic women had subjectively impaired cognitive functioning. They later reported preliminary evidence that women with multiple seizures had impaired sustained attention compared with contemporaneous normotensive controls (Postma and co-workers, 2009). Because there were no studies done before these women suffered from eclampsia, the investigators appropriately concluded that only limited conclusions are warranted.

REFERENCES

Abalos E, Duley L, Steyn DW, et al: Antihypertensive drug therapy for mild to moderate hypertension during pregnancy. Cochrane Database Syst Rev 1:CD002252, 2007

Abdul-Karim R, Assali NS: Pressor response to angiotonin in pregnant and nonpregnant women. Am J Obstet Gynecol 82:246, 1961

Abenhaim HA, Bujold E, Benjamin A, et al: Evaluating the role of bedrest on the prevention of hypertensive disease of pregnancy and growth restriction. Hypertens Pregnancy 27(2):197, 2008

Abramovici D, Friedman SA, Mercer BM, et al: Neonatal outcome in severe preeclampsia at 24 to 36 weeks' gestation: Does the HELLP (hemolysis, elevated liver enzyme, and low platelet count) syndrome matter? Am J Obstet Gynecol 180:221, 1999

Airoldi J, Weinstein L: Clinical significance of proteinuria in pregnancy. Obstet Gynecol Surv 62:117, 2007

Ajne G, Wolff K, Fyhrquist F, et al: Endothelin converting enzyme (ECE) activity in normal pregnancy and preeclampsia. Hypertens Pregnancy 22:215, 2003

Akkawi C, Kent E, Geary M, et al: The incidence of eclampsia in a single defined population with a selective use of magnesium sulfate. Abstract No 798. Presented at the 29th Annual Meeting of the Society for Maternal-Fetal Medicine, January 26-31, 2009

Alanis MC, Robinson CJ, Hulsey TC, et al: Early-onset severe preeclampsia: Induction of labor vs elective cesarean delivery and neonatal outcomes. Am J Obstet Gynecol 199:262.e1, 2008

Alexander JM, Bloom SL, McIntire DD, et al: Severe preeclampsia and the very low-birthweight infant: Is induction of labor harmful? Obstet Gynecol 93:485, 1999

Alexander JM, McIntire DD, Leveno KJ, et al: Magnesium sulfate for the prevention of eclampsia in women with mild hypertension. Am J Obstet Gynecol 189:S89, 2003

Alexander JM, McIntire DD, Leveno KJ, et al: Selective magnesium sulfate prophylaxis for the prevention of eclampsia in women with gestational hypertension. Obstet Gynecol 108:826, 2006

Alexander JM, Sarode R, McIntire DD, et al: Use of whole blood in the management of hypovolemia due to obstetric hemorrhage. Obstet Gynecol, In press, 2009

American College of Obstetricians and Gynecologists: Antepartum fetal surveillance. Practice Bulletin No. 9, October 1999

American College of Obstetricians and Gynecologists: Diagnosis and management of preeclampsia and eclampsia. Practice Bulletin No. 33, January 2002a

American College of Obstetricians and Gynecologists: Obstetric analgesia and anesthesia. Practice Bulletin No. 36, July 2002b

Amorim MMR, Santos LC, Faúndes A: Corticosteroid therapy for prevention of respiratory distress syndrome in severe preeclampsia. Am J Obstet Gynecol 180:1283, 1999

Ananth C, Basso O: Impact of pregnancy-induced hypertension on perinatal survival in first and higher order births: A population-based study. Abstract No 819. Presented at the 29th Annual Meeting of the Society for Maternal-Fetal Medicine, January 26–31, 2009

Ananth CV, Bowes WA, Savitz DA, et al: Relationship between pregnancy-induced hypertension and placenta previa: A population-based study. Am J Obstet Gynecol 177:997, 1997

Andersgaard AB, Herbst A, Johansen M, et al: Eclampsia in Scandinavia: Incidence, substandard care, and potentially preventable cases. Acta Obstet Gynecol 85:929, 2006

Arango MF, Mejia-Mantilla JH: Magnesium for acute traumatic brain injury. Cochrane Database Syst Rev 4:CD005400, 2006

Arnadottir GA, Geirsson RT, Arngrimsson Reynir, et al: Cardiovascular death in women who had hypertension in pregnancy: A case-control study. BJOG 112:286, 2005

Ascarelli MH, Johnson V, McCreary H, et al: Postpartum preeclampsia management with furosemide: A randomized clinical trial. Obstet Gynecol 105:29, 2005

Askie LM, Henderson-Smart DJ, Stewart LA: Antiplatelet agents for the prevention of preeclampsia: A meta-analysis of individual data. Lancet 369:179, 2007

Atkinson MW, Guinn D, Owen J, et al: Does magnesium sulfate affect the length of labor induction in women with pregnancy-associated hypertension? Am J Obstet Gynecol 173:1219, 1995

August P, Lindheimer MD: Chronic hypertension and pregnancy. In Lindheimer MD, Roberts JM, Cunningham FG (eds): Chesley's Hypertensive Disorders of Pregnancy, 3rd ed. New York, Elsevier, In press, 2009, p 359

Aukes AM, de Groot JC, Aarnoudse JG, et al: Brain lesions several years after eclampsia. Am J Obstet Gynecol 200(5):504.e1, 2009

Aukes AM, Wessel I, Dubois AM, et al: Self-reported cognitive functioning in formerly eclamptic women. Am J Obstet Gynecol 197(4):365.e1, 2007

Bagrov AY, Shapiro JI: Endogenous digitalis: Pathophysiologic roles and therapeutic applications. Nat Clin Pract Nephrol 4(7):378, 2008

Bainbridge SA, Sidle EH, Smith GN: Direct placental effects of cigarette smoke protect women from pre-eclampsia: The specific roles of carbon monoxide and antioxidant systems in the placenta. Med Hypotheses 64:17, 2005

Barber D, Xing G, Towner D: Expectant management of severe eclampsia between 24–32 weeks gestation: A ten year review. Abstract No 742. Presented at the 29th Annual Meeting of the Society for Maternal-Fetal Medicine, January 26-31, 2009

Barron WM, Heckerling P, Hibbard JU, et al: Reducing unnecessary coagulation testing in hypertensive disorders of pregnancy. Obstet Gynecol 94:364, 1999

Barton CR, Barton JR, O'Brien JM, et al: Mild gestational hypertension: Differences in ethnicity are associated with altered outcomes in women who undergo outpatient treatment. Am J Obstet Gynecol 186:896, 2002

Barton J, Barton L, Istwan N, et al: The frequency of elective delivery at 34.0–36.9 weeks' gestation and its impact on neonatal outcomes in women with stable mild gestational hypertension (MGHTN). Abstract No 252. Presented at the 29th Annual Meeting of the Society for Maternal-Fetal Medicine, January 26–31, 2009

Barton JR, Riely CA, Adamec TA, et al: Hepatic histopathologic condition does not correlate with laboratory abnormalities in HELLP syndrome (hemolysis, elevated liver enzymes, and low platelet count). Am J Obstet Gynecol 167:1538, 1992

Barton JR, Sibai BM: HELLP and the liver diseases of preeclampsia. Clin Liver Dis 3:31, 1999

Basso O, Rasmussen S, Weinberg CR, et al: Trends in fetal and infant survival following preeclampsia. JAMA 296(11):1357, 2006

Bdolah Y, Palomaki GE, Yaron Y, et al: Circulating angiogenic proteins in trisomy 13. Am J Obstet Gynecol 194(1):239, 2006

Belfort MA, Anthony J, Buccimazza A, et al: Hemodynamic changes associated with intravenous infusion of the calcium antagonist verapamil in the treatment of severe gestational proteinuric hypertension. Obstet Gynecol 75:970, 1990

Belfort M, Anthony J, Saade G, et al: A comparison of magnesium sulfate and nimodipine for the prevention of eclampsia. N Engl J Med 348:304, 2003

Belfort MA, Taskin O, Buhur A, et al: Intravenous nimodipine in the management of severe preeclampsia: Double blind, randomized, controlled clinical trial. Am J Obstet Gynecol 174:451, 1996

Belizan JM, Villar J: The relationship between calcium intake and edema-, proteinuria-, and hypertension-getosis: An hypothesis. Am J Clin Nutr 33: 2202, 1980

Bellamy L, Casas JP, Hingorani AD, et al: Pre-eclampsia and risk of cardiovascular disease and cancer in later life: Systematic review and meta-analysis. BMJ 335:974, 2007

Benedetti TJ, Cotton DB, Read JC, et al: Hemodynamic observations in severe preeclampsia with a flow-directed pulmonary artery catheter. Am J Obstet Gynecol 136:465, 1980

Benedetti TJ, Kates R, Williams V: Hemodynamic observations in severe preeclampsia complicated by pulmonary edema. Am J Obstet Gynecol 152: 330,1985

Benhamou D, Chassard D, Mercier FJ, et al: The seventh report of the confidential enquiries into maternal deaths in the United Kingdom: Comparison with French data. Ann Fr Anesth Reanim 28:38, 2009

Berends AL, de Groot CJ, Sijbrands EJ, et al: Shared constitutional risks for maternal vascular-related pregnancy complications and future cardiovascular disease. Hypertension 51:1034, 2008

Berg CJ, Chang J, Callaghan WM, et al: Pregnancy-related mortality in the United States 1991–1997. Obstet Gynecol 101:289, 2003

Berg CJ, Harper MA, Atkinson SM, et al: Preventability of pregnancy-related deaths. Obstet Gynecol 106:1228, 2005

Bhalla AK, Dhall GI, Dhall K: A safer and more effective treatment regimen for eclampsia. Aust NZ J Obstet Gynecol 34:14,1994

Blodi BA, Johnson MW, Gass JD, et al: Purtscher's-like retinopathy after childbirth. Ophthalmology 97(12):1654, 1990

Bloom SL, Leveno KJ: Corticosteroid use in special circumstances: Preterm ruptured membranes, hypertension, fetal growth restriction, multiple fetuses. Clin Obstet Gynecol 46:150, 2003

Bolte AC, Gafar S, van Eyck J, et al: Ketanserin, a better option in the treatment of preeclampsia? Am J Obstet Gynecol 178:S118, 1998

Bolte AC, van Eyck J, Gaffar SF, et al: Ketanserin for the treatment of preeclampsia. J Perinat Med 29:14, 2001

Bombrys AE, Barton JR, Habli M, Sibai BM: Expectant management of severe preeclampsia at 27⁰∕₇ to 33⁶∕₇ weeks' gestation: maternal and perinatal outcomes according to gestational age by weeks at onset of expectant management. Am J Perinatol 26:441, 2009

Bombrys AE, Barton JR, Nowacki EA, et al: Expectant management of severe preeclampsia at less than 27 weeks' gestation: maternal and perinatal outcomes according to gestational age by weeks at onset of expectant management. Am J Obstet Gynecol 199:247.e1, 2008

Borghi C, Esposti DD, Immordino V, et al: Relationship of systemic hemodynamics, left ventricular structure and function, and plasma natriuretic peptide concentrations during pregnancy complicated by preeclampsia. Am J Obstet Gynecol 183:140, 2000

Borowski K, Kair L, Zeng S, et al: Lack of association of FAS gene and preeclampsia. Abstract No 706. Presented at the 29th Annual Meeting of the Society for Maternal-Fetal Medicine, January 26–31, 2009

Borzychowski AM, Sargent IL, Redman CW: Inflammation and pre-eclampsia. Semin Fetal Neonatal Med 11(5), 309, 2006

Bosio PM, McKenna PJ, Conroy R, et al: Maternal central hemodynamics in hypertensive disorders of pregnancy. Obstet Gynecol 94:978, 1999

Brown CEL, Cunningham FG, Pritchard JA: Convulsions in hypertensive, proteinuric primiparas more than 24 hours after delivery: Eclampsia or some other cause? J Reprod Med 32:499, 1987

Brown MA, Gallery EDM, Ross MR, et al: Sodium excretion in normal and hypertensive pregnancy: A prospective study. Am J Obstet Gynecol 159:297, 1988

Brown MA, Zammit VC, Lowe SA: Capillary permeability and extracellular fluid volumes in pregnancy-induced hypertension. Clin Sci 77:599, 1989

Brubaker DB, Ross MG, Marinoff D: The function of elevated plasma fibronectin in preeclampsia. Am J Obstet Gynecol 166:526, 1992

Budden A, Wilkinson L, Buksh MJ, et al: Pregnancy outcomes in women presenting with pre-eclampsia at less than 25 weeks gestation. Aust NZ J Obstet Gynaecol 46(5):407, 2006

Bush KD, O'Brien JM, Barton JR: The utility of umbilical artery Doppler investigation in women with HELLP (hemolysis, elevated liver enzymes, and low platelet count) syndrome. Am J Obstet Gynecol 184:1087, 2001

Caritis S, Sibai B, Hauth J, et al: Low-dose aspirin to prevent preeclampsia in women at high risk. National Institute of Child Health and Human Development Network of Maternal–Fetal Medicine Units. N Engl J Med 338:701, 1998

Carlson KL, Bader CL: Ruptured subcapsular liver hematoma in pregnancy: A case report of nonsurgical management. Am J Obstet Gynecol 190:558, 2004

Chambers KA, Cain TW: Postpartum blindness: Two cases. Ann Emerg Med 43:243, 2004

Chames MC, Livingston JC, Ivester TS, et al: Late postpartum eclampsia: A preventable disease? Am J Obstet Gynecol 186:1174, 2002

Chavarria ME, Lara-Gonzalez L, Gonzalez-Gleason A, et al: Maternal plasma cellular fibronectin concentrations in normal and preeclamptic pregnancies: A longitudinal study for early prediction of preeclampsia. Am J Obstet Gynecol 187:595, 2002

Chavarria ME, Lara-González L, González-Gleason A, et al: Prostacyclin/thromboxane early changes in pregnancies that are complicated by preeclampsia. Am J Obstet Gynecol 188:986, 2003

Chen BA, Parviainen K, Jeyabalan A: Correlation of catheterized and clean catch urine protein/creatinine ratios in preeclampsia evaluation. Obstet Gynecol 112:606, 2008

Chesley LC: Diagnosis of preeclampsia. Obstet Gynecol 65:423, 1985

Chesley LC (ed): Hypertensive Disorders in Pregnancy. Appleton-Century-Crofts, New York, 1978

Chesley LC, Williams LO: Renal glomerular and tubular function in relation to the hyperuricemia of preeclampsia and eclampsia. Am J Obstet Gynecol 50:367, 1945

Chowdhury JR, Chaudhuri S, Bhattacharyya N, et al: Comparison of intramuscular magnesium sulfate with low dose intravenous magnesium sulfate regimen for treatment of eclampsia. J Obstet Gynaecol Res 35:119, 2009

Churchill D, Beever GD, Meher S, et al: Diuretics for preventing preeclampsia. Cochrane Database Syst Rev 1:CD004451, 2007

Cipolla MJ: Brief review: Cerebrovascular function during pregnancy and eclampsia. Hypertension 50:14, 2007

Cipolla MJ, Smith J, Kohlmeyer MM, et al: SKCa and IKCa channels, myogenic tone, and vasodilator responses in middle cerebral arteries and parenchymal arterioles: Effect of ischemia and reperfusion. Stroke 40(4): 1451, 2009

Clark BA, Halvorson L, Sachs B, et al: Plasma endothelin levels in preeclampsia: Elevation and correlation with uric acid levels and renal impairment. Am J Obstet Gynecol 166:962, 1992

Clark SL, Cotton DB: Clinical indications for pulmonary artery catheterization in the patient with severe preeclampsia. Am J Obstet Gynecol 158:453, 1988

Clark SL, Cotton DB, Wesley L, et al: Central hemodynamic assessment of normal term pregnancy. Am J Obstet Gynecol 161:1439, 1989

Clark SL, Divon MY, Phelan JP: Preeclampsia/eclampsia: Hemodynamic and neurologic correlations. Obstet Gynecol 66:337, 1985

Cnossen JS, de Ruyter-Hanhijarvi H, van der Post JA, et al: Accuracy of serum uric acid determination in predicting pre-eclampsia: A systematic review. Acta Obstet Gynecol Scand 85(5):519, 2006

Coetzee EJ, Dommisse J, Anthony J: A randomised controlled trial of intravenous magnesium sulphate versus placebo in the management of women with severe pre-eclampsia. Br J Obstet Gynaecol 105(3):300, 1998

Conde-Agudelo A, Belizan JM: Risk factors for pre-eclampsia in a large cohort of Latin American and Caribbean women. Br J Obstet Gynaecol 107:75, 2000

Conde-Agudelo A, Romero R, Lindheimer MD: Tests to predict preeclampsia. In Lindheimer MD, Roberts JM, Cunningham FG (eds): Chesley's Hypertensive Disorders of Pregnancy, 3rd ed. New York, Elsevier, In press, 2009, p 191

Conrad KP, Gaber LW, Lindheimer MD: The kidney in normal pregnancy and preeclampsia. In Lindheimer MD, Roberts JM, Cunningham FG (eds):

Chesley's Hypertensive Disorders of Pregnancy, 3rd ed. New York, Elsevier, In press, 2009, p 297

Conrad KP, Vernier KA: Plasma level, urinary excretion and metabolic production of cGMP during gestation in rats. Am J Physiol 257:R847, 1989

Cotton DB, Jones MM, Longmire S, et al: Role of intravenous nitroglycerine in the treatment of severe pregnancy-induced hypertension complicated by pulmonary edema. Am J Obstet Gynecol 154:91, 1986a

Cotton DB, Longmire S, Jones MM, et al: Cardiovascular alterations in severe pregnancy-induced hypertension: Effects of intravenous nitroglycerin coupled with blood volume expansion. Am J Obstet Gynecol 154:1053, 1986b

Crowther C: Magnesium sulphate versus diazepam in the management of eclampsia: A randomized controlled trial. Br J Obstet Gynaecol 97(2):110, 1990

Crowther CA, Bouwmeester AM, Ashurst HM: Does admission to hospital for bed rest prevent disease progression or improve fetal outcome in pregnancy complicated by non-proteinuric hypertension? Br J Obstet Gynaecol 99:13, 1992

Cunningham FG: Liver disease complicating pregnancy. Williams Obstetrics, 19th ed. (Suppl 1). Norwalk, CT, Appleton & Lange, 1993

Cunningham FG: Severe preeclampsia and eclampsia: Systolic hypertension is also important. Obstet Gynecol 105(2):237, 2005

Cunningham FG, Fernandez CO, Hernandez C: Blindness associated with preeclampsia and eclampsia. Am J Obstet Gynecol 172:1291, 1995

Cunningham FG, Lowe T, Guss S, et al: Erythrocyte morphology in women with severe preeclampsia and eclampsia. Am J Obstet Gynecol 153:358, 1985

Cunningham FG, Pritchard JA: How should hypertension during pregnancy be managed? Experience at Parkland Memorial Hospital. Med Clin North Am 68:505, 1984

Cunningham FG, Pritchard JA, Hankins GDV, et al: Peripartum heart failure: Idiopathic cardiomyopathy or compounding cardiovascular events? Obstet Gynecol 67:157, 1986

Cunningham FG, Twickler D: Cerebral edema complicating eclampsia. Am J Obstet Gynecol 182:94, 2000

D'Anna R, Baviera G, Corrado F, et al: Plasma homocysteine in early and late pregnancy complicated with preeclampsia and isolated intrauterine growth restriction. Acta Obstet Gynecol Scand 83:155, 2004

Dashe JS, Ramin SM, Cunningham FG: The long-term consequences of thrombotic microangiopathy (thrombotic thrombocytopenic purpura and hemolytic uremic syndrome) in pregnancy. Obstet Gynecol 91:662, 1998

De Paco C, Kametas N, Rencoret G, et al: Maternal cardiac output between 11 and 13 weeks of gestation in the prediction of preeclampsia and small for gestational age. Obstet Gynecol 111:292, 2008

De Snoo K: The prevention of eclampsia. Am J Obstet Gynecol 34:911, 1937

De Wolf F, De Wolf-Peeters C, Brosens I, et al: The human placental bed: Electron microscopic study of trophoblastic invasion of spiral arteries. Am J Obstet Gynecol 137:58, 1980

DiFederico E, Genbacev O, Fisher SJ: Preeclampsia is associated with widespread apoptosis of placental cytotrophoblasts within the uterine wall. Am J Pathol 155:293, 1999

Doyle LW, Crowther CA, Middleton S, et al: Magnesium sulfate for women at risk of preterm birth for neuroprotection of the fetus. Cochrane Database of Systemic Reviews 1:CD004661, 2009

Drakeley AJ, Le Roux PA, Anthony J, et al: Acute renal failure complicating severe preeclampsia requiring admission to an obstetric intensive care unit. Am J Obstet Gynecol 186:253, 2002

Dürr JA, Lindheimer MD: Control of volume and body tonicity. In Lindheimer MD, Roberts JM, Cunningham FG (eds): Chesley's Hypertensive Disorders in Pregnancy, 2nd ed. Stamford, CT, Appleton & Lange, 1999, p 103

Dyer RA, Els I, Farbas J, et al: Prospective, randomized trial comparing general with spinal anesthesia for cesarean delivery in preeclamptic patients with a nonreassuring fetal heart trace. Anesthesiology 99:561, 2003

Dyer RA, Piercy JL, Reed AR, et al: Hemodynamic changes associated with spinal anesthesia for cesarean delivery in severe preeclampsia. Anesthesiology 108(5):802, 2008

Easterling TR, Benedetti TJ, Schmucker BC, et al: Maternal hemodynamics in normal and preeclamptic pregnancies: A longitudinal study. Obstet Gynecol 76:1061, 1990

Eclampsia Trial Collaborative Group: Which anticonvulsant for women with eclampsia? Evidence from the collaborative eclampsia trial. Lancet 345:1455, 1995

Ehrenberg HM, Mercer BM: Abbreviated postpartum magnesium sulphate therapy for women with mild preeclampsia: A randomized controlled trial. Obstet Gynecol 108(4):833, 2006

Eremina V, Baelde HJ, Quaggin SE: Role of the VEGF—A signaling pathway in the glomerulus: Evidence for crosstalk between components of the glomerular filtration barrier. Nephron Physiol 106(2):32, 2007

Faas MM, Schuiling GA, Linton EA, et al: Activation of peripheral leukocytes in rat pregnancy and experimental preeclampsia. Am J Obstet Gynecol 182:351, 2000

Facchinetti F, Marozio L, Frusca T, et al: Maternal thrombophilia and the risk of recurrence of preeclampsia. Am J Obstet Gynecol 200:46.e1, 2009

Finnerty FA, Buchholz JH, Tuckman J: Evaluation of chlorothiazide (Diuril) in the toxemias of pregnancy. JAMA 166:141, 1958

Fisher SJ, McMaster M, Roberts JM: The placenta in normal pregnancy and preeclampsia. In Lindheimer MD, Roberts JM, Cunningham FG (eds): Chesley's Hypertensive Disorders of Pregnancy, 3rd ed. New York, Elsevier, In press, 2009, p 73

Fleischer A, Schulman H, Farmakides G, et al: Uterine artery Doppler velocimetry in pregnant women with hypertension. Am J Obstet Gynecol 154:806, 1986

Flowers CE, Grizzle JE, Easterling WE, et al: Chlorothiazide as a prophylaxis against toxemia of pregnancy. A double blind study. Am J Obstet Gynecol 84:919, 1962

Fonseca JE, Méndez F, Cataño C, et al: Dexamethasone treatment does not improve the outcome of women with HELLP syndrome: A double-blind, placebo-controlled, randomized clinical trial. Am J Obstet Gynecol 193:1591, 2005

Förster JG, Peltonen S, Kaaja R, et al: Plasma exchange in severe postpartum HELLP syndrome. Acta Anaesthesiol Scand 46:955, 2002

Gamzu R, Rotstein R, Fusman R, et al: Increased erythrocyte adhesiveness and aggregation in peripheral venous blood of women with pregnancy-induced hypertension. Obstet Gynecol 98:307, 2001

Gant NF, Chand S, Worley RJ, et al: A clinical test useful for predicting the development of acute hypertension in pregnancy. Am J Obstet Gynecol 120:1, 1974

Ganzevoort W, Rep A, Bonsel GJ, et al: Plasma volume and blood pressure regulation in hypertensive pregnancy. J Hypertens 22:1235, 2004

Ganzevoort W, Rep A, PERTA investigators, et al: A randomized controlled trial comparing two temporizing management strategies, one with and one without plasma volume expansion, for severe and early onset pre-eclampsia. BJOG 112:1337, 2005a

Ganzevoort W, Rep A, Bonsel GJ, et al: A randomized trial of plasma volume expansion in hypertensive disorders of pregnancy: Influence on the pulsatile indices of the fetal umbilical artery and middle cerebral artery. Am J Obstet Gynecol 192:233, 2005b

Garovic VD, Wagner SJ, Turner ST, et al: Urinary podocyte excretion as a marker for preeclampsia. Am J Obstet Gynecol 196:320.e1, 2007

Gaugler-Senden IP, Huijssoon AG, Visser W, et al: Maternal and perinatal outcome of preeclampsia with an onset before 24 weeks' gestation. Audit in a tertiary referral center. Eur J Obstet Gynecol Reprod Biol 128:216, 2006

Gebb J, Landsberger E, Merkatz I, et al: First trimester uterine artery Doppler, PAPP-A and 3D power Doppler of the intervillous space in patients at risk for preeclampsia. Abstract No 251. Presented at the 29th Annual Meeting of the Society for Maternal-Fetal Medicine, January 26–31, 2009a

Gebb J, Einstein F, Merkatz IR, et al: First trimester 3D power Doppler of the intervillous space in patients with decreased PAPP-A levels and increased uterine artery pulsatility index. Abstract No 279. Presented at the 29th Annual Meeting of the Society for Maternal-Fetal Medicine, January 26–31, 2009b

Gervasi MT, Chaiworapongsa T, Pacora P, et al: Phenotypic and metabolic characteristics of monocytes and granulocytes in preeclampsia. Am J Obstet Gynecol 185:792, 2001

Getahun D, Ananth CV, Oyeese Y, et al: Primary preeclampsia in the second pregnancy. Obstet Gynecol 110:1319, 2007

Ghidini A, Locatelli A: Monitoring of fetal well-being: Role of uterine artery Doppler. Semin Perinatol 32:258, 2008

Gilstrap LC, Cunningham FG, Whalley PJ: Management of pregnancy-induced hypertension in the nulliparous patient remote from term. Semin Perinatol 2:73, 1978

Gortzak-Uzan L, Mezad D, Smolin A: Increasing amniotic fluid magnesium concentrations with stable maternal serum levels. A prospective clinical trial. J Reprod Med 50:817, 2005

Grisaru D, Zwang E, Peyser MR, et al: The procoagulant activity of red blood cells from patients with severe preeclampsia. Am J Obstet Gynecol 177:1513, 1997

Groom KM, North RA, Stone PR, et al: Patterns of change in uterine artery Doppler studies between 20 and 24 weeks of gestation and pregnancy outcomes. Obstet Gynecol 113(2):332, 2009

Grundmann M, Woywodt A, Kirsch T, et al: Circulating endothelial cells: A marker of vascular damage in patients with preeclampsia. Am J Obstet Gynecol 198:317.e1, 2008

Gutsche BB, Cheek TG: Anesthesia considerations in preeclampsia-eclampsia. In Shnider SM, Levinson G (eds): Anesthesia for Obstetrics, 3rd ed. Baltimore, Williams & Wilkins, 1993, p 321

Habek D, Bobic MV, Habek JC: Oncotic therapy in management of preeclampsia. Arch Med Res 37:619, 2006

Habli M, Eftekhari N, Wiebrach E, et al: Long term outcome of HELLP syndrome. Abstract No 763. Presented at the 29th Annual Meeting of the Society for Maternal-Fetal Medicine, January 26–31, 2009

Haddad B, Barton JR, Livingston JC, et al: Risk factors for adverse maternal outcomes among women with HELLP (hemolysis, elevated liver enzymes, and low platelet count) syndrome. Am J Obstet Gynecol 183:444, 2000

Haddad B, Deis S, Goffinet F, et al: Maternal and perinatal outcomes during expectant management of 239 preeclamptic women between 24 and 33 weeks' gestation. Am J Obstet Gynecol 190(6):1590, 2004

Haddad B, Kayem G, Deis S, et al: Are perinatal and maternal outcomes different during expectant management of severe preeclampsia in the presence of intrauterine growth restriction? Am J Obstet Gynecol 196:237.e1, 2007

Hall DR, Odendaal HJ, Steyn DW: Expectant management of severe preeclampsia in the mid-trimester. Eur J Obstet Gynecol Reprod Biol 96(2): 168, 2001

Hallak M, Berry SM, Madincea F, et al: Fetal serum and amniotic fluid magnesium concentrations with maternal treatment. Obstet Gynecol 81:185, 1993

Hallak M, Hotca JW, Evans JB: Magnesium sulfate affects the N-methyl-D-aspartate receptor binding in maternal rat brain. Am J Obstet Gynecol 178:S112, 1998

Hallak M, Kupsky WJ, Hotra JW, et al: Fetal rat brain damage caused by maternal seizure activity: Prevention by magnesium sulfate. Am J Obstet Gynecol 181:828, 1999a

Hallak M, Martinez-Poyer J, Kruger ML, et al: The effect of magnesium sulfate on fetal heart rate parameters: A randomized, placebo-controlled trial. Am J Obstet Gynecol 181:1122, 1999b

Hankins GDV, Wendel GW Jr, Cunningham FG, et al: Longitudinal evaluation of hemodynamic changes in eclampsia. Am J Obstet Gynecol 150:506, 1984

Harskamp RE, Zeeman GG: Preeclampsia: At risk for remote cardiovascular disease. Am J Med Sci 334(4):291, 2007

Hauser RA, Lacey DM, Knight MR: Hypertensive encephalopathy. Arch Neurol 45:1078, 1988

Hauth JC, Cunningham FG, Whalley PJ: Management of pregnancy-induced hypertension in the nullipara. Obstet Gynecol 48:253, 1976

Hay JE: Liver disease in pregnancy. Hepatology 47:1067, 2008

Head BB, Owen J, Vincent RD Jr, et al: A randomized trial of intrapartum analgesia in women with severe preeclampsia. Obstet Gynecol 99:452, 2002

Hefler LA, Tempfer CB, Gregg AR: Polymorphisms within the interleukin-1β gene cluster and preeclampsia. Obstet Gynecol 97:664, 2001

Heilmann L, Rath W, Pollow K: Hemostatic abnormalities in patients with severe preeclampsia. Clin Appl Thromb Hemost 13: 285, 2007

Heller PJ, Scheider EP, Marx GF: Pharyngo-laryngeal edema as a presenting symptom in preeclampsia. Obstet Gynecol 62:523, 1983

Hertig AT: Vascular pathology in the hypertensive albuminuric toxemias of pregnancy. Clinics 4:602, 1945

Hibbard JU, Shroff SG, Lindheimer MD: Cardiovascular alterations in normal and preeclamptic pregnancies. In Lindheimer MD, Roberts JM, Cunningham FG (eds): Chesley's Hypertensive Disorders of Pregnancy, 3rd ed. New York, Elsevier, In press, 2009, p 251

Hinchey J, Chaves C, Appignani B, et al: A reversible posterior leukoencephalopathy syndrome. N Engl J Med 334(8):494, 1996

Hinselmann H: Die Eklampsie. Bonn, F Cohen, 1924

Hjartardottir S, Leifsson BG, Geirsson RT, et al: Recurrence of hypertensive disorder in second pregnancy. Am J Obstet Gynecol 194:916, 2006

Hnat MD, Sibai BM, Caritis S, et al: Perinatal outcome in women with recurrent preeclampsia compared with women who develop preeclampsia as nulliparas. Am J Obstet Gynecol 186:422, 2002

Hogg B, Hauth JC, Caritis SN, et al: Safety of labor epidural anesthesia for women with severe hypertensive disease. Am J Obstet Gynecol 181:1096, 1999

Holzgreve W, Ghezzi F, Di Naro E, et al: Disturbed feto-maternal cell traffic in preeclampsia. Obstet Gynecol 91:669, 1998

Horsager R, Adams M, Richey S, et al: Outpatient management of mild pregnancy induced hypertension. Am J Obstet Gynecol 172:383, 1995

Hubel CA, McLaughlin MK, Evans RW, et al: Fasting serum triglycerides, free fatty acids, and malondialdehyde are increased in preeclampsia, are positively correlated, and decrease within 48 hours postpartum. Am J Obstet Gynecol 174:975, 1996

Hunter SK, Martin M, Benda JA, et al: Liver transplant after massive spontaneous hepatic rupture in pregnancy complicated by preeclampsia. Obstet Gynecol 85:819, 1995

Hupuczi P, Nagy B, Sziller I, et al: Characteristic laboratory changes in pregnancies complicated by HELLP syndrome. Hypertens Pregnancy 26: 389, 2007

Isler CM, Barrilleaux PS, Magann EF, et al: A prospective, randomized trial comparing the efficacy of dexamethasone and betamethasone for the treatment of antepartum HELLP (hemolysis, elevated liver enzymes, and low platelet count) syndrome. Am J Obstet Gynecol 184:1332, 2001

Ito T, Sakai T, Inagawa S, et al: MR angiography of cerebral vasospasm in preeclampsia. AJNR Am J Neuroradiol 16(6):1344, 1995

Jenkins SM, Head BB, Hauth JC: Severe preeclampsia at < 25 weeks of gestation: Maternal and neonatal outcomes. Am J Obstet Gynecol 186:790, 2002

Jeyabalan A, Stewart DR, McGonigal SC, et al: Low relaxin concentrations in the first trimester are associated with increased risk of developing preeclampsia. Reprod Sci 16:101A, 2009

John JH, Ziebland S, Yudkin P, et al: Effects of fruit and vegetable consumption on plasma antioxidant concentrations and blood pressure: A randomized controlled trial. Lancet 359:1969, 2002

Kanasaki K, Palmsten K, Sugimoto H, et al: Deficiency in catechol-O-methyltransferase and 2-methoxyoestradiol is associated with pre-eclampsia. Nature 453:1117, 2008

Karumanchi SA, Stillman IE, Lindheimer MD: Angiogenesis and preeclampsia. In Lindheimer MD, Roberts JM, Cunningham FG (eds): Chesley's Hypertensive Disorders of Pregnancy, 3rd ed. New York, Elsevier, In press, 2009, p 87

Katz L, de Amorim MMR, Figueroa JN, et al: Postpartum dexamethasone for women with hemolysis, elevated liver enzymes, and low platelets (HELLP) syndrome: A double-blind, placebo-controlled, randomized clinical trial. Am J Obstet Gynecol 198:283.e1, 2008

Keiser S, Owens M, Parrish M, et al: HELLP syndrome II. Concurrent eclampsia in 70 cases. Abstract No 781. Presented at the 29th Annual Meeting of the Society for Maternal-Fetal Medicine, January 26–31, 2009

Kenny L, Baker P, Cunningham FG: Platelets, coagulation and the liver. In Lindheimer MD, Roberts JM, Cunningham FG (eds): Chesley's Hypertensive Disorders of Pregnancy, 3rd ed. New York, Elsevier, In press, 2009, p 335

Kenny LC, Broadhurst DI, Dunn W, et al: Early pregnancy prediction of preeclampsia using metabolomic biomarkers. Reprod Sci 16:102A, 2009

Khan KS, Wojdyla D, Say L, et al: WHO analysis of causes of maternal death: A systematic review. Lancet 367:1066, 2006

Khong TY: Acute atherosis in pregnancies complicated by hypertension, small-for-gestational age infants, and diabetes mellitus. Arch Pathol Lab Med 115:722, 1991

Kirshon B, Lee W, Mauer MB, et al: Effects of low-dose dopamine therapy in the oliguric patient with preeclampsia. Am J Obstet Gynecol 159:604, 1988

Knight M on behalf of UKOSS: Eclampsia in the United Kingdom 2005. BJOG 114:1072, 2007

Knuist M, Bonsel GJ, Zondervan HA, et al: Low sodium diet and pregnancy-induced hypertension: A multicentre randomized controlled trial. Br J Obstet Gynaecol 105:430, 1998

Kyle PM, Fielder JN, Pullar B, et al: Comparison of methods to identify significant proteinuria in pregnancy in the outpatient setting. BJOG 115:523, 2008

Labarrere C: Acute atherosis. A histopathological hallmark of immune aggression? Placenta 9:108, 1988

Lachmeijer AMA, Crusius JBA, Pals G, et al: Polymorphisms in the tumor necrosis factor and lymphotoxin-α gene region and preeclampsia. Obstet Gynecol 98:612, 2001

Lam DS, Chan W: Images in clinical medicine. Choroidal ischemia in preeclampsia. N Engl J Med 344(10):739, 2001

Landesman R, Douglas RG, Holze E: The bulbar conjunctival vascular bed in the toxemias of pregnancy. Am J Obstet Gynecol 68:170, 1954

Lang RM, Pridjian G, Feldman T, et al: Left ventricular mechanics in preeclampsia. Am Heart J 121:1768, 1991

Lara-Torre E, Lee MS, Wolf MA, et al: Bilateral retinal occlusion progressing to long-lasting blindness in severe preeclampsia. Obstet Gynecol 100:940, 2002

Lavies NG, Meiklejohn BH, May AE, et al: Hypertensive and catecholamine response to tracheal intubation in patients with pregnancy-induced hypertension. Br J Anaesth 63:429, 1989

Lawlor DA, Morton SM, Nitsch D, Leon DA: Association between childhood and adulthood socioeconomic position and pregnancy induced hypertension: Results from the Aberdeen children of the 1950s cohort study. J Epidemiol Community Health 59:49, 2005

Leduc L, Wheeler JM, Kirshon B, et al: Coagulation profile in severe preeclampsia. Obstet Gynecol 79:14, 1992

Leeflang MM, Cnossen JS, van der Post JA, et al: Accuracy of fibronectin tests for the prediction of pre-eclampsia: A systematic review. Eur J Obstet Gynecol Reprod Biol 133(1):12, 2007

Le Ray C, Wavrant S, Rey E, et al: Induction or elective caesarean in severe early-onset preeclampsia: A meta-analysis of observational studies. Abstract No 724. Presented at the 29th Annual Meeting of the Society for Maternal-Fetal Medicine, January 26–31, 2009

Leveno KJ, Alexander JM, McIntire DD, et al: Does magnesium sulfate given for prevention of eclampsia affect the outcome of labor? Am J Obstet Gynecol 178:707, 1998

Leveno KJ, Cunningham FG: Management. In Lindheimer MD, Roberts JM, Cunningham FG (eds): Chesley's Hypertensive Disorders of Pregnancy, 3rd ed. New York, Elsevier, In press, 2009, p 395

Levine RJ, Ewell MG, Hauth JC, et al: Should the definition of preeclampsia include a rise in diastolic blood pressure of >/= 15 mm Hg to a level < 90 mm Hg in association with proteinuria? Am J Obstet Gynecol 183:787, 2000

Levine RJ, Hauth JC, Curet LB, et al: Trial of calcium to prevent preeclampsia. N Engl J Med 337:69, 1997

Levine RJ, Lam C, Qian C et al: Soluble endoglin and other circulating antiangiogenic factors in preeclampsia. N Engl J Med 355:992, 2006

Levine RJ, Lindheimer MD: First-trimester prediction of early preeclampsia: A possibility at last! Hypertension 53(5):747, 2009

Li H, Gudnason H, Olofsson P, et al: Increased uterine artery vascular impedance is related to adverse outcome of pregnancy but is present in only one-third of late third-trimester pre-eclampsia women. Ultrasound Obstet Gynecol 25:459, 2005

Lindheimer MD, Conrad K, Karumanchi SA: Renal physiology and disease in pregnancy. In Alpern RJ, Hebert SC, (eds): Seldin and Giebisch's The Kidney: Physiology and Pathophysiology, 4th ed. New York, Elsevier, 2008a, p 2339

Lindheimer MD, Taler SJ, Cunningham FG: Hypertension in pregnancy [Invited Am Soc Hypertension position paper]. J Am Soc Hypertens 2:484, 2008b

Lindheimer MD, Taler S, Cunningham FG: Hypertensive disorders in pregnancy. J Am Soc Hyper 6:484, 2009

Livingston JC, Park V, Barton JR, et al: Lack of association of severe preeclampsia with maternal and fetal mutant alleles for tumor necrosis factor α and lymphotoxin α genes and plasma tumor necrosis α levels. Am J Obstet Gynecol 184:1273, 2001

Lo C, Taylor RS, Gamble G, et al: Use of automated home blood pressure monitoring in pregnancy: Is it safe? Am J Obstet Gynecol 187:1321, 2002

Lo YM, Corbetta N, Chamberlain PF, et al: Presence of fetal DNA in maternal plasma and serum. Lancet 350:485, 1997

López-Jaramillo P, Narváez M, Weigel RM, et al: Calcium supplementation reduces the risk of pregnancy-induced hypertension in an Andes population. Br J Obstet Gynaecol 96:648, 1989

López-Llera M: Complicated eclampsia: Fifteen years' experience in a referral medical center. Am J Obstet Gynecol 142:28, 1982

Loureiro R, Leite CC, Kahhale S, et al: Diffusion imaging may predict reversible brain lesions in eclampsia and severe preeclampsia: Initial experience. Am J Obstet Gynecol 189:1350, 2003

Lucas MJ, Leveno KJ, Cunningham FG: A comparison of magnesium sulfate with phenytoin for the prevention of eclampsia. N Engl J Med 333:201, 1995

Lucas MJ, Sharma S, McIntire DD, et al: A randomized trial of the effects of epidural analgesia on pregnancy-induced hypertension. Am J Obstet Gynecol 185:970, 2001

Luft FC, Gallery EDM, Lindheimer MD: Normal and abnormal volume homeostasis. In Lindheimer MD, Roberts JM, Cunningham FG (eds): Chesley's Hypertensive Disorders of Pregnancy, 3rd ed. New York, Elsevier, In press, 2009, p 271

Lykke JA, Langhoff-Roos J, Sibai BM, et al: Hypertensive pregnancy disorders and subsequent cardiovascular morbidity and type 2 diabetes mellitus in the mother. Hypertension 53:944, 2009a

Lykke JA, Paidas MJ, Langhoff-Roos J: Recurring complications in second pregnancy. Obstet Gynecol 113:1217, 2009b

Mabie WC, Gonzalez AR, Sibai BM, et al: A comparative trial of labetalol and hydralazine in the acute management of severe hypertension complicating pregnancy. Obstet Gynecol 70:328, 1987

Madazli R, Budak E, Calay Z, et al: Correlation between placental bed biopsy findings, vascular cell adhesion molecule and fibronectin levels in preeclampsia. Br J Obstet Gynaecol 107:514, 2000

Magee LA, Cham C, Waterman EJ, et al: Hydralazine for treatment of severe hypertension in pregnancy: Meta-analysis. BMJ 327(7421):955, 2003

Magee LA, Yong PJ, Espinosa V, et al: Expectant management of severe preeclampsia remote from term: A structured systematic review. Hypertens Pregnancy 25:1, 2009

Magpie Trial Collaborative Group: Do women with pre-eclampsia, and their babies, benefit from magnesium sulphate? The Magpie Trial: A randomized placebo-controlled trial. Lancet 359:1877, 2002

Magpie Trial Follow-Up Collaborative Group: The Magpie Trial: a randomized trial comparing magnesium sulphate with placebo for pre-eclampsia. Outcome for women at 2 years. BJOG 114:300, 2007

Makrides M, Duley L, Olsen SF: Marine oil, and other prostaglandin precursor supplementation for pregnancy uncomplicated by pre-eclampsia or intrauterine growth restriction. Cochrane Database Syst Rev 3:CD003402, 2006

Manten GT, van der Hoek YY, Marko Sikkema J, et al: The role of lipoprotein (a) in pregnancies complicated by pre-eclampsia. Med Hypotheses 64:162, 2005

Márquez-Rodas I, Longo F, Rothlin RP, et al: Pathophysiology and therapeutic possibilities of calcitonin gene-related peptide in hypertension. J Physiol Biochem 62:45, 2006

Martin JA, Hamilton BE, Sutton PD, et al: Births: Final data for 2004. Natl Vital Stat Rep Vol. 55, 2006

Martin JN, Bailey AP, Rehberg JF, et al: Thrombotic thrombocytopenic purpura in 166 pregnancies: 1955-2006. Am J Obstet Gynecol 199(2), 98, 2008

Martin JN Jr, Files JC, Blake PG, et al: Postpartum plasma exchange for atypical preeclampsia–eclampsia as HELLP (hemolysis, elevated liver enzymes, and low platelets) syndrome. Am J Obstet Gynecol 172:1107, 1995

Martin JN Jr, Thigpen BD, Moore RC, et al: Stroke and severe preeclampsia and eclampsia: A paradigm shift focusing on systolic blood pressure. Obstet Gynecol 105(2):246, 2005

Martin JN Jr, Thigpen BD, Rose CH, et al: Maternal benefit of high-dose intravenous corticosteroid therapy for HELLP syndrome. Am J Obstet Gynecol 189:830, 2003

Marya RK, Rathee S, Manrow M: Effect of calcium and vitamin D supplementation on toxaemia of pregnancy. Gynecol Obstet Invest 24:38, 1987

Mastrogiannis DS, O'Brien WF, Krammer J, et al: Potential role of endothelin-1 in normal and hypertensive pregnancies. Am J Obstet Gynecol 165:1711, 1991

Matijevic R, Johnston T: In vivo assessment of failed trophoblastic invasion of the spiral arteries in pre-eclampsia. Br J Obstet Gynaecol 106:78, 1999

Mattar F, Sibai BM: Eclampsia: VIII. Risk factors for maternal morbidity. Am J Obstet Gynecol 182:307, 2000

Maxwell CV, Lieberman E, Norton M, et al: Relationship of twin zygosity and risk of preeclampsia. Am J Obstet Gynecol 185:819, 2001

Maynard SE, Min J-Y, Merchan J, et al: Excess placental soluble fms-like tyrosine kinase 1 (sFlt1) may contribute to endothelial dysfunction, hypertension, and proteinuria in preeclampsia. J Clin Invest 111(5):649, 2003

Maynard S, Epstein FH, Karumanchi SA: Preeclampsia and angiogenic imbalance. Annu Rev Med 59:61, 2008

McCubbin JH, Sibai BM, Abdella TN, et al: Cardiopulmonary arrest due to acute maternal hypermagnesemia. Lancet 1:1058, 1981

Meher S, Duely L: Rest during pregnancy for preventing pre-eclampsia and its complications in women with normal blood pressure. Cochrane Database Syst Rev 19:CD005939, 2006

Meldrum BS: Implications for neuroprotective treatments. Prog Brain Res 135:487, 2002

Melrose EB: Maternal deaths at King Edward VIII Hospital, Durban. A review of 258 consecutive cases. S Afr Med J 65:161, 1984

Mignini LE, Latthe PM, Villar J, et al: Mapping the theories of preeclampsia: The role of homocysteine. Obstet Gynecol 105: 411, 2005

Moseman CP, Shelton S: Permanent blindness as a complication of pregnancy induced hypertension. Obstet Gynecol 100:943, 2002

Mostello D, Catlin TK, Roman L, et al: Preeclampsia in the parous woman: Who is at risk? Am J Obstet Gynecol 187:425, 2002

Murphy MA, Ayazifar M: Permanent visual deficits secondary to the HELLP syndrome. J Neuro-Ophthalmol 25(2): 122, 2005

Myatt L, Brewer AS, Langdon G, et al: Attenuation of the vasoconstrictor effects of thromboxane and endothelin by nitric oxide in the human fetal–placental circulation. Am J Obstet Gynecol 166:224, 1992

Myers JE, Hart S, Armstrong S, et al: Evidence for multiple circulating factor in preeclampsia. Am J Obstet Gynecol 196(3):266.e1, 2007

Narbone MC, Musolino R, Granata F, et al: PRES: Posterior or potentially reversible encephalopathy syndrome? Neurol 27:187, 2006

National High Blood Pressure Education Program: Working Group Report on High Blood Pressure in Pregnancy. Am J Obstet Gynecol 183:51, 2000

Nelson KB, Grether JK: Can magnesium sulfate reduce the risk of cerebral palsy in very low birthweight infants? Pediatrics 95:263, 1995

Ness RB, Roberts JM: Heterogeneous causes constituting the single syndrome of preeclampsia: A hypothesis and its implications. Am J Obstet Gynecol 175(5):1365, 1996

Newsome LR, Bramwell RS, Curling PE: Severe preeclampsia: Hemodynamic effects of lumbar epidural anesthesia. Anesth Analg 65:31, 1986

Nilsson E, Ros HS, Cnattingius S, et al: The importance of genetic and environmental effects for pre-eclampsia and gestational hypertension: A family study. Br J Obstet Gynaecol 111:200, 2004

Nolan TE, Wakefield ML, Devoe LD: Invasive hemodynamic monitoring in obstetrics. A critical review of its indications, benefits, complications, and alternatives. Chest 101:1429, 1992

North RA, Taylor RS, Schellenberg J-C: Evaluation of a definition of preeclampsia. Br J Obstet Gynaecol 106:767, 1999

Nova A, Sibai BM, Barton JR, et al: Maternal plasma level of endothelin is increased in preeclampsia. Am J Obstet Gynecol 165:724, 1991

Obeidat B, MacDougall J, Harding K: Plasma exchange in a woman with thrombotic thrombocytopenic purpura or severe pre-eclampsia. Br J Obstet Gynaecol 109:961, 2002

O'Brien JM, Shumate SA, Satchwell SL, et al: Maternal benefit of corticosteroid therapy in patients with HELLP (hemolysis, elevated liver enzymes, and low platelet count) syndrome: Impact on the rate of regional anesthesia. Am J Obstet Gynecol 186:475, 2002

Oettle C, Hall D, Roux A, et a: Early onset severe pre-eclampsia: Expectant management at a secondary hospital in close association with a tertiary institution. BJOG 112(1):84, 2005

Øian P, Maltau JM, Noddleland H, et al: Transcapillary fluid balance in preeclampsia. Br J Obstet Gynaecol 93:235, 1986

Olafsdottir AS, Skuladottir GV, Thorsdottir I, et al: Relationship between high consumption of marine fatty acids in early pregnancy and hypertensive disorders in pregnancy. BJOG 113:301, 2006

Olsen SF, Secher NJ, Tabor A, et al: Randomized clinical trials of fish oil supplementation in high risk pregnancies. Br J Obstet Gynaecol 107:382, 2000

Ong SS, Moore RJ, Warren AY, et al: Myometrial and placental artery reactivity alone cannot explain reduced placental perfusion in pre-eclampsia and intrauterine growth restriction. BJOG 110(10):909, 2003

Palmer SK, Moore LG, Young DA, et al: Altered blood pressure and increased preeclampsia at high altitude (3100 meters) in Colorado. Am J Obstet Gynecol 180:1161, 1999

Papanna R, Mann LK, Kouides RW, et al: Protein/creatinine ratio in preeclampsia: A systematic review. Obstet Gynecol 112:135, 2008

Parra MC, Lees C, Mann GE, et al: Vasoactive mediator release by endothelial cells in intrauterine growth restriction and preeclampsia. Am J Obstet Gynecol 184:497, 2001

Phelan JP, Yurth DA: Severe preeclampsia. I. Peripartum hemodynamic observations. Am J Obstet Gynecol 144(1):17, 1982

Pickles CJ, Broughton Pipkin F, Symonds EM: A randomised placebo controlled trial of labetalol in the treatment of mild to moderate pregnancy induced hypertension. Br J Obstet Gynaecol 99(12):964, 1992

Poon LC, Kametas N, Bonino S, et al: Urine albumin concentration and albumin-to-creatinine ratio at 11(+0) to 13(+6) weeks in the prediction of pre-eclampsia. BJOG 115:866, 2008

Poon LC, Kametas NA, Maiz N, et al: First-trimester prediction of hypertensive disorders in pregnancy. Hypertension 53(5):812, 2009

Postma IR, Wessel I, Aarnoudse JG, Zeeman GG: Neurocognitive functioning in formerly eclamptic women: Sustained attention and executive functioning. Reprod Sci 16:175A, 2009

Poston L, Briley AL, Seed PT, et al: Vitamin C and vitamin E in pregnant women at risk for pre-eclampsia (VIP trial): Randomized placebo-controlled trial. Lancet 367:1145, 2006

Powers RW, Bodnar LM, Ness RB, et al: Uric acid concentrations in early pregnancy among preeclamptic women with gestational hyperuricemia at delivery. Am J Obstet Gynecol 194:160.e1, 2006

Powers RW, Evans RW, Ness RB, et al: Homocysteine is increased in preeclampsia but not in gestational hypertension (Abstract #375). J Soc Gynecol Investig 7(1):(Suppl), 2000

Pritchard JA: The use of magnesium ion in the management of eclamptogenic toxemias. Surg Gynecol Obstet 100:131, 1955

Pritchard JA, Cunningham FG, Mason RA: Coagulation changes in eclampsia: Their frequency and pathogenesis. Am J Obstet Gynecol 124:855, 1976

Pritchard JA, Cunningham FG, Pritchard SA: The Parkland Memorial Hospital protocol for treatment of eclampsia: Evaluation of 245 cases. Am J Obstet Gynecol 148(7):951, 1984

Pritchard JA, Cunningham FG, Pritchard SA, et al: How often does maternal preeclampsia–eclampsia incite thrombocytopenia in the fetus? Obstet Gynecol 69:292, 1987

Pritchard JA, Pritchard SA: Standardized treatment of 154 consecutive cases of eclampsia. Am J Obstet Gynecol 123(5):543, 1975

Pritchard JA, Weisman R Jr, Ratnoff OD, et al: Intravascular hemolysis, thrombocytopenia and other hematologic abnormalities associated with severe toxemia of pregnancy. N Engl J Med 250:87, 1954

Raab W, Schroeder G, Wagner R, et al: Vascular reactivity and electrolytes in normal and toxemic pregnancy. J Clin Endocrinol 16:1196, 1956

Rafferty TD, Berkowitz RL: Hemodynamics in patients with severe toxemia during labor and delivery. Am J Obstet Gynecol 138:263, 1980

Raijmakers MT, Dechend R, Poston L: Oxidative stress and preeclampsia: Rationale for antioxidant clinical trials. Hypertension 44:374, 2004

Redman CWG, Sacks GP, Sargent IL: Preeclampsia: An excessive maternal inflammatory response to pregnancy. Am J Obstet Gynecol 180:499, 1999

Redman CWG, Sargent IL: Circulating microparticles in normal pregnancy and preeclampsia. Placenta 22 (Suppl A):S73, 2008

Redman CWG, Sargent IL, Roberts JM: Immunology of abnormal pregnancy and preeclampsia. In Lindheimer MD, Roberts JM, Cunningham FG (eds): Chesley's Hypertensive Disorders of Pregnancy, 3rd ed. New York, Elsevier, In press, 2009, p 129

Richards A, Graham DI, Bullock MRR: Clinicopathological study of neurological complications due to hypertensive disorders of pregnancy. J Neurol Neurosurg Psychiatry 51:416, 1988

Rinehart BK, Terrone DA, Magann EF, et al: Preeclampsia-associated hepatic hemorrhage and rupture: Mode of management related to maternal and perinatal outcome. Obstet Gynecol Surv 54:3, 1999

Roberts JM: A randomized controlled trial of antioxidant vitamins to prevent serious complications associated with pregnancy related hypertension in low risk, nulliparous women. Abstract No 8. Presented at the 29th Annual Meeting of the Society for Maternal-Fetal Medicine, January 26–31, 2009

Rogers BB, Bloom SL, Leveno KJ: Atherosis revisited: Current concepts on the pathophysiology of implantation site disorders. Obstet Gynecol Surv 54:189, 1999

Rosen SA, Merchant SH, Vanderjagt TJ, et al: Spontaneous subcapsular liver hematoma associated with pregnancy. Arch Pathol Lab Med 127:1639, 2003

Royal College of Obstetricians and Gynaecologists: The management of severe pre-eclampsia. RCOG Guideline 10A:1, 2006

Rumbold AR, Crowther CA, Haslam RR: Vitamins C and E and the risks of preeclampsia and perinatal complications. N Engl J Med 354:17, 2006

Sagsoz N, Kucukozkan T: The effect of treatment on endothelin-1 concentration and mean arterial pressure in preeclampsia and eclampsia. Hypertens Pregnancy 22:185, 2003

Saito Y, Tano Y: Retinal pigment epithelial lesions associated with choroidal ischemia in preeclampsia. Retina 18:103, 1998

Samuels P, Main EK, Tomaski A, et al: Abnormalities in platelet antiglobulin tests in preeclamptic mothers and their neonates. Am J Obstet Gynecol 157:109, 1987

Sanchez-Ramos L, Adair CD, Todd JC, et al: Erythrocyte membrane fluidity in patients with preeclampsia and the HELLP syndrome: A preliminary study. J Matern Fetal Invest 4:237, 1994

Scardo JA, Vermillion ST, Newman RB, et al: A randomized, double-blind, hemodynamic evaluation of nifedipine and labetalol in preeclamptic hypertensive emergencies. Am J Obstet Gynecol 181:862, 1999

Schendel DE, Berg CJ, Yeargin-Allsopp M, et al: Prenatal magnesium sulfate exposure and the risk for cerebral palsy or mental retardation among very low birthweight children aged 3 to 5 years. JAMA 276:1805, 1996

Schutte JM, Schuitemaker NW, van Roosmalen J, et al: Substandard care in maternal mortality due to hypertensive disease in pregnancy in the Netherlands. BJOG 115(10):1322, 2008

Schwartz RB, Feske SK, Polak JF, et al: Preeclampsia-eclampsia: Clinical and neuroradiographic correlates and insights into the pathogenesis of hypertensive encephalopathy. Radiology 217:371, 2000

Sciscione AC, Ivester T, Largoza M, et al: Acute pulmonary edema in pregnancy. Obstet Gynecol 101:511, 2003

Sep S, Verbeek J, Spaanderman M, et al: Clinical differences between preeclampsia and the HELLP syndrome suggest different pathogeneses. Reprod Sci 16:176A, 2009

Sergis F, Clara DM, Galbriella F, et al: Prophylaxis of recurrent preeclampsia: Low molecular weight heparin plus low-dose aspirin versus low-dose aspirin alone. Hypertension Pregnancy 25:115, 2006

Shear RM, Rinfret D, Leduc L: Should we offer expectant management in cases of severe preterm preeclampsia with fetal growth restriction? Am J Obstet Gynecol 192:1119, 2005

Sheehan HL, Lynch JB (eds): Cerebral lesions. In Pathology of Toxaemia of Pregnancy. Baltimore, Williams & Wilkins, 1973

Sibai BM: Diagnosis and management of gestational hypertension and preeclampsia. Obstet Gynecol 102:181, 2003

Sibai BM: Diagnosis, controversies, and management of the syndrome of hemolysis, elevated liver enzymes, and low platelet count. Obstet Gynecol 103:981, 2004

Sibai BM: Diagnosis, prevention, and management of eclampsia. Obstet Gynecol 105:402, 2005

Sibai BM: Imitators of severe preeclampsia. Obstet Gynecol 109:956, 2007

Sibai BM, Barton JR: Expectant management of severe preeclampsia remote from term: Patient selection, treatment and delivery indications. Am J Obstet Gynecol 196:514, 2007

Sibai BM, Barton JR, Akl S, et al: A randomized prospective comparison of nifedipine and bed rest versus bed rest alone in the management of preeclampsia remote from term. Am J Obstet Gynecol 167(1):879, 1992

Sibai BM, Cunningham FG: Prevention of preeclampsia and eclampsia. In Lindheimer MD, Roberts JM, Cunningham FG (eds): Chesley's Hypertensive Disorders of Pregnancy, 3rd ed. New York, Elsevier, In press, 2009, p 215

Sibai BM, El-Nazer A, Gonzalez-Ruiz A: Severe preeclampsia–eclampsia in young primigravid women: Subsequent pregnancy outcome and remote prognosis. Am J Obstet Gynecol 155:1011, 1986

Sibai BM, Ewell M, Levine RJ, et al: Risk factors associated with preeclampsia in healthy nulliparous women. Am J Obstet Gynecol 177:1003, 1997

Sibai BM, Gonzalez AR, Mabie WC, et al: A comparison of labetalol plus hospitalization versus hospitalization alone in the management of preeclampsia remote from term. Obstet Gynecol 70:323, 1987a

Sibai BM, Graham JM, McCubbin JH: A comparison of intravenous and intramuscular magnesium sulfate regimens in preeclampsia. Am J Obstet Gynecol 150:728, 1984

Sibai BM, Hauth J, Caritis S, et al: Hypertensive disorders in twin versus singleton gestations. Am J Obstet Gynecol 182:938, 2000

Sibai BM, Mabie BC, Harvey CJ, et al: Pulmonary edema in severe preeclampsia–eclampsia: Analysis of thirty-seven consecutive cases. Am J Obstet Gynecol 156:1174, 1987b

Sibai BM, Mercer B, Sarinoglu C: Severe preeclampsia in the second trimester: Recurrence risk and long-term prognosis. Am J Obstet Gynecol 165:1408, 1991

Sibai BM, Mercer BM, Schiff E, et al: Aggressive versus expectant management of severe preeclampsia at 28 to 32 weeks' gestation: A randomized controlled trial. Am J Obstet Gynecol 171:818, 1994

Sibai BM, Ramadan MK, Chari RS, et al: Pregnancies complicated by HELLP syndrome (hemolysis, elevated liver enzymes, and low platelets): Subsequent pregnancy outcome and long-term prognosis. Am J Obstet Gynecol 172:125, 1995

Sibai BM, Spinnato JA, Watson DL, et al: Eclampsia, 4. Neurological findings and future outcome. Am J Obstet Gynecol 152:184, 1985

Sibai BM, Stella CL: Diagnosis and management of atypical preeclampsia-eclampsia. Am J Obstet Gynecol 200:481.e1-481.e7, 2009

Silver HM, Seebeck M, Carlson R: Comparison of total blood volume in normal, preeclamptic, and non-proteinuric gestational hypertensive pregnancy by simultaneous measurement of red blood cell and plasma volumes. Am J Obstet Gynecol 179:87, 1998

Singhal AB, Kimberly WT, Schaefer PW, Hedley-Whyte ET: Case 8-2009: a 36-year-old woman with headache, hypertension, and seizure 2 weeks post partum. N Engl J Med 360:1126, 2009

Smith GN, Walker MC, Liu A, et al: A history of preeclampsia identifies women who have underlying cardiovascular risk factors. Am J Obstet Gynecol 200:58.e1, 2009

Somjen G, Hilmy M, Stephen CR: Failure to anesthetize human subjects by intravenous administration of magnesium sulfate. J Pharmacol Exp Ther 154(3):652, 1966

Spaan JJ, Ekhart T, Spaanderman MEA, et al: Remote hemodynamics and renal function in formerly preeclamptic women. Obstet Gynecol 113:853, 2009

Spargo B, McCartney CP, Winemiller R: Glomerular capillary endotheliosis in toxemia of pregnancy. Arch Pathol 68:593, 1959

Spencer J, Polavarapu S, Timms D, et al: Regional and monthly variation in rates of preeclampsia at delivery among U.S. births. Abstract No 294. Presented at the 29th Annual Meeting of the Society for Maternal-Fetal Medicine, January 26–31, 2009

Spitz B, Magness RR, Cox SM: Low-dose aspirin. I. Effect on angiotensin II pressor responses and blood prostaglandin concentrations in pregnant women sensitive to angiotensin II. Am J Obstet Gynecol 159(5):1035, 1988

Staff AC, Braekke K, Johnsen GM, et al: Circulating concentration of soluble endoglin (CD105) in fetal and maternal serum and in amniotic fluid in preeclampsia. Am J Obstet Gynecol 197(2):176.e1, 2007

Strickland DM, Guzick DS, Cox K, et al: The relationship between abortion in the first pregnancy and the development of pregnancy-induced hypertension in the subsequent pregnancy. Am J Obstet Gynecol 154:146, 1986

Stubbs TM, Lazarchick J, Horger EO III: Plasma fibronectin levels in preeclampsia: A possible biochemical marker for vascular endothelial damage. Am J Obstet Gynecol 150: 885, 1984

Sunderji S, Sibai B, Wothe D et al: Differential diagnosis of preterm preeclampsia and hypertension using prototype automated assays for SVEGF R1 and PLGF: A prospective clinical study. Abstract No 249. Presented at the 29th Annual Meeting of the Society for Maternal-Fetal Medicine, January 26-31, 2009

Suzuki Y, Yamamoto T, Mabuchi Y, et al: Ultrastructural changes in omental resistance artery in women with preeclampsia. Am J Obstet Gynecol 189:216, 2003

Szal SE, Croughan-Minibane MS, Kilpatrick SJ: Effect of magnesium prophylaxis and preeclampsia on the duration of labor. Am J Obstet Gynecol 180:1475, 1999

Taber EB, Tan L, Chao CR, et al: Pharmacokinetics of ionized versus total magnesium in subjects with preterm labor and preeclampsia. Am J Obstet Gynecol 186:1017, 2002

Talledo OE, Chesley LC, Zuspan FP: Renin-angiotensin system in normal and toxemic pregnancies, 3. Differential sensitivity to angiotensin II and norepinephrine in toxemia of pregnancy. Am J Obstet Gynecol 100:218, 1968

Tan LK, de Swiet M: The management of postpartum hypertension. BJOG 109(7):733, 2002

Taufield PA, Ales KL, Resnick LM, et al: Hypocalciuria in preeclampsia. N Engl J Med 316:715, 1987

Taylor RN, Davidge ST, Roberts JM: Endothelial cell dysfunction and oxidative stress. In Lindheimer MD, Roberts JM, Cunningham FG (eds): Chesley's Hypertensive Disorders in Pregnancy, 3rd ed. Elsevier, In press, 2009, p 145

Taylor RN, Roberts JM: Endothelial cell dysfunction. In Lindheimer MD, Roberts JM, Cunningham FG (eds): Chesley's Hypertensive Disorders in Pregnancy, 2nd ed. Stamford, CT, Appleton & Lange, 1999, p 395

Thangaratinam S, Ismail KMK, Sharp S, et al: Accuracy of serum uric acid in predicting complications of pre-eclampsia: A systematic review. BJOG 113: 369, 2006

Thiagarajah S, Bourgeois FJ, Harbert GM, et al: Thrombocytopenia in preeclampsia: Associated abnormalities and management principles. Am J Obstet Gynecol 150:1, 1984

Thurnau GR, Kemp DB, Jarvis A: Cerebrospinal fluid levels of magnesium in patients with preeclampsia after treatment with intravenous magnesium sulfate: A preliminary report. Am J Obstet Gynecol 157:1435, 1987

Tihtonen K, Kööbi T, Yli-Hankala A, et al: Maternal haemodynamics in preeclampsia compared with normal pregnancy during caesarean delivery. BJOG 113(6):657, 2006

Tompkins MJ, Thiagarajah S: HELLP (hemolysis, elevated liver enzymes, and low platelet count) syndrome: The benefit of corticosteroids. Am J Obstet Gynecol 181:304, 1999

Trommer BL, Homer D, Mikhael MA: Cerebral vasospasm and eclampsia. Stroke 19:326, 1988

Trudinger BJ, Cook CM: Doppler umbilical and uterine flow waveforms in severe pregnancy hypertension. Br J Obstet Gynaecol 97:142, 1990

Tuffnell DJ, Lilford RJ, Buchan PC, et al: Randomized controlled trial of day care for hypertension in pregnancy. Lancet 339:224, 1992

Turnbull DA, Wilkinson C, Gerard K, et al: Clinical, psychosocial, and economic effects of antenatal day care for three medical complications of pregnancy: A randomized controlled trial of 395 women. Lancet 363:1104, 2004

Umans JG, Abalos EJ, Lindheimer MD: Antihypertensive treatment. In Lindheimer MD, Roberts JM, Cunningham FG (eds): Chesley's Hypertensive Disorders in Pregnancy, 3rd ed. Elsevier, In press, 2009, p 375

Urban G, Vergani P, Ghindini A, et al: State of the art: Non-invasive ultrasound assessment of the uteroplacental circulation. Semin Perinatol 31(4), 232, 2007

Venkatesha S, Toporsian M, Lam C, et al: Soluble endoglin contributes to the pathogenesis of preeclampsia. Nat Med 12:642, 2006

Ventura SJ, Martin JA, Curtin SC, et al: Births: Final data for 1998. National Vital Statistics Reports, Vol. 48, No. 3. Hyattsville, Md, National Center for Health Statistics, 2000

Vermillion ST, Scardo JA, Newman RB, et al: A randomized, double-blind trial of oral nifedipine and intravenous labetalol in hypertensive emergencies of pregnancy. Am J Obstet Gynecol 181:858, 1999

Vigil-De Gracia P, Montufar-Rueda C, Ruiz J: Expectant management of severe preeclampsia and preeclampsia superimposed on chronic hypertension between 24 and 34 weeks' gestation. Eur J Obstet Gynecol Reprod Biol 107:24, 2003

Vigil-De Gracia P, Ruiz E, Lopez JC, et al: Management of severe hypertension in the postpartum period with intravenous hydralazine or labetalol: A randomized clinical trial. Hypertens Pregnancy 26(2):163, 2007

Vikse BE, Irgens LM, Leivestad T, et al: Preeclampsia and the risk of end-stage renal disease. N Engl J Med 359:800, 2008

Villar J, Hany AA, Merialdi M, et al: World Health Organization randomized trial of calcium supplementation among low calcium intake pregnant women. Am J Obstet Gynecol 194:639, 2006

Villar J, Purwar M, Merialdi M, et al: WHO randomised trial if vitamin C & E supplementation among women at high risk for preeclampsia and nutritional deficiency. Society of Maternal-Fetal Medicine Abstract #8. Am J Obstet Gynecol 197:S4, 2007

Virchow R: Gesammette Abhandlungen zur Wissenschaftlichen Medicin. Frankfurt AM, Meidinger Sohn, 1856, p 778

Volhard F: Die doppelseitigen haematogenen Nierenerkrankungen. Berlin, Springer, 1918

Vollebregt K, Van Leijden L, Westerhof B, et al: Arterial stiffness is higher in early pregnancy in women, who will develop preeclampsia. Abstract No 712. Presented at the 29th Annual Meeting of the Society for Maternal-Fetal Medicine, January 26–31, 2009

von Dadelszen P, Magee LA: Fall in mean arterial pressure and fetal growth restriction in pregnancy hypertension: An updated metaregression analysis. J Obstet Gynaecol Can 24(12):941, 2002

von Dadelszen P, Ornstein MP, Bull SB, et al: Fall in mean arterial pressure and fetal growth restriction in pregnancy hypertension: A meta-analysis. Lancet 355:87, 2000

von Mandach U, Lauth D, Huch R: Maternal and fetal nitric oxide production in normal and abnormal pregnancy. J Matern Fetal Neonatal Med 13:22, 2003

Walker JJ: Pre-eclampsia. Lancet 356:1260, 2000

Wallace DH, Leveno KJ, Cunningham FG, et al: Randomized comparison of general and regional anesthesia for cesarean delivery in pregnancies complicated by severe preeclampsia. Obstet Gynecol 86:193, 1995

Wallace K, Wells A, Bennett W: African-Americans, preeclampsia and future cardiovascular disease: Is nitric oxide the missing link? Abstract No 827. Presented at the 29th Annual Meeting of the Society for Maternal-Fetal Medicine, January 26–31, 2009

Wallenburg HC, Makovitz JW, Dekker GA, et al: Low-dose aspirin prevents pregnancy-induced hypertension and preeclampsia in angiotensin-sensitive primigravidae. Lancet 327:1, 1986

Walsh SC: Lipid peroxidation in pregnancy. Hypertens Pregnancy 13:1, 1994

Walsh SW: Plasma from preeclamptic women stimulates transendothelial migration of neutrophils. Reprod Sci 16(3):320, 2009

Wang Y, Gu Y, Granger DN, et al: Endothelial junctional protein redistribution and increased monolayer permeability in human umbilical vein endothelial cells isolated during preeclampsia. Am J Obstet Gynecol 186:214, 2002

Ward K, Lindheimer MD: Genetic factors in the etiology of preeclampsia/eclampsia. In Lindheimer MD, Roberts JM, Cunningham FG (eds): Chesley's Hypertensive Disorders in Pregnancy, 3rd ed. Elsevier, In press, 2009, p 51

Watt-Morse ML, Caritis SN, Kridgen PL: Magnesium sulfate is a poor inhibitor of oxytocin-induced contractility in pregnant sheep. J Matern Fetal Med 4:139, 1995

Weiner CP, Thompson LP, Liu KZ, et al: Endothelium derived relaxing factor and indomethacin-sensitive contracting factor alter arterial contractile responses to thromboxane during pregnancy. Am J Obstet Gynecol 166: 1171, 1992

Weinstein L: Syndrome of hemolysis, elevated liver enzymes and low platelet count: A severe consequence of hypertension in pregnancy. Am J Obstet Gynecol 142:159, 1982

Weinstein L: Preeclampsia-eclampsia with hemolysis, elevated liver enzymes, and thrombocytopenia. Obstet Gynecol 66:657, 1985

Wicke C, Pereira PL, Neeser E, et al: Subcapsular liver hematoma in HELLP syndrome: Evaluation of diagnostic and therapeutic options—a unicenter study. Am J Obstet Gynecol 190:106, 2004

Wide-Swensson DH, Ingemarsson I, Lunell NO, et al: Calcium channel blockade (isradipine) in treatment of hypertension in pregnancy: A randomized placebo-controlled study. Am J Obstet Gynecol 173(1):872, 1995

Widmer M, Villar J, Benigni A, et al: Mapping the theories of preeclampsia and the role of angiogenic factors. Obstet Gynecol 109:168, 2007

Wikström AK, Haglund B, Olovsson M, et al: The risk of maternal ischaemic heart disease after gestational hypertensive disease. BJOG 112:1486, 2005

Wilson ML, Desmond DH, Goodwin TM, et al: Transforming growth factor-3 polymorphisms are associated with preeclampsia (PE). Abstract No 47. Presented at the 29th Annual Meeting of the Society for Maternal-Fetal Medicine, January 26–31, 2009

Winkel CA, Milewich L, Parker CR Jr, et al: Conversion of plasma progesterone to deoxycorticosterone in men, nonpregnant and pregnant women, and adrenalectomized subjects. J Clin Invest 66:803, 1980

Witlin AG, Friedman SA, Egerman RS, et al: Cerebrovascular disorders complicating pregnancy beyond eclampsia. Am J Obstet Gynecol 176:1139, 1997a

Witlin AG, Friedman SA, Sibai BA: The effect of magnesium sulfate therapy on the duration of labor in women with mild preeclampsia at term: A randomized, double-blind, placebo-controlled trial. Am J Obstet Gynecol 176:623, 1997b

Worley LC, Hnat MD, Cunningham FG: Advanced extrauterine pregnancy: Diagnostic and therapeutic challenges. Am J Obstet Gynecol 198(3):297.e1, 2008

Zeeman GG, Alexander JM, McIntire DD, et al: Homocysteine plasma concentration levels for the prediction of preeclampsia in women with chronic hypertension. Am J Obstet Gynecol 189:574, 2003

Zeeman GG, Cipolla MJ, Cunningham FG: Cerebrovascular pathophysiology in preeclampsia/eclampsia. In Lindheimer MD, Roberts JM, Cunningham FG (eds): Chesley's Hypertensive Disorders in Pregnancy, 3rd ed. Elsevier, In press, 2009b, p 227

Zeeman GG, Cunningham FG, Pritchard JA: The magnitude of hemoconcentration with eclampsia. Hypertens Pregnancy 28(2):127, 2009a

Zeeman GG, Fleckenstein JL, Twickler DM, et al: Cerebral infarction in eclampsia. Am J Obstet Gynecol 190:714, 2004a

Zeeman GG, Hatab M, Twickler DM: Increased large-vessel cerebral blood flow in severe preeclampsia by magnetic resonance (MR) evaluation. Presented at the 24th Annual Meeting of the Society for Maternal-Fetal Medicine, New Orleans, LA, February 2, 2004b

Zhang C, Williams MA, King IB, et al: Vitamin C and the risk of preeclampsia—results from dietary questionnaire and plasma assay. Epidemiology 13:382, 2002

Zhang J, Klebanoff MA, Levine RJ, et al: The puzzling association between smoking and hypertension during pregnancy. Am J Obstet Gynecol 181:1407, 1999

Zinaman M, Rubin J, Lindheimer MD: Serial plasma oncotic pressure levels and echoencephalography during and after delivery in severe preeclampsia. Lancet 1:1245, 1985

Zondervan HA, Oosting J, Smorenberg-Schoorl ME, et al: Maternal whole blood viscosity in pregnancy hypertension. Gynecol Obstet Invest 25:83, 1988

Zwart JJ, Richters A, Öry F, et al: Eclampsia in The Netherlands. Obstet Gynecol 112:820, 2008

Obstetrical Hemorrhage

Obstetrics is "bloody business." Although medical advances have dramatically reduced the dangers of childbirth, death from hemorrhage still remains a leading cause of maternal mortality. Hemorrhage was a direct cause of more than 17 percent of 4200 pregnancy-related maternal deaths in the United States as ascertained from the Pregnancy Mortality Surveillance System of the Centers for Disease Control and Prevention (Gerberding, 2003). Hemorrhage was the major factor for maternal deaths in the United Kingdom reported in the Confidential Enquiry into Maternal and Child Health (2008). In a private-sector report from the Hospital Corporation of America, Clark and co-workers (2008) reported that 12 percent of maternal deaths were caused by obstetrical hemorrhage. Finally, in many developed countries, hemorrhage is a leading reason for admission of pregnant women to intensive care units (Gilbert, 2003; Hazelgrove, 2001; Zeeman, 2003; Zwart, 2008, and all their associates).

In countries with fewer resources, the contribution of hemorrhage to maternal mortality rates is even more striking (Jegasothy, 2002; Rahman and co-workers, 2002). Indeed, hemorrhage is the single most important cause of maternal death worldwide. Obstetrical hemorrhage accounts for almost half of all postpartum deaths in developing countries (Lalonde and colleagues, 2006; McCormick and associates, 2002).

A number of reports exemplify the great improvement in mortality rates from hemorrhage with modernization of American obstetrics. Maternal deaths from hemorrhage in Massachusetts declined tenfold from the mid-1950s to the mid-1980s (Sachs and co-workers, 1987). Similarly, at Grady Memorial Hospital in Atlanta, maternal mortality rates from hemorrhage decreased from 13 percent between 1949 and 1971 to 6 percent between 1972 and 2000 (Ho and associates, 2002).

OVERVIEW, IMPLICATIONS, AND CLASSIFICATION

Some causes of severe obstetrical hemorrhage and their contribution to maternal mortality are shown in Figure 35-1. Fatal hemorrhage is most likely in circumstances in which blood or components are not available immediately. Moreover, Singla and associates (2001) reported that women who are Jehovah's Witnesses have a 44-fold increased risk of maternal death because of hemorrhage. Establishment and maintenance of facilities that allow prompt administration of blood are absolute requirements for acceptable obstetrical care.

Generally speaking, obstetrical hemorrhage may be *antepartum*—such as with placenta previa or placental abruption, or more commonly it is *postpartum*—from uterine atony or genital tract lacerations.

Incidence and Predisposing Conditions

The exact incidence of obstetrical hemorrhage is not known because of its imprecise definition as well as difficulty in its recognition and thus its diagnosis. One indicator is the number of women transfused, and this has likely decreased because of prevailing conservative attitudes towards blood replacement. For example, in older studies, the incidence of postpartum hemorrhage was cited to be 3.9 percent in women delivered vaginally and 6 to 8 percent in those undergoing cesarean delivery (Combs and associates, 1991a, b; Naef and colleagues, 1994). In a recent 24-center investigation from Argentina and

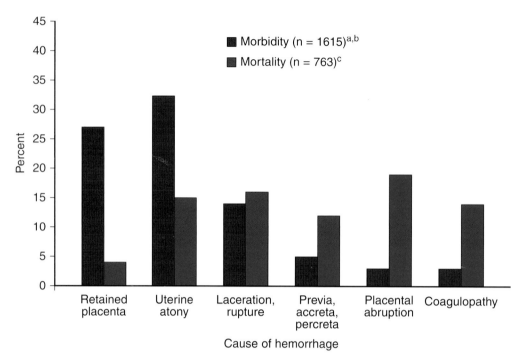

FIGURE 35-1 Incidences of some causes of obstetrical hemorrhage and their contribution to maternal death from hemorrhage. Percentages are approximations because of different classification schemata used. (Data from Al-Zirqi, 2008[a]; Chichakli, 1999[c]; Zwart, 2008[b], and all their colleagues.)

Uruguay, Sosa and colleagues (2009) used especially made plastic sheets to collect blood shed at delivery. They reported that 10.8 percent of women lost more than 500 mL, and 1.9 percent lost greater than 1000 mL. In another recent population-based study of more than 66,000 women delivered at Parkland Hospital from 2002 to 2006, Alexander and colleagues (2009) reported that 2.3 percent were given blood transfusions for hypovolemia. Half of these had undergone cesarean delivery, and this is related to the substantively increased maternal mortality and severe morbidity rate with cesarean compared with vaginal delivery (Alexander, 2009; Clark, 2008; Pallasmaa, 2008, and all their colleagues).

When these prospective audits are compared with evaluations using discharge statistics, it is apparent that hemorrhage is underreported. Recently, Berg and colleagues (2009) from the Centers for Disease Control and Prevention sampled nearly 185,000 hospitalizations for delivery in the National Hospital Discharge Summary database representing more than 40 million deliveries in the United States from 1993–1997 and 2001–2005. For these two epochs, the incidence of postpartum hemorrhage by ICD-9-CM codes was 2.0 and 2.6 percent, respectively. The rate for transfusions in these women between 1991 and 2003 increased from 3 per 1000 deliveries to 5 per 1000. These incidences are far below those reported in the studies above.

Table 35-1 lists the many clinical circumstances in which risk of hemorrhage is appreciably increased. It is apparent that serious hemorrhage may occur at any time throughout pregnancy and the puerperium. Although the timing of bleeding is widely used to classify obstetrical hemorrhage, the term *third-trimester* bleeding is imprecise, and its use is not recommended.

One factor not generally considered as "predisposing" to exsanguination is the lack of adequate obstetrical and anesthetic services. According to the 2002 Confidential Enquiry into Maternal and Child Health (CEMACH), however, most maternal deaths from hemorrhage in the United Kingdom were associated with substandard care. Moreover, from Japan, Nagaya and associates (2000) concluded that many hemorrhage-related maternal deaths were preventable and were associated with inadequate facilities. Zwart and co-workers (2008) provided similar observation from the Netherlands.

Antepartum Hemorrhage

Slight vaginal bleeding is common during active labor. This "bloody show" is the consequence of effacement and dilatation of the cervix, with tearing of small vessels. Uterine bleeding, however, coming from above the cervix, is cause for concern. It may follow some separation of a placenta implanted in the immediate vicinity of the cervical canal—*placenta previa*. It may come from separation of a placenta located elsewhere in the uterine cavity—*placental abruption*. Rarely, there may be velamentous insertion of the umbilical cord, and involved placental vessels may overlie the cervix—*vasa previa* (see Figs. 27-6 and 27-7, p. 583). In such cases, hemorrhage may follow laceration of these vessels at the time of membrane rupture.

The source of uterine bleeding is not always identified. In that circumstance, antepartum bleeding typically begins with few, if any, symptoms and then stops. At delivery no anatomical cause is identified. In many of these cases, bleeding likely is the consequence of slight marginal placental separation. *A pregnancy with such bleeding remains at increased risk for a poor*

TABLE 35-1. Causes and Predisposing Factors of Obstetrical Hemorrhage

Abnormal Placentation
Placenta previa
Placental abruption
Placenta accreta/increta/percreta
Ectopic pregnancy
Hydatidiform mole

Trauma During Labor and Delivery
Episiotomy
Complicated vaginal delivery
Low- or midforceps delivery
Cesarean delivery or hysterectomy
Uterine rupture-risk increased by:
  Previously scarred uterus
  High parity
  Hyperstimulation
  Obstructed labor

  Intrauterine manipulation
  Midforceps rotation

Small Maternal Blood Volume
Small women
Pregnancy hypervolemia not yet maximal
Pregnancy hypervolemia constricted
  Severe preeclampsia
  Eclampsia
Sepsis syndrome
Chronic renal insufficiency

Other Factors
Obesity
Previous postpartum hemorrhage

Uterine Atony
Overdistended uterus
  Large fetus
  Multiple fetuses
  Hydramnios
  Distension with clots
Labor induction
Anesthesia or analgesia
  Halogenated agents
  Conduction analgesia with hypotension
Exhausted myometrium
  Rapid labor
  Prolonged labor
  Oxytocin or prostaglandin stimulation
  Chorioamnionitis
Previous uterine atony

Coagulation Defects—Intensify Other Causes
Massive transfusions
Placental abruption
Sepsis syndrome
Severe preeclampsia and eclampsia
Anticoagulant treatment
Congenital coagulopathies
Amnionic fluid embolism
Prolonged retention of dead fetus
Saline-induced abortion

outcome even though the bleeding soon stops and placenta previa appears to have been excluded by sonography. Lipitz and colleagues (1991) studied 65 consecutive women with uterine bleeding between 14 and 26 weeks and found that a fourth had placental abruption or previa. Total fetal loss rates including abortions and perinatal deaths were 32 percent. Leung and colleagues (2001) found that unexplained antepartum hemorrhage before 34 weeks was associated with a 62-percent risk of delivery within 1 week when associated with uterine contractions and with a 13-percent risk even in the absence of contractions. In pregnancies with hemorrhage after 26 weeks not explained by placental abruption or previa, Ajayi and associates (1992) reported adverse outcomes in a third. For this reason, delivery should be considered in any woman at term with unexplained vaginal bleeding.

Postpartum Hemorrhage

Postpartum hemorrhage describes an event rather than a diagnosis, and when encountered, its etiology must be determined. Common causes include bleeding from the placental implantation site, trauma to the genital tract and adjacent structures, or both (Table 35-2).

Definition

Traditionally, postpartum hemorrhage has been defined as the loss of 500 mL of blood or more after completion of the third stage of labor. This is problematic because half of all women delivered vaginally shed that amount of blood or more when losses are measured quantitatively (Fig. 35-2). Pritchard and associates (1962) used precise methods and found that approximately 5 percent of women delivering vaginally lost more than 1000 mL of blood. **They also reported that estimated blood loss is commonly only approximately half the actual loss.** Because of this, estimated blood loss in excess of 500 mL should call attention to mothers who are bleeding excessively. Toledo and colleagues (2007) have shown that calibrated drape markings improve estimation accuracy. Still, as shown by the study of Sosa and associates (2009) cited above, even this technique underestimates blood loss when compared with more precise methods described by Pritchard and colleagues (1962).

The blood volume of a pregnant woman with normal pregnancy-induced hypervolemia usually increases by 30 to 60 percent. This amounts to 1500 to 2000 mL for an average-sized woman (Pritchard, 1965). The equation that determines this is

TABLE 35-2. Predisposing Factors and Causes of Immediate Postpartum Hemorrhage

Bleeding from Placental Implantation Site
Hypotonic myometrium—uterine atony
    Some general anesthetics—halogenated hydrocarbons
    Poorly perfused myometrium—hypotension
        Hemorrhage
        Conduction analgesia
    Overdistended uterus: large fetus, twins, hydramnios
    Prolonged labor
    Very rapid labor
    Induced or augmented labor
    High parity
    Uterine atony in previous pregnancy
    Chorioamnionitis
Retained placental tissue
    Avulsed lobule, succenturiate lobe
    Abnormally adhered: accreta, increta, percreta

Trauma to the Genital Tract
Large episiotomy, including extensions
Lacerations of perineum, vagina, or cervix
Ruptured uterus

Coagulation Defects
Intensify all of the above

shown in Table 35-3. This computation was constructed by studying blood volumes and blood losses in more than 100 women using chromium-51 labeled erythrocytes. A normally pregnant woman tolerates, without any remarkable decrease in postpartum hematocrit, a blood loss at delivery that approaches the volume of blood that she added during pregnancy. Thus, if blood loss is less than the amount added by pregnancy, the hematocrit stays the same acutely and during the first several days. It eventually increases as normal plasma volume shrinks postpartum.

Any time the postpartum hematocrit is lower than one obtained on admission for delivery, blood loss can be estimated as the sum of the calculated pregnancy hypervolemia plus 500 mL for each 3 volumes percent drop in the hematocrit. In the study by Combs and colleagues (1991b), the mean postpartum hematocrit declined from 2.6 to 4.3 volumes percent. Only a third of women had no decline or had an actual increase. The same investigators found that women undergoing cesarean delivery had a mean decrease in hematocrit of 4.2 volumes percent—only 20 percent had no decline (Combs and co-workers, 1991a).

Late Postpartum Hemorrhage. Bleeding after the first 24 hours is designated *late postpartum hemorrhage* and is discussed in Chapter 30 (p. 648).

Hemostasis at the Placental Site

Near term, it is estimated that at least 600 mL/min of blood flows through the intervillous space (see Chap. 5, p. 108). This flow is carried by the spiral arteries—which average 120 in number—and their accompanying veins. With separation of the placenta, these vessels are avulsed (see Chap. 3, p. 46). Hemostasis at the placental implantation site is achieved first by contraction of the myometrium that compresses this formidable number of relatively large vessels (Fig. 2-14, p. 25). This is followed by subsequent clotting and obliteration of their lumens. Thus, adhered pieces of placenta or large blood clots that prevent effective myometrial contraction can impair hemostasis at the implantation site.

It is therefore readily apparent that fatal postpartum hemorrhage can result from uterine atony despite normal coagulation. Conversely, if the myometrium within and adjacent to the denuded implantation site contracts vigorously, fatal hemorrhage *from the placental implantation site* is unlikely even in circumstances when coagulation may be severely impaired.

Clinical Characteristics

Postpartum bleeding may begin before or after placental separation. Instead of sudden massive hemorrhage, there usually is steady bleeding. At any given instant, it appears to be only moderate, but may persist until serious hypovolemia develops. Especially with hemorrhage after placental delivery, constant seepage can lead to enormous blood loss.

The effects of hemorrhage depend to a considerable degree on the nonpregnant blood volume and the corresponding magnitude of pregnancy-induced hypervolemia. A treacherous feature of postpartum hemorrhage is the failure of the pulse and blood pressure to undergo more than moderate alterations until large amounts of blood have been lost. The normotensive woman initially may actually become somewhat hypertensive in response to hemorrhage. Moreover, the already hypertensive woman may be interpreted to be normotensive although remarkably hypov-

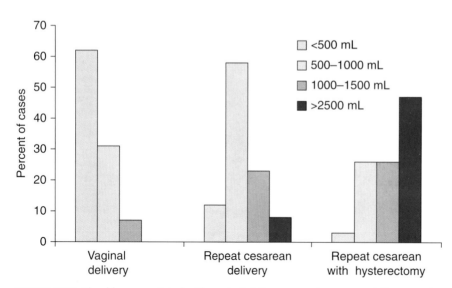

FIGURE 35-2 Blood loss associated with vaginal delivery, repeat cesarean delivery, and repeat cesarean delivery plus hysterectomy. (Data from Pritchard and associates, 1962.)

TABLE 35-3. Calculation of Maternal Total Blood Volume

Nonpregnant blood volume:

$$\frac{[\text{Height (inches)} \times 50] + [\text{Weight (pounds)} \times 25]}{2} = \text{Blood volume (mL)}$$

Pregnant blood volume:
- Varies from 30 to 60 percent of calculated nonpregnant volume
- Increases across gestational age and plateaus at approximately 34 weeks
- Usually larger with low normal-range hematocrit (~30) and smaller with high normal-range hematocrit (~38)
- Average increase is 40 to 80 percent with multifetal gestation
- Average increase is less with preeclampsia—volumes vary inversely with severity

Postpartum blood volume with serious hemorrhage
  Assume acute return to nonpregnant total volume—with fluid resuscitation—because pregnancy hypervolemia will not be attained again

Modified from Leveno and colleagues (2003).

olemic. Accordingly, hypovolemia may not be recognized until very late.

The woman with severe preeclampsia or eclampsia does not have normally expanded blood volume. Zeeman and colleagues (2009) documented a mean increase above nonpregnant volume of only 10 percent in 29 eclamptic women at delivery. Thus, these women are very sensitive to, or even intolerant of, what may be considered normal blood loss (see Chap. 34, p. 717). **When excessive hemorrhage is suspected in the woman with severe preeclampsia, efforts should be made immediately to identify those clinical and laboratory findings that would prompt vigorous crystalloid and blood administration to resuscitate hypovolemia.**

In some women after delivery, blood may not escape vaginally but instead may collect within the uterine cavity, which can become distended by 1000 mL or more of blood. In some, the attendant may massage a roll of abdominal fat mistaken for the postpartum uterus. Thus, observation of the uterus postpartum must not be left to an inexperienced person (see Chap. 17, p. 398).

Diagnosis

Except possibly when intrauterine and intravaginal accumulation of blood is not recognized, or in some instances of uterine rupture with intraperitoneal bleeding, the diagnosis of postpartum hemorrhage should be obvious. The differentiation between bleeding from uterine atony and that from genital tract lacerations is tentatively determined by predisposing risk factors and the condition of the uterus (see Table 35-2). If bleeding persists despite a firm, well-contracted uterus, the cause of the hemorrhage most likely is from lacerations. Bright red blood also suggests arterial blood from lacerations. *To confirm that lacerations are a cause of bleeding, careful inspection of the vagina, cervix, and uterus is essential.*

Sometimes bleeding may be caused by both atony and trauma, especially after major operative delivery. If easily accessible, such as with conduction analgesia, inspection of the cervix

and vagina should be performed after every delivery to identify hemorrhage from lacerations. Palpation of the uterine cavity and inspection of the cervix and entire vagina is essential after internal podalic version and breech extraction. The same is true when unusual bleeding is identified during the second stage of labor.

CAUSES OF OBSTETRICAL HEMORRHAGE

Placental Abruption

Placental separation from its implantation site before delivery has been variously called *placental abruption, abruptio placentae,* and in Great Britain, *accidental hemorrhage.* The Latin term *abruptio placentae* means "rending asunder of the placenta" and denotes a sudden accident, which is a clinical characteristic of most cases. The cumbersome term *premature separation of the normally implanted placenta* is most descriptive. It differentiates the placenta that separates prematurely but is implanted some distance beyond the cervical internal os from one that is implanted over the cervical internal os—that is, *placenta previa.*

The bleeding of placental abruption typically insinuates itself between the membranes and uterus, ultimately escaping through the cervix, causing *external hemorrhage* (Fig. 35-3). Less often, the blood does not escape externally but is retained between the detached placenta and the uterus, leading to *concealed hemorrhage* (Fig. 35-3). As shown in Figures 35-4 and 35-5, placental abruption may be *total* or *partial.* Concealed hemorrhage carries much greater maternal and fetal hazards. This is not only because of possible consumptive coagulopathy, but also because the extent of the hemorrhage is not readily appreciated, and the diagnosis typically is delayed (Chang and co-workers, 2001).

Significance and Frequency

Abruption severity often depends on how quickly the woman is seen following symptom onset. With delay, the likelihood of extensive separation causing fetal death is increased remarkably.

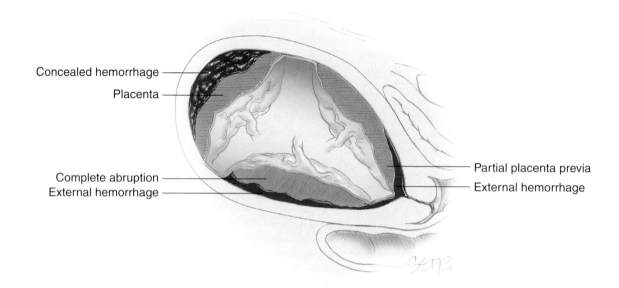

FIGURE 35-3 Hemorrhage from extensive placental abruption. **External hemorrhage:** the placenta has detached peripherally, and the membranes between the placenta and cervical canal are detached from the underlying decidua. This allows blood egress through the vagina. **Concealed hemorrhage:** the periphery of the placenta and the membranes are still adhered and blood remains within the uterus. **Partial placenta previa:** there is placental separation and external hemorrhage.

The frequency with which placental abruption is diagnosed varies because of different criteria, but the reported frequency averages 1 in 200 deliveries. In the 15-million delivery database of the National Center for Health Statistics, Salihu and associates (2005) reported an incidence in singleton births of 1 in 160. Using birth certificate data for the United States for 2003, the incidence of placental abruption was found to be 1 in 190 deliveries (Martin and co-workers, 2005). At Parkland Hospital from 1988 through 2006, the incidence of placental abruption in more than 280,000 deliveries has been approximately 1 in 290 (Fig. 35-6).

At least at Parkland Hospital, both incidence and severity have decreased over time. Applying the criterion of placental separation so extensive as to kill the fetus, the incidence was 1 in 420 deliveries from 1956 through 1967 (Pritchard and Brekken, 1967). As the number of high-parity women giving birth decreased and as availability of prenatal care and emergency transportation improved, the frequency of abruption causing fetal death dropped to approximately 1 in 830 deliveries from 1974 through 1989 (Pritchard and colleagues, 1991). Between 1996 and 2003, it decreased further to approximately 1 in 1600.

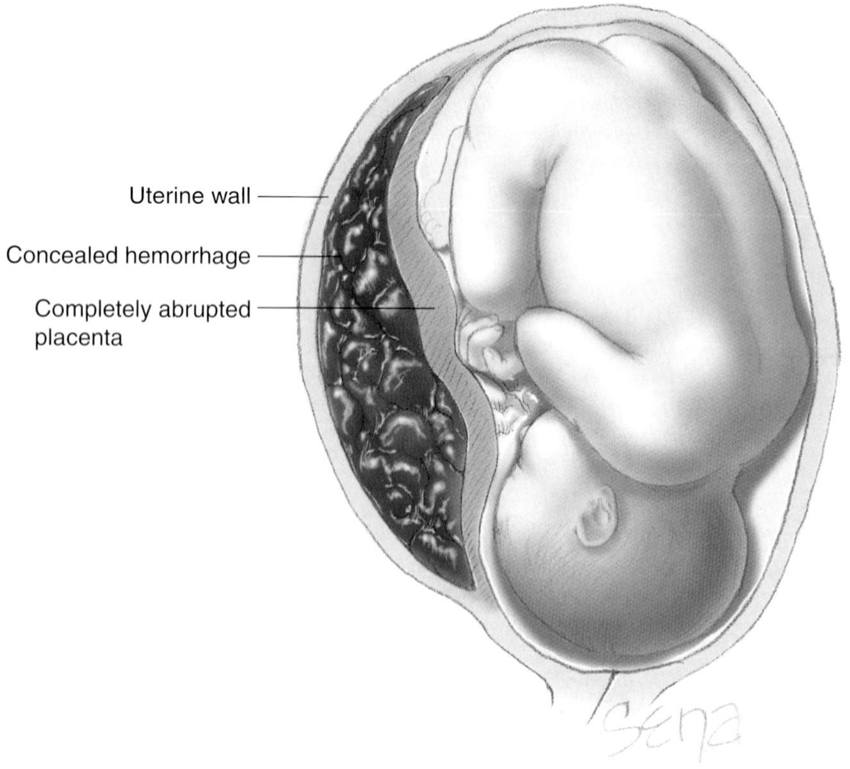

Perinatal Morbidity and Mortality

Although the rates of fetal death from abruption have declined, they remain especially prominent as stillbirth rates from other causes have decreased. For example, since the early 1990s, 10 to 12 percent of all third-trimester stillbirths at Parkland Hospital have been the consequence of placental abruption. This is similar to the rate reported by Fretts and Usher (1997) for the Royal Victoria Hospital in Montreal

FIGURE 35-4 Total placental abruption with concealed hemorrhage and fetal death.

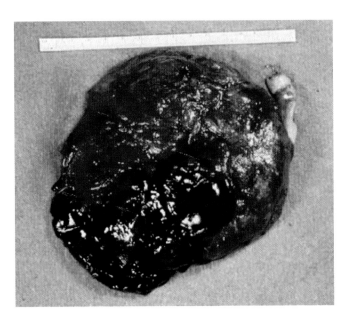

FIGURE 35-5 Partial placental abruption with adhered clot.

during the 18-year period ending in 1995 (see Chap. 29, p. 630).

Excessive perinatal mortality rates from placental abruption have been documented in several reports. Salihu and colleagues (2005) analyzed more than 15 million singletons in the United States between 1995 and 1998. They reported that the perinatal mortality rate associated with placental abruption was 119 per 1000 births compared with 8 per 1000 for those without this complication. Importantly, they emphasized that the high perinatal mortality rate was not due solely to placental abruption, but also to the associated increased incidence of preterm delivery and fetal-growth restriction. Nath and co-workers

(2008), however, reported that preterm birth was the overriding association with these low-birthweight perinates.

There are also increased serious adverse sequelae in infants who survive. In the study by Abdella and associates (1984), approximately 15 percent of 182 surviving infants were identified to have significant neurological deficits within the first year of life. Similarly, Matsuda and co-workers (2003) reported that approximately 20 percent of 39 survivors delivered between 26 and 36 weeks developed cerebral palsy compared with only 1 percent of gestational age–matched controls.

Etiology and Associated Factors

The primary cause of placental abruption is unknown, but several associated conditions are listed in Table 35-4.

Age, Parity, Race, and Familial Factors. As is shown in Figure 35-6, the incidence of abruption increases with *maternal age*. In the First- and Second-Trimester Evaluation of Risk (FASTER) trial, women older than 40 years were 2.3 times more likely to experience abruption compared with those 35 years or younger (Cleary-Goldman and co-workers, 2005). Although Pritchard and colleagues (1991) reported the incidence to be higher in women of *great parity*, Toohey and associates (1995) did not find this. *Race* or ethnicity appears to be important. Of the almost 170,000 deliveries reported by Pritchard and co-workers (1991) from Parkland Hospital, abruption was more common in African-American and Caucasian women (1 in 200) than in Asian (1 in 300) or Latin-American women (1 in 450). A familial association was recently reported by Rasmussen and Irgens (2009), who analyzed outcomes in the Norwegian population-based registry that included almost 378,000 sisters with more than 767,000 pregnancies. If a woman had a severe abruption, then the risk for her sister was doubled, and the

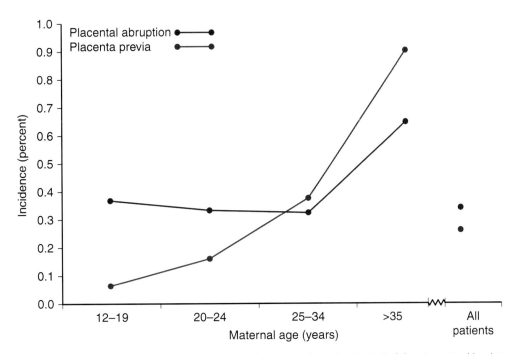

FIGURE 35-6 Incidence of placental abruption and placenta previa by maternal age in 280,960 deliveries at Parkland Hospital from 1988 through 2006. (Data courtesy of Dr. Don McIntire.)

TABLE 35-4. Risk Factors for Placental Abruption

Risk Factor	Relative Risk
Increased age and parity	1.3–1.5
Preeclampsia	2.1–4.0
Chronic hypertension	1.8–3.0
Preterm ruptured membranes	2.4–4.9
Multifetal gestation	2.1
Low birthweight	14.0
Hydramnios	2.0
Cigarette smoking	1.4–1.9
Thrombophilias	3–7
Cocaine use	NA
Prior abruption	10–25
Uterine leiomyoma	NA

NA = not available.
Adapted from Cunningham and Hollier (1997); risk data from Ananth (1999a,b, 2001b), Eskes (2001), Kramer (1997), Kupferminc (1999), Nath (2008), and all their associates.

heritability risk was estimated to be 16 percent. There was no increase in their sisters-in-law's risk.

Hypertension. By far the most common condition associated with placental abruption is some type of *hypertension*—gestational hypertension, preeclampsia, chronic hypertension, or combinations of these. In the Parkland Hospital report of 408 women with placental abruption and fetal demise, hypertension was apparent in approximately half of the women once the depleted intravascular compartment was adequately refilled (Pritchard and co-workers, 1991). Half of these women—a fourth of all 408—had chronic hypertension. Looked at another way, Sibai and co-workers (1998) reported for the Maternal–Fetal Medicine Units Network that 1.5 percent of pregnant women with chronic hypertension suffered placental abruption. Ananth and associates (2007) reported a 2.4-fold increased incidence of abruption with chronic hypertension, and this was increased further if there was superimposed preeclampsia or fetal-growth restriction. Zetterstrom and colleagues (2005) reported a twofold increased incidence of abruption in women with chronic hypertension compared with normotensive women—an incidence of 1.1 versus 0.5 percent.

The severity of hypertension does not necessarily correlate with the incidence of abruption (Witlin and colleagues, 1999; Zetterstrom and co-workers, 2005). Also, observations from the Magpie Trial Collaborative Group (2002) suggest that women with preeclampsia may have a reduced risk of abruption when treated with magnesium sulfate.

Prematurely Ruptured Membranes and Preterm Delivery. There is no doubt that there is an increased incidence of abruption when the membranes rupture before term. Major and colleagues (1995) reported that 5 percent of 756 women with ruptured membranes between 20 and 36 weeks developed an abruption. Kramer and co-workers (1997) found an incidence of 3.1 percent in all women if membranes were ruptured for longer than 24 hours. Ananth and associates

(2004) studied data from the 1988 National Maternal and Infant Health Survey and reported a threefold risk of abruption with prematurely ruptured membranes. This risk was further increased with infection. This same group has suggested that inflammation and infection may be the primary cause of placental abruption (Nath and co-workers, 2007). They also reported a strong association with low birthweight principally due to perterm delivery, but not growth restriction (2008).

Smoking. Early studies from the Collaborative Perinatal Project linked *cigarette smoking* with an increased risk for abruption (Misra and Ananth, 1999; Naeye, 1980). In a meta-analysis of 1.6 million pregnancies, Ananth and colleagues (1999a, b) found a twofold risk for abruption in smokers. This was increased to five- to eightfold if smokers had chronic hypertension, severe preeclampsia, or both. Similar findings have been reported by Mortensen (2001), Hogberg (2007), Kaminsky (2007), and all their associates.

Cocaine. Women who used cocaine have an alarming frequency of placental abruption. In the report from Bingol and colleagues (1987) of 50 women who abused cocaine during pregnancy, there were eight stillbirths caused by placental abruption. In their systematic review of 15 studies of cocaine-using women, Addis and associates (2001) reported that placental abruption was more common in women who used cocaine than in those who did not.

Thrombophilias. Over the past decade, a number of inherited or acquired *thrombophilias* have been associated with thromboembolic disorders during pregnancy. Some of these disorders—for example factor V Leiden or prothrombin gene mutation—are associated with placental abruption and infarction as well as preeclampsia. These have been reviewed recently by Kenny and colleagues (2009) and are discussed further in Chapter 47 (p. 1014).

Traumatic Abruption. In some cases of external trauma, usually associated with motor vehicle accidents or physical violence, placental separation may follow. In earlier studies from Parkland Hospital, only approximately 2 percent of placental abruptions causing fetal death were due to trauma (see Chap. 42, p. 938). However, as placental abruption incidence has declined over the years, traumatic abruptions have become relatively more common. Kettel (1988) and Stafford (1988) and their co-workers have appropriately stressed that abruption can be caused by relatively minor trauma. Moreover, a nonreassuring fetal heart rate tracing is not always immediately associated with evidence of placental separation.

Leiomyomas. These tumors, especially if located behind the placental implantation site, predispose to abruption (see Chap. 40, p. 901). Rice and associates (1989) reported that eight of 14 women with retroplacental leiomyomas developed placental abruption, and four women had stillborns. In contrast, abruption developed in only two of 79 women whose leiomyomas were not retroplacental.

Recurrent Abruption

A woman who has suffered a placental abruption—especially that caused fetal death—has a high recurrence rate. Pritchard and co-workers (1970) identified this to be 12 percent in a subsequent pregnancy. Importantly, eight of 14 recurrent abruptions caused a second fetal death. Tikkanen and colleagues (2006) looked at this another way and found that of 114 parous women who experienced an abruption, 9 percent had a prior abruption. Furuhashi and colleagues (2002) analyzed subsequent pregnancy outcomes in 27 women with one prior placental abruption. There was a 22-percent recurrence rate, and four of six recurrences were at a gestational age 1 to 3 weeks earlier than the first abruption. In a population-based study of 767,000 pregnancies, Rasmussen and Irgens (2009) reported an odds ratio of 6.5 for recurrent mild abruption and 11.5 for recurrent severe abruption. For women who had two severe placental abruptions, the risk became 50-fold for a third.

Management of a pregnancy subsequent to an abruption is thus difficult because another separation may suddenly recur, even remote from term. In many of these recurrences, fetal well-being is reassuring beforehand. Thus, antepartum fetal testing is usually not predictive (Toivonen and colleagues, 2002).

Pathology

Placental abruption is initiated by hemorrhage into the decidua basalis. The decidua then splits, leaving a thin layer adhered to the myometrium. Consequently, the process in its earliest stages consists of the development of a decidual hematoma that leads to separation, compression, and ultimate destruction of the placenta adjacent to it. Nath and colleagues (2007) found histological evidence of inflammation more commonly in cases of placental abruption than in normal controls. As discussed above, they suggested that inflammation—infection—may be a contributor to causal pathways.

In its early stage, there may be no clinical symptoms, and the separation is discovered upon examination of the freshly delivered placenta. In these cases, there is a circumscribed depression on the placenta's maternal surface. It usually measures a few centimeters in diameter and is covered by dark, clotted blood. Because several minutes are required for these anatomical changes to materialize, a very recently separated placenta may appear to be totally normal at delivery. According to Benirschke and Kaufmann (2000) and also our experiences, the "age" of the retroplacental clot cannot be determined exactly. In the example shown in Figure 35-5, a substantive-sized dark clot is well formed, it has depressed the placental bulk, and it likely is several hours old.

In some instances, a decidual spiral artery ruptures to cause a retroplacental hematoma, which as it expands, disrupts more vessels to separate more placenta (see Fig. 27-3, p. 579). The area of separation rapidly becomes more extensive and reaches the margin of the placenta. Because the uterus is still distended by the products of conception, it is unable to contract sufficiently to compress the torn vessels that supply the placental site. The escaping blood may dissect the membranes from the uterine wall and eventually appear externally or may be completely retained within the uterus (see Figs. 35-3 and 35-4).

Concealed Hemorrhage. Retained or concealed hemorrhage is likely when:

- There is an effusion of blood behind the placenta, but its margins still remain adhered

- The placenta is completely separated, yet the membranes retain their attachment to the uterine wall
- Blood gains access to the amnionic cavity after breaking through the membranes
- The fetal head is so closely applied to the lower uterine segment that blood cannot make its way past.

Most often, however, the membranes are gradually dissected off the uterine wall, and blood sooner or later escapes.

Chronic Placental Abruption. In some women, hemorrhage with retroplacental hematoma formation is somehow arrested completely without delivery. We have been able to document this phenomenon by labeling maternal red cells with chromium-51. In one case, red blood cells were concealed as a 400-mL clot, which was found within the uterus at delivery 3 weeks later. The clot contained no radiochromium, whereas peripheral blood at that time did. The blood in the clot therefore had accumulated before the erythrocytes were labeled.

Some cases of abruption first develop very early in pregnancy. Dugoff and colleagues (2004) observed an association between abnormally elevated maternal serum markers in the first trimester and subsequent abruption. Ananth (2006) and Weiss (2004) and their many associates have correlated first- and second-trimester bleeding with placental abruption in the third trimester.

Fetal-to-Maternal Hemorrhage. Bleeding with placental abruption is almost always maternal. This is logical because the separation is within the maternal decidua. In 78 women with a nontraumatic placental abruption, we found evidence of fetal-to-maternal hemorrhage in 20 percent. In all, the volume of fetal blood was less than 10 mL (Stettler and colleagues, 1992). Conversely, significant fetal bleeding is much more likely with traumatic abruption. *In this circumstance, fetal bleeding results from a tear or fracture in the placenta rather than from the placental separation itself.* Traumatic abruption is considered further in Chapter 42 (p. 938), and an example of a placental tear is shown in Figure 42-9. Pearlman and associates (1990) documented fetal bleeding that averaged 12 mL in a third of women with a traumatic abruption. Stettler and colleagues (1992) reported that there was fetal-to-maternal hemorrhage of 80 to 100 mL in three of eight cases of traumatic placental abruption.

Clinical Diagnosis

The signs and symptoms of placental abruption can vary considerably. For example, external bleeding can be profuse, yet placental separation may not be so extensive as to compromise the fetus. Rarely, there may be no external bleeding, but the placenta may be completely sheared off and the fetus dead as the direct consequence. In one unusual case, a multiparous woman near term presented to Parkland Hospital because of a nosebleed. There was no abdominal or uterine pain or tenderness and no vaginal bleeding, but her fetus was dead. Her blood did not clot, and the plasma fibrinogen level was 25 mg/dL. Labor was induced, and at delivery a total abruption with fresh clots was found.

In a prospective study of 59 women with a placental abruption, Hurd and co-workers (1983) reported vaginal bleeding in 78 percent, uterine tenderness or back pain in 66 percent, and fetal distress in 60 percent. *In 22 percent, preterm labor was initially diagnosed until subsequent fetal death or distress developed.* Other findings included frequent uterine contractions and persistent uterine hypertonus.

Sonography infrequently confirms the diagnosis of placental abruption at least acutely, because the placenta and fresh clot have similar sonographic appearances. In an early study, Sholl (1987) used sonography and confirmed the clinical diagnosis in only 25 percent of women. In a later study, Glantz and Purnell (2002) reported 24-percent sensitivity in 149 consecutive women who underwent sonography to exclude placental abruption. *Importantly, negative findings with sonographic examination do not exclude placental abruption.*

Differential Diagnosis. With severe placental abruption, the diagnosis generally is obvious. Milder and more common forms of abruption may be difficult to recognize with certainty, and the diagnosis is often made by exclusion. Unfortunately, neither laboratory tests nor diagnostic methods are available to detect lesser degrees of placental separation accurately. Therefore, with vaginal bleeding in a pregnancy with a live fetus, it often becomes necessary to exclude placenta previa and other causes of bleeding by clinical and sonographic evaluation.

Clinically, it has long been taught—perhaps with some justification—that *painful* uterine bleeding signifies placental abruption, whereas *painless* uterine bleeding is indicative of placenta previa. The differential diagnosis is usually not this straightforward, and labor accompanying previa may cause pain suggestive of placental abruption. On the other hand, pain from abruption may mimic normal labor, or it may be painless, especially with a posterior placenta. At times, the cause of the vaginal bleeding remains obscure even after delivery.

Shock. It was once held that the shock sometimes seen with placental abruption was disproportionate to the amount of hemorrhage. Supposedly, placental thromboplastin enters the maternal circulation and incites intravascular coagulation and other features of the amnionic fluid embolism syndrome (see p. 788). This rarely happens, and hypovolemic shock is instead directly due to maternal blood loss. In 141 women with abruption so severe as to kill the fetus, Pritchard and Brekken (1967) proved that blood loss often amounted to at least half of the pregnant blood volume. Conversely, neither hypotension nor anemia is obligatory even with extreme concealed hemorrhage. Oliguria from inadequate renal perfusion that is observed in these circumstances is responsive to vigorous intravenous fluid and blood infusion.

Consumptive Coagulopathy. Placental abruption is one of the most common causes of clinically significant consumptive coagulopathy in obstetrics. In approximately a third of women with an abruption severe enough to kill the fetus, there are measurable changes in coagulation factors. Specifically, clinically significant hypofibrinogenemia—plasma levels less than 150 mg/dL—is found. This is coupled with elevated levels of fibrinogen-fibrin degradation products and/or D-dimers, which are specific degradation products of fibrin. Other coagulation factors are also variably decreased. Consumptive coagulopathy is more likely with a concealed abruption because intrauterine pressure is higher, thus forcing more thromboplastin into the

maternal venous system. In those cases in which the fetus survives, severe coagulation defects are seen less commonly. Our experience has been that if serious coagulopathy develops, it is usually evident by the time abruption symptoms appear.

The major mechanism is activation of intravascular coagulation with varying degrees of defibrination (see p. 785). Procoagulants are also consumed in the retroplacental clots, although the amounts recovered are insufficient to account for all of the missing fibrinogen (Pritchard and Brekken, 1967). Moreover, Bonnar and co-workers (1969) have observed, and we have confirmed, that the levels of fibrin degradation products are higher in serum from peripheral blood than in serum from blood contained in the uterine cavity. The reverse would be anticipated in the absence of significant intravascular coagulation.

An important consequence of intravascular coagulation is the activation of plasminogen to plasmin, which lyses fibrin microemboli to maintain microcirculatory patency. With placental abruption severe enough to kill the fetus, there are always pathological levels of fibrinogen–fibrin degradation products and/or D-dimers in maternal serum.

Overt thrombocytopenia may or may not accompany severe hypofibrinogenemia initially, but becomes common after repeated blood transfusions.

Renal Failure. Acute renal failure may be seen with severe placental abruption. It is more common if treatment of hypovolemia is delayed or incomplete. It is unclear if abruption contributes significantly to the increasing incidence of obstetric-related acute kidney injury in this country as recently reported by Kuklina and co-workers (2009). Drakeley and colleagues (2002) described 72 pregnant women with acute renal failure, and a third had suffered an abruption. Fortunately, most cases of acute kidney injury are reversible, however, according to Lindheimer and associates (2007), *acute cortical necrosis,* when it occurs in pregnancy, is usually caused by placental abruption. In older reports, such as the one by Grünfeld and Pertuiset (1987), a third of women with this lesion had suffered an abruption.

Seriously impaired renal perfusion is the consequence of massive hemorrhage. Because preeclampsia frequently coexists with placental abruption, renal vasospasm and hypoperfusion are likely intensified (Hauth and Cunningham, 1999). Even when abruption is complicated by severe intravascular coagulation, prompt and vigorous treatment of hemorrhage with blood and crystalloid solution usually prevents clinically significant renal dysfunction. For unknown reasons, even without preeclampsia, *proteinuria* is initially common, especially with more severe forms of placental abruption. It usually clears soon after delivery.

Sheehan Syndrome. Severe intrapartum or early postpartum hemorrhage rarely is followed by pituitary failure or *Sheehan syndrome.* It is characterized by failure of lactation, amenorrhea, breast atrophy, loss of pubic and axillary hair, hypothyroidism, and adrenal cortical insufficiency. The exact pathogenesis is not well understood, and such endocrine abnormalities develop infrequently even in women who hemorrhage severely. In some but not all instances of Sheehan syndrome, there may be varying degrees of anterior pituitary necrosis and impaired secretion of one or more trophic hormones. It is discussed further in

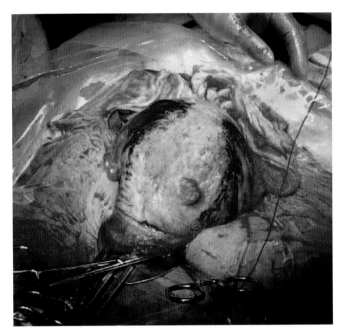

FIGURE 35-7 Couvelaire uterus from total placental abruption after cesarean delivery. Blood markedly infiltrates the myometrium to reach the serosa, especially at the cornua. It gives the myometrium a bluish-purple tone as shown. After the hysterotomy incision was closed, the uterus remained well contracted despite extensive extravasation of blood into the uterine wall. The small serosal leiomyoma seen on the lower anterior uterine surface is an incidental finding. (Courtesy of Dr. Allison Smith).

Chapter 53 (p. 1140), and its diagnosis by magnetic resonance (MR) imaging is shown in Figure 53-5.

Couvelaire Uterus. There may be widespread extravasation of blood into the uterine musculature and beneath the uterine serosa (Fig. 35-7). First described by Couvelaire in the early 1900s as *uteroplacental apoplexy,* it is now termed *Couvelaire uterus.* Such effusions of blood are also occasionally seen beneath the tubal serosa, between the leaves of the broad liga-

ments, in the substance of the ovaries, and free in the peritoneal cavity. Its precise incidence is unknown because it can be demonstrated conclusively only at laparotomy. These myometrial hemorrhages seldom interfere with myometrial contraction to cause atony, and they are not an indication for hysterectomy.

Management

Treatment for placental abruption varies depending on gestational age and the status of the mother and fetus. With a fetus of viable age, and if vaginal delivery is not imminent, then emergency cesarean delivery is chosen by most clinicians. As discussed on page 791, with massive external bleeding, intensive resuscitation with blood plus crystalloid and prompt delivery to control hemorrhage are lifesaving for the mother and hopefully, for the fetus. If the diagnosis is uncertain and the fetus is alive but without evidence of compromise, then close observation can be practiced in facilities capable of immediate intervention.

Expectant Management in Preterm Pregnancy. Delaying delivery may prove beneficial when the fetus is immature. Bond and associates (1989) expectantly managed 43 women with placental abruption before 35 weeks, and 31 of them were given tocolytic therapy. The mean time to delivery in all 43 was approximately 12 days, and there were no stillborns. Cesarean delivery was performed in 75 percent of cases.

Women with evidence of very early abruption frequently develop oligohydramnios, either with or without premature membrane rupture. In one report by Elliott and associates (1998), four women with an abruption at a mean of 20 weeks also developed oligohydramnios. They were delivered at an average gestational age of 28 weeks.

Lack of ominous decelerations does not guarantee the safety of the intrauterine environment. The placenta may further separate at any instant and seriously compromise or kill the fetus unless delivery is performed immediately. Some of the immediate causes of fetal distress from placental abruption are shown in Figure 35-8. Importantly, for the welfare of the distressed fetus,

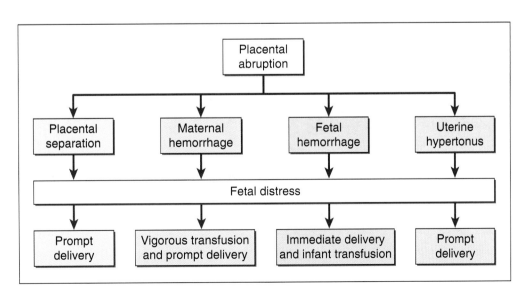

FIGURE 35-8 Various causes of fetal distress from placental abruption and their treatment. Fetal hemorrhage usually is seen only with traumatic abruption and placental tear.

steps should be initiated immediately to correct maternal hypovolemia, anemia, and hypoxia to restore and maintain function of any placenta that is still implanted. Little can be done to favorably modify the other causes that contribute to fetal distress except delivery.

Tocolysis. Some—but certainly not all—advocate tocolysis for the preterm pregnancy complicated by suspected abruption but with no fetal compromise. In an early study, Hurd and associates (1983) reported that abruption went unrecognized for dangerously long periods if tocolysis was initiated. Conversely, Sholl (1987) as well as Combs and co-workers (1992) provided data showing that tocolysis improved outcome in a highly selected group of preterm pregnancies complicated by partial abruption. In another supportive study, Towers and co-workers (1999) administered magnesium sulfate, terbutaline, or both to 95 of 131 women with placental abruption diagnosed before 36 weeks. The perinatal mortality rate of 5 percent in these women did not differ from the nontreated group. The investigators concluded that a randomized clinical trial could be safely conducted. Until then, we are of the view that clinically evident placental abruption should be considered a contraindication to tocolytic therapy.

Cesarean Delivery. Rapid delivery of the fetus who is alive but in distress practically always means cesarean delivery. Kayani and colleagues (2003) studied the relationship between the speed of delivery and neonatal outcome in 33 singleton pregnancies with a clinically overt placental abruption and fetal bradycardia. Of the 22 neurologically intact survivors, 15 were delivered within 20 minutes of the decision to operate. Of the 11 infants who died or developed cerebral palsy, eight were delivered beyond 20 minutes of the decision time. This suggests that the speed of response is an important factor in neonatal outcome.

It is important to note that an electrode applied directly to the fetus may rarely provide misleading information, as in the case illustrated in Figure 35-9. At first impression, fetal bradycardia of 80 to 90 beats/min, with some beat-to-beat variability,

seemed evident. In this case, however, the fetus was dead, and the maternal pulse rate was identical to that recorded through the fetal scalp electrode. Cesarean delivery at this time would likely have proved dangerous for the mother because she was profoundly hypovolemic and had severe consumptive coagulopathy. Serious coagulation defects are likely to prove especially troublesome with cesarean delivery. The abdominal and uterine incisions are prone to bleed excessively when coagulation is impaired.

Vaginal Delivery. If placental separation is so severe that the fetus has died, then vaginal delivery is usually preferred. Hemostasis at the placental implantation site depends primarily on myometrial contraction. Therefore, with vaginal delivery, stimulation of the myometrium pharmacologically and by uterine massage causes placental site vessels to be compressed and constricted so that serious hemorrhage is avoided even though coagulation defects may be present.

One exception to vaginal delivery includes hemorrhage that is so brisk that it cannot be successfully managed even by vigorous blood replacement. A second is presence of other obstetrical complications that prevent vaginal delivery.

Labor. With extensive placental abruption, the uterus is likely to be persistently hypertonic. The baseline intra-amnionic pressure may be 50 mm Hg or higher, with rhythmic increases up to 75 to 100 mm Hg. Because of persistent hypertonus, it may be difficult at times to determine by palpation whether the uterus is contracting and relaxing to any degree (Fig. 35-10).

Amniotomy. Rupture of the membranes as early as possible has long been championed in the management of placental abruption. The rationale for amniotomy is that diminished amnionic fluid volume might allow better spiral artery compression and serve to both decrease bleeding from the implantation site and reduce entry of thromboplastin into the maternal circulation. There is no evidence, however, that either is accomplished by amniotomy. If the fetus is reasonably mature, rupture

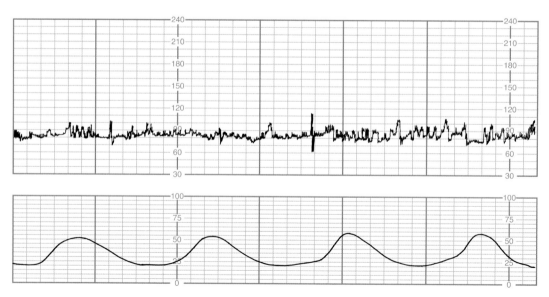

FIGURE 35-9 Placental abruption with dead fetus. Lower panel: Intrauterine pressure monitoring shows tachysystole and increased uterine basal tone. Upper panel: The scalp electrode conducted the maternal ECG signal, which could be mistaken for fetal bradycardia.

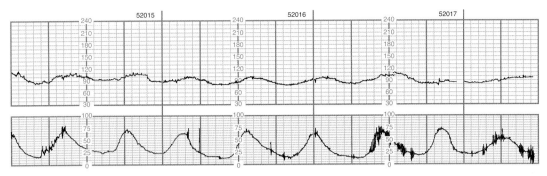

FIGURE 35-10 Lower panel: Placental abruption causing uterine hypertonus with a baseline pressure of 20 to 25 mm Hg and frequent contractions peaking at approximately 75 mm Hg. Upper panel: The fetal heart rate demonstrates baseline bradycardia with repetitive late decelerations.

of the membranes may hasten delivery. If the fetus is immature, the intact sac may be more efficient in promoting cervical dilatation than a small fetal part poorly applied to the cervix.

Oxytocin. Although baseline hypertonus characterizes myometrial function in most cases of severe placental abruption, if no rhythmic uterine contractions are superimposed, and there has been no previous uterine surgery, then oxytocin is given in standard doses. Uterine stimulation to effect vaginal delivery usually provides benefits that override risks. The use of oxytocin has been challenged on the basis that it might enhance the escape of thromboplastin into the maternal circulation and thereby initiate or enhance consumptive coagulopathy or amnionic fluid embolism syndrome. There is no evidence to support this fear (Clark and colleagues, 1995; Pritchard and Brekken, 1967).

Timing of Delivery after Severe Placental Abruption. When the fetus is dead or previable, there is no evidence that establishing an arbitrary time limit for delivery is necessary. Experiences indicate that maternal outcome depends on the diligence with which adequate fluid and blood replacement therapy is pursued, rather than on the interval to delivery. At the University of Virginia Hospital, women with severe placental abruption who were transfused for 18 hours or more before delivery experienced complications that were neither more numerous nor greater in severity than did the group in which delivery was accomplished sooner (Brame and associates, 1968). Our observations from Parkland Hospital described by Pritchard and Brekken (1967) are similar.

Placenta Previa

Placenta previa is used to describe a placenta that is implanted over or very near the internal cervical os. There are several possibilities:

- *Total placenta previa*—the internal os is covered completely by placenta (Fig. 35-11)
- *Partial placenta previa*—the internal os is partially covered by placenta (Fig. 35-12)
- *Marginal placenta previa*—the edge of the placenta is at the margin of the internal os
- *Low-lying placenta*—the placenta is implanted in the lower uterine segment such that the placental edge does not reach the internal os, but is in close proximity to it

- *Vasa previa*—the fetal vessels course through membranes and present at the cervical os (see Chap. 27, p. 583).

The relationships and definitions used for classification in some cases of placenta previa depend on cervical dilatation at the time of assessment. For example, a low-lying placenta at 2-cm dilatation may become a partial placenta previa at 8-cm dilatation because the dilating cervix has uncovered placenta. Conversely, a placenta previa that appears to be total before cervical dilatation may become partial at 4-cm dilatation because the cervix dilates beyond the edge of the placenta (see Fig. 35-12). **Digital palpation in an attempt to ascertain these changing relations between the placental edge and internal os as the cervix dilates usually causes severe hemorrhage!**

With both total and partial placenta previa, a certain degree of spontaneous placental separation is an inevitable consequence of lower uterine segment formation and cervical dilatation. Such separation is usually associated with hemorrhage. And although technically this constitutes a placental abruption, it usually is not termed such.

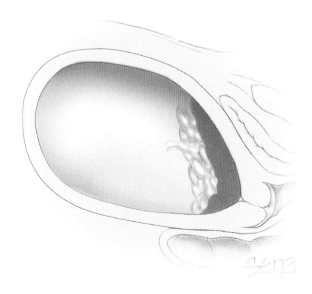

FIGURE 35-11 Total placenta previa showing that copious hemorrhage could be anticipated even with modest cervical dilatation.

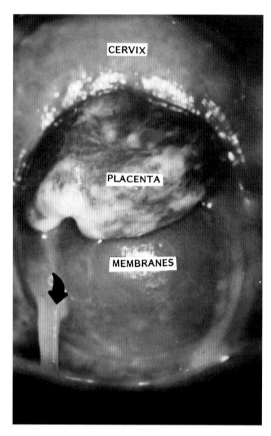

FIGURE 35-12 Partial placenta previa with a 22-week pregnancy. On speculum examination, the cervix appears 3- to 4-cm dilated. The arrow points to mucus dripping from the cervix. Uterine cramping continued, and a 410-g fetus was delivered vaginally the next day with minimal blood loss. (Photograph courtesy of Dr. Rigoberto Santos.)

Incidence

According to 2003 birth certificate data in the United States, placenta previa complicated almost 1 in 300 deliveries (Martin and co-workers, 2005). From Nova Scotia, Crane and associates (1999) found the incidence to be 1 in 300 of almost 93,000 deliveries. At Parkland Hospital, the incidence was 1 in 390 for more than 280,000 deliveries from 1998 through 2006. These prevalences are remarkably similar considering the lack of precision in definition and identification for reasons already discussed.

Associated Factors

Advancing *maternal age* increases the risk of placenta previa. As shown in Figure 35-6, the incidence of previa increased significantly with each advancing maternal age group. It is 1 in 1500 for women 19 years or younger and is 1 in 100 for women older than 35. Increasing maternal age in this country has caused an increased overall incidence of previa from 0.3 percent in 1976 to 0.7 percent in 1997 (Frederiksen and colleagues, 1999). In more than 36,000 women enrolled in the FASTER trial, those older than 35 years had a 1.1-percent risk for previa compared with that of 0.5 percent for women less than 35 (Cleary-Goldman and associates, 2005).

Multiparity is also associated with an increased risk for placenta previa. Babinszki and colleagues (1999) reported that the 2.2-percent incidence in women para 5 or greater was increased significantly compared with that of women with lower parity. Ananth and associates (2003a) reported the rate of placenta previa to be 40 percent higher in *multifetal gestations* compared with singletons.

For unknown reasons, *prior cesarean delivery* increases the risk for placenta previa. In a study of 30,132 women in labor undergoing cesarean delivery, Silver and associates (2006) cited an increased risk of previa in women who had prior cesarean delivery. The incidence was 1.3 percent for those with one prior cesarean delivery and 3.4 percent in women who had six or more cesarean deliveries (see also Chap. 26, p. 574, and Fig. 26-4). Miller and associates (1996) cited a threefold increased risk for previa in women with a prior cesarean delivery in more than 150,000 deliveries at Los Angeles County Women's Hospital. And the risk for previa increases progressively as parity and number of prior cesarean deliveries increases. Gesteland and co-workers (2004) and Gilliam and colleagues (2002) calculated that the likelihood of previa was increased more than eightfold in women with parity greater than four and more than four prior cesareans. Finally, a prior uterine incision with a previa increases the likelihood that *cesarean hysterectomy* will be necessary to control bleeding from a placenta accreta, increta, or percreta (see p. 776). Frederiksen and co-workers (1999) reported a 25-percent hysterectomy rate in women undergoing repeat cesarean delivery with a coexistent previa compared with only 6 percent in those undergoing primary cesarean for placenta previa.

The relative risk of placenta previa was reported by Williams and colleagues (1991) to be increased twofold in women who *smoked cigarettes*. These findings were confirmed by Ananth (2003a), Handler (1994), Usta (2005), and all their associates. It was theorized that carbon monoxide hypoxemia caused compensatory placental hypertrophy. Perhaps related, defective decidual vascularization, the possible result of inflammatory or atrophic changes, is implicated in the development of previa.

Women with otherwise unexplained elevated screening levels of *maternal serum alpha-fetoprotein* (*MSAFP*) are at greater risk for previa. Butler and co-workers (2001) reported that women with a placenta previa who also had increased MSAFP levels of ≥ 2.0 MoM at 16-week screening were at increased risk for late-pregnancy bleeding and preterm birth. (see also Chap. 13, p. 290).

Clinical Findings

The most characteristic event in placenta previa is painless hemorrhage, which usually does not appear until near the end of the second trimester or after. However, bleeding may begin earlier, and some abortions may result from such an abnormal location of the developing placenta.

With many previas, bleeding begins without warning and without pain in a woman who has had an uneventful prenatal course. Fortunately, the initial bleeding is rarely so profuse as to prove fatal. Usually it ceases, only to recur. In some women, particularly those with a placenta implanted near but not over the cervical os, bleeding does not appear until the onset of labor.

Then, it may vary from slight to profuse and clinically may mimic placental abruption.

The cause of hemorrhage is reemphasized: when the placenta is located over the internal os, the formation of the lower uterine segment and the dilatation of the internal os result inevitably in tearing of placental attachments. The bleeding is augmented by the inherent inability of myometrial fibers of the lower uterine segment to contract and thereby constrict the avulsed vessels.

Hemorrhage from the implantation site in the lower uterine segment may continue after placental delivery because the lower uterine segment contracts poorly. Bleeding may also result from lacerations in the friable cervix and lower uterine segment, especially following manual removal of a somewhat adhered placenta.

Placenta Accreta, Increta, and Percreta. Placenta previa may be associated with *placenta accreta* or one of its more advanced forms, *placenta increta* or *placenta percreta*. Such abnormally firm attachment of the placenta might be anticipated because of poorly developed decidua in the lower uterine segment. Almost 7 percent of 514 cases of previa reported by Frederiksen and associates (1999) had an associated abnormal placental attachment. Biswas and co-workers (1999) performed placental bed biopsies at cesarean delivery in 50 women with a previa and in 50 control women. Although approximately half of specimens from previas showed myometrial spiral arterioles with trophoblastic giant-cell infiltration, only 20 percent from normally implanted placentas had these changes. Placenta accreta and its more severe forms are discussed in detail on page 776.

Coagulation Defects. In our experience, coagulopathy is rare with placenta previa, even when there is extensive separation from the implantation site. Wing and colleagues (1996b) studied 87 antepartum women with bleeding from placenta previa and found no evidence of coagulopathy. Presumably thromboplastin, which incites intravascular coagulation that commonly characterizes placental abruption, readily escapes through the cervical canal rather than being forced into the maternal circulation.

Diagnosis

Placenta previa or abruption should always be suspected in women with uterine bleeding during the latter half of pregnancy. The possibility of placenta previa should not be dismissed until sonographic evaluation has clearly proved its absence. The diagnosis can seldom be established firmly by clinical examination unless a finger is passed through the cervix and the placenta is palpated. **Such digital cervical examination is never permissible unless the woman is in an operating room with all the preparations for immediate cesarean delivery— even the gentlest digital examination can cause torrential hemorrhage.** Furthermore, this type of examination should not be performed unless delivery is planned, for it may cause bleeding that necessitates immediate delivery. This "double set-up" examination is rarely necessary because placental location can almost always be ascertained by sonography.

Sonographic Localization. The simplest, safest, and most accurate method of placental localization is provided by *transabdominal sonography* (Fig. 35-13A). According to Laing (1996), the average accuracy is 96 percent, and rates as high as 98 percent have been obtained. *False-positive results are often a result of bladder distension. Therefore, scans in apparently positive cases should be repeated after emptying the bladder.* An uncommon source of error has been identification of abundant placenta implanted in the uterine fundus but failure to appreciate that the placenta was large and extended downward all the way to the internal cervical os.

The use of *transvaginal sonography* has substantively improved diagnostic accuracy of placenta previa (Figs. 35-13B and 35-14). Although it may appear dangerous to introduce an ultrasound probe into the vagina in suspected cases, the technique has been shown to be safe (Timor-Tritsch and Yunis, 1993).

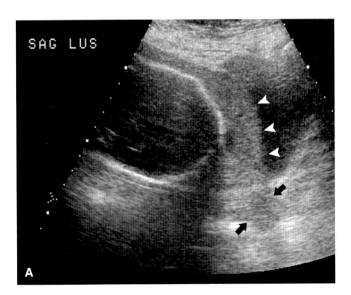 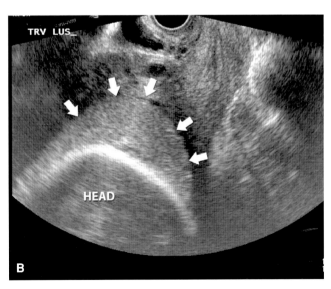

FIGURE 35-13 Total placenta previa. **A.** Transabdominal sonogram of the placenta (*white arrowheads*) behind the bladder covering the cervix (*black arrows*). **B.** Transvaginal sonographic image of the placenta (*arrows*) completely covering the cervix adjacent to the fetal head.

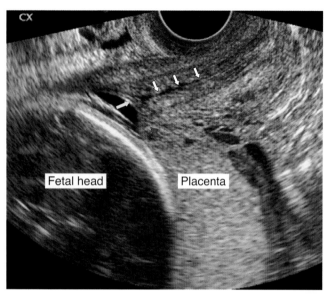

FIGURE 35-14 Partial anterior placenta previa at 36 weeks' gestation. The placental margin (*red arrow*) extends downward toward the cervix. The internal os (*yellow arrow*) and cervical canal (*short white arrows*) are marked to show their relationship to the leading edge of the placenta.

Farine and associates (1988) were able to visualize the internal cervical os in all cases using the transvaginal technique, in contrast to only 70 percent using transabdominal equipment. In studies comparing abdominal with transvaginal imaging, Smith (1997) and Taipale (1998) and their colleagues found the transvaginal technique to be superior.

Transperineal sonography was reported accurate to localize placenta previa by Hertzberg and colleagues (1992). More recently, Rani and associates (2007) demonstrated its accuracy in 75 women in whom placenta previa was visualized using transabdominal sonography. Previa was correctly identified in 69 of the 70 women in which it was confirmed at delivery. The positive-predictive value was 98 percent and negative-predictive value was 100 percent.

Magnetic Resonance (MR) Imaging. A number of investigators have used MR imaging to visualize placental abnormalities, including previa. Although there are many positive attributes to its use, it is unlikely that MR imaging will replace sonographic scanning for routine evaluation in the near future. As discussed on page 779, MR imaging may prove useful for diagnosis of placenta accreta (Palacios Jaraquemada and Bruno, 2005).

Placental "Migration." Since its description by King (1973), the apparent peripatetic nature of the placenta has been well established. Sanderson and Milton (1991) studied 4300 women at 18 to 20 weeks and found that 12 percent of placentas were "low lying." Of those not covering the internal os, previa did not persist and hemorrhage was not encountered. Conversely, of those covering the os at midpregnancy, approximately 40 percent persisted as a previa. Thus, placentas that lie close to the internal os—but not over it—during the second trimester or early third trimester are unlikely to persist as a previa by term.

As shown in Figure 35-15, the likelihood that placenta previa persists after being identified sonographically before 28 weeks is greater in women who have had a prior cesarean delivery (Chama, 2004; Dashe, 2002; Laughon, 2005, and all their associates). In the absence of any other abnormality, sonography need not be frequently repeated simply to follow placental position. Restriction of activity is not necessary unless a previa persists beyond 28 weeks or becomes clinically apparent before that time.

The mechanism of apparent placental movement is not completely understood. That said, *migration* is clearly a misnomer because decidual invasion by chorionic villi on either side of the cervical os persists. The apparent movement of the low-lying placenta relative to the internal os probably results from inability to precisely define this relationship in a three-dimensional manner using two-dimensional sonography in early pregnancy. This difficulty is coupled with differential growth of lower and upper myometrial segments as pregnancy progresses. Thus, those placentas that "migrate" most likely never had actual circumferential villus invasion that reached the internal cervical os in the first place.

Management of Placenta Previa

Women with a previa may be considered in one of the following categories:

- The fetus is preterm and there are no other indications for delivery
- The fetus is reasonably mature
- Labor has ensued
- Hemorrhage is so severe as to mandate delivery despite gestational age.

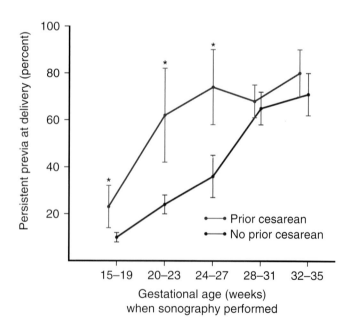

FIGURE 35-15 Percentage of women with persistent placenta previa at delivery according to gestational age at diagnosis and with and without a prior cesarean delivery. Shown as means with error bars that represent 95-percent confidence intervals. (Asterisks note that $p < .05$ comparing women with prior cesarean delivery with multiparous women with no prior cesarean delivery.) (Data from Dashe and colleagues, 2002.)

Management with a preterm fetus, but without persistent active uterine bleeding, consists of close observation. For some women, prolonged hospitalization may be ideal. However, a woman is usually discharged after bleeding has ceased and her fetus judged to be healthy. The woman and her family must fully appreciate the possibility of complications and be prepared to transport her to the hospital immediately. In properly selected patients, there appears to be no benefit to inpatient versus outpatient management of placenta previa (Mouer, 1994; Neilson, 2003). And Drost and Keil (1994) demonstrated a 50-percent reduction in hospitalization and maternal costs, as well as a 40-percent reduction in costs for mother–infant pairs when outpatient was compared with inpatient management.

Importantly, there are no differences in maternal or fetal morbidity rates with outpatient versus inpatient observation. Wing and colleagues (1996a) reported preliminary results from their randomized clinical trial of inpatient versus home management of 53 women with a bleeding previa from 24 to 36 weeks. Maternal and perinatal morbidities were similar in each group, but home management saved $15,000 per case in 1996 dollars. Despite this, 62 percent of these 53 women had recurrent bleeding, and 52 percent required expeditious cesarean delivery.

Delivery

Cesarean delivery is necessary in practically all women with placenta previa. Most often, a transverse uterine incision is possible. However, because fetal bleeding may result from a transverse incision into an anterior placenta, a vertical incision is sometimes employed. But, even when the incision extends through the placenta, maternal or fetal outcomes are rarely compromised.

Ward (2003) described an alternative surgical technique in which a cleavage plane is developed following the uterine incision. The operator undermines the placenta toward the closest edge until the membranes are palpable and they are then ruptured with the fetus delivered *around* the intact placenta. This approach has not yet been evaluated in controlled studies.

Because of the poorly contractile nature of the lower uterine segment, there may be uncontrollable hemorrhage following placental removal. When bleeding from the placental bed cannot be controlled by conservative means, other methods can be attempted. Oversewing the implantation site with 0-chromic sutures may provide hemostasis. In some women, bilateral uterine or internal iliac artery ligation described on page 796 may provide hemostasis. Cho and colleagues (1991) described placing interrupted 0-chromic sutures one centimeter apart and forming a sutured circle around the bleeding portion of the lower segment. This method controlled hemorrhage in all eight women in whom it was employed. Druzin (1989) described four cases in which the lower uterine segment was tightly packed with gauze that successfully arrested hemorrhage. The pack was removed transvaginally 12 hours later. Pelvic artery embolization as discussed on page 797 also has gained acceptance.

If such conservative methods fail, and bleeding is brisk, then hysterectomy is necessary (see Chap. 25, p. 555). *For women whose placenta previa is implanted anteriorly in the site of a prior hysterotomy incision, there is an increased likelihood of associated placenta accreta and need for hysterectomy.* During the year ending in February 2006, 40 percent of 318 peripartum hysterec-

tomies in the United Kingdom were done for abnormally adhered placentation (Knight, 2007).

Maternal and Perinatal Outcomes

A marked reduction in maternal mortality rates from placenta previa was achieved during the last half of the 20th century. Still, as shown in Figure 35-1, placenta previa is an important cause of maternal morbidity and mortality. In their recent review, Oyelese and Smulian (2006) cite an approximately threefold increased maternal mortality ratio of 30 per 100,000.

Preterm delivery as a result of placenta previa is a major cause of perinatal death. Using 1997 linked birth and infant death data sets for the United States, Salihu and associates (2003) reported the neonatal mortality rate to be threefold increased in pregnancies complicated by placenta previa. This was primarily because of increased preterm birth rates. In another large series, Ananth and associates (2003b) reported a comparably increased risk of neonatal death even for those fetuses delivered at term. Some of this risk appears related to fetal-growth restriction and limited prenatal care. And although suspected by some investigators, an association of increased congenital malformations and previa was not confirmed until relatively recently by Crane and co-workers (1999). Importantly, they controlled for maternal age, and for reasons that are unclear, fetal anomalies were increased 2.5-fold in pregnancies complicated by placenta previa.

The association of fetal-growth restriction with placenta previa is less certain. Brar and colleagues (1988) reported the incidence to be nearly 20 percent, but Crane and co-workers (1999) found no increased incidence after controlling for gestational age. Ananth and associates (2001a) examined this relationship in a population-based cohort of more than 500,000 singleton births. They found that most of the association between placenta previa and low birthweight was from preterm birth, and only to a lesser extent from growth impairment.

Third-Stage Bleeding

Some bleeding is inevitable during the third stage of labor as the result of transient partial separation of the placenta. As the placenta separates, blood from the implantation site may escape into the vagina immediately—the *Duncan mechanism* of placental separation. Alternately, it may be concealed behind the placenta and membranes until the placenta is delivered—the *Schultze mechanism*.

In the presence of any external hemorrhage during the third stage, the uterus should be massaged if it is not contracted firmly. If the signs of placental separation have appeared, expression of the placenta should be attempted by manual fundal pressure as described in Chapter 17 (p. 398). Descent of the placenta is indicated by the cord becoming slack. If bleeding continues, manual removal of the placenta may be necessary. *Delivery of the placenta by cord traction, especially when the uterus is atonic, may cause uterine inversion.* Prevention and management of this complication are discussed in detail on page 780.

Bleeding with Prolonged Third Stage

In some cases, the placenta does not separate promptly. There is still no definite answer to the question concerning the length of time that should elapse in the absence of bleeding before the placenta is removed manually. Obstetrical tradition has set somewhat arbitrary limits on third-stage duration in attempts to define *abnormally retained placenta* and thus, to reduce blood loss from prolonged placental separation. Combs and Laros (1991) studied 12,275 singleton vaginal deliveries and reported the median third-stage duration to be 6 minutes, and for 3.3 percent of these women, it was more than 30 minutes. Several measures of hemorrhage, including curettage or transfusion, increased when the third stage was approximately 30 minutes or longer. Prolonged third-stage labor is discussed in Chapter 17 (p. 397).

Technique of Manual Placental Removal

Adequate analgesia is mandatory, and aseptic surgical technique should be used. After grasping the fundus through the abdominal wall with one hand, the other hand is introduced into the vagina and passed into the uterus, along the umbilical cord. As soon as the placenta is reached, its margin is located, and the border of the hand is insinuated between it and the uterine wall (Fig. 35-16). Then with the back of the hand in contact with the uterus, the placenta is peeled off its uterine attachment by a motion similar to that used in separating the leaves of a book. After its complete separation, the placenta should be grasped with the entire hand, which is then gradually withdrawn. Membranes are removed at the same time by carefully teasing them from the decidua, using ring forceps to grasp them as necessary. Another method is to wipe out the uterine cavity with a laparotomy sponge.

Management after Placental Delivery

The fundus should always be palpated following either spontaneous or manual placental delivery to confirm that the uterus is well contracted. If it is not firm, vigorous fundal massage is indicated. Most evidence suggests that uterine massage prevents postpartum hemorrhage from atony (Hofmeyr and associates,

2008). Typically, 20 U of oxytocin in 1000 mL of lactated Ringer or normal saline proves effective when administered intravenously at approximately 10 mL/min—200 mU of oxytocin per minute—simultaneously with effective uterine massage. Oxytocin should never be given as an undiluted bolus dose, because serious hypotension or cardiac arrhythmias may occur (see Chap. 17, p. 399).

Uterine Atony

Failure of the uterus to contract properly following delivery is the most common cause of obstetrical hemorrhage. In many women, uterine atony can at least be anticipated well in advance of delivery (Table 35-2). Although risk factors are well known, the ability to identify which individual woman will experience atony is limited. Rouse and colleagues (2006) studied 23,900 women undergoing primary cesarean delivery and reported that half of those women experiencing atony had no risk factors.

The *overdistended uterus* is prone to be hypotonic after delivery. Thus, women with a large fetus, multiple fetuses, or hydramnios are prone to uterine atony. The woman whose labor is characterized by *uterine activity* that is either remarkably vigorous or barely effective is also likely to bleed excessively from postpartum atony. Similarly, labor either initiated or augmented with *oxytocics* is more likely to be followed by atony and hemorrhage.

High parity may be a risk factor for uterine atony. Fuchs and colleagues (1985) described outcomes of nearly 5800 women para 7 or greater. They reported that the 2.7-percent incidence of postpartum hemorrhage was increased fourfold compared with that of the general obstetrical population. Babinszki and colleagues (1999) reported the incidence of postpartum hemorrhage to be 0.3 percent in women of low parity, but it was 1.9 percent in those para 4 or greater.

Another risk is if the woman has had a *prior postpartum hemorrhage*. Finally, attempts to *hasten placental delivery* may incite

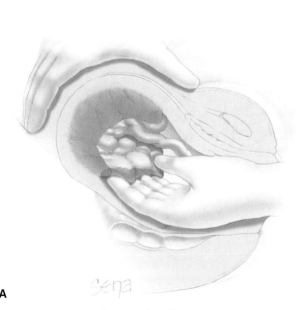

A

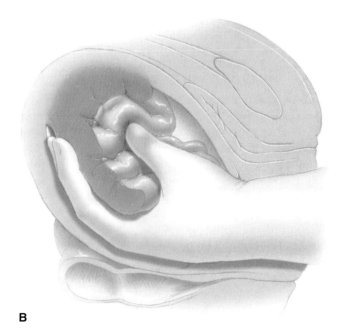

B

FIGURE 35-16 Manual removal of placenta is accomplished as the fingers are swept from side to side and advanced **(A)** until the placenta is detached, grasped, and removed **(B)**.

atony. *Constant kneading and squeezing of the uterus that already is contracted likely impedes the physiological mechanism of placental detachment, causing incomplete placental separation and increased blood loss.*

Retained Placental Fragments

Immediate postpartum hemorrhage is seldom caused by retained placental fragments, but a remaining piece of placenta is a common cause of bleeding late in the puerperium. Inspection of the placenta after delivery should be routine. If a portion is missing, the uterus should be explored and the fragment removed, particularly with continuing postpartum bleeding. Retention of a *succenturiate lobe* is an occasional cause of postpartum hemorrhage (see Chap. 27, p. 577). The late bleeding that may result from a placental polyp is discussed in Chapter 30 (p. 648).

Uterotonic Agents

A number of compounds are used to cause the postpartum uterus to contract.

Oxytocin. In most units, after placental delivery is accomplished, oxytocin is given intravenously or intramuscularly, as described in Chapter 17 (p. 399). This or other oxytocics will prevent most cases of uterine atony.

Ergot Derivatives. If oxytocin does not prove effective to reverse uterine atony, we usually administer 0.2 mg of methylergonovine intramuscularly. This may stimulate the uterus to contract sufficiently to control hemorrhage. Any superior therapeutic effects of ergot derivatives compared with those of oxytocin are speculative. Importantly, if ergot agents are intravenously administered, they may cause dangerous hypertension, especially in women with preeclampsia.

Prostaglandin Analogs. The 15-methyl derivative of prostaglandin $F_{2\alpha}$–carboprost tromethamine–has been approved since the mid-1980s for treatment of uterine atony. The initial recommended dose is 250 μg (0.25 mg) given intramuscularly. This is repeated if necessary at 15- to 90-minute intervals up to a maximum of eight doses. Oleen and Mariano (1990) studied its use for postpartum hemorrhage at 12 obstetrical units. Arrest of bleeding was considered successful in 88 percent of 237 women treated. Another 7 percent required other oxytocics for control of hemorrhage. The remaining 5 percent required surgical intervention.

Carboprost is associated with side effects in approximately 20 percent of women (Oleen and Mariano, 1990). In descending order of frequency, these include diarrhea, hypertension, vomiting, fever, flushing, and tachycardia. We have encountered serious hypertension in a few women so treated. And Hankins and colleagues (1988) observed that intramuscular carboprost was followed within 15 minutes by arterial oxygen desaturation that averaged 10 percent. They concluded that this was due to pulmonary airway and vascular constriction.

Rectally administered prostaglandin E_2 20-mg suppositories are used for uterine atony but have not been studied in clinical trials. A few reports have suggested that synthetic prostaglandin E_1 analog—misoprostol or Cytotec—may be effective for the

treatment of atony (Abdel-Aleem and associates, 2001; O'Brien and colleagues, 1998). In a recent Cochrane review, however, Mousa and Alfirevic (2007) reported no benefit to misoprostol compared with standard therapy with oxytocin and ergometrine. Only three studies met the stringent criteria for inclusion, and all dosing regimens were different.

Misoprostol has also been evaluated for prophylaxis of postpartum hemorrhage. In a randomized trial, Derman and coworkers (2006) compared a 600-μg oral dose with placebo given at delivery. Postpartum hemorrhage was significantly reduced from 12 to 6 percent, and severe hemorrhage from 1.2 to 0.2 percent with misoprostol use. However, based on their study of 325 women, Gerstenfeld and Wing (2001) concluded that 400 μg of misoprostol administered rectally was no more effective than intravenous oxytocin in preventing postpartum hemorrhage. And in their systematic review, Villar and coworkers (2002) reported that oxytocin and ergot preparations administered during third-stage labor were more effective than misoprostol for prevention of postpartum hemorrhage.

Bleeding Unresponsive to Oxytocics

Continued bleeding after multiple administrations of oxytocics may be from unrecognized genital tract lacerations, including in some cases uterine rupture. Thus, if bleeding persists, no time should be lost in haphazard efforts to control hemorrhage, but the following management steps should be initiated immediately:

1. Initiate bimanual uterine compression, a simple procedure that controls most uterine hemorrhage (Fig. 35-17). This technique consists of massage of the posterior aspect of the uterus with a hand on the abdomen and massage through the vagina of the anterior uterine wall with the other hand made into a fist.
2. Call for help!

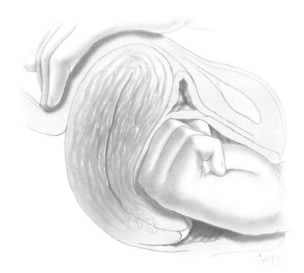

FIGURE 35-17 Bimanual compression of the uterus between the fist in the anterior fornix and the abdominal hand, which is also used for uterine massage. This usually controls hemorrhage from uterine atony.

3. Add a second large-bore intravenous catheter so that crystalloid with oxytocin may be continued at the same time blood is given.

4. Begin blood transfusions. The blood group of every obstetrical patient should be known, if possible, before labor, and an indirect Coombs test done to detect erythrocyte antibodies. If the latter is negative, then crossmatching of blood is not necessary (see p. 793). In an extreme emergency, type O, D-negative "universal donor" blood is given.

5. Explore the uterine cavity manually for retained placental fragments or lacerations.

6. Thoroughly inspect the cervix and vagina for lacerations after adequate exposure.

7. Insert a Foley catheter to monitor urine output, which is a good measure of renal perfusion.

8. Begin volume resuscitation as described subsequently on page 791.

Blood transfusion should be considered in any woman with postpartum hemorrhage in whom abdominal uterine massage and oxytocic agents fail to control bleeding. With transfusion and simultaneous manual uterine compression and intravenous oxytocin, additional measures are rarely required.

Surgical Management of Uterine Atony

With intractable atony unresponsive to the above measures, surgical intervention can be lifesaving. In our experience, *uterine artery ligation*—discussed on page 795—is less helpful for hemorrhage from uterine atony compared with its use for hysterotomy extensions at cesarean delivery. It is also debatable whether *internal iliac artery ligation* is beneficial for uterine atony (Clark and colleagues, 1985). From India, Joshi and co-workers (2007) described 36 women who had the procedure for postpartum atony—a third of those required hysterectomy. Our concern, in addition to an inherently high failure rate, is that the procedure, discussed on page 796, is technically difficult and consumes valuable time if hysterectomy is necessary.

Uterine Compression Sutures. In 1997, B-Lynch and colleagues described a surgical technique for severe postpartum atony in which a pair of vertical brace, #2-chromic sutures were secured around the uterus. When tightened and tied, they give the appearance of suspenders—or braces—that compress the anterior and posterior walls together (Fig. 35-18). Price and B-Lynch (2005) summarized 17 reports in which 44 of 46 procedures were successful. In another preliminary report, B-Lynch (2005) cited 948 cases with only seven failures. Our experiences are not nearly so successful, but the technique certainly is effective in some cases. A number of modifications of the B-Lynch technique have been described (Bhal, 2005; Cho, 2000; Ghezzi, 2007; Hayman, 2002; Pereira, 2005, and all their colleagues).

Reports of complications from compression sutures have been slowly emerging. At this time, their incidence is unknown but is likely low. Uterine ischemic necrosis with peritonitis has been described in several case reports (Gottlieb, 2008; Joshi, 2004; Ochoa, 2002; Treloar, 2006, and all their colleagues). The

women described by Akoury and Sherman (2008) had one B-Lynch suture and two Cho sutures and were found to have one large triangular and two smaller defects in the uterine wall in a subsequent pregnancy. Total ischemic uterine necrosis developed in a woman described by Friederich and associates (2007). In addition to B-Lynch compression sutures, the woman also had bilateral ligation of uterine, uterovarian, and round ligament arteries.

Uterine Packing

This technique should be considered in women with refractory postpartum hemorrhage related to uterine atony who wish to preserve fertility. Popular during the first half of the 20th century, uterine packing subsequently fell from favor because of concerns about concealed bleeding and infection (Hsu and co-workers, 2003). Newer techniques, however, have allayed some of these concerns (Roman and Rebarber, 2003). In one technique, the tip of a 24F Foley catheter with a 30-mL balloon is guided into the uterine cavity and filled with 60 to 80 mL of saline. The open tip permits continuous drainage from the uterus. If bleeding subsides, the catheter is typically removed after 12 to 24 hours. Alternatively, the uterus or pelvis may be packed directly with gauze (Gilstrap, 2002).

Placenta Accreta, Increta, and Percreta

In most instances, the placenta separates spontaneously from its implantation site during the first few minutes after delivery of the infant. Infrequently, detachment is delayed because the placenta is unusually adhered to the implantation site. In these cases, the decidua is scanty or absent, and the physiological line of cleavage through the decidual spongy layer is lacking. As a consequence, one or more placental lobules, also termed *cotyledons*, are firmly bound to the defective decidua basalis or even to the myometrium. When the placenta is densely anchored in this fashion, the condition is called placenta accreta. Varying degrees of accreta cause significant morbidity and at times, mortality from severe hemorrhage, uterine perforation, and infection.

Definitions

The term *placenta accreta* is used to describe any implantation in which there is abnormally firm adherence to the uterine wall. As the consequence of partial or total absence of the decidua basalis and imperfect development of the fibrinoid or *Nitabuch layer*, placental villi are attached to the myometrium in placenta accreta (Fig. 35-19A). With *placenta increta*, villi actually invade into the myometrium (Fig. 35-19B). Finally, with *placenta percreta*, villi penetrate through the myometrium (Fig. 35-19C). The abnormal adherence may involve all lobules—*total placenta accreta*—as was the case in Figure 35-20A. Or, it may involve only a few to several lobules—*partial placenta accreta*—such as shown in Figure 35-20B. All or part of a single lobule may be attached—*focal placenta accreta*. According to Benirschke and colleagues (2006), histological diagnosis cannot be made from the placenta alone, and the entire uterus or curettings with myometrium are necessary for histopathological confirmation.

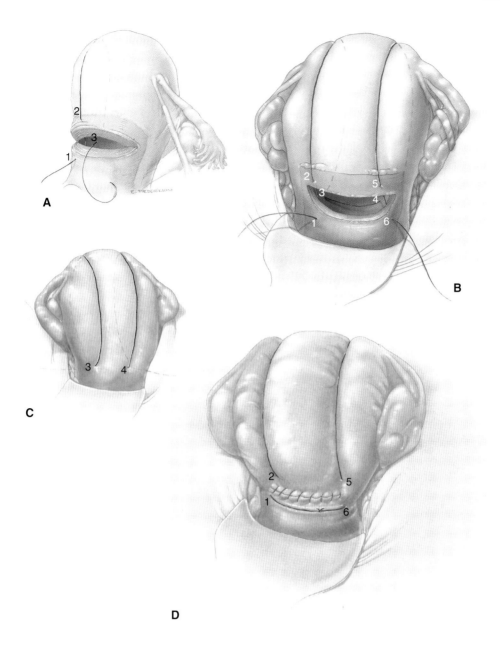

FIGURE 35-18 The B-Lynch uterine compression suture technique. Figures **(A)**, **(B)**, and **(D)** demonstrate an anterior view of the uterus. Figure **(C)** is a posterior view. Numbers denote the sequential path of the suture and are shown in more than one figure. In step 1, beginning below the incision, the needle pierces the lower uterine segment to enter the uterine cavity. In step 2, the needle exits the cavity above the incision. The suture then loops up and around the fundus to the posterior uterine surface. Here, in step 3, the needle pierces the posterior uterine wall to reenter the uterine cavity. The suture then traverses from left to right within the cavity. In step 4, the needle exits the uterine cavity through the posterior uterine wall. From the back of the uterus, the suture loops up and around the fundus to the front of the uterus. In step 5, the needle pierces the myometrium above the incision to reenter the uterine cavity. In step 6, the needle exits below the incision. Finally, the sutures at points 1 and 6 are tied below the incision.

Incidence

Over the past few decades, the incidences of placenta accreta, increta, and percreta have increased. This is because of the increasing cesarean delivery rate (see Chap. 25, p. 544). The American College of Obstetricians and Gynecologists (2002) estimated that placenta accreta complicates 1 in 2500 deliveries. From their review, Stafford and Belfort (2008) cite the incidence of approximately 1 in 2500 in the 1980s, 1 in 535 in 2002, and 1:210 in 2006. For some time, it has been a leading cause of intractable postpartum hemorrhage requiring emer-

gency peripartum hysterectomy (Zelop and colleagues, 1993). And as shown in Figure 35-1, various forms of accreta are a substantive cause of maternal deaths from hemorrhage.

Associated Conditions

Decidual formation is commonly defective in the lower uterine segment over a previous cesarean delivery scar or after uterine curettage. In a review of 622 cases of placenta accreta collected between 1945 and 1969, Fox (1972) reported that: (1) a third of cases had placenta previa, (2) a fourth had a prior cesarean delivery,

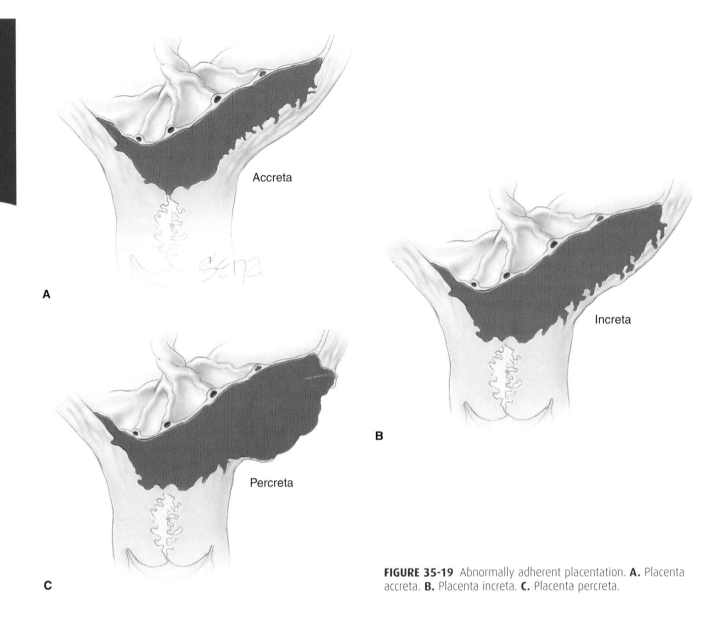

FIGURE 35-19 Abnormally adherent placentation. **A.** Placenta accreta. **B.** Placenta increta. **C.** Placenta percreta.

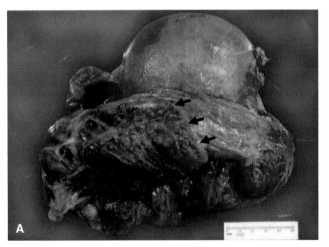
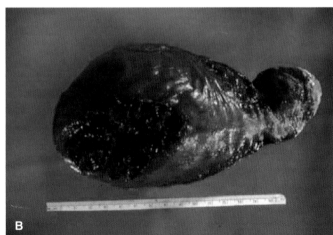

FIGURE 35-20 Cesarean hysterectomy specimens with placenta percreta. **A.** Total placenta previa with percreta involving the lower uterine segment and cervical canal. Black arrows show the invading line of the placenta through the myometrium (Courtesy of Dr. Thomas R. Dowd). **B.** Lateral fundal percreta caused hemoperitoneum in late pregnancy.

(3) nearly a fourth had previously undergone curettage, and (4) a fourth were gravida 6 or more. Zaki and associates (1998) found that 10 percent of 112 consecutive cases of placenta previa had associated accreta. Hardardottir and colleagues (1996) observed that almost 50 percent of placentas in women with a prior cesarean delivery had adhered myometrial fibers detected microscopically.

There are risk factors for placenta accreta that have come to light with MSAFP screening for neural-tube defects and aneuploidies (see Chap. 13, p. 289). Hung and co-workers (1999) analyzed outcomes of more than 9300 women screened for Down syndrome at 14 to 22 weeks. They reported a 54-fold increased risk for accreta in women with placenta previa. The risk for accreta was increased eightfold when MSAFP levels exceeded 2.5 MoM; it was increased fourfold when maternal free β-hCG levels were greater than 2.5 MoM; and it was increased threefold when maternal age was 35 years or older.

Clinical Course and Diagnosis

In the first trimester, as discussed in Chapter 10 (p. 253), abnormal myometrial invasion may manifest as a *cesarean scar pregnancy* (Ash and associates, 2007). According to their review, Rotas and colleagues (2006) reported this type of ectopic pregnancy to be increasing in frequency and cited an incidence of approximately 1 in 2000 pregnancies. If pregnancy advances, placental villi at the site of a previous cesarean scar may lead to uterine rupture before labor (Liang and co-workers, 2003). Antepartum hemorrhage with placenta accreta is common and usually the consequence of coexisting placenta previa. In many cases, placenta accreta is not identified until third-stage labor. In this setting, an adhered placenta, as described on page 775, is encountered.

Perioperative Evaluation

Efforts are ongoing to better identify placental ingrowth antepartum. Lam and colleagues (2004) found that sonography was only 33-percent sensitive for detecting placenta accreta. With sonographic Doppler color flow mapping-such as shown in Figure 35-21, Twickler and colleagues (2000) reported that

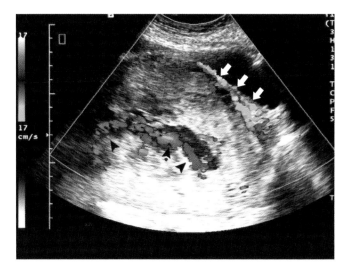

FIGURE 35-21 Transabdominal sonogram of placental invasion. Retroplacental vessels (*white arrows*) invade the myometrium and obscure the bladder-serosal interface. Abnormal intraplacental venous lakes (*black arrows*) are commonly seen in this setting.

two factors were highly predictive of myometrial invasion: (1) a distance less than 1 mm between the uterine serosa-bladder interface and the retroplacental vessels, and (2) identification of large intraplacental lakes. These had a sensitivity of 100 percent and positive-predictive value of 78 percent. Chou and co-workers (2001) also described successful use of three-dimensional color Doppler imaging for diagnosis of placenta percreta.

Magnetic resonance (MR) imaging is used as an adjunct to sonography when there is strong clinical suspicion of an accreta. Warshak and colleagues (2006) described a two-step protocol in which MR imaging was used if sonography was inconclusive. They reported that 23 of 26 cases of placenta accreta were accurately predicted, and 14 of 14 were correctly excluded. Lax and co-workers (2007) identified three MR imaging findings that suggested accreta: (1) uterine bulging, (2) heterogeneous signal intensity within the placenta, and (3) presence of dark intraplacental bands on T2-weighted imaging.

Baxi and associates (2004) found that elevated serum D-dimer levels may predict significant blood loss and morbidity in women with placenta accreta. This perhaps reflects trophoblastic invasion into the myometrium and adjacent tissues.

Management

Thorough preoperative assessment allows better planning. Exigencies to be considered are appropriate surgical and blood banking facilities, as well as availability of gynecological oncological, surgical, or urological consultation (Bauer and Bonanno, 2009; Stafford and Belfort, 2008). Transfer to a level III facility should be considered (Worley and colleagues, 2008).

Preoperative Arterial Catheter Placement. Experience has accrued with preoperative placement of pelvic arterial catheters. Balloon-tipped catheters are placed before surgery into the internal iliac arteries and are inflated after the fetus is delivered to decrease blood loss during placental delivery and hysterectomy, if indicated. Alternatively, the catheters can be injected with a substance to embolize the arterial sites. Yu and colleagues (2009) presented data from 11 women with abnormal placentation during late gestation in whom uterine artery embolization was done after fetal but before placental delivery. They reported favorable outcomes. From France, Sentilhes and co-workers (2009) described successes in four of 17 women. Oyelese and Smulian (2006) reviewed the limited reported results in the literature and reached no firm conclusions concerning efficacy. Greenburg and colleagues (2007) described a woman who developed thrombolic occlusion of the common and left iliac arteries and advise caution with embolization use.

Delivery of the Placenta. Problems associated with delivery of the placenta and subsequent developments vary appreciably, depending on the site of implantation, depth of myometrial penetration, and number of lobules involved. It is likely that focal placenta accreta with implantation in the upper uterine segment develops more often than recognized. Either the involved lobule is pulled off the myometrium with perhaps somewhat excessive bleeding, or the lobule is torn from the placenta and adheres to the implantation site with increased bleeding, immediately or later. According to Benirschke and Kaufmann (2006), this may be one mechanism for formation of a so-called *placental polyp* (see Chap. 30, p. 648).

With more extensive involvement, hemorrhage becomes profuse as delivery of the placenta is attempted. Successful treatment depends on immediate blood replacement therapy as subsequently described, and nearly always prompts hysterectomy. *This may be aided by fully developing the bladder flap and dissecting it around the percreta if possible prior to delivery.* Other measures include uterine or internal iliac artery ligation, balloon occlusion, or embolization as discussed above. Karam and colleagues (2003) described use of argon beam coagulation for hemostasis in a woman with placenta percreta and bladder invasion.

With total placenta accreta, there may be very little or no bleeding, at least until manual placental removal is attempted. At times, traction on the umbilical cord inverts the uterus. Mostly, however, usual attempts at manual removal do not succeed because a cleavage plane between the placenta and uterine wall cannot be developed. In the past, "conservative" management included manual removal of as much placenta as possible followed by uterine packing. Unfortunately, 25 percent of women managed conservatively died (Fox, 1972). Thus, the safest treatment in this circumstance is hysterectomy.

At cesarean delivery, another option for a woman who is not bleeding significantly is to leave the entire placenta in place without attempts to extract it and to close the cesarean hysterotomy incision. Leaving the placenta in situ has also been attempted with advanced gestational-age extrauterine pregnancies (Worley and associates, 2008). Currently, there is minimal experience with this approach, and these are chronicled in case reports. Several scenarios have been described. In most, methotrexate was given at the time of surgery. In some, pelvic arterial embolization was also performed (Kayem and colleagues, 2002; Lee and co-workers, 2008). In a few cases, the placenta spontaneously resorbed (Henrich and co-workers, 2002; Kayem and associates, 2002). Subsequent hysterectomy—either planned or prompted by bleeding or infection—is performed several weeks postpartum when blood loss may be less torrential (Hays, 2008; Lee, 2008; Nijman, 2002, and all their colleagues).

Management Outcomes. Most reported outcomes with abnormal placentation are retrospective observational studies of limited size. These are usually reported to describe successes with one particular management method such as some of the ones cited above. Eller and co-workers (2009) reviewed outcomes in 76 cases of placenta accreta cared for at the University of Utah. They found that preoperative identification with scheduled cesarean hysterectomy without placental removal was associated with significantly reduced morbidity—36 versus 67 percent—compared with those of attempted placental removal. They also reported that preoperative bilateral ureteral stenting significantly reduced morbidity—18 versus 55 percent—compared with no stenting. Finally, internal iliac artery ligation did not lower morbidity. Although such a primary surgical approach can be technically difficult in some cases, at Parkland Hospital we have found this management to be preferable, except that we do not routinely perform preoperative ureteral catheterization, and instead, place such catheters transvesically

during surgery if necessary. The use of preoperative arterial catheterization as described may be useful in some cases.

Leaving the placenta in situ may prevent massive hemorrhage requiring hysterectomy with the goal of fertility preservation and potential damage to pelvic structures. Timmermans and co-workers (2007) reviewed 48 publications from 1985 through 2006 and described so-called conservative management in 60 such women. Initially, the placenta was either only partially removed or left completely intact. Approximately half were treated with either adjuvant methotrexate or uterine artery embolization. The overall success rate—defined as fertility prevention—was 80 percent. The most common complication was vaginal bleeding in a third that began hours to 3 months' postpartum. A third of these—15 percent of the whole group—required hysterectomy to arrest hemorrhage. Of 11 women with puerperal infection, two required hysterectomy. Serial serum β-hCG measurements were not found to be predictive, and the authors recommend serial imaging with sonography or MR imaging.

Inversion of the Uterus

Complete uterine inversion after delivery of the infant is almost always the consequence of strong traction on an umbilical cord attached to a placenta implanted in the fundus (Fig. 35-22). Incomplete uterine inversion may also occur (Fig. 35-23). Contributing to uterine inversion is a sturdy cord that does not readily break away from the placenta, combined with fundal pressure and a relaxed uterus, including the lower segment and cervix. Placenta accreta may be implicated as in the case in Figure 35-22, although uterine inversion can occur without a firmly adhered placenta.

The incidence of uterine inversion varies, and in three reports totaling approximately 116,500 deliveries, it averaged 1 in 3000 (Achanna and colleagues, 2006; Baskett, 2002; Platt and Druzin, 1981). This is consistent with experiences from the obstetrical service at Parkland Hospital, in which we encounter several cases annually among approximately 15,000 deliveries. Perhaps ironically, most are seen with "low-risk" deliveries.

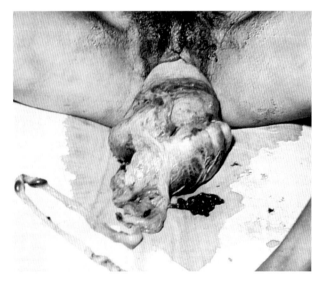

FIGURE 35-22 Uterine inversion associated with a fundal placenta accreta during a home delivery was fatal for this woman.

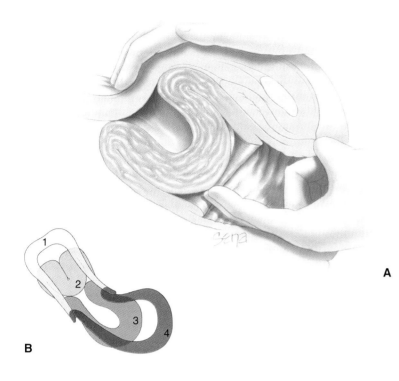

A

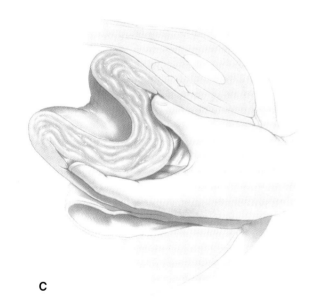

C

FIGURE 35-23 A. Incomplete uterine inversion is diagnosed by abdominal palpation of a crater-like depression and vaginal palpation of the fundal wall in the lower segment and cervix. **B.** Progressive degrees of inversion are shown in the inset. **C.** To replace the uterus, the palm is placed on the center of the inverted fundus, while fingers identify the cervical margins. Upward pressure by the palm restores the uterus and elevates it past the level of the cervix.

Management

Uterine inversion is most often associated with immediate life-threatening hemorrhage. In the past, it was taught that shock was disproportionate to blood loss, possibly mediated by parasympathetic stimulation caused by stretching of tissues. Careful evaluation of the need in many cases for transfusion of large volumes of blood, however, illustrates that blood loss is usually massive and greatly underestimated (Watson and associates, 1980).

Delay in treatment increases the mortality rate appreciably. It is imperative that a number of steps be taken urgently and simultaneously:

- Immediate assistance is summoned to include anesthesia personnel and other physicians
- The recently inverted uterus with placenta already separated from it may often be replaced simply by pushing up on the fundus with the palm of the hand and fingers in the direction of the long axis of the vagina
- Adequate large-bore intravenous infusion systems are established, and crystalloid and blood are given to treat hypovolemia
- If still attached, the placenta is not removed until infusion systems are operational, fluids are being given, and a uterine-relaxing anesthetic such as a halogenated inhalation agent has been administered. Other tocolytic drugs such as terbutaline, ritodrine, magnesium sulfate, and nitroglycerin have been used successfully for uterine relaxation and repositioning (Hong and colleagues, 2006; You and Zahn, 2006). In the meantime, if the inverted uterus has prolapsed beyond the vagina, it is replaced within the vagina
- After removing the placenta, steady pressure with the fist is applied to the inverted fundus in an attempt to push it up into the dilated cervix. Alternatively, two fingers are rigidly extended and are used to push the center of the fundus upward. *Care is taken not to apply so much pressure as to perforate the uterus with the fingertips.* As soon as the uterus is restored to its normal configuration, the tocolytic agent is stopped. An oxytocin infusion is begun while the operator maintains the fundus in its normal anatomical position.

Initially, bimanual compression as shown in Figure 35-17 aids in control of further hemorrhage until uterine tone is recovered. After the uterus is well contracted, the operator continues to monitor the uterus transvaginally for any evidence of subsequent inversion.

Surgical Intervention

Most often, the inverted uterus can be restored to its normal position by the techniques described. Occasionally, the uterus cannot be reinverted by vaginal manipulation because of a dense constriction ring (Kochenour, 2002). In this case, laparotomy is imperative. The configuration seen at surgery is shown in Figure 35-24. The fundus may be simultaneously pushed upward from below and pulled from above. A deep traction suture well placed in the inverted fundus may be of aid. If the constriction ring still prohibits reposition, it is carefully incised posteriorly to expose the fundus (Van Vugt and associates, 1981). A variant using tissue forceps to grasp the top of the fundus has been described by Robson and colleagues (2005). After replacement of the fundus, the

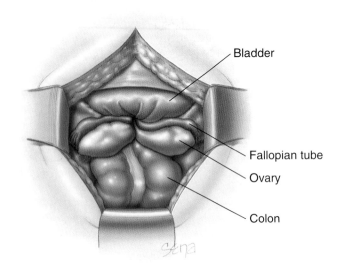

FIGURE 35-24 Completely inverted uterus viewed from above at laparotomy and showing pelvic viscera and landmarks.

Labels: Bladder, Fallopian tube, Ovary, Colon

anesthetic agent used to relax the myometrium is stopped, oxytocin infusion is begun, and the uterine incision is repaired.

Genital Tract Lacerations

Perineal Lacerations

All except the most superficial perineal lacerations are accompanied by varying degrees of injury to the lower portion of the vagina. Such tears may reach sufficient depth to involve the anal sphincter and may extend to varying depths through the vaginal walls. Bilateral lacerations into the vagina are usually unequal in length and separated by a tongue-shaped portion of vaginal mucosa.

Vaginal Lacerations

Isolated lacerations involving the middle or upper third of the vagina, but unassociated with lacerations of the perineum or cervix, are encountered less commonly. These are usually longitudinal and frequently result from injuries sustained during a forceps or vacuum delivery. However, they may even develop with spontaneous delivery. Such lacerations frequently extend deep into the underlying tissues and may give rise to significant hemorrhage, which usually is controlled by appropriate suturing. They may be missed unless thorough inspection of the upper vagina is performed. *Bleeding while the uterus is firmly contracted is strong evidence of genital tract laceration, retained placental fragments, or both.*

Lacerations of the anterior vaginal wall in close proximity to the urethra are relatively common. They are often superficial with little to no bleeding, and repair is usually not indicated. If such lacerations are large enough to require extensive repair, difficulty in voiding can be anticipated, and an indwelling catheter is placed.

Injuries to Levator Ani Muscles

These result from overdistension of the birth canal (see Figs. 2-25 and 2-26, p. 33). Muscle fibers are separated, and diminu-

tion in their tonicity may be sufficient to interfere with pelvic diaphragm function. In such cases, pelvic relaxation may develop. If the injuries involve the pubococcygeus muscle, urinary incontinence also may result (see Chap. 30, p. 649).

Injuries to the Cervix

The cervix is lacerated in more than half of all vaginal deliveries (Fahmy and associates, 1991). Most of these are less than 0.5 cm, although deep cervical tears may extend to the upper third of the vagina. In rare instances, the cervix may be entirely or partially avulsed from the vagina. Such colporrhexis may occur in the anterior, posterior, or lateral fornices. These injuries sometimes follow difficult forceps rotations or deliveries performed through an incompletely dilated cervix with the forceps blades applied over the cervix. Rarely, cervical tears may reach to involve the lower uterine segment and uterine artery and its major branches, and even extend through the peritoneum. They may be totally unsuspected, but more often, they manifest as excessive external hemorrhage or as hematomas.

Extensive tears of the vaginal vault should be explored carefully. If there is question of peritoneal perforation or of retroperitoneal or intraperitoneal hemorrhage, laparotomy should be considered. With damage of this severity, intrauterine exploration for possible rupture is also indicated. Surgical repair is usually required, and effective analgesia or anesthesia, vigorous blood replacement, and capable assistance are mandatory.

Cervical lacerations up to 2 cm must be regarded as inevitable in childbirth. Such tears heal rapidly and are rarely the source of complications. In healing, they cause a significant change in the round shape of the external os, from circular before labor to appreciably widened after delivery (see Fig. 2-12, p. 24). As the consequence of such tears, there may be eversion with exposure of the mucus-producing endocervical epithelium.

Occasionally, the edematous anterior lip of the cervix may be caught during labor and compressed between the fetal head and maternal symphysis pubis. If ischemia is severe, the cervical lip may necrose and separate. Rarely, the entire vaginal portion may be avulsed from the rest of the cervix—termed *annular* or *circular detachment of the cervix.*

Diagnosis. A deep cervical tear should always be suspected in women with profuse hemorrhage during and after third-stage labor, particularly if the uterus is firmly contracted. Thorough examination is necessary, and the flabby cervix often makes digital examination alone unsatisfactory. Thus, the extent of the injury can be fully appreciated only after adequate exposure and visual inspection of the cervix. Visualization is best accomplished when an *assistant* applies firm downward pressure on the uterus while the operator exerts traction on the lips of the cervix with ring forceps. Right-angle vaginal wall retractors are often helpful.

In view of the frequency with which deep tears follow major operative vaginal deliveries, the cervix should be inspected routinely at the conclusion of the third stage after all difficult deliveries, even if there is no bleeding.

Management. Deep cervical tears usually require surgical repair. When the laceration is limited to the cervix, or even when it extends somewhat into the vaginal fornix, satisfactory results

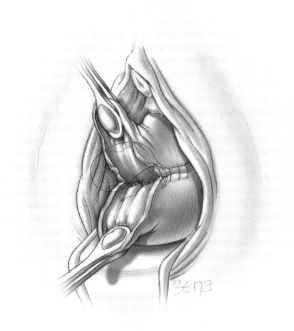

FIGURE 35-25 Repair of cervical laceration with appropriate surgical exposure.

are obtained by suturing the cervix after bringing it into view at the vulva (Fig. 35-25). Because the hemorrhage usually comes from the upper angle of the wound, the first suture is placed proximal to the angle. Suturing proceeds outward toward the operator. Associated vaginal lacerations may be tamponaded with gauze packs to retard hemorrhage while cervical lacerations are repaired. Either interrupted or running absorbable sutures are suitable. Overzealous suturing in an attempt to restore the normal cervical appearance may lead to subsequent stenosis during uterine involution. Alternatively, Lichtenberg (2003) described the successful use of angiographic embolization for treatment of a high cervical tear after failed surgical repair.

Puerperal Hematomas

In a review of seven series, the incidence of puerperal hematomas was found to vary from 1 in 300 to 1 in 1000 deliveries (Cunningham, 2002). Nulliparity, episiotomy, and forceps delivery are the most commonly associated risk factors (Propst and Thorp, 1998; Ridgway, 1995). In other cases, hematomas may develop following rupture of a blood vessel without laceration of superficial tissues. These may occur with spontaneous or operative delivery, and hemorrhage may be delayed. Finally, coagulopathies, such as von Willebrand disease, are rarer causes.

Puerperal hematomas may be classified as vulvar, vulvovaginal, paravaginal, or retroperitoneal. Vulvar hematomas most often involve branches of the pudendal artery, including the posterior rectal, transverse perineal, or posterior labial artery (see Fig. 2-5, p. 20). Paravaginal hematomas may involve the descending branch of the uterine artery (Zahn and Yeomans, 1990). Infrequently, a torn vessel lies above the pelvic fascia. In that event, the hematoma develops above it. In its early stages,

the hematoma forms a rounded swelling that projects into the upper portion of the vaginal canal and may almost occlude its lumen. If the bleeding continues, it dissects retroperitoneally, and thus, may form a tumor palpable above the inguinal ligament. Alternatively, it may dissect upward, eventually reaching the lower margin of the diaphragm.

Vulvar Hematomas

These hematomas, such as the one shown in Figure 35-26, and particularly those that develop rapidly, may cause excruciating pain. This often is the first symptom noticed. Moderate-sized hematomas may be absorbed spontaneously. The tissues overlying the hematoma may rupture as a result of pressure necrosis, and profuse hemorrhage may follow. In others, the contents of the hematoma may be discharged in the form of large clots. In the subperitoneal variety, extravasation of blood beneath the peritoneum may be massive and occasionally fatal. Some of these dissect behind the ascending colon up to the hepatic flexure.

Diagnosis. A vulvar hematoma is readily diagnosed by severe perineal pain and usually rapid appearance of a tense, fluctuant, and sensitive swelling of varying size covered by discolored skin. When the mass develops adjacent to the vagina, it may escape detection temporarily. Symptoms of pressure, if not pain or inability to void, should prompt a vaginal examination with discovery of a round, fluctuant mass encroaching on the lumen. When a hematoma extends upward between the folds of the broad ligament, it may escape detection unless a portion of the hematoma can be felt on abdominal palpation or unless hypovolemia develops. These are worrisome because they can be fatal. Sonographic or CT imaging may be helpful to assess the location and extent of these hematomas.

Treatment. Smaller vulvar hematomas identified after leaving the delivery room may be treated expectantly (Propst and Thorp, 1998). But if pain is severe or the hematoma continues

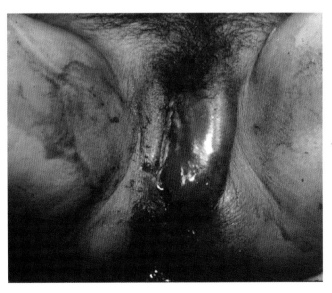

FIGURE 35-26 Right-sided vulvar hematoma associated with a vaginal laceration following spontaneous delivery in a woman with consumptive coagulopathy from fatty liver of pregnancy.

to enlarge, the best treatment is prompt incision and drainage. This is done at the point of maximal distension along with evacuation of blood and clots and ligation of bleeding points. The cavity may then be obliterated with mattress sutures. Often, no sites of bleeding are identified after the hematoma has been drained. In such cases, the cavity is surgically closed, and the vagina is packed for 12 to 24 hours. **With hematomas of the genital tract, blood loss is nearly always considerably more than the clinical estimate.** Hypovolemia and severe anemia should be prevented by adequate blood replacement. Half of women with hematomas requiring surgical repair also require transfusions (Zahn and Yeomans, 1990).

Subperitoneal and supravaginal hematomas are more difficult to treat because of difficult surgical access. Some can be evacuated by vulvar or vaginal incision, but unless there is complete hemostasis, laparotomy is advisable.

Angiographic Embolization. This technique has become popular for management of intractable puerperal hematomas. Embolization can be used primarily or most often when hemostasis is not obtained by surgical methods. It is described further on page 797. Ojala and co-workers (2005) described three women with a vulvovaginal hematoma in which it was used.

Rupture of the Uterus

Uterine rupture may develop as a result of preexisting injury or anomaly, it may be associated with trauma, or it may complicate labor in a previously unscarred uterus. A classification of the etiology of uterine rupture is presented in Table 35-5.

The most common cause of uterine rupture is separation of a previous cesarean hysterotomy scar. With decreasing interest in a trial of labor following a prior cesarean delivery, rupture of an unscarred uterus may now be associated with up to half of cases of uterine rupture (Porrecco and co-workers, 2009). This is discussed in detail in Chapter 26 (p. 573). Other common predisposing factors to uterine rupture are previous traumatizing operations or manipulations such as curettage, perforation, or myomectomy (Kieser and Baskett, 2002; Pelosi and Pelosi, 1997). Excessive or inappropriate uterine stimulation with oxytocin, a previously frequent cause, has become uncommon. Mishra and colleagues (1995) described a 43-year-old woman who suffered a ruptured vertical cesarean incision associated with inhaled crack cocaine that produced tetanic contractions.

Morbidity and Mortality

Prenatal morbidity and mortality rates can be substantive with rupture of a prior uterine incision during labor (see Chap. 26, p. 573). Rachagan and colleagues (1991) reported the fetal mortality rate to be almost 70 percent with either spontaneous or traumatic uterine rupture. In 24 women with uterine rupture principally unassociated with prior incisions, Eden and associates (1986) reported one maternal death and a 46-percent perinatal loss rate. As discussed above, Porrecco and co-workers (2009) reported a 46-percent incidence of perinatal mortality or severe morbidity in 37 women who suffered a uterine rupture with a viable-aged fetus. Hysterectomy may be necessary to control hemorrhage.

Traumatic Rupture

Although the uterus is surprisingly resistant to blunt trauma, pregnant women sustaining such trauma to the abdomen should be watched carefully for signs of a ruptured uterus (see

TABLE 35-5. Classification of Causes of Uterine Rupture

Uterine Injury or Anomaly Sustained before Current Pregnancy	Uterine Injury or Abnormality During Current Pregnancy
Surgery involving the myometrium: Cesarean delivery or hysterotomy / Previously repaired uterine rupture / Myomectomy incision through or to the endometrium / Deep cornual resection of interstitial oviduct / Metroplasty	**Before delivery:** Persistent, intense, spontaneous contractions / Labor stimulation—oxytocin or prostaglandins / Intra-amnionic instillation—saline or prostaglandins / Perforation by internal uterine pressure catheter / External trauma—sharp or blunt / External version / Uterine overdistension—hydramnios, multifetal pregnancy
Coincidental uterine trauma: Abortion with instrumentation—curette, sounds / Sharp or blunt trauma—accidents, bullets, knives / Silent rupture in previous pregnancy	**During delivery:** Internal version / Difficult forceps delivery / Rapid tumultuous labor and delivery / Breech extraction / Fetal anomaly distending lower segment / Vigorous uterine pressure during delivery / Difficult manual removal of placenta
Congenital anomaly: Pregnancy in undeveloped uterine horn	**Acquired:** Placenta increta or percreta / Gestational trophoblastic neoplasia / Adenomyosis / Sacculation of entrapped retroverted uterus

Chap. 42, p. 938) as well as a placental abruption, described on page 761. Miller and Paul (1996) found that trauma accounted for a ruptured uterus in only 3 of more than 150 women. In the past, internal podalic version and extraction often caused traumatic rupture during delivery. Other causes of traumatic rupture include difficult forceps delivery, unusual fetal enlargement such as hydrocephaly, and breech extraction.

Spontaneous Rupture

In the study by Miller and Paul (1996), the incidence of spontaneous uterine rupture was only approximately 1 in 15,000 deliveries. The investigators also found that spontaneous rupture is more likely in women of high parity (Miller and colleagues, 1997). Oxytocin stimulation of labor has been commonly associated with uterine rupture, especially in women of high parity (Fuchs and co-workers, 1985; Rachagan and associates, 1991). Other uterotonic agents are also implicated. Uterine rupture has resulted from labor induction with prostaglandin E_2 gel or E_1 vaginal tablets (Bennett, 1997; Maymon and associates, 1991). For these reasons, all uterotonic agents should be given with great caution to induce or stimulate labor in women of high parity. Similarly, in women of high parity, a trial of labor with suspected cephalopelvic disproportion, high cephalic presentation, or abnormal presentation, such as a brow, must be undertaken with caution.

Pathological Anatomy

Rupture of the previously intact uterus at the time of labor most often involves the thinned-out lower uterine segment. The rent, when it is in the immediate vicinity of the cervix, frequently extends transversely or obliquely. Usually, the tear is longitudinal when it occurs in the portion of the uterus adjacent to the broad ligament (Fig. 35-27). Although developing primarily in the lower uterine segment, it is not unusual for the laceration to extend further upward into the body of the uterus or downward through the cervix into the vagina. At times, the bladder may also be lacerated (Rachagan and colleagues, 1991). After complete rupture, the uterine contents escape into the peritoneal cavity. In cases in which the presenting part is firmly engaged, however, then only a portion of the fetus may be extruded from the uterus. In uterine rupture in which the peritoneum remains intact, hemorrhage frequently extends into the broad ligament. This may result in a large retroperitoneal hematoma and exsanguination.

Clinical Course and Treatment

A discussion of the various clinical presentations of uterine rupture as well as treatment approaches is covered in detail in Chapter 26 (p. 573).

CONSUMPTIVE COAGULOPATHY

In 1901, DeLee reported that "temporary hemophilia" developed in a woman with a placental abruption and in another with a long-dead macerated fetus. Observations that extensive placental abruption and other accidents of pregnancy were frequently associated with hypofibrinogenemia stimulated interest in causes of intense intravascular coagulation. Although these observations were initially almost totally confined to obstetrical cases, subsequently they were made for almost all areas of medicine (Baglin, 1996). These syndromes are commonly termed *consumptive coagulopathy* or *disseminated intravascular coagulation (DIC)*.

Pregnancy Hypercoagulability

Pregnancy normally induces appreciable increases in the concentrations of coagulation factors I (fibrinogen), VII, VIII, IX, and X (see Chap. 5, p. 116). Many of these are shown in the Appendix. Other plasma factors and platelets do not change so remarkably. Plasminogen levels are increased considerably, yet plasmin activity antepartum is normally decreased compared with that of nonpregnancy. At the same time, in pregnancy, there does appear to be increased activation of platelet, clotting, and fibrinolytic mechanisms (Baker and associates, 2009). Specifically, there are significant increases in fibrinopeptide A, β-thromboglobulin, platelet factor 4, and fibrinogen-fibrin degradation products. Gerbasi and colleagues (1990) concluded that this compensated, accelerated intravascular coagulation may serve to maintain the uteroplacental interface.

Pathological Activation of Coagulation

In pathological states, an abnormal cycle of coagulation and fibrinolysis may be initiated. Coagulation may be activated via the extrinsic pathway by thromboplastin from tissue destruction and perhaps via the intrinsic pathway by collagen and other tissue components when there is loss of endothelial integrity (Fig. 35-28). Tissue factor is released and complexes with factor VII. This in turn activates tenase (factor IX) and prothrombinase (factor X) complexes. As a result, fibrin is deposited in

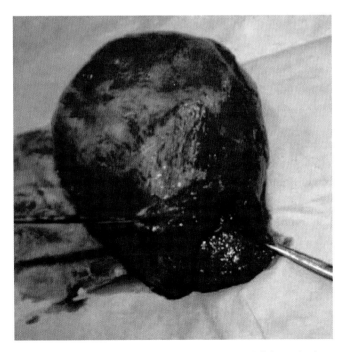

FIGURE 35-27 Spontaneously ruptured uterus at left lateral edge of lower uterine segment.

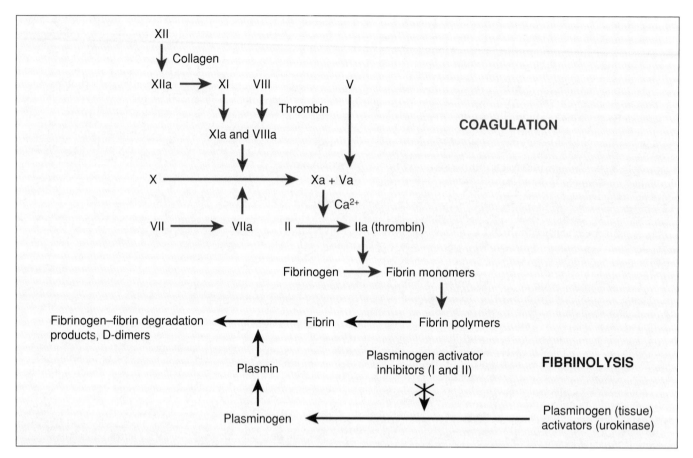

FIGURE 35-28 The coagulation and fibrinolysis cascades.

small vessels of virtually every organ system. However, this seldom causes organ failure. Small vessels are protected because of fibrinolysis. Coagulation releases fibrin monomers. These monomers combine with tissue plasminogen activator and plasminogen, which releases plasmin as shown in Figure 35-28. In turn, plasmin lyses fibrinogen, fibrin monomer, and fibrin polymers to form a series of fibrinogen-fibrin derivatives. Measured by immunoassay, these are known as *fibrin degradation products* or *fibrin split products* that include D-dimers. With this pathological cycle of consumption and fibrinolysis, there is depletion of platelets and coagulation factors in variable quantities. As a consequence, bleeding results.

Common inciting factors for consumptive coagulation in obstetrics include thromboplastin from placental abruption as well as endotoxin and exotoxins. Another mechanism is direct activation of factor X by proteases, for example, as present in mucin or as produced by neoplasms. Amnionic fluid contains abundant mucin from fetal squames, and this likely causes the rapid defibrination found with amnionic fluid embolism. Zhou and associates (2009) have presented evidence that in addition to tissue factor, phosphatidylserine expressed by the amnionic cell membrane is an inciting factor.

Consumptive coagulopathy is almost always seen as a complication of an identifiable, underlying pathological process against which treatment must be directed to reverse defibrination. Thus, identification and prompt elimination of the coagulopathy source is the first priority.

Significance

In addition to bleeding and circulatory obstruction, which may cause ischemia from hypoperfusion, consumptive coagulopathy may be associated with microangiopathic hemolysis. This is caused by mechanical disruption of the erythrocyte membrane within small vessels in which fibrin has been deposited. Varying degrees of hemolysis with anemia, hemoglobinemia, hemoglobinuria, and erythrocyte morphological changes are produced. According to Pritchard and colleagues (1976), this likely causes or contributes to the hemolysis encountered with the so-called *HELLP syndrome—hemolysis, elevated liver enzymes, low platelets* (see Chap. 34, p. 720).

In obstetrical syndromes involving consumptive coagulopathy, the importance of vigorous restoration and maintenance of the circulation to treat hypovolemia and persistent intravascular coagulation cannot be overemphasized. With adequate perfusion of vital organs, activated coagulation factors and circulating fibrin and fibrin degradation products are promptly removed by the reticuloendothelial system. At the same time, hepatic and endothelial synthesis of procoagulants is promoted.

The likelihood of life-threatening hemorrhage in obstetrical situations complicated by defective coagulation depends not only on the extent of the coagulation defects but—of great importance—on whether the vasculature is intact or disrupted. With gross derangement of blood coagulation, there may be fatal hemorrhage when vascular integrity is disrupted, yet no hemorrhage as long as all blood vessels remain intact.

Clinical and Laboratory Evidence of Defective Hemostasis

Bioassay is an excellent method to clinically detect or suspect significant coagulopathy. *Excessive bleeding at sites of modest trauma characterizes defective hemostasis.* Persistent bleeding from venipuncture sites, nicks from shaving the perineum or abdomen, trauma from insertion of a catheter, and spontaneous bleeding from the gums or nose are signs of possible coagulation defects. Purpuric areas at pressure sites such as blood pressure cuffs may indicate incoagulable blood, or more commonly, clinically significant thrombocytopenia. A surgical procedure provides the ultimate bioassay for coagulation. Continuous generalized oozing from the skin, subcutaneous and fascial tissues, the retroperitoneal space, or episiotomy site should at least suggest coagulopathy.

Hypofibrinogenemia

In late pregnancy, plasma fibrinogen levels typically are 300 to 600 mg/dL. With consumptive coagulopathy, these high levels may sometimes serve to protect against clinically significant hypofibrinogenemia. To promote clinical coagulation, fibrinogen levels must be approximately 150 mg/dL. If serious *hypofibrinogenemia* is present, the clot formed from whole blood in a glass tube may initially be soft but not necessarily remarkably reduced in volume. Then, over the next half hour or so, as platelet-induced clot retraction develops, it becomes quite small, so that many of the erythrocytes are extruded, and the volume of liquid clearly exceeds that of clot.

Fibrin and Fibrinogen Derivatives

Serum fibrin degradation products may be detected by a number of sensitive test systems. Monoclonal antibodies to detect D-dimers are commonly used. With clinically significant consumption coagulopathy, these measurements are always abnormally high.

Thrombocytopenia

Serious thrombocytopenia is likely if petechiae are abundant, if clotted blood fails to retract over a period of an hour or so, or if platelets are rare in a stained blood smear. Confirmation is provided by platelet count. With severe preeclampsia and eclampsia, there may also be *qualitative platelet dysfunction* (see Chap. 34, p. 717).

Prothrombin and Partial Thromboplastin Times

Prolongation of these standard coagulation tests may result from appreciable reductions in those coagulants essential for generating thrombin, from fibrinogen concentrations below a critical level—approximately 100 mg/dL, or from appreciable amounts of circulating fibrinogen-fibrin degradation products. Prolongation of the prothrombin time and partial thromboplastin time need not be the consequence of consumptive coagulopathy.

Coagulation- and Fibrinolysis-Directed Agents

Heparin

The infusion of heparin to try to block disseminated intravascular coagulation associated with placental abruption or other situations in which the integrity of the vascular system is compromised is mentioned only to condemn its use.

Epsilon-Aminocaproic Acid

This agent has been administered in an attempt to control fibrinolysis by inhibiting the conversion of plasminogen to plasmin. Epsilon-aminocaproic acid inhibits the proteolytic action of plasmin on fibrinogen, fibrin monomer, and fibrin polymer (clot). Failure to clear fibrin polymer from the microcirculation could result in organ ischemia and infarction, such as renal cortical necrosis. Its use in most types of obstetrical coagulopathy has not been efficacious and is not recommended.

Placental Abruption

This is the most common cause of severe consumptive coagulopathy in obstetrics and is discussed on page 761.

Fetal Death and Delayed Delivery

In the past, in most women with fetal death, spontaneous labor eventually ensued, most often within 2 weeks. Studies indicated that gross disruption of the maternal coagulation mechanism rarely developed within 1 month after fetal death (Pritchard, 1959, 1973). If the fetus was retained longer, however, approximately 25 percent of the women developed a coagulopathy. Today, because of certainty with which fetal death can be confirmed with sonography and because highly effective methods are available to induce labor, coagulopathy from a retained dead fetus is unusual.

Coagulopathy

The fibrinogen concentration typically falls over 6 weeks or more to levels that are normal for the nonpregnant state—and in some cases, it falls to critical concentrations of 100 mg/dL or less. Simultaneously, fibrin degradation product levels become elevated in serum (Pritchard, 1973). These changes are presumably mediated by thromboplastin from the dead products of conception (Jimenez and Pritchard, 1968; Lerner and associates, 1967). The platelet count tends to decrease in these instances, but severe thrombocytopenia is uncommon even if the fibrinogen level is quite low. Although coagulation defects may correct spontaneously before evacuation, this is unusual and happens slowly (Pritchard, 1959).

Heparin

Correction of coagulation defects in this circumstance has been accomplished using low doses of heparin—5000 U, two to three times daily—under carefully controlled conditions *in women with an intact circulation* (Pacheco and colleagues, 2004). Heparin appropriately administered can block further pathological consumption of fibrinogen and other clotting factors, thereby slowing or temporarily reversing the cycle of consumption and fibrinolysis. Such correction should be undertaken only if the patient is not actively bleeding and with simultaneous steps to effect delivery.

Fetal Death in Multifetal Pregnancy

It is uncommon that an obvious coagulation derangement develops in a multifetal pregnancy complicated by the death of at least one fetus and survival of another (Landy and Weingold, 1989). Petersen and Nyholm (1999) followed 22 women with a multifetal pregnancy with one fetal death after the first trimester and did not detect a coagulopathy in any of these cases.

Chescheir and Seeds (1988) reported a woman in whom, following the death of one twin fetus, there was a progressive but transient fall in the plasma fibrinogen concentration and rise in the level of fibrin degradation products. Most cases are seen in monochorionic twins with vascular anastomoses (see Chap. 39, p. 878). We have encountered a few such cases at Parkland Hospital, and one is shown in Figure 35-29. Coagulation changes ceased spontaneously, and the surviving fetus, when delivered near term, was healthy. The placenta of the long-dead fetus was filled with fibrin.

Amnionic Fluid Embolism

This is a complex disorder classically characterized by the abrupt onset of hypotension, hypoxia, and consumptive coagulopathy. There is great individual variation in its clinical manifestation. Thus, women are encountered in whom one of these three clinical hallmarks dominates or is entirely absent. Although uncommon in an absolute sense, amnionic fluid embolism was implicated as the cause of death in 9 percent of the 3201 pregnancy-related maternal deaths ascertained by the Centers for Disease Control and Prevention from 1991 through 1997 (Berg and colleagues, 2003). Similarly, Clark and associates (2008) reported that 14 percent of 95 maternal deaths in a 1.46-million delivery database were due to amnionic fluid embolism.

Using data from 3 million deliveries in the United States from 1999 and 2003, Abenhaim and colleagues (2008) estimated a frequency of approximately 7.7 cases per 100,000 births. Risk factors included advanced maternal age, minority race, placenta previa, preeclampsia, and forceps or cesarean delivery. The case-fatality rate was 22 percent.

In obvious cases, the clinical picture is dramatic. Classically, a woman in the late stages of labor or immediately postpartum begins gasping for air, and then rapidly suffers seizure or cardiorespiratory arrest complicated by consumptive coagulopathy, massive hemorrhage, and death. These are unquestionably the most dramatic cases. But there appears to be variation in the clinical presentation of this condition. For example, we have managed a number of women in whom otherwise uncomplicated vaginal delivery was followed by severe acute consumptive coagulopathy without cardiorespiratory symptoms. Thus, in some women, consumptive coagulopathy appears to be the *forme fruste* of amnionic fluid embolism (Awad and Shorten, 2001; Davies, 1999; Porter and colleagues, 1996). Other features common to amnionic fluid embolism are meconium staining and rapid labor.

Pathogenesis

Amnionic fluid embolism was originally described in 1941 by Steiner and Lushbaugh. Subsequent studies by Adamsons and associates (1971) and Stolte and co-workers (1967) demon-

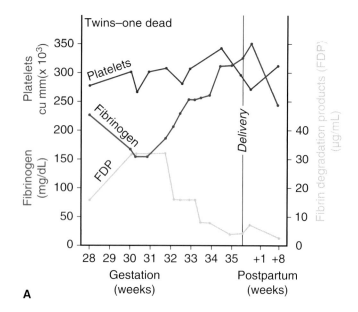

A

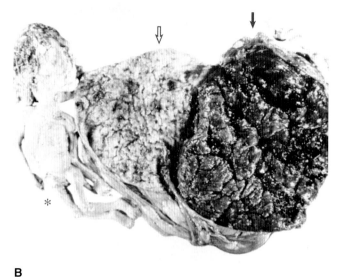

B

FIGURE 35-29 A. Death of one twin was confirmed sonographically at 28 weeks' gestation. Serial studies then demonstrated decreasing plasma fibrinogen concentration and abnormally elevated serum fibrin degradation products that reached a nadir 4 weeks later. After this, spontaneously, the fibrinogen concentration rose, and the fibrin degradation product levels fell in mirror-like fashion. When delivered at 36 weeks, the liveborn co-twin was healthy and had normal coagulation studies and normal appearing placenta (*blue arrow*). **B.** The fibrin-filled placenta of the long-dead fetus is apparent (*clear arrow*). Presumably, the fibrin curtailed the escape of thromboplastin from the dead products into the maternal circulation. FDP = fibrin degradation products.

strated that amnionic fluid is innocuous, even when infused in large amounts.

Amnionic fluid enters the circulation as a result of a breach in the physiological barrier that normally exists between maternal and fetal compartments. Such events appear to be common, if not universal, with both squames of presumed fetal origin and trophoblasts being commonly found in the maternal circulation (Clark and colleagues, 1986; Lee and co-workers, 1986). There may be maternal exposure to various fetal elements during pregnancy termination, following amniocentesis or trauma, or more

TABLE 35-6. Clinical Findings in 84 Women with Amnionic Fluid Embolism

Clinical Findings	Clark et al (1995) (n = 46)	Weiwen (2000) (n = 38)
Hypotension	43	38
Fetal distress	30/30	NS
Pulmonary edema or ARDS	28/30	11
Cardiopulmonary arrest	40	38
Cyanosis	38	38
Coagulopathy	38	12/16
Dyspnea	22/45	38
Seizure	22	6

ARDS = acute respiratory distress syndrome; NS = not stated.

commonly during labor or delivery as small lacerations develop in the lower uterine segment or cervix. Alternatively, cesarean delivery affords ample opportunity for mixture of maternal blood and fetal tissue.

In most cases, these events are innocuous. In certain women, however, such exposure initiates a complex series of physiological reactions that are listed in Table 35-6. A similar process has been shown for traumatic fat embolism (Peltier, 1984). A complete understanding of the precise pathophysiological cascade remains elusive. In a case-controlled study of nine women with presumed amnionic fluid embolism, Benson and associates (2001) found that levels of some indicators of anaphylaxis—serum tryptase and urinary histamine—were increased in some of the women, yet none had evidence of mast cell degranulation. Of note, complement levels were decreased uniformly, suggesting that complement activation may play an important role. Because such activation also occurs in seriously ill patients with acute respiratory distress syndrome, however, it is not known whether complement activation is a primary or secondary result of amnionic fluid embolism. A number of chemokines and cytokines likely are also important in the pathogenesis. For example, Khong (1998) found intense expression of endothelin-1 in fetal squames recovered from the lungs of two fatal cases.

Pathophysiology

Studies in primates using homologous amnionic fluid injection, as well as a carefully performed study in the goat model, have provided important insights into central hemodynamic aberrations (Adamsons and co-workers, 1971; Hankins and colleagues, 1993; Stolte and colleagues, 1967). The initial phase consists of pulmonary and systemic hypertension. Indeed, in a remarkable case report, Stanten and associates (2003) described the results of a transesophageal echocardiogram performed within 10 minutes of circulatory collapse related to amnionic fluid embolism. The findings included a massively dilated akinetic right ventricle and a small, vigorously contracting, cavity-obliterated left ventricle. These were all consistent with failure to transfer blood from the right to the left heart because of catastrophic pulmonary vasoconstriction. Transient but profound oxygen desaturation is often seen in the initial phase, resulting in neurological injury in most survivors (Harvey and associates, 1996).

Decreased systemic vascular resistance and left ventricular stroke work index occur following this initial phase (Clark and colleagues, 1988). In women who live beyond the initial cardiovascular collapse, a secondary phase of lung injury and coagulopathy often ensues.

The association of uterine hypertonus with cardiovascular collapse appears to be the effect of amnionic fluid embolism rather than the cause (Clark and co-workers, 1995). Indeed, uterine blood flow ceases completely when intrauterine pressures exceed 35 to 40 mm Hg (Towell, 1976). Thus, a hypertonic contraction is the *least* likely time for fetal–maternal exchange to take place. Similarly, there is no causal association between oxytocin use and amnionic fluid embolism (American College of Obstetricians and Gynecologists, 1993).

Diagnosis

In the past, the detection of squamous cells or other debris of fetal origin in the central pulmonary circulation was believed to be pathognomonic for amnionic fluid embolism. Indeed, in fatal cases, histopathological findings may be dramatic, especially in those involving meconium-stained amnionic fluid (Fig. 35-30). The detection of such debris, however, may require extensive special staining, and even then it is often not seen. For example, Hankins and colleagues (2002) injected raw amnionic fluid into eight goats. Using special staining, there was microscopic evidence of pulmonary embolization in only 25 percent. Interestingly, of seven other animals who were injected with fluid stained with *meconium*, all had histopathological evidence of embolization.

In a study by Clark and associates (1995), fetal elements were detected in 75 percent of autopsies and in 50 percent of specimens prepared from concentrated buffy coat aspirates taken antemortem from a pulmonary artery catheter. Further, several studies have demonstrated that squamous cells, trophoblasts, and other debris of fetal origin may commonly be found in the central circulation of women with conditions other than amnionic fluid embolism. Thus, this finding is neither sensitive nor specific, and the diagnosis is generally made by identifying clinically characteristic signs and symptoms. In

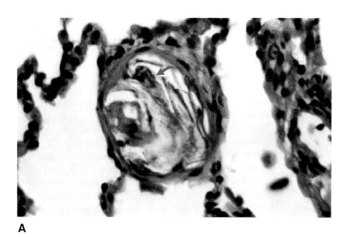

A

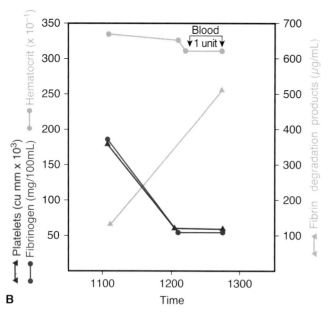

B

FIGURE 35-30 Fatal amnionic fluid embolism. **A.** Fetal squames (*arrow*) packed into a small pulmonary artery. Most of the empty spaces within the vessel were demonstrated by special lipid stains to be filled with vernix caseosa. **B.** Acute and rapid defibrination in the same woman showing levels of fibrinogen, fibrinogen–fibrin degradation products, and platelets.

less typical cases, diagnosis is contingent on careful exclusion of other causes.

Management

Although an initial period of systemic and pulmonary hypertension appears to be involved in amnionic fluid embolism, this phase is transient. Women who survive long enough to receive any treatment other than cardiopulmonary resuscitation should receive therapy directed at oxygenation and support of the failing myocardium. Circulatory support and blood and component replacement are paramount. *There are no data that any type of intervention improves maternal prognosis with amnionic fluid embolism.* In undelivered women suffering cardiac arrest, consideration should be given to emergency perimortem cesarean delivery in an effort to improve newborn outcome. Such decision making is more complex in a woman who is hemodynamically unstable, but who has not suffered cardiac arrest (see Chap. 42, p. 942).

Prognosis

The dismal outcomes with amnionic fluid embolism are undoubtedly related to reporting biases. Also, the syndrome likely is underdiagnosed in all but the most severe cases. In the report by Clark and co-workers (1995), there was a 60-percent maternal mortality rate. In the California database of 1.1 million deliveries by Gilbert and Danielsen (1999), only 25 percent of reported cases were fatal. Weiwen (2000) has provided preliminary data from 38 cases in the Suzhou region of China, and almost 90 percent of these women died. Death can be amazingly rapid, and of the 34 women who died in the series from China, 12 died within 30 minutes.

Profound neurological impairment is common in survivors. *In the cases reported by Clark and colleagues (1995), only 8 percent of women who had a cardiac arrest in conjunction with initial symptoms survived neurologically intact.* Outcome is also poor for fetuses and is related to the cardiac arrest-to-delivery interval. Overall, the neonatal survival rate is 70 percent, but almost half suffer residual neurological impairment.

Sepsis Syndrome

Infections that lead to bacteremia and septic shock in obstetrics are most commonly due to septic abortion, antepartum pyelonephritis, or puerperal sepsis. Other aspects of sepsis syndrome and septic shock are discussed in Chapter 42 (p. 932).

Abortion

Remarkable blood loss may occur as the consequence of abortion. Hemorrhage during early pregnancy is less likely to be severe unless abortion was induced and the procedure was traumatic. When pregnancy is more advanced, the mechanisms responsible for hemorrhage are most often the same as those described for placental abruption and placenta previa—that is, the disruption of a large number of maternal blood vessels at the site of placental implantation.

Coagulopathy

Serious disruption of the coagulation mechanism as the consequence of abortion may develop in the following circumstances:

- Prolonged retention of a dead fetus
- Sepsis syndrome—a notorious cause
- Labor induction with a prostaglandin
- Instrumented termination of the pregnancy
- Intrauterine instillation of hypertonic saline or urea solutions

The kinds of changes in coagulation that have been identified with abortion induced with *hypertonic solutions* imply at least that thromboplastin is released from placenta, fetus, decidua, or all three by the necrobiotic effect of the hypertonic solutions, which then initiates coagulopathy within the maternal circulation (Burkman and associates, 1977). Coagulation defects have been observed to develop rarely during induction of abortion with prostaglandin. Saraiya and colleagues (1999) reviewed 62 spontaneous abortion–related deaths reported to the Pregnancy Mortality Surveillance System. Almost 60 percent of the deaths were caused by infection, and half of these women had consumptive coagulopathy.

Consumptive coagulopathy has been an uncommon but serious complication among women with *septic abortion*. The incidence of coagulation defects in the past at Parkland Hospital was highest in those with *Clostridium perfringens* sepsis and intense intravascular hemolysis (Pritchard and Whalley, 1971). Management consists of prompt restoration and maintenance of the circulation, and appropriate steps to control the infection, including evacuation of the infected products (see Chap. 9, p. 222).

MANAGEMENT OF HEMORRHAGE

Hypovolemic Shock

Shock from hemorrhage evolves through several stages. Early in the course of massive bleeding, there are decreases in mean arterial pressure, stroke volume, cardiac output, central venous pressure, and pulmonary capillary wedge pressure. Increases in arteriovenous oxygen content difference reflect a relative increase in tissue oxygen extraction, although overall oxygen consumption falls.

Blood flow to capillary beds in various organs is controlled by arterioles, which are resistance vessels that in turn are partially controlled by the central nervous system. At least 70 percent of total blood volume is contained in venules, which are passive resistance vessels controlled by humoral factors. Catecholamine release during hemorrhage causes a generalized increase in venular tone, resulting in an autotransfusion from this capacitance reservoir (Barber and colleagues, 1999). These changes are accompanied by compensatory increases in heart rate, systemic and pulmonary vascular resistance, and myocardial contractility. In addition, there is redistribution of cardiac output and blood volume by selective, centrally mediated arteriolar constriction. This results in diminished perfusion to the kidneys, splanchnic beds, skin, and uterus, but relative maintenance of blood flow to the heart, brain, adrenal glands, and organs that autoregulate their own flow.

As the blood volume deficit exceeds 25 percent, compensatory mechanisms usually are inadequate to maintain cardiac output and blood pressure. At this point, additional small losses of blood result in rapid clinical deterioration. Despite an initial increase in *total oxygen extraction* by maternal tissue, maldistribution of blood flow results in *local* tissue hypoxia and metabolic acidosis, producing a vicious cycle of vasoconstriction, organ ischemia, and cellular death. Hemorrhage also activates lymphocytes and monocytes, which in turn cause endothelial cell activation. As with sepsis syndrome, these events lead to loss of capillary membrane integrity and additional loss of intravascular volume. There is also increased platelet aggregation in hypovolemic shock, resulting in the release of a number of vasoactive mediators that cause small vessel occlusion and further impairment of microcirculatory perfusion.

Often overlooked is the importance of extracellular fluid and electrolyte shifts in both the pathophysiology and successful treatment of hypovolemic shock. This involves changes in the cellular transport of various ions, in which sodium and water enter skeletal muscles and cellular potassium is lost to the extracellular fluid. Replacement of extracellular fluid is thus an important component of therapy in hypovolemic shock. *Survival is reduced in acute hemorrhagic shock when blood alone, compared with blood and lactated Ringer solution, is administered.*

Estimation of Blood Loss

Visual inspection is notoriously inaccurate, and clinical estimates can average half the measured loss. Importantly, in obstetrics, part or all of the hemorrhage may be concealed. It is important to realize that in a situation of acute hemorrhage, the immediate hematocrit may not reflect actual blood loss. After the loss of 1000 mL, the hematocrit typically falls only 3 volume percent in the first hour. When resuscitation is given with rapid infusion of intravenous crystalloids, there is prompt equilibration. **During an episode of acute significant hemorrhage, the initial hematocrit is always the highest.** This is true whether it is measured in the delivery room, operating room, or recovery room.

Urine output is one of the most important "vital signs" to follow in the woman with obstetrical hemorrhage. *Renal blood flow is especially sensitive to changes in blood volume. Thus, in the absence of diuretics, the rate of urine formation, when carefully measured, reflects the adequacy of renal perfusion and in turn, the perfusion of other vital organs.* Urine flow of at least 30 mL, and preferably 60 mL per hour, should be maintained. With potentially serious hemorrhage, an indwelling bladder catheter should be inserted promptly to measure urine flow. Potent diuretics such as furosemide invalidate the relationship between urine flow and renal perfusion. This need not be a problem in the management of the woman who is hemorrhaging, because diuretics should be avoided in a hypovolemic patient. Another effect of furosemide is venodilation, which further reduces cardiac venous return, thereby further compromising cardiac output.

Resuscitation and Acute Management

Whenever there is any suggestion of excessive blood loss after delivery, it is essential to immediately identify uterine atony, retained placental fragments, or genital tract lacerations. It is imperative that at least one or two intravenous infusion systems of large caliber be established promptly to allow rapid administration of crystalloid solutions and blood. An operating room, surgical team, and anesthesiologist should always be immediately available. Specific causes of postpartum hemorrhage are managed as discussed earlier in this chapter.

Fluid Replacement

Treatment of serious hemorrhage demands prompt and adequate refilling of the intravascular compartment. Crystalloid solutions typically are used for initial volume resuscitation. Such solutions rapidly equilibrate into the extravascular space and only 20 percent of crystalloid remains in the circulation of critically ill patients after 1 hour (Shoemaker and Kram, 1991). Because of such equilibration, initial fluid infusion should involve about three times as much crystalloid as the estimated blood loss.

There is debate concerning fluid resuscitation of hypovolemic shock with colloid versus crystalloid solutions. Perel and Roberts (2007) performed a Cochrane review for resuscitation of nonpregnant critically ill patients. They found equivalent benefits but concluded that colloid solutions were more expensive. The Saline versus Albumin Fluid Evaluation (SAFE) trial of almost 7000 randomized nonpregnant patients reported similar results (Finfer and co-workers, 2004). Because of this, we concur with Bonnar (2000) that fluid resuscitation should be with crystalloid and blood.

Blood Replacement

Considerable debate also surrounds the hematocrit level or hemoglobin concentration that mandates blood transfusion. According to deliberations of a Consensus Development Conference (1988), cardiac output does not substantively decrease until the hemoglobin concentration falls to approximately 7 g/dL or hematocrit of 20 volumes percent. Although the committee reported that otherwise healthy anesthetized animals survived isovolemic anemia with hematocrit decreases to 5 volumes percent, they further cited that there was significant functional deterioration well before that point. It is difficult to define a universal hematocrit or hemoglobin value below or above which transfusion is either mandatory or contraindicated. That said, recommendations of the Consensus Conference should be considered in clinical decision making. According to these guidelines, red blood cells are not infused for moderate anemia in stable women.

For the woman acutely bleeding, we recommend rapid blood infusion if the hematocrit is less than 25 volumes percent. This decision is obviously dependent on whether there is imminent surgery, acute operative blood loss, acute hypoxia, vascular collapse, or other factors present. In Iraq, U.S. Military Combat Trauma Units aim for a hematocrit of 21 volumes percent (Barbieri, 2007).

Hebert and associates (1999) reported results from the Canadian Critical Care Trials Group. A total of 838 critically ill nonpregnant patients were randomly assigned to restrictive red cell transfusions to maintain hemoglobin concentration above 7 g/dL or to liberal transfusions to maintain the hemoglobin 10 to 12 g/dL. The 30-day mortality rate was similar—19 versus 23 percent in the restrictive versus liberal groups, respectively. In patients who were not as ill—defined by Acute Physiology and Chronic Health Evaluation (APACHE) scores of 20 or less—the 30-day mortality rate was significantly lower in the restrictive group—9 versus 26 percent. Morrison and colleagues (1991) reported no benefits of red cell transfusions given to women who had suffered postpartum hemorrhage and who were *isovolemic but anemic* with a hematocrit between 18 and 25 volumes percent. *Clearly, the level to which a woman is transfused depends not only on the present red cell mass, but also on the likelihood of additional blood loss.*

Whole Blood and Blood Components

Contents and effects of transfusion of various blood components are shown in Table 35-7. *Compatible whole blood is ideal for treatment of hypovolemia from catastrophic acute hemorrhage.* It has a shelf life of 40 days, and 70 percent of the transfused red cells function for at least 24 hours following transfusion. One unit raises the hematocrit by 3 to 4 volume percent. Whole blood replaces many coagulation factors, especially fibrinogen, and its plasma expands hypovolemia. Importantly, women with severe hemorrhage are resuscitated with fewer blood donor exposures than with packed red cells and components. For example, after their review, Shaz and co-workers (2009) recommended that plasma, platelets, and red cells be given in a 1:1:1 ratio for trauma patients undergoing massive transfusions. Drawbacks of such a scheme are exposure to many more donors. In a randomized study of 33 nonpregnant patients undergoing liver transplantation, Laine and colleagues (2003) found that whole blood, compared with component therapy, was associated with fewer donor exposures yet provided equally

TABLE 35-7. Blood Products Commonly Transfused in Obstetrical Hemorrhage

Product	Volume per Unit	Contents per Unit	Effect(s) in Obstetrical Hemorrhage
Whole blood	About 500 mL; Hct ~ 40 percent	RBCs, plasma, 600–700 mg of fibrinogen, no platelets	Restores blood volume and fibrinogen, increases Hct 3–4 volume percent per unit
Packed RBCs ("packed cells")	About 250 mL plus additive solutions; Hct ~ 55–80 percent	RBCs only, no fibrinogen, no platelets	Increases Hct 3–4 volume percent per unit
Fresh-frozen plasma (FFP)	About 250 mL; 30-minute thaw needed before use	Colloid plus 600–700 mg fibrinogen, no platelets	Restores circulating volume and fibrinogen
Cryoprecipitate	About 15 mL, frozen	About 200 mg fibrinogen plus other clotting factors, no platelets	About 3000–4000 mg total is needed to restore fibrinogen to > 150 mg/dL
Platelets	About 50 mL, stored at room temperature	One unit raises platelet count about 5000/μL (single-donor apheresis "6-pack" is preferable)	6–10 units usually transfused (single-donor 6-pack preferable)

Hct = hematocrit; RBCs = red blood cells.
Modified from Leveno and colleagues (2003).

effective therapy for blood loss. Freshly donated whole blood has also been used for casualties with life-threatening massive hemorrhage at combat support hospitals in Iraq (Spinella and co-workers, 2008).

Our experiences at Parkland Hospital also favor whole blood for massive hemorrhage. In a recent audit of more than 66,000 women delivered at Parkland Hospital, Alexander and associates (2009) reported significantly decreased incidences of renal failure, adult respiratory distress syndrome, pulmonary edema, hypofibrinogenemia, admission to an intensive care unit, and maternal death when whole blood transfusions were compared with packed red cell transfusions or combinations of blood products.

For women who are more stable and do not have massive blood loss, packed red blood cell transfusions are suitable. According to the National Institutes of Health (1993), component therapy provides better treatment because only the specific component needed is given. Accordingly, the infusion of whole banked blood is usually not necessary and is rarely available.

Dilutional Coagulopathy

When blood loss is massive, replacement with crystalloid solutions and packed red blood cells usually results in a relative depletion of platelets and soluble clotting factors. This leads to a dilutional coagulopathy that clinically is indistinguishable from disseminated intravascular coagulopathy (see p. 785). Such dilution impairs hemostasis and further contributes to blood loss.

The most frequent coagulation defect found in women with blood loss and multiple transfusions is thrombocytopenia (Counts and colleagues, 1979). Stored whole blood is deficient in platelets and in factors V, VIII, and XI. Moreover, all soluble clotting factors are absent from packed red blood cells. Thus, severe hemorrhage without factor replacement may also cause hypofibrinogenemia and prolongation of the prothrombin and partial thromboplastin times. In some women, frank consumptive coagulopathy may accompany shock and confuse the distinction between dilutional and consumptive coagulopathy. Fortunately, in most situations encountered in obstetrics, treatment of both types of coagulopathy is the same.

The impact of massive transfusion with resultant coagulopathy has been studied recently by both civilian trauma groups and military combat hospitals (Bochicchio, 2008; Borgman, 2007; Gonzalez, 2007; Johansson, 2007, and all their co-workers). Patients undergoing massive transfusion—defined as 10 or more units of blood—had much higher survival rates as the ratio of plasma:red cell units was closer to 1:1.4, that is, one unit of plasma for each unit of packed red cells. The highest mortality group had a 1:8 ratio. *Component replacement is rarely necessary with acute replacement of 5 to 10 units of packed red blood cells or less.* When blood loss exceeds this amount, consideration should be given to evaluation of platelet count, clotting studies, and plasma fibrinogen concentration.

In the woman with obstetrical hemorrhage, the platelet count should be maintained above 50,000/μL with the infusion of platelet concentrates. A fibrinogen level of less than 100 mg/dL or sufficiently prolonged prothrombin or partial thromboplastin times in a woman with surgical bleeding is an indication for fresh-frozen plasma administration in doses of 10 to 15 mL/kg.

Type and Screen versus Crossmatch

In any woman at significant risk for hemorrhage, typing and screening or crossmatching is essential. The screening procedure involves mixing the maternal serum with standard reagent red cells that carry the antigens with which most of the common clinically significant antibodies react. A crossmatch, on the other hand, involves the use of actual donor erythrocytes rather than standard red cells.

Only 0.03 to 0.07 percent of patients who are determined not to have antibodies in a type-and-screen procedure subsequently have antibodies as determined by crossmatch (Boral and colleagues, 1979). Thus, administration of screened blood rarely results in adverse clinical sequelae. Not performing a crossmatch also decreases blood bank costs. Moreover, blood that is crossmatched is held exclusively for that single potential recipient. With type-and-screening, blood is available for any potential recipient and blood wastage is reduced. For all of these reasons, type and screen is preferred in most obstetrical situations.

Packed Red Blood Cells

Cells packed from a unit of whole blood have a hematocrit of 55 to 80 volumes percent, depending on the method used for preparation and storage. A unit of packed red blood cells contains the same volume of erythrocytes as whole blood and also raises the hematocrit by 3 to 4 volumes percent. Packed red blood cell and crystalloid infusion are the mainstays of transfusion therapy for most cases of obstetrical hemorrhage.

Platelets

When needed, it is preferable to transfuse platelets obtained by apheresis from one donor. In this scheme, the equivalent of platelets from six individual donors is given as a one-unit one-donor transfusion. Such units generally cannot be stored more than 5 days.

If single-donor platelets are not available, random donor platelet packs are used. These are prepared from individual units of whole blood by centrifugation, and then resuspended in 50 to 70 mL of plasma. One unit of random donor platelets contains about 5.5×10^{10} platelets, and 6 to 10 such units are generally transfused. Each unit transfused should raise the platelet count by 5000/μL (National Institutes of Health, 1993). The donor plasma must be compatible with recipient erythrocytes. Further, because some red blood cells are invariably transfused along with the platelets, only platelets from D-negative donors should be given to D-negative recipients. Even so, Lin and colleagues (2002) found that transfusion of ABO-nonidentical platelets in nonpregnant patients undergoing cardiovascular surgery was not associated with adverse effects. Platelet transfusion is considered in a bleeding patient with a platelet count below 50,000/μL. In the *nonsurgical patient*, bleeding is rarely encountered if the platelet count exceeds 5000 to 10,000/μL (Sachs, 1991).

Fresh-Frozen Plasma

This component is prepared by separating plasma from whole blood and then freezing it. Approximately 30 minutes are required for the frozen plasma to thaw. It is a source of all stable and labile clotting factors, including fibrinogen. Thus, it is often used in the acute treatment of women with consumptive or dilutional coagulopathy as discussed previously. Fresh-frozen plasma is not appropriate for use as a volume expander in the absence of specific clotting factor deficiency. It should be considered in a bleeding woman with a fibrinogen level below 100 mg/dL or with abnormal prothrombin and partial thromboplastin times.

Cryoprecipitate

This component is prepared from fresh-frozen plasma. Cryoprecipitate is composed of factor VIII:C, factor VIII:von Willebrand factor, 200 mg of fibrinogen, factor XIII, and fibronectin, all combined in less than 15 mL of the plasma from which it was derived (American Association of Blood Banks, 1994). Cryoprecipitate is an ideal source of fibrinogen if levels are dangerously low and there is oozing from surgical incisions. There is no advantage to the use of cryoprecipitate for general clotting factor replacement in the bleeding woman instead of fresh-frozen plasma. The exception to this is in states of general factor deficiency where potential volume overload is a problem, and in a few conditions involving deficiency of specific factors.

Recombinant Activated Factor VII

This synthetic vitamin K-dependent protein was approved by the Food and Drug Administration (FDA) principally for treatment of bleeding in individuals with hemophilia. Recombinant activated factor VII—*rFVIIa* or *NovoSeven*—acts by binding to exposed tissue factor at the site of tissue and vascular injury. Thrombin so generated activates platelets and the coagulation cascade. Over the past 10 years, rFVIIa has been used successfully to help control hemorrhage from surgery, trauma, and other causes (Mannucci and Levi, 2007). A number of reports of successful treatment for obstetrical hemorrhage in women with hemophilia have accrued.

Recombinant FVIIa has also been used to control severe obstetrical hemorrhage in women *without* hemophilia who have severe hemorrhage from complications of pregnancy. In their review of 65 published cases, Franchini and associates (2007) reported that two thirds of women underwent cesarean delivery, and in a third of treated women, postpartum atony was the cause of bleeding. Overall, half of all 65 women also underwent hysterectomy. Alfirevic and co-workers (2007) described 113 women with postpartum hemorrhage treated with rFVIIa and reported to the Northern European Registry. Over half had uterine atony, a third lacerations, and a fourth had placenta previa or abruption. Almost 35 percent underwent hysterectomy and 10 percent had uterine artery embolization. Bleeding was diminished or arrested in over 80 percent with no complications due to rFVIIa. Lewis and co-workers (2009) caution that rFVIIa administration will not be effective if plasma fibrinogen is depleted and levels are around 50 mg/dL or less.

The specter of thrombosis with rFVIIa use is of concern (Mannucci and Levi, 2007). In a review of the FDA adverse event reporting system by O'Connell and associates (2006), there were 185 thrombotic events in 168 nonpregnant patients, and most were with off-label use of rFVIIa, mainly for hemorrhage. These events may affect as many as 7 percent of treated patients, but appear so far to be uncommon in obstetrical patients.

Autotransfusion

There are no convincing data that intraoperative blood salvage and autotransfusion is safe in obstetrical patients. A few small studies have uncovered no obvious problems (Rainaldi and colleagues, 1998). In their contemporary review, Allam and associates (2008) document the lack of prospective trials, but found no serious reported complications.

Autologous Transfusion

Under some circumstances, autologous blood storage for transfusion may be considered. In general, however, this has been disappointing. For example, McVay and colleagues (1989) reported observations from 273 pregnant women in whom blood was drawn in the third trimester. Minimal requirements were a hemoglobin concentration 11 g/dL or a hematocrit of 34 volumes percent. Unfortunately, almost three fourths of these women donated only one unit, a volume of questionable value.

In many cases, the need for transfusion cannot be predicted. Sherman and colleagues (1992) studied 27 women given two or more transfusions in more than 16,000 deliveries. In only 40 percent was an antepartum risk factor identified. Similar findings were reported by Reyal and associates (2004). Andres and co-workers (1990) and Etchason and associates (1995) concluded that autologous transfusions were not cost effective.

Complications of Blood Transfusion

Each unit of blood or any component is associated with risk of exposure to blood-borne infections. During the past several decades, substantial advances have been achieved in blood transfusion safety. Currently, the most serious known risks are administrative error leading to ABO-incompatible blood transfusion, transfusion-related acute lung injury (TRALI), and bacterial and viral transmission (Goodnough, 2003).

Hemolytic Transfusion Reaction. The transfusion of an incompatible blood component may result in acute hemolysis characterized by disseminated intravascular coagulation, acute renal failure, and death. Preventable errors, such as mislabeling of a specimen or transfusing an incorrect patient, are responsible for most reactions. Although the rate of such errors in the United States is estimated to be 1 in 14,000 units, it is likely greater due to underreporting (Goodnough, 2003; Linden and co-workers, 2001).

Signs and symptoms of a transfusion reaction include fever, hypotension, tachycardia, dyspnea, chest or back pain, flushing, severe anxiety, and hemoglobinuria. Immediate supportive measures include stopping the transfusion, treating hypotension and hyperkalemia, administering a diuretic, and alkalinizing the urine. Assays for urine and plasma hemoglobin concentration and an antibody screen help confirm the diagnosis.

Transfusion-Related Acute Lung Injury (TRALI). This is a life-threatening complication characterized by severe dyspnea, hypoxia, and noncardiogenic pulmonary edema that develops within 6 hours of transfusion (Silliman and associates, 2003). It is estimated to complicate at least 1 in 5000 transfusions. Although the pathogenesis of TRALI is incompletely understood, the mechanisms of injury to the pulmonary capillaries appear to involve lipid products from stored components as well as leukocyte reactions (Kopko and co-workers, 2002; Silliman and associates, 2003). More recently, the delayed TRALI syndrome has been described as having an onset 6 to 72 hours following transfusion (Marik and Corwin, 2008). Management is discussed in Chapter 42 (p. 930).

Bacterial Contamination. The transfusion of a contaminated blood component is associated with a 60-percent mortality rate. The most commonly implicated contaminant of red cells is *Yersinia enterocolitica*. In the United States, the risk of bacterial contamination is less than 1 per million units. Currently, the greatest risk of transfusion-transmitted disease is bacterial contamination of platelets, which is estimated to affect as many as 1 in 2000 units (Goodnough, 2003).

Viral Transmission. Fortunately, the most feared infection— *human immunodeficiency virus (HIV)*—is the least common. With current screening methods using nucleic acid amplification testing, the time between infection and the first appearance of viral RNA is 11 days for HIV-1 and 8 to 10 days for hepatitis C (Busch and colleagues, 2003). As a result, the risk of HIV infection in screened blood is currently estimated to be less than 1 per 2 million units transfused. Only four transfusion-transmitted HIV infections have been identified since 1999 (Dodd, 2003). Similarly, the risk of hepatitis C infection is approximately 1 in 2 million units transfused (Stramer and associates, 2004).

The likelihood of *HIV-2* infection is even less. After implementation of a combined HIV-1/HIV-2 screening of blood donors in 1992, only three units of 74 million tested through 1995 were positive for HIV-2 (Centers for Disease Control and Prevention, 1995). The risk of *hepatitis B* transmission is higher, although it is estimated to be less than 1 per 100,000 units transfused (Jackson and colleagues, 2003). The risk of transmitting other infectious diseases with transfusion, such as malaria and cytomegalovirus, is estimated to be less than 1 in 1 million (National Institutes of Health, 1993). There have been reports of West Nile virus infection acquired via transfusion. Pealer and colleagues (2003) identified 23 confirmed cases between August 2002 and April 2003.

Red-Cell Substitutes

There are three varieties of these substitutes, and their history and development have been recently reviewed by Ness and Cushing (2007) as well as by Spiess (2009).

- Perfluorochemicals are fluoridated hydrocarbons that are biologically inert liquids with relatively high oxygen solubility. The use of such emulsions allows oxygen to be transported and delivered to tissues by simple diffusion. The only approved substitute, *Fluosol*, was removed from the market. *Oxygant* is a second-generation perfluorochemical that was suspended from Phase III studies.

- Liposome-encapsulated hemoglobin has not proved promising.
- Hemoglobin-based oxygen carriers are still in development. One is *diaspirin cross-linked hemoglobin (DCLHb)*, which proved to be dangerous (Sloan and colleagues, 1999).

SURGICAL MANAGEMENT OF HEMORRHAGE

Uterine Artery Ligation

Used primarily for lacerations at the lateral part of the hysterotomy incision, this technique is shown in Figure 35-31.

Uterine Compression Sutures

Several modifications of the vertical brace suture described by B-Lynch and colleagues (1997) have been described for intractable postpartum atony. These are discussed on page 777 and shown in Figure 35-18.

Internal Iliac Artery Ligation

Ligation of the internal iliac arteries can reduce hemorrhage appreciably (Allahbadia, 1993; Joshi and colleagues, 2007). The procedure may be technically difficult, however, and is successful in only approximately half of patients in whom it is attempted (American College of Obstetricians and Gynecologists, 1998).

Technique

With adequate exposure, ligation is accomplished by opening the peritoneum over the common iliac artery and dissecting

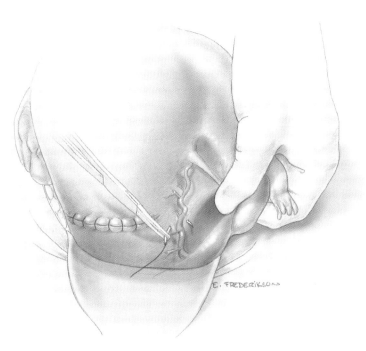

FIGURE 35-31 Uterine artery ligation. The suture goes through the lateral uterine wall anteriorly, curves around posteriorly, then re-enters anteriorly. When tied, it encompasses the uterine artery.

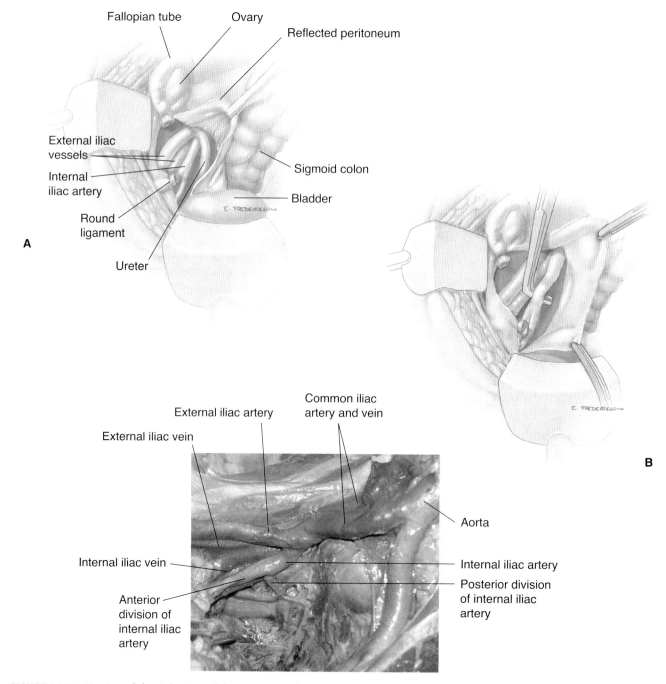

FIGURE 35-32 Ligation of the right internal iliac artery. **A.** The peritoneum covering the right iliac vessels is opened and reflected. **Inset.** Unembalmed cadaveric dissection shows the most common location of the internal iliac vein, which lies lateral to the artery. Ideally, the ligature is place around the anterior division of the internal iliac artery to spare tissues supplied by its posterior division. (Inset, reprinted from *American Journal of Obstetrics & Gynecology*, Vol. 197, No. 6, AT Bleich, DD Rahn, CK Wieslander, et al., Posterior division of the internal iliac artery: Anatomic variations and clinical applications, pp. 658.e1–658.e5, Copyright 2007, with permission from Elsevier.) **B.** Ligation of the right internal iliac artery. A ligature is carried beneath the artery from laterally to medially with a right-angle clamp and firmly tied.

down to the bifurcation of the external and internal iliac arteries as shown in Figure 35-32. Bleich and associates (2007) have shown in dissections of nonpregnant female cadavers that ligation of the internal iliac artery 5 cm distal to the common iliac bifurcation should avoid the posterior division branches. The areolar sheath covering the internal iliac artery is incised longitudinally, and a right-angle clamp is carefully passed just beneath the artery from the lateral side to the medial side. Care must be taken not to perforate contiguous large veins, especially the internal iliac vein. Suture, usually nonabsorbable, is then in-

serted into the open clamp, the jaws are locked, and the suture is carried around the vessel. The vessel is then securely ligated. Pulsations in the external iliac artery, if present before tying the ligature, should be present afterward as well. If not, pulsations must be identified after arterial hypotension has been successfully treated to ensure that the blood flow through the external iliac artery has not been compromised by the ligature.

The most important mechanism of action with internal iliac artery ligation is an 85-percent reduction in pulse pressure in those arteries distal to the ligation (Burchell, 1968). This converts an arterial pressure system into one with pressures approaching those in the venous circulation and more amenable to hemostasis via simple clot formation. Fortunately, bilateral ligation of these arteries does not appear to interfere with subsequent reproduction. Nizard and associates (2003) documented 21 pregnancies in 17 women after bilateral internal iliac artery ligation including three abortions, three miscarriages, two ectopic pregnancies, and 13 normal pregnancies.

Angiographic Embolization

Perhaps used most commonly for puerperal hematomas, angiographic embolization may be used if surgical access to bleeding pelvic vessels is difficult (Fig. 35-33). These techniques have been advanced over the past 10 years, and a number of reports describe their use for various causes of intractable hemorrhage (Bodner, 2006; Chung, 2003; Sentilhes, 2009; Steinauer, 2008, and all their colleagues). In these cited, embolization was successful in 90 percent of 180 women. Fertility is not impaired, and many of these women have had subsequent successful pregnancies (Chauleur, 2008; Fiori, 2009; Goldberg, 2002; Kolomeyevskaya, 2009; Ornan, 2003, and all their associates).

Its use has even been described during pregnancy by Rebarber and co-workers (2009), who used it to embolize a large lower uterine segment arteriovenous malformation at 20 weeks. In most of these reports, complications were few, but at least two cases of ischemic necrosis have been described (Cottier and colleagues, 2002; Sentilhes and associates, 2009).

Preoperative Arterial Catheter Placement

Balloon-tipped catheters are inserted into the iliac arteries preoperatively, and they can be inflated or embolization performed when heavy blood loss is encountered (Oyelese and Smulian, 2006; Yu and co-workers, 2009). In addition to their use for placenta percreta and its variants, it has been described for abdominal pregnancy (see Chap. 10, p. 249). Adverse effects are limited, but one case each of associated postoperative iliac and popliteal artery thrombosis has been described (Greenberg and associates, 2007; Sewell and colleagues, 2006).

Pelvic Umbrella Pack

Described by Logothetopulos (1926), the umbrella or parachute pack is placed for continuing pelvic hemorrhage following

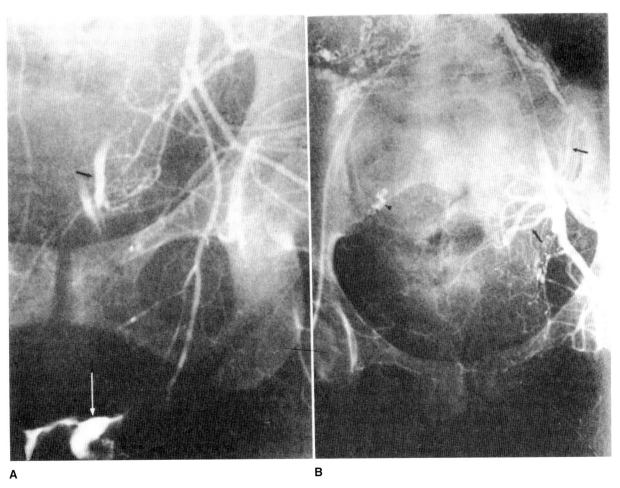

A   **B**

FIGURE 35-33 A. Selective left internal iliac arteriogram before embolization. Note marked extravasation from vaginal artery (*black arrow*) and vulvar branches (*white arrow*) of the left internal pudendal artery. **B.** After embolization, the branches of the left internal pudendal artery are occluded. Patency of the left uterine artery (*arrows*) and coils in the right internal iliac artery (*arrowhead*) are noted. (This figure was published in *American Journal of Obstetrics & Gynecology*, Vol. 160, No. 2, HG Chin, DR Scott, R Resnik, et al., Angiographic embolization of intractable puerperal hematomas, pp. 434–438, Copyright Elsevier 1989)

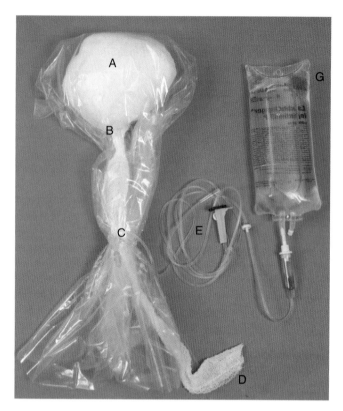

FIGURE 35-34 Assembly of a pelvic pressure pack to control hemorrhage. A sterile x-ray cassette cover drape (plastic bag) is filled with gauze rolls tied end-to-end. The length of gauze is then folded into a ball **(A)** and placed within the cassette bag in such a way that the gauze can be unwound eventually with traction on the tail **(D)**. Intravenous tubing **(E)** is tied to the exiting part of the neck **(C)** and connected to a 1-liter bag **(G)**. Once in place, the gauze pack **(A)** fills the pelvis to tamponade vessels and the narrow upper neck **(B)** passes to exit the vagina **(C)**. The IV bag is suspended off the foot of the bed to sustain pressure of the gauze pack on bleeding sites.

hysterectomy (Howard and associates, 2002). It more commonly has been used for gynecological surgery, and usually internal iliac artery ligation or pelvic artery embolization was also used. The pack is constructed of a sterile x-ray cassette bag, filled with gauze rolls knotted together to provide enough volume to fill the pelvis as shown in Figure 35-34. The pack is introduced transabdominally with the stalk exiting the vagina. Mild traction is applied by tying the stalk to a 1-liter fluid bag which is hung over the foot of the bed. An indwelling urinary catheter is used to monitor urinary output and to prevent urinary obstruction. Placement of percutaneous pelvic drains should be considered to monitor ongoing bleeding within the peritoneal cavity. Broad-spectrum antimicrobials should be administered, and the umbrella pack is removed vaginally after 24 hours.

Dildy and colleagues (2006) presented their results with 11 women in whom the pack was used to arrest hemorrhage following hysterectomy. These women were given 7 to 77 units of packed red cells. The pack was successful to stop bleeding in nine of 11 women. Over the years, we have had mixed results with this technique but recommend it as a "last-ditch" attempt.

REFERENCES

Abdel-Aleem H, El-Nashar I, Abdel-Aleem A: Management of severe postpartum hemorrhage with misoprostol. Int J Gynaecol Obstet 72:75, 2001
Abdella TN, Sibai BM, Hays JM Jr, et al: Perinatal outcome in abruptio placentae. Obstet Gynecol 63:365, 1984
Abenhaim HA, Azoulay L, Kramer MS, et al: Incidence and risk factors of amniotic fluid embolisms: A population-based study on 3 million births in the United States. Am J Obstet Gynecol 199:49.e1, 2008
Achanna S, Mohamed Z, Krishman M: Puerperal uterine inversion: A report of four cases. J Obstet Gynaecol 32:341, 2006
Adamsons K, Mueller-Heubach E, Myers RE: The innocuousness of amniotic fluid infusion in the pregnant rhesus monkey. Am J Obstet Gynecol 109:977, 1971
Addis A, Moretti ME, Ahmed Syed F, et al: Fetal effects of cocaine: An updated meta-analysis. Reprod Toxicol 15:341, 2001
Ajayi RA, Soothill PW, Campbell S, et al: Antenatal testing to predict outcome in pregnancies with unexplained antepartum haemorrhage. Br J Obstet Gynaecol 99:122, 1992
Akoury H, Sherman C: Uterine wall partial thickness necrosis following combined B-Lynch and Cho square sutures for the treatment of primary postpartum hemorrhage. J Obstet Gynaecol Can 30:421, 2008
Al-Zirqi I, Vangen S, Forsen L, et al: Prevalence and risk factors of severe obstetric haemorrhage. BJOG 115:1265, 2008
Alexander JM, Sarode R, McIntire DD, et al: Use of whole blood in the management of hypovolemia due to obstetric hemorrhage. Obstet Gynecol 113:1320, 2009
Alfirevic Z, Elbourne D, Pavord S, et al: Use of recombinant activated factor VII in primary postpartum hemorrhage: The North European Registry 2000-2004. Obstet Gynecol 110:1270, 2007
Allahbadia G: Hypogastric artery ligation: A new perspective. J Gynecol Surg 9:35, 1993
Allam J, Cox M, Yentis SM: Cell salvage in obstetrics. Int J Obstet Anesth 17(1):37, 2008
American Association of Blood Banks: Circular of information for the use of human blood and blood components. American Red Cross 1751, March 1994
American College of Obstetricians and Gynecologists: PROLOG Obstetrics, 3rd ed. Washington, DC, American College of Obstetricians and Gynecologists, 1993, p 94
American College of Obstetricians and Gynecologists: Postpartum hemorrhage. Educational Bulletin No. 243, January 1998
American College of Obstetricians and Gynecologists: Placenta accreta. Committee Opinion No. 266, January 2002
Ananth CV, Berkowitz GS, Savitz DA, et al: Placental abruption and adverse perinatal outcomes. JAMA 282:1646, 1999a
Ananth CV, Demissie K, Smulian JC, et al: Placenta previa in singleton and twin births in the United States, 1989 through 1998: A comparison of risk factor profiles and associated conditions. Am J Obstet Gynecol 188:275, 2003a
Ananth CV, Demissie K, Smulian JC, et al: Relationship among placenta previa, fetal growth restriction, and preterm delivery: A population-based study. Obstet Gynecol 98:299, 2001a
Ananth CV, Getahun D, Peltier MR, et al: Placental abruption in term and preterm gestations. Obstet Gynecol 107:785, 2006
Ananth CV, Oyelese Y, Srinivas N, et al: Preterm premature rupture of membranes, intrauterine infection, and oligohydramnios: Risk factors for placental abruption. Obstet Gynecol 104:71, 2004
Ananth CV, Peltier MR, Kinzler WL, et al: Chronic hypertension and risk of placental abruption: Is the association modified by ischemic placental disease? Am J Obstet Gynecol 197:273.e1, 2007
Ananth CV, Smulian JC, Demissie K, et al: Placental abruption among singleton and twin births in the United States: Risk factor profiles. Am J Epidemiol 153:771, 2001b
Ananth CV, Smulian JC, Vintzileos AM: Incidence of placental abruption in relation to cigarette smoking and hypertensive disorders during pregnancy: A meta-analysis of observational studies. Obstet Gynecol 93:622, 1999b
Ananth CV, Smulian JC, Vintzileos AM: The effect of placenta previa on neonatal mortality: A population-based study in the United States, 1989 through 1997. Am J Obstet Gynecol 188:1299, 2003b
Andres RL, Piacquadio KM, Resnik R: A reappraisal of the need for autologous blood donation in the obstetric patient. Am J Obstet Gynecol 163:1551, 1990
Ash A, Smith A, Maxwell D: Caesarean scar pregnancy. BJOG 114:253, 2007
Awad IT, Shorten GD: Amniotic fluid embolism and isolated coagulopathy: Atypical presentation of amniotic fluid embolism. Eur J Anaesthesiol 18:410, 2001

Babinszki A, Kerenyi T, Torok O, et al: Perinatal outcome in grand and great-grand multiparity: Effects of parity on obstetric risk factors. Am J Obstet Gynecol 181:669, 1999

Baglin T: Disseminated intravascular coagulation: Diagnosis and treatment. BMJ 312:683, 1996

Barber A, Shires GT III, Shires GT: Shock. In Schwartz SI, Shires GT, Spencer FC, et al (eds): Principles of Surgery, 7th ed. New York, McGraw-Hill, 1999, p 101

Barbieri RL: Control of massive hemorrhage: Lessons from Iraq reach the U.S. labor and delivery suite. OBG Management 19:8, 2007

Baskett TF: Acute uterine inversion: A review of 40 cases. J Obstet Gynaecol Can 24:953, 2002

Bauer ST, Bonanno C: Abnormal placentation. Semin Perinatol 33:88, 2009

Baxi LV, Liwanpo LI, Fink DJ: D-dimer as a predictor of morbidity in patients with ultrasonographic evidence of placental previa accreta, Abstract 424. J Soc Gynecol Investig 11:215A, 2004

Benirschke K, Kaufmann P (eds): Pathology of the Human Placenta, 4th ed. New York, Springer, 2000, p 554

Benirschke K, Kaufmann P, Baergen R: Pathology of the Human Placenta, 5th ed. New York, Springer, 2006, p 61

Bennett BB: Uterine rupture during induction of labor at term with intravaginal misoprostol. Obstet Gynecol 89:832, 1997

Benson MD, Kobayashi H, Silver RK, et al: Immunologic studies in presumed amniotic fluid embolism. Obstet Gynecol 97:510, 2001

Berg CJ, Chang J, Callaghan WM, et al: Pregnancy-related mortality in the United States, 1991–1997. Obstet Gynecol 101:289, 2003

Berg CJ, MacKay AP, Qin C, et al: Overview of maternal morbidity during hospitalizations for labor and delivery in the United States. 1993–1997 and 2001–2005. Obstet Gynecol 113:1075, 2009

Bhal K, Bhal N, Mulik V, et al: The uterine compression suture—a valuable approach to control major haemorrhage at lower segment caesarean section. J Obstet Gynaecol 24:10, 2005

Bingol N, Fuchs M, Diaz V, et al: Teratogenicity of cocaine in humans. J Pediatr 110:93, 1987

Biswas R, Sawhney H, Dass R, et al: Histopathological study of placental bed biopsy in placenta previa. Acta Obstet Gynecol Scand 78:173, 1999

Bleich AT, Rahn DD, Wieslander CK, et al: Posterior division of the internal iliac artery: Anatomic variations and clinical applications. Am J Obstet Gynecol 197:658.e1, 2007

B-Lynch C: Partial ischemic necrosis of the uterus following a uterine brace compression suture. BJOG 112:126, 2005

B-Lynch CB, Coker A, Laval AH, et al: The B-Lynch surgical technique for control of massive postpartum hemorrhage: An alterative to hysterectomy? Five cases reported. Br J Obstet Gynaecol 104:372, 1997

Bochicchio GV, Napolitano L, Joshi M, et al: Outcome analysis of blood product transfusion in trauma patients: A prospective, risk-adjusted study. World J Surg 32(10):2185, 2008

Bodner LJ, Nosher JL, Grivvin C, et al: Balloon-assisted occlusion of the internal iliac arteries in patients with placenta accreta/percreta. Cardiovasc Intervent Radiol 29:354, 2006

Bond AL, Edersheim TG, Curry L, et al: Expectant management of abruptio placentae before 35 weeks gestation. Am J Perinatol 6:121, 1989

Bonnar J: Massive obstetric haemorrhage. Baillieres Best Pract Res Clin Obstet Gynaecol 14:1, 2000

Bonnar J, McNicol GP, Douglas AS: The behavior of the coagulation and fibrinolytic mechanisms in abruptio placentae. J Obstet Gynaecol Br Commonw 76:799, 1969

Boral LI, Hill SS, Apollon CJ, et al: The type and antibody screen, revisited. Am J Clin Pathol 71:578, 1979

Borgman MA, Spinella PC, Perkins JC, et al: The ratio of blood products transfused affects mortality in patients receiving massive transfusions at a combat support hospital. J Trauma 63:805, 2007

Brame RG, Harbert GM Jr, McGaughey HS Jr, et al: Maternal risk in abruption. Obstet Gynecol 31:224, 1968

Brar HS, Platt LD, DeVore GR, et al: Fetal umbilical velocimetry for the surveillance of pregnancies complicated by placenta previa. J Reprod Med 33:741, 1988

Burchell RC: Physiology of internal iliac artery ligation. J Obstet Gynaecol Br Commonw 75:642, 1968

Burkman RT, Bell WR, Atienza MF, et al: Coagulopathy with midtrimester induced abortion: Association with hyperosmolar urea administration. Am J Obstet Gynecol 127:533, 1977

Busch MP, Kleinman SH, Nemo GJ: Current and emerging infectious risks of blood transfusions. JAMA 289:959, 2003

Butler EL, Dashe JS, Ramus RM: Association between maternal serum alpha-fetoprotein and adverse outcomes in pregnancies with placenta previa. Obstet Gynecol 97:35, 2001

Centers for Disease Control and Prevention: Update: HIV-2 infection among blood and plasma donors—United States, June 1992–June 1995. MMWR 44:603, 1995

Chama CM, Wanonyi IK, Usman JD: From low-lying implantation to placenta praevia: A longitudinal ultrasonic assessment. J Obstet Gynaecol 24:516, 2004

Chang YL, Chang SD, Cheng PJ: Perinatal outcome in patients with placental abruption with and without antepartum hemorrhage. Int J Gynaecol Obstet 75:193, 2001

Chauleur C, Fanget C, Tourne G, et al: Serious primary post-partum hemorrhage, arterial embolization and future fertility: A retrospective study of 46 cases. Hum Reprod 23:1553, 2008

Chescheir NC, Seeds JW: Spontaneous resolution of hypofibrinogenemia associated with death of a twin in utero: A case report. Am J Obstet Gynecol 159:1183, 1988

Chichakli LO, Atrash HK, Mackay AP, et al: Pregnancy-related mortality in the United States due to hemorrhage: 1979–1992. Obstet Gynecol 94:721, 1999

Cho JH, Jun HS, Lee CN: Haemostatic suturing technique or uterine bleeding during cesarean delivery. Obstet Gynecol 96:129, 2000

Cho JY, Kim SJ, Cha KY, et al: Interrupted circular suture: Bleeding control during cesarean delivery in placenta previa accreta. Obstet Gynecol 78:876, 1991

Chou MM, Tseng JJ, Ho ES, et al: Three-dimensional color power Doppler imaging in the assessment of uteroplacental neovascularization in placenta previa increta/percreta. Am J Obstet Gynecol 185:1257, 2001

Chung JW, Jeong HJ, Joh JH, et al: Percutaneous transcatheter angiographic embolization in the management of obstetric hemorrhage. J Reprod Med 48:268, 2003

Clark SL, Belfort MA, Dildy GA, et al: Maternal death in the 21st century: Causes, prevention, and relationship to cesarean delivery. Am J Obstet Gynecol 199:36.e1, 2008

Clark SL, Cotton DB, Gonik B, et al: Central hemodynamic alterations in amniotic fluid embolism. Am J Obstet Gynecol 158:1124, 1988

Clark SL, Hankins GDV, Dudley DA, et al: Amniotic fluid embolism: Analysis of the National Registry. Am J Obstet Gynecol 172:1158, 1995

Clark SL, Pavlova Z, Greenspoon J, et al: Squamous cells in the maternal pulmonary circulation. Am J Obstet Gynecol 154:104, 1986

Clark SL, Phelan JP, Yeh S-Y: Hypogastric artery ligation for obstetric hemorrhage. Obstet Gynecol 66:353, 1985

Cleary-Goldman J, Malone FD, Vidaver J, et al: Impact of maternal age on obstetric outcome. Obstet Gynecol 105:983, 2005

Combs CA, Laros RK Jr: Prolonged third stage of labor: Morbidity and risk factors. Obstet Gynecol 77:863, 1991

Combs CA, Murphy EL, Laros RK Jr: Factors associated with hemorrhage in cesarean deliveries. Obstet Gynecol 77:77, 1991a

Combs CA, Murphy EL, Laros RK Jr: Factors associated with postpartum hemorrhage with vaginal birth. Obstet Gynecol 77:69, 1991b

Combs CA, Nyberg DA, Mack LA, et al: Expectant management after sonographic diagnosis of placental abruption. Am J Perinatol 9:170, 1992

Confidential Enquiry into Maternal and Child Health (CEMACH): Haemorrhage. In Why Mothers Die 2000-2002 report. 2005. Available at http://www.cemach.org.ul/getdoc/b69706f0-5c40-480b-89ea-5ecad87b68e4/Chapter4.aspx. Accessed October 6, 2008

Consensus Development Conference: Perioperative red cell transfusion. Bethesda, MD, National Institutes of Health, Vol 7, No. 4, June 27–29, 1988

Cottier JP, Fignon A, Tranquart F, et al: Uterine necrosis after arterial embolization for postpartum hemorrhage. Obstet Gynecol 100:1074, 2002

Counts RB, Haisch C, Simon TL, et al: Hemostasis in massively transfused trauma patients. Ann Surg 190:91, 1979

Crane JMG, Van Den Hof MC, Dodds L, et al: Neonatal outcomes with placenta previa. Obstet Gynecol 93:541, 1999

Cunningham FG: Genital tract lacerations and puerperal hematomas. In Gilstrap LC III, Cunningham FG, Van Dorsten JP (eds): Operative Obstetrics, 2nd ed. New York, McGraw-Hill, 2002, p 223

Cunningham FG, Hollier LM: Fetal death. In: Williams Obstetrics, 20th ed (Suppl 4). Norwalk, CT, Appleton & Lange, August/September 1997

Dashe JS, McIntire DD, Ramus RM, et al: Persistence of placenta previa according to gestational age at ultrasound detection. Obstet Gynecol 99:692, 2002

Davies S: Amniotic fluid embolism and isolated disseminated intravascular coagulation. Can J Anaesth 46:456, 1999

DeLee JB: A case of fatal hemorrhagic diathesis, with premature detachment of the placenta. Am J Obstet Gynecol 44:785, 1901

Derman RJ, Kodkany BS, Gaudar SS, et al: Oral misoprostol in preventing postpartum haemorrhage in resource-poor communities: A randomized controlled trial. Lancet 368:1248, 2006

Dildy GA, Scott AR, Saffer CS: An effective pressure pack for severe pelvic hemorrhage. Obstet Gynecol 108(5):1222, 2006

Dodd RY: Emerging infections, transfusion safety, and epidemiology. N Engl J Med 349:1205, 2003

Drakeley AJ, Le Roux PA, Anthony J, et al: Acute renal failure complicating severe preeclampsia requiring admission to an obstetric intensive care unit. Am J Obstet Gynecol 186:253, 2002

Drost S, Keil K: Expectant management of placenta previa: Cost-benefit analysis of outpatient treatment. Am J Obstet Gynecol 170:1254, 1994

Druzin ML: Packing of lower uterine segment for control of postcesarean bleeding in instances of placenta previa. Surg Gynecol Obstet 169:543, 1989

Dugoff L, Hobbins JC, Malone FD, et al: First trimester maternal serum PAPP-A and free-beta subunit human chorionic gonadotropin concentrations and nuchal translucency are associated with obstetric complications: A population-based screening study (The FASTER Trial). Am J Obstet Gynecol 191:1446, 2004

Eden RD, Parker RT, Gall SA: Rupture of the pregnant uterus: A 53-year review. Obstet Gynecol 68:671, 1986

Eller AG, Porter TF, Soisson P, et al: Optimal management strategies for placenta accreta. BJOG 116:648, 2009

Elliott JP, Gilpin B, Strong TH Jr, et al: Chronic abruption–oligohydramnios sequence. J Reprod Med 43:418, 1998

Eskes TK: Clotting disorders and placental abruption: Homocysteine—a new risk factor. Eur J Obstet Gynecol Reprod Biol 95:206, 2001

Etchason J, Petz L, Keeler E, et al: The cost effectiveness of preoperative autologous blood donations. N Engl J Med 332:719, 1995

Fahmy K, el-Gazar A, Sammour M, et al: Postpartum colposcopy of the cervix: Injury and healing. Int J Gynaecol Obstet 34:133, 1991

Farine D, Fox HE, Jakobson S, et al: Vaginal ultrasound for diagnosis of placenta previa. Am J Obstet Gynecol 159:566, 1988

Finfer S, Bellomo R, Boyce N, et al: A comparison of albumin and saline for fluid resuscitation in the intensive care unit. N Engl J Med 350:2247, 2004

Fiori O, Deux JF, Kambale JC, et al: Impact of pelvic arterial embolization for intractable postpartum hemorrhage on fertility. Am J Obstet Gynecol 200:384.e1, 2009

Fox H: Placenta accreta, 1945–1969. Obstet Gynecol Surv 27:475, 1972

Franchini M, Lippi G, Franchi M: The use of recombinant activated factor VII in obstetric and gynaecological haemorrhage. BJOG 114:8, 2007

Frederiksen MC, Glassenberg R, Stika CS: Placenta previa: A 22-year analysis. Am J Obstet Gynecol 180:1432, 1999

Fretts RC, Usher RH: Causes of fetal death in women of advanced maternal age. Obstet Gynecol 89:40, 1997

Friederich L, Roman H, Marpeau L: A dangerous development. Am J Obstet Gynecol 196:92, 2007

Fuchs K, Peretz B-A, Marcovici R, et al: The "grand multipara"–is it a problem? A review of 5785 cases. Int J Gynaecol Obstet 23:321, 1985

Furuhashi M, Kurauchi O, Suganuma N: Pregnancy following placental abruption. Arch Gynecol Obstet 267:11, 2002

Gerbasi FR, Bottoms S, Farag A, et al: Increased intravascular coagulation associated with pregnancy. Obstet Gynecol 75:385, 1990

Gerberding JL: Centers for Disease Control and Prevention: Update: Pregnancy-related mortality ratios, by year of death—United States, 1991-1999. MMWR 52:1, 2003

Gerstenfeld TS, Wing DA: Rectal misoprostol versus intravenous oxytocin for the prevention of postpartum hemorrhage after vaginal delivery. Am J Obstet Gynecol 185:878, 2001

Gesteland K, Oshiro B, Henry E, et al: Rates of placenta previa and placental abruption in women delivered only vaginally or only by cesarean section. Abstract No. 403. J Soc Gynecol Investig 11:208A, 2004

Ghezzi F, Cromi A, Uccella S, et al: The Hayman technique: A simple method to treat postpartum haemorrhage. BJOG 114:362, 2007

Gilbert TT, Smulian JC, Martin AA, et al: Obstetric admission to the intensive care unit: Outcomes and severity of illness. Obstet Gynecol 102:897, 2003

Gilbert WM, Danielsen B: Amniotic fluid embolism: Decreased mortality in a population-based study. Obstet Gynecol 93:973, 1999

Gilliam M, Rosenberg D, Davis F: The likelihood of placenta previa with greater number of cesarean deliveries and higher parity. Obstet Gynecol 99:976, 2002

Gilstrap LC III: Management of postpartum hemorrhage. In Gilstrap LC III, Cunningham FG, Van Dorsten JP (eds): Operative Obstetrics, 2nd ed. New York, McGraw-Hill, 2002, p 397

Glantz C, Purnell L: Clinical utility of sonography in the diagnosis and treatment of placental abruption. J Ultrasound Med 21:837, 2002

Goldberg J, Pereira L, Berghella V: Pregnancy after uterine artery embolization. Obstet Gynecol 100:869, 2002

Gonzalez EA, Moore FA, Holcomb JB, et al: Fresh frozen plasma should be given earlier to patients requiring massive transfusion. J Trauma 62:112, 2007

Goodnough LT: Risks of blood transfusion. Crit Care Med 31:S678, 2003

Gottlieb AG, Pandipati S, Davis KM, et al: Uterine necrosis. A complication of uterine compression sutures. Obstet Gynecol 112:429, 2008

Greenberg JI, Suliman A, Iranpour P, et al: Prophylactic balloon occlusion of the internal iliac arteries to treat abnormal placentation: A cautionary case. Am J Obstet Gynecol 197:470.e1, 2007

Grünfeld JP, Pertuiset N: Acute renal failure in pregnancy: 1987. Am J Kidney Dis 4:359, 1987

Handler AS, Mason ED, Rosenberg DL, et al: The relationship between exposure during pregnancy to cigarette smoking and cocaine use and placenta previa. Am J Obstet Gynecol 170:884, 1994

Hankins GDV, Berryman GK, Scott RT Jr, et al: Maternal arterial desaturation with 15-methyl prostaglandin F2 alpha for uterine atony. Obstet Gynecol 72:367, 1988

Hankins GDV, Snyder RR, Clark SL, et al: Acute hemodynamic and respiratory effects of amniotic fluid embolism in the pregnant goat model. Am J Obstet Gynecol 168:1113, 1993

Hankins GDV, Snyder R, Dinh T, et al: Documentation of amniotic fluid embolism via lung histopathology: Fact or fiction? J Reprod Med 47:1021, 2002

Hardardottir H, Borgida AF, Sanders MM, et al: Histologic myometrial fibers adherent to the placenta: Impact of method of placental removal. Am J Obstet Gynecol 174:358, 1996

Harvey C, Hankins G, Clark S: Amniotic fluid embolism and oxygen transport patterns. Am J Obstet Gynecol 174:304, 1996

Hauth JC, Cunningham FG: Preeclampsia-eclampsia. In Lindheimer ML, Roberts JM, Cunningham FG (eds): Chesley's Hypertensive Disorders in Pregnancy, 2nd ed. Stamford, CT, Appleton & Lange, 1999, p 179

Hayman RG, Arulkumaran S, Steer PJ: Uterine compression sutures: Surgical management of postpartum hemorrhage. Obstet Gynecol 99:502, 2002

Hays AME, Worley KC, Roberts SR: Conservative management of placenta percreta. Experience in two cases. Obstet Gynecol 112:1, 2008

Hazelgrove JF, Price C, Pappachan VJ, et al: Multicenter study of obstetric admissions to 14 intensive care units in southern England. Crit Care Med 29:770, 2001

Hebert PC, Wells G, Blajchman MA, et al: A multicenter, randomized, controlled clinical trial of transfusion requirements in critical care. N Engl J Med 340:409, 1999

Henrich W, Fuchs I, Ehrenstein T, et al: Antenatal diagnosis of placenta percreta with planned *in situ* retention and methotrexate therapy in a woman infected with HIV. Ultrasound Obstet Gynecol 20:90, 2002

Hertzberg BS, Bowie JD, Carroll BA, et al: Diagnosis of placenta previa during the third trimester: Role of transperineal sonography. AJR Am J Roentgenol 159:83, 1992

Ho EM, Brown J, Graves W, et al: Maternal death at an inner-city hospital, 1949–2000. Am J Obstet Gynecol 187:1213, 2002

Hofmeyr GJ, Abdel-Aleem H, Abdel-Aleem MA: Uterine massage for preventing postpartum haemorrhage. Cochrane Database Syst Rev CD006431 Jul 16, 2008

Hogberg V, Rasmussen S, Irgens L: The effect of smoking and hypertensive disorders on abruptio placentae in Norway 1999-2002. Acta Obstet Gynecol Scand 86:304, 2007

Hong RW, Greenfield ML, Polley LS: Nitroglycerin for uterine inversion in the absence of placental fragments. Anesth Anal 103:511, 2006

Howard RJ, Straughn JM Jr, Huh WK, et al: Pelvic umbrella pack for refractory obstetric hemorrhage secondary to posterior uterine rupture. Obstet Gynecol 100:1061, 2002

Hsu S, Rodgers B, Lele A, et al: Use of packing in obstetric hemorrhage of uterine origin. J Reprod Med 48:69, 2003

Hung T-H, Shau W-Y, Hsieh C-C, et al: Risk factors for placenta accreta. Obstet Gynecol 93:545, 1999

Hurd WW, Miodovnik M, Hertzberg V, et al: Selective management of abruptio placentae: A prospective study. Obstet Gynecol 61:467, 1983

Jackson BR, Busch MP, Stramer SL, et al: The cost-effectiveness of NAT for HIV, HCV, and HBV in whole-blood donations. Transfusion 43:721, 2003

Jegasothy R: Sudden maternal deaths in Malaysia: A case report. J Obstet Gynaecol Res 28:186, 2002

Jimenez JM, Pritchard JA: Pathogenesis and treatment of coagulation defects resulting from fetal death. Obstet Gynecol 32:449, 1968

Johansson PI, Stensballe J, Rosenberg I, et al: Proactive administration of platelets and plasma for patients with a ruptured abdominal aortic aneurysm: Evaluating a change in transfusion practice. Transfusion 47:593, 2007

Joshi VM, Otiv SR, Majumder R, et al: Internal iliac artery ligation for arresting postpartum haemorrhage. BJOG 114:356, 2007

Joshi VM, Shrivastava M: Partial ischemic necrosis of the uterus following a uterine brace compression suture. BJOG 111:279, 2004

Kaminsky LM, Ananth CV, Prasad V, et al: The influence of maternal cigarette smoking on placental pathology in pregnancies complicated by abruption. Am J Obstet Gynecol 197:275.e1, 2007

Karam AK, Bristow RE, Bienstock J, et al: Argon beam coagulation facilitates management of placenta percreta with bladder invasion. Obstet Gynecol 102:555, 2003

Kayani SI, Walkinshaw SA, Preston C: Pregnancy outcome in severe placental abruption. Br J Obstet Gynaecol 110:679, 2003

Kayem G, Pannier E, Goffinet F, et al: Fertility after conservative treatment of placenta accreta. Fertil Steril 78:637, 2002

Kenny L, Baker P, Cunningham FG: Platelets, coagulation, and the liver. In Lindheimer MD, Roberts JM, Cunningham FG (eds) Chesley's Hypertension in Pregnancy, 3rd ed. New York, Elsevier, 2009, p 335

Kettel LM, Branch DW, Scott JR: Occult placental abruption after maternal trauma. Obstet Gynecol 71:449, 1988

Khong TY: Expression of endothelin-1 in amniotic fluid embolism and possible pathophysiological mechanism. Br J Obstet Gynaecol 105:802, 1998

Kieser KE, Baskett TF: A 10-year population-based study of uterine rupture. Obstet Gynecol 100:749, 2002

King DL: Placental migration demonstrated by ultrasonography. Radiology 109:167, 1973

Knight M, UKOSS: Peripartum hysterectomy in the UK: management and outcomes of the associated haemorrhage. BJOG 114:1380, 2007

Kochenour N: Diagnosis and management of uterine inversion. In Gilstrap LG III, Cunningham FG, VanDorsten JP (eds): Operative Obstetrics. New York, McGraw-Hill, 2002, p 241

Kolomeyevskaya NV, Tanyi JL, Coleman NM, et al: Balloon tamponade of hemorrhage after uterine curettage for gestational trophoblastic disease. Obstet Gynecol 113:557, 2009

Kopko PM, Marshal CS, MacKenzie MR, et al: Transfusion-related acute lung injury: Report of a clinical look-back investigation. JAMA 287:1968, 2002

Kramer MS, Usher RH, Pollack R, et al: Etiologic determinants of abruptio placentae. Obstet Gynecol 89:221, 1997

Kuklina EV, Meikle SG, Jamieson DJ, et al: Severe obstetric morbidity in the United States: 1998–2005. Obstet Gynecol 113:298, 2009

Kupferminc MJ, Eldor A, Steinman N, et al: Increased frequency of genetic thrombophilia in women with complications of pregnancy. N Engl J Med 340:9, 1999

Laine E, Steadman R, Calhoun L, et al: Comparison of RBCs and FFP with whole blood during liver transplant surgery. Transfusion 43:322, 2003

Laing FC: Ultrasound evaluation of obstetric problems relating to the lower uterine segment and cervix. In Fleischer AC, Manning FA, Jeanty P, et al (eds): Sonography in Obstetrics and Gynecology: Principles and Practice, 5th ed. Stamford, CT, Appleton & Lange, 1996, p 720

Lalonde A, Daviss BA, Acosta A, et al: Postpartum hemorrhage today: ICM/FIGO initiative 2004-2006. Int J Obstet Gynaecol 94:243, 2006

Lam H, Pun TC, Lam PW: Successful conservative management of placenta previa accreta during cesarean section. Int J Obstet Gynecol 86:31, 2004

Landy HJ, Weingold AB: Management of a multiple gestation complicated by an antepartum fetal demise. Obstet Gynecol Surv 44:171, 1989

Laughon SK, Wolfe HM, Visco AG: Prior cesarean and the risk for placenta previa on second-trimester ultrasonography. Obstet Gynecol 105:962, 2005

Lax A, Prince MR, Mennitt KW, et al: The value of specific MRI features in the evaluation of suspected placental invasion. Magn Reson Imaging 25:87, 2007

Lee PS, Bakelaar R, Fitpatrick CB, et al: Medical and surgical treatment of placenta percreta to optimize bladder preservation. Obstet Gynecol 112:421, 2008

Lee W, Ginsburg KA, Cotton DB, et al: Squamous and trophoblastic cells in the maternal pulmonary circulation identified by invasive hemodynamic monitoring during the peripartum period. Am J Obstet Gynecol 155:999, 1986

Lerner R, Margolin M, Slate WG, et al: Heparin in the treatment of hypofibrinogenemia complicating fetal death in utero. Am J Obstet Gynecol 97:373, 1967

Leung TY, Chan LW, Tam WH, et al: Risk and prediction of preterm delivery in pregnancies complicated by antepartum hemorrhage of unknown origin before 34 weeks. Gynecol Obstet Invest 52:227, 2001

Leveno KJ, Cunningham FG, Gant NF, et al: Williams Manual of Obstetrics, 1st ed. New York, McGraw-Hill, 2003

Lewis NH, Brunker P, Lemire SJ, et al: Failure of recombinant factor VIIa to correct the coagulopathy in a case of severe postpartum hemorrhage. Transfusion 49:689, 2009

Liang H-S, Jeng C-J, Sheen T-C, et al: First-trimester uterine rupture from a placenta percreta. J Reprod Med 48:474, 2003

Lichtenberg ES: Angiography as treatment for a high cervical tear—a case report. J Reprod Med 48:287, 2003

Lin Y, Callum JL, Coovadia AS, et al: Transfusion of ABO-nonidentical platelets is not associated with adverse clinical outcomes in cardiovascular surgery patients. Transfusion 42:166, 2002

Linden JV, Wagner K, Voytovich AE, et al: Transfusion errors in New York State: An analysis of 10 years' experience. Transfusion 40:1207, 2001

Lindheimer MD, Conrad KP, Karumanchi SA: Renal physiology and disease in pregnancy. In Alpern R (ed): Seldin and Greisch's The Kidney. New York, Elsevier, 2007, p 2361

Lipitz S, Admon D, Menczer J, et al: Midtrimester bleeding: Variables which affect the outcome of pregnancy. Gynecol Obstet Invest 32:24, 1991

Logothetopulos K: Eine absolut sichere Blutstillungsmethode bei vaginalen und abdominalen gynakologischen Operationen. Zentralbl Gynakol 50:3202, 1926

Magpie Trial Collaborative Group: Do women with pre-eclampsia, and their babies, benefit from magnesium sulphate? The Magpie Trial: A randomised placebo-controlled trial. Lancet 359:1877, 2002

Major CA, deVeciana M, Lewis DF, et al: Preterm premature rupture of membranes and abruptio placentae: Is there an association between these pregnancy complications? Am J Obstet Gynecol 172:672, 1995

Mannucci PM, Levi M: Prevention and treatment of major blood loss. N Engl J Med 356:2301, 2007

Marik PE, Corwin HL: Acute lung injury following blood transfusion: Expanding the definition. Crit Care Med 36(11):3080, 2008

Martin JA, Hamilton BE, Sutton PD, et al: Births: Final data for 2003. National Vital Statistics Reports, Vol 54, No 2. Hyattsville, MD, National Center for Health Statistics, 2005

Matsuda Y, Maeda T, Kouno S: Comparison of neonatal outcome including cerebral palsy between abruption placentae and placenta previa. Eur J Obstet Gynecol Reprod Biol 106:125, 2003

Maymon R, Shulman A, Pomeranz M, et al: Uterine rupture at term pregnancy with the use of intracervical prostaglandin E_2 gel for induction of labor. Am J Obstet Gynecol 165:368, 1991

McCormick ML, Sanghvi HC, McIntosh N: Preventing postpartum hemorrhage in low-resource settings. Int J Gynaecol Obstet 77:267, 2002

McVay PA, Hoag RW, Hoag MS, et al: Safety and use of autologous blood donation during the third trimester of pregnancy. Am J Obstet Gynecol 160:1479, 1989

Miller DA, Diaz FG, Paul RH: Incidence of placenta previa with previous cesarean. Am J Obstet Gynecol 174:345, 1996

Miller DA, Goodwin TM, Gherman RB, et al: Intrapartum rupture of the unscarred uterus. Obstet Gynecol 89:671, 1997

Miller DA, Paul RH: Rupture of the unscarred uterus. Am J Obstet Gynecol 174:345, 1996

Mishra A, Landzberg BR, Parente JT: Uterine rupture in association with alkaloidal ("crack") cocaine abuse. Am J Obstet Gynecol 173:243, 1995

Misra DP, Ananth CV: Risk factor profiles of placental abruption in first and second pregnancies: Heterogeneous etiologies. J Clin Epidemiol 52:453, 1999

Morrison JC, Martin RW, Dodson MK, et al: Blood transfusions after postpartum hemorrhage due to uterine atony. J Matern Fetal Invest 1:209, 1991

Mortensen JT, Thulstrup AM, Larsen H, et al: Smoking, sex of the offspring, and risk of placental abruption, placenta previa, and preeclampsia: A population-based cohort study. Acta Obstet Gynecol Scand 80:894, 2001

Mouer JR: Placenta previa: Antepartum conservative management, inpatient versus outpatient. Am J Obstet Gynecol 170:1683, 1994

Mousa HA, Alfirevic Z: Treatment for primary postpartum haemorrhage. Cochrane Database Syst Rev 1: CD003249, 2007

Naef RW III, Chauhan SP, Chevalier SP, et al: Prediction of hemorrhage at cesarean delivery. Obstet Gynecol 83:923, 1994

Naeye RL: Abruptio placentae and placenta previa: Frequency, perinatal mortality, and cigarette smoking. Obstet Gynecol 55:701, 1980

Nagaya K, Fetters MD, Ishikawa M, et al: Causes of maternal mortality in Japan. JAMA 283:2661, 2000

Nath CA, Ananth CV, DeMarco C, et al: Low birthweight in relation to placental abruption and maternal thrombophilia status. Am J Obstet Gynecol 198:293.e1, 2008

Nath CA, Ananth CV, Smulian JC, et al: Histologic evidence of inflammation and risk of placental abruption. Am J Obstet Gynecol 197:319.e1, 2007

National Institutes of Health: Indications for the use of red blood cells, platelets and fresh frozen plasma. Washington, DC, U.S. Department of Health and Human Services, Pub. No. 89-2974A, August 1993

Neilson JP: Interventions for suspected placenta praevia. Cochrane Database Syst Rev 2: CD001998, 2003

Ness PM, Cushing M: Oxygen therapeutics: Pursuit of an alternative to the donor red blood cell. Arch Pathol Lab Med 131(5):734, 2007

Nijman RG, Mantingh A, Aarnoudse JG: Persistent retained placenta percreta: Methotrexate treatment and Doppler flow characteristics. Br J Obstet Gynaecol 109:587, 2002

Nizard J, Barrinque L, Frydman R, et al: Fertility and pregnancy outcomes following hypogastric artery ligation for severe post-partum haemorrhage. Hum Reprod 18:844, 2003

O'Brien P, El-Refaey H, Gordon A, et al: Rectally administered misoprostol for the treatment of postpartum hemorrhage unresponsive to oxytocin and ergometrine: A descriptive study. Obstet Gynecol 92:212, 1998

Ochoa M, Allaire AD, Stitely ML: Pyometra after hemostatic square suture technique. Obstet Gynecol 99:506, 2002

O'Connell KA, Wood JJ, Wise RP, et al: Thromboembolic adverse events after use of recombinant human coagulation Factor VIIa. JAMA 295:293, 2006

Ojala K, Perala J, Kariniemi J, et al: Arterial embolization and prophylactic catheterization for the treatment for severe obstetric hemorrhage. Acta Obstet Gynecol Scand 84:1075, 2005

Oleen MA, Mariano JP: Controlling refractory atonic postpartum hemorrhage with Hemabate sterile solution. Am J Obstet Gynecol 162:205, 1990

Ornan D, White R, Pollak J, et al: Pelvic embolization for intractable postpartum hemorrhage: Long-term follow-up and implications for fertility. Obstet Gynecol 102:904, 2003

Oyelese Y, Smulian JC: Placenta previa, placenta accreta, and vasa previa. Obstet Gynecol 107:927, 2006

Pacheco LD, Van Hook JW, Gei AF: Disseminated intravascular coagulopathy. In Dildy GA, Belfort MA, Saade GR, et al (eds): Critical Care Obstetrics, 4th ed. Malden, MA, Blackwell Science, 2004, p 404

Palacios Jaraquemada JM, Bruno CH: Magnetic resonance imaging in 300 cases of placenta accreta: Surgical correlation of new findings. Acta Obstet Gynecol Scand 84:716, 2005

Pallasmaa N, Ekblad U, Gissler M: Severe maternal morbidity and the mode of delivery. Acta Obstet Gynecol Scand 87:662, 2008

Pealer LN, Marfin AA, Petersen LR, et al: Transmission of West Nile virus through blood transfusion in the United States in 2002. N Engl J Med 349:1236, 2003

Pearlman MD, Tintinalli JE, Lorenz RP: A prospective controlled study of outcome after trauma during pregnancy. Am J Obstet Gynecol 162:1502, 1990

Pelosi MA III, Pelosi MA: Spontaneous uterine rupture at thirty-three weeks subsequent to previous superficial laparoscopic myomectomy. Am J Obstet Gynecol 177:1547, 1997

Peltier LF: Fat embolism: A reappraisal of the problem. Clin Orthop 187:3, 1984

Pereira A, Nunes F, Pedroso S, et al: Compressive uterine sutures to treat postpartum bleeding secondary to uterine atony. Obstet Gynecol 106:569, 2005

Perel P, Roberts I: Colloids versus crystalloids for fluid resuscitation in critically ill patients. Cochrane Database Syst Rev 17:CD000567, 2007

Petersen IR, Nyholm HCJ: Multiple pregnancies with single intrauterine demise. Description of twenty-eight pregnancies. Acta Obstet Gynecol Scand 78:202, 1999

Platt LD, Druzin ML: Acute puerperal inversion of the uterus. Am J Obstet Gynecol 141:187, 1981

Porreo RP, Clark SL, Belfort MA, et al: The changing specter of uterine rupture. Am J Obstet Gynecol 200:269.e1, 2009

Porter TF, Clark SL, Dildy GA, et al: Isolated disseminated intravascular coagulation and amniotic fluid embolism. Am J Obstet Gynecol 174:486, 1996

Price N, B-Lynch C: Technical description of the B-Lynch brace suture for treatment of massive postpartum hemorrhage and review of published cases. Int J Fertil 50:148, 2005

Pritchard JA: Fetal death in utero. Obstet Gynecol 14:573, 1959

Pritchard JA: Changes in the blood volume during pregnancy and delivery. Anesthesiology 26:393, 1965

Pritchard JA: Haematological problems associated with delivery, placental abruption, retained dead fetus, and amniotic fluid embolism. Clin Haematol 2:563, 1973

Pritchard JA, Baldwin RM, Dickey JC, et al: Blood volume changes in pregnancy and the puerperium, 2. Red blood cell loss and changes in apparent blood volume during and following vaginal delivery, cesarean section, and cesarean section plus total hysterectomy. Am J Obstet Gynecol 84:1271, 1962

Pritchard JA, Brekken AL: Clinical and laboratory studies on severe abruptio placentae. Am J Obstet Gynecol 97:681, 1967

Pritchard JA, Cunningham FG, Mason RA: Coagulation changes in eclampsia: Their frequency and pathogenesis. Am J Obstet Gynecol 124:855, 1976

Pritchard JA, Cunningham FG, Pritchard SA, et al: On reducing the frequency of severe abruptio placentae. Am J Obstet Gynecol 165:1345, 1991

Pritchard JA, Mason R, Corley M, et al: Genesis of severe placental abruption. Am J Obstet Gynecol 108:22, 1970

Pritchard JA, Whalley PJ: Abortion complicated by Clostridium perfringens infection. Am J Obstet Gynecol 111:484, 1971

Propst AM, Thorp JM Jr: Traumatic vulvar hematomas: Conservative versus surgical management. South Med J 91:144, 1998

Rachagan SP, Raman S, Balasundram G, et al: Rupture of the pregnant uterus—a 21-year review. Aust NZ J Obstet Gynaecol 31:37, 1991

Rahman MH, Akhter HH, Khan Chowdhury ME, et al: Obstetric deaths in Bangladesh, 1996–1997. Int J Gynaecol Obstet 77:161, 2002

Rainaldi MP, Tazzari PL, Scagliarini G, et al: Blood salvage during caesarean section. Br J Anesth 81(5):825, 1998

Rani PR, Haritha PH, Gowri R: Comparative study of transperineal and transabdominal sonography in the diagnosis of placenta previa. J Obstet Gynaecol 33:134, 2007

Rasmussen S, Irgens LM: Occurrence of placental abruption in relatives. BJOG 116:693, 2009

Rebarber A, Fox NS, Eckstein DA, et al: Successful bilateral uterine artery embolization during an ongoing pregnancy. Obstet Gynecol 113:554, 2009

Reyal F, Sibony O, Oury JF, et al: Criteria for transfusion in severe postpartum hemorrhage: Analysis of practice and risk factors. Eur J Obstet Gynecol Reprod Biol 112:61, 2004

Rice JP, Kay HH, Mahony BS: The clinical significance of uterine leiomyomas in pregnancy. Am J Obstet Gynecol 160:1212, 1989

Ridgway LE: Puerperal emergency: Vaginal and vulvar hematomas. Obstet Gynecol Clin North Am 22:275, 1995

Robson S, Adair S, Bland P: A new surgical technique for dealing with uterine inversion. Aust NZ J Obstet Gynaecol 45:250, 2005

Roman AS, Rebarber A: Seven ways to control postpartum hemorrhage. Contemp Ob/Gyn, March 2003, p 34

Rotas MA, Haberman S, Luvgur M: Cesarean scar ectopic pregnancies: Etiology, diagnosis, and management. Obstet Gynecol 107:1373, 2006

Rouse DJ, MacPherson C, Landon M, et al: Blood transfusion and cesarean delivery. Obstet Gynecol 108:891, 2006

Sachs BP, Brown DA, Driscoll SG, et al: Maternal mortality in Massachusetts. Trends and prevention. N Engl J Med 316:667, 1987

Sachs DA: Blood and component therapy in obstetrics. In Clark SL, Cotton DB, Hankins GDV, et al (eds): Critical Care Obstetrics, 2nd ed. Boston, Blackwell, 1991, p 599

Salihu HM, Bekan B, Aliyu MH, et al: Perinatal mortality associated with abruptio placenta in singletons and multiples. Am J Obstet Gynecol 193:198, 2005

Salihu HM, Li Q, Rouse DJ, et al: Placenta previa: Neonatal death after live births in the United States. Am J Obstet Gynecol 188:1305, 2003

Sanderson DA, Milton PJD: The effectiveness of ultrasound screening at 18–20 weeks gestational age for predication of placenta previa. J Obstet Gynaecol 11:320, 1991

Saraiya M, Green CA, Berg CJ, et al: Spontaneous abortion-related deaths among women in the United States—1981–1991. Obstet Gynecol 94:172, 1999

Sentilhes L, Gromez A, Clavier E, et al: Predictors of failed pelvic arterial embolization for severe postpartum hemorrhage. Obstet Gynecol 113:992, 2009

Sewell MF, Rosenblum D, Ehrenberg H: Arterial embolus during common iliac balloon catheterization at cesarean hysterectomy. Obstet Gynecol 108:746, 2006

Shaz BH, Dente CJ, Harris RS, et al: Transfusion management of trauma patients. Anesth Analg 108:1760, 2009

Sherman SJ, Greenspoon JS, Nelson JM, et al: Identifying the obstetric patient at high risk of multiple-unit blood transfusions. J Reprod Med 37:649, 1992

Shoemaker WC, Kram HB: Comparison of the effects of crystalloids and colloids on hemodynamic oxygen transport, mortality and morbidity. In Simmons RS, Udeko AJ (eds): Debates in General Surgery. Chicago, Year Book, 1991

Sholl JS: Abruptio placentae: Clinical management in nonacute cases. Am J Obstet Gynecol 156:40, 1987

Sibai BM, Lindheimer M, Hauth J, et al: Risk factors for preeclampsia, abruptio placentae, and adverse neonatal outcomes among women with chronic hypertension. N Engl J Med 339:667, 1998

Silliman CC, Boshkov LK, Mehdizadehkashi Z, et al: Transfusion-related acute lung injury: Epidemiology and a prospective analysis of etiologic factors. Blood 101:454, 2003

Silver RM, Landon MB, Rouse DJ, et al: Maternal morbidity associated with multiple repeat cesarean deliveries. Obstet Gynecol 107:1226, 2006

Singla AK, Lapinski RH, Berkowitz RL, et al: Are women who are Jehovah's Witnesses at risk of maternal death? Am J Obstet Gynecol 185:893, 2001

Sloan EP, Koenigsberg M, Gens D, et al: Diaspirin cross-linked hemoglobin (DCLHb) in the treatment of severe traumatic hemorrhagic shock: A randomized controlled efficacy trial. JAMA 282:1857, 1999

Smith RS, Lauria MR, Comstock CH, et al: Transvaginal ultrasonography for all placentas that appear to be low-lying or over the internal cervical os. Ultrasound Obstet Gynecol 9:22, 1997

Sosa CG, Alathabe F, Belizan JM, et al: Risk factors for postpartum hemorrhage in vaginal deliveries in a Latin-American population. Obstet Gynecol 113:1313, 2009

Spiess BD: Perfluorocarbon emulsions as a promising technology: A review of tissue and vascular gas dynamics. J Appl Physiol 106:1444, 2009

Spinella PC, Perkins JC, Grathwohl KW, et al: Fresh whole blood transfusions in coalition military, foreign national, and enemy combatant patients during Operation Iraqi Freedom at a U.S. combat support hospital. World J Surg 32:2, 2008

Stafford I, Belfort MA: Placenta accrete, increta, and percreta: A team-based approach starts with prevention. Contemp Ob/Gyn April:77, 2008

Stafford PA, Biddinger PW, Zumwalt RE: Lethal intrauterine fetal trauma. Am J Obstet Gynecol 159:485, 1988

Stanten RD, Iverson LI, Daugharty TM, et al: Amniotic fluid embolism causing catastrophic pulmonary vasoconstriction: Diagnosis by transesophageal echocardiogram and treatment by cardiopulmonary bypass. Obstet Gynecol 102:496, 2003

Steinauer JE, Diedrich JT, Wilson MW, et al: Uterine artery embolization in postabortion hemorrhage. Obstet Gynecol 11:881, 2008

Steiner PE, Lushbaugh CC: Maternal pulmonary embolism by amniotic fluid. JAMA 117:1245, 1941

Stettler RW, Lutich A, Pritchard JA, et al: Traumatic placental abruption: A separation from traditional thought. Presented at the American College of Obstetricians and Gynecologists Annual Clinical Meeting, Las Vegas, April 27, 1992

Stolte L, van Kessel H, Seelen J, et al: Failure to produce the syndrome of amniotic fluid embolism by infusion of amniotic fluid and meconium into monkeys. Am J Obstet Gynecol 98:694, 1967

Stramer SL, Glynn SA, Kleinman SH, et al: Detection of HIV-I and HCV infections among antibody-negative blood donors by nucleic acid–amplification testing. N Engl J Med 351:760, 2004

Taipale P, Hiilesmaa V, Ylostalo P: Transvaginal ultrasonography at 18–23 weeks in predicting placenta previa at delivery. Ultrasound Obstet Gynecol 12:422, 1998

Tikkanen M, Nuutila M, Hiilesmaa V, et al: Prepregnancy risk factors for placental abruption. Acta Obstet Gynecol Scand 85:40, 2006

Timmermans S, van Hof AC, Duvekot JJ: Conservative management of abnormally invasive placentation. Obstet Gynecol 62:529, 2007

Timor-Tritsch IE, Yunis RA: Confirming the safety of transvaginal sonography in patients suspected of placenta previa. Obstet Gynecol 81:742, 1993

Toivonen S, Heinonen S, Anttila M, et al: Reproductive risk factors, Doppler findings, and outcome of affected births in placental abruption: A population-based analysis. Am J Perinatol 19:451, 2002

Toledo P, McCarthy RJ, Hewlett BJ, et al: The accuracy of blood loss estimation after simulated vaginal delivery. Anesth Analg 105:1736, 2007

Toohey JS, Keegan KA Jr, Morgan MA, et al: The "dangerous multipara": Fact or fiction? Am J Obstet Gynecol 172:683, 1995

Towell ME: Fetal acid–base physiology and intrauterine asphyxia. In Goodwin JW, Godden JO, Chance GW (eds): Perinatal Medicine. Baltimore, Williams & Wilkins, 1976, p 200

Towers CV, Pircon RA, Heppard M: Is tocolysis safe in the management of third-trimester bleeding? Am J Obstet Gynecol 180:1572, 1999

Treloar EJ, Anderson RS, Andrews HG, et al: Uterine necrosis following B-Lynch suture for primary postpartum haemorrhage. BJOG 113:486, 2006

Twickler DM, Lucas MJ, Balis AB, et al: Color flow mapping for myometrial invasion in women with a prior cesarean delivery. J Matern Fetal Med 9:330, 2000

Usta IM, Hobeika EM, Abu Musa AA, et al: Placenta previa-accreta: Risk factors and complications. Am J Obstet Gynecol 193:1045, 2005

Van Vugt PJH, Baudoin P, Blom VM, et al: Inversio uteri puerperalis. Acta Obstet Gynecol Scand 60:353, 1981

Villar J, Gülmezoglu AM, Hofmeyr GJ, et al: Systematic review of randomized controlled trials of misoprostol to prevent postpartum hemorrhage. Obstet Gynecol 100:1301, 2002

Ward CR: Avoiding an incision through the anterior previa at cesarean delivery. Obstet Gynecol 102:552, 2003

Warshak CR, Eskander R, Hull AD, et al: Accuracy of ultrasonography and magnetic resonance imaging in the diagnosis of placenta accreta. Obstet Gynecol 108:573, 2006

Watson P, Besch N, Bowes WA Jr: Management of acute and subacute puerperal inversion of the uterus. Obstet Gynecol 55:12, 1980

Weiss JL, Malone FD, Vidaver J, et al: Threatened abortion: A risk factor for poor pregnancy outcome, a population-based screening study. Am J Obstet Gynecol 190:745, 2004

Weiwen Y: Study of the diagnosis and management of amniotic fluid embolism: 38 cases of analysis. Obstet Gynecol 95:385, 2000

Williams MA, Mittendorf R, Lieberman E, et al: Cigarette smoking during pregnancy in relation to placenta previa. Am J Obstet Gynecol 165:28, 1991

Wing DA, Paul RH, Millar LK: Management of the symptomatic placenta previa: A randomized, controlled trial of inpatient versus outpatient expectant management. Am J Obstet Gynecol 174:305, 1996a

Wing DA, Paul RH, Millar LK: The usefulness of coagulation studies and blood banking in the symptomatic placenta previa. Am J Obstet Gynecol 174:346, 1996b

Witlin AG, Saade GR, Mattar F, et al: Risk factors for abruptio placentae and eclampsia: Analysis of 445 consecutively managed women with severe preeclampsia and eclampsia. Am J Obstet Gynecol 180:1322, 1999

Worley KC, Hnat MD, Cunningham FG: Advanced extrauterine pregnancy: Diagnostic and therapeutic challenges. Am J Obstet Gynecol 198:297.e1, 2008

You WB, Zahn CM: Postpartum hemorrhage: Abnormally adherent placenta, uterine inversion, and puerperal hematomas. Clin Obstet Gynecol 49:184, 2006

Yu PC, Ou HY, Tsang LC, et al: Prophylactic intraoperative uterine artery embolization to control hemorrhage in abnormal placentation during late gestation. Fertil Steril 91(5):1951, 2009

Zahn CM, Yeomans ER: Postpartum hemorrhage: Placenta accreta, uterine inversion and puerperal hematomas. Clin Obstet Gynecol 33:422, 1990

Zaki ZM, Bahar AM, Ali ME, et al: Risk factors and morbidity in patients with placenta previa accreta compared to placenta previa non-accreta. Acta Obstet Gynecol Scand 77:391, 1998

Zeeman GG, Cunningham FG, Pritchard JA: The magnitude of hemocontration with eclampsia. Hypertension Preg, 28(2):127, 2009

Zeeman GG, Wendel Jr GD, Cunningham FG: A blueprint for obstetric critical care. Am J Obstet Gynecol 188:532, 2003

Zelop CM, Harlow BL, Frigoletto FD Jr, et al: Emergency peripartum hysterectomy. Am J Obstet Gynecol 168:1443, 1993

Zetterstrom K, Lindeberg SN, Haglund B, et al: Maternal complications in women with chronic hypertension: A population-based cohort study. Acta Obstet Gynecol Scand 84:419, 2005

Zhou J, Liu S, Ma M, et al: Procoagulant activity and phosphatidylserine of amniotic fluid cells. Thromb Haemost 101:795, 2009

Zwart JJ, Richters JM, Öry F, et al: Severe maternal morbidity during pregnancy, delivery and puerperium in the Netherlands: A nationwide population-based study of 371,000 pregnancies. BJOG 115:842, 2008

Preterm Birth

Low birthweight defines neonates who are born too small. *Preterm or premature births* are terms used to define neonates who are born too early. With respect to gestational age, a newborn may be preterm, term, or postterm. With respect to size, a newborn may be normally grown and *appropriate for gestational age*; small in size, thus, *small for gestational age*; or overgrown and consequently, *large for gestational age*. In recent years, the term *small for gestational age* has been widely used to categorize newborns whose birthweight is usually below the 10th percentile for gestational age. Other frequently used terms have included *fetal-growth restriction* or *intrauterine growth restriction*. The term *large for gestational age* has been widely used to categorize newborns whose birthweight is above the 90th percentile for gestational age. The term *appropriate for gestational age* designates newborns whose weight is between the 10th and 90th percentiles. Thus, infants born before term can be small or large for gestational age but still fit the definition of preterm. *Low birthweight* refers to

births 500 to 2500 g; *very low birthweight* refers to births 500 to 1500 g; and *extremely low birthweight* refers to births 500 to 1000 g. In 1960, a neonate weighing 1000 g had a 95-percent risk of death. Today, a neonate with the same birthweight has a 95-percent chance of surviving (Ingelfinger, 2007). This remarkable improvement in survival is due to the widespread application of neonatal intensive care in the early 1970s.

MORTALITY RATES OF PRETERM INFANTS

In the United States in 2005, 28,384 infants died in their first year of life (Table 36-1). *Preterm birth*, which is defined as delivery before 37 completed weeks, was implicated in approximately two thirds of these deaths. As shown in Table 36-1, *late preterm births*, defined as those 34 to 36 weeks' gestation, composed approximately 70 percent of all preterm births. As discussed in Chapter 1 (p. 4), although the infant mortality rate for the United States has declined substantively over the past century, it has remained static from 2000 to 2005 (MacDorman and Matthews, 2008). Thus, the issue of preterm birth remains a major health problem.

The rates of preterm birth—the largest contributor to infant mortality—began to increase in the United States in 1996. As shown in Figure 36-1, medically indicated preterm births are largely responsible for this rise. Equally disturbing is the persistent racial disparity such that black infants are twice as likely to die within the first year of life, and almost two thirds of this disparity can be attributed to preterm birth (Schempf and colleagues, 2007). Some investigators attribute this inequity to class (racial) disparities in health related to socioeconomic issues (Collins and co-workers, 2007). Rates of preterm birth in the United States are also higher compared with those of other industrialized countries (Ananth and associates, 2009; Joseph and colleagues, 2007). For example, the preterm birth rate was 12.3 percent in the United States in 2003 compared with 7.7 percent in Canada. Part of this difference has been attributed

TABLE 36-1. Infant Mortality Rates in the United States in 2005

	Live Births No. (%)	Infant Deaths No. (%)
Total infants	4,138,573 (100)	28,384 (100)
Gestational age at birth		
<32 weeks	83,428 (2)	15,287 (54)
32–33 weeks	65,853 (1.6)	1099 (4)
34–36 weeks	373,663 (9)	1727 (10)
37–41 weeks	3,346,237 (81)	8116 (29)
≥42 weeks	239,850 (6)	637 (2)
Unknown	29,542 (0.7)	516 (2)

Adapted from Mathews and MacDorman (2008).

to the use of menstrual dates for calculation of gestational age in the United States compared with the use of clinical estimates in Canada.

MORBIDITY IN PRETERM INFANTS

A variety of morbidities, largely due to organ system immaturity, are significantly increased in infants born before 37 weeks' gestation compared with those delivered at term (Table 36-2). For

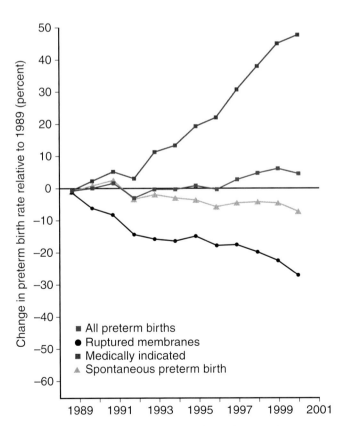

FIGURE 36-1 Rates of births < 37 weeks in the United States from 1989 to 2001. (Reprinted from Ananth CV, Joseph KS, Oyelese Y, et al: Trends in preterm birth and perinatal mortality among singletons: United States, 1989 through 2000, *Obstetrics & Gynecology,* 2005, vol. 105, no. 5, pt. 1, pp. 1084–1091, with permission.)

approximately 40 years, complications in infants born before 34 weeks have been the primary focus. Only recently, *late preterm* infants—34 to 36 weeks—have gained attention because of increased morbidity rates compared with those of term infants. Attention has also been given to increasingly small preterm infants—very low-birthweight and extremely low-birthweight. These infants predominantly suffer not only the immediate complications of prematurity but also long-term sequelae such as neurodevelopmental disability. Indeed, live births once considered "abortuses" because they weighed less than 500 g are now classified as live births. There were 6666 such births recorded in the United States in 2006 (Martin and colleagues, 2009). Remarkable strides have been made in neonatal survival for infants born preterm. This is especially true for those born after 28 weeks. Shown in Figure 36-2 are survival rates for more than 18,000 infants born between 400 and 1500 g or between 22 and 32 weeks' gestation (Fanaroff and associates, 2007). Importantly, the results are shown as a function of both birthweights *and* gestational age. After achieving a birthweight of ≥ 1000 g or a gestational age of 28 weeks (for females) to 30 weeks (for males), survival rates reach 95 percent.

Resources used to care for low-birthweight infants are a measure of the societal burden of preterm birth. The immediate economic costs of preterm birth alone were estimated to exceed $18 billion in 2003. This represented half of all hospital charges for newborn care in the United States (Behrman and Butler, 2007). The economic consequences of preterm birth that reach beyond the newborn period into infancy, adolescence, and adulthood have not been estimated but must be enormous when the effects of adult diseases associated with prematurity such as hypertension and diabetes are considered (Hofman, 2004; Hovi, 2007; Ingelfinger, 2007; Kaijser, 2009, and all their co-workers).

MORTALITY AND MORBIDITY AT THE LOWER AND UPPER EXTREMES OF PREMATURITY

The tremendous advances in the perinatal and neonatal care of the preterm infant have been found predominantly in those infants delivered at ≤ 33 weeks. With survival of increasingly very immature infants in the 1990s, there has been uncertainty and controversy as to the lower limit of fetal maturation compatible

TABLE 36-2. Major Short- and Long-Term Problems in Very-Low-Birthweight Infants

Organ or System	Short-Term Problems	Long-Term Problems
Pulmonary	Respiratory distress syndrome, air leak, bronchopulmonary dysplasia, apnea of prematurity	Bronchopulmonary dysplasia, reactive airway disease, asthma
Gastrointestinal or nutritional	Hyperbilirubinemia, feeding intolerance, necrotizing enterocolitis, growth failure	Failure to thrive, short-bowel syndrome, cholestasis
Immunological	Hospital-acquired infection, immune deficiency, perinatal infection	Respiratory syncytial virus infection, bronchiolitis
Central nervous system	Intraventricular hemorrhage, periventricular leukomalacia, hydrocephalus	Cerebral palsy, hydrocephalus, cerebral atrophy, neurodevelopmental delay, hearing loss
Ophthalmological	Retinopathy of prematurity	Blindness, retinal detachment, myopia, strabismus
Cardiovascular	Hypotension, patent ductus arteriosus, pulmonary hypertension	Pulmonary hypertension, hypertension in adulthood
Renal	Water and electrolyte imbalance, acid–base disturbances	Hypertension in adulthood
Hematological	Iatrogenic anemia, need for frequent transfusions, anemia of prematurity	
Endocrinological	Hypoglycemia, transiently low thyroxine levels, cortisol deficiency	Impaired glucose regulation, increased insulin resistance

From Eichenwald and Stark (2008) with permission.

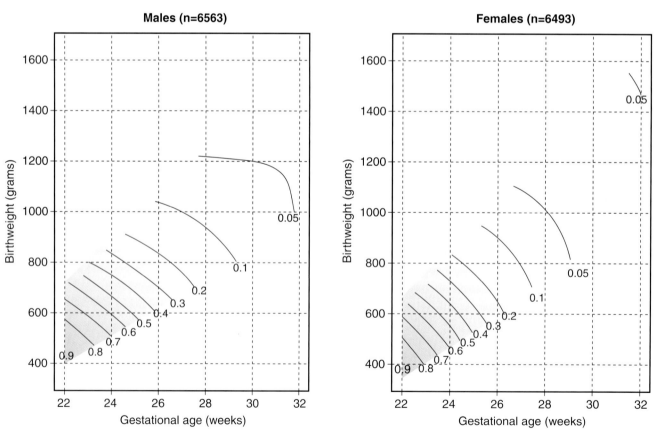

FIGURE 36-2 Mortality rates by birthweight, gestational age, and gender. The limits of the colored area indicate the upper 95th and lower 5th percentiles of birthweight for each gestational age. The curved lines indicate combinations of birthweight and gestational age with the same estimated probability of mortality from 10 to 90 percent. The gradation of color denotes the change in estimated probability of death—green indicates infants of lower gestational age and birthweight who are more likely to die; yellow indicates infants of higher gestational ages and birthweights who are less likely to die. The methods used underestimate mortality rates in those at 22 and 23 weeks with a birthweight up to 600 g. (From Fanaroff and associates, 2007, with permission.)

TABLE 36-3. Overall Survival and Survival with Selected Complications among Very-Low-Birthweight Infants

| Outcome | Birthweight Groups | | | |
	501–750 g (n = 4046)	751–1000 g (n = 4266)	1001–1250 g (n = 4557)	1251–1500 g (n = 5284)
Overall survival (percent)	55	88	94	96
Survival with complications (percent)	65	43	22	11
Bronchopulmonary dysplasia alone	42	25	11	4
Severe intraventricular hemorrhage alone	5	6	5	4
Necrotizing enterocolitis alone	3	3	3	2
Bronchopulmonary dysplasia and severe intraventricular hemorrhage	10	4	2	<1

Data from National Institute of Child Health and Human Development Neonatal Research Network, 1997 to 2002. From Fanaroff and colleagues (2007) as adapted by Eichenwald and Stark (2008), with permission.

with extrauterine survival. This has resulted in continual re-assessment of the *threshold of viability.*

Threshold of Viability

It appears generally accepted that births before 26 weeks, especially those weighing less than 750 g, are at the current threshold of viability and that these preterm infants pose a variety of complex medical, social, and ethical considerations (American College of Obstetricians and Gynecologists, 2002, 2008c). For example, Sidney Miller is a child who was born at 23 weeks, weighed 615 g, and survived but developed severe physical and mental impairment (Annas, 2004). At age 7 years, she was described as a child who "could not walk, talk, feed herself, or sit up on her own . . . was legally blind, suffered from severe mental retardation, cerebral palsy, seizures and spastic quadriparesis in her limbs." An important issue for her family was the need for a lifetime of medical care estimated to cost tens of millions of dollars.

According to current guidelines developed by the American Academy of Pediatrics (Braner and co-workers, 2000), it is considered appropriate not to initiate resuscitation for infants younger than 23 weeks or those whose birthweight is less than 400 g. The involvement of the family is considered critical to the decision-making process with regard to resuscitation. Thus, infants now considered to be at the threshold of viability are those born at 22, 23, 24, or 25 weeks. These infants have been described as fragile and vulnerable because of their immature organ systems (Vohr and Allen, 2005). Moreover, they are at high risk for brain injury from hypoxic-ischemia injury and sepsis (Stoll and associates, 2004). In this setting, hypoxia and sepsis start a cascade of events that lead to brain hemorrhage, white-matter injury that causes periventricular leukomalacia, and poor subsequent brain growth eventuating in neurodevelopmental impairment (see Chap. 29, p. 610). It is thought that because active brain development normally occurs throughout the second and third trimesters, those infants born at 22 to 25 weeks are especially vulnerable to brain injury because of their extreme immaturity.

Considerable outcome data for preterm live births between 22 and 25 weeks have become available since the last edition of

this textbook. Shown in Table 36-3 are rates of overall survival as well as survival with selected complications in 250-g birthweight increments for very-low-birthweight infants. Of those with birthweights 500 to 750 g, only 55 percent survived, and most had severe complications. Survival, even with no complications apparent at initial hospital discharge, does not preclude serious developmental impairment at age 8 to 9 years (Fig. 36-3). Importantly, survival of very low-birthweight infants with and without complications of prematurity was not substantially improved when two epochs—1997 to 2002 and 1995 to 1996 are compared (Eichenwald and Stark, 2008). Saigal and Doyle (2008) collated 16 reports based on geographically defined cohorts from Australia and several European countries. Survival increased progressively from 1.7 percent at 22 weeks to 54 percent at 25 weeks. Overall, 25 percent of infants born at 22 to 25 weeks had severe neurological disabilities, and 72 percent of those with birthweights < 750 g experienced difficulty in school. Marlow and colleagues (2005) identified all infants born between 22 and 25 weeks in the United Kingdom and Ireland between March and December 1995 and examined the children at age 6 years. As shown in Table 36-4, survival was

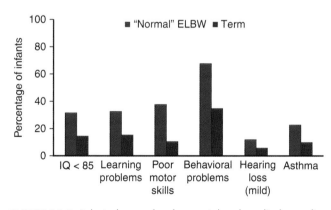

FIGURE 36-3 Selected neurodevelopmental and medical complications at age 8 to 9 years in children with extremely low birthweight (ELBW) but with no apparent neurosensory abnormalities at initial hospital discharge. IQ = intelligence quotient. (Data from Hack and colleagues, 2005, as adapted by Eichenwald and Stark, 2008, with permission.)

TABLE 36-4. 6-Year Outcomes of Surviving Infants Born from 22 to 25 Weeks in the United Kingdom in 1995

Outcomes	Gestational Age (weeks)			
	22	23	24	25
Live births	138	241	382	424
Surviving infants	2 (1)	25 (10)	98 (26)	183 (43)
Without moderate to severe disability at age 6 years	1 (0.7)	8 (3)	36 (9)	86 (20)

Data shown as number (percent).
Adapted from Marlow and colleagues (2005).

rare at 22 weeks—only 2 of 138 infants lived. This rate increased to 10 percent, 26 percent, and 43 percent, at 23, 24 and 25 weeks, respectively. Moderate to severe disability at age 6 years was identified in more than 90 percent of infants surviving following birth at 22 to 24 weeks. As shown in Figure 36-4, cognitive scores were much lower for infants born at 22 to 25 weeks compared with those of normal term births.

The reported results from the Neonatal Research Network were made available by Tyson and associates (2008). A total of 4192 infants born at 22 to 25 weeks and undergoing neurodevelopmental testing at age 18 to 22 months were studied prospectively. A total of 61 percent died or had profound impairment. Interestingly, only 23 percent of infants born at 22 weeks received intensive care compared with 99 percent at 25 weeks. Importantly, female gender, singleton pregnancy, corticosteroids given for lung maturation, and higher gestational age improved the prognosis for these infants born at the threshold of viability.

Cesarean delivery at the threshold of viability is controversial. For example, if the fetus-infant is perceived to be too immature for aggressive support, then cesarean delivery for common indications such as breech presentation or nonreassuring fetal heart rate patterns might be preempted. This aside, national data clearly show a high frequency of cesarean delivery for the smallest infants (Fig. 36-5). Moreover, neonatal mortality rates in the very smallest infants—500 to 700 g—are approximately half if cesarean delivery is used compared with vaginal birth (Fig. 36-6). But this apparent advantage of cesarean delivery vis-à-vis survival is not the whole story. Louis and colleagues (2004) compared outcomes by route of delivery for infants born at 23 to 26 weeks during two epochs. Deliveries from 1990 through 1995 were compared with births between 1996 and 2001. There were 31 percent cesarean deliveries in the first epoch for malpresentation or nonreassuring fetal heart rate, and this increased significantly to 47 percent in the later epoch. Although this increase in cesarean use was associated with increased survival, it was not associated with a reduction in the short-term serious morbidities in infants born at the threshold of viability. Cazan-London and co-workers (2005) analyzed willingness or unwillingness to perform cesarean delivery at 24 weeks. They found that although survival increased with willingness, so too did survival with major morbidity. They stressed that both absolute survival and long-term handicaps must be considered when proceeding with aggressive intervention in extremely preterm pregnancies.

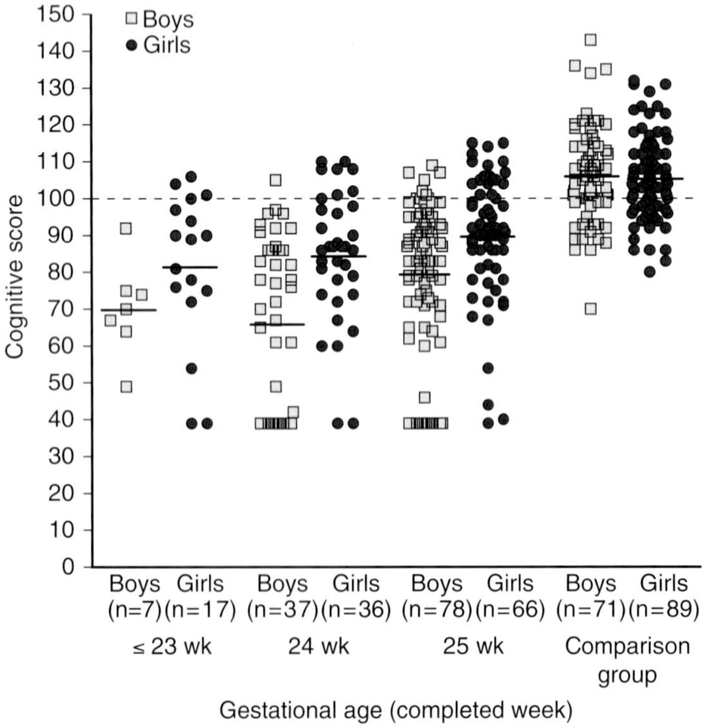

FIGURE 36-4 Cognitive scores for infants born at 22 to 23 weeks, 24 weeks, and 25 weeks compared with those for normal infants delivered at term. (From Marlow and colleagues, 2005, with permission).

Policy for Threshold of Viability at Parkland Hospital

Policies were developed in conjunction with the Neonatology Service. We must emphasize that the decision not to perform cesarean delivery does not necessarily imply

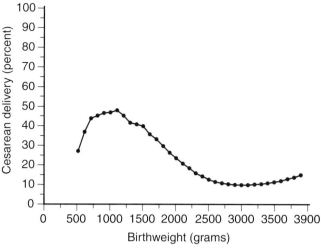

FIGURE 36-5 U.S. cesarean delivery rates by birthweight from 1999 to 2000. (Reprinted from Lee HC, Gould JB: Survival advantage associated with cesarean delivery in very low birth weight vertex neonates, *Obstetrics & Gynecology,* 2006, vol. 107, no. 1, pp. 97–105, with permission.)

that the fetus is "nonviable" or "written off." Neonatologists are consulted before delivery, and there is discussion of survival and morbidity with the woman and her family. A neonatologist attends each delivery and determines subsequent management.

From an obstetrical standpoint, all fetal indications for cesarean delivery in more advanced pregnancies are practiced in women at 25 weeks. Cesarean delivery is not offered for fetal indications at 23 weeks. At 24 weeks, cesarean delivery is not offered unless fetal weight is estimated at 750 g or greater. Aggressive obstetrical management is practiced in cases of growth restriction.

Late Preterm Birth

Infants between 34 and 36 weeks account for approximately 75 percent of all preterm births, as shown in Figure 36-7, and are the fastest increasing and largest proportion of singleton preterm births in the United States (Raju and colleagues, 2006).

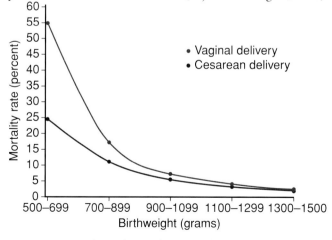

FIGURE 36-6 Birthweight-specific neonatal mortality rate by mode of delivery in the United States from 1999 to 2000. (Reprinted from Lee HC, Gould JB: Survival advantage associated with cesarean delivery in very low birth weight vertex neonates, *Obstetrics & Gynecology,* 2006, vol. 107, no. 1, pp. 97–105, with permission.)

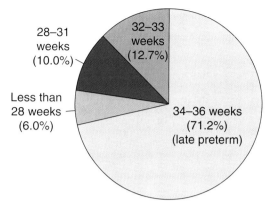

FIGURE 36-7 Percent distribution of preterm births in the United States for 2004. (From Martin and colleagues, 2006.)

As such, late preterm birth is receiving increased attention as to optimal obstetrical and neonatal management.

To estimate the risks associated with late preterm births, we analyzed neonatal mortality and morbidity rates at 34, 35, and 36 weeks compared with those of births at term between 1988 and 2005 at Parkland Hospital (McIntire and Leveno, 2008). We were particularly interested in obstetrical complications during this time, because if modified, rates of late preterm birth can possibly be decreased. Approximately 3 percent of births during the study period occurred between 24 and 32 weeks, and 9 percent were during the late preterm weeks. Thus, late preterm births accounted for three fourths of all preterm births. Approximately 80 percent of late preterm births were due to idiopathic spontaneous preterm labor or prematurely ruptured membranes (Fig. 36-8). Complications such as hypertension or placental accidents were implicated in approximately 20 percent of cases.

Neonatal mortality rates were significantly increased in each late preterm week compared with those at 39 weeks as the referent and as shown in Figure 36-9. Similarly, Tomashek and co-workers (2007) analyzed all United States births between 1995 and 2002 and also found increased neonatal mortality rates for late preterm infants. Importantly, indices of neonatal morbidity shown in Table 36-5 are increased in late preterm infants born

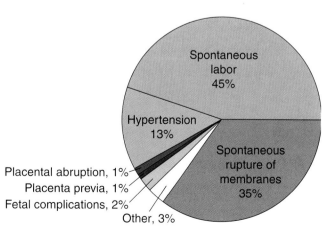

FIGURE 36-8 Obstetrical complications associated with 21,771 late preterm births at Parkland Hospital. (Adapted from McIntire and Leveno, 2008.)

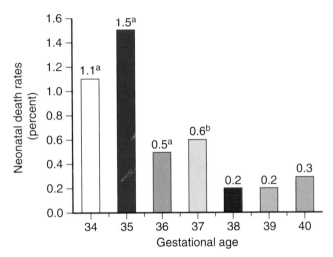

FIGURE 36-9 Neonatal death rates at Parkland Hospital from 34 to 40 weeks' gestation in singleton infants without malformations. [a]$p < .001$ compared with 39 weeks as the referent. [b]$p = .02$ compared with 39 weeks as the referent. (Reprinted from McIntire DD, Leveno KJ: Neonatal mortality and morbidity rates in late preterm births compared with births at term, *Obstetrics & Gynecology*, 2008, vol. 111, no. 1, pp. 35–41, with permission.)

at Parkland. Fuchs and colleagues (2009) reported similar results regarding respiratory morbidity in 722 infants. Specifically, the frequency of respiratory morbidity decreased by approximately 50 percent per week from 34 to 37 completed weeks. Increased rates of adverse neurodevelopment have also been found in late preterm infants compared with term newborns (Petrini and co-workers, 2009).

These findings from Parkland Hospital suggest that the healthcare focus on prematurity should be expanded to include late preterm births. Even so, because approximately 80 percent of these women begin labor spontaneously—similar to births before 32 weeks—attempts to interrupt preterm labor have not been satisfactory. Specifically, the Institute of Medicine report *Preterm Birth: Causes, Consequences, and Prevention* (2006) acknowledges that treatment of preterm labor has not prevented preterm birth. Thus, we are of the view that a national strategy aimed at prevention of late preterm births is unlikely to provide discernible benefit without new developments in the prevention and management of preterm labor. In the meantime, the Maternal-Fetal Medicine Units Network is preparing a study of corticosteroid efficacy in late preterm births. The American College of Obstetricians and Gynecologists (2008a) has emphasized that late preterm deliveries should occur only when an accepted maternal or fetal indication for delivery exists.

REASONS FOR PRETERM DELIVERY

There are four main direct reasons for preterm births in the United States:

1. Delivery for maternal or fetal indications in which labor is induced or the infant is delivered by prelabor cesarean delivery
2. Spontaneous unexplained preterm labor with intact membranes

TABLE 36-5. Neonatal Morbidity Rates at Parkland Hospital in Live Births Delivered Late Preterm Compared with 39 Weeks

Morbidity[a]	Preterm Births			Term Births
	34 weeks (n = 3498)	35 weeks (n = 6571)	36 weeks (n = 11,702)	39 Weeks (n = 84,747)
Respiratory distress				
Ventilator	116 (3.3)[b]	109 (1.7)[b]	89 (0.8)[b]	275 (0.3)
Transient tachypnea	85 (2.4)[b]	103 (1.6)[b]	130 (1.1)[b]	34 (0.4)
Intraventricular hemorrhage				
Grades 1,2	16 (0.5)[b]	13 (0.2)[b]	7 (0.06)[c]	13 (0.01)
Grades 3,4	0	1 (0.02)	1 (0.01)	3 (0.004)
Sepsis				
Work-up	1073 (31)[b]	1443 (22)[b]	1792 (15)[b]	10,588 (12)
Culture proven	18 (0.5)[b]	23 (0.4)[b]	26 (0.2)[c]	97 (0.1)
Phototherapy	13 (6.1)[b]	227 (3.5)[b]	36 (2.0)[b]	857 (1)
Necrotizing enterocolitis	3 (0.09)[b]	1 (0.02)[c]	1 (0.001)	1 (0.001)
Apgar ≤3 at 5 min	5 (0.1)	12 (0.2)[b]	10 (0.9)	54 (0.06)
Intubation in delivery room	49 (1.4)[b]	55 (0.8)[c]	36 (0.6)	477 (0.6)
One or more of the above	1175 (34)[b]	1565 (24)[b]	1993 (17)[b]	11,513 (14)

[a]Data presented as number (percent).
[b]$p < .001$ compared with 39 weeks referent.
[c]$p < .05$ compared with 39 weeks referent.
Reprinted from McIntire DD, Leveno KJ: Neonatal mortality and morbidity rates in late preterm births compared with births at term, *Obstetrics & Gynecology*, 2008, vol. 111, no. 1, pp. 35–41, with permission.

3. Idiopathic preterm premature rupture of membranes (PPROM)
4. Twins and higher-order multifetal births.

Of preterm births, 30 to 35 percent are indicated, 40 to 45 percent are due to spontaneous preterm labor, and 30 to 35 percent follow preterm rupture of membranes (Goldenberg and colleagues, 2008b). Indeed, much of the increase in the singleton preterm birth rate in the United States is explained by rising numbers of indicated preterm births (Ananth and colleagues, 2005).

Reasons for preterm birth have multiple, often interacting, antecedents and contributing factors. This complexity has greatly confounded efforts to prevent and manage this complication. This is particularly true for preterm ruptured membranes and spontaneous preterm labor, which together lead to 70 to 80 percent of preterm births. Lastly, according to data from Martin and co-workers (2006), approximately one in six preterm births in the United States are from twins or higher-order multifetal pregnancies (see Chap. 39, p. 859). For example, in 2004, there were 508,356 preterm births, and of these, 86,116 or 17 percent were from multifetal pregnancies. Many of these pregnancies were achieved using ovulation-inducing drugs and assisted reproductive technologies.

Medical and Obstetrical Indications

Ananth and Vintzileos (2006) used Missouri birth data from 1989 to 1997 to analyze factors leading to indicated birth before 35 weeks. Preeclampsia, fetal distress, small for gestational age, and placental abruption were the most common indications for medical intervention resulting in preterm birth. Other less common causes were chronic hypertension, placenta previa, unexplained bleeding, diabetes, renal disease, Rh isoimmunization, and congenital malformations.

Preterm Prematurely Ruptured Membranes

Defined as rupture of the membranes before labor and prior to 37 weeks, preterm premature rupture of membranes can result from a wide array of pathological mechanisms, including intra-amnionic infection. Other factors implicated include low socioeconomic status, low body mass index—less than 19.8, nutritional deficiencies, and cigarette smoking. Women with prior preterm ruptured membranes are at increased risk for recurrence during a subsequent pregnancy (Bloom and associates, 2001). Most cases of preterm rupture, however, occur without risk factors.

Spontaneous Preterm Labor

Most commonly, preterm birth—up to 45 percent of cases—follows spontaneous labor. Goldenberg and colleagues (2008b) reviewed the pathogenesis of preterm labor and implicated: (1) progesterone withdrawal, (2) oxytocin initiation, and (3) decidual activation. Deviations from normal fetal growth have also been noted in spontaneous preterm labor and suggest a fetal role (Morken and co-workers, 2006).

The progesterone withdrawal theory stems from studies in sheep. As parturition nears, the fetal-adrenal axis becomes more sensitive to adrenocorticotropic hormone, increasing the secretion of cortisol (see Chap. 6, p. 157). Fetal cortisol stimulates placental 17-α-hydroxylase activity, which decreases progesterone secretion and increases estrogen production. The reversal in the estrogen/progesterone ratio results in increased prostaglandin formation, which initiates a cascade that culminates in labor. In human beings, serum progesterone concentrations do not fall as labor approaches. Even so, because progesterone antagonists such as RU486 initiate preterm labor and progestational agents prevent preterm labor, decreased local progesterone concentrations may play a role.

Because intravenous oxytocin increases the frequency and intensity of uterine contractions, oxytocin is assumed to play a part in labor initiation. But serum concentrations of oxytocin do not rise before labor, and the clearance of oxytocin remains constant. Accordingly, oxytocin is an unlikely initiator.

An important pathway leading to labor initiation implicates inflammatory decidual activation. At term, such activation seems to be mediated at least in part by the fetal-decidual paracrine system and perhaps through localized decreases in progesterone concentration. In many cases of early preterm labor, however, decidual activation seems to arise in the context of intrauterine bleeding or occult intrauterine infection.

ANTECEDENTS AND CONTRIBUTING FACTORS

Threatened Abortion

Vaginal bleeding in early pregnancy is associated with increased adverse outcomes later. Weiss and associates (2004) reported outcomes with vaginal bleeding at 6 to 13 weeks in nearly 14,000 women. Both light and heavy bleeding were associated with subsequent preterm labor, placental abruption, and subsequent pregnancy loss prior to 24 weeks.

Lifestyle Factors

Cigarette smoking, inadequate maternal weight gain, and illicit drug use have important roles in both the incidence and outcome of low-birthweight neonates (see Chap. 14, p. 329). In addition, Ehrenberg and colleagues (2009) found that overweight women at risk for preterm birth had lower rates of preterm delivery before 35 weeks than at-risk women with normal weight. Some of these effects are undoubtedly due to restricted fetal growth, but Hickey and colleagues (1995) linked prenatal weight gain specifically with preterm birth. Other maternal factors implicated include young or advanced maternal age, poverty, short stature, vitamin C deficiency, and occupational factors such as prolonged walking or standing, strenuous working conditions, and long weekly work hours (Casanueva, 2005; Gielchinsky, 2002; Kramer, 1995; Luke, 1995; Meis, 1995; Satin, 1994, and all their colleagues).

Psychological factors such as depression, anxiety, and chronic stress have been reported in association with preterm birth (Copper, 1996; Li, 2008; Littleton, 2007; Mercer, 2002, and all their associates). Neggers and co-workers (2004) found a significant link between low birthweight and preterm birth in women injured by physical abuse (see Chap. 42, p. 936).

Racial and Ethnic Disparity

In the United States and in the United Kingdom, women classified as black, African-American, and Afro-Caribbean are consistently reported to be at higher risk of preterm birth (Goldenberg and colleagues, 2008b). Other associations include low socioeconomic status and educational status. Lu and Chen (2004) used the federal-state cooperative survey, *Pregnancy Risk Assessment Monitoring System (PRAMS)*, to study stressful life events in minority populations of pregnant women and found these to be unrelated to preterm birth. Kistka and colleagues (2007) used Missouri state data to analyze racial disparity independent of medical and socioeconomic risk factors and found black women to have an increased risk of recurrent preterm birth. The authors implied evidence of an intrinsic increased risk of preterm birth in this population.

Work During Pregnancy

Studies of work and physical activity related to preterm birth have produced conflicting results (Goldenberg and colleagues, 2008b). There is some evidence, however, that working long hours and hard physical labor are probably associated with increased risk of preterm birth.

Genetic Factors

The recurrent, familial, and racial nature of preterm birth has led to the suggestion that genetics may play a causal role (Anum, 2009; Lie, 2006; Ward, 2005, and all their co-workers). There is an accumulating literature on genetic variants that buttresses this concept (Gibson, 2007; Hampton, 2006; Li, 2004; Macones, 2004, and all their associates). Several such studies have also implicated immunoregulatory genes in potentiating chorioamnionitis in cases of preterm delivery due to infection (Varner and Esplin, 2005).

Periodontal Disease

Gum inflammation is a chronic anaerobic inflammation that affects as many as 50 percent of pregnant women in the United States (Goepfert and co-workers, 2004). Vergnes and Sixou (2007) performed a meta-analysis of 17 studies and concluded that periodontal disease was significantly associated with preterm birth—odds ratio 2.83 (CI 1.95–4.10). In an accompanying editorial, Stamilio and colleagues (2007) concluded that the data used were not robust enough to recommend screening and treatment of pregnant women.

To better study the relationship with periodontitis, Michalowicz and associates (2006) randomly assigned 813 pregnant women between 13 and 17 weeks with periodontal disease to treatment during pregnancy or postpartum. They found that treatment during pregnancy improved periodontal disease and that it is safe, but it did not significantly alter rates of preterm birth.

Birth Defects

In a secondary analysis of data from the First- and Second-Trimester Evaluation of Risk (FASTER) Trial, Dolan and col-

TABLE 36-6. Recurrent Spontaneous Preterm Births According to Prior Outcome

Birth Outcome[a]	Second Birth ≤ 34 Weeks Percent
First birth ≥ 35 weeks	5
First birth ≤ 34 weeks	16
First and second birth ≤ 34 weeks	41

[a]Data from 15,863 women delivering their first and subsequent pregnancies at Parkland Hospital.
Adapted from Bloom and associates (2001) with permission.

leagues (2007) found after controlling for multiple confounding factors that birth defects were associated with preterm birth and low birthweight.

Interval between Pregnancies and Preterm Birth

Short intervals between pregnancies have been known for some time to be associated with adverse perinatal outcomes. In a recent meta-analysis, Conde-Agudelo and co-workers (2006) reported that intervals shorter than 18 months and longer than 59 months were associated with increased risks for both preterm birth and small-for-gestational age infants.

Prior Preterm Birth

A major risk factor for preterm labor is prior preterm delivery (Spong, 2007). Shown in Table 36-6 is the incidence of recurrent preterm birth in nearly 16,000 women delivered at Parkland Hospital (Bloom and associates, 2001). The risk of recurrent preterm delivery for women whose first delivery was preterm was increased threefold compared with that of women whose first neonate was born at term. More than a third of women whose first two newborns were preterm subsequently delivered a third preterm newborn. Most—70 percent—of the recurrent births in this study occurred within 2 weeks of the gestational age of the prior preterm delivery. Importantly, the causes of prior preterm delivery also recurred.

Although women with prior preterm births are clearly at risk for recurrence, they contributed only 10 percent of the total preterm births in this study. Expressed another way, 90 percent of the preterm births at Parkland Hospital cannot be predicted based on a history of preterm birth. Extrapolating data from the new United States birth certificate, which was updated in 2003, it is estimated that approximately 2.5 percent of women delivered in 2004 had a history of prior preterm birth (Martin and Menacker, 2007). Self-reported coitus during early pregnancy was not associated with an increased risk of recurrent preterm birth (Yost and co-workers, 2006).

Infection

Goldenberg and colleagues (2008b) have reviewed the role of infection in preterm birth. It is hypothesized that intrauterine infections trigger preterm labor by activation of the innate immune system. In this hypothesis, microorganisms elicit release of inflammatory cytokines such as interleukins and tumor necrosis factor (TNF), which in turn stimulate the production of prostaglandin and/or matrix-degrading enzymes. Prostaglandins stimulate uterine contractions, whereas degradation of extracellular matrix in the fetal membranes leads to preterm rupture of membranes. It is estimated that 25 to 40 percent of preterm births result from intrauterine infection. Potential routes of intrauterine infection are shown in Figure 36-10.

Two microorganisms, *Ureaplasma urealyticum* and *Mycoplasma hominis*, have emerged as important perinatal pathogens. Goldenberg and colleagues (2008a) reported that 23 percent of neonates born between 23 and 32 weeks have positive umbilical blood cultures for these genital mycoplasmas. Similar results were reported earlier by the research group at the Perinatology Research Branch of the National Institute of Child Health and Human Development (NICHD). In one study, amnionic fluid was aspirated by amniocentesis from 219 Korean women with prematurely ruptured membranes before 25 weeks. A positive culture result, primarily for *U. urealyticum*, was found in 23 percent (Shim and associates, 2004). Similarly, Gomez and co-workers (2005) performed amniocentesis in 401 Chilean women and found microbial invasion in 7 percent—the most common organism was *U. urealyticum*. A sonographically measured short cervix was associated with microbial invasion suggesting ascent from the lower genital tract (see Fig. 36-10).

There have been several studies in which antimicrobial treatment was given to prevent preterm labor due to microbial invasion. Because of the above-cited data, these strategies especially targeted mycoplasma species. Morency and Bujold (2007) performed a meta-analysis of 61 articles and suggested that antimicrobials given in the second trimester may prevent subsequent preterm birth. Andrews and colleagues (2006) reported results of a double-blind interconceptional trial from the University of Alabama in Birmingham. A course of azithromycin plus metronidazole was given every 4 months to 241 nonpregnant women whose last pregnancy resulted in spontaneous delivery before 34 weeks. Approximately 80 percent of the women with subsequent pregnancies had received study drug within 6 months of their subsequent conception. Such interconceptional antimicrobial treatment did not reduce the rate of recurrent preterm birth. Tita and co-workers (2007) performed a subgroup analysis of these same data and concluded that such use of antimicrobials may be harmful. In another study, Goldenberg and colleagues (2006) randomized 2661 women at four African sites to placebo or metronidazole plus erythromycin between 20 and 24 weeks followed by ampicillin plus metronidazole during labor. This antimicrobial regimen did not reduce the rate of preterm birth nor that of histological chorioamnionitis.

Bacterial Vaginosis

In this condition, normal, hydrogen peroxide-producing, lactobacillus-predominant vaginal flora is replaced with anaerobes that include *Gardnerella vaginalis, Mobiluncus* species, and *Mycoplasma hominis* (Hillier and colleagues, 1995; Nugent and co-workers, 1991). Its diagnosis and management are discussed in Chapter 59 (see p. 1246). Using Gram staining, relative concentrations of the bacterial morphotypes characteristic of bacterial vaginosis are determined and graded as the *Nugent score*.

Bacterial vaginosis has been associated with spontaneous abortion, preterm labor, preterm rupture of membranes, chorioamnionitis, and amnionic fluid infection (Hillier, 1995; Kurki, 1992; Leitich, 2003a, b, and all their colleagues). Environmental factors appear to be important in the development of bacterial vaginosis. Exposure

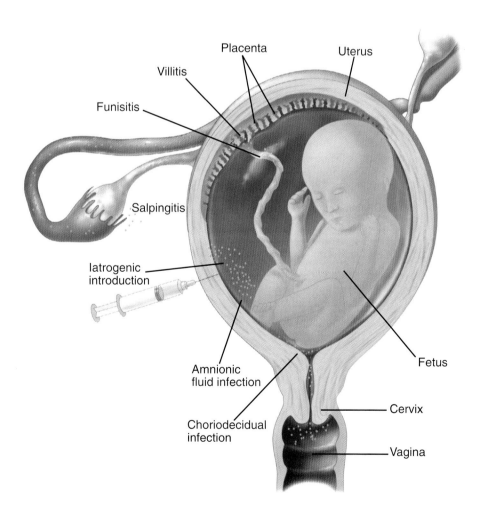

FIGURE 36-10 Potential routes of intrauterine infection.

to chronic stress, ethnic differences, and frequent or recent douching have all been associated with increased rates of the condition (Culhane and co-workers, 2002; Ness and associates, 2002). A gene-environment interaction was identified by Macones and colleagues (2004). Women with bacterial vaginosis and a susceptible TNF-α genotype had a ninefold increased incidence of preterm birth.

From all of these studies, there seems no doubt that adverse vaginal flora is associated in some way with spontaneous preterm birth. Unfortunately, to date, screening and treatment have not been shown to prevent preterm birth. Indeed, microbial resistance or antimicrobial-induced change in the vaginal flora has been reported as a result of regimens intended to eliminate bacterial vaginosis (Beigi and colleagues, 2004; Carey and Klebanoff, 2005). Okun and associates (2005) performed a systematic review of reports on the use of antibiotics given for bacterial vaginosis and for *Trichomonas vaginalis*. They found no evidence to support such use for the prevention of preterm birth in either low-risk or high-risk women.

Screening Methods for Prevention of Preterm Birth

Risk-Scoring Systems

There has been considerable interest in risk-scoring systems to identify women at greatest risk for preterm birth. In their review, Hueston and associates (1995) found no benefits of this programmatic approach. Mercer and colleagues (1996) concluded that risk assessment failed to identify most women who deliver preterm neonates. In another study, Klerman and co-workers (2001) randomly assigned 619 women with a modified risk assessment score for preterm delivery of 10 or higher to receive augmented or customary prenatal care. Mean birthweight and incidences of preterm delivery and low birthweight were similar in both groups and in the general obstetrical population. Recommendations from the American College of Obstetricians and Gynecologists (2008a) are listed in Table 36-7.

TABLE 36-7. Recommended Screening Strategies to Prevent Preterm Birth

---

- No current data support use of home uterine-activity monitoring or bacterial vaginosis screening.
- Screening for risk of preterm labor, other than historical risk factors, is not beneficial in the general obstetrical population.
- Sonography to determine cervical length and/or fetal fibronectin level measurement may be useful in determining women at risk for preterm labor. However, their value may rest primarily with their negative-predictive value given the lack of proven treatment options.

Compiled from American College of Obstetricians and Gynecologists (2001, 2008a).

DIAGNOSIS

Patient Symptoms

Early differentiation between true and false labor is difficult before there is demonstrable cervical effacement and dilatation. Uterine activity alone can be misleading because of *Braxton Hicks contractions,* which are discussed in detail in Chapter 18 (p. 437). These contractions, described as irregular, nonrhythmical, and either painful or painless, can cause considerable confusion in the diagnosis of true preterm labor. Not infrequently, women who deliver before term have uterine activity that is attributed to Braxton Hicks contractions, prompting an incorrect diagnosis of false labor. Because uterine contractions alone may be misleading, the American Academy of Pediatrics and the American College of Obstetricians and Gynecologists (1997) had earlier proposed the following criteria to document preterm labor:

1. Contractions of four in 20 minutes or eight in 60 minutes plus progressive change in the cervix
2. Cervical dilatation greater than 1 cm
3. Cervical effacement of 80 percent or greater.

Currently, however, such clinical findings are now considered inaccurate predictors of preterm delivery (American College of Obstetricians and Gynecologists, 2003). Thus, such explicit criteria do not appear in more recent guidelines (American Academy of Pediatrics and the American College of Obstetricians and Gynecologists, 2008).

In addition to painful or painless uterine contractions, symptoms such as pelvic pressure, menstrual-like cramps, watery vaginal discharge, and lower back pain have been empirically associated with impending preterm birth. Such complaints are thought by some to be common in normal pregnancy and are therefore often dismissed by patients, clinicians, and nurses. The importance of these symptoms as a harbinger of labor has been emphasized by some but not all investigators (Copper and colleagues, 1990; Iams and associates, 1990; Kragt and Keirse, 1990). Iams and colleagues (1994) found that the signs and symptoms signaling preterm labor, including uterine contractions, appeared only within 24 hours of preterm labor.

Cervical Changes

Cervical Dilatation

Asymptomatic cervical dilatation after midpregnancy is suspected as a risk factor for preterm delivery, although some clinicians consider it to be a normal anatomical variant, particularly in parous women. Studies, however, have suggested that parity alone is not sufficient to explain cervical dilatation discovered early in the third trimester. Cook and Ellwood (1996) longitudinally evaluated cervical status with transvaginal sonography between 18 and 30 weeks in both nulliparous and parous women who all subsequently gave birth at term. Cervical length and diameter were identical in both groups throughout these critical weeks. At Parkland Hospital, routine cervical examinations were performed between 26 and 30 weeks in 185 women. Approximately 25 percent of women whose cervices were dilated 2 or 3 cm delivered prior to 34 weeks. Other investigators have verified cervical dilatation as a predictor of increased preterm delivery risk (Copper and associates, 1995; Pereira and colleagues, 2007).

Although women with dilatation and effacement in the third trimester are at increased risk for preterm birth, detection does not improve pregnancy outcome. Buekens and co-workers (1994) randomly assigned 2719 women to undergo routine cervical examinations at each prenatal visit and compared them with 2721 women in whom serial examinations were not performed. Knowledge of antenatal cervical dilatation did not affect any pregnancy outcome related to preterm birth or the frequency of interventions for preterm labor. The investigators also reported that cervical examinations were not related to preterm membrane rupture. It seems, therefore, that prenatal cervical examinations are neither beneficial nor harmful.

Cervical Length

Vaginal-probe sonographic cervical assessment has been evaluated extensively over the past decade. Technique is important, and Yost and colleagues (1999) have cautioned that special expertise is needed. Iams and co-workers (1996) measured cervical length at approximately 24 weeks and again at 28 weeks in 2915 women not at risk for preterm birth. The mean cervical length at 24 weeks was approximately 35 mm, and those women with progressively shorter cervices experienced increased rates of preterm birth.

In women with a previous birth before 32 weeks, Owen and associates (2001) reported a significant correlation of cervical length at 16 to 24 weeks and subsequent preterm birth before 35 weeks. In their review, Owen and colleagues (2003) concluded that the value of cervical length to predict birth before 35 weeks is apparent only in women at high risk for preterm birth. De Carvalho and co-workers (2005) reported an interesting study of sonographic examination of the cervix in 1958 women attending a routine prenatal clinic at the University of São Paulo. These investigators correlated sonographic cervical length, funneling, and prior history of preterm birth with delivery before 35 weeks. Funneling was defined as bulging of the membranes into the endocervical canal and protruding at least 25 percent of the entire cervical length (Fig. 36-11). As shown in Figure 36-12, a short cervix by itself was the poorest predictor of preterm birth, whereas funneling plus a history of prior preterm birth was highly predictive.

Incompetent Cervix

Cervical incompetence is a clinical diagnosis characterized by recurrent, painless cervical dilatation and spontaneous midtrimester birth in the absence of spontaneous membrane rupture, bleeding, or infection. It is considered in detail in Chapter 9 (see p. 218).

Ambulatory Uterine Monitoring

An external tocodynamometer belted around the abdomen and connected to an electronic waist recorder allows a woman to ambulate while uterine activity is recorded. Results are transmitted via telephone daily. Women are educated concerning

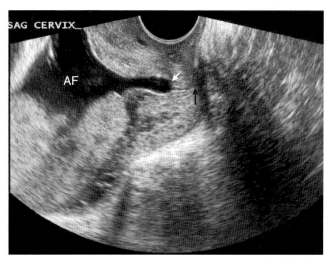

FIGURE 36-11 Transvaginal sonogram of a cervix and funneling. The amnionic sac is seen to bulge into the endocervical canal (*white arrow*). The cervix is markedly shortened. Its length is measured between the leading edge of the protruding amnionic sac and the ectocervix. The ectocervix is marked by a blue arrow. AF = amnionic fluid. (Courtesy of Dr. Irene Stafford.)

signs and symptoms of preterm labor, and clinicians are kept apprised of their progress. The 1985 approval of this monitor by the Food and Drug Administration prompted its widespread clinical use. Subsequently, the American College of Obstetricians and Gynecologists (1995) concluded that the use of this expensive, bulky, and time-consuming system does not reduce preterm birth rates. Studies that followed confirmed this conclusion. In the Collaborative Home Uterine Monitoring Study Group (1995), sham transducers were used in 655 women and outcomes compared with those of 637 women with functioning monitors. The rate of preterm birth was similar in both groups.

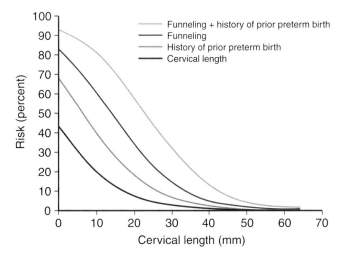

FIGURE 36-12 The probability of delivery at or before 34 weeks' gestation according to cervical length, presence of funneling, previous history of prematurity, and presence of funneling combined with a previous history of prematurity. (Modified from de Carvalho and colleagues, 2005, with permission.)

Iams and colleagues (2002) analyzed data from almost 35,000 hours of daily home monitoring from 306 women. They verified that contraction frequency increased with gestational age but that no pattern efficiently predicted preterm birth.

In a study by Dyson and associates (1998), women were randomly assigned to receive weekly contact with a nurse or to use home contraction monitoring. There were no differences in the rates of preterm delivery before 35 weeks or in the incidence of birthweights less than 1500 g or less than 2500 g. Moreover, women who used home monitoring had a significant increase in the number of unscheduled visits, and women with twins had increased use of tocolytic therapy.

Fetal Fibronectin

This glycoprotein is produced in 20 different molecular forms by a variety of cell types, including hepatocytes, fibroblasts, endothelial cells, and fetal amnion. Present in high concentrations in maternal blood and in amnionic fluid, it is thought to play a role in intercellular adhesion during implantation and in the maintenance of placental adhesion to uterine decidua (Leeson and colleagues, 1996). Fetal fibronectin is detected in cervicovaginal secretions in women who have normal pregnancies with intact membranes at term. It appears to reflect stromal remodeling of the cervix prior to labor.

Lockwood and co-workers (1991) reported that fibronectin detection in cervicovaginal secretions prior to membrane rupture was a possible marker for impending preterm labor. Fetal fibronectin is measured using an enzyme-linked immunosorbent assay, and values exceeding 50 ng/mL are considered positive. Sample contamination by amnionic fluid and maternal blood should be avoided.

A positive value for cervical or vaginal fetal fibronectin assay, even as early as 8 to 22 weeks, has been found to be a powerful predictor of subsequent preterm birth (Goldenberg and co-workers, 2000). In a randomized trial, a negative fibronectin assay in women with threatened preterm labor was associated with fewer admissions and decreased hospital stay (Lowe and associates, 2004). In contrast, Grobman and colleagues (2004) in a randomized trial of open versus blinded fetal fibronectin test results in 100 women found that this test did not affect physician behavior or healthcare costs associated with preterm contractions.

Andrews and associates (2003) studied the effectiveness of antimicrobial treatment to reduce the incidence of preterm birth in women with positive cervicovaginal fetal fibronectin tests. Of 16,317 women screened between 21 and 26 weeks, 6.6 percent had a positive result. In women given antimicrobial treatment or placebo, no differences were observed in rates of spontaneous preterm birth before 37 weeks—14.4 versus 12.4 percent; before 35 weeks—6.9 versus 7.5 percent; or before 32 weeks—4.3 versus 2.2 percent.

PREVENTION OF PRETERM BIRTH

Prevention of preterm birth has been an elusive goal. Recent reports, however, suggest that prevention in selected populations may be achievable.

Progesterone

Maternal plasma progesterone levels increase throughout pregnancy (see Chap. 3, p. 67). Accordingly, the use of progesterone to maintain uterine quiescence and "block" labor initiation, as espoused by Csapo (1956), has stimulated several studies. A pivotal study was done in the NICHD Maternal-Fetal Medicine Units Network (Meis and colleagues, 2003). In this trial, 310 women with prior preterm births were randomized to receive 17-hydroxyprogesterone caproate, while another 153 received placebo. Weekly intramuscular injections of either inert oil or 17-hydroxyprogesterone caproate were given from 16 through 36 weeks. Rates of delivery before 37, 35, and 32 weeks were all significantly reduced by progestin therapy. But similar studies of 17-hydroxyprogesterone caproate in both twins and triplets done by the Network showed no improvement in preterm birth rates (Caritis and associates, 2009; Rouse and co-workers, 2007).

There have also been two large studies by da Fonseca and colleagues (2003, 2007) of vaginal progesterone suppositories. In the first study, 142 women with a prior preterm birth, prophylactic cervical cerclage, or uterine malformation were randomly assigned to daily 100-mg progesterone or placebo suppositories. Progesterone suppositories were associated with a significant reduction in births before 34 weeks. In the second study, 413 women with sonographically short cervices—15 mm or less—were identified during routine prenatal care. They were randomly assigned to be given nightly 200-mg progesterone vaginal suppositories or placebo from 24 to 34 weeks. Spontaneous delivery before 34 weeks was significantly reduced by progesterone therapy. In contrast, O'Brien and colleagues (2007) randomized 659 women with a prior preterm birth to treatment with vaginal progesterone gel (90 mg) or placebo, and they found no differences in preterm birth rates. A study of the efficacy of 17-hydroxyprogesterone caproate in nulliparous women with sonographically short cervices is under way in the Maternal-Fetal Medicine Units Network.

Recommendations for Progesterone Use

Given the conflicting results surrounding progesterone use for prevention of preterm birth, there have been several meta-analyses of published studies. All investigators identified evidence of some benefits in terms of reducing preterm birth in specific populations. At the same time, all also called for more study, primarily because there was insufficient information regarding potential harms (Dodd, 2008; Mackenzie, 2006; Sanchez-Ramos, 2005; Tita and Rouse, 2009, and all their associates). At this time, the American College of Obstetricians and Gynecologists (2008c) has concluded that progesterone therapy should be limited to women with a documented history of a previous spontaneous birth at less than 37 weeks. Further studies are needed as to optimal preparation, dosage, and route of administration.

Cervical Cerclage

There are at least three circumstances when cerclage placement may be used to prevent preterm birth. First, cerclage may be used in women who have a history of recurrent midtrimester losses and who are diagnosed with an incompetent cervix

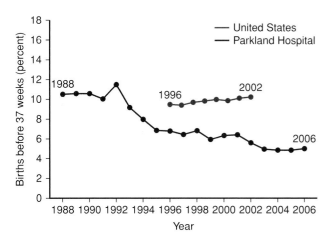

FIGURE 36-13 Number of births before 37 weeks' gestation at Parkland Hospital from 1988 to 2006 compared with that in the United States from 1995 to 2002. Analysis in both cohorts was limited to singleton live births ≥ 500 g who received prenatal care. (Reprinted from Leveno KJ, McIntire DD, Bloom SL, et al: Decreased preterm births in an inner-city public hospital, *Obstetrics & Gynecology*, 2009, vol. 113, no. 3, pp. 578–584, with permission.)

(see Chap. 9, p. 218). A second circumstance is in women identified during sonographic examination to have a short cervix. The third indication is "rescue" cerclage, done emergently when cervical incompetence is recognized in the women with threatened preterm labor (see p. 822).

Regarding the second indication, Berghella and colleagues (2005) reviewed several small trials of cerclage in this group and concluded that cerclage may reduce preterm birth rates in those women with a prior preterm birth. Owen and co-workers (2009) randomly assigned 302 women with prior preterm birth from 16 centers with a short cervix—defined as length < 25 mm—to cerclage or no procedure. Women with a cervical length < 15 mm delivered before 35 weeks significantly less often following cerclage compared with women with no cerclage—30 versus 65

percent. This study suggests that recurrent preterm birth can be prevented in a subset of women who have a history of prior preterm births.

Geographic-Based Public Healthcare Program

The decreasing rate of preterm births at Parkland Hospital between 1988 and 2006 shown in Figure 36-13 coincided with a substantial increase in prenatal care utilization as shown in Figure 36-14. In the early 1990s, a concerted effort was made to improve access to and use of prenatal care. The intention was to develop a program of seamless care beginning with enrollment during the prenatal period and extending through delivery and into the puerperium. Prenatal clinics are placed strategically throughout Dallas County to provide convenient access for indigent women. When possible, these clinics were co-located with comprehensive medical and pediatric clinics that enhance patient use. Because the entire clinic system is operated by Parkland Hospital, administrative and medical oversight is seamless. For example, prenatal protocols are used by nurse practitioners at all clinic sites to guarantee homogeneous care. Women with high-risk pregnancy complications are referred to the hospital-based central clinic system. Here, high-risk pregnancy clinics operate each weekday, with specialty clinics for women with prior preterm birth, gestational diabetes, infectious diseases, multifetal pregnancy, and hypertensive disorders. Clinics are staffed by residents and midwives supervised by maternal-fetal medicine fellows and faculty. Because Parkland Hospital has a closed medical staff, all attending physicians are employed by the University of Texas Southwestern Department of Obstetrics and Gynecology. These faculty members adhere to agreed-upon practice guidelines using an evidence-based outcomes approach. Thus, prenatal care is considered one component of a comprehensive and orchestrated public health care system that is community-based. Putting this together, we hypothesize that the decrease in preterm births experienced at our inner-city hospital was attributable to a geographically based public healthcare program specifically targeting minority populations of pregnant women.

MANAGEMENT OF PRETERM RUPTURE OF MEMBRANES AND PRETERM LABOR

Women identified as being at risk for preterm birth and those who present with signs and symptoms of preterm labor have become candidates for a number of interventions intended to improve neonatal outcomes. In the absence of maternal or fetal indications warranting intentional delivery, interventions are intended to forestall preterm birth. Although many of these interventions are described in the following sections, they are not necessarily recommended. Some may produce borderline improvement at best, and others are unproven. For example, the American College of

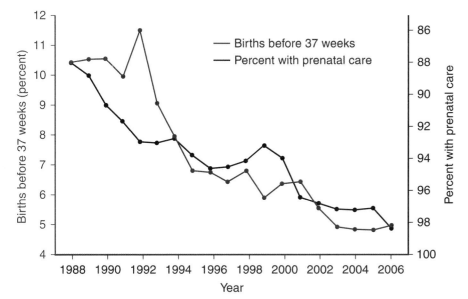

FIGURE 36-14 Relationship of increased prenatal care rates to decreased preterm birth rates at Parkland Hospital from 1988 to 2006. (Reprinted from Leveno KJ, McIntire DD, Bloom SL, et al: Decreased preterm births in an inner-city public hospital, *Obstetrics & Gynecology*, 2009, vol. 113, no. 3, pp. 578–584, with permission.)

Obstetricians and Gynecologists (2003, 2008b), in its review of preterm labor management, has concluded: "Despite the numerous management methods proposed, the incidence of preterm birth has changed little over the past 40 years. Uncertainty persists about the best strategies for managing preterm labor."

Diagnosis of Preterm Prematurely Ruptured Membranes

Diagnosis of ruptured membranes is detailed in Chapter 17 (see p. 392). A history of vaginal leakage of fluid, either as a continuous stream or as a gush, should prompt a speculum examination to visualize gross vaginal pooling of amnionic fluid, clear fluid from the cervical canal, or both. Confirmation of ruptured membranes is usually accompanied by sonographic examination to assess amnionic fluid volume, to identify the presenting part, and if not previously determined, to estimate gestational age. Amnionic fluid is slightly alkaline (pH 7.1–7.3) compared with vaginal secretions (pH 4.5–6.0), and this is the basis of frequently used pH testing for ruptured membranes. Blood, semen, antiseptics, or bacterial vaginosis, however, are all also alkaline and can give false-positive results.

Natural History of Preterm Ruptured Membranes

Cox and associates (1988) described pregnancy outcomes of 298 consecutive women who gave birth following spontaneously ruptured membranes between 24 and 34 weeks. Although this complication was identified in only 1.7 percent of pregnancies, it contributed to 20 percent of all perinatal deaths. By the time they presented, 75 percent of the women were already in labor, 5 percent were delivered for other complications, and another 10 percent were delivered within 48 hours. In only 7 percent was delivery delayed 48 hours or more after membrane rupture. This latter subgroup, however, appeared to benefit from delayed de-

livery, because there were no neonatal deaths. This contrasted with a neonatal death rate of 80 per 1000 in preterm newborns delivered within 48 hours of membrane rupture. Nelson and co-workers (1994) reported similar results.

The time from preterm ruptured membranes to delivery is inversely proportional to the gestational age when rupture occurs (Carroll and associates, 1995). As shown in Figure 36-15, very few days were gained when membranes ruptured during the third trimester compared with midpregnancy.

Hospitalization

Most clinicians hospitalize women with preterm ruptured membranes. Concerns about the costs of lengthy hospitalizations are usually moot, because most women enter labor within a week or less after membrane rupture. Carlan and co-workers (1993) randomly assigned 67 women with ruptured membranes to home or hospital management. No benefits were found for hospitalization, and maternal hospital stays were reduced by 50 percent in those sent home—14 versus 7 days. Importantly, the investigators emphasized that this study was too small to conclude that home management was safe.

Intentional Delivery

Prior to the mid-1970s, labor was usually induced in women with preterm ruptured membranes because of fears of sepsis. Two randomized trials compared labor induction with expectant management in such pregnancies. Mercer and colleagues (1993) randomly assigned 93 women with pregnancies between 32 and 36 weeks to undergo delivery or expectant management. Fetal lung maturity, as evidenced by mature surfactant profiles, was present in all cases. Intentional delivery reduced the length of maternal hospitalization and also reduced infection rates in both mothers and neonates. Cox and Leveno (1995) similarly apportioned 129 women between 30 and 34 weeks. Fetal lung maturity was not assessed. One fetal death resulted from sepsis in the pregnancies managed expectantly. Among those intentionally delivered, there were three neonatal deaths—two from sepsis and one from pulmonary hypoplasia. Thus, neither management approach proved to be superior.

Expectant Management

Despite extensive literature concerning expectant management of preterm ruptured membranes, tocolysis has been used in few studies. In randomized studies, women were assigned to receive either tocolysis or expectant management. The investigators concluded that active interventions did not improve perinatal outcomes (Garite and associates, 1981, 1987; Nelson and co-workers, 1985).

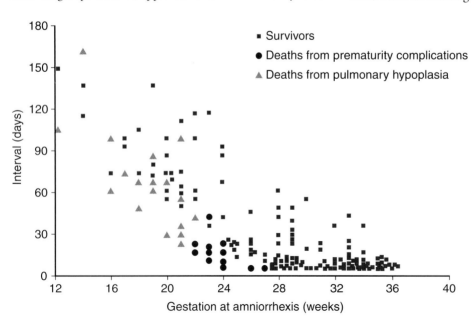

FIGURE 36-15 Relationship of time between preterm membrane rupture and delivery in 172 singleton pregnancies. (Reprinted from Carroll SG, Blott M, Nicolaides KH: Preterm prelabor amniorrhexis: Outcome of live births, *Obstetrics & Gynecology,* 1995, vol. 86, no. 1, pp. 18–25, with permission.)

Other considerations with expectant management involve the use of digital cervical examination and cerclage. Alexander and colleagues (2000) analyzed findings in women expectantly managed between 24 and 32 weeks. They compared those who had one or two digital cervical examinations with women who were not examined digitally. Women who were examined had a rupture-to-delivery interval of 3 days compared with 5 days in those who were not examined. This difference did not worsen maternal or neonatal outcomes. McElrath and associates (2002) studied 114 women with cerclage in place who later had ruptured membranes prior to 34 weeks. They were compared with 288 controls who had not received a cerclage. Pregnancy outcomes were equivalent in both groups. As discussed in Chapter 9 (see p. 219), such management is controversial.

Risks of Expectant Management

Maternal and fetal risks vary with the gestational age at membrane rupture. Morales and Talley (1993b) expectantly managed 94 singleton pregnancies with ruptured membranes prior to 25 weeks. The average time gained was 11 days. *Although 41 percent of infants survived to age 1 year, only 27 percent were neurologically normal.* Similar results were reported by Farooqi (1998) and Winn (2000) and their associates. Lieman and colleagues (2005) found no improved neonatal outcomes with expectant management beyond 33 weeks. In contrast, McElrath and co-workers (2003) found that prolonged latency after membrane rupture was not associated with an increased incidence of fetal neurological damage.

The volume of amnionic fluid remaining after rupture appears to have prognostic importance in pregnancies before 26 weeks. Hadi and associates (1994) described 178 pregnancies with ruptured membranes between 20 and 25 weeks. Forty percent of women developed oligohydramnios defined by the absence of fluid pockets 2 cm or larger. Virtually all women with oligohydramnios delivered before 25 weeks, whereas 85 percent with adequate amnionic fluid volume were delivered in the third trimester. Carroll and colleagues (1995) observed no cases of pulmonary hypoplasia in fetuses born after membrane rupture at 24 weeks or beyond. This suggests that 23 weeks or less is the threshold for development of lung hypoplasia. Further, when contemplating early expectant management, consideration is also given to oligohydramnios and resultant limb compression deformities (see Chap. 21, p. 495).

Other risk factors have also been evaluated. In neonates born to women with active herpetic lesions who were expectantly managed, the infectious morbidity risk appeared to be outweighed by risks associated with preterm delivery (Major and associates, 2003). Lewis and colleagues (2007) found that expectant management of women with preterm ruptured membranes and noncephalic presentation had an increased rate of umbilical cord prolapse, especially before 26 weeks.

Clinical Chorioamnionitis

Most authors report that prolonged membrane rupture is associated with increased fetal and maternal sepsis (Ho and colleagues, 2003). If chorioamnionitis is diagnosed, prompt efforts to effect delivery, preferably vaginally, are initiated. Fever is the only reliable indicator for this diagnosis, and temperature of 38°C (100.4°F) or higher accompanying ruptured membranes implies infection. Maternal leukocytosis alone has not been found to be reliable. During expectant management, monitoring for sustained maternal or fetal tachycardia, for uterine tenderness, and for a malodorous vaginal discharge is warranted.

With chorioamnionitis, fetal and neonatal morbidity is substantively increased. Alexander and co-workers (1998) studied 1367 very-low-birthweight neonates delivered at Parkland Hospital. Approximately 7 percent were born to women with overt chorioamnionitis, and their outcomes were compared with similar newborns without clinical infection. Those in the infected group had a higher incidence of sepsis, respiratory distress syndrome, early-onset seizures, intraventricular hemorrhage, and periventricular leukomalacia. The investigators concluded that these very-low-birthweight neonates were vulnerable to neurological injury attributable to chorioamnionitis.

Although Locatelli and colleagues (2005) have challenged this finding, there is other evidence that very small newborns are at increased risk for sepsis. Yoon and associates (2000) found that intra-amnionic infection in preterm neonates was related to increased rates of cerebral palsy at 3 years. Petrova and co-workers (2001) studied more than 11 million singleton live births from 1995 to 1997 who were in the database of the National Center for Health Statistics. During labor, 1.6 percent of all women had fever, and this was a strong predictor of infection-related death in both term and preterm neonates. Bullard and associates (2002) reported similar results.

Accelerated Pulmonary Maturation

A variety of clinical events—some well defined—were once proposed to accelerate fetal surfactant production (Gluck, 1979). These included chronic renal or cardiovascular disease, hypertensive disorders, heroin addiction, fetal-growth restriction, placental infarction, chorioamnionitis, and preterm ruptured membranes. Although this view was widely held for many years, subsequent observations do not support this association (Hallak and Bottoms, 1993; Owen and associates, 1990).

Antimicrobial Therapy

The proposed microbial pathogenesis for spontaneous preterm labor or ruptured membranes has prompted investigators to give various antimicrobials in an attempt to forestall delivery. Mercer and Arheart (1995) reviewed 13 randomized trials performed before 35 weeks. Meta-analysis indicated that only three of 10 outcomes were *possibly* benefited: (1) fewer women developed chorioamnionitis, (2) fewer newborns developed sepsis, and (3) pregnancy was more often prolonged 7 days in women given antimicrobials. Neonatal survival, however, was unaffected, as was the incidence of necrotizing enterocolitis, respiratory distress, or intracranial hemorrhage.

To further address this issue, the Maternal-Fetal Medicine Units Network designed a trial to study expectant management combined with a 7-day treatment of ampicillin, amoxicillin plus erythromycin, or placebo. The women had membrane rupture between 24 and 32 weeks. Neither tocolytics nor corticosteroids were given. Antimicrobial-treated women had significantly fewer newborns with respiratory distress syndrome, necrotizing entero-colitis, and composite adverse outcomes (Mercer and colleagues, 1997). The latency period was significantly longer. Specifically, 50 percent of women given an antimicrobial regimen remained undelivered after 7 days of treatment compared with only 25 percent of those given placebo. There was also significant prolongation of pregnancy at 14 and 21 days. Cervicovaginal group B streptococcal colonization did not alter these results.

More recent studies have examined the efficacy of shorter treatment lengths and other antimicrobial combinations. Three-day treatment compared with 7-day regimens using either ampicillin or ampicillin-sulbactam appeared equally effective in regard to perinatal outcomes (Lewis and associates, 2003; Segel and co-workers, 2003). Similarly, erythromycin compared with placebo offered a range of significant neonatal benefits. The amoxicillin-clavulanate regimen was not recommended, however, because of its association with an increased incidence of necrotizing enterocolitis (Kenyon and colleagues, 2004).

Some predicted that prolonged antimicrobial therapy in such pregnancies might have unwanted consequences. Carroll and co-workers (1996) and Mercer and associates (1999) cautioned that such therapy potentially increased the risk for resistant bacteria. Stoll and colleagues (2002) studied 4337 neonates weighing from 400 to 1500 g and born from 1998 to 2000 at centers of the Neonatal Research Network. Their outcomes were compared with those of 7606 neonates of similar birthweight born from 1991 to 1993. The overall rate of early-onset sepsis did not change between these two epochs. But the rate of group B streptococcal sepsis decreased from 5.9 per 1000 births in the 1991 to 1993 group to 1.7 per 1000 births in the 1998 to 2000 group. Comparing these same epochs, the rate of *Escherichia coli* sepsis increased—from 3.2 to 6.8 per 1000 births. Almost 85 percent of coliform isolates from the more recent cohort were ampicillin resistant. Neonates with early-onset sepsis were more likely to die, especially if they were infected with coliforms. Kenyon and co-workers (2008a) found that the prescription of antimicrobials for women with preterm rupture of membranes had no effect on the health of the children at age 7 years.

Corticosteroids

The National Institutes of Health Consensus Development Conference (2000) recommended a single course of antenatal corticosteroids for women with preterm membrane rupture before 32 weeks and in whom there was no evidence of chorioamnionitis. Since then, a number of meta-analyses have addressed this issue, and according to the American College of Obstetricians and Gynecologists (2007), single-dose therapy is recommended from 24 to 32 weeks. There is no consensus regarding treatment between 32 and 34 weeks. They are not recommended prior to 24 weeks.

Membrane Repair

Tissue sealants have been used for a variety of purposes in medicine and have become important in maintaining surgical hemostasis and stimulating wound healing. Devlieger and colleagues (2006) have reviewed the efficacy of sealants in the repair of fetal membrane defects such as in preterm ruptured membranes.

Recommended Management

The management scheme recommended by the American College of Obstetricians and Gynecologists (2007) is summarized in Table 36-8. This management is similar to that practiced at Parkland Hospital and the University of Alabama Hospital at Birmingham.

TABLE 36-8. Recommended Management of Preterm Ruptured Membranes

Gestational Age	Management
34 weeks or more	• Proceed to delivery, usually by induction of labor • Group B streptococcal prophylaxis is recommended
32 weeks to 33 completed weeks	• Expectant management unless fetal pulmonary maturity is documented • Group B streptococcal prophylaxis is recommended • Corticosteroids—no consensus, but some experts recommend • Antimicrobials to prolong latency if no contraindications
24 weeks to 31 completed weeks	• Expectant management • Group B streptococcal prophylaxis is recommended • Single-course corticosteroids use is recommended • Tocolytics—no consensus • Antimicrobials to prolong latency if no contraindications
Before 24 weeks[a]	• Patient counseling • Expectant management or induction of labor • Group B streptococcal prophylaxis is not recommended • Corticosteroids are not recommended • Antimicrobials—there are incomplete data on use in prolonging latency

[a]The combination of birthweight, gestational age, and sex provide the best estimate of chances of survival and should be considered in individual cases.
Reprinted, with permission, from American College of Obstetricians and Gynecologists. Preterm rupture of membranes. ACOG Practice Bulletin 80. Washington, DC:ACOG; 2007.

PRETERM LABOR WITH INTACT MEMBRANES

Women with signs and symptoms of preterm labor with intact membranes are managed much the same as described above for those with preterm ruptured membranes. The cornerstone of treatment is to avoid delivery prior to 34 weeks, if possible. Drugs used to abate or suppress preterm uterine contractions are subsequently discussed.

Amniocentesis to Detect Infection

Several tests have been used to diagnose intra-amnionic infection. Romero and co-workers (1993) evaluated the diagnostic value of amnionic fluid containing an elevated leukocyte count, a low glucose level, a high interleukin-6 concentration, or a positive Gram stain result in 120 women with preterm labor and intact membranes. Women with positive amnionic fluid culture results were considered infected. These investigators found that a negative Gram stain result was 99-percent specific to exclude amnionic fluid bacteria. A high interleukin-6 level was 82-percent sensitive for detection of amnionic fluids containing bacteria. Other investigators have also found good correlation between amnionic fluid interleukin-6 or leukocyte levels and chorioamnionic infection (Andrews and colleagues, 1995; Yoon and associates, 1996). Despite these associations, it has not been shown that amniocentesis to diagnose infection is associated with improved pregnancy outcomes in women with or without membrane rupture (Feinstein and colleagues, 1986). The American College of Obstetricians and Gynecologists (2003) has concluded that there is no evidence to support routine amniocentesis to identify infection.

Corticosteroid Therapy to Enhance Fetal Lung Maturation

Glucosteroids will accelerate lung maturation in preterm sheep fetuses, and thus Liggins and Howie (1972) evaluated them to treat women. Corticosteroid therapy was effective in lowering the incidence of respiratory distress and neonatal mortality rates if birth was delayed for at least 24 hours after *initiation* of betamethasone. Remarkably, infants exposed to corticosteroids in these early studies have been now followed to age 31 years with no ill effects detected. The work by Liggins and Howie (1972) has stimulated more than 35 years of fetal lung research. In 1995, a National Institutes of Health Consensus Development Panel recommended corticosteroids for fetal lung maturation in threatened preterm birth.

In a follow-up meeting, the National Institutes of Health Consensus Development Conference (2000) concluded that data were insufficient to assess the effectiveness of corticosteroids in pregnancies complicated by hypertension, diabetes, multifetal gestation, fetal-growth restriction, and fetal hydrops. It concluded, however, that it was reasonable to administer corticosteroids for these complications. Roberts and Dalziel (2006) reviewed antenatal corticosteroids for accelerating fetal lung maturation.

The issue of the fetal and infant safety with single versus repeat courses of corticosteroids for lung maturation has been the topic of two major trials. Although both found repeated courses to be beneficial in reducing neonatal respiratory morbidity rates, the long-term consequences were much different. Specifically, Crowther and colleagues (2007) studied outcomes in 982 women from the Australian Collaborative Study. These women were given a single weekly dose of 11.4 mg of betamethasone. These investigators found no adverse effects in the infants followed to age 2 years. Wapner and colleagues (2007) studied infants born to 495 women in a Network study who were randomized to receive two weekly 12-mg betamethasone doses given 24 hours apart. They were concerned by their finding of a nonsignificant increase in cerebral palsy rates in infants exposed to repeated courses. The twice-as-large betamethasone dose in the Network study was worrisome because there is some experimental evidence to support the view that adverse corticosteroid effects are dose dependent. Bruschettini and colleagues (2006) studied the equivalent of 12-mg versus 6-mg betamethasone given to pregnant cats. They reported that the lower dose had less severe effects on somatic growth without affecting cell proliferation in the fetal brain.

Stiles (2007) summarized the Australian and American studies as "early gain, long-term questions." We agree, and at Parkland Hospital, we follow the recommendation for single-course therapy by the American College of Obstetricians and Gynecologists (2008a).

"Rescue" Therapy

This refers to administration of a repeated corticosteroid dose when delivery becomes imminent and more than 7 days have elapsed since the initial dose. The 2000 Consensus Development Conference recommended that rescue therapy should not be routinely used and that it should be reserved for clinical trials. The first randomized trial reported by Peltoniemi and colleagues (2007) allocated 326 women to placebo or 12-mg betamethasone single-dose rescue regimens. Paradoxically, they found that the rescue dose of betamethasone increased the risk of respiratory distress syndrome! Subsequently, the American College of Obstetricians and Gynecologists (2008a) also recommended such therapy for trials. Most recently, in a multicenter study of 437 women < 33 weeks who were randomized to rescue therapy or placebo, Kurtzman and associates (2009) reported significantly decreased rates of respiratory complications and neonatal composite morbidity with rescue corticosteroids. There were, however, no differences in perinatal mortality rates and other morbidities. In another trial, McEvoy and co-workers (2009) showed that treated infants had improved respiratory compliance.

Which Corticosteroid?

As summarized by Murphy (2007), there is a 10-year question as to whether betamethasone is superior to dexamethasone for fetal lung maturation. Elimian and co-workers (2007) randomized 299 women between 24 and 33 weeks in a double-blinded trial of betamethasone versus dexamethasone. These two drugs were comparable in reducing the rates of major neonatal morbidities in preterm infants.

Antimicrobials

As with preterm ruptured membranes, antimicrobials have been given to arrest preterm labor. Here too, results have been disappointing. A Cochrane meta-analysis by King and Flenady (2000) of 10 randomized trials found no difference in the rates of newborn respiratory distress syndrome or of sepsis between placebo- and antimicrobial-treated groups. They did find, however, increased perinatal morbidity in the antimicrobial-treated group. Kenyon and associates (2001) reported the OR-ACLE Collaborative Group study of 6295 women with spontaneous preterm labor, intact membranes, and without evidence of infection. Women were randomly assigned to receive antimicrobial or placebo therapy. The primary outcomes of neonatal death, chronic lung disease, and major cerebral abnormality were similar in both groups. In his review, Goldenberg (2002) also concluded that antimicrobial treatment of women with preterm labor for the sole purpose of preventing delivery is generally not recommended. In a recent follow-up of the ORACLE II trial, Kenyon and colleagues (2008b) reported that fetal exposure to antimicrobials in this clinical setting was associated with an increased cerebral palsy rate at age 7 years compared with that of nonexposed infants.

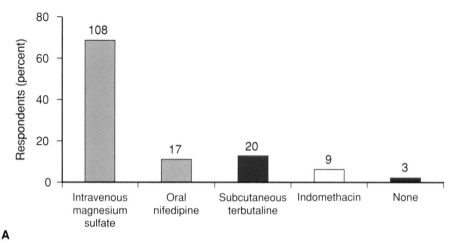

A

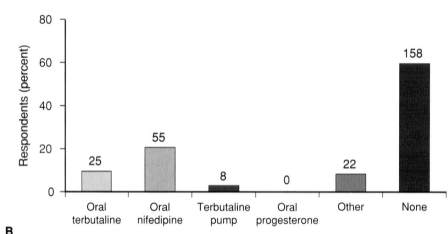

B

FIGURE 36-16 Results from an interactive questionnaire that surveyed use of tocolytic therapy for preterm labor. **A.** Tocolytic agent used by 157 respondents for initial treatment of a woman in preterm labor at 31 weeks 2 days of gestation. **B.** Maintenance tocolytic agent chosen by 268 respondents for this same woman when discharged 2 days later with no further contractions or cervical change. (From Norwitz and associates, 2004, with permission.)

Emergency or Rescue Cerclage

There is support for the concept that cervical incompetence and preterm labor are part of a spectrum leading to preterm delivery. Consequently, investigators have evaluated the role of cerclage done after preterm labor begins to manifest clinically. Harger (1983) concluded that if cervical incompetence is recognized with threatened preterm labor, emergency cerclage can be attempted, albeit with an appreciable risk of infection and pregnancy loss. Althuisius and associates (2003) randomly assigned 23 women with cervical incompetence prior to 27 weeks to bed rest, with or without emergency McDonald cerclage. Delivery delay was significantly greater in the cerclage group compared with that of bed rest alone—54 versus 24 days. Terkildsen and co-workers (2003) studied 116 women who underwent second-trimester emergency cerclage. Nulliparity, membranes extending beyond the external cervical os, and cerclage prior to 22 weeks were associated with a significantly decreased chance of pregnancy continuation to 28 weeks or beyond. Cerclage is discussed further on page 816 as well as in Chapter 9 (p. 218).

Inhibition of Preterm Labor

Although a number of drugs and other interventions have been used to prevent or inhibit preterm labor, none has been shown to be completely effective. The American College of Obstetricians and Gynecologists (2007) has concluded that tocolytic agents do not markedly prolong gestation, but may delay delivery in some women for at least 48 hours. This may facilitate transport to a regional obstetrical center and allow time for administration of corticosteroid therapy. It is estimated that 72,733 women giving birth in the United States in 2006 received tocolytic drugs (Martin and colleagues, 2009). The rate of tocolysis use was 1.7 percent in 2006, a rate that has fluctuated only slightly since 1996. Norwitz and co-workers (2004) performed an interactive survey of tocolytic treatment at the 2004 Annual Meeting of the Society of Maternal-Fetal Medicine. As shown in Figure 36-16, intravenous magnesium sulfate was the most commonly used tocolytic—about 70 percent of respondents. Approximately the same proportion of respondents would not prescribe *maintenance* therapy.

Bed Rest

This is one of the most often prescribed interventions during pregnancy, yet one of the least studied. In 1994, Goldenberg and colleagues reviewed the available literature on bed rest in pregnancy and concluded that they could find no evidence supporting or refuting the benefit of either bed rest or hospitalization in women threatening preterm delivery. More recently, Sosa and associates (2004) searched the Cochrane Database for randomized trials done to assess the efficacy of bed rest at home or with hospitalization. They concluded that the available evidence neither supported nor refuted the use of bed rest to prevent preterm birth.

Goulet and colleagues (2001) randomized 250 Canadian women to either home care or hospitalization after treatment of an acute episode of preterm labor and also found no benefits. Yost and colleagues (2005) attempted a randomized study at Parkland Hospital but terminated the study after 6 years due to low recruitment. In this study, bed rest in the hospital compared with bed rest at home had no effect on pregnancy duration in women with threatened preterm labor before 34 weeks. Bed rest was not enforced—that is, women were permitted ambulation *ad lib* either in the hospital or at home. Kovacevich and associates (2000) reported that bed rest for 3 days or more increased thromboembolic complications to 16 per 1000 women compared with only 1 per 1000 with normal ambulation. Promislow and co-workers (2004) observed significant bone loss in pregnant women prescribed outpatient bed rest.

Hydration and Sedation

Helfgott and associates (1994) compared hydration and sedation with bed rest in a randomized trial of 119 women with threatened preterm labor. Women who were randomly selected to receive 500 mL of crystalloid over 30 minutes and 8 to 12 mg of intramuscular morphine sulfate had outcomes similar to those prescribed bed rest. Although women with preterm contractions treated with 0.25-mg subcutaneous terbutaline may have contractions that cease more quickly and may be discharged significantly earlier compared with women not treated, pregnancy outcomes are similar (Guinn and co-workers, 1997).

β-Adrenergic Receptor Agonists

A number of compounds react with β-adrenergic receptors to reduce intracellular ionized calcium levels and prevent activation of myometrial contractile proteins (see Chap. 6, p. 148). In the United States, ritodrine and terbutaline have been used in obstetrics, but only ritodrine had been approved for preterm labor by the Food and Drug Administration.

Ritodrine. In a multicenter trial, neonates whose mothers were treated with ritodrine for threatened preterm labor had lower rates of death and respiratory distress. They also achieved a gestational age of 36 weeks or a birthweight of 2500 g more often than did those of untreated mothers (Merkatz and colleagues, 1980). In a randomized trial at Parkland Hospital, Leveno and associates (1986) allocated 106 women between 24 and 33 weeks to receive either intravenous ritodrine or no tocolysis. Al-

though drug treatment delayed delivery for 24 hours, there were no other benefits. The transient tocolytic effects of ritodrine and its ultimate failure to arrest labor may be due to β-adrenergic receptor desensitization (Hausdorff and co-workers, 1990).

The infusion of β-agonists has resulted in frequent and at times, serious and fatal side effects. Pulmonary edema is a special concern, and its contribution to morbidity is discussed in Chapter 42 (see p. 929). Tocolysis was the third most common cause of acute respiratory distress and death in pregnant women during a 14-year period in Mississippi (Perry and associates, 1996). *The cause of pulmonary edema is multifactorial, and risk factors include tocolytic therapy with β-agonists, multifetal gestation, concurrent corticosteroid therapy, tocolysis for more than 24 hours, and large intravenous crystalloid volume infusion.* Because β-agonists cause retention of sodium and water, with time—usually 24 to 48 hours, these can cause volume overload (Hankins and colleagues, 1988). The drugs have been implicated as a cause of increased capillary permeability, disturbance of cardiac rhythm, and myocardial ischemia. Finally, maternal sepsis—a relatively common occurrence with preterm labor—appreciably increases this risk (see Chap. 42, p. 932).

Schiff and co-workers (1993) challenged the efficacy of oral ritodrine on pharmacokinetic grounds, and its manufacturer discontinued distribution of tablets in 1995. According to the *Federal Register*, ritodrine was withdrawn voluntarily in 2003 by its manufacturer and is not available in the United States.

Terbutaline. This β-agonist is commonly used to forestall preterm labor. Like ritodrine, it can cause pulmonary edema (Angel and associates, 1988). Long-term low-dose terbutaline given by subcutaneous pump in nine pregnancies was described by Lam and colleagues (1988). The Tokos Corporation promptly marketed this approach, and between 1987 and 1993, these pumps were used in nearly 25,000 women with suspected preterm labor (Perry and co-workers, 1995). Adverse reports concerning terbutaline pumps describe a sudden maternal death and a newborn with myocardial necrosis after the mother used the pump for 12 weeks (Fletcher and colleagues, 1991; Hudgens and Conradi, 1993). Elliott and co-workers (2004) have used continuous terbutaline subcutaneous infusion in 9359 patients and reported that only 12 women experienced severe adverse events—primarily pulmonary edema.

Two randomized trials found no benefit for terbutaline pump therapy. In one, Wenstrom and colleagues (1997) randomly assigned 42 women with preterm labor to a terbutaline pump, to a saline pump, or to oral terbutaline. In the other, Guinn and associates (1998) randomly treated 52 women with terbutaline or with saline pump therapy. Terbutaline did not significantly prolong pregnancy, prevent preterm delivery, or improve neonatal outcomes in either of these studies.

Oral terbutaline therapy to prevent preterm delivery has also not been effective (How and associates, 1995; Parilla and co-workers, 1993). In a double-blind trial, Lewis and colleagues (1996) studied 203 women with arrested preterm labor at 24 to 34 weeks. They were randomly assigned to receive 5-mg terbutaline tablets or placebo every 4 hours. Delivery rates at 1 week were similar in both groups, as was median latency, mean gestational age at delivery, and the incidence of recurrent preterm labor.

Overview of Beta-Adrenergic Drugs to Inhibit Preterm Labor.

Analyses of *parenteral* β-agonists to prevent preterm birth have confirmed a delay of delivery for at least 48 hours (Canadian Preterm Labor Investigators Group, 1992). Unfortunately, this delay has not proven to be beneficial. Macones and colleagues (1995) used meta-analysis to assess the efficacy of *oral* β-agonist therapy and found no benefits. Keirse (1995b) suggests that this brief delay may aid maternal transport to tertiary care or effect fetal lung maturation with corticosteroids. Although this intuitive reasoning is logical, there are no data to support this viewpoint.

Magnesium Sulfate

Ionic magnesium in a sufficiently high concentration can alter myometrial contractility. Its role is presumably that of a calcium antagonist. Clinically, magnesium in pharmacological doses may inhibit labor. Steer and Petrie (1977) concluded that intravenously administered magnesium sulfate—a 4-g loading dose followed by a continuous infusion of 2 g/hr—usually arrests labor. Women given magnesium sulfate must be monitored closely for evidence of hypermagnesemia. The pharmacology and toxicology of magnesium are considered in more detail in Chapter 34 (p. 738). Samol and Lambers (2005) found 67 cases—8.5 percent—of pulmonary edema among 789 women given tocolysis with magnesium sulfate at their hospital.

There have been only two randomized placebo-controlled studies of tocolysis with magnesium sulfate. Cotton and associates (1984) compared magnesium sulfate, ritodrine, and placebo in 54 women in preterm labor. They identified few differences in outcomes. Cox and co-workers (1990) randomly assigned 156 women to receive magnesium sulfate or normal saline infusions. These women were at appreciable risk, and few reached 33 weeks. Magnesium-treated women and their fetuses had identical outcomes compared with those given placebo. Because of these findings, this method of tocolysis was abandoned at Parkland Hospital. Grimes and Nanda (2006) reviewed the use of magnesium sulfate for tocolysis and concluded it was "Time to Quit" on the basis that this therapy was ineffective and potentially harmful to infants.

Neonatal Effects of Magnesium.

In intriguing reports, very-low-birthweight neonates whose mothers were treated with magnesium sulfate for preterm labor or preeclampsia were found to have a reduced incidence of cerebral palsy at 3 years (Grether and associates, 2000; Nelson and Grether, 1995). This was logical, as magnesium has been shown in adults to stabilize intracranial tone, minimize fluctuations in cerebral blood flow, reduce reperfusion injury, and block calcium-mediated intracellular damage (Aslanyan and colleagues, 2007; Marret and associates, 1995). Magnesium reduces synthesis of cytokines and bacterial endotoxins and thus, also may minimize the inflammatory effects of infection (Nelson and Grether, 1997).

Because epidemiological evidence suggested that maternal magnesium sulfate therapy had a fetal neuroprotective effect, randomized trials were designed to investigate this hypothesis. An Australian randomized trial by Crowther and colleagues (2003) included 1063 women at imminent risk of delivery before 30 weeks and who were given magnesium sulfate or placebo. These investigators showed that magnesium exposure improved some perinatal outcomes. Rates of both neonatal death and cerebral palsy were lower in the magnesium-treated group—but the study was not sufficiently powered. The multicenter French trial reported by Marret and associates (2008) had similar problems. This trial included 573 pregnancies at <33 weeks, and the investigators showed improvements of magnesium-treated infants at 2 years compared with infants not exposed to magnesium.

More convincing evidence for magnesium neuroprotection then came from the NICHD Maternal-Fetal Medicine Units Network study reported by Rouse and colleagues (2008). The *Beneficial Effects of Antenatal Magnesium Sulfate—BEAM—Study* was a placebo-controlled trial in 2241 women at imminent risk for preterm birth between 24 and 31 weeks. Almost 87 percent had preterm ruptured membranes, and almost a fifth had previously received magnesium sulfate for tocolysis. Women randomized to magnesium sulfate were given a 6-g bolus over 20 to 30 minutes followed by a maintenance infusion of 2 g per hour. A 2-year follow-up was available for 96 percent of the children. Selected results are shown in Table 36-9. This

---

TABLE 36-9. Magnesium Sulfate for the Prevention of Cerebral Palsy[a]

Perinatal Outcome[a]	Treatment		
	Magnesium Sulfate No. (%)	Placebo No. (%)	Relative Risk (95% CI)
Infants with 2-year follow-up	1041 (100)	1095 (100)	—
Fetal or infant death	99 (9.5)	93 (8.5)	1.12 (0.85–1.47)
Moderate or severe cerebral palsy:			
Overall	20/1041 (1.9)	3/1095 (3.4)	0.55 (0.32–0.95)
<28–31 weeks[b]	12/442 (2.7)	30/496 (6)	0.45 (0.23–0.87)
≥24–27 weeks[b]	8/599 (1.3)	8/599 (1.3)	1.00 (0.38–2.65)

[a]Selected results from the *Beneficial Effects of Antenatal Magnesium Sulfate—BEAM—Study*.
[b]Weeks' gestation at randomization.
Data from Rouse and colleagues (2008).

trial was interpreted differently depending upon statistical philosophy. Those who disdain subgroup analysis opted to interpret these findings to mean that magnesium sulfate infusion prevents cerebral palsy regardless of the gestational age at which the therapy is given. Those with a differing view concluded that this trial only supports use of magnesium sulfate for prevention of cerebral palsy before 28 weeks. What is certain, however, is that maternally administered magnesium sulfate infusions cannot be implicated in increased perinatal deaths as reported by Mittendorf and colleagues (1997).

Subsequent to these studies, Doyle and co-workers (2009) performed a Cochrane review of the five randomized trials dose to assess neuroprotective effects of magnesium sulfate. A total of 6145 infants were available, and as expected, the vast majority came from larger Australian, French, and Network multicenter studies. These reviewers reported that magnesium exposure compared with no exposure significantly decreased risks for cerebral palsy—RR 0.68 (0.54 to 0.87) and substantial gross motor function—RR 0.61 (0.44 to 0.85). There were no significant effects on rates of pediatric mortality or other neurological impairments or disabilities. These reviewers calculated that treatment given to 63 women would prevent one case of cerebral palsy.

Because of these findings, at Parkland Hospital, our policy is to give magnesium sulfate for threatened preterm delivery from 24 to 28 completed weeks. At the University of Alabama at Birmingham Hospital, we administer neuroprotection magnesium from 23 to 32 completed weeks. In both, a 6-g loading dose is followed by an infusion of 2 g per hour for at least 12 hours.

Prostaglandin Inhibitors

Drugs that inhibit prostaglandins have been of considerable interest because prostaglandins are intimately involved in contractions of normal labor (see Chap. 6, p. 153). Antagonists act by inhibiting prostaglandin synthesis or by blocking their action on target organs. A group of enzymes collectively termed *prostaglandin synthase* is responsible for the conversion of free arachidonic acid to prostaglandins. A number of drugs block this system, including acetylsalicylate and indomethacin.

Indomethacin was first used as a tocolytic for 50 women by Zuckerman and associates (1974). Studies that followed reported the efficacy of indomethacin in halting contractions and delaying preterm birth (Muench and colleagues, 2003; Niebyl and associates, 1980). Morales and co-workers (1989, 1993a), however, compared indomethacin with either ritodrine or magnesium sulfate and found no difference in their efficacy to forestall preterm delivery. Berghella and colleagues (2006) reviewed four trials of indomethacin given to women with sonographically short cervices and found such therapy to be ineffective.

Indomethacin is administered orally or rectally. A dose of 50 to 100 mg is followed at 8-hour intervals not to exceed a total 24-hour dose of 200 mg. Serum concentrations usually peak 1 to 2 hours after oral administration, whereas levels after rectal administration peak slightly sooner. Most studies have limited indomethacin use to 24 to 48 hours because of concerns of oligohydramnios, which can develop with these doses.

If amnionic fluid is monitored, oligohydramnios can be detected early, and it is reversible with discontinuation of indomethacin.

Case-control studies have been performed to assess neonatal effects of indomethacin exposure given for preterm labor. In a study of neonates born before 30 weeks, Norton and associates (1993) identified necrotizing enterocolitis in 30 percent of 37 indomethacin-exposed newborns compared with 8 percent of 37 control newborns. Higher incidences of intraventricular hemorrhage and patent ductus arteriosus were also documented in the indomethacin group. The impact of treatment duration and its timing in relation to delivery were not reported. In contrast, several investigators have challenged the association between indomethacin exposure and necrotizing enterocolitis (Muench and co-workers, 2001; Parilla and colleagues, 2000). Finally, Gardner and associates (1996) and Abbasi and co-workers (2003) showed no link between indomethacin use and intraventricular hemorrhage, patent ductus arteriosus, sepsis, necrotizing enterocolitis, or neonatal death.

Schmidt and colleagues (2001) followed 574 newborns who were randomly assigned to receive either indomethacin or placebo to prevent pulmonary hypertension from patent ductus arteriosus. The infants, who weighed 500 to 1000 g, were followed to a corrected age of 18 months. Those given indomethacin had a significantly *reduced* incidence of both patent ductus as well as severe intraventricular hemorrhage. Survival without impairment, however, was similar in both groups. Peck and Lutheran (2003) reported that indomethacin therapy for 7 or more days prior to 33 weeks does not increase the risk of neonatal or childhood medical problems. There have been two meta-analyses of the effects of antenatal indomethacin on neonatal outcomes with conflicting findings (Amin and colleagues, 2007; Loe and associates, 2005).

Calcium-Channel Blockers

Myometrial activity is directly related to cytoplasmic free calcium, and a reduction in its concentration inhibits contractions. Calcium-channel blockers act to inhibit, by a variety of mechanisms, the entry of calcium through channels in the cell membrane. Although they were developed to treat hypertension, their use to arrest preterm labor has been the subject of research since the late 1970s.

Using the Cochrane Database, Keirse (1995a) compared nifedipine and β-agonists and concluded that although nifedipine treatment reduced births of neonates weighing less than 2500 g, significantly more of these were admitted for intensive care. Other investigators have also concluded that calcium-channel blockers, especially nifedipine, are safer and more effective tocolytic agents than are β-agonists (King and colleagues, 2003; Papatsonis and co-workers, 1997). Lyell and colleagues (2007) randomized 192 women at 24 to 33 weeks to either magnesium sulfate or nifedipine and found no substantial differences in efficacy or adverse effects. Finally, oral nifedipine does not significantly prolong pregnancy in women initially treated with intravenous magnesium sulfate for preterm labor (Carr and colleagues, 1999).

The combination of nifedipine with magnesium for tocolysis is potentially dangerous. Ben-Ami and co-workers (1994) and

Kurtzman and associates (1993) reported that nifedipine enhances neuromuscular blocking effects of magnesium that can interfere with pulmonary and cardiac function. How and colleagues (2006) randomized 54 women between $32^{0/7}$ and $34^{6/7}$ weeks to magnesium sulfate plus nifedipine or no tocolytic and found neither benefit nor harm.

Atosiban

This nonapeptide oxytocin analog is a competitive antagonist of oxytocin-induced contractions. Goodwin and colleagues (1995) described its pharmacokinetics in pregnant women. In randomized clinical trials, however, atosiban failed to improve relevant neonatal outcomes and was linked with significant neonatal morbidity (Moutquin and co-workers, 2000; Romero and associates, 2000). The Food and Drug Administration has denied approval of atosiban because of concerns regarding efficacy and fetal-newborn safety. Goodwin (2004) has reviewed the history of atosiban both in the United States and in Europe, where this drug is approved for use and is widely used as a tocolytic.

Nitric Oxide Donors

These potent smooth-muscle relaxants affect the vasculature, gut, and uterus. In randomized clinical trials, nitroglycerin administered orally, transdermally, or intravenously was not effective or showed no superiority to other tocolytics. In addition, maternal hypotension was a common side effect (Bisits, 2004; Buhimschi, 2002; Clavin, 1996; El-Sayed, 1999; Lees, 1999, and all their colleagues).

Summary of Tocolytic Use for Preterm Labor

In many women, tocolytics stop contractions temporarily but rarely prevent preterm birth. In a meta-analysis of tocolytic therapy, Gyetvai and colleagues (1999) concluded that although delivery may be delayed long enough for administration of corticosteroids, treatment does not result in improved perinatal outcome. Berkman and associates (2003) reviewed 60 reports and concluded that tocolytic therapy can prolong gestation, but that β-agonists are not better than other drugs and pose potential maternal danger. They also concluded that there are no benefits of maintenance tocolytic therapy.

As a general rule, if tocolytics are given, they should be given concomitantly with corticosteroids. The gestational age range for their use is debatable, but because corticosteroids are not generally used after 33 weeks and because the perinatal outcomes in preterm neonates are generally good after this time, most practitioners do not recommend use of tocolytics at or after 33 weeks (Goldenberg, 2002).

Recommended Management of Preterm Labor

The following considerations should be given to women in preterm labor:

1. Confirmation of preterm labor as detailed on p. 814
2. For pregnancies less than 34 weeks in women with no maternal or fetal indications for delivery, close observation with monitoring of uterine contractions and fetal heart rate is appropriate. Serial examinations are done to assess cervical changes
3. For pregnancies less than 34 weeks, corticosteroids are given for enhancement of fetal lung maturation
4. Consideration is given for maternal magnesium sulfate infusion for 12 to 24 hours to afford fetal neuroprotection
5. For pregnancies less than 34 weeks in women who are not in advanced labor, some practitioners believe it is reasonable to attempt inhibition of contractions to delay delivery while the women are given corticosteroid therapy and group B streptococcal prophylaxis. Although tocolytic drugs are not used at Parkland Hospital, they are given at University of Alabama at Birmingham Hospital
6. For pregnancies at 34 weeks or beyond, women with preterm labor are monitored for labor progression and fetal well-being
7. For active labor, an antimicrobial is given for prevention of neonatal group B streptococcal infection.

Intrapartum Management

In general, the more immature the fetus, the greater the risks of labor and delivery.

Labor

Whether labor is induced or spontaneous, abnormalities of fetal heart rate and uterine contractions should be sought. We prefer continuous electronic monitoring. Fetal tachycardia, especially with ruptured membranes, is suggestive of sepsis. There is some evidence that intrapartum acidemia may intensify some of the neonatal complications usually attributed to preterm delivery. For example, Low and colleagues (1995) observed that intrapartum acidosis—umbilical artery blood pH less than 7.0—had an important role in neonatal complications (see Chap. 29, p. 614). Similarly, Kimberlin and colleagues (1996) found that increasing umbilical artery blood acidemia was related to more severe respiratory disease in preterm neonates. Despite this, no effects were found in short-term neurological outcomes that included intracranial hemorrhages.

Group B streptococcal infections are common and dangerous in the preterm neonate. Accordingly, as discussed in Chapter 58 (see p. 1220), prophylaxis should be provided.

Delivery

In the absence of a relaxed vaginal outlet, an episiotomy for delivery may be necessary once the fetal head reaches the perineum. Perinatal outcome data do not support routine forceps delivery to protect the "fragile preterm fetal head." Staff proficient in resuscitative techniques commensurate with the gestational age and fully oriented to any specific problems should be present at delivery. Principles of resuscitation described in Chapter 28 are applicable. The importance of the availability of specialized personnel and facilities in the care of preterm newborns is underscored by the improved survival of these neonates when they are delivered in tertiary care centers.

Prevention of Neonatal Intracranial Hemorrhage

Preterm newborns frequently have intracranial germinal matrix bleeding that can extend to more serious intraventricular hemorrhage (see Chap. 29, p. 607). It was hypothesized that cesarean delivery to obviate trauma from labor and vaginal delivery might prevent these complications. This has not been validated by most subsequent studies. Malloy and colleagues (1991) analyzed 1765 newborns with birthweights less than 1500 g and found that cesarean delivery did not lower the risk of mortality or intracranial hemorrhage. Anderson and co-workers (1988), however, made an interesting observation regarding the role of cesarean delivery in the prevention of neonatal intracranial hemorrhages. These hemorrhages related to whether or not the fetus had been subjected to the active phase of labor. They emphasized that avoidance of active-phase labor is impossible in most preterm births because the route of delivery cannot be decided until the active phase of labor is firmly established.

REFERENCES

Abbasi S, Gerdes JS, Sehdev HM, et al: Neonatal outcomes after exposure to indomethacin in utero: A retrospective case cohort study. Am J Obstet Gynecol 189:782, 2003

Alexander JM, Gilstrap LC, Cox SM, et al: Clinical chorioamnionitis and the prognosis for very low birthweight infants. Obstet Gynecol 91:725, 1998

Alexander JM, Mercer BM, Miodovnik M, et al: The impact of digital cervical examination on expectantly managed preterm ruptured membranes. Am J Obstet Gynecol 183:1003, 2000

Althuisius SM, Dekker G, Hummel P, et al: Cervical incompetence prevention randomized cerclage trial: Emergency cerclage with bed rest versus bed rest alone. Am J Obstet Gynecol 189:907, 2003

American Academy of Pediatrics and the American College of Obstetricians and Gynecologists: Guidelines for Perinatal Care, 4th ed. Elk Grove Village, IL, 1997, p 100

American Academy of Pediatrics (AAP) Committee on Fetus and Newborn and the American College of Obstetricians and Gynecologists (ACOG) Committee on Obstetric Practice. Guidelines for Perinatal Care, 6th ed. Elk Grove Village, IL, 2008

American College of Obstetrician and Gynecologists: Preterm labor. Technical Bulletin No. 206, June 1995

American College of Obstetrician and Gynecologists: Assessment of risk factors for preterm birth. Practice Bulletin No. 31, October 2001

American College of Obstetrician and Gynecologists: Perinatal care at the threshold of viability. Practice Bulletin No. 38, September 2002

American College of Obstetricians and Gynecologists: Management of preterm labor. Practice Bulletins No. 43, May 2003

American College of Obstetricians and Gynecologists: Premature rupture of membranes. Practice Bulletin No. 80, April 2007

American College of Obstetricians and Gynecologists: Antenatal corticosteroid therapy for fetal maturation. Committee Opinion No. 402, March 2008a

American College of Obstetricians and Gynecologists: Late-preterm infants. Committee Opinion No. 404, April 2008b

American College of Obstetricians and Gynecologists: Use of progesterone to reduce preterm birth. Committee Opinion No. 419, October 2008c

Amin SB, Sinkin RA, Glantz C: Metaanalysis of the effect of antenatal indomethacin on neonatal outcomes. Am J Obstet Gynecol 197:486, 2007

Ananth CV, Joseph KS, Oyelese Y, et al: Trends in preterm birth and perinatal mortality among singletons: United States, 1989 through 2000. Obstet Gynecol 105:1084, 2005

Ananth CV, Liu S, Joseph KS, et al: A comparison of foetal and infant mortality in the United States and Canada. Int J Epidemiol 38(2):480, 2009

Ananth CV, Vintzileos AM: Maternal-fetal conditions necessitating a medical intervention resulting in preterm birth. Am J Obstet Gynecol 195:1557, 2006

Anderson GD, Bada HS, Sibai BM, et al: The relationship between labor and route of delivery in the preterm infant. Am J Obstet Gynecol 158:1382, 1988

Andrews WW, Goldenberg RL, Hauth JC, et al: Interconceptional antibiotics to prevent spontaneous preterm birth: A randomized clinical trial. Am J Obstet Gynecol 194:617, 2006

Andrews WW, Hauth JC, Goldenberg RL, et al: Amniotic fluid interleukin-6: Correlation with upper genital tract microbial colonization and gestational age in women delivered after spontaneous labor versus indicated delivery. Am J Obstet Gynecol 173:606, 1995

Andrews WW, Sibai BM, Thom EA, et al: Randomized clinical trial of metronidazole plus erythromycin to prevent spontaneous preterm delivery in fetal fibronectin-positive women. Obstet Gynecol 101:847, 2003

Angel JL, O'Brien WF, Knuppel RA, et al: Carbohydrate intolerance in patients receiving oral tocolytics. Am J Obstet Gynecol 159:762, 1988

Annas GJ: Extremely preterm birth and parental authority to refuse treatment—the case of Sidney Miller. N Engl J Med 35:2118, 2004

Anum EA, Springel EH, Shriver MD, et al: Genetic contributions to disparities in preterm birth. Pediatr Res 65(1):1, 2009

Aslanyan S, Weir CJ, Muir KW, et al: Magnesium for treatment of acute lacunar stroke syndromes: Further analysis of the IMAGES trial. Stroke 38(4):1269, 2007

Behrman RE, Butler S, eds: Preterm birth: Causes, consequences, and prevention. Washington, DC, National Academics Press, 2007

Beigi RH, Austin MN, Meyn LA, et al: Antimicrobial resistance associated with the treatment of bacterial vaginosis. Am J Obstet Gynecol 191:1124, 2004

Ben-Ami M, Giladi Y, Shalev E: The combination of magnesium sulphate and nifedipine: A cause of neuromuscular blockade. Br J Obstet Gynaecol 101:262, 1994

Berghella V, Odibo AO, To MS, et al: Cerclage for short cervix on ultrasonography: Meta-analysis of trials using individual patient-level data. Obstet Gynecol 106(1):181, 2005

Berghella V, Rust OA, Althuisius SM: Short cervix on ultrasound: Does indomethacin prevent preterm birth? Am J Obstet Gynecol 195:809, 2006

Berkman ND, Thorp JM, Lohr KN, et al: Tocolytic treatment for the management of preterm labor: A review of the evidence. Am J Obstet Gynecol 188:1648, 2003

Bisits A, Madsen G, Knox M, et al: The randomized nitric oxide tocolysis trial (RNOTT) for the treatment of preterm labor. Am J Obstet Gynecol 191:683, 2004

Bloom SL, Yost NP, McIntire DD, et al: Recurrence of preterm birth in singleton and twin pregnancies. Obstet Gynecol 98:379, 2001

Braner D, Kattwinkel J, Denson S, et al: Textbook of Neonatal Resuscitations, 4th ed. Elk Grove Village, IL, American Academy of Pediatrics, 2000

Bruschettini M, van den Hove DL, Gazzolo D, et al: Lowering the dose of antenatal steroids: The effects of a single course of betamethasone on somatic growth and brain cell proliferation in the rat. Am J Obstet Gynecol 194:1341, 2006

Buekens P, Alexander S, Boutsen M, et al: Randomised controlled trial of routine cervical examinations in pregnancy. Lancet 344:841, 1994

Buhimschi CS, Buhimschi IA, Malinow AM, et al: Effects of sublingual nitroglycerin on human uterine contractility during the active phase of labor. Am J Obstet Gynecol 187:235, 2002

Bullard I, Vermillion S, Soper D: Clinical intraamniotic infection and the outcome for very low birth weight neonates [Abstract]. Am J Obstet Gynecol 187:S73, 2002

Canadian Preterm Labor Investigators Group: Treatment of preterm labor with the beta-adrenergic agonist ritodrine. N Engl J Med 327:308, 1992

Carey JC, Klebanoff MA: Is a change in the vaginal flora associated with an increased risk of preterm birth? Am J Obstet Gynecol 192(4):1341, 2005

Caritis SN, Rouse DJ, Peaceman AM, et al: Prevention of preterm birth in triplets using 17 alpha-hydroxyprogesterone caproate. Obstet Gynecol 113:285, 2009

Carlan SJ, O'Brien WF, Parsons MT, et al: Preterm premature rupture of membranes: A randomized study of home versus hospital management. Obstet Gynecol 81:61, 1993

Carr DB, Clark AL, Kernek K, et al: Maintenance oral nifedipine for preterm labor: A randomized clinical trial. Am J Obstet Gynecol 181:822, 1999

Carroll SG, Blott M, Nicolaides KH: Preterm prelabor amniorrhexis: Outcome of live births. Obstet Gynecol 86:18, 1995

Carroll SG, Papaionnou S, Ntumazah IL, et al: Lower genital tract swabs in the prediction of intrauterine infection in preterm prelabour rupture of the membranes. Br J Obstet Gynaecol 103:54, 1996

Casanueva E, Ripoll C, Meza-Camacho C, et al: Possible interplay between vitamin C deficiency and prolactin in pregnant women with premature rupture of membranes: Facts and hypothesis. Med Hypotheses 64:241, 2005

Cazan-London G, Mozurkewich EL, Xu X, et al: Willingness or unwillingness to perform cesarean section for impending preterm delivery at 24 weeks' gestation: A cost-effectiveness analysis. Am J Obstet Gynecol 193(3):1187, 2005

Clavin DK, Bayhi DA, Nolan TE, et al: Comparison of intravenous magnesium sulfate and nitroglycerin for preterm labor: Preliminary data. Am J Obstet Gynecol 174:307, 1996

Collaborative Home Uterine Monitoring Study Group: A multicenter randomized controlled trial of home uterine monitoring: Active versus sham device. Am J Obstet Gynecol 173:1170, 1995

Collins JW Jr, David RJ, Simon DM, et al: Preterm birth among African American and white women with a lifelong residence in high-income Chicago neighborhoods: An exploratory study. Ethn Dis 17(1):113, 2007

Conde-Agudelo A, Rosas-Bermúdez A, Kafury-Goeta AC: Birth spacing and risk of adverse perinatal outcomes: A meta-analysis. JAMA 295:1809, 2006

Cook CM, Ellwood DA: A longitudinal study of the cervix in pregnancy using transvaginal ultrasound. Br J Obstet Gynaecol 103:16, 1996

Copper RL, Goldenberg RL, Das A, et al: The preterm prediction study: Maternal stress is associated with spontaneous preterm birth at less than thirty-five weeks' gestation. Am J Obstet Gynecol 175:1286, 1996

Copper RL, Goldenberg RL, Davis RO, et al: Warning symptoms, uterine contractions, and cervical examination findings in women at risk of preterm delivery. Am J Obstet Gynecol 162:748, 1990

Copper RL, Goldenberg RL, Dubard MB, et al: Cervical examination and tocodynamometry at 28 weeks' gestation: Prediction of spontaneous preterm birth. Am J Obstet Gynecol 172:666, 1995

Cotton DB, Strassner HT, Hill LM, et al: Comparison between magnesium sulfate, terbutaline and a placebo for inhibition of preterm labor: A randomized study. J Reprod Med 29:92, 1984

Cox SM, Leveno KJ: Intentional delivery versus expectant management with preterm ruptured membranes at 30–34 weeks' gestation. Obstet Gynecol 86:875, 1995

Cox SM, Sherman ML, Leveno KJ: Randomized investigation of magnesium sulfate for prevention of preterm birth. Am J Obstet Gynecol 163:767, 1990

Cox SM, Williams ML, Leveno KJ: The natural history of preterm ruptured membranes: What to expect of expectant management. Obstet Gynecol 71:558, 1988

Crowther CA, Doyle LW, Haslam RR, et al: Outcomes at 2 years of age after repeat doses of antenatal corticosteroids. N Engl J Med 357:1179, 2007

Crowther CA, Hiller JE, Doyle LW, et al: Effect of magnesium sulfate given for neuroprotection before preterm birth: A randomized controlled trial. JAMA 290:2669, 2003

Csapo AI: Progesterone "block." Am J Anat 98:273, 1956

Culhane JF, Rauh V, McCollum KF, et al: Exposure to chronic stress and ethnic differences in rates of bacterial vaginosis among pregnant women. Am J Obstet Gynecol 187:1272, 2002

da Fonseca EB, Bittar RE, de Carvalho MH, et al: Prophylactic administration of progesterone by vaginal suppository to reduce the incidence of spontaneous preterm birth in women at increased risk: A randomized placebo-controlled double-blind study. Am J Obstet Gynecol 188:419, 2003

da Fonseca EB, Celik E, Parra M, et al: Progesterone and the risk of preterm birth among women with a short cervix. N Engl J Med 357:462, 2007

de Carvalho MH, Bittar RE, Brizot Mde L, et al: Prediction of preterm delivery in the second trimester. Obstet Gynecol 105:532, 2005

Devlieger R, Millar LK, Bryant-Greenwood G, et al: Fetal membrane healing after spontaneous and iatrogenic membrane rupture: A review of current evidence. Am J Obstet Gynecol 195:1512, 2006

Dodd JM, Flenady VJ, Cincotta R, et al: Progesterone for the prevention of preterm birth: A systematic review. Obstet Gynecol 112:127, 2008

Dolan SM, Gross SJ, Merkatz IR, et al: The contribution of birth defects to preterm birth and low birth weight. Obstet Gynecol 110:318, 2007

Doyle LW, Crowther CA, Middleton S, et al: Magnesium sulfate for women at risk of preterm birth for neuroprotection of the fetus. Cochrane Database of Syst Rev 1:CD004661, 2009

Duhig KE, Chandiramani M, Seed PT, et al: Fetal fibronectin as a predictor of spontaneous preterm labour in asymptomatic women with a cervical cerclage. BJOG 116(6):799, 2009

Dyson DC, Danbe KH, Bamber JA, et al: Monitoring women at risk for preterm labor. N Engl J Med 338:15, 1998

Ehrenberg HM, Iams JD, Goldenberg RL, et al: Maternal obesity, uterine activity, and the risk of spontaneous preterm birth. Obstet Gynecol 113(1):48, 2009

Eichenwald EC, Stark AR: Management and outcomes of very low birth weight. N Engl J Med 358:1700, 2008

Elimian A, Garry D, Figueroa R, et al: Antenatal betamethasone compared with dexamethasone (Betacode Trial): A randomized controlled trial. Obstet Gynecol 110:26, 2007

Elliott JP, Istwan NB, Rhea D, et al: The occurrence of adverse events in women receiving continuous subcutaneous terbutaline therapy. Am J Obstet Gynecol 191:1277, 2004

El-Sayed Y, Riley ET, Holbrook RH, et al: Randomized comparison of intravenous nitroglycerin and magnesium sulfate for treatment of preterm labor. Obstet Gynecol 93:79, 1999

Fanaroff AA, Stoll BJ, Wright LL, et al: Trends in neonatal morbidity and mortality for very low birthweight infants. Am J Obstet Gynecol 196:e1.147, 2007

Farooqi A, Holmgren PA, Engberg S, et al: Survival and 2-year outcome with expectant management of second trimester rupture of membranes. Obstet Gynecol 92:895, 1998

Feinstein SJ, Vintzileos AM, Lodeiro JG, et al: Amniocentesis with premature rupture of membranes. Obstet Gynecol 68:147, 1986

Fletcher SE, Fyfe DA, Case CL, et al: Myocardial necrosis in a newborn after long-term maternal subcutaneous terbutaline infusion for suppression of preterm labor. Am J Obstet Gynecol 165:1401, 1991

Fuchs K, Albright C, Scott K, et al: Obstetric factors affecting respiratory morbidity among late preterm infants. Am J Obstet Gynecol, In press, 2009

Gardner MO, Owen J, Skelly S, et al: Preterm delivery after indomethacin: A risk factor for neonatal complications? J Reprod Med 41:903, 1996

Garite TJ, Freeman RK, Linzey EM, et al: Prospective randomized study of corticosteroids in the management of premature rupture of the membranes and the premature gestation. Am J Obstet Gynecol 141:508, 1981

Garite TJ, Keegan KA, Freeman RK, et al: A randomized trial of ritodrine tocolysis versus expectant management in patients with premature rupture of membranes at 25 to 30 weeks of gestation. Am J Obstet Gynecol 157:388, 1987

Gibson CS, MacLennan AH, Dekker GA, et al: Genetic polymorphisms and spontaneous preterm birth. Obstet Gynecol 109:384, 2007

Gielchinsky Y, Mankuta D, Samueloff A, et al: First pregnancy in women over 45 years of age carries increased obstetrical risk [Abstract]. Am J Obstet Gynecol 187:S87, 2002

Gluck L: Fetal lung maturity. Paper presented at the 78th Ross Conference on Pediatric Research, San Diego, May 1979

Goepfert AR, Jeffcoat MK, Andrews W, et al: Periodontal disease and upper genital tract inflammation in early spontaneous preterm birth. Obstet Gynecol 104:777, 2004

Goldenberg RL: The management of preterm labor. Obstet Gynecol 100:1020, 2002

Goldenberg RL, Andrews WW, Goepfert AR, et al: The Alabama Preterm Birth Study: Umbilical cord blood *Ureaplasma urealyticum* and *Mycoplasma hominis* cultures in very preterm newborn infants. Am J Obstet Gynecol 198:43, 2008a

Goldenberg RL, Cliver SP, Bronstein J, et al: Bed rest in pregnancy. Obstet Gynecol 84:131, 1994

Goldenberg RL, Culhane JF, Iams JD, et al: Preterm birth 1: Epidemiology and causes of preterm birth. Lancet 371:75, 2008b

Goldenberg RL, Klebanoff M, Carey JC, et al: Vaginal fetal fibronectin measurements from 8 to 22 weeks' gestation and subsequent spontaneous preterm birth. Am J Obstet Gynecol 183:469, 2000

Goldenberg RL, Mwatha A, Read JS, et al: The HPTN 024 Study: The efficacy of antibiotics to prevent chorioamnionitis and preterm birth. Am J Obstet Gynecol 194:650, 2006

Gomez R, Romero R, Nien JK, et al: A short cervix in women with preterm labor and intact membranes: A risk factor for microbial invasion of the amniotic cavity. Am J Obstet Gynecol 192:678, 2005

Goodwin TM: The Gordian knot of developing tocolytics. J Soc Gynecol Investig 11(6)339, 2004

Goodwin TM, Millar L, North L, et al: The pharmacokinetics of the oxytocin antagonist atosiban in pregnant women with preterm uterine contractions. Am J Obstet Gynecol 173:913, 1995

Goulet C, Gevry H, Lemay M, et al: A randomized clinical trial of care for women with preterm labour: Home management versus hospital management. CMAJ 164:985, 2001

Grether JK, Hoogstrate J, Walsh-Greene E, et al: Magnesium sulfate for tocolysis and risk of spastic cerebral palsy in premature children born to women without preeclampsia. Am J Obstet Gynecol 183:717, 2000

Grimes DA, Nanda K: Magnesium sulfate tocolysis: Time to quit. Obstet Gynecol 108:986, 2006

Grobman WA, Welshman EE, Calhoun EA: Does fetal fibronectin use in the diagnosis of preterm labor affect physician behavior and health care costs? A randomized trial. Am J Obstet Gynecol 191:235, 2004

Guinn DA, Goepfert AR, Owen J, et al: Management option in women with preterm uterine contractions: A randomized clinical trial. Am J Obstet Gynecol 177:814, 1997

Guinn DA, Goepfert AR, Owen J, et al: Terbutaline pump maintenance therapy for prevention of preterm delivery: A double-blind trial. Am J Obstet Gynecol 179:874, 1998

Gyetvai K, Hannah ME, Hodnett ED, et al: Tocolytics for preterm labor: A systematic review. Obstet Gynecol 94:869, 1999

Hack M, Taylor M, Drotar D, et al: Chronic conditions, functional limitations, and special health care needs of school-aged children born with extremely low-birth-weight in the 1990s. JAMA 294:318, 2005

Hadi HA, Hodson CA, Strickland D: Premature rupture of the membranes between 20 and 25 weeks' gestation: Role of amniotic fluid volume in perinatal outcome. Am J Obstet Gynecol 170:1139, 1994

Hallak M, Bottoms SF: Accelerated pulmonary maturation from preterm premature rupture of membranes: A myth. Am J Obstet Gynecol 169:1045, 1993

Hampton T: Genetic link found for premature birth risk. JAMA 296:1713, 2006

Hankins GD, Hauth JC, Cissik JH, et al: Effects of ritodrine hydrochloride on arteriovenous blood gas and shunt in healthy pregnant yellow baboons. Am J Obstet Gynecol 158:658, 1988

Harger JM: Cervical cerclage: Patient selection morbidity, and success rates. Clin Perinatol 10: 321, 1983

Hausdorff WP, Caron MG, Lefkowitz RJ: Turning off the signal: Desensitization of beta-adrenergic receptor function. FASEB J 4:2881, 1990

Helfgott AW, Willis DC, Blanco JD: Is hydration and sedation beneficial in the treatment of threatened preterm labor? A preliminary report. J Matern Fetal Med 3:37, 1994

Hickey CA, Cliver SP, McNeal SF, et al: Prenatal weight gain patterns and spontaneous preterm birth among non-obese black and white women. Obstet Gynecol 85:909, 1995

Hillier SL, Nugent RP, Eschenbach DA, et al: Association between bacterial vaginosis and preterm delivery of a low-birthweight infant. N Engl J Med 333:1737, 1995

Ho M, Ramsey P, Brumfield C, et al: Changes in maternal and neonatal infectious morbidity as latency increases after preterm premature rupture of membranes [Abstract]. Obstet Gynecol 101:41S, 2003

Hofman PL, Regan F, Jackson WE, et al: Premature birth and later insulin resistance. N Engl J Med 351:2179, 2004

Hovi P, Andersson S, Eriksson JG, et al: Glucose regulation in young adults with very low birth weight. N Engl J Med 356:2053, 2007

How HY, Hughes SA, Vogel RL, et al: Oral terbutaline in the outpatient management of preterm labor. Am J Obstet Gynecol 173:1518, 1995

How HY, Zafaranchi L, Stella CL, et al: Tocolysis in women with preterm labor between $32^{0/7}$ and $34^{6/7}$ weeks of gestation: A randomized controlled pilot study. Am J Obstet Gynecol 194:976, 2006

Hudgens DR, Conradi SE: Sudden death associated with terbutaline sulfate administration. Am J Obstet Gynecol 169:120, 1993

Hueston WJ, Knox MA, Eilers G, et al: The effectiveness of preterm-birth prevention educational program for high-risk women: A meta-analysis. Obstet Gynecol 86:705, 1995

Iams JD, Goldenberg RL, Meis PJ, et al: The length of the cervix and the risk of spontaneous premature delivery. N Engl J Med 334:567, 1996

Iams JD, Johnson FF, Parker M: A prospective evaluation of the signs and symptoms of preterm labor. Obstet Gynecol 84:227, 1994

Iams JD, Newman RB, Thom EA, et al: Frequency of uterine contractions and the risk of spontaneous preterm birth. N Engl J Med 346:250, 2002

Iams JD, Stilson R, Johnson FF, et al: Symptoms that precede preterm labor and preterm premature rupture of the membranes. Am J Obstet Gynecol 162:486, 1990

Ingelfinger JR: Prematurity and the legacy of intrauterine stress. N Engl J Med 356:2093, 2007

Institute of Medicine, Committee on Understanding Premature Birth and Assuring Healthy Outcomes Board on Health Sciences Policy, Behrman RE, Butler AS, eds. Preterm Birth: Causes, Consequences, and Prevention. Washington, DC: National Academics Press, 2006

Joseph KS, Huang L, Liu S, et al: Reconciling the high rates of preterm and postterm birth in the United States. Obstet Gynecol 109:813, 2007

Kaijser M, Bonamy AK, Akre O, et al: Perinatal risk factors for diabetes in later life. Diabetes 58(3):523, 2009

Keirse MJNC: Calcium antagonists vs. betamimetics in preterm labour. In Neilson JP, Crowther C, Hodnett ED, et al (eds): Pregnancy and Childbirth Module. Cochrane Database of Systematic Reviews, Issue 2. Oxford, Update Software, 1995a

Keirse MJNC: New perspectives for the effective treatment of preterm labor. Am J Obstet Gynecol 173:618, 1995b

Kenyon S, Boulvain M, Neilson J: Antibiotics for preterm rupture of the membranes: A systematic review. Obstet Gynecol 104:1051, 2004

Kenyon S, Pike K, Jones DR, et al: Childhood outcomes after prescription of antibiotics to pregnant women with preterm rupture of the membranes: 7-year follow-up of the ORACLE I trial. Lancet 372:1310, 2008a

Kenyon S, Pike K, Jones DR, et al: Childhood outcomes after prescription of antibiotics to pregnant women with spontaneous preterm labour: 7-year follow-up of the ORACLE II trial. Lancet 372:1319, 2008b

Kenyon SL, Taylor DJ, Tarnow-Mordi, et al: Broad-spectrum antibiotics for spontaneous preterm labour: The ORACLE II randomized trial. Lancet 357:989, 2001

Kimberlin DF, Hauth JC, Goldenberg RL, et al: Relationship of acid–base status and neonatal morbidity in 1000 g infants. Am J Obstet Gynecol 174:382, 1996

King J, Flenady V: Antibiotics for preterm labour with intact membranes. Cochrane Database Syst Rev 2:CD000246, 2000

King JF, Flenady V, Papatsonis D, et al: Calcium channel blockers for inhibiting preterm labour: A systematic review of the evidence and a protocol for administration of nifedipine. Aust NZ J Obstet Gynaecol 43:192, 2003

Kistka ZA, Palomar L, Lee KA, et al: Racial disparity in the frequency of recurrence of preterm birth. Am J Obstet Gynecol 196:131, 2007

Klerman LV, Ramey SL, Goldenberg RL, et al: A randomized trial of augmented prenatal care for multiple-risk, Medicaid-eligible African American women. Am J Public Health 91:105, 2001

Kovacevich GJ, Gaich SA, Lavin JP, et al: The prevalence of thromboembolic events among women with extended bed rest prescribed as part of the treatment for premature labor or preterm premature rupture of membranes. Am J Obstet Gynecol 182:1089, 2000

Kragt H, Keirse MJ: How accurate is a woman's diagnosis of threatened preterm delivery? Br J Obstet Gynaecol 97:317, 1990

Kramer MS, Coates AL, Michoud MC, et al: Maternal anthropometry and idiopathic preterm labor. Obstet Gynecol 86:744, 1995

Kurki T, Sivonen A, Renkonen OV, et al: Bacterial vaginosis in early pregnancy and pregnancy outcome. Obstet Gynecol 80:173, 1992

Kurtzman J, Garite T, Clark R, et al: Impact of a "rescue course" of antenatal corticosteroids (ACS): A multi-center randomized placebo controlled trial. Am J Obstet Gynecol, In press, 2009

Kurtzman JL, Thorp JM Jr, Spielman FJ, et al: Do nifedipine and verapamil potentiate the cardiac toxicity of magnesium sulfate? Am J Perinatol 10:450, 1993

Lam F, Gill P, Smith M, et al: Use of the subcutaneous terbutaline pump for long-term tocolysis. Obstet Gynecol 72:810, 1988

Lee HC, Gould JB: Survival advantage associated with cesarean delivery in very low birth weight vertex neonates. Obstet Gynecol 107:97, 2006

Lees CC, Lojacono A, Thompson C, et al: Glyceryl trinitrate and ritodrine in tocolysis: An international multicenter randomized study. Obstet Gynecol 94:403, 1999

Leeson SC, Maresh MJA, Martindale EA, et al: Detection of fetal fibronectin as a predictor of preterm delivery in high risk symptomatic pregnancies. Br J Obstet Gynaecol 103:48, 1996

Leitich H, Bodner-Adler B, Brunbauer M, et al: Bacterial vaginosis as a risk factor for preterm delivery: A meta-analysis. Am J Obstet Gynecol 189:139, 2003a

Leitich H, Brunbauer M, Bodner-Adler B, et al: Antibiotic treatment of bacterial vaginosis in pregnancy: A meta-analysis. Am J Obstet Gynecol 188:752, 2003b

Leveno KJ, Klein VR, Guzick DS, et al: Single-centre randomised trial of ritodrine hydrochloride for preterm labour. Lancet 1:1293, 1986

Leveno KJ, McIntire DD, Bloom SL, et al: Decreased preterm births in an inner-city public hospital. Obstet Gynecol 113(3):578, 2009

Lewis DF, Adair CD, Robichaux AG, et al: Antibiotic therapy in preterm premature rupture of membranes: Are seven days necessary? A preliminary, randomized clinical trial. Am J Obstet Gynecol 188:1413, 2003

Lewis DF, Robichaux AG, Jaekle RK, et al: Expectant management of preterm premature rupture of membranes and nonvertex presentation: What are the risks? Am J Obstet Gynecol 196:566, 2007

Lewis R, Mercer BM, Salama M, et al: Oral terbutaline after parenteral tocolysis: A randomized, double-blind, placebo-controlled trial. Am J Obstet Gynecol 175:834, 1996

Li D, Liu L, Odouli R: Presence of depressive symptoms during early pregnancy and the risk of preterm delivery: A prospective cohort study. Hum Reprod 24:146, 2008

Li D-K, Odouli R, Liu L, et al: Transmission of parentally shared human leukocyte antigen alleles and the risk of preterm delivery. Obstet Gynecol 104:594, 2004

Lie RT, Wilcox AJ, Skjaerven R: Maternal and paternal influences on length of pregnancy. Obstet Gynecol 107:880, 2006

Lieman JM, Brumfield CG, Carlo W, et al: Preterm premature rupture of membranes: Is there an optimal gestational age for delivery? Obstet Gynecol 105:12, 2005

Liggins GC, Howie RN: A controlled trial of antepartum glucocorticoid treatment for prevention of the respiratory distress syndrome in premature infants. Pediatrics 50:515, 1972

Littleton HL, Breitkopf CR, Berenson AB: Correlates of anxiety symptoms during pregnancy and association with perinatal outcomes: A meta-analysis. Am J Obstet Gynecol 196:424, 2007

Locatelli A, Ghidini A, Paterlini G, et al: Gestational age at preterm premature rupture of membranes: A risk factor for neonatal white matter damage. Am J Obstet Gynecol 193:947, 2005

Lockwood CJ, Senyei AE, Dische MR, et al: Fetal fibronectin in cervical and vaginal secretions as a predictor of preterm delivery. N Engl J Med 325:669, 1991

Loe SM, Sanchez-Ramos L, Kaunitz AM: Assessing the neonatal safety of indomethacin tocolysis: A systematic review with meta-analysis. Obstet Gynecol 106:173, 2005

Louis JM, Ehrenberg HM, Collin MF, et al: Perinatal intervention and neonatal outcomes near the limit of viability. Am J Obstet Gynecol 191:1398, 2004

Low JA, Panagiotopoulos C, Derrick EJ: Newborn complication after intrapartum asphyxia with metabolic acidosis in the preterm fetus. Am J Obstet Gynecol 172:805, 1995

Lowe MP, Zimmerman B, Hansen W: Prospective randomized controlled trial of fetal fibronectin on preterm labor management in a tertiary care center. Am J Obstet Gynecol 190:358, 2004

Lu MC, Chen B: Racial and ethnic disparities in preterm birth: The role of stressful life events. Am J Obstet Gynecol 191:691, 2004

Luke B, Mamelle N, Keith L, et al: The association between occupational factors and preterm birth: A United States nurses study. Am J Obstet Gynecol 173:849, 1995

Lyell DJ, Pullen K, Campbell L, et al: Magnesium sulfate compared with nifedipine for acute tocolysis of preterm labor: A randomized controlled trial. Obstet Gynecol 1108:61, 2007

MacDorman MF, Mathews TJ: Recent trends in infant mortality in the United States. NCHS Data Brief, No. 9. Hyattsville, MD, National Center for Health Statistics, 2008

Mackenzie R, Walker M, Armson A, et al: Progesterone for the prevention of preterm birth among women at increased risk: A systematic review and meta-analysis of randomized controlled trials. Am J Obstet Gynecol 194:1234, 2006

Macones GA, Berlin M, Berlin JA: Efficacy of oral beta-agonist maintenance therapy in preterm labor: A meta-analysis. Obstet Gynecol 85:313, 1995

Macones GA, Parry S, Elkousy M, et al: A polymorphism in the promoter region of TNF and bacterial vaginosis: Preliminary evidence of gene-environment interaction in the etiology of spontaneous preterm birth. Am J Obstet Gynecol 190:1504, 2004

Major CA, Towers CW, Lewis DF, et al: Expectant management of preterm premature rupture of membranes complicated by active recurrent genital herpes. Am J Obstet Gynecol 188:1551, 2003

Malloy MH, Onstad L, Wright E: The effect of cesarean delivery on birth outcome in very low birth weight infants. Obstet Gynecol 77:498, 1991

Marlow N, Wolke D, Bracewell MA, et al: Neurologic and developmental disability at six years of age after extremely preterm birth. N Engl J Med 352:9, 2005

Marret S, Gressens P, Gadisseux JF, et al: Prevention by magnesium of excitotoxic neuronal death in the developing brain: An animal model for clinical intervention studies. Dev Med Child Neurol 37(6):473, 1995

Marret S, Marpeau L, Bénichou J: Benefit of magnesium sulfate given before very preterm birth to protect infant brain. Pediatrics 121(1):225, 2008

Martin JA, Hamilton BE, Sutton PD, et al: Births: Final data for 2004. National Vital Statistics Reports, vol 55, no 1. Hyattsville, MD, National Center for Health Statistics, 2006

Martin JA, Hamilton BE, Sutton PD, et al: Births: Final data for 2005. National Vital Statistics Reports, vol 56, no 6. Hyattsville, MD, National Center for Health Statistics, 2007

Martin JA, Hamilton BE, Sutton PD, et al: Births: Final Data for 2006. National Vital Statistics Reports, Vol 57, No 7. Hyattsville, MD, National Center for Health Statistics, 2009

Martin JA, Menacker F: Expanded health data from the new birth certificate, 2004. National Vital Statistics Reports, vol 55, no 12. Hyattsville, MD, National Center for Health Statistics, 2007

Mathews TJ, MacDorman MF: Infant mortality statistics from the 2005 period linked birth/infant death data set. National Vital Statistics Reports, vol 57, no 2. Hyattsville, MD, National Center for Health Statistics, 2008

McElrath TF, Allred E, Leviton A: Prolonged latency after preterm premature rupture of membranes: An evaluation of histologic condition and intracranial ultrasonic abnormality in the neonate born at <28 weeks of gestation. Am J Obstet Gynecol 189:794, 2003

McElrath TF, Norwitz ER, Lieberman ES, et al: Perinatal outcome after preterm premature rupture of membranes with in situ cervical cerclage. Am J Obstet Gynecol 187:1147, 2002

McEvoy C, Schilling D, Segel S, et al: Improved respiratory compliance in preterm infants after a single rescue course of antenatal steroids: A randomized trial. Am J Obstet Gynecol [In Press] 2009

McIntire DD, Leveno KJ: Neonatal mortality and morbidity rates in late preterm births compared with births at term. Obstet Gynecol 111:35, 2008

Meis PJ, Klebanoff M, Thom E, et al: Prevention of recurrent preterm delivery by 17 alpha-hydroxyprogesterone caproate. National Institute of Child Health and Human Development Maternal-Fetal Medicine Units Network. N Engl J Med 348:2379, 2003

Meis PJ, Michielutte R, Peters TJ, et al: Factors associated with preterm birth in Cardiff, Wales, I. Univariable and multivariable analysis. Am J Obstet Gynecol 173:590, 1995

Mercer BM, Ahokas R, Beazley D, et al: Corticol, ACTG, and psychosocial stress in women at high risk for preterm birth [Abstract]. Am J Obstet Gynecol 187:S72, 2002

Mercer BM, Arheart KL: Antimicrobial therapy in expectant management of preterm premature rupture of the membranes. Lancet 346:1271, 1995

Mercer BM, Carr TL, Beazley DD, et al: Antibiotic use in pregnancy and drug-resistant infant sepsis. Am J Obstet Gynecol 181:816, 1999

Mercer BM, Crocker LG, Boe NM, et al: Induction versus expectant management in premature rupture of the membranes with mature amniotic fluid at 32 to 36 weeks: A randomized trial. Am J Obstet Gynecol 169:775, 1993

Mercer BM, Goldenberg RL, Das A, et al: The preterm prediction study: A clinical risk assessment system. Am J Obstet Gynecol 174:1885, 1996

Mercer BM, Miodovnik M, Thurnau GR, et al: Antibiotic therapy for reduction of infant morbidity after preterm premature rupture of the membranes. JAMA 278:989, 1997

Merkatz IR, Peter JB, Barden TP: Ritodrine hydrochloride: A betamimetic agent for use in preterm labor, II. Evidence of efficacy. Obstet Gynecol 56:7, 1980

Michalowicz BS, Hodges JS, DiAngelis AJ, et al: Treatment of periodontal disease and the risk of preterm birth. N Engl J Med 355:1885, 2006

Mittendorf R, Covert R, Boman J, et al: Is tocolytic magnesium sulfate associated with increased total paediatric mortality? Lancet 350:1517, 1997

Morales WJ, Madhav H: Efficacy and safety of indomethacin compared with magnesium sulfate in the management of preterm labor: A randomized study. Am J Obstet Gynecol 169:97, 1993a

Morales WJ, Smith SG, Angel JL, et al: Efficacy and safety of indomethacin versus ritodrine in the management of preterm labor: A randomized study. Obstet Gynecol 74:567, 1989

Morales WJ, Talley T: Premature rupture of membranes <25 weeks: A management dilemma. Am J Obstet Gynecol 168:503, 1993b

Morency AM, Bujold E: The effect of second-trimester antibiotic therapy on the rate of preterm birth. J Obstet Gynaecol Can 29:35, 2007

Morken N-H, Källen K, Jacobsson B: Fetal growth and onset of delivery: A nationwide population-based study of preterm infants. Am J Obstet Gynecol 195:154, 2006

Moutquin JM, Sherman D, Cohen H, et al: Double-blind, randomized, controlled trial of atosiban and ritodrine in the treatment of preterm labor: A multicenter effectiveness and safety study. Am J Obstet Gynecol 183:1191, 2000

Muench MV, Baschat AA, Kopelman J, et al: Indomethacin therapy initiated before 24 weeks of gestation for the prevention of preterm birth [Abstract]. Obstet Gynecol 101:65S, 2003

Muench V, Harman CR, Baschat AA, et al: Early fetal exposure to long term indomethacin therapy to prevent preterm delivery: Neonatal outcome. Am J Obstet Gynecol 185:S149, 2001

Murphy KE: Betamethasone compared with dexamethasone for preterm birth: A call for trials. Obstet Gynecol 110:7, 2007

National Institutes of Health Consensus Development Conference: Statement on Repeat Courses of Antenatal Corticosteroids. Bethesda, MD. August 17–18, 2000. Available at: http://consensus.nih.gov/2000/2000Antenatal-CorticosteroidsRevisted112html.htm. Accessed January 25, 2009

Neggers Y, Goldenberg R, Cliver S, et al: Effects of domestic violence on preterm birth and low birth weight. Acta Obstet Gynecol Scand 83:455, 2004

Nelson KB, Grether JK: Can magnesium sulfate reduce the risk of cerebral palsy in very-low-birthweight infants? Pediatrics 95:263, 1995

Nelson KB, Grether JK: More on prenatal magnesium sulfate and risk of cerebral palsy. JAMA 278(18):1493, 1997

Nelson LH, Anderson RL, O'Shea M, et al: Expectant management of preterm premature rupture of the membranes. Am J Obstet Gynecol 171:350, 1994

Nelson LH, Meis PJ, Hatjis CG, et al: Premature rupture of membranes: A prospective, randomized evaluation of steroids, latent phase, and expectant management. Obstet Gynecol 66:55, 1985

Ness RB, Hillier SL, Richter HE: Douching in relation to bacterial vaginosis, lactobacilli, and facultative bacteria in the vagina. Obstet Gynecol 100:765, 2002

Niebyl JR, Blake DA, White RD, et al: The inhibition of premature labor with indomethacin. Am J Obstet Gynecol 136:1014, 1980

Norton ME, Merrill J, Cooper BA, et al: Neonatal complications after the administration of indomethacin for preterm labor. N Engl J Med 329:1602, 1993

Norwitz ER, Bahtiyar MO, Sibai BM: Defining standards of care in maternal-fetal medicine. Am J Obstet Gynecol 191:1491, 2004

Nugent RP, Krohn MA, Hillier SL: Reliability of diagnosing bacterial vaginosis by a standardized method of gram stain interpretation. J Clin Microbiol 29:297, 1991

O'Brien JM, Adair CD, Lewis DF, et al: Progesterone vaginal gel for the reduction of recurrent preterm birth: Primary results from a randomized, double-blind, placebo-controlled trial. Ultrasound Obstet Gynecol 30:687, 2007

Okun N, Gronau KA, Hannah ME: Antibiotics for bacterial vaginosis or *Trichomonas vaginalis* in pregnancy: A systematic review. Obstet Gynecol 105:857, 2005

Owen J: Multicenter randomized trial of cerclage for preterm birth prevention in high-risk women with shortened mid-trimester cervical length, Abstract #4. Am J Obstet Gynecol, In press, 2009

Owen J, Baker SL, Hauth JC, et al: Is indicated or spontaneous preterm delivery more advantageous for the fetus? Am J Obstet Gynecol 163:868, 1990

Owen J, Iams JD, Hauth JC: Vaginal sonography and cervical incompetence. Am J Obstet Gynecol 188:586, 2003

Owen J, Yost N, Berghella V, et al: Mid-trimester endovaginal sonography in women at high risk for spontaneous preterm birth. JAMA 286:1340, 2001

Papatsonis DN, Van Geijn HP, Ader HJ, et al: Nifedipine and ritodrine in the management of preterm labor: A randomized multicenter trial. Obstet Gynecol 90:230, 1997

Parilla BV, Dooley SL, Minogue JP, et al: The efficacy of oral terbutaline after intravenous tocolysis. Am J Obstet Gynecol 169:965, 1993

Parilla BV, Grobman WA, Holtzman RB, et al: Indomethacin tocolysis and risk of necrotizing enterocolitis. Obstet Gynecol 96:120, 2000

Peck T, Lutheran G: Long-term and short-term childhood health after long-term use of indomethacin in pregnancy. Am J Obstet Gynecol 189:S168, 2003

Peltoniemi OM, Kari MA, Tammela O, et al: Randomized trial of a single repeat dose of prenatal betamethasone treatment in imminent preterm birth. Pediatrics, 119:290, 2007

Pereira L, Cotter A, Gómez R, et al: Expectant management compared with physical examination-indicated cerclage (EM-PEC) in selected women with a dilated cervix at 14$^{0/7}$-25$^{6/7}$ weeks: Results from the EM-PEC international cohort study. Am J Obstet Gynecol 197:483, 2007

Perry KG, Martin RW, Blake PC, et al: Maternal outcome associated with adult respiratory distress syndrome. Am J Obstet Gynecol 174:391, 1996

Perry KG Jr, Morrison JC, Rust OA, et al: Incidence of adverse cardiopulmonary effects with low-dose continuous terbutaline infusion. Am J Obstet Gynecol 173:1273, 1995

Petrini JR, Dias T, McCormick MC, et al: Increased risk of adverse neurological development for late preterm infants. J Pediatr 154(2):169, 2009

Petrova A, Demissie K, Rhoads GG, et al: Association of maternal fever during labor with neonatal and infant morbidity and mortality. Obstet Gynecol 98:20, 2001

Promislow JH, Hertz-Picciotto I, Schramm M, et al: Bed rest and other determinants of bone loss during pregnancy. Am J Obstet Gynecol 191:1077, 2004

Raju TN, Higgins RD, Stark AR, et al: Optimizing care and outcome for late-preterm (near-term) infants: A summary of the workshop sponsored by the National Institute of Child Health and Human Development. Pediatrics 118:1207, 2006

Roberts D, Dalziel SR: Antenatal corticosteroids for accelerating fetal lung maturation for women at risk of preterm birth. Cochrane Database Syst Rev 3: CD004454, 2006

Romero R, Sibai BM, Sanchez-Ramos L, et al: An oxytocin receptor antagonist (atosiban) in the treatment of preterm labor: A randomized, double-blind, placebo-controlled trial with tocolytic rescue. Am J Obstet Gynecol 182:1173, 2000

Romero R, Yoon BH, Mazor M, et al: The diagnostic and prognostic value of amniotic fluid white blood cell count, glucose, interleukin-6 and gram stain in patients with preterm labor and intact membranes. Am J Obstet Gynecol 169:805, 1993

Rouse DJ, Caritis SN, Peaceman AM, et al: A trial of 17 alpha-hydroxyprogesterone caproate to prevent prematurity in twins. National Institute of Child Health and Human Development Maternal-Fetal Medicine Units Network. N Engl J Med 357:454, 2007

Rouse DJ, Hirtz DG, Thom E, et al: A randomized, controlled trial of magnesium sulfate for the prevention of cerebral palsy. N Engl J Med 359:895, 2008

Saigal S, Doyle LW: Preterm births: An overview of mortality and sequelae of preterm birth from infancy to childhood. Lancet 371:261, 2008

Samol JM, Lambers DS: Magnesium sulfate tocolysis and pulmonary edema: The drug or the vehicle? Am J Obstet Gynecol 192:1430, 2005

Sanchez-Ramos L, Kaunitz AM, Delke I: Progestational agents to prevent preterm birth: A meta-analysis of randomized controlled trials. Obstet Gynecol 105:273, 2005

Satin AJ, Leveno KJ, Sherman ML, et al: Maternal youth and pregnancy outcomes: Middle school versus high school age groups compared to women beyond the teen years. Am J Obstet Gynecol 171:184, 1994

Schempf AH, Branum AM, Lukacs SL, et al: The contribution of preterm birth to the Black –White infant mortality gap, 1990 and 2000. Am J Public Health 97:1255, 2007

Schiff E, Sivan E, Terry S, et al: Currently recommended oral regimen for ritodrine tocolysis result in extremely low plasma levels. Am J Obstet Gynecol 169:1059, 1993

Schmidt B, Davis P, Moddemann D, et al: Long-term effects of indomethacin prophylaxis in extremely-low-birth-weight infants. N Engl J Med 344:1966, 2001

Segel SY, Miles AM, Clothier B, et al: Duration of antibiotic therapy after preterm premature rupture of fetal membranes. Am J Obstet Gynecol 189:799, 2003

Shim S-S, Romero R, Hong J-S, et al: Clinical significance of intra-amniotic inflammation in patients with preterm premature rupture of membranes. Am J Obstet Gynecol 191:1339, 2004

Sosa C, Althabe F, Belizan J, et al: Bed rest in singleton pregnancies for preventing preterm birth. Cochrane Database Syst Rev 1:CD003581, 2004

Spong CY: Prediction and prevention of recurrent spontaneous preterm birth. Obstet Gynecol 110:405, 2007

Stamilio DM, Chang JJ, Macones GA: Periodontal disease and preterm birth: Do the data have enough teeth to recommend screening and preventive treatment? Am J Obstet Gynecol 196:93, 2007

Steer CM, Petrie RH: A comparison of magnesium sulfate and alcohol for the prevention of premature labor. Am J Obstet Gynecol 129:1, 1977

Stiles AD: Prenatal corticosteroids—Early gain, long-term questions. N Engl J Med 357:1248, 2007

Stoll BJ, Hansen NI, Adams-Chapman I, et al: Neurodevelopmental and growth impairment among extremely-low-birth-weight infants with neonatal infection. JAMA 292:2353, 2004

Stoll BJ, Hansen N, Fanaroff AA, et al: Changes in pathogens causing early-onset sepsis in very-low-birth-weight infants. N Engl J Med 347:240, 2002

Terkildsen MFC, Parilla BV, Kumar P, et al: Factors associated with success of emergent second-trimester cerclage. Obstet Gynecol 101:565, 2003

Tita AT, Cliver SP, Goepfert AR, et al: Clinical trial of interconceptional antibiotics to prevent preterm birth: Subgroup analyses and possible adverse antibiotic-microbial interaction. Am J Obstet Gynecol 196:367, 2007

Tita AT, Rouse DJ: Progesterone for preterm birth prevention: an evolving intervention. Am J Obstet Gynecol 200(3):219, 2009

Tomashek KM, Shapiro-Mendoza CK, Davidoff MJ, et al: Differences in mortality between late-preterm and term singleton infants in the United States, 1995-2002. J Pediatr 151:450, 2007

Tyson JE, Parikh NA, Langer J, et al: Intensive care for extreme prematurity—moving beyond gestational age. N Engl J Med 358:1672, 2008

Varner MW, Esplin MS: Genetic factors in preterm birth—the future. BJOG 112(Suppl 1):28, 2005

Vergnes J-N, Sixou M: Preterm low birthweight and maternal periodontal status: A meta-analysis. Am J Obstet Gynecol 196:135.e1, 2007

Vohr BR, Allen M: Extreme prematurity—the continuing dilemma. N Engl J Med 352:71, 2005

Wapner RJ, Sorokin Y, Mele L, et al: Long-term outcomes after repeat doses of antenatal corticosteroids. N Engl J Med 357:1190, 2007

Ward K, Argyle V, Meade M, et al: The heritability of preterm delivery. Obstet Gynecol 106:1235, 2005

Weiss JL, Malone FD, Vidaver J, et al: Threatened abortion: A risk factor for poor pregnancy outcome, a population-based screening study. Am J Obstet Gynecol 190:745, 2004

Wenstrom K, Weiner CP, Merrill D, et al: A placebo controlled randomized trial of the terbutaline pump for prevention of preterm delivery. Am J Perinatol 14:87, 1997

Winn HN, Chen M, Amon E, et al: Neonatal pulmonary hypoplasia and perinatal mortality in patients with mid-trimester rupture of amniotic membranes—a critical analysis. Am J Obstet Gynecol 182:1638, 2000

Yoon BH, Romero R, Park JS, et al: Fetal exposure to an intra-amniotic inflammation and the development of cerebral palsy at the age of three years. Am J Obstet Gynecol 182:675, 2000

Yoon BH, Yang SH, Jun JK, et al: Maternal blood C-reactive protein, white blood cell count, and temperature in preterm labor: A comparison with amniotic fluid white blood cell count. Obstet Gynecol 87:231, 1996

Yost NP, Bloom SL, McIntire DD, et al: Hospitalization for women with arrested preterm labor: A randomized trial. Obstet Gynecol 106:14, 2005

Yost NP, Bloom SL, Twickler DM, et al: Pitfalls in ultrasonic cervical length measurement for predicting preterm birth. Obstet Gynecol 93:510, 1999

Yost NP, Owen J, Berghella V, et al: Effect of coitus on recurrent preterm birth. Obstet Gynecol 107:793, 2006

Zuckerman H, Reiss U, Rubinstein I: Inhibition of human premature labor by indomethacin. Obstet Gynecol 44:787, 1974

CHAPTER 36

Postterm Pregnancy

The adjectives *postterm, prolonged, postdates,* and *postmature* are often loosely used interchangeably to describe pregnancies that have exceeded a duration considered to be the upper limit of normal. We do not use the term *postdates* because the real issue in many postterm pregnancies is "post-*what* dates?" *Postmature* is reserved for the relatively uncommon specific clinical fetal syndrome in which the infant has recognizable clinical features indicating a pathologically prolonged pregnancy. Therefore, *postterm* or *prolonged* pregnancy is our preferred expression for an extended pregnancy.

The international definition of prolonged pregnancy, endorsed by the American College of Obstetricians and Gynecologists (2004), is 42 completed weeks (294 days) or more from the first day of the last menstrual period. It is important to emphasize the phrase "42 completed weeks." Pregnancies between 41 weeks 1 day and 41 weeks 6 days, although in the 42nd week, do not complete 42 weeks until the seventh day has elapsed. Thus, technically speaking, prolonged pregnancy could begin either on day 294 or on day 295 following the onset of the last menses. Which is it? Day 294 or 295? We cannot resolve this question, and emphasize this dilemma only to ensure that

litigators and others understand that some imprecision is inevitable when there is biological variation such as with prolonged pregnancy. Amersi and Grimes (1998) have cautioned against use of ordinal numbers such as "42nd week" because of imprecision. For example, "42nd week" refers to 41 weeks and 1 through 6 days, whereas the cardinal number "42 weeks" refers to precisely 42 completed weeks.

ESTIMATED GESTATIONAL AGE USING MENSTRUAL DATES

The definition of postterm pregnancy as one that persists for 42 weeks or more from the onset of a menstrual period assumes that the last menses was followed by ovulation 2 weeks later. This said, some pregnancies may not actually be postterm, but rather are the result of an error in gestational age estimation because of faulty recall of menstrual dates or delayed ovulation. Thus, there are two categories of pregnancies that reach 42 completed weeks: (1) those truly 40 weeks past conception, and (2) those of less advanced gestation but with inaccurately estimated gestational age.

Even with precisely recalled menstrual dates, there is still not precision. Specifically, Munster and associates (1992) reported that large variations in menstrual cycle lengths are common in normal women. Boyce and associates (1976) studied 317 French women with periconceptional basal body temperature profiles. They found that 70 percent who completed 42 postmenstrual weeks had a less advanced gestation based on ovulation dates. These variations in menstrual cycle may partially explain why a relatively small proportion of fetuses delivered postterm have evidence of *postmaturity*. Even so, because there is no accurate method to identify the truly prolonged pregnancy, all those judged to be 42 completed weeks should be managed as if abnormally prolonged.

Sonographic evaluation of gestational age during pregnancy has been used to add precision. Blondel and colleagues (2002) studied 44,623 women delivered at the Royal Victoria Hospital in

Montreal. They analyzed postterm pregnancy rates according to six algorithms for gestational age estimates based on either the last menstrual period, sonographic evaluation at 16 to 18 weeks, or both. The proportion of births at 42 weeks or longer was 6.4 percent when based on the last menstrual period alone, but was 1.9 percent when based on sonographic measurements alone. Sonographic pregnancy dating at 12 weeks or less resulted in a 2.7-percent incidence of postterm gestation compared with 3.7 percent in a group assessed at 13 to 24 weeks (Caughey and co-workers, 2008). These findings suggest that menstrual dates are frequently inaccurate in predicting postterm pregnancy. Subsequent clinical studies have confirmed these observations (Bennett, 2004; Joseph, 2007; Wingate, 2007, and all their colleagues).

INCIDENCE

From their review, Divon and Feldman-Leidner (2008) report that the incidence of postterm pregnancy ranges from 4 to 19 percent. Using criteria that likely overestimate the incidence, approximately 6 percent of 4 million infants born in the United States during 2006 were estimated to have been delivered at 42 weeks or more (Martin and colleagues, 2009). The trend toward fewer births at 42 weeks suggests earlier intervention. Specifically, in 2000, 7.2 percent of births in this country were 42 weeks or beyond, compared with 5.6 percent in 2006.

There are contradictory findings concerning the significance of maternal demographic factors such as parity, prior postterm birth, socioeconomic class, and age. Olesen and colleagues (2006) analyzed a variety of risk factors in 3392 participants in the 1998 to 2001 Danish Birth Cohort. They reported that only prepregnancy body mass index (BMI) ≥ 25 and nulliparity were significantly associated with prolonged pregnancy. Denison (2008) and Caughey (2009) and their co-workers also reported similar associations.

The tendency for some mothers to have repeated postterm births suggests that some prolonged pregnancies are biologically determined. In 27,677 births in Norway, Bakketeig and Bergsjø (1991) reported that the incidence of a subsequent postterm birth increased from 10 to 27 percent if the first birth was postterm. This was increased to 39 percent if there had been two previous, successive postterm deliveries. Similar results were reported from Missouri by Kistka and colleagues (2007). And Mogren and colleagues (1999) reported that prolonged pregnancy recurred across generations in Swedish women. When mother and daughter had a prolonged pregnancy, the risk for the daughter to have a subsequent postterm pregnancy was increased two- to threefold. In another Swedish study, Laursen and associates (2004) found that maternal, but not paternal, genes influenced prolonged pregnancy. Rare fetal–placental factors that have been reported as predisposing to postterm pregnancy include anencephaly, adrenal hypoplasia, and X-linked placental sulfatase deficiency (MacDonald and Siiteri, 1965; Naeye, 1978; Rabe and colleagues, 1983).

PERINATAL MORTALITY

The historical basis for the concept of an upper limit of human pregnancy duration was the observation that perinatal mortality

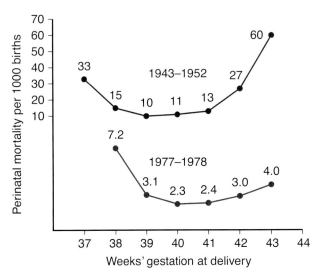

FIGURE 37-1 Perinatal mortality rates in late pregnancy according to gestational age in Sweden of all births during 1943–1952 compared with those during 1977–1978. The logarithmic scale is used for convenience in depiction. (Adapted from Bakketeig and Bergsjø, 1991, and Lindell, 1956.)

rates increased after the expected due date was passed. This is best seen when perinatal mortality rates are analyzed from times before widespread intervention for postterm pregnancies. In two large Swedish studies shown in Figure 37-1, after reaching a nadir at 39 to 40 weeks, the perinatal mortality rate increased as pregnancy exceeded 41 weeks. More recently, MacDorman and Kirmeyer (2009) noted this trend also in the U.S. Similar observations were recently reported by Cheng and associates (2008), who described more than 2.5 million births in the United States in 2003. The major causes of death included gestational hypertension, prolonged labor with cephalopelvic disproportion, "unexplained anoxia," and malformations. Similar outcomes were reported by Olesen and colleagues (2003) in their analysis of 78,022 women with postterm pregnancies delivered before routine labor induction was adopted in Denmark. Lindstrom and colleagues (2005) performed developmental tests at age 4 to 5½ years in 354 consecutive infants born at 42 weeks or more in a Swedish hospital in 1991. Children born postterm had more developmental abnormalities compared with those born before 42 weeks.

Alexander and colleagues (2000a) reviewed 56,317 consecutive singleton pregnancies delivered at 40 or more weeks between 1988 and 1998 at Parkland Hospital. As shown in Table 37-1, labor was induced in 35 percent of pregnancies completing 42 weeks. The rate of cesarean delivery for dystocia and fetal distress was significantly increased at 42 weeks compared with earlier deliveries. More infants of postterm pregnancies were admitted to intensive care units. Finally, the incidence of neonatal seizures and deaths doubled at 42 weeks. Tita and co-workers (2009) evaluated outcomes in women undergoing elective repeat cesarean delivery. They reported a 19.5-percent incidence of adverse neonatal outcomes in pregnancies ≥ 42 weeks. Caughey and colleagues (2007) compared 119,254 low-risk pregnancies delivered at 39 weeks versus 40, 41, and 42 weeks. They reported a continuum of increasing risk in successive epochs for cesarean delivery as well as maternal complications of labor and delivery.

TABLE 37-1. Pregnancy Outcomes in 56,317 Consecutive Singleton Pregnancies Delivered at or Beyond 40 Weeks at Parkland Hospital from 1988 through 1998

	Weeks' Gestation			
Outcome	40 (n = 29,136)	41 (n = 16,386)	42 (n = 10,795)	p value[a]
Maternal Outcomes (percent)				
Labor induction	2	7	35	<.001
Cesarean delivery				
Dystocia	7	6	9	<.001
Fetal distress	2	3	4	<.001
Perinatal outcomes (per 1000)				
Neonatal ICU	4	5	6	<.001
Neonatal seizures	1	1	2	.12
Stillbirth	2	1	2	.84
Neonatal death	0.2	0.2	0.6	.17

[a]p value is for the trend using 42 weeks as the referent.
ICU = intensive care unit.
Adapted from Alexander and colleagues (2000a).

Smith (2001) has challenged analyses such as these because the population at risk for perinatal mortality rate in a given week consists of all ongoing pregnancies rather than just the births in a given week. Figure 37-2 shows perinatal mortality rates calculated using only births in a given week of gestation from 37 to 43 completed weeks compared with the cumulative probability—the perinatal index—of death when all ongoing pregnancies are included in the denominator. As shown, delivery at 38 weeks had the lowest risk index for perinatal death.

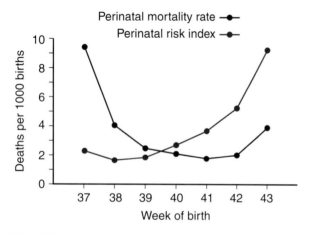

FIGURE 37-2 Perinatal risk index and perinatal mortality rate for births between 37 and 43 weeks in Scotland from 1985 through 1996, and expressed as deaths per 1000 births. The perinatal risk index is the cumulative probability of perinatal death multiplied by 1000. The perinatal mortality rate is the number of perinatal deaths with delivery in a given gestational week divided by the total number of births in that week multiplied by 1000. (Modified from *American Journal of Obstetrics & Gynecology*, Vol. 184, No. 3, GCS Smith, Life-table analysis of the risk of perinatal death at term and post term in singleton pregnancies, pp. 489–496, Copyright 2001, with permission from Elsevier.)

PATHOPHYSIOLOGY

Clifford (1954) described a recognizable clinical syndrome that did much to dispel the prevailing obstetrical opinion that prolonged human pregnancy did not exist (Calkins, 1948). Infants, either live or stillborn, demonstrating these clinical characteristics are now diagnosed to be pathologically *postmature*, or to have the *postmaturity syndrome*. Many of the postmature infants described by Clifford died, and many were seriously ill due to birth asphyxia and meconium aspiration. Several survivors were brain damaged. Interestingly, Ballantyne (1902) had reported this postmature syndrome more than 50 years before Clifford did.

Postmaturity Syndrome

The postmature infant presents a unique and characteristic appearance such as shown in Figure 37-3. Features include wrinkled, patchy, peeling skin; a long, thin body suggesting wasting; and advanced maturity because the infant is open-eyed, unusually alert, and appears old and worried. Skin wrinkling can be particularly prominent on the palms and soles. The nails are typically long. Most such postmature infants are not technically growth restricted because their birthweight seldom falls below the 10th percentile for gestational age. On the other hand, severe growth restriction—which logically must have preceded completion of 42 weeks—may be present.

The incidence of postmaturity syndrome in infants at 41, 42, or 43 weeks, respectively, has not been conclusively determined. In one of the rare contemporary reports that chronicle postmaturity, Shime and colleagues (1984) found this syndrome in approximately 10 percent of pregnancies between 41 and 43 weeks. The incidence increased to 33 percent at 44 weeks. Associated oligohydramnios substantially increases the

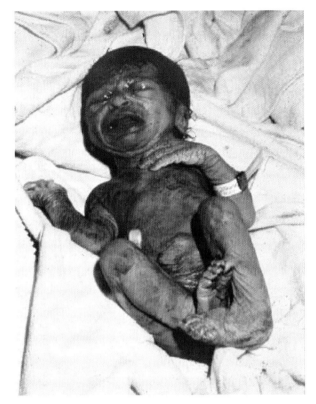

FIGURE 37-3 Postmature infant delivered at 43 weeks' gestation. Thick, viscous meconium coated the desquamating skin. Note the long, thin appearance and wrinkling of the hands.

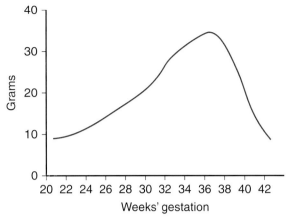

FIGURE 37-4 Mean daily fetal growth during previous week of gestation. (From Jazayeri and co-workers, 1998, with permission.)

likelihood of postmaturity. Trimmer and colleagues (1990) diagnosed oligohydramnios when the sonographic maximum-vertical amnionic fluid pocket measured 1 cm or less at 42 weeks, and 88 percent of the infants were postmature.

Placental Dysfunction

Clifford (1954) proposed that the skin changes of postmaturity were due to loss of the protective effects of vernix caseosa. He also attributed the postmaturity syndrome to placental senescence, although he did not find placental degeneration histologically. Still, the concept that postmaturity is due to placental insufficiency has persisted despite an absence of morphological or significant quantitative findings (Larsen and co-workers, 1995; Rushton, 1991). Of interest, Smith and Baker (1999) reported that placental apoptosis—programmed cell death—was significantly increased at 41 to 42 completed weeks compared with that at 36 to 39 weeks. The clinical significance of such apoptosis is currently unclear.

Jazayeri and co-workers (1998) investigated cord blood erythropoietin levels in 124 appropriately grown newborns delivered from 37 to 43 weeks. The only known stimulator of erythropoietin is decreased partial oxygen pressure. Thus, they sought to assess whether fetal oxygenation was compromised due to placental aging in postterm pregnancies. All women had an uncomplicated labor and delivery. These investigators reported that cord blood erythropoietin levels were significantly increased in pregnancies reaching 41 weeks or more. Although Apgar scores and acid-base studies were normal, these researchers

concluded that there was decreased fetal oxygenation in some postterm gestations.

Another scenario is that the postterm fetus may continue to gain weight and thus be unusually large at birth. This at least suggests that placental function is not severely compromised. Indeed, continued fetal growth—albeit at a slower rate—is characteristic beginning at 37 completed weeks (Fig. 37-4). Nahum and colleagues (1995) confirmed that fetal growth continues until at least 42 weeks. Despite this, Link and associates (2007) showed that umbilical blood flow did not increase concomitantly.

Fetal Distress and Oligohydramnios

The principal reasons for increased risks for postterm fetuses were described by Leveno and associates (1984). They reported that both antepartum fetal jeopardy and intrapartum fetal distress were the consequence of cord compression associated with oligohydramnios. In their analysis of 727 postterm pregnancies, intrapartum fetal distress detected with electronic monitoring was not associated with late decelerations characteristic of uteroplacental insufficiency. Instead, one or more prolonged decelerations such as shown in Figure 37-5 preceded three fourths of emergency cesarean deliveries for nonreassuring fetal heart rate tracings. In all but two cases, there were also variable decelerations (Fig. 37-6). Another common fetal heart rate pattern, although not ominous by itself, was the saltatory baseline shown in Figure 37-7. As described in Chapter 18 (p. 423), these findings are consistent with cord occlusion as the proximate cause of the nonreassuring tracings. Other correlates found were oligohydramnios and viscous meconium. Schaffer and colleagues (2005) implicated a nuchal cord in abnormal intrapartum fetal heart rate patterns, meconium, and compromised newborn condition in prolonged pregnancies.

The volume of amnionic fluid normally continues to decrease after 38 weeks and may become problematic (Fig. 37-8). Moreover, meconium release into an already reduced amnionic fluid volume causes thick, viscous meconium that may cause *meconium aspiration syndrome* (see Chap. 29, p. 628).

Trimmer and co-workers (1990) sonographically measured hourly fetal urine production using sequential bladder volume

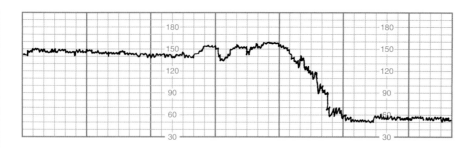

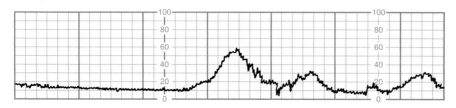

FIGURE 37-5 Upper panel: Prolonged fetal heart rate deceleration prior to emergency cesarean delivery in a postterm pregnancy with oligohydramnios. (This figure was published in *American Journal of Obstetrics & Gynecology*, Vol. 150, No. 5, pt. 1, KJ Leveno, JG Quirk, Jr., FG Cunningham, et al., Prolonged pregnancy. I. Observations concerning the causes of fetal distress, pp. 465–473, Copyright Elsevier 1984.)

measurements in 38 pregnancies of 42 weeks or more. Diminished urine production was found to be associated with oligohydramnios. They hypothesized, however, that decreased fetal urine flow was likely the result of preexisting oligohydramnios that limited fetal swallowing. Oz and co-workers (2002), using Doppler waveforms, concluded that fetal renal blood flow is reduced in those postterm pregnancies complicated by oligohydramnios. Mentioned above was the study by Link and associates (2007), which showed that umbilical blood flow did not increase past term.

Fetal-Growth Restriction

It was not until the late 1990s that the clinical significance of fetal-growth restriction in the otherwise uncomplicated pregnancy

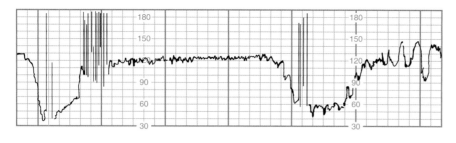

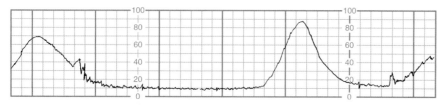

FIGURE 37-6 Upper panel: Severe—less than 70 bpm for 60 seconds or longer—variable decelerations in a postterm pregnancy with oligohydramnios. (This figure was published in *American Journal of Obstetrics & Gynecology*, Vol. 150, No. 5, pt. 1, KJ Leveno, JG Quirk, Jr., FG Cunningham, et al., Prolonged pregnancy. I. Observations concerning the causes of fetal distress, pp. 465–473, Copyright Elsevier 1984.)

became more fully appreciated. Divon and associates (1998) and Clausson and co-workers (1999) analyzed births between 1991 and 1995 in the National Swedish Medical Birth Registry. As shown in Table 37-2, stillbirths were more common among growth-restricted infants who were delivered after 42 weeks. Indeed, a third of postterm stillborn infants were growth restricted. During this time in Sweden, labor induction and antenatal fetal testing usually commenced at 42 weeks.

In a study from Parkland Hospital, Alexander and colleagues (2000d) analyzed outcomes for 355 infants who were 42 weeks or greater and whose birthweights were at or below the 3rd percentile. They compared these with outcomes of 14,520 similarly aged infants above the 3rd percentile and found that morbidity and mortality rates were significantly increased in the growth-restricted infants. Notably, a fourth of all stillbirths associated with prolonged pregnancy were in this comparatively small number of growth-restricted infants.

COMPLICATIONS

Oligohydramnios

The aggregate of most clinical studies is consistent with the view that diminished amnionic fluid determined by various sonographic methods identifies a postterm fetus with increased risks. Indeed, decreased amnionic fluid in any pregnancy signifies increased fetal risk (see Chap. 21, p. 496). Unfortunately, lack of an exact quantification method to define "decreased amnionic fluid" has limited investigators, and many different criteria for sonographic diagnosis have been proposed. Fischer and colleagues (1993) attempted to determine which criteria were most predictive of normal versus abnormal outcomes in postterm pregnancies. As shown in Figure 37-9, the smaller the amnionic fluid pocket, the greater the likelihood that there was clinically significant oligohydramnios. Importantly, normal amnionic fluid volume did not preclude abnormal outcomes. Alfirevic and co-workers (1997) randomly assigned 500 women with postterm pregnancies to assessment of amnionic fluid volume using either the amnionic fluid index (AFI) or the deepest vertical pocket (see Chap. 21, p. 490). They concluded that the AFI overestimated the number of abnormal outcomes in postterm pregnancies.

Regardless of the criteria used to diagnose oligohydramnios in postterm pregnancies, most investigators have found an increased incidence of "fetal distress" during labor. Thus, oligohydramnios by most definitions is a clinically meaningful finding. Conversely, reassurance of continued fetal well-being in the presence of "normal" amnionic fluid volume is tenuous. This may be related to how quickly pathological oligohydramnios develops. For example, Clement and co-workers (1987) described six postterm pregnancies in which amnionic fluid volume diminished abruptly over 24 hours—in one of these, the fetus died.

Macrosomia

The velocity of fetal weight gain peaks at approximately 37 weeks as shown in Figure 37-4. Although growth velocity slows at that time, most fetuses continue to gain weight. For example, the percentage of fetuses born in 2006 whose birthweight exceeded 4000 g was 8.5 percent at 37 to 41 weeks and increased to 11.2 percent at 42 weeks or more (Martin and colleagues, 2009). Intuitively at least, it seems that both maternal and fetal morbidity associated with macrosomia would be mitigated with timely induction to preempt further growth. This does not appear to be the case, however, and the American College of Obstetricians and Gynecologists (2000) has concluded that current evidence does not support such a practice in women at term with suspected fetal macrosomia. Moreover, the College concluded that in the absence of diabetes, vaginal delivery is not contraindicated for women with an estimated fetal weight up to 5000 g. Cesarean delivery was recommended for estimated fetal weights greater than 4500 g if there is prolonged

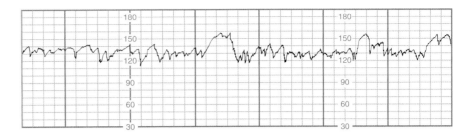
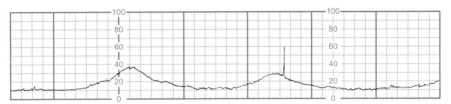

FIGURE 37-7 Saltatory baseline fetal heart rate showing oscillations exceeding 20 bpm and associated with oligohydramnios in a postterm pregnancy. (This figure was published in *American Journal of Obstetrics & Gynecology*, Vol. 150, No. 5, pt. 1, KJ Leveno, JG Quirk, Jr., FG Cunningham, et al., Prolonged pregnancy. I. Observations concerning the causes of fetal distress, pp. 465–473, Copyright Elsevier 1984.)

second-stage labor or arrest of descent. Obvious problems with all such recommendations are substantive normal variations of fetal weight estimation (see Chap. 38, p. 854).

Medical or Obstetrical Complications

In the event of a medical or other obstetrical complication, it is generally unwise to allow a pregnancy to continue past 42 weeks. Indeed, in many such instances, *earlier* delivery is indicated. Common examples include gestational hypertensive disorders, prior cesarean delivery, and diabetes.

MANAGEMENT

It is generally accepted that some form of intervention is indicated for prolonged pregnancies. The types of interventions and timing of their use, however, are not unanimous (Divon and Feldman-Leidner, 2008). After this decision is reached, the second issue is whether labor induction is warranted or if expectant management with fetal surveillance is best. Although hindered by the biases of surveys, Cleary-Goldman and colleagues (2006) reported that 73 percent of members of the American College of Obstetricians and Gynecologists responding to a 2004 poll routinely induced women at 41 weeks. Most of the remainder performed twice weekly fetal testing until 42 weeks.

Prognostic Factors for Successful Induction

Unfavorable Cervix

Although all obstetricians know what an "unfavorable cervix" is, the term unfortunately defies precise definition. Thus, various investigators have used different criteria for studies of prolonged pregnancies. For example, Harris and colleagues (1983) defined an unfavorable cervix by a Bishop score of less than 7 and reported this in 92 percent of women at 42 weeks. Hannah and

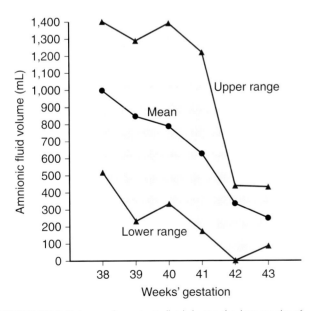

FIGURE 37-8 Volume of amnionic fluid during the last weeks of pregnancy. (Adapted from *The Lancet*, Vol. 278, PM Elliott and WHW Inman, Volume of liquor amnii in normal and abnormal pregnancy, pp. 835–840, Copyright 1961, with permission from Elsevier.)

TABLE 37-2. Effects of Fetal-Growth Restriction on Stillbirth Rates in 537,029 Swedish Women Delivered before and after 42 Weeks

	Pregnancy Duration	
Outcome	37–41 Weeks	≥ 42 Weeks
Births (number)	469,056	40,973
Fetal-growth restriction[a] (%)	10,312 (2)	1,558 (4)
Stillbirths (per 1000)		
Appropriate growth	650 (1.4)	69 (1.8)
Fetal-growth restriction	116 (11)	23 (15)

[a]Defined as birthweight two standard deviations below mean birthweights for fetal gender and gestational age.
From Clausson and colleagues (1999), with permission.

colleagues (1992) found that only 40 percent of 3407 women with a 41-week pregnancy had an undilated cervix. Alexander and associates (2000b) evaluated 800 women undergoing induction for postterm pregnancy at Parkland Hospital. Women in whom there was no cervical dilatation had a twofold increased cesarean delivery rate for "dystocia." Yang and co-workers (2004) found that cervical length of 3 cm or less measured with transvaginal ultrasonography was predictive of successful induction. In a similar study, Vankayalapati and associates (2008) found that cervical length of 25 mm or less was predictive of spontaneous labor or successful induction.

Cervical Ripening. A number of investigators have evaluated prostaglandin E_2 (PGE_2) for induction in women with an unfa-

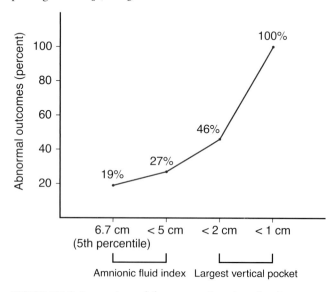

FIGURE 37-9 Comparison of the prognostic value of various sonographic estimates of amnionic fluid volume in prolonged pregnancies. Abnormal outcomes include cesarean or operative vaginal delivery for fetal jeopardy, 5-minute Apgar score of 6 or less, umbilical arterial blood pH less than 7.1, or admission to the neonatal intensive care unit. (Adapted from Fischer RL, McDonnell M, Bianculli KW, et al: Amniotic fluid volume estimation in the postdate pregnancy: A comparison of techniques, *Obstetrics & Gynecology*, 1993, vol. 81, no. 5, part 1, pp. 698–704, with permission.)

vorable cervix and prolonged pregnancies. The National Institute of Child Health and Human Development Network of Maternal-Fetal Medicine Units (1994) reported that PGE_2 gel was not more effective than placebo. Alexander and associates (2000c) treated 393 women with a postterm pregnancy with PGE_2, even if the cervix was "favorable." They reported that almost half of the 84 women with cervical dilatation of 2 to 4 cm entered labor with prostaglandin E_2 use alone. The American College of Obstetricians and Gynecologists (2004) has concluded that prostaglandin gel can be used safely in postterm pregnancies. Fasset and Wing (2008) reported that mifepristone increased uterine activity without uterotonic agents in women beyond 41 weeks. Prostaglandins and other agents used for cervical ripening are discussed in Chapter 22 (p. 502).

Sweeping or stripping of the membranes to induce labor and thereby prevent postterm pregnancy was studied in 15 randomized trials during the 1990s. Boulvain and co-workers (1999) performed a meta-analysis of these and found that membrane stripping at 38 to 40 weeks decreased the frequency of postterm pregnancy. This, however, did not modify the risk for cesarean delivery. They also found that maternal and neonatal infection rates were not increased by cervical manipulation. Since then, randomized trials by Wong (2002), Kashanian (2006), Hill (2008), and their colleagues found that sweeping membranes did not reduce the need to induce labor (see Chap. 22, p. 504). Drawbacks of membrane stripping included pain, vaginal bleeding, and irregular contractions without labor.

Station of Vertex

The station of fetal head in the pelvis is another important predictor of successful postterm pregnancy induction. Shin and colleagues (2004) studied 484 nulliparas who underwent induction after 41 weeks. The cesarean delivery rate was directly related to station. It was 6 percent if the vertex prior to induction was at −1 station; 20 percent at −2; 43 percent at −3; and 77 percent at −4.

Induction versus Fetal Testing

Because of marginal benefits for induction with an unfavorable cervix as discussed above, some clinicians prefer to use the alternative strategy of fetal testing beginning at 41 completed weeks.

CHAPTER 37

There now have been a number of quality studies designed to resolve these important questions.

Hannah and colleagues (1992) randomly assigned 3407 Canadian women at 41 or more weeks to induction or to fetal testing. In the latter group, evaluation included: (1) counting fetal movements during a 2-hour period each day, (2) nonstress testing three times weekly, and (3) amnionic fluid volume assessment two to three times weekly with pockets less than 3 cm considered abnormal. Labor induction resulted in a small, albeit significantly lower, cesarean delivery rate compared with fetal testing—21 versus 24 percent, respectively. This difference was due to fewer procedures for fetal distress. Importantly, the only two stillbirths were in the fetal testing group.

The Maternal–Fetal Medicine Network performed a randomized trial of induction versus fetal testing beginning at 41 weeks (Gardner and associates, 1996). Fetal surveillance included nonstress testing and sonographic estimation of amnionic fluid volume performed twice weekly in 175 women. Their perinatal outcomes were compared with those of 265 women randomized to induction with or without cervical ripening. There were no perinatal deaths, and the cesarean delivery rate was not different between management groups. Thus, this study supported the validity of these management schemes, and similar results were subsequently reported from a Norwegian randomized trial of 508 women (Heimstad and colleagues, 2007).

These and similar findings caused Menticoglou and Hall (2002) to lament that labor induction at 41 weeks had become the standard of care in Canada. They termed this a *nonsensus consensus* resulting in "ritual induction at 41 weeks." They opined that this practice is based on seriously flawed evidence and that it constituted "an abuse of biological norms." They called for its discontinuation because it had potential to do more harm than good, and with staggering resource implications.

In an analysis of 19 trials in the Cochrane Pregnancy and Childbirth Trials Registry, Gulmezoglu and colleagues (2006) found that induction after 41 weeks was associated with fewer perinatal deaths without significantly increasing the cesarean delivery rate. Similar findings were reported by Mozurkewich and co-workers (2009) in their review of 2 meta-analyses and a recent randomized controlled study.

In a study to "lower" the number of postterm pregnancies, Harrington and colleagues (2006) randomized 463 women to pregnancy dating with sonography between 8 and 12 weeks versus no first-trimester sonographic evaluation. Their primary endpoint was the labor induction rate for prolonged pregnancy, and they found no advantages to early sonographic pregnancy dating.

At 42 weeks, labor induction has a higher cesarean delivery rate compared with spontaneous labor. From Parkland Hospital, Alexander and colleagues (2001) evaluated pregnancy outcomes in 638 such women in whom labor was induced and compared them with those of 687 women who had spontaneous labor. Cesarean delivery rates were significantly increased—19 versus 14 percent—in the induced group because of failure to progress. When these investigators corrected for risk factors, however, they concluded that intrinsic maternal factors, rather than the induc-

tion itself, led to the higher rate. These factors included nulliparity, an unfavorable cervix, and epidural analgesia.

Evidence to substantiate intervention—whether induction or fetal testing—commencing at 41 versus 42 weeks is limited. Most evidence used to justify intervention at 41 weeks is from the randomized Canadian and American investigations cited earlier. No randomized studies have specifically assessed intervention at 41 weeks versus an identical intervention used at 42 weeks. But there have been observational studies. In one, Usher and colleagues (1988) analyzed outcomes in 7663 pregnancies in women determined to be 40, 41, or 42 weeks confirmed by early sonographic evaluation. After correction for malformations, perinatal death rates were 1.5, 0.7, and 3.0 per 1000 at 40, 41, and 42 weeks, respectively. These results could be used to challenge the concept of routine intervention at 41 instead of 42 weeks.

Management Recommendations

American College of Obstetricians and Gynecologists

Because of the studies discussed above, the American College of Obstetricians and Gynecologists (2004) defines postterm pregnancies as having completed 42 weeks. There is insufficient evidence to recommend a management strategy between 40 and 42 completed weeks. Thus, although not considered mandatory, initiation of fetal surveillance at 41 weeks is a reasonable option. After completing 42 weeks, recommendations are for either antenatal testing or labor induction. These are summarized in Figure 37-10.

Parkland Hospital

Based on results discussed above, we consider 41-week pregnancies without other complications to be normal. Thus, no interventions are practiced solely based on fetal age until 42

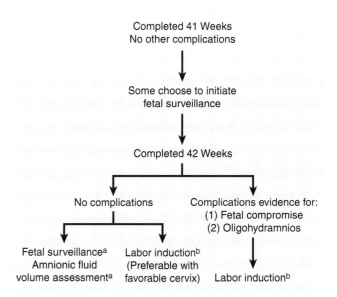

FIGURE 37-10 Management of postterm pregnancy—summary of recommendations of the American College of Obstetricians and Gynecologists (2004). [a]See text for options; [b]prostaglandins may be used for cervical ripening or induction.

completed weeks. If there are complications such as hypertension, decreased fetal movements, or oligohydramnios, then labor induction, with cervical ripening if indicated, is carried out at 41 weeks. It is our view that large, randomized trials should be performed before otherwise uncomplicated 41-week gestations are routinely considered pathologically prolonged.

In women in whom a *certain* gestational age is known, labor is induced at the completion of 42 weeks. Almost 90 percent of such women are induced successfully or enter labor within 2 days of induction. For those who do not deliver with the first induction, a second induction is performed within 3 days. Almost all women are delivered using this management plan, but in the unusual few who are not delivered, management decisions involve a third—or even more—induction versus cesarean delivery.

Women classified as having *uncertain* postterm pregnancies are managed with weekly nonstress fetal testing and assessment of amnionic fluid volume. Women with an AFI $\leq$ 5 cm or with reports of diminished fetal movement undergo labor induction.

INTRAPARTUM MANAGEMENT

Labor is a particularly dangerous time for the postterm fetus. Therefore, women whose pregnancies are known or suspected to be postterm should come to the hospital as soon as they suspect labor. While being evaluated for active labor, we recommend that fetal heart rate and uterine contractions be monitored electronically for variations consistent with fetal compromise (American College of Obstetricians and Gynecologists, 2005).

The decision to perform amniotomy is problematic. Further reduction in fluid volume following amniotomy can certainly enhance the possibility of cord compression. Conversely, amniotomy aids identification of thick meconium, which may be dangerous to the fetus if aspirated. And also, after membranes rupture, a scalp electrode and intrauterine pressure catheter can be placed. These usually provide more precise data concerning fetal heart rate and uterine contractions.

Identification of *thick meconium* in the amnionic fluid is particularly worrisome. The viscosity probably signifies the lack of liquid and thus oligohydramnios. Aspiration of thick meconium may cause severe pulmonary dysfunction and neonatal death (see Chap. 29, p. 628). Because of this, Wenstrom and Parsons (1989) proposed *amnioinfusion* during labor as a way of diluting meconium to decrease the incidence of aspiration syndrome. As discussed in Chapter 18 (p. 433), the benefits of amnioinfusion remain controversial. In a large randomized trial by Fraser and colleagues (2005), amnioinfusion did not reduce the risk of meconium aspiration syndrome or perinatal death. According to the American College of Obstetricians and Gynecologists (2005, 2006), amnioinfusion does not prevent meconium aspiration, however, it remains a reasonable treatment approach for repetitive variable decelerations, regardless of meconium status.

The likelihood of a successful vaginal delivery is reduced appreciably for the nulliparous woman who is in early labor with thick, meconium-stained amnionic fluid. Therefore, when the woman is remote from delivery, strong consideration should be given to prompt cesarean delivery, especially when cephalopelvic disproportion is suspected or either hypotonic or hypertonic dysfunctional labor is evident. Some practitioners choose to avoid oxytocin use in these cases.

Until recently, it was taught—including here—that aspiration of meconium could be minimized but not eliminated by suctioning the pharynx as soon as the head was delivered. According to the American Heart Association (2006) guidelines, there is no evidence that such practices prevent or alter the meconium aspiration syndrome. The American College of Obstetricians and Gynecologists (2007) does not recommend routine intrapartum suctioning. However, if the depressed newborn has meconium-stained fluid, then intubation is done with tracheal suctioning.

REFERENCES

Alexander JM, McIntire DD, Leveno KJ: Forty weeks and beyond: Pregnancy outcomes by week of gestation. Obstet Gynecol 96:291, 2000a

Alexander JM, McIntire DD, Leveno KJ: Postterm pregnancy: Does induction increase cesarean rates? J Soc Gynecol Invest 7:79A, 2000b

Alexander JM, McIntire DD, Leveno KJ: Postterm pregnancy: Is cervical "ripening" being used in the right patients? J Soc Gynecol Invest 7:247A, 2000c

Alexander JM, McIntire DD, Leveno KJ: The effect of fetal growth restriction on neonatal outcome in postterm pregnancy. Abstract No. 463. Am J Obstet Gynecol 182:S148, 2000d

Alexander JM, McIntire DD, Leveno KJ: Prolonged pregnancy: Induction of labor and cesarean births. Obstet Gynecol 97:911, 2001

Alfirevic Z, Luckas M, Walkinshaw SA, et al: A randomized comparison between amniotic fluid index and maximum pool depth in the monitoring of postterm pregnancy. Br J Obstet Gynaecol 104:207, 1997

American College of Obstetricians and Gynecologists: Fetal macrosomia. Practice Bulletin No. 22, November 2000

American College of Obstetricians and Gynecologists: Management of postterm pregnancy. Practice Bulletin No. 55, September 2004

American College of Obstetrics and Gynecologists: Intrapartum fetal heart rate monitoring. Practice Bulletin No. 70, December 2005

American College of Obstetricians and Gynecologists: Amnioinfusion does not prevent meconium aspiration syndrome. Committee Opinion No. 346, October 2006

American College of Obstetrics and Gynecologists: Management of delivery of a newborn with meconium-stained amniotic fluid. Committee Opinion No. 379, September 2007

American Heart Association: 2005 American Heart Association (AHA) guidelines for cardiopulmonary resuscitation (CPR) and emergency cardiovascular care (ECC) of pediatric and neonatal patients: Pediatric basic life support. Pedi 117:e989, 2006

Amersi S, Grimes DA: The case against using ordinal numbers for gestational age. Obstet Gynecol 91:623, 1998

Bakketeig LS, Bergsjø P: Post-term pregnancy: Magnitude of the problem. In Chalmers I, Enkin M, Keirse M (eds): Effective Care in Pregnancy and Childbirth. Oxford, Oxford University Press, 1991, p 765

Ballantyne JW: The problem of the postmature infant. J Obstet Gynaecol Br Emp 2:522, 1902

Bennett KA, Crane JM, O'Shea P, et al: First trimester ultrasound screening is effective in reducing postterm labor induction rates: A randomized controlled trial. Am J Obstet Gynecol 190:1077, 2004

Blondel B, Morin I, Platt RW, et al: Algorithms for combining menstrual and ultrasound estimates of gestational age: Consequences for rates of preterm and postterm birth. Br J Obstet Gynaecol 109:718, 2002

Boulvain M, Irion O, Marcoux S, et al: Sweeping of the membranes to prevent post-term pregnancy and to induce labour: A systematic review. Br J Obstet Gynaecol 106:481, 1999

Boyce A, Magaux MJ, Schwartz D: Classical and "true" gestational post maturity. Am J Obstet Gynecol 125:911, 1976

Calkins LA: Postmaturity. Am J Obstet Gynecol 56:167, 1948

Caughey AB, Nicholson JM, Washington AE: First- vs second-trimester ultrasound: The effect on pregnancy dating and perinatal outcomes. Am J Obstet Gynecol 198(6):703.e1, 2008

Caughey AB, Stotland NE, Washington E, et al: Maternal and obstetric complications of pregnancy are associated with increasing gestational age at term. Am J Obstet Gynecol 15:156, 2007

Caughey AB, Stotland NE, Washington AE, et al: Who is at risk for prolonged and postterm pregnancy? Am J Obstet Gynecol 200(6):683.e1, 2009

Cheng YW, Nicholson JM, Nakagawa S, et al: Perinatal outcomes in low-risk term pregnancies: Do they differ by week of gestation? Am J Obstet Gynecol 199(4):370.e1, 2008

Clausson B, Cnattingus S, Axelsson O: Outcomes of postterm births: The role of fetal growth restriction and malformations. Obstet Gynecol 94:758, 1999

Cleary-Goldman J, Bettes B, Robinon JN, et al: Postterm pregnancy: Practice patterns of contemporary obstetricians and gynecologists. Am J Perinatol 23:15, 2006

Clement D, Schifrin BS, Kates RB: Acute oligohydramnios in postdate pregnancy. Am J Obstet Gynecol 157:884, 1987

Clifford SH: Postmaturity with placental dysfunction. Clinical syndromes and pathologic findings. J Pediatr 44:1, 1954

Denison FC, Price J, Graham C, et al: Maternal obesity, length of gestation, risk of postdates pregnancy and spontaneous onset of labour at term. BJOG 115(6):720, 2008

Divon MY, Feldman-Leidner N: Postdates and antenatal testing. Semin Perinatol 32(4):295, 2008

Divon MY, Haglund B, Nisell H, et al: Fetal and neonatal mortality in the postterm pregnancy: The impact of gestational age and fetal growth restriction. Am J Obstet Gynecol 178:726, 1998

Elliott PM, Inman WH: Volume of liquor amnii in normal and abnormal pregnancy. Lancet 2:835, 1961

Fasset MJ, Wing DA: Uterine activity after oral mifepristone administration in human pregnancies beyond 41 weeks' gestation. Gynecol Obstet Invest 65(2):112, 2008

Fischer RL, McDonnell M, Bianculli KW, et al: Amniotic fluid volume estimation in the postdate pregnancy: A comparison of techniques. Obstet Gynecol 81:698, 1993

Fraser WD, Hofmeyr J, Lede R, et al: Amnionfusion for the prevention of the meconium aspiration syndrome. New Eng J Med 353:909, 2005

Gardner M, Rouse D, Goldenberg R, et al: Cost comparison of induction of labor at 41 weeks versus expectant management in the postterm pregnancy. Am J Obstet Gynecol 174:351, 1996

Gulmezoglu AM, Crowther CA, Middleton P: Induction of labour for improving birth outcomes for women at or beyond term. Cochrane Database System Rev 4:CD004945, 2006

Hannah ME, Hannah WJ, Hellman J, et al: Induction of labor as compared with serial antenatal monitoring in post-term pregnancy. N Engl J Med 326:1587, 1992

Harrington DJ, MacKenzie IZ, Thompson K, et al: Does a first trimester data scan using crown rump length measurement reduce the rate of induction of labour for prolonged pregnancy? BJOG 113:171, 2006

Harris BA Jr, Huddleston JF, Sutliff G, et al: The unfavorable cervix in prolonged pregnancy. Obstet Gynecol 62:171, 1983

Heimstad R, Skogvoll E, Mattsson LK, et al: Induction of labor or serial antenatal fetal monitoring in postterm pregnancy: A randomized controlled trial. Obstet Gynecol 109:609, 2007

Hill MJ, McWilliams GC, Garcia-Sur, et al: The effect of membrane sweeping on prelabor rupture of membranes: A randomized controlled trial. Obstet Gynecol 111(6):1313, 2008

Jazayeri A, Tsibris JC, Spellacy WN: Elevated umbilical cord plasma erythropoietin levels in prolonged pregnancies. Obstet Gynecol 92:61, 1998

Joseph KS, Huang L, Liu S, et al: Reconciling the high rates of preterm and postterm birth in the United States. Obstet Gynecol 109(4):798, 2007

Kashanian M, Aktarian A, Baradaron H, et al: Effect of membrane sweeping at term pregnancy on duration of pregnancy and labor induction: A randomized trial. Gynecologic and Obstetric Investigation 62:41, 2006

Kistka Z-F, Palomar L, Boslaugh, SE, et al: Risk for postterm delivery after previous postterm deliveries. Am J Obstet Gynecol 196:241, 2007

Larsen LG, Clausen HV, Andersen B, et al: A stereologic study of postmature placentas fixed by dual perfusion. Am J Obstet Gynecol 172:500, 1995

Laursen M, Bille C, Olesen AW, et al: Genetic influence on prolonged gestation: A population-based Danish twin study. Am J Obstet Gynecol 190:489, 2004

Leveno KJ, Quirk JG, Cunningham FG, et al: Prolonged pregnancy, I. Observations concerning the causes of fetal distress. Am J Obstet Gynecol 150:465, 1984

Lindell A: Prolonged pregnancy. Acta Obstet Gynecol Scand 35:136, 1956

Lindstrom K, Fernell E, Westgren M: Developmental data in preschool children born after prolonged pregnancy. Acta Paediatrica 94:1192, 2005

Link G, Clark KE, Lang U: Umbilical blood flow during pregnancy: Evidence for decreasing placental perfusion. Am J Obstet Gynecol 196(5)489.e1, 2007

MacDorman MF, Kirmeyer S: Fetal and perinatal mortality, United States, 2005. Natl Vital Stat Rep 57(8):1, 2009

MacDonald PC, Siiteri PK: Origin of estrogen in women pregnant with an anencephalic fetus. J Clin Invest 44:465, 1965

Martin JA, Hamilton BE, Sutton PD, et al: Births: Final data for 2004. National Vital Statistics Reports, Vol 55, No 1. Hyattsville, MD: National Center for Health Statistics, 2006

Martin JA, Hamilton BE, Sutton PD, et al: Births: Final Data for 2006. National Vital Statistics Reports, Vol 57, No 7. Hyattsville, Md, National Center for Health Statistics, 2009

Menticoglou SM, Hall PF: Routine induction of labour at 41 weeks' gestation: Nonsensus consensus. Br J Obstet Gynaecol 109:485, 2002

Mogren I, Stenlund H, Högberg U: Recurrence of prolonged pregnancy. Int J Epidemiol 28:253, 1999

Mozurkewich E, Chilimigras J, Koepke E, et al: Indications for induction of labour: A best-evidence review. BJOG 116(5):626, 2009

Munster K, Schmidt L, Helm P: Length and variation in the menstrual cycle—a cross-sectional study from a Danish county. Br J Obstet Gynaecol 99:422, 1992

Naeye RL: Causes of perinatal mortality excess in prolonged gestations. Am J Epidemiol 108:429, 1978

Nahum GG, Stanislaw H, Huffaker BJ: Fetal weight gain at term: Linear with minimal dependence on maternal obesity. Am J Obstet Gynecol 172:1387, 1995

National Institute of Child Health and Human Development Network of Maternal–Fetal Medicine Units: A clinical trial of induction of labor versus expectant management in postterm pregnancy. Am J Obstet Gynecol 170:716, 1994

Olesen AW, Westergaard JG, Olsen J: Perinatal and maternal complications related to postterm delivery: A national register-based study, 1978–1993. Am J Obstet Gynecol 189:227, 2003

Olesen AW, Westergaard JG, Olsen J: Prenatal risk indicators of a prolonged pregnancy. The Danish Birth Cohort 1998-2001. Acta Obstet Gynecol Scand 85:1338, 2006

Oz AU, Holub B, Mendilcioglu I, et al: Renal artery Doppler investigation of the etiology of oligohydramnios in postterm pregnancy. Obstet Gynecol 100:715, 2002

Rabe T, Hosch R, Runnebaum B: Sulfatase deficiency in the human placenta: Clinical findings. Biol Res Pregnancy Perinatol 4:95, 1983

Rushton DI: Pathology of placenta. In Wigglesworth JS, Singer DB (eds) Textbook of Fetal and Perinatal Pathology. Boston, Blackwell, 1991, p 171

Schaffer L, Burkhardt T, Zimmerman R, et al: Nuchal cords in term and postterm deliveries—Do we need to know? Obstet Gynecol 106:23, 2005

Shime J, Gare DJ, Andrews J, et al: Prolonged pregnancy: Surveillance of the fetus and the neonate and the course of labor and delivery. Am J Obstet Gynecol 148:547, 1984

Shin KS, Brubaker KL, Ackerson LM: Risk of cesarean delivery in nulliparous women at greater than 41 weeks' gestational age with an unengaged vertex. Am J Obstet Gynecol 190:129, 2004

Smith GC: Life-table analysis of the risk of perinatal death at term and post term in singleton pregnancies. Am J Obstet Gynecol 184:489, 2001

Smith SC, Baker PN: Placental apoptosis is increased in postterm pregnancies. Br J Obstet Gynaecol 106:861, 1999

Tita AT, Landon MB, Spong CY, et al: Timing of elective repeat cesarean delivery at term and neonatal outcomes. N Engl J Med 360(2):111, 2009

Trimmer KJ, Leveno KJ, Peters MT, et al: Observation on the cause of oligohydramnios in prolonged pregnancy. Am J Obstet Gynecol 163:1900, 1990

Usher RH, Boyd ME, McLean FH, et al: Assessment of fetal risk in postdate pregnancies. Am J Obstet Gynecol 158:259, 1988

Vankayalapati P, Sethna F, Roberts N, et al: Ultrasound assessment of cervical length in prolonged pregnancy: Prediction of spontaneous onset of labor and successful vaginal delivery. Ultrasound Obstet Gynecol 31(3):328, 2008

Wenstrom KD, Parsons MT: The prevention of meconium aspiration in labor using amnioinfusion. Obstet Gynecol 73:647, 1989

Wingate MS, Alexander GR, Buekens, et al: Comparison of gestational age classifications: Date of last menstrual period vs clinical estimate. Ann Epidemiol 17(6):425, 2007

Wong SF, Hui SK, Choi H, et al: Does sweeping of membranes beyond 40 weeks reduce the need for formal induction of labour? Br J Obstet Gynaecol 109:632, 2002

Yang SH, Roh CR, Kim JH: Transvaginal ultrasonography for cervical assessment before induction of labor. Obstet Gynecol Surv 59:577, 2004

CHAPTER 38

Fetal Growth Disorders

Each year, approximately 20 percent of the almost 4 million infants in the United States are born at the low and high extremes of fetal growth. Although most low-birthweight infants are preterm, approximately 3 percent are term. In 2006, 8.3 percent of infants weighed less than 2500 g at birth, whereas 7.8 percent weighed more than 4000 g. The proportion of those < 2500 g has increased by 22 percent since 1984 and by 8 percent since 2000. At the same time, the incidence of macrosomia—defined as birthweight > 4000 g—continues to decline as the distribution has shifted toward lower weights (Martin and colleagues, 2007, 2009).

NORMAL FETAL GROWTH

Human fetal growth is characterized by sequential patterns of tissue and organ growth, differentiation, and maturation. Development is determined by maternal provision of substrate, placental transfer of these substrates, and fetal-growth potential governed by the genome. Steer (1998) has summarized the potential effects of evolutionary pressures on human fetal growth. In humans, there is an increasing conflict between the need to walk—requiring a narrow pelvis—and the need to think—requiring a large brain. Humans may be resolving this dilemma by acquiring the ability to restrict growth late in pregnancy. Thus, the ability to *growth restrict* may be adaptive rather than pathological.

Lin and Santolaya-Forgas (1998) have divided cell growth into three consecutive phases. The initial phase of hyperpla-sia occurs in the first 16 weeks and is characterized by a rapid increase in cell number. The second phase, which extends up to 32 weeks, includes both cellular hyperplasia and hypertrophy. After 32 weeks, fetal growth is by cellular hypertrophy, and it is during this phase that most fetal fat and glycogen deposition takes place. The corresponding fetal-growth rates during these three phases are 5 g/day at 15 weeks, 15 to 20 g/day at 24 weeks, and 30 to 35 g/day at 34 weeks (Williams and co-workers, 1982). As shown in Figure 38-1, there is considerable biological variation in the velocity of fetal growth.

Although many factors have been implicated, the precise cellular and molecular mechanisms by which normal fetal growth occurs are not well understood. In early fetal life, the major determinant is the fetal genome, but later in pregnancy, environmental, nutritional, and hormonal influences become increasingly important (Holmes and colleagues, 1998). For example, there is considerable evidence that insulin and insulin-like growth factor-I (IGF-I) and II (IGF-II) have a role in the regulation of fetal growth and weight gain (Chiesa and associates, 2008; Forbes and Westwood, 2008). These growth factors are produced by virtually all fetal organs beginning early in development. They are potent stimulators of cell division and differentiation.

Since the discovery of the *obesity gene* and its protein product, *leptin*, there has been interest in maternal and fetal serum leptin levels. Fetal concentrations increase during the first two trimesters, and they correlate with birthweight (Catov, 2007; Sivan, 1998; Tamura, 1998; and all their colleagues). This relationship, however, is controversial in growth-restricted fetuses (Kyriakakou, 2008; Mise, 2007; Savvidou, 2006, and all their associates). Angiogenic factors have also been studied. For example, higher levels of sFlt-1 at 10 to 14 weeks are associated with small-for-gestational age infants (Smith and co-workers, 2007).

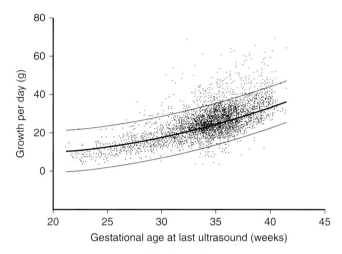

FIGURE 38-1 Increments in fetal weight gain in grams per day from 24 to 42 weeks' gestation. The black line represents the mean and the outer blue lines depict ±2 standard deviations. (Data courtesy of Dr. Don McIntire.)

Fetal growth is also dependent on an adequate supply of nutrients. As discussed in Chapter 4 (p. 87), glucose transfer has been extensively studied during pregnancy. Both excessive and diminished maternal glucose availability affect fetal growth. Excessive glycemia produces macrosomia, whereas diminished glucose levels have been associated with fetal-growth restriction. The Hyperglycemia and Adverse Pregnancy Outcomes (HAPO) Study Cooperative Research Group (2008) found that elevated cord c-peptide levels, which reflect fetal hyperinsulinemia, have been associated with increased birthweight even in women with maternal glucose levels below the threshold for diabetes.

There is less information concerning the physiology of maternal-fetal transfer of other nutrients such as amino acids and lipids. Ronzoni and colleagues (1999) studied maternal-fetal concentrations of amino acids in 26 normal pregnancies. These investigators reported that an increase in maternal amino acid levels led to an increase in fetal levels. In growth-restricted fetuses, amino acid disturbance similar to the biochemical changes seen in postnatal protein-starvation states has also been detected (Economides and colleagues, 1989b). In a study of 38 growth-restricted infants, Jones and colleagues (1999) found impaired use of circulating triglycerides consistent with peripheral adipose depletion.

FETAL-GROWTH RESTRICTION

Low-birthweight infants who are small-for-gestational age are often designated as having *fetal-growth restriction*. The term fetal-growth retardation has been discarded because "retardation" implies abnormal mental function, which is not the intent. It is estimated that 3 to 10 percent of infants are growth restricted.

Definition

In 1963, Lubchenco and co-workers published detailed comparisons of gestational ages with birthweights in an effort to derive norms for expected fetal size at a given gestational week. Battaglia and Lubchenco (1967) then classified *small-for-gestational-age* (*SGA*) infants as those whose weights were below the 10th percentile for their gestational age. Such infants were shown to be at increased risk for neonatal death. For example, the neonatal mortality rate of SGA infants born at 38 weeks was 1 percent compared with 0.2 percent in those with appropriate birthweights.

Many infants with birthweights less than the 10th percentile, however, are not pathologically growth restricted but are small simply because of normal biological factors. Indeed, Manning and Hohler (1991) and Gardosi and colleagues (1992) concluded that 25 to 60 percent of SGA infants were in fact appropriately grown when maternal ethnic group, parity, weight, and height were considered.

Because of these disparities, other classifications have been developed. Seeds (1984) suggested a definition based on birthweight below the 5th percentile. Usher and McLean (1969) suggested that fetal-growth standards should be based on mean weights-for-age with normal limits defined by ±2 standard deviations. This definition would limit SGA infants to 3 percent of births instead of 10 percent. As demonstrated from their analysis of 122,754 pregnancies, McIntire and colleagues (1999) showed this definition to be clinically meaningful. Also, as shown in Figure 38-2, most adverse outcomes are in infants below the 3rd percentile. Lastly, individual fetal-growth potential has been proposed in place of a population-based cutoff. In this model, a fetus who deviates from its individual optimal size at a given gestational age is considered either overgrown or growth restricted (Bukowski and associates, 2008).

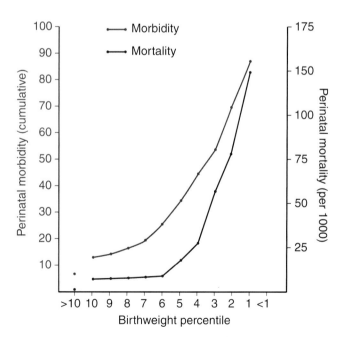

FIGURE 38-2 Relationship between birthweight percentile and perinatal mortality and morbidity rates in 1560 small-for-gestational age fetuses. A progressive increase in both mortality and morbidity rates is observed as birthweight percentile falls. (Data from Manning, 1995.)

TABLE 38-1. Smoothed Percentiles of Birthweight (g) for Gestational Age in the United States Based on 3,134,879 Singleton Live Births

Age (wk)	Percentile				
	5th	10th	50th	90th	95th
20	249	275	412	772	912
21	280	314	433	790	957
22	330	376	496	826	1023
23	385	440	582	882	1107
24	435	498	674	977	1223
25	480	558	779	1138	1397
26	529	625	899	1362	1640
27	591	702	1035	1635	1927
28	670	798	1196	1977	2237
29	772	925	1394	2361	2553
30	910	1085	1637	2710	2847
31	1088	1278	1918	2986	3108
32	1294	1495	2203	3200	3338
33	1513	1725	2458	3370	3536
34	1735	1950	2667	3502	3697
35	1950	2159	2831	3596	3812
36	2156	2354	2974	3668	3888
37	2357	2541	3117	3755	3956
38	2543	2714	3263	3867	4027
39	2685	2852	3400	3980	4107
40	2761	2929	3495	4060	4185
41	2777	2948	3527	4094	4217
42	2764	2935	3522	4098	4213
43	2741	2907	3505	4096	4178
44	2724	2885	3491	4096	4122

From Alexander and associates (1996), with permission.

Normal Birthweight

Normative data for fetal growth based on birthweight vary with ethnic and regional differences. For example, infants born to women who reside at high altitudes are smaller than those born to women who live at sea level. Term infants average 3400 g at sea level, 3200 g at 5000 feet, and 2900 g at 10,000 feet. Accordingly, researchers have developed fetal-growth curves using various populations and geographic locations throughout the United States (Brenner and co-workers, 1976; Ott, 1993; Overpeck and colleagues, 1999; Williams, 1975). These curves are based on specific ethnic or regional groups and therefore are not representative of the entire population.

To address this, data such as those shown in Table 38-1 were derived on a nationwide basis in both the United States and Canada (Alexander and co-workers, 1996; Arbuckle and colleagues, 1993). Data from more than 3.1 million mothers with singleton liveborn infants in the United States during 1991 were used to derive the growth curve shown in Figure 38-3. In general, the previously published fetal-growth curve data underestimated birthweights compared with national data. Impor-

tantly, there are significant ethnic or racial variations in neonatal mortality rates within the national neonatal mortality rate as well as within birthweight and gestational age categories (Alexander and associates, 1999, 2003).

Birthweight versus Growth

Most of what is known about normal and abnormal human fetal growth is actually based on standards for birthweight, which is the end point of fetal growth. These standards do not define the *rate* of fetal growth. Indeed, such birthweight curves reveal compromised growth only at the extreme of impaired growth. Thus, they cannot be used to identify the fetus who fails to achieve an expected or potential size but whose birthweight is above the 10th percentile. For example, a fetus with a birthweight in the 40th percentile may not have achieved its genomic growth potential for a birthweight in the 80th percentile. The rate or *velocity* of fetal growth can be estimated by serial sonographic anthropometry. Reports suggest that a diminished growth velocity is related to perinatal morbidity (Owen and co-workers, 1997; Owen and Khan, 1998).

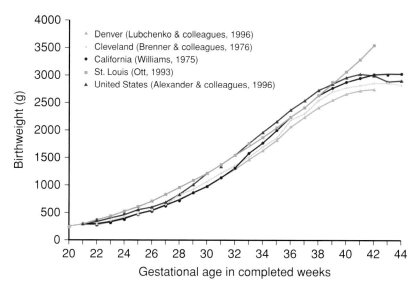

FIGURE 38-3 Comparison of fetal-growth curves for infants born in different regions of the United States and compared with those of the nation at large. (Modified from Alexander and colleagues, 1996.)

Metabolic Abnormalities

Several disturbances in fetal metabolism have been implicated in abnormal fetal growth. Economides and Nicolaides (1989a) found that the major cause of hypoglycemia in SGA fetuses was reduced supply rather than increased fetal consumption or diminished fetal glucose production. These fetuses had hypoinsulinemia along with hypoglycemia (Economides and co-workers, 1989c). The degree of fetal-growth restriction, however, did not correlate with plasma insulin levels, suggesting that glycemia is not the primary determinant of poor fetal growth.

In children with *kwashiorkor*—dietary protein malnutrition—the ratio of nonessential to essential amino acids is increased. This ratio presumably results from a decreased intake of essential amino acids. By comparison, Economides and colleagues (1989b) measured the glycine:valine ratio in cord blood from growth-restricted fetuses and found ratios similar to those observed in older children with kwashiorkor. Moreover, protein deprivation correlated with fetal hypoxemia. Economides and associates (1990) then measured plasma triglyceride concentrations in SGA fetuses and compared those with the concentrations of appropriately grown fetuses. Growth-restricted fetuses demonstrated hypertriglyceridemia that was correlated with the degree of fetal hypoxemia. They hypothesized that hypoglycemic, growth-restricted fetuses mobilize adipose tissue and that hypertriglyceridemia is the result of lipolysis of their fat stores. Beltrand and colleagues (2008) calculated growth velocity in 235 pregnancies at risk for low birthweight and found higher cord triglyceride levels, lower insulin levels, and greater insulin sensitivity in those infants with the most diminished growth velocity. They concluded that these changes represented adaptive mechanisms in fetal metabolism in response to a deleterious fetal environment.

Elevated plasma concentrations of interleukin-10, placental atrial natriuretic peptide, and endothelin-1, as well as a defect in epidermal growth factor function, have also been described in growth-restricted fetuses (Varner and colleagues, 1996). Some of these may be effect and not cause. But at the same time, these findings suggest a possible role for abnormal immune activation and abnormal placentation in the genesis of growth-restricted fetuses as well as preeclampsia syndrome (Gabriel, 1994; Heyborne, 1994; Kingdom, 1994; McQueen, 1993; Neerhof, 1995, and all their associates). These interactions are discussed further in Chapter 34 (p. 710).

In animals, chronic *reduction* in nitric oxide—an endothelium-derived, locally acting vasorelaxant—has been shown to result in diminished fetal growth (Diket and associates, 1994). Conversely, Giannubilo and co-workers (2008) showed that placenta-induced nitric oxide synthase was significantly *increased* in growth restriction, possibly representing an adaptive response to placental insufficiency.

Morbidity and Mortality

As shown in Figure 38-2, fetal-growth restriction is associated with substantive perinatal morbidity and mortality rates. Fetal demise, birth asphyxia, meconium aspiration, and neonatal hypoglycemia and hypothermia are all increased, as is the prevalence of abnormal neurological development (Jacobsson and colleagues, 2008; Paz and associates, 1995). This is true for both term and preterm growth-restricted infants (McIntire and colleagues, 1999; Minior and Divon, 1998; Wu and co-workers, 2006). Smulian and colleagues (2000) reported that growth-restricted infants had a higher 1-year infant mortality rate compared with normal infants. Boulet and associates (2006) demonstrated that for a fetus at the 10th percentile, the risk of neonatal death is increased but variably across gestational age. Risk is increased threefold at 26 weeks compared with only a 1.13-fold increased risk at 40 weeks.

Postnatal growth and development of the growth-restricted fetus depends on the cause of restriction, nutrition in infancy, and the social environment (Kliegman, 1997). Infants with growth restriction due to congenital, viral, chromosomal, or maternal size typically remain small throughout life. Fetal umbilical blood sampling for karyotyping of severely growth-restricted fetuses has permitted remarkable insights into the pathophysiology of diminished fetal growth (see Chap. 13, p. 301). If growth restriction is due to placental insufficiency, affected infants often have increased postnatal growth, and they approach their inherited growth potential.

Accelerated Maturation

There have been numerous reports describing accelerated fetal pulmonary maturation in complicated pregnancies associated with growth restriction (Perelman and colleagues, 1985). One explanation is that the fetus responds to a stressed environment by increasing adrenal glucocorticoid secretion, which leads to earlier or accelerated fetal lung maturation (Laatikainen and associates, 1988). Although this concept pervades modern perinatal thinking, there is negligible evidence to support it (see also Chap. 29, p. 605).

To examine this hypothesis, Owen and associates (1990) analyzed perinatal outcomes in 178 women delivered because of hypertension. They compared these with outcomes in infants of 159 women delivered because of spontaneous preterm labor or ruptured membranes. They concluded that a "stressed" pregnancy did not confer an appreciable survival advantage. Similar findings were reported by Friedman and coworkers (1995) in women with severe preeclampsia. Two studies from Parkland Hospital also substantiate that the preterm infant accrues no apparent advantages from fetal-growth restriction (McIntire and associates, 1999; Tyson and colleagues, 1995).

Symmetrical Versus Asymmetrical Growth Restriction

Campbell and Thoms (1977) described the use of the sonographically determined *head-to-abdomen circumference ratio* (*HC/AC*) to differentiate growth-restricted fetuses. Those who were *symmetrical* were proportionately small, and those who were *asymmetrical* had disproportionately lagging abdominal growth.

The onset or etiology of a particular fetal insult has been hypothetically linked to either type of growth restriction. In the instance of *symmetrical growth restriction*, an early insult could result in a relative decrease in cell number and size. For example, global insults such as from chemical exposure, viral infection, or cellular maldevelopment with aneuploidy may cause a proportionate reduction of both head and body size.

Asymmetrical growth restriction might follow a late pregnancy insult such as placental insufficiency from hypertension. Resultant diminished glucose transfer and hepatic storage would primarily affect cell size and not number, and fetal abdominal circumference—which reflects liver size—would be reduced. Such somatic growth restriction is proposed to result from preferential shunting of oxygen and nutrients to the brain, which allows normal brain and head growth—so-called *brain sparing*. The fetal brain is normally relatively large and the liver relatively small. Accordingly, the ratio of brain weight to liver weight during the last 12 weeks—usually about 3 to 1—may be increased to 5 to 1 or more in severely growth-restricted infants.

Because of brain-sparing effects, asymmetrical fetuses were thought to be preferentially protected from the full effects of growth restriction. Considerable evidence has since accrued that fetal-growth patterns are much more complex. Nicolaides and co-workers (1991) found that fetuses with aneuploidy typically had disproportionately large head sizes and thus were *asymmetrically* growth restricted, which was contrary to thinking at that time. Moreover, most preterm infants with growth restriction due to preeclampsia and associated uteroplacental insufficiency were found to have symmetrical growth impair-

ment—again, a departure from contemporaneous thinking (Salafia and associates, 1995).

More evidence was presented by Dashe and colleagues (2000), who analyzed 8722 consecutive liveborn singletons who had undergone sonographic examination within 4 weeks of delivery. Although only 20 percent of growth-restricted fetuses demonstrated sonographic head-to-abdomen asymmetry, these fetuses were at increased risk for intrapartum and neonatal complications. Symmetrically growth-restricted fetuses were not at increased risk for adverse outcomes compared with those appropriately grown. These researchers concluded that asymmetrical fetal-growth restriction represented significantly disordered growth, whereas symmetrical growth restriction more likely represented normal, genetically determined small stature.

Finally, recent data from Holland further challenges the concept of "brain sparing." Roza and associates (2008) provided follow-up of 935 toddlers enrolled between 2003 and 2007 in the Generation R Study in Rotterdam. Using the Child Behavior Checklist at 18 months of age, they found that infants with circulatory redistribution—brain sparing—had a higher incidence of behavioral problems.

Risk Factors

Constitutionally Small Mothers

It is not disputed that small women typically have smaller infants. If a woman begins pregnancy weighing less than 100 pounds, the risk of delivering an SGA infant is increased at least twofold (Simpson and colleagues, 1975). Moreover, intergenerational effects on birthweight are transmitted through the maternal line such that reduced intrauterine growth of the mother is a risk factor for reduced intrauterine growth of her offspring (Emanuel and associates, 1992; Klebanoff and co-workers, 1997).

Whether the phenomenon of a small mother giving birth to a small infant is nature or nurture is unclear. Brooks and colleagues (1995) analyzed 62 births after ovum donation to examine the relative influence of the donor versus the recipient on birthweight. They concluded that the environment provided by the recipient mother was more important than the genetic contribution to birthweight.

Poor Maternal Nutrition

In the woman of average or low body mass index (BMI), poor weight gain throughout pregnancy may be associated with fetal-growth restriction (Rode and colleagues, 2007). Lack of weight gain in the second trimester especially correlates with decreased birthweight (Abrams and Selvin, 1995). As perhaps expected, eating disorders are associated with up to a ninefold increase in fetal-growth restriction (Bansil and associates, 2008). This is discussed further in Chapter 55 (p. 1180).

Marked restriction of weight gain after midpregnancy should not be encouraged (see Chap. 43, p. 949). Even so, it appears that caloric restriction to less than 1500 kcal/day adversely affects fetal growth only minimally (Lechtig and co-workers, 1975). The best documented effect of famine on fetal growth was in the "hunger winter" of 1944 in Holland. The German

Occupation Army restricted dietary intake to 600 kcal/day for civilians, including pregnant women. The famine persisted for 28 weeks. Although this resulted in an average birthweight decrease of only 250 g, fetal mortality rates increased significantly (Stein and colleagues, 1975).

Undernourished women may benefit from micronutrient supplementation as shown in the study by the Supplementation with Multiple Micronutrients Intervention Trial (SUMMIT) Study Group (2008). Almost 32,000 Indonesian women were randomized to receive micronutrient supplementation or only iron and folate tablets. Infants of those receiving the supplement had lower risks of early infant mortality and low birthweight. A smaller trial done in West Africa was less convincing (Roberfroid and associates, 2008).

Social Deprivation

The effect of social deprivation on birthweight is interconnected to the effects of associated lifestyle factors such as smoking, alcohol or other substance abuse, and poor nutrition. In a study of 7493 British women, Wilcox and associates (1995) found that the most socially deprived mothers had the smallest infants. Similarly, Dejin-Karlsson and colleagues (2000) prospectively studied a cohort of Swedish women and found that lack of psychosocial resources increased the risk of growth-restricted infants.

Maternal and Fetal Infections

Viral, bacterial, protozoan, and spirochetal infections have been implicated in up to 5 percent of cases of fetal-growth restriction and are discussed in Chapters 58 and 59. The best known of these are infections caused by rubella and cytomegalovirus (Lin and Evans, 1984; Stagno and associates, 1977). Mechanisms affecting fetal growth appear to be different with each. *Cytomegalovirus* is associated with direct cytolysis and loss of functional cells. *Rubella* infection causes vascular insufficiency by damaging the endothelium of small vessels, and it also reduces cell division (Pollack and Divon, 1992).

Hepatitis A and B are associated with preterm delivery but may also adversely affect fetal growth (Waterson, 1979). *Listeriosis, tuberculosis,* and *syphilis* have also been reported to cause fetal-growth restriction. Paradoxically, with syphilis, the placenta is almost always increased in weight and size due to edema and perivascular inflammation (Varner and Galask, 1984). *Toxoplasmosis* is the protozoan infection most often associated with compromised fetal growth (Klein and Remington, 1995). Despite this, an analysis by Freeman and colleagues (2005) of 386 pregnant women who seroconverted due to toxoplasma infection found no association between congenital toxoplasmosis and low birthweight. *Congenital malaria* has also been implicated (Varner and Galask, 1984).

Congenital Malformations

In a study of more than 13,000 infants with major structural anomalies, 22 percent had accompanying growth restriction (Khoury and associates, 1988). In their study of 84 pregnancies complicated by fetal gastroschisis, Towers and Carr (2008) identified birthweights less than the 10th percentile in 38

percent of newborns and less than the 3rd percentile in 19 percent. As a general rule, the more severe the malformation, the more likely the fetus is to be SGA. This is especially evident in fetuses with chromosomal abnormalities or those with serious cardiovascular malformations.

Chromosomal Aneuploidies

Fetuses with *autosomal trisomies* have a placenta with reduced numbers of small muscular arteries in the tertiary stem villi (Rochelson and associates, 1990). Depending on which chromosome is extra, there may be associated growth restriction. For example, in *trisomy 21*, fetal-growth restriction is generally mild. Both shortened femur length and hypoplasia of the middle phalanx occur with increased frequency with this aneuploidy.

By contrast, fetal growth in *trisomy 18* is virtually always significantly restricted. Growth failure has been documented as early as the first trimester. Bahado-Singh (1997) and Schemmer (1997) and their colleagues found that crown-rump length in fetuses with trisomy 18 and 13, unlike that with trisomy 21, was shorter than expected. By the second trimester, long-bone measurements typically fall below the 3rd percentile for age, and the upper extremity is even more severely affected (Droste and co-workers, 1990). Visceral organ growth is also abnormal (Droste, 1992). Fetuses with *trisomy 13* and *trisomy 22* have some degree of growth restriction, but generally not as severe as those with trisomy 18 (Schwendemann and co-workers, 2009).

Trisomy 16 is the most common trisomy in spontaneous miscarriage and is usually lethal in the nonmosaic state (Lindor and associates, 1993). As discussed in Chapter 12 (p. 275), patches of trisomy 16 (or others) in the placenta—*confined placental mosaicism*—can cause placental insufficiency that may account for many cases of previously unexplained growth-restricted fetuses (Kalousek and colleagues, 1993; Towner and co-workers, 2001).

According to Droste (1992), significant fetal-growth restriction is not seen with *Turner syndrome* (45,X) or *Klinefelter syndrome* (47,XXY).

First-trimester prenatal screening programs to identify women at risk for aneuploidy may incidentally identify pregnancies at risk for fetal-growth restriction unrelated to karyotype. In their analysis of 8012 women, Krantz and associates (2004) identified an increased risk for growth restriction in those with extremely low free β-human chorionic gonadotropin (β-hCG) and pregnancy-associated plasma protein-A (PAPP-A) levels despite normal chromosomes. Similar findings have also been reported for second-trimester quad screening by the First- and Second-Trimester Evaluation of Risk (FASTER) Trial Research Consortium (Dugoff and colleagues, 2005). Abnormalities in two or more markers were more strongly associated with diminished growth than any single marker. Nuchal translucency, however, has not been shown to be predictive of fetal-growth restriction. These are discussed further in Chapter 13 (p. 292).

Disorders of Cartilage and Bone

Numerous inherited syndromes such as *osteogenesis imperfecta* and various chondrodystrophies are associated with fetal-growth restriction.

Drugs with Teratogenic and Fetal Effects

A number of drugs and chemicals are capable of adversely affecting fetal growth. Some are teratogenic and affect the fetus before organogenesis is complete. Some exert—or continue to exert—fetal effects after embryogenesis ends at 8 weeks. Many of these are considered in detail in Chapter 14, and examples include anticonvulsants and antineoplastic agents. Some antirejection immunosuppression drugs used for organ transplantation maintenance are implicated as a cause of restricted fetal growth (Mastrobattista and associates, 2008). In addition, cigarette smoking, opiates and related drugs, alcohol, and cocaine may cause growth restriction, either primarily or by decreasing maternal food intake. Finally, caffeine use throughout pregnancy has recently been linked to fetal-growth restriction. Diminished growth may be related to a phenotypic enzyme expression that slows caffeine metabolism (CARE Study Group, 2008).

Vascular Disease

Especially when complicated by superimposed preeclampsia, chronic vascular disease commonly causes growth restriction (see Chap. 34, p. 708). Preeclampsia may cause fetal-growth failure and is an indicator of its severity, especially when the onset is before 37 weeks (Gainer, 2005; Odegard, 2000; Xiong, 1999, and all their colleagues). In a study of more than 2000 women, vascular disease as evidenced by abnormal uterine artery Doppler velocimetry early in pregnancy was associated with increased rates of preeclampsia, small-for-gestational age neonates, and delivery before 34 weeks (Groom and co-workers, 2009).

Renal Disease

Chronic renal insufficiency is often associated with underlying hypertension and vascular disease (see Chap. 48, p. 1039). Chronic nephropathies are commonly accompanied by restricted fetal growth (Cunningham and colleagues, 1990; Vidaeff and associates, 2008).

Pregestational Diabetes

Fetal-growth restriction in women with diabetes may be related to congenital malformations or may follow substrate deprivation from advanced maternal vascular disease (see Chap. 52, p. 1113). As mentioned previously, the degree of growth restriction is related to malformation severity. Also, the likelihood of growth restriction increases with development of nephropathy and proliferative retinopathy—especially in combination (Haeri and co-workers, 2008).

Chronic Hypoxia

Conditions associated with chronic uteroplacental hypoxia include preeclampsia, chronic hypertension, asthma, smoking, and high altitude. When exposed to a chronically hypoxic environment, some fetuses have significantly reduced birthweight. Bahtiyar and colleagues (2007) induced growth restriction in pregnant rats using conditions of chronic hypoxia and by inhibiting nitric oxide synthase, a pathway implicated in hyper-

tension-related growth abnormalities. They concluded that each restrictive etiology was independent but failed to demonstrate that they were synergistic. As discussed in Chapter 44 (p. 969), severe hypoxia from maternal cyanotic heart disease frequently is associated with severely growth-restricted fetuses (Patton and co-workers, 1990).

Anemia

In most cases, maternal anemia does not cause fetal-growth restriction. Exceptions include sickle-cell disease and some other inherited anemias (Chakravarty and colleagues 2008; Tongsong and associates, 2009). Conversely, curtailed maternal blood-volume expansion has been linked to fetal-growth restriction (Duvekot and colleagues, 1995). This is further discussed in Chapter 51 (p. 1079).

Placental and Cord Abnormalities

A number of placental abnormalities may cause fetal-growth restriction. These are discussed further throughout Chapter 27 and include chronic placental abruption, extensive infarction, chorioangioma, marginal or velamentous cord insertion, circumvallate placenta, placenta previa, and umbilical artery thrombosis. Growth failure in these cases is presumed to be due to *uteroplacental insufficiency*. Some pregnancies with otherwise unexplained fetal-growth restriction and a grossly normal placenta have reduced uteroplacental blood flow compared with that of normally grown fetuses (Kotini and colleagues, 2003; Lunell and Nylund, 1992; Papageorghiou and co-workers, 2001). Similar blood flow reductions have also been reported in growth-restricted fetuses with congenital malformations. These results suggest that maternal blood flow may in part be regulated by the fetus (Howard, 1987; Rankin and McLaughlin, 1979). It is interesting that the converse is likely not the case. There is no evidence that macrosomic infants have increased uteroplacental blood flow.

Abnormal placental implantation with endothelial dysfunction may also result in fetal-growth restriction (Ness and Sibai, 2006). This pathology has been implicated in pregnancies complicated by preeclampsia as discussed in Chapter 34 (p. 710) and recently reviewed by Fisher and colleagues (2009).

Infertility

Pregnancies in women with a history of infertility have an increased risk of small-for-gestational age infants with or without infertility treatments (Zhu and colleagues, 2007).

Extrauterine Pregnancy

If the placenta is implanted outside the uterus, the fetus is usually growth restricted (see Chap. 10, p. 249). Also, some uterine malformations have been linked to impaired fetal growth (see Chap. 40, p. 890).

Antiphospholipid Antibody Syndrome

Two classes of antiphospholipid antibodies—*anticardiolipin antibodies* and *lupus anticoagulant*—have been associated with fetal-growth restriction. Pathophysiological mechanisms appear to be caused by maternal platelet aggregation and placental thrombosis. These syndromes are considered in detail in Chapter 47 (p. 1017) and Chapter 54 (p. 1151). Pregnancy outcome in women with these antibodies may be poor and include early-onset preeclampsia and fetal demise (Levine and associates, 2002; Lockwood, 2002). Not all have reported these adverse outcomes, and Infante-Rivard (2002) and Rodger (2008) and their colleagues found no association between maternal or newborn thrombophilia polymorphisms and fetal-growth restriction.

Genetics

Several studies have been done to evaluate the role of genetic polymorphisms in the mother or fetus and their relationship to growth-restricted infants. Engel and colleagues (2006) suggest a possible role for the *SHMT1(1420)T* variant in the folate metabolism pathway that affects homocysteine levels and results in SGA infants. Similarly, Stonek and associates (2007) identified *MTHFR C677T* as a marker for growth restriction. Other maternal metabolic gene polymorphisms—*CYP1A1, STT1, GSTM1*—have also been shown to modulate the risk of growth restriction in mothers who smoke (Delpisheh and co-workers, 2009). Others have evaluated microRNAs (Pineles and colleagues, 2007). Larger studies are needed to confirm and quantify the role of heredity.

Multiple Fetuses

As shown in Figure 38-4, pregnancy with two or more fetuses is more likely to be complicated by diminished growth of one or more fetuses compared with that of normal singletons (see Chap. 39, p. 868).

Identification of Fetal-Growth Restriction

Early establishment of gestational age, attention to maternal weight gain, and careful measurement of uterine fundal growth

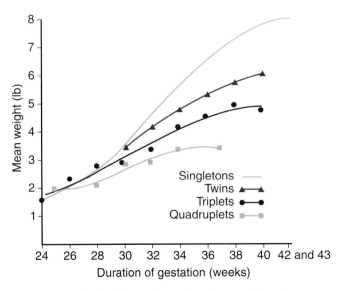

FIGURE 38-4 Birthweight and gestational age relationships in multifetal gestations. (From McKeown and Record, 1952, with permission.)

throughout pregnancy will identify many cases of abnormal fetal growth in low-risk women. Risk factors, including a *previous growth-restricted fetus,* increase the possibility of recurrence. Specifically, the rate of recurrence is believed to be nearly 20 percent (Berghella, 2007). In women with risk factors, consideration should be given to serial sonographic evaluation. Although frequency of examinations varies depending on indications, an initial early dating examination followed by a second examination at 32 to 34 weeks, or when otherwise clinically indicated, will identify many cases of growth restriction. Even so, *definitive diagnosis* frequently cannot be made until delivery.

Identification of the inappropriately growing fetus remains a challenge. There are, however, both simple clinical techniques and more complex technologies that may prove useful.

Uterine Fundal Height

Carefully performed serial fundal height measurements are a simple, safe, inexpensive, and reasonably accurate *screening* method to detect SGA fetuses (Gardosi and Francis, 1999). As a screening tool, its principal drawback is imprecision (Jelks and colleagues, 2007). For example, Jensen and Larsen (1991) and Walraven and co-workers (1995) found that this method helped to correctly identify only 40 percent of such infants. Thus, SGA fetuses were both overlooked and overdiagnosed. Despite this, these results do not diminish the importance of carefully performed fundal measurements as a simple screening technique.

Technique. The method used by most for fundal height measurement was described by Jimenez and colleagues (1983). Briefly, a tape calibrated in centimeters is applied over the abdominal curvature from the upper edge of the symphysis to the upper edge of the uterine fundus, which is identified by palpation or percussion. The tape is applied with the markings apposed to the maternal abdomen and away from the examiner's view to avoid bias. Between 18 and 30 weeks, the uterine fundal height in centimeters coincides within 2 weeks of gestational age. Thus, if the measurement is more than 2 to 3 cm from the expected height, inappropriate fetal growth may be suspected.

Sonographic Measurements

Central to the debate over whether all pregnancies should routinely undergo sonographic evaluation is the potential for diagnosis of growth restriction (Ewigman and colleagues, 1993). Typically, such routine screening incorporates an initial sonographic examination at 16 to 20 weeks to establish gestational age and identify anomalies. This is repeated at 32 to 34 weeks to evaluate fetal growth (see Chap. 16, p. 352). Ironically, Gardosi and Geirsson (1998) found that accurate gestational dating at the initial examination resulted in a lower diagnosis rate of fetal-growth restriction. In a study of 8313 pregnancies, Verburg and co-workers (2008) found that sonography prior to 24 weeks—optimally at 10 to 12 weeks—provides a better prediction of gestational age than the last menstrual period.

With sonography, the most common method for establishing the diagnosis of fetal-growth restriction is the estimation of fetal weight using multiple fetal biometric measurements. Combining head, abdomen, and femur dimensions has been

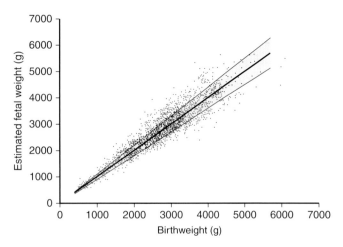

FIGURE 38-5 Correlation of sonographic fetal weight estimation using abdominal circumference (AC) with actual birthweight. (Data courtesy of Dr. Don McIntire.)

shown to optimize accuracy with little incremental improvement by addition of other biometric measurements (Platz and Newman, 2008). These are considered separately:

1. Femur length (FL) measurement is technically the easiest and the most reproducible
2. Biparietal diameter (BPD) and head circumference (HC) measurements are dependent on the plane of section and may also be affected by deformative pressures on the skull
3. Abdominal circumference (AC) measurement is more variable, but it is most commonly abnormal in cases of fetal-growth restriction because mostly soft tissue is involved (Fig. 38-5).

An abdominal circumference within the normal range for gestational age reliably excludes growth restriction, whereas a measurement less than the 5th percentile is highly suggestive of growth restriction (American College of Obstetricians and Gynecologists, 2000b). And as shown in Figure 38-6, such small circumferences are linked to decreased fetal pO₂ and pH.

Despite its accuracy, sonography used for detection of fetal-growth restriction has false-negative findings. Dashe and colleagues (2000) studied 8400 live births at Parkland Hospital in which fetal sonographic evaluation had been performed within 4 weeks of delivery. They reported that 30 percent of growth-restricted fetuses were not detected. In a study of 1000 high-risk fetuses, Larsen and associates (1992) performed serial sonographic examinations beginning at 28 weeks and then every 3 weeks. Reporting results to clinicians significantly increased the diagnosis of SGA fetuses. And although elective deliveries in this group were increased, there was no overall improvement in neonatal outcome.

Amnionic Fluid Measurement. An association between pathological fetal-growth restriction and oligohydramnios has long been recognized (see Chap. 21, p. 495). Chauhan and coworkers (2007) found oligohydramnios in less than 10 percent of pregnancies suspected of growth restriction, but this group of women was two times more likely to undergo cesarean delivery for nonreassuring fetal heart rate patterns. As shown in Figure 38-7, the smaller the pocket of amnionic fluid, the greater the perinatal mortality rate. One likely explanation for oligohydramnios is diminished fetal urine production caused by hypoxia and diminished renal blood flow (Nicolaides and associates, 1990).

Doppler Velocimetry

Abnormal umbilical artery Doppler velocimetry—characterized by absent or reversed end-diastolic flow—has been uniquely

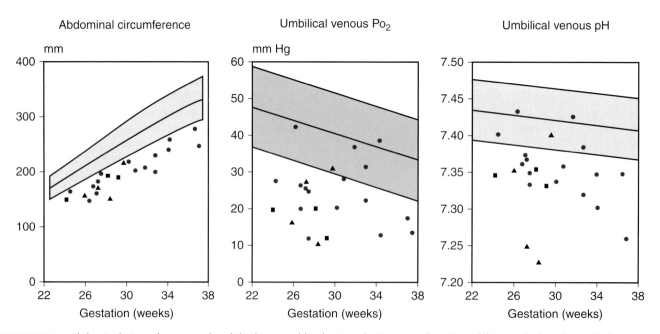

FIGURE 38-6 Abdominal circumference and umbilical venous blood pO₂ and pH in growth-restricted fetuses (red circles = liveborns; black triangles = fetal deaths; black squares = neonatal deaths). The lines within and bordering the shaded areas are the mean and the 5th and 95th percentiles, respectively, for gestational age. (From Hecher and colleagues, 1995, with permission.)

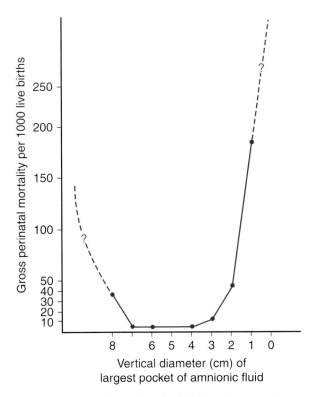

FIGURE 38-7 Relationship of amnionic fluid volume, as determined by the largest vertical pocket, to perinatal mortality rates. Mortality rates rise significantly when the largest pocket of fluid falls below 2 cm. (Data from Manning, 1995.)

associated with fetal-growth restriction (see Chap. 16, p. 363). The use of Doppler velocimetry in the management of fetal-growth restriction has been recommended as a possible adjunct to techniques such as nonstress testing or biophysical profile (American College of Obstetricians and Gynecologists, 2000b). Abnormalities in Doppler flow characterize early versus severe fetal-growth restriction and represent the transition from fetal adaptation to failure. Early changes in placenta-based growth restriction are detected in peripheral vessels such as the umbilical and middle cerebral arteries. Late changes are characterized by abnormal flow in the ductus venosus and aortic and pulmonary outflow tracts, as well as by reversal of umbilical artery flow (Pardi and Cetin, 2006). An example of this is shown in Figure 38-8.

In a series of 604 neonates < 33 weeks who had an abdominal circumference < 5th percentile, Baschat and colleagues (2007) found that the ductus venosus Doppler parameters were the primary cardiovascular factor in predicting neonatal outcome. These late changes are felt to reflect myocardial deterioration and acidemia, which are major contributors to adverse perinatal and neurological outcome. In their longitudinal evaluation of 46 growth-restricted fetuses, Figueras and colleagues (2009) determined that Doppler flow abnormalities at the aortic isthmus preceded those in the ductus venosus by one week. Similarly, Towers and co-workers (2008) prospectively observed 104 fetuses with abdominal circumference < 5th percentile. They broadly identified two patterns of progression of Doppler abnormalities: (1) *mild placental dysfunction*, which remained

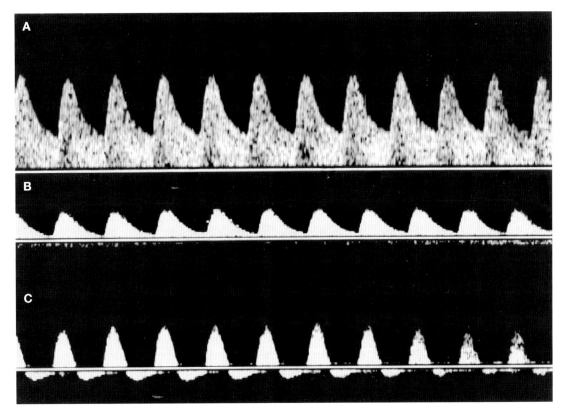

FIGURE 38-8 Umbilical arterial Doppler velocimetry studies, ranging from normal to markedly abnormal. **A.** Normal velocimetry pattern with a systolic to diastolic (S/D) ratio of < 30. **B.** The diastolic velocity approaching zero reflects increased placental vascular resistance. **C.** During diastole, arterial flow is reversed (negative S/D ratio), which is an ominous sign that may precede fetal demise.

confined to umbilical and middle cerebral arteries, and (2) *progressive placental dysfunction,* which progressed from peripheral vessels to the ductus venosus at variable intervals depending on gestational age. Both groups of investigators stressed that knowledge of these patterns of progression is critical for planning subsequent fetal surveillance and timing of delivery.

Prevention

Prevention of fetal-growth restriction ideally begins preconceptionally with optimization of maternal medical conditions, medications, and nutrition as discussed throughout Chapter 7. Smoking cessation is critical. Other risk factors should be tailored to the maternal condition, such as antimalarial prophylaxis for women living in endemic areas and correction of nutritional deficiencies. Studies have shown that treatment of mild to moderate hypertension does not reduce the incidence of SGA infants (see Chap. 45, p. 988).

During early pregnancy, accurate pregnancy dating is essential. In pregnancies at risk for fetal-growth restriction, for example, those in women with hypertension or prior fetal-growth restriction, prophylaxis with low-dose aspirin beginning early in gestation has been shown to reduce growth restriction by only 10 percent (Berghella, 2007).

Management

Once fetal-growth restriction is suspected, efforts should be made to confirm the diagnosis, assess fetal condition, and evaluate for anomalies. Growth restriction near term is easier to manage but often missed. As aptly stated by Miller and associates (2008), although growth restriction before 34 weeks is readily recognized, it presents a management challenge. Cordocentesis allows rapid karyotyping for detection of a lethal aneuploidy, which may simplify management. The American College of Obstetricians and Gynecologists (2000b) has concluded that there are not enough data to warrant routine cord blood sampling in this situation. The timing of delivery is crucial, and the risks of fetal death versus the hazards of preterm delivery must be assessed as reported in the Growth Restriction Intervention Trial (GRIT) by Thornton and colleagues (2004).

Growth Restriction Near Term

Prompt delivery is likely best for the fetus at or near term who is considered growth restricted. In fact, most clinicians recommend delivery at 34 weeks or beyond if there is clinically significant oligohydramnios. With a reassuring fetal heart rate pattern, vaginal delivery may be attempted. Some of these fetuses do not tolerate labor, and cesarean delivery is necessary.

Uncertainty about the diagnosis should preclude intervention until fetal lung maturity is assured. Expectant management can be guided using antepartum fetal surveillance techniques described in Chapter 15.

Growth Restriction Remote from Term

When growth restriction is identified in an anatomically normal fetus prior to 34 weeks, and amnionic fluid volume and fetal surveillance are normal, observation is recommended. Screening

for toxoplasmosis, rubella, cytomegalovirus, herpes, and other infections is recommended by some, however, we have not found this to be productive.

As long as fetal growth continues and fetal health remains normal, pregnancy is allowed to continue until fetal maturity is reached. In some cases, amniocentesis may be helpful to assess pulmonary maturity. Although the development of oligohydramnios is highly suggestive of fetal-growth failure, it is important to recognize that normal amnionic fluid volume does not preclude growth restriction. Owen and colleagues (2001) reported that 4- and 6-week evaluation intervals were superior to 2-week intervals for predicting growth restriction. Depending on the gestational age when fetal-growth restriction is first suspected, this interval may be impractical clinically, and sonography is usually repeated more frequently.

With growth restriction remote from term, no specific treatment ameliorates the condition. For example, there is no evidence that bed rest results in accelerated growth or improved outcome. Despite this, many clinicians intuitively advise a program of modified rest. Nutrient supplementation, attempts at plasma volume expansion, oxygen therapy, antihypertensive drugs, heparin, and aspirin have all been shown to be ineffective (American College of Obstetricians and Gynecologists, 2000b).

In most cases diagnosed prior to term, neither a precise etiology nor a specific therapy is apparent. Management decisions hinge on an assessment of the relative risks of fetal death with expectant management versus the risks from preterm delivery. Although reassuring fetal testing may allow observation with continued maturation, there is concern regarding long-term neurological outcome as discussed later (Blair and Stanley, 1992; Thornton and colleagues, 2004).

Some authorities believe that various tests of fetal well-being are unnecessary to reduce risks for stillbirth. Weiner and associates (1996) performed nonstress tests, biophysical profiles, and umbilical artery velocimetry within 3 days of delivery in 135 fetuses confirmed at birth to have growth restriction. Other than metabolic acidosis at delivery, which was predicted by absent or reversed end-diastolic umbilical blood flow, morbidity and mortality were determined primarily by gestational age and birthweight and not by abnormal fetal testing. According to the American College of Obstetricians and Gynecologists (2000a), there is no convincing evidence that such testing schemes reduce the risk of long-term neurological deficits. And recently, Baschat and colleagues (2009) provided data that substantiated this opinion. Specifically, they showed that neurodevelopmental outcome at 2 years in growth-restricted fetuses was best predicted by birthweight and gestational age.

A review of the status of Doppler velocimetry to aid in delivery timing was provided by Baschat (2004). It is clear that serial changes in Doppler flow represent a new and promising frontier in the management of pregnancies complicated by growth restriction. *Nonetheless, the optimal management of the preterm growth-restricted fetus remains problematic.*

Labor and Delivery

Fetal-growth restriction is commonly the result of placental insufficiency due to faulty maternal perfusion, ablation of functional placenta, or both. If present, these conditions are likely aggravated by labor. Equally important, diminished amnionic fluid volume increases the likelihood of cord compression during labor. For these reasons, a woman with a suspected growth-restricted fetus should undergo "high-risk" intrapartum monitoring (see Chap. 18, p. 436). For these and other reasons, the incidence of cesarean delivery is increased.

The risk of being born hypoxic or with aspirated meconium is increased. Care for the newborn should be provided immediately by an attendant who can skillfully clear the airway and ventilate the infant as needed (see Chap. 28, p. 591). The severely growth-restricted newborn is particularly susceptible to hypothermia and may also develop other metabolic derangements such as hypoglycemia, polycythemia, and hyperviscosity. In addition, low-birthweight infants are at increased risk for motor and other neurological disabilities. Risk is highest at the lowest extremes of birthweight (Baschat and colleagues, 2007, 2009; Nelson and Grether, 1997).

Long-Term Sequelae

In his book *Fetal and Infant Origins of Adult Disease,* Barker (1992) hypothesizes that adult mortality and morbidity are related to fetal and infant health. In the context of fetal-growth restriction, there are numerous reports of a relationship between suboptimal fetal nutrition and an increased risk of subsequent adult hypertension and atherosclerosis (Skilton, 2008). Low birthweight has also been implicated in subsequent development of type 2 diabetes, however, some challenge this hypothesis (Hubinette and colleagues, 2001; Huxley and co-workers, 2002). In their systematic review of 30 reports they considered relevant, Whincup and associates (2008) found that in most populations, birthweight was inversely related to type 2 diabetes risk.

Smith and colleagues (2001) found that pregnancy complications resulting in low-birthweight infants were associated with increased risk of subsequent ischemic heart disease in the mother. This suggests that common genetic risk factors might explain the link between low birthweight and risk of heart disease in both the developing fetus and the mother. In addition to risk to long-term maternal health, epidemiological studies have found that delivery of a small-for-gestational age infant increases the risk for a subsequent pregnancy complicated by stillbirth (Salihu and associates, 2006; Surkan and co-workers, 2004).

MACROSOMIA

The term *macrosomia* is used rather imprecisely to describe a very large fetus or neonate. Although there is general agreement among obstetricians that newborns weighing < 4000 g are not excessively large, a similar consensus has not been reached for the definition of macrosomia.

Newborn weight rarely exceeds 11 pounds (5000 g), and excessively large infants are a curiosity. The birth of a 16lb (7300 g) infant in the United States in 1979 was widely publicized. The largest newborn cited in the *Guinness Book of World Records* was a 23lb 12-oz (10,800 g) infant boy born to a Canadian woman, Anna Bates, in 1879 (Barnes, 1957). In the United States in 2006, of more than 4 million births, 6.7 percent weighed 4000

to 4499 g; 1 percent weighed 4500 to 4999 g; and 0.1 percent were born weighing 5000 g or more (Martin and colleagues, 2009). To be sure, the incidence of excessively large infants increased during the 20th century. According to Williams (1903), at the beginning of the 20th century, the incidence of birthweight > 5000 g was 1 to 2 per 10,000 births. This compares with 15 per 10,000 at Parkland Hospital from 1988 through 2002 and 11 per 10,000 in the United States in 2005.

The influence of increasing maternal obesity is overwhelming. The Parkland mothers with infants born weighing > 5000 g had a mean BMI of 37.8 kg/cm², and 20 percent were diabetic. Henriksen (2008) searched the Cochrane Database and reported that the rapid increase in prevalence of large infants was due to maternal obesity and type 2 diabetes. Importantly however, review of national vital statistics from the National Center for Health Statistics (2009a, b) indicates that the rate of birthweight ≥ 4000 g has steadily declined since 1994 from 10.4 percent to less than 9 percent in 2003. This is discussed further in Chapters 43 (p. 952) and 52 (p. 1109).

Definition

As noted, there are no precise definitions of macrosomia on which all authorities agree. Thus, there are several definitions in general clinical use. A common scheme includes use of empirical birthweights. In another, macrosomia is viewed as those weights that exceed certain percentiles for populations.

Birthweight Distribution

Commonly, macrosomia is defined based on mathematical distributions of birthweight. Those infants exceeding the 90th percentile for a given gestational week are usually used as the threshold for macrosomia. For example, the 90th percentile at 39 weeks is 4000 g. If, however, birthweights 2 standard deviations above the mean are used, then thresholds lie at the 97th and 99th percentile. Thus, substantially larger infants are considered macrosomic compared with those at the 90th percentile. Specifically, the birthweight threshold at 39 weeks would be approximately 4500 g for the 97th percentile rather than 4000 g for the 90th percentile.

Empirical Birthweight

Newborn weight exceeding 4000 g—8 lb 13 oz—is a frequently used threshold to define macrosomia. Others use 4250 g or even 4500 g—10 lb. As shown in Table 38-2, birthweights of 4500 g or more are uncommon. During a 10-year period at Parkland Hospital, during which there were more than 171,000 singleton births, only 1.5 percent of newborns weighed 4500 g or more. We are of the view that the upper limit of fetal growth, above which growth can be deemed abnormal, is likely two standard deviations above the mean, representing perhaps 3 percent of births. At 40 weeks such a threshold would correspond to approximately 4500 g. This definition of excessive growth is clearly more restrictive than using the upper 10 percent to define macrosomia. The American College of Obstetricians and Gynecologists (2000a) concluded that the term

TABLE 38-2. Birthweight Distribution of 171,755 Liveborn Infants at Parkland Hospital between 1998 and 2008

Birthweight (g)	Births		Maternal Diabetes
	Number	Percent	Percent
500–3999	154,906	90.2	5
4000–4249	9897	5.8	6
4250–4499	4349	2.5	7
4500–4649	1693	1.0	9
4750–4999	606	0.4	12
5000–5249	202	0.1	12
5250–5499	71	.0	25
5500–5749	22	.0	23
5750–5999	7	.0	0
6000–6249	1	.0	0
6250–6499	0	.0	—
6500 or more	1	.0	0
Total	171,755		5.4

Data courtesy of Dr. Don McIntire.

macrosomia was an appropriate designation for fetuses who weigh 4500 g or more at birth.

Risk Factors

A number of factors associated with fetal macrosomia are listed in Table 38-3. Some of these are interrelated, and in many cases they are additive. For example, advancing age is usually related to multiparity and diabetes. Obesity is obviously related to diabetes. And among women who are simultaneously diabetic, obese, and postterm, the incidence of fetal macrosomia ranges from 5 to 15 percent (Arias, 1987; Catalano 2007; Chervenak, 1992). Maternal diabetes is an important risk factor for development of fetal macrosomia (see Chap. 52, p. 1109). As shown in Table 38-2, the incidence of maternal diabetes increases as birthweight > 4000 g increases. It should be emphasized, however, that maternal diabetes is associated with only a small percentage of such large infants.

TABLE 38-3. Some Factors Associated with Fetal Macrosomia

Obesity
Diabetes—gestational and type 2
Postterm gestation
Multiparity
Large size of parents
Advancing maternal age
Previous macrosomic infant
Racial and ethnic factors

Diagnosis

Because there are no current methods to estimate excessive fetal size accurately, the diagnosis of macrosomia cannot be definitively made until delivery. Inaccuracy in clinical estimates of fetal weight by physical examination is often attributable, at least in part, to maternal obesity. Numerous attempts have been made to improve the accuracy of sonographic fetal weight estimations. A number of formulas have been proposed to estimate fetal weight using measurements of the head, femur, and abdomen. The estimates provided by these computations, although reasonably accurate for predicting the weight of small, preterm fetuses, are less valid in predicting the weight of large fetuses. For example, as shown in Figure 38-9, an infant predicted to weigh 4000 g can actually weigh considerably more or less than predicted. Rouse and associates (1996) reviewed 13 studies completed between 1985 and 1995 to assess the accuracy of sonographic prediction of macrosomic fetuses. They found only fair sensitivity—60 percent—in the accurate diagnosis of macrosomia but higher specificity—90 percent—in excluding excessive fetal size.

We can only conclude that the estimation of fetal weight from sonographic measurements is not reliable. Certainly, its routine use to identify macrosomia cannot be recommended. Indeed, the findings of several studies are indicative that clinical estimates of fetal weight are as reliable as, or even superior to, those made from sonographic measurements (O'Reilly-Green and Divon, 2000; Sherman and colleagues, 1998).

Controversies

"Prophylactic" Labor Induction

Some clinicians have proposed labor induction when fetal macrosomia is diagnosed in nondiabetic women. This approach

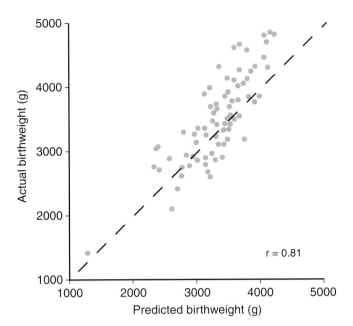

FIGURE 38-9. Relationship between actual birthweight and that predicted from sonographic measurement of abdominal circumference within 7 days of delivery. (From Johnstone and colleagues, 1996, with permission.)

is suggested to obviate further fetal growth and thereby reduce potential delivery complications. Such prophylactic induction should theoretically reduce the risk of shoulder dystocia and cesarean delivery. Gonen and colleagues (1997) randomized 273 nondiabetic women with sonographic fetal weight estimates of 4000 to 4500 g to either induction or expectant management. Labor induction did not decrease the rate of cesarean delivery or shoulder dystocia. Similar results were reported by Leaphart and associates (1997), who also found that induction unnecessarily increased the rate of cesarean delivery. In their systematic review of 11 studies of expectant management versus labor induction for suspected macrosomia, Sanchez-Ramos and colleagues (2002) found that labor induction results in increased cesarean delivery rates without improved perinatal outcomes. We agree with the American College of Obstetricians and Gynecologists (2000a) that current evidence does not support a policy for early induction for suspected macrosomia.

Elective Cesarean Delivery

Rouse and colleagues (1996, 1999) analyzed the potential effects of a policy of elective cesarean delivery for sonographically diagnosed fetal macrosomia compared with standard obstetrical management. They concluded that for women who are not diabetic, a policy of elective cesarean delivery was medically and economically unsound. Conversely, in *diabetic* women with macrosomic fetuses, such a policy of elective cesarean delivery was tenable. Conway and Langer (1998) described a protocol of routine cesarean delivery for sonographic estimates of 4250 g or greater in diabetic women. This management significantly reduced the rate of shoulder dystocia from 2.4 to 1.1 percent.

Prevention of Shoulder Dystocia

A major concern in the delivery of macrosomic infants is shoulder dystocia and attendant risks of permanent brachial plexus palsy. Such dystocia occurs when the maternal pelvis is of sufficient size to permit delivery of the fetal head but not large enough to allow delivery of the larger-diameter fetal shoulders. In this circumstance, the anterior shoulder becomes impacted against the maternal symphysis pubis (see Chap. 20, p. 481). Even with expert obstetrical assistance at delivery, stretching and injury of the brachial plexus may be inevitable (see Chap. 29, p. 636). According to the American College of Obstetricians and Gynecologists (1997), fewer than 10 percent of all shoulder dystocia cases result in a persistent brachial plexus injury.

Planned cesarean delivery on the basis of suspected macrosomia to prevent brachial plexopathy is an unreasonable strategy in the *general population* (Chauhan and colleagues, 2005). Ecker and co-workers (1997) analyzed 80 cases of brachial plexus injury in 77,616 consecutive infants born at Brigham and Women's Hospital. They concluded that an excessive number of otherwise unnecessary cesarean deliveries would be needed to prevent a single brachial plexus injury in infants born to women without diabetes. Conversely, planned cesarean delivery may be a reasonable strategy for diabetic women with an estimated fetal weight exceeding 4250 to 4500 g.

REFERENCES

Abrams B, Selvin S: Maternal weight gain pattern and birth weight. Obstet Gynecol 86:163, 1995

Alexander GR, Himes JH, Kaufman RB, et al: A United States national reference for fetal growth. Obstet Gynecol 87:163, 1996

Alexander GR, Kogan M, Bader D, et al: U.S. birthweight/gestational age-specific neonatal mortality: 1995–1997 rates for whites, Hispanics and blacks. Pediatrics 111:e61, 2003

Alexander GR, Kogan MD, Himes JH, et al: Racial differences in birthweight for gestational age and infant mortality in extremely-low-risk U.S. populations. Paediatr Perinat Epidemiol 13:205, 1999

American College of Obstetricians and Gynecologists: Shoulder dystocia. Practice Bulletin No. 7, October 1997

American College of Obstetricians and Gynecologists: Fetal macrosomia. Practice Bulletin No. 22, November 2000a

American College of Obstetricians and Gynecologists: Intrauterine growth restriction. Practice Bulletin No. 12, January 2000b

Arbuckle TE, Wilkins R, Sherman GJ: Birth weight percentiles by gestational age in Canada. Obstet Gynecol 81:39, 1993

Arias F: Predictability of complications associated with prolongation of pregnancy. Obstet Gynecol 70:101, 1987

Bahado-Singh RO, Lynch L, Deren O, et al: First-trimester growth restriction and fetal aneuploidy: The effect of type of aneuploidy and gestational age. Am J Obstet Gynecol 176(5):976, 1997

Bahtiyar MO, Buhimschi C, Ravishankar V, et al: Contrasting effects of chronic hypoxia and nitric oxide synthase inhibition on circulating angiogenic factors in a rat model of growth restriction. Am J Obstet Gynecol 196:72.e1-6, 2007

Bansil P, Kuklina EV, Whiteman MK, et al: Eating disorders among delivery hospitalizations: Prevalence and outcomes. J Womens Health 17:1523, 2008

Barker DJP (ed): Fetal and Infant Origins of Adult Disease. London, BMJ Publishing, 1992

Barnes AC: An obstetric record from the medical record. Obstet Gynecol 9:237, 1957

Baschat AA: Doppler application in the delivery timing of the preterm growth-restricted fetus: Another step in the right direction. Ultrasound Obstet Gynecol 23:111, 2004

Baschat AA, Cosmi E, Bilardo CM, et al: Predictors of neonatal outcome in early-onset placental dysfunction. Obstet Gynecol 109:253, 2007

Baschat AA, Viscardi RM, Hussey-Gardner B, et al: Infant neurodevelopment following fetal growth restriction: Relationship with antepartum surveillance parameters. Ultrasound Obstet Gynecol 33(1):44, 2009

Battaglia FC, Lubchenco LO: A practical classification of newborn infants by weight and gestational age. J Pediatr 71:159, 1967

Beltrand J, Verkauskiene R, Nicolescu R, et al: Adaptive changes in neonatal hormonal and metabolic profiles induced by fetal growth restriction. J Clin Endocrinol Metab 93:4027, 2008

Berghella V: Prevention of recurrent fetal growth restriction. Obstet Gynecol 110:904, 2007

Blair E, Stanley F: Intrauterine growth and spastic cerebral palsy, 2. The association with morphology at birth. Early Hum Dev 28:91, 1992

Boulet SL, Alexander GR, Salihu HM, et al: Fetal growth risk curves: Defining levels of fetal growth restriction by neonatal death risk. Am J Obstet Gynecol 195:1571; 2006

Brenner WE, Edelman DA, Hendricks CH: A standard of fetal growth for the United States of America. Am J Obstet Gynecol 126:555, 1976

Brooks AA, Johnson MR, Steer PJ, et al: Birthweight: Nature or nurture? Early Hum Dev 2:29, 1995

Bukowski R, Uchida T, Smith GC, et al: Individualized norms of optimal fetal growth. Obstet Gynecol 111:1065, 2008

Campbell S, Thoms A: Ultrasound measurement of the fetal head to abdomen circumference ratio in the assessment of growth retardation. Br J Obstet Gynaecol 84:165, 1977

CARE Study Group: Maternal caffeine intake during pregnancy and risk of fetal growth restriction: A large prospective observational study. BMJ 337:a2332, 2008

Catalano P: Management of obesity in pregnancy. Obstet Gynecol 109:419, 2007

Catov JM, Patrick TE, Powers RW, et al: Maternal leptin across pregnancy in women with small-for-gestational-age infants. Am J Obstet Gynecol 196:558.e1-8, 2007

Chakravarty EF, Khanna D, Chung L: Pregnancy outcomes in systemic sclerosis, primary pulmonary hypertension, and sickle cell disease. Obstet Gynecol 111:927, 2008

Chauhan SP, Grobman WA, Gherman RA, et al: Suspicion and treatment of the macrosomic fetus: A review. Am J Obstet Gynecol 193:332, 2005

Chauhan SP, Taylor M, Shields D, et al: Intrauterine growth restriction and oligohydramnios among high risk patients. Am J Perinat 24:215, 2007

Chiesa C, Osborn JF, Haass C, et al: Ghrelin, leptin, IGF-1, IGFBP-3, and insulin concentrations at birth: Is there a relationship with fetal growth and neonatal anthropometry? Ped Clin Chem 54(3):550, 2008

Chervenak JL: Macrosomia in the postdates pregnancy. Clin Obstet Gynecol 35:161, 1992

Conway DL, Langer O: Elective delivery of infants with macrosomia in diabetic women: Reduced shoulder dystocia versus increased cesarean deliveries. Am J Obstet Gynecol 178:922, 1998

Cunningham FG, Cox SM, Harstad TW, et al: Chronic renal disease and pregnancy outcome. Am J Obstet Gynecol 163:453, 1990

Dashe JS, McIntire DD, Lucas MJ, et al: Impact of asymmetric versus symmetric fetal growth restriction on pregnancy outcomes. SGI abstract 96:321, 2000

Dejin-Karlsson E, Hanson BS, Ostergren PO, et al: Association of a lack of psychosocial resources and the risk of giving birth to small for gestational age infants: A stress hypothesis. Br J Obstet Gynaecol 107:89, 2000

Delpisheh A, Brabin L, Topping J, et al: A case-control study of CYP1A1, GSTT1, and GSTM1 gene polymorphisms, pregnancy smoking and fetal growth restriction. Eur J Obstet Gynecol Reprod Biol 143(1):38, 2009

Diket AL, Pierce MR, Munshi UK, et al: Nitric oxide inhibition causes intrauterine growth retardation and hind-limb disruptions in rats. Am J Obstet Gynecol 171:1243, 1994

Droste S: Fetal growth in aneuploid conditions. Clin Obstet Gynecol 35:119, 1992

Droste S, Fitzsimmons J, Pascoe-Mason J, et al: Growth of linear parameters in trisomy 18 fetuses. Am J Obstet Gynecol 163:158, 1990

Dugoff L, Hobbins JC, Malone FD, et al: Quad screen as a predictor of adverse pregnancy outcome. Obstet Gynecol 106:260, 2005

Duvekot JJ, Cheriex EC, Pieters FAA, et al: Maternal volume homeostasis in early pregnancy in relation to fetal growth restriction. Obstet Gynecol 85:361, 1995

Ecker JL, Greenberg JA, Norwitz ER, et al: Birthweight as a predictor of brachial plexus injury. Obstet Gynecol 89:643, 1997

Economides DL, Crook D, Nicolaides KH: Hypertriglyceridemia and hypoxemia in small-for-gestational-age fetuses. Am J Obstet Gynecol 162:387, 1990

Economides DL, Nicolaides KH: Blood glucose and oxygen tension levels in small-for-gestational-age fetuses. Am J Obstet Gynecol 160:385, 1989a

Economides DL, Nicolaides KH, Gahl WA, et al: Cordocentesis in the diagnosis of intrauterine starvation. Am J Obstet Gynecol 161:1004, 1989b

Economides DL, Proudler A, Nicolaides KH: Plasma insulin in appropriate- and small-for-gestational-age fetuses. Am J Obstet Gynecol 160:1091, 1989c

Engel SM, Olshan AF, Siega-Ruiz AM et al: Polymorphisms in folate metabolizing genes and risk for spontaneous preterm and small-for-gestational age birth. Am J Obstet Gynecol 195:1231, 2006

Emanuel I, Alberman HFE, Evans SJ: Intergenerational studies of human birthweight from the 1958 birth cohort, 1. Evidence for a multi-generational effect. Br J Obstet Gynaecol 99:67, 1992

Ewigman BG, Crane JP, Frigoletto FD, et al: Effect of prenatal ultrasonic screening on perinatal outcome. N Engl J Med 329:821, 1993

Figueras F, Benavides A, Del Rio M, et al: Monitoring of fetuses with intrauterine growth restriction: Longitudinal changes in ductus venosus and aortic isthmus flow. Ultrasound Obstet Gynecol 33:39, 2009

Fisher SJ, McMaster M, Roberts, JM: The Placenta in Normal Pregnancy and Preeclampsia. In Lindheimer MD, Roberts JM, Cunningham FG (eds): Chesley's Hypertension in Pregnancy, 3rd ed. Elsevier, New York, 2009, p 73

Forbes K, Westwood M: The IGF axis and placental function. Horm Res 69:129, 2008

Freeman K, Oakley L, Pollak A, et al: Association between congenital toxoplasmosis and preterm birth, low birthweight and small for gestational age birth. BJOG 112:31, 2005

Friedman SA, Schiff E, Kao L, et al: Neonatal outcome after preterm delivery for preeclampsia. Am J Obstet Gynecol 172:1785, 1995

Gabriel R, Alsat E, Evion-Brion D: Alteration of epidermal growth factor receptor in placental membranes of smokers: Relationship with intrauterine growth retardation. Am J Obstet Gynecol 170:1238, 1994

Gainer J, Alexander J, McIntire D, et al: Fetal growth velocity in women who develop superimposed preeclampsia. Presented at the 25th Annual Meeting of the Society for Maternal-Fetal Medicine, Reno, Nevada, February 7–12, 2005

Gardosi J, Chang A, Kalyan B, et al: Customized antenatal growth charts. Lancet 339:283, 1992

Gardosi J, Francis A: Controlled trial of fundal height measurement plotted on customized antenatal growth charts. Br J Obstet Gynaecol 106:309, 1999

Gardosi J, Geirsson RT: Routine ultrasound is the method of choice for dating pregnancy. Br J Obstet Gynaecol 105:933, 1998

Giannubilo SR, Menegazzi M, Tedeschi E, et al: Doppler analysis and placental nitric oxide synthase expression during fetal growth restriction. J Matern Fetal Neonatal Med 21:617, 2008

Gonen O, Rosen DJD, Dolfin Z, et al: Induction of labor versus expectant management in macrosomia: A randomized study. Obstet Gynecol 89:913, 1997

Groom KM, North RA, Stone PR, et al: Patterns of change in uterine artery Doppler studies between 20 and 24 weeks of gestation and pregnancy outcomes. Obstet Gynecol 113:332, 2009

HAPO Study Cooperative Research Group: Hyperglycemia and adverse pregnancy outcomes. N Eng J Med 358:1991, 2008

Haeri S, Khoury J, Kovilam O, et al: The association of intrauterine growth abnormalities in women with type 1 diabetes mellitus complicated by vasculopathy. Am J Obstet Gynecol 199:278, 2008

Hecher K, Snijder R, Campbell S, et al: Fetal venous, intracardiac, and arterial blood flow measurements in intrauterine growth retardation: Relationship with fetal blood gases. Am J Obstet Gynecol 173:10, 1995

Henriksen T: The macrosomic fetus: A challenge in current obstetrics. Acta Obstet Gynecol Scand 87:134, 2008

Heyborne KD, McGregor JA, Henry G, et al: Interleukin-10 in amniotic fluid at midtrimester: Immune activation and suppression in relation to fetal growth. Am J Obstet Gynecol 171:55, 1994

Holmes RP, Holly JMP, Soothill PW: A prospective study of maternal serum insulin-like growth factor-I in pregnancies with appropriately grown or growth restricted fetuses. Br J Obstet Gynaecol 105:1273, 1998

Howard RB: Control of human placental blood flow. Med Hypotheses 23:51, 1987

Hubinette A, Cnattingius S, Ekbom A, et al: Birthweight, early environment, and genetics: A study of twins discordant for acute myocardial infarction. Lancet 357:1997, 2001

Huxley R, Neil A, Collins R: Unraveling the fetal origins hypothesis: Is there really an inverse association between birthweight and subsequent blood pressure? Lancet 360:659, 2002

Infante-Rivard C, Rivard GE, Yotov WV, et al: Absence of association of thrombophilia polymorphisms with intrauterine growth restriction. N Engl J Med 347:19, 2002

Jacobsson B, Ahlin K, Francis A, et al: Cerebral palsy and restricted growth status at birth: Population-based case-control study. BJOG 115:1250, 2008

Jelks A, Cifuentes R, Ross MG: Clinician bias in fundal height measurement. Obstet Gynecol 110:892, 2007

Jensen OH, Larsen S: Evaluation of symphysis fundus measurements and weighing during pregnancy. Acta Obstet Gynecol Scand 70:13, 1991

Jimenez JM, Tyson JE, Reisch J: Clinical measurements of gestational age in normal pregnancies. Obstet Gynecol 61:438, 1983

Johnstone FD, Prescott RJ, Steel JM, et al: Clinical and ultrasound prediction of macrosomia in diabetic pregnancy. Br J Obstet Gynaecol 103:747, 1996

Joncs JW, Gercel Taylor C, Taylor DD: Altered cord serum lipid levels associated with small for gestational age infants. Obstet Gynecol 93:527, 1999

Kalousek DK, Langlois S, Barrett I, et al: Uniparental disomy for chromosome 16 in humans. Am J Hum Genet 52:8, 1993

Khoury MJ, Erickson JD, Cordero JF, et al: Congenital malformations and intrauterine growth retardation: A population study. Pediatrics 82:83, 1988

Kingdom JCP, McQueen J, Ryan G, et al: Fetal vascular atrial natriuretic peptide receptors in human placenta: Alteration in intrauterine growth retardation and preeclampsia. Am J Obstet Gynecol 170:142, 1994

Klebanoff MA, Schulsinger C, Mednick BR, et al: Preterm and small-for-gestational-age birth across generations. Am J Obstet Gynecol 176:521, 1997

Klein JO, Remington JS: Current concepts of infections of the fetus and newborn infant. In Remington JS, Klein JO (eds): Infectious Diseases of the Fetus and Newborn Infant, 4th ed. Philadelphia, Saunders, 1995, p 1

Kliegman RM: Intrauterine growth retardation. In Fanroff AA, Martin RJ (eds): Neonatal-Perinatal Medicine, 6th ed. New York, Mosby, 1997, p 203

Kotini A, Avgidou K, Koutlaki N, et al: Correlation between biomagnetic and Doppler findings of umbilical artery in fetal growth restriction. Prenat Diagn 23:325, 2003

Krantz D, Goetzl L, Simpson J, et al: Association of extreme first-trimester free human chorionic gonadotropin-β, pregnancy-associated plasma protein A, and nuchal translucency with intrauterine growth restriction and other adverse pregnancy outcomes. Am J Obstet Gynecol 191:1452, 2004

Kyriakakou M, Malamitsi-Puchner A, Militsi H, et al: Leptin and adiponectin concentrations in intrauterine growth restricted and appropriate for gestational age fetuses, neonates and their mothers. Eur J Endocrinol 158:343, 2008

Laatikainen TJ, Raisanen IJ, Salminen KR: Corticotrophin-releasing hormone in amnionic fluid during gestation and labor and in relation to fetal lung maturation. Am J Obstet Gynecol 59:891, 1988

Larsen T, Larsen JF, Petersen S, et al: Detection of small-for-gestation-age fetuses by ultrasound screening in a high risk population: A randomized controlled study. Br J Obstet Gynaecol 99:469, 1992

Leaphart WL, Meyer MC, Capeless EL: Labor induction with a prenatal diagnosis of fetal macrosomia. J Matern Fetal Med 6:99, 1997

Lechtig A, Delgado H, Lasky RE, et al: Maternal nutrition and fetal growth in developing societies. Am J Dis Child 129:434, 1975

Levine JS, Branch DW, Rauch J: The antiphospholipid syndrome. N Engl J Med 346:752, 2002

Lin CC, Evans MI: Introduction. In Lin CC, Evans MI (eds): Intrauterine Growth Retardation. New York, McGraw-Hill, 1984

Lin CC, Santolaya-Forgas J: Current concepts of fetal growth restriction: Part I. Causes, classification, and pathophysiology. Obstet Gynecol 92:1044, 1998

Lindor NM, Jalal SM, Thibedeau SM, et al: Mosaic trisomy 16 in a thriving infant: Maternal heterodisomy for chromosome 16. Clin Genet 44:185, 1993

Lockwood CJ: Inherited thrombophilias in pregnant patients: Detection and treatment paradigm. Obstet Gynecol 99:333, 2002

Lubchenco LO, Hansman C, Dressler M, et al: Intrauterine growth as estimated from liveborn birth-weight data at 24 to 42 weeks of gestation. Pediatrics 32:793, 1963

Lunell NO, Nylund L: Uteroplacental blood flow. Clin Obstet Gynecol 35:108, 1992

Manning FA: Intrauterine growth retardation. In: Fetal Medicine. Principles and Practice. Norwalk, CT, Appleton & Lange, 1995, p 317

Manning FA, Hohler C: Intrauterine growth retardation: Diagnosis, prognostication, and management based on ultrasound methods. In Fleischer AC, Romero R, Manning FA, et al (eds): The Principles and Practices of Ultrasonography in Obstetrics and Gynecology, 4th ed. Norwalk, CT, Appleton & Lange, 1991, p 331

Martin JA, Hamilton BE, Sutton PD, et al: Births: Final data for 2005. National Vital Statistics Reports Vol. 56, No. 6, 2007

Martin JA, Hamilton BE, Sutton PD, et al: Births: Final Data for 2006. National Vital Statistics Reports, Vol 57, No 7. Hyattsville, Md, National Center for Health Statistics, 2009

Mastrobattista JM, Gomez-Lobo V, Society for Maternal-Fetal Medicine: Pregnancy after solid organ transplantation. Obstet Gynecol 112:919, 2008

McIntire DD, Bloom SL, Casey BM, et al: Birthweight in relation to morbidity and mortality among newborn infants. N Engl J Med 340:1234, 1999

McKeown T, Record RG: Observations on foetal growth in multiple pregnancy in man. Endocrinology 8:386, 1952

McQueen J, Kingdom JCP, Connell JMC, et al: Fetal endothelin levels and placental vascular endothelin receptors in intrauterine growth retardation. Obstet Gynecol 82:992, 1993

Miller J, Turan S, Baschat AA: Fetal growth restriction. Semin Perinatol 32:274, 2008

Minior VK, Divon MY: Fetal growth restriction at term: Myth or reality? Obstet Gynecol 92:57, 1998

Mise H, Yura S, Itoh H, et al: The relationship between maternal plasma leptin levels and fetal growth restriction. Endocr J 54(6) 945, 2007

National Center for Health Statistics: Vital statistics of the United States, 1994 volume I, natality. Available at: http://www.cdc.gov/nchs/data/statab/t941x26.pdf. Accessed March 2, 2009a

National Center for Health Statistics: Vital statistics of the United States, 2003 volume I, natality. Available at: http://www.cdc.gov/nchs/data/statab/natfinal2003.annvol1_26.pdf. Accessed March 2, 2009b

Neerhof MG: Causes of intrauterine growth restriction. Clin Perinatol 22:375, 1995

Nelson KB, Grether JK: Cerebral palsy in low-birthweight infants: Etiology and strategies for prevention. Men Ret Dev Dis Res Rev 3:112, 1997

Ness RB, Sibai BM: Shared and disparate components of the pathophysiologies of fetal growth restriction and preeclampsia. Am J Obstet Gynecol 195:40, 2006

Nicolaides KH, Peters MT, Vyas S, et al: Relation of rate of urine production to oxygen tension in small-for-gestational-age infants. Am J Obstet Gynecol 162:387, 1990

Nicolaides KH, Snijders RJM, Noble P: Cordocentesis in the study of growth-retarded fetuses. In Divon MY (ed): Abnormal Fetal Growth. New York, Elsevier, 1991

O'Reilly-Green C, Divon M: Sonographic and clinical methods in the diagnosis of macrosomia. Clin Obstet Gynecol 43:309, 2000

Odegard RA, Vatten LJ, Nilsen ST, et al: Preeclampsia and fetal growth. Obstet Gynecol 96:950, 2000

Ott W: Intrauterine growth retardation and preterm delivery. Am J Obstet Gynecol 168:710, 1993

Overpeck MD, Hediger ML, Zhang J, et al: Birthweight for gestational age of Mexican American infants born in the United States. Obstet Gynecol 93:943, 1999

Owen J, Baker SL, Hauth JC: Is indicated or spontaneous preterm delivery more advantageous for the fetus? Am J Obstet Gynecol 163:868, 1990

Owen P, Harrold AJ, Farrell T: Fetal size and growth velocity in the prediction of intrapartum cesarean section for fetal distress. Br J Obstet Gynaecol 104:445, 1997

Owen P, Khan KS: Fetal growth velocity in the prediction of intrauterine growth restriction in a low risk population. Br J Obstet Gynaecol 105:536, 1998

Owen P, Maharaj S, Khan KS, et al: Interval between fetal measurements in predicting growth restriction. Obstet Gynecol 97:499, 2001

Papageorghiou AT, Yu CKH, Bindra R, et al: Multicenter screening for preeclampsia and fetal growth restriction by transvaginal uterine artery Doppler at 23 weeks of gestation. Ultrasound Obstet Gynecol 18:441, 2001

Pardi G, Cetin I: Human fetal growth and organ development: 50 years of discoveries. Am J Obstet Gynecol 194:1088, 2006

Patton DE, Lee W, Cotton DB, et al: Cyanotic maternal heart disease in pregnancy. Obstet Gynecol Surv 45:594, 1990

Paz I, Gale R, Laor A, et al: The cognitive outcome of full-term small-for-gestational age infants at late adolescence. Obstet Gynecol 85:452, 1995

Perelman RH, Farrell PM, Engle MJ, et al: Development aspects of lung lipids. Annu Rev Physiol 47:803, 1985

Pineles BL, Romero R, Montenegro D: Distinct subsets of microRNAs are expressed differentially in the human placentas of patients with preeclampsia. Am J Obstet Gynecol 196:261.e1-6, 2007

Platz E, Newman R: Diagnosis of IUGR: Traditional biometry. Semin Perinatol 32:140, 2008

Pollack RN, Divon MY: Intrauterine growth retardation: Definition, classification and etiology. Clin Obstet Gynecol 35:99, 1992

Rankin JHG, McLaughlin MK: The regulation of the placental blood flows. J Dev Physiol 1:3, 1979

Roberfroid D, Huybregts L, Lanou H, et al: Effects of maternal multiple micronutrient supplementation on fetal growth: A double-blinded randomized controlled trial in rural Burkina Faso. Am J Clin Nutr 88:1330, 2008

Rochelson B, Kaplan C, Guzman E, et al: A quantitative analysis of placental vasculature in the third trimester fetus with autosomal trisomy. Obstet Gynecol 75:59, 1990

Rode L, Hegaard HK, Kjoergaard H, et al: Association between maternal weight gain and birth weight. Obstet Gynecol 109:1309, 2007

Rodger MA, Paidas M, Claire M, et al: Inherited thrombophilia and pregnancy complications revisited. Obstet Gynecol 112:320, 2008

Ronzoni S, Marconi AM, Cetin I, et al: Umbilical amino acid uptake at increasing maternal amino acid concentrations: Effect of a maternal amino acid infusate. Am J Obstet Gynecol 181:477, 1999

Roza SJ, Steegers EA, Verburg BO, et al: What is spared by fetal brain-sparing? Fetal circulatory redistribution and behavioral problems in the general population. Am J Epidemiol 168:1145, 2008

Rouse DJ, Owen J: Prophylactic cesarean delivery for fetal macrosomia diagnosed by means of ultrasonography—a Faustian bargain? Am J Obstet Gynecol 181:332, 1999

Rouse DJ, Owen J, Goldenberg RL, et al: The effectiveness and costs of elective cesarean delivery for fetal macrosomia diagnosed by ultrasound. JAMA 276:1480, 1996

Savvidou MD, Yu CK, Harland LC, et al: Maternal serum concentration of soluble fms-like tyrosine kinase 1 and vascular endothelial growth factor in women with abnormal uterine artery Doppler and in those with fetal growth restriction. Am J Obstet Gynecol 195:1668, 2006

Salafia CM, Minior VK, Pezzullo JC, et al: Intrauterine growth restriction in infants of less than 32 weeks' gestation: Associated placental pathologic features. Am J Obstet Gynecol 173:1049, 1995

Salihu HM, Sharma PP, Aliyu MH, et al: Is small for gestational age a marker of future fetal survival in utero? Obstet Gynecol 107:851, 2006

Sanchez-Ramos L, Bernstein S, Kaunitz AM: Expectant management versus labor induction for suspected fetal macrosomia: A systematic review. Obstet Gynecol 100:997, 2002

Schemmer G, Wapner RJ, Johnson A, et al: First-trimester growth patterns of aneuploid fetuses. Prenat Diagn 17(2):155, 1997

Schwendemann WD, Contag SA, Koty PP, et al: Ultrasound findings in trisomy 22. Am J Perinatol 26(2):135, 2009

Seeds JW: Impaired fetal growth: Definition and clinical diagnosis. Obstet Gynecol 64:303, 1984

Sherman DJ, Arieli S, Tovbin J, et al: A comparison of clinical and ultrasonic estimations of fetal weight. Obstet Gynecol 91:212, 1998

Simpson JW, Lawless RW, Mitchell AC: Responsibility of the obstetrician to the fetus, 2. Influence of prepregnancy weight and pregnancy weight gain on birth weight. Obstet Gynecol 45:481, 1975

Sivan E, Whittaker PG, Sinha D, et al: Leptin in human pregnancy: The relationship with gestation hormones. Am J Obstet Gynecol 179:1128, 1998

Skilton MR: Intrauterine risk factors for precocious atherosclerosis. Pediatrics 121:570, 2008

Smith GCS, Crossley JA, Aitken DA, et al: Circulating angiogenic factors in early pregnancy and the risk of preeclampsia, intrauterine growth restriction, spontaneous preterm birth, and stillbirth. Obstet Gynecol 109:1316, 2007

Smith GCS, Pell JP, Walsh D: Pregnancy complications and maternal risk of ischaemic heart disease: A retrospective cohort study of 129,290 births. Lancet 357:2002, 2001

Smulian JC, Anauth CV, Martins ME, et al: Timing of infant death by gestational age at delivery in pregnancies complicated by intrauterine growth-restriction: A population based study. Am J Obstet Gynecol 182:S68, 2000

Stagno S, Reynolds DW, Hwang ES: Congenital cytomegalovirus infection. N Engl J Med 296:1254, 1977

Steer P: Fetal growth. Br J Obstet Gynaecol 105:1133, 1998

Stein Z, Susser M, Saenger G, et al: In Famine and Human Development: The Dutch Hunger Winter of 1944–1945. New York, Oxford University Press, 1975

Stonek F, Hafner E, Philipp K, et al: Methylenetetrahydrofolate reductase C677T polymorphism and pregnancy complications. Obstet Gynecol 110:363, 2007

Surkan PJ, Stephansson O, Dickman PW, et al: Previous preterm and small-for-gestational-age births and the subsequent risk of stillbirth. N Engl J Med 350:777, 2004

Supplementation with Multiple Micronutrients Intervention Trial (SUMMIT) Study Group: Effect of maternal multiple micronutrient supplementation on fetal loss and infant death in Indonesia: A double-blind cluster-randomized trial. Lancet 371:215, 2008

Tamura T, Goldenberg RL, Johnston KE, et al: Serum leptin concentrations during pregnancy and their relationship to fetal growth. Obstet Gynecol 91:389, 1998

Thornton JG, Hornbuckle J, Vail A, et al, GRIT study group: Infant well-being at 2 years of age in the Growth Restriction Intervention Trial (GRIT): Multicentred randomized controlled trial. Lancet 364:483, 2004

Tongsong T, Srisupundit K, Luewan S: Outcomes of pregnancies affected by hemoglobin H disease. Int J Gynaecol Obstet 104(3):206, 2009

Towers C, Carr M: Antenatal fetal surveillance in pregnancies complicated by fetal gastroschisis. Am J Obstet Gynecol 198:686.e1, 2008

Towner DR, Shaffer LG, Yang SP, et al: Confined placental mosaicism for trisomy 14 and maternal uniparental disomy in association with elevated second trimester maternal serum human chorionic gonadotrophin and third trimester fetal growth restriction. Prenat Diag 21: 395, 2001

Tyson JE, Kennedy K, Broyles S, et al: The small for gestational age infant: Accelerated or delayed pulmonary maturation? Increased or decreased survival? Pediatrics 95:534, 1995

Usher R, McLean F: Intrauterine growth of live-born Caucasian infants at sea level: Standards obtained from measurements in 7 dimensions of infants born between 25 and 44 weeks' gestation. J Pediatr 74:901, 1969

Varner MW, Dildy GA, Hunter BS, et al: Amniotic fluid epidermal growth factor levels in normal and abnormal pregnancies. J Soc Gynecol Investing 3:17, 1996

Varner MW, Galask RP: Infectious causes. In Linc CC, Evans MI (eds): Intrauterine Growth Retardation. New York, McGraw-Hill, 1984

Verburg BO, Steegers EAP, Ridder M, et al: New charts for ultrasound dating of pregnancy and assessment of fetal growth: Longitudinal data from a population-based cohort study. Ultrasound Obstet Gynecol 31:388, 2008

Vidaeff AC, Yeomans ER, Ramin SM: Pregnancy in women with renal disease. Part I: General principles. Am J Perinatol 25:385, 2008

Walraven GEL, Mkanje RJB, van Roosmalen J, et al: Single pre-delivery symphysis-fundal height measurement as a predictor of birthweight and multiple pregnancy. Br J Obstet Gynaecol 102:525, 1995

Waterson AP: Viral infections (other than rubella) during pregnancy. BMJ 2:564, 1979

Weiner Z, Divon MY, Katz VK, et al: Multivariate analysis of antepartum fetal tests in predicting neonatal outcome of growth retarded fetus. Am J Obstet Gynecol 174:339, 1996

Whincup PH, Kaye SK, Owen CG, et al: Birth weight and risk of type 2 diabetes: A systematic review. JAMA 300:2886, 2008

Wilcox MA, Smith SJ, Johnson IR, et al: The effect of social deprivation on birthweight, excluding physiological and pathological effects. Br J Obstet Gynaecol 102:918, 1995

Williams JW: Obstetrics: A Text-Book for Students and Practitioners, 1st ed. New York, Appleton, 1903, p 133

Williams RL: Intrauterine growth curves. Intra- and international comparisons with different ethnic groups in California. Prev Med 4:163, 1975

Williams RL, Creasy RK, Cunningham GC, et al: Fetal growth and perinatal viability in California. Obstet Gynecol 59:624, 1982

Wu YW, Croen LA, Shah SJ, et al: Cerebral palsy in term infants. Pediatrics 118:690, 2006

Xiong X, Mayes D, Demianczuk N, et al: Impact of pregnancy-induced hypertension on fetal growth. Am J Obstet Gynecol 180:207, 1999

Zhu JL, Obel C, Bech BH, et al: Infertility, infertility treatment and fetal growth restriction. Obstet Gynecol 110:1326, 2007

Multifetal Gestation

Fueled largely by infertility therapy, over the past 25 years, both the rate and the number of twin and higher-order multifetal births have increased in the United States at an unprecedented pace. Between 1980 and 2005, the twinning rate rose from 18.9 to 32.1 per 1000 live births (Martin and colleagues, 2009). Over the same time period, the number of live births from twin deliveries rose nearly 50 percent, and the number of higher-order multifetal births increased more than 400 percent (Fig. 39-1). However, as discussed later, changing infertility therapy has led to slight decreases in rates of higher-order multifetal births.

This extraordinary increase in multifetal births is a public health concern. The higher rate of preterm delivery of these neonates compromises their survival chances and increases their risk of lifelong disability. More than a fourth of very-low-birthweight (<1500 g) neonates born in the United States are the product of a multifetal gestation, as is one in every seven infants who die (Martin and colleagues, 2006; Mathews and MacDorman, 2006). Data comparing singleton and twin outcomes at Parkland Hospital are found in Table 39-1. Comparing twins with triplets or quadruplets, Luke and Brown (2008) found lower risks with twins for preterm prematurely ruptured membranes, preterm delivery, and perinatal mortality.

Multifetal gestations are at higher risk of fetal malformations, and also twin-twin transfusion syndrome may develop. Maternal complications are also increased. Walker and colleagues (2004) studied more than 44,000 multifetal gestations and found that, compared with singletons, risks for preeclampsia, postpartum hemorrhage, and maternal death were increased twofold or more. Wen and co-workers (2004) reported that these maternal risks correlated with fetal number. Francois and associates (2005) reported that compared with women who delivered singletons, those who delivered twins were three times as likely to undergo emergent peripartum hysterectomy, and those who delivered triplets or quadruplets were 24 times as likely. Maternal risks of multifetal gestation are not exclusively acute or physical. Choi and associates (2009) reported that at 9 months postpartum, mothers of multifetal births were almost 50 percent more likely to have moderate to severe depressive symptoms than mothers of singletons.

ETIOLOGY OF MULTIFETAL GESTATIONS

Twin fetuses usually result from fertilization of two separate ova–*dizygotic* or *fraternal twins*. Less often, twins arise from a single fertilized ovum that subsequently divides–*monozygotic* or *identical twins*. Either or both processes may be involved in the formation of higher numbers. Quadruplets, for example, may arise from as few as one to as many as four ova.

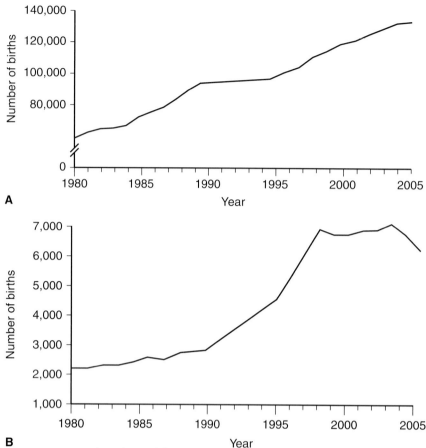

FIGURE 39-1 Number of twin **(A)** and triplet or higher-order multifetal births **(B)** in the United States, 1980-2005. (From Martin and colleagues, 1999, 2007.)

Fraternal versus Identical Twins

Dizygotic twins are not in a strict sense true twins because they result from the maturation and fertilization of two ova during a single ovulatory cycle. Also, monozygotic or identical twins are usually not identical. As discussed subsequently, the division of one fertilized zygote into two does not necessarily result in equal sharing of protoplasmic materials. Monozygotic twins may actually be discordant for genetic mutations as the result of a postzygotic mutation, or may have the same genetic disease but with marked variability in expression. In female fetuses, skewed lyonization can produce differential expression of X-linked traits or diseases. Furthermore, the process of monozygotic twinning is in a sense a teratogenic event, and monozygotic twins have an increased incidence of often discordant malformations (Glinianaia and co-workers, 2008). For example, Machin (1996) found that monozygotic twins may be discordant for malformations that involve asymmetrical organs such as the heart. For these reasons, dizygotic or fraternal twins of the same sex may appear more nearly identical at birth than monozygotic twins, and growth of monozygotic twin fetuses may be discordant, at times dramatically so. Accordingly, determination of zygosity frequently requires sophisticated genetic testing.

Genesis of Monozygotic Twins

The developmental mechanisms underlying monozygotic twinning are poorly understood. Minor trauma to the blastocyst during assisted reproductive technology (ART) may lead to the increased incidence of monozygotic twinning observed in pregnancies conceived in this manner (Wenstrom and co-workers, 1993).

The outcome of the monozygotic twinning process depends on when division occurs. If zygotes divide within the first 72 hours after fertilization, two embryos, two amnions, and two chorions develop, and a diamnionic, dichorionic twin pregnancy evolves (Fig. 39-2). Two distinct placentas or a single, fused placenta may develop. If division occurs between the fourth and eighth day, a diamnionic, monochorionic twin pregnancy results. By approximately 8 days after fertilization, the chorion and the amnion have already differentiated, and division results in two embryos within a common amnionic sac, that is, a monoamnionic, monochorionic twin pregnancy. Conjoined twins result if twinning is initiated later.

It has long been accepted that monochorionicity incontrovertibly indicated monozygosity. Rarely, however, monochorionic twins may in fact be dizygotic (Souter and colleagues,

TABLE 39-1. Selected Outcomes in Singleton and Twin Pregnancies Delivered at Parkland Hospital from 2002 through 2006

Outcome	Singletons	Twins
Pregnancies	78,879	850
Births[a]	78,879	1700
Stillbirths	406 (5.1)	24 (14.1)
Neonatal deaths	253 (3.2)	38 (22.4)
Perinatal deaths	659 (8.4)	62 (36.5)
Very-low-birthweight (<1500 g)	895 (1.0)	196 (11.6)

[a]Birth data are represented as number (per 1000).

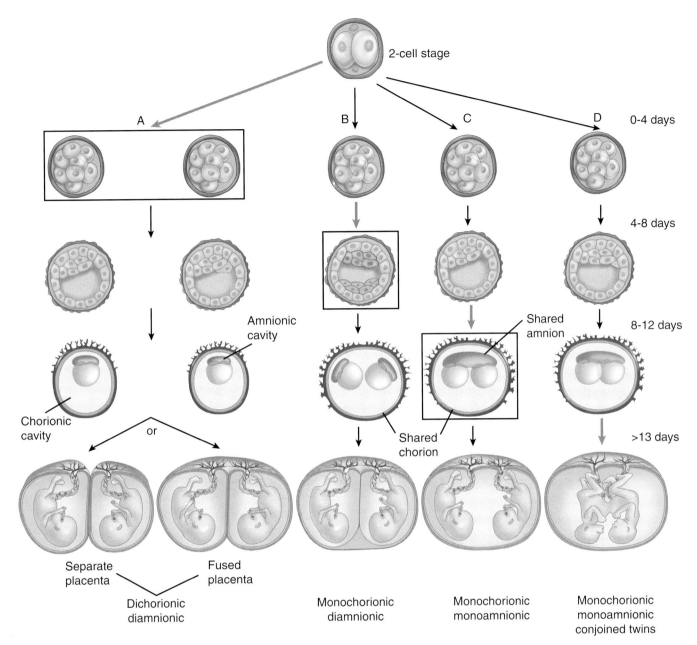

2-cell stage

A

B   C   D   0-4 days

4-8 days

Amnionic
cavity   Shared
                                          amnion   8-12 days

Chorionic
cavity   or   >13 days

                                          Shared
                                          chorion

Separate   Fused
placenta   placenta

Dichorionic   Monochorionic   Monochorionic   Monochorionic
diamnionic   diamnionic   monoamnionic   monoamnionic
                                                          conjoined twins

FIGURE 39-2 Mechanism of monozygotic twinning. Black boxing and blue arrows in columns A, B, and C indicates timing of division. **A.** At 0 to 4 days postfertilization, an early conceptus may divide into two. Division at this early stage creates two chorions and two amnions (dichorionic, diamnionic). Placentas may be separate or fused. **B.** Division between 4 to 8 days leads to formation of a blastocyst with two separate embryoblasts (inner cell masses). Each embryoblast will form its own amnion within a shared chorion (monochorionic, diamnionic). **C.** Between 8 and 12 days, the amnion and amnionic cavity form above the germinal disc. Embryonic division leads to two embryos with a shared amnion and shared chorion (monochorionic, monoamnionic). **D.** Differing theories explain conjoined twin development. One describes an incomplete splitting of one embryo into two. The other describes fusion of a portion of one embryo from a monozygotic pair onto the other.

2003). Mechanisms for this are speculative, and zygotic manipulations that accompany ART have been implicated (Redline, 2003).

Superfetation and Superfecundation

In *superfetation*, an interval as long as or longer than a menstrual cycle intervenes between fertilizations. Superfetation requires ovulation and fertilization during the course of an established preg-

nancy, which is theoretically possible until the uterine cavity is obliterated by fusion of the decidua capsularis to the decidua parietalis. Although known to occur in mares, superfetation is as yet unproven in humans. Most authorities believe that the alleged cases of human superfetation result from markedly unequal growth and development of twin fetuses with the same gestational age.

Superfecundation refers to fertilization of two ova within the same menstrual cycle but not at the same coitus, nor necessarily by sperm from the same male. An instance of superfecundation,

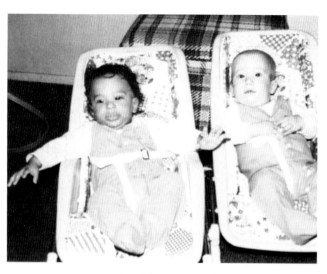

FIGURE 39-3 An example of dizygotic twin boys as the consequence of superfecundation. (Used with permission from Dr. David W. Harris.)

documented by Harris (1982), is demonstrated in Figure 39-3. The mother was sexually assaulted on the 10th day of her menstrual cycle and had intercourse 1 week later with her husband. She was delivered of a black neonate whose blood type was A and a white neonate whose blood type was O. The blood type of the mother and her husband was O.

Frequency of Twins

The frequency of monozygotic twin births is relatively constant worldwide—approximately one set per 250 births, and is largely independent of race, heredity, age, and parity. There is now evidence that the incidence of zygotic splitting is also increased following ART (Aston and colleagues, 2008). In contrast, the incidence of dizygotic twinning is influenced remarkably by race, heredity, maternal age, parity, and, especially, fertility treatment.

The "Vanishing Twin"

The incidence of twins in the first trimester is much greater than the incidence of twins at birth. Studies in which fetuses were evaluated with sonography in the first trimester have shown that one twin is lost or "vanishes" before the second trimester in up to 20 to 60 percent of spontaneous twin conceptions (Dickey, 2002; Kol, 1993; Landy, 1986; Parisi, 1983, and all their co-workers).

Monochorionic twins have a significantly greater risk of abortion than dichorionic twins (Sperling and colleagues, 2006). In some cases, the entire pregnancy aborts. In many cases, however, only one fetus dies, and the remaining fetus delivers as a singleton. Undoubtedly, some threatened abortions have resulted in death and resorption of one embryo from an unrecognized twin gestation, whereas the other embryo continued its growth and development (Jauniaux and co-workers, 1988).

Dickey and colleagues (2002) described spontaneous reduction in 709 women with a multifetal pregnancy. Prior to

12 weeks, one or more embryos died in 36 percent of twin pregnancies, 53 percent of triplet pregnancies, and 65 percent of quadruplet pregnancies. Interestingly, pregnancy duration and birthweight were inversely related to the initial gestational sac number regardless of the final number of fetuses at delivery. This effect was most pronounced in twins who started as quadruplets. Chasen and colleagues (2006) reported that spontaneous reduction of an in-vitro fertilization (IVF) twin pregnancy to a singleton pregnancy was associated with perinatal outcomes intermediate between IVF singleton pregnancies and IVF twin pregnancies that did not undergo spontaneous reduction.

A vanishing twin may cause an elevated maternal serum alpha-fetoprotein level, an elevated amnionic fluid alpha-fetoprotein level, and a positive amnionic fluid acetylcholinesterase assay result (Winsor and associates, 1987). Therefore, the diagnosis of vanishing twin should be excluded to avoid confusion during maternal serum screening for Down syndrome or neural-tube defects (see Chap. 13, p. 292). Similarly, a vanishing twin can cause a discrepancy between the karyotype established by chorionic villus sampling and the karyotype of a surviving twin when tissue from a vanished twin is inadvertently sampled. For these reasons, amniocentesis for karyotype may be preferable if a vanishing twin is suspected (Reddy and associates, 1991).

Factors That Influence Twinning

Race

The frequency of multifetal births varies significantly among different races and ethnic groups (Table 39-2). In one rural community in Nigeria, Knox and Morley (1960) found that twinning occurred once in every 20 births! These marked differences in twinning frequency may be the consequence of racial variations in levels of follicle-stimulating hormone (FSH) (Nylander, 1973).

Heredity

As a determinant of twinning, the family history of the mother is much more important than that of the father. In a study of 4000 genealogical records, White and Wyshak (1964) found that women who themselves were a dizygotic twin gave birth to twins at a rate of 1 set per 58 births. Women who were not a twin, but whose husbands were a dizygotic twin, gave birth to twins at a rate of 1 set per 116 pregnancies. Genetic studies are beginning to identify genes that increase the rate of dizygotic twinning. That said, the contribution of these variants to the overall incidence of twinning is likely small (Hoekstra and associates, 2008).

Maternal Age and Parity

The rate of natural twinning peaks at age 37 years, when maximal FSH stimulation increases the rate of multiple follicles developing (Beemsterboer and co-workers, 2006). The fall in incidence thereafter probably reflects physiological follicle depletion.

Increasing parity has also been shown to increase the incidence of twinning independently in all populations studied. In Sweden, Pettersson and associates (1976) determined that the frequency of multiple fetuses in first pregnancies was 1.3 percent, compared

TABLE 39-2. Twinning Rates per 1000 Births by Zygosity

Country	Monozygotic	Dizygotic	Total
Nigeria	5.0	49	54
United States			
Black	4.7	11.1	15.8
White	4.2	7.1	11.3
England and Wales	3.5	8.8	12.3
India (Calcutta)	3.3	8.1	11.4
Japan	3.0	1.3	4.3

This table was published in *Seminars in Perinatology*, Vol. 10, I MacGillivray, Epidemiology of twin pregnancy, pp. 4–8, Copyright Elsevier 1986.

with 2.7 percent in the fourth pregnancy. In Nigeria, Azubuike (1982) showed that the frequency of twinning increased from 1 in 50–2 percent–among nulliparous women to 1 in 15–6.6 percent–for women pregnant six or more times!

Nutritional Factors

In animals, litter size increases in proportion to nutritional sufficiency. Evidence from a variety of sources indicates that this occurs in humans as well. Nylander (1971) showed a definite increasing gradient in the twinning rate related to greater nutritional status as reflected by maternal size. Taller, heavier women had a twinning rate 25- to 30-percent greater than short, nutritionally deprived women. MacGillivray (1986) also found that dizygotic twinning is more common in large and tall women than in small women. Evidence acquired during and after World War II showed that twinning correlated more with nutrition than body size. Widespread undernourishment in Europe during those years was associated with a marked fall in the dizygotic twinning rate (Bulmer, 1959). Haggarty and associates (2006) reported that higher folate intake and plasma folate concentrations were associated with an increased rate of twinning in women undergoing IVF.

Pituitary Gonadotropin

The common factor linking race, age, weight, and fertility to multifetal gestation may be FSH levels (Benirschke and Kim, 1973). This theory is supported by the fact that increased fecundity and a higher rate of dizygotic twinning have been reported in women who conceive within 1 month after stopping oral contraceptives, but not during subsequent months (Rothman, 1977). This may be due to the sudden release of pituitary gonadotropin in amounts greater than usual during the first spontaneous cycle after stopping hormonal contraception.

Infertility Therapy

Ovulation induction with FSH plus chorionic gonadotropin or clomiphene citrate remarkably enhances the likelihood of multiple ovulations. The incidence of multifetal gestation following conventional gonadotropin therapy is 16 to 40 percent, of which 75 percent are twins (Schenker and co-workers, 1981). Tuppin and colleagues (1993) reported that in France, the incidence of twin and triplet deliveries and the sale of human menopausal gonadotropin (hMG) rose in parallel between 1972 and 1989. By 1989, half of triplet pregnancies resulted from ovulation induction. Superovulation therapy, which increases the chance of pregnancy by recruiting multiple follicles, results in multifetal gestation rates of 25 to 30 percent (Bailey-Pridham and associates, 1990).

Risk factors for multiple fetuses after ovarian stimulation with hMG include increased estradiol levels on the day of chorionic gonadotropin injection and sperm characteristics such as increased concentration and motility (Dickey and associates, 1992; Pasqualotto and colleagues, 1999). With recognition of these factors, plus the ability to monitor follicular growth and size sonographically, physicians may cancel cycles likely to lead to a multifetal gestation. This approach has reduced the incidence of multifetal births.

Assisted Reproductive Technology (ART)

These techniques are designed to increase the probability of pregnancy. But they also increase the probability of multifetal gestation. In general with IVF, the greater the number of embryos that are transferred, the greater the risk of twins and multiple fetuses. In 2005, 1 percent of infants born in the United States were conceived through ART, and these infants accounted for 17 percent of multiple births (Wright and colleagues, 2008).

Reducing Multifetal Gestation

The American Society for Reproductive Medicine (1999) initiated a concerted effort to reduce the incidence of higher-order multifetal gestation. By this time, some practitioners of ART had already begun to modify their practices to reduce the rate of multifetal gestations. In their review of IVF practices in the United States from 1995 to 2001, Jain and colleagues (2004) found that the number of embryos transferred per cycle decreased steadily *after* 1997, as did the percentage of pregnancies with three or more fetuses (see Fig. 39-1B). Paradoxically, there was a consistent increase in the percentage of live births per cycle. Improved ART techniques explain this paradox. For

TABLE 39-3. Overview of the Incidence of Twin Pregnancy Zygosity and Corresponding Twin-Specific Complications

Type of Twinning	Twins	Rates of Twin-Specific Complication in Percent			
		Fetal-Growth Restriction	Preterm Delivery[a]	Placental Vascular Anastomosis	Perinatal Mortality
Dizygous	80	25	40	0	10–12
Monozygous	20	40	50		15–18
Diamnionic/dichorionic	6–7	30	40	0	18–20
Diamnionic/monochorionic	13–14	50	60	100	30–40
Monoamnionic/monochorionic	<1	40	60–70	80–90	58–60
Conjoined	0.002 to 0.008	—	70–80	100	70–90

[a]Delivery before 37 weeks.
Modified from Manning FA: Fetal biophysical profile scoring. In *Fetal Medicine: Principles and Practices,* 1995. Copyright © The McGraw-Hill Companies, Inc.

example, culturing embryos for 5 days to the blastocyst stage as opposed to culturing for 3 days results in improved live birth rates (Papanikolaou and associates, 2006).

Sex Ratios with Multiple Fetuses

In humans, as the number of fetuses per pregnancy increases, the percentage of male conceptuses decreases. Strandskov and co-workers (1946) found the percentage of males in 31 million singleton births in the United States was 51.6 percent. For twins, it was 50.9 percent; for triplets, 49.5 percent; and for quadruplets, 46.5 percent. Females predominate even more in twins from late twinning events. For example, 70 percent of monochorionic–monoamnionic twins and 75 percent of conjoined twins are female (Machin, 1996). Two explanations have been offered. First, beginning in utero and extending throughout the life cycle, mortality rates are lower in females. Nutritional and space limitations associated with multiple fetuses in utero may exaggerate this biological tendency. Second, female zygotes have a greater tendency to divide.

Determination of Chorionicity

This determination can aid obstetrical risk assessment and guide management of multifetal gestation. The rate of twin-specific complications varies in relation to zygosity and chorionicity, with the latter being the more important determinant (Table 39-3). There are increased rates of perinatal mortality and neurological injury in monochorionic diamnionic twins compared with dichorionic pairs (Hack and co-workers, 2008; Lee and colleagues, 2008). In a study of 146 sets of twins in which zygosity and chorionicity were carefully assessed, monozygotic dichorionic twins had perinatal outcomes equivalent to those of dizygotic twins (Carroll and colleagues, 2005).

Sonographic Evaluation

Chorionicity can sometimes be determined sonographically in the first trimester. The presence of two separate placentas and a thick—generally 2 mm or greater—dividing membrane supports a presumed diagnosis of dichorionicity (Fig. 39-4). Fetuses of opposite gender are almost always dizygotic, thus dichorionic (Mahony and co-workers, 1985).

In pregnancies in which a single placental mass is identified, it may be difficult to distinguish one large placenta from two placentas lying side by side. Examining the point of origin of the dividing membrane on the placental surface may clarify this situation. If as shown in Figure 39-4, a triangular projection of placental tissue is seen to extend beyond the chorionic surface between the layers of the dividing membrane, then there are two fused placentas—the *twin-peak sign.*

In contrast, monochorionic pregnancies have a dividing membrane that is so thin it may not be seen until the second trimester. The membrane is generally less than 2 mm thick, and magnification reveals only two layers (Scardo and associates, 1995). This right-angle relationship between the membranes and placenta with no apparent extension of placenta between the dividing membrane is called the *T sign* (Fig. 39-5). Sonographic evaluation of the dividing membrane is easiest and most accurate in the first half of pregnancy when fetuses are smaller (Stagiannis and colleagues, 1995).

Lee and colleagues (2006) used the combination of placental location, presence or absence of the twin-peak sign, and fetal gender to determine chorionicity in 410 consecutive twins at midgestation. Compared with the pathological diagnosis determined by examining the placenta after delivery, the sonographic determination had 96-percent accuracy. They also reported improved sensitivity and specificity of sonography to determine chorionicity if performed during the first trimester compared with second-trimester imaging.

Placental Examination

A carefully performed visual examination of the placenta and membranes following delivery serves to establish zygosity and chorionicity promptly in approximately two thirds of cases. The following system for examination is recommended: As the first neonate is delivered, one clamp is placed on a portion of its

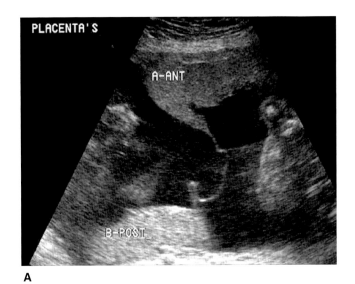

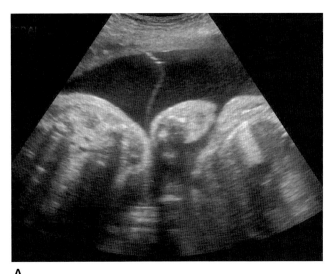

A

A

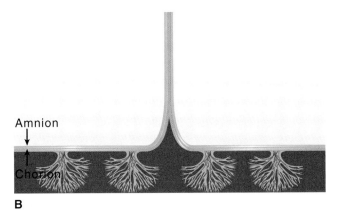

Amnion

Chorion

B

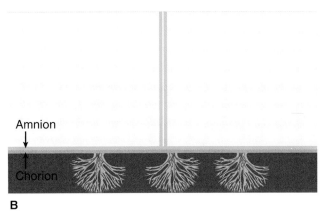

Amnion

Chorion

B

FIGURE 39-4 A. Sonographic image of the "twin-peak" sign, also termed the "lambda sign," in a 24-week gestation. At the top of this sonogram, tissue from the anterior placenta is seen extending downward between the amnion layers. This sign confirms dichorionic twinning. **B.** Schematic diagram of the "twin-peak" sign. A triangular portion of placenta is seen insinuating between the amniochorion layers.

FIGURE 39-5 A. Sonographic image of the "T" sign in a monochorionic diamnionic gestation at 30 weeks. **B.** Schematic diagram of the "T" sign. Twins are separated only by a membrane created by the juxtaposed amnion of each twin. A "T" is formed at the point at which amnions meet the placenta.

cord. Cord blood is not collected until after delivery of the other twin, unless it has been clearly shown prior to delivery that there are two placentas. As the second neonate is delivered, two clamps are placed on that cord. Three clamps are used to mark the cord of a third neonate, and so on as necessary. Until the delivery of the last fetus, each cord segment must remain clamped to prevent fetal hypovolemia and anemia caused by blood leaving the placenta via anastomoses and then through an unclamped cord.

The placenta should be carefully delivered to preserve the attachment of the amnion and chorion, because identification of the relationship of the membranes to each other is critical. With one common amnionic sac, or with juxtaposed amnions not separated by chorion arising between the fetuses, the fetuses are monozygotic. If adjacent amnions are separated by chorion, then the fetuses could be either dizygotic or monozygotic, but dizygosity is more common (see Figs. 39-2 and 39-6). If the neonates are of the same sex, blood typing of cord blood samples may be helpful. Different blood types confirm dizygosity,

although demonstrating the same blood type in each fetus does not confirm monozygosity. For definitive diagnosis, more complicated techniques such as DNA fingerprinting can be used, but these tests are generally not performed at birth unless there is a pressing medical indication (St. Clair and associates, 1998).

Infant Sex and Zygosity

Twins of opposite sex are almost always dizygotic. Rarely, monozygotic twins may be discordant for phenotypic sex. This occurs if one twin is phenotypically female due to Turner syndrome (45,X) and her sibling is 46,XY.

DIAGNOSIS OF MULTIPLE FETUSES

History and Clinical Examination

A maternal personal or family history of twins, advanced maternal age, high parity, and large maternal size are weakly associated with multifetal gestation. Recent administration of either clomiphene citrate or gonadotropins or pregnancy accomplished by ART are much stronger associates.

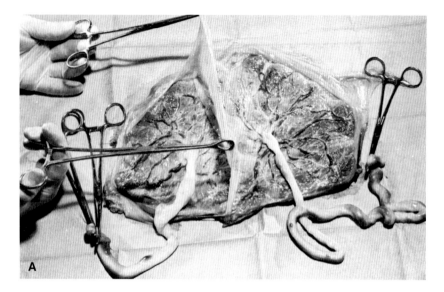

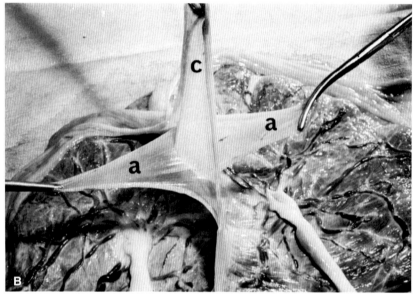

FIGURE 39-6 A. The membrane partition that separated twin fetuses is elevated. **B.** The membrane partition consists of chorion (**c**) between two amnions (**a**).

Clinical examination with accurate measurement of fundal height, as described in Chapter 8 (p. 199), is essential. With multiple fetuses, uterine size is typically larger during the second trimester than expected. Rouse and co-workers (1993) reported fundal heights in 336 well-dated twin pregnancies. Between 20 and 30 weeks, fundal heights were on average approximately 5 cm greater than expected for singletons of the same fetal age.

In women with a uterus that appears large for gestational age, the following possibilities are considered:

1. Multiple fetuses
2. Elevation of the uterus by a distended bladder
3. Inaccurate menstrual history
4. Hydramnios
5. Hydatidiform mole
6. Uterine leiomyomas
7. A closely attached adnexal mass
8. Fetal macrosomia (late in pregnancy)

In general, it is difficult to diagnose twins by palpation of fetal parts before the third trimester. Even late in pregnancy, it may be difficult to identify twins by abdominal palpation, especially if one twin overlies the other, if the woman is obese, or if there is hydramnios. If uterine palpation leads to the diagnosis of twins, it is most often because two fetal heads have been detected, often in different uterine quadrants.

Late in the first trimester, fetal heart action may be detected with Doppler ultrasonic equipment. Thereafter, it becomes possible to identify two fetal heartbeats if their rates are clearly distinct from each other and from that of the mother. Careful examination with an aural fetal stethoscope can identify fetal heart sounds in twins as early as 18 to 20 weeks.

Sonography

By careful sonographic examination, separate gestational sacs can be identified early in twin pregnancy (Fig. 39-7). Subsequently, each fetal head should be seen in two perpendicular planes so as not to mistake a cross section of the fetal trunk for a second fetal head. Ideally, two fetal heads or two abdomens should be seen in the same image plane, to avoid scanning the same fetus twice and interpreting it as twins. Sonographic examination should detect practically all sets of twins. Indeed, one argument in favor of sonographic screening is earlier detection of multiple fetuses (see Chap. 16, p. 350). In a large randomized trial, LeFevre and co-workers (1993) demonstrated that routine midgestation sonographic examinations detected 99 percent of multifetal gestations before 26 weeks, whereas if performed just for specific indications, only 62 percent were detected before this time. Higher-order multifetal gestations are more difficult to evaluate. Even in the first trimester, it can be difficult to determine the actual number of fetuses and their position, which is important for nonselective pregnancy reduction and essential for selective termination (see p. 884).

Other Diagnostic Aids

Radiological Examination

An x-ray of the maternal abdomen can be helpful if the number of fetuses in a higher-order multifetal gestation is uncertain. Radiographs, however, are generally not useful and may lead to an incorrect diagnosis if there is hydramnios, obesity, fetal movement during the exposure, or inappropriate exposure time. Additionally, fetal skeletons before 18 weeks' gestation are insufficiently radiopaque and may be poorly seen. Although not typically used to diagnose multifetal pregnancy, magnetic resonance (MR)

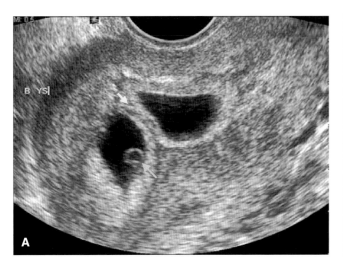 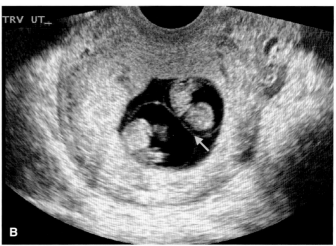

FIGURE 39-7 Sonograms of first-trimester twins. **A.** Dichorionic diamnionic twin pregnancy at 6 weeks' gestation. Note the thick dividing chorion (*yellow arrow*). One of the yolk sacs is indicated (*blue arrow*). **B.** Monochorionic diamnionic twin pregnancy at 8 weeks' gestation. Note the thin amnion encircling each embryo, resulting in a thin dividing membrane (*blue arrow*).

imaging may help delineate complications in monochorionic twins (Hu and associates, 2006).

Biochemical Tests

There is no biochemical test that reliably identifies multiple fetuses. Levels of human chorionic gonadotropin in plasma and in urine, on average, are higher than those found with a singleton pregnancy. These levels, however, are not so high as to allow a definite diagnosis. Twins are frequently diagnosed during evaluation for an elevated maternal serum alpha-fetoprotein level (see Chap. 13, p. 292).

MATERNAL ADAPTATION TO MULTIFETAL PREGNANCY

In general, the degree of maternal physiological change is greater with multiple fetuses than with a single fetus. Beginning in the first trimester, and temporarily associated with higher serum β-hCG levels, women with multifetal gestation often have nausea and vomiting in excess of women with a singleton pregnancy. Normal maternal blood volume expansion is greater (Pritchard, 1965). Whereas the average increase in late pregnancy is 40 to 50 percent with a single fetus, it is 50 to 60 percent with twins–an additional 500 mL. The red cell mass increases as well, but proportionately less in twin pregnancies than in singletons. Both the remarkable increase in maternal blood volume and the increased iron and folate requirements predispose to a greater prevalence of maternal anemia. Average blood loss with vaginal delivery of twins is 1000 mL, or twice that with a single fetus.

Kametas and associates (2003) used two-dimensional and M-mode echocardiography to assess cardiac function in 119 women with a twin pregnancy from 10 to 40 weeks. Cardiac output was increased 20 percent compared with that of women with a singleton pregnancy. This was predominantly due to greater stroke volume, and to a much lesser degree, increased heart rate. At the same time, pulmonary function tests do not differ between women with twins and those with singletons (McAuliffe and colleagues, 2002).

Women carrying twins also have a typical pattern of arterial blood pressure change. Compared with the diastolic blood pressure of mothers carrying singletons, theirs is lower at 20 weeks but increases more by delivery. The increase is at least 15 mm Hg in 95 percent of women carrying twins compared with only 54 percent of women pregnant with singleton pregnancies (Campbell, 1986).

Uterine growth in multifetal gestation is substantively greater than with singleton pregnancy. The uterus and its nonfetal contents may achieve a volume of 10 L or more and weigh in excess of 20 pounds! Especially with monozygotic twins, rapid accumulation of excessive amounts of amnionic fluid may develop. In these circumstances, maternal abdominal viscera and lungs may be appreciably compressed and displaced by the expanding uterus. As a result, the size and weight of the large uterus may preclude more than a sedentary existence for these women.

If hydramnios develops, maternal renal function may become seriously impaired, most likely as the consequence of obstructive uropathy. Quigley and Cruikshank (1977) described two women each carrying twins in whom acute and severe hydramnios led to maternal oliguria and azotemia. Maternal urine output and plasma creatinine levels promptly returned to normal after delivery. In severe hydramnios, therapeutic amniocentesis may be used to provide relief for the mother, to improve obstructive uropathy, and possibly to lower the risk of preterm delivery from preterm labor or prematurely ruptured membranes (see Chap. 21, p. 494). Unfortunately, hydramnios is often characterized by acute onset remote from term and by rapid reaccumulation following amniocentesis.

The various physiological burdens of pregnancy and the likelihood of serious maternal complications are almost invariably greater with multiple fetuses than with a singleton. This should be considered, especially when counseling a woman whose health is compromised and whose multifetal gestation is recognized early. The same is true for a woman who is not pregnant but is considering infertility treatment by ovulation induction or ART.

PREGNANCY OUTCOME

Abortion

Spontaneous abortion is more likely with multiple fetuses. Detailed reviews have identified three times more twins among aborted than among term pregnancies (Livingston and Poland, 1980; Uchida and co-workers, 1983). Monochorionic greatly outnumber dichorionic abortuses with an 18:1 ratio, thus implicating monozygosity as the risk factor.

Malformations

The incidence of congenital malformations is appreciably increased in multifetal gestations compared with singletons. These rates are not increased in twins conceived by ART compared with those spontaneously conceived (McDonald and associates, 2005). Major malformations develop in 2 percent and minor malformations in 4 percent of twins (Cameron and colleagues, 1983; Kohl and Casey, 1975). This increase is almost entirely due to the high incidence of structural defects in monozygotic twins. According to Schinzel and associates (1979), anomalies in monozygotic twins generally fall into one of three categories:

1. Defects resulting from twinning itself, a process that some consider to be a teratogenic event. This category includes conjoined twinning, acardiac anomaly, neural-tube defects, holoprosencephaly, and sirenomelia, which involves fusion of the lower extremities.
2. Defects resulting from vascular interchange between monochorionic twins. Vascular anastomoses can give rise to reverse flow with acardia in one twin (p. 872). Alternatively, if one twin dies and intravascular coagulation develops, emboli to the living twin may traverse these connections. These anastomoses may also transmit dramatic blood pressure fluctuations, causing defects such as microcephaly, hydranencephaly, intestinal atresia, aplasia cutis, or limb amputation.
3. Defects may develop from fetal crowding–examples include talipes equinovarus (clubfoot) or congenital hip dislocation. Dizygotic twins are also subject to these.

Baldwin (1991) comprehensively reviewed anomalies that develop in twins. Persistent hydramnios is associated with anomalies of one or both twins. Hashimoto and colleagues (1986) subjectively identified increased amnionic fluid in a fourth of 75 twin pregnancies. In nine pregnancies, hydramnios was transient, and all of these fetuses were normal. Conversely, there were fetal anomalies in nine of 10 pregnancies in which hydramnios persisted.

Birthweight

Multifetal gestations are more likely to be low birthweight than singleton pregnancies, due to restricted fetal growth and preterm delivery (Buekens and Wilcox, 1993). When more than 500,000 singleton neonates were compared with over 10,000 twin neonates, birthweights in twin infants closely paralleled those of singletons until 28 to 30 weeks. Thereafter, twin birthweights progressively lagged as shown in Figure 39-8. Beginning at 34 to

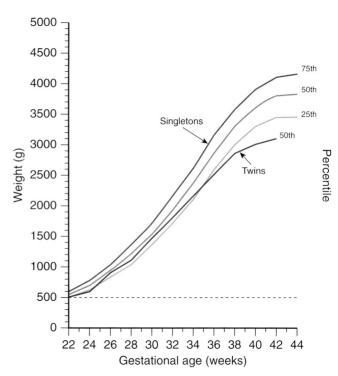

FIGURE 39-8 Birthweight percentiles (25 to 75) for singleton male newborns compared with the 50th birthweight percentile for twin males, Canada, 1986–1988. (Modified from Arbuckle TE, Wilkins R, and Sherman GJ: Birth weight percentiles by gestational age in Canada, *Obstetrics & Gynecology*, 1993, vol. 81, no. 1, pp. 39–48, with permission.)

35 weeks, twin birthweights clearly diverge from those of singletons. At 38 weeks or later, the incidence of overt growth restriction is quadrupled, and almost half of twins are affected.

In general, the more fetuses, the greater the degree of growth restriction. The caveat is that this assessment is based on growth curves established for singletons. Several authorities argue that fetal growth in twins is different from that of singleton pregnancies, and thus abnormal growth should be diagnosed only when fetal size is less than expected for *multifetal gestation.* Accordingly, twin and triplet growth curves have been developed (Ong and associates, 2002; Rodis and colleagues, 1999).

In the third trimester, the larger fetal mass leads to accelerated placental maturation and relative placental insufficiency. In dizygotic pregnancies, marked size discordancy usually results from unequal placentation, with one placental site receiving more perfusion than the other. Size differences may also reflect different genetic fetal-growth potentials. Discordancy can also result from fetal malformations, genetic syndromes, infection, or umbilical cord abnormalities such as velamentous insertion, marginal insertion, or vasa previa (see Chap. 27, p. 582).

The degree of growth restriction in monozygotic twins is likely to be greater than that in dizygotic pairs (Fig. 39-9). With monochorionic embryos, allocation of blastomeres may not be equal, vascular anastomoses within the placenta may cause unequal distribution of nutrients and oxygen, and discordant structural anomalies resulting from the twinning event itself may affect growth. For example, the quintuplets shown in Figure 39-10 represent three dizygotic and two monozygotic fetuses. When delivered at 31 weeks, the three neonates from separate ova

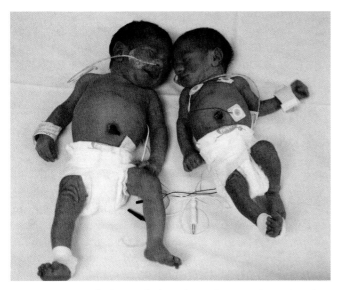

FIGURE 39-9 Marked growth discordance in monochorionic twins. (Courtesy of Dr. Laura Greer).

weighed 1420, 1530, and 1440 g, whereas the two derived from the same ovum weighed 990 and 860 g.

Multiple fetuses may overtax the capacity of the mother, the uterus, or both to provide nutrients. Selective reduction of triplets to twins before 12 weeks results in a growth pattern typical of twins rather than triplets (Lipitz, 1996; Smith-Levitin, 1996; Yaron, 1999, and all their associates). Somewhat related, Casele and co-workers (1996) reported that women with twins were more vulnerable to starvation ketosis after fasting compared with women with singleton pregnancies.

Duration of Gestation

As the number of fetuses increases, the duration of gestation decreases (Fig. 39-11). According to Martin and colleagues (2009), 60 percent of twins and 93 percent of triplets born in the United States in 2006 were delivered preterm.

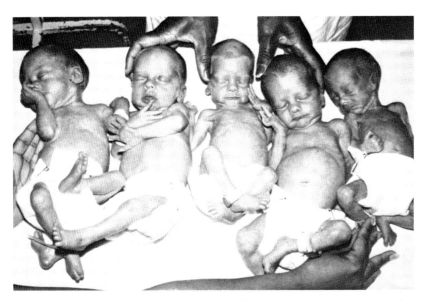

FIGURE 39-10 Davis quintuplets at 3 weeks following delivery. The first, second, and fourth newborns from the left each arose from separate ova, whereas the third and fifth neonates are from the same ovum.

Preterm Birth

Delivery before term is the major reason for increased neonatal morbidity and mortality rates in twins. Gardner and associates (1995) found that the causes of preterm birth differed between twins and singletons. Spontaneous preterm labor accounted for a larger and preterm ruptured membranes for a smaller proportion of twin preterm birth. Indicated preterm delivery accounted for equal proportions of prematurely delivered twins and singletons.

The rate of preterm birth among multifetal gestations has increased over the past two decades. In an analysis of nearly 350,000 twin births, Kogan and colleagues (2002) showed that during the 16-year period ending in 1997, the rate of term birth among twins declined by 22 percent. Joseph and colleagues (2001) attributed this decline to an increased rate of indicated preterm deliveries. This trend is not necessarily negative, as it was associated with decreased perinatal morbidity and mortality rates among twins that reached 34 weeks. Similarly, twin gestations in women receiving more than the recommended number of prenatal visits showed higher rates of preterm birth but lower neonatal mortality rates (Kogan and colleagues, 2000). Although the causes of preterm delivery in twins and singletons may be different, once delivered, neonatal outcome is generally the same at similar gestational ages (Gardner and co-workers, 1995; Kilpatrick and colleagues, 1996; Ray and Platt, 2009).

The previous statements apply to twins who are essentially concordant. As perhaps expected, outcomes for preterm twins who are markedly discordant may not be comparable with that of singletons because whatever caused the discordance may have long-lasting effects.

Prolonged Pregnancy

More than 40 years ago, Bennett and Dunn (1969) suggested that a twin pregnancy of 40 weeks or more should be considered postterm. Twin stillborn neonates delivered at 40 weeks or beyond had features similar to those of postmature singletons (Chap. 37, p. 834). From an analysis of almost 300,000 twin births from 1995 to 1998, Kahn and colleagues (2003) calculated that at and beyond 39 weeks, the risk of subsequent stillbirth was greater than the risk of neonatal mortality. At Parkland Hospital, twin gestations have empirically been considered to be prolonged at 40 weeks.

Long-Term Infant Development

In a study in Norway, Nilsen and associates (1984) evaluated the physical and intellectual development of male twins at age 18 years. Compared with singletons, twice as many twins were found to be physically unfit for military service. These investigators attributed this to sequelae of preterm delivery, such as visual impairment, rather than to twinning. General intelligence did not appear to differ, a finding confirmed in a Danish cohort of 3411 twins and 7796 singletons born from 1986 to 1988 who were assessed in the ninth grade (Christensen and colleagues, 2006).

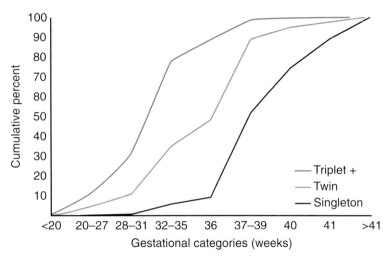

FIGURE 39-11 Cumulative percent of singleton, twin, and triplet or higher-order multifetal births according to gestational age at delivery in the United States during 1990. (Redrawn from Luke B: The changing pattern of multiple births in the United States: Maternal and infant characteristics, 1973 and 1990, *Obstetrics & Gynecology,* 1994, vol. 84, no. 1, pp. 101–106, with permission.)

Birthweight and anthropomorphic discordancy may persist. For example, Babson and Phillips (1973) reported that in monozygotic twins whose birthweights differed on average 35 percent, the smaller twin at birth remained so into adulthood. Height, weight, head circumference, and intelligence often remained greater in the twin who weighed more at birth.

UNIQUE COMPLICATIONS

A number of unique complications develop in multifetal pregnancies. Although these have been best described in twins, they also occur in higher-order multifetal gestation.

Monoamnionic Twins

Approximately 1 percent of monozygotic twins are monoamnionic (Hall, 2003). Their associated high fetal death rate may result from cord entanglement, congenital anomaly, preterm birth, or twin–twin transfusion syndrome, which is described subsequently (Cordero and colleagues, 2006). In a comprehensive review, Allen and colleagues (2001) reported that monoamnionic twins diagnosed antenatally and that are still alive at 20 weeks have an approximately 10-percent risk of subsequent fetal demise. In a report of 98 monoamnionic twin pregnancies from 10 Dutch centers, the perinatal mortality rate was 17 percent (Hack and associates, 2009). Umbilical cord intertwining, a common cause of death, is estimated to complicate at least half of cases (Fig. 39-12). Diamnionic twins can become monoamnionic if the dividing membrane ruptures, and they then have similar associated morbidity and mortality rates (Gilbert and colleagues, 1991).

Management

Once diagnosed, management of monoamnionic twins is somewhat problematic due to the unpredictability of fetal death resulting from cord entan-

glement and to the lack of an effective means of monitoring for it. Some data suggest that morbid cord entanglement is likely to occur early, and that monoamnionic pregnancies that have successfully reached 30 to 32 weeks are at greatly reduced risk (Carr and co-workers, 1990; Demaria and associates, 2004; Tessen and Zlatnik, 1991). But based on their review, Roqué and colleagues (2003) dispute this.

Although umbilical cords frequently entangle, factors that lead to pathological umbilical vessel constriction during entanglement are unknown. Belfort and colleagues (1993) and Aisenbrey and co-workers (1995) used color-flow Doppler sonography to diagnose umbilical cord entanglement in 10 monoamnionic twin pregnancies. The recognition of cord entanglement in seven of these prompted admission, increased fetal surveillance, or both. Interestingly, only one set of twins with entangled cords required immediate delivery. In fact, the remaining six pregnancies continued for an average of 6 weeks after the diagnosis, and one of these continued for 12 weeks!

Evidence to guide management is observational, retrospective, and subject to biased reporting. At the University of Alabama at Birmingham, management is based in large part on the report of Heyborne and co-workers (2005). There were no stillbirths in 43 twin pregnancies in women admitted at 26 to 27 weeks for daily fetal surveillance. Conversely, there were 13 stillbirths in twin pregnancies in 44 women who were managed as outpatients and admitted only for an obstetrical indication. Because of this report, women with monoamnionic twins are managed with 1 hour of daily fetal heart rate monitoring, either as outpatients or as inpatients, beginning at 26 to 28 weeks. With initial testing, a course of betamethasone is given to promote pulmonary maturation (see Chap. 36, p. 821). If fetal testing remains reassuring, cesarean delivery is performed at 34 weeks after a second course of betamethasone.

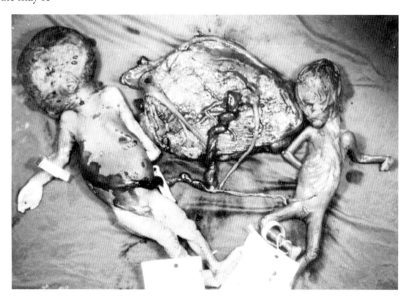

FIGURE 39-12 Monozygotic twins in a single amnionic sac. The smaller fetus apparently died first, and the second subsequently succumbed when umbilical cords entwined.

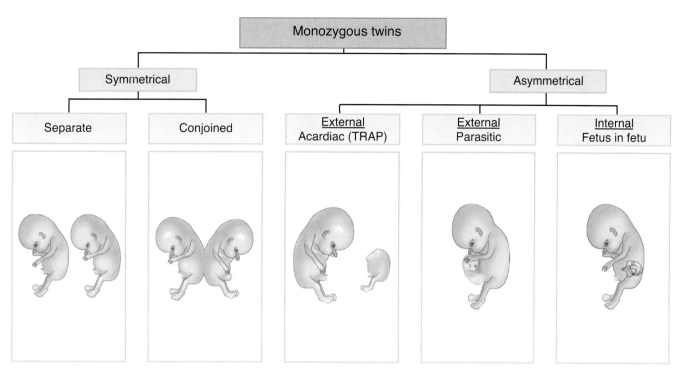

FIGURE 39-13 Possible outcomes of monozygotic twinning.

Abnormal Twinning

Conjoined twins may result from aberrations in the twinning process, traditionally ascribed to incomplete splitting of an embryo into two separate twins (Kaufman, 2004). An alternative hypothesis describes early secondary fusion of two originally separated embryos (Spencer, 2000a, b). As shown in Figure 39-13, aberrant twinning encompasses a spectrum of abnormalities that includes not only conjoined twins but also *external parasitic twins* and *fetus in fetu*.

Conjoined Twins

In the United States, united or conjoined twins (see Fig. 39–2) are commonly referred to as *Siamese twins*—after Chang and Eng

Bunker of Siam (Thailand), who were displayed worldwide by P.T. Barnum. Joining of the twins may begin at either pole and may produce characteristic forms (Fig. 39-14). Of these, *parapagus* is the most common (Spencer, 2001). The frequency of conjoined twins is not well established. At Kandang Kerbau Hospital in Singapore, Tan and co-workers (1971) identified seven cases of conjoined twins among more than 400,000 deliveries—an incidence of 1 in 60,000.

As reviewed by McHugh and associates (2006), conjoined twins can frequently be identified using sonography at midpregnancy, time enough for parents to decide whether to continue the pregnancy. A targeted examination, including a careful evaluation of the point of connection and the organs involved, is necessary before counseling can be provided (Fig. 39-15). In

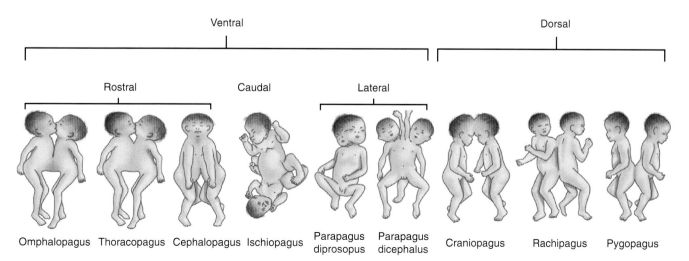

FIGURE 39-14 Types of conjoined twins. (Redrawn from Spencer, 2000a.)

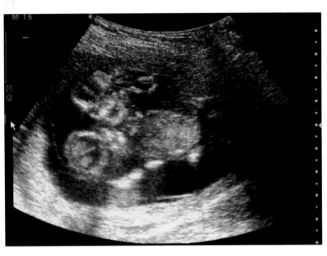

FIGURE 39-15 Sonogram of a conjoined twin pregnancy at 13 weeks' gestation. Twins with two heads but only one torso are termed parapagus dicephalus.

later pregnancy, when there is diminished amnionic fluid and increased fetal crowding, MR imaging may provide necessary anatomical information.

Surgical separation of nearly completely joined twins may be successful if essential organs are not shared (Spitz and Kiely, 2003). Consultation with a pediatric surgeon often assists parental decision making. Conjoined twins may have discordant structural anomalies that further complicate decisions about whether to continue the pregnancy. For example, one of the conjoined twins shown in Figure 39-16 was anencephalic.

Viable conjoined twins should be delivered by cesarean. For the purpose of pregnancy termination, however, vaginal delivery is possible because the union is most often pliable. Still, dystocia is common, and if the fetuses are mature, vaginal delivery may be traumatic to the uterus or cervix.

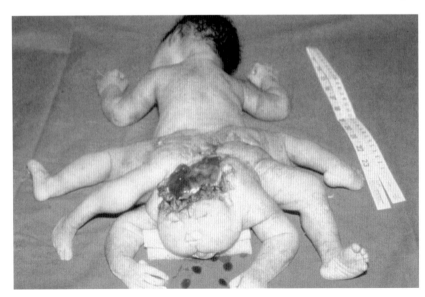

FIGURE 39-16 Conjoined twins in which one was anencephalic. (Courtesy of Dr. Craig Syrop, University of Iowa.)

External Parasitic Twins

This is a grossly defective fetus or merely fetal parts, attached externally to a relatively normal twin. A parasitic twin usually consists of externally attached supernumerary limbs, often with some viscera. Classically, however, a functional heart or brain is absent. Attachment mirrors those sites described earlier for conjoined twins (see Fig. 39-13). Parasites are believed to result from demise of the defective twin, with its surviving tissues attached to and vascularized by its normal twin (Spencer, 2001).

Fetus-in-Fetu

Early in development, one embryo may be enfolded inside its twin. Normal development of this rare parasitic twin usually arrests at the first trimester. As a result, normal spatial arrangement of and presence of many organs is lost. Classically, vertebral or axial bones are found in these fetiform masses, whereas heart and brain are lacking. These masses are typically supported by their host by a few large parasitic vessels (Spencer, 2000a).

Vascular Anastomoses between Fetuses

With rare exceptions, vascular anastomoses between twins are present only in monochorionic twin placentas (Baldwin, 1991; Hall, 2003). And although nearly all of these have anastomoses, there are marked variations in the number, size, and direction of these seemingly haphazard connections (Fig. 39-17). Artery-to-artery anastomoses are most common and are found on the chorionic surface of the placenta in up to 75 percent of monochorionic twin placentas. Vein-to-vein and artery-to-vein communications are each found in approximately half. One vessel may have several connections, sometimes to both arteries and veins. In contrast to these superficial vascular connections on the surface of the chorion, deep artery-to-vein communications extend through the capillary bed of the villous tissue. These deep arteriovenous anastomoses create a common villous compartment or third circulation that has been identified in approximately half of monochorionic twin placentas (Fig. 39-18).

Most of these vascular communications are hemodynamically balanced and of little fetal consequence. In others, however, hemodynamically significant shunts develop between fetuses. Two such significant patterns include *acardiac twinning* and *twin-twin transfusion syndrome*. The incidence of the latter syndrome is unclear, but approximately one fourth of monochorionic twins have some of its clinical features (Sperling and co-workers, 2007).

Acardiac Twin

Twin reversed-arterial-perfusion (TRAP) sequence is a rare—1 in 35,000 births, but serious complication of monochorionic multifetal gestation. In the TRAP sequence, there is usually a normally formed donor twin who has features of heart failure as well as a recipient twin who lacks a heart (acardius) and other structures. It has been hypothesized that the

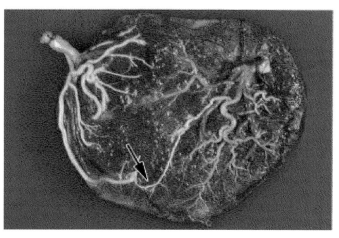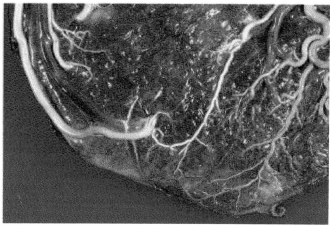

FIGURE 39-17 Placenta from pregnancy complicated by twin-twin transfusion syndrome. The following color code was applied for injection. Left twin: yellow = artery, blue = vein; right twin: red = artery, green = vein. **A.** Part of the arterial network of the right twin is filled with yellow dye, due to the presence of a small artery-to-artery anastomosis (*arrow*). **B.** Close-up of the lower portion of the placenta displays the yellow dye-filled anastomosis (Reprinted from Placenta, Vol. 26, ME De Paepe, P DeKoninck, and RM Friedman, Vascular distribution patterns in monochorionic twin placentas, pp. 471–475, Copyright 2005, with permission from Elsevier.)

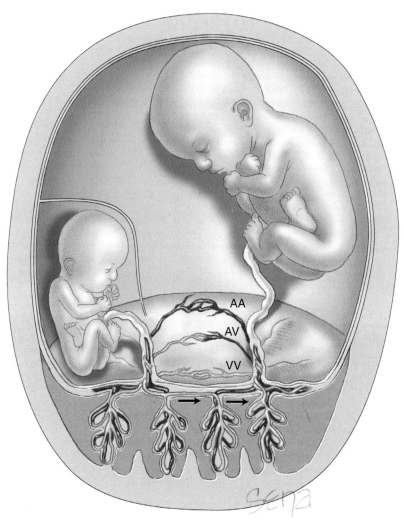

FIGURE 39-18 Anastomoses between twins may be artery-to-venous (AV), artery-to-artery (AA), or vein-to-vein (VV). Schematic representation of an AV anastomosis in twin-twin transfusion syndrome that forms a "common villous district" or "third circulation" deep within the villous tissue. Blood from a donor twin may be transferred to a recipient twin through this shared circulation. This transfer leads to a growth-restricted discordant donor twin with markedly reduced amnionic fluid, causing it to be "stuck."

TRAP sequence is caused by a large artery-to-artery placental shunt, often also accompanied by a vein-to-vein shunt (Fig. 39-19). Within the single, shared placenta, arterial perfusion pressure of the donor twin exceeds that in the recipient twin, who thus receives reverse blood flow of deoxygenated arterial blood from its co-twin (Jones, 1997). This "used" arterial blood reaches the recipient twin through its umbilical arteries and preferentially goes to its iliac vessels. Thus, only the lower body is perfused, and disrupted growth and development of the upper body results. Failure of head growth is called *acardius acephalus*; a partially developed head with identifiable limbs is called *acardius myelacephalus*; and failure of any recognizable structure to form is *acardius amorphous* shown in Figure 39-20 (Faye-Petersen and colleagues, 2006). Because of this vascular connection, the normal donor twin must not only support its own circulation but also pump its blood through the underdeveloped acardiac recipient. This may lead to cardiomegaly and high-output heart failure in the normal twin (Fox and Sebire, 2007).

Without treatment, the death rates of a donor or "pump" twin range from 50 to 75 percent (Moore and colleagues, 1990). Quintero and colleagues (1994, 2006) have reviewed methods of in utero treatment of acardiac twinning in which the goal is interruption of aberrant vascular communication between the twins. Of these methods, Livingston (2007) and Lee (2007), with their colleagues, found an approximately 90-percent survival rate with radiofrequency ablation, which cauterizes umbilical vessels in the malformed recipient twin so as to terminate blood flow from the donor.

Conversely, survival has been reported for nine of 10 donor twins managed expectantly (Sullivan

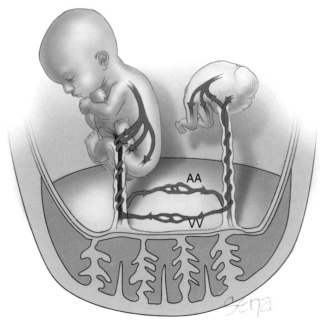

FIGURE 39-19 In the TRAP sequence, there is usually a normally formed donor twin, who has features of heart failure, and a recipient twin, who lacks a heart. It has been hypothesized that the TRAP sequence is caused by a large artery-to-artery placental shunt, often also accompanied by a vein-to-vein shunt. Within the single, shared placenta, perfusion pressure of the donor twin overpowers that in the recipient twin, who thus receives reverse blood flow from its twin sibling. The "used" arterial blood that reaches the recipient twin preferentially goes to its iliac vessels and thus perfuses only the lower body. This disrupts growth and development of the upper body.

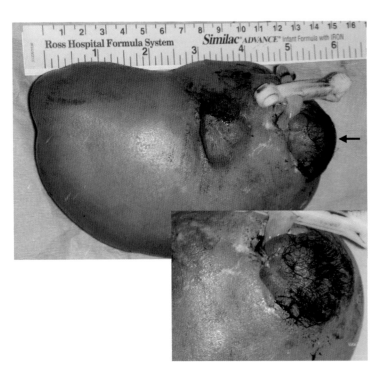

FIGURE 39-20 Photograph of an acardiac twin weighing 475 grams. The underdeveloped head is indicated by the black arrow, and its details are shown in the inset. A yellow clamp is seen on this twin's umbilical cord. Its viable donor co-twin was delivered vaginally at 36 weeks and weighed 2325 grams. (Courtesy of Dr. Michael D. Hnat.)

and associates, 2003). These authors advocate that expectant management with close fetal surveillance as a management option.

Twin-Twin Transfusion Syndrome (TTTS)

In this syndrome, blood is transfused from a donor twin to its recipient sibling such that the donor becomes anemic and its growth may be restricted. In contrast, the recipient becomes polycythemic and may develop circulatory overload manifest as hydrops. The donor twin is pale, and its recipient sibling is plethoric (Fig. 39-21). Similarly, one portion of the placenta often appears pale compared with the remainder.

In the recipient twin, the neonatal period may be complicated by circulatory overload with heart failure, if severe hypervolemia and hyperviscosity are not identified promptly and treated. Occlusive thrombosis is also much more likely to develop in this setting. During the neonatal period, polycythemia in the recipient twin may lead to severe hyperbilirubinemia and kernicterus (see Chap. 29, p. 625).

Pathophysiology. Any of the different types of vascular anastomoses discussed before may be found with monochorionic placentas. Classically, chronic TTTS results from unidirectional flow through arteriovenous anastomoses. Deoxygenated blood from a donor placental artery is pumped into a cotyledon shared by the recipient (see Fig. 39-18). Once oxygen exchange is completed in the chorionic villus, the oxygenated blood leaves the cotyledon via a placental vein of the recipient twin. Unless compensated, this unidirectional flow leads to an imbalance in blood volumes (Lopriore and Oepkes, 2008; Machin and co-workers, 2000).

Clinically important twin-twin transfusion syndrome frequently is chronic and results from significant vascular volume differences between the twins. The syndrome typically presents in midpregnancy when the donor fetus becomes oliguric from decreased renal perfusion (Mari and co-workers, 1993). This fetus develops oligohydramnios, and the recipient fetus develops severe hydramnios, presumably due to increased urine production. Virtual absence of amnionic fluid in the donor sac prevents fetal motion, giving rise to the descriptive term *stuck twin* or *hydramnios-oligohydramnios–"poly-oli"–syndrome.* This amnionic fluid imbalance is associated with growth restriction, contractures, and pulmonary hypoplasia in one twin, and premature rupture of the membranes and heart failure in the other.

Fetal Brain Damage. Cerebral palsy, microcephaly, porencephaly, and multicystic encephalomalacia are serious complications associated with placental vascular anastomoses in multifetal gestation. Neurological damage is most likely caused by ischemic necrosis leading to cavitary brain lesions (Fig. 39-22). In the donor twin, ischemia results from hypotension, anemia, or both. In the recipient, ischemia develops from blood pressure instability and episodes of severe hypotension (Larroche and associates, 1990). Quarello and colleagues (2007) reviewed data from 315 liveborn fetuses from

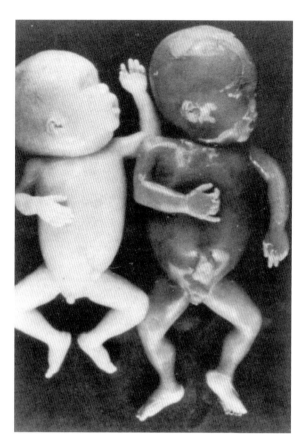

FIGURE 39-21 Twin-twin transfusion syndrome at 23 weeks. Pale donor twin (690 g) is shown on the left. The plethoric recipient twin (730 g) on the right also had hydramnios. The donor twin had oligohydramnios. (This figure was published in *American Journal of Obstetrics & Gynecology*, Vol. 169, PR Mahone, DM Sherer, JS Abramowicz, and JR Woods, Twin-twin transfusion syndrome: Rapid development of severe hydrops of the donor following selective feticide of the hydropic recipient, pp. 166–168, Copyright Elsevier 1993.)

onic twins were calculated, however, it was soon appreciated that in many cases, these were later clinical findings. Harkness and Crombleholme (2005) propose the following sonographic findings as being suggestive of this diagnosis: (1) monochorionicity, (2) same-sex gender, (3) hydramnios defined if the largest vertical pocket is > 8 cm in one twin and oligohydramnios defined if the largest vertical pocket is < 2 cm in the other twin, (3) umbilical cord size discrepancy, (4) cardiac dysfunction in the recipient twin with hydramnios, (5) abnormal umbilical vessel or ductus venosus Doppler velocimetry, and (6) significant growth discordance.

Once identified, TTTS is typically staged by the Quintero staging system (Quintero and colleagues, 1999). These are defined as follows:

- Stage I–discordant amnionic fluid volumes as described above, but urine still visible sonographically within the donor twin's bladder
- Stage II–criteria of stage I, but urine is not visible within the donor's bladder
- Stage III–criteria of stage II and abnormal Doppler studies of the umbilical artery, ductus venosus, or umbilical vein
- Stage IV–ascites or frank hydrops in either twin; and
- Stage V–demise of either fetus.

In addition to these criteria, there is now evidence that cardiac function of the recipient twin correlates with fetal outcome (Crombleholme and associates, 2007). Thus, many also assess cardiovascular function of TTTS twins with echocardiography (Rychik and co-workers, 2007). One scoring system–the *cardiovascular profile score or CVPS*–evaluates presence or absence of hydrops, abnormal venous and arterial Doppler findings, cardiomegaly, atrioventricular valve regurgitation, and cardiac dysfunction (Shah and colleagues, 2008). Cardiac function is measured by the Doppler *myocardial performance index or MPI*, which is an index of global ventricular function and calculated for each ventricle (Michelfelder and associates, 2007).

Prior to treatment at Parkland Memorial Hospital, our protocol includes anatomical and neurological fetal assessment using echocardiography, MPI calculation, Doppler velocimetry, and MR imaging; genetic counseling and amniocentesis; and placental mapping.

Therapy and Outcome. The prognosis for multifetal gestations complicated by TTTS is extremely guarded. Unfortunately, the most serious form of TTTS, with acute hydramnios in one sac and a stuck twin with anhydramnios in the other sac, usually presents between 18 and 26 weeks. The survival rate for those diagnosed before 28 weeks varies widely, from 7 to 75 percent (Berghella and Kaufmann, 2001).

Several therapies are currently used for TTTS, including amnioreduction, laser ablation of vascular anastomoses, selective feticide, and septostomy (intentional creation of a communication in the dividing amnionic membrane). Recently, comparative data from randomized trials for some of these techniques have become available.

In a randomized trial of 142 women with severe TTTS diagnosed before 26 weeks, Senat and colleagues (2004) reported increased survival of at least one twin to age 6 months with laser ablation of vascular anastomoses compared with serial amnioreduction–76 versus 51 percent, respectively. Moreover, analyses

pregnancies with twin-twin transfusion syndrome. They found that cerebral abnormalities developed in 8 percent.

If one twin of an affected pregnancy dies, cerebral pathology in the survivor most likely results from acute hypotension (Benirschke, 1993). A less likely cause is emboli of thromboplastic material originating from the dead fetus. Fusi and co-workers (1990, 1991) observed that with the death of one twin, acute twin-twin anastomotic transfusion from the high-pressure vessels of the living twin to the low-resistance vessels of the dead twin leads rapidly to hypovolemia and ischemic antenatal brain damage in the survivor. Pharoah and Adi (2000) surveyed 348 survivors whose twin sibling had died in utero. The prevalence of cerebral palsy was 83 per 1000 live births–a 40-fold increased risk over baseline.

The acute nature of the twin-twin transfusion and subsequent hypotension following the death of one twin makes successful intervention for the survivor nearly impossible. Even with delivery immediately after the co-twin demise is recognized, the hypotension that occurs at the moment of death has likely already caused irreversible damage (Langer and associates, 1997; Wada and co-workers, 1998).

Diagnosis. There have been dramatic changes in the criteria used to diagnose and classify varying severities of TTTS. Classically, weight discordancy and hemoglobin differences in monochori-

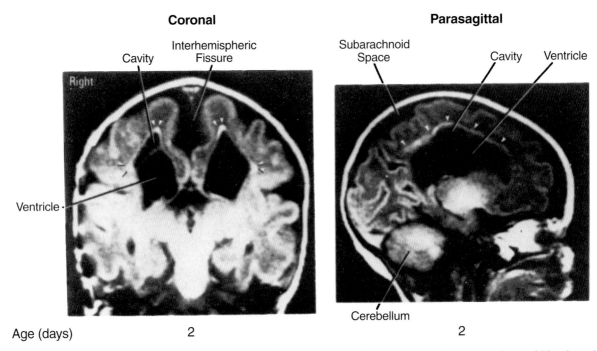

Coronal

Cavity — Interhemispheric Fissure

Ventricle·

Parasagittal

Subarachnoid Space — Cavity — Ventricle

Cerebellum

Age (days)   2   2

FIGURE 39-22 Cranial magnetic resonance imaging study of a diamnionic–monochorionic twin performed on day 2 of life. The subarachnoid space and lateral ventricles are markedly enlarged. There are large cavitary lesions in the white matter adjacent to the ventricles. The bright signals (*arrowheads*) in the periphery of the cavitary lesions most probably correspond to gliosis. (This figure was published in *American Journal of Obstetrics & Gynecology*, Vol. 162, R Bejar, G Vigliocco, H Gramajo, et al., Antenatal origin of neurological damage in newborn infants. II. Multiple gestations, pp. 1230–1236, Copyright Elsevier 1990.)

of randomized studies by Roberts and colleagues (2008) and Rossi and D'Addario (2008) showed better neonatal outcomes with laser therapy compared with selective amnioreduction. In contrast, Crombleholme and colleagues (2007), in a randomized trial of 42 women, found equivalent rates of 30-day survival of one or both twins treated with either amnioreduction or selective fetoscopic laser ablation–75 versus 65 percent, respectively.

At this time, laser ablation of anastomoses is preferred for severe TTTS, although optimal therapy for Stage I and Stage II disease is controversial. Even after laser therapy, however, close ongoing surveillance is necessary. Robyr and associates (2006) reported that a fourth of 101 pregnancies treated with laser required additional invasive therapy because of recurrent TTTS–14, or middle cerebral artery Doppler evidence of anemia or polycythemia–13.

Moise and colleagues (2005) compared amnioreduction and septostomy in a multicentered randomized trial of 73 women. Repeated procedures were performed for symptoms or if the greatest vertical pocket of amnionic fluid met the original inclusion criteria of > 8 to 12 cm, depending on gestational age. Perinatal outcomes were the same in each group, with at least one survivor in 80 percent of pregnancies. The average number of additional procedures was two in each group.

Selective reduction has generally been considered if severe amnionic fluid and growth disturbances develop before 20 weeks. In such cases, both fetuses typically will die without intervention. Selection of which twin is to be terminated is based on evidence of damage to either fetus and comparison of their prognoses. Any substance injected into one twin may affect the other twin because of shared circulations. Therefore, feticidal techniques may include injection of an occlusive substance into the selected twin's umbilical vein or radiofrequency ablation, fe-

toscopic ligation, laser coagulation, monopolar coagulation, or bipolar cautery of one umbilical cord (Challis, 1999; Donner, 1997; Weiner, 1987; Wittmann, 1986, and all their colleagues). Even after these procedures, however, the risks to the remaining fetus are still appreciable (Rossi and D'Addario, 2009).

DISCORDANT TWINS

Size inequality of twin fetuses, which can be a sign of pathological growth restriction in one fetus, is calculated using the larger twin as the index. Generally, as the weight difference within a twin pair increases, perinatal mortality rates increase proportionately. As discussed further in Chapter 38 (p. 846), restricted growth of one twin fetus usually develops late in the second and early third trimester and is often asymmetrical (Leveno and coworkers, 1979). Earlier discordancy is usually symmetrical and indicates higher risk for fetal demise. Generally, the earlier discordancy in pregnancy develops, the more serious the sequelae. In an extreme example, Weissman and colleagues (1994) identified weight discordancy between 6 and 11 weeks in five twin gestations, and all of the smaller twins had major malformations.

Pathology

The cause of birthweight inequality in twin fetuses is often unclear, but we assume that the etiology differs in monochorionic compared with dichorionic twins. Discordancy in monochorionic twins is usually attributed to placental vascular anastomoses that cause hemodynamic imbalance between the twins. Reduced pressure and perfusion of the donor twin likely cause diminished placental and fetal growth (Benirschke, 1993).

Occasionally, monochorionic twins are discordant in size because they are discordant for structural anomalies.

Discordancy in dichorionic twins is likely due to a variety of factors. Importantly, dizygotic fetuses may have different genetic growth potential, especially if they are of opposite genders. Alternatively, because the placentas are separate and require more implantation space, there is a greater chance that one of the placentas would have a suboptimal implantation site. Mordel and colleagues (1993) observed that the incidence of discordancy is twice as great in triplets as it is in twins. This finding lends additional credence to the view that in utero crowding plays a role in fetal-growth restriction. Placental pathology may also play a role. Eberle and co-workers (1993) evaluated placental abnormalities in 147 twin gestations. They quantified placental lesions that are usually associated with singleton growth restriction. Placentas from the smaller fetus in discordant dichorionic twin pairs demonstrated these typical lesions, whereas these lesions were not found in discordant monochorionic twin pairs.

Diagnosis

Size discordancy between twins can be determined in several ways. One common method of determining discordancy uses all fetal measurements to compute the estimated weight of each twin and then to compare the weight of the smaller twin with that of the larger twin. Thus, percent discordancy = weight of larger twin minus weight of smaller twin, divided by weight of larger twin. Alternatively, considering that growth restriction is the primary concern and that abdominal circumference reflects fetal nutrition, some authors diagnose discordancy when abdominal circumferences differ by more than 20 mm (Brown and associates, 1987; Hill and colleagues, 1994).

Several different weight disparities between twins have been used to define discordancy. Accumulated data suggest that weight discordancy greater than 25 to 30 percent most accurately predicts an adverse perinatal outcome. Hollier and co-workers (1999) retrospectively evaluated 1370 twin pairs delivered at Parkland Hospital and stratified twin weight discordancy in 5-percent increments within a range of 15 to 40 percent. They found that the incidence of respiratory distress, intraventricular hemorrhage, seizures, periventricular leukomalacia, sepsis, and necrotizing enterocolitis increased directly with the degree of weight discordancy. These conditions increased substantially if discordancy was greater than 25 percent. The relative risk of fetal death increased significantly to 5.6 if there was more than 30-percent discordancy. It increased to 18.9 if there was greater than 40-percent discordancy.

Management

Sonographic monitoring of growth within a twin pair and calculating discordancy has become a mainstay in management. Other sonographic findings, such as oligohydramnios, may be helpful in gauging fetal risk. Depending on the degree of discordancy and the gestational age, fetal surveillance may be indicated, especially if one or both fetuses exhibit growth restriction. Delivery is usually not performed for size discordancy alone, except occasionally at advanced gestational ages.

TWIN DEMISE

Death of One Fetus

On occasion, one fetus dies remote from term, but pregnancy continues with one living fetus. Rydhström (1994) reviewed fetal death in 15,066 twin pairs weighing 500 g or more. One or both twins died in 1.1 percent of opposite-sex twins and 2.6 percent of same-sex twins. Weight discordancy also increased the risk of death. In opposite-sex twins, however, the risk of death remained constant at 1.2 percent until weight discordancy exceeded 40 to 50 percent or 1000 g. In same-sex twins, discordancy of only 20 percent or 250 g increased the risk. After the death of one twin, the risk of subsequent death in the surviving twin was sixfold greater in same-sex twins. Although chorionicity was not known in all cases, the authors estimated that the death rate for same-sex dizygotic twins was the same as for opposite-sex twins–0.8 percent, and that monochorionic twins had the greatest risk of death–3 percent.

At delivery, a dead fetus may be identifiable but may be compressed appreciably–*fetus compressus*. In others, it may be flattened remarkably through loss of fluid and most of the soft tissue–*fetus papyraceous* (Fig. 39-23).

The prognosis for the surviving twin depends on the gestational age at the time of the demise, the chorionicity, and the length of time between the demise and delivery of the surviving twin. Early demise such as a "vanishing twin" does not appear to increase the risk of death in the surviving fetus after the first trimester. Afterwards, however, the neurological prognosis for a surviving co-twin depends almost exclusively on chorionicity. In their comprehensive review, Ong and colleagues (2006) found an 18-percent rate of neurological abnormality with

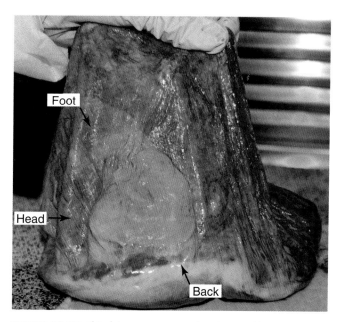

FIGURE 39-23 This fetus papyraceous is a tan ovoid mass compressed against the fetal membranes. Anatomical parts can be identified as marked. Demise of this twin had been noted during sonographic examination performed at 17 weeks' gestation. Its viable co-twin delivered at 40 weeks' gestation. (Courtesy of Dr. Michael V. Zaretsky.)

monochorionic placentation compared with only 1 percent with dichorionic placentation.

Later in gestation, the death of one of multiple fetuses could theoretically trigger coagulation defects in the mother. Only a few cases of maternal coagulopathy after a single fetal death in a twin pregnancy have been reported, probably because the surviving twin is usually delivered within a few weeks of the demise (see Chap. 35, p. 788). That said, we have observed transient, spontaneously corrected consumptive coagulopathy in multifetal gestations in which one fetus died and was retained in utero along with its surviving twin. The plasma fibrinogen concentration initially decreased but then increased spontaneously, and the level of serum fibrinogen-fibrin degradation products increased initially but then returned to normal levels. At delivery, the portions of the placenta that supplied the living fetus appeared normal. In contrast, the part that had once provided for the dead fetus was the site of massive fibrin deposition.

Management decisions should be based on the cause of death and the risk to the surviving fetus. Most cases of a single fetal death in twin pregnancy involve monochorionic placentation. Evidence indicates that morbidity in the monochorionic twin survivor is almost always due to vascular anastomoses, which first cause the demise of one twin followed by sudden hypotension in the other.

Occasionally, death of one but not all fetuses results from a maternal complication such as diabetic ketoacidosis or severe preeclampsia with abruption. Pregnancy management is based on the diagnosis and the status of both mother and surviving fetus. If the death of one dichorionic twin is due to a discordant congenital anomaly, its death should not affect its surviving twin. Santema and co-workers (1995b) assessed the cause and outcome of 29 consecutive twin pregnancies in which one of the fetuses died after 20 weeks. The causes of fetal death were not clear in all cases. The most common associations were monochorionic placentation and severe preeclampsia. These investigators concluded that in most cases, the benefit derived from continuation of a multifetal pregnancy exceeded the risks of preterm delivery after diagnosis of fetal death. They recommended conservative management of the living fetus.

Impending Death of One Fetus

Abnormal antepartum test results of fetal health in one twin fetus, but not the other, pose a particular dilemma. Delivery may be the best option for the compromised fetus yet may result in death from immaturity of the second. If fetal lung maturity is confirmed, salvage of both the healthy fetus and its jeopardized sibling is possible. Unfortunately, ideal management if twins are immature is problematic but should be based on the chances of intact survival for both fetuses. Often the compromised fetus is severely growth restricted or anomalous. Thus, performing amniocentesis for fetal karyotyping in women of advanced maternal age carrying twin pregnancies is advantageous, even for those who would continue their pregnancies regardless of the diagnosis. Aneuploidy identification in one fetus allows rational decisions about interventions.

Death of Both Twin Fetuses

Rydhström (1996) reported that, excluding abortions, both fetuses died in 0.5 percent of twin pregnancies. Causes implicated in these deaths were monochorionic placentation and discordant fetal growth.

COMPLETE HYDATIDIFORM MOLE AND COEXISTING FETUS

This entity is different from a partial molar pregnancy because there are two separate conceptuses. A normal placenta supplies nutrition to one twin, and the co-pregnancy is a complete molar gestation. Optimal management is uncertain, but preterm delivery is frequently required because of bleeding or severe preeclampsia. Bristow and colleagues (1996) reviewed 26 cases and found that 73 percent required evacuation before fetal viability. The remainder continued without serious complications until fetal viability was reached. Sebire and colleagues (2002) reported a live-birth rate of almost 40 percent in 53 such pregnancies. Any pregnancy consisting of a complete mole carries significant risk for subsequent gestational trophoblastic neoplasia, but Niemann and colleagues (2007) did not find rates of persistent trophoblastic disease following a twin gestation complicated by a complete mole to be higher than those following a singleton complete mole (see Chap. 11, p. 258).

ANTEPARTUM MANAGEMENT OF TWIN PREGNANCY

To reduce perinatal mortality and morbidity rates in pregnancies complicated by twins, it is imperative that:

1. Delivery of markedly preterm neonates be prevented
2. Fetal-growth restriction be identified and afflicted fetuses be delivered before they become moribund
3. Fetal trauma during labor and delivery be avoided, and
4. Expert neonatal care be available.

Diet

The requirements for calories, protein, minerals, vitamins, and essential fatty acids are further increased in women with multiple fetuses. The Recommended Dietary Allowances made by the Food and Nutrition Board of the National Research Council for uncomplicated pregnancy should not only be met but in most instances exceeded (see Chap. 8, p. 200). Caloric consumption should be increased by another 300 kcal/day. Brown and Carlson (2000) have recommended that weight gain be based in part on prepregnancy weight but that women with triplet pregnancies should gain at least 50 pounds. Supplementation with 60 to 100 mg/day of iron and with 1 mg/day of folic acid is preferred.

Hypertension

Hypertensive disorders due to pregnancy are more likely to develop with multiple fetuses. The exact incidence attributable to twin gestation is difficult to determine, because twin pregnancies are more likely to deliver preterm before preeclampsia can develop, and because women with twin pregnancies are often older and multiparous. For example, the incidence of pregnancy-related hypertension in women with twins is 20 percent at Parkland Hospital. Santema and co-workers (1995a) performed a case-control study in which 187 twin and 187 singleton pregnancies were matched for maternal age, parity, and gestational age at delivery. The incidence of hypertension was significantly higher in women carrying twin pregnancies–15 versus 6 percent. Mastrobattista and colleagues (1997) compared 53 triplet with 53 twin pregnancies and observed that the rate of severe preeclampsia was significantly higher in women with triplets–23 versus 6 percent.

These data suggest that fetal number and placental mass are involved in the pathogenesis of preeclampsia. With multifetal gestation, hypertension not only develops more often but also tends to develop earlier and to be more severe.

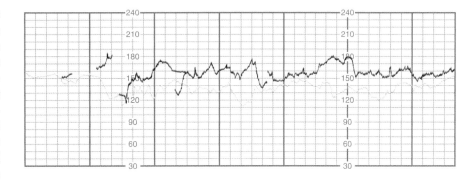
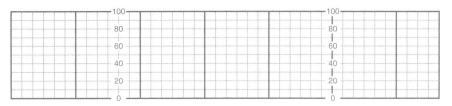

FIGURE 39-24 Simultaneous antepartum fetal heart rate recordings from twin fetuses showing that accelerations are not necessarily synchronous.

Antepartum Surveillance

Serial sonographic examinations are usually performed throughout the third trimester to monitor fetal growth. Assessment of amnionic fluid volume is also important. Associated oligohydramnios may indicate uteroplacental pathology and should prompt further evaluation of fetal well-being. That said, quantifying amnionic fluid volume in multifetal gestation is sometimes difficult. Some measure the deepest vertical pocket in each sac or assess the fluid subjectively. If sacs are side by side, as opposed to one on top of the other, measurement of the amnionic fluid index (AFI) may be helpful. Using data from 405 uncomplicated twin pregnancies, Porter and associates (1996) described a protocol for measuring the AFI in twin gestations and provided normal values. As in singletons, the deepest vertical pocket in each quadrant was measured, regardless of the dividing membrane location. An AFI of < 8 cm–below the 5th percentile or > 24 cm–above the 95th percentile–was considered abnormal at gestational ages of 28 to 40 weeks. If the overall AFI is abnormal, a determination should be made as to which sac is involved and how quantitatively severe the abnormality is. Subjective assessment may be required but is not always accurate. Magann and co-workers (1995) reported that oligohydramnios, defined as less than 500 mL, is poorly identified by any sonographic method in twin gestations.

Tests of Fetal Well-Being

As described throughout Chapter 15, there are several methods of assessing fetal health in singleton pregnancies. The nonstress test or biophysical profile is commonly used in management of twin or higher-order multifetal gestations. Because of the complexity of complications associated with multifetal gestations, and the potential technical difficulties in differentiating fetuses

during antepartum testing, the usefulness of these methods appears limited. For example, Elliott and Finberg (1995) used the biophysical profile as the primary method for monitoring higher-order multifetal gestations. They reported that four of 24 monitored pregnancies had a poor outcome despite reassuring biophysical profile scores. In a randomized trial of 526 twin pregnancies, the addition of umbilical artery Doppler velocimetry to management compared with fetal testing based on fetal-growth parameters alone resulted in no improvement in perinatal outcome (Giles and associates, 2003).

Whatever method is used, care must be taken to evaluate each fetus separately. Gallagher and colleagues (1992) analyzed fetal heart rate accelerations, fetal movement, and other behavioral states in 15 twin pairs. If one twin of a pair was awake or asleep, so was its sibling, however, accelerations and movements were usually not coincidental (Fig. 39-24).

Doppler Velocimetry

As discussed in Chapters 15 and 16, Doppler evaluation of vascular resistance may provide a measure of fetal well-being. Increased resistance with diminished diastolic flow velocity often accompanies restricted fetal growth. Doppler values in twins and triplets are the same as in singletons and can thus be used in a similar manner (Akiyama and co-workers, 1999). As in singletons, however, the clinical utility of this technology is controversial.

Gerson and co-workers (1987) used duplex Doppler ultrasound to measure umbilical venous blood flow and arterial systolic–diastolic velocity ratios to predict concordant and discordant growth in twins. Normal studies correctly predicted concordancy in 44 of 45 concordant twin pairs. Abnormal values, especially those from the umbilical artery, correctly predicted discordancy in nine of 11 sets of discordant twins. Conversely, DiVou and co-workers (1989) reported that velocimetry alone was not consistently useful in identifying twin discordancy. Ezra and colleagues (1999) found that in triplets and quadruplets, as in singletons, absent end-diastolic blood flow in the umbilical artery was associated with low birthweight and increased perinatal mortality rates.

Prevention of Preterm Delivery

Preterm labor is common in multifetal pregnancies and may complicate up to 50 percent of twin, 75 percent of triplet, and 90 percent of quadruplet pregnancies (Elliott, 2007). Several techniques have been applied in attempts to prolong these multifetal gestations. These include bed rest—especially through hospitalization, prophylactic administration of beta-mimetic drugs or progestins, and prophylactic cervical cerclage.

Bed Rest

Most evidence suggests that routine hospitalization is not beneficial in prolonging multifetal pregnancy. In one study, Crowther and co-workers (1990) randomly chose hospitalization or routine care for 139 Zimbabwean women with twin pregnancies. They found that hospitalized bed rest did not prolong pregnancy or improve neonatal survival, although it did improve fetal growth. At Parkland Hospital, elective hospitalization at 26 weeks was compared with outpatient management, and no advantages were found (Andrews and colleagues, 1991). Importantly, however, almost half of the women required admission for specific indications such as hypertension or threatened preterm delivery.

Limited physical activity, early work leave, more frequent health care visits and sonographic examinations, and structured maternal education on preterm delivery risks have been advocated to reduce preterm births in women with multiple fetuses. Unfortunately, there is little evidence that these measures substantially change outcome. For example, Pons and co-workers (1998) found virtually no difference in outcomes of 70 triplet pregnancies managed intensively from 1987 to 1993 and compared with 21 triplet pregnancies managed routinely between 1975 and 1986. The only major difference between these two periods was that neonates born in the later period group had significantly less hyaline membrane disease—13 versus 31 percent—which these investigators attributed to the use of corticosteroids.

Tocolytic Therapy

As for singleton pregnancies, there is no valid evidence that tocolytic therapy improves neonatal outcomes in multifetal gestation (Gyetvai and co-workers, 1999). Importantly, tocolytic therapy in these women entails a higher risk than in singletons. This is in part because twin-induced maternal increased blood volume and cardiovascular demands increase susceptibility to hydration-associated pulmonary edema. Gabriel and colleagues (1994) compared outcomes of 26 twin and six triplet pregnancies with those of 51 singletons—all treated with a beta-mimetic for preterm labor without ruptured membranes. Women with a multifetal gestation had significantly more cardiovascular complications—43 versus 4 percent—including three with pulmonary edema.

Progesterone Therapy

Weekly injections of 17-α hydroxyprogesterone caproate fail to reduce birth rates in women carrying twins or triplets (Caritis and associates, 2009; Rouse and colleagues, 2007).

Corticosteroids for Lung Maturation

Although corticosteroids are less studied in multifetal gestations than in singletons, there is no biological reason that these drugs would not benefit multiple fetuses (Roberts and Dalziel, 2006). Therefore, guidelines for the use of corticosteroids are not different from those for singleton gestation (American College of Obstetricians and Gynecologists, 2004).

Cervical Cerclage

Prophylactic cerclage has not been shown to improve perinatal outcome in women with multifetal pregnancies. Studies have included women who were not specially selected as well as those who were selected because of a shortened cervix as assessed by transvaginal sonography (Dor, 1982; Elimian, 1999; Newman, 2002; Rebarber, 2005, and all their colleagues). In fact, cerclage my actually worsen outcomes in the latter group (Berghella and colleagues, 2005).

PRETERM LABOR PREDICTION

Goldenberg and colleagues (1996) prospectively screened 147 twin pregnancies for more than 50 potential risk factors for preterm birth and found that only cervical length and fetal fibronectin levels predicted preterm birth (see Chap. 36, p. 814). At 24 weeks, a cervical length of 25 mm or less was the best predictor of birth before 32 weeks. At 28 weeks, an elevated fetal fibronectin level was the best predictor. Similarly, To and co-workers (2006) sonographically measured the cervical length in 1163 twin pregnancies at 22 to 24 weeks. Rates of preterm delivery before 32 weeks were 66 percent in those with cervical lengths of 10 mm; 24 percent for lengths of 20 mm; 12 percent for 25 mm; and only 1 percent for 40 mm. Conversely, McMahon and colleagues (2002) found that women with multifetal gestation at 24 weeks who had a closed internal os on digital cervical examination, a normal cervical length by sonographic examination, and a negative fetal fibronectin test result were at *low* risk to deliver before 32 weeks. Interestingly, a closed internal os by digital examination was as predictive as the combination of normal measured cervical length and negative fetal fibronectin test results.

Pulmonary Maturation

As measured by determination of the lecithin-sphingomyelin ratio, pulmonary maturation is usually synchronous in twins (Leveno and associates, 1984). Moreover, although this ratio usually does not exceed 2.0 until 36 weeks in singleton pregnancies, it often does so by approximately 32 weeks in multifetal pregnancies. In some cases, however, pulmonary function may be markedly different, with the smallest, most stressed fetus being more mature.

Preterm Premature Membrane Rupture

Twin gestations with preterm ruptured membranes are managed expectantly much like singleton pregnancies (see Chap. 36, p. 817). Mercer and colleagues (1993) compared outcomes of twin and singleton pregnancies, both with ruptured membranes at 19 to 36 weeks. They found that labor ensued earlier in twins.

Specifically, the median time from rupture to delivery was 1.1 days in twins compared with 1.7 days in singletons. More than 90 percent in both groups delivered within 7 days of membrane rupture.

Delayed Delivery of Second Twin

Infrequently, after preterm birth of the presenting fetus, it may be advantageous for undelivered fetus(es) to remain in utero. Trivedi and Gillett (1998) reviewed the English literature and found 45 case reports of asynchronous birth in multifetal gestation. Although likely biased, those pregnancies with a surviving retained twin or triplet continued for an average of 49 days. Management with tocolytics, prophylactic antimicrobials, and cerclage appeared to make no difference. Oyelese and associates (2005), in their retrospective cohort study of 258 twins with delayed delivery of the second fetus, found no improvement in rates of second-twin mortality if the first delivered between 24 to 28 weeks. Reduced rates were seen if the first twin delivered between 22 to 23 weeks, and the second delivery was delayed for 1 to 3 weeks. Livingston and colleagues (2004) described 14 pregnancies in which an active attempt was made to delay delivery of 19 fetuses after delivery of the first neonate. Only one fetus survived without major sequelae, and one mother developed sepsis syndrome with shock. Arabin and van Eyck (2009) reported better outcomes in the minority of 93 twin and 34 triplet pregnancies that qualified for delayed delivery in their center over a 17-year period.

If asynchronous birth is attempted, there must be careful evaluation for infection, abruption, and congenital anomalies. The mother must be thoroughly counseled, particularly about the potential for serious, even life-threatening infection. The range of gestational age in which the benefits outweigh the risks for delayed delivery is likely narrow. Avoidance of delivery from 23 to 26 weeks would seem most beneficial. In our experience, good candidates for delayed delivery are rare.

LABOR AND DELIVERY

Labor

Many complications of labor and delivery are encountered more often with multiple fetuses than with singletons. These include preterm labor, uterine contractile dysfunction, abnormal presentation, umbilical cord prolapse, premature separation of the placenta, and immediate post-partum hemorrhage. For these reasons, certain precautions and special arrangements are prudent. Recommendations for intrapartum management include:

1. An appropriately trained obstetrical attendant should remain with the mother throughout labor. Continuous external electronic monitoring is employed. If membranes are ruptured and the cervix dilated, then simultaneous evaluation of both the presenting fetus by internal electronic monitoring and the remaining sibling(s) by external monitors is typically used
2. Blood transfusion products are readily available

3. An intravenous infusion system capable of delivering fluid rapidly is established. In the absence of hemorrhage, lactated Ringer or an aqueous dextrose solution is infused at a rate of 60 to 125 mL/hr
4. An obstetrician skilled in intrauterine identification of fetal parts and in intrauterine manipulation of a fetus should be present
5. A sonography machine is made readily available to help evaluate position and status of the remaining fetus(es) after delivery of the first
6. Experienced anesthesia personnel are immediately available in the event that intrauterine manipulation or cesarean delivery is necessary
7. For each fetus, two attendants, one of whom is skilled in resuscitation and care of newborns, are appropriately informed of the case and remain immediately available
8. The delivery area should provide adequate space for all team members to work effectively. Moreover, the site must be appropriately equipped to provide maternal and neonatal resuscitation.

Presentation and Position

With twins, all possible combinations of fetal positions may be encountered. The most common presentations at admission for delivery are cephalic-cephalic, cephalic-breech, and cephalic-transverse (Fig. 39-25). Importantly, these presentations, especially those other than cephalic–cephalic, are unstable before and during labor and delivery. Compound, face, brow, and footling breech presentations are relatively common, especially if fetuses are small, amnionic fluid is excessive, or maternal parity is high. Cord prolapse is also common in these circumstances. The presentation can often be ascertained by sonography. If any confusion about the relationship of the twins to each other or to the maternal pelvis persists, a single anteroposterior radiograph of the abdomen may be helpful.

Induction or Stimulation of Labor

Although labor is generally shorter with twins, it can be desultory (Schiff and associates, 1998). If women meet all criteria for

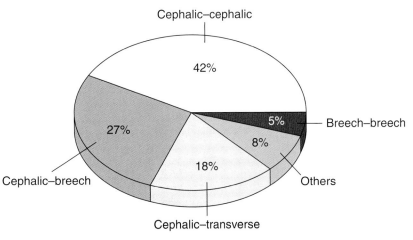

FIGURE 39-25 Presentations of twin fetuses on admission for delivery. (Data from Divon and colleagues, 1993.)

the administration of oxytocin, it may be used as described in Chapter 22 (see p. 505).

Analgesia and Anesthesia

During labor and delivery of multiple fetuses, decisions regarding analgesia and anesthesia may be complicated by problems imposed by preterm labor, preeclampsia, desultory labor, need for intrauterine manipulation, and postpartum uterine atony and hemorrhage.

Epidural analgesia is recommended by many because it provides excellent pain relief and can be rapidly extended cephalad if internal podalic version or cesarean delivery is required (Koffel, 1999). Special care must be taken in hypertensive women or in those who have hemorrhaged because epidural analgesia may cause hypotension with inadequate perfusion of vital organs, especially the placenta (see Chap. 19, p. 455). Therefore, placement and maintenance of continuous epidural analgesia should be performed by anesthesia personnel knowledgeable in obstetrics. It should be preceded by adequate hydration and administered slowly. Because women pregnant with multiple fetuses are especially vulnerable to supine hypotension during labor and delivery, they should be placed in full lateral position during and after induction of epidural analgesia. Left uterine displacement is maintained for cesarean delivery.

If general anesthesia is used, the increased maternal oxygen demand associated with multifetal gestation increases the risk of hypoxemia, thus making adequate preoxygenation essential. Pudendal blockade if administered with nitrous oxide plus oxygen can provide pain relief for spontaneous delivery. If intrauterine manipulation is necessary, as with internal podalic version, uterine relaxation can be accomplished rapidly with the inhalation anesthetic isoflurane. Such agents provide effective relaxation for intrauterine manipulation, but they also cause an increase in blood loss during the third stage of labor. Some clinicians use intravenous or sublingual nitroglycerin to achieve uterine relaxation yet avoid the aspiration and hypoxia risks associated with general anesthetics (Vinatier and associates, 1996).

Vaginal Delivery

Cephalic-Cephalic Presentation

During labor, the presenting twin typically dilates the cervix. If a first twin is cephalic, delivery can usually be accomplished spontaneously or with forceps. Hogle and colleagues (2003) performed an extensive literature review and concluded that planned cesarean delivery does not improve neonatal outcome when both twins are cephalic. Muleba and associates (2005) identified increased rates of respiratory distress in the second twin of preterm pairs regardless of the mode of delivery or corticosteroid use.

Cephalic-Noncephalic Presentation

The optimal delivery route for cephalic–noncephalic twins is controversial. Several reports attest to the safety of vaginal delivery of second noncephalic twins who weigh more than 1500 g (Blickstein, 1987; Chervanak, 1985; Gocke, 1989, and all their associates). Thus, when the estimated fetal weight is greater than 1500 g, vaginal delivery of a nonvertex second twin is rea-

sonable. If the estimated fetal weight is less than 1500 g, the issue is less clear, although comparable or even improved fetal outcomes have been reported with vaginal delivery (Caukwell and Murphy, 2002; Davidson and co-workers, 1992; Rydhström, 1990). Mauldin and colleagues (1998) retrospectively reviewed the delivery courses of 84 cephalic–noncephalic twins. They found that vaginal delivery of the presenting twin followed by breech extraction of the second twin resulted in significantly shorter maternal and neonatal hospital stays, in part because vaginally extracted breech twins had less respiratory disease and fewer infections.

Breech Presentation

As in singletons, if a first fetus presents as a breech, major problems may develop if:

1. The fetus is unusually large, and the aftercoming head is larger than the birth canal
2. The fetus is sufficiently small. The extremities and trunk may deliver through an inadequately effaced and dilated cervix, but the head may become trapped above the cervix
3. The umbilical cord prolapses.

If these problems are anticipated or identified, cesarean delivery is often preferred except in those instances in which the fetuses are so immature that they will not survive. Even without these problems, if the first twin is breech, many obstetricians perform cesarean delivery. However, Blickstein and colleagues (2000) reported the collective experience from 1990 to 1997 of 13 European centers that attempted vaginal delivery in 374 of 613 twin pairs when the presenting twin was breech. In their report, vaginal delivery did not increase the mortality rate of breech-presenting first twins who weighed at least 1500 g. Fetuses with breech presentation may be delivered as described in Chapter 24.

The phenomenon of locked twins is rare. According to Cohen and co-workers (1965), it occurred only once in 817 twin gestations. For twins to lock, the first fetus must present breech and the second, cephalic. With descent of the breech through the birth canal, the chin of the first fetus locks between the neck and chin of the second. Cesarean delivery is recommended when the potential for locking is identified.

Vaginal Delivery of the Second Twin

Following delivery of the first twin, the presenting part of the second twin, its size, and its relationship to the birth canal should be quickly and carefully ascertained by combined abdominal, vaginal, and at times, intrauterine examination. Sonography may be a valuable aid. If the fetal head or the breech is fixed in the birth canal, moderate fundal pressure is applied and membranes are ruptured. Immediately afterward, digital examination of the cervix is repeated to exclude prolapse of the cord. Labor is allowed to resume. If contractions do not resume within approximately 10 minutes, dilute oxytocin may be used to stimulate contractions.

In the past, the safest interval between delivery of the first and second twins was commonly cited as less than 30 minutes. Subsequently, as shown by Rayburn and colleagues (1984), as well as others, if continuous fetal monitoring is used, a good outcome is achieved even if this interval is longer. Leung and colleagues (2002) demonstrated a direct correlation between worsening umbilical cord blood gas values and increasing time between delivery of first and second twins. Thus, vigilant monitoring for nonreassuring fetal heart rate or bleeding is required. Hemorrhage may indicate placental abruption.

If the occiput or breech presents immediately over the pelvic inlet, but is not fixed in the birth canal, the presenting part can often be guided into the pelvis by one hand in the vagina, while a second hand on the uterine fundus exerts moderate pressure caudally. Alternatively, with abdominal manipulation, an assistant can guide the presenting part into the pelvis. Sonography can add guidance and allow heart rate monitoring. Intrapartum external version of a noncephalic second twin has also been described (Chervanak and co-workers, 1983).

A presenting shoulder may be gently converted into a cephalic presentation. If the occiput or breech is not over the pelvic inlet and cannot be so positioned by gentle pressure, or if appreciable uterine bleeding develops, delivery of the second twin can be problematic.

To obtain a favorable outcome, it is essential to have an obstetrician skilled in intrauterine fetal manipulation and anesthesia personnel skilled in providing anesthesia to effectively relax the uterus for vaginal delivery of a noncephalic second twin. To take maximum advantage of the dilated cervix before the uterus contracts and the cervix retracts, delay must be avoided. Prompt cesarean delivery of the second fetus is preferred if no one present is skilled in the performance of internal podalic version or if anesthesia that will provide effective uterine relaxation is not immediately available.

Internal Podalic Version

With this maneuver, a fetus is turned to a breech presentation using the hand placed into the uterus (Fig. 39-26). The obstetrician grasps the fetal feet to then effect delivery by breech extraction. Chauhan and colleagues (1995) compared outcomes of 23 second twins delivered by podalic version and breech extraction with those of 21 who underwent external cephalic version. Breech extraction was considered superior to external version, because less fetal distress developed. The technique of breech extraction is described in Chapter 24 (p. 536).

Vaginal Birth after Cesarean

There are studies that support an attempt at vaginal birth after cesarean for selected women with twins. With this situation, there is approximately the same risk for uterine rupture as an attempt at vaginal birth with a singleton gestation (Cahill, 2005; Ford, 2006; Varner, 2005, and all their co-workers).

Cesarean Delivery

Twin fetuses create unusual intraoperative problems. Hypotension commonly develops in women carrying twins when they are placed supine. Therefore, these women should be positioned in a left lateral tilt to deflect uterine weight off the aorta (see Chap. 5, p. 119). The uterine incision should be large enough to allow atraumatic delivery of both fetuses. In some cases, a vertical incision in the lower uterine segment may be advantageous. For example, if a fetus is transverse with its back down, and the arms are inadvertently delivered first, it is much easier and safer to extend a vertical uterine incision upward than to extend a transverse incision. If a second twin is breech and delivery of the head is obstructed, Piper forceps can be used just as for a vaginal delivery (see Fig. 24-16, p. 539).

At times, attempts to deliver a second twin vaginally after delivery of a first twin are not only unwise but also impossible. In these cases, prompt cesarean delivery is required. Cesarean delivery of the second twin may be necessary, for example, when the second fetus is much larger than the first and is breech or transverse. Even more perplexing, cesarean delivery may be required if the cervix promptly contracts and thickens after delivery of the first twin and does not dilate subsequently or if a nonreassuring fetal heart rate pattern develops.

TRIPLET OR HIGHER-ORDER GESTATION

Fetal heart rate monitoring during labor is challenging. A scalp electrode can be attached to the presenting fetus, but it is difficult to ensure that the other two triplets are each being monitored separately. With vaginal delivery, the first neonate is usually born spontaneously or with little manipulation. Subsequent fetuses, however, are delivered according to the presenting part. This often requires complicated obstetrical maneuvers such as total breech extraction with or without internal podalic version or even cesarean delivery. Associated with malposition of fetuses is an increased incidence of cord prolapse. Moreover, reduced

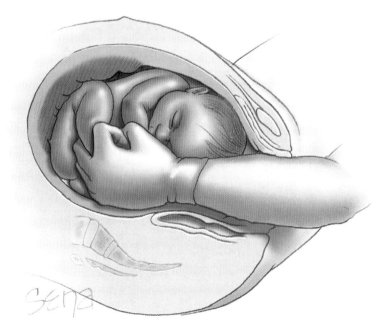

FIGURE 39-26 Internal podalic version. Upward pressure on the head by an abdominal hand is applied as downward traction is exerted on the feet.

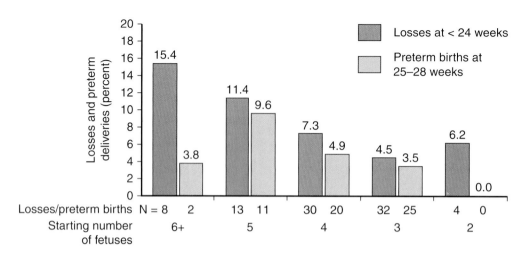

FIGURE 39-27 Histogram showing the rate of pregnancy losses at less than 24 weeks and preterm birth at 25 to 28 weeks as a function of the initial number of multiple fetuses in more than 1000 women who underwent selective reduction of pregnancy from 1995 to 1998. (Modified from *American Journal of Obstetrics & Gynecology*, Vol. 184, No. 2, MI Evans, RL Berkowitz, RJ Wapner, et al., Improvement in outcomes of multifetal pregnancy reduction with increased experience, pp. 97–103, Copyright 2001, with permission from Elsevier.)

placental perfusion and hemorrhage from separating placentas are more likely during delivery.

For all these reasons, many clinicians believe that pregnancies complicated by three or more fetuses are best delivered by cesarean. Vaginal delivery is reserved for those circumstances in which survival is not expected because fetuses are markedly immature or maternal complications make cesarean delivery hazardous to the mother. Other clinicians believe that vaginal delivery is safe under certain circumstances. For example, Alamia and colleagues (1998) evaluated a protocol for vaginal delivery of triplet pregnancies in which the presenting fetus was cephalic. A total of 23 sets of triplets were analyzed, and a third of these were delivered vaginally. Neonatal outcomes were the same in the vaginal and cesarean delivery groups, with no morbidity and 100-percent fetal survival. Grobman and colleagues (1998) and Alran and co-workers (2004) reported vaginal delivery completion rates of 88 and 84 percent, respectively, in women carrying triplets who underwent a trial of labor. Neonatal outcomes did not differ from those of a matched group of triplet pregnancies delivered by elective cesarean. As in any obstetrical procedure, the safety of vaginal triplet delivery depends on the skill and experience of the operator.

SELECTIVE REDUCTION OR TERMINATION

In some cases of higher-order multifetal gestation, reduction in the number of fetuses to two or three improves survival of the remaining fetuses. Selective reduction implies early pregnancy intervention, whereas selective termination is performed later.

Selective Reduction

Reduction of a selected fetus or fetuses in a multichorionic multifetal gestation may be chosen as a therapeutic intervention to enhance survival of the other fetuses. Pregnancy reduction can be performed transcervically, transvaginally, or transabdominally, but the transabdominal route is usually easiest. Transabdominal fetal reductions are typically performed between 10

and 13 weeks. This gestational age is chosen because most spontaneous abortions have already occurred, the remaining fetuses are large enough to be evaluated sonographically, the amount of devitalized fetal tissue remaining after the procedure is small, and the risk of aborting the entire pregnancy as a result of the procedure is low. The smallest fetuses and any anomalous fetuses are chosen for reduction. Potassium chloride is then injected into the heart or thorax of each selected fetus under sonographic guidance, taking care not to enter or traverse the sacs of fetuses selected for retention. In most cases, pregnancies are reduced to twins to increase the chances of delivering at least one viable fetus.

Evans and associates (2005) reported continued improvement in fetal outcomes with this procedure. They analyzed more than 1000 pregnancies managed in 11 centers from 1995 to 1998 (Fig. 39-27). The pregnancy loss rate varied from a low of 4.5 percent for triplets who were reduced to twins, and increased with each addition to the starting number of fetuses, peaking at 15 percent for six or more fetuses (Evans and colleagues, 2001). Operator skill and experience are believed responsible for the low and declining rates of pregnancy loss.

Selective Termination

With the identification of multiple fetuses discordant for structural or genetic abnormalities, three options are available: abortion of all fetuses, selective termination of the abnormal fetus, or continuation of the pregnancy. Because anomalies are typically not discovered until the second trimester, selective termination is performed later in gestation than selective reduction and entails greater risk. This procedure is therefore usually not performed unless the anomaly is severe but not lethal, meaning that the anomalous fetus would survive and require lifetime care, or the estimated risk of continuing the pregnancy is greater than the risk of the procedure.

Thus, a triplet pregnancy in which one fetus has Down syndrome might be a candidate for selective termination, whereas a twin pregnancy in which one has trisomy 18 might not. In some cases, termination is considered because the abnormal fetus may jeopardize the normal one. For example, pathological hydramnios in a twin with esophageal atresia could lead to preterm birth of its sibling. Audibert and colleagues (2003) reported the selective termination of a severely growth-restricted twin fetus at 32 weeks, with marked improvement in the severity of maternal preeclampsia and subsequent delivery of a healthy sibling twin at 38 weeks. Prerequisites to selective termination include a precise diagnosis for the anomalous fetus and absolute certainty of fetal location. Thus, if genetic amniocentesis is performed on a multifetal gestation, a map of the uterus with locations of all the fetuses clearly labeled should be made at the time of the diagnostic procedure. Unless a special procedure such as umbilical cord interruption is used, selective termination should be performed only in multichorionic multifetal gestations to avoid damaging the surviving fetus(es) (Lewi and associates, 2006).

Evans and co-workers (1999) have provided the most comprehensive results to date on second-trimester selective termination for fetal abnormalities. A total of 402 cases were analyzed from eight centers worldwide. Included were 345 twin, 39 triplet, and 18 quadruplet pregnancies. Selective termination using potassium chloride resulted in delivery of a viable neonate or neonates in more than 90 percent of cases, with a mean age at delivery of 35.7 weeks. Loss of the entire pregnancy was 7.1 percent of pregnancies reduced to singletons and 13 percent of those reduced to twins. The gestational age at the time of the procedure did not appear to affect pregnancy loss. Several losses occurred because the pregnancy was actually monochorionic and potassium chloride also killed the normal fetus through placental vascular anastomoses.

Ethics

The ethical issues associated with these techniques are almost limitless. The interested reader is referred to the excellent reviews by Evans and co-workers (1996, 2004) and Simpson and Carson (1996).

Informed Consent

Prior to selective termination or reduction, a discussion should include the morbidity and mortality rates expected if the pregnancy is continued; the morbidity and mortality rates expected with surviving twins or triplets; and the risks of the procedure itself.

With couples seeking infertility treatment, the issue of selective reduction should ideally be discussed *prior* to conception. Grobman and associates (2001) reported that these couples were generally unaware of the risks associated with multifetal gestation, and they were less desirous of having a multifetal gestation once apprised of the risks.

Specific risks that are common to selective termination or reduction include:

1. Abortion of the remaining fetuses
2. Abortion of the wrong (normal) fetus(es)
3. Retention of genetic or structurally abnormal fetuses after a reduction in number

4. Damage without death to a fetus
5. Preterm labor
6. Discordant or growth-restricted fetuses
7. Maternal infection, hemorrhage, or possible disseminated intravascular coagulopathy because of retained products of conception.

The procedure should be performed by an operator skilled and experienced in sonographically guided procedures. Because selective reduction increases the maternal serum alpha-fetoprotein level, a couple should be informed that this screening test will not be useful after the procedure (Lynch and Berkowitz, 1993). Instead, a second-trimester targeted sonographic evaluation or possibly amniocentesis may be offered.

Psychological Reaction

Women and their spouses who elect to undergo selective termination or reduction find this decision highly stressful. Schreiner-Engel and associates (1995) retrospectively studied the emotional reactions of 100 women following selective reduction. Although 70 percent of the women mourned for their dead fetus(es), most grieved only for 1 month. Persistent depressive symptoms were mild, although moderately severe sadness and guilt continued for many for them. Fortunately, most were reconciled to the termination of some fetuses to preserve the lives of a remaining few. Indeed, 93 percent of the women would have made the same decision again.

REFERENCES

Aisenbrey GA, Catanzarite VA, Hurley TJ, et al: Monoamniotic and pseudomonoamniotic twins: Sonographic diagnosis, detection of cord entanglement, and obstetric management. Obstet Gynecol 86:218, 1995

Akiyama M, Kuno A, Tanaka Y, et al: Comparison of alterations in fetal regional arterial vascular resistance in appropriate-for-gestational-age singleton, twin and triplet pregnancies. Hum Reprod 14:2635, 1999

Alamia V Jr, Royek AB, Jaekle RK, et al: Preliminary experience with a prospective protocol for planned vaginal delivery of triplet gestations. Am J Obstet Gynecol 179:1133, 1998

Allen VM, Windrim R, Barrett J, et al: Management of monoamniotic twin pregnancies: A case series and systematic review of the literature. Br J Obstet Gynaecol 108:931, 2001

Alran S, Sibony O, Luton D, et al: Maternal and neonatal outcome of 93 consecutive triplet pregnancies with 71% vaginal delivery. Acta Obstet Gynec Scand 83:554, 2004

American College of Obstetricians and Gynecologists: Multiple gestation: Complicated twin, triplet, and high-order multifetal pregnancy. Practice Bulletin No. 56, October 2004

American Society for Reproductive Medicine: A Practice Committee Report: Guidelines on number of embryos transferred. Birmingham, Alabama, November 1999

Andrews WW, Leveno KJ, Sherman ML, et al: Elective hospitalization in the management of twin pregnancies. Obstet Gynecol 77:826, 1991

Arabin B, van Eyck J: Delayed-interval delivery in twin and triplet pregnancies: 17 years of experience in 1 perinatal center. Am J Obstet Gynecol 200(2):154.e1, 2009

Arbuckle TE, Wilkins R, Sherman GJ: Birth weight percentiles by gestational age in Canada. Obstet Gynecol 81:39, 1993

Aston K, Peterson C, Carrell D: Monozygotic twinning associated with assisted reproductive technologies: A review. Reproduction June 24, 2008

Audibert F, Salomon LJ, Castaigne-Meary V, et al: Selective termination of a twin pregnancy as a treatment of severe pre-eclampsia. Br J Obstet Gynaecol 110:68, 2003

Azubuike JC: Multiple births in Igbo women. Br J Obstet Gynaecol 89:77, 1982

Babson SG, Phillips DS: Growth and development of twins dissimilar in size at birth. N Engl J Med 289:937, 1973

Bailey-Pridham DD, Reshef E, Drury K, et al: Follicular fluid lidocaine levels during transvaginal oocyte retrieval. Fertil Steril 53:171, 1990

Baldwin VJ: Pathology of multiple pregnancy. In Wigglesworth JS, Singer J (eds): Textbook of Fetal and Perinatal Pathology. Boston, Blackwell, 1991, p 238

Beemsterboer SN, Homburg R, Gorter NA, et al: The paradox of declining fertility but increasing twinning rates with advancing maternal age. Hum Reprod 21:1531, 2006

Bejar R, Vigliocco G, Gramajo H, et al.: Antenatal origin of neurological damage in newborn infants, 2. Multiple gestations. Am J Obstet Gynecol 162:1230, 1990

Belfort MA, Moise KJ, Kirshon B, et al: The use of color flow Doppler ultrasonography to diagnose umbilical cord entanglement in monoamniotic twin gestations. Am J Obstet Gynecol 168:601, 1993

Benirschke K: Intrauterine death of a twin: Mechanisms, implications for surviving twin, and placental pathology. Semin Diagn Pathol 10:222, 1993

Benirschke K, Kim CK: Multiple pregnancy. N Engl J Med 288:1276, 1973

Bennett D, Dunn LC: Genetical and embryological comparisons of semilethal t-alleles from wild mouse populations. Genetics 61:411, 1969

Berghella V, Kaufmann M: Natural history of twin-twin transfusion syndrome. J Reprod Med 46:480, 2001

Berghella V, Odibo AO, To MS, et al: Cerclage for short cervix on ultrasonography: Meta-analysis of trials using individual patient-level data. Obstet Gynecol 106(1):181, 2005

Blickstein I, Goldman RD, Kupferminc M: Delivery of breech first twins: A multicenter retrospective study. Obstet Gynecol 95:37, 2000

Blickstein I, Schwartz-Shoham Z, Lancet M, et al: Vaginal delivery of the second twin in breech presentation. Obstet Gynecol 68:774, 1987

Bristow RE, Shumway JB, Khouzami AN, et al: Complete hydatidiform mole and surviving coexistent twin. Obstet Gynecol Surv 51:705, 1996

Brown CEL, Guzick DS, Leveno KJ, et al: Prediction of discordant twins using ultrasound measurement of biparietal diameter and abdominal perimeter. Obstet Gynecol 70:677, 1987

Brown JE, Carlson M: Nutrition and multifetal pregnancy. J Am Diet Assoc 100:343, 2000

Buekens P, Wilcox A: Why do small twins have a lower mortality rate than small singletons? Am J Obstet Gynecol 168:937, 1993

Bulmer MG: The effect of parental age, parity, and duration of marriage on the twinning rate. Hum Genet 23:454, 1959

Cahill A, Stamilio DM, Paré E, et al: Vaginal birth after cesarean (VBAC) attempt in twin pregnancies: Is it safe? Am J Obstet Gynecol 193:1050, 2005

Cameron AH, Edwards JH, Derom R, et al: The value of twin surveys in the study of malformation. Eur J Obstet Gynecol Reprod Biol 14:347, 1983

Campbell DM: Maternal adaptation in twin pregnancy. Semin Perinatol 10:14, 1986

Caritis SN, Rouse DJ, Peaceman AM, et al: Prevention of preterm birth in triplets using 17 alpha-hydroxyprogesterone caproate: A randomized controlled trial. Obstet Gynecol 113(2 Pt 1):285, 2009

Carr SR, Aronson MP, Coustan DR: Survival rates of monoamnionic twins do not decrease after 30 weeks gestation. Am J Obstet Gynecol 163:719, 1990

Carroll SGM, Tyfield L, Reeve L, et al: Is zygosity or chorionicity the main determinant of fetal outcome in twin pregnancies? Am J Obstet Gynecol 193:757, 2005

Casele H, Daley S, Metzger B: Metabolic response to meal eating and extended overnight fasting in twin gestation. Am J Obstet Gynecol 174:375, 1996

Caukwell S, Murphy DJ: The effect of mode of delivery and gestational age on neonatal outcome of the non-cephalic-presenting second twin. Am J Obstet Gynecol 187:1356, 2002

Challis D, Gratacos E, Deprest JA: Cord occlusion techniques for selective termination in monochorionic twins. J Perinat Med 27:327, 1999

Chasen ST, Luo G, Perni SC, et al: Are in vitro fertilization pregnancies with early spontaneous reduction high risk? Am J Obstet Gynecol 195:814, 2006

Chauhan SP, Roberts WE, McLaren RA, et al: Delivery of the nonvertex second twin: Breech extraction versus external cephalic version. Am J Obstet Gynecol 173:1015, 1995

Chervanak FA, Johnson RE, Berkowitz RL, et al: Intrapartum external version of the second twin. Obstet Gynecol 62:160, 1983

Chervanak FA, Johnson RE, Youcha S, et al: Intrapartum management of twin gestation. Obstet Gynecol 65:119, 1985

Choi Y, Bishai D, Minkovitz CS: Multiple births are a risk factor for postpartum maternal depressive symptoms. Pediatrics 123(4):1147, 2009

Christensen K, Petersen I, Skythe A, et al: Comparison of academic performance of twins and singletons in adolescence: Follow-up study. BMJ 333:1095, 2006

Cohen M, Kohl SG, Rosenthal AH: Fetal interlocking complicating twin gestation. Am J Obstet Gynecol 91:407, 1965

Cordero L, Franco A, Joy SD: Monochorionic monoamniotic twins: Neonatal outcome. J Perinatol 26:170, 2006

Cromleholme TM, Shera D, Lee H, et al: A prospective, randomized, multicenter trial of amnioreduction vs selective fetoscopic laser photocoagulation for the treatment of severe twin-twin transfusion syndrome. Am J Obstet Gynecol 197:396.e1, 2007

Crowther CA, Neilson JP, Ashurst HM, et al: The effects of hospitalization for rest on fetal growth, neonatal morbidity and length of gestation in twin pregnancy. Br J Obstet Gynaecol 97:872, 1990

Davidson L, Easterling TR, Jackson JC, et al: Breech extraction of low-birth-weight second twins. Am J Obstet Gynecol 166:497, 1992

Demaria F, Goffinet F, Kayem G, et al: Monoamniotic twin pregnancies: Antenatal management and perinatal results of 19 consecutive cases. BJOG 111:22, 2004

De Paepe ME, DeKoninck P, Friedman RM: Vascular distribution patterns in monochorionic twin placentas. Placenta 26(6):471, 2005

Dickey RP, Olar TT, Taylor SN, et al: Relationship of follicle number and other factors to fecundability and multiple pregnancy in clomiphene citrate–induced intrauterine insemination cycles. Fertil Steril 57:613, 1992

Dickey RP, Taylor SN, Lu PY, et al: Spontaneous reduction of multiple pregnancy: Incidence and effect on outcome. Am J Obstet Gynecol 186:77, 2002

Divon MY, Marin MJ, Pollack RN, et al: Twin gestation: Fetal presentation as a function of gestational age. Am J Obstet Gynecol 168:1500, 1993

DiVou MY, Girz BA, Sklar A, et al: Discordant twins–a prospective study of the diagnostic value of real time ultrasonography combined with umbilical artery velocimetry. Am J Obstet Gynecol 161:757, 1989

Donner C, Shahabi S, Thomas D, et al: Selective feticide by embolization in twin-twin transfusion syndrome. A report of two cases. J Reprod Med 42:747, 1997

Dor J, Shalev J, Mashiach S, et al: Elective cervical suture of twin pregnancies diagnosed ultrasonically in the first trimester following induced ovulation. Gynecol Obstet Invest 13:55, 1982

Eberle AM, Levesque D, Vintzileos AM, et al: Placental pathology in discordant twins. Am J Obstet Gynecol 169:931, 1993

Elimian A, Figueroa R, Nigam S, et al: Perinatal outcome of triplet gestation: Does prophylactic cerclage make a difference? J Matern Fetal Med 8:119, 1999

Elliott JP: Preterm labor in twins and high-order multiples. Clin Perinatol 34:599, 2007

Elliott JP, Finberg HJ: Biophysical profile testing as an indicator of fetal well-being in high-order multiple gestations. Am J Obstet Gynecol 172:508, 1995

Evans MI, Berkowitz RL, Wapner RJ, et al: Improvement in outcomes of multifetal pregnancy reduction with increased experience. Am J Obstet Gynecol 184:97, 2001

Evans MI, Ciorica D, Britt DW, et al: Update on selective reduction. Prenat Diagn 25:807, 2005

Evans MI, Goldberg JD, Horenstein J, et al: Elective termination for structural, chromosomal, and mendelian anomalies: International experience. Am J Obstet Gynecol 181:893, 1999

Evans MI, Johnson MP, Quintero RA, et al: Ethical issues surrounding multifetal pregnancy reduction and selective termination. Clin Perinatol 23:437, 1996

Evans MI, Kaufman MI, Urban AJ, et al: Fetal reduction from twins to a singleton: A reasonable consideration? Obstet Gynecol 104:1423, 2004

Ezra Y, Jones J, Farine D: Umbilical artery waveforms in triplet and quadruplet pregnancies. Gynecol Obstet Invest 47:239, 1999

Faye-Petersen OM, Heller DS, Joshi VV: Handbook of Placental Pathology, 2nd ed, London, Taylor & Francis, 2006

Ford AA, Bateman BT, Simpson LL: Vaginal birth after cesarean delivery in twin gestations: A large, nationwide sample of deliveries. Am J Obstet Gynecol 195:1138, 2006

Fox H, Sebire NJ: Pathology of the Placenta, 3rd ed. Philadelphia, Saunders, 2007

Francois K, Ortiz J, Harris C, et al: Is peripartum hysterectomy more common in multiple gestations? Obstet Gynecol 105:1369, 2005

Fusi L, Gordon H: Twin pregnancy complicated by single intrauterine death. Problems and outcome with conservative management. Br J Obstet Gynaecol 97:511, 1990

Fusi L, McParland P, Fisk N, et al: Acute twin-twin transfusion: A possible mechanism for brain-damaged survivors after intrauterine death of a monochorionic twin. Obstet Gynecol 78:517, 1991

Gabriel R, Harika G, Saniez D, et al: Prolonged intravenous ritodrine therapy: A comparison between multiple and singleton pregnancies. Eur J Obstet Gynecol Reprod Biol 57:65, 1994

Gallagher MW, Costigan K, Johnson TRB: Fetal heart rate accelerations, fetal movement, and fetal behavior patterns in twin gestations. Am J Obstet Gynecol 167:1140, 1992

CHAPTER 39

Gardner MO, Goldenberg RL, Cliver SP, et al: The origin and outcome of preterm twin pregnancies. Obstet Gynecol 85:553, 1995

Gerson AG, Wallace DM, Bridgens NK, et al: Duplex Doppler ultrasound in the evaluation of growth in twin pregnancies. Obstet Gynecol 70:419, 1987

Gilbert WM, Davis SE, Kaplan C, et al: Morbidity associated with prenatal disruption of the dividing membrane in twin gestations. Obstet Gynecol 78:623, 1991

Giles W, Bisits A, O'Callaghan S, et al: The Doppler assessment in multiple pregnancy randomized controlled trial of ultrasound biometry versus umbilical artery Doppler ultrasound and biometry in twin pregnancy. Br J Obstet Gynaecol 110:593, 2003

Glinianaia SV, Rankin J, Wright C: Congenital anomalies in twins: A register-based study. Hum Reprod 23:1306, 2008

Gocke SE, Nageotte MP, Garite T, et al: Management of the non-vertex second twin: Primary cesarean section, external version, or primary breech extraction. Am J Obstet Gynecol 161:111, 1989

Goldenberg RL, Iams JD, Miodovnik M, et al: The preterm prediction study: Risk factors in twin gestations. Am J Obstet Gynecol 175:1047, 1996

Grobman WA, Milad MP, Stout J, et al: Patient perceptions of multiple gestations: An assessment of knowledge and risk aversion. Am J Obstet Gynecol 185:920, 2001

Grobman WA, Peaceman AM, Haney EI, et al: Neonatal outcomes in triplet gestations after a trial of labor. Am J Obstet Gynecol 179:942, 1998

Gyetvai K, Hannah ME, Hodnett ED, et al: Tocolytics for preterm labor: A systematic review. Obstet Gynecol 94:869, 1999

Hack KE, Derks JB, Elias SG, et al: Increased perinatal mortality and morbidity in monochorionic versus dichorionic twin pregnancies: Clinical implications of a large Dutch cohort study. BJOG 115:58, 2008

Hack KE, Derks JB, Schaap AH: Placental characteristics of monoamniotic twin pregnancies in relation to perinatal outcome. Obstet Gynecol 113(2 Pt 1):353, 2009

Haggarty P, McCallum H, McBain H, et al: Effect of B vitamins and genetics on success of in-vitro fertilisation: Prospective cohort study. Lancet 367(9521):1513, 2006

Hall JG: Twinning. Lancet 362:735, 2003

Harkness UF, Crombleholme TM: Twin-twin transfusion syndrome: Where do we go from here? Semin Perinatol 29:296, 2005

Harris DW: Superfecundation: Letter. J Reprod Med 27:39, 1982

Hashimoto B, Callen PW, Filly RA, et al: Ultrasound evaluation of polyhydramnios and twin pregnancy. Am J Obstet Gynecol 154:1069, 1986

Heyborne KD, Porreco RP, Garite TJ, et al: Improved perinatal survival of monoamniotic twins with intensive inpatient monitoring. Am J Obstet Gynecol 192(1):96, 2005

Hill LM, Guzick D, Chenevey P, et al: The sonographic assessment of twin discordancy. Obstet Gynecol 84:501, 1994

Hoekstra C, Zhao ZZ, Lambalk CB, et al: Dizygotic twinning. Hum Reprod Update 14:37, 2008

Hogle KL, Hutton EK, McBrien KA, et al: Cesarean delivery for twins: A systematic review and meta-analysis. Am J Obstet Gynecol 188:220, 2003

Hollier LM, McIntire DD, Leveno KJ: Outcome of twin pregnancies according to intrapair birth weight differences. Obstet Gynecol 94:1006, 1999

Hu LS, Caire J, Twickler DM: MR findings of complicated multifetal gestations. Pediatr Radiol 36:76, 2006

Jain T, Missmer SA, Hornstein MD: Trends in embryo-transfer practice and in outcomes of the use of assisted reproductive technology in the United States. N Engl J Med 350:1639, 2004

Jauniaux E, Elkazen N, Leroy F, et al: Clinical and morphologic aspects of the vanishing twin phenomenon. Obstet Gynecol 72:577, 1988

Jones KL: Smith's Recognizable Patterns of Human Malformation, 5th ed. Philadelphia, Saunders, 1997, p 658

Joseph KS, Allen AC, Dodds L, et al: Causes and consequences of recent increases in preterm birth among twins. Obstet Gynecol 98:57, 2001

Kahn B, Lumey LH, Zybert PA, et al: Prospective risk of fetal death in singleton, twin, and triplet gestations: Implications for practice. Obstet Gynecol 102:685, 2003

Kametas NA, McAuliffe F, Krampl E, et al: Maternal cardiac function in twin pregnancy. Obstet Gynecol 102:806, 2003

Kaufman, MH: The embryology of conjoined twins. Childs Nerv Syst 20:508, 2004

Kilpatrick SJ, Jackson R, Croughan-Minihane MS: Perinatal mortality in twins and singletons matched for gestational age at delivery at > or = 30 weeks. Am J Obstet Gynecol 174:66, 1996

Knox G, Morley D: Twinning in Yoruba women. J Obstet Gynaecol Br Emp 67:981, 1960

Koffel B: Abnormal presentation and multiple gestation. In Chestnut DH (ed): Obstetrical Anesthesia, 2nd ed. St Louis, Mosby, 1999, p 694

Kogan MD, Alexander GR, Kotelchuck M: Trends in twin birth outcomes and prenatal care utilization in the United States, 1981–1997. JAMA 283:335, 2000

Kohl SG, Casey G: Twin gestation. Mt Sinai J Med 42:523, 1975

Kol S, Levron J, Lewit N, et al: The natural history of multiple pregnancies after assisted reproduction: Is spontaneous fetal demise a clinically significant phenomenon? Fertil Steril 60:127, 1993

Landy HJ, Weiner S, Corson SL, et al: The "vanishing twin": Ultrasonographic assessment of fetal disappearance in the first trimester. Am J Obstet Gynecol 150:14, 1986

Langer B, Boudier E, Gasser B, et al: Antenatal diagnosis of brain damage in the survivor after the second trimester death of a monochorionic monoamniotic co-twin: Case report and literature review. Fetal Diagn Ther 12:286, 1997

Larroche JC, Droulle P, Delezoide AL, et al: Brain damage in monozygous twins. Biol Neonate 57:261, 1990

Lee H, Wagner AJ, Sy E, et al: Efficacy of radiofrequency ablation for twin-reversed arterial perfusion sequence. Am J Obstet Gynecol 196:459.e1, 2007

Lee YM, Cleary-Goldman J, Thaker HM, et al: Antenatal sonographic prediction of twin chorionicity. Am J Obstet Gynecol 195:863, 2006

Lee YM, Wylie BJ, Simpson LL, et al: Twin chorionicity and the risk of stillbirth. Obstet Gynecol 111:301, 2008

LeFevre ML, Bain RP, Ewigman BG, et al: A randomized trial of prenatal ultrasonographic screening: Impact on maternal management and outcome. RADIUS (Routine Antenatal Diagnostic Imaging with Ultrasound) study group. Am J Obstet Gynecol 169:483, 1993

Leung TY, Tam WH, Leung TN, et al: Effect of twin-to-twin delivery interval on umbilical cord blood gas in the second twins. Br J Obstet Gynaecol 109:63, 2002

Leveno KJ, Quirk JG, Whalley PJ, et al: Fetal lung maturation in twin gestation. Am J Obstet Gynecol 148:405, 1984

Leveno KJ, Santos-Ramos R, Duenhoelter JH, et al: Sonar cephalometry in twins: A table of biparietal diameters for normal twin fetuses and a comparison with singletons. Am J Obstet Gynecol 135:727, 1979

Lewi L, Gratacos E, Ortibus E, et al: Pregnancy and infant outcome of 80 consecutive cord coagulations in complicated monochorionic multiple pregnancies. Am J Obstet Gynecol 194(3):782, 2006

Lipitz S, Uval J, Achiron R, et al: Outcome of twin pregnancies reduced from triplets compared with nonreduced twin gestations. Obstet Gynecol 87:511, 1996

Livingston JC, Lim FY, Polzin W, et al: Intrafetal radiofrequency ablation for twin reversed arterial perfusion (TRAP): A single-center experience. Am J Obstet Gynecol 197:399.e1, 2007

Livingston JC, Livingston LW, Ramsey R, et al: Second-trimester asynchronous multifetal delivery results in poor perinatal outcome. Obstet Gynecol 103:77, 2004

Livingston JE, Poland BJ: A study of spontaneously aborted twins. Teratology 21:139, 1980

Lopriore E, Oepkes D: Fetal and neonatal haematological complications in monochorionic twins. Semin Fetal Neonatal Med 13(4):231, 2008

Luke B: The changing pattern of multiple births in the United States: Maternal and infant characteristics, 1973 and 1990. Obstet Gynecol 84:101, 1994

Luke B, Brown MB: Maternal morbidity and infant death in twin vs triplet and quadruplet pregnancies. Am J Obstet Gynecol 198:401.e1, 2008

Lynch L, Berkowitz RL: Maternal serum alpha-fetoprotein and coagulation profiles after multifetal pregnancy reduction. Am J Obstet Gynecol 169:987, 1993

MacGillivray I: Epidemiology of twin pregnancy. Semin Perinatol 10:4, 1986

Machin GA: Some causes of genotypic and phenotypic discordance in monozygotic twin pairs. Am J Med Genet 61:216, 1996

Machin GA, Feldstein VA, van Gemert JM, et al: Doppler sonographic demonstration of arterio-venous anastomosis in monochorionic twin gestation. Ultrasound Obstet Gynecol 16(3):214, 2000

Mahone PR, Sherer DM, Abramowicz JS, et al: Twin-twin transfusion syndrome: Rapid development of severe hydrops of the donor following selective feticide of the hydropic recipient. Am J Obstet Gynecol 169:166, 1993

Magann EF, Chauhan SP, Martin JN, et al: Ultrasound assessment of the amniotic fluid volume in diamniotic twins. J Soc Gynecol Investig 2:609, 1995

Mahony BS, Filly RA, Callen PW: Amnionicity and chorionicity in twin pregnancies: Prediction using ultrasound. Radiology 155:205, 1985

Manning FA: Fetal biophysical profile scoring. In: Fetal Medicine: Principles and Practices. Norwalk, CT, Appleton & Lange, 1995, p 288

Mari G, Kirshon B, Abuhamad A: Fetal renal artery flow velocity waveforms in normal pregnancies and pregnancies complicated by polyhydramnios and oligohydramnios. Obstet Gynecol 81:560, 1993

Martin JA, Hamilton BE, Sutton PD, et al: Births: Final data for 2004. Natl Vital Stat Rep 55:1, 2006

Martin JA, Hamilton BE, Sutton PD, et al: Births: Final data for 2005. Natl Vital Stat Rep 56:1, 2007

Martin JA, Hamilton BE, Sutton PD, et al: Births: Final Data for 2006. National Vital Statistics Reports, Vol 57, No 7. Hyattsville, MD, National Center for Health Statistics, 2009

Martin JA, Kung HC, Mathews TJ, et al: Annual summary of vital statistics: 2006. Pediatrics 121:788, 2008

Martin JA, Park MM: Trends in twin and triplet births: 1980-97. Natl Vital Stat Rep 47:1, 1999

Mastrobattista JM, Skupski DW, Monga M, et al: The rate of severe preeclampsia is increased in triplet as compared to twin gestations. Am J Perinatol 14:263, 1997

Mathews TJ, MacDorman FM: Infant mortality statistics from the 2003 period linked birth/infant death data set. Natl Vital Stat Rep 54:1, 2006

Mauldin JG, Newman RB, Mauldin PD: Cost-effective delivery management of the vertex and nonvertex twin gestation. Am J Obstet Gynecol 179:864, 1998

McAuliffe F, Kametas N, Costello J, et al: Respiratory function in singleton and twin pregnancy. Br J Obstet Gynaecol 109:765, 2002

McDonald S, Murphy K, Beyene J, et al: Perinatal outcomes of in vitro fertilization twins: A systematic review and meta-analyses. Am J Obstet Gynecol 193:141, 2005

McHugh K, Kiely EM, Spitz L: Imaging of conjoined twins. Pediatr Radiol 36:899, 2006

McMahon KS, Neerhof MG, Haney EI, et al: Prematurity in multiple gestations: Identification of patients who are at low risk. Am J Obstet Gynecol 186:1137, 2002

Mercer B, Crocker LG, Pierce WF, et al: Clinical characteristics and outcome of twin gestation complicated by preterm premature rupture of the membranes. Am J Obstet Gynecol 168:467, 1993

Michelfelder E, Gottliebson W, Border W, et al: Early manifestations and spectrum of recipient twin cardiomyopathy in twin-twin transfusion syndrome: Relation to Quintero stage. Ultrasound Obstet Gynecol 30:965, 2007

Moise KJ, Dorman K, Lamvu G, et al: A randomized trial of amnioreduction versus septostomy in the treatment of twin-twin transfusion syndrome. Am J Obstet Gynecol 193:701, 2005

Moore TR, Gale S, Benirschke K: Perinatal outcome of forty nine pregnancies complicated by acardiac twinning. Am Obstet Gynecol 163:907, 1990

Mordel N, Benshushan A, Zajicek G, et al: Discordancy in triplets. Am J Perinatol 10:224, 1993

Muleba N, Dashe N, Yost D, et al: Respiratory morbidity among second-born twins. Presented at the 25th Annual Meeting of the Society for Maternal Fetal Medicine, Reno, Nevada, February 7–12, 2005

Newman RB, Krombach S, Myers MC, et al: Effect of cerclage on obstetrical outcome in twin gestations with a shortened cervical length. Am J Obstet Gynecol 186:634, 2002

Niemann I, Sunde L, Petersen LK: Evaluation of the risk of persistent trophoblastic disease after twin pregnancy with diploid hydatidiform mole and coexisting normal fetus. Am J Obstet Gynecol 197:45.e1, 2007

Nilsen ST, Bergsjo P, Nome S: Male twins at birth and 18 years later. Br J Obstet Gynaecol 91:122, 1984

Nylander PP: Biosocial aspects of multiple births. J Biosoc Sci 3:29, 1971

Nylander PP: Serum levels of gonadotropins in relation to multiple pregnancy in Nigeria. Br J Obstet Gynaecol 80:651, 1973

Ong SS, Zamora J, Khan KS, et al: Prognosis for the co-twin following single-twin death: A systematic review. BJOG 113:992, 2006

Oyelese Y, Ananth CV, Smulian JC, et al: Delayed interval delivery in twin pregnancies in the United States: Impact on perinatal mortality and morbidity. Am J Obstet Gynecol 192:439, 2005

Papanikolaou EG, Camus M, Kolibianakis EM, et al: In vitro fertilization with single blastocyst-stage versus single cleavage-stage embryos. N Engl J Med 354:1139, 2006

Parisi P, Gatti M, Prinzi G, et al: Familial incidence of twinning. Nature 304:626, 1983

Pasqualotto EB, Falcone T, Goldberg JM, et al: Risk factors for multiple gestation in women undergoing intrauterine insemination with ovarian stimulation. Fertil Steril 72:613, 1999

Pettersson F, Smedby B, Lindmark G: Outcome of twin birth: Review of 1636 children born in twin birth. Acta Paediatr Scand 64:473, 1976

Pharoah PO, Adi Y: Consequences of in-utero death in twin pregnancy. Lancet 355:1597, 2000

Pons JC, Charlemaine C, Dubreuil E, et al: Management and outcome of triplet pregnancy. Eur J Obstet Gynecol Reprod Biol 76:131, 1998

Porter TF, Dildy GA, Blanchard JR, et al: Normal values for amnionic fluid index during uncomplicated twin pregnancy. Obstet Gynecol 87:699, 1996

Pritchard JA: Changes in blood volume during pregnancy. Anesthesiology 26:393, 1965

Quarello E, Molho M, Ville Y: Incidence, mechanisms, and patterns of fetal cerebral lesions in twin-to-twin transfusion syndrome. J Matern Fetal Neonatal Med 20:589, 2007

Quigley MM, Cruikshank DP: Polyhydramnios and acute renal failure. J Reprod Med 19:92, 1977

Quintero RA, Chmait RH, Murakoshi T, et al: Surgical management of twin reversed arterial perfusion sequence. Am J Obstet Gynecol 194:982, 2006

Quintero RA, Morales WJ, Allen MH, et al: Staging of twin-twin transfusion syndrome. J Perinatol 19:550, 1999

Quintero RA, Reich H, Puder KS, et al: Brief report: Umbilical-cord ligation in an acardiac twin by fetoscopy at 19 weeks gestation. N Engl J Med 330:469, 1994

Ray B, Platt MP: Mortality of twin and singleton livebirths under 30 weeks' gestation: a population-based study. Arch Dis Child Fetal Neonatal Ed 94(2):F140, 2009

Rayburn WF, Lavin JP Jr, Miodovnik M, et al: Multiple gestation: Time interval between delivery of the first and second twins. Obstet Gynecol 63:502, 1984

Rebarber A, Roman AS, Istwan N, et al: Prophylactic cerclage in the management of triplet pregnancies. Am J Obstet Gynecol 193:1193, 2005

Reddy KS, Petersen MB, Antonarakis SE, et al: The vanishing twin: An explanation for discordance between chorionic villus karyotype and fetal phenotype. Prenat Diagn 11:679, 1991

Redline RW: Nonidentical twins with a single placenta–disproving dogma in perinatal pathology. N Engl J Med 349:111, 2003

Roberts D, Dalziel S: Antenatal corticosteroids for accelerating fetal lung maturation for women at risk of preterm birth. Cochrane Database Syst Rev 19:3:CD004454, 2006

Roberts D, Gates S, Kilby M, et al: Interventions for twin-twin transfusion syndrome: A Cochrane review. Ultrasound Obstet Gynecol 31:701, 2008

Robyr R, Lewi L, Salomon LJ, et al: Prevalence and management of late fetal complications following successful selective laser coagulation of chorionic plate anastomoses in twin-to-twin transfusion syndrome. Am J Obstet Gynecol 194:796, 2006

Rodis JF, Lawrence A, Egan JF, et al: Comprehensive fetal ultrasonographic growth measurements in triplet gestations. Am J Obstet Gynecol 181:1128, 1999

Roqué H, Gillen-Goldstein J, Funai E, et al: Perinatal outcomes in monoamniotic gestations. J Matern Fetal Neonatal Med 13:414, 2003

Rossi AC, D'Addario V: Laser therapy and serial amnioreduction as treatment for twin-twin transfusion syndrome: A metaanalysis and review of literature. Am J Obstet Gynecol 198:147, 2008

Rossi AC, D'Addario V: Umbilical cord occlusion for selective feticide in complicated monochorionic twins: a systematic review of literature. Am J Obstet Gynecol 200(2):123, 2009

Rothman KJ: Fetal loss, twinning and birthweight after oral contraceptive use. N Engl J Med 297:468, 1977

Rouse DJ, Caritis SN, Peaceman AM, et al: A trial of 17 alpha-hydroxyprogesterone caproate to prevent prematurity in twins. N Engl J Med 357:454, 2007

Rouse DJ, Skopec GS, Zlatnik FJ: Fundal height as a predictor of preterm twin delivery. Obstet Gynecol 81:211, 1993

Rychik J, Tian Z, Bebbington M, et al: The twin-twin transfusion syndrome: Spectrum of cardiovascular abnormality and development of a cardiovascular score to assess severity of disease. Am J Obstet Gynecol 197(4):392.e1, 2007

Rydhström H: Prognosis for twins with birthweight < 1,500 g: The impact of cesarean section in relation to fetal presentation. Am J Obstet Gynecol 163:528, 1990

Rydhström H: Discordant birthweight and late fetal death in like-sexed and unlike-sexed twin pairs: A population-based study. Br J Obstet Gynaecol 101:765, 1994

Rydhström H: Pregnancy with stillbirth of both twins. Br J Obstet Gynaecol 103:25, 1996

Santema JG, Koppelaar I, Wallenburg HC: Hypertensive disorders in twin pregnancy. Eur J Obstet Gynecol Reprod Biol 58:9, 1995a

Santema JG, Swaak AM, Wallenburg HCS: Expectant management of twin pregnancy with single fetal death. Br J Obstet Gynaecol 102:26, 1995b

Scardo JA, Ellings JM, Newman RB: Prospective determination of chorionicity, amnionicity, and zygosity in twin gestations. Am J Obstet Gynecol 173:1376, 1995

Schenker JG, Yarkoni S, Granat M: Multiple pregnancies following induction of ovulation. Fertil Steril 35:105, 1981

Schiff E, Cohen SB, Dulitzky M, et al: Progression of labor in twins versus singleton gestations. Am J Obstet Gynecol 179:1181, 1998

Schinzel AA, Smith DW, Miller JR: Monozygotic twinning and structural defects. J Pediatr 95:951, 1979

Schreiner-Engel P, Walther VN, Mindes J, et al: First-trimester multifetal pregnancy reduction: Acute and persistent psychologic reactions. Am J Obstet Gynecol 172:544, 1995

Sebire NJ, Foskett M, Paradinas FJ, et al: Outcome of twin pregnancies with complete hydatidiform mole and healthy co-twin. Lancet 359:2165, 2002

Senat M-V, Deprest J, Boulvain M, et al: Endoscopic laser surgery versus serial amnioreduction for severe twin-to-twin transfusion syndrome. N Engl J Med 351:136, 2004

Shah AD, Border WL, Crombleholme TM, et al: Initial fetal cardiovascular profile score predicts recipient twin outcome in twin-twin transfusions syndrome. J Am Soc Echocardiogr 21(10):1105, 2008

Simpson JL, Carson SA: Multifetal reduction in high-order gestations: A non-elective procedure? J Soc Gynecol Invest 3:1, 1996

Smith-Levitin M, Kowalik A, Birnholz J, et al: Comparison of birthweight of twin gestations resulting from embryo reduction of higher order gestations to birthweights of twin and triplet gestations using a novel way to correct for gestational age at delivery. Am J Obstet Gynecol 174:346, 1996

Souter VL, Kapur RP, Nyholt DR, et al: A report of dizygous monochorionic twins. N Engl J Med 349:154, 2003

Spencer R: Theoretical and analytical embryology of conjoined twins: Part I: Embryogenesis. Clin Anat 13:36, 2000a

Spencer R: Theoretical and analytical embryology of conjoined twins: Part II: Adjustments to union. Clin Anat 13:97, 2000b

Spencer R: Parasitic conjoined twins: External, internal (fetuses in fetu and teratomas), and detached (acardiacs). Clin Anat 14:428, 2001

Sperling L, Kiil C, Larsen LU, et al: Naturally conceived twins with monochorionic placentation have the highest risk of fetal loss. Ultrasound Obstet Gynecol 28:644, 2006

Sperling L, Kiil C, Larsen LU, et al: Detection of chromosomal abnormalities, congenital abnormalities and transfusion syndrome in twins. Ultrasound Obstet Gynecol 29:517, 2007

Spitz L, Kiely EM: Conjoined twins. JAMA 289:1307, 2003

St. Clair DM, St. Clair JB, Swainson CP, et al: Twin zygosity testing for medical purposes. Am J Med Genet 77:412, 1998

Stagiannis KD, Sepulveda W, Southwell D, et al: Ultrasonic measurement of the dividing membrane in twin pregnancy during the second and third trimesters: A reproducibility study. Am J Obstet Gynecol 173:1546, 1995

Strandskov HH, Edelen EW, Siemens GJ: Analysis of the sex ratios among single and plural births in the total white and colored U.S. populations. Am J Phys Anthropol 4:491, 1946

Sullivan AE, Varner MW, Ball RH, et al: The management of acardiac twins: A conservative approach. Am J Obstet Gynecol 189:1310, 2003

Tan KL, Goon SM, Salmon Y, et al: Conjoined twins. Acta Obstet Gynecol Scand 50:373, 1971

Tessen JA, Zlatnik FJ: Monoamniotic twins: A retrospective controlled study. Obstet Gynecol 77:832, 1991

To MS, Fonseca EB, Molina FS, et al: Maternal characteristics and cervical length in the prediction of spontaneous early preterm delivery in twins. Am J Obstet Gynecol 194(5):1360, 2006

Trivedi AN, Gillett WR: The retained twin/triplet following a preterm delivery–an analysis of the literature. Aust NZ J Obstet Gynaecol 38:461, 1998

Tuppin P, Blondel B, Kaminski M: Trends in multiple deliveries and infertility treatments in France. Br J Obstet Gynaecol 100:383, 1993

Uchida IA, Freeman VCP, Gedeon M, et al: Twinning rate in spontaneous abortions. Am J Hum Genet 35:987, 1983

Varner MW, Leindecker S, Spong CY, et al: The maternal-fetal medicine unit cesarean registry: Trial of labor with a twin gestation. Am J Obstet Gynecol 193:135, 2005

Vinatier D, Dufour P, Beard J: Utilization of intravenous nitroglycerin for obstetrical emergencies. Int J Gynecol Obstet 55:129, 1996

Wada H, Nunogami K, Wada T, et al: Diffuse brain damage caused by acute twin-twin transfusion during late pregnancy. Acta Paediatr Jpn 40:370, 1998

Walker MC, Murphy KE, Pan S, et al: Adverse maternal outcomes in multifetal pregnancies. BJOG 111:1294, 2004

Weiner CP: Diagnosis and treatment of twin to twin transfusion in the mid-second trimester of pregnancy. Fetal Ther 2:71, 1987

Weissman A, Achiron R, Lipitz S, et al: The first-trimester growth-discordant twin: An ominous prenatal finding. Obstet Gynecol 84:110, 1994

Wen SW, Demissie K, Yang Q, et al: Maternal morbidity and obstetric complications in triplet pregnancies and quadruplet and higher-order multiple pregnancies. Am J Obstet Gynecol 191:254, 2004

Wenstrom KD, Syrop CH, Hammitt DG, et al: Increased risk of monochorionic twinning associated with assisted reproduction. Fertil Steril 60:510, 1993

White C, Wyshak G: Inheritance in human dizygotic twinning. N Engl J Med 271:1003, 1964

Winsor EJ, Brown BS, Luther ER, et al: Deceased co-twin as a cause of false positive amniotic fluid AFP and AChE. Prenat Diagn 7:485, 1987

Wittmann BK, Farquharson DF, Thomas WD, et al: The role of feticide in the management of severe twin transfusion syndrome. Am J Obstet Gynecol 155:1023, 1986

Wright VC, Chang J, Jeng G, et al: Assisted reproductive technology surveillance–United States, 2005. MMWR Surveill Summ 57:1, 2008

Yaron Y, Bryant-Greenwood PK, Dave N, et al: Multifetal pregnancy reductions of triplets to twins: Comparison with nonreduced triplets and twins. Am J Obstet Gynecol 180:1268, 1999

CHAPTER 40

Reproductive Tract Abnormalities

In some cases, pregnancy is complicated by preexisting abnormalities of the reproductive tract. Most of these are developmental anomalies formed during embryogenesis, but they may be acquired during adulthood and sometimes during pregnancy.

DEVELOPMENTAL REPRODUCTIVE TRACT ABNORMALITIES

Due to abnormal embryogenesis, a number of sporadic genitourinary defects may occur. Serious defects are hazardous for the fetus and mother. Even minor maternal defects may result in an increased incidence of miscarriage, preterm labor, and abnormal fetal presentation.

Embryogenesis of the Reproductive Tract

To understand the etiology of developmental abnormalities of the vagina, cervix, and uterus, it is important to first understand their embryogenesis. This is discussed in further detail in Chapter 4 (p. 98) and summarized in Figure 40-1. The proper temporal sequence of gene expression and appropriate spatial relationships of developing tissues are crucial to normal development.

Development of the reproductive organs from intermediate mesodermal elements begins between the third and fifth gestational weeks. Differentiation of the urinary system begins as the mesonephric ducts emerge and connect with the cloaca. Between the fourth and fifth weeks, two ureteric buds develop

from the mesonephric (Wolffian) ducts and begin to grow cephalad toward the mesonephros. As each bud lengthens, it induces differentiation of the metanephros, which will become the kidney. The genital system begins development when the müllerian (paramesonephric) ducts form bilaterally between the developing gonad and the mesonephros. The müllerian ducts extend downward and laterally to the mesonephric ducts. They finally turn medially to meet and fuse together in the midline. The fused müllerian duct descends to the urogenital sinus to join the müllerian tubercle behind the cloaca. The close association between the müllerian and mesonephric ducts has clinical relevance. Damage to either duct system is often associated with anomalies that involve the uterine horn, kidney, and ureter.

The uterus is formed by the union of the two müllerian ducts at about the 10th week. Fusion begins in the middle and then extends caudally and cephalad. The characteristic uterine shape is then formed, with cellular proliferation at the upper portion and a simultaneous dissolution of cells at the lower pole, thus establishing the first uterine cavity. This cavity is formed at the lower pole, whereas a thick wedge of tissue lies above it, which is the septum. As the septum is slowly resorbed, it creates the uterine cavity, which is usually completed by the 20th week. Failure of fusion of the two müllerian ducts leads to separate uterine horns, whereas failure of cavitation between them results in some degree of persistent uterine septum. Uncommonly, there is cervical and vaginal duplication associated with a septate uterus. This supports Müller's alternative hypothesis that fusion and absorption begin at the isthmus and progress in both cranial and caudad directions simultaneously.

The uterovaginal canal is the distal end of the fused müllerian ducts. The vagina forms between the urogenital sinus and the müllerian tubercle by a dissolution of the cell cord between the two structures. It is believed that this dissolution starts at the hymen and moves upward toward the cervix. Failure of this process is associated with persistence of the cell cord. *Vaginal*

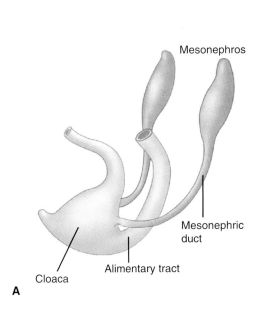

A

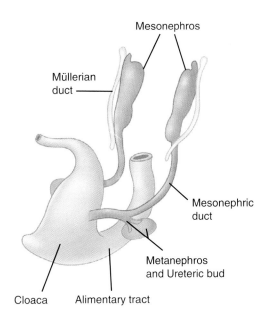

B

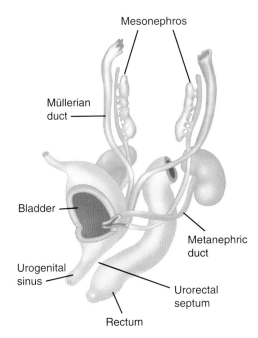

C

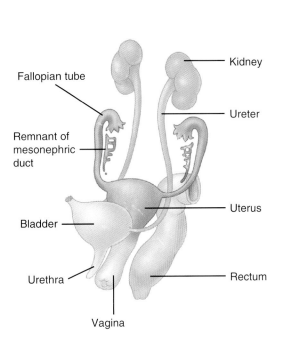

D

FIGURE 40-1 Development of the female reproductive systems from the genital ducts and urogenital sinus. Vestigial structures are also shown. **A.** Reproductive system at 6 weeks before differentiation. **B.** In the female, the müllerian (paramesonephric) ducts grow downward and extend to enter the urogenital sinus, after which they become fused. **C.** Uterine cavitation occurs at site of fused müllerian ducts and the uterus continues downward growth. **D.** Cavitation is complete and the lower segment and cervix, along with the upper vagina, are formed. (Reprinted from Schorge J, Schaffer J, Halvorson L, et al: *Williams Gynecology*, p. 403. Copyright © 2008 The McGraw-Hill Companies, Inc.)

agenesis is the result of either failed caudal migration of the fused müllerian duct or incomplete cell cord resorption. The latter may result in complete vaginal obstruction, or, if less severe, partial persistence and a *vaginal septum.*

The cephalad portion of the urogenital sinus forms the bladder. The caudal portion of the mesonephric ducts penetrates the trigone area. Later, metanephric ducts penetrate nearby and will become the ureters. The close association of the mesonephric–Wolffian and paramesonephric-müllerian ducts explains why there are commonly simultaneous abnormalities involving these

structures. *Bladder exstrophy* is likely caused by abnormalities from failure of ingrowth of supporting mesoderm. For a more detailed discussion, see Bradshaw (2008) in *Williams Gynecology.*

Genesis and Classification of Müllerian Abnormalities

Because fusion of the two müllerian ducts forms the upper two thirds of the vagina as well as the cervix and uterus, the principal groups of deformities arising from three types of embryological defects can be classified as follows:

TABLE 40-1. American Fertility Society Classification of Müllerian Anomalies

I.	**Segmental müllerian hypoplasia or agenesis**
	a. Vaginal
	b. Cervical
	c. Uterine fundus
	d. Tubal
	e. Combined anomalies
II.	**Unicornuate uterus**
	a. Communicating rudimentary horn
	b. Noncommunicating horn
	c. No endometrial cavity
	d. No rudimentary horn
III.	**Uterine didelphys**
IV.	**Bicornuate uterus**
	a. Complete—division to internal os
	b. Partial
V.	**Septate uterus**
	a. Complete—septum to internal os
	b. Partial
VI.	**Arcuate**
VII.	**Diethylstilbestrol related**

Adapted from the American Fertility Society (1988).

1. Defective canalization of the vagina resulting in a transverse septum, or in the most extreme form, vaginal agenesis
2. Unilateral maturation of the müllerian duct with incomplete or absent development of the opposite duct resulting in defects associated with upper urinary tract abnormalities
3. Absent or faulty midline fusion of the müllerian ducts–the most common defect. Complete lack of fusion results in two entirely separate uteri, cervices, and vaginas. Incomplete tissue resorption between the two fused müllerian ducts results in a uterine septum. Fusion anomalies are thought to be polygenic or multifactorial (see Chap. 12, p. 280).

Various classifications of these anomalies have been proposed. As shown in Table 40-1, the American Fertility Society uses one suggested by Buttram and Gibbons (1979), which is based on failure of normal development. It separates a diversity of anomalies into groups with similar clinical characteristics, prognosis for pregnancy, and treatment. It includes a category for abnormalities associated with fetal exposure to diethylstilbestrol (DES). Vaginal anomalies have not been classified because they are not associated with fetal loss. In the current classification, they are most often associated with uterine didelphys and bicornuate anomalies. Class I segmental defects as shown in Figure 40-2 can affect the vagina, cervix, uterus, or tubes.

Vulvar Abnormalities

Complete *vulvar atresia* involves the introitus and lower third of the vagina. In most cases, however, atresia is incomplete and re-

sults from adhesions or scars following injury or infection. The defect may present a considerable obstacle to vaginal delivery, and although the resistance usually is overcome, deep perineal tears may result.

Labial fusion in adult women is most commonly due to classical congenital adrenal hyperplasia (see Chap. 4, p. 102). Other causes include fetal exogenous androgen exposure or abdominal wall defects. *Imperforate hymen* is persistence of the fusion between the sinovaginal bulbs at the vestibules. Typically, it is associated with primary amenorrhea and hematocolpos and is not encountered often during pregnancy.

Vaginal Abnormalities

Developmental abnormalities of the normal single vagina include:

1. Vaginal agenesis
2. Vaginal atresia
3. Double vagina
4. Longitudinal vaginal septum
5. Transverse vaginal septum

Obstetrical Significance

With complete müllerian agenesis, pregnancy is impossible because the uterus and vagina are absent. **About one third of women with vaginal atresia have associated urological abnormalities.** *Complete vaginal atresia*, unless corrected operatively, obviously precludes pregnancy by vaginal intercourse (American College of Obstetricians & Gynecologists, 2006). *Incomplete atresia* can be a manifestation of faulty development, as shown in Figure 40-2, or the result of scarring from injury or inflammation as discussed subsequently. In most cases of partial atresia, because of pregnancy-induced tissue softening, obstruction during labor is gradually overcome.

A *complete longitudinal vaginal septum* usually does not cause dystocia because half of the vagina through which the fetus descends dilates satisfactorily. An incomplete septum, however, occasionally interferes with descent. Sometimes the upper vagina is separated from the rest of the canal by a *transverse septum* with a small opening. Some of these are associated with in utero exposure to DES and are discussed on page 897. Such strictures may be mistaken for the upper limit of the vaginal vault. If so, at the time of labor, the septal opening is misidentified as an undilated cervical os. After the external os has dilated completely, the head impinges on the septum and causes it to bulge downward. If the septum does not yield, slight pressure on its opening usually leads to further dilatation, but occasionally cruciate incisions are required to permit delivery (Blanton and Rouse, 2003).

Cervical Abnormalities

There are a number of anatomical and developmental anomalies of the normal single cervix:

1. *Atresia.* The entire cervix may fail to develop. This may be combined with incomplete development of the upper vagina or lower uterus (see Fig. 40-2)

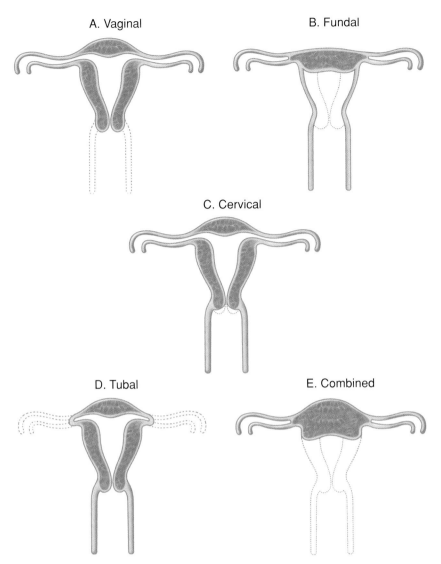

A. Vaginal

B. Fundal

C. Cervical

D. Tubal

E. Combined

FIGURE 40-2 Class I müllerian anomaly: Segmental müllerian agenesis or hypoplasia (*hatched areas*).

2. *Double cervix.* Both septate and true double cervices are frequently associated with a longitudinal vaginal septum. Many septate cervices are erroneously classified as double

3. *Single hemicervix*

4. *Septate cervix.* This consists of a single muscular ring partitioned by a septum. The septum may be confined to the cervix, or more often, it may be the downward continuation of a uterine septum or the upward extension of a vaginal septum.

Obstetrical Significance

Uncorrected complete cervical atresia is incompatible with natural conception. Deffarges and colleagues (2001) reported six successful pregnancies in four women with cervical atresia after creation of a uterovaginal anastomosis.

Uterine Malformations

Some of the large variety of congenital uterine malformations are listed in Table 40-1, and examples shown in Figure 40-3.

Although some are simply innocuous oddities, others may preclude normal procreation. Their incidence in all women is about 0.5 percent. Nahum (1998) reviewed 22 studies with more than 573,000 women who were screened for these malformations. Overall, the incidence was 1 in 200—it was about 1 in 600 for fertile women and 1 in 30 for those who were infertile. The distribution of uterine anomalies was as follows: bicornuate, 39 percent; septate, 24 percent; didelphic, 11 percent; arcuate, 7 percent; and hypo- or aplastic, 4 percent. Müllerian anomalies associated with recurrent pregnancy loss are discussed in Chapter 9 (p. 218).

Diagnosis

Some uterine anomalies are discovered by routine pelvic examination. Frequently, they are discovered at cesarean delivery. Others are first discovered at laparoscopy, for example, at the time of tubal sterilization. Several radiological modalities can aid diagnosis. However, each has diagnostic limitations, and thus they may be used in combination to completely define anatomy (Olpin and Heilbrun, 2009). Sonographic screening for uterine anomalies, while specific, is not sensitive (Nicolini and associates, 1987). Sonohysterography can be used to differentiate septate and bicornuate uteri (Alborzi and associates, 2002). In some cases, hysteroscopy and hysterosalpingography (HSG) are of value in ascertaining the configuration of the uterine cavity. In yet other cases, magnetic resonance (MR) imaging may be necessary to delineate müllerian duct anomalies and their extent. Although MR imaging is more expensive, it has a reported accuracy of up to 100 percent in evaluation of müllerian duct anomalies (Fedele and co-workers, 1989; Pellerito and colleagues, 1992).

Urological Defects

Asymmetrical reproductive tract abnormalities are frequently associated with urinary tract anomalies. When unilateral uterine atresia is present or when one side of a double vagina terminates blindly, an ipsilateral urological anomaly is common (Fedele and associates, 1987; Heinonen, 1983, 1984).

Auditory Defects

Up to a third of women with müllerian defects will have auditory defects (Letterie and Vauss, 1991). Typically these are sensorineural hearing deficits in the high-frequency range.

Uterine Anomalies in Wilms Tumor Survivors

This rare malignancy appears to be associated with an increased incidence of congenital urinary and reproductive tract anomalies

A-1a. Communicating   A-1b. Noncommunicating

A-2. No cavity   B. No horn

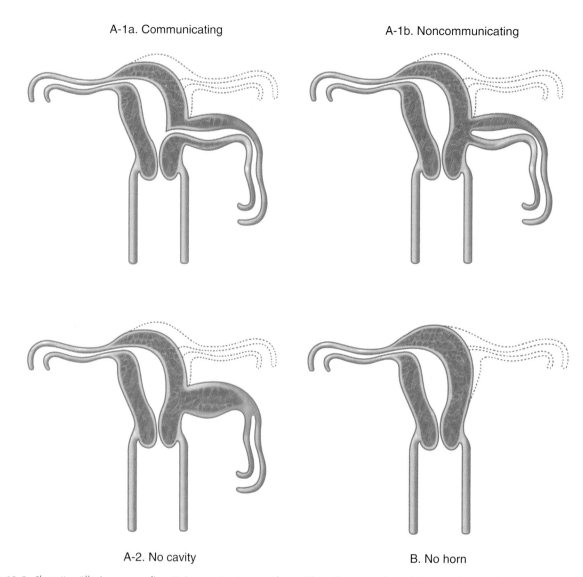

FIGURE 40-3 Class II müllerian anomalies: Unicornuate uterus either with rudimentary horn (**A**) or without rudimentary horn (**B**). Those with a rudimentary horn are divided into groups with an endometrial cavity (**A-1**) or without an endometrial cavity (**A-2**). Those with an endometrial cavity either have a communication with the opposite uterine horn (**A-1-a**) or do not have a communication with the opposite horn (**A-1-b**). Hatching reflects the expected normal anatomy that is absent in these anomalies.

(Nicholson and colleagues, 1996). This might partially explain the increased rate of infertility reported in female survivors.

Obstetrical Significance

Major difficulties arise from many uterine anomalies. Defects that result from development of only one müllerian duct, or from lack of fusion, often give rise to a hemiuterus that fails to dilate and hypertrophy appropriately (Fig. 40-3). This may result in miscarriage, ectopic pregnancy, rudimentary horn pregnancy, preterm delivery, fetal growth restriction, abnormal fetal lie, uterine dysfunction, or uterine rupture (Ben-Rafael and associates, 1991; Michalas, 1991). In 64 women with a variety of uterine anomalies, Airoldi and associates (2005) found that midtrimester sonographic assessment of cervical length was fairly accurate for predicting preterm birth.

Valli and colleagues (2001) reported a 32-percent recurrent miscarriage rate in 344 women with a septate or unicornuate uterus compared with 6 percent in 922 control women. Miscarriage is even increased in women whose only anomaly is a uterine septum (Buttram and Gibbons, 1979; Raga and associates, 1997). That said, the American College of Obstetricians and Gynecologists (2001) cautions that repair of such defects may not prevent miscarriage. Anomalies may cause late pregnancy complications as well. Ravasia and colleagues (1999) reported that two of 25 women–8 percent–with a müllerian anomaly who underwent a trial of labor after cesarean delivery experienced uterine rupture. Tikkanen and associates (2006) found an eight-fold increased incidence of placental abruption in women with uterine anomalies.

Unicornuate Uterus (Class II). In a series of 1160 uterine anomalies, Zanetti and associates (1978) reported the incidence of unicornuate uterus diagnosed by HSG to be 14 percent. HSG, however, cannot be used to identify a noncommunicating rudimentary horn–by far the more common type.

TABLE 40-2. Pregnancy Outcomes in Women with a Unicornuate Uterus

Outcome	Heinonen 1983	Moutos 1992	Acien 1993	Fedele 1995	Total
Patients	15	20	24	26	85
Pregnancies	35	36[a]	55	57	183
Spontaneous abortions (%)[b]	4 (11)	13 (36)	12 (22)	33 (58)	62 (34)
Ectopic pregnancies (%)[b]	4 (11)	1 (2.8)	1 (1.8)	3 (5.2)[c]	9 (5)
Deliveries (%)[b]	27 (77)	22 (61)	42 (76)	21 (37)	112 (61)
Breech presentations[d]	9 (33)	—	13 (31)	—	
Cesarean deliveries[d]	8 (30)	8 (36)	—	—	
Preterm deliveries[d]	4 (15)	3 (14)	9 (21)	5 (24)	21 (19)
Term deliveries[d]	23 (85)	19 (86)	33 (79)	16 (76)	91 (81)
Fetal survival (%)[b]	25 (71)	21 (58)	39 (71)	20 (35)	105 (57)

[a]Excludes four elective abortions.
[b]Of all pregnancies.
[c]Includes one blind-horn pregnancy.
[d]Excludes abortions and ectopic pregnancies.

Women with a unicornuate uterus have an increased incidence of infertility, endometriosis, and dysmenorrhea (Fedele and associates, 1987, 1995; Heinonen, 1983). Obstetrical outcomes from a number of studies are shown in Table 40-2. Implantation in the normal-sized hemiuterus is associated with increased incidences of spontaneous abortion, preterm delivery, and intrauterine fetal demise (Reichman and co-workers, 2009).

Pregnancies in the rudimentary horn are usually disastrous (Fig. 40-4). Rolen and associates (1966) reported that uterine rupture occurred prior to 20 weeks in most of 70 rudimentary horn pregnancies. Nahum (2002) reviewed the literature from 1900 to 1999 and identified 588 such pregnancies. Half had uterine rupture, and 80 percent of these were before the third trimester. Of the total 588, neonatal survival was only 6 percent. Most of the 23 maternal deaths were before 1950. More liberal use of high-resolution sonography and MR imaging may result in an earlier diagnosis of rudimentary horn pregnancy, allowing surgical or medical therapy before rupture (Edelman, 2003; Vo, 2003; Worley, 2008, and all their colleagues).

Uterine Didelphys (Class III). This anomaly is distinguished from bicornuate and septate uteri by the presence of complete nonfusion of the cervix and hemiuterine cavity (Fig. 40-5). Heinonen (1984) reported that all 26 women with a uterine didelphys had a longitudinal vaginal septum as well. Occasionally, one hemivagina is obstructed by an oblique or transverse vaginal septum (Asha, 2008; Coskun, 2008; Hinckley, 2003, and all their associates).

Except for ectopic and rudimentary horn pregnancies, problems associated with uterine didelphys are similar but less frequent than those seen with unicornuate uterus. Heinonen (1984) reported 70 percent successful pregnancy outcomes. There was preterm delivery in 20 percent, fetal-growth restriction in 10 percent, and breech presentation in 43 percent. The cesarean delivery rate was 82 percent. Multifetal gestation is unusual in these women (Oláh, 2002).

An increasing number of cases have been described in which there is a septate uterus—instead of two hemiuteri—along with a duplicated cervix and longitudinal

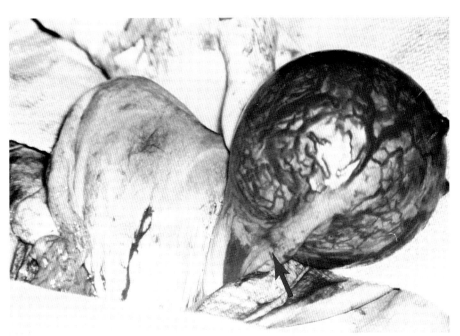

FIGURE 40-4 A 15-week pregnancy in a woman with three prior vaginal breech deliveries. As seen at laparotomy, the pregnancy is in the left noncommunicating rudimentary uterine horn. The attached fallopian tube (*arrow*) was patent.

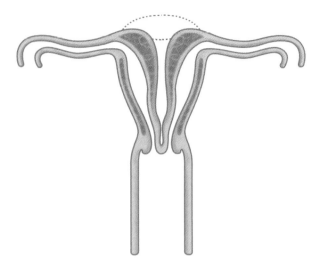

FIGURE 40-5 Class III müllerian anomaly: Uterine didelphys.

vaginal septum (Patton, 2004; Pavone, 2006; Saygili-Yilmaz, 2004, and all their colleagues). And Varras and colleagues (2007) described such duplication with a single, nonseptate uterine cavity. These constellations of features do not fit into the standard classification scheme (Table 40-1).

Bicornuate and Septate Uteri (Classes IV and V). In both of these types of anomalies–shown in Figures 40-6 and 40-7, there is a marked increase in miscarriages that is likely due to the abundant muscle tissue in the septum (Dabirashrafi and colleagues, 1995). In addition, abnormal endometrium overlying the uterine septum may lead to abnormal implantation or defective early embryo development and subsequent miscarriage (Candiani and co-workers, 1983; Fedele and colleagues, 1996). Of the two defects, miscarriage with a septate uterus is more common (Proctor and Haney, 2003). Pregnancy losses in the first 20 weeks were reported by Buttram and Gibbons (1979) to be 70 percent for bicornuate and 88 percent for septate uteri. Woelfer and colleagues (2001) reported a first-trimester loss rate for septate uteri of 42 percent. The majority of women with müllerian anomalies

A. Complete   B. Partial

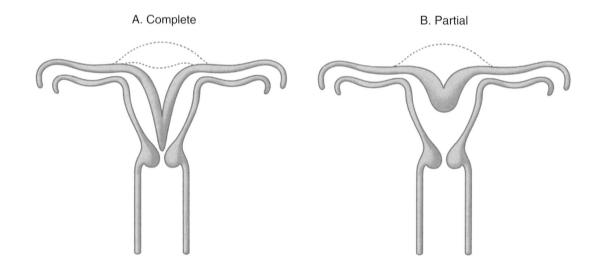

C. Arcuate

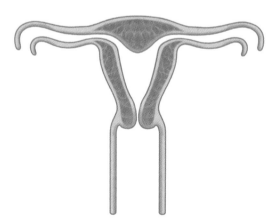

FIGURE 40-6 Class IV müllerian anomaly: Complete bicornuate uterus **(A)** and partial **(B)**. Class VI arcuate uterus **(C)**.

A. Complete   B. Partial

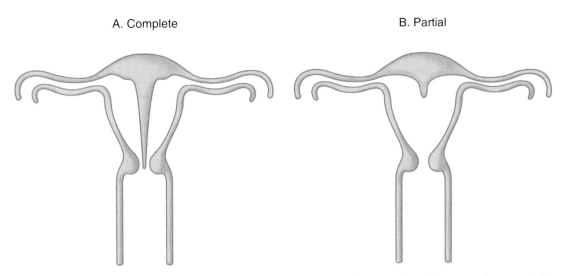

FIGURE 40-7 Class V müllerian anomaly: Septate uterus with complete septum to the cervical os **(A)** or partial septum **(B)**.

have lateral placental implantation with poor perinatal outcomes (Leible and associates, 1998). There also is an increased incidence of preterm delivery, abnormal fetal lie, and cesarean delivery. Heinonen (1999) described three newborns with a limb-reduction defect born to women with a septate uterus.

Arcuate Uterus (Class VI). This malformation is only a mild deviation from the normally developed uterus. Raga and associates (1997) reported no impact on reproductive outcomes. Conversely, Woelfer and colleagues (2001) found excessive second-trimester losses and preterm labor.

Management

Women with nonobstructive defects such as uterine didelphys and unicornuate uterus usually do not need surgical correction (Stenchever, 2001). Although abnormal fetal presentation is common, external cephalic version is less likely to be successful.

Cerclage. A number of investigators have reported that cervical cerclage in women with some of these anomalies and repetitive pregnancy losses may improve outcomes (Golan, 1990b, 1992; Golan and Caspi, 1992; Maneschi, 1988; Seidman, 1991, and all their co-workers). Transabdominal cerclage may offer the best prognosis for women with partial cervical atresia or hypoplasia (Hampton and colleagues, 1990; Mackey and co-workers, 2001). Transvaginal cerclage has been used successfully in DES-exposed women with cervical hypoplasia (Ludmir and co-workers, 1991).

Cerclage should not be done simply because a uterine septum has been resected. It probably should still be used following abdominal metroplasties for uterine didelphys and bicornuate uteri. If active labor supervenes, the cervical ligature is removed to prevent uterine rupture. Cerclage is discussed in detail in Chapter 9 (p. 219).

Metroplasty. Women with septate or bicornuate anomalies and poor reproductive outcomes may benefit from uterine surgery (Lolis and associates, 2005; Papp and co-workers, 2006). Repair of a bicornuate uterus is by transabdominal metroplasty

involving septal resection and fundal recombination (Candiani and associates, 1990).

Repair of a septate uterus is usually by hysteroscopic septal resection (Grimbizis and colleagues, 1998; Pabuccu and Gomel, 2004). Some prefer transabdominal surgery (Papp and colleagues, 2006). In a review of pregnancy outcomes following repair of a septate uterus, Stenchever (2001) reported that about half of 351 pregnancies resulted in a liveborn infant. Preterm labor is common (Litta and colleagues, 2004). Despite minimal operative uterine wall invasion, disastrous fundal rupture has been reported (Angell and co-workers, 2002).

Diethylstilbestrol-Induced Reproductive Tract Abnormalities

Through the early 1960s, diethylstilbestrol (DES), a synthetic nonsteroidal estrogen, was prescribed for an estimated 3 million pregnant women in the United States to treat abortion, preeclampsia, diabetes, and preterm labor. Although the drug was remarkably *ineffective* for these indications, Herbst and co-workers (1971) discovered that fetal DES exposure was linked to the later development of rare vaginal clear cell adenocarcinoma. Subsequently, it was found that women exposed as fetuses also had an increased risk of developing cervical intraepithelial neoplasia, small-cell cervical carcinoma, vaginal adenosis, and several non-neoplastic structural abnormalities. Although most, if not all, of women exposed as fetuses have passed childbearing age, a summary of this pharmaceutical debacle follows.

About a fourth of women exposed to DES in utero have identifiable structural variations in the cervix and vagina (Swan, 2000). These are in class VII of the American Fertility Society (1988) and include transverse septa, circumferential ridges involving the vagina and cervix, and cervical collars. Smaller uterine cavities, shortened upper uterine segments, and T-shaped and irregular cavities have also been described, as well as oviduct abnormalities (Barranger and associates, 2002).

In general, DES-exposed women have impaired conception rates possibly associated with cervical hypoplasia and atresia (Palmer and colleagues, 2001; Senekjian and co-workers, 1988). Their incidences of miscarriage, ectopic pregnancy, and preterm delivery are also increased, especially in women with structural abnormalities (Goldberg and Falcone, 1999; Kaufman and associates, 1984, 2000). Exposed women enter menopause slightly earlier than nonexposed controls (Hatch and co-workers, 2006). Spontaneous uterine rupture with pregnancy is more likely and was reported as early as 12 weeks (Porcu and colleagues, 2003). The risk of ectopic pregnancy is increased at least fourfold. Finally, an increased incidence of cervical incompetence is associated with midpregnancy losses and preterm delivery (Ludmir and colleagues, 1987).

Transgenerational Anomalies

Genital tract anomalies have been described in the offspring of women exposed to DES *when they were a fetus*. Felix and colleagues (2007) recently discussed a possible transgenerational association with tracheoesophageal anomalies (see Chap. 14, p. 322).

ACQUIRED REPRODUCTIVE TRACT ABNORMALITIES

Vulvar Abnormalities

A number of acute and chronic vulvar conditions may prove vexing to both the woman and her obstetrician.

Edema

Many women have some degree of vulvar edema during pregnancy. At times, it can be impressive and without an identifiable pathological cause. In women with the nephrotic syndrome and hypoproteinemia, vulvar edema may be problematic as early as midpregnancy (see Fig. 48-6, p. 1044). During labor, the vulva may become edematous, especially in women with severe preeclampsia. Venous thromboses and hematomas occasionally cause edema and significant pain. In postpartum women, edema associated with a paravaginal, vulvar, or perineal hematoma arising from lacerations or an episiotomy may be extensive (see Chap. 35, p. 783).

Inflammatory Lesions

Extensive perineal inflammation and scarring from *hidradenitis suppurativa*, *lymphogranuloma venereum*, or *Crohn disease* may create difficulty with vaginal delivery, episiotomy, and repair. A mediolateral episiotomy may prevent some of these difficulties. McCarthy-Keith and Coggins (2008) described a woman with a known perineal endometrioma that grew slightly but became more painful during pregnancy.

Bartholin Gland Lesions

Cysts of the Bartholin gland duct are usually sterile and need no treatment during pregnancy. If the cysts are large enough to cause difficulty at delivery, then needle aspiration as a temporary measure is sufficient. If the gland is infected, there is ten-

derness accompanying vulvar edema. Treatment is given with broad-spectrum antimicrobials, and if there is an abscess, drainage is established. Cultures for *Neisseria gonorrhoeae* and *Chlamydia trachomatis* are obtained. For a large abscess with extensive cellulitis, drainage is best performed in the operating room. The cut edges of the abscess cavity are marsupialized and packed with gauze, which is removed the next day. Alternatively, a Word catheter may be used. In some cases, especially in diabetic or immunocompromised women, life-threatening *necrotizing fasciitis* may develop (see Chap. 31, p. 669).

Urethral and Bladder Lesions

Infections may cause periurethral abscesses that usually resolve spontaneously, but some become asymptomatic cysts. Urethral diverticula are associated with recurrent urinary infections. From their review, Patel and Chapple (2006) recommend MR imaging for evaluation. Drainage may be necessary, but in general, excision of cysts or diverticula is not performed during pregnancy.

Bladder lesions are uncommon, but obstructed labor by stones has been reported (Penning and associates, 1997; Rai and Ramesh, 1998). Occasionally, *bladder tumors* may require cesarean delivery (Hendry, 1997).

Condyloma Acuminata

Genital infection with the sexually transmitted human papillomavirus (HPV) results in condyloma acuminata–also called *venereal warts*. Rarely, they are so extensive that they preclude vaginal or vulvar distension and prohibit vaginal delivery (see Chap. 59, p. 1245). The newly approved quadrivalent HPV vaccines are expected to prevent some of these (Garland and colleagues, 2007).

Female Genital Mutilation

Inaccurately called female circumcision, mutilation refers to medically unnecessary vulvar and perineal modification. According to the World Health Organization (2006), forms of female genital mutilation are practiced in countries throughout Africa, the Middle East, and Asia. As many as 130 million women have undergone one of these procedures, and approximately 230,000 live in the United States (Nour and colleagues, 2006). Cultural sensitivity is imperative, because many women may be offended by the suggestion that they have been mutilated (American College of Obstetricians and Gynecologists, 2002).

The World Health Organization (2000) classifies genital mutilations into four types shown in Table 40-3. Other commonly used terms include *sunna* for type I, *excision* for type II, and *infibulation* or *pharaonic circumcision* for type III. A type I procedure performed under sterile conditions, which is often not the case, rarely has long-term adverse physical consequences (Toubia, 1994). A type III extreme form of mutilation consists of the removal of the entire clitoris and labia minora, and at least two thirds of the labia majora (Fig. 40-8). The procedure is typically performed on girls 7 years of age without anesthesia by midwives or village women. Commonly used instruments are razor blades, kitchen knives, scissors, glass, and even the teeth of the midwife. The two vulvar edges are stitched together by silk or catgut or are held together by thorns. A small open-

TABLE 40-3. World Health Organization Classification of Female Genital Mutilation

Type I	Excision of the prepuce with or without excision of the clitoris
Type II	Excision of the clitoris and partial or total excision of the labia minora
Type III	Excision of part or all of the external genitalia and infibulation
Type IV	Unclassified and includes pricking, piercing, incision, stretching, and introduction of corrosive substances into the vagina

Adapted from the World Health Organization, 1997.

ing—usually made by the insertion of a matchstick—is left for the passage of menstrual blood and urine. The legs of the girl are then bound from hip to ankle for as many as 40 days so that scar tissue will form. Immediate dangers are exsanguination and severe infections. Urinary retention is common.

Long-term sequelae depend on the severity of mutilation. Okonofua and associates (2002) reported that half of women attending clinics in Nigeria had been mutilated. Of these, 70 percent had undergone type I and 25 percent type II procedures. These women had normal sexual function but a threefold risk of vaginal infection or genital ulcers. Complications of type III procedures include sterility, dysmenorrhea, dyspareunia, and propensity to HIV infection (Almroth and co-workers, 2005; Chen and

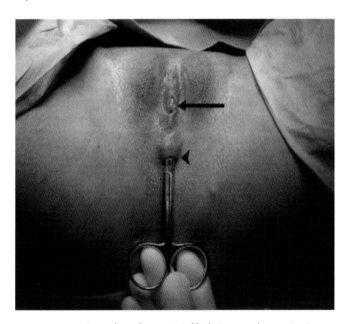

FIGURE 40-8 Sequelae of type III infibulation or pharaonic circumcision. This ritual mutilation procedure included clitoridectomy, excision of labia minora, and incision of labia majora. Remnant labia majora have been approximated, leaving a small neointroitus (*arrowhead*) into which scissors are inserted. The arrow points to the clitoris. (Reprinted from Nour NM, Michels KB, and Bryant AE: Defibulation to treat female genital cutting: Effect on symptoms and sexual function, *Obstetrics & Gynecology*, 2006, vol. 108, no. 1, pp. 55–60, with permission.)

associates, 2004; Nour, 2004, 2006). Neuroma formation after clitoral amputation has also been described (Fernández-Aguilar and Noël, 2003). In another case, a urinary calculus formed under an infibulation scar from urine stagnation (Nour, 2006).

In general, women with significant symptoms following type III procedures are candidates for surgical defibulation, also referred to as deinfibulation.

Legislation to Prohibit Mutilations. The American College of Obstetricians and Gynecologists (2002), along with the International Federation of Gynecology and Obstetrics, the American Medical Association, the United Nations International Children's Emergency Fund, and the World Health Organization, has supported legislation to eliminate female genital mutilation. The American Academy of Pediatrics (1998) encourages development of community educational programs for immigrant populations. In the United States it is a federal crime to perform unnecessary genital surgery on a girl younger than 18 years. In some countries where female genital mutilation has been routinely performed, laws are being enacted to prohibit such mutilation (Ciment, 1999; Cook and colleagues, 2002; Eke and Nkanginieme, 1999).

Pregnancy Complications. There are a number of associated adverse maternal and neonatal complications, and the degree of mutilation correlates with their incidence. The World Health Organization (2006) estimated that these procedures *increased* perinatal morbidity rates by 10 to 20 per 1000.

For those women who do not desire deinfibulation until they become pregnant, the procedure can be done at midpregnancy using spinal analgesia (Nour and colleagues, 2006). Another option is to wait until delivery, at which time scarred tissue is incised between the index and middle fingers inserted between the crowning fetal head and the scar. In our experiences, in many cases, intrapartum deinfibulation allows successful vaginal delivery without major complications.

Vaginal Abnormalities

Acquired vaginal abnormalities are uncommon. Even after major trauma, long-term sexual and reproductive function is usually normal (Fallat and colleagues, 1998). Vaginal stenosis may develop as a result of mucositis from graft-versus-host reaction following organ transplantation (Louis-Sylvestre and associates, 2003).

Partial Atresia

Incomplete atresia may result from infection or trauma that leads to extensive scarring. During labor, this is usually overcome by pressure from the presenting part, but occasionally incisions or even cesarean delivery are necessary.

Genital Tract Fistulas

Fistulas found during pregnancy likely existed previously, but in rare cases they develop during pregnancy. McKay and Hanlon (2003) described a *vesicovaginal fistula* following a McDonald cerclage done at 20 weeks. In prolonged obstructed labor, the genital tract may be compressed between the fetal head and the bony pelvis. Brief pressure is not significant, but prolonged pressure may result in necrosis with subsequent fistula formation. Miklos and colleagues (1995) described a *vesicouterine fistula* that developed following vaginal delivery after prior cesarean delivery. Rarely, the anterior cervical lip is compressed against the symphysis pubis with development of a *vesicocervical fistula*. In an unusual case, after 5 days of obstructed labor at home, a psychotic woman presented with sepsis from necrosis of the bladder and uterus (Korell and co-workers, 2007).

In some cases, these fistulas heal spontaneously, but subsequent repair may be necessary. Murray and associates (2002) report a high rate of successful closures performed in more than 15,000 cases at The Fistula Hospital in Addis Ababa, Ethiopia. Unfortunately, urinary incontinence persisted in 55 percent. Wall (2002) has provided a poignant chronicle of the societal impact of obstetrical fistulas on Nigerian culture.

Cervical Abnormalities

Cicatricial *cervical stenosis* is uncommon, but it may follow cervical trauma such as conization. Cryotherapy occasionally produces stenosis, but the loop electrosurgical excision procedure (LEEP) and laser surgery usually do not (Mathevet and associates, 2003a). Overall, both surgical and laser conization or loop excision for cervical intraepithelial neoplasia increase preterm delivery (Albrechtsen, 2008; Kyrgiou, 2006; Samson, 2005, and all their co-workers). Cervical stenosis almost always yields during labor. A so-called *conglutinated cervix* may undergo almost complete effacement without dilation, with the presenting part separated from the vagina by only a thin layer of cervical tissue. Dilatation usually promptly follows pressure with a fingertip, although manual dilatation or cruciate incisions may be required. Incompetent cervix is discussed in Chapter 36. Finally, extensive *cervical carcinoma* may impair vaginal delivery (see Chap. 57, p. 1201).

Uterine Abnormalities

A number of acquired uterine abnormalities may adversely affect pregnancy as well as fertility.

Anteflexion

Exaggerated degrees of anteflexion frequently observed in early pregnancy are without significance. In later months, particularly when the abdominal wall is very lax, the uterus may fall forward. This may be so exaggerated that the fundus lies below the lower margin of the symphysis. Marked anteflexion usually is associated with *diastasis recti* and a pendulous abdomen. The abnormal uterine position sometimes prevents proper transmission of contractions, however, this is usually overcome by repositioning and application of an abdominal binder.

Retroflexion

The growing normally retroflexed uterus will occasionally remain incarcerated in the hollow of the sacrum. Symptoms include abdominal discomfort, pelvic pressure, and voiding

disorders. As pressure from the full bladder increases, small amounts of urine are passed involuntarily, but the bladder never empties entirely—so called *paradoxical incontinence*. Acute urinary retention is common in our experience and was described by Myers and Scotti (1995). Such blockage also can cause severe obstructive nephropathy. The diagnosis is usually made on the basis of symptoms and examination. The cervix will be behind the symphysis pubis and the uterus is appreciated as a mass in the pelvis. If the diagnosis is not clear, sonography or MR imaging may clarify it (Beekhuizen and co-workers, 2003).

Incarceration is managed by repositioning the uterus (Özel, 2005). After bladder catheterization, the uterus can usually be pushed out of the pelvis when the woman is placed in the knee-chest position. Often, this is best accomplished by digital pressure applied through the rectum. Occasionally spinal analgesia or general anesthesia is necessary. Following repositioning, the catheter is left in place until bladder tone returns. Insertion of a soft pessary for a few weeks usually prevents reincarceration. Lettieri and colleagues (1994) described seven cases of uterine incarceration not amenable to these simple procedures. In two women, laparoscopy was used at 13 to 14 weeks to reposition the uterus using the round ligaments for traction. Seubert and associates (1999) used colonoscopy to dislodge an incarcerated uterus in five women. Hamoda and co-workers (2002) simply observed one woman and performed cesarean delivery of a healthy infant at 36 weeks. In a similar case described by Rose and colleagues (2008) in which a large myoma became incarcerated, there was spontaneous reduction at 20 weeks.

Sacculation

Persistent entrapment of the pregnant uterus in the pelvis may result in an anterior uterine sacculation (Fig. 40-9). Extensive dilatation of the lower uterine segment takes place to accommodate the fetus (Jackson and associates, 1988; Lettieri and co-workers, 1994). Sonography and MR imaging are typically required to define anatomy (Gottschalk and colleagues, 2008; Lee and associates, 2008). Cesarean delivery is necessary in these cases, and Spearing (1978) stressed the importance of identifying the distorted anatomy. An elongated vagina passing above the level of a fetal head that is deeply placed into the pelvis is suggestive of a sacculation or an abdominal pregnancy. The Foley catheter is frequently palpated above the level of the umbilicus! Spearing (1978) recommended extending the abdominal incision to above the umbilicus and delivery of the entire uterus from the abdomen before an attempt is made to incise it. **This procedure will restore anatomy to the correct relationships and prevent inadvertent incisions into and through the vagina and bladder.** Unfortunately, this may not always be possible to accomplish (Singh and colleagues, 2007).

Friedman and associates (1986) described a rare case of posterior uterine sacculation following aggressive treatment for intrauterine adhesions, or *Asherman syndrome*. Uterine retroversion and a true uterine diverticulum have been mistaken for uterine sacculations (Engel and Rushovich, 1984; Hill and associates, 1993; Rajiah and co-workers, 2009).

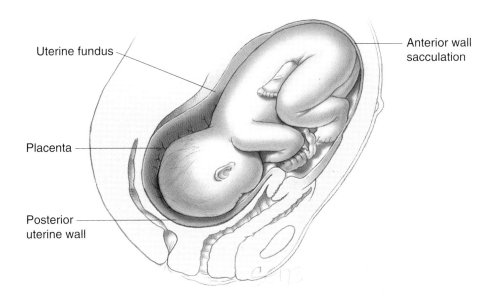

Anterior wall
sacculation

Uterine fundus

Placenta

Posterior
uterine wall

FIGURE 40-9 Anterior sacculation of a pregnant uterus. Note the markedly attenuated anterior uterine wall and atypical location of the true uterine fundus.

Uterine Prolapse

The cervix, and occasionally a portion of the uterine body, may protrude to a variable extent from the vulva during early pregnancy (Fig. 40-10). With further growth, the uterus usually rises above the pelvis and may draw the cervix up with it. If the uterus persists in its prolapsed position, symptoms of incarceration may develop from 10 to 14 weeks. To prevent this, the uterus is replaced early in pregnancy and held in position with a suitable pessary. Successful pregnancy and vaginal deliveries have been reported following sacrospinous uterosacral fixation done before

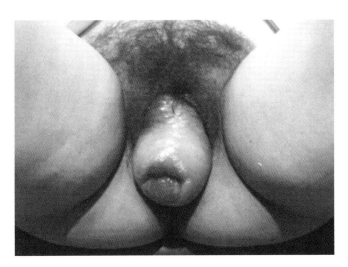

FIGURE 40-10 Uterine procidentia in a parous woman at 27 weeks. The cervix was easily reduced and was held in place by a ring pessary. Spontaneous preterm labor and uncomplicated vaginal delivery followed at 30 weeks. There was no prolapse at the postpartum examination 2 weeks later. (Courtesy of Dr. Charles P. Read.)

pregnancy (Kovac and Cruikshank, 1993).

Cystocele and Rectocele

Attenuation of fascial support between the vagina and the bladder can lead to prolapse of the bladder into the vagina, that is, a cystocele. Urinary stasis with a cystocele predisposes to infection. Pregnancy may worsen associated *urinary stress incontinence* because urethral closing pressures do not increase sufficiently to compensate for the progressively increased bladder pressure (Iosif and Ulmsten, 1981). Attenuation of rectovaginal fascia results in a rectocele. A large defect may fill with feces that occasionally can be evacuated only manually. During labor, cystocele and rectocele can block fetal descent unless they are emptied and pushed out of the way.

Enterocele

In rare instances, an enterocele of considerable size may complicate pregnancy. If symptomatic, the protrusion should be replaced, and the woman kept in a recumbent position. If the mass interferes with delivery, it should be pushed up or held out of the way.

Uterine Torsion

Rotation of the uterus, most often to the right, is common during pregnancy. Conversely, complete torsion is rare and is usually not sufficient to cause infarction. One exception reported by Cook and Jenkins (2005) was a 270-degree torsion in a 36-week pregnancy. Oláh (2002) described a case in which one horn of a bicornuate uterus became ischemic from torsion. There are other problems. In a case of severe levotorsion necessitating cesarean delivery, the hysterotomy incision was inadvertently made in the posterior uterine wall (Bakos and Axelson, 1987). Thus, as with uterine incarceration, the severely malpositioned uterus should be repositioned anatomically prior to hysterotomy. Torsion can be confused with abdominal pregnancy, and in some but not all cases, sonography or MR imaging may allow correct identification (Sherer and colleagues, 1994; Worley and associates, 2008). The vagina normally appears as an H-shaped structure but with torsion it appears X-shaped—the "X sign."

Uterine Leiomyomas

Also known as *myomas* and somewhat erroneously called *fibroids*, uterine leiomyomas are common benign smooth muscle tumors. Their incidence during pregnancy is probably about 2 percent and depends on population characteristics and the frequency of routine sonography. For example, Sheiner and co-workers (2004) cited an incidence of 0.65 percent in nearly 106,000 pregnancies. But with midtrimester sonographic screening in nearly 15,000 women, Qidwai and associates (2006) identified 2.7 percent to have at least one myoma. In a recent study of 4271 women, Laughlin and co-workers (2009) reported a first-trimester myoma prevalence of 11 percent. The prevalence was highest in black women—18 percent—and lowest in whites—8 percent.

Symptoms from leiomyomas depend principally on their location. They may be located immediately beneath the endometrial or decidual lining of the uterine cavity–*submucous*, immediately beneath the uterine serosa–*subserous*, or they may be confined within the myometrium–*intramural*. As an intramural myoma grows, it may develop a significant subserous or submucosal component, or both. Submucous and subserous myomas may be pedunculated and can undergo torsion with necrosis. At times, a subserous myoma becomes *parasitic* and derives its blood supply through the highly vascularized omentum. In one case, a large myoma was incarcerated until it spontaneously reduced at 20 weeks (Rose and colleagues, 2008).

Myomas during pregnancy occasionally undergo *red* or *carneous degeneration*, which is in actuality hemorrhagic infarction. Findings include focal pain, tenderness on palpation, and sometimes low-grade fever and leukocytosis. On occasion, the parietal peritoneum overlying the infarcted myoma becomes inflamed and a peritoneal friction rub develops. Myoma degeneration may be difficult to differentiate from appendicitis, placental abruption, ureteral stone, or pyelonephritis, and imaging techniques aid in discrimination. Treatment of symptomatic myomas consists of analgesia and observation. Most often, signs and symptoms abate within a few days, but inflammation may stimulate labor. Surgery is rarely necessary during pregnancy. An unusual exception was described by MacDonald and colleagues (2004) of small bowel obstruction due to degeneration of a pedunculated myoma. The rare form of *cotyledonoid leiomyoma* may involve bowel with fibrous adhesions (Mathew and co-workers, 2007).

Subfertility

In spite of the relatively high prevalence of myomas in young women, it is not clear whether they diminish fertility, other than by possibly causing early miscarriage (Stewart, 2001). In a review of 11 studies, Pritts (2001) concluded that only submucous myomas had a significant negative impact on fertility. He also reported that hysteroscopic myomectomy improved infertility and early miscarriage rates in women with submucous tumors. For a more detailed review, see Chapter 9 in *Williams Gynecology* (Hoffman, 2008).

Uterine Artery Embolization

Data on pregnancy outcomes following arterial embolization of uterine myomas are inconsistent despite a number of studies. Pron and colleagues (2005) described two cases of placenta previa and one of placenta accreta among 18 pregnancies following embolization. Walker and McDowell (2006) reported 56 completed pregnancies in a group of 1200 women who had undergone myoma embolization. Thirty-three women—60 percent— had successful outcomes including six preterm deliveries. However, the cesarean delivery rate was almost 75 percent, and nearly 20 percent of women had postpartum hemorrhage. In their most recent review, Goldberg and Pereira (2006) compared pregnancy outcomes following laparoscopic myomectomy versus embolization techniques. They found that miscarriage, abnormal placentation, preterm delivery, and postpartum hemorrhage were uniformly increased in women undergoing embolization procedures. The American College of Obstetricians and Gynecologists (2004) considers embolization for leiomyoma investigational or relatively contraindicated in women wishing to retain fertility. Interestingly, Rebarber and associates (2009) reported use of embolization at 20 weeks' gestation to treat a large arteriovenous malformation followed by delivery of a healthy infant at 35 weeks.

Effects of Pregnancy on Myomas

The stimulatory effects of pregnancy on the growth of uterine myomas is sometimes quite impressive. These tumors respond differently in individual women, and thus, accurate prediction of their growth is not possible. For example, in the study summarized in Table 40-4, only half of myomas changed significantly in size during pregnancy. During the first trimester, myomas of all sizes either remained unchanged or increased in size–a possible early response to increased estrogen. During the second trimester, smaller myomas–2 to 6 cm–usually remained unchanged or increased in size, whereas those larger than 6 cm became smaller–probably from initiation of estrogen receptor downregulation. Regardless of initial myoma size, during the third trimester, myomas usually remained unchanged or decreased,

TABLE 40-4. Sonographically Measured Changes in Myomas During Pregnancy—Percentage of Myomas with Change

Trimester	Small Myomas (2–6 cm) (n = 111)			Large Myomas (6–12 cm) (n = 51)		
	No Change	Increase	Decrease	No Change	Increase	Decrease
First	60	40	0	20	80	0
Second	55	30	15	40	15	50
Third	60	5	35	30	10	60

Modified from Lev-Toaff and co-workers (1987), with permission. Percentages are rounded to nearest 5 percent.

TABLE 40-5. Pregnancy Complications by Location of Myomas to Placenta

Investigators	Complication	No Contact with Placenta	Contact with Placenta
		Myoma No. (%)	
Winer-Muram et al (1984)	Bleeding and pain	5/54 (9)	8/35 (23)
	Major complications		
	Abortion	1/54 (2)	9/35 (26)
	Preterm labor	0	5/35 (14)
	Postpartum hemorrhage	0	4/35 (11)
Rice et al (1989)	Major complications		
	Preterm labor	19/79 (24)	1/14 (7)
	Abruption	2/79 (3)	8/14 (57)
	Total	48/133 (36)	35/49 (71)

reflecting estrogen receptor downregulation. Other studies have also reported increased growth of myomas in early pregnancy, but not later. The study by Neiger and co-workers (2006), who followed 72 women with 137 myomas longitudinally across pregnancy, does not reflect the findings of most others. They found no increase in mean myoma volume as pregnancy progressed.

Effects of Myomas on Pregnancy

These common tumors are associated with a number of obstetrical complications including preterm labor, placental abruption, fetal malpresentation, obstructed labor, cesarean delivery, and postpartum hemorrhage (Davis, 1990; Klatsky, 2008; Qidwai, 2006; Sheiner, 2004, and all their colleagues). In a review of pregnancy outcomes in 2065 women with leiomyoma, Coronado and co-workers (2000) reported that placental abruption and breech presentation were increased fourfold, first-trimester bleeding and dysfunctional labor twofold, and cesarean delivery sixfold. Salvador and associates (2002) reported an eightfold increased second-trimester abortion risk in women with myomas but found that genetic amniocentesis did not increase this risk.

The two factors most important in determining morbidity in pregnancy are myoma size and location (Fig. 40-11). As shown in Table 40-5, proximity of myomas to the placental implantation site is important. Specifically, abortion, placental abruption, preterm labor, and postpartum hemorrhage all are increased if the placenta is adjacent to or implanted over a myoma. Tumors in the cervix or lower uterine segment are particularly troublesome because they may obstruct labor (Fig. 40-12). In addition, cervical myomas displace the ureters laterally, and hysterectomy can be technically difficult. Large myomas may also distort anatomy, and a woman with complete vena caval obstruction by a large myoma at 17 weeks was described by Greene and colleagues (2002).

Despite these complications, Qidwai and colleagues (2006) reported a 70 percent vaginal delivery rate in women with uterine myomas that measured at least 10 cm. These data argue against empirical cesarean delivery when myomas are present. At our hos-

pitals, unless myomas clearly obstruct the birth canal, or there is another indication for cesarean delivery, we allow a trial of labor.

Imaging Studies

Sonography is indispensable to correctly identify myomas (see Fig. 40-11). Myomas can be confused with ovarian masses—both benign and malignant—as well as with molar and ectopic pregnancy, missed abortion, and bowel abnormalities (Exacoustos and Rosati, 1993). In some cases the use of color Doppler may be beneficial (Kessler and colleagues, 1993).

Magnetic resonance imaging serves as an adjunct to sonography. In comparative studies, MR-imaging techniques have been described that markedly improve the reliability of identifying uterine myomas (Schwartz and associates, 1998; Torashima and colleagues, 1998).

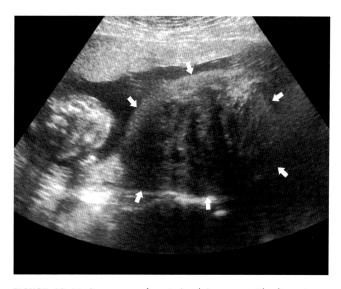

FIGURE 40-11 Sonogram of a uterine leiomyoma. The large inhomogeneous mass (*arrows*) lies beside the fetus (seen in cross section) and shows the classic appearance of a leiomyoma in pregnancy. The mass originates from the lower uterine segment and occupies greater than half of the total uterine volume.

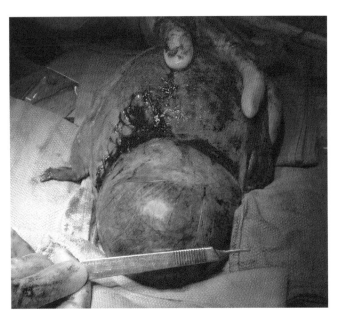

FIGURE 40-12 Cesarean delivery complicated by a large leiomyoma in the lower uterine segment. The location of the mass prompted a classical vertical uterine incision for delivery of the fetus.

Myomectomy

Resection of myomas during pregnancy is generally contraindicated. In some cases, unrelenting pain from infarction and degeneration prompts surgical treatment. We agree with most authorities that surgery should be limited to tumors with a discrete pedicle that can be clamped and easily ligated. Resection of intramural myomas during pregnancy or at the time of delivery usually stimulates profuse bleeding.

Limited data concerning indicated myomectomy during pregnancy are encouraging. De Carolis and colleagues (2001) and Celik and associates (2002) described good outcomes in 23 women. Most were between 14 and 20 weeks, and in almost half, the surgery was performed because of pain. In some of these cases, an intramural myoma was in contact with the implantation site. Except for one loss immediately following surgery at 19 weeks, most women had cesarean delivery at term. These investigators emphasize that such management is for highly selected cases. Joó and co-workers (2001) described resection at 25 weeks of a 940-g degenerating fundal myoma that caused fetal postural deformity and oligohydramnios. Postoperatively, amnionic fluid volume became normal, and later, the woman underwent cesarean delivery of a normal infant.

Intramural myomectomy in nonpregnant women can be hazardous for subsequent pregnancy. When myoma resection results in a defect into or immediately adjacent to the endometrial cavity, uterine rupture may occur remote from labor and sometimes even early in pregnancy (Golan and associates, 1990a). Prevention depends on cesarean delivery before active labor begins.

Infection of Myomas Postpartum

Although puerperal pelvic infections and myomas are both fairly common, myomas rarely become infected (Genta and col-

leagues, 2001). Most infections occur postpartum especially if the myoma is located immediately adjacent to the placental implantation site (Lin and associates, 2002). They also may become infected with a septic abortion or with myoma perforation by a sound or curette during dilatation and curettage.

Leiomyomatosis Peritonealis Disseminata

These are numerous subperitoneal smooth muscle tumors that at first appear to be disseminated carcinomatosis. The tumors are likely caused by estrogen stimulation of multicentric subcoelomic mesenchymal cells to become smooth muscle cells. From their review of 45 cases, Lashgari and colleagues (1994) found that half were discovered during pregnancy. Marom and associates (1998) as well as Ling and colleagues (2000) have described women who had tumors extending up the vena cava into the heart. Although surgical excision has been recommended, these tumors usually regress after pregnancy. Thomas and co-workers, (2007) described leiomyomatosis associated with uterine rupture and bone metastases that regressed spontaneously. Tanaka and colleagues (2009) reported two cases associated with assisted reproductive technology and accompanying high maternal estrogen concentrations.

ENDOMETRIOSIS AND ADENOMYOSIS

Although almost never symptomatic during pregnancy, occasionally endometriosis is problematic. For example, a ruptured endometrioma may cause bizarre clinical symptoms or labor dystocia. More commonly, symptoms subsequently develop from endometrial implants at the time of cesarean delivery or episiotomy (Bumpers and associates, 2002).

Adenomyosis is found in older women. Its acquisition may be at least partially related to disruption of the endometrial-myometrial border during sharp curettage for abortion (Curtis and co-workers, 2002). Although problems during pregnancy are rare, in an 80-year review, Azziz (1986) reported adenomyosis to be associated with uterine rupture, ectopic pregnancy, uterine atony, and placenta previa. Successful pregnancy may follow treatment of adenomyosis with gonadotropin-releasing hormone agonists or MR-guided focused ultrasound surgery (Rabinovici and colleagues, 2006; Silva and colleagues, 1994).

Ovarian Abnormalities

The incidence of ovarian masses during pregnancy varies depending on whether the population studied is from referral or primary care sources, the frequency with which prenatal sonography is used, and the threshold for the size of tumor. The studies listed in Table 40-6 show a variable incidence from about 1 in 100 pregnancies to 1 in 2000. Whitecar and associates (1999) described only those masses requiring laparotomy. The highest incidence was in the prospective population-based Italian study by Zanetta and associates (2003). They included almost 6650 pregnancies and found at least one mass larger than 3 cm in every 85 women.

Any type of ovarian mass can be encountered, but the most common are cystic (Table 40-6). Because pregnant women are usually young, malignant tumors, including those of low-

TABLE 40-6. Ovarian Masses Complicating Pregnancy

Investigators	No.	Size (cm)	Incidence	Pathology (Percent)				
				Teratoma	Cystadenoma	Corpus Luteum	Other Benign	Malignant[a]
Whitecar (1999)	130[b]	NS	1:1300	30	28	13	7	5
Sherard (2003)	60[c]	3+	1:630	50	20	13	—	13
Zanetta (2003)	78[d]	>3	1:85	10	—	—	50	4
Schmeler (2005)	63[c]	5+	1:2020	42	15	—	32	9
Hoffman and Sayer (2007)	1678[c]	NS	NS	27	33	14	21	4

[a]Includes tumors of low malignant potential.
[b]All managed surgically.
[c]Regional referral hospital.
[d]Population-based study.
NS = Not stated.

malignant potential, are relatively uncommon. That said, the proportion of malignant tumors in the studies shown in Table 40-6 varied from 4 to 13 percent. In our large obstetrical services in Dallas and Birmingham, the incidences are not so high. They are similar to those reported by Leiserowitz and colleagues (2006), who analyzed California hospital discharge data from 1991 through 1999. They found that only 1 percent of 9375 ovarian masses in pregnant women were frankly malignant, and another 1 percent were of low-malignant potential.

Tumors Unique to Pregnancy

Luteomas are unique to pregnancy and may be virilizing (Mazza and colleagues, 2002; Wang and associates, 2005). *Theca-lutein cysts* can be large and appear complex. They are usually seen in pregnancies with inordinately high hCG secretion–gestational trophoblastic disease, twins, and other situations with increased placental mass. The entity of *ovarian hyperstimulation syndrome* is usually caused by ovulation-induction therapy, but it may develop spontaneously in pregnancy. This phenomenon is thought to be caused by a mutation in the FSH receptor (Kaiser, 2003; Vasseur and associates, 2003).

Complications

Acute complications of ovarian masses during pregnancy include torsion or hemorrhage. Their incidence depends on tumor size and whether laparotomy is done preemptively for tumors more likely to undergo torsion. Whitecar (1999) and Zanetta (2003) and their colleagues identified torsion in 5 percent of their cases.

Management

Ovarian enlargement less than 6 cm found early in pregnancy usually represents corpus luteum formation. When high-resolution

sonography became available, Thornton and Wells (1987) proposed a conservative management approach based on sonographic characteristics. They recommended resection of all cysts suspected of rupture or torsion, those capable of obstructing labor, and those measuring more than 10 cm in diameter because of the increased risk of cancer in large cysts. Cysts 5 cm or less could be simply observed, and indeed, most undergo spontaneous resolution.

Management of masses between 5 and 10 cm diameter is controversial. Some recommend that they be managed expectantly if they have a simple cystic appearance. Whitecar and co-workers, (1999) caution against this approach, but most recent studies support it (Schmeler and colleagues, 2005). Importantly, if cysts contain septae, nodules, papillary excrescences, or solid components, then resection is recommended (Caspi and co-workers, 2000; Fleischer and associates, 1990). Women with these 5- to 10-cm cysts who are observed have been reported to require emergency exploration for rupture, torsion, or infarction in as many as half of cases (Hess and colleagues, 1988; Platek and colleagues, 1995). In our experiences, the rate is not nearly so high.

Laparoscopy is used with increased frequency to evaluate and resect intermediate-sized cysts (see Chap. 41, p. 913). The major concern is for the unrecognized malignant tumor rupturing with intraperitoneal spillage. Soriano and colleagues (1999) described maternal and fetal outcomes in 39 women undergoing laparoscopic adnexal surgery in the first trimester and in 54 who had either first- or second-trimester laparotomy and found comparable results. Akira and associates (1999) compared gasless laparoscopy with laparotomy for ovarian cystectomy in 35 women at 12 to 16 weeks and reported advantages to the laparoscopic approach. Parker and co-workers (1996) described laparoscopic resection between 9 and 17 weeks for a benign cystic teratoma in 12 women. It is worrisome that all but two of these 5- to 13-cm tumors ruptured intraoperatively, although there were no complications. Mathevet and associates (2003b) reported generally good outcomes for 47 pregnant women whose adnexal masses were resected via laparoscopy.

The major questions to be answered once a pelvic mass is discovered during pregnancy include the following:

1. What is the mass and what is the likelihood that it is malignant?
2. Is there a good possibility that the mass will regress?
3. If observed, will the mass undergo torsion or rupture, or will it be an obstruction to vaginal delivery?

Only time, serial sonographic surveillance, and labor will provide answers to the last two questions. As for the first question, Kier and associates (1990) reported that MR imaging correctly identified the origin of unknown pelvic masses in 17 of 17 women compared with 12 of 17 women in whom sonography was used. With the high-resolution equipment currently available, expectant management has become more common (Sherard and colleagues, 2003; Zanetta and co-workers, 2003). In some cases, transvaginal color Doppler assessment of tumor vascularity can be used for better characterization of adnexal tumors (Kurjak and Zalud, 1990).

Recommendations

It seems reasonable to remove all ovarian masses larger than 10 cm because of the substantive risk of malignancy and torsion. Tumors from 6 to 10 cm should be carefully evaluated for the possibility of neoplastic disease by sonography with color Doppler or MR imaging or both. If evaluation suggests a neoplasm, then resection is indicated. If the corpus luteum is removed before 10 weeks, then 17α-OH-progesterone, 250 mg intramuscularly, is given weekly until 10 weeks' gestation. Cystic masses that are thought to be benign or are less than 6 cm are imaged serially and are resected if they grow, begin to display malignant qualities, or become symptomatic. In general, we perform elective surgery at 14 to 20 weeks because most masses that will regress will have done so by this time.

Ovarian Carcinoma

Malignant ovarian neoplasms are unusual during pregnancy simply because of the young population involved. Measurement of ovarian tumor serum markers is rarely helpful during pregnancy (Zanetta and colleagues, 2003). Ovarian malignancies are discussed in Chapter 57 (see p. 1204).

REFERENCES

Acien P: Reproductive performance of women with uterine malformations. Hum Reprod 8:122, 1993

Airoldi J, Berghella V, Sehdev H, et al: Transvaginal ultrasonography of the cervix to predict preterm birth in women with uterine anomalies. Obstet Gynecol 106:553, 2005

Akira S, Yamanaka A, Ishihara T, et al: Gasless laparoscopic ovarian cystectomy during pregnancy: Comparison with laparotomy. Am J Obstet Gynecol 180:554, 1999

Alborzi S, Dehbashi S, Parsanezhad ME: Differential diagnosis of septate and bicornuate uterus by sonohysterography eliminates the need for laparoscopy. Fertil Steril 78:176, 2002

Albrechtsen S, Rasmussen S, Thoresen S, et al: Pregnancy outcome in women before and after cervical conisation: population based cohort study. BMJ 337:a1343, 2008

Almroth L, Elmusharaf S, El Hadi N, et al: Primary infertility after genital mutilation in girlhood in Sudan: A case-control study. Lancet 366:385, 2005

American Academy of Pediatrics, Committee on Bioethics: Female genital mutilation. Pediatrics 102:153, 1998

American College of Obstetricians and Gynecologists: Guidelines for Women's Health Care, 2nd ed. Washington, DC, 2002, p 305

American College of Obstetricians and Gynecologists: Management of early pregnancy loss. Practice Bulletin No. 24, February 2001

American College of Obstetricians and Gynecologists: Uterine artery embolization. Committee Opinion No. 293, February 2004

American College of Obstetricians and Gynecologists: Vaginal agenesis: Diagnosis, management, and routine care. Committee Opinion No. 355, December 2006

American Fertility Society: The American Fertility Society classifications of adnexal adhesions, distal tubal occlusion, tubal occlusion secondary to tubal ligation, tubal pregnancies, Müllerian anomalies and intrauterine adhesions. Fertil Steril 49:944, 1988

Angell NF, Domingo JT, Siddiqi N: Uterine rupture at term after uncomplicated hysteroscopic metroplasty. Obstet Gynecol 100:1098, 2002

Asha B, Manila K: An unusual presentation of uterus didelphys with obstructed hemivagina with ipsilateral renal agenesis. Fertil Steril 90(3):849.e9, 2008

Azziz R: Adenomyosis in pregnancy: A review. J Reprod Med 31:223, 1986

Bakos O, Axelsson O: Pathologic torsion of the pregnant uterus. Acta Obstet Gynecol Scand 66:85, 1987

Barranger E, Gervaise A, Doumerc S, et al: Reproductive performance after hysteroscopic metroplasty in the hypoplastic uterus: A study of 29 cases. Br J Obstet Gynaecol 109:1331, 2002

Beekhuizen van HJ, Bodewes HW, Tepe EM, et al: Role of magnetic resonance imaging in the diagnosis of incarceration of the gravid uterus. Obstet Gynecol 102:1134, 2003

Ben-Rafael Z, Seidman DS, Recabi K, et al: Uterine anomalies. A retrospective, matched-control study. J Reprod Med 36:723, 1991

Blanton EN, Rouse DJ: Trial of labor in women with transverse vaginal septa. Obstet Gynecol 101:1110, 2003

Bradshaw KB: Anatomical disorders. In Schorge JO, Schaffer JI, Halvorson LM, et al (eds): Williams Gynecology, 1st ed. New York, McGraw-Hill, 2008, p 402

Bumpers HL, Butler KL, Best IM: Endometrioma of the abdominal wall. Am J Obstet Gynecol 187:1709, 2002

Buttram VC, Gibbons WE: Müllerian anomalies: A proposed classification (an analysis of 144 cases). Fertil Steril 32:40, 1979

Candiani GB, Fedele L, Parazzini F, et al: Reproductive prognosis after abdominal metroplasty in bicornuate or septate uterus: A life table analysis. Br J Obstet Gynaecol 97:613, 1990

Candiani GB, Fedele L, Zamberletti D, et al: Endometrial patterns in malformed uteri. Acta Eur Fertil 14:311, 1983

Caspi B, Levi R, Appelman Z, et al: Conservative management of ovarian cystic teratoma during pregnancy and labor. Am J Obstet Gynecol 182:503, 2000

Celik C, Acar A, Cicek N, et al: Can myomectomy be performed during pregnancy? Gynecol Obstet Invest 53:79, 2002

Chen G, Dharia SP, Steinkampf MP, et al: Infertility from female circumcision. Fertil Steril 81:1692, 2004

Ciment J: Senegal outlaws female genital mutilation. BMJ 318:318, 1999

Coskun A, Okur N, Ozdemir O, et al: Uterus didelphys with an obstructed unilateral vagina by a transverse vaginal septum associated with ipsilateral renal agenesis, duplication of inferior vena cava, high-riding aortic bifurcation, and intestinal malrotation: a case report. Fertil Steril 90(5):2006.e9, 2008

Cook KE, Jenkins SM: Pathological uterine torsion associated with placental abruption, maternal shock, and intrauterine fetal demise. Am J Obstet Gynecol 92:2082, 2005

Cook RJ, Dickens BM, Fathalla MF: Female genital cutting (mutilation/circumcision): Ethical and legal dimensions. Int J Gynaecol Obstet 79:281, 2002

Coronado GD, Marshall LM, Schwartz SM: Complications in pregnancy, labor, and delivery with uterine leiomyomas: A population-based study. Obstet Gynecol 95:764, 2000

Curtis KM, Hillis SD, Marchbanks PA, et al: Disruption of the endometrial-myometrial border during pregnancy as a risk factor for adenomyosis. Am J Obstet Gynecol 187:543, 2002

Dabirashrafi H, Bahadori M, Mohammad K, et al: Septate uterus: New idea on the histologic features of the septum in this abnormal uterus. Am J Obstet Gynecol 172:105, 1995

Davis JL, Ray-Mazumder S, Hobel CJ, et al: Uterine leiomyomas in pregnancy: A prospective study. Obstet Gynecol 75:41, 1990

De Carolis S, Fatigante G, Ferrazzani S, et al: Uterine myomectomy in pregnant women. Fetal Diagn Ther 16:116, 2001

Deffarges JV, Haddad B, Musset R, et al: Utero-vaginal anastomosis in women with uterine cervix atresia: Long-term follow-up and reproductive performance. Hum Reprod 16:1722, 2001

Edelman AB, Jensen JT, Lee DM, et al: Successful medical abortion of a pregnancy within a noncommunicating rudimentary uterine horn. Am J Obstet Gynecol 189:886, 2003

Eke N, Nkanginieme KE: Female genital mutilation: A global bug that should not cross the millennium bridge. World J Surg 23:1082, 1999

Engel G, Rushovich AM: True uterine diverticulum: A partial Müllerian duct duplication? Arch Pathol Lab Med 108:734, 1984

Exacoustos C, Rosati P: Ultrasound diagnosis of uterine myomas and complications in pregnancy. Obstet Gynecol 82:97, 1993

Fallat ME, Weaver JM, Hertweck SP, et al: Late follow-up and functional outcome after traumatic reproductive tract injuries in women. Am Surg 64:858, 1998

Fedele L, Bianchi S, Marchini M, et al: Ultrastructural aspects of endometrium in infertile women with septate uterus. Fertil Steril 65:750, 1996

Fedele L, Bianchi S, Tozzi L, et al: Fertility in women with unicornuate uterus. Br J Obstet Gynaecol 102:1007, 1995

Fedele L, Dorta M, Brioschi D, et al: Magnetic resonance evaluation of double uteri. Obstet Gynecol 74:844, 1989

Fedele L, Zamberletti D, Vercellini P, et al: Reproductive performance of women with unicornuate uterus. Fertil Steril 47:416, 1987

Felix JF, Steegers-Theunissen RPM, de Walle HEK, et al: Esophageal atresia and tracheoesophageal fistula in children of women exposed to diethylstilbestrol in utero. Am J Obstet Gynecol 197:38.e1, 2007

Fernández-Aguilar S, Noël JC: Neuroma of the clitoris after female genital cutting. Obstet Gynecol 101:1053, 2003

Fleischer AC, Dinesh MS, Entman SS: Sonographic evaluation of maternal disorders during pregnancy. Radiol Clin North Am 28:51, 1990

Friedman A, DeFazio J, DeCherney A: Severe obstetric complications after aggressive treatment of Asherman syndrome. Obstet Gynecol 67:864, 1986

Garland SM, Hernandez-Avila M, Wheeler CM, et al: Quadrivalent vaccine against human papillomavirus to prevent anogenital diseases. N Engl J Med 356:1928, 2007

Genta PR, Dias ML, Janiszewski TA, et al: *Streptococcus agalactiae* endocarditis and giant pyomyoma simulating ovarian cancer. South Med J 94:508, 2001

Golan D, Aharoni A, Gonen R, et al: Early spontaneous rupture of the post myomectomy gravid uterus. Int J Gynaecol Obstet 31:167, 1990a

Golan A, Caspi E: Congenital anomalies of the müllerian tract. Contemp Obstet Gynecol 37:39, 1992

Golan A, Langer R, Neuman M, et al: Obstetric outcome in women with congenital uterine malformations. J Reprod Med 37:233, 1992

Golan A, Langer R, Wexler S, et al: Cervical cerclage–its role in the pregnant anomalous uterus. Int J Fertil 35:164, 1990b

Goldberg J, Pereira L: Pregnancy outcomes following treatment for fibroids: Uterine fibroid embolization versus laparoscopic myomectomy. Curr Opin Obstet Gynecol 18:402, 2006

Goldberg JM, Falcone T: Effect of diethylstilbestrol on reproductive function. Fertil Steril 72:1, 1999

Gottschalk EM, Siedentopf JP, Schoenborn I, et al: Prenatal sonographic and MRI findings in a pregnancy complicated by uterine sacculation: case report and review of the literature. Ultrasound Obstet Gynecol 32(4):582, 2008

Greene JF, DeRoche ME, Ingardia C, et al: Large myomatous uterus resulting in complete obstruction of the inferior vena cava during pregnancy. Br J Obstet Gynaecol 107:1189, 2002

Grimbizis G, Camus H, Clasen K, et al: Hysteroscopic septum resection in patients with recurrent abortions or infertility. Hum Reprod 13 (5):1188, 1998

Hamoda H, Chamberlain PF, Moore NR, et al: Conservative treatment of an incarcerated gravid uterus. Br J Obstet Gynaecol 109:1074, 2002

Hampton HL, Meeks GR, Bates GW, et al: Pregnancy after successful vaginoplasty and cervical stenting for partial atresia of the cervix. Obstet Gynecol 76:900, 1990

Hatch EE, Troisi R, Wise LA, et al: Age at natural menopause in women exposed to diethylstilbestrol in utero. Am J Epidemiol 164:682, 2006

Heinonen PK: Clinical implications of the unicornuate uterus with rudimentary horn. Int J Gynaecol Obstet 21:145, 1983

Heinonen PK: Uterus didelphys: A report of 26 cases. Eur J Obstet Gynecol Reprod Biol 17:345, 1984

Heinonen PK: Limb anomalies among offspring of women with a septate uterus: Report of three cases. Early Hum Dev 56:179, 1999

Hendry WF: Management of urological tumours in pregnancy. Br J Urol 1:24, 1997

Herbst AL, Ulfelder H, Poskanzer DC: Adenocarcinoma of the vagina. N Engl J Med 284:878, 1971

Hess LW, Peaceman A, O'Brien WF, et al: Adnexal mass occurring with intrauterine pregnancy: Report of fifty-four patients requiring laparotomy for definitive management. Am J Obstet Gynecol 158:1029, 1988

Hill LM, Chenevey P, DiNofrio D: Sonographic documentation of uterine retroversion mimicking uterine sacculation. Am J Perinatol 10:398, 1993

Hinckley MD, Milki AA: Management of uterus didelphys, obstructed hemivagina and ipsilateral renal agenesis. A case report. J Reprod Med 48:649, 2003

Hoffman BL: Pelvic masses. In Schorge JO, Schaffer JI, Halvorson LM, et al (eds): Williams Gynecology, 1st ed. New York, McGraw-Hill, 2008, p 287

Hoffman MS, Sayer RA: Adnexal masses in pregnancy: A guide to management. OBG Management, p 27, March 2007

Iosif S, Ulmsten U: Comparative urodynamic studies of continent and stress incontinent women in pregnancy and in the puerperium. Am J Obstet Gynecol 140:645, 1981

Jackson D, Elliott JP, Pearson M: Asymptomatic uterine retroversion at 36 weeks' gestation. Obstet Gynecol 71:466, 1988

Joó JG, Inovay J, Silhavy M, et al: Successful enucleation of a necrotizing fibroid causing oligohydramnios and fetal postural deformity in the 25th week of gestation: A case report. J Reprod Med 46:923, 2001

Kaiser UB: The pathogenesis of the ovarian hyperstimulation syndrome. N Engl J Med 349:729, 2003

Kaufman RH, Adam E, Hatch EE, et al: Continued follow-up of pregnancy outcomes in diethylstilbestrol-exposed offspring. Obstet Gynecol 96:483, 2000

Kaufman RH, Noller K, Adam E, et al: Upper genital tract abnormalities and pregnancy outcome in DES-exposed progeny. Am J Obstet Gynecol 148:973, 1984

Kessler A, Mitchell DG, Kuhlman K, et al: Myoma vs. contraction in pregnancy: Differentiation with color Doppler imaging. J Clin Ultrasound 21:241, 1993

Kier R, McCarthy SM, Scoutt LM, et al: Pelvic masses in pregnancy: MR imaging. Radiology 176:709, 1990

Klatsky PC, Tran ND, Caughey AB, et al: Fibroids and reproductive outcomes: a systematic literature review from conception to delivery. Am J Obstet Gynecol 198(4):357, 2008

Korell AN, Argenta PA, Strathy JH: Prolonged obstructed labor causing a severe obstetric fistula. J Reprod Med 52:555, 2007

Kovac SR, Cruikshank SH: Successful pregnancies and vaginal deliveries after sacrospinous uterosacral fixation in five of nineteen patients. Am J Obstet Gynecol 168:1778, 1993

Kurjak A, Zalud I: Transvaginal color Doppler for evaluating gynecologic pathology of the pelvis. Ultraschall Med 11:164, 1990

Kyrgiou M, Koliopoulos G, Martin-Hirsch P: Obstetric outcomes after conservative treatment for intraepithelial or early invasive cervical lesions: Systematic review and meta-analysis. Lancet 367:489, 2006

Lashgari M, Behmaram B, Ellis M: Leiomyomatosis peritonealis disseminata: A report of two cases. J Reprod Med 39:652, 1994

Laughlin SK, Baird DD, Savitz DA, et al: Prevalence of uterine leiomyomas in the first trimester of pregnancy: an ultrasound-screening study. Obstet Gynecol 113(3):630, 2009

Lee SW, Kim MY, Yang JH, et al: Sonographic findings of uterine sacculation during pregnancy. Ultrasound Obstet Gynecol 32(4):595, 2008

Leible S, Munoz H, Walton R, et al: Uterine artery blood flow velocity waveforms in pregnant women with müllerian duct anomaly: A biologic model for uteroplacental insufficiency. Am J Obstet Gynecol 178:1048, 1998

Leiserowitz GS, Xing G, Cress R, et al: Adnexal masses in pregnancy: How often are they malignant? Gynecol Oncol 101:315, 2006

Letterie GS, Vauss N: Müllerian tract abnormalities and associated auditory defects. J Reprod Med 36:765, 1991

Lettieri L, Rodis JF, McLean DA, et al: Incarceration of the gravid uterus. Obstet Gynecol Surv 49:642, 1994

Lev-Toaff AS, Coleman BG, Arger PH, et al: Leiomyomas in pregnancy: Sonographic study. Radiology 164:375, 1987

Lin YH, Hwang JL, Huang LW, et al: Pyomyoma after a cesarean section. Acta Obstet Gynecol Scand 81:571, 2002

Ling FT, David TE, Merchant N, et al: Intracardiac extension of intravenous leiomyomatosis in a pregnant woman: A case report and review of the literature. Can J Cardiol 16:73, 2000

Litta P, Pozzan C, Merlin F, et al: Hysteroscopic metroplasty under laparoscopic guidance in infertile women with septate uteri: Follow-up of reproductive outcome. J Reprod Med 49:274, 2004

Lolis DE, Paschopoulos M, Makrydimas G, et al: Reproductive outcome after Strassman metroplasty in women with a bicornuate uterus. J Reprod Med 50:297, 2005

Louis-Sylvestre C, Haddad B, Paniel BJ: Treatment of vaginal outflow tract obstruction in graft-versus-host reaction. Am J Obstet Gynecol 188:943, 2003

Ludmir J, Jackson GM, Samuels P: Transvaginal cerclage under ultrasound guidance in cases of severe cervical hypoplasia. Obstet Gynecol 78:1067, 1991

Ludmir J, Landon MB, Gabbe SG, et al: Management of the diethylstilbestrol-exposed pregnant patient: A prospective study. Am J Obstet Gynecol 157:665, 1987

MacDonald DJM, Popli K, Byrne D, et al: Small bowel obstruction in a twin pregnancy due to fibroid degeneration. Scott Med J 49:159, 2004

Mackey R, Geary M, Dornan J, et al: A successful pregnancy following transabdominal cervical cerclage for cervical hypoplasia. Br J Obstet Gynaecol 108:1111, 2001

Maneschi M, Maneschi F, Fuca G: Reproductive impairment of women with unicornuate uterus. Acta Eur Fertil 19:273, 1988

Marom D, Pitlik S, Sagie A, et al: Intravenous leiomyomatosis with cardiac involvement in a pregnant woman. Am J Obstet Gynecol 178:620, 1998

Marrocco-Trischitta MM, Nicodemi EM, Nater C, et al: Management of congenital venous malformations of the vulva. Obstet Gynecol 98:789, 2001

Mathevet P, Chemali E, Roy M, et al: Long-term outcome of a randomized study comparing three techniques of conization: Cold knife, laser, and LEEP. Eur J Obstet Gynecol Reprod Biol 106:214, 2003a

Mathevet P, Nessah K, Dargent D, et al: Laparoscopic management of adnexal masses in pregnancy: A case series. Eur J Obstet Gynecol Reprod Biol 108:217, 2003b

Mathew M, Gowri V, Hamdani AA, et al: Cotyledonoid leiomyoma in pregnancy. Obstet Gynecol 109:509, 2007

Mazza V, Di Monte I, Ceccarelli PL, et al: Prenatal diagnosis of female pseudo-hermaphroditism associated with bilateral luteoma of pregnancy. Hum Reprod 17:821, 2002

McCarthy-Keith DM, Coggins A: Perineal endometrioma occurring during pregnancy. J Reprod Med 53:57, 2008

McKay HA, Hanlon K: Vesicovaginal fistula after cervical cerclage: Repair by transurethral suture cystorrhaphy. J Urol 169:1086, 2003

Michalas SP: Outcome of pregnancy in women with uterine malformation: Evaluation of 62 cases. Int J Gynaecol Obstet 35:215, 1991

Miklos JR, Sze E, Parobeck D, et al: Vesicouterine fistula: A rare complication of vaginal birth after cesarean. Obstet Gynecol 86:638, 1995

Moutos DM, Damewood MD, Schlaff WD, et al: A comparison of the reproductive outcome between women with a unicornuate uterus and women with a didelphic uterus. Fertil Steril 58:88, 1992

Murray C, Goh JT, Fynes M, et al: Urinary and faecal incontinence following delayed primary repair of obstetric genital fistula. Br J Obstet Gynaecol 109:828, 2002

Myers DL, Scotti RJ: Acute urinary retention and the incarcerated, retroverted, gravid uterus. A case report. J Reprod Med 40:487, 1995

Nahum GG: Uterine anomalies. How common are they, and what is their distribution among subtypes? J Reprod Med 43 (10):877, 1998

Nahum GG: Rudimentary uterine horn pregnancy: The 20th-century worldwide experience of 588 cases. J Reprod Med 47:151, 2002

Neiger R, Sonek JD, Croom CS, et al: Pregnancy-related changes in the size of uterine leiomyomas. J Reprod Med 51:671, 2006

Nicholson HS, Blask AN, Markle BM, et al: Uterine anomalies in Wilms' tumor survivors. Cancer 78:887, 1996

Nicolini V, Bellotti M, Bannazzi B, et al: Can ultrasound be used to screen uterine malformations? Fertil Steril 47:89, 1987

Nour NM: Female genital cutting: Clinical and cultural guidelines. Obstet Gynecol Surv 59:272, 2004

Nour NM: Urinary calculus associated with female genital cutting. Obstet Gynecol 107:520, 2006

Nour NM, Michels KB, Bryant AE: Defibulation to treat female genital cutting–Effect on symptom and sexual function. Obstet Gynecol 108:55, 2006

Okonofua FE, Larsen U, Oronsaye F, et al: The association between female genital cutting and correlates of sexual and gynaecological morbidity in Edo State, Nigeria. Br J Obstet Gynaecol 109:1089, 2002

Oláh KS: Uterine torsion and ischaemia of one horn of a bicornute uterus: A rare cause of failed second trimester termination of pregnancy. Br J Obstet Gynaecol 109:585, 2002

Olpin JD, Heilbrun M: Imaging of Müllerian duct anomalies. Clin Obstet Gynecol 52(1):40, 2009

Özel B: Incarceration of a retroflexed, gravid uterus from severe uterine prolapse. J Reprod Med 50:624, 2005

Pabuccu R, Gomel V: Reproductive outcome after hysteroscopic metroplasty in women with septate uterus and otherwise unexplained infertility. Fertil Steril 81:1675, 2004

Palmer JR, Hatch EE, Rao RS, et al: Infertility among women exposed prenatally to diethylstilbestrol. Am J Epidemiol 154:316, 2001

Papp Z, Mezei G, Gávai M, et al: Reproductive performance after transabdominal metroplasty. J Reprod Med 51:544, 2006

Parker WH, Childers JM, Canis M, et al: Laparoscopic management of benign cystic teratomas during pregnancy. Am J Obstet Gynecol 174:1499, 1996

Patel AK, Chapple CR: Female urethral diverticula. Curr Opin Urol 16:248, 2006

Patton PE, Novy MJ, Lee DM, et al: The diagnosis and reproductive outcome after surgical treatment of the complete septate uterus, duplicated cervix and vaginal septum. Am J Obstet Gynecol 190:1669, 2004

Pavone ME, King JA, Vlahos N: Septate uterus with cervical duplication and a longitudinal vaginal septum: A müllerian anomaly without a classification. Fertil Steril 85:494.e9, 2006

Pellerito JS, McCarthy SM, Doyle MB, et al: Diagnosis of uterine anomalies: Relative accuracy of MR imaging, endovaginal sonography, and hysterosalpingography. Radiology 183:795, 1992

Penning SR, Cohen B, Tewari D, et al: Pregnancy complicated by vesical calculus and vesicocutaneous fistula. Obstet Gynecol 176:728, 1997

Platek DN, Henderson CE, Goldberg GL: The management of a persistent adnexal mass in pregnancy. Am J Obstet Gynecol 173:1236, 1995

Porcu G, Courbiere B, Sakr R, et al: Spontaneous rupture of a first-trimester gravid uterus in a woman exposed to diethylstilbestrol in utero: A case report. J Reprod Med 48:744, 2003

Pritts EA: Fibroids and infertility: A systematic review of the evidence. Obstet Gynecol Surv 56:483, 2001

Proctor JA, Haney AF: Recurrent first trimester pregnancy loss is associated with uterine septum but not with bicornuate uterus. Fertil Steril 80:1212, 2003

Pron G, Mocarski E, Bennett J, et al: Pregnancy after uterine artery embolization for leiomyomata: The Ontario multicenter trial. Obstet Gynecol 105:67, 2005

Qidwai II, Caughey AB, Jacoby AF: Obstetric outcomes in women with sonographically identified uterine leiomyomata. Obstet Gynecol 107:376, 2006

Rabinovici J, Inbar Y, Eylon SC, et al: Pregnancy and live birth after focused ultrasound surgery for symptomatic focal adenomyosis: A case report. Hum Reprod 21:1255, 2006

Raga F, Bauset C, Remohi J, et al: Reproductive impact of congenital Müllerian anomalies. Hum Reprod 12:2277, 1997

Rai L, Ramesh K: Obstructed labour due to a vesical calculus. Aust NZ J Obstet Gynaecol 38:474, 1998

Rajiah P, Eastwood KL, Gunn ML, et al: Uterine diverticulum. Obstet Gynecol 113(2 Pt 2):525, 2009

Ravasia DJ, Brain PH, Pollard JK: Incidence of uterine rupture among women with mullerian duct anomalies who attempt vaginal birth after cesarean delivery. Am J Obstet Gynecol 181:877, 1999

Rebarber A, Fox NS, Eckstein DA, et al: Successful bilateral uterine artery embolization during an ongoing pregnancy. Obstet Gynecol 113(2 Pt 2):554, 2009

Reichman D, Laufer MR, Robinson BK: Pregnancy outcomes in unicornuate uteri: a review. Fertil Steril 91(5): 1886, 2009

Rice JP, Kay HH, Mahony BS: The clinical significance of uterine leiomyomas in pregnancy. Am J Obstet Gynecol 160:1212, 1989

Rolen AC, Choquette AJ, Semmens JP: Rudimentary uterine horn: Obstetric and gynecologic implications. Obstet Gynecol 27:806, 1966

Rose CH, Brost BC, Watson WJ, et al: Expectant management of uterine incarceration from an anterior uterine myoma. J Reprod Med 53:65, 2008

Salvador E, Bienstock J, Blakemore KJ, et al: Leiomyomata uteri, genetic amniocentesis, and the risk of second-trimester spontaneous abortion. Am J Obstet Gynecol 186:913, 2002

Samson SA, Bentley JR, Fahey TJ, et al: The effect of loop electrosurgical excision procedure on future pregnancy outcome. Obstet Gynecol 105:325, 2005

Saygili-Yilmaz ES, Erman-Akar M, Bayar D, et al: Septate uterus with a double cervix and longitudinal vaginal septum. J Reprod Med 49:833, 2004

Schmeler KM, Mayo-Smith WW, Peipert JF, et al: Adnexal masses in pregnancy: Surgery compared with observation. Obstet Gynecol 105:1098, 2005

Schwartz LB, Zawin M, Carcangiu ML, et al: Does pelvic magnetic resonance imaging differentiate among the histologic subtypes of uterine leiomyomata? Fertil Steril 70:580, 1998

Seidman DS, Ben-Rafael Z, Bider D, et al: The role of cervical cerclage in the management of uterine anomalies. Surg Gynecol Obstet 173:384, 1991

Senekjian EK, Potkul RK, Frey K, et al: Infertility among daughters either exposed or not exposed to diethylstilbestrol. Am J Obstet Gynecol 158:493, 1988

Seubert DE, Puder KS, Goldmeier P, et al: Colonoscopic release of the incarcerated gravid uterus. Obstet Gynecol 94:792, 1999

Sheiner E, Bashiri A, Levy A, et al: Obstetric characteristics and perinatal outcome of pregnancies with uterine leiomyomas. Obstet Gynecol Surv 59:647, 2004

Sherard GB III, Hodson CA, Williams HJ, et al: Adnexal masses and pregnancy: A 12-year experience. Am J Obstet Gynecol 189:358, 2003

Sherer DM, Smith SA, Sanko SR: Uterine sacculation sonographically mimicking an abdominal pregnancy at 20 weeks' gestation. Am J Perinatol 11:350, 1994

Silva PD, Perkins HE, Schauberger CW: Live birth after treatment of severe adenomyosis with a gonadotropin-releasing hormone agonist. Fertil Steril 61:171, 1994

Singh MN, Payappagoudar J, Lo J: Incarcerated retroverted uterus in the third trimester complicated by postpartum pulmonary embolism. Obstet Gynecol 109:498, 2007

Soriano D, Yefet Y, Seidman DS, et al: Laparoscopy versus laparotomy in the management of adnexal masses during pregnancy. Fertil Steril 71:955, 1999

Spearing GJ: Uterine sacculation. Obstet Gynecol 51:11S, 1978

Stenchever MA: Congenital abnormalities of the female reproductive tract. In Stenchever MA, Droegemueller W, Herbst AL, et al (eds): Comprehensive Gynecology, 4th ed. St. Louis, Mosby, 2001, p 253

Stewart EA: Uterine fibroids. Lancet 357:293, 2001

Swan SH: Intrauterine exposure to diethylstilbestrol: Long-term effects in humans. APMIS 108:793, 2000

Tanaka YO, Tsunoda H, Sugano M, et al: MR and CT findings of leiomyomatosis peritonealis disseminata with emphasis on assisted reproductive technology as a risk factor. Br J Radiol 82(975):e44, 2009

Thomas EO, Gordon J, Smith-Thomas S, et al: Diffuse uterine leiomyomatosis with uterine rupture and benign metastatic lesions of the bone. Obstet Gynecol 109:528, 2007

Thornton JG, Wells M: Ovarian cysts in pregnancy: Does ultrasound make traditional management inappropriate? Obstet Gynecol 69:717, 1987

Tikkanen M, Nuutila M, Hilesmaa V, et al: Prepregnancy risk factors for placental abruption. Acta Obstet Gynecol 85:40, 2006

Torashima M, Yamashita Y, Matsuno Y, et al: The value of detection of flow voids between the uterus and the leiomyoma with MRI. J Magn Reson Imaging 8:427, 1998

Toubia N: Female circumcision as a public health issue. N Engl J Med 331:712, 1994

Valli E, Zupi E, Marconi D, et al: Hysteroscopic findings in 344 women with recurrent spontaneous abortion. J Am Assoc Gynecol Laparosc 8:398, 2001

Varras M, Christodoulos A, Demos A, et al: Double vagina and cervix communicating bilaterally with a single uterine cavity. J Reprod Med 52:238, 2007

Vasseur C, Rodien P, Beau I, et al: A chorionic gonadotropin-sensitive mutation in the follicle-stimulating hormone receptor as a cause of familial gestational spontaneous ovarian hyperstimulation syndrome. N Engl J Med 349:753, 2003

Vo CV, Dinh TV, Hankins GDV: Value of ultrasound in the early diagnosis of prerupture uterine horn pregnancy. J Reprod Med 48:471, 2003

Walker WJ, McDowell SJ: Pregnancy after uterine artery embolization for leiomyomata: A series of 56 completed pregnancies. Am J Obstet Gynecol 195:1266, 2006

Wall LL: Fitsari'Dan Duniya: An African (Hausa) praise song about vesicovaginal fistulas. Obstet Gynecol 100:1328, 2002

Wang YC, Su HY, Liu JY, et al: Maternal and female fetal virilization caused by pregnancy luteomas. Fertil Steril 84:509.e15, 2005

Whitecar P, Turner S, Higby K: Adnexal masses in pregnancy: A review of 130 cases undergoing surgical management. Am J Obstet Gynecol 181:19, 1999

Winer-Muram HT, Muram D, Gillieson MS: Uterine myomas in pregnancy. J Can Assoc Radiol 35:168, 1984

Woelfer B, Salim R, Banerjee S, et al: Reproductive outcomes in women with congenital uterine anomalies detected by three-dimensional ultrasound screening. Obstet Gynecol 98:1099, 2001

World Health Organization: Female genital mutilation: A joint WHO/UNICEF/UNFPA statement. Geneva: World Health Organization, 1997

World Health Organization Study Group: Female genital mutilation and obstetric outcome: WHO collaborative prospective study in six African countries. Lancet 367:1835, 2006

World Health Organization: Female genital mutilation. 2000. http://www.who.int/mediacentre/factsheets/fs241/en/index.html. Retrieved May 1, 2006

Worley KC, Hnat MD, Cunningham FG: Advanced extrauterine pregnancy: Diagnostic and therapeutic challenges. Am J Obstet Gynecol 198:287.e1, 2008

Zanetti E, Ferrari LR, Rossi G: Classification and radiographic features of uterine malformations: Hysterosalpingographic study. Br J Radiol 51:161, 1978

Zanetta G, Mariani E, Lissoni A, et al: A prospective study of the role of ultrasound in the management of adnexal masses in pregnancy. Br J Obstet Gynaecol 110:578, 2003

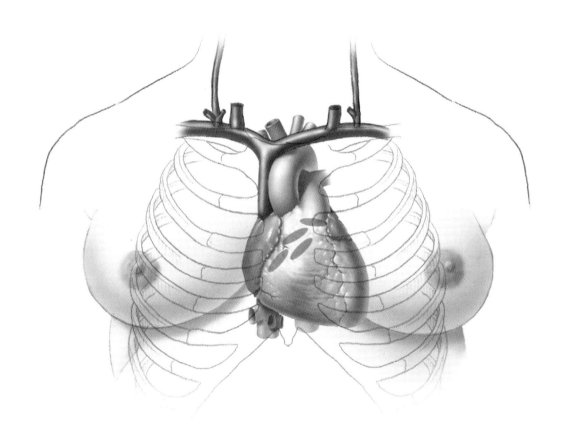

General Considerations and Maternal Evaluation

It is difficult to accurately quantify the incidence and types of medical and surgical illnesses that complicate pregnancy. Estimates have been derived from other indices of hospitalization as well as birth certificate data (Lydon-Rochelle and associates, 2005). For example, Gazmararian and colleagues (2002) reported an overall antenatal hospitalization rate of 10.1 per 100 deliveries in their managed-care population of more than 46,000 pregnant women. About a third of these were for nonobstetrical conditions such as renal, gastrointestinal, pulmonary, and infectious diseases. In a study from the 2002 Nationwide Inpatient Sample of the Healthcare Cost and Utilization Project, Kuo and associates (2007) used the International Classification of Diseases, Ninth Revision, Clinical Modification (ICD-9-CM) injury and concurrent pregnancy diagnosis codes. From these, they found the injury hospitalization rate to be 4.1 women per 1000 deliveries.

The care for some of these women with medical or surgical disorders will warrant a team effort between obstetricians and maternal-fetal medicine specialists, or with internists, surgeons, anesthesiologists, and other disciplines (American College of Obstetricians and Gynecologists, 2003). It is important that obstetricians have a working knowledge of medical and surgical diseases common to women of childbearing age. Likewise, nonobstetricians who see these women in consultation should be familiar with pregnancy-induced physiological changes that affect various diseases.

A number of generalizations concern the rational approach to management of these nonobstetrical disorders:

- A woman should never be penalized because she is pregnant.
- What management plan would be recommended if the woman was not pregnant?
- If a proposed medical or surgical management plan is altered because the woman is pregnant, what are the justifications for this?

Such an approach should allow individualization of care for most medical and surgical disorders. Moreover, it may be especially helpful when dealing with nonobstetrical consultants.

MATERNAL PHYSIOLOGY AND ALTERATIONS IN LABORATORY VALUES

Pregnancy induces physiological changes in most organ systems. Some of these are profound and may amplify or obfuscate evaluation of coexisting conditions. Results of laboratory tests can also be altered, and some of these would, in the nonpregnant woman, be considered abnormal. Conversely, some may appear to be normal but are not so in the pregnant woman. The wide ranges of pregnancy effects on normal physiology and on laboratory values are discussed in Chapter 5, in the chapters that follow, and in the Appendix.

MEDICATIONS DURING PREGNANCY

Antepartum management of nonobstetrical disorders includes administration of various drugs. Fortunately, the vast majority necessary to treat the most commonly encountered complications can be used with relative safety. However, there are a few notable exceptions, which are considered in detail in Chapter 14, as well as with the discussions of specific disorders for which these drugs are given.

SURGERY DURING PREGNANCY

The risk of an adverse pregnancy outcome is not appreciably increased in women who undergo most uncomplicated surgical procedures. With complications, however, risks may be increased. For example, perforative appendicitis with feculent peritonitis has significant maternal and perinatal morbidity and mortality rates even if surgical and anesthetic techniques are flawless. Conversely, procedure-related complications may adversely affect outcomes. For example, a woman who has uncomplicated removal of an inflamed appendix may suffer aspiration of acidic gastric contents at the time of tracheal extubation (see Chap. 19, p. 460).

Effect of Surgery and Anesthesia on Pregnancy Outcome

The most extensive experiences regarding anesthetic and surgical risks to pregnancy are from the Swedish Birth Registry reported by Mazze and Källén (1989). The effects of 5405 nonobstetrical surgical procedures performed in 720,000 pregnant women were analyzed from 1973 to 1981 (Fig. 41-1). Surgery was performed in 41 percent of women in the first trimester, 35 percent in the second, and 24 percent in the third. Of the total, 25 percent were abdominal operations, another 20 percent were gynecological and urological procedures, and 15 percent were laparoscopic procedures. Laparoscopy was the most commonly performed first-trimester operation, and appendectomy was the most common second-trimester procedure.

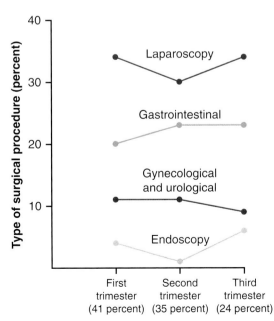

FIGURE 41-1 Selected types of surgical procedures by trimester in 3615 women. (Data from Mazze and Källén, 1989.)

TABLE 41-1. Birth Outcomes in 5405 Pregnant Women Undergoing Nonobstetrical Surgery

Outcome	Rate	p Value[a]
Major malformation	1.9 percent	NS
Stillbirth	7 per 1000	NS
Neonatal death by 7 days	10.5 per 1000	< 0.05
Preterm birth (< 37 wk)	7.5 percent	< 0.05
Birthweight < 1500 g	1.2 percent	< 0.05
Birthweight < 2500 g	6.6 percent	< 0.05

[a]Compared with 720,000 pregnancies in women without surgery.
NS = not significant
Data from Mazze and Källén (1989).

General anesthesia was used for 54 percent of procedures in the 5405 women in the Swedish report. This commonly involved nitrous oxide supplemented by another inhalation agent or intravenous medications.

Perinatal Outcomes

Excessive perinatal morbidity associated with nonobstetrical surgery is attributable to the disease itself rather than to adverse effects of surgery and anesthesia. Mazze and Källén (1989) compared pregnancy outcomes in the 5405 women undergoing surgery as described with perinatal outcomes in the other 720,000 pregnancies. As shown in Table 41-1, the incidence of neonates with congenital malformations or those stillborn was not significantly different from that of nonexposed newborns. There were, however, significantly increased incidences of low birthweight, preterm birth, and neonatal death in infants born to women who had undergone surgery. Increased neonatal mortality rates resulted in large part from preterm birth. These investigators concluded that these likely were due to a synergistic effect of the illness in concert with the surgical procedures. Similarly, Hong (2006) reported increased preterm delivery in 235 women undergoing adnexal mass surgery.

Källén and Mazze (1990) scrutinized 572 operations performed at 4 to 5 weeks and found a nonsignificant relationship with neural-tube defects. From the Hungarian database, Czeizel and colleagues (1998) found no evidence that anesthetic agents were teratogenic. Sylvester and co-workers (1994) performed a case-control study from the Metropolitan Atlanta Congenital Defects Program. They found an increased risk of hydrocephaly—but not neural-tube defects—in conjunction with other major defects in newborns of women exposed to general anesthesia. The study was based on questionnaire data, and we agree with Kuczkowski (2006) that there is no robust evidence that anesthetic agents are harmful to the fetus.

Laparoscopic Surgery During Pregnancy

During the past decade, laparoscopic techniques have become commonly used for diagnosis and management of a number of surgical disorders complicating pregnancy. The obvious example is management of ectopic pregnancy (see Chap. 10, p. 246). From his review, Kuczkowski (2007) reported that laparoscopy is the most common first-trimester surgical procedure. It is used preferentially for exploration and treatment of adnexal masses (Chap. 40, p. 905), for appendectomy (Chap. 49, p. 1059), and for cholecystectomy (Chap. 50, p. 1074). In 2008, the Guidelines Committee of the Society of American Gastrointestinal and Endoscopic Surgeons (SAGES) published its recommendations concerning the use of laparoscopy in pregnant women. These guidelines are reasonable and are generally followed by most obstetricians and surgeons.

Lachman and colleagues (1999) and Fatum and Rojansky (2001) reviewed more than 800 laparoscopic procedures performed during pregnancy. The most common were cholecystectomy, adnexal surgery, and appendectomy. These generally had good outcomes, and these researchers concluded that 26 to 28 weeks was the upper gestational age limit for successful laparoscopy. Predictably, some centers are now describing laparoscopic surgery performed in the third trimester. For example, Rollins and colleagues (2004) described 59 pregnant women managed with laparoscopic procedures—31 cholecystectomies and 28 appendectomies. Of these 59 women, 30 percent underwent surgery after 26 weeks. There were no serious adverse sequelae to these procedures. There are also a number of reports of laparoscopic splenectomy, adrenalectomy, and nephrectomy done in pregnant women (Felbinger, 2007; Gernsheimer and McCrae, 2007; Kosaka, 2006; Stroup, 2007, and all their colleagues).

Maternal Effects

Hemodynamic changes from abdominal insufflation for laparoscopy are similar in pregnant and nonpregnant women as summarized in Table 41-2. Reedy and colleagues (1995) studied baboons at the human equivalent of 22 to 26 weeks' gestation. Although they found no substantive physiological changes with 10 mm Hg insufflation pressures, 20 mm Hg caused significant maternal cardiovascular and respiratory changes after 20 minutes. These included increased respiratory rate, respiratory acidosis, diminished cardiac output, and increased pulmonary artery and wedge pressures.

In women, cardiorespiratory changes are generally not severe if insufflation pressures are kept below 20 mm Hg. Steinbrook and Bhavani-Shankar (2001) performed noninvasive hemodynamic monitoring in women at midpregnancy and reported that the cardiac index decreased 26 percent by 5 minutes of insufflation and 21 percent by 15 minutes. The mean arterial pressures, systemic vascular resistance, and heart rate did not change significantly.

Perinatal Outcomes

Because precise effects of laparoscopy in the human fetus are unknown, animal studies are informative. Pregnancy outcomes in women are limited to observations.

Animal Studies

In early studies of pregnant ewes, Barnard and associates (1995) and Hunter and colleagues (1995) reported that uteroplacental blood flow decreased when intraperitoneal pressure from insufflation exceeded 15 mm Hg. This was caused by decreased perfusion pressure and increased placental vessel resistance (Table 41-2). Studies in sheep since that time have corroborated these findings, which were reviewed by Reynolds and associates (2003) and O'Rourke and Kodali (2006). And the previously cited baboon study by Reedy and colleagues (1995) produced similar results. Importantly, severity of adverse effects was related to insufflation pressures greater than 15 mm Hg.

Human Data

To study the impact of laparoscopy on perinatal outcomes, Reedy and colleagues (1997) used the updated Swedish Birth Registry described earlier. Between 1973 and 1993, data accrued from more

TABLE 41-2. Physiological Effects of CO_2 Insufflation of the Peritoneal Cavity

System	Effects	Mechanisms	Possible Maternal-Fetal Effects
Respiratory	pCO_2 increases, pH decreases	CO_2 absorption	Hypercarbia and acidosis
Cardiovascular	Increased—heart rate; systemic vascular resistance; pulmonary, central venous, and mean arterial pressures	Hypercarbia and increased intra-abdominal pressure	Uteroplacental hypoperfusion—possible fetal hypoxia, acidosis, and hypoperfusion[a]
	Decreased—cardiac output	Decreased venous return	
Blood Flow	Decreased splanchnic flow with hypoperfusion of liver, kidneys, and gastrointestinal organs	Increased intra-abdominal pressure	As above
	Decreased venous return from lower extremities	Increased intra-abdominal pressure	As above
	Increased cerebral blood flow	Hypercarbia possibly from shunting due to splanchnic tamponade	Increased CSF pressure[a]

[a]Data primarily from animal studies.
CO_2 = carbon dioxide; CSF = cerebrospinal fluid; pCO_2 = partial pressure of CO_2.
Data from reviews by O'Rourke and Kodali (2006) and Reynolds and co-workers (2003).

than 2 million deliveries. There were 2181 laparoscopic procedures, which were performed primarily during the first trimester. The perinatal outcomes in these pregnancies were compared with those of all women, and the findings confirmed previous studies. Specifically, there was an increased risk of low birthweight, preterm delivery, and fetal-growth restriction in pregnancies of women in the operative group. There were no differences when outcomes of women having laparoscopy versus laparotomy were compared.

Technique

Preparation for laparoscopy differs little from that commonly used for laparotomy. Bowel cleansing empties the large intestine and may aid visualization. Nasogastric or orogastric decompression reduces the risk of stomach trocar puncture and aspiration. Aortocaval compression is avoided by a left-lateral tilt. Positioning of the lower extremities in boot-type stirrups maintains access to the vagina for fetal sonographic assessment or *manual* uterine displacement.

Most reports describe general anesthesia after tracheal intubation and monitoring of end-tidal carbon dioxide ($EtCO_2$) (Hong, 2006; Ribic-Pucelj and associates, 2007). With controlled ventilation, $EtCO_2$ is maintained at 30 to 35 mm Hg.

Beyond the first trimester, technical modifications of standard pelvic laparoscopic entry are required to avoid uterine puncture or laceration. Many recommend *open entry* techniques to avoid perforations of the uterus, pelvic vessels, and adnexa (Akira and co-workers, 1999). The abdomen is incised at or above the umbilicus and the peritoneal cavity entered under direct visualization. At this point, the cannula is then connected to the insufflation systems, and a 10-mm Hg pneumoperitoneum is created. The initial insufflation should be conducted slowly to allow for prompt assessment and reversal of any untoward pressure-related effects. Gas leakage around the cannula is managed by tightening the surrounding skin with a towel clamp. Insertion of secondary trocars is most safely performed under direct laparoscopic visual observation through the primary port.

In more advanced pregnancies, direct entry through a left upper quadrant port in the midclavicular line, 2 cm beneath the costal margin, has been described by Stepp and Falcone (2004). Known as *Palmer Point*, this entry site is used in gynecological laparoscopy because visceroparietal adhesions uncommonly form here (Vilos and colleagues, 2007).

Gasless Laparoscopy. This alternative approach involves use of a rod with fan-blade-shaped retractors, which when opened allow the abdominal wall to be lifted in an upward direction. It avoids the cardiovascular changes with pneumoperitoneum (Phupong and Bunyavejchewin, 2007).

Complications

Risks inherent to any abdominal endoscopy are *probably* not increased during pregnancy. The obvious unique complication is perforation of the pregnant uterus with either a trocar or Veress needle. Certainly, reported complications are uncommon (Fatum and Rojansky, 2001; Lachman and colleagues, 1999; Oelsner and associates, 2003). After a Cochrane Registry review, Bunyavejchewin and Phupong (2006) concluded that randomized trials would be necessary to deduce comparative

benefits and risks of laparoscopy versus laparotomy during pregnancy. Pragmatically, this seems unfeasible and common sense should dictate the approach used.

IMAGING TECHNIQUES

Imaging modalities that are used as adjuncts for diagnosis and therapy during pregnancy include sonography, radiography, and magnetic resonance imaging. Of these, radiography is the most worrisome. Inevitably, some radiographic procedures are performed prior to recognition of early pregnancy, usually because of trauma or serious illness. Fortunately, most diagnostic radiographic procedures are associated with *minimal* fetal risks. As with drugs and medications, however, these procedures may lead to litigation if there is an adverse pregnancy outcome. And x-ray exposure may lead to a needless therapeutic abortion because of patient or physician anxiety.

Ionizing Radiation

The term *radiation* is poorly understood. Literally it refers to transmission of energy, and thus it is often applied not only to x-rays, but also to microwaves, ultrasound, diathermy, and radio waves. Of these, x-rays and gamma rays have short wavelengths with very high energy and are forms of ionizing radiation. The other four energy forms have rather long wavelengths and low energy (Brent, 1999a, 2009).

The biological effects of x-rays are caused by an electrochemical reaction that can cause tissue damage. According to Brent (1999b, 2009), x- and gamma-radiation at high doses can create biological effects and reproductive risks in the fetus:

1. Deterministic effects, which may cause congenital malformations, fetal-growth restriction, mental retardation, and abortion
2. Stochastic effects—randomly determined probabilities—which may cause genetic diseases and carcinogenesis.

In this sense, ionizing radiation refers to waves or particles—photons—of significant energy that can change the structure of molecules such as those in DNA, or that can create free radicals or ions capable of causing tissue damage (Hall, 1991; National Research Council, 1990). Methods of measuring the effects of x-rays are summarized in Table 41-3. The standard terms used are *exposure* (in air), *dose* (to tissue), and *relative effective dose* (to tissue). In the range of energies for diagnostic x-rays, the dose is now expressed in gray (Gy), and the relative effective dose is now expressed in sievert (Sv). These can be used interchangeably. For consistency, all doses discussed subsequently are expressed in contemporaneously used units of gray (1 Gy = 100 rad) or sievert (1 Sv = 100 rem). To convert, 1 Sv = 100 rem = 100 rad.

X-Ray Dosimetry

When calculating the dose of ionizing radiation such as that from x-rays, according to Wagner and colleagues (1997) several factors to be considered include:

1. Type of study
2. Type and age of equipment

TABLE 41-3. Some Measures of Ionizing Radiation

Exposure	The number of ions produced by x-rays per kg of air Unit: roentgen (R)
Dose	The amount of energy deposited per kg of tissue Modern unit: gray (Gy) (1 Gy = 100 rad) Traditional unit: rad[a]
Relative effective dose	The amount of energy deposited per kg of tissue normalized for biological effectiveness Modern unit: sievert (Sv) (1 Sv = 100 rem) Traditional unit: rem[a]

[a] For diagnostic x-rays, 1 rad = 1 rem.

3. Distance of target organ from radiation source
4. Thickness of the body part penetrated
5. Method or technique used for the study.

Estimates of dose to the uterus and embryo for a variety of commonly used radiographic examinations are summarized in Table 41-4. Studies of maternal body parts farthest from the uterus, such as the head, result in a very small dose of radiation scatter to the embryo or fetus. Because the size of the woman, radiographic technique, and equipment performance are variable factors, data in the table serve only as a guideline. When the radiation dose for a specific individual is required, a medical physicist should be consulted. In his most recent review, Brent (2009) recommends consulting the Health Physics Society web-site (www.hps.org) to view some examples of questions and answers posed by patients exposed to radiation (Click on ATE—ask the expert).

Deterministic Effects of Ionizing Radiation

One potential harmful effect of radiation exposure is deterministic, which may result in abortion, growth restriction, congenital malformations, microcephaly, and mental retardation. These deterministic effects are threshold effects, and the level below which they are induced is the *NOAEL—no-adverse-effect level* (Brent, 2009).

The harmful deterministic effects of ionizing radiation have been extensively studied for cell damage with resultant dysfunction of embryogenesis. These have been assessed in animal models, as well as Japanese atomic bomb survivors and the Oxford Survey of Childhood Cancers (Sorahan and colleagues, 1995). Additional sources have confirmed previous observations and provided more information. One is the 2003 International Commission on Radiological Protection (ICRP) publication of biological fetal effects from prenatal irradiation. Another is the BEIR VII Phase 2 report of the National Research Council (2006) that discusses health risks from exposure to low levels of ionizing radiation.

Animal Studies. In the mouse model, the risk of lethality is highest during the preimplantation period—up to 10 days postconception. This is likely due to blastomere destruction caused by chromosomal damage (Hall, 1991). The NOAEL for lethality is 0.15 to 0.2 Gy. Genomic instability can be induced in some mouse models at levels of 0.5 Gy (50 rad), which greatly exceeds levels with diagnostic studies (International Commission on Radiological Protection, 2003).

During organogenesis, high-dose radiation—1 gray or 100 rad—is more likely to cause malformations and growth restriction, and less likely to have lethal effects in the mouse. Studies

TABLE 41-4. Dose to the Uterus for Common Radiological Procedures

Study	View	Dose[a] View (mGy)	Films/Study[b]	Dose/Study (mGy)
Skull[c]	AP, PA Lat	<0.0001	4.1	<0.0005
Chest	AP, PA[c] Lat[d]	<0.0001–0.0008	1.5	0.0002–0.0007
Mammogram[d]	CC Lat	<0.0003–0.0005	4.0	0.0007–0.002
Lumbosacral spine[e]	AP, Lat	1.14–2.2	3.4	1.76–3.6
Abdomen[e]	AP		1.0	0.8–1.63
Intravenous pyelogram[e]	3 views		5.5	6.9–14
Hip[b] (single)	AP	0.7–1.4		
	Lat	0.18–0.51	2.0	1–2

[a] Calculated for x-ray beams with half-value layers ranging from 2 to 4 mm aluminum equivalent using the methodology of Rosenstein (1988).
[b] Based on data and methods reported by Laws and Rosenstein (1978).
[c] Entrance exposure data from Conway (1989).
[d] Estimates based on compilation of above data.
[e] Based on NEXT data reported in National Council on Radiation Protection and Measurements (1989).
AP = anterior-posterior; CC = cranial-caudal; Lat = lateral; PA = posterior-anterior.

of brain development suggest that there are effects on neuronal development and a "window of cortical sensitivity" in early and midfetal periods with a threshold in the range of 0.1 to 0.3 Gy or 10 to 30 rad (International Commission on Radiological Protection, 2003).

Human Data. Adverse human effects of high-dose ionizing radiation are most often quoted in atomic bomb survivors from Hiroshima and Nagasaki (Greskovich and Macklis, 2000; Otake and co-workers, 1987). The International Commission on Radiological Protection (2003) confirmed initial studies showing that the increased risk of severe mental retardation was greatest between 8 and 15 weeks (Fig. 41-2). There may be a lower threshold dose of 0.3 Gy—30 rad—a similar range of the "window of cortical sensitivity" in the mouse model discussed above. The mean decrease in intelligence quotient (IQ) scores was 25 points per Gy or 100 rad. There appears to be linear dose response, but it is not clear whether there is a threshold dose. Most estimates err on the conservative side by assuming a linear nonthreshold (LNT) hypothesis. From their review, Strzelczyk and colleagues (2007) conclude that limitations of epidemiological studies at low-level exposures, along with recent new radiobiological findings, challenge the hypothesis that any amount of radiation causes adverse effects.

Finally, there is no documented increased risk of mental retardation in humans less than 8 weeks' or greater than 25 weeks' gestation, even with doses exceeding 0.5 Gy or 50 rad (Committee on Biological Effects, BEIR V, 1990; International Commission on Radiological Protection, 2003).

There are also reports that describe high-dose radiation given to treat women for malignancy, menorrhagia, and uterine myomas. In one, Dekaban (1968) described 22 infants with microcephaly, mental retardation, or both, following exposure in the first half of pregnancy to an estimated 2.5 Gy or 250 rad. Malformations in other organs were not found unless they were accompanied by microcephaly, eye abnormalities, or growth restriction (Brent, 1999a).

The implications of these findings seem straightforward. From 8 to 15 weeks, the embryo is most susceptible to radiation-induced mental retardation. It has not been resolved whether this is a threshold or nonthreshold linear function of dose. The Committee on Biological Effects (1990) estimates the risk of severe mental retardation to be low as 4 percent for 0.1 Gy (10 rad) and as high as 60 percent for 1.5 Gy (150 rad). But recall that these doses are 2 to 100 times higher than those from diagnostic radiation. Importantly, *cumulative doses from multiple procedures* may reach the harmful range, especially at 8 to 15 weeks. At 16 to 25 weeks, the risk is less. And again, there is no proven risk before 8 weeks or after 25 weeks.

Embryofetal risks from low-dose diagnostic radiation appear to be minimal. Current evidence suggests that there are no increased risks for malformations, growth restriction, or abortion from a radiation dose of less than 0.05 Gy (5 rad). Indeed, Brent (2009) concluded that gross congenital malformations would not be increased with exposure to less than 0.2 Gy (20 rad). Because diagnostic x-rays seldom exceed 0.1 Gy (10 rad), Strzelczyk and associates (2007) concluded that these procedures are unlikely to cause deterministic effects.

Stochastic Effects of Ionizing Radiation

This refers to random, presumably unpredictable oncogenic or mutagenic effects of radiation exposure. They concern associations between fetal diagnostic radiation exposure and increased risk of childhood cancers or genetic diseases. According to Doll and Wakeford (1997), as well as the National Research Council (2006) BEIR VII Phase 2 report, excess cancers can result from in utero exposure to doses as low as 0.01 Sv or 1 rad. Stated another way by Hurwitz and colleagues (2006), the estimated risk of childhood cancer following fetal exposure to 0.03 Gy or 3 rad doubles the background risk of 1 in 600 to that of 2 in 600.

In one report, in utero radiation exposure was determined for 10 solid cancers in adults from 17 to 45 years of age. There was a dose-response relationship as previously noted at the 0.1 Sv or 10 rem threshold. Intriguingly, nine of 10 cancers were found in females (National Research Council, 2006). These likely are associated with a complex series of interactions between DNA and ionizing radiation. They also make it more problematic to predict cancer risk from low-dose radiation of less than 0.1 Sv or 10 rem. Importantly, below doses of 0.1 to 0.2 Sv, there is no convincing evidence of a carcinogenic effect (Brent, 2009; Preston and colleagues, 2008; Strzelczyk and co-workers, 2007).

Therapeutic Radiation

In an earlier report, the Radiation Therapy Committee Task Group of the American Association of Physics in Medicine found that about 4000 pregnant women annually undergo cancer

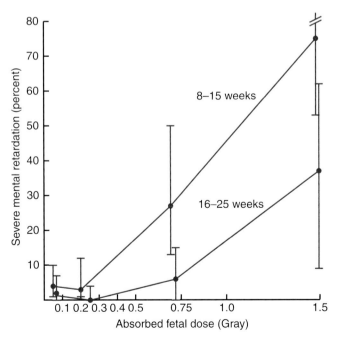

FIGURE 41-2 Follow-up of subjects from Hiroshima and Nagasaki after the atomic bomb explosion in 1945: Subsequent severe mental retardation caused by exposure to ionizing in utero radiation at two gestational age epochs to 1 Gy—or 100 rad. Mean values and 90-percent confidence levels are estimated from dosimetry calculated by two methods—T65DR and D586—used by the Radiation Effects Research Foundation of the Japanese Ministry of Health and National Academy of Sciences of the United States. (Data from Otake and associates, 1987, with permission.)

therapy in the United States (Stovall and colleagues, 1995). Their recommendations, however, stand to date. The Task Group emphasizes careful individualization of radiotherapy for the pregnant woman (see Chap. 57, p. 1193). For example, in some cases, shielding of the fetus and other safeguards can be taken (Fenig and colleagues, 2001; Nuyttens and colleagues, 2002). In other cases, the fetus will be exposed to dangerous doses of radiation, and a carefully designed plan must be improvised (Prado and colleagues, 2000). One example is the model to estimate fetal dosage with maternal brain radiotherapy, and another is the model to calculate fetal dose with tangential breast irradiation developed by Mazonakis and colleagues (1999, 2003). The impact of radiotherapy on future fertility and pregnancy outcomes was recently reviewed by Wo and Viswanathan (2009) and is discussed in detail in Chapter 57 (p. 1194).

Diagnostic Radiation

To estimate fetal risk, approximate x-ray dosimetry must be known. According to the American College of Radiology (Hall, 1991), no single diagnostic procedure results in a radiation dose significant enough to threaten embryofetal well-being.

Radiographs. Dosimetry for standard radiographs is presented in Table 41-4. In pregnancy, the two-view chest radiograph is the most commonly used study, and fetal exposure is exceptionally small—0.0007 Gy or *0.07 mrad*. With one abdominal radiograph, because the embryo or fetus is directly in the x-ray beam, the dose is higher—0.001 Gy or 100 mrad. The standard intravenous pyelogram may exceed 0.005 Gy or 500 mrad because of several films. The one-shot pyelogram described in Chapter 48 (p. 1038) is useful when urolithiasis or other causes of obstruction are suspected but unproven by sonography. Most "trauma series," such as radiographs of an extremity, skull, or rib series, deliver low doses because of the fetal distance from the target area.

Fetal indications for radiographic studies are limited. Perhaps the most common is pelvimetry with a breech presentation (see Chap. 24, p. 529 and Fig. 20-4, p. 473).

Fluoroscopy and Angiography. Dosimetry calculations are much more difficult with these procedures because of variations in the number of radiographs obtained, total fluoroscopy time, and fluoroscopy time in which the fetus is in the radiation field. As shown in Table 41-5, the range is quite variable. Although the Food and Drug Administration limits exposure rate for conventional fluoroscopy such as barium studies, special-purpose systems such as angiography units have potential for much higher exposure.

Endoscopy is the preferred method of gastrointestinal tract evaluation in pregnancy. Occasionally, an upper gastrointestinal series or barium enema may be done before the woman realizes that she is pregnant. Most would likely be performed during the period of preimplantation or early organogenesis.

Angiography may occasionally be necessary for serious maternal disorders, and especially for trauma. As before, the greater the distance from the embryo or fetus, the less the exposure and risk.

Computed Tomography. Most computed tomography (CT) imaging is now performed by obtaining a spiral of 360-degree images that are postprocessed in multiple planes. Of these, the axial image remains the most commonly obtained. Multidetector CT (MDCT) images are now standard for common clinical indications. The most recent detectors have 16 or 64 channels. MDCT protocols may result in increased dosimetry compared with traditional CT imaging. A number of imaging parameters have an effect on exposure (Brenner and colleagues, 2007). These include pitch, kilovoltage, tube current, collimation,

TABLE 41-5. Estimated X-Ray Doses to the Uterus/Embryo from Common Fluoroscopic Procedures

Procedure	Dose to Uterus (mrad)	Fluoroscopic Exposure Time (sec)	Cinegraphic Exposure Time (sec)
Cerebral angiography[a]	< 0.1	—	—
Cardiac angiography[b,c]	0.65	223 (SD = 118)	49 (SD = 9)
Single-vessel PTCA[b,c]	0.60	1023 (SD = 952)	32 (SD = 7)
Double-vessel PTCA[b,c]	0.90	1186 (SD = 593)	49 (SD = 13)
Upper gastrointestinal series[d]	0.56	136	—
Barium swallow[b,e]	0.06	192	—
Barium enema[b,f,g]	20–40	289–311	—

[a] Wagner and associates (1997).
[b] Calculations based on data of Gorson and colleagues (1984).
[c] Finci and co-workers (1987).
[d] Suleiman and colleagues (1991).
[e] Based on female data from Rowley and associates (1987).
[f] Assumes embryo in radiation field for entire examination.
[g] Bednarek and co-workers (1983).
PTCA = percutaneous transluminal coronary angioplasty; SD = standard deviation.

TABLE 41-6. Estimated Radiation Dosimetry with 16-Channel Multidetector-Imaging Protocols

	Dosimetry (mGy)	
Protocol	**Preimplantation**	**3 Months' Gestation**
Pulmonary embolism	0.20–0.47	0.61–0.66
Renal stone	8–12	4–7
Appendix	15–17	20–40

Data from Hurwitz and co-workers (2006).

number of slices, tube rotation, and total acquisition time. If a study is performed with and without contrast, the dose is doubled because twice as many images are obtained. Fetal exposure is also dependent on factors such as maternal size as well as fetal size and position. And as with plain radiography, the closer the target area is to the fetus, the greater the dosimetry.

Hurwitz and colleagues (2006) employed a 16-MDCT to calculate fetal exposure at 0 and 3 months' gestation using a phantom model (Table 41-6). Calculations were made for three commonly requested procedures in pregnant women. The pulmonary embolism protocol has the same dosimetry exposure as the ventilation-perfusion (V/Q) lung scan discussed below. Because of the pitch used, the appendicitis protocol has the highest radiation exposure, however, it is very useful clinically (Fig. 41-3). For imaging suspected urolithiasis, the MDCT scan protocol is used if sonography is nondiagnostic (Fig. 41-4). Using a similar protocol in 67 women with suspected appendicitis, Lazarus and co-workers (2007) reported sensitivity of 92 percent, specificity of 99 percent, and a negative-predictive value of 99 percent. Here dosimetry is markedly decreased compared with appendiceal imaging because of a different pitch. Using a similar protocol, White and co-workers (2007) identified urolithiasis in 13 of 20 women at an average of 26.5 weeks. Finally, abdominal tomography should be performed if indicated in the pregnant woman with severe trauma (American College of Obstetricians and Gynecologists, 1998).

Cranial CT scanning is the most commonly requested study in pregnant women. Its use in women with neurological disorders is discussed in Chapter 55 (p. 1164) and with eclampsia in Chapter 34 (p. 723). Nonenhanced CT scanning is commonly used to detect acute hemorrhage within the epidural, subdural, or subarachnoid spaces.

Pelvimetry is used by some before attempting breech vaginal delivery (see Chap. 24, p. 529). The fetal dose approaches 0.015 Gy or 1.5 rad, but use of a low-exposure technique may reduce this to 0.0025 Gy or 0.25 rad.

Most experience with chest CT scanning is with suspected pulmonary embolism. The most recent recommendations for its use in pregnancy from the Prospective Investigation of Pulmonary Embolism Diagnosis—PIOPED—II investigators were summarized by Stein and co-workers (2007). They found that pulmonary scintigraphy—the V/Q scan—was recommended for pregnant women by 70 percent of radiologists and chest CT angiography by 30 percent. But most agree that MDCT angiography has improved accuracy because of increasingly faster acquisition times. Others have reported a higher use-rate for CT angiography and emphasize that dosimetry is similar to that with V/Q scintigraphy (Brenner, 2007; Hurwitz, 2006; Matthews, 2006, and their many colleagues). At both Parkland Hospital and the University of Alabama Hospital at Birmingham, we use MDCT scanning initially for suspected pulmonary embolism (see Chap. 47, p. 1026).

Nuclear Medicine Studies

These studies are performed by "tagging" a radioactive element to a carrier that can be injected, inhaled, or swallowed. For

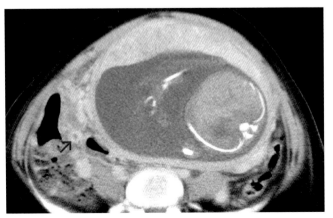

FIGURE 41-3 CT-protocol for appendix shows an enlarged, enhancing—and thus inflamed appendix (*arrow*) next to the 25-week pregnancy. (Used with permission from Dr. Jeffrey H. Pruitt.)

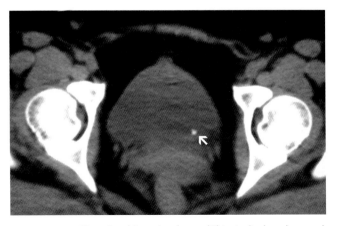

FIGURE 41-4 CT-protocol imaging for urolithiasis disclosed a renal stone in the distal ureter (*arrow*) at its junction with the bladder. (Used with permission from Dr. Jeffrey H. Pruitt.)

example, the radioisotope technetium-99m may be tagged to red blood cells, sulfur colloid, or pertechnetate. The method used to tag the agent determines fetal radiation exposure. The amount of placental transfer is obviously important, but so is renal clearance because of fetal proximity to the maternal bladder. Measurement of radioactive technetium is based on its decay, and the units used are the curie (Ci) or the becquerel (Bq). Dosimetry is usually expressed in millicuries (mCi). As shown in Table 41-3, the effective tissue dose is expressed in sievert units (Sv). As discussed, to convert: 1 Sv = 100 rem = 100 rad.

Depending on the physical and biochemical properties of a radioisotope, an average fetal exposure can be calculated (Wagner and co-workers, 1997; Zanzonico, 2000). Commonly used radiopharmaceuticals and estimated absorbed fetal doses are given in Table 41-7. The radionuclide dose should be kept as

low as possible (Adelstein, 1999). Exposures vary with gestational age and are greatest earlier in pregnancy for most radiopharmaceuticals. One exception is the later effect of [131]iodine on the fetal thyroid (Wagner and associates, 1997). The International Commission on Radiological Protection (2001) has compiled dose coefficients for radionuclides. Stather and colleagues (2002) detailed the biokinetic and dosimetric models used by the Commission to estimate fetal radiation doses from maternal radionuclide exposure.

As discussed above, MDCT-angiography is being used preferentially for suspected pulmonary embolism during pregnancy. Until recently, the imaging modality was the *ventilation-perfusion lung scan* in this setting. It is used if CT angiography is nondiagnostic (see Chap. 47, p. 1026). Perfusion is measured with injected ^{99}Tc-macroaggregated albumin, and ventilation is meas-

TABLE 41-7. Radiopharmaceuticals Used in Nuclear Medicine Studies

Study	Estimated Activity Administered per Examination in Millicuries (mCi)	Weeks' Gestation[a]	Dose to Uterus/Embryo per Pharmaceutical (mSv)[b]
Brain	20 mCi ^{99m}Tc DTPA	<12	8.8
		12	7[c]
Hepatobiliary	5 mCi ^{99m}Tc sulfur colloid	12	0.45
	5 mCi ^{99m}Tc HIDA		1.5
Bone	20 mCi ^{99m}Tc phosphate	<12	4.6
Pulmonary			
Perfusion	3 mCi ^{99m}Tc-macroaggregated albumin	Any	0.45–0.57
Ventilation	10 mCi ^{133}Xe gas		(combined)
Renal	20 mCi ^{99m}Tc DTPA	<12	8.8
Abscess or tumor	3 mCi ^{67}Ga citrate	<12	7.5
Cardiovascular	20 mCi ^{99m}Tc-labeled red blood cells	<12	5
	3 mCi [210]Tl chloride	<12	11
		12	6.4
		24	5.2
		36	3
Thyroid	5 mCi [99m]TcO$_4$	<8	2.4
	0.3 mCi [123]I (whole body)	1.5–6	0.10
	0.1 mCi [131]I[d]		
	Whole body	2–6	0.15
	Whole body	7–9	0.88
	Whole body	12–13	1.6
	Whole body	20	3
	Thyroid-fetal	11	720
	Thyroid-fetal	12–13	1300
	Thyroid-fetal	20	5900
Sentinel lymphoscintigram	5 mCi ^{99m}Tc sulfur colloid (1–3 mCi)		5

[a]To convert to mrad multiply x 100.
[b]Exposures are generally greater prior to 12 weeks compared with increasing gestational ages.
[c]Some measurements account for placental transfer.
[d]The uptake and exposure of ^{131}I increases with gestational age.
DPTA = diethylenetriaminepentaacetic acid; Ga = gallium; HIDA = hepatobiliary iminodiacetic acid; I = iodine; mCi = millicurie; mSv = millisievert; Tc = technetium; TcO$_4$ = pertechnetate; Tl = thallium. Compiled from data from Adelstein (1999), Schwartz (2003), Stather (2002), Wagner (1997), Zanzonico (2000), and all their colleagues.

ured with inhaled xenon-127 or xenon-133. Fetal exposure with either is negligible (Chan and colleagues, 2002; Mountford, 1997).

Thyroid scanning with iodine-123 or iodine-131 seldom is indicated in pregnancy. With trace doses used, however, fetal risk is minimal. **Importantly, therapeutic radioiodine in doses to treat Graves disease or thyroid cancer may cause fetal thyroid ablation and cretinism.**

The *sentinel lymphoscintigram,* which uses ^{99m}Tc-sulfur colloid to detect the axillary lymph node most likely to have metastases from breast cancer, is a commonly used preoperative study in non-pregnant women (Newman and Newman, 2007; Spanheimer and associates, 2009; Wang and co-workers, 2007). As shown in Table 41-7, the calculated dose is approximately 0.014 mSv or 1.4 mrad, which should not preclude its use during pregnancy.

SONOGRAPHY

Of all of the major advances in obstetrics, the development of sonography for study of the fetus and mother certainly is one of the greater achievements. The technique has become virtually indispensable in everyday practice. The wide range of clinical uses of sonography in pregnancy is further discussed in Chapter 16 and in most other sections of this book.

Safety

Diagnostic sonography uses sound wave transmission at certain frequencies. Recall that ultrasound is a form of radiation that transmits energy. At very high intensities, there is a *potential* for tissue damage from heat and cavitation (Callen, 2000). That said, with the low-intensity range of real-time imaging, no fetal risks have been demonstrated in more than 35 years of use (Maulik, 1997; Miller and colleagues, 1998). An example is the study done by Naumburg and associates (2000). They performed a case-control study of 578 children with leukemia compared with healthy controls. In each cohort, a third of the children had been exposed to ultrasound in utero.

Advances in technology have introduced Doppler-shift imaging coupled with gray-scale imaging to localize spectral waveforms and superimpose color mapping. Higher energy intensities are used with this duplex Doppler imaging. Again, however, these should have no embryo or fetal effects if low-level pulses are used (Kossoff, 1997).

Ultrasound equipment must have a video display of acoustic output to safeguard against exceeding standards set by a number of organizations including the American College of Obstetricians and Gynecologists (2009). Acoustic outputs are displayed as an index. The *thermal index* is an estimate of temperature increases from acoustic output. If the index is below 1.0, then no potential risk is expected (Miller and associates, 1998). Adverse effects reflected in thermal index changes have not been demonstrated with Doppler use in clinical applications (Maulik, 1997). The *mechanical index* is used to estimate the potential risk of cavitation from heat generated by real-time imaging.

As long as sonographic contrast agents are not used, there is no hypothetical fetal risk. Prolonged exposure of animal fetuses suggest that it is possible to induce cellular alterations. For example, prolonged exposure to ultrasound impeded migration of brain cells in fetal mice (Ang and co-workers, 2007). At this time, the American Institute of Ultrasound in Medicine (2007) and other organizations agree that these findings should not alter the use of ultrasound in pregnant women.

MAGNETIC RESONANCE (MR) IMAGING

Like sonography, magnetic resonance technology has proven extremely useful for maternal and fetal imaging studies because it does not use ionizing radiation. Its application is cited throughout this book. Advantages include high soft-tissue contrast, ability to characterize tissue, and acquisition of images in any plane—particularly axial, sagittal, and coronal. With MR imaging, powerful magnets are used to temporarily alter the state of protons. The hydrogen proton is used for imaging because of its abundance, especially in water and fat. Radio waves are then used to deflect the magnetic vector. When the radiofrequency source is turned off, hydrogen protons return to their normal state. In doing so, they emit radio waves of different frequencies, which are received by radio coils wrapped around the body part. The relative intensity of these signals is plotted on a gray scale. A series of pulse sequences in all planes can be obtained, and each acquisition includes information about the location and characteristics of the sequences. From this, an image is constructed. Technological advances have significantly reduced scan times and improved image quality.

Safety

The most recent update of the Blue Ribbon Panel on MR safety of the American College of Radiology was summarized by Kanal and colleagues (2007). The panel concluded that there are no reported harmful human effects from MR imaging. Chew and colleagues (2001) found no differences in blastocyst formation exposure of early murine embryos to MR imaging with 1.5 tesla strength. Vadeyar and associates (2000) noted no demonstrable fetal heart rate pattern changes during MR imaging in women. Chung (2002) has reviewed these safety issues.

In their report, the Panel described above decided that each request for MR imaging in a pregnant woman should be approved by the attending radiologist. Indicated imaging should be performed at any gestational age if no other imaging studies can be performed, or if MR imaging would provide information that would otherwise require radiation exposure. Contraindications to MR imaging include internal cardiac pacemakers, neurostimulators, implanted defibrillators and infusion pumps, cochlear implants, shrapnel or other metal in biologically sensitive areas, some intracranial aneurysm clips, and any metallic foreign body in the eye. Of more than 51,000 non-pregnant patients scheduled for MR imaging, Dewey and colleagues (2007) found that only 0.4 percent had an absolute contraindication to the procedure.

Contrast Agents

A number of elemental *gadolinium chelates* are used to create paramagnetic contrast. Some are gadopentetate, gadodiamide, gadoteridol, and gadoterate. These cross the placenta and are found in

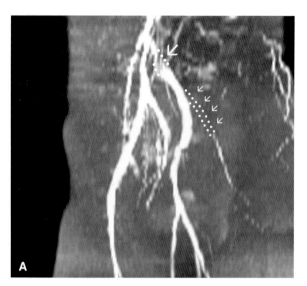
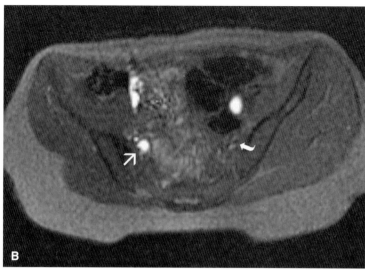

FIGURE 41-5 MR images of a pelvic vein thrombosis in a 15-week pregnant woman who presented with left leg pain but no symptoms of a pulmonary embolus. **A.** Reconstructed magnetic resonance venogram demonstrates partial chronic occlusion of the left common iliac vein (*large arrow*) and thrombosis and complete occlusion of the left internal iliac vein (*small arrows*). **B.** From the axial images, there is normal flow in the right (*arrow*) and no flow in the left internal iliac vein (*curved arrow*). (Courtesy of Dr. R. Douglas Sims.)

amnionic fluid. In doses approximately 10 times the human dose, gadopentetate caused slight developmental delay in rabbit fetuses. De Santis and associates (2007) described 26 women given a gadolinium derivative in the first trimester without adverse fetal effects. According to Briggs and colleagues (2005), as well as the Panel, these contrast agents currently are not recommended unless there are overwhelming benefits. This is because of the uncertain nature of the gadolinium ion in amnionic fluid.

Maternal Indications

With maternal disorders unrelated to pregnancy, MR imaging technology has advantages over CT scanning because there is no ionizing radiation. In some cases, MR imaging may be complementary to CT, and in others, MR imaging is preferable. Maternal central nervous system abnormalities, such as brain tumors or spinal trauma, are more clearly seen with MR imaging. As discussed in Chapter 34 (p. 723), MR imaging has provided valuable insights into the pathophysiology of eclampsia (Twickler and Cunningham, 2007; Zeeman and associates, 2003, 2009). *Magnetic-resonance angiography* provides imaging of the cerebral vasculature and can also be used to calculate flow of the middle and posterior cerebral arteries (Zeeman and colleagues, 2004a, b).

MR imaging is a superb technique to evaluate the maternal abdomen and retroperitoneal space in a pregnant woman. It has

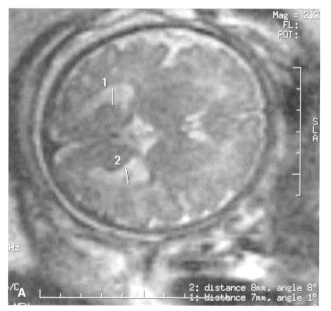
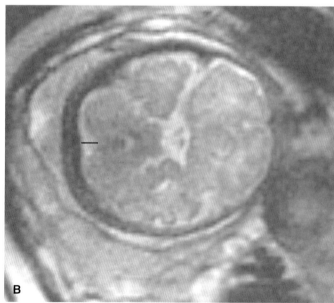

FIGURE 41-6 Magnetic resonance imaging of a normal 36-week fetal cranium. **A.** Cursors show ventricular atrial measurement. **B.** Line measurement (*red line*) of the cisterna magna.

TABLE 41-8. Guidelines for Diagnostic Imaging During Pregnancy

1. Women should be counseled that x-ray exposure from a single diagnostic procedure does not result in harmful fetal effects. Specifically, exposure to less than 5 rads has not been associated with an increase in fetal anomalies or pregnancy loss.
2. Concern about possible effects of high-dose ionizing radiation exposure should not prevent medically indicated diagnostic X-ray procedures from being performed on a pregnant woman. During pregnancy, other imaging procedures not associated with ionizing radiation (e.g., ultrasonography, MRI) should be considered instead of x-rays when appropriate.
3. Ultrasonography and MRI are not associated with known adverse fetal effects.
4. Consultation with an expert in dosimetry calculation may be helpful in calculating estimated fetal dose when multiple diagnostic x-rays are performed on a pregnant patient.
5. The use of radioactive isotopes of iodine is contraindicated for therapeutic use during pregnancy.
6. Radiopaque and paramagnetic contrast agents are unlikely to cause harm and may be of diagnostic benefit, but these agents should be used during pregnancy only if the potential benefit justifies the potential risk to the fetus.

(Reprinted, with permission, from Guidelines for diagnostic imaging during pregnancy. ACOG Committee Opinion No. 299. American College of Obstetricians and Gynecologists. *Obstet Gynecol* 2004; 104: 647–654.)

been used for detection and localization of adrenal tumors, renal lesions, gastrointestinal lesions, and pelvic masses in pregnancy. It has particular value in evaluating neoplasms of the chest, abdomen, and pelvis in pregnancy (Oto and co-workers, 2007). MR imaging may be used to confirm pelvic and vena caval thrombosis—a common source of pulmonary embolism in pregnant women (Fig. 41-5). As discussed in Chapter 31 (p. 666), CT and MR imaging is useful for evaluation of puerperal infections, but MR imaging provides better visualization of the bladder flap area following cesarean delivery (Brown and associates, 1999; Twickler and colleagues, 1997). Recently, MR imaging use has been expanded to include evaluation of right lower quadrant pain in pregnancy, specifically appendicitis (Pedrosa and co-workers, 2007, 2009; Singh and colleagues, 2007). Investigators have found disorders of the gastrointestinal tract, especially appendicitis, to be easily diagnosed with MR imaging (see Chap. 49, p. 1058).

Fetal Indications

Fetal MR imaging as a complement to sonography has been used with increasing frequency (De Wilde, 2005; Laifer-Narin, 2007; Sandrasegaran, 2006, and all their colleagues). According to Zaretsky and associates (2003a), MR imaging can be used to image almost all elements of the standard fetal anatomical survey. Bauer (2009), Reichel (2003), Twickler (2002), Weisz (2009) and their associates have validated its use for fetal central nervous system anomalies and biometry (Fig. 41-6). Caire and associates (2003) described its merits for fetal genitourinary anomalies. Hawkins and colleagues (2008) reported use of MR imaging in 21 fetuses with renal anomalies and oligohydramnios. Zaretsky and co-workers (2003b) reported that fetal weight estimation was more accurate using MR imaging than with sonography. Fast acquisition sequencing has solved problems with fetal movement to improve imaging. The technique is termed *HASTE—Half-Fourier Acquisition Single slow Turbo spin Echo*, or *SSFSE—Single Shot Fast Spin Echo*. Levine and colleagues (2001) reported that HASTE protocols do not generate significant heat in the uterus or fetus of pigs. The most common fetal indications for

MR imaging are for evaluation of complex abnormalities of the brain, chest, and genitourinary system. A more extensive discussion of fetal indications and findings of MR imaging are discussed in Chapter 16 and throughout the book.

GUIDELINES FOR DIAGNOSTIC IMAGING DURING PREGNANCY

The American College of Obstetricians and Gynecologists (2004) has reviewed the effects of radiographic, sonographic, and magnetic-resonance exposure during pregnancy. Its suggested guidelines are shown in Table 41-8.

REFERENCES

Adelstein SJ: Administered radionuclides in pregnancy. Teratology 59:236, 1999

Akira S, Yamanaka A, Ishihara T, et al: Gasless laparoscopic ovarian cystectomy during pregnancy: Comparison with laparotomy. Am J Obstet Gynecol 180:554, 1999

American College of Obstetricians and Gynecologists: Obstetric aspects of trauma management. Educational Bulletin No. 251, September 1998

American College of Obstetricians and Gynecologists: Nonobstetric surgery in pregnancy. Committee Opinion No. 284, August 2003

American College of Obstetricians and Gynecologists: Guidelines for diagnostic imaging during pregnancy. Committee Opinion No. 299, September 2004

American College of Obstetricians and Gynecologists: Ultrasonography in Pregnancy. Practice Bulletin No. 101, February 2009

American Institute of Ultrasound Medicine: AIUM practice guidelines for the performance of obstetric ultrasound examinations. AIUM, October 1, 2007

Ang ES, Gluncic V, Duque A, et al: Prenatal exposure to ultrasound waves impacts neuronal migration in mice. Proc Natl Acad Sci USA 103(34):12903, 2006

Barnard JM, Chaffin D, Droste S, et al: Fetal response to carbon dioxide pneumoperitoneum in the pregnant ewe. Obstet Gynecol 85:669, 1995

Baschat AA, Viscardi RM, Hussey-Gardner B, et al: Infant neurodevelopment following fetal growth restriction: Relationship with antepartum surveillance parameters. Ultrasound Obstet Gynecol 33(1):44, 2009

Bauer S, Mirza F, Pri-Paz S, et al: Dandy-Walker malformations: A comparison of prenatal ultrasound and magnetic resonance imaging. Abstract No. 396 Presented at the 29th Annual Meeting of the Society for Maternal-Fetal Medicine. 26-31 January 2009

Bednarek DR, Rudin S, Wong, et al: Reduction of fluoroscopic exposure for the air-contrast barium enema. Br J Radiol 56:823, 1983

Brenner DJ, Hall JH, Phil D: Computed tomography—an increasing source of radiation exposure. N Engl J Med 357:2277, 2007

Brent RL: Utilization of developmental basic science principles in the evaluation of reproductive risks from pre- and postconception environmental radiation exposures. Teratology 59:182, 1999a

Brent RL: Developmental and reproductive risks of radiological procedures utilizing ionizing radiation during pregnancy. Proceedings No. 21 in Radiation Protection in Medicine: Contemporary Issues. Proceedings of the thirty-fifth annual meeting of the National Council on Radiation Protection and Measurements. Arlington, VA, 7-8 April 1999b

Brent RL: Saving lives and changing family histories: Appropriate counseling of pregnant women and men and women of reproductive age, concerning risk of diagnostic radiation exposure during and before pregnancy. Am J Obstet Gynecol 200(1):4, 2009

Briggs GG, Freeman RK, Yaffe SJ: Drugs in Pregnancy and Lactation, 7th ed. Philadelphia, Lippincott Williams & Wilkins, 2005, p 710

Brown CE, Stettler RW, Twickler D, et al. Puerperal septic pelvic thrombophlebitis: Incidence and response to heparin therapy. Am J Obstet Gynecol 181:143, 1999

Bunyavejchevin S, Phupong V: Laparoscopic surgery for presumed benign ovarian tumor during pregnancy. Cochrane Database Systic Rev 4: CD005459, 2006.

Caire JT, Ramus RM, Magee KP, et al: MRI of fetal genitourinary anomalies. AJR Am J Roentgenol 181:1381, 2003

Callen PW: The obstetric ultrasound examination, Chap. 1. In Callen PW (ed): Ultrasonography in Obstetrics and Gynecology, 4th ed. Philadelphia, WB Saunders, 2000, p 1

Chan WS, Ray JG, Murray S, et al: Suspected pulmonary embolism in pregnancy. Arch Intern Med 152:1170, 2002

Chew S, Ahmadi A, Goh PS, et al: The effects of 1.5T magnetic resonance imaging on early murine in-vitro embryo development. J Magn Reson Imaging 13:417, 2001

Chung SM: Safety issues in magnetic resonance imaging. J Neuroophthalmol 22:35, 2002

Committee on Biological Effects of Ionizing Radiation, National Research Council: Other somatic and fetal effects. In BEIR V: Effects of Exposure to Low Levels of Ionizing Radiation. Washington, National Academy Press, 1990

Conway BJ: Nationwide evaluation of x-ray trends: Tabulation and graphical summary of surveys 1984 through 1987. Frankfort, KY, Conference of Radiation Control Program Directors, 1989

Czeizel AE, Pataki T, Rockenbauer M: Reproductive outcome after exposure to surgery under anesthesia during pregnancy. Arch Gynecol Obstet 261:193, 1998

Dekaban AS: Abnormalities in children exposed to x-irradiation during various stages of gestation: Tentative timetable of radiation injury to the human fetus. J Nucl Med 9:471, 1968

De Santis M, Straface G, Cavaliere AF, et al: Gadolinium periconceptional exposure: Pregnancy and neonatal outcome. Acta Obstet Gynecol Scand 86:99, 2007

De Wilde JP, Rivers AW, Price DL: A review of the current use of magnetic resonance imaging in pregnancy and safety implications for the fetus. Prog Biophys Mol Biol 87:335, 2005

Dewey M, Schink T, Dewey CF: Frequency of referral of patients with safety-related contraindications to magnetic resonance imaging. Eur J Radiol March 22, 2007

Doll R, Wakeford R: Risk of childhood cancer from fetal irradiation. Br J Radiol 70:130, 1997

Fatum M, Rojansky N: Laparoscopic surgery during pregnancy. Obstet Gynecol Surv 56:50, 2001

Felbinger TW, Posner M, Eltzschig HK et al: Laparoscopic splenectomy in a pregnant patient with immune thrombocytopenic purpura. Int J Obstet Anesth 16:281, 2007

Fenig E, Mishaeli M, Kalish Y, et al: Pregnancy and radiation. Cancer Treat Rev 27:1, 2001

Finci L, Meier B, Steffenino G, et al: Radiation exposure during diagnostic catheterization and single- and double-vessel percutaneous transluminal coronary angioplasty. Am J Cardiol 60:1401, 1987

Gazmararian JA, Petersen R, Jamieson DJ, et al: Hospitalizations during pregnancy among managed care enrollees. Obstet Gynecol 100:94, 2002

Gernsheimer T, McCrae KR: Immune thrombocytopenic purpura in pregnancy. Curr Opin Hematol 14:574, 2007

Gorson RO, Lassen M, Rosenstein M: Patient dosimetry in diagnostic radiology. In Waggener RG, Kereiakes JG, Shalek R (eds): Handbook of Medical Physics, Vol II. Boca Raton, FL, CRC Press, 1984

Greskovich JF, Macklis RM: Radiation therapy in pregnancy: Risk calculation and risk minimization. Semin Oncol 27:633, 2000

Guidelines Committee of the Society of American Gastrointestinal and Endoscopic Surgeons: Guidelines for diagnosis, treatment, and use of laparoscopy for surgical problems during pregnancy. Surg Endosc 22:849, 2008

Hall EJ: Scientific view of low-level radiation risks. RadioGraphics 11:509, 1991

Hawkins JS, Dashe JS, Twickler DM: Magnetic resonance imaging diagnosis of severe fetal renal anomalies. Am J Obstet Gynecol 198:328.e1, 2008

Hong J-Y: Adnexal mass surgery and anesthesia during pregnancy: A 10-year retrospective review. Intl J Obstet Anesth 15:212, 2006

Hunter JG, Swanstrom L, Thornburg K: Carbon dioxide pneumoperitoneum induces fetal acidosis in a pregnant ewe model. Surg Endosc 9:272, 1995

Hurwitz LM, Yoshizumi T, Reiman RE, et al: Radiation dose to the fetus from body MDCT during early gestation. Am J Roentgenol 186:871, 2006

International Commission on Radiological Protection: Doses to the embryo and fetus from intakes of radionuclides by the mother. Ann ICRP 31:19, 2001

International Commission on Radiological Protection: Biological effects after prenatal irradiation (embryo and fetus). IRCP Publication 90. Ann IRCP: September/December 2003

Källén B, Mazze RI: Neural tube defects and first trimester operations. Teratology 41:717, 1990

Kanal E, Barkovich AJ, Bell C, et al: ACR guidance document for safe MR practices: 2007. Am J Roentgenol 188:1, 2007

Kosaka K, Onoda N, Ishikawa T, et al: Laparoscopic adrenalectomy on a patient with primary aldosteronism during pregnancy. Endo J 53:461, 2006

Kossoff G: Contentious issues in safety of diagnostic ultrasound. Ultrasound Obstet Gynecol 10:151, 1997

Kuczkowski KM: The safety of anaesthetics in pregnant women. Expert Opin Surg Saf 5:251, 2006

Kuczkowski KM: Laparoscopic procedures during pregnancy and the risks of anesthesia: What does an obstetrician need to know? Arch Gynecol Obstet March 13, 2007

Kuo C, Jamieson DJ, McPheeters ML, et al: Injury hospitalizations of pregnant women in the United States, 2002. Am J Obstet Gynecol 196:161, 2007:

Lachman E, Schienfeld A, Voss E, et al: Pregnancy and laparoscopic surgery. J Am Assoc Gynecol Laparosc 6:347, 1999

Laifer-Narin S, Budorick NE, Simpson LL, et al: Fetal magnetic resonance imaging: A review. Curr Opin Obstet Gynecol 19:151, 2007

Laws PW, Rosenstein M: A somatic index for diagnostic radiology. Health Phys. 35:629, 1978

Lazarus E, Mayo-Smith WW, Mainiero MB, et al: CT in the evaluation of non-traumatic abdominal pain in pregnant women. Radiology 244:784, 2007

Levine D, Zuo C, Faro CB, et al: Potential heating effect in the gravid uterus during MR HASTE imaging. J Magn Reson Imaging 13:856, 2001

Lydon-Rochelle MT, Holt VL, Cárdenas V, et al: The reporting of pre-existing maternal medical conditions and complications of pregnancy on birth certificates and in hospital discharge data. Am J Obstet Gynecol 193:125, 2005

Matthews S: Imaging pulmonary embolism in pregnancy: What is the most appropriate imaging protocol? B J Radiol 79(941):441, 2006

Maulik D: Biosafety of diagnostic Doppler ultrasonography. In: Doppler Ultrasound in Obstetrics and Gynecology. New York, Springer Verlag, 1997

Mazonakis M, Damilakis J, Varveris H, et al: A method of estimating fetal dose during brain radiation therapy. Int J Radiat Oncol Biol Phys 44:455, 1999

Mazonakis M, Varveris H, Damilakis J, et al: Radiation dose to concepts resulting from tangential breast irradiation. Int J Radiat Oncol Biol Phys 55:386, 2003

Mazze RI, Källén B: Reproductive outcome after anesthesia and operation during pregnancy: A registry study of 5405 cases. Am J Obstet Gynecol 161:1178, 1989

McCollough CH, Schueler BA, Atwell, TD, et al: Radiation exposure and pregnancy: When should we be concerned? RadioGraphics 27:909, 2007

Miller MW, Brayman AA, Abramowicz JS: Obstetric ultrasonography: A biophysical consideration of patient safety—the "rules" have changed. Am J Obstet Gynecol 179:241, 1998

Mountford PJ: Risk assessment of the nuclear medicine patient. Br J Radiol 100:671, 1997

National Research Council: Health effects of exposure to low levels of ionizing radiation BEIR V. Committee on the Biological Effects of Ionizing Radiations. Board on Radiation Effects Research Commission on Life Sciences. National Academy Press, Washington, DC, 1990

National Research Council: Health risks from exposure to low levels of ionizing radiation BEIR VII Phase 2. Committee to assess health risks from exposure to low levels of ionizing radiation. Board on Radiation Effects Research Division on Earth and Life Studies. National Academies Press, Washington, DC, 2006

Naumburg E, Bellocco R, Cnattingius S, et al: Prenatal ultrasound examinations and risk of childhood leukaemia: Case-control study. BMJ 320:282, 2000

Newman EA, Newman LA: Lymphatic mapping techniques and sentinel lymph node biopsy in breast cancer. Surg Clin North Am 87:353, 2007

Nuyttens JJ, Prado KL, Jenrette JM, et al: Fetal dose during radiotherapy: Clinical implementation and review of the literature. Cancer Radiother 6:352, 2002

Oelsner G, Stockheim D, Soriano D, et al: Pregnancy outcome after laparoscopy or laparotomy in pregnancy. J Am Assoc Gynecol Laparosc 10:200, 2003

O'Rourke N, Kodali B-S: Laparoscopic surgery during pregnancy. Curr Opin Anaesthesiol 19:254, 2006

Otake M, Yoshimaru H, Schull WJ: Severe mental retardation among the prenatally exposed survivors of the atomic bombing of Hiroshima and Nagasaki: A comparison of the old and new dosimetry systems. Radiation Effects Research Foundation, Technical Report No. 16-87, 1987

Oto A, Ernst R, Jesse MK, et al: Magnetic resonance imaging of the chest, abdomen, and pelvis in the evaluation of pregnant patients with neoplasms. Am J Perinatol 24:243, 2007

Pedrosa I, Lafornara M, Pandharipande PV, et al: Pregnant patients suspected of having acute appendicitis: Effect of MR imaging on negative laparotomy rate and appendiceal rate. Radiology 250(3):749, 2009

Pedrosa I, Zeikus EA, Deborah L, et al: MR imaging of acute right lower quadrant pain in pregnant and nonpregnant patients. RadioGraphics 27:721, 2007

Phupong V, Bunyavejchewin S: Gasless laparoscopic surgery for ovarian cyst in a second trimester pregnant patient with a ventricular septal defect. Surg Laparosc Endosc Percutan Tech 17:565, 2007

Prado KL, Nelson SJ, Nuyttens JJ, et al: Clinical implementation of the AAPM Task Group 36 recommendations on fetal dose from radiotherapy with photon beams: A head and neck irradiation case report. J Appl Clin Med Phys 1:1–7, 2000

Preston DL, Cullings H, Suyama A, et al: Solid cancer incidence in atomic bomb survivors exposed in utero or as young children. J Natl Cancer Inst 100:428, 2008

Reedy MB, Galan HL, Bean-Lijewski JD, et al: Maternal and fetal effects of laparoscopic insufflation in the gravid baboon. J Am Assoc Gynecol Laparosc 2:399, 1995

Reedy MB, Källén B, Kuehl TJ: Laparoscopy during pregnancy: A study of five fetal outcome parameters with use of the Swedish Health Registry. Am J Obstet Gynecol 177:673, 1997

Reichel TF, Ramus RM, Caire JT, et al: Fetal central nervous system biometry on MR imaging. AJR Am J Roentgenol 180:1155, 2003

Reynolds JD, Booth JV, de la Fuente S, et al: A review of laparoscopy for non-obstetric-related surgery during pregnancy. Curr Surg 60:164, 2003

Ribic-Pucelj M, Kobal B, Peternelj-Marinsek S: Surgical treatment of adnexal masses in pregnancy: Indications, surgical approach and pregnancy outcome. J Reprod Med 52:273, 2007

Rollins MD, Chan KJ, Price RR: Laparoscopy for appendicitis and cholelithiasis during pregnancy. Surg Endosc 18:237, 2004

Rosenstein M: Handbook of selected tissue doses for projections common in diagnostic radiology. Rockville, MD, Department of Health and Human Services, Food and Drug Administration. DHHS Pub No. (FDA) 89-8031, 1988

Rowley KA, Hill SJ, Watkins RA, et al: An investigation into the levels of radiation exposure in diagnostic examinations involving fluoroscopy. Br J Radiol 60:167, 1987

Sandrasegaran K, Lall CG, Aisen AA: Fetal magnetic resonance imaging. Curr Opin Obstet Gynecol 18:605, 2006

Schwartz JL, Mozurkewich EL, Johnson TM: Current management of patients with melanoma who are pregnant, want to get pregnant, or do not want to get pregnant. Cancer 97:2130, 2003

Singh A, Danrad R, Hahn PF, et al: MR imaging of the acute abdomen and pelvis: Acute appendicitis and beyond. Radiographics 27:1419, 2007

Sorahan T, Lancashire RJ, Temperton DH, et al: Childhood cancer and paternal exposure to ionizing radiation: A second report from the Oxford Survey of Childhood Cancers. Am J Ind Med 28(1):71, 1995

Spanheimer PM, Graham MM, Sugg SL, et al: Measurement of uterine radiation exposure from lymphoscintigraphy indicates safety of sentinel lymph node biopsy during pregnancy. Ann Surg Oncol 16(5):1143, 2009

Stather JW, Phipps AW, Harrison JD, et al: Dose coefficients for the embryo and fetus following intakes of radionuclides by the mother. J Radiol Prot 22:1, 2002

Stein, PD, Woodard PK, Weg JG, et al: Diagnostic pathways in acute pulmonary embolism: Recommendations of the PIOPED II investigators. Radiology 242(1):15, 2007

Steinbrook RA, Bhavani-Shankar K: Hemodynamics during laparoscopic surgery in pregnancy. Anesth Analg 93:1570, 2001

Stepp K, Falcone T: Laparoscopy in the second trimester of pregnancy. Obstet Gynecol Clin North Am 31:485, 2004

Stovall M, Blackwell CR, Cundif J, et al: Fetal dose from radiotherapy with photon beams: Report of AAPM radiation therapy Committee Task Group No. 36. Med Phys 22:63, 1995

Stroup SP, Altamar HO, L'Esperance JO, et al: Retroperitoneoscopic radical nephrectomy for renal-cell carcinoma during twin pregnancy. J Endourol 21:735, 2007

Strzelczyk, J, Damilakis J, Marx MV, et al: Facts and controversies about radiation exposure, Part 2: Low-level exposures and cancer risk. J Am Coll Radiol 4:32, 2007

Suleiman OH, Anderson J, Jones B, et al: Tissue doses in the upper gastrointestinal examination. Radiology 178:653, 1991

Sylvester GC, Khoury MJ, Lu X, et al: First-trimester anesthesia exposure and the risk of central nervous system defects: A population-based case-control study. Am J Public Health 84: 1757, 1994

Twickler DM, Cunningham FG: Central nervous system findings in preeclampsia and eclampsia. In Lyall F, Belfort M (eds): Pre-eclampsia—Etiology, and Clinical Practice. Cambridge, UK, Cambridge University Press, 2007, p 424

Twickler DM, Magee KP, Caire J, et al: Second-opinion magnetic resonance imaging for suspected fetal central nervous system abnormalities. Am J Obstet Gynecol 188:492, 2003

Twickler DM, Reichel T, McIntire DD, et al: Fetal central nervous system ventricle and cisterna magna measurements by magnetic resonance imaging. Am J Obstet Gynecol 187:927, 2002

Twickler DM, Setiawan AT, Evans R, et al: Imaging of puerperal septic thrombophlebitis: A prospective comparison of MR imaging, CT, and sonography. AJR Am J Roentgenol 169:1039, 1997

Vadeyar SH, Moore RJ, Strachan BK, et al: Effect of fetal magnetic resonance imaging on fetal heart rate patterns. Am J Obstet Gynecol 182:666, 2000

Vilos GA, Ternamian A, Dempster J, et al: Laparoscopic entry: A review of techniques, technologies, and complications. J Obstet Gynaecol Can 29:433, 2007

Wagner LK, Lester RG, Saldana LR: Exposure of the Pregnant Patient to Diagnostic Radiation. Philadelphia, Medical Physics Publishing, 1997

Wang L, Yu JM, Wang YS, et al: Preoperative lymphoscintigraphy predicts the successful identification but is not necessary in sentinel lymph nodes biopsy in breast cancer. Ann Surg Oncol May 24, 2007

Weisz B, Hoffman C, Chayenn B, et al: Diffusion MRI findings in monochorionic twin pregnancies after intrauterine fetal death. Abstract No. 399 Presented at the 29th Annual Meeting of the Society for Maternal-Fetal Medicine. 26-31 January 2009

White WM, Zite NB, Gash J, et al: Low-dose computer tomography for the evaluation of flank pain in the pregnant population. J Endourol 21:1255, 2007

Wo JY, Viswanathan AN: Impact of radiotherapy on fertility, pregnancy, and neonatal outcomes in female cancer patients. Int J Radiat Oncol Biol Phys 73(5):1304, 2009

Zanzonico PB: Internal radionuclide radiation dosimetry: A review of basic concepts and recent developments. J Nucl Med 41:297, 2000

Zaretsky M, McIntire D, Twickler DM: Feasibility of the fetal anatomic and maternal pelvic survey by magnetic resonance imaging at term. Am J Obstet Gynecol 189:997, 2003a

Zaretsky M, Reichel TF, McIntire DD, et al: Comparison of magnetic resonance imaging to ultrasound in the estimation of birth weight at term. Am J Obstet Gynecol 189:1017, 2003b

Zeeman GG, Hatab M, Twickler D: Maternal cerebral blood flow changes in pregnancy. Am J Obstet Gynecol 189:968, 2003

Zeeman GG, Fleckenstein JL, Twickler DM, et al: Cerebral infarction in eclampsia. Am J Obstet Gynecol 190:714, 2004a

Zeeman G, Hatab M, Twickler D: Increased large vessel cerebral blood flow in severe preeclampsia by magnetic resonance evaluation. Am J Obstet Gynecol 191:2148, 2004b

Zeeman GG, Cipolla MJ, Cunningham FG: Cerebrovascular (patho)physiology in preeclampsia. In Lindheimer MD, Roberts JM, Cunningham FG (eds): Chesley's Hypertensive Disorders in Pregnancy. 3rd Ed. New York, Elsevier, 2009, p 229

CHAPTER 42

Critical Care and Trauma

Women with a broad spectrum of pathophysiological conditions—some of which in the past precluded pregnancy—benefit from the technology and expertise of *critical care obstetrics*. Common medical and surgical problems such as serious heart disease, acute or chronic pulmonary disorders, and trauma complicating pregnancy are just a few examples. Included also are severe obstetrical complications such as preeclampsia, hemorrhage, and sepsis syndrome. It is imperative that obstetricians and other members of the healthcare team have a working knowledge of the unique considerations for pregnant women. Because these women are usually young and in good health, their prognosis should be better than that of many other patients admitted to an intensive care unit.

OBSTETRICAL INTENSIVE CARE

Depending on methods and protocols at various institutions, approximately 1 percent of obstetrical patients need some type of intensive observation and management. Women with complications specific to pregnancy have the greatest need for obstetrical intensive care (Kuklina and associates, 2009;

Madan and co-workers, 2008). As shown in Table 42-1, nearly half of these women need critical care for hypertensive disorders, hemorrhage, sepsis, or cardiopulmonary complications. With life-threatening hemorrhage, surgical procedures may be necessary, and close proximity to a delivery-operating room is advantageous. When admitted, a fourth of these women with serious medical or surgical disorders are still pregnant, and concerns for fetal well-being are usually better served by this close proximity. In our experiences from Parkland Hospital, Zeeman and colleagues (2003) reported that the most common nonobstetrical reasons for intensive care were usually encountered antepartum and included patients with diabetes, pneumonia or asthma, heart disease, chronic hypertension, pyelonephritis, or thyrotoxicosis.

Organization of Critical Care

The concept and development of critical care began in the 1960s. In 1983, the National Institutes of Health had its first Consensus Conference on this subject, and in 1988, the Society for Critical Care Medicine promulgated definitions and established guidelines for intensive care units (ICUs). These continue to be refined by certifying organizations (Manthous, 2004).

Because of high costs incurred by medical and surgical ICUs, a step-down *intermediate care unit* evolved. These units were designed for patients who did not require intensive care, but who needed a higher level of care than provided on a general ward. In 1998, the American College of Critical Care Medicine and the Society of Critical Care Medicine published guidelines for intermediate care units (Table 42-2).

Obstetrical Critical Care

Although the evolution of critical care for obstetrical patients has generally followed developments described above, there are no specific guidelines. Most hospitals employ a blend of

TABLE 42-1. Indications for Admission to Intensive Care Units for Obstetrical Patients

Factor	Dallas, Texas[a]	Houston, Texas[b]	Leiden, The Netherlands[c]	Weighted Average
Number	483	58	142	683
Antepartum	20%	30%	31%	23%
Postpartum	80%	70%	69%	77%
Diagnosis[d]				
Hypertensive disorders	45%	24%	62%	47%
Hemorrhage	18%	16%	18%	18%
Sepsis	5%	12%	3%	5%
Cardiopulmonary	12%	24%	4%	11%
Pregnancy-related mortality	0.2%	5.2%	4.9%	1.6%

[a]Zeeman and colleagues (2003): Obstetrical Intensive Care Unit.
[b]Stevens and co-workers (2006): Medical or Surgical Intensive Care Unit.
[c]Keizer and associates (2006): Multidisciplinary Intensive Care Unit.
[d]Columns do not total 100 percent–other diagnoses not listed.

these concepts, and in general, those can be divided into three types:

1. Medical or surgical ICU—in most hospitals, severely ill women are transferred to a unit operated by medical and surgical "intensivists." Triage to one of these depends on the acuity of care needed and the ability of that facility to provide it. In most obstetrical units, women who require ventilatory support, invasive monitoring, or pharmacological support of circulation are transferred to a specialized ICU. In her review of reports from more than 25 tertiary-care referral institutions, Zeeman (2006) found that about 0.5 percent of obstetrical patients are transferred to these types of ICUs.

2. Obstetrical Intermediate Care Unit—sometimes referred to as High-Dependency Care Unit (HDU)—examples of this system have been developed at both Parkland and at the University of Alabama at Birmingham Hospitals. These units are within the labor and delivery suites in specialized areas with experienced personnel available. The two-tiered system incorporates the guidelines for intermediate and intensive care. Care is provided by specially trained maternal-

fetal medicine specialists and nurses with experience in critical care obstetrics. The team should include clinicians with special expertise sufficient to deal with all problem areas. These typically include other obstetricians and anesthesiologists with readily available pulmonologists, cardiologists, and other medical and surgical specialists. Many tertiary-care centers have developed such intermediate care units and use selected triage to other ICUs. For smaller hospitals, transfer to a medical or surgical ICU is preferable, and sometimes transfer to another hospital is necessary. In either case, there must be collaboration between obstetricians, intensivists, and other specialists.

3. Obstetrical Intensive Care Unit—these units are full-care ICUs as described above, but are operated by obstetrical and anesthesia personnel in labor and delivery. Very few units have these capabilities (Zeeman, 2006).

Recently the American College of Obstetricians and Gynecologists (2009) summarized implementation of concepts of critical obstetrical care depending on hospital size and technical facilities. Somewhat related, Gosman and colleagues (2008)

TABLE 42-2. Guidelines for Conditions That Could Qualify for Intermediate Care

Cardiac: exclude infarction, stable infarction, stable arrhythmias, mild-to-moderate congestive heart failure, hypertensive urgency without end-organ damage
Pulmonary: stable patients for weaning and chronic ventilation, patients with potential for respiratory failure who are otherwise stable
Neurological: stable central nervous system, neuromuscular, or neurosurgical conditions that require close monitoring
Drug overdose: hemodynamically stable
Gastrointestinal: stable bleeding, liver failure with stable vital signs
Endocrine: diabetic ketoacidosis, thyrotoxicosis that requires frequent monitoring
Surgical: postoperative from major procedures or complications that require close monitoring
Miscellaneous: early sepsis, patients who require closely titrated intravenous fluids, pregnant women with severe preeclampsia or other medical problems

Reprinted from Nasraway SA, Cohen IL, Dennis RC, et al: Guidelines on admission and discharge for adult intermediate care units, *Critical Care Medicine*, 1998, vol. 26, no. 3, pp. 607–610, with permission.

TABLE 42-3. Formulas for Deriving Various Cardiopulmonary Parameters

Mean arterial pressure (MAP) (mm Hg) = [SBP + 2 (DBP)] ÷ 3
Cardiac output (CO) (L/min) = heart rate × stroke volume
Stroke volume (SV) (mL/beat) = CO/HR
Stroke index (SI) (mL/beat/m^2) = stroke volume/BSA
Cardiac index (CI) (L/min/m^2) = CO/BSA
Systemic vascular resistance (SVR) (dynes × sec × cm^{-5}) = [(MAP − CVP)/CO] × 80
Pulmonary vascular resistance (PVR) (dynes × sec × cm^{-5}) = [(MPAP − PCWP)/CO] × 80

BSA = body surface area (m^2); CO = cardiac output (L/min); CVP = central venous pressure (mm Hg); DBP = diastolic blood pressure; HR = heart rate (beats/min); MAP = mean systemic arterial pressure (mm Hg); MPAP = mean pulmonary artery pressure (mm Hg); PCWP = pulmonary capillary wedge pressure (mm Hg); SBP = systolic blood pressure.

have explored the concept of a *medical emergency team— MET*—for rapid response to emergent obstetrical critical care situations.

Pulmonary Artery Catheter (PAC)

Use of the pulmonary artery catheter has contributed immensely to understanding of normal pregnancy hemodynamics as well as pathophysiology of common obstetrical conditions. These include severe preeclampsia-eclampsia, acute respiratory distress syndrome (ARDS), and amnionic fluid embolism (Clark, 1988, 1995, 1997; Cunningham, 1986, 1987; Hankins, 1984, 1985, and all their co-workers). That said, in our extensive experiences, invasive hemodynamic monitoring is seldom necessary for critically ill obstetrical patients.

After years of use, randomized trials of more than 3700 medical and surgical patients described no benefits with pulmonary artery catheter monitoring (Harvey, 2005; Richard, 2003; Sandham, 2003, and their numerous colleagues). A recent randomized trial conducted by the National Heart, Lung, and Blood Institute (2006b) assessed catheter-guided therapy in 1000 patients with acute respiratory distress syndrome (ARDS). PAC monitoring did not improve survival or organ function,

and there were more complications than with central venous pressure monitoring. A retrospective analysis of the National Trauma Data Bank by Friese and co-workers (2006) showed a survival advantage for catheter monitoring in patients with the highest injury severity scores (ISS). Its uses in obstetrics are limited (Martin and Foley, 2006). One example might be sepsis syndrome complicated by pulmonary edema and hypotension.

Hemodynamic Changes in Pregnancy

Formulas for deriving some hemodynamic parameters are shown in Table 42-3. These measurements can be corrected for body size by dividing by body surface area (BSA) to obtain *index values.* Nomograms for nonpregnant adults are used. As emphasized by Van Hook and Hankins (1997), this information does not always reflect uteroplacental perfusion.

In a landmark investigation, Clark and colleagues (1989) used PAC to obtain cardiovascular measurements in healthy pregnant women and again in these same women when nonpregnant, to serve as their own controls (Table 42-4). When plotted on a *ventricular function curve,* performance remains unchanged during pregnancy because increased blood volume and cardiac output are compensated by decreased vascular resistance and increased pulse rate (Fig. 42-1). A working knowledge of these changes is

TABLE 42-4. Hemodynamic Changes in Normal Nonpregnant Women Compared with Those When Pregnant at Term

Measurement	Nonpregnant	Term Pregnant	Change (%)
Cardiac output (L/min)	4.3 ± 0.9	6.2 ± 1.0	+44
Heart rate (beats/min)	71 ± 10	83 ± 10	+17
Mean arterial pressure (mm Hg)	86 ± 7.5	90 ± 5.8	+4
Systemic vascular resistance (dynes/cm/sec^{-5})	1530 ± 520	1210 ± 266	−21
Pulmonary vascular resistance (dynes/cm/sec^{-5})	199 ± 47	78 ± 22	−35
Pulmonary capillary wedge pressure (mm Hg)	6.3 ± 2.1	7.5 ± 1.8	+18
Central venous pressure (mm Hg)	3.7 ± 2.6	3.6 ± 2.5	−2
Left ventricular stroke work index (g/m/m^{-2})	41 ± 8	48 ± 6	+17
Colloid oncotic pressure (mm Hg)	20.8 ± 1.0	18.0 ± 1.5	−14
Colloid oncotic/wedge pressure gradient (mm Hg)	14.5 ± 2.5	10.5 ± 2.7	−28

This table was published in *American Journal of Obstetrics & Gynecology,* Vol. 161, No. 6, pt. 1, SL Clark, DB Cotton, W Lee, et al., Central hemodynamic assessment of normal term pregnancy, pp. 1439–1442, Copyright Elsevier 1989.

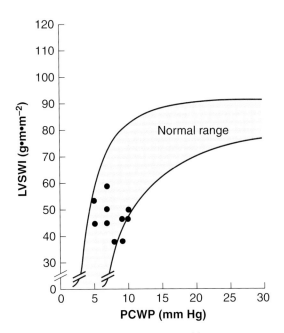

FIGURE 42-1 Ventricular function in 10 healthy pregnant women at term. Individual values are plotted and all but one fall between the lines that define normal function. (LVSWI = left ventricular stroke work index; PCWP = pulmonary capillary wedge pressure.) (Plotted data points from Clark and colleagues, 1989.)

paramount to understanding the pathophysiology of pregnancy complications discussed throughout this book.

ACUTE PULMONARY EDEMA

The incidence of pulmonary edema complicating pregnancy averages about 1 in 500 to 1000 deliveries at tertiary referral centers. The two general causes are: (1) *cardiogenic*—hydrostatic edema caused by high pulmonary capillary hydraulic pressures and (2) *noncardiogenic*—permeability edema caused by capillary endothelial and alveolar epithelial damage. In pregnancy, pulmonary edema frequently is due to a combination of these two. Taken in toto, studies in pregnant women indicate that more than half who develop pulmonary edema have some degree of sepsis syndrome in conjunction with tocolysis, severe preeclampsia, or obstetrical hemorrhage combined with vigorous fluid therapy.

Cardiogenic pulmonary edema is involved in fewer than half of cases, but resuscitation for hemorrhage and vigorous treatment for preterm labor are common precipitating causes. Sciscione and colleagues (2003) reported that among 51 cases of pulmonary edema, approximately one fourth each were due to cardiac failure, tocolytic therapy, iatrogenic fluid overload, or preeclampsia. In 25 cases described by Hough and Katz (2007), more than half were associated with preeclampsia, and there was equal distribution of the other three causes. DiFederico and associates (1998) reported that 40 percent of 84 cases of pulmonary edema were associated with tocolytic therapy. And in the report by Jenkins and colleagues (2003), tocolytic therapy caused 15 percent of cases of pulmonary edema and one maternal death in 51 women who required assisted ventilation.

Noncardiogenic Increased Permeability Edema

Endothelial activation associated with preeclampsia, sepsis syndrome, or acute hemorrhage—or more likely combinations of these—are the most common predisposing factors to pulmonary edema in pregnant women (Table 42-5). As discussed, these are often associated with vigorous fluid replacement and tocolytic therapy for preterm labor. Parenteral β-agonists such as terbutaline are undisputedly related to pulmonary edema. And although Samol and Lambers (2005) reported that pulmonary edema developed in 8 percent of 789 women given magnesium sulfate for preterm labor, half of these were also given terbutaline. In our extensive experiences with the use of magnesium sulfate for treatment of severe preeclampsia, we are dubious that magnesium *per se* causes pulmonary edema. Martin and Foley (2006) arrived at a similar conclusion after their review.

Cardiogenic Hydrostatic Edema

Most cases of cardiogenic pulmonary edema during pregnancy are associated with some form of gestational hypertension. Acute systolic hypertension exacerbates diastolic dysfunction, causing pulmonary edema (Gandhi and associates, 2001). Common causes of diastolic heart failure are chronic hypertension and obesity with left ventricular hypertrophy (Jessup and Brozena, 2003; Kenchaiah and colleagues, 2002). And such hypertrophy is two- to threefold more common in black women compared with white women (Drazner and co-workers, 2005). Other causes are congenital or acquired anatomical defects (see Chap. 44, p. 963, and Appendix). Even so, heart failure is commonly precipitated acutely by preeclampsia, hemorrhage and anemia, and puerperal sepsis (Cunningham and associates, 1986; Sibai and colleagues, 1987). In many of these, when echocardiography is done later, there is a normal ejection fraction, and evidence for diastolic dysfunction can be found (Aurigemma and Gaasch, 2004). Determination of serum levels of *brain natriuretic peptide (BNP)* has not been reported extensively in pregnancy (see Chap. 5, p. 121). This is a cardiac neurohormone that is secreted from cardiac ventricle myocytes and fibroblasts, and its plasma concentrations are increased in congestive

TABLE 42-5. Some Causes and Associated Factors for Pulmonary Edema in Pregnancy

Noncardiogenic permeability edema—endothelial activation with capillary-alveolar leakage:
  Preeclampsia syndrome
  Acute hemorrhage
  Sepsis syndrome
  Tocolytic therapy—β-mimetics,? MgSO₄

Cardiogenic pulmonary edema—myocardial failure with hydrostatic edema from excessive pulmonary capillary pressure:
  Hypertensive cardiomyopathy
  Obesity—*cordis adipositus*
  Left-sided valvular disease

heart failure. In general, values less than 100 pg/mL have an excellent negative-predictive value, and levels exceeding 500 pg/mL have an excellent positive-predictive value. But those often recorded—100 to 500 pg/mL—are nondiagnostic (Ware and Matthay, 2005). Assays for both N-terminal BNP and atrial natriuretic peptide (ANP) are elevated with preeclampsia compared with normotensive pregnancy (Tihtonen and co-workers, 2007).

ACUTE RESPIRATORY DISTRESS SYNDROME

The most common cause of respiratory failure in pregnancy is from severe permeability pulmonary edema—the acute respiratory distress syndrome (ARDS). This pathophysiological manifestation of acute lung injury is a continuum from clinical pulmonary edema with mild pulmonary insufficiency as discussed earlier to dependence on high-inspired oxygen concentrations and mechanical ventilation. Because there are no uniform criteria for the diagnosis of ARDS, its incidence is variably reported. In a review, Catanzarite and associates (2001) computed it to be 1 in 3000 to 6000 deliveries. Severe disease requiring ventilatory support has a mortality rate for all patients of 45 percent, which has remained constant since the mid-1990s (Phua and co-workers, 2009). It is as high as 90 percent if caused or complicated by sepsis. Although they are younger and healthier than the overall population, pregnant women still have mortality rates of 25 to 40 percent (Catanzarite and co-workers, 2001; Cole and associates, 2005). Women who are still pregnant with ARDS have correspondingly high perinatal mortality rates.

Definitions

Physiological criteria required for diagnosis of ARDS differ, but clinically it is important to remember that the syndrome covers a wide spectrum. For studies, most investigators define ARDS as radiographically documented pulmonary infiltrates, a ratio of arterial oxygen tension to the fraction of inspired oxygen (PaO_2:FiO_2) of less than 200, and no evidence of heart failure (Martin and Foley, 2006). For most interventional studies, a working diagnosis of *acute lung injury* is made when the PaO_2:FiO_2 ratio is less than 300 along with dyspnea, tachypnea, oxygen desaturation, and radiographic pulmonary infiltrates (Wheeler and Bernard, 2007).

Pathophysiology

ARDS is a pathophysiological description and not necessarily a diagnosis. With acute lung injury from a variety of causes, there is recruitment of neutrophils to the site of inflammation by chemokines. As neutrophils accumulate, they initiate further tissue injury by cytokine elaboration. There is widespread injury to microvascular endothelium, including the pulmonary vasculature, and there is also alveolar epithelial injury. These result in increased pulmonary capillary permeability, surfactant loss or inactivation, diminished lung volume, and vascular shunting with resultant arterial hypoxemia. The second phase of the syndrome usually begins 3 to 4 days later. It involves development of *fibrosing alveolitis* and subsequent repair. Despite

this, the long-term prognosis for pulmonary function is surprisingly good (Herridge and colleagues, 2003). This subject has been reviewed by Wheeler and Bernard (2007).

Etiology

A number of disorders have been associated with acute pulmonary injury and permeability edema during pregnancy (Table 42-6). Although many are coincidental, others are unique to pregnancy. For example, in nonpregnant patients, sepsis and diffuse infectious pneumonia are the two most common single-agent causes and together account for 60 percent of cases. In pregnancy, however, pyelonephritis, chorioamnionitis, and puerperal pelvic infection are the most frequent causes of sepsis. Severe preeclampsia and obstetrical hemorrhage are also commonly found with ARDS. Importantly, more than half of pregnant women have some combination of sepsis, shock, trauma, and fluid overload. The contribution of *transfusion-related acute lung injury (TRALI),* as described by Kopko and colleagues (2002), is unclear in obstetrical patients (see Chap. 35, p. 794). This subject has been reviewed by Bux and Sachs (2007) and by Stroncek (2007).

Clinical Course

With pulmonary injury, the clinical condition depends largely on the magnitude of the insult, the ability to compensate for it, and the stage of the disease. For example, soon after the initial injury, there commonly are no physical findings except perhaps hyperventilation. And at first, arterial oxygenation usually is adequate. Pregnancy-induced mild metabolic alkalosis may be accentuated by hyperventilation. With worsening, clinical and radiological evidence for pulmonary edema, decreased lung compliance,

TABLE 42-6. Some Causes of Acute Lung Injury and Respiratory Failure in Pregnant Women

• Pneumonia	• Tocolytic therapy
Bacterial	• Embolism
Viral	Amnionic fluid
Aspiration	Trophoblastic disease
• Sepsis syndrome	Air
Chorioamnionitis	• Connective-tissue disease
Pyelonephritis	• Substance abuse
Puerperal infection	• Irritant inhalation and
Septic abortion	burns
• Hemorrhage	• Pancreatitis
Shock	• Drug overdose
Massive transfusion	• Fetal surgery
Transfusion-related	• Trauma
acute lung injury	• Sickle-cell disease
(TRALI)	• Miliary tuberculosis
• Preeclampsia syndrome	

From Catanzarite (2001), Cole (2005), Golombeck (2006), Jenkins (2003), Lapinsky (2005), Martin and Foley (2006), Oram (2007), Sheffield and Cunningham (2005), Zeeman (2003, 2006), and all their associates.

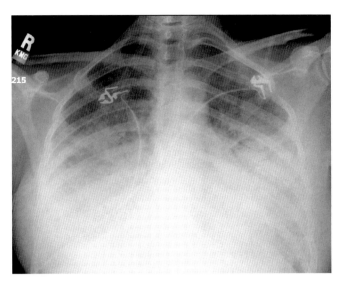

FIGURE 42-2 Anterior-posterior projection chest radiograph of a second-trimester pregnant woman. Marked bilateral parenchymal and pleural opacification secondary to acute respiratory distress syndrome (ARDS) are seen.

and increased intrapulmonary blood shunting become apparent. Progressive alveolar and interstitial edema develop with extravasation of inflammatory cells and erythrocytes.

Ideally, pulmonary injury is identified at this early stage, and specific therapy is directed at the insult if possible. Further progression to acute respiratory failure is characterized by marked dyspnea, tachypnea, and hypoxemia. Further loss of lung volume results in worsening of pulmonary compliance and increased shunting. There are now diffuse abnormalities by auscultation, and a chest radiograph characteristically demonstrates bilateral lung involvement (Fig. 42-2). At this phase, the injury ordinarily would be lethal in the absence of high inspired-oxygen concentrations and positive airway pressure by mask or by intubation. When shunting exceeds 30 percent, severe refractory hypoxemia develops along with metabolic and respiratory acidosis that can result in myocardial irritability, dysfunction, and cardiac arrest.

Management

In acute and severe lung injury, attempts are made to provide adequate oxygenation of peripheral tissues while ensuring that therapeutic maneuvers do not further aggravate lung injury. At least intuitively, increasing oxygen delivery should produce a corresponding increase in tissue uptake, but this is difficult to measure (Evans and Smithies, 1999). Support of systemic perfusion with intravenous crystalloid and blood is imperative. In this regard, a randomized trial by the National Heart, Lung, and Blood Institute (2006b) showed that pulmonary artery catheterization did not improve outcomes. Because sepsis is commonplace in lung injury, vigorous antimicrobial therapy is given for infection. Oxygen delivery can be greatly improved by correction of anemia—each gram of hemoglobin carries 1.25 mL of oxygen when 90-percent saturated. By comparison, increasing the arterial PO_2 from 100 to 200 mm Hg results in the transport of only 0.1 mL of additional oxygen for each 100 mL of blood.

Reasonable goals in caring for the woman with severe lung injury are to obtain a PaO_2 of 60 mm Hg or 90-percent saturation at an inspired oxygen content of less than 50 percent, and with positive end-expiratory pressures less than 15 mm Hg. It remains controversial whether delivery of the fetus improves maternal oxygenation (Cole and associates, 2005; Jenkins and co-workers, 2003). Further discussion of the possible effects of delivery during cardiopulmonary resuscitation is found on p. 942).

Oxyhemoglobin Dissociation Curve

The propensity of the hemoglobin molecule to release oxygen is described by the oxyhemoglobin dissociation curve. Simplistically, the curve can be divided into an upper oxygen association curve representing the alveolar-capillary environment and a lower oxygen dissociation portion representing the tissue-capillary environment (Fig. 42-3). Shifts of the curve have their greatest impact at the steep portion because they affect oxygen delivery. A rightward shift is associated with decreased hemoglobin affinity for oxygen and hence increased tissue-capillary oxygen interchange. Rightward shifts are produced by hypercapnia, metabolic acidosis, fever, and increased 2,3-diphosphoglycerate levels. During pregnancy, the erythrocyte concentration of 2,3-diphosphoglycerate is increased by approximately 30 percent. This favors oxygen delivery to both the fetus and peripheral maternal tissues (Rorth and Bille-Brahe, 1971).

Fetal hemoglobin has a higher oxygen affinity than adult hemoglobin. As seen in Figure 42-3, its curve is positioned to the left of the adult curve. To achieve 50-percent hemoglobin saturation in the mother, the PaO_2 must be 27 mm Hg compared with only 19 mm Hg in the fetus. Under normal physiological conditions, the fetus is constantly on the dissociation, or tissue,

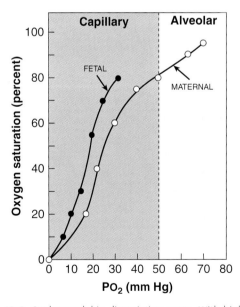

FIGURE 42-3 Oxyhemoglobin dissociation curve. With higher oxygen tension (Pao_2) in the pulmonary alveoli, adult hemoglobin is maximally saturated compared with that at the lower oxygen tension in the tissue capillaries. Note that at any given oxygen tension, fetal hemoglobin carries more oxygen than adult hemoglobin, as indicated by percent saturation.

portion of the curve. Even with severe maternal lung disease and very low PaO₂ levels, oxygen displacement to fetal tissues is favored. This has been confirmed by studies of pregnant women and their fetuses at high altitude, where despite a maternal PaO_2 of only 60 mm Hg, the fetal PaO_2 is equivalent to that at sea level (Subrevilla and colleagues, 1971).

Mechanical Ventilation

In some patients, positive pressure ventilation by face mask may be effective in early stages of pulmonary insufficiency (Roy and colleagues, 2007). In an attempt to maximize the fetal environment, early intubation is preferred in the pregnant woman if respiratory failure is more likely than not, and especially if it appears to be imminent. The use of *low tidal volume ventilation*—≤ 6 mL/kg body weight—with plateau pressures of < 30 cm H_2O has been proven most beneficial to survival (Girard and Bernard, 2007). Ventilation is adjusted to obtain a PaO_2 greater than 60 mm Hg, or a hemoglobin saturation of 90 percent and a $PaCO_2$ of 35 to 45 mm Hg. Lower levels for PaO_2 should be avoided, because placental perfusion may be impaired (Levinson and co-workers, 1974).

Across the board, the maternal mortality rate is about 20 percent for pregnant women who require ventilation for any length of time. Jenkins and associates (2003) described 51 such women, of whom almost half had severe preeclampsia. Most were intubated postpartum, but 11 were delivered while being ventilated, and another six were discharged undelivered. The maternal mortality rate was 14 percent, and this included a woman who died as a complication of tocolytic treatment. Schneider and colleagues (2003) described a 17-percent maternal mortality rate in 53 women who delivered while receiving ventilatory support. Chen and co-workers (2003) reported four maternal deaths among 16 pregnant women—25 percent—who required mechanical ventilation. None of these investigators concluded that delivery improved maternal outcome.

Positive End-Expiratory Pressure

With severe lung injury and high intrapulmonary shunt fractions, it may not be possible to provide adequate oxygenation with usual ventilatory pressures, even with 100-percent oxygen. Positive end-expiratory pressure is usually successful in decreasing the shunt by recruiting collapsed alveoli. At low levels of 5 to 15 mm Hg, positive pressure can typically be used safely. At higher levels, impaired right-sided venous return can result in decreased cardiac output, decreased uteroplacental perfusion, alveolar overdistension, falling compliance, and barotrauma.

Extracorporeal Membrane Oxygenation (ECMO)

This is not usually used in adults. But in a few pregnant women with respiratory failure, ECMO has been used successfully to allow time for lung healing. Cunningham and colleagues (2006) reviewed outcomes in five such women. The duration of support in the four survivors was 2 to 28 days.

Intravenous Fluids

Some pregnancy-induced physiological changes may predispose to greater risk of permeability edema from fluid therapy. For example, colloid oncotic pressure (COP) is determined by serum albumin concentration, and 1 g/dL exerts about 6 mm Hg pressure. As discussed in Chapter 5 (p. 126), serum albumin concentrations normally decrease in pregnancy. This results in a decline from 28 mm Hg in the nonpregnant woman to 23 mm Hg at term and to 17 mm Hg in the puerperium (Benedetti and Carlson, 1979; Robertson, 1969). With preeclampsia, endothelial activation with leakage causes extravascular albumin loss and decreased serum albumin levels. As a result, oncotic pressure averages only 16 mm Hg antepartum and 14 mm Hg postpartum (Zinaman and co-workers, 1985). These changes have a significant clinical impact on the *colloid oncotic pressure/wedge pressure gradient*. Normally, this gradient exceeds 8 mm Hg: however, when it is 4 mm Hg or less, there is an increased risk for pulmonary edema.

Other Therapy

There were no benefits from *artificial or replacement surfactant therapy* in 725 nonpregnant patients with sepsis-induced lung failure reported by Anzueto and colleagues (1996). Although inhalation of *nitric oxide* was found to cause early improvement, mortality rates were unchanged in two studies (Taylor and co-workers, 2004; Wheeler and Bernard, 2007). In a randomized trial conducted by the National Heart, Lung, and Blood Institute (2006), *prolonged methylprednisolone* therapy did not reduce mortality rates when begun in patients who had no improvement by day 7.

SEPSIS SYNDROME

The sepsis syndrome is induced by a systemic inflammatory response to bacteria or their by-products such as endotoxins or exotoxins. The severity of the syndrome is a continuum or spectrum (Fig. 42-4). Infections that most commonly cause the sepsis syndrome in obstetrics are pyelonephritis (see Chap. 48, p. 1036), chorioamnionitis and puerperal sepsis (see Chap. 31, p. 661), septic abortion (see Chap. 9, p. 220), and necrotizing fasciitis (see Chap. 31, p. 669). In more than 4000 nonpregnant patients, the mortality rate at 28 days with severe sepsis was 30 to 40 percent (Abraham and colleagues, 1997; Bernard and associates, 2001). When there is septic shock, mortality rates are higher regardless of the etiology. Mabie and associates (1997) reported a 28-percent mortality rate in 18 pregnant women with sepsis and shock.

Etiopathogenesis

The sepsis syndrome in obstetrics may be caused by a number of pathogens. Although pelvic infections are usually polymicrobial, bacteria that cause severe sepsis syndrome are frequently endotoxin-producing Enterobacteriaceae, most commonly *Escherichia coli*. Other pathogens are aerobic and anaerobic streptococci, *Bacteroides* species, and *Clostridium* species. As recently reviewed by Filbin and colleagues (2009), some strains of group A β-hemolytic streptococci and *Staphylococcus aureus*—including community-acquired methicillin-resistant strains (CA-MRSA)—produce virulent exotoxins that can rapidly cause all features of

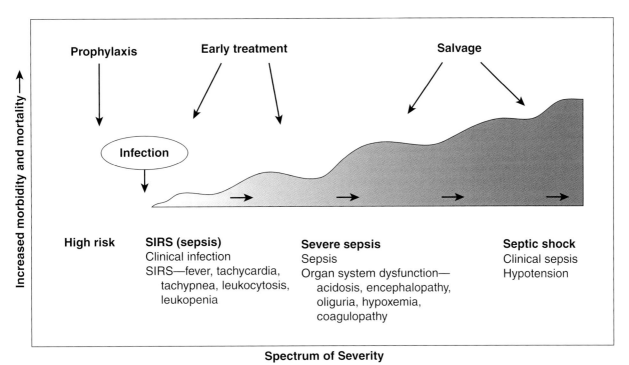

FIGURE 42-4 The sepsis syndrome begins with a systemic inflammatory response syndrome (SIRS) in response to infection that may progress to septic shock. (Redrawn with permission from Dr. Robert S. Munford.)

the sepsis syndrome, which is then termed the *toxic shock syndrome* (see Chap. 31, p. 670). Other virulent streptococci produce proteases that degrade interleukin-8 (IL-8) (Hidalgo- Grass and associates, 2004). Pyelonephritis complicating pregnancy caused by *E. coli* and *Klebsiella* species commonly is associated with bacteremia and sepsis syndrome (Cunningham and associates, 1987; Mabie and colleagues, 1997).

Endotoxin is a lipopolysaccharide released upon lysis of the cell walls of gram-negative bacteria. A number of potent bacterial *exotoxins* can also cause severe sepsis syndrome. Examples include exotoxins from *Clostridium perfringens*, toxic shock syndrome toxin (TSST-1) from *S. aureus*, and toxic shock-like exotoxin from group A β-hemolytic streptococci (Adem and associates, 2005; Daif and co-workers, 2009). As described by Nathan and colleagues (1993), these exotoxins cause rapid and extensive tissue necrosis and gangrene, especially of the postpartum uterus, and may cause profound cardiovascular collapse and maternal death.

Sequelae of the sepsis syndrome begin with an inflammatory response that is directed against microbial endotoxins and exotoxins. These and other toxins stimulate CD4 T cells and leukocytes to produce proinflammatory compounds that include tumor necrosis factor-α (TNF-α), a number of interleukins, other cytokines, proteases, oxidants, and bradykinin (Russell, 2006). For example, a very small amount of TSST-1 activates 5 to 30 percent of T cells that result in a "cytokine storm" (Que and associates, 2005). A myriad of cellular reactions follow that include stimulation of pro- and anti-inflammatory compounds, procoagulant activity, gene activation, receptor regulation, and immune suppression (Filbin and colleagues, 2009; Hotchkiss and Karl, 2003). It is also likely that IL-6 mediates myocardial suppression (Pathan and associates, 2004).

The pathophysiological response to this cascade is selective vasodilation with maldistribution of blood flow. Leukocyte and platelet aggregation causes capillary plugging. Vascular endothelial injury causes profound capillary leakage and interstitial fluid accumulation. Depending on the injury and inflammatory response, which are likely related to the virulence and dose of toxin, there is a spectrum of clinical response (see Fig. 42-4). Thus, sepsis syndrome is a clinical as well as pathophysiological continuum, the most severe result of which is *septic shock*. In its early stages, clinical shock results primarily from decreased systemic vascular resistance that is not compensated fully by increased cardiac output. Hypoperfusion results in lactic acidosis, decreased tissue oxygen extraction, and end-organ dysfunction such as renal failure (Schrier and Wang, 2004). Ultimately, *multiple organ failure* may follow (Table 42-7).

Hemodynamic Changes with Sepsis

The pathophysiology of the sepsis syndrome has been elucidated by Parker (1987) and Parrillo (1990) and their colleagues from the National Institutes of Health. They observed that capillary leakage initially causes hypovolemia. If circulating volume is restored with intravenous crystalloid at this point, sepsis is a high cardiac output, low systemic vascular resistance condition. Concomitantly, pulmonary hypertension develops. This is often referred to as the *warm phase* of septic shock. These findings are the most common cardiovascular manifestations of early sepsis, and they often have prognostic significance. Paradoxically, despite the high cardiac output, patients with severe sepsis likely have myocardial depression (Ognibene and co-workers, 1988).

Most previously healthy pregnant women with sepsis at this stage respond well to fluid resuscitation, intensive antimicrobial

TABLE 42-7. Multiple Organ Effects with Sepsis and Shock

Central nervous system	
Cerebral	Confusion, somnolence, coma, combativeness
Hypothalamic	Fever, hypothermia
Cardiovascular	
Blood pressure	Hypotension (vasodilation)
Cardiac	Increased cardiac output with fluid replacement; myocardial depression with diminished cardiac output
Pulmonary	Shunting with dysoxia and hypoxemia; diffuse infiltrates from endothelial and epithelial damage
Gastrointestinal	Gastritis, toxic hepatitis, hyperglycemia
Renal	Hypoperfusion with oliguria; acute tubular necrosis
Hematological	Thrombocytopenia, leukocytosis, activation of coagulation

therapy, and if indicated, removal of infected tissue. Conversely, if hypotension is not corrected following vigorous fluid infusion, then the prognosis is more guarded. At this juncture, if there also is no response to β-adrenergic inotropic agents, this indicates severe and unresponsive extracellular fluid extravasation with vascular insufficiency, overwhelming myocardial depression, or both. Oliguria and continued peripheral vasoconstriction characterize a secondary, *cold phase* of septic shock, survival of which is uncommon. Another poor prognostic sign is continued renal, pulmonary, and cerebral dysfunction once hypotension has been corrected. The average risk of death increases by 15 to 20 percent with failure of each organ system (Wheeler and Bernard, 1999). If three systems are involved, mortality rates are 70 percent (Martin and colleagues, 2003).

Management

In the early 2000s, after a review of various protocols for managing sepsis, an internationally directed consortium launched the Surviving Sepsis Campaign. The cornerstone of management was termed *early goal-directed management* and patterned after the protocol of Rivers and colleagues (2001). The protocol, recently updated by Dellinger and colleagues (2008), stresses prompt recognition of serious bacterial infection and close monitoring of vital signs and urine flow. In obstetrics, hypotension or oliguria should immediately prompt consideration for septicemia or hemorrhage.

One algorithm for management of sepsis syndrome is shown in Figure 42-5. The three steps are performed as simultaneously as possible. Prompt and aggressive evaluation and treatment are initiated. Rapid infusion with 2 L and sometimes as many as 4 to 6 L of crystalloid fluids may be required to restore renal perfusion in severely affected women. Because of the cap-

illary leak, there is hemoconcentration. To combat this, blood is given along with crystalloid to maintain the hematocrit at approximately 30 percent (Rivers and colleagues, 2001). According to Ware and Matthay (2000), the use of colloid solution such as 5-percent human albumin is controversial. We do not recommend its use.

If aggressive volume replacement is not promptly followed by urinary output of at least 30 and preferably 50 mL/hr, as well as other indicators of improved perfusion, then consideration is given for vasoactive drug therapy. Mortality rates are high when sepsis is further complicated by respiratory or renal failure. With severe sepsis, damage to pulmonary capillary endothelium and alveolar epithelium causes alveolar flooding and pulmonary edema. This may occur even with low or normal pulmonary capillary wedge pressures. With continued inflammation, this progresses to the *acute respiratory distress syndrome* as discussed on page 930.

Broad-spectrum antimicrobials are administered in maximal doses after appropriate cultures are taken of blood, urine, or exudates not contaminated by normal flora. In severe sepsis, appropriate empirical coverage results in better survival rates (MacArthur and colleagues, 2004). For women with an infected abortion or deep fascial infections, a Gram-stained smear may be helpful in identifying *Clostridium perfringens* or group A streptococcal organisms. Generally, empirical coverage with regimens such as ampicillin plus gentamicin plus clindamycin suffices for pelvic infections (see Chap. 31, p. 664). Wound and other soft-tissue infections are increasingly likely to be caused by methicillin-resistant *S. aureus* (Klevens and associates, 2007; Rotas and colleagues, 2007).

Surgical Treatment

Continuing sepsis may prove fatal, and debridement of necrotic tissue or drainage of purulent material is crucial. Of 18 pregnant women with septic shock, Mabie and colleagues (1997) reported that eight required surgical therapy to control the source of infection. A meticulous search is made for such foci. With an infected abortion, uterine contents must be removed promptly by curettage. Hysterectomy is seldom indicated unless gangrene has resulted, such as in the case shown in Figure 42-6.

For women with pyelonephritis, continuing sepsis should prompt a search for obstruction caused by calculi or a perinephric or intrarenal phlegmon or abscess. Renal sonography or "one-shot" pyelography may be used to diagnose obstruction and calculi, whereas computed tomography (CT) may be helpful to diagnose a phlegmon or abscess. With obstruction, ureteral catheterization, percutaneous nephrostomy, or flank exploration may be lifesaving (see Chap. 48, p. 1038).

Most cases of puerperal sepsis are clinically manifested in the first several days postpartum, and tissue debridement is not usually indicated this early. There are several exceptions:

- Necrotizing fasciitis of the episiotomy site or abdominal surgical incision. As described by Gallup and colleagues (2002), this is a surgical emergency, and aggressive management is discussed in Chapter 31 (pp. 665 and 669).
- Massive uterine myonecrosis caused by group A β-hemolytic streptococcal infections (Fig. 42-6). The mortality rate in

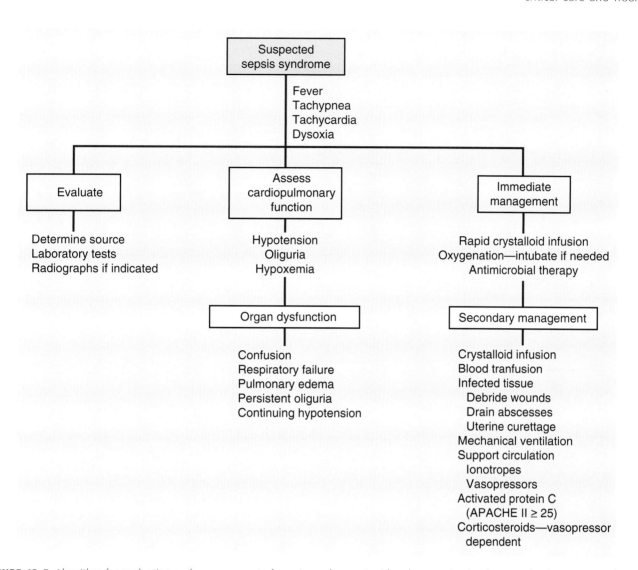

FIGURE 42-5 Algorithm for evaluation and management of sepsis syndrome. Rapid and aggressive implementation is paramount for success. The three steps—Evaluate, Assess, and Immediate management—are done as simultaneously as possible.

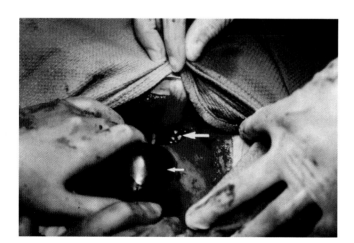

FIGURE 42-6 Group A β-hemolytic *Streptococcus pyogenes* puerperal infection that caused uterine gangrene, overwhelming sepsis syndrome, and maternal death. Arrows point to overtly "ballooned-out" gangrenous areas of postpartum uterus.

these women is high, and prompt hysterectomy may be lifesaving (Mabie and co-workers, 1997; Nathan and colleagues, 1993). Other overwhelmingly infected tissues or other virulent organisms can produce similar findings (Clad and associates, 2003; Daif and co-workers, 2009).

• Persistent or aggressive uterine infection with necrosis and dehiscence of the uterine incision with severe peritonitis (see Chap. 31, p. 666). **Any woman with infection following cesarean delivery who is suspected of having peritonitis should be carefully evaluated for uterine incisional necrosis or bowel perforation.** Prompt surgical exploration, and frequently hysterectomy, may be necessary. An abdominopelvic CT scan of the pelvis is useful to characterize these infections.

Peritonitis and sepsis much less commonly may result from a ruptured parametrial, intra-abdominal, or ovarian abscess (see Chap. 31, p. 665).

Adjunctive Therapy

Vasoactive drugs are not given unless aggressive fluid treatment fails to correct hypotension and perfusion abnormalities. First-line agents are norepinephrine, epinephrine, dopamine, dobutamine, or phenylephrine. Russell and colleagues (2008) recently showed that low-dose vasopressin combined with norepinephrine infusion did not lower 28-day mortality rates.

The use of corticosteroids is controversial. Serum cortisol levels are typically elevated in sepsis, and higher levels are associated with increased mortality rates (Sam and associates, 2004). Some but not all studies have shown a salutary effect of steroid administration, and these drugs are considered for use in patients who are vasopressor dependent (Dellinger and co-workers, 2008).

Endotoxin stimulates endothelial cells to upregulate tissue factor and thus procoagulant production. At the same time, it decreases the anticoagulant action of activated protein C. Because of this, agents were developed that block coagulation, however, *antithrombin III* and *tissue factor pathway inhibitor* did not improve outcomes (Abraham and co-workers, 2003; Warren and colleagues, 2001).

In a landmark study by Bernard and associates (2001), recombinant activated protein C—*drotrecogin alfa*—was shown to improve 28-day mortality rates from sepsis. This effect was limited to the subset of patients with severe sepsis and a high risk of death as determined by an Acute Physiology and Chronic Health Evaluation II (APACHE II) score of 25 or greater. The APACHE II score is computed from 12 physiological assessments in the ICU—scores range from 0 to 71. Subsequent trials confirmed this and again showed no advantages for patients with severe sepsis and an APACHE II score of less than 25 (Abraham and colleagues, 2005; Payen and associates, 2007). The Surviving Sepsis campaign guidelines call for recombinant human activated protein C infusion for 96 hours in patients whose APACHE II score is 25 or higher (Dellinger and colleagues, 2008). A major drawback is a 10-percent risk of serious hemorrhage (Kanji and co-workers, 2007). Importantly, its use in pregnancy is limited, although Medve and associates (2005) described its use in a woman with urosepsis at 18 weeks.

There are a number of other therapies that have proven ineffective. Some of these include *antiendotoxin antibody* and *E5 murine monoclonal IgM antiendotoxin antibody; anticytokine antibodies* and *competitive blockers of TNF-α binding;* and a *nitric oxide synthase inhibitor* (Russell, 2006). Active searches focused on novel targets continue.

TRAUMA

Trauma, homicide, and similar violent events are a leading cause of death in young women. As many as 10 to 20 percent of pregnant women suffer physical trauma (American College of Obstetricians and Gynecologists, 1998; Rickert and associates, 2003). Injury-related deaths are the most commonly identified cause of maternal morbidity in Maryland, Utah, and North Carolina (Harper and Parsons, 1997; Horon and Cheng, 2001; Jacob and colleagues, 1998). And in a California study of 4.8 million pregnancies by El Kady and co-workers (2004, 2005), almost 1 in 350 women were hospitalized for injuries from as-

saults. In an audit from Parkland Hospital, Hawkins and associates (2007) studied 1682 pregnant women who presented to the trauma service. Motor vehicle accidents and falls accounted for 85 percent of injuries, whereas 10 percent were due to assaults.

A number of reports of pregnancy-associated deaths have established homicide as a major cause of maternal deaths (Chang and associates, 2005; Christiansen and Collins, 2006; Shadigian and Bauer, 2005). In the 10-city case-control study by McFarlane and associates (2002), 5 percent of female homicide victims were pregnant. Finally, there is evidence that intimate partner violence may be linked to suicide in pregnancy (Martin and associates, 2007).

Blunt Trauma

Many forms of blunt trauma are encountered in pregnancy. Their common theme concerns immediate assessment of maternal effects of trauma, emergency treatment, and then evaluation of collateral effects on the fetus.

Physical Abuse—Intimate Partner Violence

According to the Department of Justice, women who are aged 16 to 24 years have the highest per capita rates of intimate partner violence—19.4 per 1000 (Rennison and Welchans, 2000). It is estimated that 5 million women each year are physically assaulted by their male partners (American College of Obstetricians and Gynecologists, 2006a). One goal in violence prevention for Healthy People 2010 is reduction of physical abuse directed at women by male partners. The *Pregnancy Risk Assessment Monitoring Systems—PRAMS*—report from 2000 to 2003 showed some improvement in these areas (Suellentrop and co-workers, 2006).

Even more appalling is that pregnant women are not immune to this physical violence. Most supporting data have been accrued by public institutions, and according to the American College of Obstetrics and Gynecology (2006a), abuse rates range from 1 to 20 percent during pregnancy. In Phoenix, more than 13 percent of women who enrolled for prenatal services had a history of physical or sexual abuse (Coonrod and colleagues, 2007). Abuse is linked to poverty, poor education, and use of tobacco, alcohol, and illicit drugs (Centers for Disease Control and Prevention, 2008). Unfortunately, abused women tend to remain with their abusers, and the major risk factor for intimate partner homicide is prior domestic violence (Campbell and colleagues, 2007). Finally, women seeking pregnancy termination have a higher incidence of intimate partner violence (Bourassa and Bérubé, 2007).

The woman who is physically abused tends to present late, if at all, for prenatal care. For pregnant women hospitalized in California as a result of assault, perinatal morbidity rates were significantly increased (El Kady and co-workers, 2005). Immediate sequelae included uterine rupture, maternal death, fetal death, and preterm delivery. Later, there were increased rates of placental abruption, preterm and low-birthweight infants, and other adverse outcomes. Similar results were reported by Silverman and colleagues (2006) from PRAMS, which included more than 118,000 pregnancies in 26 states. Importantly, Rodrigues

TABLE 42-8. Guidelines for Prophylaxis against Sexually Transmitted Disease in Victims of Sexual Assault

Prophylaxis Against	Regimen	Alternative
Neisseria gonorrhoeae	Ceftriaxone 125 mg IM single dose	Cefixime 400 mg orally single dose *or* Ciprofloxacin 500 mg orally single dose
Chlamydia trachomatis	Azithromycin 1 g orally single dose[a]	Erythromycin-base 500 mg orally four times daily for 7 days *or* Ofloxacin 300 mg orally twice daily for 7 days
Bacterial vaginosis	Metronidazole 500 mg orally twice daily for 7 days	Metronidazole gel, 0.75% 5 g intravaginally daily for 5 days *or* Clindamycin cream, 2%, 5 g intravaginally daily for 7 days
Trichomonas vaginalis	Metronidazole as given above	Tinidazole 2 g orally single dose[b]
Hepatitis B (HBV)	If not previously vaccinated, give first dose HBV vaccine, repeat at 1–2 and 4–6 months	
Human immunodeficiency virus (HIV)	Consider retroviral prophylaxis if risk for HIV exposure is high	

[a]For nonpregnant women, doxycycline, 100 mg orally twice daily for 7 days, can be given instead.
[b]Pregnancy category C.
From Centers for Disease Control and Prevention (2006).

and associates (2008) found that preterm delivery was increased three- to fivefold in abused women, but that it was not related to the severity of abuse. Women who are abused are also twice as likely to be depressed than unabused women—41 versus 19 percent (Rodriguez and co-workers, 2008).

Screening and Prevention. A case-finding approach based on clinical suspicion of *intimate partner violence* is recommended by some (Wathen and MacMillan, 2003). Others take a more aggressive approach, and the American College of Obstetricians and Gynecologists (2005a, 2006a) recommends universal screening at the initial prenatal visit, during each trimester, and again at the postpartum visit (see Chap. 8, p. 197).

Sexual Assault

According to the U.S. Department of Justice (2006), 17 percent of adult women will be sexually assaulted sometime during their lives. More than 90 percent of the nearly 200,000 rape victims in the United States in 2006 were women; 80 percent were younger than 30 years; and 44 percent were younger than 18. Satin and co-workers (1992) reviewed more than 5700 female sexual assault victim cases in Dallas County during 6 years and reported that 2 percent of victims were pregnant. Associated physical trauma occurs in approximately half of all women (Sugar and colleagues, 2004). From a forensic standpoint, evidence collection protocol is not altered.

The importance of psychological counseling for the rape victim and her family cannot be overemphasized. In addition to attention to physical and psychological injuries, exposure to

sexually transmitted diseases must be considered. The current recommendations for prophylaxis are shown in Table 42-8. If the woman is not pregnant, another very important aspect is emergency contraception as recommended by the American College of Obstetricians and Gynecologists (2005b) and discussed in detail in Chapter 32 (p. 692).

Automobile Accidents

At least 3 percent of pregnant women are involved in motor vehicle accidents each year in the United States. Using PRAMS, Sirin and colleagues (2007) estimated that 92,500 pregnant women are injured annually. Motor-vehicle crashes are the most common causes of serious, life-threatening, or fatal blunt trauma during pregnancy (Patteson and co-workers, 2007; Schiff and Holt, 2005). They are also the leading cause of traumatic fetal deaths (Mattox and Goetzl, 2005). Between 1995 and 2008, 10 of 12 fetal deaths from maternal trauma were caused by motor-vehicle accidents at Parkland Hospital (Hawkins and colleagues, 2007). Up to half of accidents are associated with lack of seat belt use, and many of these deaths might be preventable with use of three-point restraints shown in Figure 42-7 (Duma and associates, 2006; Metz and Abbott, 2006). Another associated risk factor is alcohol use.

Effects of airbag deployment in pregnant drivers or passengers have not been widely studied. Sims and associates (1996) reported no injuries in three women in their third trimester whose driver-side airbag deployed in 10- to 25-mph collisions. Metz and Abbott (2006) described 30 such women from 20 to 37 weeks whose airbag deployed in accidents with a median speed of 35 mph. A third were not using seat belts, and there

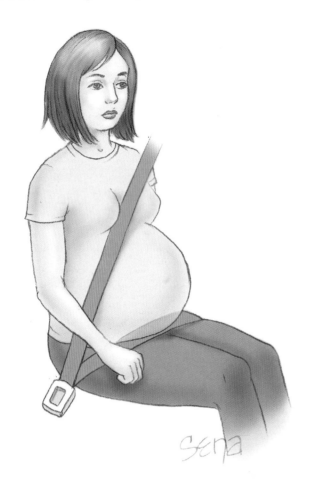

FIGURE 42-7 Illustration showing correct use of three-point automobile restraint. The upper belt is *above* the uterus and the lower belt fits snugly across the upper thighs and well *below* the uterus.

was one fetal death from the single case of placental abruption. Almost 75 percent had contractions, half had abdominal pain, and in 20 percent, there were abnormal fetal heart rate tracings. Even less is known about passenger-side bags or door bags (Moorcroft and co-workers, 2003).

Other Blunt Trauma

Some other common causes of blunt trauma are falls and aggravated assaults. In the California reports by El Kady and co-workers (2004, 2005), intentionally inflicted injuries were present in approximately one third of pregnant women who were hospitalized for trauma. Less common are blast or crush injury (Schoenfeld and colleagues, 1995). With blunt trauma, there can be serious intra-abdominal injuries. Even so, bowel injuries are less frequent because of the protective effect of the large uterus. Still, diaphragmatic, splenic, liver, and kidney injuries may also be sustained. Particularly worrisome is the specter of amnionic fluid embolism, which has been reported even with mild trauma (Ellingsen and co-workers, 2007; Pluymakers and colleagues, 2007). Retroperitoneal hemorrhage is encountered more commonly than usual.

Orthopedic injuries are also encountered with some regularity (Desai and Suk, 2007). In the experiences from the Parkland Hospital trauma unit, 6 percent of 1682 pregnant women eval-

uated had orthopedic injuries. This subset was also at increased risk for placental abruption, preterm delivery, and perinatal mortality (Cannada and associates, 2008). Leggon and associates (2002) reviewed 101 pelvic fractures during pregnancy and found a 9-percent maternal and 35-percent fetal mortality rate. Almog and co-workers (2007) described their experience with pelvic and acetabular fractures during 15 pregnancies. There was one maternal death, and four of 16 fetuses died.

Finally, head trauma and neurosurgical care is an issue with some cases (Qaiser and Black, 2007).

Fetal Injury and Death

As expected, fetal mortality rates increase with the severity of maternal injuries. Specifically, fetal death is more likely when there is direct fetoplacental injury, maternal shock, pelvic fracture, maternal head injury, or hypoxia (Ikossi and co-workers, 2005; Pearlman and colleagues, 2008). In a 16-state review of fetal deaths from trauma, Weiss and associates (2001) found that motor vehicle accidents caused 82 percent. There was placental injury in almost half, and uterine rupture in 4 percent of these fetal deaths. Patteson and colleagues (2007) reported similar findings.

Although uncommon, fetal skull and brain injuries are more likely if the head is engaged and the maternal pelvis is fractured (Palmer and Sparrow, 1994). Conversely, fetal head injuries, presumably from a *contrecoup* effect, may be sustained in unengaged vertex or nonvertex presentations. Sequelae include intracranial hemorrhage (Green-Thompson and Moodley, 2005). A newborn with paraplegia and contractures associated with a motor vehicle accident sustained several months before birth was described by Weyerts and colleagues (1992). Other injuries include fetal decapitation and another of incomplete midabdominal fetal transection at midpregnancy (Rowe and associates, 1996; Weir and colleagues, 2008).

Placental Abruption and Uterine Rupture

Two catastrophic events from blunt trauma are placental abruption and uterine rupture. These often are life-threatening to both mother and fetus. Another is a placental tear or "fracture" that can result in fetal hemorrhage and exsanguination, either into the amnionic sac or as fetomaternal hemorrhage.

Traumatic Placental Abruption. Placental separation from trauma is likely caused by deformation of the elastic myometrium around the relatively inelastic placenta (Crosby and associates, 1968). This may result from a deceleration injury as the large uterus meets the immovable steering wheel or seat belt (Fig. 42-8). Some degree of abruption complicates 1 to 6 percent of "minor" injuries and up to 50 percent of "major" injuries (Pearlman and co-workers, 1990; Schiff and associates, 2002). In one study, Reis and colleagues (2000) reported that abruption was more likely if vehicle speed exceeded 30 mph.

Clinical findings with traumatic abruption may be similar to those for spontaneous placental abruption (see Chap. 35, p. 761). Kettel and co-workers (1988) emphasized that traumatic abruption may be occult and unaccompanied by uterine pain, tenderness, or bleeding. Stettler and associates (1992) reviewed our experiences with 13 such women at Parkland Hospital and

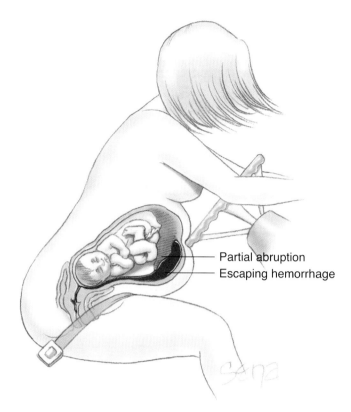

FIGURE 42-8 Acute deceleration injury when the elastic uterus meets the steering wheel, and as it stretches, the inelastic placenta shears from the decidua basalis. Intrauterine pressures as high as 550 mm Hg are generated.

reported that 11 had uterine tenderness, but only five had vaginal bleeding. Because traumatic abruption is more likely to be concealed and generate higher intrauterine pressures, associated coagulopathy is more likely than with nontraumatic abruption. Other common findings are uterine contractions; evidence of fetal compromise such as fetal tachycardia, late decelerations, and acidosis; and fetal death.

Another indication of partial separation is uterine activity. Pearlman and associates (1990) found that if contractions were fewer than every 10 minutes during 4 hours of electronic monitoring, then an abruption is unlikely. Women with contractions of greater frequency, however, have a 20-percent chance of an abruption. If tocolytics are used, they may obfuscate these findings, and we do not recommend them.

Uterine Rupture. Blunt trauma results in uterine rupture in less than 1 percent of severe cases (American College of Obstetricians and Gynecologists, 1998). Rupture is more likely in a previously scarred uterus and is usually associated with a direct impact of substantive force. Decelerative forces following a 25-mph collision can generate up to 500 mm Hg of intrauterine pressure in a properly restrained woman (Crosby and associates, 1968). Findings may be identical to those for placental abruption with an intact uterus, and maternal and fetal deterioration are soon inevitable. Pearlman and Cunningham (1996) described uterine fundal "blow out" with fetal decapitation in a 20-week pregnancy following a high-speed collision. Similarly, Weir and colleagues (2008) described supracervical uterine

avulsion and fetal transection at 22 weeks. It may be particularly difficult to diagnose uterine rupture with a dead fetus even using CT scanning (Dash and Lupetin, 1991).

Fetal-Maternal Hemorrhage

If there is considerable abdominal force associated with trauma, and especially if the placenta is lacerated, or "fractured," then life-threatening fetal-maternal hemorrhage may be encountered (Pritchard and associates, 1991). If there is ABO compatibility, fetomaternal hemorrhage can be estimated using a Kleihauer-Betke stain of maternal blood. A small amount of fetal-maternal bleeding has been described in up to one third of trauma cases, but in 90 percent of these, the volume is less than 15 mL (Goodwin and Breen, 1990; Pearlman and associates, 1990). Nontraumatic placental abruption is seldom associated with fetomaternal hemorrhage because there is no fetal bleeding into the intervillous space. Still, massive fetomaternal hemorrhage may coexist with traumatic abruption (Stettler and associates, 1992). In these cases, fetomaternal hemorrhage associated with trauma is caused by a placental tear or "fracture" caused by stretching of the inelastic placenta (Fig. 42-9). Muench and colleagues (2004) reported a 20-fold risk of associated uterine contractions and preterm labor if there is evidence for a fetomaternal bleed.

Penetrating Trauma

Knife and gunshot wounds are the most common penetrating injuries and may be associated with aggravated assaults, suicide attempts, or attempts to cause abortion. The incidence of maternal visceral injury with penetrating trauma is only 15 to 40 percent compared with 80 to 90 percent in nonpregnant individuals (Stone, 1999). When the uterus sustains penetrating wounds, the fetus is more likely than the mother to be seriously injured. Indeed, although the fetus sustains injury in two thirds of such cases, maternal visceral injuries are seen in only 20 percent.

Awwad and colleagues (1994) reported unique experiences with high-velocity penetrating wounds of the pregnant uterus during 16 years of civil war in Lebanon. Two of 14 women died, but neither as a direct result of intra-abdominal injury. They concluded that:

1. When the entrance wound was in either the upper abdomen or back, there were visceral injuries
2. When the entry wound site was anterior and below the uterine fundus, six of women had no visceral injuries
3. The perinatal mortality rate was 50 percent and due to maternal shock, uteroplacental injury, or direct fetal injury.

Management of Trauma

Maternal and fetal outcomes are directly related to the severity of injury. That said, commonly used methods of severity scoring do not take into account significant morbidity and mortality rates related to placental abruption and thus to pregnancy outcomes. For example, Schiff and Holt (2005) evaluated 582 pregnant women hospitalized for injuries. The injury severity score did not accurately predict adverse pregnancy outcomes.

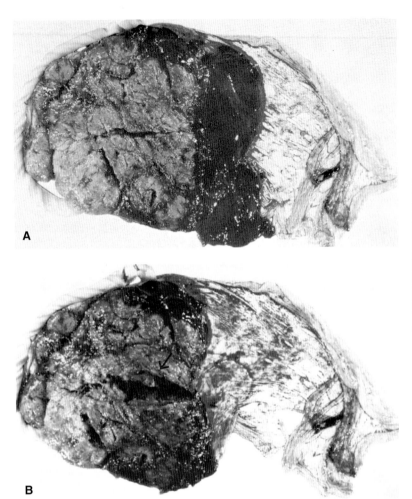

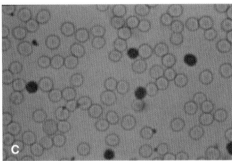

FIGURE 42-9 A. Partial placental abruption with adherent blood clot. The fetus died from massive hemorrhage, chiefly into the maternal circulation. **B.** The adherent blood clot has been removed. Note the laceration of the placenta *(arrow)*. **C.** Kleihauer–Betke stain of a smear of maternal blood after fetal death. The dark cells that constituted 4.5 percent of peripheral cells are fetal in origin, whereas the empty cells are of maternal origin.

Importantly, relatively minor injuries were associated with preterm labor and placental abruption. Biester and co-workers (1997) reached similar conclusions with the revised trauma score. Ikossi and colleagues (2005) found that scores indicating severe trauma did correlate with fetal death. But Cahill and associates (2008) studied 317 pregnant women 24 weeks or more who had "minor trauma." Only 14 percent had clinically significant uterine contractions requiring extended fetal evaluation past 4 hours. Adverse perinatal outcomes for all women were not increased. The problem, of course, is that there is no agreed-upon definition for "minor trauma."

With few exceptions, treatment priorities in injured pregnant women are directed as they would be in nonpregnant patients (Meroz and associates, 2007; Petrone and Asensio, 2006). Primary goals are evaluation and stabilization of maternal injuries. Attention to fetal assessment during the acute evaluation may divert attention from life-threatening maternal injuries (American College of Obstetricians and Gynecologists, 1998). Basic rules are applied to resuscitation, including establishing ventilation, arrest of hemorrhage, and treatment of hypovolemia with crystalloid and blood products. **An important aspect of management is repositioning of the large uterus**

away from the great vessels to diminish its effect on decreased cardiac output.

Following emergency resuscitation, evaluation is continued for fractures, internal injuries, bleeding sites, and placental, uterine, and fetal injuries. Overall, Ylagan and co-workers (2009) reported that pregnant trauma victims have less radiation exposure than nonpregnant controls. Brown and colleagues (2005) advocate screening abdominal sonography followed by CT scanning for positive sonographic findings. In some cases, open peritoneal lavage may be informative (Tsuei, 2006). Penetrating injuries in most cases must be evaluated using radiography. Because clinical response to peritoneal irritation is blunted during pregnancy, an aggressive approach to exploratory laparotomy is pursued. Whereas exploration is mandatory for abdominal gunshot wounds, some clinicians advocate close observation for selected stab wounds.

Cesarean Delivery

The necessity for cesarean delivery of a live fetus depends on several factors. Laparotomy itself is not an indication for hysterotomy. Some considerations include gestational age, fetal condition, extent of uterine injury, and whether the large uterus hinders adequate treatment or evaluation of other intra-abdominal injuries (Tsuei, 2006).

Electronic Monitoring

As for many other acute or chronic maternal conditions, fetal well-being may reflect the status of the mother, and thus, fetal monitoring is another "vital sign" that helps evaluate the extent of maternal injuries. Even if the mother is stable, electronic monitoring may be predictive of placental abruption. In the study by Pearlman and associates (1990), no woman had an abruption if uterine contractions were less often than every 10 minutes within the 4 hours after trauma was sustained. **Almost 20 percent of women who had contractions more frequently than every 10 minutes in the first 4 hours had an associated placental abruption.** In these cases, abnormal tracings were common and included fetal tachycardia and late decelerations. Connolly and co-workers (1997) reported no adverse outcomes in women who had normal monitor tracings.

Because placental abruption usually develops early following trauma, fetal monitoring is begun as soon as the mother is stabilized. The duration for which posttrauma monitoring should be performed is not precisely known. From data cited above, an observation period of 4 hours is reasonable with a normal tracing and no other sentinel findings such as contractions, uterine tenderness, or bleeding. Certainly, monitoring should be continued as long as there are uterine contractions, nonreassuring fetal heart patterns, vaginal bleeding, uterine tenderness or irritability, serious maternal injury, or ruptured membranes (American College of Obstetricians and Gynecologists, 1998). In very rare cases, placental abruption has developed days after trauma (Higgins and Garite, 1984).

Fetal-Maternal Hemorrhage

Routine use of the Kleihauer-Betke or an equivalent test in pregnant trauma victims is controversial (Pak and associates, 1998). It is unclear if their routine use will modify adverse outcomes associated with fetal anemia, cardiac arrhythmias, and death. In a retrospective review of 125 pregnant women with blunt injuries, Towery and co-workers (1993) reported that the Kleihauer-Betke test had a sensitivity of 56 percent, a specificity of 71 percent, and an accuracy of 27 percent. They concluded that the test was of little use with acute trauma management. They also concluded that electronic fetal monitoring or sonography, or both, are more useful in detecting fetal or pregnancy-associated complications. Although Dupre and associates (1993) found evidence for fetal-maternal hemorrhage in 22 percent of women studied, it was of no prognostic significance. Connolly and co-workers (1997) reached similar conclusions. According to Muench and colleagues (2003, 2004), however, a Kleihauer-Betke test showing fetal cells of 0.1 percent or greater was predictive of uterine contractions or preterm labor.

For the woman who is D-negative, administration of anti-D immunoglobulin should be considered. This may be omitted if the test for fetal bleeding is negative. Isoimmunization may still develop if the fetal-maternal hemorrhage exceeds 15 mL of fetal cells.

Another important aspect of care for the pregnant trauma patient is to ensure that her tetanus immunization is current. It is recommended that pregnant women receive a tetanus and diphtheria toxoids vaccine (Td) for protection when indicated (Murphy and colleagues, 2008).

THERMAL INJURY

Although Parkland Hospital is a major burn center for the United States, we have not seen a large number of pregnant women with severe burns. Fetal prognosis is poor with severe burns. Usually the woman enters labor spontaneously within a few days to a week and often delivers a stillborn infant. Contributory factors are hypovolemia, pulmonary injury, septicemia, and the intensely catabolic state associated with burns. Treatment of burned pregnant women is similar to that for nonpregnant patients and was reviewed by Pacheco and associates (2005).

Prognosis

It is generally agreed that pregnancy does not alter maternal outcome from thermal injury compared with that of nonpregnant women of similar age. As perhaps expected, maternal and fetal survival parallels the percentage of burned surface area. Karimi and colleagues (2009) reported higher rates for both with suicidal attempts and with inhalational injuries. In the 211 pregnant burned victims shown in Figure 42-10, as the burn area reaches or exceeds 50 percent, both maternal and fetal morbidity become formidable.

Skin Contractures

Following serious abdominal burns, skin contractures that develop may be painful during a subsequent pregnancy and may even necessitate surgical decompression and split skin autografts (Matthews, 1982). Widgerow and colleagues (1991) described two women in whom surgical release of contractures without covering the resulting defect was sufficient. McCauley and colleagues (1991) followed seven women with severe circumferential truncal burns sustained at a mean age of 7.7 years. All of 14 subsequent pregnancies were delivered at term without major complications. Loss or distortion of nipples may cause problems

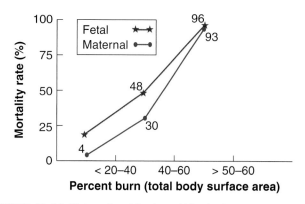

FIGURE 42-10 Maternal and fetal morbidity by burn severity in 211 women. (Data from Akhtar, 1994; Amy, 1985; Mabrouk and el-Feky, 1997; Maghsoudi, 2006; Rayburn, 1984; Rode, 1990, and all their colleagues.)

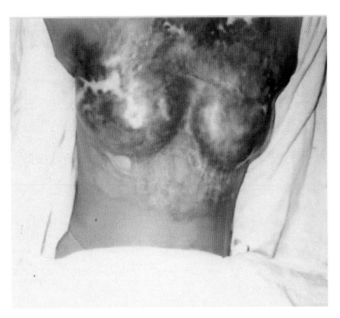

FIGURE 42-11 This 22-year-old nullipara sustained severe burns at age 12 years, and massive scarring followed. Both breasts were replaced by scar tissue. Following delivery, a few drops of colostrum were expressed from the left nipple, but no breast engorgement was detected. (Photo courtesy of Drs. A. R. Mahale and A. P. Sakhare, Maharashtra, India.)

in breast feeding (Fig. 42-11). Interestingly, normal abdominal tissue expansion due to pregnancy appears to be an excellent source for obtaining skin grafts postpartum to correct scar deformities at other body sites (Del Frari and colleagues, 2004).

Electrical Injury and Burns

Earlier case reports were suggestive of a high fetal mortality rate with electric shock (Fatovich, 1993). In a prospective cohort study, however, Einarson and colleagues (1997) showed similar perinatal outcomes in 31 injured women compared with those of pregnant controls. They concluded that traditional 110-volt North American electrical current likely is less dangerous than 220-volt currents available in Europe. Sozen and Nesin (2004) described a woman with iliofemoral thrombosis at 29 weeks that *may* have been related to a mild electrical shock at 22 weeks. Thermal burns may be extensive and require expert wound care.

Lightning Injuries

The pathophysiological effects of lightning injuries can be devastating. García Gutiérrez and associates (2005) found 12 case reports of injuries during pregnancy. They described another case and reviewed the effects of lightning injuries on the mother and fetus.

CARDIOPULMONARY RESUSCITATION

Cardiac arrest is rare during pregnancy. General considerations regarding planning and equipment were reviewed by the American College of Obstetricians and Gynecologists (2006b). There are special considerations for cardiopulmonary resuscitation (CPR) conducted in the second half of pregnancy. In nonpregnant women, external chest compression results in a cardiac output of only about 30 percent of normal (Clark and colleagues, 1997). In late pregnancy, however, cardiac output may be even less with CPR because uterine aortocaval compression may diminish forward flow as well as venous return. **Thus, uterine displacement is paramount to accompany other resuscitative efforts.** Left lateral displacement can be accomplished manually by tilting the operating table laterally, by placing a wedge under the right hip—an example is the Cardiff resuscitation wedge. Rees and Willis (1988) showed with a manikin that resuscitation with the Cardiff wedge was as efficient as resuscitation in the supine position. If no equipment is available, such as in an out-of-hospital arrest, an individual kneels on the floor with the woman's back on the thighs to form a "human wedge" (Whitty, 2002).

Over the past few years, the recommendation by many authors is to perform cesarean delivery within 4 to 5 minutes of beginning CPR if the fetus is viable (Moise and Belfort, 1997). Certainly, there is an inverse correlation between neurologically intact neonatal survival and the cardiac arrest-to-delivery interval in women delivered by perimortem cesarean. According to Clark and co-workers (1997), of newborns delivered within 5 minutes of arrest, 98 percent are neurologically intact; within 6 to 15 minutes, 83 percent are intact; within 16 to 25 minutes, 33 percent are intact; and within 26 to 35 minutes, only 25 percent are intact.

Because delivery *may* also enhance maternal resuscitative efforts, the American College of Obstetricians and Gynecologists (2009) advises *consideration* for cesarean delivery within 4 minutes of cardiac arrest in third-trimester pregnancy. Katz and associates (2005) reviewed the literature that included 38 perimortem cesarean deliveries with a "large selection bias." They concluded that these reports supported—but "fell far from proving"—that perimortem cesarean delivery within 4 minutes of maternal cardiac arrest improves maternal and fetal outcomes. Even so, as emphasized by Clark and associates (1997), and in our experiences, these goals rarely can be met in actual practice. Whitten and Irvine (2000) and Whitty (2002) have reviewed indications for postmortem and perimortem cesarean delivery.

Maternal Brain Death

Occasionally a pregnant woman with a supposedly healthy intact fetus will be kept on somatic support to await fetal viability or maturity. This is discussed in Chapter 55 (p. 1175).

REFERENCES

Abraham E, Glauser MP, Butler T, et al: p55 tumor necrosis factor receptor fusion protein in the treatment of patients with severe sepsis and septic shock. A randomized controlled multicenter trial. JAMA 277:1531, 1997

Abraham E, Laterre P-F, Garg R, et al: Drotrecogin alfa (activated) for adults with severe sepsis and a low risk of death. N Engl J Med 353:1332, 2005

Abraham E, Reinhart K, Opal S, et al: Efficacy and safety of tifacogin (recombinant tissue factor pathway inhibitor) in severe sepsis: A randomized controlled trial. JAMA 290:238, 2003

Adem PV, Montgomery CP, Husain AN, et al: *Staphylococcus aureus* sepsis and the Waterhouse-Friderichsen syndrome in children. N Engl J Med 353:1245, 2005

Akhtar MA, Mulawkar PM, Kulkarni HR: Burns in pregnancy: Effect on maternal and fetal outcomes. Burns 20:351, 1994

Almog G, Liebergall M, Tsafrir A, et al: Management of pelvic fractures during pregnancy. Am J Orthop 36:E153, 2007

American College of Critical Care Medicine and the Society of Critical Care Medicine: Guidelines on admission and discharge for adult intermediate care units. Guidelines/Practice Parameters Committee of the American College of Critical Care Medicine and the Society of Critical Care Medicine. Crit Care Med 26:607, 1998

American College of Obstetricians and Gynecologists: Obstetric aspects of trauma management. Educational Bulletin No. 251, September 1998

American College of Obstetricians and Gynecologists: Intimate partner violence and domestic violence. In special issue in Women's Health. Washington, ACOG, 2005a, p 169

American College of Obstetricians and Gynecologists: Emergency contraception. Practice Bulletin No. 69, December 2005b

American College of Obstetricians and Gynecologists: Psychosocial risk factors: Perinatal screening and intervention. Committee Opinion No. 343, August 2006a

American College of Obstetricians and Gynecologists: Medical Emergency Preparedness. Committee Opinion No. 353, December 2006b

American College of Obstetricians and Gynecologists: Critical care in pregnancy. Practice Bulletin No. 100, February 2009

Amy BW, McManus WF, Goodwin CW, et al: Thermal injury in the pregnant patient. Surg Gynecol Obstet 161:209, 1985

Anzueto A, Baughman RP, Guntupalli KK, et al: Aerosolized surfactant in adults with sepsis-induced acute respiratory distress syndrome. N Engl J Med 334:1417, 1996

Aurigemma GP, Gaasch WH: Diastolic heart failure. N Engl J Med 351:1097, 2004

Awwad JT, Azar GB, Seoud MA, et al: High-velocity penetrating wounds of the gravid uterus: Review of 16 years of civil war. Obstet Gynecol 83:259, 1994

Benedetti TJ, Carlson RW: Studies of colloid osmotic pressure in pregnancy-induced hypertension. Am J Obstet Gynecol 135:308, 1979

Bernard GR, Vincent JL, Laterre PF, et al: Efficacy and safety of recombinant human activated protein C for severe sepsis. N Engl J Med 344:699, 2001

Biester EM, Tomich PG, Esposito TJ, et al: Trauma in pregnancy: Normal Revised Trauma Score in relation to other markers of maternofetal status—a preliminary study. Am J Obstet Gynecol 176:1206, 1997

Bourassa D, Bérubé J: The prevalence of intimate partner violence among women and teenagers seeking abortion compared with those continuing pregnancy. J Obstet Gynaecol Can 29:415, 2007

Brown MA, Sirlin CB, Farahmand N, et al: Screening sonography in pregnant patients with blunt abdominal trauma. J Ultrasound Med 24:175, 2005

Bux J, Sachs UJ: The pathogenesis of transfusion-related acute lung injury (TRALI). Br J Haematol 136:788, 2007

Cahill AG, Bastek JA, Stamilio DM. et al: Minor trauma in pregnancy—is the evaluation unwarranted? Am J Obstet Gynecol 198:208.e1, 2008

Campbell JC, Glass N, Sharps PW, et al: Intimate partner homicide: Review and implications of research and policy. Trauma Violence Abuse 8:246, 2007

Cannada LK, Hawkins JS, Casey BM, et al: Outcomes in pregnant trauma patients with orthopedic injuries. Submitted for Fall Meeting of American Academy of Orthopaedic Surgeons; Dallas, TX, October 2008

Catanzarite V, Willms D, Wong D, et al: Acute respiratory distress syndrome in pregnancy and the puerperium: Causes, courses, and outcomes. Obstet Gynecol 97:760, 2001

Centers for Disease Control and Prevention: Sexually transmitted diseases. Guidelines treatment. MMWR 55(RR-11):1, 2006

Centers for Disease Control and Prevention: Adverse health conditions and health risk behaviors associated with intimate partner violence – United States, 2005. MMWR 57(5):113 2008

Chang J, Berg CJ, Saltzman LE, et al: Homicide: A leading cause of injury deaths among pregnant and postpartum women in the United States, 1991–1999. Am J Public Health 95:471, 2005

Chen C-Y, Chen C-P, Wang K-G, et al: Factors implicated in the outcome of pregnancies complicated by acute respiratory failure. J Reprod Med 48:641, 2003

Christiansen LR, Collins KA: Pregnancy-associated deaths: A 15-year retrospective study and overall review of maternal pathophysiology. Am J Forensic Med Pathol 27:11, 2006

Clad A, Orlowska-Volk M, Karck U: Fatal puerperal sepsis with necrotising fasciitis due to Streptococcus pneumoniae. BJOG 110:213, 2003

Clark SL, Cotton DB: Clinical indications for pulmonary artery catheterization in the patient with severe preeclampsia. Am J Obstet Gynecol 158:453, 1988

Clark SL, Cotton DB, Hankins GDV, et al: Critical Care Obstetrics, 3rd ed. Boston, Blackwell Science, 1997

Clark SL, Cotton DB, Lee W, et al: Central hemodynamic assessment of normal term pregnancy. Am J Obstet Gynecol 161:1439, 1989

Clark SL, Hankins GD, Dudley DA, et al: Amniotic fluid embolism: Analysis of a national registry. Am J Obstet Gynecol 172:1158, 1995

Cole DE, Taylor TL, McCullough DM, et al: Acute respiratory distress syndrome in pregnancy. Crit Care Med 33:S269, 2005

Connolly AM, Katz VL, Bash KL, et al: Trauma and pregnancy. Am J Perinatol 14:331, 1997

Coonrod DV, Bay RC, Mills TE, et al: Asymptomatic bacteriuria and intimate partner violence in pregnant women. Am J Obstet Gynecol 196:581.e1, 2007

Crosby WM, Snyder RG, Snow CC, et al: Impact injuries in pregnancy, 1. Experimental studies. Am J Obstet Gynecol 101:100, 1968

Cunningham FG, Lucas MJ, Hankins GD: Pulmonary injury complicating antepartum pyelonephritis. Am J Obstet Gynecol 156:797, 1987

Cunningham FG, Pritchard JA, Hankins GDV, et al: Peripartum heart failure: A specific pregnancy-induced cardiomyopathy or the consequence of coincidental compounding cardiovascular events? Obstet Gynecol 67:157, 1986

Cunningham JA, Devine PC, Jelic S: Extracorporeal membrane oxygenation in pregnancy. Obstet Gynecol 108:792, 2006

Daif JL, Levie M, Chudnoff S, et al: Group A Streptococcus causing necrotizing fasciitis and toxic shock syndrome after medical termination of pregnancy. Obstet Gynecol 113:504, 2009

Dash N, Lupetin AR: Uterine rupture secondary to trauma: CT findings. J Comput Assist Tomogr 15:329, 1991

Del Frari B, Pulzl P, Schoeller T, et al: Pregnancy as a tissue expander in the correction of a scar deformity. Am J Obstet Gynecol 190:579, 2004

Dellinger RP, Levy MM, Carlet JM, et al: Surviving Sepsis Campaign: International guidelines for management of severe sepsis and septic shock: 2008. Crit Care Med 36(1):296, 2008

Desai P, Suk M: Orthopedic trauma in pregnancy. Am J Orthop 36:E160, 2007

DiFederico EM, Burlingame JM, Kilpatrick SJ, et al: Pulmonary edema in obstetric patients is rapidly resolved except in the presence of infection or of nitroglycerine tocolysis after open fetal surgery. Am J Obstet Gynecol 179:925, 1998

Drazner MH, Dries DI, Peshock RM, et al: Left ventricular hypertrophy is more prevalent in blacks than whites in the general population. The Dallas heart study. Hypertension 45:124, 2005

Duma SF, Moorcroft DM, Stitzel JD, et al: Biomechanical modeling of pregnant occupants in far-side vehicle crashes. Biomed Sci Instrum 42:154, 2006

Dupre AR, Morrison JC, Martin JN Jr, et al: Clinical application of the Kleihauer-Betke test. J Reprod Med 38:621, 1993

Einarson A, Bailey B, Inocencion G, et al: Accidental electric shock in pregnancy: A prospective cohort study. Am J Obstet Gynecol 176:678, 1997

El Kady D, Gilbert WM, Anderson J, et al: Trauma during pregnancy: An analysis of maternal and fetal outcomes in a large population. Am J Obstet Gynecol 190:1661, 2004

El Kady D, Gilbert WM, Xing G, et al: Maternal and neonatal outcomes of assaults during pregnancy. Obstet Gynecol 105:357, 2005

Ellingsen CL, Eggebo TM, Lexow K: Amniotic fluid embolism after blunt abdominal trauma. Resuscitation, April 28, 2007

Evans TW, Smithies M: ABC of intensive care. Organ dysfunction. BMJ 318:1606, 1999

Fatovich DM: Electric shock in pregnancy. J Emerg Med 11:175, 1993

Filbin MR, Ring DC, Wessels MR, et al: Case 2-2009: A 25-year-old man with pain and swelling of the right hand and hypotension. N Engl J Med 360:281, 2009

Friese RS, Shafi S, Gentilello LM: Pulmonary artery catheter use is associated with reduced mortality in severely injured patients: A National Trauma Data Bank analysis of 53,312 patients. Crit Care Med 34:1597, 2006

Gallup DG, Freedman MA, Meguiar RV, et al: Necrotizing fasciitis in gynecologic and obstetric patients: A surgical emergency. Am J Obstet Gynecol 187:305, 2002

Gandhi SK, Powers JC, Nomeir A-M, et al: The pathogenesis of acute pulmonary edema associated with hypertension. N Engl J Med 344:17, 2001

García Gutiérrez JJ, Meléndez J, Torrero JV, et al: Lightning injuries in a pregnant woman: A case report and review of the literature. Burns 31:1045, 2005

Girard TD, Bernard GR: Mechanical ventilation in ARDS: A state-of-the-art review. Chest 131:921, 2007

Golombeck K, Ball RH, Lee H, et al: Maternal morbidity after maternal-fetal surgery. Am J Obstet Gynecol 194:834, 2006

Goodwin TM, Breen MT: Pregnancy outcome and fetomaternal hemorrhage after noncatastrophic trauma. Am J Obstet Gynecol 162:665, 1990

Gosman GG, Baldisseri MR, Stein KL, et al: Introduction of an obstetrics-specific medical emergency team for obstetric crises: Implementation and experience. Am J Obstet Gynecol 198:367.e1, 2008

Green-Thompson R, Moodley J: In-utero intracranial haemorrhage probably secondary to domestic violence: Case report and literature review. J Obstet Gynaecol 25:816, 2005

Hankins GD, Wendel GD, Cunningham FG, et al: Longitudinal evaluation of hemodynamic changes in eclampsia. Am J Obstet Gynecol 150:506, 1984

Hankins GD, Wendel GD, Leveno KJ, et al: Myocardial infarction during pregnancy. A review. Obstet Gynecol 65:139, 1985

Harper M, Parsons L: Maternal deaths due to homicide and other injuries in North Carolina: 1992–1994. Obstet Gynecol 90:920, 1997

Harvey S, Harrison DA, Singer M, et al: Assessment of the clinical effectiveness of pulmonary artery catheters in management of patients in intensive care (PAC-Man): A randomized controlled trial. Lancet 366:472, 2005

Hawkins JS, Casey BM, Minei J, et al: Outcomes after trauma in pregnancy. Am J Obstet Gynecol 197:S92, 2007

Herridge MS, Cheung AM, Tansey CM, et al: One-year outcomes in survivors of the acute respiratory distress syndrome. N Engl J Med 348:683, 2003

Hidalgo-Grass C, Dan-Goor M, Maly A, et al: Effect of a bacterial pheromone peptide on host chemokine degradation in group A streptococcal necrotising soft-tissue infections. Lancet 363:696, 2004

Higgins SD, Garite TJ: Late abruptio placentae in trauma patients: Implications for monitoring. Obstet Gynecol 63:10S, 1984

Horon IL, Cheng D: Enhanced surveillance for pregnancy-associated mortality—Maryland, 1993–1998. JAMA 285:1455, 2001

Hotchkiss RS, Karl IE: The pathophysiology and treatment of sepsis. N Engl J Med 348:138, 2003

Hough ME, Katz V: Pulmonary edema a case series in a community hospital. Obstet Gynecol 109:115S, 2007

Ikossi DG, Lazar AA, Morabito D, et al: Profile of mothers at risk: An analysis of injury and pregnancy loss in 1,195 trauma patients. J Am Coll Surg 200:49, 2005

Jacob S, Bloebaum L, Shah G, et al: Maternal mortality in Utah. Obstet Gynecol 91:187, 1998

Jenkins TM, Troiano NH, Graves CR, et al: Mechanical ventilation in an obstetric population: Characteristics and delivery rates. Am J Obstet Gynecol 188:439, 2003

Jessup M, Brozena S: Heart failure. N Engl J Med 348:2007, 2003

Kanji S, Perreault MM, Chant C, et al: Evaluating the use of drotrecogin alfa (activated) in adult severe sepsis: A Canadian multicenter observation study. Intensive Care Med 33:517, 2007

Karimi H, Momeni M, Momeni M, et al: Burn injuries during pregnancy in Iran. Int J Gynaecol Obstet 104(2):132, 2009

Katz V, Balderston K, DeFreest M: Perimortem cesarean delivery: Were our assumptions correct? Am J Obstet Gynecol 192:1916, 2005

Keizer JL, Zwart JJ, Meerman RH, et al: Obstetric intensive care admission: A 12-year review in a tertiary care centre. Eur J Obstet Gynecol Reprod Biol 128:152, 2006

Kenchaiah S, Evans JC, Levy D, et al: Obesity and the risk of heart failure. N Engl J Med 347:305, 2002

Kettel LM, Branch DW, Scott JR: Occult placental abruption after maternal trauma. Obstet Gynecol 71:449, 1988

Klevens RM, Morrison MA, Nadle J, et al: Invasive methicillin-resistant Staphylococcus aureus infections in the United States. JAMA 298 (15):1763, 2007

Kopko PM, Marshall CS, MacKenzie MR, et al: Transfusion-related acute lung injury: Report of a clinical look-back investigation. JAMA 287:1968, 2002

Kuklina EV, Meikle SF, Jamieson DJ, et al: Severe obstetric morbidity in the United States: 1996-2006. Obstet Gynecol 113:293, 2009

Lapinsky SE: Cardiopulmonary complications of pregnancy. Crit Care Med 33:1616, 2005

Leggon RE, Wood GC, Indeck MC: Pelvic fractures in pregnancy: Factors influencing maternal and fetal outcomes. J Trauma 53:796, 2002

Levinson G, Shnider SM, DeLorimier AA, et al: Effects of maternal hyperventilation on uterine blood flow and fetal oxygenation and acid-base status. Anesthesiology 40:340, 1974

Mabie WC, Barton JR, Sibai BM: Septic shock in pregnancy. Obstet Gynecol 90:553, 1997

Mabrouk AR, el-Feky AEH: Burns during pregnancy: A gloomy outcome. Burns 23:596, 1997

MacArthur RD, Miller M, Albertson T, et al: Adequacy of early empiric antibiotic treatment and survival in severe sepsis: Experience from the MONARCS trial. Clin Infect Dis 38:284, 2004

Madan I, Puri I, Jain NJ, et al: Intensive care unit admissions among pregnant patients. Presented at the 56th Annual Clinical Meeting of the American College of Obstetricians and Gynecologists, New Orleans, LA, May 2008.

Maghsoudi H, Samnia R, Garadaghi A, et al: Burns in pregnancy. Burns 32:246, 2006

Manthous CA: Leapfrog and critical care: Evidence- and reality-based intensive care for the 21st century. Am J Med 116:188, 2004

Martin SR, Foley MR: Intensive care in obstetrics: An evidence-based review. Am J Obstet Gynecol 195:673, 2006

Martin GS, Mannino DM, Eaton S, et al: The epidemiology of sepsis in the United States from 1979 through 2000. N Engl J Med 348:1546, 2003

Martin SL, Macy RJ, Sullivan K, et al: Pregnancy-associated violent deaths: The role of intimate partner violence. Trauma Violence Abuse 8:135, 2007

Matthews RN: Old burns and pregnancy. Br J Obstet Gynaecol 89:610, 1982

Mattox KL, Goetzl L: Trauma in pregnancy. Crit Care Med 33:S385, 2005

McCauley RL, Stenberg BA, Phillips LG, et al: Long-term assessment of the effects of circumferential truncal burns in pediatric patients on subsequent pregnancies. J Burn Care Rehabil 12:51, 1991

McFarlane J, Campbell JC, Sharps P, et al: Abuse during pregnancy and femicide: Urgent implications for women's health. Obstet Gynecol 100:27, 2002

Medve L, Csitári IK, Molnár Z, et al: Recombinant human activated protein C treatment of septic shock syndrome in a patient at 18th week of gestation: A case report. Am J Obstet Gynecol 193:864, 2005

Meroz Y, Elchalal U, Ginosar Y: Initial trauma management in advanced pregnancy. Anesthesiol Clin 25:117, 2007

Metz TD, Abbott JT: Uterine trauma in pregnancy after motor vehicle crashes with airbag deployment: A 30-case series. J Trauma 61:658, 2006

Moise KJ Jr, Belfort MA: Damage control for the obstetric patient. Surg Clin North Am 77:835, 1997

Moorcroft DM, Stitzel JD, Duma GG, et al: Computational model of the pregnant occupant: Predicting the risk of injury in automobile crash. Am J Obstet Gynecol 189:540, 2003

Muench M, Baschat A, Kush M, et al: Maternal fetal hemorrhage of greater than or equal to 0.1 percent predicts preterm labor in blunt maternal trauma. Am J Obstet Gynecol 189:S119, 2003

Muench MV, Baschat AA, Reddy UM, et al: Kleihauer-Betke testing is important in all cases of maternal trauma. J Trauma 57:1094, 2004

Murphy TV, Slade BA, Broder KR, et al: Prevention of pertussis, tetanus, and diphtheria among pregnant and postpartum women and their infants—recommendations of the Advisory Committee on Immunization Practices (ACIP). MMWR Recomm Rep 57(RR-4):1, 2008

Nathan L, Peters MT, Ahmed AM, et al: The return of life-threatening puerperal sepsis caused by group A streptococci. Am J Obstet Gynecol 169:571, 1993

National Heart, Lung, and Blood Institute Acute Respiratory Distress Syndrome (ARDS) Clinical Trials Network: Efficacy and safety of corticosteroids for persistent acute respiratory distress syndrome. N Engl J Med 354:1671, 2006a

National Heart, Lung, and Blood Institute Acute Respiratory Distress Syndrome (ARDS) Clinical Trials Network: Pulmonary-artery versus central venous catheter to guide treatment of acute lung injury. N Engl J Med 354:2213, 2006b

National Institutes of Health: Critical Care Medicine Consensus Conference. JAMA 250:798, 1983

Ognibene FP, Parker MM, Natanson C, et al: Depressed left ventricular performance. Response to volume infusion in patients with sepsis and septic shock. Chest 93:903, 1988

Oram MP, Seal P, McKinstry CE: Severe acute respiratory distress syndrome in pregnancy. Caesarean section in the second trimester to improve maternal ventilation. Anaesth Intensive Care 35(6):975, 2007

Pacheco LD, Gei AF, VanHook JW, et al: Burns in pregnancy. Obstet Gynecol 106:1210, 2005

Pak LL, Reece EA, Chan L: Is adverse pregnancy outcome predictable after blunt abdominal trauma? Am J Obstet Gynecol 179:1140, 1998

Palmer JD, Sparrow OC: Extradural haematoma following intrauterine trauma. Injury 25:671, 1994

Parker MM, Shelmamer JH, Natanson C, et al: Serial cardiovascular variables in survivors and nonsurvivors of human septic shock: Heart rate as an early predictor of prognosis. Crit Care Med 15:923, 1987

Parrillo JE, Parker MM, Natanson C, et al: Septic shock in humans: Advances in the understanding of pathogenesis, cardiovascular dysfunction, and therapy. Ann Intern Med 113:227, 1990

Pathan N, Hemingway CA, Alizadeh AA, et al: Role of interleukin 6 in myocardial dysfunction of meningococcal septic shock. Lancet 363:203, 2004

Patteson SK, Snider CC, Meyer DS, et al: The consequences of high-risk behaviors: Trauma during pregnancy. J Trauma 62:1015, 2007

Payen D, Sablotzki A, Barie PS, et al: International integrated database for the evaluation of severe sepsis and drotrecogin alfa (activated) therapy: Analysis of efficacy and safety data in a large surgical cohort. Surgery 141:548, 2007

Pearlman MD, Cunningham FG: Trauma in pregnancy. In Cunningham FG, MacDonald PC, Gant NF, Leveno KJ, Gilstrap LC (eds): Williams Obstetrics, 19th ed. Supplement No. 21, October/November 1996

Pearlman MD, Klinch KD, Flannagan CAC: Fetal outcome in motor-vehicle crashes: Effects of crash characteristics and maternal restraint. Am J Obstet Gynecol, 198(4):450.e1, 2008

Pearlman MD, Tintinalli JE, Lorenz RP: A prospective controlled study of outcome after trauma during pregnancy. Am J Obstet Gynecol 162:1502, 1990

Petrone P, Asensio JA: Trauma in pregnancy: Assessment and treatment. Scand J Surg 95:4, 2006

Phua J, Badia JR, Adhikari NK, et al: Has mortality from acute respiratory stress syndrome decreased over time?: A systematic review. Am J Respir Crit Care Med 179(3):220, 2009

Pluymakers C, De Weerdt A, Jacquemyn Y, et al: Amniotic fluid embolism after surgical trauma: Two case reports and review of the literature. Resuscitation 72:324, 2007

Pritchard JA, Cunningham G, Pritchard SA, et al: On reducing the frequency of severe abruptio placentae. Am J Obstet Gynecol 165:1345, 1991

Qaiser R, Black P: Neurosurgery in pregnancy. Semin Neurol 27:476, 2007

Que YA, Haefliger JA, Piroth L, et al: Fibrinogen and fibronectin binding cooperate for valve infection and invasion in *Staphylococcus aureus* experimental endocarditis. J Experimental Med 20:1627, 2005

Rayburn W, Smith B, Feller I, et al: Major burns during pregnancy: Effects on fetal well being. Surg Gynecol Obstet 63:392, 1984

Rees GAD, Willis BA: Resuscitation in late pregnancy. Anaesthesia 43:347, 1988

Reis PM, Sander CM, Pearlman MD: Abruptio placentae after auto accidents. A case control study. J Reprod Med 45:6, 2000

Rennison CM, Welchans S: Intimate partner violence. U.S. Department of Justice, Office of Justice Programs. NCJ-178247, 2000

Richard C, Warszawski J, Anguel N, et al: Early use of the pulmonary artery catheter and outcomes in patients with shock and acute respiratory distress syndrome. JAMA 290:2713, 2003

Rickert VI, Vaughan RD, Wiemann CM: Violence against young women: Implications for clinicians. Contemp Ob/Gyn 48:30, 2003

Rivers E, Nguyen B, Havstad S, et al: Early goal-directed therapy in the treatment of severe sepsis and septic shock. N Engl J Med 345:1368, 2001

Robertson EG: Edema in normal pregnancy. J Reprod Fertil 9:27, 1969

Rode H, Millar AJ, Cywes S, et al: Thermal injury in pregnancy—the neglected tragedy. S Afr Med J 77:346, 1990

Rodrigues T, Rocha L, Barros H: Physical abuse during pregnancy and preterm delivery. Am J Obstet Gynecol 198:171.e1, 2008

Rodriguez MA, Heilemann MV, Fielder E, et al: Intimate partner violence, depression, and PTSD among pregnant Latina women. Ann Fam Med 6:44, 2008

Rorth M, Bille-Brahe NE: 2,3-Diphosphoglycerate and creatine in the red cells during pregnancy. Scand J Clin Lab Invest 28:271, 1971

Rotas M, McCalla S, Liu C, et al: Methicillin-resistant *Staphylococcus aureus* necrotizing pneumonia arising from an infected episiotomy site. Obstet Gynecol 109:533, 2007

Rowe TF, Lafayette S, Cox S: An unusual fetal complication of traumatic uterine rupture. J Emerg Med 14:173, 1996

Roy B, Cordova FC, Travaline JM, et al: Full face mask for noninvasive positive-pressure ventilation in patients with acute respiratory failure. JAOA 107(4):148, 2007

Russell JA: Management of sepsis. N Engl J Med 355:1699, 2006

Russell JA, Walley KR, Singer J, et al: Vasopressin versus norepinephrine infusion in patients with septic shock. N Engl J Med 358:877, 2008

Sam S, Corbridge TC, Mokhlesi B: Cortisol levels and mortality in sepsis. Clin Endocrinol (Oxf) 60:29, 2004

Samol JM, Lambers DS: Magnesium sulfate tocolysis and pulmonary edema: The drug or the vehicle? Am J Obstet Gynecol 192:1430, 2005

Sandham JD, Hull RD, Brant RF, et al: A randomized, controlled trial of the use of pulmonary-artery catheters in high-risk surgical patients. N Engl J Med 348:5, 2003

Satin AJ, Ramin JM, Paicurich J, et al: The prevalence of sexual assault: A survey of 2404 puerperal women. Am J Obstet Gynecol 167:973, 1992

Schiff MA, Holt VL: Pregnancy outcomes following hospitalization for motor vehicle crashes in Washington State from 1989 to 2001. Am J Epidemiol 161:503, 2005

Schiff MA, Holt VL, Daling JR: Maternal and infant outcomes after injury during pregnancy in Washington State from 1989 to 1997. J Trauma 53:939, 2002

Schneider MB, Ivester TS, Mabie WC, et al: Maternal and fetal outcomes in women requiring antepartum mechanical ventilation. Obstet Gynecol [abstract] 101:69S, 2003

Schoenfeld A, Warchaizer S, Royburt M, et al: Crush injury in pregnancy: An unusual experience in obstetrics. Obstet Gynecol 86:655, 1995

Schrier RW, Wang W: Acute renal failure and sepsis. N Engl J Med 351:159, 2004

Sciscione A, Invester T, Largoza M, et al: Acute pulmonary edema in pregnancy. Obstet Gynecol 101:511, 2003

Shadigian EM, Bauer ST: Pregnancy-associated death: A qualitative systematic review of homicide and suicide. Obstet Gynecol Surv 60:183, 2005

Sheffield JS, Cunningham FG: Urinary tract infection in women. Obstet Gynecol 106:1085, 2005

Sibai BM, Mabie BC, Harvey CJ, et al: Pulmonary edema in severe preeclampsia–eclampsia: Analysis of thirty-seven consecutive cases. Am J Obstet Gynecol 156:1174, 1987

Silverman JG, Decker MR, Reed E, et al: Intimate partner violence victimization prior to and during pregnancy among women residing in 26 U.S. states: Associations with maternal and neonatal death. Am J Obstet Gynecol 195:140, 2006

Sims CJ, Boardman CH, Fuller SJ: Airbag deployment following a motor vehicle accident in pregnancy. Obstet Gynecol 88:726, 1996

Sirin H, Weiss HB, Sauber-Schatz EK, et al: Seat belt use, counseling and motor-vehicle injury during pregnancy: Results from a multi-state population-based survey. Matern Child Health J 11:505, 2007

Sozen I, Nesin N: Accidental electric shock in pregnancy and antenatal occurrence of maternal deep vein thrombosis. A case report. J Reprod Med 49:58, 2004

Stettler RW, Lutich A, Pritchard JA, et al: Traumatic placental abruption: A separation from traditional thought. Presented at the annual clinical meeting of the American College of Obstetricians and Gynecologists, Las Vegas, May 1992

Stevens TA, Carroll MA, Promecene PA, et al: Utility of acute physiology, age, and chronic health evaluation (APACHE III) score in maternal admissions to the intensive care unit. Am J Obstet Gyneocl 194:e13, 2006

Stone IK: Trauma in the obstetric patient. Obstet Gynecol Clin North Am 26:459, 1999

Stroncek DF: Pulmonary transfusion reactions. Semin Hematol 44:2, 2007

Subrevilla LA, Cassinelli MT, Carcelen A, et al: Human fetal and maternal oxygen tension and acid-base status during delivery at high altitude. Am J Obstet Gynecol 111:1111, 1971

Suellentrop K, Morrow B, Williams L, et al: Monitoring progress toward achieving maternal and infant Healthy People 2010 objectives—19 states, Pregnancy Risk Assessment Monitoring System (PRAMS), 2000–2003. MMWR Surveill Summ 55:1, 2006

Sugar NF, Fine DN, Eckert LO: Physical injury after sexual assault: Findings of a large case series. Am J Obstet Gynecol 190:71, 2004

Taylor RW, Zimmerman JL, Dellinger RP, et al: Inhaled Nitric Oxide in ARDS Study Group: Low-dose inhaled nitric oxide in patients with acute lung injury: A randomized controlled trial. JAMA 291:1603, 2004

Tihtonen KM, Kööbi, T, Vuolteenaho O, et al: Natriuretic peptides and hemodynamics in preeclampsia. Am J Obstet Gynecol 196:328, 2007

Towery R, English TP, Wisner D: Evaluation of pregnant women after blunt injury. J Trauma 35:731, 1993

Tsuei BJ: Assessment of the pregnant trauma patient. Injury Int J Care Injured 37:367, 2006

United States Department of Justice: Bureau of Justice Statistics: 2005 National Crime Victimization Survey. Criminal Victimization, 2005. NCJ 214644, September 2006

Van Hook JW, Hankins GDV: Invasive hemodynamic monitoring. Prim Care Update Ob/Gyn 4:39, 1997

Ware LB, Matthay MA: Acute pulmonary edema. N Engl J Med 353:2788, 2005

Ware LB, Matthay MA: The acute respiratory distress syndrome. N Engl J Med 342:1334, 2000

Warren BL, Eid A, Singer P, et al: Caring for the critically ill patient: High-dose antithrombin III in severe sepsis: A randomized controlled trial. JAMA 286:1869, 2001

Wathen CN, MacMillan HL: Interventions for violence against women: Scientific review. JAMA 289:589, 2003

Weir LF, Pierce BT, Vazquez JO: Complete fetal transection after a motor vehicle collision. Obstet Gynecol 111(2):530, 2008

Weiss HB, Songer TJ, Fabio A: Fetal deaths related to maternal injury. JAMA 286:1863, 2001

Weyerts LK, Jones MC, James HE: Paraplegia and congenital contractures as a consequence of intrauterine trauma. Am J Med Genet 43:751, 1992

Wheeler AP, Bernard GR: Acute lung injury and the acute respiratory distress syndrome: A clinical review. Lancet 369:1553, 2007

Wheeler AP, Bernard GR: Treating patients with severe sepsis. N Engl J Med 340:207, 1999

Whitten M, Irvine LM: Postmortem and perimortem caesarean section: What are the indications? J R Soc Med 93:6, 2000

Whitty JE: Maternal cardiac arrest in pregnancy. Clin Obstet Gynecol 45:377, 2002

Widgerow AD, Ford TD, Botha M: Burn contracture preventing uterine expansion. Ann Plast Surg 27:269, 1991

Ylagan MV, Trivedi N, Basu T, et al: Radiation exposure in the pregnant trauma patient: Implications for fetal risk counseling. Abstract No. 320. Presented at the 29th Annual Meeting of the Society for Maternal-Fetal Medicine, San Diego, January 2009

Zeeman GG: Obstetric critical care: A blueprint for improved outcomes. Crit Care Med 34:S208, 2006

Zeeman GG, Wendel GD Jr, Cunningham FG: A blueprint for obstetric critical care. Am J Obstet Gynecol 188:532, 2003

Zinaman M, Rubin J, Lindheimer MD: Serial plasma oncotic pressure levels and echoencephalography during and after delivery in severe preeclampsia. Lancet 1:1245, 1985

Obesity

Excessive weight has become one of the major health problems in affluent societies. Because of its medical importance and its multifaceted effects on pregnancy, it is discussed separately in this chapter. The prevalence of obesity in the United States has increased steadily as economic prosperity has increased. For a number of years, obesity has been termed *epidemic*—strictly defined, this implies a *temporary* widespread outbreak of greatly increased frequency and severity. Unfortunately, obesity more correctly is *endemic*—a condition that is habitually present. Moreover, its prevalence has continued to increase since 1960. By 1991, approximately a third of adults in the United States were overweight, and almost 300,000 deaths were attributed annually to obesity (Allison and co-workers, 1999). Sadly, the problem is not limited to adults, and 15 percent of children aged 6 through 11 years are reported to be overweight (Ogden and associates, 2002). The prevalence in adolescents is similar.

Public health authorities began to address the problem of obesity in the late 1980s. A stated goal of *Healthy People 2000* was to reduce the prevalence of overweight people to 20 percent or less by the end of the 20th century (Public Health Service, 1990). Not only was this goal not achieved, but by 2000, more than half of the population was overweight, and nearly a third of adults were obese (Flegal and colleagues, 2002; Hedley and associates, 2004).

There are many obesity-related diseases, including diabetes, heart disease, hypertension, stroke, and osteoarthritis. Together they result in a decreased life span. The worldwide diabetes epidemic that Bray (2003) predicted would follow the worldwide obesity epidemic has already begun. Obese women who become pregnant—and their fetuses—are predisposed to a variety of serious pregnancy-related complications. Long-term maternal effects include significant and increased rates of morbidity and mortality. Moreover, recent studies show that the offspring of obese women also suffer long-term morbidity.

DEFINITIONS

A number of systems have been used to define and classify obesity. The *body mass index* (*BMI*), also known as the *Quetelet index,* is currently in use. The BMI is calculated as weight in kilograms divided by height in square meters (kg/m^2). Calculated BMI values are available in various chart and graphic forms, such as the one shown in Figure 43-1. According to the National Heart, Lung, and Blood Institute (1998), a *normal* BMI is 18.5 to 24.9 kg/m^2; *overweight* is a BMI of 25 to 29.9 kg/m^2; and *obesity* is a BMI of 30 kg/m^2 or greater. According to Freedman and colleagues (2002), obesity is further categorized as class I (BMI: 30 to 34.9 kg/m^2), class II (BMI: 35 to 39.9 kg/m^2), and class III (BMI: 40-plus kg/m^2).

Prevalence

Pleis and colleagues (2003) reported that by 2000, 34 percent of adults in the United States were overweight, and another 27 percent were obese. This is an increase of 75 percent compared with 1980 statistics. **Thus, by 2000, more than half of adults in the United States were either overweight or obese.** Moreover, 2.8 percent of women and 1.7 percent of men were extremely obese (class III), with a BMI of 40 kg/m^2 or more (Mokdad and associates, 2003). Prevalence data through 2004 for women aged 20 to 39 are shown in Figure 43-2. As shown in Figure 43-3, there is a disparate prevalence of obesity in Mexican-American and

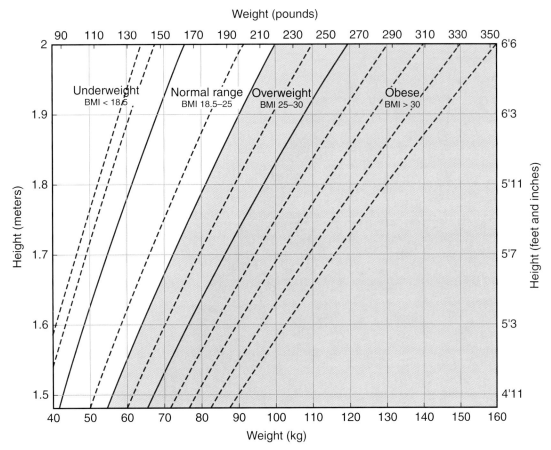

FIGURE 43-1 Chart for estimating body mass index (BMI). To find the BMI category for a particular subject, locate the point at which the height and weight intersect.

black women ages 20 to 39. This is also true among indigent individuals (Drewnowski and Specter, 2004). The prevalence of obese adults in 2006 was less than 20 percent in only four states (Centers for Disease Control and Prevention, 2007, 2008).

The Metabolic Syndrome

In some people, obesity interacts with inherited factors and leads to the onset of *insulin resistance*. This metabolic abnormality in turn is responsible for altered glucose metabolism and a predisposition to type 2 diabetes. In addition, it causes a number of subclinical abnormalities that predispose to cardiovascular disease and accelerate its onset. The most important among these are type 2 diabetes, dyslipidemia, and hypertension. When clustered together with other insulin resistance–related subclinical abnormalities, these are referred to as the *metabolic syndrome* (Abate, 2000). Virtually all obese women with hypertension demonstrate elevated plasma insulin levels. Levels are even higher in women with excessive fat in the abdomen—an apple shape, compared with those whose fat is in the hips and thighs—a pear shape (American College of Obstetricians and Gynecologists, 2003).

In fact, Gus and associates (2004) reported that for women, a waist circumference greater than 88 cm was more predictive of hypertension than a BMI greater than 30 kg/m^2.

Criteria used by the National Institutes of Health (2001) to define the metabolic syndrome are shown in Table 43-1. Of interest, the American Diabetes Association eschews the

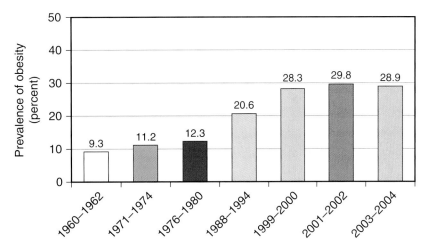

FIGURE 43-2 Prevalence (percent) of obesity among 20- to 39-year-old nonpregnant U.S. women. Obesity is defined as a body mass index of greater than 30 kg/m^2 (Redrawn with permission from *Influence of Pregnancy Weight on Maternal and Child Health Workshop Report,* 2007, by the National Academy of Sciences, Courtesy of the National Academies Press, Washington, D.C.)

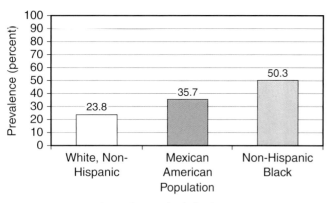

FIGURE 43-3 Prevalence (percent) of obesity among U.S. non-pregnant women, aged 20 to 39, by race/ethnicity for 2003-2004. Obesity is defined as a body mass index of greater than 30 kg/m². (Redrawn with permission from *Influence of Pregnancy Weight on Maternal and Child Health Workshop Report,* 2007, by the National Academy of Sciences, Courtesy of the National Academies Press, Washington, D.C.)

"syndrome" designation and urges consideration for these and other cardiovascular-disease risk factors that occur singly or in combination (Kahn and colleagues, 2005).

Prevalence

Because the metabolic syndrome is newly defined, prevalence data have been calculated from a study in progress. Ford and colleagues (2002) did a follow-up study of men and women enrolled in the Third National Health and Nutrition Survey (NHANES III). They found an overall prevalence of the metabolic syndrome in 24 percent of women and 22 percent of men. As expected, prevalence increased with age. For women, prevalence was about 6 percent in those 20 to 29 years of age; 14 percent in those 30 to 39 years of age; 20 percent in those 40 to 49 years of age; and 30 percent for women older than 50 years.

MORBIDITY AND MORTALITY ASSOCIATED WITH OBESITY

Obesity is costly—not only in morbidity and mortality, but also in healthcare dollars. Colditz (1999) estimated that 300,000

TABLE 43-1. Adult Treatment Panel III (ATP III): Criteria for Diagnosis of the Metabolic Syndrome

Patients with three or more of the following:

1. Abdominal obesity: waist circumference > 88 cm (34.7 in) in women or > 102 cm (40.2 in) in men

2. Hypertriglyceridemia: $\geq$ 150 mg/dL

3. High-density lipoprotein (HDL): < 50 mg/dL in women or < 40 mg/dL in men

4. High blood pressure: $\geq$ 130/85 mm Hg[a]

5. High fasting glucose: $\geq$ 110 mg/dL[a]

[a]Those with normal values while taking medications are considered to meet these criteria.
From the National Institutes of Health (2001).

TABLE 43-2. Long-term Complications of Obesity

Disorder	Possible Cause(s)
Type 2 diabetes mellitus	Insulin resistance
Hypertension	Increased blood volume and cardiac output
Coronary heart disease	Hypertension, dyslipidemia, type 2 diabetes
Obesity cardiomyopathy	Eccentric left ventricular hypertrophy
Sleep apnea/pulmonary dysfunction	Pharyngeal fat deposition
Ischemic stroke	Atherosclerosis, decreased cerebral blood flow
Gallbladder disease	Hyperlipidemia
Liver disease—nonalcoholic steatohepatitis (NASH)	Increased visceral adiposity; elevated serum, free fatty acids; hyperinsulinemia
Osteoarthritis	Stress on weight-bearing joints
Subfertility	Hyperinsulinemia
Cancer—endometrium, colon, breast	Hyperestrogenemia
Carpal tunnel syndrome	
Deep-venous thrombosis	
Poor wound healing	

Compiled from Alpert (2001); Calle (2003); Chinali (2004); Flegal (2007); Kenchaiah (2002); Mokdad (2003); Must (1999); Ninomiya (2004), and all their colleagues; National Task Force on the Prevention and Treatment of Obesity (2000).

adults die each year from obesity-related causes. He estimated direct costs of obesity and physical inactivity to be 9.4 percent of annual healthcare expenditures in the United States.

Individuals who are overweight are at increased risk for an imposing number of complications (Table 43-2). The direct link between obesity and type 2 diabetes mellitus is well known (Mokdad and associates, 2003). According to Hossain and colleagues (2007), 90 percent of type 2 diabetes is attributable to excess weight. Heart disease due to obesity—*adipositas cordis*—is caused by hypertension, hypervolemia, and dyslipidemia. Higher rates of abnormal left ventricular function, heart failure, myocardial infarction, and stroke have been noted (Chinali, 2004; Kenchaiah, 2002; Ninomiya, 2004, and all their colleagues).

Excessive weight is associated with increased early mortality rates, as shown by Peeters (2003) and Fontaine (2003) and their colleagues in follow-up studies from both the Framingham Heart Study and the NHANES III cohort. Results from a prospective study conducted by the American Cancer Society are shown in Figure 43-4. In this and other studies, mortality risk from cardiovascular disease and cancer increased directly with increasing BMI.

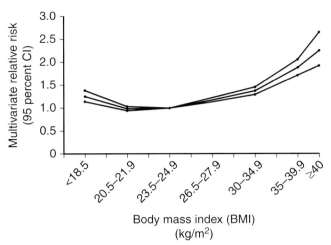

FIGURE 43-4 Relative risk of death from all causes from 1998 to 2002 in 317,875 persons entered into the Cancer Prevention Study II begun in 1982 by the American Cancer Society (Calle and colleagues, 1999, 2003). Relative risks were adjusted for age, race, sex, education, physical activity, alcohol use, marital status, aspirin use, fat and vegetable consumption, and estrogen use. The tan area represents the 95-percent confidence intervals. (Data from Calle and associates, 2005.)

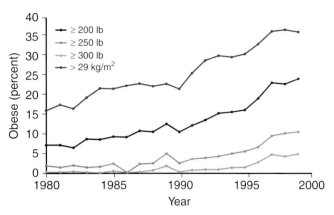

FIGURE 43-5 Increasing prevalence of obesity during 20 years in pregnant women classified at the time of their first prenatal visit at the University of Alabama at Birmingham. All women were classified into the first three categories shown on the graph. In approximately half of the women, height was available, and they were classified by body mass index. (Reprinted from *American Journal of Obstetrics & Gynecology*, Vol. 185, No. 4, GC Lu, DJ Rouse, M DuBard, et al., The effect of the increasing prevalence of maternal obesity on perinatal morbidity, pp. 845–849, Copyright 2001, with permission from Elsevier.)

TREATMENT OF OBESITY

Weight loss is tremendously difficult for obese individuals to accomplish. If achieved, long-term maintenance poses equivalent or even more daunting difficulties. There are innumerable methods espoused to help or even directly cause weight loss. Most are charlatan schemes designed to extract money from overweight individuals. That said, even the most legitimate nonsurgical methods are fraught with frequent failure. If they are successful, slow and inexorable return to preintervention weight usually follows (Yanovski, 2005). Legitimate weight loss approaches include behavioral, pharmacological, and surgical techniques, or a combination of these methods. The American College of Obstetricians and Gynecologists (2005b) encourages the role of obstetrician-gynecologists in assessment and management of obesity in adult women.

PREGNANCY AND OBESITY

Obesity is associated with subfertility due to increased insulin resistance (see Table 43-2). In their review, Neill and Nelson-Piercy (2001) linked impaired fecundity in women with a BMI in excess of 30 kg/m². In 6500 in vitro fertilization-intracytoplasmic sperm injection cycles, Bellver and associates (2009) found that implantation, pregnancy, and live-birth rates were progressively and significantly reduced with each unit of maternal BMI. In a case-control study, Lashen and colleagues (2004) found that obesity is associated with increased risk of first-trimester and recurrent miscarriage. In the many overweight and obese women who achieve pregnancy, there are a number of increased and interrelated adverse perinatal outcomes. **Marked obesity is unequivocally hazardous to the pregnant woman and her fetus**. Moreover, Chu and colleagues (2008) have provided evidence that obese pregnant women have a disparately increased use of healthcare services.

Prevalence

Obesity complicating pregnancy has also increased along with the overall prevalence of obesity. Before adoption of the BMI, investigators used a variety of definitions of obesity to assess risks during pregnancy. For example, in the study shown in Figure 43-5, four definitions were used. But, regardless of how obesity was defined, all groups showed substantive increases in its prevalence during the 20-year period. Ehrenberg and colleagues (2002) reported similar findings in a 15-year study in Cleveland.

Maternal Weight Gain and Energy Requirement

The 2007 National Research Council and Institute of Medicine (IOM) Workshop Report provides a current and comprehensive review of the determinants of maternal weight gain in relation to biological, metabolic, and social predictors. This report was a follow-up that supported the 1990 IOM recommendations for gestational weight gain, which are based on the prepregnancy BMI as shown in Table 43-3. The IOM (2009) recently amended these guidelines slightly. Fat deposition is greater in women with high BMI, and thus, energy costs are significantly lower (Butte and colleagues, 2004). Kinoshita and Itoh (2006) studied regional fat distribution changes across pregnancy using sonography. They found that during the third trimester increases were predominantly in visceral fat. Despite these stores, maternal catabolism is—at least intuitively—not good for fetal growth and development. Thus, it is recommended that even obese women should not attempt weight loss during pregnancy but should limit weight gain to 20 pounds (see also Chap. 8, p. 200).

Cogswell and associates (2006) reviewed gestational weight gain across BMI categories from 1990 through 2003. They reported that a third of pregnant women gained weight within the IOM recommendations, and these patterns were stable over

TABLE 43-3. Institute of Medicine Recommended Total Weight Gain Ranges for Pregnant Women by Prepregnancy Body Mass Index (BMI)

Category	Recommended Total Gain[a]	
	Kilograms	Pounds
Underweight—BMI <18.5 kg/m²	12.5 to 18	28 to 40
Normal—BMI 18.5 to 24.9 kg/m²	11.5 to 16	25 to 35
Overweight—BMI 25 to 29.9 kg/m²	7 to 11.5	15 to 25
Obese—BMI >30 kg/m²	5 to 9.1	11 to 20

[a]Young adolescents and black women should strive for gains at the upper end of the recommended range. Short women (<157 cm or 62 in) should strive for gains at the lower end of this range.

Redrawn with permission from *Influence of Pregnancy Weight on Maternal and Child Health Workshop Report*, 2007, and *Weight Gain During Pregnancy: Reexamining the Guidelines, 2009*, both by the National Academy of Sciences, Courtesy of the National Academies Press, Washington, D.C.

time. Similar to the overall U.S. trend from 1990, Chu and associates (2009) reported in the U.S. in 2004-2005 that 40 percent of normal-weight and 60 percent of overweight women gained excessive weight during pregnancy. Rooney and Schauberger (2002) followed 540 women after delivery for a mean of 8.5 years, during which time, the average weight gained was 6.3 kg. Women who had gained less pregnancy weight than the recommended amount were on average 4.1 kg heavier at the end of the follow-up period. Women who gained the recommended amount were 6.5 kg heavier. Finally, women who gained more than the recommended amount were 8.4 kg heavier.

Maternal Morbidity

Obesity causes excess maternal morbidity (Table 43-4). Various definitions have included more than 150 percent of ideal body weight, BMI > 35 kg/m², BMI > 40 kg/m², and >150 pounds over ideal body weight (Bianco, 1998; Cedergren, 2004; Denison, 2008; Isaacs, 1994; Kabiru and Raynor, 2004; Kumari, 2001, and all their colleagues). The significantly increased incidences of many disorders are listed in Table 43-4. Weiss and associates (2004) reported similar adverse outcomes and maternal morbidity in a prospective multicenter study of more than 16,000 women with class I—BMI 30–35—and class II—BMI

TABLE 43-4. Adverse Pregnancy Effects in Overweight and Obese Women

Complication	Prevalence in Percent in Women With Normal BMI 20–24.9 (n = 176,923)	Increased Complications (Odds Ratio[a])	
		Overweight BMI 25–29.9 (n = 79,014)	Obese BMI > 30 (n = 31,27)
Gestational diabetes	0.8	1.7	3.6
Preeclampsia	0.7	1.5	2.1
Postterm pregnancy	0.13	1.2[b]	1.7
Emergency cesarean	7.8	1.3	1.8
Elective cesarean	4.0	1.2	1.4
Postpartum hemorrhage	10.4	1.2	1.4
Pelvic infection	0.7	1.2	1.3
Urinary infection	0.7	1.2	1.4
Wound infection	0.4	1.3	2.2
Macrosomia	9.0	1.6	2.4
Stillbirth	0.4	1.1[b]	1.4

[a]Odds ratios (99% CI) are significant except when denoted.
[b]Not significantly different.
Data from Sebire and colleagues (2001).

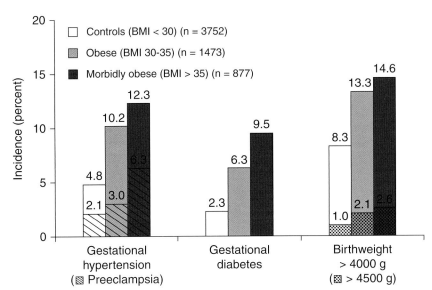

FIGURE 43-6 Incidence of selected pregnancy outcomes in 16,102 women enrolled in the FASTER (First and Second trimester Evaluation of Risk) trial according to body mass index (BMI) status. (Data from Weiss and colleagues, 2004.)

35–40—obesity within the FASTER—First- and Second-Trimester Evaluation of Risk trial. Some of these are shown in Figure 43-6. Especially striking are the marked increases in gestational hypertension and diabetes. Not shown are the cesarean delivery risks of 33.8 percent for obese and 47.4 for morbidly obese women compared with 20.7 percent for the control group. Haeri and co-workers (2009) also found increased rates of cesarean delivery and gestation diabetes in obese adolescents. More worrisome is that obese women also have increased rates of *emergency* cesarean delivery. (Lynch and associates, 2008; Poobalan and colleagues, 2009).

There are also reports of increased adverse pregnancy outcomes in overweight women whose BMI is 25 to 29.9 kg/m^2 (Hall and Neubert, 2005). Results of the study by Sebire and associates (2001) that included more than 285,000 singleton pregnancies are shown in Table 43-4. Almost all complications are significantly increased in women whose BMI is above normal.

Other morbidity associated with maternal obesity includes a higher incidence of failed trial of labor with a prior cesarean delivery (Bujold, 2005; Goodall, 2005; Hibbard, 2006; Robinson, 2005, and all their colleagues). Obesity and hypertension are common cofactors in causing peripartum heart failure (Cunningham and associates, 1986). And obese women present anesthesia challenges that include difficult epidural and spinal analgesia placement and complications from failed or difficult intubations (Hood and Dewan, 1993). Second-trimester dilatation and evacuation was reported to take longer and be more difficult in women whose BMI was 30 kg/m^2 or greater (Dark and co-workers, 2002).

Obese women are less likely to breast feed than normal-weight women (Li and colleagues, 2003). They also have greater weight retention 1 year after delivery (Catalano, 2007; National Research Council and Institute of Medicine, 2007; Rode and colleagues, 2005). Finally, there is evidence that quality-of-life measures are negatively affected by obesity during pregnancy (Amador and co-workers, 2008). LaCoursiere and Varner

(2009) found that postpartum depression was significantly increased in obese women and also in relation to the degree of obesity—class 1 (22.6 percent), class 2 (32.4 percent), and class 3 (40 percent).

Preeclampsia

There is no doubt that obesity is a consistent risk factor for preeclampsia (Cedergren, 2004; Jensen, 2003; Sebire, 2001; Weiss, 2004, and all their colleagues). In a review of studies that included more than 1.4 million women, O'Brien and associates (2003) found that the preeclampsia risk doubled with each 5 to 7 kg/m^2 increase in prepregnancy BMI.

Obesity is also associated with low-grade inflammation and endothelial activation. Endothelial activation also plays an integral role in preeclampsia (see Chap. 34, p. 712). Wolf and co-workers (2001) linked these two conditions by providing intriguing evidence that inflammation may explain, at least partly, the association of obesity with preeclampsia. Ramsay and co-workers (2002) confirmed that obese pregnant women had significantly elevated serum levels of interleukin-6 and C-reactive protein as well as evidence of impaired endothelial function. These investigators found that obese gravid women had significantly higher levels of triglycerides, very-low-density lipoprotein cholesterol, insulin, and leptin compared with normal-weight pregnant woman.

Contraception

Most studies report that oral contraceptive failure is more likely in overweight women. In reviewing general studies on hormonal contraceptive efficacy, it is apparent that the typical study subject is not representative of the average American woman. As discussed earlier, at least 50 percent of American women are overweight with a BMI > 25 kg/m^2. In contraceptive studies, however, most subjects have a BMI between 18 and 28 kg/m^2 (Holt and co-workers, 2002; Zieman and colleagues, 2002).

Holt and colleagues (2002) studied oral contraceptive use and found that women in the highest weight quartile—70.5 kg—had a 1.6-fold increased pregnancy risk. Importantly, women in this quartile who used very-low-dose oral contraceptives had a four- to fivefold increased pregnancy rate (see Chap. 32, p. 673). A recent report from the National Survey of Family Growth did not find an increased rate of unintended pregnancy (Kaneshiro and associates, 2008). Zieman and colleagues (2002) studied efficacy of the Ortho-Evra patch and found a significant association between increasing body weight and contraceptive failure.

Perinatal Mortality

An increased incidence of otherwise inexplicable late-pregnancy stillbirths has been associated with obesity. Cnattingius and colleagues (1998) found a significant 1.6-fold increase in the stillbirth rate in women whose BMI was 25 to 29.9 kg/m^2. The rate increased 2.6-fold for women with a BMI $\geq$ 30 kg/m^2. In addition, the early neonatal death rate was nearly doubled in nulliparous women with a BMI $\geq$ 30 kg/m^2. With the same database, Stephansson and associates (2001) confirmed an almost threefold late-stillbirth rate in women with a BMI $>$ 25 kg/m^2. From their meta-analysis, Chu and co-workers (2007) found 1.5-fold increased risks for stillbirth in overweight and 2.1-fold in obese women. The recent Scottish study of more than 186,000 nulliparas described an almost fourfold increased stillbirth rate in women with a BMI $\geq$ 35 kg/m^2 compared with women whose BMI was 20 to 25 kg/m^2 (Denison and colleagues, 2008).

Huang and colleagues (2000) found increased prepregnancy weight to be the factor most strongly associated with 196 unexplained fetal deaths even after adjusting for maternal age and excluding women with diabetes and hypertensive disorders. Nohr and associates (2005) confirmed this association in 54,000 births from 1998 to 2001. Compared with normal-weight women, the fetal death rate among obese women increased with gestational age. The hazard ratio was 2.1 at 28 to 36 weeks, 3.5 at 37 to 39 weeks, and 4.6 at 40 or more weeks. The stillbirth rate was 240-percent greater in obese compared with normal-weight women.

Perinatal Morbidity

Both fetal and neonatal complications are increased in obese women. Earlier studies by Shaw and colleagues (1996, 2000) reported that women with a BMI $>$ 30 kg/m^2 had a twofold increased incidence of neural-tube defects compared with that of control women. In their recent meta-analysis, Rasmussen and associates (2008) found 1.2-, 1.7-, and 3.1-fold increased risks in overweight, obese, and severely obese women compared with controls of normal weight (see also Chap. 13, p. 287). In addition to increased neural-tube defects, in a case-control study from the Atlantic Birth Defects Risk Factor Surveillance Study, Watkins and associates (2003) reported a 3.5-fold increase in rates of neural-tube defects in obese women. They also found a two- to threefold increased incidence in omphalocele, heart defects, and multiple anomalies in obese women. The last two were also increased twofold in overweight women whose BMI was 25 to 29.9 kg/m^2. In a meta-analysis, Stothard and colleagues (2009) found that maternal obesity was significantly associated with an increased risk of a wide range of fetal/newborn structural anomalies. Of appreciable concern are the many reports of unreliable fetal anatomy sonographic screening in obese gravidas (Dashe, 2009; Grace, 2009; Hendler, 2005; Thornburn, 2009, and all their co-workers).

Two important and interrelated cofactors that contribute to excessive rates of perinatal morbidity and mortality are chronic hypertension and diabetes mellitus, both of which are associated with obesity. Chronic hypertension is a well-known cause of fetal-growth restriction (see Chap. 45, p. 987). Pregestational diabetes increases the rate of birth defects, and gestational diabetes is complicated by excessive numbers of large-for-gestational age and macrosomic fetuses (see Chap. 52, p. 1104). And even without diabetes, the prevalence of macrosomic newborns is increased in obese women (Bianco and co-workers, 1998; Cedergren, 2004; Isaacs and associates, 1994).

The group from MetroHealth Medical Center in Cleveland has conducted studies of prepregnancy obesity, gestational weight gain, and prepregnancy and gestational diabetes and their relationship to newborn weight and fat mass (Catalano, 2005, 2007; Ehrenberg, 2004; Sewell, 2006, and all their co-workers). They concluded that although each of these variables is associated with larger and more corpulent newborns, prepregnancy BMI exhibits the strongest influence on the prevalence of these neonates. They attributed this increased prevalence of macrosomic infants to the marked frequency of overweight or obese women in pregnancy—46.7 percent—compared with only 4 percent of pregnant women with diabetes.

Maternal obesity is linked with increased childhood obesity. Combined with sociological and dietary factors, Armstrong and colleagues (2002) reported that breast feeding decreases the risk of childhood obesity. At the same time, recall that Ruowei and co-workers (2003) reported that obese women were less likely to breast feed.

Morbidity in Children Born to Obese Women

There seems to be no doubt that obese women beget obese children, who themselves become obese adults. Just a few studies are cited that confirm this association. Whitaker (2004) studied low-income children in the Special Supplemental Food Program for Women, Infants, and Children (WIC) and found a linear association between early pregnancy maternal BMI and prevalence of overweight children at 2, 3, and 4 years. From Denmark, Schack-Nielson and colleagues (2005) found a direct association between maternal, newborn, and childhood BMI. This association strengthened as offspring progressed to adulthood. Catalano and colleagues (2005) studied offspring at a median age of 7 and found a direct association with maternal prepregnancy obesity and childhood obesity. They also reported associations with central obesity, elevated systolic blood pressure, increased insulin resistance, and decreased high-density lipoprotein (HDL) cholesterol levels—all elements of the metabolic syndrome discussed on page 947. Boney and co-workers (2005) studied 84 large-for-gestational age (LGA) and 95 appropriate-for-gestational age (AGA) offspring of women with or without gestational diabetes. These investigators followed these cohorts longitudinally from age 6 to 11 years. They observed that children who were LGA at birth and whose mothers were either obese or had gestational diabetes had significantly increased risks for subsequently developing metabolic syndrome.

It also appears that excessive maternal weight gain in pregnancy may prognosticate adulthood obesity. Schack-Nielsen and colleagues (2005) found a linear association of maternal weight gain with the subsequent BMI in their study children. Analyzing data from Project Viva, Oken (2006) suggests a linear association between maternal weight gain and the risk of an overweight child at age 3. Not all studies concur. For example, Whitaker and colleagues (2004) analyzed a large population of children in the WIC program and found no obvious linear association between gestational weight gain and childhood obesity.

Fetal Programming and Childhood Morbidity

Epidemiological studies have addressed the association of childhood, adolescent, and even adult adverse health outcomes in relation to the fetal environment. Adverse health outcomes include obesity, diabetes, hypertension, and the metabolic syndrome. Variables studied have included maternal prepregnancy BMI, obesity, gestational weight gain, and pregestational or gestational diabetes. The most robust evidence suggests a direct association between children born to women who had prepregnancy obesity or gestational diabetes and the occurrence of a higher BMI in childhood and adulthood.

The potential biological causes and mechanisms of these associations are not clear at this time. It is a complex issue greatly confounded by insufficient data with consideration for all potential maternal—including genetic—predisposing factors. There also is insufficient data regarding the environment of the infant and child in relation to diet and activity. The science of *epigenetics* has provided some support for the possibility that perturbations of the maternal-fetal environment can adversely alter postdelivery events. For example, Aagard-Tillery and colleagues (2006) reported that diet supplementation with essential nutrients, unaltered in caloric content, prevented adult obesity and insulin resistance in a heritable transgenerational model of fetal-growth restriction. Perhaps more likely is the contributions of the maternal-child environment subsequent to birth. Gluck and colleagues (2009) found that maternal influence, not diabetic intrauterine environment, predicts children's energy intake. This is further discussed in Chapters 38 (p. 842) and 52 (p. 1109).

Management

A program of weight reduction is probably unrealistic during pregnancy. If such a regimen is chosen, however, it is mandatory that the quality of the diet be monitored closely and that ketosis be avoided (Rizzo and associates, 1991). It is more pragmatic to *limit* weight gain in obese or overweight women. The goal of 15 pounds, discussed previously, is an ideal target.

Polley and colleagues (2002) randomized women to an intensive behavioral intervention versus usual obstetrical care to prevent excessive pregnancy weight gain. For normal-weight women randomized to usual prenatal care, 58 percent exceeded the guidelines shown in Table 43-3, compared with 33 percent of those randomized to behavioral intervention. Among overweight women, however, this difference was just the opposite. Specifically, 59 percent of women in the intervention group gained excessive weight compared with only 32 percent in the usual-care group. Thus, behavioral modification programs to limit excessive weight gain require intensive efforts, and they have had only modest success (Olson and colleagues, 2004). Asbee and associates (2009) randomized 100 women to receive either additional intensive dietary and lifestyle counseling during gestation or to receive routine prenatal care. Women assigned to routine prenatal care had significantly more weight gain during pregnancy and higher cesarean delivery rates.

Close prenatal surveillance detects most early signs of diabetes or hypertension. Standard screening tests for fetal anomalies are sufficient. However, several investigators caution that detection of fetal anomalies in obese women is more difficult (Dashe and colleagues, 2009; Hendler and associates, 2005). Accurate assessment of fetal growth usually requires serial sonography. Antepartum and intrapartum fetal heart rate monitoring are likewise more difficult, and sometimes these are even impossible.

Surgical and Anesthetic Concerns

Evaluation by anesthesia personnel is performed at a prenatal visit or on arrival at the labor unit (American College of Obstetricians and Gynecologists, 2002). Anesthetic risks and complications faced by obese women are discussed in Chapter 19 (p. 460). Special attention is given to complications that might arise during labor and delivery.

For cesarean delivery, forethought is given to optimal placement and type of abdominal incision to allow access the fetus and to effect the best wound closure with the least intervening tissue (Alexander and Liston, 2006). One technique is shown in Figure 43-7. Individual differences in maternal body habitus preclude naming any one approach as superior (Gilstrap and colleagues, 2002). Wall and colleagues (2003) reported a four-fold wound complication rate when a vertical abdominal incision was compared with a transverse incision—31 versus 8 percent. Conversely, Houston and Raynor (2000) reported similar wound complications with either incision.

Attention to closure of the subcutaneous layer is important. Chelmow and associates (2004) performed a meta-analysis of subcutaneous closure in 887 women undergoing cesarean delivery and whose wound thickness was greater than 2 centimeters. Subcutaneous closure resulted in a modest but significant 6-percent decrease in wound disruption. Walsh and colleagues (2009) have reviewed the prevention and management of surgical site infections in morbidly obese women.

Graduated compression stockings, hydration, and early mobilization after cesarean delivery in obese women is recommended by the American College of Obstetricians and Gynecologists (2005a). Some recommend "mini-dose" heparin prophylaxis, but we do not routinely use this.

Pregnancy Following Surgical Procedures for Obesity

A number of surgical procedures have been designed to treat morbid obesity by either decreasing gastric volume or bypassing gastrointestinal absorption (Adams and co-workers, 2007; Saber and colleagues, 2008). In a meta-analysis of these procedures in nonpregnant patients, Buchwald and associates (2007) found them to improve or resolve diabetes, hyperlipidemia, hypertension, and obstructive sleep apnea. Kini and associates (2007) reported that the metabolic syndrome also improves.

Indeed, these procedures are common, and Catalano (2007) estimates that more than 150,000 are done annually in this country. Although these are not performed during pregnancy, many women are becoming pregnant following weight-reduction surgery (Abodeely and associates, 2008). Guelinckx and co-workers (2009) found improved fertility and reduced risks of obstetrical complications in those following bariatric surgery compared with morbidly obese controls. The three procedures commonly performed currently are vertical gastroplasty, gastric banding, and Roux-en-Y gastric bypass. Older procedures no longer in use include the jejunoileal bypass and upper gastrojejunostomy bypass.

SECTION 8

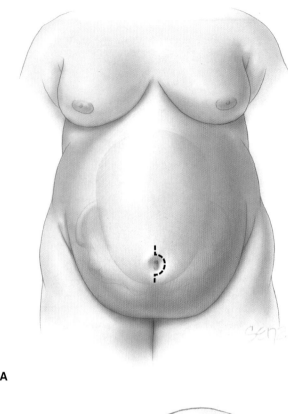

A

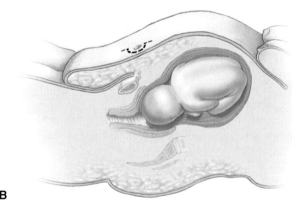

B

FIGURE 43-7 Abdominal incision for the obese woman. **A.** Frontal view. The dotted line indicates an appropriate skin incision for abdominal entry relative to panniculus. As shown by the uterus in the background, selection of this periumbilical site permits access to the lower uterine segment. **B.** Sagittal view.

Vertical Gastroplasty. A narrow channel is created through the stomach using stapling devices. The small gastric pouch empties through a narrow outlet into the remainder of the stomach. Subsequent pregnancy outcomes were described by Bilenka and colleagues (1995). There were 14 pregnancies in nine women who had undergone the procedure. Their mean weight loss was 80 pounds, and the women had fewer complications compared with their preprocedure pregnancies.

Gastric Banding. An adjustable band is placed 2 cm below the gastroesophageal junction to create a small pouch, as described above. Of 23 pregnancies in women subsequent to the procedure, Martin and co-workers (2000) reported that in three there was excessive nausea and vomiting, and band adjustment to decrease

obstruction was successful. Dixon and associates (2005) described the outcomes in 79 women following laparoscopic adjustable banding. Pregnancy outcomes were compared with those in 40 pregnancies delivered of these women preprocedure, as well as with a matched cohort of 79 obese women. In the 79 pregnancies following banding, the incidences of gestational hypertension—10 versus 45 percent—and gestational diabetes—6 versus 15 percent—were significantly lower compared with preprocedure pregnancies. Incidences in banded patients were also significantly lower than those in the obese cohort, whose rates for hypertension were 38 percent, and for diabetes, 19 percent. The results from these and other studies are shown in Table 43-5.

Roux-en-Y Bypass. This type of bypass is the most effective bariatric procedure currently in use (Brunicardi and associates, 2001). It most often is performed laparoscopically (Dao and colleagues, 2006). The proximal stomach is completely transected to leave a 30-mL pouch. A gastroenterotomy is then created by connecting the proximal end of the distal jejunum to the pouch. A Roux-en-Y enteroenterostomy is also completed 60 cm distal to this gastrojejunostomy to allow drainage of the unused stomach and proximal small intestine.

Brunicardi and colleagues (2001) summarized four series totaling almost 400 men and nonpregnant women. Mean weight loss at 1 year in the four series ranged from 21 to 43 kg. In the largest study, at 1 year, 300 patients had lost a mean of 80 percent of their excessive weight. At 5 years, 50 to 75 percent of the weight loss had been maintained, and at 14 years, maintenance of lost weight still exceeded 50 percent (American Society for Bariatric Surgery, 2003).

As with other bariatric procedures, pregnancy outcomes are changed remarkably following Roux-en-Y bypass. Wittgrove and associates (1998) described 49 pregnancies in 36 women after these procedures. When 17 prior pregnancy outcomes were compared with those after bypass, there was a dramatic reduction in hypertension—40 versus 0 percent, diabetes—24 versus 0 percent, and infant weight > 4000 g—30 versus 5 percent. Results of pregnancy outcomes from studies summarized by Abodeely and co-workers (2008) are shown in Table 43-5. Serious complications are uncommon, but intussusception occurs, and at least one maternal death from herniation and obstruction has been reported (Moore and colleagues, 2004; Wax and associates, 2007).

Recommendations. The American College of Obstetricians and Gynecologists (2005a) recommends the following counseling before and during pregnancy in women who have undergone bariatric surgery:

- Patients with adjustable gastric banding should be advised that they are at risk of becoming pregnant unexpectedly after weight loss following surgery
- All patients are advised to delay pregnancy for 12 to 18 months after surgery to avoid pregnancy during the rapid-weight-loss phase
- Women with a gastric band should be monitored by their bariatric team during pregnancy because adjustments of the band may be necessary
- Patients should be evaluated for nutritional deficiencies, and vitamin supplementation should be given when indicated.

CHAPTER 43

TABLE 43-5. Pregnancy Outcomes Following Gastric Banding Surgery and Roux-en-Y Gastric Bypass

Outcome	Gastric Banding[a] (n = 227)	Roux-en-Y Gastric Bypass[b] (n = 164)
Hypertension	~8%	6%
Gestational diabetes	~12%	4%
Cesarean delivery	~25%	23%
Mean birthweight	—	~3300 g
Small for gestational age	8%	—
Stillbirth	4/1000	6/1000

[a]Data from Bar-Zohar (2006), Dixon (2001), Martin (2000), Skull (2004), and all their colleagues.
[b]From review by Abodeely and associates (2008).

REFERENCES

Aagard-Tillery K, Holland W, McKnight R, et al: Fetal origins of disease: Essential nutrient supplementation prevents adult metabolic disease in a transgenerational model of IUGR. Am J Obstet Gynecol 195:S3, 2006

Abate N: Obesity and cardiovascular disease: Pathogenetic role of the metabolic syndrome and therapeutic implications. J Diabetes Complications 14:154, 2000

Abodeely A, Roye GD, Harrington DT, et al: Pregnancy outcomes after bariatric surgery: Maternal, fetal, and infant implications. Surg Obes Relat Dis 4(3):464, 2008

Adams TD, Gress RE, Smith SC, et al: Long-term mortality after gastric bypass surgery. N Engl J Med 357(8):753, 2007

Alexander CI, Liston WA: Operating on the obese woman—A review. BJOG 113(10):1167, 2006

Allison DB, Fontaine KR, Manson JE, et al: Annual deaths attributable to obesity in the United States. JAMA 282:1530, 1999

Alpert MA: Obesity cardiomyopathy: Pathophysiology and evolution of the clinical syndrome. Am J Med Sci 321:225, 2001

Amador N, Juárez JM, Guizar JM, et al: Quality of life in obese pregnant women: A longitudinal study. Am J Obstet Gynecol 198:203.e1, 2008

American College of Obstetricians and Gynecologists: Obstetric analgesia and anesthesia. Practice Bulletin No. 36, July 2002

American College of Obstetricians and Gynecologists: Weight Control: Assessment and management. Clinical updates in women's health care. Vol II, No. 3, 2003

American College of Obstetricians and Gynecologists: Obesity in pregnancy. Committee Opinion No. 315, September 2005a

American College of Obstetricians and Gynecologists: The role of the obstetrician-gynecologist in the assessment of and management of obesity. Committee Opinion No. 319, October 2005b

American Society for Bariatric Surgery, 2003. Available at: http://www.asbs.org/html/rationale/rationale.html. Accessed July 21, 2008

Armstrong J, Reilly JJ; Child Health Information Team: Breastfeeding and lowering the risk of childhood obesity. Lancet 359:2003, 2002

Asbee SM, Jenkins TR, Butler JR, et al: Preventing excessive weight gain during pregnancy through dietary and lifestyle counseling. Obstet Gynecol 113:305, 2009

Bar-Zohar D, Azem F, Klausner J, et al: Pregnancy after laparoscopic adjustable gastric banding: Perinatal outcome is favorable also for women with relatively high gestational weight gain. Surg Endosc 20(10):1580, 2006

Bellver J, Ayllón Y, Verrando M, et al: Female obesity impairs in vitro fertilization outcome without affecting embryo quality. Fertil Steril [In press], 2009

Bianco AT, Smilen SW, Davis Y, et al: Pregnancy outcome and weight gain recommendations for the morbidly obese woman. Obstet Gynecol 91:97, 1998

Bilenka B, Ben-Shlomo I, Cozacov C, et al: Fertility, miscarriage and pregnancy after vertical banded gastroplasty operation for morbid obesity. Acta Obstet Gynecol Scand 74:42, 1995

Boney CM, Verma A, Tucker R, et al: Metabolic syndrome in childhood: Association with birth weight, maternal obesity, and gestational diabetes mellitus. Pediatrics 115:e290, 2005

Bray GA: Low-carbohydrate diets and realities of weight loss. JAMA 289:1853, 2003

Brunicardi FC, Reardon PR, Matthews BD: The surgical treatment of obesity. In Townsend CM, Beauchamp RD, Evers BM, et al (eds): Sabiston Textbook of Surgery, 16th ed. Philadelphia, WB Saunders, 2001, p 247

Buchwald H, Estok R. Fahrbach K, et al: Trends in mortality in bariatric surgery: A systematic review and meta-analysis. Surgery 142(4):621, 2007

Bujold E, Hammoud A, Schild C, et al: The role of maternal body mass index in outcomes of vaginal births after cesarean. Am J Obstet Gynecol 193(4):1517, 2005

Butte NF, Wong WW, Treuth MS, et al: Energy requirements during pregnancy based on total energy expenditure and energy deposition. Am J Clin Nutr 79:1078, 2004

Calle EE, Rodriguez C, Walker-Thurmond K, et al: Overweight, obesity, and mortality from cancer in a prospectively studied cohort of U.S. adults. N Engl J Med 348:1625, 2003

Calle EE, Teras LR, Thun MJ: Obesity and mortality. N Engl J Med 353:20, 2005

Calle EE, Thun MJ, Petrelli JM, et al: Body-mass index and mortality in a prospective cohort of US adults. N Engl J Med 341:1097, 1999

Catalano P, Farrell K, Presley L, et al: Long-term follow-up of infants of women with normal glucose tolerance (NGT) and gestational diabetes (GDM): Risk factors for obesity and components of the metabolic syndrome in childhood. Am J Obstet Gynecol 193:S3, 2005

Catalano PM: Management of obesity in pregnancy. Obstet Gynecol 109:419, 2007

Cedergren MI: Maternal morbid obesity and the risk of adverse pregnancy outcome. Obstet Gynecol. 103:219, 2004

Centers for Disease Control and Prevention: National Center for Chronic Disease Prevention and Health Promotion. Obesity and Overweight: U.S. Obesity Trends 1985-2006. Available at: http://www.cdc.gov/nccdphp/dnpa/obesity/trend/maps/index.htm. Accessed July 27, 2007

Centers for Disease Control and Prevention: State-specific prevalence of obesity among adults—United States, 2007. 57:766, 2008

Chelmow D, Rodriquez EJ, Sabatini MM: Suture closure of subcutaneous fat and wound disruption after cesarean delivery: A meta-analysis. Obstet Gynecol 103:974, 2004

Chinali M, Devereux RB, Howard BV, et al: Comparison of cardiac structure and function in American Indians with and without the metabolic syndrome (the Strong Heart Study). Am J Cardiol 93:40, 2004

Chu SY, Bachman DJ, Callaghan WM, et al: Association between obesity during pregnancy and increased use of health care. N Engl J Med 358:1444, 2008

Chu SY, Callaghan WM, Bish CL, et al: Gestational weight gain by body mass index among US women delivering live births, 2004-2005: Fueling future obesity. Am J Obstet Gynecol 200:271.e1, 2009

Chu SY, Kim SY, Lau J, et al: Maternal obesity and risk of stillbirth: A meta-analysis. Am J Obstet Gynecol 197(3):223, 2007

Cnattingius S, Bergstrom R, Lipworth L, et al: Prepregnancy weight and the risk of adverse pregnancy outcomes. N Engl J Med 338: 147, 1998

Cogswell ME, Dietz PM, Branum AM: Maternal weight before, during, and after pregnancy in the United States. Presentation at the Workshop on the Impact of Pregnancy Weight on Maternal and Child Health, Washington, DC, May 30, 2006

Colditz G: Economic costs of obesity and inactivity. Med Sci Sports Exerc 31:S663, 1999

Cunningham FG, Pritchard JA, Hankins GVD, et al: Idiopathic cardiomyopathy or compounding cardiovascular events? Obstet Gynecol 67:157, 1986

Dao T, Juhn J, Ehmer D, et al: Pregnancy outcomes after gastric-bypass surgery. Am J Surg 192(6):762, 2006

Dark AC, Miller L, Kothenbeutel RL, et al: Obesity and second-trimester abortion by dilation and evacuation. J Reprod Med 47:226, 2002

Dashe JS, McIntire DD, Twickler DM: Effect of maternal obesity on the ultrasound detection of anomalous fetuses. Obstet Gynecol 113:1, 2009

Denison FC, Price J, Graham C, et al: Maternal obesity, length of gestation, risk of postdates pregnancy and spontaneous onset of labour at term. BJOG 115(6):720, 2008

Dixon JB, Dixon ME, O'Brien PE: Birth outcomes in obese women after laparoscopic adjustable gastric banding. Obstet Gynecol 106:965, 2005

Dixon JB, Dixon ME, O'Brien PE: Pregnancy after Lap-Band surgery: Management of the band to achieve healthy weight outcomes. Obes Surg 11:59, 2001

Drewnowski A, Specter SE: Poverty and obesity: The role of energy density and energy costs. Am J Clin Nutr 79:6, 2004

Ehrenberg HM, Dierker L, Milluzzi C, et al: Prevalence of maternal obesity in an urban center. Am J Obstet Gynecol 187:1189, 2002

Ehrenberg HM, Mercer BM, Catalano PM: The influence of obesity and diabetes on the prevalence of macrosomia. Am J Obstet Gynecol 191:964, 2004

Flegal KM, Carroll MD, Ogden CL, Johnson CL: Prevalence and trends in obesity among U.S. adults, 1999-2000. JAMA 288:1723-7, 2002

Flegal KM, Graubard BI, Williamson DF, et al: Cause-specific excess deaths associated with underweight, overweight, and obesity. JAMA 298:2028, 2007

Fontaine KR, Redden DT, Wang C, et al: Years of life lost due to obesity. JAMA 289:187, 2003

Ford ES, Giles WH, Dietz WH: Prevalence of the metabolic syndrome among U.S. adults. Findings from the Third National Health and Nutrition Examination Survey. JAMA 287:356, 2002

Freedman DS, Khan LK, Serdula MK, et al: Trends and correlates of Class 3 obesity in the United States from 1990 through 2000. JAMA 288:1758, 2002

Gilstrap LC, Cunningham FG, VanDorsten JP (eds): Anatomy, incisions, and closures. In Operative Obstetrics, 2nd ed. New York, McGraw-Hill, 2002, p 55

Gluck ME, Venti CA, Lindsay RS, et al: Maternal influence, not diabetic intrauterine environment, predicts children's energy intake. Obesity 17:772, 2009

Goodall PT, Ahn JT, Chapa JB, et al: Obesity as a risk factor for failed trial of labor in patients with previous cesarean delivery. Am J Obstet Gynecol 192:1423, 2005

Grace D, Zastrow A, Pressman E, et al: Completion rate of screening fetal echocardiography in the obese gravida. Abstract No. 471. Presented at the 29th Annual Meeting of the Society for Maternal-Fetal Medicine. 26-31 January 2009

Guelinckx I, Devlieger R, Vansant G: Reproductive outcome after bariatric surgery: a critical review. Hum Reprod Update 15(2):189, 2009

Gus M, Fuchs SC, Moreira LB, et al: Association between different measurements of obesity and the incidence of hypertension. Am J Hypertens 17:50, 2004

Haeri S, Guichard I, Baker AM, et al: The effect of teenage maternal obesity on perinatal outcomes. Obstet Gynecol. 113:300, 2009

Hall LF, Neubert AG: Obesity and pregnancy. Obstet Gynecol Surv 60(4):253, 2005

Hedley AA, Ogeden CL, Johnson CL, et al: Prevalence of overweight and obesity among U.S. children, adolescents, and adults, 1999–2002. JAMA 291:2847, 2004

Hendler I, Blackwell SC, Bujold E, et al: Suboptimal second-trimester ultrasonographic visualization of the fetal heart in obese women. Should we repeat the examination? J Ultrasound Med 24:1205, 2005

Hibbard JU, Gilbert S, Landon MB, et al: Trial of labor or repeat cesarean delivery in women with morbid obesity and previous cesarean delivery. Obstet Gynecol 108(1):125, 2006

Holt VL, Cushing-Haugen KL, Daling J: Body weight and risk of oral contraceptive failure. Obstet Gynecol 99:820, 2002

Hood DD, Dewan DM: Anesthetic and obstetric outcome in morbidly obese parturients. Anesthesiology 79:1210, 1993

Hossain P, Kawar B, El Nahas M: Obesity and diabetes in the developing world—a growing challenge. N Engl J Med 356(9):973, 2007

Houston MC, Raynor BD: Postoperative morbidity in the morbidly obese parturient woman: Supraumbilical and low transverse abdominal approaches. Am J Obstet Gynecol 182(5):1033, 2000

Huang DY, Usher RH, Kramer MS, et al: Determinants of unexplained antepartum fetal deaths. Obstet Gynecol 95:215, 2000

Institute of Medicine: Nutrition During Pregnancy. Washington, DC, National Academy Press, 1990

Institute of Medicine: The development of DRIs 1994–2004: lessons learned and new challenges. Workshop summary. November 30, 2007

Institute of Medicine: Weight gain during pregnancy: reexamining the guidelines. National Academy of Sciences. 28 May 2009

Isaacs JD, Magann EF, Martin RW, et al: Obstetric challenges of massive obesity complicating pregnancy. J Perinatol 14:10, 1994

Jensen DM, Damm P, Sorensen B et al: Pregnancy outcome and prepregnancy body mass index in 2459 glucose-tolerant Danish women. Am J Obstet Gynecol 189:239, 2003

Kabiru W, Raynor BD: Obstetric outcomes associated with increase in BMI category during pregnancy. Am J Obstet Gynecol 191:928, 2004

Kahn R, Buse J, Ferrannini E, et al: The metabolic syndrome: Time for a critical appraisal. Diabetes Care 28(9):2289, 2005

Kaneshiro B, Edelman A, Carlson N, et al: The relationship between body mass index and unintended pregnancy: Results from the 2002 National Survey of Family Growth. Contraception 77(4):234, 2008

Kenchaiah S, Evans JC, Levy D, et al: Obesity and the risk of heart failure. N Engl J Med 347:305, 2002

Kini S, Herron DM, Yanagisawa RT: Bariatric surgery for morbid obesity—a cure for metabolic syndrome? Med Clin North Am 91(6):1255, 2007

Kinoshita T, Itoh M: Longitudinal variance of fat mass deposition during pregnancy evaluated by ultrasonography: The ratio of visceral fat to subcutaneous fat in the abdomen. Gynecol Obstet Invest 61:115, 2006

Kumari AS: Pregnancy outcome in women with morbid obesity. Int J Gynaecol Obstet 73:101, 2001

LaCoursiere Y, Varner M: The association between prepregnancy obesity and postpartum depression, supported by NIH grant R03-HD-048865. Abstract No. 92. Presented at the 29th Annual Meeting of the Society for Maternal-Fetal Medicine. 26-31 January 2009

Lashen H, Fear K, Sturdee DW: Obesity is associated with increased risk of first trimester and recurrent miscarriage: Matched case-control study. Hum Reprod 19:1644, 2004

Li R, Jewell S, Grummer-Strawn L: Maternal obesity and breast-feeding practices. Am J Clin Nutr 77:931, 2003

Lu GC, Rouse DJ, DuBard MA, et al: The effect of the increasing prevalence of maternal obesity on perinatal morbidity. Am J Obstet Gynecol 185:845, 2001

Lynch CM, Sexton DJ, Hession M, et al: Obesity and mode of delivery in primigravid and multigravid women. Am J Perinatol 25(3):163, 2008

Martin LF, Finigan KM, Nolan TE: Pregnancy after adjustable gastric banding. Obstet Gynecol 95:927, 2000

Mokdad AH, Ford ES, Bowman BA, et al: Prevalence of obesity, diabetes, and obesity-related health risk factors, 2001. JAMA 289:76, 2003

Moore KA, Ouyang DW, Whang EE: Maternal and fetal deaths after gastric bypass surgery for morbid obesity. N Engl J Med. 351:721, 2004

Must A, Spadano J, Coakley EH, et al: The disease burden associated with overweight and obesity. JAMA 282:1523, 1999

National Heart, Lung, and Blood Institute. Clinical Guidelines on the Identification, Evaluation and Treatment of Overweight and Obesity in Adults: The Evidence Report. Washington, DC: Government Printing Office, 1998

National Institutes of Health. Third Report of the National Cholesterol Education Program Expert Panel on detection, evaluation, and treatment of high blood cholesterol in adults (Adult Treatment Panel III), NIH Publication 01-3670. Bethesda, MD, National Institutes of Health, 2001

National Research Council and Institute of Medicine. Influence of Pregnancy Weight on Maternal and Child Health. Workshop Report. Committee on the Impact of Pregnancy Weight on Maternal and Child Health. Board on Children, Youth, and Families, Division of Behavioral and Social Sciences and Education and Food and Nutrition Board, Institute of Medicine. Washington, DC, The National Academies Press, 2007

National Task Force on the Prevention and Treatment of Obesity: Overweight, obesity, and health risk. Arch Intern Med 160:898, 2000

Neill AM, Nelson-Piercy C: Hazards of assisted conception in women with severe medical disease. Hum Fertil (Camb) 4:239, 2001

Ninomiya JK, L'Italien G, Criqui MH, et al: Association of the metabolic syndrome with history of myocardial infarction and stroke in the third national health and nutrition examination survey. Circulation 109:42, 2004

Nohr EA, Bech BH, Davies MJ, et al: Pregnancy obesity and fetal death: A study within the Danish National Birth Cohort. Obstet Gynecol 106:250, 2005

O'Brien TE, Ray JG, Chan WS: Maternal body mass index and the risk of preeclampsia: A systematic overview. Epidemiology 14:368, 2003

Ogden CL, Flegal KM, Carroll MD, et al: Prevalence and trends in overweight among US children and adolescents, 1999–2000. JAMA 288:1728, 2002

Oken E: Maternal weight and gestational weight gain as predictors of long-term off-spring growth and health. Presentation at the Workshop on the Impact of

Pregnancy Weight on Maternal and Child Health, May 30, Washington DC, 2006

Olson CM, Strawderman MS, Reed R: Efficacy of an intervention to prevent excessive gestational weight gain. Am J Obstet Gynecol 191:530, 2004

Peeters A, Barendregt JJ, Willekens F, et al: Obesity in adulthood and its consequences for life expectancy: A life-table analysis. Ann Intern Med 138:24, 2003

Pleis JR, Senson V, Schiller JS: Summary health statistics for US Adults: National Health Interview Survey, 2000. National Center for Health Statistics. Vital Health Stat 10, 2003

Polley BA, Wing RR, Sims CJ: Randomized controlled trial to prevent excessive weight gain in pregnant women. Int J Obesity 26:1494, 2002

Poobalan AS, Aucott LS, Gurung T, et al: Obesity as an independent risk factor for elective and emergency caesarean delivery in nulliparous women—systematic review and meta-analysis of cohort studies. Obes Rev 10:28, 2009

Public Health Service: Healthy People 2000: National Health Promotion and Disease Prevention Objectives. Washington, DC, U.S. Department of Health and Human Services, Public Health Service, DHHS Publication No. (PHS) 90-50212, 1990

Ramsay JE, Ferrell WR, Crawford L, et al: Maternal obesity is associated with dysregulation of metabolic, vascular, and inflammatory pathways. J Clin Endocrinol Metab 87:4231, 2002

Rasmussen SA, Chu SY, Kim SY, et al: Maternal obesity and risk of neural tube defects; a metaanalysis. Am J Obstet Gynecol 198(6):611, 2008

Rizzo T, Metzger BE, Burns WJ, et al: Correlations between antepartum maternal metabolism and intelligence of offspring. N Engl J Med 325:911, 1991

Robinson HE, O'Connell CM, Joseph KS, et al: Maternal outcomes in pregnancies complicated by obesity. Obstet Gynecol 106(6):1357, 2005

Rode L, Nilas L, Wøjdemann K, et al: Obesity-related complications in Danish single cephalic term pregnancies. Obstet Gynecol 105:537, 2005

Rooney BL, Schauberger CW: Excess pregnancy weight gain and long-term obesity: One decade later. Obstet Gynecol 100:245, 2002

Ruowei L, Jewell S, Grummer-Strawn L: Maternal obesity and breast-feeding practices. Am J Clin Nutr 77:931, 2003

Saber AA, Elgamal MH, McLeod MK: Bariatric surgery: The past, present, and future. Obes Surg 18(1):121, 2008

Schack-Nielsen L, Mortensen EL, Sorensen TIA: High maternal pregnancy weight gain is associated with an increased risk of obesity in childhood and adulthood independent of maternal BMI. Pediatric Res 58:1020, 2005

Sebire NJ, Jolly M, Harris JP, et al: Maternal obesity and pregnancy outcome: A study of 287,213 pregnancies in London. Int J Obes Relat Metab Disord 25:1175, 2001

Sewell MF, Huston-Presley L, Super DM, Catalano PM: Increased neonatal fat mass, not lean body mass, is associated with maternal obesity. Am J Obstet Gynecol 195:1100, 2006

Shaw GM, Todoroff K, Schaffer DM, et al: Maternal height and prepregnancy body mass index as risk factors for selected congenital anomalies. Paediatr Perinat Epidemiol 14:234, 2000

Shaw GM, Velie EM, Schaffer D: Risk of neural tube defect–affected pregnancies among obese women. JAMA 275:1093, 1996

Skull AJ, Slater GH, Duncombe JE, et al: Laparoscopic adjustable banding in pregnancy: Safety, patient tolerance and effect on obesity-related pregnancy outcomes. Obes Sur 14:230, 2004

Steinbrook R: Surgery for severe obesity. N Engl J Med 350:1075, 2004

Stephansson O, Dickman PW, Johansson A, et al: Maternal weight, pregnancy weight gain, and the risk of antepartum stillbirth. Am J Obstet Gynecol 184:463, 2001

Stothard KJ, Tennant PW, Bell R, et al: Maternal overweight and obesity and the risk of congenital anomalies: a systematic review and meta-analysis. JAMA 301:636, 2009

Thornburg L, Mulconry M, Grace M, et al: Nuchal translucency measurements in the obese gravida. Abstract No. 456. Presented at the 29th Annual Meeting of the Society for Maternal-Fetal Medicine. 26-31 January 2009

Wall PD, Deucy EE, Glantz JC, et al: Vertical skin incisions and wound complications in the obese parturient. Obstet Gynecol 102:952, 2003

Walsh C, Scaife C, Hopf H: Prevention and management of surgical site infection in morbidly obese women. Obstet Gynecol 113:411, 2009

Watkins ML, Rasmussen SA, Honein MA, et al: Maternal obesity and risk for birth defects. Pediatrics 111:1152, 2003

Wax JR, Wolff R, Cobean R, et al: Intussusception complicating pregnancy following laparoscopy Roux-en-Y gastric bypass. Obes Surg 17(7):977, 2007

Weiss JL, Malon FD, Emig D, et al: Obesity, obstetric complications and cesarean delivery rate—a population based screening study. FASTER Research Consortium. Am J Obstet Gynecol 190:1091, 2004

Whitaker RC: Predicting preschooler obesity at birth: The role of maternal obesity in early pregnancy. Pediatrics 114:e29, 2004

Wittgrove AC, Jester L, Wittgrove P, et al: Pregnancy following gastric bypass for morbid obesity. Obes Surg 8:461, 1998

Wolf M, Kettyle E, Sandler L, et al: Obesity and preeclampsia: The potential role of inflammation. Obstet Gynecol 98:757, 2001

Wolfe HM, Sokol RJ, Martier SM, et al: Maternal obesity: A potential source of error in sonographic prenatal diagnosis. Obstet Gynecol 76:339, 1990

Yanovski SZ: Pharmacotherapy for obesity—promise and uncertainty. N Engl J Med 353(20):2187, 2005

Zieman M, Guillebaud J, Weisberg E, et al: Contraceptive efficacy and cycle control with the Ortho Evra/Evra transdermal system: The analysis of pooled data. Fertil Steril 77:S13, 2002

CHAPTER 44

Cardiovascular Disease

According to the Centers for Disease Control and Prevention, heart disease is the leading cause of death in women who are 25 to 44 years old (Kung and colleagues, 2008). Cardiac disorders of varying severity complicate approximately 1 percent of pregnancies and contribute significantly to maternal morbidity and mortality rates. For example, Chang and co-workers (2003) reported that cardiomyopathy alone was responsible for 8 percent of 4200 pregnancy-related deaths in the United States from 1991 to 1999. From Brazil, Avila and associates (2003) reported the maternal mortality rate to be 2.7 percent in 1000 pregnancies complicated by heart disease. In addition to maternal mortality, cardiac disorders accounted for 7.6 percent of severe obstetrical morbidities diagnosed during hospitalization for delivery in the United States from 1991 to 2003 (Callaghan and associates, 2008).

PHYSIOLOGICAL CONSIDERATIONS IN PREGNANCY

The marked pregnancy-induced hemodynamic alterations can have a profound effect on underlying heart disease. These are further detailed in Chapter 5 (p. 118). The most important is that cardiac output is increased by as much as 50 percent during pregnancy. Capeless and Clapp (1989) have shown that almost half of this total increase takes place by 8 weeks, and it is maximized by midpregnancy. The early increase stems from augmented stroke volume that results from decreased vascular resistance. Later in pregnancy, resting pulse and stroke volume increase even more because of increased diastolic filling from pregnancy hypervolemia. These changes are even more profound in multifetal pregnancy (Kametas and colleagues, 2003).

An important study by Clark and colleagues (1989) contributed greatly to the understanding of cardiovascular physiology during pregnancy. Using right-sided heart catheterization, these investigators measured hemodynamic function in 10 healthy primigravid women. Pregnancy values were compared with those measured again at 12 weeks postpartum. As shown in Table 44-1, near term the cardiac output in the lateral recumbent position increased 43 percent because of increased pulse rate and augmented stroke volume as the result of ventricular dilatation. Systemic and pulmonary vascular resistance were concomitantly decreased. Importantly, there was no change in intrinsic left ventricular contractility. Despite these changes, normal left ventricular function is maintained during pregnancy—specifically, hyperdynamic function or a high cardiac-output state does not develop (see Fig. 5-10, p. 120).

Recent noninvasive studies have elucidated further the maternal adaptation to the "natural volume overload state." For example, possible controlling-gene expression/function of signaling molecules that mediate reversible eccentric hypertrophy have been described (Eghbali and co-workers, 2006). These may be

TABLE 44-1. Hemodynamic Changes in 10 Normal Pregnant Women at Term Compared with Their 12-Week Postpartum Values

Parameter	Change (Percent)
Cardiac output	+43
Heart rate	+17
Left ventricular stroke work index	+17
Vascular resistance	
Systemic	−21
Pulmonary	−34
Mean arterial pressure	+4
Colloid osmotic pressure	−14

Data from Clark and colleagues (1989).

activated by estrogens or other G-protein-coupled receptor agonists such as endothelin-1 or angiotensin II (see Chap. 5, p. 120).

Women with underlying cardiac disease may not accommodate these changes, and ventricular dysfunction leads to cardiogenic heart failure. A few women with severe cardiac dysfunction may experience evidence of heart failure before midpregnancy. In others, heart failure may develop after 28 weeks when pregnancy-induced hypervolemia and cardiac output reach their maximum. In most, however, heart failure develops peripartum when a number of common obstetrical conditions place undue burdens on cardiac function. In the 542 women with heart disease reported by Etheridge and Pepperell (1977), eight of 10 maternal deaths were during the puerperium.

DIAGNOSIS OF HEART DISEASE

The physiological adaptations of normal pregnancy can induce symptoms and alter clinical findings that may confound the diagnosis of heart disease. For example, in normal pregnancy, functional systolic heart murmurs are common; respiratory effort is accentuated and at times suggests dyspnea; edema in the lower extremities after midpregnancy is common; and fatigue and exercise intolerance develop in most women. Some systolic flow murmurs may be loud, and normal changes in the various heart sounds depicted in Figure 44-1 may suggest cardiac disease. Listed in Table 44-2 are a number of clinical findings that may suggest heart disease. Pregnant women who have none of these rarely have serious heart disease.

Diagnostic Studies

In most women, noninvasive cardiovascular studies such as electrocardiography, echocardiography, and chest radiography will provide data necessary for evaluation. In some situations, for example, suspected pulmonary embolism with biventricular dysfunction, CT angiography has become commonplace. Albumin or red cells tagged with technicium-99 are rarely needed during pregnancy to evaluate ventricular function. Even so, the estimated fetal radiation exposure for a 20-mCi dose is only about 200 mrad, well below the accepted level (see Chap. 41, p. 920). Regional coronary perfusion is measured with thallium-201 chloride with a typical fetal exposure of 300 to 1100 mrad that is inversely proportional to gestational age. If indicated, right-sided heart catheterization can be performed with limited fluoroscopy. On rare occasions, it may be necessary to perform left-sided heart catheterization. In women with clear indications, any minimal theoretical risk is outweighed by maternal benefits.

Electrocardiography

As the diaphragm is elevated in advancing pregnancy, there is an average 15-degree left-axis deviation in the electrocardiogram (ECG), and mild ST changes may be seen in the inferior leads. Atrial and ventricular premature contractions are relatively frequent (Carruth and colleagues, 1981). Pregnancy does not alter voltage findings.

Chest Radiography

Anteroposterior and lateral chest radiographs are useful, and when a lead apron shield is used, fetal radiation exposure is minimal (see Chap. 41, p. 918). Gross cardiomegaly can usually be excluded, but slight heart enlargement cannot be detected accurately because the heart silhouette normally is larger in pregnancy.

Echocardiography

The widespread use of echocardiography has allowed accurate diagnosis of most heart diseases during pregnancy. It allows noninvasive evaluation of structural and functional cardiac factors. Some normal pregnancy-induced changes include slightly but significantly increased tricuspid regurgitation, left atrial end-diastolic dimension, and left ventricular mass. Normal morphological and functional echocardiographic parameters associated with pregnancy have been provided by Yuan and associates (2006).

Clinical Classification of Heart Disease

There is no clinically applicable test for accurately measuring functional cardiac capacity. The clinical classification of the New York Heart Association (NYHA) was first published in 1928, and it was revised for the eighth time in 1979. This classification is based on past and present disability and is uninfluenced by physical signs.

- **Class I.** *Uncompromised—no limitation of physical activity:* These women do not have symptoms of cardiac insufficiency or experience anginal pain.
- **Class II.** *Slight limitation of physical activity:* These women are comfortable at rest, but if ordinary physical activity is undertaken, discomfort in the form of excessive fatigue, palpitation, dyspnea, or anginal pain results.
- **Class III.** *Marked limitation of physical activity:* These women are comfortable at rest, but less than ordinary activity causes excessive fatigue, palpitation, dyspnea, or anginal pain.
- **Class IV.** *Severely compromised—inability to perform any physical activity without discomfort:* Symptoms of cardiac insufficiency or angina may develop even at rest. If any physical activity is undertaken, discomfort is increased.

Siu and associates (2001) expanded the NYHA classification and developed a scoring system for predicting cardiac

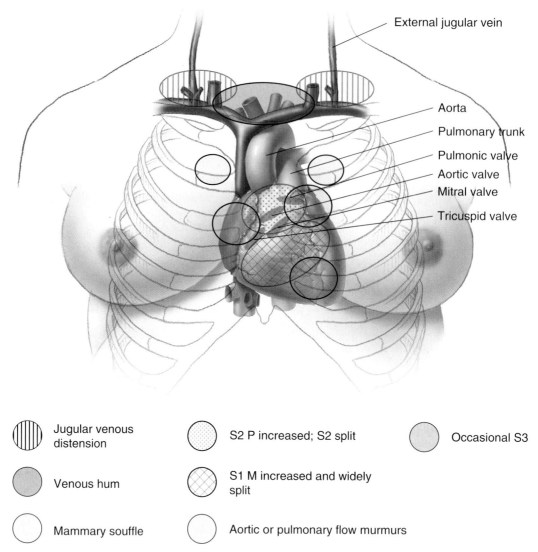

	Jugular venous distension		S2 P increased; S2 split		Occasional S3
	Venous hum		S1 M increased and widely split		
	Mammary souffle		Aortic or pulmonary flow murmurs		

FIGURE 44-1 Normal cardiac examination findings in the pregnant woman. S_1 = first sound, M_1 = mitral first sound, S_2 = second sound, P_2 = pulmonary second sound. (From Gei and Hankins, 2001; Hytten and Chamberlain, 1991.)

TABLE 44-2. Clinical Indicators of Heart Disease During Pregnancy

Symptoms
Progressive dyspnea or orthopnea
Nocturnal cough
Hemoptysis
Syncope
Chest pain

Clinical Findings
Cyanosis
Clubbing of fingers
Persistent neck vein distension
Systolic murmur grade 3/6 or greater
Diastolic murmur
Cardiomegaly
Persistent arrhythmia
Persistent split second sound
Criteria for pulmonary hypertension

complications during pregnancy. The system is based on their prospective analysis of 562 consecutive pregnant women with heart disease during 617 pregnancies in 13 Canadian teaching hospitals. Predictors of cardiac complications included the following:

- Prior heart failure, transient ischemic attack, arrhythmia, or stroke.
- Baseline NYHA class III or IV or cyanosis.
- Left-sided obstruction defined as mitral valve area less than 2 cm^2, aortic valve area less than 1.5 cm^2, or peak left ventricular outflow tract gradient above 30 mm Hg by echocardiography.
- Ejection fraction less than 40 percent.

The risk of pulmonary edema, sustained arrhythmia, stroke, cardiac arrest, or cardiac death was substantively increased with one of these factors and even more so with two or more factors.

At lease two studies have been done using these risk criteria. Khairy and colleagues (2006) reviewed 90 pregnancies in

TABLE 44-3. Approximated Risks for Cardiac Complications During 1712 Pregnancies in Women with Preexisting Heart Disease

Type of Cardiac Lesion	No.	Complication No. (%)			
		Heart Failure	Arrhythmia	Thrombosis	Death
Congenital	804	52 (6.5)	26 (3.2)	2 (0.3)	11 (1.4)
Acquired	820	116 (14)	35 (4.3)	18 (2.2)	11 (1.3)
Arrhythmia	88	2 (23)	22 (25)	0	0

Data from Avila (2003), Ford (2008), Madazli (2009), Siu (2001), Stangl (2008), and all their co-workers.

53 women with congenital heart disease at Brigham and Women's Hospital. There were no maternal deaths, and heart failure and symptomatic arrhythmias occurred in 16.7 and 2.8 percent of the women, respectively. Similar to the Canadian study cited above, the most important predictors of complications were prior congestive heart failure, depressed ejection fraction, and smoking. In a German study, Stangl and co-workers (2008) also used the predefined risk predictors and found them to be accurate in assessing outcomes in most of the 93 pregnancies in women with congenital or acquired heart disease.

Preconceptional Counseling

Women with severe heart disease will benefit immensely from counseling before deciding to become pregnant (see Chap. 7, p. 177). Maternal mortality rates generally vary directly with functional classification, however, this relationship may change as pregnancy progresses. In the Canadian study cited earlier, Siu and colleagues (2001) observed significant worsening of NYHA class in 26 of 579 pregnancies—4.4 percent—in which the baseline class was I or II. Their experiences, however, as well as those of McFaul and co-workers (1988), were that there were no maternal deaths in 1041 women with class I or II disease.

In some women, life-threatening cardiac abnormalities can be reversed by corrective surgery, and subsequent pregnancy is less dangerous. In other cases, such as women with mechanical valves taking warfarin, fetal considerations predominate. Shown in Table 44-3 are cardiac complications during pregnancy compiled from five recent reports. In most of these, about 15 percent of all pregnant women with heart disease suffered one or more of these complications.

Congenital Heart Disease in Offspring

Many congenital heart lesions appear to be inherited as polygenic characteristics (see Chap. 12, p. 281). Thus, some women with congenital lesions give birth to similarly affected infants, the risk of which varies widely as shown in Table 44-4.

GENERAL MANAGEMENT

In most instances, management involves a team approach with an obstetrician, cardiologist, anesthesiologist, and other specialists as needed. Cardiovascular changes likely to be poorly tolerated by an individual woman are identified, and a plan is formulated to minimize these. Four changes that affect management are emphasized by the American College of Obstetricians and Gynecologists (1992):

- The 50-percent increase in blood volume and cardiac output by the early third trimester
- Further fluctuations in volume and cardiac output in the peripartum period

TABLE 44-4. Congenital Heart Disease Risks in the Fetus with Affected Family Members

Maternal Heart Disease	Congenital Heart Disease in Fetus (Percent)		
Cardiac Lesion	Previous Sibling Affected	Father Affected	Mother Affected
Marfan syndrome	NS	50	50
Aortic stenosis	2	3	15–18
Pulmonary stenosis	2	2	6–7
Ventricular septal defect	3	2	10–16
Atrial septal defect	2.5	1.5	5–11
Patent ductus arteriosus	3	2.5	4
Coarctation of the aorta	NS	NS	14
Fallot tetralogy	2.5	1.5	2–3

NS = not stated.
From Lupton and colleagues (2002), with permission.

- A decline in systemic vascular resistance, reaching a nadir in the second trimester, and then rising to 20 percent below normal by late pregnancy
- Hypercoagulability, which is of special importance in women requiring anticoagulation before pregnancy with coumarin derivatives.

Within this framework, both prognosis and management are influenced by the nature and severity of the specific lesion in addition to the functional classification.

Management of NYHA Class I and II Disease

With rare exceptions, women in NYHA class I and most in class II proceed through pregnancy without morbidity. Special attention should be directed toward both prevention and early recognition of heart failure. As reviewed by Jessup and Brozena (2003), the onset of congestive heart failure is generally gradual. The first warning sign is likely to be persistent basilar rales, frequently accompanied by a nocturnal cough. A sudden diminution in ability to carry out usual duties, increasing dyspnea on exertion, or attacks of smothering with cough are symptoms of serious heart failure. Clinical findings may include hemoptysis, progressive edema, and tachycardia.

Infection with sepsis syndrome is an important factor in precipitating cardiac failure. Moreover, bacterial endocarditis is a deadly complication of valvular heart disease. Each woman should receive instructions to avoid contact with persons who have respiratory infections, including the common cold, and to report at once any evidence for infection. Pneumococcal and influenza vaccines are recommended.

Cigarette smoking is prohibited, both because of its cardiac effects and its propensity to cause upper respiratory infections. Illicit drug use may be particularly harmful, an example being the cardiovascular effects of cocaine or amphetamines. In addition, intravenous drug use increases the risk of infective endocarditis.

Labor and Delivery

In general, vaginal delivery is preferred unless there are obstetrical indications for cesarean delivery. Induction is generally safe (Oron and colleagues, 2004). In some women, *pulmonary artery catheterization* may be indicated for hemodynamic monitoring (see Chap 42, p. 928). In our experience, however, invasive monitoring is rarely indicated.

During labor, the mother with significant heart disease should be kept in a semirecumbent position with lateral tilt. Vital signs are taken frequently between contractions. Increases in pulse rate much above 100 bpm or respiratory rate above 24 per minute, particularly when associated with dyspnea, may suggest impending ventricular failure. If there is any evidence of cardiac decompensation, intensive medical management must be instituted immediately. It is essential to remember that delivery itself does not necessarily improve the maternal condition. Moreover, emergency operative delivery may be particularly hazardous. Clearly, both maternal and fetal status must be considered in the decision to hasten delivery under these circumstances.

Analgesia and Anesthesia. Relief from pain and apprehension is important. Although intravenous analgesics provide satisfactory pain relief for some women, continuous epidural analgesia is recommended in most cases. The major problem with conduction analgesia is maternal hypotension (see Chap. 19, p. 455). This is especially dangerous in women with intracardiac shunts in whom flow may be reversed. Blood passes from right to left within the heart or aorta and thereby bypasses the lungs. Hypotension can also be life-threatening with pulmonary hypertension or aortic stenosis because ventricular output is dependent on adequate preload. In women with these conditions, narcotic conduction analgesia or general anesthesia may be preferable.

For vaginal delivery in women with only mild cardiovascular compromise, epidural analgesia given with intravenous sedation often suffices. This has been shown to minimize intrapartum cardiac output fluctuations and allows forceps or vacuum-assisted delivery. Subarachnoid blockade is not generally recommended in women with significant heart disease. For cesarean delivery, epidural analgesia is preferred by most clinicians with caveats for its use with pulmonary hypertension (see p. 971). Finally, general endotracheal anesthesia with thiopental, succinylcholine, nitrous oxide, and at least 30-percent oxygen has also proved satisfactory (see Chap. 19, p. 459).

Intrapartum Heart Failure. Cardiovascular decompensation during labor may manifest as pulmonary edema with hypoxia or as hypotension, or both. The proper therapeutic approach depends on the specific hemodynamic status and the underlying cardiac lesion. For example, decompensated mitral stenosis with pulmonary edema due to fluid overload is often best approached with aggressive diuresis. If precipitated by tachycardia, heart rate control with β-blocking agents is preferred. Conversely, the same treatment in a woman suffering decompensation and hypotension due to aortic stenosis could prove fatal. Unless the underlying pathophysiology is understood and the cause of the decompensation clear, empirical therapy may be hazardous.

Puerperium

Women who have shown little or no evidence of cardiac distress during pregnancy, labor, or delivery may still decompensate postpartum. Therefore, it is important that meticulous care be continued into the puerperium (Keizer and colleagues, 2006; Zeeman, 2006). Postpartum hemorrhage, anemia, infection, and thromboembolism are much more serious complications in those with heart disease. Indeed, these factors often act in concert to precipitate postpartum heart failure (Cunningham and associates, 1986). In many of these—for example, sepsis and severe preeclampsia—pulmonary edema is caused by or worsened by permeability edema resulting from endothelial activation and capillary-alveolar leakage (see Chap. 42, p. 929).

Sterilization and Contraception

If tubal sterilization is to be performed after vaginal delivery, it is best to delay the procedure until the mother has become

TABLE 44-5. Outcomes Reported Since 1990 in Pregnancies Complicated by a Heart-Valve Replacement

Type of Valve	Total	Complications[a]	
		Maternal	**Perinatal**
Mechanical	499[b]	34 thromboses 17 emboli 14 hemorrhages 12 deaths	94 miscarriages/abortions 34 stillbirths
Porcine	265[c]	32 valve failure or deterioration	9 abortions 3 stillbirths

[a]Numbers estimated in some because definitions are not consistent.
[b]Data from Cotrufo (2002), Hanania (1994), Kawamata (2007), Nassar (2004), Sadler (2000), Sbarouni (1994), Suri (1999), and their many colleagues.
[c]Data from Hanania (1994), Lee (1994), Sadler (2000), Sbarouni (1994), and all their colleagues.

hemodynamically near normal, and when she is afebrile, not anemic, and ambulates normally. Other women are given detailed contraceptive advice. Special considerations for contraception in women with various cardiac disorders are discussed in some of the following sections and throughout Chapter 32.

Management of Class III and IV Disease

These severe cases are uncommon today. In the Canadian study by Siu and associates (2001), only 3 percent of approximately 600 pregnancies were complicated by NYHA class III heart disease, and no women had class IV when first seen. An important question in these women is whether pregnancy should be undertaken. If women make that choice, they must understand the risks and cooperate fully with planned care. If feasible, women with some types of severe cardiac disease should consider pregnancy interruption. If the pregnancy is continued, prolonged hospitalization or bed rest is often necessary.

Epidural analgesia for labor and delivery is usually recommended. Vaginal delivery is preferred in most cases, and labor induction can usually be done safely (Oron and associates, 2004). Cesarean delivery is usually limited to obstetrical indications, and considerations are given for the specific cardiac lesion, overall maternal condition, and availability of experienced anesthesia personnel and general support facilities. These women often tolerate major surgical procedures poorly and are best delivered in a unit facile with management of complicated cardiac disease.

SURGICALLY CORRECTED HEART DISEASE

Most clinically significant lesions are repaired during childhood. Examples of defects not diagnosed until adulthood include atrial septal defects, pulmonic stenosis, bicuspid aortic valve, and aortic coarctation (Brickner and colleagues, 2000). In some cases, the defect is mild and surgery is not required. In others, a significant structural anomaly is amenable to surgical correction. With successful repair, many women attempt preg-

nancy. In some instances, surgical corrections have been performed during pregnancy.

Valve Replacement before Pregnancy

A number of reproductive-aged women have had a prosthesis implanted to replace a severely damaged mitral or aortic valve. Reports of subsequent pregnancy outcomes are now numerous, and indeed, successful pregnancies have followed prosthetic replacement of even three heart valves (Nagorney and Field, 1981).

Effects on Pregnancy

Pregnancy is undertaken only after serious consideration. Women with a *mechanical valve prosthesis* must be anticoagulated, and when not pregnant, warfarin is recommended. As shown in Table 44-5, a number of serious complications can develop, especially with mechanical valves. Thromboembolism involving the prosthesis and hemorrhage from anticoagulation are of extreme concern (Nassar and co-workers, 2004). There also may be deterioration in cardiac function. **Overall, the maternal mortality rate is 3 to 4 percent with mechanical valves, and fetal loss is common.**

Porcine tissue valves are much safer during pregnancy, primarily because anticoagulation is not required as thrombosis is rare (see Table 44-5). To the contrary, valvular dysfunction, deterioration, or failure are common, and develop in 5 to 25 percent of pregnancies. Another drawback is that bioprostheses are not as durable as mechanical ones, and valve replacement averages every 10 to 15 years. Although some reports suggest that pregnancy may accelerate structural deterioration of bioprosthetic valves, this could simply reflect normal deterioration (Elkayam and Bitar, 2005).

Management

The critical issue for women with mechanical prosthetic valves is anticoagulation, and there is a suggestion that heparin may be less effective than warfarin in preventing thromboembolic events.

Warfarin. Although most effective to prevent mechanical valve thrombosis, warfarin is teratogenic and can cause miscarriage,

SECTION 8

TABLE 44-6. American College of Chest Physicians Guidelines for Anticoagulation of Pregnant Women with Mechanical Prosthetic Valves

For pregnant women with mechanical heart valves, any one of the following anticoagulant regimens is recommended:

- Adjusted-dose *LMWH* twice daily throughout pregnancy. The doses should be adjusted to achieve the manufacturer's peak anti-Xa level 4 hours after subcutaneous injection.
- Adjusted-dose *UFH* administered every 12 hours throughout pregnancy. The doses should be adjusted to keep the midinterval aPTT at least twice control or attain an anti-Xa heparin level of 0.35 to 0.70 U/mL.
- LMWH or UFH as above until 13 weeks' gestation with warfarin substitution until close to delivery when LMWH or UFH is resumed.

In women judged to be at very high risk of thromboembolism and in whom concerns exist about the efficacy and safety of LMWH or UFH as dosed above—some examples include older-generation prosthesis in the mitral position or history of thromboembolism. Warfarin is suggested throughout pregnancy with replacement by UFH or LMWH (as above) close to delivery. In addition, low-dose aspirin—75 to 100 mg daily—should be orally administered.

aPTT = activated partial thromboplastin time; LMWH = low-molecular-weight heparin; UFH = unfractionated heparin.
Adapted from Bates and colleagues (2008).

stillbirths, and fetal malformation (see Chap. 14, p. 325). For example, Cotrufo and colleagues (2002) described 71 pregnancies in women given warfarin for a mechanical valve prosthesis throughout pregnancy. Although there were no serious maternal complications, the rates of miscarriage were 32 percent; stillbirth, 7 percent; and embryopathy, 6 percent. The risk was highest when the mean daily dose of warfarin exceeded 5 mg. From their review, Chan and co-workers (2000) concluded that the best maternal outcomes were achieved with warfarin anticoagulation with the tradeoff of a 6.4-percent embryopathy rate. And although heparin substituted before 12 weeks eliminated embryopathy, thromboembolic complications increased significantly.

Low-Dose Heparin. Prophylaxis using low-dose unfractionated heparin is definitely inadequate. Iturbe-Alessio and colleagues (1986) reported that three of 35 women on such therapy suffered massive thrombosis of a mitral prosthesis—two of these died. Similarly, Chan and co-workers (2000) found that two of five women treated solely with low-dose heparin during pregnancy died.

Anticoagulation with Heparin. Full anticoagulation with either unfractionated heparin (UFH) or one of the low-molecular-weight heparins (LMWH) is also problematic because of reports of valvular thrombosis in patients. This has been especially problematic with LMWH given to pregnant women, who were apparently adequately anticoagulated (Leyh and colleagues, 2002, 2003; Rowan and associates, 2001). Following such reports and a warning issued by Aventis Pharmaceuticals, the American College of Obstetricians and Gynecologists (2002) advised against use of low-molecular-weight heparins during pregnancy for those with prosthetic valves. On the other hand, the American College of Chest Physicians has recommended use of any of several regimens that include adjusted-dose UFH or LMWH heparin given throughout pregnancy as subsequently discussed.

Recommendations for Anticoagulation. A number of different treatment options—none of which are completely ideal—have been proposed and are principally based on consensus opinion. For this reason, they differ and allow more than one scheme. For example, and as shown in Table 44-6, the most recent guidelines of the American College of Chest Physicians for the management of pregnant women with mechanical prosthetic valves offer several different treatment options.

Similar to one of the American College of Chest Physicians recommendations, Reimold and Rutherford (2003) suggest unfractionated heparin from 6 to 12 weeks, and again after 36 weeks. Throughout the rest of pregnancy, they recommend warfarin therapy to achieve a target international normalized ratio (INR) of 2.0 to 3.0. The European Society of Cardiology favors warfarin anticoagulation until 36 weeks, at which time heparin is given until delivery (Butchart and associates, 2005).

Heparin is discontinued just before delivery. If delivery supervenes while the anticoagulant is still effective, and extensive bleeding is encountered, then *protamine sulfate* is given intravenously. Anticoagulant therapy with warfarin or heparin may be restarted 6 hours following vaginal delivery, usually with no problems. Following cesarean delivery, full anticoagulation is withheld, but the duration is not exactly known. It is our practice to wait at least 24 hours—and preferably 48 hours—following a major surgical procedure. Clark and colleagues (2000) reviewed the use of warfarin derivatives and concluded they are safe for breast-feeding women because of minimal transfer to milk.

Contraception

Because of their possible thrombogenic action, estrogen-progestin oral contraceptives are relatively contraindicated in women with prosthetic valves (see Chap. 32, p. 680). These women are generally fully anticoagulated, and thus any increased risk is speculative. Sterilization should be considered because of the serious pregnancy risks faced by women with significant heart disease.

Valve Replacement During Pregnancy

Although usually postponed until after delivery, valve replacement during pregnancy may be lifesaving. A number of reviews all confirm that surgery on the heart or great vessels is associated with major maternal and fetal morbidity and mortality. For example, Sutton and associates (2005) found that maternal mortality rates with cardiopulmonary bypass are between 1.5 and 5 percent. Although these are similar to rates for nonpregnant women, the fetal mortality rate approaches 20 percent. In a study from Brazil, Arnoni and associates (2003) described 58 such women in whom the maternal mortality rate was 8 percent. Almost 20 percent of the fetuses died as a direct result of the surgery. To minimize these bad outcomes, Chandrasekhar and co-workers (2009) recommend that surgery is done electively when possible, pump flow rate is maintained >2.5 L/min/m^2, normothermic perfusion pressure is >70 mm Hg, pulsatile flow is used, and hematocrit is >28 percent.

Mitral Valvotomy During Pregnancy

Tight mitral stenosis that requires intervention during pregnancy was previously treated by closed mitral valvotomy (Pavankumar and associates, 1988). In the past two decades, however, percutaneous transcatheter balloon dilatation of the mitral valve has largely replaced surgical valvotomy during pregnancy (Fawzy, 2007). To compare these two, de Souza and colleagues (2001a) studied 24 consecutive pregnant women who underwent open mitral commissurotomy between 1985 and 1990 and compared them with 21 women who underwent percutaneous valvuloplasty between 1990 and 1995. The balloon procedure was more than 90-percent successful, and functional outcomes in the two groups were similar. There was one maternal death in the open-repair group. Importantly, perinatal mortality rate was sixfold higher in the open repair group—33 versus 5 percent.

More recently, Rahimtoola (2006) summarized outcomes of 36 women—25 of whom were NYHA class III or IV—who underwent balloon commissurotomy at an average gestational age of 26 weeks. The procedure was successful in 35. Left atrial and pulmonary artery pressures were reduced and associated with an increased mitral valve area from 0.74 to 1.59 cm^2. Esteves and associates (2006) described similarly good outcomes in 71 pregnant women with tight mitral stenosis and heart failure who underwent percutaneous valvuloplasty. At delivery, 98 percent were in either NYHA Class I or II. At a mean of 44 months, their total event-free maternal survival rate was 54 percent. One woman died from transfusion-acquired hepatitis, and eight required another surgical intervention. The 66 infants who were delivered at term all had normal growth and development.

Pregnancy after Heart Transplantation

The first successful pregnancy in a heart transplant recipient was reported more than 20 years ago by Löwenstein and associates (1988). Since that time, more than 50 pregnancies in heart-transplant recipients have been described. Key (1989) and Kim (1996) and their colleagues provided detailed data to show that the transplanted heart responds normally to pregnancy-induced

changes. Despite this, complications are common during pregnancy (Dashe and associates, 1998). Armenti and associates (2002) from the National Transplantation Pregnancy Registry and Miniero and colleagues (2004) described outcomes of 53 pregnancies in 37 heart recipients. Almost half developed hypertension, and 22 percent suffered at least one rejection episode during pregnancy. They were delivered—usually by cesarean—at a mean of 37 to 38 weeks, and three fourths of infants were liveborn. At follow-up, at least five women had died more than 2 years postpartum. A scholarly review of pregnancy in solid-organ transplant recipients is provided by McKay and Josephson (2006). Ethical considerations of counseling and caring for such women regarding pregnancy were summarized by Ross (2006).

VALVULAR HEART DISEASE

Rheumatic fever is uncommon in the United States because of less crowded living conditions, availability of penicillin, and evolution of nonrheumatogenic streptococcal strains. Still, it remains the chief cause of serious mitral valvular disease (O'Shea and Braunwald, 2008).

Mitral Stenosis

Rheumatic endocarditis causes three fourths of mitral stenosis cases. The normal mitral valve surface area is 4.0 cm^2. When stenosis narrows this to less than 2.5 cm^2, symptoms usually develop (Desai and colleagues, 2000). The contracted valve impedes blood flow from the left atrium to the ventricle. The most prominent complaint is dyspnea due to pulmonary venous hypertension and edema. Fatigue, palpitations, cough, and hemoptysis are also common.

With tight stenosis, the left atrium is dilated, left atrial pressure is chronically elevated, and significant passive pulmonary hypertension can develop (Table 44-7). The increased preload of normal pregnancy, as well as other factors that increase cardiac output, may cause ventricular failure with pulmonary edema in these women who have a relatively fixed cardiac output. Indeed, a fourth of women with mitral stenosis have cardiac failure for the first time during pregnancy (Caulin-Glaser and Setaro, 1999). Because the murmur may not be heard in some women, this clinical picture may be confused with idiopathic peripartum cardiomyopathy (Cunningham and colleagues, 1986).

With significant stenosis, tachycardia shortens ventricular diastolic filling time and increases the mitral gradient. This increase raises left atrial and pulmonary venous and capillary pressures and may result in pulmonary edema. Thus, sinus tachycardia is often treated prophylactically with β-blocking agents. Atrial tachyarrhythmias, including fibrillation, are common in mitral stenosis and are treated aggressively. Atrial fibrillation also predisposes to mural thrombus formation and cerebrovascular embolization that can cause stroke (see Chap. 55, p. 1168). Hameed and associates (2005) described three pregnant women with tight mitral stenosis—valve area of 0.9 cm^2—who each developed an atrial thrombus despite a sinus rhythm. One suffered an embolic stroke, and another had pulmonary edema and maternal hypoxemia that caused fetal encephalopathy.

TABLE 44-7. Major Cardiac Valve Disorders

Type	Cause	Pathophysiology	Pregnancy
Mitral stenosis	Rheumatic valvulitis	LA dilation and passive pulmonary hypertension Atrial fibrillation	Heart failure from fluid overload, tachycardia
Mitral insufficiency	Rheumatic valvulitis Mitral-valve prolapse LV dilatation	LV dilatation and eccentric hypertrophy	Ventricular function improves with afterload decrease
Aortic stenosis	Congenital Bicuspid valve	LV concentric hypertrophy, decreased cardiac output	Moderate stenosis tolerated; severe is life-threatening with decreased preload, e.g., obstetrical hemorrhage or regional analgesia
Aortic insufficiency	Rheumatic valvulitis Connective-tissue disease Congenital	LV hypertrophy and dilatation	Ventricular function improves with afterload decrease
Pulmonary stenosis	Congenital Rheumatic valvulitis	Severe stenosis associated with RA and RV enlargement	Mild stenosis usually well tolerated; severe stenosis associated with right heart failure and atrial arrhythmias

LA = left atrium, LV = left ventricle, RA = right atrium, RV = right ventricle.

Pregnancy Outcomes

In general, complications are directly associated with the degree of valvular stenosis. Recall that investigators from the large Canadian study found that women with a mitral-valve area $<2 \text{ cm}^2$ were at greatest risk for complications. In another study from the University of Southern California Medical Center between 1979 and 1998, Hameed and associates (2001) cared for 46 pregnant women with mitral stenosis. Complications included heart failure in 43 percent and arrhythmias in 20 percent. Fetal-growth restriction was more common in those women with a mitral valve area less than 1.0 cm^2.

The maternal prognosis is also related to functional capacity. Among 486 pregnancies complicated by rheumatic heart disease—predominantly mitral stenosis—Sawhney and associates (2003) reported that eight of 10 maternal deaths were in women in NYHA classes III or IV.

Management

Limited physical activity is generally recommended. If symptoms of pulmonary congestion develop, activity is further reduced, dietary sodium is restricted, and diuretic therapy is started (Siva and Shah, 2005). A β-blocker drug is usually given to blunt the cardiac response to activity and anxiety (Al Kasab and associates, 1990). If new-onset atrial fibrillation develops, intravenous verapamil, 5 to 10 mg, is given, or electrocardioversion is performed. For chronic fibrillation, digoxin, a β-blocker, or a calcium-channel blocker is given to slow ventricular

response. Therapeutic anticoagulation with heparin is indicated with persistent fibrillation. Hameed and co-workers (2005) recommend heparinization with severe stenosis even if there is a sinus rhythm.

Labor and delivery are particularly stressful for women with symptomatic mitral stenosis. Pain, exertion, and anxiety cause tachycardia, with possible rate-related heart failure. Epidural analgesia for labor is ideal, but with strict attention to avoid fluid overload. Abrupt increases in preload may increase pulmonary capillary wedge pressure and cause pulmonary edema. The cardiovascular effects of labor in women with mitral stenosis are shown in Figure 44-2. Wedge pressures increase even more immediately postpartum. Clark and colleagues (1985) hypothesize that this is likely due to loss of the low-resistance placental circulation along with the venous "autotransfusion" from the lower extremities, pelvis, and the now-empty uterus.

Most consider vaginal delivery to be preferable in women with mitral stenosis. Elective induction is reasonable so that labor and delivery are attended by a scheduled, experienced team. With severe stenosis and chronic heart failure, insertion of a pulmonary artery catheter may help guide management decisions. Consideration for endocarditis prophylaxis is discussed on page 974.

Mitral Insufficiency

When there is improper coaptation of mitral valve leaflets during systole, some degree of mitral regurgitation develops. This is

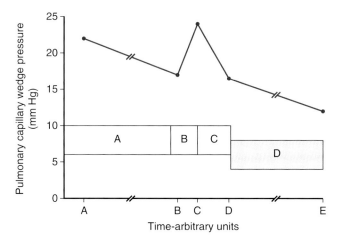

FIGURE 44-2 Mean pulmonary capillary wedge pressure measurements in eight women with mitral valve stenosis (*red graph line*). **A.** First-stage labor. **B.** Second-stage labor 15 to 30 minutes before delivery. **C.** Postpartum 5 to 15 minutes. **D.** Postpartum 4 to 6 hours. **E.** Postpartum 18 to 24 hours. Shaded yellow and blue boxes are mean (±1 SD) pressures in nonlaboring normal women at term. (Data from Clark and colleagues, 1985, 1989.)

eventually followed by left ventricular dilatation and eccentric hypertrophy (see Table 44-7). *Chronic mitral regurgitation* has a number of causes, including rheumatic fever, mitral valve prolapse, or left ventricular dilatation of any etiology—for example, dilated cardiomyopathy. Less common causes include a calcified mitral annulus, possibly some appetite suppressants, and in older women, ischemic heart disease. Mitral valve vegetations—*Libman-Sacks endocarditis*—are relatively common in women with antiphospholipid antibodies (Roldan and colleagues, 1996). These sometimes coexist with systemic lupus erythematosus (see Chap. 54, p. 1152). *Acute mitral insufficiency* is caused by rupture of a chorda tendineae, infarction of papillary muscle, or leaflet perforation from infective endocarditis.

In nonpregnant patients, symptoms from mitral valve incompetence are rare, and valve replacement is seldom indicated unless infective endocarditis develops. Likewise, mitral regurgitation is well tolerated during pregnancy, probably because decreased systemic vascular resistance results in less regurgitation. Heart failure only rarely develops during pregnancy, and occasionally tachyarrhythmias need to be treated. Intrapartum prophylaxis against bacterial endocarditis may be indicated (see p. 974).

Aortic Stenosis

This is a disease of aging, and in women younger than 30 years, it is most likely due to a congenital lesion. Aortic stenosis itself is less common since the decline in incidences of rheumatic diseases. In the United States, the most common lesion is a bicuspid valve (Friedman and co-workers, 2008). Stenosis reduces the normal 2- to 3-cm^2 aortic orifice and creates resistance to ejection. Reduction in the valve area to a fourth its normal size produces severe obstruction to flow and a progressive pressure overload on the left ventricle (Carabello, 2002). Concentric left ventricular hypertrophy follows, and if severe, end-diastolic pressures become elevated, ejection fraction declines, and cardiac output is reduced (see Table 44-7). Characteristic clinical manifestations develop late and include chest pain, syncope, heart failure, and sudden death from arrhythmias. Life expectancy averages only 5 years after exertional chest pain develops, and valve replacement is indicated for symptomatic patients.

Clinically significant aortic stenosis is uncommonly encountered during pregnancy. Although mild to moderate degrees of stenosis are well tolerated, severe disease is life threatening. The principal underlying hemodynamic problem is the fixed cardiac output associated with severe stenosis. During pregnancy, a number of factors commonly decrease preload further and thus aggravate the fixed cardiac output. These include regional analgesia, vena caval occlusion, and hemorrhage. Importantly, these also decrease cardiac, cerebral, and uterine perfusion. It follows that severe aortic stenosis may be extremely dangerous during pregnancy. From the large Canadian multicenter study by Siu and co-workers (2001) cited above, there were increased complications when aortic valve area was < 1.5 cm^2. And in the report described earlier by Hameed and associates (2001), the maternal mortality rate with aortic stenosis was 8 percent. Women with valve gradients exceeding 100 mm Hg appear to be at greatest risk.

Management

For the asymptomatic woman with aortic stenosis, no treatment except close observation is required. Management of the symptomatic woman includes strict limitation of activity and prompt treatment of infections. If symptoms persist despite bed rest, valve replacement or valvotomy using cardiopulmonary bypass must be considered. In general, balloon valvotomy for aortic valve disease is avoided because of serious complications, which exceed 10 percent. These include stroke, aortic rupture, aortic valve insufficiency, and death (Carabello and Crawford, 1997; Reich and co-workers, 2004). In rare cases, it may be preferable to perform valve replacement during pregnancy (Angel and colleagues, 1988; Lao and associates, 1993).

For women with critical aortic stenosis, intensive monitoring during labor is important. Pulmonary artery catheterization may be helpful because of the narrow margin separating fluid overload from hypovolemia. Women with aortic stenosis are dependent on adequate end-diastolic ventricular filling pressures to maintain cardiac output and systemic perfusion. Abrupt decreases in end-diastolic volume may result in hypotension, syncope, myocardial infarction, and sudden death. Thus, the key to management is the avoidance of decreased ventricular preload and the maintenance of cardiac output. During labor and delivery, such women should be managed on the "wet" side, maintaining a margin of safety in intravascular volume in anticipation of possible hemorrhage. In women with a competent mitral valve, pulmonary edema is rare, even with moderate volume overload.

During labor, narcotic epidural analgesia seems ideal, thus avoiding potentially hazardous hypotension, which may be encountered with standard conduction analgesia techniques. Easterling and colleagues (1988) studied the effects of epidural analgesia in five women with severe stenosis and demonstrated immediate and profound effects of decreased filling pressures. Camann and Thornhill (1999) and Xia and associates (2006) emphasize slow administration of dilute local anesthetics into the epidural space. Forceps or vacuum delivery are used for standard obstetrical indications in hemodynamically stable women. Tzemos and co-workers (2009) reported that late cardiac events that included pulmonary edema, arrhythmias, cardiac interventions, and death were identified within 1 year of delivery in 70 pregnancies.

Aortic Insufficiency

Aortic regurgitation is the diastolic flow of blood from the aorta into the left ventricle. Common causes of aortic valvular incompetence are rheumatic fever, connective-tissue abnormalities, and congenital lesions. With Marfan syndrome, the aortic root may dilate, resulting in regurgitation (see p. 976). Acute insufficiency may develop with bacterial endocarditis or aortic dissection. Aortic and mitral valve insufficiency have been linked to the appetite suppressants fenfluramine and dexfenfluramine and to ergot-derived dopamine agonists (Gardin, 2000; Khan, 1998; Schade, 2007; Zanettini, 2007, and all their associates). With chronic disease, left ventricular hypertrophy and dilatation develop (see Table 44-7). This is followed by slow-onset fatigue, dyspnea, and edema, although rapid deterioration usually follows.

Aortic insufficiency is generally well tolerated during pregnancy. Like mitral valve incompetence, diminished vascular resistance is thought to improve the lesion. If symptoms of heart failure develop, diuretics are given and bed rest is encouraged. Epidural analgesia is used for labor and delivery, and bacterial endocarditis prophylaxis may be required (see p. 974).

Pulmonic Stenosis

The pulmonary artery valve is affected by rheumatic fever far less often than the other valves. Instead, pulmonic stenosis is usually congenital and also may be associated with Fallot tetralogy or Noonan syndrome. The clinical diagnosis is typically identified by auscultating a systolic ejection murmur over the pulmonary area that is louder during inspiration.

Increased hemodynamic burdens of pregnancy can precipitate right-sided heart failure or atrial arrhythmias in women with severe stenosis (see Table 44-7). Siu and Colman (2001) recommend consideration for surgical correction before or during pregnancy if symptoms progress. Drenthen and co-workers (2006a) studied outcomes of 81 pregnancies in 51 Dutch women with pulmonary stenosis. Cardiac complications were infrequent. However, NYHA classification worsened in two women, and nine experienced palpitations or arrhythmias. No changes in pulmonary valvular function or other adverse cardiac events were reported. Noncardiac complications were increased—17 percent had preterm delivery; 15 percent, hypertension; and 3.7 percent, thromboembolism. Interestingly, two of the offspring were diagnosed with pulmonary stenosis, and another had complete transposition and anencephaly.

CONGENITAL HEART DISEASE

The incidence of congenital heart disease in the United States is approximately 8 per 1000 liveborn infants. About a third of these have critical disease that requires cardiac catheterization or surgery during the first year of life. Others require surgery in childhood, and it is currently estimated that there are nearly 1 million adults in this country with congenital heart disease (Bashore, 2007). With the decline in rheumatic heart disease, congenital lesions are now responsible for most heart disease during pregnancy (Iserin, 2001). Morbidity depends largely on the individual lesion. Khairy and colleagues (2006) reported 90 pregnancies complicated by maternal congenital heart disease. Almost 20 percent of mothers and 30 percent of neonates experienced complications. Ford and co-workers (2008) reported similar findings in 74 pregnancies in 69 women with a congenital heart lesion. Almost half suffered at least one adverse obstetrical event. Those with abnormal shunts had the most serious complications.

Septal Defects

Atrial Septal Defects

After bicuspid aortic valve, these are the most commonly encountered adult congenital cardiac lesions. Indeed, a fourth of all adults have a patent foremen ovale (Kizer and Devereux, 2005). Most are asymptomatic until the third or fourth decade. The secundum-type defect accounts for 70 percent, and associated mitral valve myxomatous abnormalities with prolapse are common. Most recommend repair if discovered in adulthood. Pregnancy is well tolerated unless pulmonary hypertension has developed, but this is rare because pulmonary artery pressures are usually low (Zuber and associates, 1999). If congestive heart failure or an arrhythmia develops, treatment is given. Bacterial endocarditis prophylaxis has been recommended in certain circumstances with unrepaired defects (see p. 974). Based on their review, Aliaga and associates (2003) concluded that the risk of endocarditis with an atrial septal defect is negligible.

The potential to shunt blood right to left makes possible a *paradoxical embolism*—entry of a venous thrombus through the septal defect and into the systemic circulation. This may result in an embolic stroke (see Chap. 55, p. 1169). Erkut and associates (2006) described a postpartum woman who developed an entrapped thrombus in a patent foramen ovale. In an asymptomatic woman, prophylaxis against thromboembolism is problematic, and recommendations for a septal defect alone are either observation or antiplatelet therapy (Kizer and Devereux, 2005). Compression stockings and prophylactic heparin in the pregnant woman with a septal defect in the presence of immobility or other risk factors for thromboembolism has been recommended (Head and Thorne, 2005).

Ventricular Septal Defects

These defects close spontaneously during childhood in 90 percent of cases. Most defects are paramembranous, and physiological derangements are related to the size of the defect. In general, if the defect is less than 1.25 cm^2, pulmonary hypertension and heart failure do not develop. When the effective size of the defect exceeds that of the aortic valve orifice, symptoms rapidly develop. For these reasons, most children undergo surgical repair before pulmonary hypertension develops. Adults with unrepaired large defects develop left ventricular failure and pulmonary hypertension, as well as a high incidence of bacterial endocarditis (Brickner and colleagues, 2000).

Pregnancy is well tolerated with small to moderate left-to-right shunts. When pulmonary arterial pressures reach systemic levels, however, there is reversal or bidirectional flow—*Eisenmenger syndrome* (see p. 970). When this develops, the maternal mortality rate is 30 to 50 percent. Thus, pregnancy is not generally advisable. Bacterial endocarditis is more common with unrepaired defects, and antimicrobial prophylaxis is often required (see p. 974). About 10 to 15 percent of offspring born to these women also have a ventricular septal defect (see Table 44-4).

Atrioventricular Septal Defect

These account for approximately 3 percent of all congenital cardiac malformations and are distinct from isolated atrial or ventricular septal defects. An atrioventricular (AV) septal defect is characterized by a common, ovoid-shaped AV junction. Although this defect is associated with aneuploidy, Eisenmenger syndrome, and other malformations, some of these women become pregnant. Compared with simple septal defects, complications are more frequent during pregnancy. Drenthen and associates (2005b) reviewed outcomes in 48 pregnancies of 29 such women. Complications included persistent deterioration of NYHA class in 23 percent, significant arrhythmias in 19 percent, and heart failure in 2 percent. Congenital heart disease was identified in 15 percent of the offspring.

Persistent Ductus Arteriosus

Physiological consequences of this lesion are related to its size, as is the case for other shunts. Most significant lesions are repaired in childhood, but for individuals who do not undergo repair, the mortality rate is high after the fifth decade (Brickner and colleagues, 2000). With an unrepaired persistent ductus, some women develop pulmonary hypertension, heart failure, or cyanosis if systemic blood pressure falls with reversal of blood flow from the pulmonary artery into the aorta. A sudden blood pressure decrease at delivery—such as with conduction analgesia or hemorrhage—may lead to fatal collapse. Therefore, hypotension should be avoided whenever possible and treated vigorously if it develops. Prophylaxis for bacterial endocarditis may be indicated at delivery for unrepaired defects (see p. 974). The incidence of inheritance is approximately 4 percent (see Table 44-4).

Cyanotic Heart Disease

When congenital heart lesions are associated with right-to-left shunting of blood past the pulmonary capillary bed, cyanosis develops. The classical and most commonly encountered lesion in pregnancy is the *Fallot tetralogy*. This is characterized by a large ventricular septal defect, pulmonary stenosis, right ventricular hypertrophy, and an overriding aorta that receives blood from both the right and left ventricles. The magnitude of the

shunt varies inversely with systemic vascular resistance. Hence, during pregnancy, when peripheral resistance decreases, the shunt increases and cyanosis worsens. Women who have undergone repair, and in whom cyanosis did not reappear, do well in pregnancy.

Some women with *Ebstein anomaly* of the tricuspid valve may reach reproductive age. Right ventricular failure from volume overload and appearance or worsening of cyanosis are common during pregnancy. In the absence of cyanosis, these women usually tolerate pregnancy well.

Effects on Pregnancy

Women with cyanotic heart disease generally do poorly during pregnancy. With uncorrected Fallot tetralogy, for example, maternal mortality rates approach 10 percent. Moreover, any disease complicated by severe maternal hypoxemia is likely to lead to miscarriage, preterm delivery, or fetal death. There is a relationship between chronic hypoxemia, polycythemia, and pregnancy outcome. When hypoxemia is intense enough to stimulate a rise in hematocrit above 65 percent, pregnancy wastage is virtually 100 percent.

Pregnancy after Surgical Repair

With satisfactory surgical correction before pregnancy, maternal and fetal outcomes are much improved. Gelson (2008) and Singh (1982) and their associates described 66 pregnancies in 43 women with surgically corrected tetralogy. Pregnancy was usually well tolerated in those with no major residual defects. Similarly, Meijer and co-workers (2005) reported generally good perinatal outcomes, however, six of 50 pregnancies were complicated by symptomatic right-sided heart failure or arrhythmias, or both. Two women with heart failure had severe pulmonary regurgitation. For those with a pulmonary valve replacement, Oosterhof and co-workers (2006) reported that pregnancy did not adversely affect graft function.

Pregnancy following surgical correction of *transposition of the great vessels* also has risks. Canobbio and colleagues (2006) and Drenthen and co-workers (2005a) described the outcomes of 119 pregnancies in 68 women—90 percent had a *Mustard procedure* and 10 percent a *Senning procedure*. A fourth had arrhythmias, and 12 percent developed heart failure—one of these subsequently required cardiac transplantation. One woman died suddenly a month after delivery, and another died 4 years later. A third of the newborns were delivered preterm, but no infant had heart disease.

Successful—although eventful—pregnancies in women with previously repaired *truncus arteriosus* and *double-outlet right ventricle* have been described by Hoendermis and colleagues (2008) and Drenthen and associates (2008), respectfully. Hoare and Radford (2001) described four pregnancies in three women who had previously undergone a *Fontan repair* for a congenital *single functional ventricle*. There were no maternal deaths, but complications were frequent. All were delivered preterm, two had supraventricular arrhythmias, and two developed ventricular failure. In a comprehensive review, Drenthen and co-workers (2006b) also found no reports of maternal mortality, but they described similarly high complication rates.

Labor and Delivery

Vaginal delivery is preferred. Pulmonary artery catheter monitoring has limitations because of the sometimes bizarre anatomical abnormalities. Care must be taken to avoid sudden hypotension. For labor pain, epidural opiates may suffice. There is controversy regarding epidural analgesia versus general anesthesia for cesarean delivery in these women (Camann and Thornhill, 1999).

Eisenmenger Syndrome

This is secondary pulmonary hypertension that develops from any cardiac lesion. The syndrome develops when pulmonary vascular resistance exceeds systemic resistance, with concomitant right-to-left shunting. The most common underlying defects are atrial or ventricular septal defects and persistent ductus arteriosus. Patients are asymptomatic for years, but eventually pulmonary hypertension becomes severe enough to cause right-to-left shunting. After it develops, survival is 20 to 30 years (Makaryus and associates, 2006).

The prognosis for pregnancy depends on the severity of pulmonary hypertension. In a review of 44 cases through 1978, Gleicher and associates (1979) reported maternal and perinatal mortality rates to approximate 50 percent. In a later review of 73 pregnancies, Weiss and co-workers (1998) cited a 36-percent maternal death rate. Only three of the 26 deaths were antepartum, and the remainder died intrapartum or within a month of delivery. Women with Eisenmenger syndrome tolerate hypotension poorly, and the cause of death usually is right ventricular failure with cardiogenic shock. Management is discussed subsequently.

PULMONARY HYPERTENSION

Normal resting mean pulmonary artery pressure is 12 to 16 mm Hg. In the study by Clark and colleagues (1989), pulmonary vascular resistance was approximately 80 dyne/sec/cm^{-5} in late pregnancy—a 34-percent decrease compared with the nonpregnant value of 120 dyne/sec/cm^{-5}. Pulmonary hypertension—*a hemodynamic observation and not a diagnosis*—is defined in nonpregnant individuals as a mean pulmonary pressure >25 mm Hg. Some causes of pulmonary hypertension are shown in Table 44-8. Currently, classification of the World Health Organization is used, and this has been adopted by the American College of Cardiology and the American Heart Association (McLaughlin and co-workers, 2009).

There are important prognostic and therapeutic distinctions between class I pulmonary hypertension and all the other conditions. Class I indicates a *specific disease that affects pulmonary arterioles*. It includes idiopathic or "primary" pulmonary hypertension as well as those cases secondary to a known cause such as connective-tissue disease. Approximately one third of women with scleroderma and 10 percent with systemic lupus erythematosus have pulmonary hypertension (Rich and McLaughlin, 2005). Other causes in young women are sickle-cell disease and thyrotoxicosis (Sheffield and Cunningham, 2004). Moreover, Sigel and colleagues (2007) described a maternal death from

TABLE 44-8. Clinical Classification of Some Causes of Pulmonary Hypertension in Pregnancy

I Pulmonary arterial hypertension
   Idiopathic—previously "primary" pulmonary hypertension
   Familial—e.g., chromosome 2 gene in TGF superfamily
   Associated with: collagen-vascular disorders, congenital left-to-right cardiac shunts, HIV infection, thyrotoxicosis, sickle hemoglobinopathies, antiphospholipid antibody syndrome, diet drugs, portal hypertension
   Persistent pulmonary hypertension of the newborn
   Other
II Pulmonary hypertension with left-sided heart disease
   Left-sided atrial or ventricular disease
   Left-sided valvular disease
III Pulmonary hypertension associated with lung disease
   Chronic obstructive pulmonary disease
   Interstitial lung disease
   Other
IV Pulmonary hypertension due to chronic thromboembolic disease
V Miscellaneous

HIV = Human immunodeficiency virus; TGF = transforming growth factor.
Adapted from the World Health Organization classification of pulmonary hypertension reported by Simmoneau and co-workers (2004).

plexogenic pulmonary arteriopathy associated with cirrhosis and portal hypertension.

Class II disorders are more commonly encountered in pregnant women. These are secondary to pulmonary *venous* hypertension caused by left-sided atrial, ventricular, or valvular disorders. A typical example is mitral stenosis discussed on page 965. Although cardiac catheterization remains the standard criterion for the measurement of pulmonary artery pressures, noninvasive echocardiography is often used to provide an estimate.

Diagnosis

Symptoms may be vague, and dyspnea with exertion is the most common. With class II disorders, orthopnea and nocturnal dyspnea are usually also present. Angina and syncope occur when right ventricular output is fixed, and they suggest advanced disease. Chest radiography commonly shows enlarged pulmonary hilar arteries and attenuated peripheral markings. It also may disclose parenchymal causes of hypertension. Diagnosis is by echocardiography and is confirmed by right-sided catheterization, which usually may be deferred during pregnancy. In their review of 33 pregnant women who underwent both echocardiography and cardiac catheterization, Penning and colleagues

CHAPTER 44

(2001) cautioned that pulmonary artery pressures were significantly overestimated by echocardiography in a third of cases.

Prognosis

Longevity depends on the cause and severity at discovery. For example, although invariably fatal, idiopathic pulmonary hypertension has a 3-year survival rate of 60 percent, whereas for collagen-vascular diseases, this rate is only 35 percent (McLaughlin and colleagues, 2004). Some disorders respond to pulmonary vasodilators, calcium-channel blockers, prostacyclin analogs, or endothelin-receptor blockers, all which may improve quality of life. The prostacyclin analogs, epoprostenol and trepostinil, significantly lower pulmonary vascular resistance but must be given parenterally (Humbert and colleagues, 2004; Roeleveld and co-workers, 2004). Preconceptional counseling is imperative as emphasized by Easterling and associates (1999).

Pulmonary Hypertension and Pregnancy

Maternal mortality is appreciable, especially with idiopathic pulmonary hypertension. In the past, there were usually poor distinctions between causes and severity of hypertension. The most severe cases—usually idiopathic—had the worst prognosis, and it was erroneously assumed that all types of pulmonary hypertension were equally dangerous. With widespread use of echocardiography, the less-severe better-prognosis lesions were identified. Kiss and colleagues (1995) reported maternal mortality in seven of 11 women—65 percent—with primary disease. Weiss and associates (1998) reviewed 27 cases of assorted causes reported from 1978 through 1996 and found a 30-percent mortality rate. After their recent review, Bedard and co-workers (2009) reported that mortality statistics improved during the decade ending in 2007 compared with those for the decade ending 1996—it was 25 vs 38 percent, respectively. Importantly, almost 80 percent of the deaths were during the first month postpartum.

Pregnancy is contraindicated with severe disease, especially those with pulmonary arterial changes—most class I. With milder degrees of other causes—class II being common—the prognosis is much better. For example, with the more common use of echocardiography and pulmonary artery catheterization in young women with heart disease, we have identified women with mild to moderate pulmonary hypertension who tolerate pregnancy, labor, and delivery well. Sheffield and Cunningham (2004) described pulmonary hypertension that develops with thyrotoxicosis but is reversible with its treatment (see Chap. 53, p. 1128). Boggess and colleagues (1995) described nine women with interstitial and restrictive lung disease with varying degrees of pulmonary hypertension, and all tolerated pregnancy reasonably well.

Treatment of symptomatic pregnant women includes limitation of activity and avoidance of the supine position in late pregnancy. Diuretics, supplemental oxygen, and vasodilator drugs are standard therapy for symptoms. In addition, there are several reports describing the successful use of direct pulmonary artery vasodilators such as epoprostenol (prostacyclin) in both singleton and twin gestations (Badalian, 2000; Easterling, 1999; Nahapetian, 2008, and all their associates).

Management of labor and delivery is particularly problematic. These women are at greatest risk when there is diminished venous return and right ventricular filling, which is associated with most maternal deaths. To avoid hypotension, careful attention is given to epidural analgesia induction and to preventing blood loss at delivery. Pollack and colleagues (1990), as well as others, have reported successful labor analgesia without significant cardiovascular effects from morphine administered intrathecally. Parneix and co-workers (2009) describe low-dose spinal-epidural analgesia for cesarean delivery. Lam and colleagues (2001) have described intubation and inhaled nitric oxide during labor and forceps delivery of a nullipara with severe primary pulmonary hypertension. Weiss and co-workers (2000) described a woman with severe primary pulmonary hypertension who had a successful cesarean delivery with epidural analgesia and inhalation of 20 mg of aerosolized iloprost, a prostacyclin analog. Successful intrapartum use of inhaled epoprostenol has also been described (Bildirici and Shumway, 2004).

OTHER CARDIOVASCULAR CONDITIONS

Mitral Valve Prolapse

This diagnosis implies the presence of a pathological connective tissue disorder—often termed *myxomatous degeneration*—which may involve the valve leaflets themselves, the annulus, or the chordae tendineae. Mitral insufficiency may develop. Most women with mitral valve prolapse are asymptomatic and are diagnosed by routine examination or while undergoing echocardiography. The small percentage of women with symptoms have anxiety, palpitations, atypical chest pain, and syncope. Those with redundant or thickened mitral valve leaflets are at increased risk for sudden death, infective endocarditis, or cerebral embolism (Braunwald, 2005). Looking at this another way, of 213 young women with documented ischemic strokes, only 1.9 percent had mitral valve prolapse compared with 2.7 percent of controls (Gilon and co-workers, 1999).

Effects on Pregnancy

Pregnant women with mitral valve prolapse rarely have cardiac complications. In fact, pregnancy-induced hypervolemia may improve alignment of the mitral valve (Rayburn and colleagues, 1987). Women without evidence of pathological myxomatous change may in general expect excellent pregnancy outcome (Chia and associates, 1994; Leśniak-Sobelga and co-workers, 2004). For women who are symptomatic, β-blocking drugs are given to decrease sympathetic tone, relieve chest pain and palpitations, and reduce the risk of life-threatening arrhythmias. Mitral valve prolapse with regurgitation or valvular damage is considered to be a moderate risk for bacterial endocarditis (see p. 974).

Peripartum Cardiomyopathy

Currently, this disorder is a diagnosis of exclusion following a contemporaneous cardiac evaluation of peripartum heart failure. In most aspects, it is similar to idiopathic dilated cardiomyopathy encountered in nonpregnant adults. Although the term peripartum cardiomyopathy has been used widely, there is very little evidence to support a unique pregnancy-induced cardiomyopathy. In 1997, the National Heart, Lung, and Blood Institute and the Office of Rare Diseases convened a workshop that established the following diagnostic criteria (Pearson and associates, 2000):

1. Development of cardiac failure in the last month of pregnancy or within 5 months after delivery,
2. Absence of an identifiable cause for the cardiac failure,
3. Absence of recognizable heart disease prior to the last month of pregnancy, and
4. Left ventricular systolic dysfunction demonstrated by classic echocardiographic criteria such as depressed shortening fraction or ejection fraction.

Although the workshop panel concluded that the disease is acute, rather than a preexisting one preceding pregnancy, at least three reports do not support idiopathic pregnancy-induced cardiomyopathy. Cunningham and associates (1986) carefully evaluated 28 women at Parkland Hospital with peripartum heart failure of obscure etiology who were initially thought to have idiopathic peripartum cardiomyopathy. In 21 of these, heart failure was found to be caused by hypertensive heart disease, clinically silent mitral stenosis, obesity, or viral myocarditis. Particularly important were the silent cardiomyopathic effects that even intermediate-duration chronic hypertension may have on ventricular function.

Felker and colleagues (2000) performed endomyocardial biopsies in 1230 nonpregnant patients who had unexplained cardiomyopathy. In half of these, a cause for cardiomyopathy was found—the most common was myocarditis. And in the subset of 51 women with peripartum cardiomyopathy, 26 had histological evidence for myocarditis. Bültmann and co-workers (2005) studied endomyocardial biopsy specimens from 26 women with peripartum cardiomyopathy and reported that 16—over half—had histological evidence of "borderline myocarditis." Half of these 16 also had viral genomic material for parvovirus B19, human herpesvirus 6, Epstein-Barr virus, and human cytomegalovirus. The researchers attributed these findings to reactivation of latent viral infection that triggered an autoimmune response.

Chronic hypertension with superimposed preeclampsia is likely the most common cause of heart failure during pregnancy (see Chap. 45, p. 987). In some cases, mild antecedent hypertension is undiagnosed, and when superimposed preeclampsia develops, it may cause otherwise inexplicable peripartum heart failure. As discussed throughout Chapter 43, obesity is a common cofactor with chronic hypertension, and it can cause or contribute to underlying ventricular hypertrophy. In the Framingham Heart Study, obesity alone was associated with a doubling of the risk of heart failure in nonpregnant individuals (Kenchaiah and colleagues, 2002). Dilated cardiomyopathy is also found in human immunodeficiency virus (HIV) infection (Barbaro and associates, 1998).

Regardless of the underlying condition that causes cardiac dysfunction, women who develop peripartum heart failure often have obstetrical complications that either contribute to or precipitate heart failure. For example, preeclampsia is common and may precipitate afterload failure. Acute anemia from blood loss magnifies the physiological effects of compromised ventricular function. Similarly, infection and accompanying fever increase cardiac output and oxygen utilization.

It seems probable that specific human pregnancy-related cardiomyopathies are yet undiscovered. For example, Hilfiker-Kleiner and associates (2007) recently described mice that developed peripartum cardiomyopathy associated with a cardiomyocyte-specific deletion of the *stat 3* gene. Ultimately, a biologically active prolactin derivative serves to mediate development of the cardiomyopathy.

Idiopathic Cardiomyopathy in Pregnancy

After exclusion of an underlying cause for heart failure, the default diagnosis is idiopathic or peripartum cardiomyopathy. Thus, its incidence is highly dependent upon the diligence of the search for a cause. Because of this, the cited incidence varies from 1 in 1500 to 1 in 15,000 pregnancies. In a review of the National Hospital Discharge Survey database, Mielniczuk and co-workers (2006) screened 3.6 million discharges of all patients from 1990 to 2002. Those coded with diagnoses consistent with peripartum cardiomyopathy had an incidence of 1 in 3200. Unfortunately, this figure ignores overdiagnosis, which is common in our experiences. Specifically, after careful evaluation of women with peripartum heart failure at Parkland Hospital, we identified idiopathic cardiomyopathy in approximately 1 in 15,000 deliveries—an incidence similar to that of idiopathic cardiomyopathy in young nonpregnant women (Cunningham and colleagues, 1986).

Women with cardiomyopathy present with signs and symptoms of congestive heart failure. Dyspnea is universal, and other symptoms include orthopnea, cough, palpitations, and chest pain (Sheffield and Cunningham, 1999). The hallmark finding usually is impressive cardiomegaly (**Fig. 44-3**). Echocardiographic findings include an ejection fraction less than 45 percent or a fractional shortening less than 30 percent, or both, and an end-diastolic dimension greater than 2.7 cm/m^2 (Hibbard and colleagues, 1999).

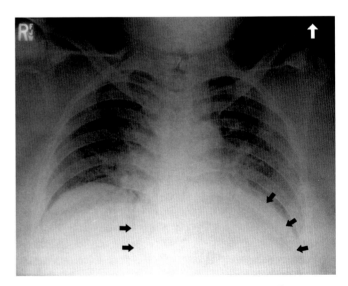

FIGURE 44-3 Cardiomyopathy with mild pulmonary edema. Anterior-posterior projection chest radiograph of a woman with an abnormally enlarged heart (*black arrows*) and mild perihilar opacification consistent with dilated cardiomyopathy.

Management. Therapy consists of treatment for heart failure (Ro and Frishman, 2006). Diuretics are given to reduce preload, and afterload reduction is accomplished with hydralazine or another vasodilator. Because of marked fetal effects, angiotensin-converting enzyme inhibitors are withheld until the woman is delivered (see Chap. 14, p. 319). Digoxin is given for its inotropic effects unless complex arrhythmias are identified. Because there is a high incidence of associated thromboembolism, prophylactic heparin is often recommended. Smith and Gillham (2009) reported that extracorporeal membranous oxygenation was lifesaving in a woman with fulminating cardiomyopathy.

Acute mortality rate varies, depending again on the accuracy of the diagnosis. In the database survey by Mielniczuk and associates (2006), the immediate mortality rate was approximately 2 percent.

Long-Term Prognosis

The distinction between peripartum heart failure from an identifiable cause versus idiopathic cardiomyopathy is of primary importance. In a follow-up study from the Albert Schweitzer Hospital in Haiti, Fett and co-workers (2009) performed echocardiography every 6 months in 116 women with peripartum cardiomyopathy. Using a left ventricular ejection fraction >.50 as recovery, only 28 percent of these women recovered, and three fourths took more than 12 months to attain this level of function. These data indicate that long-term mortality rates are significant. As shown in Figure 44-4, the 5- and 10-year survival rates are substantially lower in nonpregnant patients with idiopathic cardiomyopathy. That said, these mortality statistics are optimistic compared with other reports. There seems to be no doubt that women with peripartum cardiomyopathy who regain ventricular function within 6 months have a good prognosis (Lampert and associates, 1997). But those who do not, however, have high morbidity and mortality rates. With a mean follow-up of 39 months, de Souza and colleagues (2001b) reported that eight of 44 such women—18 percent—had died from end-stage heart failure. Of the others, two women had a nonfatal pulmonary embolism, one had a cerebral ischemic stroke, and another underwent heart transplantation at 14

months. Of eight women with NYHA class IV heart failure, only five improved to class I or II, and two to class III.

Elkayam and co-workers (2001) reported similar long-term outcomes obtained by a survey of members of the American College of Cardiology. There were 60 subsequent pregnancies in 44 women who had peripartum cardiomyopathy. In 28 of 44 women—63 percent—in whom left ventricular function had returned to normal, 20 percent developed heart failure during pregnancy, but none died. In the remaining 16 with persistent left ventricular dysfunction, 44 percent developed heart failure, and three women died between 2 and 24 months postpartum. Thus, although a return to normal ventricular function does not guarantee a problem-free pregnancy, these studies certainly indicate that another pregnancy is undertaken with reservations in women with an ejection fraction persistently less than 50 percent.

Hypertrophic Cardiomyopathy

Concentric left ventricular hypertrophy may be familial, and there also is a sporadic form not related to hypertension, termed *idiopathic hypertrophic subaortic stenosis.* Epidemiological studies suggest that the disorder is common, affecting approximately 1 in 500 adults (Maron, 2004). The condition—characterized by cardiac hypertrophy, myocyte disarray, and interstitial fibrosis—is caused by mutations in any one of more than a dozen genes that encode proteins of the cardiac sarcomere. Inheritance is autosomal dominant, and genetic screening is complex and not currently clinically available (Osio and associates, 2007; Spirito and Autore, 2006). The abnormality is in the myocardial muscle, and it is characterized by left ventricular myocardial hypertrophy with a pressure gradient to left ventricular outflow (Wynne and Braunwald, 2008). Diagnosis is established by echocardiographic identification of a hypertrophied and nondilated left ventricle in the absence of other cardiovascular conditions.

Most affected women are asymptomatic, but dyspnea, anginal or atypical chest pain, syncope, and arrhythmias may develop. Complex arrhythmias may progress to sudden death, which is the most common form of death. Asymptomatic patients with runs of ventricular tachycardia are especially prone to sudden death. Symptoms are usually worsened by exercise. Nishimura and Holmes (2004) have provided an excellent review.

Pregnancy

Although limited reports suggest that pregnancy is well tolerated, congestive heart failure is common (Benitez, 1996). Thaman and co-workers (2003) reviewed 271 pregnancies in 127 affected women. Although there were no maternal deaths, more than 25 percent experienced at least one adverse cardiac symptom, including dyspnea, chest pain, or palpitations.

Management is similar to that for aortic stenosis. Strenuous exercise is prohibited during pregnancy. Abrupt positional changes are avoided to prevent reflex vasodilation and decreased preload. Likewise, drugs that evoke diuresis or diminish vascular resistance are generally not used. If symptoms develop, especially angina, β-adrenergic or calcium-channel blocking drugs are given. The route of delivery is determined by obstetrical indications. Spinal analgesia is contraindicated, and even carefully administered epidural analgesia is controversial (Camann and

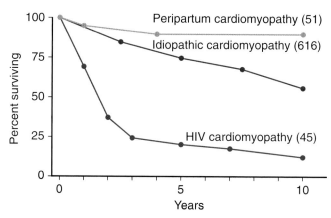

FIGURE 44-4 Survival according to underlying cause of cardiomyopathy. (HIV = human immunodeficiency virus.)(Data from Felker and colleagues, 2000.)

Thornhill, 1999). Endocarditis prophylaxis is given if bacteremia is suspected. Infants rarely demonstrate inherited lesions at birth.

Infective Endocarditis

This infection involves cardiac endothelium and produces vegetations that usually deposit on a valve. Infective endocarditis can involve a native or a prosthetic valve, and it may be associated with intravenous drug abuse. Children and adults who have had corrective surgery for congenital heart disease are at greatest risk (Morris and co-workers, 1998). Approximately half of affected adults have a known preexisting heart lesion (Hoen and colleagues, 2002).

Subacute bacterial endocarditis usually is due to a low-virulence bacterial infection superimposed on an underlying structural lesion. These are usually native valve infections. Organisms that cause indolent endocarditis are most commonly viridans-group streptococci or *Enterococcus* species. Historically, *acute endocarditis* was usually caused by coagulase-positive staphylococci. Two large and more recent epidemiological studies, however, indicate that the most common causative organisms are streptococci—especially viridans—followed by *Staphylococcus aureus* and *Enterococcus* species (Hasbun and associates, 2003; Hoen and colleagues, 2002). Among intravenous drug abusers, *S. aureus* is the predominant organism. *Staphylococcus epidermidis* commonly causes prosthetic valve infections. *Streptococcus pneumoniae* and *Neisseria gonorrhoeae* may occasionally cause acute, fulminating disease (Bataskov and colleagues, 1991). Antepartum endocarditis has been described with *Neisseria sicca* and *Neisseria mucosa*, the latter causing maternal death (Cox and associates, 1988; Deger and Ludmir, 1992). Only a few cases of group B streptococcal endocarditis have been described (Kangavari and co-workers, 2000). Kulaš and Habek (2006) reported a case of endocarditis due to *Escherichia coli* following cesarean delivery in an otherwise healthy young woman.

Diagnosis

Symptoms of endocarditis are variable and often develop insidiously. Fever is virtually universal, and a murmur ultimately is heard in 80 to 85 percent of cases (Karchmer, 2005). Anorexia, fatigue, and other constitutional symptoms are common, and the illness is frequently described as "flulike." Other findings are anemia, proteinuria, and manifestations of embolic lesions, including petechiae, focal neurological manifestations, chest or abdominal pain, and ischemia in an extremity. In some cases, heart failure develops. Symptoms may persist for several weeks before the diagnosis is found, and a high index of suspicion is necessary. Diagnosis is made using the *Duke criteria,* which include positive blood cultures for typical organisms and evidence of endocardial involvement (Karchmer, 2005). Echocardiography is useful, but lesions less than 2 mm in diameter or those on the tricuspid valve may be missed. A negative echocardiographic study does not exclude endocarditis.

Management

Treatment is primarily medical with appropriate timing of surgical intervention if necessary. Knowledge of the infecting or-

ganism is imperative for sensible antimicrobial selection. Most viridans streptococci are sensitive to penicillin G given intravenously with gentamicin for 2 weeks (Karchmer, 2005). Complicated infections are treated longer, and women allergic to penicillin are either desensitized or given intravenous ceftriaxone or vancomycin for 4 weeks. Staphylococci, enterococci, and other organisms are treated according to microbial sensitivity for 4 to 6 weeks (Darouiche, 2004). Prosthetic valve infections are treated for 6 to 8 weeks. Persistent native valve infection may require replacement, and this is even more commonly indicated with an infected prosthetic valve. Right-sided infections caused by *methicillin-resistant S. aureus (MRSA)* are treated with vancomycin (see Chap. 58, p. 1223). Fowler and colleagues (2006) have presented promising findings for treatment of MRSA endocarditis with *daptomycin*—a cyclic lipopeptide.

Endocarditis in Pregnancy

Infective endocarditis is uncommon during pregnancy and the puerperium. During a 7-year period, the incidence of endocarditis at Parkland Hospital was approximately 1 in 16,000 deliveries (Cox and associates, 1988). Two of seven women died. Treatment is the same as that described earlier. From their reviews, Seaworth and Durack (1986) and Cox and Leveno (1989) cited a maternal mortality rate of 25 to 35 percent.

Antimicrobial Prophylaxis

The efficacy of antimicrobial prophylaxis to prevent bacterial endocarditis is questionable. Only 13 percent of cases arising in patients with high-risk cardiac lesions do so after a procedure (Van der Meer and associates, 1992). The American Heart Association recommends prophylaxis based on risk stratification (Table 44-9). These recommendations have

---

TABLE 44-9. American Heart Association Guidelines for Endocarditis Prophylaxis with Dental Procedures

Prophylaxis is recommended for all dental procedures that involve manipulation of gingival tissue or the periapical tooth region or perforation of oral mucosa in patients with any of the following cardiac conditions:

(1) Prosthetic heart valve or prosthetic material used for valve repair
(2) Previous infective endocarditis
(3) Certain forms of congenital heart lesions:
- Unrepaired cardiac lesions causing cyanotic heart disease, including palliative shunts and conduits
- Repaired defect with prosthetic material or device—placed surgically or by catheter—for 6 months following repair procedure and before endothelialization
- Repaired defect with residual defects at or adjacent to the site of a prosthetic part or device that inhibit endothelialization

From Wilson and colleagues, 2007.

been endorsed by the American College of Obstetricians and Gynecologists (2003).

Obstetrical Procedures. The current recommendations of the American College of Cardiology and the American Heart Association are shown in Table 44-9. These guidelines suggest that prophylaxis for bacterial endocarditis be administered intrapartum to women at risk only in the presence of suspected bacteremia or active infection. They estimate that the incidence of transient bacteremia at delivery is 1 to 5 percent. Antimicrobial prophylaxis is considered optional for women undergoing an uncomplicated delivery who are at high risk for endocarditis (American College of Obstetricians and Gynecologists, 2003). Prophylaxis is overused, likely because of previously liberal recommendations. In a study from one busy institution, Pocock and Chen (2006) reported that only six of 50 women who received antibiotics for endocarditis prophylaxis had an appropriate indication.

Only a few regimens are recommended by the American College of Obstetricians and Gynecologists (2008) for prophylaxis, which is given preferably 30 to 60 minutes before the procedure. Either ampicillin, 2 g, or cefazolin or ceftriaxone, 1 g, is given intravenously. For penicillin-sensitive patients, one of the latter regimens is given, or if there is a history of anaphylaxis, then clindamycin, 600 mg is given intravenously. The recommended oral regimen is 2 g of amoxicillin. If enterococcus infection is of concern, vancomycin is also given.

Arrhythmias

Both new and preexisting cardiac arrhythmias are commonly encountered during pregnancy, labor, delivery, and the puerperium (Gowda and associates, 2003). In a study of 73 women with a history of prepregnant supraventricular tachycardia, paroxysmal atrial flutter or fibrillation, or ventricular tachycardia, Silversides and associates (2006) observed recurrence rates of 50, 52, and 27 percent, respectively. The mechanism(s) responsible for the increased incidence of arrhythmias during pregnancy is not well elucidated. According to Eghbali and associates (2006), adaptive electric cardiac remodeling of K^+-channel genes may be key. Perhaps the normal but mild hypokalemia of pregnancy and/or the physiological increase in heart rate serve to induce arrhythmias (see Chap. 5, p. 118). Alternatively, their detection may be increased because of more frequent visits during prenatal care.

Bradyarrhythmias, including complete heart block, are compatible with a successful pregnancy outcome. Some women with complete heart block have syncope during labor and delivery, and occasionally temporary cardiac pacing is necessary (Hidaka and colleagues, 2006). In our experiences, as well as those of Jaffe and associates (1987), women with permanent artificial pacemakers usually tolerate pregnancy well. With fixed-rate devices, cardiac output apparently is increased by augmented stroke volume.

Tachyarrhythmias are relatively common and should prompt consideration of underlying cardiac disease. *Paroxysmal supraventricular tachycardia* is encountered most frequently. Siu and associates (1997) followed 25 women who had supraventricular tachycardia diagnosed before pregnancy. Half of these

women had *Wolff-Parkinson-White (WPW) syndrome.* Three of 12 women with WPW syndrome and six of 13 without the condition had supraventricular tachycardia during pregnancy. If vagal maneuvers do not stimulate conversion, treatment consists of adenosine followed by calcium-channel or β-blocking drugs (Delacrétez, 2006). Our experiences are similar to those of others that adenosine is safe and effective for cardioversion in hemodynamically stable pregnant women (Chakhtoura and coworkers, 1998; Robins and Lyons, 2004). Although these drugs do not appear to harm the fetus, fetal bradycardia with adenosine has been described (Dunn and Brost, 2000).

Electrical cardioversion is not contraindicated in pregnancy, but vigilance is important. Barnes and associates (2002) described a case in which direct current cardioversion led directly to a sustained uterine contraction and fetal bradycardia. In some patients, accessory pathway ablation may be indicated (Pappone and colleagues, 2003). The typical fluoroscopic procedure-related fetal radiation dose is less than 1 cGy (Damilakis and associates, 2001).

Atrial flutter or fibrillation are more likely associated with underlying disease, such as thyrotoxicosis or mitral stenosis. Major complications include stroke (Ezekowitz and Levine, 1999). Thus, heparin is recommended by some if fibrillation is chronic and persists during pregnancy, especially if there is mitral stenosis (O'Gara and Braunwald, 2008). If atrial fibrillation is associated with mitral stenosis, pulmonary edema may develop in late pregnancy if the ventricular rate is increased.

Ventricular tachycardia is uncommon in healthy young women without underlying heart disease. Brodsky and associates (1992) described seven pregnant women with new-onset ventricular tachycardia and reviewed 23 reports. Most of these women were not found to have structural heart disease—in 14 tachycardia was precipitated by physical exercise or psychological stress. Abnormalities found included two cases of myocardial infarction, two of prolonged QT interval, and anesthesia-provoked tachycardia in another. They concluded that pregnancy events precipitated tachycardia and recommended β-blocker therapy for control. Occasionally *arrhythmogenic right ventricular dysplasia* will result in ventricular tachyarrhythmias (Lee and co-workers, 2006). For pregnant women requiring defibrillation for ventricular arrhythmias, Nanson and associates (2001) found that standard adult energy settings were adequate.

QT-interval prolongation may predispose individuals to a potentially fatal ventricular arrhythmia known as *torsades de pointes* (Roden, 2008). Two studies involving a combined total of 502 pregnant women with *long QT syndrome* both reported a significant increase in cardiac events postpartum but not during pregnancy (Rashba and colleagues, 1998; Seth and associates, 2007). They hypothesized that the normal increase in heart rate during pregnancy may be partially protective. Paradoxically, β-blocker therapy has been shown to decrease the risk of torsades de pointes in patients with long QT syndrome and should be continued during pregnancy and postpartum (Gowda and colleagues, 2003; Seth and associates, 2007). Importantly, many medications, including some used during pregnancy such as erythromycin and clarithromycin, may predispose to QT prolongation (Al-Khatib and associates, 2003; Roden, 2004).

DISEASES OF THE AORTA

Aortic Dissection

Marfan syndrome and coarctation are two aortic diseases that place the pregnant woman at increased risk for *aortic dissection.* Half of cases of dissection in young women are related to pregnancy (O'Gara and associates, 2004). Other risk factors are bicuspid aortic valve and Turner or Noonan syndrome. Pepin and colleagues (2000) reported a high rate of aortic dissection or rupture in patients with *Ehlers-Danlos syndrome* (see Chap. 54, p. 1159). Although the mechanism(s) involved is unclear, the initiating event is an aortic intimal tear, and rupture may follow medial hemorrhage.

In most cases, aortic dissection presents with severe chest pain described as ripping, tearing, or stabbing in nature. Diminution or loss of peripheral pulses in conjunction with a recently acquired murmur of aortic insufficiency are important physical findings. The differential diagnosis of aortic dissection includes myocardial infarction, pulmonary embolism, pneumothorax, and aortic valve rupture. Lang and Borow (1991) rightfully add obstetrical catastrophes to the list, especially placental abruption and uterine rupture.

More than 90 percent of affected patients have an abnormal chest radiograph. Aortic angiography is the most definitive method for confirming the diagnosis, however, noninvasive imaging—sonography, computed tomography, and magnetic resonance (MR) imaging—is used more frequently. The urgency of the clinical situation frequently dictates which procedure is best.

Initial medical treatment is given to lower blood pressure. Proximal dissections most often need to be resected, and the aortic valve replaced if necessary. Distal dissections are more complex, and many may be treated medically. Lederle and colleagues (2002) have shown that survival in nonpregnant patients is not improved by elective repair of abdominal aortic aneurysms smaller than 5.5 cm. Lee and associates (2001) described a successful vaginal delivery in a woman with a 4.5-cm thoracic aortic aneurysm.

Marfan Syndrome

This syndrome is usually inherited as an autosomal dominant trait with a high degree of penetrance. The incidence is 2 to 3 per 10,000 individuals and is without racial or ethnic predilection (Ammash and associates, 2008). Prenatal diagnosis is usually possible using linkage analysis (see Chap. 12, p. 283). The syndrome is caused by abnormal *fibrillin*—a constituent of elastin—caused by any of dozens of mutations in the *FBN1* gene located on chromosome 15q21 (Biggin and co-workers, 2004). Thus, Marfan syndrome is a connective-tissue disorder characterized by generalized weakness that can result in dangerous cardiovascular complications. Because all tissues are involved, other defects are frequent and include joint laxity and scoliosis. Progressive aortic dilatation causes aortic valve insufficiency, and there may be infective endocarditis and mitral valve prolapse with insufficiency. Aortic dilatation and dissecting aneurysm are the most serious abnormalities. Early death is due either to valvular insufficiency and heart failure or to a dissecting aneurysm. Long-term benefits

from β-blocker therapy have been described for nonpregnant adults (Shores and colleagues, 1994).

Effect of Pregnancy

In the past, case reports reflected biased outcomes, and the maternal mortality rate was magnified (Elkayam and associates, 1995). In a prospective evaluation of 21 women during 45 pregnancies cared for at the Johns Hopkins Hospital, only two had dissection, and one died postpartum from graft infection (Rossiter and colleagues, 1995). Although there were no maternal deaths among 14 women followed by Rahman and co-workers (2003), two required surgical correction of an aortic aneurysm.

Both latter groups of investigators concluded that aortic dilatation of more than 40 mm or mitral valve dysfunction are high-risk factors for life-threatening cardiovascular complications during pregnancy. Conversely, women with minimal or no dilatation and those with normal cardiac function by echocardiography are counseled regarding the small but serious potential risk of aortic dissection. Elkayam and colleagues (1995) also concluded that pregnancy was safer in women with Marfan syndrome who had no cardiovascular manifestations or aortic arch dilatation. They recommended prophylactic β-blocker therapy during pregnancy.

The aortic root usually measures about 20 mm, and during normal pregnancy it increases slightly (Easterling and colleagues, 1991). If dilatation reaches 40 mm, then dissection is more likely (Simpson and D'Alton, 1997). If it reaches 50 to 60 mm, then elective surgery should be considered before pregnancy (Gott and associates, 1999; Williams and co-workers, 2002). Successful cases of aortic root replacement during pregnancy have been described, but it has also been associated with fetal hypoxic-ischemic cerebral damage (Mul and co-workers, 1998; Seeburger and associates, 2007). And Papatsonis and co-workers (2009) described emergency cesarean delivery at term in a woman with an acute type A dissection that was repaired successfully during the same operation. Although Marfan syndrome itself is not an indication, some recommend cesarean delivery if there is aortic involvement. Otherwise, obstetrical indications for delivery are followed.

Perinatal Outcomes

Obstetrical outcomes of 63 women with Marfan syndrome with a total of 142 pregnancies were reviewed by Meijboom and colleagues (2006). There were 111 delivered after 20 weeks; 15 percent had preterm delivery; and 5 percent, preterm prematurely ruptured membranes. Two infants were stillborn, and there were six neonatal deaths. As expected, half of the survivors were subsequently diagnosed with Marfan syndrome.

Aortic Coarctation

This is a relatively rare lesion often accompanied by abnormalities of other large arteries. A fourth of affected patients have a bicuspid aortic valve, and another 10 percent have cerebral artery aneurysms. Other associated lesions are persistent ductus arteriosus, septal defects, and Turner syndrome. The collateral circulation arising above the coarctation expands, often to a striking extent, to cause localized erosion of rib margins by hypertrophied intercostal arteries. Typical findings include hypertension in the upper extremities but normal or reduced pressures in the lower extremities. Sherer (2002), Dizon-Townson (1995), Zwiers (2006), and their colleagues have described diagnoses during pregnancy using MR imaging.

Effects on Pregnancy

Major complications are congestive heart failure after long-standing severe hypertension, bacterial endocarditis of the bicuspid aortic valve, and aortic rupture. Maternal mortality rates average 3 percent (McAnulty and co-workers, 1990). Because hypertension may worsen in pregnancy, antihypertensive therapy using β-blocking drugs is usually required. Aortic rupture is more likely late in pregnancy or early postpartum. Cerebral hemorrhage from *circle of Willis aneurysms* may also develop. Beauchesne and associates (2001) described the outcomes of 188 pregnancies from the Mayo Clinic in 50 such women. A third had hypertension that was related to significant coarctation gradients, and one woman died from dissection at 36 weeks.

Congestive heart failure demands vigorous efforts to improve cardiac function and may warrant pregnancy interruption. Some authors have recommended that resection of the coarctation be undertaken during pregnancy to protect against the possibility of a dissecting aneurysm and aortic rupture. This poses significant risk, especially for the fetus, because all the collaterals must be clamped for variable periods of time.

Some authors recommend cesarean delivery to prevent transient blood pressure elevations that might lead to rupture of the aorta or coexisting cerebral aneurysms. Available evidence, however, suggests that cesarean delivery should be limited to obstetrical indications. Intrapartum endocarditis prophylaxis is given if bacteremia is suspected.

ISCHEMIC HEART DISEASE

Mortality from coronary artery disease and *myocardial infarction* is a rare complication of pregnancy. In fact, the overall incidence appears to be declining due to reductions in major risk factors and better medical therapies (Ford and co-workers, 2007). That said, evidence suggests that the incidence in pregnancy may be increasing. In a review of California hospital discharge records between 1991 and 2000, Ladner and co-workers (2005) reported myocardial infarction to complicate 1 in 37,500 deliveries. In a similar review of Canadian hospitals between 1970 and 1998, MacArthur and co-workers (2006) reported the incidence of peripartum myocardial ischemia to be 1.1 per 100,000 deliveries. James and co-workers (2006) used the Nationwide Inpatient Sample database for 2000 to 2002 and reported acute myocardial infarction in 6.2 per 100,000 deliveries. Collectively, these epidemiological studies are consistent with mortality statistics from the United States that indicate that the mortality rate from coronary heart disease among all women aged 35 to 44 years has been increasing by an average of 1.3 percent per year since 1997 (Ford and Capewell, 2007).

Pregnant women with coronary artery disease commonly have classic risk factors such as diabetes, smoking, hypertension, hyperlipidemia, and obesity (James and co-workers, 2006). Bagg and colleagues (1999) reviewed the course of 22 diabetic pregnant women with ischemic heart disease—class H diabetes (see Chap. 52, p. 1105). These authors, as well as Pombar (1995) and Reece (1986) and their colleagues, documented unusually high mortality rates in those who suffered myocardial infarction. Mousa (2000) and Sutaria (2000) and their associates each described coronary artery occlusion in two pregnant smokers with hypercholesterolemia following a routine intramuscular injection of 0.5-mg ergometrine. Schulte-Sasse (2000) described myocardial ischemia associated with prostaglandin E_1 vaginal suppositories for labor induction. Karpati and co-workers (2004) reported that half of 55 otherwise healthy normal women with shock from postpartum hemorrhage developed myocardial ischemia.

Diagnosis during pregnancy is not different from the nonpregnant patient. Measurement of serum levels of the cardiac-specific contractile protein, *troponin I*, is accurate for diagnosis (Shade and associates, 2002). Troponin I was reported by Shivvers and colleagues (1999) to be undetectable across normal pregnancy. Moreover, Koscica and colleagues (2002) found that levels do not increase following either vaginal or cesarean delivery. Finally, Atalay (2005) and Yang (2006) and their associates found that levels of troponin I are higher in preeclamptic women than in normotensive controls.

Pregnancy with Prior Ischemic Heart Disease

The advisability of pregnancy after a myocardial infarction is unclear. Ischemic heart disease is characteristically progressive, and because it is usually associated with hypertension or diabetes, pregnancy in most of these women seems inadvisable. Vinatier and associates (1994) reviewed 30 pregnancies in women who had sustained an *infarction remote from pregnancy*. Although none of these women died, four had congestive heart failure and four had worsening angina during pregnancy. Pombar and co-workers (1995) reviewed outcomes of women with diabetes-associated ischemic heart disease and infarction. Three had undergone coronary artery bypass grafting before pregnancy. Of 17 women, eight died during pregnancy. Certainly, pregnancy increases cardiac workload, and all of these investigators concluded that ventricular performance should be assessed using ventriculography, radionuclide studies, echocardiography, or coronary angiography prior to conception. If there is no significant ventricular dysfunction, pregnancy will likely be tolerated.

For the woman who becomes pregnant before these studies are performed, echocardiography should be done. Exercise tolerance testing may be indicated, and radionuclide ventriculography results in minimal radiation exposure for the fetus (see Chap. 41, p. 920). Zaidi and co-workers (2008) have described the use of serial T2-weighted cardiovascular MR imaging in a woman with suffered a myocardial infarction during the first trimester to better define the extent and severity of infarction.

Myocardial Infarction During Pregnancy

In this setting, most agree that the mortality rate in pregnancy is increased compared with age-matched nonpregnant women.

Hankins and co-workers (1985) reviewed 68 cases and reported an overall maternal mortality rate of approximately 35 percent. Hands and colleagues (1990) found an overall mortality rate of 30 percent. The mortality rate was 40 percent in the third trimester compared with 20 percent before then. Recent studies are more reassuring. In the Nationwide Inpatient Sample study totaling 859 pregnancies complicated by acute infarction during 2000 to 2002, James and associates (2006) cited a 5.1-percent death rate. Women who sustain an infarction less than 2 weeks prior to labor are at especially high risk of death (Esplin and Clark, 1999).

Treatment is similar to that for nonpregnant patients (Roth and Elkayam, 2009). Acute management includes administration of nitroglycerin and morphine with close blood pressure monitoring (Esplin and Clark, 1999). Lidocaine is used to suppress malignant arrhythmias. Calcium-channel blockers or β-blockers are given if indicated. *Tissue plasminogen activator* has been used in pregnant women remote from delivery (Schumacher and associates, 1997). In some women, invasive or surgical procedures may be indicated because of acute or unrelenting disease. Balmain (2007) and Dwyer (2005) and their associates recently reported successful percutaneous transluminal coronary angioplasty and stent placement during pregnancy.

If the infarct has healed sufficiently, cesarean delivery is reserved for obstetrical indications, and epidural analgesia is ideal for labor (Esplin and Clark, 1999). Epidural analgesia or general anesthesia may be used for cesarean delivery (Smith and associates, 2008). Camann and Thornhill (1999) recommend pulmonary artery catheter monitoring if an infarction occurs within 6 months of delivery or if there is ventricular dysfunction. Others, including us, recommend such monitoring only if there is cardiac dysfunction.

REFERENCES

Al Kasab SM, Sabag T, Al Zaibag M, et al: β-Adrenergic receptor blockade in the management of pregnant women with mitral stenosis. Am J Obstet Gynecol 163:37, 1990

Al-Khatib SM, LaPointe NM, Kramer JM, et al: What clinicians should know about the QT interval. JAMA 289:2120, 2003

Aliaga L, Santiago FM, Marti J, et al: Right-sided endocarditis complicating an atrial septal defect. Am J Med Sci 325:282, 2003

American College of Obstetricians and Gynecologists: Cardiac disease in pregnancy. Technical Bulletin No. 168, June 1992

American College of Obstetricians and Gynecologists: Safety of Lovenox in pregnancy. Committee Opinion No. 276, October 2002

American College of Obstetricians and Gynecologists: Antibiotic prophylaxis for infective endocarditis. Committee Opinion No. 421. November 2008

Ammash NM, Sundt TM, Connolly HM: Marfan syndrome—Diagnosis and management. Curr Probl Cardiol 33:7, 2008

Angel JL, Chapman C, Knuppel RA, et al: Percutaneous balloon aortic valvuloplasty in pregnancy. Obstet Gynecol 72:438, 1988

Armenti VT, Radomski JS, Moritz MJ, et al: Report from the National Transplantation Pregnancy Registry (NTPR): Outcomes of pregnancy after transplantation. In Cecka JM, Terasaki PI (eds): Clinical Transplants. Los Angeles, UCLA Immunogenetics Center, 121:30, 2002

Arnoni RT, Arnoni AS, Bonini R, et al: Risk factors associated with cardiac surgery during pregnancy. Ann Thorac Surg 76:1605, 2003

Atalay C, Erden G, Turhan T, et al: The effect of magnesium sulfate treatment on serum cardiac troponin I levels in preeclamptic women. Acta Obstet Gynecol Scand 84:617, 2005

Avila WS, Rossi EG, Ramires JA, et al: Pregnancy in patients with heart disease: Experience with 1,000 cases. Clin Cardiol 26:135, 2003

Badalian SS, Silverman RK, Aubry RH, et al: Twin pregnancy in a woman on long-term epoprostenol therapy for primary pulmonary hypertension: A case report. J Reprod Med 45:149, 2000

Bagg W, Henley PG, Macpherson P, et al: Pregnancy in women with diabetes and ischemic heart disease. Aust N Z J Obstet Gynaecol 39:99, 1999

Balmain S, McCullough CT, Love C, et al: Acute myocardial infarction during pregnancy successfully treated with primary percutaneous coronary intervention. Intl J Cardiol 116:e85, 2007

Barbaro G, di Lorenzo G, Grisorio B, et al: Incidence of dilated cardiomyopathy and detection of HIV in myocardial cells of HIV-positive patients. N Engl J Med 339:1093, 1998

Barnes EJ, Eben F, Patterson D: Direct current cardioversion during pregnancy should be performed with facilities available for fetal monitoring and emergency caesarean section. Br J Obstet Gynaecol 109:1406, 2002

Bashore TM: Adult congenital heart disease: Right ventricular outflow tract lesions. Circulation 115:1933, 2007

Bataskov KL, Hariharan S, Horowitz MD, et al: Gonococcal endocarditis complicating pregnancy: A case report and literature review. Obstet Gynecol 78:494, 1991

Bates SM, Greer IA, Pabinger I, et al: Venous thromboembolism, thrombophilia, antithrombotic therapy, and pregnancy: American College of Chest Physicians Evidence-Based Clinical Practice Guidelines (8th ed). Chest 133:844, 2008

Beauchesne LM, Connolly HM, Ammash NM, et al: Coarctation of the aorta: Outcome of pregnancy. J Am Coll Cardiol 38:1728, 2001

Bédard E, Dimopoulos K, Gatzoulis MA: Has there been any progress made on pulmonary outcomes among women with pulmonary arterial hypertension? Eur Heart J 30:256, 2009

Benitez RM: Hypertrophic cardiomyopathy and pregnancy: Maternal and fetal outcomes. J Matern Fetal Invest 6:51, 1996

Biggin A, Holman K, Brett M, et al: Detection of thirty novel FBN1 mutations in patients with Marfan syndrome or a related fibrillinopathy. Hum Mutat 23:99, 2004

Bildirici I, Shumway JB: Intravenous and inhaled epoprostenol for primary pulmonary hypertension during pregnancy and delivery. Obstet Gynecol 103:1102, 2004

Boggess KA, Easterling TR, Raghu G: Management and outcome of pregnant women with interstitial and restrictive lung disease. Am J Obstet Gynecol 173:1007, 1995

Braunwald E: Valvular heart disease. In Kasper DL, Braunwald E, Fauci AS, et al (eds): Harrison's Principles of Internal Medicine, 16th ed. New York, McGraw-Hill, 2005, p 1390

Brickner ME, Hillis LD, Lange RA: Congenital heart disease in adults. First of two parts. N Engl J Med 342:256, 2000

Brodsky M, Doria R, Allen B, et al: New-onset ventricular tachycardia during pregnancy. Am Heart J 123:933, 1992

Bültmann BD, Klingel K, Näbauer M, et al: High prevalence of viral genomes and inflammation in peripartum cardiomyopathy. Am J Obstet Gynecol 193:363, 2005

Butchart EG, Gohlke-Bärwolf C, Antunes MJ, et al: Recommendations for the management of patients after heart valve surgery. Eur Heart J 26:2463, 2005

Camann WR, Thornhill ML: Cardiovascular disease. In Chestnut DH (ed): Obstetric Anesthesia, 2nd ed. St. Louis, Mosby, 1999, p 776

Canobbio MM, Morris CD, Graham TP, et al: Pregnancy outcomes after atrial repair for transposition of the great arteries. Am J Cardiol 98:668, 2006

Capeless EL, Clapp JF: Cardiovascular changes in early phase of pregnancy. Am J Obstet Gynecol 161:1449, 1989

Carabello BA: Aortic stenosis. N Engl J Med 346:677, 2002

Carabello BA, Crawford FA: Valvular heart disease. N Engl J Med 337:32, 1997

Carruth JE, Mirvis SB, Brogan DR, et al: The electrocardiogram in normal pregnancy. Am Heart J 102:1075, 1981

Caulin-Glaser T, Setaro JF: Pregnancy and cardiovascular disease. In Burrow GN, Duffy TP (eds): Medical Complications During Pregnancy, 5th ed. Philadelphia, Saunders, 1999, p 111

Chakhtoura N, Angioli R, Yasin S: Use of adenosine for pharmacological cardioversion of SVT in pregnancy. Prim Care Update Ob Gyns 5:154, 1998

Chan WS, Anand S, Ginsberg JS: Anticoagulation of pregnant women with mechanical heart valves: A systematic review of the literature. Arch Intern Med 160:191, 2000

Chandrasekhar S, Cook CR, Collard CD: Cardiac surgery in the parturient. Anesth Analg 108:777, 2009

Chia YT, Yeoh SC, Lim MCL, et al: Pregnancy outcome and mitral valve prolapse. Asia-Oceania J Obstet Gynaecol 20:383, 1994

Clark SL, Cotton DB, Lee W, et al: Central hemodynamic assessment of normal term pregnancy. Am J Obstet Gynecol 161:1439, 1989

Clark SL, Phelan JP, Greenspoon J, et al: Labor and delivery in the presence of mitral stenosis: Central hemodynamic observations. Am J Obstet Gynecol 152:984, 1985

Clark SL, Porter TF, West FG: Coumarin derivatives and breast-feeding. Obstet Gynecol 95:938, 2000

Cotrufo M, De Feo M, De Santo LS, et al: Risk of warfarin during pregnancy with mechanical valve prostheses. Obstet Gynecol 99:35, 2002

Cox SM, Hankins GDV, Leveno KJ, et al: Bacterial endocarditis: A serious pregnancy complication. J Reprod Med 33:671, 1988

Cox SM, Leveno KJ: Pregnancy complicated by bacterial endocarditis. Clin Obstet Gynecol 32:48, 1989

Cunningham FG, Pritchard JA, Hankins GDV, et al: Peripartum heart failure: Idiopathic cardiomyopathy or compounding cardiovascular events? Obstet Gynecol 67:157, 1986

Damilakis J, Theocharopoulos N, Perisinakis K, et al: Conceptus radiation dose and risk from cardiac catheter ablation procedures. Circulation 104:893, 2001

Darouiche RO: Treatment of infections associated with surgical implants. N Engl J Med 350:1422, 2004

Dashe JS, Ramin KD, Ramin SM: Pregnancy following cardiac transplantation. Prim Care Update Ob Gyns 5:257, 1998

Deger R, Ludmir J: *Neisseria sicca* endocarditis complicating pregnancy. J Reprod Med 37:473, 1992

Delacrétaz E: Supraventricular tachycardia. N Engl J Med 354:1039, 2006

Desai DK, Adanlawo M, Naidoo DP, et al: Mitral stenosis in pregnancy: A four-year experience at King Edward VIII Hospital, Durban, South Africa. Br J Obstet Gynaecol 107:953, 2000

de Souza JA, Martinez Jr EE, Ambrose JA, et al: Percutaneous balloon mitral valvuloplasty in comparison with open mitral valve commissurotomy for mitral stenosis during pregnancy. J Am Coll Cardiol 37:900, 2001a

de Souza JL Jr, Frimm CD, Nastari L, et al: Left ventricular function after a new pregnancy in patients with peripartum cardiomyopathy. J Card Fail 7:30, 2001b

Dizon-Townson D, Magee KP, Twickler DM, et al: Coarctation of the abdominal aorta in pregnancy: Diagnosis by magnetic resonance imaging. Obstet Gynecol 85:817, 1995

Drenthen W, Pieper PG, Ploeg M, et al: Risk of complications during pregnancy after Senning or Mustard (atrial) repair of complete transposition of the great arteries. Eur Heart J 26:2588, 2005a

Drenthen W, Pieper PG, Roos-Hesselink JW, et al: Non-cardiac complications during pregnancy in women with isolated congenital pulmonary valvar stenosis. Heart 92:1838, 2006a

Drenthen W, Pieper PG, Roos-Hesselink JW, et al: Pregnancy and delivery in women after Fontan palliation. Heart 92:1290, 2006b

Drenthen W, Pieper PG, van der Tuuk K, et al: Cardiac complications relating to pregnancy and recurrence of disease in the offspring of women with atrioventricular septal defects. Eur Heart J 26:2581, 2005b

Drenthen W, Pieper PG, van der Tuuk K, et al: Fertility, pregnancy and delivery in women after biventricular repair for double outlet right ventricle. Cardiology 109:105, 2008

Dunn JS Jr, Brost BC: Fetal bradycardia after IV adenosine for maternal PSVT. Am J Emerg Med 18:234, 2000

Dwyer BK, Taylor L, Fuller A, et al: Percutaneous transluminal coronary angioplasty and stent placement in pregnancy. Obstet Gynecol 106:1162, 2005

Easterling TR, Benedetti TJ, Schmucker BC, et al: Maternal hemodynamics and aortic diameter in normal and hypertensive pregnancies. Obstet Gynecol 78:1073, 1991

Easterling TR, Chadwick HS, Otto CM, et al: Aortic stenosis in pregnancy. Obstet Gynecol 72:113, 1988

Easterling TR, Ralph DD, Schmucker BC: Pulmonary hypertension in pregnancy: Treatment with pulmonary vasodilators. Obstet Gynecol 93:494, 1999

Eghbali M, Wang Y, Toro L, et al: Heart hypertrophy during pregnancy: A better functioning heart? Trends Cardiovasc Med 16:285, 2006

Elkayam U, Akhter MW, Singh H, et al: Pregnancy-associated cardiomyopathy clinical characteristics and a comparison between early and late presentation. Circ 111:2050, 2005

Elkayam U, Bitar F: Valvular heart disease and pregnancy: Part II: Prosthetic valves. J Am Coll Cardiol 46:403, 2005

Elkayam U, Ostrzega E, Shotan A, et al: Cardiovascular problems in pregnant women with Marfan syndrome. Ann Intern Med 123:117, 1995

Elkayam U, Tummala PP, Rao K, et al: Maternal and fetal outcomes of subsequent pregnancies in women with peripartum cardiomyopathy. N Engl J Med 344:1567, 2001

Erkut B, Kocak H, Becit N, et al: Massive pulmonary embolism complicated by a patent foramen ovale with straddling thrombus: Report of a case. Surg Today 36:528, 2006

Esplin S, Clark SL: Ischemic heart disease and myocardial infarction during pregnancy. Contemp Ob/Gyn 44:27, 1999

Esteves CA, Munoz JS, Braga S, et al: Immediate and long-term follow-up of percutaneous balloon mitral valvuloplasty in pregnant patients with rheumatic mitral stenosis. Am J Cardiol 98:812, 2006

Etheridge MJ, Pepperell RJ: Heart disease and pregnancy at the Royal Women's Hospital. Med J Aust 2:277, 1977

Ezekowitz MD, Levine JA: Preventing stroke in patients with atrial fibrillation. JAMA 281:1830, 1999

Fawzy ME: Percutaneous mitral balloon valvotomy. Cathet Cardio Interv 69:313, 2007

Felker GM, Thompson RE, Hare JM, et al: Underlying causes and long-term survival in patients with initially unexplained cardiomyopathy. N Engl J Med 342:1077, 2000

Fett JD, Sannon H, Thélisma E, et al: Recovery from severe heart failure following peripartum cardiomyopathy. Int J Obstet Gynecol 104:125, 2009

Ford AA, Wylie BJ, Waksmonski CA, et al: Maternal congenital cardiac disease. Outcomes of pregnancy in a single tertiary care center. Obstet Gynecol 112:828, 2008

Ford ES, Ajan UA, Croft JB, et al: Explaining the decrease in U.S. deaths from coronary disease, 1980-2000. N Engl J Med 356:2388, 2007

Ford ES, Capewell S: Coronary heart disease mortality among young adults in the U.S. from 1980 through 2002. J Am Coll Cardiol 50:2128, 2007

Fowler VG, Boucher HW, Corey GR, et al: Daptomycin versus standard therapy for bacteremia and endocarditis caused by *Staphylococcus aureus*. N Engl J Med 355:653, 2006

Friedman T, Mani A, Elefteriades JA: Bicuspid aortic valve: Clinical approach and scientific review of a common clinical entity. Expert Rev Cardiovasc Ther 6:235, 2008

Gardin J, Schumacher D, Constantine G, et al: Valvular abnormalities and cardiovascular status following exposure to dexfenfluramine or phentermine/fenfluramine. JAMA 283:1703, 2000

Gei AF, Hankins GDV: Cardiac disease and pregnancy. Obstet Gynecol Clin North Am 28:465, 2001

Gelson E, Gatzoulis M, Steer PJ, et al: Tetralogy of Fallot: Maternal and neonatal outcomes. BJOG 115:398, 2008

Gilon D, Buonanno FS, Joffe MM, et al: Lack of evidence of an association between mitral-valve prolapse and stroke in young patients. N Engl J Med 341:8, 1999

Gleicher N, Midwall J, Hochberger D, et al: Eisenmenger's syndrome and pregnancy. Obstet Gynecol Surv 34:721, 1979

Gott VL, Greene PS, Alejo DE, et al: Replacement of the aortic root in patients with Marfan's syndrome. N Engl J Med 340:1307, 1999

Gowda RM, Khan IA, Mehta NJ, et al: Cardiac arrhythmias in pregnancy: Clinical and therapeutic considerations. Int J Cardiol 88:129, 2003

Hameed A, Akhter M, Bitar F, et al: Left atrial thrombosis in pregnant women with mitral stenosis and sinus rhythm. Am J Obstet Gynecol 193:501, 2005

Hameed A, Karaalp IS, Tummala PP, et al: The effect of valvular heart disease on maternal and fetal outcome of pregnancy. J Am Coll Cardiol 37:893, 2001

Hanania G, Thomas D, Michel PL, et al: Pregnancy and prosthetic heart valves: A French cooperative retrospective study of 155 cases. Eur Heart J 15:1651, 1994

Hands ME, Johnson MD, Saltzman DH, et al: The cardiac, obstetric, and anesthetic management of pregnancy complicated by acute myocardial infarction. J Clin Anesth 2:258, 1990

Hankins GDV, Wendel GD Jr, Leveno KJ, et al: Myocardial infarction during pregnancy: A review. Obstet Gynecol 65:138, 1985

Hasbun R, Vikram HR, Barakat LA, et al: Complicated left-sided native valve endocarditis in adults: Risk classification for mortality. JAMA 289:1933, 2003

Head CEG, Thorne SA: Congenital heart disease in pregnancy. Postgrad Med J 81:292, 2005

Heron MP, Smith BL: Deaths: Leading causes for 2003. National Vital Statistics Reports, Vol 55, No 10. Hyattsville, MD, National Center for Health Statistics, 2007

Hibbard JU, Lindheimer M, Lang RM: A modified definition for peripartum cardiomyopathy and prognosis based on echocardiography. Obstet Gynecol 94:311, 1999

Hidaka N, Chiba Y, Kurita T, et al: Is intrapartum temporary pacing required for women with complete atrioventricular block? An analysis of seven cases. BJOG 113:605, 2006

Hilfiker-Kleiner D, Kaminski K, Podewski E, et al: A cathepsin D-cleaved 16 kDa form of prolactin mediates postpartum cardiomyopathy. Cell 128:589, 2007

Hoare JV, Radford D: Pregnancy after Fontan repair of complex congenital heart disease. Aust N Z J Obstet Gynaecol 41:464, 2001

Hoen B, Alla F, Selton-Suty C, et al: Changing profile of infective endocarditis: Results of a 1-year survey in France. JAMA 288:75, 2002

Hoendermis ES, Drenthen W, Sollie KM, et al: Severe pregnancy-induced deterioration of truncal valve regurgitation in an adolescent patient with repaired truncus arteriosus. Cardiology 109:177, 2008

Humbert M, Sitbon O, Simonneau G: Treatment of pulmonary arterial hypertension. N Engl J Med 351:1425, 2004

Hytten FE, Chamberlain G: Clinical Physiology in Obstetrics. Oxford, Blackwell, 1991

Iserin L: Management of pregnancy in women with congenital heart disease. Heart 85:493, 2001

Iturbe-Alessio I, Fonseca MDC, Mutchinik O, et al: Risks of anticoagulant therapy in pregnant women with artificial heart valves. N Engl J Med 315:1390, 1986

Jaffe R, Gruber A, Fejgin M, et al: Pregnancy with an artificial pacemaker. Obstet Gynecol Surv 42:137, 1987

James AH, Jamison MG, Biswas MS, et al: Acute myocardial infarction in pregnancy: A United States population-base study. Circulation 113:1564, 2006

Jessup M, Brozena S: Heart failure. N Engl J Med 348:2007, 2003

Kametas NA, McAuliffe F, Krampl E, et al: Maternal cardiac function in twin pregnancy. Obstet Gynecol 102:806, 2003

Kangavari S, Collins J, Cercek B, et al: Tricuspid valve group B streptococcal endocarditis after an elective termination of pregnancy. Clin Cardiol 23:301, 2000

Karchmer AW: Infective endocarditis. In Kasper DL, Braunwald E, Fauci AS, et al (eds): Harrison's Principles of Internal Medicine, 16th ed. New York, McGraw-Hill, 2005, p 731

Karpati PCJ, Rossignol M, Pirot M, et al: High incidence of myocardial ischemia during postpartum hemorrhage. Anesthesiology 100:30, 2004

Kawamata K, Neki R, Yamanaka K, et al: Risks and pregnancy outcome in women with prosthetic mechanical heart valve replacement. Circ J 71:211, 2007

Keizer JL, Zwart JJ, Meerman RH, et al: Obstetric intensive care admission: A 12-year review in a tertiary care centre. Eur J Obstet Gynecol Reprod Biol 128:152, 2006

Kenchaiah S, Evans JC, Levy D, et al: Obesity and the risk of heart failure. N Engl J Med 347:305, 2002

Key TC, Resnik R, Dittrich HC, et al: Successful pregnancy after cardiac transplantation. Am J Obstet Gynecol 160:367, 1989

Khairy P, Ouyang DW, Fernandes SM, et al: Pregnancy outcomes in women with congenital heart disease. Circulation 113:517, 2006

Khan MA, Herzog CA, St. Peter JV, et al: The prevalence of cardiac valvular insufficiency assessed by transthoracic echocardiography in obese patients treated with appetite-suppressant drugs. N Engl J Med 339:713, 1998

Kim KM, Sukhani R, Slogoff S, et al: Central hemodynamic changes associated with pregnancy in a long-term cardiac transplant recipient. Am J Obstet Gynecol 174:1651, 1996

Kiss H, Egarter C, Asseryanis E, et al: Primary pulmonary hypertension in pregnancy: A case report. Am J Obstet Gynecol 172:1052, 1995

Kizer JR, Devereux RB: Patent foramen ovale in young adults with unexplained stroke. N Engl J Med 353:2361, 2005

Koscica KL, Anyaogu C, Bebbington M, et al: Maternal levels of troponin I in patients undergoing vaginal and cesarean delivery. Obstet Gynecol 99:83S, 2002

Kulas T, Habek D: Infective puerperal endocarditis caused by Escherichia coli. J Perinat Med 34:342, 2006

Kung HC, Hoyert DL, Xu J, et al: Deaths: Final data for 2005. NVSR 56(10):121, 2008

Ladner HE, Danielser B, Gilbert WM: Acute myocardial infarction in pregnancy and the puerperium: A population-based study. Obstet Gynecol 105:480, 2005

Lam GK, Stafford RE, Thorp J, et al: Inhaled nitric oxide for primary pulmonary hypertension in pregnancy. Obstet Gynecol 98:895, 2001

Lampert MB, Weinert L, Hibbard J, et al: Contractile reserve in patients with peripartum cardiomyopathy and recovered left ventricular function. Am J Obstet Gynecol 176:189, 1997

Lang RM, Borow KM: Heart disease. In Barron WM, Lindheimer MD (eds): Medical Disorders During Pregnancy. St. Louis, Mosby Yearbook, 1991, p 148

Lao TT, Adelman AG, Sermer M, et al: Balloon valvuloplasty for congenital aortic stenosis in pregnancy. Br J Obstet Gynaecol 100:1141, 1993

Lederle FA, Wilson SE, Johnson GR, et al: Immediate repair compared with surveillance of small abdominal aortic aneurysms. N Engl J Med 346:1437, 2002

Lee C-N, Wu C-C, Lin P-Y, et al: Pregnancy following cardiac prosthetic valve replacement. Obstet Gynecol 83:353, 1994

Lee LC, Bathgate SL, Macri CJ: Arrhythmogenic right ventricular dysplasia in pregnancy. A case report. J Reprod Med 51:725, 2006

Lee MJ, Huang A, Gillen-Goldstein J, et al: Labor and vaginal delivery with maternal aortic aneurysm. Obstet Gynecol 98:935, 2001

Lesniak-Sobelga A, Tracz W, Kostkiewicz M, et al: Clinical and echocardiographic assessment of pregnant women with valvular heart disease—maternal and fetal outcome. Intl J Cardiol 94:15, 2004

Leyh RG, Fischer S, Ruhparwar A, et al: Anticoagulant therapy in pregnant women with mechanical heart valves. Arch Gynecol Obstet 268:1, 2003

Leyh RG, Fischer S, Ruhparwar A, et al: Anticoagulation for prosthetic heart valves during pregnancy: Is low-molecular-weight heparin an alternative? Eur J Cardiothorac Surg 21:577, 2002

Löwenstein BR, Vain NW, Perrone SV, et al: Successful pregnancy and vaginal delivery after heart transplantation. Am J Obstet Gynecol 158:589, 1988

Lupton M, Oteng-Ntim E, Ayida G, et al: Cardiac disease in pregnancy. Curr Opin Obstet Gynecol 14:137, 2002

MacArthur A, Cook L, Pollard JK, et al: Peripartum myocardial ischemia: A review of Canadian deliveries from 1970 to 1998. Am J Obstet Gynecol 194:1027, 2006

MacKay AP, Berg CJ, Duran C, et al: An assessment of pregnancy-related mortality in the United States. Paediat Perinat Epidemiol 19:206, 2005

Madazli R, Şal V, Çift T, et al: Pregnancy outcomes in women with heart disease. Arch Gynecol Obstet [Epub ahead of print], 2009

Makaryus AN, Forouzesh A, Johnson M: Pregnancy in the patient with Eisenmenger's syndrome. Mount Sinai J Med 73:1033, 2006

Maron BJ: Hypertrophic cardiomyopathy: An important global disease. Am J Med 116:63, 2004

McAnulty JH, Metcalfe J, Ueland K: Heart disease and pregnancy. In Hurst JW, Schlant RC, Rackley CE, et al (eds): The Heart, 7th ed. New York, McGraw-Hill, 1990, p 1465

McFaul PB, Dornan JC, Lamki H, et al: Pregnancy complicated by maternal heart disease: A review of 519 women. Br J Obstet Gynaecol 95:861, 1988

McKay DB, Josephson MA: Pregnancy in recipients of solid organs—Effects on mother and child. N Engl J Med 354:1281, 2006

McLaughlin VV, Presberg KW, Doyle RL, et al: Prognosis of pulmonary arterial hypertension: ACCP evidence-based clinical practice guidelines. Chest 126:78S, 2004

Meijboom LJ, Drenthen W, Pieper PG, et al: Obstetric complications in Marfan syndrome. Intl J Cardiol 110:53, 2006

Meijer JM, Pieper PG, Drenthen W, et al: Pregnancy, fertility, and recurrence risk in corrected tetralogy of Fallot. Heart 91:801, 2005

Mielniczuk LM, Williams K, Davis DR, et al: Peripartum cardiomyopathy: Frequency of peripartum cardiomyopathy. Am J Cardiol 97:1765, 2006

Miniero R, Tardivo I, Centofanti P, et al: Pregnancy in heart transplant recipients. J Heart Lung Transplant 23:898, 2004

Morris CD, Reller MD, Menashe VD: Thirty-year incidence of infective endocarditis after surgery for congenital heart defect. JAMA 279:599, 1998

Mousa HA, McKinley CA, Thong J: Acute postpartum myocardial infarction after ergometrine administration in a woman with familial hypercholesterolaemia. Br J Obstet Gynaecol 107:939, 2000

Mul TFM, van Herwerden LA, Cohen-Overbeek TE, et al: Hypoxic–ischemic fetal insult resulting from maternal aortic root replacement, with normal fetal heart rate at term. Am J Obstet Gynecol 179:825, 1998

Nagorney DM, Field CS: Successful pregnancy 10 years after triple cardiac valve replacement. Obstet Gynecol 57:386, 1981

Nahapetian A, Oudiz RJ: Serial hemodynamics and complications of pregnancy in severe pulmonary arterial hypertension. Cardiology 109:237, 2008

Nanson J, Elcock D, Williams M, et al: Do physiological changes in pregnancy change defibrillation energy requirements? Br J Anaesth 87:237, 2001

Nassar AH, Hobeika EM, Abd Essamad HM, et al: Pregnancy outcome in women with prosthetic heart valves. Am J Obstet Gynecol 191:1009, 2004

Nishimura RA, Holmes Jr DR: Hypertrophic obstructive cardiomyopathy. N Engl J Med 350:1320, 2004

O'Gara P, Braunwald E: Valvular Heart Disease. In Fauci AS, Braunwald E, Kasper KL, et al (eds): Harrison's Principles of Internal Medicine, 17th ed, New York, McGraw-Hill, 2008, p 1465

O'Gara PT, Greenfield AJ, Afridi NA, et al: Case 12-2004: A 38-year-old woman with acute onset of pain in the chest. N Engl J Med 350:16, 2004

Oosterhof T, Meijboom FJ, Vliegen HW, et al: Long-term follow-up of homograft function after pulmonary valve replacement in patients with tetralogy of Fallot. Eur Heart J 27:1478, 2006

Oron G, Hirsch R, Ben-Haroush A, et al: Pregnancy outcome in women with heart disease undergoing induction of labour. BJOG 111:669, 2004

Osio A, Tan L, Chen SN, et al: Myozenin 2 is a novel gene for human hypertrophic cardiomyopathy. Circ Res 100:766, 2007

Ozer O, Cebesoy FM, Sari I, et al: A case of Salmonella typhi endocarditis in pregnancy. Am J Med Sci 337(3):210, 2009

Papatsonis DNM, Heetkamp A, van den Hombergh C, et al: Acute type A aortic dissection complicating pregnancy at 32 weeks: Surgical repair after cesarean section. Am J Perinatol 26(2):153, 2009

Pappone C, Santinelli V, Manguso F, et al: A randomized study of prophylactic catheter ablation in asymptomatic patients with the Wolff-Parkinson-White syndrome. N Engl J Med 349:1803, 2003

Parneix M, Fanou L, Morau E, et al: Low-dose combined spinal-epidural anaesthesia for caesarean section in a patient with Eisenmenger's syndrome. Int J Obstet Anesth 18:81, 2009

Pavankumar P, Venugopal P, Kaul U, et al: Closed mitral valvotomy during pregnancy: A 20 year experience. Scand J Thorac Cardiovasc Surg 22:11, 1988

Pearson GD, Veille JC, Rahimtoola S, et al: Peripartum cardiomyopathy. National Heart, Lung, and Blood Institute and Office of Rare Diseases (National Institutes of Health) Workshop Recommendations and Review. JAMA 283:1183, 2000

Penning S, Robinson KD, Major CA, et al: A comparison of echocardiography and pulmonary artery catheterization for evaluation of pulmonary artery pressures in pregnant patients with suspected pulmonary hypertension. Am J Obstet Gynecol 184:1568, 2001

Pepin M, Schwarze U, Superti-Furga A, et al: Clinical and genetic features of Ehlers–Danlos syndrome type IV, the vascular type. N Engl J Med 342:673, 2000

Pocock SB, Chen KT: Inappropriate use of antibiotic prophylaxis to prevent infective endocarditis in obstetric patients. Obstet Gynecol 108:280, 2006

Pollack KL, Chestnut DH, Wenstrom KD: Anesthetic management of a parturient with Eisenmenger's syndrome. Anesth Analg 70:212, 1990

Pombar X, Strassner HT, Fenner PC: Pregnancy in a woman with class H diabetes mellitus and previous coronary artery bypass graft: A case report and review of the literature. Obstet Gynecol 85:825, 1995

Rahimtoola SH: The year in valvular heart disease. J Am Coll Cardiol 47:427, 2006

Rahman J, Rahman FZ, Rahman W, et al: Obstetric and gynecologic complications in women with Marfan syndrome. J Reprod Med 48:723, 2003

Rashba EJ, Zareba W, Moss AJ, et al: Influence of pregnancy on the risk for cardiac events in patients with hereditary long QT syndrome. Circulation 97:451, 1998

Rayburn WF, LeMire MS, Bird JL, et al: Mitral valve prolapse: Echocardiographic changes during pregnancy. J Reprod Med 32:185, 1987

Reece EA, Egan JFX, Coustan DR, et al: Coronary artery disease in diabetic pregnancies. Am J Obstet Gynecol 154:150, 1986

Reich O, Tax P, Marek J, et al: Long term results of percutaneous balloon valvoplasty of congenital aortic stenosis: Independent predictors of outcome. Heart 90:70, 2004

Reimold SC, Rutherford JD: Valvular heart disease in pregnancy. N Engl J Med 349:52, 2003

Rich S, McLaughlin VV: Pulmonary hypertension. In Zipes (ed): Brauwald's Heart Disease: A Textbook of Cardiovascular Medicine, 7th ed. Saunders, 2005, p 1817

Ro A, Frishman WH: Peripartum cardiomyopathy. Cardiol Rev 14:35, 2006

Robins K, Lyons G: Supraventricular tachycardia in pregnancy. Br J Anaesth 92:140, 2004

Roden DM: Drug-induced prolongation of the QT interval. N Engl J Med 350:1013, 2004

Roden DM: Long-QT syndrome. N Engl J Med 358:169, 2008

Roeleveld RJ, Vonk-Noordegraaf A, Marcus JT, et al: Effects of epoprostenol on right ventricular hypertrophy and dilatation in pulmonary hypertension. Chest 125:572, 2004

Roldan CA, Shively BK, Crawford MH: An echocardiographic study of valvular heart disease associated with systemic lupus erythematosus. N Engl J Med 335:1424, 1996

Ross LF: Ethical considerations related to pregnancy in transplant recipients. N Engl J Med 354:1313, 2006

Rossiter JP, Repke JT, Morales AJ, et al: A prospective longitudinal evaluation of pregnancy in the Marfan syndrome. Am J Obstet Gynecol 173:1599, 1995

Roth A, Elkayam U: Acute myocardial infarction associated with pregnancy. J Am Coll Cardiol 52:171, 2008

Rowan JA, McCowan LM, Raudkivi PJ, et al: Enoxaparin treatment in women with mechanical heart valves during pregnancy. Am J Obstet Gynecol 185:633, 2001

Sadler L, McCowan L, White H, et al: Pregnancy outcomes and cardiac complications in women with mechanical, bioprosthetic and homograft valves. Br J Obstet Gynaecol 107:245, 2000

Sawhney H, Aggarwal N, Suri V, et al: Maternal and perinatal outcome in rheumatic heart disease. Int J Gynaecol Obstet 80:9, 2003

Sbarouni E, Oakley CM: Outcome of pregnancy in women with valve prostheses. Br Heart J 71:196, 1994

Schade R, Andersohn F, Suissa S, et al: Dopamine agonists and the risk of cardiac-valve regurgitation. N Engl J Med 356:29, 2007

Schulte-Sasse U: Life threatening myocardial ischaemia associated with the use of prostaglandin E_1 to induce abortion. Br J Obstet Gynaecol 107:700, 2000

Schumacher B, Belfort MA, Card RJ: Successful treatment of acute myocardial infarction during pregnancy with tissue plasminogen activator. Am J Obstet Gynecol 176:716, 1997

Seaworth BJ, Durack DT: Infective endocarditis in obstetric and gynecologic practice. Am J Obstet Gynecol 154:180, 1986

Seeburger J, Wilhelm-Mohr F, Falk V: Acute type A dissection at 17 weeks of gestation in a Marfan patient. Ann Thorac Surg 83:674, 2007

Seth R, Moss AJ, McNitt S, et al: Long QT syndrome and pregnancy. J Am Coll Cardiol 49:1092, 2007

Shade GH Jr, Ross G, Bever FN, et al: Troponin I in the diagnosis of acute myocardial infarction in pregnancy, labor, and postpartum. Am J Obstet Gynecol 187:1719, 2002

Sheffield JS, Cunningham FG: Diagnosing and managing peripartum cardiomyopathy. Contemp Ob/Gyn 44:74, 1999

Sheffield JS, Cunningham FG: Thyrotoxicosis and heart failure that complicate pregnancy. Am J Obstet Gynecol 190:211, 2004

Sherer DM: Coarctation of the descending thoracic aorta diagnosed during pregnancy. Obstet Gynecol 100:1094, 2002

Shivvers SA, Wians FH Jr, Keffer JH, et al: Maternal cardiac troponin I levels during normal labor and delivery. Am J Obstet Gynecol 180:122, 1999

Shores J, Berger KR, Murphy EA, et al: Progression of aortic dilatation and the benefit of long-term β-adrenergic blockade in Marfan's syndrome. N Engl J Med 330:1335, 1994

Sigel CS, Harper TC, Thorne LB: Postpartum sudden death from pulmonary hypertension in the setting of portal hypertension. Obstet Gynecol 110:501, 2007

Silversides CK, Harris L, Haberer K, et al: Recurrence rates of arrhythmias during pregnancy in women with previous tachyarrhythmia and impact on fetal and neonatal outcomes. Am J Cardiol 97:1206, 2006

Simmoneau G, Galie N, Rubin LJ, et al: Clinical classification of pulmonary hypertension. J Am Coll Cardiol 43:55, 2004

Simpson LL, D'Alton ME: Marfan syndrome: An update on pregnancy. Prim Care Update Ob Gyns 4:1, 1997

Singh H, Bolton PJ, Oakley CM: Pregnancy after surgical correction of tetralogy of Fallot. BMJ 285:168, 1982

Siu SC, Colman JM: Congenital heart disease: Heart disease and pregnancy. Heart 85:710, 2001

Siu SC, Sermer M, Colman JM, et al: Prospective multicenter study of pregnancy outcomes in women with heart disease. Circulation 104:515, 2001

Siu SC, Sermer M, Harrison DA, et al: Risk and predictors for pregnancy-related complications in women with heart disease. Circulation 96:2789, 1997

Siva A, Shah AM: Moderate mitral stenosis in pregnancy: The haemodynamic impact of diuresis. Heart 91:e3, 2005

Smith IJ, Gillham MJ: Fulminant peripartum cardiomyopathy rescue with extracorporeal membranous oxygenation. Int J Obstet Anesthe 18:186, 2009

Smith RL, Young SJ, Greer IA: The parturient with coronary heart disease. Int J Obstet Anesth 17:46, 2008

Spirito P, Autore C: Management of hypertrophic cardiomyopathy. BMJ 332:1251, 2006

Stangl V, Schad J, Gossing G, et al: Maternal heart disease and pregnancy outcome: A single-centre experience. Eur J Heart Fail 10:855, 2008

Suri V, Sawhney H, Vasishta K, et al: Pregnancy following cardiac valve replacement surgery. Int J Gynaecol Obstet 64:239, 1999

Sutaria N, O'Toole L, Northridge D: Postpartum acute MI following routine ergometrine administration treated successfully by primary PTCA. Heart 83:97, 2000

Sutton SW, Duncan MA, Chase VA, et al: Cardiopulmonary bypass and mitral valve replacement during pregnancy. Perfusion 20:359, 2005

Thaman R, Varnava A, Hamid MS, et al: Pregnancy related complications in women with hypertrophic cardiomyopathy. Heart 89:752, 2003

Tzemos N, Silversides CK, Colman JM, et al: Late cardiac outcomes after pregnancy in women with congenital aortic stenosis. Am Heart J 157:474, 2009

Van der Meer JTM, Van Wijk W, Thompson J, et al: Efficacy of antibiotic prophylaxis for prevention of native-valve endocarditis. Lancet 339:135, 1992

Vinatier D, Virelizier S, Depret-Mosser S, et al: Pregnancy after myocardial infarction. Eur J Obstet Gynecol Reprod Biol 56:89, 1994

Weiss BM, Maggiorini M, Jenni R, et al: Pregnant patient with primary pulmonary hypertension: Inhaled pulmonary vasodilators and epidural anesthesia for cesarean delivery. Anesthesiology 92:1191, 2000

Weiss BM, Zemp L, Seifert B, et al: Outcome of pulmonary vascular disease in pregnancy: A systematic overview from 1978 through 1996. J Am Coll Cardiol 31:1650, 1998

Wilson W, Taubert KA, Gewitz M, et al: Prevention of infective endocarditis: guidelines from the American Heart Association: a guideline from the American Heart Association Rheumatic Fever, Endocarditis and Kawasaki Disease Committee, Council on Cardiovascular Disease in the Young, and the Council on Clinical Cardiology, Council on Cardiovascular Surgery and Anesthesia, and the Quality of Care and Outcomes Research Interdisciplinary Working Group. Circulation 116:1736, 2007

Wynne J, Braunwald E: Cardiomyopathy and Myocarditis. In Fauci AS, Braunwald E, Kasper KL, et al (eds): Harrison's Principles of Internal Medicine, 17th ed, New York, McGraw-Hill, 2008, p. 1481

Williams A, Child A, Rowntree J, et al: Marfan's syndrome: Successful pregnancy after aortic root and arch replacement. Br J Obstet Gynaecol 109:1187, 2002

Xia V.W, Messerlian AK, Mackley J, et al: Successful epidural anesthesia for cesarean section in a parturient with severe aortic stenosis and a recent history of pulmonary edema—A case report. J Clin Anesth 18:142, 2006

Yang X, Wang H, Wang Z, et al: Alteration and significance of serum cardiac troponin I and cystatin C in preeclampsia (Letter). Clin Chim Acta 374:168, 2006

Yuan L, Duan Y, Cao T: Echocardiographic study of cardiac morphological and functional changes before and after parturition in pregnancy-induced hypertension. Echocardiography 23:177, 2006

Zaidi AN, Raman SV, Cook SC: Acute myocardial infarction in early pregnancy: Definition of myocardium at risk with noncontrast T2-weighted cardiac magnetic resonance. Am J Obstet Gynecol e9, March 2008

Zanettini R, Antonini A, Gatto G, et al: Valvular heart disease and the use of dopamine agonists for Parkinson's disease. N Engl J Med 356:39, 2007

Zeeman GG: Obstetric critical care: A blueprint for improved outcomes. Crit Care Med 34:S208, 2006

Zuber M, Gautschi N, Oechslin E, et al: Outcome of pregnancy in women with congenital shunt lesions. Heart 81:271, 1999

Zwiers WJ, Blodgett TM, Vallejo MC, et al: Successful vaginal delivery for a parturient with complete aortic coarctation. J Clin Anesth 18:300, 2006

CHAPTER 45

Chronic Hypertension

Worldwide, it is estimated that hypertension affected 972 million adults in 2000, and it was further predicted this would increase to 1.56 billion by 2025 (Kearney and colleagues, 2005). The prevalence of chronic hypertension in American women has been chronicled since 1960 by the National Center for Health Statistics (1964). The ongoing study—the National Health and Nutrition Examination Survey (NHANES)—still provides periodic information. The average prevalence of hypertension in women 18 to 39 years of age was 7.2 percent for the 1999–2000 biennium (Hajjar and Kotchen, 2003). This is a substantive increase when compared with 6 percent for the previous decade. Importantly, a third of these patients are unaware of their hypertension, and its importance in relation to women's healthcare was highlighted in the Clinical Update by the American College of Obstetricians and Gynecologists (2005).

Chronic hypertension is also one of the most common medical complications encountered during pregnancy. For example, Podymow and August (2007) cite a 3-percent incidence from their review. Its variable incidence and severity, along with the well-known proclivity for pregnancy to induce or aggravate hypertension, has caused confusion concerning its management.

Most women with antecedent hypertension demonstrate improved blood-pressure control during pregnancy. In others, however, there is worsening of hypertension that may be accompanied by proteinuria, symptoms, and convulsions. These latter women in whom hypertension antedates pregnancy are indistinguishable from an otherwise normotensive woman who develops preeclampsia in her first pregnancy.

DEFINITIONS

There is a wide range of blood pressures in normal adults as well as in those with chronic hypertension. Categorization therefore relates to acute or long-term adverse effects associated with sustained levels of those blood pressures. These associations with normal or abnormal blood pressures are primarily based on morbidity and mortality in men. A useful categorization is that provided by the Joint National Committee on Prevention, Detection, Evaluation, and Treatment of High Blood Pressure. In its seventh report—JNC-7—the Joint National Committee (2003) used the classification and management scheme summarized in Table 45-1. A newly added significant change is the category termed *prehypertension*, which was intended to convey that cardiovascular risk begins to increase at levels of 115 mm Hg systolic and 75 mm Hg diastolic. Within each of these categories shown in Table 45-1, morbidity or mortality rates are further influenced by age, gender, race, and personal behaviors that include smoking, excessive alcohol, obesity, and physical activity.

Proven benefits accrue with treatment of chronic hypertension at sustained diastolic pressures of 90 mm Hg or greater using Korotkoff phase, systolic pressures of 160 mm Hg or more, or both. Benefits are apparent even in otherwise healthy adults. Treatment at even lower levels may benefit patients with evidence of renal or cardiac dysfunction, those who have had a cerebrovascular thrombosis or hemorrhage, elderly patients, or patients with appreciable underlying atherosclerotic disease or

TABLE 45-1. Classification and Management of Blood Pressure for Adults

| | Blood Pressure | | | Management[a] | |
| | | | | Initial Drug Therapy | |
Classification	Systolic mm Hg	Diastolic mm Hg	Lifestyle Modification	Without Compelling Indication	With Compelling Indications[b]
Normal	<120	and <80	Encourage	Treatment not indicated	Chronic renal disease or diabetes
Prehypertension	120–139	or 80–90	Yes		
Stage 1 Hypertension	140–159	or 90–99	Yes	Thiazide-type diuretics for most. May consider ACE inhibitor, ARB, β-blocker, CCB, or combination	Chronic renal disease or diabetes. Other drugs as needed: diuretics, ACE inhibitors, ARB, β-blocker, CCB
Stage 2 Hypertension	≥160	or ≥100	Yes	Two-drug combination for most[c]: usually thiazide-type diuretic and ACEI, or ARB, or β-blocker, or CCB[c]	

[a]Treatment determined by highest blood pressure category.
[b]Treat patients with chronic kidney disease or diabetes to a goal of blood pressure < 130/80 mm Hg.
[c]Initial combined therapy should be used cautiously in those at risk for orthostatic hypotension.
ACEI = angiotensin-converting enzyme inhibitor; ARB = angiotensin-receptor blocker; CCB = calcium-channel blocker.
From the Joint National Committee (2003).

postmyocardial infarction. The Seventh Joint National Committee report (2003) recommends:

1. In persons older than 50 years, systolic pressures >140 mm Hg are a more important cardiovascular disease risk factor than diastolic pressure
2. Individuals with a systolic blood pressure of 120 to 139 mm Hg, or a diastolic blood pressure of 80 to 89 mm Hg, should be considered as *prehypertensive* and require health-promoting lifestyle modifications to prevent cardiovascular disease
3. Thiazide-type diuretics should be used in drug treatment for most patients with uncomplicated hypertension, either alone or combined with drugs from other classes
4. Most adults with hypertension require two or more medications to achieve a blood pressure less than 140/90 mm Hg or less than 130/80 mm Hg in patients with diabetes or renal disease.

Throughout middle and old age, blood pressure is strongly and directly related to vascular as well as overall mortality rates and with values down to at least 115/75 mm Hg (Prospective Studies Collaboration, 2002; Qureshi and colleagues, 2002).

DIAGNOSIS

Chronic hypertension precedes pregnancy or may be apparent prior to 20 weeks (see Chap. 34, p. 709). Some women without overt chronic hypertension have repeated pregnancies in which *transient hypertension* appears only late in pregnancy and regresses postpartum. It is considered evidence of latent chronic hypertension, and thus it is analogous to gestational diabetes. Long-term follow-up studies of Chesley and co-workers (1976) and Sibai and colleagues (1986b, 1992) support this view.

In most women with hypertension antedating pregnancy, elevated blood pressure is the only demonstrable finding. Some, however, have complications that increase the risks during pregnancy and may shorten life expectancy. These include hypertensive or ischemic cardiac disease, renal insufficiency, or a prior cerebrovascular event. These are encountered more frequently in older women.

Obesity is an important factor predisposing to chronic hypertension (see Chap. 43). Specifically, the prevalence of hypertension may be increased as much as tenfold in obese women, and these women also are more likely to develop superimposed preeclampsia. Diabetes mellitus is also prevalent in chronically hypertensive women, and its interplay with obesity is overwhelming. Heredity has an important role, and according to the review by Cowley (2006), there are hundreds of blood pressure–related phenotypes and genomic regions that have been identified. In some cases, candidate genes for preeclampsia and chronic hypertension have been described (Levesque and associates, 2004). Hypertension is common in African- and Latino-Americans, and frequently many members of the same family are hypertensive. Wang and colleagues (2006) observed significant ethnic and gender differences in a 15-year longitudinal study of blood pressures in African- and European-American young adults. They reported that the nocturnal blood-pressure decline was blunted and also exacerbated with age in African-American patients.

Chronic hypertension all too frequently remains undetected. Even if detected, therapy is not universal, not always adequate, and not always monitored appropriately. For example, Roumie and colleagues (2006) reported poor blood-pressure control in 65 percent of hypertensive patients. This is worsened by the alarming frequency reported with medication noncompliance (Simpson, 2006).

Pregnancy

In most women with chronic hypertension, blood pressure falls in early pregnancy and then rises during the third trimester to levels somewhat above those in early pregnancy (Fig. 45-1). According to studies by Tihtonen and associates (2007), women with chronic hypertension have persistently elevated vascular resistance and possibly reduced intravascular volume increase. There is no doubt that adverse outcomes in these women are dependent largely on whether superimposed preeclampsia develops. This may be related to observations reported by Hibbard and colleagues (2005) that arterial mechanical properties are most marked in women with superimposed preeclampsia.

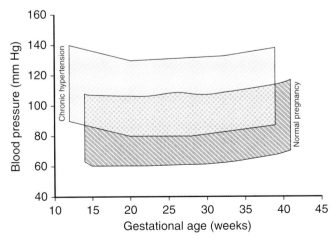

FIGURE 45-1 Mean systolic and diastolic blood pressures across pregnancy in 90 untreated chronically hypertensive women (*yellow*). Compared with mean blood pressures across pregnancy in 4589 healthy nulliparous women (*blue*). (Data from Levine and associates, 1997; Sibai and colleagues, 1990a.)

TREATMENT FOR NONPREGNANT ADULTS

Even with mildly elevated blood pressures shown in Table 45-1, interventions to reduce pressure are beneficial. Almost 30 trials involving nearly 162,000 participants have established that antihypertensive treatment of adults with mild to moderate hypertension will decrease mortality rates, stroke, and major cardiac events (Blood Pressure Lowering Treatment Trialists' Collaboration, 2003; Psaty and colleagues, 2003). Reductions in stroke average approximately 35 percent, myocardial infarction about 25 percent, and heart failure more than 50 percent (Neal and colleagues, 2000). In patients with stage 1 hypertension who have additional cardiovascular risk factors, a sustained 12-mm Hg reduction in systolic pressure will decrease 10-year mortality rates by 10 percent (Ogden and colleagues, 2000).

Most women with stage 1 hypertension would ideally have been prescribed lifestyle modifications and antihypertensive medications (Table 45-2). Low-dose diuretics are very effective for first-line treatment. In the ALLHAT Trial (2002) of 33,357 adults 55 years or older, thiazide-type diuretics were superior to and less expensive than angiotensin-converting enzyme (ACE) inhibitors or calcium-channel blockers to prevent cardiovascular disease. These results were similar for women treated in the Second Australian National Blood Pressure Study Group (Wing and associates, 2003). In the CONVINCE Trial reported by Black and colleagues (2003), 16,602 hypertensive adults with one or more risk factors for cardiovascular disease were randomized to verapamil, atenolol, or hydrochlorothiazide. Over a 3-year period, verapamil was the least effective to reduce cardiovascular disease.

In older adults, daily *low-dose aspirin* is recommended for the prevention of myocardial infarction. Hermida and colleagues (2005) reported significant lowering of blood pressure in 328 untreated hypertensive patients given 100 mg of aspirin at bedtime—but not on awakening. Further data are obviously needed. Abbott and Bakris (2004) have provided a useful summary of treatment trials done to study essential hypertension.

From the foregoing, it is clear that antihypertensive therapy in nonpregnant reproductive-aged women with sustained diastolic pressures of 90 mm Hg or greater would be considered standard. In women identified to have chronic hypertension prior to midpregnancy, the benefits and safety of instituting antihypertensive therapy are less clear, as subsequently discussed.

PRECONCEPTIONAL AND EARLY PREGNANCY EVALUATION

Women with chronic hypertension should ideally be counseled prior to pregnancy (see Chap. 7, p. 177). The duration of hypertension, degree of blood-pressure control, and current therapy are ascertained. Women with average pressures greater than 135/85 mm Hg measured at home are considered to be hypertensive. Home measurement devices should be checked for accuracy (American Heart Association, 2004). General health, daily activities, diet, and adverse behaviors are also assessed.

TABLE 45-2. Lifestyle Modifications to Manage Hypertension

Modification[a]	Recommendation	Systolic Blood Pressure Reduction (Range)
Weight reduction	Maintain normal body weight: BMI 18.5–24.9 kg/m²	5–20 mm Hg/10 kg weight loss
DASH eating plan	Diet rich in fruits, vegetables, and low-fat dairy products with a reduced content of saturated and total fat	8–14 mm Hg
Dietary sodium reduction	Reduce dietary sodium intake to no more than 100 mmol per day: 2.4 g sodium or 6 g sodium chloride	2–8 mm Hg
Physical activity	Engage in regular aerobic physical activity such as brisk walking, at least 30 min per day, most days of the week	4–9 mm Hg
Alcohol consumption moderation	Limit consumption to no more than 2 drinks—1-oz or 30-mL ethanol, e.g., 24-oz beer, 10-oz wine, or 3-oz 80-proof whiskey—per day in most men and to no more than 1 drink per day in women and lighter weight persons	2–4 mm Hg

[a]The effects of implementing these modifications are dose and time dependent, and could be greater for some individuals.
BMI = body mass index; DASH = dietary approaches to stop hypertension.
From the Joint National Committee (2003).

Women with prior adverse events such as a cerebrovascular accident or myocardial infarction, as well as cardiac or renal dysfunction, are at markedly increased risk for a recurrence or worsening during pregnancy. Those who require multiple medications for control, or those who are poorly controlled, are also at increased risk for adverse pregnancy outcomes.

Renal and cardiovascular function should be assessed. Ophthalmological evaluation and echocardiography are indicated in women with any prior adverse outcome or in those with long-term hypertension. Gainer and co-workers (2005) found that pregnant women with treated chronic hypertension commonly have underlying heart lesions such as left ventricular hypertrophy determined by echocardiography. Cardiac dysrhythmias or evidence of left ventricular hypertrophy indicate long-standing or poorly controlled hypertension, or both. Women with these conditions are at increased risk for heart failure during pregnancy (see Chap. 42, p. 929).

Renal function is assessed by serum creatinine measurement and quantification of proteinuria. If either is abnormal, there is further increased risk for adverse pregnancy outcomes. The Working Group Report on High Blood Pressure in Pregnancy (2000) of the National Heart, Lung, and Blood Institute concluded that the risks of fetal loss and accelerated deterioration of renal disease are increased if serum creatinine is above 1.4 mg/dL around the time of conception. It can be difficult to separate the effects of the pregnancy from progression of renal disease (Cunningham, 1990; Lindheimer, 2007; Ramin, 2006, and all their associates). Severity of renal insufficiency is proportional to the risk of hypertensive complications during pregnancy, although the relationship is not linear (see Chap. 48, p. 1040). Most clinicians believe that pregnancy is relatively contraindicated in women who maintain persistent diastolic pressures of ≥110 mm Hg despite therapy, require multiple antihypertensives, or have a serum creatinine level of >2 mg/dL. Stronger contraindications are prior cerebrovascular thrombosis or hemorrhage, myocardial infarction, or cardiac failure. Symptoms at rest and with activity should be determined.

Of interest, Poyares and colleagues (2007) recommend use of nasal continuous positive airway pressure (CPAP) at night in women with chronic hypertension and who chronically snore. They reported better blood-pressure control and improved pregnancy outcomes with CPAP use.

EFFECTS OF CHRONIC HYPERTENSION ON PREGNANCY

Maternal Morbidity/Mortality

Most women taking monotherapy whose hypertension is well controlled prior to pregnancy do well. That said, even these women are at increased risk for superimposed preeclampsia and placental abruption. Jain (1997) reported a maternal mortality rate of 230 per 100,000 live births in women with chronic hypertension. Complications were more likely with severe baseline maternal disease, especially with documented end-organ damage. More recently, Gilbert and colleagues (2007) reported pregnancy outcomes in 29,842 chronically hypertensive California women from 1991 to 2001. In addition to markedly increased fetal, neonatal, and in-hospital maternal mortality rates, there was also markedly increased maternal morbidity including stroke and renal failure.

Pregnancy-aggravated hypertension manifests as an increase in blood pressure. Systolic pressures >200 mm Hg or diastolic pressures >130 mm Hg may rapidly result in renal or cardiopulmonary dysfunction. When there is superimposed severe preeclampsia or eclampsia, the maternal prognosis is poor unless the pregnancy is terminated. Placental abruption is a common and serious complication (see Chap. 35, p. 761). Aortic dissection at term has been described by Weissman-Brenner and associates (2004) and is discussed in Chapter 44 (p. 976).

Hypertensive disorders contribute appreciably to maternal mortality rates. This is especially of concern in less developed countries. The World Health Organization (2004) reported the maternal mortality rate in 2000 to be 440 per 100,000 in developing countries compared with 20 per 100,000 in developed countries. Moodley (2007) reported that 18 percent of 3406 maternal deaths from 2002 to 2004 in South Africa were associated with hypertensive disorders. Of these 628 deaths, cerebrovascular complications were responsible for half.

Superimposed Preeclampsia

There is no precise definition of superimposed preeclampsia in women with chronic hypertension. In their review, August and Lindheimer (1999) reported that superimposed preeclampsia developed in 4 to 40 percent of women. The risk of superimposed preeclampsia is directly related to the severity of baseline hypertension, especially early in pregnancy, as well as the need for treatment to achieve control. In a Maternal-Fetal Medicine Units Network trial, Caritis and co-workers (1998) used predefined criteria to diagnose preeclampsia in 774 women with chronic hypertension. They identified superimposed preeclampsia in 25 percent. The incidence of superimposed preeclampsia was similar whether or not the women had baseline proteinuria (Sibai and co-workers, 1998). It was, however, significantly increased in those who had hypertension for at least 4 years or who had preeclampsia during a prior pregnancy.

There is evidence that women destined to develop superimposed preeclampsia may be identified early. Zeeman and colleagues (2003) found that uterine artery Doppler velocimetry findings of increased impedance at 16 to 20 weeks were predictive of superimposed preeclampsia at 28 to 32 weeks. Riskin-Mashiah and Belfort (2004, 2005) reported that pregnant women with mild chronic hypertension had normal cerebral vasomotor reactivity to carbon dioxide (CO_2) breathing and isometric handgrip testing. They then studied 17 such women during midpregnancy. The seven women who subsequently developed superimposed preeclampsia demonstrated increased Doppler-determined perfusion pressure when they inhaled 5 percent CO_2 or when exposed to a 2-minute isometric handgrip test.

More recently, there has been interest in the use of circulating angiogenic factor levels to discriminate among chronic hypertension, gestational hypertension, and preeclampsia (Moore Simas, 2007; Sibai, 2008; Woolcock, 2008, and all their associates). This is discussed further in Chapter 34 (p. 714).

Prevention of Superimposed Preeclampsia. Trials of low-dose aspirin to prevent preeclampsia in women with chronic hypertension have shown little tangible benefits. In the Network study by Caritis and associates (1998) cited above, the incidence of superimposed preeclampsia, fetal-growth restriction, or both

was similar in women given low-dose aspirin or placebo. Reduced maternal serum levels of thromboxane B_2 were also not predictive of improved pregnancy outcomes in women given low-dose aspirin (Hauth and colleagues, 1998).

The efficacy of low-dose aspirin is not entirely settled. Both Duley (2007) and Meads (2008) and their colleagues performed Cochrane reviews and reported that low-dose aspirin was beneficial in high-risk women. Askie and associates (2007) also reported minimal benefits from their meta-analysis. To the contrary, the PARIS Collaborative Group (2007) reviewed individual data from 33,897 pregnant women enrolled in 33 randomized trials of low-dose aspirin. They found a 10-percent significant reduction in women randomized to aspirin for the incidence of preeclampsia, delivery before 34 weeks, and serious adverse outcomes, however, women with chronic hypertension had no derived benefits.

Spinnato and colleagues (2007) randomized 311 women with chronic hypertension to antioxidant treatment with vitamins C and E or to a placebo. A similar number in both groups developed preeclampsia—17 versus 20 percent, respectively.

Placental Abruption

In all women, premature placental separation complicates about 1 in 200 to 300 pregnancies (see Chap. 35, p. 761). This incidence is substantively increased to 1 in 60 to 120 pregnancies in women with chronic hypertension (Hogberg, 2007; Ananth, 2007; Sibai, 1998, and all their colleagues). This risk is increased further if the woman smokes or if she develops superimposed preeclampsia. The likelihood of abruption is also increased with severe hypertension. Vigil-De Gracia and colleagues (2004) reported that 8.4 percent of 154 women with severe chronic hypertension suffered a placental abruption. Data from the Norwegian Birth Registry showed a slightly decreased incidence when adjusted for chronic hypertension of abruption if women took supplemental folic acid (Nilsen and co-workers, 2008).

Perinatal Outcomes

Almost all adverse perinatal outcomes are increased in pregnancies complicated by chronic hypertension. Shown in Table 45-3 are three comparisons that exemplify this. From the University of Alabama at Birmingham, all pregnant women with chronic hypertension were included. Perinatal outcomes were similar to those from the Network study that included all women. In the latter study, however, development of superimposed preeclampsia doubled the rates of preterm delivery and NICU admission. The Parkland study shows the affects of more severe chronic hypertension on fetal growth.

Fetal-Growth Restriction

In a population-based study from Sweden, Zetterström and associates (2006) reported a 2.4-fold risk for fetal-growth restriction in 2754 chronically hypertensive women. The incidence and severity of restricted fetal growth are directly related to the severity of hypertension. Chappell and associates (2007) recently reported that almost half of women with superimposed preeclampsia had fetal-growth restriction compared with 21 percent in women without

TABLE 45-3. Selected Pregnancy Outcomes in Women with Chronic Hypertension, Superimposed Preeclampsia, or Who Required Antihypertensive Treatment Early in Pregnancy

Data	Category of Chronic Hypertension	N	Pregnancy Outcomes in Percent			
			Delivery <35 weeks[a]	Birthweight <10th Percentile	NICU Admission	Perinatal Mortality Rate
University of Alabama at Birmingham (1991–1995)[b]	All patients	568	20	—	21	9
Maternal-Fetal Medicine Units Network (1991–1995)[c]	All patients	763	18	11	24	5
	No Preeclampsia	570	12	11	19	4
	Preeclampsia	193	36	13	40	8
Parkland Hospital (1997–2002)[d]	R_x BP >150/100 mm Hg before 20 weeks	117	—	20	17	5

[a]At UAB delivery was <34 weeks.
[b]Data courtesy of Cherry Neely and Rachel Copper.
[c]From Sibai and colleagues, 1998.
[d]Data courtesy of Dr. Gerda Zeeman.
BP = blood pressure; NICU = neonatal intensive care unit.

preeclampsia. Growth restriction is also dependent on other maternal factors such as age and hypertension control to include the need for additional antihypertensive medications. Moreover, fetal-growth restriction is more prevalent and severe in women who develop superimposed preeclampsia (Table 45-3). If there is end-organ damage such as renal or cardiac dysfunction, the risk is also increased. In the Network trial, the 81 women who also had proteinuria early in pregnancy had a 23-percent incidence of fetal-growth restriction (Sibai and colleagues, 1998).

Preterm Delivery and Perinatal Mortality

Preterm delivery is often indicated in women with chronic hypertension. As seen in Table 45-3, in all women with chronic hypertension, almost a fifth were delivered prior to 35 weeks and there was a correspondingly high NICU admission rate. These numbers were almost doubled if superimposed preeclampsia developed. Importantly, perinatal mortality rate is increased three- to fourfold in women with chronic hypertension when compared with either normotensive controls or the general obstetrical population (Ferrer and colleagues, 2000). Finally, if diabetes coexists with chronic hypertension, then preterm delivery, fetal-growth restriction, and perinatal mortality rates are increased even more (Gonzalez-Gonzalez and co-workers, 2008).

MANAGEMENT DURING PREGNANCY

Diagnosis of chronic hypertension in pregnancy should be confirmed. For example, Brown and associates (2005) reported "white-coat" hypertension in a third of 241 women diagnosed in early pregnancy. Within this third, pregnancy outcomes were good, and only 8 percent developed preeclampsia. Confirmation of abnormal blood pressures with home self-measurements

may be beneficial as well as to optimize blood-pressure control (Staessen and co-workers, 2004).

The goal is to reduce adverse maternal or perinatal outcomes discussed in the preceding section. Management is targeted toward prevention of moderate or severe hypertension and delay or amelioration of pregnancy-aggravated hypertension. To some extent, these goals can be achieved pharmacologically. Blood-pressure self-monitoring is encouraged with caveats for the accuracy of automated devices (Brown and colleagues, 2004). Personal health behavioral modifications include dietary counseling and reduction of behaviors such as smoking, alcohol, cocaine, or other substance abuse (see Table 45-2).

Blood Pressure Control

Pregnant women with *severe hypertension* must be treated for maternal indications regardless of pregnancy status (American College of Obstetricians and Gynecologists, 2001). These are women with prior adverse outcomes to include cerebrovascular events, myocardial infarction, and cardiac or renal dysfunction. We agree with the philosophy of beginning antihypertensive treatment in otherwise healthy pregnant women with persistent diastolic pressures of 100 mm Hg or greater (August and Lindheimer, 1999; Working Group Report, 2000). With end-organ dysfunction, treatment of pregnant women with diastolic pressures of 90 mm Hg or higher is reasonable.

There are no data indicating salutary effects on pregnancy outcomes with simply lowering blood pressure. For example, it seems certain that the incidence of superimposed preeclampsia is not appreciably affected. And although there is minimal evidence that outcomes are improved by such treatment, the same evidence attests to the apparent safety of antihypertensive therapy. Exclusions are angiotensin-converting enzyme (ACE) inhibitors, angiotensin-receptor blockers, and possibly atenolol. Despite lack of scientific data that treatment improves maternal or perinatal outcomes, some clinicians recommend empirical antihypertensive therapy. As emphasized by the Working Group Report (2000), there is a need for further trials in these women.

"Tight Control"

Recently the concept has been espoused that "tight control" of blood pressure—similar to that of glycemic control of pregnant diabetic women—will improve pregnancy outcome. El Guindy and Nabhan (2008) randomized 125 women with mild chronic essential hypertension or gestational hypertension to tight or to less strict blood pressure control during pregnancy. More women in the less tightly controlled group had severe hypertension during follow-up, and antenatal hospitalization was also significantly higher in this group. The gestational age at delivery was significant better in the tightly controlled group. At this time, there are no data to support this theory.

Antihypertensive Drugs

The following summary of antihypertensive drugs is abstracted from several sources, including the *2007 Physicians' Desk Reference*. In nonpregnant adults with chronic hypertension, results of large trials of single-drug therapy cited earlier support conclusions of Frohlich (2003) and August (2003) that antihypertensive use should be based on proven efficacy in persons with equivalent degrees of hypertension.

Diuretics. Thiazide and loop-acting diuretics such as furosemide are commonly used in nonpregnant hypertensives. In the short term, they provide sodium and water diuresis with volume depletion, but with time, there is *sodium escape,* and volume depletion is corrected. Some aspect of lowered peripheral vascular resistance likely contributes to their effectiveness in reducing long-term morbidity and mortality rates (Williams, 2001).

Volume reexpansion may not occur in pregnant women. Sibai and colleagues (1984) assessed plasma volume during pregnancy in 20 chronically hypertensive women. Plasma volume expanded only about 20 percent in the half who continued diuretic therapy throughout pregnancy compared with 50 percent in the other half who discontinued treatment early in pregnancy. Despite this, perinatal outcomes were similar in both groups. Largely due to concerns regarding their effect on maternal plasma volume expansion, diuretics are usually not given as first-line therapy during pregnancy, particularly after 20 weeks (Working Group Report, 2000). Even so, in their recent Cochrane review, Churchill and colleagues (2007) reported no differences in perinatal outcomes in 1836 nonhypertensive women randomized to a thiazide diuretic or placebo for primary preeclampsia prevention.

Adrenergic-Blocking Agents. Some of these drugs act *centrally* by reducing sympathetic outflow to effect a generalized decreased vascular tone. Central-acting agents include clonidine and α-methyldopa. *Peripherally* acting β-adrenergic receptor blockers also cause a generalized decrease in sympathetic tone. Examples are propranolol, metoprolol, and atenolol. Labetalol is a commonly used α/β-adrenergic blocker. Peripheral blockers are

thought to have more potential for postural hypotension than centrally acting agents. The most commonly used drugs in pregnancy to treat hypertension are methyldopa or a β- or α/β-receptor blocker.

Vasodilators. Hydralazine relaxes arterial smooth muscle and has been used parenterally for decades to safely treat severe peripartum hypertension (see Chap. 34, p. 740). Oral hydralazine monotherapy for chronic hypertension is not recommended because of its weak antihypertensive effects and resultant tachycardia. It may be an effective adjunct for long-term use with other antihypertensives, especially if there is chronic renal insufficiency.

Calcium-Channel Blockers. These agents are divided into three subclasses based on their modification of calcium entry into cells and interference with binding sites on voltage-dependent calcium channels. Common agents include nifedipine—a dihydropyridine, and verapamil—a phenylalkyl amine derivative. These agents have negative inotropic effects and thus can worsen ventricular dysfunction and congestive heart failure. Pahor and associates (2000) concluded that they are inferior to other first-line drugs in nonpregnant hypertensives. There is minimal published experience with these agents during pregnancy (Smith and colleagues, 2000).

The safety of acute peripartum nifedipine treatment has been questioned by various authors. In obstetrics, the drug is used by some for rapid control of severe hypertension, and is becoming widely used for tocolysis in preterm labor (see Chap. 36, p. 825). Oei (2006) reviewed the use of nifedipine for tocolysis and concluded that calcium-channel blockers should not be combined with intravenous β-agonists. He also recommended that intravenous nicardipine or high doses of oral nifedipine not be given to women with cardiovascular compromise or those with multifetal gestation. Finally, he recommended that blood pressure be monitored and cardiotocography recorded during the administration of immediate release tablets which should not be chewed. Van Geijn and colleagues (2005) expressed similar concerns.

Myocardial infarction during nifedipine therapy for preterm labor has been reported (Oei and colleagues, 1999; Verhaert and Van Acker, 2004). Its use has also been associated with pulmonary edema (Abbas, 2006; Bal, 2004; Vaast, 2004, and all their colleagues). Severe maternal hypotension with resultant fetal compromise necessitating cesarean delivery and fetal death have also been reported (Johnson and Mason, 2005; Kandysamy and Thomson, 2005; van Veen and colleagues, 2005).

Angiotensin-Converting Enzyme Inhibitors. These drugs inhibit the conversion of angiotensin-I to the potent vasoconstrictor angiotensin-II. They can cause severe fetal malformations that include hypocalvaria when given in the second and third trimesters (Chap. 14, p. 319). Because of this, they are not recommended during pregnancy (Briggs and colleagues, 2005).

Angiotensin-receptor blockers act in a similar manner, but instead of blocking the production of angiotensin-II, they inhibit binding to its receptor. They are presumed to have the same fetal effects as ACE inhibitors and are also contraindicated.

Drug Treatment During Pregnancy

As discussed, continuation of prepregnancy antihypertensive treatment when women become pregnant is debated. Although blood-pressure reduction is certainly beneficial to the mother in the long term, it at least theoretically can decrease uteroplacental perfusion. Older observational reports in general described that most pregnancy outcomes were good without treatment (Chesley, 1978). In general, perinatal mortality rates were acceptable unless superimposed preeclampsia developed.

Some randomized trials of drug therapy in pregnant women with mild chronic hypertension reported after 1975 are shown in Table 45-4. Only two of three trials reported during the 1990s were of appreciable size. Thus, data are not sufficient to provide a definitive answer regarding whether to treat women with mild or even moderate hypertension in pregnancy. An important observation of the two largest recent studies was that no adverse outcomes were found in women given treatment. Thus, it is not unreasonable to treat women with uncomplicated mild or moderate sustained chronic hypertension who would be prescribed antihypertensive therapy when not pregnant.

The concern over fetal-growth restriction from reduced placental perfusion from lowering maternal blood pressure is confounded because worsening blood pressure itself is associated with abnormal fetal growth. Breart and colleagues (1982) found that women with chronic hypertension whose diastolic pressure was less than 90 mm Hg had a 3-percent risk of fetal-growth restriction, those with 90 mm Hg had a 6-percent risk, and those with 110 mm Hg or more had a 16-percent risk. Again, in the two most recent large randomized trials shown in Table 45-4, the incidence of growth restriction did not change when women were randomized to treatment.

Other findings of these two trials are worthy of mention. In the Memphis trial reported by Sibai and colleagues (1990a), the goal of therapy was to maintain pressures less than 140/90 mm Hg. Although women treated throughout pregnancy had significantly lower blood pressures than those randomized to no treatment, adverse outcomes were not altered by treatment. The important clinical difference was that more women who initially were not treated eventually required antihypertensive therapy for pressures >160/110 mm Hg—11 versus 6 percent compared with women treated with either labetalol or methyldopa.

In the study by the Gruppo di Studio Ipertensione in Raviana (1998), 283 women were randomized to treatment with slow-release nifedipine, 10 mg twice daily, or to no treatment. After this, all women were treated with nifedipine if diastolic pressure exceeded 110 mm Hg. The investigators found neither benefits nor harm in either group. The 45-percent preterm delivery rate in treated women was not significant from that of 37 percent in those not treated. Birthweight and the incidence of fetal-growth restriction were similar in each group.

Severe Chronic Hypertension

All available data suggest that the prognosis for pregnancy outcome with chronic hypertension is dependent on the severity of disease before pregnancy. This may be related to findings that many women with severe hypertension have underlying renal disease (Cunningham and colleagues, 1990). In the study by Sibai and co-workers (1986a), there were 44 pregnancies in women whose blood pressure at 6 to 11 weeks was 170/110 mm Hg or higher. They all were given treatment with α-methyldopa and oral hydralazine to maintain pressures less than 160/110 mm Hg. Afterward, they were hospitalized and

TABLE 45-4. Randomized Trials of Antihypertensive Drug Therapy in Pregnancies Complicated by Mild Chronic Hypertension

Study	No.	Mean Gestation at Entry (weeks)	Mean DBP at Entry (mm Hg)	Treatment	Principal Findings
Redman (1976)	208	21–22	88–90	Methyldopa ± hydralazine vs no drug	Fewer midpregnancy losses in treated women
Arias and Zamora (1979)	58	15–16	90–99	Methyldopa, diuretics, or hydralazine vs no drug	Compromised infants born to mothers in whom severe hypertension developed despite treatment
Butters et al. (1990)	29	16	86	Atenolol vs placebo	Poor fetal growth in treated women
Sibai et al. (1990a)	263	<11	91–92	Methyldopa vs labetalol vs no drug	No differences in outcomes
Gruppo di Studio Ipertensione in Gravidanza (1998)	283	24	95–96	Slow-release nifedipine vs no drug	No differences in outcomes

DBP = diastolic blood pressure.
Adapted from Haddad B, Sibai BM: Chronic hypertension in pregnancy, *Ann Med* 31(4):246, 1999, with permission.

treated with parenteral hydralazine if pressures exceeded 180/120 mm Hg. Half developed superimposed preeclampsia, and all adverse perinatal outcomes were in this group. Specifically, all infants born to women with superimposed preeclampsia were preterm, and nearly 80 percent were growth restricted. The perinatal mortality rate was 48 percent. Women with severe chronic hypertension who did not develop superimposed preeclampsia, however, had much better outcomes—only 5 percent of fetuses were growth restricted, and there were no perinatal deaths.

Antihypertensive Therapy Selection

Mulrow and colleagues (2000) performed an extensive review for the Agency for Healthcare Research and Quality and summarized the risks and benefits of antihypertensive agents given during pregnancy. They found no evidence of major adverse fetal or maternal events.

Because of its long-standing record of safety, α-methyldopa is frequently used to control chronic hypertension during pregnancy. The drug has been extensively studied during pregnancy (Cockburn and associates, 1982; Montan and colleagues, 1992, 1993). In their review, Ferrer and colleagues (2000) concluded that its use in the first trimester has not been associated with any pattern of fetal anomalies. Various adrenergic-blocking drugs have been used extensively in England, Scotland, and Australia (Redman, 1982; Rubin and colleagues, 1983; Walker and associates, 1983). The results of treatment with labetalol are consistent with the view that the drug offers no advantages over α-methyldopa (Sibai and colleagues, 1990a). Khalil and colleagues (2009) found that vascular stiffness was significantly improved by treatment with alpha methyldopa in women with preeclampsia but remained higher than in normotensive controls.

The β-blocker atenolol has especial considerations. Butters and colleagues (1990) reported that atenolol treatment resulted in a higher incidence of growth-restricted neonates compared with those born to untreated mothers. In another study of 223 women, Lydakis and colleagues (1999) observed that atenolol treatment was associated with lower birthweight and ponderal indices—birthweight/length[3]. There was also a trend toward more preterm births compared with the effects of other antihypertensives or of no treatment. Easterling and associates (1999) also concluded that atenolol therapy was associated with reduced infant birthweight. Montan and Ingemarsson (1989) reported ominous intrapartum fetal heart rate patterns in 20 percent of women receiving β-blocker therapy for hypertension. Ominous patterns were increased even more in growth-restricted fetuses as well as in half of women given epidural analgesia. Because of these findings, the American College of Obstetricians and Gynecologists (2001) recommends that atenolol not be given during pregnancy.

Experiences and newer safety concerns are not sufficient to permit recommendations to be made about routine use of nifedipine for pregnant women with chronic hypertension. Bartolus and associates (2000) reported the effects of maternal nifedipine on child development at 18 months. Outcomes were similar in 94 infants whose hypertensive mothers were treated compared with those of 161 similar women who were not exposed. Malformations were identified in 5.3 percent of nifedipine-exposed women compared with 1.2 percent of controls, however, the study was underpowered to determine significance.

Therapy Recommendations

The Working Group on High Blood Pressure in Pregnancy (2000) concluded that there were limited data from which to draw conclusions concerning any decision to treat mild chronic hypertension in pregnancy. The Group did recommend empirical therapy in women whose blood pressures exceed threshold levels of 150 to 160 mm Hg systolic or 100 to 110 mm Hg diastolic or when there is target-organ damage such as left ventricular hypertrophy or renal insufficiency. They also concluded that early treatment of hypertension would probably reduce subsequent hospitalization during pregnancy. Recall the study by Sibai and associates (1990a) in which subsequent treatment was needed for dangerous hypertension in 11 percent of women not given treatment beginning early in pregnancy. This compared with only 6 percent in women initially randomized to either α-methyldopa or labetalol earlier in pregnancy.

Resistant Hypertension

In some women, worrisome hypertension persists despite usual therapy. For nonpregnant patients, Moser and Setaro (2006) provided a comprehensive review of resistant hypertension. Considerations include inaccurate blood-pressure measurements, suboptimal treatment, and antagonizing substances. In pregnant women, consideration is always given for possible pregnancy-aggravated hypertension, with or without superimposed preeclampsia. Again in nonpregnant patients, Garg and colleagues (2005) confirmed that a suboptimal medication regimen was the most common reason for resistant hypertension. Sowers and colleagues (2005) reported destabilization of hypertension control from simultaneous administration of nonsteroidal anti-inflammatory drugs including cyclooxygenase-2 inhibitors. And ideally not often seen in pregnant women is worsening blood-pressure control from alcohol consumption (Xin and associates, 2001).

Pregnancy-Aggravated Hypertension or Superimposed Preeclampsia

As discussed, the incidence of superimposed preeclampsia for women with chronic hypertension varies depending on severity. A reasonable average is about 25 percent as determined in the Network study reported by Caritis and co-workers (1998). The incidence of superimposed preeclampsia may be underreported in some studies because diagnosis is based solely on urine protein dipstick testing. Lai and colleagues (2006) and Gangaram and associates (2005) found appreciable false-negative rates—39 and 25 percent—when dipstick testing of a single voided urine sample was compared with a 24-hour collection.

The diagnosis may be difficult to make, especially in women with hypertension who have underlying renal disease with chronic proteinuria (Cunningham and associates, 1990). Conditions that support the diagnosis of superimposed preeclampsia include new-onset proteinuria; neurological symptoms such as severe headaches and visual disturbances; generalized edema; oliguria; and certainly, convulsions or pulmonary edema. Laboratory abnormalities that support the diagnosis include increasing serum creatinine, thrombocytopenia, appreciable serum hepatic transaminase elevations, or combinations of the three.

Some women with chronic hypertension have worsening during pregnancy with no other findings of superimposed preeclampsia. This is most commonly encountered near the end of the second trimester. In the absence of other supporting criteria for superimposed preeclampsia, including fetal-growth restriction or decreased amnionic fluid volume, this likely represents the higher end of the normal blood-pressure curve shown in Figure 45-1. In such women, it is reasonable to begin or to increase the dose of antihypertensive therapy.

Fetal Assessment

Women with well-controlled chronic hypertension and who have no complicating factors can generally be expected to have a good pregnancy outcome. Because even those with mild hypertension have an increased risk of superimposed preeclampsia and fetal-growth restriction, serial antepartum assessment of fetal well-being as detailed in Chapter 15 (p. 337) is recommended by some. According to the American College of Obstetricians and Gynecologists (2001), there are no conclusive data to address either benefit or harm associated with various monitoring strategies.

Delivery

In women with uncomplicated and well-controlled chronic hypertension who have documented normal fetal growth and amnionic fluid volume, it is our practice to await labor at term. Special consideration for delivery prior to term for women with a multifetal gestation may be advisable. In women with complications or in those in whom fetal testing becomes abnormal, delivery is considered. Superimposed severe preeclampsia prompts delivery even with markedly preterm pregnancy. These women are at increased risk for placental abruption and cerebral hemorrhage (Cunningham, 2005; Martin and colleagues, 2005). And, as discussed in Chapter 42 (p. 926), pulmonary edema from peripartum heart failure is common at this time.

In general, management of these women is the same as for preeclampsia described in Chapter 34 (p. 728). Tenets of this management are summarized:

1. Magnesium sulfate prophylaxis is recommended for prevention of eclampsia in women with chronic hypertension who develop severe gestational hypertension with or without other evidence for preeclampsia (Alexander and colleagues, 2006). The optimal duration to continue prophylaxis postpartum is not known. That said, the safety and efficacy of its empirical use for 24 hours is well documented. For women with mild preeclampsia, Ehrenberg and Mercer (2006) provided preliminary evidence that 12 hours may be sufficient. We are of the view that further data are needed before changing current management guidelines.

2. Severe hypertension—diastolic blood pressure 110 mm Hg or higher or systolic pressure 160 mm Hg or higher—is treated with either intravenous hydralazine or labetalol. Some prefer to treat women with a diastolic pressure of 100 to 105 mm Hg as detailed in Chapter 34 (p. 740). Vigil-De Gracia and colleagues (2006) randomized 200 women to intravenous hydralazine or labetalol to acutely lower severe blood pressure in pregnancy. Outcomes were similar except for significantly more maternal palpitations and tachycardia with hydralazine and significantly more neonatal hypotension and bradycardia with labetalol.

3. Vaginal delivery is usually preferable, and cesarean delivery performed for usual obstetrical indications. Most women can be induced successfully and delivered vaginally (Alexander and colleagues, 1999; Atkinson and associates, 1995). Conduction analgesia for labor and delivery, including cesarean delivery, is appropriate in these women and as described in Chapter 19 (p. 454). Importantly, labor epidural analgesia does not serve to treat hypertension (Lucas and colleagues, 2001).

Some recommend glucocorticoid therapy ostensibly to improve the clinical response of women with chronic hypertension and superimposed hemolysis, elevated liver enzymes, low platelet count (HELLP) syndrome (see Chap. 34, p. 734). In a randomized trial, however, Fonseca and colleagues (2005) reported no benefit from dexamethasone treatment. Thus, we agree with Sibai and Barton (2005) that high-dose dexamethasone for women with HELLP syndrome after 34 weeks or postpartum should be considered experimental.

Postpartum Considerations

In many respects, postpartum observation and prevention and management of adverse complications are similar in women with severe chronic hypertension and in those with severe preeclampsia–eclampsia. The development of cerebral or pulmonary edema, heart failure, renal dysfunction, or cerebral hemorrhage is especially high within the first 48 hours after delivery (Benedetti, 1980, 1985; Cunningham, 1986, 2005; Martin, 2005; Sibai, 1990b, and all their co-workers). Following delivery, as maternal peripheral resistance increases, left ventricular workload also increases. This increase is further aggravated by appreciable amounts of interstitial fluid that are mobilized for excretion as endothelial damage is repaired. In these women, sudden hypertension—either moderate or severe—exacerbates diastolic dysfunction and may cause pulmonary edema (Cunningham and colleagues, 1986; Gandhi and associates, 2001). Prompt hypertension control, along with diuretic therapy, usually quickly resolves pulmonary edema. In some cases, this clinical situation can be forestalled by the administration of intravenous furosemide to augment the normal diuresis that develops postpartum. Ascarelli and colleagues (2005) reported that 20-mg oral furosemide given daily to postpartum women with severe preeclampsia aided in blood-pressure control.

CHAPTER 45

Contraception

Women with chronic hypertension have especial consideration for contraceptive choices. These are discussed in detail throughout Chapter 32. In addition, these women are at ultimate high risk for lifetime cardiovascular complications which are increased if preeclampsia and diabetes coexist (Berends and colleagues, 2008).

REFERENCES

Abbas OM, Nassar AH, Kanj N, et al: Acute pulmonary edema during tocolytic therapy with nifedipine. Am J Obstet Gynecol 195:e3, 2006

Abbott KC, Bakris GL: What have we learned from the current trials? Med Clin North Am 88:189, 2004

Alexander JM, Bloom SL, McIntire DD, et al: Severe preeclampsia and the very low birth weight infant: Is induction of labor harmful? Obstet Gynecol 93:485, 1999

Alexander JM, McIntire DD, Leveno KJ, et al: Selective magnesium sulfate prophylaxis for the prevention of eclampsia in women with gestational hypertension. Obstet Gynecol 108:826, 2006

ALLHAT (Antihypertensive and Lipid-Lowering Treatment to Prevent Heart Attack Trial): Major outcomes in high-risk hypertensive patients randomized to angiotensin-converting enzyme inhibitor or calcium channel blocker vs. diuretic. JAMA 288:2981, 2002

American College of Obstetricians and Gynecologists: Chronic hypertension in pregnancy. Practice Bulletin No. 29, July 2001

American College of Obstetricians and Gynecologists: Hypertension. Clinical Updates in Women's Health Care. Vol IV, No. 5, November 2005

American Heart Association: Home monitoring of high blood pressure. Available at: http://www.americanheart.org/presenter.jhtml?identifier=576. Accessed January 9, 2004

Ananth CV, Peltier MR, Kinzler WL: Chronic hypertension and risk of placental abruption: Is the association modified by ischemic placental disease? Am J Obstet Gynecol 197:273, 2007

Arias F, Zamora J: Antihypertensive treatment and pregnancy outcome in patients with mild chronic hypertension. Obstet Gynecol 53:489, 1979

Ascarelli MH, Johnson V, McCreary H, et al: Postpartum preeclampsia management with furosemide: A randomized clinical trial. Obstet Gynecol 105:29, 2005

Askie LM, Duley L, Henderson-Smart DJ, et al: Antiplatelet agents for prevention of pre-eclampsia: A meta-analysis of individual patient data. Lancet 369:1791, 2007

Atkinson MW, Guinn D, Owen J, et al: Does magnesium sulfate affect the length of labor induction in women with pregnancy-associated hypertension? Am J Obstet Gynecol 173:1219, 1995

August P: Initial treatment of hypertension. N Engl J Med 348:610, 2003

August P, Lindheimer MD: Chronic hypertension in pregnancy. In Lindheimer MD, Roberts JM, Cunningham FG (eds): Chesley's Hypertensive Disorders in Pregnancy, 2nd ed. Stamford, CT, Appleton & Lange, 1999, p 605

Bal L, Thierry S, Brocas E, et al: Pulmonary edema induced by calcium-channel blockade for tocolysis. Anesth Analg 99:910, 2004

Bartolus R, Ricci E, Chatenoud L, et al: Nifedipine administration in pregnancy: Effect on the development of children at 18 months. Br J Obstet Gynaecol 107:792, 2000

Benedetti TJ, Kates R, Williams V: Hemodynamic observations in severe preeclampsia complicated by pulmonary edema. Am J Obstet Gynecol 152:330, 1985

Benedetti TJ, Quilligan EJ: Cerebral edema in severe pregnancy-induced hypertension. Am J Obstet Gynecol 137:860, 1980

Berends AL, deGroo CJ, Sijbrands EJ, et al: Shared constitutional risks for maternal vascular-related pregnancy complications and future cardiovascular disease. Hypertension 51:1034,2008

Black HR, Elliott WJ, Grandits G, et al: Principal results of the controlled onset verapamil investigation of cardiovascular end points (CONVINCE) Trial. JAMA 289:2073, 2003

Blood Pressure Lowering Treatment Trialists' Collaboration: Effects of different blood-pressure-lowering regimens on major cardiovascular events: Results of prospectively-designed overviews of randomised trials. Lancet 362:1527, 2003

Breart G, Rabarison Y, Plouin PF, et al: Risk of fetal growth retardation as a result of maternal hypertension: Preparation to a trial on antihypertensive drugs. Dev Pharmacol Ther 4:116, 1982

Briggs GG, Freeman RK, Yaffe SJ: Drugs in Pregnancy and Lactation, 7th ed. Philadelphia, Lippincott Williams & Wilkins, 2005, p 549

Brown M, McHugh L, Mangos G, et al: Automated self-initiated blood pressure or 24-hour ambulatory blood pressure monitoring in pregnancy? Br J Obstet Gynaecol 111:38, 2004

Brown MA, Mangos G, Homer C: The natural history of white coat hypertension during pregnancy. Br J Obstet Gynaecol 112:601, 2005

Butters L, Kennedy S, Rubin PC: Atenolol in essential hypertension during pregnancy. BMJ 301:587, 1990

Caritis S, Sibai B, Hauth J, et al: Low-dose aspirin to prevent preeclampsia in women at high risk. N Engl J Med 338:701, 1998

Chappell LC, Enye S, Seed P, et al: Adverse perinatal outcomes and risk factors for preeclampsia in women with chronic hypertension: A prospective study. Hypertension 51:1002, 2008

Chesley LC: Superimposed preeclampsia or eclampsia. In Chesley LC (ed): Hypertensive Disorders in Pregnancy. New York, Appleton-Century-Crofts, 1978, pp 14, 302, 482

Chesley LC, Annitto JE, Cosgrove RA: Long-term follow-up study of eclamptic women: Sixth periodic report. Am J Obstet Gynecol 124:446, 1976

Churchill D, Beevers GD, Meher S, et al: Diuretics for preventing pre-eclampsia. Cochran Database Syst Rev 1:CD004451, 2007

Cockburn J, Moar VA, Ounsted M, et al: Final report of study on hypertension during pregnancy: The effects of specific treatment on the growth and development of the children. Lancet 1:647, 1982

Cowley AW Jr: The genetic dissection of essential hypertension. Natl Rev Genet 7:829, 2006

Cunningham FG: Severe preeclampsia and eclampsia: Systolic hypertension is also important. Obstet Gynecol 105:237-38, 2005

Cunningham FG, Cox SM, Harstad TW, et al: Chronic renal disease and pregnancy outcome. Am J Obstet Gynecol 163:453, 1990

Cunningham FG, Pritchard JA, Hankins GDN, et al: Idiopathic cardiomyopathy or compounding cardiovascular events? Obstet Gynecol 67:157, 1986

Duley L, Henderson-Smart DJ, Meher S, et al: Antiplatelet agents for preventing pre-eclampsia and its complications. Cochrane Database Syst Rev. 2:CD004659, 2007

Easterling TR, Brateng D, Schmuchker B, et al: Prevention of preeclampsia: A randomized trial of atenolol in hyperdynamic patients before onset of hypertension. Obstet Gynecol 93:725, 1999

Ehrenberg HM, Mercer BM: Abbreviated postpartum magnesium sulfate therapy for women with mild preeclampsia. Obstet Gynecol 108:833, 2006

Ferrer RL, Sibai BM, Mulrow CD, et al: Management of mild chronic hypertension during pregnancy: A review. Obstet Gynecol 96:849, 2000

Fonseca JE, Méndez F, Cataño C, et al: Dexamethasone treatment does not improve the outcome of women with HELLP syndrome: A double-blind, placebo-controlled, randomized clinical trial. Am J Obstet Gynecol 193:1591, 2005

Frohlich ED: Treating hypertension—what are we to believe? N Engl J Med 348:639, 2003

Gainer J, Alexander J, Mcintire D, et al: Maternal echocardiogram findings in pregnant patients with chronic hypertension. Presented at the 25th Annual Meeting of the Society for Maternal-Fetal Medicine, Reno, Nevada, February 7–12, 2005

Gandhi SK, Powers JC, Nomeir A, et al: The pathogenesis of acute pulmonary edema associated with hypertension. N Engl J Med 344:17, 2001

Gangaram R, Ojwang PJ, Moodley J, et al: The accuracy of urine dipstick as a screening test for proteinuria in hypertensive disorders of pregnancy. Hypertens Pregnancy 24:117, 2005

Garg JP, Elliott WJ, Folker A, et al: Resistant hypertension revisited: A comparison of two university-based cohorts. Am J Hypertens 18:619, 2005

Gilbert WM, Young AL, Danielsen B: Pregnancy-outcomes in women with chronic hypertension: A population-based study. J Reprod Med 52:1046, 2007

Gonzalez-Gonzalez NL, Ramirez O, Mozas J, et al: Factors influencing pregnancy outcomes in women with type 2 versus type 1 diabetes mellitus. Acta Obstet Gynecol Scand. 87(1):43, 2008

Gruppo di Studio Ipertensione in Gravidanza: Nifedipine versus expectant management in mild to moderate hypertension in pregnancy. Br J Obstet Gynaecol 105:718, 1998

Gueyffier F, Boutitie F, Boissel J, et al: Effect of antihypertensive drug treatment on cardiovascular outcomes in women and men. A meta-analysis of individual patient data from randomized controlled trials. The INDANA Investigators. Ann Intern Med 126:761, 1997

Haddad B, Sibai BM: Chronic hypertension in pregnancy. Ann Med 31:246, 1999

Hajjar I, Kotchen TA: Trends in prevalence, awareness, treatment, and control of hypertension in the United States, 1988–2000. JAMA 290:199, 2003

Hauth JC, Sibai B, Caritis S, et al: Maternal serum thromboxane B₂ concentrations do not predict improved outcomes in high risk pregnancies in a low-dose aspirin trial. Am J Obstet Gynecol 179:1193, 1998

Hermida RC, Ayala DE, Calvo C, et al: Aspirin administered at bedtime, but not on awakening, has an effect on ambulatory blood pressure in hypertensive patients. J Am Coll Cardiol 46(6):975, 2005

Hibbard JU, Korcarz CE, Nendaz GG, et al: The arterial system in pre-eclampsia and chronic hypertension with superimposed pre-eclampsia. BJOG 112:897, 2005

Hogberg V, Rasmussen S, Irgens LM: The effect of smoking and hypertensive disorders on abruptio placentae in Norway 1999-2002. Acta Obstet Gynecol 86:304, 2007

Jain L: Effect of pregnancy-induced and chronic hypertension on pregnancy outcome. J Perinatol 17:425, 1997

Joint National Committee: The seventh report of the Joint National Committee on prevention, detection, evaluation, and treatment of high blood pressure. National Institutes of Health Publication No. 03-5233, May 2003

Johnson KA, Mason GC: Severe hypotension and fetal death due to tocolysis with nifedipine. BJOG 112:1583, 2005

Kandysamy V, Thomson AJ: Severe hypotension and fetal death due to tocolysis with nifedipine. BJOG 112:1583, 2005

Kearney PM, Whelton M, Reynolds K, et al: Global burden of hypertension: Analysis of worldwide data. Lancet 365:217, 2005

Lai J, Tan J, Moore T, et al: Comparing urine dipstick to protein/creatinine ratio in the setting of suspected preeclampsia. Am J Obstet Gynecol 195:S148, 2006

Levesque S, Moutquin JM, Lindsay C, et al: Implication of an AGT haplotype in a multigene association study with pregnancy hypertension. Hypertension 43:71, 2004

Levine RJ, Hauth JC, Curet LB, et al: Trial of calcium to prevent preeclampsia. N Engl J Med 337:69, 1997

Lindheimer MD, Conrad KP, Karumanchi SA: Renal physiology and disease in pregnancy. In Alpern R and Hebert S (eds): Seldin and Giebisch's The Kidney, 4th ed. New York, Academic Press, 2008, p 2339

Lucas MJ, Sharma SK, McIntire DD, et al: A randomized trial of labor analgesia in women with pregnancy-induced hypertension. Am J Obstet Gynecol 185:970, 2001

Lydakis C, Lip GYH, Beevers M, et al: Atenolol and fetal growth in pregnancies complicated by hypertension. Am J Hypertension 12:541, 1999

Martin JN Jr, Thigpen BD, Moore RC, et al: Stroke and severe preeclampsia and eclampsia: A paradigm shift focusing on systolic blood pressure. Obstet Gynecol 105:246, 2005

Meads CA, Cnossen JS, Meher S, et al: Methods of prediction and prevention of pre-eclampsia: Systematic reviews of accuracy and effectiveness literature with economic modelling. Health Technol Assess 12(6):1, 2008

Montan S, Anandakumar C, Arulkeurnaran S, et al: Effects of methyldopa on uteroplacental and fetal hemodynamics in pregnancy-induced hypertension. Am J Obstet Gynecol 168:152, 1993

Montan S, Ingemarsson I: Intrapartum fetal heart rate patterns in pregnancies complicated by hypertension. Am J Obstet Gynecol 160:283, 1989

Montan S, Ingemarsson I, Marsal K, et al: Randomized controlled trial of atenolol and pindolol in human pregnancy: Effects on fetal hemodynamics. BMJ 304:946, 1992

Moodley J: Maternal deaths due to hypertensive disorders in pregnancy: Saving Mothers report 2002-2004. Cardiovasc J Afr 18:358, 2007

Moore Simas TA, Crawford SL, Solitro MJ, et al: Angiogenic factors for the prediction of preeclampsia in high-risk women. Am J Obstet Gynecol 197:244, 2007

Moser M, Setaro JF: Resistant or difficult-to-control hypertension. N Engl J Med 355:385, 2006

Mulrow CD, Chiquette E, Ferrer RL, et al: Evidence Report/Technology Assessment No. 14. AHRQ publication No. 00-E011. Rockville, MD, Agency for Healthcare Research and Quality, August 2000

National Center for Health Statistics: Blood pressure of adults by age and sex, United States, 1960–1962. Vital Health Stat 11:4, 1964

Neal B, MacMahon S, Chapman N: Effects of ACE inhibitors, calcium antagonists, and other blood-pressure-lowering drugs: Results of prospectively designed overviews of randomised trials. Lancet 356:1955, 2000

Nilsen RM, Vollset SE, Rasmussen SA, et al: Folic acid and multivitamin supplement use and risk of placental abruption: A population-based registry study. Am J Epidemiol, Jan 10, 2008

Oei SG: Calcium channel blockers for tocolysis: A review of their role and safety following reports of serious adverse events. Eur J Obstet Gynecol Repro Biol 126:137, 2006

Oei SG, Oei SK, Brolmann HA: Myocardial infarction during nifedipine therapy for preterm labour. N Engl J Med 340:154, 1999

Ogden LG, He J, Lydick E, et al: Long-term absolute benefit of lowering blood pressure in hypertensive patients according to the JNC VI risk stratification. Hypertension 35:539, 2000

Pahor M, Psaty BM, Alderman MH, et al: Health outcomes associated with calcium antagonists compared with other firstline antihypertensive therapies: A meta-analysis of randomized controlled trials. Lancet 356:1949, 2000

PARIS: Perinatal Anteplatelet Review of International Studies (PARIS) Collaborative Group: Antiplatelet agents prevent pre-eclampsia, and its consequences: An individual patient data review. Lancet, 369:1791, 2007

Physicians' Desk Reference, 61st ed. Montvale, NJ, Thomson PDR, 2007

Podymow T, August P: Hypertension in pregnancy. Adv Chronic Kid Dis 14:178, 2007

Poyares D, Guilleminault C, Hachul H, et al: Pre-eclampsia and nasal CPAP: Part 2. Hypertension during pregnancy, chronic snoring, and early nasal CPAP intervention. Sleep Med 9:15, 2007

Prospective Studies Collaboration: Age-specific relevance of usual blood pressure to vascular mortality: A meta-analysis of individual data for one million adults in 61 prospective studies. Lancet 360:1903, 2002

Psaty BM, Lumley T, Furberg CD: Health outcomes associated with various antihypertensive therapies used as first-line agents. JAMA 289:2534, 2003

Qureshi AI, Suri FK, Mohammad Y, et al: Isolated and borderline isolated systolic hypertension relative to long-term risk and type of stroke: A 20-year follow-up of the National Health and Nutrition Survey. Stroke 33:2781, 2002

Ramin SM, Vidaeff AC, Yeomans ER, et al: Chronic renal disease in pregnancy. Obstet Gynecol 108:1531, 2006

Redman CWG: Fetal outcome in trial of antihypertensive treatment in pregnancy. Lancet 2:753, 1976

Redman CWG: Controlled trials of treatment of hypertension during pregnancy. Obstet Gynecol Surv 37:523, 1982

Riskin-Mashiah S, Belfort MA: Cerebrovascular hemodynamics in pregnant women with mild chronic hypertension. Obstet Gynecol 103:294, 2004

Riskin-Mashiah S, Belfort MA: Cerebrovascular hemodynamics in chronic hypertensive pregnant women who later develop superimposed preeclampsia. J Soc Gynecol Investig 12:282, 2005

Roumie CL, Elasy TA, Greevy R, et al: Improving blood pressure control through provider education, provider alerts, and patient education. Ann Intern Med 145: 165, 2006

Rubin PC, Butters L, Clark DM, et al: Placebo-controlled trial of atenolol in treatment of pregnancy-associated hypertension. Lancet 1:431, 1983

Sibai BM, Anderson GD: Pregnancy outcome of intensive therapy in severe hypertension in first trimester. Obstet Gynecol 67:517, 1986a

Sibai BM, Barton JR: Dexamethasone to improve maternal outcome in women with hemolysis, elevated liver enzymes, and low platelets syndrome. Am J Obstet Gynecol 193:1587, 2005

Sibai BM, El-Nazer A, Gonzalez-Ruiz A: Severe preeclampsia–eclampsia in young primigravid women: Subsequent pregnancy outcome and remote prognosis. Am J Obstet Gynecol 155:1011, 1986b

Sibai BM, Grossman RA, Grossman HG: Effects of diuretics on plasma volume in pregnancies with long-term hypertension. Am J Obstet Gynecol 150:831, 1984

Sibai BM, Lindheimer M, Hauth JC, et al: Risk factors for preeclampsia, abruptio placentae, and adverse neonatal out-comes among women with chronic hypertension. N Engl J Med 339:667, 1998

Sibai BM, Mabie WC, Shamsa F, et al: A comparison of no medication versus methyldopa or labetalol in chronic hypertension during pregnancy. Am J Obstet Gynecol 162:960, 1990a

Sibai BM, Sarinoglu C, Mercer BM: Eclampsia, VII. Pregnancy outcome after eclampsia and long-term prognosis. Am J Obstet Gynecol 166:1757, 1992

Sibai BM, Villar MA, Mabie BC: Acute renal failure in hypertensive disorders of pregnancy. Pregnancy outcome and remote prognosis in thirty-one consecutive cases. Am J Obstet Gynecol 162:777, 1990b

Simpson RJ Jr: Challenges for improving medication adherence. JAMA 296:2614, 2006

Smith P, Anthony J, Johanson R: Nifedipine in pregnancy. Br J Obstet Gynaecol 107:299, 2000

Sowers JR, White WB, Pitt B, et al: The effects of cyclooxygenase-2 inhibitors and nonsteroidal anti-inflammatory therapy on 24-hour blood pressure in patients with hypertension, osteoarthritis, and type 2 diabetes mellitus. Arch Intern Med 165:161, 2005

Spinnato JA, Freire S, Pinto e Silva JL, et al: Antioxidant therapy to prevent preeclampsia. Obstet Gynecol 110:1311, 2007

Staessen JA, Hond ED, Celis H, et al: Antihypertensive treatment based on blood pressure measurement at home or in the physician's office: A randomized controlled trial. JAMA 291:955, 2004

Tihtonen K, Kööbi T, Huhtala H, et al: Hemodynamic adaptation during pregnancy in chronic hypertension. Hypertens Pregnancy. 26(3):315, 2007

Vaast P, Dubreucq-Fossaert S, Houfflin-Debarge V, et al: Acute pulmonary oedema during nicardipine therapy for preterm labour: Report of five cases. Eur J Obstet Gynecol Reprod Biol 113:98, 2004 van Geijn HP, Lenglet JE, Bolte AC: Nifedipine trials: Effectiveness and safety aspects. Br J Obstet Gynaecol 112:79, 2005

van Veen AJ, Pelinck MJ, van Pampus MG, et al: Severe hypotension and fetal death due to tocolysis with nifedipine. BJOG 112:509, 2005

Verhaert D, Van Acker R: Acute myocardial infarction during pregnancy. Acta Cardiol 59:331, 2004

Vigil-De Gracia P, Lasso M, Montufar-Rueda C: Perinatal outcome in women with severe chronic hypertension during the second half of pregnancy. Int J Gynaecol Obstet 85:139, 2004

Vigil-De Gracia P, Lasso M, Ruiz E, et al: Severe hypertension in pregnancy: Hydralazine or labetalol a randomized clinical trial. Eur J Obstet Gynecol Repro Biol 128:157, 2006

Walker JJ, Bonduelle M, Greer I: Antihypertensive therapy in pregnancy. Lancet 1:932, 1983

Wang Z, Poole JC, Treiber FA, et al: Ethnic and gender differences in ambulatory blood pressure trajectories: Results from a 15-year longitudinal study in youth and young adults. Circulation 114:2780, 2006

Weissman-Brenner A, Schoen R, Divon MY: Aortic dissection in pregnancy. Obstet Gynecol 103:1110, 2004

Williams GH: Hypertensive vascular disease. In Braunwald E, Fauci AS, Kasper DL, et al (eds): Harrison's Principles of Internal Medicine, 15th ed. New York, McGraw-Hill, 2001, p 1421

Wing LMH, Reid CM, Ryan P, et al: A comparison of outcomes with angiotensin-converting-enzyme inhibitors and diuretics for hypertension in the elderly. N Engl J Med 348:583, 2003

Woolcock J, Hennessy A, Xu B, et al: Soluble Flt-1 as a diagnostic marker of pre-eclampsia. Aust NZ J Obstet Gynaecol 48(1):64, 2008

World Health Organization: Maternal mortality in 2000: estimates developed by WHO, UNICEF, and UNFPA. 2004

Working Group Report on High Blood Pressure in Pregnancy: National Institutes of Health. NIH Publication No. 00-3029, 2000

Xin X, He J, Frontini MG, et al: Effects of alcohol reduction on blood pressure: A meta-analysis of randomized controlled trials. Hypertension 38: 1112, 2001

Zeeman GG, McIntire DD, Twickler DM: Maternal and fetal artery Doppler findings in women with chronic hypertension who subsequently develop superimposed pre-eclampsia. J Matern Fetal Neonatal Med 14:1, 2003

Zetterström K, Lindeberg SN, Haglund B, et al: Chronic hypertension as a risk factor for offspring to be born small for gestational age. Acta Obstet Gynecol 85:1046, 2006

Pulmonary Disorders

A number of acute and chronic pulmonary disorders are encountered during pregnancy. The most common is asthma, which affects up to 4 percent of women. Together with community-acquired pneumonia, it accounted for almost 10 percent of nonobstetrical antepartum hospitalizations in one managed care plan (Gazmararian and colleagues, 2002). Acute and chronic lung disorders are superimposed upon several important adaptive changes of pulmonary physiology and function during pregnancy. And although there is no evidence that pulmonary function is impaired because of pregnancy, advanced pregnancy may intensify the pathophysiological effects of some lung diseases. One example is the disparate number of maternal deaths during the influenza pandemics of 1918 and 1957. Another is the poor tolerance for pregnancy of women with severe chronic lung disease.

PULMONARY PHYSIOLOGY

The important and sometimes marked changes in the respiratory system induced by pregnancy are found in Chapter 5 (p. 121) and the Appendix. Lung volumes and capacities that are measured directly to describe pulmonary pathophysiology may be significantly altered. In turn, these change the results of gas concentrations and acid-base values in blood. Some of the physiological changes induced by pregnancy were recently summarized by Wise and associates (2006):

1. *Vital capacity* and *inspiratory capacity* increase by approximately 20 percent by late pregnancy
2. *Expiratory reserve volume* decreases from 1300 mL to approximately 1100 mL
3. *Tidal volume* increases approximately 40 percent as a result of the respiratory stimulant properties of progesterone
4. *Minute ventilation* increases about 30 to 40 percent due to increased tidal volume. Arterial pO_2 also increases from 100 to 105 mm Hg
5. Carbon dioxide production increases approximately 30 percent, but diffusion capacity also increases, and with alveolar hyperventilation, the pCO_2 decreases from 40 to 32 mm Hg
6. *Residual volume* decreases approximately 20 percent from 1500 mL to approximately 1200 mL
7. The expanding uterus and increased abdominal pressure cause chest wall compliance to be reduced by a third. Thus, the *functional residual capacity*—the sum of expiratory reserve and residual volumes—decreases by 10 to 25 percent.

The sum of these changes is substantively increased ventilation due to deeper but not more frequent breathing. These changes presumably are induced by basal oxygen consumption, which increases incrementally by 20 to 40 mL/min in the second half of pregnancy. The kidney increases bicarbonate excretion and serum levels decrease to approximately 15 to 20 meq/L, while pH is slightly alkalotic at 7.45.

ASTHMA

Asthma is common in young women and therefore is seen frequently during pregnancy. Asthma prevalence increased steadily in many countries beginning in the mid-1970s but may have plateaued in the United States during the past decade (Eder and colleagues, 2006). According to Fanta (2009) and the National Center for Health Statistics (2007), almost 8 percent of the general population has asthma. Kwon and associates (2006) estimated asthma prevalence during pregnancy to range between 4 and 8 percent. Moreover, Namazy and Schatz (2005) reported that the prevalence in pregnant women appears to be increasing.

Pathophysiology

Asthma is a chronic inflammatory airway disorder with a *major hereditary component*. Increased airway responsiveness and persistent subacute inflammation have been associated with genes on chromosomes 5, 11, and 12 that include cytokine gene clusters, β-adrenergic and glucocorticoid receptor genes, and the T-cell antigen receptor gene (McFadden, 2005). There inevitably is an *environmental allergic stimulant* such as influenza or cigarette smoke in susceptible individuals (Hartert and colleagues, 2003).

The hallmarks of asthma are reversible airway obstruction from bronchial smooth muscle contraction, vascular congestion, tenacious mucus, and mucosal edema. There is airway inflammation and increased responsiveness to a number of stimuli including irritants, viral infections, aspirin, cold air, and exercise. Inflammation is caused by response of mast cells, eosinophils, lymphocytes, and bronchial epithelium. A number of inflammatory mediators by these and other cells include histamine, leukotrienes, prostaglandins, cytokines, and many others. IgE also plays a central role in pathophysiology (Strunk and Bloomberg, 2006). **Because F-series prostaglandins and ergonovine exacerbate asthma, these commonly used obstetrical drugs should be avoided if possible.**

Clinical Course

Asthma represents a broad spectrum of clinical illness ranging from mild wheezing to severe bronchoconstriction. The functional result of acute bronchospasm is airway obstruction and decreased airflow. The work of breathing progressively increases, and patients present with chest tightness, wheezing, or breathlessness. Subsequent alterations in oxygenation primarily reflect ventilation–perfusion mismatching, because the distribution of airway narrowing is uneven.

The variations of asthma manifestations have led to a simple classification that considers severity as well as onset and duration of symptoms (Table 46-1). With persistent or worsening bronchial obstruction, stages progress as shown in Figure 46-1. Hypoxia initially is well compensated by hyperventilation, normal arterial pO_2, decreased pCO_2, and resultant respiratory alkalosis. As airway narrowing worsens, ventilation–perfusion defects increase, and arterial hypoxemia ensues. With severe obstruction, ventilation becomes impaired because fatigue causes early CO_2 retention. Because of hyperventilation, this may only be seen initially as an arterial pCO_2 returning to the normal range. With continuing obstruction, respiratory failure follows from fatigue.

Although these changes are generally reversible and well tolerated by the healthy nonpregnant individual, even early stages of asthma may be dangerous for the pregnant woman and her fetus. This is because smaller functional residual capacity and

TABLE 46-1. Classification of Asthma Severity

	Severity			
	Intermittent	**Persistent**		
Component		**Mild**	**Moderate**	**Severe**
Symptoms	≤2 day/wk	>2 day/wk, not daily	Daily	Throughout day
Nocturnal awakenings	≤2×/mo	3–4×/mo	>1/wk, not nightly	Often 7×/wk
Short-acting β-agonist for symptoms	≤2 day/wk	≥2 day/wk, but not >1×/day	Daily	Several times daily
Interference with normal activity	None	Minor limitation	Some limitation	Extremely limited
Lung function	Normal between exacerbations			
• FEV₁	>80% predicted	≥80% predicted	60–80% predicted	<60% predicted
• FEV₁/FVC	Normal	Normal	Reduced 5%	Reduced >5%

FEV = forced expiratory volume, FVC = forced vital capacity.
From National Institutes of Health, National Heart, Lung, and Blood Institute. National Asthma Education Program (2007).

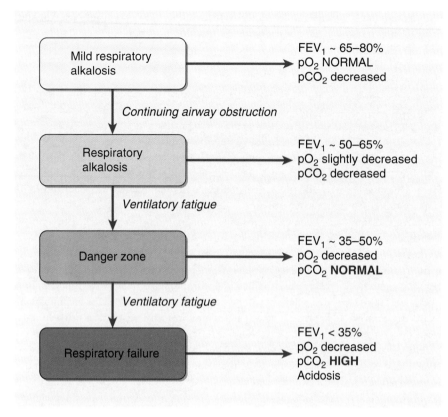

FIGURE 46-1 Clinical stages of asthma.

unchanged, or clearly worsened. In a study by Schatz and associates (2003), baseline severity correlated with asthma morbidity during pregnancy. With mild disease, 13 percent of women had an exacerbation and 2.3 percent required admission; with moderate disease, these numbers were 26 and 7 percent; and for severe asthma, 52 and 27 percent. Murphy and colleagues (2005) reported similar observations. Hendler and co-workers (2006) reported that women with severe disease were more likely to have an exacerbation during pregnancy. And Carroll and associates (2005) reported disparate morbidity in black compared with white women.

Approximately 20 percent of women with mild or moderate asthma have been reported to have an intrapartum exacerbation (Schatz and associates, 2003). Conversely, Wendel and associates (1996) reported exacerbations at the time of delivery in only 1 percent of women. Mabie and co-workers (1992) reported an 18-fold increased risk of exacerbation following cesarean versus vaginal delivery.

increased effective shunt render the woman more susceptible to hypoxia and hypoxemia.

Effects of Pregnancy on Asthma

There is no evidence that pregnancy has a predictable effect on underlying asthma. In their review of six prospective studies of more than 2000 pregnant women, Gluck and Gluck (2006) reported that approximately one third each improved, remained

Pregnancy Outcome

Pregnancy outcomes in asthmatics have improved during the past 20 years. From his scholarly review of some recent studies, Dombrowski (2006) concluded that, unless there is severe disease, pregnancy outcomes are generally excellent. Maternal and perinatal outcomes for more than 9000 pregnancies in asthmatic women are shown in Table 46-2. However, findings are not consistent between the studies. In some studies, there is a slightly increased incidence of preeclampsia, preterm labor,

TABLE 46-2. Maternal and Perinatal Outcomes in Pregnancies Complicated by Asthma

Study	No.	Perinatal Outcomes (Percent)		
		Gestational Hypertension	Growth Restriction	Preterm Delivery
Demissie et al (1998)	2289	8	15	18
Liu et al (2001)	2193	13	12	10
Bracken et al (2003)	872	NS[a]	8.5	8.5
Ramsey et al (2003)	1381	NS	1.7	Not ↑[b]
Dombrowski et al (2004a)	1739	12.2[b]	7.1[b]	16[b]
Mihrshahi et al (2003)	340	7[c]	—	3.2[b]
Schatz et al (2006)	384	8.1	7	18
Approximate average	9291	11	12	12

[a]NS = not stated.
[b]Incidence not significantly different compared with control group or general obstetrical population.
[c]Incidence significantly greater than control group.

low-birthweight infants, or perinatal mortality. In another report, Getahun and associates (2006) found a small increase in the incidence of placental abruption and an increase in preterm rupture of membranes (Getahun and co-workers, 2007). But, in a recent European report, 37,585 pregnancies of women with asthma were compared with pregnant nonasthmatics. Risks of most obstetrical complications were not higher in asthmatic women, except depression, miscarriages, and cesarean delivery (Tata and co-workers, 2007).

It appears that significantly increased morbidity is linked to progressively more severe disease, poor control, or both (Källén and Otterblad Olausson, 2007). For example, in the study by the Maternal-Fetal Medicine Units (MFMU) Network, delivery before 37 weeks was not increased among the 1687 pregnancies of asthmatics compared with 881 controls (Dombrowski and colleagues, 2004a). But for women with severe asthma, the rate was increased about twofold. In a prospective evaluation of 656 asthmatic pregnant women and 1052 pregnant controls, Triche and co-workers (2004) found that women with moderate to severe asthma, regardless of treatment, are at increased risk of preeclampsia. Finally, the MFMU Network study suggests a direct relationship of baseline pregnancy *forced expiratory volume at 1 second (FEV$_1$)* with birthweight and an inverse relationship with rates of gestational hypertension and preterm delivery (Schatz and associates, 2006).

Life-threatening complications from *status asthmaticus* include muscle fatigue with respiratory arrest, pneumothorax, pneumomediastinum, acute cor pulmonale, and cardiac arrhythmias. Maternal and perinatal mortality rates are substantively increased when mechanical ventilation is required.

Fetal Effects. With reasonable control of asthma, perinatal outcomes are generally good. For example, in the MFMU Network study cited above, there were no significant adverse neonatal sequelae from asthma (Dombrowski and co-workers, 2004a). The caveat is that severe asthma was uncommon in this closely monitored group. But when respiratory alkalosis develops, both animal and human studies suggest that fetal hypoxemia develops well before the alkalosis compromises maternal oxygenation (Rolston and associates, 1974). It is hypothesized that the fetus is jeopardized from decreased uterine blood flow, decreased maternal venous return, and an alkaline-induced leftward shift of the oxyhemoglobin dissociation curve.

The fetal response to maternal hypoxemia is decreased umbilical blood flow, increased systemic and pulmonary vascular resistance, and decreased cardiac output. Observations by Bracken and colleagues (2003) confirm that the incidence of fetal-growth restriction increases with asthma severity. The realization that the fetus may be seriously compromised as asthma severity increases underscores the need for aggressive management. Monitoring the fetal response is, in effect, an indicator of maternal status.

Possible teratogenic or adverse fetal effects of drugs given to control asthma have been a concern. Fortunately, and as discussed in Chapter 14 (p. 315), considerable data have accrued with no evidence that commonly used anti-asthmatic drugs are harmful (Blais and colleagues, 2007; Källén, 2007; Namazy and Schatz, 2006). Despite this, Enriquez and co-workers (2006) reported a 13- to 54-percent patient-generated decrease in β-agonist and corticosteroid use between 5 to 13 weeks of pregnancy.

Clinical Evaluation

The subjective severity of asthma frequently does not correlate with objective measures of airway function or ventilation. Clinical examination also is inaccurate as a predictor of severity. Useful clinical signs include labored breathing, tachycardia, pulsus paradoxus, prolonged expiration, and use of accessory muscles. Signs of a potentially fatal attack include central cyanosis and altered consciousness.

Arterial blood gas analysis provides objective assessment of maternal oxygenation, ventilation, and acid–base status. With this information, the severity of an acute attack can be assessed (see Fig. 46-1). That said, in a prospective evaluation, Wendel and associates (1996) found that *routine* arterial blood gas analysis did not help to manage most pregnant women who required admission for asthma control. If used, the results must be interpreted in relation to normal values for pregnancy. For example, a $pCO_2 > 35$ mm Hg with a pH < 7.35 is consistent with hyperventilation and CO_2 retention in a pregnant woman.

Pulmonary function testing should be routine in the management of chronic and acute asthma. Sequential measurement of the FEV$_1$ or the *peak expiratory flow rate—PEFR—*are the best measures of severity. An FEV$_1$ less than 1 L, or less than 20 percent of predicted value, correlates with severe disease defined by hypoxia, poor response to therapy, and a high relapse rate (Noble and colleagues, 1988). The PEFR correlates well with the FEV$_1$, and it can be measured reliably with inexpensive portable meters. Each woman determines her own baseline when asymptomatic—*personal best*—to compare with values when symptomatic. Brancazio and associates (1997) showed that the PEFR did not change during the course of pregnancy in normal women.

Management of Chronic Asthma

The most recent management guidelines of the Working Group on Asthma and Pregnancy include:

1. Patient education—general asthma management and its effect on pregnancy.
2. Environmental precipitating factors—avoidance or control.
3. Objective assessment of pulmonary function and fetal well-being—monitor with PEFR or FEV$_1$.
4. Pharmacological therapy—in appropriate combinations and doses to provide baseline control and treat exacerbations (National Heart, Lung and Blood Institute, 2004).

In general, women with moderate to severe asthma should measure and record either their FEV$_1$ or PEFR twice daily. The FEV$_1$ ideally is >80 percent of predicted. For PEFR, predicted values range from 380 to 550 L/min. Each woman has her own baseline value, and therapeutic adjustments can be made using this (American College of Obstetricians and Gynecologists, 2008; Rey and Boulet, 2007).

TABLE 46-3. Stepwise Therapy of Chronic Asthma During Pregnancy

Severity	Stepwise Therapy
Mild intermittent	Inhaled β-agonists as needed[a]
Mild persistent	Low-dose inhaled corticosteroids[b] Alternative—cromolyn, leukotriene antagonists, or theophylline
Moderate persistent	Low-dose inhaled corticosteroids and long-acting β-agonists[c] *or* medium-dose inhaled steroids and long-acting β-agonist if needed Alternative—low-dose (or medium if needed) inhaled steroids *and* either theophylline or leukotriene antagonists
Severe persistent	High-dose inhaled corticosteroids and long-acting β-agonist and oral steroids if needed Alternative—high-dose inhaled corticosteroids and theophylline and oral steroids

[a]Albuterol preferred because of more human data on safety in pregnancy.
[b]Budesonide preferred because of more experience in pregnancy.
[c]Salmeterol preferred because of its long availability in this country.
From Dombroski (2006); Fanta (2009); Namazy and Schatz (2006); National Heart, Lung and Blood Institute, National Asthma Education and Prevention Program Working Group Report (2004).

Treatment depends on the severity of disease. Although β-agonists help to abate bronchospasm, corticosteroids treat the inflammatory component. Regimens recommended for outpatient management are listed in Table 46-3. For mild asthma, inhaled *β-agonists* as needed are usually sufficient. For persistent asthma, *inhaled corticosteroids* are administered every 3 to 4 hours. The goal is to reduce the use of β-agonists for symptomatic relief. A case-control study from Canada with a cohort of more than 15,600 nonpregnant women with asthma showed that inhaled corticosteroids reduced hospitalizations by 80 percent (Blais and associates, 1998). And Wendel and colleagues (1996) achieved a 55-percent reduction in readmissions for severe exacerbations in pregnant asthmatics given maintenance inhaled corticosteroids along with β-agonist therapy.

Theophylline is a methylxanthine, and its various salts are bronchodilators and possibly anti-inflammatory agents. They have been used less frequently since inhaled corticosteroids became available. Some theophylline derivatives are considered useful for oral maintenance therapy if the initial response is not optimal to inhaled corticosteroids and β-agonists (see Table 46-3). Dombrowski and colleagues (2004b) conducted a randomized trial with nearly 400 pregnant women with moderate asthma. Oral theophylline was compared with inhaled beclomethasone for maintenance. In both groups, about 20 percent had exacerbations. Women taking theophylline had a significantly higher discontinuation rate because of side effects. Pregnancy outcomes were similar in the two groups.

Leukotriene modifiers inhibit their synthesis and include *zileuton, zafirinkast,* and *montelukast.* These drugs are given orally or by inhalation for prevention, but they are not effective for acute disease. For maintenance, they are used in conjunction with inhaled corticosteroids to allow minimal dosing. About half of asthmatics will improve with these drugs (McFadden, 2005). They are not as effective as inhaled corticosteroids (Fanta, 2009). Finally, there is little experience with their use in pregnancy (Bakhireva and colleagues, 2007).

Cromolyn and *nedocromil* inhibit mast cell degranulation. They are ineffective for acute asthma and are taken chronically for prevention. They likely are not as effective as inhaled corticosteroids and have generally been replaced by leukotriene modifiers (Fanta, 2009).

There is no experience in pregnant women with *omalizumab,* a recombinant humanized monoclonal anti-IgE antibody. It binds circulating IgE to deactivate it.

Management of Acute Asthma

Treatment of acute asthma during pregnancy is similar to that for the nonpregnant asthmatic. An exception is a significantly lowered threshold for hospitalization. Intravenous hydration may help clear pulmonary secretions, and supplemental oxygen is given by mask. The therapeutic aim is to maintain the pO_2 greater than 60 mm Hg, and preferably normal, along with 95-percent oxygen saturation. Baseline pulmonary function testing includes FEV_1 or PEFR. Continuous pulse oximetry and electronic fetal monitoring may provide useful information.

First-line therapy for acute asthma includes a *β-adrenergic agonist,* such as terbutaline, albuterol, isoetharine, epinephrine, isoproterenol, or metaproterenol, which is given subcutaneously, taken orally, or inhaled. These drugs bind to specific cell-surface receptors and activate adenylyl cyclase to increase intracellular cyclic AMP and modulate bronchial smooth muscle relaxation. Long-acting preparations are used for outpatient therapy.

If not previously given for maintenance, inhaled corticosteroids are commenced along with intensive β-agonist therapy. For severe exacerbations, inhaled ipratropium bromide is given. *Corticosteroids* should be given early to all patients with severe acute asthma. Unless there is a timely response to treatment, oral or parenteral preparations are given. Intravenous methylprednisolone, 40 to 60 mg, every 6 hours is commonly used. Equipotent doses of hydrocortisone by infusion or prednisone orally can be given instead. **Because their onset of action is several hours, corticosteroids are given initially along with β-agonists for acute asthma.**

Further management depends on the response to therapy. If initial therapy with β-agonists is associated with improvement of FEV$_1$ or PEFR to above 70 percent of baseline, then discharge can be considered. Some women may benefit from observation. Alternatively, for the woman with obvious respiratory distress, or if the FEV$_1$ or PEFR is less than 70 percent of predicted after three doses of β-agonist, admission is advisable. Intensive therapy includes inhaled β-agonists, intravenous corticosteroids, and close observation for worsening respiratory distress or fatigue in breathing (Wendel and colleagues, 1996). The woman is cared for in the delivery unit or an intermediate or intensive care unit (Dombrowski, 2006).

Status Asthmaticus and Respiratory Failure

Severe asthma of any type not responding after 30 to 60 minutes of intensive therapy is termed *status asthmaticus*. Braman and Kaemmerlen (1990) have shown that management of nonpregnant patients with status asthmaticus in an intensive care setting results in a good outcome in most cases. Consideration should be given to early intubation when maternal respiratory status worsens despite aggressive treatment (see Fig. 46-1). Fatigue, carbon dioxide retention, and hypoxemia are indications for mechanical ventilation.

Labor and Delivery

Maintenance medications are continued through delivery. Stress-dose corticosteroids are administered to any woman given systemic steroid therapy within the preceding 4 weeks. The usual dose is 100 mg of hydrocortisone given intravenously every 8 hours during labor and for 24 hours after delivery. The PEFR or FEV$_1$ should be determined on admission, and serial measurements are taken if symptoms develop.

Oxytocin or prostaglandins E$_1$ or E$_2$ are used for cervical ripening and induction. A nonhistamine-releasing narcotic such as fentanyl may be preferable to meperidine for labor, and epidural analgesia is ideal. For surgical delivery, conduction analgesia is preferred because tracheal intubation can trigger severe bronchospasm. Postpartum hemorrhage is treated with oxytocin or prostaglandin E$_2$. **Prostaglandin F$_{2\alpha}$ or ergotamine derivatives are contraindicated because they may cause significant bronchospasm.**

ACUTE BRONCHITIS

Infection of the large airways is manifest by cough without pneumonitis. It is common in adults, especially in winter months. Infections are usually caused by viruses, and of these, influenza A and B, parainfluenza, respiratory syncytial, coronavirus, adenovirus, and rhinovirus are common isolates (Wenzel and Fowler, 2006). Bacterial agents causing community-acquired pneumonia are rarely implicated. The cough of acute bronchitis persists for 10 to 20 days (mean 18 days) and occasionally lasts for a month or longer. According to the 2006 guidelines of the American College of Chest Physicians, routine antibiotic treatment is not justified (Braman, 2006). Influenza bronchitis is managed as discussed below.

PNEUMONIA

According to Anand and Kollef (2009), current classification includes several types of pneumonia. *Community-acquired pneumonia (CAP)* is typically encountered in otherwise healthy young women, including during pregnancy. *Healthcare-associated pneumonia (HCAP)* develops in patients in outpatient care facilities and more closely resembles *hospital-acquired pneumonia (HAP)*. Other types are *nursing home-acquired pneumonia (NHAO)* and *ventilator-associated pneumonia (VAP)*. Community-acquired pneumonia in pregnant women is relatively common and is caused by a number of bacterial or viral pathogens (Sheffield and Cunningham, 2009). Gazmararian and colleagues (2002) reported that pneumonia accounts for 4.2 percent of antepartum admissions for nonobstetrical complications. During influenza season, admissions for respiratory illnesses double compared with the remaining months (Cox and colleagues, 2006). Mortality from pneumonia is infrequent in young women, but during pregnancy severe pneumonitis with appreciable loss of ventilatory capacity is not as well tolerated (Laibl and Sheffield, 2006). This generalization seems to hold true regardless of the etiology of the pneumonia. Hypoxemia and acidosis are also poorly tolerated by the fetus and frequently stimulate preterm labor after midpregnancy. Because many cases of pneumonia follow viral upper respiratory illnesses, worsening or persistence of symptoms may represent developing pneumonia. **Any pregnant woman suspected of having pneumonia should undergo chest radiography.**

Bacterial Pneumonia

Many bacteria that cause community-acquired pneumonia, such as *Streptococcus pneumoniae*, are part of the normal resident flora (Bogaert and co-workers, 2004). Some factors that perturb the symbiotic relationship between colonizing bacteria and mucosal phagocytic defenses include acquisition of a virulent strain or bacterial infections following a viral infection. Cigarette smoking and chronic bronchitis favor colonization with *S. pneumoniae, Haemophilus influenzae,* and *Legionella* species. Other risk factors include asthma, binge drinking, and human immunodeficiency virus (HIV) infection (Goodnight and Soper, 2005; Sheffield and Cunningham, 2009).

Incidence and Causes

Pregnancy itself does not predispose to pneumonia. From Alberta, Jin and colleagues (2003) reported the rate of antepartum hospitalization for pneumonia to be 1.5 per 1000 deliveries—almost identical to the rate of 1.47 per 1000 for nonpregnant women. Likewise, Yost and associates (2000) reported an incidence of 1.5 per 1000 for pneumonia complicating 75,000 pregnancies cared for at Parkland Hospital.

More than half of adult pneumonias are bacterial, and *S. pneumoniae* is the most common cause. Lim and colleagues (2001) studied 267 nonpregnant inpatients with pneumonia and identified a causative agent in 75 percent—*S. pneumoniae* in 37 percent; influenza A, 14 percent; *Chlamydophila pneumoniae,* 10 percent; *H. influenzae,* 5 percent; and *Mycoplasma pneumoniae* and *Legionella pneumophila,* 2 percent each.

Community-acquired methicillin-resistant *Staphylococcus aureus* has recently been reported as causing a necrotizing pneumonia (Rotas and colleagues, 2007).

Diagnosis

Typical symptoms include cough, dyspnea, sputum production, and pleuritic chest pain. Mild upper respiratory symptoms and malaise usually precede these symptoms, and mild leukocytosis is usually present. Chest radiography is essential for diagnosis but does not accurately predict the etiology (Fig. 46-2). The responsible pathogen is identified in less than half of cases. According to the Infectious Diseases Society of

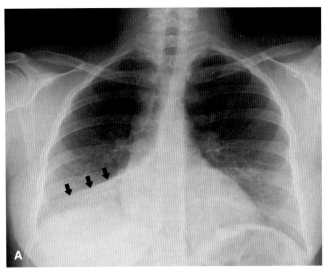

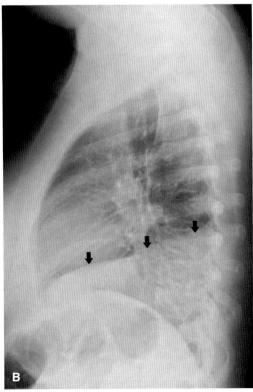

FIGURE 46-2 Chest radiographs in a pregnant woman with right lower lobe pneumonia. **A.** Complete opacification of the right lower lobe (*arrows*) is consistent with the clinical suspicion of pneumonia. **B.** Opacification (*arrows*) is also seen on the lateral projection.

TABLE 46-4. Criteria for Severe Community-Acquired Pneumonia

Respiratory rate ≥30/min
PaO_2/FiO_2 ratio ≤250
Multilobular infiltrates
Confusion/disorientation
Uremia
Leukopenia—WBC <4000/μL
Thrombocytopenia—platelets <100,000/μL
Hypothermia—core temperature <36°C
Hypotension requiring aggressive fluid resuscitation

The Infectious Diseases Society of America/American Thoracic Society (Adapted from Mandell and colleagues, 2007).

America (IDSA) and the American Thoracic Society (ATS), tests to identify a specific agent are optional. Thus, sputum cultures, serological testing, cold agglutinin identification, and tests for bacterial antigens are not recommended. At Parkland Hospital, the one exception to this is rapid serological testing for influenza A and B (Sheffield and Cunningham, 2009).

Management

Although many otherwise healthy young adults can be safely treated as outpatients, at Parkland Hospital we hospitalize all pregnant women with radiographically proven pneumonia. Outpatient therapy or 23-hour observation is reasonable with optimal follow-up. Risk factors shown in Table 46-4 should prompt hospitalization.

With severe disease, admission to an intensive care or intermediate care unit is advisable. Approximately 20 percent of pregnant women admitted to Parkland Hospital for pneumonia require this level of care (Zeeman and associates, 2003). Severe pneumonia is a relatively common cause of acute respiratory distress syndrome during pregnancy, and mechanical ventilation may become necessary. Indeed, of the 51 pregnant women who required mechanical ventilation in the review by Jenkins and co-workers (2003), 12 percent had pneumonia.

Antimicrobial treatment is empirical. Because most adult pneumonias are caused by pneumococci, mycoplasma, or chlamydophilia, monotherapy initially is with a macrolide—azithromycin, clarithromycin, or erythromycin. Yost and colleagues (2000) reported that erythromycin monotherapy, given intravenously and then orally, was effective in all but one of 99 pregnant women with uncomplicated pneumonia.

For women with severe disease according to criteria in Table 46-4, the IDSA/ATS guidelines call for either: (1) a respiratory fluoroquinolone—levofloxacin, moxifloxacin, or gemifloxacin; or (2) a β-lactam *plus* a macrolide—high-dose amoxicillin or amoxicillin-clavulanate are preferred β-lactams, and alternatives include ceftriaxone, cefpodoxime, or cefuroxime. Levofloxacin is also acceptable. In areas in which 25 percent or more of pneumococcal isolates are resistant to macrolides, these latter regimens are preferred. The teratogenicity risk of fluoroquinolones is low, and these should be given if indicated (Briggs and colleagues, 2005). If community-acquired methicillin-resistant *S. aureus* is suspected, then vancomycin is added (Sheffield and Cunningham, 2009).

Clinical improvement is usually evident in 48 to 72 hours with resolution of fever in 2 to 4 days. Radiographic abnormalities may take up to 6 weeks to completely resolve (Torres and Menéndez, 2008). Worsening disease is a poor prognostic feature, and follow-up radiography is recommended if fever persists. Even with improvement, however, about 20 percent of women develop a pleural effusion. Therapy is recommended for a minimum of 5 days. Treatment failure may occur in up to 15 percent of cases, and a wider microbial antibiotic regimen is warranted in these cases (Menedez and Torres, 2008).

Pregnancy Outcome with Pneumonia

During the pre-antimicrobial era, as many as a third of pregnant women with pneumonia died (Finland and Dublin, 1939). Although much improved, maternal and perinatal mortality rates both remain formidable. In five studies published after 1990, the maternal mortality rate was 0.8 percent of 632 women. Importantly, almost 7 percent of the women required intubation and mechanical ventilation.

Prematurely ruptured membranes and preterm delivery are common complications and are reported in up to a third of cases (Getahun and associates, 2007; Shariatzadeh and Marrie, 2006). Likely related are older studies reporting a twofold increase in low-birthweight infants (Sheffield and Cunningham, 2009).

Prevention

Pneumococcal vaccine is 60- to 70-percent protective against its 23 included serotypes. Its use has been shown to decrease emergence of drug-resistant pneumococci (Kyaw and associates, 2006). The vaccine is not recommended for otherwise healthy pregnant women (American College of Obstetricians and Gynecologists, 2003). It is recommended for those who are immunocompromised, including those with HIV infection; significant smoking history; diabetes or cardiac, pulmonary, or renal disease; and asplenia, such as with sickle-cell disease.

Influenza Pneumonia

Respiratory infection, including pneumonitis, is caused by RNA viruses of which influenza A and B form one genus (see Chap. 58, p. 1212). Influenza infection can be serious, and it is epidemic in the winter months. The virus is spread by aerosolized droplets and quickly infects ciliated columnar epithelium, alveolar cells, mucus gland cells, and macrophages. Disease onset is 1 to 4 days following exposure (Longman and Johnson, 2007). In most healthy adults, infection is self-limited. Pneumonia is the most common complication, and it is difficult to distinguish from bacterial pneumonia. At Parkland Hospital during the 2003–2004 influenza season, pneumonia developed in 12 percent of pregnant women with influenza (Laibl and Sheffield, 2006).

Primary influenza pneumonitis is the most severe and is characterized by sparse sputum production and radiographic interstitial infiltrates (Fig. 46-3). More commonly, secondary pneumonia develops from bacterial superinfection by streptococci or staphylococci after 2 to 3 days of initial clinical

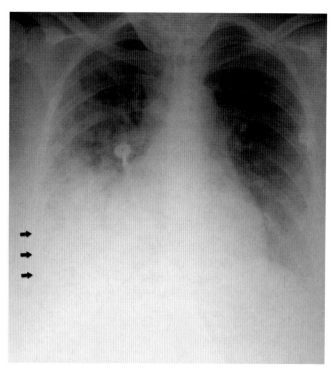

FIGURE 46-3 Chest radiograph of a 30-week pregnant woman with confirmed influenza A pneumonia. Extensive right lower lung field opacification (*arrows*), which represents parenchymal infiltrate and pleural effusion, obscures the right hemidiaphragm. (Used with permission from Dr. Vanessa Laibl Rogers.)

improvement. The Centers for Disease Control and Prevention (2007a) reported a number of cases in which community-acquired methicillin-resistant staphylococci caused influenza-associated pneumonitis with a case-fatality rate of 25 percent.

Management

Hospitalizations for influenza during late pregnancy are increased compared with nonpregnant women (Dodds and colleagues, 2007; Schanzer and associates, 2007). Supportive treatment with antipyretics and bed rest is recommended for uncomplicated influenza. Rapid resistance of influenza A (H3N2) strains to *amantadine* or *rimantadine* in 2005 prompted the Centers for Disease Control and Prevention (2006) to recommend against their use. Instead, *neuraminidase inhibitors* were given within 2 days of symptoms onset for chemoprophylaxis and treatment of influenza A and B (see Chap. 58, p. 1212). The drugs interfere with the release of progeny virus from infected host cells and thus prevent infection of new host cells (Moscona, 2005). *Oseltamivir* is given orally, 75 mg twice daily, or *zanamivir* is given by inhalation, 10 mg twice daily. The drugs shorten the course of illness by 1 to 2 days, and they may reduce the risk for pneumonitis. Our practice is to treat all pregnant women who are admitted for severe influenza whether or not pneumonitis is identified. There are few data on the use of these agents in pregnant women, but the drugs were not teratogenic in animal studies and are considered low risk (Briggs and colleagues, 2005).

The concerns that resistance to oseltamivir would develop proved correct, and there was sudden and rapid resistance by influenza A (H1N1) strains during the 2007–2008 flu season

(Gooskens and colleagues, 2009). In December 2008, a CDC Health Advisory was issued with recommendations for treatment of influenza A with oseltamivir *and* amantadine or rimantadine. If the predominate strain in the community is known do be H1N1, then an adamantane is used. However, with the H3N2 strain, oseltamivir is given instead. Local isolates can be determined by visiting the website for the Centers for Disease Control and Prevention.

Other concerns for viral resistance are for avian H5N1 strain isolated in Southeast Asia, which is a candidate virus for an influenza pandemic with a projected mortality rate that exceeds 50 percent (Beigi, 2007; World Health Organization, 2008). Currently, international efforts are being made to produce a vaccine effective against this strain (World Health Organization, 2007).

Prevention

Vaccination for influenza A is recommended and is discussed in detail in Chapter 58 (p. 1213). Prenatal vaccination also affords protection for a third of infants for at least 6 months (Zaman and colleagues, 2008).

Effects on Pregnancy

Severe viral pneumonitis is life-threatening during pregnancy. Other possible adverse effects of influenza A and B on pregnancy outcome are discussed in Chapter 58 (p. 1212).

Varicella Pneumonia

Infection with varicella-zoster virus—chicken pox—results in pneumonitis in 5 percent of pregnant women (Harger and colleagues, 2002). Diagnosis and management are considered in Chapter 58 (p. 1211).

Fungal and Parasitic Pneumonia

Fungal and parasitic pulmonary infections are usually of greatest consequence in immunocompromised hosts, especially in women with acquired immunodeficiency syndrome (AIDS).

Pneumocystis Pneumonia

Lung infection with *Pneumocystis jiroveci*, formerly called *Pneumocystis carinii*, is a common complication in women with AIDS. The opportunistic fungus causes interstitial pneumonia characterized by dry cough, tachypnea, dyspnea, and diffuse radiographic infiltrates. Although this organism can be identified by sputum culture, bronchoscopy with lavage or biopsy may be necessary.

In a report from the AIDS Clinical Trials Centers, Stratton and colleagues (1992) described pneumocystis pneumonia as the most common HIV-related disorder in pregnant women. Ahmad and co-workers (2001) reviewed 22 cases during pregnancy and cited a 50-percent mortality rate. Treatment is with trimethoprim-sulfamethoxazole or the more toxic pentamidine (Walzer, 2005). Experience with dapsone or atovaquone is limited. In some cases, tracheal intubation and mechanical ventilation may be required.

Prophylaxis. A number of international health agencies recommend prophylaxis with one double-strength trimethoprim-sulfamethoxazole tablet daily for some HIV-infected pregnant women. These include women with CD4$^+$ T-lymphocyte counts less than 200/μL, those whose CD4$^+$ T lymphocytes constitute less than 14 percent, or if there is an AIDS-defining illness, particularly oropharyngeal candidiasis (Centers for Disease Control and Prevention, 2008a). After their systematic review, Forna and colleagues (2006) concluded that the benefits of prophylaxis outweighed any risks.

Fungal Pneumonia

Any of a number of fungi can cause pneumonia, and in pregnancy, these are usually seen in women with HIV infection or who are otherwise immunocompromised. Infection is usually mild and self-limited. It is characterized initially by cough and fever, and dissemination is infrequent.

Histoplasmosis and *blastomycosis* do not appear to be more common or more severe during pregnancy. Data concerning *coccidioidomycosis* are conflicting. In a case-control study from an endemic area, Rosenstein and co-workers (2001) reported that pregnancy was a significant risk factor for disseminated disease. In another study, however, Caldwell and colleagues (2000) identified 32 serologically confirmed cases during pregnancy and documented dissemination in only three cases. Arsura (1998) and Caldwell (2000) and their associates reported that pregnant women with symptomatic infection had a better overall prognosis if there was associated *erythema nodosum*. Crum and Ballon-Landa (2006) recently reviewed 80 cases of coccidioidomycosis complicating pregnancy. Almost all women diagnosed in the third trimester had disseminated disease. Although the overall maternal mortality rate was 40 percent, it was only 20 percent for 29 cases reported since 1973. Spinello and colleagues (2007) have recently reviewed coccidioidomycosis in pregnancy.

Most cases of *cryptococcosis* reported during pregnancy were manifest as meningitis. Ely and co-workers (1998) described four otherwise healthy pregnant women with cryptococcal pneumonia. Diagnosis is difficult, because clinical presentation is similar to that of other community-acquired pneumonias.

The 2007 IDSA/ATS guidelines recommend itraconazole as preferred therapy for disseminated fungal infections (Mandell and colleagues, 2007). Pregnant women with disseminated fungal infections have also been given intravenous *amphotericin B* or *ketoconazole* (Hooper and associates, 2007; Paranyuk and colleagues, 2006). Amphotericin B has been used extensively in pregnancy with no embryofetal effects. Because of evidence that fluconazole, itraconazole, and ketoconazole may be embryotoxic in large doses in early pregnancy, Briggs and colleagues (2005) recommend that use at this time should be avoided if possible. Later in pregnancy, however, use of itraconazole seems reasonable.

There are three echinocandin derivatives—*caspofungin, micafungin,* and *anidulafungin*—that are effective for invasive candidiasis (Medical Letter, 2006; Reboli and colleagues, 2007). They are embryotoxic and teratogenic in laboratory animals, but use in human pregnancies has not been reported (Briggs and associates, 2005).

Severe Acute Respiratory Syndrome (SARS)

This coronaviral respiratory infection was first identified in China in 2002. It causes atypical pneumonitis with a case-fatality rate of approximately 5 percent (Centers for Disease Control and Prevention, 2003b). Most cases were reported from Asia with an outbreak in Canada (Yudin and associates, 2005). Experience with SARS in pregnancy comes mostly from Wong (2004) and Lam (2004) and their colleagues from Hong Kong. From their review, Longman and Johnson (2007) reported a case-fatality rate in pregnancy of up to 25 percent. Ng and associates (2006) reported that the placentas from seven of 19 cases showed abnormal intervillous or subchorionic fibrin deposition in three, and extensive fetal thrombotic vasculopathy in two. One recent report noted improvement in maternal respiratory function when a pregnant woman with SARS underwent cesarean delivery (Oram and colleagues, 2007).

TUBERCULOSIS

Although tuberculosis is still a major worldwide concern, it is uncommon in the United States. As shown in Figure 46-4, the incidence of *active tuberculosis* decreased by almost half in the decade ending in 2003. Because the incidence in foreign-born persons did not change, over half of active cases in this country are in immigrants (Centers for Disease Control and Prevention, 2009a). Importantly, from 10 to 15 million persons in the United States have *latent tuberculosis* manifest by a positive tuberculin skin test. U.S.-born persons have newly acquired infection, whereas foreign-born persons usually have reactivation of latent infection (Geng and co-workers, 2002). In this country, tuberculosis is a disease of the elderly, the urban poor, minority groups, and patients with AIDS.

Infection is via inhalation of *Mycobacterium tuberculosis*, which incites a granulomatous pulmonary reaction. In more than 90 percent of patients, infection is contained and is dormant for long periods. In some patients, especially those who are immunocompromised or who have other diseases, tuberculosis becomes reactivated to cause clinical disease. Manifestations usually include cough with minimal sputum production, low-grade fever, hemoptysis, and weight loss. A variety of infiltrative patterns are seen on chest radiograph, and there may be associated cavitation or mediastinal lymphadenopathy. Acid-fast bacilli are seen on stained smears of sputum in about two thirds of culture-positive patients. Extrapulmonary tuberculosis may occur in any

organ, and almost 40 percent of affected HIV-positive patients have disseminated disease (Weinberger and Weiss, 1999).

Treatment

Cure rates with 6-month short-course *directly observed therapy*—DOT—approach 90 percent for new infections. Resistance to antituberculosis drugs was first manifest in the United States in the early 1990s following the epidemic from 1985 through 1992 (Centers for Disease Control and Prevention, 2007b). Strains of *multidrug-resistant tuberculosis (MDR-TB)* increased rapidly as TB incidence fell during the 1990s (Fig. 46-4). Because of this, the Centers for Disease Control and Prevention (2003a) now recommends a four-drug regimen for initial empirical treatment of patients with symptomatic tuberculosis. Isoniazid, rifampin, pyrazinamide, and ethambutol are given until susceptibility studies are performed. Other second-line drugs may need to be added. Drug susceptibility is performed on all first isolates.

In 2005, there was a worldwide emergence of *extensively drug-resistant tuberculosis—XDR-TB.* This is defined as resistance in vitro to at least the first-line drugs isoniazid and rifampin as well as to three or more of the six main classes of second-line drugs—aminoglycosides, polypeptides, fluoroquinolones, thioamides, cycloserine, and para-aminosalicylic acid (Centers for Disease Control and Prevention, 2009b). Like their predecessor MDR-TB, these extensively resistant strains predominate in foreign-born persons (Tino and associates, 2007).

Tuberculosis and Pregnancy

The considerable influx of women into the United States from Asia, Africa, Mexico, and Central America has been accompanied by an increased frequency of tuberculosis in pregnant women. Sackoff and co-workers (2006) reported positive-tuberculin tests in half of 678 foreign-born women attending perinatal clinics in New York City. Almost 60 percent were newly diagnosed. Pillay and co-workers (2004) stress the prevalence of tuberculosis in HIV-positive pregnant women. Margono and colleagues (1994) reported that for two New York City hospitals, more than half of pregnant women with active tuberculosis were HIV positive. At Jackson Memorial Hospital in Miami, Schulte and associates (2002) reported that 21 percent of 207 HIV-infected pregnant women had a positive skin test.

Without antituberculosis therapy, pregnancy likely has adverse effects on the course of active tuberculosis (Anderson, 1997). Contemporaneous experiences are few, because chemotherapy has diminished severe disease. Outcomes are dependent on the site of infection and timing of diagnosis in relation to delivery. Jana and colleagues (1994) from India and Figueroa-Damian and Arrendondo-Garcia (1998) from Mexico City reported that active pulmonary tuberculosis was associated with increased incidences of preterm delivery, low-birthweight and growth-restricted infants, and perinatal mortality. From her review, Efferen (2007) cited twofold increased rates of low-birthweight and preterm infants as well as preeclampsia. The perinatal mortality rate was increased almost tenfold. Adverse outcomes correlate with late diagnosis, incomplete or irregular treatment, and advanced pulmonary lesions.

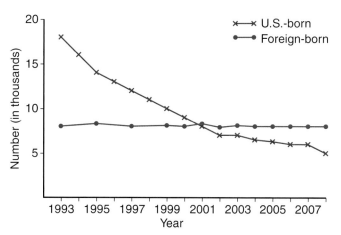

FIGURE 46-4 Number of cases of active tuberculosis reported in the United States from 1993 through 2006. (Adapted from Centers for Disease Control and Prevention, 2009a)

TABLE 46-5. Groups at High Risk for Having Latent
Tuberculosis Infection

Healthcare workers
Contact with infectious person(s)
Foreign-born
HIV-infected
Working or living in homeless shelters
Alcoholics
Illicit drug use
Detainees and prisoners

From Centers for Disease Control and Prevention (2005a).

Extrapulmonary tuberculosis is less common. Jana and co-workers (1999) reported outcomes in 33 pregnant women with renal, intestinal, and skeletal tuberculosis, and a third had low-birthweight newborns. Llewelyn and associates (2000) reported that 9 of 13 pregnant women had extrapulmonary disease associated with delayed diagnoses. Prevost and Fung Kee Fung (1999) reviewed 56 cases of tuberculous meningitis, which were associated with maternal death in a third. Other presentations have included cervical spine tuberculosis with paraplegia, widespread intraperitoneal tuberculosis simulating ovarian carcinomatosis and degenerating leiomyoma, and hyperemesis gravidarum from tubercular meningitis (Kutlu, 2007; Moore, 2008; Nanda, 2002; Sherer, 2005, and all their colleagues).

Diagnosis

Current guidelines from the Centers for Disease Control and Prevention (2005a) include skin testing of pregnant women who are in any of the high-risk groups shown in Table 46-5. The preferred antigen is purified protein derivative (PPD) of intermediate strength of 5 tuberculin units. If the intracutaneously applied test is negative, no further evaluation is needed. A positive skin test measures ≥5 mm in diameter and requires evaluation for active disease, including a chest radiograph (Centers for Disease Control and Prevention, 2005b). It also may be interpreted according to risk factors proposed by the American Thoracic Society/Centers for Disease Control and Prevention (1990). For *very high-risk* patients—that is, those who are HIV-positive, those with abnormal chest radiography, or those who have a recent contact with an active case—5 mm or greater is considered treatable. For those at *high risk*—foreign-born individuals, intravenous drug users who are HIV-negative, low-income populations, or those with medical conditions that increase the risk for tuberculosis—10 mm or greater is considered treatable. For persons with none of these risk factors, 15 mm or greater is defined as requiring treatment.

The in vitro *QuantiFERON-TB Gold test* is recommended by the Centers for Disease Control and Prevention (2005a, b) for the same indications as skin testing to diagnose latent infection. It has not been evaluated as extensively as tuberculin skin testing. Both the QuantiFERON-TB Gold test and the new T-Spot *TB* have been extensively reviewed by Lalvani (2007) and shown to be useful in identifying patients with latent TB and at risk for progression to active disease. They also distinguish between immune responses due to infection and responses resulting from bacille Calmette-Guérin (BCG) vaccination (Ernst and colleagues, 2007).

Essential laboratory methods for detection or verification of infection—both active and latent—include microscopy, culture, nucleic acid amplification assay, and drug-susceptibility testing (Centers for Disease Control and Prevention, 2009b).

Treatment

Different schemes are recommended for latent and active tuberculosis.

Latent Infection. In nonpregnant tuberculin-positive patients who are younger than 35 years and who have no evidence of active disease, isoniazid, 300 mg orally daily, is given for 1 year. Isoniazid has been used for decades, and it is considered safe in pregnancy (Briggs and colleagues, 2005). Compliance is a major problem, and Sackoff (2006) and Cruz (2005) and their associates reported a disappointing 10-percent treatment completion. One obvious disconnect is that care for tuberculosis is given in health systems different from prenatal care. These observations are important because most recommend that isoniazid therapy be delayed until after delivery. Because of possibly increased isoniazid-induced hepatitis risk in postpartum women, some recommend withholding treatment until 3 to 6 months after delivery. That said, neither method is as effective as antepartum treatment to prevent active infection. Boggess and colleagues (2000) reported that only 42 percent of 167 tuberculin-positive asymptomatic women delivered at San Francisco General Hospital completed 6-month therapy that was not given until the first postpartum visit.

There are exceptions to delayed treatment in pregnancy. Known recent skin-test convertors are treated antepartum because the incidence of active infection is 3 percent in the first year. Skin-test-positive women exposed to active infection are treated because the incidence of infection is 0.5 percent per year. Finally, HIV-positive women are treated because they have an 8-percent annual risk of active disease (Brost and Newman, 1997).

Active Infection. Recommended initial treatment for active tuberculosis in pregnant patients is a three-drug regimen with isoniazid, rifampin, and ethambutol. In areas in which the prevalence of isoniazid-resistant tuberculosis is high, pyrazinamide is added to the initial regimen until susceptibility testing is completed. If the organism is susceptible, the regimen is given for 9 months. Reports of MDR-TB during pregnancy are few, and Lessnau and Qarah (2003) and Shin and colleagues (2003) have reviewed treatment options. Breast feeding is not prohibited during antituberculous therapy. Pregnant women receiving isoniazid should also be given pyridoxine, 25 mg/day orally, to decrease hepatic toxicity.

For HIV-infected women, the use of rifampin or rifabutin may be contraindicated if certain protease inhibitors or nonnucleoside reverse transcriptase inhibitors are being administered. If there is resistance to rifabutin or rifampin, then pyrazinamide therapy is given. Of the second-line regimens, the aminoglycosides—streptomycin, kanamycin, amikacin, and capreomycin—are ototoxic to the fetus and are contraindicated (Briggs and associates, 2005).

Neonatal Tuberculosis

Tubercular bacillemia can infect the placenta, but in only a few of these, the fetus is also infected to cause *congenital tuberculosis*. The term also applies to newborns who are infected by aspiration of infected secretions at delivery. Each route of infection constitutes about half of the cases. Neonatal tuberculosis simulates other congenital infections and manifests with hepatosplenomegaly, respiratory distress, fever, and lymphadenopathy (Smith, 2002).

Cantwell and associates (1994) reviewed 29 cases of congenital tuberculosis reported since 1980. Only 12 of the mothers had active infection, and tuberculosis was commonly demonstrated by postpartum endometrial biopsy. Adhikari and colleagues (1997) described 11 South African postpartum women whose endometrial biopsy was culture-positive. Six of their neonates had congenital tuberculosis.

Neonatal infection is unlikely if the mother with active disease has been treated before delivery or if her sputum culture is negative. Because the newborn is susceptible to tuberculosis, most authors recommend isolation from the mother suspected of having active disease. If untreated, the risk of disease in the infant born to a woman with active infection is 50 percent in the first year (Jacobs and Abernathy, 1988).

SARCOIDOSIS

Sarcoidosis is a chronic, multisystem disease of unknown etiology characterized by an accumulation of T lymphocytes and phagocytes within noncaseating granulomas (Noor and Knox, 2007; Rossman and Kreider, 2007). Predisposition to the disease is genetically determined and characterized by an exaggerated response of helper T lymphocytes to environmental triggers (Grunewald and Eklund, 2007; Moller, 2007; Spagnolo and du Bois, 2007). Pulmonary involvement is most common, followed by skin, eyes, and lymph nodes. The prevalence of sarcoid in the United States is 10 to 40 per 100,000, with equal sex distribution, but it is 10 times more common for black compared with white persons (Crystal, 2005). Most patients are between 20 and 40 years. Clinical presentation varies, but more than half of patients have dyspnea and a dry cough without constitutional symptoms that develop insidiously over months. Disease onset is abrupt in about 25 percent of patients, and 10 to 20 percent are asymptomatic at discovery.

Pulmonary symptoms are dominant, and more than 90 percent of patients have an abnormal chest radiograph at some point (Lynch and associates, 2007). *Interstitial pneumonitis* is the hallmark of pulmonary involvement. Approximately 50 percent of affected patients develop permanent radiological changes. *Lymphadenopathy,* especially of the mediastinum, is present in 75 to 90 percent of cases, and 25 percent have *uveitis.* A fourth have skin involvement, usually manifest as *erythema nodosum.* In women, sarcoid causes about 10 percent of cases of erythema nodosum (Mert and colleagues, 2007). Finally, any other organ system may be involved. Confirmation of diagnosis is with biopsy, and because the lung may be the only obviously involved organ, tissue acquisition is often difficult.

The overall prognosis for sarcoidosis is good, and it resolves without treatment in 50 percent of patients. Still, there is dimin-

ished quality of life (de Vries and Drent, 2007). In the other 50 percent, permanent organ dysfunction, albeit mild and nonprogressive, persists. About 10 percent die because of their disease.

Glucocorticoids are the most widely used treatment, and methotrexate is second-line medication. Permanent organ derangement is seldom reversed by their use (Paramothayan and Jones, 2002). Thus, the decision to treat is based on symptoms, physical findings, chest radiograph, and pulmonary function tests. Unless respiratory symptoms are prominent, therapy is usually withheld for a several-month observation period. If inflammation does not subside, then prednisone, 1 mg/kg, is given daily for 4 to 6 weeks (Crystal, 2005).

Sarcoidosis and Pregnancy

Because sarcoidosis is uncommon and is frequently benign, it is not seen often in pregnancy. De Regt (1987) described 14 cases in 20,000 pregnancies over a 12-year period—almost 1 in 1500. Although sarcoidosis seldom affects pregnancy adversely, serious complications such as meningitis, heart failure, and neurosarcoidosis have been described (Cardonick, 2000; Maisel, 1996; Seballos, 1994, and all their colleagues).

In general, perinatal outcomes are unaffected by sarcoidosis. Selroos (1990) reviewed 655 patients with sarcoidosis referred to the Mjölbolsta Hospital District in Finland. Of 252 women between 18 and 50 years, 15 percent had sarcoidosis during pregnancy or within 1 year postpartum. There was no evidence for disease progression in the 26 pregnancies in women with active disease. Three aborted spontaneously, and the other 23 women were delivered at term. In 18 pregnancies in 12 women with inactive disease, pregnancy outcome was good. Agha and colleagues (1982) reported similar experiences with 35 pregnancies at the University of Michigan.

Active sarcoidosis is treated using the same guidelines as for the woman who is not pregnant. Severe disease warrants serial determination of pulmonary function. Symptomatic uveitis, constitutional symptoms, and pulmonary symptoms are treated with prednisone, 1 mg/kg orally per day.

CYSTIC FIBROSIS

One of the most common fatal genetic disorders in Caucasians, cystic fibrosis is caused by one of more than 1000 mutations in a 230-kb gene on the long arm of chromosome 7 that encodes a 1480–amino acid polypeptide (Rowe and co-workers, 2005). This peptide functions as a chloride channel and is termed the *cystic fibrosis transmembrane conductance receptor regulator (CFTR).* There is a wide phenotypic variation, even among homozygotes for the common ΔF508 mutation (Rowntree and Harris, 2003). This is discussed in greater detail in Chapter 13 (p. 298). Currently, nearly 80 percent of females with cystic fibrosis now survive to adulthood (Gillet and associates, 2002). Their median survival is about 30 years.

Pathophysiology

The mutations in the chloride channel cause altered epithelial cell membrane transport of electrolytes. This affects all organs that express CFTR—secretory cells, sinuses, lung, pancreas, liver, and reproductive tract. Severity of the disease depends on which two alleles are inherited, and homozygosity for ΔF508 is one of the most severe (McKone and colleagues, 2003).

Exocrine gland ductal obstruction develops from thick, viscid secretions (Rowe and colleagues, 2005). In the lung, submucosal glandular ducts are affected. Eccrine sweat gland abnormalities are the basis for the diagnostic *sweat test*, characterized by elevated sodium, potassium, and chloride levels in sweat.

Lung involvement is commonplace and is frequently the cause of death. Bronchial gland hypertrophy with mucous plugging and small-airway obstruction lead to subsequent infection that ultimately causes chronic bronchitis and bronchiectasis. For complex and not completely explicable reasons, chronic inflammation from *Pseudomonas aeruginosa* occurs in more than 90 percent of patients. *Staphylococcus aureus, Haemophilus influenzae,* and *Burkholderia cepacia* are recovered in a minority (Rowe and associates, 2005). Colonization with the last has been reported to signify a worse prognosis, especially in pregnancy (Gillet and colleagues, 2002). Acute and chronic parenchymal inflammation ultimately causes extensive fibrosis, and along with airway obstruction, there is a ventilation–perfusion mismatch. Pulmonary insufficiency is the end result. Lung or heart–lung transplantation has a 5-year survival rate of 33 percent (Aurora and associates, 1999). A few women have successfully undergone pregnancy following lung transplantation (Kruszka and Gherman, 2002).

Preconceptional Counseling

Infertility

Women with cystic fibrosis are subfertile because of tenacious cervical mucus. Males have oligospermia or aspermia from vas deferens obstruction, and 98 percent are infertile (Boyd and co-workers, 1999). Despite this, the North American Cystic Fibrosis Foundation estimates that 4 percent of affected women become pregnant every year (Edenborough and colleagues, 1995). The endometrium and tubes express some CFTR but are normal functionally, and the ovaries do not express the *CFTR* gene (Edenborough, 2001). Both intrauterine insemination and in vitro fertilization have been used successfully in affected women (Rodgers and colleagues, 2000). A number of ethical considerations of undertaking pregnancy by these women were reviewed recently by Wexler and colleagues (2007). For male infertility, Sobczyńska-Tomaszewska and associates (2006) have emphasized the importance of molecular diagnosis.

Screening

The American College of Obstetricians and Gynecologists (2005) recommends that carrier screening be offered to at-risk couples. This is discussed in detail in Chapter 13 (p. 298). The Centers for Disease Control and Prevention have also recently added cystic fibrosis to newborn screening programs (Comeau and colleagues, 2007). This is discussed also in Chapter 28 (p. 598 and Table 28-5) and was recently the subject of a Cochrane Database review by Southern and associates (2009).

Pregnancy with Cystic Fibrosis

Pregnancy outcome is inversely related to severity of lung dysfunction. Severe chronic lung disease, hypoxia, and frequent infections may prove deleterious. At least in the past, *cor pulmonale* was common, but even that does not preclude successful pregnancy (Cameron and Skinner, 2005). In some women, *pancreatic dysfunction* may cause poor maternal nutrition. Normal pregnancy-induced insulin resistance frequently results in gestational diabetes after midpregnancy (Hardin and associates, 2005; McMullen and co-workers, 2006).

Cystic fibrosis per se is not affected by pregnancy (Edenborough, 2001). Early reports of a deleterious effect on the course of cystic fibrosis were related to severe disease (Olson, 1997). An important factor to be considered in childbearing is the long-term prognosis for the mother. When matched with nonpregnant women by disease severity, recent reports indicate no deleterious effects on long-term survival (Goss and co-workers, 2003; McMullen and associates, 2006).

Management

Prepregnancy counseling is imperative as discussed in Chapter 7 (p. 178). Women who choose to become pregnant should have close surveillance for development of superimposed infection, diabetes, and heart failure. They are followed closely with serial pulmonary function testing, for management as well as for prognosis. When the FEV_1 is at least 70 percent, women usually tolerate pregnancy well. Emphasis is placed on postural drainage, bronchodilator therapy, and control of infection.

β-adrenergic bronchodilators help to control airway constriction. Inhaled recombinant human deoxyribonuclease I improves lung function by reducing sputum viscosity (Boucher, 2005). Inhaled 7-percent saline has been shown to produce short- and long-term benefits (Donaldson and colleagues, 2006; Elkins and co-workers, 2006). Nutritional status is assessed and appropriate dietary counseling given. Pancreatic insufficiency is treated with replacement of oral pancreatic enzyme.

Infection is heralded by increasing cough and mucus production. Oral semisynthetic penicillins or cephalosporins usually suffice to treat staphylococcal infections. *Pseudomonas* is most problematic in adults. Inhaled tobramycin and colistin have been used successfully to control this organism (Ratjen and Döring, 2003).

Immediate hospitalization and aggressive therapy are warranted for serious pulmonary infections. The threshold for hospitalization with other complications is low. For labor and delivery, epidural analgesia is recommended.

Pregnancy Outcome

When Cohen and colleagues (1980) conducted the first major survey of cystic fibrosis centers, severity was assessed by the *Schwachman-Kulezycki* or *Taussig* scores based on radiological and clinical criteria. Although pregnancy outcomes were not disastrous, 18 percent of 129 women died within 2 years of giving birth. In a later review through 1991, Kent and Farquharson (1993) described similar outcomes in 215 pregnancies in 160 women.

More recent reports describe better outcomes, but there still are serious complications (Tonelli and Aitken, 2007). Severity of disease is now quantified by pulmonary function studies, which are the best predictor of pregnancy and long-term maternal outcome. Edenborough and colleagues (2000) reported 69 pregnancies from 11 cystic fibrosis centers in the United Kingdom. If prepregnancy FEV_1 was less than 60 percent of predicted, there was substantive risk of preterm delivery, respiratory complications, and death of the mother within a few years of childbirth.

Fitzsimmons and co-workers (1996) performed a case-control study of 258 women with cystic fibrosis who had a live birth. The 889 matched controls were women with cystic fibrosis who had not been pregnant. Pregnancy had no effect on worsening of any serious complications, and 8 percent in both groups had died by 2 years. Gillet and co-workers (2002) reported 75 pregnancies from the French Cystic Fibrosis Registry. Almost 20 percent of infants were delivered preterm, and 30 percent had growth restriction. The one maternal death was due to pseudomonas sepsis in a woman whose prepregnancy FEV_1 was 60 percent. Long-term, however, 17 percent of women died and four infants had confirmed cystic fibrosis.

Lung Transplantation

Cystic fibrosis is a common antecedent disease leading to lung transplantation. Gyi and colleagues (2006) reviewed 10 pregnancies in such women and reported successful outcomes with nine liveborn infants. Maternal outcomes were less favorable—three developed rejection during pregnancy, and all had progressively declining pulmonary function and died of chronic rejection by 38 months after delivery.

CARBON MONOXIDE POISONING

Carbon monoxide is a ubiquitous gas, and most nonsmoking adults have a carbon monoxyhemoglobin saturation of 1 to 3 percent. In cigarette smokers, levels may be as high as 5 to 10 percent. Carbon monoxide is the most common cause of poisoning worldwide (Stoller, 2007). Toxic levels are frequently encountered in inadequately ventilated areas warmed by space heaters.

Carbon monoxide is particularly toxic because it is odorless and tasteless and has a high affinity for hemoglobin binding. Thus, it displaces oxygen and impedes its transfer with resultant hypoxia. Besides acute sequelae including death and anoxic encephalopathy, cognitive defects develop in as many as half of patients following loss of consciousness or in those with carbon monoxide levels greater than 25 percent (Weaver and colleagues, 2002). Hypoxic brain damage has a predilection for the cerebral cortex and white matter and for the basal ganglia (Lo and co-workers, 2007; Prockop and Chichkova, 2007).

Pregnancy and Carbon Monoxide Poisoning

Through a number of physiological alterations, the rate of endogenous carbon monoxide production almost doubles in normal pregnancy (Longo, 1977). Although the pregnant woman is not more susceptible to carbon monoxide poisoning, the fetus does not tolerate excessive exposure. With chronic exposure, maternal symptoms usually appear when the carboxyhemoglobin concentration is 5 to 20 percent. Symptoms include headache, weakness, dizziness, physical and visual impairment, palpitations, and nausea and vomiting. With acute exposure, concentrations of 30 to 50 percent produce symptoms of impending cardiovascular collapse. Levels greater than 50 percent may be fatal for the mother.

Because hemoglobin F has an even higher affinity for carbon monoxide, fetal carboxyhemoglobin levels are 10 to 15 percent higher than those in the mother. This may be due to facilitated diffusion (Longo, 1977). Importantly, the half-life of carboxyhemoglobin is 2 hours in the mother but 7 hours in the fetus. Because carbon monoxide is bound so tightly to hemoglobin F, the fetus may be hypoxic even before maternal carbon monoxide levels are appreciably elevated. A number of anomalies are associated with embryonic exposure, and anoxic encephalopathy is the primary sequela of later fetal exposure (Alehan and colleagues, 2007; Aubard and Magne, 2000).

Treatment

For all victims, treatment of carbon monoxide poisoning is supportive along with immediate administration of 100-percent inspired oxygen. Indications for hyperbaric oxygen treatment in nonpregnant individuals are unclear (Kao and Nañagas, 2005). Weaver and co-workers (2002) reported that hyperbaric oxygen treatment minimized the incidence of cognitive defects in adults at both 6 weeks and 1 year compared with that of normobaric oxygen. Hyperbaric oxygen is generally recommended in pregnancy if there has been "significant" carbon monoxide exposure (Aubard and Magne, 2000; Ernst and Zibrak, 1998). The problem is how to define significant exposure. Although maternal carbon monoxide levels are not accurately predictive of those in the fetus, some clinicians recommend hyperbaric therapy if maternal levels exceed 15 to 20 percent. Treatment of the affected newborn with hyperbaric oxygen is also controversial (Bar and co-workers, 2007).

Elkharrat and colleagues (1991) reported successful hyperbaric treatments in 44 pregnant women. Silverman and Montano (1997) reported successful management of a woman whose abnormal neurological and cardiopulmonary findings abated in a parallel fashion with resolution of associated fetal heart rate variable decelerations. Greingor and colleagues (2001) used 2.5-atm hyperbaric 100-percent oxygen for 90 minutes in a 21-week pregnant woman who was delivered of a healthy infant at term. According to the Divers Alert Network (DAN) at Duke University (2009), there are 700 chambers in North and Central America and the Caribbean. Consultation from DAN is available at 919-684-8111.

REFERENCES

Adhikari M, Pillay T, Pillay DG: Tuberculosis in the newborn: An emerging disease. Pediatr Infect Dis J 16:1108, 1997
Agha FP, Vade A, Amendola MA, et al: Effects of pregnancy on sarcoidosis. Surg Gynecol Obstet 155:817, 1982
Ahmad H, Mehta NJ, Manikal VM, et al: *Pneumocystis carinii* pneumonia in pregnancy. Chest 120:666, 2001

Alehan F, Erol I, Onay OS: Cerebral palsy due to nonlethal maternal carbon monoxide intoxication. Birth Defects Res A Clin Mol Teratol 79(8):614, 2007

American College of Obstetricians and Gynecologists: Immunization during pregnancy. Committee Opinion No. 282, January 2003

American College of Obstetricians and Gynecologists: Update on carrier screening for cystic fibrosis. Committee Opinion No. 325, December 2005

American College of Obstetricians and Gynecologists: Asthma in Pregnancy. ACOG Practice Bulletin No. 90, February 2008

American Thoracic Society/Centers for Disease Control and Prevention: Diagnostic standards and classification of tuberculosis. Am Rev Respir Dis 142:725, 1990

Anand N, Kollef MH: The alphabet soup of pneumonia: CAP, HAP, HCAP, NHAP, and VAP. Semin Respir Crit Care Med 30(1):3, 2009

Anderson GD: Tuberculosis in pregnancy. Semin Perinatol 21:328, 1997

Annapureddy SR, Masterson SW, David HG, et al: Postpartum osteomyelitis due to *Cryptococcus neoformans*. Scand J Infect Dis 39(4):354, 2007

Arsura EL, Kilgore WB, Ratnayake SN: Erythema nodosum in pregnant patients with coccidioidomycosis. Clin Infect Dis 27:1201, 1998

Aubard Y, Magne I: Carbon monoxide poisoning in pregnancy. Br J Obstet Gynaecol 107:833, 2000

Aurora P, Whitehead B, Wade A, et al: Lung transplantation and life extension in children with cystic fibrosis. Lancet 354:1594, 1999

Bakhireva LN, Jones KL, Schatz M, et al: Safety of leukotriene receptor antagonists in pregnancy. J Allergy Clin Immunol 119 (3):618, 2007

Bar R, Cohen M, Bentur Y, et al: Pre-labor exposure to carbon monoxide: Should the neonate be treated with hyperbaric oxygenation? Clin Toxicol 45(5):579, 2007

Beigi RH: Pandemic influenza and pregnancy. Obstet Gynecol 109:1193, 2007

Blais L, Beauchesne MF, Malo RE, et al: Use of inhaled corticosteroids during the first trimester of pregnancy and the risk of congenital malformations among women with asthma. Thorax 62(4):320, 2007

Blais L, Suissa S, Boivin JF, et al: First treatment with inhaled corticosteroids and the prevention of admissions to hospital for asthma. Thorax 53:1025, 1998

Bogaert D, De Groot R, Hermans PW: *Streptococcus pneumoniae* colonisation: The key to pneumococcal disease. Lancet Infect Dis 4:144, 2004

Boggess KA, Myers ER, Hamilton CD: Antepartum or postpartum isoniazid treatment of latent tuberculosis infection. Obstet Gynecol 96:747, 2000

Boucher RC: Cystic fibrosis. In Kasper DL, Fauci AS, Longo DL, et al (eds): Harrison's Principles of Internal Medicine, 16th ed. New York, McGraw-Hill, 2005, p 1543

Boyd JM, Mehta A, Murphy DJ: Fertility and pregnancy outcomes in men and women with cystic fibrosis in the United Kingdom. Hum Reprod 19:2238, 1999

Bracken MB, Triche EW, Belanger K, et al: Asthma symptoms, severity, and drug therapy: A prospective study of effects on 2205 pregnancies. Obstet Gynecol 102:739, 2003

Braman SS: Chronic cough due to acute bronchitis: ACCP evidence-based clinical practice guidelines. Chest 129:95S, 2006

Braman SS, Kaemmerlen JT: Intensive care of status asthmaticus. A 10-year experience. JAMA 264:366, 1990

Brancazio LR, Laifer SA, Schwartz T: Peak expiratory flow rate in normal pregnancy. Obstet Gynecol 89:383, 1997

Briggs GG, Freeman RK, Yaffe SJ (eds): Drugs in Pregnancy and Lactation, 7th ed. Baltimore, Williams & Wilkins, 2005

Brost BC, Newman RB: The maternal and fetal effects of tuberculosis therapy. Obstet Gynecol Clin North Am 24:659, 1997

Caldwell JW, Asura EL, Kilgore WB, et al: Coccidioidomycosis in pregnancy during an epidemic in California. Obstet Gynecol 95:236, 2000

Cameron AJ, Skinner TA: Management of a parturient with respiratory failure secondary to cystic fibrosis. Anaesthesia 60:77, 2005

Cantwell MF, Shehab ZM, Costello AM, et al: Congenital tuberculosis. N Engl J Med 330:1051, 1994

Cardonick EH, Naktin J, Berghella V: Neurosarcoidosis diagnosed during pregnancy by thoracoscopic lymph node biopsy. J Reprod Med 45:585, 2000

Carroll KN, Griffin MR, Gebretsadik T, et al: Racial differences in asthma morbidity during pregnancy. Obstet Gynecol 106(1):66, 2005

Centers for Disease Control and Prevention: Treatment of tuberculosis. American Thoracic Society, CDC, and Infection Disease Society of America. MMWR 52:RR1, 2003a

Centers for Disease Control and Prevention: Update: Severe acute respiratory syndrome—United States, 2003. MMWR 52:388, 2003b

Centers for Disease Control and Prevention: Guidelines for using the QuantiFERON®-TB gold test for detecting *Mycobacterium tuberculosis* infection, United States. MMWR 54/RR-15:29, 2005a

Centers for Disease Control and Prevention: Controlling tuberculosis in the United States. Recommendations from the American Thoracic Society, CDC, and the Infectious Disease Society of America. MMWR 54:RR-12, 2005b

Centers for Disease Control and Prevention: Prevention and control of influenza. Recommendations of the Advisory Committee on Immunization Practices (ACIP). MMWR 55 (RR-10):1, 2006

Centers for Disease Control and Prevention: Severe methicillin-resistant *Staphylococcus aureus* community-acquired pneumonia associated with influenza—Louisiana and Georgia—December 2006–January 2007. MMWR 56:325, 2007a

Centers for Disease Control and Prevention: Extensively drug-resistant tuberculosis—United States, 1993–2006. MMWR 56(11):250, 2007b

Centers for Disease Control and Prevention: Trends in tuberculosis incidence—United States, 2006. MMWR 56:247, 2007c

Centers for Disease Control and Prevention: Guidelines for prevention and treatment of opportunistic infections in HIV-infected adults and adolescents, June 31, 2008. Available at: http://aidsinfo.nih.gov/contentfiles/Adult_OI.pdf. Accessed July 31, 2008b

Centers for Disease Control and Prevention: CDC issues interim recommendations for the use of influenza antiviral medications in the setting of oseltamivir resistance among circulating influenza A (H1N1) viruses, 2008–09 influenza season. December 19, 2008a

Centers for Disease Control and Prevention: Trends in tuberculosis – United States, 2008. MMWR 58(10):1, 2009a

Centers for Disease Control and Prevention: Plan to combat extensively drug-resistant tuberculosis. MMWR 58(RR-3):1, 2009b

Cohen LF, di Sant Agnese PA, Friedlander J: Cystic fibrosis and pregnancy: A national survey. Lancet 2:842, 1980

Comeau AM, Accurso FJ, White TB, et al: Guidelines for implementation of cystic fibrosis newborn screening programs: Cystic Fibrosis Foundation workshop report. Pediatrics 119:e495, 2007

Cox S, Posner SF, McPheeters M, et al: Hospitalizations with respiratory illness among pregnant women during influenza season. 107:1315, 2006

Crum NF, Ballon-Landa G: Coccidioidomycosis in pregnancy: Case report and review of the literature. Am J Med 119:993, 2006

Cruz CA, Caughey AB, Jasmer R: Postpartum follow-up of a positive purified protein derivative (PPD) among an indigent population. Am J Obstet Gynecol 192:1455, 2005

Crystal RG: Sarcoidosis. In Kasper DL, Braunwald E, Fauci AS, et al (eds): Harrison's Principles of Internal Medicine, 16th ed. New York, McGraw-Hill, 2005, p 2017

de Jong MD, Thanh TT, Khanh TH, et al: Oseltamivir resistance during treatment of influenza A (H5N1) infection. N Engl J Med 353:25, 2005

de Regt RH: Sarcoidosis and pregnancy. Obstet Gynecol 70:369, 1987

de Vries J, Drent M: Quality of life and health status in sarcoidosis: A review. Semin Respir Crit Care Med 28:121, 2007

Demissie K, Breckenridge M, Rhoads G: Infant and maternal outcomes in the pregnancies of asthmatic women. Am J Respir Crit Care Med 158:1091, 1998

Divers Alert Network: Chamber location and availability. Available at: http://www.diversalertnetwork.org/medical/chamberlocations.asp. Accessed March 12, 2009

Dodds L, McNeil SA, Fell DB, et al: Impact of influenza exposure on rates of hospital admissions and physician visits because of respiratory illness among pregnant women. CMAJ 17:463, 2007

Dombrowski MP: Asthma and pregnancy. Obstet Gynecol 108:667, 2006

Dombrowski MP, Schatz M, Wise R, et al: Asthma during pregnancy. Obstet Gynecol 103:5, 2004a

Dombrowski MP, Schatz M, Wise R, et al: Randomized trial of inhaled beclomethasone dipropionate versus theophylline for moderate asthma during pregnancy. Am J Obstet Gynecol 190:737, 2004b

Donaldson SH, Bennett WD, Zeman KL, et al: Mucus clearance and lung function in cystic fibrosis with hypertonic saline. N Engl J Med 354:241, 2006

Edenborough FP: Women with cystic fibrosis and their potential for reproduction. Thorax 56:648, 2001

Edenborough FP, Mackenzie WE, Stableforth DE: The outcome of 72 pregnancies in 55 women with cystic fibrosis in the United Kingdom 1977–1996. Br J Obstet Gynaecol 107:254, 2000

Edenborough FP, Stableforth DE, Webb AK, et al: The outcome of pregnancy in cystic fibrosis. Thorax 50:170, 1995

Eder W, Ege MJ, von Mutius E: The asthma epidemic. N Engl J Med 355:2226, 2006

Efferen LS: Tuberculosis and pregnancy. Curr Opin Pulm Med 13:205, 2007

Elkharrat D, Raphael JC, Korach JM, et al: Acute carbon monoxide intoxication and hyperbaric oxygen in pregnancy. Intensive Care Med 17:289, 1991

Elkins MR, Robinson M, Rose BR, et al: A controlled trial of long-term inhaled hypertonic saline in patients with cystic fibrosis. N Engl J Med 354:229, 2006

Ely EW, Peacock JE, Haponik EF, et al: Cryptococcal pneumonia complicating pregnancy. Medicine 77:153, 1998

Enriquez R, Pingsheng W, Griffin MR, et al: Cessation of asthma medication in early pregnancy. Am J Obstet Gynecol 195:149, 2006

Ernst A, Zibrak JD: Carbon monoxide poisoning. N Engl J Med 339:1603, 1998

Ernst JD, Trevejo-Nuñez G, Banaiee N: Genomics and the evolution, pathogenesis, and diagnosis of tuberculosis. J Clin Invest 117:1738, 2007

Fanta CH: Asthma. N Engl J Med 360:1002, 2009

Figueroa-Damian R, Arrendondo-Garcia JL: Pregnancy and tuberculosis: Influence of treatment on perinatal outcome. Am J Perinatol 15:303, 1998

Finland M, Dublin TD: Pneumococcic pneumonias complicating pregnancy and the puerperium. JAMA 112:1027, 1939

Fitzsimmons SC, Fitzpatrick S, Thompson D, et al: A longitudinal study of the effects of pregnancy on 325 women with cystic fibrosis. Ped Pulmono l13:99, 1996

Forna F, McConnell M, Kitabire FN: Systematic review of the safety of trimethoprim-sulfamethoxazole for prophylaxis in HIV-infected pregnant women: Implications for resource-limited settings. AIDS Rev 8:24, 2006

Gazmararian JA, Petersen R, Jamieson DJ, et al: Hospitalizations during pregnancy among managed care enrollees. Obstet Gynecol 100:94, 2002

Geng E, Kreiswirth B, Driver C, et al: Changes in the transmission of tuberculosis in New York City from 1990 to 1999. N Engl J Med 346:1453, 2002

Getahun D, Ananth CV, Peltier MR: Acute and chronic respiratory disease in pregnancy: Association with placental abruption. Am J Obstet Gynecol 195:1180, 2006

Getahun D, Ananth CV, Oyelese MR: Acute and chronic respiratory diseases in pregnancy: Associations with spontaneous premature rupture of membranes. J Matern Fetal Neonatal Med 20(9):669, 2007

Gillet D, de Brackeleer M, Bellis G, et al: Cystic fibrosis and pregnancy. Report from French data (1980–1999). Br J Obstet Gynaecol 109:912, 2002

Gluck JC, Gluck PA: The effect of pregnancy on the course of asthma. Immunol Allergy Clin N AM 26:63, 2006

Goodnight WH, Soper DE: Pneumonia in pregnancy. Crit Care Med 33(10):S390, 2005

Gooskens J, Jonges M, Claas ED, et al: Morbidity and mortality associated with nosocomial transmission of oseltamivir-resistant influenza A (H1N1) virus. JAMA 301(10):1066, 2009

Goss CH, Rubenfeld GD, Otto K, et al: The effect of pregnancy on survival in women with cystic fibrosis. Chest 124:1460, 2003

Greingor JL, Tosi JM, Ruhlmann S, et al: Acute carbon monoxide intoxication during pregnancy. One case report and review of the literature. Emerg Med J 18:399, 2001

Grunewald J, Eklund A: Role of CD4$^+$ T cell in sarcoidosis. Proc Am Thorac Soc 4:461, 2007

Gyi KM, Hodson ME, Yacoub MY: Pregnancy in cystic fibrosis lung transplant recipients: Case series and review. J Cyst Fibros 5(3):171, 2006

Hardin DS, Rice J, Cohen RC, et al: The metabolic effects of pregnancy in cystic fibrosis. Obstet Gynecol 106(2):367, 2005

Harger JH, Ernest JM, Thurnau GR, et al: Risk factors and outcome of varicella-zoster virus pneumonia in pregnant women. J Infect Dis 185:422, 2002

Hartert TV, Neuzil KM, Shintani AK, et al: Maternal morbidity and perinatal outcomes among pregnant women with respiratory hospitalizations during influenza season. Am J Obstet Gynecol 189:1705, 2003

Hendler I, Schatz M, Momirova V, et al: Association of obesity with pulmonary and nonpulmonary complications of pregnancy in asthmatic women. Obstet Gynecol 108(1):77, 2006

Hooper JE, Lu Q, Pepkowitz SH: Disseminated coccidioidomycosis in pregnancy. Arch Pathol Lab Med 131:652, 2007

Jacobs RF, Abernathy RS: Management of tuberculosis in pregnancy and the newborn. Clin Perinatol 15:305, 1988

Jana N, Vasishta K, Jindal SK, et al: Perinatal outcome in pregnancies complicated by pulmonary tuberculosis. Int J Gynecol Obstet 44:119, 1994

Jana N, Vasishta K, Saha SC, et al: Obstetrical outcomes among women with extrapulmonary tuberculosis. N Engl J Med 341:645, 1999

Jenkins TM, Troiano NH, Grave CR, et al: Mechanical ventilation in an obstetric population: Characteristics and delivery rates. Am J Obstet Gynecol 188:549, 2003

Jin Y, Carriere KC, Marrie TJ, et al: The effects of community-acquired pneumonia during pregnancy ending with a live birth. Am J Obstet Gynecol 188:800, 2003

Källén B: The safety of asthma medications during pregnancy. Expert Opin Drug Saf 6:15, 2007

Källén B, Otterblad Olausson PO: Use of anti-asthmatic drugs during pregnancy. 2. Infant characteristics excluding congenital malformations. Eur J Clin Pharmacol 63(4):375, 2007

Kao LW, Nañagas KA: Carbon monoxide poisoning. Med Clin North Am 89(6):1161, 2005

Kent NE, Farquharson DF: Cystic fibrosis in pregnancy. Can Med Assoc J 149:809, 1993

Kruszka SJ, Gherman RB: Successful pregnancy outcome in a lung transplant recipient with tacrolimus immunosuppression. A case report. J Reprod Med 47:60, 2002

Kutlu T, Tugrul S, Aydin A, et al: Tuberculosis meningitis in pregnancy presenting as hyperemesis gravidarum. J Matern Fetal Neonatal Med 20:357, 2007

Kwon HL, Triche EW, Belander K, et al: The epidemiology of asthma during pregnancy: Prevalence, diagnosis, and symptoms. Immunol Allergy Clin North Am 26:29, 2006

Kyaw MH, Lynfield R, Schaffner W, et al: Effect of introduction of the pneumococcal conjugate vaccine on drug-resistant *Streptococcus pneumoniae*. N Engl J Med 354:1455, 2006

Laibl V, Sheffield J: The management of respiratory infections during pregnancy. Immunol Allergy Clin North Am 26: 155, 2006

Lam CM, Wong SF, Leung TN, et al: A case-controlled study comparing clinical course and outcomes of pregnant and non-pregnant women with severe acute respiratory syndrome. BJOG 111:771, 2004

Lalvani A: Diagnosing tuberculosis infection in the 21st century: New tools to tackle an old enemy. Chest 131:1898, 2007

Lessnau KD, Qarah S: Multidrug-resistant tuberculosis in pregnancy: Case report and review of the literature. Chest 123:953, 2003

Lim WS, Macfarlane JT, Boswell TC, et al: Study of community acquired pneumonia etiology (SCAPA) in adults admitted to hospital: Implications for management guidelines. Thorax 56:296, 2001

Liu S, Wen SW, Demissie K, et al: Maternal asthma and pregnancy outcomes: A retrospective cohort study. Am J Obstet Gynecol 184:90, 2001

Llewelyn M, Cropley I, Wilkinson RJ, et al: Tuberculosis diagnosed during pregnancy: A prospective study from London. Thorax 55:129, 2000

Lo CP, Chen SY, Lee KW, et al: Brain injury after acute carbon monoxide poisoning: Early and late complications. Am J Roentgenol 189(4):W205, 2007

Longman RE, Johnson TRB: Viral respiratory disease in pregnancy. Curr Opin Obstet Gynecol 18:120, 2007

Longo L: The biologic effects of carbon monoxide on the pregnant woman, fetus and newborn infant. Am J Obstet Gynecol 129:69, 1977

Lynch III JP, Ma YL, Koss MN, et al: Pulmonary sarcoidosis. Semin Respir Crit Care Med 28:53, 2007

Mabie WC, Barton JR, Wasserstrum N, et al: Clinical observations on asthma in pregnancy. J Matern Fetal Med 1:45, 1992

Maisel JA, Lynam T: Unexpected sudden death in a young pregnant woman: Unusual presentation of neurosarcoidosis. Ann Emerg Med 28:94, 1996

Mandell LA, Wunderink RG, Anzueto A, et al: Infectious Diseases Society of America/American Thoracic Society consensus guidelines on the management of community-acquired pneumonia in adults. Clin Infect Dis 44:S27, 2007

Margono F, Mroueh J, Garely A, et al: Resurgence of active tuberculosis among pregnant women. Obstet Gynecol 83:911, 1994

McFadden ER: Asthma. In Kasper DL, Fauci AS, Longo DL, et al (eds): Harrison's Principles of Internal Medicine, 16th ed. New York, McGraw-Hill, 2005, p 1508

McKone EF, Emerson SS, Edwards KL, et al: Effect of genotype on phenotype and mortality in cystic fibrosis: A retrospective cohort study. Lancet 361:1671, 2003

McMullen AH, Past DJ, Frederick PD: Impact of pregnancy on women with cystic fibrosis. Chest 129(3):706, 2006

Medical Letter: Anidulafungin (Eraxis) for candida infections. 48:1235, 2006

Mert A, Kumbasar H, Ozaras R, et al: Erythema nodosum: An evaluation of 100 cases. Clin Exp Rheumatol 25:563, 2007

Mihrshahi S, Belousova E, Marks GB, et al: Pregnancy and birth outcomes in families with asthma. J Asthma 40:181, 2003

Moller DR: Potential etiologic agents in sarcoidosis. Proc Am Thorac Soc 4:465, 2007

Moore AR, Rogers FM, Dietrich D, et al: Extrapulmonary tuberculosis in pregnancy masquerading as a degenerating leiomyoma. Obstet Gynecol 111(2): 551, 2008

Moscona A: Neuraminidase inhibitors for influenza. N Engl J Med 353(13): 1363, 2005

Murphy VE, Gibson P, Talbot P, et al: Severe asthma exacerbations during pregnancy. Obstet Gynecol 106(5):1046, 2005

Namazy JA, Schatz M: Pregnancy and asthma: Recent developments. Curr Opin Pulm Med 11:56, 2005

Namazy JA, Schatz M: Current guidelines for the management of asthma during pregnancy. Immunol Allergy Clin North Am 26:93, 2006

Nanda S, Agarwal U, Sangwan K: Complete resolution of cervical spinal tuberculosis with paraplegia in pregnancy. Acta Obstet Gynecol Scand 81:569, 2002

National Center for Health Statistics: Asthma prevalence, health care use and morbidity: United States, 2003-05. www.cdc.gov/nchs/products/pubs/hestats/asthma03-05 (last reviewed January 11, 2007). Accessed October 13, 2007

National Institutes of Health, National Heart, Lung, and Blood Institute. National Asthma Education Program (2007). www.nhbli.nih.gov/guidelines/asthma/index.htm. Retrieved August 30, 2007

National Heart, Lung and Blood Institute. National Asthma Education and Prevention Program. Working group report on managing asthma during pregnancy: Recommendations for pharmacologic treatment, update 2004. Available at: http://www.nhbli.nih.gov/health/prof/lung/asthma/astpreg.htm. Accessed June 28, 2006

Ng WF, Wong SF, Lam A, et al: The placentas of patients with severe acute respiratory syndrome: A pathophysiological evaluation. Pathology 38:210, 2006

Noble PW, Lavee AE, Jacobs NM: Respiratory diseases in pregnancy. Obstet Gynecol Clin North Am 15:391, 1988

Noor A, Knox KS: Immunopathogenesis of sarcoidosis. Clin Dermatol 25:250, 2007

Olson GL: Cystic fibrosis in pregnancy. Semin Perinatol 21:307, 1997

Oram MP, Seal P, McKinstry CE: Severe acute respiratory distress syndrome in pregnancy. Cesarean section in the second trimester to improve maternal ventilation. Anaesth Intensive Care 35:975, 2007

Paramothayan S, Jones PW: Corticosteroid therapy in pulmonary sarcoidosis. A systematic review. JAMA 287:1301, 2002

Paranyuk Y, Levine G, Figueroa R: Candida septicemia in a pregnant woman with hyperemesis receiving parenteral nutrition. Obstet Gynecol 107:535, 2006

Pillay T, Khan M, Moodley J, et al: Perinatal tuberculosis and HIV-1: Considerations for resource-limited settings. Lancet Infect Dis 4:155, 2004

Prevost MR, Fung Kee Fung KM: Tuberculous meningitis in pregnancy—implications for mother and fetus: Case report and literature review. J Matern Fetal Med 8:289, 1999

Prockop LD, Chichkova RI: Carbon monoxide intoxication: An updated review. J Neurol Sci 262(1-2):122, 2007

Ramsey PS, Maddox DE, Ramin KD, et al: Asthma: Impact on maternal morbidity and adverse perinatal outcome [Abstract]. Obstet Gynecol 101:40S, 2003

Ratjen F, Döring G: Cystic fibrosis. Lancet 361:681, 2003

Reboli AC, Rotstein C, Pappas PG, et al: Anidulafungin versus fluconazole for invasive candidiasis. N Engl J Med 356:2472, 2007

Rey E, Boulet LP: Asthma in pregnancy. BMJ 334:582, 2007

Rodgers HC, Knox AJ, Toplis PH, et al: Successful pregnancy and birth after IVF in a woman with cystic fibrosis. Human Reprod 15:2152, 2000

Rolston DH, Shnider SM, de Lorimer AA: Uterine blood flow and fetal acid–base changes after bicarbonate administration to the pregnant ewe. Anesthesiology 40:348, 1974

Rosenstein NE, Emery KW, Werner SB, et al: Risk factors for severe pulmonary and disseminated coccidioidomycosis: Kern County, California, 1995–1996. Clin Infect Dis 32:708, 2001

Rossman MD, Kreider ME: Lesson learned from ACCESS (A case controlled etiologic study of sarcoidosis). Proc Am Thorac Sec, 4:453, 2007

Rotas M, McCalla S, Liu C, et al: Methicillin-resistant *Staphylococcus aureus* necrotizing pneumonia arising from an infected episiotomy site. Obstet Gynecol 109(2):533, 2007

Rowe SM, Miller S, Sorscher EJ: Cystic fibrosis. N Engl J Med 353:1992, 2005

Rowntree RK, Harris A: The phenotypic consequences of *CFTR* mutations. Ann Hum Genet 67(5):471, 2003

Sackoff JE, Pfieffer MR, Driver CR, et al: Tuberculosis prevention for non-U.S.-born pregnant woman. Am J Obstet Gynecol 194:451, 2006

Schanzer DL, Langley JM, Tam TW: Influenza-attributed hospitalization rates among pregnant women in Canada 1994–2000. J Obstet Gynaecol Can 29:622, 2007

Schatz M, Dombrowski MP, Wise R, et al: Asthma morbidity during pregnancy can be predicted by severity classification. J Allergy Clin Immunol 112:283, 2003

Schatz M, Dombrowski MP, Wise R, et al: Spirometry is related to perinatal outcomes in pregnant women with asthma. Am J Obstet Gynecol 194:120, 2006

Schulte JM, Bryan P, Dodds S, et al: Tuberculosis skin testing among HIV-infected pregnant women in Miami, 1995 to 1996. J Perinatol 22:159, 2002

Seballos RJ, Mendel SG, Mirmiran-Yazdy A, et al: Sarcoid cardiomyopathy precipitated by pregnancy with cocaine complications. Chest 105:303, 1994

Selroos O: Sarcoidosis and pregnancy: A review with results of a retrospective survey. J Intern Med 227:221, 1990

Shariatzadeh MR, Marrie TJ: Pneumonia during pregnancy. Am J Med 119:872, 2006

Sheffield JS, Cunningham FG: Management of community-acquired pneumonia in pregnancy. Obstet Gynecol, In Press, 2009

Sherer DM, Osho, JA, Zinn H, et al: Peripartum disseminated extrapulmonary tuberculosis simulating ovarian carcinoma. Am J Perinatol 22:383, 2005

Shin S, Guerra D, Rich M, et al: Treatment of multidrug-resistant tuberculosis during pregnancy: A report of 7 cases. Clin Infect Dis 36:996, 2003

Silverman RK, Montano J: Hyperbaric oxygen treatment during pregnancy in acute carbon monoxide poisoning. A case report. J Reprod Med 42:309, 1997

Smith KC: Congenital tuberculosis: A rare manifestation of a common infection. Curr Opin Infect Dis 15:269, 2002

Sobczynska-Tomaszewska A, Bak D, Wolski JK, et al: Molecular analysis of defects in the *CFTR* gene and *AZF* locus of the Y chromosome in male infertility. J Reprod Med 51(2):120, 2006

Southern KW, Mérelle MM, Dankert-Roelse JE, et al: Newborn screening for cystitis fibrosis. Cochrane Database Syst Rev 21(1):CD001402

Spagnolo P, du Bois RM: Genetics of sarcoidosis. Clin Dermatol 25:242, 2007

Spinello IM, Johnson RH, Baqi S: Coccidioidomycosis and pregnancy: A review. Ann N Y Acad Sci 1111:358, 2007

Stoller KP: Hyperbaric oxygen and carbon monoxide poisoning: A critical review. Neurol Res 29(2):146, 2007

Stratton P, Mofenson LM, Willoughby AD: Human immunodeficiency virus infection in pregnant women under care at AIDS Clinical Trials Centers in the United States. Obstet Gynecol 79:364, 1992

Strunk RC, Bloomberg GR: Omalizumab for asthma. N Engl J Med 354(24):2689, 2006

Tata LJ, Lewis SA, McKeever TM, et al: A comprehensive analysis of adverse obstetric and pediatric complications in women with asthma. Am J Respir Crit Care Med 175:991, 2007

Tino G, Ware LB, Moss M: Clinical Year in Review IV: chronic obstructive pulmonary disease, nonpulmonary critical care, diagnostic imaging, and mycobacterial disease. Proc Am Thorac Soc 4(6):494, 2007

Tonelli MR, Aitken ML: Pregnancy in cystic fibrosis. Curr Opin Pulm Med 13(6):437, 2007

Torres A, Menéndez R: Hospital admission in community-acquired pneumonia [Spanish]. Med Clin (Barc) 131(6):216, 2008

Triche EW, Saftlas AF, Belanger K, et al: Association of asthma diagnosis, severity, symptoms, and treatment with risk of preeclampsia. Obstet Gynecol 104:585, 2004

Walzer PD: Pneumocystis infection. In Kasper DL, Fauci AS, Longo DL, et al (eds): Harrison's Principles of Internal Medicine, 16th ed. New York, McGraw-Hill, 2005, p 1194

Weaver LK, Hopkins RO, Chan KJ, et al: Hyperbaric oxygen for acute carbon monoxide poisoning. N Engl J Med 347:1057, 2002

Weinberger SE, Weiss ST: Pulmonary diseases. In Duffy TP, Burrow GN (eds): Medical Complications During Pregnancy, 5th ed. Philadelphia, Saunders, 1999, p 363

Wendel PJ, Ramin SM, Hamm CB, et al: Asthma treatment in pregnancy: A randomized controlled study. Am J Obstet Gynecol 175:150, 1996

Wenzel RP, Fowler III AA: Acute bronchitis. N Engl J Med355:2125, 2006

Wexler ID, Johnnesson M, Edenborough FP, et al: Pregnancy and chronic progressive pulmonary disease. Am J Respir Crit Care Med 175:330, 2007

Wise RA, Polito AJ, Krishnan V: Respiratory physiologic changes in pregnancy. Immunol Allergy Clin N Am 26:1, 2006

Wong SF, Chow KM, Leung TN, et al: Pregnancy and perinatal outcomes of women with severe acute respiratory syndrome. Am J Obstet Gynecol 191:292, 2004

World Health Organization: Cumulative number of confirmed human cases of avian influenza A/(H5N1) reported to WHO. Available at: www.who.int/csr/disease/avian_influenza. Accessed January 15, 2007

World Health Organization: Update on avian influenza A (H%N1) virus infection in humans. N Engl J Med 358:261, 2008

Yost NP, Bloom SL, Richey SD, et al: An appraisal of treatment guidelines for antepartum community-acquired pneumonia. Am J Obstet Gynecol 183:131, 2000

Yudin MH, Steele DM, Sgro MD, et al: Severe acute respiratory syndrome in pregnancy. Obstet Gynecol 105:124, 2005

Zaman K, Roy E, Arifeen SE, et al: Effectiveness of maternal influenza immunization in mothers and infants. N Engl J Med 359(15):1555, 2008

Zeeman GG, Wendel GD, Cunningham FG: A blueprint for obstetrical critical care. Am J Obstet Gynecol 188:532, 2003

Thromboembolic Disorders

The risk of venous thrombosis and pulmonary embolism in otherwise healthy women is considered highest during pregnancy and the puerperium. Indeed, the risk of pulmonary embolism has been estimated to be as much as four- to six-fold higher during pregnancy (Christiansen and Collins, 2006; Marik and Plante, 2008). The incidence of all thromboembolic events averages about 1 per 1000 pregnancies, and about an equal number are identified antepartum and in the puerperium. In a recent study from Norway of more than 600,000 pregnancies, Jacobsen and colleagues (2008) reported that deep-venous thrombosis alone was more common antepartum whereas pulmonary embolism was more common in the first 6 weeks postpartum. The frequency of venous thromboembolic disease during the puerperium has decreased remarkably as early ambulation has become more widely practiced. Even so, there is evidence that it has increased 50 percent from 1999 to 2005 (Kuklina and associates, 2009). Importantly, pulmonary embolism still remains a leading cause of maternal death in the United States (see Table 1-2). By way of example, pulmonary embolism caused approximately 9 percent of the 623 pregnancy-related deaths in the United States in 2005 (Kung and co-workers, 2008).

PATHOPHYSIOLOGY

In 1856, Rudolf Virchow postulated the conditions that predispose to the development of venous thrombosis: (1) stasis, (2) local trauma to the vessel wall, and (3) hypercoagulability. The risk for each increases during normal pregnancy. For example, compression of the pelvic veins and inferior vena cava by the enlarging uterus renders the venous system of the lower extremities particularly vulnerable to stasis (see Chap. 5, p. 119). From their review, Marik and Plante (2008) cite a 50-percent reduction in venous flow velocity in the legs that lasts from the early third trimester until 6 weeks postpartum. This stasis is the most constant predisposing risk factor for venous thrombosis. Venous stasis and delivery may also contribute to endothelial cell injury. Lastly, marked increases in the synthesis of most clotting factors during pregnancy favor coagulation.

As shown in Table 47-1, there are a number of factors associated with an increased risk of developing thromboembolism during pregnancy. Using data from the Agency for Healthcare Research and Quality that included 90 percent of all hospital discharges during 2000 and 2001, James and co-workers (2006) identified the diagnosis of venous thromboembolism in 7177 women during pregnancy and 7158 during the postpartum period. They calculated that risks for thromboembolism were approximately doubled in women with multifetal gestation, anemia, hyperemesis, hemorrhage, and cesarean delivery. The risk was even greater in pregnancies complicated by postpartum infection. These data are consistent with those reported by Ros and associates (2002), who studied a population-based cohort of more than 1 million deliveries in Sweden. Compared with uncomplicated delivery, they calculated the relative risk of pulmonary embolism to be 4.8 with severe preeclampsia, 3.8 with cesarean delivery, 2.7 with diabetes, and 2.3 with multifetal gestation. By contrast, analyzing data from the United Kingdom Obstetrical Surveillance System, Knight (2008) found significantly increased risk with a body mass index (BMI) ≥ 30 kg/m^2 or with multiparity.

TABLE 47-1. Some Risk Factors Associated with an Increased Risk for Thromboembolism.

Risk Factor	Chapter Referral
Obstetrical	
Cesarean delivery	25
Diabetes	52
Hemorrhage and anemia	35
Hyperemesis	49
Immobility—prolonged bed rest	47
Multifetal gestation	39
Multiparity	
Preeclampsia	34
Puerperal infection	31
General	
Age 35 years or older	12
Cancer	57
Connective-tissue disease	54
Dehydration	
Immobility—long-distance travel	8
Infection and inflammatory disease	58
Myeloproliferative disease	51
Nephrotic syndrome	48
Obesity	43
Oral contraceptive use	32
Orthopedic surgery	42
Paraplegia	
Prior thromboembolism	47
Sickle cell disease	51
Smoking	8
Thrombophilia	47

The likelihood of developing a thrombosis during pregnancy is especially increased in women with certain genetic risk factors. Indeed, the American College of Chest Physicians now estimates that approximately half of pregnant women with thrombosis have an identifiable underlying genetic disorder (Bates and co-workers, 2008). Importantly, 50 to 60 percent of patients with a hereditary basis for thrombosis probably do not experience a thrombotic event until one of the other risk factors is present (American College of Obstetricians and Gynecologists, 2007).

THROMBOPHILIAS

Several important regulatory proteins act as inhibitors in the coagulation cascade. Normal values for many of these proteins during pregnancy are found in the Appendix. Inherited or acquired deficiencies of these inhibitory proteins are collectively referred to as *thrombophilias*. These can lead to hypercoagulability and recurrent venous thromboembolism. Although these disorders are collectively present in about 15 percent of white European populations, they are responsible for more than 50 percent of all thromboembolic events during pregnancy (Lock-

wood, 2002). Some aspects of the more common inherited thrombophilias are summarized in Table 47-2 and Figure 47-1. Recommendations for antepartum and postpartum thromboprophylaxis for women diagnosed with a thrombophilia are discussed later in this chapter (p. 1018).

There is a considerable variety of opinion concerning which patients should be advised to undergo thrombophilia testing (Scifres and Malone, 2008). Lockwood (2007) concluded that it would be prudent to test pregnant women with a history of venous thromboembolism associated with temporary and reversible risk factors because the presence of a thrombophilic state would be an indication for antepartum thromboprophylaxis. The current recommendation of the American Academy of Pediatrics and the American College of Obstetricians and Gynecologists (2007) is that women with a personal or family history of venous thromboembolic disease be evaluated for hereditary and acquired thrombophilic disorders. In addition to these indications, a consensus panel organized by Aventis Pharmaceuticals—the manufacturer of enoxaparin (see p. 1022)—listed additional indications. They concluded that women with unexplained fetal loss at 20 weeks' gestation or later; severe preeclampsia or hemolysis, elevated liver enzymes, low platelet count (HELLP) syndrome before 34 weeks; or severe fetal-growth restriction may also benefit from thrombophilia screening (Duhl and associates, 2007). The American College of Chest Physicians takes a more conservative stance (Bates and colleagues, 2008). Because of uncertainty associated with the magnitude of risk as well as uncertainty associated with any benefits of prophylaxis given to prevent pregnancy complications in women with heritable thrombophilias, it remains unproven that screening is in the best interests of these women. We agree with this position.

Antithrombin Deficiency

This protein, previously known as antithrombin III, is one of the most important inhibitors of thrombin in clot formation. Antithrombin functions as a natural anticoagulant by binding to, and inactivating, thrombin and the activated coagulation factors IXa, Xa, XIa, and XIIa (Franchini and co-workers, 2006). Antithrombin deficiency may result from numerous mutations that are almost always autosomal dominant. Homozygous antithrombin deficiency is lethal (Katz, 2002).

Antithrombin deficiency is rare—it affects about 1 in 5000 individuals, and it is the most thrombogenic of the heritable coagulopathies. Indeed, the risk of thrombosis during pregnancy among antithrombin-deficient women *without* a personal or family history is 3 to 7 percent, and it is 11 to 40 percent with such a history (Lockwood, 2007). Given this risk, many recommend that these women be treated during pregnancy with heparin regardless of whether a prior thrombosis has occurred.

Seguin and colleagues (1994) reviewed the outcomes of 23 newborns with antithrombin deficiency. There were 11 cases of thrombosis and 10 deaths.

TABLE 47-2. Inherited Thrombophilias and Their Association with Venous Thromboembolism (VTE) in Pregnancy

Thrombophilia	Percentage of VTE During Pregnancy	Relative Risk (95% CI) of VTE During Pregnancy	Probability of VTE During Pregnancy and Postpartum in Patients Without Personal or Family History (Percent)
Factor V Leiden (homozygous)	<1[a]	25.4 (8.8–66)	1.5
Factor V Leiden (heterozygous)	44	6.9 (3.3–15.2)	0.26
Prothrombin G20201A (homozygous)	<1[a]	NA	2.8
Prothrombin G20201A (heterozygous)	17	9.5 (2.1–66.7)	0.37
Factor V Leiden and prothrombin G20201A (compound heterozygous)	<1[a]	84 (19–369)	4.7
Hyperhomocyste-inemia			
Antithrombin deficiency[b] (heterozygous)	1–8	119 (N/A)	3–7.2
Protein S deficiency[c] (heterozygous)	12.4	NA	<1–6.6
Protein C deficiency[d] (heterozygous)	<14	13 (1.4–123)	0.8–1.7

[a] = Calculated based on Hardy-Weinbery equation.
[b] = Less than 60-percent activity.
[c] = Less than 55-percent activity.
[d] = Less than 50-percent activity.
CI = confidence interval; NA = not available; VTE = venous thromboembolism.
Adapted from Lockwood (2007).

Protein C Deficiency

When thrombin is bound to thrombomodulin on endothelial cells of small vessels, its procoagulant activities are neutralized. It also activates protein C, a natural anticoagulant that in the presence of protein S controls thrombin generation, in part, by inactivating factors Va and VIIIa (see Fig. 47-1). Activated protein C also inhibits the synthesis of plasminogen-activator inhibitor 1.

More than 160 different protein C gene mutations have been described. The prevalence of protein C deficiency is 2 to 3 per 1000, and inheritance is autosomal dominant. These prevalence estimates correspond with functional activity cutoff values of 50 to 60 percent, which are used by most laboratories and which are associated with a six- to 12-fold increased risk for venous thromboembolism (Lockwood, 2007).

Protein S Deficiency

This circulating anticoagulant is activated by protein C to decrease thrombin generation. Protein S deficiency may be caused by more than 130 different mutations with an aggregate preva-

lence of about 2 per 1000 (Lockwood, 2007). Protein S deficiency is measured by antigenically determined free, functional, and total S levels. All three of these levels decline substantively during normal gestation, thus the diagnosis in pregnant women—as well as in those taking certain oral contraceptives—is difficult (Archer and associates, 1999). Detection of free protein S antigen levels of less than 55 percent in nonpregnant patients and less than 30 percent in pregnant women appears to most closely correlate with a mutated gene. Using such criteria, the prevalence of free protein S deficiency is low—0.03 to 0.13 percent—and as shown in Table 47-2, its degree of thrombogenicity is modest (Lockwood, 2007).

Conard and colleagues (1990) described thrombosis in 5 of 29 pregnant women with protein S deficiency. One woman had a cerebral vein thrombosis. Similarly, Burneo and associates (2002) reported cerebral venous thrombosis at 14 weeks. Neonatal homozygous protein C or S deficiency is usually associated with a severe clinical phenotype known as *purpura fulminans*, which is characterized by extensive thromboses in the microcirculation soon after birth leading to skin necrosis (Salonvaara and colleagues, 2004).

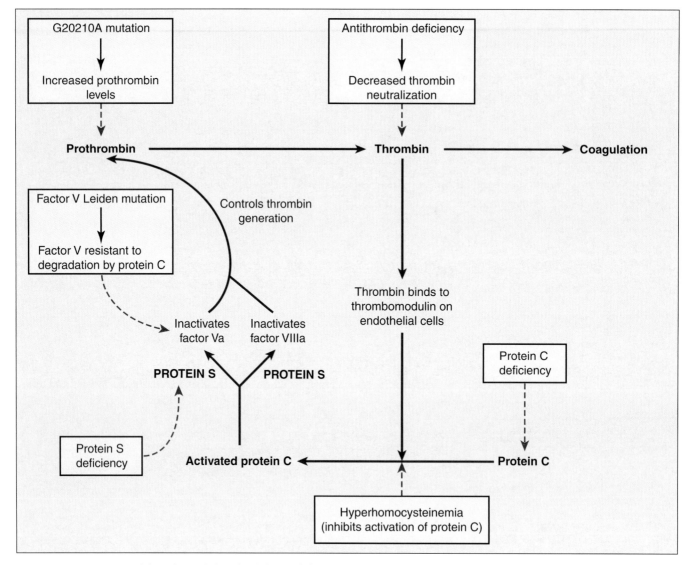

FIGURE 47-1 Overview of the inherited thrombophilias and their effect(s) on the coagulation cascade. (Adapted from Seligsohn and Lubetsky, 2001.)

Activated Protein C Resistance (Factor V Leiden Mutation)

The most prevalent of the known thrombophilic syndromes, this condition is characterized by resistance of plasma to the anticoagulant effects of activated protein C. A number of mutations have been described, but the most common is the factor V Leiden mutation, which was named after the city where it was described. This missense mutation in the factor V gene results in a substitution of glutamine for arginine at position 506 in the factor V polypeptide, which confers resistance to degradation by activated protein C (Kalafatis and colleagues, 1994). The unimpeded abnormal factor V protein retains its procoagulant activity and predisposes to thrombosis (see Fig. 47-1).

Heterozygous inheritance for factor V Leiden is the most common heritable thrombophilia. It is found in 3 to 15 percent of select European populations, 3 percent of African Americans, and it is virtually absent in African blacks and Asians (Lockwood, 2007). Moreover, factor V Leiden mutation is found in up to half of nonpregnant individuals with thromboembolic

disease. Homozygous inheritance of two aberrant copies is rare and increases the risk of thrombosis during pregnancy by more than tenfold (Lockwood, 2007).

Diagnosis is made in one of two ways. In the bioassay, resistance to activated protein C is measured (Bloomenthal and colleagues, 2002). One caveat is that activated protein C resistance can also be caused by the antiphospholipid antibody syndrome (Eldor, 2001). More importantly, and as discussed in Chapter 5 (p. 117), resistance is normally increased after early pregnancy because of alterations in other coagulation proteins (Walker and associates, 1997). Thus, during pregnancy, DNA analysis for the mutant factor V gene is used to confirm the diagnosis.

In a comprehensive review of 63 studies, Biron-Andreani and associates (2006) reported that the Leiden mutation was associated with a four- to eightfold increased risk of a first-episode venous thromboembolism during pregnancy. Despite the large number of publications, however, they cautioned that data remain limited. One of the more meticulously executed studies was a prospective observational study of approximately 5000 women conducted by the Maternal-Fetal Medicine Units Network (Dizon-Townson and associates, 2005). These investigators found that the heterozygous mutant gene incidence was 2.7 percent. Of the three pulmonary emboli and one deep-venous thrombosis—a rate of 0.8 per 1000 pregnancies—none were among these carriers. There was no increased risk of preeclampsia, placental abruption, fetal-growth restriction, or pregnancy loss in heterozygous women. The investigators concluded that universal prenatal screening for the Leiden mutation and prophylaxis for carriers without a prior venous thromboembolism is not indicated. Clark and colleagues (2002) concluded that such routine prenatal screening was not cost effective.

Prothrombin G20210A Mutation

This missense mutation in the prothrombin gene leads to excessive accumulation of prothrombin, which then may be converted to thrombin. Found in approximately 2 percent of the white population, it is extremely uncommon in nonwhites (Federman and Kirsner, 2001). Case-control studies suggest that the relative risk of thromboembolism is increased 3- to 15-fold during pregnancy (Gerhardt and associates, 2000; Martinelli and colleagues, 2002).

Homozygous patients and those who co-inherit a G20210A mutation with a factor V Leiden mutation have an even greater risk of thromboembolism. Stefano and associates (1999) performed a retrospective cohort study of 624 nonpregnant patients with one prior episode of deep-venous thrombosis. They found that those doubly heterozygous individuals had a 2.6-fold increased risk of recurrence relative to those with the homozygous Leiden mutation alone. They concluded that carriers of both mutations are candidates for lifelong anticoagulation after a first thrombotic episode.

Hyperhomocysteinemia

The most common cause of elevated homocysteine is the C667T thermolabile mutation of the enzyme 5,10-methylene-tetrahydrofolate reductase (MTHFR). Inheritance is autosomal recessive, and Kupferminc and co-workers (1999) found a homozygote prevalence of 8 percent in normally pregnant women. Elevated levels of homocysteine may also result from deficiency of one of several enzymes involved in methionine metabolism and from correctible nutritional deficiencies of folic acid, vitamin B_6, or vitamin B_{12} (Hague, 2003; McDonald and Walker, 2001). During normal pregnancy, mean homocysteine plasma concentrations are decreased (López-Quesada and colleagues, 2003; McDonald and Walker, 2001). Thus, to make a diagnosis in pregnancy, Lockwood (2002) recommends a fasting cutoff level of >12 μmol/L to define hyperhomocysteinemia.

The precise pathological mechanism(s) by which high levels of homocysteine increase the risk of thromboembolism remains undefined. Possible pathways include decreased activation of protein C as well as interference with the ability of activated protein C to inactivate factor Va (Gatt and Makris, 2007). Although hyperhomocysteinemia is associated with an increased risk of venous thromboembolism in nonpregnant patients, it is

unclear whether MTHFR C667T homozygotes have an increased risk during pregnancy. It may be that reduced risk is related to physiologically lower homocysteine levels during pregnancy and/or that most pregnant women take folic acid supplements (Bates and co-workers, 2008). Recall that folic acid serves as a cofactor in the remethylation reaction of homocysteine to methionine. Also of note, hyperhomocysteinemia increases the lifetime risk of having a fetus with a neural-tube defect as well as premature atherosclerosis (see Chap. 12, p. 281).

Other Thrombophilia Mutations

A number of potentially thrombophilic polymorphisms are being discovered at an ever-increasing rate. Unfortunately, information regarding the prognostic significance of such newly discovered rare mutations is limited.

Protein Z Deficiency

This vitamin K-dependent protein serves as a cofactor in the inactivation of factor Xa (see Chap. 5, p. 117). Studies in nonpregnant patients have found that low levels of protein Z are associated with an increased risk of thromboembolism (Santacroce and associates, 2006). Preliminary studies in pregnant women have suggested that low protein Z levels may be associated with early pregnancy losses, preterm labor, fetal-growth restriction, and late-pregnancy fetal demise (Bretelle and co-workers, 2005; Kusanovic and associates, 2007; Vasse, 2008).

Antiphospholipid Antibodies

These autoantibodies are detected in about 2 percent of patients who have nontraumatic venous thrombosis. The antibodies are directed against cardiolipin(s) or against phospholipid-binding proteins such as β_2-glycoprotein I. They are commonly found in patients with systemic lupus erythematosus and are described in Chapter 54 (see p. 1151). Women with moderate-to-high levels of these antibodies may have *antiphospholipid syndrome,* which is defined by a number of clinical features such as thromboembolism or certain obstetrical complications that include.

1. at least one otherwise unexplained fetal death at or beyond 10 weeks;
2. at least one preterm birth before 34 weeks; or
3. at least three consecutive spontaneous abortions before 10 weeks.

In these patients, thromboembolism—either venous or arterial—most commonly involves the lower extremities. Importantly, the syndrome also should be considered in women with thromboses in unusual sites, such as the portal, mesenteric, splenic, subclavian, and cerebral veins (American College of Obstetricians and Gynecologists, 2005). Antiphospholipid antibodies are also a predisposing factor for arterial thromboses. In fact, they account for up to 5 percent of arterial strokes in otherwise healthy young women (see Chap. 55, p. 1168). Thromboses may occur in relatively unusual locations, such as the retinal, subclavian, brachial, or digital arteries.

Branch and Khamashta (2003) and Levine and colleagues (2002) have reviewed a number of hypotheses proposed to

TABLE 47-3. Obstetrical Complications Associated with Some Inherited and Acquired Thrombophilias

Thrombophilia	Early Pregnancy Loss	Stillbirth	Preeclampsia	Placental Abruption	Fetal-Growth Restriction
FVL—homozygous	**2.7 (1.3–5.6)**	2.0 (0.4–9.7)	1.9 (0.4–7.9)	8.4 (0.4–171.2)	4.6 (0.2–115.7)
FVL—heterozygous	**1.7 (1.1–2.6)**	**2.1 (1.1–3.9)**	**2.2 (1.5–3.3)**	**4.7 (1.1–19.6)**	2.7 (0.6–12.1)
Prothrombin—heterozygous	**2.5 (1.2–5.0)**	**2.7 (1.3–5.5)**	**2.5 (1.5–4.2)**	**7.7 (3.0–19.8)**	2.9 (0.6–13.7)
MTHFR—homozygous	1.4 (0.8–2.6)	1.3 (0.9–1.1)	**1.4 (1.1–1.8)**	1.5 (0.4–5.4)	1.2 (0.8–1.8)
Hyperhomocysteinemia	**6.3 (1.4–28.4)**	1.0 (0.2–5.6)	**3.5 (1.2–10.1)**	2.4 (0.4–15.9)	N/A
Antithrombin deficiency	0.9 (0.2–4.5)	7.6 (0.3–196.4)	3.9 (0.2–97.2)	1.1 (0.1–18.1)	N/A
Protein C deficiency	2.3 (0.2–26.4)	3.1 (0.2–38.5)	5.2 (0.3–102.2)	5.9 (0.2–151.6)	N/A
Protein S deficiency	3.6 (0.4–35.7)	**20.1 (3.7–109.2)**	2.8 (0.8–10.6)	2.1 (0.5–9.3)	N/A
Acquired activated protein C resistance	**4.0 (1.7–9.8)**	0.9 (0.2–3.9)	1.8 (0.7–4.6)	1.3 (0.4–4.4)	N/A
Anticardiolipin antibody	**3.4 (1.3–8.7)**	**3.3 (1.6–6.7)**	**2.7 (1.7–4.5)**	1.4 (0.4–4.8)	**6.9 (2.7–17.7)**
Lupus anticoagulant	**3.0 (1.0–8.6)**	2.4 (0.8–7.0)	1.5 (0.8–2.8)	N/A	N/A

Data presented as odds ratios (95-percent confidence intervals). Bolded numbers are statistically significant.
FVL = factor V Leiden, MTHFR = methylenetetrahydrofolate reductase, N/A = data not available.
Data from Robertson and associates (2005).

explain mechanism(s) by which antiphospholipid antibodies promote thrombosis. For example, they may interfere with the normal function of phospholipids or phospholipid-binding proteins involved in coagulation regulation, including prothrombin, protein C, annexin V, and tissue factor. Many of these antibodies are directed against β₂-glycoprotein I, which may itself function as a natural anticoagulant (see Chap. 54, p. 1151). Another proposed mechanism is that these antibodies promote thrombosis through augmented platelet and/or complement activation.

Thrombophilias and Pregnancy Complications

Considerable attention has been directed recently toward a possible relationship between thrombophilias and certain pregnancy complications other than venous thrombosis (De Santis and associates, 2006). Table 47-3 summarizes the findings of 79 studies systematically reviewed by Robertson and associates (2005). The heterogeneity of these findings is apparent. For example, only heterozygous factor V Leiden and prothrombin gene mutations are consistently associated with most of these adverse outcomes. Recent investigations continue to underscore the heterogeneity of results. For example, Kahn and co-workers (2009) found no increased risk for early-onset or severe preeclampsia in women with factor V Leiden mutation, prothrombin G20210A mutation, MTHFR C677T polymorphism, or hyperhomocysteinemia. Falcao and associates (2009) found no association between the latter thrombophilia and the development of preeclampsia in an animal model. Conversely, Facchinetti and colleagues (2009) found that recurrent preeclampsia was significantly more common in Italian women diagnosed with a thrombophilia. The associations between thrombophilias and certain pregnancy complications are discussed in greater detail in other chapters: preeclampsia and

HELLP syndrome (see Chap. 34, p. 748), fetal-growth restriction (see Chap. 38, p. 848), placental abruption (see Chap. 35, p. 764), recurrent miscarriage (see Chap. 9, p. 224), stillbirth (see Chap. 29, p. 631), and placental findings of intervillous or spiral artery thrombosis (see Chap. 27, p. 579).

Thrombophilia Prophylaxis to Prevent Adverse Pregnancy Outcomes

There are no randomized trials to guide prophylaxis to prevent recurrent adverse pregnancy outcomes in women with any of the inherited thrombophilias. Even so, some recommend consideration for empirical aspirin and/or low-molecular-weight heparin (Lockwood, 2002). There are a few observational studies designed to assess the efficacy of treatment during pregnancy. De Carolis and co-workers (2006) treated 38 women with an inherited thrombophilia and a prior thromboembolic event and/or poor obstetrical outcome during 39 consecutive pregnancies. Among the previous pregnancies, only 18 resulted in a live birth, and only 12 neonates survived. In general, treatment during subsequent pregnancies consisted of enoxaparin, 40 mg daily in those with previous pregnancy complications, and 60 mg daily in those with a prior thromboembolic event. Among the 39 subsequent pregnancies, 32 resulted in a term delivery, six delivered preterm, and there was one spontaneous abortion. There were no thromboembolic events. In another observational study, Folkeringa and associates (2007) observed that thromboprophylaxis resulted in a significant reduction in the rate of historical fetal loss in women with hereditary deficiencies of antithrombin, protein C, or protein S. Similarly, Leduc and colleagues (2007) in a retrospective chart review found that the combination of dalteparin (see p. 1022) and low-dose aspirin given to women with an inherited thrombophilia and a prior pregnancy complicated by fetal death, placental abruption, early-onset severe preeclampsia, or fetal-growth restriction decreased the risks of the latter two in a subsequent pregnancy. Other observational studies have not found improved perinatal outcomes with heparin (Warren and co-workers, 2009).

DEEP-VENOUS THROMBOSIS

Clinical Presentation

Most cases of venous thrombosis during pregnancy are probably confined to the deep veins of the lower extremity. The frequency and extent to which they involve the pelvic veins is not known precisely, but preliminary observations indicate that iliac vein thrombosis may be frequent in those after cesarean delivery (Rodger and colleagues, 2006). The signs and symptoms vary greatly and depend in large measure on the degree of occlusion and the intensity of the inflammatory response. Interestingly, most cases during pregnancy occur in the left leg. Ginsberg and colleagues (1992) reported that 58 of 60 antepartum women—97 percent—had left leg thromboses. Blanco-Molina and co-workers (2007) reported that 78 percent were diagnosed in the left leg. Our experiences at Parkland Hospital are similar—90 percent of lower extremity thromboses involved the left leg. Greer (2003) hypothesizes that this may result from compression of the left iliac vein by the right iliac artery and ovarian artery, both of which cross the vein only on the left side. Yet, as described in Chapter 5 (p. 124), the ureter is compressed more on the right side!

Classical thrombosis involving the lower extremity is abrupt in onset, and there is pain and edema of the leg and thigh. The lower-extremity thrombus typically involves much of the deep venous system to the iliofemoral region. Occasionally, reflex arterial spasm causes a pale, cool extremity with diminished pulsations. Conversely, there may be appreciable clot, yet little pain, heat, or swelling. Importantly, calf pain, either spontaneous or in response to squeezing or to stretching the Achilles tendon—*Homans sign*—may be caused by a strained muscle or a contusion.

A fourth of untreated cases have an associated pulmonary embolism. Anticoagulation reduces this risk to less than 5 percent as discussed subsequently.

Diagnosis

Because clinical diagnosis of deep-venous thrombosis is difficult, other methods are imperative for confirmation. For example, in one study of pregnant women, clinical diagnosis was confirmed in only 10 percent of patients (Hull and co-workers,

1990). Shown in Figure 47-2 is one algorithm promulgated by the American College of Obstetricians and Gynecologists that can be used for evaluation of pregnant women. With a few modifications, we follow a similar evaluation at Parkland Hospital. Importantly, many of the tests used commonly in various diagnostic algorithms that have been extensively investigated in nonpregnant patients have not been validated in pregnant women. These include compression ultrasonography (CUS), ventilation-perfusion scintigraphy, and helical computed tomography-angiography (Nijkeuter and co-workers, 2006).

Venography

Invasive contrast venography remains the standard to exclude lower extremity deep-venous thrombosis (Chunilal and Ginsberg, 2001). It has a negative-predictive value of 98 percent, and as discussed in Chapter 41 (p. 921), fetal radiation exposure without shielding is only about 300 mrad (Nijkeuter and co-workers, 2006). But venography is associated with significant

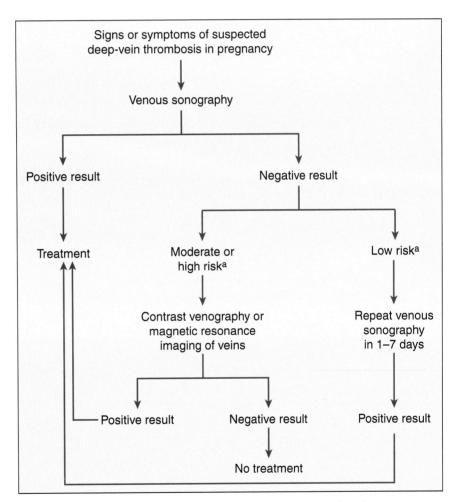

FIGURE 47-2 Algorithm for evaluation of suspected deep-venous thrombosis in pregnancy. *Pretest risk score calculated by assigning 1 point for each of the nine following characteristics: active cancer, immobilization, bed rest more than 3 days or surgery within 12 weeks, local tenderness, entire leg swollen, asymmetric calf swelling greater than 3 cm when measured 10 cm below tibial tuberosity, pitting edema only in symptomatic leg, collateral nonvaricose superficial veins, or prior deep-venous thrombosis. Two points are subtracted if an alternative diagnosis is at least as likely as deep-venous thrombosis. [a] High risk = 3 or more points, moderate risk = 1 or 2 points, low risk = 0 or less points. (From Lockwood, 2007, with permission.)

complications, including thrombosis, and it is time consuming and cumbersome. Thus, noninvasive methods are usually used to confirm the clinical diagnosis.

Impedance Plethysmography

This is an extremely accurate test to assess thromboses in the lower iliac, femoral, and popliteal veins. It is based on the observation that alterations in venous return in the calf, produced by inflation and deflation of a pneumatic thigh cuff, result in changes in electrical resistance detected at the skin surface. These changes occur when the popliteal or more proximal veins are obstructed (Chunilal and Ginsberg, 2001). Impedance plethysmography, however, is only 50-percent sensitive for detection of clots in the small calf veins (Davis, 2001). Moreover, because of decreased venous return of the lower extremities, it is associated with increased false-positive results during pregnancy (Andres and Miles, 2001). Given these limitations as well as the wide availability of ultrasonography, it is seldom used today.

Compression Ultrasonography

This noninvasive technique is currently the most-used first-line test to detect deep-venous thrombosis (Greer, 2003). The diagnosis is based on the noncompressibility and typical echoarchitecture of a thrombosed vein (Davis, 2001). In symptomatic nonpregnant patients, examination of the femoral, popliteal, and calf trifurcation veins is more than 90-percent sensitive and more than 99-percent specific for proximal thrombosis. Moreover, it has a negative-predictive value of 98 percent (American College of Obstetricians and Gynecologists, 2000a, b).

For *nonpregnant* patients with suspected thrombosis, the safety of withholding anticoagulation has been established for those who have normal serial compression examinations over a week (Birdwell and co-workers, 1998; Heijboer and associates, 1993). Specifically, in these nonpregnant patients, isolated calf thromboses extend into the proximal veins in up to a fourth of cases. They do so within 1 to 2 weeks of presentation and are usually detected by serial ultrasonographic compression.

In *pregnant* women, the important caveat is that normal findings with venous ultrasonography results do not always exclude a pulmonary embolism. This is because the thrombosis may have already embolized or because it arose from deep pelvic veins inaccessible to ultrasound evaluation (Goldhaber and colleagues, 2004). **In pregnant women, thrombosis associated with pulmonary embolism frequently originates in the iliac veins.** Moreover, the natural history of calf deep-venous thrombosis during pregnancy is unknown. Thus, the safety of withholding anticoagulation with negative compression ultrasonography has not been evaluated in pregnant women who may have an isolated iliac vein thrombosis that is less accessible for imaging (Bates and Ginsberg, 2002).

Computed Tomography

Spiral computed tomography (CT) scanning is widely available and very useful for detecting lower extremity deep-venous thrombosis as well as those within the vena cava and iliac and pelvic venous systems. Although radiation and contrast agents are required, the benefits of CT outweigh any theoretical risks if lead shielding is used. Fetal radiation exposure is negligible unless the pelvic veins are imaged (see Chap. 41, p. 918).

Magnetic Resonance (MR) Imaging

This imaging technique allows excellent delineation of anatomical detail above the inguinal ligament. Thus, in many cases, MR imaging is immensely useful for diagnosis of iliofemoral and pelvic vein thrombosis. The venous system can also be reconstructed using MR venography as discussed in Chapter 41 (see p. 921 and Fig. 41-5). Erdman and co-workers (1990) reported that MR imaging was 100-percent sensitive and 90-percent specific for detection of venographically proven deep-venous thrombosis in nonpregnant patients. Importantly, almost half of those without deep-venous thrombosis had detectable nonthrombotic conditions to explain the clinical findings. These included cellulitis, myositis, edema, hematomas, and superficial phlebitis. More recent studies have confirmed the high levels of sensitivity and specificity as well as the additional advantage of low interobserver variability (Palareti and associates, 2006).

D-Dimer Screening Tests

These specific fibrin degradation products are generated when fibrinolysin degrades fibrin, as occurs in thromboembolism. Their measurement is frequently incorporated into diagnostic algorithms for venous thromboembolism in nonpregnant patients (Kelly and Hunt, 2002; Wells and co-workers, 2003). Screening with the D-dimer test in pregnancy, however, is problematic for a number of reasons. Depending on assay sensitivity, D-dimer serum levels increase with gestational age along with substantively elevated plasma fibrinogen concentrations (Kenny and associates, 2009). In a serial study of 50 healthy women, Kline and colleagues (2005) found not only that D-dimer levels increased progressively during pregnancy, but that 22 percent of women in midpregnancy and no women in the third trimester had a D-dimer concentration below 0.50 mg/L—a conventional cut-off used to exclude thromboembolism. D-Dimer concentrations can also be elevated in certain pregnancy complications such as placental abruption, preeclampsia, and sepsis syndrome. For these reasons, their use during pregnancy remains uncertain, but a negative D-dimer test should be considered reassuring (Lockwood, 2007; Marik and Plante, 2008).

Management

Optimal management of venous thromboembolism during pregnancy has not undergone major clinical studies to provide evidence-based practices (Copplestone and colleagues, 2004). There is, however, consensus for treatment with anticoagulation and limited activity. If thrombophilia testing is performed, it is done before anticoagulation because heparin induces a decline in antithrombin levels, and warfarin decreases protein C and S concentrations (Lockwood, 2002).

Anticoagulation is initiated with either unfractionated or low-molecular-weight heparin. During pregnancy, heparin therapy is continued, and for postpartum women, anticoagulation is begun simultaneously with warfarin. Recall that pulmonary embolism develops in about 25 percent of patients with untreated venous thrombosis, and anticoagulation decreases this risk to less than 5 percent. In nonpregnant patients, the mortality rate is less than 1 percent (Douketis and co-workers, 1998; Weiss and Bernstein, 2000).

Over several days, leg pain dissipates. After symptoms have abated, graded ambulation should be started. Elastic stockings are fitted and anticoagulation is continued. Recovery to this stage usually takes 7 to 10 days.

Heparinization

Treatment of thromboembolism during pregnancy is with either unfractionated or low-molecular-weight heparin. Although either type is acceptable, most recommend one of the low-molecular-weight heparins. In its recently revised guidelines, the American College of Chest Physicians suggests preferential use of this heparin class during pregnancy but scores this recommendation a Grade 2C level of evidence—the lowest quality (Bates and colleagues, 2008; Guyatt and co-workers, 2008).

Unfractionated Heparin (UFH)

Treatment is with an intravenous heparin bolus followed by continuous infusion titrated to achieve full anticoagulation. The American Academy of Pediatrics and the American College of Obstetricians and Gynecologists (2007) recommend an initial bolus of intravenous unfractionated heparin at a dose of 80 units/kg. This is followed by continuous infusion of at least 30,000 IU for 24 hours, titrated to achieve an activated partial thromboplastin time (aPTT) of 1.5 to 2.5 times control values. There are a number of protocols to accomplish this, and the one used at Parkland Hospital is shown in Table 47-4. Intravenous anticoagulation should be maintained for at least 5 to 7 days, after which, treatment is converted to subcutaneous heparin. Injections are then given every 8 hours to maintain the aPTT to at least 1.5 to 2.5 times control throughout the dosing interval. For women with antiphospholipid syndrome, aPTT does not accurately assess heparin anticoagulation, and thus anti-factor Xa levels are preferred.

The duration of full anticoagulation varies, and there are several acceptable schemes. The American Academy of Pediatrics

and the American College of Obstetricians and Gynecologists (2007) recommend therapeutic anticoagulation for at least 3 months after the acute event. The American College of Chest Physicians (Bates and colleagues, 2008) recommends anticoagulation throughout pregnancy and for 6 weeks postpartum but for a minimum total duration of 6 months. Lockwood (2007) recommends full anticoagulation be continued for at least 20 weeks followed by prophylactic doses if the woman is still pregnant. Prophylactic doses of subcutaneous unfractionated heparin can range from 5000 to 10,000 units every 12 hours titrated to maintain an antifactor Xa level of 0.1 to 0.2 units, measured 6 hours after the last injection. If the venous thromboembolism occurs during the postpartum period, Lockwood (2007) recommends a minimum of 6 months of anticoagulation treatment.

Low-Molecular-Weight Heparin

This is a family of derivatives of unfractionated heparin, and their molecular weights average 4000 to 5000 daltons compared with 12,000 to 16,000 daltons for conventional heparin. None of these heparins cross the placenta, and all exert their anticoagulant activity by activating antithrombin. The primary difference is in their relative inhibitory activity against factor Xa and thrombin (Garcia and Spyropoulos, 2008). Specifically, unfractionated heparin has equivalent activity against factor Xa and thrombin, but low-molecular-weight heparins have greater activity against factor Xa than thrombin. They also have a more predictable anticoagulant response and fewer bleeding complications than unfractionated heparin because of their better bioavailability, longer half-life, dose-independent clearance, and decreased interference with platelets (Tapson, 2008). Their major drawback is expense.

A number of studies have shown that venous thromboembolism is treated effectively with low-molecular-weight heparin (Quinlan and colleagues, 2004; Tapson, 2008). Using serial venograms, Breddin and co-workers (2001) observed that low-molecular-weight heparins were more effective than the unfractionated form in reducing thrombus size without increasing mortality rates or major bleeding complications.

Pharmacokinetics in Pregnancy. Several low-molecular-weight heparins are available for use in pregnancy and include

---

TABLE 47-4. Parkland Hospital Protocol for Continuous Heparin Infusion for Patients with Venous Thromboembolism

Initial Heparin Dose:

☐ units IV push (recommended 80 units/kg rounded to nearest 100, maximum 7500 units), then

☐ units/hr by infusion (recommended 18 units/kg/hr rounded to nearest 50).

Infusion Rate Adjustments—based on partial thromboplastin time (PTT):

PTT (sec)[a]	Intervention[b]	Baseline Infusion Rate Change[c]
<45	80 units/kg bolus	↑ by 4 units/kg/hr
45–54	40 units/kg bolus	↑ by 2 units/kg/hr
55–84	None	None
85–100	None	↓ by 2 units/kg/hr
>100	Stop infusion 60 minutes	↓ by 3 units/kg/hr

[a]PTT goal 55–84; [b]Rounded to nearest 100; [c]Rounded to nearest 50.

enoxaparin, dalteparin, and tinzaparin. *Enoxaparin (Lovenox)* pharmacokinetics were studied by Casele and colleagues (1999) in 13 pregnant women. They were given 40 mg subcutaneously daily, and serial measurements of anti-factor Xa activity were determined during early pregnancy, the third trimester, and then postpartum. They concluded that, likely because of increased renal clearance, twice-daily dosing may be necessary to maintain anti-factor Xa activity above 0.1 U/mL. They also suggested that optimal dosing was best achieved with periodic monitoring of peak activity—about 3.5 hours after a dose—and predose anti-factor Xa activity.

Rodie and co-workers (2002) studied 36 women with venous thromboembolism during pregnancy or immediately postpartum who were treated with enoxaparin. The dose was approximately 1 mg/kg given twice daily based on early pregnancy weight. Treatment was monitored by peak anti-factor Xa activity 3 hours postinjection, with a target therapeutic range of 0.4–1.0 U/mL. In 33 women, enoxaparin provided satisfactory anticoagulation. In the other three women, dose reduction was necessary. None developed recurrent thromboembolism or bleeding complications.

Dalteparin (Fragmin) pharmacokinetics were studied by Sephton and associates (2003) in a longitudinal investigation of 24 pregnant women. Those given once-daily dalteparin subcutaneously had mean anti-factor Xa levels that were significantly lower across pregnancy compared with levels measured 6 weeks' postpartum.

Smith and co-workers (2004) reported similar results with *tinzaparin (Innohep)* given as a once-daily 50 U/kg dose. They found that a dosage of 75 to 175 U/kg/day was necessary to achieve peak anti-factor Xa levels of 0.1 to 1.0 U/mL.

The American Academy of Pediatrics and the American College of Obstetricians and Gynecologists (2007) recommend that anti-factor Xa levels be periodically reevaluated during pregnancy in a woman fully anticoagulated with these agents. Monitoring anti-Xa levels during pregnancy is especially important in women who also have impaired renal or hepatic function, weigh less than 50 kg or greater than 100 kg, or have risk factors for bleeding (Duhl and associates, 2007). Dosing should be enough to achieve a peak anti-factor Xa level of 0.5 to 1.2 U/mL. Importantly, each low-molecular-weight heparin compound has a somewhat different pharmacodynamic pattern. Thus, a peak concentration of 1.0 U/mL may be appropriate in an enoxaparin-treated patient but may be an overdose in a dalteparin-treated patient (Gris and associates, 2006).

For women given thromboprophylaxis, most authorities do not recommend monitoring anti-factor Xa levels. Fox and colleagues (2008) reviewed anti-factor Xa levels in 77 women given "pregnancy-adjusted" doses of either dalteparin or enoxaparin for thromboprophylaxis. They reported that a fourth of 321 determinations showed "subtherapeutic" levels defined as less than 0.2 to 0.4 units/mL. They called for consideration of such monitoring. At this time, however, this is considered unnecessary for prophylactic dosing because the "therapeutic range" is uncertain (Bates and associates, 2008).

Safety in Pregnancy. Early reviews by Sanson and associates (1999) and Lepercq and co-workers (2001) concluded that low-molecular-weight heparins were safe and effective. Despite this, in 2002, the manufacturer of Lovenox warned that its use in pregnancy had been associated with congenital anomalies and an increased risk of hemorrhage. After its own extensive review, the American College of Obstetricians and Gynecologists (2002) concluded that these risks were rare, that their incidence was not higher than expected, and that no cause-and-effect relationship had been established. The committee further concluded that enoxaparin and dalteparin could be given safely during pregnancy. A subsequent review by Deruelle and Coulon (2007) also confirmed their safety.

Caveats are that low-molecular-weight heparins should not be used in women with prosthetic heart valves because of reports of valvular thrombosis (see Chap. 44, p. 964). They also should be avoided in women with renal failure (Krivak and Zorn, 2007). When given within 2 hours of cesarean delivery, these agents increase the risk of wound hematoma (van Wijk and co-workers, 2002). Lee and Goodwin (2006) described development of a massive subchorionic hematoma associated with enoxaparin use. Frosnes and associates (2009) reported a woman who developed a spontaneous thoracolumbar epidural hematoma that required surgical drainage.

As discussed in Chapter 19 (p. 457), use of low-molecular-weight heparins may also increase the risk of *spinal hematoma* associated with regional analgesia. As a result, the American Academy of Pediatrics and American College of Obstetricians and Gynecologists (2007) advise that women receiving once-daily prophylactic low-dose low-molecular-weight heparin not be offered regional analgesia until at least 10 to 12 hours after the last injection. In addition, low-molecular-weight heparin should be withheld for at least 2 hours after the removal of an epidural catheter. The safety of regional analgesia in women receiving twice-daily therapeutic low-molecular-weight heparin has not been studied sufficiently, and it is not known whether delaying regional techniques for 24 hours after the last injection is adequate. Of note, *protamine sulfate* (see p. 1024) may help partially reverse the effects of low-molecular-weight heparin.

Anticoagulation with Warfarins

Warfarin derivatives are generally contraindicated because they readily cross the placenta and cause fetal death and malformations from hemorrhages (see Chap. 14, p. 325). Like unfractionated and low-molecular-weight heparin, however, they are safe during breast feeding (American Academy of Pediatrics and American College of Obstetricians and Gynecologists, 2007; Bates and associates, 2004).

Postpartum venous thrombosis is usually treated with intravenous heparin and oral warfarin initiated simultaneously. To avoid paradoxical thrombosis and skin necrosis from the early anti-protein C effect of warfarin, these women are maintained on therapeutic doses of unfractionated or low-molecular-weight heparin for 5 days and until the international normalized ratio (INR) is in a therapeutic range (American Academy of Pediatrics and American College of Obstetricians and Gynecologists, 2007). The initial dose of warfarin is usually 5 to 10 mg for the first 2 days. Subsequent doses are titrated to achieve an INR of 2 to 3.

Brooks and colleagues (2002) compared anticoagulation in postpartum women with that of age-matched nonpregnant controls. Recently delivered women required a significantly larger median total dose of warfarin—45 versus 24 mg—and a longer time—7 versus 4 days—to achieve the target INR. Moreover, the mean maintenance dose was higher in postpartum women compared with that in the control group—4.9 versus 4.3 mg.

Duration of Therapy

The optimal duration of continued anticoagulation after delivery is uncertain, but anticoagulation with warfarin is continued for at least 4 to 6 weeks. Most recommendations have been extrapolated from studies in nonpregnant patients (Kearon and colleagues, 1999; Ridker and co-workers, 2003). This is problematic because most studies in nonpregnant patients included bedridden older patients with medical complications. The current consensus of the American College of Chest Physicians is that warfarin anticoagulation be given for at least 6 weeks postpartum, but to complete a minimum 6-month course following the initial episode (Bates and colleagues, 2008). Lockwood (2007) recommends a minimum of 6 weeks. As previously mentioned (see p. 1021), most agree that deep-venous thrombosis that develops postpartum requires a minimum of 6 months of anticoagulation (Lockwood, 2007).

Complications of Anticoagulation

Three significant complications associated with anticoagulation are hemorrhage, thrombocytopenia, and osteoporosis. The latter two are unique to heparin, and their risk may be reduced with low-molecular-weight heparins (American College of Obstetricians and Gynecologists, 2000). The most serious complication is hemorrhage, which is more likely if there has been recent surgery or lacerations. Troublesome bleeding also is more likely if the heparin dosage is excessive. Unfortunately, management schemes using laboratory testing to identify when a heparin dosage is sufficient to inhibit further thrombosis, yet not cause serious hemorrhage, have been discouraging.

Heparin-Induced Thrombocytopenia

There are two types of *heparin-induced thrombocytopenia*—commonly referred to as *HIT*. The most common is a *nonimmune*, benign, reversible form that occurs within the first few days of therapy and resolves in about 5 days without cessation of therapy (American College of Obstetricians and Gynecologists, 2000). The second is the more severe form of HIT, which results from an *immune* reaction involving IgG antibodies directed against complexes of platelet factor 4 and heparin. When most severe, HIT paradoxically causes thrombosis, which is the most common presentation. The American College of Chest Physicians advises that the diagnosis of HIT be considered when the platelet count decreases by 50 percent between 5 and 14 days after the initiation of heparin therapy (Greinacher and Warkentin, 2006).

The incidence of HIT is approximately 3 to 5 percent in nonpregnant individuals. Interestingly, however, Fausett and colleagues (2001) reported no cases of HIT among 244 heparin-treated pregnant women compared with 10 among 244 nonpregnant controls. The American College of Obstetricians and Gynecologists (2000) recommends that platelet counts be measured on day 5 and then periodically for the first 2 weeks of heparin therapy. If unchanged, further platelet counts are not indicated because most cases manifest within 15 days of standard heparin initiation.

If thrombocytopenia is severe, heparin therapy must be stopped and alternative anticoagulation initiated. Low-molecular-weight heparin may not be an entirely safe alternative because it has some cross reactivity with unfractionated heparin. In these cases, many recommend *danaparoid*—a sulfated glycosaminoglycan heparinoid. In a review of approximately 50 pregnant women with either HIT or skin rashes, Lindhoff-Last and associates (2005) also concluded that danaparoid was a reasonable alternative, however, *two fatal maternal hemorrhages and three fetal deaths were recorded.*

Direct thrombin inhibitors—examples include *hirudin, argatroban,* and *lepirudin*—also have been used as a heparin alternative (Chapman and associates, 2008; Tapson, 2008). There are reports, however, that hirudin crosses the placenta and is fetotoxic (Gris and associates, 2006; Mazzolai and co-workers, 2006). Lockwood (2007) recommends the use of *fondaparinux*—a pentasaccharide factor Xa inhibitor—in pregnant women for whom there are no alternatives. Successful use in pregnancy has been reported, including a case report describing a woman with an intolerance to both heparin and danaparoid (Mazzolai and colleagues, 2006). At least one recent report suggests that fondaparinux can rarely cause a disorder that resembles HIT (Warkentin and co-workers, 2007). Interestingly, heparin-dependent antibodies do not invariably reappear with subsequent heparin use (Warkentin and Kelton, 2001).

Heparin-Induced Osteoporosis

Bone loss may develop with long-term heparin administration—usually 6 months or longer—and is more prevalent in cigarette smokers (see Chap. 53, p. 1136). Low-molecular-weight heparins can cause osteopenia (Deruelle and Coulon, 2007), although such a result is less likely than with unfractionated heparin. Women treated with any heparin should be encouraged to take a daily supplement of 1500 mg of calcium (Cunningham, 2005; Lockwood, 2007). Low-molecular-weight heparins may cause less adverse effects. Rodger and colleagues (2007) found that longer-term use with a mean of 212 days with dalteparin, 5000 units subcutaneously given daily until 20 weeks and 5000 units twice daily thereafter, was not associated with a significant decrease in bone mineral density.

Anticoagulation and Abortion

The treatment of deep-venous thrombosis with heparin does not preclude termination of pregnancy by careful curettage. After the products are removed without trauma to the reproductive tract, full-dose heparin can be restarted in several hours.

Anticoagulation and Delivery

The effects of heparin on blood loss at delivery depend on a number of variables:

- Dose, route, and time of administration
- Number and severity of incisions and lacerations
- Intensity of postpartum myometrial contractions
- Presence of other coagulation defects.

Blood loss should not be greatly increased with vaginal delivery if the midline episiotomy is modest in depth, there are no lacerations, and the uterus promptly contracts. Unfortunately, such ideal circumstances do not always prevail. For example, Mueller and Lebherz (1969) described 10 women with antepartum thrombophlebitis treated with heparin. Three women who continued to receive heparin during labor and delivery bled remarkably and developed large hematomas. Thus, heparin therapy generally is stopped during labor and delivery. If the uterus is well contracted and there has been negligible trauma to the lower genital tract, it can be restarted after about 12 hours. Otherwise, a delay of 1 or 2 days may be prudent.

Protamine sulfate administered slowly intravenously generally reverses the effect of heparin promptly and effectively. It should not be given in excess of the amount needed to neutralize the heparin, because it also has an anticoagulant effect. Serious bleeding is likely when heparin in usual therapeutic doses is administered to a woman who has undergone cesarean delivery within the previous 24 to 48 hours.

SUPERFICIAL VENOUS THROMBOPHLEBITIS

Thrombosis limited strictly to the superficial veins of the saphenous system is treated with analgesia, elastic support, and rest. If it does not soon subside, or if deep-venous involvement is suspected, appropriate diagnostic measures are performed. Heparin is given if deep-venous involvement is confirmed. Superficial thrombophlebitis is typically seen in association with varicosities or as a sequela to an indwelling intravenous catheter.

PULMONARY EMBOLISM

Although it causes about 10 percent of maternal deaths, pulmonary embolism is relatively uncommon during pregnancy and the puerperium. The incidence averages about 1 in 7000 pregnancies. There is an almost equal prevalence for antepartum and postpartum embolism, but those developing postpartum have a higher mortality rate. According to Marik and Plante (2008), 70 percent of women presenting with a pulmonary embolism have associated clinical evidence of deep-venous thrombosis. In women presenting with a deep-venous thrombosis, almost half will have a silent pulmonary embolism.

Clinical Presentation

Findings from the international cooperative pulmonary embolism registry were reported by Goldhaber and colleagues (1999). Over a 2-year period, almost 2500 nonpregnant patients with a proven pulmonary embolism were enrolled.

Common symptoms included dyspnea in 82 percent, chest pain in 49 percent, cough in 20 percent, syncope in 14 percent, and hemoptysis in 7 percent. Other predominant clinical findings typically include tachypnea, apprehension, and tachycardia. In some cases, there is an accentuated pulmonic closure sound, rales, and/or friction rub.

Right axis deviation and T-wave inversion in the anterior chest leads may be evident on the electrocardiogram. On chest radiography, there may be loss of vascular markings in the region of the lungs supplied by the obstructed artery. Although most women are hypoxemic, it is emphasized that a normal arterial blood gas analysis does not exclude pulmonary embolism. Approximately a third of patients younger than 40 years will have pO_2 values >80 mm Hg. In contrast, the alveolar-arterial oxygen tension difference is a more useful indicator of disease, as more than 86 percent of patients with acute pulmonary embolism will have an alveolar-arterial difference of more than 20 mm Hg (Lockwood, 2007). Even with massive pulmonary embolism, signs, symptoms, and laboratory data to support the diagnosis may be deceptively nonspecific.

Massive Pulmonary Embolism

This is defined as embolism causing hemodynamic instability (Tapson, 2008). Acute mechanical obstruction of the pulmonary vasculature causes increased vascular resistance and pulmonary hypertension. Acute right ventricular dilatation follows. In otherwise healthy patients, significant pulmonary hypertension does not develop until 60 to 75 percent of the pulmonary vascular tree is occluded (Guyton and colleagues, 1954). Moreover, circulatory collapse requires 75- to 80-percent obstruction. This is depicted schematically in Figure 47-3 and emphasizes that most acutely symptomatic emboli are large and likely a saddle embolism. These are suspected when pulmonary artery pressure is substantively increased as estimated by echocardiography.

If there is evidence of right ventricular dysfunction, the mortality rate approaches 25 percent, compared with 1 percent without such dysfunction (Kinane and co-workers, 2008). It is important in these cases to infuse crystalloids carefully and to support blood pressure with vasopressors. Oxygen treatment, tracheal intubation, and mechanical ventilation are carried out preparatory to thrombolysis, filter placement, or embolectomy (Tapson, 2008).

Diagnosis

As with deep-venous thrombosis, the diagnosis of pulmonary embolism requires an initial high index of suspicion followed by objective testing (Chunilal and colleagues, 2003). As shown in Figure 47-4, the initial imaging evaluation for suspected pulmonary embolism during pregnancy generally includes ventilation-perfusion scintigraphy, computed tomography, or bilateral compression ultrasonography. Of note, a chest radiograph should be performed if there is underlying suspicion for other diagnoses. The current opinion of the American Academy of Pediatrics and American College of Obstetricians and Gynecologists (2007) is that, in contemporary practice, pulmonary embolism is commonly diagnosed with multidetector-row spiral computed tomography pulmonary angiography (MDCT).

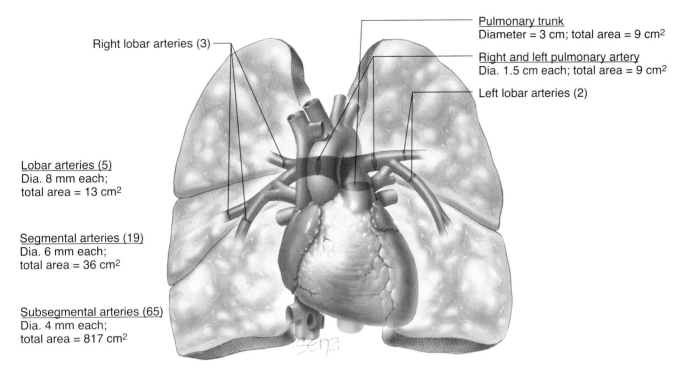

Right lobar arteries (3)

Pulmonary trunk
Diameter = 3 cm; total area = 9 cm²

Right and left pulmonary artery
Dia. 1.5 cm each; total area = 9 cm²

Left lobar arteries (2)

Lobar arteries (5)
Dia. 8 mm each;
total area = 13 cm²

Segmental arteries (19)
Dia. 6 mm each;
total area = 36 cm²

Subsegmental arteries (65)
Dia. 4 mm each;
total area = 817 cm²

FIGURE 47-3 Schematic of pulmonary arterial circulation. Note that the cross-sectional area of the pulmonary trunk and the combined pulmonary arteries is 9 cm². A large saddle embolism could occlude 50 to 90 percent of the pulmonary tree causing hemodynamic instability. As the arteries give off distal branches, the total surface area rapidly increases, that is, 13 cm² for the combined five lobar arteries, 36 cm² for combined 19 segmental arteries, and more than 800 cm² for the total 65 subsegmental arterial branches. Thus, hemodynamic instability is less likely with emboli past the lobar arteries. (Data from Singhal and colleagues, 1973.)

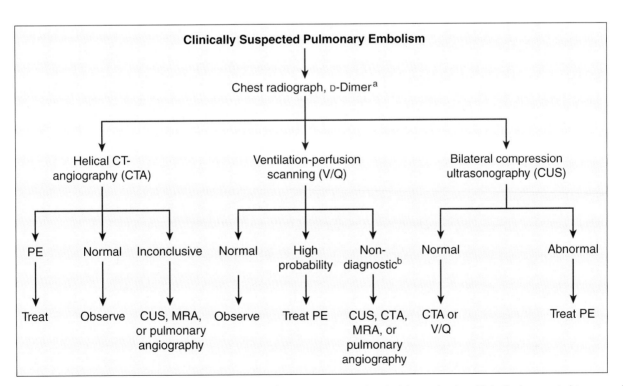

FIGURE 47-4 Evaluation of suspected pulmonary embolism during pregnancy. The decision to begin with helical computed tomography (CT), ventilation/perfusion (V/Q) scan, or bilateral CUS depends on local availability and expertise. CTA = CT angiography; CUS = compression ultrasonography; MRA = magnetic resonance angiography; PE = pulmonary embolism. [a]See text (p. 1020) for discussion. [b]Nondiagnostic results are those that indicate an intermediate or low probability of pulmonary embolism, or that do not indicate a high probability. (Adapted from Nijkeuter and colleagues, 2006, and Tapson, 2008.)

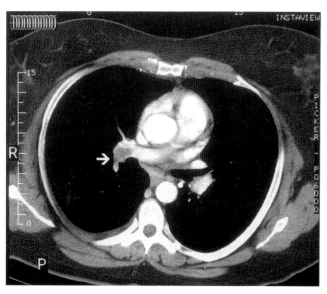

FIGURE 47-5 Axial image of the chest from a four-channel multi-detector spiral computed tomographic scan performed after administration of intravenous contrast. There is enhancement of the pulmonary artery with a large thrombus on the right (*arrow*) consistent with pulmonary embolism. (Courtesy of Dr. Michael Landay.)

Computed Tomographic Pulmonary Angiography

It is likely that *multidetector spiral CT* will replace pulmonary angiography as the gold standard for diagnosis of pulmonary embolism (Goldhaber, 2004; Srivastava and colleagues, 2004). The technique is described further in Chapter 41 (p. 918), and an imaging example is shown in Figure 47-5. Except in late pregnancy, fetal x-ray exposure is less than with V/Q scanning (Table 47-5). In a prospective study of 102 consecutive non-pregnant patients with suspected pulmonary embolism who underwent multidetector spiral CT, Kavanagh and co-workers (2004) found that during a mean follow-up period of 9 months, only one patient had a false-negative scan. Stein and colleagues (2006) reported that combined MDCT angiography and venography was even more sensitive.

We now use multidetector spiral CT as first-line evaluation of pregnant women both at Parkland Hospital and at the University of Alabama at Birmingham Hospital. Although the technique has many advantages, we have found that the better resolution allows detection of previously inaccessible smaller distal emboli that have uncertain clinical significance. Similar observations have been reported by Anderson and associates (2007). Others have found that the hyperdynamic circulation and increased plasma volume associated with pregnancy lead to a higher number of nondiagnostic studies compared with non-pregnant patients (Scarsbrook and associates, 2006).

Ventilation–Perfusion Scintigraphy—Lung Scan

Although used less commonly in the past 5 years, ventilation–perfusion (V/Q) lung scanning is still used by some centers. As seen in Figure 47-4, V/Q scintigraphy may be used if compression ultrasonography results are negative. The technique involves a small dose of radiotracer such as intravenously administered ^{99m}technetium-macroaggregated albumin. As shown in Table 47-5, there is negligible fetal radiation exposure. The scan may not provide a definite diagnosis because many other conditions—for example, pneumonia or local bronchospasm—can cause perfusion defects. Ventilation scans with inhaled xenon-133 or technetium-99m were added to perfusion scans to detect abnormal areas of ventilation in areas with normal perfusion such as with pneumonia or hypoventilation. The method is not precise, and although ventilation scanning increased the probability of an accurate diagnosis with large perfusion defects and ventilation mismatches, normal V/Q scan findings do not exclude pulmonary embolism.

Because of these uncertainties, the National Heart, Lung and Blood Institute commissioned the Prospective Investigation of Pulmonary Embolism Diagnosis to determine sensitivities and specificities of V/Q lung scans (PIOPED, 1990). The investigators concluded that a high-probability scan usually indicates pulmonary embolism, but that only a small number of patients with emboli have a high-probability scan. A low-probability scan, combined with a strong clinical impression that embolism is unlikely, makes the possibility of pulmonary embolism remote.

TABLE 47-5. Estimated Mean Fetal Radiation Dosimetry from Ventilation-Perfusion (V/Q) Lung Scanning Compared with 4-Channel Multidetector Spiral Computed Tomography (CT) Scanning

Pregnancy Duration	V/Q Scintigraphy		Spiral CT Scanning	
	mGy	mrem	mGy	mrem
Early	0.46	46	0.04	4
First trimester	0.46	46	0.04	4
Second trimester	0.57	57	0.11	11
Third trimester[a]	0.45	45	0.31	31

[a]In late pregnancy, the maximum exposure with spiral CT scanning may exceed the estimated mean by a factor of 5 to 7 due to increased proximity of the fetus to the primary beam.
Data courtesy of Dr. Jon Anderson.

Similarly, near-normal or normal scans make the diagnosis very unlikely. Finally, an intermediate-probability scan is of no help in establishing the diagnosis. Thus, the V/Q lung scan combined with clinical assessment permits a noninvasive diagnosis or exclusion of pulmonary embolism for only a minority of patients. Indeed, two thirds of nonpregnant patients with a suspected pulmonary embolism have a nondiagnostic scan and require additional testing (Raj, 2003). In our experience, this proportion is smaller in pregnant women, probably because they are younger and usually healthy and less likely to have coexisting pulmonary disease. Similarly, Chan and associates (2002) reported that only 25 percent of 120 pregnant women had a nondiagnostic scan.

Magnetic Resonance Angiography (MRA)

Although conventional magnetic resonance angiography has a high sensitivity for detection of central pulmonary emboli, the sensitivity for detection of subsegmental emboli is less precise (Scarsbrook and associates, 2006). In a study of 141 nonpregnant patients with suspected pulmonary embolism, Oudkerk and co-workers (2002) performed MRA before conventional angiography. About a third of patients were found to have an embolus, and the sensitivity of MRA for isolated subsegmental, segmental, and central or lobar pulmonary embolism was 40, 84, and 100 percent, respectively. There are no currently published reports specifically involving magnetic resonance angiography during pregnancy.

Pulmonary Angiography

This requires catheterization of the right side of the heart and is the most definitive study for pulmonary embolism. In addition to being invasive, it is also time consuming, uncomfortable, and associated with dye-induced allergy and renal failure. The procedure-related mortality rate is about 1 in 200 (Stein and colleagues, 1992). If absolutely necessary for confirmation when less invasive tests are equivocal, angiography should be considered.

Management

Immediate treatment for pulmonary embolism is full anticoagulation similar to that for deep-venous thrombosis as discussed on page 1021. A number of complementary procedures may be indicated.

Vena Caval Filters

The woman who has very recently suffered a pulmonary embolism and who must undergo cesarean delivery presents a particularly serious problem. Reversal of anticoagulation may be followed by another embolus, and surgery while fully anticoagulated frequently results in life-threatening hemorrhage or troublesome hematomas. In these, placement of a vena caval filter should be considered before surgery (Marik and Plante, 2008). Routine filter placement has no added advantage to heparin given alone (Decousus and associates, 1998). In the very infrequent circumstances in which heparin therapy fails to prevent recurrent pulmonary embolism from the pelvis or legs, or when embolism develops from these sites despite heparin treatment, a vena caval filter may be indicated. Such filters can also be used with massive emboli in patients who are not candidates for

thrombolysis (Deshpande and colleagues, 2002). The device may be inserted through either the jugular or femoral vein.

Retrievable filters may be used as short-term protection against embolism. These may be removed before they become endothelialized, or they can be left in place permanently (Tapson, 2008). Neill and colleagues (1997) placed a *Gunther Tulip filter* at 37 weeks, and it was removed 5 days postcesarean delivery at 38 weeks. Jamjute and co-workers (2006) described successful placement in a woman during labor.

Thrombolysis

Compared with heparin, thrombolytic agents provide more rapid lysis of pulmonary clots and improvement of pulmonary hypertension (Tapson, 2008). Konstantinides and colleagues (2002) studied 256 nonpregnant patients heparinized for an acute submassive pulmonary embolism. They also were assigned randomly to a placebo or the recombinant tissue plasminogen activator, *alteplase*. Those given the placebo had a threefold increased risk of death or treatment escalation compared with those given alteplase. Agnelli and associates (2002) performed a meta-analysis of nine randomized trials involving 461 nonpregnant patients. They reported that the risk of recurrence or death was significantly lower in patients given thrombolytic agents compared with those given heparin alone—10 versus 17 percent. Importantly, there were five—2 percent—fatal bleeding episodes in the thrombolysis group and none in the heparin-only group.

There are very few studies of thrombolysis during pregnancy. In their review of the literature, Leonhardt and associates (2006) identified 28 reports of thrombolytic therapy using tissue plasminogen activator during pregnancy. Ten of these cases were for thromboembolism. Complication rates were similar compared with reports from nonpregnant patients, and the authors concluded that such therapy should not be withheld during pregnancy if indicated. Tissue plasminogen activator does not cross the placenta. Our anecdotal experiences with these drugs has been favorable.

Embolectomy

Surgical embolectomy is uncommonly indicated with use of thrombolysis and filters. Published experience with emergency embolectomy during pregnancy is limited to case reports such as those by Funakoshi (2004) and Taniguchi (2008) and their co-workers. Based on their review, Ahearn and associates (2002) found that although the operative risk to the mother is reasonable, the stillbirth rate is 20 to 40 percent.

THROMBOPROPHYLAXIS

Thromboembolism Antedating Pregnancy

Optimal management of women with firm evidence of a prior thromboembolism is unclear. Most recommendations represent consensus guidelines, and some are diametrically opposed to others. The confusion that has ensued has provided fertile ground for the plaintiff bar to plow. Cleary-Goldman and colleagues (2007) surveyed 151 fellows of the American College of Obstetricians and Gynecologists and reported that intervention without firm indications is common. In Table 47-6 are listed a

SECTION 8

TABLE 47-6. Various Recommendations for Thromboprophylaxis During Pregnancy

Clinical Scenario	Pregnancy[a]	Postpartum[b]
Prior single-episode VTE[c]		
Associated with a risk factor that is no longer present	Surveillance only[1,2,4] or prophylactic UFH or LMWH[4]	Warfarin or prophylactic LMWH 4[1] to 6[1,2,4] weeks
VTE in a prior pregnancy, estrogen-related, or with additional risk factors (such as obesity)	Surveillance only[1] or prophylactic or intermediate-dose UFH[1,2,4] or LMWH[1,2,3,4]	Prophylactic UFH or LMWH[1,3,4]
Idiopathic—no known associations	Surveillance only[1]; prophylactic UFH[1,2,4] or LMWH[1,2,3,4]	Postpartum anticoagulants[1,3] or postpartum UFH or LMWH prophylaxis[2,4]
Associated with a heterozygous thrombophilia trait or strong family history of thrombosis	Surveillance only[1]; prophylactic[1,2,3] or intermediate-dose[1] LMWH or UFH[1]	Postpartum anticoagulants[1,3] or postpartum UFH or LMWH prophylaxis[2]
Women with AT deficiency not receiving long-term anticoagulation; compound heterozygotes for prothrombin G20210A and FVL; FVL homozygous; or prothrombin G20210A homozygous	Prophylactic or intermediate-dose[1] or adjusted-dose[2,4] LMWH; or prophylactic or intermediate-dose[1] or adjusted-dose[2,4] UFH	Postpartum anticoagulants[1] or warfarin for 12 months[2](AT deficiency may require lifetime anticoagulation
Two or more prior episodes of VTE and/or women receiving long-term anticoagulation[c]	Adjusted-dose UFH or adjusted-dose LMWH[1,4]	Warfarin 6 weeks[4] or resumption of long-term anticoagulation[1]
No prior VTE and:		
Require prolonged bed rest and are at an increased risk for VTE due to obesity, thrombophilia, or strong family history	Graduated elastic compression stockings[2]	Graduated elastic compression stockings[2]
Delivery by elective cesarean		Risk assessment—see Table 47–7
Known thrombophilia and no prior VTE and:		
AT deficiency not receiving long-term anticoagulation	Prophylactic UFH or LMWH[1]; or adjusted-dose UFH or LMWH throughout pregnancy[2]	Prophylactic UFH or LMWH[1]; or warfarin 6 weeks or longer[4]; or adjusted-dose UFH or LMWH[2]
Compound heterozygotes for prothrombin G20210A and FVL; FVL homozygous; or prothrombin G20210A homozygous	Surveillance only[1]; prophylactic UFH or LMWH[1]; or adjusted-dose UFH or LMWH throughout pregnancy[2]	Prophylactic UFH or LMWH[1]; warfarin 6 weeks or longer[4]; or adjusted-dose UFH or LMWH[2]
Less thrombogenic thrombophilias—heterozygous FVL or heterozygous prothrombin gene mutations; protein C, S, or Z deficiencies	Surveillance only[1,2] or prophylactic UFH or LMWH[1]	Prophylactic UFH or LMWH[1]; or postpartum anticoagulation with cesarean delivery or with an affected first-degree relative[2]
Homozygous for thermolabile variant (C677T) of MTHFR	Folic acid supplementation prior to and throughout pregnancy	Consider warfarin for 6 weeks if homocysteine serum levels abnormally high(?)[2]
Antiphospholipid antibodies and:		
History of 3 or more early pregnancy losses; one or more late pregnancy loss	Prophylactic or intermediate-dose UFH or prophylactic LMWH combined with low-dose aspirin[1]	Prophylactic UFH or LMWH[1] for 6–8 weeks[5]
History of VTE	Prophylactic or intermediate-dose LMWH or UFH[1]; adjusted-dose LMWH or adjusted-dose UFH[5] plus low-dose aspirin after 1st trimester[1]	Full anticoagulation for 6–8 weeks and referral to specialist[5] or long-term anticoagulation[1,2]

(Continued)

TABLE 47-6. Various Recommendations for Thromboprophylaxis During Pregnancy (*Continued*)

Clinical Scenario	Pregnancy[a]	Postpartum[b]
No prior VTE or pregnancy loss	Surveillance only[1] or prophylactic LMWH[1,5] or UFH[1,5] and [5] low-dose aspirin	Prophylactic heparin and low-dose aspirin for 6–8 weeks[5]

AT = antithrombin; FVL = factor V Leiden; LMWH = low-molecular-weight heparin; UFH = unfractionated heparin; VTE = venous thromboembolism.

Various UFH and LMWH regimens:

- Prophylactic UFH—5000 units SC q 12h[1]; 5000 to 10,000 units SC q 12h to maintain anti-Xa level of 0.1-0.2 units, 6h after the last injection[2]; or 5000 to 7500 units q 12h during the 1st trimester, 7500 to 10,000 units q 12 hours during the 2nd trimester, and 10,000 units q 12h during the 3rd trimester unless the aPTT is elevated[4]; or 5000 to 10,000 units q 12h throughout pregnancy[4].
- Intermediate-dose UFH-SC q 12h in doses adjusted to target anti-Xa level of 0.1-0.3 U/mL[1].
- Adjusted-dose UFH-SC q 12h in doses adjusted to target a mid-interval aPTT in the therapeutic range[1] or UFH SC q 8–12h to maintain the aPTT value at 1.5-2.0 times control, 6h after the injection[2].
- Prophylactic LMWH-dalteparin 5000 U SC q 12[4] or q 24h[1,4] or enoxaparin 40 mg SC q 12[4] or q 24h[1] or enoxaparin 40 mg SC q 12h adjusted to maintain anti-Xa levels at 0.12-0.2 unit/mL, 4h after an injection.[2] (At extremes of body weight, dose modification may be required.)
- Intermediate-dose—dalteparin 5000 units SC q 12h or enoxaparin 40 mg SC q 12h[1].
- Adjusted-dose LMWH—weight-adjusted, therapeutic doses of LMWH administered once or twice daily—dalteparin 200 units/kg q 12h or enoxaparin 1 mg/kg q 12h[1]. The anti-Xa level is maintained at 0.6–1 unit/mL, 4–6h after an injection[2].

[a]Suggest LMWH over UFH for all pregnant patients[1].

[b]Postpartum anticoagulation—initial UFH or LMWH until the INR is ≥ 2.0 to overlap with warfarin for 4[1] to 6[1,3,4] weeks with a target INR of 2.0 to 3.0[1]; or prophylactic LMWH for 4 to 6 weeks[1].

[c]Graduated elastic compression stockings both ante- and postpartum[1].

Recommendations from the:

- [1] American College of Chest Physicians (Bates and co-workers, 2008).
- [2] Lockwood (2007).
- [3] American Academy of Pediatrics and American College of Obstetricians and Gynecologists (2007).
- [4] American College of Obstetricians and Gynecologists (2000b).
- [5] American College of Obstetricians and Gynecologists (2005).

number of consensus recommendations for thromboprophylaxis from recognized experts. In some cases, a number of different options are listed, thus illustrating the confusion that currently reigns.

In general, and as shown in Table 47-6, either antepartum surveillance or heparin prophylaxis is recommended for women without a recurrent risk factor, including no known thrombophilia. The study by Tengborn and colleagues (1989) suggested that such prophylaxis is not effective. They reported outcomes in 87 pregnant Swedish women who had prior thromboembolic disease. Despite heparin prophylaxis which was usually 5000 U twice daily, three of 20—15 percent—of women developed antepartum recurrence, compared with eight of 67—12 percent—of women not given heparin. These women were not tested for thrombophilia.

Brill-Edwards and associates (2000) prospectively studied 125 pregnant women with a single previous episode of venous thromboembolism. Antepartum heparin was not given, but anticoagulant therapy was given for 4 to 6 weeks postpartum. A total of six women had a recurrent venous thrombosis—three antepartum and three postpartum. There were no recurrences in the 44 women without a known thrombophilia or whose

prior thrombosis was associated with a temporary risk factor. These findings imply that prophylactic heparin may not be required for these two groups of women. In contrast, women with a prior thrombosis in association with a thrombophilia or in the absence of a temporary risk factor generally should be given both antepartum and postpartum prophylaxis (see Table 47-6).

More recently, De Stefano and co-workers (2006) studied 1104 women who had a first-episode venous thromboembolism before the age of 40 years. After excluding those with antiphospholipid antibodies, 88 women were identified who subsequently had a total of 155 pregnancies and who were not given antithrombotic prophylaxis. There were 19 women—22 percent—who had a subsequent pregnancy- or puerperium-related venous thromboembolism. Of 20 women whose original thrombosis was associated with a transient risk factor—not including pregnancy or oral contraceptive use—there were no recurrences during pregnancy, but two during the puerperium. Like the findings by Brill-Edwards and associates (2000), these data suggest that for women with a prior venous thromboembolism, antithrombotic prophylaxis during pregnancy could be tailored according to the circumstances of the original event. It is emphasized that more data are needed.

TABLE 47-7. Risk Assessment to Determine Thromboprophylaxis Following Uncomplicated Cesarean Delivery

Risk	Intervention
Low	Early ambulation In hospital, consider compression stockings
Medium or high Age older than 35 yrs BMI > 30 Multiparity (? 3) Varicosities Preeclampsia Postpartum hemorrhage Emergency delivery Hysterectomy	Early ambulation In hospital, consider compression or pneumatic stockings *or* In hospital, consider prophylactic LMWH or UFH (see Table 47-6)
Very high Multiple risk factors	Consider stockings as above and prophylactic heparin. For persistent risks, consider prophylactic heparin for 4-6 wks

BMI = body mass index; LMWH = low-molecular-weight heparin; UFH = unfractionated heparin.
From Bates and colleagues (2008), Marik and Plante (2008), and the Royal College of Obstetricians and Gynecologists (2004).

Our practice at Parkland Hospital for many years for women with a history of prior thromboembolism has been to administer subcutaneous unfractionated heparin, 5000 to 7500 units two to three times daily. With this regimen, the recurrence of documented deep-venous thrombosis embolization has been rare. More recently, we have successfully used 40-mg enoxaparin given subcutaneously daily.

Cesarean Delivery and Antepartum Bed Rest

Currently in the United States, use of thromboprophylaxis for women undergoing cesarean delivery or antepartum bed rest is not widely employed. In a survey of 157 members of the Society for Maternal-Fetal Medicine, for example, Casele and Grobman (2007) found that only 8 percent of respondents routinely used thromboprophylaxis—defined as compression boots, stockings, or heparin—for women undergoing cesarean delivery. And only 25 percent routinely used such measures for pregnant women placed on bed rest for more than 72 hours.

The risk for deep-venous thrombosis and especially for fatal thromboembolism is increased manyfold in women following cesarean compared with vaginal delivery. When considering that a third of women giving birth in the United States yearly undergo cesarean delivery, it is easily understandable that pulmonary embolism is a major cause of maternal mortality (see Chap. 1, (p. 5). Because of this, the Royal College of Obstetricans and Gynaecologists (2004) now recommends risk assessment for women undergoing uncomplicated cesarean delivery. The American College of Chest Physicians (Bates and colleagues, 2008) *suggests* risk assessment with thromboprophylaxis—mechanical, pharmacological, or both—for factors such as those shown in Table 47-7. They note this to be Grade 2C level of recommendation because of "low- or very-low quality evidence." According to Clark and associates (2008), some prophylaxis scheme for all women undergoing cesarean delivery in the Hospital Corporation of America system likely would result in a substantively lower maternal mortality rate from pulmonary embolism.

REFERENCES

Agnelli G, Becattini C, Kirschstein T: Thrombolysis vs heparin in the treatment of pulmonary embolism. Arch Intern Med 162: 2537, 2002
Ahearn GS, Hadjiliadis D, Govert JA, et al: Massive pulmonary embolism during pregnancy successfully treated with recombinant tissue plasminogen activator. Arch Intern Med 162:1221, 2002
American Academy of Pediatrics and American College of Obstetricians and Gynecologists: Guidelines for Perinatal Care, 6th ed. 2007
American College of Obstetricians and Gynecologists: Prevention of deep vein thrombosis and pulmonary embolism. Practice Bulletin No. 21, October 2000a
American College of Obstetricians and Gynecologists: Thromboembolism in pregnancy. Practice Bulletin No. 19, August 2000b
American College of Obstetricians and Gynecologists: Safety of Lovenox in pregnancy. Committee Opinion No. 276, October 2002
American College of Obstetricians and Gynecologists: Antiphospholipid syndrome. Practice Bulletin No. 68, November 2005
Anderson DR, Kahn SR, Rodger MA, et al: Computed tomographic pulmonary angiography vs ventilation-perfusion lung scanning in patients with suspected pulmonary embolism: A randomized controlled trial. JAMA 298:2743, 2007
Andres RL, Miles A: Venous thromboembolism and pregnancy. Obstet Gynecol Clin North Am 28:613, 2001
Archer DF, Mammen EF, Grubb GS: The effects of a low-dose monophasic preparation of levonorgestrel and ethinyl estradiol on coagulation and other hemostatic factors. Am J Obstet Gynecol 181:S63, 1999
Bates SM, Ginsberg JS: How we manage venous thromboembolism during pregnancy. Blood 100:3470, 2002
Bates SM, Ginsberg JS: Treatment of deep-vein thrombosis. N Engl J Med 351:268, 2004
Bates SM, Greer IA, Hirsh J, et al: Use of antithrombotic agents during pregnancy: The Seventh ACCP Conference on antithrombotic and thrombolytic therapy. Chest 126:627S, 2004
Birdwell BG, Raskob GE, Whitsett TL, et al: The clinical validity of normal compression ultrasonography in outpatients suspected of having deep venous thrombosis. Ann Intern Med 128:1, 1998
Biron-Andreani C, Schved JF, Daures JP: Factor V Leiden mutation and pregnancy-related venous thromboembolism: What is the exact risk? Results from a meta analysis. Thromb Haemost 96:14, 2006
Blanco-Molina A, Trujillo-Santos J, Criado J, et al: Venous thromboembolism during pregnancy or postpartum: Findings from the RIETE Registry. Thromb Haemost 97:186, 2007
Bloomenthal D, Delisle MF, Tessier F, et al: Obstetric implications of the factor V Leiden mutation: A review. Am J Perinatal 19:37, 2002
Branch DW, Khamashta MA: Antiphospholipid syndrome: Obstetric diagnosis, management, and controversies. Obstet Gynecol 101:1333, 2003
Breddin HK, Hach-Wunderle V, Nakov R, et al: Effects of a low-molecular-weight heparin on thrombus regression and recurrent thromboembolism in patients with DVT. N Engl J Med 344:626, 2001

Bretelle F, Arnoux D, Shojai R, et al: Protein Z in patients with pregnancy complications. Am J Obstet Gynecol 193:1698, 2005

Brill-Edwards P, Ginsberg JS, Gent M, et al: Safety of withholding heparin in pregnant women with a history of venous thromboembolism. N Engl J Med 343:1439, 2000

Brooks C, Rutherford JM, Gould J, et al: Warfarin dosage in postpartum women: A case-control study. Br J Obstet Gynaecol 109:187, 2002

Burneo JG, Elias SB, Barkley GL: Cerebral venous thrombosis due to protein S deficiency in pregnancy. Lancet 359:892, 2002

Casele HL, Grobman WA: Management of thromboprophylaxis during pregnancy among specialists in maternal—fetal medicine. J Reprod Med 52:1085, 2007

Casele HL, Laifer SA, Woelkers DA, et al: Changes in the pharmacokinetics of the low-molecular-weight heparin enoxaparin sodium during pregnancy. Am J Obstet Gynecol 181:1113, 1999

Chan WS, Ray JG, Murray S, et al: Suspected pulmonary embolism in pregnancy. Arch Intern Med 162:1170, 2002

Chapman ML, Martinez-Borges AR, Mertz HL: Lepirudin for treatment of acute thrombosis during pregnancy. Obstet Gynecol 112:432, 2008

Christiansen LR, Collins KA: Pregnancy-associated deaths: A 15-year retrospective study and overall review of maternal pathophysiology. Am J Forensic Med Pathol 27:11, 2006

Chunilal SD, Eikelboom JW, Attia J, et al: Does this patient have pulmonary embolism? JAMA 290:2849, 2003

Chunilal SD, Ginsberg JS: Advances in the diagnosis of venous thromboembolism—A multimodal approach. J Thromb Thrombolysis 12:53, 2001

Clark P, Twaddle S, Walker ID, et al: Cost-effectiveness of screening for the factor V Leiden mutation in pregnant women. Lancet 359:1919, 2002

Clark SL, Belfort MA, Dildy GA, et al: Maternal death in the 21st century: Causes, prevention, and relationship to cesarean delivery. Am J Obstet Gynecol 199(1):36.e1, 2008

Cleary-Goldman J, Bettes B, Robinson JN, et al: Thrombophilia and the obstetric patient. Obstet Gynecol 110:669, 2007

Conard J, Horellou MH, Van Dreden P, et al: Thrombosis and pregnancy in congenital deficiencies in AT III, protein C or protein S: Study of 78 women. Thromb Haemost 63:319, 1990

Copplestone JA, Pavord S, Hunt BJ: Anticoagulation in pregnancy: A survey of current practice [Letter]. Br J Haematol 124:124, 2004

Cunningham FG: Screening for osteoporosis. N Engl J Med 353:1975, 2005

Davis JD: Prevention, diagnosis, and treatment of venous thromboembolic complications of gynecologic surgery. Am J Obstet Gynecol 184:759, 2001

De Carolis S, Ferrazzani S, de Stefano, et al: Inherited thrombophilia: Treatment during pregnancy. Fetal Diagn Therapy 21:281, 2006

Decousus H, Leizorovicz A, Parent F, et al: A clinical trial of vena caval filters in the prevention of pulmonary embolism in patients with proximal deep-vein thrombosis. N Engl J Med 338:409, 1998

De Santis M, Cavaliere AF, Straface G, et al: Inherited and acquired thrombophilia: Pregnancy outcome and treatment. Reprod Toxicol 22:227, 2006

Deruelle P, Coulon C: The use of low-molecular-weight heparins in pregnancy—How safe are they? Curr Opin Obstet Gynecol 19:573, 2007

Deshpande KS, Hatem C, Karwa M, et al: The use of inferior vena cava filter as a treatment modality for massive pulmonary embolism. A case series and review of pathophysiology. Respir Med 96:984, 2002

De Stefano V, Martinelli I, Rossi E, et al: The risk of recurrent venous thromboembolism in pregnancy and puerperium without antithrombotic prophylaxis. Br J Haematol 135:386, 2006

Dizon-Townson D, Miller C, Sibai B, et al: The relationship of the Factor V Leiden mutation and pregnancy outcomes for mother and fetus. Obstet Gynecol 106:517, 2005

Douketis JD, Kearon C, Bates S, et al: Risk of fatal pulmonary embolism in patients with treated venous thromboembolism. JAMA 279:458, 1998

Duhl AJ, Paidas MJ, Ural SH, et al: Antithrombotic therapy and pregnancy: Consensus report and recommendations for prevention and treatment of venous thromboembolism and adverse pregnancy outcomes. Am J Obstet Gynecol 197:457.e1, 2007

Eldor A: Thrombophilia, thrombosis and pregnancy. Thromb Haemost 86:104, 2001

Erdman WA, Jayson HT, Redman HC, et al: Deep venous thrombosis of extremities: Role of MR imaging in the diagnosis. Radiology 174:425, 1990

Facchinetti F, Marozio L, Frusca T, et al: Maternal thrombophilia and the risk of recurrence of preeclampsia. Am J Obstet Gynecol 200:46.e1, 2009

Falcoa S, Bisotto S, Gutkowska J, et al: Hyperhomocysteinemia is not sufficient to cause preeclampsia in an animal model: The importance of folate intake. Am J Obstet Gynecol 200:198.e1, 2009

Fausett MB, Vogtlander M, Lee RM, et al: Heparin-induced thrombocytopenia is rare in pregnancy. Am J Obstet Gynecol 185:148, 2001

Federman DG, Kirsner RS: An update on hypercoagulable disorders. Arch Intern Med 161:1051, 2001

Folkeringa N, Bronwer JL, Korteweg FJ, et al: Reduction of high fetal loss rate by anticoagulant treatment during pregnancy in antithrombin, protein C or protein S deficient women. Br J Haematol 136:656, 2007

Fox NS, Laughon K, Bender SD, et al: Anti-factor Xa plasma levels in pregnant women receiving low molecular weight heparin thromboprophylaxis. Obstet Gynecol 112:884, 2008

Forsnes E, Occhino A, Acosta R: Spontaneous spinal epidural hematoma in pregnancy associated with low molecular weight heparin. Obstet Gynecol 113:532, 2009

Franchini M, Veneri D, Salvagno GL, et al: Inherited thrombophilia. Crit Rev Clin Lab Sci 43:249, 2006

Funakoshi Y, Kato M, Kuratani T, et al: Successful treatment of massive pulmonary embolism in the 38th week of pregnancy. Ann Thorac Surg 77:694, 2004

Garcia DA, Spyropoulos AC: Update in the treatment of venous thromboembolism. Semin Respir Crit Care Med 29:40, 2008

Gatt A, Makris M: Hyperhomocysteinemia and venous thrombosis. Semin Hematol 44:70, 2007

Gerhardt A, Scharf RE, Beckmann MW, et al: Prothrombin and factor V mutations in women with a history of thrombosis during pregnancy and the puerperium. N Engl J Med 342:374, 2000

Ginsberg JS, Brill-Edwards P, Burrows RF, et al: Venous thrombosis during pregnancy: Leg and trimester of presentation. Thromb Haemost 67:519, 1992

Goldhaber SZ: Pulmonary embolism. Lancet 363:1295, 2004

Goldhaber SZ, Tapson VF, DVT FREE Steering Committee: A prospective registry of 5,451 patients with ultrasound-confirmed deep vein thrombosis. Am J Cardiol 93:259, 2004

Goldhaber SZ, Visani L, De Rosa M: Acute pulmonary embolism: Clinical outcomes in the International Cooperative Pulmonary Embolism Registry (ICOPER). Lancet 353:1386, 1999

Greer IA: Prevention and management of venous thromboembolism in pregnancy. Clin Chest Med 24:123, 2003

Greinacher A, Warkentin TE: Recognition, treatment, and prevention of heparin-induced thrombocytopenia: Review and update. Thromb Res 118:165, 2006

Gris J-C, Lissalde-Lavigne G, Quéré I, et al: Monitoring the effects and managing the side effects of anticoagulation during pregnancy. Obstet Gynecol Clin N Am 33:397, 2006

Guyatt GH, Cook DJ, Jaeschke R, et al: Grades of recommendation for antithrombotic agents. Chest 133:1238, 2008

Guyton AC, Lindsey AW, Gilluly JJ: The limits of right ventricular compensation following acute increase in pulmonary circulatory resistance. Circ Res 2:326, 1954

Hague WM: Homocysteine and pregnancy. Best Pract Res Clin Obstet Gynaecol 17:459, 2003

Heijboer H, Buller HR, Lensing AW, et al: A comparison of real-time compression ultrasonography with impedance plethysmography for the diagnosis of deep-vein thrombosis in symptomatic outpatients. N Engl J Med 329:1365, 1993

Hull RD, Raskob GF, Carter CJ: Serial IPG in pregnancy patients with clinically suspected DVT: Clinical validity of negative findings. Ann Intern Med 112:663, 1990

Jacobsen AF, Skjeldstad FE, Sandset PM: Incidence and risk patterns of venous thromboembolism in pregnancy and puerperium—A register-based case-control study. Am J Obstet Gynecol 198:233.e1, 2008

James AH, Jamison MG, Brancazio LR, et al: Venous thromboembolism during pregnancy and the postpartum period: Incidence, risk factors, and mortality. Am J Obstet Gynecol 194:1311, 2006

Jamjute P, Reed N, Hinwood D: Use of inferior vena cava filters in thromboembolic disease during labor: Case report with a literature review. J Mat Fet Neonat Med 19:741, 2006

Kahn SR, Platt R, McNamara H, et al: Inherited thrombophilia and preeclampsia within a multicenter cohort: The Montreal Preeclampsia Study. Am J Obstet Gynecol 200:151.e1, 2009

Kalafatis M, Rand MD, Mann KG: The mechanism of inactivation of human factor V and human factor Va by activated protein C. J Biol Chem 269:31869, 1994

Katz VL: Detecting thrombophilia in OB/GYN patients. Contemp Ob/Gyn October 2002, p 68

Kavanagh EC, O'Hare A, Hargaden G, et al: Risk of pulmonary embolism after negative MDCT pulmonary angiography findings. Am J Roentgenol 182:499, 2004

Kearon C, Gent M, Hirsh J, et al: A comparison of three months of anticoagulation with extended anticoagulation for a first episode of idiopathic venous thromboembolism. N Engl J Med 340:901, 1999

Kelly J, Hunt BJ: Role of D-dimers in diagnosis of venous thromboembolism. Lancet 359:456, 2002

Kenny L, Baker P, Cunningham FG: Platelets, coagulation, and the liver. In Lindheimer MD, Roberts JM, Cunningham FG (eds): Chesley's Hypertensive Disorders in Pregnancy, 3rd Edition, Elsevier, New York, 2009, p. 335

Kinane TB, Grabowski EF, Sharma A, et al: Case 7-2008: A 17-year-old girl with chest pain and hemoptysis. N Engl J Med 358:941, 2008

Kline JA, Williams GW, Hernandez-Nino J: D-Dimer concentrations in normal pregnancy: New diagnostic thresholds are needed. Clin Chem 51:825, 2005

Knight, UKOSS: Antenatal pulmonary embolism: Risk factors, management, and outcomes. BJOG 115(4):453, 2008

Konstantinides S, Geibel A, Heusel G, et al: Heparin plus alteplase compared with heparin alone in patients with submassive pulmonary embolism. N Engl J Med 347:1143, 2002

Krivak TC, Zorn KK: Venous thromboembolism in obstetrics and gynecology. Obstet Gynecol 109:761, 2007

Kuklina EV, Meikle SF, Jamieson DJ, et al: Severe obstetric morbidity in the United States: 1998-2005. Obstet Gynecol 113:293, 2009

Kung HC, Hoyert DL, Xu JQ, et al: Deaths: Final data for 2005. National Vital Statistics Reports; Vol. 56, No. 10. Hyattsville, MD: National Center for Health Statistics, 2008

Kupferminc MJ, Eldor A, Steinman N, et al: Increased frequency of genetic thrombophilia in women with complications of pregnancy. N Engl J Med 340:9, 1999

Kusanovic JP, Espinoza J, Romero R, et al: Plasma protein Z concentrations in pregnant women with idiopathic intrauterine bleeding and in women with spontaneous preterm labor. J Matern Fetal Neonatal Med 20:453, 2007

Leduc L, Dubois E, Takser L, et al: Dalteparin and low-dose aspirin in the prevention of adverse obstetric outcomes in women with inherited thrombophilia. J Obstet Gynaecol Can 29:787, 2007

Lee RH, Goodwin TM: Massive subchorionic hematoma associated with enoxaparin. Obstet Gynecol 108:787, 2006

Leonhardt G, Gaul C, Nietsch HH, et al: Thrombolytic therapy in pregnancy. J Thromb Thrombolysis 21:271, 2006

Lepercq J, Conard J, Borel-Derlon A, et al: Venous thromboembolism during pregnancy: A retrospective study of enoxaparin safety in 624 pregnancies. Br J Obstet Gynaecol 108:1134, 2001

Levine JS, Branch DW, Rauch J: The antiphospholipid syndrome. N Engl J Med 346:752, 2002

Lindhoff-Last E, Kreutzenbeck HJ, Magnani HN: Treatment of 51 pregnancies with danaparoid because of heparin intolerance. Thromb Haemost 93:63, 2005

Lockwood CJ: Inherited thrombophilias in pregnant patients: Detection and treatment paradigm. Obstet Gynecol 99:333, 2002

Lockwood C: Thrombosis, thrombophilia, and thromboembolism: Clinical updates in women's health care. American College of Obstetricians and Gynecologists Vol. VI, No. 4, October 2007

López-Quesada E, Vilaseca MA, Lailla JM: Plasma total homocysteine in uncomplicated pregnancy and in preeclampsia. Eur J Obstet Gynecol Reprod Biol 108:45, 2003

Marik PE, Plante LA: Venous thromboembolic disease and pregnancy. N Engl J Med 359(19):2025, 2008

Martinelli I, De Stefano V, Taioli E, et al: Inherited thrombophilia and first venous thromboembolism during pregnancy and puerperium. Thromb Haemost 87:791, 2002

Mazzolai L, Hohlfeld P, Spertini F, et al: Fondaparinux is a safe alternative in case of heparin intolerance during pregnancy. Blood 108:1569, 2006

McDonald SD, Walker MC: Homocysteine levels in pregnant women who smoke cigarettes. Med Hypotheses 57:792, 2001

Mueller MJ, Lebherz TB: Antepartum thrombophlebitis. Obstet Gynecol 34:867, 1969

Neill AM, Appleton DS, Richards P: Retrievable inferior vena caval filter for thromboembolic disease in pregnancy. Br J Obstet Gynaecol 104:1416, 1997

Nijkeuter M, Ginsberg JS, Huisman MV: Diagnosis of deep vein thrombosis and pulmonary embolism in pregnancy: A systematic review. J Thromb Haemost 4:496, 2006

Oudkerk M, van Beek JR, Wielopolski P, et al: Comparison of contrast-enhanced magnetic resonance angiography and conventional pulmonary angiography for the diagnosis of pulmonary embolism: A prospective study. Lancet 359:1643, 2002

Palareti G, Cosmi B, Legnani C: Diagnosis of deep vein thrombosis. Semin Thromb Hemost 32:659, 2006

PIOPED Investigators: Value of the ventilation/perfusion scan in acute pulmonary embolism: Results of the Prospective Investigation of Pulmonary Embolism Diagnosis (PIOPED). JAMA 263:2753, 1990

Quinlan DJ, McQuillan A, Eikelboom JW: Low-molecular-weight heparin compared with intravenous unfractionated heparin for treatment of pulmonary embolism: A meta-analysis of randomized, controlled trials. Ann Intern Med 140:143, 2004

Raj G: Non-invasive strategies for the diagnosis of pulmonary embolism: Their role and limitations. Internal Medicine Grand Rounds, University of Texas Southwestern Medical Center, Dallas, Texas, June 12, 2003

Ridker PM, Goldhaber SZ, Danielsone E, et al: Long-term, low-intensity warfarin therapy for the prevention of recurrent venous thromboembolism. N Engl J Med 348:1425, 2003

Robertson L, Wu O, Langhorne P, et al: Thrombophilia in pregnancy: A systematic review. Br J Haematol 132:171, 2005

Rodger MA, Avruch LI, Howley HE, et al: Pelvic magnetic resonance venography reveals high rate of pelvic vein thrombosis after cesarean section. Am J Obstet Gynecol 194:436, 2006

Rodger MA, Kahn SR, Cranney A, et al: Long-term dalteparin in pregnancy not associated with a decrease in bone mineral density: Substudy of a randomized controlled trial. J Thromb Haemost 5:1600, 2007

Rodie VA, Thomson AJ, Stewart FM, et al: Low molecular weight heparin for the treatment of venous thromboembolism in pregnancy: A case series. Br J Obstet Gynaecol 109:1020, 2002

Ros SH, Lichtenstein P, Bellocco R, et al: Pulmonary embolism and stroke in relation to pregnancy: How can high-risk women be identified? Am J Obstet Gynecol 186:198, 2002

Salonvaara M, Kuismanen K, Mononen T, et al: Diagnosis and treatment of a newborn with homozygous protein C deficiency. Acta Paediatr 93:137, 2004

Sanson BJ, Lensing AW, Prins MH, et al: Safety of low-molecular-weight heparin in pregnancy: A systematic review. Thromb Haemost 81:668, 1999

Santacroce R, Sarno M, Cappucci F, et al: Low protein Z levels and risk of occurrence of deep vein thrombosis. J Thromb Haemost 4:2417, 2006

Scarsbrook AF, Evans AL, Owen AR, et al: Diagnosis of suspected venous thromboembolic disease in pregnancy. Clin Radiol 61:1, 2006

Scifres CM, Macones GA: The ultility of thrombophilia testing in pregnant women with thrombosis: Fact or fiction? Am J Obstet Gynecol 199:344.e1, 2008

Seguin J, Weatherstone K, Nankervis C: Inherited antithrombin III deficiency in the neonate. Arch Pediatr Adolesc Med 148:389, 1994

Seligsohn U, Lubetsky A: Genetic susceptibility to venous thrombosis. N Engl J Med 344:1222, 2001

Sephton V, Farquharson RG, Topping J, et al: A longitudinal study of maternal dose response to low molecular weight heparin in pregnancy. Obstet Gynecol 101:1307, 2003

Singhal S, Henderson R, Horsfield K, et al: Morphometry of the human pulmonary arterial tree. Cir Res 33:190, 1973

Smith MP, Norris LA, Steer PJ, et al: Tinzaparin sodium for thrombosis treatment and prevention during pregnancy. Am J Obstet Gynecol 190:495, 2004

Srivastava SD, Eagleton MJ, Greenfield LJ: Diagnosis of pulmonary embolism with various imaging modalities. Semin Vasc Surg 17:173, 2004

Stefano VD, Martinelli I, Mannucci PM, et al: The risk of recurrent deep venous thrombosis among heterozygous carriers of both factor V Leiden and the G20210A prothrombin mutation. N Engl J Med 341:801, 1999

Stein PD, Athanasoulis C, Alavi A, et al: Complications and validity of pulmonary angiography in acute pulmonary embolism. Circulation 85:462, 1992

Stein PD, Fowler SE, Goodman LR, et al: Multidetector computed tomography for acute pulmonary embolism. N Engl J Med 354:2317, 2006

Taniguchi S, Fukuda I, Minakawa M, et al: Emergency pulmonary embolectomy during the second trimester of pregnancy: Report of a case. Surg Today 38:59, 2008

Tapson VF: Acute pulmonary embolism. N Engl J Med 358:1037, 2008

Tengborn L, Bergqvist D, Matzsch T, et al: Recurrent thromboembolism in pregnancy and puerperium: Is there a need for thromboprophylaxis? Am J Obstet Gynecol 160:90, 1989

van Wijk FH, Wolf H, Piek JM, et al: Administration of low molecular weight heparin within two hours before caesarean section increases the risk of wound haematoma. Br J Obstet Gynaecol 109:955, 2002

Vasse M: Protein Z, a protein seeking a pathology. Thromb Haemost 100(4):548, 2008

Virchow R: Gesammelte Abhandlungen zur wissenschaftlichen Medizin. Frankfurt: Medinger Sohn & Co., 1856, p 219

Walker MC, Garner PR, Keely EJ, et al: Changes in activated protein C resistance during normal pregnancy. Am J Obstet Gynecol 177:162, 1997

Warkentin TE, Kelton JG: Temporal aspects of heparin-induced thrombocytopenia. N Engl J Med 344:1286, 2001

Warkentin TE, Maurer BT, Aster RH: Heparin-induced thrombocytopenia associated with fondaparinux, N Engl J Med 356:2653, 2007

Warren JE, Simonsen SE, Branch W, et al: Thromboprophylaxis and pregnancy outcomes in asymptomatic women with inherited thrombophilias. Am J Obstet Gynecol 200:281.e1, 2009

Weiss N, Bernstein PS: Risk factor scoring for predicting venous thromboembolism in obstetric patients. Am J Obstet Gynecol 182:1073, 2000

Wells PS, Anderson DR, Rodger M, et al: Evaluation of D-dimer in the diagnosis of suspected deep-vein thrombosis. N Engl J Med 349:1227, 2003

CHAPTER 48

Renal and Urinary Tract Disorders

Renal and urinary tract disorders are commonly encountered in pregnancy. Some precede pregnancy—one example being nephrolithiasis. In some women, pregnancy-induced changes may predispose to development or worsening of urinary tract disorders—an example is the markedly increased risk of pyelonephritis. Finally, there may be complications unique to pregnancy such as preeclampsia. With good prenatal care, most women with these disorders will likely develop no long-term serious consequences.

PREGNANCY-INDUCED URINARY TRACT CHANGES

Significant changes in both structure and function that take place in the urinary tract during normal pregnancy are discussed in Chapter 5 (p. 123). The kidneys become larger, and as shown in Figure 48-1, dilatation of the renal calyces and ureters can be striking. Some dilatation develops before 14 weeks and likely is due to progesterone-induced relaxation of the muscular

layers. More marked dilatation is apparent beginning in mid-pregnancy because of ureteral compression, especially on the right side (Faúndes and associates, 1998). There is also some *vesicoureteral reflux* during pregnancy. An important consequence of these physiological changes is an increased risk of upper urinary infection, and occasionally erroneous interpretation of studies done to evaluate obstruction.

Evidence of functional hypertrophy becomes apparent very soon after conception. Glomeruli are larger, although cell numbers do not increase (Strevens and colleagues, 2003). Pregnancy-induced intrarenal vasodilatation increases effective renal plasma flow and glomerular filtration. By 12 weeks' gestation, the glomerular filtration rate is already increased 20 percent above nonpregnant values (Hladunewich and colleagues, 2004). Ultimately, plasma flow and glomerular filtration increase by 40 and 65 percent, respectively. Consequently, serum concentrations of creatinine and urea decrease substantively across pregnancy, and values within a nonpregnant normal range may be abnormal in pregnancy (see Appendix). Other alterations include those related to maintaining normal acid-base homeostasis, osmoregulation, and fluid and electrolyte retention.

Assessment of Renal Function During Pregnancy

The *urinalysis* is essentially unchanged during pregnancy, except for occasional glucosuria. Although *protein excretion* normally is increased, it seldom reaches levels that are detected by usual screening methods. Higby and colleagues (1994) reported 24-hour protein excretion to be 115 mg with a 95-percent confidence level at 260 mg/day (see Appendix). There were no significant differences by trimester. Albumin constitutes only a small part of total protein excretion and ranges from 5 to 30 mg/day. From their review, Airoldi and Weinstein (2007) concluded that proteinuria must exceed 300 mg/day to be considered abnormal. Most consider 500 mg/day to be important with gestational hypertension.

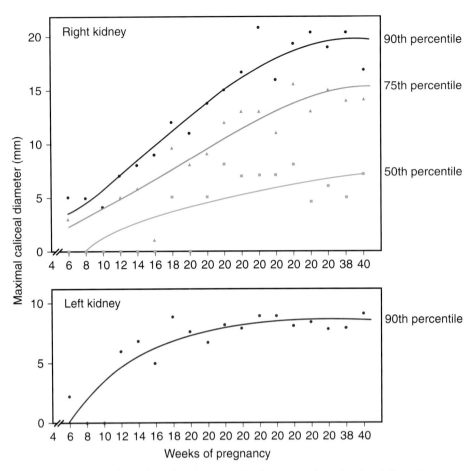

FIGURE 48-1 The 50th, 75th, and 90th percentiles for maternal renal caliceal diameters measured using sonography in 1395 pregnant women from 4 to 42 weeks. (Reprinted from *American Journal of Obstetrics & Gynecology*, Vol. 178, No. 5, A Faúndes, M Bricola-Filho, JC Pinto e Silva, Dilatation of the urinary tract during pregnancy: Proposal of a curve of maximal caliceal diameter by gestational age, pp. 1082–1086, Copyright 1998, with permission from Elsevier.)

sideration for rapid deterioration of renal function with no obvious cause or for symptomatic nephrotic syndrome. We have found biopsy helpful in a few cases, and Chen and co-workers (2001) described 15 women in whom biopsy helped to direct management. Strevens and associates (2003) performed renal biopsy in 12 *normal* pregnant volunteers and reported that five had slight to moderate glomerular endotheliosis. In contrast, all 27 women with proteinuric hypertension had endotheliosis, and in all but one, it was moderate to severe.

Pregnancy after Unilateral Nephrectomy

In general, the excretory capacity of two kidneys exceeds ordinary needs. In addition, after nephrectomy, the surviving kidney undergoes pregnancy-induced hypertrophy of function (Fig. 48-2). Therefore, women with one normal kidney most often have no difficulty in pregnancy (Baylis and Davison, 1991). Thorough functional evaluation of the remaining kidney is essential. There are no long-term adverse consequences of kidney donation (Ibrahim and associates, 2009).

Stehman-Breen and associates (2002) found that 3 percent of 4589 nulliparas had *idiopathic hematuria* defined as 1+ or greater blood on urine dipstick when screened before 20 weeks. They also reported that these women had a twofold risk of preeclampsia. In another study of 1000 women screened during pregnancy, Brown and colleagues (2005) reported a 15-percent incidence of dipstick hematuria. Most women had trace levels of hematuria, and the false-positive rate was 40 percent.

If the serum creatinine persistently exceeds 0.9 mg/dL (75 μmol/L), then intrinsic renal disease should be suspected. In these cases, some determine the creatinine clearance as an estimate of the glomerular filtration rate. *Sonography* provides imaging of renal size and relative consistency, as well as elements of obstruction (see Fig. 48-1). Full-sequence *intravenous pyelography* is not done routinely, but injection of contrast media with one or two abdominal radiographs may be indicated by the clinical situation (see Chap. 41, p. 918). The usual clinical indications for *cystoscopy* are followed. Semins and associates (2009) described an 8-percent complication rate in their review of 14 reports of *ureteroscopy* done for stone removal in 108 pregnancies.

Although *renal biopsy* is relatively safely performed during pregnancy, biopsy usually is postponed unless it would change therapy. Lindheimer and colleagues (2008) recommend its con-

Orthostatic Proteinuria

Orthostatic or *postural proteinuria* has been observed in up to 5 percent of normal young adults. Without other evidence of renal disease, the pregnant woman with orthostatic proteinuria should be evaluated for bacteriuria, abnormal urinary sediment, reduced glomerular filtration, and hypertension. In the absence of these, orthostatic proteinuria is probably inconsequential.

URINARY TRACT INFECTIONS

These are the most common bacterial infections during pregnancy. Although *asymptomatic bacteriuria* is the most common, symptomatic infection includes *cystitis*, or it may involve the renal calyces, pelvis, and parenchyma—*pyelonephritis*.

Organisms that cause urinary infections are those from the normal perineal flora. Approximately 90 percent of *Escherichia coli* strains that cause nonobstructive pyelonephritis have *adhesins* such as *P-* and *S-fimbriae* that enhance their virulence (Dodson and co-workers, 2001; Lügering and associates, 2003). These adhesins promote binding to vaginal and uroepithelial cells through expression of the *PapG gene* that encodes the P-fimbriae tip, as well as by production of hemolysin (Hooton and

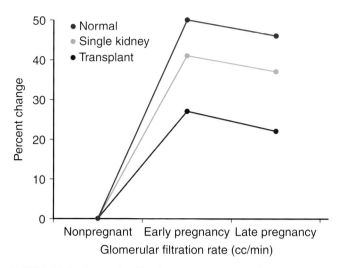

FIGURE 48-2 Glomerular filtration rate changes with pregnancy in normal women, those stable after unilateral nephrectomy, and those with a successful renal transplant. (Data from Newcastle-upon-Tyne, 1974–2006, courtesy of Dr. John Davison.)

co-workers, 2000). The expression of the *dra gene cluster* has been associated with ampicillin-resistant *E. coli* (Hart and colleagues, 2001). Although pregnancy itself does not enhance these virulence factors, urinary stasis and vesicoureteral reflux predispose to symptomatic upper urinary infections (Twickler and associates, 1994). Diabetics are especially susceptible to developing pyelonephritis (Czaja and colleagues, 2009).

In the puerperium, several risk factors exist that predispose a woman to urinary infections. Bladder sensitivity to intravesical fluid tension is often decreased as a consequence of the trauma of labor as well as conduction analgesia (see Chap. 30, p. 655). Sensation of bladder distension can also be diminished by discomfort caused by an episiotomy, periurethral lacerations, or vaginal wall hematomas. Normal postpartum diuresis may worsen bladder overdistension. Catheterization to relieve retention and distension commonly leads to urinary infection, however, there appear to be no long-term sequelae (Yip and colleagues, 2002).

Asymptomatic Bacteriuria

This refers to persistent, actively multiplying bacteria within the urinary tract in asymptomatic women. Its prevalence in nonpregnant women is 5 to 6 percent and depends on parity, race, and socioeconomic status (Hooton and colleagues, 2000). The highest incidence is in African-American multiparas with sickle-cell trait, and the lowest incidence is in affluent white women of low parity. Because most women have recurrent or persistent bacteriuria, it frequently is discovered during prenatal care. The incidence during pregnancy is similar to that in nonpregnant women and varies from 2 to 7 percent.

Bacteriuria is typically present at the time of the first prenatal visit, and if an initial positive urine culture is treated, fewer than 1 percent of women develop urinary infection (Whalley, 1967). A clean-voided specimen containing more than 100,000 organisms per milliliter is diagnostic. It may be prudent to treat when lower concentrations are identified, because pyelonephritis develops in some women with colony counts of 20,000 to 50,000 organisms/mL (Lucas and Cunningham, 1993).

Significance

If asymptomatic bacteriuria is not treated, approximately 25 percent of infected women will develop symptomatic infection during pregnancy. Eradication of bacteriuria with antimicrobial agents prevents most of these. The American Academy of Pediatrics and the American College of Obstetricians and Gynecologists (2007), as well as a U.S. Preventative Task Force (2006), recommend screening for bacteriuria at the first prenatal visit (see Chap. 8, p. 194). The dipstick culture technique has excellent positive- and negative-predictive values (Mignini and co-workers, 2009). Standard urine cultures may not be cost-effective when the prevalence is low, but less expensive screening tests such as the leukocyte esterase-nitrite dipstick are when the prevalence is 2 percent or less (Rouse and colleagues, 1995). Because of a high prevalence—5 to 8 percent—at Parkland and the University of Alabama at Birmingham Hospitals, culture screening is done in most women. Susceptibility determination is not necessary because initial treatment is empirical, and these tests have variable sensitivity (Bachman and co-workers, 1993).

In some, but not all studies, covert bacteriuria has been associated with preterm or low-birthweight infants (Kass, 1962). It is even more controversial whether eradication of bacteriuria decreases these complications. Using multivariate analysis for a perinatal registry cohort of 25,746 mother-infant pairs, Schieve and colleagues (1994) reported increased risks for low-birthweight infants, preterm delivery, pregnancy-associated hypertension, and anemia. These findings are at variance with those of Gilstrap and colleagues (1981b) and Whalley (1967). In most studies, asymptomatic infection is not evaluated separately from acute renal infection (Banhidy and associates, 2007). Cochrane reviews by Vasquez and Villar (2006) found that benefits of treatment for asymptomatic bacteria are limited to the reduction of the incidence of pyelonephritis. In our opinion, it seems unlikely that asymptomatic bacteriuria has any significant impact on pregnancy outcome except for potentially serious urinary infections.

Bacteriuria that persists or recurs after delivery has been associated with pyelographic evidence of chronic infection, obstructive lesions, and congenital abnormalities (Kincaid-Smith and Bullen, 1965; Whalley and associates, 1965).

Treatment

Bacteriuria responds to empirical treatment with any of several antimicrobial regimens listed in Table 48-1. Although selection can be based on in vitro susceptibilities, in our extensive experience, empirical oral treatment for 10 days with nitrofurantoin macrocrystals, 100 mg at bedtime, is usually effective. Lumbiganon and colleagues (2009) reported satisfactory results with a 7-day course of nitrofurantoin, 100 mg given twice daily. Single-dose antimicrobial therapy has also been used with success for bacteriuria. The important caveat is that, regardless of regimen given, the recurrence rate is approximately 30 percent. This may indicate covert upper tract infection and the need for longer therapy. For recurrences, we have had success with nitrofurantoin, 100 mg orally at bedtime for 21 days (Lucas and Cunningham, 1994). For women with persistent or frequent bacteriuria recurrences, suppressive therapy for the

TABLE 48-1. Oral Antimicrobial Agents Used for Treatment of Pregnant Women with Asymptomatic Bacteriuria

Single-dose treatment
  Amoxicillin 3 g
  Ampicillin 2 g
  Cephalosporin 2 g
  Nitrofurantoin 200 mg
  Trimethoprim-sulfamethoxazole 320/1600 mg

3-day course
  Amoxicillin 500 mg three times daily
  Ampicillin 250 mg four times daily
  Cephalosporin 250 mg four times daily
  Ciprofloxacin 250 mg twice daily
  Levofloxacin 250 mg daily
  Nitrofurantoin 50 to 100 mg four times daily; 100 mg twice daily
  Trimethoprim-sulfamethoxazole 160/800 mg two times daily

Other
  Nitrofurantoin 100 mg four times daily for 10 days
  Nirofurantoin 100 mg twice daily fo 7 days
  Nitrofurantoin 100 mg at bedtime for 10 days

Treatment failures
  Nitrofurantoin 100 mg four times daily for 21 days

Suppression for bacterial persistence or recurrence
  Nitrofurantoin 100 mg at bedtime for remainder of pregnancy

remainder of pregnancy can be given. We routinely use nitrofurantoin, 100 mg orally at bedtime. This drug may rarely cause an acute pulmonary reaction that dissipates on its withdrawal (Boggess and colleagues, 1996).

Cystitis and Urethritis

Lower urinary infection during pregnancy may develop without antecedent covert bacteriuria (Harris and Gilstrap, 1981). Cystitis is characterized by dysuria, urgency, and frequency, but with few associated systemic findings. Pyuria and bacteriuria are usually found. Microscopic hematuria is common, and occasionally there is gross hematuria from hemorrhagic cystitis (Fakhoury and co-workers, 1994). Although cystitis is usually uncomplicated, the upper urinary tract may become involved by ascending infection. Almost 40 percent of pregnant women with acute pyelonephritis have preceding symptoms of lower tract infection (Gilstrap and associates, 1981a).

Treatment

Women with cystitis respond readily to any of several regimens. Most of the three-day regimens listed in Table 48-1 are usually 90-percent effective (Fihn, 2003). Single-dose therapy is less effective, and if it is used, concomitant pyelonephritis must be confidently excluded.

Lower urinary tract symptoms with pyuria accompanied by a sterile urine culture may be from urethritis caused by *Chlamydia trachomatis*. Mucopurulent cervicitis usually coexists, and erythromycin therapy is effective.

Acute Pyelonephritis

Renal infection is the most common serious medical complication of pregnancy. In a study of the California Pregnancy Complication Surveillance System by Scott and associates (1997), genitourinary infection was the second most common reason for a nondelivery admission. The rate was 4 per 100 for nearly 150,000 pregnancies. In a study of more than 70,000 pregnancies in a managed care organization, Gazmararian and colleagues (2002) reported that 3.5 percent of antepartum admissions were for urinary infections. The potential seriousness is underscored by the observations of Mabie and associates (1997) that pyelonephritis was the leading cause of septic shock during pregnancy. And in a 2 year audit of admissions to the Parkland Hospital Obstetrical Intensive Care Unit, 12 percent of antepartum admissions were for sepsis syndrome caused by pyelonephritis (Zeeman and co-workers, 2003). There is also concern that urosepsis may be related to an increased incidence of cerebral palsy in preterm infants (Jacobsson and colleagues, 2002). Fortunately, there appear to be no serious long-term maternal sequelae (Raz and co-workers, 2003).

Clinical Findings

Renal infection develops more frequently in the second trimester, and nulliparity and young age are associated risk factors (Hill and associates, 2005). It is unilateral and right-sided in more than half of cases, and it is bilateral in a fourth. There is usually a rather abrupt onset with fever, shaking chills, and aching pain in one or both lumbar regions. Anorexia, nausea, and vomiting may worsen dehydration. Tenderness usually can be elicited by percussion in one or both costovertebral angles. The urinary sediment contains many leukocytes, frequently in clumps, and numerous bacteria. Bacteremia is demonstrated in 15 to 20 percent of these women. *E. coli* is isolated from urine or blood in 70 to 80 percent of infections, *Klebsiella pneumoniae* in 3 to 5 percent, *Enterobacter* or *Proteus* in 3 to 5 percent, and gram-positive organisms including group B *Streptococcus* in up to 10 percent of cases (Hill and co-workers, 2005; Wing and colleagues, 2000). The differential diagnosis includes, among others, labor, chorioamnionitis, appendicitis, placental abruption, or infarcted leiomyoma. Evidence of the *sepsis syndrome* is common, and this is discussed in detail in Chapter 42 (p. 932).

Plasma creatinine is monitored because early studies reported that 20 percent of pregnant women developed renal dysfunction. More recent findings, however, show this to be only 5 percent with aggressive fluid resuscitation (Hill and colleagues, 2005). Follow-up studies have demonstrated that this endotoxin-induced damage is reversible in the long term. Varying degrees of respiratory insufficiency from endotoxin-induced alveolar injury are manifest in up to 10 percent of women and may result in frank pulmonary edema (Hill and colleagues, 2005; Sheffield and Cunningham, 2005). In some cases, pulmonary injury may be so severe that it causes *acute respiratory distress syndrome* (*ARDS*) as shown in **Figure 48-3.**

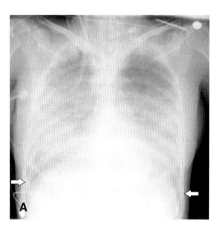 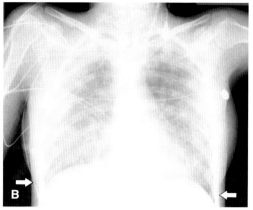 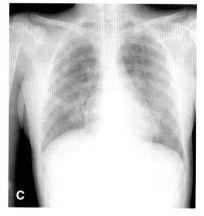

FIGURE 48-3 A series of anterior-posterior projection chest radiographs of improving acute respiratory distress syndrome (ARDS) in a second-trimester pregnant woman with severe pyelonephritis. **A.** An extensive infiltrative process and complete obliteration of the diaphragm (*white arrows*) is seen. **B.** Improved aeration of lung fields bilaterally is noted as pleural disease resolves (*arrows*). **C.** Markedly improved visualization of the lungs fields with residual platelike atelectasis and normal appearance of the diaphragm.

Uterine activity from endotoxin is common and is related to the severity of fever (Graham and associates, 1993). In the study by Millar and colleagues (2003), women with pyelonephritis averaged 5 contractions per hour at admission, and this decreased to 2 per hour within 6 hours of intravenous fluid and antimicrobial administration. As discussed in Chapter 42 (p. 929), β-agonist therapy for tocolysis increases the likelihood of respiratory insufficiency from permeability edema because of the sodium- and fluid-retaining properties of those agents (Lamont, 2000). The incidence of pulmonary edema in women with pyelonephritis who were given β-agonists was reported to be 8 percent—a fourfold increase over that expected (Towers and co-workers, 1991).

Endotoxin-induced *hemolysis* is common, and approximately a third of patients with pyelonephritis develop anemia (Cox and colleagues, 1991). With recovery, hemoglobin regeneration is normal because acute infection does not affect erythropoietin production (Cavenee and colleagues, 1994).

Management

One scheme for management of acute pyelonephritis is shown in Table 48-2. Although we routinely obtain urine and blood cultures, prospective trials show them to be of limited clinical utility (Wing and co-workers, 2000). **Intravenous hydration to ensure adequate urinary output is the cornerstone of treatment.** Antimicrobials are also begun promptly, however, their administration may initially worsen endotoxemia from bacterial lysis. Ongoing surveillance for worsening of sepsis syndrome is monitored by serial determinations of urinary output, blood pressure, pulse, and temperature. High fever should be lowered with a cooling blanket or acetaminophen. This is especially important in early pregnancy because of possible teratogenic effects of hyperthermia (see Chap. 12, p. 281).

Antimicrobial therapy usually is empirical, and ampicillin plus gentamicin; cefazolin or ceftriaxone; or an extended-spectrum antibiotic was 95-percent effective in randomized trials (Sanchez-Ramos and associates, 1995; Wing and colleagues, 1998, 2000). Fewer than half of *E. coli* strains are sensitive to ampicillin in vitro, but cephalosporins and gentamicin gener-

ally have excellent activity. Serum creatinine is monitored if nephrotoxic drugs are given. Initial treatment at Parkland Hospital is ampicillin plus gentamicin, and at the University of Alabama at Birmingham Hospital, cefotetan is given. Some recommend suitable substitutes if bacterial studies show in vitro resistance. With any of the regimens discussed, response is relatively prompt in most cases, and 95 percent of women are afebrile by 72 hours (Hill and associates, 2005; Sheffield and Cunningham, 2005; Wing and colleagues, 2000). After discharge, most recommend oral therapy for a total of 7 to 10 days.

Outpatient Management of Pyelonephritis. Wing and associates (1999) have described outpatient management in 92 women who were first given in-hospital intramuscular ceftriaxone, two 1-g doses 24 hours apart. At this point, a third were

---

TABLE 48-2. Management of the Pregnant Woman with Acute Pyelonephritis

1. Hospitalize patient
2. Obtain urine and blood cultures
3. Evaluate hemogram, serum creatinine, and electrolytes
4. Monitor vital signs frequently, including urinary output—consider indwelling catheter
5. Establish urinary output to ≥ 50 mL/hr with intravenous crystalloid
6. Administer intravenous antimicrobial therapy (see text)
7. Obtain chest radiograph if there is dyspnea or tachypnea
8. Repeat hematology and chemistry studies in 48 hours
9. Change to oral antimicrobials when afebrile
10. Discharge when afebrile 24 hours, consider antimicrobial therapy for 7 to 10 days
11. Repeat urine culture 1 to 2 weeks after antimicrobial therapy completed

Modified from Lucas and Cunningham (1994) and Sheffield and Cunningham (2005).

considered candidates for outpatient therapy and were randomized either to discharge and oral antimicrobials or to continued hospitalization with intravenous therapy. A third of the outpatient management group were unable to adhere to their treatment regimen and were admitted. These findings suggest that outpatient management is applicable to very few women.

Management of Nonresponders. If there is no clinical improvement by 48 to 72 hours, then sonography is recommended to look for urinary tract obstruction manifest by abnormal ureteral or pyelocaliceal dilatation (Seidman and co-workers, 1998). Although most women with continuing infection have no evidence of obstruction, some are found to have calculi. Even though renal sonography will detect hydronephrosis, stones are not always visualized in pregnancy (Butler and associates, 2000; Maikranz and colleagues, 1987). If stones are strongly suspected despite a nondiagnostic sonographic examination, a plain abdominal radiograph will identify nearly 90 percent. Intravenous pyelography is another option. The modified *one-shot pyelogram*—a single radiograph obtained 30 minutes after contrast injection—almost always provides adequate imaging (Butler and colleagues, 2000). Finally, magnetic resonance urography may be used (Spencer and associates, 2004). Other causes of persistent infection are an intrarenal or perinephric abscess or phlegmon (Cox and Cunningham, 1988).

Obstruction can be relieved by cystoscopic placement of a double-J ureteral stent (Rodriguez and Klein, 1988). Because these stents tend to become encrusted, we have found percutaneous nephrostomy to be a better option as the stents are easier to replace. Surgical removal of stones may be required in some cases.

Follow-Up

Recurrent infection—either covert or symptomatic—is common and develops in 30 to 40 percent of women following completion of treatment for pyelonephritis (Cunningham and associates, 1973). Unless other measures are taken to ensure urine sterility, nitrofurantoin, 100 mg orally at bedtime, is given for the remainder of the pregnancy. Van Dorsten and co-workers (1987) reported that this regimen reduces recurrence of bacteriuria.

Reflux Nephropathy

This is chronic interstitial nephritis that classically was thought to be due to infection, that is, *chronic pyelonephritis*. Because radiologically identified scarring is frequently accompanied by ureteral reflux with voiding, it is termed *reflux nephropathy*. Long-term complications include hypertension, which may be quite severe if there is demonstrable renal damage (Köhler and associates, 2003). In most cases, childhood renal infections are documented to precede these lesions. After surgical correction, half of these women have bacteriuria when pregnant (Mor and colleagues, 2003). That said, fewer than half of women have a clear history of preceding cystitis, acute pyelonephritis, or obstructive disease. Certainly, only a very few individuals with recurrent urinary infections develop progressive renal involvement.

Maternal and fetal prognosis depends on the extent of renal destruction. El-Khatib (1994), Jungers (1996), Köhler (2003), and their associates reported outcomes of 939 pregnancies in 379 women with reflux nephropathy. Impaired renal function

and bilateral renal scarring were associated with increased maternal complications.

NEPHROLITHIASIS

Kidney stones develop in 7 percent of women during their lifetime with an average age of onset in the third decade (Asplin and colleagues, 2008). Calcium salts comprise approximately 80 percent of stones, and up to a half of affected women have polygenic *familial idiopathic hypercalciuria*. Hyperparathyroidism should be excluded. Although calcium oxalate stones in young nonpregnant women are most common, Ross and co-workers (2008) found that 75 percent of stones in pregnancy were calcium phosphate (hydroxyapatite). Patients who have a stone typically form another stone every 2 to 3 years.

Contrary to past teachings, a low-calcium diet *promotes* stone formation. Prevention of recurrences with hydration and a diet low in sodium and protein is currently recommended (Asplin and co-workers, 2008). Thiazide diuretics also diminish stone formation. In general, obstruction, infection, intractable pain, and heavy bleeding are indications for stone removal. Removal by a flexible basket via cystoscopy, although used less often than in the past, is still a reasonable consideration for pregnant women. In nonpregnant patients, stone destruction by *lithotripsy* is preferred to surgical therapy in most cases. There is limited information on the use of these procedures during pregnancy, and they are not recommended.

Stone Disease During Pregnancy

In a population-based study from Washington state, Swartz and colleagues (2007) reported that admissions for nephrolithiasis were 1.7 per 1000 pregnancies. Butler and colleagues (2000) found a 1 per 3300 incidence in more than 186,000 deliveries at Parkland Hospital. Lewis and associates (2003) reported an unprecedented incidence of 4 per 1000 deliveries that they attributed to their geographic location and predominantly Caucasian population.

Although it is generally accepted that stone disease does not have any adverse effects on pregnancy outcome—except for infection—Swartz and colleagues (2007) also reported an association with preterm delivery. In their case-control study of 2239 pregnant women with stone disease, the incidence of preterm delivery was 10.6 percent compared with 6.4 percent for matched controls. In the case-control Hungarian study, Banhidy and associates (2007) found similar outcomes in women with stones and normal controls. Pregnant women may have fewer symptoms with stone passage because of urinary tract dilatation (Hendricks and colleagues, 1991).

Diagnosis

More than 90 percent of pregnant women with nephrolithiasis present with pain. Gross hematuria was a presenting symptom in 23 percent of women described by Butler and associates (2000). In the report by Lewis and co-workers (2003), however, only 2 percent had hematuria. As discussed, sonography may confirm a suspected stone, but pregnancy hydronephrosis may obscure these findings (McAleer and Loughlin, 2004). If there is abnormal dilatation without stone visualization, then the one-shot pyelogram may be useful. Transabdominal color Doppler sonography to detect *absence* of ureteral "jets" of urine into the bladder has been used to exclude obstruction (Asrat and colleagues, 1998).

In nonpregnant patients, helical computed tomographic (CT) scanning is the initial imaging method of choice (Asplin and associates, 2008). White and colleagues (2006) recommend unenhanced helical-CT in pregnancy, citing an average fetal dose to be 700 mrad (see Chap. 42, p. 918).

Management

Treatment depends on symptoms and gestational age. Intravenous hydration and analgesics are always given. Half of pregnant women with symptomatic stones have associated infection, which is treated vigorously. **Although calculi infrequently cause symptomatic obstruction during pregnancy, persistent pyelonephritis should prompt a search for obstruction due to nephrolithiasis.**

In approximately two thirds of women with symptoms, there is improvement with conservative therapy, and the stone usually passes spontaneously. The other third require an invasive procedure such as ureteral stenting, ureteroscopy, percutaneous nephrostomy, transurethral laser lithotripsy, or basket extraction (Butler, 2000; Carlan, 1995; Lewis, 2003, and all their co-workers). Of 623 procedures in the 2239 women with stones described by Swartz and associates (2007), only 1 to 2 percent underwent surgical exploration. In the report by Watterson and colleagues (2002), holmium:YAG laser lithotripsy was successful in nine of 10 women. The need for fluoroscopy limits the utility of percutaneous nephrolithotomy (Toth and colleagues, 2005).

CHRONIC RENAL DISEASE

Chronic renal disease is a pathophysiological process that ultimately results in end-stage renal disease (ESRD) through a progressive loss of nephron number and function. It can be caused by multiple etiologies and must be present for at least 3 months to be considered chronic. According to Skorecki and colleagues (2005), the most common causes of ESRD are diabetes—33 percent, hypertension—24 percent, glomerulonephritis—17 percent, and polycystic kidney disease—15 percent.

In most young women with these diseases, there is usually some renal insufficiency, proteinuria, or both. For counseling regarding fertility and pregnancy outcome, it is important to determine the degree of renal functional impairment and associated hypertension. Successful pregnancy outcome in general may be more related to these two factors than to the specific underlying disorder. A general prognosis can be estimated by considering women in arbitrary categories of renal function (Lindheimer and associates, 2008). These include normal or *mild impairment,* defined as a serum creatinine of less than 1.5 mg/dL; *moderate impairment,* defined as a serum creatinine of 1.5 to 3.0 mg/dL; and *severe renal insufficiency,* defined as a serum creatinine greater than 3.0 mg/dL.

Pregnancy and Chronic Renal Disease

Most women with chronic renal disease have relatively mild insufficiency, and the degrees of hypertension and renal insufficiency are prognostic of pregnancy outcome. Renal disease as

part of a systemic disorder—diabetes and connective-tissue disorders—as well as other co-morbidities portend a worse prognosis (Fischer and colleagues, 2004; Lindheimer and Davison, 2007). For all women with chronic renal disease, despite the high incidence of hypertension and preeclampsia, preterm and growth-restricted infants, and other problems, the National High Blood Pressure Education Working Group (2000) has concluded that the prognosis has substantively improved over the past decades. This was verified in recent reviews by Hou (2007) and Ramin and colleagues (2006).

Physiological Changes

Loss of renal tissue is associated with compensatory intrarenal vasodilation and hypertrophy of the surviving nephrons. Eventually this compensation fails and the surviving nephrons sclerose, resulting in worsening renal function. With mild renal insufficiency, pregnancy causes greater augmentation of renal plasma flow and glomerular filtration (Baylis, 2003). With progressively worse degrees of renal function, augmented renal plasma flow becomes diminished to absent. For example, only half of pregnant women with moderate renal insufficiency demonstrate augmented glomerular filtration, and there is no increase in those with severe disease (Cunningham and colleagues, 1990).

Nonpregnant women with chronic renal insufficiency have blood volumes similar to those of healthy women. Blood volume expansion during pregnancy, however, is dependent on disease severity and correlates inversely with serum creatinine concentration. As shown in Figure 48-4, women with mild to moderate dysfunction have normal pregnancy-induced hypervolemia that averages 55 percent. In women with severe renal insufficiency, however, volume expansion averages only 25 percent—a degree of volume attenuation similar to women with eclampsia. Finally, because there is only minimal pregnancy-induced erythropoiesis in these women, preexisting anemia is intensified.

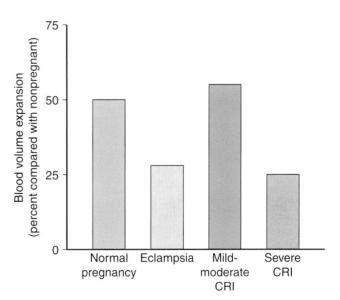

FIGURE 48-4 Comparison of blood volume expansion in 44 normally pregnant women at term with 29 who had eclampsia; 10 with moderate chronic renal insufficiency (CRI)—serum creatinine 1.5 to 2.9 mg/dL; and 4 with severe CRI—serum creatinine ≥3.0 mg/dL. (Data from Zeeman and colleagues, 2009, and Cunningham and associates, 1990.)

TABLE 48-3. Complications Associated with Chronic Renal Disease During Pregnancy

	Incidence in Percent		
	Preserved Renal Function	**Renal Insufficiency**	
Complication		**Moderate and Severe**	**Severe**
Chronic hypertension	25	30–70	50
Gestational hypertension	20–50	30–50	75
Worsening renal function	8–15	20–43	35
Permanent dysfunction	4–5	10–20	35
Preterm delivery	7	35–60	73
Fetal-growth restriction	8–14	30–37	57
Perinatal mortality	5–14	4–7	0

Data from Cunningham (1990), Hou (1985), Imbasciati (2007), Jones and Hayslett (1996), Packham (1989), Stettler and Cunningham (1992), Surian (1984), Trevisan (2004), and all their colleagues.

Chronic Renal Disease with Preserved Function

As emphasized, chronic renal disease is problematic in pregnancy even for women with preserved renal function. Reported complications and their incidences are shown in Table 48-3. Surian and colleagues (1984) described 123 pregnancies in 86 women with biopsy-proven glomerular disease in whom only a few had renal dysfunction. Forty percent developed obstetrical or renal complications, or both.

Packham and co-workers (1989) reported 395 pregnancies in 238 women with preexisting glomerulonephritis and minimal renal insufficiency. During pregnancy, 15 percent of these women developed impaired renal function, and 60 percent had worsening proteinuria. Although only 12 percent had hypertension antedating pregnancy, more than 50 percent of all these women developed gestational hypertension. These pregnancies were complicated by a high incidence of gestational hypertension—50 percent, irreversibly worsened renal function—5 percent, and perinatal mortality—140 per 1000. In the absence of early or severe hypertension or nephrotic-range proteinuria, the perinatal mortality rate was still 50 per 1000.

Chronic Renal Insufficiency

Overall, pregnancy complication rates in women with chronic renal disease who have renal insufficiency are greater than in women with preserved renal function (see Table 48-3). In general, adverse outcomes are directly related to the degree of renal impairment. Of the more recent reports shown in Table 48-3, outcomes of women with moderate versus severe renal insufficiency, as previously defined, are usually not separated. That said, Hou and colleagues (1985) described 25 pregnancies complicated by mild to moderate renal insufficiency—serum creatinine from 1.2 to 1.7 mg/dL. Gestational-induced or aggravated hypertension developed in slightly more than 50 percent of pregnancies. Primarily because of hypertension, 60 percent were delivered preterm.

Cunningham and associates (1990), Jones and Hayslett (1996), and Imbasciati and colleagues (2002) described pregnancies complicated by moderate or severe renal insufficiency. Despite a high incidence of chronic hypertension, anemia, preeclampsia, preterm delivery, and fetal-growth restriction, perinatal outcomes were generally good. As shown in Figure 48-5, fetal growth is, in general, impaired and related to severity of renal dysfunction.

Management

Frequent prenatal visits are scheduled to monitor blood pressure. Serial serum creatinine values are measured and protein excretion is quantified if indicated. Bacteriuria is treated to decrease the risk of pyelonephritis. Protein-restricted diets are not

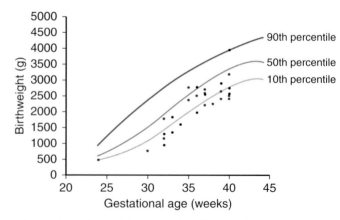

FIGURE 48-5 Birthweight percentiles of infants born to 29 women at Parkland Hospital with mild to moderate renal insufficiency—serum creatinine 1.4–2.4 mg/dL (*black points*) and severe renal insufficiency—serum creatinine ≥2.5 mg/dL (*red points*). (Data are from Cunningham and colleagues, 1990; and Stettler and Cunningham, 1992. Growth curves are those reported by Alexander and co-workers, 1996.)

recommended (Lindheimer and colleagues, 2000; Ruggenenti and associates, 2001). Anemia from chronic renal insufficiency responds to recombinant erythropoietin, however, hypertension is a well-documented side effect. Suspected fetal-growth restriction is managed as discussed in Chapter 38 (p. 843). If hypertension develops, it is managed as described in Chapter 34 (p. 708).

Follow-Up

At least in some women, pregnancy appears to accelerate chronic renal disease. Theoretically, renal hyperperfusion and increased glomerular blood pressure could accelerate nephrosclerosis (Baylis, 2003). In 360 women with chronic glomerulonephritis who mostly had normal renal function, there was little adverse long-term effect of pregnancy (Jungers and associates, 1995). In women with severe chronic renal insufficiency, however, pregnancy may worsen function (Abe, 1991; Jones and Hayslett, 1996). Imbasciati and colleagues (2007) reported that this was more likely to develop in women with a serum creatinine ≥1.4 mg/dL and proteinuria >1 g/day. It seems reasonable to conclude that, in the absence of superimposed preeclampsia or severe hemorrhage and hypovolemia, pregnancy does not usually accelerate renal insufficiency.

Even if there is no pregnancy-induced renal dysfunction in the short term, the natural history of many chronic renal disorders is one of long-term progression. Cunningham and associates (1990) reported that at least 20 percent of pregnant women with moderate to severe insufficiency developed end-stage renal failure by a mean of 4 years. In the report by Jones and Hayslett, 10 percent of pregnancies were followed by end-stage disease within 1 year. Imbasciati and co-workers (2007) reported that with a median follow-up of 3 years, 30 percent of women whose serum creatinine was ≥1.4 mg/dL and proteinuria >1 g/day had developed end-stage disease. Similarly, Stettler and Cunningham (1992) reported that at least 20 percent of women with chronic proteinuria discovered during pregnancy developed end-stage renal failure within several years.

Dialysis During Pregnancy

Significantly impaired renal function is accompanied by subfertility that may be corrected with chronic hemodialysis or peritoneal dialysis. Not unexpectedly, these pregnancies can be complicated. Okundaye and associates (1998) surveyed dialysis units between 1992 and 1995 listed by the Health Care Financing Administration. A total of 241 women became pregnant—60 percent were undergoing hemodialysis and 40 percent peritoneal dialysis. Almost 80 percent were hypertensive and 95 percent were anemic. Pregnancy outcomes included early losses in 42 percent, preterm births in 26 percent, and stillbirths in 8 percent. Infant survival was 40 percent in women who conceived during dialysis compared with 75 percent in those who commenced dialysis after becoming pregnant. The type of dialysis did not influence pregnancy outcome. Chou and colleagues (2008) reviewed 131 cases reported since 1990. They found that mean birthweight was higher in women who conceived while undergoing dialysis—1530 g versus 1245 g in women who conceived prior to starting dialysis. A number of reports from single centers since 1999 and shown in Table 48-4 have described similar outcomes.

Indications for Dialysis

Both hemodialysis and peritoneal dialysis are feasible. If peritoneal dialysis is ongoing, this can be continued during pregnancy. Lindheimer and colleagues (2008) recommend initiation of dialysis when serum creatinine levels are between 5 and 7 mg/dL. Abrupt volume changes that cause hypotension should be avoided. To accomplish this, dialysis frequency likely is extended to five to six times weekly (Reddy and Holley, 2007). Calciferol and erythropoietin doses may require increases. Maternal complications are common and include severe hypertension, placental abruption, heart failure, and sepsis.

TABLE 48-4. Pregnancy Outcomes in 118 Women Undergoing Dialysis During Pregnancy

		Pregnancies		**Pregnancy Outcomes (Percent)**			
Study (Year)	N	Delivery (wks)	Birthweight (g)	Hypertension	Hydramnios	Perinatal Mortality	Surviving Infants
Toma et al (1999)	54	31.9	1545	35	44	33	67
Luciani et al (2002)	5	28.6	1430	20	100	20	80
Chao et al (2002)	13	32	1540	72	46	31	69
Kazancioglu et al (2002)	3	31	1250	67	67	3	67
Eroğlu et al (2004)	7	32	1400	67	29	14	86
Haase et al (2005)	5	33	1765	—	40	0	100
Tan et al (2006)	11	31	1390	36	18	18	82
Barua et al (2008)	6	36.2	2420	33	0	0	100
Chou et al (2008)	13	30.8	1510	57	71	50	50
Approximate averages	118	31–32	1500	40–50	40	25–30	70–80

PREGNANCY AFTER RENAL TRANSPLANTATION

In 2007, there were approximately 75,000 registrants on the waiting list for renal transplantations through the Organ Procurement and Transplantation Network (OPTN) (2007). The 1-year graft survival rate is 95 percent for grafts from living donors and 89 percent from deceased donors (Carpenter and associates, 2008). Survival rates approximately doubled between 1988 and 1996, due in large part to the introduction of cyclosporine and muromonab-CD3 (OKT3 monoclonal antibody) to prevent and treat organ rejection. Since then, mycophenolate mofetil and tacrolimus have further reduced acute rejection episodes. Experience with these newer drugs during pregnancy is limited (Alston, 2001; Briggs, 2005; Le Ray, 2004, and all their co-workers). Importantly, resumption of renal function after transplantation promptly restores fertility in reproductive-aged women (Lessan-Pezeshki and associates, 2004).

Pregnancy Outcomes

Armenti and colleagues (2004) reviewed the outcomes of 1418 pregnancies in 919 transplant recipients as reported to the National Transplantation Pregnancy Registry. Most were treated with cyclosporine and tacrolimus. The incidence of miscarriage and therapeutic abortion was 20 percent. Overall, 76 percent of pregnancies resulted in a live birth. Preterm births were common, and half of the women were delivered before 37 weeks. Similarly, half of the infants were low birthweight—because of preterm birth as well as fetal-growth restriction. Importantly, the incidence of fetal malformations was not increased.

In the Registry results presented by Armenti and co-workers (2004), the incidence of preeclampsia was 30 percent. In some cases, rejection is difficult to distinguish from preeclampsia. That said, the incidence of rejection episodes was only 3 percent. Infections that developed in 22 percent and diabetes in 10 percent were thought to be likely related to immunosuppression therapy. Since that time, similar outcomes have been reported by Al Duraihimh (2008), Ghafari and Sanadgol (2008), Cruz Lemini (2007), Gutierrez (2005), and all their co-workers.

Lindheimer and colleagues (2008) and Hou (2003) recommend that women who have undergone transplantation satisfy the following requisites before attempting pregnancy:

1. They should be in good general health for at least 2 years after transplantation
2. There should be stable renal function without severe renal insufficiency—serum creatinine <2 mg/dL and preferably <1.5 mg/dL, none to minimal proteinuria, no evidence of graft rejection, and absence of pyelocalyceal distension by urography
3. Absent or easily controlled hypertension
4. Drug therapy reduced to maintenance levels.

Cyclosporine or tacrolimus is given routinely to renal transplantation recipients (Jain and associates, 2004). Cyclosporine blood levels decline during pregnancy, although this was not reported to be associated with rejection episodes (Thomas and co-workers, 1997). Unfortunately, these agents are nephrotoxic and also may cause renal hypertension. In fact, they likely contribute substantively to chronic renal disease that develops in 10 to 20 percent of patients with nonrenal solid-organ transplantation (Goes and Colvin, 2007).

Concern persists over the possibility of late effects in offspring subjected to immunosuppressive therapy in utero. These include malignancy, germ cell dysfunction, and malformations in the children of the *offspring*. In addition, cyclosporine is secreted in breast milk, and in at least one instance, it produced *therapeutic* serum levels in the nursing child (Moretti and associates, 2003).

Finally, although pregnancy-induced renal hyperfiltration theoretically may impair long-term graft survival, Sturgiss and Davison (1995) found no evidence for this in a case-control study of 34 allograft recipients followed for a mean of 15 years.

Management

Close surveillance is necessary. Covert bacteriuria is treated, and if it is recurrent, suppressive treatment is given for the remainder of pregnancy. Serial hepatic enzyme concentrations and blood counts are monitored for toxic effects of azathioprine and cyclosporine. Some recommend measurement of serum cyclosporine levels. Gestational diabetes is more common if corticosteroids are taken. Overt diabetes must be excluded, and glucose tolerance testing is done at approximately 26 weeks. Surveillance for opportunistic infections from herpesvirus, cytomegalovirus, and toxoplasmosis is important because they are more common.

Renal function is monitored, and as shown in Figure 48-2 the glomerular filtration rate usually increases 20 to 25 percent. If a significant increase in serum creatinine is detected, then its cause must be determined. Possibilities include acute rejection, cyclosporine toxicity, preeclampsia, infection, and urinary tract obstruction. Evidence of pyelonephritis or graft rejection should prompt admission for aggressive management. Imaging studies and kidney biopsy may be indicated. The woman is carefully monitored for development or worsening of underlying hypertension, and especially superimposed preeclampsia. Management of hypertension during pregnancy is the same as for nontransplanted patients.

Because of increased incidences of fetal-growth restriction and preterm delivery, vigilant fetal surveillance is indicated. Although cesarean delivery is reserved for obstetrical indications, occasionally the transplanted kidney obstructs labor. In all women with renal transplant, the cesarean delivery rate approaches 50 percent (Armenti and co-workers, 2004).

POLYCYSTIC KIDNEY DISEASE

This usually autosomally dominant systemic disease primarily affects the kidneys. The disease is found in 1 in 800 live births and causes approximately 10 percent of end-stage renal disease in the United States (Wilson, 2004). Although genetically heterogeneous, almost 85 percent of cases are due to *PKD1* gene mutations on chromosome 16, and the other 15 percent to *PKD2* mutations on chromosome 4 (Salant and Patel, 2008). Genetic and environmental influences on disease progression were reviewed by Peters and Breuning (2001). Prenatal diagnosis is available if the mutation has been identified in a family member or if linkage has been established in the family.

Renal complications are more common in men than in women, and symptoms usually appear in the third or fourth decade. Flank pain, hematuria, nocturia, proteinuria, and associated calculi and infection are common findings. Hypertension develops in 75 percent, and progression to renal failure is a major problem. Superimposed acute renal failure may also develop from infection or obstruction from ureteral angulation by cyst displacement.

Other organs are commonly involved. Hepatic involvement is more common and more aggressive in women than in men (Chapman, 2003). Asymptomatic *hepatic cysts* coexist in a third of patients with polycystic kidneys. Hossack and colleagues (1988) reported a substantively increased incidence of *cardiac valvular lesions* with excessive rates of mitral, aortic, and tricuspid incompetence. The incidence of *mitral valve prolapse* was increased 13-fold. Importantly, approximately 10 percent of patients with polycystic kidney disease die from rupture of an associated *intracranial berry aneurysm*.

Polycystic Kidney Disease and Pregnancy

Pregnancy outcome depends on the degree of associated hypertension and renal insufficiency. Upper urinary tract infections are common. Chapman and co-workers (1994) compared pregnancy in 235 affected women who had 605 pregnancies with those of 108 unaffected family members who had 244 pregnancies. Composite perinatal complication rates were similar—33 versus 26 percent—but hypertension, including preeclampsia, was more common in women with polycystic kidneys. Pregnancy does not seem to accelerate the natural disease course (Lindheimer and colleagues, 2007).

GLOMERULOPATHIES

The kidney, especially the glomerulus and its capillaries, is subject to a large number and variety of acute and chronic diseases. They may result from a single stimulus such as poststreptococcal glomerulonephritis, or from a multisystem disease such as systemic lupus erythematosus or diabetes. Many first become apparent when chronic renal insufficiency is discovered. According to Lewis and Neilsen (2008), there are several distinct clinical glomerulopathic syndromes: acute nephritic, pulmonary-renal, nephrotic, basement membrane, glomerulovascular, and infectious-disease syndromes. The majority of these diseases are encountered in young women of childbearing age and thus are encountered during pregnancy.

Acute Nephritic Syndrome

Acute glomerulonephritis may result from any of several causes as shown in Table 48-5. They present with hypertension, hematuria, red-cell casts, pyuria, and proteinuria. There are varying degrees of renal insufficiency and salt and water retention, which causes edema, hypertension, and circulatory congestion (Lewis and Neilsen, 2008).

TABLE 48-5. Causes of Acute Nephritic Syndrome

Poststreptococcal infection
Subacute bacterial endocarditis
Systemic lupus erythematosus
Antiglomerular basement membrane disease
IgA nephropathy
ANCA small vessel vasculitis
Henoch-Schönlein purpura
Cryoglobulinemia
Membranoproliferative glomerulonephritis
Mesangioproliferative glomerulonephritis

ANCA = antineutrophil cytoplasmic antibodies.
Adapted from Lewis and Neilsen (2008).

Acute poststreptococcal glomerulonephritis is prototypical of these syndromes. Although it rarely develops during pregnancy, it is of historical interest because it was confused with eclampsia until the mid-1800s. In 1843, Lever discovered that the proteinuria of eclampsia was different from that due to *Bright disease* because it disappeared after delivery.

The prognosis and treatment of the other acute nephritic syndromes listed in Table 48-5 depend on their etiology. Renal biopsy may be necessary to determine etiology as well as to direct management (Lindheimer and colleagues, 2007; Ramin and colleagues, 2006). One relatively common example is systemic lupus erythematosus (Germain and Nelson-Piercy, 2006). As discussed in Chapter 54 (p. 1148), differentiation between lupus flare and preeclampsia is problematic. We have occasionally encountered *Goodpasture syndrome,* characterized by antibasement membrane autoantibodies, pulmonary hemorrhage, and glomerulonephritis. Vasilou and colleagues (2005) described maternal and neonatal morbidity in a woman in whom the diagnosis was established by renal biopsy performed at 18 weeks. In some patients, *rapidly progressive glomerulonephritis* leads to end-stage renal failure. In others, *chronic glomerulonephritis* develops with slowly progressive renal disease.

IgA Nephropathy

This condition, which is also known as *Berger disease*, is the most common form of acute glomerulonephritis worldwide. Its primary form is an immune-complex disease. *Henoch-Schönlein purpura* may be a systemic form of the disease (Donadio and Grande, 2002). In a review of more than 300 pregnancies complicated by IgA nephropathy, Lindheimer and colleagues (2000) concluded that pregnancy outcome depended on the degree of renal insufficiency and hypertension. Ronkainen and associates (2005) reported long-term outcomes in a cohort of patients with childhood IgA nephritis. During an average follow-up of 19 years, there were 22 pregnancies. Half had hypertension and a third delivered preterm.

Effect of Glomerulonephritis on Pregnancy

Whatever the underlying etiology, acute glomeruloncphritis has profound effects on pregnancy outcome. Packham and colleagues (1989) described 395 pregnancies in 238 women with *primary* glomerulonephritis diagnosed before pregnancy. The most common lesions on biopsy were membranous glomerulonephritis, IgA glomerulonephritis, and diffuse mesangial glomerulonephritis. Most of these women had normal renal function, but still overall fetal loss was 25 percent, and the perinatal mortality rate after 28 weeks was 80 per 1000 (see Table 48-3). A fourth were delivered preterm, and 15 percent of fetuses were growth restricted. Overall, approximately half of these women developed hypertension, and it was severe in the majority who did. Proteinuria worsened in 60 percent of all women. The worst perinatal outcomes were in women with impaired renal function, early or severe hypertension, and nephrotic-range proteinuria.

Chronic Glomerulonephritis

Primary renal lesions that cause chronic nephritis shown in Table 48-5 are frequently not identified. Chronic disease is characterized by progressive renal destruction over years or decades, eventually producing ESRD. Persistent proteinuria and hematuria commonly accompany a gradual decline in renal function. Microscopically, the renal lesions are categorized as proliferative, sclerosing, or membranous. In most cases, proteinuria, anemia, or elevated creatinine is detected by screening in symptomatic patients, or it is found during evaluation for chronic hypertension. In some women, "typical" preeclampsia-eclampsia does not resolve postpartum, and they subsequently are found to have chronic glomerulonephritis. Its prognosis depends on its etiology, and renal biopsy may be helpful. In some patients, 10 to 20 years may elapse before end-stage renal failure supervenes.

Nephrotic Syndrome

This is a spectrum of renal disorders in which proteinuria is the hallmark. Some of the causes are shown in Table 48-6. Nephrotic syndrome is characterized by proteinuria in excess of 3 g/day, hypoalbuminemia, hyperlipidemia, and edema. There may be accompanying evidence of renal dysfunction. Most patients who undergo biopsy have microscopic renal abnormalities. The defects in the barriers of the glomerular capillary wall that allow excessive filtration of plasma proteins are caused by primary glomerular disease. These lesions may follow immunological or toxic injury, or they are from diabetes or vascular diseases.

Management depends on etiology. Edema is managed cautiously, especially during pregnancy. Jakobi and associates (1995) have described problems associated with massive vulvar edema that may complicate the nephrotic syndrome caused by diabetes. Another cause is viral, bacterial, or protozoal infections—the woman shown in Figure 48-6 had nephrosis due to secondary syphilis. Normal amounts of dietary protein of high biological value are encouraged—high-protein diets only increase proteinuria. The incidence of thromboembolism is increased and varies in relation to the severity of hypertension, proteinuria, and renal insufficiency (Stratta and associates, 2006). Although both arte-

TABLE 48-6. Causes of the Nephrotic Syndrome in Adults

Minimal change disease (MCD) (10–15%): primary idiopathic (most cases), drug-induced (NSAIDs), allergies, viral infections

Focal segmental glomerulosclerosis (FSGS) (33%): viruses, hypertension, reflux nephropathy, sickle-cell disease

Membranous glomerulonephritis (30%): idiopathic (majority), malignancy, infection, connective-tissue diseases

Diabetic nephropathy: most common cause of ESRD

Amyloidosis

ESRD = end-stage renal disease; NSAIDs = nonsteroidal anti-inflammatory drugs.
Adapted from Lewis and Neilsen (2008).

rial and venous thrombosis occur, renal vein thrombosis is particularly worrisome. The value, if any, of prophylactic anticoagulation is unclear. Some cases of nephrosis from primary glomerular disease respond to corticosteroid or cytotoxic drug therapy. In most of those cases caused by infection or drugs, proteinuria recedes when the underlying cause is corrected.

Nephrotic-Range Proteinuria in Pregnancy

When nephrosis complicates pregnancy, the maternal and fetal prognosis, as well as appropriate treatment, depends on the underlying cause and severity of the disease. Whenever possible, the specific cause should be ascertained, and renal biopsy may be indicated.

Approximately half of women with the nephrotic-range proteinuria have increased protein excretion during pregnancy (Packham and colleagues, 1989). In two thirds of women, protein excretion exceeds 3 g/day (Stettler and Cunningham, 1992). Despite this, pregnant women without appreciably diminished renal function usually have an augmented glomerular filtration rate (Cunningham and colleagues, 1990).

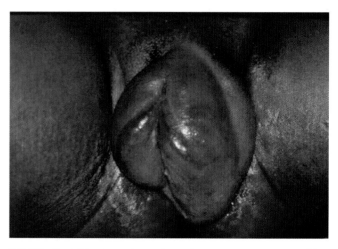

FIGURE 48-6 Massive vulvar edema in a pregnant woman with the nephrotic syndrome due to secondary syphilis.

TABLE 48-7. Causes and Outcomes of Obstetrical Acute Renal Failure

		Causes and Associated Factors (Percent)				
Study	N	Preeclampsia-Eclampsia	Obstetrical Hemorrhage	Abortion	Dialysis	Maternal Mortality Rate (Percent)
Turney (1989) Leeds, UK	142	50	35	25	NR	20
Sibai (1990)[a] Memphis, TN	31	100	Abruption (50) Postpartum (90)		15/31	10
Nzerue (1998) Atlanta, GA	21	38 (50% HELLP)	14	14	2/21	16
Drakeley (2002) Cape Town, SA	72	93	32 Abruption (10)		10/72	0

[a]Review was limited to women with hypertension.
NR = not reported.

Most women with nephrosis who do not have severe hypertension or renal insufficiency have a successful pregnancy outcome. With renal insufficiency, moderate to severe hypertension, or both, the prognosis is much worse. Our experience from Parkland Hospital indicates that women with proteinuria before pregnancy frequently develop a number of complications during pregnancy (Stettler and Cunningham, 1992). Protein excretion in 65 pregnancies averaged 4 g/day, and 33 percent of these women had classic nephrotic syndrome. Some degree of renal insufficiency was found in 75 percent, chronic hypertension in 40 percent, and persistent anemia in 25 percent. Importantly, preeclampsia developed in 60 percent, and 45 percent had preterm deliveries. Excluding abortions, however, 53 of 57 infants were born alive. A third of these infants are reported to be growth restricted (Stratta and associates, 2006).

Long-term follow-up in women with chronic proteinuria during pregnancy is important. In the 21 women who subsequently underwent renal biopsy reported by Stettler and Cunningham (1992), histological evidence of renal disease was found. Long-term follow-up indicated that at least 20 percent of women had progressed to end-stage renal failure. Similarly, Chen and colleagues (2001) reported that eight of 15 women undergoing biopsy during pregnancy for the nephrotic syndrome either had died (three), had developed chronic renal failure (three), or had end-stage disease (two) by 2 years following delivery. In the report by Imbasciati and associates (2007), women whose serum creatinine was >1.4 mg/dL and whose 24-hour protein excretion exceeded 1 g/day had the shortest renal survival times after pregnancy.

ACUTE RENAL FAILURE

Defined as a rapid decrease in the glomerular filtration rate over minutes to days, acute renal failure is termed *acute kidney injury* by the American Society of Nephrology (2005). Fortunately, the incidence of renal failure associated with pregnancy has decreased substantively over the past 30 years. Despite this, it remains a significant source of obstetrical morbidity in this country (Kuklina and co-workers, 2009). Associated mortality depends on its sever-

ity and whether dialysis is needed (Singri and colleagues, 2003). Pregnancy outcomes from four studies are shown in Table 48-7. Except for a decreased incidence of abortion-related renal failure, the etiology has not changed dramatically over the past several decades. Turney and colleagues (1989) described findings from the Renal Unit in Leeds, England. Whereas in earlier years obstetrical cases composed 33 percent of all patients requiring dialysis, more recently these accounted for only 10 percent.

Today, renal failure is most often associated with severe preeclampsia-eclampsia. Frangieh and co-workers (1996) reported that 3.8 percent of eclamptic women from the University of Tennessee had acute renal failure. From the same institution, Audibert and colleagues (1996) reported that 3 percent of 69 women with hemolysis, elevated liver enzymes, and low platelets (*HELLP syndrome*) developed renal failure. Obstetrical hemorrhage, notably placental abruption, alone or in concert with severe preeclampsia, is strongly linked to severe renal failure (Drakeley and co-workers, 2002). Septicemia is another common co-morbidity (Zeeman and colleagues, 2003). From his review, Sibai (2007) reported a 44-percent increase of acute renal failure with acute fatty liver of pregnancy (see Chap. 50, p. 1065). In one unusual case, Hill and associates (2002) described a woman managed at Parkland Hospital with acute renal failure caused by hyperemesis gravidarum at 15 weeks. Her serum creatinine level was 10.7 mg/dL and she required hemodialysis for 5 days.

Management

In most women, renal failure develops postpartum, thus management is not complicated by fetal considerations. An acute increase in serum creatinine is usually due to renal ischemia (Abuelo, 2007). Oliguria is an important sign of acutely impaired renal function. In obstetrical cases, both prerenal and intrarenal factors are commonly operative. For example, with total placental abruption, severe hypovolemia is common from massive hemorrhage. Superimposed preeclampsia may cause oliguria.

When azotemia is evident and severe oliguria persists, some form of hemofiltration or dialysis is initiated before marked deterioration occurs. Medication dose adjustments are imperative

(Singri and associates, 2003). Early dialysis appears to reduce the mortality rate appreciably and may enhance the extent of recovery of renal function. With time, renal function usually returns to normal or near normal.

Prevention

Acute tubular necrosis may often be prevented by the following means:

1. Prompt and vigorous replacement of blood in instances of massive hemorrhage, such as in placental abruption, placental previa, uterine rupture, and postpartum uterine atony
2. Termination of pregnancies complicated by severe preeclampsia or eclampsia and careful blood replacement if loss is excessive
3. Close observation for early signs of sepsis syndrome and shock in women with pyelonephritis, septic abortion, chorioamnionitis, or sepsis from other pelvic infections
4. Avoidance of potent diuretics to treat oliguria before initiating appropriate efforts to ensure that cardiac output is adequate for renal perfusion
5. Avoidance of vasoconstrictors to treat hypotension, unless pathological vasodilation is unequivocally the cause of the hypotension.

Renal cortical necrosis has become exceedingly uncommon. Before widespread availability of dialysis, it complicated a fourth of cases of obstetrical renal failure (Grünfeld and Pertuiset, 1987; Turney and colleagues, 1989). Most cases followed placental abruption, preeclampsia-eclampsia, and endotoxin-induced shock. Histologically, the lesion appears to result from thrombosis of segments of the renal vascular system. The lesions may be focal, patchy, confluent, or gross. Clinically, renal cortical necrosis follows the course of acute renal failure, and its differentiation from acute tubular necrosis is not possible during the early phase. The prognosis depends on the extent of the necrosis. There is variable recovery of function and stable renal insufficiency results (Lindheimer and colleagues, 2007).

Obstructive Renal Failure

Rarely, bilateral ureteral compression by a very large pregnant uterus is greatly exaggerated, causing ureteral obstruction and in turn, severe oliguria and azotemia. Brandes and Fritsche (1991) reviewed 13 cases that were the consequence of a markedly overdistended uterus. They described a woman with twins who developed anuria and a serum creatinine level of 12.2 mg/dL at 34 weeks. After amniotomy, urine flow resumed at 500 mL/hr and was followed by rapid return to normal of the serum creatinine. Eckford and Gingell (1991) described 10 women in whom ureteral obstruction was relieved by stenting. The stents were left in place for a mean of 15.5 weeks and removed 4 to 6 weeks postpartum. Sadan and associates (1994) reported a similar experience in eight such women who underwent stent placement at a mean of 29 weeks for moderate to severe hydronephrosis. The stents remained in situ for a mean of 9 weeks, during which time renal function remained normal.

We have observed this phenomenon on several occasions (Satin and colleagues, 1993). Partial ureteral obstruction may be accompanied by fluid retention and significant hypertension.

When the obstructive uropathy is relieved, diuresis ensues and hypertension dissipates. In one woman with massive hydramnios (9.4 L) and an anencephalic fetus, amniocentesis and removal of some of the amnionic fluid was followed promptly by diuresis, decreasing plasma creatinine concentration, and improvement of hypertension. In our experience, women with previous urinary tract surgery are more likely to have such obstructions. Even so, the phenomenon appears uncommon. Vordermark and associates (1990) reviewed pregnancy following major urinary reconstruction and found minimal complications.

REFERENCES

Abe S: An overview of pregnancy in women with underlying renal disease. Am J Kidney Dis 17:112, 1991

Abuelo JG: Normotensive ischemic acute renal failure. N Engl J Med 357:797, 2007

Airoldi J, Weinstein L: Clinical significance of proteinuria in pregnancy. Obstet Gynecol Surv 62(2):117, 2007

Al Duraihimh H, Ghamdi G, Moussa D, et al: Outcome of 234 pregnancies in 140 renal transplant recipients from five Middle Eastern countries. Transplantation 85:840, 2008

Alexander GR, Himes JH, Kaufman RB, et al: A United States national reference for fetal growth. Obstet Gynecol 87:163, 1996

Alston PK, Kuller JA, McMahon MJ: Pregnancy in transplant recipients. Obstet Gynecol Surv 56:289, 2001

American Academy of Pediatrics and American College of Obstetricians and Gynecologists: Guidelines for perinatal care, 6th ed. Washington, DC, 2007, p 101

American Society of Nephrology Renal Research Report. J Am Soc Nephrol 16:1886, 2005

Armenti VT, Radomski JS, Moritz MJ, et al: Report from the National Transplantation Pregnancy Registry (NTPR): Outcomes of pregnancy after transplantation. Clin Transpl 103, 2004

Asplin JR, Coe FL, Favus MJ: Nephrolithiasis. In Fauci AS, Braunwald E, Kasper DL, et al (eds): Harrison's Principles of Internal Medicine, 17th ed. New York, McGraw-Hill, 2008, p 1815

Asrat T, Roossin M, Miller EI: Ultrasonographic detection of ureteral jets in normal pregnancy. Am J Obstet Gynecol 178:1194, 1998

Audibert F, Friedman SA, Frangieh AY, et al: Diagnostic criteria for HELLP syndrome: Tedious or "helpful"? Am J Obstet Gynecol 174:454, 1996

Bachman JW, Heise RH, Naessens JM, et al: A study of various tests to detect asymptomatic urinary tract infections in an obstetric population. JAMA 270:1971, 1993

Banhidy F, Acs N, Puho EH, et al: Pregnancy complications and birth outcomes of pregnant women with urinary tract infections and related drug treatments. Scand J Infect Dis 39:390, 2007

Barua M, Hladunewich M, Keunen J, et al: Successful pregnancies on nocturnal home hemodialysis. Clin J Am Soc Nephrol 3:312, 2008

Baylis C: Impact of pregnancy on underlying renal disease. Adv Ren Replace Ther 10:31, 2003

Baylis C, Davison J: The urinary system. In Hytten F, Chamberlain G (eds): Clinical Physiology in Obstetrics, 2nd ed. London, Blackwell, 1991, p 245

Boggess KA, Benedetti TJ, Raghu G: Nitrofurantoin-induced pulmonary toxicity during pregnancy: A report of a case and review of the literature. Obstet Gynecol Surv 41:367, 1996

Brandes JC, Fritsche C: Obstructive acute renal failure by a gravid uterus: A case report and review. Am J Kidney Dis 18:398, 1991

Briggs GG, Freeman RK, Yaffe SJ: Drugs in Pregnancy and Lactation, 7th ed. Philadelphia, Lippincott Williams and Wilkins, 2005

Brown MA, Holt JL, Mangos GK, et al: Microscopic hematuria in pregnancy: Relevance to pregnancy outcome. Am J Kidney Dis 45:667, 2005

Butler EL, Cox SM, Eberts E, et al: Symptomatic nephrolithiasis complicating pregnancy. Obstet Gynecol 96:753, 2000

Carlan SJ, Schorr SJ, Ebenger MF, et al: Laser lithotripsy in pregnancy: A case report. J Reprod Med 40:74, 1995

Carpenter CB, Milford EL, Sayegh MH: Transplantation in the treatment of renal failure. In Harrison's Principles of Internal Medicine, 17th ed. New York, McGraw-Hill, 2008, p 1776

Cavenee MR, Cox SM, Mason R, et al: Erythropoietin in pregnancies complicated by pyelonephritis. Obstet Gynecol 84:252, 1994

Chao AS, Huang JY, Lien R, et al: Pregnancy in women who undergo long-term hemodialysis. Am J Obstet Gynecol 187(1):152, 2002

Chapman AB: Cystic disease in women: Clinical characteristics and medical management. Adv Ren Replace Ther 10:24, 2003

Chapman AB, Johnson AM, Gabow PA: Pregnancy outcome and its relationship to progression of renal failure in autosomal dominant polycystic kidney disease. J Am Soc Nephrol 5:1178, 1994

Chen HH, Lin HC, Yeh JC, et al: Renal biopsy in pregnancies complicated by undetermined renal disease. Acta Obstet Gynecol Scand 80:888, 2001

Chou CY, Ting IW, Lin TH, et al: Pregnancy in patients on chronic dialysis: A single center experience and combined analysis of reported results. Eur J Obstet Gynecol Reprod Biol 136:165, 2008

Cox SM, Cunningham FG: Acute focal pyelonephritis (lobar nephronia) complicating pregnancy. Obstet Gynecol 71:510, 1988

Cox SM, Shelburne P, Mason R, et al: Mechanisms of hemolysis and anemia associated with acute antepartum pyelonephritis. Am J Obstet Gynecol 164:587, 1991

Cruz Lemini MC, Ibarguengoitia Ochoa F, Villanueva Gonzalez MA: Perinatal outcome following renal transplantation. Int J Gynaecol Obstet 95:76, 2007

Cunningham FG, Cox SM, Harstad TW, et al: Chronic renal disease and pregnancy outcome. Am J Obstet Gynecol 163:453, 1990

Cunningham FG, Morris GB, Mickal A: Acute pyelonephritis of pregnancy: A clinical review. Obstet Gynecol 42:112, 1973

Czaja CA, Rutledge BN, Cleary PA, et al: Urinary tract infections in women with type 1 diabetes mellitus: Survey of female participants in the epidemiology of diabetes interventions and complications study cohort. J Urol 181(3):1129, 2009

Dodson KW, Pinkner JS, Rose T, et al: Structural basis of the interaction of the pyelonephritic *E. coli* adhesin to its human kidney receptor. Cell 105:733, 2001

Donadio JV, Grande JP: IgA nephropathy. N Engl J Med 347:738, 2002

Drakeley AJ, Le Roux PA, Anthony J, et al: Acute renal failure complicating severe preeclampsia requiring admission to an obstetric intensive care unit. Am J Obstet Gynecol 186:253, 2002

Eckford SD, Gingell JC: Ureteric obstruction in pregnancy—diagnosis and management. Br J Obstet Gynaecol 98:1137, 1991

El-Khatib M, Packham DK, Becker GJ, et al: Pregnancy-related complications in women with reflux nephropathy. Clin Nephrol 41:50, 1994

Eroğlu D, Lembet A, Ozdemir FN, et al: Pregnancy during hemodialysis: Perinatal outcome in our cases. Transplant Proc 36(1):53, 2004

Fakhoury GF, Daikoku NH, Parikh AR: Management of severe hemorrhagic cystitis in pregnancy: A report of two cases. J Reprod Med 39:485, 1994

Faúndes A, Bricola-Filho M, Pinto e Silva JC: Dilatation of the urinary tract during pregnancy: Proposal of a curve of maximal caliceal diameter by gestational age. Am J Obstet Gynecol 178:1082, 1998

Fihn SD: Acute uncomplicated urinary tract infection in women. N Engl J Med 349:259, 2003

Fischer MJ, Lehnerz SD, Hebert JR, et al: Kidney disease is an independent risk factor for adverse fetal and maternal outcomes in pregnancy. Am J Kidney Dis 43:415, 2004

Frangieh SA, Friedman SA, Audibert F, et al: Maternal outcome in women with eclampsia. Am J Obstet Gynecol 174:453, 1996

Galvagno SM Jr, Camann W: Sepsis and acute renal failure in pregnancy. Anesth Analg 108(2):572, 2009

Gazmararian JA, Petersen R, Jamieson DJ, et al: Hospitalizations during pregnancy among managed care enrollees. Obstet Gynecol 100:94, 2002

Germain S, Nelson-Piercy C: Lupus nephritis and renal disease in pregnancy. Lupus 15:148, 2006

Ghafari A, Sanadgol H: Pregnancy after renal transplantation: Ten-year single-center experience. Transp Proc 40:251, 2008

Gilstrap LC III, Cunningham FG, Whalley PJ: Acute pyelonephritis in pregnancy: An anterospective study. Obstet Gynecol 57:409, 1981a

Gilstrap LC III, Leveno KJ, Cunningham FG, et al: Renal infection and pregnancy outcome. Am J Obstet Gynecol 141:708, 1981b

Goes NB, Calvin RB: Case 12-2007: A 56-year-old woman with renal failure after heart–lung transplantation. N Engl J Med 356:1657, 2007

Graham JM, Oshiro BT, Blanco JD, et al: Uterine contractions after antibiotic therapy for pyelonephritis in pregnancy. Am J Obstet Gynecol 168:577, 1993

Grünfeld JP, Pertuiset N: Acute renal failure in pregnancy: 1987. Am J Kidney Dis 9:359, 1987

Gutierrez MJ, Acebedo-Ribo M, Garcia-Donaire JA, et al: Pregnancy in renal transplant recipients. Transplant Proc 37:3721, 2005

Harris RE, Gilstrap LC III: Cystitis during pregnancy: A distinct clinical entity. Obstet Gynecol 57:578, 1981

Hart A, Nowicki BJ, Reisner B, et al: Ampicillin-resistant *Escherichia coli* in gestational pyelonephritis: Increased occurrence and association with the colonization factor Dr adhesin. J Infect Dis 183:1526, 2001

Haase M, Morgera S, Bamberg C, et al: A systematic approach to managing pregnant dialysis patients-the importance of an intensified haemodiafiltration protocol. Nephrol Dial Transplant 20(11):2537, 2005

Hendricks SK, Ross SO, Krieger JN: An algorithm for diagnosis and therapy of management and complications of urolithiasis during pregnancy. Surg Gynecol Obstet 172:49, 1991

Higby K, Suiter CR, Phelps JY, et al: Normal values of urinary albumin and total protein excretion during pregnancy. Am J Obstet Gynecol 171:984, 1994

Hill JB, Sheffield JS, McIntire DD, et al: Acute pyelonephritis in pregnancy. Obstet Gynecol 105:38, 2005

Hill JB, Yost NP, Wendel GD Jr: Acute renal failure in association with severe hyperemesis gravidarum. Obstet Gynecol 100:1119, 2002

Hladunewich MA, Lafayette RA, Derby GC, et al: The dynamics of glomerular filtration in the puerperium. Am J Physiol Renal Physiol 286:F496, 2004

Hooton TM, Scholes D, Stapleton AE, et al: A prospective study of asymptomatic bacteriuria in sexually active young women. N Engl J Med 343:992, 2000

Hossack KF, Leddy CL, Johnson AM, et al: Echocardiographic findings in autosomal dominant polycystic kidney disease. N Engl J Med 319:907, 1988

Hou S: Pregnancy in renal transplant recipients. Adv Ren Replace Ther 10:40, 2003

Hou S: Historical perspective of pregnancy in chronic kidney disease. Adv Chronic Kidney Dis 14:116, 2007

Hou SH, Grossman SD, Madias NE: Pregnancy in women with renal disease and moderate renal insufficiency. Am J Med 78:185, 1985

Ibrahim HN, Foley R, Tan L, et al: Long-term consequences of kidney donation. N Engl J Med 360:459, 2009

Imbasciati E, Gregorini G, Cabiddu G, et al: Pregnancy in CKD stages 3 to 5: Fetal and maternal outcomes. Am J Kidney Dis 49:753, 2007

Jacobsson B, Hagberg G, Hagberg B, et al: Cerebral palsy in preterm infants: A population-based case-control study of antenatal and intrapartal risk factors. Acta Paediatr 91:946, 2002

Jain AB, Shapiro R, Scantlebury VP, et al: Pregnancy after kidney and kidney-pancreas transplantation under tacrolimus: A single center's experience. Transplantation 77:897, 2004

Jakobi P, Friedman M, Goldstein I, et al: Massive vulvar edema in pregnancy: A case report. J Reprod Med 40:479, 1995

Jones DC, Hayslett JP: Outcome of pregnancy in women with moderate or severe renal insufficiency. N Engl J Med 335:226, 1996

Jungers P, Houillier P, Chauveau D, et al: Pregnancy in women with reflux nephropathy. Kidney Int 50:593, 1996

Jungers P, Houillier P, Forget D, et al: Influence of pregnancy on the course of primary chronic glomerulonephritis. Lancet 346:1122, 1995

Kass EH: Pyelonephritis and bacteriuria. Ann Intern Med 56:46, 1962

Kazancioglu R, Sahin S, Has R, et al: The outcome of pregnancy among patients receiving hemodialysis treatment. Clin Nephrol 59(5):379, 2003

Kincaid-Smith P, Bullen M: Bacteriuria in pregnancy. Lancet 1:395, 1965

Köhler JR, Tencer J, Thysell H, et al: Long-term effects of reflux nephropathy on blood pressure and renal function in adults. Nephron Clin Pract 93:c35, 2003

Kuklina EV, Meikle SF, Jamieson DJ, et al: Severe obstetric morbidity in the United States: 1998-2005. Obstet Gynecol 113:293, 2009

Lamont RF: The pathophysiology of pulmonary edema with the use of beta-agonists. Br J Obstet Gynaecol 107:439, 2000

Le Ray C, Coulomb A, Elefant E, et al: Mycophenolate mofetil in pregnancy after renal transplantation: A case of major fetal malformations. Obstet Gynecol 103:1091, 2004

Lessan-Pezeshki M, Ghazizadeh S, Khatami MR, et al: Fertility and contraceptive issues after kidney transplantation in women. Transplant Proc 36:1405, 2004

Lewis DF, Robichaux AG III, Jaekle RK, et al: Urolithiasis in pregnancy: Diagnosis, management and pregnancy outcome. J Reprod Med 48:28, 2003

Lewis JB, Neilsen EG: Glomerular diseases. In Harrison's Principles of Internal Medicine, 17th ed. New York, McGraw-Hill, 2008, p 1782

Lindheimer MD, Conrad KP, Karumanchi SA: Renal physiology and diseases in pregnancy. In Alpern R, Hebert S (eds): Seldin and Giebisch's The Kidney, Elsevier, San Diego, 2007, p 2339

Lindheimer MD, Davison JM: Pregnancy and CKD: Any progress? Am J Kidney Dis 49:729, 2007

Lindheimer MD, Grünfeld JP, Davison JM: Renal disorders. In Barron WM, Lindheimer MD (eds): Medical Disorders During Pregnancy, 3rd ed. St. Louis, Mosby, 2000, p 39

Lucas MJ, Cunningham FG: Urinary infection in pregnancy. Clin Obstet Gynecol 36:855, 1993

Lucas MJ, Cunningham FG: Urinary tract infections complicating pregnancy. Williams Obstetrics, 19th ed. (Suppl 5). Norwalk, CT, Appleton & Lange, February/March 1994

Luciani G, Bossola M, Tazza L, et al: Pregnancy during chronic hemodialysis: A single dialysis-unit experience with five cases. Ren Fail 24:853, 2002

Lügering A, Benz I, Knochenhauer S, et al: The Pix pilus adhesin of the uropathogenic *Escherichia coli* strain X2194 (O2:K(-): H6) is related to Pap pili but exhibits a truncated regulatory region. Microbiology 149:1387, 2003

Lumbiganon P, Villar J, Laopaiboon M, et al: One-day compared with 7-day nitrofurantoin for asymptomatic bacteriuria in pregnancy. Obstet Gynecol 113:339, 2009

Mabie WC, Barton JR, Sibai B: Septic shock in pregnancy. Obstet Gynecol 90:553, 1997

Maikranz P, Coe FL, Parks J, et al: Nephrolithiasis in pregnancy. Am J Kidney Dis 9:354, 1987

McAleer SJ, Loughlin KR: Nephrolithiasis and pregnancy. Curr Opin Urol 14:123, 2004

Mignini L, Carroli G, Abalos E, et al: Accuracy of diagnostic tests to detect asymptomatic bacteriuria during pregnancy. Obstet Gynecol 113(1):346, 2009

Millar LK, DeBuque L, Wing DA: Uterine contraction frequency during treatment of pyelonephritis in pregnancy and subsequent risk of preterm birth. J Perinat Med 31:41, 2003

Mor Y, Leibovitch I, Zalts R, et al: Analysis of the long-term outcome of surgically corrected vesicoureteric reflux. BJU Int 92:97, 2003

Moretti ME, Sgro M, Johnson DW, et al: Cyclosporine excretion into breast milk. Transplantation 75:2144, 2003

National High Blood Pressure Education Program Working Group on High Blood Pressure in Pregnancy: Report of the National High Blood Pressure Education Program Working Group on High Blood Pressure in Pregnancy. Am J Obstet Gynecol 183:S1, 2000

Nzerue CM, Hewan-Lowe K, Nwawka C: Acute renal failure in pregnancy: A review of clinical outcomes at an inner city hospital from 1986–1996. J Natl Med Assoc 90:486, 1998

Okundaye I, Abrinko P, Hou S: Registry of pregnancy in dialysis patients. Am J Kidney Dis 31:766, 1998

Organ Procurement and Transplantation Network. Available at: www.optn.oprg/latestdata/rptdata.asp. Accessed April 21, 2007

Packham DK, North RA, Fairley KF, et al: Primary glomerulonephritis and pregnancy. Q J Med 71:537, 1989

Peters DJM, Breuning MH: Autosomal dominant polycystic kidney disease: Modification of disease progression. Lancet 358:1439, 2001

Ramin SM, Vidaeff AC, Yeomans ER, et al: Chronic renal disease in pregnancy. Obstet Gynecol 108(6):1531, 2006

Raz R, Sakran W, Chazan B, et al: Long-term follow-up of women hospitalized for acute pyelonephritis. Clin Infect Dis 37:1014, 2003

Reddy SS, Holley JL: Management of the pregnant chronic dialysis patient. Adv Chronic Kidney Dis 14:146, 2007

Rodriguez PN, Klein AS: Management of urolithiasis during pregnancy. Surg Gynecol Obstet 166:103, 1988

Ronkainen J, Ala-Houhala M, Autio-Harmainen H, et al: Long-term outcome 19 years after childhood IgA nephritis: A retrospective cohort study. Pediatr Nephrol 21:1266, 2006

Ross AE, Handa S, Lingeman JE, et al: Kidney stones during pregnancy: An investigation into stone composition. Urol Res 36:99, 2008

Rouse DJ, Andrews WW, Goldenberg RL, et al: Screening and treatment of asymptomatic bacteriuria of pregnancy to prevent pyelonephritis. A cost-effectiveness and cost benefit analysis. Obstet Gynecol 86:119, 1995

Ruggenenti P, Schieppati A, Remuzzi G: Progression, remission, regression of chronic renal diseases. Lancet 357:1601, 2001

Sadan O, Berar M, Sagiv R, et al: Ureteric stent in severe hydronephrosis of pregnancy. Eur J Obstet Gynecol Reprod Biol 56:79, 1994

Salant DJ, Patel PS: Polycystic kidney disease and other inherited tubular disorders. In Harrison's Principles of Internal Medicine, 17th ed. New York, McGraw-Hill, 2008, p 1797

Sanchez-Ramos L, McAlpine KJ, Adair CD, et al: Pyelonephritis in pregnancy: Once a day ceftriaxone versus multiple doses of cefazolin. A randomized double-blind trial. Am J Obstet Gynecol 172:129, 1995

Satin AJ, Seiken GL, Cunningham FG: Reversible hypertension in pregnancy caused by obstructive uropathy. Obstet Gynecol 81:823, 1993

Schieve LA, Handler A, Hershow R, et al: Urinary tract infection during pregnancy: Its association with maternal morbidity and perinatal outcome. Am J Public Health 84:405, 1994

Scott CL, Chavez GF, Atrash HK, et al: Hospitalizations for severe complications of pregnancy 1987–1992. Obstet Gynecol 90:225, 1997

Seidman DS, Soriano D, Dulitzki M, et al: Role of renal ultrasonography in the management of pyelonephritis in pregnant women. J Perinatol 18:98, 1998

Semins MJ, Trock BJ, Matlaga BR: The safety of ureteroscopy during pregnancy: A systematic review and meta-analysis. J Urol 181(1):139, 2009

Sheffield JS, Cunningham FG: Urinary tract infection in women. Obstet Gynecol 106:1085, 2005

Sibai BM: Imitators of severe preeclampsia. Obstet Gynecol 109:956, 2007

Sibai BM, Villar MA, Mabie BC: Acute renal failure in hypertensive disorders of pregnancy. Pregnancy outcome and remote prognosis in thirty-one consecutive cases. Am J Obstet Gynecol 162(3):777, 1990

Singri N, Ahya SN, Levin ML: Acute renal failure. JAMA 289:747, 2003

Skorecki K, Green J, Brenner BM: Chronic renal failure. In Braunwald E, Fauci AS, Martin JB, et al (eds): Harrison's Principles of Internal Medicine, 16th ed. New York, McGraw-Hill, 2005, p 1653

Spencer JA, Chahal R, Kelly A, et al: Evaluation of painful hydronephrosis in pregnancy: Magnetic resonance urographic patterns in physiological dilatation versus calculous obstruction. J Urol 171:256, 2004

Stehman-Breen CO, Levine RJ, Qian C, et al: Increased risk of preeclampsia among nulliparous pregnant women with idiopathic hematuria. Am J Obstet Gynecol 187:703, 2002

Stettler RW, Cunningham FG: Natural history of chronic proteinuria complicating pregnancy. Am J Obstet Gynecol 167:1219, 1992

Stratta P, Canavese C, Quaglia M: Pregnancy in patients with kidney disease. Nephrol 19:135, 2006

Strevens H, Wide-Swensson D, Hansen A, et al: Glomerular endotheliosis in normal pregnancy and pre-eclampsia. Br J Obstet Gynaecol 110:831, 2003

Sturgiss SN, Davison JM: Effect of pregnancy on long-term function of renal allografts. Am J Kidney Dis 26:54, 1995

Surian M, Imbasciati E, Cosci P, et al: Glomerular disease and pregnancy: A study of 123 pregnancies in patients with primary and secondary glomerular diseases. Nephron 36:101, 1984

Swartz MA, Lydon-Rochelle MT, Simon D, et al: Admission for nephrolithiasis in pregnancy and risk of adverse birth outcomes. Obstet Gynecol 109(5):1099, 2007

Tan LK, Kanagalingam D, Tan HK, et al: Obstetric outcomes in women with end-stage renal failure requiring renal dialysis. Int J Gynaecol Obstet 94:17, 2006

Thomas AG, Burrows L, Knight R, et al: The effect of pregnancy on cyclosporine levels in renal allograft patients. Obstet Gynecol 90:916, 1997

Toma H, Tanabe K, Tokumoto T, et al: Pregnancy in women receiving renal dialysis or transplantation in Japan: A nationwide survey. Nephrol Dial Transplant 14(6):1511, 1999

Toth C, Toth G, Varga A, et al: Percutaneous nephrolithotomy in early pregnancy. Int Urol Nephrol 37:1, 2005

Towers CV, Kaminskas CM, Garite TJ, et al: Pulmonary injury associated with antepartum pyelonephritis: Can patients at risk be identified? Am J Obstet Gynecol 164:974, 1991

Trevisan G, Ramos JG, Martins-Costa S, et al: Pregnancy in patients with chronic renal insufficiency at Hospital de Clinicas of Porto Alegre, Brazil. Ren Fail 26:29, 2004

Turney JH, Ellis CM, Parsons FM: Obstetric acute renal failure 1956–1987. Br J Obstet Gynaecol 96:679, 1989

Twickler DM, Lucas MJ, Bowe L, et al: Ultrasonographic evaluation of central and end-organ hemodynamics in antepartum pyelonephritis. Am J Obstet Gynecol 170:814, 1994

U.S. Preventive Services Task Force. Guide to Clinical Preventive Services 2006. Available at: www.ahrq.gov. Accessed September 16, 2008

Van Dorsten JP, Lenke RR, Schifrin BS: Pyelonephritis in pregnancy: The role of in-hospital management and nitrofurantoin suppression. J Reprod Med 32:897, 1987

Vasilou DM, Maxwell C, Prakesykumar S, et al: Goodpasture syndrome in a pregnant woman. Obstet Gynecol 106:1196, 2005

Vasquez JC, Villar J. Treatments for symptomatic urinary tract infections during pregnancy Cochrane Database Syst Rev 3: CD002256, 2006

Vordermark JS, Deshon GE, Agee RE: Management of pregnancy after major urinary reconstruction. Obstet Gynecol 75:564, 1990

Watterson JD, Girvan AR, Beiko DT, et al: Management strategy for ureteral calculi in pregnancy. Urology 60:383, 2002

Whalley PJ: Bacteriuria of pregnancy. Am J Obstet Gynecol 97:723, 1967

Whalley PJ, Martin FG, Peters PC: Significance of asymptomatic bacteriuria detected during pregnancy. JAMA 198:879, 1965

Wilson PD: Polycystic kidney disease. N Engl J Med 350:151, 2004

White WM, Klein FA, Loughlin KR: Urinary stone disease during pregnancy: Evolving management strategies. Contemp Urol 18.6:34, 2006

Wing DA, Hendershott CM, Debuque L, et al: A randomized trial of three antibiotic regimens for the treatment of pyelonephritis in pregnancy. Am J Obstet Gynecol 92:249, 1998

Wing DA, Hendershott CM, Debuque L, et al: Outpatient treatment of acute pyelonephritis in pregnancy after 24 weeks. Obstet Gynecol 94:683, 1999

Wing DA, Park AS, DeBuque L, et al: Limited clinical utility of blood and urine cultures in the treatment of acute pyelonephritis during pregnancy. Am J Obstet Gynecol 182:1437, 2000

Yip S-K, Sahota D, Chang AMZ, et al: Four-year follow-up of women who were diagnosed to have postpartum urinary retention. Am J Obstet Gynecol 187:648, 2002

Zeeman GG, Cunningham FG, Pritchard JA: The magnitude of hemoconcentration with eclampsia. Hypertens Preg 28:127, 2009

Zeeman GG, Wendel GD Jr, Cunningham FG: A blueprint for obstetric critical care. Am J Obstet Gynecol 188:532, 2003

Gastrointestinal Disorders

During normal pregnancy, the gastrointestinal tract and its appendages undergo remarkable anatomical, physiological, and functional changes. These changes, which are discussed in detail in Chapter 5 (p. 125), can appreciably alter clinical findings normally relied on for diagnosis and treatment of gastrointestinal disorders. One example is nausea and vomiting, which is frequent early in normal pregnancy. If these symptoms persist or develop later, they may be erroneously attributed to normal physiological changes, and a serious pregnancy complication or nonobstetrical problem may be overlooked. In another example, most obstetricians, but not most internists or gastroenterologists, are aware that epigastric or right upper quadrant pain can be an ominous sign of severe preeclampsia. Finally, as pregnancy progresses, gastrointestinal symptoms become more difficult to assess, and physical findings are often obscured by the large uterus, which displaces abdominal organs and can alter the location and intensity of pain and tenderness.

GENERAL CONSIDERATIONS

Diagnostic Techniques

In general, gastrointestinal tract evaluation can be completed without reliance on radiological techniques.

Endoscopy

Fiberoptic endoscopic instruments have revolutionized diagnosis and management of most gastrointestinal conditions. They are particularly well suited for use during pregnancy. Cappell (2006) estimates that nearly 20,000 pregnant women annually have indications for endoscopy to evaluate the esophagus, stomach, duodenum, and colon. The proximal jejunum can also be studied, and the ampulla of Vater cannulated to perform *endoscopic retrograde cholangiopancreatography—ERCP* (Al-Hashem and colleagues, 2008). Experience in pregnancy with *videocapsule endoscopy* for small-bowel evaluation is limited (Storch and Barkin, 2006). In most endoscopies, sedation is required, and especial considerations are given to complications unique to pregnancy.

Upper gastrointestinal endoscopy is used for management as well as diagnosis of a number of problems. Common bile duct exploration and drainage are used for choledocholithiasis as described in Chapter 50 (p. 1073). It is also used for sclerotherapy as well as placement of *percutaneous endoscopic gastrostomy (PEG)* tubes. A number of concise reviews have been provided (Bruno and Kroser, 2006; Cappell, 2006; Gilinsky and Muthunayagam, 2006).

Flexible sigmoidoscopy can be used safely in pregnant women (Siddiqui and Denise-Proctor, 2006). *Colonoscopy* is used to view the entire colon and distal ileum for diagnosis and management of inflammatory bowel disease. Bowel preparation is completed using polyethylene glycol electrolyte or sodium phosphate solutions with care to avoid serious maternal dehydration. Reports of colonoscopy during pregnancy are limited, but preliminary results are encouraging, and it should be performed if indicated (Cappell, 2003).

Noninvasive Imaging Techniques

The obvious technique for gastrointestinal evaluation is abdominal sonography. Because computed tomography (CT) use is limited in pregnancy due to radiation exposure, magnetic resonance (MR) imaging is now commonly used for evaluating the abdomen and retroperitoneal space. These and other imaging modalities, and their safety for use in pregnancy, are considered in detail in Chapter 41 (p. 915).

Laparotomy and Laparoscopy

Surgery is lifesaving for certain gastrointestinal conditions—perforative appendicitis being the most common example. In the first study using the Swedish Registry database through 1981, Mazze and Källén (1989) reported that abdominal exploration by laparotomy or laparoscopy was performed in 1331 of 720,000 pregnancies—approximately 1 in every 500. Kort and associates (1993) reported a similar incidence of 1 in 635 in nearly 50,000 pregnancies. In both studies, the most common indications for surgery were appendicitis, an adnexal mass, and cholecystitis.

Laparoscopic procedures have replaced traditional surgical techniques for many abdominal disorders during pregnancy (Carter and Soper, 2004). In the updated report from the Swedish Registry database, Reedy and associates (1997) described 2181 pregnant women who underwent laparoscopy and 1522 who had laparotomy for nonobstetrical indications. The incidence for all procedures was similar to their first study—approximately 1 in every 800 pregnancies. Both were mostly performed before 20 weeks, and they were found to be safe. Finally, long-term surveillance studies suggest no deleterious effects for either mother or child (Rizzo, 2003).

The most common nongynecological procedures performed during pregnancy are cholecystectomy and appendectomy (Fatum and Rojansky, 2001; Rollins and associates, 2004). For more details and for descriptions of surgical technique, see Chapter 41 (p. 913) as well as *Operative Obstetrics*, 2nd edition (Gilstrap and colleagues, 2002). Guidelines for diagnosis, treatment, and use of laparoscopy for surgical problems during pregnancy have been provided by the Society of American Gastrointestinal and Endoscopic Surgeons (2008).

Nutritional Support

Specialized nutritional support can be delivered *enterally*, usually via nasogastric tube feedings, or intravenously with peripheral or central venous access. When possible, enteral alimentation is preferable because it has fewer serious complications (Hamaoui and Hamaoui, 2003; Vaisman and co-workers, 2004). In obstetrical patients, very few conditions prohibit enteral nutrition as a first effort to prevent catabolism.

The purpose of *parenteral feeding*, or *hyperalimentation*, is to provide nutrition when the intestinal tract must be kept quiescent. Peripheral venous access may be adequate for short-term supplemental nutrition, which derives calories from isotonic fat solutions. Central venous access is necessary for total parenteral nutrition because its hyperosmolarity requires rapid dilution in a high-flow vascular system. These solutions provide 24 to 40 kcal/kg/day, principally as a hypertonic glucose solution. Heyland and colleagues (1998) reviewed 26 randomized trials involving more than 2200 critically ill nonpregnant patients and reported that overall mortality rates were not influenced by parenteral nutrition.

Parenteral Nutrition During Pregnancy

There have been a variety of conditions for which total parenteral nutrition was employed during pregnancy (Table 49-1). Gastrointestinal disorders are the most common indication, and in the many studies cited, duration of feeding averaged 33 days. **It is imperative to emphasize that complications of par-**

TABLE 49-1. Some Conditions Treated with Parenteral Nutrition During Pregnancy

Anorexia nervosa	Jejunoileal bypass
Appendiceal rupture	Malignancies
Bowel obstruction	Pancreatitis
Burns	Preeclampsia syndrome
Cholecystitis	Preterm labor/ruptured
Crohn disease	membranes
Diabetic gastropathy	Short bowel syndrome
Esophageal injury	Small bowel obstruction
Hyperemesis gravidarum	Stroke

From Kirby (1988), Ogura (2003), and Russo-Stieglitz (1999), and all their colleagues.

enteral nutrition are frequent and they may be severe. The myriad gastrointestinal complications were recently reviewed by Guglielmi and colleagues (2006). And Russo-Stieglitz and associates (1999) described 26 pregnancies with a 50-percent rate of complications, which include pneumothorax, hemothorax, and brachial plexus injury. The most frequent serious complication is catheter sepsis, and Folk and co-workers (2004) described a 25-percent incidence in 27 women with hyperemesis gravidarum. Although bacterial sepsis is most common, *Candida* septicemia has been described (Paranyuk and associates, 2006). The Centers for Disease Control and Prevention (2002) has published detailed guidelines for management to prevent catheter-related sepsis. Perinatal complications are uncommon, however, fetal subdural hematoma caused by maternal vitamin K deficiency was described by Sakai and colleagues (2003).

There is also appreciable morbidity from a *peripherally inserted central catheter (PICC)*. Ogura and colleagues (2003) reported infection with long-term access in 31 of 52 pregnant women. Holmgren and co-workers (2008) reported complications in 21 of 33 women in whom a PICC line was placed for hyperemesis. Infections were the most common, and half of infected women also had bacteremia. From their review of 48 reports of nonpregnant adults, Turcotte and associates (2006) concluded that there were no advantages to peripherally placed catheters compared with centrally placed ones.

DISORDERS OF THE UPPER GASTROINTESTINAL TRACT

Hyperemesis Gravidarum

In most women, mild to moderate nausea and vomiting are especially common until approximately 16 weeks (see Chap. 8, p. 210). In some women, however, it is severe and unresponsive to simple dietary modification and antiemetics. In an attempt to quantify the severity of nausea and vomiting, Lacasse and colleagues (2008) have proposed a PUQE scoring index—Pregnancy-Unique Quantification of Emesis and Nausea. *Hyperemesis gravidarum* is defined variably as vomiting sufficiently severe to produce weight loss, dehydration, alkalosis from loss of hydrochloric acid, and hypokalemia. Acidosis develops from partial starvation (Chihara and co-workers, 2003). In some women, transient hepatic dysfunction develops (see Chap. 50, p. 1063).

Population incidences vary, and there appears to be an ethnic or familial predilection (Grjibovski and co-workers, 2008). In population-based studies from California and Nova Scotia, the hospitalization rate for hyperemesis was 0.5 to 0.8 percent (Bailit, 2005; Fell and co-workers, 2006). Hospitalization is less common in obese women (Cedergren and associates, 2008). In women hospitalized in a previous pregnancy for hyperemesis, up to 20 percent require hospitalization in a subsequent pregnancy (Dodds and associates, 2006; Trogstad and co-workers, 2005).

Hyperemesis appears to be related to high or rapidly rising serum levels of pregnancy-related hormones. Although the exact stimulus is unknown, putative culprits include human chorionic gonadotropin (hCG), estrogens, progesterone, leptin, placental growth hormone, prolactin, thyroxine, and adrenocortical hormones (Verberg and associates, 2005). Studies by Goodwin and co-workers (2008) implicate the vestibular system. There seems to be no doubt that in some but not nearly all severe cases, there are interrelated psychological components (Buckwalter and Simpson, 2002). In some, hyperemesis is given as a reason for elective termination (Poursharif and colleagues, 2007). Other factors that increase the risk for admission include hyperthyroidism, previous molar pregnancy, diabetes, gastrointestinal illnesses, and asthma (Fell and co-workers, 2006). And for unknown reasons, a female fetus increases the risk by 1.5-fold (Schiff and colleagues, 2004; Tan and co-workers, 2006).

Helicobacter pylori Infection

An association of *H. pylori* infection has been proposed, but evidence is not conclusive. Goldberg and colleagues (2007) performed a scholarly systematic review of 14 case-control studies. Although the analysis indicated an association between *H. pylori* and hyperemesis, heterogenicity between study groups was extensive. At this time, we do not test for or treat for gastric infection in women with hyperemesis. Certainly, the "cocktail(s)" required for eradication would most likely *cause* vomiting in most pregnant women.

Somewhat unrelated, Ponzetto and colleagues (2006) reported that *H. pylori* seropositivity was linked to an increased risk for preeclampsia. In the population-based California study by Dodds and associates (2006), however, the incidence of gestational hypertension was not different from that in control women. *H. pylori* infection has also been linked to iron deficiency in pregnancy (Weyermann and associates, 2005).

Complications

Vomiting may be prolonged, frequent, and severe. Plasma zinc levels are increased, copper levels decreased, and magnesium levels unchanged (Dokmeci and associates, 2004). Preliminary findings are that a third of women with hyperemesis have an abnormal electroencephalogram (EEG) (Vaknin and colleagues, 2006). A list of potentially fatal complications is given in Table 49-2. Various degrees of acute renal failure from dehydration are encountered, and we have cared for a number of women with markedly impaired renal function. The extreme example, which was described by Hill and colleagues (2002), is a woman who required 5 days of dialysis when her serum crea-

TABLE 49-2. Some Life-Threatening Complications of Recalcitrant Hyperemesis Gravidarum

Depression—cause versus effect?
Esophageal rupture—Boerhaave syndrome
Hypoprothrombinemia—vitamin K
Hyperalimentation complications
Mallory-Weiss tears—bleeding, pneumothorax, pneumomediastinum, pneumopericardium
Renal failure—may require dialysis
Wernicke encephalopathy—thiamine deficiency

tinine level rose to 10.7 mg/dL. Life-threatening complications of continuous retching include *Mallory-Weiss tears,* such as shown in Figure 49-1. Others are *esophageal rupture, pneumothorax,* and *pneumomediastinum* (Schwartz and Rossoff, 1994; Yamamoto and colleagues, 2001).

At least two serious vitamin deficiencies have been reported with hyperemesis in pregnancy. *Wernicke encephalopathy* from thiamine deficiency is not uncommon. Chiossi and colleagues (2006) reviewed 49 cases and reported that only half had the triad of confusion, ocular findings, and ataxia. Usually, there are MR imaging findings. At least three maternal deaths have been described, and long-term sequelae are common and include blindness, convulsions, and coma (Selitsky and co-workers, 2006). *Vitamin K deficiency* has been reported causing maternal coagulopathy and fetal intracranial hemorrhage (Kawamura, 2008; Robinson, 1998; Sakai, 2003, and all their colleagues).

Management

Methods to control nausea and vomiting of early pregnancy are discussed in Chapter 8 (see p. 210). A Cochrane Database review by Jewell and Young (2000) confirmed a salutary effect from a number of antiemetics given orally or by rectal suppository as first-line agents. When simple measures fail, intravenous

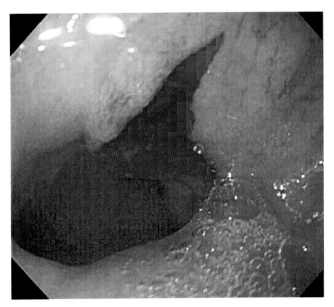

FIGURE 49-1 Endoscopic view of Mallory-Weiss tear. (From Michel and co-workers, 2008, with permission.)

crystalloid solutions are given to correct dehydration, ketonemia, electrolyte deficits, and acid-base imbalances. Thiamine, 100 mg, is given to prevent Wernicke encephalopathy previously discussed.

If vomiting persists after rehydration and failed outpatient management, hospitalization is recommended (American College of Obstetricians and Gynecologists, 2004). Antiemetics such as promethazine, prochlorperazine, chlorpromazine, or metoclopramide are given parenterally. There is little evidence that treatment with *glucocorticosteroids* is effective. Two small trials found no benefits of *methylprednisolone* compared with placebo, but the steroid-treated group had significantly fewer readmissions (Duggar and Carlan, 2001; Safari and co-workers, 1998). In a study of 110 women at Parkland Hospital, Yost and colleagues (2003) compared placebo with intravenous methylprednisolone plus tapered oral steroids. A third in each group required readmission. In a study by Bondok and co-workers (2006), pulsed hydrocortisone therapy was superior to metoclopramide to reduce vomiting and readmissions. *Serotonin antagonists* are the most effective agents for controlling chemotherapy-induced nausea and vomiting (Hesketh, 2008). When used in one trial for hyperemesis gravidarum, however, *ondansetron* was not superior to promethazine (Sullivan and associates, 1996). Reports of serotonin antagonist use in pregnancy are limited, but there is no evidence of teratogenicity (Briggs and associates, 2005; Mahadevan and Kane, 2006).

With persistent vomiting after hospitalization, appropriate steps should be taken to exclude possible underlying diseases as a cause of hyperemesis. Endoscopy did not change management in 49 women reported by Debby and co-workers (2008). Examples include gastroenteritis, cholecystitis, pancreatitis, hepatitis, peptic ulcer, and pyelonephritis. In addition, severe preeclampsia and fatty liver are considerations after midpregnancy. And although clinical thyrotoxicosis has been implicated as a cause of hyperemesis, it is more likely that abnormally elevated serum thyroxine levels are a surrogate for higher-than-average serum hCG levels (see Chap. 3, p. 63). Tan and colleagues (2002) have described this as "chemical hyperthyroidism." And of interest, Panesar and associates (2006) showed that a cohort of women with hyperemesis had lower serum thyrotropin levels. In our experiences, serum free thyroxine levels normalize quickly with hydration.

Following treatment, most women have had a salutary response and may be sent home with antiemetic therapy. Their readmission rate is 25 to 35 percent in most prospective studies.

If associated psychiatric and social factors contribute to the illness, the woman usually improves remarkably while hospitalized, but may relapse after discharge. In these women, assistance with psychosocial problems is beneficial (Swallow and co-workers, 2004).

Nutritional Support

In the small percentage of women who continue to have recalcitrant vomiting, consideration is given for enteral nutrition as discussed on page 1050. Vaisman and co-workers (2004) described successful use of nasojejunal feeding for up to 21 days in 11 such women. *Percutaneous endoscopic gastrostomy with a jejunal port—PEG (J) tube*—was described by Schrag and co-workers (2007).

In our experiences, only a very few women will require parenteral nutrition. In their study of 166 women, Folk and colleagues (2004) reported that in 16 percent, central venous access was established for nutrition. The litany of complications included line sepsis in 25 percent and thrombosis and infective endocarditis in one woman each.

Reflux Esophagitis

Heartburn, or *pyrosis*, is common in late pregnancy. The retrosternal burning sensation is caused by esophagitis from gastroesophageal reflux related to relaxation of the lower esophageal sphincter (Hytten, 1991). Common folklore has held that women with excessive heartburn give birth to infants with more hair. And although this may seem strange, Costigan and associates (2006) recently confirmed this! They proposed a shared biological mechanism. Pregnancy hormones caused both relaxation of the esophageal sphincter—thus more reflux, more heartburn, and they also modulated hair growth.

Symptoms usually respond to raising the head of the bed and treatment with oral antacids. If severe symptoms persist, an H_2-receptor antagonist such as *cimetidine* or *ranitidine* is prescribed. These are considered safe, but *misoprostol* is contraindicated because it may stimulate labor (see Chap. 22, p. 503). The commonly used proton-pump inhibitor, *omeprazole*, is also safe for use in pregnancy (Diav-Citrin and associates, 2005; Mahadevan and Kane, 2006). If there still is no relief, then endoscopy should be considered.

Biertho and associates (2006) described 25 women who had undergone laparoscopic Nissen fundoplication for reflux prior to pregnancy. Only 20 percent had reflux symptoms requiring antacids during pregnancy.

Hiatal Hernia

The older literature is informative here. Rigler and Eneboe (1935) performed upper gastrointestinal radiographs in 195 women in late pregnancy. Almost 20 percent of 116 multiparas and 5 percent of 79 nulliparas had a hiatal hernia. Notably, in only three of 10 women, a hernia persisted for 1 to 18 months postpartum.

The relationship of hiatal hernia with reflux esophagitis, and thus symptoms, is not clear. Cohen and Harris (1971) demonstrated no relationship between reflux and hernia and showed that the lower esophageal sphincter functioned effectively even when displaced intrathoracically. Nevertheless, during pregnancy, these hiatal hernias may cause vomiting, epigastric pain, and bleeding from ulceration. Curran and colleagues (1999) described a 30-week pregnancy complicated by gastric outlet obstruction from a paraesophageal hernia, which they subsequently successfully repaired. Biertho and associates (2006) reported a woman with a prior Nissen fundoplication whose pregnancy was complicated by gastric herniation into the thoracic cavity. Emergency surgical intervention was followed by spontaneous abortion.

Diaphragmatic Hernia

These are caused by herniations of abdominal contents through either the foramen of Bochdalek or foramen of Morgagni. Fortunately, they rarely complicate pregnancy. Kurzel and associates

(1988) reviewed the outcomes of 18 pregnant women with such a hernia and who developed acute obstruction. Because the maternal mortality rate was 45 percent, they recommend repair during pregnancy even if a woman is asymptomatic. Flick and co-workers (1999) reported a 23-week pregnancy complicated by maternal intrathoracic bowel herniation through an old traumatic diaphragmatic defect. Finally, several case reports describe spontaneous diaphragmatic rupture from increased intra-abdominal pressure during delivery (Ortega-Carnicer, 1998; Sharifah, 2003; Watkin, 1993, and all their colleagues).

Achalasia

The word literally means "failure to relax." Achalasia is a motility disorder in which the lower esophageal sphincter fails to relax properly with swallowing, and there are nonperistaltic contractions of the esophageal muscularis (Khudyak and colleagues, 2006). The defect is caused by inflammatory destruction of the myenteric, that is, Auerbach plexus, of smooth muscle of the lower esophagus and its sphincter. Postganglionic cholinergic neurons are unaffected; thus, there is unopposed sphincter stimulation. Symptoms are dysphagia, chest pain, and regurgitation. Barium swallow radiography demonstrates "bird beak" or "ace of spades" narrowing at the distal esophagus. Endoscopy is performed to exclude gastric carcinoma, and manometry is confirmatory. If dilatation of the esophagus and medical therapy does not provide relief, myotomy is considered (Torquati and associates, 2006).

Pregnancy

Normal relaxation of the lower esophageal sphincter during pregnancy theoretically should not occur with achalasia. Even so, in most women, pregnancy does not seem to worsen achalasia. Mayberry and Atkinson (1987) interviewed 20 affected women who reported no excessive reflux esophagitis. In their review of 35 pregnancies, Khudyak and colleagues (2006) described most as symptom free, although esophageal dilatation was needed in a few. A maternal death at 24 weeks associated with a 14-cm diameter megaesophagus was described by Fassina and Osculati (1995).

Management includes soft diet and anticholinergic drugs. With persistent symptoms, other options include nitrates, calcium-channel antagonists, and botulinum toxin injection (Khudyak and co-workers, 2006). Balloon dilatation of the sphincter may be necessary, and 85 percent of nonpregnant patients respond to this. Satin and colleagues (1992) and Fiest and associates (1993) reported successful use of pneumatic dilatation in pregnancy. It is important to remember that esophageal perforation is a serious complication of dilatation.

Peptic Ulcer

Erosive ulcer disease more often involves the duodenum rather than the stomach in young women. Gastroduodenal ulcers in nonpregnant women may be caused by chronic gastritis from *H. pylori*, or they develop from use of aspirin or other nonsteroidal anti-inflammatory drugs. Neither is common in pregnancy (McKenna and colleagues, 2003; Weyermann and asso-

ciates, 2003). Acid secretion is also important, and thus the efficacy of antisecretory agents (Suerbaum and Michetti, 2002).

Gastroprotection during pregnancy is probably due to reduced gastric acid secretion, decreased motility, and considerably increased mucus secretion (Hytten, 1991). Despite this, Cappell and Garcia (1998) theorize that ulcer disease may be underdiagnosed because of frequent treatment for reflux esophagitis. In the past 40 years at Parkland Hospital, during which time we have cared for more than 400,000 pregnant women, we have encountered very few who had symptomatic ulcer disease. Before appropriate therapy was commonplace, Clark (1953) studied 313 pregnancies in 118 women with proven ulcer disease and reported a clear remission during pregnancy in almost 90 percent. Benefits were short lived, however, and symptoms recurred in over half by 3 months postpartum and in almost all by 2 years.

Management

Antacids are first-line therapy, and H_2-receptor blockers are prescribed for those who do not respond. Proton-pump inhibitors are effective, and at least two studies have shown no apparent teratogenic effects (Diav-Citrin and co-workers, 2005; Mahadevan and Kane, 2006). *Sucralfate* is the aluminum salt of sulfated sucrose that provides a protective coating at the ulcer base. Only approximately 10 percent of the aluminum salt is absorbed, and it is considered safe for pregnant women.

With active ulcers, a search for *H. pylori* is undertaken. Diagnostic aids include the urea breath test, serological testing, or endoscopic biopsy. If any of these are positive, antimicrobial therapy is indicated. There are a number of effective oral treatment regimens that do not include tetracycline and that can be used during pregnancy. These include amoxicillin, 1000 mg twice daily; clarithromycin, 500 mg twice daily; or metronidazole, 500 mg twice daily, used in paired combination for 7 days (Dzieniszewski and Jarosz, 2006).

Upper Gastrointestinal Bleeding

Occasionally, persistent vomiting is accompanied by worrisome upper gastrointestinal bleeding (see p. 1051). Occasionally, there is a bleeding peptic ulceration. However, most of these women have small linear mucosal tears near the gastroesophageal junction—*Mallory-Weiss tears* (see Fig. 49-1). Bleeding usually responds promptly to conservative measures, including iced saline irrigations, topical antacids, and intravenously administered H_2-blockers. Transfusions may be needed, and if there is persistent bleeding, then endoscopy is indicated (O'Mahony, 2007). With persistent retching, the less common, but more serious, esophageal rupture—*Boerhaave syndrome*—may develop from greatly increased esophageal pressure.

DISORDERS OF THE SMALL BOWEL AND COLON

The small bowel has diminished motility during pregnancy. Using a nonabsorbable carbohydrate, Lawson and colleagues (1985) showed that small bowel mean transit times were 99, 125, and 137 minutes in each trimester, compared with 75 minutes when nonpregnant. In a study cited by Everson (1992), mean transit time for a mercury-filled balloon from the stomach to the cecum was 58 hours in term pregnant women compared with 52 hours in nonpregnant women.

Muscular relaxation of the colon is accompanied by increased absorption of water and sodium that predisposes to constipation, which is reported by almost 40 percent of women at some time during pregnancy (Everson, 1992). Such symptoms are usually only mildly bothersome, and preventive measures include a high-fiber diet and bulk-forming laxatives. Treatment options have been reviewed by Wald (2003). We have encountered several pregnant women who developed megacolon from impacted stool. These women almost invariably had chronically abused stimulatory laxatives.

Infectious Diarrhea

The large variety of viruses, bacteria, helminths, and protozoa that cause diarrhea in adults inevitably afflict pregnant women.

For example, the incidence of *Clostridium difficile* pseudomembranous colitis has tripled in the past decade (Kelly and LaMont, 2008). Travelers diarrhea is usually mild and responds to loperamide (Medical Letter, 2008). These are discussed in Chapter 58.

Inflammatory Bowel Disease

The two presumably noninfectious forms of intestinal inflammation are *ulcerative colitis* and *Crohn disease*. The latter also is known as regional enteritis, Crohn ileitis, and granulomatous colitis. Differentiation between the two is important because treatment is not the same. That said, they both share common factors, and sometimes it is impossible to distinguish them if Crohn disease involves the colon. The salient clinical and laboratory features shown in Table 49-3 permit a reasonably confident diagnostic differentiation in most cases. The etiopathogenesis of both disorders is enigmatic, but there is genetic predisposition toward either. Inflammation is thought to result

TABLE 49-3. Some Differentiating Characteristics of Ulcerative Colitis and Crohn Disease

Characteristic	Ulcerative Colitis	Crohn Disease
Genetics and heredity	Polygenic; 6–20% monozygous twin concordance; HLA Bw35, B27, DR2; chromosomes 3,5,7,12,16	Polygenic; 50–58% monozygous twins; HLA A2, B27, DR5, DQ1; chromosome 16 (*IBD1–IBD9*)
Natural History		
Bowel involvement	Large bowel mucosa and submucosa; continuous involvement beginning at rectum (40% proctitis only)	Small and large bowel mucosa and deeper layers; transmural involvement common; may affect small or large bowel only, or both; discontinuous and segmental involvement; strictures or fistulas common
Colonoscopy	Mucosal erythema with granularity and friability with superficial ulceration; rectal involvement almost always	Patchy involvement; rectum usually spared; perianal involvement common
Symptoms	Diarrhea with blood or mucus; tenesmus	Cramping abdominal pain and watery diarrhea; vomiting; malnutrition; low-grade fever; weight loss
Clinical course	Exacerbations and remission; acute and intermittent common; may be chronic and unremitting	Exacerbations and remission; surgery commonly required
Extraintestinal manifestations	Arthritis; erythema nodosum; pyoderma gangrenosum; uveitis	Arthritis; erythema nodosum; uveitis; anemia; carcinoma
Serum antibodies	Antineutrophil cytoplasm-antibody (pANCA) ~70%	Anti-*Saccharomyces cerevisiae* ~50%
Complications	Toxic megacolon (5%); strictures; reactive arthritis; sclerosing cholangitis; cancer (3–5%)	Fistulas; reactive arthritis; toxic megacolon
Management	Medical; proctocolectomy curative	Medical; segmental resection if indicated

HLA = human leukocyte antigen; IBD = inflammatory bowel disease.
From Farrell and Peppercorn (2002), Friedman and Blumberg (2008), Lichtenstein and colleagues, 2009; and Podolsky (2002).

from inappropriate response of the mucosal immune system to normal bacterial flora, with or without an autoimmune component (Friedman and Blumberg, 2008).

Ulcerative Colitis

Inflammation is confined to the superficial luminal layers of the colon, typically beginning at the rectum and extending proximally for a variable distance. Half of afflicted patients have disease confined to the rectum and rectosigmoid. Endoscopic findings include mucosal granularity and friability interspersed with mucosal ulcerations and a mucopurulent exudate. The extent of inflammation is proportional to symptoms, and bloody diarrhea is the cardinal presenting finding. The disease is characterized by exacerbations and remissions. For unknown reasons, prior appendectomy protects against development of ulcerative colitis (Selby and colleagues, 2002). *Toxic megacolon* is a particularly dangerous complication that frequently necessitates colectomy. *Extraintestinal manifestations* include arthritis, uveitis, and erythema nodosum. Another serious problem is that the risk of cancer approaches 1 percent per year.

Management. Ulcerative colitis is treated medically. Drugs that deliver 5-aminosalicyclic acid (5-ASA) or mesalamine are used for active colitis as well as maintenance therapy. *Sulfasalazine* is the prototype, and its 5-ASA moiety inhibits prostaglandin synthase in the colon. Glucocorticoids are given orally, parenterally, or by enema for more severe disease that does not respond to 5-ASA. Immunomodulating drugs, including *azathioprine, 6-mercaptopurine, cyclosporine,* and *methotrexate,* are used in conjunction with prednisone in nonpregnant patients for maintenance. High-dose intravenous cyclosporine may be beneficial for severely ill patients and used in lieu of colectomy. For recalcitrant disease, proctocolectomy is performed, and a permanent ileostomy or an ileoanal anastomosis with a continent ileal pouch is created. Within the past few years, the anti-tumor necrosis factor (TNF) antibody *infliximab* has been reported to be modestly effective for treatment and maintenance of moderate to severe active disease (Rutgeerts and colleagues, 2005, 2009).

Crohn Disease

This disorder has more protean manifestations than ulcerative colitis. It involves not only the bowel mucosa but also the deeper layers, and sometimes there is transmural involvement. The disease is typically segmental. Approximately 30 percent of patients have small-bowel involvement, 25 percent have isolated colon involvement, and 40 percent have both, usually with the terminal ileum and colon involved.

Symptoms depend on which bowel segment(s) is involved. Thus, complaints may include cramping abdominal pain, diarrhea, weight loss, low-grade fever, and obstructive symptoms. The disease is chronic with exacerbations and remissions and importantly, it cannot be cured medically or surgically (Lichtenstein and associates, 2009). Almost 30 percent of patients require surgery during the first year after diagnosis, and thereafter, 5 percent per year require surgery. Reactive arthritis is common, and the risk of cancer, although not as great as with ulcerative colitis, is increased substantively.

Management. There is no regimen that is universally effective for maintenance during asymptomatic periods. *Sulfasalazine* is effective for some, but the newer 5-ASA formulations are better tolerated. As a class, they appear to be safe in pregnancy (Rahimi and associates, 2008). *Prednisone* therapy may control moderate to severe flares, but is less effective for small-bowel involvement. Immunomodulators such as *azathioprine, 6-mercaptopurine, methotrexate,* and *cyclosporine* are used for active disease and for maintenance (Prefontaine and colleagues, 2009). With the exception of methotrexate, most of these drugs appear relatively safe during pregnancy (Briggs and co-workers, 2005; Moskovitz and associates, 2004). Methotrexate is category X as discussed in Chapter 14 (p. 320). In the past few years, anti-TNF-α antibodies, which include *infliximab, adatimumab,* and *certolizumab,* have been found effective for active Crohn disease and maintenance (Sandborn, 2007; Sands, 2004; Schreiber, 2007, and all their colleagues). This class of immunomodulators is considered category B, but data supporting safety in pregnancy are limited (Roux and colleagues, 2007).

Conservative surgery is indicated for complications. Patients with small-bowel involvement more likely will require surgery for complications that include fistulas, strictures, abscesses, and intractable disease. Some develop perineal communications that interfere with vaginal delivery (Forsnes and co-workers, 1999).

Inflammatory Bowel Disease and Fertility

Subfertility is commonly linked to any chronic medical disease (Bradley and Rosen, 2004). Despite this, Mahadevan (2006) cited a normal fertility rate unless surgery is performed for bowel disease. It may also be partially due to sulfasalazine, which causes reversible sperm abnormalities (Feagins and Kane, 2009). Alstead and Nelson-Piercy (2003) reported that decreased female fertility from active Crohn disease returned to normal with remission. After ileal pouch-anal anastomosis, however, up to half of women with ulcerative colitis are infertile (Waljee and associates, 2006). Thus, subfertility may be associated with active or severe disease.

Inflammatory Bowel Disease and Pregnancy

Both disorders are relatively common in young women and thus are encountered during pregnancy. In this regard, a few generalizations can be made. The consensus is that pregnancy does not increase the likelihood of an inflammatory bowel disease flare. Pertinent to this, Riis and colleagues (2006) performed a 10-year surveillance of women in the European Collaborative on Inflammatory Bowel Disease. The likelihood of a flare during pregnancy was decreased compared with their preconceptional course. This diminished rate persisted for years after pregnancy and was attributed to close attention and monitoring of enrolled patients. Although most women with quiescent disease in early pregnancy uncommonly have relapses, when a flare develops, it may be severe. Conversely, active disease in early pregnancy increases the likelihood of poor pregnancy outcome. In general, most usual treatment regimens may be continued during pregnancy. If needed to direct management, diagnostic evaluations should be undertaken, and if indicated, surgery should be performed.

Regarding effects on pregnancy, it is likely that overall, adverse perinatal outcomes are increased. Kornfeld and co-workers (1997) described outcomes in a population-based cohort study of 756 Swedish women with preexisting ulcerative colitis or Crohn disease. Rates of preterm birth, low birthweight, fetal-growth restriction, and cesarean delivery were all increased 1.5- to 2-fold. According to Reddy and associates (2008), these are more likely in women with multiple recurrences. Mahadevan and colleagues (2005) reported similar findings from a population-based Northern California study. Bush (2004) and Elbaz (2005) and their co-workers also confirmed these observations. Importantly, despite these results, perinatal mortality rates were not increased in either study. Also, there is evidence that much of this excessive morbidity is attributable to Crohn disease (Dominitz and associates, 2002; Fonager and co-workers, 1998).

Ulcerative Colitis and Pregnancy. There is no evidence to suggest that pregnancy has any significant effects on ulcerative colitis. In a meta-analysis of 755 pregnancies, Fonager and colleagues (1998) reported that ulcerative colitis quiescent at conception worsened in approximately a third of pregnancies. In women with active disease at the time of conception, approximately 45 percent worsened, 25 percent remained unchanged, and only 25 percent improved. These observations were similar to those previously described in an extensive review by Miller (1986).

Management for colitis for the most part is the same as for nonpregnancy. Flares may be caused by psychogenic stress and reassurance is important. *Calcium supplementation* is provided because osteoporosis is common. Maintenance of colitis is continued with 5-ASA derivatives, and flares are treated with corticosteroids. Recalcitrant disease is treated with immunomodulators as discussed on page 1055. Okada and associates (2006) described a dramatic response in a 13-week pregnant woman treated with *leukocytapheresis*. Parenteral nutrition may be necessary for women with prolonged exacerbations (see p. 1050).

Colorectal endoscopy is performed as indicated (Katz, 2002). Colectomy for fulminant colitis may be lifesaving, and it has been performed during each trimester. Dozois and colleagues (2005) reviewed 42 such cases and found that, in general, outcomes have been good in reports published after 1980. Most women underwent partial or complete colectomy, but decompression colostomy with ileostomy was described by Ooi and co-workers (2003) in a 10- and a 16-week pregnancy.

Proctocolectomy improves sexual function and fertility (Cornish and co-workers, 2007). Women who have had a colectomy and ileal pouch–anal anastomosis can safely deliver vaginally. Hahnloser and colleagues (2004) reviewed routes of delivery in women with 235 pregnancies before and 232 pregnancies after continent pouch surgery. Functional outcomes were similar, and these researchers concluded that cesarean delivery should be for obstetrical indications. In at least one case, however, adhesions to the growing uterus led to pouch perforation (Aouthmany and Horattas, 2004). *Pouchitis* is an inflammatory condition of the ileoanal pouch, probably due to bacterial proliferation, stasis, and endotoxin release. It usually responds to cephalosporins or metronidazole.

By most accounts, ulcerative colitis has minimal adverse effects on pregnancy outcome. Modigliani (2000) reviewed outcomes in 2398 pregnancies in women with colitis. Perinatal outcomes were not substantively different from those in the general obstetrical population. Specifically, the incidences of spontaneous abortion, preterm delivery, and stillbirths were remarkably low. In a population-based cohort study from Washington state, Dominitz and co-workers (2002) described pregnancy outcomes in 107 women with ulcerative colitis. With two exceptions, perinatal outcomes were similar to those of 1308 normal pregnancies. One exception was an inexplicably increased incidence of congenital malformations, and the other was a the cesarean delivery rate that was increased from 20 to 29 percent compared with controls.

Crohn Disease and Pregnancy. There is no evidence that pregnancy affects Crohn disease. One report suggested that disease activity might even be decreased (Agret and colleagues, 2005). In general, disease activity is related to its status around the time of conception. In their cohort study, Fonager and associates (1998) analyzed outcomes in 279 pregnancies based on disease activity at conception. For 186 women whose disease was inactive at conception, only a fourth relapsed during pregnancy. In contrast, of the 93 with active disease at conception, two thirds either worsened or had no change. Miller (1986) had described similar findings from his earlier review.

Maintenance therapy is similar to that for nonpregnant women. Oral or topical 5-ASA derivatives, usually with azathioprine, 6-mercaptopurine, or cyclosporine, are continued as they appear to be safe during pregnancy (Briggs and colleagues, 2005). Methotrexate is contraindicated, and recently mycophenolate mofetil and mycophenolic acid have been reported to cause serious congenital anomalies (Food and Drug Administration, 2008). These are discussed further in Chapter 14 (p. 317). Katz and co-workers (2004) described treatment with the monoclonal antibody infliximab in 96 pregnancies. In 31 of these, treatment was given in the first trimester with no adverse sequelae. Calcium supplementation is given to combat osteoporosis. Parenteral hyperalimentation has been used successfully during severe recurrences (Russo-Stieglitz and colleagues, 1999). Endoscopy or surgery is performed as indicated. An abdominal surgical procedure was required during 5 percent of pregnancies described by Woolfson and colleagues (1990). In one instance, a woman with known Crohn disease at 32 weeks underwent emergent cesarean delivery for a presumed abruption. Instead, an abscess was found around the hepatic flexure (Panayotidis and Triantafyllidis, 2006).

As discussed previously, Crohn disease is associated with increased adverse perinatal outcomes usually related to disease activity. Based on a 20-year review, Korelitz (1998) concluded that perinatal outcomes were generally good with quiescent disease. That said, in the case-control Danish study, Norgård and colleagues (2007) reported a twofold risk of preterm neonates. Dominitz and co-workers (2002) reported a two- to threefold increase in preterm delivery, low birthweight, and fetal-growth restriction in fetuses of 149 women with Crohn disease. The rate of cesarean delivery in this study was also increased compared with normal controls—28 versus 20 percent. As discussed subsequently, women with an ileal loop colostomy may have significant problems. Women with perianal fistula—unless these are rectovaginal—usually can undergo vaginal delivery without complications (Takahashi and colleagues, 2007).

Ostomy and Pregnancy

A colostomy or an ileostomy can be problematic during pregnancy because of its location. Gopal and colleagues (1985) described 82 pregnancies in 66 women with an ostomy. Although stomal dysfunction was common, it responded to conservative management in all cases. But surgical intervention was necessary in three of six women who developed bowel obstruction and in another four with ileostomy prolapse—almost 10 percent overall. Although only a third of 82 women underwent cesarean delivery, Takahashi and associates (2007) described six of seven cesarean deliveries in women with enterostoma created for Crohn disease.

Colectomy with mucosal proctectomy and ileal pouch-anal anastomosis is the preferred surgical procedure for ulcerative colitis and familial colonic polyposis. As discussed on page 1056, Hahnloser (2004) and Ravid (2002) and their colleagues have described pregnancies in such women. Disadvantages include frequent bowel movements, fecal incontinence including nocturnal soilage in almost half of patients, and pouchitis. Although these disadvantages temporarily worsened during pregnancy, they abated postpartum. Importantly, Farouk and associates (2000) reported that pregnancy did not worsen long-term ostomy function. Most have concluded that vaginal delivery is acceptable in these women.

Intestinal Obstruction

The incidence of bowel obstruction is not increased during pregnancy, although it generally is more difficult to diagnose. Meyerson and colleagues (1995) reported a 20-year incidence of 1 in 17,000 deliveries at two Detroit hospitals. As shown in Table 49-4, approximately half of cases are due to adhesions from previous pelvic surgery that includes cesarean delivery. When

women of all ages are considered, small-bowel obstruction eventually develops in only 1 per 1000 cesarean deliveries performed (Al-Sunaidi and Tulandi, 2006). Another 25 percent of bowel obstruction is caused by volvulus—sigmoid, cecal, or small bowel. These have been reported in late pregnancy or early puerperium (Alshawi, 2005; Biswas, 2006; Lal, 2006, and all their colleagues). Intussusception is occasionally encountered (Gould and co-workers, 2008). A degenerating uterine leiomyoma causing small-bowel obstruction was described by MacDonald and associates, (2004).

Etiopathogenesis

Most cases of intestinal obstruction during pregnancy result from pressure of the growing uterus on intestinal adhesions. According to Davis and Bohon (1983), this more likely occurs: (1) around midpregnancy, when the uterus becomes an abdominal organ; (2) in the third trimester, when the fetal head descends; or (3) immediately postpartum, when there is an acute change in uterine size. Perdue and colleagues (1992) reported that 80 percent of pregnant women had nausea and vomiting. Importantly, 98 percent of all women had either continuous or colicky abdominal pain. Abdominal tenderness was found in 70 percent and abnormal bowel sounds in only 55 percent. Plain abdominal radiographs following soluble contrast showed evidence of obstruction in 90 percent of women. Plain radiographs are less accurate for diagnosing small-bowel obstruction, and CT and MR imaging are useful (Biswas, 2006; Essilfie, 2007; McKenna, 2007, and all their associates).

Pregnancy Outcomes

Mortality rates with obstruction during pregnancy can be excessive because of difficult and thus delayed diagnosis, reluctance to operate during pregnancy, and the need for emergency surgery (Firstenberg and Malangoni, 1998). Of 66 pregnancies, Perdue and associates (1992) described a 6-percent maternal mortality rate and 26-percent fetal mortality rate. Perforation from massively dilated bowel such as shown in Figure 49-2 causes sepsis. Two of the four women who died had sigmoid or cecal volvulus caused by adhesions late in pregnancy.

| **TABLE 49-4.** Causes of Intestinal Obstruction During Pregnancy and the Puerperium ||
Cause of Obstruction	**Percent**
Adhesions:	~60
1st and 2nd trimester ~10–15%	
3rd trimester ~2%	
Postpartum ~10%	
Volvulus:	~25
Midgut ~2%	
Cecal ~5%	
Sigmoid ~10%	
Intussusception	~5
Hernia, carcinoma, other	~5

Data from Connolly (1995) and Redlich (2007) and all their colleagues.

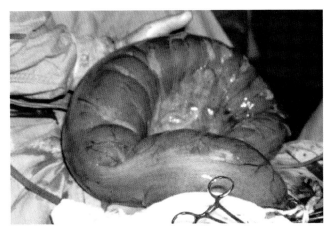

FIGURE 49-2 Massively dilated colon in a pregnant woman with colonic volvulus. (Courtesy of Dr. Lowell Davis.)

Colonic Pseudo-obstruction

Also known as *Ogilvie syndrome,* pseudo-obstruction is caused by adynamic colonic ileus. Approximately 10 percent of all cases are associated with pregnancy. The syndrome usually develops post-partum, but it has been reported occasionally antepartum (Tung and associates, 2008). It is characterized by massive abdominal distension with cecal dilatation. Although unusual, the large bowel may rupture (Singh and colleagues, 2005). In most cases, intravenous infusion of neostigmine, 2 mg, results in prompt decompression (Ponec and associates, 1999). In some cases, colonoscopic decompression is performed, but laparotomy is done for perforation. (De Giorgio and Knowles, 2009).

Appendicitis

Suspected appendicitis is one of the most common indications for abdominal exploration during pregnancy. Mazze and Källén (1991) reported this in approximately 1 in 1000 pregnant women in the Swedish registry of 720,000 pregnancies. Appendicitis was confirmed in 65 percent for an incidence of approximately 1 in 1500 pregnancies. It is interesting—and inexplicable—that the incidence was much lower in the Danish registry of more than 320,000 pregnancies. Hée and Viktrup (1999) reported the confirmed appendicitis rate of only 1 per 5500 pregnancies. There is some evidence that appendicitis is less common during pregnancy compared with its incidence in age-matched nonpregnant controls (Andersson and Lambe, 2001).

It is repeatedly—and appropriately—emphasized that pregnancy makes diagnosis of appendicitis more difficult. This is partly because nausea and vomiting accompany normal pregnancy. In addition, as the uterus enlarges, the appendix commonly moves upward and outward so that pain and tenderness are "displaced" (Baer and colleagues, 1932). These latter findings have been challenged (Mourad and associates, 2000). Another oft-stated reason is that some degree of leukocytosis accompanies normal pregnancy.

For all of these reasons, pregnant women—and especially those late in gestation—frequently do not have clinical findings "typical" for appendicitis. It commonly is confused with chole-cystitis, preterm labor, pyelonephritis, renal colic, placental abruption, or degeneration of a uterine leiomyoma.

Most reports indicate increasing morbidity and mortality rates with increasing gestational age. And as the appendix is progressively deflected upward by the growing uterus, omental containment of infection becomes increasingly unlikely. It is indisputable that appendiceal perforation is more common during later pregnancy. In the studies by Andersson and Lambe (2001) and Ueberrueck and associates (2004), the incidence of perforation averaged approximately 8, 12, and 20 percent in successive trimesters.

Diagnosis

Persistent abdominal pain and tenderness are the most reproducible findings. As discussed, although most have reported

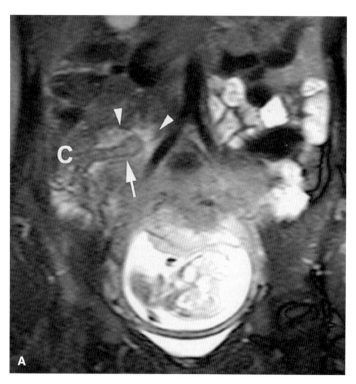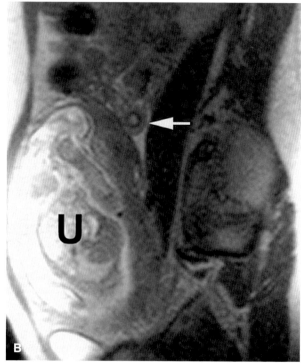

FIGURE 49-3 Magnetic resonance (MR) imaging in a woman with appendicitis at 20 weeks' gestation. **A.** The left coronal image shows an enlarged appendix (*arrow*) with high signal intensity within the lumen. Increased periappendiceal signal intensity (*arrowheads*) is due to inflammation. C = cecum. **B.** The right sagittal image demonstrates the high-intensity signal due to fluid in the distended, obstructed appendix (*arrow*) and the thickened wall. Nonperforative appendicitis was confirmed at surgery. U = uterus. (Reproduced from I Pedrosa, D Levine, AD Eyvazzadeh, et al., MR imaging evaluation of acute appendicitis in pregnancy, *Radiology,* 2006;238:891–899, with permission from The Radiological Society of North America (RSNA) and Dr. Ivan Pedrosa)

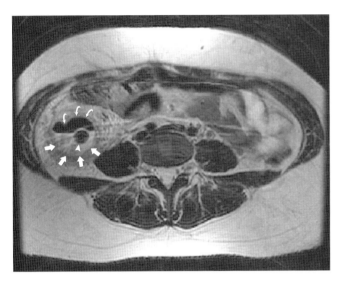

FIGURE 49-4 Appendiceal abscess in a pregnant woman at 14 weeks' gestation. Axial magnetic resonance (MR) image of the abdomen and pelvis shows air (*curved arrows*)-fluid (*arrows*) levels of the abscess surrounding the appendix (*arrowhead*). (Courtesy of Dr. R. Douglas Sims.)

that pain migrates upward with appendiceal displacement, this has been disputed.

Graded compression sonography during pregnancy is difficult because of cecal displacement and uterine imposition (Pedrosa and co-workers, 2009). *Appendiceal computed tomography* is more sensitive and accurate than sonography to confirm suspected appendicitis (Gearhart, 2008; Paulson, 2003; Raman, 2008, and all their colleagues). Specific views can be designed to decrease fetal radiation exposure (see Chap. 41, p. 918). In one study, Wallace and co-workers (2008) reported that the negative appendectomy rate was 54 percent with clinical diagnosis alone, but only 8 percent if sonography and CT scanning were used. *MR imaging* may be preferable, and we and others have had good results with its use (Israel and associates, 2008). Shown in Figure 49-3 is an example of nonperforative appendicitis, whereas a periappendiceal phlegmon/abscess is shown in Figure 49-4. Although not as accurate as preliminary findings suggested, Pedrosa and associates (2009) reported no false-negative diagnoses with MR imaging, but a 30-percent false-positive rate in 140 pregnant women with suspected appendicitis. Finally, appendiceal scanning following administration of native leukocytes tagged with technetium-99 was not successful in 13 pregnant women reported by Stewart and associates (2006).

Management

When appendicitis is suspected, treatment is prompt surgical exploration. Although diagnostic errors sometimes lead to removal of a normal appendix, surgical evaluation is superior to postponed intervention and generalized peritonitis. In most reports, the diagnosis is verified in 60 to 70 percent of pregnant women who undergo surgical exploration. Related to the successive perforation rate by trimester discussed above, the accuracy of diagnosis is inversely proportional to gestational age. Mazze and Källén (1991) reported that 77 percent of first-

trimester diagnoses were correct. In the latter two trimesters, however, only 57 percent were verified.

During the first half of pregnancy, laparoscopy for suspected appendicitis has become the norm. From the Swedish database, Reedy and colleagues (1997) reported similar perinatal outcomes in nearly 2000 laparoscopic appendectomies compared with those of more than 1500 laparotomies done before 20 weeks. In many centers, laparoscopic appendectomy is performed in the third trimester (Barnes and colleagues, 2004; Rollins and associates, 2004). Parangi and co-workers (2007) are less enthusiastic about this approach, and we are of the opinion that laparoscopic surgery in pregnancy past 26 to 28 weeks should be performed only by the most experienced surgeons. For laparotomy most surgeons prefer a McBurney incision.

Before exploration, intravenous antimicrobial therapy is begun, usually with a second-generation cephalosporin or third-generation penicillin. Unless there is gangrene, perforation, or a periappendiceal phlegmon, antimicrobial therapy can usually be discontinued after surgery. Without generalized peritonitis, the prognosis is excellent. Seldom is cesarean delivery indicated at the time of appendectomy. Uterine contractions are common, and although some clinicians recommend tocolytic agents, we do not. De Veciana and colleagues (1994) reported that tocolytic use increased the risk for maternal pulmonary-permeability edema with sepsis syndrome (see Chap. 42, p. 929).

If appendicitis is undiagnosed before delivery, often when the large uterus rapidly empties, walled-off infection is disrupted, causing an acute surgical abdomen. New-onset appendicitis during the immediate puerperium is uncommon. **However, it is important to remember that puerperal pelvic infections typically do not cause peritonitis**.

Effects on Pregnancy

Appendicitis increases the likelihood of abortion or preterm labor, especially if there is peritonitis. Mazze and Källén (1991) and Cohen-Kerem and associates (2005) reported that spontaneous labor ensued with greater frequency following surgery for appendicitis compared with other indications after 23 weeks. In the former study, fetal loss was 22 percent if surgery was performed after 23 weeks. McGory and colleagues (2007) surveyed the California Inpatient File of 3133 pregnant women undergoing surgery for suspected appendicitis. Overall, the fetal loss rate was 23 percent. The rate was doubled—6 versus 11 percent with simple versus complicated disease. Interestingly, it was higher in those with negative appendiceal pathology compared with those with simple appendicitis—4 versus 10 percent.

Mays and colleagues (1995) have suggested a link between sepsis and neonatal neurological injury. Viktrup and Hée (1998) found that appendicitis during pregnancy was not associated with subsequent infertility.

REFERENCES

Agret F, Cosnes J, Hassani Z, et al: Impact of pregnancy on the clinical activity of Crohn's disease. Aliment Pharmacol Ther 21:509, 2005

Al-Hashem H, Muralidharan V, Cohen H, et al: Biliary disease in pregnancy with an emphasis on role of ERCP. J Clin Gastroenterol Nov 15, 2008

Alshawi JS: Recurrent sigmoid volvulus in pregnancy: Report of a case and review of the literature. Dis Colon Rectum 48:1811, 2005

Alstead EM, Nelson-Piercy C: Inflammatory bowel disease in pregnancy. Gut 52:159, 2003

Al-Sunaidi M, Tulandi T: Adhesion-related bowel obstruction after hysterectomy for benign conditions. Obstet Gynecol 108:1162, 2006

American College of Obstetricians and Gynecologists: Nausea and vomiting of pregnancy. Practice Bulletin No. 52, April 2004

Andersson RE, Lambe M: Incidence of appendicitis during pregnancy. Int J Epidemiol 30:1281, 2001

Aouthmany A, Horattas MC: Ileal pouch perforation in pregnancy: Report of a case and review of the literature. Dis Colon Rectum 47:243, 2004

Baer JL, Reis RA, Arens RA: Appendicitis in pregnancy with changes in position and axis of normal appendix in pregnancy. JAMA 98:1359, 1932

Bailit JL: Hyperemesis gravidarum: Epidemiologic findings from a large cohort. Am J Obstet Gynecol 193:811, 2005

Barnes SL, Shane MD, Schoemann MB, et al: Laparoscopic appendectomy after 30 weeks pregnancy: Report of two cases and description of technique. Am Surg 70:733, 2004

Biertho L, Sebajang H, Bamehriz F, et al: Effect of pregnancy on effectiveness of laparoscopic Nissen fundoplication. Surg Endosc 20:385, 2006

Biswas S, Gray KD, Cotton BA: Intestinal obstruction in pregnancy: A case of small bowel volvulus and review of the literature. Am Surg 72:1218, 2006

Bondok RS, Sharnouby NM, Eid HE, et al: Pulsed steroid therapy is an effective treatment for intractable hyperemesis gravidarum. Crit Care Med 34:2781, 2006

Bradley RJ, Rosen MP: Subfertility and gastrointestinal disease: "Unexplained" is often undiagnosed. Obstet Gynecol Surv 59:108, 2004

Briggs GG, Freeman RK, Yaffee SJ: Drugs in Pregnancy and Lactation, 7th ed. Baltimore, Williams & Wilkins, 2005

Bruno JM, Kroser J: Efficacy and safety of upper endoscopy procedures during pregnancy. Gastrointest Endosc Clin N Am 16:33, 2006

Buckwalter JG, Simpson SW: Psychological factors in the etiology and treatment of severe nausea and vomiting in pregnancy. Am J Obstet Gynecol 186:S210, 2002

Bush MC, Patel S, Lapinski RH, et al: Perinatal outcomes in inflammatory bowel disease. J Matern Fetal Neonatal Med 15:237, 2004

Cappell MS: Sedation and analgesia for gastrointestinal endoscopy during pregnancy. Gastrointest Endosc Clin N Am 16:1, 2006

Cappell MS: The fetal safety and clinical efficacy of gastrointestinal endoscopy during pregnancy. Gastroenterol Clin North Am 32:123, 2003

Cappell MS, Garcia A: Gastric and duodenal ulcers during pregnancy. Gastroenterol Clin North Am 27:169, 1998

Carter JF, Soper DE: Operative laparoscopy in pregnancy. J Soc Laparoendosc Surg 8:57, 2004

Cedergren M, Brynhildsen, Josefsson A, et al: Hyperemesis gravidarum that requires hospitalization and the use of antiemetic drugs in relation to maternal body composition. Am J Obstet Gynecol 198:412.e1, 2008

Centers for Disease Control and Prevention: Guidelines for the prevention of intravascular catheter-related infections. MMWR 51:RR-10, 2002

Chihara H, Otsubo Y, Yoneyama Y, et al: Basal metabolic rate in hyperemesis gravidarum: Comparison to normal pregnancy and response to treatment. Am J Obstet Gynecol 188:434, 2003

Chiossi G, Neri I, Cavazzuti M, et al: Hyperemesis gravidarum complicated by Wernicke encephalopathy: Background, case report, and review of the literature. Obstet Gynecol Surv 61:255, 2006

Clark DH: Peptic ulcer in women. BMJ 1:1254, 1953

Cohen S, Harris LD: Does hiatus hernia affect competence of the gastroesophageal sphincter? N Engl J Med 284(19):1053, 1971

Cohen-Kerem R, Railton C, Oren D, et al: Pregnancy outcome following non-obstetric surgical intervention. Am J Surg 190:467, 2005

Connolly MM, Unti JA, Nora PF: Bowel obstruction in pregnancy. Surg Clin North Am 75:101, 1995

Cornish JA, Tan E, Teare J, et al: The effect of restorative proctocolectomy on sexual function, urinary function, fertility, pregnancy and delivery: A systematic review. Dis Colon Rectum 50:1128, 2007

Costigan KA, Sipsma HL, DiPietro JA: Pregnancy folklore revisited: The case of heartburn and hair. Birth 33:311, 2006

Curran D, Lorenz R, Czako P: Gastric outlet obstruction at 30 weeks' gestation. Obstet Gynecol 93:851, 1999

Davis MR, Bohon CJ: Intestinal obstruction in pregnancy. Clin Obstet Gynecol 26:832, 1983

de Veciana M, Towers CV, Major CA, et al: Pulmonary injury associated with appendicitis in pregnancy: Who is at risk? Am J Obstet Gynecol 171:1008, 1994

Debby A, Golan A, Sadan O, et al: Clinical utility of esophagogastroduodenoscopy in the management of recurrent and intractable vomiting in pregnancy. J Reprod Med 53:347, 2008

DeGiorgio R, Knowles CH: Acute colonic pseudo-obstruction. Br J Surg 96(3):229, 2009

Diav-Citrin O, Arnon J, Shechtman S, et al: The safety of proton pump inhibitors in pregnancy: A multicentre prospective controlled study. Aliment Pharmacol Ther 21:269, 2005

Dodds L, Fell DB, Joseph KS, et al: Outcomes of pregnancies complicated by hyperemesis gravidarum. Obstet Gynecol 107:285, 2006

Dokmeci F, Engin-Ustun Y, Ustun Y, et al: Trace element status in plasma and erythrocytes in hyperemesis gravidarum. J Reprod Med 49:200, 2004

Dominitz JA, Young JC, Boyko EJ: Outcomes of infants born to mothers with inflammatory bowel disease: A population-based cohort study. Am J Gastroenterol 97:641, 2002

Dozois EJ, Wolff BG, Tremaine WJ, et al: Maternal and fetal outcome after colectomy for fulminant ulcerative colitis during pregnancy: Case series and literature review. Dis Colon Rectum 49:64, 2005

Duggar CR, Carlan SJ: The efficacy of methylprednisolone in the treatment of hyperemesis gravidarum: A randomized double-blind controlled study [Abstract]. Obstet Gynecol 97:45S, 2001

Dzieniszewski J, Jarosz M: Guidelines in the medical treatment of Helicobacter pylori infection. J Physiol Pharmacol 57 (Suppl 3):143, 2006

Elbaz G, Fich A, Levy A: Inflammatory bowel disease and preterm pregnancy. Int J Gynecol Obstet 90:193, 2005

Essilfie P, Hussain M, Stokes IM: Small bowel infarction secondary to volvulus during pregnancy: A case report. J Reprod Med 52:553, 2007

Everson GT: Gastrointestinal motility in pregnancy. Gastroenterol Clin North Am 21:751, 1992

Food and Drug Administration (FDA) MedWatch: FDA alert and healthcare profession information sheet issued for mycophenolate mofetil (CellCept) and mycophenolic acid (Myfortic), 2008. Available at: http://www.feda.gov/medwatch/safety/2008/safety08. htm#MMF. Accessed January 31, 2009

Farouk R, Pemberton JH, Wolff BG, et al: Functional outcomes after ileal pouch–anal anastomosis for chronic ulcerative colitis. Ann Surg 231:919, 2000

Farrell RJ, Peppercorn MA: Ulcerative colitis. Lancet 359:331, 2002

Fassina G, Osculati A: Achalasia and sudden death: A case report. Forensic Sci Int 75:133, 1995

Fatum M, Rojansky N: Laparoscopic surgery during pregnancy. Obstet Gynecol Surv 56:50, 2001

Feagins LA, Kane SV: Sexual and reproductive issues for men with inflammatory bowel disease. Am J Gastroenterol 104(3):768, 2009

Fell DB, Dodds L, Joseph KS, et al: Risk factors for hyperemesis gravidarum requiring hospital admission during pregnancy. Obstet Gynecol 107:277, 2006

Fiest TC, Foong A, Chokhavatia S: Successful balloon dilation of achalasia during pregnancy. Gastrointest Endosc 39:810, 1993

Firstenberg MS, Malangoni MA: Gastrointestinal surgery during pregnancy. Gastroenterol Clin North Am 27:73, 1998

Flick RP, Bofill JA, King JC: Pregnancy complicated by traumatic diaphragmatic rupture. A case report. J Reprod Med 44:127, 1999

Folk JJ, Leslie-Brown HF, Nosovitch JT, et al: Hyperemesis gravidarum: Outcomes and complications with and without total parenteral nutrition. J Reprod Med 49:497, 2004

Fonager K, Sorensen HT, Olsen J, et al: Pregnancy outcome for women with Crohn's disease: A follow-up study based on linkage between national registries. Am J Gastroenterol 93:2426, 1998

Forsnes EV, Eggleston MK, Heaton JO: Enterovesical fistula complicating pregnancy: A case report. J Reprod Med 44:297, 1999

Friedman S, Blumberg RS: Inflammatory bowel disease. In Fauci AS, Braunwald E, Kasper DL, et al (eds): Harrison's Principles of Internal Medicine, 17th ed. New York, McGraw-Hill, 2008, p 1886

Gearhart SL, Silen W: Acute appendicitis and peritonitis. In Fauci AS, Braunwald E, Kasper DL, et al (eds): Harrison's Principles of Internal Medicine, 17th ed. New York, McGraw-Hill, 2008, p 1914

Gilinsky NH, Muthunayagam N: Gastrointestinal endoscopy in pregnant and lactating women: Emerging standard of care to guide decision-making. Obstet Gynecol Surv 61:791, 2006

Gilstrap LC, Van Dorsten PV, Cunningham FG (eds): Diagnostic and operative laparoscopy. In Operative Obstetrics, 2nd ed. New York, McGraw-Hill, 2002, p 453

Goldberg D, Szilagyi A, Graves L: Hyperemesis gravidarum and Helicobacter pylori infection. Obstet Gynecol 110:695, 2007

Goodwin TM, Nwankwo OA, O'Leary LD, et al: The first demonstration that a subset of women with hyperemesis gravidarum has abnormalities in the vestibuloocular reflex pathway. Am J Obstet Gynecol 199:417.e1, 2008

Gopal KA, Amshel AL, Shonberg IL, et al: Ostomy and pregnancy. Dis Colon Rectum 28:912, 1985

Gould CH, Maybee GJ, Leininger B, et al: Primary intussusception in pregnancy: a case report. J Reprod Med 53:703, 2008

Grjibovski AM, Vikanes A, Stoltenberg C, et al: Consanguinity and the risk of hyperemesis gravidarum in Norway. Acta Obstet Gynecol Scand 87:20, 2008

Guglielmi FW, Baggio-Bertinet D, Federico A, et al: Total parenteral nutrition-related gastroenterological complications. Digest Liver Dis 38:623, 2006

Hahnloser D, Pemberton JH, Wolff BG, et al: Pregnancy and delivery before and after ileal pouch-anal anastomosis for inflammatory bowel disease: Immediate and long-term consequences and outcomes. Dis Colon Rectum 47:1127, 2004

Hamaoui E, Hamaoui M: Nutritional assessment and support during pregnancy. Gastroenterol Clin North Am 32:59, 2003

Hée P, Viktrup L: The diagnosis of appendicitis during pregnancy and maternal and fetal outcome after appendectomy. Int J Gynaecol Obstet 65:129, 1999

Hesketh PJ: Chemotherapy-induced nausea and vomiting. N Engl J Med 358:2482, 2008

Heyland DK, MacDonald S, Keefe L, et al: Total parenteral nutrition in the critically ill patient. JAMA 280:2013, 1998

Hill JB, Yost NP, Wendel GW Jr: Acute renal failure in association with severe hyperemesis gravidarum. Obstet Gynecol 100:1119, 2002

Holmgren C, Aagaard-Tillery KM, Silver RM, et al: Hyperemesis in pregnancy: An evaluation of treatment strategies with maternal and neonatal outcomes. Am J Obstet Gynecol 198:56.e1, 2008

Hytten FE: The alimentary system. In Hytten F, Chamberlain G (eds): Clinical Physiology in Obstetrics. London, Blackwell, 1991, p 137

Israel GM, Malguira N, McCarthy S, et al: MRI vs. ultrasound for suspected appendicitis during pregnancy. J Magn Reson Imaging 28:428, 2008

Jewell D, Young G: Interventions for nausea and vomiting in early pregnancy. Cochrane Database Syst Rev 2: CD000145, 2000

Katz JA: Endoscopy in the pregnant patient with inflammatory bowel disease. Gastrointest Endosc Clin N Am 12:635, 2002

Katz JA, Antonio C, Keenan GF, et al: Outcome pregnancy in women receiving infliximab for the treatment of Crohn's disease and rheumatoid arthritis. Am J Gastroenterol 99:2385, 2004

Kawamura Y, Kawamata K, Shinya M, et al: Vitamin K deficiency in hyperemesis gravidarum as a potential cause of fetal intracranial hemorrhage and hydrocephalus. Prenat Diagn 28:59, 2008

Kelly CP, LaMont JT: Clostridium difficile—More difficult than ever. N Engl J Med 359:1932, 2008

Khudyak V, Lysy J, Mankuta D: Achalasia in pregnancy. Obstet Gynecol Surv 61:207, 2006

Kirby DF, Fiorenza V, Craig RM: Intravenous nutritional support during pregnancy. JPEN J Parenter Enteral Nutr 12:72, 1988

Korelitz BI: Inflammatory bowel disease and pregnancy. Gastroenterol Clin North Am 27:214, 1998

Kornfeld D, Cnattingius S, Ekbom A: Pregnancy outcomes in women with inflammatory bowel disease—a population based cohort study. Am J Obstet Gynecol 177:942, 1997

Kort B, Katz VL, Watson MJ: The effect of nonobstetric operation during pregnancy. Surg Gynecol Obstet 177:371, 1993

Kurzel RB, Naunheim KS, Schwartz RA: Repair of symptomatic diaphragmatic hernia during pregnancy. Obstet Gynecol 71:869, 1988

Lacasse A, Rey E, Ferreira E, et al: Validity of a modified Pregnancy-Unique Quantification of Emesis and Nausea (PUQE) scoring index to assess severity of nausea and vomiting of pregnancy. Am J Obstet Gynecol 198:71.e1, 2008

Lal SK, Morgenstern R, Vinjirayer EP, et al: Sigmoid volvulus: An update. Gastrointest Endosc Clin N Am 16:175, 2006

Lawson M, Kern F, Everson GT: Gastrointestinal transit time in human pregnancy: Prolongation in the second and third trimesters followed by postpartum normalization. Gastroenterology 89:996, 1985

Lichtenstein GC, Hanauer SB, Sandborn WJ, et al: Management of Crohn's disease in adults. Am J Gastroenterol 104(2):465, 2009

MacDonald DJ, Popli K, Byrne D, et al: Small bowel obstruction in a twin pregnancy due to fibroid degeneration. Scott Med J 49:159, 2004

Mahadevan U: Fertility and pregnancy in the patient with inflammatory bowel disease. Gut 55:1198, 2006

Mahadevan U, Kane S: American Gastroenterological Association Institute technical review on the use of gastrointestinal medications in pregnancy. Gastroenterology 131(1):283, 2006

Mahadevan US, Sandborn W, Hakimian S: Pregnancy outcomes in women with inflammatory bowel disease: A population based cohort study. Gastroenterology 128(Suppl 2):A322, 2005

Mayberry JF, Atkinson M: Achalasia and pregnancy. Br J Obstet Gynaecol 94:855, 1987

Mays J, Verma U, Klein S, et al: Acute appendicitis in pregnancy and the occurrence of major intraventricular hemorrhage and periventricular leukomalacia. Obstet Gynecol 86:650, 1995

Mazze RI, Källén B: Appendectomy during pregnancy: A Swedish registry study of 778 cases. Obstet Gynecol 77:835, 1991

Mazze RI, Källén B: Reproductive outcome after anesthesia and operation during pregnancy: A registry study of 5405 cases. Am J Obstet Gynecol 161:1178, 1989

McGory ML, Zingmond DS, Tillou A, et al: Negative appendectomy in pregnant women is associated with a substantial risk of fetal loss. J Am Coll Surg 205:534, 2007

McKenna DA, Meehan CP, Alhajeri AN, et al: The use of MRI to demonstrate small bowel obstruction during pregnancy. Br J Radiol 80:e11, 2007

McKenna D, Watson P, Dornan J: Helicobacter pylori infection and dyspepsia in pregnancy. Obstet Gynecol 102:845, 2003

Medical Letter: Drugs for travelers' diarrhea. 50(1291):226, 2008

Meyerson S, Holtz T, Ehrinpresis M, et al: Small bowel obstruction in pregnancy. Am J Gastroenterol 90:299, 1995

Michel L, Song WK, Topazian M: Gastrointestinal endoscopy. In Fauci AS, Braunwald E, Kasper DL, et al (eds): Harrison's Principles of Internal Medicine, 17th ed. New York, McGraw-Hill, 2008, p 1841

Miller JP: Inflammatory bowel disease in pregnancy: A review. J R Soc Med 79:221, 1986

Modigliani RM: Gastrointestinal and pancreatic disease. In Barron WM, Lindheimer MD, Davison JM (eds): Medical Disorders of Pregnancy, 3rd ed. St. Louis, Mosby, 2000, p 316

Moskovitz DN, Bodian C, Chapman ML, et al: The effect on the fetus of medications used to treat pregnant inflammatory bowel-disease patients. Am J Gastroenterol 99:656, 2004

Mourad J, Elliott JP, Erickson L, et al: Appendicitis in pregnancy: New information that contradicts long-held clinical beliefs. Am J Obstet Gynecol 185:1027, 2000

Norgård B, Hundborg HH, Jacobsen BA, et al: Disease activity in pregnant women with Crohn's disease and birth outcomes: A regional Danish cohort study. Am J Gastroenterol 102:1947, 2007

Ogura JM, Francois KE, Perlow JH, et al: Complications associated with peripherally inserted central catheter use during pregnancy. Am J Obstet Gynecol 188:1223, 2003

Okada H, Makidona C, Takenaka R, et al: Therapeutic efficacy of leukocytapheresis in a pregnant woman with severe active ulcerative colitis. Digestion 74:15, 2006

O'Mahony S: Endoscopy in pregnancy. Best Pract Res Clin Gastroenterol 21:893, 2007

Ooi BS, Remzi FH, Fazio VW: Turnbull-blowhole colostomy for toxic ulcerative colitis in pregnancy: Report of two cases. Dis Colon Rectum 46:111, 2003

Ortega-Carnicer J, Ambrós A, Alcazar R: Obstructive shock due to labor-related diaphragmatic hernia. Crit Care Med 26:616, 1998

Panayotidis c, Triantafyllidis S: Acute abdomen in Crohn's disease mimicking concealed placental abruption in pregnancy. J Obstet Gynaecol 26:166, 2006

Panesar NS, Chan KW, Li CY, et al: Status of anti-thyroid peroxidase during normal pregnancy and in patients with hyperemesis gravidarum. Thyroid 16:481, 2006

Parangi S, Levine D, Henry A, et al: Surgical gastrointestinal disorders during pregnancy. Am J Surg 193:223, 2007

Paranyuk Y, Levin G, Figueroa R: Candida septicemia in a pregnant woman with hyperemesis receiving parenteral nutrition. Obstet Gynecol 107:535, 2006

Paulson EK, Kalady MF, Pappas TN: Suspected appendicitis. N Engl J Med 348:236, 2003

Pedrosa I, Lafornara M, Pandharipande PV, et al: Pregnant patients suspected of having acute appendicitis: effect of MR imaging on negative laparotomy rate and appendiceal perforation rate. Radiology 250(3):749, 2009

Pedrosa I, Levine D, Eyvazzadeh AD, et al: MR imaging evaluation of acute appendicitis in pregnancy. Radiology 238:891, 2006

Perdue PW, Johnson HW Jr, Stafford PW: Intestinal obstruction complicating pregnancy. Am J Surg 164:384, 1992

Podolsky DK: Inflammatory bowel disease. N Engl J Med 347:417, 2002

Ponec RJ, Saunders MD, Kimmey MB: Neostigmine for the treatment of acute colonic pseudo-obstruction. N Engl J Med 341:137, 1999

Ponzetto A, Cardaropoli S, Piccoli E, et al: Pre-eclampsia is associated with Helicobacter pylori seropositivity in Italy. J Hyperten 24:2445, 2006

Poursharif B, Korst LM, Macgibbon KW, et al: Elective pregnancy termination in a large cohort of women with hyperemesis gravidarum. Contraception 76:451, 2007

Prefontaine E, Sutherland LR, Macdonald JK, et al: Azathioprine or 6-mercaptopurine for maintenance of remission in Crohn's disease. Cochrane Database Syst Rev 1:CD000067, 2009

Rahimi R, Nikfar S, Rezaie A, et al: Pregnancy outcome in women with inflammatory bowel disease following exposure to 5-aminosalicylic acid drugs: A meta-analysis. Reprod Toxicol 25:271, 2008

Raman SS, Osuagwu FC, Kadell B, et al: Effect of CE on false positive diagnosis of appendicitis and perforation. N Engl J Med 358:972, 2008

Ravid A, Richard CS, Spencer LM, et al: Pregnancy, delivery, and pouch function after ileal pouch-anal anastomosis for ulcerative colitis. Dis Colon Rectum 45:1283, 2002

Reddy D, Murphy SJ, Kane SV, et al: Relapses of inflammatory bowel disease during pregnancy: In-hospital management and birth outcomes. Am J Gastroenterol 103:1203, 2008

Redlich A, Rickes S, Costa SD: Small bowel obstruction in pregnancy. Arch Gynecol Obstet 275:381, 2007

Reedy MB, Källén B, Kuehl TJ: Laparoscopy during pregnancy: A study of five fetal outcome parameters with use of the Swedish Health Registry. Am J Obstet Gynecol 177:673, 1997

Rigler LG, Eneboe JB: Incidence of hiatus hernia in pregnant women and its significance. J Thorac Surg 4:262, 1935

Riis L, Vind I, Politi P, et al: Does pregnancy change the disease course? A study in a European cohort of patients with inflammatory bowel disease. Am J Gastroenterol 101:1539, 2006

Rizzo AG: Laparoscopic surgery in pregnancy: Long-term follow-up. J Laparoendosco Adv Surg Tech A 13:11, 2003

Robinson JN, Banerjee R, Thiet MP: Coagulopathy secondary to vitamin K deficiency in hyperemesis gravidarum. Obstet Gynecol 92:673, 1998

Rollins MD, Chan KJ, Price RR: Laparoscopy for appendicitis and cholelithiasis during pregnancy: A new standard of care. Surg Endosc 18:237, 2004

Roux CH, Brocq O, Breuil V, et al: Pregnancy in rheumatology patients exposed to anti-tumour necrosis factor (TNF)-α therapy. Rheumatology 46:695, 2007

Russo-Stieglitz KE, Levine AB, Wagner BA, et al: Pregnancy outcome in patients requiring parenteral nutrition. J Matern Fetal Med 8:164, 1999

Rutgeerts P, Sandborn WJ, Feagan BG, et al: Infliximab for induction and maintenance therapy for ulcerative colitis. N Engl J Med 353:2462, 2005

Rutgeerts P, Vermeire S, Van Assche G: Biological therapies for inflammatory bowel diseases. Gastroenterology 136(4):1182, 2009

Safari HR, Fassett MJ, Souter IC, et al: The efficacy of methylprednisolone in the treatment of hyperemesis gravidarum: A randomized, double-blind, controlled study. Am J Obstet Gynecol 179:921, 1998

Sakai M, Yoneda S, Sasaki Y, et al: Maternal total parenteral nutrition and fetal subdural hematoma. Obstet Gynecol 101:1142, 2003

Sandborn WJ, Feagan BG, Stoinov S, et al: Certolizumab pegol for the treatment of Crohn's disease. N Engl J Med 357:228, 2007

Sands BE, Anderson FH, Bernstein CN, et al: Infliximab maintenance therapy for fistulizing Crohn's disease. N Engl J Med 350:876, 2004

Satin AJ, Twickler D, Gilstrap LC: Esophageal achalasia in late pregnancy. Obstet Gynecol 79:812, 1992

Schiff MA, Reed SD, Daling JR: The sex ratio of pregnancies complicated by hospitalisation for hyperemesis gravidarum. Br J Obstet Gynaecol 111:27, 2004

Schrag SP, Sharma R, Jaik NP, et al: Complications related to percutaneous endoscopic gastrostomy (PEG) tubes: A comprehensive clinical review. J Gastrointestin Liver Dis 16:407, 2007

Schreiber S, Khaliq-Kareemi M, Lawrance IC, et al: Maintenance therapy with certolizumab pegol for Crohn's disease. N Engl J Med 357:239, 2007

Schwartz M, Rossoff L: Pneumomediastinum and bilateral pneumo-thoraces in a patient with hyperemesis gravidarum. Chest 106:1904, 1994

Selby WS, Griffin S, Abraham N, et al: Appendectomy protects against the development of ulcerative colitis but does not affect its course. Am J Gastroenterol 97:2834, 2002

Selitsky T, Chandra P, Schiavello HJ: Wernicke's encephalopathy with hyperemesis and ketoacidosis. Obstet Gynecol 107:486, 2006

Sharifah H, Naidu A, Vimal K: Diaphragmatic hernia: An unusual cause of postpartum collapse. Br J Obstet Gynaecol 110:701, 2003

Siddiqui U, Denise-Proctor D: Flexible sigmoidoscopy and colonoscopy during pregnancy. Gastrointest Endosc Clin N Am 16:59, 2006

Singh S, Nadgir A, Bryan RM: Post-cesarean section acute colonic pseudo-obstruction with spontaneous perforation. Int J Gynaecol Obstet 89:144, 2005

Society of American Gastrointestinal and Endoscopic Surgeons: Guidelines for diagnosis, treatment, and use of laparoscopy for surgical problems during pregnancy. Surg Endosc 22:849, 2008

Stewart D, Grewal N, Choi R, et al: The use of tagged white blood cell scans to diagnose appendicitis in pregnant patients. Am Surg 72:894, 2006

Storch I, Barkin JS: Contraindications to capsule endoscopy: Do any still exist? Gastrointest Endosc Clin N Am 16:329, 2006

Suerbaum S, Michetti P: Helicobacter pylori infection. N Engl J Med 347:1175, 2002

Sullivan CA, Johnson CA, Roach H, et al: A pilot study of intravenous ondansetron for hyperemesis gravidarum. Am J Obstet Gynecol 174:1565, 1996

Swallow BL, Lindow SW, Masson EA, et al: Psychological health in early pregnancy: Relationship with nausea and vomiting. J Obstet Gynaecol 24:28, 2004

Takahashi K, Funayama Y, Fukushima K, et al: Pregnancy and delivery in patients with enterostomy due to anorectal complications from Crohn's disease. Int J Colorectal Dis 22:313, 2007

Tan JY, Loh KC, Yeo GS, et al: Transient hyperthyroidism of hyperemesis gravidarum. Br J Obstet Gynaecol 109:683, 2002

Tan PC, Jacob R, Quek KF, et al: The fetal sex ratio and metabolic, biochemical, haematological and clinical indicators of severity of hyperemesis gravidarum. BJOG 113:733, 2006

Torquati A, Lutfi R, Khaitan L, et al: Heller myotomy vs Heller myotomy plus Dor fundoplication: Cost-utility analysis of a randomized trial. Surg Endosc 20:389, 2006

Trogstad LI, Stoltenberg C, Magnus P, et al: Recurrence risk in hyperemesis gravidarum. BJOG 112:1641, 2005

Tung CS, Zighelboim I, Gardner MO: Acute colonic pseudoobstruction complicating twin pregnancy. J Reprod Med 53:52, 2008

Turcotte S, Dubé S, Beauchamp G: Peripherally inserted central venous catheters are not superior to central venous catheters in the acute care of surgical patients on the ward. World J Surg 30:1603, 2006

Ueberrueck T, Koch A, Meyer L, et al: Ninety-four appendectomies for suspected acute appendicitis during pregnancy. World J Surg 28:508, 2004

Vaisman N, Kaidar R, Levin I, et al: Nasojejunal feeding in hyperemesis gravidarum—a preliminary study. Clin Nutr 23:53, 2004

Vaknin Z, Halperin R, Schneider D, et al: Hyperemesis gravidarum and nonspecific abnormal EEG findings. J Reprod Med 51:623, 2006

Verberg MF, Gillott JD, Fardan NA, et al: Hyperemesis gravidarum, a literature review. Hum Reprod Update 11:527, 2005

Viktrup L, Hée P: Fertility and long-term complications four to nine years after appendectomy during pregnancy. Acta Obstet Gynecol Scand 77:746, 1998

Wald A: Constipation, diarrhea, and symptomatic hemorrhoids during pregnancy. Gastroenterol Clin North Am 32:309, 2003

Waljee A, Waljee J, Morris AM, et al: Threefold increased risk of infertility: A meta-analysis of infertility after ileal pouch anal anastomosis in ulcerative colitis. Gut 55:1575, 2006

Wallace CA, Petrov MS, Soybel DI, et al: Influence of imaging on the negative appendectomy rate in pregnancy. J Gastrointest Surg 12:46, 2008

Watkin DS, Hughes S, Thompson MH: Herniation of colon through the right diaphragm complicating the puerperium. J Laparoendosc Surg 3:583, 1993

Weyermann M, Brenner H, Adler G, et al: Helicobacter pylori infection and the occurrence and severity of gastrointestinal symptoms during pregnancy. Am J Obstet Gynecol 189:526, 2003

Weyermann M, Rothenbacher D, Gayer L, et al: Role of Helicobacter pylori infection in iron deficiency during pregnancy. Am J Obstet Gynecol 192:548, 2005

Woolfson K, Cohen Z, McLeod RS: Crohn's disease and pregnancy. Dis Colon Rectum 33:869, 1990

Yamamoto T, Suzuki Y, Kojima K, et al: Pneumomediastinum secondary to hyperemesis gravidarum during early pregnancy. Acta Obstet Gynecol Scand 80:1143, 2001

Yost NP, McIntire DD, Wians FH Jr, et al: A randomized, placebo-controlled trial of corticosteroids for hyperemesis due to pregnancy. Obstet Gynecol 102:1250, 2003

CHAPTER 50

Hepatic, Gallbladder, and Pancreatic Disorders

Disorders of the liver, gallbladder, and pancreas together comprise a formidable list of complications that may arise in pregnancy, including some unique to pregnancy. Their relationships with pregnancy can be fascinating, intriguing, and challenging.

HEPATIC DISORDERS

It is customary to divide liver diseases complicating pregnancy into three general categories. The first includes those specifically related to pregnancy that resolve either spontaneously or following delivery. Examples are hepatic dysfunction from hyperemesis gravidarum, intrahepatic cholestasis, acute fatty liver, and hepatocellular damage with preeclampsia—the "HELLP syndrome" (Hay, 2008). The second category includes acute hepatic disorders that are coincidental to pregnancy, such as acute viral hepatitis. The third category includes chronic liver diseases that predate pregnancy, such as chronic hepatitis, cirrhosis, or esophageal varices.

Hepatic Physiology in Pregnancy

Pregnancy may induce appreciable changes in some clinical and laboratory manifestations related to the liver (see Chap. 5, p. 126 and Appendix). Findings such as elevated serum alkaline phosphatase, palmar erythema, and spider angiomas, which might suggest liver disease, are commonly found during normal pregnancy. However, histological liver findings with uncomplicated pregnancies are unchanged compared with those of nonpregnant subjects (Ingerslev and Teilum, 1945).

Hyperemesis Gravidarum

Pernicious nausea and vomiting are discussed in detail in Chapter 49 (p. 1050). The liver may be involved, and there may be mild hyperbilirubinemia with serum transaminase levels elevated in up to half of women hospitalized (Table 50-1). Levels, however, seldom exceed 200 U/L. Liver biopsy may show some fatty changes (Knox and Olans, 1996).

Intrahepatic Cholestasis of Pregnancy

This disorder also has been referred to as recurrent jaundice of pregnancy, cholestatic hepatosis, and icterus gravidarum. It is characterized clinically by pruritus, icterus, or both. It may be more common in multifetal pregnancy (Lausman and colleagues, 2008). There is a significant genetic influence, and thus the incidence of this disorder varies by population. For example, cholestasis is uncommon in North America, with an incidence of approximately 1 in 500 to 1000 pregnancies. In Israel, the incidence reported by Sheiner and associates (2006) is approximately 1 in 400. In Italy, the incidence is 1 percent; in Sweden, it is 1.5 percent; and in Chile, it is 4 percent (Glantz, 2004; Paternoster, 2002; Reyes, 1997, and all their colleagues).

Pathogenesis

The cause of obstetrical cholestasis is unknown, but it probably occurs in genetically susceptible women. Leslie and colleagues (2000) reported that plasma estrogen levels are *decreased* in affected women. Diminished secretion of sulfated progesterone metabolites

TABLE 50-1. Clinical and Laboratory Findings with Acute Liver Diseases in Pregnancy

			Hepatic		Renal	Hematological and Coagulation					
Disorder	Onset in Pregnancy	Clinical Findings	AST μ/L	Bili mg/dL	Cr mg/dL	Hct	Plat	Fib	DD	PT	Hemolysis
Hyperemesis	Early	Severe N&V	NL-300	NL-4	↑	↑↑	NL	NL	NL	NL	No
Cholestasis	Late	Pruritus, jaundice	NL-200	1–5	NL	NL	NL	NL	NL	NL	No
Fatty liver	Late	Moderate N&V, ± HTN, liver failure	200–800	4–10	↑↑↑	↑↑↑	↓↓	↓↓↓	↑	↑↑	↑↑↑
Preeclampsia	Mid to late	HA, HTN	NL-300	2–4	↑	↑	↓↓	NL	↑	NL	↑–↑↑
Hepatitis	Variable	Jaundice	2000+	5–20	NL	↑	↓	NL	NL	↑	No

↑ = increased levels; ↓ = decreased levels; AST = aspartate aminotransferase; Bili = bilirubin; Cr = creatinine; DD = D-dimers; Fib = fibrinogen; HA = headache; Hct = hematocrit; HTN = hypertension; N&V = nausea and vomiting; NL = normal; Plat = platelets; PT = prothrombin time.

may play a role (Mullally and Hansen, 2001; Reyes and Sjovall, 2000). At least some cases are related to the many gene mutations that control hepatocellular transport systems (Germain and associates, 2002; Hay, 2008). One example is mutation of the *multidrug resistance 3 (MDR3) gene* found with *progressive familial intrahepatic cholestasis.* (Gonzales and co-workers, 2009). Some drugs that similarly decrease canalicular transport of bile acids aggravate the disorder. For example, we have encountered impressive cholestatic jaundice in pregnant women taking azathioprine following renal transplantation.

Whatever the inciting cause(s), bile acids are cleared incompletely and accumulate in plasma. Of note, total bile acid concentration may already be elevated 10- to 100-fold in normal pregnancy (Lunzer and associates, 1986). Even *before* bile acid levels increase, associated dyslipidemia is apparent (Dann and colleagues, 2006). These researchers found that total cholesterol levels are significantly higher compared with those of normal pregnancy, and low-density lipoprotein (LDL) cholesterol levels become elevated earliest. Hyperbilirubinemia results from retention of conjugated pigment, but total plasma concentrations rarely exceed 4 to 5 mg/dL. Alkaline phosphatase is usually elevated even more so than in normal pregnancy. Serum transaminase levels are normal to moderately elevated but seldom exceed 250 U/L (see Table 50-1). Liver biopsy shows mild cholestasis with bile plugs in the hepatocytes and canaliculi of the centrilobular regions, but without inflammation or necrosis. These changes disappear after delivery but often recur in subsequent pregnancies or with estrogen-containing contraceptives.

Clinical Presentation

Pruritus develops in late pregnancy, although it occasionally begins in the late second trimester. Occasionally, it manifests even earlier, and Kirkinen and Ryynänen (1995) described a woman at 13 weeks with cholestasis associated with hyperplacentosis and a triploid fetus. There are no constitutional symptoms, and generalized pruritus develops with predilection for the soles of

the feet. Skin changes are limited to excoriations from scratching. Biochemical tests may be abnormal at presentation, but pruritus usually precedes laboratory findings by a mean of 3 weeks and sometimes by months (Kenyon and colleagues, 2001, 2002). Approximately 10 percent of women develop jaundice.

With normal liver enzymes, the differential diagnosis of pruritus includes other skin disorders (see Chap. 56, p. 1187). Findings are unlikely to be due to preeclamptic liver disease if there are no blood pressure changes and proteinuria. Sonography may be warranted to exclude cholelithiasis and biliary obstruction. *Acute* viral hepatitis is an unlikely diagnosis because of the usually low serum transaminase levels seen with cholestasis. Conversely, asymptomatic *chronic* hepatitis C is associated with a 20-fold increased incidence of cholestasis (Locatelli and colleagues, 1999; Paternoster and associates, 2002).

Management

Pruritus may be troublesome and is thought to result from elevated serum bile salts. *Antihistamines* and *topical emollients* may provide some relief. Based on their review, Kroumpouzos and Cohen (2003) estimated that *cholestyramine* may be effective in 50 to 70 percent of women. This compound also causes further decreased absorption of fat-soluble vitamins, which may lead to vitamin K deficiency. Fetal coagulopathy may develop, and there are reports of intracranial hemorrhage and stillbirth (Matos and colleagues, 1997; Sadler and associates, 1995). Finally, the opioid antagonist *naltrexone* was found to be superior to placebo for pruritus (Terg and colleagues, 2002).

Some reports suggest that *ursodeoxycholic acid* quickly relieves pruritus and lowers serum enzyme levels (Germain and co-workers, 2002; Mazzella and associates, 2001). Lucangioli and colleagues (2009) documented an especially profound decrease in serum levels of lithocholic acid. Kondrackiene and colleagues (2005) randomized 84 symptomatic women to ursodeoxycholic acid (8 to 10 mg/kg/d) versus cholestyramine

(8 g/d) and reported superior relief with ursodeoxycholic acid—67 versus 19 percent, respectively. Glantz and co-workers (2005), however, found no benefits to women randomly assigned to ursodeoxycholic acid versus dexamethasone. The American College of Obstetricians and Gynecologists (2006) has concluded that ursodeoxycholic acid both relieves pruritus and improves fetal outcomes, although evidence for the latter is not compelling. Finally, Warren and associates (2005) reported dramatic relief in a woman with refractory pruritus who was treated by plasmapheresis and 5-percent albumin replacement.

Cholestasis and Pregnancy Outcomes

Most earlier reports described excessive adverse pregnancy outcomes in women with cholestatic jaundice. Data accrued over the past two decades are ambiguous concerning increased perinatal mortality rates and whether close fetal surveillance is preventative. A review of a few studies illustrates this. Rioseco and co-workers (1994) compared outcomes in 320 affected women with those of normal controls. They observed that rates of meconium-stained amnionic fluid—25 versus 16 percent, and preterm delivery—12 versus 4 percent, were significantly increased with cholestasis. They attributed equivalent perinatal mortality rates in these two groups to close pregnancy surveillance. In a prospective investigation of 70 women with cholestasis, Kenyon and co-workers (2002) found that weekly amnionic fluid assessment, every-other-day antepartum fetal testing, and elective delivery at 37 to 38 weeks resulted in zero perinatal mortalities. Glantz and associates (2004) described outcomes in 693 Swedish women. Perinatal mortality rates were slightly increased, but death was limited to infants of mothers with severe disease characterized by total bile acid levels ≥ 40 μmol/L. More recently, Sheiner and co-workers (2006) described no differences in perinatal outcomes in 376 affected pregnancies compared with their overall obstetrical population. There was, however, a significant increase in labor inductions and cesarean deliveries in affected women. Finally, Lee and associates (2009) described two cases of sudden fetal death not predicted by nonstress testing.

Gorelik and colleagues (2006) suggest that bile acids may cause fetal cardiac arrest after entering cardiomyocytes in abnormal amounts. Using fetal myocyte cultures, they showed expression of several genes that may play a role in bile transport.

Acute Fatty Liver of Pregnancy

The most common cause of acute liver failure during pregnancy is acute fatty liver—also called *acute fatty metamorphosis* or *acute yellow atrophy*. In its worst form, the incidence is probably approximately 1 in 10,000 pregnancies.

Fatty liver is characterized by accumulation of microvesicular fat that literally "crowds out" normal hepatocytic function (Fig. 50-1). Grossly, the liver is small, soft, yellow, and greasy.

Etiopathogenesis

Although much has been learned about this disorder, interpretation of conflicting data has led to incomplete but intriguing observations. For example, some if not most cases of maternal fatty liver are associated with recessively inherited mitochondrial abnormalities of fatty acid oxidation. These are similar to those in children with Reye-like syndromes. A number of mutations have been described for the mitochondrial trifunctional protein enzyme complex that catalyzes the last oxidative steps in the pathway. The most common are the G1528C and E474Q mutations of the gene on chromosome 2 that code for long-chain-3-hydroxyacyl-CoA-dehydrogenase—known as LCHAD.

There are other mutations for medium- and short-chain dehydrogenase—MCHAD and SCHAD (Dann and colleagues, 2006). Similar findings have been reported with autosomal recessive carnitine palmitoyltransferase 1 (CPT1) deficiency (Ylitalo and co-workers, 2005).

Sims and co-workers (1995) observed that some *homozygous* LCHAD-deficient children with Reye-like syndromes had *heterozygous* mothers with fatty liver. This was also seen in women with a compound heterozygous fetus. Although some conclude that heterozygous LCHAD-deficient mothers are at risk *only* if their fetus is homozygous, this is not always the case (Blish and Ibdah, 2005; Tyni and colleagues, 1998).

There is a controversial association between fatty acid β-oxidation enzyme defects and

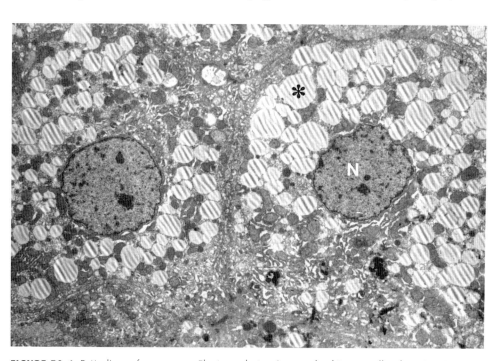

FIGURE 50-1 Fatty liver of pregnancy. Electron photomicrograph of two swollen hepatocytes containing numerous microvesicular fat droplets (*). The nuclei (N) remain centered within the cells, unlike with the case of macrovesicular fat deposition. (Used with permission from Dr. Donald A. Wheeler.)

severe preeclampsia—especially in women with *HELLP syndrome*—hemolysis, elevated serum liver transaminase levels, and low platelet counts (see Chap. 34, p. 720). Most of these observations have been arrived at by retrospectively studying mothers delivered of a child who later developed Reye-like syndrome. In the study by Tyni and associates (1998), 29 of 63 women with a clinically affected and presumably homozygous fetus had increased incidences of preeclampsia, HELLP syndrome, acute fatty liver, and cholestasis. More recently, Browning and co-workers (2006) performed a case-control study of 50 mothers of children with a fatty-acid oxidation defect and 1250 mothers of matched control infants. During their pregnancy, 16 percent of mothers with an affected child developed liver problems compared with only 0.9 percent of control women. These included HELLP syndrome in 12 percent and fatty liver in 4 percent. Despite these findings, the clinical, biochemical, and histopathological findings are sufficiently disparate to suggest that severe preeclampsia, with or without HELLP syndrome, and fatty liver are distinct syndromes (American College of Obstetricians and Gynecologists, 2006; Sibai, 2007).

Recurrence. Fatty liver recurring in subsequent pregnancy is uncommon, but a few cases have been described (Usta and colleagues, 1994). Recurrence appears to be more likely if the woman has a homozygous enzyme-deficient fetus (Tyni and colleagues, 1998).

Clinical and Laboratory Findings

Acute fatty liver almost always manifests late in pregnancy. Castro and colleagues (1996a) reported 28 women with a mean gestational age of 37.5 weeks—range 31 to 42. In 45 cases at Parkland Hospital, the earliest onset was at 31 weeks and a fourth of women presented at 34 weeks or earlier. Fatty liver is more common in nulliparas with a male fetus, and in 10 to 20 percent of cases there is a multifetal gestation (Davidson and associates, 1998; Fesenmeier and co-workers, 2005).

Fatty liver has a clinical spectrum of severity. In the worst cases, symptoms usually develop over several days. Persistent nausea and vomiting are major symptoms, and there are varying degrees of malaise, anorexia, epigastric pain, and progressive jaundice. Perhaps half of affected women have hypertension, proteinuria, and edema, alone or in combination—signs suggestive of preeclampsia. As shown in Tables 50-1 and 50-2, there are variable degrees from moderate to severe liver dysfunction manifest with hypofibrinogenemia, hypoalbuminemia, hypocholesterolemia, and prolonged clotting times. Serum bilirubin levels usually are less than 10 mg/dL, and serum transaminase levels are modestly elevated and usually less than 1000 U/L.

In almost all severe cases, there is profound endothelial cell activation with capillary leakage causing hemoconcentration, hepatorenal syndrome, ascites, and sometimes permeability pulmonary edema. Fetal death is more common in cases with severe hemoconcentration. Stillbirth possibly follows diminished uteroplacental perfusion, but is also related to more severe disease and acidosis. There is maternal leukocytosis and thrombocytopenia. Hemolysis can be severe, and it is likely caused by the effects of hypocholesterolemia on erythrocyte membranes (Cunningham and colleagues, 1985). As a consequence, lactic acid dehydrogenase (LDH) levels are elevated, and the peripheral blood smear demonstrates echinocytosis and nucleated red cells.

Various liver imaging techniques have been used to confirm the diagnosis, however, none are particularly reliable. Specifically, Castro and associates (1996b) reported poor sensitivity with sonography—three of 11 patients, computed tomography (CT)—five of 10, and magnetic resonance imaging—none of five. Our experiences are similar.

The syndrome typically continues to worsen after diagnosis. Hypoglycemia is common, and obvious hepatic encephalopathy, severe coagulopathy, and some degree of renal failure each develop in approximately half of women. Fortunately, delivery arrests deterioration of liver function.

We have encountered a number of women with a *forme fruste* of this disorder. Clinical involvement is relatively minor and laboratory aberrations—usually only hemolysis and

TABLE 50-2. Laboratory Findings in 131 Women with Acute Fatty Liver of Pregnancy

Series	No.	Most Abnormal Laboratory Values Mean ± 1 SD (range)			
		Fibrinogen (mg/dL)	Platelets (10³/μL)	Creatinine (mg/dL)	AST (U/L)
Castro et al (1996a)	28	125 (32–446)	113 (11–186)	2.5 (1.1–5.2)	210 (45–1200)
Pereira et al (1997)	32	ND	123 (26–262)	2.7 (1.1–8.4)	99 (25–911)
Vigil-De Gracia (2001)	10	136 ± 120	76 ± 50	ND	444 ± 358
Fesenmeier et al (2005)	16	—	88 (22–226)	3.3 (0.5–8.6)	692 (122–3195)
Parkland Hospital (2007)[a]	45	157 ± 110	105 ± 72	1.9 ± 0.8	552 ± 343
		(27–700)	(9–385)	(0.7–5.0)	(25–2245)
Estimated weighted average		145	109	2.5	370

[a]Data courtesy of Dr. Nicole Yost.
AST = aspartate aminotransferase; ND = not done.

decreased plasma fibrinogen—signify the problem. Thus, the spectrum of liver involvement varies from milder cases that go unnoticed or are attributed to preeclampsia, to overt hepatic failure with encephalopathy.

Coagulopathy. The degree of clotting dysfunction is also variable and can be serious and life threatening, especially if operative delivery is undertaken. Coagulopathy is caused by diminished hepatic procoagulant synthesis, although there is also some evidence for increased consumption. As shown in Table 50-2, hypofibrinogenemia sometimes is profound. Of 45 women with fatty liver cared for at Parkland Hospital, more than half had a plasma fibrinogen nadir <100 mg/dL. Modest elevations of serum D-dimers or fibrin split product levels indicate an element of consumptive coagulopathy. Although usually modest, occasionally there is profound thrombocytopenia (Table 50-2). The mean platelet count was 105,000/μL in 45 women from Parkland Hospital—in a fourth of these, the platelet nadir was less than 50,000/μL.

Management

The key to a good outcome is intensive supportive care and good obstetrical management. Spontaneous resolution usually follows delivery. In some cases, the fetus may be already dead when the diagnosis is made, and the route of delivery less problematic. Many viable fetuses tolerate labor poorly. Because significant procrastination in effecting delivery may increase maternal and fetal risks, we prefer a trial of labor induction with close fetal surveillance. Although some recommend cesarean delivery to hasten hepatic healing, this increases maternal risk when there is a severe coagulopathy. Transfusions with whole blood or packed red cells, along with fresh-frozen plasma, cryoprecipitate, and platelets, are usually necessary if surgery is performed or if obstetrical lacerations complicate vaginal delivery (see Chap. 35, p. 791).

Hepatic dysfunction begins to resolve postpartum. It usually normalizes within a week, and in the interim, intensive medical support may be required. There are two associated conditions that may develop around this time. Perhaps a fourth of women have evidence for *transient diabetes insipidus.* This presumably is due to elevated vasopressinase concentrations caused by diminished hepatic production of its inactivating enzyme. Another problem is *acute pancreatitis,* which develops in up to half of women.

With supportive care, recovery usually is complete. Maternal deaths are caused by sepsis, hemorrhage, aspiration, renal failure, pancreatitis, and gastrointestinal bleeding. In some women, heroic measures have included plasma exchange and even liver transplantation (Fesenmeier, 2005; Franco, 2000; Martin, 2008, and all their colleagues). In our now extensive experience, we have not found these necessary.

Maternal and Perinatal Outcomes

Although maternal mortality rates in the past approached 75 percent, the contemporaneous outlook is much better. From his review, Sibai (2007) cites an average mortality rate of 7 percent. He also cited a 70-percent preterm delivery rate and a perinatal mortality rate of approximately 15 percent, which in the past was nearly 90 percent.

The Liver in Preeclampsia–Eclampsia

Hepatic involvement is relatively common in women with severe preeclampsia and eclampsia (see Table 50-1). These changes are discussed in detail in Chapter 34 (p. 720).

Viral Hepatitis

Acute symptomatic hepatitis has become less common in the United States over the past 25 years (Centers for Disease Control and Prevention, 2008c). There are at least five distinct types of viral hepatitis: A (HAV), B (HBV), D (HDV) caused by the hepatitis B–associated delta agent, C (HCV), and E (HEV). During their acute phases, these disorders are similar, and the viruses themselves probably are not hepatotoxic, but rather the immune response to them causes hepatocellular necrosis (Dienstag, 2008a).

Acute infections are most often subclinical and *anicteric.* Annual rates of *new* infections in the United States for hepatitis A, B, and C are shown in Figure 50-2. When clinically apparent, nausea and vomiting, headache, and malaise may precede jaundice by 1 to 2 weeks. Low-grade fever is more common with hepatitis A. By the time jaundice develops, symptoms are usually improving. Serum transaminase levels vary, and their peaks do not correspond with disease severity (see Table 50-1). Peak levels that range from 400 to 4000 U/L are usually reached by the time jaundice develops. Serum bilirubin typically continues to rise, despite falling aminotransferase levels, and peaks at 5 to 20 mg/dL.

Any evidence for severe disease should prompt hospitalization. These include prolonged prothrombin time, low serum albumin level, hypoglycemia, high serum bilirubin level, or central nervous system symptoms. In most cases, however, there is complete clinical and biochemical recovery within 1 to 2 months in all cases of hepatitis A, in most cases of hepatitis B, but in only a small proportion of cases of hepatitis C.

When patients are hospitalized, their feces, secretions, bedpans, and other articles in contact with the intestinal tract should be handled with glove-protected hands. Extra precautions, such as double gloving during delivery and surgical procedures, are recommended. Due to significant exposure of healthcare personnel to hepatitis B, the Centers for Disease Control and Prevention (2006a, b) recommend active and passive vaccination. There is no vaccine for hepatitis C, so recommendations are for postexposure serosurveillance only.

Complications and Sequelae

Acute hepatitis has a case-fatality rate of 0.1 percent. For patients ill enough to be hospitalized, it is as high as 1 percent. Most fatalities are due to *fulminant hepatic necrosis,* which in later pregnancy may resemble acute fatty liver. Hepatic encephalopathy is the usual presentation, and the mortality rate is 80 percent. Approximately half of patients with fulminant disease have hepatitis B infection, and co-infection with the delta agent is common.

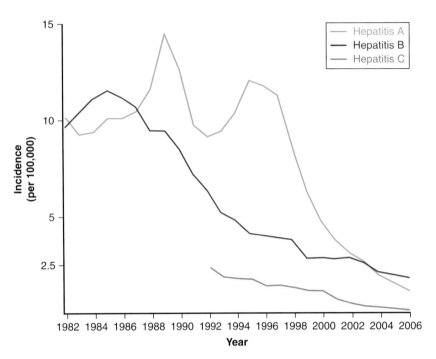

FIGURE 50-2 Annual incidence in the United States of new hepatitis A and B infection for 1982 through 2006, and for hepatitis C from 1991 through 2006. (Hepatitis C was reported as non-A, non-B hepatitis until 1995.) (Data from the Centers for Disease Control and Prevention, 2008c).

leagues, 2009). There are two *interferons*—standard and pegylated—these are *cytokines* with antiviral, antiproliferative, and immunoregulatory effects. There are five antiviral agents approved for 6-month treatment. They have been shown to decrease viremia and improve histological findings in approximately 20 percent of patients per year. Their cure rate ranges from 30 to 40 percent. The nucleoside analog *lamivudine* is better tolerated than interferon, however, a major problem is viral resistance. The nucleotide analog *adefovir dipivoxil* has been used successfully for both e antigen– negative as well as antigen-positive hepatitis B (Hadziyannis and colleagues, 2003; Marcellin and associates, 2003). The guanosine analog *entecavir* was recently found to be superior to lamivudine for patients with hepatitis B—either HBeAg-negative or -positive (Chang and associates, 2006; Lai and co-workers, 2006). And, *telbivudine* is an L-nucleoside with potent anti-HBV activity. (Lai and colleagues, 2007). Finally, *tenofovir disoproxil fumarate* is another recently available nucleotide derivative.

Chronic hepatitis is by far the most common complication of hepatitis B and C. It is diagnosed serologically in most cases (Table 50-3). Chronic infection follows acute hepatitis B in approximately 10 percent of cases in adults. Most become asymptomatic carriers, but a small percentage have low-grade chronic persistent hepatitis or chronic active hepatitis with or without cirrhosis. With acute hepatitis C, however, chronic hepatitis develops in the *majority* of patients. With persistently abnormal biochemical tests, liver biopsy usually discloses active inflammation, continuing necrosis, and fibrosis that may lead to cirrhosis. Chronic hepatitis is classified by cause; grade, defined by histological activity; and stage, that is, degree of progression (Dienstag and Isselbacher, 2005b). There is evidence that a cellular immune reaction is interactive with a genetic predisposition.

Although most chronically infected persons are asymptomatic, approximately 20 percent develop cirrhosis within 10 to 20 years (Dienstag, 2008a). When present, symptoms are nonspecific and usually include fatigue. Diagnosis can be confirmed by liver biopsy, however, treatment is usually given to patients after serological or virological diagnosis. In some patients, cirrhosis with liver failure or bleeding varices may be the presenting findings.

Treatment of Chronic Hepatitis

There is now considerable experience with treatment of chronic hepatitis B and C in nonpregnant patients. At least seven agents are approved for therapy of chronic hepatitis B (Sorrell and col-

Chronic Hepatitis and Pregnancy. Most young women with chronic hepatitis either are asymptomatic or have only mild liver disease. For seropositive asymptomatic women, there usually is no problem with pregnancy. With symptomatic chronic active hepatitis, pregnancy outcome depends primarily on the intensity of the disease and fibrosis, and especially whether there is portal hypertension. The few women who we

TABLE 50-3. Simplified Diagnostic Approach in Patients with Hepatitis

Diagnosis	HBsAg	IgM Anti-HAV	IgM Anti-HBc	Anti-HCV
Acute hepatitis A	−	+	−	−
Acute hepatitis B	+	−	+	−
Chronic hepatitis B	+	−	−	−
Acute hepatitis A with chronic B	+	+	−	−
Acute hepatitis A and B	+	+	+	−
Acute hepatitis C	−	−	−	+

HAV = hepatitis A virus; HBc = hepatitis B core; HbsAg = hepatitis B surface antigen; HCV = hepatitis C virus.
From the Centers for Disease Control and Prevention (2006a) and Dienstag and Isselbacher (2005a, b).

have managed have done well, but their long-term prognosis is poor. Accordingly, they should be counseled regarding possible liver transplantation as well as abortion and sterilization options.

Hepatitis A (HAV)

Because of vaccination programs, the incidence of hepatitis A has decreased 88 percent since 1995 (see Fig. 50-2). This 27-nm RNA picornavirus is transmitted by the fecal–oral route, usually by ingestion of contaminated food or water. The incubation period is approximately 4 weeks. Individuals shed virus in their feces, and during the relatively brief period of viremia, their blood is also infectious. Signs and symptoms are nonspecific, and most cases are anicteric and usually mild. Early serological detection is by identification of IgM anti-HAV antibody that may persist for several months. During convalescence, IgG antibody predominates, and it persists and provides subsequent immunity.

Pregnancy. Management of hepatitis A in pregnant women consists of a balanced diet and diminished physical activity. Women with less severe illness may be managed as outpatients. In developed countries, the effects of hepatitis A on pregnancy outcomes are not dramatic (American College of Obstetricians and Gynecologists, 2006, 2007). Both perinatal and maternal mortality rates, however, are substantively increased in third-world countries. There is no evidence that hepatitis A virus is teratogenic, and transmission to the fetus is negligible. Preterm birth may be increased, and neonatal cholestasis has been reported (Urganci and co-workers, 2003).

Immunization and Postexposure Prophylaxis. Childhood immunization with formalin-inactivated viral vaccine is more than 90-percent effective. HAV vaccination is recommended by the American College of Obstetricians and Gynecologists (2007) for high-risk adults, a category that includes behavioral and occupational risk populations and travelers to high-risk countries. These countries are listed by the Centers for Disease Control and Prevention (2008a) at www.cdc.gov/travel/contentdiseases.aspx. Passive immunization for the pregnant woman recently exposed by close personal or sexual contact with a person with hepatitis A is provided by a 0.02 mL/kg dose of immune globulin (Centers for Disease Control and Prevention, 2006b). Recently, Victor and colleagues (2007) reported that HAV vaccine given in the usual dosage to exposed persons was equally as effective as immune serum globulin to prevent HAV. In both groups, HAV developed in 3 to 4 percent.

Hepatitis B (HBV)

This infection is found worldwide but is endemic in some regions, especially in Asia and Africa. As shown in Figure 50-2, its annual incidence has decreased in the United States by approximately 80 percent since vaccination was introduced in the 1980s (Centers for Disease Control and Prevention, 2008c; Hoffnagle, 2006). Despite this, there are an estimated 1.2 million chronic carriers in the United States and 400 million worldwide. Hepatitis B is caused by a hepadnavirus whose

DNA codes for four viral products. Its serious sequelae include chronic hepatitis, cirrhosis, and hepatocellular carcinoma. *The World Health Organization considers hepatitis B to be second only to tobacco among human carcinogens.* Chronic infection follows in 5 to 10 percent of acutely infected adults and in 70 to 90 percent of infants.

According to the American College of Obstetricians and Gynecologists (2006), maternal-fetal transmission is the principal mode of transmission throughout the world. Other groups at high risk for hepatitis B infection are intravenous drug abusers, spouses of acutely infected individuals, sexually promiscuous persons—especially homosexual men, healthcare personnel, and patients who frequently receive blood products. HBV can be transmitted by any body fluid, but exposure to virus-laden serum is the most efficient mode of transmission. It is also sexually transmitted by saliva, vaginal secretions, and semen. Ye and co-workers (2006) have presented evidence that the virus infects the ova and may be transmitted to the fetus by that route. Because of similar modes of transmission, co-infection with human immunodeficiency virus type 1 (HIV-1) is common and has increased liver-related morbidity (Thio and colleagues, 2002).

At least half of initial HBV infections are asymptomatic. A variety of immunological serum markers have been identified in those with acute or chronic hepatitis B, in those previously infected but now immune, and in chronic carriers (see Table 50-3). The hepatitis B virus—the Dane particle, hepatitis B core antigen (HBcAg), hepatitis B surface antigen (HBsAg), hepatitis B e antigen (HBeAg), and their corresponding antibodies are all detectable by various techniques. Concentrations of viral antigen and particles in serum and other body fluids may reach 10^{12}/mL.

After infection, the first serological marker is HBsAg (Fig. 50-3). HBeAg signifies intact viral particles that invariably are present during early acute hepatitis. However, antigen persistence indicates chronic infection. After acute hepatitis, approximately 90 percent of persons recover completely. The

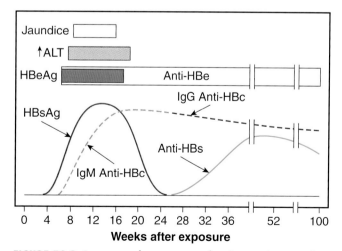

FIGURE 50-3 Sequence of appearance of various antigens and antibodies in acute hepatitis B. ALT = alanine aminotransferase; anti-HBc = antibody to hepatitis B core antigen; anti-HBe = antibody to hepatitis B e antigen; anti-HBs = antibody to hepatitis B surface antigen; HBeAg = hepatitis B e antigen; HBsAg = hepatitis B surface antigen. (Redrawn from Dienstag, 2008a.)

10 percent who remain chronically infected are considered to have chronic hepatitis B. Approximately a fourth of these develop chronic liver disease as subsequently discussed. Those seropositive for HBeAg are at greatest risk for hepatocellular carcinoma (Yang and co-workers, 2002).

Pregnancy. The clinical course of acute HBV is similar to that of HAV and is not altered by pregnancy in developed countries. Treatment is supportive, and the likelihood of preterm delivery is increased. Most HBV infections identified during pregnancy are chronic, asymptomatic, and diagnosed by routine prenatal serological screening as recommended by the American College of Obstetricians and Gynecologists (2007) and discussed in Chapter 8 (p. 194). Although these women have chronic hepatitis, most are asymptomatic, and antiviral treatment is generally not given until after pregnancy. The prevalence of prenatal seropositivity in inner-city groups is approximately 1 percent. It is somewhat lower for military populations and private patients.

Transplacental viral infection is uncommon, and Towers and associates (2001) reported that viral DNA is rarely found in amnionic fluid or cord blood. Thus, most neonatal infection is vertically transmitted by peripartum exposure. There is no evidence, however, that cesarean delivery lowers the risk (American College of Obstetricians and Gynecologists, 2007). Although virus is present in breast milk, the incidence of transmission is not lowered by formula feeding. Mothers with hepatitis B surface and e antigens are more likely to transmit infection to their infants, whereas those positive for anti-HBe antibody are usually not infective. *Infants infected with hepatitis B are generally asymptomatic, but 85 percent become chronically infected.*

Prevention of Neonatal Infection. Along with successful vaccination programs that began in 1982, perinatal infection has declined dramatically. For example, from 1990 through 2005, the incidence of HBV in the United States in children younger than 15 years declined by 98 percent (Centers for Disease Control and Prevention, 2006a). Passive three-dose immunization with hepatitis immune globulin does not decrease this further (Yuan and associates, 2006). Neonatal infection can usually be prevented by prenatal screening, by passive and active immunization for newborns of seropositive mothers, and by active vaccination during pregnancy of seronegative women. Results of a study from China indicate that lamivudine added to neonatal immunoprophylaxis will decrease infection rates even more. Xu and colleagues (2009) decreased perinatal infection rates from 40 to 20 percent in highly viremic women by administering lamivudine from 32 weeks' gestation until 4 weeks postpartum.

Infants born to seropositive mothers are given hepatitis B immune globulin—HBIG—very soon after birth. This is accompanied by the first of a three-dose hepatitis B recombinant vaccine. Hill and colleagues (2002) applied this strategy in 369 infants and reported that the 2.4-percent transmission rate was not increased with breast feeding if vaccination was completed. As discussed in Chapter 8 (p. 208), concern over adverse vaccine effects is unfounded according to the Institute of Medicine and the Food and Drug Administration (Centers for Disease Control and Prevention, 2006a).

For high-risk mothers who are seronegative, vaccine can be given during pregnancy. Ingardia and colleagues (2004) reported that women immunized during one pregnancy had an 85-percent seropositivity rate in a subsequent pregnancy. After the first dose, vaccination is repeated at 1 and 6 months, at 1 and 4 months, or at 2 and 4 months (see Table 8-10, p. 208). Sheffield and colleagues (2006) reported that the three-dose regimen given prenatally—initially and at 1 and 4 months—resulted in seroconversion rates of 56, 77, and 90 percent, respectively. This compares with the 96-percent rate reported by Jurema and associates (2001) for postpartum women given all three doses.

Hepatitis D (HDV)

Also called *delta hepatitis*, this is a defective RNA virus that is a hybrid particle with an HBsAg coat and a delta core. The virus must co-infect with hepatitis B either simultaneously or secondarily. It cannot persist in serum longer than hepatitis B virus. Transmission is similar to hepatitis B. Chronic co-infection with B and D hepatitis is more severe and accelerated than HBV alone, and up to 75 percent of affected patients develop cirrhosis. Neonatal transmission is unusual because neonatal HBV vaccination usually prevents delta hepatitis.

Hepatitis C (HCV)

This is a single-stranded RNA virus of the family *Flaviviridae*. Transmission is similar to that of hepatitis B except that sexual transmission of the virus is less efficient. A third of anti-HCV–positive persons have no risk factors (Dienstag, 2008a). Acute HCV infection is usually asymptomatic or with mild symptoms, and chronic infection is identified through various screening programs. Prenatal screening has been recommended for women in high-risk categories by the American College of Obstetricians and Gynecologists (2007). As shown in Figure 50-2, the incidence of new cases decreased by 92 percent from 1992 to 2005, probably because of risk-reduction strategies in high-risk groups (Centers for Disease Control and Prevention, 2008c). Screening of blood donors for hepatitis C virus has markedly decreased the incidence of posttransfusion hepatitis (Lauer and Walker, 2001).

When there is acute or initial infection, anti-HCV antibody is not detected for an average of 15 weeks and in some cases as long as a year. Antibody usually does not prohibit transmission if viral RNA coexists as it does in 75 to 85 percent of anti-HCV–positive persons (Mast and associates, 2005). After initial infection, nearly 75 percent of patients have chronic viremia, and half of these have abnormal liver tests for more than a year (Lauer and Walker, 2001). In two thirds of these with transaminase elevations, liver biopsy shows chronic active hepatitis. Approximately a third of these progress to cirrhosis within 20 to 30 years. Despite this, long-term mortality rates are not appreciably increased (Dienstag, 2008b). Chronic hepatitis C does not worsen the prognosis of patients who have HIV co-infection (Sulkowski and colleagues, 2002).

Pregnancy. The incidence of anti-HCV seropositivity during pregnancy varies with the population studied. The American College of Obstetricians and Gynecologists (2006) cites a 0.14- to

2.4-percent pregnancy seroprevalence. It is higher in women who are HIV positive, and Santiago-Munoz and associates (2005) found that 6.3 percent of HIV-infected pregnant women at Parkland Hospital were co-infected with hepatitis B or C.

Almost 80 percent of seropositive women will have chronic hepatitis. Despite this, hepatitis C infection—acute or chronic—has no apparent adverse effects on pregnancy. For example, serum transaminase levels are not different from those in infected nonpregnant individuals. There are conflicting reports concerning changes in RNA viral load in pregnancy (Gervais and associates, 2000; Paternoster and co-workers, 2001). As discussed on page 1068, Locatelli and co-workers (1999) observed a 16-percent incidence of cholestatic jaundice in seropositive women compared with only 0.8 percent in controls. This is not surprising—recall that almost two thirds of anti-HCV–positive individuals have chronic liver disease. At this time, antiviral treatment is not advised during pregnancy (Hoffnagle and Seeff, 2006).

Perinatal Transmission. The primary adverse perinatal outcome is vertical transmission of HCV infection to the fetus-infant. Vertical transmission is higher in mothers with viremia. From their review, Airoldi and Berghella (2006) cited a rate of 1 to 3 percent in HCV-positive, RNA-negative women compared with 4 to 6 percent in those RNA-positive. In a more recent report from Dublin, McMenamin and colleagues (2008) described transmission rates in 545 HCV-positive women. They found a 7.1-percent vertical transmission rate in RNA-positive women compared with none in those who were RNA-negative. Some have found an even greater risk when the mother is co-infected with HIV (Ferrero and associates, 2003). Other outcomes are not usually affected even when the viral load exceeds 500,000 copies/mL (Laibl and associates, 2005). That said, Pergam and colleagues (2008) recently reported an association with HCV-infected women and low-birthweight infants who had increased risk for ventilation.

At this time, there are no methods to prevent perinatal transmission, including cesarean delivery (American College of Obstetricians and Gynecologists, 2006). Because of this, the Centers for Disease Control and Prevention (2008b) do not recommend routine prenatal screening. Infants delivered of known HCV-positive mothers should be tested and followed clinically.

Hepatitis E (HEV)

This water-borne RNA virus usually is enterically transmitted by contaminated water supplies. It causes epidemic outbreaks in third-world countries with substantive morbidity and mortality rates. Boccia and associates (2006) cited a case-fatality rate of 30 percent in 61 pregnant women refugees admitted to a hospital in Darfur, Sudan. Hepatitis E has features resembling those of hepatitis A, and it is not easily communicable by person-to-person contact. There are four HEV genotypes, and type 1 causes most human disease. Shrestha and co-workers (2007) recently reported 95-percent preventive efficacy with a recombinant HEV vaccine in Nepal, although there is currently no FDA-approved vaccine available.

Hepatitis G (HGV)

This blood-borne infection with flavivirus-like RNA virus does not actually cause hepatitis (Dienstag, 2008a). Its seroprevalence in a Scottish study was 0.08 percent (Jarvis and associates, 1996). Infant transmission has been described by Feucht (1996) and Inaba (1997) and all their colleagues.

Autoimmune Hepatitis

This is a generally progressive chronic hepatitis that is important to distinguish from chronic viral hepatitis because treatments are markedly different. According to Krawitt (2006), an environmental agent—a virus or drug—triggers events that mediate T-cells to destroy liver antigens in genetically susceptible patients. Type 1 hepatitis is more common and is characterized by multiple autoimmune antibodies such as antinuclear antibodies (ANA) as well as certain human leukocyte genes. Treatment employs corticosteroids, alone or combined with azathioprine. In some patients, cirrhosis or hepatocellular carcinoma develops.

In general, pregnancy outcomes of women with autoimmune hepatitis are poor, but the prognosis is good with well-controlled disease (Uribe and associates, 2006). In one study, Schramm and colleagues (2006) described 42 pregnancies in 22 German women with autoimmune hepatitis. A fifth had a flare antepartum and half had a flare postpartum. One woman underwent liver transplantation at 18 weeks, and another died of sepsis at 19 weeks. In their 38-year review, Candia and associates (2005) found 101 pregnancies in 58 women. They reported that preeclampsia developed in approximately a fourth, and there were two maternal deaths. As with other autoimmune disorders, chronic autoimmune hepatitis is more common in women and frequently co-exists with thyroiditis, ulcerative colitis, type 1 diabetes, and rheumatoid arthritis. Hepatitis is usually subclinical, but exacerbations can cause fatigue and malaise that can be debilitating.

Nonalcoholic Fatty Liver Disease

Steatohepatitis is an increasingly recognized condition that may occasionally progress to hepatic cirrhosis. As a macrovesicular fatty liver condition, it resembles alcohol-induced liver injury but is seen without alcohol abuse. Obesity, type 2 diabetes, and hyperlipidemia—*syndrome X*—frequently coexist and likely are etiological agents or "triggers" (McCullough, 2006). Fatty liver is common in obese persons and as many as 50 percent of the morbidly obese are affected (see Chap. 43, p. 948). Moreover, half of persons with type 2 diabetes have steatohepatitis. According to Bacon (2008a), there is a continuum or spectrum of liver damage in which *fatty liver progresses to nonalcoholic steatohepatitis—NASH,* and then *hepatic fibrosis* develops that may progress to cirrhosis.

In most persons, the disease is usually asymptomatic, and it is a common explanation for elevated transaminase levels found in blood donors and other routine screening testing. Indeed, it is the cause of elevated asymptomatic aminotransferase levels in up to 90 percent of cases in which other liver disease is excluded. It also is the most common cause of abnormal liver tests among adults in this country. Currently, weight loss along with diabetes and dyslipidemia control is the only recommended treatment.

Pregnancy

Fatty liver infiltration is probably much more common than realized in obese and diabetic pregnant women. We have encountered a number of cases in women in later pregnancy. Once severe liver injury, that is, acute fatty liver of pregnancy, was excluded, they were observed with no adverse outcomes relative to liver involvement. As the obesity endemic worsens, any adverse effects of pregnancy will eventually surface.

Cirrhosis

Irreversible chronic liver injury with extensive fibrosis and regenerative nodules is the final common pathway for several disorders. *Laënnec cirrhosis* from chronic alcohol exposure is the most common cause in the general population. But in young women—including pregnant women, most cases are caused by *postnecrotic cirrhosis* from chronic hepatitis B and C. Many cases of *cryptogenic cirrhosis* are now known to be caused by nonalcoholic fatty liver disease (Bacon, 2008b). Clinical manifestations of cirrhosis include jaundice, edema, coagulopathy, metabolic abnormalities, and portal hypertension with gastroesophageal varices and splenomegaly. The incidence of deep-venous thromboembolism is increased (Søgaard and colleagues, 2009). The prognosis is poor, and 75 percent have progressive disease leading to death in 1 to 5 years.

Cirrhosis and Pregnancy

Women with symptomatic cirrhosis frequently are infertile. Those who become pregnant generally have poor outcomes. Common complications include transient hepatic failure, variceal hemorrhage, preterm delivery, fetal-growth restriction, and maternal death (Aggarwal and associates, 1999; Tan and colleagues, 2008). In older studies, outcome generally was worse if there were coexisting esophageal varices. Schreyer and associates (1982) reviewed 69 pregnancies in 60 women with cirrhosis without hepatic shunts and 28 pregnancies in another 23 women who had undergone portal decompression shunting. Severe variceal hemorrhage was increased sevenfold in nonshunted women compared with that in those who had undergone such procedures—24 versus 3 percent.

Portal Hypertension and Esophageal Varices in Pregnancy

Hypertension of the hepatic portal system with resultant esophageal varices may result either from cirrhosis or from extrahepatic portal vein obstruction. Varices in pregnant women are caused by equal numbers of each cause. Some extrahepatic cases follow portal vein thrombosis associated with one of the *thrombophilia syndromes* (see Chap. 47, p. 1014). Others follow thrombosis from umbilical vein catheterization when the woman was a neonate, especially if preterm.

With either intrahepatic or extrahepatic resistance to flow, portal vein pressure rises from its normal range of 5 to 10 mm Hg, and values may exceed 30 mm Hg. Collateral circulation develops that carries portal blood to the systemic circulation. Drainage is via the gastric, intercostal, and other veins to the esophageal system, where varices develop. Bleeding is usually from varices near the gastroesophageal junction, and hemorrhage can be torrential. Bleeding during pregnancy from varices occurs in a third to half of affected women and is the major cause of maternal mortality (Aggarwal and colleagues, 2001; Britton, 1982).

Maternal prognosis is largely dependent on whether there is variceal hemorrhage. Mortality rates are higher if varices are associated with cirrhosis than for varices without cirrhosis—18 versus 2 percent, respectively. Perinatal mortality rates are high in women with esophageal varices. And like maternal outcomes, those of the neonate are worse if cirrhosis caused the varices.

Management

Treatment is the same as for nonpregnant patients. Preventatively, consideration should be given to determining the extent of variceal dilatation by endoscopy or multidector CT esophagography (Kim and colleagues, 2007). Beta-blocking drugs such as propranolol are given to reduce portal pressure and hence the risk of bleeding (Groszmann and co-workers, 2005).

For acute bleeding, endoscopic band ligation is preferred according to Bacon (2008b). Zeeman and Moise (1999) described a pregnant woman who underwent *prophylactic* banding at 15, 26, and 31 weeks' gestation to prevent bleeding. Sclerotherapy can also be used and in some cases may aid banding (Aggarwal and co-workers, 2001). Acute medical management for bleeding varices verified by endoscopy includes intravenous vasopressin or octreotide and somatostatin (Chung and Podolsky, 2005). *Balloon tamponade* of severe bleeding using a triple-lumen tube can be lifesaving if endoscopy is not available. Emergency shunting is used in 10 to 20 percent of patients in whom hemorrhage cannot be controlled by endoscopy. The interventional radiology procedure—*transjugular intrahepatic portosystemic stent shunting* (*TIPSS*)—can also control bleeding from gastric varices (Khan and associates, 2006; Sharara and Rockey, 2001). TIPSS can be done electively in patients with previous variceal hemorrhage.

Acute Acetaminophen Overdose

Nonsteroidal anti-inflammatory drugs (NSAIDs) are commonly used in suicide attempts. In a study from Denmark, Flint and associates (2002) reported that more than half of such attempts by 122 pregnant women were with either acetaminophen or aspirin. In the United States, acetaminophen is much more commonly used during pregnancy, and overdose may lead to hepatocellular necrosis and acute liver failure (Lee and colleagues, 2008). Massive necrosis causes a *cytokine storm* and multi-organ dysfunction. Early symptoms of overdose are nausea, vomiting, diaphoresis, malaise, and pallor. After a latent period of 24 to 48 hours, liver failure ensues and usually begins to resolve in 5 days. For patients with liver failure, mortality rates are 20 to 40 percent (Hay, 2008).

The antidote is *N-acetylcysteine*, which must be given promptly. The drug is thought to act by increasing glutathione levels, which aid metabolism of the toxic metabolite, *N-acetyl-para*-benzoquinoneimine. The need for treatment is based on projections of possible plasma hepatotoxic levels as a function of the time from acute ingestion. Many poison control centers use the nomogram established by Rumack and Matthew (1975). A plasma level is measured 4 hours after ingestion, and if the level is greater than 120 μg/mL, treatment is given. If plasma determinations are not available, empirical treatment is given if the ingested amount exceeded 7.5 g. An oral loading dose of 140 mg/kg of *N*-acetylcysteine is followed by 17 maintenance doses of 70 mg/kg every 4 hours for 72 hours of total treatment time. The drug reaches therapeutic concentrations in the fetus, but its protective effects are unknown (Heard, 2008).

Effects on Pregnancy

After 14 weeks, the fetus has some cytochrome P$_{450}$ activity necessary for metabolism of acetaminophen to the toxic metabolite. Riggs and colleagues (1989) reported follow-up data from the Rocky Mountain Poison and Drug Center in 60 such women. The likelihood of maternal and fetal survival was better if the antidote was given soon after overdose. At least one 33-week fetus appears to have died as a direct result of hepatotoxicity 2 days after ingestion. In another case, Wang and associates (1997) confirmed acetaminophen placental transfer with maternal and cord blood levels of 41 μg/mL. Both mother and infant died from hepatorenal failure.

Liver Transplantation

According to the Organ Procurement and Transplantation Network (OPTN), as of late 2008, liver transplant patients comprised 16 percent of all proposed waiting organ recipients. A fourth of these are childbearing-aged women. Almost 30 years after the first liver transplantation, McKay and Josephson (2006) reviewed experiences from the National Transplantation Pregnancy Registry and described 182 pregnancies in 106 liver recipients. Approximately a third of pregnancies were complicated by hypertension, a fourth had preeclampsia, and 5 percent had a rejection episode (Table 50-4). Live-birth rates for pregnancies in women who underwent liver transplantation approximate 70 percent (Dei Malatesta and associates, 2006; Sibanda and colleagues, 2007). Importantly, however, 5 percent of mothers had died within 28 months after delivery. This rate is

TABLE 50-4. Pregnancy Complications in More Than 400 Women with a Liver Transplant

Complication	Percent
Maternal	
Preeclampsia	13–33
Hypertension	20–40
Liver dysfunction	27
Rejection	0–17
Perinatal	
Preterm birth	31
Fetal-growth restriction	23

Data from Bonanno and Dove (2007), Christopher and associates (2006), Dei Malatesta and colleagues (2006), Mastrobattista and Gomez-Lobo (2008), and McKay and Josephson (2006).

comparable with nonpregnant liver transplantation patients, and pregnancy does not appear to worsen survival.

In pregnant women who have undergone transplantation, close surveillance is mandatory to detect hypertension, renal dysfunction, preeclampsia, and graft rejection. Management considerations, including immunosuppressive therapy, were recently reviewed by Mastrobattista and Gomez-Lobo (2008) and by McKay and Josephson (2006). Because of increased metabolic clearance, serum levels of some antirejection drugs should be determined. Ethical considerations of pregnancy in transplant recipients were reviewed by Ross (2006).

GALLBLADDER DISORDERS

Cholelithiasis and Cholecystitis

In the United States, 20 percent of women older than 40 years have gallstones. Most stones contain cholesterol, and its oversecretion into bile is thought to be a major factor in stone formation. Biliary sludge, which may increase during pregnancy, is an important precursor to gallstone formation. The incidence of sonographically identified asymptomatic gallstones in more than 1500 pregnant or postpartum women was 2.5 to 10 percent (Maringhini and colleagues, 1987; Valdivieso and co-workers, 1993). Moreover, the cumulative risk of all patients with silent gallstones to require surgery for symptoms or complications is 10 percent at 5 years, 15 percent at 10 years, and 18 percent at 15 years (Greenberger and Paumgartner, 2008). For these reasons, prophylactic cholecystectomy is not warranted for *asymptomatic* stones.

For *symptomatic* gallstone disease, nonsurgical approaches have been used and include oral bile acid therapy with ursodeoxycholic acid and extracorporeal shock wave lithotripsy. There is no experience with these during pregnancy.

Acute cholecystitis usually develops when there is obstruction of the cystic duct. Bacterial infection plays a role in 50 to 85 percent of cases. In more than half of patients with acute cholecystitis, a history of previous right upper quadrant pain from cholelithiasis is elicited. With acute disease, pain is accompanied by anorexia, nausea and vomiting, low-grade fever, and mild leukocytosis. As shown in Figure 50-4, sonography can be used to see stones as small as 2 mm, and false-positive and false-negative rates are 2 to 4 percent (Greenberger and Paumgartner, 2008).

Symptomatic gallbladder diseases in young women include acute cholecystitis, biliary colic, and acute pancreatitis. Rarely, a gallbladder undergoes torsion or a neoplasm is found (Kleiss and co-workers, 2003; Wiseman and associates, 2008). In most symptomatic patients, cholecystectomy is warranted. Although acute cholecystitis responds to medical therapy, contemporary consensus is that early cholecystectomy is indicated (Greenberger and Paumgartner, 2008). In acute cases, medical therapy consisting of nasogastric suction, intravenous fluids, antimicrobials, and analgesics is instituted before surgical therapy. Laparoscopic cholecystectomy has become the treatment of choice for most patients.

Gallbladder Disease During Pregnancy

During pregnancy, approximately 1 in 1000 women develops cholecystitis. There is no doubt that pregnancy is "lithogenic." After the first trimester, both gallbladder volume during fasting

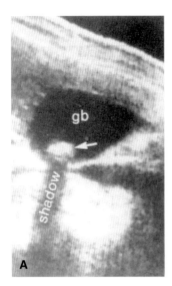
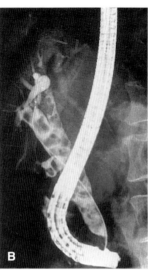

FIGURE 50-4 Gallstones. **A.** Visualization of a lone large gallstone by sonography. Note acoustic shadowing. **B.** Endoscopic retrograde cholangiopancreatogram (ERCP) showing multiple common-duct stones. (From Greenberger and Paumgartner, 2008, with permission.)

and residual volume after contracting in response to a test meal are doubled (Braverman and colleagues, 1980). Incomplete emptying may result in retention of cholesterol crystals, a prerequisite for cholesterol gallstones. Biliary sludge, which can be a forerunner to gallstones, develops in 30 percent of women during pregnancy (Maringhini and co-workers, 1987). After delivery, hospitalization for gallbladder disease within a year is relatively common. Ko (2006) studied Washington state discharge databases and documented that 0.5 percent of postpartum women were hospitalized within a year for a variety of conditions. Of these 6211 women, 76 had uncomplicated cholecystitis—55 underwent cholecystectomy.

Management

Acute cholecystitis during pregnancy or the puerperium is usually associated with gallstones or biliary sludge. Symptomatic cholecystitis is initially managed in a manner similar to that for nonpregnant women. In the past, most favored medical therapy, however, 25 to 50 percent of women ultimately require cholecystectomy for persistent symptoms (Cosenza and associates, 1999; Glasgow and co-workers, 1998). In an observational study of 44 pregnant women, Dixon and colleagues (1987) performed cholecystectomies in 18 with symptomatic acute cholecystitis or cholelithiasis. These women did well. Conversely, 15 of the 26 managed medically had recurrent symptoms during pregnancy. Similarly, Davis (1995) and Lee (2000) and their associates described a total of 77 cases of cholecystitis during pregnancy and cited better outcomes with primary surgical management.

These reports led to current management favoring surgical therapy during pregnancy. If treated conservatively, there is a high recurrence rate during the same pregnancy. Moreover, if cholecystitis recurs later in gestation, preterm labor is more likely and cholecystectomy technically more difficult. Man-

agement at Parkland Hospital has evolved to a more aggressive surgical approach, especially if there is concomitant biliary pancreatitis as subsequently discussed.

Laparoscopic Cholecystectomy. Reasonable experiences have been reported from several centers to indicate that laparoscopic surgery is as acceptable as open cholecystectomy in pregnant women (Barone, 1999; Cosenza, 1999; Glasgow, 1998, and all their colleagues). After their review of 213 cases, Lachman and co-workers (1999) concluded that laparoscopic cholecystectomy was safe throughout pregnancy. This procedure is discussed in Chapter 41 (p. 913).

Endoscopic Retrograde Cholangiopancreatography. Relief from symptomatic biliary duct gallstones during pregnancy has been greatly aided by use of endoscopic retrograde cholangiopancreatography—ERCP (Menees and Elta, 2006). The procedure is performed if there is suspected common duct obstruction, usually from stones (see Fig. 50-4). Approximately 10 percent of patients with symptomatic stone disease have common duct stones (Greenberger and Paumpartner, 2008). ERCP can be modified in many cases so that radiation exposure from fluoroscopy is avoided (Shelton and co-workers, 2008; Simmons and colleagues, 2004).

Results from 68 ERCP procedures performed in 65 pregnant women at Parkland Hospital were recently reported by Tang and associates (2009). All but two women had gallstones, and sphincterotomy was performed in all but one woman. Common-duct stones were identified in half of these 65 women, and in all but one, the stones were successfully removed. A biliary stent was placed in 22 percent and removed after delivery. Complications were minimized and post-ERCP pancreatitis developed in 16 percent. Pregnancy outcomes were not different than the general obstetrical population.

PANCREATIC DISORDERS

Pancreatitis

Pathogenesis and Incidence

Acute pancreatic inflammation is triggered by activation of pancreatic trypsinogen followed by autodigestion. It is characterized by cellular membrane disruption and proteolysis, edema, hemorrhage, and necrosis (Whitcomb, 2006). Approximately 20 percent have severe pancreatitis, and mortality rates in these patients reach up to 25 percent (Swaroop and associates, 2004).

In nonpregnant patients, acute pancreatitis is almost equally associated with gallstones and alcohol abuse. During pregnancy, however, cholelithiasis is almost always the predisposing condition. Other causes are hyperlipidemias, usually hypertriglyceridemia; hyperparathyroidism; congenital ductal anomalies; and rarely autoimmune pancreatitis (Crisan and colleagues, 2008; Finkelberg and associates, 2006). Nonbiliary pancreatitis occasionally develops postoperatively, or it is associated with trauma, drugs, or some viral infections. Certain metabolic conditions, including acute fatty liver of pregnancy and familial hypertriglyceridemia, also predispose to pancreatitis. Acute and chronic pancreatitis have been linked to the more than 1000

TABLE 50-5. Laboratory Values in 43 Pregnant Women with Pancreatitis

Test	Mean	Range	Normal
Serum amylase (IU/L)	1392	111–4560	30–110
Serum lipase (IU/L)	6929	36–41,824	23–208
Total bilirubin (mg/dL)	1.7	0.1–4.9	0.2–1.3
Aspartate transferase(U/L)	120	11–498	3–35
Leukocytes (per μL)	12,000	1000–14,600	4100–10,900

Reprinted from *American Journal of Obstetrics & Gynecology*, Vol. 173, No. 7, KD Ramin, SM Ramin, SD Richey, et al., Acute pancreatitis in pregnancy, pp. 187–191, Copyright 1995, with permission from Elsevier.

mutations of the cystic fibrosis transmembrane conductance regulator gene (Rowntree and Harris, 2003).

At Parkland Hospital, with a predominate Mexican-American population, acute pancreatitis complicated approximately 1 in 3300 pregnancies (Ramin and colleagues, 1995). At Brigham and Women's Hospital, with a more diversely ethnic population, Hernandez and co-workers (2007) reported an incidence of 1 in 4450. In a multi-institution Midwestern three-state review of more than 305,000 pregnancies, Eddy and associates (2008) found the incidence to be 1 in 3450 for acute pancreatitis.

Diagnosis

Acute pancreatitis is characterized by mild to incapacitating epigastric pain, nausea and vomiting, and abdominal distension. Patients are usually in distress and have low-grade fever, tachycardia, hypotension, and abdominal tenderness. As many as 10 percent have systemic inflammatory response syndrome, which causes endothelial activation and can lead to *acute respiratory distress syndrome* (see Chap. 42, p. 930).

Laboratory confirmation is from serum amylase levels three times upper normal values. As shown in Table 50-5, the mean amylase value in 43 pregnant women with pancreatitis was approximately 1400 IU/L, and the mean lipase value approximated 7000 IU/L. Importantly, there is no correlation between their degree of elevation and disease severity. Indeed, by 48 to 72 hours, amylase levels may return to normal despite other evidence for continuing pancreatitis. Serum lipase activity is also increased and usually remains elevated with continued inflammation. There is usually leukocytosis, and 25 percent of patients have hypocalcemia. Elevated serum bilirubin and aspartate aminotransferase levels usually signify gallstone disease.

A number of prognostic factors may be used to predict disease severity (Whitcomb, 2006). Some of these are respiratory failure, shock, need for massive colloid replacement, hypocalcemia of <8 mg/dL, and dark hemorrhagic fluid on paracentesis. If three of the first four features are documented, survival is only 30 percent.

Management

Medical treatment mirrors that for nonpregnant patients and includes analgesics, intravenous hydration, and measures to de-

crease pancreatic secretion by interdiction of oral intake. Other than supportive therapy, no particular treatment schemes have improved outcomes (Whitcomb, 2006). In the series by Ramin and colleagues (1995), all 43 affected pregnant women responded to conservative treatment and were hospitalized for a mean of 8.5 days. Nasogastric suction does not improve outcomes of mild to moderate disease, but enteral feeding may be helpful once pain improves and associated ileus resolves. Although we try to avoid parenteral nutrition, in 65 women with acute pancreatitis described by Eddy and co-workers (2008), a fourth had total parenteral nutrition. With bacterial superinfection of necrotizing pancreatitis, antimicrobials are indicated. For pregnant patients with gallstone pancreatitis, ERCP for removal of common duct stones and papillotomy has been used successfully (Simmons and co-workers, 2004; Tang and colleagues, 2009). Cholecystectomy should be considered after inflammation subsides if there is gallbladder disease. Hernandez and associates (2007) reported that half of such women who did not undergo cholecystectomy had recurrent pancreatitis during the same pregnancy. Severe necrotizing pancreatitis can be life threatening, and laparotomy for debridement and drainage may be required (Gosnell and colleagues, 2001; Robertson and associates, 2006).

Pregnancy outcomes appear to be related to the severity of acute pancreatitis. Eddy and associates (2008) reported a 30-percent preterm delivery rate—11 percent delivered before 35 weeks. There were only two pancreatitis-related deaths. Importantly, almost a third of 73 women had recurrent pancreatitis during pregnancy.

Pancreatic Transplantation

According to the United Network for Organ Sharing, the 5-year graft survival for pancreatic transplantation is 80 percent. Because there is improved survival when a combined pancreas and kidney are grafted for those with type 1 diabetes and renal failure, most operations include both organs.

Tydén and colleagues (1989) described four women in whom pancreas-kidney transplantation was followed in 1 to 2 years by pregnancy. Pelvic placement of the graft was not problematic. Glucose homeostasis was well maintained throughout pregnancy. Successful vaginal deliveries have been described by Allenby and colleagues (1998). Mastrobattista and Gomez-Lobo (2008) reported results from the National Transplantation Pregnancy Registry. Of 44 pregnancies in 73 women following pancreas-kidney transplantation, outcomes have been encouraging. Although the incidence of hypertension, preeclampsia, preterm delivery, and fetal-growth restriction was high, there was only one perinatal death. There were four rejection episodes during pregnancy, which were treated successfully.

Pancreatic islet autotransplantation may be performed to prevent diabetes following pancreatectomy, and at least three successful pregnancies have been described (Jung, 2007; Teuscher, 1994; Wahoff, 1995, and all their colleagues).

REFERENCES

Aggarwal SH, Suril V, Vasishta K, et al: Pregnancy and cirrhosis of the liver. Aust NZ J Obstet Gynaecol 39:503, 1999

Aggarwal N, Sawhney H, Vasishta K, et al: Non-cirrhotic portal hypertension in pregnancy. Int J Gynaecol Obstet 72:1, 2001

Airoldi J, Berghella V: Hepatitis C and pregnancy. Obstet Gynecol Surv 61:666, 2006

Allenby K, Campbell DJ, Lodge JPA: Vaginal delivery following combined pelvic renal and pancreatic transplant. Br J Obstet Gynaecol 105:1036, 1998

American College of Obstetricians and Gynecologists: Liver disease. Clinical Updates in Women's Health Care, Vol. V, No. 4, 2006

American College of Obstetricians and Gynecologists: Viral hepatitis in pregnancy. Practice Bulletin No. 86, October 2007

Armenti VY, Radomski JS, Moritz MJ, et al: Report from the National Transplantation Pregnancy Registry (NTPR): Outcomes of pregnancy after transplantation, Chapter 7. In Cecka JM, Terasaki PI (eds): Clinical Transplants 2001. Los Angeles, UCLA Immunogenetics Center, 2001, p 97

Bacon BR: Cirrhosis and its complications. In Fauci A, Braunwald E, Kasper DL, et al (eds): Harrison's Principles of Internal Medicine, 17th ed. New York, McGraw-Hill, 2008b, p 1971

Bacon BR: Genetic, metabolic, and infiltrative diseases affecting the liver. In Fauci A, Braunwald E, Kasper DL, et al (eds): Harrison's Principles of Internal Medicine, 17th ed. New York, McGraw-Hill, 2008a, p 1980

Barone JE, Bears S, Chen S, et al: Outcome study of cholecystectomy during pregnancy. Am J Surg 177:232, 1999

Blish KR, Ibdah JA: Maternal heterozygosity for a mitochondrial trifunctional protein mutation as a cause for liver disease in pregnancy. Med Hypotheses 64:96, 2005

Boccia D, Guthmann JP, Klovstad H, et al: High mortality associated with an outbreak of hepatitis E among displaced persons in Darfur, Sudan. Clin Infect Dis 42:1679, 2006

Bonanno C, Dove L: Pregnancy after liver transplantation. Semin Perinatol 31:348, 2007

Braverman DZ, Johnson ML, Kern F Jr: Effects of pregnancy and contraceptive steroids on gallbladder function. N Engl J Med 302:362, 1980

Britton RC: Pregnancy and esophageal varices. Am J Surg 143:421, 1982

Browning MF, Levy HL, Wilkins-Haug LE, et al: Fetal fatty acid oxidation defects and maternal liver disease in pregnancy. Obstet Gynecol 107:115, 2006

Candia L, Marquez J, Espinoza LR: Autoimmune hepatitis and pregnancy: A rheumatologist's dilemma. Semin Arthritis Rheum 35:49, 2005

Castro MA, Goodwin TM, Shaw KJ, et al: Disseminated intravascular coagulation and antithrombin III depression in acute fatty liver of pregnancy. Am J Obstet Gynecol 174:211, 1996a

Castro MA, Ouzounian JG, Colletti PM, et al: Radiologic studies in acute fatty liver of pregnancy. A review of the literature and 19 new cases. J Reprod Med 41:839, 1996b

Centers for Disease Control and Prevention: A comprehensive immunization strategy to eliminate transmission of hepatitis B virus infection in the United States. MMWR 55(No. RR-16):13, 2006a

Centers for Disease Control and Prevention: General recommendations on immunization: Recommendations of the Advisory Committee on Immunization Practice (ACIP). MMWR 50 (No. 44-15):32, 2006b

Centers for Disease Control and Prevention: Diseases related to travel. Available at: http://wwwn.cdc.gov/travel/contentdiseases.aspx Accessed June 18, 2008a

Centers for Disease Control and Prevention: Hepatitis C FAQs for health professionals. Available at: www.cdc.gov/hepatitis/hcv/hcvfaq.htm#section7 Accessed October 19, 2008b

Centers for Disease Control and Prevention: Surveillance for acute viral hepatitis—United States, 2006. MMWR 57 (No. SS 2), 2008c

Chang TT, Gish RG, de Man R, et al: A comparison of entecavir and lamivudine for HBeAg-positive chronic hepatitis B. N Engl J Med 354:1001, 2006

Christopher V, Al-Chalabi T, Richardson PD, et al: Pregnancy outcome after liver transplantation: A single-center experience of 71 pregnancies in 45 recipients. Liver Transpl 12:1037, 2006

Chung RT, Podolsky DK: Cirrhosis and its complications. In Kasper DL, Braunwald E, Fauci AS, et al (eds): Harrison's Principles of Internal Medicine, 16th ed. New York, McGraw-Hill, 2005, p 1858

Cosenza CA, Saffari B, Jabbour N, et al: Surgical management of biliary gallstone disease during pregnancy. Am J Surg 178:545, 1999

Crisan LS, Steidl ET, Rivera-Alsina ME: Acute hyperlipidemic pancreatitis in pregnancy. Am J Obstet [Epub ahead of print], 2008

Cunningham FG, Lowe TW, Guss S, et al: Erythrocyte morphology in women with severe preeclampsia and eclampsia. Am J Obstet Gynecol 153:358, 1985

Dann AT, Kenyon AP, Wierzbicki AS, et al: Plasma lipid profiles of women with intrahepatic cholestasis of pregnancy. Obstet Gynecol 107:106, 2006

Davidson KM, Simpson LL, Knox TA, et al: Acute fatty liver of pregnancy in triplet gestation. Obstet Gynecol 91:806, 1998

Davis A, Katz VL, Cox R: Gallbladder disease in pregnancy. J Reprod Med 40:759, 1995

Dei Malatesta MF, Rossi M, Rocca B, et al: Pregnancy after liver transplantation: Report of 8 new cases and review of the literature. Transpl Immunol 15:297, 2006

Dienstag JL: Acute viral hepatitis. In Fauci AS, Braunwald E, Kasper DL, et al (eds): Harrison's Principles of Internal Medicine, 17th ed. New York, McGraw-Hill, 2008a, p 1955

Dienstag JL: Chronic hepatitis. In Fauci AS, Braunwald E, Kasper DL, et al (eds): Harrison's Principles of Internal Medicine, 17th ed. New York, McGraw-Hill, 2008b

Dienstag JL, Isselbacher KJ: Acute viral hepatitis. In Kasper DL, Braunwald E, Fauci AS, et al (eds): Harrison's Principles of Internal Medicine, 16th ed. New York, McGraw-Hill, 2005a

Dienstag JL, Isselbacher KJ: Chronic hepatitis. In Kasper DL, Braunwald E, Fauci AS, et al (eds): Harrison's Principles of Internal Medicine, 16th ed. New York, McGraw-Hill, 2005b, p 1932

Dixon NP, Faddis DM, Silberman H: Aggressive management of cholecystitis during pregnancy. Am J Surg 154:294, 1987

Eddy JJ, Gideonsen MD, Song JY, et al: Pancreatitis in pregnancy. Obstet Gynecol 112:1075, 2008

Ferrero S, Lungaro P, Bruzzone BM, et al: Prospective study of mother-to-infant transmission of hepatitis C virus: A 10-year survey (1990–2000). Acta Obstet Gynecol Scand 82:229, 2003

Fesenmeier MF, Coppage KH, Lambers DS, et al: Acute fatty liver of pregnancy in 3 tertiary care centers. Am J Obstet Gynecol 192:1416, 2005

Feucht HH, Zollner B, Polywka S, et al: Vertical transmission of hepatitis G. Lancet 347:615, 1996

Finkelberg DL, Sahani D, Deshpande V, et al: Autoimmune pancreatitis. N Engl J Med 355:2670, 2006

Flint C, Larsen H, Nielsen GL, et al: Pregnancy outcome after suicide attempt by drug use: A Danish population-based study. Acta Obstet Gynecol Scand 81:516, 2002

Franco J, Newcomer J, Adams M, et al: Auxiliary liver transplant in acute fatty liver of pregnancy. Obstet Gynecol 95:1042, 2000

Germain AM, Carvajal JA, Glasinovic JC, et al: Intrahepatic cholestasis of pregnancy: An intriguing pregnancy-specific disorder. J Soc Gynecol Invest 9:10, 2002

Gervais A, Bacq Y, Bernuau J, et al: Decrease in serum ALT and increase in serum HCV RNA during pregnancy in women with chronic hepatitis C. J Hepatol 32:293, 2000

Glantz A, Marschall H, Mattsson L: Intrahepatic cholestasis of pregnancy: Relationships between bile acid levels and fetal complication rates. Hepatology 40:467, 2004

Glantz A, Marschall H, Lammert F, et al: Intrahepatic Cholestasis of pregnancy: A randomized controlled trial comparing dexamethasone and ursodeoxycholic acid. Hepatology 42:1399, 2005

Glasgow RE, Visser BC, Harris HW, et al: Changing management of gallstone disease during pregnancy. Surg Endosc 12:241, 1998

Gonzales E, Davit-Spraul A, Baussan C: Liver disease related to MDR3 (ABCB4) gene deficiency. Front Biosci 14:4242, 2009

Gorelik J, Patel P, Ng'andwe C, et al: Genes encoding bile acid, phospholipid and anion transporters are expressed in a human fetal cardiomyocyte culture. BJOG 113:552, 2006

Gosnell FE, O'Neill BB, Harris HW: Necrotizing pancreatitis during pregnancy: A rare case and review of the literature. J Gastrointest Surg 5:371, 2001

Greenberger NJ, Paumgartner G: Diseases of the gallbladder and bile ducts. In Fauci AS, Braunwald E, Kasper DL, et al (eds): Harrison's Principles of Internal Medicine, 17th ed. New York, McGraw-Hill, 2008, p 1991

Groszmann RJ, Garcia-Tsao G, Bosch J, et al: Beta-blockers to prevent gastroesophageal varices in patients with cirrhosis. N Engl J Med 353:2254, 2005

Hadziyannis SJ, Tassopoulos NC, Heathcote EJ, et al: Adefovir dipivoxil for the treatment of hepatitis B e antigen-negative chronic hepatitis B. N Engl J Med 348:800, 2003

Hay JE: Liver disease in pregnancy. Hepatology 47(3):1067, 2008

Heard KJ: Acetylcysteine for acetaminophen poisoning. N Engl J Med 359:285, 2008

Hernandez A, Petrov MS, Brooks DC, et al: Acute pancreatitis and pregnancy: A 10-year single center experience. J Gastrointest Surg 11:1623, 2007

Hill JB, Sheffield JS, Kim MJ, et al: Risk of hepatitis B transmission in breast-fed infants of chronic hepatitis B carriers. Obstet Gynecol 99;1049, 2002

Hoffnagle JH: Hepatitis B—Preventable and now treatable. N Engl J Med 354:1074, 2006

Hoffnagle JH, Seeff LB: Peginterferon and ribavirin for chronic hepatitis C. N Engl J Med 355:2444, 2006

Horowitz RS, Dart RC, Jarvie DR, et al: Placental transfer of N-acetylcysteine following human maternal acetaminophen toxicity. Clin Toxicol 35:447, 1997

Inaba N, Okajima Y, Kang XS, et al: Maternal–infant transmission of hepatitis G virus. Am J Obstet Gynecol 177:1537, 1997

Ingardia C, Morgan M, Feldman D, et al: Hepatitis B vaccination in pregnancy—factors associated with immunity in subsequent pregnancy. Abstract 137. Presented at the 24th Annual Meeting of the Society for Maternal–Fetal Medicine, 2–7 February 2004

Ingerslev M, Teilum G: Biopsy studies on the liver in pregnancy, 2. Liver biopsy on normal pregnant women. Acta Obstet Gynecol Scand 25:352, 1945

Jarvis LM, Davidson F, Hanley JP, et al: Infection with hepatitis G virus among recipients of plasma products. Lancet 348:1352, 1996

Jung HS, Choi SH, Noh JH, et al: Healthy twin birth after autologous islet transplantation in a pancreatectomized patient due to a benign tumor. Transplant Proc 39(5):1723, 2007

Jurema MW, Polaneczky M, Ledger WJ: Hepatitis B immunization in postpartum women. Am J Obstet Gynecol 185:355, 2001

Kenyon AP, Piercy CN, Girling J, et al: Pruritus may precede abnormal liver function tests in pregnant women with obstetric cholestasis: A longitudinal analysis. Br J Obstet Gynaecol 108:1190, 2001

Kenyon AP, Piercy CN, Girling J, et al: Obstetric cholestasis, outcome with active management: A series of 70 cases. Br J Obstet Gynaecol 109:282, 2002

Khan S, Tudur Smith C, Williamson P, et al: Portosystemic shunts versus endoscopic therapy for variceal rebleeding in patients with cirrhosis. Cochrane Database Syst Rev 4:CD000553, 2006

Kim SH, Kim YJ, Lee JM, et a: Esophageal varices in patients with cirrhosis: Multidetector CT esophagography—Comparison with endoscopy. Radiology January 17, 2007

Kirkinen P, Ryynänen M: First-trimester manifestation of intrahepatic cholestasis of pregnancy and high fetoplacental hormone production in a triploid fetus. J Reprod Med 40:471, 1995

Kleiss K, Choy-Hee L, Fogle R, et al: Torsion of the gallbladder in pregnancy: A case report. J Reprod Med 48:206, 2003

Knox TA, Olans LB: Liver disease in pregnancy. N Engl J Med 335:568, 1996

Ko CW: Risk factors for gallstone-related hospitalization during pregnancy and the postpartum. Am K Gastroenterol 101:2263, 2006

Kondrackiene J, Beuers U, Kupcinskas L: Efficacy and safety of ursodeoxycholic acid versus cholestyramine in intrahepatic cholestasis of pregnancy. Gastroenterology 129:894, 2005

Krawitt EL: Autoimmune hepatitis. N Engl J Med 354:54, 2006

Kroumpouzos G, Cohen LM: Specific dermatoses of pregnancy: An evidence-based systematic review. Am J Obstet Gynecol 188:1083, 2003

Lachman E, Schienfeld A, Voss E, et al: Pregnancy and laparoscopic surgery. J Am Assoc Gynecol Laparosc 6:347, 1999

Lai CL, Gane E, Liaw YF, et al: Telbivudine versus lamivudine in patients with chronic hepatitis B. N Engl J Med 357(25):2576, 2007

Lai CL, Shouval D, Lok AS, et al: Entecavir versus lamivudine for patients with HBeAg-negative chronic hepatitis B. N Engl J Med 354:1011, 2006

Laibl V, Sheffield J, Robert S, et al: Hepatitis C quantitative viral load as a predictor of pregnancy outcome. Presented at the 25th Annual Meeting of the Society for Maternal–Fetal Medicine, Reno, Nevada, February 7, 2005

Lauer GM, Walker BD: Hepatitis C virus infection. N Engl J Med 345:41, 2001

Lausman AY, Al-Yaseen E, Sam E, et al: Intrahepatic cholestasis of pregnancy in women with a multiple pregnancy: An analysis of risks and pregnancy outcomes. J Obstet Gynaecol Can 30(11):1008, 2008

Lee RH, Incerpi MH, Miller DA, et al: Sudden death in intrahepatic cholestasis of pregnancy. Obstet Gynecol 113(2):528, 2009

Lee S, Bradley JP, Mele MM, et al: Cholelithiasis in pregnancy: Surgical versus medical management. Obstet Gynecol 95:S70, 2000

Lee WM, Squires RH Jr, Nyberg SL, et al: Acute liver failure: Summary of a workshop. Hepatology 47:1401, 2008

Leslie KK, Reznikov L, Simon FR, et al: Estrogens in intrahepatic cholestasis of pregnancy. Obstet Gynecol 95:372, 2000

Lin HM, Kauffman HM, McBride MA, et al: Center-specific graft and patient survival rates. 1997 United Network for Organ Sharing (UNOS) report. JAMA 280:1153, 1998

Locatelli A, Roncaglia N, Arreghini A, et al: Hepatitis C virus infection is associated with a higher incidence of cholestasis of pregnancy. Br J Obstet Gynaecol 106:498, 1999

Lucangioli SE, Castaño G, Contin MD, et al: Lithocholic acid as a biomarker of intrahepatic cholestasis of pregnancy during ursodeoxycholic acid treatment. Ann Clin Biochem 46(1):44, 2009

Lunzer M, Barnes P, Byth K, et al: Serum bile acid concentrations during pregnancy and their relationship to obstetric cholestasis. Gastroenterology 91:825, 1986

Marcellin P, Chang TT, Lim SG, et al: Adefovir dipivoxil for the treatment of hepatitis B e antigen-positive chronic hepatitis B. N Engl J Med 348:808, 2003

Maringhini A, Marcenó MP, Lanzarone F, et al: Sludge and stones in gallbladder after pregnancy: Prevalence and risk factors. J Hepatol 5:218, 1987

Martin JN Jr, Briery CM, Rose CH, et al: Postpartum plasma exchange as adjunctive therapy for severe acute fatty liver of pregnancy. J Clin Apher Jul 16, 2008

Mast EE, Hwang LY, Seto DS, et al: Risk factors for perinatal transmission of hepatitis C virus (HCV) and the natural history of HCV infection acquired in infancy. J Infect Dis 192:1880, 2005

Mastrobattista JM, Gomez-Lobo V: Pregnancy after solid organ transplantation. Obstet Gynecol 112:919, 2008

Matos A, Bernardes J, Ayres-de-Campos D, et al: Antepartum fetal cerebral hemorrhage not predicted by current surveillance methods in cholestasis of pregnancy. Obstet Gynecol 89:803, 1997

Mazzella G, Nicola R, Francesco A, et al: Ursodeoxycholic acid administration in patients with cholestasis of pregnancy: Effects on primary bile acids in babies and mothers. Hepatology 33:504, 2001

McCullough AJ: Thiazolidinediones for nonalcoholic steatohepatitis—promising but not ready for prime time. N Engl J Med 355:2361, 2006

McKay DB, Josephson MA: Pregnancy in recipients of solid organs—Effects on mother and child. N Engl J Med 354:1281, 2006

McMenamin MB, Jackson AD, Lambert J, et al: Obstetric management of hepatitis C-positive mothers: Analysis of vertical transmission in 559 mother-infant pairs. Am J Obstet Gynecol 199:315.e1, 2008

Menees S, Elta G: Endoscopic retrograde cholangiopancreatography during pregnancy. Gastrointest Endoscopy Clin N Am 16:41, 2006

Mullally B, Hansen W: Intrahepatic cholestasis of pregnancy: Review of the literature. Obstet Gynecol Surv 57:47, 2001

Organ Procurement and Transplantation Network: Data. Available at: http://www.optn.org/data/. Accessed April 9, 2008

Paternoster DM, Fabris F, Palù G, et al: Intra-hepatic cholestasis of pregnancy in hepatitis C virus infection. Acta Obstet Gynecol Scand 81:99, 2002

Paternoster, Santarossa C, Grella P, et al: Viral load in HCV RNA-positive pregnant women. Am J Gastroenterol 96:2751, 2001

Pereira SP, O'Donohue J, Wendon J, et al: Maternal and perinatal outcome in severe pregnancy-related liver disease. Hepatology 26:1258, 1997

Pergam SA, Wang CC, Gardella CM, et al: Pregnancy complications associated with hepatitis C: Data from a 2003–2005 Washington state birth cohort. Am J Obstet Gynecol 199:38.e1, 2008

Ramin KD, Ramin SM, Richey SD, et al: Acute pancreatitis in pregnancy. Am J Obstet Gynecol 173:187, 1995

Reyes H: Intrahepatic cholestasis. A puzzling disorder of pregnancy. J Gastroenterol Hepatol 12:211, 1997

Reyes H, Sjovall J: Bile acids and progesterone metabolites in intrahepatic cholestasis of pregnancy. Ann Med 32:94, 2000

Riggs BS, Bronstein AC, Kulig K, et al: Acute acetaminophen overdose during pregnancy. Obstet Gynecol 74:247, 1989

Rioseco AJ, Ivankovic MB, Manzur A, et al: Intrahepatic cholestasis of pregnancy: A retrospective case-control study of perinatal outcome. Am J Obstet Gynecol 170:890, 1994

Robertson KW, Stewart IS, Imrie CW: Severe acute pancreatitis and pregnancy. Pancreatology 6:309, 2006

Ross LF: Ethical considerations related to pregnancy in transplant recipients. N Engl J Med 354:1313, 2006

Rowntree RK, Harris A: The phenotypic consequences of CFTR mutations. Ann Hum Genet 67:471, 2003

Rumack BH, Matthew H: Acetaminophen poisoning and toxicity. Pediatrics 55:871, 1975

Sadler LC, Lane M, North R: Severe fetal intracranial haemorrhage during treatment with cholestyramine for intrahepatic cholestasis of pregnancy. Br J Obstet Gynaecol 102:169, 1995

Santiago-Munoz P, Roberts S, Sheffield J, et al: Prevalence of hepatitis B and C in pregnant women who are infected with human immunodeficiency virus. Am J Obstet Gynecol 193:1270, 2005

Schramm C, Herkel J, Beuers U, et al: Pregnancy in autoimmune hepatitis: Outcome and risk factors. Am J Gastroenterol 101:556, 2006

Schreyer P, Caspi E, El-Hindi JM, et al: Cirrhosis—pregnancy and delivery: A review. Obstet Gynecol Surv 37:304, 1982

Sharara AI, Rockey DC: Gastroesophageal variceal hemorrhage. N Engl J Med 345:669, 2001

Sheffield J, Roberts S, Laibl V, et al: The efficacy of an accelerated hepatitis B vaccination program during pregnancy [Abstract No. 212]. Am J Obstet Gynecol 195:S73, 2006

Sheiner E, Ohel I, Levy A, et al: Pregnancy outcome in women with pruritus gravidarum. J Reprod Med 51:394, 2006

Shelton J, Linder JD, Rivera-Alsina ME, et al: Commitment, confirmation, and clearance: New techniques for nonradiation ERCP during pregnancy (with videos). Gastrointest Endosc 67:364, 2008

Shrestha MP, Scott RM, Joshi DM, et al: Safety and efficacy of recombinant hepatitis E vaccine. N Engl J Med 356:895, 2007

Sibai BM: Imitators of severe preeclampsia. Obstet Gynecol 109:956, 2007

Sibanda N, Briggs JD, Davison JM, et al: Pregnancy after organ transplantation: A report from the UK Transplant pregnancy registry. Transplantation 83:1301, 2007

Simmons DC, Tarnasky PR, Rivera-Alsina ME, et al: Endoscopic retrograde cholangiopancreatography (ERCP) in pregnancy without the use of radiation. Am J Obstet Gynecol 190:1467, 2004

Sims HF, Brackett JC, Powell CK, et al: The molecular basis of pediatric long chain 3-hydroxyacyl-CoA dehydrogenase deficiency associated with maternal acute fatty liver of pregnancy. Proc Natl Acad Sci USA 92:841, 1995

Søgaard KK, Horváth-Puhó E, Grønback H, et al: Risk of venous thromboembolism in patients with liver disease: A nationwide population-based case-control study. Am J Gastroenterol 104(1):96, 2009

Sorrell MF, Belongia EA, Costa J, et al: National Institutes of Health Consensus Development Conference Statement: Management of hepatitis B. Ann Intern Med 150:104, 2009

Sulkowski MS, Moore RD, Mehta SH, et al: Hepatitis C and progression of HIV disease. JAMA 288:199, 2002

Swaroop VS, Chari ST, Clain JE: Severe acute pancreatitis. JAMA 291:2865, 2004

Swisher SG, Hunt KK, Schmit PJ, et al: Management of pancreatitis complicating pregnancy. Am Surg 60:759, 1994

Tan J, Surti B, Saab S: Pregnancy and cirrhosis. Liver Transpl 14(8):1081, 2008

Tang S, Mayo MJ, Rodriguez-Frias E, et al: Safety and utility of ERCP during pregnancy. Gastrointest Endosc 69:453, 2009

Terg R, Coronel E, Sorda J, et al: Efficacy and safety of oral naltrexone treatment for pruritus of cholestasis, a crossover, double blind, placebo-controlled study. J Hepatol 37:717, 2002

Teuscher AU, Sutherland DER, Robertson RP: Successful pregnancy after pancreatic islet autotransplantation. Transplant Proc 26:3520, 1994

Thio CL, Seaberg EC, Skolasky R, et al: HIV-1, hepatitis B virus, and risk of liver-related mortality in the multicenter cohort study (MACS). Lancet 360:1921, 2002

Towers CV, Asrat T, Rumney P: The presence of hepatitis B surface antigen and deoxyribonucleic acid in amniotic fluid and cord blood. Am J Obstet Gynecol 184:1514, 2001

Tydén G, Brattstrom C, Bjorkman U, et al: Pregnancy after combined pancreas-kidney transplantation. Diabetes 38 Suppl 1:43, 1989

Tyni T, Ekholm E, Pihko H: Pregnancy complications are frequent in long-chain 3-hydroxyacyl-coenzyme A dehydrogenase deficiency. Am J Obstet Gynecol 178:603, 1998

Urganci N, Arapoglu M, Akyildiz B, et al: Neonatal cholestasis resulting from vertical transmission of hepatitis A infection. Pediatr Infect Dis J 22(4):381, 2003

Uribe M, Chavez-Tapia NC, Mendez-Sanchez N: Pregnancy and autoimmune hepatitis. Ann Hepatol 5(3):187, 2006

Usta IM, Barton JR, Amon EA, et al: Acute fatty liver of pregnancy: An experience in the diagnosis and management of fourteen cases. Am J Obstet Gynecol 171:1342, 1994

Valdivieso V, Covarrubias C, Siegel F, et al: Pregnancy and cholelithiasis: Pathogenesis and natural course of gallstones diagnosed in early puerperium. Hepatology 17:1, 1993

Victor JC, Monto AS, Surdina TY, et al: Hepatitis A vaccine versus immune globulin for postexposure prophylaxis. N Engl J Med 357:1685, 2007

Vigil-De Gracia P, Lavergne JA: Acute fatty liver of pregnancy. Int J Gynaecol Obstet 72(2):193, 2001

Wahoff DC, Leone JP, Farney AC, et al: Pregnancy after total pancreatectomy and autologous islet transplantation. Surgery 117:353, 1995

Wang PH, Yang MJ, Lee WL, et al: Acetaminophen poisoning in late pregnancy. A case report. J Reprod Med 42:367, 1997

Warren JE, Blaylock RC, Silver RM: Plasmapheresis for the treatment of intrahepatic cholestasis of pregnancy refractory to medical treatment. Am J Obstet Gynecol 192:2088, 2005

Whitcomb DC: Acute pancreatitis. N Engl J Med 354:2142, 2006

Wiseman JE, Yamamoto M, Nguyen TD, et al: Cystic pancreatic neoplasm in pregnancy: A case report and review of the literature. Arch Surg 143(1):84, 2008

Xu WM, Cui YT, Wang L, et al: Lamivudine in late pregnancy to prevent perinatal transmission of hepatitis B virus infection: A multicentre, randomized, double-blind, placebo-controlled study. J Viral Hepat 16(2):94, 2009

Yang HI, Lu SN, Liaw YF, et al: Hepatitis B e antigen and the risk of hepatocellular carcinoma. N Engl J Med 347:168, 2002

Ye F, Yue Y, Li S, et al: Presence of HBsAg, HBcAg, and HBVDNA in ovary and ovum of the patients with chronic hepatitis B virus infection. Am J Obstet Gynecol 194:387, 2006

Ylitalo K, Vänttinen T, Halmesmäki E, et al: Serious pregnancy complications in a patient with previously undiagnosed carnitine palmitoyltransferase 1 deficiency. Am J Obstet Gynecol 192:2060, 2005

Yuan J, Lin J, Xu A, et al: Antepartum immunoprophylaxis of three doses of hepatitis B immunoglobulin is not effective: A single-centre randomized study. J Viral Hepat 13:597, 2006

Zeeman GG, Moise KJ: Prophylactic banding of severe esophageal varices associated with liver cirrhosis in pregnancy. Obstet Gynecol 94:842, 1999

Hematological Disorders

Pregnancy induces physiological changes that often confuse the diagnosis of hematological disorders and assessment of their treatment. This is especially true for anemia. A number of pregnancy-induced hematological changes are discussed in detail in Chapter 5 (p. 114). One of the most significant changes is blood volume expansion with a disproportionate plasma volume increase, resulting in a normally decreased hematocrit.

Pregnant women are susceptible to hematological abnormalities that may affect any woman of childbearing age. These include chronic disorders such as hereditary anemias, immunological thrombocytopenia, and malignancies, including leukemias and lymphomas. Other disorders arise during pregnancy because of pregnancy-induced demands, two examples being iron-deficiency and megaloblastic anemias. Pregnancy may also unmask underlying hematological disorders such as compensated hemolytic anemias caused by hemoglobinopathies or red cell membrane defects. Finally, any hematological disease may first arise during pregnancy, such as autoimmune hemolysis or aplastic anemia.

ANEMIAS

Extensive hematological measurements have been made in healthy nonpregnant women. Concentrations of many cellular elements that are normal during pregnancy are listed in the Appendix. As shown in Table 51-1, anemia is defined as hemoglobin concentration less than 12 g/dL in nonpregnant women and less than 10 g/dL during pregnancy or the puerperium. The Centers for Disease Control and Prevention (1998) defined anemia in iron-supplemented pregnant women using a cutoff of the 5th percentile—11 g/dL in the first and third trimesters, and 10.5 g/dL in the second trimester.

The modest fall in hemoglobin levels during pregnancy is caused by a relatively greater expansion of plasma volume compared with the increase in red cell volume (Fig. 51-1). The disproportion between the rates at which plasma and erythrocytes are added to the maternal circulation is greatest during the second trimester. Late in pregnancy, plasma expansion essentially ceases, while hemoglobin mass continues to increase.

After delivery, the hemoglobin level fluctuates and then rises to and usually exceeds the nonpregnant level. The rate and magnitude of increase early in the puerperium result from the amount of hemoglobin added during pregnancy and the amount of blood loss at delivery modified by normally decreasing plasma volume postpartum.

Incidence and Causes of Anemia

The frequency of anemia during pregnancy depends primarily on preexisting iron states and prenatal supplementation. It is more common among indigent women and influenced by dietary customs (American College of Obstetricians and Gynecologists, 2008). For example, Ren and colleagues (2007) found that 22 percent of 88,149 Chinese women were anemic in the first trimester. In studies from the United States, Taylor and associates (1982) reported that hemoglobin levels at term averaged 12.7 g/dL among women who took supplemental iron compared with 11.2 g/dL for those who did not. Bodnar and associates (2001) studied a cohort of 59,248 pregnancies and found a prevalence of 27 percent for postpartum anemia. Although this was strongly correlated with prenatal anemia, 20 percent of women with normal prenatal hemoglobin levels had postpartum anemia that was caused by hemorrhage at delivery.

TABLE 51-1. Hemoglobin Concentrations in 85 Healthy Women with Proven Iron Stores

Hemoglobin (g/dL)	Nonpregnant	Midpregnancy	Late Pregnancy
Mean	13.7	11.5	12.3
Less than 12.0	1%	72%	36%
Less than 11.0	None	29%	6%
Less than 10.0	None	4%	1%
Lowest	11.7	9.7	9.8

From Scott and Pritchard (1967), with permission.

The etiology of the more common anemias encountered in pregnancy are listed in Table 51-2. The specific cause of anemia is important when evaluating effects on pregnancy outcome. For example, maternal and perinatal outcomes are seldom affected by moderate iron-deficiency anemia, yet they are altered markedly in women with sickle-cell anemia.

Effects of Anemia on Pregnancy

Most studies of the effects of anemia on pregnancy, such as those discussed in Chapter 8 (p. 202), describe large populations. As indicated, these likely deal with nutritional anemias and specifically those due to iron deficiency. Klebanoff and co-workers (1991) studied nearly 27,000 women and found a slightly increased risk of preterm birth with midtrimester anemia. Ren and colleagues (2007) found that a low first-trimester hemoglobin concentration increased the risk of low birthweight, preterm birth, and small-for-gestational age infants. In a study from Tanzania, Kidanto and co-workers (2009) reported that the incidence of preterm delivery and low birthweight was increased as the severity of anemia increased. They did not, however, take into account the cause(s) of anemia, which was diagnosed in almost 80 percent of their obstetrical population. Kadyrov and co-workers (1998) have provided evidence that maternal anemia influences placental vascularization by altering angiogenesis during early pregnancy.

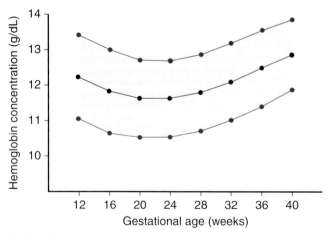

FIGURE 51-1 Mean hemoglobin concentrations (*black line*) and 5th and 95th percentiles (*blue lines*) for healthy pregnant women taking iron supplements. (Data from Centers for Disease Control and Prevention, 1989.)

A seemingly paradoxical finding is that healthy pregnant women with a higher hemoglobin concentration are also at increased risk for adverse perinatal outcomes (von Tempelhoff and colleagues, 2008). This may result from lower than average plasma volume expansion of pregnancy concurrent with normal red cell mass increase. Murphy and colleagues (1986) described more than 54,000 singleton pregnancies in the Cardiff Birth Survey and reported excessive perinatal morbidity with *high* maternal hemoglobin concentrations. Scanlon and associates (2000) studied the relationship between maternal hemoglobin levels and preterm or growth-restricted infants in 173,031 pregnancies. Women whose hemoglobin concentration was three standard deviations *above* the mean at 12 or 18 weeks had 1.3- to 1.8-fold increases in the incidence of fetal-growth restriction. These findings have led some to the illogical conclusion that withholding iron supplementation to cause iron-deficiency anemia will improve pregnancy outcomes (Ziaei and colleagues, 2007).

Iron-Deficiency Anemia

The two most common causes of anemia during pregnancy and the puerperium are iron deficiency and acute blood loss. The Centers for Disease Control and Prevention (1989) estimated that as many as 8 million American women of childbearing age were iron deficient. In a typical singleton gestation, the maternal need for iron averages close to 1000 mg. Of this, 300 mg is for the fetus and placenta; 500 mg for maternal hemoglobin mass expansion; and 200 mg that is shed normally through the gut, urine, and skin. The total amount of 1000 mg considerably exceeds the iron stores

TABLE 51-2. Causes of Anemia During Pregnancy

Acquired
  Iron-deficiency anemia
  Anemia caused by acute blood loss
  Anemia of inflammation or malignancy
  Megaloblastic anemia
  Acquired hemolytic anemia
  Aplastic or hypoplastic anemia
Hereditary
  Thalassemias
  Sickle-cell hemoglobinopathies
  Other hemoglobinopathies
  Hereditary hemolytic anemias

of most women and results in iron-deficiency anemia unless iron supplementation is given.

With the expansion of blood volume during the second trimester, iron deficiency is often manifested by an appreciable drop in hemoglobin concentration. In the third trimester, additional iron is needed to augment maternal hemoglobin and for transport to the fetus. Because the amount of iron diverted to the fetus is similar in a normal and in an iron-deficient mother, the newborn infant of a severely anemic mother does not suffer from iron-deficiency anemia. As discussed in Chapter 17 (p. 397), neonatal iron stores are related to maternal iron status and to timing of cord clamping.

Diagnosis

Classical morphological evidence of iron-deficiency anemia—erythrocyte hypochromia and microcytosis—is less prominent in the pregnant woman compared with that in the nonpregnant woman. Moderate iron-deficiency anemia during pregnancy usually is not accompanied by obvious morphological changes in erythrocytes. Serum ferritin levels, however, are lower than normal, and there is no stainable bone marrow iron. *Iron-deficiency anemia during pregnancy is the consequence primarily of expansion of plasma volume without normal expansion of maternal hemoglobin mass.*

The initial evaluation of a pregnant woman with moderate anemia should include measurements of hemoglobin, hematocrit, and red cell indices; careful examination of a peripheral blood smear; a sickle-cell preparation if the woman is of African origin; and measurement of serum iron, ferritin, or both. Expected values in pregnancy are found in the Appendix. Serum ferritin levels normally decline during pregnancy (Goldenberg and colleagues, 1996). Levels less than 10 to 15 mg/L confirm iron-deficiency anemia (American College of Obstetricians and Gynecologists, 2008). Ferritin concentrations across pregnancy, as well as other measurements used to assess this, are shown in the Appendix. Pragmatically, the diagnosis of iron deficiency in moderately anemic pregnant women usually is presumptive and based largely on exclusion.

When pregnant women with moderate iron-deficiency anemia are given adequate iron therapy, a hematological response is detected by an elevated reticulocyte count. The rate of increase of hemoglobin concentration or hematocrit is typically slower than in nonpregnant women due to the increasing and larger blood volumes during pregnancy.

Treatment

Correction of anemia and restitution of iron stores can be accomplished with simple iron compounds—ferrous sulfate, fumarate, or gluconate—that provide approximately 200 mg daily of *elemental iron*. If a woman cannot or will not take oral iron preparations, then parenteral therapy is given. Although both are administered intravenously, ferrous sucrose has been shown to be safer than iron-dextran (American College of Obstetricians and Gynecologists, 2008). There are equivalent increases in hemoglobin levels in women treated with either oral or parenteral iron therapy (Bayouneu and colleagues, 2002; Sharma and co-workers, 2004).

Transfusions of red cells or whole blood seldom are indicated unless hypovolemia from blood loss coexists or an emergency operative procedure must be performed on a *severely* anemic woman. To replenish iron stores, oral therapy should be continued for 3 months after anemia has been corrected.

Anemia from Acute Blood Loss

In early pregnancy, anemia caused by acute blood loss is common in instances of abortion, ectopic pregnancy, and hydatidiform mole. Anemia is much more common postpartum from obstetrical hemorrhage. Massive hemorrhage demands immediate treatment as described in Chapter 35 (p. 791). If a moderately anemic woman—defined by a hemoglobin value $\geq$ 7 g/dL—is hemodynamically stable, is able to ambulate without adverse symptoms, and is not septic, then blood transfusions are not indicated, and instead iron therapy is given for at least 3 months (Krafft and colleagues, 2005). In a randomized trial, Van Wyck and associates (2007) reported that intravenous ferric carboxymaltose given weekly was as effective as thrice-daily oral ferrous sulfate tablets for hemoglobin regeneration with postpartum anemia.

Anemia Associated with Chronic Disease

Weakness, weight loss, and pallor have been recognized since antiquity as characteristics of chronic disease. A wide variety of disorders, such as chronic renal failure, cancer and chemotherapy, human immunodeficiency virus (HIV) infection, and chronic inflammation, result in moderate and sometimes severe anemia, usually with slightly hypochromic and microcytic erythrocytes (Weiss and Goodnough, 2005).

In nonpregnant patients with chronic inflammatory diseases, the hemoglobin concentration is rarely less than 7 g/dL; bone marrow cellular morphology is not altered; and serum iron concentration is decreased, whereas ferritin levels usually are elevated. Thus, although slightly different from each other mechanistically, these anemias share similar features that include alterations in reticuloendothelial function, iron metabolism, and decreased erythropoiesis (Andrews, 1999).

During pregnancy, a number of chronic diseases may cause anemia, including renal insufficiency, suppuration, inflammatory bowel disease, systemic lupus erythematosus, granulomatous infections, malignant neoplasms, and rheumatoid arthritis. Chronic anemia is typically intensified as plasma volume expands disproportionately to red cell mass expansion.

Chronic Renal Disease

Chronic renal insufficiency may be accompanied by anemia, usually due to erythropoietin deficiency with an element of anemia of chronic disease. During pregnancy, the degree of red cell mass expansion is inversely related to renal impairment (see Fig. 48-4, p. 1039). Because plasma volume expansion usually is normal, however, anemia is intensified (Cunningham and associates, 1990).

Women who have acute *pyelonephritis* with sepsis often develop overt anemia. This is caused by acute red cell destruction from endotoxin-mediated sepsis, but with normal erythropoietin production (Cavenee and colleagues, 1994).

Treatment. Adequate iron stores must be ensured. Treatment with *recombinant erythropoietin* has been used successfully to treat chronic anemia (Weiss and Goodnough, 2005). In pregnancies complicated by chronic renal insufficiency, recombinant erythropoietin is usually considered when the hematocrit approximates 20 percent (Ramin and colleagues, 2006). One worrisome side effect is hypertension, which is already prevalent in women with renal disease. In addition, Casadevall and colleagues (2002) reported pure red cell aplasia and anti-erythropoietin antibodies in 13 nonpregnant patients given erythropoietin.

Megaloblastic Anemia

These anemias are characterized by blood and bone-marrow abnormalities from impaired DNA synthesis. Worldwide, the prevalence of megaloblastic anemia during pregnancy varies considerably, and in the United States, it is rare.

Folic Acid Deficiency

In the United States, megaloblastic anemia beginning during pregnancy almost always results from folic acid deficiency. In the past, this condition was referred to as *pernicious anemia of pregnancy*. It usually is found in women who do not consume fresh green leafy vegetables, legumes, or animal protein. As folate deficiency and anemia worsen, anorexia often becomes intense, further aggravating the dietary deficiency. In some instances, excessive ethanol ingestion either causes or contributes to folate deficiency.

In nonpregnant women, the folic acid requirement is 50 to 100 μg/day. During pregnancy, requirements are increased, and 400 μg/day is recommended (see Chap. 8, p. 204). The earliest biochemical evidence is low plasma folic acid concentrations. (see Appendix). Early morphological changes usually include neutrophils that are hypersegmented and newly formed erythrocytes that are macrocytic. With preexisting iron deficiency, macrocytic erythrocytes cannot be detected by measurement of the mean corpuscular volume. Careful examination of a peripheral blood smear, however, usually demonstrates some macrocytes. As the anemia becomes more intense, peripheral nucleated erythrocytes appear and examination of the bone marrow discloses megaloblastic erythropoiesis. Anemia may then become severe, and thrombocytopenia, leukopenia, or both may develop. The fetus and placenta extract folate from maternal circulation so effectively that the fetus is not anemic despite severe maternal anemia. There have been instances in which newborn hemoglobin levels were 18 g/dL or more whereas maternal values were as low as 3.6 g/dL (Pritchard and Scott, 1970).

Treatment. The treatment of pregnancy-induced megaloblastic anemia should include folic acid, a nutritious diet, and iron. As little as 1 mg of folic acid administered orally once daily produces a striking hematological response. By 4 to 7 days after the beginning of treatment, the reticulocyte count is increased, and leukopenia and thrombocytopenia are corrected.

Prevention. A diet sufficient in folic acid prevents megaloblastic anemia. A great deal of attention has been devoted to the role

of folate deficiency in the genesis of neural-tube defects (see Chap. 8, p. 204, and Chap. 12, p. 281). Since the early 1990s, governmental nutrition experts, as well as the American College of Obstetricians and Gynecologists (2003), have recommended that all women of childbearing age consume at least 400 μg of folic acid daily. Additional folic acid is given in circumstances in which folate requirements are increased, such as in multifetal pregnancy, hemolytic anemia, Crohn disease, alcoholism, and inflammatory skin disorders. There is evidence that women who previously have had infants with neural-tube defects have a lower recurrence rate if daily 4-mg folic acid is given prior to and throughout early pregnancy.

Vitamin B₁₂ Deficiency

Megaloblastic anemia during pregnancy caused by lack of vitamin B_{12}, that is, cyanocobalamin, is exceedingly rare. In *Addisonian pernicious anemia,* a lack of intrinsic factor results in failure to absorb vitamin B_{12}. It is an extremely uncommon autoimmune disease in women of reproductive age and typically has its onset after age 40 years. Unless treated with vitamin B_{12}, infertility may be a complication. In our limited experience, vitamin B_{12} deficiency in pregnant women is more likely encountered following partial or total gastric resection. Other causes are Crohn disease, ileal resection, and bacterial overgrowth in the small bowel.

During pregnancy, vitamin B_{12} levels are lower than nonpregnant values because of decreased levels of binding proteins that include haptocorrin (transcobalamins I and III) and transcobalamin II (Morkbak and colleagues, 2007). Women who have had a total gastrectomy require 1000 μg of vitamin B_{12} intramuscularly at monthly intervals. Those with a partial gastrectomy usually do not need such therapy, but vitamin B_{12} levels during pregnancy should be measured (see Appendix).

Acquired Hemolytic Anemias

Autoimmune Hemolytic Anemia

This is an uncommon condition, and the cause of aberrant antibody production is unknown. Typically, both the direct and indirect antiglobulin (Coombs) tests are positive. Anemias caused by these factors may be due to warm-active autoantibodies—80 to 90 percent, cold-active antibodies, or a combination. These syndromes also may be classified as primary (idiopathic) or secondary due to underlying diseases or other factors. Examples of the latter include lymphomas and leukemias, connective-tissue diseases, infections, chronic inflammatory diseases, and drug-induced antibodies (Provan and Weatherall, 2000). *Cold-agglutinin disease* may be induced by infectious etiologies like *Mycoplasma pneumoniae* or Epstein-Barr viral mononucleosis (Dhingra and colleagues, 2007).

Hemolysis and positive antiglobulin test results may be the consequence of either IgM or IgG anti-erythrocyte antibodies. Spherocytosis and reticulocytosis are characteristic of the peripheral blood smear. IgM antibodies do not cross the placenta, and thus, fetal red cells are not affected.

With autoimmune hemolytic anemia, there may be marked acceleration of hemolysis during pregnancy. Glucocorticoids usually are effective, and treatment is with prednisone, 1 mg/kg orally per day, or its equivalent. Coincidental thrombocytopenia usually is corrected by therapy. Transfusion of red cells is complicated by the presence of circulating anti-erythrocyte antibodies. Warming the donor cells to body temperature, however, decreases their destruction by cold agglutinins.

Drug-Induced Hemolytic Anemia

This must be differentiated from other forms of autoimmune hemolytic anemia. Hemolysis typically is mild, resolves with drug withdrawal, and can be prevented by avoidance of the drug. Mechanisms of action generally are through drug-mediated immunological injury to red cells. The drug may act as a high-affinity hapten with a red cell protein to which antidrug antibodies attach—for example, IgM antipenicillin or anticephalosporin antibodies. Other drugs become low-affinity haptens and adhere to cell membrane proteins. Examples include probenecid, quinidine, rifampin, and thiopental.

The severity of symptoms depends on the degree of hemolysis. Usually there is mild to moderate chronic hemolysis, but some drugs that act as low-affinity haptens may precipitate severe acute hemolysis. Garratty and associates (1999) described seven cases of severe direct Coombs-positive hemolytic anemia caused by cefotetan prophylaxis for obstetrical procedures. In most cases, withdrawing the offending drug results in reversal of symptoms. Corticosteroids are of questionable efficacy. Drug-induced hemolysis is much more often related to a congenital erythrocyte enzymatic defect, such as *glucose-6-phosphate dehydrogenase (G6PD) deficiency*, especially in African-American women (see p. 1084).

Pregnancy-Induced Hemolytic Anemia

Unexplained hemolytic anemia during pregnancy is a rare but distinct entity in which severe hemolysis develops early in pregnancy and resolves within months after delivery. There is no evidence of an immune mechanism or intraerythrocytic or extraerythrocytic defects (Starksen and associates, 1983). Because the fetus-infant also may demonstrate transient hemolysis, an immunological cause is suspected. Maternal corticosteroid treatment is often but not always effective (Kumar and colleagues, 2001). We have observed one woman with recurrent hemolysis during several pregnancies. In each instance, intense severe hemolytic anemia was controlled by prednisone given until delivery.

Paroxysmal Nocturnal Hemoglobinuria

Although commonly regarded as a hemolytic anemia, this hemopoietic stem cell disorder is characterized by formation of defective platelets, granulocytes, and erythrocytes. Paroxysmal nocturnal hemoglobinuria is acquired and arises from one abnormal clone of cells, much like a neoplasm (Nguyen and associates, 2006). One mutated X-linked gene responsible for this condition is termed *PIG-A* because it codes for phosphatidylinositol glycan protein A. Resultant abnormal anchor proteins of the erythrocyte and granulocyte membrane make these cells unusually susceptible to lysis by complement (Provan and Weatherall, 2000).

Chronic hemolytic anemia has an insidious onset, and its severity ranges from mild to lethal. Hemoglobinuria develops at irregular intervals and is not necessarily nocturnal. Hemolysis may be initiated by transfusions, infections, or surgery. Almost 40 percent of patients suffer venous thromboses, as well as renal failure, hypertension, and Budd-Chiari syndrome. Because of the thrombotic risk, prophylactic anticoagulation is recommended (Parker and colleagues, 2005). Median survival after diagnosis is 10 years, and bone marrow transplantation is the definitive treatment. Successful treatment of nonpregnant patients has been reported with eculizumab, an antibody that inhibits complement activation (Hillmen and associates, 2006; Parker, 2009). There is no published experience with this drug in pregnant women.

Effects on Pregnancy. Paroxysmal nocturnal hemoglobinuria is a serious and unpredictable disease. During pregnancy, complications are reported in up to three fourths of affected women (De Gramont and colleagues, 1987). Maternal mortality is reported in 10 to 20 percent. Maternal complications are more common postpartum, and venous thrombosis is reported in 50 percent (Fieni, 2006; Greene, 1983; Ray, 2000, and all their colleagues).

Severe Preeclampsia and Eclampsia

Fragmentation or microangiopathic hemolysis with thrombocytopenia is relatively common with severe preeclampsia and eclampsia (Kenny and co-workers, 2009; Pritchard and associates, 1976). Mild degrees are likely present in most cases of severe disease and may be referred to as *HELLP syndrome*—hemolysis, elevated liver enzymes, and low platelet (see Chap. 34, p. 718).

Bacterial Toxins

The most fulminant acquired hemolytic anemia encountered during pregnancy is caused by the exotoxin of *Clostridium perfringens* (see Chap. 42, p. 932) or by group A β-hemolytic streptococcus (see Chap. 31, p. 662). Gram-negative bacterial endotoxin—lipopolysaccharide—especially with bacteremia from severe pyelonephritis may be accompanied by hemolysis and mild to moderate anemia (Cox and colleagues, 1991).

Hemolytic Anemias Caused by Inherited Erythrocyte Defects

The normal erythrocyte shape is a biconcave disc, and its membrane surface area is redundant relative to its volume. This allows numerous cycles of reversible deformations as the erythrocyte withstands shearing forces within arteries and negotiates through splenic slits half the width of its cross-sectional diameter. Several inherited red cell membrane defects or enzyme deficiencies result in destabilization of the membrane lipid bilayer. The loss of lipids from the erythrocyte membrane causes a surface area deficiency and poorly deformable cells that undergo hemolysis (Fig. 51-2). There are varying degrees of anemia that depend upon the degree of rigidity or decreased distensibility. Three examples of inherited membrane defects that cause accelerated destruction are *hereditary spherocytosis, pyropoikilocytosis,* and *ovalocytosis.*

Hereditary Spherocytosis. Several inherited molecular deficits in erythrocyte membrane proteins give rise to the syndrome of hereditary spherocytosis. Most are due to an autosomally

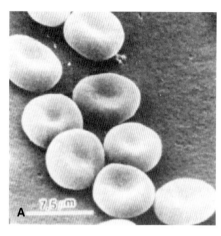

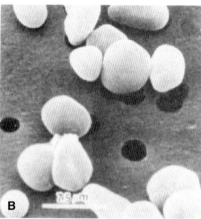

FIGURE 51-2 Scanning electron micrograph showing **(A)** normal-appearing erythrocytes from a heterozygous carrier of recessive spherocytosis, and **(B)** her daughter, a homozygote with severe anemia. (From Agre, 1989, with permission.)

dominant, variably penetrant *spectrin* deficiency. Others are autosomally recessive or de novo gene mutations and may be caused by deficiency of *ankyrin, protein 4.2, moderate band 3,* or combinations thereof (Bunn and Rosse, 2001; Yawata and colleagues, 2000). These disorders are characterized by varying degrees of anemia and jaundice as the consequence of hemolysis. The diagnosis is confirmed by identification of spherocytes on peripheral smear, reticulocytosis, and increased osmotic fragility.

So-called *crisis* is characterized by severe anemia from accelerated red cell destruction and develops in patients with a functioning spleen, which is usually enlarged. The balance between bone marrow production and hemolysis can be disrupted by infection, which may either increase hemolysis or suppress bone marrow production—one example is parvovirus B19 infection (see Chap. 58, p. 1215). For many patients, splenectomy reduces hemolysis, anemia, and jaundice.

Pregnancy. In general, women with hereditary spherocytosis do well during pregnancy. Folic acid supplementation is recommended. Maberry and associates (1992) reported the Parkland Hospital experience with 50 pregnancies in 23 women with spherocytosis. In late pregnancy, the mean hematocrit was 31 volumes percent and ranged from 23 to 41. Reticulocyte counts

ranged from 1 to 23 percent. Eight women miscarried and four of 42 infants were born preterm, but none were growth restricted. Infection in four women intensified hemolysis, and three required transfusions. Similar results were reported by Pajor and colleagues (1993) in 19 pregnancies in eight women. The newborn who has inherited hereditary spherocytosis may have hyperbilirubinemia and anemia. We observed the hemoglobin level to fall to as low as 5.0 g/dL by 5 weeks of age in one infant.

Red Cell Enzyme Deficiencies. A deficiency of erythrocyte enzymes that permit anaerobic glucose use may cause *hereditary nonspherocytic anemia.* Most are inherited as autosomal recessive traits. *Glucose-6-phosphate dehydrogenase (G6PD) deficiency,* by far the most common, is a well-known exception that is X-linked. There are more than 400 variants of G6PD, predominantly due to a base substitution that leads to an amino acid replacement and to a broad range of clinical severity (Beutler, 1991). In the homozygous or A variant, both X chromosomes are affected, and erythrocytes are markedly deficient in normal enzyme activity. This condition is inherited by approximately 2 percent of African-American women. In the heterozygous variant, only one X chromosome is affected. This condition occurs in 10 to 15 percent of African-American women and may confer some degree of protection against malaria (Mockenhaupt and colleagues, 2003). Random X-chromosome inactivation, or *lyonization,* results in a variable deficiency of enzyme activity. Newborn screening for G6PD deficiency is not included in the American College of Medical Genetics (2006) recommendations for the United States (see Table 28-5, p. 599). That said, the World Health Organization (1989) recommends screening all newborns in countries with a high prevalence.

Infections or drugs may induce hemolysis in both heterozygous and homozygous women. Anemia is usually episodic, although some variants induce chronic nonspherocytic hemolysis. Because young erythrocytes contain more enzyme activity than older erythrocytes, in the absence of bone marrow depression, anemia ultimately stabilizes and is corrected soon after the drug is discontinued or the infection clears.

Pyruvate kinase deficiency, although uncommon, is probably the next most common enzyme deficiency. It is inherited as an autosomal recessive trait and is associated with variable anemia and hypertensive complications (Wax and associates, 2007). Due to recurrent transfusions in homozygous carriers, iron overload is common, and associated myocardial dysfunction should be monitored (Dolan and colleagues, 2002). Conservative management without transfusions can be accomplished (Ghidini and Korker, 1998). Recurrent hydrops fetalis due to homozygously affected fetuses has been described, and fetal anemia and pyruvate kinase deficiency were confirmed using funipuncture (Gilsanz and colleagues, 1993).

Other rare enzyme abnormalities may cause hemolysis. Although the degree of chronic hemolysis varies, most episodes of severe anemia with enzyme deficiencies are induced by drugs or infections. During pregnancy, iron and folic acid are given, oxidant drugs are avoided, and bacterial infections are treated promptly.

Aplastic and Hypoplastic Anemia

Although rarely encountered during pregnancy, aplastic anemia is a grave complication. It is characterized by pancytopenia and markedly hypocellular bone marrow (Young, 2008). There may be more than one form, and there is evidence that one is linked to persons with autoimmune diseases (Stalder and co-workers, 2009). The etiology can be identified in approximately a third of cases, and causes include drugs and other chemicals, infection, irradiation, leukemia, immunological disorders, and inherited conditions such as *Fanconi anemia* and *Diamond-Blackfan syndrome* (Green and Kupfer, 2009; Lipton and Ellis, 2009). The functional defect appears to be a marked decrease in committed marrow stem cells. The condition is likely immunologically mediated (Young and Maciejewski, 1997).

Hematopoietic stem-cell transplantation is optimal therapy in a young patient (Young, 2008). Immunosuppressive therapy is given with bone marrow transplantation, and approximately three fourths of patients have a good response and long-term survival when treated with antithymocyte globulin and cyclosporine (Rosenfeld and colleagues, 2003). There is a potential for transplantation with umbilical cord blood-derived stem cells (Moise, 2005; Pinto and Roberts, 2008). Previous blood transfusions and even pregnancy enhance the risk of graft rejection, which is the most common serious complication. It causes two thirds of deaths within the first 2 years (Socié and co-workers, 1999).

Aplastic Anemia During Pregnancy

In most cases, aplastic anemia and pregnancy simultaneously occur by chance. In a few women, hypoplastic anemia has been identified first during a pregnancy and then improved or even resolved when the pregnancy terminated, only to recur with a subsequent pregnancy (Bourantas and associates, 1997; Choudhry and colleagues, 2002).

Of 64 pregnancies with *Diamond-Blackfan anemia,* two thirds had complications that stemmed from placental vascular etiologies and that included abortion, preeclampsia, stillbirth, fetal-growth restriction, and preterm birth (Faivre and colleagues, 2006). This rare form of pure red cell aplasia may be inherited in an autosomal recessive pattern. Some patients respond to glucocorticoid therapy, but most are transfusion- dependent.

Gaucher disease is an autosomally recessive lysosomal enzyme deficiency that has multisystem involvement. When these women are pregnant, anemia and thrombocytopenia usually worsen (Granovsky-Grisaru and associates, 1995). In another report, *alglucerase* enzyme replacement improved pregnancy outcomes in six affected women (Elstein and colleagues, 1997).

The major risks to the pregnant woman with aplastic anemia are hemorrhage and infection. Overall mortality rates reported since 1960 during or after pregnancy have been 50 percent (Choudhry and co-workers, 2002). More recent case series report better outcomes (Kwon and associates, 2006). *Fanconi anemia* appears to be associated with a better prognosis (Alter and colleagues, 1991).

Management depends on gestational age, severity of disease, and whether treatment has been given. Supportive care includes continuous infection surveillance and prompt antimicrobial therapy. Granulocyte transfusions are given only during infections. Red cell transfusions are given to improve symptomatic anemia, and routinely to maintain the hematocrit at approximately 20 volumes percent. Platelet transfusions may be needed to control hemorrhage. Even when thrombocytopenia is intense, the risk of severe hemorrhage can be minimized by vaginal rather than cesarean delivery.

Bone Marrow Transplantation. There have been several case reports of successful pregnancies in women who had undergone bone marrow transplantation (Borgna-Pignatti and associates, 1996; Eliyahu and Shalev, 1994). Sanders and colleagues (1996) reviewed outcomes in 41 women with 72 pregnancies following bone marrow transplantation. Excluding spontaneous and induced abortions, 52 resulted in liveborn infants, however, almost half of these pregnancies were complicated by preterm delivery or hypertension. Our experiences with a few of these women indicate that they have normal pregnancy-augmented erythropoiesis and total blood volume expansion.

HEMOGLOBINOPATHIES

Sickle-Cell Hemoglobinopathies

Sickle hemoglobin (hemoglobin S) results from a single β-chain substitution of glutamic acid by valine because of an A for T substitution at codon 6 of the β-globin gene. Sickle-cell diseases include sickle-cell anemia—Hgb SS; sickle cell-hemoglobin C disease—Hgb SC; sickle cell-β-thalassemia disease—either Hb S/B° or Hb S/B$^+$, and sickle-cell E disease—Hgb SE (Stuart and Nagel, 2004). All are also associated with increased rates of maternal and perinatal morbidity and mortality.

Pathophysiology

Red cells with hemoglobin S undergo sickling when they are deoxygenated and the hemoglobin aggregates. Constant sickling and de-sickling cause membrane damage, and the cell may become irreversibly sickled. Events that slow erythrocyte transit through the microcirculation contribute to vaso-occlusion. These include endothelial cell adhesion, erythrocytic dehydration, and vasomotor dysregulation. Clinically, the hallmark of sickling episodes are periods during which there is ischemia and infarction in various organs. These produce clinical symptoms, predominately pain, which is often severe—the *sickle-cell crises.* There may be aplastic, megaloblastic, sequestration, and hemolytic crises.

Chronic and acute changes from sickling include bony abnormalities such as osteonecrosis of femoral and humeral heads, renal medullary damage, autosplenectomy in homozygous SS patients and splenomegaly in other variants, hepatomegaly, ventricular hypertrophy, pulmonary infarctions, pulmonary hypertension, cerebrovascular accidents, leg ulcers, and a propensity to infection and sepsis (Driscoll and colleagues, 2003; Gladwin and associates, 2004; Stuart and Nagel, 2004). Of increasing importance is acquisition of pulmonary hypertension, which can be demonstrated in 20 percent of adults with SS hemoglobin (Gladwin and Vichinsky, 2008). Depending on its severity, it increases the relative risk for death from four- to 11-fold. The median age at death for women is 48 years. Even so, Serjeant and colleagues (2008) described a cohort of 102 patients followed since birth in which 40 were still alive at 60 to 87 years!

Inheritance

Sickle-cell anemia results from the inheritance of the gene for S hemoglobin from each parent. In the United States, 1 of 12 African Americans has the sickle-cell trait, which results from inheritance of one gene for hemoglobin S and one for normal hemoglobin A. The computed incidence of sickle-cell anemia among African Americans is 1 in 576 ($1/12 \times 1/12 \times 1/4 = 1/576$). But, the disease is less common in adults and therefore during pregnancy because of earlier mortality, especially during early childhood.

Approximately 1 in 40 African Americans has the gene for hemoglobin C. The theoretical incidence for co-inheritance of the gene for hemoglobin S and an allelic gene for hemoglobin C in an African-American child is about 1 in 2000 ($1/12 \times 1/40 \times 1/4$). Similarly, because the incidence of β-thalassemia minor is approximately 1 in 40, S-β-thalassemia also is found in about 1 in 2000 ($1/12 \times 1/40 \times 1/4$).

Pregnancy and Sickle-Cell Syndrome

Pregnancy is a serious burden to women with any of the major sickle hemoglobinopathies, particularly those with hemoglobin SS disease. Two large cohorts of pregnant women with sickle-cell syndromes were described recently using the Nationwide Inpatient Sample of the Healthcare Cost and Utilization Project of the Agency for Healthcare Research and Quality. The study by Villers and colleagues (2008) included 17,952 deliveries of women with sickle-cell syndromes from 2000 through 2003. The other reported by Chakravarty and associates (2008) was from 2002 through 2004 and included 4352 pregnancies. Common complications and their frequencies were compared with the cohort of more than 18 million pregnancies of women without sickle hemoglobin and their relative risks are shown in Table 51-3. In addition, Chakravarty and co-workers (2008) reported that sickle-cell disease was associated with significantly increased odds ratios for renal failure, various forms of gestational hypertension, and fetal-growth restriction. The risk of complications shown in Table 51-3 is increased in affected pregnant women compared with unaffected pregnant controls. Additionally, data from another four studies are compiled in Table 51-4.

Other morbidity includes ischemic necrosis of multiple organs, especially bone marrow, that causes episodes of severe pain, which usually becomes more frequent in pregnancy. Pyelonephritis and pneumonia are common, as are other pulmonary complications. The latter manifest by the *acute chest syndrome*—the radiological appearance of a new pulmonary infiltrate accompanied by fever and respiratory symptoms. There are four precipitants of this—infection, marrow emboli, thromboembolism, and atelectasis (Medoff and colleagues, 2005). Of these, infection stimulates about half of cases, with most caused by atypical bacteria and viruses. When the chest syndrome develops, the mean duration of hospitalization is 10.5 days, mortality rate is about 3 percent, and mechanical ventilation is required in about 15 percent (Gladwin and Vichinsky, 2008).

Pregnancy outcomes in women with the sickle syndromes have improved substantively in the past 25 to 30 years. Powars and colleagues (1986) reported a 6-percent maternal mortality rate before 1972 and only 1 percent after 1972. In the series shown in Table 51-4, there was only one pregnancy-related maternal death, and the average perinatal mortality rate was approximately 9 percent.

TABLE 51-3. Increased Rates for Maternal Complications in Pregnancies Complicated by Sickle-Cell Syndromes

Complications	OR[a]	*p* value
Preexisting Medical Disorders		
Cardiomyopathy	3.7	<.001
Pulmonary hypertension	6.3	<.001
Renal failure	3.5	.09
Pregnancy Complications		
Cerebral vein thrombosis	4.9	<.001
Pneumonia	9.8	<.001
Pyelonephritis	1.3	0.5
Deep-venous thrombosis	2.5	<.001
Pulmonary embolism	1.7	.08
Sepsis syndrome	6.8	<.001
Delivery Complications		
Gestational hypertension/preeclampsia	1.2	.01
Eclampsia	3.2	<.001
Placental abruption	1.6	<.001
Preterm delivery	1.4	<.001
Fetal-growth restriction	2.2	<.001

[a] OR = odds ratios.
Data from Villers and colleagues (2008).

TABLE 51-4. Maternal and Perinatal Outcomes in Women with Hemoglobin SS and SC Disease

Study	Pregnancies[a]	Maternal Outcomes (Percent)			Perinatal Outcome (Percent)			
		ACS	Pyelo	Death	FGR	SB	NND	PMR
Sun et al (2001)								
SS Hgb	69	NS	7	0	45	4	7	11
SC Hgb	58	NS	5	0	21	2	0	2
Serjeant et al (2004, 2005)[b]								
SS Hgb	54	20	15	1	42	11	1.9	12.9
SC Hgb	70	6	10	0	NS	3	1.4	4.4
Thame et al (2007)[b]								
SS Hgb	126	8	6	NS	33	10	1.6	11.6
Total/Weighted Average	**377**	**~10**	**~8**	**-**	**~35**	**6.4**	**2.3**	**8.7**

[a]Excludes spontaneous and induced abortions.
[b]Study periods overlap and may contain some duplicated pregnancy outcomes.
ACS = acute chest syndrome; Pyelo = pyelonephritis; FGR = fetal-growth restriction; SB = stillborn; NND = neonatal death; NS = not stated; PMR = perinatal mortality rate.

Hemoglobin SC. In nonpregnant women, morbidity and mortality rates from SC disease are appreciably lower than those from sickle-cell anemia. Indeed, fewer than half of women with SC disease have symptoms prior to pregnancy. In our experiences, affected pregnant and puerperal women suffer attacks of severe bone pain and episodes of pulmonary infarction and embolization—acute chest syndrome—more commonly compared with when they are not pregnant (Cunningham and associates, 1983). It is arguable whether SC disease has an equivalent maternal mortality rate with hemoglobin SS disease (Pritchard and co-workers, 1973; Serjeant and associates, 2005). In the reports shown in Table 51-4, the perinatal mortality rate is somewhat greater than that of the general obstetrical population, but nowhere as great as with sickle-cell anemia (Tita and colleagues, 2007).

Management During Pregnancy

Adequate management of pregnant women with sickle-cell hemoglobinopathies necessitates close observation. These women maintain hemoglobin mass by intense hemopoiesis to compensate for the markedly shortened erythrocyte life span. Thus, any factor that impairs erythropoiesis or increases red cell destruction, or both, aggravates the anemia. Prenatal folic acid supplementation with 4 mg/day is needed to support the rapid turnover of red blood cells (American College of Obstetricians and Gynecologists, 2007).

One common danger is that a symptomatic woman may categorically be considered to be suffering from a sickle-cell crisis. As a result, serious obstetrical or medical problems that cause pain, anemia, or both may be overlooked. Some examples are ectopic pregnancy, placental abruption, pyelonephritis, or appendicitis. *The term "sickle-cell crisis" should be applied only after all other possible causes of pain or fever or worsening anemia have been excluded.*

Pain is from intense sequestration of sickled erythrocytes with infarction in various organs. These episodes may develop acutely, especially late in pregnancy, during labor and delivery,

and early in the puerperium. Acute infarction is usually accompanied by severe pain, and because the bone marrow is frequently involved, intense bone pain is common. A system for care of these women has been appropriately stressed by Rees and colleagues (2003). Marti-Carvajal and co-workers (2009) performed a Cochrane Review and reported that there have been no randomized trials to evaluate treatments during pregnancy for these episodes. At the minimum, intravenous fluids are given and opioids administered promptly for severe pain. Oxygen via nasal cannula may decrease the intensity of sickling at the capillary level. We have found that red cell transfusions after the onset of severe pain do not dramatically improve the intensity of the current pain crisis and may not shorten its duration. Conversely, as discussed later, prophylactic transfusions almost always prevent further vaso-occlusive episodes and pain crises.

Rates of covert bacteriuria and acute pyelonephritis are increased substantively, and screening and treatment for bacteriuria are essential. If pyelonephritis develops, sickle cells are extremely susceptible to bacterial endotoxin, which can cause dramatic and rapid red cell destruction while simultaneously suppressing erythropoiesis. Pneumonia, especially due to *Streptococcus pneumoniae,* is common. The Centers for Disease Control and Prevention (2008 a, b, c) recommends the following vaccines for sickle cell—and all asplenic—patients: polyvalent pneumococcal, *Haemophilus influenzae* type B, and meningococcal vaccine.

As many as 40 percent of patients suffer from pulmonary complications—the acute chest syndrome. Described above, it is characterized by pleuritic chest pain, fever, cough, lung infiltrates, and hypoxia (Vichinsky and colleagues, 2000). And the spectrum of its pathology includes infection, infarction, pulmonary sequestration, and fat embolization from bone marrow (Fig. 51-3). At least for nonpregnant adults, some recommend rapid simple or exchange transfusions to remove the 'trigger' for acute chest syndromes (Gladwin and Vichinsky, 2009). In a

SECTION 8

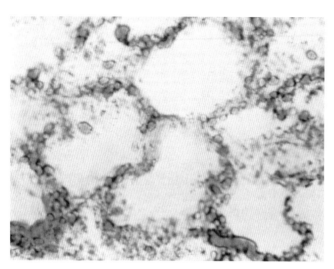

FIGURE 51-3 Photomicrograph of a section of lung from a 21-year-old primipara with hemoglobin SC who died 36 hours post-partum after developing acute dyspnea. Massive amounts of fat and bone marrow have embolized to both lungs. (From Maberry and Cunningham, 1993.)

cohort study of nonpregnant patients, Turner and colleagues (2009) reported that there were no increased benefits of exchange versus simple transfusions, and the former were associated with fourfold increased blood usage. Recurrent episodes may lead to restrictive chronic lung disease or arteriolar vasculopathy and pulmonary hypertension.

Pregnant women with sickle-cell anemia usually have some degree of *cardiac dysfunction* from ventricular hypertrophy. There is increased preload and decreased afterload with a normal ejection fraction and a high cardiac output. Chronic hypertension worsens this (Gandhi and colleagues, 2000). During pregnancy, the basal hemodynamic state characterized by high cardiac output and increased blood volume is augmented (Veille and Hanson, 1994). Although most women tolerate pregnancy without problems, complications such as severe preeclampsia or serious infections may result in ventricular failure (Cunningham and associates, 1986). As discussed in Chapter 44 (p. 970), heart failure caused by pulmonary hypertension must also be considered (Chakravarty and associates, 2008; Stuart and Nagel, 2004).

In a review of 4352 pregnancies in women with sickle-cell syndromes, Chakravarty and colleagues (2008) reported significantly increased pregnancy complications compared with the total population of 11.2 million women. Compared with controls, women with sickling disorders had a 63-percent rate of nondelivery-related admissions. They had a 1.8-fold increased incidence of hypertensive disorders—19 percent; a 2.9-fold increased rate of fetal-growth restriction—6 percent; and a 1.7-fold increased cesarean delivery rate—45 percent.

Assessment of Fetal Health. Because of the high incidence of fetal-growth restriction and perinatal mortality, serial fetal assessment is necessary. According to the American College of Obstetricians and Gynecologists (2007), a plan for serial sonographic examinations and antepartum fetal surveillance is rea-

sonable. Anyaegbunam and colleagues (1991) evaluated fetal well-being during 39 sickling crises in 24 women. Almost 60 percent had nonreactive stress tests, which became reactive with crisis resolution, and all had an increased uterine artery systolic-diastolic (S/D) ratio. At the same time, there were no changes in umbilical artery S/D ratios (see Chap. 16, p. 362). These investigators concluded that transient effects of sickle-cell crisis do not compromise umbilical, and hence fetal, blood flow. At Parkland Hospital, we serially assess these women with sonography for fetal growth and amnionic fluid volume changes. Non-stress or contraction stress tests are not done routinely unless complications such as fetal-growth restriction develop or fetal movement is reported to be diminished.

Labor and Delivery. Management is essentially identical to that for women with cardiac disease (see Chap. 44, p. 961). Women should be kept comfortable but not oversedated. Labor epidural analgesia is ideal, and conduction analgesia seems preferable for operative delivery (Camous and associates, 2008). Compatible blood should be available. If a difficult vaginal or cesarean delivery is contemplated, and the hematocrit is less than 20 volumes percent, then packed erythrocyte transfusions are administered. Care must be taken to prevent circulatory overload and pulmonary edema from ventricular failure.

Prophylactic Red Cell Transfusions. These have been shown to decrease morbidity in sickle-cell syndromes when given perioperatively and during pregnancy or to prevent strokes in high-risk children. The use of routine prophylactic transfusions during pregnancy remains controversial (American College of Obstetricians and Gynecologists, 2007). Their most dramatic impact has been on maternal morbidity. In a 10-year prospective study at Parkland Hospital, we offered prophylactic transfusions to all pregnant women with sickle-cell syndromes. Red cell transfusions were given throughout pregnancy to maintain the hematocrit greater than 25 volumes percent and hemoglobin S no greater than 60 percent (Cunningham and Pritchard, 1979). There was minimal maternal morbidity such as pain, fever, and suppression of erythropoiesis. In a later study, these women were compared with historical controls not given blood, and there was a significant reduction in maternal morbidity and hospitalizations in the transfused groups (Cunningham and associates, 1983). A comparative study by Howard and colleagues (1995) produced similar data.

In a multicenter trial, Koshy and colleagues (1988) randomized 72 pregnant women with sickle-cell disease to prophylactic or indicated transfusions. They reported a significant decrease in the incidence of painful sickle-cell crises with prophylactic transfusions but no differences in perinatal outcomes. Because of risks inherent with blood administration, they concluded that prophylactic transfusions were not necessary.

Current consensus is that management should be individualized. Some clinicians choose prophylactic transfusions in women with a history of multiple vaso-occlusive episodes and poor obstetrical outcomes (Castro and colleagues, 2003).

Complications. Morbidity from multiple transfusions is significant. Delayed hemolytic transfusion reactions occur in as many as 10 percent of patients (Garratty, 1997). Hepatitis is a major concern. At Parkland Hospital, the incidence of red cell isoimmunization was 3 percent per unit of blood transfused (Cox and associates, 1988). In 12 studies reviewed by Garratty (1997), a mean of 25 percent of chronically transfused sickle-cell patients had become isoimmunized. Although the specter of iron overload and transfusion hemochromatosis is worrisome, we found no evidence for this or for chronic hepatitis in liver biopsies from 40 women transfused during pregnancy (Yeomans and co-workers, 1990).

Other Therapy

There are several therapeutic schemes for sickle-cell patients, some of which are still experimental (Stuart and Nagel, 2004). Hemoglobin F induction has been studied for sickling and thalassemia syndromes. There are drugs that stimulate gamma-chain synthesis and thus hemoglobin F, which inhibits polymerization of hemoglobin S and resultant sickling. For patients with moderate to severe disease, *hydroxyurea* increases hemoglobin F production with fewer clinical sickling episodes (Platt, 2008). It may also reduce red cell membrane damage and decrease adherence to endothelium with less vascular damage. At this time, it is unknown if hydroxyurea increases long-term survival (Brawley and co-workers, 2008). Experience with hydroxyurea in pregnancy is limited, but it is teratogenic in animals (Briggs and colleagues, 2005).

Another cancer drug, *decitabine*, has been used in patients who are unresponsive to hydroxyurea (DeSimone and colleagues, 2002). Findings from a placebo-controlled trial of *inhaled nitric oxide* versus placebo suggested benefit for acute vaso-occlusive crises (Weiner and colleagues, 2003).

Hemopoietic cell transplantation as been used as a "cure" for patients with sickle-cell syndromes as well as with thalassemia major. Oringanje and co-workers (2009) performed a Cochrane Review and found that only observational studies have been reported. *Bone marrow transplantation*, as discussed on page 1085, has been used to provide normal hemoglobin A erythrocyte precursors in pediatric or adult patients with severe disease, and 5-year survival rates exceed 90 percent (Bhatia and Walters, 2008). *Cord blood stem cell transplantation* from related donors has shown great promise (Pinto and Roberts, 2008). Prenatal diagnosis of sickle-cell disease may allow for in utero *stem cell therapy* with hemoglobin A cells (Shaaban and Flake, 1999). Perhaps even more intriguing is the possibility that cells taken for prenatal diagnosis from a fetus destined to have sickle-cell anemia can be conditioned to produce hemoglobin A and used for replacement after birth (Ye and co-workers, 2009). Other experimental therapies include a gene therapy technique using a modified β-globin gene that encodes a sickling-resistant protein, which corrected the globin chain in transgenic hemoglobin SS knock-out mice (Pawliuk and colleagues, 2001).

Contraception and Sterilization

Because of chronic debility, complications caused by pregnancy, and the predictably shortened life span of women with sickle-cell anemia, contraception and possibly sterilization are important considerations. According to the American College of Obstetricians and Gynecologists (2000), estrogen-progesterone oral contraceptives have not been assessed well in women with sickle hemoglobinopathies. Many clinicians do not recommend their use because of potential adverse vascular and thrombotic effects (see Chap. 32, p. 679).

Progesterone has been long known to prevent painful sickle-cell crises. Because of this, low-dose oral progesterone, progesterone injections, or implants seem ideal. In one study, de Abood and associates (1997) reported significantly fewer and less intense pain crises in women given depot medroxyprogesterone intramuscularly. Some advise against the use of intrauterine contraceptive devices because of possibly increased risk of infection, but this has not been proven clinically. The safest contraceptives are unfortunately those with the highest failure rates—condoms with foam and diaphragms. Permanent sterilization is also an option (see Chap. 33, p 698).

Sickle-Cell Trait

The heterozygous inheritance of the gene for hemoglobin S results in sickle-cell trait, or AS hemoglobin. Hemoglobin A is most abundant, and the amount of hemoglobin S averages only approximately 30 percent in each red cell. The frequency of sickle-cell trait among African-Americans is approximately 8 percent. There is evidence that carriers have occasional hematuria, renal papillary necrosis, and hyposthenuria (Tsaras and co-workers, 2009). And although controversial, we are of the view that sickle trait is not associated with increased rates of abortion, perinatal mortality, low birthweight, or pregnancy-induced hypertension (Pritchard, 1973; Tita, 2007; Tuck, 1983, and all their associates). One unquestioned relationship is the twofold increased incidence of asymptomatic bacteriuria and urinary infection. ***Sickle-cell trait therefore should not be considered a deterrent to pregnancy on the basis of increased maternal risks.*** Finally, preliminary findings from a cohort study by Lally and colleagues (2009) suggested that African-American women with sickle trait may have a higher incidence of venous thromboembolism when using hormonal contraceptives compared with women without the trait. More data is needed before these effective contraceptive methods are withheld from trait-positive women.

Inheritance is a concern for the infant of a mother with sickle trait whenever the father carries a gene for abnormal hemoglobins that include S, C, and D or for β-thalassemia trait. Prenatal diagnosis through amniocentesis or chorionic villus sampling as well as preimplantation genetic screening is available (see Chap. 13, p. 299).

Other Hemoglobinopathies

Hemoglobin C and C-β-Thalassemia

The single β-chain substitution of glutamic acid by lysine at position 6 results in production of hemoglobin C. About 2 percent of African-Americans have C trait, which does not cause anemia or adverse pregnancy outcomes. However, when co-inherited with sickle-cell trait, hemoglobin SC causes the problems previously discussed.

Pregnancy and homozygous hemoglobin CC disease or hemoglobin C-β-thalassemia are relatively benign associations.

TABLE 51-5. Outcomes in 72 Pregnancies Complicated by Hemoglobin CC and C-β-Thalassemia

	Hemoglobin CC	C-β-Thalassemia
Women	15	5
Pregnancies	49	23
Hematocrit (range)	27 (21–23)	30 (28–33)
Birthweight (g)		
Mean	2990	2960
Range	1145–4770	2320–3980
Perinatal deaths	1	2
Surviving infants	42	20

Data from Maberry and colleagues (1990).

Maberry and colleagues (1990) reported our experiences from Parkland Hospital as shown in Table 51-5. Other than mild to moderate anemia, pregnancy outcomes were not different compared with those of the general obstetrical population. When severe anemia is identified, iron or folic acid deficiency or some other superimposed cause should be suspected. Supplementation with folic acid and iron is indicated.

Hemoglobin E

The second most common hemoglobin variant worldwide, is hemoglobin E, although it is uncommon in the United States. Hemoglobin E results from a single β-chain substitution of lysine for glutamic acid at codon 26. The hemoglobin is susceptible particularly to oxidative stress. The heterozygous E trait is common in Southeast Asia. Hurst and co-workers (1983) identified homozygous hemoglobin E, hemoglobin E plus β-thalassemia, or hemoglobin E trait in 36 percent of Cambodians and 25 percent of Laotians. In addition, α- and β-thalassemia traits were prevalent in all groups.

Homozygous hemoglobin EE is associated with little or no anemia, hypochromia, marked microcytosis, and erythrocyte targeting. In our limited experience, pregnant women do not appear to be at increased risk. Conversely, doubly heterozygous *hemoglobin E-β-thalassemia* is a common cause of childhood anemia in Southeast Asia (Fucharoen and Winichagoon, 2000). In a retrospective cohort study of 54 women with singleton pregnancies, Luewan and associates (2009) reported a threefold increased risk of preterm birth and fetal-growth restriction in affected women compared with normal controls. It is not clear if *hemoglobin SE* disease is as ominous during pregnancy as hemoglobin SC or S-β-thalassemia disease (Ramahi and colleagues, 1988).

Hemoglobinopathy in the Newborn

Infants with homozygous SS, SC, and CC disease can be identified accurately at birth by cord blood electrophoresis. The Maternal and Child Health Bureau (2005) recommends that all newborn infants be tested for sickle-cell disease. In most states, such screening is mandated by law and performed routinely on blood submitted for phenylketonuria

and hypothyroidism testing (see Chap. 28, p. 599). Screening for sickle hemoglobinopathies leads to clearly decreased mortality rates in children with sickle-cell disease identified at birth.

Prenatal Diagnosis

There are many tests to detect sickle-cell disease prenatally. Most are DNA based and can be done using CVS samples or amnionic fluid specimens obtained by amniocentesis at 15 weeks (American College of Obstetricians and Gynecologists, 2007). A number of mutations that encode hemoglobin S as well as other abnormal hemoglobins can be detected by targeted mutation analysis as well as PCR-based techniques (see Chap. 12, p. 283).

Thalassemias

These genetically determined hemoglobinopathies are characterized by impaired production of one or more of the normal globin peptide chains. Abnormal synthesis rates may result in ineffective erythropoiesis, hemolysis, and varying degrees of anemia. Thalassemias are classified according to the globin chain that is deficient, and several hundred syndromes have been identified. The two major forms involve impaired production or instability either of α-peptide chains—causing α-thalassemia or of β-chains—causing β-thalassemia. The incidence of these traits during pregnancy for all races is 1 in 300 to 500 (Gehlbach and Morgenstern, 1988).

α-Thalassemias

Because there are four α-globin genes, the inheritance of α-thalassemia is more complicated than for β-thalassemia (Leung and associates, 2008). Possible genotypes and phenotypes arising from these mutations are shown in Table 51-6. For each, a close correlation has been established between clinical severity and the degree of α-globin chains synthesis impairment. In most populations, the α-globin chain "cluster" or gene loci are doubled on chromosome 16. Thus, the normal genotype for diploid cells can be expressed as αα/αα. There are two main groups of α-thalassemia determinants: α°-thalassemia is characterized by the deletion of both loci from one chromosome (−−/αα), whereas α⁺-thalassemia is characterized by the loss of a single locus from one allele (−α/αα heterozygote) or a loss from each allele alleles (−α/−α homozygote).

There are two major phenotypes. The deletion of all four α-globin chain genes (−−/−−) characterizes *homozygous* α-thalassemia. Because α chains are contained in fetal hemoglobin, the fetus is affected. With none of the four genes expressed, there are no α-globin chains, and instead, hemoglobin Bart (γ_4) and hemoglobin H (β_4) are formed as abnormal tetramers (see Chap. 4, p. 92).

Hemoglobin Bart has an appreciably increased affinity for oxygen, and *hemoglobin Bart disease* is a common cause of stillbirths in Southeast Asia. Hsieh and associates (1989) studied 20 such hydropic fetuses by funipuncture and reported that blood contained 65 to 98 percent Bart hemoglobin. The fetus dies

TABLE 51-6. Genotypes and Phenotypes of α-Thalassemia Syndromes

Genotype	Genotype	Phenotype
Normal	$\alpha\alpha/\alpha\alpha$	--
α^+-thalassemia heterozygote	$-\alpha/\alpha\alpha$ $\alpha\alpha/-\alpha$	Silent carrier
α^+-thalassemia homozygote[a] α^0-thalassemia heterozygote[b]	$-\alpha/-\alpha$ $--/\alpha\alpha$	α-thalassemia minor—mild hypochromic microcytic anemia
Compound heterozygous α^0/α^+	$--/-\alpha$	Hgb H (β^4) with moderate to severe hemolytic anemia
Homozygous α-thalassemia	$--/--$	Hgb Bart (γ^4) disease, hydrops fetalis

[a]More common in African-Americans.
[b]More common in Asian-Americans.

either in utero or very soon after birth and demonstrates the typical features of nonimmune hydrops fetalis as shown in Figure 51-4 (see also Chap. 29, p. 626). Lam and associates (1999) reported that sonography at 12 to 13 weeks was 100-percent sensitive and specific for identifying affected fetuses by measuring the cardiothoracic ratio. Carr and colleagues (1995) transfused a fetus with α-thalassemia at 25, 26, and 32 weeks and reversed its ascites. The transfusion-dependent infant was delivered at 34 weeks. Fetal anemia can be detected using Doppler flow measurement of middle cerebral artery velocity as described in Chapter 16 (p. 364).

The compound heterozygous state for α^0- and α^+-thalassemia results in the deletion of three of four genes ($--/-\alpha$). There is only one functional α-globin gene per diploid genome. This is referred to as *hemoglobin H disease* (β_4) and is compatible with extrauterine life. The abnormal red cells at birth contain a mixture of hemoglobin Bart (γ_4), hemoglobin H (β_4), and hemoglobin A. The neonate appears well at birth but soon develops hemolytic anemia. Most of the hemoglobin Bart present at birth is replaced postnatally by hemoglobin H. The disease is characterized by hemolytic anemia, which may be severe and similar to β-thalassemia major in children and adults. Anemia in these women usually is worsened during pregnancy.

A deletion of two genes results clinically in α-*thalassemia minor*, which is characterized by minimal to moderate hypochromic microcytic anemia. This may be due to α^0- or α^+-thalassemia traits. Thus, genotypes may be $-\alpha/-\alpha$ or $--/\alpha\alpha$, and differentiation can be made only by DNA analysis (Weatherall and Provan, 2000). Other than mild anemia, there are no associated clinical abnormalities with α-thalassemia minor, and it often goes unrecognized. Hemoglobin Bart is present at birth, but as its levels drop, it is replaced by hemoglobin H. Red cells are hypochromic and microcytic, and the hemoglobin concentration is normal to slightly depressed. Women with α-thalassemia minor tolerate pregnancy well.

The single gene deletion ($-\alpha/\alpha\alpha$) is the silent carrier state. No clinical abnormality is evident in the individual with a single gene deletion.

Frequency. The relative frequency of α-thalassemia minor, hemoglobin H disease, and hemoglobin Bart disease varies remarkably among racial groups. All of these variants are encountered in Asians. In individuals of African descent, however, even though α-thalassemia minor is demonstrated in approximately 2 percent, hemoglobin H disease is rare and hemoglobin Bart disease is unreported. This is because Asians usually have α^0-thalassemia minor with both gene deletions typically from the same chromosome ($--/\alpha\alpha$), whereas in blacks with α^+-thalassemia minor, one gene is deleted from each chromosome ($-\alpha/-\alpha$). The α-thalassemia syndromes appear sporadically in other racial and ethnic groups. Diagnosis of α-thalassemia minor as well as α-thalassemia major in the fetus can be accomplished by

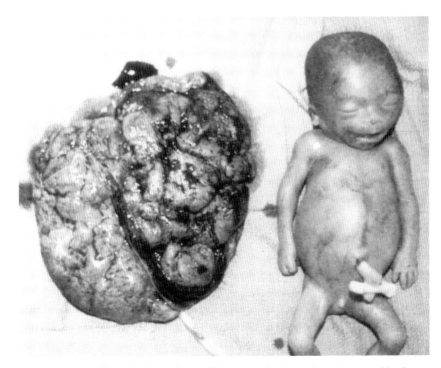

FIGURE 51-4 Stillborn hydropic fetus with extremely large placenta caused by homozygous α-thalassemia. (From Hsia, 1991, with permission.)

DNA analysis using molecular techniques (American College of Obstetricians and Gynecologists, 2007). Fetal diagnosis of hemoglobin Bart has been described using capillary electrophoresis or HPLC techniques (Sirichotiyakul, 2009; Srivorakun, 2009, and all their colleagues).

Beta-Thalassemias

These are the consequences of impaired production of β-globin chains or instability of α chains (Benz, 2008). More than 150 point mutations in the β-globin gene have been described (Weatherall, 2000). Most are single-nucleotide substitutions that produce transcription or translation defects, RNA splicing or modification, or frameshifts that result in highly unstable hemoglobins. Thus, deletional and nondeletional mutations affect β-globin RNA. The δγβ-gene "cluster" is on chromosome 11 (see Fig. 4-14, p. 92).

In β-thalassemia, there is decreased β-chain production, and excess α chains precipitate to cause cell membrane damage. In addition, β-thalassemia may be due to α-chain instability. Kihm and colleagues (2002) described a molecular chaperone that regulates α-globin subunit stability—*α-hemoglobin-stabilizing protein (AHSP)*—which forms a stable complex with free α-globin and prevents precipitation. Mutations in the AHSP gene may modify the clinical picture of β-thalassemia. For example, an overexpression of AHSP may convert β-thalassemia major to β-thalassemia intermedia. These basic defects lead to the panorama of pathology that characterizes homozygous β-thalassemia, so-called *β-thalassemia major* or *Cooley anemia*. With heterozygous β-thalassemia minor, hypochromia, microcytosis, and slight to moderate anemia develop without the intense hemolysis that characterizes the homozygous state. The hallmark of the common β-thalassemias is an elevated hemoglobin A₂ level.

In the typical case of thalassemia major, the neonate is healthy at birth, but as the hemoglobin F level falls, the infant becomes severely anemic and fails to thrive. A child who is entered into an adequate transfusion program develops normally until the end of the first decade. Then, effects of iron loading become apparent. Prognosis is improved by iron chelation therapy with deferoxamine (Olivieri and associates, 1998).

Prior to chelation and transfusions, pregnancy in women with severe thalassemia was rare. Aessopos (1999), Daskalakis (1998), and Kumar (1997) and their colleagues reported a total of 63 pregnancies without severe complications. Pregnancy is recommended only if there is normal maternal cardiac function and prolonged hypertransfusion to maintain the hemoglobin concentration at 10 g/dL. This is coupled with surveillance and monitoring of fetal growth (American College of Obstetricians and Gynecologists, 2007; Sheiner and colleagues, 2004).

With *β-thalassemia minor*, hemoglobin A₂, which is composed of two α- and two δ-globin chains, is increased to more than 3.5 percent. Simultaneously, hemoglobin F, which is composed of two α- and two γ-globin chains, is usually increased to more than 2 percent. Anemia is mild, and the red cells are hypochromic and microcytic. There is usually pregnancy-induced augmentation of erythropoiesis, and using erythrocytes tagged with chromium-51, we have documented normal

blood volume expansion with slightly subnormal red cell mass expansion.

There is no specific therapy for β-thalassemia minor during pregnancy. Prophylactic iron and folic acid are given. Sheiner and associates (2004) reported that fetal-growth restriction and oligohydramnios were increased twofold in 261 affected women.

Prenatal diagnosis of β-thalassemia major is more difficult than detecting abnormal hemoglobins because of the large number of mutations. To diagnose a particular mutation, targeted mutation analysis is done that requires prior identification of the disease-causing mutation for that particular family (American College of Obstetricians and Gynecologists, 2007). Most of these are done using samples obtained by CVS. Preimplantation blastomere biopsy has been described by Galvani (2000) and Kanavakis (1999) and their associates. Isolation of single nucleated red blood cells from maternal circulation is being explored for prenatal diagnosis of β-thalassemia (Kolialexi and colleagues, 2007).

Polycythemia

Excessive erythrocytosis during pregnancy is usually related to chronic hypoxia due to maternal congenital cardiac disease or a pulmonary disorder. Occasionally, it is from heavy cigarette smoking. We have encountered otherwise healthy young pregnant women who were heavy smokers with chronic bronchitis and with a hematocrit from 55 to 60 volumes percent! Brewer and colleagues (1992) described a woman with persistent erythrocytosis associated with a placental site tumor. If polycythemia is severe, the probability of a successful pregnancy outcome is low.

Polycythemia vera is a myeloproliferative hemopoietic stem cell disorder characterized by excessive proliferation of erythroid, myeloid, and megakaryocytic precursors. It is uncommon and likely an acquired genetic disorder of stem cells (Spivak, 2008). Measurement of serum erythropoietin by radioimmunoassay differentiates polycythemia vera—low values—from secondary polycythemia—high values. Symptoms are related to increased blood viscosity, and thrombotic complications are common. Fetal loss has been reported to be high in women with polycythemia vera and pregnancy outcome may be improved with aspirin therapy (Deruelle, 2005; Griesshammer, 2006; Robinson, 2005; Tefferi, 2000, and all their associates).

PLATELET DISORDERS

Thrombocytopenia in pregnant women may be inherited or idiopathic. It is often associated with acquired hemolytic anemia, severe preeclampsia or eclampsia, severe hemorrhage with blood transfusions, consumptive coagulopathy from placental abruption or similar hypofibrinogenemic states, sepsis syndrome, systemic lupus erythematosus, antiphospholipid antibody syndrome, aplastic anemia, and megaloblastic anemia from severe folate deficiency. It also may result from viral infection, exposure to a variety of drugs, allergic reaction, and irradiation (Konkle, 2008). Drug-induced thrombocytopenia was reviewed by Aster and Bougie (2007).

Gestational Thrombocytopenia

Normal pregnancy may be accompanied by a physiological decrease in platelet concentration. This is usually evident in the third trimester and is thought to be predominantly due to hemodilution (see Appendix). Most evidence shows that platelet life span is unchanged in normal pregnancy (Kenny and colleagues, 2009).

Thus, some degree of *gestational thrombocytopenia* is considered normal. Obviously, the definition used for thrombocytopenia is important. In their review, Rouse and associates (1998) cite an incidence of 4 to 7 percent for gestational thrombocytopenia, defined by platelet counts $< 150,000/\mu L$. Burrows and Kelton (1993a) reported that 6.6 percent of 15,471 pregnant women had platelet counts $< 150,000/\mu L$, and in 1.2 percent, they were $< 100,000/\mu L$. They reported that almost 75 percent of 1027 women whose platelet counts were $< 150,000/\mu L$ were found to have normal-variant incidental thrombocytopenia. Of the remainder, 21 percent had a hypertensive disorder of pregnancy, and 4 percent had an immunological disorder. In another study, Boehlen and associates (2000) found that 11.6 percent of 6770 pregnant women had platelet counts $< 150,000/\mu L$. In this study, $116,000/\mu L$ was 2.5 standard deviations below the mean. Al-Kouatly and colleagues (2003) found a much higher rate of thrombocytopenia in triplet gestations, affecting nearly a third of cases. In contrast to thrombocytopenia in singletons, more than 70 percent of cases were due to hypertensive disorders.

Inherited Thrombocytopenias

The *Bernard-Soulier syndrome* is characterized by lack of platelet membrane glycoprotein (GPIb/IX), which causes severe dysfunction. Maternal antibodies against fetal GPIb/IX antigen can cause isoimmune fetal thrombocytopenia. Peng and colleagues (1991) described an affected woman who during four pregnancies had episodes of postpartum hemorrhage, gastrointestinal hemorrhage, and fetal thrombocytopenia. Fujimori and associates (1999) described a similarly affected woman whose neonate died from thrombocytopenic intracranial hemorrhage. Close monitoring through pregnancy and 6 weeks postpartum is critical due to the possibility of life-threatening hemorrhage (Prabu and Parapia, 2006).

Chatwani and associates (1992) reported a woman with autosomally dominant *May-Hegglin anomaly* whose infant was not affected. This condition is characterized by thrombocytopenia, giant platelets, and leukocyte inclusions. Urato and Repke (1998) also described such a woman who was delivered vaginally. Despite a platelet count of $16,000/\mu L$, she did not bleed excessively. The neonate inherited the anomaly, but also had no bleeding despite a platelet count of $35,000/\mu L$. Fayyad and colleagues (2002) managed three pregnancies in a woman with May-Hegglin anomaly. In the first, the mother had a term cesarean delivery of an unaffected infant; in the second, she had a fetal demise with multiple placental infarcts; and in the third, she received low-dose aspirin (75 mg/d) and gave birth to an unaffected infant.

Immune Thrombocytopenic Purpura

This is also called *idiopathic thrombocytopenic purpura (ITP)* and usually results from a cluster of IgG antibodies directed against one or more platelet glycoproteins (Schwartz, 2007). Antibody-coated platelets are destroyed prematurely in the reticuloendothelial system, especially the spleen. The mechanism of production of these platelet-associated immunoglobulins—PAIgG, PAIgM, and PAIgA—is not known, but most investigators consider them to be autoantibodies.

The American Society of Hematology formulated guidelines for the diagnosis and management of ITP, which are still in effect (George and colleagues, 1996). Acute ITP is most often a childhood disease that follows a viral infection. Most cases resolve spontaneously, although perhaps 10 percent become chronic. Conversely, in adults, immune thrombocytopenia is primarily a chronic disease of young women and rarely resolves spontaneously.

Secondary forms of chronic thrombocytopenia appear in association with systemic lupus erythematosus, lymphomas, leukemias, and a number of systemic diseases. For example, about 2 percent of thrombocytopenic patients have positive serological tests for lupus, and in some cases, there are high levels of anticardiolipin antibodies. As many as 10 percent of HIV-positive patients have associated thrombocytopenia (Konkle, 2008; Scaradavou, 2002).

Only a small number of adults with primary ITP recover spontaneously, and for those who do not, platelet counts usually range from 10,000 to $100,000/\mu L$ (George and associates, 1996). Those whose platelet counts remain less than $30,000/\mu L$ or those with significant bleeding at higher levels are treated. Prednisone, 1 to 2 mg/kg orally daily, raises the platelet count in approximately two thirds of cases. Unfortunately, relapse is common. Glucocorticoids suppress the phagocytic activity of the splenic monocyte-macrophage system. Also, intravenous immunoglobulin (IVIG) given in a total dose of 2 g/kg over 2 to 5 days is usually effective (Konkle, 2008). Godeau and colleagues (2002) reported results of a randomized trial of intravenous immunoglobulin or high-dose methylprednisolone given for 3 days. These were followed by either oral prednisone or placebo. Intravenous immunoglobulin plus oral prednisone was most effective, although methylprednisolone with prednisone was effective and well tolerated. Therapy is expensive, and IVIG currently costs $40 to $55 per gram with a typical course of therapy averaging 150 to 200 grams (Medical Letter, 2006).

For patients with no response to corticosteroid therapy in 2 to 3 weeks, those in whom massive doses are needed to sustain remission, or those with frequent recurrences, splenectomy is indicated. In approximately 60 percent, there is substantive improvement as the consequence of decreased removal of platelets and reduced antibody production. Massive doses described above of immunoglobulin given intravenously over 5 days result in satisfactory platelet count elevation in two thirds of patients. Such therapy may be useful for those with life-threatening thrombocytopenia refractory to other therapy or for patients preoperatively before splenectomy.

Therapy is problematic for the 30 percent of adults who do not respond to corticosteroids or splenectomy. Immunosuppressive drugs, including azathioprine, cyclophosphamide, and cyclosporine, have been used with some success. Danazol, vinca alkaloids, plasma exchange, and high-dose dexamethasone pulse therapy have also been described. Thrombopoietin agonists, such as *eltrombopag,* have shown promise but are considered experimental (Bussel and co-workers, 2007).

Immune Thrombocytopenia and Pregnancy

There is no evidence that pregnancy increases the risk of relapse in women with previously diagnosed immune thrombocytopenia. Nor does it worsen thrombocytopenia in women with active disease. That said, it is certainly not unusual for women who have been in clinical remission for several years to have recurrent thrombocytopenia during pregnancy. Although this may be from closer surveillance, hyperestrogenemia has also been suggested as a cause.

Treatment is considered if the platelet count is less than 30,000 to 50,000/μL (George and associates, 1996; Konkle, 2008). Prednisone in a dose of 1 mg/kg orally per day may be required for improvement, and most likely treatment will have to be continued throughout pregnancy. Corticosteroid therapy usually produces amelioration. With steroid-refractory disease, high-dose immunoglobulin is given intravenously and may be considered as first-line therapy in the third trimester (Gernsheimer and McCrae, 2007). Clark and Gall (1997) reviewed 16 reports of 21 pregnancies in which ITP was treated with immunoglobulin. All but four responded with posttreatment platelet counts greater than 50,000/μL, and in 11 cases, counts exceeded 100,000/μL.

In pregnant women with no response to steroid or immunoglobulin therapy, open or laparoscopic splenectomy may be effective. In late pregnancy, surgery is technically more difficult, and cesarean delivery may be necessary for exposure. Intravenous anti-D IgG 50 to 75 μg/kg has been described for treatment of resistant ITP in D-positive patients with a spleen (Konkle, 2008). There usually is improvement by 1 to 3 days with a peak at approximately 8 days. Sieunarine and colleagues (2007) reported such therapy in a pregnant woman.

Fetal and Neonatal Effects

Platelet-associated IgG antibodies cross the placenta and may cause thrombocytopenia in the fetus-neonate. Fetal death from hemorrhage occurs occasionally (Webert and associates, 2003). The severely thrombocytopenic fetus is at increased risk for intracranial hemorrhage with labor and delivery. This fortunately is unusual. Payne and colleagues (1997) reviewed studies of maternal ITP published since 1973 and added their experiences with 55 cases. Of 601 newborns, 12 percent had severe thrombocytopenia defined as a platelet count < 50,000/μL. Six infants had intracranial hemorrhage, and in three, their initial platelet count was > 50,000/μL.

Considerable attention has been directed at identifying the fetus with potentially dangerous thrombocytopenia. All investigators have concurred that there is not a strong correlation between fetal and maternal platelet counts (George and associates, 1996; Payne and co-workers, 1997). Because of this, there have been attempts to quantify the relationships among maternal IgG free platelet antibody levels, platelet-associated antibody levels, and fetal platelet count. Again, there is little concurrence. Kaplan (1990) and Samuels (1990) and their colleagues reported conflicting results in using indirect platelet immunoglobulin for identification of high-risk neonates.

Investigators have also examined the association between the specific maternal cause of thrombocytopenia and the risk of a thrombocytopenic fetus. Four causes investigated include gestational thrombocytopenia, hypertension-associated thrombocytopenia, ITP, and isoimmune thrombocytopenia. Burrows and Kelton (1993a) reported neonatal umbilical cord platelet counts of < 50,000/μL in 19 of 15,932 consecutive newborns (0.12 percent). Of all of these pregnancies, only one of 756 mothers with gestational thrombocytopenia had an affected infant. Of 1414 hypertensive women with thrombocytopenia, five infants had thrombocytopenia. In contrast, of 46 mothers with ITP, four infants had thrombocytopenia. Finally, isoimmune thrombocytopenia was associated with profound thrombocytopenia and cord platelet counts < 20,000/μL. One of these fetuses died, and two others had intracranial hemorrhage.

In a similar population study to the one above, Boehlen and associates (1999) determined antiplatelet antibody levels in 430 pregnant women whose platelet counts were < 150,000/μL. Antibodies were detected in 9 percent but had no predictive value. In another study, Sainio and co-workers (2000) performed cord platelet counts in almost 4500 neonates. Approximately 2 percent were < 150,000/μL, and only 0.2 percent (1 in 410) were < 50,000/μL. Once again, bleeding in all infants was due to isoimmune thrombocytopenia.

Detection of Fetal Thrombocytopenia

From the foregoing, it is apparent that there are no clinical characteristics or laboratory tests that accurately predict fetal platelet count. This led Scott and associates (1983) to recommend intrapartum fetal scalp platelet determinations once the cervix was 2 cm dilated and the membranes were ruptured. Cesarean delivery was performed for fetuses with platelet counts < 50,000/μL. Daffos and colleagues (1985) subsequently reported a high complication rate with percutaneous umbilical cord blood sampling—PUBS—for platelet quantification (see Chap. 13, p. 300). Berry and associates (1997) reported no complications but found a high negative-predictive value. Payne and colleagues (1997) summarized six such studies reported since 1988. Of 195 cases, severe neonatal thrombocytopenia of < 50,000/μL was found in 7 percent, however, there were serious complications from cordocentesis in 4.6 percent of the fetuses.

Because of the low incidence of severe neonatal thrombocytopenia and morbidity, Burrows and Kelton (1993b), Silver and colleagues (1995), Payne and associates (1997), and the American Society of Hematology (George and co-workers, 1996) all concluded that fetal platelet determinations and cesarean delivery are not necessary.

Isoimmune Thrombocytopenia

Platelet isoimmunization can develop in a manner identical to erythrocyte antigen isoimmunization. This disorder is discussed in detail in Chapter 29 (p. 629).

Thrombocytosis

Also called *thrombocythemia,* thrombocytosis generally is defined as persistent platelet counts > 450,000/μL. Common causes of *secondary* or *reactive thrombocytosis* are iron deficiency, infection, inflammatory diseases, and malignant tumors (Konkle, 2008). Platelet counts seldom exceed 800,000/μL in these secondary disorders, and prognosis depends on the underlying disease. On the other hand, *essential thrombocytosis* is a myeloproliferative disorder that accounts for most cases in which platelet counts exceed 1 million/μL. Thrombocytosis usually is asymptomatic, but arterial and venous thromboses may develop (Rabinerson and associates, 2007). In one study, Cortelazzo and colleagues (1995) reported that myelosuppression with hydroxyurea for nonpregnant patients with essential thrombocytosis decreased thrombotic episodes from 24 to 4 percent compared with those of untreated controls.

Thrombocytosis in Pregnancy

In 40 pregnancies of 16 women with essential thrombocythemia, 45 percent were complicated by spontaneous abortion, fetal demise, and preeclampsia (Niittyvuopio and colleagues, 2004). Experiences from the Mayo Clinic with 63 pregnancies in 36 women were described recently by Gangat and co-workers (2009). Again, abortion was common, and 35 percent of pregnancies miscarried, most in the first trimester. Aspirin therapy was associated with a significantly lower abortion rate than that in untreated women—1 vs. 75 percent. Other pregnancy complications were uncommon. Normal pregnancies have been described in women whose mean platelet counts were > 1.25 million/μL (Beard and co-workers, 1991; Randi and colleagues, 1994). Treatment that has been suggested during pregnancy includes aspirin, dipyridamole, heparin, platelet pheresis, or combinations thereof (Griesshammer and associates, 2003). Delage and co-workers (1996) reviewed 11 cases in which interferon-α was given during pregnancy with successful outcomes. They also described a woman at midpregnancy who had a platelet count of 2.3 million/μL and transient blindness. Thrombocytapheresis and interferon-α were used to keep the platelets at approximately 1 million/μL until delivery.

Thrombotic Microangiopathies

Although not proven a primary platelet disorder, there almost always is some degree of thrombocytopenia with the thrombotic microangiopathies. Their similarities to the preeclampsia syndrome underlie their obstetrical ramifications.

Moschcowitz (1925) originally described *thrombotic thrombocytopenic purpura* by the pentad of thrombocytopenia, fever, neurological abnormalities, renal impairment, and hemolytic anemia. Gasser and colleagues (1955) later described the similar *hemolytic uremic syndrome*, which had more profound renal involvement and fewer neurological aberrations. Allford and associates (2003) provided guidelines for the British Committee for Standards in Haematology for the diagnosis and management of thrombotic microangiopathic hemolytic anemias. The syndromes have an incidence of 2 to 6 per million persons per year (Miller and colleagues, 2004).

Although it is likely that different causes account for the variable findings within these syndromes, they frequently are clinically indistinguishable in adults. Thrombotic thrombocytopenic purpura—TTP—is thought to be caused by a plasma deficiency of a von Willebrand factor-clearing protease termed ADAMTS-13 (Crowther and George, 2008; Mayer and Aledort, 2005). Conversely, hemolytic uremic syndrome—HUS—is usually due to endothelial damage incited by viral or bacterial infections. There is no evidence that postpartum renal failure is a separate syndrome (Robson and associates, 1968).

Pathogenesis

Microthrombi of hyaline material consisting of platelets and small amounts of fibrin develop within arterioles and capillaries. These aggregates produce ischemia or infarctions in various organs. The general consensus is that intravascular platelet aggregation stimulates the cascade of events leading to end-organ failure. Although there is endothelial activation and damage, it is unclear whether this is a consequence or a cause. Elevated levels of unusually large multimers of von Willebrand factor are identified with active TTP. The endothelium-derived protease responsible for cleaving von Willebrand factor is neutralized by antibodies during an acute episode (Furlan and colleagues, 1998; Tsai and Lian, 1998). The *ADAMTS13 gene* encodes this protease (Levy and colleagues, 2001). Defects in this gene result in various clinical presentations of thrombotic microangiopathy (Camilleri and colleagues, 2007; Moake, 2002, 2004).

Clinical Presentation

Thrombotic microangiopathies are characterized by thrombocytopenia, fragmentation hemolysis, and variable organ dysfunction. A viral prodrome may precede up to 40 percent of cases. Neurological symptoms develop in up to 90 percent and include headache, altered consciousness, convulsions, fever, or stroke. Because renal involvement is common, the two syndromes are difficult to separate clinically. Renal failure is thought to be more severe with the hemolytic uremic syndrome, and in half of the cases, dialysis is required.

Hematological Abnormalities

Thrombocytopenia is usually severe. Fortunately, even with very low platelet counts, spontaneous severe hemorrhage is uncommon. Microangiopathic hemolysis is associated with moderate to marked anemia, and transfusions are frequently necessary. The blood smear is characterized by erythrocyte fragmentation with schizocytosis. The reticulocyte count is high, and nucleated red blood cells are numerous. Consumptive coagulopathy, although common, is usually subtle and clinically insignificant.

Treatment

Plasmapheresis with fresh-frozen plasma replacement has remarkably improved the outcome for patients with these formerly fatal diseases (Michael and co-workers, 2009). Red cell transfusions are imperative for life-threatening anemia. Rock and colleagues (1991) found plasma exchange to be superior to plasma infusion in nonpregnant patients, but mortality rates were still 30 percent. Bell and co-workers (1991) reported their experiences with 108 patients treated at Johns Hopkins Hospital, of which 10 percent were pregnant. Those with mild neurological symptoms were given prednisone, 200 mg orally daily. If there were neurological abnormalities or rapid clinical deterioration, plasmapheresis and plasma exchange were performed daily. Approximately a fourth of patients with mild disease responded to prednisone alone. Of those requiring plasmapheresis, relapses were common, but the overall survival rate was 91 percent. According to Konkle (2008), 25 to 40 percent have a relapse within 30 days, whereas up to 40 percent have a later relapse. In addition, there may be long-term sequelae, such as renal impairment (Dashe and colleagues, 1998).

Pregnancy and Thrombotic Microangiopathy

It has been shown that ADAMTS-13 enzyme activity decreases almost 50 percent across pregnancy (Sanchez-Luceros and co-workers, 2004). At least intuitively, this is consonant with prevailing opinions that TTP is more common in pregnant women. We, however, are of the contrary view. This is because of observations over a 25-year period, during which Dashe and co-workers (1998) reported 11 pregnancies complicated by these syndromes among nearly 275,000 obstetrical patients within our well-defined catchment area for Parkland Hospital. This frequency of 1 in 25,000 approximates that in our general hospital population.

It is not surprising that severe preeclampsia and eclampsia complicated further by thrombocytopenia and overt hemolysis have been confused with thrombotic thrombocytopenic purpura and vice versa (Hsu and colleagues, 1995; Magann and co-workers, 1994). One constant feature of thrombotic microangiopathies is hemolytic anemia, which is rarely severe with preeclampsia, even with the *HELLP syndrome* (see Chap. 34, p. 718). Although deposition of hyaline microthrombi within the liver is seen with thrombotic microangiopathy, hepatocellular necrosis characteristic of preeclampsia has not been described. In addition, whereas delivery is imperative to treat preeclampsia in women with the HELLP syndrome, there is no evidence that thrombotic microangiopathy is improved by delivery (Letsky, 2000). Finally, microangiopathic syndromes are usually recurrent and unassociated with pregnancy. For example, 7 of 11 women described by Dashe and colleagues (1998) had recurrent disease either when not pregnant or within the first trimester of a subsequent pregnancy. George (2009) reported recurrent TTP in only five of 36 subsequent pregnancies.

Unless the diagnosis is unequivocally one of these thrombotic microangiopathies, rather than severe preeclampsia, the response to pregnancy termination should be evaluated before resorting to plasmapheresis and exchange transfusion, massive-dose glucocorticoid therapy, or other therapy. Measurement of ADAMTS-13 enzyme activity may not be helpful because it decreases with HELLP syndrome to levels lower that those for normal pregnancy (Franchini and co-workers, 2007). *Plasmapheresis is not indicated for preeclampsia-eclampsia complicated by hemolysis and thrombocytopenia.*

Paralleled with improved survival of nonpregnant patients treated with plasmapheresis and plasma exchange, maternal survival rates from thrombotic microangiopathy have increased appreciably with these treatments. Egerman and co-workers (1996) described 11 pregnant women so treated and noted two maternal and three fetal deaths. In our experiences at Parkland Hospital, five of eight women treated by plasmapheresis had a dramatic salutary response, although one woman died (Dashe and associates, 1998).

Long-Term Prognosis. Pregnant women with thrombotic microangiopathy have a number of long-term complications. In the study by Dashe and associates (1998), 9-year surveillance disclosed multiple recurrences; renal disease requiring dialysis, transplantation, or both; severe hypertension; and transfusion-acquired infectious diseases. Two women died remote from pregnancy—one from dialysis complications and one from HIV infection transmitted by blood or plasma transfusions. Egerman and colleagues (1996) reported similar observations. And for nonpregnant patients who have recovered from TTP, there are persistent cognitive defects as well as physical disabilities in most of those assessed at a median duration of 4 years (Kennedy and associates, 2009; Lewis and colleagues, 2009). These cognitive defects are intriguingly similar to those reported years later in eclamptic women as described by The Netherlands group (Aukes and co-workers, 2009) and discussed in further detail in Chapter 34 (p. 749).

INHERITED COAGULATION DEFECTS

Obstetrical hemorrhage is common, but it rarely is the consequence of an inherited defect in the coagulation mechanism. Several syndromes, however, are particularly important.

Hemophilias

There are two types of hemophilias, which are seen in varying degrees. They are considered mild, moderate, or severe, corresponding to plasma factor levels of 6 to 30, 2 to 5, or < 1 percent, respectively (Mannucci and Tuddenham, 2001).

Hemophilia A is an X-linked recessively transmitted disease characterized by a marked deficiency of *small component* antihemophilic factor (factor VIII:C). It is rare among women compared with men, in whom the heterozygous state is responsible for the disease. Although heterozygous women have diminished factor VIII levels, almost invariably the homozygous state is the requisite for hemophilia A. In a few instances, it appears in women spontaneously from a newly mutant gene.

The genetic and clinical features of severe deficiency of factor IX—*Christmas disease* or *hemophilia B*—are similar to those of hemophilia A. Guy and associates (1992) reviewed five cases in pregnancy, all with a favorable outcome. They recommended administration of factor IX when levels are below 10 percent.

Clinical Manifestations

The degree of risk for each hemophilia is influenced markedly by the level of circulating factor VIII:C or factor IX. If the level is at or very close to zero, the risk is major. In female carriers, activity is expected to average 50 percent, but there is a range due to lyonization (Letsky, 2000). If levels fall below 10 to 20 percent, hemorrhage may occur. Both of these clotting factors increase appreciably during normal pregnancy and in pregnant women who are carriers of hemophilia A and B (see Appendix).

Desmopressin may also stimulate factor VIII:C release. The risk of hemorrhage is reduced by avoiding lacerations, by minimizing episiotomy use and size, and by maximizing postpartum myometrial contractions and retraction. Kadir and co-workers (1997) reported that 20 percent of carriers had postpartum hemorrhage, and in two, it was massive.

An affected male fetus may develop hematomas with either vaginal or cesarean delivery (Kadir and associates, 1997). After delivery, the risk of hemorrhage in the neonate increases, especially if circumcision is attempted.

Inheritance

Whenever the mother has hemophilia A or B, all of her sons will have the disease, and all of her daughters will be carriers. If she is a carrier, half of her sons will inherit the disease and half of her daughters will be carriers. Prenatal diagnosis of hemophilia is possible in some families using chorionic villus biopsy (see Chap. 13, p. 300). Premiplantation genetic diagnosis for hemophilia was recently reviewed by Lavery (2009).

Factor VIII or IX Inhibitors

Rarely, antibodies directed against factor VIII or IX are acquired and may lead to life-threatening hemorrhage. Patients with hemophilia A or B, because of prior treatment with factor VIII or IX, more commonly develop such antibodies. In contrast, acquisition of these antibodies in nonhemophiliacs is rare. This phenomenon has also been identified rarely in women during the puerperium (Santoro and Prejano, 2009). In these cases, the prominent clinical feature is severe, protracted, repetitive hemorrhage from the reproductive tract starting a week or so after an apparently uncomplicated delivery (Reece and associates, 1988). The activated partial thromboplastin time is markedly prolonged. Treatment has included multiple transfusions of whole blood and plasma; huge doses of cryoprecipitate; large volumes of an admixture of activated coagulation factors, including porcine factor VIII; immunosuppressive therapy; and attempts at various surgical procedures, especially curettage and hysterectomy. Another treatment involves bypassing factor VIII or IX by the use of activated forms of factors VII, IX, and X. A recombinant activated factor VII (NovoSeven) stops bleeding in up to 75 percent of patients with inhibitors (Mannucci and Tuddenham, 2001). As discussed in Chapter 35 (p. 794), NovoSeven has also been used in nonhemophilic patients in cases of intractable obstetrical hemorrhage caused by uterine atony and by dilutional effects of multiple transfusions.

Von Willebrand Disease

Clinically, von Willebrand disease (vWD) is a heterogenous group of approximately 20 functional disorders involving aberrations of factor VIII complex and platelet dysfunction. These abnormalities are the most commonly inherited bleeding disorders, and their prevalence is as high as 1 to 2 percent (Mannucci, 2004). Most von Willebrand variants are inherited as autosomal dominant traits. Examples are types I and II, which are the most common variants. Type III, which is the most severe, is phenotypically recessive. These and other aspects of vWD were re-

cently reviewed by an expert panel of the National Heart, Lung, and Blood Institute (Nichols and co-workers, 2008).

Fewer than 300 cases of *acquired vWD (AvWD)* have been reported in the literature. Most symptoms include rapid onset of subcutaneous bruising or mucous membrane bleeding in those with no prior personal or family history of clotting abnormalities. Etiologies include benign and malignant hematological conditions, solid tumors, autoimmune disorders, and medications. For example, autoantibodies against von Willebrand factor (vWF) lead to rapid clearance from the circulation or interference with its function. Alternatively, lymphoid or other tumors can express specific vWF receptors and selectively adsorb vWF onto their surfaces, thereby nullifying its function. Additionally, decreased synthesis of vWF has been found in those with hypothyroidism and valproate-induced vWD. Lastly, the vWF shows increased degradation in those with poorly controlled diabetes mellitus, congenital or acquired cardiac defects, and ciprofloxacin-induced vWD (Shau and colleagues, 2002). Although most cases of AvWD develop in those older than 50 years, management of AvWD in pregnancy has been described (Lipkind and colleagues, 2005).

Pathogenesis

The *von Willebrand factor* is a series of large plasma multimeric glycoproteins that form part of the factor VIII complex. It is essential for normal platelet adhesion to subendothelial collagen and formation of a primary hemostatic plug at the site of blood vessel injury. It also plays a major role in the stabilization of the coagulant properties of factor VIII. The procoagulant component is the antihemophilic factor or factor VIII:C, which is a glycoprotein synthesized by the liver. Conversely, von Willebrand precursor, which is present in platelets as well as plasma, is synthesized by endothelium and megakaryocytes under the control of autosomal genes on chromosome 12. The von Willebrand factor antigen (vWF:Ag) is the antigenic determinant measured by immunoassays.

Clinical Presentation

Symptomatic patients usually present with evidence of a platelet defect. The possibility of vWD is usually considered in women with bleeding suggestive of a chronic disorder of coagulation. The classical autosomal dominant form usually is symptomatic in the heterozygous state. The less common but clinically more severe autosomal recessive form is manifest when inherited from both parents, both of whom typically demonstrate little or no disease. Type I, which accounts for 75 percent of von Willebrand variants, is characterized clinically by easy bruising; epistaxis; mucosal hemorrhage; and excessive bleeding with trauma, including surgery. Its laboratory features are usually a prolonged bleeding time, prolonged partial thromboplastin time, decreased vWF antigen levels, decreased factor VIII immunological as well as coagulation-promoting activity, and inability of platelets in plasma from an affected person to react to a variety of stimuli.

Pregnancy and vWD

During normal pregnancy, maternal levels of both factor VIII as well as vWF antigen increase substantively (see Appendix).

Because of this, pregnant women with vWD often develop normal levels of factor VIII coagulant activity as well as vWF antigen, although the bleeding time still may be prolonged. If factor VIII activity is very low or if there is bleeding, treatment is recommended. Desmopressin by infusion may transiently increase factor VIII and vWF factor levels, especially in patients with type I disease (Kujovich, 2005; Mannucci, 2004). With significant bleeding, 15 or 20 units or "bags" of cryoprecipitate are given every 12 hours. Alternatively, factor VIII concentrates may be given that contain high-molecular-weight vWF multimers (Alfanate, Hemate-P). These concentrates are highly purified and are heat treated to destroy HIV. Lubetsky and associates (1999) have described continuous infusion with Hemate-P in nonpregnant patients during nine surgical procedures and in another woman during a vaginal delivery. According to Chi and associates (2009), conduction analgesia can be given safely if coagulation defects have normalized or if hemostatic agents are given prophylactically.

Pregnancy outcomes in women with von Willebrand disease are generally good, but postpartum hemorrhage is encountered in up to 50 percent of cases. Of 38 cases summarized by Conti and associates (1986), bleeding was reported with abortion, with delivery, or in the puerperium in a fourth. Greer and colleagues (1991) reported that 8 of 14 pregnancies were complicated by postpartum hemorrhage. Kadir and co-workers (1998) reported their experiences from the Royal Free Hospital in London with 84 pregnancies. They described a 20-percent incidence of immediate postpartum hemorrhage and another 20-percent incidence of late hemorrhage. Most cases were associated with low vWF levels in untreated women, and none given treatment peripartum had hemorrhage. In our experiences, levels of coagulant factors within the normal range do not always protect against such bleeding.

Inheritance

Although most patients with von Willebrand disease have heterozygous variants with a mild bleeding disorder, the disease can be severe. Certainly when both parents have the disorder, their homozygous offspring develop a serious bleeding disorder. Mullaart and colleagues (1991) reported periventricular hemorrhage in a 32-week fetus who inherited type IIa vWD from her father. Chorionic villus biopsy with DNA analysis to detect the missing genes has been described (see Chap. 13, p. 300). Some authorities recommend cesarean delivery to avoid trauma to a possibly affected fetus if the mother has severe disease.

Other Inherited Coagulation Factor Deficiencies

In general, the activity of most procoagulant factors in maternal plasma rise across pregnancy (see Appendix). A number of rare coagulopathies may be inherited in a manner similar to the hemophilias. *Factor VII deficiency* is a rare autosomal recessive disorder. The gene that codes for factor VII is on chromosome 13. Normally, factor VII increases during pregnancy, but it may do so only mildly in women with factor VII deficiency (Fadel and Krauss, 1989). Treatment with factor VIIa has been reported during labor, delivery, and the puerperium (Eskandari and associates, 2002).

Factor X or *Stuart-Prower factor* deficiency is rare and is inherited as an autosomal recessive trait. Factor X levels typically rise by 50 percent during normal pregnancy. Konje and colleagues (1994) described a woman with 2-percent activity who was given prophylactic treatment with plasma-derived factor X, which raised plasma levels to 37 percent. Despite this, she suffered an intrapartum placental abruption. Bofill and co-workers (1996) gave intrapartum fresh-frozen plasma to a woman with less than 1-percent factor X activity. She delivered spontaneously without incident. Beksac and associates (2009) described a woman with severe factor X deficiency who was successfully managed with prophylactic prothrombin complex concentrate.

Factor XI—plasma thromboplastin antecedent—deficiency is inherited as an autosomal trait that is manifest as severe disease in homozygotes but only as a minor defect in heterozygotes. It is most prevalent in Ashkenazi Jews, and it is rarely seen in pregnancy. Musclow and colleagues (1987) described 41 deliveries in 17 affected women with factor XI deficiency, none of whom required transfusions. They also described a woman who developed a spontaneous hemarthrosis at 39 weeks. Kadir and associates (1998) described 29 pregnancies in 11 affected women. In none of these did factor XI levels increase; 15 percent had immediate postpartum hemorrhage; and another 25 percent had delayed hemorrhage. Myers and colleagues (2007) reported 105 pregnancies in 33 affected women with uneventful pregnancy and delivery in 70 percent. They recommend peripartum treatment with factor XI concentrate if cesarean delivery is performed, and advise against epidural analgesia unless factor XI is given. From their review, Martin-Salces and associates (2008) found that there was poor correlation between factor XI levels and bleeding in women with severe deficiency.

Factor XII deficiency is another autosomal recessive disorder that rarely complicates pregnancy. An increased incidence of thromboembolism is encountered in nonpregnant patients with this deficiency. Lao and colleagues (1991) reported an affected pregnant woman in whom placental abruption developed at 26 weeks.

Factor XIII deficiency is autosomal recessive and may be associated with maternal intracranial hemorrhage (Letsky, 2000). According to their review, Kadir and co-workers (2009) cited an increased risk of recurrent miscarriage and placental abruption. Treatment is given with fresh frozen plasma.

Autosomally inherited abnormalities of fibrinogen usually involve the formation of a functionally defective fibrinogen and are commonly referred to as *dysfibrinogenemias* (Edwards and Rijhsinghani, 2000). Familial *hypofibrinogenemia,* and sometimes *afibrinogenemia*, are infrequent recessive disorders. In some cases, both are found—*hypodysfibrinogenemia* (Deering and colleagues, 2003). Our experience suggests that hypofibrinogenemia represents a heterozygous autosomal dominant state with 50 percent of the offspring affected. Typically, the thrombin-clottable protein level in these patients ranges from 80 to 110 mg/dL when nonpregnant, and this increases by 40 or 50 percent in normal pregnancy. Those pregnancy complications that give rise to acquired hypofibrinogenemia, for example, placental abruption, are more common with fibrinogen deficiency. Trehan and Fergusson (1991) and Funai and associates

(1997) described successful outcomes in two affected women in whom fibrinogen or plasma infusions were given weekly or bi-weekly throughout pregnancy.

Conduction Analgesia for Labor and Cesarean Delivery

Most serious bleeding disorders would logically preclude the use of epidural or subarachnoid space injections for obstetrical analgesia. If the bleeding disorder is controlled, either spontaneously or with therapy, then these methods may be considered. Chi and colleagues (2009) reviewed intrapartum outcomes in 80 pregnancies in 63 women with an inherited bleeding disorder. These included 19 with factor XI deficiency, 16 hemophilia carriers, 15 with von Willebrand disease, and the remainder with platelet disorders or a deficiency of factor VII, XI, and X. Regional block was used in 41, of whom 35 had spontaneously normalized hemostatic dysfunction and 10 were given prophylactic replacement therapy. They encountered no unusual complications and concluded that such practices were safe. Singh and associates (2009) reviewed 13 women with factor XI deficiency delivered at Brigham and Women's Hospital. Nine of the 11 women were given neuraxial analgesia without complications, but only after fresh-frozen plasma was given to most of them to correct the activated partial thromboplastin time.

Thrombophilias

Several important regulatory proteins inhibit clotting. There are physiological antithrombotic proteins that act as inhibitors at strategic sites in the coagulation cascade to maintain blood fluidity under normal circumstances. Inherited deficiencies of these inhibitory proteins are caused by mutations of genes influencing their control. Because they may be associated with recurrent thromboembolism, they are collectively referred to as *thrombophilias*. Examples include deficiencies of antithrombin III, protein C, or of its co-factor, protein S; activated protein C resistance from factor V single-gene mutations; a function-enhancing mutation in the prothrombin gene (G20210A); and hyperhomocystinemia. Because these deficiencies may be associated with thromboembolism, they are discussed in detail in Chapter 47 (p. 1014).

REFERENCES

Aessopos A, Karabatsos F, Farmakis D, et al: Pregnancy in patients with well-treated β-thalassemia: Outcome for mothers and newborn infants. Am J Obstet Gynecol 180:360, 1999

Agre P: Hereditary spherocytosis. JAMA 262:2887, 1989

Al-Kouatly HB, Chasen ST, Kalish RB, et al: Causes of thrombocytopenia in triplet gestations. Am J Obstet Gynecol 189:177, 2003

Allford SL, Hunt BJ, Rose P, et al: Guidelines on the diagnosis and management of the thrombotic microangiopathic haemolytic anaemias. Br J Haematol 120:556, 2003

Alter BP, Frissora CL, Halpérin DS, et al: Fanconi's anaemia and pregnancy. Br J Haematol 77:410, 1991

American College of Medical Genetics Newborn Screening Expert Group: Newborn screening: Toward a uniform screening panel and system—executive summary. Pediatrics 117:S296, 2006

American College of Obstetricians and Gynecologists: Neural tube defects. Practice Bulletin No. 44, July 2003

American College of Obstetricians and Gynecologists: The use of hormonal contraception in women with coexisting medical conditions. Practice Bulletin No. 18, July 2000

American College of Obstetricians and Gynecologists: Hemoglobinopathies in pregnancy. Practice Bulletin No. 78, January 2007

American College of Obstetricians and Gynecologists: Anemia in pregnancy. Committee Opinion No. 95, July 2008

Andrews NC: Disorders of iron metabolism. N Engl J Med 341:1986, 1999

Anyaegbunam A, Morel MIG, Merkatz IR: Antepartum fetal surveillance tests during sickle cell crisis. Am J Obstet Gynecol 165:1081, 1991

Aster RH, Bougie DW: Drug-induced immune thrombocytopenia. N Engl J Med 357:580, 2007

Aukes AM, de Groot JC, Aarnoudse JG, et al: Brain lesions several years after eclampsia. Am J Obstet Gynecol 200:504.e1, 2009

Austin H, Lally C, Benson JM, et al: Hormonal contraception, sickle cell trait, and risk for venous thromboembolism among African American women. Am J Obstet Gynecol 200(6):620.e1, 2009

Barker DJP, Bull AR, Osmond C, et al: Fetal and placental size and risk of hypertension in adult life. BMJ 301:259, 1990

Bayouneu F, Subiran-Buisset C, Baka NE, et al: Iron therapy in iron deficiency anemia in pregnancy: Intravenous route versus oral route. Am J Obstet Gynecol 186:518, 2002

Beard J, Hillmen P, Anderson CC, et al: Primary thrombocythaemia in pregnancy. Br J Haematol 77:371, 1991

Beksaç MS, Atak Z, Ozlü T: Severe factor X deficiency in a twin pregnancy. Arch Gynecol Obstet Apr 26, 2009 [Epub ahead of print]

Bell WR, Braine HG, Ness PM, et al: Improved survival in thrombotic thrombocytopenic purpura–hemolytic uremic syndrome. Clinical experience in 108 patients. N Engl J Med 325:398, 1991

Benz EJ: Disorder of hemoglobin. In Fauci AS, Braunwald E, Kasper DL, et al (eds): Harrison's Principles of Internal Medicine, 17th ed. New York, Mc-Graw-Hill, 2008, p 635

Berry SM, Leonardi MR, Wolfe HM, et al: Maternal thrombocytopenia. Predicting neonatal thrombocytopenia with cordocentesis. J Reprod Med 42:276, 1997

Beutler E: Glucose-6-phosphate dehydrogenase deficiency. N Engl J Med 324:169, 1991

Bhatia M, Walters MC: Hematopoietic cell transplantation for thalassemia and sickle cell disease: Past, present, and future. Bone Marrow Transplant 41(2):109, 2008

Bodnar LM, Scanlon KS, Freedman DS, et al: High prevalence of postpartum anemia among low-income women in the United States. Am J Obstet Gynecol 185:438, 2001

Boehlen F, Hohlfeld P, Extermann P, et al: Maternal antiplatelet antibodies in predicting risk of neonatal thrombocytopenia. Obstet Gynecol 93:169, 1999

Boehlen F, Hohlfeld P, Extermann P, et al: Platelet count at term pregnancy: A reappraisal of the threshold. Obstet Gynecol 95:29, 2000

Bofill JA, Young RA, Perry KG Jr: Successful pregnancy in a woman with severe factor X deficiency. Obstet Gynecol 88:723, 1996

Borgna-Pignatti C, Marradi P, Rugolotto S, et al: Successful pregnancy after bone marrow transplantation for thalassaemia. Bone Marrow Transplant 18:235, 1996

Bourantas K, Makrydimas G, Georgiou I, et al: Aplastic anemia: Report of a case with recurrent episodes in consecutive pregnancies. J Reprod Med 42:672, 1997

Brawley OW, Cornell LJ, Edwards LR, et al: National Institutes of Health Consensus Development Conference Statement: Hydroxyurea treatment for sickle cell disease. Ann Intern Med 148:1, 2008

Brewer CA, Adelson MD, Elder RC: Erythrocytosis associated with a placental-site trophoblastic tumor. Obstet Gynecol 79:846, 1992

Briggs GG, Freeman RK, Yaffe SJ: Drugs in Pregnancy and Lactation, 7th ed. Philadelphia, Lippincott, Williams & Wilkins, 2005, p 791

Bunn HF, Rosse W: Hemolytic anemias and acute blood loss. In Braunwald E, Fauci AS, Kasper DL, et al (eds): Harrison's Principles of Internal Medicine, 15th ed. New York, McGraw-Hill, 2001, p 681

Burrows RF, Kelton JG: Fetal thrombocytopenia and its relation to maternal thrombocytopenia. N Engl J Med 329:1463, 1993a

Burrows RF, Kelton JG: Pregnancy in patients with idiopathic thrombocytopenic purpura: Assessing the risks for the infant at delivery. Obstet Gynecol Surv 48:781, 1993b

Bussel JB, Cheng G, Saleh MN, et al: Eltrombopag for the treatment of chronic idiopathic thrombocytopenic purpura. N Engl J Med 357:2237, 2007

Camilleri RS, Cohen H, Mackie I, et al: Prevalence of the ADAMTS13 missense mutation R1060W in late onset adult TTP. J Thromb Haemost 2007

Camous J, N'da A, Etienne-Julan M, et al: Anesthetic management of pregnant women with sickle cell diseases—Effect on postnatal sickling complications. Can J Anaesth 55:276, 2008

Carr S, Dixon D, Star J, et al: Intrauterine therapy for homozygous αλπηα-thalassemia. Obstet Gynecol 85:876, 1995

Casadevall N, Natataf J, Viron B, et al: Pure red-cell aplasia and antierythropoietin antibodies in patients treated with recombinant erythropoietin. N Engl J Med 346:469, 2002

Castro O, Hogue M, Brown BD: Pulmonary hypertension in sickle cell disease: Cardiac catheterization results and survival. Blood 101:4, 2003

Cavenee MR, Cox SM, Mason R, et al: Erythropoietin in pregnancies complicated by pyelonephritis. Obstet Gynecol 84:252, 1994

Centers for Disease Control and Prevention: CDC criteria for anemia in children and childbearing-aged women. MMWR 38:400, 1989

Centers for Disease Control and Prevention: Recommendations for the use of folic acid to reduce the number of cases of spina bifida and other neural tube defects. MMWR 41:1, 1992

Centers for Disease Control and Prevention: Recommendations to prevent and control iron deficiency in the United States. MMWR 47:1, 1998

Centers for Disease Control and Prevention: Vaccines. Available at: http://www.cdc.gov/vaccines/pubs/vis-text-files.htm#hib. Accessed September 17, 2008a

Centers for Disease Control and Prevention: Vaccines. Available at: http://www.cdc.gov/vaccines/pubs/vis-text-files.htm#ppv. Accessed October 8, 2008b

Centers for Disease Control and Prevention: Meningococcal vaccines. Available at: http://www.cdc.gov/vaccines/pubs/vis/downloads/vis-mening.pdf. Accessed January 28, 2008c

Chakravarty EF, Khanna D, Chung L: Pregnancy outcomes in systemic sclerosis, primary pulmonary hypertension, and sickle cell disease. Obstet Gynecol 111:927, 2008

Chatwani A, Bruder N, Shapiro T, et al: May–Hegglin anomaly: A rare case of maternal thrombocytopenia in pregnancy. Am J Obstet Gynecol 166:143, 1992

Chi C, Lee CA, England A, et al: Obstetric analgesia and anaesthesia in women with inherited bleeding disorders. Thromb Haemost 101(6):1104, 2009

Choudhry VP, Gupta S, Gupta M, et al: Pregnancy associated aplastic anemia—A series of 10 cases with review of literature. Hematol 7:233, 2002

Clark AL, Gall SA: Clinical uses of intravenous immunoglobulin in pregnancy. Am J Obstet Gynecol 176:241, 1997

Conti M, Mari D, Conti E, et al: Pregnancy in women with different types of von Willebrand disease. Obstet Gynecol 68:282, 1986

Cortelazzo S, Finazzi G, Ruggeri M, et al: Hydroxyurea for patients with essential thrombocythemia and a high risk of thrombosis. N Engl J Med 332:1132, 1995

Cox JV, Steane E, Cunningham G, et al: Risk of alloimmunization and delayed hemolytic transfusion reactions in patients with sickle cell disease. Arch Intern Med 148:2485, 1988

Cox SM, Shelburne P, Mason R, et al: Mechanisms of hemolysis and anemia associated with acute antepartum pyelonephritis. Am J Obstet Gynecol 164:587, 1991

Crowther MA, George JN: Thrombotic thrombocytopenic purpura: 2008 update. Cleve Clin J Med 75:369, 2008

Cunningham FG, Cox SM, Harstad TW, et al: Chronic renal disease and pregnancy outcome. Am J Obstet Gynecol 163:453, 1990

Cunningham FG, Pritchard JA: Prophylactic transfusions of normal red blood cells during pregnancies complicated by sickle cell hemoglobinopathies. Am J Obstet Gynecol 135:994, 1979

Cunningham FG, Pritchard JA, Hankins GDV, et al: Idiopathic cardiomyopathy or compounding cardiovascular events. Obstet Gynecol 67:157, 1986

Cunningham FG, Pritchard JA, Mason R: Pregnancy and sickle hemoglobinopathy: Results with and without prophylactic transfusions. Obstet Gynecol 62:419, 1983

Daffos F, Capella-Pavlovsky M, Forestier F: Fetal blood sampling during pregnancy with the use of a needle guided by ultrasound: A study of 606 consecutive cases. Am J Obstet Gynecol 153:655, 1985

Dashe JS, Ramin SM, Cunningham FG: The long-term consequences of thrombotic microangiopathy (thrombotic thrombocytopenic purpura and hemolytic uremic syndrome) in pregnancy. Obstet Gynecol 91:662, 1998

Daskalakis GJ, Papageorgiou IS, Antsaklis AJ, et al: Pregnancy and homozygous beta thalassaemia major. Br J Obstet Gynaecol 105:1028, 1998

de Abood M, de Castillo Z, Guerrero F, et al: Effect of Depo-Provera or Microgynon on the painful crises of sickle cell anemia patients. Contraception 56:313, 1997

De Gramont A, Krulik M, Debray J: Paroxysmal nocturnal haemoglobinuria and pregnancy. Lancet 1:868, 1987

Deering SH, Landy HL, Tchabo N, et al: Hypodysfibrinogenemia during pregnancy, labor, and delivery. Obstet Gynecol 101:1092, 2003

Delage R, Demers C, Cantin G, et al: Treatment of essential thrombocythemia during pregnancy with interferon-α. Obstet Gynecol 87:814, 1996

Deruelle P, Bouhassoun J, Trillot N, et al: Polycythemia vera and pregnancy: Difficulties for diagnosis and treatment. Gynecol Obstet Fertil 33:331, 2005

DeSimone J, Koshy M, Dorn L, et al: Maintenance of elevated fetal hemoglobin levels by decitabine during dose interval treatment of sickle cell anemia. Blood 99:3905, 2002

Dhingra S, Wiener JJ, Jackson H: Management of cold agglutinin-immune hemolytic anemia in pregnancy. Obstet Gynecol 110:485, 2007

Dolan LM, Ryan M, Moohan J: Pyruvate kinase deficiency in pregnancy complicated by iron overload. Br J Obstet Gynaecol 109:844, 2002

Driscoll MC, Hurlet A, Styles L, et al: Stroke risk in siblings with sickle cell anemia. Blood 101:2401, 2003

Edwards RZ, Rijhsinghani A: Dysfibrinogenemia and placental abruption. Obstet Gynecol 95:1043, 2000

Egerman RS, Witlin AG, Friedman SA, et al: Thrombotic thrombocytopenic purpura and hemolytic uremic syndrome in pregnancy: Review of 11 cases. Am J Obstet Gynecol 195:950, 1996

Eliyahu S, Shalev E: A successful pregnancy after bone marrow transplantation for severe aplastic anaemia with pretransplant conditioning of total lymph-node irradiation and cyclophosphamide. Br J Haematol 86:649, 1994

Elstein D, Granovsky-Grisaru S, Rabinowitz R, et al: Use of enzyme replacement therapy for Gaucher disease during pregnancy. Am J Obstet Gynecol 177:1509, 1997

Eskandari N, Feldman N, Greenspoon JS: Factor VII deficiency in pregnancy treated with recombinant factor VIIa. Obstet Gynecol 99:935, 2002

Fadel HE, Krauss JS: Factor VII deficiency and pregnancy. Obstet Gynecol 73:453, 1989

Faivre L, Meerpohl J, Da Costa L, et al: High-risk pregnancies in Diamond-Blackfan anemia: A survey of 64 pregnancies from the French and German registries. Haematologica 91:530, 2006

Fayyad AM, Brummitt DR, Barker HF, et al: May-Hegglin anomaly: The role of aspirin in the treatment of this rare platelet disorder in pregnancy. Br J Obstet Gynaecol 109:223, 2002

Fieni S, Bonfanti L, Gramellini D, et al: Clinical management of paroxysmal nocturnal hemoglobinuria in pregnancy: A case report and updated review. Obstet Gyn Surv 61:593, 2006

Franchini M, Montagnana M, Targher G, et al: Reduced von Willebrand factor-cleaving protease levels in secondary thrombotic microangiopathies and other diseases. Sem Thromb Hemost 33(8):787, 2007

Fucharoen S, Winichagoon P: Clinical and hematologic aspects of hemoglobin E beta-thalassemia. Curr Opin Hematol 7:106, 2000

Fujimori K, Ohto H, Honda S, et al: Antepartum diagnosis of fetal intracranial hemorrhage due to maternal Bernard–Soulier syndrome. Obstet Gynecol 94:817, 1999

Funai EF, Klein SA, Lockwood CJ: Successful pregnancy outcome in a patient with both congenital hypofibrinogenemia and protein S deficiency. Obstet Gynecol 90:858, 1997

Furlan M, Robles R, Galbusera M, et al: Von Willebrand factor–cleaving protease in thrombotic thrombocytopenic purpura and the hemolytic-uremic syndrome. N Engl J Med 339:1578, 1998

Galvani DW, Jayakumar KS, Jordan A, et al: Antenatal testing for haemoglobinopathies [Letter]. Br J Haematol 108:198, 2000

Gandhi SK, Powers JC, Nomeir A-M, et al: The pathogenesis of acute pulmonary edema associated with hypertension. N Engl J Med 344:17, 2000

Gangat N, Wolanskij AP, Schwager S, et al: Predictors of pregnancy outcomes in essential thrombocythemia: A single institution study of 63 pregnancies. Eur J Haematol 82(5):350, 2009

Garratty G: Severe reactions associated with transfusion of patients with sickle cell disease. Transfusion 37:357, 1997

Garratty G, Leger RM, Arndt PA: Severe immune hemolytic anemia associated with prophylactic use of cefotetan in obstetric and gynecologic procedures. Am J Obstet Gynecol 181:103, 1999

Gasser C, Gautier E, Steck A, et al: Haemolytisch-uramisch Syndrome: Bilaterale Nierenrindennekrosen bei akuten erworbenin haemolytischen Anamien. Schweiz Med Wochenschr 85:905, 1955

Gehlbach DL, Morgenstern LL: Antenatal screening for thalassemia minor. Obstet Gynecol 71:801, 1988

George JN: The thrombotic thrombocytopenic purpura and hemolytic uremic syndromes: Overview of pathogenesis (Experience of The Oklahoma TTP-HUS Registry, 1989–2007). Kidney Int 75(112):S8, 2009

George JN, Woolf SH, Raskob GE, et al: Idiopathic thrombocytopenic purpura: A practice guideline developed by explicit methods for The American Society of Hematology. Blood 88:3, 1996

Gernsheimer T, McCrae KR: Immune thrombocytopenic purpura in pregnancy. Curr Opin Hematol 14:574, 2007

Ghidini A, Korker VL: Severe pyruvate kinase deficiency anemia. A case report. J Reprod Med 43:713, 1998

Gilsanz F, Vega MA, Gomez-Castillo E, et al: Fetal anaemia due to pyruvate kinase deficiency. Arch Dis Child 69:523, 1993

Gladwin MT, Sachdev V, Jison ML, et al: Pulmonary hypertension as a risk factor for death in patients with sickle cell disease. N Engl J Med 350:886, 2004

Gladwin MT, Vichinsky E: Pulmonary complications of sickle cell disease. N Engl J Med 359:2254, 2008

Godeau B, Chevret S, Varet B, et al: Intravenous immunoglobulin or high-dose methylprednisolone, with or without oral prednisone, for adults with untreated severe autoimmune thrombocytopenic purpura: A randomized, multicenter trial. Lancet 359:23, 2002

Goldenberg RL, Tamura T, DuBard M, et al: Plasma ferritin and pregnancy outcome. Am J Obstet Gynecol 175:1356, 1996

Granovsky-Grisaru S, Aboulafia Y, Diamant YZ, et al: Gynecologic and obstetric aspects of Gaucher's disease: A survey of 53 patients. Am J Obstet Gynecol 172:1284, 1995

Green AM, Kupfer GM: Fanconi anemia. Hematol Oncol Clin North Am 23(2):193, 2009

Greene MF, Frigoletto FD Jr, Claster SZ, et al: Pregnancy and paroxysmal nocturnal hemoglobinuria: Report of a case and review of the literature. Obstet Gynecol Surv 38:591, 1983

Greer IA, Lowe GDO, Walker JJ, et al: Haemorrhagic problems in obstetrics and gynaecology in patients with congenital coagulopathies. Br J Obstet Gynaecol 98:909, 1991

Griesshammer M, Grunewald M, Michiels JJ: Acquired thrombophilia in pregnancy: Essential thrombocythemia. Semin Thromb Hemost 29:205, 2003

Griesshammer M, Struve S, Harrison CM: Essential thrombocythemia/polycythemia vera and pregnancy: The need for an observational study in Europe. Semin Thromb Hemost 32:422, 2006

Guy GP, Baxi LV, Hurlet-Jensen A, et al: An unusual complication in a gravida with factor IX deficiency: Case report with review of the literature. Obstet Gynecol 80:502, 1992

Hillmen P, Young NS, Schubert J, et al: The complement inhibitor eculizumab in paroxysmal nocturnal hemoglobinuria. N Engl J Med 355:1233, 2006

Howard RJ, Tuck SM, Pearson TC: Pregnancy in sickle cell disease in the UK: Results of a multicentre survey of the effect of prophylactic blood transfusion on maternal and fetal outcome. Br J Obstet Gynaecol 102:947, 1995

Hsia YE: Detection and prevention of important α-thalassemia variants. Semin Perinatol 15:35, 1991

Hsieh FJ, Chang FM, Ko TM, et al: The antenatal blood gas and acid–base status of normal fetuses and hydropic fetuses with Bart hemoglobinopathy. Obstet Gynecol 74:722, 1989

Hsu HW, Belfort MA, Vernino S, et al: Postpartum thrombotic thrombocytopenic purpura complicated by Budd–Chiari syndrome. Obstet Gynecol 85:839, 1995

Hurst D, Little B, Kleman KM, et al: Anemia and hemoglobinopathies in Southeast Asian refugee children. J Pediatric 102:692, 1983

Kadir R, Chi C, Bolton-Maggs P: Pregnancy and rare bleeding disorders. Haemophilia Feb 27, 2009 [Epub ahead of print]

Kadir RA, Economides DL, Braithwaite J, et al: The obstetric experience of carriers of haemophilia. Br J Obstet Gynaecol 104:803, 1997

Kadir RA, Lee CA, Sabin CA, et al: Pregnancy in women with von Willebrand's disease or factor XI deficiency. Br J Obstet Gynaecol 105:314, 1998

Kadyrov M, Kosanke G, Kingdom J, et al: Increased fetoplacental angiogenesis during first trimester in anaemic women. Lancet 352:1747, 1998

Kanavakis E, Vrettou C, Palmer G, et al: Preimplantation genetic diagnosis in 10 couples at risk for transmitting beta-thalassaemia major: Clinical experience including the initiation of six singleton pregnancies. Prenat Diagn 19:1217, 1999

Kaplan C, Daffos F, Forestier F, et al: Fetal platelet counts in thrombocytopenic pregnancy. Lancet 336:979, 1990

Kennedy AS, Lewis QF, Scott JG, et al: Cognitive deficits after recovery from thrombotic thrombocytopenic purpura. Transfusion Feb 12, 2009 [Epub ahead of print]

Kenny L, Baker P, Cunningham FG: Platelets, coagulation, and the liver. In Lindheimer MD, Roberts JM, Cunningham FG (eds) Chesley's Hypertension in Pregnancy, 3rd ed. Elsevier, New York, 2009, p 335

Kidanto HL, Mogren I, Lindmark G, et al: Risks for preterm delivery and low birth weight are independently increased by severity of maternal anaemia. S Afr Med J 99(2):98, 2009

Kihm AJ, Kong Y, Hong W, et al: An abundant erythroid protein that stabilizes free a haemoglobin. Nature 417:758, 2002

Klebanoff MA, Shiono PH, Selby JV, et al: Anemia and spontaneous preterm birth. Am J Obstet Gynecol 164:59, 1991

Kolialexi A, Vrettou C, Traeger-Synodinos J, et al: Noninvasive prenatal diagnosis of β-thalassemia using individual fetal erythroblasts isolated from maternal blood after enrichment. Prenat Diag 27:1228, 2007

Konje JC, Murphy P, de Chazal R, et al: Severe factor X deficiency and successful pregnancy. Br J Obstet Gynaecol 101:910, 1994

Konkle BA: Disorder of platelets and vessel wall. In Fauci AS, Braunwald E, Kasper DL, et al (eds): Harrison's Principles of Internal Medicine, 17th ed. New York, McGraw-Hill, 2008, p 718

Koshy M, Burd L, Wallace D, et al: Prophylactic red-cell transfusions in pregnant patients with sickle cell disease: A randomized cooperative study. N Engl J Med 319:1447, 1988

Krafft A, Perewusnyk G, Hänseler E, et al: Effect of postpartum iron supplementation on red cell and iron parameters in non-anaemic iron-deficient women: A randomized placebo-controlled study. BJOG 112:445, 2005

Kujovich JL: Von Willebrand disease and pregnancy. J Thromb Haemostasis 3:246, 2005

Kumar R, Advani AR, Sharan J, et al: Pregnancy induced hemolytic anemia: an unexplained entity. Ann Hematol 80:623, 2001

Kumar RM, Rizk DEE, Khuranna A: β-Thalassemia major and successful pregnancy. J Reprod Med 42:294, 1997

Kwon JY, Lee Y, Shin JC, et al: Supportive management of pregnancy-associated aplastic anemia. Int J Gynecol Obstet 95:115, 2006

Lam YH, Tang MHY, Lee CP, et al: Prenatal ultrasonographic prediction of homozygous type 1 alpha-thalassemia at 12 to 13 weeks of gestation. Am J Obstet Gynecol 180:148, 1999

Lao TT, Lewinsky RM, Ohlsson A, et al: Factor XII deficiency and pregnancy. Obstet Gynecol 78:491, 1991

Letsky EA: Hematologic disorders. In Barron WM, Lindheimer MD (eds): Medical Disorders During Pregnancy, 3rd ed. St. Louis, Mosby, 2000, p 267

Leung WC, Leung KY, Lau ET, et al: Alpha-thalassemia. Semin Fetal Neonatal Med 13:215, 2008

Levy GG, Nichols WC, Lian EC, et al: Mutations in a member of the ADAMTS gene family cause thrombotic thrombocytopenic purpura. Nature 413:488, 2001

Lewis QF, Lanneau MS, Mathias SD, et al: Long-term deficits in health-related quality of life after recovery from thrombotic thrombocytopenia purpura. Transfusion 49(1):118, 2009

Lipkind HS, Kurtis JD, Powrie R, et al: Acquired von Willebrand disease: Management of labor and delivery with intravenous dexamethasone, continuous factor concentrate, and immunoglobulin infusion. Am J Obstet Gynecol 192:2067, 2005

Lipton JM, Ellis SR: Diamond-Blackfan anemia: Diagnosis, treatment, and molecular pathogenesis. Hematol Oncol Clin North Am 23(2):261, 2009

Lubetsky A, Schulman S, Varon D, et al: Safety and efficacy of continuous infusion of a combined factor VIII–von Willebrand factor (vWF) concentrate (Haemate-P) in patients with von Willebrand disease. Thromb Haemost 81:229, 1999

Luewan S, Srisupundit K, Tongsong T: Outcomes of pregnancies complicated by beta-thalassemia/hemoglobin E disease. Int J Gynaecol Obstet 104(3): 203, 2009

Maberry MC, Cunningham FG: Sickle cell hemoglobinopathies complicating pregnancy. In Williams Obstetrics, 19th ed. Norwalk, CT, Appleton & Lange, Suppl 2, August/September 1993

Maberry MC, Mason RA, Cunningham FG, et al: Pregnancy complicated by hemoglobin CC and C–beta-thalassemia disease. Obstet Gynecol 76:324, 1990

Maberry MC, Mason RA, Cunningham FG, et al: Pregnancy complicated by hereditary spherocytosis. Obstet Gynecol 79:735, 1992

Magann EF, Bass D, Chauhan SP, et al: Antepartum corticosteroids: Disease stabilization in patients with the syndrome of hemolysis, elevated liver enzymes, and low platelets (HELLP). Am J Obstet Gynecol 171:1148, 1994

Mannucci PM: Treatment of von Willebrand's Disease. N Engl J Med 351:683, 2004

Mannucci PM, Tuddenham EGD: The hemophilias—from royal genes to gene therapy. N Engl J Med 344:1773, 2001

Marti-Carvajal AJ, Peña-Marti GE, Comunián-Carrasco G, et al: Interventions for treating painful sickle cell crisis during pregnancy. Cochrane Database Syst Rev 1:CD006786, 2009

Martin-Salces M, Jimenez-Yuste V, Alvarez MT, et al: Factor XI deficiency: Review and management in pregnant women. Clin Appl Thromb Hemost Dec 1, 2008 [Epub ahead of print)

Maternal and Child Health Bureau: Newborn screening: Toward a uniform screening panel and system. Executive Summary, Rockville, MD: MCHB, 2005, available at: http://mchb.hrsa.gov/screening/summary.htn. Accessed April 27, 2009

Mayer SA, Aledort LM: Thrombotic microangiopathy: Differential diagnosis, pathophysiology and therapeutic strategies. Mt Sinai J Med 72:166, 2005

Medical Letter: Intravenous immunoglobulin (IVIG). Vol 48, Issue 1249/1250, December 4–18, 2006

Medoff BD, Shepard JO, Smith RN, et al: Case 17-2005: A 22-year-old woman with back and leg pain and respiratory failure. N Engl J Med 352:2425, 2005

Michael M, Elliott EJ, Ridley GF, et al: Interventions for haemolytic uraemic syndrome and thrombotic thrombocytopenic purpura. Cochrane Database Sys Rev 1:CDE003595, 2009

Miller DP, Kaye JA, Shea K, et al: Incidence of thrombotic thrombocytopenic purpura/hemolytic uremic syndrome. Epidemiology 15:208, 2004

Moake JL: Thrombotic microangiopathies. N Engl J Med 347:589, 2002

Moake JL: Von Willebrand factor, ADAMTS-13, and thrombotic thrombocytopenic purpura. Semin Hematol 41:4, 2004

Mockenhaupt FP, Mandelkow J, Till H, et al: Reduced prevalence of *Plasmodium falciparum* infection and of concomitant anaemia in pregnant women with heterozygous G6PD deficiency. Trop Med Int Health 8:118, 2003

Moise KJ Jr: Umbilical cord stem cells. Obstet Gynecol 106:1393, 2005

Monni G, Ibba RM, Lai R, et al: Early transabdominal chorionic villus sampling in couples at high genetic risk. Am J Obstet Gynecol 168:170, 1993

Morkbak AL, Hvas AM, Milman N, et al: Holotranscobalamin remains unchanged during pregnancy. Longitudinal changes of cobalamins and their binding proteins during pregnancy and postpartum. Haematol 92:1711, 2007

Moschcowitz E: An acute febrile pleiochromic anemia with hyaline thrombosis of the terminal arterioles and capillaries. Arch Intern Med 36:89, 1925

Mullaart RA, Van Dongen P, Gabreëls FJM, et al: Fetal periventricular hemorrhage in von Willebrand's disease: Short review and first case presentation. Am J Perinatol 8:190, 1991

Murphy JF, O'Riordan J, Newcombe RG, et al: Relation of haemoglobin levels in first and second trimester to outcome of pregnancy. Lancet 1:992, 1986

Musclow CE, Goldenberg H, Bernstein EP, et al: Factor XI deficiency presenting as hemarthrosis during pregnancy. Am J Obstet Gynecol 157:178, 1987

Myers B, Pavorod S, Kean L, et al: Pregnancy outcome in Factor XI deficiency: Incidence of miscarriage, antenatal and postnatal haemorrhage in 33 women with Factor XI deficiency. BJOG 114:643, 2007

Nichols WL, Hultin MB, James AH, et al: von Willebrand disease (VWD): Evidence-based diagnosis and management guidelines, the National Heart, Lung, and Blood Institute (NHLBI) Expert Panel report (USA). Haemophilia 14(2):171, 2008

Niittyvuopio R, Juvonen E, Kaaja R, et al: Pregnancy in essential thrombocythaemia: Experience with 40 pregnancies. Eur J Haematol 73:431, 2004

Nguyen JS, Marinopoulos SS, Ashar BH, et al: More than meets the eye. N Engl J Med 355:1048, 2006

Olivieri NF, Brittenham GM, McLaren CE, et al: Long-term safety and effectiveness of iron-chelation therapy with deferiprone for thalassemia major. N Engl J Med 339:417, 1998

Oringanje C, Nemecek E, Oniyangi O: Hematopoietic stem cell transplantation for children with sickle cell disease. Cochrane Database Syst Rev 1:CD007001

Pajor A, Lehoczky D, Szakács Z: Pregnancy and hereditary spherocytosis. Arch Gynecol Obstet 253:37, 1993

Parker C: Eculizumab for paroxysmal nocturnal haemoglobinuria. Lancet 373(9665):759, 2009

Parker C, Omine M, Richards S, et al: Diagnosis and management of paroxysmal nocturnal hemoglobinuria. Blood 106:3699, 2005

Pawliuk R, Westerman KA, Fabry ME, et al: Correction of sickle cell disease in transgenic mouse models by gene therapy. Science 294:2368, 2001

Payne SD, Resnik R, Moore TR, et al: Maternal characteristics and risk of severe neonatal thrombocytopenia and intracranial hemorrhage in pregnancies complicated by autoimmune thrombocytopenia. Am J Obstet Gynecol 177:149, 1997

Peng TC, Kickler TS, Bell WR, et al: Obstetric complications in a patient with Bernard–Soulier syndrome. Am J Obstet Gynecol 165:425, 1991

Pinto FO, Roberts I: Cord blood stem cell transplantation for haemoglobinopathies. Br J Haematol 141:309, 2008

Platt OS: Hydroxyurea for the treatment of sickle cell anemia. N Engl J Med 358:1362, 2008

Powars DR, Sandhu M, Niland-Weiss J, et al: Pregnancy in sickle cell disease. Obstet Gynecol 67:217, 1986

Prabu P, Parapia LA: Bernard-Soulier syndrome in pregnancy. Clin Lab Haem 28:198, 2006

Pritchard JA, Cunningham FG, Mason RA: Coagulation changes in eclampsia: Their frequency and pathogenesis. Am J Obstet Gynecol 124:855, 1976

Pritchard JA, Scott DE: Iron demands in pregnancy. In Hallberg L, Harwerth HG, Vanotti A (eds): Iron Deficiency Pathogenesis, Clinical Aspects, Therapy. New York, Academic Press, 1970

Pritchard JA, Scott DE, Whalley PJ, et al: The effects of maternal sickle cell hemoglobinopathies and sickle cell trait on reproductive performance. Am J Obstet Gynecol 117:662, 1973

Provan D, Weatherall D: Red cells II: Acquired anaemias and polycythaemia. Lancet 355:1260, 2000

Rabinerson D, Fradin Z, Zeidman A, et al: Vulvar hematoma after cunnilingus in a teenager with essential thrombocythemia: A case report. J Reprod Med 52:458, 2007

Ramahi AJ, Lewkow LM, Dombrowski MP, et al: Sickle cell E hemoglobinopathy and pregnancy. Obstet Gynecol 71:493, 1988

Ramin SM, Vidaeff AC, Yeomans ER, et al: Chronic renal disease in pregnancy. Obstet Gynecol 108:1531, 2006

Randi ML, Barbone E, Rossi C, et al: Essential thrombocythemia and pregnancy. A report of six normal pregnancies in five untreated patients. Obstet Gynecol 83:915, 1994

Ray JG, Burrows RF, Ginsberg JS, et al: Paroxysmal nocturnal hemoglobinuria and the risk of venous thrombosis: Review and recommendations for management of the pregnant and nonpregnant patient. Haemostasis 30(3):103, 2000

Reece EA, Coustan DR, Hayslett JP, et al: Diabetic nephropathy: Pregnancy performance and fetomaternal outcome. Am J Obstet Gynecol 159:56, 1988

Rees DC, Olujohungbe AD, Parker NE, et al: Guidelines for the management of the acute painful crisis in sickle cell disease. Br J Haematol 120:744, 2003

Ren A, Wang J, Ye RW, et al: Low first-trimester hemoglobin and low birth weight, preterm birth and small for gestational age newborns. Int J Gynaecol Obstet 98:124, 2007

Robinson S, Bewley S, Hunt BJ, et al: The management and outcome of 18 pregnancies in women with polycythemia vera. Haematol 90: 1477, 2005

Robson JS, Martin AM, Ruckley VA, et al: Irreversible postpartum renal failure. Q J Med 37:423, 1968

Rock GA, Shumak KH, Buskard NA, et al: Comparison of plasma exchange with plasma infusion in the treatment of thrombotic thrombocytopenic purpura. N Engl J Med 325:393, 1991

Rosenfeld S, Follmann D, Nunez O, et al: Antithymocyte globulin and cyclosporine for severe aplastic anemia: Association between hematologic response and long-term outcome. JAMA 289:1130, 2003

Rouse DJ, Owen J, Goldenberg RL: Routine maternal platelet count: An assessment of a technologically driven screening practice. Am J Obstet Gynecol 179:573, 1998

Sainio S, Järvenpää AL, Renlund M, et al: Thrombocytopenia in term infants: A population-based study. Obstet Gynecol 95:441, 2000

Samuels P, Bussel JB, Braitman LE, et al: Estimation of the risk of thrombocytopenia in the offspring of pregnant women with presumed immune thrombocytopenic purpura. N Engl J Med 323:229, 1990

Sánchez-Luceros A, Farias CE, Amaral MM, et al: von Willibrand factor-cleaving protease (ADAMTS13) activity in normal non-pregnant women, pregnant and post-delivery women. Thromb Haemost 92(6):1320, 2004

Sanders JE, Hawley J, Levy W, et al: Pregnancies following high-dose cyclophosphamide with or without high-dose busulfan or total body irradiation and bone marrow transplantation. Blood 87:3045, 1996

Scanlon KS, Yip R, Schieve LA, et al: High and low hemoglobin levels during pregnancy: Differential risk for preterm birth and small for gestational age. Obstet Gynecol 96:741, 2000

Scaradavou A: HIV-related thrombocytopenia. Blood Rev 16:73, 2002

Schwartz RS: Immune thrombocytopenic purpura—From agony to agonist. N Engl J Med 357:2299, 2007

Scott DE, Pritchard JA: Iron deficiency in healthy young college women. JAMA 199:147, 1967

Scott JR, Rote NS, Cruikshank DP: Antiplatelet antibodies and platelet counts in pregnancies complicated by autoimmune thrombocytopenic purpura. Am J Obstet Gynecol 145:932, 1983

Serjeant GR, Hambleton I, Thame M: Fecundity and pregnancy outcome in a cohort with sickle cell-haemoglobin C disease followed from birth. BJOG 112:1308, 2005

Serjeant GR, Loy LL, Crowther M, et al: Outcome of pregnancy in homozygous sickle cell disease. Obstet Gynecol 103:1278, 2004

Serjeant GR, Serjeant BE, Mason KP, et al: The changing face of homozygous sickle cell disease: 102 patients over 60 years. Int J Lab Hematol [Epub ahead of print], 2008

Shaaban AF, Flake AW: Fetal hematopoietic stem cell transplantation. Semin Perinatol 23:515, 1999

Sharma JB, Jain S, Mallika V, et al: A prospective, partially randomized study of pregnancy outcomes and hematologic responses to oral and intramuscular iron treatment in moderately anemic pregnant women. Am J Clin Nutr 79:116, 2004

Shau WY, Hsieh CC, Hsieh TT, et al: Factors associated with endometrial bleeding in continuous hormone replacement therapy. Menopause 9:188, 2002

Sheiner E, Levy A, Yerushalmi R, et al: Beta-thalassemia minor during pregnancy. Obstet Gynecol 103:1273, 2004

Sieunarine K, Shapiro S, Al Obaidi MJ, et al: Intravenous anti-D immunoglobulin in the treatment of resistant immune thrombocytopenic purpura in pregnancy. BJOG 114(4):505, 2007

Silver RM, Branch W, Scott JR: Maternal thrombocytopenia in pregnancy: Time for a reassessment. Am J Obstet Gynecol 173:479, 1995

Singh A, Harnett MJ, Connors JM, et al: Factor XI deficiency and obstetrical anesthesia. Anesth Analg 108:1882, 2009

Sirichotiyakul S, Saetung R, Sanguansermsri T: Prenatal diagnosis of beta-thalassemia/Hb E by hemoglobin typing compared to DNA analysis. Hemoglobin 33(1):17, 2009

Socié G, Stone JV, Wingard JR, et al: Long-term survival and late deaths after allogeneic bone marrow transplantation. N Engl J Med 341:14, 1999

Spivak JL: Polycythemia vera and other myeloproliferative diseases. In Fauci AS, Braunwald E, Kasper DL, et al (eds): Harrison's Principles of Internal Medicine, 17th ed. New York, McGraw-Hill, 2008, p 671

Srivorakun H, Fucharoen G, Sae-Ung N, et al: Analysis of fetal blood using capillary electrophoresis system: A simple method for prenatal diagnosis of severe thalassemia diseases. Eur J Haematol 83(1):79, 2009

Stalder MP, Rovó A, Halter J, et al: Aplastic anemia and concomitant autoimmune diseases. Ann Hematol 88(7):659, 2009

Starksen NF, Bell WR, Kickler TS: Unexplained hemolytic anemia associated with pregnancy. Am J Obstet Gynecol 146:617, 1983

Stuart MJ, Nagel RL: Sickle-cell disease. Lancet 364:1343, 2004

Sun PM, Wilburn W, Raynor D, et al: Sickle cell disease in pregnancy: Twenty years of experience at Grady Memorial Hospital, Atlanta, Georgia. Am J Obstet Gynecol 184:1127, 2001

Taylor DJ, Mallen C, McDougal N, et al: Effect of iron supplementation on serum ferritin levels during and after pregnancy. Br J Obstet Gynaecol 89:1011, 1982

Tefferi A, Soldberg LA, Silverstein MN: A clinical update in polycythemia vera and essential thrombocythemia. Am J Med 109:141, 2000

Thame M, Lewis J, Trotman H, et al: The mechanisms of low birth weight in infants of mothers with homozygous sickle cell disease. Pediatrics 120:e677, 2007

Tita ATN, Biggio JR, Chapman V, et al: Perinatal and maternal outcomes in women with sickle or hemoglobin C trait. Obstet Gynecol 110:1113, 2007

Trehan AK, Fergusson ILC: Congenital afibrinogenaemia and successful pregnancy outcome. Case report. Br J Obstet Gynaecol 98:722, 1991

Tsai HM, Lian ECY: Antibodies to Von Willebrand factor–cleaving protease in acute thrombotic thrombocytopenic purpura. N Engl J Med 339:1585, 1998

Tsaras G, Owusu-Ansah, Boateng FO, et al: Complications associated with sickle cell trait: A brief narrative review. Am J Med 122(6):507, 2009

Tuck SM, Studd JWW, White JM: Pregnancy in women with sickle cell trait. Br J Obstet Gynaecol 90:108, 1983

Turner JM, Kaplan JB, Cohen HW, et al: Exchange versus simple transfusion for acute chest syndrome in sickle cell anemia adults. Transfusion 49(5):863, 2009

Urato AC, Repke JT: May-Hegglin anomaly: A case of vaginal delivery when both mother and fetus are affected. Am J Obstet Gynecol 179:260, 1998

Van Wyck DB, Martens MG, Seid MH, et al: Intravenous ferric carboxymaltose compared with oral iron in the treatment of postpartum anemia: A randomized controlled trial. Obstet Gynecol 110:267, 2007

Veille J, Hanson R: Left ventricular systolic and diastolic function in pregnant patients with sickle cell disease. Am J Obstet Gynecol 170:107, 1994

Vichinsky EP, Neumayr LD, Earles AN, et al: Causes and outcomes of the acute chest syndrome in sickle cell disease. N Engl J Med 342:1855, 2000

Villers MS, Jamison MG, De Castro LM, et al: Morbidity associated with sickle cell disease in pregnancy. Am J Obstet Gynecol 199:125.e1, 2008

Von Tempelhoff GF, Heilmann L, Rudig L, et al: Mean maternal second-trimester hemoglobin concentration and outcome of pregnancy: A population based study. Clin Appl Thromb/Hemost 14:19, 2008

Wax JR, Pinette MG, Cartin A, et al: Pyruvate kinase deficiency complicating pregnancy. Obstet Gynecol 109:553, 2007

Weatherall DJ: Single gene disorders or complex traits: Lessons from the thalassemias and other monogenic diseases. BMJ 321:1117, 2000

Weatherall DJ, Provan AB: Red cell I: Inherited anaemias. Lancet 355:1169, 2000

Webert KE, Mittal R, Sigouin C, et al: A retrospective 11-year analysis of obstetric patients with idiopathic thrombocytopenic purpura. Blood 102:4306, 2003

Weiner DL, Hibberd PL, Betit P, et al: Preliminary assessment of inhaled nitric oxide for acute vaso-occlusive crisis in pediatric patients with sickle cell disease. JAMA 289:1136, 2003

Weiss G, Goodnough LT: Anemia of chronic disease. N Engl J Med 352:1011, 2005

World Health Organization Working Group. Glucose-6-phosphate dehydrogenase deficiency. Bull World Health Organ 67:601, 1989

Yawata Y, Kanzaki A, Yawata A, et al: Characteristic features of the genotype and phenotype of hereditary spherocytosis in the Japanese population. Int J Hematol 71:118, 2000

Ye L, Chang JC, Lin C, et al: Induced pluripotent stem cells offer new approach to therapy in thalassemia and sickle cell anemia and option in prenatal diagnosis in genetic diseases. Proc Natl Acad Sci USA 16(24):9826, 2009

Yeomans E, Lowe TW, Eigenbrodt EH, et al: Liver histopathologic findings in women with sickle cell disease given prophylactic transfusion during pregnancy. Am J Obstet Gynecol 163:958, 1990

Young NS: Aplastic anemia. In Fauci AS, Braunwald E, Kasper DL, et al (eds): Harrison's Principles of Internal Medicine, 17th ed. New York, McGraw-Hill, 2008, p 663

Young NS, Maciejewski J: The pathophysiology of acquired aplastic anemia. N Engl J Med 336:1365, 1997

Ziaei S, Norrozi M, Faghihzadeh S, et al: A randomized placebo-controlled trial to determine the effect of iron supplementation on pregnancy outcome in pregnant women with haemoglobin ≥ 13.2 g/dl. BJOG 114:684, 2000

CHAPTER 52

Diabetes

The prevalence of diagnosed diabetes among American adults has increased by 40 percent in 10 years and rose from 4.9 percent in 1990 to 6.9 percent in 1999 (Narayon and colleagues, 2003). More worryingly, it is estimated that this incidence will increase another 165 percent by 2050. To put this into perspective, the lifetime risk of diabetes in individuals born in 2000 is 33 percent for males and 39 percent for females! This increase primarily is due to type 2 diabetes, which is also referred to as *diabesity.* As discussed in Chapter 43, this term reflects the strong relationship of diabetes with the current epidemic of obesity in the United States and other countries (Gale, 2003; Mokdad and associates, 2003).

The increasing prevalence of type 2 diabetes in general, and in younger people in particular, has led to an increasing number of pregnancies with this complication (Ferrara and co-workers, 2004). Many women found to have gestational diabetes are likely to have type 2 diabetes that has previously gone undiagnosed (Feig and Palda, 2002). Indeed, the incidence of diabetes complicating pregnancy has increased approximately 40 percent between 1989 and 2004 (Getahun and colleagues, 2008). In Los Angeles County, Baraban and co-workers (2008) reported that the age-adjusted prevalence tripled from 14.5 cases per 1000 women in 1991 to 47.9 cases per 1000 in 2003.

There is keen interest in events that precede diabetes, and this includes the *mini-environment of the uterus,* where it is believed that early imprinting can have effects later in life (Saudek, 2002). For example, in utero exposure to maternal hyperglycemia leads to fetal hyperinsulinemia, causing an increase in fetal fat cells, which leads to obesity and insulin resistance in childhood (Feig and Palda, 2002). This in turn leads to impaired glucose tolerance and diabetes in adulthood. Thus, a cycle of fetal exposure to diabetes leading to childhood obesity and glucose intolerance is set in motion. This sequence has been reported in Pima Indians as well as a heterogeneous Chicago population (Silverman and colleagues, 1995).

CLASSIFICATION

Diabetes is now classified based on the pathogenic processes involved (Powers, 2008). Absolute insulin deficiency characterizes *type 1 diabetes,* whereas defective insulin secretion or insulin resistance characterizes *type 2 diabetes* (Table 52-1). The terms insulin-dependent diabetes mellitus (IDDM) and noninsulin-dependent diabetes mellitus (NIDDM) are no longer used. Age is also no longer used in classification, because pancreatic β-cell destruction can begin at any age. Most commonly, its onset is before age 30, but in 5 to 10 percent of affected individuals, onset is after age 30 years. Type 2 diabetes, although most typical with increasing age, also develops in obese adolescents.

Classification During Pregnancy

Diabetes is the most common medical complication of pregnancy. Women can be separated into those who were known to have diabetes before pregnancy—*pregestational* or *overt,* and those diagnosed during pregnancy—*gestational.* In 2006, slightly more than 179,898 American women had pregnancies complicated by some form of diabetes, representing 4.2 percent of all live births (Martin and associates, 2009). In the United States, African-Americans, Native Americans, Asians, and Hispanic women are at higher risk for gestational diabetes compared

TABLE 52-1. Etiological Classification of Diabetes Mellitus

I. Type 1: β-Cell destruction, usually absolute insulin deficiency
   A. Immune-mediated
   B. Idiopathic

II. Type 2: Ranges from predominantly insulin resistance to predominantly an insulin secretory defect with insulin resistance

III. Other types
   A. Genetic mutations of β-cell function
   B. Genetic defects in insulin action
   C. Genetic syndromes—e.g., Down, Klinefelter, Turner
   D. Diseases of the exocrine pancreas—e.g., pancreatitis, cystic fibrosis
   E. Endocrinopathies—e.g., Cushing syndrome, pheochromocytoma, others
   F. Drug or chemical induced—e.g., glucocorticosteroids, thiazides, β-adrenergic agonists, others
   G. Infections—congenital rubella, cytomegalovirus, coxsackievirus

IV. Gestational diabetes (GDM)

Adapted from Fauci AS, Braunwald E, Kasper DL, et al: *Harrison's Principles of Internal Medicine,* 17th ed., pp. 2275–2304. Copyright © 2008 The McGraw-Hill Companies, Inc.

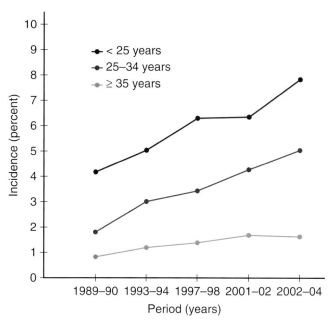

FIGURE 52-1 Age-specific incidence of gestational diabetes from National Hospital Discharge Survey Data (NHDS) of nearly 59 million births in the United States from 1989 to 2004. (Redrawn from *American Journal of Obstetrics & Gynecology,* Vol. 198, No. 5, D Getahun, C Nath, CV Ananth, et al., Gestational diabetes in the United States: temporal trends 1989 through 2004, pp. 525.e1–525.e5, Copyright 2008, with permission from Elsevier.)

with white women (Ferrara, 2007). The increasing incidence of gestational diabetes over the past 15 years shown in **Figure 52-1** is reminiscent of similar statistics for obesity discussed in Chapter 43 (p. 946).

White Classification in Pregnancy

It is important to describe the evolution of diabetes classification during pregnancy over the past 20 years because many older terms continue to be used. For example, frequent reference is made to the classification by White (1978). And because most literature currently cited contains data from these older classifications, the one recommended by the American College of Obstetricians and Gynecologists in 1986 is shown in **Table 52-2**. This was replaced in 1994 because, according to the College, "a single classification based on the presence or absence of good maternal metabolic control and the presence or absence of maternal diabetic vasculopathy is more helpful."

In the 1986 classification, women diagnosed with gestational diabetes were subdivided, and those with fasting hyperglycemia of 105 mg/dL or greater were placed into class A₂. Approximately 15 percent of women with gestational diabetes exhibit fasting hyperglycemia (Sheffield and co-workers, 1999). Women in classes B to H, corresponding to the White classification (1978), have overt diabetes antedating pregnancy. The White system emphasized that end-organ derangements, espe-

cially involving the eyes, kidneys, and heart, have significant effects on pregnancy outcome.

For several years now, the American College of Obstetricians and Gynecologists (2001, 2005) has no longer used a classification according to the White scheme. Instead, the focus is now on whether diabetes is first diagnosed during pregnancy or antedates pregnancy.

DIAGNOSIS OF DIABETES DURING PREGNANCY

Overt Diabetes

Women with high plasma glucose levels, glucosuria, and ketoacidosis present no problem in diagnosis. Similarly, women with a random plasma glucose level greater than 200 mg/dL plus classic signs and symptoms such as polydipsia, polyuria, and unexplained weight loss or a fasting glucose exceeding 125 mg/dL are considered by the American Diabetes Association (2004) to have overt diabetes. The diagnostic cutoff value for overt diabetes is a fasting plasma glucose of 126 mg/dL or higher. This is used because data indicate the risk of retinopathy rises dramatically at that fasting level. Women at the opposite end of the spectrum or those with only minimal metabolic derangement may be difficult to identify. The likelihood of impaired carbohydrate metabolism is increased appreciably in women who have a strong familial

TABLE 52-2. Classification Scheme Used from 1986 through 1994 for Diabetes Complicating Pregnancy

Class	Onset	Fasting	2-hour Postprandial	Therapy
A₁	Gestational	<105 mg/dL	<120 mg/dL	Diet
A₂	Gestational	>105 mg/dL	>120 mg/dL	Insulin

Class	Age of Onset (yr)	Duration (yr)	Vascular Disease	Therapy
B	Over 20	<10	None	Insulin
C	10 to 19	10 to 19	None	Insulin
D	Before 10	>20	Benign retinopathy	Insulin
F	Any	Any	Nephropathy[a]	Insulin
R	Any	Any	Proliferative retinopathy	Insulin
H	Any	Any	Heart	Insulin

[a]When diagnosed during pregnancy: proteinuria ≥ 500 mg/24 h before 20 weeks' gestation.

history of diabetes, have given birth to large infants, demonstrate persistent glucosuria, or have unexplained fetal losses.

Reducing substances are commonly found in the urine of pregnant women. Commercially available dipsticks may be used to identify glucosuria while avoiding a positive reaction from lactose. Even then, glucosuria most often does not reflect impaired glucose tolerance, but rather augmented glomerular filtration (see Chap. 5, p. 123). Nonetheless, the detection of glucosuria during pregnancy warrants further investigation (Gribble and associates, 1995).

Gestational Diabetes

This is defined as carbohydrate intolerance of variable severity with onset or first recognition during pregnancy. This definition applies whether or not insulin is used for treatment. Undoubtedly, some women with gestational diabetes have previously unrecognized overt diabetes. Sheffield and co-workers (1999) studied outcomes in 1190 diabetic women delivered at Parkland Hospital between 1991 and 1995. They found that women with fasting hyperglycemia diagnosed before 24 weeks had pregnancy outcomes similar to those for women with overt diabetes. Bartha (2000) and Most (2009) with their colleagues reported similar results. Thus, fasting hyperglycemia early in pregnancy almost invariably represents overt diabetes.

Screening

Despite more than 40 years of research, there is no consensus regarding the optimal approach to screening for gestational diabetes (American College of Obstetricians and Gynecologists, 2001). The major issues include whether universal or selective screening should be used and which plasma glucose level after a 50-g glucose test threshold is best to identify women at risk for gestational diabetes (Bonomo and colleagues, 1998; Danilenko-Dixon and associates, 1999).

Since 1980, there have been five International Workshop Conferences on gestational diabetes, and participants have attempted to provide consensus statements on screening. Those at the Fifth Conference endorsed use of the definition, classification criteria, and strategies for detection and diagnosis of gestational diabetes recommended at the Fourth Workshop Conference in 1997 (Metzger and co-workers, 2007). Instead of *universal screening*, recommendations are now for *selective screening* using the guidelines shown in Table 52-3. Screening should be performed between 24 and 28 weeks in those women not known to have glucose intolerance earlier in pregnancy. This evaluation is usually done in two steps. In the two-step procedure, a 50-g oral glucose challenge test is followed by a diagnostic 100-g oral glucose tolerance test (OGTT) if initial results exceed a predetermined plasma glucose concentration.

Plasma glucose level is measured 1 hour after a 50-g glucose load without regard to the time of day or time of last meal. A value of ≥ 140 mg/dL (7.8 mmol/L) identifies 80 percent of all women with gestational diabetes. Using a value of ≥ 130 mg/dL (7.2 mmol/L) increases the yield to greater than 90 percent. However, 20 to 25 percent of women will have false positive test results compared with only 14 to 18 percent when the ≥ 140 mg/dL cutoff value is used.

The day-to-day reproducibility of the 50-g screening test has been evaluated by Espinosa de los Monteros and co-workers (1993). Although 90 percent of normal results were reproducible the next day, only 83 percent of abnormal test results were reproducible. Murphy and colleagues (1994) studied the accuracy and precision of reflectance photometers—*Accu-Check III*—for screening. Because this required redefining the circumstances for testing and threshold values for abnormal results, it seems best to avoid these devices for screening.

Gabbe and associates (2004) surveyed practicing obstetricians-gynecologists in 2003 and reported that 96 percent used universal screening for gestational diabetes. Integral to justifying this practice is the requirement to show that women who screen

TABLE 52-3. Fifth International Workshop-Conference on Gestational Diabetes: Recommended Screening Strategy Based on Risk Assessment for Detecting Gestational Diabetes (GDM)

GDM risk assessment: Should be ascertained at the first prenatal visit
- **Low Risk:** Blood glucose testing not routinely required if all the following are present:
  - Member of an ethnic group with a low prevalence of GDM
  - No known diabetes in first-degree relatives
  - Age < 25 years
  - Weight normal before pregnancy
  - Weight normal at birth
  - No history of abnormal glucose metabolism
  - No history of poor obstetrical outcome
- **Average Risk:** Perform blood glucose testing at 24 to 28 weeks using either:
  - Two-step procedure: 50-g oral glucose challenge test (GCT), followed by a diagnostic 100-g oral glucose tolerance test for those meeting the threshold value in the GCT.
  - One-step procedure: Diagnostic 100-g oral glucose tolerance test performed on all subjects.
- **High Risk:** Perform blood glucose testing as soon as feasible, using the procedures described above if one or more of these are present:
  - Severe obesity
  - Strong family history of type 2 diabetes
  - Previous history of GDM, impaired glucose metabolism, or glucosuria. If GDM is not diagnosed, blood glucose testing should be repeated at 24 to 28 weeks or at any time there are symptoms or signs suggestive of hyperglycemia.

Modified from Metzger and Colleagues (2007); Copyright © 2007 American Diabetes Association. From Diabetes Care®, Vol. 30; 2007, S251–S260. Reprinted with permission from The American Diabetes Association.

positive are benefited by the treatment. The justification for screening, and by extension, treatment of women with gestational diabetes, was given considerable impetus by a study reported by Crowther and colleagues (2005). They assigned 1000 women with gestational diabetes between 24 and 34 weeks' gestation to receive dietary advice with blood glucose monitoring plus insulin therapy—intervention group—versus routine prenatal care. Women were diagnosed to have gestational diabetes if their blood glucose was < 100 mg/dL after an overnight fast and between 140 and 198 mg/dL 2 hours after ingesting a 75-g glucose solution. Women in the intervention group had a significantly reduced risk of a composite adverse outcome that included one or more of perinatal death, shoulder dystocia, bone fracture, and nerve palsy. Macrosomia defined by birthweight ≥ 4000 g complicated 10 percent of deliveries in the intervention group compared with 21 percent in the routine prenatal care group ($p <$ .001). Cesarean delivery rates were almost identical in the two study groups. In an editorial accompanying this report, Greene and Solomon (2005) concluded that the study provided important evidence that identifying and treating gestational diabetes can substantially reduce the risk of adverse perinatal outcomes.

Slightly different results were recently reported by the Maternal Fetal Medicine Units Network randomized trial of 958 women (Landon and colleagues, 2009). This study was designed to compare whether dietary counseling and glucose monitoring in women with mild gestational diabetes would reduce the incidence of perinatal morbidity compared with standard obstetrical care. Mild gestational diabetes was identified in women with fasting glucose < 95 mg/dL. They reported no dif-

ferences in rates of composite morbidity that included stillbirth; neonatal hypoglycemia, hyperinsulinemia, and hyperbilirubinemia; and birth trauma. Importantly, though, secondary analyses did reveal a 50-percent reduction in macrosomia, fewer cesarean deliveries, and a significant decrease in shoulder dystocia—1.5 versus 4 percent—in treated versus control women.

From the foregoing, it is easy to understand why some of these issues are often contentious. Indeed, the U.S. Preventive Services Task Force (2008) recently again concluded that evidence is insufficient to assess the balance of benefits versus harms of screening, either before or after 24 weeks.

Diagnosis

There is not international agreement as to the optimal glucose tolerance test to identify gestational diabetes. The World Health Organization (1985) has recommended the 75-g 2-hour oral glucose tolerance test, which is often used in Europe (Weiss and colleagues, 1998). In the United States, the *100-g 3-hour oral glucose tolerance test* performed after an overnight fast remains the standard recommended by the American College of Obstetricians and Gynecologists (2001). Even so, Catalano and coworkers (1993) found that the 100-g 3-hour test was not reproducible in 25 percent of women when repeated 1 week after the initial test. They attributed this to increased norepinephrine-mediated gluconeogenesis from maternal stress at initial testing.

Recommended criteria for interpretation of the 100-g diagnostic glucose tolerance test are shown in Table 52-4. Also shown are the criteria for the 75-g test most often used outside the United States, but increasingly used in this country.

TABLE 52-4. Fifth International Workshop Conference on Gestational Diabetes: Diagnosis of Gestational Diabetes by Oral Glucose Tolerance Testing[a]

	Oral Glucose Load			
Time	100-g Glucose[b]		75-g Glucose[b]	
Fasting	95 mg/dL	5.3 mmol/L	95 mg/dL	5.3 mmol/L
1-h	180 mg/dL	10.0 mmol/L	180 mg/dL	10.0 mmol/L
2-h	155 mg/dL	8.6 mmol/L	155 mg/dL	8.6 mmol/L
3-h	140 mg/dL	7.8 mmol/L	—	—

[a]The test should be performed in the morning after an overnight fast of at least 8 h but not more than 14 h and after at least 3 days of unrestricted diet ($\geq$ 150 g carbohydrate/d) and physical activity. The subject should remain seated and should not smoke during the test.
[b]Two or more of the venous plasma glucose concentrations indicated below must be met or exceeded for a positive diagnosis.
From Metzger and colleagues (2007), with permission.

The Hyperglycemia and Adverse Pregnancy Outcome (HAPO) Study

This was a seven-year international epidemiological study of 23,325 pregnant women at 15 centers in nine countries that comprised the HAPO Study Cooperative Research Group (2008). The investigation was designed to determine the association of various levels of glucose intolerance during the third trimester with adverse infant outcomes in women with gestational diabetes. Between 24 and 32 weeks, the general population of pregnant women underwent 75-g oral glucose tolerance testing after overnight fasting. Blood glucose levels were measured pretest fasting and again, 1 and 2 hours after glucose ingestion. Caregivers were blinded to results except for women whose glucose levels exceeded values that required treatment and removal from the study. Values at each of three time posts were stratified into seven categories and analyzed for birthweight > 90th percentile (LGA), primary cesarean delivery, clinical neonatal hypoglycemia, and cord-serum C-peptide levels > 90th percentile. Odds of each outcome were calculated using the lowest category—for example, fasting plasma glucose < 75 mg/dL—as the referent group. Their findings in general supported the supposition that increasing plasma glucose levels at each epoch were associated with increasing adverse outcomes. One example is shown in Figure 52-2.

In an editorial accompanying publication of the HAPO trial, Ecker and Greene (2008) posed the question: "Given the results of the HAPO study, should we lower our threshold for the diagnosis and treatment of gestational diabetes?" It was concluded that it will be difficult to show that treating lesser degrees of carbohydrate intolerance—as suggested in the HAPO study—would provide any meaningful improvements in clinical outcomes. Ecker and Greene (2008) concluded, and we agree, that changes of criteria are not justified until clinical trials prove benefits.

GESTATIONAL DIABETES

The word *gestational* implies that diabetes is induced by pregnancy—ostensibly because of exaggerated physiological changes in glucose metabolism (see Chap. 5, p. 113). Another explanation is that gestational diabetes is type 2 diabetes unmasked or discovered during pregnancy. As the incidence of type 2

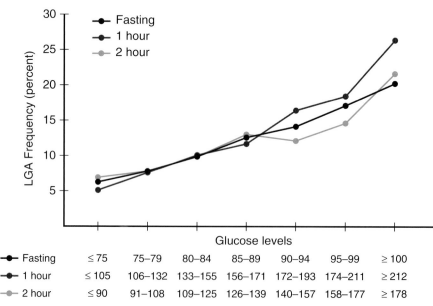

	≤75	75–79	80–84	85–89	90–94	95–99	≥100
Fasting	≤75	75–79	80–84	85–89	90–94	95–99	≥100
1 hour	≤105	106–132	133–155	156–171	172–193	174–211	≥212
2 hour	≤90	91–108	109–125	126–139	140–157	158–177	≥178

FIGURE 52-2 Hyperglycemia and Adverse Pregnancy Outcome (HAPO) Study. The frequency of infant birthweight ≥ 90th percentile for gestational age plotted against glucose levels fasting and at 1- and 2-hr intervals following a 75-g oral glucose load. LGA = large for gestational age. (Adapted from The HAPO Study Cooperative Research Group: Hyperglycemia and adverse pregnancy outcomes. *N Engl J Med* 358(19):1991–2002, with permission. Copyright © 2008 Massachusetts Medical Society. All rights reserved.)

diabetes accrues with age and is unmasked by other diabetogenic factors, that is, obesity, it is likely that *both* pregnancy aggravation and impending insulinopenia are involved. For example, Harris (1988) found that the prevalence of undiagnosed glucose intolerance in nonpregnant women between ages 20 and 44 years was virtually identical to the prevalence of gestational diabetes. Catalano and associates (1999) compared longitudinal changes in insulin sensitivity, insulin response, and endogenous glucose production in women who had normal glucose tolerance with changes identified in women with gestational diabetes. The latter women had abnormalities in glucose metabolism that are hallmarks of type 2 diabetes.

Use of the diagnostic term *gestational diabetes* has been encouraged to communicate the need for increased surveillance and to stimulate women to seek care for further testing postpartum. The likelihood of fetal death with appropriately treated gestational diabetes is not different than in the general population (Metzger and Coustan, 1998). The most important perinatal concern is excessive fetal growth, which may result in both maternal and fetal birth trauma. *More than half of women with gestational diabetes ultimately develop overt diabetes in the ensuing 20 years, and there is mounting evidence for long-range complications that include obesity and diabetes in their offspring.*

Maternal and Fetal Effects

There is an important difference concerning adverse fetal consequences of gestational diabetes. Unlike in women with overt diabetes, fetal anomalies are not increased (Sheffield and colleagues, 2002). Similarly, whereas pregnancies in women with overt diabetes are at greater risk for fetal death, this danger is not apparent for those who have diet-treated postprandial hyperglycemia (Lucas and co-workers, 1993; Sheffield and associates, 2002).

In contrast, women with *elevated* fasting glucose levels have increased rates of unexplained stillbirths similar to women with pregestational diabetes (Johnstone and colleagues, 1990). Specifically, the American Diabetes Association (1999a) has concluded that fasting hyperglycemia > 105 mg/dL may be associated with an increased risk of fetal death during the last 4 to 8 weeks of gestation. Adverse maternal effects include an increased frequency of hypertension and cesarean delivery.

Macrosomia

Excessive fetal size can be problematic, and macrosomia is defined variably by different authors. The American College of Obstetricians and Gynecologists (2000) defines macrosomic infants as those whose birthweight exceeds 4500 g. Approximately a third of women delivered of such infants give birth to another in their next pregnancy (Mahony and associates, 2006). The perinatal goal is avoidance of difficult delivery due to macrosomia, with concomitant birth trauma associated with shoulder dystocia. Except for the brain, most fetal organs are affected by the macrosomia that commonly characterizes the fetus of a diabetic woman.

Macrosomic infants of diabetic mothers are described as anthropometrically different from other large-for-gestational age infants (Durnwald and colleagues, 2004; McFarland and associ-

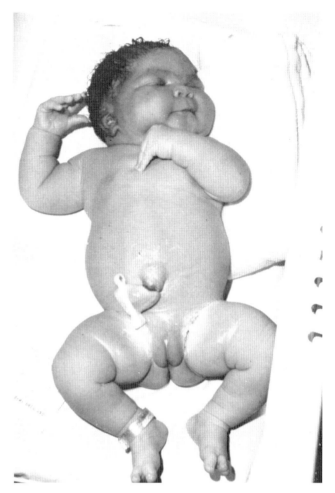

FIGURE 52-3 This 6050-g macrosomic infant was born to a woman with gestational diabetes.

ates, 2000). Specifically, those whose mothers are diabetic have excessive fat deposition on the shoulders and trunk, which predisposes them to shoulder dystocia or cesarean delivery (Fig. 52-3). Fortunately, shoulder dystocia is uncommon, even in women with gestational diabetes. For example, Magee and co-workers (1993) diagnosed shoulder dystocia in 3 percent of women with class A₁ diabetes. None of these infants sustained brachial plexus injuries.

Maternal hyperglycemia prompts fetal hyperinsulinemia particularly during the second half of gestation, which in turn stimulates excessive somatic growth. Macrosomia results. Similarly, neonatal hyperinsulinemia may provoke hypoglycemia within minutes of birth. The incidence varies greatly depending on the threshold used to define significant neonatal hypoglycemia. For example, the American Diabetes Association (1995) defines values < 35 mg/dL as abnormal in a term infant and lower values for preterm infants because glycogen stores are less. Infants described by the HAPO Study Cooperative Research Group (2008) had an incidence of clinical neonatal hypoglycemia that increased with increasing maternal OGTT values defined in Figure 52-2. The frequency varied from 1 to 2 percent, but was as high as 4.6 percent in women with fasting glucose levels ≥ 100 mg/dL. Likewise, cord-blood insulin levels are related to maternal glucose control (Leipold and colleagues, 2004).

There is extensive evidence that insulin-like growth factors I (IGF-I) and II (IGF-II) also play a role in the regulation of fetal growth (see Chap. 38, p. 842). These growth factors, which structurally are proinsulin-like polypeptides, are produced by virtually all fetal organs and are potent stimulators of cell differentiation and division. Verhaeghe and co-workers (1993) measured cord IGFs and insulin (C-peptide) concentrations throughout gestation in women without diabetes and found that levels correlated with birthweight. Large-for-gestational age infants had significantly increased levels of these factors. The HAPO investigators also reported dramatic increases of cord serum C-peptide levels with increasing maternal glucose levels following a 75-g OGTT. Levels > 90th percentile were found in almost a third of newborns in the highest glucose categories. Other factors implicated in macrosomia include epidermal growth factor, leptin, and adiponectin (Loukovaara, 2004; Mazaki-Tovi, 2005; Okereke, 2002, and all their colleagues).

Maternal obesity is an independent and more important risk factor for large infants in women with gestational diabetes than is glucose intolerance (Ehrenberg and colleagues, 2004; Lucas and associates, 1993). Moreover, maternal obesity is an important confounding factor in the diagnosis of gestational diabetes. Johnson and co-workers (1987) reported that 8 percent of 588 women who weighed more than 250 pounds had gestational diabetes compared with less than 1 percent of women who weighed less than 200 pounds. Weight distribution also seems to play a role because Landon (1994) and Zhang (1995) and their colleagues found that the risk of gestational diabetes was increased with truncal obesity.

Management

Women with gestational diabetes can be divided into two functional classes using fasting glucose levels. Insulin therapy is usually recommended when standard dietary management does not consistently maintain the fasting plasma glucose at < 95 mg/dL or the 2-hour postprandial plasma glucose < 120 mg/dL (American College of Obstetricians and Gynecologists, 2001). Whether insulin should be used in women with lesser degrees of fasting hyperglycemia—105 mg/dL or less before dietary intervention—is unclear because there have been no controlled trials to identify ideal glycemia targets for prevention of fetal risks. The Fifth International Workshop Conference on Gestational Diabetes, however, recommended that maternal capillary glucose levels be kept ≤ 95 mg/dL in the fasting state (Metzger and colleagues, 2007).

Diet. As discussed previously, recent reports by Crowther and colleagues (2005) and Landon and associates (2009) describe the benefits of dietary counseling and monitoring in women with gestational diabetes. The American Diabetes Association (ADA) (2000) has recommended nutritional counseling with individualization based on height and weight and a diet that provides an average of 30 kcal/kg/d based on prepregnant body weight for nonobese women. Although the most appropriate diet for women with gestational diabetes has not been established, the ADA has suggested that obese women with a body mass index (BMI) > 30 kg/m^2 may benefit from a 30-percent caloric restriction. This should be monitored with weekly tests for ketonuria,

because maternal ketonemia has been linked with impaired psychomotor development in offspring (Rizzo and co-workers, 1995). That said, Langer and colleagues (2005a, b) found that insulin was necessary to achieve glucose control in obese women.

Exercise. Because exercise is known to be important in nonpregnant patients, the American College of Obstetricians and Gynecologists (2001) reviewed three randomized trials of exercise in women with gestational diabetes (Avery, 1997; Bung, 1993; Jovanovic-Peterson, 1989, and all their colleagues). The results suggested that exercise improved cardiorespiratory fitness without improving pregnancy outcome. Dempsey and co-workers (2004) found that physical activity during pregnancy reduced the risk of gestational diabetes. Brankston and associates (2004) reported that resistance exercise diminished the need for insulin therapy in overweight women with gestational diabetes.

Glucose Monitoring. Hawkins and colleagues (2009) compared outcomes in 315 women with diet-treated gestational diabetes who used personal glucose monitors with those of 615 gestational diabetics who were also diet-treated but who underwent intermittent fasting glucose evaluation during semiweekly obstetrical visits. Women using daily self blood-glucose monitoring had fewer macrosomic infants and gained less weight after diagnosis—median 0.56 compared with 0.74 pounds per week—than women evaluated during clinic visits only. These researchers' findings support the common practice of self blood-glucose monitors for women with gestational diabetes who are treated with diet alone.

Postprandial surveillance for gestational diabetes has been shown to be superior to preprandial surveillance. DeVeciana and colleagues (1995) studied 66 pregnant women with class A$_2$ diabetes in whom insulin was initiated for fasting hyperglycemia. The women were randomized to glucose surveillance using either preprandial or 1-hour postprandial capillary blood-glucose concentrations measured by glucometer. Postprandial surveillance was shown to be superior in that blood-glucose control was significantly improved and was associated with fewer cases of neonatal hypoglycemia—3 versus 21 percent, less macrosomia—12 versus 42 percent, and fewer cesarean deliveries for dystocia—24 versus 39 percent.

Insulin. Insulin given to decrease complications related to macrosomia in women with gestational diabetes and fasting euglycemia has long been controversial. Langer and co-workers (1994) reviewed 23 reports from 1979 through 1993 and found that none demonstrated improved perinatal outcomes related to any management approach, including prophylactic insulin treatment. Four randomized studies reported between 1989 and 2001 showed that intensive therapy had little effect on birthweight, birth trauma, operative delivery, or neonatal complications (Garner, 1997; Kjos, 2001; Nordlander, 1989; Thompson, 1990, and all their associates).

Most practitioners—93 percent according to Owen and colleagues (1995)—initiate insulin therapy in women with gestational diabetes if fasting glucose levels exceeding 105 mg/dL persist despite diet therapy. At Parkland Hospital, this is accomplished in a specialized outpatient clinic, but occasionally hospitalization is necessary. Experts differ in their approach to insulin therapy in gestational diabetes. A total dose of 20 to 30 units given once daily, before breakfast, is commonly used to initiate therapy. The total dose is usually divided into two-thirds intermediate-acting insulin and a third short-acting insulin. Alternatively, weight-based split-dose insulin is administered twice daily. Once therapy has been initiated, it must be recognized that the level of glycemic control to reduce fetal and neonatal complications has not been established.

Oral Hypoglycemic Agents. The American College of Obstetricians and Gynecologists (2001) has not recommended these agents during pregnancy. Langer and colleagues (2000, 2005a) randomized 404 women with gestational diabetes to *insulin versus glyburide* therapy. Near normoglycemic levels were achieved equally well with either regimen, and there were no apparent neonatal complications attributable to glyburide. In a follow-up study, Conway and co-workers (2004) reported that women with fasting glucose levels > 110 mg/dL did not adequately respond to glyburide therapy. Similar results were reported by Chmait (2004) and Kahn (2006) and their associates. Until recently, glyburide was thought not to cross the placenta. Hebert and colleagues (2008), however, sampled 20 paired maternal and umbilical specimens and found umbilical cord concentrations were half that of maternal concentrations in women treated with glyburide.

There is increasing support for the use of glyburide as an alternative to insulin in the management of gestational diabetes (Durnwald and Landon, 2005; Saade, 2005). A survey of almost 1400 fellows of the American College of Obstetricians and Gynecologists found that 13 percent of respondents were using glyburide as first-line therapy for diet failure with gestational diabetes (Gabbe and co-workers, 2004). Further evidence of expanding use of glyburide was provided by Kremer (2004) and Jacobson (2005) and their colleagues. They reported retrospective studies of glyburide as an alternative to insulin in a combined total of 309 women who failed diet therapy. Most of these women required daily glyburide doses < 7.5 mg to achieve glucose control (Table 52-5). Hypoglycemia was reported to be less frequent when glyburide was compared with insulin (Yogev and co-workers, 2004). In a recent meta-analysis, Moretti and associates (2008) reported no increased perinatal risks with glyburide therapy and recommended further randomized trials.

Metformin has been used as treatment for polycystic ovarian disease and has been reported to reduce the incidence of gestational diabetes in women who use the drug throughout pregnancy (Glueck and colleagues, 2004). Even so, it is usually recommended that metformin be discontinued once pregnancy is diagnosed because it is long known to reach the fetus (Harborne and associates, 2003). The Fifth International Workshop Conference recommended that metformin treatment for gestational diabetes be limited to clinical trials with long-term infant follow-up (Metzger and co-workers, 2007).

Subsequently, Rowan and colleagues (2008) reported results of a study in which they randomized 751 women with gestational diabetes to metformin or insulin treatment. The primary outcome was a composite of one or more of neonatal hypoglycemia, respiratory distress, phototherapy, birth trauma, 5-minute Apgar score of 7 or less, and preterm birth. Similarities in the composite outcome between metformin and insulin led the investigators to conclude that metformin was not associated with increased perinatal complications. As expected, women preferred metformin to insulin treatment. It is noteworthy that 46 percent of women in the metformin trial required supplemental insulin compared with only 4 percent of women treated with glyburide by Langer and colleagues (2000).

Obstetrical Management

In general, women with gestational diabetes who do not require insulin seldom require early delivery or other interventions. Elective cesarean delivery to avoid brachial plexus injuries in macrosomic infants is an important issue. The American College of Obstetricians and Gynecologists (2001) has suggested that cesarean delivery should be considered in women with a sonographically estimated fetal weight ≥ 4500 g. Effects of such a policy were retrospectively analyzed by Gonen and colleagues (2000) in a general obstetrical population of more than 16,000 women. *Elective cesarean delivery had no significant effect on the incidence of brachial plexus injury.*

Elective induction to prevent shoulder dystocia in women with sonographically diagnosed fetal macrosomia, compared with spontaneous labor, is also controversial. Conway and Langer (1996) found that elective delivery reduced the rate of shoulder dystocia from 2.2 to 0.7 percent. In contrast, Combs and colleagues (1993b) and Adasheck (1996) and their associates reported no advantages. Chauhan and co-workers (2005) reviewed the literature and concluded that sonographic suspicion of macrosomia was too inaccurate to recommend induction or primary cesarean delivery without a trial of labor.

There is no consensus regarding whether antepartum fetal testing is necessary, and if so, when to begin such testing in women without severe hyperglycemia (American College of Obstetricians and Gynecologists, 2001; Metzger and associates,

TABLE 52-5. Glyburide Treatment Regimen for Women with Gestational Diabetes Who Fail Diet Therapy

1. Glucometer blood glucose measurements fasting and 1 or 2 hours following breakfast, lunch, and dinner.
2. Glucose level goals (mg/dL): Fasting < 100, 1-h < 155, and 2-h < 130.
3. Glyburide starting dose 2.5 mg orally with morning meal.
4. If necessary, increase daily glyburide dose by 2.5-mg/wk increments until 10 mg/d, then switch to twice-daily dosing until maximum of 20 mg/d reached. Switch to insulin if 20 mg/d does not achieve glucose goals.

Adapted from Jacobson and colleagues (2005).

TABLE 52-6. Fifth International Workshop-Conference: Metabolic Assessments Recommended after Pregnancy with Gestational Diabetes

Time	Test	Purpose
Postdelivery (1–3 d)	Fasting or random plasma glucose	Detect persistent, overt diabetes
Early postpartum (6–12 wks)	75-g 2-h OGTT	Postpartum classification of glucose metabolism
1 yr postpartum	75-g 2-h OGTT	Assess glucose metabolism
Annually	Fasting plasma glucose	Assess glucose metabolism
Tri-annually	75-g 2-h OGTT	Assess glucose metabolism
Prepregnancy	75-g 2-h OGTT	Classify glucose metabolism

Classification of the American Diabetes Association (2003)

Normal	Impaired Fasting Glucose or Impaired Glucose Tolerance	Diabetes Mellitus
Fasting < 110 mg/dL	110–125 mg/dL	≥ 126 mg/dL
2 hr < 140 mg/dL	2 hr ≥ 140–199 mg/dL	2 hr ≥ 200 mg/dL

Copyright © 2007 American Diabetes Association. From Diabetes Care®, Vol. 30; 2007, S251–S260. Reprinted with permission from The American Diabetes Association.

2007). This is because of the low risk of fetal death with gestational diabetes. Those women who require insulin therapy for fasting hyperglycemia, however, typically undergo fetal testing and are managed as if they had overt diabetes.

Postpartum Evaluation

The Fifth International Workshop Conference on Gestational Diabetes recommended that women diagnosed with gestational diabetes undergo evaluation with a 75-g oral glucose tolerance test at 6 to 12 weeks postpartum and other intervals thereafter (Metzger and associates, 2007). These recommendations are shown in Table 52-6 along with the classification scheme of the American Diabetes Association (2003).

Although postpartum follow-up of women diagnosed with gestational diabetes was recommended throughout the 1990s, reports on compliance have only recently become available. Smirnakis and co-workers (2005) reviewed electronic medical records in 197 women diagnosed with gestational diabetes in 2000 and 2001 and found that only 37 percent underwent postpartum screening tests. In a more recent study, Almario and colleagues (2008) reported a 33-percent compliance rate at an academic medical center. At Parkland Hospital, after discharge, women with insulin-treated gestational diabetes undergo evaluation of fasting plasma glucose at 2 and 6 weeks postpartum.

Recommendations for postpartum follow-up are based on the 50-percent likelihood of women with gestational diabetes developing overt diabetes within 20 years (O'Sullivan, 1982). If fasting hyperglycemia develops during pregnancy, then diabetes is more likely to persist postpartum. For example, in women with fasting glucose levels of 105 to 130 mg/dL, 43 percent were found to be overtly diabetic (Metzger and associates, 1985). When fasting glucose exceeded 130 mg/dL during pregnancy, 86 percent became overtly diabetic. Likewise, insulin therapy during pregnancy, and especially before 24 weeks, is a powerful predictor of persistent diabetes (Dacus and co-workers, 1994; Greenberg and colleagues, 1995).

Women with a history of gestational diabetes are also at risk for cardiovascular complications associated with dyslipidemia, hypertension, and abdominal obesity—the *metabolic syndrome* (see Chap. 43, p. 947). Pallardo and colleagues (1999) evaluated cardiovascular disease risk factors 3 to 6 months' postpartum in 788 women with gestational diabetes. They found that the degree of postpartum glucose intolerance was significantly associated with these risk factors. A recent Canadian study by Shah and co-workers (2008) documented excessive cardiovascular disease even by 10 years in these women compared with nondiabetic controls. Finally, Akinci and associates (2009) reported that a fasting glucose level ≥ 100 mg/dL with the index OGTT was an independent predictor of the metabolic syndrome.

Recurrence of gestational diabetes in subsequent pregnancies was documented in 40 percent of 344 primiparous women analyzed by Holmes and colleagues (2003). Obese women were more likely to have impaired glucose tolerance in subsequent pregnancies. Thus, lifestyle behavioral changes, including weight control and exercise between pregnancies, likely would prevent recurrence of gestational diabetes as well as modify onset and severity of type 2 diabetes later in life (Kim and co-workers, 2008; Pan and associates, 1997). Interestingly, perinatal outcomes in women with previous gestational diabetes but with normal glucose tolerance tests during a subsequent pregnancy were not improved with regard to birthweight, macrosomia, route of delivery, and neonatal complications (Danilenko-Dixon and colleagues, 2000). Finally, Lu and co-workers (2002) found that women *without* gestational diabetes in their first pregnancy were unlikely to have gestational diabetes when screened in a second pregnancy.

Contraception

Low-dose hormonal contraceptives may be used safely by women with recent gestational diabetes (see Chap. 32, p. 678). The rate of subsequent diabetes in oral contraceptive users is not significantly different from that in those who did not use hormonal contraception (Kjos and colleagues, 1990a).

TABLE 52-7. Pregnancy Outcomes of Births in Nova Scotia from 1988 to 2002 in Women with and without Pregestational Diabetes

Factor	Diabetic (n = 516) Percent	Nondiabetic (n = 150,589) Percent	p value
Gestational hypertension	28	9	< .001
Preterm birth	28	5	< .001
Macrosomia	45	13	< .001
Fetal-growth restriction	5	10	< .001
Stillbirths	1.0	0.4	.06
Perinatal deaths	1.7	0.6	.004

Adapted from Yang and colleagues (2006).

Gestational Diabetes at Parkland Hospital

Prior to 1997, selective glucose screening was employed. For women with risk factors, a standard 50-g oral glucose tolerance test was performed between 24 and 28 weeks without regard to recent meal status. For screen-positive women, the standard 100-g 3-hour OGTT was used. Women identified with diet-treated gestational diabetes were seen weekly in a specific clinic designed to provide dietary counseling. Fasting plasma-glucose measurements were obtained at each visit. Women without other complications such as hypertension or postterm gestation were permitted to enter spontaneous labor, and antepartum testing was not used. Women identified with insulin-treated gestational diabetes were managed as overt diabetics, as described later.

Beginning in 1997, women at high risk for gestational diabetes underwent immediate glucose screening at their first prenatal clinic visit. All other women without risk factors underwent universal screening at 24 to 28 weeks using a standard 1-hour, 50-g oral glucose challenge test. Obstetrical management practices previously used during selective screening were continued. Casey and colleagues (1999) found that obstetrical outcomes attributable to the diagnosis of gestational diabetes were not different after the change in screening. In a subsequent analysis, Hawkins and associates (2008) found that women with diet-treated gestational diabetes identified during early pregnancy with risk-based screening had an increased risk for preeclampsia, shoulder dystocia, and macrosomic infants compared with women identified using universal screening at 24 to 28 weeks' gestation.

PREGESTATIONAL DIABETES

It is unquestioned that pregestational—or overt—diabetes has a significant impact on pregnancy outcome. The embryo, the fetus, and the mother commonly experience serious complications directly attributable to diabetes. The likelihood of successful outcomes with overt diabetes is related somewhat to the degree of glycemic control, but more importantly, to the degree of underlying cardiovascular or renal disease. Therefore, as the alphabetical classification shown in Table 52-2 worsens, the likelihood of good pregnancy outcomes lessens.

Yang and associates (2006) chronicled the effects of overt diabetes on pregnancy outcomes in Nova Scotia from 1998 through

2002. They compared outcomes in 516 overtly diabetic women with those of 150,589 pregnancies in nondiabetic women. As shown in Table 52-7, women with diabetes experienced significantly worse pregnancy outcomes. The incidence of chronic and gestational hypertension—and especially preeclampsia—are remarkably increased. As shown in Figure 52-4, women with type 1 diabetes who are in the more advanced white classes of overt diabetes increasingly developed preeclampsia. Similar results have been reported for the United Kingdom and Australia (MacIntosh and colleagues, 2006; Shand and co-workers, 2008).

Fetal Effects

Improved fetal surveillance, neonatal intensive care, and maternal metabolic control have reduced perinatal losses with overt diabetes to 2 to 4 percent. From Edinburgh, Johnstone and colleagues (2006) assessed pregnancy outcomes in women with type 1 diabetes and reported a dramatic reduction in perinatal mortality rates—from 22 percent in the 1960s to 1 percent in the 1990s—but no change in fetal overgrowth. One reason that perinatal mortality rates have seemingly plateaued is that the two major causes of fetal death—congenital malformations and

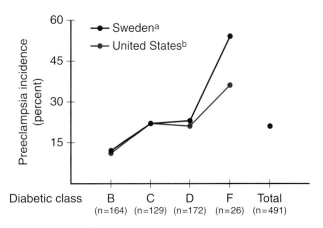

FIGURE 52-4 Incidence of preeclampsia in 491 type 1 diabetic women in Sweden and the United States reported by the National Institute of Child Health and Human Development Maternal-Fetal Medicine Units Network. (Data from Hanson and Persson, 1993; Sibai and colleagues, 2000.)

unexplained fetal death—remain unchanged by medical intervention (Garner, 1995a).

Miscarriage

Several studies have shown that early abortion is associated with poor glycemic control (Greene and co-workers, 1989; Mills and associates, 1988a). In 215 women with type 1 diabetes enrolled for prenatal care before 9 weeks, 24 percent had a miscarriage (Rosenn and colleagues, 1994). Only those whose initial glycohemoglobin A1c concentrations were > 12 percent or whose persistent preprandial glucose concentrations were > 120 mg/dL were at increased risk (see also Chap. 9, p. 226).

Preterm Delivery

Overt diabetes is an undisputed risk factor for preterm birth. The Maternal-Fetal Medicine Units Network analyzed pregnancy outcomes in 461 such women (Sibai and associates, 2000). Almost 9 percent of these women spontaneously delivered before 35 weeks compared with 4.5 percent of nondiabetic women. Moreover, another 7 percent of diabetic women underwent indicated preterm delivery compared with 2 percent of nondiabetic women. In the Canadian study shown in Table 52-7, the incidence of preterm birth was 28 percent—a fivefold increase compared with that of their normal population.

Malformations

The incidence of major malformations in women with type 1 diabetes is approximately 5 percent (Sheffield and co-workers, 2002). These account for almost half of perinatal deaths in diabetic pregnancies. Specific types of anomalies linked to maternal diabetes and their relative incidence are summarized in Table 52-8. *Diabetes is not associated with increased risk for fetal chromosomal abnormalities.*

TABLE 52-8. Congenital Malformations in Infants of Women with Overt Diabetes

Anomaly	Ratios of Incidence[a]
Caudal regression	252
Situs inversus	84
Spina bifida, hydrocephaly, or other central nervous system defects	2
Anencephaly	3
Cardiac anomalies	4
Anal/rectal atresia	3
Renal anomalies	5
Agenesis	4
Cystic kidney	4
Duplex ureter	23

[a]Ratio of incidence is in comparison with the general population. Cardiac anomalies include transposition of the great vessels and ventricular or atrial septal defects. Adapted from Mills and colleagues (1979) and the American Diabetes Association (1995).

It is generally believed that the increased risk of severe malformations is the consequence of poorly controlled diabetes, both preconceptionally and early in pregnancy. Eriksson (2009) concluded that the etiology was multifactorial. One proposed mechanism for cardiac defects is that of hyperglycemia-induced oxidative stress that inhibits expression of cardiac neural crest migration (Morgan and associates, 2008). Miller and co-workers (1981) suggested that women with lower glycosylated hemoglobin values at the time of conception had fewer fetuses with anomalies compared with women with abnormally high values. The Diabetes in Early Pregnancy Study did not totally corroborate these findings. Specifically, Mills and colleagues (1988b) enrolled more than 600 diabetic women in this investigation, and they concluded that a normal glycosylated hemoglobin distribution did not guarantee avoidance of all diabetes-associated anomalies. Conversely, not all women with elevated levels had poor outcomes. It appeared, however, that women in whom periconceptional glucose control was optimized had a 5-percent fetal malformation rate compared with a 9-percent rate in the group who presented after organogenesis was completed. Ray and co-workers (2001) performed a meta-analysis of seven studies addressing preconceptional care published between 1970 and 2000. They concluded that such care was associated with a lower risk of congenital anomalies, and this was further linked to lower glycosylated hemoglobin values (see Chap. 7, p. 175).

Altered Fetal Growth

The incidence of macrosomia rises significantly when mean maternal blood glucose concentrations exceed 130 mg/dL (Willman and co-workers, 1986). Some authors have objected to classification of these infants as either "macrosomic" or "nonmacrosomic," because this ignores the observation that virtually all are *growth promoted* (Bradley and associates, 1988). This is discussed further in Chapter 38 (p. 853). As shown in Figure 52-5, the birthweight distribution of infants of diabetic mothers is skewed toward consistently heavier birthweights compared with that of normal pregnancies. In contrast, fetal-growth restriction in women with diabetes may be seen and may be related to substrate deprivation from advanced maternal vascular disease or to congenital malformations.

Landon and co-workers (1989) performed serial sonographic examinations during the third trimester in 79 women with diabetes and observed that excessive fetal abdominal circumference growth was detectable by 32 weeks (Fig. 52-6). Ben-Haroush and colleagues (2007) analyzed fetal sonographic measurements between 29 and 34 weeks in 423 diabetic pregnancies and found that accelerated fetal growth was particularly evident in women with poor glycemic control.

Unexplained Fetal Demise

Stillbirths without identifiable causes are a phenomenon relatively unique to pregnancies complicated by overt diabetes. They are "unexplained" because factors such as obvious placental insufficiency, abruption, fetal-growth restriction, or oligohydramnios are not apparent. These infants are typically large-for-gestational age and die before labor, usually at 35 weeks or later (Garner, 1995b). Studies employing cordocentesis have

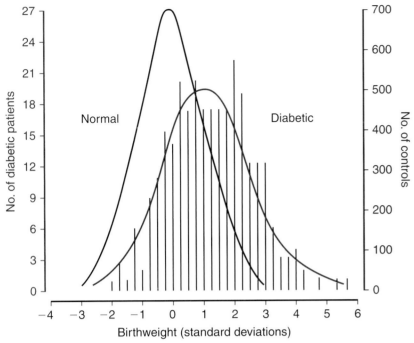

FIGURE 52-5 Distribution of birthweights—standard deviation from the normal mean for gestational age—for 280 infants of diabetic mothers and 3959 infants of nondiabetic mothers. (From Bradley and co-workers, 1988; redrawn from *British Medical Journal*, 1988, Vol. 297, No. 6663, pp. 1583–1584, with permission from the BMJ Publishing Group.)

levels in some of these fetuses. Such findings lend credence to the long-held hypothesis that hyperglycemia-mediated chronic aberrations in transport of oxygen and fetal metabolites may account for unexplained fetal deaths (Pedersen, 1977).

Two observations also lend some insight into these deaths. Richey and co-workers (1995) at Parkland Hospital were at the bedsides of two diabetic women whose pregnancies were complicated by a macrosomic fetus and hydramnios. Otherwise unexplained fetal deaths were seemingly in progress. In both of these rare clinical instances, both fetuses were acidemic before labor, and both placentas were hydropic due to edema of the chorionic villi. These features were linked to maternal hyperglycemia, and it was hypothesized that osmotically induced villous edema led to impaired fetal oxygen transport. The observations of Daskalakis and associates (2008), who found microscopic evidence of placental dysfunction in 40 consecutive placentas from pregnancies in women with gestational diabetes, also corroborate this hypothesis.

Explicable stillbirths due to placental insufficiency also occur with increased frequency in women with overt diabetes, usually in association with severe preeclampsia. This, in turn, is increased in women with advanced diabetes and vascular complications. Similarly, ketoacidosis can cause fetal death.

provided some insights into acid-base metabolism in fetuses of diabetic women. Salvesen and colleagues (1992, 1993) reported decreased pH and increased P_{CO_2}, lactate, and erythropoietin

Hydramnios

Although diabetic pregnancies are often complicated by hydramnios, the cause is unclear. A likely—albeit unproven—explanation is that fetal hyperglycemia causes polyuria (see Chap. 21, p. 493). In a study from Parkland Hospital, Dashe and co-workers (2000) found that the amnionic fluid index parallels the amnionic fluid glucose level among women with diabetes. This finding suggests that the hydramnios associated with diabetes is a result of increased amnionic fluid glucose concentration. Further support for this hypothesis was provided by Vink and colleagues (2006), who linked poor maternal glucose control to macrosomia and hydramnios.

Neonatal Mortality and Morbidity

Before tests of fetal health and maturity became available, preterm delivery was deliberately effected to avoid unexplained fetal deaths. Although this practice has been abandoned, there is still an increased frequency of preterm delivery in women with diabetes (see Table 52-7). Most preterm

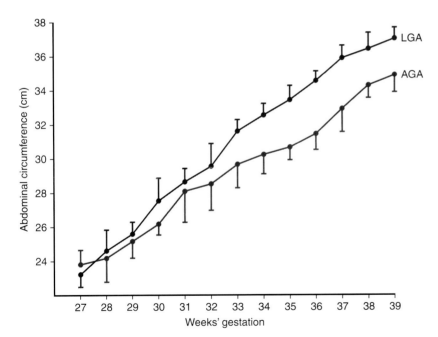

FIGURE 52-6 Comparison of abdominal circumference growth curve for appropriate-for-gestational age (AGA) and large-for-gestational age (LGA) fetuses of diabetic mothers. Growth is accelerated at 32 weeks in the LGA group. (This figure was published in *American Journal of Obstetrics & Gynecology*, Vol. 160, No. 1, MB Landon, MC Mintz, and SG Gabbe, Sonographic evaluation of fetal abdominal growth: Predictor of the large-for-gestational-age infant in pregnancies complicated by diabetes mellitus, pp. 115–121, Copyright Elsevier 1989.)

births are associated with advanced diabetes and superimposed preeclampsia.

Modern neonatal care has largely eliminated neonatal deaths due to immaturity. More than 15 years ago, Cnattingius and colleagues (1994) reported only one neonatal death due to immaturity in 914 singleton births to overtly diabetic women. Conversely, neonatal *morbidity* due to preterm birth continues to be a serious consequence. Indeed, some of the morbidities in these infants are considered to be uniquely related to aberrations in maternal glucose metabolism.

Respiratory Distress Syndrome

Conventional obstetrical teaching through the late 1980s generally held that fetal lung maturation was delayed in diabetic pregnancies (see Chap. 29, p. 607). Thus, it was taught that these infants were at increased risk for respiratory distress (Gluck and Kulovich, 1973). Subsequent observations have challenged this concept, and gestational age rather than overt diabetes is likely the most significant associated factor with respiratory distress (Berkowitz and colleagues, 1996; Kjos and associates, 1990b).

Hypoglycemia

A rapid decrease in plasma glucose concentration after delivery is characteristic of the infant of a diabetic mother. This is attributed to hyperplasia of the fetal β-islet cells induced by chronic maternal hyperglycemia. Taylor and associates (2002) found that neonatal hypoglycemia—blood glucose levels < 45 mg/dL before the second feeding—was related to maternal blood glucose levels > 145 mg/dL during labor. Prompt recognition and treatment of the hypoglycemic infant has minimized adverse sequelae.

Hypocalcemia

Defined as a total serum calcium concentration < 8 mg/dL in term infants, hypocalcemia is one of the major metabolic derangements in infants of diabetic mothers. Its cause has not been explained. Theories include aberrations in magnesium–calcium economy, asphyxia, and preterm birth (Cruikshank and co-workers, 1980). In the randomized study by DeMarini and colleagues (1994), 137 pregnant women with type 1 diabetes were managed with strict versus customary glucose control. Almost a third of infants in the customary control group developed hypocalcemia compared with only 18 percent of those in the strict control group. Gestational age and preeclampsia were also implicated.

Hyperbilirubinemia and Polycythemia

The pathogenesis of hyperbilirubinemia in infants of diabetic mothers is uncertain. Factors implicated have included preterm birth and polycythemia with hemolysis (see Chap. 29, p. 625). Venous hematocrits of 65 to 70 volume percent have been observed in up to 40 percent of these infants (Salvesen and associates, 1992). Renal vein thrombosis is also reported to result from polycythemia.

Cardiomyopathy

Infants of diabetic pregnancies may have hypertrophic cardiomyopathy that occasionally progresses to congestive heart failure (Gandhi and co-workers, 1995; Reller and Kaplan, 1988). These infants typically have macrosomia, and fetal hyperinsulinemia has been implicated in the pathogenesis of heart disease. Girsen and colleagues (2008) reported that 32 neonates born to women with type 1 diabetes had higher mean cord-blood levels of N-terminal proatrial natriuretic peptide (NT-proANP) and probrain natriuretic peptide (proBNP) compared with those of control infants. They also found that NT-proANP levels were higher in those fetuses of diabetic mothers whose glycemic control was poor. Way (1979) reported that the cardiomyopathy generally disappears by 6 months of age.

Long-Term Cognitive Development

Rizzo and colleagues (1995) used multiple tests of intelligence and psychomotor development to assess 196 children of diabetic women up to age 9 years. They concluded that maternal diabetes had a negligible impact on cognitive development.

Inheritance of Diabetes

Offspring born to women with overt diabetes have a 1- to 3-percent risk of developing type 1 diabetes (Garner, 1995a). The risk is 6 percent if only the father has diabetes. If both parents have type 1 diabetes, the risk is 20 percent. McKinney and associates (1999) studied 196 children with type 1 diabetes and found that older maternal age and maternal type 1 diabetes are important risk factors. Plagemann and colleagues (2002) have implicated breast feeding by diabetic mothers in the genesis of childhood diabetes.

Maternal Effects

Diabetes and pregnancy interact significantly such that maternal welfare can be seriously jeopardized. With the possible exception of diabetic retinopathy, however, the long-term course of diabetes is not affected by pregnancy.

Although maternal death is uncommon, rates in women with diabetes are still increased tenfold (Cousins, 1987). Deaths most often result from ketoacidosis, hypertension, preeclampsia, and pyelonephritis. Especially ominous is ischemic heart disease. Pombar and colleagues (1995) reviewed 17 women with coronary artery disease—class H diabetes—and reported that only half survived pregnancy.

Diabetic Nephropathy

Diabetes is the leading cause of end-stage renal disease in the United States (see Chap. 48, p. 1039). The incidence of renal failure is nearly 30 percent in individuals with type 1 diabetes and ranges from 4 to 20 percent in those with type 2 diabetes. Importantly, the incidence of nephropathy in individuals with type 1 diabetes declined during the 1980s, presumably from improved glucose control. Investigators for the Diabetes Control and Complications Trial (2002) reported that there was a 25-percent decrease in the rate of nephropathy for each 10-percent decrease in hemoglobin A1c levels.

Clinically detectable nephropathy in type 1 disease begins with microalbuminuria—30 to 300 mg/24 h of albumin. This may manifest as early as 5 years after the onset of diabetes

(Nathan, 1993). After another 5 to 10 years, overt proteinuria—more than 300 mg/24 h—develops in patients destined to have end-stage renal disease. Hypertension almost invariably develops during this period, and renal failure ensues typically in the next 5 to 10 years.

Approximately 5 percent of pregnant women with diabetes already have renal involvement—White class F (Hanson and Persson, 1993; Siddiqi and associates, 1991). Recall that as shown in Figure 52-4, these women are at significantly increased risk for preeclampsia and for indicated preterm delivery. Combs and co-workers (1993a) reported that 38 percent of 311 women with proteinuria > 500 mg/day before 20 weeks developed preeclampsia. They also found that women with microproteinuria—190 to 500 mg/d—had an increased risk of preeclampsia. Conversely, in an analysis of 460 women with classes B through F-R diabetes, How and colleagues (2004) found no association between preeclampsia and microproteinuria. However, chronic hypertension with diabetic nephropathy increased the risk of preeclampsia to 60 percent. Gordon and associates (1996) reported that chronic renal insufficiency and heavy proteinuria before 20 weeks were predictive of preeclampsia.

There appear to be no long-term sequelae of pregnancy on diabetic nephropathy. Chaturvedi and associates (1995) provided long-term follow-up studies in 1358 European women with type 1 diabetes, of whom 582 had been pregnant. The incidence of either micro- or macroalbuminuria was not increased in women with prior pregnancies compared with that of nulliparas. That said, renal involvement carries a guarded long-term prognosis for these women. Miodovnik and colleagues (1996) found that a fourth of 46 women with class F diabetes developed end-stage renal failure at a mean of 6 years after pregnancy. This is similar to pregnant women with nondiabetic glomerulopathies reported by Stettler and Cunningham (1992) and discussed in Chapter 48 (p. 1043).

Diabetic Retinopathy

Retinal vasculopathy is a highly specific complication of both type 1 and type 2 diabetes. Its prevalence is related to duration of diabetes. Almost 8 percent of persons with impaired glucose tolerance already have retinopathy, and 13 percent of those newly identified with diabetes in the Diabetes Prevention Project (2007) were already affected. In the United States, diabetic retinopathy is the most important cause of visual impairment in persons younger than age 60 years (Frank, 2004).

The first and most common visible lesions are small microaneurysms followed by blot hemorrhages that form when erythrocytes escape from the aneurysms. These areas leak serous fluid that creates hard exudates. Such features are termed *benign* or *background* or *nonproliferative retinopathy*. With increasingly severe retinopathy, the abnormal vessels of background eye disease become occluded, leading to retinal ischemia and infarctions that appear as *cotton wool exudates*. These are considered *preproliferative retinopathy*. In response to ischemia, there is neovascularization on the retinal surface and out into the vitreous cavity. Vision is obscured when there is hemorrhage. Laser photocoagulation before hemorrhage, as shown in Figure 52-7, reduces the rate of visual loss progression and blindness by half. The procedure is performed during pregnancy when indicated.

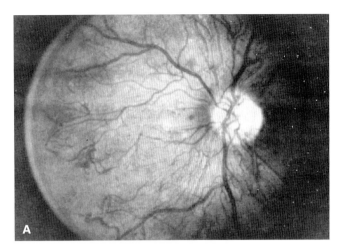
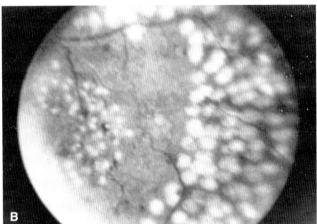

FIGURE 52-7 Retinal photographs from a 30-year-old diabetic woman. **A.** Optic nerve head showing severe proliferative retinopathy characterized by extensive networks of new vessels surrounding the optic disc. **B.** A portion of the acute photocoagulation full "scatter" pattern following argon laser treatment. (From Elman and colleagues, 1990, with permission.)

Siddiqi and colleagues (1991) reported that almost a third of 175 insulin-dependent pregnant women examined by 10 weeks had background retinal changes—class D, or proliferative retinopathy—class R. The effects of pregnancy on proliferative retinopathy are controversial (Garner, 1995a). It has been long taught that this complication is a rare example of a long-term adverse effect of pregnancy. Whereas Klein and co-workers (1990) concluded that pregnancy worsened proliferative retinopathy, Chaturvedi and associates (1995) found an equivalent prevalence of retinopathy in multiparous and nulliparous women. In a prospective postpartum 5-year follow-up of 59 type 1 diabetic women, Arun and Taylor (2008) confirmed that baseline retinopathy was the only independent risk factor for progression. Currently, most agree that laser photocoagulation and good glycemic control during pregnancy minimize the potential for deleterious effects of pregnancy.

Ironically, there are case reports that link "acute" rigorous metabolic control during pregnancy to acute worsening of retinopathy (Dahl-Jørgensen and co-workers, 1985; Van Ballegooie and associates, 1984). In a study of 201 women with retinopathy, McElvy and associates (2001) found that almost 30 percent suffered

SECTION 8

progression of eye disease during pregnancy despite intensive glucose control. That said, Wang and co-workers (1993) have observed that retinopathy worsened during the critical months of rigorous glucose control, but in the longer term, deterioration of eye disease slowed. In the report by McElvy and co-workers (2001), progression of retinopathy was associated with reduced fetal growth. Lauszus and colleagues (1998), however, reported that proliferative retinopathy, per se, did not worsen perinatal outcome.

In a preliminary report, Kitzmiller and colleagues (1999) implicated insulin lispro, that is, short-acting insulin, in the development of proliferative retinopathy during pregnancy. Conversely, Buchbinder and associates (2000) found no evidence that such therapy was linked to the development or progression of diabetic retinopathy. Also, Durnwald and Landon (2008) reported no such complications with lispro insulin.

Diabetic Neuropathy

Peripheral symmetrical sensorimotor diabetic neuropathy is uncommon in pregnant women. But a form of this, known as *diabetic gastropathy*, is troublesome in pregnancy because it causes nausea and vomiting, nutritional problems, and difficulty with glucose control. Treatment with metoclopramide and H_2-receptor antagonists is sometimes successful. *Hyperemesis gravidarum* is further discussed in Chapter 49 (p. 1050).

Preeclampsia

Hypertension that is induced or exacerbated by pregnancy is the major complication that most often forces preterm delivery in diabetic women. According to Garner (1995a), the perinatal mortality rate is increased 20-fold for preeclamptic women with diabetes compared with that for those who remain normotensive. Special risk factors for preeclampsia include any vascular complications and preexisting proteinuria, with or without chronic hypertension. Referring back to Figure 52-4, the risk of preeclampsia is 11 to 12 percent in class B, 21 to 22 percent in class C, 21 to 23 percent in class D, and 36 to 54 percent in classes F-R. Savvidou and colleagues (2002) described impaired vascular reactivity in pregnant women with type 1 diabetes. Temple and co-workers (2006) prospectively studied HbA1c levels at 24 weeks in 290 women with type 1 diabetes and found that preeclampsia was related to glucose control. Management of preeclampsia is discussed in Chapter 34 (p. 728).

Diabetic Ketoacidosis

Although it affects only approximately 1 percent of diabetic pregnancies, ketoacidosis remains one of the most serious complications (Garner, 1995a). It is unique to type 1 diabetes, and it may develop with hyperemesis gravidarum, β-mimetic drugs given for tocolysis, infection, and corticosteroids given to induce fetal lung maturation. Kent and colleagues (1994) found that only half of young women with recurrent ketoacidosis had successful pregnancies compared with 95 percent of women without ketoacidosis.

The incidence of fetal loss is about 20 percent with ketoacidosis. Noncompliance is a prominent factor, and this and ketoacidosis have long been considered prognostically bad signs in pregnancy (Pedersen and co-workers, 1974). Pregnant women usually have ketoacidosis with lower blood glucose levels than when non-

pregnant. In a study from China, the mean glucose level for pregnant women with DKA was 293 mg/dL compared with 495 mg/dL for nonpregnant women (Guo and co-workers, 2008). These investigators described one woman whose plasma glucose was only 124 mg/dL. Chico and associates (2008) reported ketoacidosis in a pregnant woman whose plasma glucose was only 87 mg/dL! A management protocol is shown in Table 52-9.

Infections

Almost all types of infections are increased in diabetic pregnancies. Stamler and associates (1990) reported that almost 80 percent of women with type 1 diabetes develop at least one infection during pregnancy compared with only 25 percent in those without diabetes. Takoudes and colleagues (2004) found that pregestational diabetes is associated with a two- to threefold increase in wound complications after cesarean delivery. Common infections include candida vulvovaginitis, urinary infections, respiratory tract infections, and puerperal pelvic infections. Cousins (1987) observed that antepartum pyelonephritis developed in

TABLE 52-9. Protocol Recommended by the American College of Obstetricians and Gynecologists (2005) for Management of Diabetic Ketoacidosis During Pregnancy

Laboratory assessment
Obtain arterial blood gases to document degree of acidosis present; measure glucose, ketones, and electrolyte levels at 1- to 2-hour intervals
Insulin
Low-dose, intravenous
Loading dose: 0.2–0.4 U/kg
Maintenance: 2–10 U/h
Fluids
Isotonic sodium chloride
Total replacement in first 12 hours of 4–6 L
1 L in first hour
500–1000 mL/h for 2–4 hours
250 mL/h until 80 percent replaced
Glucose
Begin 5-percent dextrose in normal saline when glucose plasma level reaches 250 mg/dL (14 mmol/L)
Potassium
If initially normal or reduced, an infusion rate up to 15–20 mEq/h may be required; if elevated, wait until levels decrease into the normal range, then add to intravenous solution in a concentration of 20–30 mEq/L
Bicarbonate
Add one ampule (44 mEq) to 1 L of 0.45 normal saline if pH is < 7.1

This table was published in Landon MB, Catalano PM, and Gabbe SG, Diabetes mellitus complicating pregnancy, in *Obstetrics: Normal and Problem Pregnancies*, 5th ed., SG Gabbe, JR Niebyl, and JL Simpson (eds.), pp. 977–1011, Copyright Elsevier/Saunders 2007, with permission.

TABLE 52-10. Action Profiles of Commonly Used Insulins

Insulin Type	Onset	Peak (hours)	Duration (hours)
Short-acting, SC			
Lispro	<15 min	0.5–1.5	3–4
Aspart	<15 min	0.5–1.5	3–4
Regular	30–60 min	2–3	4–6
Long-acting			
Isophane insulin suspension	1–3 hr	5–7	13–18
Insulin zinc suspension	1–3 hr	4–8	13–20
Extended insulin zinc suspension	2–4 hr	8–14	18–30
Insulin glargine	1–4 hr	Minimal peak activity	24

SC = subcutaneous.
Reprinted from Fauci AS, Braunwald E, Kasper DL, et al: *Harrison's Principles of Internal Medicine,* 17th ed., pp. 2275–2304. Copyright © 2008 The McGraw-Hill Companies, Inc.

4 percent of women with type 1 diabetes compared with 1 percent in those without diabetes. Importantly, renal infection was associated with increased preterm delivery. Fortunately, these latter infections can be minimized by screening and eradication of asymptomatic bacteriuria (see Chap. 48, p. 1035).

Management of Diabetes in Pregnancy

The goals of management are tailored somewhat uniquely for pregnant women. Management preferably should begin before pregnancy and include specific goals during each trimester.

Preconceptional Care

To minimize early pregnancy loss and congenital malformations in infants of diabetic mothers, optimal medical care and education are recommended before conception (see Chap. 7, p. 175). Unfortunately, up to 60 percent of pregnancies in these women are unplanned (Holing and co-workers, 1998). Thus, diabetic women frequently begin pregnancy with suboptimal glucose control (Casele and Laifer, 1998; Kim and colleagues, 2005).

The American Diabetes Association (1999a) has defined optimal preconceptional glucose control using insulin to include self-monitored preprandial glucose levels of 70 to 100 mg/dL and postprandial values < 140 mg/dL and < 120 mg/dL at 1 and 2 hours, respectively. Glycosylated hemoglobin measurement, which expresses an average of circulating glucose for the past 4 to 8 weeks, is useful to assess early metabolic control. The Association further defines optimal preconceptional glycosylated hemoglobin values as those within or near the upper limit of normal for a specific laboratory or within three standard deviations of the normal mean. The most significant risk for malformations is with levels exceeding 10 percent (American College of Obstetricians and Gynecologists, 1994). Finally, folate, 400 μg/d, is given periconceptionally and during early pregnancy to decrease the risk of neural-tube defects.

First Trimester

Careful monitoring of glucose control is essential. For this reason, many clinicians hospitalize overtly diabetic women during

early pregnancy to institute an individualized glucose control program and to provide education concerning the ensuing months of pregnancy. It also provides an opportunity to assess the extent of vascular complications of diabetes and to precisely establish gestational age.

Insulin Treatment

Insulin is used for overtly diabetic pregnant women. Although oral hypoglycemic agents have been used successfully for gestational diabetes (p. 1111), these agents are not currently recommended for overt diabetes except on an investigational basis (American College of Obstetricians and Gynecologists, 2005). Maternal glycemic control can usually be achieved with *multiple daily insulin injections* and adjustment of dietary intake. The action profiles of commonly used insulins are shown in Table 52-10.

Subcutaneous insulin infusion by a calibrated pump may be used during pregnancy. It has both advantages and disadvantages, but, as demonstrated in a Cochrane Database review by Farrar and associates (2007), there is scarce robust evidence for any salutary pregnancy effects. Kernaghan and co-workers (2007) in a retrospective study of 42 pregnant women failed to show improved glycemic control or reduced infant birthweight comparing those using a pump with those treated with conventional insulin therapy. Women who use an insulin pump must be highly motivated and compliant to minimize the risk of nocturnal hypoglycemia (Gabbe and Graves, 2003).

Self-monitoring of capillary glucose levels using a glucometer is recommended because this involves the woman in her own care. The goals of glucose control recommended during pregnancy are shown in Table 52-11. Parretti and colleagues (2001) measured maternal capillary glucose responses to meals throughout 51 normal pregnancies to better characterize glucose goals for management of diabetic women (Table 52-12).

Noninvasive Monitoring. Technology under development may provide methods for noninvasive glucose monitoring. Such an automatic and painless means to obtain blood glucose information would undoubtedly greatly aid patient compliance. Tamada and colleagues (1999) reported clinical results in

TABLE 52-11. Self-Monitored Capillary Blood Glucose Goals

Specimen	Level (mg/dL)
Fasting	≤95
Premeal	≤100
1-hr postprandial	≤140
2-hr postprandial	≤120
0200–0600	≥60
Mean (average)	100
Hb A1c	≤6

Reprinted, with permission, from American College of Obstetricians and Gynecologists. Pregestational Diabetes Mellitus. ACOG Practice Bulletin 60. Washington, DC: ACOG; 2005.

nonpregnant diabetics with such a monitoring device (Cygnus, Inc., Redwood City, California). It extracts glucose through the skin by iontophoresis, which uses electrical potentials. It then measures glucose concentrations in the extracted sample. The device provides up to three glucose readings per hour and causes only transient mild skin irritation at the sensor site. These investigators found close agreement between noninvasive glucose measurements and those obtained by standard fingersticks.

Diet

For women of normal weight, the American Diabetes Association (1999b) recommends a caloric intake of 30 to 35 kcal/kg, taken as three meals and three snacks daily (Franz and colleagues, 2004; Garner, 1995a). For underweight women, this is increased to 40 kcal/kg/d. For those more than 120 percent above ideal

TABLE 52-12. Average Diurnal Capillary Blood Glucose Levels in 51 Normal Pregnant Women During the Third Trimester

Time of Day	Blood Glucose Range of Values, mg/dL
0800 hr	51–65
← Breakfast	
0900 hr	87–112
1000 hr	73–100
1200 hr	58–75
← Lunch	
1400 hr	77–102
2000 hr	59–73
← Dinner	
0400 hr	57–70

Approximate glucose based on the range of mean value ± SD between 28 and 38 weeks' gestation.
Adapted from Parretti and colleagues (2001); Copyright © 2001 American Diabetes Association. From Diabetes Care®, Vol. 24; 2001, 1319–1323. Modified with permission from The American Diabetes Association.

weight, it is decreased to 24 kcal/kg/d. An ideal dietary composition is 55 percent carbohydrate, 20 percent protein, and 25 percent fat with less than 10 percent as saturated fat.

Hypoglycemia

Diabetes tends to be unstable in the first trimester. Rosenn and colleagues (1995) assessed the impact of maternal hypoglycemia in 84 pregnant women with overt diabetes. Clinically significant hypoglycemia with glucometer values less than 35 mg/dL was documented in 70 percent of the women, with a peak incidence between 10 and 15 weeks. Almost 25 percent of these 84 women experienced unconsciousness, and 15 percent developed seizures as a result of hypoglycemia. These investigators recommended caution in attempting euglycemia in women with recurrent episodes of hypoglycemia.

We have reported that good pregnancy outcomes can be achieved in women with mean preprandial plasma glucose values up to 143 mg/dL (Leveno and associates, 1979). In women with diabetes who are not pregnant, the Diabetes Control and Complications Trial Research Group (1993) found that similar glucose values—intensive control was defined as mean values < 155 mg/dL—delayed and slowed diabetic retinopathy, nephropathy, and neuropathy. Thus, women with overt diabetes who have glucose values considerably above those defined as normal both during and after pregnancy can expect good outcomes.

Second Trimester

Maternal serum alpha-fetoprotein determination at 16 to 20 weeks is used in association with targeted sonographic examination at 18 to 20 weeks in an attempt to detect neural-tube defects and other anomalies (see Chap. 13, p. 288). Maternal alpha-fetoprotein levels may be lower in diabetic pregnancies, and interpretation is altered accordingly. Targeted sonography is important, and Albert and co-workers (1996) identified 72 percent of 29 fetal anomalies in 289 diabetic pregnancies. That said, Dashe and colleagues (2009) cautioned that detection of fetal anomalies in obese diabetic women is more difficult than in similarly sized women without diabetes.

Euglycemia with self-monitoring continues to be the goal in management. Individualized programs are necessary to avoid both excessive hyperglycemia and frequent episodes of hypoglycemia. After the first-trimester instability, a stable period ensues. This is followed by an increased insulin requirement after approximately 24 weeks (Steel and co-workers, 1994). This rise results from the increased production of pregnancy hormones, which are insulin antagonists (see Chap. 3, p. 65, and Chap. 5, p. 113). These investigators reported the absolute increase in mean insulin requirement to be 52 units in 237 women with type 1 diabetes—importantly, however, there was wide variation. The magnitude of increase was directly related to maternal weight and inversely related to the duration of diabetes.

Third Trimester and Delivery

In a woman with White class B or C diabetes, cesarean delivery has commonly been used to avoid traumatic birth of a large infant at or near term. In women with more advanced diabetes, especially those with vascular disease, the reduced likelihood of

TABLE 52-13. Insulin Management During Labor and Delivery Recommended by the American College of Obstetricians and Gynecologists (2005)

- Usual dose of intermediate-acting insulin is given at bedtime.
- Morning dose of insulin is withheld.
- Intravenous infusion of normal saline is begun.
- Once active labor begins or glucose levels decrease to < 70 mg/dL, the infusion is changed from saline to 5-percent dextrose and delivered at a rate of 100–150 mL/hr (2.5 mg/kg/min) to achieve a glucose level of approximately 100 mg/dL.
- Glucose levels are checked hourly using a bedside meter allowing for adjustment in the insulin or glucose infusion rate.
- Regular (short-acting) insulin is administered by intravenous infusion at a rate of 1.25 U/hr if glucose levels exceed 100 mg/dL.

Reprinted, with permission, from American College of Obstetricians and Gynecologists. Pregestational Diabetes Mellitus. ACOG Practice Bulletin 60. Washington, DC: ACOG; 2005.

successfully inducing labor remote from term has also contributed appreciably to an increased cesarean delivery rate. Labor induction may be attempted when the fetus is not excessively large and the cervix is considered favorable (see Chap. 22, p. 500). Cesarean delivery rates range from 50 to 80 percent (Gabbe, 1977; Kitzmiller, 1978; Leveno, 1979; Martin, 1987; Schneider, 1980, and all their associates). The rate for women with overt diabetes has remained at approximately 80 percent for the past 30 years at Parkland Hospital.

It is important to considerably reduce or delete the dose of long-acting insulin given on the day of delivery. Regular insulin should be used to meet most or all of the insulin needs of the mother at this time, because insulin requirements typically drop markedly after delivery. We have found that continuous insulin infusion by calibrated pump is most satisfactory (Table 52–13). During labor and after delivery, the woman should be adequately hydrated intravenously and given glucose in sufficient amounts to maintain normoglycemia. Capillary or plasma glucose levels should be checked frequently, and regular insulin should be administered accordingly. It is not unusual for a woman to require virtually no insulin for the first 24 hours or so postpartum and then for insulin requirements to fluctuate markedly during the next few days. Infection must be promptly detected and treated.

CONTRACEPTION

There is no single contraceptive method appropriate for all women with diabetes. Because of the risk of vascular disease, hormonal contraceptives may be problematic. Many clinicians are reluctant to recommend intrauterine devices in women with diabetes, primarily because of a possible increased risk of pelvic infections. All of these concerns, along with available options, are discussed in Chapter 32 (p. 673). For many of these reasons, and because of frequent associated morbidity with chronic diseases, many overtly diabetic women elect puerperal sterilization as discussed in Chapter 33 (p. 698). This option should be made readily available. Schwarz and colleagues (2006) compared counseling provided to nonpregnant, diabetic and nondiabetic, women during 40,304 ambulatory visits. Only 4 percent of diabetic women received contraception counseling. They concluded that this was inevitably implicated in diabetic women conceiving before optimal periconceptional glucose control was obtained.

REFERENCES

Adasheck JA, Lagrew DC, Iriye BK, et al: The influence of ultrasound examination at term on the rate of cesarean section. Am J Obstet Gynecol 174:328, 1996

Akinci B, Celtik A, Yener S, et al: Prediction of developing metabolic syndrome after gestational diabetes mellitus. Fertil Steril January 13, 2009 [Epub ahead of print]

Albert TJ, Landon MB, Wheller JJ, et al: Prenatal detection of fetal anomalies in pregnancies complicated by insulin-dependent diabetes mellitus. Am J Obstet Gynecol 174:1424, 1996

Almario CV, Ecker T, Moroz LA, et al: Obstetricians seldom provide postpartum diabetes screening for women with gestational diabetes. Am J Obstet Gynecol 198:528.e1, 2008

American College of Obstetricians and Gynecologists: Management of diabetes mellitus in pregnancy. Technical Bulletin No. 92, May 1986

American College of Obstetricians and Gynecologists: Diabetes and pregnancy. Technical Bulletin No. 200, December 1994

American College of Obstetricians and Gynecologists: Fetal macrosomia. Practice Bulletin No. 22, November 2000

American College of Obstetricians and Gynecologists: Gestational diabetes. Practice Bulletin No. 30, September 2001

American College of Obstetricians and Gynecologists: Pregestational diabetes mellitus. Practice Bulletin No. 60, March 2005

American Diabetes Association: Medical Management of Pregnancy Complicated by Diabetes, 2nd ed. Jovanovic-Peterson L (ed). Alexandria, VA, American Diabetes Association, 1995

American Diabetes Association: Clinical practice recommendations, 1999. Diabetes Care 23:S10, 1999a

American Diabetes Association: Report of the Expert Committee on the Diagnosis and Classification of Diabetes Mellitus. Diabetes Care 22:512, 1999b

American Diabetes Association: Nutritional management during pregnancy in preexisting diabetes. In Medical Management of Pregnancy Complicated by Diabetes, 3rd ed. Alexandria, VA, American Diabetes Association, 2000, p 70

American Diabetes Association: Gestational diabetes mellitus. Diabetes Care 26:S103, 2003

American Diabetes Association: Report of the Expert Committee on the Diagnosis and Classification of Diabetes Mellitus. Diabetes Care 27:5, 2004

Arun CS, Taylor R: Influence of pregnancy on long-term progression of retinopathy in patients with type 1 diabetes. Diabetologia 51:1041, 2008

Avery MD, Leon AS, Kopher RA: Effects of a partially home-based exercise program for women with gestational diabetes. Obstet Gynecol 89:10, 1997

Baraban E, McCoy L, Simon P: Increasing prevalence of gestational diabetes and pregnancy-related hypertension in Los Angeles County, California, 1991–2003. Prev Chronic Dis 5:A77, 2008

Bartha JL, Martinez-Del-Fresno P, Comino-Delgado R: Gestational diabetes mellitus diagnosed during early pregnancy. Am J Obstet Gynecol 182:346, 2000

Ben-Haroush A, Chen R, Hadar E, et al: Accuracy of a single fetal weight estimation at 29–34 weeks in diabetic pregnancies: Can it predict large-for-gestational-age infants at term? Am J Obstet Gynecol 197:497, 2007

Berkowitz K, Reyes C, Sadaat P, et al: Comparison of fetal lung maturation in well dated diabetic and non-diabetic pregnancies. Am J Obstet Gynecol 174:373, 1996

Bernstein IM, Catalano PM: Examination of factors contributing to the risk of cesarean delivery in women with gestational diabetes. Obstet Gynecol 83:462, 1994

Bonomo M, Gandini ML, Mastropasqua A, et al: Which cutoff level should be used in screening for glucose intolerance in pregnancy? Am J Obstet Gynecol 179:179, 1998

Bradley RJ, Nicolaides KH, Brudenell JM: Are all infants of diabetic mothers "macrosomic"? BMJ 297:1583, 1988

Brankston GH, Mitchell BF, Ryan EA, et al: Resistance exercise decreases the need for insulin in overweight women with gestational diabetes mellitus. Am J Obstet Gynecol 190:188, 2004

Buchbinder A, Miodovnik M, McElvy S, et al: Is insulin lispro associated with the development or progression of diabetic retinopathy during pregnancy? Am J Obstet Gynecol 183:1162, 2000

Bung P, Bung C, Artal R, et al: Therapeutic exercise for insulin-requiring gestational diabetes: Effects on the fetus—results of a randomized prospective longitudinal study. J Perinat Med 21:125, 1993

Casele HL, Laifer SA: Factors influencing preconception control of glycemia in diabetic women. Arch Intern Med 158:1321, 1998

Casey BM, Lucas MJ, McIntire DD, et al: Population impact of universal screening for gestational diabetes. Am J Obstet Gynecol 180:536, 1999

Catalano PM, Avallone DA, Drago BS, et al: Reproducibility of the oral glucose tolerance test in pregnant women. Am J Obstet Gynecol 169:874, 1993

Catalano PM, Huston L, Amini SB, et al: Longitudinal changes in glucose metabolism during pregnancy in obese women with normal glucose tolerance and gestational diabetes mellitus. Am J Obstet Gynecol 180:903, 1999

Chaturvedi N, Stephenson JM, Fuller JH: The relationship between pregnancy and long-term maternal complications in the EURODIAB IDDM complications study. Diabetic Med 12:494, 1995

Chauhan SP, Grobman WA, Gherman RA, et al: Suspicion and treatment of the macrosomic fetus: A review. Am J Obstet Gynecol 193:332, 2005

Chico M, Levine SN, Lewis DF: Normoglycemic diabetic ketoacidosis in pregnancy. J Perinatol 28:310, 2008

Chmait R, Dinise T, Moore T: Prospective observational study to establish predictors of glyburide success in women with gestational diabetes mellitus. J Perinatol 24:617, 2004

Cnattingius C, Berne C, Nordstrom ML: Pregnancy outcome and infant mortality in diabetic patients in Sweden. Diabetic Med 11:696, 1994

Combs CA, Rosenn B, Kitzmiller JL, et al: Early-pregnancy proteinuria in diabetes related to preeclampsia. Obstet Gynecol 82:802, 1993a

Combs CA, Singh NB, Khoury JC: Elective induction versus spontaneous labor after sonographic diagnosis of fetal macrosomia. Obstet Gynecol 81:492, 1993b

Conway D, Langer O: Elective delivery for macrosomia in the diabetic pregnancy: A clinical cost-benefit analysis. Am J Obstet Gynecol 174:331, 1996

Conway DL, Gonzales O, Skiver D: Use of glyburide for the treatment of gestational diabetes: The San Antonio experience. J Matern Fetal Neonatal Med 15:51, 2004

Cousins L: Pregnancy complications among diabetic women: Review 1965–1985. Obstet Gynecol Surv 42:140, 1987

Crowther CA, Hiller JE, Moss JR, et al: Effect of treatment of gestational diabetes mellitus on pregnancy outcomes. N Engl J Med 352:2477, 2005

Cruikshank DP, Pitkin RM, Reynolds WA, et al: Altered maternal calcium homeostasis in diabetic pregnancy. J Clin Endocrinol Metab 50:264, 1980

Dacus JV, Meyer NL, Muram D, et al: Gestational diabetes: Postpartum glucose tolerance testing. Am J Obstet Gynecol 171:927, 1994

Dahl-Jørgensen K, Brinchmann-Hansen O, Hanssen KF, et al: Rapid tightening of blood glucose control leads to transient deterioration of retinopathy in insulin-dependent diabetes mellitus: The Oslo study. BMJ 290:811, 1985

Danilenko-Dixon D, Annamalai A, Mattson L, et al: Perinatal outcomes in consecutive pregnancies discordant for gestational diabetes. Am J Obstet Gynecol 182:S80, 2000

Danilenko-Dixon DR, Van Winter JT, Nelson RL, et al: Universal versus selective gestational diabetes screening: Application of 1997 American Diabetes Association recommendations. Am J Obstet Gynecol 181:798, 1999

Dashe JS, McIntire DD, Twickler DM: Effect of maternal obesity on the ultrasound detection of anomalous fetuses. Obstet Gynecol 113(5):1001, 2009

Dashe JS, Nathan L, McIntire DD, et al: Correlation between amniotic fluid glucose concentration and amniotic fluid volume in pregnancy complicated by diabetes. Am J Obstet Gynecol 182:901, 2000

Daskalakis G, Marinopoulos s, Krielesi V, et al: Placental pathology in women with gestational diabetes. Acta Obstet Gynecol Scand 87:403, 2008

DeMarini S, Mimouni F, Tsang RC, et al: Impact of metabolic control of diabetes during pregnancy on neonatal hypocalcemia: A randomized study. Obstet Gynecol 83:918, 1994

Dempsey JC, Sorensen TK, Williams MA, et al: Prospective study of gestational diabetes mellitus in relation to maternal recreational physical activity before and during pregnancy. Am J Epidemiol 159:663, 2004

DeVeciana M, Major CA, Morgan M, et al: Postprandial versus preprandial blood glucose monitoring in women with gestational diabetes mellitus requiring insulin therapy. N Engl J Med 333:1237, 1995

Diabetes Control and Complications Trial Research Group: The effect of intensive treatment of diabetes on the development and progression of long-term complications in insulin-dependent diabetes mellitus. N Engl J Med 329:977, 1993

Diabetes Prevention Project: The prevalence of retinopathy in impaired glucose tolerance and recent-onset diabetes in the Diabetes Prevention Program. Diabet Med 24:451, 2007

Durnwald C, Huston-Presley L, Amini S, et al: Evaluation of body composition of large-for-gestational-age infants of women with gestational diabetes mellitus compared with women with normal glucose levels. Am J Obstet Gynecol 191:804, 2004

Durnwald C, Landon MB: Glyburide: The new alternative for treating gestational diabetes? Am J Obstet Gynecol 193:1, 2005

Durnwald CP, Landon MB: A comparison of lispro and regular insulin for the management of type 1 and type 2 diabetes in pregnancy. J Matern Fetal Neonatal Med 21:309, 2008

Ecker JL, Greene MF: Gestational diabetes—setting limits, exploring treatment. N Eng J Med 358(19):2061, 2008

Ehrenberg HM, Mercer BM, Catalano PM: The influence of obesity and diabetes on the prevalence of macrosomia. Am J Obstet Gynecol 191:964, 2004

Elman KD, Welch RA, Frank RN, et al: Diabetic retinopathy in pregnancy: A review. Obstet Gynecol 75:119, 1990

Eriksson UJ: Congenital anomalies in diabetic pregnancy. Semin Fetal Neonatal Med 14(2):85, 2009

Espinosa de los Monteros A, Parra A, Carino N, et al: The reproducibility of the 50-g, 1-hour glucose screen for diabetes in pregnancy. Obstet Gynecol 82:515, 1993

Farrar D, Tufnell DJ, West J: Continuous subcutaneous insulin infusion versus multiple daily injections of insulin for pregnant women with diabetes. Cochrane Database Syst Rev 3:CD005542, 2007

Feig DS, Palda VA: Type 2 diabetes in pregnancy: A growing concern. Lancet 359:1690, 2002

Ferrara A: Increasing prevalence of gestational diabetes. Diabetes Care 30:S141, 2007

Ferrara A, Kahn HS, Quesenberry CP, et al: An increase in the incidence of gestational diabetes mellitus: Northern California, 1991–2000. Obstet Gynecol 103:526, 2004

Frank RN: Diabetic retinopathy. N Engl J Med 350:48, 2004

Franz MJ, Bantle JP, Beebe CA, et al: Nutrition principles and recommendations in diabetes. Diabetes Care 27(Suppl 1):S36, 2004

Gabbe S, Gregory R, Power M, et al: Management of diabetes mellitus by obstetricians-gynecologists. Obstet Gynecol 103:1229, 2004

Gabbe SG, Graves CR: Management of diabetes mellitus complicating pregnancy. Obstet Gynecol 102:857, 2003

Gabbe SG, Mestman JH, Freeman RK, et al: Management and outcome of diabetes mellitus, classes B–R. Am J Obstet Gynecol 129:723, 1977

Gale EAM: Is there really an epidemic of type 2 diabetes? Lancet 362:503, 2003

Gandhi JA, Zhang Y, Maidman JE: Fetal cardiac hypertrophy and cardiac function in diabetic pregnancies. Am J Obstet Gynecol 173:1132, 1995

Garner P: Type 1 diabetes mellitus and pregnancy. Lancet 346:157, 1995a

Garner P, Okun N, Keely E, et al: A randomized controlled trial of strict glycemic control and tertiary level obstetric care versus routine obstetric care in the management of gestational diabetes: A pilot study. Am J Obstet Gynecol 177:190, 1997

Garner PR: Type 1 diabetes and pregnancy. Correspondence. Lancet 346:966, 1995b

Getahun D, Nath C, Ananth CV, et al: Gestational diabetes in the United States: Temporal trends 1989 through 2004. Am J Obstet Gynecol 198: 525.e1, 2008

Girsen A, Ala-Kopsala M, Mäkikallio K, et al: Increased fetal cardiac natriuretic peptide secretion in type-1 diabetic pregnancies. Acta Obstet Gynecol Scand 87:307, 2008

Gluck L, Kulovich MV: Lecithin:sphingomyelin ratios in amniotic fluid in normal and abnormal pregnancy. Am J Obstet Gynecol 115:539, 1973

Glueck CJ, Goldenberg N, Wang P, et al: Metformin during pregnancy reduces insulin, insulin resistance, insulin secretion, weight, testosterone and development of gestational diabetes: Prospective longitudinal assessment of women with polycystic ovary syndrome from preconception throughout pregnancy. Hum Reprod 19:510, 2004

Gonen R, Bader D, Ajami M: Effects of policy of elective cesarean delivery in cases of suspected fetal macrosomia on the incidence of brachial plexus injury and the rate of cesarean delivery. Am J Obstet Gynecol 183:1296, 2000

Van Ballegooie E, Hooymans JMM, Timmerman Z, et al: Rapid deterioration of diabetic retinopathy during treatment with continuous subcutaneous insulin infusion. Diabetes Care 7:236, 1984

Verhaeghe J, Van Bree B, Van Herck E, et al: C-peptide, insulin-like growth factor I and II, and insulin-like growth factor binding protein-1 in umbilical cord serum: Correlations with birthweight. Am J Obstet Gynecol 169:89, 1993

Vink JY, Poggi SH, Ghidini A: Amniotic fluid index and birth weight: Is there a relationship in diabetics with poor glycemic control? Am J Obstet Gynecol 195:848, 2006

Wang PH, Lau J, Chalmers TC: Meta-analysis of effects of intensive blood-glucose control on late complications of type 1 diabetes. Lancet 341:1306, 1993

Way GL: The natural history of hypertrophic cardiomyopathy in infants of diabetic mothers. J Pediatr 95:1020, 1979

Weiss PAM, Haeusler M, Kainer F, et al: Toward universal criteria for gestational diabetes: Relationships between seventy-five and one hundred gram glucose loads and between capillary and venous concentrations. Am J Obstet Gynecol 178:830, 1998

White P: Classification of obstetric diabetes. Am J Obstet Gynecol 130:228, 1978

Willman SP, Leveno KJ, Guzick DS, et al: Glucose threshold for macrosomia in pregnancy complicated by diabetes. Am J Obstet Gynecol 154:470, 1986

World Health Organization: Diabetes Mellitus: Report of a WHO Study Group. Technical Report Series No. 727, Geneva, WHO, 1985

Yang J, Cummings EA, O'Connell C, et al: Fetal and neonatal outcomes of diabetic pregnancies. Obstet Gynecol 108:644, 2006

Yogev Y, Ben-Haroush AB, Chen R, et al: Undiagnosed asymptomatic hypoglycemia: Diet, insulin and glyburide for gestational diabetic pregnancy. Obstet Gynecol 104:88, 2004

Zhang S, Folsom AR, Flack JM, et al: Body fat distribution before pregnancy and gestational diabetes: Findings from Coronary Artery Risk Development in Young Adults (CARDIA) study. BMJ 311:1139, 1995

CHAPTER 53

Thyroid and Other Endocrine Disorders

A variety of endocrine disorders can complicate pregnancy and vice versa. Diabetes mellitus is the most prevalent and is discussed in Chapter 52 (p. 1104). Thyroid disorders are also common, and a number of less common endocrinopathies—for example, pheochromocytoma—can have devastating effects on pregnancy outcome. The pathogenesis of many endocrinopathies is disordered autoimmunity. And as with most organ-specific autoimmune disorders, clinical manifestations of endocrinopathies result from a complex interplay among genetic, environmental, and endogenous factors that activate the immune system against target cells (Weetman, 2004). In many cases, a nonspecific event such as a viral infection initiates an organ-specific response with subsequent immune-mediated glandular destruction. Also, studies implicating cells transferred between mother and fetus during pregnancy in development of autoimmune disease decades later represent a new investigative frontier (Muraji and associates, 2008; Rust and Bianchi, 2009).

THYROID DISORDERS

Taken in aggregate, thyroid disorders are common in young women. There is an intimate relationship between maternal and fetal thyroid function, and drugs that affect the maternal thyroid also affect the fetal gland. Thyroid autoantibodies have been associated with increased early pregnancy wastage, and uncontrolled thyrotoxicosis and untreated hypothyroidism are both associated with adverse pregnancy outcomes (Männistö and colleagues, 2009). Finally, there is evidence that the severity of autoimmune thyroid disorders is ameliorated during pregnancy, only to be exacerbated postpartum.

Thyroid Physiology and Pregnancy

The impact of pregnancy on maternal thyroid physiology is substantial. Changes in the structure and function of the gland sometimes cause confusion in the diagnosis of thyroid abnormalities. These are discussed in greater detail in Chapter 5 (p. 126), and normal hormone level changes are found in the Appendix. Maternal serum concentration of thyroid-binding globulin is increased concomitantly with total or bound thyroid hormone levels (Fig. 5-16). *Thyrotropin,* or *thyroid-stimulating hormone (TSH),* currently plays a central role in screening and diagnosis of many thyroid disorders. Serum thyrotropin levels in early pregnancy decrease because of thyroid stimulation from the weak TSH effects of human chorionic gonadotropin (hCG) (Grossman and associates, 1997). TSH does not cross the placenta. At the same time, hCG serum levels are maximal for the first 12 weeks, free thyroxine levels increase to suppress pituitary thyrotropin secretion (Fig. 53-1). Accordingly, *thyrotropin-releasing hormone (TRH)* is undetectable in maternal serum. Fetal serum TRH is detectable beginning at midpregnancy, but does not increase.

Throughout pregnancy, maternal thyroxine is transferred to the fetus (Calvo and associates, 2002; Vulsma and colleagues, 1989). Maternal thyroxine is important for normal fetal brain development, especially prior to development of fetal thyroid gland function (Bernal, 2007). And even though the fetal gland begins concentrating iodine and synthesizing thyroid hormone after 12 weeks, maternal thyroxine contribution remains important. In fact, maternal thyroxine accounts for 30 percent of thyroxine in fetal serum at term (Thorpe-Beeston and colleagues, 1991; Vulsma and co-workers, 1989). Developmental risks associated with maternal hypothyroidism after midpregnancy remain poorly understood (Morreale de Escobar and colleagues, 2004).

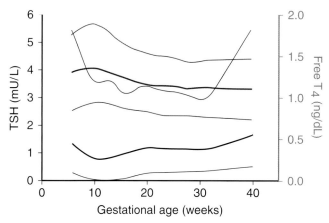

FIGURE 53-1 Gestational age-specific values for serum thyroid-stimulating hormone (TSH) levels (*black lines*) and free thyroxine (T$_4$) levels (*blue lines*). Data were derived from 17,298 women tested during pregnancy. For each color, the dark solid lines represent the 50th percentile, whereas the upper and lower light lines represent the 2.5th and 97.5th percentiles, respectively. (Data from Casey and colleagues, 2005; Dashe and co-workers, 2005.)

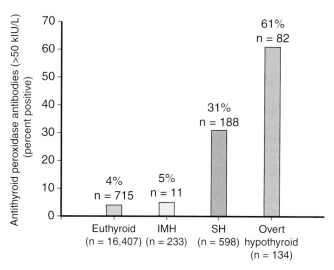

FIGURE 53-2 Incidence of antithyroid peroxidase antibodies in women who are euthyroid; in those with isolated maternal hypothyroxinemia (IMH), defined by a normal serum thyroid-stimulating hormone (TSH) value and serum free thyroxine (T$_4$) level < 0.86 ng/dL; in those with subclinical hypothyroidism (SH), defined as serum TSH value ≥ 3.0 mU/L with a normal reference range serum free T$_4$ level; and in those with overt hypothyroidism defined by an abnormally high serum TSH value with an abnormally low serum free T$_4$ level. (Data from Casey and associates, 2007.)

Autoimmunity and Thyroid Disease

Most thyroid disorders are inextricably linked to the presence of autoantibodies to various cell components. A number of these antibodies variably stimulate thyroid function, block function, or cause thyroid inflammation that may lead to follicular cell destruction. Oftentimes, these effects overlap or even coexist.

Thyroid-stimulating autoantibodies, also called *thyroid-stimulating immunoglobulins (TSI)*, bind to the thyrotropin receptor and activate it, causing thyroid hyperfunction and growth. Although these antibodies are identified in most patients with classic Graves disease, simultaneous production of *thyroid-stimulating blocking antibodies* may blunt this effect (Weetman, 2000). *Thyroid peroxidase antibodies*, previously called thyroid *microsomal autoantibodies,* have been identified in 5 to 15 percent of all pregnant women as shown in Figure 53-2 (Casey and colleagues, 2007; Kuijpens and co-workers, 2001). These antibodies have been associated with early pregnancy loss (Abramson and Stagnaro-Green, 2001). Conversely, women with antibodies identified in the first half of pregnancy did not have increased rates of poor pregnancy outcomes (Casey and colleagues, 2008). These women are, however, at high risk for postpartum thyroid dysfunction and at lifelong risk for permanent thyroid failure (Hidaka and associates, 1994; Premawardhana and co-workers, 2000).

Autoimmune thyroid disease is much more common in women than in men. One intriguing explanation for this disparity is fetal-to-maternal cell trafficking. When fetal lymphocytes enter the maternal circulation, they can live for more than 20 years. Stem cell interchange also seems likely with engraftment in a number of maternal tissues to include the thyroid (Bianchi and Romero, 2003; Khosrotehrani and associates, 2004). Such maternal *microchimerism* with male fetuses has been identified in some women who have the *SRY* sex-determining gene. Up to a third of women who have borne a male fetus have *SRY*-positive lymphocytes in their peripheral blood. Specimens from women with thyroiditis or Graves disease also have *SRY*-positive thyrocyte microchimerism with a greater frequency and intensity than euthyroid controls (Ando and associates, 2002; Klintschar and colleagues, 2001). A high prevalence of Y-chromosome-positive cells has also been identified using fluorescent in situ hybridization in thyroid glands of women with Hashimoto thyroiditis—60 percent, or Graves disease—40 percent (Renné and co-workers, 2004). These are presumed to have arisen from stem cells acquired from a male fetus.

Hyperthyroidism

Symptomatic thyrotoxicosis or hyperthyroidism complicates 1 in 1000 to 2000 pregnancies as shown in Table 53-1 (Casey and Leveno, 2006; Mestman and colleagues, 1995). Because normal pregnancy simulates some clinical findings similar to thyroxine (T$_4$) excess, mild thyrotoxicosis may be difficult to diagnose. Suggestive findings include tachycardia that exceeds that usually seen with normal pregnancy, thyromegaly, exophthalmos, and failure to gain weight despite adequate food intake. Laboratory confirmation is by a markedly depressed thyrotropin (TSH) level along with an elevated serum free T$_4$ (fT$_4$) level. Rarely, hyperthyroidism is caused by abnormally high serum triiodothyronine (T$_3$) levels—so-called *T$_3$-toxicosis.*

Thyrotoxicosis and Pregnancy

The overwhelming cause of thyrotoxicosis in pregnancy is *Graves disease,* an organ-specific autoimmune process usually associated with thyroid-stimulating antibodies as previously discussed. Such antibody activity declines during pregnancy, and it

TABLE 53-1. Incidence of Hyper- and Hypothyroidism in Two Large Cohorts of Pregnant Women Undergoing Serum Thyrotropin Screening

Thyroid Activity	Casey et al (2005, 2007) (n = 17,298)[a]	Cleary-Goldman et al (2008) (n = 10,990)[b]
Hyperthyroidism	1.7%	
Overt	0.5/1000	
Subclinical	1.7%	
Hypothyroidism	2.5%	2.5%
Overt	2/1000	3/1000
Subclinical	2.3%	2.2%

[a]Before 20 weeks.
[b]First trimester.

may become undetectable in the third trimester (Kung and Jones, 1998; Smyth and co-workers, 2005). Amino and colleagues (2003) have found that levels of blocking antibodies are also decreased during pregnancy.

Treatment. Thyrotoxicosis during pregnancy can nearly always be controlled by thionamide drugs. Some clinicians prefer *propylthiouracil (PTU)* because it partially inhibits the conversion of T_4 to T_3 and crosses the placenta less readily than *methimazole*. Although not definitely proven, methimazole use in early pregnancy has been associated with a rare methimazole embryopathy characterized by *esophageal* or *choanal atresia* as well as *aplasia cutis*, which is a congenital skin defect (Diav-Citrin and Ornoy, 2002; Di Gianantonio and colleagues, 2001). Although these malformations are uncommon in women treated with methimazole, and despite the lack of epidemiological studies that PTU is safer, PTU still is the preferred thionamide in the United States (Brent, 2008).

Transient leukopenia can be documented in up to 10 percent of women taking antithyroid drugs but does not require cessation of therapy. In 0.3 to 0.4 percent, *agranulocytosis* develops suddenly and mandates discontinuance of the drug. It is not dose related, and because of its acute onset, serial leukocyte counts during therapy are not helpful. Thus, if fever or sore throat develop, women are instructed to discontinue medication immediately and report for a complete blood count (Brent, 2008). Hepatotoxicity is another potentially serious side effect that occurs in 0.1 to 0.2 percent. Approximately 20 percent of patients treated with PTU develop *antineutrophil cytoplasmic antibodies (ANCA)*, but only a small percentage of these go on to develop serious vasculitis (Helfgott, 2002). Finally, although thionamides have the potential to cause fetal complications, these are uncommon. In some cases, thionamides may even be therapeutic, because thyrotropin receptor antibodies cross the placenta and can stimulate the fetal thyroid gland to cause thyrotoxicosis and goiter.

The initial propylthiouracil dose is empirical. For nonpregnant patients, the American Thyroid Association recommends an initial daily dose of 100 to 600 mg for PTU or 10 to 40 mg

for methimazole (Singer and colleagues, 1995). At Parkland Hospital, we usually start with 300 or 450 mg of PTU daily for our pregnant patients. In our experience, overt thyrotoxicosis in pregnant women requires higher doses than are recommended by most (Davis and colleagues, 1989). With a PTU dose that averaged 600 mg daily, only half of women had a remission, and in these, the dose was decreased to less than 300 mg daily within 8 weeks. In a third, however, it was necessary to increase the dose. Serum free T_4 is considered a better indicator of thyroid status than TSH during the first 2 to 3 months of treatment for hyperthyroidism (National Academy of Clinical Biochemistry Guidelines, 2002).

Subtotal thyroidectomy can be performed after thyrotoxicosis is medically controlled. This seldom is done during pregnancy but may be appropriate for the very few women who cannot adhere to medical treatment or in whom drug therapy proves toxic (Davison and co-workers, 2001). **Ablation with therapeutic radioactive iodine is contraindicated during pregnancy.** Therapeutic doses for maternal thyroid disease may also cause fetal thyroid gland destruction. Thus, when given unintentionally, most clinicians recommend abortion. Any exposed infant must be carefully evaluated for hypothyroidism (Berg and colleagues, 1998). The incidence of fetal hypothyroidism depends on gestational age and radioiodine dose (Berlin, 2001). There is no evidence that therapeutic radioiodine given before pregnancy causes fetal anomalies if enough time has passed to allow radiation effects to dissipate and the woman is euthyroid (Ayala and associates, 1998; Casara and colleagues, 1993). The International Commission on Radiological Protection has recommended that women avoid pregnancy for 6 months after radioablative therapy (Brent, 2008).

Pregnancy Outcome

Women with thyrotoxicosis have pregnancy outcomes that largely depend on whether metabolic control is achieved. For example, excess thyroxine may cause miscarriage (Anselmo and associates, 2004). In untreated women or in those who remain hyperthyroid despite therapy, there is a higher incidence of

TABLE 53-2. Pregnancy Outcomes in 239 Women with Overt Thyrotoxicosis

Factor	Treated and Euthyroid (n = 149)	Uncontrolled Thyrotoxicosis (n = 90)
Maternal outcome		
Preeclampsia	17 (11%)	15 (17%)
Heart failure	1	7 (8%)
Death	—	1
Perinatal outcome		
Preterm delivery	12 (8%)	29 (32%)
Growth restriction	11 (7%)	15 (17%)
Stillbirth	0/59	6/33 (18%)
Thyrotoxicosis	1	2
Hypothyroidism	4	0
Goiter	2	0

Data from Davis (1989), Kriplani (1994), Millar (1994), and all their colleagues.

preeclampsia, heart failure, and adverse perinatal outcomes (Table 53-2). Perinatal mortality rates varied from 6 to 12 percent in several studies.

Fetal and Neonatal Effects

In most cases, the perinate is euthyroid. In some, however, hyper- or hypothyroidism can develop with or without a goiter (Fig. 53-3). Clinical hyperthyroidism occurs in approximately 1 percent of neonates born to women with Graves disease (Luton and colleagues, 2005). If fetal thyroid disease is suspected, nomograms are available for sonographically measured thyroid

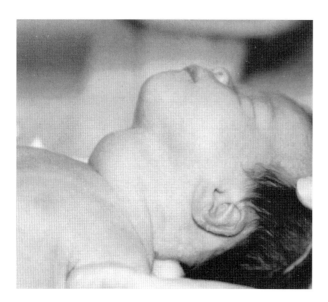

FIGURE 53-3 Term neonate delivered of a woman with a 3-year history of thyrotoxicosis that recurred at 26 weeks' gestation. The mother was given methimazole, 30 mg orally daily, and she was euthyroid at delivery. Laboratory studies showed that the infant was hypothyroid.

volume (Ranzini and co-workers, 2001). Newborns exposed to excessive maternal thyroxine may have any of several clinical presentations.

1. The fetus or newborn may manifest goitrous thyrotoxicosis caused by placental transfer of thyroid-stimulating immunoglobulins. *Nonimmune hydrops* and fetal demise have been reported with fetal thyrotoxicosis (Nachum and co-workers, 2003; Stulberg and Davies, 2000). In a study of 72 pregnant women with Graves disease, Luton and colleagues (2005) reported that none of the fetuses in 31 low-risk mothers had a goiter, and all were euthyroid at delivery. Low risk was defined by no antithyroid medications during the third trimester or absence of antithyroid antibodies. Conversely, in a group of 41 women who either were taking antithyroid medication at delivery or had thyroid receptor antibodies, 11 fetuses—27 percent—had sonographic evidence of a goiter at 32 weeks. Seven of these 11 were determined to be hypothyroid, and the remainder were hyperthyroid. If the fetus is thyrotoxic, treatment is by adjustment of maternal thionamide drugs (Duncombe and Dickinson, 2001). Occasionally, neonatal thyrotoxicosis may also require short-course antithyroid drug treatment.

2. Fetal exposure to maternally administered thionamides as described above may cause goitrous hypothyroidism (Fig. 53-3). Although there are theoretical neurological implications of fetal hypothyroidism, reports of adverse fetal effects seem to have been exaggerated. Available data indicate that thionamides carry an extremely small risk for causing neonatal hypothyroidism (Momotani and associates, 1997; O'Doherty and colleagues, 1999). For example, of the 239 treated thyrotoxic women shown in Table 53-1, there was evidence of hypothyroidism in only four infants despite relatively high maternal doses of propylthiouracil. Furthermore, at least four long-term studies report no abnormal

intellectual and physical development of these children (Mestman, 1998). If hypothyroidism is identified, the fetus can be treated by a reduction in maternal antithyroid medication and injection of intra-amnionic thyroxine if necessary.

3. The fetus may develop nongoitrous hypothyroidism from transplacental passage of maternal thyrotropin-receptor blocking antibodies (Gallagher and associates, 2001).

4. Even after maternal thyroid gland ablation, usually with ^{131}I radioiodine, fetal thyrotoxicosis may result from transplacental thyroid-stimulating antibodies.

Fetal Diagnosis. Fetal thyroid function evaluation is somewhat controversial. Although fetal thyroid sonographic assessment has been reported in women taking thionamide drugs or those with thyroid-stimulating antibodies, most investigators do not currently recommend routine evaluation (Cohen and associates, 2003; Luton and colleagues, 2005). For example, Kilpatrick (2003) recommends fetal antibody testing only if the mother has previously undergone ^{131}I ablation. Because fetal hyper- or hypothyroidism may cause hydrops, growth restriction, goiter, or tachycardia, fetal blood sampling seems appropriate if these conditions develop during pregnancy complicated by Graves disease (Brand and co-workers, 2005).

Thyroid Storm and Heart Failure

Thyroid storm is an acute, life-threatening, hypermetabolic state and is rare in pregnancy. In contrast, pulmonary hypertension and heart failure from cardiomyopathy caused by the profound myocardial effects of thyroxine is common in pregnant women (Sheffield and Cunningham, 2004). As shown in Table 53-2, heart failure developed in 8 percent of 90 women with uncontrolled thyrotoxicosis. In these women, cardiomyopathy is characterized by a high-output state, which may lead to a dilated cardiomyopathy (Fadel and colleagues, 2000; Klein and Ojamaa, 1998). The pregnant woman with thyrotoxicosis has minimal cardiac reserve, and decompensation is usually precipitated by preeclampsia, anemia, sepsis, or a combination of these. Fortunately, thyroxine-induced cardiomyopathy and pulmonary hypertension are frequently reversible (Sheffield and Cunningham, 2004; Siu and associates, 2007; Vydt and colleagues, 2006).

Management. Treatment for thyroid storm or heart failure is similar and should be carried out in an intensive care unit (Zeeman and colleagues, 2003). Specific treatment consists of 1000 mg of PTU given orally or crushed and placed through a nasogastric tube. PTU is continued in 200-mg doses every 6 hours. An hour after initial PTU administration, iodide is given to inhibit thyroidal release of T_3 and T_4. It is given intravenously as 500 to 1000 mg of sodium iodide every 8 hours; orally as 5 drops of supersaturated solution of potassium iodide (SSKI) every 8 hours; or as Lugol solution, 10 drops orally every 8 hours. With a history of iodine-induced anaphylaxis, lithium carbonate, 300 mg every 6 hours, is given instead (Burch and Wartofsky, 1993). Most authorities recommend dexamethasone, 2 mg intravenously every 6 hours for four doses, to further

block peripheral conversion of T_4 to T_3. If a β-blocker drug is given to control tachycardia, its effect on heart failure must be considered. Propranolol, labetalol, and esmolol have all been used successfully intrapartum (Bowman and colleagues, 1998). Coexisting severe preeclampsia, infection, or anemia should be aggressively managed.

Hyperemesis Gravidarum and Gestational Thyrotoxicosis

Many women with hyperemesis gravidarum have abnormally high serum thyroxine levels and low thyrotropin levels (see Chap. 49, p. 1050). This results from thyrotropin receptor stimulation from massive—but normal for pregnancy—concentrations of hCG. This transient condition is also termed *gestational thyrotoxicosis*. Even if associated with hyperemesis, antithyroid drugs are not warranted (American College of Obstetricians and Gynecologists, 2002). Serum thyroxine and thyrotropin values become more normal by midpregnancy.

Gestational Trophoblastic Disease

Thyroxine levels in women with molar pregnancy usually are appreciably elevated. As discussed, abnormally high hCG levels lead to overstimulation of the TSH receptor. Because these tumors are now usually diagnosed early, clinically apparent hyperthyroidism has become less common (Goodwin and Hershman, 1997). With definitive treatment, serum free-T_4 levels usually normalize in parallel with the decline in hCG concentrations. This is discussed further in Chapter 11 (p. 260).

Subclinical Hyperthyroidism

Introduction into clinical practice of third-generation thyrotropin assays with an analytical sensitivity of 0.002 mU/mL makes it possible to identify subclinical thyroid disorders. These biochemically defined extremes usually represent normal biological variations but may herald the earliest stages of thyroid dysfunction. *Subclinical hyperthyroidism* is characterized by an abnormally low serum thyrotropin concentration in concert with thyroxine hormone levels within the normal reference range (Surks and associates, 2004). Long-term effects of persistent subclinical thyrotoxicosis include osteoporosis, cardiovascular morbidity, and progression to overt thyrotoxicosis or thyroid failure. Casey and Leveno (2006) identified subclinical hyperthyroidism in 1.7 percent of pregnant women (Table 53-1). Importantly, these investigators showed that subclinical hyperthyroidism was not associated with adverse pregnancy outcomes.

Management

Currently there is no convincing evidence that subclinical hyperthyroidism should be treated in nonpregnant individuals. Thus, it seems especially unwarranted in pregnancy because antithyroid drugs reach the fetus. Women identified with subclinical hyperthyroidism may benefit from periodic surveillance, and approximately half eventually have normal thyrotropin concentrations.

Hypothyroidism

Overt hypothyroidism complicates from 2 to 3 pregnancies per 1000 (Casey and colleagues, 2005; Cleary-Goldman and associates, 2008). It is characterized by insidious nonspecific clinical findings that include fatigue, constipation, cold intolerance, muscle cramps, and weight gain. A pathologically enlarged thyroid gland depends on the etiology of hypothyroidism and is more likely in women in areas of endemic iodine deficiency or those with Hashimoto thyroiditis. Other findings include edema, dry skin, hair loss, and prolonged relaxation phase of deep tendon reflexes. *Clinical* or *overt hypothyroidism* is diagnosed when an abnormally high serum thyrotropin level is accompanied by an abnormally low thyroxine level. *Subclinical hypothyroidism* is defined by an elevated serum thyrotropin level and *normal* serum thyroxine concentration (Surks and associates, 2004).

Overt Hypothyroidism and Pregnancy

The most common cause of hypothyroidism in pregnancy is Hashimoto thyroiditis, characterized by glandular destruction from autoantibodies, particularly antithyroid peroxidase antibodies. Clinical identification of hypothyroidism is especially difficult during pregnancy because many of the signs or symptoms are also common to pregnancy itself. Thyroid testing should be performed on symptomatic women or those with a history of thyroid disease (American College of Obstetricians and Gynecologists, 2002). *Severe* hypothyroidism with pregnancy is uncommon, probably because it is often associated with infertility and increased miscarriage rates (Abalovich and colleagues, 2002).

Treatment. Replacement therapy for hypothyroidism is with levothyroxine in doses of 1 to 2 μg/kg/day or approximately 100 μg daily. Serum thyrotropin levels are measured at 4- to 6-week intervals, and the thyroxine dose is adjusted by 25- to 50-μg increments until normal TSH values between 0.5 and 2.5 mU/L are reached. Pregnancy is associated with an increase in thyroxine requirements in approximately a third of supplemented women (Alexander and associates, 2004). Because a similar increased requirement is seen in women with postmenopausal hypothyroidism after estrogen replacement, the increased demand in pregnancy is believed to be related to increased estrogen production (Alexander and colleagues, 2004; Arafah, 2001).

Increased thyroxine requirements begin as early as 5 weeks. Thus, significant hypothyroidism may develop early in women without thyroid reserve such as those with a previous thyroidectomy, history of radioiodine ablation, or those undergoing assisted reproductive techniques (Alexander, 2004; Loh, 2009; Rotondi, 2004, and all their colleagues). Increasing thyroxine replacement by 25 percent at pregnancy confirmation will reduce this likelihood. All other women with hypothyroidism should undergo TSH testing at initiation of prenatal care.

Pregnancy Outcome with Overt Hypothyroidism. Observational studies, although limited, indicate that there are excessive adverse perinatal outcomes associated with overt thyroxine deficiency (Table 53-3). With appropriate replacement therapy however, several recent studies show no increase in perinatal morbidity rates (Matalon, 2006; Tan, 2006; Wolfberg, 2005; and all their co-workers). However, Wikner and co-workers (2008) found an increased risk for some pregnancy complications even in those taking replacement therapy. Most experts agree that adequate hormone replacement during pregnancy minimizes the risk of adverse outcomes and most complications (Abalovich and associates, 2002).

Fetal and Neonatal Effects. There is no doubt that maternal and fetal thyroid abnormalities are related. In both, thyroid function is dependent on adequate iodide intake, and its deficiency early in pregnancy can cause both maternal and fetal hypothyroidism. And as discussed, maternal TSH-receptor-blocking antibodies can cross the placenta and cause fetal thyroid dysfunction. The more common antithyroid peroxidase and antithyroglobulin antibodies, however, have little or no effect on

TABLE 53-3. Pregnancy Complications in 112 Women with Hypothyroidism

Complications	Hypothyroidism (Percent)	
	Overt (n = 49)	Subclinical (n = 63)
Preeclampsia	31	16
Placental abruption	8	0
Cardiac dysfunction	3	2
Birthweight less than 2000 g[a]	31	19
Stillbirths	8	2[b]

[a]Preterm or term delivery were the only outcomes reported by Abalovich and colleagues (2002).
[b]One infant died from syphilis.
Modified from Abalovich (2002), Davis (1988), and Leung (1993), and all their associates.

fetal thyroid function even though they too cross the placenta (Fisher, 1997). Maternal Hashimoto thyroiditis is not typically associated with fetal thyroid dysfunction. In fact, prevalence of fetal hypothyroidism in women with Hashimoto thyroiditis is estimated to be only 1 in 180,000 neonates (Brown and co-workers, 1996).

Subclinical Hypothyroidism

The incidence of subclinical hypothyroidism in women between 18 and 45 years of age is about 5 percent (Canaris and colleagues, 2000). In two large studies totaling more than 25,000 pregnant women screened in the first half of pregnancy, subclinical hypothyroidism was identified in 1.7 and 2.3 percent of women (Table 53-1). The rate of progression to overt thyroid failure is impacted by TSH level, age, other disorders such as diabetes, and presence of antithyroid antibodies. Diez and Iglesias (2004) prospectively followed 93 nonpregnant women with subclinical hypothyroidism for 5 years and reported that in a third, TSH values became normal. In the other two thirds, those women whose TSH levels were 10 to 15 mU/L developed overt disease at a rate of 19 per 100 patient-years. Those women whose TSH levels were < 10 mU/L developed overt hypothyroidism at a rate of 2 per 100 patient-years. The U.S. Preventative Services Task Force on screening for subclinical hypothyroidism also reported that nearly all patients who develop overt hypothyroidism within 5 years have an initial TSH level greater than 10 mU/L (Helfand, 2004; Karmisholt and associates, 2008). TSH analyses have a much higher variance at these higher levels. Consequently, the likelihood of development of overt hypothyroidism during pregnancy in otherwise healthy women with subclinical hypothyroidism seems unlikely.

Subclinical Hypothyroidism and Pregnancy

Small observational studies shown in Table 53-3 were suggestive that subclinical hypothyroidism might be associated with adverse pregnancy outcomes. Interest was further heightened by two studies that suggested that undiagnosed maternal thyroid hypofunction may impair fetal neuropsychological development. In one study, Pop and associates (1999) described 22 women who had free T_4 levels below the 10th percentile in early pregnancy whose offspring were at increased risk for impaired psychomotor development. In the other study, Haddow and colleagues (1999) retrospectively evaluated children born to 48 untreated women whose serum thyrotropin values exceeded the 98th percentile. Some had diminished school performance, reading recognition, and IQ scores. Although described as "subclinically hypothyroid," these women had an abnormally low mean serum free thyroxine level and thus likely had overt hypothyroidism.

To further evaluate any adverse effects, Casey and co-workers (2005) identified subclinical hypothyroidism in 2.3 percent of 17,298 women screened before midpregnancy. As shown in Table 53-4, these women had higher incidences of preterm birth, placental abruption, and admission of infants to the intensive care nursery compared with control women. In the study of 10,990 First- and Second-Trimester Evaluation of Risk (FASTER) Trial participants, Cleary-Goldman and associates (2008) did not find a link with these adverse obstetrical outcomes.

In a subsequent study of these 17,298 women with subclinical hypothyroidism, Casey and colleagues (2008) showed that 31 percent had antithyroid peroxidase antibodies compared with 4 percent of euthyroid controls. The cohort with TPO antibodies had a significant threefold risk for placental abruption. Cleary-Goldman and associates (2008) measured antithyroglobulin and antithyroid peroxidase antibodies in the FASTER Trial cohort of 10,990 women and reported an incidence of approximately 15 percent of either antibodies present. When both were present, risk for preterm prematurely ruptured membranes was increased by almost threefold.

Thyrotropin Screening in Pregnancy. Because of the 1999 studies cited above, some organizations have recommended routine prenatal screening and treatment for subclinical hypothyroidism (Gharib and associates, 2005). The American College of Obstetricians and Gynecologists (2002) concluded

TABLE 53-4. Pregnancy Outcomes in Women with Untreated Subclinical Hypothyroidism and Isolated Maternal Hypothyroxinemia Compared with Pregnant Women with Normal Thyroid Function Studies

Outcome	Normal TSH and Free T_4 (n = 16,011)	Subclinical Hypothyroidism (n = 598)	P value	Isolated Hypothyroxinemia (n = 233)	P value
Hypertension (%)	9	9	.68	11	.53
Placental abruption (%)	0.3	1.0	.03	0.4	.75
Gestational age delivered (%)					
≤36 weeks	6.0	7.0	.09	6.0	.84
≤34 weeks	2.5	4.3	.005	2.0	.44
≤32 weeks	1.0	2.2	.13	1.0	.47
RDS—ventilator (%)	1.5	2.5	.05	1.3	.78
Neonatal intensive care (%)	2.2	4.0	.005	1.3	.32

RDS = Respiratory distress syndrome; T_4 = thyroxine; TSH = thyroid-stimulating hormone.
Data from Casey and colleagues (2007).

that although observational data were consistent with the *possibility* that subclinical hypothyroidism was associated with adverse neuropsychological development, there have been no interventional trials to demonstrate improvement. The College thus recommended against implementation of screening until further studies were done to validate or refute these findings. One major concern is that it seems unlikely that treatment given *after* the period of early cerebral development would be totally efficacious to prevent neurological damage (Utiger, 1999).

These issues continue to be the source of debate. At least two consensus conferences were held to reconcile differing viewpoints. Two major groups recommended against routine prenatal thyrotropin screening (Surks and associates, 2004). Subsequently, however, representatives of the American Thyroid Association, American Association of Clinical Endocrinologists, and Endocrine Society published dissenting opinions and recommended routine screening and treatment (Gharib and colleagues, 2005). More recently, following a 2-year development process by an international task force, evaluation of high-risk pregnant women was recommended because current evidence does not justify routine pregnancy screening (Abalovich and co-workers, 2007). Finally, the American College of Obstetricians and Gynecologists (2007) also continues to recommend against routine screening.

Isolated Maternal Hypothyroxinemia

Women with low serum free-T_4 values but a normal range TSH level are considered to have *isolated maternal hypothyroxinemia.* This was identified by Casey and colleagues (2007) in 1.3 percent of more than 17,000 pregnant women screened before 20 weeks. Cleary-Goldman and associates (2008) found a 2.1-percent incidence in the FASTER Trial cohort. As discussed previously, offspring of women with isolated hypothyroxinemia have been reported to have neurodevelopmental difficulties at 3 weeks, 10 months, and 2 years of age (Kooistra and colleagues, 2006; Pop and associates 1999, 2003). These findings have not stimulated recommendations for prenatal serum thyroxine screening. Additionally, free T_4 estimates by crudely available immunoassays may not be accurate during pregnancy because of sensitivity to alterations in binding proteins (Lee and co-workers, 2009).

In a study of 233 women with isolated maternal hypothyroxinemia, Casey and colleagues (2007) reported that there were no increased adverse perinatal outcomes (see Table 53-4). And unlike subclinical hypothyroidism, these women had a low prevalence of antithyroid antibodies (see Fig. 53-2). Moreover, there was no correlation between their TSH and free T_4 levels. Cleary-Goldman and co-workers (2008) reported a twofold incidence of fetal macrosomia in these women. Taken together, these findings indicate the isolated maternal hypothyroxinemia has no apparent serious adverse effects on pregnancy outcome and may simply be a biochemical finding (Casey and co-workers, 2007). Because of this, routine screening for isolated hypothyroxinemia is not recommended.

Iodine Deficiency

Decreasing iodide fortification of table salt and bread products in the United States over the past 25 years resulted in occasional identification of iodide deficiency (Caldwell and colleagues,

2005; Hollowell and associates, 1998). At this time, however, general maternal iodine intake has stabilized. The most recent National Health and Nutrition Examination survey indicated that, overall, the population is again iodine sufficient (Caldwell and co-workers, 2005; Haddow and associates, 2007). Even so, experts agree that iodine nutrition in vulnerable populations such as pregnant women requires continued monitoring.

Iodine and Pregnancy

Adequate iodine is requisite for fetal neurological development beginning soon after conception, and abnormalities are dependent on the degree of deficiency. The World Health Organization (WHO) estimates at least 50 million people worldwide have varying degrees of preventable brain damage due to iodine deficiency (Brundtland, 2002). Although it is doubtful that *mild deficiency* causes intellectual impairment, supplementation does prevent fetal goiter (Fadeyev and colleagues, 2003). Conversely, *severe deficiency* is frequently associated with damage typically encountered with *endemic cretinism* (Delange and co-workers, 2001). Although not quantified, it is presumed that *moderate deficiency* has intermediate and variable effects on intellectual and psychomotor function (Glinoer, 2001).

The Institute of Medicine (2001) recommended daily iodine intake during pregnancy of 220 µg/day and 290 µg/day for lactating women. Iodine supplementation before pregnancy prevents neurological morbidity from severe deficiency and partially does so even if given after pregnancy is established (Cao and colleagues, 1994). The American Thyroid Association has recommended supplementation of pregnant or lactating women with 150 µg of iodine added to prenatal vitamins (Becker and colleagues, 2006). It has even been suggested that because most cases of maternal hypothyroxinemia world wide are related to relative iodine deficiency, suppplementation may obviate the need to consider thyroxine treatment in such women (Gyamfi and associates, 2009). Teng and co-workers (2006) have suggested that excessive iodine intake—defined as > 300 mg/day—may lead to subclinical hypothyroidism and autoimmune thyroiditis.

Congenital Hypothyroidism

Because the clinical diagnosis of hypothyroidism in neonates is usually missed, universal newborn screening was introduced in 1974 and is now required by law. According to the National Newborn Screening and Genetics Resource Center (2008), 1 in 2500 newborns in the United States in 2007 had confirmed hypothyroidism. Developmental disorders of the thyroid gland such as agenesis and hypoplasia account for 80 to 90 percent of these cases (Topaloglu, 2006). The list of identified gene mutations that cause hypothyroidism continues to grow rapidly (Moreno and co-workers, 2008).

Early and aggressive thyroxine replacement is critical for infants with congenital hypothyroidism. Still some infants identified by screening programs with severe congenital hypothyroidism who were treated promptly will exhibit cognitive deficits into adolescence (Song and associates 2001). Therefore, the severity of congenital hypothyroidism, rather than timing of treatment, is an important factor in long-term cognitive outcomes

(Kempers and colleagues, 2006). Olivieri and colleagues (2002) reported that 8 percent of 1420 infants with congenital hypothyroidism also had other major congenital malformations.

Postpartum Thyroiditis

Transient autoimmune thyroiditis is consistently found in 5 to 10 percent of women during the first year after childbirth (Amino and colleagues, 2000; Dayan and Daniels, 1996). The propensity for thyroiditis antedates pregnancy and is directly related to increasing serum levels of thyroid autoantibodies. Women with high antibody titers in early pregnancy commonly are affected (Pearce and co-workers, 2003). Up to 25 percent of women with type 1 diabetes develop postpartum thyroid dysfunction (Alvarez-Marfany and associates, 1994). In some women with quiescent Graves disease, recurrent postpartum hyperthyroxinemia may be stimulated by thyroid destruction (Iitaka and co-workers, 2004).

Clinical Manifestations

In clinical practice, postpartum thyroiditis is diagnosed infrequently because it typically develops months after delivery and has vague and nonspecific symptoms. They often may be ascribed to the stresses of motherhood (Stagnaro-Green and Glinoer, 2004). The two recognized clinical phases of postpartum thyroiditis are summarized in Table 53-5. Between 1 and 4 months after delivery, approximately 4 percent of all women develop transient *destruction-induced thyrotoxicosis* from excessive release of hormone from glandular disruption (Lucas and colleagues, 2000). The onset is abrupt, and a small, painless goiter is commonly found. Although there may be many symptoms, only fatigue and palpitations are more frequent in thyrotoxic women compared with normal controls. The time course of this thyrotoxic phase usually is no longer than a few months and thionamides are ineffective. If symptoms are severe, a β-blocker may be given. Lucas and colleagues (2005) reported that all women with a purely hyperthyroid form of postpartum thyroiditis normalized and remained euthyroid.

Between 4 and 8 months postpartum, 2 to 5 percent of all women develop *hypothyroidism* from thyroiditis (Amino and colleagues, 2000). From thyroiditis onset, hypothyroidism can develop within one month. Thyromegaly and other symptoms are common and more prominent than during the thyrotoxic phase. Thyroxine replacement is typically given for 6 to 12 months, and the dose ranges from 25 to 75 μg/day.

Overall, women who experience either type of postpartum thyroiditis have approximately a 30-percent risk of eventually developing permanent hypothyroidism with an annual progression rate of 3.6 percent (Lucas, 2005; Muller, 2001; Premawardhana, 2000, and all their associates). Others may develop subclinical disease, but half of those with thyroiditis who are positive for peroxidase antibodies develop permanent hypothyroidism by 6 to 7 years.

An association between postpartum thyroiditis and postpartum depression has been proposed but remains unresolved. Lucas and co-workers (2001) found a 1.7-percent incidence of postpartum depression at 6 months in women with thyroiditis as well as in controls. Pederson and colleagues (2007) found a significant correlation between abnormal scores on the Edinburgh Postnatal Depression Scale and total thyroxine values in the low normal range during pregnancy in 31 women. Kuijpens and associates (2001) reported that thyroid peroxidase antibodies were a marker for postpartum depression in euthyroid women.

Nodular Thyroid Disease

Management of a palpable thyroid nodule during pregnancy depends on the stage of gestation. Small nodules detected by sensitive sonographic methods are common during pregnancy in some populations. For example, Kung and associates (2002) used high-resolution sonography and found that 15 percent of Chinese women had nodules larger than 2 mm. Almost half were multiple, and the nodules usually enlarged modestly across pregnancy and did not regress postpartum. Biopsy of those > 5 mm³ that persisted at 3 months usually showed nodular hyperplasia, and none was malignant. In some studies, however, up to 40 percent of solitary nodules were malignant (Doherty and

---

TABLE 53-5. Clinical Phases of Postpartum Thyroid

	Phase of Postpartum Thyroiditis	
Factor	**Thyrotoxicosis**	**Hypothyroidism**
Onset	1–4 months	4–8 months
Incidence	4 percent	2–5 percent
Mechanism	Destruction-induced hormone release	Thyroid insufficiency
Symptoms	Small, painless goiter; fatigue, palpitations	Goiter, fatigue, inability to concentrate
Treatment	β-Blockers for symptoms	Thyroxine for 6–12 months
Sequelae	2/3 become euthyroid 1/3 develop hypothyroidism	1/3 permanently hypothyroid

co-workers, 1995; Rosen and Walfish, 1986). Even so, the majority were low-grade neoplasms.

Most recommend against *radioiodine scanning* in pregnancy, although tracer doses used are associated with minimal fetal irradiation (see Chap. 41, p. 921). *Sonographic* examination reliably detects nodules larger than 0.5 cm, and their solid or cystic nature also is determined. *Fine-needle aspiration* is an excellent method for assessment, and tumor markers and immunostaining are reliable to evaluate for malignancy (Bartolazzi and associates, 2001; Hegedüs, 2004).

Evaluation of thyroid cancer involves a multidisciplinary approach (American College of Obstetricians and Gynecologists, 2002). Most thyroid carcinomas are well differentiated and pursue an indolent course. Thus, some recommend that surgery be postponed until after delivery. Moosa and Mazzaferri (1997) studied 61 women with thyroid cancer diagnosed during pregnancy. In 75 percent, thyroidectomy was delayed until after delivery, and outcomes were similar to those in nonpregnant controls. In their reviews, Driggers and co-workers (1998) and Morris (1998) reported minimal fetal loss attributed to thyroid cancer surgery. We are of the view that thyroid surgery can be safely performed before 24 to 26 weeks. Surgery after this time *might* stimulate preterm labor.

PARATHYROID DISEASES

The function of *parathyroid hormone (PTH)* is to maintain extracellular fluid calcium concentration. This 115-amino acid hormone acts directly on bone and kidney and indirectly on small intestine through its effects on synthesis of vitamin D $(1,25(OH_2)D)$ to increase serum calcium. Secretion is regulated by serum ionized calcium concentration through a negative feedback system. *Calcitonin* is a potent hypocalcemic parathyroid hormone that acts as a physiological parathyroid hormone antagonist. The interrelationships between these hormones and calcium metabolism, as well as *PTH-related protein* produced by fetal tissue, are discussed in Chapter 4 (p. 88).

Fetal calcium needs—300 mg/day in late pregnancy and a total of 30 g—as well as increased renal calcium loss from augmented glomerular filtration, substantively increase maternal calcium demands. Pregnancy is associated with a twofold increase in serum concentrations of 1,25-dihydroxyvitamin D, which increases gastrointestinal calcium absorption. This hormone is probably of placental and decidual origin because PTH levels are low normal or decreased during pregnancy (Molitch, 2000; Seely and colleagues, 1997). Total serum calcium levels decline with serum albumin concentrations, but ionized calcium levels remain unchanged (Dahlman and colleagues, 1994; Power and associates, 1999). Vargas Zapata and colleagues (2004), as well as others, have suggested a role for insulin-like growth factor-1 (IGF-1) in maternal calcium homeostasis and bone turnover, especially in mothers with low calcium intake.

Hyperparathyroidism

Hypercalcemia is caused by hyperparathyroidism or cancer in 90 percent of cases. Primary hyperparathyroidism is reported most often in women older than 50 (Miller and colleagues, 2008). Because many automated laboratory systems include serum calcium measurement, more cases are being detected (Mestman, 2002). It has a reported prevalence of 2 to 3 per 1000 women, but some have estimated the rate to be as high as 14 per 1000 when asymptomatic cases are included (Farford and colleagues, 2007; Schnatz and Thaxton, 2005). Almost 80 percent are caused by a solitary adenoma and another 15 percent by hyperfunction of all four glands. In the remainder, a malignancy and the cause of increased serum calcium are obvious. PTH produced by tumors is not identical to the natural hormone and may not be detected by routine assays.

In most patients, the serum calcium level is only elevated to within 1 mg/dL over the upper normal limit. This may help to explain why only 20 percent of those who have abnormally elevated levels are symptomatic (Bilezikian and Silverberg, 2004). In a fourth, however, symptoms become apparent when the serum calcium level continues to rise. *Hypercalcemic crisis* manifests as stupor, nausea, vomiting, weakness, fatigue, and dehydration.

Guidelines for management of asymptomatic hyperparathyroidism in nonpregnant patients were updated after a 2002 National Institutes of Health Workshop, reported by Bilezikian and Silverberg (2004). Based on long-term follow-up, indications for parathyroidectomy include a serum calcium level 1.0 mg/dL above the upper normal range, daily urine calcium excretion of 400 mg or more, reduced bone density, or age less than 50. Those not meeting these criteria should undergo semiannual calcium measurement.

Hyperparathyroidism in Pregnancy

In their review, Schnatz and Thaxton (2005) found fewer than 200 reported cases complicating pregnancy. As in nonpregnant patients, hyperparathyroidism is usually caused by a parathyroid adenoma. Cases of ectopic parathyroid hormone production and rare cases of parathyroid carcinoma have been reported (Montoro and colleagues, 2000). Symptoms include hyperemesis, generalized weakness, renal calculi, and psychiatric disorders. Occasionally, pancreatitis is the presenting finding (Dahan and Chang, 2001).

Pregnancy theoretically improves hyperparathyroidism because of significant calcium shunting to the fetus and augmented renal excretion (Power and colleagues, 1999). When the "protective effects" of pregnancy are withdrawn, however, there is significant danger of postpartum hypercalcemic crisis. Early reports described excessive stillbirths and preterm deliveries in pregnancies complicated by hyperparathyroidism (Shangold and associates, 1982). The more recent review by Schnatz and Thaxton (2005) cited above reported a 25-percent incidence of preeclampsia, however, other adverse effects were much less common.

Management in Pregnancy. If symptomatic, surgical removal of the parathyroid adenoma is preferable (Mestman, 2002). Elective neck exploration during pregnancy is usually well tolerated, even in the third trimester (Graham, 1998; Kort, 1999; Schnatz, 2005, and all their co-workers). In one woman, a mediastinal adenoma was removed at 23 weeks (Rooney and co-workers, 1998).

If pregnant women are asymptomatic, they may be treated with oral phosphate, 1 to 1.5 g daily in divided doses. Serum calcium levels may decrease so that parathyroidectomy can be postponed until after delivery. For women with dangerously elevated serum calcium levels or those who are mentally obtunded with *hypercalcemic crisis,* emergency treatment is instituted. Diuresis with intravenous normal saline is begun so that urine flow exceeds 150 mL/hr. *Furosemide* is given in conventional doses to block tubular calcium reabsorption. Careful attention to prevent hypokalemia and hypomagnesemia is important. Adjunctive therapy includes *mithramycin,* which inhibits bone resorption; *calcitonin,* which decreases skeletal calcium release; and oral phosphorus.

Neonatal Effects. Normally, cord blood calcium levels are higher than maternal levels. With maternal hyperparathyroidism, abnormally elevated maternal and thence fetal levels further suppress fetal parathyroid function. Because of this, after birth, there is a rapidly decreasing newborn calcium level and 15 to 25 percent of these infants develop severe hypocalcemia with or without tetany (Molitch, 2000). Neonatal tetany or seizures should stimulate a search for maternal hyperparathyroidism (Beattie, 2000; Ip, 2003; Jaafar, 2004, and all their associates).

Hypoparathyroidism

The most common cause of hypocalcemia is hypoparathyroidism that usually follows parathyroid or thyroid surgery. Hypoparathyroidism is estimated to follow up to 7 percent of total thyroidectomies (Shoback, 2008). It is a rare condition, characterized by spasms of the facial muscles, muscle cramps, and paresthesias of the lips, tongue, fingers and feet. Chronically hypocalcemic pregnant women may have a fetus with skeletal demineralization resulting in multiple bone fractures in the neonatal period (Alikasifoglu and colleagues, 2005). Maternal treatment includes 1,25-dihydroxyvitamin D_3 (calcitriol), dihydrotachysterol, or large doses of vitamin D of 50,000 to 150,000 U/day; calcium gluconate or calcium lactate in doses of 3 to 5 g/day; and a diet low in phosphates. The fetal risks from large doses of vitamin D have not been established.

Pregnancy-Associated Osteoporosis

Even with remarkably increased calcium requirements, it is uncertain whether pregnancy causes osteopenia in most women (Kaur and associates, 2003; To and co-workers, 2003). In one study, Naylor and colleagues (2000) evaluated longitudinal bone mineral density change in 16 women during pregnancy. They documented loss of bone density in trabecular bone, but an increase in cortical bone sites. From their review, Thomas and Weisman (2006) cite a 3-to 4-percent average reduction in bone-mineral density during pregnancy. Feigenberg and associates (2008) found cortical bone mass reductions using ultrasound in young primiparas in the puerperium compared with nulligravid controls. Rarely, some women develop idiopathic osteoporosis while pregnant or lactating. Its incidence is estimated to be 4 per million women (Hellmeyer and colleagues, 2007).

The most common symptom of osteoporosis is back pain in late pregnancy or postpartum. Other symptoms are hip pain, either unilateral or bilateral, and difficulty in weight bearing (Dunne and colleagues, 1993; Smith and associates, 1995). In more than half of women, no apparent reason for osteopenia is found. Some known causes include heparin, prolonged bed rest, and corticosteroid therapy (Cunningham, 2005; von Mandach and co-workers, 2003). In a few cases, overt hyperparathyroidism or thyrotoxicosis eventually develops.

Treatment is problematical, but most clinicians recommend calcium and vitamin D supplementation. Long-term follow-up indicates that although bone density improves, these women, as well as their offspring, may have chronic osteopenia (Carbone and colleagues, 1995).

ADRENAL GLAND DISORDERS

Pregnancy has profound effects on adrenal cortical secretion and its control or stimulation. These interrelationships are discussed in detail in Chapter 5 (p. 129).

Pheochromocytoma

These tumors are common findings at autopsy but are infrequently diagnosed. Only 0.1 percent of hypertensive patients have a pheochromocytoma. These chromaffin tumors secrete catecholamines and usually are located in the adrenal medulla, although 10 percent are located in sympathetic ganglia. They are called the *10-percent tumor* because approximately 10 percent are bilateral, 10 percent are extra-adrenal, and 10 percent are malignant. There is an association with medullary thyroid carcinoma and hyperparathyroidism in some of the autosomally dominant or recessive *multiple endocrine neoplasia syndromes* as well as in neurofibromatosis and von Hippel-Lindau disease.

Symptoms are usually paroxysmal and manifest as hypertensive crisis, seizure disorders, or anxiety attacks. Hypertension is sustained in 60 percent of patients, but half of these also have paroxysmal crises. Other symptoms during paroxysmal attacks are headaches, profuse sweating, palpitations, chest pain, nausea and vomiting, and pallor or flushing.

The standard screening test is quantification of catecholamine metabolites in a 24-hour urine specimen (Keely, 1998). Diagnosis is established by measurement of a 24-hour urine collection with at least two of three assays for free catecholamines, metanephrines, or vanillylmandelic acid (VMA). Determination of plasma catecholamine levels may be accurate but is associated with technical difficulties (Conlin, 2001; Lenders and associates, 2002). Boyle and colleagues (2007) determined that measurement of urinary free metanephrine was superior to assessment of a VMA or urinary or plasma catecholamine level in 159 outpatients undergoing evaluation for pheochromocytoma. In nonpregnant patients, adrenal localization is usually successful with either computed tomography (CT) or magnetic resonance (MR) imaging. Occasionally ^{131}I-metaiodobenzylguanidine (MIBG) scanning is necessary to locate extra-adrenal tumors. For most cases, preferred treatment is laparoscopic adrenalectomy (Lal and Duh, 2003).

TABLE 53-6. Outcomes of Pregnancies Complicated by Pheochromocytoma and Reported in Two Contiguous Epochs

	Incidence in Percent	
Factor	1980–1987[a] (n = 48)	1988–1997[b] (n = 42)
Diagnosis		
Antepartum	51	83
Postpartum	36	14
Autopsy	12	2
Maternal mortality	16	4
Fetal wastage	26	11

[a]Data from Harper and colleagues (1989).
[b]Data from Ahlawat and associates (1999).

Pheochromocytoma Complicating Pregnancy

These tumors are rare but dangerous complications of pregnancy. Geelhoed (1983) cited an earlier review of 89 cases in which 43 mothers died. Maternal death was much more common if the tumor was not diagnosed antepartum—58 versus 18 percent. As seen in Table 53-6, with modern management, maternal mortality rates decreased from 16 to 4 percent, and maternal deaths are rare when the diagnosis is made antepartum.

Diagnosis is similar to that for nonpregnant patients. MR imaging is considered the radiological technique of choice during pregnancy because it almost always locates adrenal and extra-adrenal pheochromocytomas, such as that shown in Figure 53-4 (Manger, 2005). In many cases, the principal challenge is to differentiate preeclampsia from the hypertensive crisis caused by pheochromocytoma. Also, as in nonpregnant patients, there are individual considerations. For example, one postpartum woman described by Ahn and associates (2003) presented with dilated cardiomyopathy. Grimbert and colleagues (1999) diagnosed two pheochromocytomas during 56 pregnancies in 30 women with *von Hippel-Lindau disease*. Bassoon-Zaltzman and associates (1995) described a normotensive 20-week pregnant woman with intermittent ventricular tachycardia caused by a bladder pheochromocytoma.

Management. Immediate control of hypertension and symptoms with an α-adrenergic blocker such as *phenoxybenzamine* is imperative. The dose is 10 to 30 mg, two to four times daily. After α-blockade is achieved, β-blockers may be given for tachycardia if necessary. In many cases, surgical exploration and tumor removal are performed during pregnancy (Miller and associates, 2005). Successful laparoscopic removal of adrenal tumors prior to 24 weeks has been reported (Janetschek, 1998; Junglee, 2007; Kim, 2006, and all their colleagues). When diagnosed later in pregnancy, either planned cesarean delivery with excision or postpartum tumor resection is appropriate.

Recurrent tumors are troublesome, and even with good blood pressure control, dangerous peripartum hypertension may develop. We have cared for three women in whom recurrent pheochromocytoma was identified during pregnancy. Hypertension was managed with phenoxybenzamine in all three. Two infants were healthy, but a third was stillborn in a mother with a massive tumor burden who was receiving phenoxybenzamine, 100 mg daily. In all three women, tumor resection was done postpartum. One woman died of persistent metastases several years later.

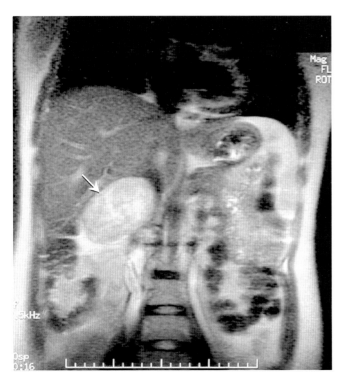

FIGURE 53-4 Coronal magnetic resonance image taken in a 32-week pregnant woman shows a right-sided pheochromocytoma (*arrow*) and its position relative to the liver.

Cushing Syndrome

The most common cause of Cushing syndrome is long-term corticosteroid treatment. Cases of endogenous Cushing syndrome are typically due to *Cushing disease*, which is bilateral adrenal hyperplasia stimulated by corticotropin-producing pituitary adenomas. Most are microadenomas smaller than 1 cm, and half are 5 mm or less. Rarely, abnormal secretion of hypothalamic corticotropin-releasing factor may cause corticotropic hyperplasia. Hyperplasia may also be caused by nonendocrine tumors that produce polypeptides similar to either corticotropin-releasing factor or corticotropin. Approximately a fourth of cases of Cushing syndrome are corticotropin-independent, and most of these are caused by an adrenal adenoma. Tumors are usually bilateral, and half are malignant. Occasionally, androgen excess may lead to severe virilization (Danilowicz and colleagues, 2002).

The typical body habitus is caused by adipose tissue deposition that characteristically results in *moon facies,* a *buffalo hump,* and *truncal obesity.* Fatigability and weakness, hypertension, hirsutism, and amenorrhea are each encountered in 75 to 85 percent of nonpregnant patients (Williams and Dluhy, 2001). Personality changes, cutaneous striae, and easy bruisability are common, and approximately 20 percent have nephrolithiasis. Diagnosis is verified by elevated plasma cortisol levels that cannot be suppressed by dexamethasone or by elevated 24-hour urine free cortisol excretion (Boscaro and colleagues, 2001). Neither test is totally accurate, and both are more difficult to interpret in obese patients. CT and MR imaging are used to localize pituitary and adrenal tumors or hyperplasia.

Pregnancy

Because most women have corticotropin-dependent Cushing syndrome, associated androgen excess may cause anovulation, and pregnancy is rare. In their review, Lindsay and colleagues (2005) identified fewer than 150 cases of Cushing syndrome in pregnancy. Kamiya and colleagues (1998) summarized 97 cases from the Japanese literature. The distribution of causes is different in pregnant women, and corticotropin-independent adrenal lesions account for approximately half of cases (Klibanski and co-workers, 2006). Indeed, most cases in the reviews cited were caused by adrenal tumors, of which 80 percent were benign. These reports stressed difficulties in diagnosis because of pregnancy-induced increases in plasma cortisol, corticotropin, and corticotropin-releasing factor. Measurement of 24-hour urinary free cortisol excretion is recommended, with consideration for normal elevation in pregnancy.

Pregnancy outcomes in women with Cushing syndrome are listed in Table 53-7. Heart failure is common during pregnancy and is a major cause of maternal mortality (Buescher and associates, 1992).

Management

Long-term medical therapy for Cushing syndrome usually is ineffective, and definitive therapy is resection of the pituitary or adrenal adenoma or bilateral adrenalectomy for hyperplasia. During pregnancy, management of hypertension in mild cases may suffice until delivery. In their review, Lindsay and associates (2005) described primary medical therapy in 20 women with Cushing syndrome. Most were successfully treated with *metyrapone* as an interim treatment until definitive surgery was possible after delivery. A few cases were treated with oral *keto-*

TABLE 53-7. Perinatal Complications in Pregnancies Complicated by Cushing Syndrome

Complication	Approximate Incidence in Percent
Maternal	
Hypertension	68
Diabetes	25
Preeclampsia	15
Osteoporosis/fracture	5
Psychiatric disorders	4
Cardiac failure	3
Mortality	2
Perinatal	
Fetal-growth restriction	21
Preterm delivery	43
Stillbirth	6
Neonatal death	2

Data from Lindsay and colleagues (2005).

conazole, but because it also blocks testicular steroidogenesis, treatment during pregnancy with a male fetus is worrisome. *Mifepristone,* the norethindrone derivative used for abortion and labor induction, has shown promise for treating Cushing disease but should not be used in pregnancy. If necessary, pituitary adenomas can be treated by transsphenoidal resection (Boscaro and colleagues, 2001; Lindsay and associates, 2005). Removal of an adrenal adenoma in pregnancy can also be curative (Kamiya and colleagues, 1998; Keely, 1998).

Adrenal Deficiency

Primary adrenocortical insufficiency—*Addison disease*—is rare. More than 90 percent of the glands must be destroyed for symptoms to develop. *Idiopathic autoimmune adrenalitis* has surpassed tuberculosis and histoplasmosis as the most frequent cause. There is an increased incidence of concurrent Hashimoto thyroiditis, premature ovarian failure, type 1 diabetes, and Graves disease. These *polyglandular autoimmune syndromes* also include pernicious anemia, vitiligo, alopecia, nontropical sprue, and myasthenia gravis.

Adrenal Insufficiency and Pregnancy

Untreated adrenal hypofunction frequently causes infertility, but with replacement therapy, ovulation is restored. If untreated, common symptoms include weakness, fatigue, nausea and vomiting, and weight loss (Mestman, 2002). Because serum cortisol levels are increased during pregnancy, the finding of a low value should prompt an adrenocorticotropic hormone (ACTH) stimulation test to document the lack of response to infused corticotropin (Salvatori, 2005).

There are a few reports of hypoadrenalism complicating pregnancy. Successful pregnancy outcomes have been described in women diagnosed with adrenal insufficiency and treated before conception (Adonakis and colleagues, 2005; Ozdemir and associates, 2004). Most pregnant women with Addison disease are already taking cortisone-like drugs. These should be continued, and women are observed for evidence of either inadequate or excessive steroid replacement. During labor, delivery, and postpartum, or after a surgical procedure, corticosteroid replacement must be increased appreciably to approximate the normal adrenal response—so-called *stress doses*. Hydrocortisone, 100 mg, is usually given intravenously every 8 hours. It is important that shock from causes other than adrenocortical insufficiency—for example, hemorrhage or sepsis—be recognized and treated promptly.

Primary Aldosteronism

Hyperaldosteronism is caused by an adrenal aldosteronoma in approximately 75 percent of cases, and idiopathic bilateral adrenal hyperplasia in the remainder (Ganguly, 1998). Findings include hypertension, hypokalemia, and muscle weakness. High serum or urine levels of aldosterone confirm the diagnosis.

Pregnancy and Hyperaldosteronism

Progesterone blocks aldosterone action, thus, there are very high levels of aldosterone in normal pregnancy (see Chap. 5, p. 129 and Appendix). Accordingly, there may be amelioration of symptoms and of electrolyte abnormalities during pregnancy (Murakami and associates, 2000). Medical management includes potassium supplementation and antihypertensive therapy. In many cases, hypertension responds to *spironolactone*, but β-blockers or calcium-channel blockers may be preferred because of the potential fetal antiandrogenic effects of the diuretic. Deruelle and colleagues (2004) reported successful use of *amiloride* in a pregnant woman. Tumor resection is curative, and laparoscopic adrenalectomy during the second trimester has been shown to be safe (Baron and associates, 1995; Kosaka and colleagues, 2006). Two women described by Nezu and co-workers (2000) were normotensive throughout pregnancy but were found to have an aldosteronoma postpartum after severe hypertension developed.

PITUITARY DISEASES

There is normal pituitary enlargement during pregnancy, predominately from lactotrophic cellular hyperplasia induced by estrogen stimulation (see Chap. 5, p. 126).

Prolactinomas

These adenomas are found relatively commonly since the advent of widely available assays for serum prolactin. Symptoms and findings include amenorrhea, galactorrhea, and hyperprolactinemia. Tumors are classified arbitrarily by their size measured by CT or MR imaging. A microadenoma is ≤ 10 mm, and a macroadenoma is > 10 mm. Treatment for microadenomas is usually with bromocriptine, a dopamine agonist and powerful prolactin inhibitor, which frequently restores ovulation. For suprasellar macroadenomas, most recommend surgical resection before pregnancy is attempted (Schlechte, 2007).

Prolactinomas and Pregnancy

In almost 250 pregnant women with previously untreated *microadenomas*, only four developed symptomatic enlargement during pregnancy (Molitch, 1985). Another 11 who remained asymptomatic had radiographic evidence of enlargement. Although the risk of tumor enlargement during pregnancy is less than 2 percent with microadenomas, symptomatic enlargement of *macroadenomas* is more common. For example, 15 to 35 percent of suprasellar macroadenomas have tumor enlargement that causes visual disturbances, headaches, and diabetes insipidus (Schlechte, 2007). Visual loss during pregnancy was described by Kupersmith and colleagues (1994) in six of eight women with macroadenomas.

Gillam and colleagues (2006) recommend that pregnant women with microadenomas be queried regularly for headaches and visual symptoms. Those with macroadenomas should have visual field testing during each trimester. CT or MR imaging is recommended only if symptoms develop. Serial serum prolactin levels are not recommended because of normal increases during pregnancy. Symptomatic tumor enlargement is treated immediately with bromocriptine, but macroprolactinomas may be relatively resistant (Shanis and Check, 1996). More than 6000 pregnant women have taken bromocriptine at some time during pregnancy, and there have been no adverse effects (Molitch, 2001). Surgery is recommended for women with no response. Gondim and colleagues (2003) have described transnasal transseptal endoscopic resection.

Acromegaly

This is caused by excessive growth hormone, usually from an acidophilic or a chromophobic pituitary adenoma. In normal pregnancy, pituitary growth hormone levels decrease as placental epitopes are secreted. Diagnosis is confirmed by the failure of an oral glucose tolerance test to suppress pituitary growth hormone (Melmed, 2006). Pregnancy is rare in women with acromegaly, possibly because half are hyperprolactinemic.

Management is similar to that for prolactinomas, with close monitoring for symptoms of tumor enlargement. Bromocriptine is not as effective as it is for prolactinomas, and surgery may be necessary for symptomatic tumor enlargement during pregnancy (Prager and Braunstein, 1995). Guven and associates (2006) reported a case of pituitary apoplexy necessitating emergent transsphenoidal adenomectomy and cesarean delivery at 34 weeks. Successful treatment of pregnant women with the somatostatin-receptor ligand, *octreotide,* and with the GH-analog, *pegvisomant,* has been reported (Brian, 2007; Herman-Bonert, 1998; Neal, 2000, and all their colleagues).

Diabetes Insipidus

The vasopressin deficiency evident in diabetes insipidus is usually due to a hypothalamic or pituitary stalk disorder rather than to a pituitary lesion (Lamberts and associates, 1998). True diabetes insipidus is a rare complication of pregnancy. Only a few cases have been cared for in the last 50 years at Parkland Hospital, during which time there were nearly 400,000 deliveries.

Therapy for diabetes insipidus is intranasal administration of *desmopressin,* the synthetic analog of vasopressin—1-deamino-8-D-arginine vasopressin (DDAVP). Ray (1998) reviewed 53 cases in which DDAVP was used during pregnancy with no adverse sequelae. Most women require increased doses during pregnancy because of an increased metabolic clearance rate stimulated by placental vasopressinase (Lindheimer and Barron, 1994). By this same mechanism, *subclinical diabetes insipidus* may become symptomatic or cases of *transient diabetes insipidus* may be encountered during pregnancy (Brewster and Hayslett, 2005; Krege and associates, 1989).

In our experience, transient secondary diabetes insipidus is more likely encountered with *acute fatty liver of pregnancy* (see Chap. 50, p. 1064). This probably is due to altered vasopressinase clearance because of hepatic dysfunction. Harper and associates (1987) described transient disease in a 38-week pregnant woman with biopsy-proven viral hepatitis. Another cause of diabetes insipidus is pituitary infarction with severe obstetrical hemorrhage as described below.

Sheehan Syndrome

Sheehan (1937) reported that pituitary ischemia and necrosis associated with obstetrical blood loss could result in hypopituitarism. With modern methods of treatment for hemorrhagic shock, Sheehan syndrome is now seldom encountered (Feinberg and associates, 2005; Vaphiades and colleagues, 2003). It has also been reported with infarction of a macroadenoma (Kaiser, 2001). A recently encountered case at Parkland Hospital is shown in Figure 53-5. Another case caused by hemorrhage and necrosis of lymphocytic hypophysitis was described by Lee and Pless (2003). With acute hemorrhage, affected women may have persistent hypotension, tachycardia, hypoglycemia, and failure of lactation. Subsequent deficiencies of some or all pituitary responsive hormones may develop. For example, as discussed above, diabetes insipidus with or without anterior pituitary deficiency has been described following massive obstetrical hemorrhage and prolonged shock (Kan and Calligerous, 1998). In 20 cases of Sheehan syndrome from Turkey reported by Dökmetas and associates (2006), latency between hemorrhage and onset of symptoms varied from 2 to 40 years.

Lymphocytic Hypophysitis

This autoimmune pituitary disorder is characterized by massive infiltration by lymphocytes and plasma cells with parenchymal destruction of the gland. Most cases are temporarily linked to pregnancy (Caturegli and associates, 2005; Madsen, 2000). There are varying degrees of hypopituitarism or symptoms of mass effect, including headaches and visual field defects. A sellar mass is seen with CT or MR imaging. A mass accompanied by a modestly elevated serum prolactin level—usually < 100 pg/mL—suggests lymphocytic hypophysitis, whereas levels > 200 pg/mL are encountered with a prolactinoma. Associated hypothyroidism is common. Pressman and colleagues (1995) reviewed 44 cases and found that 25 percent had other autoimmune diseases. Treatment is with hormone replacement, but the disease may be self-limited (Gagneja and associates, 1999). Surgery during pregnancy is war-

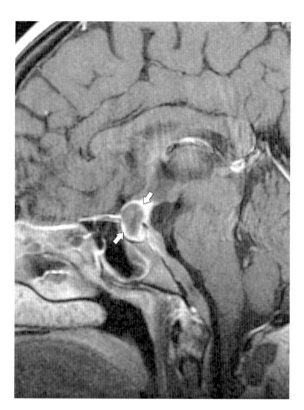

FIGURE 53-5 Sheehan syndrome in 23-year-old primipara who had major postpartum hemorrhage and hypotension intraoperatively with cesarean delivery. Magnetic resonance imaging was obtained because she failed to lactate, and her serum prolactin level was 18 ng/mL. Sagittal magnetic resonance (MR) image shows a large pituitary gland mass (*arrows*) consistent with hemorrhage. Follow-up MR imaging showed complete involution of the hematoma.

ranted only in cases of severe chiasmal compression unresponsive to corticosteroid therapy (Lee and Pless, 2003).

REFERENCES

Abalovich M, Amino N, Barbour L, et al: Management of thyroid dysfunction during pregnancy and postpartum: An Endocrine Society Clinical Practice Guideline. J Clin Endocrinol Metab 92(8 Suppl):S1, 2007

Abalovich M, Gutierrez S, Alcaraz G, et al: Overt and subclinical hypothyroidism complicating pregnancy. Thyroid 12:63, 2002

Abramson J, Stagnaro-Green A: Thyroid antibodies and fetal loss: An evolving story. Thyroid 11:57, 2001

Adonakis G, Georgopoulos N, Michail G, et al: Successful pregnancy outcome in a patient with primary Addison's disease. Gynecol Endocrinol 21:90, 2005

Ahlawat SK, Jain S, Kumari S, et al: Pheochromocytoma associated with pregnancy: Case report and review of the literature. Obstet Gynecol Surv 54:728, 1999

Ahn JT, Hibbard JU, Chapa JB: Atypical presentation of pheochromocytoma as part of multiple endocrine neoplasia IIa in pregnancy. Obstet Gynecol 102:1202, 2003

Alexander EK, Marquesee E, Lawrence J, et al: Timing and magnitude of increases in levothyroxine requirements during pregnancy in women with hypothyroidism. N Eng J Med 351:241, 2004

Alikasifoglu A, Gonc EN, Yalcin E, et al: Neonatal hyperparathyroidism due to maternal hypoparathyroidism and vitamin D deficiency: A cause of multiple bone fractures. Clin Pediatr 44:267, 2005

Alvarez-Marfany M, Roman SH, Drexler AJ, et al: Long-term prospective study of postpartum thyroid dysfunction in women with insulin dependent diabetes mellitus. J Clin Endocrinol Metab 79:10, 1994

American College of Obstetricians and Gynecologists: Thyroid disease in pregnancy. Practice Bulletin No. 37, August 2002

American College of Obstetricians and Gynecologists: Subclinical hypothyroidism in pregnancy. Committee Opinion No. 381, October 2007

Amino N, Izumi Y, Hidaka Y, et al: No increase of blocking type antithyrotropin receptor antibodies during pregnancy in patients with Graves' disease. J Clin Endocrinol Metab 88(12):5871, 2003

Amino N, Tada H, Hidaka Y, et al: Postpartum autoimmune thyroid syndrome. Endocr J 47:645, 2000

Ando T, Imaizumi M, Graves PN, et al: Intrathyroidal fetal microchimerism in Graves' disease. J Clin Endocrinol Metab 87:3315, 2002

Anselmo J, Cao D, Karrison T, et al: Fetal loss associated with excess thyroid hormone exposure. JAMA 292:691, 2004

Arafah BM: Increased need for thyroxine in women with hypothyroidism during estrogen therapy. N Engl J Med 344:1743, 2001

Ayala C, Navarro E, Rodríguez JR, et al: Conception after iodine-131 therapy for differentiated thyroid cancer. Thyroid 8:1009, 1998

Baron F, Sprauve ME, Huddleston JF, et al: Diagnosis and surgical treatment of primary aldosteronism in pregnancy: A case report. Obstet Gynecol 86:644, 1995

Bartolazzi A, Gasbarri A, Papotti M, et al: Application of an immunodiagnostic method for improving reoperative diagnosis of nodular thyroid lesions. Lancet 357:1644, 2001

Bassoon-Zaltzman C, Sermer M, Lao TT, et al: Bladder pheochromocytoma in pregnancy without hypertension. J Reprod Med 40:149, 1995

Beattie GC, Ravi NR, Lewis M, et al: Rare presentation of maternal primary hyperparathyroidism. BMJ 321:223, 2000

Becker DV, Braverman LE, Delange F, et al: Iodine supplementation for pregnancy and lactation—United States and Canada: Recommendations of the American Thyroid Association. Thyroid 16:949, 2006

Berg GEB, Nyström EH, Jacobsson L, et al: Radioiodine treatment of hyperthyroidism in a pregnant woman. J Nucl Med 39:357, 1998

Berlin L: Malpractice issues in radiology: Iodine-131 and the pregnant patient. AJR 176:869, 2001

Bernal J: Thyroid hormone receptors in brain development and function. Nat Clin Pract Endocrinol Metab 3(3):249, 2007

Bianchi DW, Romero R: Biological implications of bi-directional fetomaternal cell trafficking summary of a National Institute of Child Health and Human Development-sponsored conference. J Matern Fetal Neonatal Med 14:123, 2003

Bilezikian JP, Silverberg SJ: Asymptomatic primary hyperparathyroidism. N Engl J Med 350:1746, 2004

Boscaro M, Barzon L, Fallo F, et al: Cushing's syndrome. Lancet 357:783, 2001

Bowman ML, Bergmann M, Smith JF: Intrapartum labetalol for the treatment of maternal and fetal thyrotoxicosis. Thyroid 8:795, 1998

Boyle JG, Davidson DF, Perry CG, et al: Comparison of diagnostic accuracy of urinary free metanephrines, vanillyl mandelic acid, and catecholamines and plasma catecholamines for diagnosis of pheochromocytoma. J Clin Endocrinol Metab 92:4602, 2007

Brand F, Liegeois P, Langer B: One case of fetal and neonatal variable thyroid dysfunction in the context of Graves' disease. Fetal Diagn Ther 20:12, 2005

Brent GA: Graves' disease. N Eng J Med 358:2594, 2008

Brewster UC, Hayslett JP: Diabetes insipidus in the third trimester of pregnancy. Obstet Gynecol 105:1173, 2005

Brian SR, Bidlingmaier M, Wajnrajch MP, et al: Treatment of acromegaly with pegvisomant during pregnancy: Maternal and fetal effects. J Clin Endocrinol Metab 92:3374, 2007

Brown RS, Bellisario RL, Botero D, et al: Incidence of transient congenital hypothyroidism due to maternal thyrotropin receptor-blocking antibodies in over one million babies. J Clin Endocrinol Metab 81:1147, 1996

Brundtland GH: United Nations General Assembly special session on children sustained elimination of iodine deficiency disorders. World Health Organization 2002. Available at: http://www.who.int/director-general/speeches/2002/english/20020508_UNGASSSustainedeliminationofIodineDeficiencyDisorders.html. Accessed September 27, 2008

Buescher MA, McClamrock HD, Adashi EY: Cushing syndrome in pregnancy. Obstet Gynecol 79:130, 1992

Burch HB, Wartofsky L: Life-threatening thyrotoxicosis. Endocrinol Metab Clin North Am 22:263, 1993

Caldwell KL, Jones R, Hollowell JG: Urinary Iodine Concentration: United States National Health and Nutrition Examination Survey 1001–2002. Thyroid 15(7):692, 2005

Calvo RM, Jauniaux E, Gulbis B, et al: Fetal tissues are exposed to biologically relevant free thyroxine concentrations during early phases of development. J Clin Endocrinol Metab 87:1768, 2002

Canaris GJ, Manowitz NR, Mayor G, et al: The Colorado Thyroid Disease Prevalence Study. Arch Intern Med 160:526, 2000

Cao XY, Jiang XM, Dou ZH, et al: Timing of vulnerability of the brain to iodine deficiency in endemic cretinism. N Engl J Med 331:1739, 1994

Carbone LD, Palmieri GMA, Graves SC, et al: Osteoporosis of pregnancy: Long-term follow-up of patient and their offspring. Obstet Gynecol 86:664, 1995

Casara D, Rubello D, Saladini G, et al: Pregnancy after high therapeutic doses of iodine-131 in differentiated thyroid cancer: Potential risks and recommendations. Eur J Nucl Med 20:192, 1993

Casey BM, Dashe JS, Spong CY, et al: Perinatal significance of isolated maternal hypothyroxinemia identified in the first half of pregnancy. Obstet Gynecol 109:1129, 2007

Casey BM, Dashe JS, Wells CE, et al: Subclinical hypothyroidism pregnancy outcomes. Obstet Gynecol 105:38, 2005

Casey BM, Leveno KJ: Thyroid disease in pregnancy. Obstet Gynecol 108:1283, 2006

Casey B, Spong C, McIntire D, et al: Pregnancy outcomes in women with antithyroid peroxidase antibodies. Am J Obstet Gynecol 197(6):S126, 2008

Caturegli P, Lupi I, Landek-Salgado M, et al: Pituitary autoimmunity: 30 years later. Autoimmun Rev 7:631, 2008

Cleary-Goldman J, Malone FD, Lambert-Messerlian G, et al: Maternal thyroid hypofunction and pregnancy outcome. Obstet Gynecol 112(1):85, 2008

Cohen O, Pinhas-Hamiel O, Sivian E, et al: Serial in utero ultrasonographic measurements of the fetal thyroid: A new complimentary tool in the management of maternal hyperthyroidism in pregnancy. Prenat Diagn 23:740, 2003

Conlin PR: Case 13-2001. Case records of the Massachusetts General Hospital. N Eng J Med 344:1314, 2001

Cunningham FG: Screening for osteoporosis. N Engl J Med 353:1975, 2005

Dahan M, Chang RJ: Pancreatitis secondary to hyperparathyroidism during pregnancy. Obstet Gynecol 98:923, 2001

Dahlman T, Sjberg H, Bucht E: Calcium homeostasis in normal pregnancy and puerperium. Acta Obstet Gynecol Scand 73:393, 1994

Danilowicz K, Albiger N, Vanegas M, et al: Androgen-secreting adrenal adenomas. Obstet Gynecol 100:1099, 2002

Dashe JS, Casey BM, Wells CE, et al: Thyroid-stimulating hormone in singleton and twin pregnancy: Importance of gestational age-specific reference ranges. Obstet Gynecol 107(1):205, 2005

Davis LE, Leveno KL, Cunningham FG: Hypothyroidism complicating pregnancy. Obstet Gynecol 72:108-112, 1988

Davis LE, Lucas MJ, Hankins GDV, et al: Thyrotoxicosis complicating pregnancy. Am J Obstet Gynecol 160:63, 1989

Davison S, Lennard TWJ, Davison J, et al: Management of a pregnant patient with Graves' disease complicated by thionamide-induced neutropenia in the first trimester. Clin Endocrin 54:559, 2001

Dayan CM, Daniels GH: Chronic autoimmune thyroiditis. N Engl J Med 335:99, 1996

Delange F: Iodine deficiency as a cause of brain damage. Postgrad Med J 77:217, 2001

Deruelle P, Dufour P, Magnenant E, et al: Maternal Bartter's syndrome in pregnancy treated by amiloride. Eur J Obstet Gynecol Reprod Biol 115:106, 2004

Diav-Citrin O, Ornoy A: Teratogen update: Antithyroid drugs-methimazole, carbimazole, and propylthiouracil. Teratology 65:38, 2002

Diez JJ, Iglesias P: Spontaneous subclinical hypothyroidism in patients older than 55 years: An analysis of natural course and risk factors for the development of overt thyroid failure. J Clin Endocrinol Metab 89:4890, 2004

Di Gianantonio E, Schaefer C, Mastroiacovo PP, et al: Adverse effects of prenatal methimazole exposure. Teratology 64(5):262, 2001.

Doherty CM, Shindo ML, Rice DH, et al: Management of thyroid nodules during pregnancy. Laryngoscope 105:251, 1995

Dökmetas HS, Kilicli F, Korkmaz S, et al: Characteristic features of 20 patients with Sheehan's syndrome. Gynecol Endocrinol 22:279, 2006

Driggers RW, Kopelman JN, Satin AJ: Delaying surgery for thyroid cancer in pregnancy. A case report. J Reprod Med 43:909, 1998

Duncombe GJ, Dickinson JE: Fetal thyrotoxicosis after maternal thyroidectomy. Aust NZ J Obstet Gynaecol 41: 2:224, 2001

Dunne F, Walters B, Marshall T, et al: Pregnancy associated osteoporosis. Clin Endocrinol 39:487, 1993

Fadel BM, Ellahham S, Ringel MD, et al: Hyperthyroid heart disease. Clin Cardiol 23:402, 2000

Fadeyev V, Lesnikova S, Melnichenko G: Prevalence of thyroid disorders in pregnant women with mild iodine deficiency. Gynecol Endocrinol 17:413, 2003

Farford B, Presutti RJ, Moraghan TJ: Nonsurgical management of primary hyperparathyroidism. Mayo Clin Proc 82:351, 2007

Feigenberg T, Ben-Shushan A, Daka K, et al: Ultrasound-diagnosed puerperal osteopenia in young primiparas. J Reprod Med 53(4):287, 2008

Feinberg EC, Molitch ME, Endres LK, et al: The incidence of Sheehan's syndrome after obstetric hemorrhage. Fertil Steril 84:975, 2005

Fisher DA: Fetal thyroid function: Diagnosis and management of fetal thyroid disorders. Clin Obstet Gynecol 40:16, 1997

Gagneja H, Arafah B, Taylor HC: Histologically proven lymphocytic hypophysitis: Spontaneous resolution and subsequent pregnancy. Mayo Clin Proc 74:150, 1999

Gallagher MP, Schachner HC, Levine LS, et al: Neonatal thyroid enlargement associated with propylthiouracil therapy of Graves' diseases during pregnancy: A problem revisited. J Pediatr 139:896, 2001

Ganguly A: Primary aldosteronism. N Engl J Med 339:1828, 1998

Geelhoed GW: Surgery of the endocrine glands in pregnancy. Clin Obstet Gynecol 26:865, 1983

Gharib H, Tuttle RM, Baskin HJ, et al: Subclinical thyroid dysfunction: A joint statement on management from the American Association of Clinical Endocrinologists, the American Thyroid Association, and The Endocrine Society. J Clin Endocrinol Metab 90:581, 2005

Gillam MP, Molitch ME, Lombardi G, et al: Advances in the treatment of prolactinomas. Endocr Rev 27:485, 2006

Glinoer D: Pregnancy and iodine. Thyroid 11:471, 2001

Gondim J, Ramos JF, Pinheiro I, et al: Minimally invasive pituitary surgery in a hemorrhagic necrosis adenoma during pregnancy. Minim Invasive Neurosurg 46(3):173, 2003

Goodwin TM, Hershman JM: Hyperthyroidism due to inappropriate production of human chorionic gonadotropin. Clin Obstet Gynecol 40:32, 1997

Graham EM, Freedman LJ, Forouzan I: Intrauterine growth retardation in a woman with primary hyperparathyroidism. J Reprod Med 43:451, 1998

Grimbert P, Chauveau D, Richard S, et al: Pregnancy in von Hippel–Lindau disease. Am J Obstet Gynecol 180:110, 1999

Grossman M, Weintraub BD, Szkudlinski MW: Novel insights into the molecular mechanisms of human thyrotropin action: Structural, physiological, and therapeutic implications for the glycoprotein hormone family. Endocr Rev 18:476, 1997

Guven S, Durukan T, Berker M, et al: A case of acromegaly in pregnancy: Concomitant transsphenoidal adenomectomy and cesarean section. J Matern Fetal Neonatal Med 19:69, 2006

Gyamfi C, Wapner RJ, D'Alton ME: Thyroid dysfunction in pregnancy. The basic science and clinical evidence surrounding the controversy in management. Obstet Gynecol 113:702, 2009

Haddow JE, McClain MR, Palomaki GE, et al: Urine iodine measurements, creatinine adjustment, and thyroid deficiency in an adult United States population. J Clin Endocrinol Metab 92:1019, 2007

Haddow JE, Palomaki GE, Allan WC, et al: Maternal thyroid deficiency during pregnancy and subsequent neuropsychological development of the child. N Engl J Med 341:549, 1999

Harper M, Hatjis CG, Appel RG, et al: Vasopressin resistant diabetes insipidus, liver dysfunction, and hyperuricemia and decreased renal function. J Reprod Med 32:862, 1987

Harper MA, Murnaghan GA, Kennedy L, et al: Pheochromocytoma in pregnancy. Five cases and a review of the literature. Br J Obstet Gynaecol 96:594, 1989

Hegedüs L: The thyroid nodule. N Eng J Med 351:1764, 2004

Helfand M: Screening for subclinical thyroid dysfunction in nonpregnant adults: A summary of the evidence for the U.S. Preventive Services Task Force. Ann Intern Med 140:128, 2004

Helfgott SM: Weekly clinicopathological exercises: Case 21-2002. N Engl J Med 347:122, 2002

Hellmeyer L, Kühnert M, Ziller V, et al: The use of I.V. bisphosphonate in pregnancy-associated osteoporosis—Case study. Exp Clin Endocrinol Diabetes 115:139, 2007

Herman-Bonert V, Seliverstov M, Melmed S: Pregnancy in acromegaly: Successful therapeutic outcome. J Clin Endocrinol Metab 83:727, 1998

Hidaka Y, Tamaki H, Iwatani Y, et al: Prediction of postpartum Graves thyrotoxicosis by measurement of thyroid stimulating antibody in early pregnancy. Clin Endocrinol 41:15, 1994

Hollowell JG, Staehling NW, Hannon WH, et al: Iodine nutrition in the United States. Trends and public health implications: Iodine excretion data from National Health and Nutrition Examination Surveys I and III (1971–1974 and 1988–1994). J Clin Endocrinol Metab 83:3401, 1998

Iitaka M, Morgenthaler NG, Momotani N, et al: Stimulation of thyroid-stimulating hormone (TSH) receptor antibody production following painless thyroiditis. Clin Endocrinol 60:49, 2004

Institute of Medicine: Dietary Reference Intakes for vitamin A, vitamin K, arsenic, boron, chromium, copper, iodine, manganese, molybdenum, nickel, silicon, vanadium, and zinc. Washington, DC, National Academies Press, 2001

Ip P: Neonatal convulsion revealing maternal hyperparathyroidism: An unusual case of late neonatal hypoparathyroidism. Arch Gynecol Obstet 268:227, 2003

Jaafar R, Boo NY, Rasat R, et al: Neonatal seizures due to maternal primary hyperparathyroidism. Letters to the Editor. J Paediatr, Child Health 40:329, 2004

Janetschek G, Finkenstedt G, Gasser R, et al: Laparoscopic surgery for pheochromocytoma: Adrenalectomy, partial resection, excision of paragangliomas. J Urol 150:330, 1998

Junglee N, Harries SE, Davies N, et al: Pheochromocytoma in pregnancy: When is operative intervention indicated? J Womens Health 16:1362, 2007

Kaiser UB: Weekly clinicopathological exercises: Case 15-2001. N Engl J Med 344:1536, 2001

Karmisholt J, Andersen S, Laurberg P: Variation in thyroid function tests in patients with stable untreated subclinical hypothyroidism. Thyroid 18(3):303, 2008

Kamiya Y, Okada M, Yoneyama A, et al: Surgical successful treatment of Cushing's syndrome in a pregnant patient complicated with severe cardiac involvement. Endocr J 45:499, 1998

Kan AKS, Calligerous D: A case report of Sheehan syndrome presenting with diabetes insipidus. Aust NZ J Obstet Gynaecol 38:224, 1998

Kaur M, Pearson D, Godber I, et al: Longitudinal changes in bone mineral density during normal pregnancy. Bone 32:449, 2003

Keely E: Endocrine causes of hypertension in pregnancy—when to start looking for zebras. Semin Perinatol 22:471, 1998

Kempers MJE, van der Sluijs Veer, Nijhuis-van der Sanden MWG, et al: Intellectual and motor development of young adults with congenital hypothyroidism diagnosed by neonatal screening. J Clin Endocrinol Metab 91:418, 2006

Khosrotehrani K, Johnson KL, Cha DH, et al: Transfer of fetal cells with multilineage potential to maternal tissue. JAMA 292:75, 2004

Kilpatrick S: Umbilical blood sampling in women with thyroid disease in pregnancy: Is it necessary? Am J Obstet Gynecol 189:1, 2003

Kim PTW, Kreisman SH, Vaughn R, et al: Laparoscopic adrenalectomy for pheochromocytoma in pregnancy. J Can Chir 49:62, 2006

Klein I, Ojamaa K: Thyrotoxicosis and the heart. Endocrinol Metab Clin North Am 27:51, 1998

Klibanski A, Stephen AE, Green MF, et al: Case records of the Massachusetts General Hospital. Case 36-2006, A 35-year old pregnant woman with new hypertension. N Engl J Med 355:2237, 2006

Klintschar M, Schwaiger P, Mannweiler S, et al: Evidence of fetal microchimerism in Hashimoto's thyroiditis. J Clin Endocrinol Metab 86:2494, 2001

Kooistra L, Crawford S, van Baar AL, et al: Neonatal effects of maternal hypothyroxinemia during early pregnancy. Pediatrics 117:161, 2006

Kort KC, Schiller HJ, Numann PJ: Hyperparathyroidism and pregnancy. Am J Surg 177:66, 1999

Kosaka K, Onoda N, Ishikawa T, et al: Laparoscopic adrenalectomy on a patient with primary aldosteronism during pregnancy. Endocr J 53:461, 2006

Krege J, Katz VL, Bowes WA Jr: Transient diabetes insipidus of pregnancy. Obstet Gynecol Surv 44:789, 1989

Kriplani A, Buckshee K, Bhargava VL, et al: Maternal and perinatal outcome in thyrotoxicosis complicating pregnancy. Eur J Obstet Gynecol Reprod Biol 54:159, 1994

Kuijpens JL, Vader HL, Drexhage HA, et al: Thyroid peroxidase antibodies during gestation are a marker for subsequent depression postpartum. Euro J Endocrinol 145:579, 2001

Kung AWC, Chau MT, LAO TT, et al: The effect of pregnancy on thyroid nodule formation. J Clin Endocrinol Metab 87:1010, 2002

Kung AWC, Jones BM: A change from stimulatory to blocking antibody activity in Graves' disease during pregnancy. J Clin Endocrinol Metab 83:514, 1998

Kupersmith MJ, Rosenberg C, Kleinberg D: Visual loss in pregnant women with pituitary adenomas. Ann Intern Med 121:473, 1994

Lal G, Duh QY: Laparoscopic adrenalectomy—indications and technique. Surg Oncol 12:105, 2003

Lamberts SWJ, de Herder WW, van der Lely AJ: Pituitary insufficiency. Lancet 352:127, 1998

Lee MS, Pless M: Apoplectic lymphocytic hypophysitis: Case report. J Neurosurg 98:183, 2003

Lee RH, Spencer CA, Mestman JH, et al: Free T_4 immunoassays are flawed during pregnancy. Am J Obstet Gynecol 200:260.e1, 2009

Lenders JWM, Pacak K, Walther MM, et al: Biochemical diagnosis of pheochromocytoma: Which test is best? JAMA 287:1427, 2002

Leung AS, Millar LE, Koonings PP, et al: Perinatal outcome in hypothyroid pregnancies. Obstet Gynecol 81:349, 1993

Lindheimer MD, Barron WM: Water metabolism and vasopressin secretion during pregnancy. Baillieres Clin Obstet Gynaecol 8:311, 1994

Lindsay JR, Jonklaas J, Oldfield EH, et al: Cushing's syndrome during pregnancy: Personal experience and review of literature. J Clin Endocrinol Metab 90:3077, 2005

Loh JA, Wartofsky L, Jonklass J, et al: The magnitude of increased levothyroxine requirements in hypothyroid pregnant women depends upon the etiology of the hypothyroidism. Thyroid 19(3):269, 2009

Lucas A, Pizarro E, Granada ML, et al: Postpartum thyroiditis: Epidemiology and clinical evolution in a nonselected population. Thyroid 10:71, 2000

Lucas A, Pizarro E, Granada ML, et al: Postpartum thyroid dysfunction and postpartum depression: Are they two linked disorders? Clin Endocrinol 55:809, 2001

Lucas A, Pizarro E, Granada ML, et al: Postpartum thyroiditis: Long-term follow up. Thyroid 15:1177, 2005

Luton D, Le Gac I, Vuillard E, et al: Management of Graves' disease during pregnancy: The key role of fetal thyroid gland monitoring. J Clin Endocrinol Metab 90:6093, 2005

Madsen JR: Case records of the Massachusetts General Hospital: Case 34-2000. N Engl J Med 343:1399, 2000

Manger WM: The vagaries of pheochromocytomas. Am J Hypertens 18:1266, 2005

Männistö, T, Vääräsmäki M, Pouta A, et al: Perinatal outcome of children born to mothers with thyroid dysfunction or antibodies: A prospective population-based cohort study. J Clin Endocrinol Metab 94:772, 2009

Matalon S, Sheiner E, Levy A, et al: Relationship of treated maternal hypothyroidism and perinatal outcome. J Reprod Med 51:59, 2006

Melmed S: Acromegaly. N Engl J Med 355(24):2558, 2006

Mestman JH: Hyperthyroidism in pregnancy. Endocrinol Metab Clin North Am 27:127, 1998

Mestman JH: Endocrine diseases in pregnancy. In: Gabbe S, Niebyl JR, Simpson JL (eds): Obstetrics: Normal and Problem Pregnancies, 4th ed. New York, Churchill Livingstone, 2002, p 1117

Mestman JH, Goodwin TM, Montoro MM: Thyroid disorders of pregnancy. Endocrinol Metab Clin North Am 24:41, 1995

Millar LK, Wing DA, Leung AS, et al: Low birth weight and preeclampsia in pregnancies complicated by hyperthyroidism. Obstet Gynecol 84:946, 1994

Miller BS, Dimick J, Wainess R, et al: Age- and sex-related incidence of surgically treated primary hyperparathyroidism. World J Surg 32:795, 2008

Miller C, Bernet V, Elkas JC, et al: Conservative management of extra-adrenal pheochromocytoma during pregnancy. Obstet Gynecol 105:1185, 2005

Molitch ME: Pregnancy and the hyperprolactinemic woman. N Engl J Med 312:1364, 1985

Molitch ME: Pituitary, thyroid, adrenal, and parathyroid disorders. In: Barron WM, Lindheimer MD (eds): Medical Disorders During Pregnancy, 3rd ed. St. Louis, Mosby, 2000, p 101

Molitch ME: Disorders of prolactin secretions. Endocrinol Metab Clin North Am 30:585, 2001

Momotani N, Noh JH, Ishikawa N, et al: Effects of propylthiouracil and methimazole on fetal thyroid status in mothers with Graves' hyperthyroidism. J Clin Endocrinol Metab 82:3633, 1997

Montoro MN, Paler RJ, Goodwin TM, et al: Parathyroid carcinoma during pregnancy. Obstet Gynecol 96: 841, 2000

Moosa M, Mazzaferri EL: Outcome of differentiated thyroid cancer diagnosed in pregnant women. J Clin Endocrinol Metab 82:2862, 1997

Moreno JC, Klootwijk W, van Toor H, et al: Mutations in the iodotyrosine deiodinase gene and hypothyroidism. N Engl J Med 358(17):1811, 2008

Morreale De Escobar G, Obregon MJ, Escobar Del Rey F: Role of thyroid hormone during early brain development. Eur J Endocrinol 151:U25, 2004

Morris PC: Thyroid cancer complicating pregnancy. Obstet Gynecol Clin North Am 25:401, 1998

Muller AF, Drexhage HA, Berghout A: Postpartum thyroiditis and autoimmune thyroiditis in women of childbearing age: Recent insights and consequences for antenatal and postnatal care. Endocr Rev 22:605, 2001

Muraji T, Hosaka N, Irie N, et al: Maternal microchimerism in underlying pathogenesis of biliary atresia: Quantification and phenotypes of maternal cells in the liver. Pediatrics 121:517, 2008

Murakami T, Ogura EW, Tanaka Y, et al: High blood pressure lowered by pregnancy. Lancet 356:1980, 2000

Nachum Z, Rakover Y, Weiner E, Shalev E: Graves' disease in pregnancy: Prospective evaluation of a selective invasive treatment protocol. Am J Obstet Gynecol 189:159, 2003

National Academy of Clinical Biochemistry: NACB: Laboratory support for the diagnosis and monitoring of thyroid disease. Washington, National Academy of Clinical Biochemistry, 2002, p 125

National Newborn Screening and Genetics Resource Center. Available at: http://genes-r-us.uthscsa.edu/. Accessed September 27, 2008

Naylor KE, Iqbal P, Fledelius C, et al: The effect of pregnancy on bone density and bone turnover. J Bone Miner Res 15:129, 2000

Neal JM: Successful pregnancy in a woman with acromegaly treated with octreotide: Case report. Endocr Prac 6:148, 2000

Nezu M, Miura Y, Noshiro T, et al: Primary aldosteronism as a cause of severe postpartum hypertension in two women. Am J Obstet Gynecol 182:745, 2000

O'Doherty MJ, McElhatton PR, Thomas SHL: Treating thyrotoxicosis in pregnant or potentially pregnant women. BMJ 318:5, 1999

Olivieri A, Stazi MA, Mastroiacovo P, et al: A population-based study on the frequency of additional congenital malformations in infants with congenital hypothyroidism: Data from the Italian Registry for Congenital hypothyroidism (1991–1998). J Clin Endocrinol Metab 87:557, 2002

Ozdemir I, Demirci F, Yücel O, et al: A case of primary Addison's disease with hyperemesis gravidarum and successful pregnancy. Eur J Obstet Gynecol Reprod Biol 113:100, 2004

Pearce EN, Farwell AP, Braverman LE: Thyroiditis. N Engl J Med 348:2646, 2003

Pederson CA, Johnson JL, Silva S, et al: Antenatal thyroid correlates of postpartum depression. Psychoneuroendocrinology 32:235, 2007

Pop VJ, Brouwers EP, Vader HL, et al: Maternal hypothyroxinemia during early pregnancy and subsequent child development: A 3-year follow-up study. Clin Endocrinol 59:282, 2003

Pop VJ, Kujipens JL, van Baar AL, et al: Low maternal free thyroxine concentrations during early pregnancy are associated with impaired psychomotor development in infancy. Clin Endocrinol 50:149, 1999

Power ML, Heaney RP, Kalkwarf HJ, et al: The role of calcium in health and disease. Am J Obstet Gynecol 181:1560, 1999

Prager D, Braunstein GD: Pituitary disorders during pregnancy. Endocrinol Metab Clin North Am 24:1, 1995

Premawardhana LD, Parkes AB, Ammari F, et al: Postpartum thyroiditis and longterm thyroid status: Prognostic influence of thyroid peroxidase antibodies and ultrasound echogenicity. J Clin Endocrinol Metab 85:71, 2000

Pressman EK, Zeidman SM, Reddy UM, et al: Differentiating lymphocytic adenohypophysitis from pituitary adenoma of the peripartum patient. J Reprod Med 40:251, 1995

Ranzini AC, Ananth CV, Smulian JC, et al: Ultrasonography of the fetal thyroid: Nomograms based on biparietal diameter and gestational age. J Ultrasound Med 20:613, 2001

Ray JG: DDAVP use during pregnancy: An analysis of its safety for mother and child. Obstet Gynecol Surv 53:450, 1998

Renné C, Lopez ER, Steimle-Grauer SA, et al: Thyroid fetal male microchimerisms in mothers with thyroid disorders: Presence of Y-chromosomal immunofluorescence in thyroid-infiltrating lymphocytes is more prevalent in Hashimoto's thyroiditis and Graves' disease than in follicular adenomas. J Clin Endocrinol Metab 89:5810, 2004

Rooney DP, Traub AI, Russell CFJ, et al: Cure of hyperparathyroidism in pregnancy by sternotomy and removal of a mediastinal parathyroid adenoma. Postgrad Med J 74:233, 1998

Rosen IB, Walfish PG: Pregnancy as a predisposing factor in thyroid neoplasia. Arch Surg 121:1287, 1986

Rotondi M, Mazziotti G, Sorvillo F, et al: Effects of increased thyroxine dosage pre-conception on thyroid function during early pregnancy. Eur J Endocrinol 151:695, 2004

Rust DW, Bianchi DW: Microchimerism in endocrine pathology. Endocr Pathol 20(1):11, 2009

Salvatori R: Adrenal insufficiency. JAMA 294:2481, 2005

Schlechte JA: Long-term management of prolactinomas. J Clin Endocrinol Metab 92:2861, 2007

Schnatz PF, Thaxton S: Parathyroidectomy in the third trimester of pregnancy. Obstet Gynecol Surv 60:672, 2005

Seely EW, Brown EM, DeMaggio DM, et al: A prospective study of calciotropic hormones in pregnancy and postpartum: Reciprocal changes in serum intact parathyroid hormone and 1,25-dihydroxyvitamin D. Am J Obstet Gynecol 176:214, 1997

Shangold MM, Dor N, Welt SI, et al: Hyperparathyroidism and pregnancy: A review. Obstet Gynecol Surv 37:217, 1982

Shanis BS, Check JH: Relative resistance of a macroprolactinoma to bromocriptine therapy during pregnancy. Gynecol Endocrinol 10:91, 1996

Sheehan HL: Post-partum necrosis of the anterior pituitary. J Path Bact 45:189, 1937

Sheffield JS, Cunningham FG: Thyrotoxicosis and heart failure that complicate pregnancy, Am J Obstet Gynecol 190:211, 2004

Shoback D: Hypoparathyroidism. N Engl J Med 359:391, 2008

Singer PA, Cooper DS, Levy EG, et al: Treatment guidelines for patients with hyperthyroidism and hypothyroidism. JAMA 273:808, 1995

Siu CW, Zhang XH, Yung C, et al: Hemodynamic changes in hyperthyroidism-related pulmonary hypertension: A prospective echocardiographic study. J Clin Endocrinol Metab 92:1736, 2007

Smith R, Athanasou NA, Ostlere SJ, et al: Pregnancy associated osteoporosis. Q J Med 88:865, 1995

Smyth PP, Wijeyaratne CN, Kaluarachi WN, et al: Sequential studies on thyroid antibodies during pregnancy. Thyroid 15:474, 2005

Song SI, Daneman D, Rovet J: The influence of etiology and treatment factors on intellectual outcome in congenital hypothyroidism. J Dev Behav Pediatr 22:376, 2001

Stagnaro-Green A, Glinoer D: Thyroid autoimmunity and the risk of miscarriage: Baillieres Best Pract Res Clin Endocrinol Metab 18:167, 2004

Stulberg RA, Davies GAL: Maternal thyrotoxicosis and fetal nonimmune hydrops. Obstet Gynecol 95:1036, 2000

Surks MI, Ortiz E, Daniels GH, et al: Subclinical thyroid disease: Scientific review and guidelines for diagnosis and management. JAMA (291)2:228, 2004

Tan TO, Cheng YW, Caughey AB: Are women who are treated for hypothyroidism at risk for pregnancy complications? Am J Obstet Gynecol 194:e1, 2006

Teng W, Shan Z, Teng X, et al: Effect of iodine intake on thyroid diseases in China. N Engl J Med 354:2783, 2006

Thomas M, Weisman SM: Calcium supplementation during pregnancy and lactation: Effects on the mother and the fetus. Am J Obstet Gynecol 194:937, 2006

Thorpe-Beeston JG, Nicolaides KH, Snijders RJM, et al: Thyroid function in small for gestational age fetuses. Obstet Gynecol 77:701, 1991

To WW, Wong MW, Leung TW: Relationship between bone mineral density changes in pregnancy and maternal and pregnancy characteristics: A longitudinal study. Acta Obstet Gynecol Scand 82:820, 2003

Topaloglu AK: Athyreosis, dysgenesis, and dyshormonogenesis in congenital hypothyroidism. Pediatr Endocrinol Rev 3:498, 2006

Utiger RD: Maternal hypothyroidism and fetal development. N Engl J Med 341:601, 1999

Utiger RD: Iodine nutrition—more is better. N Engl J Med 354:2819, 2006

Vaphiades MS, Simmons D, Archer RL, et al: Sheehan syndrome: A splinter of the mind. Surv Ophthalmol 48(2):230, 2003

Vargas Zapata CL, Donangelo CM, Woodhouse LR, et al: Calcium homeostasis during pregnancy and lactation in Brazilian women with low calcium intakes: A longitudinal study. Am J Clin Nutri 80:417, 2004

von Mandach U, Aebersold F, Huch R, et al: Short-term low-dose heparin plus bedrest impairs bone metabolism in pregnant women. Eur J Obstet Gynecol Reprod Biol 106:25, 2003

Vulsma T, Gons M, De Vijilder JJM: Maternal–fetal transfer of thyroxine in congenital hypothyroidism due to a total organification defect or thyroid agenesis. N Engl J Med 321:13, 1989

Vydt T, Verhelst J, De Keulenaer G: Cardiomyopathy and thyrotoxicosis: Tachycardiomyopathy or thyrotoxic cardiomyopathy? Acta Cardiol 61:115, 2006

Weetman AP: Graves' disease. N Engl J Med 343:1236, 2000

Weetman JP: Cellular immune responses in autoimmune thyroid disease. Clin Endocrin 61:405, 2004

Wikner BN, Sparre LS, Stiller CO, et al: Maternal use of thyroid hormones in pregnancy and neonatal outcome. Acta Obstet Gynecol Scand 87(6):617, 2008

Williams DH, Dluhy RG: Diseases of the adrenal cortex. In Braunwald E, Fauci AS, Kasper DL, et al (eds): Harrison's Principles of Internal Medicine, 15th ed. New York, McGraw-Hill, 2001, p 2084

Wolfberg AJ, Lee-Parritz A, Peller AJ, et al: Obstetric and neonatal outcomes associated with maternal hypothyroid disease. J Maternal-Fetal Neonatal Med 17(1):35, 2005

Zeeman GG, Wendel G, Cunningham FG: A blueprint for obstetric critical care. Am J Obstet Gynecol 188:532, 2003

CHAPTER 54

Connective-Tissue Disorders

Connective-tissue disorders, also referred to as *collagen-vascular disorders*, cause a variety of generalized clinical findings and are characterized by autoantibody-mediated connective-tissue abnormalities. These are also called *immune-complex diseases* because many involve deposition of immune complexes in specific organ or tissue sites. Some of these disorders are characterized by sterile inflammation, especially of the skin, joints, blood vessels, and kidneys, and are referred to as *rheumatic diseases*. For inexplicable reasons, many rheumatic diseases primarily affect women. Another major category of connective-tissue diseases includes inherited disorders of bone, skin, cartilage, blood vessels, and basement membranes. Examples include Marfan syndrome, osteogenesis imperfecta, and Ehlers-Danlos syndrome.

Relative to future pregnancies, hemopoietic stem-cell transplantation is becoming accepted therapy for severe autoimmune diseases that include systemic lupus erythematosus, systemic sclerosis, rheumatoid arthritis, and vasculitis. According to Marmont (2008), randomized clinical trials have been launched by the European Group of Blood and Marrow Transplantation

(EBMT). At this time, however, even tentative conclusions are not yet available.

IMMUNE-MEDIATED CONNECTIVE-TISSUE DISEASES

Although the pathogenesis has not been elucidated, immune-mediated disorders can be separated into those clearly associated with and those without autoantibody formation. So-called *rheumatoid factor* is an autoantibody found in many autoimmune inflammatory conditions. Those associated with rheumatoid factor include systemic lupus erythematosus, rheumatoid arthritis, systemic sclerosis (scleroderma), mixed connective-tissue disease, dermatomyositis, polymyositis, and a variety of vasculitis syndromes. In contrast, the *seronegative spondyloarthropathies* do not display rheumatoid factor, but are strongly associated with the presence of the HLA-B27 antigen (Benjamin and Parham, 1992; Moll, 1994). These include ankylosing spondylitis, psoriatic arthritis, Reiter disease, and likely the arthritis syndromes associated with ulcerative colitis and Crohn disease.

Because renal involvement is common and often adversely affects pregnancy, a search for coexisting renal involvement is paramount. Hypertension likewise is common, and exacerbation during pregnancy frequently forces early delivery (Wolfberg and colleagues, 2004). In some of these immune-mediated diseases, *antiphospholipid antibodies* are formed that can cause injury to maternal vasculature and to the placenta.

Immunological Aspects

The immune system is designed to protect cells, tissues, and organs perceived as *self*, and to attack and destroy foreign or *nonself* antigenic material by the production of antibodies. This protection has two phases. The first is the *innate phase*, which is broad and rapid and is mediated through neutrophils, macrophages, and complement. The second is the *adaptive phase*, which is precise and is caused by antigen-specific reactions through T and B lymphocytes that result in memory for future exposures (Parkin and Cohen, 2001).

For some as yet unknown reason, the immune system may be stimulated to begin producing antibodies directed against self or normal tissues. These "misdirected" antibodies are called *autoantibodies*. The stimulus responsible for their production is unknown, but may be due to bacterial or viral injury to genetically susceptible tissues.

Autoantibodies induce destruction by at least two mechanisms. The *cytotoxic mechanism* involves direct antibody attachment to a specific surface antigen, which results in cell injury or destruction. The *immune-complex mechanism* results in tissue damage when an antigen-antibody complex attaches to a susceptible tissue. The complex may then incite a complement response or *cascade*, resulting in the release of chemotactic substances that attract polymorphonuclear cells.

The *major histocompatibility complex (MHC)* is a series of 40 to 50 genes located on the short arm of chromosome 6, and is known as the *human leukocyte antigen (HLA)* complex. These genetic loci code for distinct cell-surface glycoproteins, including transplantation antigens, and are involved in self and nonself recognition. Class I antigens include HLA-A, -B, and -C. Class II antigens include HLA-DR, -DQ, and –DP. Through complex interactions that include T- and B-cell stimulation and interaction with immunoglobulins and the complement system, nonself antigens or, in the abnormal state, self antigens in normal tissue are destroyed.

Immune-Mediated Disease and Pregnancy

Very few immune disorders arise only during pregnancy. Maternal isoimmunization from fetal red cell or platelet antigens is the most common (see Chap. 29, p. 618). Some theories of the causes of preeclampsia-eclampsia (see Chap. 34, p. 709) and recurrent abortion (see Chap. 9, p. 225) implicate an immunological basis.

Some pregnancy-induced immune alterations may modulate connective-tissue disorders (see Chap. 5, p. 116). For example, one considered important is the predominance of T2 helper cells over the cytokine-producing T1 helper cells (Keeling and Oswald, 2009). Although it is generally thought that these immunological changes have negligible effects on immune-mediated collagen-vascular disorders, the effects of large amounts of estrogen, progesterone, and prolactin must be considered. For example, estrogens upregulate and androgens downregulate T-cell response, and a number of cytokines are regulated by sex hormones (Häupl and associates, 2008a; Refojo and colleagues, 2003). Progesterone is an immunosuppresive (Cutolo and co-workers, 2006). In addition, given that autoimmune rheumatic diseases mostly affect women, Lockshin (2002) postulates a modulating effect of hormones rather than a causative role. Østensen and Villiger (2007) suggest that the hormonal and immunological alterations in pregnancy may correct the altered immunoregulation in rheumatoid arthritis.

Fetal Cell Microchimerism

Fetal cells and DNA are present in maternal blood starting in the first trimester (Sitar and associates, 2005; Waldorf

and Nelson, 2008). *Fetal cell microchimerism* is an intriguing phenomenon that has been used to help explain the predilection of autoimmune disorders for women (Adams and Nelson, 2004). By this putative mechanism, persistent fetal cells in the maternal circulation stimulate the production of autoantibodies that underlie some autoimmune conditions. In this scheme, fetal cells such as thymocytes become engrafted in maternal tissues, and "immortal" long-lived lymphocytes circulate. Lupus may therefore represent a chronic graft-versus-host response to transplacentally acquired fetal cells, which is also suggested for some thyroid diseases and systemic sclerosis (Artlett and associates, 1998; Jimenez and Artlett, 2005; Srivatsa and associates, 2001).

Women with lupus who have given birth to a male(e) have also been found to have male cells in every histologically abnormal tissue type, but not in normal tissue. Although this suggests that fetal cells may be associated with lupus, it is unclear if this causes or is an effect of disease progression or if it even is unrelated (Johnson and colleagues, 2001). Microchimerism with rheumatoid arthritis-associated HLA alleles has also been described in women with rheumatoid arthritis compared with nonaffected controls (Rak and co-workers, 2009). Interestingly, microchimeric cells may play a beneficial role by helping to repair damaged or diseased tissue (Barinaga, 2002).

SYSTEMIC LUPUS ERYTHEMATOSUS (SLE)

Lupus is a heterogeneous autoimmune disease with a complex pathogenesis that results in interactions between susceptibility genes and environmental factors that cause an abnormal immune response (Hahn, 2008). Immune system abnormalities include overactive B lymphocytes that are responsible for autoantibody production. These result in tissue and cellular damage when autoantibodies or immune complexes are directed at one or more cellular nuclear components (Tsokos, 2001). Some autoantibodies produced in patients with lupus are shown in Table 54-1.

Almost 90 percent of cases of lupus are in women, and its prevalence in those of childbearing age is about 1 in 500 (Lockshin and Sammaritano, 2000). Because of this, the disease is encountered relatively frequently during pregnancy. The 15-year survival rate is 80 percent (Rahman and Isenberg, 2008). Infection, lupus flares, end-organ failure, hypertension, strokes, and cardiovascular disease account for most deaths.

Genetic influences are implicated by a higher concordance with monozygotic compared with dizygotic twins—25 versus 2 percent, respectively, and a 10-percent frequency in patients with one affected family member. The relative risk of disease is increased if there is inheritance of the "autoimmunity gene" on chromosome 16 that predisposes to SLE, rheumatoid arthritis, Crohn disease, and psoriasis (Hahn, 2008). Other susceptibility genes include HLA-A1, B8, DR3, and DRB1; IRF5; and STAT 4 as well as others (Hom and associates, 2008; Rahman and Isenberg, 2008).

Clinical Findings

Lupus is notoriously variable in its presentation, course, and outcome (Rahman and Isenberg, 2008). Clinical manifestations may be confined initially to one organ system, with others

TABLE 54-1. Some Autoantibodies Produced in Patients with Systemic Lupus Erythematosus (SLE)

Antibody	Prevalence (percent)	Clinical Associations
Antinuclear (ANA)	84–98	Best screening test, multiple antibodies; a second negative test makes SLE unlikely
Anti-double-stranded (ds)-DNA	62–70	High titers SLE-specific; may correlate with nephritis and vasculitis activity
Anti-Sm	30–38	Specific for SLE
Anti-RNP	33–40	Not SLE specific, correlates with myositis, esophageal dysmotility; a defining antibody for mixed-connective tissue disease
Anti-Ro (SS-A)	30–49	Not SLE specific; associated with Sjögren syndrome, cutaneous lupus, ANA-negative lupus, neonatal lupus with heart block
Anti-La (SS-B)	10–35	Present in SLE—possibly decreased risk of nephritis; Sjögren syndrome, neonatal lupus with heart block
Antihistone	70	Common in drug-induced lupus (95%)
Antiphospholipid	21–50	Lupus anticoagulant and anticardiolipin antibodies associated with thrombosis, fetal loss, thrombocytopenia, valvular heart disease; false-positive test for syphilis
Antierythrocyte	60	Overt hemolysis uncommon
Antiplatelet	30	Thrombocytopenia in 15%; poor clinical test

Data from Arbuckle and colleagues (2003), Hahn (2008), and Shmerling (2003).

becoming involved as the disease progresses (Table 54-2). Alternatively, lupus may initially manifest by multisystem involvement. Common findings are malaise, fever, arthritis, rash, pleuropericarditis, photosensitivity, anemia, and cognitive dysfunction. At least half of patients have renal involvement. *Libman-Sacks endocarditis* was described with lupus but likely is due to presence of subsequently discussed anticardiolipin antibodies (Hojnik and associates, 1996). These valvular lesions may cause thromboembolic seeding but uncommonly lead to hemodynamic dysfunction (Moyssakis and colleagues, 2002).

There is also evidence that lupus is associated with decline in attention, memory, and reasoning (Kozora and associates, 2008).

Laboratory Findings

Identification of antinuclear antibodies (ANA) is the best screening test, however, a positive test result is not specific for lupus. For example, low titers are found in normal individuals, other autoimmune diseases, acute viral infections, and chronic inflammatory processes. Several drugs can also cause a positive

TABLE 54-2. Clinical Manifestations of Systemic Lupus Erythematosus

Organ System	Clinical Manifestations	Percent
Systemic	Fatigue, malaise, fever, weight loss	95
Musculoskeletal	Arthralgias, myalgias, polyarthritis, myopathy	95
Hematological	Anemia, hemolysis, leukopenia, thrombocytopenia, lupus anticoagulant, splenomegaly	85
Cutaneous	Malar (butterfly) rash, discoid rash, photosensitivity, oral ulcers, alopecia, skin rashes	80
Neurological	Cognitive dysfunction, mood disorder, headache, seizures	60
Cardiopulmonary	Pleuritis, pericarditis, myocarditis, pneumonitis, Libman-Sacks endocarditis, pulmonary hypertension	60
Renal	Proteinuria, casts, nephrotic syndrome, renal failure	30–50
Gastrointestinal	Anorexia, nausea, pain, diarrhea	40
Vascular	Thrombosis: venous (10%), arterial (5%)	15
Ocular	Conjunctivitis	15

Modified from Hahn (2008), with permission.

reaction. Antibodies to double-stranded DNA (dsDNA) and to Smith (Sm) antigens are relatively specific for lupus, whereas other antibodies are not (see Table 54-1). More than 100 antigen-autoantibody pairs have been described in SLE (Sherer and co-workers, 2004).

Anemia is common, and there may be leukopenia and thrombocytopenia. Proteinuria and casts are found in the half of patients with glomerular lesions, and there may be renal insufficiency. Nephropathy is more common when antiphospholipid antibodies are found (Moroni and colleagues, 2004). Other laboratory findings include false-positive syphilis serology, prolonged partial thromboplastin time, and positive serum rheumatoid factor assay. Elevated serum D-dimer levels commonly follow a flare or infection, but unexplained persistent elevations are associated with a high risk for thrombosis (Wu and associates, 2008).

Diagnosis

The revised criteria of the American Rheumatism Association for diagnosis of systemic lupus are listed in Table 54-3. If any four or more of these 11 criteria are present, serially or simultaneously, the diagnosis of lupus is made.

Drug-Induced Lupus

Numerous drugs have been reported to induce a lupus-like syndrome. These include procainamide, quinidine, hydralazine, α-methyldopa, phenytoin, and phenobarbital. Drug-induced lupus is rarely associated with glomerulonephritis and usually regresses when the medication is discontinued (Rubin, 1997).

Lupus and Pregnancy

Of nearly 16.7 million pregnancies in the United States from 2000 to 2003, 13,555 were complicated by lupus—an incidence of approximately 1 in 1250 pregnancies (Clowse and associates, 2008). Over the past several decades, pregnancy outcomes in women with SLE have improved remarkably. Important factors for pregnancy outcome include whether disease is active at the beginning of pregnancy, age and parity, coexistence of other medical or obstetrical disorders, and whether antiphospholipid antibodies are detected (see p. 1151).

During pregnancy, lupus improves in a third of women, remains unchanged in a third, and worsens in the remaining third. Thus, in any given pregnancy, the clinical condition can worsen or *flare* without warning (Khamashta and colleagues, 1997). Petri (1998) reported a 7-percent risk of major morbidity during pregnancy. Common complications in a cohort of 13,555 women with SLE during pregnancy are shown in Table 54-4. The maternal mortality and morbidity rate was 325 per 100,000—a massively increased rate. **It is certain that lupus can be life threatening to both the mother and her fetus-infant.** In general, pregnancy outcome is better if:

- Lupus activity has been quiescent for at least 6 months before conception
- There is no active renal involvement manifest by proteinuria or renal dysfunction
- Superimposed preeclampsia does not develop
- There is no evidence of antiphospholipid antibody activity.

TABLE 54-3. The 1997 Revised Criteria of the American Rheumatism Association for Systemic Lupus Erythematosus (SLE)

Criteria[a]	Comments
Malar rash	Malar erythema
Discoid rash	Erythematous patches, scaling, follicular plugging
Photosensitivity	Exposure to UV light causes rash
Oral ulcers	Usually painless oral and nasopharyngeal ulcers
Arthritis	Nonerosive involving two or more peripheral joints
Serositis	Pleuritis or pericarditis
Renal disorder	Proteinuria greater than 0.5 g/day or > 3+ dipstick, or cellular casts
Neurological disorders	Seizures or psychosis without other cause
Hematological disorders	Hemolytic anemia, leukopenia, lymphopenia, or thrombocytopenia
Immunological disorders	Anti-dsDNA or anti-Sm antibodies, or false-positive VDRL, abnormal level of IgM or IgG anticardiolipin antibodies, or lupus anticoagulant
Antinuclear antibodies	Abnormal titer of ANAs

[a]If four or more criteria are present at any time during disease course, SLE can be diagnosed with 75-percent specificity and 95-percent sensitivity.
ANAs = antinuclear antibodies; dsDNA = double-stranded DNA; Sm = Smith; UV = ultraviolet; VDRL = Venereal Disease Research Laboratory.
From Hochberg (1997), with permission.

Lupus Nephritis

The prognosis for women with SLE and glomerulonephritis has improved remarkably over the past 30 years (Moroni and Ponticelli, 2005). Women with renal disease have a high incidence of gestational hypertension and preeclampsia, but if their disease remains in remission, they usually have good pregnancy outcomes (Huong, 2001; Moroni, 2002; Packham, 1992, and all their colleagues). Of the 125 pregnancies reported by Lockshin (1989), 63 percent of women with preexisting renal disease developed preeclampsia compared with only 14 percent of those without underlying renal disease. Moroni and Ponticelli (2005) reviewed results published between 1980 and 2003. Of a total of 309 pregnancies complicated by established lupus

TABLE 54-4. Complications in 13,555 Pregnancies in Women with Systemic Lupus Erythematosus

Complications	Percent
Comorbid illness	
Pregestational diabetes	5.6
Thrombophilia	4.0
Hypertension	3.9
Renal failure	0.2
Pulmonary hypertension	0.2
Pregnancy complications	
Preeclampsia	22.5
Preterm labor	20.8
Fetal-growth restriction	5.6
Eclampsia	0.5
Medical complications	
Anemia	12.6
Thrombocytopenia	4.3
Thrombotic—stroke, pulmonary embolism, deep-vein thrombosis	1.7
Infections—pneumonia, sepsis syndrome	2.2
Maternal morbidity-mortality rate	325/100,000

Data from Clowse and colleagues (2008).

nephritis, 30 percent suffered a flare, and 40 percent of these had associated renal insufficiency. The maternal mortality rate was 1.3 percent.

There are two recent studies describing pregnancy outcomes in women with lupus nephritis. Wagner and co-workers (2009) compared outcomes of 58 women cared for during 90 pregnancies at the Mayo Clinic. Active nephritis was associated with a significantly higher incidence of maternal complications—57 versus 11 percent—compared with women without nephritis. Quiescent nephritis had a nonsignificant effect on preeclampsia rates compared with lupus patients without renal impairment. The fetal death rate with active maternal nephritis was 35 compared with 9 percent in those with quiescent nephritis. Imbasciati and associates (2009) described outcomes in 113 pregnancies in 81 women with known lupus nephritis. During a third of pregnancies, there was a renal flare. Nine pregnancy were excluded to due miscarriage. Of the 104 remaining pregnancies, a third were delivered preterm, a third of infants weighed < 2500 g, and the perinatal mortality rate was 6 percent.

Most authorities recommend continuation of immunosuppressive therapy for nephritis during pregnancy. It is not clear whether the dosage should be increased peripartum. Although it is often stated that this is the time that activation or exacerbations are most likely to develop, the evidence is not conclusive.

Lupus versus Preeclampsia-Eclampsia

Chronic hypertension complicates up to 30 percent of pregnancies in women with SLE (Egerman and colleagues, 2005). Moreover, preeclampsia is common, and superimposed preeclampsia is encountered even more often in those with nephropathy and in women with antiphospholipid antibodies (Bertsias and associates, 2008). It may be difficult, if not impossible, to differentiate lupus nephropathy from severe preeclampsia if organs other than the kidney are not involved (Petri, 2007). We are of the view that decreased complement values or increased anti-DNA titers are not useful to identify worsening lupus activity in this setting. If identified, however, they reportedly support the diagnosis of a reactivation of lupus nephritis, termed *renal flare*. Central nervous system involvement with lupus may culminate in convulsions similar to those of eclampsia. Thrombocytopenia, with or without hemolysis, may further confuse the diagnosis because of its similarity to the hemolysis, elevated liver enzymes, low platelet count (HELLP) syndrome. Management is identical to that for preeclampsia-eclampsia, described in Chapter 34 (p. 728).

Management During Pregnancy

Management consists primarily of monitoring the maternal clinical and laboratory conditions as well as fetal well-being. Pregnancy-induced thrombocytopenia and proteinuria resemble lupus disease activity, and the identification of a lupus flare is confounded by the increase in facial and palmar erythema of normal pregnancy (Lockshin and Sammaritano, 2003). Some authorities have advocated a number of numerical scales to emphasize ongoing disease activity. Components are weighted for severity, both with the SLE-Pregnancy Disease Activity Index (SLEPDAI) and the Lupus Activity Index (Buyon and colleagues, 1999; Ruiz-Irastorza and associates, 2004).

Monitoring of lupus activity and identification of pending lupus flares by a variety of laboratory techniques has been recommended. The sedimentation rate may be misleading because of pregnancy-induced hyperfibrinogenemia. Serum complement levels are also normally increased in pregnancy (see Chap. 5, p. 116 and the Appendix.). And although falling or low levels of complement components C_3, C_4, and CH_{50} are more likely to be associated with active disease, higher levels provide no assurance against disease activation. Our experiences, as well as those of Varner and co-workers (1983) and Lockshin and Druzin (1995), are that there is no correlation between clinical manifestations of disease and complement levels.

Serial hematological studies may detect changes in disease activity. Hemolysis is characterized by a positive Coombs test, anemia, reticulocytosis, and unconjugated hyperbilirubinemia. Thrombocytopenia, leukopenia, or both may develop. According to Lockshin and Druzin (1995), chronic thrombocytopenia in early pregnancy may be due to *antiphospholipid antibodies*. Later, thrombocytopenia may indicate the onset of preeclampsia.

Serum transaminase activity reflects hepatic involvement, as does a rise in serum bilirubin. Azathioprine therapy also may induce enzyme elevations. Urine is tested frequently to detect new-onset or worsening proteinuria. Overt proteinuria that persists is an ominous sign, even more so if accompanied by other evidence of the nephrotic syndrome or abnormal serum creatinine levels.

The fetus should be closely observed for adverse effects. Fetal growth is monitored, and careful attention is given to the development of hypertension. Singsen and colleagues (1985) and Petri (1998) recommend screening for anti-SS-A and anti-SS-B antibodies, and if found, fetal cardiac function should be evaluated. Although we routinely evaluate the fetus for arrhythmias, we do not screen for these antibodies. As discussed in Chapter 15 (p. 345), antepartum fetal surveillance is done as outlined by the American College of Obstetricians and Gynecologists (2007a). Unless hypertension develops or there is evidence of fetal compromise or growth restriction, pregnancy is allowed to progress to term. Peripartum corticosteroids in "stress doses" are given to women who are taking these drugs or who recently have done so.

Pharmacological Treatment

There is no cure, and complete remissions are rare. Approximately a fourth of patients have mild disease, which is not life threatening, but may be disabling because of pain and fatigue. Arthralgia and serositis are managed by *nonsteroidal anti-inflammatory drugs*, including aspirin. Because of the risk of premature closure of the fetal ductus arteriosus, therapeutic doses probably should not be used after 24 weeks (Briggs and colleagues, 2005). Low-dose aspirin, however, can be used safely throughout gestation. Severe disease is managed with *corticosteroids* such as prednisone, 1 to 2 mg/kg per day. After the disease is controlled, this dose is tapered to a daily dose of 10 to 15 mg each morning. Corticosteroid therapy can result in the development of gestational or even type 1 diabetes. Long-term antibody-based immunoadsorption has been used in pregnancy for removal of autoantibodies and lipoproteins in women with serious complications who did not respond to conventional therapy (Dittrich and colleagues, 2002).

Immunosuppressive agents such as *azathioprine* are beneficial in controlling active disease (Contreras and colleagues, 2004; Hahn, 2008). In nonpregnant patients, these are usually reserved for lupus nephritis or disease that is steroid resistant. Azathioprine has a good safety record during pregnancy (Petri, 2007). Its recommended daily oral dose is 2 to 3 mg/kg. According to Buhimschi and Weiner (2009), *cyclophosphamide* is teratogenic, and although not usually recommended during pregnancy, severe disease may be treated after 12 weeks. As discussed in Chapter 14 (pp. 320 and 322), other medications to be avoided include *mycophenolate mofetil* and *methotrexate* (Anderka and colleagues, 2009; FDA Alert, 2008).

Antimalarials help control skin disease. Although these agents cross the placenta, *hydroxychloroquine* has not been associated with congenital malformations. Because of the long half life of antimalarials and because discontinuing therapy can precipitate a lupus flare, most authors recommend their continuation (Borden and Parke, 2001; Harris, 2002). Levy and colleagues (2001) randomly assigned 20 pregnant women to hydroxychloroquine or placebo and reported improvement in SLEPDAI scores with drug use compared with placebo administration.

When severe disease supervenes—usually a lupus flare—high-dose glucocorticoid therapy is given. Petri (2007) recommends pulse therapy consisting of methylprednisolone, 1000 mg given intravenously over 90 minutes daily for 3 days, then a return to maintenance doses if possible.

Perinatal Mortality and Morbidity

Adverse perinatal outcomes are increased significantly in pregnancies complicated by lupus. These include preterm delivery, fetal-growth restriction, stillbirths, and neonatal lupus. Outcomes are worse with a lupus flare; significant proteinuria; renal impairment; and with chronic hypertension, development of preeclampsia, or both (Aggarwal, 1999; Scott, 2002; Wagner, 2009, and all their associates). The recent observations of Lee and co-workers (2009) are worrisome. In a mouse SLE model, they showed that autoantibodies directed against the *N*-methyl-D-aspartate neuroreceptor caused fetal neurotoxicity and speculate that this might account for the high incidence of learning disorders in children of affected mothers.

The reasons at least partially responsible for adverse fetal consequences include decidual vasculopathy with placental infarction and decreased perfusion (Hanly and colleagues, 1988; Lubbe and Liggins, 1984). Anti-SS-A (Ro) and anti-SS-B (La) antibodies may damage the fetal heart and conduction system, causing neonatal death (Alexander and co-workers, 1992; Tseng and Buyon, 1997). Women with livedo reticularis and lupus or a lupus-like illness, but who do not produce antiphospholipid antibodies, display increased rates of pregnancy complications (Sangle and associates, 2005).

Neonatal Lupus

This unusual syndrome is characterized by skin lesions, or *lupus dermatitis*; a variable number of hematological and systemic derangements; and occasionally congenital heart block (Boh, 2004; Lee, 2009). Although usually associated with anti-SS-A and -SS-B antibodies, McGeachv and Lam (2009) described an affected infant in whom only anti-RNP antibodies were found. Thrombocytopenia and hepatic involvement is seen in 5 to 10 percent. One report suggests that neonatal lupus may appear up to 4 weeks after birth (Stirnemann and associates, 2002). Lockshin and co-workers (1988) prospectively followed 91 infants born to women with lupus. Four had definite neonatal lupus and four had possible disease. Clinical manifestations, which include cutaneous lupus, thrombocytopenia, and autoimmune hemolysis, are transient and clear within a few months (Lee and Weston, 1984). The recurrence risk in subsequent offspring for neonatal lupus is 25 percent (Julkunen and colleagues, 1993).

Congenital Heart Block

This fetal complication results from diffuse myocarditis and fibrosis in the region between the atrioventricular (AV) node and bundle of His. Buyon and colleagues (1993) reported that congenital heart block occurred almost exclusively in fetuses of women with antibodies to the SS-A or SS-B antigens. These antibodies may also cause otherwise unexplained stillbirths (Ottaviani and co-workers, 2004). Even in the presence of such antibodies, however, the incidence of arrhythmia is only 3 percent (Lockshin and associates, 1988). The cardiac lesion is permanent, and a pacemaker is generally necessary. Long-term prognosis is poor, and a third of affected infants die within 3 years (Waltuck and Buyon, 1994). The risk of recurrence in subsequent offspring is 10 to 15 percent (Julkunen and colleagues, 1993).

Maternal corticosteroid administration to treat fetal heart block is controversial. Shinohara and colleagues (1999) reported no heart block in 26 neonates whose mothers received corticosteroid maintenance therapy before 16 weeks. By contrast, 15 of 61 neonates with heart block were born to women in whom corticosteroid therapy was begun after 16 weeks. In an intriguing observational study from Israel, Rein and colleagues (2009) followed 70 fetuses of mothers positive for anti-SS-A or -SS-B antibodies prospectively with serial kinetocardiography (FKCG) to measure AV conduction time. In six fetuses, first-degree block developed at 21 to 34 weeks, and maternal dexamethasone treatment was associated with normalization of AV conduction in all within 3 to 14 days. There were no recurrences, and the infants all were well at a median follow-up of 4 years.

Long-Term Prognosis and Contraception

In general, women with lupus and chronic vascular or renal disease should limit family size because of morbidity associated with the disease as well as increased adverse perinatal outcomes. Two large multicenter clinical trials have shown that combination oral contraceptives (COCs) did not increase the incidence of lupus flares (Sánchez-Guerrero and colleagues, 2005; Petri and co-workers, 2005). Still, the American College of Obstetricians and Gynecologists (2006) recommends that COC use be avoided in women who have nephritis, antiphospholipid anti-

bodies, or a vascular disease. Progestin-only implants and injections also provide effective contraception with no known effects on lupus flares. Concerns that intrauterine device (IUD) use and immunosuppressive therapy lead to increased infection rates in these patients are not evidenced based. Tubal sterilization may be advantageous and is performed with greatest safety postpartum or whenever the disease is quiescent.

ANTIPHOSPHOLIPID ANTIBODIES

Phospholipids are the main lipid constituents of cell and organelle membranes. Several antibodies directed against these various phospholipids and to proteins bound to phospholipids have been described. These antibodies include *lupus anticoagulant (LAC)* and *anticardiolipin antibodies (ACAs)*. They may be of IgG, IgM, and IgA classes, alone or in combination. Cardiolipin is but one of many phospholipids and is found in mitochondrial membranes and platelets.

The term *lupus anticoagulant* was introduced by Feinstein and Rapaport (1972) in a review of acquired inhibitors of coagulation. They described that certain patients with lupus had some coagulation tests that were prolonged and thus suggested anticoagulant activity. Paradoxically, the so-called anticoagulant is powerfully thrombotic in vivo, although LAC prolongs all phospholipid-dependent coagulation tests, including the prothrombin time, partial thromboplastin time, and Russell viper venom time. Each of these tests requires a phospholipid surface to which other clotting factors attach and combine (Fig. 54-1).

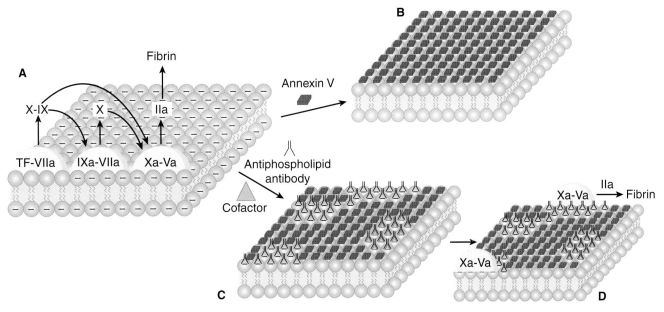

FIGURE 54-1 A. Negatively charged anionic phospholipids (*light blue circles*), as part of the cell-membrane bilayer, serve as potent cofactors for assembly of three coagulation complexes. These complexes include: tissue factor–VIIa (TF-VIIa) complex (*first, yellow half circle*), IXa-VIIIa complex (*second, yellow half circle*), and Xa-Va complex (*third*). The phospholipids thus accelerate blood coagulation by generating factors IXa and Xa. Factor Xa yields factor IIa (thrombin), which in turn cleaves fibrinogen to form fibrin. **B.** When antiphospholipid antibodies are absent, annexin V (*green squares*) forms clusters that bind to the surface of anionic phospholipids. Coagulation complexes are unable to bind to the surface phospholipids, and coagulation is inhibited. **C.** Through direct binding to surface phospholipids or through an interaction with protein-phospholipid cofactors, antiphospholipid antibodies disrupt the ability of annexin V to cluster on the phospholipid surface. **D.** These unbound areas, free of annexin V, permit more anionic phospholipids to be available to coagulation complexes. Coagulation is thus accelerated, and thrombosis promoted. (Adapted from Rand and colleagues, 1997a, 2008.)

Clinical Features

Antiphospholipid antibodies may be found in asymptomatic patients with or without lupus, or they may be associated with the *antiphospholipid antibody syndrome (APS)*. This syndrome is characterized by recurrent arterial or venous thromboses, thrombocytopenia, and fetal losses—especially stillbirths—during the second half of pregnancy (Branch and Khamashta, 2003; Oshiro and associates, 1996; Warren and Silver, 2004).

Antiphospholipid antibody syndrome may develop alone or in association with lupus or other autoimmune disorders. Central nervous system involvement is one of the most prominent clinical manifestations and includes arterial and venous thrombotic events, psychiatric features, and other nonthrombotic neurological syndromes (Sanna and co-workers, 2003). Renovascular involvement may lead to renal failure, and it may be difficult to differentiate from lupus nephritis (D'Cruz, 2009). Interestingly, APS may mimic the presentation of multiple sclerosis (Ruiz-Irastorza and associates, 2001). Finally, Ahmed and associates (2009) reported a woman who developed spontaneous cecal perforation postpartum presumably from antibody induced infarction.

Pathophysiology

Many patients with lupus have circulating antibodies specifically directed either against phospholipids or against phospholipid-binding proteins such as β_2-glycoprotein I (apolipoprotein H). Anticardiolipin antibodies apparently bind directly to β_2-glycoprotein I, and this protein acts as a co-factor in this antigen-antibody reaction (Chamley and co-workers, 1999). There is evidence that complement activation may contribute to pathogenesis (Avalos and Tsokos, 2009).

β_2-Glycoprotein I

The major activity of this protein appears to be its phospholipid-dependent anticoagulant inhibition of prothrombinase activity of platelets and ADP-induced platelet aggregation (Shi and colleagues, 1993). β_2-Glycoprotein I competitively inhibits the binding of coagulation factors, especially factor XII, and the prothrombinase complex to phospholipid surfaces. This prevents activation of the coagulation cascade. An antibody directed against β_2-glycoprotein I would bind and prevent it from acting as a phospholipid-dependent anticoagulant. β_2-Glycoprotein I is found in high concentrations on the surface of the syncytiotrophoblast. This seems intuitive because the decidua is a critical area in which to prevent coagulation. In addition, β_2-glycoprotein I may be involved in implantation because it is known that this protein binds heparin. Moreover, trophoblastic cells have heparin-like binding sites. Thus, a local loss of β_2-glycoprotein I by an antibody directed against it might prevent implantation or result in intervillous space thrombosis, or both (Chamley and associates, 1999).

Lupus Anticoagulant

LAC appears to require a cofactor for its in vitro anticoagulant function. Specifically, it does not bind directly to negatively charged phospholipids, but instead, LAC binds to phospholipid-bound prothrombin (Galli and Bevers, 1994). Other phospho-lipid-binding proteins may be involved in the pathophysiology of the antiphospholipid antibody syndrome. These include *protein C* and *protein S*, which are both endogenous anticoagulants, and *annexin V* (Robertson and Greaves, 2006). The last is also known as *placental anticoagulant protein I* or *lipocortin V*, and annexin V coats the syncytiotrophoblast in high concentration (Chamley and associates, 1999). Thus, an antibody that binds protein C or S would result in venous, arterial, or decidual thrombosis, whereas binding of annexin V would result in coagulation and thrombosis in the intervillous space (see Fig. 54-1).

Rand and co-workers (1997b) reported that placental tissue from pregnancy complicated by APS had significantly less apical membrane-associated annexin V than normal placenta. Exposure of placental villous cultures to five antiphospholipid IgGs also resulted in a significant reduction in apical membrane annexin V. In another study, there was a reduction in annexin V in endothelial cell tissue cultures exposed to antiphospholipid antibodies (Rand and colleagues, 1997a).

These discoveries led to the development of direct assays to measure antibodies against β_2-glycoprotein I and prothrombin. A number of investigators have found these to be increased in and associated with pregnancies complicated by APS (Destefano, 2009; Falcón, 1997; Yamada, 2009, and all their co-workers). Conversely, others have not observed a clinically significant association with these antibodies (Lee, 1999; Lynch, 1999; Manuck, 2009, and all their associates).

Association of Antiphospholipid Antibodies with Lupus

Patients with clinical lupus frequently also have lupus anticoagulant or antiphospholipid antibodies, or both. Love and Santoro (1990) reviewed 29 series that included more than 1000 patients with lupus and reported an average frequency of 34 percent for LAC and 44 percent for ACAs. In nearly half of those with positive testing, both antibodies were found.

In general, patients with LAC have higher levels of antiphospholipid antibodies, and about a third of those with biological false-positive tests for syphilis have ACAs (Branch, 1991). Only about 20 percent of patients with identifiable ACAs also have LAC. Importantly, in patients with lupus, documentation of either ACA or LAC is a risk factor for thrombosis, neurological disorders, and thrombocytopenia (Hahn, 2008). As discussed in Chapter 9 (p. 225), these antibodies have also been associated with excessive pregnancy loss (Robertson and Greaves, 2006). *Libman-Sacks endocarditis* is much more prevalent in patients with lupus who have antiphospholipid antibodies (Hojnik and colleagues, 1996). These antibodies have been associated with the development of "primary" vaso-occlusive disease involving different organs such as the kidney as discussed previously.

Antiphospholipid Antibodies and Normal Pregnancy

About 5 percent of all otherwise healthy *nonpregnant* individuals screened have nonspecific antiphospholipid antibodies in low titers. Lockwood and colleagues (1989) studied 737 normal pregnant women and found that two–0.3 percent–had lupus anticoagulant and 16–2.2 percent–had elevated concentrations of either IgM- or IgG-ACAs. Harris and Spinnato (1991) studied 1449 consecutive pregnant women and found 1.8 percent were positive for IgG-ACAs and 4.3 percent for IgM-ACAs. Pattison and co-workers (1993) studied 933 consecutive prenatal patients and found nine–0.1 percent–with ACAs, 11–1.2 percent–with LACs, and two women with both. Yasuda and associates (1995) found that 7 percent of 860 pregnant Japanese women had ACAs. Taken together, these studies totalling almost 4000 normal pregnancies reported an average prevalence of 4.7 percent—the same as normal nonpregnant individuals.

Diagnosis of Antiphospholipid Antibody Syndrome (APS)

By international consensus, the syndrome is diagnosed on the basis of clinical and laboratory criteria (Levine and co-workers, 2002; Robertson and Greaves, 2006). These are shown in Table 54-5, and one of two clinical criteria, which include vascular thrombosis or certain pregnancy morbidity, must be present. In addition, at least two laboratory criteria that include LAC activity or medium- to high-positive specific IgG- or IgM-ACAs must be confirmed on two occasions 6 weeks apart.

Classification criteria shown in Table 54-5 also provide indications for testing. Branch and Khamashta (2003) recommend conservative interpretation of results based on repeated tests from a reliable laboratory that are consistent with each clinical case. Because only approximately 20 percent of patients with APS have a positive LAC reaction alone, both the clotting test to identify the LAC and the anticardiolipin enzyme-linked immunosorbent assay (ELISA) test must be performed. Giannakopoulos and associates (2009) describe a beta(2)GPI enzyme-linked immunosorbent assay in addition.

Efforts have been made to standardize ACA assays by using ELISA, and values are reported in units and expressed as *negative, low-positive, medium-positive,* or *high-positive* (Harris and colleagues, 1987a, b). Despite this, there still is no totally accurate standardization for these assays (Branch and Khamashta, 2003). Interlaboratory variation can be large, and agreement between commercial kits is also poor.

Tests for the LAC are nonspecific coagulation tests. The *partial thromboplastin time* is generally prolonged because the anticoagulant interferes with conversion of prothrombin to thrombin in vitro. Tests considered most specific are the *dilute Russell viper venom test (dRVVT)* and the *platelet neutralization procedure.* There is currently disagreement as to which of these is best for screening. If either is positive after addition of normal plasma, the diagnosis is confirmed.

Pathophysiology of Antiphospholipid Antibodies in Pregnancy

The combination of lupus anticoagulant and high levels of ACAs is strongly associated with decidual vasculopathy, placental infarction, fetal-growth restriction, early-onset preeclampsia, and recurrent fetal death. Some of these women, like those with lupus, also have a high incidence of venous and arterial thromboses, cerebral thrombosis, hemolytic anemia, thrombocytopenia, and pulmonary hypertension (American College of Obstetricians and Gynecologists, 2007b; Clowse and co-workers, 2008).

Mechanism of Action

It is not precisely known how these antibodies cause damage, but it is likely that their actions are multifactorial. According to Chamley and co-workers (1999), platelets may be damaged directly by antiphospholipid antibody or indirectly by binding β_2-glycoprotein I, which causes platelets to be susceptible to aggregation. Rand and colleagues (1997a, b, 1998) propose that phospholipid-containing endothelial cell or syncytiotrophoblast membranes may be damaged directly by the antiphospholipid antibody or indirectly by antibody binding to either β_2-glycoprotein I or annexin V (see Fig. 54-1). This prevents the cell membranes from protecting the syncytiotrophoblast and endothelium and results in exposure of basement membrane. It is known that damaged platelets adhere to exposed basement membrane of endothelium and syncytiotrophoblast and result in thrombus formation (Lubbe and Liggins, 1984).

There are other proposed mechanisms. Pierro and co-workers (1999) reported that antiphospholipid antibodies decreased

---

TABLE 54-5. Classification Criteria for the Antiphospholipid Antibody Syndrome

Criteria	
Clinical	
Thrombosis	Unexplained venous, arterial, or small vessel thrombosis in any organ or tissue
Pregnancy	One or more unexplained fetal losses after 10 weeks; three or more consecutive miscarriages before 10 weeks; or preterm delivery for severe preeclampsia or placental insufficiency before 34 completed weeks
Laboratory	
Anticardiolipin antibodies	IgG or IgM isotypes in medium to high titers at least 6 weeks apart
Lupus anticoagulant	Identified twice, at least 6 weeks apart

From International Consensus Statement (Wilson and colleagues, 1999) and the American College of Obstetricians and Gynecologists (2007b).

decidual production of the vasodilating prostaglandin E_2. Decreased protein C or S activity and increased prothrombin activation have been reported (Ogunyemi and associates, 2002; Zangari and colleagues, 1997). Amengual and co-workers (2003) presented evidence that thrombosis with APS is due to activation of the tissue factor pathway. Finally, there is evidence that uncontrolled placental complement activation by antiphospholipid antibodies may play a role in fetal loss and growth restriction (Holers and colleagues, 2002).

Adverse Pregnancy Outcomes

There is no doubt that antiphospholipid antibodies are associated with increased rates of fetal wastage (see Chap. 9, p. 225). In most early reports, however, women were usually included *because* they had repeated adverse outcomes. Moreover, as previously discussed, the incidence of antiphospholipid antibodies in the general obstetrical population is about 5 percent. Accordingly, data currently are too limited to draw precise conclusions concerning the impact of these antibodies on adverse pregnancy outcomes. Fetal deaths, however, are more characteristic than first-trimester miscarriages (Oshiro and co-workers, 1996; Roque and colleagues, 2001). It has also been shown that women with higher antibody titers have worse outcomes compared with those with low titers (Nodler and colleagues, 2009; Simchen and associates, 2009).

Looking at the issue another way, the incidence of these antibodies may be increased in adverse obstetrical outcomes associated with these syndromes. Polzin and colleagues (1991) identified antiphospholipid antibodies in a fourth of 37 women with growth-restricted fetuses, however, none had evidence for LAC. Approximately a third of women with APS will develop preeclampsia during pregnancy (Clark and colleagues, 2007b). And Branch and co-workers (1989) found a 16-percent incidence of antiphospholipid antibodies in 43 women with severe preeclampsia before 34 weeks. Six of the seven women with antibodies also had LAC, and one woman had multiple cerebral infarctions. Similarly, Moodley and associates (1995) found antibodies in 11 percent of 34 women with severe preeclampsia before 30 weeks.

When otherwise unexplained fetal deaths are examined, ACAs do not appear to play a significant role. Haddow and co-workers (1991) measured ACAs in 309 pregnancies with fetal death and found no differences compared with 618 normal pregnancies. In women with a history of recurrent pregnancy loss, those with antiphospholipid antibodies had a higher rate of preterm delivery (Clark and colleagues, 2007a). Despite a worse pregnancy outcome, there was no evidence of greater endothelial cell activation during pregnancy in women who were receiving treatment for APS (Stone and colleagues, 2003).

Treatment Guidelines

Because of the heterogeneity of studies, current treatment recommendations may be confusing to the clinician (Branch and Khamashta, 2003; Robertson and Greaves, 2006). The schema discussed on page 1153 is used to semiquantify antibody levels that bind immunoglobulins G, M, and A. Thus, GPL, MPL, and APL binding units are expressed as negative, low-positive, medium-positive, or high-positive (American College of Obste-

tricians and Gynecologists, 2007b). Low-positive titers of GPL or MPL anticardiolipin antibodies are of questionable clinical significance. And *any titer* of APL antibodies has no known relevance at this time.

As discussed in Chapter 47 (see p. 1017), women with prior thromboembolic events who have antiphospholipid antibodies are at risk for recurrence in subsequent pregnancies. Recommendations for management from the American College of Obstetricians and Gynecologists (2007b) and the American College of Chest Physicians (Baker and colleagues, 2008) are varied and listed in Table 47-6 (p. 1028). Some acceptable schemes include close antepartum observation with or without prophylactic- or intermediate-dose heparin, and some form of postpartum anticoagulation for 4 to 6 weeks. Less clear, some recommend that women with medium- or high-positive ACA titers or those with LAC activity and a previous second- or third-trimester fetal death not attributable to other causes should also be treated (Dizon-Townson and Branch, 1998; Lockshin and Druzin, 1995). Similarly, as discussed in Chapter 9 (p. 225), some report that women with recurrent early pregnancy loss and medium- or high-positive titers of antibodies may benefit from therapy (Robertson and Greaves, 2006).

Aspirin

Given in doses of 60 to 80 mg daily, aspirin blocks the conversion of arachidonic acid to thromboxane A_2 while sparing prostacyclin production. This results in reduced thromboxane A_2, which may cause platelet aggregation and vasoconstriction, while sparing prostacyclin, which has the opposite effect. There appear to be no major side effects from low-dose aspirin other than a slight risk of small-vessel bleeding during surgical procedures.

Heparin

Unfractionated heparin is given subcutaneously in dosages of 5000 to 10,000 units every 12 hours. Some prefer low-molecular-weight heparin. With therapeutic dosing, some recommend measurement of heparin levels because clotting tests may be altered by LAC (Cowchock, 1998). The rationale for heparin therapy is to prevent venous and arterial thrombotic episodes. Heparin therapy also prevents thrombosis in the microcirculation, including the decidual-trophoblastic interface (Toglia and Weg, 1996). As discussed, heparin binds to β_2-glycoprotein I, which coats the syncytiotrophoblast. This prevents binding of anticardiolipin and anti-β_2-glycoprotein I antibodies to their surfaces, which likely prevents cellular damage (Chamley and colleagues, 1999; Schousboe and Rasmussen, 1995). Heparin also binds to antiphospholipid antibodies in vitro and likely in vivo (Ermel and associates, 1995).

It is problematic that heparin therapy is associated with a number of complications that include bleeding, thrombocytopenia, osteopenia, and osteoporosis. A detailed description of the use of various heparins and their doses and adverse effects is found in Chapter 47 (p. 1021).

Immunotherapy

Glucocorticoids likely should not be used with *primary APS*—that is, without an associated connective-tissue disorder. Even so, some patients with these conditions can be expected to develop an associated disorder such as lupus over time (Carbone and colleagues, 1999). In instances of *secondary APS* seen with lupus, the dose of prednisone should be maintained at the lowest effective level to prevent flares. Steroid therapy has significant adverse effects, including osteopenia, osteoporosis, and pathological fractures. Steroids also impede wound healing, and they induce gestational and overt diabetes (Laskin and co-workers, 1997).

Immunoglobulin therapy has usually been reserved for women with overt disease, heparin-induced thrombocytopenia, or both. It is used when other first-line therapies have failed, especially in the setting of preeclampsia and fetal-growth restriction (Cowchock, 1996, 1998; Heilmann and colleagues, 2003; Silver and Branch, 1997). Immunoglobulin is administered intravenously in doses of 0.4 g/kg daily for 5 days—total dose of 2 g/kg. This is repeated monthly, or it is given as a single dose of 1 g/kg each month. Treatment is expensive—at $50 per gram, one course for a 70-kg woman costs $7000 (Medical Letter, 2006). Immunoglobulin has been evaluated in a preliminary placebo-controlled study by Branch and colleagues (2000). In a retrospective study, Heilmann and associates (2008) treated 121 women with the syndrome with low-molecular-weight heparin plus aspirin, but only 43 additionally received IVIG in the dose described. This latter group had fewer late complications, but randomized trials are needed before its widespread application.

Immunosuppressive therapy has also not been well evaluated, but azathioprine and cyclosporine do not appear to improve standard therapies (Silver and Branch, 1997). As previously discussed, methotrexate, cyclophosphamide, and mycophenolate mofetil are contraindicated because of teratogenic potential (Briggs and associates, 2005; Buhimschi and Weiner, 2009).

Low-Dose Aspirin Plus Heparin

Current data suggest the most efficacious therapy to be low-dose heparin—7500 to 10,000 units administered subcutaneously, twice daily—given concurrently with low-dose aspirin, 60 to 80 mg once daily (American College of Obstetricians and Gynecologists, 2007b). If active lupus coexists, then prednisone is usually also given.

Effect of Treatment on Perinatal Loss

Regarding perinatal outcomes, Branch and Khamashta (2003) caution that recurrent fetal loss is still 20 to 30 percent even with treatments described above. In one study, Lockshin and co-workers (1989) reported that 23 of 32 women with a prior fetal death and antiphospholipid antibody levels greater than 40 IgG units had a recurrent fetal death despite treatment with prednisone, aspirin, or both. Conversely, some women with lupus and antiphospholipid antibodies have normal pregnancy outcomes without treatment. In addition, women with LAC and prior bad pregnancy outcomes have had liveborns without treatment (Trudinger and associates, 1988).

Because 30 percent of neonates demonstrate passively acquired antiphospholipid antibodies, there is concern for any adverse effects. According to Tincani and co-workers (2009), some findings suggest possible increased learning disabilities. And Simchen and colleagues (2009) reported a fourfold

TABLE 54-6. American College of Rheumatology Revised 1987 Criteria for Classification of Rheumatoid Arthritis[a]

1. Morning joint stiffness
2. Arthritis of three or more joint areas
3. Arthritis of wrist, metacarpophalangeal joint, or proximal interphalangeal joint
4. Symmetrical arthritis
5. Rheumatoid nodules
6. Serum rheumatoid factor
7. Radiographic changes

[a] Four of seven criteria required for diagnosis. Criteria 1-4 must be present for at least 6 weeks. Criteria 2-5 must be observed by a physician. Adapted from Lipsky (2008).

increased risk for perinatal strokes in these infants. More data are needed before firm conclusions can be drawn.

RHEUMATOID ARTHRITIS

This is a chronic multisystem disease of unknown cause with an immunologically mediated pathogenesis. Infiltrating T cells secrete cytokines that mediate inflammation and systemic symptoms. Its prevalence is about 0.8 percent, and women are affected three times more often than men (Lipsky, 2008). The cardinal feature is inflammatory synovitis that usually involves the peripheral joints. The disease has a propensity for cartilage destruction, bony erosions, and joint deformities. Onset is generally between 35 and 50 years. Diagnostic criteria are shown in Table 54-6.

There is a genetic predisposition, and the results of several studies have shown a higher disease concordance among monozygotic than dizygotic twins—15 versus 4 percent (Lee and Weinblatt, 2001). There is an association with the class II major histocompatibility complex molecule HLA-DR4 and HLA-DRB1 alleles (Harney and colleagues, 2003). Cigarette smoking also appears to increase the risk of rheumatoid arthritis in women (Papadopoulos and colleagues, 2005). As discussed subsequently, a protective effect of pregnancy has been reported for the development of rheumatoid arthritis (Hazes and colleagues, 1990).

Clinical Manifestations

Rheumatoid arthritis is a chronic polyarthritis with symptoms of synovitis, fatigue, anorexia, weakness, weight loss, depression, and vague musculoskeletal symptoms. The hands, wrists, knees, and feet are commonly involved. Pain, aggravated by movement, is accompanied by swelling and tenderness. Extra-articular manifestations include rheumatoid nodules, vasculitis, and pleuropulmonary symptoms. The 1987 revised criteria of the American College of Rheumatology shown in Table 54-6 have a 90-percent specificity and sensitivity for the diagnosis (Lipsky, 2008).

Management

Treatment is directed at pain relief, reduction of inflammation, protection of articular structures, and preservation of function. Physical and occupational therapy and self-management instructions are essential. Aspirin or nonsteroidal anti-inflammatory drugs (NSAIDs) are the cornerstone of symptomatic therapy. However, they do not retard progression of disease. Conventional NSAIDs nonspecifically inhibit both cyclooxygenase-1 (COX-1)—an enzyme critical to normal platelet function, and COX-2—an enzyme which mediates inflammatory response mechanisms. Gastritis with acute bleeding is an unwanted side effect common to conventional NSAIDs. Specific COX-2 inhibitors have been used to avert this complication. There are now concerns, however, that long-term use of COX-2 inhibitors is associated with increased myocardial infarction, stroke, and heart failure (Solomon and associates, 2005). Thus, risks versus benefits of these medications must be considered.

Glucocorticoid therapy may be added to NSAIDs, and 7.5 mg of prednisone daily for the first 2 years of active disease substantively reduces progressive joint erosions (Kirwan and colleagues, 1995). Thus, corticosteroids are avoided if possible, but low-dose therapy is used by some, along with salicylates.

Because NSAIDs and glucocorticoids are primarily for symptomatic relief, the American College of Rheumatology (2002) recommends disease-modifying antirheumatic drugs (DMARDs). These have the potential to reduce or prevent joint damage and are given within 3 months of diagnosis. There are a variety of DMARDs, and many have considerable toxicity. These include hydroxychloroquine, sulfasalazine, leflunomide, and methotrexate (Vroom and colleagues, 2006). More recently, the tumor necrosis factor alpha (TNF-α) inhibitors, which include etanercept (*Enbrel*), adalimumab (*Humira*), and infliximab (*Remicade*), have been approved. Experience with these agents in pregnancy has been accruing. Berthelot and colleagues (2009) found more than 300 reported cases in their review with no fetal effects. In addition, the interleukin-1 receptor antagonist, anakinra (*Kineret*), and the antagonist to the B-cell CD20 antigen, rituximab (*Rituxan*), are now available. Drugs used less frequently include azathioprine, penicillamine, gold salts, minocycline, and cyclosporine. Orthopedic surgery for joint deformities, including replacement, is commonly performed.

Pregnancy and Rheumatoid Arthritis

Rheumatoid arthritis improves in up to 90 percent of affected women during pregnancy (de Man and associates, 2008). That said, some women develop disease during pregnancy, and others become worse (Nelson and Østensen, 1997). In addition, postpartum exacerbation is common (Østensen and Villiger, 2007). Barrett and co-workers (2000a) reported that a flare was more common if women were breast feeding. Barrett and co-workers (2000b) performed a prospective study in the United Kingdom, and 140 women recruited during the last trimester were seen at 1 and 6 months postpartum. There was only a modest fall in objective disease activity. Only 16 percent had complete remission. At least 25 percent had substantive levels of disability. Thus, although overall disease actually did not exacerbate postpartum, the mean number of inflamed joints increased significantly.

There are some studies that report a protective effect of pregnancy for women developing subsequent new-onset rheumatoid arthritis. Silman and associates (1992) performed a case-control study of 88 affected women. They found that although there was a protective effect of pregnancy in the long term, the likelihood of new-onset rheumatoid arthritis was increased sixfold during the first 3 postpartum months. Pikwer and colleagues (2009) reported a significant reduction in the risk of subsequent arthritis in women who breastfed longer than 12 months. Finally, Mandl and co-workers (2009) described long-term follow-up of more than 87,000 women followed in the Nurses' Health Study. From 1976 through 2002, 619 women developed rheumatoid arthritis—a prevalence of 0.7 percent. They found a twofold increased risk for its development in women with infants born weighing more than 4540 g—10 pounds. Other problems for macrosomic infants are discussed further in Chapter 38 (p. 853).

As an explanation, and as discussed previously, sex hormones supposedly interfere with a number of putative processes involved in arthritis pathogenesis, including immunoregulation and interactions with the cytokine system (Häupl and associates, 2008a, b). First, Unger and associates (1983) reported that amelioration of rheumatoid arthritis correlated with serum levels of *pregnancy-associated* α_2*-glycoprotein*. This compound has immunosuppressive properties. Second, Nelson and co-workers (1993) reported that amelioration of disease was associated with a disparity in HLA class II antigens between mother and fetus. They suggested that the maternal immune response to paternal HLA antigens may play a role in pregnancy-induced remission of arthritis. In addition to monocytes, there may be T-lymphocyte activation (Förger and co-workers, 2008).

Juvenile Rheumatoid Arthritis

This is a group of diseases that are the most common cause of chronic arthritis in children. They persist into adulthood. Østensen (1991) reviewed outcomes of 76 pregnancies in 51 affected Norwegian women. Pregnancy had no effects on presentation of disease, but disease activity became quiescent or remained so during pregnancy. Postpartum flares were common, as discussed for rheumatoid arthritis. Joint deformities were common in these women, and 15 of 20 cesarean deliveries were done for contracted pelves or joint prostheses. These observations are supported by the summary of similar results in 39 Polish women with a history of juvenile rheumatoid arthritis (Musiej-Nowakowska and Ploski, 1999).

Perinatal Outcome

There are no obvious adverse effects of rheumatoid arthritis on pregnancy outcome, including preterm labor (Klipple and Cecere, 1989). In a national population-based cohort study in Norway, however, Skomsvoll and colleagues (2002) reported that women with rheumatic disease with two previous poor pregnancy outcomes were at high risk for recurrent adverse outcomes. Although Kaplan (1986) reported that women who later develop the disease have had a higher-than-expected incidence of spontaneous abortion, Nelson and colleagues (1992) did not corroborate this.

Management During Pregnancy

Treatment of symptomatic women during pregnancy is with aspirin and NSAIDs, but with appropriate concerns for impaired hemostasis, prolonged gestation, and premature closure of the ductus arteriosus (Briggs and co-workers, 2005). Low-dose corticosteroids are also used as indicated. Gold compounds have been used in pregnancy, and of 14 women experiencing 20 pregnancies on gold therapy, 75 percent delivered healthy liveborns (Almarzouqi and colleagues, 2007).

Immunosuppressive therapy with azathioprine, cyclophosphamide, or methotrexate is not routinely used during pregnancy. Of these, only azathioprine should be considered during early pregnancy because the other agents are teratogenic as discussed previously (Buhimschi and Weiner, 2009). (Ramsey-Goldman and Shilling, 1997). TNF-α drugs are considered category B for pregnancy, although data with regard to safety for a developing human fetus are limited (Roux and associates, 2007). Leflunomide is a pyrimidine synthesis inhibitor used for rheumatoid arthritis in nonpregnant patients. It is teratogenic in animals, and it is detectable up to 2 years in plasma after discontinuation (Briggs and associates, 2005). It has not been shown to be teratogenic for humans, but it should be avoided (Chambers and colleagues, 2007).

If cervical spine involvement exists, particular attention is warranted during pregnancy. Subluxation is common, and pregnancy, at least theoretically, predisposes to this because of joint laxity, as discussed in Chapter 5 (p. 129). In addition, there are anesthesia concerns regarding endotracheal intubation.

Contraception

Combination oral contraceptives are a logical choice because of their effectiveness and the possibility that they might improve rheumatoid arthritis (Bijlsma and Van Den Brink, 1992). In fact, all reversible methods of contraception discussed in Chapter 32 are appropriate.

SYSTEMIC SCLEROSIS (SCLERODERMA)

This is a chronic multisystem disorder of unknown etiology characterized by microvascular damage, immune system activation leading to inflammation, and excessive deposition of collagen in the skin and often in the lungs, heart, gastrointestinal tract, and kidneys. It is uncommon, displays a 3-to-1 female dominance and typically affects those aged 30 to 50 years (Varga, 2008).

This strong prevalence of scleroderma for women and its increased incidence in the years following childbirth contribute much to the hypothesis that *microchimerism* may be involved in the pathogenesis as discussed on page 1146. Artlett and co-workers (1998) demonstrated Y-chromosomal DNA in almost half—32 of 69 women—with systemic sclerosis compared with only 4 percent of controls. Rak and colleagues (2009) identified male microchimerism in peripheral blood mononuclear cells more frequently in women with limited versus diffuse disease—20 versus 5 percent. Fetal cells are likely present long before fibrosis develops (Sawaya and associates, 2004).

Clinical Course

The hallmark of the disease is overproduction of normal collagen. In the more benign form—*limited cutaneous systemic sclerosis*—progression is slow. With *diffuse cutaneous systemic sclerosis*, skin thickening progresses rapidly, and skin fibrosis is followed by gastrointestinal tract fibrosis, especially the distal esophagus (Varga, 2008). Pulmonary interstitial fibrosis along with vascular changes may cause pulmonary hypertension. Antinuclear antibodies are found in 95 percent of patients, and immunoincompetence is common.

Common symptoms are Raynaud phenomenon, which includes cold-induced episodic digital ischemia—in 95 percent, as well as swelling of the distal extremities and face. Half of patients have symptoms from esophageal involvement, especially fullness and epigastric burning pain. Pulmonary involvement is common and causes dyspnea. Mortality rates are high with renal or pulmonary involvement, and the 10-year survival rate is less than 50 percent. Renal failure causes half of the deaths. Women with limited cutaneous disease such as the *CREST syndrome—calcinosis, Raynaud phenomenon, esophageal involvement, sclerodactyly, and telangiectasia*—have milder disease.

Overlap syndrome refers to the presence of systemic sclerosis with features of other connective-tissue disorders. *Mixed-connective-tissue disease* is a term used for the syndrome involving features of lupus, systemic sclerosis, polymyositis, rheumatoid arthritis, and high titers of anti-RNP antibodies (see Table 54-1).

Although systemic sclerosis cannot be cured, treatment directed at end-organ involvement can relieve symptoms and improve function (Varga, 2008). Corticosteroids are helpful only for inflammatory myositis, pericarditis, and hemolytic anemia. Renal involvement and hypertension are common, and angiotensin-converting enzyme (ACE) inhibitors are usually effective treatment. As reviewed recently by Buhimschi and Weiner (2009), these agents are associated with severe fetal abnormalities (see also Chap. 14, p. 319). *Scleroderma renal crisis* develops in up to a fourth of these patients and is characterized by obliterative vasculopathy of the renal cortical arteries resulting in renal failure and malignant hypertension. Interstitial restrictive lung disease is common and becomes life-threatening. Cyclophosphamide provides some improvement (Tashkin and co-workers, 2006). As discussed in Chapter 44 (p. 970), associated pulmonary hypertension is usually fatal.

Pregnancy and Systemic Sclerosis

The prevalence of scleroderma in pregnancy can be estimated from the study of nearly 11.2 million pregnant women registered in the Nationwide Inpatient Sample. In this report, Chakravarty and colleagues (2008) reported that 504 women suffered from systemic sclerosis—a prevalence of about 1 in 22,000 pregnancies. These women usually have stable disease during gestation if their baseline function is good. As perhaps expected, dysphagia and reflux esophagitis are aggravated by pregnancy (Steen, 1999). Dysphagia results from loss of esophageal motility due to neuromuscular dysfunction. A decrease in amplitude or disappearance of peristaltic waves in the lower two thirds of the esophagus is seen using manometry. Symptomatic treatment for reflux is described in Chapter 49

(p. 1052). Chin and colleagues (1995) described a woman with scleroderma who developed a Mallory-Weiss tear from persistent vomiting.

Women with renal insufficiency and malignant hypertension have an increased incidence of superimposed preeclampsia. In the presence of rapidly worsening renal or cardiac disease, pregnancy termination should be considered. As discussed, renal crisis is life threatening and is treated with ACE inhibitors, but it does not improve with delivery (Gayed and Gordon, 2007) Pulmonary hypertension usually contraindicates pregnancy (see Chap. 44, p. 970).

Vaginal delivery may be anticipated, unless the soft tissue thickening wrought by scleroderma produces dystocia requiring abdominal delivery. Tracheal intubation for general anesthesia has special concerns because of limited ability of these women to open their mouths widely (Black and Stevens, 1989). Because of esophageal dysfunction, aspiration is also more likely, and epidural analgesia is preferable.

Pregnancy Outcomes

Maternal and fetal outcomes are related to the severity of underlying disease. In the past, a high cited incidence of maternal deaths was due to biased case reporting. In a review of 94 pregnancies, Maymon and Fejgin (1989) found that a third of women had exacerbations of symptoms during pregnancy. The maternal mortality rate was 15 percent and was due to hypertension, renal failure, or cardiopulmonary complications. The fetal mortality rate was 20 percent.

Steen and colleagues (1989, 1999) reported more optimistic outcomes in 214 women with systemic sclerosis, 45 percent of whom had had diffuse disease. Major complications included renal crisis in three women. There were increased rates of preterm birth. Chung and colleagues (2006) also reported increased rates of preterm delivery, fetal-growth restriction, and perinatal mortality. These are likely related to placental abnormalities that include decidual vasculopathy, acute atherosis, and infarcts. These reduce placental blood flow and are found in many cases (Doss and co-workers, 1998; Papakonstantinou and associates, 2007).

Contraception

Scleroderma may be associated with subfertility (Bernatsky and co-workers, 2008; Lambe and colleagues, 2004). For those who do not choose pregnancy, several reversible contraceptive methods are acceptable. That said, hormonal agents, especially combination oral contraceptives, probably should not be used, especially in women with pulmonary, cardiac, or renal involvement. Due to the progressive and often unrelenting nature of progressive systemic sclerosis, permanent sterilization should also be considered (see Chap. 33, p. 698).

VASCULITIS SYNDROMES

Inflammation and damage to blood vessels may be primary or due to another disease. Most cases are presumed to be caused by immunopathogenic mechanisms, specifically, immune-complex deposition (Langford and Fauci, 2008). These syndromes are difficult to classify because of overlap. Primary causes include polyarteritis nodosa, Wegener granulomatosis, Churg-Strauss syndrome, temporal or giant cell arteritis, Takayasu arteritis, Henoch-Schönlein purpura, Behçet syndrome, and cutaneous or hypersensitivity arteritis.

Polyarteritis Nodosa

This type of vasculitis is an uncommon disease with protean manifestations. The pathological lesion is necrotizing vasculitis of small and medium-sized arteries. The classical variety is one of the progressive vasculitis syndromes characterized clinically by myalgia, neuropathy, gastrointestinal disorders, hypertension, and renal disease. About a third of cases are associated with hepatitis B antigenemia (Langford and Fauci, 2008).

Symptoms are nonspecific and vague. Fever, weight loss, and malaise are present in more than half of cases. Renal failure, hypertension, and arthralgias are common. Diagnosis is made by biopsy, and treatment consists of high-dose prednisone plus cyclophosphamide. Vasculitis due to hepatitis B antigenemia responds to lamivudine (see Chap. 50, p. 1069).

Pregnancy

Only a few documented cases of polyarteritis nodosa in association with pregnancy have been reported. Although definitive conclusions are unclear, certainly if active arteritis is identified during pregnancy, mortality rates are high. Owen and Hauth (1989) reviewed the courses of 12 such pregnant women. In seven, polyarteritis first manifested during pregnancy, and it was rapidly fatal by 6 weeks postpartum. The diagnosis was not made until autopsy in six of the seven women. Four women continued pregnancy, resulting in one stillborn and three successful outcomes.

Wegener Granulomatosis

This is a necrotizing granulomatous vasculitis of the upper and lower respiratory tract and kidney. Common lesions include sinusitis and nasal disease—90 percent, pulmonary infiltrates or nodules—85 percent, glomerulonephritis—75 percent, and musculoskeletal lesions—65 percent (Sneller, 1995). It is uncommon and usually encountered after 50 years of age. The few cases reported in association with pregnancy were reviewed recently by Koukoura and colleagues (2008). Corticosteroids are the standard treatment. For moderate and severe cases in the late second or third trimester, the use of cyclophosphamide in combination with prednisolone is acceptable. Azathioprine, cyclosporine, and intravenous immunoglobulin can also be used.

Takayasu Arteritis

So-called *pulseless disease,* this syndrome is most prevalent in young women. It is a chronic inflammatory arteritis affecting large vessels. Unlike *temporal arteritis,* which occurs almost exclusively after 55 years of age, the onset of Takayasu arteritis is almost exclusively before age 40. It is associated with abnormal angiography of the upper aorta and its main branches, resulting in upper extremity vascular impairment. Death usually results from congestive heart failure or cerebrovascular events. Computed tomography or magnetic resonance angiography can be used to detect this disorder prior to the development of severe vascular compromise (Numano and Kobayashi, 1999). Takayasu arteritis may respond symptomatically to corticosteroid therapy, however, it is not curative. Selection of surgical bypass or angioplasty has improved survival.

Severe renovascular hypertension, cardiac involvement, or pulmonary hypertension worsen pregnancy prognosis. Despite this, from their review of 14 cases, Nagey and colleagues (1983) reported good outcomes. Subsequent reports and reviews support this (Johnston and colleagues, 2002; Kraemer and coworkers, 2008). When the abdominal aorta is involved, however, pregnancy outcome may be disastrous (Sharma and associates, 2000). Blood pressure is taken in the lower extremity. Vaginal delivery is preferred, and epidural analgesia has been advocated for labor and delivery (Langford and Kerr, 2002). *Polymyalgia rheumatica*, closely related to giant-cell arteritis, was described in one case as developing at 34 weeks and responding to prednisone (Sasaki and colleagues, 2005).

Other Vasculitides

Vasculitis caused by *Henoch-Schönlein purpura* is uncommon after childhood, and Kalmantis and associates (2008) reviewed 15 pregnancies complicated by this vasculitis. Cutaneous lesions were found in three fourths. About half had arthralgias, and half had nephritis that included cases of nephrotic syndrome and acute renal failure. Despite this, all but one woman had a successful pregnancy outcome. Jadaon and colleagues (2005) described 135 pregnancies in 31 women with *Behçet disease* compared with matched nonaffected controls. Although there were no deleterious effects of pregnancy on the underlying disease, the miscarriage rate was significantly increased threefold. Hwang and coworkers (2009) described necrotizing villitis and decidual vasculitis in a placenta from a first-trimester pregnancy termination and another from a term delivery. *Churg-Strauss vasculitis* is rare in pregnancy. Hot and associates (2007) described a pregnant woman who responded to intravenous immune globulin (IVIG) therapy. Corradi and co-workers (2009) described an affected 35-year-old woman at term whose necrotizing vasculitis involved the heart, and she subsequently underwent heart transplantation.

DERMATOMYOSITIS AND POLYMYOSITIS

These are uncommon acute, subacute, or chronic inflammatory diseases of unknown cause that involve mainly skin and muscle. Polymyositis is a subacute inflammatory myopathy that is frequently associated with one of the autoimmune connective-tissue disorders. Dermatomyositis manifests as a characteristic rash accompanying or preceding weakness. Laboratory findings include elevated muscle enzyme levels in serum and an abnormal electromyogram. Confirmation is by biopsy, which shows perivascular and perimysial inflammatory infiltrates, vasculitis, and muscle fiber degeneration. It usually develops alone but can overlap with scleroderma or mixed connective-tissue disease.

Prevailing theories are that the syndromes are caused by viral infections, autoimmune disorders, or both. *About 15 percent of adults who develop dermatomyositis have an associated malignant tumor.* The time of appearance of the two diseases may be separated by several years. The most common sites of associated cancer are breast, lung, stomach, and ovary. The disease usually responds to high-dose corticosteroid therapy, immunosuppressive drugs such as azathioprine or methotrexate, or intravenous immune globulin (Dalakas, 2008; Williams and colleagues, 2007).

Experiences in pregnancy are garnered mostly from case series and reviews. Gutierrez and colleagues (1984) reviewed outcomes in 10 pregnancies among seven women with active disease and described three abortions, three perinatal deaths, and five preterm deliveries. Rosenzweig and colleagues (1989) reviewed 24 pregnancy outcomes in 18 women with primary polymyositis-dermatomyositis. In half, the diagnosis preceded pregnancy. Of these, a fourth had an exacerbation in the second or third trimester. Excluding abortions, there were two perinatal deaths and two growth-restricted neonates. In the other half in whom disease became manifest first during pregnancy, outcomes were less favorable. One woman died 6 weeks postpartum. Excluding abortions, half of the eight pregnancies resulted in perinatal death. Ohno and associates (1992) and Papapetropoulos and co-workers (1998) described similar cases. From their review, Doria and colleagues (2004) concluded that pregnancy outcome was related to disease activity and that new-onset disease was particularly aggressive.

INHERITED CONNECTIVE-TISSUE DISORDERS

These are among the most common genetic diseases and may involve bone, skin, cartilage, blood vessels, and basement membranes. Among others, they include Marfan and Ehlers-Danlos syndromes, osteogenesis imperfecta, chondrodysplasia, and epidermolysis bulla.

Marfan Syndrome

Marfan syndrome is a common autosomal dominant connective-tissue disorder and has a prevalence of 1 in 3000 to 5000 (Prockop and Czarny-Ratajczak, 2008). It affects both sexes equally. The syndrome is caused by mutation of the fibrillin-1 (*FBN1*) gene on the long arm of chromosome 15 (Loeys and colleagues, 2002). The *FBN1* gene has a high mutation rate, and there are many mild, subclinical cases. In severe disease, there is degeneration of the elastic lamina in the media of the aorta. This weakness predisposes to aortic dilatation or dissecting aneurysm that appears more likely in pregnancy (Mor-Yosef and colleagues, 1988; Savi and associates, 2007). Aortic dissection may occur after elective cesarean delivery. Marfan syndrome complicating pregnancy is discussed in detail in Chapter 44 (p. 976).

Ehlers-Danlos Syndrome

This disease is characterized by a variety of changes in connective tissue, including hyperelasticity of the skin. In the more severe types, there is a strong tendency for rupture of any of several arteries to cause either strokes or bleeding. Rupture of the colon or uterus has been described. There are several types of disease based on skin, joint, or other tissue involvement. Some are autosomal dominant, some recessive, and some X-linked. Their aggregate prevalence is about 1 in 5000 (Prockop and Czarny-Ratajczak, 2008). Types I, II, and III are autosomally dominant, and each accounts for about 30 percent of cases. Type IV is uncommon, but is known to predispose to preterm delivery, maternal great-vessel rupture, postpartum bleeding, and uterine rupture (Pepin and co-workers, 2000). In most, the underlying molecular defect is that of collagen or procollagen.

In general, women with Ehlers-Danlos syndrome have an increased frequency of preterm rupture of membranes, preterm delivery, and antepartum and postpartum hemorrhage (Volkov and associates, 2006). Tissue fragility makes episiotomy repair and cesarean delivery difficult. Sorokin and colleagues (1994) surveyed female members of the Ehlers-Danlos National Foundation. They reported a stillbirth rate of 3 percent, a preterm delivery rate of 23 percent, a cesarean delivery rate of 8 percent, and problematic postpartum bleeding in 15 percent. A number of cases of spontaneous uterine rupture have been described (Rudd and associates, 1983; Walsh and co-workers, 2007). A maternal and fetal death from spontaneous rupture of the right iliac artery was described by Esaka and colleagues (2009). Finally, Bar-Yosef and colleagues (2008) described a newborn with multiple congenital skull fractures and intracranial hemorrhage caused by Ehlers-Danlos type VIIC.

REFERENCES

Adams KM, Nelson JL: Microchimerism: An investigative frontier in autoimmunity and transplantation. JAMA 291:1127, 2004

Aggarwal N, Sawhney H, Vasishta K, et al: Pregnancy in patients with systemic lupus erythematosus. Aust NZ J Obstet Gynaecol 39:28, 1999

Ahmed K, Darakhshan A, Au E, et al: Postpartum spontaneous colonic perforation due to antiphospholipid syndrome. World J Gastroenterol 15(4):502, 2009

Alexander E, Buyon JP, Provost TT, et al: Anti-Ro/SSA antibodies in the pathophysiology of congenital heart block in neonatal lupus syndrome: An experimental model. Arthritis Rheum 35:176, 1992

Almarzouqi M, Scarsbrook D, Klinkhoff A: Gold therapy in women planning pregnancy: Outcomes in one center. J Rheumatol 34:1827, 2007

Amengual O, Atsumi T, Khamashta MA: Tissue factor in antiphospholipid syndrome: Shifting the focus from coagulation to endothelium. Rheumatology 42:1029, 2003

American College of Obstetricians and Gynecologists: Use of hormonal contraception in women with coexisting medical conditions. Obstet Gynecol 107:1453, 2006

American College of Obstetricians and Gynecologists: Antepartum fetal surveillance. Practice Bulletin No. 9, October 1999, Reaffirmed 2007a

American College of Obstetricians and Gynecologists: Antiphospholipid syndrome. Practice Bulletin No. 68, November 2005, Reaffirmed 2007b

American College of Rheumatology: Guidelines for the management of rheumatoid arthritis. Arthritis Rheumat 46(2):328, 2002

Anderka MT, Lin AE, Abuelo DN: Reviewing the evidence for mycophenolate mofetil as a new teratogen: Case report and review of the literature. Am J Med Genet A [Epub ahead of print], 2009

Arbuckle MF, McClain MT, Rubertone MV, et al: Development of autoantibodies before the clinical onset of systemic lupus erythematosus. N Engl J Med 349:1526, 2003

Artlett CM, Smith B, Jimenez SA: Identification of fetal DNA and cells in skin lesions from women with systemic sclerosis. N Engl J Med 338:1186, 1998

Avalos I, Tsokos GC: The role of complement in the antiphospholipid syndrome-associated pathology. Clin Rev Allergy Immunol 34(2-3):141, 2009

Bar-Yosef O, Polak-Charcon S, Hoffman C, et al: Multiple congenital skull fractures as a presentation of Ehlers-Danlos syndrome type VIIC. Am J Med Genet A 146A:3054, 2008

Barinaga M: Cells exchanged during pregnancy live on. Science 296:2169, 2002

Barrett JH, Brennan P, Fiddler M, et al: Breast-feeding and postpartum relapse in women with rheumatoid and inflammatory arthritis. Arthritis Rheum 43:1010, 2000a

Barrett JH, Brennan P, Fiddler M, et al: Does rheumatoid arthritis remit during pregnancy and relapse postpartum? Results from a nationwide study in the United Kingdom performed prospectively from late pregnancy. Arthritis Rheum 42:1219, 2000b

Benjamin R, Parham P: HLA-B27 and diseases: A consequence of inadvertent antigen presentation? Rheum Dis Clin North Am 18:11, 1992

Bernatsky S, Hudson M, Pope J, et al: Assessment of reproductive history in systemic sclerosis. Arthritis Rheum 59:1661, 2008

Berthelot JM, De Bandt M, Goupille P, et al: Exposition to anti-TNF drugs during pregnancy: Outcome of 15 cases and review of the literature. Joint Bone Spine 76(1):28, 2009

Bertsias G, Ionnidis JPA, Boletis J, et al: EULAR recommendations for the management of systemic lupus erythematosus (SLE). Ann Rheum Dis 67(2):195, 2008

Bijlsma JWJ, Van Den Brink HR: Estrogens and rheumatoid arthritis. Am J Reprod Immunol 28:231, 1992

Black CM, Stevens WM: Scleroderma. Rheum Dis Clin North Am 15:193, 1989

Boh EE: Neonatal lupus erythematosus. Clin Dermatol 22:125, 2004

Borden M, Parke A: Antimalarial drugs in systemic lupus erythematosus. Drug Saf 24:1055, 2001

Branch DW: Antiphospholipid syndrome—laboratory concerns, fetal loss, and pregnancy management. Semin Perinatol 15:230, 1991

Branch DW, Andres R, Digre KB, et al: The association of antiphospholipid antibodies with severe preeclampsia. Obstet Gynecol 73:541, 1989

Branch DW, Khamashta M: Antiphospholipid syndrome: Obstetric diagnosis, management, and controversies. Obstet Gynecol 101:1333, 2003

Branch DW, Peaceman AM, Druzin M, et al: A multicenter, placebo-controlled pilot study of intravenous immune globulin treatment of antiphospholipid syndrome during pregnancy. Am J Obstet Gynecol 182:122, 2000

Briggs GG, Freeman RK, Yaffe SJ: Drugs in Pregnancy and Lactation, 7th ed. Philadelphia, Lippincott Williams & Wilkins, 2005

Buhimschi CS, Weiner CP: Medications in pregnancy and lactation. Part 1. Teratology Obstet Gynecol 113:166, 2009

Buyon J, Kalunian K, Ramsey-Goldman R, et al: Assessing disease activity in SLE patients during pregnancy. Lupus 8:677, 1999

Buyon JP, Winchester RJ, Slade SG, et al: Identification of mothers at risk for congenital heart block and other neonatal lupus syndromes in their children. Comparison of enzyme-linked immunoabsorbent assay and immunoblot for measurement of anti SSA/Ro and anti SSB/La antibodies. Arthritis Rheum 36:1263, 1993

Carbone J, Orera M, Rodriguez-Mahou M, et al: Immunological abnormalities in primary APS evolving into SLE: 6 years' follow-up in women with repeated pregnancy loss. Lupus 8:274, 1999

Chakravarty EF, Khanna D, Chung L: Pregnancy outcomes in systemic sclerosis, primary pulmonary hypertension, and sickle cell disease. Obstet Gynecol 111(4):927, 2008

Chambers C, Koren G, Tutuncu ZN, et al: Are new agents used to treat rheumatoid arthritis safe to take during pregnancy? Motherisk Update 53:409, 2007

Chamley LW, Duncalf AM, Konarkowska B, et al: Conformationally altered beta(2)-glycoprotein I is the antigen for anti-cardiolipin autoantibodies. Clin Exp Immunol 115:571, 1999

Chin KAJ, Kaseba CM, Weaver JB: Mallory–Weiss syndrome complicating pregnancy in a patient with scleroderma: Diagnosis and management. Br J Obstet Gynaecol 102:498, 1995

Chung L, Flyckt RL, Colon I, et al: Outcome of pregnancies complicated by systemic sclerosis and mixed connective tissue disease. Lupus 15:595, 2006

Clark CA, Spitzer KA, Crowther MA, et al: Incidence of postpartum thrombosis and preterm delivery in women with antiphospholipid antibodies and recurrent pregnancy loss. J Rheumatol 34:992, 2007a

Clark EAS, Silver RM, Branch DW: Do antiphospholipid antibodies cause preeclampsia and HELLP syndrome? Curr Rheum Reports 9:219, 2007b

Clowse ME, Jamison M, Myers E, et al: A national study of the complications of lupus in pregnancy. Am J Obstet Gynecol 199:127.e1, 2008

Contreras G, Pardo V, Leclercq B, et al: Sequential therapies for proliferative lupus nephritis. N Engl J Med 350:971, 2004

Corradi D, Maestri R, Facchetti F: Postpartum Churg-Strauss syndrome with severe cardiac involvement: Description of a case and review of the literature. Clin Rheumatol, February 24, 2009 [Epub ahead of print]

Cowchock S: Prevention of fetal death in the antiphospholipid antibody syndrome. Lupus 5:467, 1996

Cowchock S: Treatment of antiphospholipid syndrome in pregnancy. Lupus 7:S95, 1998

Cutolo M, Capellino S, Sulli A, et al: Estrogens and autoimmune diseases. Ann NY Acad Sci 1089:538, 2006

Dalakas MC: Polymyositis, dermatomyositis, and inclusion body myositis. In Fauci AS, Braunwald E, Kasper DL, et al (eds): Harrison's Principles of Internal Medicine, 17th ed, New York, McGraw-Hill, 2008, p 2696

D'Cruz D: Renal manifestations of the antiphopholipid syndrome. Curr Rheumatol Rep 11(1):52, 2009

de Man YA, Dolhain RJ, van de Geijn FE, et al: Disease activity of rheumatoid arthritis during pregnancy: Results from a nationwide prospective study. Arthritis Rheum 59:1241, 2008

Destefano K, Belogolovkin V, Salihu H, et al: Does anti β₂-glycoprotein I improve the detection rate of antiphospholipid syndrome in pregnancy? Abstract no 521. Presented at the 29th Annual Meeting of the Society for Maternal-Fetal Medicine, January 26-31, 2009

Dittrich E, Schamaldienst S, Langer M, et al: Immunoadsorption and plasma exchange in pregnancy. Kidney Blood Press Res 25:232, 2002

Dizon-Townson D, Branch DW: Anticoagulant treatment during pregnancy: An update. Semin Thromb Hemost 24:55S, 1998

Doria A, Iaccarino L, Ghirardello A, et al: Pregnancy in rare autoimmune rheumatic diseases: UCTD, MCTD, myositis, systemic vasculitis and Behçet disease. Lupus 13:690, 2004

Doss BJ, Jacques SM, Mayes MD, et al: Maternal scleroderma: Placental findings and perinatal outcome. Hum Path 29(12):1524, 1998

Egerman RS, Ramsey RD, Kao LW, et al: Hypertensive disease in pregnancies complicated by systemic lupus erythematosus. Am J Obstet Gynecol 193:1676, 2005

Ermel LD, Marshburn PB, Kutteh WH: Interaction of heparin with antiphospholipid antibodies (APA) from the sera of women with recurrent pregnancy loss (RPL). Am J Reprod Immunol 33:14, 1995

Esaka EJ, Golde SH, Stever MR, et al: A maternal and perinatal mortality in pregnancy complicated by the kyphoscoliotic form of Ehlers-Danlos syndrome. Obstet Gynecol 113(2):515, 2009

Falcón CR, Martinuzzo ME, Forastiero RR, et al: Pregnancy loss and autoantibodies against phospholipid-binding proteins. Obstet Gynecol 89:975, 1997

FDA Alert: Inosine monophosphate dehydrogenase inhibitors (IMPDH). Center for Drug Education and Research, U.S. Food and Drug Administration. May 16, 2009

Feinstein DI, Rapaport SI: Acquired inhibitors of blood coagulation. In Spaet TH (ed): Progress in Hemostasis and Thrombosis, Vol 1. New York, Grune & Stratton, 1972, p 75

Förger F, Marcoli N, Gadola S, et al: Pregnancy induces numerical and functional changes of CD4+CD25 high regulatory T cells in patients with rheumatoid arthritis. Ann Rheum Dis 67(7):984, 2008

Galli M, Bevers EM: Inhibition of phospholipid-dependent coagulation reactions by antiphospholipid antibodies—possible modes of action. Lupus 3:223, 1994

Gayed M, Gordon C: Pregnancy and rheumatic diseases. Rheumatology 46:1634, 2007

Giannakopoulos B, Passam F, Ioannou Y, et al: How we diagnose the antiphospholipid syndrome. Blood 113(5):985, 2009

Gutierrez G, Dagnino R, Mintz G: Polymyositis/dermatomyositis and pregnancy. Arthritis Rheum 27:291, 1984

Haddow JE, Rote NS, Dostaljohnson D, et al: Lack of an association between late fetal death and antiphospholipid antibody measurements in the 2nd trimester. Am J Obstet Gynecol 165:1308, 1991

Hahn BH: Systemic lupus erythematosus. In Fauci AS, Braunwald E, Kasper DL, et al (eds): Harrison's Principles of Internal Medicine, 17th ed, New York, McGraw-Hill, 2008, p 2075

Hanly JG, Gladman DD, Rose TH, et al: Lupus pregnancy: A prospective study of placental changes. Arthritis Rheum 31:358, 1988

Harney S, Newton J, Milicic A, et al: Non-inherited maternal HLA alleles are associated with rheumatoid arthritis. Rheumatology 42:171, 2003

Harris EN: Antirheumatic drugs in pregnancy. Lupus 11:683, 2002

Harris EN, Gharavi AE, Patel SP, et al: Evaluation of the anti-cardiolipin antibody test: Report of an international workshop. Clin Exp Immunol 68:215, 1987a

Harris EN, Hughes GRV: Standardizing the anticardiolipin antibody-test. Lancet 1:277, 1987b

Harris EN, Spinnato JA: Should anticardiolipin tests be performed in otherwise healthy pregnant women? Am J Obstet Gynecol 165:1272, 1991

Häupl T, Østensen M, Grützkau A, et al: Interaction between rheumatoid arthritis and pregnancy: Correlation of molecular data with clinical disease activity measures. Rheumatology (Oxford) 47(Supp l):19, 2008a

Häupl T, Østensen M, Grützkau A, et al: Reactivation of rheumatoid arthritis after pregnancy: Increased phagocyte and recurring lymphocyte gene activity. Arthritis Rheum 58(10):2981, 2008b

Hazes JMW, Dijkmans BAC, Vandenbroucke JP, et al: Pregnancy and the risk of developing rheumatoid arthritis. Arthritis Rheum 33:1770, 1990

Heilmann L, Schorch M, Hahn T, et al: Pregnancy outcome in women with antiphospholipid antibodies: Report on a retrospective study. Semin Thromb Hemost 34(8):794, 2008

Heilmann L, von Tempelhoff GF, Pollow K: Antiphospholipid syndrome in obstetrics. Clin Appl Thromb Hemost 9:143, 2003

Hochberg MC: Updating the American College of Rheumatology revised criteria for the classification of systemic lupus erythematosus. Arthritis Rheum 40:1725, 1997

Hojnik M, George J, Ziporen L, et al: Heart valve involvement (Libman–Sacks endocarditis) in the antiphospholipid syndrome. Circulation 93:1579, 1996

Holers VM, Girardi G, Mo L, et al: Complement C3 activation is required for antiphospholipid antibody-induced fetal loss. J Exp Med 195:211, 2002

Hom G, Graham RR, Modrek B, et al: Association of systemic lupus erythematosus with C8orf13—BLK and ITGAM—ITGAX. N Engl J Med 358:900, 2008

Hot A, Perard L, Coppere B, et al: Marked improvement of Churg-Strauss vasculitis with intravenous gamma globulins during pregnancy. Clin Rheumatol 26(12):2149, 2007

Huong DLT, Wechsler B, Vauthier-Brouzes D, et al: Pregnancy in past or present lupus nephritis: A study of 32 pregnancies from a single centre. Ann Rheum Dis 60:599, 2001

Hwang I, Lee CK, Yoo B, et al: Necrotizing villitis and decidual vasculitis in the placentas of mothers with Behçet disease. Hum Pathol 40(1):135, 2009

Imbasciati E, Tincani A, Gregorini G, et al: Pregnancy in women with pre-existing lupus nephritis: predictors of fetal and maternal outcome. Nephrol Dial Transplant 24(2):519, 2009

Jadaon J, Shushan A, Ezra Y, et al: Behçet's disease and pregnancy. Acta Obstet Gynecol Scand 84:939, 2005

Jimenez SA, Artlett CM: Microchimerism and systemic sclerosis. Curr Opin Rheumatol 17:86, 2005

Johnson KL, McAlindon TE, Mulcahy E, et al: Microchimerism in a female patient with systemic lupus erythematosus. Arthritis Rheum 44:2107, 2001

Johnston SL, Lock RJ, Gompels MM: Takayasu arteritis: A review. J Clin Pathol 55:481, 2002

Julkunen H, Jouhikainen T, Kaaja R, et al: Fetal outcomes in lupus pregnancy: A retrospective case control study of 242 pregnancies in 112 patients. Lupus 2:125, 1993

Kalmantis K, Daskalakis G, Iavazzo C, et al: Henoch Schonlein purpura in pregnancy. Obstet Gynaecol 28(4):403, 2008

Kaplan D: Fetal wastage in patients with rheumatoid arthritis. J Rheumatol 13:875, 1986

Keeling SO, Oswald AE: Pregnancy and rheumatic disease: "By the book" or "by the doc." Clin Rheumatol 28(1):1, 2009

Khamashta MA, Ruiz-Irastorza G, Hughes GRV: Systemic lupus erythematosus flares during pregnancy. Rheum Dis Clin North Am 23:15, 1997

Kirwan JR: The Arthritis and Rheumatism Council Low-Dose Glucocorticoid Study Group: The effect of glucocorticoids on joint destruction in rheumatoid arthritis. N Engl J Med 333:142, 1995

Klipple GL, Cecere FA: Rheumatoid arthritis and pregnancy. Rheum Dis Clin North Am 15:213, 1989

Koukoura O, Mantas N, Linardakis H, et al: Successful term pregnancy in a patient with Wegener's granulomatosis: Case report and literature review. Fertil Steril 89:457.e1, 2008

Kozora E, Arciniegas DB, Filley CM, et al: Cognitive and neurologic status in patients with systemic lupus erythematosus without major neuropsychiatric syndromes. Arthritis Rheum 59:1639, 2008

Kraemer B, Abele H, Hahn M, et al: A successful pregnancy in a patient with Takayasu's arteritis. Hypertens Pregnancy 27(3):247, 2008

Lambe M, Bjornadal L, Neregard P, et al: Childbearing and the risk of scleroderma: A population-based study in Sweden. Am J Epidemiol 159:162, 2004

Langford CA, Fauci AS: The vasculitis syndromes. In Fauci AS, Braunwald E, Kasper DL, et al (eds): Harrison's Principles of Internal Medicine, 17th ed, New York, McGraw-Hill, 2008, p 2119

Langford C, Kerr G: Pregnancy in vasculitis. Curr Opin Rheumatol 14:36, 2002

Laskin CA, Bombardier C, Hannah ME, et al: Prednisone and aspirin in women with autoantibodies and unexplained recurrent fetal loss. New Engl J Med 337:148, 1997

Lee DM, Weinblatt ME: Rheumatoid arthritis. Lancet 358:903, 2001

Lee JY, Huerta PT, Zhang J, et al: Neurotoxic autoantibodies mediate congenital cortical impairment of offspring in maternal lupus. Nat Med 15(1):91, 2009

Lee LA: The clinical spectrum of neonatal lupus. Arch Dermatol Res 301(1):107, 2009

Lee LA, Weston WL: New findings in neonatal lupus syndrome. Am J Dis Child 138:233, 1984

Lee RM, Emlen W, Scott JR, et al: Anti-β_2 glycoprotein I antibodies in women with recurrent spontaneous abortion, unexplained fetal death, and antiphospholipid syndrome. Am J Obstet Gynecol 181:642, 1999

Levine JS, Branch W, Rauch J: The antiphospholipid syndrome. N Engl J Med 346:752, 2002

Levy RA, Vilela VS, Cataldo MJ, et al: Hydroxychloroquine (HCQ) in lupus pregnancy: Double-blind and placebo-controlled study. Lupus 10:401, 2001

Lipsky PE: Rheumatoid arthritis. In Fauci AS, Braunwald E, Kasper DL, et al (eds): Harrison's Principles of Internal Medicine, 17th ed. New York, McGraw-Hill, 2008, p 2083

Lockshin MD: Pregnancy does not cause systemic lupus erythematosus to worsen. Arthritis Rheum 32:665, 1989

Lockshin MD: Sex ratio and rheumatic disease: Excerpts from an Institute of Medicine reports. Lupus 11:662, 2002

Lockshin MD, Bonfa E, Elkon K, et al: Neonatal lupus risk to newborns of mothers with systemic lupus erythematosus. Arthritis Rheum 31:697, 1988

Lockshin MD, Druzin ML: Rheumatic disease. In Barron WM, Lindheimer JD (eds): Medical Disorders During Pregnancy, 2nd ed. St. Louis, Mosby, 1995, p 307

Lockshin MD, Druzin ML, Qamar T: Prednisone does not prevent recurrent fetal death in women with antiphospholipid antibody. Am J Obstet Gynecol 160:439, 1989

Lockshin MD, Sammaritano LR: Rheumatic disease. In Barron WM, Lindheimer MD (eds): Medical Disorders During Pregnancy, 3rd ed. St. Louis, Mosby, 2000, p 355

Lockshin M, Sammaritano L: Lupus pregnancy. Autoimmunity 36:33, 2003

Lockwood CJ, Romero R, Feinberg RF, et al: The prevalence and biologic significance of lupus anticoagulant and anticardiolipin antibodies in a general obstetric population. Am J Obstet Gynecol 161:369, 1989

Loeys B, Nuytinck L, Van Acker P, et al: Strategies for prenatal and preimplantation genetic diagnosis in Marfan syndrome (MFS). Prenat Diagn 22:22, 2002

Love PE, Santoro SA: Antiphospholipid antibodies: Anticardiolipin and the lupus anticoagulant in systemic lupus erythematosus (SLE) and in non-SLE disorders. Ann Intern Med 112:682, 1990

Lubbe WF, Liggins GC: The lupus-anticoagulant: Clinical and obstetric complications. NZ Med J 97:398, 1984

Lynch A, Byers T, Emlen W, et al: Association of antibodies to beta$_2$-glycoprotein 1 with pregnancy loss and pregnancy-induced hypertension: A prospective study in low-risk pregnancy. Obstet Gynecol 93:193, 1999

Mandl LA, Costenbader KH, Simard JF: Is birthweight associated with risk of rheumatoid arthritis? Data from a large cohort study. Ann Rheum Dis 86(4):514, 2009

Manuck T: Do antiphospholipid antibodies affect pregnancy outcomes in women heterozygous for factor V leiden? Abstract no 519. Presented at the 29th Annual Meeting of the Society for Maternal-Fetal Medicine, January 26-31, 2009

Marmont AM: Will hematopoietic stem cell transplantation cure human autoimmune diseases? J Autoimmun 30(3):145, 2008

Maymon R, Fejgin M: Scleroderma in pregnancy. Obstet Gynecol Surv 44:530, 1989

McGeachy C, Lam J: Anti-RNP neonatal lupus in a female newborn. Lupus 18(2):172, 2009

Medical Letter: Intravenous immunoglobulin (IVIG). 1249:101, 2006

Moll JMH: The place of psoriatic arthritis in the spondarthritides. Baillières Clin Rheumatol 8:395, 1994

Moodley J, Ramphal SR, Duursma J, et al: Antiphospholipid antibodies in eclampsia. Hypertens Preg 14:179, 1995

Moroni G, Ponticelli C: Pregnancy after lupus nephritis. Lupus 14:89, 2005

Moroni G, Quaglini S, Banfi G, et al: Pregnancy in lupus nephritis. Am J Kidney Dis 40:713, 2002

Moroni G, Ventura D, Riva P, et al: Antiphospholipid antibodies are associated with an increased risk for chronic renal insufficiency in patients with lupus nephritis. Am J Kidney Dis 43:28, 2004

Mor-Yosef S, Younis J, Granat M, et al: Marfan's syndrome in pregnancy. Obstet Gynecol Surv 43:382, 1988

Moyssakis I, Tzioufas A, Triposkiadis F, et al: Severe aortic stenosis and mitral regurgitation in a woman with systemic lupus erythematosus. Clin Cardiol 25:194, 2002

Musiej-Nowakowska E, Ploski R: Pregnancy and early onset pauciarticular juvenile chronic arthritis. Ann Rheum Dis 58:475, 1999

Nagey DA, Fortier KJ, Hayes BA, et al: Takayasu's arteritis in pregnancy: A case presentation demonstrating the absence of placental pathology. Am J Obstet Gynecol 147:463, 1983

Nelson JL, Hughes KA, Smith AG, et al: Maternal–fetal disparity in HLA class II alloantigens and the pregnancy-induced amelioration of rheumatoid arthritis. N Engl J Med 329:466, 1993

Nelson JL, Østensen M: Pregnancy and rheumatoid arthritis. Rheum Dis Clin North Am 23:195, 1997

Nelson JL, Voigt LF, Koepsell TD, et al: Pregnancy outcome in women with rheumatoid arthritis before disease onset. J Rheumatol 19:18, 1992

Nochy D, Daugas E, Droz D, et al: The intrarenal vascular lesions associated with primary antiphospholipid syndrome. J Am Soc Nephrol 10:507, 1999

Nodler J, Moolamalla SR, Ledger EM, et al: Elevated antiphospholipid antibody titers and adverse pregnancy outcomes: Analysis of a population-based hospital dataset. BMC Pregnancy Childbirth 9(1):11, 2009

Numano F, Kobayashi Y: Takayasu arteritis—beyond pulselessness. Intern Med 38:226, 1999

Ogunyemi D, Ku W, Arkel Y: The association between inherited thrombophilia, antiphospholipid antibodies and lipoprotein A levels with obstetrical complications in pregnancy. J Thromb Thrombolysis 14:157, 2002

Ohno T, Imai A, Tamaya T: Successful outcomes of pregnancy complicated with dermatomyositis. Gynecol Obstet Invest 33:187, 1992

Oshiro BT, Silver RM, Scott JR, et al: Antiphospholipid antibodies and fetal death. Obstet Gynecol 87:489, 1996

Østensen M: Pregnancy in patients with a history of juvenile rheumatoid arthritis. Arthritis Rheum 34:881, 1991

Østensen M, Villiger PM: The remission of rheumatoid arthritis during pregnancy. Semin Immunopathol 29:185, 2007

Ottaviani G, Lavezzi AM, Rossi L, et al: Sudden unexpected death of a term fetus in an anticardiolipin-positive mother. Am J Perinatol 21:79, 2004

Owen J, Hauth JC: Polyarteritis nodosa in pregnancy: A case report and brief literature review. Am J Obstet Gynecol 160:606, 1989

Packham DK, Lam SS, Nicholls K, et al: Lupus nephritis and pregnancy. QJM 83:315, 1992

Papadopoulos NG, Alamanos Y, Voulgari PV, et al: Does cigarette smoking influence disease expression, activity and severity in early rheumatoid arthritis patients? Clin Exp Rheumatol 23(6):861, 2005

Papakonstantinou K, Hasiakos D, Kondi-Paphiti A: Clinicopathology of maternal scleroderma. Int J Gynaecol Obstet 99(3):248, 2007

Papapetropoulos T, Kanellakopoulou N, Tsibri E, et al: Polymyositis and pregnancy: Report of a case with three pregnancies. J Neurol Neurosurg Psychiatry 64:406, 1998

Parkin J, Cohen B: An overview of the immune system. Lancet 357:1777, 2001

Pattison NS, Chamley LW, McKay EJ, et al: Antiphospholipid antibodies in pregnancy—prevalence and clinical associations. Br J Obstet Gynecol 100:909, 1993

Pepin M, Schwarze U, Superti-Furga A, et al: Clinical and genetic features of Ehlers-Danlos syndrome type IV, the vascular type. N Engl J Med 342:673, 2000

Petri M: Pregnancy in SLE. Baillières Clin Rheumatol 12:449, 1998

Petri M: The Hopkins Lupus Pregnancy Center: Ten key issues in management. Rheum Dis Clin N Am 33:227, 2007

Petri M, Kim MY, Kalunian KC, et al: Combined oral contraceptives in women with systemic lupus erythematosus. N Engl J Med 353:2550, 2005

Pierro E, Cirino G, Bucci MR, et al: Antiphospholipid antibodies inhibit prostaglandin release by decidual cells of early pregnancy: Possible involvement of extracellular secretory phospholipase A2. Fertil Steril 71:342, 1999

Pikwer M, Bergström U, Nilsson JA, et al: Breast feeding, but not use of oral contraceptives, is associated with a reduced risk of rheumatoid arthritis. Ann Rheum Dis 68(4):526, 2009

Polzin WJ, Kopelman JN, Robinson RD, et al: The association of antiphospholipid antibodies with pregnancies complicated by fetal growth restriction. Obstet Gynecol 78:1108, 1991

Prockop DJ, Czarny-Ratajczak M: Heritable disorders of connective tissue. In Fauci AS, Braunwald E, Kasper DL, et al (eds): Harrison's Principles of Internal Medicine, 17th ed, New York, McGraw-Hill, 2008, p 2461

Rahman A, Isenberg DA: Systemic lupus erythematosus. N Engl J Med 358:929, 2008

Rak JM, Maestroni L, Balandraud C, et al: Transfer of the shared epitope through microchimerism in women with rheumatoid arthritis. Arthritis Rheum 60(1):73, 2009

Rak JM, Pagni PP, Tiev K, et al: Male microchimerism and HLA compatibility in French women with scleroderma: A different profile in limited and diffuse subset. Rheumatology 48(4):363, 2009

Ramsey-Goldman R, Schilling E: Immunosuppressive drug use during pregnancy. Rheum Dis Clin North Am 23:149, 1997

Rand JH, Wu XX, Andree HAM, et al: Pregnancy loss in the antiphospholipid antibody syndrome—a possible thrombogenic mechanism. N Engl J Med 337:154, 1997a

Rand JH, Wu XX, Andree HAM, et al: Antiphospholipid antibodies accelerate plasma coagulation by inhibiting annexin-V binding to phospholipids: A "lupus procoagulant" phenomenon. Blood 92:1652, 1998

Rand JH, Wu XX, Guller S, et al: Antiphospholipid immunoglobulin G antibodies reduce annexin-V levels on syncytiotrophoblast apical membranes and in culture media of placental villi. Am J Obstet Gynecol 177:918, 1997b

Rand JH, Wu XX, Quinn AS, et al: Resistance to annexin A5 anticoagulant activity: A thrombogenic mechanism for the antiphospholipid syndrome. Lupus 17:922, 2008

Refojo D, Liberman AC, Giacomini D: Integrating systemic information at the molecular level. Ann NY Acad Sci 922:196, 2003

Rein AJ, Mevorach D, Perles Z, et al: Early diagnosis and treatment of atrioventricular block in the fetus exposed to maternal anti-SSA/Ro-SSB/La antibodies: A prospective, observational, fetal kinetocardiogram-based study. Circulation 119(14):1867, 2009

Robertson B, Greaves M: Antiphospholipid syndrome: An evolving story. Blood Reviews 20:201, 2006

Roque H, Paidas M, Rebarber A, et al: Maternal thrombophilia is associated with second- and third-trimester fetal death. Am J Obstet Gynecol 184:S27, 2001

Rosenzweig BA, Rotmensch S, Binette SP, et al: Primary idiopathic polymyositis and dermatomyositis complicating pregnancy: Diagnosis and management. Obstet Gynecol Surv 44:162, 1989

Roux CH, Brocq O, Breuil V, et al: Pregnancy in rheumatology patients exposed to anti-tumour necrosis factor (TNF)-alpha therapy. Rheumatology (Oxford) 46:695, 2007

Rubin RL: Drug induced lupus. In Wallace DJ, Hahn BH (eds): Dubois' Lupus Erythematosus, 5th ed. Baltimore, Williams & Wilkins, 1997, p 871

Rudd NL, Nimrod C, Holbrook KA, et al: Pregnancy complications in type IV Ehlers-Danlos Syndrome. Lancet 1:50, 1983

Ruiz-Irastorza G, Khamashta MA, Gordon C, et al: Measuring systemic lupus erythematosus activity during pregnancy: Validation of the lupus activity index in pregnancy scale. Arthritis Rheum 51:78, 2004

Ruiz-Irastorza G, Khamashta MA, Hughes G: Systemic lupus erythematosus. Lancet 358:586, 2001

Saleeb S, Copel J, Friedman D, et al: Comparison of treatment with fluorinated glucocorticoids to the natural history of autoantibody-associated congenital heart block. Arthritis Rheum 42:2335, 1999

Sánchez-Guerrero J, Uribe AG, Jiménez-Santana L, et al: A trial of contraceptive methods in women with systemic lupus erythematosus. N Engl J Med 353:2539, 2005

Sangle S, D'Cruz DP, Hughes GR: Livedo reticularis and pregnancy morbidity in patients negative for antiphospholipid antibodies. Ann Rheum Dis 64:147, 2005

Sanna G, Bertolaccini ML, Cuadrado MJ: Central nervous system involvement in the antiphospholipid (Hughes) syndrome. Rheumatology 42:200, 2003

Sasaki H, Washio M, Ohara N, et al: Acute onset of polymyalgia rheumatica in pregnancy. Obstet Gynecol 106:1194, 2005

Savi C, Villa L, Civardi L, et al: Two consecutive cases of type A aortic dissection after delivery. Minerva Anestesiol 73:381, 2007

Sawaya HH, Jimenez SA, Artlett CM: Quantification of fetal microchimeric cells in clinically affected and unaffected skin of patients with systemic sclerosis. Rheumatology 43:965, 2004

Schousboe I, Rasmussen MS: Synchronized inhibition of the phospholipid mediated autoactivation of factor XII in plasma by β_2 glycoprotein I and anti-β_2 glycoprotein I. Thromb Haemost 73:798, 1995

Scott JR: Risks to the children born to mothers with autoimmune diseases. Lupus 11:655, 2002

Sharma BK, Jain S, Vasishta K: Outcome of pregnancy in Takayasu arteritis. Int J Cardiol 75:S159, 2000

Sherer Y, Gorstein A, Fritzler MJ, et al: Autoantibody explosion in systemic lupus erythematosus: More than 100 different antibodies found in SLE patients. Semin Arthri Rheum 34:501, 2004

Shi W, Chong BH, Hogg PJ: Anticardiolipin antibodies block the inhibition by β_2 glycoprotein I of the factor Xa generating activity of platelets. Thromb Haemost 70:342, 1993

Shinohara K, Miyagawa S, Fujita T, et al: Neonatal lupus erythematosus: Results of maternal corticosteroid therapy. Obstet Gynecol 93:952, 1999

Shmerling RH: Autoantibodies in systemic lupus erythematosus—there before you know it. N Engl J Med 349:1499, 2003

Silman A, Kay A, Brennan P: Timing of pregnancy in relation to the onset of rheumatoid arthritis. Arthritis Rheum 35:152, 1992

Silver RM, Branch DW: Autoimmune diseases in pregnancy: Systemic lupus erythematosus and antiphospholipid syndrome. Clin Perinatol 24:91, 1997

Simchen MJ, Goldstein G, Lubetsky A, et al: Factor V Leiden and antiphospholipid antibodies in either mothers or infants increase the risk for perinatal arterial ischemic stroke. Stroke 40(1):65, 2009

Simchen MJ, Pauzner R, Rofe G, et al: High antiphospholipid antibody titers are associated with adverse pregnancy outcome in women with antiphospholipid antibody syndrome. Abstract No 462. Presented at the 29th Annual Meeting of the Society for Maternal-Fetal Medicine, January 26-31, 2009

Singsen BH, Akhter JE, Weinstein MM, et al: Congenital complete heart block and SSA antibodies: Obstetric implications. Am J Obstet Gynecol 153:495, 1985

Sitar G, Brambati B, Baldi M, et al: The use of non-physiological conditions to isolate fetal cells from maternal blood. Exp Cell Res 302:153, 2005

Skomsvoll JF, Baste V, Irgens LM, et al: The recurrence risk of adverse outcome in the second pregnancy in women with rheumatic disease. Obstet Gynecol 100:1196, 2002

Sneller MC: Wegener's granulomatosis. JAMA 273:1288, 1995

Solomon SD, McMurray JJ, Pfeffer MA, et al: Cardiovascular risk associated with celecoxib in a clinical trial for colorectal adenoma prevention. N Engl J Med 352(11):1071, 2005

Sorokin Y, Johnson MP, Rogowski N, et al: Obstetric and gynecologic dysfunction in the Ehlers–Danlos syndrome. J Reprod Med 39:281, 1994

Srivatsa B, Srivatsa S, Johnson K, et al: Microchimerism of presumed fetal origin in thyroid specimens from women: A case-control study. Lancet 358:2034, 2001

Steen VD: Pregnancy in women with systemic sclerosis. Obstet Gynecol 94:15, 1999

Steen VD, Conte C, Day N, et al: Pregnancy in women with systemic sclerosis. Arthritis Rheum 32:151, 1989

Stirnemann J, Fain O, Lachassinne E, et al: Neonatal lupus erythematosus. Presse Med 31:1407, 2002

Stone S, Hunt BJ, Seed PT: Longitudinal evaluation of markers of endothelial cell dysfunction and hemostasis in treated antiphospholipid syndrome and in healthy pregnancy. Am J Obstet Gynecol 188:454, 2003

Tashkin DP, Elashoff R, Clements PJ, et al: Cyclophosphamide versus placebo in scleroderma lung disease. N Engl J Med 354:2655, 2006

Tincani A, Rebaioli CB, Andreoli L, et al: Neonatal effects of maternal antiphospholipid syndrome. Curr Rheumatol Rep 11(1):70, 2009

Toglia MR, Weg JG: Venous thromboembolism during pregnancy. N Engl J Med 335:108, 1996

Trudinger BJ, Stewart GJ, Cook C, et al: Monitoring lupus anticoagulant-positive pregnancies with umbilical artery flow velocity waveforms. Obstet Gynecol 72:215, 1988

Tsokos G: A disease with a complex pathogenesis. Lancet 358:S65, 2001

Unger A, Kay A, Griffin AJ, et al: Disease activity and pregnancy associated β_2-glycoprotein in rheumatoid arthritis. BMJ 286:750, 1983

Varga J: Systemic sclerosus (scleroderma) and related disorders. In Fauci AS, Braunwald E, Kasper DL, et al (eds): Harrison's Principles of Internal Medicine, 17th ed, New York, McGraw-Hill, 2008, p 2096

Varner MW, Meehan RT, Syrop CH, et al: Pregnancy in patients with systemic lupus erythematosus. Am J Obstet Gynecol 145:1025, 1983

Volkov N, Nisenblat V, Ohel G, et al: Ehlers-Danlos syndrome: Insight on obstetric aspects. Obstet Gynecol Surv 62:51, 2006

Vroom F, de Walle HE, van de Laar MA, et al: Disease-modifying antirheumatic drugs in pregnancy: Current status and implications for the future. Drug Safety 29:845, 2006

Wagner S, Craici I, Reed D, et al: Maternal and foetal outcomes in pregnant patients with active lupus nephritis. Lupus 18(4)342, 2009

Waldorf KM, Nelson JL: Autoimmune disease during pregnancy and the microchimerism legacy of pregnancy. Immunol Invest 37:631, 2008

Walsh CA, Reardon W, Foley ME: Unexplained prelabor uterine rupture in a term primigravida. Obstet Gynecol 109:455, 2007

Waltuck J, Buyon JP: Autoantibody-associated congenital heart block: Outcome in mothers and children. Ann Intern Med 120:544, 1994

Warren JB, Silver RM: Autoimmune disease in pregnancy: Systemic lupus erythematosus and antiphospholipid syndrome. Obstet Gynecol Clin North Am 31:345, 2004

Williams L, Chang PY, Park E, et al: Successful treatment of dermatomyositis during pregnancy with intravenous immunoglobulin monotherapy. Obstet Gynecol 109:561, 2007

Wilson WA, Gharavi AE, Koike T, et al: International consensus statement on preliminary classification criteria for definite antiphospholipid syndrome: Report of an international workshop. Arthritis Rheum 42:1309, 1999

Wolfberg AJ, Lee-Parritz A, Peller AJ, et al: Association of rheumatologic disease with preeclampsia. Obstet Gynecol 103:1190, 2004

Wu H, Birmingham DJ, Rovin B, et al: D-Dimer level and the risk for thrombosis in systemic lupus erythematosus. Clin J Am Soc Nephrol 3:1628, 2008

Yamada H, Atsumi T, Kobashi G, et al: Antiphospholipid antibodies increase the risk of pregnancy-induced hypertension and adverse pregnancy outcomes. J Reprod Immunol 79(2):188, 2009

Yasuda M, Takakuwa K, Okinaga A, et al: Prospective studies of the association between anticardiolipin antibody and outcome of pregnancy. Obstet Gynecol 86:555, 1995

Zangari M, Lockwood CJ, Scher J, et al: Prothrombin activation fragment (F1.2) is increased in pregnant patients with antiphospholipid antibodies. Thromb Res 85:177, 1997

CHAPTER 55

Neurological and Psychiatric Disorders

Neurological and psychiatric disorders encountered during pregnancy are those that are common to reproductive-aged women. Some may be even more common in pregnancy. Examples are Bell palsy, some types of stroke, and depression.

NEUROLOGICAL DISORDERS

A number of neurological diseases are relatively common in women of childbearing age. Many of these once precluded childbearing, but less so now. Somewhat related, neurological disorders can profoundly disrupt normal sexual function (Rees and colleagues, 2007). That said, many women with chronic neurological disease become pregnant and have successful pregnancy outcomes. Conversely, neurological diseases do contribute to maternal mortality rates, and there are specific risks with which the clinician should be familiar.

Diagnosis of Neurological Disease During Pregnancy

Many women with chronic neurological disease have been diagnosed before pregnancy. In others, neurological symptoms appear for the first time and must be distinguished from pregnancy complications. Because these symptoms may involve cognitive as well as neuromuscular functions, they must also be distinguished from psychiatric disorders. In general, pregnant women should receive the same evaluation as any other patient.

Central Nervous System Imaging

Computed tomography (CT) and *magnetic resonance (MR) imaging* have opened new vistas for the diagnosis, classification, and management of many neurological and psychiatric disorders (Dineen and colleagues, 2005). As discussed in Chapter 41 (p. 918), both imaging methods can be used safely during pregnancy. Computed tomography is commonly used whenever rapid diagnosis is necessary. However, in less acute situations, MR imaging is often preferred because of its low radiation exposure. It is particularly helpful to diagnose demyelinating diseases, screen for arteriovenous malformations, evaluate congenital and developmental nervous system abnormalities, identify posterior fossa lesions, and diagnose spinal cord diseases. MR imaging is superior for detecting acute ischemia and acute and chronic hemorrhage, and therefore, is preferable for stroke evaluation (Chalela and associates, 2007). For either test, the woman should be positioned in a left lateral tilt with a wedge under one hip to prevent hypotension as well as to diminish aortic pulsations, which may degrade the image.

Cerebral angiography with contrast injection, usually via the femoral artery, is a valuable adjunct to the diagnosis and treatment of some cerebrovascular diseases. *Fluoroscopy* involves more radiation but can be performed if necessary with careful abdominal shielding.

Headache

According to the National Health Interview Survey updated annually by the Centers for Disease Control and Prevention (2006a, b), a fourth of women aged 18 to 44 years report a severe headache or migraine within the past 3 months. And the most common neurological complaint during pregnancy is headache. The classification of headaches by the International Headache Society (2004) is shown in Table 55-1. *Cluster headaches* are not commonly reported in pregnancy and were reviewed by Giraud and Chauvet (2009). *Thunderclap headaches*

TABLE 55-1. Classification of Headache

Primary
 Tension-type
 Migraine
 Cluster and other trigeminal cephalgias
 Other
Secondary
 Head or neck trauma
 Cranial or cervical vascular disorders
 Intracranial nonvascular
 Substance use
 Infection
 Head and neck disorders
 Psychiatric cranial neuralgias

Adapted from the International Headache Society (2004).

can be primary or may be due to other causes in Table 55-1 (Singhal and colleagues, 2009).

Tension-Type Headache

These are common, and characteristic features include muscle tightness and mild to moderate pain that can persist for hours in the back of the neck and head. There are no associated neurological disturbances or nausea. The pain usually responds to rest, massage, application of heat or ice, anti-inflammatory medications, or mild tranquilizers. In 95 women with a headache postpartum, 39 percent were tension-type headaches (Stella and colleagues, 2007). Headaches from depression may be attributed to tension headaches.

Migraine Headache

The term *migraine* describes a periodic, sometimes incapacitating neurological disorder characterized by episodic attacks of severe headache and autonomic nervous system dysfunction. The International Headache Society (2004) classifies three migraine types based on the presence or absence of an aura as well as chronicity:

1. Migraine without aura—formerly common migraine—is characterized by a unilateral throbbing headache, nausea and vomiting, or photophobia
2. Migraine with aura—formerly classical migraine—has similar symptoms preceded by premonitory neurological phenomena such as visual scotoma or hallucinations. A third of patients have this type of migraine, which sometimes can be averted if medication is taken at the first premonitory sign
3. Chronic migraine is defined by headache occurring at least 15 days each month, for more than 3 months, and without obvious cause.

Migraines may begin in childhood, peak in adolescence, and tend to diminish in both frequency and severity with advancing years. The annual prevalence is 17 percent in women and

6 percent in men (Lipton and colleagues, 2007). Another 5 percent of women have *probable migraine*—they have all criteria but one (Silberstein and co-workers, 2007). Migraines are especially common in young women and have been linked to hormone levels in an as yet unclear relationship. For example, migraine headaches are worsened in at least half of women at the time of menstruation (Brandes, 2006).

The exact pathophysiology of migraines is uncertain, but they occur when neuronal dysfunction leads to decreased cortical blood flow, activation of vascular and meningeal nociceptors, and stimulation of trigeminal sensory neurons (Brandes and associates, 2007; Silberstein, 2004a). A predilection for the posterior circulation has been described by Kruit and co-workers (2004). Migraines—especially those with aura in young women—are associated with increased risk for ischemic strokes. The risk is greater in those who smoke or use oral contraceptives.

Migraine in Pregnancy. At least two comprehensive reviews document that 50 to 70 percent of *migraineurs* have improvement of headaches during pregnancy (Adeney and Williams, 2006; Silberstein, 2004b). However, migraines—usually with an aura—occasionally appear for the first time during pregnancy. Pregnant women with preexisting migraine symptoms may have other symptoms suggestive of a more serious disorder. Thus, the onset of new neurological symptoms should prompt a complete evaluation (Detsky and colleagues, 2006; Marcus, 2007).

Banhidy and associates (2006) reported preliminary data that possibly link severe migraine in the first 8 weeks with a slightly increased risk for a fetus with limb-reduction defects. Data has accrued linking migraine headaches with other serious pregnancy complications such as preeclampsia and other cardiovascular morbidities (Adeney and Williams, 2006; Faccinetti and colleagues, 2009; Scher and associates, 2005). In a case-control study done from nearly 18.5 million pregnancy-related discharges from 2000 through 2003, Bushnell and co-workers (2009) identified ICD-9 (International Classification of Disease, 9th edition) migraine codes in 185 per 100,000 discharges. Associated diagnoses and significant odds ratios were found for migraines and stroke—15; migraines and myocardial infarction or heart disease—2.1; and venous thromboembolism—3.2; hypertension—8.6; smoking—2.9; and gestational hypertension including preeclampsia—2.3.

Management. Most migraine headaches respond to simple analgesics such as aspirin, ibuprofen, or acetaminophen, especially if given early. Severe headaches should be treated aggressively with intravenous hydration, parenteral antiemetics, and opioids if necessary (American College of Obstetricians and Gynecologists, 2002a). Antiemetics such as promethazine, prochlorperazine, or metoclopramide are frequently needed and are commonly given with meperidine.

Ergotamine derivatives are potent vasoconstrictors that should be avoided in pregnancy, although inadvertent use in early pregnancy does not appear to pose significant risk (Briggs and colleagues, 2005).

Triptans are serotonin 5-HT$_{1B/2D}$-receptor agonists that are highly effective to relieve headaches by causing intracranial vasoconstriction (Silberstein, 2004a). They also relieve nausea and vomiting and greatly reduce the need for analgesics. They can be given orally, by injection, as a rectal suppository, or as a nasal spray. The greatest experience is with sumatriptan, and although not studied extensively in pregnancy, it appears to be safe (Briggs and co-workers, 2005). In nonpregnant adults, Brandes and colleagues (2007) showed superior efficacy of sumatriptan 85 mg plus naproxen 500 mg—about 60-percent of migraineurs gained relief at 2 hours—compared with either drug given alone. The manufacturer's Sumatriptan and Naratriptan Pregnancy Registry (2004) of 414 prospectively enrolled pregnancies has reported no adverse effects. There is correspondingly less experience with other triptans in pregnancy.

For women with frequent migraine headaches, prophylactic therapy is indicated (American College of Obstetricians and Gynecologists, 2002a). Amitriptyline, 10 to 150 mg/day; propranolol, 20 to 80 mg three times daily; atenolol, 50 to 100 mg/day; or labetalol, 50 to 150 mg two times daily, are safe in pregnancy and have been used with success (Dey and associates, 2002; Marcus, 2007).

Seizure Disorders

The Centers for Disease Control and Prevention reported that the prevalence of epilepsy in adults in 2005 was 1.65 percent (Kobau and colleagues, 2008). This is estimated to include 1.1 million American women of childbearing age, and seizure disorders complicate 1 in 200 pregnancies (Brodie and Dichter, 1996; Yerby, 1994). After headaches, these are the second most prevalent—and a more serious—neurological condition encountered in pregnant women. Epilepsy itself can alter fetal development and can affect the course of pregnancy, labor, and delivery. Importantly, the teratogenic effects of several anticonvulsant medications are unquestioned.

Pathophysiology

A seizure is defined as a paroxysmal disorder of the central nervous system characterized by an abnormal neuronal discharge with or without loss of consciousness. Epilepsy encompasses a number of different syndromes whose cardinal feature is a predisposition to recurrent unprovoked seizures (Chang and Lowenstein, 2003). Epileptic syndromes fit into two broad categories—*partial* or *generalized seizures*. Accurate classification is important when therapy is selected.

Partial Seizures. These originate in one localized area of the brain and affect a correspondingly localized area of neurological function. They are believed to result from trauma, abscess, tumor, or perinatal factors, although a specific lesion is rarely demonstrated. *Simple motor seizures* start in one region of the body and progress toward other ipsilateral areas of the body, producing tonic and then clonic movements. Simple seizures can affect sensory function or produce autonomic dysfunction or psychological changes. Consciousness is usually not lost, and recovery is rapid. *Partial seizures* can secondarily generalize, producing loss of consciousness and convulsions. *Complex partial seizures,* also called *temporal lobe* or *psychomotor seizures,* usually involve clouding of consciousness.

Generalized Seizures. These involve both brain hemispheres simultaneously and may be preceded by an aura before an abrupt loss of consciousness. There is a strong hereditary component. In grand mal seizures, loss of consciousness is followed by tonic contraction of the muscles and rigid posturing, and then by clonic contractions of all extremities while the muscles gradually relax. Return to consciousness is gradual, and the patient may remain confused and disoriented for several hours. *Absence* seizures, also called *petit mal seizures,* are a form of generalized epilepsy that involve a brief loss of consciousness without muscle activity and are characterized by immediate recovery of consciousness and orientation.

Causes of Seizures

Some identifiable causes of convulsive disorders in young adults include trauma, alcohol- and other drug-induced withdrawals, brain tumors, biochemical abnormalities, and arteriovenous malformations. A search for these is prudent with a new-onset seizure disorder in a pregnant woman. The diagnosis of idiopathic epilepsy is one of exclusion.

Epilepsy During Pregnancy

The major pregnancy-related threats to women with epilepsy are increased seizure rates and risks for fetal malformations. Although earlier studies described a worsening of seizure activity during pregnancy, this is not so now because of better prenatal management. In a recent community-based, prospective study from Finland, Viinikainen and co-workers (2006) reported that epilepsy either was better controlled or showed no change in 83 percent of pregnant women. Meador and co-workers (2006) reported an 81-percent seizure-free rate in pregnancy for 333 women enrolled in multicenter observational studies. Prepregnancy control seems important too. From the Australian Registry, Vajda and colleagues (2008) reported that the risk of seizures during pregnancy was decreased by 50 to 70 percent if the year before was seizure free.

Increased seizure frequency is often associated with lowered and thus subtherapeutic anticonvulsant levels, a lower seizure threshold, or both. Subtherapeutic levels can be caused by nausea and vomiting; decreased gastrointestinal motility and use of antacids that diminish drug absorption; pregnancy hypervolemia offset by protein binding; induction of hepatic, plasma, and placental enzymes that increase drug metabolism; and increased glomerular filtration that hastens drug clearance. Importantly, some women discontinue medication because of teratogenicity concerns. Finally, the seizure threshold can be affected by pregnancy-related sleep deprivation as well as hyperventilation and pain during labor.

Embryofetal Malformations. Recent evidence suggests that untreated epilepsy is not associated with increased malformations (Thomas and co-workers, 2008; Viinikainen and colleagues, 2006). *But the fetus of an epileptic mother who takes anticonvulsant medications has an indisputably increased risk of congenital malformations.* Monotherapy is associated with a lower birth defect rate compared with multiagent therapy. And if necessary, increasing monotherapy dosage initially is preferable to adding another agent (Buhimschi and Weiner, 2009). When given alone, therapy with phenytoin, carbamazepine, and probably phenobarbital increases the major malformation rate two- to threefold above baseline (Perucca, 2005; Thomas and associates, 2008). Early data indicate a similar risk with lamotrigine. The major exception is valproate, which is dose dependent and increases the risk to as high as four- to eightfold (Eadie, 2008; Wyszynski and colleagues, 2005). Fetal exposure to monotherapy with valproate—but not phenytoin, carbamazepine, or lamotrigine—was recently linked with impaired cognitive function at age 3 years (Meador and co-workers, 2009). When polytherapy is used, the risk increases with each drug used. These are discussed in greater detail in Chapter 14 (p. 317).

Pregnancy Complications. Women with epilepsy have a small increased risk of some pregnancy complications other than seizures (Harden and associates, 2009). Olafsson and colleagues (1998) performed a population-based study and found that Icelandic epileptic women had a twofold increased cesarean delivery rate. In a cohort study from Montreal, Richmond and co-workers (2004) reported an increased incidence of nonproteinuric hypertension and labor induction. From a Swedish study of 1207 epileptic women, Pilo and colleagues (2006) reported a 1.5-fold increased incidence of cesarean delivery, preeclampsia, and postpartum hemorrhage. Postpartum depression has also been reported as increased (Turner and associates, 2009). Finally, children of epileptic mothers have a 10-percent risk of developing a seizure disorder.

Preconceptional Counseling. Women with epilepsy should benefit from preconceptional counseling (see Chap. 7, p. 176). According to findings in their Cochrane review, however, Winterbottom and associates (2009) found no objective evidence of its effectiveness. Topics addressed include optimal anticonvulsant management, preferably monotherapy with the least teratogenic drug, or at least a reduction in the number of drugs taken. Although some recommend that these be limited to the older and more traditional anticonvulsants—phenytoin, carbamazepine, and phenobarbital—there are newer drugs that may actually have less teratogenic potential. For example, Cunnington and Tennis (2005) described outcomes from the International Lamotrigine Pregnancy Registry. When used as monotherapy, *lamotrigine* was associated with a 2.9-percent rate of malformations, and as polytherapy with other drugs, except valproate, the risk was 2.7 percent. Hunt and associates (2006) presented preliminary data that *levetiracetam* use was associated with a 2.7-percent birth defect rate. Other new anticonvulsants were reviewed by Stefan and Feuerstein (2007).

Physical activity should exclude driving during early pregnancy if associated vomiting prevents drug ingestion. Folic acid supplementation is emphasized, and it likely decreases malformation rates in women taking anticonvulsants (Kjaer and associates, 2008). Plans for fetal evaluation and optimal pregnancy management are outlined.

Contraception should be discussed. Anticonvulsants such as phenobarbital, primidone, phenytoin, and carbamazepine may cause breakthrough bleeding and hormonal contraceptive failure (Table 32-5, p. 678). They do this by induction of hepatic P_{450} microsomal enzyme systems, which increase estrogen metabolism. For these reasons, some recommend that oral contraceptives containing 50 μg of estrogen be used with anticonvulsants (Harden and Leppik, 2006). Conversely, anticonvulsants may adversely affect both male and female fertility (Artama and co-workers, 2006).

Management in Pregnancy. The major goal is seizure prevention. To accomplish this, treatment for nausea and vomiting should be provided, seizure-provoking stimuli should be avoided, and medication compliance should be emphasized. Anticonvulsants should be maintained at the lowest dosage associated with seizure control. Although some routinely monitor serum drug levels during pregnancy, these may be unreliable because of altered protein binding. Free or unbound drug levels, although more helpful, are not widely available. And also, there is no evidence that such monitoring improves seizure control (Adab, 2006). For these reasons, drug levels may be measured only following seizures or if noncompliance is suspected. Exceptions may be newer agents such as lamotrigine and oxcarbazepine (Battino and Tomson, 2007; Pennell and associates, 2007).

At midpregnancy, specialized sonographic examination may aid in identifying anomalies (see Chap. 16, p. 351). Tests of fetal well-being are generally not performed for uncomplicated epilepsy.

Cerebrovascular Diseases

Most malformations of blood vessels of the brain involve the arterial system. They can cause a *stroke*, defined as an abrupt neurological deficit caused by embolization or occlusion. Embolization causes an *ischemic stroke*, and rupture of a cerebral vessel causes a *hemorrhagic stroke* (Smith and colleagues, 2008a). The Centers for Disease Control and Prevention (2007) estimates that in 2005, 0.8 percent of all women aged 18 to 44 years had a history of a stroke.

Stroke is relatively uncommon in pregnant women, but contributes disparately to maternal mortality. The reported incidence ranges from 15 to 35 per 100,000 pregnancies (James, 2005; Liang, 2006; Simolke, 1994, and all their co-workers). According to data from the Centers for Disease Control and Prevention reported by Chang and colleagues (2003), stroke caused 5 percent of 4200 pregnancy-related maternal deaths in the United States from 1991 through 1999. From indicators of severe obstetrical morbidity described in two reports from the Centers for Disease Control and Prevention, strokes were responsible for 2.5 percent of hospitalizations for severe maternal morbidity in the United States from 1991 through 2003 (Callaghan and co-workers, 2008). Importantly, the prevalence of stroke-related hospitalization did not increase from 1998 through 2005 (Kuklina and associates, 2009).

Risk Factors

Various risk factors—unrelated and related to pregnancy—from three large studies that included more than 10 million pregnancies are shown in Table 55-2. By far, in aggregate, the most common risk factor is some form of hypertension—chronic, gestational, or preeclampsia. In their study of 2850 pregnancy-related strokes, James and co-workers (2005) reported that about 10 percent of

TABLE 55-2. Risk Factors for Strokes During Pregnancy

Not Pregnancy Related	Pregnancy Related
Age	Gestational hypertension
Migraine headaches	Preeclampsia
Thrombophilias	Hemorrhage
Heart disease	Transfusions
Valve prosthesis	Cesarean delivery
Patent foramen ovale	Puerperal sepsis
Lupus erythematosus	
Sickle-cell disease	
Hypertension	

From De La Vega (2007); James (2005); Lanska and Kryscio (2000); Lin (2008); Ros (2002), and all their associates.

all strokes developed antepartum, 40 percent intrapartum, and almost 50 percent postpartum. Ros and associates (2002) computed a 100-fold risk of stroke at the time of delivery. Peripartum stroke is about 1.5-fold more common in cesarean compared with vaginal delivery (Lin and colleagues, 2008).

Types of Stroke

Causes of the two major types of stroke are shown in Table 55-3. Their distribution differs depending on definition and classification, but they are almost equal in incidence.

Ischemic Stroke

These are most common in older patients. In young pregnant women, however, they constitute a relatively smaller proportion of the total number of strokes. Ischemic strokes usually result from arterial or venous thrombosis or arterial embolism.

TABLE 55-3. Types of Strokes During Pregnancy or Puerperium

Type	Comments
Ischemic Strokes	
Preeclampsia-eclampsia	Common
Arterial thrombosis	Common
Venous thrombosis	Uncommon
Others—vasculopathy, arterial dissection, metastatic malignancy, unknown	Uncommon
Hemorrhagic Strokes	
Hypertension	Common
Arteriovenous malformation	Common
Saccular aneurysm	Less common
Others—cocaine, angioma, vasculopathy, unknown	Uncommon

From Ishimori (2006); Jaigobin (2000); James (2005); Jeng (2004); Kittner (1996); Liang (2006); Pervulov, 2009; Saad (2006); Sharshar (1995); Simolke (1991); Witlin (2000), and all their colleagues.

Particular to pregnancy, evidence has accrued in the past 10 years that some women with eclampsia suffer from areas of cerebral infarction (Zeeman and colleagues, 2004a). Aukes and associates (2007, 2009) have shown that such women may have increased white-matter lesions that persist at follow-up several years later, and some suffer residual cognitive dysfunction (see Chap. 34, p. 749). A few women with eclampsia will suffer symptomatic strokes from larger cortical infarctions (see Chap. 34, p. 721 and Fig. 34-14). The *reversible cerebral vasoconstriction syndrome*—also termed *postpartum angiopathy*—can cause extensive cerebral edema with necrosis and widespread infarction with areas of hemorrhage (Ramnarayan and Sriganesh, 2009; Singhal and colleagues, 2009).

Cerebral Artery Thrombosis. Most thrombotic strokes occur in older individuals. They are caused by atherosclerosis, and the internal carotid artery is the most commonly affected site. Most cases are preceded by one or more transient ischemic attacks. With stroke, patients usually present with sudden onset of severe headache, hemiplegia or other neurological deficits, or seizures. In contrast, focal neurological symptoms accompanied by an aura usually signify a first-episode migraine (Liberman and co-workers, 2008). Evaluation includes serum lipid profile, echocardiography, and cranial imaging with CT, MR imaging, or angiography. Because antiphospholipid antibodies cause up to a third of ischemic strokes in otherwise healthy young patients, pregnant women with this stroke type are usually evaluated for these (see Chap. 54, p. 1151). In some, vasculopathy such as Moyamoya disease may be found (Ishimori and colleagues, 2006).

Over the past decade, thrombolytic therapy has become standard care for ischemic stroke seen within the first 3 hours (Khaja and Grotta, 2007). Recombinant tissue plasminogen activator—rt-PA or alteplase—is recommended if the patient is within the 3-hour window, if there is measurable neurological deficit, and if neuroimaging has excluded hemorrhage. A principal risk is hemorrhagic transformation of an ischemic stroke in about 5 percent of treated patients (van der Worp and van Gijn, 2007). There is limited experience with thrombolytic treatment for ischemic stroke in pregnancy. Leonhardt (2006) and Murugappan (2006) and their associates found only three case reports and added another eight. Outcomes were similar to those in nonpregnant patients. One woman at 12 weeks' gestation developed an "intrauterine hematoma" and elected pregnancy termination.

The recurrence risk for ischemic stroke in association with pregnancy is low unless a specific, persistent cause is identified. Lamy and colleagues (2000) studied 489 consecutive women of reproductive age with stroke. There were 37 women with an ischemic stroke during pregnancy or the puerperium, and none of their 24 subsequent pregnancies was complicated by recurrent stroke. Coppage and associates (2004) described 23 women with strokes before pregnancy due to a variety of causes. They had 35 subsequent pregnancies without a recurrent stroke. This may even be the case if antiphospholipid antibodies are detected. For example, the Antiphospholipid Antibodies and Stroke Study observed 1770 nonpregnant patients with ischemic stroke (APASS Investigators, 2004). In these subjects, there was no difference in the recurrence risk whether anticardiolipin or antiphospholipid antibodies were present as long as preventative treatment was given with warfarin or aspirin. Currently, there are no firm guidelines regarding prophylaxis in pregnant women with a stroke history (Helms and co-workers, 2009).

Cerebral Embolism. This usually involves the middle cerebral artery and is more common during the latter half of pregnancy or early puerperium (Lynch and Nelson, 2001). The diagnosis can be made with confidence only after thrombosis and hemorrhage have been excluded. The latter can be difficult to distinguish because cerebral artery embolization and thrombosis are both followed by infarction. The diagnosis of thromboembolism is more certain if an embolic source is identified. Paradoxical embolism is thought to be a common cause because more than a fourth of adults have a patent foramen ovale. This allows right-sided venous thromboemboli to bypass filtration by the lungs (Kizer and Devereux, 2005). Foraminal closure prevents recurrences, and Schrale and co-workers (2007) described percutaneous closure in three women in their third trimester. Other causes of embolism include an arrhythmia—especially atrial fibrillation, rheumatic valvular damage, or mitral valve prolapse. Finally, emboli from infective endocarditis must be considered (Cox and associates, 1988).

Management of embolic stroke consists of supportive measures and antiplatelet therapy. Anticoagulation is controversial (Kizer and Devereux, 2005).

Cerebral Venous Thrombosis. In a 10-center study in the United States, 7 percent of cerebral venous thromboses were associated with pregnancy (Wasay and co-workers, 2008). Even so, pregnancy-associated cerebral venous thrombosis is rare in developed countries—reported incidences range from 1 in 11,000 to 1 in 45,000 pregnancies (Cross, 1968; Lanska and Kryscio, 1997; Simolke, 1991, and all their colleagues). In the Nationwide Inpatient Sample of more than 8 million deliveries, James and associates (2005) observed that venous thrombosis caused only 2 percent of strokes during pregnancy. According to Ehtisham and Stern (2006), more than 100 causes have been documented.

Lateral or superior sagittal venous sinus thrombosis usually occurs in the puerperium, and often in association with preeclampsia, sepsis, or thrombophilias. It is more common in patients with inherited thrombophilias, lupus anticoagulant, or antiphospholipid antibodies (see Chap. 54, p. 1151). Headache is the most common presenting symptom, neurological deficits are common, and up to a third of patients have convulsions (Wasay and colleagues, 2008). MR imaging is the preferred radiological procedure (Ehtisham and Stein, 2006).

Management includes anticonvulsants for seizures, and antimicrobials if septic thrombophlebitis is suspected. Heparin anticoagulation is recommended by most, but its efficacy is controversial (de Freitas and Bogousslavsky, 2008; Smith and co-workers, 2008a). Thrombolytic therapy as discussed above has also been used. The clinical course is unpredictable and the prognosis guarded. Mortality rates are 15 to 30 percent, and survivors have a recurrence rate of 1 to 2 percent, including during subsequent pregnancy (Mehraein and colleagues, 2003).

Hemorrhagic Stroke

The two distinct categories of spontaneous intracranial bleeding are *intracerebral* and *subarachnoid hemorrhage*. Trauma-associated subdural and epidural hemorrhage are not considered.

Intracerebral Hemorrhage. Bleeding into the substance of the brain most commonly is caused by spontaneous rupture of small vessels damaged by chronic hypertension (Qureshi and colleagues, 2001; Takebayashi and Kaneko, 1983). In pregnancy-associated hemorrhagic strokes such as the one shown in **Figure 55-1**, there often is chronic hypertension with superimposed preeclampsia (Cunningham, 2005). Intracerebral hemorrhage has much higher morbidity and mortality rates than subarachnoid hemorrhage because of its location. And chronic hypertension is associated with *Charcot-Bouchard microaneurysms* of the penetrating branches of the middle cerebral artery. Pressure-induced rupture causes bleeding in the putamen, thalamus, adjacent white matter, pons, and cerebellum. In the 28 women described by Martin and associates (2005), half died and most survivors had permanent disabilities. They underscored the importance of proper management for gestational hypertension—especially systolic hypertension—to prevent cerebrovascular pathology (see Chap. 34, p. 721).

Subarachnoid Hemorrhage. These bleeds are more likely caused by an underlying cerebrovascular malformation in an otherwise normal patient. Ruptured saccular or "berry" aneurysms cause 80 percent of all subarachnoid hemorrhages, and ruptured arteriovenous malformations (AVMs), coagulopathies, angiopathies, venous thromboses, infections, drug abuse, tumors, and trauma cause the remainder. Rupture of a cerebral aneurysm or angioma or bleeding from a vascular malformation occurs in 1 in 75,000 pregnancies. This incidence does not differ from that in

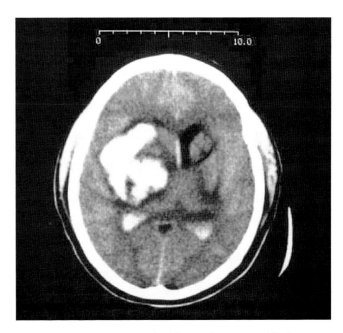

FIGURE 55-1 Large intracerebral hemorrhage caused by hypertensive stroke in a nulliparous woman whose blood pressure was recorded at 270/140 mm Hg.

the general nonobstetrical population, but the mortality rate during pregnancy is reported to be as high as 35 percent (Dias and Sekhar, 1990). Case-control studies from Japan and New Zealand found that nulligravidity significantly increased the risk of subarachnoid hemorrhage (Mhurchu and co-workers, 2001; Okamoto and colleagues, 2001).

Pregnancy-induced effects on cerebrovascular hemodynamics are unclear as related to intracranial hemorrhage. For example, Zeeman and co-workers (2003) reported that cerebral blood flow *decreased* by 20 percent from midpregnancy until term. Intuitively, this would "protect" against bleeding from vascular malformations. With gestational hypertension, however, Zeeman and colleagues (2004b) showed that cerebral blood flow *increased* significantly. Although such hyperperfusion is assumed to be dangerous with vascular anomalies, most saccular aneurysm ruptures are not associated with preeclampsia.

Intracerebral Aneurysm. Approximately 2 percent of adults have an intracranial aneurysm. Only a small percentage of these rupture—approximately 0.1 percent for aneurysms <10 mm and 1 percent for those >10 mm (Smith and colleagues, 2008a). Aneurysms are not more likely to bleed during pregnancy (Groenestege and co-workers, 2009). Still, during pregnancy, bleeding from aneurysms is more common than that from AVMs. Aneurysms are more likely to bleed during the second half of pregnancy—only about 20 percent bleed during the first half (Dias and Sekhar, 1990). As in the nonpregnant population, most aneurysms identified during pregnancy are in the circle of Willis and 20 percent are multiple (Stoodley and co-workers, 1998). The cardinal symptom is sudden severe headache, accompanied by visual changes, cranial nerve abnormalities, focal neurological deficits, or altered consciousness. Patients typically have signs of meningeal irritation, tachycardia, transient hypertension, low-grade fever, leukocytosis, and proteinuria.

Prompt diagnosis and treatment may prevent potentially lethal complications. A recent comparative study showed MR imaging to be superior to CT scanning for all varieties of stroke (Chalela and associates, 2007). If the initial study is normal but the clinical picture strongly suggests subarachnoid hemorrhage, the cerebrospinal fluid should be examined, and if it is bloody, angiography is done to locate the lesion (Roman and associates, 2004).

Treatment includes bed rest, analgesia, and sedation, with neurological monitoring and strict control of blood pressure. The decision to attempt repair of a potentially accessible aneurysm during pregnancy depends in part on the risk of recurrent hemorrhage and the risks of surgery. In nonpregnant patients, with conservative treatment only, the risk of subsequent bleeding from the aneurysm is 20 to 30 percent for the first month and then 3 percent per year. Recurrent hemorrhage leads to death in 70 percent. Early repair is done with clipping of the aneurysm or by endovascular coil placement. It seems reasonable that for women near term, cesarean delivery followed by either method is a consideration. There appears to be no advantage to pregnancy termination unless there is associated preeclampsia.

It also seems reasonable to allow vaginal delivery if labor occurs remote from aneurysmal repair. A problem is what "remote" implies—although some say 2 months, the time for healing is unknown. For women who survive subarachnoid hemorrhage, but in whom surgical repair is not done, we agree with Cartlidge (2000) and recommend against bearing down—put another way, we favor cesarean delivery.

Arteriovenous Malformations (AVMs). When these congenital vascular anomalies bleed, half do so into the subarachnoid space and half are intraparenchymal hemorrhage with subarachnoid extension (Smith and colleagues, 2008a). The incidence of bleeding from cerebral AVMs probably is not increased during pregnancy (Finnerty and co-workers, 1999; Horton and associates, 1990). Thus, they are very uncommon, and in the study from Parkland Hospital, Simolke and associates (1991) reported only one case in nearly 90,000 deliveries (Fig. 55-2). Although some suggest that AVMs bleed with similar frequency throughout gestation, Dias and Sekhar (1990) reported an increase with gestational age. Karlsson and colleagues (1997) reported that the risk of bleeding from an AVM increases with maternal age.

In nonpregnant patients, there is no consensus on whether all of these lesions should be resected, even when accessible. Whether or not the lesion has bled is also a factor. After hemorrhage, the risk of recurrent bleeding in unrepaired lesions is almost 20 percent within the first year and 2 to 3 percent per year thereafter (Smith and associates, 2008a). The mortality rate with bleeding AVMs is 10 to 20 percent. In pregnancy, the decision to operate is usually based on neurosurgical considerations (Finnerty and associates, 1999). Citing a *possible* higher risk of rebleeding during pregnancy, Friedlander

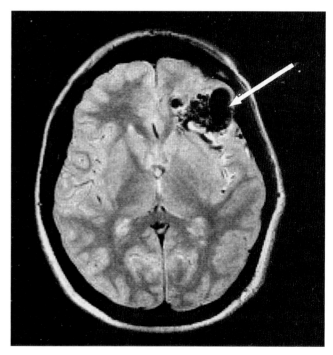

FIGURE 55-2 Magnetic resonance imaging of a left-sided frontal lobe atriovenous malformation. The lesion caused subarachnoid bleeding at 29 weeks in a 24-year-old primigravida who presented with severe headache, nausea, and vomiting. (From Simolke and colleagues, 1991, with permission.)

(2007) recommends strong consideration for treatment during pregnancy. Because of the high risk of recurrent hemorrhage from an unresected or inoperable lesion, we favor cesarean delivery.

Demyelinating or Degenerative Diseases

Demyelinating diseases compose a group of neurological disorders that involve focal or patchy destruction of central nervous system myelin sheaths accompanied by an inflammatory response. The degenerative diseases are multifactorial and are characterized by progressive neuronal death.

Multiple Sclerosis (MS)

In the United States, multiple sclerosis is second to trauma as a cause of neurological disability in middle adulthood (Hauser and Goodin, 2008). Because MS affects women twice as often as men and usually begins in the 20s and 30s, women of reproductive age are most susceptible. The familial recurrence rate of MS is 15 percent, and the incidence in offspring is increased 15-fold.

The demyelinating characteristic of this disorder results from predominately T cell-mediated autoimmune destruction of oligodendrocytes that synthesize myelin. There is a genetic susceptibility and likely an environmental trigger such as exposure to certain bacteria and viruses, for example, *Chlamydophilia pneumoniae,* human herpesvirus 6, or Epstein-Barr virus (Frohman and associates, 2006).

There are four clinical types of MS (Hauser and Goodin, 2008):

1. *Relapsing-remitting MS* accounts for initial presentation in 85 percent of affected individuals. It is characterized by unpredictable recurrent episodes of focal or multifocal neurological dysfunction usually followed by full recovery. Over time, however, relapses lead to persistent deficits.
2. *Secondary progressive MS* disease is when relapsing-remitting disease begins to pursue a progressive downhill course after each relapse. It is likely that all patients eventually develop this type.
3. *Primary progressive MS* accounts for 15 percent of cases. It is characterized by gradual progression of disability from the time of initial diagnosis.
4. *Progressive-relapsing MS* refers to primary progressive MS with apparent relapses.

Classical symptoms include sensory loss, visual symptoms from optic neuritis, weakness, paresthesias, and a host of other neurological symptoms. Almost 75 percent of women with isolated optic neuritis develop multiple sclerosis within 15 years. Clinical diagnosis is confirmed by MR imaging and cerebrospinal fluid analysis. In greater than 95 percent of cases, MR imaging shows characteristic multifocal white matter *plaques* that represent discrete areas of demyelination. Their appearance and extent are less helpful for treatment response. Similarly, Kuhle and colleagues (2007) reported that identification of serum antibodies against myelin oligodendrocyte glycoprotein (MOG) and myelin basic protein (MBP) is not predictive of recurrent disease activity.

Management. Some treatments of MS may need to be modified during pregnancy. Goals are to arrest acute or initial attacks, employ disease modifying agents, and provide symptomatic relief. Acute or initial attacks are treated with high-dose intravenous methylprednisolone—500 to 1000 mg daily for 3 to 5 days, followed by oral prednisone for 2 weeks. Plasma exchange may be considered. Symptomatic relief can be provided by analgesics; carbamazepine, phenytoin, or amitriptyline for neurogenic pain; baclofen for spasticity; α_2-adrenergic blockade to relax the bladder neck; and cholinergic and anticholinergic drugs to stimulate or inhibit bladder contractions.

Several immunomodulators can be used for relapsing MS or exacerbations. These include interferons β1a and β1b, glatiramer acetate, and mitoxantrone (Frohman and colleagues, 2006). Other medications sometimes used include azathioprine, methotrexate, cyclophosphamide, and intravenous immunoglobulin G. Recent clinical trials show that treatment with *natalizumab*—alpha 4 integrin antagonist—especially when combined with interferon B1a, significantly reduced MS clinical relapses (Polman and colleagues, 2006; Rudick and co-workers, 2006).

Data concerning the safety of some of these drugs in pregnancy are limited (Sandberg-Wollheim and associates, 2005). Interferon appears to be safe however, methotrexate and cyclophosphamide should not be given during fetal organogenesis (Briggs and co-workers, 2005; Buhimschi and Weiner, 2009).

Effects of Pregnancy on MS. The *Pregnancy In Multiple Sclerosis (PRIMS)* study is a European prospective multicenter effort. From this study, findings from 254 pregnancies that were complicated by MS were reported by Vukusic and Confavreux (2006). They confirmed a decreased relapse rate during pregnancy and significantly increased relapses postpartum (Fig. 55-3). This may be related to increased T helper type 2: type 1 cell ratios during pregnancy (Airas and colleagues, 2008). In an earlier review of eight studies including

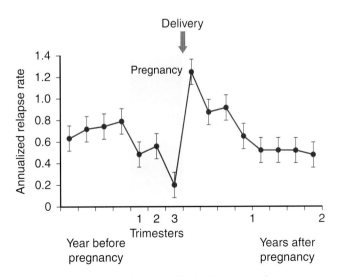

FIGURE 55-3 PRIMS study: Annualized relapse rates for women with multiple sclerosis in the year before, during, and the 2 years after pregnancy. (Data from Vukusic and Confavreux, 2006.)

more than 1000 pregnancies, Abramsky (1994) found that MS worsened during pregnancy in only 10 percent.

Effects of MS on Pregnancy. Uncomplicated MS usually has no adverse effects on pregnancy outcome. Women may become fatigued more easily, and those with bladder dysfunction are prone to urinary infection. Dahl and co-workers (2006) described 449 pregnancies in women with MS. From 1991 through 2002, they reported a higher induction rate and longer second-stage labors. The increased cesarean delivery rate was due to these inductions as well as elective planned operations. It is reasonable to use usual obstetrical indicators for cesarean delivery. Vaginal delivery does not worsen voiding problems (Durufle and associates, 2006). Women with spinal lesions at or above T6 are at risk for autonomic dysreflexia and epidural analgesia is recommended (see p. 1174). Dahl and associates (2005) studied perinatal outcomes in 649 women with MS and reported that despite a lower mean birthweight than controls, neonatal mortality rates were not increased.

There is evidence that intravenous immune globulin (IVIG) therapy—0.4 g/kg for 5 days—given during postpartum weeks 1, 6, and 12 reduces relapse rates (Argyriod and Makris, 2008). Postpartum exacerbations may prevent women from breast feeding. These may also inhibit the ability to provide general newborn care, and the need for assistance during this period should be anticipated.

Huntington Disease

This adult-onset neurodegenerative disease results from an autosomal dominant mutation that encodes the protein *huntingtin* (Walker, 2007). The disorder is characterized by a combination of choreoathetotic movements and progressive dementia. Because the mean age of onset is 40 years, Huntington disease rarely complicates pregnancy. Prenatal diagnosis is discussed in Chapter 12 (p. 276). Prenatal screening is controversial because this usually is a late-onset adult disease (Richards and Rea, 2005).

Myasthenia Gravis (MG)

This autoimmune-mediated neuromuscular disorder affects about 1 in 7500 persons. It is more common in women, and its incidence peaks when they are in their 20s and 30s. The etiology is unknown, but genetic factors likely play a role. The pathological basis of the disease is IgG-mediated damage to acetylcholine receptors. This leads to diminished end-plate action potentials that result in weakened muscle contractions (Conti-Fine and associates, 2006).

Cardinal features of MG are weakness and easy fatigability of facial, oropharyngeal, extraocular, and limb muscles. Deep tendon reflexes are preserved. Cranial muscles are involved early and disparately, and diplopia and ptosis are common. Facial muscle weakness causes difficulty in smiling, chewing, and speaking. In 85 percent of patients, the weakness becomes generalized. Other autoimmune diseases may coexist, and hypothyroidism should be excluded. The clinical course of MG is marked by exacerbations and remissions, especially when it first becomes clinically apparent. Remissions are not always complete and are seldom permanent. Systemic diseases, concurrent infections, and even emotional upset may precipitate exacerbations, of which there are three types:

1. *Myasthenic crises,* characterized by severe muscle weakness, inability to swallow, and respiratory muscle paralysis
2. *Refractory crises,* characterized by the same symptoms but unresponsive to the usual therapy
3. *Cholinergic crises,* in which excessive cholinergic medication leads to nausea, vomiting, muscle weakness, abdominal pain, and diarrhea.

All three of these can be life threatening, but a refractory crisis is a medical emergency. Those with bulbar myasthenia are at particular risk because they may be unable to swallow or even ask for help.

Management. Myasthenia is manageable but not curable. About 75 percent of patients have thymic hyperplasia or a thymoma that can be seen with CT or MR imaging. In these individuals, thymectomy is generally recommended because of long-term benefits (Drachman, 2008). Anticholinesterase medications such as *pyridostigmine,* an analog of neostigmine, bring about improvement by impeding acetylcholine degradation. They seldom produce normal muscle function, and ironically, overdose is manifest by increased weakness that may be difficult to differentiate from myasthenic symptoms. For those refractory to medical therapy, most respond to immunosuppressive therapy with glucocorticoids, azathioprine, cyclosporine, and mycophenolate mofetil. Cyclophosphamide is reserved for refractory cases. When short-term rapid clinical improvement is needed—for example, a surgical procedure or a myasthenic crisis—high-dose immunoglobulin G or plasmapheresis, and possibly methylprednisolone, can be used (Gajdos and colleagues, 2006).

Myasthenia and Pregnancy. Because the greatest period of risk is within the first year following diagnosis, it seems reasonable to postpone pregnancy until there is sustained symptomatic improvement. Antepartum management includes close observation with liberal bed rest and prompt treatment of any infections (Kalidindi and associates, 2007). Most patients respond well to pyridostigmine administered every 3 to 4 hours. Those in remission who become pregnant while taking corticosteroids or azathioprine should continue these. *Thymectomy* has been successfully performed during pregnancy in refractory cases (Ip and colleagues, 1986). Acute onset of myasthenia or its exacerbation demands prompt hospitalization and supportive care. *Plasmapheresis* and high-dose immunoglobulin therapy should be used for emergency situations, taking care not to provoke maternal hypotension or hypovolemia (Drachman, 2008).

Although pregnancy does not appear to affect the overall course of MG, the expanding uterus may compromise respiration, and fatigue common to most pregnancies may be tolerated poorly. The clinical course during pregnancy is unpredictable, and frequent hospitalizations are the norm. In three observational studies of 136 women, about 20 percent worsened during pregnancy (Batocchi, 1999; Djelmis, 2002; Podciechowski, 2005, and all their colleagues). Maternal deaths are usually due to complications of myasthenia or its treatment.

Labor and Delivery. MG does not affect smooth muscle, and most women have normal labor. Oxytocin is given as necessary. Cesarean delivery is reserved for obstetrical indications. Close observation and prompt respiratory support are essential. Narcotics may cause respiratory depression. Any drug with a curare-like effect should be avoided—examples include magnesium sulfate, muscle relaxants used with general anesthesia, and aminoglycosides. Amide-type local anesthetic agents should be used for epidural analgesia. Regional analgesia is preferred unless there is significant bulbar involvement or respiratory compromise. During second-stage labor, some women may have impaired voluntary expulsive efforts, and forceps delivery may be indicated.

Neonatal Effects. Anti-acetylcholine-receptor IgG antibodies can be found in 85 percent of MG patients. These can cross the placenta and affect the fetus. About 10 to 20 percent of exposed neonates develop symptoms (Podciechowski and associates, 2005). Neonatal symptoms are most likely if the mother produces autoantibodies directed against embryonic rather than adult acetylcholine receptors (Vernet-der Garabedian and colleagues, 1994). Transient symptomatic myasthenia gravis in an affected neonate typically results in a feeble cry, poor suckling, and respiratory distress. All of these can be corrected by parenteral neostigmine or small doses of edrophonium, and symptoms usually resolve within 2 to 6 weeks.

Neuropathies

Peripheral neuropathy is a general term used to describe disorders of peripheral nerve(s) of any cause. Because neuropathy can result from a variety of causes, its discovery should prompt a search for an etiology. *Polyneuropathies* can be axonal or demyelinating as well as acute, subacute, or chronic (Chaudhry, 2008). They are often associated with systemic diseases such as diabetes, with drug or environmental toxin exposure, or with genetic diseases. *Mononeuropathies* signify focal involvement of a single nerve trunk and imply local causation such as trauma, compression, or entrapment—an example is carpal-tunnel syndrome (England and Asbury, 2004).

Guillain-Barré Syndrome (GBS)

In 75 percent of cases, this acute demyelinating polyradiculoneuropathy has clinical or serological evidence of an acute infection. Commonly associated are *Campylobacter jejuni*, cytomegalovirus, and Epstein-Barr virus (Hauser and Asbury, 2008). Some cases follow surgical procedures or immunizations. The syndrome is thought to be immune-mediated from antibodies formed against infective agents. Demyelination causes sensory and motor conduction blockade, but is restored with remyelination.

Clinical features include areflexic paralysis with mild sensory disturbances and at times, autonomic dysfunction. The full syndrome develops after 1 to 3 weeks. Management is supportive, but in the worsening phase, patients should be hospitalized because approximately 25 percent need ventilatory assistance. If begun within 1 to 2 weeks of motor symptoms, intravenous high-dose immunoglobulin or plasmapheresis is beneficial but does not decrease mortality rates (Hughes and colleagues, 2007). Almost 85 percent of patients recover fully, but the remainder are disabled or have one or more late relapses.

Pregnancy. The incidence of Guillain-Barré syndrome is not increased antepartum. Although it is said to be increased threefold postpartum, data are sparse (Cheng and co-workers, 1998). When GBS develops during pregnancy, its clinical course does not seem to be changed. After an insidious onset, paresis and paralysis most often continue to ascend, and respiratory insufficiency can then become a common and serious problem. Hurley and colleagues (1991) reported that a third of affected pregnant women ultimately required ventilatory support, and the overall mortality rate was 13 percent. Treatment of acute GBS in pregnancy is with either high-dose immunoglobulin or plasmapheresis (Chan, 2004; Kuller, 1995; Rockel, 1994, and all their co-workers).

Bell Palsy

This acute idiopathic peripheral facial paralysis of unknown etiology is relatively common, especially in women of reproductive age. Reactivation of herpes-virus infection may cause it, and there is some evidence to link neural damage with acute HIV-1 retroviral infections (Serrano and associates, 2007). Women are affected two to four times more often than men of the same age, and pregnant women are affected three to four times more often than nonpregnant women (Cohen and colleagues, 2000). The onset is usually abrupt and painful, with maximum weakness within 48 hours. In some cases, hyperacusis and loss of taste accompany varying degrees of facial muscle paralysis (Beal and Hauser, 2008).

Increased extracellular fluid, viral inflammation, and the relative immune suppression of pregnancy are thought to be predisposing factors. Data from five Canadian centers suggest that women who developed Bell palsy had a fivefold increase incidence of gestational hypertension compared with their general obstetrical population (Shmorgun and colleagues, 2002).

Sullivan and colleagues (2007) reported a randomized trial of nearly 500 nonpregnant patients enrolled within 72 hours of symptom onset. Those given prednisolone had better outcomes than those given acyclovir or placebo. At 3 months, 83 percent given steroids had recovery of facial function, compared with only 64 percent of those not given prednisolone. At 9 months, these were 95 versus 82 percent, respectively. The addition of acyclovir to prednisolone did not improve outcomes. Importantly, supportive care includes facial muscle massage, prevention of injury to the constantly exposed cornea, and reassurance.

Effects of Pregnancy. It is uncertain if pregnancy alters the prognosis for spontaneous recovery from facial palsy. Gillman and colleagues (2002) found that only half of pregnant women recovered to a satisfactory level after 1 year—this compares with about 80 percent of nonpregnant women and men. Bilateral palsies, recurrence in a subsequent pregnancy, greater percentage of nerve function loss, and a faster rate of loss are prognostic markers for incomplete recovery (Cohen and associates, 2000; Gilden, 2004). Electroneurography may also be helpful in determining prognosis. As discussed, corticosteroid therapy given early in the course of the disease significantly improves outcomes. Supportive treatment is given, and measures taken to prevent corneal injury.

Carpal Tunnel Syndrome

This syndrome results from pressure on the median nerve. There are a variety of associated conditions, and pregnancy is a common one (Smith and colleagues, 2008b). Symptoms include burning, numbness, or tingling in the inner half of one or both hands, and wrist pain and numbness extending into the forearm and sometimes into the shoulder (Katz and Simmons, 2002). Symptoms are bilateral in 80 percent of pregnant women, and 10 percent have signs of severe denervation (Seror, 1998). Carpal tunnel syndrome should be distinguished from *De Quervain tendonitis* caused by swelling of the conjoined tendons and sheaths near the distal radius. Nerve conduction studies may be helpful in distinguishing these two.

Pregnancy. The incidence in pregnancy varies greatly and is reported to range from 1 to 17 percent (Bahrami, 2005; Finsen and Zeitlmann, 2006; Stolp-Smith, 1998, and all their co-workers). In a multicenter Italian study, the incidence of the syndrome diagnosed clinically during the third trimester was an astounding 63 percent. In more than half of these, diagnosis was confirmed by neurophysiological evaluation (Pazzaglia and colleagues, 2005). Importantly, one year later, half of affected women still had some symptoms. This high incidence has not been observed by others, and it is far less common in our large services at Parkland and the University of Alabama at Birmingham Hospitals.

Carpal tunnel syndrome is usually self-limited, and in most cases, symptomatic treatment is sufficient. A splint applied to a slightly flexed wrist and worn during sleep relieves pressure to provide relief for most women. Occasionally, surgical decompression and corticosteroid injections are necessary (Dammers and associates, 1999; Gerritsen and co-workers, 2002).

Spinal Cord Injury

Of the 11,000 spinal cord injuries each year, at least 50 percent are in patients of reproductive age, and 18 percent of these are women (American College of Obstetricians and Gynecologists, 2002b). Management guidelines are available for impaired sexual functioning (Elliott, 2006; Rees and colleagues, 2007). In a survey of 472 reproductive-aged women with such injuries, Jackson and Wadley (1999) found that two thirds resumed intercourse after the injury, and almost 14 percent became pregnant. Although fertility in women is probably not affected, pregnancy rates are only 50 percent in partners of injured men (De Forge and co-workers, 2005).

Women with spinal cord injury have increased frequencies of preterm and low-birthweight infants, and they experience more pregnancy complications compared with unaffected women. The majority have either asymptomatic bacteriuria or symptomatic urinary infection. Serum creatinine levels are used to detect renal damage from repeated infection. Significant bowel dysfunction and constipation develop in more than half of women. Anemia and pressure necrosis skin lesions are also common. There are two serious and life-threatening complications that can develop:

1. If the spine is transected above T10, the cough reflex is impaired, and respiratory function may be compromised. Pneumonitis triggered by covert aspiration can be serious. Pulmonary function tests may be indicated, and some women with high lesions may need ventilatory support in late pregnancy or in labor.

2. In women with lesions above T5–T6, *autonomic dysreflexia* can develop. With this complication, stimuli from structures innervated below the level of the lesion—usually the bowel, bladder, or uterus—lead to massive disordered sympathetic stimulation. Vasoconstriction and sudden catecholamine release can cause severe hypertension and a range of symptoms including a throbbing headache, facial flushing, sweating, bradycardia, tachycardia, arrhythmia, and respiratory distress. Dysreflexia can be precipitated by a variety of stimuli, including urethral, bladder, rectal, or cervical distension; catheterization; cervical dilatation; uterine contractions; or manipulation of pelvic structures (American College of Obstetricians and Gynecologists, 2002b). In a report by Westgren and colleagues (1993), 12 of 15 women at risk for dysreflexia suffered at least one episode during pregnancy.

Uterine contractions are not affected by cord lesions, and labor is usually easy, even precipitous, and comparatively painless. If the lesion is below T12, uterine contractions are felt normally. For lesions above T12, the risk of delivery at home can be minimized by teaching women to palpate for uterine contractions. Up to 20 percent of women deliver preterm (Westgren and co-workers, 1993). Because of this, some investigators recommend tocodynamometry and weekly cervical examinations beginning at approximately 28 weeks. Hughes and associates (1991) recommend elective hospitalization between 36 and 37 weeks until delivery.

Spinal or epidural analgesia extending to T10 prevents autonomic dysreflexia and should be instituted at the start of labor. If severe symptoms begin before epidural placement, the first step is to stop whatever stimulus provoked the episode. Then, an antihypertensive agent or a peripheral vasodilator should be given. Vaginal delivery is preferred with epidural or spinal analgesia to minimize autonomic dysreflexia (Kuczkowski, 2006). Prolonged second-stage labor may be expedited with forceps or vacuum extraction with adequate conduction analgesia.

Shunts for Maternal Hydrocephalus

Pregnancies in women with ventriculoperitoneal, ventriculoatrial, or ventriculopleural shunts for hydrocephalus usually have satisfactory outcomes (Landwehr and colleagues, 1994). Partial shunt obstruction is common, typically late in pregnancy. Wisoff and associates (1991) reported neurological complications in 13 of 17 such pregnancies—these included headaches in 60 percent, nausea and vomiting in 35 percent, lethargy in 30 percent, and ataxia or gaze paresis, each in 20 percent. Most responded to conservative management. If CT scanning discloses acute hydrocephaly, the shunt can be tapped or pumped several times daily. In some cases, surgical revision is necessary.

More recently *endoscopic third ventriculostomy* has been used for hydrocephalus in children as well as adults (de Ribaupierre and associates, 2007). In the report by Riffaud and co-workers (2006), five pregnant women underwent successful ventriculostomy placement for either obstructive hydrocephalus or a malfunctioning ventriculopheritoneal shunt.

Vaginal delivery is preferred in women with shunts, and unless there is a meningomyelocele, conduction analgesia is permitted. Antimicrobial prophylaxis is indicated if the peritoneal cavity is entered for cesarean delivery or tubal sterilization.

Maternal Brain Death

There are now at least six case reports describing *maternal brain death with somatic support.* Life-support systems and parenteral alimentation were used 1 to 15 weeks to gain fetal maturity (Hussein and colleagues, 2006; Souza and associates, 2006). Aggressive tocolysis and antimicrobial therapy were used by some. Chiossi and co-workers (2006) reviewed the clinical course of 17 women with *persistent vegetative state* given various levels of support during pregnancy. At least five died after delivery, and most of the remainder continue to be in the vegetative state. The ethical, financial, and legal implications, both civil and criminal, that arise from attempting or not attempting such care are profound (Farragher and Laffey, 2005; Feldman and colleagues, 2000). Perimortem cesarean delivery is discussed in Chapter 42 (p. 942).

Benign Intracranial Hypertension—Pseudotumor Cerebri

This condition is characterized by increased intracranial pressure without hydrocephalus, possibly as the result of either overproduction or underabsorption of cerebrospinal fluid. Symptoms include headache in at least 90 percent of cases and visual disturbances—loss of a visual field or central visual acuity—in 70 percent (Evans and Friedman, 2000). Other complaints are stiff neck, back pain, pulsatile tinnitus, facial palsy, ataxia, or paresthesias. The syndrome is commonly found in young women, and it is prevalent in those who are obese, who recently gained weight, or both (Daniels and associates, 2007). Along with symptoms, other criteria for diagnosis include elevated intracranial pressure—> 200 mm H_2O or > 250 mm H_2O if obese—and normal composition of cerebrospinal fluid (CSF), normal cranial CT or MR imaging findings, and no evidence for systemic disease (International Headache Society, 2004).

Benign intracranial hypertension is usually self-limited. Visual defects can be prevented by lowering the CSF pressure. Drugs given to lower pressure include acetazolamide, furosemide, topiramate, or corticosteroids such as dexamethasone. In some cases, lumboperitoneal shunting of spinal fluid or optic nerve sheath decompression is necessary.

Effects of Pregnancy

Although once taught, the incidence of benign intracranial hypertension is not increased during pregnancy. The onset of symptoms, however, may first appear in pregnancy, and women previously diagnosed may become symptomatic. Symptoms usually develop by midpregnancy, tend to be self-limited, and usually resolve postpartum.

Pregnancy does not alter treatment. Some recommend serial visual field testing because visual loss can become permanent. In 16 pregnant women, Huna-Baron and Kupersmith (2002) reported that visual field loss developed in four, and it was permanent in one. Visual field loss is often coincident with the development of papilledema. Acetazolamide is given as described above, and Lee and associates (2005) reported successful treatment of 12 pregnant women. Although outmoded for treatment of nonpregnant individuals, repeated lumbar punctures are generally successful in providing temporary relief throughout pregnancy. Surgical options are lumboperitoneal shunting, endoscopic third ventriculostomy, or optic nerve sheath fenestration (Thambisetty and co-workers, 2007).

Pregnancy complications are likely due to the associated obesity, not to intracranial hypertension. In their review of 54 pregnancies, Katz and associates (1989) reported no excessive adverse perinatal outcomes. The route of delivery is decided by obstetrical indications. Conduction analgesia is permitted, and Aly and Lawther (2007) described a woman with an intrathecal catheter placed to control intracranial hypertension as well as to provide labor analgesia.

Chorea Gravidarum

Involuntary writhing of the limbs or facial muscles—chorea—may develop during pregnancy. In the past, most cases were linked to rheumatic fever in association with group A streptococcal infection (Brockington, 2006). Currently, pregnancy-related chorea is rare (Palanivelu, 2007). According to Branch (1990), chorea in pregnancy is usually caused by collagen-vascular disease, especially if there are antiphospholipid antibodies (see Chap. 54, p. 1151).

PSYCHIATRIC DISORDERS

Pregnancy and the puerperium are at times sufficiently stressful to provoke mental illness. Such illness may represent recurrence or exacerbation of a preexisting psychiatric disorder, or may signal the onset of a new disorder. In a Swedish population-based study, Andersson and associates (2003) reported a 14-percent point prevalence of psychiatric disorders during pregnancy. Unfortunately, they also found that only 5.5 percent of this fraction had some form of treatment. Importantly, Borri and co-workers (2008) found that many disorders preceded pregnancy and were detected by screening at 12 weeks.

In both the United Kingdom and Australia, where late maternal deaths—those between 43 and 365 days postpartum—are considered, psychiatric illness is a leading cause of mortality (Austin and colleagues, 2007). Suicide by violent means was responsible for 65 percent of these deaths. In a 10-year review of Washington state hospitalizations, Comtois and associates (2008) studied 355 women with a postpartum suicide attempt. In a case-control analysis, significantly increased risk factors included prior hospitalization for a psychiatric diagnosis—27 fold, for substance abuse—sixfold, and both together—11 fold. All these rates were further increased if there were multiple hospitalizations.

Adjustment to Pregnancy

Biochemical factors—including effects of hormones—and life stressors can markedly influence mental illness. It is thus intuitive that pregnancy would affect some coexisting mental disorders. Women respond in a variety of ways to stressors of pregnancy, and some express persistent concerns about fetal health, child care, lifestyle changes, or fear of childbirth pain. Anxiety and functional impairment are common (Morewitz, 2003; Vythilingum, 2008). But, according to Littleton and co-workers (2007), anxiety symptoms in pregnancy are associated with psychosocial variables similar to those for nonpregnant women. The level of perceived stress is significantly higher for women whose fetus is at high risk for a malformation, for those with preterm labor or delivery, and for those with other medical complications (Alder and associates, 2007; Ross and McLean, 2006). For example, Hippman and co-workers (2009) screened 81 women at increased risk for a fetus with aneuploidy. Half of these had a positive screening score compared with only 2.4 percent of normal pregnant controls. A number of steps can be taken to diminish psychological stress in the event of a poor obstetrical outcome. For example, following a stillbirth, Gold and colleagues (2007) encourage parental contact with the newborn and provision of photos and other memorabilia of the infant.

The Puerperium

Because psychological stress often increases postpartum, there is increased risk for mental illness. For example, approximately 15 percent of women develop a nonpsychotic postpartum depressive disorder within 6 months of delivery (Tam and Chung, 2007). Others have a severe, psychotic illness following delivery that usually is manic-depressive (Wisner and associates, 2002). This likely is more common in women with obstetrical complications such as severe preeclampsia or fetal-growth restriction, especially if associated with early delivery (Rep and co-workers, 2007).

Maternity Blues

Also called *postpartum blues*, this is a transient state of heightened emotional reactivity experienced by half of women within approximately the first week after parturition (Miller, 2002). The predominant mood is happiness, but they are more emotionally labile with insomnia, weepiness, depression, anxiety, poor concentration, irritability, and affective lability. They may be transiently tearful for several hours and then recover completely, only to be tearful again the next day. Symptoms are mild and usually last only between a few hours to a few days. Supportive treatment is indicated, and sufferers can be reassured that the dysphoria is transient and most likely due to biochemical changes. They should be monitored for development of depression and other severe psychiatric disturbances as discussed above.

Prenatal Evaluation

Screening for mental illness is done at the first prenatal visit. Factors include a search for any psychiatric disorders, including hospitalizations, outpatient care, prior or current use of psychoactive medications, and current symptoms. Risk factors should be evaluated. For example, a prior personal or family history of depression is a significant risk for depression. Women with a history of sexual, physical, or verbal abuse; substance abuse; and personality disorders are also at greater risk for depression (Akman and colleagues, 2007; Tam and Chung, 2007). And smoking and nicotine dependence have been associated with an increase in *all* mental disorders in pregnancy (Goodwin and co-workers, 2007). Finally, because eating disorders may be exacerbated by pregnancy, affected women should be followed closely.

Treatment Considerations

A large number of psychotropic medications may be used for management of the myriad mental disorders encountered in pregnancy. Their application is discussed with respective disorders. Women taking psychotropic medication should be informed of likely side effects. Dell and O'Brien (2003) advocate a risk-benefit model of drug selection that factors the concerns of both mother and fetus. Many of these drugs are discussed in more detail throughout Chapter 14 as well as by the American College of Obstetricians and Gynecologists (2007).

Pregnancy Outcomes

There are only a few reports of psychiatric disorders and pregnancy outcomes. In a population-based cohort of more than 500,000 California births, Kelly and colleagues (2002) assessed the perinatal effects of a psychiatric diagnosis that included all *ICD-9-CM* diagnostic codes. Women with these diagnoses had up to a threefold increased incidence of very-low- or low-birthweight neonates or preterm delivery. Conversely, Littleton and associates (2007) reviewed 50 studies and concluded that anxiety symptoms had no adverse effect on outcomes.

Classification of Mental Disorders

The *Diagnostic and Statistical Manual-IV-TR* is the most recent updated version by the American Psychiatric Association (2000b). Its purpose is to assist in the classification of mental disorders, and it specifies criteria for each diagnosis. Shown in Table 55-4 are 12-month prevalences for adults.

Major Mood Disorders

These include major depression—a unipolar disorder—and manic-depression—a bipolar disorder with both manic and depressive episodes. It also includes dysthymia, which is chronic, mild depression. Major mood disorders as a group contribute to two thirds of all suicides.

Major Depression

This is the most common mood disorder, and the National Mental Health Association (2004) estimates that each year 12 million women are affected. The lifetime incidence is 12 percent, but only half ever seek care. The diagnosis is arrived at by identifying symptoms listed in Table 55-5.

Major depression is multifactorial and prompted by genetic and environmental factors. First-degree relatives have a 25-percent risk, and female relatives are at even higher risk. Families of affected individuals often have members with alcohol abuse and anxiety disorders. Provocative conditions leading to depression include life events that prompt grief reactions, substance abuse, use of certain medications, and other medical disorders. Although life events can trigger depression, genes influence the liability to life events, making the distinction between genetic and environmental factors difficult.

TABLE 55-4. The 12-Month Prevalence of Mental Disorders in Adults in the United States

Disorder[a]	1-Year Prevalence (Percent)	Adults Affected[b]	Comments
All disorders	26.2	58 million	1 in 4 adults affected annually
Mood disorders	9.5	21 million	Median onset age 30 years
Major depression—6.7%		15 million	Leading cause of disability in the United States
Dysthymia—1.5%		3.3 million	Chronic, mild depression
Bipolar disorder—2.6%		5.7 million	
Suicide		32,400	90% have mental disorder; depression most common
Schizophrenia	1.1	18 million	Men = women; onset women 20s or early 30s
Anxiety disorders	18	40 million	Frequent co-occurrence with depression or substance abuse
Panic—2.7%			
Obsessive-compulsive—1%			
Posttraumatic stress—3.5%			
Generalized anxiety—3.1%			
Social phobias—6.8%			
Eating disorders			
Anorexia nervosa	Lifetime: 0.5–3.7		Females = 85–95%; mortality rate 0.56% per year
Bulimia nervosa	Lifetime: 1.1–5		
Binge eating	6–month: 2–5		

[a]Based on *Diagnostic and Statistical Manual-IV-R (DSM-IV-R)* of the American Psychiatric Association (2000b).
[b]Based on 2004 census data.
From the National Institute of Mental Health (2006).

Pregnancy. It is unquestionable that pregnancy is a major life stressor that can precipitate or exacerbate depressive tendencies. In addition, there are likely a variety of pregnancy-induced effects. Hormones certainly affect mood as evidenced by premenstrual syndrome and menopausal depression. Estrogen modu-

TABLE 55-5. Symptoms of Depressive Illness[a]

Persistent sad, anxious, or "empty" feelings
Feelings of hopelessness and/or pessimism
Feelings of guilt, worthlessness, and/or helplessness
Irritability, restlessness
Loss of interest in activities or hobbies once pleasurable, including sex
Fatigue and decreased energy
Difficulty concentrating, remembering detail, and making decisions
Insomnia, early-morning wakefulness, or excessive sleeping
Overeating or appetite loss
Thoughts of suicide, suicide attempts
Persistent aches or pains, headaches, cramps, or digestive problems that do not ease even with treatment

[a]Not all patients experience the same symptoms and their severity, frequency, and duration will vary among individuals.
From the National Institute of Mental Health (2007).

lates serotonergic function, and women who experience postpartum depression often have higher predelivery serum estrogen and progesterone levels and experience a greater decline postpartum (Ahokas and co-workers, 1999).

Dennis and associates (2007) reviewed the Cochrane Database and reported the prevalence of antenatal depression to average 10.7 percent. And although Gavin and co-workers (2005) found it to range from 6 to 12 percent in their systematic review, others have reported the incidence to be as high as 30 percent (Lee and colleagues, 2007; Westdahl and associates, 2007). The higher estimates may be closer, as Cooper and associates (2007) reported that 13 percent of pregnant women in the Tennessee Medicaid program were prescribed antidepressants. Conversely, Wichman and colleagues (2009) reported that only 3.2 percent of more than 25,000 prenatal patients at the Mayo Clinic took selective serotonin-reuptake inhibitors (SSRIs) during pregnancy.

Postpartum depression—major or minor—develops in 10 to 20 percent of parturients (Centers for Disease Control and Prevention, 2008; National Mental Health Association, 2004). These incidences are slightly higher than the usual 6-month prevalence for depression among nonpregnant women. In addition to antenatal depression, postpartum depression has been associated with young maternal age, unmarried status, smoking or drinking, substance abuse, hyperemesis gravidarum, preterm birth, and high utilization of sick leave during pregnancy (Josefsson, 2002; Lee, 2007; Marcus, 2009, and all their colleagues).

Depression is frequently recurrent. At least 60 percent of women taking antidepressant medication before pregnancy have symptoms during pregnancy. For those who discontinue treatment, almost 70 percent have a relapse compared with 25 percent who continue therapy. Up to 70 percent of women with previous postpartum depression have a subsequent episode. Women with both a previous puerperal depression episode and a current episode of "maternity blues" described on page 1176 are at inordinately high risk for major depression. Indeed, the need for help for postpartum depression was the fourth most common challenge identified at 2 to 9 months postpartum identified by the Pregnancy Risk Assessment Monitoring System—PRAMS (Kanotra and colleagues, 2007).

Without treatment, the natural course of depression is one of gradual improvement in the 6 months after delivery (Fleming and colleagues, 1992). As the duration of depression increases, however, so do the number of sequelae and their severity. In addition, maternal depression during the first weeks and months after delivery can lead to insecure attachment and later behavioral problems in the child.

Treatment. Antidepressant medications, along with some form of psychotherapy, are indicated for severe depression during pregnancy or the puerperium (American College of Obstetricians and Gynecologists, 2007). An SSRI should be tried initially (Table 55-6). If depressive symptoms improve during a 6-week trial, the medication should be continued for a minimum of 6 months to prevent relapse (Wisner and associates,

2002). If the response is suboptimal or a relapse occurs, psychiatric referral is considered.

And again, recurrence some time after medication is stopped is common and develops in 50 to 85 percent of women with an initial postpartum depression. Women with a history of more than one depressive episode are at greater risk (American Psychiatric Association, 2000a). Surveillance should also include monitoring for thoughts of suicide or infanticide, emergence of psychosis, and response to therapy. For some women, the course of illness is severe enough to warrant hospitalization.

Fetal Effects of Therapy. Some known and possible fetal and neonatal effects are listed in Table 55-6. These were reviewed recently by the American College of Obstetricians and Gynecologists (2007) and Way (2007) and are detailed in Chapter 14 (p. 323). Although some psychotropic medications pass into breast milk, in most cases, the levels are very low or undetectable. The possible exception is lithium (Buhimschi and Weiner, 2009). Importantly, there have been no reports of adverse events in breast-fed infants of these women.

Electroconvulsive Therapy. Treatment of depression with electroconvulsive therapy (ECT) during pregnancy is occasionally necessary for women with major mood disorders unresponsive to pharmacological therapy. With proper preparation, the risks to both mother and fetus appear to be reasonable (Pinette

TABLE 55-6. Some Drugs Used for Treatment of Major Mental Disorders in Pregnancy

Indication of Class	Examples	Comments
Antidepressants		
Selective serotonin-reuptake inhibitors[a]	Citalopram, fluoxetine, paroxetine, sertraline	*Possible* link with heart defects; neonatal withdrawal syndrome; *possible* persistent pulmonary hypertension[a]; paroxetine use avoided by some
Others	Buproprion, duloxetine, nefazodone, venlafaxine	
Tricyclics	Amitryptyline, desipramine, doxepin, imipramine, nortryptyline	Not commonly used currently; no evidence of teratogenicity
Antipsychotics		
Typical	Chlorpromazine, fluphenazine, haloperidol, thiothixene	
Atypical	Aripiprazole, clozapine, olanzapine, risperidone, ziprasidone	
Bipolar Disorders		
Lithium	Lithium carbonate	Treatment of manic episodes; definite teratogen—heart defects, *viz.*, Ebstein anomaly; little data after 12 weeks
Antipsychotics	See above	

[a] See Chapter 14 (p. 323).
Data from American College of Obstetricians and Gynecologists (2007); Briggs and colleagues (2005); Buhimschi and Weiner (2009); Physicians' Desk Reference (2008).

and co-workers, 2007). That said, adverse maternal and perinatal outcomes have been described. For example, Balki and associates (2006) reported a pregnancy in which fetal brain damage likely was caused by sustained maternal hypotension associated with treatment of status epilepticus stimulated by ECT.

Women undergoing ECT should be fasting for at least 6 hours. They are given a rapid-acting antacid before the procedure, and their airway protected to decrease the likelihood of aspiration. A wedge should be placed under one hip to prevent sudden maternal hypotension from aortocaval compression. Other important preparatory steps include cervical assessment, discontinuation of nonessential anticholinergic medication, uterine and fetal heart rate monitoring, and intravenous hydration. During the procedure, excessive hyperventilation should be avoided. In most cases, maternal and fetal heart rate and maternal blood pressure and oxygen saturation remain normal throughout the procedure.

There have been at least two reviews of ECT outcomes in pregnancy. In the earlier one, Miller (1994) found 300 cases and reported complications in 10 percent. These included fetal arrhythmias, vaginal bleeding, abdominal pain, and self-limited contractions. Women not adequately prepared had increased risks for aspiration, aortocaval compression, and respiratory alkalosis. In the recent review, Anderson and Reti (2009) found 339 cases, undoubtedly with some homology with the earlier study. In most cases, ECT was done to treat depression, and it was 78-percent effective in this regard. They reported a 5-percent maternal ECT-related complication rate and a 3-percent associated perinatal complication rate that included two fetal deaths. For all of these reasons, we agree with Richards (2007) that ECT in pregnancy is not "low risk" and that it should be reserved for women whose depression is recalcitrant to intensive pharmacotherapy.

Bipolar Disorder

Manic-depressive illness has a strong genetic component and has been linked to possible mutations on chromosomes 16 and 8 (Jones and associates, 2007). The risk that monozygotic twins are both affected is 40 to 70 percent, and the risk for first-degree relatives is 5 to 10 percent (Muller-Oerlinghausen and colleagues, 2002). Periods of depression last at least 2 weeks. At other times, there are manic episodes-distinct periods during which there is an abnormally raised, expansive, or irritable mood. Potential organic causes of mania include substance abuse, hyperthyroidism, and central nervous system tumors. Up to 20 percent of patients with manic-depression commit suicide. Treatment is with drugs listed in Table 55-6, with special caution for lithium during fetal organogenesis.

Postpartum Psychosis. This severe mental disorder is usually a bipolar disorder, but it may be due to major depression (American Psychiatric Association, 2000b). It is more common in primiparas, especially those with obstetrical complications (Blackmore and colleagues, 2006). In most cases, it manifests within 2 weeks of delivery. In their experiences with 101 cases, Heron and associates (2007, 2008) reported that a fourth were symptomatic on the first day and half by the third day postpartum. Manic symptoms—excited, elated, "high"; not needing sleep or unable to sleep; feeling active or energetic; and "chatty"—were common early. Affected women

have signs of confusion and disorientation but may also have episodes of lucidity. Because women with underlying disease have a 10- to 15-fold risk for recurrence postpartum, close monitoring is imperative. Postpartum psychosis has a 50-percent recurrence risk in the next pregnancy. In most instances, these women ultimately develop relapsing, chronic psychotic manic-depression.

The clinical course of bipolar illness with postpartum psychosis is comparable with that for nonpregnant women. They usually require hospitalization, pharmacological treatment, and long-term psychiatric care. Psychotic women may have delusions leading to thoughts of self-harm or harm to their infants. Unlike women with nonpsychotic depression, these women commit infanticide, albeit uncommonly (Kim and associates, 2008).

Schizophrenia

This major form of mental illness affects 1.1 percent of adults (Table 55-4). Four major subtypes of schizophrenia are recognized: catatonic, disorganized, paranoid, and undifferentiated. The hallmarks of paranoid schizophrenia are delusions, hallucinations, flat or blunted affect, and confused or impoverished speech. Brain scanning techniques such as positron emission tomography and functional magnetic resonance imaging have shown that schizophrenia is a degenerative brain disorder. Subtle anatomical abnormalities are present early in life and worsen with time.

The disorder has a major genetic component with 50-percent concordance in monozygotic twins. If one parent has schizophrenia, the risk to offspring is 5 to 10 percent. Some data, including a strong association between schizophrenia and the velocardiofacial syndrome, suggest that associated genes are located on chromosome 22q11 (Murphy, 2002). Other putative risk factors for subsequent schizophrenia in a fetus include maternal iron-deficiency anemia, diabetes, and acute maternal stress (Insel and colleagues, 2008; Malaspina and associates, 2008; Van Lieshout and Voruganti, 2008). These remain unproven as does the association with maternal influenza A infection, which is discussed further in Chapter 58 (p. 1212).

Signs of illness begin approximately at age 20 years, and commonly, work and psychosocial functioning deteriorate over time. Because women have a slightly later onset than men and are less susceptible to autism and other neurodevelopmental abnormalities, many investigators theorize that estrogen has a protective effect. Affected women may marry and become pregnant before symptoms manifest. With appropriate treatment, patients may experience a decrease or cessation of symptoms. Within 5 years from the first signs of illness, 60 percent have social recovery, 50 percent are employed, 30 percent are mentally handicapped, and 10 percent require continued hospitalization (American Psychiatric Association, 2000b).

Patients with *schizoaffective disorder* have a chronic deteriorating psychotic disorder similar to schizophrenia but combined with prominent mood symptoms. Although the psychosis rarely abates, the mood symptoms often improve with therapy.

Pregnancy

There has been an increase in relative fertility in schizophrenic women (Solari and co-workers, 2009). Adverse maternal outcomes do not appear to be increased in most studies. There is a link, however, to increased adverse perinatal outcomes in Swedish studies to include low birthweight, fetal-growth restriction, and preterm delivery (Bennedsen and colleagues, 1999). In the Australian study by Jablensky and associates (2005) of more than 3000 pregnancies in schizophrenic women, placental abruption was increased threefold and "fetal distress"—vaguely defined, was increased 1.4-fold.

Treatment. Because schizophrenia has a high recurrence if medications are discontinued, it is advisable to continue therapy during pregnancy. After 40 years of use, there is no evidence that conventional or "typical" antipsychotic drugs cause adverse fetal or maternal sequelae (McKenna and colleagues, 2005; Yaeger and associates, 2006). Because less is known about "atypical" antipsychotics, the American College of Obstetricians and Gynecologists (2007) recommends against their *routine* use in pregnant and breast feeding women.

Anxiety Disorders

These relatively common disorders include panic attack, panic disorder, social anxiety disorder, specific phobia, obsessive-compulsive disorder, posttraumatic stress disorder, and generalized anxiety disorder. All are characterized by irrational fear, tension, and worry, which are accompanied by physiological changes such as trembling, nausea, hot or cold flashes, dizziness, dyspnea, insomnia, and frequent urination (Schneier, 2006). They are treated with psychotherapy and medication, including selective serotonin-reuptake inhibitors, tricyclic antidepressants, monoamine oxide inhibitors, and others.

Pregnancy

Despite their relative high prevalence in childbearing-aged women as shown in Table 55-4, little specific attention has been directed to anxiety disorders in pregnancy. Older studies indicate increased risks for adverse pregnancy outcomes with some of these disorders (American College of Obstetricians and Gynecologists, 2007). From their review, Ross and McLean (2006) concluded that some of the anxiety disorders may have important maternal-fetal implications, but that there are limited data to guide antenatal treatment. Conversely, Littleton and associates (2007) found no excessive adverse pregnancy outcomes with "anxiety symptoms." One important exception is their link with postpartum depression (Vythilingum, 2008).

Eating Disorders

These severe disturbances in eating behavior largely affect adolescent females and young adults with a lifetime prevalence of 2 to 3 percent each (Table 55-4). They include *anorexia nervosa*, in which the patient refuses to maintain minimally normal body weight. With *bulimia nervosa,* there usually is binge eating followed by purging or by excessive fasting to maintain normal body weight (Zerbe and Rosenberg, 2008). Bulik and co-workers (2009) studied pregnancy outcomes in almost 36,000 Norwegian women screened for eating disorders. About 0.1 percent—1 in 1025—had anorexia nervosa; 0.85 percent—1 in

120—had bulimia nervosa; and 5.1 percent reported a binge-eating disorder—a pregnancy prevalence similar to the 6-month prevalence for nonpregnant individuals (see Table 55-4). The last group had a higher risk for large-for-gestational age infants with a concomitantly increased cesarean delivery rate.

Pregnancy

A high miscarriage rate is characteristic of both eating disorders (Sollid and colleagues, 2004). As perhaps expected, anorexia is associated with low-birthweight infants, and it likely is related to small body mass (Micali and associates, 2007). According to Ekéus and associates (2006), women with a prior history of anorexia do well without special surveillance.

Personality Disorders

These disorders are characterized by the chronic use of certain coping mechanisms in an inappropriate, stereotyped, and maladaptive manner. They are rigid and unyielding personality traits. The American Psychiatric Association (2000b) recognizes three clusters of personality disorders:

1. Paranoid, schizoid, and schizotypal personality disorders, which are characterized by oddness or eccentricity
2. Histrionic, narcissistic, antisocial, and borderline disorders, which are all characterized by dramatic presentations along with self-centeredness and erratic behavior
3. Avoidant, dependent, compulsive, and passive-aggressive personalities, which are characterized by underlying fear and anxiety.

Genetic and environmental factors are important in the genesis of these disorders, whose prevalence may be as high as 20 percent. Although management is through psychotherapy, most affected individuals do not recognize their problem, and thus only 20 percent seek help.

Pregnancy

Problems during pregnancy are probably no different than in nonpregnant women. Management may be vexing with some of these disorders. Akman and colleagues (2007) reported that avoidant, dependent, and obsessive-compulsive disorders are associated with an excessive prevalence of postpartum major depression. Magnusson and associates (2007) found a link between some *personality traits*—not disorders—and excessive alcohol consumption, but not necessarily addiction or dependence.

REFERENCES

Abramsky O: Pregnancy and multiple sclerosis. Ann Neurol 36:S38, 1994

Adab N: Therapeutic monitoring of antiepileptic drugs during pregnancy and in the postpartum period: Is it useful? CNS Drugs 20:791, 2006

Adeney KL, Williams MA: Migraine headaches and preeclampsia: An epidemiologic review. Headache 46:794, 2006

Ahokas A, Kaukoranta J, Aito M: Effect of oestradiol on postpartum depression. Psychopharmacology 146:108, 1999

Airas L, Saraste M, Rinta S, et al: Immunoregulatory factors in multiple sclerosis patients during and after pregnancy: Relevance of natural killer cells. Clin Exp Immunol 151:235, 2008

Akman C, Uguz F, Kaya N: Postpartum-onset major depression is associated with personality disorders. Compr Psychiatry 48:343, 2007

Alder J, Fink N, Bitzer J, et al: Depression and anxiety during pregnancy: A risk factor for obstetric, fetal and neonatal outcome? A critical review of the literature. J Matern Fetal Neonatal Med 20:189, 2007

Aly EE, Lawther BK: Anaesthetic management of uncontrolled idiopathic intracranial hypertension during labour and delivery using an intrathecal catheter. Anaesthesia 62:178, 2007

American College of Obstetricians and Gynecologists: Migraine and other headache disorders. Clinical Updates in Women's Health Care, Vol I, No. 3, Summer 2002a

American College of Obstetricians and Gynecologists: Obstetric management of patients with spinal cord injuries. Committee Opinion No. 275, September 2002b

American College of Obstetricians and Gynecologists: Use of psychiatric medications during pregnancy and lactation. Practice Bulletin No. 87, November 2007

American Psychiatric Association: Guidelines for the treatment of patients with major depressive disorder (Revision). Am J Psychiatry 157:1, 2000a

American Psychiatric Association: The Diagnostic and Statistical Manual of Mental Disorders, 4th ed, Text Revision (DSM-IV-TR) Washington, DC, 2000b

Andersson L, Sundström-Poromaa I, Bixo M, et al: Point prevalence of psychiatric disorders during the second trimester of pregnancy: A population-based study. Am J Obstet Gynecol 189:148, 2003

APASS Investigators: Antiphospholipid antibodies and subsequent thrombo-occlusive events in patients with ischemic stroke. JAMA 291:576, 2004

Argyriou AA, Makris N: Multiple sclerosis and reproductive risks in women. Reprod Sci 15(8):755, 2008

Artama M, Isojärvi J, Auvinen A: Antiepileptic drug use and birth rate in patients with epilepsy—a population-based cohort study in Finland. Hum Reprod 21:2290, 2006

Aukes AM, de Groot JC, Aarnoudse JG, et al: Brain lesions several years after eclampsia. Am J Obstet Gynecol 200(5):504.e1, 2009

Aukes AM, Wessel I, Dubois AM, et al: Self-reported cognitive functioning in formerly eclamptic women. Am J Obstet Gynecol 197:365.e1, 2007

Austin M-P, Kildea S, Sullivan E: Maternal mortality and psychiatric morbidity in the perinatal period: Challenges and opportunities for prevention in the Australian setting. MJA 186:364, 2007

Bahrami MH, Rayegani SM, Fereidouni M, et al: Prevalence and severity of carpal tunnel syndrome (CTS) during pregnancy. Electromyogr Clin Neurophysiol 45:123, 2005

Balki M, Castro C, Ananthanarayan C: Status epilepticus after electroconvulsive therapy in a pregnant patient. Int J Obstet Anest 15:325, 2006

Banhidy F, Acs N, Horvath-Puho E, et al: Maternal severe migraine and risk of congenital limb deficiencies. Birth Defects Res A Clin Mol Teratol 76:592, 2006

Batocchi AP, Majolini L, Evoli A, et al: Course and treatment of myasthenia gravis during pregnancy. Neurology 52:447, 1999

Battino D, Tomson T: Management of epilepsy during pregnancy. Drugs 67(18):2727, 2007

Beal MF, Hauser SL: Trigeminal neuralgia, Bell's palsy, and other cranial nerve disorders. In Fauci AS, Braunwald E, Kasper DL, et al (eds): Harrison's Principles of Internal Medicine, 17th ed. McGraw-Hill, New York, 2008, p 2583

Bennedsen BE, Mortensen PB, Olesen Av, et al: Preterm birth and intra-uterine growth retardation among children of women with schizophrenia. Br J Psychiatry 175:239, 1999

Blackmore ER, Jones I, Doshi M, et al: Obstetric variables associated with bipolar affective puerperal psychosis. British Journal of Psychiatry 188:12, 2006

Borri C, Mauri M, Oppo A, et al: Axis I psychopathology and functional impairment at the third month of pregnancy: Results from the Perinatal Depression-Research and Screening Unit (PND-ReScU) study. J Clin Psychiatry 69(10):1617, 2008

Branch DW: Antiphospholipid antibodies and pregnancy: Maternal implications. Semin Perinatol 14:139, 1990

Brandes JL: The influence of estrogen on migraine: A systematic review. JAMA 295:1824, 2006

Brandes JL, Kudrow D, Stark SR, et al: Sumatriptan-naproxen for acute treatment of migraine. JAMA 297:1443, 2007

Briggs GG, Freeman RK, Yaffe SJ: Drugs in pregnancy and lactation, 7th ed. Philadelphia, Lippincott Williams & Wilkins, 2005

Brodie MJ, Dichter MA: Antiepileptic drugs. N Engl J Med 334:168, 1996

Brockington I: Psychosis complicating chorea gravidarum. Arch Womens Ment Health 9:113, 2006

Buhimschi CS, Weiner CP: Medication in pregnancy and lactation: Part 1. Teratology. Obstet Gynecol 113:166, 2009

Bulik CM, Von Holle A, Siega-Riz AM, et al: Birth outcomes in women with eating disorders in the Norweigian mother and child cohort (MoBa). Int J Eat Disord 42(1):9, 2009

Bushnell CD, Jamison M, James AH: Migraines during pregnancy linked to stroke and vascular diseases: US population based case-control study. BMJ 338:b664, 2009

Callaghan WM, MacKay AP, Berg CJ: Identification of severe maternal morbidity during delivery hospitalizations, United States, 1991–2003. 199:133.e1, 2008

Cartlidge NEF: Neurologic disorders. In Barron WM, Lindheimer MD (eds): Medical Disorders During Pregnancy, 3rd ed. St. Louis, Mosby, 2000, p 516

Centers for Disease Control and Prevention: National Health Interview Survey. Health, United States, 2006a

Centers for Disease Control and Prevention: QuickStats: Percentage of persons aged ≥ 18 years reporting severe headache or migraine during the preceding 3 months, by sex and age groups—United States, 2004. MMWR 55:77, 2006b

Centers for Disease Control and Prevention: Prevalence of stroke—United States, 2005. MMWR 56:469, 2007

Centers for Disease Control and Prevention: Prevalence of self-reported postpartum depressive symptoms—17 states, 2004–2005. MMWR 57(14):361, 2008

Chalela JA, Kidwell CS, Nentwich LM, et al: Magnetic resonance imaging and computed tomography in emergency assessment of patients with suspected acute stroke: A prospective comparison. Lancet 369:293, 2007

Chan LY, Tsui MH, Leung TN: Guillain-Barré syndrome in pregnancy. Acta Obstet Gynecol Scand 83:319, 2004

Chang BS, Lowenstein DH: Epilepsy. N Engl J Med 349:1257, 2003

Chang J, Elam-Evans LD, Berg CJ, et al: Pregnancy-related mortality surveillance—United States, 1991–1999. MMWR Surveillance Summaries. 52(5502):1, 2003

Chaudhry V: Peripheral neuropathy. In Fauci AS, Braunwald E, Kasper DL, et al (eds): Harrison's Principles of Internal Medicine, 17th ed. McGraw-Hill, New York, 2008, p 2651

Cheng Q, Jiang GX, Fredrikson S, et al: Increased incidence of Guillain-Barré syndrome postpartum. Epidemiology 9:601, 1998

Chiossi G, Novic K, Celebrezze JU, et al: Successful neonatal outcome in 2 cases of maternal persistent vegetative state treated in a labor and delivery suite. Am J Obstet Gynecol 195:316, 2006

Cohen Y, Lavie O, Granoxsky-Grisaru S, et al: Bell palsy complicating pregnancy: A review. Obstet Gynecol Surv 55:184, 2000

Comtois KA, Schiff MA, Grossman DC: Psychiatric risk factors associated with postpartum suicide attempt in Washington state, 1992–2001. Am J Obstet Gynecol 199:120.e1, 2008

Conti-Fine BM, Milani M, Kaminski HJ: Myasthenia gravis: Past, present, and future. J Clin Invest 116:2843, 2006

Cooper WO, Willy ME, Pont SJ, et al: Increasing use of antidepressants in pregnancy. Am J Obstet Gynecol 196:544.e1, 2007

Coppage KH, Hinton AC, Moldenhauer J, et al: Maternal and perinatal outcome in women with a history of stroke. Am J Obstet Gynecol 190:1331, 2004

Cox SM, Hankins GDV, Leveno KJ, et al: Bacterial endocarditis: A serious pregnancy complication. J Reprod Med 33:671, 1988

Cross JN, Castro PO, Jennett WB: Cerebral strokes associated with pregnancy and the puerperium. BMJ 3:214, 1968

Cunningham FG: Severe preeclampsia and eclampsia: Systolic hypertension is also important. Obstet Gynecol 105:237, 2005

Cunnington M, Tennis P, and the International Lamotrigine Pregnancy Registry Scientific Advisory Committee. Lamotrigine and the risk of malformations in pregnancy. Neurology 64:955, 2005

Dahl J, Myhr KM, Daltveit AK, et al: Pregnancy, delivery, and birth outcome in women with multiple sclerosis. Neurology 65:1961, 2005

Dahl J, Myhr KM, Daltveit AK, et al: Planned vaginal births in women with multiple sclerosis: Delivery and birth outcome. Acta Neurol Scand Suppl 183:51, 2006

Daniels AB, Liu GT, Volpe NJ, et al: Profiles of obesity, weight gain, and quality of life in idiopathic intracranial hypertension (pseudotumor cerebri). Am J Ophthalmol 143:683, 2007

Dammers JWHH, Veering MM, Vermeulen M: Injection with methylprednisolone proximal to the carpal tunnel: Randomised double blind trial. BMJ 319:884, 1999

De Forge D, Blackmer J, Garrity C, et al: Fertility following spinal cord injury: A systematic review. Spinal Cord 43:693, 2005

De Freitas GR, Bogousslavsky J: Risk factors of cerebral vein and sinus thrombosis. Front Neurol Neurosci 23:23, 2008

De La Vega GA, Debbs R, Sehdev H, et al: Cerebrovascular accidents in women of reproductive age. Obstet Gynecol 109:35S, 2007

De Ribaupierre S, Rilliet B, Vernet O, et al: Third ventriculostomy vs ventriculoperitoneal shunt in pediatric obstructive hydrocephalus: Results from a Swiss series and literature review. Childs Nerv Syst 23:527, 2007

Dell DL, O'Brien BW: Suicide in pregnancy. Obstet Gynecol 102:1306, 2003

Dennis CL, Ross LE, Grigoriadis S: Psychosocial and psychological interventions for treating antenatal depression. Cochrane Database Syst Rev 3:CD006309, 2007

Dey R, Khan S, Akhouri V, et al: Labetalol for prophylactic treatment of intractable migraine during pregnancy. Headache 42:642, 2002

Detsky ME, McDonald DR, Baerlocher MO: Does this patient with headache have a migraine or need neuroimaging? JAMA 296(10):1274, 2006

Dias MS, Sekhar LN: Intracranial hemorrhage from aneurysms and arteriovenous malformations during pregnancy and the puerperium. Neurosurgery 27:855, 1990

Dineen R, Banks A, Lenthall R: Imaging of acute neurological conditions in pregnancy and the puerperium. Clin Radiol 60:1156, 2005

Djelmis J, Sostarko M, Mayer D, et al: Myasthenia gravis in pregnancy: Report on 69 cases. Eur J Obstet Gynecol Reprod Biol 104:21, 2002

Drachman DB: Myasthenia gravis and other diseases of the neuromuscular junction. In Fauci AS, Braunwald E, Kasper DL, et al (eds): Harrison's Principles of Internal Medicine, 17th ed. McGraw-Hill, New York, 2008, p 2518

Durufle A, Nicolas B, Petrilli S, et al: Effects of pregnancy and childbirth on the incidence of urinary disorders in multiple sclerosis. Clin Exp Obstet Gynecol 33:215, 2006

Eadie MJ: Antiepileptic drugs as human teratogens. Expert Opin Drug Saf 7:195, 2008

Ehtisham A, Stern BJ: Cerebral venous thrombosis: A review. Neurologist 12:32, 2006

Ekéus C, Lindberg L, Lindblad F, et al: Birth outcomes and pregnancy complications in women with a history of anorexia nervosa. BJOG 113:925, 2006

Elliott SL: Problems of sexual function after spinal cord injury. Prog Brain Res 152:387, 2006

England JD, Asbury AK: Peripheral neuropathy. Lancet 363:2151, 2004

Evans J, Heron J, Francomb H, et al: Cohort study of depressed mood during pregnancy and after childbirth. BMJ 323:257, 2001

Evans RW, Friedman DI: Expert opinion: the management of pseudotumor cerebri during pregnancy. Headache 40:495, 2000

Facchinetti F, Allais G, Nappi RE: Migraine is a risk factor for hypertensive disorders in pregnancy: A prospective cohort study. Cephalagia 29(3):286, 2009

Farragher RA, Laffey JG: Maternal brain death and somatic support. Neurocrit Care 3:99, 2005

Feldman DM, Borgida AF, Rodis JF, et al: Irreversible maternal brain injury during pregnancy: A case report and review of the literature. Obstet Gynecol Surv 55:708, 2000

Finnerty JJ, Chisholm CA, Chapple H, et al: Cerebral arteriovenous malformation in pregnancy: Presentation and neurologic, obstetric, and ethical significance. Am J Obstet Gynecol 181:296, 1999

Finsen V, Zeitlmann H: Carpal tunnel syndrome during pregnancy. Scand J Plast Reconstr Hand Surg 40:41, 2006

Fleming AS, Klein E, Corter C: The effects of a social support group on depression, maternal attitudes and behavior in new mothers. J Child Psychol Psychiatry 33:685, 1992

Friedlander, RM: Arteriovenous malformations of the brain. N Engl J Med 356(26):2704, 2007

Frohman EM, Racke MK, Raine CS: Multiple sclerosis—The plaque and its pathogenesis. N Engl J Med 354:942, 2006

Gajdos P, Chevret S, Toyka K: Intravenous immunoglobulin for myasthenia gravis. Cochrane Database Syst Rev 2:CD002277, 2006

Gavin NI, Gaynes BN, Lohr KN, et al: Perinatal depression: A systematic review of prevalence and incidence. Obstet Gynecol 106:1071, 2005

Gerritsen AAM, de Vet HCW, Scholten RJPM, et al: Splinting vs surgery in the treatment of carpal tunnel syndrome. JAMA 288:1245, 2002

Gilden DH: Bell's palsy. N Engl J Med 351:1323, 2004

Gillman GS, Schaitkin BM, May M, et al: Bell's palsy in pregnancy: A study of recovery outcomes. Otolaryngol Head Neck Surg 126:26, 2002

Giraud P, Chauvet S: Cluster headache during pregnancy: Case report and literature review. Headache 49(1):136, 2009

Gold KJ, Dalton VK, Schwenk TL: Hospital care for parents after perinatal death. Obstet Gynecol 109:1156, 2007

Goodwin RD, Keyes K, Simuro N: Mental disorders and nicotine dependence among pregnant women in the United States. Obstet Gynecol 109:875, 2007

Harden CL, Hopp J, Ting TY, et al: Practice parameter update: Management issues for women with epilepsy—focus on pregnancy (an evidence-based review): Obstetrical complications and change in seizure frequency. Neurology [Epub ahead of print], 2009

Harden CL, Leppik I: Optimizing therapy of seizures in women who use oral contraceptives. Neurology 67:S56, 2006

Hauser SL, Asbury AK: Guillain-Barré syndrome and other immune-mediated neuropathies. In Kasper DL, Braunwald E, Fauci AD, et al (eds): Harrison's Principles of Internal Medicine, 17th ed. McGraw-Hill, New York, 2008, p 2667

Hauser SL, Goodin DS: Multiple sclerosis and other demyelinating diseases. In Kasper DL, Braunwald E, Fauci AD, et al (eds): Harrison's Principles of Internal Medicine, 17th ed. McGraw-Hill, New York, 2008, p 2611

Helms AK, Drogan O, Kittner SJ: First trimester stroke prophylaxis in pregnant women with a history of stroke. Stroke 40(4):1158, 2009

Heron J, Blackmore ER, McGuinnes M, et al: No "latent period" in the onset of bipolar affective puerperal psychosis. Arch Womens Ment Health 10:79, 2007

Heron J, McGuinness M, Blackmore ER, et al: Early postpartum symptoms in puerperal psychosis. BJOG 115(3):348, 2008

Hippman C, Oberlander TG, Honer WG, et al: Depression during pregnancy: The potential impact of increased risk for fetal aneuploidy on maternal mood. Clin Genet 75(1):30, 2009

Horton JC, Chambers WA, Lyons SL, et al: Pregnancy and the risk of hemorrhage from cerebral arteriovenous malformations. Neurosurgery 27:867, 1990

Hughes RA, Swan AV, Raphael JC, et al: Immunotherapy for Guillain-Barré syndrome: A systematic review. Brain, March 2, 2007

Hughes SJ, Short DJ, Usherwood MM, et al: Management of the pregnant women with spinal cord injuries. Br J Obstet Gynaecol 98:513, 1991

Huna-Baron R, Kupersmith MJ: Idiopathic intracranial hypertension in pregnancy. J Neurol 249(8):1078, 2002

Hunt S, Craig J, Russell A, et al: Levetiracetam in pregnancy: Preliminary experience from the UK Epilepsy and Pregnancy Register. Neurology 67:1876, 2006

Hurley TJ, Brunson AD, Archer RL, et al: Landry Guillain-Barre Strohl syndrome in pregnancy: Report of three cases treated with plasmapheresis. Obstet Gynecol 78:482, 1991

Hussein IY, Govenden V, Grant JM, et al: Prolongation of pregnancy in a woman who sustained brain death at 26 weeks of gestation. BJOG 113:120, 2006

Insel BJ, Schaefer CA, McKeague IW, et al: Maternal iron deficiency and the risk of schizophrenia in offspring. Arch Gen Psychiatry 65(10):1136, 2008

International Headache Society: Headache Classification Committee. The International Classification of Headache Disorders, 2nd ed. Cephalgia 24:1, 2004

Ip MSM, So SY, Lam WK, et al: Thymectomy in myasthenia gravis during pregnancy. Postgrad Med J 62:473, 1986

Ishimori ML, Cohen SN, Hallegue DS, et al: Ischemic stroke in a postpartum patient: Understanding the epidemiology, pathogenesis, and outcome of Moyamoya disease. Semin Arthritis Rheum 35:250, 2006

Jablensky AV, Morgan V, Zubrick SR, et al: Pregnancy, delivery, and neonatal complications in a population cohort of women with schizophrenia and major affective disorders. Am J Psychiatry 162:79, 2005

Jackson AB, Wadley V: A multicenter study of women's self reported reproductive health after spinal cord injury. Arch Phys Med Rehabil 80:1420, 1999

Jaigobin C, Silver FL: Stroke and pregnancy. Stroke 31:2948, 2000

James AH, Bushnell CD, Jamison MG, et al: Incidence and risk factors for stroke in pregnancy and the puerperium. Obstet Gynecol 106:509, 2005

Jeng JS, Tang SC, Yip PK: Stroke in women of reproductive age: Comparison between stroke related and unrelated to pregnancy. J Neurol Sci 221:25, 2004

Jones I, Hamshere M, Nangle JM, et al: Bipolar affective puerperal psychosis: Genome-wide significant evidence for linkage to chromosome 16. Am J Psychiatry 164:999, 2007

Josefsson A, Angelsiöö L, Berg G, et al: Obstetric, somatic and demographic risk factors for postpartum depressive symptoms. Obstet Gynecol 99:223, 2002

Kalidindi M, Ganpot S, Tahmesebi F, et al: Myasthenia gravis and pregnancy. J Obstet Gynaecol 27:30, 2007

Kanotra S, D'Angelo D, Phares TM, et al: Challenges faced by new mothers in the early postpartum period: An analysis of comment data from the 2000 Pregnancy Risk Assessment Monitoring System (PRAMS) Survey. Matern Child Health J Jun 12, 2007

Karlsson B, Lindquist C, Johansson A, et al: Annual risk for the first hemorrhage from untreated cerebral arteriovenous malformations. Minim Invasive Neurosurg 40:40, 1997

Katz JN, Simmons BP: Carpal tunnel syndrome. N Engl J Med 346: 1807, 2002

Katz VL, Peterson R, Cefalo RC: Pseudotumor cerebri and pregnancy. Am J Perinatol 6:442, 1989

Kelly RH, Russo J, Holt VL, et al: Psychiatric and substance use disorders as risk factors for low birth weight and preterm delivery. Obstet Gynecol 100:297, 2002

Khaja AM, Grotta JC: Established treatments for acute ischaemic stroke. Lancet 369:319, 2007

Kim JH, Choi SS, Ha K: A closer look at depression in mothers who kill their children: Is it unipolar or bipolar depression? J Clin Psychiatry 69(10):1625, 2008

Kittner SJ, Stern BJ, Feeser BR, et al: Pregnancy and the risk of stroke. N Engl J Med 335:768, 1996

Kizer JR, Devereux RB: Patient foramen ovale in young adults with unexplained stroke. N Engl J Med 353:2361, 2005

Kjaer D, Horvath-Puhó E, Christensen J, et al: Antiepileptic drug use, folic acid supplementation, and congenital abnormalities: A population-based case-control study. BJOG 115:98, 2008

Kobau R, Zahran H, Thurman DJ, et al: Epilepsy surveillance among adults—19 states, behavioral risk factor surveillance system, 2005. MMWR 57:1, 2008

Kruit MC, van Buchem MA, Hofman PA, et al: Migraine as a risk factor for subclinical brain lesions. JAMA 291:427, 2004

Kuczkowski KM: Labor analgesia for the parturient with spinal cord injury: What does an obstetrician need to know? Arch Gynecol Obstet 274:108, 2006

Kuhle J, Pohl C, Mehling M, et al: Lack of association between antimyelin antibodies and progression to multiple sclerosis. N Engl J Med 356:371, 2007

Kuklina EV, Meikle SF, Jamieson DJ, et al: Severe obstetric morbidity in the United States: 1998–2005. Obstet Gynecol 113:293, 2009

Kuller JA, Katz VL, McCoy MC, et al: Pregnancy complicated by Guillain Barré syndrome. South Med J 88:987, 1995

Lamy C, Hamon JB, Coste J, et al: Ischemic stroke in young women. Neurology 55:269, 2000

Landwehr JB, Isada NB, Pryde PG, et al: Maternal neurosurgical shunts and pregnancy outcome. Obstet Gynecol 83:134, 1994

Lanska DJ, Kryscio RJ: Peripartum stroke and intracranial venous thrombosis in the National Hospital Discharge Survey. Obstet Gynecol 89:413, 1997

Lanska DJ, Kryscio RJ: Risk factors for peripartum and postpartum stroke and intracranial venous thrombosis. Stroke 31:1274, 2000

Lee AG, Pless M, Falardeau J, et al: The use of acetazolamide in idiopathic intracranial hypertension during pregnancy. Am J Ophthalmol 139:855, 2005

Lee AM, Lam SK, Lau SM, et al: Prevalence, course, and risk factors for antenatal anxiety and depression. Obstet Gynecol 110:1102, 2007

Leonhardt G, Gaul C, Nietsch HH, et al: Thrombolytic therapy in pregnancy. J Thromb Thrombolysis 21:271, 2006

Liang CC, Chang SD, Lai SL, et al: Stroke complicating pregnancy and the puerperium. Eur J Neurol 13:1256, 2006

Liberman A, Karussis D, Ben-Hur T, et al: Natural course and pathogenesis of transient focal neurologic symptoms during pregnancy. Arch Neurol 65:218, 2008

Lin SY, Hu CJ, Lin HC: Increased risk of stroke in patients who undergo cesarean section delivery: A nationwide population-based study. Am J Obstet Gynecol 198:391.e1, 2008

Lipton RB, Bigal ME, Diamond M, et al: Migraine prevalence, disease burden, and the need for preventive therapy. Neurology 68:343, 2007

Littleton HL, Breitkopf CR, Berenson AB: Correlates of anxiety symptoms during pregnancy and association with perinatal outcomes: A meta-analysis. Am J Obstet Gynecol 424, May 2007

Lynch JK, Nelson KB: Epidemiology of perinatal stroke. Curr Opin Pediatr 13:499, 2001

Magnusson Å, Göransson M, Heilig M: Hazardous alcohol users during pregnancy: Psychiatric health and personality traits. Drug Alcohol Depend 89:275, 2007

Malaspina D, Corcoran C, Kleinhaus KR, et al: Acute maternal stress in pregnancy and schizophrenia in offspring: A cohort prospective. BMC Psychiatry 8:71, 2008

Marcus DA: Headache in pregnancy. Curr Treat Options Neurol 9:23, 2007

Marcus SM: Depression during pregnancy: Rates, risks and consequences—Motherisk Update 2008. Can J Clin Pharmacol 16(1):e15, 2009

Martin JN Jr, Thigpen BD, Moore RC, et al: Stroke and severe preeclampsia and eclampsia: A paradigm shift focusing on systolic blood pressure. Obstet Gynecol 105:246, 2005

McKenna K, Koren G, Tetelbaum M, et al: Pregnancy outcome of women using atypical antipsychotic drugs: A prospective comparative study. J Clin Psychiatry 66:444, 2005

Meador KJ, Baker GA, Browning N, et al: Cognitive function at 3 years of age after fetal exposure to antiepileptic drugs. N Engl J Med 360:1597, 2009

Meador KJ, Baker GA, Finnell RH, et al: In utero antiepileptic drug exposure: Fetal death and malformations. Neurology 67:407, 2006

Mehraein S, Ortwein H, Busch M, et al: Risk of recurrence of cerebral venous and sinus thrombosis during subsequent pregnancy and puerperium. J Neurol Neurosurg Psychiatry 74:814, 2003

Mhurchu CN, Anderson C, Jamrozik K, et al: Hormonal factors and risk of aneurysmal subarachnoid hemorrhage: An international population-based, case-control study. Stroke 32:606, 2001

Micali N, Simonoff E, Treasure J: Risk of major adverse perinatal outcomes in women with eating disorders. Br J Psychiatry 190:255, 2007

Miller LJ: Use of electroconvulsive therapy during pregnancy. Hosp Community Psychiatry 45:444, 1994

Miller LJ: Postpartum depression. JAMA 287:762, 2002

Morewitz SJ: Feelings of anxiety and functional impairment during pregnancy. Obstet Gynecol 101:109S, 2003

Muller-Oerlinghausen B, Berghofer A, Bauer M: Bipolar disorder. Lancet 359:241, 2002

Murphy KC: Schizophrenia and velocardiofacial syndrome. Lancet 359:426, 2002

Murugappan A, Coplin WM, Al-Sadat AN, et al: Thrombolytic therapy of acute ischemic stroke during pregnancy. Neurology 66:768, 2006

National Institute of Mental Health. The numbers count: Mental disorders in America. NIH Publication No. 06-4584, 2006

National Institute of Mental Health: Depression. www.nimh.nihgov/health/topics/depression/index. Updated November 29, 2007

National Mental Health Association: Depression in women. Available at: http://www.nmha.org/infoctr. Accessed April 15, 2004

Okamoto K, Horisawa R, Kawamura T, et al: Menstrual and reproductive factors for subarachnoid hemorrhage risk in women: A case-control study in Nagoya, Japan. Stroke 32:2841, 2001

Olafsson E, Hallgrimsson JT, Hauser WA, et al: Pregnancies of women with epilepsy: A population-based study in Iceland. Epilepsia 39:887, 1998

Palanivelu LM: Chorea gravidarum. J Obstet Gynaecol 27:310, 2007

Pazzaglia C, Caliandro P, Aprile I, et al: Multicenter study on carpal tunnel syndrome and pregnancy incidence and natural course. Acta Neurochir Suppl 92:35, 2005

Pennell PB, Peng L, Newport DJ, et al: Lamotrigine in pregnancy. Clearance, therapeutic drug monitoring, and seizure frequency. Neurology Nov 28, 2007

Perucca E: Birth defects after prenatal exposure to antiepileptic drugs. Lancet Neurol 4:781, 2005

Pervulov M, Gojnic M, Jovanovic D: Cerebrovascular diseases during pregnancy and puerperium. J Matern Fetal Neonatal Med 22(1):51, 2009

Physicians' Desk Reference 62nd Edition. Thomson Corp, Toronto, Ontario, Canada, 2008

Pilo C, Wide K, Winbladh B: Pregnancy, delivery, and neonatal complications after treatment with antiepileptic drugs. Acta Obstet Gynecol 85:643, 2006

Pinette MG, Santarpio C, Wax JR, et al: Electroconvulsive therapy in pregnancy. Obstet Gynecol 110:465, 2007

Podciechowski L, Brocka-Nitecka U, Dabrowska K, et al: Pregnancy complicated by myasthenia gravis—twelve years experience. Neuro Endocrinol Lett 26:603, 2005

Polman CH, O'Connor PW, Havrdova E, et al: A randomized, placebo-controlled trial of natalizumab for relapsing multiple sclerosis. N Engl J Med 354:899, 2006

Qureshi AI, Tuhrim S, Broderick JP, et al: Spontaneous intracerebral hemorrhage. N Engl J Med 344:1450, 2001

Ramnarayan R, Sriganesh J: Postpartum cerebral angiopathy mimicking hypertensive putaminal hematoma: A case report. Hypertens Pregnancy 28(1)34, 2009

Rees PM, Fowler CJ, Maas CP: Sexual function in men and women with neurological disorders. Lancet 369:512, 2007

Rep A, Ganzevoort W, Bonsel GJ, et al: Psychosocial impact of early-onset hypertensive disorders and related complications in pregnancy. Am J Obstet Gynecol 197:158.e1, 2007

Richards DS: Is electroconvulsive therapy in pregnancy safe? Obstet Gynecol 110:451, 2007

Richards FH, Rea G: Reproductive decision making before and after predictive testing for Huntington's disease: An Australian perspective. Clin Genet 67:404, 2005

Richmond JR, Krishnamoorthy P, Andermann E, et al: Epilepsy and pregnancy: An obstetric perspective. Am J Obstet Gynecol 190:371, 2004

Riffaud L, Ferre JC, Carsin-Nicol B, et al: Endoscopic third ventriculostomy for the treatment of obstructive hydrocephalus during pregnancy. Obstet Gynecol 108:801, 2006

Rockel A, Wissel J, Rolfs A: Guillain–Barré syndrome in pregnancy: An indication for caesarean section? J Perinat Med 22:393, 1994

Roman H, Descargues G, Lopes M, et al: Subarachnoid hemorrhage due to cerebral aneurysmal rupture during pregnancy. Acta Obstet Gynecol Scand 83:330, 2004

Ros HS, Lichtenstein P, Bellocco R, et al: Pulmonary embolism and stroke in relation to pregnancy: How can high-risk women be identified? Am J Obstet Gynecol 186:198, 2002

Ross LE, McLean LM: Anxiety disorders during pregnancy and the postpartum period: A systematic review. J Clin Psychiatry 67:1285, 2006

Rudick RA, Stuart WH, Calabresi PA, et al: Natalizumab plus interferon beta-1a for relapsing multiple sclerosis. N Engl J Med 354:911, 2006

Saad N, Tang YM, Sclavos E, et al: Metastatic choriocarcinoma: A rare cause of stroke in the young adult. Australas Radiol 50:481, 2006

Sandberg-Wollheim M, Frank D, Goodwin TM, et al: Pregnancy outcomes during treatment with interferon beta-1a in patients with multiple sclerosis. Neurology 65:802, 2005

Scher AI, Terwindt GM, Picavet HS, et al: Cardiovascular risk factors and migraine: The GEM population-based study. Neurology 64:614, 2005

Schneier FR: Social anxiety disorder. N Engl J Med 355:1029, 2006

Schrale RG, Ormerod J, Ormerod OJ: Percutaneous device closure of the patient foramen ovale during pregnancy. Catheter Cardiovasc Interv February 12, 2007

Seror P: Pregnancy-related carpal tunnel syndrome. J Hand Surg [Br] 23:98, 1998

Serrano P, Hernandez N, Arroyo JA, et al: Bilateral Bell palsy and acute HIV type 1 infection: Report of 2 cases and review. Clin Infect Dis 44:e57, 2007

Sharshar T, Lamy C, Mas JL: Incidence and causes of strokes associated with pregnancy and puerperium. A study in public hospitals of Île de France. Stroke 26:930, 1995

Shmorgun D, Chan WS, Ray JG: Association between Bell's palsy in pregnancy and pre-eclampsia. QJM 95:359, 2002

Silberstein SD: Migraine. Lancet 363:381, 2004a

Silberstein SD: Headaches in pregnancy. Neurol Clin 22:727, 2004b

Silberstein S, Loder E, Diamond S, et al: Probable migraine in the United States: Results of the American Migraine Prevalence and Prevention (AMPP) Study. Cephalalgia January 29, 2007

Simolke GA, Cox SM, Cunningham FG: Cerebrovascular accident complicating pregnancy and the puerperium. Obstet Gynecol 78:37, 1991

Singhal AB, Kimberly WT, Schaefer PW, et al: Case 8—2009—A 36-year-old woman with headache, hypertension, and seizure 2 weeks postpartum. N Engl J Med 360(11):1126, 2009

Smith WS, English JD, Johnston C: Cerebrovascular diseases. In Fauci AS, Braunwald E, Kasper DL, et al (eds): Harrison's Principles of Internal Medicine, 17th ed. McGraw-Hill, New York, 2008a, p 2513

Smith MW, Marcus PS, Wurtz LD: Orthopedic issues in pregnancy. Obstet Gynecol Surv 63:103, 2008b

Solari H, Dickson KE, Miller L: Understanding and treating women with schizophrenia during pregnancy and postpartum—Motherisk Update 2008. Can J Clin Pharmacol 16(1):e32, 2009

Sollid CP, Wisborg K, Hjort J, et al: Eating disorder that was diagnosed before pregnancy and pregnancy outcome. Am J Obstet Gynecol 190:206, 2004

Souza JP, Oliveira-Neto A, Surita FG, et al: The prolongation of somatic support in a pregnant woman with brain-death: A case report. Reprod Health 27:3, 2006

Stefan H, Feuerstein TJ: Novel anticonvulsant drugs. Pharmacol Ther 113(1):165, 2007

Stella CL, Jodicke CD, How HY, et al: Postpartum headache: Is your workup complete? Am J Obstet Gynecol 196:318, 2007

Stolp-Smith KA, Pascoe MK, Ogburn PL Jr: Carpal tunnel syndrome in pregnancy: Frequency, severity, and prognosis. Arch Phys Med Rehabil 79:1285, 1998

Stoodley MA, Macdonald RL, Weir BK: Pregnancy and intracranial aneurysms. Neurosurg Clin N Am 9:549, 1998

Sullivan FM, Swan IR, Donnan PT, et al: Early treatment with prednisolone or acyclovir in Bell's palsy. N Engl J Med 357:1598, 2007

Sumatriptan and Naratriptan Pregnancy Registry: Interim Report: 1 January 1996–30 April 2004. Glaxo Wellcome, July 2004

Takebayashi S, Kaneko M: Electron microscopic studies of ruptured arteries in hypertensive intracerebral hemorrhage. Stroke 14:28, 1983

Tam WH, Chung T: Psychosomatic disorders in pregnancy. Curr Opin Obstet Gynecol 19:126, 2007

Thambisetty M, Lavin PJ, Newman NJ, et al: Fulminant idiopathic intracranial hypertension. Neurology 68:229, 2007

Thomas SV, Ajaykumar B, Sindhu K, et al: Cardiac malformations are increased in infants of mothers with epilepsy. Pediatr Cardiol 29:604, 2008

Tiel Groenestege AT, Rinkel GJ, van der Bom JG, et al: The risk of aneurysmal subarachnoid hemorrhage during pregnancy, delivery, and the puerperium in the Utrecht population: Case-crossover study and standardized incidence ratio estimation. Stroke 40(4):1148, 2009

Turner K, Piazzini A, Franza A, et al: Epilepsy and postpartum depression. Epilepsia 50(1):24, 2009

Vajda FJ, Hitchcock A, Graham J, et al: Seizure control in antiepileptic drug-treated pregnancy. Epilepsia 49(1):172, 2008

Van der Worp HB, van Gijn J: Acute ischemic stroke. N Eng J Med 357(6):572, 2007

Van Lieshout RJ, Voruganti LP: Diabetes mellitus during pregnancy and increased risk of schizophrenia in offspring: A review of the evidence and putative mechanisms. J Psychiatry Neurosci 33(5):395, 2008

Vernet-der Garabedian B, Lacokova M, Eymard B, et al: Association of neonatal myasthenia gravis with antibodies against the fetal acetylcholine receptor. J Clin Invest 94:555, 1994

Viinikainen K, Heinonen S, Eriksson K, et al: Community-based, prospective, controlled study of obstetric and neonatal outcome of 179 pregnancies in women with epilepsy. Epilepsia 47:186, 2006

Vukusic S, Confavreux C: Pregnancy and multiple sclerosis: The children of PRIMS. Clin Neurol Neurosurg 108:266, 2006

Vythilingum B: Anxiety disorders in pregnancy. Curr Psychiatry Rep 10(4):331, 2008

Walker FO: Huntington's disease. Lancet 369:218, 2007

Wasay M, Bakshi R, Bobustuc G, et al: Cerebral venous thrombosis: Analysis of a multicenter cohort from the United States. J Stroke Cerebrovasc Dis 17:49, 2008

Way CM: Safety of newer antidepressants in pregnancy. Pharmacotherapy 37(4):546, 2007

Westdahl C, Milan S, Magriples U, et al: Social support and social conflict as predictors of prenatal depression. Obstet Gynecol 110:134, 2007

Westgren N, Hultling C, Levi R, et al: Pregnancy and delivery in women with a trauma spinal cord injury in Sweden, 1980–1991. Obstet Gynecol 81:926, 1993

Wichman CL, Moore KM, Lang TR, et al: Congenital heart disease associated with selective serotonin reuptake inhibitor use during pregnancy. May Clin Proc 84(1):23, 2009

Winterbottom J, Smyth R, Jacoby A, et al: The effectiveness of preconception to reduce adverse pregnancy outcome in women with epilepsy: What's the evidence? Epilepsy Behav 14(2):273, 2009

Wisner KL, Parry BL, Piontek CM: Postpartum depression. N Engl J Med 347:194, 2002

Wisoff JH, Kratzert KJ, Handwerker SM, et al: Pregnancy in patients with cerebrospinal fluid shunts: Report of a series and review of the literature. Neurosurgery 29:827, 1991

Witlin AG, Mattar F, Sibai BM: Postpartum stroke: A twenty year experience. Am J Obstet Gynecol 183:83, 2000

Wyszynski DF, Nambisan M, Surve T, et al: Increased rate of major malformations in offspring exposed to valproate during pregnancy. Neurology 64:961, 2005

Yaeger D, Smith HG, Altshuler LL: Atypical antipsychotics in the treatment of schizophrenia during pregnancy and the postpartum. Am J Psychiatry 163:2064, 2006

Yerby MS: Pregnancy, teratogenesis, and epilepsy. Neurol Clin 12:749, 1994

Zeeman GG, Fleckenstein JL, Twickler DM, et al: Cerebral infarction in eclampsia. Am J Obstet Gynecol 190:714, 2004a

Zeeman GG, Hatab M, Twickler DM: Maternal cerebral blood flow changes in pregnancy. Am J Obstet Gynecol 189:968, 2003

Zeeman GG, Hatab M, Twickler DM: Increased cerebral blood flow in preeclampsia with magnetic resonance imaging. Am J Obstet Gynecol 191:1425, 2004b

Zerbe KJ, Rosenberg J: Eating disorders. Clinical Updates in Women's Health Care. American College of Obstetricians and Gynecologists, Vol VII, No 1, January 2008

Dermatological Disorders

There are a number of normal pregnancy-induced skin changes that may be alarming to some women. There are also several pregnancy-specific dermatoses, and some are associated with adverse perinatal outcomes. And of course, any skin disease that affects women of childbearing age may be encountered in pregnancy.

SKIN CHANGES IN PREGNANCY

A number of factors are responsible for normal skin changes during pregnancy. These include that fetoplacental hormone production or alteration of clearance may increase plasma availability of estrogens, progesterone, and a variety of androgens. There is accumulating evidence that sex steroids have modulating influences on some skin diseases (Kanda and Watanabe, 2005). There are also profound changes in the availability or concentrations of some adrenal steroids, including cortisol, aldosterone, and deoxycorticosterone. Moreover, presumably as a result of enlargement of the intermediate lobe of the pituitary gland, plasma levels of melanocyte-stimulating hormone (MSH) become remarkably elevated by 8 weeks' gestation. Production of pro-opiomelanocortin has been demonstrated in placental extracts, and this ultimately is a source of α- and β-MSH. Neurotropins and neuropeptides, some produced by trophoblastic cells, may also play a role in skin and hair changes (Botchkarev and associates, 2006; Imperatore and colleagues, 2006).

A synopsis of these changes is shown in Table 56-1. They are also discussed in more detail in Chapter 5 (p. 111). Nguyen Huu and associates (2009) found that *fetal microchimerism*

may also involve the skin. Thus, endothelial-type fetal cells become grafted in maternal skin cells discussed with nevi. This phenomenon has been associated with maternal autoimmune diseases such as lupus, sclerosis, Hashimoto thyroiditis, and other conditions. Its mechanisms are considered further in Chapters 3 (p. 58), 53 (p. 1127) and 54 (p. 1146).

Pigmentation

Some degree of skin darkening from melanin deposition into epidermal and dermal macrophages develops in 90 percent of pregnant women. Pigmentation is more pronounced in brunettes and in women with dark complexions, especially those of Hispanic descent (Aronson and Bass, 2000). Its exact cause is not known, but it is doubtful that elevated serum levels of MSH are responsible. Estrogens play a role in melanogenesis and may be the inciting factor. Melanocytes also respond directly to corticotropin-releasing hormone (Kauser and colleagues, 2006).

Hyperpigmentation is evident beginning early in pregnancy and is more pronounced in naturally hyperpigmented areas such as the areolae, perineum, and umbilicus. Areas prone to friction, such as the axillae and inner thighs, also may become darkened. Recent scars may be involved. When the *linea alba* becomes pigmented, it is called the *linea nigra*. Pigmentation of the face, referred to as the mask of pregnancy, is also called *chloasma* or *melasma*. This is seen in about half of pregnant women. Ultraviolet (UV) light exacerbates melasma by stimulating melanogenesis. Thus, the severity of pigmentation may be mitigated by avoiding excessive sun exposure and by using sunscreens (Lakhdar and co-workers, 2007).

Although hyperpigmentation usually regresses postpartum, dermal melanosis may persist up to 10 years in a third of affected women. Oral contraceptives may aggravate melasma and should be avoided in susceptible women. Sunscreen use should be continued. If particularly disfiguring, hyperpigmentation can be treated with topical application of hydroxyquinone, tretinoin gel or cream, or azelaic acid cream (Muallem and Rubeiz, 2006).

TABLE 56-1. Some Pregnancy-Induced Skin Changes

Structure	Involved Areas
Skin	Hyperpigmentation pronounced in normally hyperpigmented areas
	Chloasma (melasma) common
	Striae gravidarum
	Linea nigra
	Acne—may improve
Connective tissue	Striae gravidarum
	Skin tags—common in neck area
Nevi	Some darken
	Only 3 percent enlarge
Hair	Scalp hair thickens
	Hirsutism—some degree in most women
	Telogen effluvium-postpartum hair loss
	Nails become soft and brittle
Vascular changes	Palmar erythema
	Spider and capillary hemangiomas
Oral cavity	Gingivitis
	Epulis
	Pyogenic granuloma

Data from Muallem and Rubiez (2006), Nussbaum and Benedetto (2006), Salter and Kimball (2006), and Torgerson and colleagues (2006).

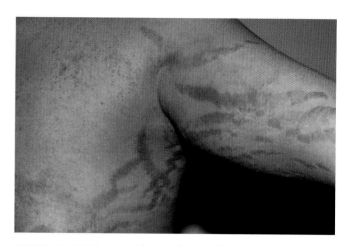

FIGURE 56-1 Striae gravidarum of the axilla and upper arm. (Reprinted from *Clinics in Dermatology*, Vol. 24, No. 2, SA Salter and AB Kimball, Striae gravidarum, pp. 97–100, Copyright 2006, with permission from Elsevier.)

sirable to most women, but unfortunately they are unpreventable. Treatment is also problematic, but some lesions respond to laser and a variety of topical preparations (Salter and Kimball, 2006).

Nevi

All persons have some form of benign melanocytic nevi. Pennoyer and colleagues (1997) found that only 6 percent of 129 nevi changed in diameter over pregnancy—3 percent increased by 1 mm, and 3 percent *decreased* by 1 mm. And although a small minority of nevi develop enlarged melanocytes and increased melanin deposition during pregnancy, there is no evidence for malignant transformation (Driscoll and Grant-Kels, 2006, 2009). Because it is uncommon during pregnancy for nevi to enlarge or become darker as shown in Figure 56-2, it is reasonable to be concerned if either occurs (MacKelfresh and associates, 2005). As discussed previously, Nguyen Huu and coworkers (2009) found engrafted endothelial-type fetal cells in 12 percent of nevi from pregnant women. Moreover, these cells were identified in 63 percent of malignant melanomas from pregnant women (see Chap. 57, p. 1199).

Striae Gravidarum

These are linear lesions that frequently appear during pregnancy and are commonly found on the abdomen and breasts. They are at least partially tension related, but there are other factors (Osman and associates, 2007). Histologically, these lesions show a decrease and reorganization of the dermal elastin fiber network (Watson and associates, 1998). During pregnancy they are reddish purple, but over time lose pigmentation and overlying skin becomes atrophic (Fig. 56-1). These "stretch marks" are unde-

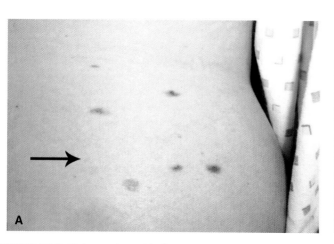
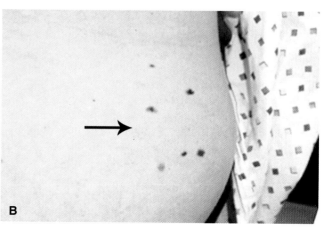

FIGURE 56-2 Melanocytic nevi before pregnancy **A.** and during pregnancy **B.** Note the darkening of all the nevi in the photograph on the right taken during pregnancy. Each arrow is placed proportionally between the six nevi in each image. (From MacKelfresh and co-workers, 2005, with permission.)

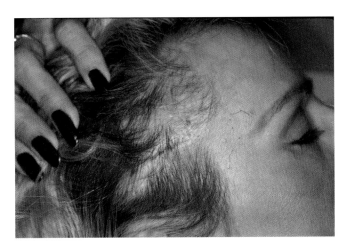

FIGURE 56-3 Telogen effluvium in a postpartum woman. (Reprinted from *Clinics in Dermatology*, Vol. 24, No. 2, R Nussbaum and AV Benedetto, Cosmetic aspects of pregnancy, pp. 133–141, Copyright 2006, with permission from Elsevier.)

Hair

During pregnancy, the *anagen*—hair-growth phase, is increased relative to the *telogen*—resting hair phase (Randall, 1994). Estrogens prolong anagen, and androgens cause enlargement of follicles in responsive areas such as the face (Paus and Cotsarelis, 1999). When these effects dissipate postpartum, hair shedding develops—*telogen effluvium* (Fig. 56-3). This rather abrupt hair loss begins approximately 1 to 4 months postpartum. It may sometimes be characterized by alarming amounts of hair shedding with brushing or washing. Fortunately, the process is self-limited, and women may be reassured that normal hair growth is usually restored in 6 to 12 months.

Because hair growth is modulated by estrogens, androgens, thyroid hormones, glucocorticoids, and prolactin, it is not surprising that mild *hirsutism* is common during pregnancy. This may be most noticeable on the face, and women who are predisposed genetically to coarse hair growth are more severely affected. Hirsutism typically regresses within several months after delivery. Severe hirsutism with other evidence of masculinization should prompt consideration for another androgen source such as adrenal tumors (see Chap. 53, p. 1138) or pregnancy luteomas and theca-lutein cysts (see Chap. 5, p. 110). A few cases of women with recurrent and regressing severe hyperandrogenism during pregnancy have been reported (Holt and co-workers, 2005).

Nail Changes

Fingernails may become soft and brittle, but treatment is not necessary. Occasionally in darker-skinned individuals, a brown pigment stripe extends the length of the nail. Termed *melanonychia*, it usually regresses postpartum (Muallem and Rubeiz, 2006).

Vascular Changes

Augmented cutaneous blood flow in pregnancy is due to a marked decrease in peripheral vascular resistance (Spetz, 1964). Pregnancy incites estrogen-induced changes in small blood vessels, and they are widely dilated in the superficial dermis (Henry

and associates, 2006). *Spider hemangiomas* are found in most white women during pregnancy, but in only 10 percent of black women. Most of these vascular lesions regress postpartum. *Palmar erythema* is noticed in two thirds of white women and a third of black women. *Capillary hemangiomas* or *glomus tumors*, especially of the head and neck, are seen in up to a third of women during pregnancy.

One vascular condition that may be distressing is *pregnancy gingivitis* caused by growth of the mucosal capillaries and fibroblasts. This swelling—*epulis of pregnancy*—is common in the gum region and usually is controlled by proper dental hygiene. It is uncertain if this exacerbates periodontal infection that is associated with adverse pregnancy outcomes (Boggess and associates, 2008). These lesions may appear on any mucosal or cutaneous surface and are termed *pyogenic granuloma or granuloma gravidarum*. Radar and co-workers (2008) described five cases in which the hand was involved. Lesions are erythematous and friable, and although treatment is usually unnecessary, large granulomas may require excision. If this is done, however, recurrences are common (Torgerson and colleagues, 2006).

DERMATOSES OF PREGNANCY

A number of dermatological conditions either are identified as unique to pregnancy or are encountered more often during gestation. Their terminology can be confusing because of differing usage in the United States and Europe and other countries. Shornick (1998) concluded that only three conditions are universally accepted as unique to pregnancy: *pruritus gravidarum* caused by cholestasis; *pruritic urticarial papules* and *plaques of pregnancy;* and *herpes gestationis*. Their gross appearance may be similar to each other or to unrelated skin disorders. Shown in Table 56-2 is one classification scheme with various international differences in nomenclature.

This classification does not include atopic eczema, recently described by Ambros-Rudolph and co-workers (2006) to comprise half of symptomatic skin disorders seen in their clinics. Fortunately, inflammatory skin diseases such as atopic dermatitis and psoriasis have no significant effects on pregnancy outcome (Seeger and associates, 2007).

Pruritus

Complaints of itching during pregnancy are common, and its cited incidence varies directly with the vigilance for which it is sought. In almost 3200 women carefully studied by Roger and colleagues (1994), 1.6 percent had significant pruritus at some time during pregnancy.

Pruritus Gravidarum

This common pregnancy-related skin condition is not primarily a dermatological disorder. It is considered to be a mild variant of *intrahepatic cholestasis of pregnancy* (see Chap. 50, p. 1063). Contributing factors include pregnancy hormones, genetics, dyslipidemia, and environmental factors (Dann and colleagues, 2006; Rutherford and Pratt, 2006). In the population-based

TABLE 56-2. Dermatoses Unique to Pregnancy

Disorder	Frequency	Clinical Characteristics	Histopathology	Effects on Pregnancy	Treatment	Comments
Pruritus gravidarum (also cholestasis of pregnancy)	Common (1–2%)	Onset third trimester; intense pruritus; generalized; excoriations common	Nonspecific; no primary lesions, but excoriations common	Perinatal morbidity increased	Antipruritics, cholestyramine, ursodeoxycholic acid	Mild form of cholestatic jaundice; recurs in subsequent pregnancies (see Chap. 50, p. 1063)
Pruritic urticarial papules and plaques of pregnancy (PUPPP) In Europe: polymorphic eruption of pregnancy (PEP)	Common (0.25–1%)	Onset usually third trimester; intense pruritus; patchy or generalized on abdomen, thighs, arms, buttocks; erythematous papules, urticarial papules, plaques	Lymphocytic perivascular infiltrate; negative immunofluorescence	No adverse effects	Antipruritics, emollients, topical steroids, oral steroids if severe	More common in white women, nulliparas, and those with twins; seldom recurs
Prurigo of pregnancy (also prurigo gestationis, papular dermatitis)	Uncommon (1:300–1:2400)	Onset late second or third trimester; localized or generalized; usually forearms and trunk; 1–5 mm commonly excoriated pruritic papules	Lymphocytic perivascular infiltrate; parakeratosis acanthosis; negative immunofluorescence	Probably unaffected	Antipruritics, topical steroids, oral steroids if severe	Prurigo gestationis localized to forearms and trunk; papular dermatitis is generalized; does not recur
Pruritic folliculitis of pregnancy (PFP) (also impetigo herpetiformis)	Rare	Onset third trimester; local, then generalized; erythema with marginal sterile pustules; mucous membranes involved; systemic symptoms	Microabscesses; spongiform pustules of Kogoj; neutrophils	Maternal sepsis common	Antibiotics, oral steroids	Possibly pustular psoriasis; persists weeks to months postpartum; usually does not recur
Herpes gestationis In Europe: pemphigoid gestationis, bullous pemphigoid of pregnancy	Rare (1:10,000)	Onset after midpregnancy, 1–2 weeks postpartum; severe pruritus; abdomen, extremities, or generalized; urticarial papules and plaques, erythema, vesicles, and bullae	Edema; infiltrate of lymphocytes, histiocytes, and eosinophils; C_3 and IgG deposition at basement membrane	Possibly increased preterm birth; transient neonatal lesions (5–10%)	Antipruritics, topical steroids, oral steroids if severe	Autoimmune HLA-related; may occur with trophoblastic disease; exacerbations and remissions common with pregnancy and postpartum; recurrence common; neonatal skin lesions in 10%

study by Sheiner and colleagues (2006), it was found in 0.2 percent of nearly 160,000 deliveries. With cholestasis, bile salt serum levels increase in most women, and they are deposited in the dermis to cause pruritus. Not all women, however, have elevated bile salt levels (Yoong and co-workers, 2008). Skin lesions develop from scratching and excoriation. Treatment of pruritis follows that for cholestasis of pregnancy.

Pruritic Urticarial Papules and Plaques of Pregnancy

This is the most common pruritic pregnancy-specific dermatosis. It is called *PUPPP* in the United States and referred to as *polymorphic eruption of pregnancy (PEP)* in much of Europe. Almost half of the 3200 reported women by Roger and co-workers (1994) with pruritus had this dermatosis. The incidence is approximately 1 in 200 pregnancies, but increases to 8 in 200 for multifetal gestations (Kroumpouzos and Cohen, 2003). PUPPP is more common in white and nulliparous women and is characterized by an intensely pruritic cutaneous eruption that usually appears late in pregnancy (see Table 56-2). It is more common with a male fetus (Regnier and colleagues, 2008). Shown in Figure 56-4 are the erythematous urticarial papules and plaques that involve the abdomen and proximal thighs in 97 percent of affected women (Rudolph and colleagues, 2005). Half of these women will develop erythema, vesicles, and targetoid lesions with eczema. Although rare, the face, palms, and soles may be affected (High and co-workers, 2005). There is no evidence that perinatal morbidity is increased with PUPPP (Kroumpouzos and Cohen, 2003; Rudolph and associates, 2005). It seldom recurs in subsequent pregnancies.

Pathophysiology

The etiopathogenesis is unknown. Histologically, there is a mild, nonspecific lymphohistiocytic perivasculitis with an eosinophilic component. There is no immunoglobulin or complement dermal deposition, and absence of a linear band of C_3 in the basement membrane differentiates it from herpes gestationis (Rudolph and co-workers, 2005). It has been hypothesized that this disorder may be stimulated by fetal cells that have

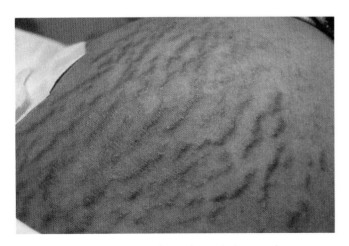

FIGURE 56-4 Pruritic urticarial papules and plaques of pregnancy (PUPPP).

invaded maternal skin (Aractingi and associates, 1998). This intriguing possibility has been linked with nevi and malignant melanoma and reviewed by Gilliam (2006). Also as discussed, similar mechanisms are proposed for lupus and systemic sclerosis (see Chap. 54, p. 1146) and postpartum thyroiditis (see Chap. 53, p. 1027).

Treatment

Most women respond to treatment with oral antihistamines, skin emollients, and topical corticosteroids. About 10 percent require systemic corticosteroids to relieve severe itching (Rudolph and colleagues, 2005; Scheinfeld, 2008). In most cases, the rash disappears quickly either before or within several days following delivery. Symptoms persist for 2 to 4 weeks postpartum in 15 to 20 percent (Vaughan Jones and co-workers, 1999). Up to 15 percent of cases will begin postpartum (Buccolo and Viera, 2005).

Prurigo of Pregnancy

This likely refers to a group of disorders previously described by a multitude of names (Dahdah and Kibbi, 2006). According to Shornick (1998), it includes *prurigo gestationis* and *papular dermatitis* as likely variants of the same disease and not pregnancy specific (see Table 56-2). They appear to share a strong component of atopic eczema.

Prurigo gestationis is the milder and more common variant, characterized by small, pruritic, rapidly excoriated lesions on the forearms and trunk. The bitelike papules may resemble scabies or other insect bites. Pruritis is usually controlled with oral antihistamines and topical corticosteroid creams. The course is protracted and lesions typically appear at 25 to 30 weeks and may persist for 3 months after delivery. Perinatal outcome does not appear to be adversely affected. Recurrence in subsequent pregnancy is common.

Pruritic Folliculitis of Pregnancy

This rare pustular eruption—also called *impetigo herpetiformis*—is seen in late pregnancy. It is uncertain if it is unique to pregnancy, or if it is a form of pustular psoriasis coincidental to pregnancy. Less than 50 cases have been reported (Green and co-workers, 2009; Kroumpouzos and Cohen, 2003). The hallmark lesions of pruritic folliculitis are sterile pustules that form around the margin of erythematous patches that characteristically begin at flexures and extend peripherally. Mucous membranes are usually involved. The characteristic histological lesion is a spongelike epidermal cavity filled with neutrophils— the *spongiform pustule of Kogoj*.

Pruritus is not severe, but constitutional symptoms are common. In addition to nausea, vomiting, diarrhea, chills, and fever, hypoalbuminemia and hypocalcemia are common. Although the pustules are initially sterile, they may become infected after rupture, and sepsis is a serious concern. Treatment is with systemic corticosteroids along with antimicrobials for secondary infection. Infliximab has also been used (Sheth and colleagues, 2009). The disease may persist for several weeks to months after delivery.

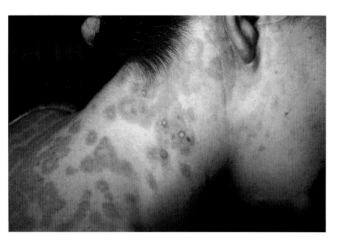

FIGURE 56-5 Herpes gestationis. (Courtesy of Dr. Amit Pandya.)

Herpes Gestationis

This uncommon noninfectious skin disorder shares an etymological but not biological connection with herpes viral infection. In Europe, it is also called *pemphigoid gestationis* (see Table 56-2). It is a rarely encountered autoimmune blistering skin eruption with a cited incidence of 1 in 10,000 to 50,000 pregnancies. It can also occur with trophoblastic disease.

It is characterized by an extremely pruritic widespread eruption that most commonly begins in the last trimester (Ambros-Rudolph and colleagues, 2006; Hon and co-workers, 2008). Lesions vary from erythematous and edematous papules to large, tense vesicles and bullae (Figs. 56-5 and 56-6). Before bullae form, these lesions may resemble PUPPP as described previously. Common sites of involvement are the abdomen and periumbilical area—70 percent, and the extremities—95 percent (Ambros-Rudolph and associates, 2006). Exacerbations and remissions throughout pregnancy are common, and up to 75 percent of women suffer intrapartum flares (Shornick, 1998). In subsequent pregnancies, the disease invariably recurs, and it usually does so earlier and is more severe (Al-Fouzan and colleagues, 2006).

There is an inherited predisposition, and more than half of affected women have HLA-DR3 and HLA-DR4 antigens com-

pared with only 3 percent of unaffected women (Al-Fouzan and colleagues, 2006). Maternal HLA-DR antigens are also associated with other autoimmune disorders to include Addison disease, type 1 diabetes, systemic lupus erythematosus, Graves disease, and Hashimoto thyroiditis. And Shornick and Black (1992) reported that 10 percent of 75 women with herpes gestationis also had Graves disease.

Etiopathogenesis

Herpes gestationis is characterized by development of an immunoglobulin G_1 antibody to the epidermal basement membrane. It is a thermostable immunoglobulin G (IgG) that reacts with the bullous pemphigoid 180-kDa (BP180) epidermal antigen (Patton and associates, 2006). BP180 is a glycoprotein integral to adhesion structures that anchor basal cells to their basement membrane (Shimanovich and colleagues, 2002). The antibody is also called *herpes gestationis serum factor,* and it both reacts with amnionic tissue and is passively transferred to the fetus.

The classical histological finding is subepidermal edema with perivascular infiltrates of lymphocytes, histocytes, and eosinophils. With immunofluorescent techniques, C_3 complement and sometimes IgG are deposited along the basement membrane zone between the epidermis and the dermis (Fig. 56-7).

Treatment

Pruritus with this condition may be severe. Topical corticosteroids and oral antihistamines are usually not effective. Orally administered prednisone, 0.5 to 1 mg/kg daily, brings relief promptly in most women and also inhibits formation of new lesions. Cyclosporine as well as plasmapheresis and high-dose intravenous immunoglobulin therapy have been used in intractable cases (Al-Fouzan and colleagues, 2006; Kroumpouzos and Cohen, 2003). Some women develop chronic disease that

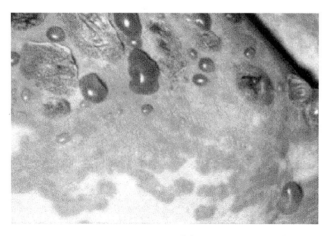

FIGURE 56-6 Herpes gestationis with large, tense generalized bullous eruptions. (From Al-Fouzan and co-workers, 2006, with permission.)

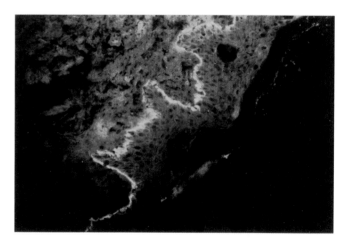

FIGURE 56-7 Herpes gestationis. Direct immunofluorescent stain of a punch biopsy of a skin vesicle in a postpartum women shows a linear pattern of C_3 staining on the basement membrane (original ×200). (Reprinted from Erickson NI, Ellis RL: Neonatal rash due to herpes gestationis. *N Engl J Med* 347(9):660, with permission. Copyright © 2002 Massachusetts Medical Society. All rights reserved.)

may be identical to bullous pemphigoid (Amato and associates, 2003).

Effect on Pregnancy

Observations from small studies have been inconclusive but suggest an association with preterm birth, stillbirths, and fetal-growth restriction (Aronson and Bass, 2000). In a recent study from Oxford, Chi and colleagues (2009) retrospectively analyzed perinatal outcomes in 63 pregnancies. They found significantly increased risks of preterm birth and low birthweight with the presence of blisters and with disease onset in the first and second trimesters. These findings lend credence to recommendations for antepartum surveillance. Up to 10 percent of neonates develop lesions similar to those of the mother (Erickson and Ellis, 2002). These lesions typically clear spontaneously within a few weeks. Chiaverini and associates (2006) described four neonates with bullous pemphigoid, but their mothers had neither skin lesions nor anti-BP180 antibodies.

PREEXISTING SKIN DISEASE

A number of chronic dermatological disorders may complicate pregnancy. These may antedate pregnancy or manifest for the first time during pregnancy. Like other chronic inflammatory disorders, their course may vary during pregnancy (Oumeish and Al-Fouzan, 2006).

Acne is unpredictably affected by pregnancy, but may improve. For nonpregnant women, treatment may include some of the highly teratogenic congeners of retinoic acid (see Chap. 14, p. 324). **Isotretinoin, etretinate, and tretinoin are strictly contradicted in pregnancy.** For severe acne, topically applied *benzoyl peroxide* appears to be safe. *Topical tretinoin* is absorbed poorly and thought to pose no significant teratogenic risk (Briggs and colleagues, 2005; Leachman and Reed, 2006).

From their review, Oumeish and Al-Fouzan (2006) reported that *psoriasis* improves in approximately 40 percent of women during pregnancy, it is unchanged in another 40 percent, and it worsens in another 20 percent. Raychaudhuri and associates (2003) theorize that improvement may be due to downregulated proinflammatory Th-1 cytokines. Ben-David and colleagues (2008) performed a case-control study of 145 pregnancies complicated by psoriasis. Perinatal outcomes were generally not different from affected women compared with 860 normal controls. There was, however, a significant two- to fourfold increase in recurrent miscarriage—OR 2.1; in chronic hypertension—OR 2.9; and cesarean delivery—OR 4.1. There are a number of regimens used in nonpregnant individuals that are contraindicated during pregnancy. Topical corticosteroids are recommended for localized disease (Tauscher and co-workers, 2002). If there is no response, then stepwise therapy is given with topical calcipotriene, anthralin, and then tacrolimus. For generalized mild disease, they recommended UVB phototherapy. Vun and colleagues (2006) reported the successful use of narrowband UVB phototherapy for pustular psoriasis in a pregnant woman. If there is no response, psoralens are given with UVB phototherapy, followed by oral cyclosporine, if unsuccessful. Topical or oral corticosteroids may

also be given for moderate or severe disease. Coal tar derivatives and some systemic immunosuppressives such as methotrexate are avoided. Recently, mycophenolate mofetil is again being used for psoriasis (Orvis and co-workers, 2009). As discussed in Chapter 14 (p. 322), the drug is teratogenic and should be avoided.

Hidradenitis suppurativa is a chronic, progressive, inflammatory and suppurative skin disorder. It is characterized by apocrine gland plugging that leads to anhidrosis and bacterial infection. The disease is hormonally responsive and thus not seen until puberty. It has been said to improve with pregnancy, but in our experiences, it is not appreciably changed. Treatment is control of acute infections with either systemic antimicrobials or clindamycin ointment. Milder inflammatory changes and maintenance are treated with oral antimicrobial agents, and more recently, with anti-inflammatory polyclonal antibodies (Alikhan and associates, 2009). Some women will require surgical drainage and debridement during pregnancy. Radical surgical resection may be necessary to control and prevent recurrences, but this can usually be done after pregnancy (Buimer and colleagues, 2009).

If *pemphigus* appears for the first time during pregnancy, it may be confused with herpes gestationis (Vaughan Jones and Black, 1999). Even with corticosteroid therapy, the mortality rate is 10 percent from sepsis caused by infection of denuded skin. Lesions of *neurofibromatosis* may increase in size and number as a result of pregnancy. According to Perez-Maldonado and Kurban (2006), both *porphyria cutanea tarda* and *acrodermatitis enteropathica* characteristically exacerbate during pregnancy.

Erythema nodosum is a cutaneous reaction associated with a number of disorders. These include sarcoidosis, drugs, connective-tissue disorders, inflammatory bowel disease, infections, and malignancies. Although pregnancy itself is reported by Requena and Sánchez (2007) to be a cause, in our experiences, this is rare.

REFERENCES

Al-Fouzan AWS, Galadari I, Oumeish I, et al: Herpes gestationis (pemphigoid gestationis). Clin Dermatol 24:109, 2006

Alikhan A, Lunch PJ, Eisen DB: Hidradenitis suppurativa: A comprehensive review. J Am Acad Dermatol 60(4):539, 2009

Amato L, Mei S, Gallerani I, et al: A case of chronic herpes gestationis: Persistent disease or conversion to bullous pemphigoid? J Am Acad Dermatol 49:302, 2003

Ambros-Rudolph CM, Müllegger RR, Vaughan-Jones SA, et al: The specific dermatoses of pregnancy revisited and reclassified: Results of a retrospective two-center study on 505 pregnant patients. J Am Acad Dermatol 54:395, 2006

Aractingi S, Berkane N, Bertheau P, et al: Fetal DNA in skin of polymorphic eruptions of pregnancy. Lancet 352:1898, 1998

Aronson IK, Bass BN: Dermatologic disease. In Barron WM, Lindheimer MD (eds): Medical Disorders During Pregnancy, 3rd ed. St Louis, Mosby, 2000, p 540

Ben-David Gila, Sheiner E, Hallak M, et al: Pregnancy outcome in women with psoriasis. J Reprod Med 53:183, 2008

Boggess KA, Society for Maternal-Fetal Medicine Publications Committee: Maternal oral health and pregnancy. Obstet Gynecol 111:976, 2008

Botchkarev VA, Yaar M, Peters EM, et al: Neurotrophins in skin biology and pathology. J Invest Dermatol 126:1719, 2006

Briggs GG, Freeman RK, Yaffe SJ (eds): Drugs in Pregnancy and Lactation. Philadelphia, Lippincott Williams & Wilkins, 2005, p 1613

Buccolo LS, Viera AJ: Pruritic urticarial papules and plaques of pregnancy presenting in the postpartum period: A case report. J Repro Med 50:61, 2005

Buimer MG, Wobbes T, Klinkenbijl JH: Hidradenitis suppurativa. Br J Surg 96(4):350, 2009

Chi CC, Wang SH, Charles-Holmes R, et al: Pemphigoid gestationis: Early onset and blister formations are associated with adverse pregnancy outcomes. Br J Dermatol 160(6):1222, 2009

Chiaverini C, Hamel-Teillac D, Gilbert D, et al: Absence of anti-BP180 antibodies in mothers of infants with bullous pemphigoid. Br J Dermatol 154:839, 2006

Dahdah MJ, Kibbi AG: Less well-defined dermatoses of pregnancy. Clin Dermatol 24:118, 2006

Dann AT, Kenyon AP, Wierzbicki AS, et al: Plasma lipid profiles of women with intrahepatic cholestasis of pregnancy. Obstet Gynecol 107:106, 2006

Driscoll MS, Grant-Keis JM: Nevi and melanoma in pregnancy. Dermatol Clin 24:199, 2006

Driscoll MS, Grant-Kels JM: Nevi and melanoma in the pregnant woman. Clin Dermatol, 27(1):116, 2009

Erickson NI, Ellis RL: Neonatal rash due to herpes gestationis. N Engl J Med 347:660, 2002

Gilliam AC: Microchimerism and skin disease: True-true unrelated? J Investigative Dermatology 126:239, 2006

Green MG, Bragg J, Rosenman KS, et al: Pustular psoriasis of pregnancy in a patient whose dermatosis showed features of acute generalized exanthematous pustulosis. Int J Dermatol 48(3):299, 2009

Henry F, Quatresooz P, Valverde-Lopez JC, et al: Blood vessel changes during pregnancy: A review. Am J Clin Dermatol 7:65, 2006

High WA, Hoang MP, Miller MD: Pruritic urticarial papules and plaques of pregnancy with unusual and extensive palmoplantar involvement. Obstet Gynecol 105:1261, 2005

Holt HB, Medbak SM Kirk D, et al: Recurrent severe hyperandrogenism during pregnancy: A case report. J Clin Pathol 58:439, 2005

Hon KL, Chiu LS, Lam MC, et al: Measurement of pruritis in a Chinese woman with pemphigoid gestationis using a wrist movement detector. Int J Dermatol 47 (1):64, 2008

Imperatore A, Florio P, Torres PB, et al: Urocortin 2 and urocortin 3 are expressed by the human placenta, deciduas, and fetal membranes. Am J Obstet Gynecol 195:288, 2006

Kanda N, Watanabe S: Regulatory roles of sex hormones in cutaneous biology and immunology. J Dermatol Sci 38:1, 2005

Kauser S, Slominski A, Wei ET, et al: Modulation of the human hair follicle pigmentary unit by corticotropin-releasing hormone and urocortin peptides. FASB J 20:882, 2006

Kroumpouzos G, Cohen LM: Specific dermatoses of pregnancy: An evidence-based systematic review. Am J Obstet Gynecol 188:1083, 2003

Lakhdar H, Zouhair K, Khadir K, et al: Evaluation of the effectiveness of a broad-spectrum sunscreen in the prevention of chloasma in pregnant women. JEADV 21(6):738, 2007

Leachman SA, Reed BR: The use of dermatologic drugs in pregnancy and lactation. Dermatol Clin 24:167, 2006

MacKelfresh J, Chen SC, Monthrope YM: Pregnancy and changes in melanocytic nevi. Obstet Gynecol 106:857, 2005

Muallem MM, Rubeiz NG: Physiological and biological skin changes in pregnancy. Clin Dermatol 24:80, 2006

Nguyen HS, Oster M, Afril M, et al: Fetal microchimeric cells participate in tumour angiogenesis in melanomas occurring during pregnancy. Am J Pathol 174(2):630, 2009

Nussbaum R, Benedetto AV: Cosmetic aspects of pregnancy. Clin Dermatol 24:133, 2006

Orvis AK, Wesson SK, Breza TS, et al: Mycophenolate mofetil in dermatology. J Am Acad Dermatol 60(2):183, 2009

Osman H, Rubeiz N, Tamim H, et al: Risk factors for the development of striae gravidarum. Am J Obstet Gynecol 196:62, 2007.

Oumeish OY, Al-Fouzan AW: Miscellaneous diseases affected by pregnancy. Clin Dermatol 24:113, 2006

Patton T, Plunkett RW, Beutner EH, et al: IgG4 as the predominant IgG subclass in pemphigoides gestationis. J Cutan Pathol 33:299, 2006

Paus R, Cotsarelis G: The biology of hair follicles. N Engl J Med 341:491, 1999

Pennoyer JW, Grin CM, Driscoll MS, et al: Changes in size of melanocytic nevi during pregnancy. J Am Acad Dermatol 36:378, 1997

Perez-Maldonado A, Kurban AK: Metabolic diseases and pregnancy. Clin Dermatol 24:88, 2006

Radar C, Piorkowski J, Bass DM, et al: Epulis gravidarum manum: Pyogenic granuloma of the hand occurring in pregnant women. J Hand Surg 33 (2):263, 2008

Randall VA: Androgens and human hair growth. Clin Endocrinol 40:439, 1994

Raychaudhuri SP, Navare T, Gross J, et al: Clinical course of psoriasis during pregnancy. Int J Dermatol 42:518, 2003

Regnier S, Fermand V, Levy P, et al: A case-control study of polymorphic eruption of pregnancy. J Am Acad Dermatol 58 (1):63, 2008

Requena L, Sánchez YE: Erythema nodosum. Semin Cutan Med Surg 26(2):114, 2007

Roger D, Vaillant L, Fignon A, et al: Specific pruritic diseases of pregnancy: A prospective study of 3192 pregnant women. Arch Dermatol 130:734, 1994

Rudolph CM, Al-Fares S, Vaughan-Jones SA, et al: Polymorphic eruption of pregnancy: Clinicopathology and potential trigger factors in 181 patients. Br J Dermatol 154:54, 2005

Rutherford AE, Pratt DS: Cholestasis and cholestatic syndromes. Curr Opin Gastroenterol 22:209, 2006

Salter SA, Kimball AB: Striae gravidarum. Clin Dermatol 24:97, 2006

Scheinfeld N: Pruritic urticarial papules and plaques of pregnancy wholly abated with one week twice daily application of fluticasone propionate lotion: A case report and review of the literature. Dermatol Online 14(11):4, 2008

Seeger JD, Lanza LL, West WA, et al: Pregnancy and pregnancy outcome among women with inflammatory skin diseases. Dermatology 214(1):32, 2007

Sheiner E, Ohel I, Levy A, et al: Pregnancy outcome in women with pruritis gravidarum. J Reprod Med 51(5):394, 2006

Sheth N, Greenblatt DT, Acland K, et al: Generlaized pustular psoriasis of pregnancy treated with infliximab. Clin Exp Dermatol [Epub ahead of print], 2009

Shimanovich I, Skrobek C, Rose C, et al: Pemphigoid gestationis with predominant involvement of oral mucous membranes and IgA autoantibodies targeting the C-terminus of BP180. J Am Acad Dermatol 47:780, 2002

Shornick JK: Dermatoses of pregnancy. Semin Cutan Med Surg 17:172, 1998

Shornick JK, Black MM: Fetal risks in herpes gestationis. J Am Acad Dermatol 26:63, 1992

Spetz S: Peripheral circulation during normal pregnancy. Acta Obstet Gynecol Scand 43:309, 1964

Tauscher AE, Fleischer AB Jr, Phelps KC, et al: Psoriasis and pregnancy. J Cutan Med Surg 6:561, 2002

Torgerson RR, Marnach ML, Bruce AJ, et al: Oral and vulvar changes in pregnancy. Clin Dermatol 24:122, 2006

Vaughan Jones SA, Black MM: Pregnancy dermatoses. J Am Acad Dermatol 40:233, 1999

Vaughan Jones SA, Hern S, Nelson-Piercy C, et al: A prospective study of 200 women with dermatoses of pregnancy correlating clinical findings with hormonal and immunopathological profiles. Br J Dermatol 141:71, 1999

Vun YY, Jones b, Al-Mudhaffer M, et al: Generalized pustular psoriasis of pregnancy treated with narrow band UVB and topical steroids. J Am Acad Dermatol 54:S28, 2006

Watson REB, Parry EJ, Humphries JD, et al: Fibrillin microfibrils are reduced in skin exhibiting striae distensae. Br J Dermatol 138(6):931, 1998

Yoong W, Memtsa M, Pus S, et al: Pregnancy outcomes of women with pruritis, normal bile salts and liver enzymes: A case control study. Acta Obstet Gynecol Scand 87(4):419, 2008

CHAPTER 57

Neoplastic Diseases

Cancer during pregnancy is uncommon but not rare. Reported rates for most cancers vary widely, reflecting not only differences in populations, but also differing methods of ascertainment and inconsistency of reporting. In a review of more than 4.8 million deliveries in California during a 9-year period, Smith and colleagues (2003) found the incidence of malignant neoplasms during pregnancy or in the subsequent 12 months to be 0.94 per 1000 live births. About a third were diagnosed in the prenatal period and the others within 12 months of delivery. Shown in Table 57-1 are some of the more common cancers associated with pregnancy. Breast, thyroid, and cervical cancers; lymphoma; and melanoma account for at least 85 percent of these malignancies. Although management of the pregnant woman with cancer is problematic, a basic tenet should be followed: she should not be penalized because she is pregnant. That said, treatment must be individualized and include consideration of the type and stage of cancer, her desire to continue the pregnancy, and risks of modifying or delaying treatment.

PRINCIPLES OF CANCER THERAPY DURING PREGNANCY

Surgery

Surgical intervention for cancer may be indicated for diagnostic, staging, or therapeutic purposes. Most procedures that do not interfere with the reproductive tract are well tolerated by both mother and fetus (see Chap. 41, p. 913). Although many operative procedures have classically been deferred until after 12 to 14 weeks to minimize abortion risks, this probably is not necessary. Specifically, visualizing a live, normal-appearing fetus with sonography between 9 and 11 weeks forecasts a 95-percent chance that pregnancy will reach viability. We are of the opinion that surgery should be performed regardless of gestational age if maternal well-being is imperiled.

Radiation Therapy

Most diagnostic radiographic procedures have very low x-ray exposure and should not be delayed if they would directly affect therapy (American College of Obstetricians and Gynecologists, 2004). Radiation dosimetry of many procedures is discussed in Chapter 41 (p. 915). Conversely, therapeutic radiation often results in significant fetal exposure. The amount depends on the dose, tumor location, and field size. Although the most susceptible period is during organogenesis, there is no gestational age considered safe for therapeutic radiation exposure. Adverse effects include cell death, carcinogenesis, and genetic effects on future generations (Brent, 1989, 1999; Hall, 1991). Characteristic adverse fetal effects are microcephaly and mental retardation. In some cases, even late exposure can cause fetal-growth restriction and brain damage.

These dangers raise very practical issues. For example, therapeutic radiation doses to the maternal abdomen are contraindicated because of a high risk of fetal death or damage, unless of

TABLE 57-1. Incidence of Malignant Tumors Associated with Pregnancy in 4.85 Million Women

| | | Incidence Per 100,000 | | |
Cancer	No.	Pregnancy	Postpartum[a]	Incidence Per Pregnancy[b]
Any	4539	34.0	59.6	1:1100
Breast	935	5.5	13.8	1:5000
Thyroid	699	3.6	10.8	1:7000
Cervix	580	4.6	7.4	1:8500
Lymphoma	425	4.1	4.6	1:12,000
Melanoma	424	3.2	5.5	1:12,000
Ovary	253	3.6	1.7	1:19,000
Gastrointestinal	225	1.2	3.5	1:21,500
Leukemia	206	2.4	1.8	1:23,500
Nervous System	175	1.5	2.2	1:28,000

[a]Cancer diagnosed within 12 months of delivery.
[b]Rounded to nearest 500.
Data from the California Cancer Registry (Smith and colleagues, 2003).

course abortion induction is one of its purposes. In some cases, such as head and neck cancers, radiotherapy to supradiaphragmatic areas can be given relatively safely with abdominal shielding. In others, such as breast cancer, significant scatter doses can accrue to the fetus.

Chemotherapy

Chemotherapy is recommended for primary treatment or as adjunctive therapy along with surgery or radiation. Although chemotherapy often improves long-term maternal outcome, there is too often a reluctance to employ it during pregnancy. To be sure, fetal concerns include malformations, growth restriction, mental retardation, and the risk of future malignancies. But the risks for these effects are dependent primarily on gestational age at exposure. For example, most antineoplastic drugs are potentially harmful to the fetus if given during organogenesis. Indeed, embryonic exposure to cytotoxic drugs causes major malformations in 10 to 20 percent of cases (Muslin and colleagues, 2001).

After the first trimester, most antineoplastic drugs are without immediate obvious adverse sequelae (Avilés and Neri, 2001; Cardonick and Iacobucci, 2004). Long-term effects, however, have not been evaluated thoroughly (Gwyn, 2005; Partridge and Garber, 2000). Late mutagenic effects on offspring of women treated during pregnancy have been of concern. In one study, Li and associates (1979) found only two childhood malignancies in offspring of 146 women treated during 286 pregnancies. In another study, Avilés and Neri (2001) found no adverse sequelae in 84 children exposed to antineoplastic drugs in utero.

Regarding specific agents, from their reviews of *alkylating agents,* Glantz (1994) and Doll and colleagues (1988) con-

cluded that these agents could be used after the first trimester. These observations also apparently apply to the two potent teratogens—*all-trans-retinoic acid* and *methotrexate*—both of which have few adverse effects after the first trimester (Briggs and co-workers, 2002).

Other Considerations

Chemotherapy is a contraindication to breast feeding. There is also concern with contact exposure of healthcare workers to chemotherapeutic agents. Selevan and colleagues (1985) and Stucker and co-workers (1990) reported a twofold increased risk of fetal loss in nurses exposed during the first trimester. They recommend caution during mixing and administration of antineoplastic drugs (see Chap. 14, p. 320).

Immunotherapy

Hybridized monoclonal antibodies directed against tumor-specific antigens are commonly used for treatment of an ever-increasing list of malignant neoplasms. A common example is *trastuzumab,* whose trade name is *Herceptin.* It is directed against human epidermal growth factor receptor type 2—*Her2/neu*—commonly found in breast cancers (Hudis, 2007). These drugs are described in more detail on page 1197 as well as with tumors for which they are used.

Fertility after Cancer Therapy

Subsequent fertility may be diminished after chemotherapy or radiotherapy in both men and women. In one example, treatment of advanced Hodgkin lymphoma with multiple-drug chemotherapy may result in azoospermia in men and in decreased follicular maturation, destruction, and ovarian fibrosis in women (Waxman, 1985). Gershenson (1988) reviewed outcomes in women successfully treated for germ cell ovarian tumors and found that a third had total or partial ablation of ovarian function. Tangir and associates (2003) reviewed women who had ovarian germ cell malignancies treated with fertility-sparing surgery, followed in most cases by chemotherapy. More than 75 percent who attempted pregnancy were successful at least once. Falconer and Ferns (2002) presented similar findings. The likelihood of fertility effects is both age- and dose-related. Interestingly, the prepubertal ovary is more resistant to chemotherapy effects.

Recently, pretherapy harvesting and cryopreservation of ovarian tissue for posttherapy autologous transplantation has been described (Falcone and Bedaiwy, 2005). This is an expensive and still experimental approach to fertility preservation that has been used in women who are to undergo chemotherapy (Patrizio and colleagues, 2005). At least one live birth using this approach was reported (Donnez and co-workers, 2004). Current methods of fertility preservation and conception options have been reviewed by Jeruss and Woodruff (2009) and Maltaris and associates (2009).

Pregnancy in Cancer Survivors

The Childhood Cancer Survivor Study (CCSS) was established in 1994 to study long-term effects of therapy on cancer survivors. In a description of more than 10,000 surviving adults, Oeffinger and colleagues (2006) reported that relative to their siblings, survivors had a threefold risk of developing a number of chronic health conditions. Problems include second malignancies and heart failure, as well as cranial radiotherapy-related cognitive dysfunction, growth hormone deficiency, and obesity. Pregnancy outcomes from 1953 women in the CCSS cohort, who had a total of 4029 pregnancies, have also been reported (Green and colleagues, 2002; Robison and associates, 2005). In general, there were no increased adverse outcomes. Signorello and associates (2006) reported similar results. In a Scottish study, Clark and co-workers (2007) reported that 917 first pregnancies in cancer survivors had slightly higher rates of preterm birth and postpartum hemorrhage.

Finally, Larsen and colleagues (2004) reported that radiotherapy, but not chemotherapy, at a young age irreversibly reduces uterine volume of childhood cancer survivors. Similarly, Wo and Viswanathan (2009) in their review concluded that abdomino-pelvic radiation impairs subsequent reproductive function. Reassuringly, however, mothers who were treated in childhood with radiotherapy did not have significantly increased risks of delivering neonates with congenital malformations (Winther and co-workers, 2009).

BREAST CARCINOMA

Breast cancer is the most common malignancy of women of all age groups. However, there is encouraging evidence from the Centers for Disease Control and Prevention (2007) that its incidence is decreasing. Despite this, the American College of Obstetricians and Gynecologists (2003b) estimates that almost 1 of every 8 women will eventually be afflicted. It is also one of

the more common malignancies encountered during pregnancy with an incidence that ranges from 1 in 5000 to 50,000 pregnancies (Smith and associates, 2003; Sorosky and Scott-Conner, 1998). As more women choose to delay childbearing until a later age, the frequency of associated breast cancer likely will increase (Woo and associates, 2003).

According to some studies, women with *BRCA1* and *BRCA2* breast cancer gene mutations, as well as those with a family history of breast cancer, are more likely to develop malignancy during pregnancy than those without mutations (Johannsson and co-workers, 1998; Shen and colleagues, 1999). Ultimately, however, parity may modify risk in women with *BRCA1* and *BRCA2* mutations. In this group, parous women older than 40 have a significantly reduced cancer risk (Andrieu and co-workers, 2006; Antoniou and colleagues, 2006). Women in this group undergoing induced abortions or those who breast feed do not have an increased risk of breast cancer (Beral and associates, 2004; Friedman and colleagues, 2006). Moreover, Jernström and associates (2004) found that breast feeding actually conveyed a protective effect against this cancer in those with *BRCA1* gene mutation, but not in those with *BRCA2* mutations. It is controversial whether diethylstilbestrol exposure in utero is associated with an increased risk (Larson and co-workers, 2006; Titus-Ernstoff and associates, 2006).

Pregnancy and Breast Cancer

The effects of pregnancy on the course of breast cancer and its prognosis are complex and not simply due to the massively increased levels of both estrogens and progestins. Certainly, some data suggest that higher estrogen levels cause excess breast cancer later in life and that progesterone may be protective (Ward and Bristow, 2002). There is intriguing evidence that higher serum levels of alpha-fetoprotein are associated with a decreased incidence of breast cancer (Melbye and colleagues, 2000). Even so, it appears that pregnancy interruption following diagnosis of pregnancy-associated cancer has no influence on its course or prognosis.

Most clinical reports maintain that when breast cancer is diagnosed during pregnancy, the regional lymph nodes are more likely to contain microscopic metastases. This is important, because the 5-year survival rate is primarily dependent on its stage at diagnosis and is comparable stage for stage with that in nonpregnant women (King and colleagues, 1985; Nugent and O'Connell, 1985; Zemlickis and associates, 1992). According to Jacob and Stringer (1990), about 30 percent of pregnant women with breast cancer have stage I disease, 30 percent have stage II, and 40 percent stages III or IV. As shown in Table 57-2, the aggregate of studies published after 1990 indicate that about 60 percent of pregnant women have concomitant axillary node involvement.

Other findings support that breast cancer is generally more advanced in pregnant women. Zemlickis and associates (1992) found that pregnant women had a two- to threefold increased risk of metastatic disease compared with nonpregnant women. Bonnier and associates (1997) found a much higher incidence of inflammatory cancer in 154 pregnant women compared with that of 308 age-matched nonpregnant controls—26 versus 9 percent.

TABLE 57-2. Axillary Node Involvement in Pregnancy-Associated Breast Cancer in Reports after 1990

		Positive Nodes	
Investigators	Patients (No.)	Patients (No.)	%
Petrek et al (1991)	56	34	61
Ishida et al (1992)	192	111	58
Souadka et al (1994)	43	34	80
Bonnier et al (1997)	114	64	56
Berry et al (1999)	22	14	67
Shousha (2000)	14	11	78
Gentilini et al (2005)	38	21	55
Total	479	289	60[α]

[α] Compared with 80 percent reported before 1980.

There are usually slight delays in clinical assessment, diagnostic procedures, and treatment of pregnant women with breast tumors (Berry and colleagues, 1999). The mean delay was found to be only 1 or 2 months by Woo and associates (2003). The delay can partially be attributed to pregnancy-induced breast changes that obscure breast masses. These changes are even more magnified during lactation, when there is lobular hyperplasia and galactostasis. Concerns that excessive nodal involvement is related to delayed diagnosis seem unlikely considering the biology of breast cancer. Nettleton and colleagues (1996) used mathematical modeling to conclude that even a 6-month delay increases the chance of axillary metastasis by only 5 percent. There is no doubt that breast cancer is more aggressive in younger women. Whether it is more aggressive during pregnancy in these same women is debatable. Beadle and co-workers (2009) found no differences in overall survival rates in young women with pregnancy-associated breast cancer compared with similarly aged and staged women whose cancer was not diagnosed during pregnancy. These findings were in contrast to Rodriguez and colleagues (2008), who reported poorer overall survival rates in those with pregnancy-associated breast cancer compared with matched controls. Both studies conclude that later disease stages seem to be more prevalent in pregnant women, and thus, overall survival is adversely affected. In the Swedish Cancer Registry, Bladström and associates (2003) reported a 5-year survival rate of 52 percent if breast cancer was diagnosed in pregnant women compared with 80 percent if detected in nonpregnant women. After an extensive review, Schedin (2006) hypothesized that postpregnancy breast remodeling contributes to tumor cell dissemination.

Placental Metastases

Malignant breast cells are occasionally found on placental microscopic examination (Dunn and co-workers, 1999). These have been confined to the intervillous space, and fetal disease has not been reported (see Chap. 27, p. 581).

Diagnosis

The diagnostic approach in pregnant women with a breast tumor should not differ significantly from that for nonpregnant women.

Any suspicious breast mass found during pregnancy should prompt an aggressive plan to determine its cause. The "triple test" for a solid breast mass consists of clinical examination, imaging, and needle biopsy. At the University of Alabama, sonography is the initial diagnostic study performed. An oval or elongated lesion with smooth borders and no shadowing is highly suggestive of a benign mass. Most masses in pregnancy have these reassuring features, and definitive diagnosis can often await the conclusion of pregnancy.

Some use mammography to evaluate a breast mass. Fetal radiation risk is negligible with appropriate shielding, and the exposure is only 0.004 cGy for the typical two-view mammogram (Nicklas and Baker, 2000). Because breast tissue is denser in pregnancy, mammography is associated with a false-negative rate of 35 to 40 percent (Woo and associates, 2003).

Finally, magnetic resonance (MR) imaging is more sensitive than mammography but has a higher false-positive rate in nonpregnant women (Leach and colleagues, 2005). Importantly, if a suspicious mass is present and imaging studies are nondiagnostic, or if there are worrisome clinical features, then biopsy is indicated. Although there are no large studies in pregnant women, core biopsy is recommended. Fine-needle aspiration for cytology has become less popular in the past few years because it has a higher insufficient tissue sample rate and findings with pregnancy-associated breast cancer are more difficult to interpret (Woo and associates, 2003).

Once malignancy is diagnosed, a chest radiograph and a limited metastatic search are performed. Although routine computed tomography (CT) scans of bone and liver are both sensitive and specific, they are usually avoided during pregnancy because of excessive radiation (Pelsang, 1998). Magnetic resonance imaging is a reasonable alternative to assess liver involvement because it is sensitive and has excellent contrast resolution.

Treatment

The best clinical approach is by a multidisciplinary team with obstetricians, surgeons, and medical oncologists. Breast conservation surgery for small tumors, with or without adjunctive chemo- or radiotherapy, is preferable in nonpregnant women (Fisher and colleagues, 2002; Veronesi and co-workers, 2002).

Surgical treatment may be definitive for breast carcinoma during pregnancy (Woo and colleagues, 2003). In the absence of metastatic disease, wide excision, modified radical mastectomy, or total mastectomy, each with axillary node staging can be performed (Rosenkranz and Lucci, 2006). During staging, sentinel lymph node biopsy appears safe to perform in pregnant women (Mondi and associates, 2007; Spanheimer and co-workers, 2009).

Chemotherapy is recommended for node-positive disease if delivery is not anticipated within several weeks. It is given for advanced disease, and termination should be considered if pregnancy is early (Shah and Saunders, 2001). Cyclophosphamide, doxorubicin, and 5-fluorouracil are currently recommended by most clinicians (García-Manero and associates, 2009). After the first trimester, methotrexate can be substituted for doxorubicin (Sorosky and Scott-Conner, 1998). Because survival is improved with chemotherapy in premenopausal women, it should be considered even if lymph nodes are cancer free.

Immunotherapy for breast cancers has become commonplace in the past decade. *Trastuzumab—Herceptin—*is a monoclonal antibody to the human epidermal growth factor receptor type 2 (HER2/neu), which is found in about a third of invasive breast cancers (Hudis, 2007). The drug is used in metastatic breast cancer and is being used more commonly as adjunct therapy for early disease in HER2-positive tumors. Experience with its use in pregnancy is limited, but it may be associated with oligohydramnios (Shrim and colleagues, 2008; Sekar and Stone, 2007).

In 22 women treated with modified radical mastectomy and followed in most by chemotherapy, Berry and colleagues (1999) reported minimal fetal risks. Moreover, Hahn and co-workers (2006) reported good short-term outcomes for the offspring of 57 women treated during pregnancy with multi-agent chemotherapy for breast cancer. Adjunctive radiotherapy is not recommended during pregnancy because abdominal scatter is considerable. Sorosky and Scott-Conner (1998) determined that when the maternal radiation dose is 5000 cGy, the fetus receives at least 100 to 150 cGy. Bradley and colleagues (2006) emphasize that fetal size and depth within the maternal abdomen (as opposed to uterine size) should be used to calculate fetal dose.

Pregnancy Following Breast Cancer

Some women are rendered infertile by chemotherapy, as discussed previously on page 1194. For those who can choose pregnancy, there is little evidence to suggest that pregnancy adversely affects survival in women who have undergone prior breast cancer treatment (Averette and colleagues, 1999). Dow and colleagues (1994) found no differences in rates of recurrence or distant metastasis in those with or without subsequent pregnancies. Reports by Kroman (1997) and Velentgas (1999) and their colleagues have since confirmed these findings.

No data suggest that lactation adversely affects the course of breast cancer. Successful lactation and breast feeding are possible after conservative surgery and radiation for breast cancer, even from the treated side (Higgins and Haffty, 1994). Recommendations for future pregnancies in women successfully treated for breast malignancy are based on several factors, including consideration of recurrence risk. It seems reasonable to advise a delay of

2 to 3 years, which is the most critical observation period. Women who conceive before this time, however, do not appear to have diminished survival (Ives and associates, 2006). Finally, it is reassuring that women who undertake pregnancy after a diagnosis of breast cancer have birth outcomes comparable with those without cancer (Langagergaard and colleagues, 2006).

LYMPHOID CELL MALIGNANCIES

Some of these present as leukemia involving bone marrow and blood, and others are solid tumors, that is, lymphomas. They may be of B- or T-cell origin.

Hodgkin Disease

This is the most common malignant lymphoma in women of childbearing age. It is *probably* B-cell derived and is distinguished from other lymphomas by Reed–Sternberg cells. It has a bimodal incidence peak at age 18 to 30 years and again after age 50. Prognosis is good, and survival is greater than 70 percent.

In more than 70 percent of Hodgkin disease cases, there is painless enlargement of lymph nodes above the diaphragm—the axillary, cervical, or submandibular chains. About a third have symptoms including fever, night sweats, malaise, weight loss, and pruritus. The World Health Organization 1999 classification, used for clinical and therapeutic applications, includes consideration of morphological, clinical, immunological, and genetic information. The most common finding is peripheral adenopathy, and neck and supraclavicular nodes are commonly involved. Diagnosis is by histological examination of involved nodes (Armitage and Longo, 2005).

Pregnancy and Hodgkin Disease

In a population-based review of approximately 4 million deliveries, Smith and associates (2003) reported this lymphoma to complicate only 1 per 34,000 live births. Our experiences are similar during the past 35 years at Parkland Hospital with more than 300,000 pregnancies.

Pregnant women with Hodgkin disease present special management considerations. A tenet of treatment is that careful staging is essential, and either local radiotherapy or systemic chemotherapy is indicated. The Ann Arbor staging system, shown in Table 57-3, was designed for Hodgkin lymphomas but is also used for other lymphomas. Although pregnancy limits the widespread application of some radiographic studies, at minimum, evaluation includes chest radiography, bone marrow biopsy, and abdominal imaging (Williams and Schilsky, 2001). Spiral CT can be used with the "pitch" set so that radiation dose approaches that of conventional scanning (see Chap. 41, p. 918). MR imaging is an excellent alternative for evaluating thoracic and abdominal para-aortic lymph nodes (Fig. 57-1). Radionuclide gallium scanning, which is being used more frequently in nonpregnant patients, emits only 0.75 to 1.0 cGy, and its use should be considered. Staging is essential when radiotherapy alone is chosen because the presence of abdominal disease significantly alters treatment.

Treatment is individualized depending on stage and pregnancy duration. In nonpregnant patients, initial chemotherapy is given with increasing frequency even in stage I disease-isolated

TABLE 57-3. Ann Arbor Staging System for Hodgkin Disease

Stage	Findings
I	Involvement in a single lymph node region or lymphoid site—e.g., spleen or thymus.
II	Involvement of two or more lymph node groups on the same side of the diaphragm—the mediastinum is a single site
III	Involvement of lymph nodes on both sides of diaphragm
IV	Extralymphatic involvement—e.g., liver or bone marrow.

Substage A = no symptoms; substage B = fever, sweats, or weight loss; substage E = extralymphatic involvement excluding liver and bone marrow.

lymph node involvement. Radiotherapy alone for stage I disease has a 90-percent cure rate. In pregnancy, radiotherapy is preferable for isolated neck adenopathy, but it is not recommended for areas that would result in significant radiation scatter to the fetus.

As discussed on page 1194, chemotherapy is best avoided during the first trimester. A course of chemotherapy to precede local disease radiation should be an individualized decision and is probably best done after 12 weeks. With obvious widespread disease, however, we recommend that chemotherapy be initiated regardless of gestational age. Postponement of therapy until fetal maturity is achieved seems justifiable only when the diagnosis is found late in pregnancy (Shulman and associates, 2008).

Pregnancy does not adversely affect the course or survival of women with Hodgkin lymphoma (Pavlidis, 2002). Moreover, adverse perinatal outcomes do not appear to be increased (Langagergaard and colleagues, 2008). Because aggressive radiation and chemotherapy are often necessary for cure, however, preg-

nancy termination is reasonable in the first half of pregnancy. Jacobs and associates (1981) reported that neither chemotherapy during the second and third trimesters nor irradiation to the mediastinum and neck adversely affected the fetus or neonate. In our experiences, pregnant women with Hodgkin disease are inordinately susceptible to infection and sepsis, and both radiotherapy and chemotherapy increase this susceptibility.

Long-Term Prognosis

Horning and co-workers (1981) reported that 55 percent of women resumed normal menses after chemotherapy. There were no birth defects in 24 neonates subsequently born to these women. The risk of second cancers, especially leukemia, in treated individuals is about 20 percent within 15 years. Kaldor and associates (1990) reported that the risk of leukemia was increased almost ninefold following chemotherapy compared with that of radiotherapy given alone. Travis and co-workers (2003) presented surveillance data from 3817 female survivors who were treated for Hodgkin disease before age 30. Women treated with radiation had an overall 3.2-fold increased risk of breast cancer. When given chemotherapy alone, the risk was significantly decreased below baseline. Other complications of therapy for Hodgkin disease include myocardial damage and infarction, pulmonary fibrosis, hypothyroidism, and marrow suppression (Armitage and Longo, 2005).

Non-Hodgkin Lymphomas

Non-Hodgkin lymphoma, although usually B-cell tumors, can also be T-cell or natural killer-cell neoplasms. Their biology, classification, and treatment are complex (Armitage and Longo, 2005; Shulman and colleagues, 2008). For example, they are associated with viral infections including human immunodeficiency virus (HIV), Epstein-Barr virus (EBV), hepatitis C virus (HCV), and human herpes virus 8 (HHV8). These lymphomas tend to be more aggressive overall than Hodgkin lymphomas, and survival varies. The incidence of non-Hodgkin lymphomas has risen sharply, partly because 5 to 10 percent of HIV-infected persons develop a lymphoma.

Non-Hodgkin lymphomas are rare during pregnancy. In an earlier review, Ward and Weiss (1989) described only 75 cases associated with pregnancy. Avilés and colleagues (1990) reported their experiences with 16 pregnant women with non-Hodgkin lymphomas, half of whom were in the first trimester.

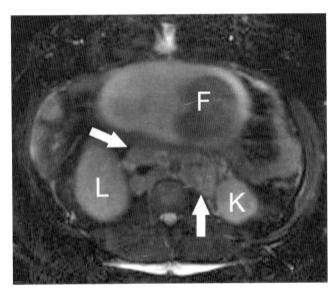

FIGURE 57-1 24-year-old woman diagnosed with Hodgkin lymphoma in the second trimester, undergoing noncontrast chest, abdomen, and pelvis MR imaging for staging. Axial T2 weighted MR image through the midabdomen demonstrates bilateral paraaortic adenopathy (*arrows*). Fetal abdomen (F), maternal inferior liver (L), maternal left kidney (K) are seen. (Used with permission of Dr. Desiree Morgan.)

They were treated with cytotoxic drugs, and there were no fetal malformations. All but one of the offspring were healthy at 3 to 11 years. Half of the mothers who had remissions were alive 4 to 9 years later. In another study, Avilés and Neri (2001) described long-term surveillance of 55 children whose mothers had received chemotherapy for lymphomas during pregnancy. They found no congenital, neurological, or psychological abnormalities at 6 to 29 years. They observed that there were also no cancers, including leukemia.

Burkitt lymphoma is an aggressive B-cell tumor associated with Epstein-Barr virus (EBV) infection. Barnes and associates (1998) reviewed the outcome of 19 women whose pregnancies were complicated by this lymphoma: 17 died within a year. Pollack and colleagues (1993) described an HIV-infected woman with a B-cell lymphoma that metastasized to the placenta. Catlin and co-workers (1999) described a fascinating case in which a maternal T-cell/natural killer-cell lymphoma metastasized transplacentally and engrafted the fetus. Both mother and infant succumbed from the malignancy. Magloire and colleagues (2006) described the removal of a 15-cm Burkitt lymphoma of the ovary at 13 weeks' gestation in a woman with stage IV disease. She was delivered vaginally at term of a healthy neonate after being given six courses of multi-agent chemotherapy.

Management

Staging for non-Hodgkin lymphomas is performed according to the Ann Arbor system shown in Table 57-3. Radiotherapy typically is used for stage I disease, whereas chemotherapy and immunotherapy with rituximab is recommended for most stage II and all stage III and IV tumors. During pregnancy at least, if the peripheral nodes are involved, the disease is often widespread and staging laparotomy has limited benefit (Peleg and Ben-Ami, 1998).

Leukemias

There are, in general, two varieties of leukemia. These malignancies arise from lymphoid tissues—lymphoblastic or lymphocytic leukemias, or they arise from bone marrow—myeloid leukemias. They can be acute or chronic. Although adult leukemias are more prevalent after age 40, they still are among the most common malignancies of young women. For this reason, they are relatively common in pregnancy. Smith and colleagues (2003) reported an incidence of leukemia of 1:40,000 from the California Cancer Registry. Caligiuri and Mayer (1989) reviewed 350 reports of pregnancy complicated by leukemia. Of 72 women reported since 1975, 44 had acute myelogenous leukemia; 20 had acute lymphocytic leukemia; and 8 had one of the chronic leukemias.

Pregnancy and Leukemia

Before 1970, the maternal mortality rate was virtually 100 percent. However, with contemporary therapy, remission during pregnancy is common. *Induction chemotherapy* is aggressively pursued with a goal to attain complete remission. Thereafter, *postremission therapy* is mandatory to prevent a relapse which, if it occurs, is usually treated with stem-cell transplantation (Wetzler and colleagues, 2005). With some chronic leukemias it may

be possible to delay therapy until after delivery (Fey and Surbeck, 2008). Combination chemotherapeutic regimes are complex and toxicity is common. The usual considerations for fetal exposure apply. More recently, monoclonal antibodies have been used to treat some leukemias. Ault and colleagues (2006) described 19 pregnancies conceived with either partner of the couple taking *imatinib—Gleevec—*for chronic myeloid leukemia. The fetal effects for this drug are unknown at this time.

There is no evidence that termination improves the prognosis. That said, abortion is a consideration in early pregnancy to avoid potential teratogenesis from chemotherapy. And because it may also simplify management of the acutely ill woman, it remains a consideration until fetal viability. Infection and hemorrhage are significant complications that should be anticipated in women with active disease. Puerperal infection is particularly problematic.

Greenlund and associates (2001) reviewed experiences with 17 women with acute leukemia during pregnancy. Of these, 13 had newly diagnosed acute myeloid leukemia, and the remission rate with induction chemotherapy was 70 percent. Importantly, three of four women who elected to delay chemotherapy until after delivery died within days of delivery and just after beginning such therapy. Survival has also improved for women with chronic myelogenous and chronic lymphocytic leukemias. Chronic hairy-cell leukemia has been reported in only six pregnancies (Stiles and colleagues, 1998).

Perinatal Outcome

There are few contemporaneous studies of leukemia treated during pregnancy. In an earlier review of 58 cases, Reynoso and colleagues (1987) reported that 75 percent were diagnosed during the second or third trimesters. Half were acute myelogenous leukemia, and they had a remission rate of 75 percent with chemotherapy. Only 40 percent of these pregnancies resulted in liveborn neonates. Caligiuri and Mayer (1989) reported preterm delivery in about half of women diagnosed during pregnancy. The stillbirth rate was also increased.

Leukemia cells may be seen in the placenta, however, these are usually in the intervillous space, and maternal-to-fetal transmission has never been authenticated (see Chap. 27, p. 581).

Fetal effects of chemotherapy are concerning. For example, treatment for acute promyelocytic leukemia may include all-trans-retinoic-acid (Carradice and associates, 2002; Celo and colleagues, 1994). Also known as tretinoin, this is a potent teratogen (see Chap. 14, p. 324). Although outcomes have been generally good, Siu and colleagues (2002) described transient dilated cardiomyopathy in a newborn exposed to tretinoin in the second trimester. Hansen and colleagues (2001) reported transient oligohydramnios in each of three cycles of intensive multi-agent chemotherapy for leukemia.

MALIGNANT MELANOMA

Melanomas are relatively common in women of childbearing age, and many of these malignancies are first recognized during pregnancy. Their general incidence has been increasing over the past several decades (Katz and associates, 2002; MacKie and co-workers, 2002). The reported incidence of melanoma in pregnancy ranges widely from 0.03 to 2.8 per 1000 live births (Wong and Strassner, 1990; Smith and associates, 2003). Because many are treated on an outpatient basis, they are not entered into a tumor registry and are thus underreported (Salopek and colleagues, 1995).

Melanomas are most common in light-skinned Caucasians. More than 90 percent originate in the skin from pigment-producing melanocytes, usually arising from a preexisting nevus. Any suspicious "behavior" in a pigmented cutaneous lesion warrants a biopsy, including changes in contour, surface elevation, discoloration, itching, bleeding, or ulceration.

Staging of Melanomas

Staging is by clinical findings: In stage I, there are no palpable lymph nodes; in stage II, lymph nodes are palpable; in stage III, there are distant metastases. Tumor thickness is the single most important predictor of survival in stage I patients. The *Clark classification* is most widely used and includes five levels of involvement by depth into the epidermis, dermis, and subcutaneous fat. Alternatively, the *Breslow scale* measures tumor thickness and size, in addition to depth of invasion.

Pregnancy and Melanoma

There is probably little interaction between pregnancy and melanomas (Lens and Bataille, 2008). Previously, it had been widely held that the prognosis was worse during pregnancy and that future pregnancies increased the recurrence risk. This was disputed by Holly (1986) in his review of 11 studies. He concluded that there were no adverse effects on survival if melanoma was diagnosed during pregnancy or if pregnancy developed in a woman with a preexisting melanoma. These findings are supported by the later observations of Lens and colleagues (2004). Somewhat related, Lea and associates (2006) reported that a change in nevi during pregnancy was a risk factor for melanoma.

Overall, prognosis is determined by the stage, and women with deep cutaneous invasion or regional node involvement have a much poorer prognosis. MacKie (1999) from the World Health Organization Melanoma Programme reported that women diagnosed during pregnancy had significantly greater tumor thickness. These women have a correspondingly higher mortality rate compared with women whose melanoma was diagnosed before or after pregnancy (**Fig. 57-2**). Survival is equivalent, however, stage-for-stage, between pregnant and non-

pregnant women (Kjems and Krag, 1993). Finally, therapeutic abortion does not appear to improve survival (Dipaola and colleagues, 1997).

Treatment

Primary surgical treatment for melanoma is determined by the stage of the disease and includes wide local resection, sometimes with extensive regional lymph node dissection. Schwartz and associates (2003) have recommended sentinel lymph node mapping and biopsy using ^{99m}Tc-sulfur colloid, which has a fetal dose of less than 100 mGy (see Chap. 41, p. 920). Cascinelli and co-workers (1998) reported that routine regional node dissection improved survival in nonpregnant patients with microscopic metastases. Although prophylactic chemotherapy or immunotherapy is usually avoided during pregnancy, chemotherapy should be given if indicated by tumor stage and maternal prognosis. In most cases of distant metastatic melanoma, treatment is at best palliative.

Sixty percent of recurrences manifest by 2 years, and 90 percent by 5 years. Thus, most recommend that pregnancy be avoided for 3 to 5 years after initial treatment. Subsequent pregnancies in woman with localized melanoma do not appear to have an adverse effect on survival (Driscoll and Grant-Kels, 2009). Importantly, there do not appear to be adverse effects from oral contraceptive use in these women (Katz and associates, 2002; Schwartz and colleagues, 2003).

Placental Metastases

Metastasis of any tumor type to the placenta or fetus is uncommon. As discussed in Chapter 27 (p. 581), a third of such cases are from malignant melanoma. In an extensive review, Alexander

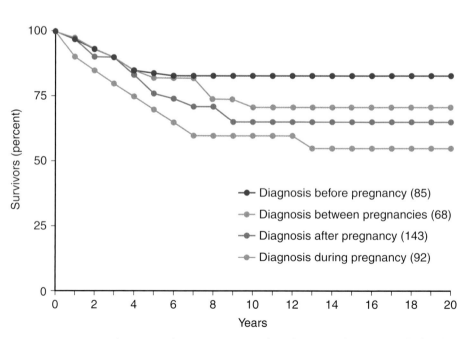

FIGURE 57-2 Disease-free survival in 388 women with malignant melanoma enrolled in the World Health Organization Melanoma Programme. Decreased survival in women diagnosed during pregnancy is due to increased thickness of tumors. (Modified from *The Lancet*, Vol. 337, No. 8742, RM MacKie, R Bufalino, A Morabito, et al., Lack of effect of pregnancy on outcome of melanoma, pp. 653–655, Copyright 1991, with permission from Elsevier.)

and colleagues (2003) found that placental metastasis had been reported in 27 cases of melanoma. Five of the six infants who were affected died of metastatic tumor. Trumble and colleagues (2005) reported transplacental melanoma metastasis to the fetal posterior cranial fossa which manifested at 7 months of age and ultimately proved fatal.

REPRODUCTIVE TRACT NEOPLASIA

Combined together, genital tract cancers are the most common malignancies encountered during pregnancy. Cervical cancer comprises almost 70 percent of these as shown in Figure 57-3. Advent of the quadrivalent HPV-6/11/16/18 vaccine—*Gardasil*—should decrease the incidence of high-grade dysplasia and thence cervical carcinoma (American College of Obstetricians and Gynecologists, 2006; FUTURE II study group, 2007). In addition, neonatal respiratory papillomatosis should also decrease (Paavonen, 2008).

Cervical Neoplasia

The effects of pregnancy and delivery on premalignant and malignant epithelial cervical lesions are not understood completely. It is well known that certain types of human papillomavirus (HPV) are associated with high-grade intraepithelial lesions and invasive cancer. Fife and colleagues (1996) found an increased incidence of high-cancer-risk viruses—HPV types 16, 18, 31, 35, 45, 51, 52 and 56—when they compared pregnant with nonpregnant women. Pregnancy provides an opportune time to screen for premalignant and malignant cervical disease, especially in women who do not seek or have access to routine healthcare (American College of Obstetricians and Gynecologists, 2002; Hunter and associates, 2008).

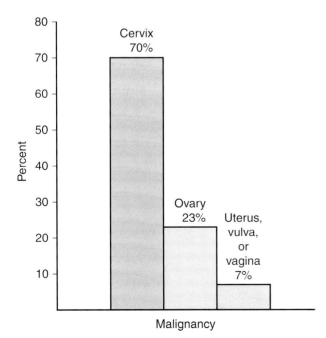

FIGURE 57-3 Frequency of reproductive-tract malignancies in 844 pregnant women. (Data from Haas, 1984; Lutz, 1977; Smith, 2003, and all their colleagues.)

Abnormal Cytological Results

The incidence of abnormal cervical cytology during pregnancy is at least as high as that reported for nonpregnant women. This is despite the fact that Papanicolaou smear evaluation is more difficult during pregnancy (Connor, 1998). Several types of pathological cellular changes may be identified with cervical cytology, and recommendations for their management have been summarized in the American Society for Colposcopy and Cervical Pathology Consensus Guidelines (Wright and colleagues, 2007a):

1. *Atypical squamous cells of undetermined significance (ASCUS)*—management mirrors that for nonpregnant women. It is acceptable to defer colposcopy until at least 6 weeks postpartum

2. *Low-grade squamous intraepithelial lesions (LSIL)*—colposcopy is preferred for pregnant, nonadolescent women. However, deferring the initial colposcopy until at least 6 weeks postpartum is acceptable. Additional colposcopic and cytological examinations during pregnancy are not encouraged unless evidence of advanced disease is noted during colposcopy

3. *High-grade squamous intraepithelial lesions (HSIL)*—it is recommended that colposcopic examination be performed by clinicians with experience in pregnancy-induced cytological changes. Lesions suspicious for high-grade disease or cancer should be biopsied. In the event of unsatisfactory colposcopy, repeat examination should be performed in 12 weeks. After delivery, repeat cytology or colposcopy should generally be delayed for at least 6 weeks to allow reparative healing

4. *Atypical glandular cells (AGC)*—initial evaluation is identical for that of nonpregnant women and colposcopy is recommended. For obvious reasons, endocervical curettage should not be performed during pregnancy.

Colposcopy and Biopsy. During pregnancy, colposcopic evaluation is easier to perform because the transformation zone is better exposed due to physiological eversion. Colposcopically directed biopsies are used liberally to assess any suspicious lesions (Palle and co-workers, 2000). Multiple biopsies need not all be taken on one occasion but rather may be obtained over time. Biopsy sites may actively bleed because of hyperemia, but this can be stopped with Monsel solution, silver nitrate, vaginal packing, or suture.

Loop electrosurgical excision procedure (LEEP) and cone biopsy usually are reserved to exclude invasive cancer. If possible, conization is avoided in pregnant women because of an increased incidence of hemorrhage, abortion, and preterm labor. Indeed, conization during pregnancy is less than satisfactory for two main reasons:

1. The epithelium and underlying stroma within the endocervical canal cannot be excised extensively because of the risk of membrane rupture. Of 376 conizations during pregnancy reviewed by Hacker and colleagues (1982), residual neoplasia was found in 43 percent of subsequent specimens

2. Blood loss is common. Averette and colleagues (1970) reported that nearly 10 percent of 180 pregnant women required transfusion after cone biopsy.

Cervical Intraepithelial Neoplasia

Women with histologically confirmed intraepithelial neoplasia may be followed with cytology and colposcopically directed biopsies, allowed to delivery vaginally, and provided definitive treatment after delivery. Therefore, colposcopic examination during pregnancy should have the exclusion of invasive cancer as its primary goal (American College of Obstetricians and Gynecologists, 2008). For pregnant women with *cervical intraepithelial neoplasia (CIN) 1*, the recommended management is reevaluation postpartum. For those with CIN 2 or 3 in the absence of invasive disease or advanced pregnancy, additional colposcopic and cytological examinations are acceptable at intervals no more frequent than every 12 weeks. Repeat biopsy is recommended only if appearance of the lesion worsens or if cytology suggests invasive cancer. Alternatively, deferring reevaluation until at least 6 weeks postpartum is acceptable (Wright and co-workers, 2007b).

In a study by Yost and colleagues (1999), there was spontaneous postpartum regression in 68 percent of women with CIN 2 and 70 percent of those with CIN 3 neoplasia. Although 7 percent of women with CIN 2 lesions progressed to CIN 3, no lesion progressed to invasive carcinoma. Ackermann and colleagues (2006) described the outcomes of 77 women with carcinoma in situ (CIS) diagnosed during pregnancy and managed conservatively. One third had postpartum regression, two thirds had persistent CIS, and only two women had microinvasive cancer diagnosed by cone biopsy after delivery. For adenocarcinoma in situ (AIS), management is similar as for CIN 3. Lacour and colleagues (2005) performed cold knife conization in five of 11 such women before 19 weeks.

Thus, unless invasive cancer is identified, treatment of these lesions antepartum is not recommended (Wright and co-workers, 2007b). A diagnostic excisional procedure is recommended only if invasion is suspected.

Invasive Cervical Cancer

The incidence of invasive carcinoma has been cited to be about 1 per 2000 pregnancies (Anderson and colleagues, 2001). In our experiences with a high-risk population both from Parkland Hospital and from the University of Alabama, invasive cervical cancer is not nearly so common. The incidence is probably closer to that of 1 in 27,000 as reported by Smith and colleagues (2003).

Pregnancy impedes both the staging and treatment of cervical carcinoma. Cervical cancer is staged clinically rather than surgically. The extent of cancer is more likely to be underestimated in pregnant women. Specifically, induration of the base of the broad ligaments, which characterizes tumor spread beyond the cervix, may be less prominent due to cervical, paracervical, and parametrial softening of pregnancy.

Diagnostically, limited use of CT scanning to evaluate the pelvis is acceptable during pregnancy. MR imaging is a useful adjunct to ascertain disease extent, including urinary tract and lymph node involvement as shown in Figure 57-4 (Gilstrap and colleagues, 2001; Oto and associates, 2007). Cystoscopy and sigmoidoscopy can be performed as necessary to ascertain mucosal involvement.

Stage-for-stage, the survival rate for invasive cervical carcinoma is not profoundly different for pregnant and nonpregnant women. Van der Vange and colleagues (1995) performed a case-

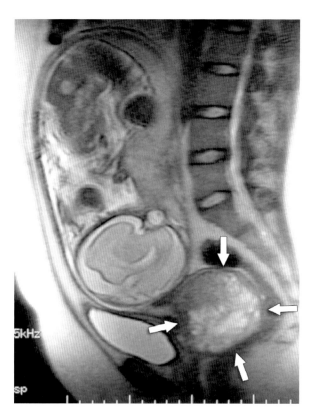

FIGURE 57-4 Sagittal T-2 weighted magnetic resonance image of a gravid uterus at 32 weeks' gestation with a large cervical mass representing carcinoma (*arrows*).

control study of 44 women with pregnancy-associated cervical cancer. The overall 5-year survival rate was approximately 80 percent in both pregnant women and nonpregnant controls.

Management. Treatment of cervical cancer in pregnant women is individualized and depends on the stage, pregnancy duration, and individual desire to continue pregnancy (Hunter and associates, 2008). The American College of Obstetricians and Gynecologists (2002) recommends a multidisciplinary approach. Treatment for microinvasive disease diagnosed by cone biopsy follows guidelines similar to those for intraepithelial disease. In general, continuation of pregnancy and vaginal delivery are considered safe, and definitive therapy is reserved until postpartum.

On the other hand, invasive cancer demands relatively prompt therapy. During the first half of pregnancy, immediate treatment is advisable but depends on the decision to continue the pregnancy. During the latter half of pregnancy, one option is to await not only fetal viability but also fetal maturity (Greer and colleagues, 1989). In a review of 12 pregnant women past 20 weeks with less than stage IIB carcinoma, van Vliet and colleagues (1998) concluded that delayed treatment was reasonable in women without bulky lesions. Takushi and associates (2002) described outcomes in 28 pregnant women, of whom 22 had stage I disease, and reached similar conclusions. Most other studies of women with early stages of cervical cancer indicate that intentional delay in treatment did not appear to worsen prognosis (American College of Obstetricians and Gynecologists, 2002;

Goff and associates, 2000). Staging using laparoscopic lymphadenopathy is another option (Alouini and associates, 2008).

Preferred treatment for invasive carcinoma in most women with stage I and early stage IIA lesions less than 3 cm is radical hysterectomy plus pelvic lymphadenectomy. Before 20 weeks, hysterectomy is usually performed with the fetus in situ. In later pregnancy, however, hysterotomy may first be necessary.

Although many elect surgery, both radical surgery and radiation result in similar cure rates for early cervical cancer during pregnancy (American College of Obstetricians and Gynecologists, 2002). Surgical treatment is favored because it preserves ovarian and sexual function as well as avoids exposure of the intestinal and urinary tracts to radiation and its adverse effects. Nisker and Shubat (1983) described 49 cases of stage IB cervical cancer complicating pregnancy and reported a 30-percent severe complication rate from radiotherapy compared with only 7 percent with surgery.

There is a growing experience with pregnancy following radical trachelectomy for fertility preservation in stage IB1 and IB2 cervical cancer. Shepherd and colleagues (2006) presented outcomes for 123 such women cared for at their institution. Of 63 women who attempted pregnancy, 19 had 28 live births. All had classical cesarean deliveries, and a fourth were before 32 weeks. Ungár and colleagues (2006) performed abdominal radical trachelectomy prior to 20 weeks for stage IB1 carcinoma in five pregnant women. Although three aborted spontaneously, the other two delivered healthy term newborns. Yahata and associates (2008) treated four women at 16 to 23 weeks for stage IA1 adenocarcinoma with KTP laser conization and all delivered at term. And Van Calsteren and co-workers (2008) reported similar success in a woman at 8 weeks with stage IB2 adenocarcinoma. It is clearly too early to conclude that this approach should be used in lieu of more definitive treatment.

Radiotherapy is given for more extensive cancer. If a woman chooses treatment early in pregnancy, external irradiation is given, and then if spontaneous abortion does not ensue, curettage is performed. During the second trimester, spontaneous abortion may be delayed and may necessitate hysterotomy in up to a fourth of cases. About a week following abortion, external beam radiation therapy is begun, followed by intracavitary radium application. After 24 weeks, the risk of delay to allow fetal pulmonary maturation is unknown, but many judge this to be a reasonable approach, especially for early-stage lesions.

Delivery. The mode of delivery is controversial, especially for small, early-stage lesions. The effect on prognosis of vaginal delivery through a cancerous cervix is unknown (American College of Obstetricians and Gynecologists, 2002). Most favor abdominal delivery based on theoretical considerations that tumor may spread when there is cervical tearing. In addition, bulky or friable lesions may bleed significantly with vaginal delivery. Finally, recurrences in the episiotomy scar have been reported (Cliby and colleagues, 1994). In their review, Goldman and Goldberg (2003) described 12 such cases. In most of these, recurrent lesions were manifest within 6 months, but one woman was asymptomatic for 5 years.

With cesarean delivery, a classical incision is preferred. An incision in the lower uterine segment increases the risk of cutting through tumor, which can cause significant blood loss.

Prognosis. The overall prognosis for all stages of cervical cancer during pregnancy is probably similar to that for nonpregnant women (Sood and Sorosky, 1998). The results from several reports suggest no difference in survival when pregnant women are compared with nonpregnant women (Table 57-4).

TABLE 57-4. Five-Year Survival Rates of Pregnant and Nonpregnant Women Treated for Cervical Cancer

| | 5-Year Survival | | | |
| | Pregnant | | Nonpregnant | |
Investigators	Number	(Percent Survivors)	Number	(Percent Survivors)
Sablinska et al (1977)				
Stage I	114	(72)	208	(76)
Stage II	116	(54)	270	(56)
Lee et al (1981)				
Stage IA	3	(100)	30	(100)
Stage IB—Surgery	17	(93)	156	(91)
Stage IB—Radiation	4	(80)	32	(88)
Nisker and Shubat (1983)				
Stage IB	49	(70)	NS[a]	(87)
Van Der Vange et al (1995)				
Stage IA, IB, IIA	21	(85)	18	(85)

[a]NS = not stated.

Endometrial Carcinoma

Because endometrial carcinoma characteristically develops in women past reproductive age, it is seen only rarely with pregnancy. Schammel and colleagues (1998) reviewed 14 cases and described an additional 5. Most are well-differentiated adenocarcinomas, and treatment usually consists primarily of abdominal hysterectomy and bilateral salpingo-oophorectomy. To preserve fertility in 19 nonpregnant women, these investigators described therapy consisting of curettage with or without progestational therapy. At least four viable newborns subsequently were delivered to these women. Gotlieb and associates (2003) reported 13 nonpregnant women treated with progestins for adenocarcinoma. Four of six women with a recurrence were retreated and responded. At least nine neonates have been delivered to these 13 women. Niwa and associates (2005) reported similar outcomes in 12 women, and Signorelli and co-workers (2009) in 21 women. However, Anderson and associates (2001) emphasized that this approach should not be encouraged as standard therapy.

Ovarian Cancer

Malignant ovarian neoplasms are the fourth most common cause of death from cancer in women. They are the leading cause of death from genital tract cancers and eclipse death rates from cervical and uterine cancers combined (American College of Obstetricians and Gynecologists, 2003a). The incidence of ovarian malignancy during pregnancy is not accurately known. From their review, Rahman and co-workers (2002) reported it to average 1 per 20,000 deliveries. A very similar incidence was reported by Smith and associates (2003) from the large California Cancer Registry database. Because most women now undergo sonography during pregnancy, the detection of adnexal masses has increased concomitantly. Certainly, sonography is indicated for women in whom there is a palpable adnexal mass. As discussed in Chapter 40 (p. 904), about 1 of every 1000 pregnant women undergoes surgical exploration for an adnexal mass. Most tumors are either mature cystic teratomas (dermoids) or benign cystadenomas (Boulay and Podczaski, 1998). Perhaps 5 percent of adnexal neoplasms diagnosed during pregnancy are malignant compared with 15 to 20 percent in nonpregnant women (Jacob and Stringer, 1990; Whitecar and associates, 1999). This is likely due to the younger age of pregnant women and due to the disparate number of corpus luteum cysts.

Pregnancy apparently does not alter the prognosis of most ovarian malignancies, but complications such as torsion and rupture may develop. Occasionally, primary or metastatic ovarian tumors cause maternal virilization during pregnancy (Pather and co-workers, 2007; Powell and associates, 2002; Tinkanen and Kuoppala, 2001).

Management

Sonography can be used to help differentiate cystic masses from solid or multiseptated masses. With simple cysts, expectant management may be acceptable, but the latter usually require surgery for diagnosis. Additional information can be obtained using either CT or MR imaging (see Chap. 40, p. 905).

Treatment of ovarian cancer in pregnant women is similar to that for nonpregnant women, but with appropriate modifications depending on gestational age. After frozen section analysis verifies malignancy, surgical staging with careful inspection of all accessible peritoneal and visceral surfaces is performed (Giuntoli and co-workers, 2006; Yazigi and associates, 1988). Malignant tumors apparently confined to one ovary require complete surgical staging, as do tumors of low malignant potential. Procedures include peritoneal washings for cytology, biopsies of the diaphragmatic surface and peritoneum, omentectomy, and biopsies of pelvic and infrarenal para-aortic lymph nodes. However, because of the gravid uterus, some of these components, especially lymphadenectomy, may not be advisable or even technically feasible. If advanced disease is discovered, bilateral adnexectomy and omentectomy would be indicated to remove most tumor burden. Hysterectomy and aggressive surgical debulking procedures such as bowel resection would rarely be indicated in a pregnant patient. Depending on the gestational age, it may be justified to simply remove the tumor and await fetal maturity. In some cases of aggressive or large-volume disease, chemotherapy can be given during pregnancy while awaiting pulmonary maturation. Although maternal CA125 serum levels may be used to monitor disease response during chemotherapy, these values may be too variable during pregnancy to provide an accurate assessment of clinical response (Aslam and associates, 2000; Spitzer and colleagues, 1998).

Prognosis

In most reports, the majority of ovarian cancers found during pregnancy are common epithelial types (Jolles, 1989). Many of the remainder are germ cell tumors, and in the report from Iran by Behtash and colleagues (2008), almost half were of this type. Any type is possible, and endodermal sinus tumors and Burkitt lymphoma of the ovary have been described (Magloire and colleagues, 2006; Motegi and co-workers, 2007). There have been at least 80 or 90 cases of invasive epithelial cell tumors reported coexistent with pregnancy (Dgani and colleagues, 1989; Rahman and associates, 2002). Because of the relatively young age of the pregnant population, tumors with low malignant potential and stage IA disease are seen more often in pregnant women than in nonpregnant women.

Vulvar Cancer

Invasive squamous cell carcinoma of the vulva is primarily a disease of postmenopausal women and thus is only rarely associated with pregnancy. Even so, any suspicious vulvar lesion detected during pregnancy should be biopsied. In their review, Heller and associates (2000) found 23 cases and described a 28-year-old woman with a 4-cm vulvar lesion noted near term. They concluded that radical surgery for stage I disease was feasible during pregnancy, even in the last trimester. Anderson and colleagues (2001) advised that definitive therapy for vulvar cancer can often be delayed because of its slow progression. This is not always the case, however, as Ogunleye and associates (2004) reported recurrence of vulvar carcinoma 11 weeks after treatment during pregnancy. Treatment is individualized according to the clinical stage and depth of invasion. Vaginal delivery is not contraindicated if the vulvar and inguinal incisions are well healed.

In young women, *vulvar intraepithelial neoplasia* is seen more often than invasive disease and is commonly associated with HPV infection. It may progress to invasive disease, the rate of which seems to have risen in younger women (Messing and Gallup, 1995).

Kuller and colleagues (1990) reviewed five cases of *vulvar sarcoma* first recognized during pregnancy. In four of these, cure was obtained by a variety of therapies. Matsuo and co-workers (2009) evaluated eight cases that were identified during pregnancy or the puerperium. Most present as painless enlarging vulvar masses. Alexander and associates (2004) described a woman with *vulvar melanoma* with placental metastases.

Uterine Leiomyomas

Benign uterine leiomyomas are common in older pregnant women, especially in black women. They are seldom malignant and are considered in detail in Chapter 40 (p. 901).

GASTROINTESTINAL TRACT CANCER

Colorectal Carcinoma

Cancers of the colon and rectum are the second most frequent malignancies in women of all age groups in the United States. Despite that, colorectal tumors seldom complicate pregnancy because they are uncommon before age 40. Smith and colleagues (2003) reported an approximate incidence of 1 per 150,000 deliveries in the California Cancer Registry. Accordingly, fewer than 250 cases of colon cancer have been reported in pregnant women (Walsh and Fazio, 1998). The majority—80 percent—of colorectal carcinomas in pregnant women arise from the rectum.

The most common symptoms of colorectal cancer are abdominal pain, distension, nausea and vomiting, constipation, and rectal bleeding. The diagnosis may be delayed because these symptoms are common in pregnancy. Certainly, if symptoms suggestive of colon disease persist, digital rectal examination, tests for occult blood, and flexible sigmoidoscopy or colonoscopy should be done. Tumors above the peritoneal reflection are uncommon in pregnancy, and Chan and associates (1999a) described only 41 cases in their review. Van Voorhis and Cruikshank (1989) reported two women with colon cancer who had persistent microcytic, hypochromic anemia from occult bleeding.

Treatment of colorectal cancer in pregnant women follows the same general guidelines as for nonpregnant women. When there is no evidence of metastatic disease, surgery is performed. Unfortunately, pregnant women usually present with advanced disease (Walsh and Fazio, 1998). During the first half of the pregnancy, hysterectomy is not necessary to perform colon or rectal resection, and thus therapeutic abortion is not mandated. During later pregnancy, delaying therapy to allow fetal maturation can be considered. Vaginal delivery is usually permitted if obstetrical conditions are favorable, but lower rectal lesions may cause dystocia. Hemorrhage, obstruction, or perforation may force surgical intervention (Minter and colleagues, 2005).

There is no evidence that pregnancy influences the usual course of colorectal cancer (Dahling and associates, 2009). Thus, prognosis is similar to that for identical stages in nonpregnant patients. Carcinoembryonic antigen (CEA) is a useful tumor marker for colon cancer, and although it may be elevated during normal pregnancy, baseline values may be useful (Minter and colleagues, 2005).

Other Gastrointestinal Neoplasms

Gastric cancer is rarely associated with pregnancy, and most reported cases are from Japan. Hirabayashi and associates (1987) reviewed outcomes in 60 pregnant women with this malignancy seen during a 70-year period from 1916 to 1985. A delay in diagnosis during pregnancy is common, and the prognosis is consistently poor (Lee and co-workers, 2009). Davis and Chen (1991) and Chan and colleagues (1999b) each described a woman with gastric cancer who attributed her continued epigastric pain during pregnancy to preexisting peptic ulcer disease. Thus, persistent unexplained upper gastrointestinal symptoms should be evaluated by endoscopy.

Stewart and colleagues (1997) reviewed their experiences with seven pregnancies in five women with *Zollinger–Ellison syndrome*. With this, tumors typically found in the duodenum or pancreas secrete excess gastrin. This leads to excess stomach acid production and gastric ulceration. These authors advise surgical resection before pregnancy, but in women with metastatic disease or in those with previously undiagnosed tumors, antacid and antisecretory treatment during pregnancy usually suffices. Radich and associates (2006) reported a 24-week pregnancy complicated by adenocarcinoma of the small bowel.

At least 21 cases of *carcinoid tumors* complicating pregnancy have been reported. In his review, Durkin (1983) found that most cases were of gastrointestinal origin, and some were incidentally diagnosed at cesarean delivery. *Pancreatic cancer* is rare during pregnancy (Kakoza and co-workers, 2009; Marinoni and associates, 2006). *Primary hepatocellular carcinoma* during pregnancy also is uncommon (Gisi and Floyd, 1999; Hsieh and associates, 1996). Bladerston and co-workers (1998) described a 23-year-old woman at 26 weeks who had a massive intrahepatic cholangiocarcinoma masquerading as HELLP syndrome—hemolysis, elevated liver enzymes, and low platelet count. She died 3 weeks postpartum. Hsu and colleagues (2001) reported spontaneous rupture of hepatocellular carcinoma at 25 weeks that was treated by packing, and pregnancy continued until term.

Gastrointestinal cancers during pregnancy may be discovered as a result of metastases to the ovaries—*Krukenberg tumors*. Obviously, the prognosis is poor in these women (Glišić and co-workers, 2006).

RENAL NEOPLASMS

Walker and Knight (1986) reviewed 71 cases of primary renal neoplasms associated with pregnancy—half were *renal cell carcinoma*. Almost 90 percent of these women had a palpable abdominal mass as the presenting finding. In half, pain was the presenting symptom, and hematuria was also found in half. Only a fourth of these women had the classical triad of hematuria, pain, and palpable mass. Diagnosis of these and other intra-abdominal or retroperitoneal tumors has been improved by CT and MR imaging studies. Smith and co-workers (1994) added nine new cases since 1986 in their updated review. They suggest that earlier diagnosis is common now because of sonography. Fazeli-Matin and co-workers (1998) described partial nephrectomy in a woman with renal carcinoma at 14 weeks, and Sainsbury and colleagues (2004) reported laparoscopic radical nephrectomy for carcinoma at 11 weeks followed by delivery at term. Two recent studies have shown a response to the kinase inhibitors *sunitinib* and *sorafenib* (Escudier and colleagues, 2007; Motzer and co-workers, 2007).

We have encountered only a small number of pregnant women with renal carcinoma during the past 35 years at Parkland Hospital. Either they presented because of painless hematuria, or the tumor was found by abdominal palpation done routinely in conjunction with cesarean delivery. Currently, because of almost universal use of regional analgesia for cesarean delivery, thorough intra-abdominal inspection is seldom routinely performed.

OTHER TUMORS

Thyroid cancers are the most common endocrine malignancies. Morris (1998) has estimated that approximately 10 percent developing during the reproductive years are diagnosed during pregnancy or within the first year after birth. Most thyroid cancers are well-differentiated and follow an indolent course. Tewari and associates (1998) described a woman with Graves thyrotoxicosis and thyroid storm who was subsequently found to also have papillary adenocarcinoma. Rossing and colleagues (2000) have presented intriguing findings suggesting that thyroid stimulation during pregnancy and lactation may result in a transient increased growth of papillary thyroid cancer. Diagnosis is usually by fine-needle aspiration. Treatment consists primarily of surgery performed during the second trimester or after delivery (Nam and associates, 2005).

Soft-tissue and *bone tumors*, although rare in pregnancy, can usually be successfully managed with surgery during pregnancy (Maxwell and associates, 2004). Cheung and co-workers (2009) detailed the difficult management of advanced tongue cancer diagnosed at 25 weeks' gestation.

Tumors of the central nervous system complicated about 1 in 67,000 deliveries in the California Cancer Registry (Smith and co-workers, 2003). Isla and colleagues (1997) described seven cases of primary brain tumors in more than 126,000 deliveries from Hospital La Paz in Madrid. According to Finfer (1991), the types of tumors are the same as for same-aged nonpregnant women, and about a third each are gliomas or meningiomas. Tewari and co-workers (2000) described eight pregnant women with a malignant brain tumor and another two with postpartum gestational choriocarcinoma metastatic to the brain. Maternal outcomes were horrific—five women died, and two survivors had significant neurological defects.

REFERENCES

Ackermann S, Gehrsitz C, Mehihorn G, et al: Management and course of histologically verified cervical carcinoma *in situ* during pregnancy. Acta Obstet Gynecol Scand 85:1134, 2006

Alexander A, Harris RM, Grossman D, et al: Vulvar melanoma: Diffuse melanosis and metastases to the placenta. J Am Acad Dermatol 50(20):293, 2004

Alexander A, Samlowski WE, Grossman D, et al: Metastatic melanoma in pregnancy: Risk of transplacental metastases in the infant. J Clin Oncol 21:2179, 2003

Alouini S, Rida K, Mathevet P: Cervical cancer complicating pregnancy: Implications of laparoscopic lymphadenectomy. Gynecol Oncol 108(3):472, 2008

American College of Obstetricians and Gynecologists: Diagnosis and treatment of cervical carcinomas. Practice Bulletin No. 35, October 2002

American College of Obstetricians and Gynecologists: Cancer of the ovary. Technical Bulletin No. 141, August 2003a

American College of Obstetricians and Gynecologists: Breast cancer screening. Practice Bulletin No. 42, April 2003b

American College of Obstetricians and Gynecologists: Guidelines for diagnostic imaging during pregnancy. Committee Opinion No. 299, September 2004

American College of Obstetricians and Gynecologists: Human papillomavirus vaccination. Committee Opinion No. 344, September 2006

American College of Obstetricians and Gynecologists: Management of abnormal cervical cytology and histology. Practice Bulletin No. 99, December, 2008

Anderson ML, Mari G, Schwartz PE: Gynecologic malignancies in pregnancy. In Barnea ER, Jauniaux E, Schwartz PE (eds): Cancer and Pregnancy. London, Springer, 2001, p 33

Andrieu N, Goldgar DE, Easton DF, et al: Pregnancies, breast-feeding, and breast cancer risk in the International BRCA1/2 Carrier Cohort Study (IBCCS). J Natl Cancer Inst 98:535, 2006

Antoniou AC, Shenton A, Maher ER, et al: Parity and breast cancer risk among BRCA1 and BRCA2. Breast Cancer Res 8:R72, 2006

Armitage JO, Longo DL: Malignancies of lymphoid cells. In Kasper DL, Brauward E, Fauci AS, et al (eds): Harrison's Principles of Internal Medicine, 15th ed, New York, McGraw-Hill, 2005, p 641

Aslam N, Ong C, Woelfer B, et al: Serum CA125 at 11–14 weeks of gestation in women with morphologically normal ovaries. Br J Obstet Gynaecol 107:689, 2000

Ault P, Kantarjian H, O'Brien S, et al: Pregnancy among patients with chronic myeloid leukemia treated with imatinib. J Clin Oncol 24(7):1204, 2006

Averette HE, Mirhashemi R, Moffat FL: Pregnancy after breast carcinoma: The ultimate medical challenge. Cancer 85:2301, 1999

Averette HE, Nasser N, Yankow SL, et al: Cervical conization in pregnancy: Analysis of 180 operations. Am J Obstet Gynecol 106:543, 1970

Avilés A, Diaz-Maqueo JC, Torras V, et al: Non-Hodgkin lymphomas and pregnancy: Presentation of 16 cases. Gynecol Oncol 37:355, 1990

Avilés A, Neri N: Hematological malignancies and pregnancy: A final report of 84 children who received chemotherapy in utero. Clin Lymphoma 2:173, 2001

Barnes MN, Barrett JC, Kimberlin DF, et al: Burkitt lymphoma in pregnancy. Obstet Gynecol 92:675, 1998

Beadle BM, Woodward WA, Middleton LP, et al: The impact of pregnancy on breast cancer outcomes in women < or = 35 years. Cancer 115(6):1174, 2009

Behtash N, Karimi Zarchi M, Modares Gilani M, et al: Ovarian carcinoma associated with pregnancy: A clinicopathologic analysis of 23 cases and review of the literature. BMC Pregnancy Childbirth 8:3, 2008

Beral V, Bull D, Doll R, et al: Breast cancer and abortion: Collaborative reanalysis of data from 53 epidemiological studies, including 83,000 women with breast cancer from 16 countries. Lancet 363:1007, 2004

Berry DL, Theriault RL, Holmes FA, et al: Management of breast cancer during pregnancy using a standardized protocol. J Clin Oncol 17:855, 1999

Bladerston KD, Tewari K, Azizi F, et al: Intrahepatic cholangiocarcinoma masquerading as the HELLP syndrome (hemolysis, elevated liver enzymes, and low platelet count) in pregnancy: Case report. Am J Obstet Gynecol 179:823, 1998

Bladström A, Anderson H, Olsson H: Worse survival in breast cancer among women with recent childbirth: Results from Swedish population-based register study. Clin Breast Cancer 4:280, 2003

Bonnier P, Romain S, Dilhuydy JM, et al: Influence of pregnancy on the outcome of breast cancer: A case-control study. Int J Cancer 72:720, 1997

Boulay R, Podczaski E: Ovarian cancer complicating pregnancy. Obstet Gynecol Clin North Am 25:3856, 1998

Bradley B, Fleck A, Osei EK: Normalized data for the estimation of fetal radiation dose from radiotherapy of the breast. Br J Radiol 79:818, 2006

Brent RL: The effect of embryonic and fetal exposure to x-ray, microwaves, and ultrasound: Counseling the pregnant and nonpregnant patient about these risks. Semin Oncol 16:347, 1989

Brent RL: Utilization of developmental basic science principles in the evaluation of reproductive risks from pre- and postconception environmental radiation exposures. Teratology 59:182, 1999

Briggs GG, Freeman RK, Yaffe SJ: Drugs in Pregnancy and Lactation, 6th ed. Philadelphia, Lippincott Williams & Wilkins, 2002

Caligiuri MA, Mayer RJ: Pregnancy and leukemia. Semin Oncol 16:388, 1989

Cardonick E, Iacobucci A: Use of chemotherapy during human pregnancy. Lancet Oncol 5:283, 2004

Carradice D, Austin N, Bayston K, et al: Successful treatment of acute promyelocytic leukaemia during pregnancy. Clin Lab Haematol 24:307, 2002

Cascinelli N, Morabito A, Santinami M, et al: Immediate or delayed dissection of regional nodes in patients with melanoma of the trunk: A randomized trial. Lancet 351:793, 1998

Catlin EA, Roberts JD Jr, Erana R, et al: Transplacental transmission of natural-killer-cell lymphoma. N Engl J Med 341:85, 1999

Celo JS, Kim EK, Houlihan C, et al: Acute promyelocytic leukemia in pregnancy: All-trans retinoic acid as a newer therapeutic option. Obstet Gynecol 83:808, 1994

Centers for Disease Control and Prevention Morbidity and Mortality Weekly Report: Decline in breast cancer incidence—United States, 1999–2003, MMWR 56:549, 2007

Chan YM, Ngai SW, Lao TT: Colon cancer in pregnancy. A case report. J Reprod Med 44:733, 1999a

Chan YM, Ngai SW, Lao TT: Gastric adenocarcinoma presenting with persistent, mild gastrointestinal symptoms in pregnancy: A case report. J Reprod Med 44:986, 1999b

Cheung EJ, Wagner H Jr, Botti JJ, et al: Advanced oral tongue cancer in a 22-year-old pregnant woman. Ann Otol Rhinol Laryngol 118(1):21, 2009

Clark H, Kurinczuk JJ, Lee AJ, et al: Obstetric outcomes in cancer survivors. Obstet Gynecol 110(4):849, 2007

Cliby WA, Dodson MK, Podratz KC: Cervical cancer complicated by pregnancy: Episiotomy site recurrences following vaginal delivery. Obstet Gynecol 84:179, 1994

Connor JP: Noninvasive cervical cancer complicating pregnancy. Obstet Gynecol Clin North Am 25:331, 1998

Dahling MT, Xing G, Cress R, et al: Pregnancy-associated colon and rectal cancer: Perinatal and cancer outcomes. J Matern Fetal Neonatal Med 22(3):204, 2009

Davis JL, Chen MD: Gastric carcinoma presenting as an exacerbation of ulcers during pregnancy: A case report. J Reprod Med 36:450, 1991

Dgani R, Shoham Z, Atar E, et al: Ovarian carcinoma during pregnancy: A study of 23 cases in Israel between the years 1960 and 1984. Gynecol Oncol 33:326, 1989

Dipaola RS, Goodin S, Ratzell M, et al: Chemotherapy for metastatic melanoma during pregnancy. Gynecol Oncol 66:526, 1997

Doll DC, Ringenberg QS, Yarbro JW: Management of cancer during pregnancy. Arch Intern Med 148:2058, 1988

Donnez J, Dolmans MM, Demylle D, et al: Livebirth after orthotopic transplantation of cryopreserved ovarian tissue. Lancet 364:1405, 2004

Dow KH, Harris JR, Roy C: Pregnancy after breast-conserving surgery and radiation therapy for breast cancer. J Natl Cancer Inst Monogr 16:131, 1994

Driscoll MS, Grant-Kels JM: Nevi and melanoma in the pregnant woman. Clin Dermatol 27(1):116, 2009

Dunn JS Jr, Anderson CD, Brost BC: Breast carcinoma metastatic to the placenta. Obstet Gynecol 94:846, 1999

Durkin JW Jr: Carcinoid tumor and pregnancy. Am J Obstet Gynecol 145:757, 1983

Escudier B, Eisen T, Stadler WM, et al: Sorafenib in advanced clear-cell renal-cell carcinoma. N Engl J Med 345(2):125, 2007

Falcone T, Bedaiwy MA: Fertility preservation and pregnancy outcome after malignancy. Curr Opin Obstet Gynecol 17(1):21, 2005

Falconer AD, Ferns P: Pregnancy outcomes following treatment of cancer. J Obstet Gynaecol 22:43, 2002

Fazeli-Matin S, Goldfarb DA, Novick AC: Renal and adrenal surgery during pregnancy. Urology 52:510, 1998

Fey MF, Surbek D: Leukaemia and pregnancy. Recent Results Cancer Res 178:97, 2008

Fife KH, Katz BP, Roush J, et al: Cancer-associated human papillomavirus types are selectively increased in the cervix of women in the first trimester of pregnancy. Am J Obstet Gynecol 174:1487, 1996

Finfer SR: Management of labour and delivery in patients with intracranial neoplasms. Br J Anaesth 67:784, 1991

Fisher B, Anderson S, Bryant J, et al: Twenty-year follow-up of a randomized trial comparing total mastectomy, lumpectomy, and lumpectomy plus irradiation for the treatment of invasive breast cancer. N Engl J Med 347:1233, 2002

Friedman E, Kotsopoulos J, Lubinski J, et al: Spontaneous and therapeutic abortions and the risk of breast cancer among BRCA mutation carriers. Breast Cancer Res 8:R15, 2006

FUTURE II Study Group: Quadrivalent vaccine against human papillomavirus to prevent high-grade cervical lesions. N Engl J Med 356:1915, 2007

García-Manero M, Royo MP, Espinos J, et al: Pregnancy associated breast cancer. Eur J Surg Oncol 35(2):215, 2009

Gentilini O, Masullo M, Rotmensz N, et al: Breast cancer diagnosed during pregnancy and lactation: Biological features and treatment options. Eur J Surg Oncol 31:232, 2005

Gershenson DM: Menstrual and reproductive function after treatment with combination chemotherapy for malignant ovarian germ cell tumors. J Clin Oncol 6:270, 1988

Gilstrap LG, Van Dorsten PV, Cunningham FG (eds): Cancer in pregnancy. In Operative Obstetrics, 2nd ed. New York, McGraw-Hill, 2001

Gisi P, Floyd R: Hepatocellular carcinoma in pregnancy: A case report. J Reprod Med 44:65, 1999

Giuntoli RL II, Vang RS, Bristow RE: Evaluation and management of adnexal masses during pregnancy. Clin Obstet Gynecol 49(3):492, 2006

Glantz JC: Reproductive toxicology of alkylating agents. Obstet Gynecol Surv 49:709, 1994

Glišić A, Atanacković J: Krukenberg tumor in pregnancy. The lethal outcome. Pathol Oncol Res 12(2):108, 2006

Goff BA, Paley PJ, Koh WJ, et al: Cancer in the pregnant patient. In Hoskins WJ, Perez CA, Young RC (eds): Principles and Practice of Gynecologic Oncology. Philadelphia: Lippincott Williams & Wilkins, 2000

Goldman NA, Goldberg GL: Late recurrence of squamous cell cervical cancer in an episiotomy site after vaginal delivery. Obstet Gynecol 101:1127, 2003

Gotlieb WH, Beiner ME, Shalmon B, et al: Outcome of fertility-sparing treatment with progestins in young patients with endometrial cancer. Obstet Gynecol 102:718, 2003

Green DM, Whitton JA, Stovall M, et al: Pregnancy outcome of female survivors of childhood cancer: A report from the Childhood Cancer Survivor Study. Am J Obstet Gynecol 187:1070, 2002

Greenlund LJ, Letendre L, Tefferi A: Acute leukemia during pregnancy: A single institutional experience in 17 cases. Leuk Lymphoma 41:571, 2001

Greer BE, Easterling TR, McLennan DA, et al: Fetal and maternal considerations in the management of stage I-B cervical cancer during pregnancy. Gynecol Oncol 34:61, 1989

Gwyn K: Children exposed to chemotherapy in utero. J Natl Cancer Inst Monogr 34:69, 2005

Haas JF: Pregnancy in association with newly diagnosed cancer: A population-based epidemiologic assessment. Int J Cancer 34:229, 1984

Hacker NF, Berek JS, Lagasse LD, et al: Carcinoma of the cervix associated with pregnancy. Obstet Gynecol 59:735, 1982

Hahn KM, Johnson PH, Gordon N, et al: Treatment of pregnant breast cancer patients and outcomes of children exposed to chemotherapy in utero. Cancer 107:1219, 2006

Hall EJ: Scientific view of low-level radiation risks. Radiographics 11:509, 1991

Hannigan EV: Cervical cancer in pregnancy. Clin Obstet Gynecol 33:837, 1990

Hansen WF, Fretz P, Hunter SK, et al: Leukemia in pregnancy and fetal response to multiagent chemotherapy. Obstet Gynecol 97:809, 2001

Heller DS, Cracchiolo B, Hameed M, et al: Pregnancy-associated invasive squamous cell carcinoma of the vulva in a 28-year-old, HIV-negative woman: A case report. J Reprod Med 45:659, 2000

Higgins S, Haffty BG: Pregnancy and lactation after breast-conserving therapy for early stage breast cancer. Cancer 73:2175, 1994

Hirabayashi M, Ueo H, Okudaira Y, et al: Early gastric cancer and a concomitant pregnancy. Am Surg 53:730, 1987

Holly EA: Melanoma and pregnancy. Recent Results Cancer Res 102:118, 1986

Horning SJ, Hoppe RT, Kaplan HS, et al: Female reproductive potential after treatment for Hodgkin's disease. N Engl J Med 304:1377, 1981

Hsieh TT, Hou HC, Hsu JJ, et al: Term delivery after hepatocellular carcinoma resection in previous pregnancy. Acta Obstet Gynecol Scand 75:77, 1996

Hsu KL, Ko SF, Cheng YF, et al: Spontaneous rupture of hepatocellular carcinoma during pregnancy. Obstet Gynecol 98:913, 2001

Hudis CA: Trastuzumab—mechanism of action and use in clinical practice. N Engl J Med 357:39, 2007

Hunter MI, Monk BJ, Tewari KS: Cervical neoplasia in pregnancy. Part 1: Screening and management of preinvasive disease. Am J Obstet Gynecol 199(1):3, 2008

Hunter MI, Tewari KS, Monk BJ: Cervical neoplasia in pregnancy. Part 2: Current treatment of invasive disease. Am J Obstet Gynecol 199(1):10, 2008

Ishida T, Yoko T, Kasumi F: Clinical pathological characteristics and progress of breast cancer patients associated with pregnancy and lactation. Analysis of case-control study in Japan. Jpn J Cancer Res 83:1143, 1992

Isla A, Alvarez F, Gonzalez A, et al: Brain tumor and pregnancy. Obstet Gynecol 89:19, 1997

Ives A, Saunders C, Bulsara M, et al: Pregnancy after breast cancer: Population based study. BMJ 334:194, 2006

Jacob JH, Stringer CA: Diagnosis and management of cancer during pregnancy. Semin Perinatol 14:79, 1990

Jacobs C, Donaldson SS, Rosenberg SA, et al: Management of the pregnant patient with Hodgkin's disease. Ann Intern Med 95:669, 1981

Jernström H, Lubinski J, Lynch HT, et al: Breast-feeding and the risk of breast cancer in BRCA1 and BRCA2 mutation carriers. J Natl Cancer Inst 96(14):1094, 2004

Jeruss JS, Woodruff TK: Preservation of fertility in patients with cancer. N Engl J Med 360(9):902, 2009

Johannsson O, Loman N, Borg A, et al: Pregnancy-associated breast cancer in BRCA1 and BRCA2 germ-line mutation carriers. Lancet 352:1359, 1998

Jolles CJ: Gynecologic cancer associated with pregnancy. Semin Oncol 16:417, 1989

Kakoza RM, Vollmer CM Jr, Stuart KE, et al: Pancreatic adenocarcinoma in the pregnant patient: A case report and literature review. J Gastrointest Surg 13(3):535, 2009

Kaldor JM, Day NE, Clarke EA, et al: Leukemia following Hodgkin's disease. N Engl J Med 322:7, 1990

Katz VL, Farmer RM, Dotters D: Focus on primary care: From nevus to neoplasm: Myths of melanoma in pregnancy. Obstet Gynecol Surv 57:112, 2002

King RM, Welch JS, Martin JK Jr, et al: Carcinoma of the breast associated with pregnancy. Surg Gynecol Obstet 160:228, 1985

Kjems E, Krag C: Melanoma and pregnancy. Acta Oncol 32:371, 1993

Kroman N, Jensen MB, Melbye M, et al: Should women be advised against pregnancy after breast-cancer treatment? Lancet 350:319, 1997

Kuller JA, Zucker PK, Peng TC: Vulvar leiomyosarcoma in pregnancy. Am J Obstet Gynecol 162:164, 1990

Lacour RA, Garner EIO, Molpus KL, et al: Management of cervical adenocarcinoma in situ during pregnancy. Am J Obstet Gynecol 192:1449, 2005

Langagergaard V, Gislum M, Skriver MV, et al: Birth outcome in women with breast cancer. Br J Cancer 94:142, 2006

Langagergaard V, Horvath-Puho E, Norgaard M, et al: Hodgkin's disease and birth outcome: A Danish nationwide cohort study. Br J Cancer 98(1):183, 2008

Larsen EC, Schmiegelow K, Rechnitzer C, et al: Radiotherapy at a young age reduces uterine volume of childhood cancer survivors. Acta Obstet Gynecol Scand 83:96, 2004

Larson PS, Ungarelli RA, de Las Morenas A, et al: In utero exposure to diethylstilbestrol (DES) does not increase genomic instability in normal or neoplastic breast epithelium. 107:212, 2006

Lea CS, Holly EA, Hartge P, et al: Reproductive risk factors for cutaneous melanoma in women: A case-control study. Am J Epidemiol 165(5):505, 2006

Leach MO, Boggis CR, Dixon AK, et al: Screening with magnetic resonance imaging and mammography of a UK population at high familial risk of breast cancer: A prospective multicentre cohort study (MARIBS) Lancet 365:1769, 2005

Lee HJ, Lee IK, Kim JW, et al: Clinical characteristics of gastric cancer associated with pregnancy. Dig Surg 26(1):31, 2009

Lee RB, Neglia W, Park RC: Cervical carcinoma in pregnancy. Obstet Gynecol 58:584, 1981

Lens M, Bataille V: Melanoma in relation to reproductive and hormonal factors in women: Current review on controversial issues. Cancer Causes Control 19(5):437, 2008

Lens MB, Rosdahl I, Ahlbom A, et al: Effect of pregnancy on survival in women with cutaneous malignant melanoma. J Clin Oncol 22:4369, 2004

Levy C, Pereira L, Dardarian T, et al: Solid pseudopapillary pancreatic tumor in pregnancy. A case report. J Reprod Med 49:61, 2004

Li FP, Fine W, Jaffe N, et al: Offspring of patients treated for cancer in childhood. J Natl Cancer Inst 62:1193, 1979

Lutz MH, Underwood PB Jr, Rozier JC, et al: Genital malignancy in pregnancy. Am J Obstet Gynecol 129:536, 1977

MacKie RM: Pregnancy and exogenous hormones in patients with cutaneous malignant melanoma. Curr Opin Oncol 11:129, 1999

MacKie RM, Bray CA, Hole DJ, et al: Incidence of and survival from malignant melanoma in Scotland: An epidemiological study. Lancet 360:587, 2002

MacKie RM, Bufalino R, Morabito A, et al: Melanoma and pregnancy. Lancet 337(8757):1607, 1991

Magloire LK, Pettker CM, Buhimschi CS, et al: Burkitt's lymphoma of the ovary in pregnancy. Obstet Gynecol 108:743, 2006

Maltaris T, Beckmann MW, Dittrich R: Review. Fertility preservation for young female cancer patients. In Vivo 23(1):123, 2009

Marinoni, E, Di Netta T, Caramanico L, et al: Metastatic pancreatic cancer in late pregnancy: A case report and review of the literature. J Matern Fetal Neonatal Med 19(4):247, 2006

Matsuo K, Eno ML, Im DD, et al: Pregnancy and genital sarcoma: A systematic review of the literature. Am J Perinatol Mar 13, (Epub ahead of print) 2009

Maxwell C, Barzilay B, Shah V, et al: Maternal and neonatal outcomes in pregnancies complicated by bone and soft-tissue tumors. Obstet Gynecol 104:344, 2004

Melbye M, Wohlfahrt J, Lei U, et al: Alpha-fetoprotein levels in maternal serum during pregnancy and maternal breast cancer incidence. J Natl Cancer Inst 92:1001, 2000

Messing MJ, Gallup DG: Carcinoma of the vulva in young women. Obstet Gynecol 86:51, 1995

Minter A, Malik R, Ledbetter L, et al: Colon cancer in pregnancy. Cancer Control 12(3):196, 2005

Mondi MM, Cuenca RE, Ollila DW, et al: Sentinel lymph node biopsy during pregnancy: Initial clinical experience. Ann Surg Oncol 14(1):218, 2007

Morris PC: Thyroid cancer complicating pregnancy. Obstet Gynecol Clin North Am 25:401, 1998

Motegi M, Takakura S, Takano H, et al: Adjuvant chemotherapy in a pregnant woman with endodermal sinus tumor of the ovary. Obstet Gynecol 109(2):537, 2007

Motzer RJ, Hutson TE, Tomczak P, et al: Sunitinib versus interferon alfa in metastatic renal-cell carcinoma. N Engl J Med 346(2):115, 2007

Muslin M, Goldberg J, Hageboutros A: Chemo and radiation therapy during pregnancy. In Barnea ER, Jauniaux E, Schwartz PE (eds): Cancer and Pregnancy. London, Springer, 2001, p 108

Nam K, Yoon JH, Chang H, et al: Optimal timing of surgery in well-differentiated thyroid carcinoma detected during pregnancy. J Surg Oncol 91:199, 2005

Nettleton J, Long J, Kuban D, et al: Breast cancer during pregnancy: Quantifying the risk of treatment delay. Obstet Gynecol 87:414, 1996

Nicklas A, Baker M: Imaging strategies in pregnant cancer patients. Semin Oncol 27:623, 2000

Nisker JA, Shubat M: Stage IB cervical carcinoma and pregnancy: Report of 49 cases. Am J Obstet Gynecol 145:203, 1983

Niwa K, Tagami K, Lian Z, et al: Outcome of fertility-preserving treatment in young women with endometrial carcinomas. Br J Obstet Gynaecol 112:317, 2005

Nugent P, O'Connell TX: Breast cancer and pregnancy. Arch Surg 120:1221, 1985

Oeffinger KC, Mertens AC, Sklar CA, et al: Chronic health conditions in adult survivors of childhood cancer. N Engl J Med 355(15):1572, 2006

Ogunleye D, Lewin SN, Huettner P, et al: Recurrent vulvar carcinoma in pregnancy. Gynecol Oncol 95:400, 2004

Oto A, Ernst R, Jesse MK, et al: Magnetic resonance imaging of the chest, abdomen, and pelvis in the evaluation of pregnant patients with neoplasms. Am J Perinatol 24(4):243, 2007

Paavonen J: Human papillomavirus infection and the development of cervical cancer and related genital neoplasias. Int J Infect Dis 11 Suppl 2:S3, 2007

Palle C, Bangsboll S, Andreasson B: Cervical intraepithelial neoplasia in pregnancy. Acta Obstet Gynecol Scand 79:306, 2000

Partridge AH, Garber JE: Long-term outcomes of children exposed to antineoplastic agents in utero. Semin Oncol 27:712, 2000

Pather S, Atkinson K, Wang I, et al: Virilization in pregnancy due to a borderline mucinous ovarian tumor. J Obstet Gynaecol Res 33(3):384, 2007

Patrizio P, Butts S, Caplan A: Ovarian tissue preservation and future fertility: Emerging technologies and ethical considerations. J Natl Cancer Inst Monogr 34:107, 2005

Pavlidis NA: Coexistence of pregnancy and malignancy. Oncologist 7:279, 2002

Peleg D, Ben-Ami M: Lymphoma and leukemia complicating pregnancy. Obstet Gynecol Clin North Am 25:365, 1998

Pelsang RE: Diagnostic imaging modalities during pregnancy. Obstet Gynecol Clin North Am 25:287, 1998

Petrek JA, Dukoff R, Rogatko A: Prognosis of pregnancy-associated breast cancer. Cancer 67:869, 1991

Pollack RN, Sklarin NT, Rao S, et al: Metastatic placental lymphoma associated with maternal human immunodeficiency virus infection. Obstet Gynecol 81:856, 1993

Powell JL, Bock KA, Gentry JK, et al: Metastatic endocervical adenocarcinoma presenting as a virilizing ovarian mass during pregnancy. Obstet Gynecol 100:1129, 2002

Radich GA, Altinok D, Adsay NV, et al: Papillary adenocarcinoma in a small-bowel duplication in a pregnant woman. Am J Roentgenol 186:895, 2006

Rahman MS, Al-Sibai MH, Rahman J, et al: Ovarian carcinoma associated with pregnancy: A review of 9 cases. Acta Obstet Gynecol Scand 81:260, 2002

Reynoso EE, Shepherd FA, Messner HA, et al: Acute leukemia during pregnancy: The Toronto Leukemia Study Group experience with long-term follow-up of children exposed in utero to chemotherapeutic agents. J Clin Oncol 5:1098, 1987

Robison LL, Green DM, Hudson M, et al: Long-term outcomes of adult survivors of childhood cancer. Results from the Childhood Cancer Survivor Study. Cancer Supplement 104(11):2557, 2005

Rodriguez AO, Chew H, Cress R, et al: Evidence of poorer survival in pregnancy-associated breast cancer. Obstet Gynecol 112(1):71, 2008

Rosenkranz KM, Lucci A: Surgical treatment of pregnancy associated breast cancer. Breast Dis 23:87, 2006

Rossing MA, Voigt LF, Wicklund KG, et al: Reproductive factors and risk of papillary thyroid cancer in women. Am J Epidemiol 151:765, 2000

Sablinska R, Tarlowska L, Stelmachow J: Invasive carcinoma of the cervix associated with pregnancy: Correlation between patient age, advancement of cancer and gestation, and result of treatment. Gynecol Oncol 5:363, 1977

Sainsbury DCG, Dorkin TJ, MacPhail S, et al: Laparoscopic radical nephrectomy in first-trimester pregnancy. Urology 64:1231.e7, 2004

Salopek TG, Marghoob AA, Slade JM, et al: An estimate of the incidence of malignant melanoma in the United States: Based on a survey of members of the American Academy of Dermatology. Dermatol Surg 21:301, 1995

Schammel DP, Mittal KR, Kaplan K, et al: Endometrial adenocarcinoma associated with intrauterine pregnancy: A report of five cases and a review of the literature. Int J Gynecol Pathol 17:327, 1998

Schedin P: Pregnancy-associated breast cancer and metastasis. Nature Reviews/Cancer 6:281, 2006

Schwartz JL, Mozurkewich EL, Johnson TM: Current management of patients with melanoma who are pregnant, want to get pregnant, or do not want to get pregnant. Cancer 97:2130, 2003

Sekar R, Stone RP: Trastuzumab use for metastatic breast cancer in pregnancy. Obstet Gynecol 110:507, 2007

Selevan SG, Lindbohm ML, Hornung RW, et al: A study of occupational exposure to antineoplastic drugs and fetal loss in nurses. N Engl J Med 313:1173, 1985

Shah E, Saunders C: Breast cancer in pregnancy. In Barnea ER, Jauniaux E, Schwartz PE (eds): Cancer and Pregnancy. London, Springer, 2001, p 21

Shen T, Vortmeyer AO, Zhuang Z, et al: High frequency of allelic loss of BRCA2 gene in pregnancy-associated breast carcinoma. J Natl Cancer Inst 91:1686, 1999

Shepherd JH, Spencer C, Herod J, et al: Radical vaginal trachelectomy as a fertility-sparing procedure in women with early-stage cervical cancer—cumulative pregnancy rate in a series of 123 women. Br J Obstet Gynaecol 113:719, 2006

Shousha S: Breast carcinoma presenting during or shortly after pregnancy and lactation. Arch Pathol Lab Med 124:1053, 2000

Shrim A, Garcia-Bournissen F, Maxwell C, et al: Trastuzumab treatment for breast cancer during pregnancy. Can Fam Physician 54(1):31, 2008

Shulman LN, Hitt RA, Ferry JA: Case records of the Massachusetts General Hospital. Case 4-2008. A 33-year-old pregnant woman with swelling of the left breast and shortness of breath. N Engl J Med 358(5):513, 2008

Signorelli M, Caspani G, Bonazzi C, et al: Fertility-sparing treatment in young women with endometrial cancer or atypical complex hyperplasia: A prospective single-institution experience of 21 cases. BJOG 116(1):114, 2009

Signorello LB, Cohen SS, Bosetti C, et al: Female survivors of childhood cancer: Preterm birth and low birth weight among their children. J Natl Cancer Inst 98:1453, 2006

Siu BL, Alonzo MR, Vargo TA, et al: Transient dilated cardiomyopathy in a newborn exposed to idarubicin and all-trans-retinoic acid (ATRA) early in the second trimester of pregnancy. Int J Gynecol Cancer 12:399, 2002

Smith DP, Goldman SM, Beggs DS, et al: Renal cell carcinoma in pregnancy: Report of three cases and review of the literature. Obstet Gynecol 83:818, 1994

Smith LH, Danielsen B, Allen ME, et al: Cancer associated with obstetric delivery: Results of linkage with the California cancer registry. Am J Obstet Gynecol 189:1128, 2003

Sood AK, Sorosky JI: Invasive cervical cancer complicating pregnancy: How to manage the dilemma? Obstet Gynecol Clin North Am 25:343, 1998

Sorosky JI, Scott-Conner CE: Breast disease complicating pregnancy. Obstet Gynecol Clin North Am 25:353, 1998

Souadka A, Zouhal A, Souadka F, et al: Breast cancer and pregnancy: Forty-three cases reported in the National Oncology Institute between 1985 and 1988. Rev Fr Gynecol Obstet 89:67, 1994

Spanheimer PM, Graham MM, Sugg SL, et al: Measurement of uterine radiation exposure from lymphoscintigraphy indicates safety of sentinel lymph node biopsy during pregnancy. Ann Surg Oncol 16(5):1143, 2009

Spitzer M, Kaushal N, Benjamin F: Maternal CA-125 levels in pregnancy and the puerperium. J Reprod Med 43:387, 1998

Stewart CA, Termanini B, Sutliff VE, et al: Management of the Zollinger–Ellison syndrome in pregnancy. Am J Obstet Gynecol 176:224, 1997

Stiles GM, Stanco LM, Saven A, et al: Splenectomy for hairy cell leukemia in pregnancy. J Perinatol 18:200, 1998

Stucker I, Caillard JF, Collin R, et al: Risk of spontaneous abortion among nurses handling antineoplastic drugs. Scand J Work Environ Health 16:102, 1990

Takushi M, Moromizato H, Sakumoto K, et al: Management of invasive carcinoma of the uterine cervix associated with pregnancy: Outcome of intentional delay in treatment. Gynecol Oncol 87:185, 2002

Tangir J, Zelterman D, Ma W, et al: Reproductive function after conservative surgery and chemotherapy for malignant germ cell tumors of the ovary. Obstet Gynecol 101:251, 2003

Tewari K, Balderston KD, Carpenter SE, et al: Papillary thyroid carcinoma manifesting as thyroid storm of pregnancy: Case report. Am J Obstet Gynecol 179:818, 1998

Tewari KS, Cappuccini F, Asrat T, et al: Obstetric emergencies precipitated by malignant brain tumors. Am J Obstet Gynecol 182:1215, 2000

Tinkanen H, Kuoppala T: Virilization during pregnancy caused by ovarian mucinous cystadenocarcinoma. Acta Obstet Gynecol Scand 80:476, 2001

Titus-Ernstoff L, Troisi R, Hatch EE, et al: Mortality in women given diethylstilbestrol during pregnancy. Br J Cancer 95:107, 2006

Travis LB, Hill DA, Dores GM, et al: Breast cancer following radiotherapy and chemotherapy among young women with Hodgkin disease. JAMA 290:465, 2003

Trumble ER, Smith RM, Pearl G, et al: Transplacental transmission of metastatic melanoma to the posterior fossa. J Neurosurg Pediatr 103:191, 2005

Ungár L, Smith JR, Pálfavli L, et al: Abdominal radical trachelectomy during pregnancy to preserve pregnancy and fertility. Obstet Gynecol 108:811, 2006

Van Calsteren K, Hanssens M, Moerman P, et al: Successful conservative treatment of endocervical adenocarcinoma stage Ib1 diagnosed early in pregnancy. Acta Obstet Gynecol Scand 87(2):250, 2008

van der Vange N, Weverling GJ, Ketting BW, et al: The prognosis of cervical cancer associated with pregnancy: A matched cohort study. Obstet Gynecol 85:1022, 1995

van Vliet W, van Loon AJ, ten Hoor KA, et al: Cervical carcinoma during pregnancy: Outcome of planned delay in treatment. Eur J Obstet Gynecol Reprod Biol 79:153, 1998

van Voorhis B, Cruikshank DP: Colon carcinoma complicating pregnancy: A report of two cases. J Reprod Med 34:923, 1989

Velentgas P, Daling JR, Malone KE, et al: Pregnancy after breast carcinoma: Outcomes and influence on mortality. Cancer 85:2424, 1999

Veronesi U, Cascinelli N, Mariani L, et al: Twenty-year follow-up of a randomized study comparing breast-conserving surgery with radical mastectomy for early breast cancer. N Engl J Med 347:1227, 2002

Walker JL, Knight EL: Renal cell carcinoma in pregnancy. Cancer 58:2343, 1986

Walsh C, Fazio VW: Cancer of the colon, rectum, and anus during pregnancy. The surgeon's perspective. Gastroenterol Clin North Am 27:257, 1998

Ward FT, Weiss RB: Lymphoma and pregnancy. Semin Oncol 16:397, 1989

Ward RM, Bristow RE: Cancer and pregnancy: Recent developments. Curr Opin Obstet Gynecol 14:613, 2002

Waxman J: Cancer, chemotherapy and fertility. Br Med J 290:1096, 1985

Wetzler M, Byrd JC, Bloomfield CD: Acute and chronic myeloid leukemia. In Kasper DL, Brauward E, Fauci AS, et al (eds): Harrison's Principles of Internal Medicine, 15th ed, New York, McGraw-Hill, 2005, p 677

Whitecar MP, Turner S, Higby MK: Adnexal masses in pregnancy: A review of 130 cases undergoing surgical management. Am J Obstet Gynecol 181:19, 1999

Williams SF, Schilsky RL: Neoplastic disorders. In Barron WM, Lindheimer MD (eds): Medical Disorders During Pregnancy, 3rd ed. St. Louis, Mosby, 2001, p. 392

Winther JF, Boice JD Jr, Frederiksen K, et al: Radiotherapy for childhood cancer and risk for congenital malformations in offspring: A population-based cohort study. Clin Genet 75(1):50, 2009

Wo JY, Viswanathan AN: Impact of radiotherapy on fertility, pregnancy, and neonatal outcome in female cancer patients. Int J Radiat Oncol Biol Phys 73(5):1304, 2009

Wong DJ, Strassner HT: Melanoma in pregnancy: A literature review. Clin Obstet Gynecol 33:782, 1990

Woo JC, Yu T, Hurd TC: Breast cancer in pregnancy. Arch Surg 138:91, 2003

Wright TC, Massad LS, Dunton CJ, et al: 2006 consensus guidelines for the management of women with abnormal cervical cancer screening tests. Am J Obstet Gynecol, October, p 346, 2007a

Wright TC, Massad LS, Dunton CJ, et al: 2006 consensus guidelines for the management of women with cervical intraepithelial neoplasia or adenocarcinoma in situ. Am J Obstet Gynecol p.340, October, 2007b

Yahata T, Numata M, Kashima K, et al: Conservative treatment of stage IA1 adenocarcinoma of the cervix during pregnancy. Gynecol Oncol 109(1):49, 2008

Yazigi R, Sandstad J, Munoz AK: Primary staging in ovarian tumors of low malignant potential. Gynecol Oncol 31:402, 1988

Yost NP, Santoso JT, McIntire DD, et al: Postpartum regression rates of antepartum cervical intraepithelial neoplasia II and III lesions. Obstet Gynecol 93:359, 1999

Zemlickis D, Lishner M, Degendorfer P, et al: Maternal and fetal outcome after breast cancer in pregnancy. Am J Obstet Gynecol 166:781, 1992

Infectious Diseases

Infections have historically been a major cause of maternal and fetal morbidity and mortality worldwide, and they remain so in the 21st century. Factors such as maternal serological status, timing of infection during pregnancy, mode of acquisition, and immunological status influence disease outcome.

MATERNAL AND FETAL IMMUNOLOGY

Pregnancy-Induced Immunological Changes

Even after intensive study, many of the maternal immunological adaptations to pregnancy are not well elucidated (see Chap. 5, p. 116). Some of the abnormal aspects of human immunity are considered in Chapter 54 (p. 1145). And finally, factors dealing with the maternal-fetal interface that allow immunological tolerance of the fetus as a graft are discussed in Chapter 3 (p. 58). Suffice it to say that these myriad changes also affect to a certain degree maternal response to infections. An under-

standing of fetal and newborn immunology is also imperative as the fetus is susceptible to many of these infections.

Fetal and Newborn Immunology

The active immunological capacity of the fetus and neonate is compromised compared with that of older children and adults. According to Stirrat (1991), fetal cell-mediated and humoral immunity begin to develop by 9 to 15 weeks. The primary fetal response to infection is immunoglobulin M (IgM). Passive immunity is provided by IgG transferred across the placenta. By 16 weeks, this transfer begins to increase rapidly, and by 26 weeks, fetal concentrations are equivalent to those of the mother. After birth, breast feeding is protective against some infections, although this protection begins to decline at 2 months of age (World Health Organization Collaborative Study Team, 2000).

Vertical transmission of infection refers to passage from the mother to her fetus of an infectious agent through the placenta, during labor or delivery, or by breast feeding. Thus, preterm rupture of membranes, prolonged labor, and obstetrical manipulations may increase the risk of neonatal infection. Those occurring less than 72 hours after delivery are usually caused by bacteria acquired in utero or during delivery, whereas infections after that time most likely were acquired afterward. Table 58-1 details specific infections by mode and timing of acquisition.

Neonatal infection, especially in its early stages, may be difficult to diagnose because neonates often fail to express classic clinical signs. If the fetus was infected in utero, there may be depression and acidosis at birth for no apparent reason. The neonate may suck poorly, vomit, or develop abdominal distension. Respiratory insufficiency may develop, which may present similarly to idiopathic respiratory distress syndrome (see Chap. 29, p. 605). The neonate may be lethargic or jittery. The response to sepsis may be hypothermia rather than hyperthermia, and the total leukocyte and neutrophil counts may be depressed.

TABLE 58-1. Specific Causes of Some Fetal and Neonatal Infections

Intrauterine
Transplacental
  Viruses: varicella-zoster, Coxsackie, human parvovirus B19, rubella, cytomegalovirus, human immunodeficiency virus
  Bacteria: listeria, syphilis, *Borrelia*
  Protozoa: toxoplasmosis, malaria
Ascending infection
  Bacteria: group B streptococcus, coliforms
  Viruses: herpes simplex

Intrapartum
Maternal exposure
  Bacteria: gonorrhea, chlamydia, group B streptococcus, tuberculosis, mycoplasmas
  Viruses: herpes simplex, papillomavirus, human immunodeficiency virus, hepatitis B, hepatitis C
External contamination
  Bacteria: staphylococcus, coliforms
  Viruses: herpes simplex, varicella zoster

Neonatal
Human transmission: staphylococcus, herpes simplex virus
Respirators and catheters: staphylococcus, coliforms

Hospital-acquired infections are dangerous for preterm neonates, and individuals who care for them are a major source of infection (Stoll and Hansen, 2003). Ventilatory systems and indwelling venous and arterial umbilical catheters may cause life-threatening infection. Thus, a very-low-birthweight infant who survives the first few days is still at considerable risk of dying from infection acquired in the intensive care nursery.

Ascending infections caused by bacteria—for example, *Escherichia coli*, group B streptococci, and *Ureaplasma urealyticum*—are the most common cause of infectious perinatal mortality from sepsis. In developed countries, 10 to 25 percent of stillbirths may be caused by infectious pathogens (Goldenberg and Thompson, 2003). In high-prevalence areas, syphilis and malaria in nonimmune women are also major causes of stillbirths.

VIRAL INFECTIONS

Varicella-Zoster Virus (VZV)

This double-stranded DNA herpesvirus is acquired predominately during childhood, and 95 percent of adults have serological evidence of immunity (Plourd and Austin, 2005). Primary infection—*varicella* or *chicken pox*—is transmitted by direct contact with an infected individual, although respiratory transmission has been reported. The incubation period is 10 to 21 days, and a nonimmune woman has a 60- to 95-percent risk of becoming infected after exposure. She is then contagious from 1 day prior to the onset of the rash until the lesions are crusted over.

Clinical Manifestations

Varicella infection presents with a 1- to 2-day flulike prodrome, which is followed by pruritic vesicular lesions that crust over in 3 to 7 days. Infection tends to be more severe in adults, and almost half of varicella deaths are within the 5 percent of nonimmune adults (Centers for Disease Control and Prevention, 1999).

Mortality is predominately due to varicella pneumonia, which is thought to be more severe during adulthood and particularly in pregnancy. Harger and associates (2002) reported that 5 percent of infected pregnant women developed pneumonitis. Maternal mortality rates with pneumonia have decreased to 1 to 2 percent (Chandra and colleagues, 1998). Symptoms of pneumonia usually appear 3 to 5 days into the course of illness. It is characterized by fever, tachypnea, dry cough, dyspnea, and pleuritic pain. Nodular infiltrates are similar to other viral pneumonias (see Chapter 46, p. 1003). Although resolution of pneumonitis parallels that of skin lesions, fever and compromised pulmonary function may persist for weeks.

Herpes Zoster. If primary varicella infection is reactivated years later, it causes *herpes zoster* or *shingles* (Gilden and coworkers, 2000). There is no evidence that zoster is more frequent or more severe in pregnant women. And from their review of 366 cases during pregnancy, Enders and associates (1994) found little evidence that zoster causes congenital malformations. Zoster is contagious if blisters are broken, although less so than primary varicella infection.

Diagnosis

Maternal varicella is usually diagnosed clinically. The virus may also be isolated by scraping the vesicle base during primary infection and performing a Tzanck smear, tissue culture, or direct fluorescent antibody testing. Also, available nucleic acid amplification techniques are very sensitive. Congenital varicella may be diagnosed using nucleic acid amplification techniques on amnionic fluid, although a positive result does not correlate well with the development of congenital infection (Mendelson and colleagues, 2006).

Fetal and Neonatal Varicella Infection

In women with chicken pox during the first half of pregnancy, the fetus may develop congenital varicella syndrome. Some features include chorioretinitis, microphthalmia, cerebral cortical atrophy, growth restriction, hydronephrosis, and skin or bone defects (Fig. 58-1) (Auriti and associates, 2009). Enders and co-workers (1994) evaluated 1373 pregnant women with varicella infection. When maternal infection developed before 13 weeks, only two of 472 pregnancies—0.4 percent—had neonates with congenital varicella. The highest risk was between 13 and 20 weeks, during which time seven of 351 exposed fetuses—2 percent—had evidence of congenital varicella. After 20 weeks' gestation, they found no clinical evidence of congenital infection. Thus, congenital infections, particularly after 20 weeks, are uncommon. At least nine case reports have reported central nervous system abnormalities and skin lesions in fetuses who developed congenital varicella in weeks 21 to 28 of gestation (Koren, 2005).

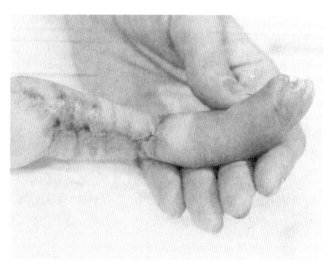

FIGURE 58-1 Atrophy of the lower extremity with bony defects and scarring in a fetus infected during the first trimester by varicella. (Reprinted from Paryani SG, Arvin AM: Intrauterine infection with varicella zoster virus after maternal varicella. *N Engl J Med* 314(24):1542–1546, with permission. Copyright © 1986 Massachusetts Medical Society. All rights reserved.)

Peripartum Infection. Perinatal varicella exposure just before or during delivery, and therefore before maternal antibody has been formed, poses a serious threat to newborns. Attack rates range from 25 to 50 percent, and mortality rates approach 25 percent. In some instances, neonates develop disseminated visceral and central nervous system disease, which is commonly fatal. For this reason, varicella-zoster immune globulin should be administered to neonates born to mothers who have clinical evidence of varicella 5 days before and up to 2 days after delivery. Varicella-zoster immune globulin—*VZIG*—production was discontinued in the United States in 2005. The Centers for Disease Control and Prevention (CDC) (2006c) recommends use of an unlicensed Canadian varicella zoster immune globulin—*VariZIG*. The sole authorized distributor for the United States is FFF Enterprises (Temecula, CA, 1-800-843-7477 or www.fffenterprises.com).

Management

Exposure to Virus

Because most adults (95 percent) are VZV seropositive, even exposed pregnant women with a negative history for chicken pox should be tested for VZV serology. At least 70 percent of these will be seropositive, and thus immune. Exposed pregnant women who are susceptible should be given VariZIG within 96 hours of exposure to prevent or attenuate varicella infection.

Infection

Pregnant women diagnosed with primary varicella infection should be isolated from other pregnant women. Because pneumonia often presents with few symptoms, a chest radiograph is considered. Most women require only supportive care, but those who require intravenous fluids and especially those with pneumonia are hospitalized. Intravenous acyclovir therapy is given—500 mg/m^2 or 10 to 15 mg/kg every 8 hours.

Vaccination

An attenuated live-virus vaccine—*Varivax*—was approved in 1995. Two doses, given 4 to 8 weeks apart, are recommended for adolescents and adults with no history of varicella. This results in 97-percent seroconversion (Centers for Disease Control and Prevention, 2007e). Importantly, vaccine-induced immunity diminishes over time, and the breakthrough infection rate is about 5 percent at 10 years (Chaves and co-workers, 2007). **The vaccine is not recommended for pregnant women and should not be given to women who may become pregnant during the month following each vaccine dose.** A registry of 362 vaccine-exposed pregnancies reports no cases of congenital varicella syndrome or other congenital associated malformations (Shields and colleagues, 2001). The attenuated vaccine virus is not secreted in breast milk. Thus, postpartum vaccination should not be delayed because of breast feeding (Bohlke and associates, 2003).

A vaccine for the prevention of herpes zoster—*Zostavax*—was licensed in 2006 but is currently not recommended for individuals younger than 60 years (Centers for Disease Control and Prevention, 2007a).

Influenza

These respiratory infections are caused by members of the family *Orthomyxoviridae. Influenza A* and *B* form one genus of these RNA viruses, and both cause epidemic human disease. Influenza A viruses are subclassified further by hemagglutinin (H) and neuraminidase (N) surface antigens. Symptoms include fever, dry cough, and systemic symptoms, and infection can be confirmed with rapid enzyme immunoassay or immunofluorescence assay (Salgado and co-workers, 2002).

Influenza A is more serious and usually develops during winter. Infection usually is not life-threatening in otherwise healthy adults, but pregnant women appear to be more susceptible to serious pulmonary involvement (Cox and associates, 2006; Neuzil and colleagues, 1998). In early 2003, widespread influenza A commonly infected pregnant women. At Parkland Hospital, more than 100 women were hospitalized for infection, and 12 percent had pulmonary infiltrates seen on chest radiograph.

Treatment

There are currently two classes of antiviral medications available. The *adamantanes* include amantadine and rimantadine, which were used for years for treatment and chemoprophylaxis of influenza A. In 2005, influenza A resistance to adamantine was reported to be more than 90 percent in the United States, up from 2 percent in 2001. Currently, the Centers for Disease Control and Prevention (2007b) recommends against adamantane use, but the drugs may again be effective for subsequent mutated strains.

The second class of anti-influenzal drugs are *neuraminidase inhibitors* that are highly effective for the treatment of early influenza A and B. *Oseltamivir* is taken orally for both treatment and chemoprophylaxis, and *zanamivir* is inhaled for treatment. During the 2007–2008 flu season, sudden and rapid resistance was detected for H1N1 strains of influenza A (Gooskens and colleagues, 2009). In December 2008, a CDC Health Advisory was issued with recommendations for treatment of influenza A with oseltamivir and amantadine or rimantadine. If the predominate strain in the community is known to be H1N1, then an adamantane derivative is given. If the strain is know to be H3N2, then oseltamivir is given instead. Local isolates can be determined by visiting the Web site for the Centers for Disease Control and Prevention.

There is limited experience with all four of these antiviral agents in pregnant women. They are category C drugs used when the potential benefits outweigh the risks. At Parkland Hospital, we recommend starting oseltamivir treatment within 48 hours of symptom onset (75 mg orally twice daily for 5 days). Prophylaxis with oseltamivir 75 mg orally once daily for 10 days is also recommended for significant exposures.

In the spring of 2009, respiratory infections caused by a novel influenza A H1N1 viral strain were identified. The Centers for Disease Control and Prevention (2009) recommends that pregnant women with confirmed or suspected H1N1 infection should be given treatment with oseltamivir for 5 days. If possible, treatment should begin within 48 hours of symptom onset. Finally, pregnant women who are in close contact with an infected or suspected infected person should receive a 10-day course of chemoprophylaxis with zanamivir or oseltamivir.

Fetal Effects

There is no firm evidence that influenza A virus causes congenital malformations (Irving and colleagues, 2000; Saxén and associates, 1990). Conversely, Lynberg and co-workers (1994) reported increased neural-tube defects in neonates born to women with influenza early in pregnancy possibly associated with early hyperthermia. Finally, there is controversial evidence that fetal exposure to influenza A may predispose to schizophrenia in later life (Kunugi and associates, 1995; McGrath and Castle, 1995).

Prevention

Vaccination against influenza throughout the influenza season, but optimally in October or November, is recommended by the Centers for Disease Control and Prevention (2007a) for all women who will be pregnant during the influenza season. This is especially important for those affected by chronic medical disorders such as diabetes, heart disease, asthma, or human immunodeficiency virus (HIV) infection. Inactivated vaccine prevents clinical illness in 70 to 90 percent of healthy adults, and importantly, there is no evidence of teratogenicity (see Chap. 8, p. 207). Moreover, Zaman and associates (2008) found decreased rates of influenza in infants up to 6 months of age whose mothers were vaccinated during pregnancy.

Only 44 percent of obstetricians who were surveyed provided influenza vaccination in pregnancy (Schrag and co-workers, 2003). Many did not offer vaccine because of reimbursement issues or availability of vaccination elsewhere. Although most

who are offered vaccine choose to be vaccinated, in 2004 only 14 percent of healthy pregnant women received it (Centers for Disease Control and Prevention, 2007a). A trivalent, cold-adapted, live attenuated-virus vaccine was approved for intranasal use in 2003 but is not recommended for pregnant women.

Mumps

This uncommon adult infection is caused by an RNA paramyxovirus. Because of childhood immunization, up to 90 percent of adults are seropositive (Haas and associates, 2005). The virus primarily infects the salivary glands and hence its name—mumps—is derived from Latin, "to grimace." It also may involve the gonads, meninges, pancreas, and other organs. It is transmitted by direct contact with respiratory secretions, saliva, or through fomites. Treatment is symptomatic, and mumps during pregnancy is no more severe than in nonpregnant adults.

The live attenuated Jeryl-Lynn vaccine strain is part of the MMR vaccine—measles, mumps, and rubella—and is contraindicated in pregnancy (American College of Obstetricians and Gynecologists, 2003). No malformations attributable to MMR vaccination in pregnancy have been reported, but pregnancy should be avoided for 30 days after mumps vaccination (Centers for Disease Control and Prevention, 1998, 2002a). The vaccine may be given to susceptible women postpartum, and breast feeding is not a contraindication.

Fetal Effects

Women who develop mumps in the first trimester may have an increased risk of spontaneous abortion. Infection in pregnancy is not associated with congenital malformations, and fetal infection is rare (Centers for Disease Control and Prevention, 1998; Siegel, 1973).

Rubeola (Measles)

Most adults are immune to measles due to childhood immunization. In a study in pregnant women, 17 percent were found to be seronegative (Haas and co-workers, 2005). The infection is highly contagious, and when measles becomes epidemic, unvaccinated women have an increased risk of pneumonia and severe diarrhea with adverse perinatal outcomes (American Academy of Pediatrics, 2006; Centers for Disease Control and Prevention, 2005). Measles occurs most often in late winter and spring and is characterized by fever, coryza, conjunctivitis, and cough. The characteristic rash—Koplik spots—develops on the face and neck and then spreads to the back, trunk, and extremities. Treatment is supportive.

Passive maternal immunization is given with immune serum globulin—0.25 mL/kg with a maximum dose of 15 mL, administered intramuscularly within 6 days of exposure. Active vaccination is not performed during pregnancy, but susceptible women can be vaccinated routinely postpartum (American College of Obstetricians and Gynecologists, 2003; Centers for Disease Control and Prevention, 1998). Breast feeding is not contraindicated with vaccination (Ohji and associates, 2009).

Fetal Effects

The virus does not appear to be teratogenic (Siegel, 1973). There is an increased frequency of abortion, preterm delivery, and low-birthweight neonates with maternal measles (American Academy of Pediatrics, 2006; Siegel and Fuerst, 1966). If a woman develops measles shortly before birth, there is considerable risk of serious infection developing in the neonate, especially in a preterm neonate.

Rubella (German Measles)

This RNA togavirus typically causes infections of minor importance in the absence of pregnancy. Infection in the first trimester, however, is directly responsible for abortion and severe congenital malformations. Transmission occurs via nasopharyngeal secretions, and the transmission rate is 80 percent to susceptible individuals. The peak incidence is late winter and spring.

Clinical Manifestations

In adults, rubella is usually a mild, febrile illness with a generalized maculopapular rash beginning on the face and spreading to the trunk and extremities. Other symptoms may include arthralgias or arthritis, head and neck lymphadenopathy, and conjunctivitis. The incubation period is 12 to 23 days. Viremia usually precedes clinical signs by about a week, and adults are infectious during viremia and through 5 to 7 days of the rash. Up to a half of maternal infections are subclinical despite viremia that may cause fetal infection with malformations.

Congenital Rubella Syndrome. Rubella is one of the most teratogenic agents known with the sequela of fetal infection being worst during organogenesis (see Chap. 4, p. 80). Miller and colleagues (1982) have shown that 80 percent of pregnant women with rubella infection and a rash during the first 12 weeks have a fetus with congenital infection. At 13 to 14 weeks, this incidence was 54 percent, and by the end of the second trimester, it was 25 percent. According to Reef and colleagues (2000), congenital rubella syndrome includes one or more of the following:

- Eye defects—cataracts and congenital glaucoma
- Heart disease—patent ductus arteriosus and pulmonary artery stenosis
- Sensorineural deafness—the most common single defect
- Central nervous system defects—microcephaly, developmental delay, mental retardation, and meningoencephalitis
- Pigmentary retinopathy
- Neonatal purpura
- Hepatosplenomegaly and jaundice
- Radiolucent bone disease

Neonates born with congenital rubella may shed the virus for many months and thus be a threat to other infants as well as to susceptible adults who come in contact with them.

The *extended rubella syndrome*, with progressive panencephalitis and type 1 diabetes, may not develop clinically until the second or third decade of life. As many as a third of neonates who are asymptomatic at birth may manifest such developmental injury (Webster, 1998).

Diagnosis

Rubella may be isolated from the urine, nasopharynx, and cerebrospinal fluid. But the diagnosis is usually made with serological analysis. Specific IgM antibody can be detected using enzyme-linked immunoassay from 4 to 5 days after onset of clinical disease, but it can persist for up to 8 weeks after appearance of the rash (American College of Obstetricians and Gynecologists, 1992). Importantly, rubella reinfection can give rise to transient low levels of IgM. Best and associates (2002) reviewed low rubella-specific IgM antibody levels in pregnant women without a rash in locales in which rubella seldom occurs. They were able to exclude recent maternal infection by detecting high rubella IgG avidity in most cases. Rubella IgG avidity assays were recently reviewed by Mubareka and associates (2007).

Nonimmune persons demonstrate peak serum IgG antibody titers 1 to 2 weeks after the onset of the rash or 2 to 3 weeks after the onset of viremia. This rapid antibody response may complicate serodiagnosis unless samples are initially collected within a few days after the onset of the rash. If, for example, the first specimen was obtained 10 days after the rash, detection of IgG antibodies would fail to differentiate between very recent disease and preexisting immunity to rubella.

Confirmation of fetal infection is possible in confirmed cases of maternal rubella in the first half of pregnancy. Sonography is not sensitive, nor specific. However, some abnormalities identified by sonography include fetal-growth restriction; ventriculomegaly, intracranial calcification, microcephaly, and microphthalmia; cardiac malformations; meconium peritonitis; and hepatosplenomegaly. Tanemura and associates (1996) found rubella RNA in chorionic villi, amnionic fluid, or fetal blood in 23 percent of 34 suspected cases. Detection of second-trimester fetal rubella infection using fetal blood has been described by Tang and colleagues (2003).

Management and Prevention

There is no specific treatment for rubella. Droplet precautions for 7 days after the onset of the rash are recommended. Primary prevention relies on comprehensive vaccination programs (Coonrod and co-workers, 2008). Although large epidemics of rubella have virtually disappeared in the United States because of immunization, up to 10 percent of women in the United States are susceptible (Haas and associates, 2005). Cluster outbreaks during the 1990s mainly involved foreign-born persons born outside the United States, as congenital rubella is still common in developing nations (Banatvala and Brown, 2004; Reef and co-workers, 2002).

To eradicate rubella and prevent congenital rubella syndrome completely, a comprehensive approach is recommended for immunizing the adult population (Centers for Disease Control and Prevention, 1998). MMR vaccine should be offered to nonpregnant women of childbearing age who do not have evidence of immunity whenever they make contact with the healthcare system.

Vaccination of all susceptible hospital personnel who might be exposed to patients with rubella or who might have contact with pregnant women is important. Rubella vaccination should be avoided 1 month before or during pregnancy because the vaccine contains attenuated live virus (Centers for Disease

Control and Prevention, 2002a). Although there is a small overall theoretical risk of about 1 percent, according to pooled data from the Centers for Disease Control and Prevention, there is no evidence that the vaccine induces malformations.

Despite native or vaccine-induced immunity, subclinical rubella maternal *reinfection* may develop during outbreaks. And although fetal infection can rarely occur, no adverse fetal effects have been described.

Respiratory Viruses

More than 200 antigenically distinct respiratory viruses cause the common cold, pharyngitis, laryngitis, bronchitis, and pneumonia. Rhinovirus, coronavirus, and adenovirus are major causes of the common cold. The RNA-containing rhinovirus and coronavirus usually produce a trivial, self-limited illness characterized by rhinorrhea, sneezing, and congestion. The DNA-containing adenovirus is more likely to produce cough and lower respiratory tract involvement, including pneumonia.

Fetal Effects

Teratogenic effects are controversial. Women with a common cold had a four- to fivefold increased risk of fetal anencephaly in a 393-woman cohort in the Finnish Register of Congenital Malformations (Kurppa and associates, 1991). In another population study, Shaw and co-workers (1998) analyzed California births from 1989 to 1991 and concluded that low attributable risks for neural-tube defects were associated with many illnesses in early pregnancy.

Adenoviral infection is a common cause of childhood myocarditis. Towbin and colleagues (1994) and Forsnes and associates (1998) used polymerase chain reaction (PCR) to identify and link adenovirus to fetal myocarditis and nonimmune hydrops.

Hantaviruses

These RNA viruses are members of the family *Bunyaviridae*. They are associated with a rodent reservoir, and transmission involves inhalation of virus excreted in rodent urine and feces. Prevention focuses on lowering exposure to infected rodents (Centers for Disease Control and Prevention, 2002b). An outbreak in the Western United States occurred in 1993 due to Sin Nombre virus. The resulting Hantavirus pulmonary syndrome was characterized by severe adult respiratory distress syndrome with a case-fatality rate of 45 percent.

Hantaviruses are a heterogenous group of viruses with low and variable rates of transplacental transmission. Howard and co-workers (1999) reported the syndrome to cause maternal death, fetal demise, and preterm birth. They found no evidence of vertical transmission of the Sin Nombre virus. Vertical transmission, however, occurred inconsistently in association with hemorrhagic fever with renal syndrome caused by another Hantavirus species, the Hantaan virus.

Enteroviruses

These viruses are a major subgroup of RNA picornaviruses that include poliovirus, coxsackievirus, and echovirus. They are trophic for intestinal epithelium but can also cause widespread maternal, fetal, and neonatal infections that may include the central nervous system, skin, heart, and lungs. Most maternal infections, however, are subclinical, yet can be fatal to the fetus-neonate (Goldenberg and Thompson, 2003). Hepatitis A is an enterovirus that is discussed in Chapter 50 (p. 1069).

Coxsackievirus

Infections with coxsackievirus group A and B are usually asymptomatic. Symptomatic infections—usually with group B—include aseptic meningitis, polio-like illness, hand foot and mouth disease, rashes, respiratory disease, pleuritis, pericarditis, and myocarditis. No treatment or vaccination is available. Coxsackievirus may be transmitted by maternal secretions to the fetus at delivery in up to half of mothers who seroconverted during pregnancy (Modlin, 1988). Transplacental passage has also been reported (Ornoy and Tenenbaum, 2006).

Congenital malformations may be increased slightly in pregnant women who had serological evidence of coxsackievirus (Brown and Karunas, 1972). Coxsackie viremia can cause fetal hepatitis, skin lesions, myocarditis, and encephalomyelitis, all of which may be fatal. Koro'lkova and associates (1989) have also described cardiac anomalies. Finally, the association between maternal coxsackievirus infection and insulin-dependent diabetes in the offspring has been rarely reported (Dahlquist, 1996; Hyoti, 1995; Viskari, 2002, and all of their associates).

Poliovirus

Most of these highly contagious but rare infections are subclinical or mild. The virus is trophic for the central nervous system, and it can cause paralytic poliomyelitis. Siegel and Goldberg (1955) demonstrated that pregnant women not only were more susceptible to polio but also had a higher death rate. Perinatal transmission has been observed, especially when maternal infection developed in the third trimester (Bates, 1955). Inactivated subcutaneous polio vaccine is recommended for susceptible pregnant women who must travel to endemic areas or are placed in other high-risk situations. Live oral polio vaccine has been used for mass vaccination during pregnancy without harmful fetal effects (Harjulehto and associates, 1989).

Parvovirus

Human parvovirus B19 causes *erythema infectiosum*, or *Fifth disease*. The B19 virus is a small, single-stranded DNA virus that replicates in rapidly proliferating cells such as erythroblast precursors (Young and Brown, 2004). This can lead to anemia, which is its central fetal effect. Only individuals with the erythrocyte membrane P antigen are susceptible. In women with severe hemolytic anemia—for example, sickle-cell disease—parvovirus infection may cause an aplastic crisis.

The main mode of parvovirus transmission is respiratory or hand-to-mouth contact, and the infection is common in spring months. The maternal infection rate is highest in women with school-age children and in day-care workers, but not usually schoolteachers. Viremia develops 4 to 14 days after exposure. By adulthood only 40 percent of women are susceptible. The annual seroconversion rate is 1 to 2 percent but is greater than 10 percent during epidemic periods (Dembinski and colleagues, 2003).

Clinical Manifestations

In 20 to 30 percent of adults, infection is asymptomatic. Fever, headache, and flulike symptoms may begin in the last few days of the viremic phase. Several days later, a bright red rash with erythroderma affects the face, giving a *slapped cheek* appearance. The rash becomes lacelike and spreads to the trunk and extremities. Adults often have milder rashes and develop symmetrical polyarthralgia that may persist several weeks. There is no evidence that parvovirus infection is altered by pregnancy (Valeur-Jensen and colleagues, 1999). Recovery includes production of IgM antibody 10 to 12 days postinfection. IgM persists for 3 to 6 months. Several days after IgM production, IgG antibody is detectable and persists for life with natural immunity.

Fetal Infection

There is vertical transmission to the fetus in about a third of maternal parvovirus infections (de Jong and associates, 2006). Fetal infection has been associated with abortion, nonimmune hydrops, and stillbirth (Goldenberg and Thompson, 2003; McClure and Goldenberg, 2009). In a review of 1089 cases of maternal B19 infection from nine studies, Crane (2002) reported an overall fetal loss rate of 10 percent. It was 15 percent for infection before 20 weeks but only 2.3 percent after 20 weeks. Its role in later unexplained stillbirths is unclear because most data are from retrospective cohorts with incomplete maternal and fetal histological evaluations (Norbeck, 2002; Skjöldebrand-Sparre, 2000; Tolfvenstam, 2001, and all their colleagues). Currently, there are no data to support evaluating asymptomatic mothers and stillborn fetuses for parvovirus infection.

Parvovirus is the most common infectious cause of nonimmune hydrops in autopsied fetuses (Rogers, 1999). That said, this complication develops only in about 1 percent of infected women and usually is caused by infection in the first half of gestation (Crane, 2002; Enders and co-workers, 2004).

Yaegashi (2000) has extensively investigated the development and pathophysiology of parvovirus B19 fetal hydrops. At least 85 percent of cases of fetal infection developed within 10 weeks of maternal infection, and the mean interval was 6 to 7 weeks. More than 80 percent of hydrops cases were found in the second trimester, with a mean gestational age of 22 to 23 weeks. The critical period for maternal infection leading to fetal hydrops was estimated to be between 13 and 16 weeks—coincident with the period in which fetal hepatic hemopoiesis is greatest.

Diagnosis

As shown in **Figure 58-2**, the diagnosis of maternal infection is generally made by serological testing for specific IgG and IgM antibodies (Butchko and Jordan, 2004; Enders and co-workers, 2006). Viral DNA may be detectable by PCR in maternal serum during the prodrome but not after the rash develops. Fetal infection can be identified by detecting viral DNA in amnionic fluid or fetal serum parvoviral IgM with cordocentesis (Schild and colleagues, 1999). Fetal and maternal viral loads do not predict fetal morbidity and mortality (de Haan and associates, 2007).

Management

The majority of parvovirus-associated hydrops develops in the first 10 weeks after infection (Enders and colleagues, 2004). Thus, serial sonography every 2 weeks should be performed in women with recent infection (see Fig. 58-2). Middle cerebral artery (MCA) Doppler evaluation can also be used to predict fetal anemia (see Chap. 16, p. 364). Delle Chiaie (2001) and Cosmi (2002) and their colleagues have shown that elevated peak systolic velocity values in the fetal middle cerebral artery accurately predict fetal anemia (Fig. 58-3). Fetal blood sampling is warranted with hydrops to assess the degree of fetal anemia. Fetal myocarditis may induce hydrops with less severe anemia.

Depending on gestational age, fetal transfusion for hydrops may improve outcome in some cases (Enders and co-workers, 2004; Schild and colleagues, 1999; von Kaisenberg and Jonat, 2001). Mortality rates as high as 30 percent have been reported in hydropic fetuses without transfusions. With transfusion, 94 percent of hydrops cases resolve within 6 to 12 weeks, and the overall mortality rate is less than 10 percent. Most fetuses require only one transfusion because hemopoiesis resumes as infection resolves. The technique for fetal transfusion is described in Chapter 13 (p. 300).

Prognosis

Long-term neurodevelopmental outcomes after fetal transfusion for B19 infection-induced anemia are conflicting. Nagel and colleagues (2007) reviewed 25 transfusions in 24 hydropic fetuses. There was abnormal neurodevelopment in 5 of 16 survivors—32 percent—at 6 months to 8 years. Outcomes were not related to severity of fetal anemia or acidemia, and these investigators hypothesized that the infection itself induced cerebral damage. Conversely, Dembinski and colleagues (2003) followed 20 children for a mean of 52 months after transfusion. They found no significant neurodevelopmental delay despite severe fetal anemia. At this time, more data are required to definitively assess long-term outcomes.

Prevention

There is currently no approved vaccine for human parvovirus B19, and there is no evidence that antiviral treatment prevents maternal or fetal infection (Broliden and colleagues, 2006). Decisions to avoid higher-risk work settings are complex and require assessment of exposure risks. Pregnant women should be counseled that risks for infection are about 5 percent for casual, infrequent contact; 20 percent for intense, prolonged work exposure such as for teachers; and 50 percent for close, frequent interaction such as in the home. Workers at day-care centers and schools need not avoid infected children because infectivity is greatest before clinical illness. Finally, infected children do not require isolation.

Cytomegalovirus

This ubiquitous DNA herpesvirus eventually infects most humans. Cytomegalovirus (CMV) is the most common perinatal

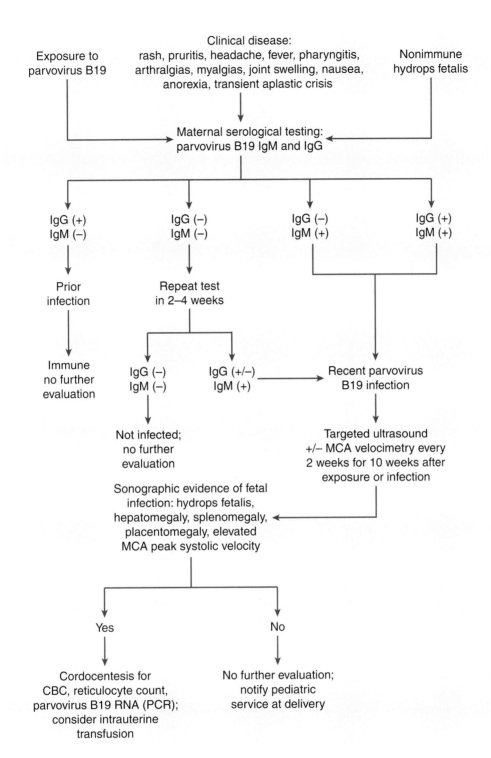

FIGURE 58-2 Algorithm for evaluation and management of human parvovirus B19 infection in pregnancy. CBC = complete blood count; IgG = immunoglobulin G; IgM = immunoglobulin M; MCA = middle cerebral artery; PCR = polymerase chain reaction; RNA = ribonucleic acid.

infection in the developed world, and evidence of fetal infection is found in from 0.2 to 2 percent of all neonates (Revello and Gerna, 2004). CMV is present in body fluids, and person-to-person transmission usually occurs by contact with infected nasopharyngeal secretions, urine, saliva, semen, cervical secretions, or blood. There may be intrauterine or intrapartum infection or neonatal infection from breast feeding. Day-care centers are a common source of infection, and by 2 to 3 years of age, children usually acquire infection from one another and may transmit it to their parents (Demmler, 1991; Pass, 1991). Fortunately, Revello and co-workers (2008) have shown that CMV DNA in maternal peripheral blood is not a risk factor for iatrogenic fetal transmission during amniocentesis.

Up to 85 percent of women from lower socioeconomic backgrounds are seropositive by the time of pregnancy, whereas only half of women in higher income groups are immune.

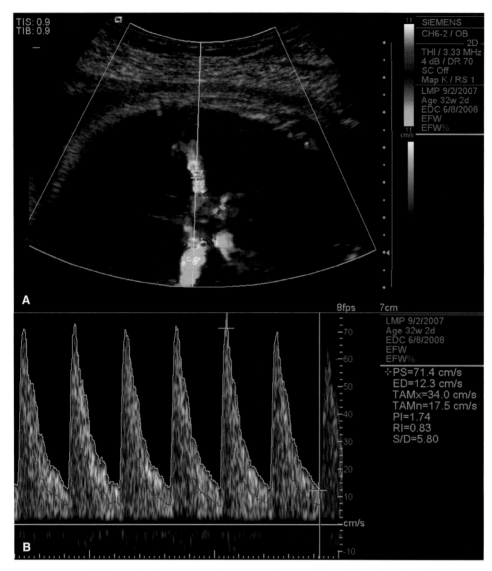

FIGURE 58-3 Middle cerebral artery Doppler images showing elevated peak systolic velocity.

Primary maternal CMV infection is transmitted to the fetus in about 40 percent of cases and can cause severe morbidity (Fowler and co-workers, 1992; Liesnard and associates, 2000). In contrast, recurrent maternal infection infects the fetus in only 0.15 to 1 percent of cases. Transplacental fetal infection is more likely during the first half of pregnancy. Naturally acquired immunity during pregnancy results in a 70-percent reduction of risk of congenital CMV infection in future pregnancies (Fowler and colleagues, 2003). And because maternal immunity does not prevent recurrences, maternal antibodies do not prevent fetal infection. Some seropositive women can also be reinfected with a different strain of virus that can cause fetal infection with symptomatic congenital disease (Boppana and associates, 2001).

Congenital Infection

Symptomatic—apparent—congenital CMV infection is a syndrome that may include growth restriction, microcephaly, intracranial calcifications, chorioretinitis, mental and motor re-tardation, sensorineural deficits, hepatosplenomegaly, jaundice, hemolytic anemia, and thrombocytopenic purpura. The pathogenesis of these outcomes have recently been reviewed by Cheeran and co-workers (2009). Of the estimated 40,000 infected neonates born each year, only 5 to 6 percent demonstrate this syndrome (Fowler and associates, 1992). Thus, most infected infants are asymptomatic at birth, but some develop late-onset sequelae such as hearing loss, neurological deficits, chorioretinitis, psychomotor retardation, and learning disabilities.

However, similar to other herpesviral infections, following primary infection, CMV becomes latent, and there is periodic reactivation with viral shedding. This occurs despite serum IgG antibody, which does not prevent recurrence-reactivation, exogenous reinfection, and does not prevent congenital infection. The risk of infection manifest by seroconversion among antibody-negative women during pregnancy is 1 to 4 percent.

Clinical Manifestations

Pregnancy does not increase the risk or severity of maternal CMV infection. Most infections are asymptomatic, but about 15 percent of infected adults have a mononucleosis-like syndrome characterized by fever, pharyngitis, lymphadenopathy, and polyarthritis. Immunocompromised women may develop myocarditis, pneumonitis, hepatitis, retinitis, gastroenteritis, or meningoencephalitis. Nigro and associates (2003) reported that most women in a cohort with primary infection had elevated serum aminotransferases or lymphocytosis. Reactivation disease usually is asymptomatic, although viral shedding is common.

Diagnosis

Routine prenatal CMV serological screening is currently not recommended (American College of Obstetricians and Gynecologists, 2000; Collinet and associates, 2004; Peckham and co-workers, 2001). *Primary infection* is diagnosed by seroconversion of CMV-specific IgG in paired acute and convalescent sera assayed simultaneously. It is preferable to document maternal CMV IgM antibody. Unfortunately, specific IgM antibody may be present with primary infection, recurrent infection, or reactivation infection, thus limiting its utility for serological diagnosis (Duff, 2007). CMV IgM is also found in only 75 to 90 percent of women with acute infection (Stagno, 1985). As shown in Figure 58-4, when CMV-specific IgG and IgM are detected, complimentary tests are used to date the infection (Grangeot-Keros and Cointe, 2001). The measurement of specific IgG avidity is valuable in confirming primary CMV infection (Lazzarotto and associates, 2004). The IgG antibody response matures from low-avidity to high-avidity production over several weeks to months (Revello and Gerna, 2004). Finally, viral culture may be useful, though a minimum of 21 days is required before culture is reported as negative.

Imaging Studies. Perinatal infection may be suspected from abnormalities seen with sonography, computed tomography (CT), or magnetic resonance (MR) imaging. Findings include microcephaly, ventriculomegaly, and cerebral calcifications; ascites, hepatomegaly, splenomegaly, and hyperechoic bowel; hydrops; and oligohydramnios (Malinger and colleagues, 2003). Abnormal sonographic findings seen in combination with positive findings in fetal blood or amnionic fluid are predictive of an approximate 75-percent risk of symptomatic congenital infection (Enders and co-workers, 2001).

Amnionic Fluid Studies. CMV nucleic acid amplification testing of amnionic fluid is considered the gold standard for the diagnosis of fetal infection (Nigro and colleagues, 2005; Revello and Gerna, 2004). Amnionic fluid testing may be coupled with sonography. Guerra and colleagues (2007) evaluated 430 fetuses of women with primary infection using targeted sonography and amnionic fluid DNA analysis. Of these, only a third were confirmed to be infected. However, as emphasized by Bodéus (1999) and Antsaklis (2000) and their associates, a negative amnionic fluid culture or PCR assay result does not always exclude fetal infection.

Management and Prevention

The management of the immunocompetent pregnant woman with primary or recurrent CMV is limited to symptomatic treatment. If recent primary CMV infection is confirmed, amnionic fluid analysis should be offered. Counseling regarding fetal outcome depends on the stage of gestation during which primary infection is documented. Even with the high infection rate with

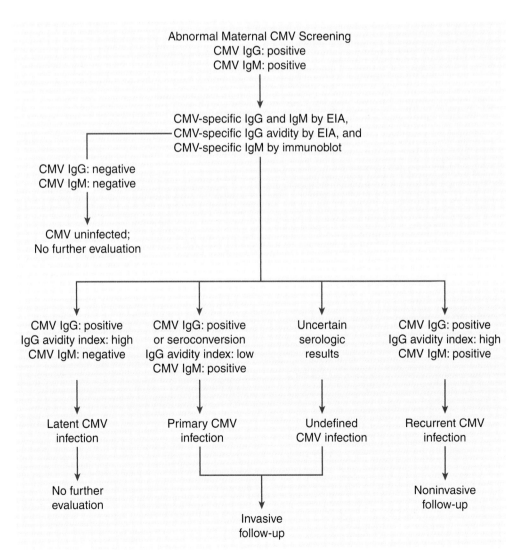

FIGURE 58-4 Algorithm for evaluation of suspected maternal primary cytomegalovirus (CMV) infection in pregnancy. EIA = enzyme immunoassay; IgG = immunoglobulin G; IgM = immunoglobulin M.

primary infection in the first half of pregnancy, most fetuses develop normally. Pregnancy termination may be an option for some.

Kimberlin and co-workers (2003) showed that intravenous ganciclovir administered for 6 weeks to neonates with symptomatic central nervous system disease prevents hearing deterioration at 6 months and possibly later. Conversely, antiviral chemotherapy given antepartum is not effective to prevent in utero CMV transmission. Passive immunization with CMV-specific hyperimmune globulin significantly lowers the risk of congenital CMV infection when given to pregnant women with primary disease (Nigro and co-workers, 2005). Further clinical trials are necessary before this becomes standard of care.

There is no CMV vaccine. Prevention of congenital infection relies on prevention of maternal primary infection, especially in early pregnancy. Basic measures such as good hygiene and hand washing have been promoted, particularly for women with toddlers in day-care settings (Fowler, 2000). Although there may be sexual transmission from infected partners, there are no data on the efficacy of preventive strategies (Nigro and co-workers, 2003).

BACTERIAL INFECTIONS

Group A Streptococcus

More specifically known as *Streptococcus pyogenes*, this bacteria remains an important cause of infection in pregnant women. It is the most frequent bacterial cause of acute pharyngitis and is associated with a number of systemic and cutaneous infections. *S. pyogenes* produces a number of toxins and enzymes, and infections especially with *M3 super antigen strains* are particularly severe (Rogers and colleagues, 2007; Sriskandan and associates, 2007).

Streptococcal pharyngitis, scarlet fever, and erysipelas are seldom life-threatening. Management is similar in pregnant and nonpregnant women, usually treatment with penicillin. Puerperal infections caused by *S. pyogenes* are rarely encountered today (see Chap. 31, p. 661) (O'Brien and colleagues, 2002). The most common postpartum group A streptococcal infections are bacteremia without a septic focus—46 percent; pelvic infection—28 percent; peritonitis—8 percent; and septic abortion—7 percent. Over the past two decades, *S. pyogenes* has acquired a toxic shock-like toxin (TSST) that produces an often fatal syndrome (Brown, 2004; Daif and associates, 2009). The case-fatality rate for postpartum group A infection is 3 to 4 percent (Chuang and associates, 2002). A mortality rate of almost 75 percent was reported by Udagawa and co-workers (1999). In addition, these infections were fatal in two of three pregnant women at Parkland Hospital in 1992 (Nathan and colleagues, 1993). Prompt penicillin treatment, often with surgical debridement, may be lifesaving (Centers for Disease Control and Prevention, 2002c).

Group B Streptococcus (GBS)

Of group B streptococci, *Streptococcus agalactiae* is a major cause of neonatal morbidity and mortality. It colonizes the gastroin-testinal and genitourinary tract in 20 to 30 percent of pregnant women, which serves as a source for perinatal transmission (Schrag and associates, 2002, 2003; Wendel and colleagues, 2002). Maisey and co-workers (2007), as well as others, showed that this gram-positive coccus has adhesive pili that confer invasiveness. Throughout pregnancy, GBS is isolated in a transient, intermittent, or chronic fashion. Most likely the organism is always present in these same women, but isolation is not always homologous.

Clinical Infection

The spectrum of maternal and fetal GBS infections range from asymptomatic colonization to septicemia. *S. agalactiae* has been implicated in adverse pregnancy outcomes, including preterm labor, prematurely ruptured membranes, clinical and subclinical chorioamnionitis, and fetal and neonatal infections. GBS can also cause maternal bacteriuria, pyelonephritis, and postpartum metritis. Maternal osteomyelitis and postpartum mastitis have also been described (Barbosa-Cesnik and associates, 2003; Berkowitz and McCaffrey, 1990).

Neonatal sepsis has received the most attention due to its devastating consequences and available effective preventative measures. Infection less than 7 days after birth is defined as *early-onset disease* (Schrag and colleagues, 2000). Many investigators use a threshold of less than 72 hours of life as most compatible with intrapartum acquisition of disease (Stoll and associates, 2002a; Wendel and co-workers, 2002). We and others have also encountered a number of unexpected intrapartum stillbirths from GBS infections. In many neonates, septicemia involves signs of serious illness that usually develop within 6 to 12 hours of birth—these include respiratory distress, apnea, and hypotension. At the outset, therefore, neonatal infection must be differentiated from respiratory distress syndrome caused by insufficient surfactant production of the preterm neonate (see Chap. 29, p. 605). The mortality rate with early-onset disease has declined to about 4 percent, and preterm newborns are affected disparately.

Late-onset disease caused by GBS usually manifests as meningitis 1 week to 3 months after birth. These cases are most often caused by serotype III organisms. The mortality rate, although appreciable, is less for late-onset meningitis than for early-onset sepsis. Unfortunately, it is not uncommon for surviving infants of both early- and late-onset disease to exhibit devastating neurological sequelae.

Neonatal Prophylaxis

As group B neonatal infections evolved beginning in the 1970s before widespread intrapartum chemoprophylaxis, rates of early-onset sepsis ranged from 2 to 3 per 1000 live births. In 2002, the Centers for Disease Control and Prevention, the American College of Obstetricians and Gynecologists, and the American Academy of Pediatrics revised guidelines for perinatal prevention of GBS disease. They recommended universal culture screening for rectovaginal GBS at 35 to 37 weeks followed by intrapartum antibiotic prophylaxis for women identified to be carriers of GBS (see p. 1221). Subsequent to implementation of these guidelines, the incidence of GBS neonatal sepsis has decreased to 0.33 cases per 1000 live births in 2003 to 2005 (Centers for Disease Control and Prevention, 2007d). It is worrisome, however, that widespread intrapartum antimicrobial prophylaxis has been associated with increased risk for non-streptococcal early-onset sepsis in preterm and especially very-low-birthweight neonates (Eschenbach, 2002; Towers and Briggs, 2002). In one example, marked reduction in group B streptococcal sepsis in preterm neonates was offset by increased *E. coli* sepsis (Stoll and associates, 2002b; Stoll and Hansen, 2003).

Late-onset neonatal GBS sepsis is less well understood. Cited rates vary from 0.5 to 2 cases per 1000 live births and account for about half of GBS disease in newborns (Lin and colleagues, 2003). The incidence of late-onset disease has remained stable despite widespread use of intrapartum antimicrobials (Centers for Disease Control and Prevention, 2009). This suggests that GBS screening and chemoprophylaxis intervention may not affect late-onset disease.

Recommended Prevention Strategies

In the absence of randomized trials, consensus opinions and guidelines for prevention strategies of neonatal GBS infection have been promulgated by the Centers for Disease Control and Prevention (2002d) and endorsed by the American College of Obstetricians and Gynecologists (2002a). These guidelines, shown in Figure 58-5, advocate a culture-based screening approach to identify women who should be given intrapartum antimicrobial prophylaxis. Their recommendations were derived from a multistate, retrospective cohort study of live births in 1998 and 1999 from the Active Bacterial Surveillance/Emerging Infections Program Network.

There are further recommendations for management of preterm labor or preterm prematurely ruptured membranes (Fig. 58-6). It is emphasized that there are insufficient data to suggest a single management scheme for GBS-positive women with arrested preterm labor or preterm prematurely ruptured

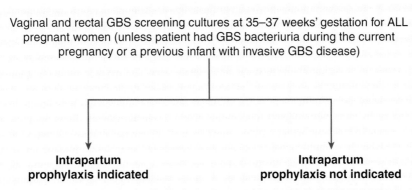

Vaginal and rectal GBS screening cultures at 35–37 weeks' gestation for ALL pregnant women (unless patient had GBS bacteriuria during the current pregnancy or a previous infant with invasive GBS disease)

Intrapartum prophylaxis indicated

- Previous infant with invasive GBS disease

- GBS bacteriuria during current pregnancy

- Positive GBS screening culture during current pregnancy (unless a planned cesarean delivery, in the absence of labor or amniotic membrane rupture, is performed)

- Unknown GBS status (culture not done, incomplete, or results unknown) and any of the following:

  - Delivery at < 37 weeks' gestation

  - Amnionic membrane rupture ≥ 18 hours

  - Intrapartum temperature ≥ 100.4°F (≥ 38.0°C)

Intrapartum prophylaxis not indicated

- Previous pregnancy with a positive GBS screening culture (unless a culture was also positive during the current pregnancy)

- Planned cesarean delivery performed in the absence of labor or membrane rupture (regardless of maternal GBS culture status)

- Negative vaginal and rectal GBS screening culture in late gestation during the current pregnancy, regardless of intrapartum risk factors

FIGURE 58-5 Indications for intrapartum prophylaxis to prevent perinatal group B streptococcal (GBS) disease under a universal prenatal screening strategy based on combined vaginal and rectal cultures taken at 35 to 37 weeks' gestation. (From Centers for Disease Control and Prevention, 2002d.)

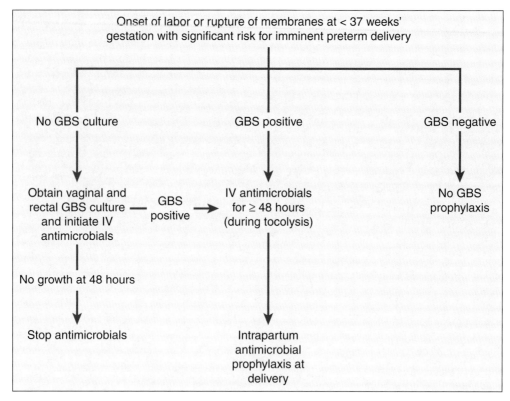

FIGURE 58-6 Sample algorithm for prophylaxis for women with group B streptococcal (GBS) disease and threatened preterm delivery. This algorithm is not an exclusive course of management, and variations that incorporate individual circumstances or institutional preferences may be appropriate. IV = intravenous. (Adapted from Centers for Disease Control and Prevention, 2002d.)

membranes (American College of Obstetricians and Gynecologists, 2002a).

With the culture-based approach, women are screened for GBS colonization at 35 to 37 weeks, and intrapartum antimicrobials are given to women with rectovaginal GBS-positive cultures. Previous siblings with GBS invasive disease and prior identification of GBS bacteriuria are also considered indications for prophylaxis. A risk-based approach is recommended for women in labor and whose GBS culture results are not known (see Fig. 58-4).

The choice of antimicrobials may be important in terms of allergic reactions; selection of resistant GBS strains; and emergence of other pathogens, including antimicrobial-resistant strains, that may cause neonatal sepsis. Treatment regimens are shown in Table 58-2. Although penicillin is recommended as the first-line agent, ampicillin is an acceptable alternative (Bloom and co-workers, 1996; Centers for Disease Control and Prevention, 2002c). For women with penicillin allergy, if the risk of anaphylaxis is low, cefazolin is recommended (Mitchell and associates, 2001). If the risk of anaphylaxis is high, selection of another agent is dependent on GBS susceptibility testing. Patients with isolates susceptible to clindamycin or erythromycin may be given either drug. Antimicrobial-resistant strains require vancomycin prophylaxis. This treatment scheme is dependent on laboratory capability to perform susceptibility testing. Awareness of the potential for worsening antibiotic resistance in the setting of more widespread use is mandatory (Chohan and

associates, 2006). The duration of intrapartum prophylaxis required for disease prevention is unknown (Illuzzi and co-workers, 2006). For ampicillin, bactericidal levels are achieved in cord blood by 30 minutes of maternal administration (Colombo and co-workers, 2006).

Risk-Based Treatment versus Universal Culture. There remains significant controversy whether GBS surveillance schemes are worthwhile. As discussed above, there are no randomized controlled trials that compare GBS screening—whether culture-based or risk-based—with no screening. There have also been no randomized trials to compare different screening strategies with no GBS screening or to evaluate any significant impact on overall neonatal sepsis. For these reasons, similar organizations in other countries conclude that there is insufficient evidence to recommend GBS screening (Canadian Task Force on Preventive Health Care, 2002; Jakobi and colleagues, 2003; Royal College of Obstetricians and Gynaecologists, 2003).

A number of alternative prevention strategies have been described with limited evidence for their recommendation. These include intramuscular benzathine penicillin G and chlorhexidine vaginal lavage (Bland and associates, 2000; Rouse and co-workers, 2003). In a preliminary study, Haberland and colleagues (2002) described the efficacy of intrapartum rapid PCR screening for GBS. Currently, real-time PCR for rapid GBS testing is still in the development phase (Bergseng and colleagues, 2007; Chan and associates, 2006).

TABLE 58-2. Regimens for Intrapartum Antimicrobial Prophylaxis for Perinatal GBS Disease

Regimen	Treatment
Recommended	Penicillin G, 5 million units IV initial dose, then 2.5 million units IV every 4 hours until delivery
Alternative	Ampicillin, 2 g IV initial dose, then 1 g IV every 4 hours or 2 g every 6 hours until delivery
If penicillin allergic	
Patients **not** at high risk for anaphylaxis	Cefazolin, 2 g IV initial dose, then 1 g IV every 8 hours until delivery
Patients at high risk for anaphylaxis and with GBS susceptible to clindamycin and erythromycin	Clindamycin, 900 mg IV every 8 hours until delivery *or* Erythromycin, 500 mg IV every 6 hours until delivery
Patients at high risk for anaphylaxis and with GBS resistant to clindamycin or erythromycin or susceptibility unknown	Vancomycin, 1 g IV every 12 hours until delivery

GBS = group B streptococcus.
Adapted from the Centers for Disease Control and Prevention (2002d).

At Parkland Hospital in 1995—and prior to consensus guidelines—we adopted the risk-based approach for intrapartum treatment of women at high risk for GBS infection. In addition, all term neonates who were not given intrapartum prophylaxis were treated in the delivery room with aqueous penicillin G, 50 to 60,000 units intramuscularly. Early-onset GBS infection and sepsis, as well as non-GBS sepsis, all decreased during the study to 0.4 per 1000 live births (Wendel and associates, 2002).

Vaccination

Some protection against serious neonatal infection is conferred by maternal antibodies. Indeed, Lin and colleagues (2001) confirmed that the susceptibility to invasive GBS disease correlates with deficiency in maternal type-specific antibody levels. Baker and co-workers (1988, 1999, 2000) reported that maternal immunization to type III antigen produces antibody in approximately 60 percent of women. Monovalent tetanus toxoid conjugate vaccines are immunogenic for common GBS disease-associated serotypes. Johri and associates (2006) and Larsen and Sever (2008) have reviewed the progress toward vaccine development.

Methicillin-Resistant *Staphylococcus aureus* (MRSA)

Staphylococcal infections are an important cause of skin and soft tissue infections. The recent National Health and Nutrition Examination Survey (NHANES) reported that a third of adults have nasal colonization with *Staphylococcus aureus* (Kuehnert and colleagues, 2006). Seventeen percent of pregnant women have vaginal colonization (Chen and associates, 2006). Unfortunately, multidrug-resistant strains of *S. aureus* are spreading, particularly *methicillin-resistant S. aureus (MRSA)*. These strains also are resistant to penicillinase-resistant penicillins and cephalosporins. There are two varieties. *Community-acquired*

MRSA strains—referred to as *CA-MRSA*—colonize healthy persons without historical risks for MRSA acquisition. Nosocomial MRSA infections are termed *healthcare-associated MRSA*.

MRSA has become the most common identifiable cause of skin and soft tissue infections in general emergency rooms (Moran and colleagues, 2006). There is also an increased frequency of CA-MRSA documented in pregnant women over the past few years (Chen, 2006; Hidron, 2005; Laibl, 2005, and all their colleagues). Beigi and co-workers (2009) reported that approximately 14,300 pregnant or postpartum women experience an invasive MRSA infection annually. Infections tend to involve skin and soft tissues. Abscesses or cellulitis form especially in HIV-infected women, injection drug users, and diabetics. Skin lesions such as that shown in Figure 58-7 appear to resemble

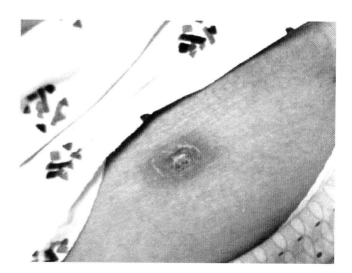

FIGURE 58-7 Typical presentation of a skin lesion caused by infection with community-acquired methicillin-resistant *S. aureus*—CA-MRSA. Patients often present with what they describe as an infected spider bite.

infected insect bites. At Parkland Hospital, we have isolated CA-MRSA from postoperative wound infections and puerperal mastitis (Laibl and co-workers, 2005).

Management

Most uncomplicated, noninvasive skin and soft tissue infections should be managed by abscess drainage. Pus is cultured and staphylococcal susceptibility testing is performed. CA-MRSA strains are usually not resistant to antistaphylococcal antimicrobials other than methicillin. Erythromycin and clindamycin resistance is variable, but most strains are sensitive to flu-oroquinolones, trimethoprim-sulfamethoxazole, gentamicin, rifampin, or vancomycin (Eady and Cove, 2003; Naimi and colleagues, 2003). Parenteral vancomycin therapy should be reserved for serious CA-MRSA infections such as wound infections and mastitis.

Pregnancy and CA-MRSA

Currently, there are no evidence-based guidelines for management. For example, it is not known if these women or their immediately families require decolonization. Careful surveillance is necessary to assure resolution of infection. Recurrences are common. The frequency and significance of intrapartum

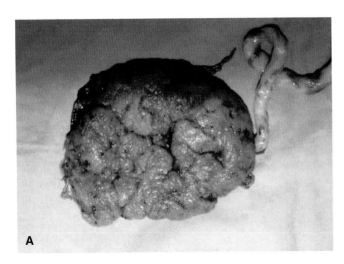

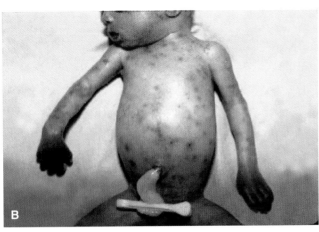

FIGURE 58-8 The pale placenta **(A)** and stillborn infant **(B)** resulted from maternal listeriosis.

transmission is unclear, and there are no recommendations regarding prophylaxis to prevent neonatal or surgical wound infections. Outbreaks of skin infections in healthy newborns have been reported by the Centers for Disease Control and Prevention (2006b). In women with culture-proven infection during pregnancy, we routinely add single-dose vancomycin to β-lactam perioperative prophylaxis for cesarean deliveries and fourth-degree perineal injury repair. Breast feeding in these women is not prohibited, but good hygiene and attention to minor skin breaks is encouraged.

Listeriosis

Listeria monocytogenes is an uncommon but probably underdiagnosed cause of neonatal sepsis. This facultative intracellular gram-positive bacillus can be isolated from the feces of 1 to 5 percent of adults. Nearly all cases of listeriosis are thought to be food-borne. Outbreaks have been caused by raw vegetables, coleslaw, apple cider, melons, milk, fresh Mexican-style cheese, smoked fish, and processed foods, such as pâté, hummus, wieners, and sliced deli meats (Janakiraman, 2008; Varma and colleagues, 2007).

Listerial infections are more common in the very old or young, pregnant women, and immunocompromised patients. Voetsch and associates (2007) recently reported data from the Foodborne Diseases Active Surveillance Network Working Group. In 2003, the overall incidence of listeria in the United States decreased to 3.1 cases per million. It is unclear why pregnant women still account for a significant number of these reported cases. One hypothesis is that pregnant women are susceptible because of decreased cell-mediated immunity (Wing and Gregory, 2002). Another is that placental trophoblasts are susceptible to *L. monocytogenes* (Le Monnier and colleagues, 2007).

Clinical Presentation

Listeriosis during pregnancy may be asymptomatic or it may cause a febrile illness that is confused with influenza, pyelonephritis, or meningitis (Mylonakis and colleagues, 2002; Silver, 1998). The diagnosis usually is not apparent until blood cultures are reported as positive. Occult or clinical infection also may stimulate labor (Boucher and Yonekura, 1986). Discolored, brownish, or meconium-stained amnionic fluid is common with fetal infection, even with preterm gestations.

Maternal listeremia causes fetal infection that characteristically produces disseminated granulomatous lesions with *microabscesses* (Topalovski and colleagues, 1993). Chorioamnionitis is common with maternal infection, and placental lesions include multiple, well-demarcated macroabscesses. The two types of neonatal infections are very similar to group B streptococcal sepsis. In a review of 222 cases by Mylonakis and associates (2002), infection resulted in abortion or stillbirth in 20 percent, and neonatal sepsis developed in 68 percent of surviving newborns. A stillbirth caused by listeriosis is shown in Figure 58-8. Voetsch and colleagues (2007) detailed similar findings.

Treatment

Ampicillin plus gentamicin is usually recommended because of synergism. Trimethoprim-sulfamethoxazole can be given to penicillin-allergic women. Maternal treatment may also be effective for fetal infection.

There is no vaccine for listeriosis. Pregnant women should thoroughly cook raw food, wash raw vegetables, and avoid the implicated foods listed previously.

Salmonella and Shigella

Salmonellosis

Infections from *Salmonella* species continue to be a major cause of food-borne illness, although significant declines in incidence have been reported in the past decade (Centers for Disease Control and Prevention, 2006a). Six serotypes account for most cases in the United States, including *Salmonella* subtypes *typhimurium* and *enteritidis*. Non-typhoid *Salmonella* gastroenteritis is contracted through contaminated food. Symptoms including diarrhea, abdominal pain, fever, chills, nausea, and vomiting start 12 to 72 hours after exposure. Diagnosis is made by stool studies. Intravenous crystalloid is given for rehydration. Antimicrobials are not given in uncomplicated infections because they do not commonly shorten illness and may prolong the convalescent carrier state. If gastroenteritis is complicated by bacteremia, antimicrobials are given as discussed below. Rare case reports have linked *Salmonella* bacteremia with abortion (Coughlin, 2002).

Typhoid fever caused by *Salmonella typhi* remains a global health problem, although uncommon in the United States. It is spread by oral ingestion of contaminated food, water, or milk. In pregnant women, the disease is more likely to be encountered during epidemics or in those with HIV infection (Hedriana and colleagues, 1995). In their review, Dildy and associates (1990) reported that antepartum typhoid fever in former years resulted in abortion, preterm labor, and maternal or fetal death.

Fluoroquinolones are the most effective treatment, but alternatives include intravenous third-generation cephalosporins or azithromycin in pregnant women, especially in areas of quinolone resistance (Parry and co-workers, 2002). Typhoid vaccines appear to exert no harmful effects when administered to pregnant women and should be given in an epidemic or before travel to endemic areas.

Shigellosis

Bacillary dysentery caused by *Shigella* is a relatively common, highly contagious cause in adults of inflammatory exudative diarrhea, frequently with bloody stools. Shigellosis is more common in children attending day-care centers and is transmitted via the fecal-oral route (Centers for Disease Control and Prevention, 2006a). Clinical manifestations range from mild diarrhea to severe dysentery, abdominal cramping, tenesmus, fever, and systemic toxicity.

Although shigellosis may be self-limited, careful attention to treatment of dehydration is essential in severe cases. We have cared for pregnant women in whom secretory diarrhea exceeded 10 L/day! Effective treatments during pregnancy include fluoroquinolones, ceftriaxone, azithromycin, or trimethoprim-sulfamethoxazole, although antimicrobial resistance is now emerging (Bhattacharya and Sur, 2003; Centers for Disease Control and Prevention, 2006a).

Hansen Disease

Also known as leprosy, this chronic infection is caused by *Mycobacterium leprae*. Diagnosis is confirmed with PCR. Multidrug therapy with dapsone, rifampin, and clofazimine are recommended for treatment and are generally safe for use during pregnancy (Britton and Lockwood, 2004). Duncan (1980) reported an excessive incidence of low-birthweight newborns born to infected women. The placenta is not involved, and neonatal infection apparently is acquired from skin-to-skin or droplet transmission (Böddinghaus and co-workers, 2007; Duncan and colleagues, 1984). Vertical transmission is common in untreated mothers (Moschella, 2004).

Lyme Disease

Caused by the spirochete *Borrelia burgdorferi*, Lyme disease is the most commonly reported vector-borne illness in the United States (Centers for Disease Control and Prevention, 2007c). Lyme borreliosis follows tick bites of the genus *Ixodes*. Early infection causes a distinctive local skin lesion, *erythema migrans*, which may be accompanied by a flulike syndrome and regional adenopathy. If untreated, disseminated infection follows in days to weeks. Multisystem involvement is common, but skin lesions, arthralgia and myalgia, carditis, and meningitis predominate. If still untreated after several weeks to months, late or persistent infection manifests in perhaps half of patients. Native immunity is acquired, and the disease enters a chronic phase. Although some patients remain asymptomatic, others in the chronic phase develop a variety of skin, joint, or neurological manifestations (Wormser and colleagues, 2006).

Clinical diagnosis is important because serological diagnosis has pitfalls. Serology yields positive results in only approximately half of patients with early disease, whereas most with late, untreated Lyme disease have a positive enzyme-linked immunosorbent assay (ELISA) and/or Western blot assay. Although transplacental transmission has been confirmed, no congenital effects of maternal borreliosis have been conclusively identified (Elliott and colleagues, 2001; Walsh and associates, 2006).

Treatment and Prevention

Optimal treatment of Lyme disease was reviewed by Wormser and associates (2006) for the Infectious Disease Society of America. For early infection, treatment with doxycycline, amoxicillin, or cefuroxime is recommended for 14 days, although doxycycline is usually avoided in pregnancy. Intravenous ceftriaxone, cefotaxime, or penicillin G is given for complicated early infections that include meningitis or carditis. Chronic arthritis and post-Lyme disease syndrome are treated with prolonged oral or intravenous regimens, however, symptoms respond poorly to treatment (Klempner and colleagues, 2001).

A vaccine was withdrawn from the market in 2002 due to low sales. Avoidance of areas in which Lyme disease is endemic and improved tick control in those areas is the most effective prevention. Self-examination with removal of unengorged ticks within 36 hours of attachment reduces risks of infection (Hayes and Piesman, 2003). For tick bites recognized within 72 hours, a single 200-mg oral dose of doxycycline may reduce the development of Lyme disease. Prompt treatment of maternal early infection should prevent most adverse pregnancy outcomes.

Tuberculosis

Diagnosis and management of tuberculosis during pregnancy is discussed in detail in Chapter 46 (p. 1005).

PROTOZOAL INFECTIONS

Toxoplasmosis

Toxoplasma gondii has a complex life cycle with three forms: (1) a *tachyzoite*, which invades and replicates intracellularly during infection, (2) a *bradyzoite*, which forms tissue cysts during latent infection, and (3) a *sporozoite*, which is found in oocysts that can be environmentally resistant (Jones and associates, 2001). This ubiquitous protozoan is transmitted by eating raw or undercooked meat that is infected with tissue cysts or through contact with oocysts from infected cat feces in contaminated litter, soil, or water. From 1988 to 1994, the seroprevalence of toxoplasmosis was found to be 15 percent in childbearing-aged women (McQuillan, 2004). Thus, 85 percent of pregnant women are likely susceptible to infection.

The incidence of congenital toxoplasmosis varies from 0.8 per 10,000 live births in the United States to 10 per 10,000 in France (Dubey, 2000). Lopez and colleagues (2000) estimate there are between 400 and 4000 cases of congenital toxoplasmosis annually in the United States.

The incidence and severity of congenital infection depend on fetal age at the time of maternal infection. The *risks* for fetal infection increase with duration of pregnancy from 6 percent at 13 weeks to 72 percent at 36 weeks (Fig. 58-9). Freeman and colleagues (2005) studied outcomes in 386 women who seroconverted during pregnancy. In those infected before 20 weeks, 11 percent of newborns had congenital toxoplasmosis. But, the rate was 45 percent if infection was documented after 20 weeks. Conversely, the *severity* of fetal infection is much greater in early pregnancy, and these fetuses are much more likely to have clinical findings of infection (Dunn and associates, 1999).

Clinical Manifestations

Most acute infections in both mothers and neonates are silent and can be detected only by prenatal or newborn serological screening. In some cases, maternal symptoms may include fatigue, fever, muscle pain, and sometimes a maculopapular rash and posterior cervical lymphadenopathy. In immunocompetent adults, initial infection confers immunity, and prepregnancy infection nearly eliminates any risk of vertical transmission. Infection in immunocompromised women, however, may be severe, with reactivation involving encephalitis or mass lesions.

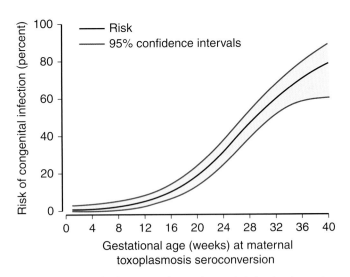

FIGURE 58-9 Risk of congenital toxoplasmosis infection by gestational age at maternal seroconversion. (From *The Lancet,* Vol. 353, No. 9167, D Dunn, M Wallon, F Peyron, et al., Mother-to-child transmission of toxoplasmosis: Risk estimates for clinical counselling, pp. 1829–1833, Copyright 1999, with permission from Elsevier.)

Maternal infection is associated with a fourfold increased preterm delivery rate before 37 weeks (Freeman and associates, 2005). Even so, growth restriction is not increased. Importantly, most infected fetuses are born without obvious stigmata of toxoplasmosis on routine examination. Clinically affected neonates usually have generalized disease with low birthweight, hepatosplenomegaly, jaundice, and anemia. Some primarily have neurological disease with intracranial calcifications such as those shown in Figure 58-10, as well as hydrocephaly or

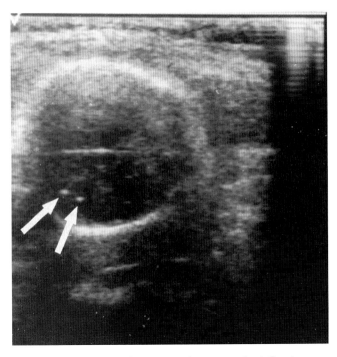

FIGURE 58-10 Sonographic image of intracranial calcifications (*arrows*) in a microcephalic fetus at approximately 30 weeks. (Courtesy of Dr. Rigoberto Santos.)

microcephaly. Many eventually develop chorioretinitis and exhibit learning disabilities. This classical triad—chorioretinitis, intracranial calcifications, and hydrocephalus—is often accompanied by convulsions. Infected neonates with clinical signs are at risk for long-term complications.

Diagnosis

The parasite is rarely detected in tissue or body fluids. Antitoxoplasma IgG develops within 1 to 2 weeks after infection, peaks at 1 to 2 months, and usually persists for life—sometimes in high titers. There is now an avidity test for toxoplasma IgG antibody used in maternal serum testing (Beghetto and colleagues, 2003; Montoya and Liesenfeld, 2004). The functional avidity of IgG antibody is low with primary infection and increases over weeks and months. If high-avidity IgG is determined, infection within the preceding 3 to 5 months is excluded. Although IgM antibodies appear by 10 days after infection and usually become negative within 3 to 4 months, they may remain detectable for years. Thus, IgM antibodies should not be used alone to diagnose acute toxoplasmosis. IgA and IgE antibodies are also useful in diagnosing acute infection. Best results are obtained with the Toxoplasma Serologic Profile performed at the Palo Alto Medical Foundation Research Institute (650-853-4828; toxolab@pamf.org). The panel includes the Sabin Feldman dye test, double-sandwich IgM ELISA, IgA and IgG ELISA, and a differential agglutination test (Montoya and Liesenfeld, 2004).

Prenatal diagnosis of toxoplasmosis is performed using DNA amplification techniques and sonographic evaluation. PCR of amnionic fluid or fetal blood has improved sensitivity over standard isolation techniques (Thalib and associates, 2005). Toxoplasma specific IgM and IgA may be present in amnionic fluid but their absence does not indicate lack of infection. Sonographic evidence of intracranial calcifications, hydrocephaly, liver calcifications, ascites, placental thickening, hyperechoic bowel, and growth restriction has all been used prenatally to help confirm diagnosis.

Management

Because of low prevalence rates, routine prenatal toxoplasma screening is not currently recommended except for women with HIV infection (American College of Obstetricians and Gynecologists, 2000). In areas of high toxoplasmosis prevalence—for example, France and Austria—routine screening has resulted in diminished congenital disease. With IgG antibody confirmed before pregnancy, there is no risk for a congenitally infected fetus (Montoya and Liesenfeld, 2004).

Treatment of pregnant women will likely reduce, but not eliminate, the risk for congenital infection (American College of Obstetricians and Gynecologists, 2000). *Spiramycin* is thought to reduce the risk of congenital infection but not to treat established fetal infection. The drug can be obtained from the Division of Special Pathogens and Immunologic Drug Products at the Food and Drug Administration (301-827-2335). Presumptive treatment with pyrimethamine and sulfonamides has been suggested for primary maternal infection in late pregnancy with negative amnionic fluid testing (Romand and associates, 2001). If fetal infection is diagnosed by prenatal testing, pyrimethamine, sulfonamides, and folinic acid are used to eradicate parasites in the placenta and fetus. The effectiveness of prenatal treatment is controversial, and Thiebart and colleagues as part of the Systematic Review on Congenital Toxoplasmosis (SYROCOT) Study Group (2007) recently performed a meta-analysis and reported a weak association of early treatment with reduced risk of congenital toxoplasmosis.

Prevention

There is no vaccine for toxoplasmosis, but congenital infection may be prevented by: (1) cooking meat to safe temperatures; (2) peeling or thoroughly washing fruits and vegetables; (3) cleaning cooking surfaces and utensils that contain raw meat, poultry, seafood, or unwashed fruits and vegetables; (4) wearing gloves when changing cat litter or delegating this duty; and (5) avoiding feeding cats raw or undercooked meat and keeping cats indoors. However, data supporting the effectiveness of such preventive steps is lacking (Di Mario and co-workers, 2009).

Malaria

The four species of *Plasmodium* that cause human malaria are *vivax, ovale, malariae,* and *falciparum.* Malaria remains the most common human parasitic disease, with nearly 300 to 500 million persons worldwide infected at any given time (Nosten and colleagues, 2007). Malaria has been effectively eradicated in Europe and most of North America except for parts of Mexico. But up to a fourth of pregnant women are infected in endemic areas such as Africa (Desai and co-workers, 2007).

Clinical findings are fever, chills, and flulike symptoms including headaches, myalgia, and malaise, which may occur at intervals. Symptoms are less severe with recurrences. Malaria may be associated with anemia and jaundice, and *falciparum* infections may cause kidney failure, coma, and death. That said, many otherwise healthy but infected adults in endemic areas are asymptomatic. Pregnant women, although often asymptomatic, are said to be more likely to develop traditional symptoms (Desai and associates, 2007; Tagbor, 2005).

Diagnosis

Identification of parasites by microscopic evaluation of a blood smear is considered the gold standard for diagnosis. In women with low parasite densities, however, the sensitivity of microscopy is poor. Malaria-specific antigens are now being used as a target for rapid diagnostic testing. Not only is their sensitivity still an issue in pregnancy, but these tests are not routinely available (Griffith and co-workers, 2007).

Effects on Pregnancy

Malaria, whether symptomatic or asymptomatic, causes a disproportionate rates of morbidity and mortality in pregnancy (Menéndez, 2007; Nosten, 2007; Rogerson, 2007, and all their colleagues). *P. falciparum* infections are more commonly associated with severe morbidity and mortality, and early infection has an increased risk for abortion (Desai and associates, 2007). The incidence of malaria increases significantly in the latter two trimesters and postpartum (Diagne and colleagues, 2000).

Infected erythrocytes as well as monocytes and macrophages accumulate in the vascular areas of the placenta (Fig. 58-11). High levels of placental parasitemia correlate with increased rates of stillbirth, preterm delivery, and fetal-growth restriction (Goldenberg and Thompson, 2003; Rogerson and co-workers, 2007). It is estimated that successful control of malaria in pregnancy would prevent 75,000 to 200,000 infant deaths worldwide every year (Steketee and collaborators, 2001).

Treatment

Most commonly used antimalarial drugs are not contraindicated during pregnancy. Some of the newer agents have antifolic acid activity and theoretically—but not pragmatically—contribute to development of megaloblastic anemia. *Chloroquine* is the treatment of choice for malaria caused by all sensitive *Plasmodium* species (Griffith and associates, 2007; Nosten and colleagues, 2007). For the woman with chloroquine-resistant infection, which constitutes the majority of *falciparum* infections, quinine plus clindamycin is currently recommended. Quinine may induce hyperinsulinemia and thus, possible maternal and fetal hypoglycemia. Mefloquine or atovaquone-proguanil are not currently recommended for treatment during pregnancy, although mefloquine is still recommended for chemoprophylaxis as subsequently discussed.

The severity of malaria, especially with *falciparum* infection, may be underestimated on initial clinical presentation. A thorough assessment of severity should precede but not delay treatment in pregnant women (Moore and associates, 2003). For severe or complicated malaria, quinidine gluconate is given parenterally. Cardiotoxicity is its major adverse effect, and women receiving this drug should have continuous electrocardiography monitoring. The Centers for Disease Control and Prevention maintains a Malaria Hotline for treatment recommendations (770-488-7788) (Thwing and associates, 2007).

Prophylaxis

Malaria control and prevention relies on chemoprophylaxis when traveling to or living in endemic areas. Vector control is also important, and insecticide-treated netting, pyrethroid insecticides, and DEET-based insect repellent have proven useful to decrease malarial rates in endemic areas. These are well tolerated in pregnancy (Menéndez and co-workers, 2007). Although not currently available, vaccine development targeting sporozoites is under study (Kanoi and Egwang, 2007). If travel is necessary, chemoprophylaxis is recommended.

Chloroquine prophylaxis is safe and well tolerated in pregnancy. It has been shown to decrease placental infection from 20 down to 4 percent in asymptomatic infected women in areas without chloroquine resistance (Cot and associates, 1992). For travelers to areas with chloroquine-resistant *P. falciparum*, mefloquine is currently the only chemoprophylaxis recommended. Primaquine and doxycycline are contraindicated in pregnancy, and there are insufficient data on atovaquone/proguanil to recommend them at this time. Likewise, amodiaquine is used in Africa, but data are limited in pregnant women.

Schwartz and associates (2003) emphasize the complexity of contemporary malaria prophylaxis due to drug resistance and the limitations of common regimens to protect against subsequent relapses from the liver stages of *P. vivax* and *P. ovale*. The latest chemoprophylaxis regimens for pregnancy can be obtained from the Centers for Disease Control and Prevention *Travelers Health* Web site at http://www.cdc.gov/travel/. The Centers for Disease Control and Prevention (2007f) also publish *Health Information for International Travel*, also called the *Yellow Book*, with detailed information.

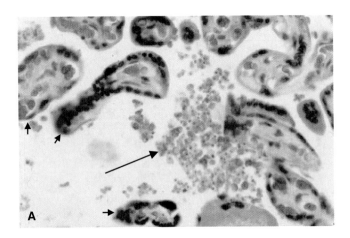

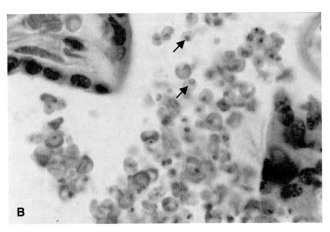

FIGURE 58-11 Photomicrograph of placental malaria. **A.** Multiple infected red blood cells (RBCs) (*long black arrow*) are seen in the intervillous space of this placenta. Multiple villi cut in cross section are shown and three are highlighted (*short arrows*). **B.** Increased magnification of image **(A).** Multiple infected RBCs are seen and two are identified (*arrows*).

Amebiasis

Most persons infected with *Entamoeba histolytica* are asymptomatic. Amebic dysentery, however, may take a fulminant course during pregnancy, with fever, abdominal pain, and bloody stools. Prognosis is worse if complicated by a hepatic abscess, which may be serious. Diagnosis is made with a stool sample and can be difficult. Therapy is similar to that for the nonpregnant woman, and metronidazole is the preferred drug for amebic colitis and invasive disease. Noninvasive infections may be treated with paromomycin (Haque and associates, 2003).

MYCOTIC INFECTIONS

Disseminated fungal infection—usually pneumonitis—during pregnancy is uncommon with coccidiomycosis, blastomycosis, cryptococcosis, or histoplasmosis. Their identification and management are considered in Chapter 46 (p. 1004).

EMERGING INFECTIONS

Infectious diseases whose incidence in humans has increased in the past two decades or has high potential to increase in the near future are termed "emerging infections" (Jamieson and colleagues, 2006a, b). They include severe acute respiratory syndrome (SARS), West Nile virus, and H1N1 influenza A (see p. 1212). They also include many of the bioterrorism agents detailed in the next section.

West Nile Virus

This mosquito-borne flavivirus is a human neuropathogen. Since 1999, reported numbers of human and animal infections have increased, and the geographical range of disease activity has expanded (Centers for Disease Control and Prevention, 2004; Morse, 2003). Infection typically is acquired through mosquito bites in late summer, or perhaps through blood transfusion (Harrington and associates, 2003). The incubation period is 3 to 14 days, and most persons have mild or no symptoms. Less than 1 percent of adults develop meningoencephalitis or acute flaccid paralysis (Granwehr and colleagues, 2004). In pregnant women, presenting symptoms are fever, mental status changes, muscle weakness, and coma (Chapa and colleagues, 2003).

The diagnosis is based on clinical symptoms and the detection of West Nile virus IgG and IgM in serum and IgM in cerebrospinal fluid. There is no known effective antiviral treatment, and management is supportive. The primary strategy for preventing exposure in pregnancy is the use of insect repellant containing *N,N*-diethyl-*m*-toluamide (DEET), which is considered safe for pregnant women (Koren and colleagues, 2003). Avoiding outdoor activity and stagnant water and wearing protective clothing is also recommended.

Pregnancy

Animal data suggest that embryos are susceptible to West Nile viral injection (Julander and associates, 2006). Human fetal infection with West Nile virus at 27 weeks resulted in a term neonate with chorioretinitis and severe temporal and occipital lobe leukomalacia (Alpert and co-workers, 2003). O'Leary and colleagues (2006) described cases reported to the West Nile Virus Pregnancy Registry. There were 77 infected pregnant women who had 72 live infants, four miscarriages, and two elective abortions. The preterm birth rate was 6 percent. Only three of 72 infants developed West Nile virus infection, although it could not be established conclusively that infection was acquired congenitally. Of three major malformations *possibly* associated with viral infection, none was definitively confirmed. Thus, any adverse fetal effects of West Nile viral infection are currently unclear.

Severe Acute Respiratory Syndrome (SARS)

Since 2002, there have been several outbreaks of SARS reported in Asia and North America. Its cause is a novel *coronavirus*—SARS-CoV—that is transmitted through droplets, close contact with infected secretions, fluids, and waste (Christian, 2004; Drosten, 2003; Ksiazek, 2003, and all their colleagues). The incubation period is 2 to 16 days, and the early clinical picture is similar to community-acquired pneumonia. SARS exposure or travel to an affected area increases the likelihood of diagnosis (Wenzel and Edmond, 2003).

There appears to be a triphasic pattern to the clinical progression of SARS. The first week is characterized by prodromal symptoms of fever, myalgias, headache, and diarrhea. During the second week, patients may suffer recurrent fever, watery diarrhea, and a dry nonproductive cough with mild dyspnea, and these are coincidental with IgG seroconversion and a declining viral load. Progression at this stage is thought to be due to an overexuberant host immune response. The third and at times lethal phase—seen in about 20 percent of patients—is progression to the acute respiratory distress syndrome (Christian and associates, 2004; Peiris and co-workers, 2003a, b).

Radiographic pulmonary manifestations of SARS include ground-glass opacities and airspace consolidations that can rapidly progress to extensive consolidation within 1 to 2 days. There also may be lymphopenia, thrombocytopenia, and elevated serum lactate dehydrogenase (Tsang and co-workers, 2003).

There currently is no proven treatment (Peiris and associates, 2003a, b; Perlman and Netland, 2009). Most patients have been given broad-spectrum antimicrobials. In pregnancy, oral therapy with clarithromycin plus amoxicillin with clavulanate have been used (So and colleagues, 2003; Wong and co-workers, 2003). Ribavirin to decrease viral replication and corticosteroids to modulate the immune response are controversial and should be reserved for severe illness (Jamieson and associates, 2006a; Mandell and co-workers, 2003).

Pregnancy

Any adverse effects of SARS on perinatal outcome is unclear because of limited published experiences. An increased incidence of miscarriage, fetal-growth restriction, and preterm delivery has been reported (Jamieson and co-workers, 2006b). Small case-control studies indicate that SARS is more severe in pregnant women compared with nonpregnant women with a case-fatality rate of 25 percent (Lam and colleagues, 2004; Wong and co-workers, 2004). There are no documented infections in neonates born to mothers with SARS (Peiris and colleagues, 2003a).

TRAVEL PRECAUTIONS DURING PREGNANCY

Pregnant travelers face obstetrical risks, general medical risks, and potentially hazardous destination risks. Some of these are discussed in detail in Chapter 8 (p. 207). The International Society for Tropical Medicines has comprehensive information available at http://www.istm.org. The Centers for Disease Control and Prevention has extensive travel information regarding pregnancy and breast feeding at its *Travelers' Health* home page at http://www.cdc.gov/travel/index.htm. There is also extensive information in the *Yellow Book* published by the Centers for Disease Control and Prevention (2007f). The American College of Obstetricians and Gynecologists (2003) also has published recommendations for active and passive immunization in pregnancy, including some vaccination issues pertinent to travel.

BIOTERRORISM

Bioterrorism involves the deliberate release of bacteria, viruses, or other infectious agents to cause illness or death. These natural agents are often altered to increase their infectivity or their resistance to medical therapy. Clinicians should be alert for significant increases in the number of persons with febrile illnesses accompanied by respiratory symptoms or with rashes not easily associated with common illnesses. Clinicians are urged to contact their state health department or bioterrorism Web sites of the Centers for Disease Control and Prevention (www.cdc.gov) for contemporary information and recommendations.

Smallpox

The variola virus is considered a serious weapon because of high transmission and overall 30-percent case-fatality rate. The last case of smallpox in the United States was reported in 1949, and worldwide it was reported in Somalia in 1977. Transmission occurs with prolonged contact, infected body fluids, or contaminated objects such as clothing. Smallpox presents with an acute onset of fever followed by a rash characterized by firm, deep-seated vesicles or pustules in the same stage of development. Nishiura (2006) and Suarez and Hankins (2002) have provided reviews addressing the severe perinatal and maternal morbidity and mortality caused by smallpox.

Because smallpox vaccine is made with live vaccinia virus, pregnancy should be delayed for 4 weeks in recipients. It is generally not given to pregnant women because of the risk of fetal vaccinia, a rare but serious complication. The Centers for Disease Control and Prevention (2003) recommends smallpox vaccination in pregnant women with emergency exposure, and it maintains a registry. Inadvertent vaccination is not ordinarily an indication for pregnancy termination.

Anthrax

Bacillus anthracis is a gram-positive, spore-forming, aerobic bacterium. It can cause three main types of clinical anthrax: inhalational, cutaneous, and gastrointestinal (Swartz, 2001; Holty and colleagues, 2006). The bioterrorist anthrax attacks of 2001 involved inhalational anthrax (Inglesby and co-workers, 2002). Spores are inhaled and deposited in the alveoli, engulfed by macrophages, and germinated in mediastinal lymph nodes. The incubation period is usually less than 1 week but may be as long as 2 months. Initial symptoms are nonspecific and include low-grade fever, nonproductive cough, malaise, and myalgias. Within 1 to 5 days of symptom onset, the second stage is heralded by the abrupt onset of severe respiratory distress and high fevers. Mediastinitis and hemorrhagic thoracic lymphadenitis

are common, and there is a widened mediastinum on chest radiograph. Case-fatality rates with inhalational anthrax are high, even with aggressive antibiotic and supportive therapy (Dixon and colleagues, 1999; Holty and associates, 2006).

There are few data regarding anthrax in pregnancy. Kadanali and associates (2003) reviewed two cases of third-trimester cutaneous anthrax treated successfully with penicillin. In both, preterm delivery followed soon after therapy was given.

The American College of Obstetricians and Gynecologists (2002b) and the Centers for Disease Control and Prevention (2001) recommend that asymptomatic pregnant and lactating women with documented exposure to *B. anthracis* be given postexposure prophylaxis with ciprofloxacin, 500 mg orally twice daily for 60 days. Amoxicillin, 500 mg orally three times daily, can be substituted if the strain is proven sensitive. In the case of ciprofloxacin allergy and either penicillin allergy or resistance, doxycycline, 100 mg orally twice daily, is given for 60 days. Risks from anthrax far outweigh any fetal risks from doxycycline.

The anthrax vaccine is an inactivated, cell-free product that requires six injections during 18 months. Vaccination is generally avoided in pregnancy because there are no safety data (Centers for Disease Control and Prevention, 2002e). That said, anthrax vaccine is an essential adjunct to postexposure antimicrobial prophylaxis, even in pregnancy (American College of Obstetricians and Gynecologists, 2002b).

Other Bioterrorism Agents

Francisella tularensis—tularemia, *Clostridium botulinum*—botulism, *Yersinia pestis*—plague, and viral hemorrhagic fevers—for example, Ebola, Marburg, Lassa, and Machupo, are also category A bioterrorism agents. There are multiple agents listed as category B and C. The guidelines for these biological agents are evolving and are detailed in the Centers for Disease Control and Prevention Bioterrorism Web site at www.bt.cdc.gov/agent.

REFERENCES

Alpert SG, Fergerson J, Noël L-P: Intrauterine West Nile Virus: Ocular and systemic findings. Am J Ophthalmol 136:722, 2003

American Academy of Pediatrics. Measles. In Pickering IK (ed). Red Book: 2006 Report of the Committee on Infections Diseases, 27th ed. Elk Grove Village, IL, American Academy of Pediatrics, 2006, p 441

American College of Obstetricians and Gynecologists: Rubella and pregnancy. Technical Bulletin No. 171, August 1992

American College of Obstetricians and Gynecologists: Perinatal viral and parasitic infections. Practice Bulletin No. 20, September 2000

American College of Obstetricians and Gynecologists: Prevention of early-onset group B streptococcal disease in newborns. Committee Opinion No. 279, December 2002a

American College of Obstetricians and Gynecologists: Management of asymptomatic pregnant or lactating women exposed to anthrax. Committee Opinion No. 268, February 2002b

American College of Obstetricians and Gynecologists: Immunization during pregnancy. Committee Opinion No. 282, January 2003

Antsaklis AJ, Daskalakis GJ, Mesogitis SA, et al: Prenatal diagnosis of fetal primary cytomegalovirus infection. Br J Obstet Gynaecol 107:84, 2000

Auriti C, Piersigilli F, De Gasperis MR, et al: Congenital Varicella Syndrome: Still a Problem? Fetal DiagnTher 25(2):224, 2009

Baker CJ, Paoletti LC, Rench MA, et al: Use of capsular polysaccharide-tetanus toxoid conjugate vaccine for Type II group B streptococcus in healthy women. J Infect Dis 182:1129, 2000

Baker CJ, Paoletti LC, Wessels MR, et al: Safety and immunogenicity of capsular polysaccharide-tetanus toxoid conjugate vaccines for group B streptococcal types Ia and Ib. J Infect Dis 179:142, 1999

Baker CJ, Rench MA, Edwards MS, et al: Immunization of pregnant women with a polysaccharide vaccine of group B streptococcus. N Engl J Med 319:1180, 1988

Banatvala JE, Brown DW: Rubella. Lancet 363:1127, 2004

Barbosa-Cesnik C, Schwartz K, Foxman B: Lactation mastitis. JAMA 289:1609, 2003

Bates T: Poliomyelitis in pregnancy, fetus and newborn. Am J Dis Child 90:189, 1955

Beghetto E, Buffolano W, Spadoni A, et al: Use of an immunoglobulin G avidity assay based on recombinant antigens for diagnosis of primary *Toxoplasma gondii* infection during pregnancy. J Clin Microbiol 41:5414, 2003

Beigi RH, Bunge K, Song Y, et al: Epidemiologic and economic effect of methicillin-resistant Staphylococcus aureus in obstetrics. Obstet Gynecol 113(5):983, 2009

Bergseng H, Bevanger L, Rygg M, et al: Real-time PCR targeting the sip gene for detection of group B *Streptococcus* colonization in pregnant women at delivery. J Med Microbiol 56:223, 2007

Berkowitz K, McCaffrey R: Postpartum osteomyelitis caused by group B streptococcus. Am J Obstet Gynecol 163:1200, 1990

Best JM, O'Shea S, Tipples G, et al: Interpretation of rubella serology in pregnancy—pitfalls and problems. BMJ 325:147, 2002

Bhattacharya SK, Sur D: An evaluation of current shigellosis treatment. Expert Opin Pharmacother 4:1315, 2003

Bland MI, Vermillion ST, Soper DE: Late third-trimester treatment of rectovaginal group B streptococci with benzathine penicillin G. Am J Obstet Gynecol 183:372, 2000

Bloom SL, Leveno KJ, Gilstrap LC, et al: Timing of intrapartum ampicillin infusion for group B streptococcus (GBS) prophylaxis. Am J Obstet Gynecol 174:407, 1996

Böddinghaus BK, Ludwig RJ, Kaufmann R, et al: Leprosy in a pregnant woman. Infection 35:37, 2007

Bodéus M, Hubinont C, Bernard P, et al: Prenatal diagnosis of human cytomegalovirus by culture and polymerase chain reaction: 98 pregnancies leading to congenital infection. Prenat Diagn 19:314, 1999

Bohlke K, Galil K, Jackson LA, et al: Postpartum varicella vaccination: Is the vaccination virus excreted in breast milk? Obstet Gynecol 102:970, 2003

Boppana SB, Rivera LB, Fowler KB, et al: Intrauterine transmission of cytomegalovirus to infants of women with preconceptional immunity. N Engl J Med 344:1366, 2001

Boucher M, Yonekura ML: Perinatal listeriosis (early onset): Correlation of antenatal manifestations and neonatal outcome. Obstet Gynecol 68:593, 1986

Britton WJ, Lockwood DN: Leprosy. Lancet 363:1209, 2004

Broliden K, Tolevenstam T, Norbeck O: Clinical aspects of parvovirus B19 infection. J Intl Med 260:285, 2006

Brown EJ: The molecular basis of streptococcal toxic shock syndrome. N Engl J Med 350:2093, 2004

Brown GC, Karunas RS: Relationship of congenital anomalies and maternal infection with selected enteroviruses. Am J Epidemiol 95:207, 1972

Butchko AR, Jordan JA: Comparison of three commercially available serologic assays used to detect human parvovirus B19-specific immunoglobulin M (IgM) and IgG antibodies in sera of pregnant women. J Clinic Microbiol 42:3191, 2004

Canadian Task Force on Preventive Health Care: Prevention of early-onset group B streptococcal (GBS) infection in the newborn. Systematic review and recommendations. CMAJ 166:928, 2002

Centers for Disease Control and Prevention: Measles, mumps, and rubella—vaccine use and strategies for elimination of measles, rubella, and congenital rubella syndrome and control of mumps. MMWR 47(RR-8):1, 1998

Centers for Disease Control and Prevention: Evaluation of varicella reporting to the National Notifiable Disease Surveillance System—United States, 1972–1997. MMWR 48:55, 1999

Centers for Disease Control and Prevention: Updated recommendations for antimicrobial prophylaxis among asymptomatic pregnant women after exposure to *Bacillus anthracis*. MMWR 50:960, 2001

Centers for Disease Control and Prevention: General recommendations on immunization. MMWR 51(RR-1):1, 2002a

Centers for Disease Control and Prevention: Hantavirus pulmonary syndrome—United States: Updated recommendations for risk reduction. MMWR 51(RR-9):1 2002b

Centers for Disease Control and Prevention: Prevention of invasive group A streptococcal disease among household contacts of case patients and among postpartum and postsurgical patients: Recommendations from the Centers for Disease Control and Prevention. Clin Infect Dis 35:950, 2002c

Centers for Disease Control and Prevention: Prevention of perinatal group B streptococci disease. Revised guidelines from the CDC. MMWR 51(RR-11):1, 2002d

Centers for Disease Control and Prevention: Status of US Department of Defense preliminary evaluation of the association of anthrax vaccination and congenital anomalies. MMWR 51:127, 2002e

Centers for Disease Control and Prevention: Women with smallpox vaccine exposure during pregnancy reported to the National Smallpox Vaccine in Pregnancy Registry—United States, 2003. MMWR 52:386, 2003

Centers for Disease Control and Prevention: West Nile virus activity: United States, September 15–21, 2004. MMWR 53:875, 2004

Centers for Disease Control and Prevention: Rubeola. MMWR 54:1229, 2005

Centers for Disease Control and Prevention: *Shigella* surveillance: Annual summary, 2005. Atlanta, GA, US Department of Health and Human Services, November 2006a

Centers for Disease Control and Prevention: Community-associated methicillin-resistant *Staphylococcus* aureus infection among healthy newborns—Chicago and Los Angeles County, 2004. MMWR 55:329, 2006b

Centers for Disease Control and Prevention: A new product (VariZIG) for postexposure prophylaxis of varicella available under an investigational new drug application expanded access protocol. MMWR 55:209 2006c

Centers for Disease Control and Prevention: Prevention and control of influenza.http://www.cdc.gov/mmwr/preview/mmwrhtml/rr5510a1.htm?s_cid = rr5510a1_e Article retrieved on July 18, 2007a

Centers for Disease Control and Prevention: High levels of adamantane resistance among influenza A (H3N2) viruses and interim guidelines for use of antiviral agents—United States, 2005–06 influenza season. http://www.cdc.gov/mmwr/preview/mmwrhtml/mm5502a7.htm?s_cid = mm5502a7_c Article retrieved on July 18, 2007b

Centers for Disease Control and Prevention: Lyme disease—United States, 2003-2005. MMWR 56:573, 2007c

Centers for Disease Control and Prevention: Perinatal group B streptococcal disease after universal screening recommendation—United States, 2003–2005. MMWR 56:701, 2007d

Centers for Disease Control and Prevention: Prevention of varicella. Recommendations of the Advisory Committee on Immunization Practices (ACIP). MMWR 56 (RR-4), 2007e

Centers for Disease Control and Prevention. Health information for International Travel 2008. Atlanta, U.S. Department of Health and Human Services. Public Health Service, 2007f

Centers for Disease Control and Prevention: Novel influenza A (H1N1) virus infections in three pregnant women—United States, April–May 2009. MMWR 58(18):497, 2009

Centers for Disease Control and Prevention: Trends in perinatal group B streptococcal disease—United States, 2000–2006. MMWR 58(5):109, 2009

Chan KL, Levi K, Towner KJ, et al: Evaluation of the sensitivity of a rapid polymerase chain reaction for detection of group B streptococcus. J Obstet Gynaecol 26:402, 2006

Chandra PC, Patel H, Schiavello HJ, et al: Successful pregnancy outcome after complicated varicella pneumonia. Obstet Gynecol 92:680, 1998

Chapa JB, Ahn JT, DiGiovanni LM, et al: West Nile virus encephalitis during pregnancy. Obstet Gynecol 102:229, 2003

Chaves SS, Gargiullo P, Zhang JX, et al: Loss of vaccine-induced immunity to varicella over time. N Engl J Med 356:1121, 2007

Cheeran MC, Lokensgard JR, Schleiss MR: Neuropathogenesis of congenital cytomegalovirus infection: Disease mechanisms and prospects for intervention. Clin Microbiol Rev 22(1):99, 2009

Chen KT, Huard RC, Della-Latta P, et al: Prevalence of methicillin-sensitive and methicillin-resistant *Staphylococcus aureus* in pregnant women. Obstet Gynecol 108:482, 2006

Chohan L, Hollier LM, Bishop K, et al: Patterns of antibiotic resistance among group B streptococcus isolates: 2001–2004. Infect Dis Obstet Gynecol 1:57472, 2006

Christian MD, Poutanen SM, Loutfy MR, et al: Severe acute respiratory syndrome. Clin Infect Dis 38:1420, 2004

Chuang I, Beneden CV, Beall B, et al: Population-based surveillance for postpartum invasive group A streptococcus infections, 1995–2000. Clin Infect Dis 35:665, 2002

Collinet P, Subtil D, Houfflin-Debarge V, et al: Routine CMV screening during pregnancy. Eur J Obstet Gynecol Reprod Biol 114(1):3, 2004

Colombo DF, Lew JL, Pedersen CA, et al: Optimal timing of ampicillin administration to pregnant women for establishing bactericidal levels in the prophylaxis of group B streptococcus. Am J Obstet Gynecol 194:466, 2006

Coonrod DV, Jack BW, Boggess KA, et al: The clinical content of preconception care: infectious diseases in preconception care. Am J Obstet Gynecol 199(6 Suppl 2):S290, 2008

Cooper NJ, Sutton AJ, Abrams KR, et al: Effectiveness of neuraminidase inhibitors in treatment and prevention and treatment of influenza A and B: Systematic review and meta-analyses of randomised controlled trials. BMJ 326:1235, 2003

Cosmi E, Mari G, Delle Chiaie L, et al: Noninvasive diagnosis by Doppler ultrasonography of fetal anemia resulting from parvovirus infection. Am J Obstet Gynecol 187:1290, 2002

Cot M, Roisin A, Barro D, et al: Effect of chloroquine chemoprophylaxis during pregnancy on birth weight: Results of a randomized trial. Am J Trop Med Hyg 46:21, 1992

Coughlin LB, McGuigan J, Haddad NG, et al: *Salmonella* sepsis and miscarriage. Clin Microbiol Infect 9:866, 2002

Cox S, Posner SF, McPheeters M, et al: Hospitalizations with respiratory illness among pregnant women during influenza season. Obstet Gynecol 107:1315, 2006

Crane J: Parvovirus B19 infection in pregnancy. J Obstet Gynaecol Can 24:727, 2002

Dahlquist G, Frisk G, Ivarsson SA, et al: Indications that maternal coxsackie B virus infection during pregnancy is a risk factor for childhood-onset IDDM. Diabetologia 38:1371, 1996

Daif JL, Levie M, Chudnoff S, et al: Group a Streptococcus causing necrotizing fasciitis and toxic shock syndrome after medical termination of pregnancy. Obstet Gynecol 113(2 Pt 2):504, 2009

de Haan TR, Beersman MF, Oepkes D, et al: Parvovirus B19 infection in pregnancy: Maternal and fetal viral load measurements related to clinical parameters. Prenat Diagn 27:46, 2007

de Jong EP, de Haan TR, Kroes AC: Parvovirus B19 infection in pregnancy. J Clin Virol 36:1, 2006

Delle Chiaie L, Buck G, Grab D, et al: Prediction of fetal anemia with Doppler measurement of the middle cerebral artery peak systolic velocity in pregnancies complicated by maternal blood group alloimmunization or parvovirus B19 infection. Ultrasound Obstet Gynecol 18:232, 2001

Dembinski J, Eis-Hübinger AM, Maar J, et al: Long term follow up of serostatus after maternofetal parvovirus B19 infection. Arch Dis Child 88:219, 2003

Demmler GJ: Summary of a workshop on surveillance for congenital cytomegalovirus disease. Rev Infect Dis 13:315, 1991

Desai M, O ter Kuile F, Nosten F, et al: Epidemiology and burden of malaria in pregnancy. Lancet Infect Dis 7:93, 2007

Diagne N, Rogier C, Sokhna CS, et al: Increased susceptibility to malaria during the early postpartum period. N Engl J Med 343:598, 2000

Dildy GA III, Martens MG, Faro S, et al: Typhoid fever in pregnancy: A case report. J Reprod Med 35:273, 1990

Di Mario S, Basevi V, Gagliotti C, et al: Prenatal education for congenital toxoplasmosis. Cochrane Database Syst Rev 1:CD006171, 2009

Dixon TC, Meselson M, Guillemin J, et al: Anthrax. N Engl J Med 341:815, 1999

Drosten C, Günther S, Preiser W, et al: Identification of a novel coronavirus in patients with severe acute respiratory syndrome. N Engl J Med 348:1967, 2003

Dubey JP: Sources of *Toxoplasma gondii* infection in pregnancy. Until rates of congenital toxoplasmosis fall, control measures are essential. BMJ 321:127, 2000

Duff P: A thoughtful algorithm for the accurate diagnosis of primary CMV infection in pregnancy. Am J Obstet Gynecol 196:221, 2007

Duncan ME: Babies of mothers with leprosy have small placentas, low birth weights and grow slowly. Br J Obstet Gynaecol 87:461, 1980

Duncan ME, Fox H, Harkness RA, et al: The placenta in leprosy. Placenta 5:189, 1984

Dunn D, Wallon M, Peyron F, et al: Mother-to-child transmission of toxoplasmosis: Risk estimates for clinical counseling. Lancet 353:1829, 1999

Eady EA, Cove JH: Staphylococcal resistance revisited: Community-acquired methicillin resistant *Staphylococcus aureus*—an emerging problem for the management of skin and soft tissue infections. Curr Opin Infect Dis 16:103, 2003

Elliott DJ, Eppes SC, Klein JD: Teratogen update: Lyme disease. Teratology 64:276, 2001

Enders G, Bäder U, Lindemann L, et al: Prenatal diagnosis of congenital cytomegalovirus infection in 189 pregnancies with known outcome. Prenat Diagn 21:362, 2001

Enders G, Miller E, Cradock-Watson J, et al: Consequences of varicella and herpes zoster in pregnancy: Prospective study of 1739 cases. Lancet 343:1548, 1994

Enders M, Schalasta G, Baisch C, et al: Human parvovirus B19 infection during pregnancy—Value of modern molecular and serological diagnostics. J Clinic Virol 35:400, 2006

Enders M, Weidner A, Zoellner I, et al: Fetal morbidity and mortality after acute human parvovirus B19 infection in pregnancy: Prospective evaluation of 1018 cases. Prenat Diagn 24:513, 2004

Eschenbach DA: Prevention of neonatal group B streptococcal infection. N Engl J Med 347:280, 2002

Forsnes EV, Eggleston MK, Wax JR: Differential transmission of adenovirus in a twin pregnancy. Obstet Gynecol 91:817, 1998

Fowler KB, Stagno S, Pass RF: Maternal immunity and prevention of congenital cytomegalovirus infection. JAMA 289:1008, 2003

Fowler KB, Stagno S, Pass RF, et al: The outcome of congenital cytomegalovirus infection in relation to maternal antibody status. N Engl J Med 326:663, 1992

Fowler SL: A light in the darkness: Predicting outcomes for congenital cytomegalovirus infections. J Pediatr 137:4, 2000

Freeman K, Oakley L, Pollak A, et al: Association between congenital toxoplasmosis and preterm birth, low birthweight and small for gestational age birth. BJOG 112:31, 2005

Gilden DH, Kleinschmidt-DeMasters BK, LaGuardia JJ, et al: Neurologic complications of the reactivation of varicella-zoster virus. N Engl J Med 342:635, 2000

Goldenberg RL, Thompson C: The infectious origins of stillbirth. Am J Obstet Gynecol 189:861, 2003

Grangeot-Keros L, Cointe D: Diagnosis and prognostic markers of HCMV infection. J Clin Virol 21:213, 2001

Granwehr BP, Lillibridge KM, Higgs S, et al: West Nile Virus: Where are we now? Lancet Infect Dis 4:547, 2004

Griffith KS, Lewis LS, Mali S, et al: Treatment of malaria in the United States: A systematic review. JAMA 297:2264, 2007

Guerra B, Simonazzi G, Banfi A, et al: Impact of diagnostic and confirmatory tests and prenatal counseling on the rate of pregnancy termination among women with positive cytomegalovirus immunoglobulin M antibody titers. Am J Obstet Gynecol 196:221.e1, 2007

Haas DM, Flowers CA, Congdon CL: Rubella, rubeola, and mumps in pregnant women. Obstet Gynecol 106:295, 2005

Haberland CA, Benitz WE, Sanders GD, et al: Perinatal screening for group B streptococci: Cost-benefit analysis of rapid polymerase chain reaction. Pediatrics 110:471, 2002

Haque R, Huston CD, Hughes M, et al: Amebiasis. N Engl J Med 348:1565, 2003

Harger JH, Ernest JM, Thurnau GR, et al: Risk factors and outcome of varicella-zoster virus pneumonia. J Infect Dis 185:422, 2002

Harjulehto T, Aro T, Hovi T, et al: Congenital malformations and oral poliovirus vaccination during pregnancy. Lancet 1:771, 1989

Harrington T, Kuehnert MJ, Lanciotti RS, et al: West Nile virus infection transmitted by blood transfusion. Transfusion 43:1018, 2003

Hayes EB, Piesman J: How can we prevent Lyme disease? N Engl J Med 348:2424, 2003

Hedriana HL, Mitchell JL, Williams SB: *Salmonella typhi* chorioamnionitis in a human immunodeficiency virus–infected pregnant woman. J Reprod Med 40:157, 1995

Hidron A, Kourbatova EV, Halvosa JS, et al: Risk factors for colonization with methicillin-resistant *Staphylococcus aureus* (MSRA) in patients admitted to an urban hospital: Emergence of community-associated MRSA nasal carriage. Clin Infect Dis 41:159, 2005

Holty JE, Bravata DM, Liu H, et al: Systemic review: A century of inhalational anthrax cases from 1900 to 2005. Ann Intern Med 144:270, 2006

Howard MJ, Doyle TJ, Koster FT, et al: Hantavirus pulmonary syndrome in pregnancy. Clin Infect Dis 29:1538, 1999

Hyoti H, Hiltunen M, Knik M, et al: Childhood diabetes in Finland (DiMe) study group: A prospective study of the role of Coxsackie B and other enterovirus infections in the pathogenesis of IDDM. Diabetes 44:652, 1995

Illuzzi JL, Bracken MB: Duration of intrapartum prophylaxis for neonatal group B streptococcal disease. Obstet Gynecol 108:1254, 2006

Inglesby TV, O'Toole T, Henderson DA, et al: Anthrax as a biological weapon, 2002. JAMA 287:2236, 2002

Irving WL, James DK, Stephenson T, et al: Influenza virus infection in the second and third trimesters of pregnancy: A clinical and seroepidemiological study. Br J Obstet Gynaecol 107:1282, 2000

Jakobi P, Goldstick O, Sujov P, et al: New CDC guidelines for prevention of perinatal group B streptococcal disease. Lancet 361:351, 2003

Jamieson DJ, Ellis JE, Jernigan DB, et al: Emerging infectious disease outbreaks: Old lessons and new challenges for obstetrician-gynecologists. Am J Obstet Gynecol 194:1546, 2006a

Jamieson DJ, Theiler RN, Rasmussen SA: Emerging infections and pregnancy. Emerg Infect Dis 12:1638, 2006b

Janakiraman V: Listeriosis in pregnancy: Diagnosis, treatment, and prevention. Rev Obstet Gynecol 1(4):179, 2008

Johri AK, Paoletti LC, Glaser P, et al: Group B *Streptococcus*: Global incidence and vaccine development. Nat Rev Microbiol 4:932, 2006

Jones JL, Lopez A, Wilson M, et al: Congenital toxoplasmosis: A review. Obstet Gynecol Surv 56:296, 2001

Julander JG, Winger QA, Rickords LF, et al: West Nile virus infection of the placenta. Virology 347:175. 2006

Kadanali A, Tasyaran MA, Kadanali S: Anthrax during pregnancy: Case reports and review. Clin Infect Dis 36:1343, 2003

Kanoi BN, Egwang TG: New concepts in vaccine development in malaria. Curr Opin Infect Dis 20:311, 2007

Kimberlin DW, Lin CY, Sanchez PJ, et al: Effect of ganciclovir therapy on hearing in symptomatic congenital cytomegalovirus disease involving the central nervous system: A randomized, controlled trial. J Pediatr 143:16, 2003

Klempner MS, Hu LT, Evans J, et al: Two controlled trials of antibiotic treatment in patients with persistent symptoms and a history of Lyme disease. N Engl J Med 345:85, 2001

Koren G: Congenital varicella syndrome in the third trimester. www.thelancet.com 366:1591, 2005

Koren G, Matsui D, Bailey B: DEET-based insect repellents: Safety implications for children and pregnant and lactating women. CMAJ 169:209, 2003

Koro'lkova EL, Lozovskaia LS, Tadtaeva LI, et al: The role of prenatal coxsackie virus infection in the etiology of congenital heart defects in children. Kardiologiia 29:68, 1989

Ksiazek TG, Erdman D, Goldsmith CS, et al. A novel coronavirus associated with severe acute respiratory syndrome. N Engl J Med 348:1953, 2003

Kuehnert MJ, Kruszon-Moran D, Hill HA, et al: Prevalence of *Staphylococcus aureus* nasal colonization in the United States, 2001–2002. J Infect Dis 193:172, 2006

Kunugi H, Nanko S, Takei N, et al: Schizophrenia following in utero exposure to the 1957 influenza epidemics in Japan. Am J Psychiatry 152:450, 1995

Kurppa K, Holmberg PC, Kuosma E, et al: Anencephaly and maternal common cold. Teratology 44:51, 1991

Laibl VR, Sheffield JS, Roberts S, et al: Clinical presentation of community-acquired methicillin-resistant *Staphylococcus aureus* in pregnancy. Obstet Gynecol 106:461, 2005

Lam CM, Wong SF, Leung TN, et al: A case-controlled study comparing clinical course and outcomes of pregnant and non-pregnant women with severe acute respiratory syndrome. BJOG 111:771, 2004

Larsen JW, Sever JL: Group B Streptococcus and pregnancy: A review. Am J Obstet Gynecol 198(4):440, 2008

Lazzarotto T, Gabrielli L, Lanari M, et al: Congenital cytomegalovirus infection: recent advances in the diagnosis of maternal infection. Hum Immunol 65:410, 2004

Le Monnier A, Autret N, Join-Lambert OF, et al: ActA is required for crossing of the fetoplacental barrier by *Listeria monocytogenes*. Infect Immun 75:950, 2007

Liesnard C, Donner C, Brancart F, et al: Prenatal diagnosis of congenital cytomegalovirus infection: Prospective study of 237 pregnancies at risk. Obstet Gynecol 95:881, 2000

Lin FYC, Philips JB III, Azimi PH, et al: Level of maternal antibody required to protect neonates against early-onset disease caused by group B streptococcus type Ia: A multicenter, seroepidemiology study. J Infect Dis 184:1022, 2001

Lin FYC, Weisman LE, Troendle J, et al: Prematurity is the major risk factor for late-onset group B streptococcus disease. J Infect Dis 188:267, 2003

Lopez A, Dietz VJ, Wilson M, et al: Preventing congenital toxoplasmosis. MMWR 49(RR02):57, 2000

Lynberg MC, Khoury MJ, Lu X, et al: Maternal flu, fever, and the risk of neural tube defects: A population-based case-control study. Am J Epidemiol 140:244, 1994

Maisey HC, Hensler M, Nizet V, et al: Group B streptococcal pilus proteins contribute to adherence to and invasion of brain microvascular endothelial cells. J Bacteriol 189:1464, 2007

Malinger G, Lev D, Zahalka N, et al: Fetal cytomegalovirus infection of the brain: The spectrum of sonographic findings. AJNR Am J Neuroradiol 24:28, 2003

Mandell LA, Bartlett JG, Dowell SF, et al: Update of practice guidelines for the management of community acquired pneumonia in immunocompetent adults. Clin Infect Dis 37:1405, 2003

McClure EM, Goldenberg RL: Infection and stillbirth. Semin Fetal Neonatal Med 14(4):182, 2009

McGrath J, Castle D: Does influenza cause schizophrenia? A five year review. Aust NZ J Psychiatry 29:23, 1995

McQuillan GM, Kruszon-Moran D, Kottiri BJ, et al: Racial and ethnic differences in the seroprevalence of 6 infectious diseases in the United States: Data from NHANES III, 1988–1994. Am J Public Health 94:1952, 2004

Mendelson E, Aboundy Y, Smetana Z, et al: Laboratory assessment and diagnosis of congenital viral infections: Rubella, cytomegalovirus (CMV), varicella-zoster virus (VZV), herpes simplex virus (HSV), parvovirus B19 and human immunodeficiency virus (HIV). Reprod Toxicol 21:350, 2006

Menéndez C, D'Alessandro U, O ter Kuile F: Reducing the burden of malaria in pregnancy by preventive strategies. Lancet Infect Dis 7:126, 2007

Miller E, Cradock-Watson JE, Pollock TM: Consequences of confirmed maternal rubella at successive stages of pregnancy. Lancet 2:781, 1982

Mitchell TF, Pearlman MD, Chapman RL, et al: Maternal and transplacental pharmacokinetics of cefazolin. Obstet Gynecol 98:1075, 2001

Modlin F: Perinatal echovirus and group B coxsackievirus infections. Clin Perinatol 15:233, 1988

Montoya JG, Liesenfeld O: Toxoplasmosis. Lancet 363:1965, 2004

Moore MR, Schrag SJ, Schuchat A: Effects of intrapartum antimicrobial prophylaxis for prevention of group B streptococcal disease on the incidence and ecology of early-onset neonatal sepsis. Lancet Infect Dis 3:201, 2003

Moran GJ, Krishnadasan A, Gorwitz RJ, et al: Methicillin-resistant *S. aureus* infections among patients in the emergency department. N Engl J Med 355:666, 2006

Morse DL: West Nile Virus—not a passing phenomenon. N Engl J Med 348:22, 2003

Moschella SL: An update on the diagnosis and treatment of leprosy. J Am Acad Dermatol 51:417, 2004

Mubareka S, Richards H, Gray M, et al: Evaluation of commercial rubella immunoglobulin G avidity assays. J Clinic Microbiol 45:231, 2007

Mylonakis E, Paliou M, Hohmann EL, et al: Listeriosis during pregnancy. Medicine 81:260, 2002

Nagel HT, de Haan TR, Vandenbussche FP, et al: Long-term outcome after fetal transfusion for hydrops associated with parvovirus B19 infection. Obstet Gynecol 109(1):42, 2007

Naimi TS, LeDell KH, Como-Sabetti K, et al: Comparison of community- and health-care associated methicillin-resistant *Staphylococcus aureus* infection. JAMA 290:2976, 2003

Nathan L, Peters MT, Ahmed AM, et al: The return of life-threatening puerperal sepsis caused by group A streptococci. Am J Obstet Gynecol 169:571, 1993

Neuzil KM, Reed GW, Mitchel EF, et al: Impact of influenza on acute cardiopulmonary hospitalizations in pregnant women. Am J Epidemiol 148:1094, 1998

Nigro G, Adler SP, La Torre R, et al: Passive immunization during pregnancy for congenital cytomegalovirus infection. N Engl J Med 353:1350, 2005

Nigro G, Anceschi MM, Cosmi EV, et al: Clinical manifestations and abnormal laboratory findings in pregnant women with primary cytomegalovirus infection. Br J Obstet Gynaecol 110:572, 2003

Nishiura H: Smallpox during pregnancy and maternal outcomes. Emerg Infect Dis 12:1119, 2006

Norbeck O, Papadogiannakis N, Petersson K, et al: Revised clinical presentation of parvovirus B19–associated intrauterine fetal death. Clin Infect Dis 35:1032, 2002

Nosten F, McGready R, Mutabingwa T: Case management of malaria in pregnancy. Lancet Infect Dis 7:118, 2007

O'Brien KL, Beall B, Barrett NL, et al: Epidemiology of invasive group A streptococcus disease in the United States, 1995–1999. Clin Infect Dis 35:268, 2002

Ohji G, Satoh H, Satoh H, et al: Congenital measles caused by transplacental infection. Pediatr Infect Dis J 28(2):166, 2009

O'Leary DR, Kuhn S, Kniss KL, et al: Birth outcomes following West Nile Virus infection of pregnant women in the United States: 2003–2004. Pediatrics 117:e537, 2006

Ornoy A, Tenenbaum A: Pregnancy outcome following infections by coxsackie, echo, measles, mumps, hepatitis, polio and encephalitis viruses. Reprod Toxicol 21:446, 2006

Parry CM, Hien TT, Dougan G, et al: Typhoid fever. N Engl J Med 347:1770, 2002

Paryani SG, Arvin AM: Intrauterine infection with varicella zoster virus after maternal varicella. N Engl J Med 314:1542, 1986

Pass RF: Day-care centers and the spread of cytomegalovirus and parvovirus B19. Pediatr Ann 20:419, 1991

Peckham C, Tookey P, Logan S, et al: Screening options for prevention of congenital cytomegalovirus infection. J Med Screen 8:119, 2001

Peiris JSM, Chu CM, Cheng VCC, et al: Clinical progression and viral load in a community outbreak of coronavirus-associated SARS pneumonia: A prospective study. Lancet 361:1767, 2003a

Peiris JSM, Yuen KY, Osterhaus ADME, et al: The severe acute respiratory syndrome. N Engl J Med 349:2431, 2003b

Perlman S, Netland J: Coronaviruses post-SARS: update on replication and pathogenesis. Nat Rev Microbiol 7(6):439, 2009

Plourd DM, Austin K: Correlation of a reported history of chickenpox with seropositive immunity in pregnant women. J Reprod Med 50:779, 2005

Reef SE, Frey TK, Theal K, et al: The changing epidemiology of rubella in the 1990s: On the verge of elimination and new challenges for control and prevention. JAMA 287:464, 2002

Reef SE, Plotkin S, Cordero JS, et al: Preparing for elimination of congenital rubella syndrome (CRS): Summary of a workshop on CRS elimination in the United States. Clin Infect Dis 31:85, 2000

Revello MG, Gerna G: Pathogenesis and prenatal diagnosis of human cytomegalovirus infection. J Clin Virol 29:71, 2004

Revello MG, Furione M, Zavattoni M, et al: Human cytomegalovirus (HCMV) DNAemia in the mother at amniocentesis as a risk factor for iatrogenic HCMF infection of the fetus. J Infect Dis 197:593, 2008

Rogers BB: Parvovirus B19: Twenty-five years in perspective. Pediatr Develop Pathol 2:296, 1999

Rogers S, Commons R, Danchin MH, et al: Strain prevalence, rather than innate virulence potential, is the major factor responsible for an increase in serious group A streptococcus infections. J Infect Dis 195:1625, 2007

Rogerson SJ, Hviid L, Duffy PE, et al: Malaria in pregnancy: Pathogenesis and immunity. Lancet Infect Dis 7:105, 2007

Romand S, Wallon M, Franck J, et al: Prenatal diagnosis using polymerase chain reaction on amniotic fluid for congenital toxoplasmosis. Obstet Gynecol 97:296, 2001

Rouse DJ, Lincoln T, Cilver S, et al: Intrapartum chlorhexidine vaginal irrigation and chorioamnion and placental microbial colonization. Int J Gynaecol Obstet 83:165, 2003

Royal College of Obstetricians and Gynaecologists: Prevention of early onset neonatal group B streptococcal disease. Guideline No. 36, November 2003

Salgado CD, Farr BM, Hall KK, et al: Influenza in the acute hospital setting. Lancet Infect Dis 2:145, 2002

Saxén L, Holmberg PC, Kurppa K, et al: Influenza epidemics and anencephaly. Am J Public Health 80:473, 1990

Schild RL, Bald R, Plath H, et al: Intrauterine management of fetal parvovirus B19 infection. Ultrasound Obstet Gynecol 13:151, 1999

Schrag SJ, Arnold KE, Mohle-Boetani JC, et al: Prenatal screening for infectious diseases and opportunities for prevention. Obstet Gynecol 102:753, 2003

Schrag SJ, Zell ER, Lynfield R, et al: A population-based comparison of strategies to prevent early-onset group B streptococcal disease in neonates. N Engl J Med 347:233, 2002

Schrag SJ, Zywicki S, Farley MM, et al: Group B streptococcal disease in the era of intrapartum antibiotic prophylaxis. N Engl J Med 342:15, 2000

Schwartz E, Parise M, Kozarsky P, et al: Delayed onset of malaria—implications for chemoprophylaxis in travelers. N Engl J Med 349:1510, 2003

Shaw GM, Todoroff K, Velie EM, et al: Maternal illness, including fever, and medication use as risk factors for neural tube defects. Teratology 57:1, 1998

Shields KE, Galil K, Seward J, et al: Varicella vaccine exposure during pregnancy: Data from the first 5 years of the Pregnancy Registry. Obstet Gynecol 98:14, 2001

Siegel M: Congenital malformations following chickenpox, measles, mumps, and hepatitis: Results of a cohort study. JAMA 226:1521, 1973

Siegel M, Fuerst HT: Low birth weight and maternal virus diseases: A prospective study of rubella, measles, mumps, chickenpox, and hepatitis. JAMA 197:88, 1966

Siegel M, Goldberg M: Incidence of poliomyelitis in pregnancy. N Engl J Med 253:841, 1955

Silver HM: Listeriosis during pregnancy. Obstet Gynecol Surv 53:737, 1998

Skjöldebrand-Sparre L, Tolfvenstam T, Papadogiannakis N, et al: Parvovirus B19 infection: Association of third-trimester intrauterine fetal death. Br J Obstet Gynaecol 107:476, 2000

So LK, Lau AC, Yam LY, et al: Development of a standard treatment protocol for severe acute respiratory syndrome. Lancet 361:1615, 2003

Sriskandan S, Faulkner L, Hopkins P: *Streptococcus pyogenes*: Insight into the function of the streptococcal superantigens. Int J Biochem Cell Biol 39:12, 2007

Stagno S, Tinker MK, Elrod C, et al: Immunoglobulin M antibodies detected by enzyme-linked immunosorbent assay and radioimmunoassay in the diagnosis of cytomegalovirus infections in pregnant women and newborn infants. J Clin Microbiol 21(6):930, 1985

Steketee RW, Nahlen BL, Parise ME, et al: The burden of malaria in pregnancy in malaria-endemic areas. Am J Trop Med Hyg 64:28, 2001

Stirrat G: The immune system. In Hytten F, Chamberlain G (eds): Clinical Physiology in Obstetrics. London, Blackwell, 1991, p 101

Stoll BJ, Hansen N: Infections in VLBW infants: Studies from the NICHD Neonatal Research Network. Semin Perinatol 27:293, 2003

Stoll BJ, Hansen N, Fanaroff AA, et al: Changes in pathogens causing early-onset sepsis in very-low-birth-weight infants. N Engl J Med 347:240, 2002a

Stoll BJ, Hansen N, Fanaroff AA, et al: Late-onset sepsis in very low birth weight neonates: The experience of the NICHD Neonatal Research Network. Pediatrics 110:285, 2002b

Suarez VR, Hankins GDV: Smallpox and pregnancy: From eradicated disease to bioterrorist threat. Obstet Gynecol 100:87, 2002

Swartz MN: Recognition and management of anthrax—an update. N Engl J Med 345:1621, 2001

SYROCOT (Systematic Review on Congenital Toxoplasmosis) Study Group: Effectiveness of prenatal treatment for congenital toxoplasmosis: A meta-analysis of individual patients' data. Lancet 369:115, 2007

Tagbor H: A randomized controlled trial of three drugs regimens for the treatment of malaria in pregnancy in Ghana. PhD thesis, University of London, 2005

Tanemura M, Suzumori K, Yagami Y, et al: Diagnosis of fetal rubella infection with reverse transcription and nested polymerase chain reaction: A study of 34 cases diagnosed in fetuses. Am J Obstet Gynecol 174:578, 1996

Tang JW, Aarons E, Hesketh LM, et al: Prenatal diagnosis of congenital rubella infection in the second trimester of pregnancy. Prenat Diagn 6:509, 2003

Thalib L, Gras L, Roman S, et al: Prediction of congenital toxoplasmosis by polymerase chain reaction analysis of amniotic fluid. BJOG 11:567, 2005

Thwing J, Skarbinski J, Newman RD, et al: Malaria surveillance—United States, 2005. MMWR Surveill Summ 56:23, 2007

Tolfvenstam T, Papadogiannakis N, Norbeck O, et al: Frequency of human parvovirus B19 infection in intrauterine fetal death. Lancet 357:1494, 2001

Topalovski M, Yang SS, Boonpasat Y: Listeriosis of the placenta: Clinicopathologic study of seven cases. Am J Obstet Gynecol 169:616, 1993

Towbin JA, Griffin LD, Martin AB, et al: Intrauterine adenoviral myocarditis presenting as nonimmune hydrops fetalis: Diagnosis by polymerase chain reaction. Pediatr Infect Dis J 13:144, 1994

Towers CV, Briggs GG: Antepartum use of antibiotics and early-onset neonatal sepsis: The next four years. Am J Obstet Gynecol 187:495, 2002

Tsang KW, Ho PL, Ooi CG, et al: A cluster of cases of severe acute respiratory syndrome in Hong Kong. N Engl J Med 348:1977, 2003

Udagawa H, Oshio Y, Shimizu Y: Serious group A streptococcal infection around delivery. Obstet Gynecol 94:153, 1999

Valeur-Jensen AK, Pedersen CB, Westergaard T, et al: Risk factors for parvovirus B19 infection in pregnancy. JAMA 281:1099, 1999

Varma JK, Samuel MC, Marcus R, et al: *Listeria monocytogenes* infection from foods prepared in a commercial establishment: A case-control study of potential sources of sporadic illness in the United States. Clin Infect Dis 44:521, 2007

Viskari HR, Roivainen M, Reunanen A, et al: Maternal first-trimester enterovirus infection and future risk of type 1 diabetes in the exposed fetus. Diabetes 51:2568, 2002

Voetsch AC, Angulo FJ, Jones TF, et al: Reduction in the incidence of invasive listeriosis in foodborne diseases active surveillance network sites, 1996–2003. Clin Infect Dis 44:513, 2007

von Kaisenberg CS, Jonat W: Fetal parvovirus B19 infection. Ultrasound Obstet Gynecol 18:280, 2001

Walsh CA, Mayer EQ, Baxi LV: Lyme disease in pregnancy: Case report and review of the literature. Obstet Gynecol Surv 62:41, 2006

Webster WS: Teratogen update: Congenital rubella. Teratology 58:13, 1998

Wendel GD Jr, Leveno KJ, Sánchez PJ, et al: Prevention of neonatal group B streptococcal disease: A combined intrapartum and neonatal protocol. Am J Obstet Gynecol 186:618, 2002

Wenzel RP, Edmond MB: Managing SARS amidst uncertainty. N Engl J Med 348:1947, 2003

Wing EJ, Gregory SH: *Listeria monocytogenes*: Clinical and experimental update. J Infect Dis 185:S18, 2002

Wong SF, Chow KM, de Swiet M: Severe acute respiratory syndrome and pregnancy. Br J Obstet Gynaecol 110:641, 2003

Wong SF, Chow KM, Leung TN, et al: Pregnancy and perinatal outcomes of women with severe acute respiratory syndrome. Am J Obstet Gynecol 191:292, 2004

World Health Organization Collaborative Study Team on the Role of Breast-feeding on the Prevention of Infant Mortality: Effect of breastfeeding on infant and child mortality due to infectious diseases in less developed countries: A pooled analysis. Lancet 355:451, 2000

Wormser GP, Dattwyler RJ, Shapiro ED, et al: The clinical assessment, treatment, and prevention of Lyme disease, human granulocytic anaplasmosis, and babesiosis: Clinical practice guidelines by the Infectious Diseases Society of America. Clin Infect Dis 43:1089, 2006

Yaegashi N: Pathogenesis of nonimmune hydrops fetalis caused by intrauterine B19 infection. Tohoku J Exp Med 190:65, 2000

Young NS, Brown KE: Mechanisms of disease: Parvovirus B19. N Engl J Med 350:586, 2004

Zaman K, Roy E, Arifeen SE, et al: Effectiveness of maternal influenza immunization in mothers and infants. N Engl J Med 359(15):1555, 2008

CHAPTER 59

Sexually Transmitted Diseases

Sexually transmitted diseases (STDs), also called sexually transmitted infections (STIs), are common during pregnancy and should be aggressively sought and treated (Coonrad and colleagues, 2008). Importantly, education, screening, treatment, and prevention are essential components of prenatal care (Piper and colleagues, 2003). STDs that affect pregnant women and potentially affect the fetus include syphilis, gonorrhea, trichomoniasis, and chlamydial, hepatitis B, human immunodeficiency virus (HIV), herpes simplex virus–1 and -2 (HSV-1, -2), and human papillomavirus (HPV) infections. Recommended treatment protocols for most adhere to the frequently updated guidelines provided by the Centers for Disease Control and Prevention (2006b). Treatment of most STDs is clearly associated with improved pregnancy outcome and prevention of perinatal mortality (Goldenberg and associates, 2003, 2009; Gray and co-workers, 2001).

SYPHILIS

Despite the availability of adequate therapy for more than 60 years, syphilis remains a major issue for both mother and fetus.

Syphilis rates reached an all time low in 2000, but from 2001 through 2006 for the United States, there has been a steady increase in primary and secondary syphilis rates (Centers for Disease Control and Prevention, 2006b). The rate of syphilis in 2006 among both sexes was 3.3 cases per 100,000 individuals, a 13.8-percent increase from the year prior. Among women for the same year, the rate of primary and secondary syphilis was 1.0 case per 100,000 population. Congenital syphilis rates were 8.5 per 100,000 live births.

Pathogenesis and Transmission

The causative agent for syphilis is *Treponema pallidum*. Minute abrasions on the vaginal mucosa provide a portal of entry for the spirochete. Cervical eversion, hyperemia, and friability increase the risk for transmission. Spirochetes replicate and then disseminate through lymphatic channels within hours to days. The incubation period averages 3 weeks—3 to 90 days—depending on host factors and inoculum size. The early stages of syphilis include primary, secondary, and early latent syphilis. These are associated with the highest spirochete loads and transmission rates of up to 30 to 50 percent. Transmission rates in late-stage disease are much lower because of smaller inoculum sizes.

The fetus acquires syphilis by several routes. Spirochetes readily cross the placenta to cause congenital infection. Because of fetal immunocompetence prior to approximately 18 weeks, the fetus generally does not manifest the immunological inflammatory response characteristic of clinical disease before this time (Silverstein, 1962). Although transplacental transmission is the most common route, neonatal infection may follow after contact with spirochetes through lesions at delivery or across the membranes.

Increased rates of maternal syphilis have been linked to substance abuse, especially crack cocaine; to inadequate prenatal care; and to inadequate screening (Johnson, 2007; Lago, 2004; Trepka, 2006; Warner, 2001; Wilson, 2007, and all their colleagues). In a study of prenatal syphilis during four decades,

Klass and associates (1994) concluded that the continued prevalence of prenatal syphilis was associated with substance abuse, HIV infection, lack of prenatal care, treatment failures, and reinfection. A report from Maricopa County, Arizona, added minority race or ethnicity as risk factors (Taylor and co-workers, 2008).

Clinical Manifestations

Antepartum syphilis can cause preterm labor, fetal death, and neonatal infection (Saloojee and associates, 2004; Watson-Jones and colleagues, 2002). Any stage of maternal syphilis may result in fetal infection, but risk is directly related to maternal spirochete load (Fiumara and colleagues, 1952; Golden and co-workers, 2003). Maternal syphilis is staged according to clinical features and disease duration:

1. Primary syphilis is diagnosed by the characteristic chancre, which develops at the site of inoculation. It is usually painless, with a raised, red, firm border and a smooth base (Fig. 59-1). Nonsuppurative lymphadenopathy may develop. A chancre will usually resolve spontaneously in 2 to 8 weeks, even if untreated. Multiple lesions may be found, predominantly in HIV-1 co-infected women

2. Secondary syphilis is diagnosed when the spirochete is disseminated and affects multiple organ systems. Manifestations develop 4 to 10 weeks after the chancre appears and include dermatological abnormalities in up to 90 percent of women. A diffuse macular rash, plantar and palmar target-like lesions, patchy alopecia, and/or mucous patches may be seen (Fig. 59-2). Condylomata lata are flesh-colored papules and nodules found on the perineum and perianal area. They are teeming with spirochetes and are highly infectious. Most women with secondary syphilis will also express

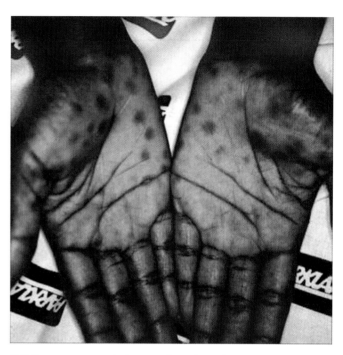

FIGURE 59-2 Target lesions on the palms of a pregnant woman with secondary syphilis.

constitutional symptoms such as fever, malaise, anorexia, headache, myalgias, and arthralgias. Up to 40 percent of women will have cerebrospinal fluid abnormalities, although only 1 to 2 percent will develop aseptic meningitis

3. *Latent syphilis* develops when primary or secondary syphilis is not treated. It is characterized by reactive serological testing, but resolved clinical manifestations. *Early latent syphilis* is latent disease acquired within the preceding 12 months. Disease diagnosed beyond 12 months is either *late latent syphilis* or *latent syphilis of unknown duration. Tertiary* or *late syphilis* is a slowly progressive disease affecting any organ system but is rarely seen in reproductive-aged women.

As noted, congenital infection is uncommon before 18 weeks. However, once fetal syphilis develops, it manifests as a continuum of involvement (Fig. 59-3). Fetal hepatic abnormalities are followed by anemia and thrombocytopenia, then ascites and hydrops (Hollier and colleagues, 2001). Stillbirth remains a major complication (Di Mario and associates, 2007). The newborn may have jaundice with petechiae or purpuric skin lesions, lymphadenopathy, rhinitis, pneumonia, myocarditis, or nephrosis.

With syphilitic infection, the placenta becomes large and pale (Fig. 59-4). Microscopically, villi lose their characteristic arborization and become thicker and clubbed (Kapur and co-workers, 2004). Sheffield and colleagues (2002c) described such large villi in more than 60 percent of placentas from 33 infected pregnancies. Blood vessels markedly diminish in number, and in advanced cases, they almost entirely disappear as a result of endarteritis and stromal cell proliferation. Perhaps related, Lucas and co-workers (1991) demonstrated increased vascular resistance in uterine and umbilical arteries of infected pregnancies. In a study of 25 untreated women, Schwartz and associates (1995) reported that necrotizing funisitis was present in a third.

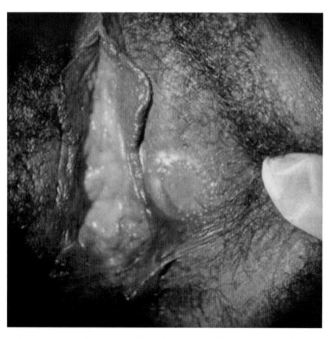

FIGURE 59-1 Primary syphilis. Photograph of a chancre with a raised, red, firm border and smooth base.

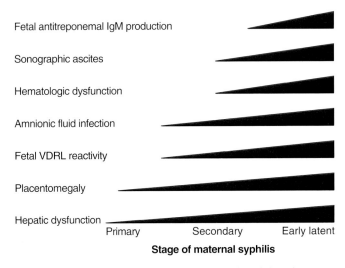

Fetal antitreponemal IgM production

Sonographic ascites

Hematologic dysfunction

Amnionic fluid infection

Fetal VDRL reactivity

Placentomegaly

Hepatic dysfunction

Primary   Secondary   Early latent

Stage of maternal syphilis

FIGURE 59-3 Hypothesized continuum of fetal syphilis infection. VDRL = Venereal Disease Research Laboratory. (Reprinted from Hollier LM, Harstad TW, Sanchez PJ, et al: Fetal syphilis: Clinical and laboratory characteristics, *Obstetrics & Gynecology*, 2001, vol. 97, no. 6, pp. 947–953, with permission.)

Spirochetes were detected in almost 90 percent using silver and immunofluorescent staining.

Diagnosis

T. pallidum cannot be cultured from clinical specimens. Definitive diagnosis of early-stage lesions is made using darkfield examination and direct fluorescent antibody testing of lesion exudates (Centers for Disease Control and Prevention, 2006b). In asymptomatic patients or for screening purposes, serological testing is used. The *Venereal Disease Research Laboratory (VDRL) slide test* or the *rapid plasma reagin (RPR) test* is performed at the first prenatal visit. Testing is required by law in many states (Connor and colleagues, 2000; Hollier and associates, 2003). Serological tests yield positive results in most women with primary syphilis and in all of those with secondary and latent syphilis. These nontreponemal tests are quantitated and expressed as titers. Titers reflect disease activity, and thus they increase during early syphilis and often exceed levels of 1:32 in secondary syphilis. Following treatment of primary and secondary syphilis, serological testing at 3 to 6 months usually confirms a fourfold drop in VDRL or RPR titers. Those with treatment failure or reinfection may lack this decline. Because

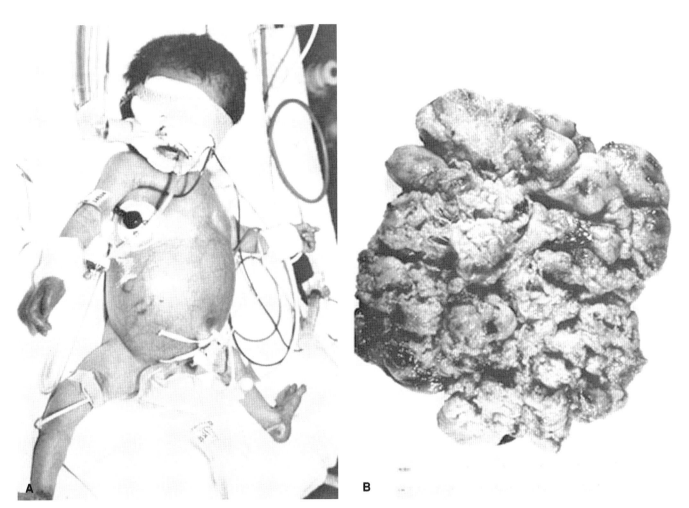

A   **B**

FIGURE 59-4 Congenital syphilis. **A.** A 29-week-old, severely ill neonate with an enlarged abdomen caused by marked hepatosplenomegaly plus ascites. **B.** The large syphilitic placenta of the same neonate weighed 1200 g, almost the birthweight of the newborn.

TABLE 59-1. Recommended Treatment for Pregnant Women with Syphilis

Category	Treatment
Early syphilis[a]	Benzathine penicillin G, 2.4 million units intramuscularly as a single injection—some recommend a second dose 1 week later
More than 1-year duration[b]	Benzathine penicillin G, 2.4 million units intramuscularly weekly for three doses
Neurosyphilis[c]	Aqueous crystalline penicillin G, 3–4 million units intravenously every 4 hours for 10–14 days *or* Aqueous procaine penicillin, 2.4 million units intramuscularly daily, plus probenecid 500 mg orally four times daily, both for 10–14 days

[a]Primary, secondary, and latent syphilis of less than 1-year duration.
[b]Latent syphilis of unknown or more than 1-year duration; tertiary syphilis.
[c]Some recommend benzathine penicillin, 2.4 million units intramuscularly after completion of the neurosyphilis treatment regimens.
From the Centers for Disease Control and Prevention (2006b).

VDRL titers do not correspond directly to RPR titers, consistent use of one test for surveillance is recommended.

Reagin tests lack specificity, and a treponemal-specific test is therefore used to confirm positive results (Pope and Fears, 2000; Young, 2000). These include the *fluorescent treponemal antibody absorption tests (FTA-ABS)*, the *microhemagglutination assay* for antibodies to *T. pallidum* (MHA-TP), or the *Treponema pallidum passive particle agglutination (TP-PA) test*. These treponemal-specific tests generally remain positive throughout life. Rapid syphilis testing for "point of care" diagnosis is currently being developed and may be useful in limited-prenatal care settings (Centers for Disease Control and Prevention, 2006b; Greer and Wendel, 2008). For women at high risk for syphilis, a nontreponemal screening test should be repeated in the third trimester and again at delivery (Centers for Disease control and Prevention, 2006b; Meyers and colleagues, 2008).

The prenatal diagnosis of congenital syphilis is difficult. Sonographic evaluation may be suggestive or even diagnostic, and hydrops fetalis, ascites, hepatomegaly, placental thickening, and hydramnios all suggest infection (see Chapter 29, p. 626). Importantly, an infected fetus often has a normal sonographic examination. Polymerase chain reaction (PCR) is specific for detection of *T. pallidum* in amnionic fluid, and treponemal DNA has been found in 40 percent of pregnancies infected before 20 weeks (Nathan and colleagues, 1997; Wendel and associates, 1991). Fetal syphilis has also been verified by amnionic fluid darkfield examination or rabbit infectivity testing in 64 percent of a cohort of women with untreated syphilis (Hollier and co-workers, 2001). Although prenatal diagnosis can be made by funipuncture or amniocentesis, its clinical utility is not yet clear.

Treatment

Syphilis therapy during pregnancy is given to eradicate maternal infection and to prevent congenital syphilis. Parenteral penicillin G remains the preferred treatment for all stages of syphilis during pregnancy. Currently recommended treatment guidelines are shown in Table 59-1 and are the same as for nonpregnant adults. Some authorities recommend a second dose of benzathine penicillin G 1 week after the initial dose.

In retrospective analyses, benzathine penicillin G has been shown to be highly effective for early maternal infection. In a study of 340 pregnant women so treated, Alexander and associates (1999) reported six cases—1.8 percent—of congenital syphilis. Four of these six neonates were from a group of 75 women with secondary syphilis. The other two were identified in those delivered from a group of 102 women with early latent syphilis. Congenital syphilis was generally confined to neonates of women treated after 26 weeks and is likely related to the duration and severity of fetal infection. Sheffield and co-workers (2002b) reported that high maternal serological titers, preterm delivery, and delivery shortly after antepartum therapy are all risks of maternal treatment failure to prevent neonatal infection.

There are no proven alternatives to penicillin therapy during pregnancy. Erythromycin may be curative for the mother, but because of limited transplacental passage, it does not prevent all - congenital disease (Berman, 2004; Wendel, 1988). The cephalosporins, such as ceftriaxone, and the newer macrolide, azithromycin, may prove useful (Augenbraun, 2002; Augenbraun and Workowski, 1999; Zhou and colleagues, 2005). Azithromycin therapy results in significant maternal and fetal serum drug levels (Ramsey and colleagues, 2003). Its efficacy in pregnancy, however, has not been adequately evaluated, and both resistance and treatment failures have been reported in adults (Centers for Disease Control and Prevention, 2004; Lukehart, 2004; Wendel, 2002; Zhou, 2007, and all their associates). Tetracyclines, including doxycycline, are effective for treatment of syphilis in the nonpregnant woman. However, these are generally not recommended during pregnancy because of the risk of yellow-brown discoloration of fetal deciduous teeth (see Chap. 14, p. 320).

TABLE 59-2. Oral Desensitization Protocol for Patients with a Positive Skin Test

Penicillin V Suspension Dose[a]	Amount[b] (units/mL)	mL	Units	Cumulative Dose (units)
1	1000	0.1	100	100
2	1000	0.2	200	300
3	1000	0.4	400	700
4	1000	0.8	800	1500
5	1000	1.6	1600	3100
6	1000	3.2	3200	6300
7	1000	6.4	6400	12,700
8	10,000	1.2	12,000	24,700
9	10,000	2.4	24,000	48,700
10	10,000	4.8	48,000	96,700
11	80,000	1.0	80,000	176,700
12	80,000	2.0	160,000	336,700
13	80,000	4.0	320,000	656,700
14	80,000	8.0	640,000	1,296,700

[a]Interval between doses: 15 minutes. Elapsed time: 3 hours and 45 minutes. Cumulative dose: 1.3 million units. Observation period: 30 minutes before parenteral administration of penicillin.
[b]The specific amount of drug was diluted in approximately 30 mL of water and administered orally.
From Wendel and colleagues (1985), with permission.

Women with a history of penicillin allergy should have skin testing performed to confirm the risk of immunoglobulin E (IgE)-mediated anaphylaxis. If confirmed, penicillin desensitization is recommended as shown in Table 59-2, and then followed by benzathine penicillin G treatment (Chisholm and associates, 1997; Wendel and co-workers, 1985).

In most women with primary syphilis and approximately half with secondary infection, penicillin treatment causes a *Jarisch-Herxheimer reaction*. Uterine contractions frequently develop with this reaction, and they may be accompanied by late fetal heart rate decelerations (Klein and co-workers, 1990). In a study of 50 pregnant women who received benzathine penicillin for syphilis, Myles and colleagues (1998) reported a 40-percent incidence of a Jarisch-Herxheimer reaction. Of the 31 women monitored electronically, 42 percent developed regular uterine contractions with a median onset of 10 hours, and 39 percent developed variable decelerations with a median onset of 8 hours. All contractions resolved within 24 hours of therapy. Lucas and associates (1991) used Doppler velocimetry and demonstrated acutely increased vascular resistance during this time.

All women with syphilis should be offered counseling and testing for HIV (Koumans and co-workers, 2000). For women with concomitant HIV infection, the Centers for Disease Control and Prevention (2006b) recommend the same treatment as for HIV-negative persons. Some authorities, however, recommend two additional weekly doses of benzathine penicillin G. Clinical and serological surveillance to detect treatment failures is also recommended at 3, 6, 9, 12, and 24 months in HIV-positive patients.

GONORRHEA

The incidence of gonorrhea in the United States for 2006 was 121 cases per 100,000 persons, an increase of 5.5 percent since 2005 (Centers for Disease Control and Prevention, 2006b). The highest rates in women of any ethnicity were in the group aged 15 to 24 years. Its prevalence in prenatal clinics in 2006 was 1.0 percent, although one inner-city STD clinic reported a prenatal prevalence of 4.8 percent (Johnson and colleagues, 2007). Risk factors include single marital status, adolescence, poverty, drug abuse, prostitution, other STDs, and lack of prenatal care. Gonococcal infection is also a marker for concomitant chlamydial infection in up to 40 percent of infected women (Christmas and co-workers, 1989; Miller and colleagues, 2004). In most pregnant women, gonococcal infection is limited to the lower genital tract—the cervix, urethra, and periurethral and vestibular glands. Acute salpingitis is rare in pregnancy, but pregnant women account for a disproportionate number of disseminated gonococcal infections (Ross, 1996; Yip and associates, 1993).

Gonococcal infection may have deleterious effects in any trimester. There is an association between untreated gonococcal cervicitis and septic abortion as well as infection after voluntary abortion (Burkman and co-workers, 1976). Preterm delivery, prematurely ruptured membranes, chorioamnionitis, and postpartum infection are more common in women infected with *Neisseria gonorrhoeae* at delivery (Alger and associates, 1988). Sheffield and colleagues (1999) reviewed outcomes of 25 pregnant women admitted at a mean gestational age of 25 weeks to Parkland Hospital for disseminated gonococcal infection. Although all of the women promptly responded to appropriate antimicrobial therapy, there was one stillbirth and one spontaneous abortion attributed to gonococcal sepsis.

Screening and Treatment

The U.S. Preventative Services Task Force (USPSTF) recommends gonorrhea screening of all sexually active women, including pregnant women, if they are at increased risk (Meyers and colleagues, 2008). Risk factors include age < 25 years, prior gonococcal infection, other STDs, prostitution, new or multiple sexual partners, drug use, and inconsistent condom use. For women who test positive, screening for syphilis, *Chlamydia trachomatis,* and HIV should precede treatment, if possible. If chlamydial testing is unavailable, presumptive therapy is given. Screening for gonorrhea in women is by culture or nucleic acid amplification tests (NAAT). Rapid tests for gonorrhea, although available, do not yet reach the sensitivity or specificity of culture or NAAT (Greer and Wendel, 2008).

Listed in Table 59-3 are recommendations for treatment of uncomplicated gonococcal infection during pregnancy. Fluoroquinolones are no longer recommended due to rapidly rising antimicrobial resistance (Centers for Disease Control and Prevention, 2007, 2008d). Cefixime tablets, previously in limited supply, are again available (Centers for Disease Control and Prevention, 2008a). In a study of 62 pregnant women with probable endocervical gonorrhea, Ramus and associates (2001) reported that intramuscular ceftriaxone, 125 mg, and oral cefixime, 400 mg, resulted in a 95- and 96-percent cure rate, respectively. Spectinomycin is recommended for women allergic to penicillin or β-lactam antimicrobials. Treatment is recommended for sexual contacts. A test-of-cure is unnecessary if symptoms resolve, but because gonococcal reinfection is common, a second screening in late pregnancy should be considered for women treated earlier during pregnancy (Centers for Disease Control and Prevention, 2006b; Miller and co-workers, 2003).

Gonococcal bacteremia may lead to disseminated gonococcal infection (DGI), which manifests as petechial or pustular skin lesions, arthralgias, septic arthritis, or tenosynovitis. The Centers for Disease Control and Prevention (2006b) have recommended ceftriaxone, 1000 mg intramuscularly or intravenously every 24 hours. Treatment should be continued for 24 to 48 hours after improvement, then therapy changed to an oral agent to complete a week of therapy.

For gonococcal *endocarditis*, antimicrobials should be continued for at least 4 weeks, and for *meningitis*, 10 to 14 days (Centers for Disease Control and Prevention, 2006b). Meningitis and endocarditis rarely complicate pregnancy, but they may be fatal (Bataskov, 1991; Burgis, 2006; Martín, 2008, and all their colleagues).

CHLAMYDIAL INFECTIONS

Chlamydia trachomatis is an obligate intracellular bacterium that has several serotypes, including those that cause *lymphogranuloma venereum (LGV)*. The most commonly encountered strains are those that attach only to columnar or transitional cell epithelium and cause cervical infection. It is the most commonly reported infectious disease in the United States with more than a million cases reported in 2006. It is estimated, however, that there are approximately 2.8 million new cases annually, although most are undiagnosed (Centers for Disease Control and Prevention, 2008c). Selective prenatal screening clinics in 2006 reported a median chlamydia infection rate of 8.1 percent (Centers for Disease Control and Prevention, 2009b).

Although most pregnant women have asymptomatic infection, a third present with urethral syndrome, urethritis, or Bartholin gland infection (Peipert, 2003). Mucopurulent cervicitis may be due to chlamydial or gonococcal infection or both. It may also represent normal, hormonally stimulated endocervical glands with abundant mucus production. Other chlamydial infections not usually seen in pregnancy are endometritis, salpingitis, peritonitis, reactive arthritis, and Reiter syndrome.

The role of chlamydial infection in pregnancy complications remains controversial. Only one study has reported a direct association between *C. trachomatis* and abortion, whereas most show no correlation (Coste, 1991; Paukku, 1999; Rastogi, 2000; Sozio and Ness, 1998; Sugiura-Ogasawara, 2005, and all their associates). It is disputed whether untreated cervical infection increases the risk of preterm delivery, preterm ruptured membranes, and perinatal mortality (Andrews, 2000, 2006; Baud, 2008; Blas, 2007, and all their colleagues).

Chlamydial infection has not been associated with an increased risk of chorioamnionitis nor with pelvic infection after cesarean delivery (Blanco and colleagues, 1985; Gibbs and Schachter, 1987). Conversely, delayed postpartum uterine metritis has been described by Hoyme and associates (1986). The syndrome, which develops 2 to 3 weeks postpartum, is distinct from early postoperative metritis. It is characterized by vaginal bleeding or discharge, low-grade fever, lower abdominal pain, and uterine tenderness.

There is vertical transmission to 30 to 50 percent of neonates delivered vaginally from infected women. Perinatal transmission to neonates can cause pneumonia, and *C. trachomatis* is the most commonly identifiable infectious cause of ophthalmia neonatorum (see Chap. 28, p. 598).

TABLE 59-3. Treatment of Uncomplicated Gonococcal Infections During Pregnancy

Ceftriaxone, 125 mg intramuscularly as a single dose
or
Cefixime, 400 mg orally in a single dose
or
Spectinomycin, 2 g intramuscularly as a single dose
plus
Treatment for chlamydial infection unless it is excluded[a]

[a]See Table 59-4.
From the Centers for Disease Control and Prevention (2006b).

TABLE 59-4. Treatment of *Chlamydia trachomatis* Infections During Pregnancy

Regimen	Drug and Dosage
Preferred choice	Azithromycin, 1000 mg orally as a single dose
	or
	Amoxicillin, 500 mg orally three times daily for 7 days
Alternatives	Erythromycin base, 500 mg orally four times daily for 7 days
	or
	Erythromycin ethylsuccinate, 800 mg orally four times daily for 7 days
	or
	Erythromycin base, 250 mg orally four times daily for 14 days
	or
	Erythromycin ethylsuccinate, 400 mg orally four times daily for 14 days

From the Centers for Disease Control and Prevention (2006b).

Screening and Treatment

Prenatal screening for *C. trachomatis* is a complex issue, although there is little evidence for its effectiveness in asymptomatic women who are not in high-risk groups (Kohl and colleagues, 2003; Meyers and co-workers, 2007; Peipert, 2003). Identification and treatment of asymptomatic infected women may prevent neonatal infections, but evidence of prevention of adverse pregnancy outcome is lacking. Currently, the U.S. Preventive Services Task Force (2007) and the CDC recommend prenatal screening at the first prenatal visit for women at increased risk for chlamydial infection and again during the third trimester if the high-risk behavior continues. In a study of 149 pregnant women with lower genital tract chlamydia, Miller (1998) found that 17 percent had recurrent chlamydial colonization after treatment. Interestingly, in another study, Sheffield and colleagues (2005) found that 44 percent of pregnant women with asymptomatic cervical chlamydia underwent spontaneous resolution of infection.

Diagnosis is made predominantly by culture or NAAT. Cultures are more expensive and less accurate than newer NAATs, including PCR (Greer and Wendel, 2008). Andrews and associates (1997) reported that a ligase chain reaction assay was both sensitive and specific for genitourinary infection in pregnant women.

Currently recommended regimens are shown in Table 59-4. Azithromycin is first-line treatment and has been found to be safe and efficacious in pregnancy (Adair, 1998; Jacobson, 2001; Kacmar, 2001; Rahangdale, 2006, and all their colleagues). The fluoroquinolones and doxycycline are avoided in pregnancy, as is erythromycin estolate because of drug-related hepatotoxicity. Subsequent chlamydial testing 3 to 4 weeks after completion of therapy is recommended.

Lymphogranuloma Venereum

Several serovars of *C. trachomatis* cause LGV. The primary genital infection is transient and seldom recognized. Inguinal adenitis may develop and at times lead to suppuration. It may be confused with chancroid. Ultimately, the lymphatics of the lower genital tract and perirectal tissues may be involved, with sclerosis and fibrosis, which can cause vulvar elephantiasis and severe rectal stricture. Fistula formation involving the rectum, perineum, and vulva also may evolve.

For treatment during pregnancy, erythromycin, 500 mg orally four times daily, is given for 21 days (Centers for Disease Control and Prevention, 2006b). Although data regarding efficacy are scarce, some authorities recommend azithromycin given in multiple doses daily for 3 weeks.

HERPES SIMPLEX VIRUS

Genital herpes simplex virus (HSV) infection is one of the most common sexually transmitted diseases—there are an estimated 50 million adolescents and adults currently affected (Centers for Disease Control and Prevention, 2006b). In 2006 alone, there were 371,000 initial office visits for genital herpes (Centers for Disease Control and Prevention, 2009b). Although most women are unaware of their infection, about one in five has serological evidence for HSV-2 infection (Xu and associates, 2006, 2007). As most cases of HSV are transmitted by persons who are asymptomatic or unaware of their disease, this has become a major public health concern. It is estimated that 0.5 to 2 percent of pregnant women acquire HSV-1 or -2 during pregnancy (Brown and colleagues, 1997).

Pathogenesis and Transmission

Two types of HSV have been distinguished based on immunological and clinical differences. Type 1 is responsible for most nongenital infections, however, more than half of new cases of genital herpes in adolescents and young adults are caused by HSV-1 infection. This is thought to be due to an increase in oral-genital sexual practices (Mertz and associates, 2003; Roberts and colleagues, 2003). Type 2 HSV is recovered almost exclusively from the genital tract and is usually transmitted by sexual contact. Most recurrences—greater than 90 percent—are secondary to HSV-2. There is a large amount of DNA sequence homology between the two viruses, and prior infection with one type attenuates a primary infection with the other type.

Neonatal transmission is by three routes: (1) intrauterine in 5 percent, (2) peripartum in 85 percent, or (3) postnatal in 10 percent (Kimberlin, 2004; Kimberlin and Rouse, 2004). The fetus becomes infected by virus shed from the cervix or lower genital tract. It either invades the uterus following membrane rupture or is transmitted by contact with the fetus at delivery. The rate of transmission is 1 in 3200 to 1 in 30,000 births depending on the population studied (Brown, 2005; Mahnert, 2007; Whitley, 2007, and all their associates). Neonatal herpes is caused by both HSV-1 and HSV-2, although HSV-2 infection predominates. Most infected infants are born to mothers with no reported history of HSV infection.

The risk of neonatal infection correlates with the presence of HSV in the genital tract, the type of HSV, invasive obstetrical procedures, and stage of maternal infection (Brown and associates, 2005, 2007). Infants born to women who acquire genital HSV near the time of delivery have a 30- to 50-percent risk of infection. This is attributed to higher viral loads and the lack of transplacental protective antibodies (Brown and co-workers, 1997). Women with recurrent HSV have less than a 1-percent risk of neonatal infection (Brown and colleagues, 1997; Prober and associates, 1987).

Clinical Manifestations

Once transmitted by genital-genital or oral-genital contact, HSV-1 or -2 replicates at the site of entry. Following mucocutaneous infection, the virus moves retrograde along sensory nerves where it then remains latent in cranial nerves or dorsal spinal ganglia. HSV infections may be categorized into three groups:

1. *First episode primary infection* describes cases in which HSV-1 or -2 is isolated from genital secretions in the absence of HSV-1 or -2 antibodies. Only a third of newly acquired HSV-2 genital infections are symptomatic (Langenberg and colleagues, 1999). The typical incubation period of 2 to 10 days may be followed by a "classic presentation," characterized by a papular eruption with itching or tingling, which then becomes painful and vesicular. Multiple vulvar and perineal lesions may coalesce, and inguinal adenopathy may be severe (Fig. 59-5). Transient systemic influenza-like symptoms are common and are presumably caused by viremia. Hepatitis, encephalitis, or pneumonia may develop, although disseminated disease is rare. Cervical involvement is common, but it may be inapparent clinically. Some cases are severe enough to require hospitalization. In 2 to 4 weeks, all signs and symptoms of infection disappear. Many women do not present with the typical lesions—instead, a pruritic or painful abraded area or knife-slit may be present.

2. *First episode nonprimary infection* is diagnosed when HSV is isolated in women who have only the other serum HSV antibody present. For example, HSV-2 is isolated from genital secretions in women already expressing serum HSV-1 antibodies. In general, these infections are characterized by fewer lesions, fewer systemic manifestations, less pain, and briefer duration of lesions and viral shedding. This is likely because of some immunity from cross-reacting antibodies,

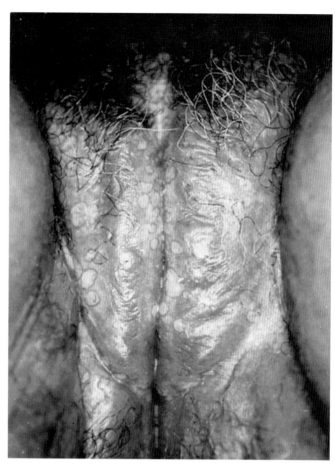

FIGURE 59-5 First-episode primary genital herpes simplex virus infection. (From Wendel and Cunningham, 1991, with permission.)

for example, from childhood-acquired HSV-1 infection. In many cases, it may be impossible to differentiate clinically between the two types of first infection. Thus, serological confirmation may be beneficial.

3. *Reactivation disease* is characterized by isolation of HSV-1 or -2 from the genital tract in women with the same serotype antibodies. During the latency period, in which viral particles reside in nerve ganglia, reactivation is common and mediated through variable but poorly understood stimuli. Reactivation is termed *recurrent infection* and results in herpesvirus shedding. Most recurrent genital herpes is caused by type 2 virus (Centers for Disease Control and Prevention, 2006b). These lesions generally are fewer in number, are less tender, and shed virus for shorter periods—2 to 5 days—than those of primary infection. Typically, they recur at the same sites. Recurrences are most common in the first year after initial infection, and rates slowly decline over several years.

Asymptomatic viral shedding is defined by HSV as detected by culture or PCR in the absence of signs or symptoms. Most infected women shed virus intermittently, and most HSV transmission to a partner occurs during periods of asymptomatic viral shedding. Gardella and colleagues (2005) reported an HSV culture-positive rate of 0.5 percent and a PCR-positive rate of 2.7 percent in asymptomatic women presenting for delivery. More data are needed to determine the effect of asymptomatic shedding on neonatal transmission.

Most primary and first-episode infections in early pregnancy are probably not associated with an increased rate of spontaneous abortion or stillbirth (Eskild and co-workers, 2002). In their review, Fagnant and Monif (1989) found only 15 cases of congenital herpetic infection that were acquired during early pregnancy. Brown and Baker (1989) reported that late-pregnancy primary infection may be associated with preterm labor.

Newborn infection may present several ways. Infection may be localized to eye or mouth disease in about 35 percent of cases. Central nervous system disease with encephalitis is seen in 30 percent of cases. Disseminated disease with involvement of multiple major organs is found in 25 percent (Fig. 59-6). Localized infection is usually associated with a good outcome. Conversely, even with acyclovir treatment, disseminated infection has a mortality rate of nearly 30 percent (Kimberlin, 2004; Kimberlin and co-workers, 2001a, b). Importantly, serious developmental and central nervous system morbidity is seen in 20 to 50 percent of survivors with disseminated or cerebral infection.

Diagnosis

According to the Centers for Disease Control and Prevention (2006b), clinical diagnosis of genital herpes is both insensitive and nonspecific and should be confirmed by laboratory testing. HSV tests available are either virological or type-specific serological tests.

Virological tests are performed on a specimen from a mucocutaneous lesion. Cell culture is preferred. However, the sensitivity of HSV isolation is relatively low as primary vesicular lesions ulcerate and then crust in recurrent lesions, and viral isolation results sometimes are not available for 1 to 2 weeks. Although PCR assays are more sensitive, and results generally

are available in 1 to 2 days, currently these are not yet approved for genital specimens by the Food and Drug Administration (FDA). The PCR assay, however, is the preferred test for HSV detection in spinal fluid. Regardless of the test performed, HSV viral type should be differentiated because HSV type influences counseling and long-term prognosis. *A negative culture or PCR result does not exclude the presence of infection. False-positive results are rare.*

Several serological assay systems are available to detect antibody to HSV glycoproteins G1 and G2 (Anzivino and co-workers, 2009). These proteins evoke type-specific antibody responses to HSV-1 and HSV-2 infection (Ashley, 2001). These tests have the potential to reliably differentiate HSV-1 from HSV-2 antibody and permit confirmation of clinical infection as well as to identify asymptomatic carriers. The FDA has approved type-specific tests that are enzyme-linked immunosorbent assay (ELISA) or blot-style tests. These include *HerpeSelect ELISA, HerpeSelect Immunoblot,* and the *Captia HSV Type Specific test kit* (Centers for Disease Control and Prevention, 2006b). The FDA has also approved two rapid or point-of-care tests—the *biokitHSV-2 Rapid Test* and the *Sure-Vue HSV-2 Rapid Test.* The reported sensitivities for all these tests are 90 to 100 percent with specificities of 91 to 100 percent (Greer, 2008; Laderman, 2008; Wald and Ashley-Morrow, 2002, and all their colleagues). Because nearly all HSV-2 infections are sexually acquired, detection of HSV-2 antibodies is virtually diagnostic of genital infection (Wald, 2004). HSV-1 antibodies may indicate prior oral HSV-1 infection or genital infection.

Prenatal Serological Screening

Brown (2000) and Wald and Ashley-Morrow (2002) have proposed prenatal serological HSV-2 antibody screening of couples. This supposedly would stimulate the need for safer sex practices and for antiviral suppression precautions if there is a discordancy, that is, one seronegative and one seropositive partner. This is controversial, and there is no clinical evidence that it may prevent HSV transmission and neonatal infection (Scoular, 2002; Wilkinson and associates, 2000). Cost-decision analysis for prenatal type-specific antibody screening and suppressive therapy for partners was judged unacceptable by Rouse and Stringer (2000), Barnabas and co-workers (2002), and Thung and Grobman (2005), but potentially cost-effective by Baker and associates (2004). Cleary and associates (2005) calculated that universal prenatal screening would reduce rates of perinatal death and severe sequelae from neonatal HSV. They also found that it would require treatment of 3849 women to prevent one case of neonatal death or disease with severe sequelae. Currently, the American College of Obstetricians and Gynecologists (2007a) does not recommend routine HSV screening of pregnant women.

Management

Antiviral therapy with acyclovir, famciclovir, or valacyclovir has been used for treatment of first-episode genital herpes in nonpregnant patients. Oral or parenteral preparations attenuate clinical infection and the duration of viral shedding. Suppressive therapy has also been given to limit recurrent infections and to

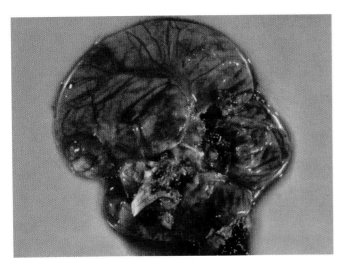

FIGURE 59-6 Cross-section showing necrotic brain tissue in a newborn who died from disseminated herpesvirus infection.

reduce heterosexual transmission (Corey and colleagues, 2004). For intense discomfort, analgesics and topical anesthetics may provide some relief, and urinary retention is treated with an indwelling bladder catheter.

Acyclovir appears to be safe for use in pregnant women (Ratanajamit and associates, 2003). The manufacturer of acyclovir and valacyclovir, in cooperation with the Centers for Disease Control and Prevention, have maintained a registry of outcomes following exposure to these drugs during pregnancy through 1999. More than 700 neonates exposed during the first trimester were evaluated, and they had no increased adverse effects (Reiff-Eldridge and co-workers, 2000; Scott, 1999). There are theoretical concerns about potential neutropenia that is similar to that seen in infants given long-term suppressive therapy (Kimberlin, 2004). At this time, there are insufficient data with famciclovir exposure, although a pregnancy registry is being maintained.

Women with a primary outbreak during pregnancy may be given antiviral therapy to attenuate and decrease the duration of symptoms and viral shedding (Table 59-5). Women with HIV coinfection may require a longer duration of treatment. Those with severe or disseminated HSV are given intravenous acyclovir, 5 to 10 mg/kg, every 8 hours for 2 to 7 days until clinical improvement is observed. This is followed by oral antiviral therapy to complete at least 10 days of total therapy (Centers for Disease Control and Prevention, 2006b). Recurrent HSV infections during pregnancy are treated for symptomatic relief only (see Table 59-5).

Peripartum Shedding Prophylaxis

A number of studies have shown that acyclovir or valacyclovir suppression initiated at 36 weeks will decrease the number of HSV outbreaks at term, thus decreasing the need for cesarean delivery (Hollier and Wendel, 2008). Such suppressive therapy will also decrease viral shedding defined by both culture and PCR techniques (Braig, 2001; Scott, 2002; Sheffield, 2006; Watts, 2003, and all their colleagues). A systemic review of studies of acyclovir prophylaxis given from 36 weeks to delivery was reported by Sheffield and colleagues (2003). They found that delivery suppressive therapy was associated with significantly decreased rates of clinical HSV recurrence, cesarean deliveries for HSV recurrences, total HSV detection, and asymptomatic shedding. Subsequent studies using valacyclovir suppression have shown similar results (Andrews and colleagues, 2006; Sheffield and associates, 2006). Because of these studies, the American College of Obstetricians and Gynecologists (2007a) recommends viral therapy at or beyond 36 weeks for women who have any recurrence during pregnancy. It is unclear whether suppression is needed for women with outbreaks before but not during pregnancy.

Upon presentation for delivery, a woman with a history of HSV should be questioned regarding prodromal symptoms such as vulvar burning or itching. A careful examination of the vulva, vagina, and cervix should be performed and suspicious lesions cultured. Cesarean delivery is indicated for women with active genital lesions or prodromal symptoms (American College of Obstetricians and Gynecologists, 2007a). Of note, 10 to 15 percent of infants with HSV are born to women undergoing cesarean delivery. Cesarean delivery is not recommended for women with a history of HSV infection but no active genital disease at the time of delivery. Moreover, an active lesion in a nongenital area is not an indication for cesarean delivery. Instead, an occlusive dressing is placed, and vaginal delivery allowed.

There is no evidence that external lesions cause ascending fetal infection with preterm ruptured membranes. Major and associates (2003) described expectant management of preterm rupture in 29 women less than 31 weeks. There were no cases of neonatal HSV, and the maximum risk of infection was calcu-

TABLE 59-5. Antiviral Medications for Herpesvirus Infection in Pregnancy

Indication	Pregnancy Recommendation
Primary or first episode infection	Acyclovir, 400 mg orally three times daily for 7–10 days *or* Valacyclovir, 1 g orally twice daily for 7–10 days
Symptomatic recurrent infection	Acyclovir, 400 mg orally three times daily for 5 days *or* Acyclovir, 800 mg orally twice daily for 5 days *or* Valacyclovir, 500 mg orally twice daily for 3 days *or* Valacyclovir, 1 g orally once daily for 5 days
Daily suppression	Acyclovir, 400 mg orally three times daily from 36 weeks until delivery *or* Valacyclovir, 500 mg orally twice daily from 36 weeks until delivery

Adapted from the Centers for Disease Control and Prevention Sexually Transmitted Diseases Treatment Guidelines (2006b).

lated to be 10 percent. The use of antiviral treatment in this setting is reasonable, but of unproven efficacy. For women with a clinical recurrence at delivery, there is not an absolute duration of membrane rupture beyond which the fetus would not benefit from cesarean delivery (American College of Obstetricians and Gynecologists, 2007b).

Women with active HSV may breast feed if there are no active HSV breast lesions. Strict hand washing is advised. Valacyclovir and acyclovir may be used during breast feeding as drug concentrations in breast milk are low. One study found the acyclovir concentration to be only 2 percent of that used for therapeutic dosing of the neonate (Sheffield and associates, 2002a).

CHANCROID

Haemophilus ducreyi can cause painful, nonindurated genital ulcers termed soft chancres that at times are accompanied by painful suppurative inguinal lymphadenopathy. Although common in some developing countries, it had become rare in the United States by the 1970s. By 1987, however, its incidence had increased tenfold during the previous decade, and drug use and sex-for-drugs were shown to be important risk factors (Schmid and co-workers, 1987). Importantly, the ulcerative lesion is a high-risk cofactor for HIV transmission (Centers for Disease Control and Prevention, 2006b).

Diagnosis by culture is difficult because appropriate media are not widely available. Instead, clinical diagnosis is made when typical painful genital ulcer(s) are darkfield negative and herpesvirus tests are negative. No FDA-cleared PCR test is yet available. Recommended treatment in pregnancy is azithromycin, 1 g orally as a single dose; erythromycin base, 500 mg orally three times daily for 7 days; or ceftriaxone, 250 mg in a single intramuscular dose (Centers for Disease Control and Prevention, 2006b).

HUMAN PAPILLOMAVIRUS

Human papillomavirus (HPV) has become one of the most common STDs with more than 30 types infecting the genital area. Most reproductive-aged women become infected within a few years of becoming sexually active, although most infections are asymptomatic and transient. High-risk HPV types 16 and 18 are associated with dysplasia and are discussed in Chapter 57. Mucocutaneous external genital warts are usually caused by HPV types 6 and 11 but may also be caused by intermediate- and high-oncogenic-risk HPV.

The most recent National Health and Nutrition Examination Survey (NHANES) 2003 to 2004 reported an overall HPV prevalence of 27 percent in the female population aged 14 to 59 years (Dunne and associates, 2007). A 27-percent seroprevalence was also reported for subjects 18 through 25 years in the National Longitudinal Study of Adolescent Health (Manhart and associates, 2006). Similar rates of HPV positivity have been reported for pregnant women (Gajewska, 2005; Hagensee,

1999; Hernandez-Giron, 2005; Smith, 2004; Worda, 2005, and all their colleagues).

External Genital Warts

For unknown reasons, genital warts frequently increase in number and size during pregnancy. Acceleration of viral replication by the physiological changes of pregnancy might explain the growth of perineal lesions and progression of some to cervical neoplasm (Fife and co-workers, 1999; Rando and colleagues, 1989). These lesions may sometimes grow to fill the vagina or cover the perineum, thus making vaginal delivery or episiotomy difficult (Fig. 59-7). Because HPV infection may be subclinical and multifocal, most women with vulvar lesions also have cervical infection, and vice versa (Ault, 2003; Spitzer and associates, 1989).

Treatment

There may be an incomplete response to treatment during pregnancy, but lesions commonly improve or regress rapidly following delivery. Consequently, eradication of warts during pregnancy is not always necessary. Therapy is directed toward minimizing treatment toxicity to the mother and fetus and debulking symptomatic genital warts. There are several agents available, but pregnancy limits their use. There is no definitive

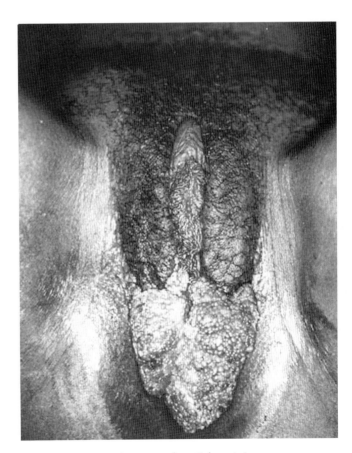

FIGURE 59-7 Extensive external genital warts in a woman near term. (From Wendel and Cunningham, 1991, with permission.)

evidence that any one of the subsequently discussed treatments is superior to another (Centers for Disease Control and Prevention, 2006b; Wiley and co-workers, 2002).

Trichloroacetic or bichloracetic acid, 80- to 90-percent solution, applied topically once a week is an effective regimen for external warts. Some prefer *cryotherapy, laser ablation,* or *surgical excision* (Arena and colleagues, 2001; Centers for Disease Control and Prevention, 2006b). *Podophyllin resin, podofilox* 0.5-percent solution or gel, *imiquimod* 5-percent cream, and *interferon* therapy are not recommended in pregnancy because of concerns for maternal and fetal safety (Centers for Disease Control and Prevention, 2006b).

Neonatal Infection

Juvenile-onset recurrent respiratory papillomatosis is a rare, benign neoplasm of the larynx. It can cause hoarseness and respiratory distress in children and is often due to HPV types 6 or 11. In some cases, maternal genital HPV infection is associated with laryngeal papillomatosis, but studies differ in their findings of neonatal transmission rates. Although some have reported rates as high as 50 percent, it is likely that these findings are from maternal contamination or transient HPV infection (Watts and associates, 1998; Winer and Koutsky, 2004). A Danish population-based study indicated a risk of neonatal transmission of 7 per 1000 infected women (Silverberg and co-workers, 2003). Prolonged rupture of membranes was associated with a twofold increased risk, but risk was not associated with the mode of delivery. This low transmission risk has been confirmed in subsequent studies (Heim and associates, 2007; Smith and colleagues, 2004). Finally, long-term follow-up studies are consistent with a very low vertical transmission risk (Manns and colleagues, 1999; Smith and associates, 2004). The benefit of cesarean delivery to decrease transmission risk is unknown, and thus it is currently not recommended solely to prevent HPV transmission (Centers for Disease Control and Prevention, 2006b).

VAGINITIS

Pregnant women commonly develop increased vaginal discharge, which in many instances is not pathological. Occasionally, however, troublesome leukorrhea is the result of vulvovaginal infections that include bacterial vaginosis, candidiasis, or trichomoniasis (Eckert, 2006).

Bacterial Vaginosis

Not an infection in the ordinary sense, bacterial vaginosis is a maldistribution of normal vaginal flora. Numbers of lactobacilli are decreased, and overrepresented species are anaerobic bacteria, including *Gardnerella vaginalis, Mobiluncus,* and some *Bacteroides* species. As many as 30 percent of nonpregnant women have vaginosis (Allsworth and Peipert, 2007; Simhan and associates, 2008). In pregnancy, it is associated with preterm birth (Denney and Culhane, 2009).

Treatment is reserved for symptomatic women, who usually complain of a fishy-smelling discharge. Preferred treatment is with metronidazole, 500 mg twice daily orally for 7 days. Alter-

natives are 0.75-percent metronidazole gel, 250-mg applicator-dose intravaginally three times daily for 7 days, or 2-percent clindamycin cream, one applicator dose inserted intravaginally at bedtime for 7 days (Centers for Disease Control and Prevention, 2006b). Unfortunately, treatment does not reduce preterm birth, and routine screening is not recommended (American College of Obstetricians and Gynecologists, 2001).

Trichomoniasis

Trichomonas vaginalis can be identified during prenatal examination in as many as 20 percent of women. Symptomatic vaginitis is much less prevalent, and it is characterized by foamy leukorrhea with pruritus and irritation. Trichomonads are demonstrated readily in fresh vaginal secretions as flagellated, pear-shaped, motile organisms that are somewhat larger than leukocytes.

Metronidazole is effective in eradicating *T. vaginalis* administered orally in a single 2-g dose (Centers for Disease Control and Prevention, 2006b). It crosses the placenta and enters the fetal circulation. Rosa and colleagues (1987) found no increased frequency of birth defects in more than 1000 women given metronidazole during early pregnancy. Even so, many recommend against its use in early pregnancy. Some studies have linked trichomonal infection with preterm birth, however, treatment has not decreased this risk (Wendel and Workowski, 2007). Thus, screening and treatment of asymptomatic women is not recommended during pregnancy (see Chap. 36, p. 814).

Candidiasis

Candida albicans can be identified by culture from the vagina during pregnancy in approximately 25 percent of women. Asymptomatic colonization requires no treatment, but the organism may sometimes cause an extremely profuse, irritating discharge associated with a pruritic, tender, edematous vulva. Effective treatment is given with a number of azole creams that include 2-percent butoconazole, 1-percent clotrimazole, 2-percent miconazole, and 0.4- or 0.8-percent terconazole (Centers for Disease control and Prevention, 2006b). Topical treatment is recommended, although oral azoles are generally considered safe (Pitsouni and colleagues, 2008). Clotrimazole, miconazole, nystatin, and terconazole are also available as vaginal tablets (see Chap. 14, p. 319). In some women, infection is likely to recur and require repeated treatment during pregnancy. In these cases, symptomatic infection usually subsides after pregnancy (Sobel, 2007).

HUMAN IMMUNODEFICIENCY VIRUS (HIV) INFECTION

Acquired immunodeficiency syndrome (AIDS) was first described in 1981 when a cluster of patients was found to have defective cellular immunity and *Pneumocystis jiroveci* (formerly *P. carinii*) pneumonia (Gallo and Montagnier, 2003). Worldwide, it was estimated in 2007 that there were 33 million infected persons with HIV/AIDS, 2.7 million new cases of HIV infection, and 2 million HIV-related deaths (United Nations

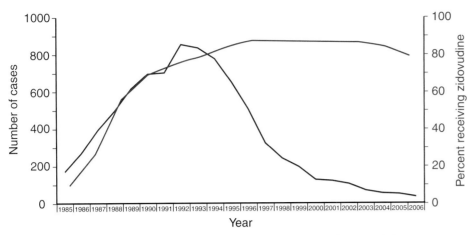

FIGURE 59-8 Estimated number of perinatally acquired AIDS cases by year of diagnosis, 1985 to 2006, in the United States and dependent areas (*blue line*). The red graph line depicts the percentage of women receiving zidovudine during pregnancy. (From the Centers for Disease Control and Prevention, 2009a.)

cells in high progesterone states such as pregnancy, possibly aiding viral entry (Sheffield and colleagues, 2009).

After initial infection, the level of viremia usually decreases to a *set-point*, and patients with the highest viral burden at this time progress more rapidly to AIDS and death (Fauci, 2007; Kahn and Walker, 1998). Over time, the number of T cells drops insidiously and progressively, resulting eventually in profound immunosuppression. Although it is thought that pregnancy has minimal effects on CD4+ T-cell counts and HIV RNA levels, the latter are often higher 6 months postpartum than during pregnancy (U.S. Public Health Service Task Force, 2008).

Programme on HIV/AIDS and World Health Organization, 2007). In the United States through 2006, the Centers for Disease Control and Prevention (2008b) estimated that there were 1.1 million infected individuals and almost a half million deaths. In 2006, women accounted for 26 percent of all HIV/AIDS cases among adults and adolescents, the vast majority of which resulted from heterosexual contact (Centers for Disease Control and Prevention, 2006a).

The estimated number of perinatally acquired AIDS cases had decreased dramatically over the last two decades. This is predominantly due to the implementation of prenatal HIV testing with antiviral therapy given to the pregnant woman and then to her neonate (Fig. 59-8). In addition, *highly active antiretroviral therapy (HAART)* has led to an increasing number of people living with chronic HIV infection (Fenton, 2007).

Etiopathogenesis

Causative agents of AIDS are RNA retroviruses termed *human immunodeficiency viruses, HIV-1 and HIV-2*. Most cases worldwide are caused by HIV-1 infection. Transmission is similar to hepatitis B virus, and sexual intercourse is the major mode. The virus also is transmitted by blood or blood-contaminated products, and mothers may infect their fetuses.

The common denominator of clinical illness with AIDS is profound immunosuppression that gives rise to a variety of opportunistic infections and neoplasms. Sexual transmission occurs when mucosal dendritic cells bind to the HIV envelope glycoprotein gp120. These dendritic cells then present the viral particle to thymus-derived lymphocytes, or *T lymphocytes*. These lymphocytes are defined phenotypically by the cluster of differentiation 4 (CD4) glycoprotein surface antigen. The CD4 site serves as a receptor for the virus. Co-receptors are necessary for viral entry into the cell, and two chemokine receptors—CCR5 and CXCR4—are the most commonly identified (Kahn and Walker, 1998; Sheffield and co-workers, 2007). The CCR5 co-receptor is found on the cell surface of CD4 positive (CD4+)

Clinical Manifestations

The incubation period from exposure to clinical disease is days to weeks. Acute HIV infection is similar to many other viral syndromes and usually lasts less than 10 days. Common symptoms include fever and night sweats, fatigue, rash, headache, lymphadenopathy, pharyngitis, myalgias, arthralgias, nausea, vomiting, and diarrhea. After symptoms abate, the set-point of chronic viremia is established. The progression from asymptomatic viremia to AIDS has a median time of approximately 10 years (Fauci and Lane, 2008). Route of infection, the pathogenicity of the infecting viral strain, the initial viral inoculum, and the immunological status of the host all affect the rapidity of progression.

A number of clinical and laboratory manifestations will herald disease progression. Generalized lymphadenopathy, oral hairy leukoplakia, aphthous ulcers, and thrombocytopenia are common. A number of opportunistic infections associated with AIDS include esophageal or pulmonary candidiasis; persistent herpes simplex or zoster lesions; condyloma acuminata; pulmonary tuberculosis; cytomegaloviral pneumonia, retinitis, or gastrointestinal disease; molluscum contagiosum; *Pneumocystis jiroveci* pneumonia; toxoplasmosis; and others. Neurological disease is common, and approximately half of patients have central nervous system symptoms. A CD4+ count <200/mm^3 is also considered definitive for the diagnosis of AIDS.

There are unique gynecological issues for women with HIV, such as menstrual abnormalities, contraceptive needs, and genital neoplasia as well as other STDs that may persist into pregnancy (Cejtin, 2003; Stuart and associates, 2005). Repeated pregnancy does not have significant effect on the clinical or immunological course of viral infection (Minkoff and colleagues, 2003).

Prenatal HIV Screening

The Center for Disease Control and Prevention (2006c), the American College of Obstetricians and Gynecologists

(2008), the American Academy of Pediatrics (2006), and the United States Preventive Services Task Force (2005) recommend prenatal screening using an *opt-out approach*. This means that the woman is notified that HIV testing is included in a comprehensive set of antenatal tests, but that testing may be declined. Women are given information regarding HIV but are not required to sign a specific consent. Through the use of such *opt-out* strategies, HIV testing rates have increased. Each provider should be aware of specific state laws concerning screening.

In areas in which the incidence of HIV or AIDS is 1 per 1000 person years or greater or in women at high risk for acquiring HIV during pregnancy, repeat testing in the third trimester is recommended (American College of Obstetricians and Gynecologists, 2008). High-risk factors include injection drug use, prostitution, a suspected or known HIV-infected sexual partner, multiple sexual partners, or a diagnosis of another sexually transmitted disease. Several states also recommend or require HIV testing at delivery.

Screening is performed using an ELISA test with a sensitivity of >99.5 percent. A positive test is confirmed with either a Western blot or immunofluorescence assay (IFA), both of which have high specificity. According to the Centers for Disease Control and Prevention (2001a, b), antibody can be detected in most patients within 1 month of infection, and thus, antibody serotesting may not exclude early infection. For acute primary HIV infection, identification of viral p24 core antigen or viral RNA or DNA is possible. False-positive confirmatory results are rare (Branson, 2007; Centers for Disease Control and Prevention, 2006c).

Women with limited prenatal care or with undocumented HIV status at delivery should have a "rapid" HIV test performed. These tests can detect HIV antibody in 60 minutes or less and have sensitivities and specificities comparable with those of conventional ELISAs. A negative rapid test result does not need to be confirmed. A positive rapid test result should be confirmed with a Western blot or IFA test. As shown in Table 59-6, peripartum and neonatal interventions to reduce perinatal transmission are based on the initial rapid testing results, and this can be discontinued if the confirmatory test is negative (American College of Obstetricians and Gynecologists, 2008; Centers for Disease Control and Prevention, 2006c).

The Mother-Infant Rapid Intervention at Delivery (MIRIAD) multicenter study indicated that rapid HIV testing can be used to identify infected women so that peripartum antiretroviral prophylaxis can be administered to mother and infant (Bulterys and colleagues, 2004). Branson (2007) reviewed the six FDA-approved rapid tests currently available—four are "point of care tests" and two require a laboratory.

Maternal and Perinatal Transmission

Transplacental HIV transmission can occur early, and the virus has even been identified in specimens from elective abortion (Lewis and co-workers, 1990). In most cases, however, mother-to-child transmission is the most common cause of pediatric HIV infections. Between 15 and 40 percent of neonates born to non-breast-feeding, untreated, HIV-infected mothers are infected. Kourtis and colleagues (2001) have proposed a model for estimation of the temporal distribution of vertical transmission. They estimate that 20 percent of transmission occurs before 36 weeks, 50 percent in the days before delivery, and 30 percent intrapartum (Fig. 59-9). Transmission rates for breast feeding may be as high as 30 to 40 percent (Kourtis and associates, 2006, 2007). Vertical transmission is more common with preterm births, especially with prolonged membrane rupture. Analyzing data from the Perinatal AIDS Collaborative Transmission Study, Kuhn and colleagues (1999) reported a 3.7 increased risk with preterm delivery. Landesman and co-workers (1996) reported that HIV-1 transmission at birth was increased from 15 to 25 percent in women whose membranes likely, for similar reasons, were ruptured for more than 4 hours.

In nonpregnant individuals, there is an association between concomitant STDs and horizontal HIV transmission. There is evidence that vertical perinatal transmission may also be increased (Koumans and colleagues, 2000; Schulte and co-workers, 2001). Recently, Cowan and associates (2008) showed that women with maternal HSV-2 antibody had a significant

---

TABLE 59-6. Strategy for Rapid HIV Testing of Pregnant Women in Labor

If the rapid HIV test result in labor and delivery is positive, the obstetrical provider should take the following steps:
1. Tell the woman she may have HIV infection and that her neonate also may be exposed
2. Explain that the rapid test result is preliminary and that false-positive results are possible
3. Assure the woman that a second test is being performed to confirm the positive rapid test result
4. To reduce the risk of transmission to the infant, immediate initiation of antiretroviral prophylaxis should be recommended without waiting for the results of the confirmatory test
5. Once the woman gives birth, discontinue maternal antiretroviral therapy pending receipt of confirmatory test results
6. Tell the women that she should postpone breast feeding until the confirmatory result is available because she should not breast feed if she is infected with HIV
7. Inform pediatric care providers (depending on state requirements) of positive maternal test results so that they may institute the appropriate neonatal prophylaxis

HIV = human immunodeficiency virus.
From American College of Obstetricians and Gynecologists (2008), with permission.

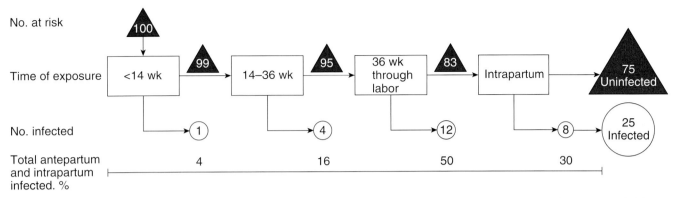

FIGURE 59-9 Estimated rates of perinatal human immunodeficiency virus (HIV) transmission for different times of gestation and delivery in non-breast-feeding populations. Estimates are based on a hypothetical cohort of 100 children born to HIV-infected women without any interventions. Numbers in blue indicated number of children at risk for infection. (From Kourtis and colleagues, 2001, with permission.)

50-percent increased risk of intrapartum HIV-1 maternal-to-child transmission. They attributed up to 25 percent of vertical transmission to maternal HSV-2 co-infection.

Perinatal HIV transmission is most accurately correlated with maternal plasma HIV RNA burden (U.S. Public Health Service Task Force, 2009; Watts, 2002). As shown in Figure 59-10, cohort neonatal infection was 1 percent with <400 copies/mL, and it was more than 30 percent when viral RNA levels were >100,000 copies/mL (Cooper and colleagues, 2002). Importantly, zidovudine (ZDV) therapy that reduced these levels to <500 copies/mL also minimized the risk of transmission, although ZDV is effective in reducing transmission across all HIV RNA levels. The investigators also reported that maternal infusions of HIV-1 hyperimmune globulin did not alter the risk of transmission. *Transmission, however, has been observed at all HIV RNA levels, including those that were nondetectable by current assays.* This may be attributed to discordance between the viral load in plasma and in the genital secretions. Because of these findings, the viral load should not be used to determine whether to initiate antiretroviral therapy in pregnancy.

Maternal and Perinatal Outcomes

Although maternal morbidity and mortality rates are not increased in seropositive asymptomatic women, it appears that adverse fetal outcomes may be increased (U.S. Public Health Service Task Force, 2009). In a review of 634 HIV-infected women, Stratton and associates (1999) reported that adverse fetal outcomes were associated with a $CD4^+$ cell proportion of <15 percent. In these otherwise asymptomatic women, the rate of preterm birth was 20 percent and that of fetal-growth restriction was 24 percent. Watts (2002) emphasized that these adverse outcomes were even more prevalent in developing countries.

Preconceptional Counseling

An important aspect of preconceptional counseling includes that of effective contraception if pregnancy is undesired. Certain antiviral medications decrease the efficacy of hormonal contraception. These drug interactions are detailed by the U.S. Public Health Service Task Force (2009) and are discussed in Chapter 32 (p. 678). These recommendations are available at http://AIDSinfo.nih.gov and are updated frequently as new data become available. Counseling should also include education for decreasing high-risk sexual behaviors to prevent transmission and to decrease the acquisition of other sexually transmitted diseases. Currently taken antiretroviral medications are reviewed to be sure that those with high teratogenic potential are avoided if the woman becomes pregnant. A specific example is efavirenz, which has significant teratogenic effects on primate fetuses (Panel on Antiretroviral Guidelines for Adults and Adolescents, 2008). Preference should also include those that decrease HIV RNA viral load effectively prior to pregnancy.

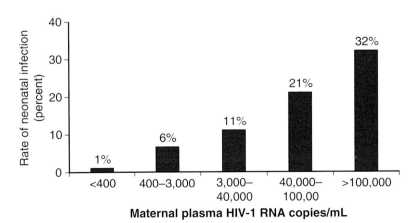

FIGURE 59-10 Incidence of perinatal human immunodeficiency virus (HIV) infection plotted against plasma HIV-1 RNA levels in 1542 neonates born to mothers in the Women and Infants Transmission Study. (Data from Cooper and colleagues, 2002.)

Management During Pregnancy

These women need special attention and are seen in consultation with physicians with special interest in this field. At Parkland Hospital, the initial assessment of an HIV-infected pregnant woman includes:

- Standard prenatal laboratory surveys that include serum creatinine, hemogram, and bacteriuria screening (see Chap. 8, p. 194)
- Plasma HIV RNA quantification—"viral load" and CD4$^+$ T-lymphocyte count as well as antiretroviral resistance testing
- Serum hepatic transaminase levels
- HSV-1 and -2, cytomegalovirus, toxoplasmosis, and hepatitis C screening
- Baseline chest radiograph
- Tuberculosis skin testing (PPD)
- Evaluation of need for pneumococcal, hepatitis B, and influenza vaccine
- Sonographic evaluation to establish gestational age.

Antiretroviral Therapy

Treatment is recommended for all HIV-infected pregnant women. This may be a departure for those not receiving treatment when nonpregnant because they did not meet certain criteria. Treatment reduces the risk of perinatal transmission regardless of CD4$^+$ T-cell count or HIV RNA level. Antiretroviral therapy is complicated, and pregnancy only adds to the complexity. In general, HAART is begun if the woman is not already receiving one of the regimens. Antiretroviral agents are grouped into several classes and used to design antiretroviral regimens (Table 59-7). The woman is counseled regarding risks and benefits of antiretroviral agents to make an informed decision as to her treatment regimen. Regardless of what regimen is begun, adherence is important because the risk of viral drug resistance is lessened.

The U.S. Public Health Service Task Force (2009) has issued guidelines that detail management of different scenarios during pregnancy (Table 59-8). Women already taking HAART at pregnancy onset are encouraged to continue the regimen if there is adequate viral suppression. The exception previously discussed is *efavirenz*, which should be discontinued in the first trimester because of teratogenicity concerns. Until recently, addition of zidovudine to all regimens was recommended. Currently, however, in women with adequate viremia suppression with a regimen not containing zidovudine, continuation of the current regimen is appropriate. In all women, zidovudine is given intravenously during labor and delivery (Table 59-9).

Women who have never received antiretroviral therapy—*antiretroviral naïve*—fall into two categories:

1. Women who meet the criteria for antiretroviral therapy initiation in nonpregnant adults are given HAART regardless of trimester, using a zidovudine-containing regimen if feasible. Because of an increased risk of hepatotoxicity, *nevirapine* is reserved for women with a CD4$^+$ cell count <250 cells/mm^3. In general, the starting HAART regimen is two nucleoside reverse transcriptase inhibitors (NRTIs) plus a non-nucleoside reverse transcriptase inhibitor (NNRTI) or

TABLE 59-7. Classes of Antiretroviral Drugs

Drug Class	Category[a]
Nucleoside and nucleotide analog	
reverse transcriptase inhibitors	
Zidovudine	C
Zalcitabine	C
Didanosine	B
Stavudine	C
Lamivudine	C
Abacavir	C
Tenofovir	B
Emtricitabine	B
Non-nucleoside reverse	
transcriptase inhibitors	
Nevirapine	B
Delavirdine	C
Efavirenz	D
Protease inhibitors	
Indinavir	C
Ritonavir	B
Saquinavir	B
Nelfinavir	B
Amprenavir	C
Atazanavir	B
Fosamprenavir	C
Lopinavir/ritonavir	C
Darunavir	B
Entry inhibitors	
Enfuvirtide	B
Maraviroc	B
Integrase Inhibitors	
Raltegravir	C

[a]Food and Drug Administration pregnancy category classification—see Chapter 14 (p. 321).
From U.S. Public Health Service (2009).

protease inhibitor(s). At Parkland Hospital as of 2009, our standard regimen in treatment-naïve women is lopinavir/ritonavir—formulated as *Kaletra*—plus zidovudine/lamivudine—formulated as *Combivir*. Nelfinavir is substituted for *Kaletra* if not tolerated.

2. Treatment-naïve HIV-infected pregnant women who do not meet nonpregnant adult indications for antiretroviral therapy are counseled regarding benefits of initiating therapy to prevent perinatal viral transmission. Because of potential teratogenic effects, they may delay therapy until the second trimester. Again, zidovudine should be a component of the regimen if feasible. Although not used at our institution, zidovudine monotherapy is an option for some women who wish to limit medication exposure. Such monotherapy is controversial but may be used for women

TABLE 59-8. Recommendations for Antiviral Drug Use During Pregnancy

Clinical Scenario	Recommendations
HIV-infected woman on antiretroviral therapy who becomes pregnant	• Continue current medication if viral suppression adequate and patient tolerating — Avoid efavirenz in the first trimester • If virus detectable, order HIV antiretroviral drug-resistance testing • If first trimester, continue medications. If stopped, stop all medications and then reinitiate in the second trimester. • If not receiving zidovudine (ZDV) antepartum, start IV ZDV in labor (see Table 59-9)
HIV-infected woman who is antiretroviral naïve and has maternal indications for HAART	• Order HIV antiretroviral drug-resistance testing • Initiate HAART: — Avoid efavirenz in the first trimester — Use ZDV-containing regimen if feasible — Avoid nevirapine in women with a CD4$^+$ count >250 cells/mm^3 • HAART should be initiated as early as possible for maternal indications • If not receiving zidovudine antepartum, start IV ZDV in labor
HIV-infected woman who is antiretroviral naïve with no maternal indication for HAART	• Order HIV antiretroviral drug-resistance testing • Initiate HAART: — Consider delaying therapy until the start of the second trimester — Use ZDV-containing regimen if feasible — Avoid nevirapine in women with a CD4$^+$ count >250 cells/mm^3 • ZDV monotherapy is controversial: — If used, use in women with HIV RNA levels <1000 copies/mL — If not receiving zidovudine antepartum, start IV ZDV in labor
HIV-infected woman previously on antiretroviral medications but not on medications currently	• Order HIV antiretroviral drug-resistance testing • Initiate HAART with regimen based on prior therapy history and resistance testing • Avoid efavirenz in the first trimester • Use ZDV-containing regimen if feasible • Avoid nevirapine in women with a CD4$^+$ count >250 cells/mm^3 • If not receiving zidovudine antepartum, start IV ZDV in labor
HIV-infected woman on no antiretroviral medication who presents in labor	• Order initial HIV laboratory assessment (see p. 1250). • Start zidovudine intravenous protocol (Table 59-9) *or* • Start intravenous zidovudine plus a single dose of nevirapine (NVP). If NVP initiated, consider adding lamivudine for 7 days postpartum to decrease NVP resistance

HAART = highly active antiretroviral therapy; HIV = human immunodeficiency virus.
Adapted from the U.S. Public Health Service Task Force (2008).

with HIV RNA levels <1000 copies/mL who are not receiving treatment.

Another group of women have previously received antiretroviral therapy but are currently not taking medications. Prior antiretroviral use increases their risk of HIV drug resistance, and thus resistance testing is imperative. Regimens may then be tailored based on prior medication use and response as well as current resistance patterns.

The last group includes women who present in labor and who are taking no medications. These women are given intravenous zidovudine intrapartum (see Table 59-9). Some

TABLE 59-9. Pediatric AIDS Clinical Trials Group (PACTG) 076 Zidovudine Regimen

Time of Administration	Zidovudine Regimen
Antepartum	100 mg orally five times daily, initiated at 14 to 34 weeks and continued throughout pregnancy.[a]
Intrapartum	During labor, intravenous zidovudine in a 1-hour initial dose of 2 mg/kg, followed by a continuous infusion of 1 mg/kg/hr until delivery.[b]
Neonate	Begin at 8 to 12 hours after birth, and give syrup at 2 mg/kg every 6 hours for 6 weeks.[c]

[a]Acceptable alternative regimens include 200 mg three times daily or 300 mg twice daily.
[b]For elective cesarean delivery, intravenous zidovudine is begun at least 3 hours prior to surgery. For premature rupture of membranes or labor with a planned operative delivery, the loading dose may be given over the half hour prior to surgery.
[c]Intravenous dosage for infants who cannot tolerate oral intake is 1.5 mg/kg intravenously every 6 hours.
AIDS = acquired immunodeficiency syndrome.
From U.S. Public Health Service (2008).

experts recommend also giving one dose of nevirapine at labor onset, and if chosen, lamivudine administered for 7 days will decrease the development of nevirapine resistance (Arrive and colleagues, 2007; U.S. Public Health Service Task Force, 2009).

Laboratory Assessment

CD4$^+$ T-lymphocyte count, HIV RNA viral load measurement, complete blood count, and liver function tests are done 4 weeks after beginning or changing therapy to assess response and evidence of toxicity. Thereafter, HIV RNA viral load and CD4$^+$ quantification are determined each trimester. If the HIV RNA viral load increases or does not decrease appropriately, then medication compliance and antiretroviral drug resistance are assessed. Poor adherence to therapy appears to be a significant problem in pregnancy. In a study of 549 women from New York by Laine and associates (2000), poor compliance was reported in a third.

Although early studies found an association with glucose intolerance and protease inhibitor use, Tang and colleagues (2006) did not corroborate this. Even so, careful surveillance is important for interactions between antiretroviral drugs as well as therapies for opportunistic infection, methadone, and tuberculosis (Piscitelli and Gallicano, 2001).

Complications of HIV

Management of some HIV complications may be altered by pregnancy. If the CD4$^+$ T-cell count is <200/mm^3, primary prophylaxis for *P. jiroveci* (formerly *P. carinii)* pneumonia is recommended with sulfamethoxazole-trimethoprim or dapsone. Pneumonitis is treated with oral or intravenous sulfamethoxazole-trimethoprim or dapsone-trimethoprim. Other symptomatic opportunistic infections that may develop are from latent or newly acquired toxoplasmosis, herpesvirus, mycobacteria, and candida. The National Institutes of Health, Infectious Diseases Society of America, and Centers for Disease Control and Prevention (2008) have published guidelines for prevention and treatment of opportunistic infections.

Perinatal Outcomes

Even with treatment, the incidence of perinatal complications in HIV-infected women is increased. Lorenzi and colleagues (1998) reported that 78 percent of women treated with two reverse transcriptase inhibitors had one or more adverse events, especially preterm delivery. Half of the neonates had adverse events. Newer drug regimens may diminish these complications. Kourtis and colleagues (2007) performed a meta-analysis of 14 studies of HIV-infected women treated with antiretroviral therapy. They did not find an overall increased risk for preterm delivery, although there was a small but significant increased risk in women who were receiving therapy before or early in pregnancy. Tuomala and associates (2002) found no association with preterm birth, low birthweight, or stillbirths when combination antiretroviral therapy was used. These investigators did report that women given combination protease-inhibitor regimens had an increased risk of very-low-birthweight infants. Despite this, combined therapy should not be withheld (Watts, 2002).

At least two follow-up studies of children from the Pediatric AIDS Clinical Trial Group (PACTG) 076 Study found no adverse effects in children at 18 months and up to a mean of 5.6 years after zidovudine exposure (Culnane and associates, 1999; Sperling and colleagues, 1998). Prenatal exposure to HAART may increase the risk for neonatal neutropenia, although no long-term hematological or hepatic toxicities have been identified (Bae and colleagues, 2008). Early data also show a possible effect on infant mitochondrial DNA proliferation and/or expression with maternal antiretroviral drug treatment (Cote and co-workers, 2008).

Prenatal HIV Transmission. Maternal HAART treatment along with intrapartum zidovudine prophylaxis has dramatically reduced the perinatal HIV transmission risk from about 25 percent to 2 percent or less in women. Optimal management of labor is uncertain, but if labor is progressing with intact membranes, artificial rupture and invasive fetal monitoring are avoided. Labor augmentation is used when needed to shorten the interval-to-delivery to further decrease the risk of transmission. Operative delivery with forceps or vacuum extractor is avoided if possible. Postpartum hemorrhage is managed with oxytocin and prostaglandin analogs because methergine and other ergot alkaloids interact with reverse transcriptase and protease inhibitors to cause severe vasoconstriction.

Cesarean delivery has been recommended to decrease HIV prenatal transmission. A meta-analysis of 15 prospective cohort studies by the International Perinatal HIV Group (1999) included 8533 mother-neonate pairs. Vertical HIV transmission was reduced by approximately half when cesarean delivery was compared with vaginal delivery. And when antiretroviral therapy was given in the prenatal, intrapartum, and neonatal periods along with cesarean delivery, the likelihood of neonatal transmission was reduced by 87 percent compared with other modes of delivery and without antiretroviral therapy. The European Mode of Delivery Collaboration (1999) and others have reported similar findings.

Based on these observations, the American College of Obstetricians and Gynecologists (2000) concluded that scheduled cesarean delivery should be discussed and recommended for HIV-infected women whose HIV-1 RNA load exceeds 1000 copies/mL. Scheduled delivery was recommended as early as 38 weeks to lessen the chances of prematurely ruptured membranes. Although data are insufficient to estimate such benefits of cesarean delivery for women whose HIV RNA levels are below 1000 copies/mL, it is unlikely that scheduled cesarean delivery would confer additional risk reduction (Jamieson and associates, 2007; Read and Newell, 2005; U.S. Public Health Service Task Force, 2009). If cesarean delivery is performed, use of standard perioperative antimicrobials for prophylaxis is recommended.

Breast Feeding

Vertical transmission is increased by breast feeding, and it generally is not recommended in HIV-positive women in this country (Read and co-workers, 2003). The probability of HIV transmission per liter of breast milk ingested is estimated to be similar in magnitude to heterosexual transmission with unsafe sex in adults (Richardson and colleagues, 2003). As with other exposures, risk is related to the maternal HIV RNA level, HIV disease status, breast health, and duration of breast feeding (De Cock and associates, 2000; John-Stewart and co-workers, 2004). Most transmission occurs in the first 6 months, and as many as two thirds of infections in breast-fed infants are from breast milk. In the Petra Study Team (2002) from Africa, the prophylactic benefits of short-course perinatal antiviral regimens were diminished considerably by 18 months of age due to breast feeding. The World Health Organization (2008) has recommended continuing breast feeding promotion with early weaning by 6 months for women living in developing countries in which infectious diseases and malnutrition are the primary causes of infant deaths.

Postpartum Management

Many otherwise healthy women with normal $CD4^+$ T-cell counts and low HIV RNA levels may discontinue treatment after delivery and be closely monitored according to adult guidelines. Psychosocial support is essential during this time, especially while awaiting diagnostic testing for pediatric infection. Contraceptive needs are complex and also may entail condoms in discordantly infected couples. As discussed in Chapter 32 (p. 678), antiretroviral drugs may affect hormone levels of oral contraceptives and possibly of injectable agents (Stuart and Cunningham, 2008). Intrauterine devices may be an acceptable choice in some women with normal immunocompetence and a low risk for STDs. Gynecological care is complex in HIV-infected women and has been comprehensively reviewed by Cejtin (2003).

REFERENCES

Adair CD, Gunter M, Stovall TG, et al: Chlamydia in pregnancy: A randomized trial of azithromycin and erythromycin. Obstet Gynecol 91:165, 1998

Alexander JM, Sheffield JS, Sanchez PJ, et al: Efficacy of treatment for syphilis in pregnancy. Obstet Gynecol 93:5, 1999

Alger LS, Lovchik JC, Hebel JR, et al: The association of *Chlamydia trachomatis, Neisseria gonorrhoeae*, and group B streptococci with preterm rupture of the membranes and pregnancy outcome. Am J Obstet Gynecol 159:397, 1988

Allsworth JE, Peipert JF: Prevalence of bacterial vaginosis: 2001–2004 National Health and Nutrition Examination Survey data. Obstet Gynecol 109(1):114, 2007

American Academy of Pediatrics and American College of Obstetricians and Gynecologists: Joint statement on human immunodeficiency virus screening. Elk Grove Village, IL, (AAP); Washington, DC, ACOG, 1999; Reaffirmed 2006

American College of Obstetricians and Gynecologists: Scheduled cesarean delivery and the prevention of vertical transmission of HIV infection. Committee Opinion No. 234, May 2000

American College of Obstetricians and Gynecologists: Assessment of risk factors for preterm birth. Practice Bulletin No. 31, October 2001

American College of Obstetricians and Gynecologists: Management of herpes in pregnancy. Practice Bulletin No. 31, June 2007a

American College of Obstetricians and Gynecologists: Premature rupture of membranes. Practice Bulletin No. 80, April 2007b

American College of Obstetricians and Gynecologists: Prenatal and perinatal human immunodeficiency virus testing: Expanded recommendations. Committee Opinion No. 418, September 2008

Andrews WW, Klebanoff MA, Thom EA, et al: Midpregnancy genitourinary tract infection with *Chlamydia trachomatis*: Association with subsequent preterm delivery in women with bacterial vaginosis and *Trichomonas vaginalis*. Am J Obstet Gynecol 194:493, 2006

Andrews WW, Goldenberg RL, Mercer B, et al: The Preterm Prediction Study: Association of second-trimester genitourinary chlamydia infection with subsequent spontaneous preterm birth. Am J Obstet Gynecol 183:662, 2000

Andrews WW, Lee H, Roden WJ, et al: Detection of genitourinary tract *Chlamydia trachomatis* infection in pregnant women by ligase chain reaction assay. Obstet Gynecol 89:556, 1997

Anzivino E, Fioriti D, Mischitelli M, et al: Herpes simplex virus infection in pregnancy and in neonate: status of art of epidemiology, diagnosis, therapy and prevention. Virol J 6:40, 2009

Arena S, Marconi M, Frega A, et al: Pregnancy and condyloma. Evaluation about therapeutic effectiveness of laser CO_2 on 115 pregnant women. Minerva Ginecol 53:389, 2001

Arrive E, Newell ML, Ekouevi DK, et al: Prevalence of resistance to nevirapine in mothers and children after single-dose exposure to prevent vertical transmission of HIV-1: A meta-analysis. Int J Epidemiology 36:1009, 2007

Ashley RL: Sorting out the new HSV type specific antibody tests. Sex Transm Infect 77:232, 2001

Augenbraun MH: Treatment of syphilis 2001: Nonpregnant adults. Clin Infect Dis 35:S187, 2002

Augenbraun M, Workowski K: Ceftriaxone therapy for syphilis: Report from the Emerging Infections Network. Clin Infect Dis 29:1337, 1999

Ault K: Human papillomavirus infections: Diagnosis, treatment and hope for a vaccine. Obstet Gynecol Clin North Am 30:809, 2003

Bae WH, Wester C, Smeaton LM, et al: Hematologic and hepatic toxicities associated with antenatal and postnatal exposure to maternal highly active antiretroviral therapy among infants. AIDS 22:1633, 2008

Baker D, Brown Z, Hollier LM, et al: Cost-effectiveness of herpes simplex virus type 2 serologic testing and antiviral therapy in pregnancy. Am J Obstet Gynecol 191:2074, 2004

Barnabas RV, Carabin H, Garnett GP: The potential role of suppressive therapy for sex partners in the prevention of neonatal herpes: A health economic analysis. Sex Transm Infect 78:425, 2002

Bataskov KL, Hariharan S, Horowitz MD, et al: Gonococcal endocarditis complicating pregnancy: A case report and literature review. Obstet Gynecol 78:494, 1991

Baud D, Regan L, Greub G: Emerging role of Chlamydia and Chlamydia-like organisms in adverse pregnancy outcomes. Curr Opin Infect Dis 21:70, 2008

Berman SM: Maternal syphilis: Pathophysiology and treatment. Bull World Health Organ 82:433, 2004

Blanco JD, Diaz KC, Lipscomb KA, et al: Chlamydia trachomatis isolation in patients with endometritis after cesarean section. Am J Obstet Gynecol 152:278, 1985

Blas MM, Canchihuaman FA, Alva IE, et al: Pregnancy outcomes in women infected with Chlamydia trachomatis: A population-based cohort study in Washington state. Sex Transm Infect 83:314, 2007

Braig S, Luton D, Sibony O, et al: Acyclovir prophylaxis in late pregnancy prevents recurrent genital herpes and viral shedding. Eur J Obstet Gynecol Reprod Biol 96:55, 2001

Branson, BM: State of the art for diagnosis of HIV infection. CID 45:S221, 2007

Brown EL, Gardella C, Malm G, et al: Effect of maternal herpes simples virus (HSV) serostatus and HSV type on risk of neonatal herpes. Acta Obstet Gynecol 86:523, 2007

Brown ZA: HSV-2 specific serology should be offered routinely to antenatal patients. Rev Med Virol 10(3):141, 2000

Brown ZA, Baker DA: Acyclovir therapy during pregnancy. Obstet Gynecol 73:526, 1989

Brown ZA, Gardella C, Wald A, et al: Genital herpes complicating pregnancy. Obstet Gynecol 106:845, 2005

Brown ZA, Selke SA, Zeh J, et al: Acquisition of herpes simplex virus during pregnancy. N Engl J Med 337:509, 1997

Bulterys M, Jamieson DJ, O'Sullivan MJ, et al: Rapid HIV-1 testing during labor: A multicenter study. JAMA 292:219, 2004

Burgis JT, Nawaz III H: Disseminated gonococcal infection in pregnancy presenting as meningitis and dermatitis. Obstet Gynecol 108:798, 2006

Burkman RT, Tonascia JA, Atienza MF, et al: Untreated endocervical gonorrhea and endometritis following elective abortion. Am J Obstet Gynecol 126:648, 1976

Cejtin HE: Gynecologic issues in the HIV-infected woman. Obstet Gynecol Clin North Am 30:711, 2003

Centers for Disease Control and Prevention: Revised guidelines for HIV counseling and testing. MMWR 50:1, 2001a

Centers for Disease Control and Prevention: Revised recommendations for HIV screening of pregnant women. MMWR 50:RR-19, 2001b

Centers for Disease Control and Prevention: Azithromycin treatment failures in syphilis infections—San Francisco, California, 2002–2003. MMWR 53:197, 2004

Centers for Disease Control and Prevention: HIV/AIDS surveillance report. Cases of HIV infection and AIDS in the United States and Dependent Areas, 2006. 18:1, 2006a

Centers for Disease Control and Prevention: Sexually transmitted diseases treatment guidelines, 2006. MMWR 55:1, 2006b

Centers for Disease Control and Prevention: Revised recommendations for HIV testing of adults, adolescents, and pregnant women in health-care settings. MMWR 55:1, 2006c

Centers for Disease Control and Prevention: Update to CDC's sexually transmitted diseases treatment guidelines, 2006: Fluoroquinolones no longer recommended for treatment of gonococcal infections. MMWR 56:332, 2007

Centers for Disease Control and Prevention: Availability of cefixime 400 mg tablets—United States, April 2008. MMWR 57:435, 2008a

Centers for Disease Control and Prevention: HIV prevalence estimates—United States. MMWR 57:1073, 2008b

Centers for Disease Control and Prevention: Sexually transmitted disease surveillance 2006 supplement, Chlamydia prevalence monitoring project annual report 2006. May 2008c

Centers for Disease Control and Prevention: Sexually transmitted disease surveillance 2006 supplement, gonococcal isolate surveillance project (GISP) annual report 2006. April 2008d

Centers for Disease Control and Prevention: Pediatrics HIV/AIDS Surveillance (through 2006). Slide set, 2008. Available at: http://www.cdc.gov/hiv/topics/surveillance/resources/slides/pediatric/index.htm. Accessed February 2, 2009a

Centers for Disease Control and Prevention: STD surveillance 2006. Trends in reportable sexually transmitted diseases in the United States. Available at: http://www.cdc.gov/std/stats/trends2006.htm. Accessed February 5, 2009b

Chisholm CA, Katz VL, McDonald TL, et al: Penicillin desensitization in the treatment of syphilis during pregnancy. Am J Perinatol 14:553, 1997

Christmas JT, Wendel GD, Bawdon RE, et al: Concomitant infection with Neisseria gonorrhoeae and Chlamydia trachomatis in pregnancy. Obstet Gynecol 74:295, 1989

Cleary KL, Oare E, Stamilio D, et al: Type-specific screening for asymptomatic herpes infection in pregnancy: A decision analysis. BJOG 112:731, 2005

Connor N, Roberts J, Nicoll A: Strategic options for antenatal screening for syphilis in the United Kingdom: A cost effectiveness analysis. J Med Screen 7:7, 2000

Coonrod DV, Jack BW, Stubblefield PG, et al: The clinical content of preconception care: infectious diseases in preconception care. Am J Obstet Gynecol 199(6 Suppl 2):S296, 2008

Cooper ER, Charurat M, Mofenson L, et al: Combination antiretroviral strategies for the treatment of pregnant HIV-1-infected women and prevention of perinatal HIV-1 transmission. J Acquir Immune Defic Syndr 29:484, 2002

Corey L, Wald A, Patel R, et al: Once-daily valacyclovir to reduce the risk of transmission of genital herpes. N Engl J Med 350:11, 2004

Coste J, Job-Spira N, Fernandez H: Risk factors for spontaneous abortion: A case-control study in France. Hum Reprod 6:1332, 1991

Cote HC, Raboud J, Bitnun A, et al: Perinatal exposure to antiretroviral therapy is associated with increased blood mitochondrial DNA levels and decreased mitochondrial gene expression in infants. J Infect Dis 198:851, 2008

Cowan FM, Humphrey JH, Ntozini R, et al: Maternal herpes simplex virus type 2 infection, syphilis and risk of intra-partum transmission of HIV-1: Results of a case control study. AIDS 22:193, 2008

Culnane M, Fowler M, Lee SS, et al: Lack of long-term effects of in utero exposure to zidovudine among uninfected children born to HIV-infected women. Pediatric AIDS Clinical Trials Group Protocol 219/076 Teams. JAMA 13:281, 1999

De Cock KM, Fowler MG, Mercier E, et al: Prevention of mother-to-child HIV transmission in resource-poor countries. JAMA 283:1175, 2000

Di Mario S, Say L, Lincetto O: Risk factors for stillbirth in developing countries: A systematic review of the literature. Sex Transm Dis 34:S11, 2007

Dunne EF, Unger ER, Sternberg M, et al: Prevalence of HPV infection among females in the United States. JAMA 297:813, 2007

Eckert LO: Clinical practice: Acute vulvovaginitis. N Engl J Med 355:1244, 2006

Eskild A, Jeansson S, Stray-Pedersen B, et al: Herpes simplex virus type-2 infection in pregnancy. No risk of fetal death: Results from a nested case-control study within 35,940 women. Br J Obstet Gynaecol 109:1030, 2002

European Mode of Delivery Collaboration: Elective caesarean-section versus vaginal delivery in prevention of vertical HIV-1 transmission: A randomized clinical trial. Lancet 353:1035, 1999

Fagnant RJ, Monif GRG: How rare is congenital herpes simplex? A literature review. J Reprod Med 34:417, 1989

Fauci AS: Pathogenesis of HIV disease: Opportunities for new prevention interventions. CID 45:S206, 2007

Fauci AS, Lane HC: Human immunodeficiency virus disease: AIDS and related disorders: Introduction. In Fauci AS, Braunwald E, Kasper DL, et al (eds): Harrison's Principles of Internal Medicine, 17th ed, New York, McGraw-Hill, 2008, p 1137

Fenton KA: Changing epidemiology of HIV/AIDS in the United States: Implications for enhancing and promoting HIV testing strategies. Clin Infect Dis 45:S213, 2007

Fife KH, Katz BP, Brizendine EJ, et al: Cervical human papillomavirus deoxyribonucleic acid persists throughout pregnancy and decreases in the postpartum period. Am J Obstet Gynecol 180:1110, 1999

Fiumara NJ, Fleming WL, Downing JG, et al: The incidence of prenatal syphilis at the Boston City Hospital. N Engl J Med 247:48, 1952

Gajewska M, Marianowski L, Wielgos M, et al: The occurrence of genital types of human papillomavirus in normal pregnancy and in pregnant women with pregestational insulin dependent diabetes mellitus. Neuroendocrinol Lett 26:766, 2005

Gallo RC, Montagnier L: The discovery of HIV as the cause of AIDS. N Engl J Med 349:2283, 2003

Gardella C, Brown ZA, Wald A, et al: Poor correlation between genital lesions and detection of herpes simplex virus in women in labor. Obstet Gynecol 106:268, 2005

Gibbs RS, Schachter J: Chlamydial serology in patients with intra-amniotic infection and controls. Sex Transm Dis 14:213, 1987

Golden MR, Marra CM, Holmes KK: Update on syphilis: Resurgence of an old problem. JAMA 290:1510, 2003

Goldenberg RL, McClure EM, Belizán JM: Commentary: reducing the world's stillbirths. BMC Pregnancy Childbirth 9 Suppl 1:S1, 2009

Goldenberg RL, Thompson C: The infectious origins of stillbirth. Am J Obstet Gynecol 189:861, 2003

Gray RH, Wabwire-Mangen F, Kigozi G, et al: Randomized trial of presumptive sexually transmitted disease therapy during pregnancy in Rakai, Uganda. Am J Obstet Gynecol 185:1209, 2001

Greer L, Wendel GD: Rapid diagnostic methods in sexually transmitted infections. Infect Dis Clin North Am 22:601, 2008

Hagensee ME, Slavinsky J 3rd, Gaffga CM, et al: Seroprevalence of human papillomavirus type 16 in pregnant women. Obstet Gynecol 94:653, 1999

Heim K, Hudelist G, Geier A, et al: Type-specific antiviral antibodies to genital human papillomavirus types in mothers and newborns. Reprod Sci 14:806, 2007

Hernandez-Giron C, Smith JS, Lorincz A, et al: High-risk human papillomavirus detection and related risk factors among pregnant and nonpregnant women in Mexico. Sex Transm Dis 32:613, 2005

Hollier LM, Harstad TW, Sanchez PJ, et al: Fetal syphilis: Clinical and laboratory characteristics. Obstet Gynecol 97:947, 2001

Hollier LM, Hill J, Sheffield JS, et al: State laws regarding prenatal syphilis screening in the United States. Am J Obstet Gynecol 189:1178, 2003

Hollier LM, Wendel GD: Third trimester antiviral prophylaxis for preventing maternal genital herpes simplex virus (HSV) recurrences and neonatal infection. Cochrane Database Syst Rev 1:CD004946, 2008

Hoyme UB, Kiviat N, Eschenbach DA: The microbiology and treatment of late postpartum endometritis. Obstet Gynecol 68:226, 1986

International Perinatal HIV Group: The mode of delivery and the risk of vertical transmission of human immunodeficiency virus type 1: A meta-analysis of 15 prospective cohort studies. N Engl J Med 340:977, 1999

Jacobson GF, Autry AM, Kirby RS, et al: A randomized controlled trial comparing amoxicillin and azithromycin for the treatment of *Chlamydia trachomatis* in pregnancy. Am J Obstet Gynecol 184:1352, 2001

Jamieson DJ, Read JS, Kourtis AP, et al: Cesarean delivery for HIV-infected women: Recommendations and controversies. Am J Obstet Gynecol 197:S96, 2007

John-Stewart G, Mbori-Ngacha D, Ekpini R, et al: Breastfeeding and transmission of HIV-1. J Acquir Immune Defic Syndr 35:196, 2004

Johnson HL, Erbelding EJ, Zenilman JM, et al: Sexually transmitted diseases and risk behaviors among pregnant women attending inner city public sexually transmitted diseases clinics in Baltimore, MD, 1996-2002. Sex Transm Dis 34:991, 2007

Kacmar J, Cheh E, Montagno A, et al: A randomized trial of azithromycin versus amoxicillin for the treatment of *Chlamydia trachomatis* in pregnancy. Infect Dis Obstet Gynecol 9:197, 2001

Kahn JO, Walker BD: Acute human immunodeficiency virus type 1 infection. N Engl J Med 339:33, 1998

Kapur P, Rakheja D, Gomez AM, et al: Characterization of inflammation in syphilitic villitis and in villitis of unknown etiology. Pediatr Dev Pathol 7:453, 2004

Kimberlin DW: Neonatal herpes simplex infection. Clin Microbiol Rev 17:1, 2004

Kimberlin DW, Lin CY, Jacobs RF, et al: Natural history of neonatal herpes simplex virus infections in the acyclovir era. Pediatrics 108:223, 2001a

Kimberlin DW, Lin CY, Jacobs RF, et al: Safety and efficacy of high-dose intravenous acyclovir in the management of neonatal herpes simplex virus infections. Pediatrics 108:230, 2001b

Kimberlin DW, Rouse DJ: Genital herpes. N Engl J Med 350:1970, 2004

Klass PE, Brown ER, Pelton SI: The incidence of prenatal syphilis at the Boston City Hospital: A comparison across four decades. Pediatrics 94:24, 1994

Klein VR, Cox SM, Mitchell MD, et al: The Jarisch–Herxheimer reaction complicating syphilotherapy in pregnancy. Obstet Gynecol 75:375, 1990

Kohl KS, Markowitz LE, Koumans EH: Developments in the screening for *Chlamydia trachomatis*: A review. Obstet Gynecol Clin North Am 30:637, 2003

Koumans EH, Sternberg M, Gwinn M, et al: Geographic variation of HIV infection in childbearing women with syphilis in the United States. AIDS 14:279, 2000

Kourtis AP, Bulterys M, Nesheim SR, et al: Understanding the timing of HIV transmission from mother to infant. JAMA 285:709, 2001

Kourtis AP, Jamieson DJ, de Vincenzi I, et al: Prevention of human immunodeficiency virus-1 transmission to the infant through breastfeeding: New developments. Am J Obstet Gynecol 197:S113, 2007

Kourtis AP, Lee FK, Abrams EJ, et al: Mother-to-child transmission of HIV-1: Timing and implications for prevention. Lancet Infect Dis 6:726, 2006

Kuhn L, Steketee RW, Weedon J, et al: Distinct risk factors for intrauterine and intrapartum human immunodeficiency virus transmission and consequences for disease progression in infected children. Perinatal AIDS Collaborative Transmission Study. J Infect Dis 179:52, 1999

Laderman EI, Whitworth E, Dumaual E, et al: Rapid, sensitive, and specific lateral-flow immunochromatographic point-of-care device for detection of herpes simplex virus type 2-specific immunoglobulin G antibodies in serum and whole blood. Clin Vaccine Immunol 15:159, 2008

Lago EG, Rodrigues LC, Fiori RM, et al: Identification of two distinct profiles of maternal characteristics associated with risk. Sex Transm Dis 31:33, 2004

Laine C, Newschaffer CJ, Zhang D, et al: Adherence to antiretroviral therapy by pregnant women infected with human immunodeficiency virus: A pharmacy claims-based analysis. Obstet Gynecol 95:167, 2000

Landesman SH, Kalish LA, Burns DN, et al: Obstetrical factors and the transmission of human immunodeficiency virus type 1 from mother to child. N Engl J Med 334:1617, 1996

Langenberg AGM, Corey L, Ashley RL, et al: A prospective study of new infections with herpes simplex virus type 1 and type 2. N Engl J Med 341:1432, 1999

Lewis SH, Reynolds-Kohler C, Fox HE, et al: HIV-1 in trophoblastic and villous Hofbauer cells, and haematological precursors in eight-week fetuses. Lancet 335:565, 1990

Lorenzi P, Spicher VM, Laubereau B, et al: Antiretroviral therapies in pregnancy: Maternal, fetal and neonatal effects. Swiss HIV Cohort Study, the Swiss Collaborative HIV and Pregnancy Study, and the Swiss Neonatal HIV Study. AIDS 12:F241, 1998

Lucas MJ, Theriot SK, Wendel GD: Doppler systolic–diastolic ratios in pregnancies complicated by syphilis. Obstet Gynecol 77:217, 1991

Lukehart SA, Godornes C, Molini BJ, et al: Macrolide resistance in *Treponema pallidum* in the United States and Ireland. N Engl J Med 351:154, 2004

Mahnert N, Roberts SW, Laibl VR, et al: The incidence of neonatal herpes infection. Am J Obstet Gynecol 196:e55, 2007

Major CA, Towers CV, Lewis DF, et al: Expectant management of preterm rupture of membranes complicated by active recurrent genital herpes. Am J Obstet Gynecol 188:1551, 2003

Manhart LE, Holmes KK, Koutsky LA, et al: Human papillomavirus infection among sexually active young women in the United States: Implications for developing a vaccination strategy. Sex Transm Dis 33:502, 2006

Manns A, Strickler HD, Wiktor SZ, et al: Low incidence of human papillomavirus type 16 antibody seroconversion in young children. Pediatr Infect Dis J 18:833, 1999

Martín MC, Pérez F, Moreno A, et al: Neisseria gonorrhoeae meningitis in pregnant adolescent. Emerg Infect Dis 14(10):1672, 2008

Mertz GJ, Rosenthal SL, Stanberry LR: Is herpes simplex virus type 1 (HSV-1) now more common than HSV-2 in first episodes of genital herpes? Sex Transm Dis 30:801, 2003

Meyers D, Wolff T, Gregory K, et al: USPSTF recommendations for STI screening. Am Fam Physician 77:819, 2008

Meyers DS, Halvorson H, Luckhaupt S: Screening for chlamydial infection: An evidence update for the U.S. Preventive Services Task Force. Ann Intern Med 147:134, 2007

Miller JM Jr: Recurrent chlamydial colonization during pregnancy. Am J Perinatol 15:307, 1998

Miller JM Jr, Maupin RT, Mestad RE, et al: Initial and repeated screening for gonorrhea during pregnancy. Sex Transm Dis 30:728, 2003

Miller WC, Ford CA, Morris M, et al: Prevalence of chlamydial and gonococcal infections among young adults in the United States. JAMA 291:2229, 2004

Minkoff HL, Hershow R, Watts H, et al: The relationship of pregnancy to human immunodeficiency virus disease progression. Am J Obstet Gynecol 189:552, 2003

Myles TD, Elam G, Park-Hwang E, et al: The Jarisch–Herxheimer reaction and fetal monitoring changes in pregnant women treated for syphilis. Obstet Gynecol 92:859, 1998

Nathan L, Bohman VR, Sanchez PJ, et al: In utero infection with *Treponema pallidum* in early pregnancy. Prenat Diagn 17:119, 1997

National Institutes of Health, the Centers for Disease Control and Prevention, and the HIV Medicine Association of the Infectious Diseases Society of America: Guidelines for Prevention and Treatment of Opportunistic Infections in HIV-Infected Adults and Adolescents. June 18, 2008. Available at: http://aidsinfo.nih.gov/contentfiles/Adult_OI.pdf. Accessed March 20, 2009

Nobbenhuis MAE, Helmerhorst TJM, van den Brule AJC, et al: High-risk human papillomavirus clearance in pregnant women: Trends for lower clearance during pregnancy with a catch-up postpartum. Br J Cancer 87:75, 2002

Panel on Antiretroviral Guidelines for Adults and Adolescents: Guidelines for the use of antiretroviral agents in HIV-1-infected adults and adolescents. Department of Health and Human Services, November 3, 2008, p 80. Available at: http://www.aidsinfo.nih.gov/ContentFiles/AdultandAdolescentGL.pdf. Accessed March 20, 2009

Paukku M, Tulppala M, Puolakkainen M, et al: Lack of association between serum antibodies to *Chlamydia trachomatis* and a history of recurrent pregnancy loss. Fertil Steril 72:427, 1999

Peipert JF: Clinical practice: Genital chlamydial infections. N Engl J Med 18:349, 2003

Petra Study Team: Efficacy of three short-course regimens of zidovudine and lamivudine in preventing early and late transmission of HIV-1 from mother to child in Tanzania, South Africa and Uganda (Petra study): A randomized, double-blind, placebo-controlled trial. Lancet 359:1178, 2002

Piper JM, Shain RN, Korte JE, et al: Behavioral interventions for prevention of sexually transmitted diseases in women: A physician's perspective. Obstet Gynecol Clin North Am 30:659, 2003

Piscitelli SC, Gallicano KD: Interactions among drugs for HIV and opportunistic infections. N Engl J Med 344:984, 2001

Pitsouni E, Iavazzo C, Falagas ME: Itraconazole vs fluconazole for the treatment of uncomplicated acute vaginal and vulvovaginal candidiasis in nonpregnant women: A metaanalysis of randomized controlled trials. Am J Obstet Gynecol 198:153, 2008

Pope V, Fears MB: Serodia *Treponema pallidum* passive particle agglutination (TP-PA) test. In Larsen SA, Pope V, Jonnson RE, et al (eds): Supplement to A Manual of Tests for Syphilis, 9th ed. Washington, DC, American Public Health Association, 2000, p 365

Prober CG, Sullender WM, Yasukawa LL, et al: Low risk of herpes simplex virus infections in neonates exposed to the virus at the time of vaginal delivery to mothers with recurrent genital herpes simplex virus infections. N Engl J Med 316:240, 1987

Rahangdale L, Guerry S, Bauer HM, et al: An observational cohort study of *Chlamydia trachomatis* treatment in pregnancy. Sex Transm Dis 33:106, 2006

Ramsey PS, Vaules MB, Vasdev GM, et al: Maternal and transplacental pharmacokinetics of azithromycin. Am J Obstet Gynecol 188:714, 2003

Ramus R, Sheffield JS, Mayfield JA, et al: A randomized trial that compared oral cefixime and intramuscular ceftriaxone for the treatment of gonorrhea in pregnancy. Am J Obstet Gynecol 185:629, 2001

Rando RF, Lindheim S, Hasty L, et al: Increased frequency of detection of human papillomavirus deoxyribonucleic acid in exfoliated cervical cells during pregnancy. Am J Obstet Gynecol 161:50, 1989

Rastogi S, Salhan S, Mittal A: Detection of *Chlamydia trachomatis* antigen in spontaneous abortions: Is this organism a primary or secondary indicator of risk? Br J Biomed Sci 57:126, 2000

Ratanajamit C, Skriver MV, Jepsen P, et al: Adverse pregnancy outcome in women exposed to acyclovir during pregnancy: A population-based observational study. Scand J Infect Dis 35:255, 2003

Read JS and the Committee on Pediatric AIDS: Human milk, breastfeeding, and transmission of human immunodeficiency virus type 1 in the United States. Pediatrics 112:1196, 2003

Read JS, Newell MK: Efficacy and safety of cesarean delivery for prevention of mother-to-child transmission of HIV-1. Cochrane Database Syst Rev (4):CD005479, 2005

Reiff-Eldridge R, Heffner CR, Ephross SA, et al: Monitoring pregnancy outcomes after prenatal drug exposure through prospective pregnancy registries: A pharmaceutical company commitment. Am J Obstet Gynecol 182:159, 2000

Richardson BA, John-Stewart GC, Hughes JP, et al: Breast milk infectivity in human immunodeficiency virus type 1-infected mothers. J Infect Dis 187:736, 2003

Roberts CW, Pfister JR, Spear SJ: Increasing proportion of herpes simplex virus type 1 as a cause of genital herpes infection in college students. Sex Transm Dis 30:797, 2003

Rosa FW, Baum C, Shaw M: Pregnancy outcomes after first-trimester vaginitis drug therapy. Obstet Gynecol 69:751, 1987

Ross JDC: Systemic gonococcal infection. Genitourin Med 72:404, 1996

Rouse DJ, Stringer JS: An appraisal of screening for maternal type-specific herpes simplex virus antibodies to prevent neonatal herpes. Am J Obstet Gynecol 183:400, 2000

Saloojee H, Velaphi S, Goga Y, et al: The prevention and management of congenital syphilis: An overview and recommendations. Bull World Health Organ 82:424, 2004

Schmid GP, Sanders LL, Blount JH, et al: Chancroid in the United States: Reestablishment of an old disease. JAMA 258:3265, 1987

Schulte JM, Burkham S, Hamaker D, et al: Syphilis among HIV-infected mothers and their infants in Texas from 1988 to 1994. Sex Transm Dis 28:316, 2001

Schwartz DA, Larsen SA, Beck-Sague C, et al: Pathology of the umbilical cord in congenital syphilis: Analysis of 25 specimens using histochemistry and immunofluorescent antibody to *Treponema pallidum*. Hum Pathol 26:784, 1995

Scott LL: Prevention of perinatal herpes: Prophylactic antiviral therapy? Clin Obstet Gynecol 42:134, 1999

Scott LL, Hollier LM, McIntire D, et al: Acyclovir suppression to prevent recurrent genital herpes at delivery. Infect Dis Obstet Gynecol 10:71, 2002

Scott LL, Sanchez PJ, Jackson GL, et al: Acyclovir suppression to prevent cesarean section after first episode genital herpes in pregnancy. Obstet Gynecol 87:69, 1996

Scoular A: Using the evidence base on genital herpes: Optimizing the use of diagnostic tests and information provision. Sex Transm Infect 78:160, 2002

Sheffield JS, Andrews WW, Klebanoff MA, et al: Spontaneous resolution of asymptomatic *Chlamydia trachomatis* in pregnancy. Obstet Gynecol 105:557, 2005

Sheffield JS, Fish DN, Hollier LM, et al: Acyclovir concentrations in human breast milk after valacyclovir administration. Am J Obstet Gynecol 186:100, 2002a

Sheffield JS, Hill JB, Hollier LM, et al: Valacyclovir prophylaxis to prevent recurrent herpes at delivery: A randomized clinical trial. Obstet Gynecol 108:141, 2006

Sheffield JS, Hollier LM, Hill JB, et al: Acyclovir prophylaxis to prevent herpes simplex virus recurrence at delivery: A systematic review. Obstet Gynecol 102:1396, 2003

Sheffield JS, Sanchez PJ, Morris G, et al: Congenital syphilis after maternal treatment for syphilis during pregnancy. Am J Obstet Gynecol 186:569, 2002b

Sheffield JS, Sanchez PJ, Wendel GD Jr, et al: Placental histopathology of congenital syphilis. Obstet Gynecol 100:126, 2002c

Sheffield JS, Sigman A, McIntire D, et al: Disseminated gonococcal infection in women: A 24-year experience, Abstract #522. Presented at the Thirteenth Annual Meeting of the International Society for Sexually Transmitted Diseases Research, Denver, July 11–14, 1999

Sheffield JS, Wendel GD, McIntire DD, et al: Effect of genital ulcer disease on HIV-1 coreceptor expression in the female genital tract. J Infect Dis 196:1509, 2007

Sheffield JS, Wendel GD Jr, McIntire DD, et al: The effect of progesterone levels and pregnancy on HIV-1 coreceptor expression. Reprod Sci 16:20, 2009

Silverberg MJ, Thorsen P, Lindeberg H, et al: Condyloma in pregnancy is strongly predictive of juvenile-onset recurrent respiratory papillomatosis. Obstet Gynecol 101:645, 2003

Silverstein AM: Congenital syphilis and the timing of immunogenesis in the human fetus. Nature 194:196, 1962

Simhan HN, Bodnar LM, Krohn MA: Paternal race and bacterial vaginosis during the first trimester of pregnancy. Am J Obstet Gynecol 198:196.e1, 2008

Smith EM, Ritchie JM, Yankowitz J, et al: Human papillomavirus prevalence and types in newborns and parents. Sex Transm Dis 31:57, 2004

Sobel JD: Vulvovaginal candidosis. Lancet 369:1961, 2007

Sozio J, Ness RB: Chlamydial lower genital tract infection and spontaneous abortion. Infect Dis Obstet Gynecol 6:8, 1998

Sperling RS, Shapiro DE, McSherry GD, et al: Safety of the maternal–infant zidovudine regimen utilized in the Pediatric AIDS Clinical Trial Group 076 Study. AIDS 12:1805, 1998

Spitzer M, Krumholz BA, Seltzer VL: The multicentric nature of disease related to human papillomavirus infection of the female lower genital tract. Obstet Gynecol 73:303, 1989

Stratton P, Tuomala RE, Abboud R, et al: Obstetric and newborn outcomes in a cohort of HIV-infected pregnant women: A report of the Women and Infants Transmission Study. J Acquir Immune Defic Syndr Hum Retrovirol 20:179, 1999

Stuart GS, Castano PM, Sheffield JS, et al: Postpartum sterilization choices made by HIV-infected women. Infect Dis Obstet Gynecol 13:217, 2005

Stuart GS, Cunningham FG: Contraception and sterilization. In Schorge JO, Schaffer JI, Halvorson LM, et al (eds): Williams Gynecology, 1st ed. New York, McGraw-Hill, 2008, p 112

Sugiura-Ogasawara M, Ozaki Y, Nakanishi T, et al: Pregnancy outcome in recurrent aborters is not influenced by *Chlamydia* IgA and/or G. Am J Reprod Immunol 53:50, 2005

Tang JH, Sheffield JS, Grimes J, et al: Effect of protease inhibitor therapy on glucose intolerance in pregnancy. Obstet Gynecol 107:1, 2006

Taylor MM, Mickey T, Browne K, et al: Opportunities for the prevention of congenital syphilis in Maricopa County, Arizona. Sex Transm Dis 35:341, 2008

Thung SF, Grobman WA: The cost-effectiveness of routine antenatal screening for maternal herpes simplex virus-1 and -2 antibodies. Am J Obstet Gynecol 192:483, 2005

Trepka MJ, Bloom SA, Zhang G, et al: Inadequate syphilis screening among women with prenatal care in a community with a high syphilis incidence. Sex Transm Dis 33:670, 2006

Tuomala RE, Shapiro DE, Mofenson LM: Antiretroviral therapy during pregnancy and the risk of an adverse outcome. N Engl J Med 346:1863, 2002

U.S. Preventive Services Task Force: Screening for HIV: Recommendation statement. Ann Intern Med 143:32, 2005

U.S. Preventive Services Task Force: Screening for chlamydial infection: A focused evidence update for the U.S. Preventive Services Task Force. Evidence synthesis No. 48. Rockville, MD: Agency for Healthcare Research and Quality. AHRQ publication No. 07-15101-EF-1, June 2007

U.S. Public Health Service Task Force: Recommendations for use of antiretroviral drugs in pregnant HIV-infected women for maternal health and interventions to reduce perinatal HIV transmission in the United States. April 2009

United Nations Programme on HIV/AIDS and World Health Organization: AIDS epidemic update. 2007. Available at: http://data.unaids.org/pub/EPISlides/2007/2007_epiupdate_en.pdf. Accessed January 28, 2009

Wald A: Herpes simplex virus type 2 transmission: Risk factors and virus shedding. Herpes 3:130A, 2004

Wald A, Ashley-Morrow R: Serological testing for herpes simplex virus (HSV)-1 and HSV-2 infection. Clin Infect Dis 35:S173, 2002

Warner L, Rohcat RW, Fichtner RR, et al: Missed opportunities for congenital syphilis prevention in an urban southeastern hospital. Sex Transm Dis 28:92, 2001

Watson-Jones D, Changalucha J, Gumodoka B, et al: Syphilis in pregnancy in Tanzania. I. Impact of maternal syphilis on outcome of pregnancy. J Infect Dis 186:940, 2002

Watts DH: Management of human immunodeficiency virus infection in pregnancy. N Engl J Med 346:1879, 2002

Watts DH, Koutsky LA, Holmes KK, et al: Low risk of perinatal transmission of human papillomavirus: Results from a prospective cohort study. Am J Obstet Gynecol 178:365, 1998

Watts DH, Brown ZA, Money D, et al: A double-blind, randomized, placebo-controlled trial of acyclovir in late pregnancy for the reduction of herpes simplex virus shedding and cesarean delivery. Am J Obstet Gynecol 188:836, 2003

Wendel GD: Gestational and congenital syphilis. Clin Perinatol 15:287, 1988

Wendel GD, Cunningham FG: Sexually transmitted diseases in pregnancy. In Williams Obstetrics, 18th ed. (Suppl 13). Norwalk, CT, Appleton & Lange, August/September 1991

Wendel GD Jr, Sanchez PJ, Peters MT, et al: Identification of *Treponema pallidum* in amniotic fluid and fetal blood from pregnancies complicated by congenital syphilis. Obstet Gynecol 78:890, 1991

Wendel GD Jr, Sheffield JS, Hollier LM, et al: Treatment of syphilis in pregnancy and prevention of congenital syphilis. Clin Infect Dis 35:S200, 2002

Wendel GD Jr, Stark BJ, Jamison RB, et al: Penicillin allergy and desensitization in serious infections during pregnancy. N Engl J Med 312:1229, 1985

Wendel KA, Workowski KA: Trichomoniasis: Challenges to appropriate management. Clin Infect Dis 44:S123, 2007

Whitley R, Davis EA, Suppapanya N: Incidence of neonatal herpes simplex virus infections in a managed-care population. Sex Transm Dis 34:704, 2007

Wiley DJ, Douglas J, Beutner K, et al: External genital warts: Diagnosis, treatment and prevention. Clin Infect Dis 35:S210, 2002

Wilkinson D, Barton S, Cowan F: HSV-2 specific serology should not be offered routinely to antenatal patients. Rev Med Virol 10:145, 2000

Wilson EK, Gavin NI, Adams EK, et al: Patterns in prenatal syphilis screening among Florida Medicaid enrollees. Sex Transm Dis 34:378, 2007

Winer RL, Koutsky LA: Delivering reassurance to parents: Perinatal human papillomavirus transmission is rare. Sex Transm Dis 31:63, 2004

Worda C, Huber A, Hudelist G, et al: Prevalence of cervical and intrauterine human papillomavirus infection in the third trimester in asymptomatic women. J Soc Gynecol Investig 12:440, 2005

World Health Organization: HIV transmission through breastfeeding: A review of available evidence: 2007 update. Geneva, WHO Press, 2008

Xu F, Markowitz LE, Gottlieb SL, et al: Seroprevalence of herpes simplex virus types 1 and 2 in pregnant women in the United States. Am J Obstet Gynecol 196:43.e1, 2007

Xu F, Sternberg MR, Kottiri BJ, et al: Trends in herpes simplex virus type 1 and type 2 seroprevalence in the United States. JAMA Aug 23/30:964, 2006

Yip L, Sweeny PJ, Bock BF: Acute suppurative salpingitis with concomitant intrauterine pregnancy. Am J Emerg Med 11:476, 1993

Young H: Guidelines for serological testing for syphilis. Sex Transm Infect 75:403, 2000

Zhou P, Gu Z, Xu J, et al: A study evaluating ceftriaxone as a treatment agent for primary and secondary syphilis in pregnancy. Sex Transm Dis 32:495, 2005

Zhou P, Qian Y, Xu J, et al: Occurrence of congenital syphilis after maternal treatment with azithromycin during pregnancy. Sex Transm Dis 34:472, 2007

APPENDIX

Reference Table of Normal Laboratory Values in Uncomplicated Pregnancies

HEMATOLOGY

	Nonpregnant Adult[a]	First Trimester	Second Trimester	Third Trimester	References
Erythropoietin[b] (U/L)	4–27	12–25	8–67	14–222	7, 10, 47
Ferritin[b] (ng/mL)	10–150[d]	6–130	2–230	0–116	7, 10, 39, 42, 45, 47, 62, 70
Folate, red blood cell (ng/mL)	150–450	137–589	94–828	109–663	45, 46, 72
Folate, serum (ng/mL)	5.4–18.0	2.6–15.0	0.8–24.0	1.4–20.7	7, 43, 45, 46, 53, 58, 72
Hemoglobin[b] (g/dL)	12–15.8[d]	11.6–13.9	9.7–14.8	9.5–15.0	10, 45, 47, 58, 62
Hematocrit[b] (%)	35.4–44.4	31.0–41.0	30.0–39.0	28.0–40.0	6, 7, 10, 42, 45 58, 66
Iron, total binding capacity (TIBC)[b] (μg/dL)	251–406	278–403	Not reported	359–609	62
Iron, serum[b] (μg/dL)	41–141	72–143	44–178	30–193	10, 62
Mean corpuscular hemoglobin (MCH) (pg/cell)	27–32	30–32	30–33	29–32	42
Mean corpuscular volume (MCV) ($\times m^3$)	79–93	81–96	82–97	81–99	6, 42, 45, 58
Platelet ($\times 10^9$/L)	165–415	174–391	155–409	146–429	4, 6, 16, 42, 45
Mean platelet volume (MPV) (μm³)	6.4–11.0	7.7–10.3	7.8–10.2	8.2–10.4	42
Red blood cell count (RBC) ($\times 10^6$/mm³)	4.00–5.20[d]	3.42–4.55	2.81–4.49	2.71–4.43	6, 42, 45, 58
Red cell distribution width (RDW) (%)	<14.5	12.5–14.1	13.4–13.6	12.7–15.3	42
White blood cell count (WBC) ($\times 10^3$/mm³)	3.5–9.1	5.7–13.6	5.6–14.8	5.9–16.9	6, 9, 42, 45, 58
Neutrophils ($\times 10^3$/mm³)	1.4–4.6	3.6–10.1	3.8–12.3	3.9–13.1	4, 6, 9, 42
Lymphocytes ($\times 10^3$/mm³)	0.7–4.6	1.1–3.6	0.9–3.9	1.0–3.6	4, 6, 9, 42
Monocytes ($\times 10^3$/mm³)	0.1–0.7	0.1–1.1	0.1–1.1	0.1–1.4	6, 9, 42
Eosinophils ($\times 10^3$/mm³)	0–0.6	0–0.6	0–0.6	0–0.6	6, 9
Basophils ($\times 10^3$/mm³)	0–0.2	0–0.1	0–0.1	0–0.1	6, 9
Transferrin (mg/dL)	200–400	254–344	220–441	288–530	39, 42
Transferrin, saturation without iron (%)	22–46[b]	Not reported	10–44	5–37	47
Transferrin, saturation with iron (%)	22–46[b]	Not reported	18–92	9–98	47

APPENDIX

COAGULATION

	Nonpregnant Adult[a]	First Trimester	Second Trimester	Third Trimester	References
Antithrombin III, functional (%)	70–130	89–114	78–126	82–116	15, 16, 74
D-Dimer (μg/mL)	0.22–0.74	0.05–0.95	0.32–1.29	0.13–1.7	16, 25, 35, 51, 74, 75
Factor V (%)	50–150	75–95	72–96	60–88	40
Factor VII (%)	50–150	100–146	95–153	149–2110	16
Factor VIII (%)	50–150	90–210	97–312	143–353	16, 40
Factor IX (%)	50–150	103–172	154–217	164–235	16
Factor XI (%)	50–150	80–127	82–144	65–123	16
Factor XII (%)	50–150	78–124	90–151	129–194	16
Fibrinogen (mg/dL)	233–496	244–510	291–538	301–696	16, 25, 42, 51, 74, 75
Homocysteine (μmol/L)	4.4–10.8	3.34–11	2.0–26.9	3.2–21.4	43, 45, 46, 53, 72
International normalized ratio (INR)	0.9–1.04[g]	0.86–1.08	0.83–1.02	0.80–1.09	15, 75
Partial thromboplastin time, activated (aPTT) (sec)	26.3–39.4	23.0–38.9	22.9–38.1	22.6–35.0	15, 16, 42, 75
Prothrombin time (PT) (sec)	12.7–15.4	9.7–13.5	9.5–13.4	9.6–12.9	16, 42, 75
Protein C, functional (%)	70–130	78–121	83–133	67–135	15, 24, 40
Protein S, total (%)	70–140	39–105	27–101	33–101	16, 24, 40
Protein S, free (%)	70–140	34–133	19–113	20–65	24, 40
Protein S, functional activity (%)	65–140	57–95	42–68	16–42	40
Tissue plasminogen activator (ng/mL)	1.6–13[h]	1.8–6.0	2.36–6.6	3.34–9.20	15, 16
Tissue plasminogen activator inhibitor-1 (ng/mL)	4–43	16–33	36–55	67–92	16
von Willebrand measurements					
von Willebrand factor antigen (%)	75–125	62–318	90–247	84–422	73, 74, 76
ADAMTS-13, von Willebrand cleaving protease (%)	40–170[i]	40–160	22–135	38–105	74, 76

BLOOD CHEMICAL CONSTITUTENTS

	Nonpregnant Adult[a]	First Trimester	Second Trimester	Third Trimester	References
Alanine transaminase (ALT) (U/L)	7–41	3–30	2–33	2–25	5, 39, 42, 70
Albumin (g/dL)	4.1–5.3[d]	3.1–5.1	2.6–4.5	2.3–4.2	3, 5, 26, 29, 39, 42, 72
Alkaline phosphatase (U/L)	33–96	17–88	25–126	38–229	3, 5, 39, 42, 70
Alpha-1 antitrypsin (mg/dL)	100–200	225–323	273–391	327–487	42
Amylase (U/L)	20–96	24–83	16–73	15–81	32, 39, 42, 68
Anion gap (mmol/L)	7–16	13–17	12–16	12–16	42
Aspartate transaminase (AST) (U/L)	12–38	3–23	3–33	4–32	5, 39, 42, 70
Bicarbonate (mmol/L)	22–30	20–24	20–24	20–24	42
Bilirubin, total (mg/dL)	0.3–1.3	0.1–0.4	0.1–0.8	0.1–1.1	5, 39
Bilirubin, unconjugated (mg/dL)	0.2–0.9	0.1–0.5	0.1–0.4	0.1–0.5	5, 42
Bilirubin, conjugated (mg/dL)	0.1–0.4	0–0.1	0–0.1	0–0.1	5
Bile acids (μmol/L)	0.3–4.8[j]	0–4.9	0–9.1	0–11.3	5, 14
Calcium, ionized (mg/dL)	4.5–5.3	4.5–5.1	4.4–5.0	4.4–5.3	26, 42, 48, 56
Calcium, total (mg/dL)	8.7–10.2	8.8–10.6	8.2–9.0	8.2–9.7	3, 29, 39, 42, 48, 56, 63
Ceruloplasmin (mg/dL)	25–63	30–49	40–53	43–78	42, 44
Chloride (mEq/L)	102–109	101–105	97–109	97–109	20, 39, 42
Creatinine (mg/dL)	0.5–0.9[d]	0.4–0.7	0.4–0.8	0.4–0.9	39, 42, 45
Gamma-glutamyl transpeptidase (GGT) (U/L)	9–58	2–23	4–22	3–26	5, 42, 39, 70
Lactate dehydrogenase (U/L)	115–221	78–433	80–447	82–524	42, 29, 39, 70
Lipase (U/L)	3–43	21–76	26–100	41–112	32
Magnesium (mg/dL)	1.5–2.3	1.6–2.2	1.5–2.2	1.1–2.2	3, 26, 29, 39, 42, 48, 63
Osmolality (mOsm/kg H_2O)	275–295	275–280	276–289	278–280	17, 63
Phosphate (mg/dL)	2.5–4.3	3.1–4.6	2.5–4.6	2.8–4.6	3, 26, 33, 39, 42
Potassium (mEq/L)	3.5–5.0	3.6–5.0	3.3–5.0	3.3–5.1	20, 26, 29, 39, 42, 63, 66
Prealbumin (mg/dL)	17–34	15–27	20–27	14–23	42
Protein, total (g/dL)	6.7–8.6	6.2–7.6	5.7–6.9	5.6–6.7	26, 29, 42
Sodium (mEq/L)	136–146	133–148	129–148	130–148	17, 26, 29, 39, 42, 63, 66
Urea nitrogen (mg/dL)	7–20	7–12	3–13	3–11	20, 39, 42
Uric acid (mg/dL)	2.5–5.6[d]	2.0–4.2	2.4–4.9	3.1–6.3	17, 39, 42

METABOLIC AND ENDOCRINE TESTS

	Nonpregnant Adult[a]	First Trimester	Second Trimester	Third Trimester	References
Aldosterone (ng/dL)	2–9	6–104	9–104	15–101	21, 34, 69
Angiotensin-converting enzyme (ACE) (U/L)	9–67	1–38	1–36	1–39	20, 54
Cortisol (μg/dL)	0–25	7–19	10–42	12–50	42, 69
Hemoglobin A_{1c} (%)	4–6	4–6	4–6	4–7	48, 49, 59
Parathyroid hormone (pg/mL)	8–51	10–15	18–25	9–26	3
Parathyroid hormone-related protein (pmol/L)	<1.3[e]	0.7–0.9	1.8–2.2	2.5–2.8	3
Renin, plasma activity (ng/mL/hr)	0.3–9.0[e]	Not reported	7.5–54.0	5.9–58.8	20, 34
Thyroid stimulating hormone (TSH) (μIU/mL)	0.34–4.25	0.60–3.40	0.37–3.60	0.38–4.04	39, 42, 57
Thyroxine-binding globulin (mg/dL)	1.3–3.0	1.8–3.2	2.8–4.0	2.6–4.2	42
Thyroxine, free (fT_4) (ng/dL)	0.8–1.7	0.8–1.2	0.6–1.0	0.5–0.8	42, 57
Thyroxine, total (T_4) (μg/dL)	5.4–11.7	6.5–10.1	7.5–10.3	6.3–9.7	29, 42
Triiodothyronine, free (fT_3) (pg/mL)	2.4–4.2	4.1–4.4	4.0–4.2	Not reported	57
Triiodothyronine, total (T_3) (ng/dL)	77–135	97–149	117–169	123–162	42

VITAMINS AND MINERALS

	Nonpregnant Adult[a]	First Trimester	Second Trimester	Third Trimester	References
Copper (μg/dL)	70–140	112–199	165–221	130–240	2 , 30, 42
Selenium (μg/L)	63–160	116–146	75–145	71–133	2, 42
Vitamin A (retinol) (μg/dL)	20–100	32–47	35–44	29–42	42
Vitamin B$_{12}$ (pg/mL)	279–966	118–438	130–656	99–526	45, 72
Vitamin C (ascorbic acid) (mg/dL)	0.4–1.0	Not reported	Not reported	0.9–1.3	64
Vitamin D, 1,25-dihydroxy (pg/mL)	25–45	20–65	72–160	60–119	3, 48
Vitamin D, 24,25-dihydroxy (ng/mL)	0.5–5.0[e]	1.2–1.8	1.1–1.5	0.7–0.9	60
Vitamin D, 25-hydroxy (ng/mL)	14–80	18–27	10–22	10–18	3, 60
Vitamin E (α-tocopherol) (μg/mL)	5–18	7–13	10–16	13–23	42
Zinc (μg/dL)	75–120	57–88	51–80	50–77	2, 42, 58

AUTOIMMUNE AND INFLAMMATORY MEDIATORS

	Nonpregnant Adult[a]	First Trimester	Second Trimester	Third Trimester	References
C3 complement (mg/dL)	83–177	62–98	73–103	77–111	42
C4 complement (mg/dL)	16–47	18–36	18–34	22–32	42
C-reactive protein (CRP) (mg/L)	0.2–3.0	Not reported	0.4–20.3	0.4–8.1	28
Erythrocyte sedimentation rate (ESR) (mm/hr)	0–20[d]	4–57	7–47	13–70	71
IgA (mg/dL)	70–350	95–243	99–237	112–250	42
IgG (mg/dL)	700–1700	981–1267	813–1131	678–990	42
IgM (mg/dL)	50–300	78–232	74–218	85–269	42

SEX HORMONES

	Nonpregnant Adult[a]	First Trimester	Second Trimester	Third Trimester	References
Dehydroepiandrosterone sulfate (DHEAS) (μmol/L)	1.3–6.8[e]	2.0–16.5	0.9–7.8	0.8–6.5	52
Estradiol (pg/mL)	<20–443[d,f]	188–2497	1278–7192	6137–3460	13, 52
Progesterone (ng/mL)	<1–20[d]	8–48		99–342	13, 52
Prolactin (ng/mL)	0–20	36–213	110–330	137–372	3, 13, 38, 49
Sex hormone binding globulin (nmol/L)	18–114[d]	39–131	214–717	216–724	1, 52
Testosterone (ng/dL)	6–86[d]	25.7–211.4	34.3–242.9	62.9–308.6	52
17-Hydroxyprogesterone (nmol/L)	0.6–10.6[d,e]	5.2–28.5	5.2–28.5	15.5–84	52

LIPIDS

	Nonpregnant Adult[a]	First Trimester	Second Trimester	Third Trimester	References
Cholesterol, total (mg/dL)	<200	141–210	176–299	219–349	8, 18, 31, 42
HDL-cholesterol (mg/dL)	40–60	40–78	52–87	48–87	8, 18, 31, 42, 55
LDL-cholesterol (mg/dL)	<100	60–153	77–184	101–224	8, 18, 31, 42, 55
VLDL-cholesterol (mg/dL)	6–40[e]	10–18	13–23	21–36	31
Triglycerides (mg/dL)	<150	40–159	75–382	131–453	8, 18, 31, 39, 42, 55
Apolipoprotein A-I (mg/dL)	119–240	111–150	142–253	145–262	18, 39, 49
Apolipoprotein B (mg/dL)	52–163	58–81	66–188	85–238	18, 39, 49

CARDIAC

	Nonpregnant Adult[a]	First Trimester	Second Trimester	Third Trimester	References
Atrial natriuretic peptide (ANP) (pg/mL)	Not reported	Not reported	28.1–70.1	Not reported	11
B-type natriuretic peptide (BNP) (pg/mL)	<167 (age and gender specific)	Not reported	13.5–29.5	Not reported	11
Creatine kinase (U/L)	39–238[d]	27–83	25–75	13–101	41, 42
Creatine kinase-MB (U/L)	<6[k]	Not reported	Not reported	1.8–2.4	41
Troponin I (ng/mL)	0–0.08	Not reported	Not reported	0–0.064 (intrapartum)	36, 65

BLOOD GAS

	Nonpregnant Adult[a]	First Trimester	Second Trimester	Third Trimester	References
Bicarbonate (HCO₃⁻) (mEq/L)	22–26	Not reported	Not reported	16–22	23
Pco₂ (mm Hg)	38–42	Not reported	Not reported	25–33	23
Po₂ (mm Hg)	90–100	93–100	90–98	92–107	23, 67
pH	7.38–7.42 (arterial)	7.36–7.52 (venous)	7.40–7.52 (venous)	7.41–7.53 (venous) 7.39–7.45 (arterial)	23, 26

RENAL FUNCTION TESTS

	Nonpregnant Adult[a]	First Trimester	Second Trimester	Third Trimester	References
Effective renal plasma flow (mL/min)	492–696[d,e]	696–985	612–1170	595–945	19, 22
Glomerular filtration rate (GFR) (mL/min)	106–132[d]	131–166	135–170	117–182	19, 22, 50
Filtration fraction (%)	16.9–24.7[l]	14.7–21.6	14.3–21.9	17.1–25.1	19, 22, 50
Osmolarity, urine (mOsm/kg)	500–800	326–975	278–1066	238–1034	61
24-hr albumin excretion (mg/24 hr)	<30	5–15	4–18	3–22	27, 61
24-hr calcium excretion (mmol/24 hr)	<7.5[e]	1.6–5.2	0.3–6.9	0.8–4.2	66
24-hr creatinine clearance (mL/min)	91–130	69–140	55–136	50–166	22, 66
24-hr creatinine excretion (mmol/24 hr)	8.8–14[e]	10.6–11.6	10.3–11.5	10.2–11.4	61
24-hr potassium excretion (mmol/24 hr)	25–100[e]	17–33	10–38	11–35	66
24-hr protein excretion (mg/24 hr)	<150	19–141	47–186	46–185	27
24-hr sodium excretion (mmol/24 hr)	100–260[e]	53–215	34–213	37–149	17, 66

[a]Unless otherwise specified, all normal reference values are from the seventeenth edition of *Harrison's Principles of Internal Medicine*. (37)

[b]Range includes references with and without iron supplementation.

[c]Reference values are from *Laboratory Reference* Handbook, Pathology Department, Parkland Hospital, 2005.

[d]Normal reference range is specific range for females.

[e]Reference values are from the fifteenth edition of *Harrison's Principles of Internal Medicine*. (12)

[f]Range is for premenopausal females and varies by menstrual cycle phase.

[g]Reference values are from Cerneca et al: Coagulation and fibrinolysis changes in normal pregnancy increased levels of procoagulants and reduced levels of inhibitors during pregnancy induce a hypercoagulable state, combined with a reactive fibrinolysis. (15)

[h]Reference values are from Cerneca et al and Choi et al: Tissue plasminogen activator levels change with plasma fibrinogen concentrations during pregnancy. (15,16)

[i]Reference values are from Mannucci et al: Changes in health and disease of the metalloprotease that cleaves von Willebrand factor. (76)

[j]Reference values are from Bacq Y et al: Liver function tests in normal pregnancy: a prospective study of 102 pregnant women and 102 matched controls. (5)

[k]Reference values are from Leiserowitz GS et al: Creatine kinase and its MB isoenzyme in the third trimester and the peripartum period. (41)

[l]Reference values are from Dunlop W: Serial changes in renal haemodynamics during normal human pregnancy. (19)

Appendix courtesy of Dr. Mina Abbassi-Ghanavati and Dr. Laura G. Greer.

APPENDIX REFERENCES

1. Acromite MT, Mantzoros CS, Leach RE, et al: Androgens in preeclampsia. Am J Obstet Gynecol 180:60, 1999
2. Álvarez SI, Castañón SG, Ruata MLC, et al: Updating of normal levels of copper, zinc and selenium in serum of pregnant women. J Trace Elem Med Biol 21(S1):49, 2007
3. Ardawi MSM, Nasrat HAN, BA'Aqueel HS: Calcium-regulating hormones and parathyroid hormone-related peptide in normal human pregnancy and postpartum: A longitudinal study. Eur J Endocrinol 137:402, 1997
4. AzizKarim S, Khurshid M, Rizvi JH, et al: Platelets and leucocyte counts in pregnancy. J Pak Med Assoc 42:86, 1992
5. Bacq Y, Zarka O, Bréchot JF, et al: Liver function tests in normal pregnancy: A prospective study of 102 pregnant women and 102 matched controls. Hepatology 23:1030, 1996
6. Balloch AJ, Cauchi MN: Reference ranges for haematology parameters in pregnancy derived from patient populations. Clin Lab Haemat 15:7, 1993
7. Beguin Y, Lipscei G, Thourmsin H, et al: Blunted erythropoietin production and decreased erythropoiesis in early pregnancy. Blood 78(1):89, 1991
8. Belo L, Caslake M, Gaffney D, et al: Changes in LDL size and HDL concentration in normal and preeclamptic pregnancies. Atherosclerosis 162:425, 2002
9. Belo L, Santos-Silva A, Rocha S, et al: Fluctuations in C-reactive protein concentration and neutrophil activation during normal human pregnancy. Eur J Obstet Gynecol Reprod Biol 123:46, 2005
10. Bianco I, Mastropietro F, D'Aseri C, et al: Serum levels of erythropoietin and soluble transferrin receptor during pregnancy in non-β-thalassemic and β-thalassemic women. Haematologica 85:902, 2000
11. Borghi CB, Esposti DD, Immordino V, et al: Relationship of systemic hemodynamics, left ventricular structure and function, and plasma natriuretic peptide concentrations during pregnancy complicated by preeclampsia. Am J Obstet Gynecol 183:140, 2000
12. Braunwald E, Fauci AS, Kasper DL, et al (eds): Harrison's Principles of Internal Medicine, 15th ed. New York, McGraw-Hill, 2001, Appendices, p A-1
13. Carranza-Lira S, Hernández F, Sánchez M, et al: Prolactin secretion in molar and normal pregnancy. Int J Gynaecol Obstet 60:137, 1998
14. Carter J: Serum bile acids in normal pregnancy. BJOG 98:540, 1991
15. Cerneca F, Ricci G, Simeone R, et al: Coagulation and fibrinolysis changes in normal pregnancy increased levels of procoagulants and reduced levels of inhibitors during pregnancy induce a hypercoagulable state, combined with a reactive fibrinolysis. Eur J Obstet Gynecol Reprod Biol 73:31, 1997
16. Choi JW, Pai SH: Tissue plasminogen activator levels change with plasma fibrinogen concentrations during pregnancy. Ann Hematol 81:611, 2002
17. Davison JB, Vallotton MB, Lindheimer MD: Plasma osmolality and urinary concentration and dilution during and after pregnancy: Evidence that lateral recumbency inhibits maximal urinary concentrating ability. BJOG 88:472, 1981
18. Desoye G, Schweditsch MO, Pfeiffer KP, et al: Correlation of hormones with lipid and lipoprotein levels during normal pregnancy and postpartum. J Clin Endocrinol Metab 64:704, 1987
19. Dunlop W: Serial changes in renal haemodynamics during normal human pregnancy. Br J Obstet Gynaecol 88:1, 1981
20. Dux S, Yaron A, Carmel A, et al: Renin, aldosterone, and serum-converting enzyme activity during normal and hypertensive pregnancy. Gynecol Obstet Invest 17:252, 1984
21. Elsheikh A, Creatsas G, Mastorakos G, et al: The renin-aldosterone system during normal and hypertensive pregnancy. Arch Gynecol Obstet 264:182, 2001
22. Ezimokhai M, Davison JM, Philips PR, et al: Non-postural serial changes in renal function during the third trimester of normal human pregnancy. Br J Obstet Gynaecol 88:465, 1981
23. Fadel HE, Northrop G, Misenhimer HR, et al: Acid-base determinations in amniotic fluid and blood of normal late pregnancy. Obstet Gynecol 53:99, 1979
24. Faught W, Garner P, Jones G, et al: Changes in protein C and protein S levels in normal pregnancy. Am J Obstet Gynecol 172:147, 1995
25. Francalanci I, Comeglio P, Liotta AA, et al: D-Dimer concentrations during normal pregnancy, as measured by ELISA. Thromb Res 78:399, 1995
26. Handwerker SM, Altura BT, Altura BM: Serum ionized magnesium and other electrolytes in the antenatal period of human pregnancy. J Am Coll Nutr 15:36, 1996
27. Higby K, Suiter CR, Phelps JY, et al: Normal values of urinary albumin and total protein excretion during pregnancy. Am J Obstet Gynecol 171:984, 1994

28. Hwang HS, Kwon JY, Kim MA, et al: Maternal serum highly sensitive C-reactive protein in normal pregnancy and pre-eclampsia. Int J Gynecol Obstet 98:105, 2007
29. Hytten FE, Lind T: Diagnostic Indices in Pregnancy. Summit, NJ, CIBA-GEIGY Corporation, 1975
30. Ilhan N, Ilhan N, Simsek M: The changes of trace elements, malondialdehyde levels and superoxide dismutase activities in pregnancy with or without preeclampsia. Clin Biochem 35:393, 2002
31. Jimenez DM, Pocovi M, Ramon-Cajal J, et al: Longitudinal study of plasma lipids and lipoprotein cholesterol in normal pregnancy and puerperium. Gynecol Obstet Invest 25:158, 1988
32. Karsenti D, Bacq Y, Bréchot JF, et al: Serum amylase and lipase activities in normal pregnancy: A prospective case-control study. Am J Gastroenterol 96:697, 2001
33. Kato T, Seki K, Matsui H, et al: Monomeric calcitonin in pregnant women and in cord blood. Obstet Gynecol 92:241, 1998
34. Kim EH, Lim JH, Kim YH, et al: The relationship between aldosterone to renin ratio and RI value of the uterine artery in the preeclamptic patient vs. normal pregnancy. Yonsei Med J 49(1):138, 2008
35. Kline JA, Williams GW, Hernandez-Nino J: D-Dimer concentrations in normal pregnancy: New diagnostic thresholds are needed. Clin Chem 51:825, 2005
36. Koscica KL, Bebbington M, Bernstein PS: Are maternal serum troponin I levels affected by vaginal or cesarean delivery? Am J Perinatol 21(1):31, 2004
37. Kratz A, Pesce MA, Fink DJ: Appendix: Laboratory values of clinical importance. In Fauci AS, Braunwald E, Kasper DL, et al (eds): Harrison's Principles of Internal Medicine, 17th ed. New York, McGraw-Hill, 2008, Appendix 1, p A-1
38. Larrea F, Méndez I, Parra A: Serum pattern of different molecular forms of prolactin during normal human pregnancy. Hum Reprod 8:1617, 1993
39. Larsson A, Palm M, Hansson L-O, et al: Reference values for clinical chemistry tests during normal pregnancy. BJOG 115:874, 2008
40. Lefkowitz JB, Clarke SH, Barbour LA: Comparison of protein S functional and antigenic assays in normal pregnancy. Am J Obstet Gynecol 175:657, 1996
41. Leiserowitz GS, Evans AT, Samuels SJ, et al: Creatine kinase and its MB isoenzyme in the third trimester and the peripartum period. J Reprod Med 37:910, 1992
42. Lockitch G: Handbook of Diagnostic Biochemistry and Hematology in Normal Pregnancy. Boca Raton, FL, CRC Press, 1993
43. López-Quesada E, Vilaseca MA, Lailla JM: Plasma total homocysteine in uncomplicated pregnancy and in preeclampsia. Eur J Obstet Gynecol Reprod Biol 108:45, 2003
44. Louro MO, Cocho JA, Tutor JC: Assessment of copper status in pregnancy by means of determining the specific oxidase activity of ceruloplasmin. Clin Chim Acta 312:123, 2001
45. Milman N, Bergholt T, Byg KE, et al: Reference intervals for haematological variables during normal pregnancy and postpartum in 434 healthy Danish women. Eur J Haematol 79:39, 2007
46. Milman N, Byg KE, Hvas AM, et al: Erythrocyte folate, plasma folate and plasma homocysteine during normal pregnancy and postpartum: A longitudinal study comprising 404 Danish women. Eur J Haematol 76:200, 2006
47. Milman N, Graudal N, Nielsen OJ: Serum erythropoietin during normal pregnancy: Relationship to hemoglobin and iron status markers and impact of iron supplementation in a longitudinal, placebo-controlled study on 118 women. Int J Hematol 66:159, 1997
48. Mimouni F, Tsang RC, Hertzbert VS, et al: Parathyroid hormone and calcitriol changes in normal and insulin-dependent diabetic pregnancies. Obstet Gynecol 74:49, 1989
49. Montelongo A, Lasunción MA, Pallardo LF, et al: Longitudinal study of plasma lipoproteins and hormones during pregnancy in normal and diabetic women. Diabetes 41:1651, 1992
50. Moran P, Baylis PH, Lindheimer, et al: Glomerular ultrafiltration in normal and preeclamptic pregnancy. J Am Soc Nephrol 14:648, 2003
51. Morse M: Establishing a normal range for D-dimer levels through pregnancy to aid in the diagnosis of pulmonary embolism and deep vein thrombosis. J Thromb Haemost 2:1202, 2004
52. O'Leary P, Boyne P, Flett P, et al: Longitudinal assessment of changes in reproductive hormones during normal pregnancy. Clin Chem 35(5):667, 1991
53. Özerol E, Özerol I, Gökdeniz R, et al: Effect of smoking on serum concentrations of total homocysteine, folate, vitamin B$_{12}$, and nitric oxide in pregnancy: A preliminary study. Fetal Diagn Ther 19:145, 2004
54. Parente JV, Franco JG, Greene LJ, et al: Angiotensin-converting enzyme: Serum levels during normal pregnancy. Am J Obstet Gynecol 135:586, 1979
55. Piechota W, Staszewski A: Reference ranges of lipids and apolipoproteins in pregnancy. Eur J Obstet Gynecol Reprod Biol 45:27, 1992

56. Pitkin RM, Gebhardt MP: Serum calcium concentrations in human pregnancy. Am J Obstet Gynecol 127:775, 1977

57. Price A, Obel O, Cresswell J, et al: Comparison of thyroid function in pregnant and non-pregnant Asian and western Caucasian women. Clin Chim Acta 208:91, 2001

58. Qvist I, Abdulla M, Jägerstad M, et al: Iron, zinc and folate status during pregnancy and two months after delivery. Acta Obstet Gynecol Scand 65:15, 1986

59. Radder JK, Van Roosmalen J: HbAIC in healthy, pregnant women. Neth J Med 63:256, 2005

60. Reiter EO, Braunstein GD, Vargas A, et al: Changes in 25-hydroxyvitamin D and 24,25-dihydroxyvitamin D during pregnancy. Am J Obstet Gynecol 135:227, 1979

61. Risberg A, Larsson A, Olsson K, et al: Relationship between urinary albumin and albumin/creatinine ratio during normal pregnancy and preeclampsia. Scand J Clin Lab Invest 64:17, 2004

62. Romslo I, Haram K, Sagen N, et al: Iron requirement in normal pregnancy as assessed by serum ferritin, serum transferring saturation and erythrocyte protoporphyrin determinations. Br J Obstet Gynaecol 90:101, 1983

63. Shakhmatova EI, Osipova NA, Natochin YV: Changes in osmolality and blood serum ion concentrations in pregnancy. Hum Physiol 26:92, 2000

64. Sharma SC, Sabra A, Molloy A, et al: Comparison of blood levels of histamine and total ascorbic acid in pre-eclampsia with normal pregnancy. Hum Nutr Clin Nutr 38C:3, 1984

65. Shivvers SA, Wians FH, Keffer JH, et al: Maternal cardiac troponin I levels during labor and delivery. Am J Obstet Gynecol 180:122, 1999

66. Singh HJ, Mohammad NH, Nila A: Serum calcium and parathormone during normal pregnancy in Malay women. J Matern Fetal Med 8:95, 1999

67. Spiropoulos K, Prodromaki E, Tsapanos V: Effect of body position on PaO_2 and $PaCO_2$ during pregnancy. Gynecol Obstet Invest 58:22, 2004

68. Strickland DM, Hauth JC, Widish J, et al: Amylase and isoamylase activities in serum of pregnant women. Obstet Gynecol 63:389, 1984

69. Suri D, Moran J, Hibbard JU, et al: Assessment of adrenal reserve in pregnancy: Defining the normal response to the adrenocorticotropin stimulation test. J Clin Endocrinol Metab 91:3866, 2006

70. Van Buul EJA, Steegers EAP, Jongsma HW, et al: Haematological and biochemical profile of uncomplicated pregnancy in nulliparous women; a longitudinal study. Neth J Med 46:73, 1995

71. van den Broek NR, Letsky EA: Pregnancy and the erythrocyte sedimentation rate. Br J Obstet Gynaecol 108:1164, 2001

72. Walker MC, Smith GN, Perkins SL, et al: Changes in homocysteine levels during normal pregnancy. Am J Obstet Gynecol 180:660, 1999

73. Wickström K, Edelstam G, Löwbeer CH, et al: Reference intervals for plasma levels of fibronectin, von Willebrand factor, free protein S and antithrombin during third-trimester pregnancy. Scand J Clin Lab Invest 64:31, 2004

74. Lattuada A, Rossi E, Calzarossa C, et al: Mild to moderate reduction of a von Willebrand factor cleaving protease (ADAMTS-13) in pregnant women with HELLP microangiopathic syndrome. Haematologica 88(9): 1029, 2003

75. Liu XH, Jiang YM, Shi H, et al: Prospective, sequential, longitudinal study of coagulation changes during pregnancy in Chinese women. Int J Gynaecol Obstet 105(3):240, 2009

76. Mannucci PM, Canciani MT, Forza I, et al: Changes in health and disease of the metalloprotease that cleaves von Willebrand factor. Blood 98(9): 2730, 2001

INDEX

Note: Page numbers followed by *f* and *t* indicate figures and tables, respectively.

Preeclampsia *(Cont.):*
inflammation in, obesity and, 951
kidneys in, 719–720
laboratory findings in, 708
labor induction in, 729
liver in, 720–721, 720*f,* 721*f,* 1067
liver involvement in, clinical and
laboratory findings in, 1064*t*
management of
expectant, *versus* aggressive, 731–732,
733*t*
hospitalization *versus* outpatient
management for, 729–731, 730*t*
maternal hyperthyroidism and, 1129,
1129*t*
maternal mortality with, 706
in multifetal gestation, 878–879
neuroanatomical lesions in, 721, 721*f,*
722*f*
nonimmune hydrops and, 627
nutrition and, 712
obesity and, 182, 709, 951
organs involved in, 708
oxidative stress and, 712
pain with, 708
pathogenesis of, 54, 121, 713–714
pathophysiology of, 715–725
persistent severe postpartum, 746–747
and placental abruption, 764, 764*t,* 766
placental CRH levels in, 157
platelets in, 717–718
polycystic kidney disease and, 1043
prediction of, 724–726
and preterm birth, 811
prevention of, 726–728
antioxidants and, 712
proteinuria in, 708, 719
in renal transplant recipient, 1042
risk factors for, 709
sequelae
cardiovascular, 748–749, 748*f*
and future pregnancies, 747–748
long-term, 747–749
neurological, 749
neurovascular, 748–749
renal, 749
severe
delayed delivery with, 731–734, 733*t,*
734*t*
early, expectant management of,
731–732
early-onset, indications for delivery in,
734*t*
magnesium sulfate for, 736–737, 737*t*
management of, expectant, 733*t*
midtrimester, expectant management of,
732
outcomes, 731–732
severity of, indicators of, 708, 708*t*
spinal block and, 453–454
and stroke, 1167
superimposed on chronic hypertension,
709, 985, 987, 991–992

Preeclampsia *(Cont.):*
and delivery, 992
diagnosis of, 707*t,* 709, 992
postpartum care for, 992
pregnancy outcome with, 988*t*
prevention of, 987
and symmetrical fetal-growth restriction,
846
systemic lupus erythematosus and, 1149
and termination of pregnancy, 729
thrombocytopenia with, 708, 1092
thrombocytosis and, 1095
and thromboembolic
disease/thromboembolism, 1013
thrombophilias and, 1018, 1018*t*
trisomy 13 and, 270
as two-stage disorder, 710, 710*f*
and two-vessel cord, 582
and uteroplacental perfusion, 724
ventricular function in, 715, 716, 716*f*
Preeclampsia syndrome, 706
superimposed on chronic hypertension, 706
Pregnancy
abdominal. *See* Ectopic pregnancy,
abdominal
adolescent. *See* Adolescent pregnancy
average number of, in American women, 4
broad-ligament. *See* Ectopic pregnancy,
broad-ligament
cervical. *See* Ectopic pregnancy, cervical
cesarean scar, 779
dating of, 47
diagnosis of, 191–193
ultrasonic, 193, 193*f*
duration of
normal, 195
terminology for, 78, 79*f*
female genital mutilation and, 899
intervals between, and preterm birth, 812
with IUD in utero, 686
luteal phase, 700
molar. *See* Hydatidiform mole
number of, 4*t*
in 2005/2006, 4
outcomes of, 4*t*
in 2005/2006, 4
ovarian. *See* Ectopic pregnancy, ovarian
postterm. *See* Postterm pregnancy
signs and symptoms of, 191–193
in teenagers. *See* Adolescent pregnancy
termination of. *See also* Abortion; Selective
termination
induced, definition of, 3
trimesters of, 78, 195
tubal. *See* Ectopic pregnancy, tubal
unintended, 174–175
prevention of, 174
by family planning programs, 10, 10*f*
vital statistics of, in U.S., 4, 4*t*
Pregnancy-associated α_2-glycoprotein,
plasma/serum level of, in
rheumatoid arthritis in pregnancy,
1156

Pregnancy-associated death, definition of, 4
Pregnancy-associated plasma protein A, in
Down syndrome screening, 293
Pregnancy failure, early, 215
management of, 223*t*
Pregnancy-induced hypertension. *See also*
Eclampsia; Gestational
hypertension; Hypertension;
Hypertensive disorder(s),
complicating pregnancy;
Preeclampsia
asthma and, 998–999, 998*t*
hydatidiform mole and, 260
Pregnancy In Multiple Sclerosis (PRIMS)
study, 1171, 1171*f*
Pregnancy loss. *See also* Abortion; Pregnancy
wastage; Stillbirth
early, 215
clinically silent, 215
dialysis during pregnancy and, 1041
management of, 223, 223*t*
thrombophilia and, 1018, 1018*t*
recurrent, 220, 224
second-trimester, prenatal consultation for,
198*t*
sporadic, 224
Pregnancy outcome
antihypertensive therapy and, 988*t*
in asthma, 998–999
in bacterial pneumonia, 1003
chronic hypertension and, 988*t*
chronic hypertension with superimposed
preeclampsia and, 988*t*
in chronic renal insufficiency, 1039
in cystic fibrosis, 1008–1009
with dialysis during pregnancy, 1041, 1041*t*
with hemoglobin CC, 1090*t*
in hereditary spherocytosis, 1084
with hydramnios, 492, 493–494, 494*t*
with hypothyroidism, 1131, 1131*t*
in inflammatory bowel disease, 1056
intrahepatic cholestasis of pregnancy and,
1065
with isolated maternal hypothyroxinemia,
1132, 1132*t*
maternal cyanotic heart disease and, 969
in multifetal gestation, 859, 860*t,*
868–870
myomas and, 903
nonobstetric surgery and, 913, 913*t*
in obesity, 950–951, 950*t,* 951*f*
with oligohydramnios, 495–496,
497–498, 497*t*
in postterm pregnancy, 833–834, 833*f,*
834*f,* 834*t*
in renal transplant recipient, 1042
with sickle cell–β-thalassemia disease,
1090*t*
with subclinical hypothyroidism, 1132,
1132*t*
thrombophilias and, 1018–1019, 1018*t*
with tuberculosis, 1005–1006
with twins, 859, 860*t*

Protein C *(Cont.)*:
  resistance to, 117, 1016–1017, 1099.
      See also Factor V Leiden mutation
      and pregnancy outcomes, 1018,
      1018*t*
  in antiphospholipid antibody syndrome,
      1152
  deficiency of, 93, 1015, 1099
    genetics of, 1015
    neonatal homozygous, 1015
    pathophysiology of, 1016*f*
    in pregnancy, 1015*t*
    and pregnancy outcomes, 1018, 1018*t*
    prevalence of, 1015
    venous thromboembolism risk in, 1015,
      1015*t*
  functional, normal laboratory values
    in nonpregnant adult, 1260
    in uncomplicated pregnancy, 1260
  in pregnancy, 117*t*
Protein 4.2 deficiency, 1084
Protein S
  in antiphospholipid antibody syndrome,
      1152
  deficiency of, 93, 1099
    diagnosis of, 1015
    genetics of, 1015
    neonatal homozygous, 1015
    pathophysiology of, 1016*f*
    in pregnancy, 1015*t*
    and pregnancy outcomes, 1018, 1018*t*
    venous thromboembolism risk in, 1015,
      1015*t*
  free, normal laboratory values
    in nonpregnant adult, 1260
    in uncomplicated pregnancy, 1260
  functional activity, normal laboratory
      values
    in nonpregnant adult, 1260
    in uncomplicated pregnancy, 1260
  levels, in pregnancy, 1015
  in pregnancy, 117, 117*t*
  total, normal laboratory values
    in nonpregnant adult, 1260
    in uncomplicated pregnancy, 1260
Proteinuria
  chronic, in pregnancy, 1044–1045
    follow-up for, 1045
  chronic glomerulonephritis and, 1044
  with chronic hypertension, 986, 991
    and superimposed preeclampsia, 991
  in chronic renal disease, 1039
  and eclampsia, 719
  and gestational hypertension, 707–708,
      719
  in hypertensive patient, 707
  measurement of, 719
  nephrotic-range, in pregnancy, 1044–1045
  orthostatic/postural, 1034
  with placental abruption, 766
  in polycystic kidney disease, 1043
  and preeclampsia, 719
  in preeclampsia, 708

Proteinuria *(Cont.)*:
  in pregnancy, 124, 124*f,* 1033
  prenatal consultation for, 199*t*
  in systemic lupus erythematosus, 1148
Protein Z
  deficiency of, 1017
  in pregnancy, 117
Proteoglycans, cervical, 140–141
Proteus, in acute pyelonephritis, 1036
Prothrombin, gene, mutation, and recurrent
      miscarriage, 225–226
Prothrombin G20210A mutation, 1099
  epidemiology of, 1017
  factor V Leiden and
    in pregnancy, 1015*t*
    venous thromboembolism risk in,
      1015*t,* 1017
  pathophysiology of, 1016*f*
  in pregnancy, 1015*t*
  and pregnancy outcomes, 1018, 1018*t*
  venous thromboembolism risk in, 1015*t,*
      1017
Prothrombin time (PT)
  with acute liver diseases of pregnancy,
      1064*t*
  in consumptive coagulopathy, 787
  normal values
    in nonpregnant adult, 1260
    in uncomplicated pregnancy, 1260
  in viral hepatitis, 1067
Proton pump inhibitors
  for peptic ulcers, 1053
  for reflux esophagitis, 1052
Protozoal infection(s), 1226–1228. *See also*
      Amebiasis; Malaria; *Pneumocystis
      jiroveci;* Toxoplasmosis
Protraction disorders, in labor, 389
Prurigo gestationis, 1188*t,* 1189. *See also*
      Prurigo of pregnancy
Prurigo of pregnancy, 1188*t,* 1189
  clinical characteristics of, 1188*t*
  effects on pregnancy, 1188*t*
  epidemiology of, 1188*t*
  histopathology of, 1188*t*
  treatment of, 1188*t*
Pruritic folliculitis of pregnancy, 1188*t,*
      1189. *See also* Impetigo
      herpetiformis
  clinical characteristics of, 1188*t*
  effects on pregnancy, 1188*t*
  epidemiology of, 1188*t*
  histopathology of, 1188*t*
  treatment of, 1188*t*
Pruritic urticarial papules and plaques of
      pregnancy (PUPPP), 1187, 1188*t*
  clinical characteristics of, 1188*t,* 1189,
      1189*f*
  effects on pregnancy, 1188*t*
  epidemiology of, 1188*t,* 1189
  histopathology of, 1188*t*
  pathophysiology of, 1189
  postpartum, 1189
  treatment of, 1188*t,* 1189

Pruritus
  in intrahepatic cholestasis of pregnancy,
      1063–1064
  in pregnancy, 1187
  regional analgesia and, 452*t,* 458
Pruritus gravidarum, 126, 1187–1188,
      1188*t. See also* Cholestasis, of
      pregnancy
  clinical characteristics of, 1188*t*
  effects on pregnancy, 1188*t*
  epidemiology of, 1188*t*
  histopathology of, 1188*t*
  treatment of, 1188*t*
Pseudocysts, of umbilical cord, 584
Pseudogestational sac, in ectopic pregnancy,
      243
Pseudohermaphroditism
  female, 102, 102*f*
  male, 102–103, 103*f*
    familial, type I, 103
Pseudohypoaldosteronism, fetal, and
      hydramnios, 492
Pseudohypoparathyroidism, genetics of, 280*t*
Pseudomonas aeruginosa, in cystic fibrosis, 1008
Pseudomosaicism, 275, 300
Pseudosac, in ectopic pregnancy, 243
Pseudosinusoidal fetal heart rate, 420
Pseudotumor cerebri, 1175
  clinical course of, 1175
  clinical features of, 1175
  diagnostic criteria for, 1175
  etiology of, 1175
  obstetric considerations with, 1175
  and pregnancy, 1175
  treatment of, 1175
    in pregnancy, 1175
Psoas abscess, 667
Psoriasis
  pregnancy and, 1191
  treatment of, in pregnancy, 1191
Psoriatic arthritis, 1145
Psychiatric disorder(s), 1175–1180
  maternal, preconceptional counseling
      about, 185*t*
  prenatal consultation for, 198*t*
  treatment of, in pregnancy, 323–324
Psychological adjustment
  to pregnancy, 1175–1176
  with selective reduction/termination in
      multifetal pregnancy, 885
Psychological factors, in hyperemesis
      gravidarum, 1051, 1052
Psychological stress, and preterm birth, 811
Psychosis
  after eclampsia, 736
  postpartum, 1179
Psychosocial screening, in prenatal care, 195,
      196*t*
Psychotropic drugs, use in pregnancy, 1176
PTH. *See* Parathyroid hormone (PTH)
PTH-related protein, 1135
PTH-rP. *See* Parathyroid hormone-related
      protein (PTH-rP)